Volume 2

TEXTBOOK OF VETERINARY INTERNAL MEDICINE

THIRD EDITION

DISEASES OF THE DOG AND CAT

STEPHEN J. ETTINGER, DVM

California Animal Hospital, Los Angeles, California

W.B. SAUNDERS COMPANY *Philadelphia, London, Toronto, Montreal, Sydney, Tokyo*
Harcourt Brace Jovanovich, Inc.

W. B. SAUNDERS COMPANY
Harcourt Brace Jovanovich, Inc.

The Curtis Center
Independence Square West
Philadelphia, PA 19106

Library of Congress Cataloging-in-Publication Data

Textbook of veterinary internal medicine.

Includes bibliographies and indexes.

1. Dogs—Diseases.   2. Cats—Diseases.   3. Veterinary
internal medicine.   I. Ettinger, Stephen J. [DNLM:
1. Cat Diseases—diagnosis.   2. Cat Diseases—therapy.
3. Dog Diseases—diagnosis.   4. Dog Diseases—therapy.
SF 991 T355]

SF991.T48   1989   636.7′0896   87–31428

ISBN 0–7216–1944–4
      0–7216–1942–8 (Vol. 1)
      0–7216–1943–6 (Vol. 2)

Listed here is the latest translated edition of this book together
with the language of the translation and the publisher.

Japanese *(first edition)*—Gakusosha Company, Tokyo, Japan
Italian *(second edition)*—Scientific Book Market, Via dei Mille 13, Parma, Italy
Italian translation, 1989

Editor: John Dyson
Production Manager: Frank Polizzano
Designer: Lorraine B. Kilmer
Manuscript Editor: Stephen J. Ettinger, DVM
Indexer: Alexandra Nickerson

Textbook of Veterinary Internal Medicine   ISBN 0–7216–1942–8 Vol. 1
                                           0–7216–1943–6 Vol. 2
                                           0–7216–1944–4 Set

Printed in the United States of America.

Last digit is the print number: 9   8   7   6   5

CONTENTS

VOLUME 1

SECTION I: MANIFESTATIONS OF CLINICAL DISEASE

iv CONTENTS

SECTION II: PROBLEMS IN VETERINARY PRACTICE

SECTION III: INFECTIOUS DISEASES

SECTION IV: THERAPEUTIC CONSIDERATIONS IN MEDICINE

SECTION V: CANCER NEOPLASIA

SECTION VI: THE NERVOUS SYSTEM

SECTION VII: THE RESPIRATORY SYSTEM

SECTION VIII: THE CARDIOVASCULAR SYSTEM

VOLUME 2

SECTION IX: THE GASTROINTESTINAL SYSTEM

SECTION X: THE ENDOCRINE SYSTEM

SECTION XI: THE REPRODUCTIVE SYSTEM

SECTION XII: THE URINARY SYSTEM

THE GASTROINTESTINAL SYSTEM

82 ORAL, DENTAL, PHARYNGEAL, AND SALIVARY GLAND DISORDERS

COLIN E. HARVEY

THE ORAL CAVITY

Anatomy and Function

The oral cavity is an open-ended tube that functions in prehension, mastication, imbibition of fluid, taste, and swallowing. Associated with the oropharyngeal tube and surrounding muscles and calcified tissues are the salivary glands.

The external opening of the oral cavity is bordered by the fleshy upper and lower lips. Between the external skin and the stratified squamous epithelium lining the lips and cheeks lie the muscles that cause changes in facial expression; these are innervated by the facial nerve (cranial nerve [C.N.] VII). The upper lips are separated rostrally by a midline fissure, the philtrum.

The fleshy, highly mobile tongue lies on the floor of the oral cavity. The root of the tongue is formed by muscles that arise from the hyoid bones, which are supplied by the hypoglossal nerves (C.N. XII). The tongue is covered by stratified squamous epithelium. On the dorsal surface, specialized areas of epithelium form the taste buds, containing the gustatory nerve endings. The dorsal surface of the tongue of the cat also contains epithelial projections, which form horny spikes. The ordinary and special sensory nerve fibers from the tongue are carried in the lingual (mandibular branch, trigeminal nerve [C.N. V]), chorda tympani (facial nerve [C.N. VII]), and glossopharyngeal (C.N. IX) nerves.

The palate forms the dorsal roof of the oral cavity, separating it from the nasal cavity. The stratified squamous epithelium that covers the rostral bony part of the palate is formed into horizontal folds. The caudal part of the palate is the soft palate, a muscular mobile structure that forms part of the nasopharyngeal closure mechanism during swallowing.

Dental Structures

The dental unit consists of the teeth and their supporting tissues, the periodontium (the gingiva, the alveolar and supporting bony portion of the mandible and maxilla, the periodontal ligament, and the cemental surfaces of the teeth). The teeth vary in size, shape, and number of roots, depending upon location and function. A tooth consists of a mass of dentin surrounding the pulpal tissues. The root portion of the dentin is covered with cementum, the crown portion with enamel (Figure 82-1).

In utero, the epithelium covering the maxilla and mandible differentiates to form the dental lamina, which gives rise to the tooth buds. The tooth bud becomes a cup-shaped dome, the enamel organ, which encapsulates invaginating mesenchymal tissue to form the dental papilla. Peripheral cells adjacent to the enamel organ differentiate into odontoblasts, which elaborate dentin. Once dentin is secreted, enamel formation starts. When enamel and dentin formation has reached the future cemento-enamel junction, root formation begins. An epithelial diaphragm directs dentin formation downward. As dentin is elaborated, the epithelial root sheath breaks up, creating the dormant epithelial cell rests of Malassez in the connective tissue. Throughout this development, the tooth bud is encased in a sac, which allows tooth formation to occur surrounded by bone. The sac condenses to become both the connective tissue of the periodontal ligament and the cells forming the thin cementum covering the dentin of the root.

Enamel, the only portion of the tooth that is of ectodermal origin, is 95 per cent mineralized inorganic substance, mostly hydroxyapatite. It provides resistance to wear and protects the underlying dentinal tissue from caries. Enamel is not permeable except in regions where cracks or defects are present.

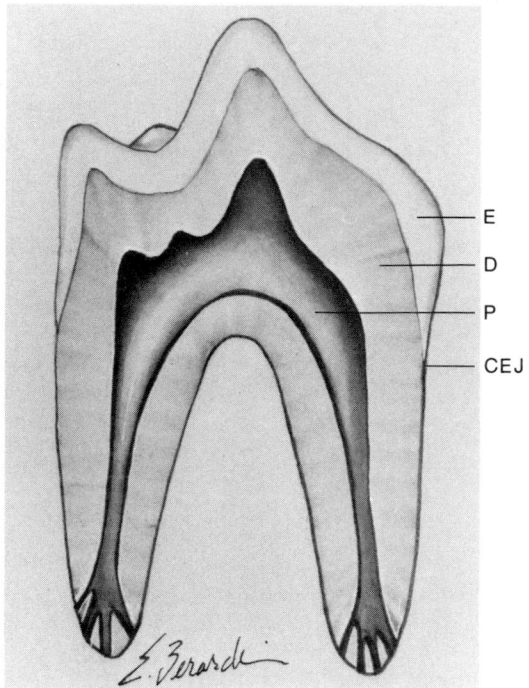

FIGURE 82–1. Diagram of the structure of a premolar tooth of a dog. CEJ, cemento-enamel junction; D, dentin; E, enamel; P, pulp.

The internal wall of dentin follows the external outline of the pulp and is lined by odontoblasts: odontoblastic processes extend through the dentinal matrix to the periphery. Dentin, which is 75 per cent mineralized hydroxyapatite and 25 per cent organic collagen, is continuously synthesized throughout the life of the dental pulp, forming a uniform layer throughout the periphery of the pulp cavity. Dentin contains pain nerve endings that are stimulated by penetration or removal of enamel.

The dental pulp is a connective tissue organ occupying the root canal. Its primary function is the development of dentin; secondary functions are nutritive, sensory, and protective. It is a highly vascular organ, having a system of arteriovenous anastomoses that can divert blood from the capillary beds and increase drainage in case of inflammation. The pulp is contiguous with the periodontal ligament at the apex of the root. A mature tooth in a dog has multiple apical foramina, forming the apical delta.[1] The apex of the canine teeth of dogs is not fully developed until about 24 to 30 months of age.[2]

Cementum is a thin, 50 per cent organic, bone-like tissue that covers the root surface. The periodontal ligament is attached to the tooth by means of collagenous Sharpey's fibers, which are embedded in it during cementum formation.

The alveolar process (the mandible and maxilla) consists of a mass of cancellous bone, the external surface of which is covered with cortical bone. The most coronal (toward the crown) aspect of the alveolar process is known as the alveolar crest (Figure 82–2). Invaginations into the mandible and maxilla form the sockets, which contain all but the most coronal one to two mm of the root. The sockets themselves are lined with cortical bone known as alveolar bone; the cancellous bone that surrounds the alveolar bone is known as the supporting

bone. Connective tissue fibers (Sharpey's fibers) insert into the alveolar bone and anastomose with similar fibers that insert into the cementum. The connective tissue attachment between the tooth and bone is the periodontal ligament, whose function is to resist the stresses placed upon the teeth.

The gingiva is the keratinized squamous epithelium that covers the bone and attaches to the tooth (Figure 82–3). The most coronal aspect of the gingiva is the free gingival margin (FGM), where the complex junction of gingiva to tooth structure occurs. The FGM approximately parallels the cemento-enamel junction (CEJ) and is located one to two mm coronal to it on the enamel surface of the crown. The junction of the gingiva with the nonkeratinized alveolar mucosa marks the most apical extent of the gingiva, the mucogingival junction (MGJ). The distance from the FGM to the MGJ is quite variable from breed to breed and from tooth to tooth: it is rarely less than one mm and may approach 10 to 20 mm.

The connective tissue underlying the gingiva is well vascularized, dense, nonelastic collagen. The deeper fibers of this connective tissue are confluent with the periosteum of the alveolar process. Connective tissue fibers (the gingival fiber apparatus) insert into the root surface, which is coronal to the alveolar crestal bone. Connective tissue fibers (transeptal fibers) also pass from the cementum of one tooth to the tooth adjacent to it. Around the circumference of each tooth is a 1- to 2-mm-deep gingival sulcus between the gingiva and enamel surface. The gingiva within the sulcus is lined by the relatively nonkeratinized sulcular epithelium. Apical to the sulcular epithelium is the junctional epithelium that forms an attachment between the connective tissue

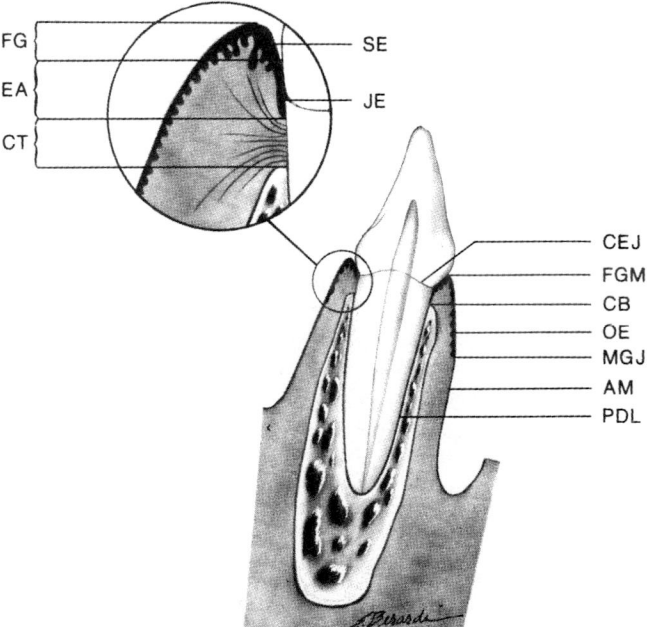

FIGURE 82–2. Diagram of a cross-section of the periodontium of the dog. AM, alveolar mucosa; CB, crestal bone; CEJ, cemento-enamel junction; CT, connective tissue attachment; EA, epithelial attachment; FGM, free gingival margin; JE, junctional epithelium; MGJ, mucogingival junction; OE, oral epithelium; SE, sulcular epithelium; PDL, periodontal ligament.

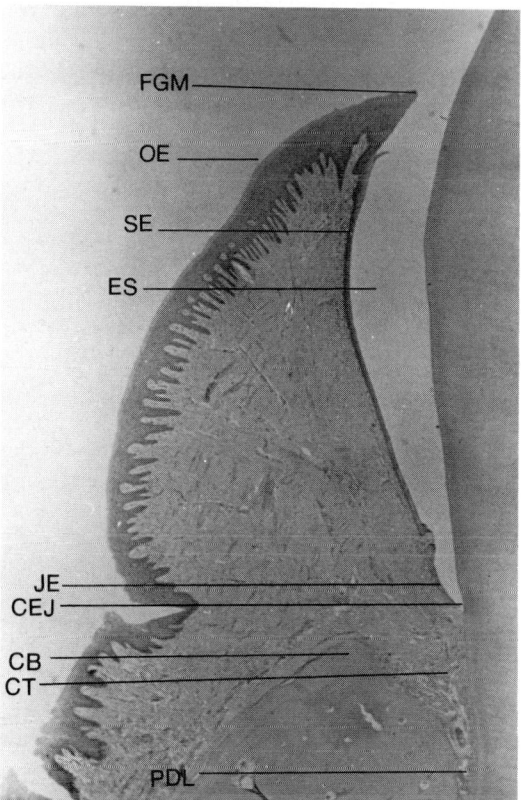

FIGURE 82–3. Histologic sections of the normal periodontium. CB, crestal bone; CEJ, cemento-enamel junction; CT, connective tissue attachment; ES, enamel space; FGM, free gingival margin; JE, junctional epithelium; OE, oral epithelium; PDL, periodontal ligament; SE, sulcular epithelium.

TABLE 82–1. DENTAL FORMULAS OF DOGS AND CATS

	Dog	Cat
Deciduous dentition	$\dfrac{3\mathrm{I},\ 1\mathrm{C},\ 3\mathrm{M}}{3\mathrm{I},\ 1\mathrm{C},\ 3\mathrm{M}}$	$\dfrac{3\mathrm{I},\ 1\mathrm{C},\ 3\mathrm{M}}{3\mathrm{I},\ 1\mathrm{C},\ 2\mathrm{M}}$
Permanent dentition	$\dfrac{3\mathrm{I},\ 1\mathrm{C},\ 4\mathrm{P},\ 2\mathrm{M}}{3\mathrm{I},\ 1\mathrm{C},\ 4\mathrm{P},\ 3\mathrm{M}}$	$\dfrac{3\mathrm{I},\ 1\mathrm{C},\ 3\mathrm{P},\ 1\mathrm{M}}{3\mathrm{I},\ 1\mathrm{C},\ 2\mathrm{P},\ 1\mathrm{M}}$

of the gingiva and the tooth surface. The junctional epithelium is a nonkeratinized stratified squamous epithelium 15 to 30 cells thick at its most coronal extent, where it meets the sulcular epithelium and tapers down to one cell at its most apical extent at or just apical to the CEJ. Hemidesmosomes attach the junctional epithelium to a cuticle-like covering on the enamel.

Eruption of the Teeth. Cats and dogs are diphyodont (they have two succeeding generations of teeth), although they are edentulous at birth. The deciduous teeth are small and can be accommodated in the developing jaws, but as the animal grows they are no longer adequate. As the tooth erupts, the root forms apical to the CEJ. Once the tooth has erupted, mechanical forces result in maturation of the alveolus into the attachment apparatus, apical calcification occurs, and the root becomes fully formed. Apical resorption of the roots of deciduous teeth starts almost immediately as the developing permanent teeth start to form.

The deciduous teeth of the dog erupt between two weeks and eight weeks after birth. Dental formulas are shown in Table 82–1, and root arrangements are shown in Figure 82–4. From two to six months of age, shedding

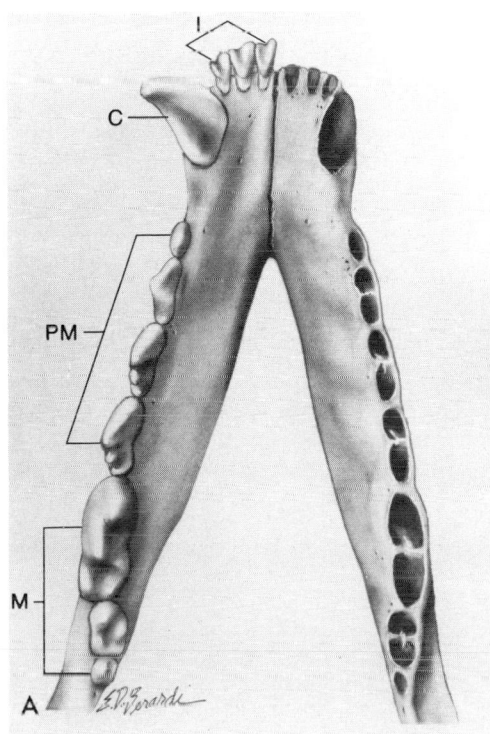

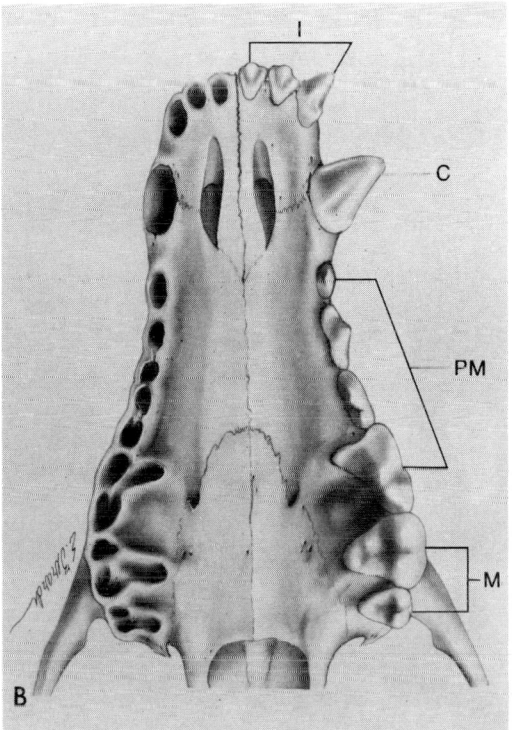

FIGURE 82–4. *A*, Drawing of a dog mandible showing tooth anatomy on the left side and the distribution of the tooth sockets on the right side. *B*, Drawing of a dog maxilla showing tooth anatomy on the right side and the distribution of the tooth sockets on the left. C, canine; I, incisors; M, molars; PM, premolars.

of the deciduous dentition occurs as the permanent teeth erupt. Eruption time appears to vary according to the breed of the dog. The larger the breed, the shorter the lifespan and the earlier the eruption sequence. Dogs seldom show signs of teething problems, except for a slight tenderness during the transition. The deciduous premolars act as molars during this period. The smaller jaw requires that the position of the functioning carnassial teeth is more rostral; shearing action is provided by the maxillary deciduous third premolar and the mandibular deciduous fourth premolar. Usually the deciduous tooth is shed before its successor erupts. Eruption of all of the permanent teeth and extrusion to full crown height is complete in most dogs by 10 to 12 months; however, the root is still immature at that age—the apex is wide open, the root is short, and the root and crown dentin are thin. The root apex of canine teeth may not close until as late as 30 months of age.[2]

The cat's deciduous dentition starts to appear within two weeks of birth. All the deciduous teeth are present by about seven weeks. Dental formulas are shown in Table 82–1. The deciduous second premolars are the carnassial teeth. The permanent teeth erupt between three and six months of age.

In both the cat and dog, the mandible is smaller than the maxilla at birth, i.e., they have a retrognathic relationship. Mandibular growth occurs in a downward and forward direction and at a faster rate than maxillary growth. The mature mandibular arch is larger than the maxillary arch; owing to the axial direction of the teeth, however, the maxillary teeth overlap the mandibular teeth.

Occlusion and Articulation. Breed selection has resulted in major variations in "normal" occlusion in the dog. The so-called "scissor bite" (see following discussion) most closely represents the occlusion of the primitive dog.

The deciduous incisors and canines of the dog closely resemble their permanent replacements, although they are somewhat smaller in size and more pointed. In the mandibular arch the deciduous first premolar is not shed, the deciduous second premolar resembles the permanent fourth premolar, and the deciduous third premolar resembles the permanent first molar. In the maxillary arch the deciduous first premolar is a short single-cusped tooth that is not shed, the deciduous second premolar is similar to the permanent fourth premolar, and the deciduous third premolar resembles the first permanent molar. Even in the short-faced breeds, there are generally spaces between the deciduous teeth. Since growth adds considerably more in arch length as opposed to arch width, the arch form in the puppy tends to appear much shorter than in the adult.

In the adult dog with the typical scissor bite, the arch form tends to be rather long and narrow. The widest portion of the maxillary arch occurs in the fourth premolar–first molar region, while the mandibular arch tends to be more V-shaped, with the widest part in the third molar region. The maxillary canine tooth is caudal to the mandibular canine, which fits between the maxillary canine and the maxillary lateral incisor (Figure 82–5B). The lingual aspect of the incisal portion of the mandibular canine may come in contact with the medial aspect of the maxillary canine. The maxillary incisors slightly overlap the mandibular incisors (Figure 82–5A). The cusp tip of each of the mandibular premolars lies just rostral and medial to its maxillary counterpart. The maxillary first, second, and third premolars make no occlusal contact with the mandibular first, second, third, and fourth premolars. The large medial cusp of the mandibular first molar (the carnassial tooth) occludes just medial to the maxillary first molar (Figure 82–5C). The caudal cusp of the mandibular first molar occludes in the central fossa of the maxillary first molar, and the caudal cusps of the mandibular second molar occlude with the central fossa of the maxillary second molar.

Variations of the scissor bite are often seen in the incisor-canine area and also occur in the premolar-molar areas, but they are less obvious there. Some of the variations are due to the eruptive pattern of the teeth, while others are secondary to alterations in jaw size. When the mandibular incisors are caudal to the maxil-

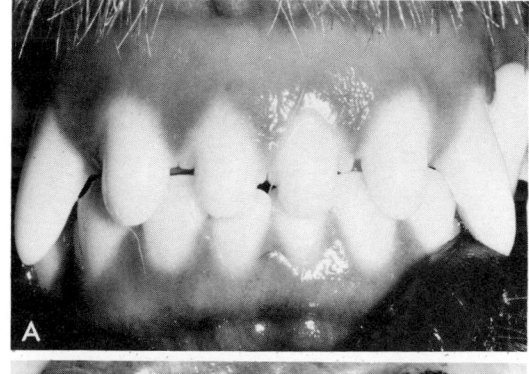
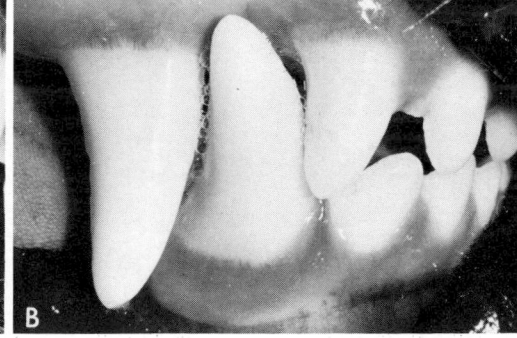
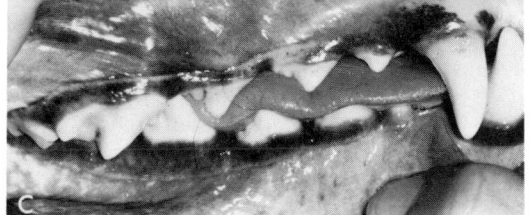

FIGURE 82–5. Normal occlusion in the dog. *A*, Incisor view. *B*, Canine-lateral incisor relationship. *C*, Canine-carnassial relationship.

lary incisors, so that they do not occlude with one another, the occlusion is termed retrognathic ("overshot"). When the incisal edge of the mandibular incisor is even with or rostral to the maxillary incisors, the occlusion is said to be prognathic ("undershot"). Short-faced (brachycephalic) breeds are often referred to as prognathic, although the abnormality is in fact brachygnathism of the upper jaw. As a result, crowding of the teeth is common. Collies and similar dolichocephalic long-nosed dogs often are retrognathic.

In the cat, the maxillary incisors slightly overlap the mandibular incisors. The mandibular canine occludes rostral to the maxillary canine, there is a large diastema between the canine and premolar teeth, and the first premolar teeth do not occlude. Shearing action occurs between the mandibular molar and the maxillary third premolar carnassial teeth.

Breeds in which a short face is desirable in the cat (such as Persian) may predispose to an undershot incisor tooth relationship.

Temporomandibular Joint. The mandible is a movable, suspended, bony component that articulates with the skull at the temporomandibular joint (TMJ). The right and left condyles of the mandible articulate with the temporal bone in the glenoid fossa. Interposed between the fossa and the condyles is the cartilaginous meniscus. The jaws are closed by the masticatory muscles (masseter, temporal, and lateral and medial pterygoid), innervated by the mandibular branch of the trigeminal nerve (C.N. V), and opened by the digastricus muscle (facial [C.N. VII] and trigeminal [C.N. V] nerves). The limits of TMJ movement are controlled by ligaments. Omnivorous animals classically have a large condyle, which permits rostral, caudal, and lateral movement. In the carnivorous dog and cat, which have shorter condyles with only limited lateral movement, the TMJ is limited largely to hinge-like movement. The condyle is cylindrical and rotates in a transversely extended glenoid cavity. The skulls of both dogs and cats show a well-developed sagittal crest and flared zygomatic arches, indicative of powerful jaw muscles. The mass of these muscles coupled with the low position of the condyle reduces the frequency of dislocation of this joint in dogs and cats.

Oropharynx

The limits of the oropharynx are poorly defined in the dog because of the length and mobility of the soft palate and the absence of well-defined arches or pillars seen in other animals. The palatine tonsils are paired lymph nodes lying on the lateral wall of the oropharynx within crypts formed by folds of the pharyngeal wall (Figure 82–6). They are elliptical in the dog, shorter and fatter in the cat. The tonsils of the dog are normally visible and in young dogs may stand out of their crypts. The tonsils of the cat are usually covered by the folds of epithelium forming the walls of the crypt.

Swallowing is a complex reflex action coordinating many muscles. The tongue is pulled caudally and dorsally, forcing the food or liquid bolus into the pharynx. The nasopharynx is constricted by the contraction of the

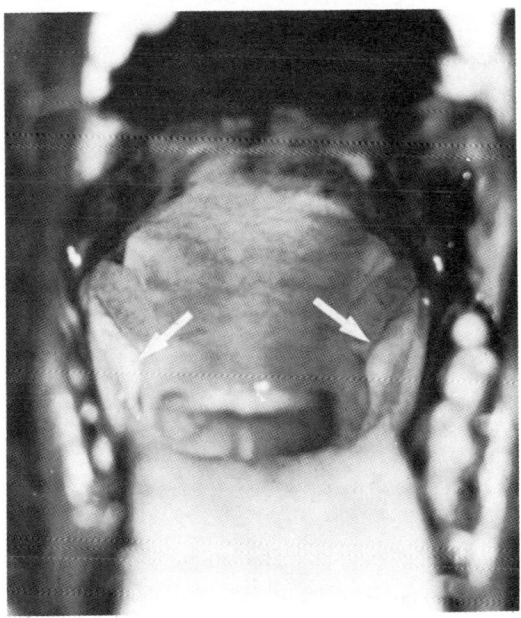

FIGURE 82–6. Pharynx of a normal dog. The tonsils are visible on the dorsolateral aspects of the oropharynx (arrows).

muscles of the soft palate and the walls and roof of the nasopharynx. The epiglottis is moved caudally while the glottis is restricted by adduction of the arytenoid cartilages and vocal folds. The muscles of the pharyngeal wall contract and the cricopharyngeal muscle relaxes, allowing the bolus to be pushed into the esophagus. The glossopharyngeal, vagus, and hypoglossal nerves are the main motor nerves involved in swallowing.

HISTORY AND METHODS OF EXAMINATION

Many factors influence the oral cavity and must be considered when evaluating signs of disease; these include high temperature, moisture, mechanical irritation, and normal oral bacterial population. The most common clinical signs of oropharyngeal disease are inappetence, halitosis, pawing at the mouth, excessive salivation, and retching. Excessive salivation, initially seromucous in consistency, often progresses to ropy, tenacious saliva, becoming blood-streaked if ulceration develops. Some animals may look at or pick up food, but they either do not swallow or have difficulty in swallowing. A slowly enlarging mass may be the only finding in more chronic diseases.

Systemic diseases may cause clinical signs related primarily to the oropharynx; therefore, a careful complete physical examination is essential in all animals with oropharyngeal disease.

Physical Examination. In a cooperative animal most of the oropharynx can be readily inspected or palpated. Examination of the oropharynx should be conducted in a consistent, systematic manner. Inspection and palpation should include the gingiva, teeth, tongue, lingual frenulum and floor of the mouth, the entire buccal surface, and the hard and soft palate. The normal oral mucosa may be pink or partially pigmented (especially

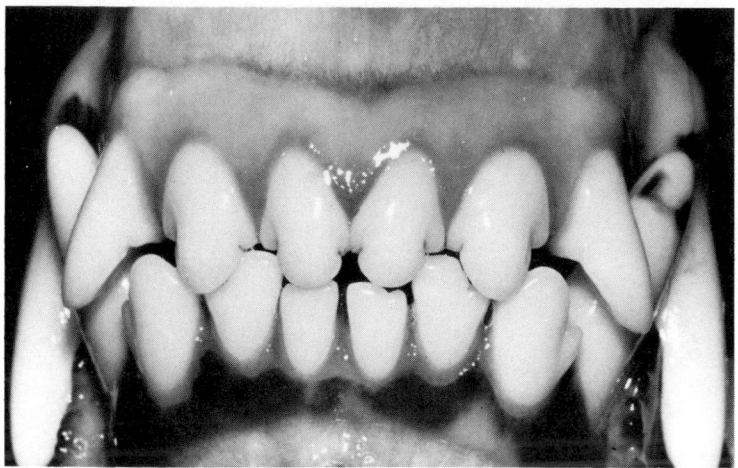

FIGURE 82–7. Normal gingiva in the mandibular arch of a dog, with a slightly hyperemic marginal gingiva in the maxillary arch. Note the pigmentation in the mandibular arch.

in dark-colored breeds) and appears smooth and glistening, with little or no accumulation of secretions (Figure 82–7). It is pliable when touched, and refill time is quick with no permanent blanching or hyperemia. Since response to touch varies with the animal's temperament, increased sensitivity is difficult to evaluate; however, a painful reaction should be obvious. It is preferable to examine the oral cavity while the animal is conscious to evaluate the function of the pertinent cranial nerves. Normally an animal will retch when the caudal pharynx is stimulated. Decreased sensitivity may be a manifestation of glossopharyngeal nerve dysfunction. In an uncooperative patient, observation of feeding, drinking, licking, and yawning must be supplemented by direct examination under anesthesia. A detailed dental examination requires a very cooperative patient or sedation. A dental explorer is used to examine crevices or other irregularities on the tooth surface for areas of softness; the use of the periodontal probe is described in the section on periodontal disease.

The breath of the dog and cat is not usually unpleasant; in the young puppy or kitten it has a characteristic milky smell. Alterations in the odor of the breath may indicate disease. In the ketoacidosis of severe diabetes and ethylene glycol poisoning, the breath may have a sweet, fruity smell. Foul-smelling breath may be caused by local disease (periodontal disease or stomatitis) or systemic disease (uremia, necrotic respiratory disease, or gastrointestinal disease). Food substances such as garlic cause halitosis. Patterns of dysphagia reported by the owner can be observed by offering the animal a small amount of highly palatable food.

Biopsy. Biopsy of oropharyngeal masses is usually a simple, quick procedure, and histopathologic examination can provide important information for treatment and prognosis. Cytologic examination of oral mucosal lesions is useful. Palpation of the cervical area, particularly lymph nodes, should be a routine part of the examination of the oropharynx.

A wide variety of bacteria as well as some fungal elements can be cultured from the oral cavity of a normal dog.[3] Bacterial or fungal smears or cultures are thus of limited value unless the specimen is taken from an area of obvious disease. *Pasteurella multocida* was present in the gingival area of 55 per cent of dogs and 80 per cent of cats studied; the strains isolated were generally sensitive to chloramphenicol and tetracycline, when treatment of an infected bite was necessary.[4]

Radiographic Examination. Lateral, ventrodorsal, and occlusal radiographs are useful to determine the presence of foreign bodies and to investigate the extent of masses in the head and neck, particularly those involving the jaws. Definitive information on the nature and location of swallowing abnormalities can be obtained from fluoroscopic visualization of a barium swallow examination.[5]

For radiographs of sections of a jaw or of individual teeth, the radiographic film should be placed parallel to the long axis of the tooth and perpendicular to the x-ray beam. However, for the upper jaw this is often not possible, and occlusal or oblique projection radiographs must be used. Dental pulp is considerably more radiolucent than dentin, which is less dense than the highly mineralized enamel covering the crown (Figure 82–8). The cementum covering the root is not sufficiently different in density from the dentin to be differentiated radiographically. The sockets of the individual teeth are

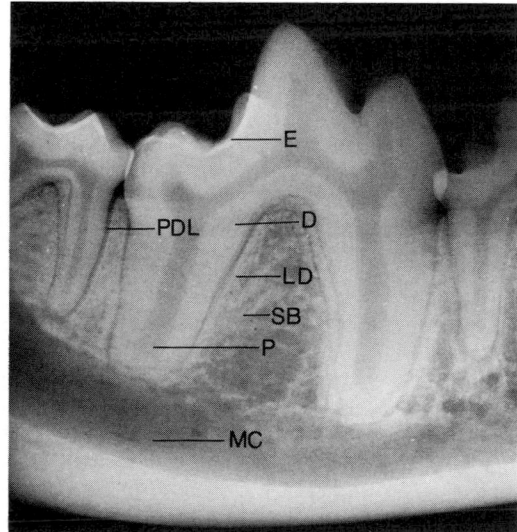

FIGURE 82–8. Radiograph of a normal tooth and mandible in a dog. D, dentin; E, enamel; LD, lamina dura; MC, mandibular canal; P, pulp; PDL, periodontal ligament; SB, supporting bone.

lined by the cortical alveolar bone (lamina dura), which is distinctly more radiopaque than the surrounding cancellous bone. Between the lamina dura and the root of the tooth is a radiolucent space, approximately 0.1 to 0.2 mm wide, containing the periodontal ligament. Between the teeth is a mass of cancellous supporting bone. The alveolar crest (the most coronal aspect of the supporting bone) is cortical and appears as a radiopaque line that is perpendicular to the lamina dura.[6]

Occasionally the roots of the teeth may be superimposed on the radiolucent mandibular canal. In the mandibular first and third premolar areas, the mental foramina can be seen; they may be confused with a periapical radiolucency but can be differentiated on an oblique projection radiograph. In radiographs of the maxillary arch, the nasal cavity and maxillary sinus recess can be seen in close proximity to the roots of the maxillary teeth. In young animals, the pulp cavity and apical foramina are large; as the animal matures, these structures decrease in relative size.[2]

DISEASES AFFECTING TOOTH STRUCTURE

Congenital Anomalies

ANODONTIA

Anodontia is the congenital absence of teeth, which is common in dogs and may be inherited.[7] The most common area for anodontia in dogs is the premolar region. Incisors are commonly absent in the cat.[8] Complete anodontia occurs very occasionally in the dog and cat. Acquired tooth loss may be confused with anodontia and is much more common, particularly in older dogs. A tooth may occasionally be buried in the gingiva, mimicking anodontia. Anodontia and acquired tooth loss do not require treatment other than providing the animals' food in a form that can be prehended and swallowed.

RETAINED DECIDUOUS TEETH

If the permanent tooth bud does not develop under the deciduous tooth, complete resorption of the roots will not occur and the deciduous tooth can be retained for the life of the animal. Retained deciduous teeth in the dog are most often seen with normal development of the permanent teeth. They occur most frequently in toy breeds and may cause displacement of the permanent teeth. Incisor and canine teeth are most commonly affected (Figure 82–9A). The retained deciduous tooth is usually rostral (incisor) or caudolateral (canine) to the erupting permanent tooth; it is narrower and has a sharper point. Extraction should be performed immediately if there is abnormal positioning of the erupting permanent tooth (Figure 82–9B). The condition is seen occasionally in the cat.[9]

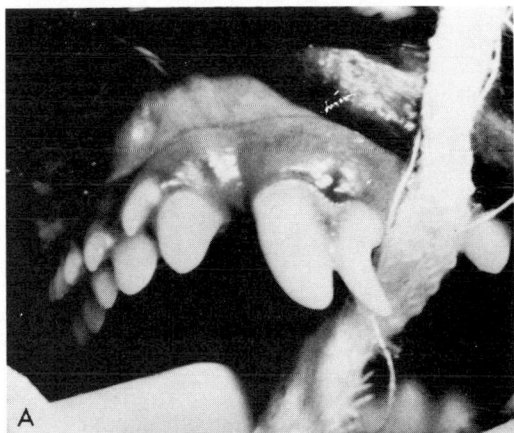
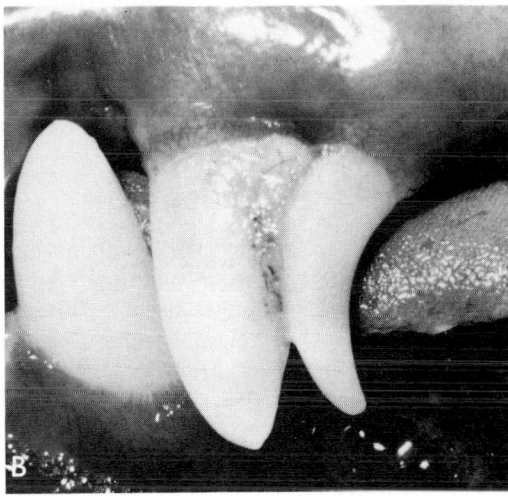

FIGURE 82–9. *A*, Retained incisor and canine teeth in the maxilla of a dog. *B*, Retained maxillary deciduous canine with accumulation of plaque and resultant soft tissue inflammation.

SUPERNUMERARY TEETH

Additional permanent teeth may erupt into occlusion and may result in crowding and rotation of teeth in the dog. This condition is common in the dog, particularly in spaniels, hounds, and greyhounds; the teeth most often involved are the premolars. The distance between the teeth may allow the presence of supernumerary teeth without secondary disease. The extra teeth should be extracted if there is crowding and periodontal health is jeopardized. Supernumerary teeth are also occasionally seen in the cat. Bizarre odontomas, with large numbers of formed or partly formed teeth (Figure 82–10), are very rare; they may cause externally obvious distortion of the jaw.

IMPACTION

Teeth that do not erupt out of the alveolar bone or the soft tissue are considered impacted. If root formation is still progressing, uncovering these teeth surgically may allow them to erupt correctly, although this situation is rarely recognized in the dog or cat. If root formation is

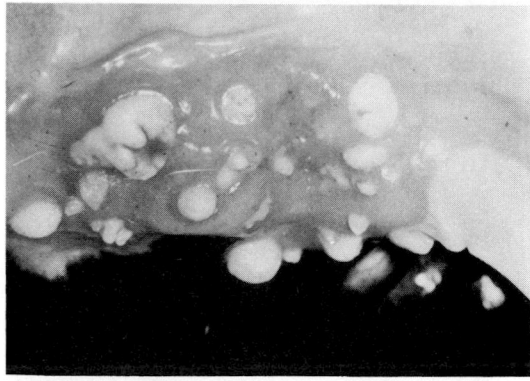

FIGURE 82–10. Multiple supernumerary teeth arising from a complex odontoma in the maxilla of a dog.

complete, no treatment is necessary. Extraction should be performed if partial impaction exists, so as to minimize the likelihood of periodontal abscess.

ABNORMALITIES IN THE SHAPE OF TEETH

Fusion of roots and abnormal crown shapes occur occasionally but are usually of no clinical significance. Dens in dente is a rare anomaly caused by invagination of the enamel organ into the dental papilla during tooth formation, forming a tooth within a tooth. There is communication between the oral environment and the enamel-lined cavity, visible directly or on radiographs as an irregular superimposed enamel density. If detected early, a restoration can be sealed into the opening so that infection will not enter the pulp cavity.

Acquired Dental Disease

ENAMEL HYPOPLASIA

Enamel hypoplasia occurs as a result of disruption during enamel formation in utero or shortly after birth, usually caused by canine distemper infection.[10, 11] The lesions appear as white opaque areas or brown-stained irregularities or depressions in the enamel of the crown (Figure 82–11). In those rare instances in which the enamel becomes soft owing to caries, it should be

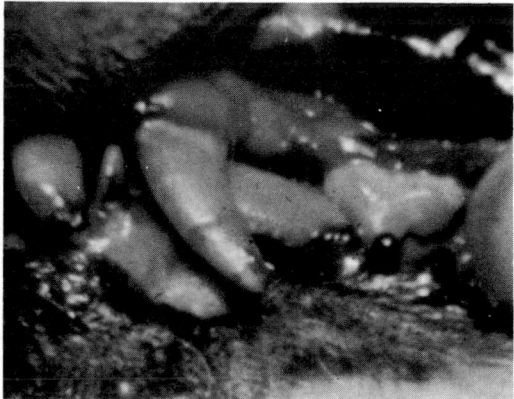

FIGURE 82–11. Enamel hypoplasia and tetracycline enamel staining in the permanent teeth of a dog.

restored before pulpal disease occurs. Enamel hypoplasia is an acquired disease; as such, it is ethical to correct the aesthetic abnormality by resin restoration.

TETRACYCLINE STAINING

If tetracycline is administered during tooth development, the tetracycline bonds with calcium in the dentin and enamel, creating a permanent discoloration of the teeth, which appear yellow-orange or brown (Figure 82–11).[12] Tetracycline should not be administered before dogs and cats are five months old or to pregnant females, as maternal transfer has been demonstrated. Although bleaching techniques have been used successfully in humans, veterinary use has not been reported.

DENTAL CARIES

Caries is the destruction of tooth structure caused by carbohydrate-fermenting bacteria, producing acids that attack the surfaces they contact. Caries, which is always initiated from the external environment, can be observed in the enamel, or if periodontal disease has caused recession, on an exposed root in the cementum. Dental caries in dogs is uncommon,[13] although not all surveys agree with this conclusion. The incidence is low because the diet is usually low in fermentable carbohydrates; the structure of the teeth is such that they are self-cleaning; the fissures of the crowns are often exposed to an abrasive diet, which keeps them clean; there are no true pits that permit retention of food and bacteria except in the maxillary molar teeth, which are the teeth most often carious; the interproximal spaces between teeth are not food traps, as is seen in species with higher caries indices; and the composition of saliva in dogs is not conducive to developing a cariogenic flora. The pH of saliva of carnivores is alkaline, which tends to neutralize oral acids.[14]

An attempt was made to develop caries in normal dogs by drilling holes in the enamel surface, placing the animals on high-sucrose diets, removing the major salivary glands, and injecting lactobacilli into the oral cavity. However, this failed to produce carious lesions.[15]

When seen in dogs, caries occurs where plaque accumulates, usually in animals that are fed soft food diets that are high in fermentable carbohydrate concentration. Plaque accumulates in the gingival sulcus of animals with periodontal disease, allowing root caries to penetrate through the cementum into dentin. Difficulty in eating, refusal of hard food, holding the head to one side, and teeth chattering are clinical signs associated with dental caries.

Careful clinical observation using a dental explorer can detect caries in its early stages. The lesion is usually dark brown and soft, which differentiates it from exposed stained dentin. Enamel and dentin cannot repair themselves; the diseased tissue must be removed and restored with an appropriate filling material. The deeper that caries extends into the dentin, the greater the inflammation in the dental pulp. Repair by the pulp can occur; however, persistent, deeper caries can directly

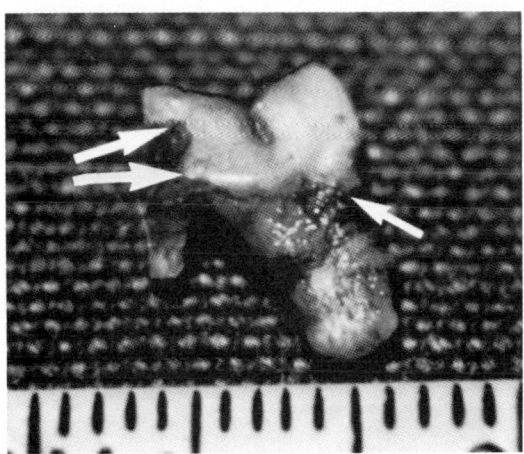

FIGURE 82–12. Lower first molar tooth of a cat with neck lesions (arrows).

infect the pulp, leading to necrosis and eventual abscess or cyst formation. At this point, endodontic therapy or extraction is indicated.

Lesions that superficially appear to be caries occur commonly in cats. These "neck lesions" (Figure 82–12) are areas of external odontoclastic resorption (see below).

TRAUMA

Fracture. Dogs and cats are both prone to fracture of the teeth. Fractures were observed in 27.4 per cent of dogs examined; the incisor teeth were most frequently involved, although canine or carnassial (Figure 82–13) tooth fractures may be more noticeable to the owner. The causes are probably external trauma or activities such as stone chewing or catching. Enamel is a crystalline structure and is easily cleaved if struck. If the fracture is only of the enamel layer, no treatment is necessary. If the fracture extends into the dentin, inflammation occurs in the pulp and odontoblasts synthesize reparative dentin, insulating the pulp. If a fracture extends into the dental pulp, endodontic treatment or extraction is indicated to prevent endodontic disease and alveolar bone abscessation.

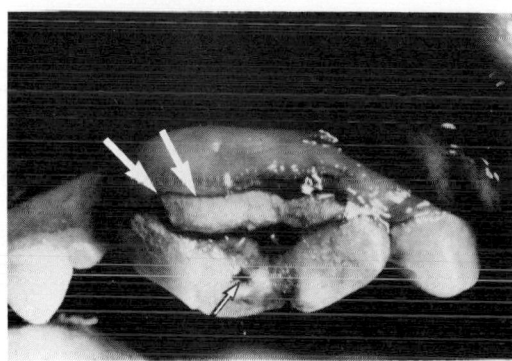

FIGURE 82–13. Fracture of a maxillary carnassial tooth, with exposure of the pulp cavity (single arrow) and a separate slab fracture of enamel (double arrow).

Avulsion. Partial or total avulsion of a tooth from the jaw results in disruption of the periodontal ligament and pulp tissue (Figure 82–14). If the owner desires it for aesthetic reasons, the tooth should be repositioned as quickly as possible to attempt to preserve the vitality of the periodontal ligament. If the tooth is firm after being replanted, no splint is necessary; an acid etch composite splint is a useful technique for splinting loose teeth. In those areas where vitality of the periodontal ligament is lost, ankylosis of the bone to the cementum may occur. The usual sequela of ankylosis is external resorption by osteoclasts, which invade the root surface from the alveolar bone.

If avulsion occurs in a tooth with an incompletely formed apical foramen, regeneration of pulpal tissue may occur; this can be monitored through radiographic examination. If avulsion occurs in a tooth with a mature root apex, endodontic therapy should be performed before the tooth is repositioned, or within two weeks of emergency splinting.

Allogenic tooth transplantation can be used for aesthetically important teeth, although external root resorption and ankylosis are likely to result in fracture after about 24 months have elapsed even if endodontic treatment has been performed.[16]

Internal and External Resorption. Either of these two phenomena may occur if the pulp is traumatized and osteoclastic cells destroy the hard tooth structure. Internal resorption occurs at the expense of dentin inside the tooth; it can be stopped by removing the pulp tissue and performing endodontic therapy. External resorption occurs by action of osteoclasts in the alveolar bone. It can sometimes be stopped by endodontic therapy, but the prognosis is not as predictable because the alveolar bone may still supply osteoclasts. Loss of the tooth will eventually occur if external resorption continues. Calcium hydroxide is used in endodontic therapy to change the environmental pH and thus eliminate osteoclasts, with some success in preventing resorption.

Attrition. Attrition or occlusal wear is caused by feeding a coarse diet, or activities such as catching or carrying a stone or stick (Figures 82–15 and 82–16). Wearing of the incisal edges or biting surfaces of the teeth is physiologic to a certain point. It is commonly seen in the incisor teeth of dogs and cats.[17] If the wear extends only into the dentin, no treatment is necessary. Wear occurs slowly enough to allow the pulp to establish reparative dentin, which is seen as a brown spot that does not accept the tip of a dental explorer. If the tooth structure is worn away and vital pulp is exposed or if the pulp dies and abscess formation occurs (Figure 82–17), extraction or endodontic therapy is indicated. Dogs that are kept in metal cages often chew on the bars; the external surface of the incisors or canines of these dogs are often stained with metal, usually aluminum.

CARNASSIAL ABSCESS (MALAR ABSCESS, FACIAL SINUS)

Carnassial abscess is a soft fluctuant swelling or draining sinus on the side of the face just below the medial canthus of the eye. The fistula occasionally drains into

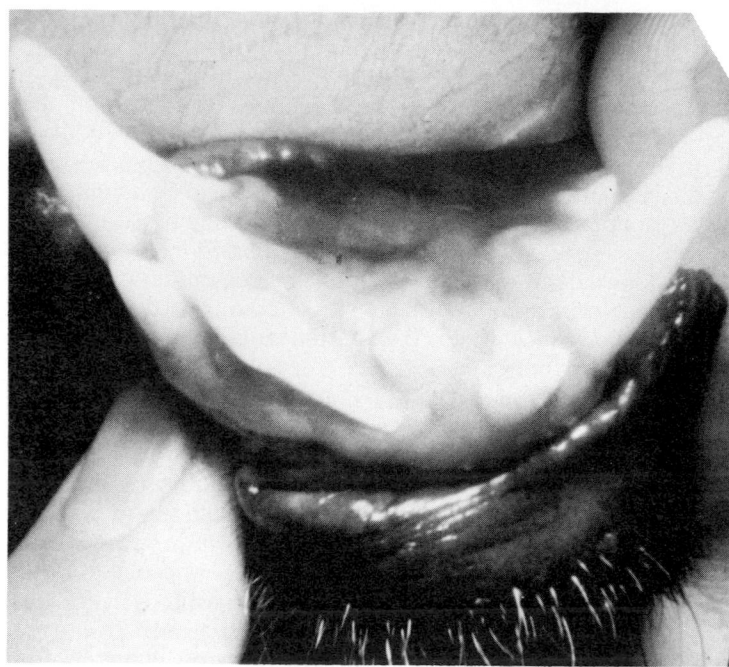

FIGURE 82–14. Effects of trauma to the mandible. Two incisor teeth are fractured, one is avulsed with the entire root exposed, and one is missing.

the oral cavity and rarely into the orbit.[18] It is a common condition in middle-aged and old dogs, and is also seen in the cat. Clinical signs are usually confined to the swelling or draining fistula. The discharge is often not purulent. Carnassial abscess is also seen, although much less frequently, in the mandible. The fistula drains onto the skin or into the oral cavity ventral to the lower carnassial tooth.[19]

The swelling or fistula is caused by necrosis of the alveolar bone over one of the roots of the upper carnassial (fourth premolar) tooth or lower carnassial (first molar) tooth. Intermittent concussion from chewing on sticks or bones, fracture of the tooth, and periodontal disease are probably contributing factors; however, the carnassial tooth and surrounding gingiva may appear normal. Radiographs usually show a radiolucent area around the root, indicating a periodontal abscess or apical cyst (Figure 82–18).

Treatment consists of either extraction of the carnassial tooth and establishment of drainage from the exter-

nal lesion to the tooth socket or endodontic treatment of the involved root. Recovery following extraction is usually uneventful, but occasionally complications occur owing to local extension of the inflammatory process, such as parotid duct injury, chronic maxillary osteomyelitis, or sinusitis. Good long-term results following endodontic treatment have been described.[20]

ENDODONTIC DISEASE

Endodontic disease results from crown fracture with pulpal exposure, carious erosion, or extension from periodontal disease, allowing infection to enter the pulp cavity. Pulpal exposure was seen in one or more teeth in ten per cent of dogs in one study.[17] With chronic diseases such as caries or periodontal disease, which stimulate the odontoblastic processes, the odontoblasts may have time to synthesize reparative dentin. When the pulp is exposed, an inflammatory process occurs,

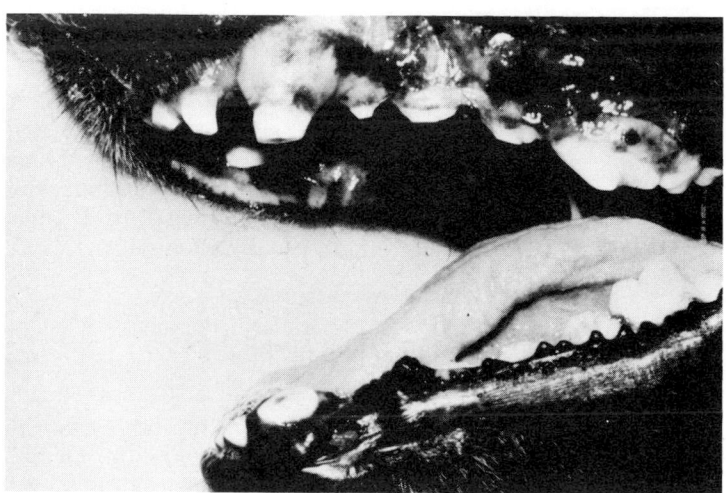

FIGURE 82–15. Severe attrition of the maxillary and mandibular incisor, canine, and premolar teeth in a dog. Brown-stained reparative dentin is visible in both canine teeth.

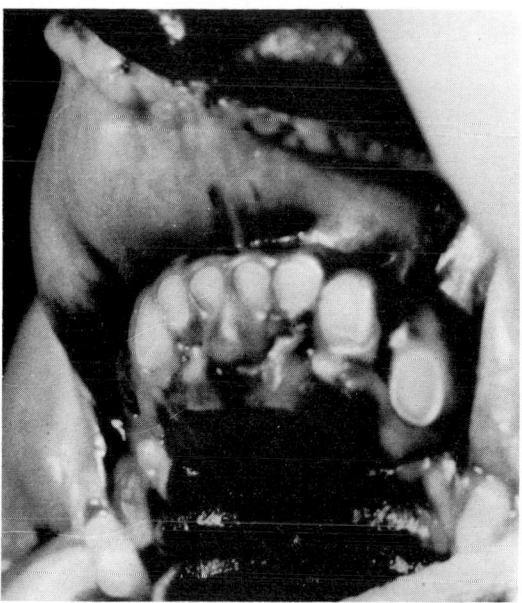

FIGURE 82–16. Extreme attrition of the maxillary incisor teeth in a dog caused by constant gnawing at hard surfaces.

which, because the pulp is contained within a noncompliant tooth structure, usually causes pulpal necrosis. Bacteria remain and their toxins spread through the apical foramina. An inflammatory response occurs around the apex of the tooth in an attempt to localize the spread of the infection.

An acute periapical abscess is associated with liquefaction necrosis and severe pain. The polymorphonuclear leukocytes release lysosomal enzymes, pus is formed quickly, and pressure builds. The purulent debris must seek release through either the root canal or fistula; otherwise, it will create local swelling as pus enters other

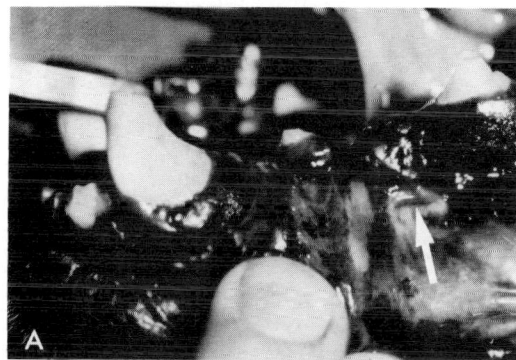

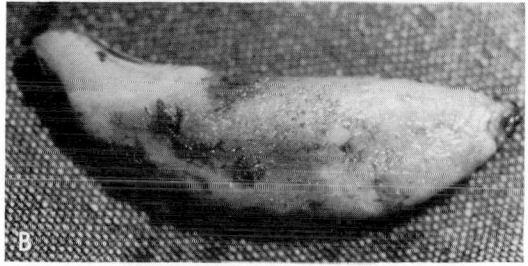

FIGURE 82–17. *A*, Fistula (arrow) from the root of a mandibular canine tooth with attritional exposure of the pulp cavity. *B*, Extracted canine tooth showing the size of the root relative to the crown

fascial planes. If a fistula forms or drainage occurs through the root canal, a chronic state is attained. Endodontic therapy or extraction of the tooth will reverse this process.

An acute abscess may enter a quiescent stage, referred to as a chronic abscess or granuloma, which is recognized by tenderness or reluctance to eat, or may be asymptomatic. Dental radiographs demonstrate the encapsulated area of periapical radiolucency. Histologically, round cell infiltration can be observed with connective tissue encapsulation of the inflamed area. Extraction or endodontic therapy is the treatment of choice. If endodontic therapy is started, a change in the equilibrium between tissue resistance and infection may cause a painful acute abscess, which can usually be controlled with antibiotic treatment.

An apical cyst may also form (Figure 82–19). The epithelial cell rests of Malassez are activated to line the fluid-filled cavity in the bone. Extraction or endodontic therapy is the treatment of choice. If endodontic treatment cannot create an environment for the body to heal, surgical removal of the cyst is necessary.

Endodontic disease can lead to cellulitis, recognized by clinical signs of fever, malaise, and pain and edema in surrounding soft tissues. Systemic antibiotics (such as ampicillin, 10 mg/lb orally four times per day) should be started immediately, with drainage of the area of infection locally if practical.

Diagnosis of an inflamed or necrotic pulp is sometimes difficult. Dogs appear to have a high pain threshold; they will often be unresponsive to situations that cause obvious pain in humans. They may first have pain with an exposed pulp, but this disappears when the pulp becomes necrotic. The pulp exposure can be observed clinically if the nerve has just been exposed or radiographically if the inflammation has reached the periapical area and developed into an abscess or cyst. The animal may become lethargic, favor one side of its mouth, stop eating, or stop performing normally. The tooth may appear discolored, loose, chipped, or cracked. If the dentin is exposed, one should look for exposure of the root canal, which appears as a dark spot or area of hemorrhage in the center of the tooth. A fistula may be present, extending to the skin or oral mucosal surface. If no discoloration or void in the enamel is noted and radiographic observation demonstrates a radiolucent area, differential diagnosis should include superimposition of a normal anatomic landmark.

ENDODONTIC THERAPY. Endodontic therapy is indicated as an alternative to extraction when disease has penetrated the dental pulp cavity and is causing pain or fistulization, or is spreading infection; or it may be used to prevent endodontic disease when the pulp cavity has been penetrated by trauma or external disease. The object is to remove the source of infection and seal off the root canal so that there is no tract from the oral environment to the bone. Infection already present in the alveolar bone is dealt with by normal body defense mechanisms.

A pulpotomy can be performed if treatment occurs immediately after traumatic exposure of the pulp. The dental pulp is removed in the coronal portion of the tooth, and a medicated dressing is placed over the tissue

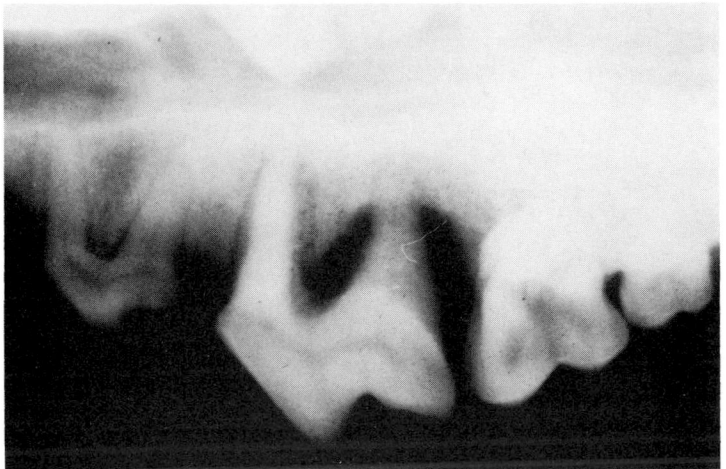

FIGURE 82–18. Radiograph showing extensive bone loss around the roots of a maxillary carnassial tooth in a dog with a carnassial abscess.

remaining in the root canal. Although it is not a procedure with predictable results, it is quick and can be performed under short-acting anesthesia or sedation. Calcium hydroxide is the material of choice to place over the remaining vital pulp tissue. If used in the form of a self-setting caulk (such as Dy-Cal), it can be covered immediately by a permanent filling.

More elaborate endodontic procedures must be carefully considered as an alternative to extraction for more chronic or severe disease, since dogs and cats can function well without their teeth. Probably the most common indication for endodontic therapy is fracture of the canine tooth in police or guard dogs. Maintaining function of these expensive dogs often requires intact canine teeth. Endodontic therapy will allow the carnassial tooth to be saved in dogs with carnassial abscess. Other patients in which extraction of teeth with acquired lesions may be contraindicated are show dogs and dogs whose owners desire to maintain their animals' dentition for aesthetic reasons. The techniques involved in performing endodontic therapy are adapted from those used for humans; general anesthesia is mandatory. Particularly for canine teeth, long endodontic files designed for veterinary use are essential.[21] The object is to cleanse the pulp cavity without irritation to the bone, using surgically clean technique to obtain an aseptic root canal.[22] Detailed descriptions of root canal treatment techniques are available elsewhere.[23]

Restorative Dentistry

Composite polymers that bond to an etched enamel surface are suitable for the repair of minor fractures, abrasions, chipped enamel surfaces, and enamel hypoplasia. The composites can also be used to splint teeth that have been loosened as a result of trauma or periodontal disease; the loose teeth can be bonded together or to adjacent firm teeth to gain stability, particularly in the incisor region. Detailed descriptions of acid-etch-composite resin bonding are available elsewhere.[23] The composites can be reinforced with pins placed into the tooth. This technique requires a dental handpiece and appropriate drills.[23, 24]

When a tooth is severely fractured and its maintenance is important for either aesthetic or functional purposes, the restoration of choice is a full crown of cast steel or, if aesthetics are a particular concern, porcelain veneer. The restoration requires two procedures. Under general anesthesia, endodontic treatment can be performed if necessary, the tooth is prepared for the crown, an impression is taken, and a temporary crown is fabricated. The temporary crown can be deleted

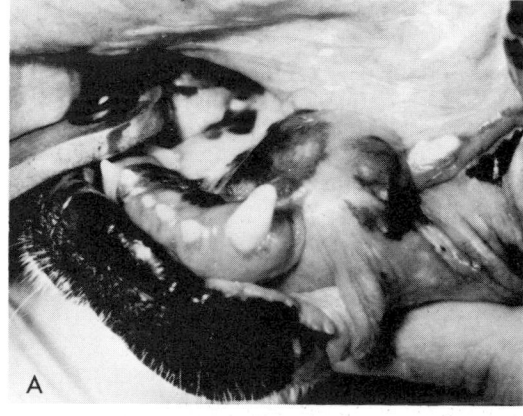
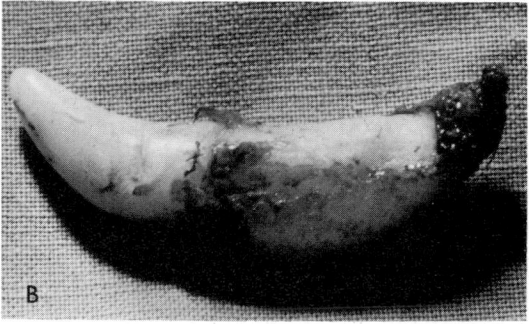

FIGURE 82–19. A, Cyst at the apex of a mandibular canine. The etiology is unknown, but the condition is most likely due to trauma and subsequent pulp death. B, The extracted canine with part of the cyst still attached to the root apex.

if the tooth is nonvital. At a second procedure, under sedation, the finished crown is fitted and cemented in place. Large canine tooth restorations are subject to considerable force and may break subsequently; restoration with a custom-made steel post and crown is recommended.

Replacement of missing teeth is possible, although rarely indicated. In most cases some type of fixed restoration can be fabricated; however, bridge techniques for replacement of an incisor tooth crown have been described.[25]

THE JAWS

The jaws are subject to conditions affecting bone in general, such as fractures resulting from trauma, neoplasms (although most neoplasms affecting the maxilla or mandible are soft tissue tumors invading bone), and disturbances in bone structure caused by nutritional deficiencies or metabolic disturbances. Bone weakness caused by renal secondary hyperparathyroidism is particularly evident in the maxilla and mandible, causing rubber jaw disease (see Hyperparathyroidism, Chapter 94).

Malocclusion

Normal occlusion was described earlier. Variations from the normal occlusal scheme for a particular dog or cat can be the result of a genetic defect or of various local factors. Local factors include deciduous teeth that have been retained, causing a displacement of the permanent teeth; malocclusion of the deciduous dentition that impedes the normal forward growth of the mandible; ectopia of one or more of the permanent teeth; and trauma to the teeth or jaws during development. Malocclusion can also result from orthopedic management of jaw fractures.[26] Correct characterization of jaw relationships requires observation of all the cuspal landmarks.

The correction of occlusal deformities to allow an animal to conform to breed specifications for breeding or show purposes is unethical. An orthodontic procedure should be performed only if there is medical need for correction or if one is convinced that the deformity is acquired. There is no satisfactory way of determining if a congenital defect is inherited in a particular animal presented for correction. Radiographs may suggest the possibility of neonatal fracture.

Very few occlusal problems are detrimental to the well-being of the animal. Although it is conceivable that severe crowding of the teeth can predispose to periodontal disease (Figure 82–20), problems of this type can be managed initially by attempting to control plaque (see Periodontal Therapy). On occasion, a tooth may be in a position that results in trauma to the soft tissues in the opposite arch when the animal closes its mouth. Depending on the functional and aesthetic significance of the tooth, it can be significantly reduced in size by grinding away tooth structure with a dental handpiece,

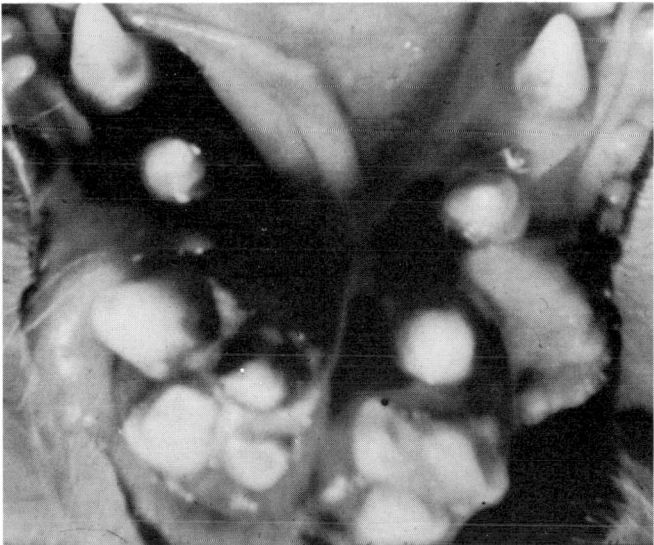

FIGURE 82–20. Crowding of the mandibular incisor teeth in a dog, contributing to an unhealthy periodontium.

it can be repositioned orthodontically, or it can be extracted.

Prevention of normal occlusion by impaction of a tooth in an abnormal position against another tooth occurs in a wide variety of breeds of dogs. The teeth most frequently involved are the canine and lateral incisors. Extraction or orthodontic therapy can be used to correct this condition. With the new dental materials that allow orthodontic brackets to bond directly to enamel surfaces, thus precluding the need for orthodontic bands, tooth movement is now much more feasible in the small animal than it was several years ago. Within the framework of skeletal patterns there is no limit to what can be accomplished orthodontically. In general, movements that require a tooth to be tipped can be done much more easily than movements that require a tooth to be moved bodily. If orthodontic treatment is attempted, it is imperative that the dentition be kept immaculately clean during therapy, since the combination of orthodontic pressures and periodontal inflammation can cause rapid periodontal breakdown.[27]

Most occlusal therapy falls within the category of interceptive orthodontics: recognition and early management of retained deciduous teeth and malocclusions of the deciduous dentition that may preclude normal growth and management of supernumerary teeth can prevent severe orthodontic problems. More severe lesions (Figure 82–21) require orthopedic correction; appropriate techniques have been described.[23, 28] Acrylic splints are particularly adaptable for repairing the mandible or maxilla.[29]

Mandibular Neuropraxia

Mandibular neuropraxia ("dropped jaw") is seen occasionally in the dog.[30, 31] These dogs present with the jaw hanging down symmetrically; the mouth can be closed easily by the owner or veterinarian, but when the jaw is released, it drops to its former position. Tongue

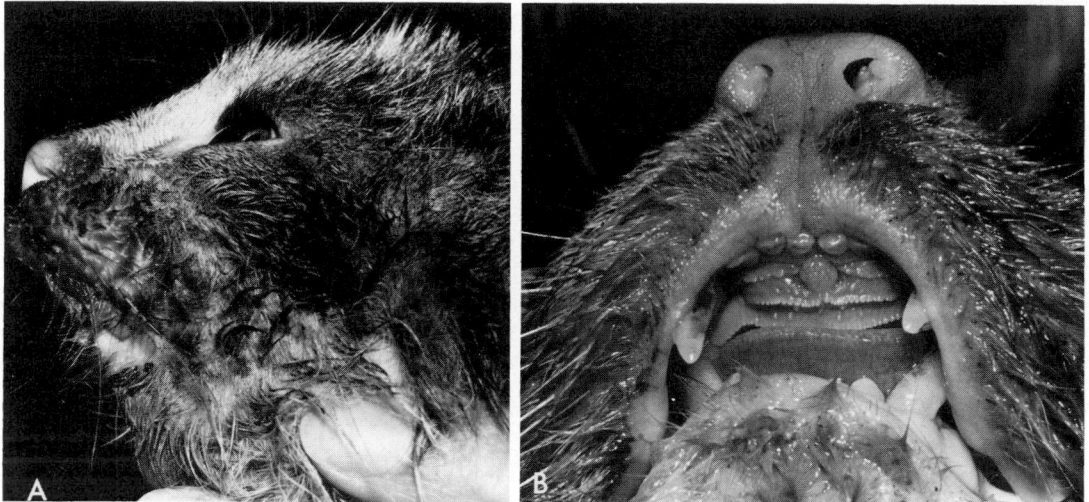

FIGURE 82–21. *A* and *B*, Cat with severe retrognathism causing constant drooling.

movement is normal, but because of the abnormal jaw position, swallowing is difficult. There is often a history of recent mechanical influences on the mouth, such as trauma or weight carrying. The condition is assumed to be due to abnormal stretching of the mandibular branch of the trigeminal nerve (C.N. V) that has caused paralysis of the masticatory muscles. Full recovery occurs over a three-week period; the only treatment necessary is to place a loose bandage around the muzzle to support the jaw while allowing imbibition of food of a soupy consistency.

Temporomandibular Joint Abnormalities

Temporomandibular joint luxation due to trauma occurs occasionally in the cat and infrequently in the dog. The animal has a dropped jaw that is painful on manipulation. The luxation is usually unilateral, causing asymmetry of position. An incorrect diagnosis of mandibular fracture may be made unless careful manipulation and radiographic examination are carried out.[32] TM luxation in a cat possibly caused by gross calculus deposition was treated successfully by teeth cleaning.[33] The luxation can usually be reduced under anesthesia by closing the jaws while placing a wooden or plastic rod across the carnassial teeth.[34] An alternative technique uses a Steinmann pin passed through the mandible at the junction of the horizontal and vertical rami; with a Jacob's chuck attached to the pin as a handle, the jaw can be manipulated as necessary.[35]

Temporomandibular subluxation or dysplasia has been reported in young Irish setters and bassett hounds, in which it has been observed in multiple members of a litter.[36, 37] It has also been described in Boxer, Labrador, and golden retriever dogs.[38] When the mouth is opened fully, the coronoid process of the mandible on one side becomes locked lateral to the zygomatic arch. In some dogs, the locking condition corrects itself spontaneously. Treatment by resecting part of the ventral aspect of the zygomatic arch avoids further locking episodes, or condylectomy can be used for permanent correction.[38]

Mandibular condylectomy has been used as treatment of dogs and cats with temporomandibular joint disease with very good clinical results.[39, 40]

Craniomandibular osteopathy (see Chapter 121) may become severe enough to prevent the jaws from opening normally. This condition, which classically occurs in young West Highland white terriers but is seen in other breeds also, is a proliferative disease of unknown cause affecting the bones of the base of the skull and mandible.[41]

PERIODONTAL DISEASE

Periodontal disease is the general term used to denote diseases of the periodontium (gingiva, periodontal ligament, alveolar bone, and cemental surface of the tooth). It includes gingivitis (acute and chronic), periodontitis, and periodontal abscess. Periodontal disease is by far the most common oral disease found in all species studied, and is arguably the most common disease condition seen in small animal practice.

There have been several studies that have examined the prevalence and severity of periodontal disease in the dog and cat,[42–46] and there is little doubt that the prevalence of periodontal disease approaches 95 per cent in animals over two years of age. Although in many cases the disease is confined to the soft tissues of the periodontium, loss of osseous support (periodontitis) is common; periodontitis was found in 50 to 80 per cent of dogs.[17, 47] Certain breeds, particularly small dogs such as poodles, had a higher incidence; others such as German shepherd dogs had a lower incidence.[45, 46] Marked differences have been found also in the incidence and severity of periodontal disease in members of a single breed, the beagle, which has been studied extensively because of its common use in dental research laboratories.[44, 48]

The severity of periodontal disease correlates with the quantity of plaque and calculus present on the teeth as well as with the age of the animal.[17] Plaque and calculus, however, have an independent effect on the severity of the disease.[43] Calculus is not seen to any great extent in animals less than nine months of age. The initial deposits of calculus occur in the region of the parotid duct (the buccal surfaces of the maxillary molars) and on the lingual surfaces of the mandibular caudal teeth.[42]

A number of studies have shown a relationship between consistency of food consumed and periodontal disease. For the most part these studies indicate that soft diet correlates positively with periodontal disease.[17, 49, 50]

The relationship between nutrition and periodontal disease is less clear. Dogs on a calcium-deficient (or low Ca:P ratio) diet can develop periodontitis at an early age and in severe form,[51-53] although there is no increased incidence of gingivitis in these animals.[52] This topic is discussed further under Periodontitis.

Periodontal disease in cats differs in some significant ways from that seen in dogs. For this reason, the disease in the two species is considered separately here.

Gingivitis

Etiology. Numerous experiments on dogs have demonstrated that dental plaque is the primary etiologic factor responsible for gingivitis. Plaque is found on the tooth surface, both subgingivally in the sulcus and supragingivally in the area coronal to the gingival margin.[54, 55]

Supragingival plaque formation begins with adhesion of bacteria to an acid glycoprotein pellicle that precipitates from the saliva onto the enamel surfaces. The plaque mass increases in size through a combination of multiplication of the original organisms and deposition of new organisms onto the plaque. Plaque consists of approximately 80 per cent water and 20 per cent organic and inorganic solids; approximately 80 per cent of the solid portion is bacteria. The organisms produce a matrix consisting largely of polysaccharide protein complexes. Plaque is not a food residue. Diet does, however, play a significant role in the formation and maturation of the plaque. A soft diet induces more plaque formation and higher levels of gingivitis than does a hard diet in dogs.[49, 57] The relative proportions of carbohydrates, protein, and fat do not quantitatively alter plaque formation.[57] Significant plaque formation occurs in dogs fed through a tube.[58]

The microbiology of plaque associated with gingivitis is complex. Various cocci, filaments, spirochetes, and rods are found, including facultative and anaerobic organisms. The specific organisms predominating in the dog are gram-negative anaerobes.[59]

Plaque is a soft, colorless mass not readily seen by the naked eye unless it either is naturally stained by dietary constituents or is extremely thick. It can be demonstrated by plaque-disclosing dyes, the most common of which are erythrosin (FDC Red #3) and fluorescein (FDC Yellow #8). The latter requires an ultraviolet light source to cause the dye to fluoresce; however, it is more specific for the bacterial components of the plaque than is erythrosin.[60]

The accumulation of plaque is enhanced by the presence of surface irregularities, the most common of which is calculus (Figure 82–22), a mass of calcium salts precipitated from saliva. Calculus appears in both supragingival and subgingival locations and is most typically off-white, yellow, or brown. The plaque-retentive characteristics of calculus are more important than its effect as a mechanical irritant. It has been shown that endotoxins from plaque may be found in calculus. In at least one study the formation of calculus in a colony of beagles was not found to be related to diet consistency.[50] Hair or food impaction in the gingival sulcus and hypoplastic or other roughened surfaces on the enamel in the vicinity of the gingival margin exacerbate plaque retention and gingivitis (Figure 82–23). When gingivitis has been present for a significant period of time, architectural changes in the gingiva, particularly hyperplasia, also aid in the retention of plaque. Not only does the deepened pocket create an area for plaque to accumulate but also it has been suggested that the environment within the pocket is more supportive of the gram-negative pathogens that are associated with subsequent periodontal breakdown.

Gingival hyperplasia caused by the anticonvulsant sodium diphenylhydantoin, which occurs in man, has been produced experimentally in the cat,[61] and has been reported in the dog.[62]

Clinical Manifestations. Gingivitis is manifested clinically by a change in the color of the marginal gingiva

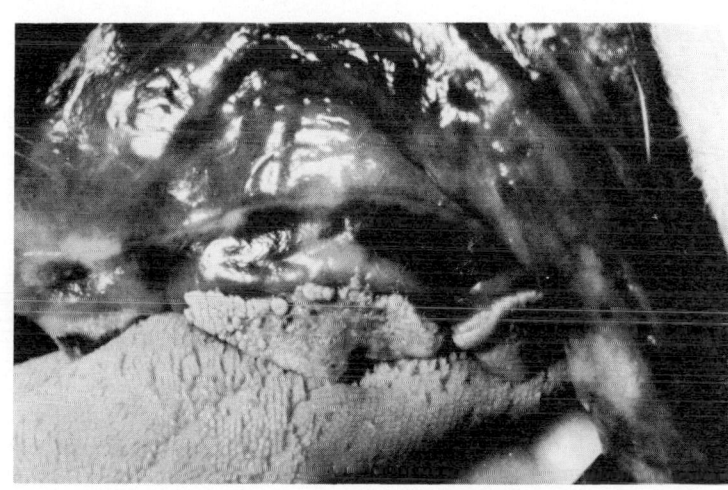

FIGURE 82–22. Calculus on the lateral aspect of a maxillary carnassial tooth in a dog.

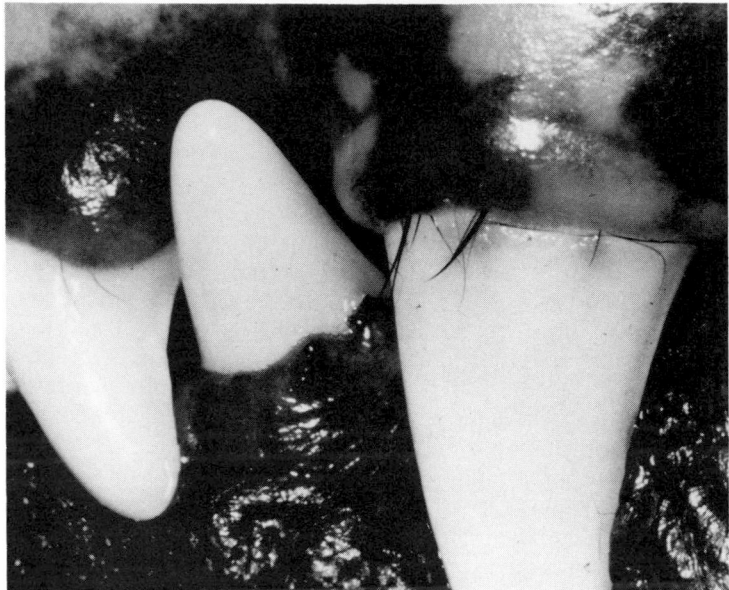

FIGURE 82–23. Hair impaction under the free gingival margin of a dog. The hair is acting as a matrix for calculus formation.

(when not masked by pigmentation) (Figure 82–24). This reddening is usually accompanied by a blunting of the free gingival margin (FGM), so that the previously knife-like FGM becomes more bulky and rolled (see Figure 82–25). In some animals the gingiva becomes hyperplastic (Figure 82–26) and the FGM may be five to six mm coronal to its normal position, covering a substantial portion of the crown (see Gingival Hyperplasia). The gentle insertion of a thin blunt-tipped periodontal probe calibrated in millimeters into the sulcus indicates the depth from the FGM to the point where the probe stops in the inflamed subsulcular connective tissue; this dimension is normally one to three mm. The increase in depth noted in an animal with gingivitis reflects the coronal movement of the FGM. Loss of soft tissue integrity of the sulcular and junctional epithelium as well as the underlying connective tissue allows the probe to pass apical to the soft tissue attach-

ment. Because the probe passes through the epithelial tissue, it is not uncommon for blood to exude from the sulcus during probing. As a result of the underlying inflammation, thin, clear gingival fluid often exudes from the sulcus. Purulent exudates may also be seen when pressure is applied to the gingiva.

Contact ulcers result from invasion of bacteria in plaque onto the buccal or lingual mucosal epithelium where the two are in contact, for example, during sleep. In an otherwise healthy dog, the oral mucosa is not affected by plaque bacteria. When contact ulcers are seen, they indicate that local or systemic immune responses are no longer functioning optimally. These contact ulcer lesions are painful; for this reason, the cheek should not be squeezed against the maxilla during physical examination.

Histopathology. The histopathologic changes that accompany early gingivitis are characteristic of an acute

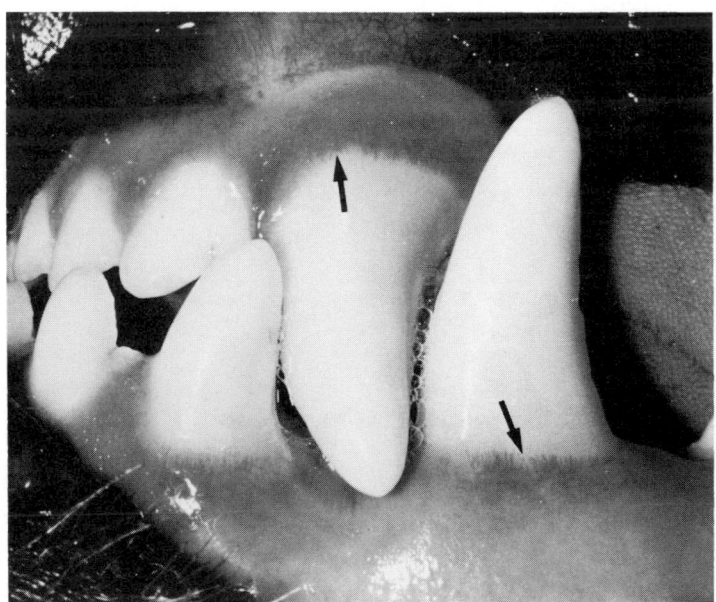

FIGURE 82–24. Early gingivitis in a dog. Note the slight color change in the marginal gingiva (arrows).

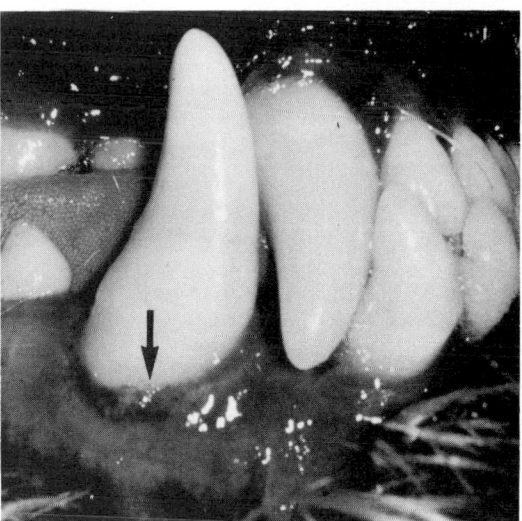

FIGURE 82–25. Established gingivitis. Note the color change (arrow) and rolled marginal gingiva.

inflammatory reaction (Figure 82–27). There is loss of perivascular collagen, vasculitis, and an influx of lymphocytes and polymorphonuclear leukocytes into the connective tissues. The polymorphs actively migrate out through the junctional and sulcular epithelium into the sulcus. After approximately four days the inflammatory changes become more chronic. Fibroblasts decrease in number, and the gingival fiber apparatus loses its integrity as collagen breakdown occurs. By the end of two weeks the inflammatory infiltrate is predominantly plasma cells, and the junctional and sulcular epithelium loses integrity as the intercellular spaces widen. In some areas, the sulcular epithelium may become ulcerated. Although the junctional epithelium loses its integrity, it does not detach from tooth surfaces.[48]

Treatment. The treatment of gingivitis is directed at the removal of bacterial plaque from the surfaces of the tooth on a consistent basis. All plaque-retentive features must be removed from the tooth surface to facilitate daily oral hygiene by the animal's owner. Positive results of removal of calculus without appropriate follow-up care will be very transient (Figure 82–28). Treatment techniques are discussed under Periodontal Therapy.

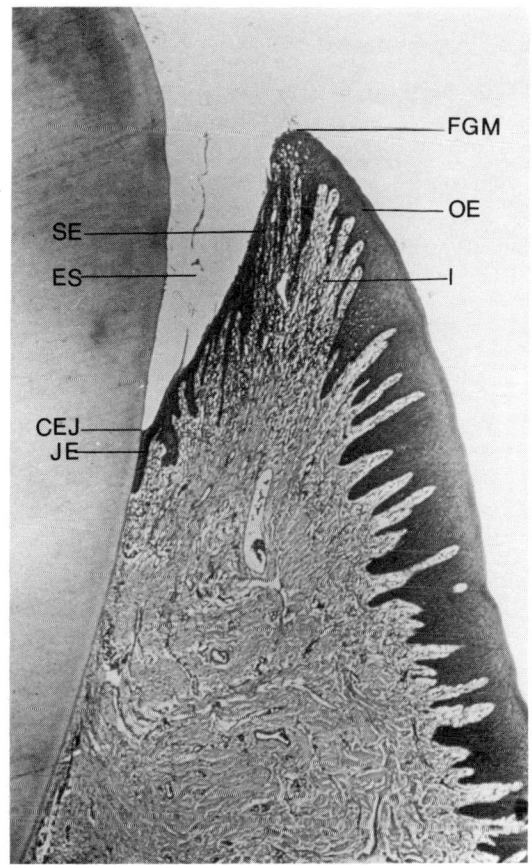

FIGURE 82–27. Histopathologic picture of gingivitis in a dog. CEJ, cemento-enamel junction; ES, enamel space; FGM, free gingival margin; I, inflammatory infiltrate; JE, junctional epithelium; OE, oral epithelium; SE, sulcular epithelium.

The consistent removal of plaque from the tooth surfaces results in a predictable diminution of clinical signs. A solution of chlorhexidine gluconate applied to the teeth cures established gingivitis;[63] however, plaque and gingivitis rapidly return when treatment is discontinued.[64] Various antibiotics, particularly clindamycin,[65] tetracycline, and metronidazole,[66, 67] have also been shown to be effective in treating gingivitis over the short term.

NECROTIZING ULCERATIVE GINGIVITIS

Necrotizing ulcerative gingivitis (NUG) is an acute infection primarily involving the marginal tissues of the gingiva. It is characterized by ulcerations of the gingival tissues, usually starting in the interdental regions. The affected areas are typically covered by a grayish mass of necrotic tissue, bacteria, and other oral debris. The tissues bleed when touched. On occasion the disease process may affect the crestal bone. The animal's breath is extremely foul, the condition causes pain, and affected animals may experience difficulty eating.[68] Necrotizing ulcerative gingivitis occurred in dogs aged 4 to 12 months in a colony of beagles.[69]

Although the etiology of this disease is not fully understood, two organisms, *Fusobacterium fusiformis* and *Borrelia vincenti*, have been associated with the

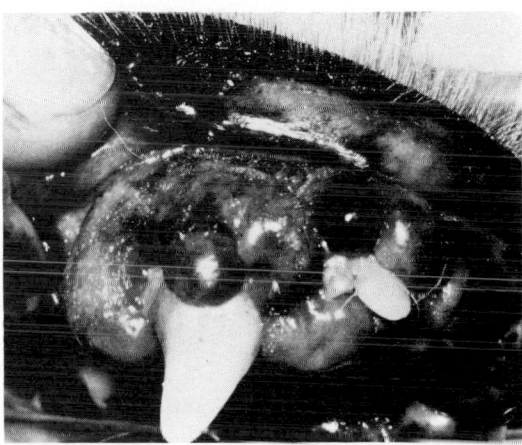

FIGURE 82–26. Nodular hyperplastic gingivitis in a dog.

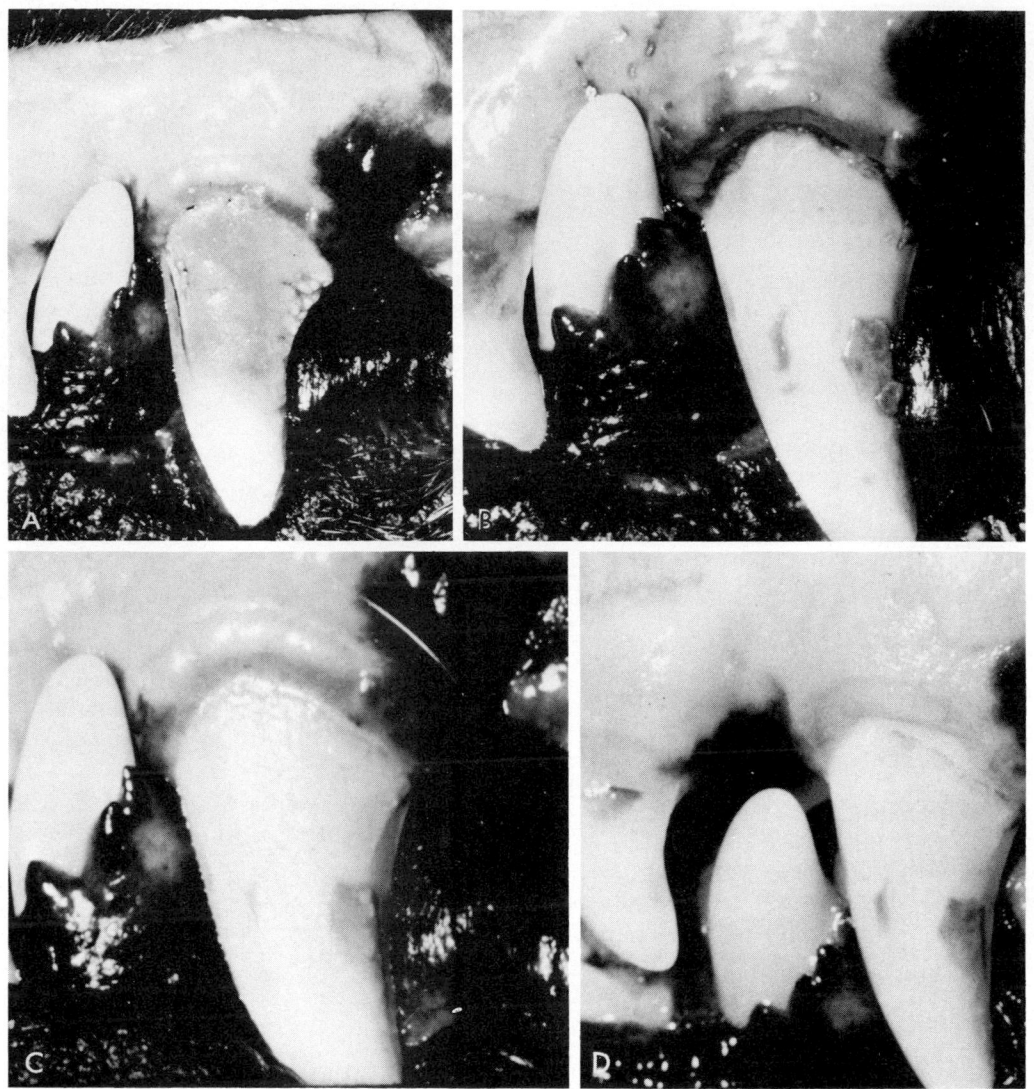

FIGURE 82–28. Canine and incisor teeth of an old dog with marginal gingivitis associated with plaque and calculus. *A,* Before treatment. *B,* Immediately after the removal of the supra- and subgingival calculus. *C,* Three weeks after calculus removal. Note the persistent gingival inflammation and associated plaque. *D,* One week after instituting tooth brushing, the gingival inflammation has subsided.

disease in humans. In addition to the bacteria, some host modifying factors seem to be necessary. The presence of elevated levels of 17-hydroxycorticosteroids in affected patients has been reported, possibly secondary to stress. Bacterial plaque from dogs with NUG was inoculated into the mouths of six healthy one-year-old beagle dogs; only the three dogs pretreated with corticosteroids contracted the disease.[70]

The disease responds to penicillin. Generally a one-week regimen of ampicillin (10 mg/lb orally four times per day) results in dramatic improvement. Debridement of the necrotic tissue accompanied by plaque and calculus removal accelerates treatment. Healing often results in a gingival deformity that may be plaque retentive and predisposes to subsequent periodontal disease; follow-up gingival surgery may be indicated to correct the soft tissue deformity after the active disease is brought under control. Recurrence is likely if the predisposing factor or stress is not recognized and corrected.

Gingival Hyperplasia

Chronic gingival hyperplasia is a firm, nonpainful swelling of the gingival epithelium (Figure 82–26). The color resembles that of normal adjacent epithelium. The extent of hyperplastic change often varies significantly within areas of the mouth. There often is little evidence of plaque or calculus accumulation or of acute gingivitis. Some of the larger protuberant lesions resemble epulides, and may be difficult to differentiate from fibromatous epulis without histologic examination. Generalized gingival hyperplasia occurs frequently in collies and some other large breeds, suggesting an inherited cause similar to that proposed for "familial epulis of Boxers."[71]

Treatment. In many dogs, gingival hyperplasia does not require treatment. When pocket depth is significantly increased, periodontitis will occur eventually because subgingival plaque is protected. Elimination of the pocket by gingivectomy is indicated. A loop-tipped electroscalpel is particularly helpful. The electroscalpel should not be applied against tooth or bone, as necrosis may result.

Periodontitis

Etiology. Periodontitis develops as a sequel to a persistent gingivitis.[48] The factors that determine whether or not gingivitis progresses to periodontitis have not been thoroughly elucidated. There is substantial evidence that the bacterial flora present in plaque is the determining factor.[48]

It is still unknown precisely which organisms actually initiate the destruction of the periodontium. There are several bacteria that, when inoculated into the mouths of gnotobiotic rats, produce extensive alveolar bone loss. Most of these organisms are found in high numbers in the plaque of human patients with active periodontitis. It has also been demonstrated in dogs that periodontitis could be produced by simply allowing plaque to accumulate on the tooth surface.[55] The control animals, which were fed identical diets but had their teeth cleaned twice daily, did not manifest periodontitis at any time during the four years of the study. It also has been demonstrated that flora associated with teeth with periodontitis is distinctly different from flora of teeth without periodontitis, even within the same mouth.[72] The former has more spirochetes and motile rods and, in general, is anaerobic gram-negative flora. The flora associated with healthy areas tends to have relatively more cocci and filamentous organisms, with proportionally fewer spirochetes and motile rods.

As in gingivitis, any factor that allows for the retention of plaque on the tooth surface is likely to contribute to the demise of the periodontium. In addition to calculus and hair or food impaction, the formation of the deepened pocket is in itself a major plaque-retentive feature. As the pocket increases in depth, significant environmental change may occur that allows the more deleterious organisms to proliferate.

As noted earlier, dogs on a calcium-deficient diet develop periodontitis earlier than do other dogs.[52] Decalcification resulting from dietary causes or from hyperparathyroidism (whether primary or secondary to renal disease) occurs selectively, developing in dogs in descending order of severity in the jaws (particularly alveolar bone surrounding the teeth), then other skull bones, ribs, vertebrae, and finally limb long bones,[53] hence the term "rubber jaw."

Clinical Manifestations. Periodontal disease does not progress beyond gingivitis in the majority of tooth surfaces in many animals. In some animals, however, there is a progression of the soft tissue inflammation into the deeper tissues of the periodontium.[73] The host factors and local factors that result in the progression of the disease are poorly understood. The loss of alveolar and supporting bone is accompanied by an apical migration of the gingival fiber apparatus and of the junctional epithelium. The loss of osseous support can occur either as a generalized horizontal loss involving all teeth on all surfaces or as isolated areas involving single teeth or even a single surface of a single tooth. Once initiated, the bone loss tends to be progressive. Typically, the soft

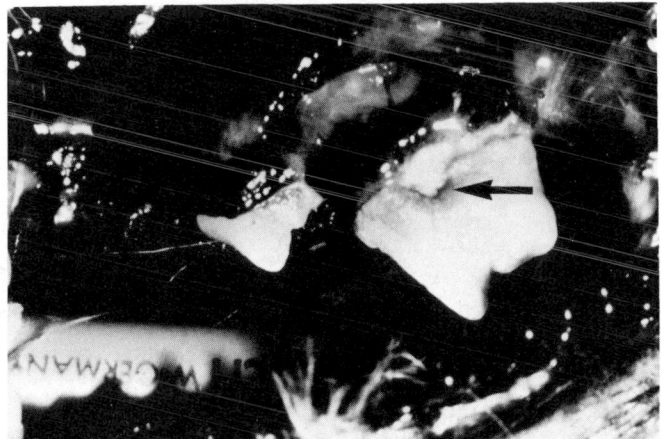

FIGURE 82–29. Carnassial tooth in a dog with gingival recession exposing the furcation (arrow).

tissues manifest the changes associated with gingivitis, with one notable exception: the free gingival margin (FGM) may recede in an apical direction as a result of the loss of osseous tissues. When this occurs the cemento-enamel junction (CEJ) and root surface will be visible. In more advanced cases, when there is excessive bone loss, the furcation area (the area between the roots of a multirooted tooth) may be exposed to the oral environment (Figures 82–29 and 82–30). Gingival recession does not always accompany the bone loss; hyperplasia of the gingiva may coexist with bone loss. Thus, the clinical diagnosis of periodontitis cannot be based only on the position of the FGM relative to the CEJ; it is also necessary to use radiographs and/or the periodontal probe. When loss of crestal height is seen on the radiograph or when the tip of a periodontal probe can be passed three or more millimeters apical to the CEJ, the diagnosis of periodontitis can be made. The probe is inserted into the sulcus parallel to the long axis of the tooth, with its tip in contact with the tooth. Bleeding will invariably accompany probing in an animal with periodontitis, and purulent discharge may exude

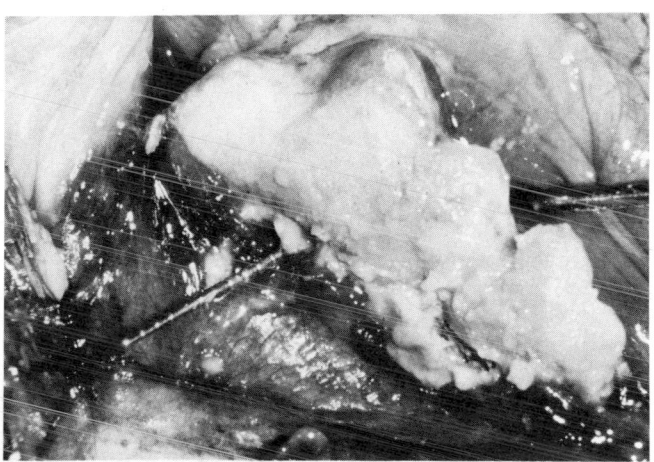

FIGURE 82–30. Extensive furcation involvement in a mandibular carnassial tooth. The periodontal probe can be passed from the medial to the lateral surface.

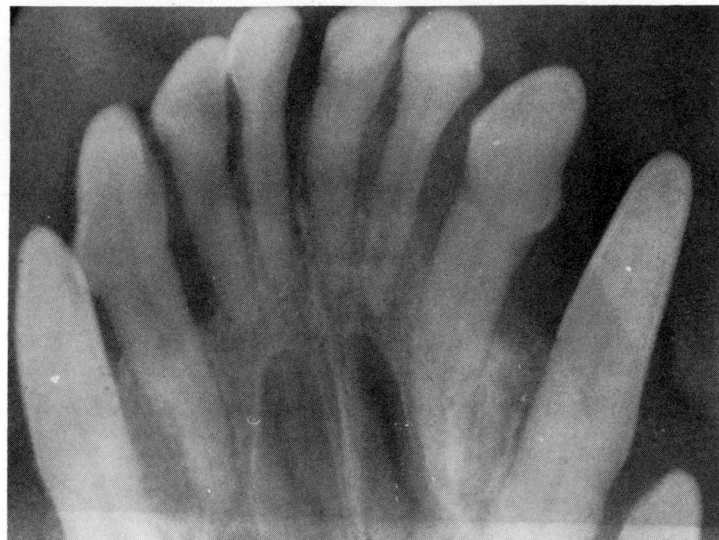

FIGURE 82–31. Radiograph of canine maxillary incisors showing generalized bone loss secondary to inflammatory periodontal disease.

out of the pocket orifice. In cases involving extreme bone loss, horizontal mobility of the teeth increases substantially. With the possible exception of incisors and first premolars in some of the smaller breeds, horizontal tooth mobility should not be seen in periodontally healthy dogs. As a result of the loss of osseous support, teeth frequently become mobile. The degree of mobility depends on root morphology, severity of the inflammatory process, and occlusal forces. The presence of mobility does not necessarily mean that the prognosis for a particular tooth is hopeless[74] provided that further bone loss is prevented.

A thorough history and physical examination are indicated for all animals with periodontal disease, as systemic disease may predispose to or manifest itself locally as periodontal disease.

Radiographic Manifestations. The earliest radiographic sign of periodontitis is loss of definition of crestal bone. In health, crestal bone appears as a radiopaque line that parallels and is one to two mm apical to an imaginary line drawn between the CEJ of two adjacent teeth. As periodontitis advances, an apical migration of the crestal bone is seen (Figure 82–31). Radiolucent areas within the furcations of multirooted teeth also become apparent. Radiographic changes correlate with clinical (probing depth) evidence of periodontitis in dogs.[75]

Histopathology. The gingival changes are the same as those in gingivitis. There is a chronic inflammatory reaction marked by a dense infiltrate of round cells; much of the gingival fiber apparatus is destroyed. Inflammatory cells are found in close proximity to the crestal bone, which may be actively reabsorbed by osteoclastic activity. The transseptal fibers, immediately coronal to the bone, are still present; the epithelial inflammatory infiltrate lies coronal to this connective tissue.

As the crestal bone resorbs, the transseptal fibers reattach at a more apical level on the root surface, which allows the junctional epithelium to move in an apical direction. The more coronal cells of the junctional epithelium detach from the tooth and become part of the sulcular epithelium, thus increasing the depth of the pocket. Bacterial plaque is seen in the pocket almost, but not quite, in contact with the most coronal cell of the junctional epithelium, although bacteria are not found within the periodontal tissues. Calculus may not be present in the pocket. Necrosis is not seen in the soft or hard tissues of the periodontium affected with periodontitis. The histopathology of periodontitis in dogs has been described in detail.[73, 76]

Treatment. The treatment of periodontitis is directed at the removal of bacterial plaque from the tooth surfaces. However, unless the disease is treated at its most incipient stage, it is almost impossible to control. Since plaque must be eliminated in the subgingival as well as the supragingival area, either the pocket must be cleaned on a more or less daily basis or the pocket must be surgically eliminated so that only supragingival areas need to be cleaned (Figures 82–32 and 82–33). Although surgical pocket elimination is possible in some cases, it is technically difficult and time-consuming. Without proper postsurgical maintenance, the therapy will almost certainly fail. The animal's age, the type of post-treatment care the owner is willing to provide, and the willingness of the animal to accept treatment are factors to consider prior to treatment. By far the easiest and most predictable way to manage advanced periodontitis is to debride the tooth surfaces thoroughly on a regular basis every two to four months as needed, based on the severity of the problem. Debridement should consist of thorough calculus and plaque removal as well as curettage of the inflamed pocket lining and the removal of the most superficial layer of cementum on the root surface within the pocket (see Periodontal Therapy). Although this treatment may not arrest the disease process, it may slow it enough to allow the teeth to remain in a relatively stable state. The long-term or intermittent use of antibiotics may be a useful adjunct. The better the follow-up care on the part of the patient's owner, the more successful the therapy. Follow-up care should include daily tooth brushing to increase the possibility of success. Switching to a totally dry food diet is also helpful.

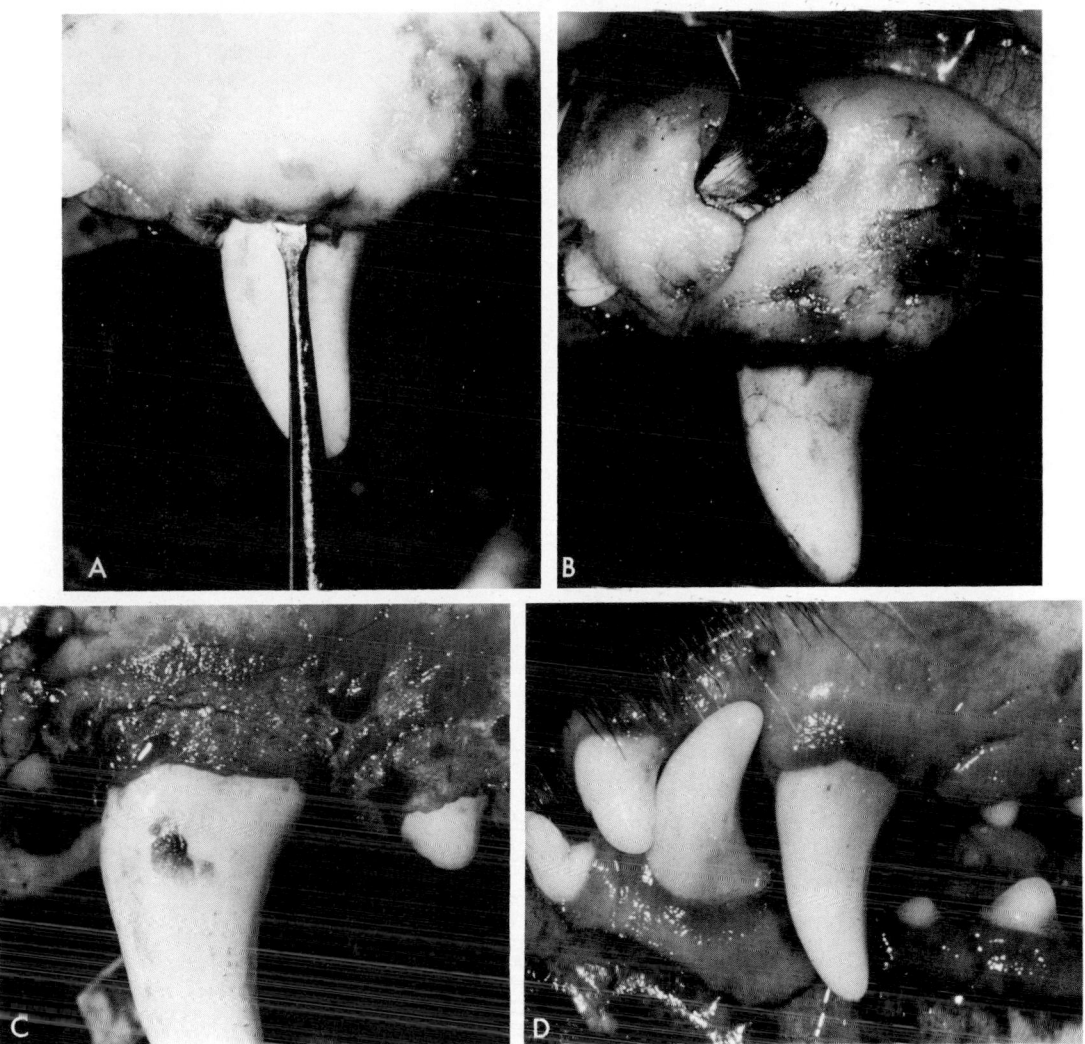

FIGURE 82–32. Gingivectomy for treatment of hyperplastic gingivitis in a dog. *A,* Maxillary canine tooth with dental instrument placed in the facial pocket. *B,* Gingivectomy knife in place for the excision of the free gingiva. *C,* The free gingiva has been excised. Note the piece of calculus that was not removed during the presurgical scaling. *D,* Postoperative healing (after four months). Note the marginal inflammation resulting from the reaccumulation of plaque.

Periodontal Abscess

Acute periodontal abscess is a localized, purulent inflammation in the periodontal tissues, generally appearing as a swelling within the gingival tissues. It may be firm or fluctuant, or if it has spontaneously drained, it may present as a mass of detached gingiva (Figure 82–34). The gingival tissues in the area of the abscess are inflamed. In most cases a probe placed into the gingival crevice easily enters the abscess, causing pus to exude out of the crevice. At times the abscess is entirely within the gingiva and not easily entered through the pocket. Tooth mobility is usually markedly increased. Periodontal abscesses are most frequently associated with deep pockets, furcation areas, or occasionally relatively shallow pockets in which a foreign body has become lodged.

The radiographic appearance of the periodontal abscess can be quite variable. It appears as a discrete area of bone loss adjacent to the root, and it may involve the more apical areas.

There is some question as to whether carnassial abscess, which is usually associated with the maxillary fourth premolar or mandibular first molar teeth, is of periodontal or endodontic origin.

Although the acute periodontal abscess responds to antibiotic therapy, it generally recurs if more vigorous treatment is not rendered. If sufficient osseous support remains around the tooth, one can thoroughly debride the abscess either by flapping the gingival tissues away from the root or curetting the lesion through the gingival crevice. In most instances, however, bony destruction precludes salvaging the tooth, and extraction is indicated.

Periodontal Therapy

Professional treatment (other than extraction) is of very transient value unless followed up by effective plaque control measures at home.

Oral Hygiene. Although it has been shown that regular

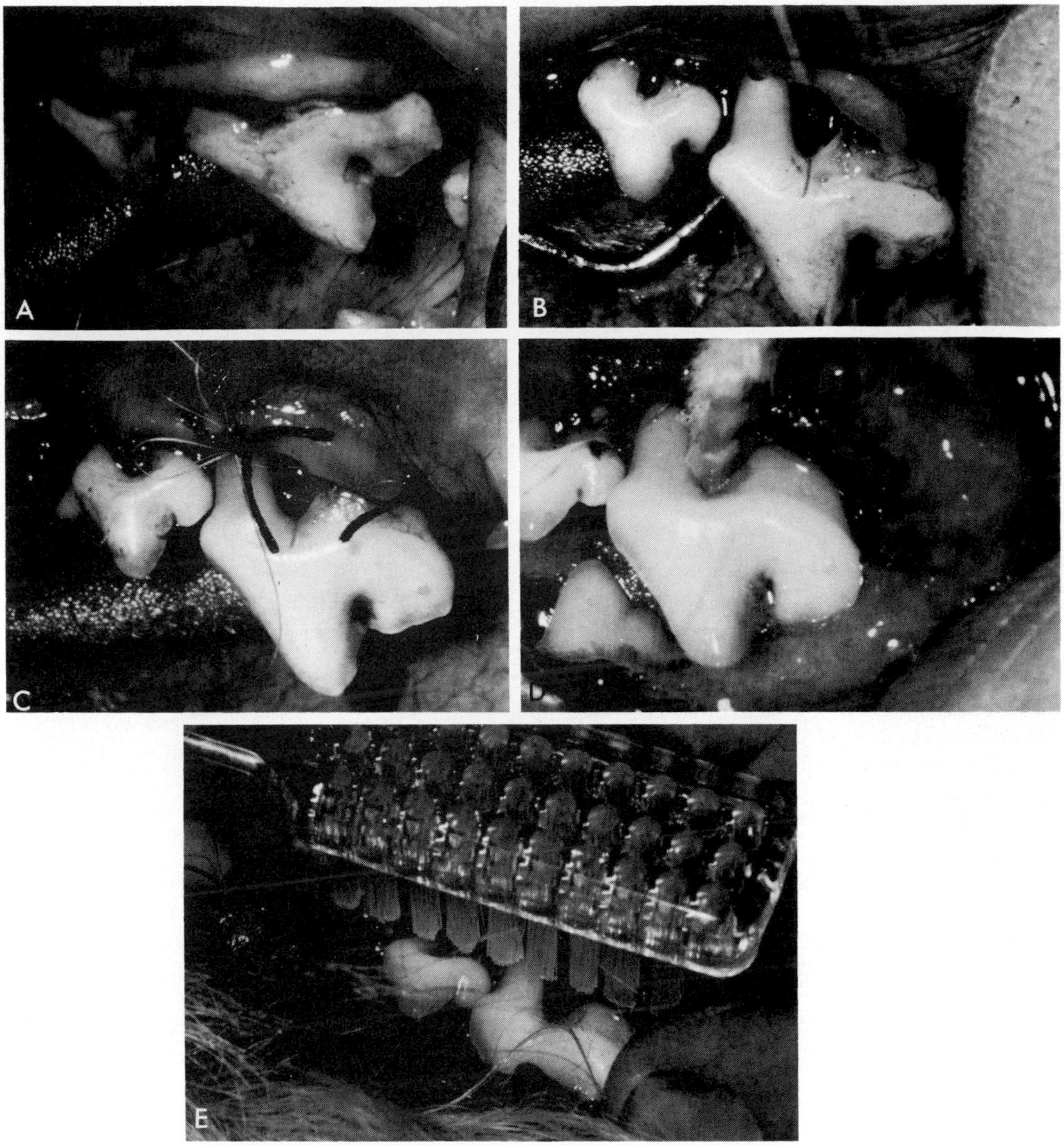

FIGURE 82–33. Apically positioned flap surgery in a dog with advanced periodontitis and furcation involvement of the maxillary fourth premolar. *A,* Pretreatment. *B,* The free gingival margin has been moved in an apical direction to expose the furcation. *C,* The facial flap has been sutured to the palatal flap. *D* and *E,* The furcation must be cleaned daily with pipe cleaners or a toothbrush. Although this treatment is feasible, it is often not practical. Prevention should be stressed.

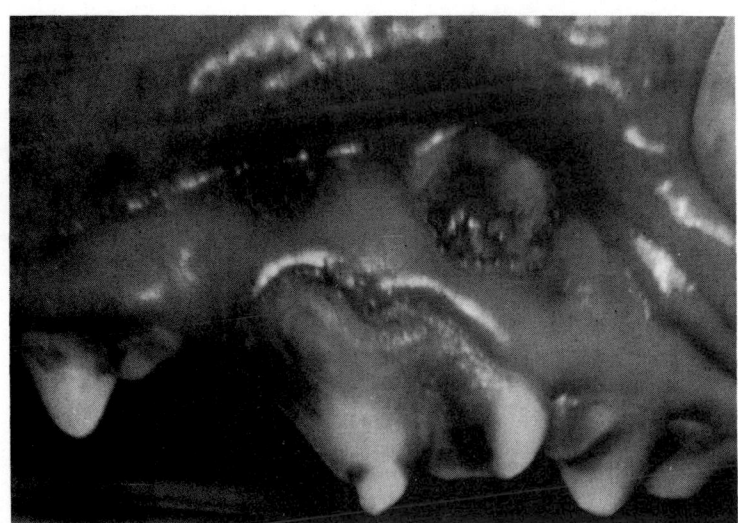

FIGURE 82–34. Gingival and bone loss caused by a periodontal abscess on the facial aspect of a maxillary carnassial tooth.

brushing of a dog's teeth may aggravate the inflammatory process in the gingiva in neutropenic dogs with gingivitis,[77] there is overwhelming evidence that a soft toothbrush with nylon bristles is the most practical implement for the daily removal of plaque. The teeth should be brushed with the toothbrush bristles aimed into the gingival sulcus, with the brush head at a 45-degree angle to the tooth surface (Figure 82–33*E*). The brush is moved with a short back and forth or circular motion. All of the facial, lingual, and palatal surfaces should be brushed. The brush should also be directed down at the occlusal surfaces of the tooth with a back and forth motion of the brush parallel to the interproximal areas. If tooth brushing is overly vigorous, or if a hard-tufted brush is used, gingival damage can result.[78] The owner should be advised that the presence of gingival bleeding during tooth brushing is evidence of gingival disease and that in most cases a week of conscientiously applied oral hygiene will cause the bleeding to stop. While a plaque-retardant dentifrice or solution can be applied with the brush, the most important consideration is the frequent application of the brush. The most effective plaque retardant identified to date is chlorhexidine, which can be applied as a 0.5 per cent gel or 0.1 to 0.2 per cent solution as a rinse or on a toothbrush.[79] In addition to its antibacterial activity, chlorhexidine is absorbed onto oral surfaces and thus retains its effectiveness for up to 24 hours.[80] The efficacy of chlorhexidine can be extended to several weeks if used with a cellulose-based sustained release device in a deep periodontal pocket.[81] Disadvantages of chlorhexidine are its bitter taste and the formation of a brown discoloration of teeth in some dogs,[64] although the discoloration is not clinically objectionable when routine brushing is provided. Palatable chlorhexidine oral solution for veterinary use is now available. Because the major concern is compliance of the animal and owner with brushing instructions, use of a dentifrice that has been shown to be particularly palatable for dogs is very beneficial. Once a dog or cat is affected by periodontitis to the extent that there is obvious pocket formation, gingival recession, or furcation involvement, tooth brushing alone is inadequate.

In order for oral hygiene to be effective in the presence of periodontitis, the oral hygiene implement must overcome the architectural deformity created by the disease. Although dental floss, toothpicks, and rubber tips could be useful, their use is impractical unless the animal is extremely cooperative and the owner is highly motivated.[83]

Scaling and Root Planing. Once calculus has formed on the crown and roots of the tooth, it is no longer possible for tooth brushing to be effective. The teeth of the animal should be scaled. This can be accomplished either by an ultrasonic device that vibrates the calculus from the tooth surface, or by dental curettes and scalers. The tip of the ultrasonic device, which should be well-cooled with a water spray, is gently moved over the tooth surfaces supra- and subgingivally. Ultrasonic dental scalers cause considerable spread of contamination,[84] and can cause bacteremia, particularly in dogs with gingivitis or periodontitis.[85, 86] When a dental curette is used, the tip should be placed apical to the calculus,

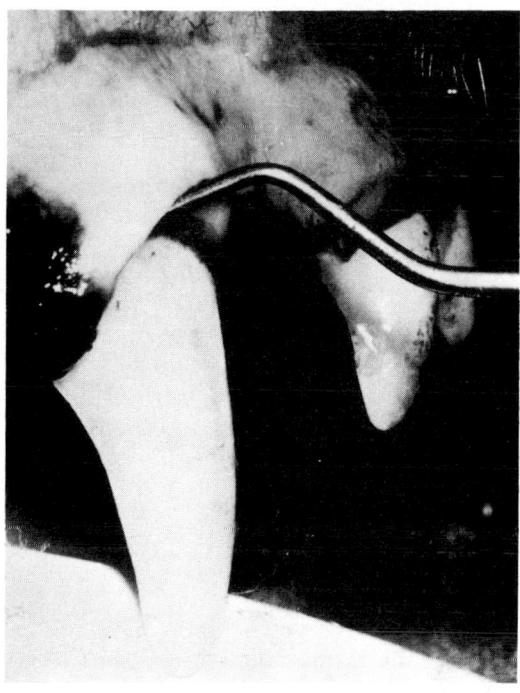

FIGURE 82–35. Use of the periodontal curette to remove calculus in a pocket apical to the free gingival margin.

with its face at a 45 to 75 degree angle to the long axis of the tooth. The curette is then pulled in a coronal direction, dislodging the calculus (Figure 82–35). It is essential that the curette be extremely sharp. If calculus was removed from the root surface of the tooth, it is necessary to plane the cemental surface of the tooth, which can also be accomplished with the curette. The purpose of root planing is to remove residual calculus as well as bacterial endotoxins that impregnate the superficial surface of the cementum. A jet of air in combination with a sharp dental explorer is useful in detecting calculus in the subgingival areas. After the teeth are scaled, they should be polished with a rotating rubber cup and mild abrasive. The value of scaling and root planing is extremely transient unless it is followed with daily oral hygiene, preferably in combination with a change to a hard food diet.

Curettage. The removal of the inflamed pocket lining and the soft tissue contents of infrabony pockets (which result from irregular resorption of bone) is useful in the control of active periodontal disease. A sharp curette, in which the cutting edge is directed toward the sulcular and junctional epithelium and the osseous tissues, is used to remove the inflamed tissue. This procedure can be accomplished at the same time as scaling and root planing.

Surgical Pocket Elimination. Some of the soft and hard tissue deformities (particularly gingival hyperplasia) created by periodontal disease are amenable to surgical treatment. The successful management of periodontal disease requires that bacterial plaque be removed on a routine, preferably daily, basis. Even with a cooperative animal and owner, however, it is impossible to successfully remove plaque from subgingival areas on a daily basis in a dog or cat. The purpose of periodontal surgery is to eliminate the pocket, thus changing a subgingival area into a cleanable supragingival one.

The two basic procedures for eliminating pockets are gingivectomy and the apically positioned flap (Figures 82–32 and 82–33). Pockets on the palatal aspect of the maxillary teeth are particularly difficult to manage because of the flatness of the palate in the dog and cat. It is beyond the scope of this chapter to describe these procedures in detail; they are described elsewhere.[23]

Extraction. Once periodontal disease has advanced to the point at which furcations have become involved or tooth mobility is excessive, the only practical modality for control of periodontitis is extraction of the involved teeth. This is not to say that such teeth cannot be salvaged; however, the techniques involved and follow-up care necessary are impractical for use in most small animals. Extraction is also a practical treatment for the earlier stages of periodontal disease if the owner is not concerned with the aesthetics of the mouth. Tooth extraction techniques have been described in detail elsewhere.[23]

Dental procedures involving the periodontium usually cause bacteremia,[86] although in the normal dog this is rapidly cleared.[87] Animals with clinical evidence of valvular heart disease or animals that are immune-suppressed or under treatment with anti-inflammatory medications should receive prophylactic antibiotic coverage. Ampicillin is appropriate (5 mg/lb once IV immediately prior to the procedure). If another surgical procedure is to be performed during the same anesthetic episode as the periodontal procedure, antibiotic coverage should be continued for several days, as infection of a clean surgical wound can result from a dental procedure.[88]

Antibiotics can be used for short-term or ancillary treatment of severe, painful oral lesions. The most effective drugs are those with activity against anaerobes, such as clindamycin, metronidazole, and tetracycline.[65–67] Clindamycin is particularly useful because, like tetracycline, it is absorbed into bone but is also concentrated in neutrophils.[65]

Periodontal Disease in Cats

The disease in cats has both similarities to and significant differences from periodontal disease in dogs and is also very common.[89, 90] Feeding exclusively soft food to male cats as a way of increasing fluid intake to avoid urethral obstruction has probably contributed to the incidence of this disease. The ranges of bacterial flora in normal and affected areas of the mouth of cats are similar to those found in dogs and humans.[91]

Significant differences between periodontal disease as seen in cats and in other species are: (1) Teeth affected by periodontal disease in cats frequently develop "neck lesions." These are cavities that form initially in the root cementum at the junction of crown and root (Figure 82–12). Although superficially similar to caries cavities, the histologic appearance indicates that the cause is external odontoclastic resorption rather than chemical decalcification.[90, 92] These cavities harbor plaque and expose the sensitive dentinal tubules of the root. This latter effect can result in pain on eating or drinking,

which is much more common in cats with periodontal disease than it is with dogs, and can lead to severe malnutrition and dehydration. (2) Soft tissue lesions affecting the cheek teeth are often very extensive. These protuberant, ulcerative lesions can spread to affect the glossopalatine arches and pharyngeal walls, with the result that this tissue cracks and reulcerates when the mouth is opened. These lesions are often the most obvious abnormality seen when opening the mouth of affected cats. Because of this, they have been regarded as areas of separate disease, which on a histopathologic basis has been described as plasmacytic-lymphocytic gingivitis-stomatitis.[93] The cheek and lingual contact ulcers that are common in dogs with advanced periodontal disease are rarely seen in cats. (3) Affected cats in general suffer more severely than do dogs or humans with periodontal disease. Unwillingness to eat and drink, emaciation, and dehydration are common in affected cats. This probably is due to a combination of items 1 and 2 above. The painful nature of these lesions in cats makes the patients less tolerant of plaque control measures. To the general reluctance to have the mouth held open and a toothbrush forcibly inserted, which makes daily brushing less than a satisfactory procedure in many dogs, is added in cats the acute pain resulting from brushing of the sensitive, eroded tooth roots.

Feline calicivirus (one of the two major viral causes of upper respiratory disease in cats) has been isolated frequently from affected feline gingival tissues.[94, 95] Feline herpes (FVR), calici-, and panleukopenia viruses cause lingual, palatal, and pharyngeal ulceration in cats (Figure 82–36). The significance of the presence of calicivirus in affected periodontal tissues in cats has not yet been established. Other associations are more controversial. The plasmacytic nature of the protuberant gingival and pharyngeal lesions has led to suggestions that this disease in cats is immune-mediated; the steroid-responsive nature of the disease in some cats adds credence to this hypothesis. The finding that many cats affected with FeLV-related diseases have periodontal disease[96, 97] is probably due to the immune-suppressive nature of FeLV infection; however, it should be noted that cats that are presented primarily because of oral signs are rarely FeLV-positive.[93–95, 98] Chronic gingivitis is a common finding in cats infected with feline T-lymphotropic virus (lentivirus).[99]

Clinical Signs. These initially consist of marginal gingivitis (a red line at the junction of the tooth crown and gingiva) and progress to salivation, reluctance or inability to eat, redness, ulceration or protuberant growths from the gingiva, weight loss, and dehydration. Diagnosis is based on inspection. Differential diagnoses include oral neoplasms and systemic causes of weight loss. FeLV and FTLV tests should be performed in cats with chronic gingival lesions.

Treatment. Therapy of periodontal disease is conservative or radical. In a severely sick cat, systemic antibiotic administration may be necessary to reduce the acute inflammation sufficiently to permit the cat to eat and drink. The antibiotics that are most effective against oral gram-negative organisms are clindamycin (5 mg/lb q12h), tetracycline (100 to 200 mg q12h), and metronidazole (50 to 100 mg q24h). Unfortunately, they all

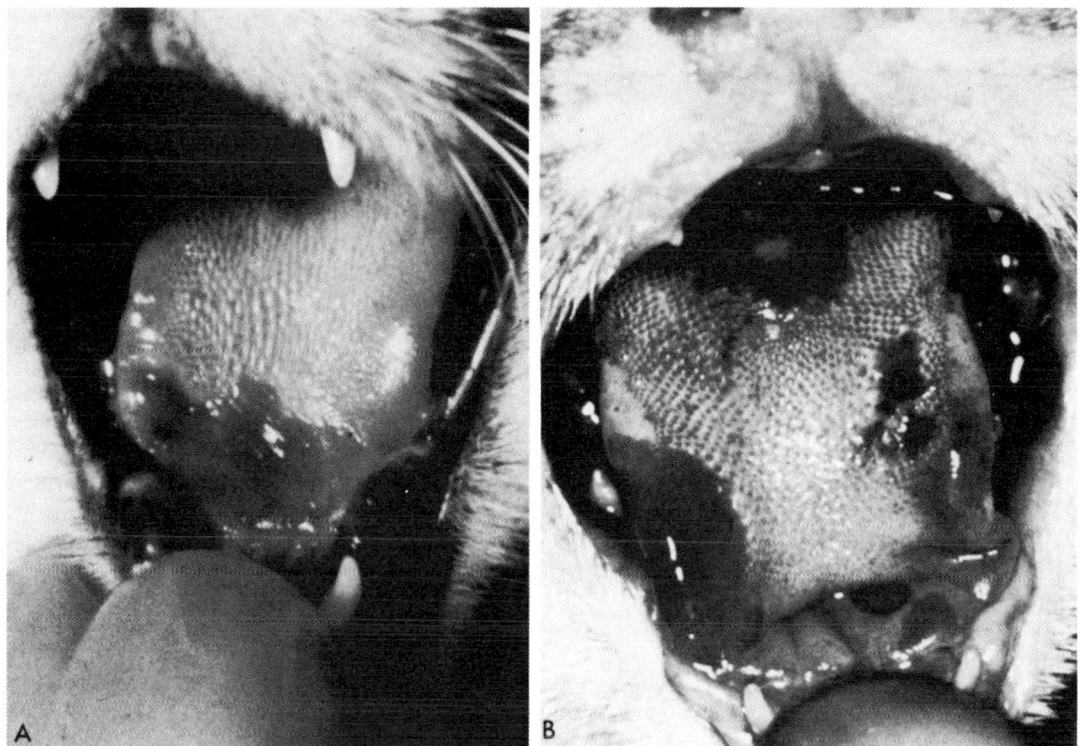

FIGURE 82–36. *A*, Glossal ulceration in a cat caused by feline calicivirus (FCV) infection. *B*, Severe glossal ulceration in a cat caused by feline viral rhinotracheitis (FVR) infection. (Courtesy of Dr. R. C. Povey).

require oral administration. Injectable antibiotic drugs such as ampicillin will have a short-term beneficial effect that may be sufficient to improve the cat's condition to the point at which it can tolerate teeth cleaning or oral medications.

Conservative treatment consists of restoring the periodontium to as near normal a condition as possible by teeth cleaning and subgingival scaling, combined with resection of protuberant gingival tissue as necessary to eliminate excessive pockets. Neck lesions can be treated as for any other area of damaged tooth structure, by resecting to clean, healthy tissue and then restoring the surface of the tooth. Amalgam and composite restoration techniques have been used but are difficult to apply correctly given the small size of the tooth and subgingival position of the lesion. Glass ionomer-silver cements are more practical options; however, preparation and restoration should be reserved for small lesions on aesthetically important teeth; other affected teeth should be extracted. To be of long-term value, conservative treatment should be combined with daily brushing or rubbing of the teeth and gingivae to eliminate plaque. Feeding a dry food diet helps maintain good oral health in cats.[100] There are no documented reports of the long-term efficacy of conservative therapy in cats; this may be due to the recognition that cats with severe periodontal disease respond poorly, as stated in most brief descriptions of results. The place of anti-inflammatory corticosteroids in the therapy of periodontal disease in cats is poorly documented. These agents would appear to be contraindicated in treatment of a disease associated with bacterial proliferation; however, the pathology of the lesions and the several unsubstantiated comments in various reports that they may be or are of benefit suggest that their use should not be ruled out.

Radical therapy consists of extraction of all of the premolar and molar teeth in severely affected cats. The rationale for this is that painful root lesions and pockets for the accumulation of plaque are eliminated. The gingiva that heals over the extraction sites should be normal tissue. The technique for extraction of teeth in cats is described elsewhere.[23] In a series of nine severely affected cats treated by premolar and molar extractions with a minimum follow-up of seven months, results were good (no continuing signs of oral disease) in six (67 per cent). One of these six was treated intermittently with a corticosteroid to control cyclic recurrences of gingival inflammation.[98]

There is a great deal that remains unknown regarding periodontal disease in cats.

STOMATITIS

Stomatitis is inflammation of the oral mucosa. The clinician examining an animal with stomatitis must consider both the general health of the patient and local factors. Any circumstances that significantly alter the dynamic replication, maturation, and exfoliation of healthy mucosa favor the development of disease. Although the oral mucosa is subject to considerable trauma and can tolerate it well, swelling, dehydration, cell death, or replication caused by disease will exaggerate the effect of normal trauma and produce injury. The saliva of carnivores is bactericidal because of the alkaline pH and lysozyme content; therefore, bacterial infection rarely becomes established unless other factors—infectious or physical—are present.

Diagnosis. A routine should be developed for the diagnosis of animals with stomatitis. When the animal is first presented, a complete history, including dietary information and thorough physical examination, is essential. Thorough examination of the oral cavity often requires sedation or anesthesia owing to the animal's temperament or to pain caused by the disease. The position, extent, symmetry, and nature of the lesions are of particular importance. Periodontal disease may be localized but is usually widespread along the gingival margins by the time that veterinary attention is sought. Usually the visible lesions are confined to the gingiva; however, ulcers are sometimes seen on the buccal mucosa that lies in contact with the diseased periodontium ("contact ulcers"). Lesions caused by viruses or poisons are usually scattered over the mucosa. In cats, ulcers caused by feline viral rhinotracheitis or calicivirus infection are seen most commonly on the tongue, palate, and fauces (Figure 82–36). Single asymmetric lesions may be neoplastic (see Oropharyngeal Neoplasia). A disclosing solution should be used to demonstrate the extent of plaque. A calibrated periodontal probe and dental explorer are very useful for examining teeth and periodontium.

Initial laboratory examination should include a complete blood count, FeLV and FTLV tests in cats, and creatinine and blood glucose determinations, particularly in older animals or in animals with polydipsia/polyuria. The next step will depend on the tentative clinical diagnosis. Observing the response to treatment is a frequent means of confirming a cause of stomatitis. Failure of the lesions to respond in the expected fashion should prompt further investigation. Cytologic examination or biopsy, histologic examination, and bacterial, fungal, or viral culture of the lesions are often helpful. Immunologic work-up may indicate an autoimmune or immune deficiency disease.

Diseases That Cause Oral Lesions

Oral changes caused by systemic diseases are important diagnostic aids to the clinician.

Uremia. The most common oral manifestation of systemic disease in the dog and cat is ulceration associated with severe uremia. Urea diffuses into all body secretions, including saliva. The irritation caused by ammonia resulting from bacterial action on urea, the dry mouth of the dehydrated uremic patient, and the clotting deficiencies that occur late in the disease all contribute to this syndrome. Local therapy can be soothing, but unless renal failure is reversed, the process is relentless. The rostral part of the tongue may undergo necrosis in dogs with acute renal failure or pancreatitis. Hyperparathyroidism secondary to chronic renal disease causes decalcification of bone, seen most severely in the jaws ("rubber jaw"), and may exacerbate mobility of periodontally involved teeth.[52]

Diabetes. Oral infections are no more common in diabetic animals than in normal animals; however, they may be more severe, progressing rapidly to periodontitis or periodontal abscess. In an animal with nonresponsive stomatitis, the possibility of diabetes should be investigated. Meticulous attention to dental hygiene is necessary in diabetic patients. There is disagreement as to whether salivary flow rates are decreased in humans with diabetes; calcium ion and immunoglobulin G are found in higher concentration in saliva from diabetics.[101, 102] The relationship between these findings, the increased incidence and severity of periodontal disease in diabetics, and the xerostomia often associated with diabetes in humans is not yet clear. The mandibular salivary gland produces a tryptic inhibitor anti-insulin factor; resection of these glands in humans with diabetes improves but does not correct the diabetic condition. A mild xerostomia persists for up to three weeks.[103]

Hematologic and Reticuloendothelial Diseases. Ulceration is uncommon, but petechiation of the palate or buccal mucosa, or blood oozing from the gingivae, may be early signs of vitamin K deficiency (as in warfarin poisoning), thrombocytopenia, or other diseases that cause a clotting defect. Any disease depressing the function of the reticuloendothelial system can predispose to oral infection.

Deficiency Diseases. Severe generalized malnutrition ("protein-calorie malnutrition") can lead to oral ulceration as a result of depressed epithelial cell turnover.[23] Documentation of specific vitamin-deficient states is now very rare. Classical niacin deficiency syndrome in the dog ("black tongue") is no longer seen as a clinical entity. In the rare animal with severe pica or a dietary idiosyncrasy that causes inadequate nutrition, replacement vitamin therapy may be justified. Dietary calcium imbalance will cause periodontal bone and tooth loss.[52]

Genetic Diseases. Stomatitis is a severe recurrent problem in silver-grey collies afflicted with the simple recessive autosomal disease that causes cyclic neutropenia ("grey collie syndrome").[104]

Poisons. All heavy metal compounds can cause oral inflammation and ulceration; thallium is the most common agent seen clinically. Warfarin and indanedione, used in rodent control, cause clotting deficiencies that may present as oral petechiation. Occasionally, other substances such as plants (e.g., Dieffenbachia) may cause oral disease when chewed by a dog or cat.

Immune System Abnormalities

Both immune deficiency disease and autoimmune disease can result in oral lesions. Immune deficiency diseases may allow local disease such as periodontal disease to worsen or secondary Candida sp. infection to become established. The severe T-cell immunodeficiency often associated with nasal aspergillosis or penicilliosis may present as oral disease by direct spread along the nasopalatine duct. Chronic gingivitis is seen in some cats infected with feline T-lymphotropic virus (lentivirus).[99]

Immune system abnormalities should be included as a possible diagnosis in intractable or recurrent stomatitis. The lymphocyte transformation test is a useful screening test for immune deficiency diseases. Immune deficiency diseases are discussed in Chapters 118 and 119.

Autoimmune Diseases. Several reports have been published detailing autoimmune disease affecting the oral cavity of the dog[105-108] and the cat.[109-110] The two forms of autoimmune disease that principally affect the oral cavity are pemphigus vulgaris and bullous pemphigoid. Both result from circulating autoantibodies to intercellular epidermal antigens, which cause acantholysis and intraepidermal bullae (pemphigus vulgaris) or epidermal connective tissue bullae (bullous pemphigoid).

PEMPHIGUS VULGARIS. This condition occurs in a wide range of ages and breeds of dogs. The oral mucosa, external nares, lips, eyelid margins, ears, anus, and prepuce or vulva are the most frequent sites of lesions. Oral lesions often appear as well-defined ulcers with scalloped edges. Diagnosis is based on careful histologic examination or direct immunofluorescence examination of a biopsy specimen. Treatment is covered in Chapter 119.

BULLOUS PEMPHIGOID. This condition appears to be somewhat less common than pemphigus vulgaris. Again, the oral mucosa is a frequent site, often with other mucocutaneous junction areas and sometimes more generalized skin lesions.

Other immune-mediated diseases documented as causing oral lesions include systemic lupus erythematosus, discoid lupus erythematosus, and drug eruption toxic epidermal necrolysis.[23]

Other autoimmune diseases may affect the skin of the lips; lesions produced by them may extend into the oral cavity as a result of self-trauma.

Xerostomia

Xerostomia (dry mouth) is an uncommon finding in dogs and cats. Removal of all of the major (mandibular, sublingual, and parotid) glands bilaterally does not cause observable abnormality.[111]

An immune-mediated xerostomia is known to occur in humans as a component of Sjögren's syndrome (xerostomia, keratoconjunctivitis sicca, and rheumatoid arthritis). Several cases of apparent Sjögren's syndrome have been reported in dogs.[112, 113] Canine Sjögren's syndrome may be widespread but subclinical, as 10 of 50 (20 per cent) dogs with keratoconjunctivitis sicca had xerostomia (severe periodontitis, loss of teeth and dry oral mucous membranes as judged by owner's report, and reduced salivary response to noxious taste stimulation); four of these ten dogs had rheumatoid factor titers of 1:16 or greater.[114] Xerostomia caused by immune-mediated disorders can be treated with immune-suppressant medications (see Chapter 119). Because of the typical microscopic appearance and frequent finding of a polyclonal hyperglobulinemia, an autoimmune basis for feline plasmacytic-lymphocytic gingivitis-stomatitis has been proposed.[93] The lesions frequently respond, at least temporarily, to prednisolone or other anti-inflammatory therapy. Treatment of recurrent or steroidal-nonresponsive chronic gingivitis-stomatitis in cats with aurothioglucose has not been successful. Treatment of

cats with a combination of pododermatitis and plasma cell stomatitis with aurothioglucose has been more successful.[110]

Local Disease That Causes Oral Lesions

Periodontal disease is the most common condition affecting the mouth of the dog and cat, as discussed previously. Other causes are described here.

INFECTION

Viral Stomatitis. In the cat, both feline rhinotracheitis virus (FVR) and feline calicivirus (FCV) (synonym: feline picornavirus) can cause ulcerative stomatitis and gingivitis (Figure 82–36).[115] Although FCV is more often responsible, the ulcerative lesions produced by FVR can be severe and extensive. Additional descriptions of these diseases are presented in Chapter 48; see also Periodontal Disease above.

Oral papillomatosis is a specific viral infection discussed under Oral Hyperplastic and Neoplastic Disease. Other viral diseases such as canine distemper and feline panleukopenia may cause stomatitis, although other organs are more severely affected.

Mycotic Infection. Candidiasis (infection with the yeast *Candida albicans*) is a rare cause of severe stomatitis in the dog and cat; it usually occurs in debilitated animals, animals that are immune-suppressed, or those that have received long-term antibiotic or corticosteroid therapy. The classic white pseudo-membrane covering the lesion ("thrush") is sometimes seen, although more often the lesions are irregular ulcerated areas surrounded by a zone of inflamed mucosa (Figure 82–37). Diagnosis is by fungal culture of the lesion. Further description is presented in Chapter 49.

Treatment with local application of antifungal drugs gives mixed results;[116] systemic antifungal therapy (ketaconazole) may be necessary, and a thorough examination should be made for causes of immune suppression.

Similar ulcerative or pseudomembranous lesions, usually associated with periodontal disease, can be

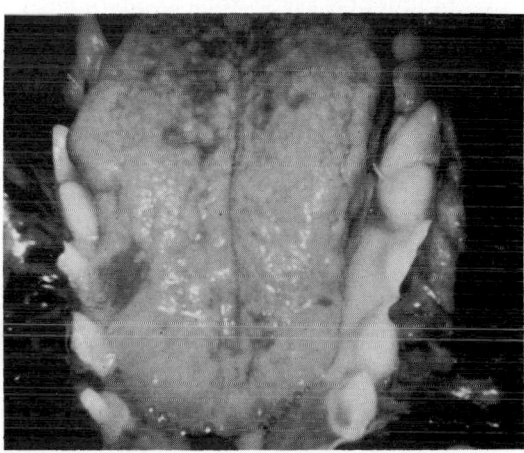

FIGURE 82–37. Tongue of a dog with *Candida albicans* infection. The tongue is almost completely covered by a thick white exudate.

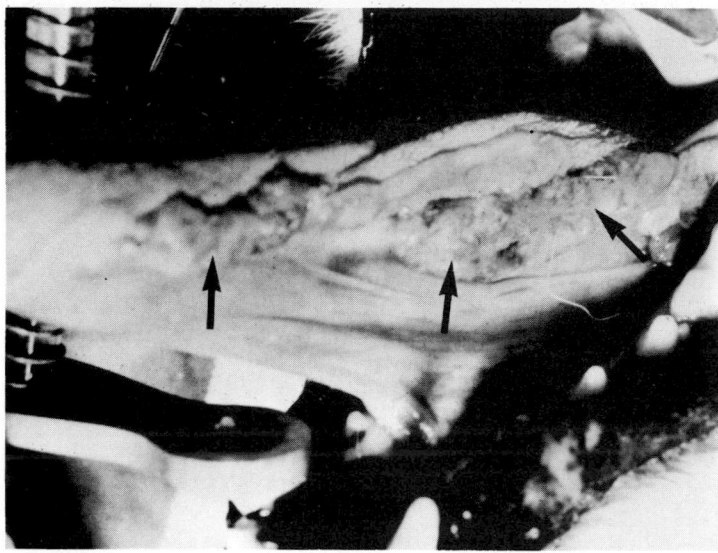

FIGURE 82–38. Eosinophilic granuloma lesions (arrows) on the tongue of a Siberian husky dog.

caused by or associated with *Nocardia* and *Actinomyces* spp.[116, 117] Rarely, nasal fungal infection (aspergillosis or penicilliosis) can spread through the nasopalatine duct and involve the oral cavity.

Oral Hyperplastic and Neoplastic Disease

The most common hyperplastic disease of the oral cavity is gingival hyperplasia, either familial or associated with periodontal disease (Figures 82–26 and 82–32) (see Periodontal Disease, above). Tumors in the oropharynx of the dog and cat are usually accompanied by some degree of stomatitis, particularly when they enlarge and impinge on normal tissue or are traumatized during mastication. A sickening halitosis caused by bacterial activity in necrotic tissue or by food trapped in crevices is frequently a major reason for presentation of an animal with neoplastic disease. Malignant neoplasms are discussed under Oropharyngeal Neoplasia. The most common benign growths are epulis and oral viral papillomatosis.

Eosinophilic granuloma lesions may be seen in the palate, fauces, or tongue of cats. Diagnosis is by cytology or biopsy; treatment is as for labial granuloma. A similar condition has been reported as occurring on the tongue or palate of Siberian husky dogs (Figure 82–38).[118, 119]

Epulis (Periodontal Fibrous Hyperplasia). Nonulcerated cauliflower-like growths at the gingival margin are frequently seen in the Boxer and bulldog and, less commonly, in other breeds (Figure 82–39). The lesions are not neoplastic, rarely causing clinical signs except when large enough to be damaged by the teeth of the other ipsilateral jaw. Treatment is rarely necessary; excessively large lesions may be removed by surgical excision or electroexcision. The exception to this is acanthomatous epulis, which often invades bone and is grossly indistinguishable from squamous cell carcinoma; this condition, while benign in the sense that it does not metastasize, behaves locally like an aggressive malignant tumor. The classification and differentiation of proliferative gingival diseases were reviewed recently with the aim of standardizing nomenclature.[120] The pathology of epulides was also reviewed recently.[121]

Oral Papillomatosis. This is a self-limiting viral disease usually seen in puppies and young dogs, consisting of wart-like growths that develop on the tongue and oral mucous membranes.[122] Clinical signs depend on the number and location of the lesions. In the severely affected animal there may be dysphagia and drooling of saliva. Treatment should be supportive and conservative; definitive treatment is difficult to evaluate, since the disease is self-limiting (disappearing in 6 to 12 weeks). Surgical removal, which may initiate regression, should be reserved for dogs in which mechanical trauma causes injury. Although the disease is known to be viral in origin, the route of transmission is unknown. Immunity is lifelong after the disease has been contracted.

Transmissible Venereal Cell Tumors. This tumor affects the mucosa of the genital organs of young, sexually mature animals. Oral lesions occasionally result from the animal's licking of the primary lesion and affect the lips, tongue, gingiva, or cheek. In most instances, these tumors regress spontaneously, although occasional metastasis is seen. The tumors appear as lobulated,

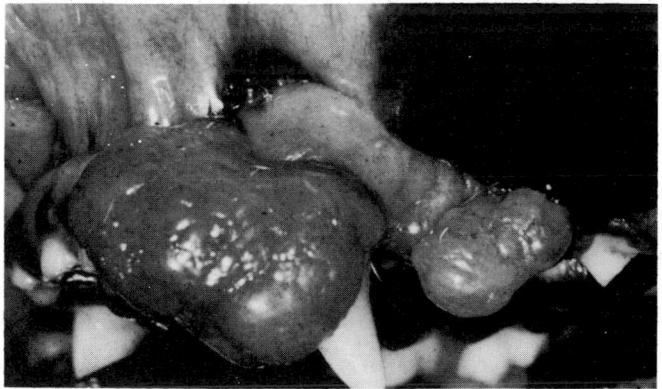

FIGURE 82–39. Maxilla of a Boxer dog with epulis. A large, nonulcerated mass is partially covering the upper canine and several incisor teeth. A smaller epulis lesion is also present caudal to the canine.

cauliflower-like sessile masses that are hyperemic and friable. Ulceration and necrosis develop later. The external genitalia should be examined. Surgical removal of lesions causing dysphagia is warranted, and treatment with cytotoxic drugs has been suggested.

Chemical, Thermal, Electric Burn, or Foreign Body Injury

Dogs and cats are occasionally presented after ingesting corrosive chemicals or chewing on electric cords. If the initial communication with the owners is by telephone, they should be instructed to flush the animal's mouth copiously with water to prevent further damage. The active ingredients should be identified from the label, but it is unlikely that specific antidotes can be used early enough to be of value. Vinegar or lemon juice may be used if the chemical is an alkaline caustic (the most common caustics readily available in the home). Acids may be counteracted by sodium bicarbonate solution.

Animals that sustain electric burn injuries of the mouth should be examined carefully for signs of shock or pulmonary edema, and appropriate treatment commenced.[123] Sustained sinus tachycardia is a complication of this problem that should not be overlooked.

Management of local injuries caused by chemical, thermal, or electric burns consists of gentle cleansing of the wounds with isotonic saline solution and careful debridement if the injury is severe. Management of specific injuries of the lips, palate, and tongue is discussed in a following section. Pharyngeal or esophageal scarring following ingestion of a caustic may require long-term steroid or surgical treatment.

PLANT AWN STOMATITIS. The most common oral locations of plant awn trauma are the tongue and gingivae, particularly the incisor and canine areas where penetration during grooming is most likely.[116] Diagnosis is made by observing the plant material in the oral tissues. When material is deeply embedded, treatment may require sedation or anesthesia to permit curettage. The lesions readily resolve once the foreign material is removed.[116]

Stomatitis of Unknown Origin

Undocumented clinical observations of Maltese terriers suggest that this breed suffers from ulcerative gingivitis/stomatitis more commonly than other breeds.[124] Although an immune-mediated cause of this condition can be demonstrated by biopsy and clinical laboratory tests in only about 20 per cent of affected dogs,[125] a combination of thorough teeth cleaning, good home oral hygiene, and intermittent or continuous prednisolone therapy is often successful in suppressing clinical signs.

Occasionally, animals with severe ulcerative or necrotic stomatitis are seen in which the search for a cause is unrewarding. If the disease does not appear to be confined to or most severe at the periodontal tissues, arbitrary removal of teeth may worsen the disease. Prolonged, intermittent antibiotic and local therapy

gives temporary relief, but signs of disease often reappear shortly after cessation of antibiotic therapy. Metronidazole (14 mg/lb orally once a day) used daily every other week is often helpful. Lesions that appear to consist of persistent, nonhealing granulation tissue may respond to oral prednisolone (0.5 mg/lb twice daily for two weeks). The use of levamisole as a nonspecific immune stimulant is effective in some cases of recurrent stomatitis in humans.[126]

Local Therapy in Oral Diseases

Gentle cleansing with cotton-wrapped applicators soaked in isotonic saline or sodium bicarbonate solution is soothing, but these can be used in only the most cooperative patient. An antiseptic (such as 0.1 to 0.2 per cent chlorhexidine solution) or antibiotic-fungicidal agent combination (such as tetracycline-amphotericin B) applied locally three to four times per day may be helpful. A soft diet and rinsing of the mouth with salt solution after feeding reduce pain and bacterial growth in diseased tissue. Occasionally, electrocautery or chemical cautery (silver nitrate or phenol) is indicated for localized, chronic, nonresponsive oral ulceration.

LIPS AND CHEEKS

Congenital Anomalies

Harelip occasionally occurs in the dog, often in association with cleft palate (Figure 82–40);[127] repair is rarely attempted because of the ethical considerations of correction of congenital abnormalities. Harelip without associated cleft palate may be midline, bilateral, or unilateral, and rarely results in clinical signs other than the obvious deformity and a slight serous discharge from the nose.

Microcheilia (reduced oral fissure) reportedly occurs, particularly in schnauzers. Contraction of the muscles of the upper lip is seen in setters occasionally.[128]

Acquired Conditions

INJURIES

The most common injuries of the lips are caused by fights or the animal's biting of an electric cord.[123] Avulsion of the lower lip from the mandible can result from blunt trauma.

Portions of lip that have been ripped from their normal attachment should be reattached as soon as possible to prevent contraction and fixation of the lip in an abnormal position, particularly in those animals in which the lower lip is separated from the mandible (Figure 82–41). A wire tension suture looped around the lower canine teeth may be used to retain the avulsed skin in a normal position.[129] Subsequent reconstructive surgery to cover a denuded mandibular symphysis is difficult, because little loose skin is available in the vicinity, which necessitates pedicle or tube grafts.

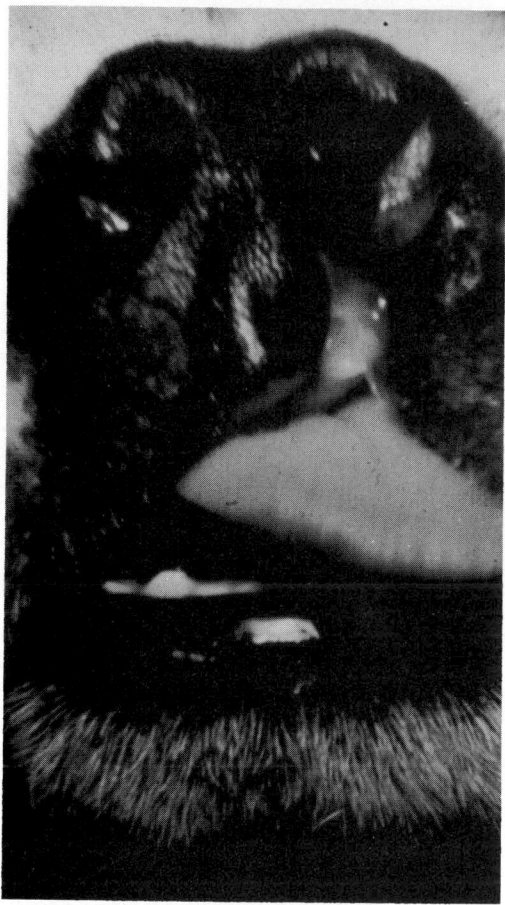

FIGURE 82–40. Nose and lips of a dog with congenital unilateral harelip.

Electric cord burn injuries affecting the commissure of the lips may require subsequent surgical treatment if sloughing and cicatrization cause reduced jaw movement.

CHEILITIS

Lip inflammation may be associated with inflammation of adjacent areas (Figure 82–42) but rarely warrants treatment other than gentle cleansing. Inflammation caused by contact with irritants such as plastic and plant material may produce a chronic cheilitis and associated dermatitis.

Firm nodules up to one cm in diameter, which are often multiple, may be felt in the lips of the dog and cat. Usually these nodules are chronically inflamed hair follicles or skin glands, or small abscesses caused by foreign body penetration. They may occasionally break open and discharge; treatment is rarely necessary.

CHRONIC LIP FOLD DERMATITIS

The hairy skin of the lips is subject to many dermatologic disorders. These conditions include immune-mediated mucocutaneous junction diseases. Skin diseases affecting the lips often are exacerbated by frequent contact with saliva or food. This is particularly true of dogs such as spaniels with lip conformation that exac-

erbates the effect of the lateral lower lip frenulum, as this results in a furrow that channels oral contents onto the skin. The result is "lip-fold dermatitis."

The clinical signs are a noxious odor, drooling from the lower lip, and pawing at the mouth. Diagnosis is made by inspection of the lip fold, since the odor can mimic that of periodontal disease or uremic halitosis (Figure 82–43).

Management consists of frequent gentle washing with an antibacterial soap and water; this is followed by application of an anti-inflammatory steroid cream. Clipping the hair around the lip fold is helpful. Surgical resection of the lip fold is curative in stubborn or recurrent cases. Coexisting periodontal disease should be treated.

LABIAL GRANULOMA

Labial granuloma (labial ulcer, eosinophilic granuloma) is a chronic granulomatous lesion of the lip of the cat. The precipitating factor is unknown. Continued licking by the hard spines of the tongue aggravates the condition. The lesion is usually located in the midline or just to one side of the midline of the upper lip (Figure 82–44). Licking may cause the lesion to spread to other areas, most often the skin of the hind limbs, although the base of the tongue, palate, and fauces of the oral cavity may also be affected. Diagnosis is made by inspection, scraping of the lesion, cytologic examination, or biopsy and histopathologic examination.

Currently the most successful methods of treatment are administration of anti-inflammatory steroids and radiation. Steroids can be given systemically (prednisolone, 1 mg/lb divided twice per day and given orally until the lesions have disappeared; the dosage is then tapered off over two weeks); locally (intralesional injection of one to two ml of repository prednisolone); or in combination.[130] The effective radiation dosage is 500 to 1000 rads given as one or two applications.[131] Alternative treatments that have been reported as successful

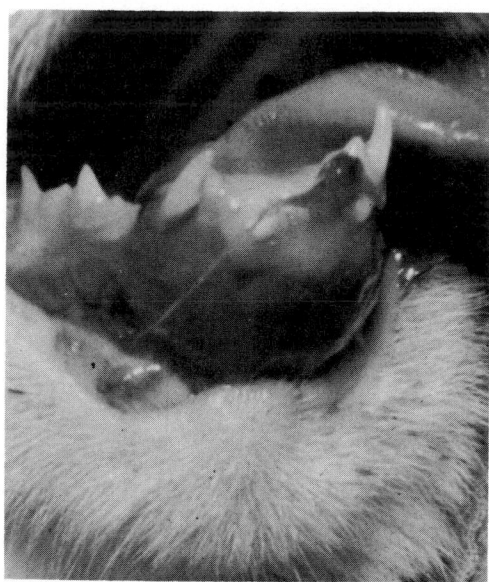

FIGURE 82–41. Mandible of a cat with an avulsed lower lip.

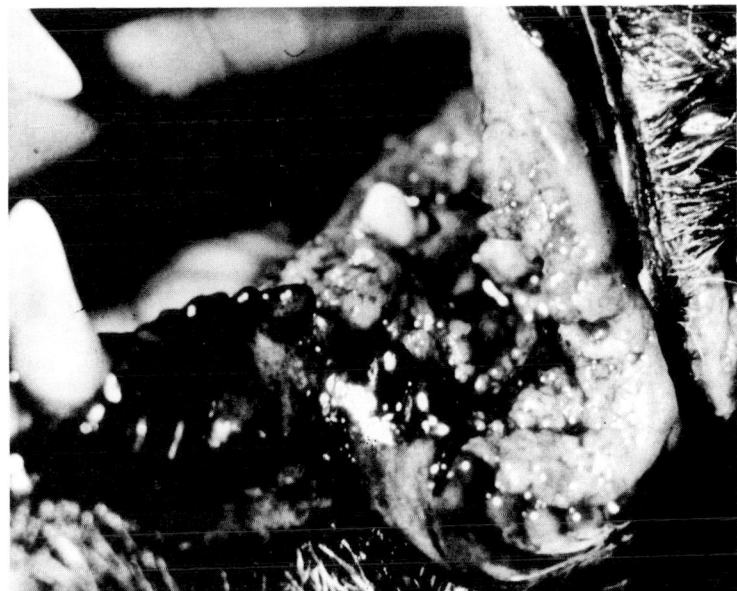

FIGURE 82–42. Extensive ulcerative and proliferative cheilitis secondary to severe periodontal disease in a dog.

include megestrol acetate (Ovaban, two mg every other day or twice weekly) and cryosurgery.[132] Recurrence is possible with any of these treatment methods.

Occasionally the disease erodes the external nares and part of the nasal bones and septum. Reconstruction following the arrest of the lesion is rarely feasible.

NEOPLASMS OF THE LIPS AND CHEEKS

Neoplasms arising from the mucosal surface of the lips and cheeks are discussed under Oropharyngeal Neoplasia. Tumors of the skin and connective tissue of the cheek occasionally occur. Treatment and prognosis are based on histopathologic diagnosis.

TONGUE

Congenital Anomalies

Abnormal narrowing of the tongue with inability to swallow has been attributed to a lethal simple recessive autosomal defect in the dog.[133] The condition (colloquially known as "bird tongue") causes the death of all affected pups a few days after birth. Lateral protrusion of the tongue has been reported in a King Charles spaniel[134] and was seen by the author in a Great Pyrenees dog.

Acquired Diseases

INJURIES

The most common tongue injuries are lacerations caused by licking sharp surfaces, ingesting caustics or foreign bodies, and biting electric cords (Figures 82–45 to 82–47). Clinical signs of lacerations or foreign body penetration of the tongue are lingual swelling, drooling of blood-tinged saliva, and pawing at the mouth.

Clean lacerations should be sutured with surgical gut to control bleeding and appose cut edges. Jagged lacerations may require debridement prior to suturing. Removal of bodies, such as fishhooks, may require

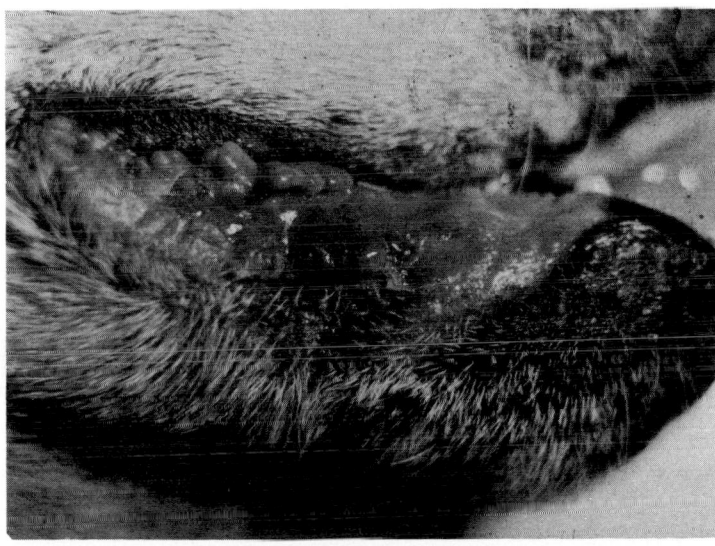

FIGURE 82–43. Lower lip of a dog with chronic lip-fold dermatitis.

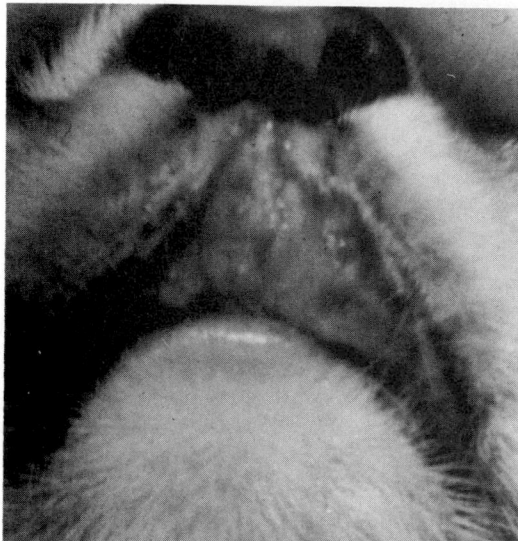

FIGURE 82–44. Upper lip of a cat with labial granuloma. The upper lip is ulcerated and thickened from the rhinarium to the lip margin.

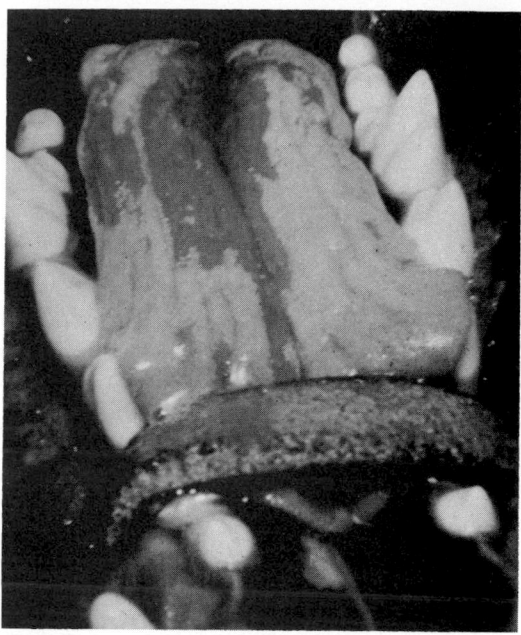

FIGURE 82–46. Tongue of a dog with superficial ulceration following lye ingestion.

incision of the tongue. If a piece of wood is embedded in the tongue, a careful check should be made to ensure that all splinters are removed. Animals with burn injuries caused by biting electric cords should be examined for signs of shock or pulmonary edema.[123] The tongue lesion is cleaned and irrigated with isotonic saline, and broad-spectrum antibiotics are administered pending sloughing of necrotic tissue. When the necrotic section has sloughed, the tongue heals by granulation. Dogs manage well if the caudal two-thirds of the tongue is intact. When more than the rostral third of the tongue sloughs, it is necessary to experiment with various types of food. Meatball-sized pieces that the dog can pick up and toss to the back of its mouth, or canned food mixed with water to a soupy consistency that the dog can suck, may be successful as management.[135] Because of an inability to groom, a cat that has lost most of its tongue may represent a problem because of hair matting or soiling.[136]

Another cause of injury is a linear foreign body such as string or thread that becomes caught around or beneath the tongue after both ends have been swallowed.[137] The animal moves its tongue constantly trying to remove the offending object, causing the string to saw its way into the frenulum. The animal shows a characteristic head-tucked-down, tongue-moving posture. A circular foreign body (tracheal rings of food animals or rubber bands) can become caught around the tongue, occasionally causing swelling and subsequent necrosis of the tongue. Foreign bodies around or caught beneath the tongue should be removed; other treatment is usually unnecessary. The granulomatous lesion seen in the frenulum caused by an embedded foreign body can be confused with a neoplasm (Figure 82–48), because this is a common site for squamous cell carcinoma in the cat.

Glossitis

Inflammation of the epithelium of the tongue can result from many causes (see Stomatitis). Sloughing of the rostral part of the tongue is seen occasionally in dogs with acute renal failure, pancreatitis, and leptospirosis; the mechanism causing the lesion is unknown. The lesions usually resolve if the primary disease can be corrected. Severe chronic renal failure causes a more intractable glossitis and glossal ulceration. An epizootic glossitis of military dogs in Southeast Asia has been reported; routine techniques for isolation of bacteria and viruses failed to suggest an etiologic agent.[138] Chronic exposure to sunlight caused a similar lesion in experimental dogs, both with and without photosensitizing medication to which clinically affected dogs may have been exposed.[139]

Ulcerative glossitis occurs in cats as a result of feline herpes (FVR), calicivirus, and panleukopenia virus infection[140] (Figure 82–36). The tongue ulcers are painful and may result in dehydration; gastrostomy or pharyn-

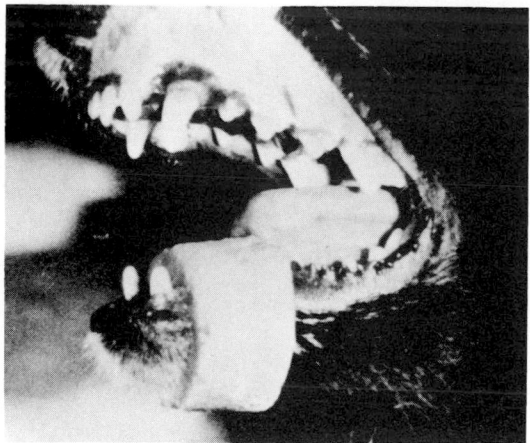

FIGURE 82–45. Oral foreign body. A section of bovine femur is trapped over the mandible and tongue.

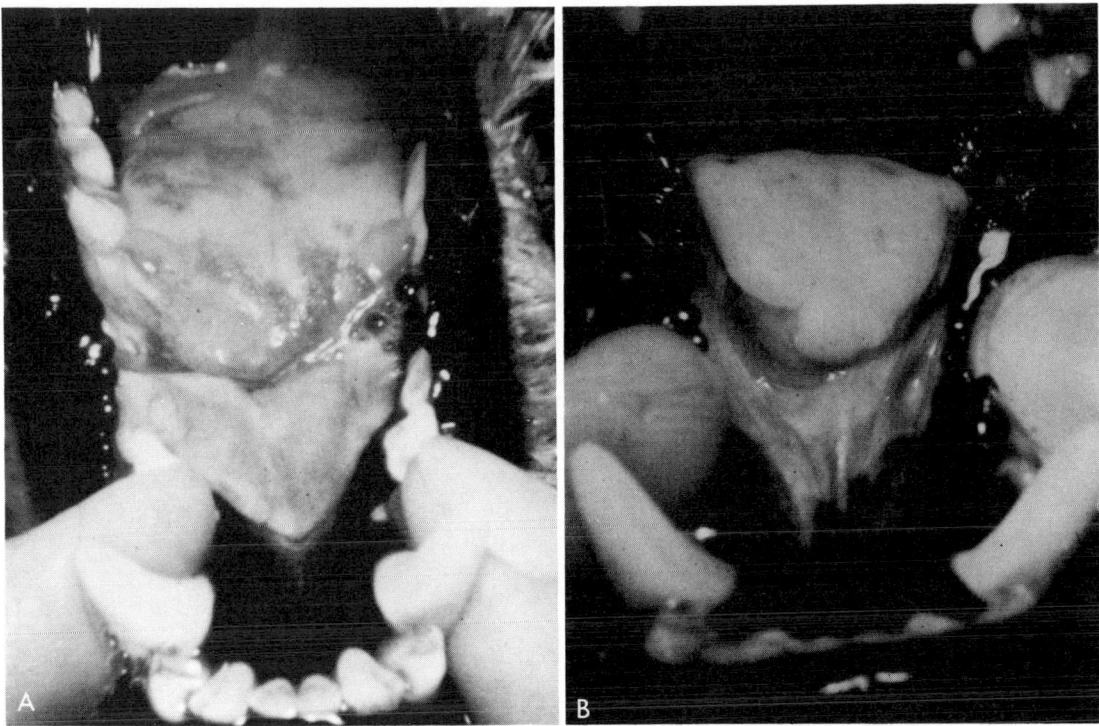

FIGURE 82-47. *A*, Tongue of a dog one day after biting an electric cord. The necrotic portion of the tongue is clearly demarcated. *B*, Eighteen days following the injury. The tongue is covered by epithelium. The dog was eating and drinking without difficulty.

gostomy intubation may be indicated for several days during the acute infection and early healing phases of the disease. These infections are described in more detail in the Infectious Diseases section.

Occasionally, chronic inflammation of the deeper tissues of the tongue occurs and may be associated with embedded foreign material (Figure 82-49) or chronic trauma from chewing on wood or metal surfaces

Secondary bacterial or fungal infections such as actinobacillosis may be superimposed. Polymyositis, which most often affects the muscles of mastication, occasionally affects the tongue. Calcinosis circumscripta occurs occasionally in the tongue of the dog[141] and has been associated with *Pasteurella multocida* infection.[4]

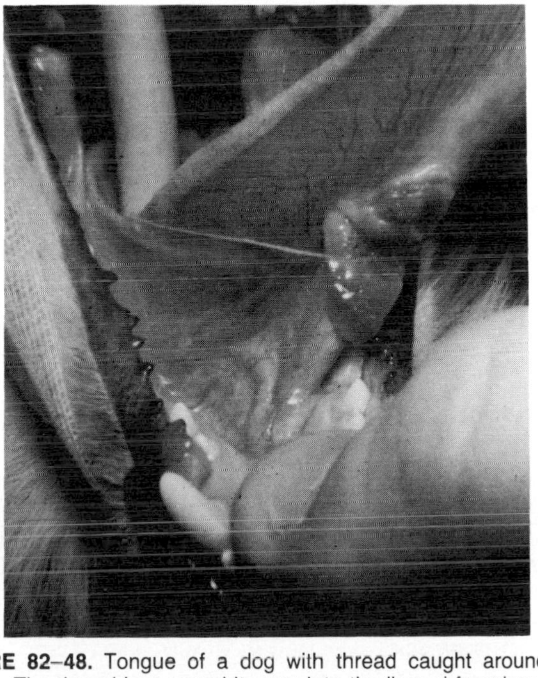

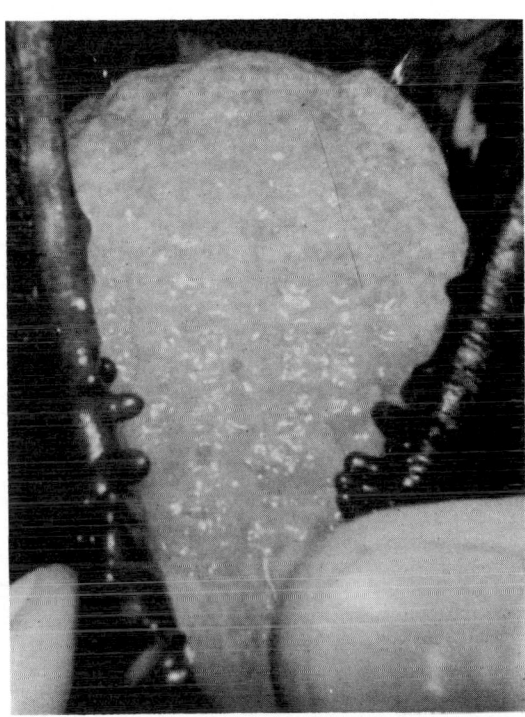

FIGURE 82-48. Tongue of a dog with thread caught around the tongue. The thread has sawed its way into the lingual frenulum.

FIGURE 82-49. Tongue of a dog with glossitis resulting from chewing cockle burrs.

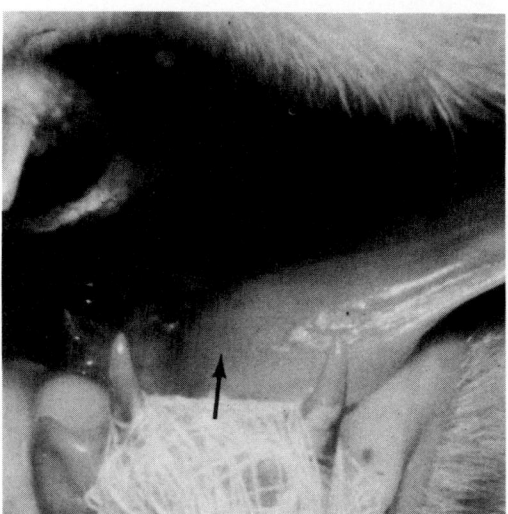

FIGURE 82–50. Mouth of a cat with abscessation of the lower jaw causing severe edema (arrow) of the sublingual tissues.

Rows of hair follicles (either a single midline row or two rows symmetrically arranged to each side of the midline) that contain long, fine hairs are occasionally seen as an incidental finding in the tongue of the dog. Rarely, a chronic granulomatous reaction may be associated with inflammation of hair follicles in the base of the tongue.

Lesions similar to labial granuloma can occasionally affect the tissues anywhere on the tongue in the cat or on the lateral edge or sublingual surface in Siberian husky dogs (Figure 82–38).[118, 119] Diagnosis and treatment are the same as that for labial granuloma.

Interference with venous drainage caused by an abscess or neoplasm of the floor of the mouth results in edema of the lingual frenulum and sublingual tissue. It may be so severe as to resemble a ranula (salivary mucocele beneath the tongue) (Figure 82–50). Differentiation is based on the grey translucent appearance, retention of pressure marks, the finding of a causative lesion for the edema, and needle aspiration of mucus from the ranula.

Neoplasia of the Tongue

Squamous cell carcinoma occurs in the tongue of cats usually as a solid mass in the root.[143] Tumors of the tongue are rare in dogs.[144] See also Oropharyngeal Neoplasia.

DISEASES OF THE PHARYNX

Congenital Anomalies and Injuries

The occurrence, diagnosis, and management of congenital anomalies and injuries of the palate and pharynx are discussed in Chapter 67.

Pharyngitis

Primary pharyngitis is not common in the dog; it is usually part of a more widespread oral or systemic disease. Viral infections of cats can cause palatal ulceration with no other obvious signs of disease, although more frequently there will be sneezing and nasal discharge. Pharyngitis in the cat is usually seen as an increase in the number and size of blood vessels on the surface of the soft palate, although the presence of obvious vessels should not automatically be regarded as indicative of inflammation.

Localized pharyngeal irritation may be caused by a foreign body. Needles, pins, and bone spicules commonly lodge in the subepiglottal or piriform fossa areas and may penetrate and migrate in soft tissue. Radiographic examination (two views) is necessary to pinpoint their location. Surgical removal of the foreign body combined with drainage of the associated abscess is curative.

Dysphagia

Difficulty in swallowing may be caused by localized diseases of the oropharynx and esophagus or by central cranial nerve disease. Clinical signs often associated with dysphagia are drooling, nasal discharge, and cough caused by airway aspiration of food or fluid.

The pain of severe inflammatory disease of the palate, pharynx, or tonsils causes dysphagia. The inflamed mucosa or tonsils are obvious on examination, and the dysphagia recedes as the animal responds to treatment for the inflammatory disease. Infiltrating tumors of the pharyngeal wall, particularly tonsillar squamous cell carcinoma, sometimes present because of dysphagia. Those diseases causing dysphagia that are insidious in onset or show no obvious cause on physical examination are a greater challenge to diagnosis and management. Several neuromuscular conditions have been recognized in the dog as causing dysphagia; differentiation by fluoroscopic contrast swallowing study has been described.[5] Similar information for the cat is unavailable.

Malfunction of the tongue can be caused by damaged hypoglossal nerves following bulla osteotomy or by sublingual salivary gland removal. Animals can usually manage well if food is provided in the form of meatballs that can be tossed to the back of the mouth.

Glossopharyngeal, vagal, and trigeminal neuropathy can cause a syndrome of dropped jaw, temporal and masseter muscle atrophy, drooling of saliva, and nasal regurgitation of fluid during drinking. The dog gags repeatedly during attempts at swallowing, and food often drops from the mouth. The pattern of dysphagia may suggest a diagnosis; however, careful neurologic examination and fluoroscopic visualization of a barium swallow is necessary to differentiate pharyngeal paralysis from cricopharyngeal (cranial esophageal sphincter) achalasia (described in Chapter 83). The etiology of this pharyngeal paralysis syndrome is unknown. Some animals recover spontaneously; in others the neural dysfunction is progressive; and in others it may respond to

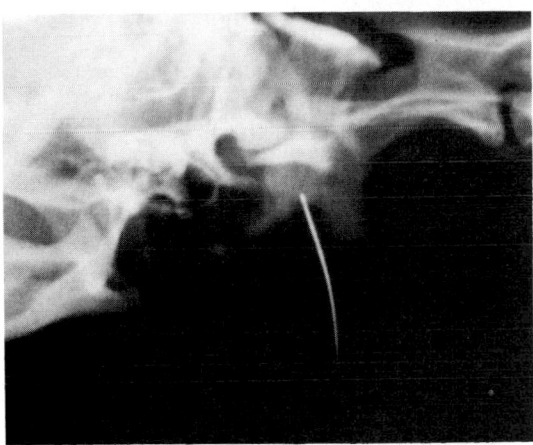

FIGURE 82–51. A sewing needle embedded in the pharyngeal soft tissues of a cat.

anti-inflammatory corticosteroid therapy.[145] Other possible causes of chronic dysphagia include temporomandibular joint disease, eosinophilic myositis, and pharyngeal space-occupying lesions or foreign bodies.

Supportive therapy maintains nutrition during the period of dysfunction. Feeding by nasogastric or pharyngostomy tube has been used, although often the owner can feed liquids using a syringe inserted into the buccal fold.

Retropharyngeal Abscess

Pharyngeal abscesses are common in the dog; evidence of external trauma is not usually found. Pins, needles, chicken bones, grass awns, and sticks are frequent causes (Figure 82–51). Often the foreign body penetrates partially and is then expelled. Clinical signs are pyrexia, anorexia, and pain and swelling of the pharyngeal area (Figure 82–52). If no foreign body is obvious on inspection and palpation of the mouth and pharynx, a therapeutic trial using a systemic orally administered antibiotic is warranted. Should clinical signs persist or localized abscess occur, lateral and dorsoventral radiographs of the head should be taken to examine for the presence of a radiopaque foreign body. If a foreign body is seen on radiographs, it should be removed and the abscess drained. If no radiopaque foreign body is present, the abscess cavity should be explored with a gloved finger in an effort to locate a nonradiopaque foreign body. A soft rubber drain is sutured in the abscess cavity and systemic antibiotics are continued. The drain is removed three to four days later. Recovery is usually uneventful. If the swelling recurs, the cavity should be laid open surgically and packed with antiseptic-soaked sponges until the wound closes by granulation-contraction.

Tonsillitis

Inflammation of the tonsils is common in the dog and, apparently, less frequent in the cat. Tonsillitis is usually bilateral, but in occasional cases a foreign body such as a grass awn caught in the tonsillar crypt causes unilateral disease.

Clinically, tonsillitis patients can often be divided into two groups. One group consists of animals with concurrent preexisting disease considered as predisposing to tonsillitis. Primary diseases causing secondary tonsillitis include those that cause chronic vomiting or regurgitation (megaesophagus, pylorospasm, gastric neoplasia), chronic productive cough (bronchitis or bronchiectasis), or chronic contamination of the nasopharynx (nasal disease causing a nasopharyngeal discharge, cleft palate, dysphagia due to pharyngeal dysfunction). The tonsillitis may be the most obvious clinical finding. Since there are many initiating causes, dogs and cats of a wide range of ages and breeds are affected.

The second group consists of animals with primary tonsillitis. Young, small breed dogs are most frequently affected. The tonsils form part of a ring of lymphoid tissue in the oropharynx that reacts to many stimuli. Dogs with primary tonsillitis retch, cough, and show malaise, fever, and inappetence. The clinical signs may be caused by inflammation of the pharyngeal mucosa, with or without tonsillar swelling. Treatment with an antibiotic usually results in clinical improvement, although tonsillar swelling is often obvious on reexamination in five to seven days. Lymphocytic hyperplasia with lymphatic infiltration of the overlying epithelium is

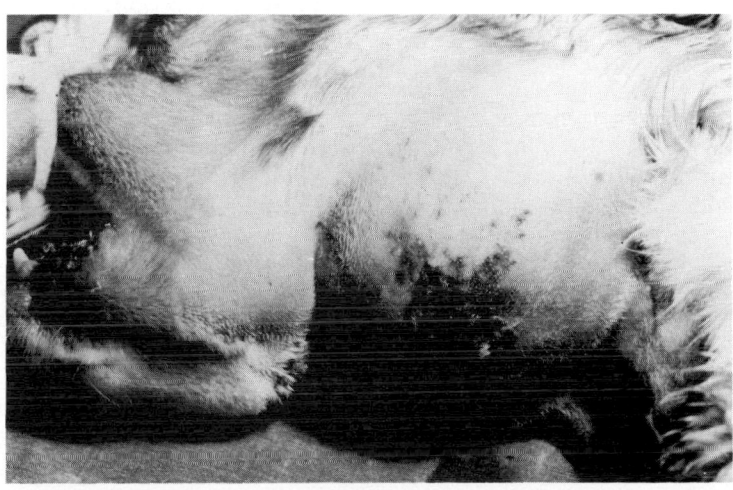

FIGURE 82–52. Retropharyngeal abscess, with necrosis of overlying skin and extensive edema of the mandibular and facial soft tissues rostral to the abscess.

TABLE 82–2. BACTERIA ISOLATED FROM THE OROPHARYNX OF DOGS

	Dogs (%)	
Organism	Healthy	With pharyngitis-tonsillitis
Streptococcus	35–100	14–60
Staphylococcus	24–89	9–45
Pasteurella	10–65	0–9
Micrococcus	30–65	0
Escherichia	15–75	0–40
Neisseria	20–100	0
Proteus	15–40	0–5
Pseudomonas	5–20	0–5
Enterobacter	0–40	0
Corynebacterium	1–15	0
Bacillus	5–40	0
Moraxella	0	0
Diphtheroids	10–35	0
Alcaligenes	25–40	0
Diplococcus	0	0–9

From Harvey, CE: Therapeutic strategies involving antimicrobial treatment of the upper respiratory tract in small animals. JAVMA 185:1159, 1984.

the most common histologic finding. Chronic or recurrent tonsillitis in young dogs is interpreted as part of the maturation of pharyngeal defense mechanisms.[146] The most common bacteria associated with tonsillitis in the dog are also bacteria that are commonly found in the tonsillar area of normal dogs, such as *Escherichia coli*, *Staphylococcus aureus*, and *S. albus*, hemolytic Streptococcus, and diplococcus, Proteus, and *Pseudomonas* spp. (Table 82–2).[147, 148]

Diagnosis of tonsillitis is made by direct inspection of the tonsils. The owner should be questioned for signs of coexistent disease that may be triggering the tonsillitis. The appearance of the tonsils in the dog varies considerably and may show little correlation with the animal's condition. Color is a more accurate indication of abnormality than size or prominence. Occasionally, the tonsils may be acutely inflamed but still be contained within the crypt; this is more likely to occur in the cat than in the dog. Acutely inflamed tonsils appear bright red, and inflammation of the surrounding mucosa may be obvious. Punctate hemorrhages may also be seen. Localized abscesses may be visible as white specks on the surface of the tonsil. The tonsil is friable and bleeds easily if touched. Other causes of tonsillar enlargement are squamous cell carcinoma and lymphosarcoma (see Neoplasia).

An inflamed, swollen tonsil is not an absolute indication for treatment. If the animal is showing clinical signs indicating pharyngeal irritation, broad-spectrum antibiotics may be administered. When pharyngeal irritation is severe, mild analgesics may offer relief.

Tonsillitis and pharyngitis may be recurrent in young dogs. Periodic attacks of retching usually cease when the dog matures. Tonsillectomy provides permanent relief from clinical signs caused by chronic, primary tonsillitis but is rarely necessary. General anesthesia and endotracheal intubation are essential. To prevent aspiration of blood, a moist gauze sponge should be placed in the pharynx around an endotracheal tube prior to removal of the tonsillar tissue by scissors or electroscal-

pel. Individual bleeding vessels are ligated, or the edges of the tonsillar crypt are sutured with fine surgical gut. The animal should be allowed to recover slowly from anesthesia to permit further checks for bleeding.

Tonsillectomy is occasionally indicated in mature animals when the enlarged tonsils stand out in their crypts, causing mechanical interference with swallowing or air flow. This is most likely to be seen in dogs with a relatively narrow oropharynx, such as cocker spaniels or Saint Bernards, or in dogs with upper airway disease when the superimposed mechanical obstruction due to the tonsillar enlargement may increase airway obstruction.

OROPHARYNGEAL NEOPLASIA

Neoplastic diseases of the mouth are important because of the high incidence (reported as 20/100,000 for the dog and 11/100,000 for the cat) and the poor prognosis.[149, 150] Male dogs are more at risk than females.[151]

The three most common malignant neoplasms of the dog's mouth are fibrosarcoma (Figure 82–53), malignant melanoma (Figure 82–54), and squamous cell carcinoma (Figure 82–55). The clinical features of a series of 361 dogs are summarized in Table 82–3.[150] The lesions usually appear both proliferative and ulcerated, although destructive lesions with little tissue proliferation are also seen. Blood-tinged saliva and halitosis are the most common clinical signs. In many cases a diagnosis cannot be made from the gross appearance and position of an oral neoplasm in the dog. Malignant melanoma (which may be amelanotic) occurs with greater frequency in cocker spaniels, and German shepherd dogs more frequently develop fibrosarcoma than other breeds. In general, malignant oropharyngeal neoplasms

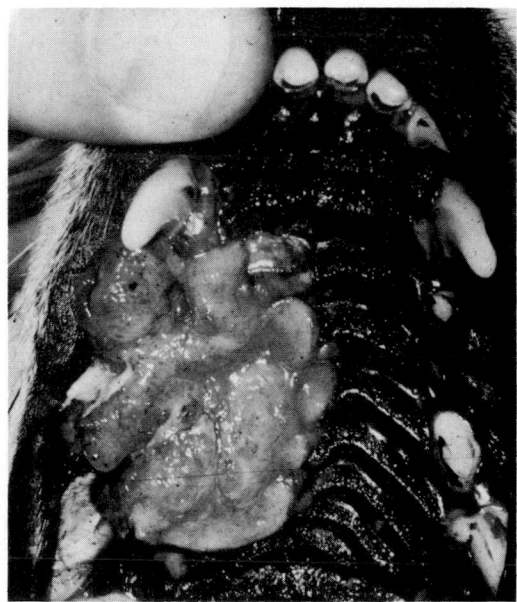

FIGURE 82–53. Hard palate of a dog with a large fibrosarcoma of the right gingival palate margin.

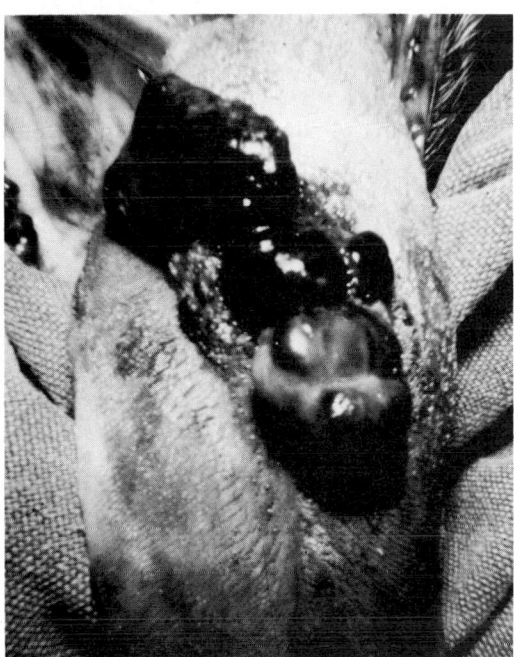

FIGURE 82–54. Tongue of a dog with melanoma of its dorsal surface.

occur in old dogs; the exception is fibrosarcoma, which occurs over a wide age range. Local invasion of bone is very frequent. Acanthomatous epulis, a benign tumor, often behaves locally as an aggressive lesion invading bone.

Because of the poor prognosis for common malignant lesions, confirmation of diagnosis by biopsy and histopathologic examination is essential. Thoracic radiographs should be examined prior to treatment.

The most common oral tumor of the cat is squamous cell carcinoma. The sites most often affected are the gingiva and the tongue, especially in the area of the lingual frenulum. As with dogs, the prognosis is poor.

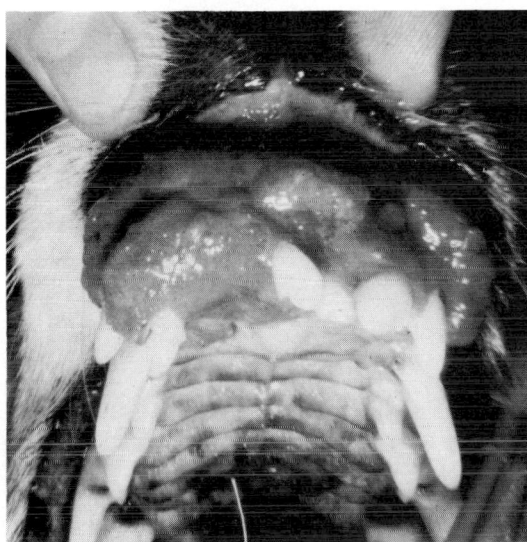

FIGURE 82–55. Upper jaw of a dog with an extensive squamous cell carcinoma of the incisive gingiva.

Management of Oropharyngeal Neoplasms

After a histopathologic diagnosis has been established, treatment and prognosis should be discussed with the owner. Conservative surgical treatment is rarely practical except as palliation, because malignant melanoma, fibrosarcoma, squamous cell carcinoma, acanthomatous epulis, and less common malignancies such as osteosarcoma all tend to invade surrounding tissue (including bone) and have a high recurrence rate after conservative resection. For maxillary and palatine lesions, radical maxillectomy is used to permit resection of the entire thickness of bone from which the tumor is arising. By using flaps of buccal mucosa, the defect created between the oral and nasal cavities is covered. The entire hemipalate and maxillary teeth on one or even both sides can be removed in this way. Detailed techniques are described elsewhere.[23] Radical surgical treatment is possible for rostral or unilateral mandibular lesions;[23] function following partial or complete hemimandibulectomy is excellent. Complex orthopedic restoration techniques are not usually necessary; however, the tongue may tend to hang out of the mouth on the operated side. To prevent this, the commissure of the lips on that side can be significantly shortened surgically.[152] Aggressive but benign lesions such as acanthomatous epulis are cured using these radical techniques.[153] For malignant lesions, prognosis depends on the lack of metastases and on resection of an adequate grossly normal zone of tissue around the lesion. Small but malignant lesions should be treated aggressively initially. Aesthetic and functional results following these major oral resections are good in dogs and cats.[153]

Radiation therapy can successfully control some malignant oral soft tissue neoplasms (Figure 82–56). The prognosis and treatment regimen depend on the type of tumor and its radiosensitivity, the type and tissue dose of radiation used, and the amount of tumor infiltration of adjacent tissues such as bone. A veterinary radiologist should be consulted, and the treatment conducted under this person's supervision. Radiation therapy combined with microwave-induced hyperthermia provides better long-term results than radiation therapy alone.[154] Results are discussed in Chapter 59. Combination therapy (surgery/radiation/chemoimmunotherapy) is likely to produce the most satisfactory results. Chemo- or immunotherapy protocols used to date for management of oropharyngeal tumors have not provided consistently satisfactory results.

Neoplasia of the Tonsils

The most common tonsillar tumor of the dog and cat is squamous cell carcinoma (Figure 82–57), a disease of old animals from an urban environment more often than a rural environment.[155] It is usually discovered because of dysphagia or a mass in the retropharyngeal lymph nodes. The tonsillar lesion often appears as a unilateral, irregular, firm ulcerated mass. In most instances, treatment is not attempted because retropharyngeal or mandibular lymph node metastasis is also frequent (see

TABLE 82–3. CLINICAL FEATURES OF MALIGNANT ORAL NEOPLASMS IN THE DOG

	Tonsillar Squamous Cell Carcinoma	Nontonsillar Squamous Cell Carcinoma	Fibrosarcoma	Malignant Melanoma
Age				
Mean (years)	10	9	8	11
Range (years)	3–17	1–14	6 mos–15	1–17
Male:Female Ratio	1.5:1	1:1	1.8:1	4.2:1
Site				
Lip		8%	4%	21%
Cheek		1%		8%
Gingiva		81%*	87%†	55%‡
Palate		1%	8%	11%
Tongue		8%	1%	3%
Tonsils	100%			
Extent of Disease§				
Local only	23%	18%	65%	15%
Local and regional lymph nodes	35%	40%	12%	15%
Distant metastasis	42%	36%	23%	67%

*Mainly rostral to canine teeth
†Mainly between canine and carnassial teeth
‡Evenly distributed rostrocaudally
§At autopsy
Data from 361 cases seen at the University of Pennsylvania recorded by Todoroff and Brodey (1979)

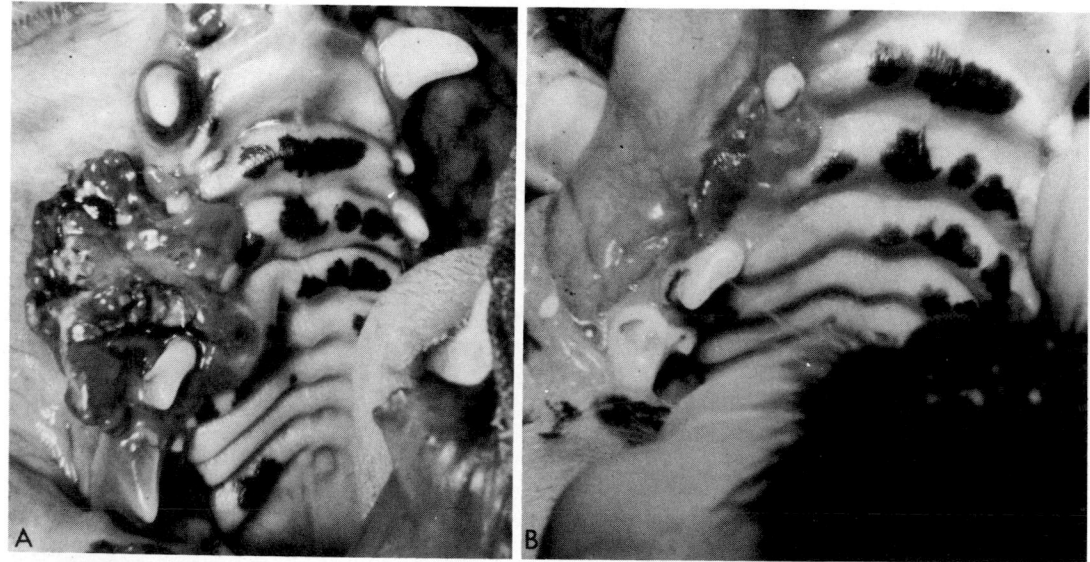

FIGURE 82–56. *A*, Palate and lip of a dog with undifferentiated sarcoma of the gingiva. *B*, The same lesion five months following radiation therapy (3800 rad total dose). No recurrence was noted for at least 18 months following initial treatment. (Courtesy of Dr. D. N. Biery.)

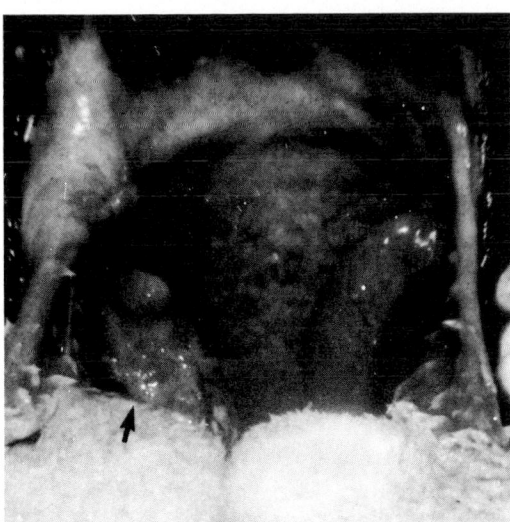

FIGURE 82–57. Pharynx of a dog with squamous cell carcinoma of the right tonsil (arrow), which is ulcerated and irregular. The left tonsil is enlarged and standing out of its crypt.

Table 82–3). Prognosis is poor, even with surgery and radiation therapy in dogs with no visible or palpable metastatic lesions. The diagnosis can be confirmed by biopsy or cytologic examination of a specimen scraped from the surface of the tonsillar lesion. On post-mortem examination, the tumor is often found in both tonsils, even if only grossly recognizable in one.

Lymphosarcoma of the tonsil occurs in middle-aged or older dogs. The lesions, usually bilateral, appear as symmetric, smooth-surfaced, creamy-pink enlarged tonsils (Figure 82–58). Treatment of lymphosarcoma is discussed in Chapter 115.

SALIVARY GLANDS

Anatomy and Physiology

The major salivary glands of the dog and cat are the paired parotid, mandibular, sublingual, and zygomatic

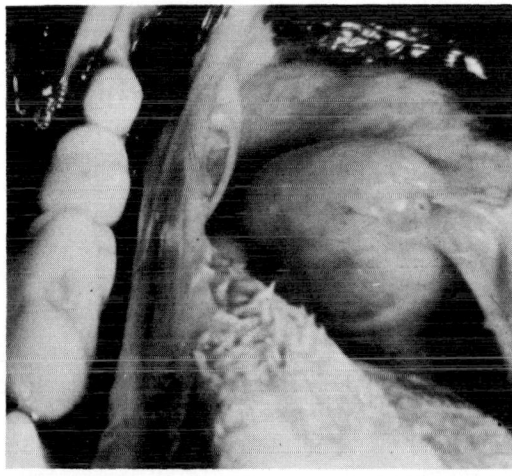

FIGURE 82–58. Pharynx of a dog with lymphosarcoma of the tonsils. A massive smooth-surface left tonsil is obvious. Part of the right tonsil is also visible.

(infraorbital) glands. The triangular parotid gland is a serous gland located below the horizontal ear canal. It is arranged in small lobules held together by connective tissue, so that the edges of the gland are irregular and poorly defined. The parotid duct runs from a branching collecting system in the gland to a prominent papilla on the mucosal surface of the cheek at the level of the upper carnassial (fourth premolar) tooth. The secretory nerve supply of the parotid gland is carried via the glossopharyngeal nerve and auriculotemporal branch of the trigeminal nerve.

The mandibular gland is a large, compact, ovoid structure lying within a strong fibrous capsule caudal and ventral to the parotid gland beneath the maxillary vein. The mandibular duct runs beside the sublingual gland on the floor of the mouth and opens on the lateral side of the sublingual frenulum. The sublingual gland is divided into several loosely connected lobules that run from the rostral surface of the mandibular gland along the root of the tongue. The sublingual duct accompanies the mandibular duct, opening either on the lingual caruncle just caudal to the mandibular duct opening, or into the mandibular duct, forming a common opening into the mouth.[156] The mandibular and sublingual glands are both mixed glands. The zygomatic gland is a mixed gland, irregularly ovoid in shape, located on the floor of the orbit ventrocaudal to the eye, medial to the zygomatic arch. Several ducts, of which the most rostral is the largest, run ventrally and open on a fold of mucosa lateral to the last upper molar tooth. The oral cavity, particularly the cheeks, also contains scattered areas of glandular tissue.

The saliva of the dog and cat has no enzymatic activity of note. Saliva softens and lubricates the passage of food to the stomach but has no other apparent function in digestion. Saliva also functions in moistening the oral mucous membrane, which is of importance for heat loss in the dog: the rate of salivation increases dramatically in the dog as the ambient temperature rises.[157]

The mandibular gland has an as yet uncertain role in the control of blood glucose concentration and diabetes.[103, 158]

History and Methods of Examination

Swelling is the most common sign of diseases of the salivary glands; it may be an accumulation of salivary secretions in an abnormal area or swelling of the salivary gland itself. "Excessive" salivation, or drooling, is usually caused by an animal's inability to swallow normally or by abnormal mouth conformation; rarely, hypersialosis is due to salivary gland abnormality or disease.[159, 160] Xerostomia (dry mouth) is uncommon because of the secretory capacity of the four major paired salivary glands and the multiple minor areas of secretory tissue in the oropharynx; it may be seen associated with kerato-conjunctivitis sicca.[113, 114]

The parotid and mandibular glands are easily palpable. In a cooperative or sedated animal, the sublingual gland can be palpated in the floor of the mouth. The zygomatic gland, located medial to the zygomatic arch, is not palpable unless grossly enlarged. Salivary gland function and duct patency can be evaluated by placing a drop of topical ophthalmic atropine solution on the tongue. In the normal animal, a copious flow of saliva ensues, particularly from the parotid papilla, from which a stream of saliva may be ejected rhythmically for one or two minutes. Pooling of saliva should also be seen in the floor of the mouth from the mandibular and sublingual glands.

Radiographic examination of the salivary glands and ducts may be performed by injecting a water-soluble radiopaque dye into the duct through a blunt-ended needle.[161] A dose of 0.20 ml/10 lb body weight of intravenous pyelogram contrast material allows good visualization of the ducts and glands in most dogs. Additional sialograms may be made five to seven minutes following each injection and radiograph to allow absorption of the dye (Figures 82–59 through 82–62).

Diseases of Salivary Glands

DROOLING

Drooling is most often caused by reluctance or inability to swallow resulting from diseases causing painful oral or pharyngeal ulcers, and less often from neurologic disease or infiltrating disease of the oropharynx. These conditions can usually be diagnosed from the history and physical examination. Some dogs show constant or intermittent drooling from an early age. The giant breeds, particularly Newfoundlands and Saint Bernards, are the worst offenders. These dogs do not have salivary gland abnormalities; rather, the drooling and frothing seen is due to conformational abnormalities of the mouth and lips. Correction of the condition should not be performed on breeding or show animals. Treatment is directed at reducing the volume of saliva produced or rerouting the flow of saliva by surgical reconstruction. If the saliva is mucoid, hanging in ropes from the corners of the mouth, bilateral ligation of the mandibular and sublingual salivary gland ducts through bilateral small incisions in the sublingual furrows eliminates most of the excessive salivation. Lip reconstruction to prevent drooling has been described.[162] Parotid gland hyperplasia and hypersialosis has been reported in a chow (Figure 82–63)[160] and a dachshund.[159] Drooling of saliva was seen in four dogs, three of which were Jack Russell terriers, which were diagnosed as having mandibular gland infarction.[163]

INJURIES

Injuries of the salivary gland are rarely recognized as acute conditions and may resolve with no long-term effects in dogs.[164] Salivary fistula or sialocele formation is caused by injury. Foreign bodies and sialoliths are rarely found in the salivary ducts of the dog or cat.[23]

Parotid Gland and Duct Injury. The superficial location of the parotid gland and duct exposes these structures to injury by superficial blows, cuts, or bite wounds of the face. Surgical procedures such as vertical ear canal resection, external ear canal ablation, and treatment of bite wounds or abscesses are potential causes of parotid damage. Another potential cause of parotid duct injury is carnassial abscess or its treatment.

Severance of the parotid duct and a resulting sialocele or fistula are occasionally seen in the dog and cat (Figures 82–64 and 82–65).[165] A previous history of trauma or surgical interference in the cheek is usually available. The fistula leads to a small skin opening oozing a clear serous fluid, which becomes more profuse while the animal is eating. Diagnosis is based on the position of the lesion, type of discharge, and the absence of saliva from the parotid papilla on the appropriate side when a drop of atropine is placed on the tongue.

The object of treatment is to reform or divert the duct or permanently obstruct the parotid flow proximal to the fistula. Parotid duct ligation is simple and effective.[165] The parotid duct is located proximal to the fistula and the duct is ligated with nonabsorbable material, using two or three ligatures, placing the rostral one more tightly than the others so as to spread out the back pressure that follows ligation.

Intermittent blockage of the parotid duct by a carnassial abscess can cause permanent dilation and secondary infection, which result in dribbling of mucopurulent discharge from the parotid papilla. As the condition progresses, the ductules within the gland and later the glandular tissue itself become involved. Diagnosis is made from a previous history of carnassial abscess and the appearance of the material milked from the parotid duct. Sialography confirms the dilation of the duct and indicates the extent of the disease (Figure 82–66). Flushing the duct and instilling antibiotics provide temporary relief from signs of disease. After the carnassial abscess is treated, acute cases may require no further treatment. Ligation of the duct proximal to the dilation is the preferred treatment of dogs with chronic disease limited to the main parotid duct. Parotidectomy is the definitive treatment for intraglandular angiectasis but is rarely necessary.

Mandibular Gland Duct Injury. Because the mandibular gland is contained within a firm fibrous capsule, long-term effects of trauma to this gland in the dog are rare.[164] The mandibular duct is larger and thicker-walled than the accompanying sublingual duct.

Sublingual Gland and Duct Injury: Salivary Mucocele. Clinically, the most common condition of the salivary glands in the dog is salivary mucocele. The sublingual gland is most frequently involved. A salivary mucocele is a collection of salivary gland mucus in a nonepithelium-lined swelling. After damage to the salivary gland or duct, saliva leaks out and follows the path of least resistance. The most frequent sites for collection of the extravasated saliva are sublingual tissues or the intermandibular or cranial cervical area. A less common site is the pharyngeal wall.[166, 167] The cause of the gland or duct damage is rarely known. Occasionally, a foreign body is found penetrating the gland in a dog with a mucocele. Sticks or bones may have been rammed into the mandible by chewing. Blunt trauma squeezing the sublingual gland is another possible cause. Poodles and German shepherds have been reported as more frequently affected than other breeds.[168, 169] Mucoceles were

Text continued on page 1249

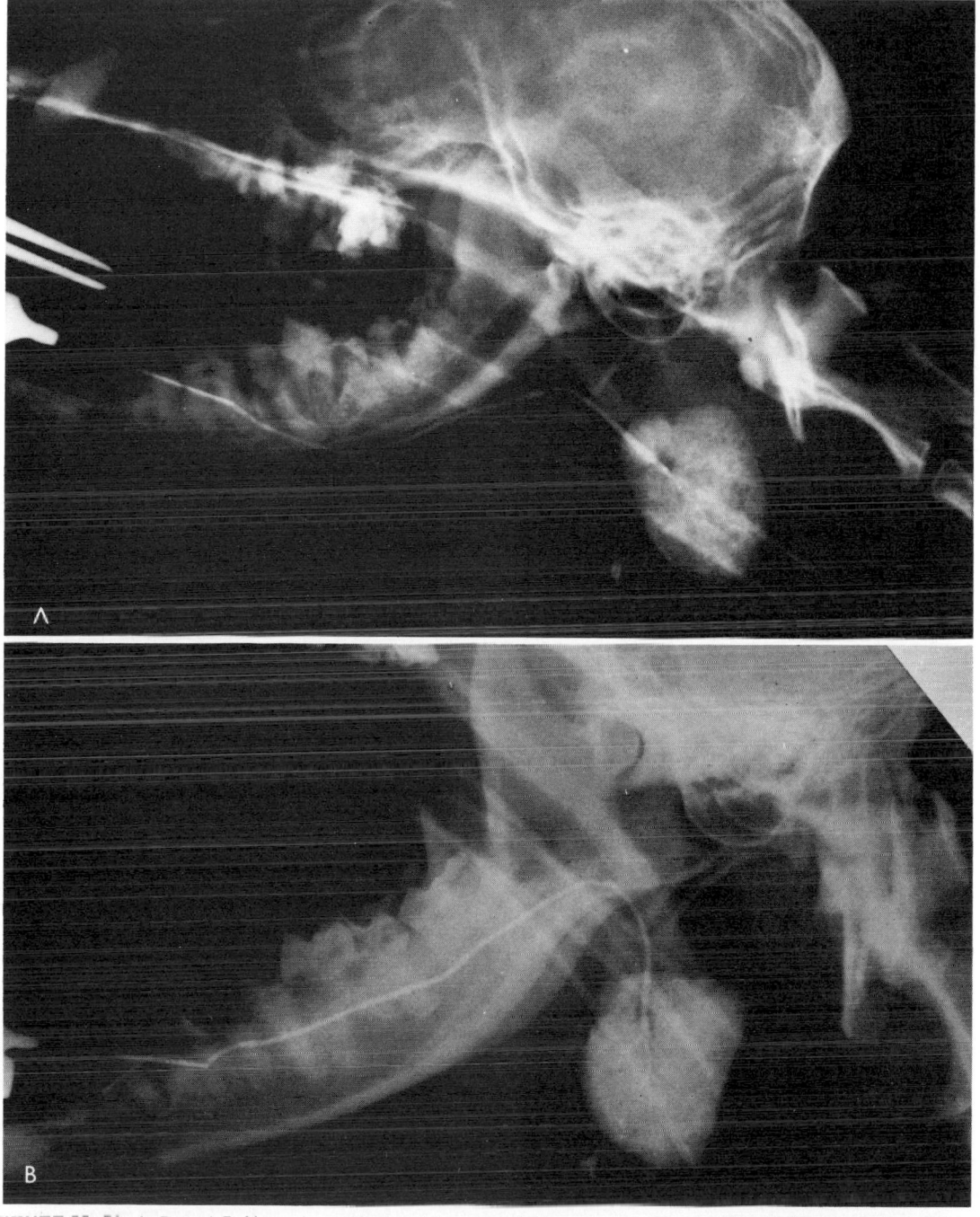

FIGURE 82–59. *A, B,* and *C,* Normal mandibular sialograms of dogs showing the variation of gland and duct pattern.

Illustration continued on following page

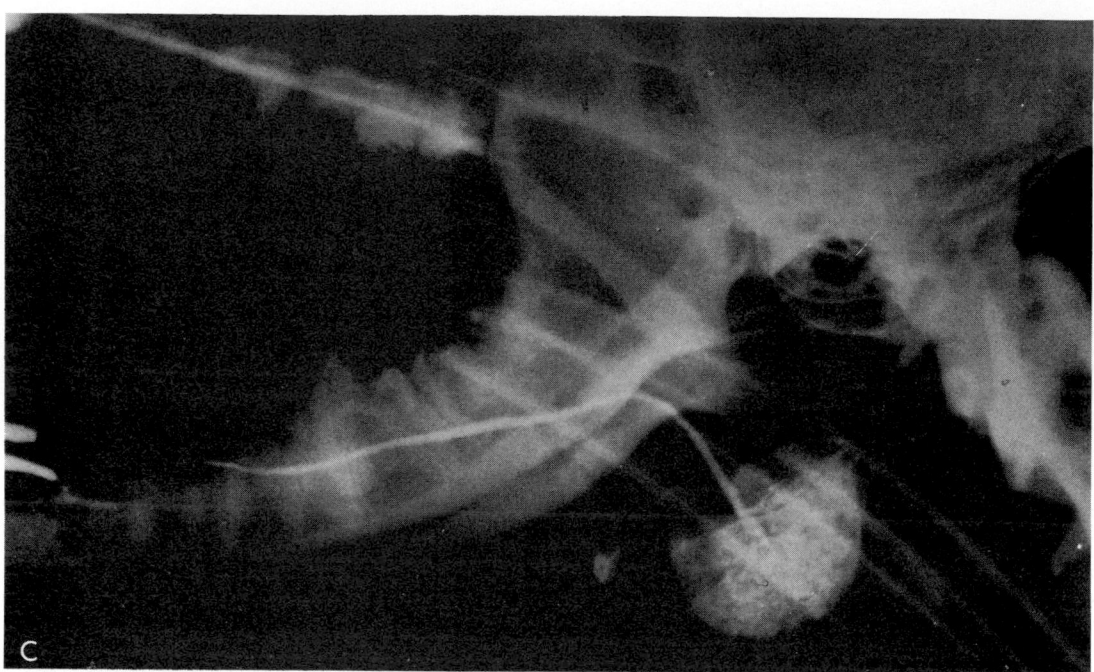

FIGURE 82–59 *Continued*

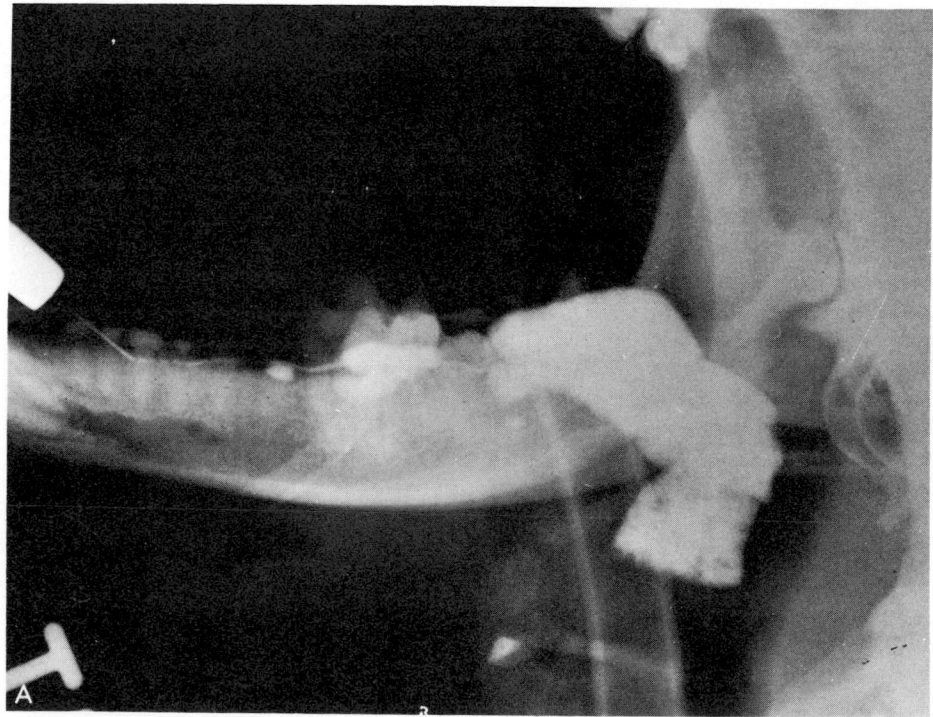

FIGURE 82–60. *A, B,* and *C,* Normal sublingual sialograms of dogs showing the variation of gland and duct pattern.

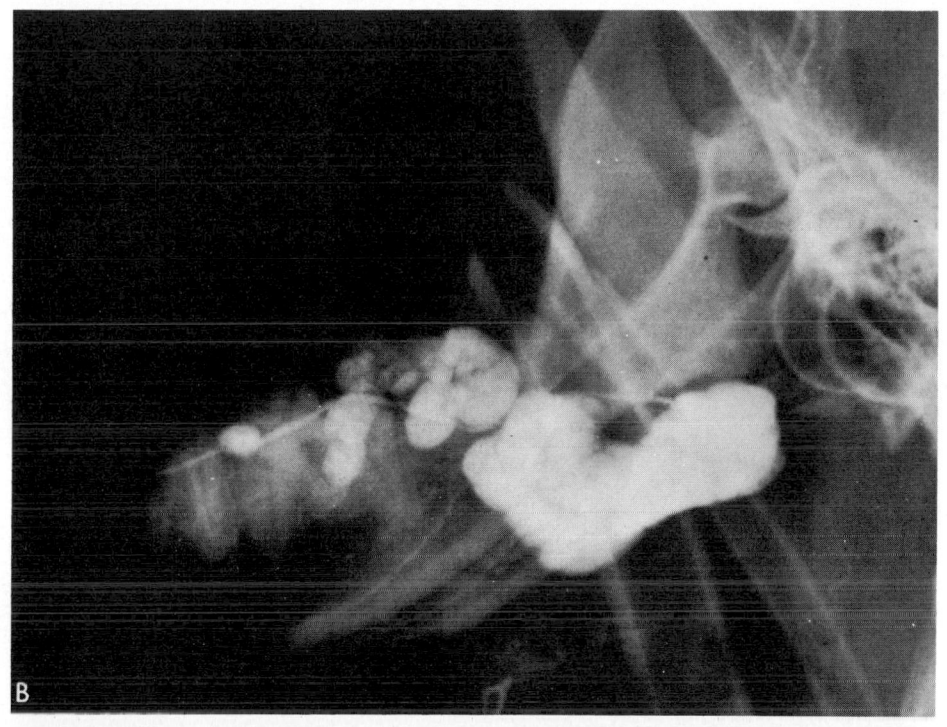

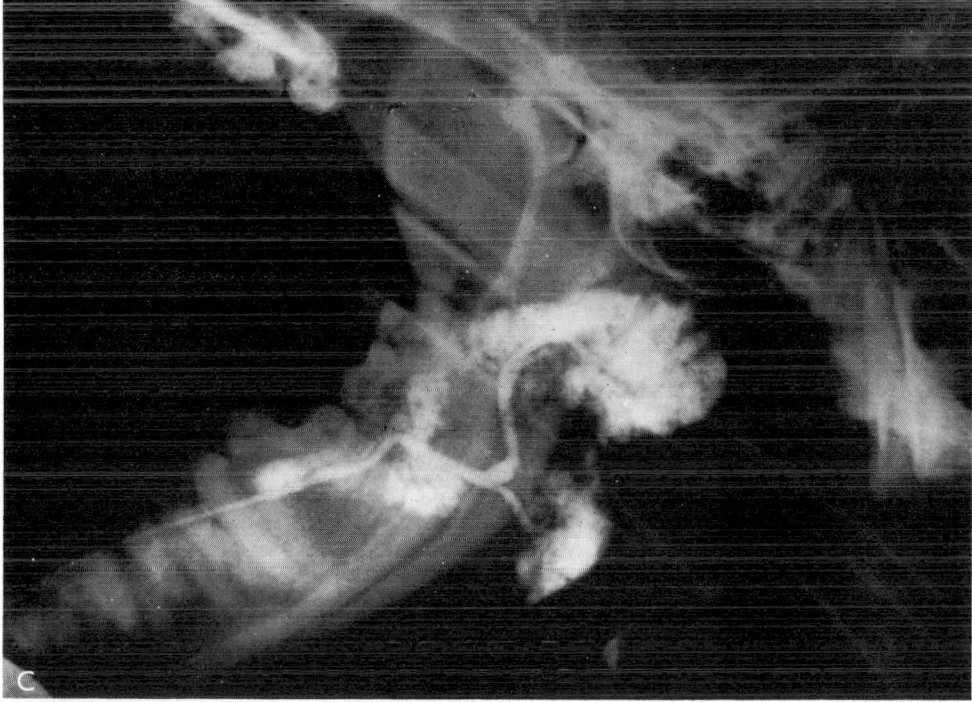

FIGURE 82–60 *Continued*

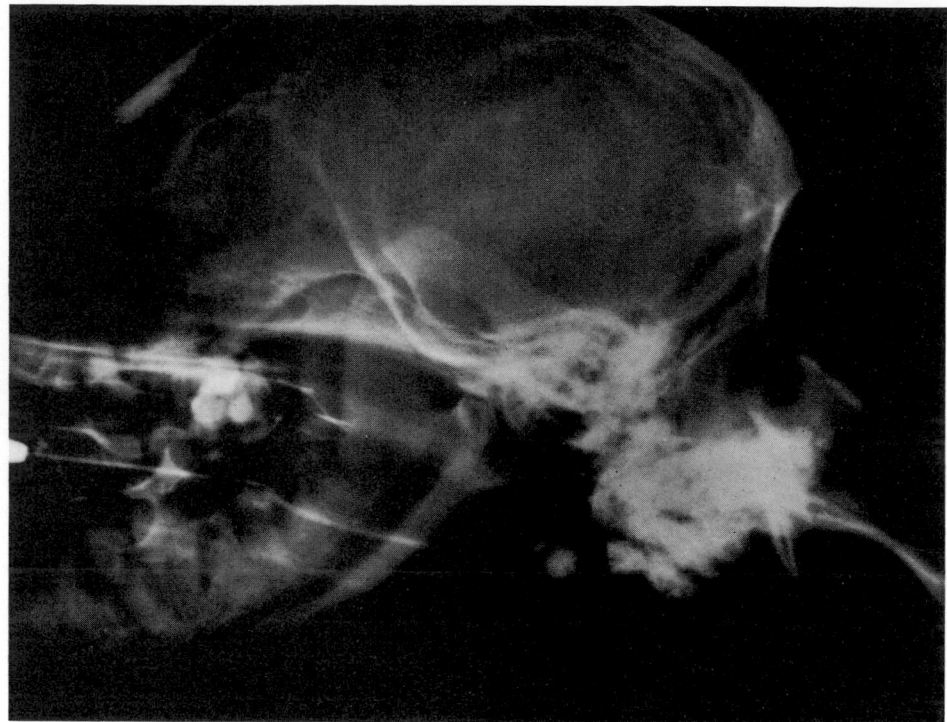

FIGURE 82–61. Normal parotid sialogram of a dog. There is some leakage of contrast medium around the duct opening.

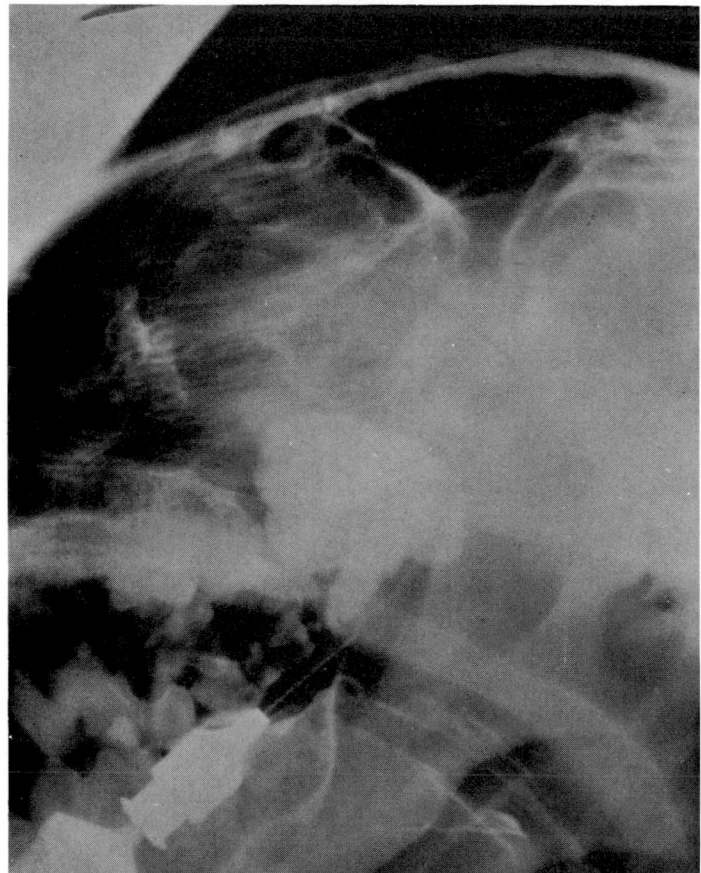

FIGURE 82–62. Normal zygomatic sialogram of a dog.

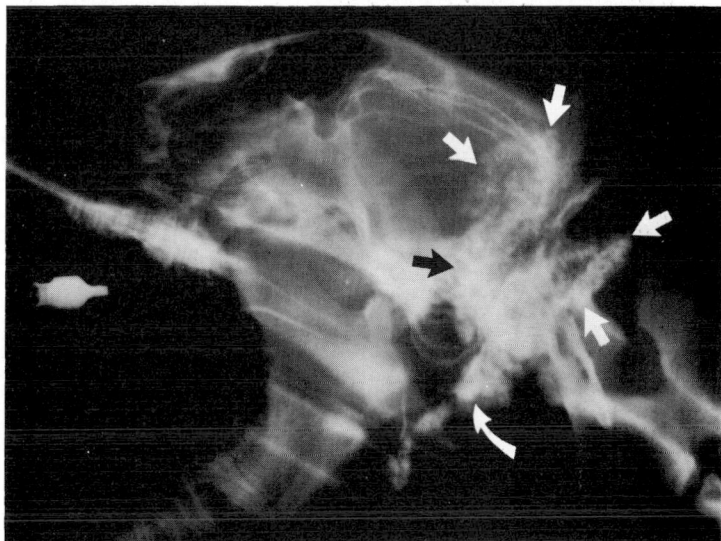

FIGURE 82–63. Sialogram of a dog with parotid gland enlargement (arrows) and hypersialosis.

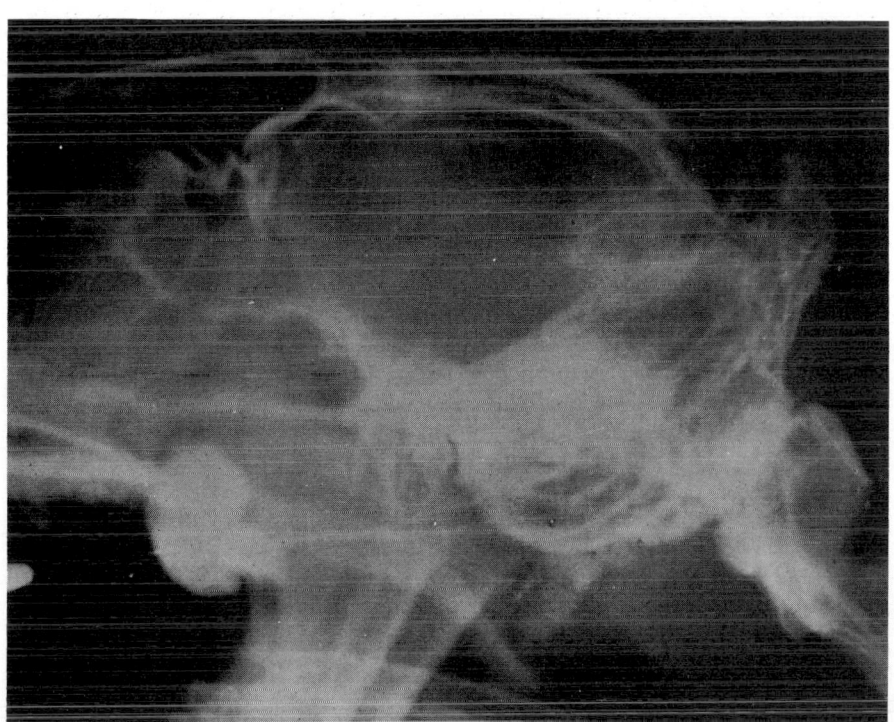

FIGURE 82–64. Parotid sialogram of a cat with parotid sialocele following surgical treatment of a superficial abscess. The parotid duct and gland are poorly filled.

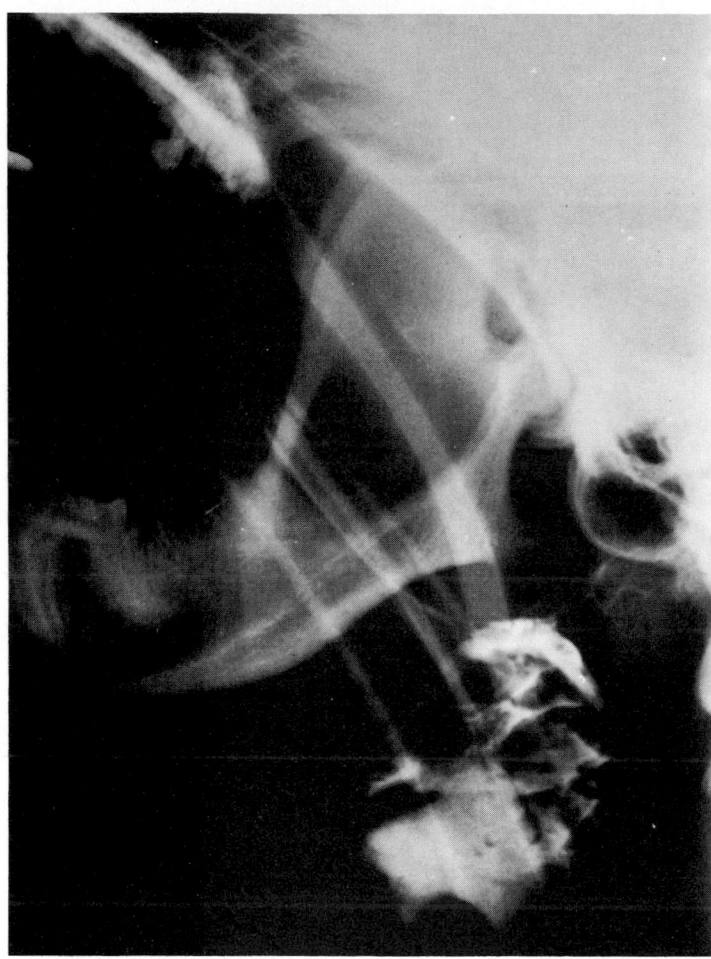

FIGURE 82–65. Parotid sialogram of a dog with a traumatic parotid fistula. The contrast material is leaking from the duct ventral to the tympanic bullae.

FIGURE 82–66. Parotid sialogram of a dog with parotid duct dilation following a carnassial tooth abscess.

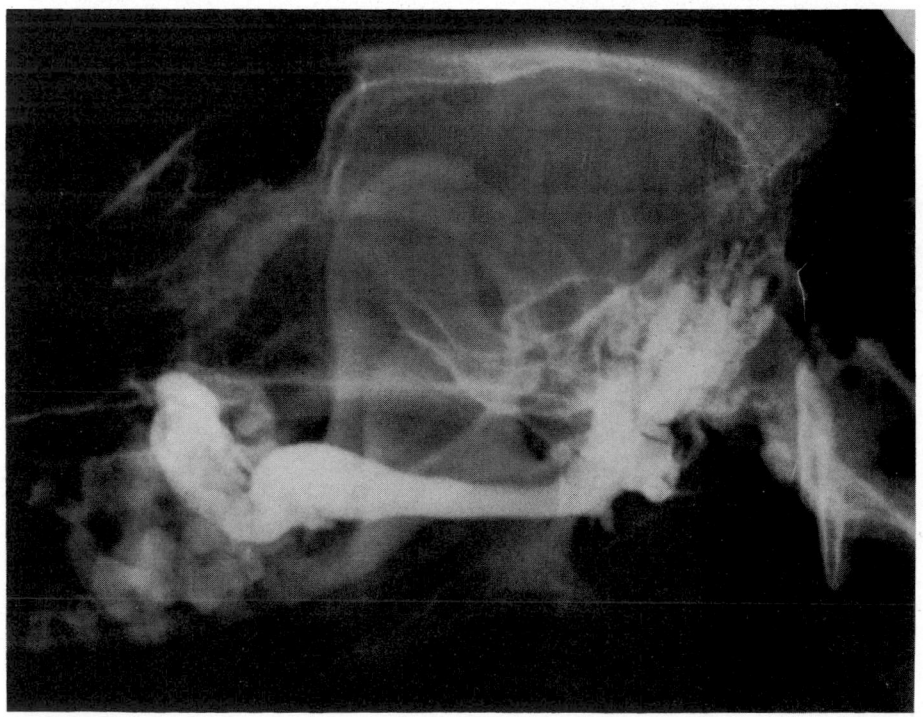

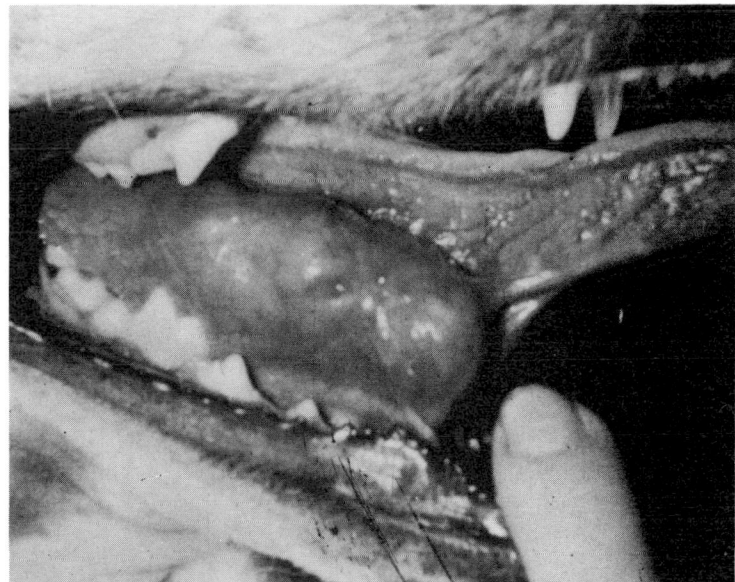

FIGURE 82–67. Mouth of a dog with a ranula (mucocele of the sublingual tissues).

produced in 12 of 27 cats in which the sublingual duct was ligated.[170]

Clinical signs of a salivary mucocele depend on the position of the mucocele. A large sublingual swelling (commonly known as a ranula) is likely to be damaged by teeth; this pushes the tongue to the opposite side, causing reluctance to eat and blood-tinged saliva. Usually the owner will have observed the lesion. A mucocele in the pharyngeal wall obstructs swallowing and respiration as it encroaches on the pharyngeal lumen.

A cervical salivary mucocele may commence with an acute period when the swelling is firm and somewhat painful; this is followed by reduction in swelling as the initial inflammatory reaction subsides. However, gradual enlargement of a soft, nonpainful mass is the most common presenting complaint.

Diagnosis of a salivary mucocele is based on palpation and aspiration of the mass, which may require sedation or anesthesia for a ranula or pharyngeal mucocele (Figures 82–67 and 82–68). The material obtained by aspiration is slightly turbid or blood-tinged mucus. Some chronic cervical mucoceles contain nodules that are free within the swelling and that resemble calculi; these are folds of the inflammatory lining sloughed into the cavity. Confirmatory tests other than aspiration are rarely needed, because there are few instances of mucus-containing nonsalivary cysts in the pharyngeal area of the dog. Although sialography confirms salivary gland or duct leakage, it is more often used as an adjunct to management (Figures 82–69 and 82–70). Histopathologic examination demonstrates the nonepithelial, nonsecretory nature of the wall of the cavity. The most common lesion with which salivary mucocele can be confused is retropharyngeal abscess. A chronic pharyngeal foreign body "abscess" may be sterile, and the fluid is serosanguineous.

Management of Salivary Mucocele. A cervical salivary mucocele causes little problem to the dog after the initial inflammatory reaction has subsided, unless the mucocele becomes large enough to cause physical discomfort. Occasionally, salivary mucoceles will not recur

after aspiration, presumably because scar tissue has sealed the gland or duct defect. Periodic aspiration as needed (usually every three to four months) to empty the mucocele may be sufficient treatment, particularly in an animal that is a poor surgical risk. Ranula (due to biting of the swelling) and pharyngeal mucocele (because of dysphagia or airway obstruction) can cause more severe problems.

Ranulae can be treated by marsupialization, which is the creation of a fistula from the mucocele to the oral cavity. A section of the mucocele wall is removed with a scalpel or scissors. The inner cell layer of a ranula, as

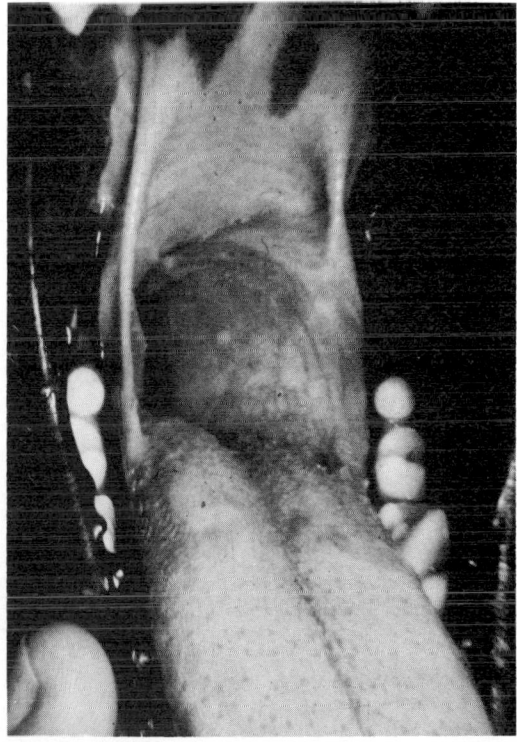

FIGURE 82–68. Pharynx of a dog with a pharyngeal mucocele of the left side.

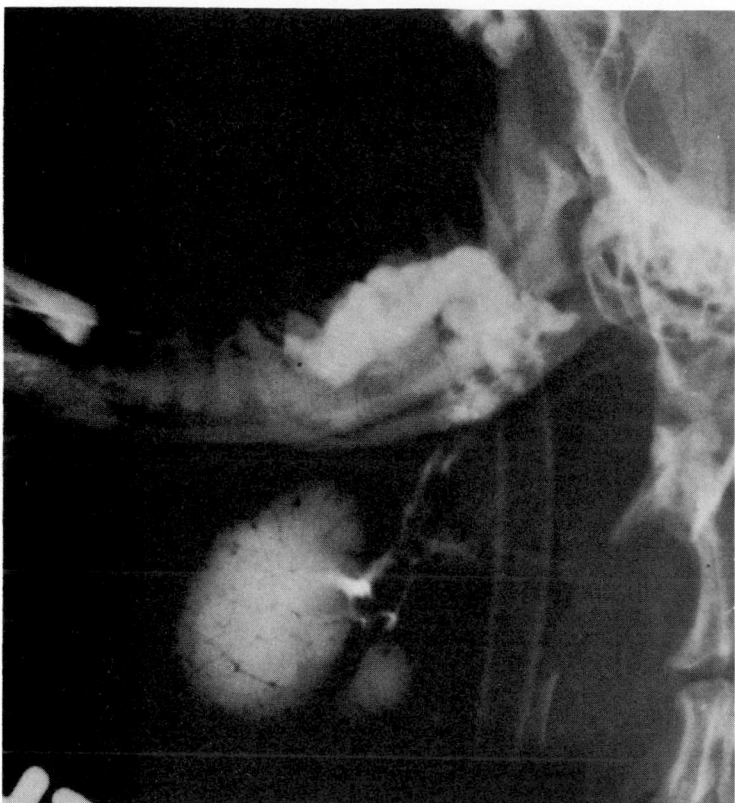

FIGURE 82–69. Sublingual sialogram of a dog with a salivary mucocele. The sublingual gland and mucocele are clearly visible.

FIGURE 82–70. Sublingual sialogram of a dog with a salivary mucocele. The sublingual gland is not well outlined, although the area of leakage and mucocele are clearly visible.

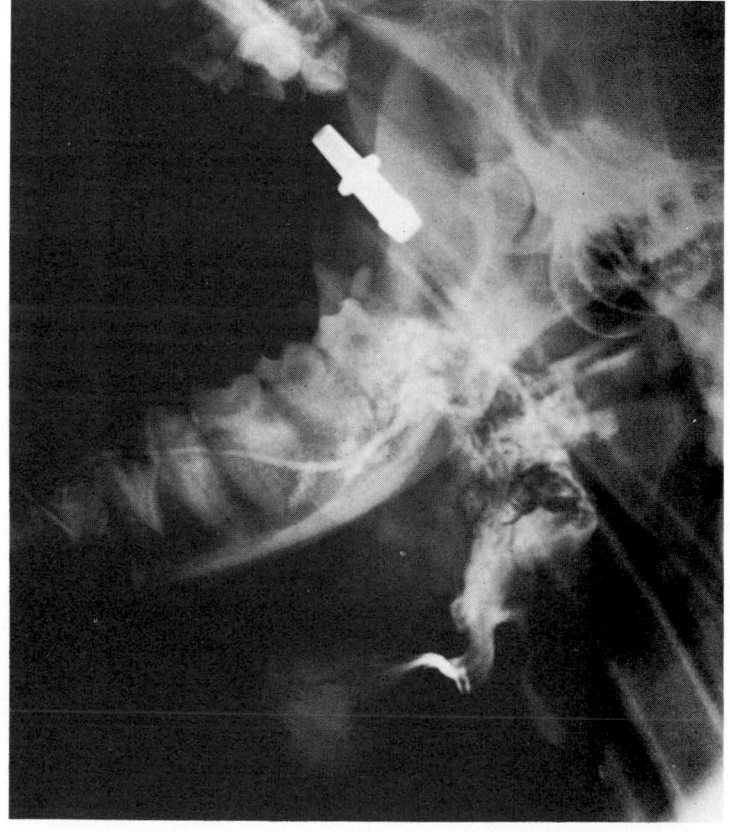

for any mucocele, is composed of inflammatory or connective tissue cells (fibroblasts) except near the site of the original trauma, where there may be some overgrowth of duct or glandular epithelium. Because of the lack of an epithelial lining, there is little point in suturing the oral mucosa to the mucocele inner lining, and recurrence following marsupialization is frequent. The use of stainless steel sutures to maintain the patency of the fistula has been suggested.[171] Ranulae can be treated satisfactorily by mandibular-sublingual gland removal.

A pharyngeal mucocele may present as an emergency because of airway obstruction. Needle aspiration alleviates such an obstruction temporarily. Marsupialization may be used, but a more satisfactory treatment to prevent recurrence is mandibular-sublingual salivary gland removal.[166, 167]

Resection of a cervical salivary mucocele is tedious. Recurrence is likely because the mucocele is merely the effect of damage to the sublingual gland or duct. Definitive treatment of cervical salivary mucocele is resection of the sublingual salivary gland. Resection of redundant skin is rarely necessary. The gland most frequently affected is the sublingual gland. It is impractical to remove the sublingual gland without removing the mandibular gland because of the close apposition of the two. The glands are often spoken of as the mandibular-sublingual gland complex. Generally, it is obvious from the history or physical examination which side is involved. When this is not the case, palpation and observation with the dog in dorsal recumbency under anesthesia may prove helpful. Sialography can determine the side involved, or the mandibular-sublingual gland complex can be removed from both sides. Mandibular and sublingual salivary gland resection has been described in detail elsewhere.[23] Following salivary gland removal, the mucocele is drained. When surgery has been performed and a mucocele recurs, the rostral part of the sublingual gland may not have been removed. Sialography delineates the remaining glandular tissue. The rostral part of the sublingual gland can be removed through an incision in the oral mucosa between the root of the tongue and the vertical ramus of the mandible. Salivary gland removal successfully prevents recurrence of the mucocele.[172, 173]

Sublingual salivary mucocele in the cat has been described.[174] Treatment by mandibular and sublingual salivary gland removal was successful.

Zygomatic salivary cyst caused by trauma to the head of a dog has been described[175] and has been seen occasionally by the author. The presenting clinical sign is exophthalmos. Zygomatic gland resection via resection of the zygomatic arch is curative.[23]

Inflammatory Diseases of the Salivary Glands. Sialoadenitis is rare in the dog and cat as a distinct clinical entity. Mild focal inflammatory changes are common incidental findings in salivary glands of dogs.[176] Sialoadenitis that severely reduces salivary secretions can result in xerostomia. Autoimmune-induced sialoadenitis producing xerostomia is seen in about 20 per cent of dogs with keratoconjunctivitis sicca.[114] Parotid or mandibular gland swelling is occasionally recognized as part of a regional or systemic disease such as distemper. Swelling of the parotid and mandibular glands in dogs and cats

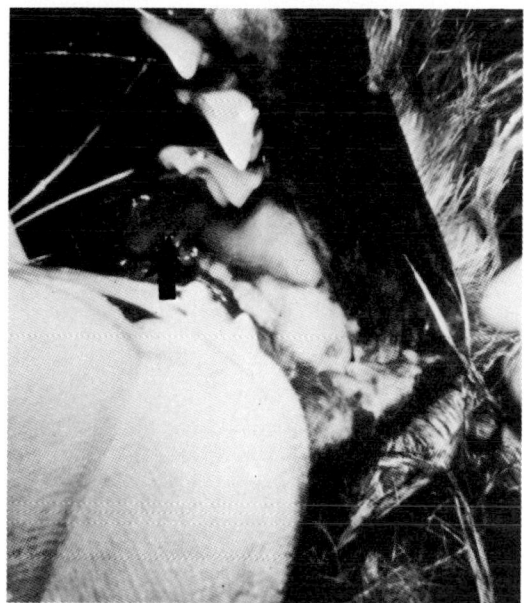

FIGURE 82–71. Mouth of a dog with a retrobulbar (zygomatic) abscess. The area of swollen, reddened oral mucosa is indicated by the arrow.

associated with the paramyxovirus causing mumps in man occurs occasionally.[177]

Idiopathic necrosis of one or both mandibular salivary glands in dogs results from constriction of the enlarging, inflamed gland within the tight, thick mandibular gland capsule.[176] This causes a clinical syndrome of very severe acute pain in the retropharyngeal area spaces—affected dogs scream when attempting to open their mouths or when the area is palpated. The inciting cause of the inflammation is not known; in one report three of four affected dogs were Jack Russell terriers.[163] Conservative (antibiotic, anti-inflammatory, and analgesic) and surgical (mandibular gland resection) therapy are both largely ineffective, and most affected dogs are euthanized.

Abscesses of the head and neck may involve the salivary glands. A syndrome of pyrexia, pain on opening the jaws, inflammation of the oral tissues lateral to the last upper molar tooth, and exophthalmos has been referred to as an abscess of the zygomatic salivary gland, although the condition is more likely to be a retrobulbar abscess secondary to a penetrating foreign body (Figure 82–71). Treatment by draining the abscess through an incision in the inflamed oral mucosa combined with systemic antibiotics is effective.

SALIVARY GLAND NEOPLASIA

Tumors of the salivary glands of the dog and cat are uncommon. The glands most often involved are the mandibular and parotid glands.[178, 179] The usual tumor type is adenocarcinoma. Affected animals are old (average age 10 to 12 years) and usually presented because of a slowly developing mass noted by the owner. Resection of the involved gland is curative for mandibular gland lesions if metastasis to the local lymph nodes or lungs has not occurred. Parotid gland lesions are more difficult to treat surgically because of the diffuse nature of the parotid gland and the many nerves and vessels that run close by or through the gland.

Tumors of the zygomatic gland occur occasionally, presenting with exophthalmos.[180] A surgical approach through the zygomatic arch allows resection of the zygomatic gland.[23, 175, 181]

Superficial Masses in the Pharyngeal Area

Animals are frequently presented with swellings in the pharyngeal area. The usual causes are retropharyngeal abscess and salivary mucocele. Other causes are lymphadenopathy (primary lymphatic, metastatic, or benign) and tumors of the skin, thyroid glands, salivary glands, or carotid body.

Of less importance because of their rarity in the dog and cat are lesions such as branchial cleft and thyroglossal duct cysts.[182, 183] In the dog, slowly developing mucus-containing swellings of the pharyngeal area should be considered as salivary in origin unless proved otherwise by histologic examination of the wall of the swelling. The rare, true branchial cyst in the dog can be satisfactorily treated by complete excision of the cyst.[184]

Foreign bodies and neoplastic infiltration of bone may be diagnosed radiographically.[185] In other conditions, radiographs confirm the presence of the mass but are not usually helpful in differentiation of the cause.

References

1. Newman, PM: Canine Teeth. Letter to the Editor. JAVMA 174:1075, 1979.
2. Harvey, CE, et al.: Development of canine teeth of dogs: A radiographic study. (Abst) J Vet Dentistry 4, 1987.
3. Snow, HD, et al.: Canine respiratory disease in an animal facility. Arch Surg 99:126, 1969.
4. Arnbjerg, J: *Pasteurella multocida* from canine and feline teeth, with a case report of glossitis calcinosa in a dog caused by *P. multocida*. Nord Vet Med 30:324, 1978.
5. Suter, PF and Watrous, BJ: Oropharyngeal dysphagias in the dog: A cinefluorographic analysis of experimentally induced and spontaneously occurring swallowing disorders. Vet Radiol 21:24, 1980.
6. Zontine, WJ: Dental radiographic technique and interpretation. Vet Clin North Am 4:741, 1974.
7. Arnall, L: Some aspects of dental development in the dog. Some common variations in dentition. J Small Anim Pract 2:195, 1961.
8. Kratochvil, Z: Oligodonty and polydonty in the domestic and wild cat. Acta Vet Brno 40:33, 1971.
9. Wisdorf, H and Hermanns, W: Persistent milk teeth (canines) in the upper jaw of a cat. Kleintierpraxis 19:14, 1974.
10. Dubielzig, RR: Effect of canine distemper virus on ameloblastic layer of developing tooth. Vet Pathol 16:268, 1979.
11. Arnbjerg, J: Schmelz- und Wurzelhypoplasien nach Staupe. Kleintierpraxis 31:313, 1986.
12. Bennett, I and Law, D: Incorporation of tetracycline in developing dog enamel and dentin. J Dent Res 44:788, 1965.
13. Schneck, GW: Caries in the dog. JAVMA 150:1142, 1967.
14. Gardner, AF, et al.: Dental caries in domesticated dogs. JAVMA 140:433, 1962.
15. Lewis, TM: Resistance of dogs to dental caries: a two-year study. J Dent Res 44:1254, 1965.
16. Runyon, CL, et al.: Allogeneic tooth transplantation in the dog. JAVMA 188:7, 1986.
17. Golden, A, et al.: A survey of oral health in small animals. JAAHA 18:891, 1982.
18. Newman, NB: Chronic ocular discharge associated with a carnassial tooth abscess. Can Vet J 15:128, 1974.
19. Holmberg, DC: Abscessation of the mandibular carnassial tooth in the dog. JAAHA 15:347, 1979.
20. Franceschini, G: Traitement des fistulaires dentaires chez le chien par obturation des canaux. Rec Med Vet 150:675, 1974.
21. Eisner, ER: Eighty sequential endodontic cases. (Abst) Am Vet Dent Soc 1985.
22. Ridgway, RL and Zielke, DR: Nonsurgical endodontic technique for dogs. JAVMA 174:82, 1979.
23. Harvey, CE: Veterinary Dentistry. Philadelphia, WB Saunders, 1985.
24. Peterson, RN and Wightman, JR: Aesthetic restoration of a fractured anterior tooth in a dog. VM/SAC 74:683, 1979.
25. Eisenmenger E and Zetner, K: Veterinary Dentistry. Philadelphia, Lea and Febiger, 1985.
26. Cechner, PE: Malocclusion in the dog caused by intramedullary pin fixation of mandibular fractures: Two case reports. JAAHA 16:79, 1980.
27. Graber, TM: Orthodontics: Principles and Practice, 3rd ed. Philadelphia, WB Saunders, 1972.
28. Brass, W: Zur korrektur von Zahnstellungs-und Kieferanomalien des Hundes mit Dehungsplatten und durch kierferchirurgische Mafnahmen. Kleintierpraxis 21:79, 1976.
29. Latimer, KS, et al.: Emergency stabilization of jaw fractures in dogs using acrylic splints. VM/SAC 72:1029, 1977.
30. Humphreys, GU: Dropped jaw in dogs. Vet Record 95:222, 1974.
31. Robins, GM: Dropped jaw—mandibular neuropraxia in the dog. J Small Anim Pract 17:753, 1976.
32. Ticer, JW and Spencer, CP: Injury of the feline temporomandibular joint: Radiographic signs. Vet Radiol 19:146, 1978.
33. Cazieux, A, et al.: Luxation de la mandibule et tarte dentaire. Rev Med Veterinaire 287, 1973.
34. Knecht, CD and Schiller, AG: Acquired lesions of the mandible. *In* Archibald, J (ed): Canine Surgery. Santa Barbara, Am Vet Pub Inc, 1974.
35. Beattie, IEJ: Treatment of dislocated feline mandible. Vet Record 110:493, 1982.
36. Stewart, WC, et al.: Temporomandibular subluxation in the dog: A case report. J Small Anim Pract 16:345, 1975.
37. Robins, G and Grandage, J: Temporomandibular joint dysplasia and open mouth jaw locking in the dog. JAVMA 171:1072, 1977.
38. Bennett, D and Prymak, C: Excision arthroplasty as a treatment for temporomandibular dysplasia. J Small Anim Pract 27:361, 1986.
39. Lantz, GC: Temporomandibular joint ankylosis: Surgical correction of three cases. JAAHA 20:1984.
40. Tomlinson, J and Presnell, KR: Mandibular condylectomy: Effects in normal dogs. Vet Surg 12:148, 1983.
41. Riser, WH, et al.: Canine craniomandibular osteopathy. J Am Vet Rad Soc 8:2331, 1967.
42. Rosenberg, HM, et al.: A method for the epidemiologic assessment of periodontal health. Disease state in a beagle hound colony. J Periodont 37:208, 1966.
43. Gad, T: Periodontal disease in dogs. I. Clinical investigation. J Periodont Res 3:268, 1968.
44. Hull, PS, et al.: Periodontal disease in a beagle dog colony. J Comp Pathol 84:143, 1974.
45. Hamp, S, et al.: A macroscopic and radiologic investigation of dental diseases of the dog. Vet Radiol 25:86, 1984.
46. Kostlin, VR: Zur Parodontopathia beim Hund. Kleintierpraxis 24:159, 1979.
47. Hamp, SE, et al.: Prevalence of periodontal disease in the dog. I. Clinical and roentgenographical observations. IADR Abstract, 119, 1975.
48. Page, RC and Schroeder, HE: Periodontitis in man and other animals. Basel, S. Karger, 1983.
49. Egelberg, J: Local effect of diet on plaque formation and development of gingivitis in dogs. I. Effect of hard and soft diets. Odont Rev 16:31, 1965.

50. Saxe, R, et al.: Debris, calculus and periodontal disease in the beagle dog. Periodontics 5:217, 1967.
51. Ghergasriu, S, et al.: Periodontopathie carencieele chez les chiens. Zbl Vet Med 22:696, 1975.
52. Henrikson, PA: Periodontal disease and calcium deficiency. Acta Odontologica Scandinavia 50:26, 1968.
53. Krook, L: Periodontal disease in dog and man. Adv Vet Sci Comp Med 20:171, 1976.
54. Lindhe, J, et al.: Experimental periodontitis in the beagle dog. J Periodont Res 8:1, 1973.
55. Lindhe, J, et al.: Plaque-induced periodontal disease in beagle dogs: A 4-year clinical, roentgenographical and histometrical study. J Peridont Res 10:235, 1975.
57. Carlson, J and Egelberg, J: Local effect of diet on plaque formation and development of gingivitis in dogs. 2. Effect of high carbohydrate versus high protein-fat diets. Odont Rev 16:42, 1965.
58. Egelberg, J: Local effect of diet on plaque formation and development of gingivitis in dogs. III. Effect of frequency of meals and tube feeding. Odont Rev 16:50, 1965.
59. Syed, SA, et al.: The predominant cultivable dental plaque flora of beagle dogs with gingivitis. J Periodont Res 15:123, 1980.
60. Lang, N and Loe, H: A fluorescent plaque disclosing agent. J Periodont Res 7:59, 1972.
61. Nuki, K and Cooper, S: The role of inflammation in the pathogenesis of gingival enlargement during the administration of diphenylhydantoin sodium in cats. J Periodont Res 7:102, 1972.
62. Rost, DR and Baker, R: Gingival hyperplasia induced by sodium diphenylhydantoin in the dog: A case report. VM/SAC 73:585, 1978.
63. Lindhe, J, et al.: Influence of topical application of chlorhexidine on chronic gingivitis and gingival wound healing in the dog. Scand J Dent Res 78:471, 1970.
64. Hull, PS and Davies, RM: The effect of a chlorhexidine gel on tooth deposits in beagle dogs. J Small Anim Pract 13:207, 1972.
65. Henke, CL and Colmery, BH: Treating canine dental infections with oral clindamycin hydrochloride. Vet Med, 1987.
66. Dean, TS, et al.: Metronidazole in the treatment of gingivitis. Vet Record 85:449, 1969.
67. Listgarten, MA, et al.: The effect of systemic antimicrobial therapy on plaque and gingivitis in dogs. J Periodont Res 14:65, 1979.
68. Kaplan, ML and Jeffcoat, MK: Acute necrotizing ulcerative gingivitis. Canine Pract 5:35, 1978.
69. Van Campen, GJ: The occurrence of acute necrotizing ulcerative gingivitis in a beagle dog colony. IADR Abs 12, 1977.
70. Wouters, SLS: Experimentally induced acute necrotizing ulcerative gingivitis in beagle dogs. IADR Abs 13, 1977.
71. Burstone, MS, et al.: Familial gingival hypertrophy in the dog (Boxer breed). Arch Pathol 54:208, 1952.
72. Heigl, L and Lindhe, J: The effect of metronidazole on the development of plaque and gingivitis in the beagle dog. J Clin Periodont 6:197, 1979.
73. Page, RC and Schroeder, HE: Spontaneous chronic periodontitis in adult dogs: A clinical and histopathological survey. J Periodont 52:60, 1981.
74. Nyman, S, et al.: The effect of progressive tooth mobility on destructive periodontitis in the dog. J Clin Periodontol 5:213, 1978.
75. Smith, MM, et al.: A correlative study of the clinical and radiographic signs of periodontal disease in dogs. JAVMA 186:12, 1985.
76. Schroeder, HE and Lindhe, J: Conditions and pathological features of rapidly destructive, experimental periodontitis in dogs. J Periodontol 51:1, 1980.
77. Schroeder, HE and Attstrom, R: Effect of mechanical plaque control on development of subgingival plaque and initial gingivitis in neutropenic dogs. Scand J Dent Res 87:279, 1979.
78. Sangnes, G: A pilot study on the effect of toothbrushing on the gingiva of a beagle dog. Scand J Dent Res 84:106, 1976.
79. Hirst, RC: Chlorhexidine: A review of the literature. J West Soc Periodont 20:52, 1972.
80. Gjermo, P: Some aspects of drug dynamics as related to oral soft tissue. J Dent Res 59 Spec No B:B44, 1975.
81. Stabholz, A, et al.: Clinical and microbiological effects of sustained release chlorhexidine in periodontal pockets. J Clin Periodontol 13:783, 1986.
83. Deitrich, U: How to incorporate an effective preventative dentistry program into the veterinary practice. California Vet 32:16, 1978.
84. Zontine, WJ, et al.: Bacterial contamination associated with ultrasonic dental procedures in dogs. JAAHA 5:150, 1969.
85. Jackson, DA, et al.: Bacteremia following ultrasonic scaling in the dog. Presented at Annual Meeting, ACVS, February 1981.
86. Black, AP, et al.: Bacteremia during ultrasonic teeth cleaning and extraction in the dog. JAAHA 16:611, 1980.
87. Silver, JG, et al.: Recovery and clearance rates of oral micro-organisms following experimental bacteremias in the dog. Arch Oral Biol 20:675, 1975.
88. Withrow, J: Dental extraction as a probable cause of septicemia in dogs. JAAHA 15:345, 1979.
89. Frost, P and Williams, C: Feline dental disease. Vet Clin North Am 16:851, 1986.
90. Reichart, PA, et al.: Periodontal disease in the domestic cat. A histopathologic study. Periodont Res 19:67, 1984.
91. Hammond, BF, et al.: Bacterial flora in cats with periodontal disease. Submitted to Arch Oral Biol 1987.
92. Schneck, GW and Osborn, JW: Neck lesions in the teeth of cats. Vet Record 99:100, 1976.
93. Johnessee, JS and Hurvitz, AI: Feline plasma cell gingivitis. JAAHA 19:179, 1983.
94. Thompson, RR, et al.: Association of calicivirus infection with chronic gingivitis and pharyngitis in cats. J Small Anim Pract 25:207, 1984.
95. Knowles, RJ, et al: Viruses in gingival fluids and tissues from cats with periodontal disease. Unpublished data, 1988.
96. Barrett, RE, et al.: Chronic relapsing stomatitis in a cat with feline leukemia virus infection. Fel Pract 5:34, 1975.
97. Cotter, SM, et al.: Association of feline leukemia virus with lymphosarcoma and other disorders in the cat. JAVMA 166:449, 1975.
98. Harvey, CE: Results following extraction of teeth in cats with severe periodontal disease. (Abst) Am Vet Dent Soc, 1986.
99. Pedersen, NC, et al.: Isolation of a T-lymphotrophic virus from cats with an immunodeficiency-like syndrome. Science 235:790, 1987.
100. Studer, E and Stapley, RB: The role of dry foods in maintaining healthy teeth and gums in the cat. VM/SAC 68:1124, 1973.
101. Conner, S, et al.: Alteration in parotid salivary flow in diabetes mellitus. Oral Surg 30:55, 1970.
102. Marder, MZ, et al.: Salivary alterations in diabetes mellitus. J Periodont 46:567, 1975.
103. Godlowski, Z and Withers, BT: Ablation of salivary glands as initial step in management of selected forms of diabetes mellitus. Laryngoscope 81:1337, 1971.
104. Cheville, NF: The gray collie syndrome. JAVMA 152:6, 1968.
105. Stannard, AA, et al.: A mucocutaneous disease in the dog resembling pemphigus vulgaris in man. JAVMA 166:575, 1975.
106. Hurvitz, AL and Feldman, E: A disease of dogs resembling human pemphigus vulgaris: Case reports. JAVMA 166:585, 1975.
107. Scott, DW: Pemphigus vegetans in a dog. Cornell Vet 67:374, 1977.
108. Bennett, D, et al.: Bullous autoimmune skin disease in the dog. 1. Clinical and pathological assessment. 2. Immunopathological assessment. Vet Record 106:497;523, 1980.
109. Brown, N and Hurvitz, AL: A mucocutaneous disease in a cat resembling human pemphigus. JAAHA 15:25, 1979.
110. Scott, DW: Feline dermatology 1979-1982: Introspective retrospections. JAAHA 19:537, 1983.
111. Richardson, RL: Effect of administering antibiotics, removing the major salivary glands, and toothbrushing on dental calculus formation in the cat. Arch Oral Biol 10:245, 1965.
112. Kaswan, RL, et al.: Keratoconjunctivitis sicca: Histopathologic study of nictitating membrane and lacrimal glands from 28 dogs. Am J Vet Res 45:1, 1984.
113. Quimby, FW, et al.: A disorder of dogs resembling Sjögren's syndrome. Clin Immunol Immunopathol 12:471, 1979.
114. Kaswan, RL, et al.: Rheumatoid factor determination in 50 dogs with keratoconjunctivitis sicca. JAVMA 10:183, 1983.
115. Povey, RC: Viral diseases of cats. Current concepts. Vet Record 98:293, 1976.

116. Mckeever, PJ and Klausner, JS: Plant awn, candidal, nocardial, and necrotizing ulcerative stomatitis in the dog. JAAHA 22, 1986.

117. Chastain, CB, et al.: Actinomycotic periodontitis in a cat. JAAHA 13, 1977.

118. Madewell, BR, et al.: Oral eosinophilic granuloma in Siberian husky dogs. JAVMA 177:701, 1980.

119. Potter, KA, et al.: Oral eosinophilic granuloma of Siberian huskies. JAAHA 16:595, 1980.

120. Dubielzig, RR: Proliferative dental and gingival diseases of dogs and cats. JAAHA 18, 1982.

121. Dubielzig, RR, et al.: The nomenclature of periodontal epulides in dogs. Vet Pathol 16:209, 1979.

122. DeMonbreun, WA and Goodpasture, EW: Infectious oral papillomatosis of dogs. Am J Pathol 8:43, 1932.

123. Kolata, RJ and Burrows, CF: The clinical features of injury by chewing electrical cords in dogs and cats. JAAHA 17, 1981.

124. Bradley, WA: Gingivitis in maltese terriers. Vet Record 110:618, 1982.

125. Verstraete, F: Unpublished data, 1986.

126. Olson, JA, et al.: Levamisole: A new treatment for recurrent aphthous stomatitis. Oral Surg 41:588, 1976.

127. Howard, DR, et al.: Primary cleft palate (harelip) and closure repair in puppies. JAAHA 12:636, 1976.

128. Clifford, DH and Clark, JJ: Mouth, lips and tongue. In Archibald, J (ed): Canine Surgery. Santa Barbara, Am Vet Pub Inc, 1965.

129. Farrow, CS: Surgical treatment of lower lip avulsion in the cat. VM/SAC 68:1418, 1973.

130. Scott, DW: Observations on the eosinophilic granuloma complex in cats. JAAHA 11:261, 1975.

131. Roenigk, WJ: Radiation Therapy. In Kirk, RW (ed): Current Veterinary Therapy, 4th ed. Philadelphia, WB Saunders, 1971.

132. Willemse, A and Lubberink, AAME: Eosinophilic ulcers in cats. Tijdschr Diergeneeskd 103:1052, 1978.

133. Hutt, FB and DeLahunta, A: A lethal glossopharyngeal defect in the dog. J Hered 62:5, 1971.

134. Dent, RSC: Operation for correction of lateral protrusion of the tongue in the dog. Vet Record 19:64, 1952.

135. Clutton, RE and Richards, DLS: The management of total tongue avulsion in a dog: A case report. J Small Anim Pract 28:307, 1987.

136. Stauffer, VD: Loss of the tongue in a cat. VM/SAC 68:1266, 1973.

137. Felts, JF, et al.: Thread and sewing needles as gastrointestinal foreign bodies in the cat: A review of 64 cases. JAVMA 184:1, 1984.

138. Stedham, MA, et al.: Glossitis of military dogs in South Vietnam. JAVMA 163:272, 1973.

139. Jennings, PB, et al.: Glossitis of military working dogs in Vietnam: Experimental production of tongue lesions. Am J Vet Res 35:1295, 1974.

140. Baker, MK: Ulcerative glossitis—a facet of feline panleukopenia. J S Afr Vet Assoc 46:295, 1975.

141. Douglas, SW and Kelly, DF: Calcinosis circumscripta of the tongue. J Small Anim Pract 7:441, 1966.

143. Cotter, SM: Oropharyngeal tumors in cats. JAAHA 17:917, 1981.

144. Beck, ER, et al.: Canine tongue tumors: A retrospective review of 57 cases. JAAHA 22, 1986.

145. Willard, MD, et al.: Progressive oropharyngeal dysfunction in a dog. JAVMA 183:9, 1983.

146. Kutschman, K and Schafer, R: Zur Tonsillitis und Tonsillektomie beim Hund. Monat Veterinarmed 30:381, 1975.

147. Dimic, J, et al.: Zur Frage der Pathologie und Therapie der tonsillener Kraukungen der Hunde. Kleintierpraxis 17:77, 1972.

148. Harvey, CE: Therapeutic strategies involving antimicrobial treatment of the upper respiratory tract in small animals. JAVMA 185:1159, 1984.

149. Brodey, RS: The biological behaviour of canine oral and pharyngeal neoplasms. J Small Anim Pract 11:45, 1970.

150. Todooroff, RJ and Brodey, RD: Oral and pharyngeal neoplasia in the dog: A retrospective study of 361 cases. JAVMA 175:567, 1979.

151. Dorn, CR and Priester, WA: Epidemiologic analysis of oral and pharyngeal cancer in dogs, cats, horses and cattle. JAVMA 169:1202, 1976.

152. Withrow, SJ and Holmberg, DL: Mandibulectomy in the treatment of oral cancer. JAAHA 19:273, 1983.

153. Harvey, CE: Radical resection of maxillary and mandibular lesions. Vet Clin North Am 16:983, 1986.

154. Thompson, JM, et al.: Hyperthermia and radiation in the management of canine tumours. J Small Anim Pract 28:457, 1987.

155. Reif, JS and Cohen, D: The environmental distribution of canine respiratory tract neoplasms. Arch Environ Health 22:136, 1971.

156. Michel, G: Beitrag zur Topographie der Aus fuhrungsgange der gl mandibularis und der gl sublingualis major des Hundes. Berl Muench Tieraerztl Wochenschr 69:132, 1956.

157. Blatt, CM, et al.: Nose sweat: A function for Steno's gland in the dog. Fed Proc 31:363, 1972.

158. Lawrence, AM, et al.: Salivary gland glucogen in man and animals. Metabolism 25:1405, 1976.

159. Bedford, PGC: Unilateral parotid hypersialation in a dachshund. Vet Record 107:557, 1980.

160. Harvey, CE: Hypersialosis and parotid gland enlargement in a dog. J Small Anim Pract 22:19, 1981.

161. Harvey, CE: Sialography in the dog. J Am Vet Rad Soc 10:18, 1969.

162. Stoll, SG: Cheiloplasty. In Bojrab, MJ (ed): Current Techniques in Small Animal Surgery. Philadelphia, Lea & Febiger, 1975.

163. Kelly, DF, et al.: Salivary gland necrosis in dogs. Vet Record 104:268, 1979.

164. DeYoung, DW, et al.: Attempts to produce salivary cysts in the dog. Am J Vet Res 39:185, 1978.

165. Harvey, CE: Parotid salivary duct rupture and fistula in the dog and cat. J Small Anim Pract 18:163, 1977.

166. Harvey, HJ: Pharyngeal mucoceles in dogs. JAVMA 178:1282, 1981.

167. Weber, WJ, et al.: Pharyngeal mucoceles in dogs. Vet Surg 15:5, 1986.

168. Harvey, CE: Letter to the editor. JAVMA 158:1454, 1971.

169. Knecht, CD and Phares, J: Characterization of dogs with salivary cyst. JAVMA 158:5, 1971.

170. Harrison, JD and Garrett, JR: Histological effects of ductal ligation of salivary glands of the cat. J Pathol 118:245, 1975.

171. Prescott, CW: Ranula in the dog: A surgical treatment. Aust Vet J 44:382, 1968.

172. Harvey, CE: Canine salivary mucocele. JAAHA 5:155, 1969.

173. Glen, JB: Canine salivary mucoceles: results of sialographic examination and surgical treatment of 50 cases. J Small Anim Pract 13:515, 1972.

174. Wallace, LJ, et al.: Anterior cervical sialocele (salivary cyst) in a domestic cat. JAAHA 8:74, 1972.

175. Knecht, CD: Treatment of diseases of the zygomatic salivary gland. JAAHA 6:1, 1970.

176. Kelly, DF, et al.: Histology of salivary gland infarction in the dog. Vet Pathol 16:438, 1979.

177. Chandler, EA: Mumps in the dog. Vet Record 96:365, 1975.

178. Karbe, E and Schiefer, B: Primary salivary gland tumors in carnivores. Can Vet J 8:212, 1967.

179. Head, KW: Tumors of the upper alimentary tract. Bull WHO 53:3427, 1976.

180. Buyukmihci, N, et al.: Exophthalmos secondary to zygomatic adenocarcinoma in a dog. JAVMA 167:162, 1975.

181. Harvey, CE: Exploration of the orbit. In Bistner, SI, et al. (eds): Atlas of Veterinary Ophthalmic Surgery. Philadelphia, WB Saunders, 1977.

182. Karbe, D: Lateral neck cysts in the dog. Am J Vet Res 26:112, 1965.

183. Dallman, MJ and Johnson, EO: Thyroglossal duct cyst in a dog. JAAHA 22:1986.

184. Karbe, D and Nielsen, SW: Branchial cyst in a dog. JAVMA 147:6, 1965.

185. Lee, R: Radiographic examination of localized and diffuse tissue swellings in the mandibular and pharyngeal area. Vet Clin North Am 4:723, 1974.

83 DISEASES OF THE ESOPHAGUS

BRENT D. JONES, ALBERT E. JERGENS, and
W. GRANT GUILFORD

The esophagus is the tubular, muscular organ that functions to transmit a bolus of material from the pharynx to the stomach. Because the esophagus is strictly an organ of transport, esophageal disease relates to impairment of only this transport function and not of digestive or absorptive processes. Even though the esophagus may be considered a relatively simple organ, we know less about the pathophysiology of esophageal diseases than about those of any other organs in the body. For this reason, treating the diseases that affect the esophagus is a therapeutic challenge.

The purpose of this chapter is to review several diseases of the esophagus and their medical therapy. Sections on anatomy, physiology, and pharmacology are also included in the hope that this will enable the reader to more completely understand the pathophysiology and treatment of esophageal diseases.

ANATOMY OF THE ESOPHAGUS

The esophagus is bounded cranially by the upper esophageal sphincter (UES) and terminates caudally with a functional sphincter called the lower esophageal sphincter (LES). The esophagus is divided into cervical, thoracic, and abdominal portions. The cervical portion extends from the caudal border of the cricoid cartilage to the thoracic inlet. The trachea lies ventral and to the right of the cervical esophagus. The thoracic esophagus includes that esophageal portion which extends from the thoracic inlet to the diaphragm. It originates on the left side of the trachea but lies dorsal at the tracheal bifurcation. A short segment of abdominal esophagus extends between the diaphragm and the stomach.

The body of the esophagus consists of four layers: the adventitia, muscularis, submucosa, and mucosa. The thin fibrous adventitia covers the esophageal muscularis. The muscularis of the esophagus of the dog is composed of two oblique layers of striated muscle throughout its entire length. The proximal portion of the muscularis of the cat esophagus consists of striated muscle. The distal third contains smooth muscle. The striated muscle of the feline esophagus consists of two layers that are oblique in the proximal portion and become spiral in the distal portion. They gradually form a distinct inner, circular layer and an outer, longitudinal layer. The muscle fiber transition from striated muscle to smooth muscle in the feline muscularis occurs gradually. The amount of smooth muscle increases distally until the final two to three cm of the esophagus, where all of the muscle fibers are smooth. The submucosal layer contains mucus glands and loosely binds the mucosal and muscular layers together. This allows the relatively inelastic mucosal coat to be thrown into prominent longitudinal folds in the dog. Transverse folds of mucosa constitute the serrated or herringbone pattern observed radiographically in the terminal thoracic esophagus of the cat.[1] The mucosal layer has a stratified squamous epithelium that contains openings for the ducts of the esophageal mucus glands. In the caudal half of the esophagus the mucosa is bounded by the muscularis mucosae.

Blood supply to the cervical esophagus is derived from the thyroid arteries. The bronchoesophageal artery supplies the cranial two-thirds of the thoracic esophagus with the remainder of the esophagus perfused by branches of the aorta, intercostals, and left gastric artery. Venous drainage of the esophagus is by satellite vessels of the arteries that supply it. Innervation of the esophagus is supplied by the vagus nerve and its associated branches. The vagus nerve contains somatic motor nerves to the esophageal striated muscle, autonomic nerves to the esophageal smooth muscle, and general visceral afferent nerves from the esophageal sensory receptors. The central nervous system organization of this innervation is discussed under Physiology of Swallowing.

Upper Esophageal Sphincter

The paired cricopharyngeal muscles and a portion of the thyropharyngeus muscle make up the upper esophageal sphincter (UES). This sphincter at rest is a high-pressure zone that serves to separate the cervical esophagus from the pharynx. Relaxation of the UES occurs in association with reflex pharyngeal peristaltic contraction; it remains open only long enough to pass a bolus of ingesta from the pharynx to the cranial esophagus. The rapid closure of the UES helps to protect against esophagopharyngeal reflux and aspiration of ingesta.

Lower Esophageal Sphincter

The lower esophageal sphincter (LES) is located at the terminal esophagus and gastroesophageal junction. In this region, the muscularis mucosae expands into a thickened layer of circular smooth muscle. It is this smooth muscle sphincter that is of primary importance in maintaining a high pressure zone at the junction of the esophagus and cardia. A number of anatomic features of the gastroesophageal junction contribute to the competency of the lower esophageal sphincter. These other structural components include: (1) interdigitating rugal folds that converge near the gastroesophageal junction and continue into the terminal esophagus; (2) the right diaphragmatic crus, which serves as a muscular sling; (3) the oblique implantation of the distal esophagus into the stomach; (4) the muscular sling provided by the smooth muscle bundles of the lesser gastric curvature around the left side of the gastroesophageal junction; and (5) the compression exerted on the short intra-abdominal terminal esophagus by the positive intra-abdominal pressure (Figure 83–1).[2]

The dog's LES consists of an outer layer of striated muscle and an inner layer of smooth muscle. In contrast, the LES in the cat is composed entirely of smooth muscle. The LES promotes unidirectional flow of ingesta between the esophagus and the stomach while preventing gastroesophageal reflux. Relaxation and contraction of the LES occurs in response to neural activity (vagal tone) but may also be influenced by hormones or local events, such as esophagitis, which results in LES relaxation.

Physiology of Swallowing

Swallowing consists of a series of sequential, well-coordinated events that transport food and liquids from the mouth to the stomach. This process has been divided into three major phases: oropharyngeal, esophageal, and gastroesophageal.[2] The oropharyngeal phase is further subdivided into oral, pharyngeal, and cricopharyngeal stages, with each stage related to the action of a particular group of structures.[2] Following the prehension of food, the voluntary *oral stage* is initiated in which a bolus is formed in the oropharynx and is passed in an aboral direction to the base of the tongue. Pharyngeal contact by the bolus next stimulates a series of rapid pharyngeal peristaltic contractions that propel the bolus from the base of the tongue to the laryngopharynx. This is the second or *pharyngeal stage* of the oropharyngeal phase. These contractions are coordinated with a simultaneous, momentary opening of the upper esophageal sphincter. Respiration is temporarily halted during the pharyngeal stage of swallowing, since the two events cannot occur simultaneously. The interval that the UES remains open is determined by the volume of the bolus propelled from the pharynx. The *cricopharyngeal stage*

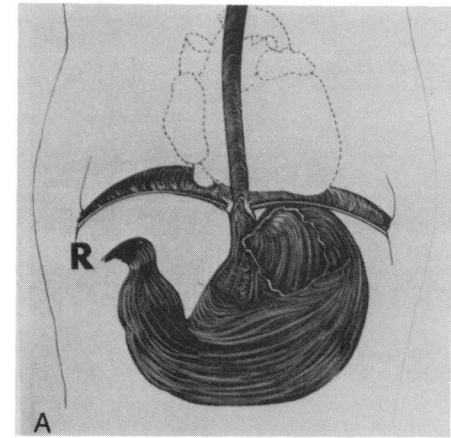

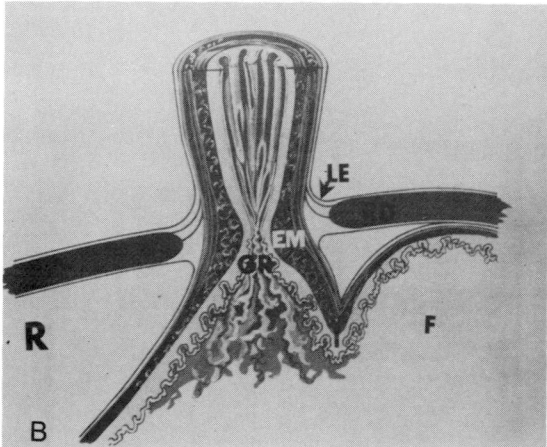

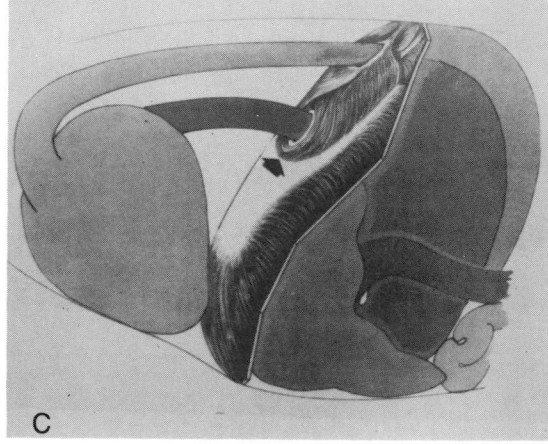

FIGURE 83–1. *A,* Ventrodorsal illustration of the oblique implantation of the esophagus into the stomach. Caudally, the esophagus is fixed via muscular fibers blending with those of the stomach and a loose pleural attachment to the esophageal hiatus located in the right crus of the diaphragm. A cut-out section shows the deep oblique muscle bundles arising from the lesser curvature of the stomach to form a muscular sling around the left side of the incisura. The incisura cardiaca is the indentation that separates the gastric fundus from the gastroesophageal opening. "R" represents the animal's right side as viewed in the ventrodorsal position. *B,* The anatomic structures that contribute to the closure of the gastroesophageal junction. These are the focal esophageal muscular thickening (EM), the gastric rugal folds (GR), the gastric fundus (F), the incisura (I), right diaphragmatic crus (RD), and ligaments of the esophagus to the diaphragm (LE). *C,* Lateral illustration of the esophagus hiatus located in the right crus of the diaphragm. A muscular sling (arrow) provided by the medial portion of the right crus of the diaphragm contributes to the closure mechanism of the LES. (From Watrous, BJ and Suter, PF: Normal swallowing in the dog: A cineradiographic study. Vet Radiol 20:99, 1979.)

is initiated by passage of the bolus through the UES into the esophagus and terminates with UES closure and relaxation of the pharynx. During closure, the UES shows phasic rather than tonic activity and generates a sphincter pressure that is higher than that on either side in the pharynx or esophagus.[3] The pressure of the UES remains highest during inspiration and predeglutition.[4]

The *esophageal phase* encompasses the passage of the bolus from the UES to the gastroesophageal junction. Several types of potential sequences between the oropharyngeal phase of swallowing and initiation of esophageal peristalsis have been described:[2] (1) a swallow followed by an immediate esophageal peristaltic wave that progresses without interruption to the gastroesophageal junction (primary peristalsis); (2) following a swallow, a bolus may remain in the proximal esophagus until a second or third swallow occurs and sweeps the combined boluses to the gastroesophageal junction (primary peristalsis); (3) a swallowed bolus may pause temporarily in the proximal esophagus, then stimulate a peristaltic wave that carries it to the gastroesophageal junction (secondary peristalsis); and (4) multiple boluses from several swallows that accumulate proximally in the esophagus may trigger a peristaltic wave that carries them all caudally (secondary peristalsis).

The majority of normal swallows induce waves of primary peristalsis that are triggered by the oropharyngeal phase of swallowing.[5] Peristaltic waves that result from esophageal luminal distention and tactile stimuli from the bolus are called secondary peristalsis and are independent of the swallowing reflex. These waves begin in the esophagus cranial to the bolus and are indistinct from primary peristalsis on manometric evaluation.[6] Progression of primary or secondary peristaltic waves is dependent upon the presence, size, and location of the bolus in the esophagus.

Functional motor activity of the esophagus is dependent on a precisely coordinated series of sequential contractions of esophageal muscle. Stimulation of sensory receptors by a bolus in the pharynx and esophagus initiates afferent impulse conduction up the vagus nerve and tractus solitarius to the nucleus of the tractus solitarius and the swallowing center in the brain stem. Efferent motor fibers to the esophageal striated muscle in the dog are somatic nerves and are carried in the vagus nerve. These fibers arise from lower motor neurons in the nucleus ambiguus. The upper motor neurons of the swallowing center act to coordinate efferent motor activity and to inhibit respiration during deglutition.[7] The smooth muscle of the esophagus receives its motor innervation by parasympathetic and sympathetic nerve fibers. Parasympathetic vagal preganglionic fibers arise from the dorsal motor nucleus in the brain stem and synapse in the intrinsic plexuses located within the smooth muscle layers.

Central nervous system lesions that disrupt the parasympathetic supply to the canine esophagus cause no discernible failure of esophageal function because the efferent motor innervation to esophageal striated muscle remains intact. In contrast, central lesions that affect the parasympathetic activity to the feline esophagus cause uncoordinated esophageal motor activity. This difference reflects the greater role that smooth muscle

plays in the feline esophagus. Normal coordinated peristalsis in the dog and cat is dependent on intact vagal innervation. Disruption of this vagal activity in the dog results in esophageal paralysis, dilation, and neurogenic atrophy of the striated muscle distal to the nervous injury.[8] Paralysis of the esophagus has also been observed following bilateral destruction of the nucleus ambiguus in the dog (see Figure 83–2).[9]

The final swallowing phase is the *gastroesophageal phase* during which the bolus passes into the stomach through the lower esophageal sphincter. Relaxation of the LES is initiated by swallowing and may be detected well in advance of the arrival of the esophageal bolus.[10, 11] Gastroesophageal reflux may occasionally occur; however, reflux is not considered abnormal if the ingesta is rapidly cleared by additional esophageal contractions. The passage of the bolus through the LES is followed by a rise in LES pressure and closure of the sphincter preventing further gastroesophageal reflux.

PHARMACOLOGIC RESPONSES OF THE ESOPHAGUS AND ITS SPHINCTERS

Optimal performance of the esophagus and the lower esophageal sphincter is dependent upon the response of these structures to a variety of hormonal, nutritional, and drug-induced stimuli. The LES has been shown to respond to numerous gastrointestinal hormones including gastrin, secretin, cholecystokinin, and glucagon. The infusion of gastrin into dogs results in increased LES pressure. However, this response appears to be related to pharmacologic and not physiologic concentrations of gastrin.[12] If gastrin does play a role in maintaining high pressure in the LES during the digestion of food, its role is less important than originally thought.[12] The effects of gastrin may be antagonized by the actions of atropine and tetrodotoxin, which suggests that gastrin's action on the LES is through a neural pathway. Secretin directly inhibits the action of gastrin on the LES and indirectly inhibits its release. This antagonism is competitive and secretin does not interact with other agents that act on esophageal neural or muscular receptors. Cholecystokinin and glucagon have a similar inhibitory effect on LES tone to that of secretin.

Dietary nutrients also affect pressure in the lower esophageal sphincter. High-protein diets cause the pressure to increase and fatty meals act to decrease LES tone. Fat in the diet also inhibits gastrin-induced increases in LES tone.

Metoclopramide and bethanechol act to increase LES tone and reduce the reflux potential in human beings.[13] The specific actions of metoclopramide on esophageal and LES function in the dog are poorly understood but appear to result in increased lower esophageal pressure and increased strength of esophageal contractions, both of which contribute to the competence of the lower esophageal sphincter.[14] Recently, four drugs with cholinergic activity (metoclopramide, atropine, bethanecol, and edrophonium) were investigated to assess their roles on esophageal peristalsis in the dog.[15] Metoclopramide was shown to enhance normal peristalsis by increasing

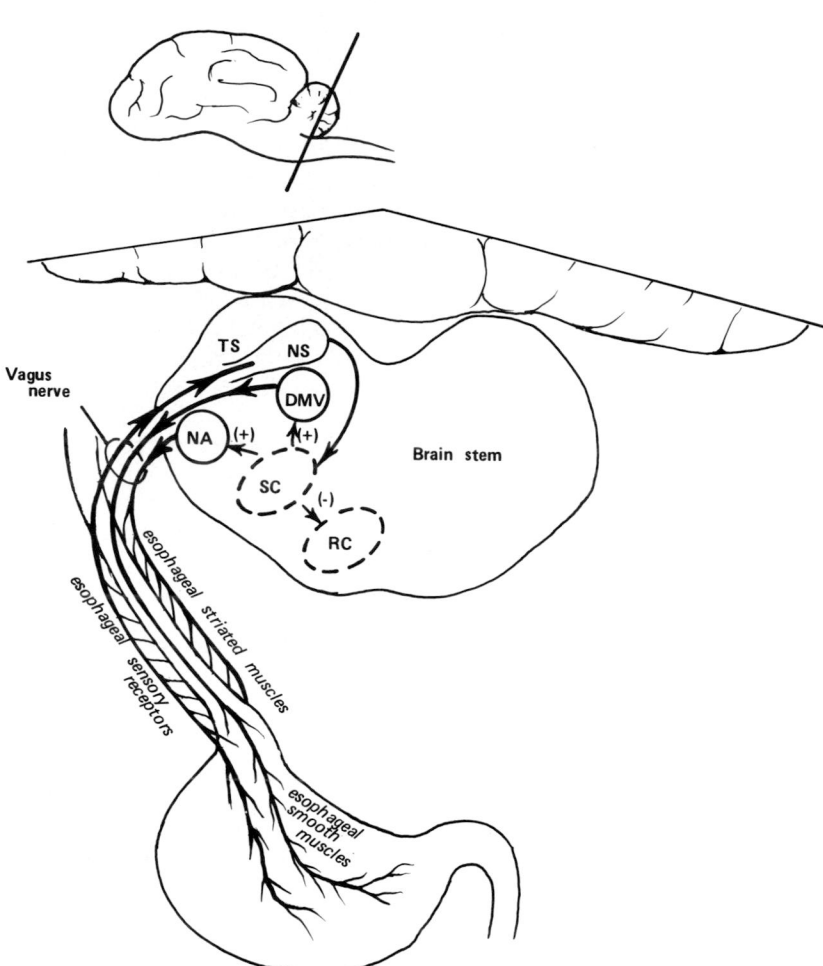

FIGURE 83–2. Schematic diagram of the regulation of esophageal motility in the dog: nucleus solitarius (NS), tractus solitarius (TS), dorsal motor nucleus of the vagus (DMV), nucleus ambiguus (NA), swallowing "center" (SC), respiratory "center" (RC).

the amplitude and duration of distal esophageal contractions. Atropine, bethanecol, and edrophonium exerted no significant effects on esophageal motility and are probably not indicated in the management of canine esophageal motility disorders. Atropine also significantly reduces LES tone and may contribute to the development of reflux esophagitis.

General anesthesia and the effects of tranquilization may strongly influence esophageal function. Deep anesthesia results in significantly decreased esophageal motility and an aberrant gag reflex. The use of certain preanesthetic drugs such as morphine sulfate, pethidine hydrochloride, and diazepam has been shown to decrease LES pressure and increase the probability of reflux in monkeys and humans.[16] The use of acepromazine at preanesthetic and higher doses (0.1 to 0.2 mg/lb or 0.2 to 0.4 mg/kg body weight) has been shown to reduce LES pressure in the dog.[17]

Study of modifiers of UES function is limited but suggests that the UES readily contracts in response to stimulation by distention or acid in the upper esophagus.[18]

DIAGNOSIS

Clinical Signs

The clinical signs of esophageal disease may be quite obvious or very subtle. The degree of esophageal in-

volvement, location of the problem, chronicity, and presence of secondary problems will influence the clinical signs. Clinical signs may be attributable to alimentary tract disease or to secondary complications, such as aspiration pneumonia, which may be mistaken for the primary problem.

Signs of esophageal disease include regurgitation through the mouth or the nares, dysphagia, odynophagia, repeated swallowing movements, and copious salivation or drooling. A common misconception is that esophageal disease causes regurgitation only immediately after eating: regurgitation may occur during and shortly after eating or may be delayed for several hours. Differentiating regurgitation from vomiting is important in distinguishing esophageal from lower gastrointestinal disease. Characteristics of vomiting include expulsion of digested and bile-stained food and retching with involuntary abdominal contractions. Gastric contents are highly acidic and pH of vomited material may be tested. However, vomiting often involves the reflux of bicarbonate-rich fluid into the stomach from the duodenum, which buffers the gastric acid. The vomited material may then have a neutral or near-neutral pH. Regurgitation involves less forceful casting-up of tubular, bile-free, undigested food. Regurgitation may involve only foam or liquid and, as stated previously, may or may not be directly related to ingestion of food. Mucoid secretions mixed with the undigested food will usually have a pH 6.5 to 7.0.[19] Copious salivation may also be a confusing sign. It may be a major sign of esophageal conditions, such as a foreign body, or it may be part of the nausea which accompanies vomiting.

Signs of esophageal disease may be attributable only to the respiratory system. Mucopurulent nasal discharge, dyspnea, or moist coughing will often accompany esophageal disease because of the high incidence of aspiration of ingesta.

Weight loss in association with either anorexia or a voracious appetite may accompany esophageal disease. For example, anorexia and dysphagia usually occur with esophageal foreign bodies or perforations, and young animals with congenital megaesophagus might have a voracious appetite accompanied by regurgitation and weight loss. Other signs include cervical cellulitis or a draining fistulous tract secondary to esophageal perforation by a foreign body. Repeated attempts at swallowing accompanied by extension, flexion, or twisting of the head and neck are also hallmarks of esophageal disease. All of these signs may be intermittent and prolonged, or acute and progressive, depending on the disease process. In summary, the major clinical signs of esophageal disease are regurgitation, dysphagia, coughing, and dyspnea.

History

As in the treatment of any medical problem, it is imperative that a complete and careful history be taken. The owner's primary complaint may be attributable to the primary esophageal signs or to extraesophageal disease. Historical details should include the exact onset and course of the problems, the type of dysphagia, and its relationship to ingestion of food. Information regarding the ability of the animal to retain liquids, soft food, or solid food may be helpful. If the animal shows signs in adulthood, the owner should be questioned regarding its possible exposure to caustic agents, foreign bodies, and traumatic incidents, previous neurologic problems, prior surgery, or anesthesia. Reports of concurrent muscle weakness or neurologic disorders should alert the clinician to an extraesophageal disease process that may underlie the esophageal disease. The clinical signs associated with congenital problems, such as vascular ring anomalies and cricopharyngeal achalasia, will be manifested in an animal that is still nursing or recently weaned to solid food. Acute onset of signs in either a young or older animal often is consistent with the presence of a foreign body. Chronic or slowly progressive regurgitation is more suggestive of gastroesophageal reflux or a developing esophageal stricture.

Physical Examination

Physical examination of patients with esophageal problems may be unrewarding but on occasion confirms the historical suspicion of esophageal disease. In addition, the physical examination may reveal the cause of the esophageal disease (e.g., palpation of a cervical mass or esophageal foreign body); it provides valuable information with regard to the presence or absence of complications (such as pneumonia) and aids in the

formulation of a prognosis. Frequently, however, special diagnostic techniques (see below) are needed to detect esophageal disease and to further evaluate any esophageal abnormalities noted on physical examination.

The physical condition of the animal may vary from normal to emaciated, depending on the severity of the disease process. Physical examination may reveal any of the clinical signs discussed above. Observation and careful palpation of the cervical and thoracic inlet region may be helpful. A dilated cervical esophagus may be visualized or palpated, especially when examined during respiration or if the animal's thorax is forcibly compressed while its nostrils are occluded. Auscultation of the cervical esophagus and thoracic inlet and thorax may be helpful. Coarse crackles (moist rales), associated with aspiration pneumonia or fluid movement in the dilated esophagus, may be detected. Watching the animal eat is often a valuable adjunct to physical examination. The type of dysphagia and regurgitation is easily observed.

The differentiation of various esophageal diseases depends on subtle differences in history and physical examination, especially in the character, duration, and time intervals between ingestion, dysphagia, and regurgitation. Definitive diagnosis and differentiation of esophageal diseases depend on various diagnostic procedures (see Table 83–4) including radiographic techniques (e.g., contrast studies and fluoroscopy), endoscopy, biopsy, and occasionally manometry, electromyography, and exploratory surgery.

Diagnostic Techniques

RADIOLOGY

The radiographic evaluation of the esophagus is a very rewarding procedure for both the diagnosis and differential diagnosis of esophageal disease. Cervical and thoracic survey films and static or dynamic contrast studies are often the cornerstone of the diagnostic workup and are indicated whenever esophageal disease is suspected. It is difficult to rule out esophageal disease without performing a dynamic contrast study,[5] and the information from such a study facilitates assessment of prognosis.

Radiographic Technique

SURVEY FILMS. Standard lateral and ventrodorsal projections should be made to survey the anatomic regions occupied by the cervical, thoracic, and abdominal esophagus. A right ventrodorsal oblique projection that reduces superimposition of the esophagus on the thoracic vertebrae may also be of value. A high MAS–low KVp abdominal technique should be used to evaluate the cervical esophagus, whereas a high KVp–low MAS thoracic technique should be used to evaluate the thoracic soft tissue structures.

ESOPHAGRAPHY. No special patient preparation is required prior to this contrast procedure. Tranquilization is normally unnecessary and should be avoided if at all possible. In particularly uncooperative patients, low-dose acetylpromazine can be used and has a minimal adverse effect on swallowing.[2] The use of a variety of contrast materials is required for adequate examination of the esophagus. Barium sulfate suspensions, pastes, and food admixtures examine the swallowing response of the esophagus to ingesta of different consistencies and have specific advantages for the diagnosis of different types of esophageal disease. Varying consistencies of ingesta may induce different swallowing responses by the esophagus. This is thought to result from changes in the sensory stimulus provided to the esophagus by the different physical properties of the ingestas and from variation in the ability of the ingestas to traverse areas of diseased esophagus. Liquid barium should be used to demonstrate esophageal luminal diameter, whereas barium paste gives better definition of the mucosal detail and barium-food admixtures better demonstrate esophageal partial obstructions. The technique described below is that recommended by Aronson et al.[20]

Liquid barium (1 to 3 ml/lb or 3 to 5 ml/kg) is administered via syringe into the buccal pouch of the animal restrained in right lateral recumbency. The contrast medium is administered at a rate that allows normal swallowing and avoids aspiration. Recumbent right lateral, ventrodorsal, and oblique right ventrodorsal radiographs are then taken immediately following administration. One to three fluid ounces of barium paste is then placed on the animal's hard palate with a tongue depressor and the radiographic sequence repeated. If no abnormalities are detected following the liquid barium and barium paste swallows, liquid barium is mixed with dog food and the radiographic series is repeated.

If fluoroscopy is available, the passage of the barium contrast agents during swallowing can be observed. The study should include recording of three to six complete swallows of liquid barium suspension followed by a similar number of barium-coated food boluses.[5]

If esophageal perforation is suspected, a water-soluble iodinated contrast material should be used. Such materials are less irritating to the periesophageal tissues. If the swallow does not identify a perforation, the study should be repeated with a liquid barium suspension because esophageal perforations may be missed with water-soluble agents.[5]

Normal Radiographic Interpretation. The esophagus of a normal animal will not be seen on survey radiography. An exception occurs following aerophagia due to excitement, nausea, dyspnea, or anesthesia. The presence of luminal air results in a radiolucency that allows visualization of part or all of the course of the esophagus and suggests some details of mucosal topography. Luminal air may also collect as a result of esophageal diseases such as luminal obstructions or motility disturbances, e.g., megaesophagus. Several radiographic features aid differentiation between benign and pathologic accumulations of gas.[20] Gas accumulations following aerophagia due to excitement or struggling are usually transient, and gas is often present in both stomach and esophagus. Esophageal gas accumulation during anesthesia is usually generalized and uniform and outlines an esophagus of normal diameter and with normal mucosal borders.

Contrast materials are rapidly cleared from the normal esophagus by a series of brisk, aboral progressive,

peristaltic waves. Any persistent pooling of contrast material in the esophagus following administration should be regarded as abnormal. Pooling usually occurs oral to the lesion, and the site at which pooling occurs, as well as the mucosal pattern revealed, provides important diagnostic information. For example, pooling of contrast material at the level of the base of the heart suggests esophageal obstruction caused by a vascular ring abnormality. An irregular mucosal border is suggestive of an intramural lesion. Following administration of barium paste, the esophageal mucosa of a normal dog is outlined as a series of parallel longitudinal folds extending the entire length of the esophagus. At the thoracic inlet the esophagus may deviate ventrally and the mucosal pattern demonstrate some irregularity. This is a normal finding in the esophagus of young dogs and should not be diagnosed as an esophageal diverticulum.[20] In cats, the barium-outlined mucosa of the cranial two-thirds of the esophagus appears as parallel longitudinal folds whereas that of the caudal third of the esophagus has a characteristic irregular herringbone pattern that should not be misinterpreted as esophagitis.[21]

The degree of dilatation revealed by the contrast medium and the amount of motility noted on fluoroscopy provides important prognostic information. Once severe esophageal dilation is present, function is unlikely to be regained.[5] Absence of motility is associated with a poor but not hopeless prognosis. It is important to realize that a hypomotile esophagus has sometimes been demonstrated in excited, dyspneic, or nauseated dogs[22] and in young dogs with no signs of regurgitation.[23] Other radiographic features suggestive of the various types of esophageal disease are detailed along with the description of the disease.

Endoscopy. Endoscopy (esophagoscopy) with either rigid or flexible fiberoptic instruments is an increasingly important tool in evaluation of esophageal diseases.

The advantage of endoscopy over the other methods of evaluating esophageal diseases is that one is able to visualize the esophagus and any of its lesions with a noninvasive procedure. Most endoscopes are equipped with an operating channel, which enables tissue specimens (biopsy, brush cytology, impression smears) to be obtained for a more definitive diagnosis. Most foreign bodies can be removed via endoscopy. The technique will be discussed completely later in this chapter. The major disadvantage is that the procedure requires anesthesia. The reader is referred to other texts for detailed information and techniques of endoscopy.[24–26]

Esophageal biopsy specimens may be obtained by three methods. The easiest method is to use alligator forceps through either the rigid or the flexible endoscope. Surgical excisional biopsy may also be utilized. Another convenient method of esophageal biopsy is use of suction biopsy equipment. Another text describes this procedure in detail.[27]

No matter which method is used to obtain a gastrointestinal biopsy specimen, one should lay or pin the specimen on a flat surface, such as a piece of thin cardboard, tongue depressor, or sliced cucumber before placing it in the formalin solution (Figure 83–3). This maneuver will enable the pathologist to orient the tissue properly and to obtain cuts at right (90°) angles to the

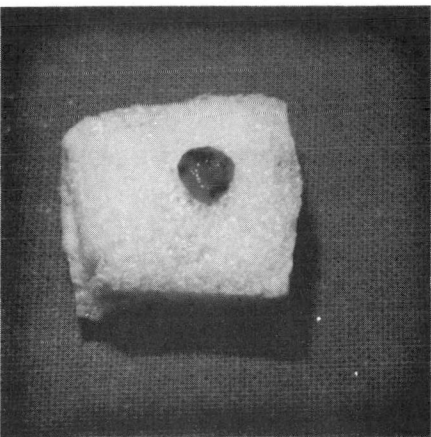

FIGURE 83–3. The esophageal biopsy specimen is laid flat on a piece of Gelfoam before it is placed in formalin. This enables the pathologist to orient the tissue properly and obtain cuts at right (90°) angles to the tissue. (From Jones, BD (ed): Canine and Feline Gastroenterology. Philadelphia, WB Saunders, 1986.)

tissues. Impression smears should also be obtained before the tissue is placed in formalin.

Intraluminal esophageal manometry is a useful clinical and investigative method for the evaluation of esophageal pressure and motor function.[17] It is currently being utilized extensively in human medicine and on research animals but is used on a limited basis in clinical veterinary medicine at this time.

ESOPHAGEAL DISEASES

Congenital Esophageal Diseases

Congenital diseases of the esophagus are uncommon. Those reported include esophageal atresia, esophageal stenosis, heterotopia of gastric mucosa in the esophagus, esophageal diverticulum, esophageal fistula, vascular anomaly, and idiopathic megaesophagus.[28] The majority of these conditions are described separately in the following discussion.

Megaesophagus

Megaesophagus is a descriptive term for the clinical sign of esophageal dilatation, a sign common to a number of distinctive disease entities of varied causes. Special care must be taken to differentiate the term megaesophagus from the diseases (or syndromes) of "idiopathic megaesophagus" and "achalasia," both of which result in megaesophagus but have stricter definitions. Idiopathic megaesophagus is a disease of the dog and cat in which esophageal dilatation and hypomotility are believed to result from primary neuromuscular dysfunction of as yet unknown cause. Achalasia is a specific disease of humans in which esophageal dilation is classically associated with a loss of primary peristalsis, the presence of a hypertonic lower esophageal sphincter (LES) that does not relax in response to a swallow, and evidence of denervation of the esophagus.[29] Acha-

lasia, so defined, has yet to be proven to exist in the dog.[5, 30–32] Table 83–1 summarizes the terms that these authors believe best reflect the current state of our knowledge of esophageal dilation. It is suggested that megaesophagus be classified according to the age of onset and according to whether a cause is identified. Thus megaesophagus may be classified as congenital idiopathic megaesophagus, adult-onset idiopathic megaesophagus, or secondary (acquired) megaesophagus.

Esophageal dilatation is the most important cause of regurgitation in the dog and cat.[31] It is seen with reasonable frequency in referral institutions. Seventy-nine and 125 dogs with generalized megaesophagus were presented to the University of Pennsylvania Veterinary Hospital, and the University of California-Davis Veterinary Teaching Hospital, respectively, over eight-year periods.[31] Over a period of eight years, fifty-three cases of canine megaesophagus were presented to the University of Missouri Veterinary Teaching Hospital, representing approximately one case per thousand of total visitations. The incidence of esophageal dilation in the cat is generally thought to be lower than in the dog. However, the increased incidence of feline dysautonomia, a condition in which megaesophagus is common,[33] is likely to make megaesophagus an important clinical entity in cats.

Cause and Pathophysiology of Idiopathic Megaesophagus (IM). In spite of considerable investigation the cause of canine idiopathic megaesophagus (IM) is unknown, the site of the lesion or lesions in IM is still unconfirmed, and the pathophysiology of the esophageal dilatation is unresolved.

The possible causes of canine IM are at present speculative. One author has suggested that the congenital form of the disease may be caused by a delay in maturation of the esophageal neuromuscular system, a theory that explains why young dogs may improve with careful feeding management.[34, 35] The finding that chronic anticholinesterase administration can cause the disease has led some authors to speculate on the possibility of a neurotoxin as the underlying cause.[36, 37] Epidemiologic evidence (see below), however, suggests that the primary defect is inherited. Karyotyping has shown no chromosomal abnormalities.[36]

The site of the lesion in canine IM is unknown. Some authors think that the lesion is in the nucleus ambiguus.[38, 39] Other authors believe that the site of the lesion is either in the afferent limb of the reflex arcs controlling esophageal motility or in the medullary connections between the tractus solitarius and the swallowing center or nucleus ambiguus.[31, 40] No lesion at these sites has been consistently demonstrated, however. The possibility of demyelinating lower motor neuron disease or

TABLE 83–1. NOMENCLATURE OF ESOPHAGEAL DILATION

Megaesophagus–A general term for esophageal dilation.
Congenital idiopathic megaesophagus–Idiopathic esophageal dilation manifested at or about the time of weaning.
Adult-onset idiopathic megaesophagus–Idiopathic esophageal dilation manifested at adulthood.
Secondary (acquired) megaesophagus–Esophageal dilation of all causes other than idiopathic megaesophagus.

neuromuscular junction defects has not been adequately examined.

The pathogenesis of canine IM is no more clear than the site of the primary lesion. Most authors do not believe that failure of the LES to relax precedes esophageal dilation in IM.[5, 13, 30–32, 36, 40–43] Instead, they describe IM as a primary neuromuscular esophageal disease in which failure of effective peristalsis is the primary reason ingesta accumulates. One author is convinced, however, that abnormal or asynchronous function of the LES and esophagus is important in the pathogenesis of IM.[44–46]

Megaesophagus of unknown cause has also been reported in the cat.[47–49] The causes may be inherited,[47] and little is known of the site of the lesion(s) or of the pathogenesis.

Cause and Pathophysiology of Secondary Megaesophagus. Numerous disease conditions have been associated with or proposed as causes for esophageal dilation (Table 83–2). Any disruption of esophageal muscle or of the central, afferent or efferent pathways that control esophageal motility (Figure 83–2) could theoretically result in megaesophagus by interference with the act of swallowing. Many such disruptions, either disease or experimentally induced, have already been shown to cause megaesophagus. For instance, myositis

TABLE 83–2. DISEASES ASSOCIATED WITH AND CAUSES OF MEGAESOPHAGUS

Neuromuscular
  Idiopathic megaesophagus (hereditary?)
  Myasthenia gravis
  SLE
  Polymyositis and polymyopathy
  Glycogen storage disease Type II
  Dermatomyositis
  Giant cell axonal neuropathy
  Polyradiculoneuritis
  Immune mediated polyneuritis
  Ganglioradiculitis
  Dysautonomia
  Spinal muscle atrophy
  Bilateral vagal damage (surgical, traumatic, neoplastic)
  Familial reflex myoclonus
  Cervical vertebral instability with leukomalacia
  Brain stem trauma, neoplasia or vascular accident
  Botulism
  Distemper
Esophageal Obstructive Diseases
  Neoplasia
  Vascular ring abnormalities
  Extraesophageal compression
  Strictures, granulomas, foreign bodies
Toxic
  Lead
  Thallium
  Anticholinesterase
  Acrylamide
Miscellaneous
  Mediastinitis
  Bronchoesophageal fistula
  Cachexia
  Pyloric stenosis
  Gastric heterotopia
  Addison's disease
  Hypothyroidism
  Pituitary dwarfism
  Trypanosoma cruzi infection
  Thymoma

and myopathy associated with a variety of diseases including SLE,[50, 51] trypanosomiasis,[52] glycogen-storage disease,[52a] polymyositis,[50, 53] advanced dermatomyositis,[54] and cachexia[5] have produced sufficient esophageal muscle damage to cause megaesophagus. Neuromuscular junction disease in botulism,[55, 56] congenital or acquired myasthenia gravis,[27, 50, 57, 58] and chronic anticholinesterase administration[59] have been shown to produce esophageal dilation. Various types of peripheral neuropathies including polyradiculoneuritis,[50] ganglioradiculitis,[60] dysautonomia,[33] demyelinating neuropathies (such as thallium toxicosis)[61] and axonopathies such as canine giant axonal neuropathy,[62] spinal muscular atrophy,[63] and polyneuritis[5] have produced megaesophagus. Megaesophagus has also been associated with lead toxicity.[64] The suggested cause was a vagal polyneuropathy. Bilateral vagal damage due to trauma, neoplasia, or surgery may cause esophageal dilation. Megaesophagus has been reported caudal to areas of mediastinitis subsequent to esophageal perforation from foreign bodies.[41] The dilatation was transient and was presumed to be caused by interference of vagal function by mediastinal cellulitis.[41] A similar finding was reported subsequent to a bronchoesophageal fistula in a dog.[65]

Central nervous system lesions have been established as causes of megaesophagus in dogs and cats. In dogs, both congenital[38] and experimental[9] lesions of the nucleus ambiguus were responsible. In cats the lesions (experimental) were in the dorsal motor nucleus of the vagus[9, 66] and the ventromedial nucleus of the hypothalamus.[67] The difference between the sites of the CNS lesions that cause megaesophagus in dogs and cats is a reflection of the difference in the proportions of the esophageal striated and smooth muscle between the species and therefore the respective importance of the somatic and autonomic nervous systems in esophageal innervation. Other CNS diseases that have been associated with megaesophagus include cervical vertebral instability with leukomalacia, stroke, and choroid plexus carcinoma with hydrocephalus.[50] Distemper has been cited as a cause of megaesophagus in two dogs.[50, 68] The pathogenesis probably relates to distemper-induced CNS lesions of the medulla or cranial nerve pathways. Familial reflex myoclonus of Labrador retrievers has been associated with megaesophagus.[69] No pathogenesis was determined.

Hypothyroidism is often cited as a possible cause of megaesophagus. However, very few dogs with hypothyroidism appear to develop megaesophagus. One hypothyroid dog with megaesophagus regained normal esophageal function following thyroid medication.[70] Addison's disease can be associated with transient megaesophagus.[71–73] Esophageal asthenia presumably occurs for the same reasons as the skeletal muscle weakness characteristic of the disease. Some authors believe that any shock-like condition can result in megaesophagus.[27] Some canine pituitary dwarves have a concurrent megaesophagus.[71]

Most obstructive esophageal diseases (neoplasia, granulomas, vascular rings, strictures, periesophageal masses, and foreign bodies) can lead to megaesophagus if they are of sufficiently chronic duration.[46] The pathogenesis probably relates to the physical overdilation of the esophagus by accumulating ingesta cranial to the obstruction. Neoplastic invasion of the esophagus may cause motility disturbances,[74] which may contribute to the pathogenesis of the dilation.

Thymomas are occasionally associated with myasthenia gravis and polymyositis in dogs and cats[75, 76] and therefore have the potential to cause megaesophagus. Difficulty swallowing and retention of barium in the esophagus (caudal and cranial to the thymoma) was reported in two cats and several dogs with myasthenia gravis.

A functional pyloric obstructive disease in cats has been associated with megaesophagus.[77] The proposed pathogenesis was an autonomic nervous system dysfunction common to both disorders. Megaesophagus associated with gastric heterotopia (gastric mucosa lining the esophagus) has also been reported in the cat.[78]

Epidemiology. Idiopathic megaesophagus is known to be inherited in the wirehaired fox terrier[68, 79] and miniature schnauzer.[80] The inheritance mode in wirehaired fox terriers is simple autosomal recessive,[68] whereas that of miniature schnauzer dogs is compatible with a simple autosomal dominant or a 60 per cent penetrance autosomal recessive pattern.[80] A breed predisposition exists for the German shepherd, Great Dane, and Irish setter.[30, 31] The high incidence of IM in these three breeds suggests a hereditary basis, as does the report of megaesophagus in litters of both German shepherds[81] and Great Danes.[82] Numerous other breeds of dogs, both large and small, have been affected by the disease,[30–32, 68] including a litter of Newfoundlands[23] and a litter of greyhounds.[83] Breeding of dogs affected by IM (or other close relatives) should be discouraged.[32] There is some evidence that idiopathic esophageal dilatation may also be inherited in the cat[47] and that Siamese related breeds are predisposed.[5] As befits the multitudinous causes of *secondary* megaesophagus, no clear breed predisposition has emerged.

No clear sex predisposition occurs in animals affected by megaesophagus. Clinical signs of megaesophagus may become evident when the animal is weaned or may not begin until adulthood. Most cases of megaesophagus have been reported in weanling dogs, but in a recent review of 50 cases, only 36 per cent of cases were classified as congenital.[50] Of the 53 cases of megaesophagus presented to the University of Missouri Veterinary Teaching Hospital over the last eight years, only one-third were less than one year of age at the time of presentation. Idiopathic megaesophagus has a higher incidence among dogs with congenital megaesophagus than among adult dogs with megaesophagus.[50]

Clinical Signs. Clinical signs of megaesophagus include regurgitation, signs of pneumonia, enlargement of the esophagus in the cervical region, and poor body condition.[27, 30–32, 50] Not all dogs with megaesophagus regurgitate[32, 68] although this is by far the most consistent clinical sign. The frequency of regurgitation varies greatly from once every two or three days to greater than ten times per day.[32] Regurgitation may be seen immediately after feeding or may occur up to 18 or more hours later. Regurgitation is delayed if the animal is inactive or if the esophageal dilation is marked.[5] Occasionally, however, regurgitation can occur during sleep.[46] Dogs with megaesophagus regurgitate both solids and fluids, in contrast with dogs with partial esophageal obstructions (caused by foreign bodies, strictures) in which fluids are often better tolerated.[46] If retained for prolonged periods, the regurgitated ingesta may ferment. Retained fermenting ingesta may cause halitosis and produce gurgling sounds detectable by the owner.[68] Profuse salivation may occur, presumably resulting from dysphagia. Such salivation may create the impression of nausea, more suggestive of nonesophageal disease. The poor body condition seen in some dogs is not a consistent finding. Up to a half of the dogs in one study were presented in good body condition.[30]

Accumulation of food in the thoracic esophagus may produce respiratory distress, especially in the presence of aspiration pneumonia. Signs of aspiration pneumonia including mucopurulent nasal discharge, respiratory crackles, dyspnea, and pyrexia may be seen. Dogs with megaesophagus may die acutely due to intussusception of the stomach into the esophagus.[52a]

Other clinical signs may reflect some of the causes of secondary rather than idiopathic megaesophagus. For instance, muscle pain and weakness may occur in dogs with megaesophagus associated with polymyositis;[53] vomiting was the predominant sign in cats in which megaesophagus was secondary to pyloric dysfunction.[77] Weakness exacerbated by exercise occurs in both cats[57] and dogs[27] with megaesophagus associated with advanced myasthenia gravis and in dogs with megaesophagus due to polymyopathy.[84] Profound depression was the predominant clinical sign in a dog with megaesophagus associated with lead poisoning;[64] ataxia and weakness were important signs in a group of dogs with megaesophagus and neuropathy.[62]

Differential Diagnosis. Megaesophagus must be differentiated from other causes of dysphagia, regurgitation and vomiting, and aspiration pneumonia. A thorough diagnostic work-up should be implemented to determine the cause of the megaesophagus. Treatment and prognosis depend on accurate diagnosis of the cause. The important differentials of regurgitation are shown in Table 83–3. At the beginning of the work-up, it is essential to differentiate regurgitation from vomiting. The history may give a clue as to the cause of the regurgitation. Foreign bodies, vascular ring abnormalities, and cricopharyngeal achalasia are more likely to become manifest in younger dogs than older dogs. A history of tolerance of fluids but not solids is more indicative of obstructive esophageal disease than megaesophagus. Regurgitation immediately after eating is suggestive of pharyngeal or early cervical esophageal disease. The physical examination may reveal dilation of the cervical esophagus diagnostic of megaesophagus and provide clues suggestive of a systemic disease that may underlie the regurgitation, e.g., muscle pain, weakness, ataxia, dilated pupils.

Survey thoracic radiographs are a high yield diagnostic procedure in the work-up of regurgitation. They may be all that is required to establish the presence of megaesophagus; however, mild degrees of dilation may not be obvious. In addition, as discussed previously, air in the esophagus as a result of aerophagia in excited, nauseated, dyspneic, or anesthetized dogs may produce

TABLE 83–3. DIFFERENTIAL DIAGNOSIS OF REGURGITATION

Pharyngeal Disorders
    Cricopharyngeal achalasia
    Rabies
    Foreign bodies and other obstructions
Esophageal Obstructive Diseases
    Foreign bodies
    Neoplasia
    Granulomas
    Strictures
    Vascular ring abnormalities
    Esophageal diverticula
    Esophageal atresia
    Extraesophageal compression
Esophageal Neuromuscular and Functional Disorders
    Megaesophagus*
    Other motility disorders
    Esophagitis
    Esophageal diverticula
    Esophageal fistula
Esophageal Hiatal Disorders

*Megaesophagus is the most common cause of regurgitation and in turn has a number of causes shown in Table 83–2.

radiographic signs suggestive of megaesophagus.[22] Particular care is necessary in anesthetized animals because anesthesia causes a significant degree of esophageal dilation.[19] In view of these difficulties, and in order to diagnose many of the obstructive esophageal diseases and functional esophageal diseases not associated with esophageal dilation, it is often necessary to utilize contrast esophagrams, fluoroscopy and esophagoscopy. Such procedures may reveal obstructions, motility disturbances, or mucosal lesions unobserved on plain radiographs. As discussed previously, it is important to realize that hypomotile esophagus has sometimes been demonstrated in excited, dyspneic, or nauseated dogs[22] and in dogs with no signs of regurgitation.[23] Therefore, as always, radiographic and other diagnostic information must be interpreted with knowledge of the clinical signs.

Once the presence of megaesophagus has been established by any of the aforementioned techniques, it is important for the clinician to attempt to determine the cause of the megaesophagus. Due to the varied nature of the possible causes of megaesophagus, the diagnostic approach must be very broad based. Useful tests are detailed in Table 83–4. Not all of these tests are necessary in the work-up of every case but some are essential and all may be useful to confirm or rule out a suspected cause. Myasthenia gravis may be detected by the acetylcholine receptor antibody test or the repetitive stimulation or Tensilon tests. Esophageal dysfunction due to myasthenia gravis can precede the weakness characteristic of the disease; therefore, at least one of these tests must be undertaken to rule out myasthenia gravis before a diagnosis of IM can be made. Botulism may be confirmed by mouse bioassay techniques. SLE may be detected by the presence of supportive systemic signs and positive LE and/or ANA tests. Neuropathies may be diagnosed by the presence of other peripheral nerve involvement and if necessary by nerve and muscle biopsies. Myositis and myopathy may be proven by EMG findings, serum chemistry results, and muscle biopsy.

Lead, thallium, and anticholinesterase toxicities may be diagnosed by history, clinical signs, and toxicologic assays. Dysautonomia is usually obvious on physical examination but can be confirmed by various ocular response tests. Obstructive esophageal diseases and miscellaneous causes such as mediastinitis may be diagnosed by esophagoscopy and radiographic procedures. It is important to re-emphasize that IM is a diagnosis of exclusion that can only be reached after an extensive work-up.

Treatment. When possible, treatment is aimed at the primary cause. Esophageal obstruction may be relieved by esophagoscopy, bougienage, or surgery.[27] SLE and immune-mediated polymyositis and polyneuritis may respond to immune suppression. Myasthenia gravis may be treated with prednisone or azathioprine and long-acting anticholinesterase agents such as neostigmine and pyridostigmine. Care is necessary when prednisone and anticholinesterases are used concurrently, as exacerbation of weakness can result during the initial phases of this combination therapy. Removal of a thymoma may result in resolution of myasthenia gravis and clinical improvement in esophageal function. Toxic causes of megaesophagus may be treated by removal of the offending agent and/or use of specific antidotes. Mega-

TABLE 83–4. DIAGNOSTIC APPROACH TO MEGAESOPHAGUS

Test	Usefulness
History, physical, and neurologic examinations	Determine direction of diagnostic work-up
CBC	Infection, immune-mediated disease, endocrinopathies, lead toxicity (NRBC, basophilic stippling)
Fecal	*Spirocerca lupi*
Urinalysis	Glomerulopathy or glomerulonephropathy
Serum chemistries including CPK	Endocrinopathy, muscle disease
LE and ANA test	SLE
ACTH stimulation test	Addison's disease
TSH stimulation test	Hypothyroidism
Distemper virus titers	Distemper
Acetylcholine receptor antibody test	Acquired myasthenia gravis
Survey radiographs	Masses, mediastinal disease, megaesophagus
Contrast esophagram and gastrogram	Obstructive diseases, megaesophagus, pyloric stenosis, esophageal fistula
Fluoroscopy	Motility
Esophagoscopy ± esophageal biopsy	Obstructive and inflammatory disease
Esophageal manometry	Achalasia, esophageal neuromuscular disease
CSF tap	Brain stem disease, distemper
Evoked potentials (auditory, somatosensory)	Brain stem disease
Electromyography	Muscle disease, polyneuropathy
Nerve conduction velocities	Polyneuropathy
Repetitive stimulation disease	Neuromuscular junction
Tensilon test	Myasthenia gravis
Muscle biopsy	Myositis, myopathy
Nerve biopsy	Polyneuropathy
Toxicology	Lead, thallium, plasma cholinesterase assays

esophagus secondary to pyloric stenosis may respond to pyloromyotomy.[77] Megaesophagus resulting from mediastinitis will improve with appropriate antibiotic therapy.

Therapy is entirely symptomatic for IM and for most cases of megaesophagus due to neurologic diseases. Symptomatic treatment is also an essential adjunct in the treatment of those cases of secondary megaesophagus for which specific treatment modalities exist. Symptomatic treatment aims at reducing the frequency and/or severity of the common complications of megaesophagus such as aspiration pneumonia, overdilatation of esophageal muscle by large amounts of retained ingesta, and esophagitis secondary to fermenting retained ingesta. The cornerstone of symptomatic therapy is the feeding and watering of the affected animal from a raised receptacle.[13, 31, 36, 85] Small amounts of sustenance should be offered frequently. If possible, the animal is maintained in an upright position for several minutes after feeding to prolong the favorable gravitation gradient.[44] Different recommendations have been made as to the best type of food to use. In general it should be energy dense and of a consistency determined by trial and error.[36] Some dogs respond best to liquid diets and others to solid diets. Liquids may pass a paralyzed portion of esophagus more easily, but they do not provide as effective a stimulation for peristalsis as does solid food.

Little attention has been paid to the use of medical therapy to improve esophageal function in animals. Drugs that improve esophageal peristalsis would have value in the treatment of megaesophagus. One author has reported that the cholinergic drug urecholine (0.01 mg/lb SQ) tends to improve the amplitude of contractions and to increase the portion of functioning esophagus in some dogs with megaesophagus.[35] Whether long-term administration of such a drug would cause improvement clinically was not determined. A second author was unable to confirm these results with the use of the cholinergic agent bethanecol.[15] The stimulatory effect of a cholinergic agent on the LES would be likely to oppose any improvement in esophageal motor function.

Another author has suggested the use of a metoclopramide trial under fluoroscopy. In this regimen, 2.5 mg of metoclopramide are given IV and, if improvement of peristalsis occurs, 5 to 10 mg of metoclopramide are given per os q8h thereafter.[15] As previously discussed, metoclopramide has been shown experimentally to enhance distal esophageal peristalsis.[15] As with the use of urecholine, the stimulatory effect of metoclopramide on the LES would oppose any improvement in esophageal motor function gained by use of this drug but may not completely negate its benefits.

Drugs that reduce LES resting pressure may also be of value in the treatment of megaesophagus. This would be especially true in any affected animal with a high resting LES pressure. In canine IM (when the LES pressure is known to be normal), reduction of the LES pressure below normal may be advantageous. The reduced LES pressure would be more easily overcome by the weak and disordered peristaltic waves of the diseased esophageal body and by the gravitational pressure developed when an animal is fed upright. Anticholinergics reduce LES tone. Use of an antispasmodic prior to feeding has been associated in a temporal fashion with improvement in several pups affected by congenital megaesophagus.[82] A clinical trial with an anticholinergic in humans suffering from achalasia produced significant improvement in the symptoms.[86] Nifedipine also decreases LES pressure in the dog[87] and may have application in the treatment of megaesophagus. Use of LES relaxants just before feeding from an elevated receptacle may be worth a clinical trial in individual animals under treatment.

The surgical treatment of IM is a controversial subject. Some authors think that it is a worthwhile procedure,[37, 44, 45, 88] whereas others, on the basis of pathophysiologic arguments and clinical experience, believe that it is of no value.[30, 31, 85] If surgery is undertaken, the modified short Heller's esophagomyotomy would appear to be the procedure of choice since it reduces LES pressure but still maintains enough LES competency to prevent esophageal reflex.[89] After surgery animals must still be fed from an elevated bowl. Surgery should not be undertaken on all patients. Criteria for selecting surgical candidates include: 1) Animals that have particularly high resting LES pressure and that show manometric evidence of failure of the LES to relax on swallowing. 2) Animals that fail to respond to feeding from an elevated bowl but that respond to elevated feeding combined with a test dose of a drug that reduces LES pressure. 3) Animals that fail to respond to feeding from an elevated bowl to the point at which euthanasia is being considered.

Surgery may also be of temporary benefit to patients with megaesophagus when used to place gastrostomy or pharyngostomy tubes.

Prognosis. The prognosis depends on the cause of the megaesophagus and the age at onset of clinical signs. In general, congenital onset IM has a better prognosis than adult-onset IM, with various authors claiming a 33 and 46 per cent[90] recovery rate and others stating a "favorable"[5] prognosis. Miniature schnauzer pups with hereditary esophageal dysfunction usually recover clinically and radiographically from their disease if they survive the first few weeks of life.[80] Several authors, however, think that congenital IM should still receive a poor prognosis with less than 20 per cent recovery.[30–32] One recent review of 18 congenital cases documented no recovery in any dog.[50] The earlier the condition is recognized and dietary management is begun, the better the prognosis.[5] Secondary and adult-onset IM have been reputed to have a hopeless prognosis for return to normality.[31, 36] However, several recent reports have indicated that both adult-onset IM and secondary megaesophagus can be transient. A return to clinical normality has been noted in some dogs affected by myasthenia gravis, polyradiculoneuritis, polymyositis, and SLE, and in five dogs with adult-onset IM.[22, 50] Megaesophagus secondary to Addison's disease, botulism, bronchoesophageal fistula, and mediastinitis has a favorable prognosis if treated early.

The prognosis of megaesophagus in cats with dysautonomia is poor. While up to 30 per cent of cats with dysautonomia return to clinical normality, the presence of significant megaesophagus in an affected cat markedly worsens its chances of recovery.[33] Similarly, the prognosis of cats with megaesophagus associated with pyloric dysfunction is poorer than those with pyloric dysfunction alone.[77] Some cats with pyloric dysfunction–associated megaesophagus did, however, show improved clinical signs and reduced esophageal diameter after pyloromyotomy.[77]

The prognosis of megaesophagus associated with obstructive esophageal diseases is poor unless the correction of the obstruction precedes significant esophageal dilation. Relief of the obstruction usually results in some clinical improvement, but the dilated esophagus rarely regains normal function.[91]

The prognosis of megaesophagus from any cause is adversely affected by evidence of concurrent inhalation pneumonia and debilitation and by the absence of esophageal motility.

In summary, the prognosis of megaesophagus with few exceptions is guarded to poor.

Esophageal Motility Abnormalities

Abnormalities of esophageal motility in the absence of concurrent megaesophagus are occasionally seen. Such motility abnormalities may be associated with the various obstructive, inflammatory, or neoplastic esophageal diseases described in this chapter. Occasionally they are idiopathic. It is possible that abnormal esophageal motility may eventually be followed by esophageal dilatation. It is suggested that animals with esophageal motility disorders receive the same diagnostic work-up recommended for animals with megaesophagus (Table 83–4).

Vascular Ring Anomalies

Congenital anomalies of the aortic arch and its branches can cause constriction of the esophagus and result in signs of esophageal obstruction. The degree of esophageal strangulation depends upon the vascular structures involved. The obstruction may range from mild to severe. The aortic arch normally develops from the fourth left aortic arch and left dorsal aortic root in the embryo. The left sixth arch forms the ductus arteriosus while the right fourth arch forms the right subclavian and brachiocephalic trunk arteries. During normal development, this arrangement causes the arch of the aorta, the ductus arteriosus, and the pulmonary artery to all position themselves to the left of the esophagus where they cause no esophageal interference. This arrangement does not occur in vascular anomalies. and the esophagus becomes constricted by vascular ring formation.

The most common vascular ring in the canine is the persistent right aortic arch (PRAA).[92] In this developmental anomaly, the embryonic right fourth arch, instead of the left fourth arch, persists as the functional aorta. This arrangement causes the esophagus to be encircled on the right by the aortic arch, ventrally by the base of the heart and pulmonary artery, and bor-

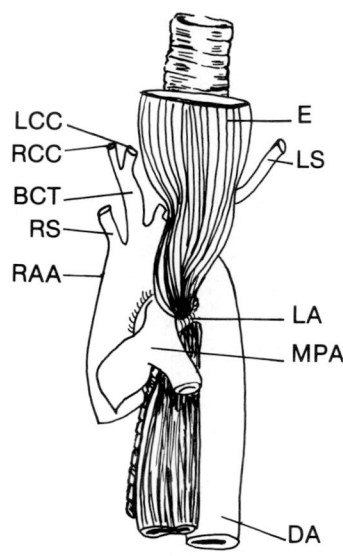

FIGURE 83–4. Vascular ring caused by a persistent right aortic arch. E, esophagus; LS, left subclavian artery; LA, ligamentum arteriosus; MPA, main pulmonary artery; DA, descending aorta; RAA, right aortic arch; RS, right subclavian arteries; BCT, bicarotid trunk; RCC, right common carotid artery; LCC, left common carotid artery. (From Jones, BD (ed): Canine and Feline Gastroenterology. Philadelphia, WB Saunders, 1986.)

dered on the left by the ductus arteriosus or ligamentum arteriosum, which passes dorsally (Figures 83–4 and 83–5). Other less common vascular anomalies include double aortic arch, anomalous left subclavian artery originating from the right aortic arch, and aberrant right subclavian artery. Irish setters, Boston terriers, and German shepherd dogs are the most commonly affected canine breeds.[93, 94] Vascular rings are considerably less common in the cat, with persistent right aortic arch and constriction by ligamentum arteriosum being described.

Clinical Signs. The most common clinical sign in affected animals is an acute onset of regurgitation at the time of weaning to solid foods. In 90 per cent of all

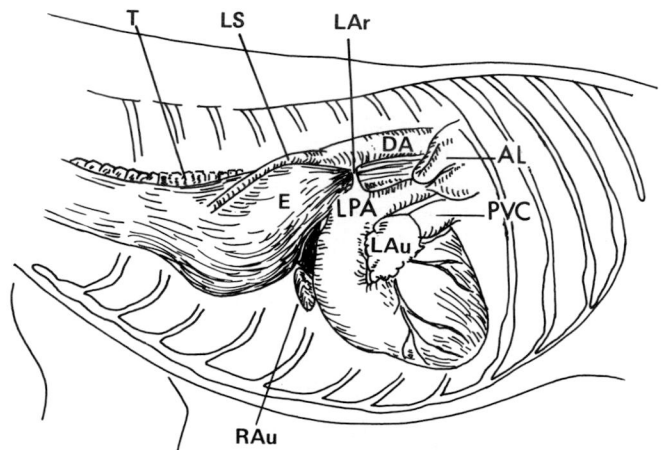

FIGURE 83–5. The vascular ring caused by persistent right aortic arch. T, trachea; LS, left subclavian artery; LAr, ligamentum arteriosum; DA, descending aorta; AL, left cranial lung lobe; PCV, posterior vena cava; LAu, left auricle; LPA, left pulmonary artery; E, esophagus; RAu, right auricle. (From Jones, BD (ed): Canine and Feline Gastroenterology. Philadelphia, WB Saunders, 1986.)

dogs with PRAA, the condition is identified before the age of six months.[95] Although regurgitation usually occurs shortly after eating in the early stages of the disease, it may occur at variable times after eating as esophageal dilation progresses. Affected puppies are malnourished and weak and demonstrate stunted growth. The food-filled esophagus may occasionally be palpated at the thoracic inlet. Coughing with respiratory distress is common and is indicative of a secondary aspiration pneumonia. In those patients, auscultation usually reveals coarse crackles.

Localized esophageal dilatation cranial to the heart visualized on survey or contrast radiographs is highly suggestive of vascular rings. The encircled esophagus will appear as a dilated air or fluid-filled saccular density that abruptly tapers over the base of the heart at the level of the sixth rib. The differential diagnoses of vascular ring anomalies should include intrinsic stricture, diverticulum, and foreign body obstruction.

Treatment. Treatment consists of surgical correction of the constricting bands forming the vascular ring. The prognosis for a complete recovery is poor. Complications are common because of the initial malnourished and debilitated condition of the animal and the high incidence of concurrent aspiration pneumonia. Permanent esophageal dilatation cranial to the constriction, as a result of irreversible degenerative changes in the esophagus itself, is common. A final possible sequela is an esophageal dilatation caudal to the vascular ring, a condition that probably occurs due to concurrent neuromuscular disease. Dogs with permanent esophageal disease following surgery should be managed with feeding procedures as described for patients with megaesophagus.

Esophagitis

Inflammation of the esophagus may result from a variety of acute or chronic insults. Causes of esophagitis include the ingestion of chemical irritants, thermal insults, acute and persistent vomiting, foreign body obstruction, and gastroesophageal reflux. Infectious causes for esophageal inflammation are uncommon. Primary infectious esophagitis has been reported in immunocompromised patients and as a sequela to systemic phycomycosis in the dog.[96] Acute esophagitis with ulcerations has been observed in some cats with caliciviral upper respiratory infections.[97] The incidence of primary acute esophagitis is thought to be relatively low; however. this is most likely an underestimation because of the obscure clinical signs, limited use of endoscopy by the practicing veterinarian, and subtle radiographic findings associated with this disorder.[27, 31, 98] The authors believe that as the use of endoscopy increases, the diagnosis of esophagitis will be made more frequently (Figures 83–6 and 83–7).

Reflux or peptic esophagitis is caused by the gastroesophageal reflux of gastric acid and enzymes. It is usually associated with LES incompetence as seen with neuromuscular disease or neoplasia, hiatal hernias, indwelling pharyngostomy tubes, or protracted vomiting. The most critical factor in canine reflux esophagitis appears to be a loss of LES tone.[99] Reduced LES pressure has been reported in dogs with concurrent megaesophagus, during inspiratory dyspnea, and following the administration of various drugs.[16, 100, 101] Occasional gastroesophageal reflux observed in normal dogs is not considered abnormal if the refluxed ingesta is rapidly returned to the stomach.

Clinical Signs. Mild esophagitis is often limited to

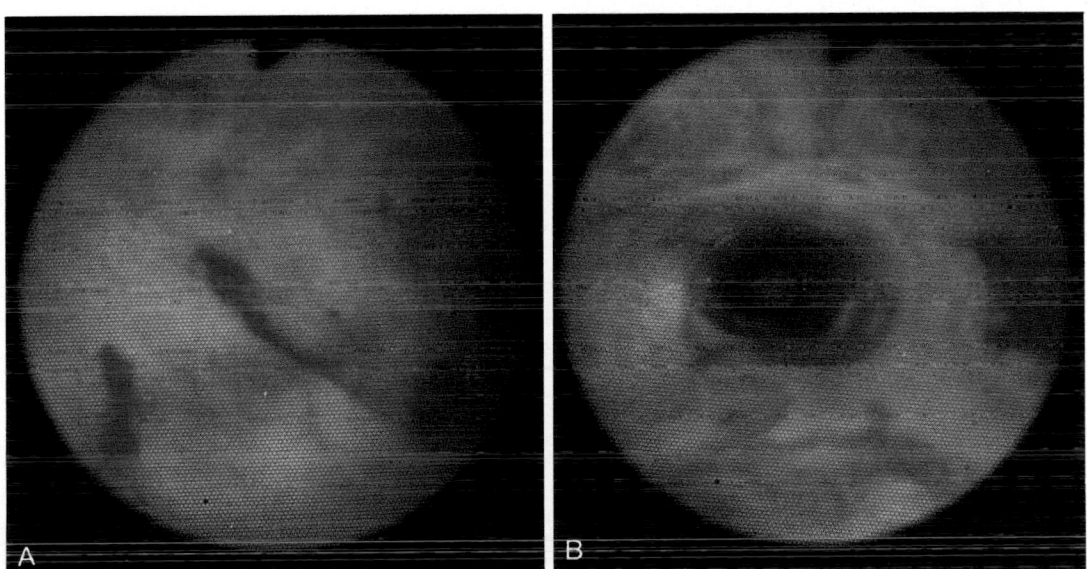

FIGURE 83–6. Views through a flexible fiberoptic endoscope of esophagitis in a two-year-old female Kerry blue terrier. Note the hemorrhagic and white-raised white plaque areas. A biopsy specimen obtained during the endoscopy examination confirmed an esophagitis. The patient developed clinical signs four days after a routine ovariohysterectomy. (From Jones, BD (ed): Canine and Feline Gastroenterology. Philadelphia, WB Saunders, 1986.)

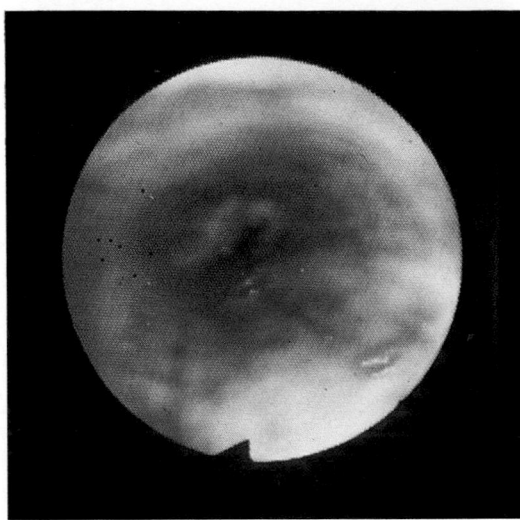

FIGURE 83–7. A view through a flexible fiberoptic endoscope of esophagitis in a three-year-old Labrador. Note the linear areas of the erythema and the cardia distally. The patient developed acute episodes of vomiting and also had a concurrent gastritis. The patient responded well with medical therapy and was clinically asymptomatic one week later. Endoscopically, all lesions had resolved by two weeks after the initial insult.

mucosal damage and is usually self-limiting when the inciting process is removed. Clinical signs are mild or nonexistent, and the esophageal mucosa heals quickly without significant fibrosis. Deep esophagitis with involvement of the muscular layers is uncommon and can lead to severe complications such as persistent ulceration, stricture formation, and esophageal perforation.

The clinical signs associated with reflux esophagitis are subtle and difficult to evaluate. They consist of esophageal discomfort leading to anorexia, weight loss, excessive salivation. and regurgitation of viscid saliva-like fluid that may contain blood. Physical examination of these animals is usually unremarkable. Radiographic procedures can be used to confirm a diagnosis of esophagitis. Unfortunately, survey radiographic evaluation of the esophagus is often normal except in severe cases that may demonstrate signs of LES achalasia, hiatal hernia, and stricture formation. Contrast radiography, such as barium contrast esophagography or fluoroscopy, may demonstrate the deleterious effects of inflammation on esophageal motility.

A definitive diagnosis of esophagitis is confirmed by endoscopic visualization of the inflamed mucosa and by obtaining biopsy specimens. Endoscopic findings in animals with superficial esophagitis include mucosal erythema, edema, and hemorrhage. A diagnosis of reflux esophagitis may be facilitated by measuring pH in the distal esophagus. Prolonged low esophageal pH, less than pH 7.0, suggests the presence of gastric reflux with poor esophageal clearance of the refluxed material.[31]

Treatment. Treatment of esophagitis is directed toward correcting the initiating cause and symptomatic therapy. Emesis should not be induced if caustic agents have been consumed. Unabsorbed acids may be neutralized with magnesium oxide solution (1:25 dilution with warm water) or milk of magnesia. A weak acid such as vinegar (1:4 diluted with water) or lemon juice

administered orally is recommended following the ingestion of caustic alkalis. Additional symptomatic therapy such as intestinal protectants, cathartics, and fluid therapy is sometimes required. Esophageal rest should follow all insults. Discontinuation of oral alimentation is recommended for a minimum of 24 hours. Subsequently, small frequent feedings of a bland diet are given until the patient can tolerate a normal diet.

Reflux esophagitis is treated by dietary modification and the use of antacids. The feeding of frequent, small high-protein, low-fat meals may significantly enhance the competency of the LES directly or indirectly by hormonal influences.[31] Antacids neutralize gastric acid secretions and reduce esophageal inflammation when reflux does occur. A disadvantage of their use, however, is that they leave the stomach rapidly; thus they must be given frequently (about every hour) to achieve maximum results.[102, 103] Cimetidine, an H_2 blocker, greatly reduces gastric acid production when given orally at a dosage of 5 mg/lb (10 mg/kg) q8h. A cimetidine analogue, ranitidine, used at 0.2 mg/lb (0.5 mg/kg) has the advantage of being required only twice daily in dogs. However, this drug is currently only available in an unscored 150 mg tablet, which limits its practical use. Clinicians should avoid the simultaneous use of oral antacids with cimetidine since impaired absorption and reduced bioavailability of cimetidine may occur. Metoclopramide is a new centrally acting antiemetic that shows great promise in the treatment of gastroesophageal reflux and gastric motility disorders. The pharmacologic actions of this drug on esophageal function include an increase in the strength of esophageal contractions and increased LES pressure.[15] A combination of cimetidine and metoclopramide is particularly effective in the management of esophagitis associated with persistent vomiting, gastroesophageal reflux, foreign body–induced trauma, and surgical manipulations.[14]

Esophageal Foreign Bodies

The ingestion of nondigestible foreign material (bones, stones, fishhooks, fabric) or pieces of food too large to pass through the esophagus may lead to intraluminal entrapment. Esophageal obstruction may be partial or complete. Obstruction usually occurs at points of minimal esophageal distensibility including the thoracic inlet, the base of the heart, and the distal esophageal hiatus. The cranial esophagus is a frequent location for nonobstructive foreign bodies bearing points or spicules. Foreign body obstruction is reported to be six times more common in dogs than in cats.[104] This species predilection appears to be related to the more discriminatory eating habits of cats. However, bones, threads with attached needles, and other small objects may cause pharyngeal or esophageal obstruction in the feline. The extent of foreign body-induced esophageal injury in the dog and cat is largely determined by the size and angularity of the foreign body as well as the duration of the obstruction. Esophageal perforation may occur following an acute tear in the esophageal wall by a sharp object or by slow pressure necrosis caused by a lodged blunt foreign body.

Clinical Signs. Clinical signs in affected animals are variable. The initial signs usually include increased salivation, labored swallowing movements, apparent discomfort, and regurgitation following food intake. Animals with partial obstructions may survive for weeks because liquids and semisolid foods may bypass the impacted object. Appetite is variable with anorexia related to esophageal pain. Respiratory embarrassment secondary to airway impingement may occur if the ingested object is very large. Clinical signs of dyspnea and wheezing will predominate in these patients. Significant airway obstruction can result in the formation of pulmonary edema. Physical examination findings will usually be supportive of the clinical findings; however, it should include careful observation of the base of the tongue for the presence of linear foreign objects that may extend into the esophagus.

Diagnosis. Diagnosis may be made on a known history that the animal has swallowed an object, clinical findings, radiographic evaluation, or endoscopy. Radiographic examination should include the entire esophagus. Radiopaque foreign objects are readily visualized, while the use of positive contrast agents is required to outline and identify radiolucent objects. Thorough review of survey radiographs should be performed prior to the initiation of a positive contrast procedure. Frequently, air in the esophagus will be visualized cranial to the foreign body if it is causing an obstruction. Perforation of the esophagus is suspected when air is visualized radiographically in the adjacent mediastinal or pulmonary structures. The use of barium sulfate as a contrast agent should be avoided in suspected cases of perforation. Esophagoscopy provides valuable information by allowing direct visualization of the foreign object and assessment of the extent of esophageal injury. Esophagoscopy is superior to radiography in recognizing inflammation, punctures, and lacerations.[51]

Treatment. Treatment consists of attempted removal of the foreign material by use of esophagoscopy. Only if esophagoscopy fails should surgery be considered. The authors prefer to use a flexible esophageal endoscope

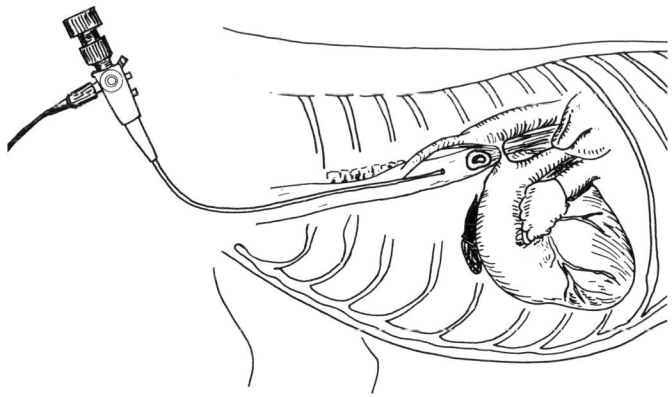

FIGURE 83–8. The use of a flexible endoscope to visualize a bone foreign body lodged at the base of the heart. (From Jones, BD (ed): Canine and Feline Gastroenterology. Philadelphia, WB Saunders, 1986.)

passed into the esophagus to directly visualize the foreign body and to inspect for possible esophageal mucosal damage (Figure 83–8). Small foreign bodies may be removed by passing flexible four-prong or basket grasping forceps through the endoscope, grasping the object, and pulling it retrograde out of the esophagus through the oral cavity (Figure 83–9). For large objects, rigid grasping forceps may be passed in conjunction with a flexible endoscope (Figure 83–10). Once the foreign body is grasped, it and the endoscope can be pulled retrograde through the mouth (Figure 83–11). If flexible endoscopes are not available, rigid endoscopes work quite nicely (Figures 83–12 to 83–14). If the foreign body cannot be removed in a retrograde manner, then attempts should be made to push the object aborally into the stomach. Once in the stomach, foreign bodies may be digested and excreted, or removed by gastrostomy. All manipulations of foreign bodies with the endoscopic equipment must be carefully performed in order to minimize further esophageal trauma and avoid laceration of thoracic vessels.

Assessment of possible esophageal damage should

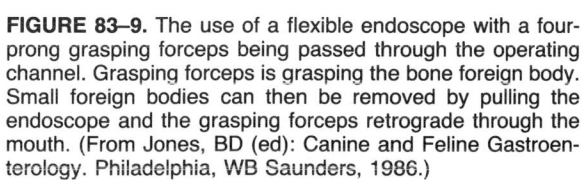
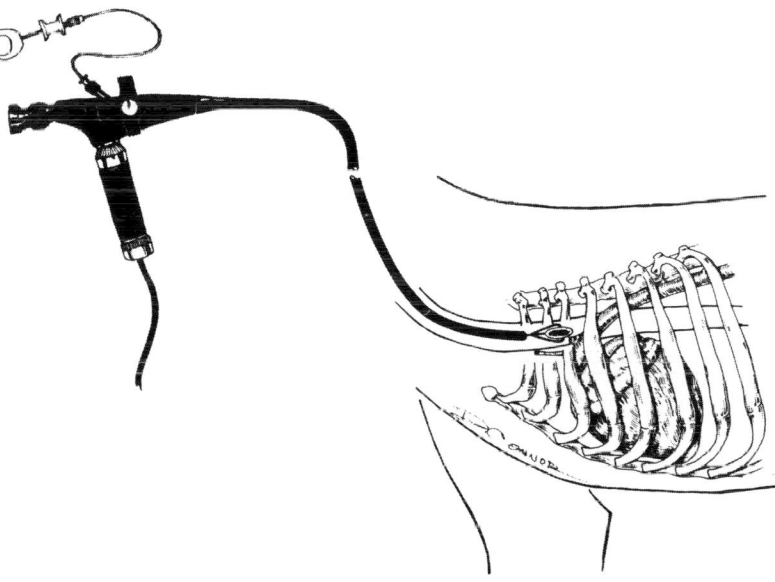

FIGURE 83–9. The use of a flexible endoscope with a four-prong grasping forceps being passed through the operating channel. Grasping forceps is grasping the bone foreign body. Small foreign bodies can then be removed by pulling the endoscope and the grasping forceps retrograde through the mouth. (From Jones, BD (ed): Canine and Feline Gastroenterology. Philadelphia, WB Saunders, 1986.)

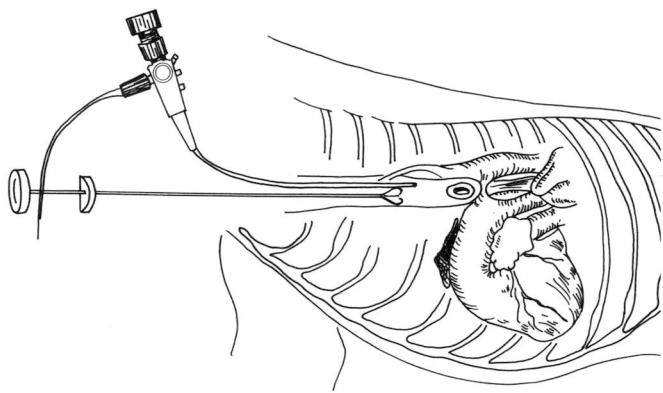

FIGURE 83–10. The use of rigid grasping forceps being passed alongside the flexible endoscope to grasp the foreign body. The foreign body can easily be grasped as one visually observes the grasping forceps and foreign body through the endoscope. (From Jones, BD (ed): Canine and Feline Gastroenterology. Philadelphia, WB Saunders, 1986.)

follow removal of the foreign body from the esophageal lumen. The esophageal mucosa should be visualized throughout its entire length. The degree of mucosal damage is usually proportional to the duration of the foreign body entrapment. Erythema and mild ulceration are common endoscopic findings. Special attention should be given to any evidence of tears, lacerations, or perforation of the esophageal wall. Survey thoracic radiographs should be performed following foreign body removal to evaluate for the presence of pneumothorax or pneumomediastinum secondary to esophageal perforation. Minor tears, lacerations, and ulcerations will heal with esophageal rest. The use of pharyngostomy or gastrostomy tubes will allow the oral alimentation of an animal while resting the esophagus. Disadvantages of the use of pharyngostomy tubes are continuing irritation of the esophagus from the tube and the necessity of maintaining an open gastroesophageal sphincter with the possible reflux of gastric contents.[105] Large defects in the esophageal wall with signs of concurrent mediastinitis or other thoracic cavity involvement require surgical exploration and repair.

Approximately one-third of the animals with esophageal foreign bodies will develop complications.[31] The

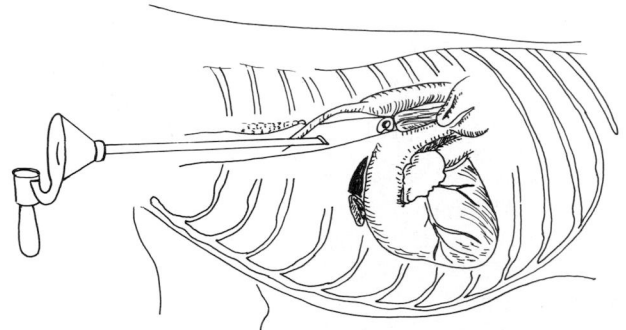

FIGURE 83–12. The use of a rigid endoscope to visualize a bone foreign body lodged at the base of the heart. A human sigmoidoscope can sometimes be used as a rigid endoscope. (From Jones, BD (ed): Canine and Feline Gastroenterology. Philadelphia, WB Saunders, 1986.)

most common complications include esophageal perforation, mediastinitis, pleuritis, esophagitis, and mucosal lacerations.[104] The incidence of complications is greatest when foreign objects become lodged between the heart and diaphragm.[98] Stricture formation may occur several weeks following the successful removal of a foreign body. Unusual chronic complications of esophageal foreign body impaction include esophagobronchial fistula formation, pericarditis, and persistent esophageal ulcers.

Esophageal Strictures

Esophageal strictures are most commonly acquired lesions and may be found in any portion of the esophagus.[31] Intraluminal stricture can develop after a variety of causes such as surgery, foreign body removal, perforating trauma, ingestion of caustic materials, and esophagitis of various causes. The most important cause of postinflammatory stricture is reflux of acidic stomach contents while an animal is under general anesthesia.[100, 106] The esophageal mucosa has extensive recuperative powers, and damage to the esophageal wall must be deep for a stricture to occur. Superficial mucosal inflammation produces a transient, mild, segmental narrowing of the esophagus without stricture formation. Severe inflammation with damage to the esophageal

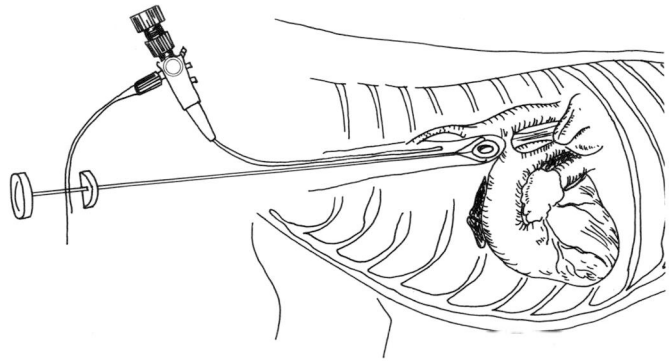

FIGURE 83–11. The grasping forceps and flexible endoscope in place. These two instruments are then both pulled retrogradely to extract the foreign body from the esophagus. (From Jones, BD (ed): Canine and Feline Gastroenterology. Philadelphia, WB Saunders, 1986.)

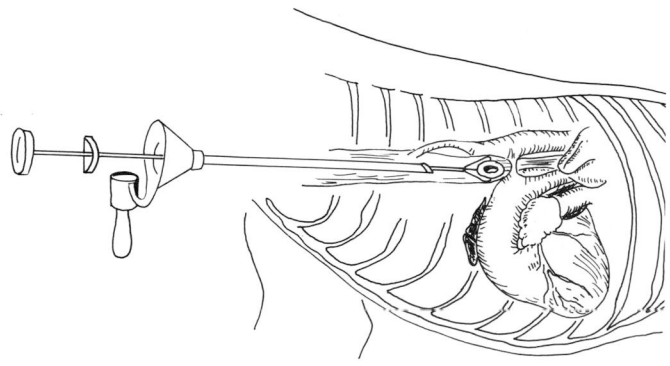

FIGURE 83–13. Grasping forceps passing through the rigid endoscope to grasp the bone esophageal foreign body. (From Jones, BD (ed): Canine and Feline Gastroenterology. Philadelphia, WB Saunders, 1986.)

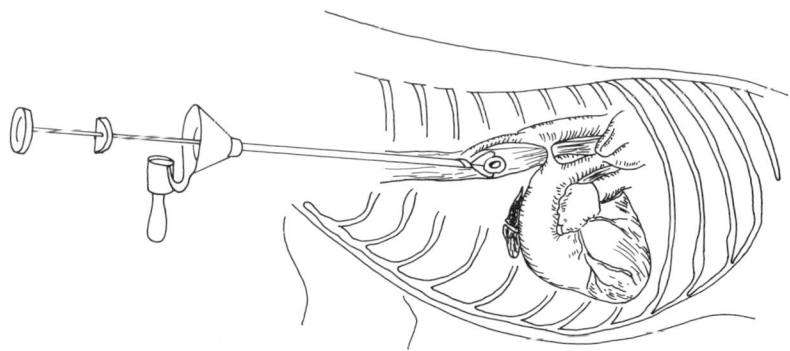

FIGURE 83–14. Grasping forceps and rigid endoscope being pulled retrograde to remove the bone foreign body. Note that the foreign body is pulled snug against the rigid endoscope to facilitate removal as the endoscope dilates the esophagus as it is pulled retrograde. (From Jones, BD (ed): Canine and Feline Gastroenterology. Philadelphia, WB Saunders, 1986.)

submucosa and muscular layers is needed to produce fibrotic changes and stricture. Strictures may develop at any point along the length of the esophagus with the extent of luminal obstruction determining the severity of the clinical signs.

Clinical Signs. The clinical signs associated with this disorder are similar to those seen with primary esophageal disease. Regurgitation is the predominant sign and is frequently observed after eating. Initially, the animal will tolerate the ingestion of both solid and liquid foods. However, as the luminal constriction progresses, dysphagia becomes more pronounced and only liquids are well tolerated. With chronic stricture formation, esophageal dilation cranial to the stricture allows for the accumulation of ingested material, and regurgitation may not immediately follow eating.

Diagnosis. Diagnosis is based on a history of recent surgery or foreign body removal, radiographic evaluation, and/or endoscopic findings. Survey radiographs usually provide little diagnostic information. Esophageal dilatation containing gas or ingesta (proximal to the stricture) is observed only with severe or chronic lesions. Contrast esophagography using liquid barium may demonstrate intraluminal retention of the contrast material or deviation and tapering around the stenotic site. Endoscopy provides the best means of identifying the presence and extent of esophageal strictures (Figure 83–15).

Treatment. Therapy of strictures can be approached from either a medical or surgical aspect. The best medical approach is the utilization of bougienage to mechanically dilate the stenotic region. The authors have used tapered, mercury-filled esophageal bougies that are supplied in a series of graded diameters. The animal is anesthetized, and the smallest well-lubricated bougie is introduced through the full esophageal length. This process is repeated by forcibly passing tubes of increasing diameter through the stenotic area. A full set of esophageal bougies can usually be borrowed from a local human hospital or is available through a surgical supply company. Balloon dilators are now available to be passed through the operating channel of an endoscope. Experience with this technique in veterinary medicine is limited. Strictures can be readily dilated if they have not been present for a long time. The bougienage procedure may need to be repeated every few months to alleviate signs of obstruction. Oral corticosteroids, at anti-inflammatory doses, for several weeks after the bougienage procedure are recommended to inhibit

the formation of new fibrous connective tissue.[41] Placement of a pharyngostomy tube beyond the stricture site is thought to reduce the recurrence of stricture formation after dilation.[31] Ideally, this tube should be of large diameter (the diameter of the trachea) and remain in place for 7 to 14 days. Unfortunately, it may not be tolerated by some patients. As stated previously, care should be taken not to position the tip of the pharyngostomy tube in the stomach such that gastric fluid can reflux around it and precipitate esophagitis. Surgical resection of the stricture site is not routinely recommended because of the difficulty of this procedure and its associated complications.

Periesophageal Obstructions

Lesions in the tissues surrounding the esophagus have the potential to mechanically obstruct normal deglutition and result in esophageal stenosis. Periesophageal masses cause esophageal dysfunction due to external compression without actually invading the esophagus. These masses include cervical neoplasms such as thyroid tumors and squamous cell carcinoma, foreign body abscesses, fungal granulomas, mediastinal masses, tumors

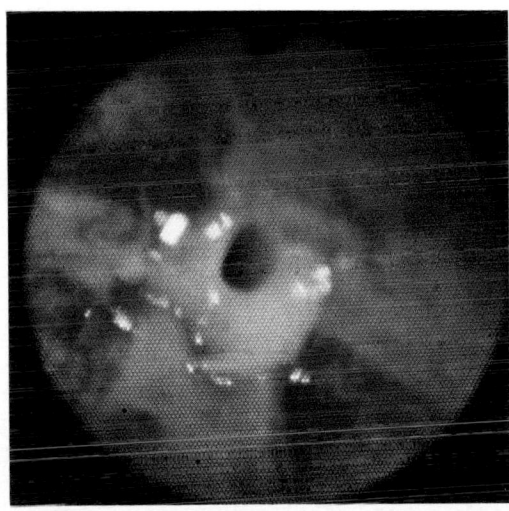

FIGURE 83–15. Viewed through a flexible endoscope is an intraluminal esophageal stricture. Note the hemorrhagic areas around the stricture. The white tissue is fibrous connective tissue. (From Jones, BD (ed): Canine and Feline Gastroenterology. Philadelphia, WB Saunders, 1986.)

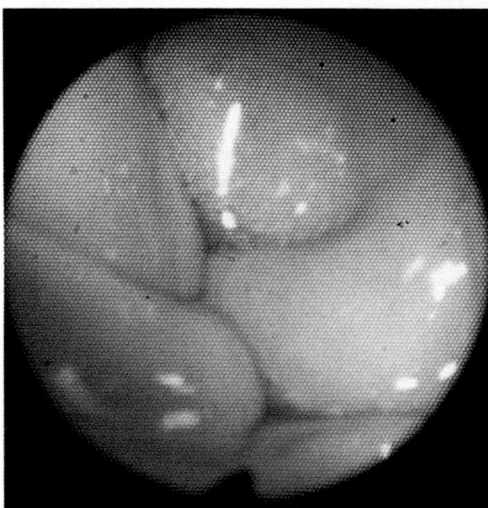

FIGURE 83–16. A view through a flexible endoscope of an extraluminal stricture. Note that the stricture is composed of normal mucosa, which is indicative of a periesophageal mass causing the stricture. This patient had a history of regurgitation for two months prior to presentation. The mass totally encircled the esophagus. Histologically the mass was a fibrosarcoma. (From Jones, BD (ed): Canine and Feline Gastroenterology. Philadelphia, WB Saunders, 1986.)

of the thoracic cavity (lymphosarcomas, thymomas, heart-base tumors), and extreme hilar lymphadenopathy. Clinical signs other than those associated with the esophagus may also be present and largely depend upon the anatomic location of the mass. The most common clinical signs of periesophageal masses include regurgitation, dysphagia, excessive salivation, respiratory distress, and reduced exercise tolerance. Survey radiographs may not demonstrate a lesion; however, radiographic studies with contrast material will usually identify the obstructive lesion. Esophagoscopy will reveal either luminal stenosis with no mucosal involvement, or stricture formation if the periesophageal mass has invaded the esophageal lumen (Figure 83–16). Treatment is directed toward the cause of the mass lesion.

Esophageal Diverticula

Esophageal diverticula are sac-like dilatations in the esophageal wall that produce a pouch. These structures may be acquired or congenital and are rarely documented in small animals.[107] They are usually found in the lower cervical esophagus cranial to the thoracic inlet or in the thoracic esophagus just cranial to the diaphragm (epiphrenic location). Congenital diverticula are thought to develop due to congenital weakness of the esophageal wall, abnormal separation of tracheal and esophageal embryonic buds, or eccentric vacuole formation in the esophagus.[98] Acquired forms are subdivided into pulsion and traction diverticula, on the basis of their etiopathogenesis.

A pulsion diverticulum is produced by exaggerated intraluminal pressure in association with abnormal regional peristalsis or when normal peristalsis is obstructed by a stenosis.[108] Pulsion diverticula can form cranial to any stenosed or diseased esophageal segment and are found most often in the epiphrenic region.[107, 108] Increased esophageal intraluminal pressure, along with

food accumulation and deep esophageal inflammation, can lead to mucosal herniation. Histologically, the wall of a pulsion diverticulum generally consists of only esophageal epithelium and connective tissue (Figure 83–17). Many causes may initiate diverticulum formation such as esophagitis, esophageal stenosis, foreign bodies, vascular ring anomalies, neuromuscular dysfunction with megaesophagus, and hiatal hernia.

Traction diverticula have been reported in humans to follow a past inflammatory process involving the trachea, bronchi, or hilar lymph nodes. This inflammation leads to the production of fibrous tissue that later contracts, pulling out an area of the esophagus to form a pouch. Traction diverticula are principally located in the cranial and midthoracic esophagus, where ample opportunity for adhesion formations exists.[98] The true incidence of traction diverticula in veterinary medicine remains unknown. In contrast to a pulsion diverticulum, the traction diverticulum histologically consists of all four esophageal layers (adventitia, muscle, submucosa, and mucosa).

Diverticula of either type should not be confused with esophageal redundancy seen at the thoracic inlet of normal young dogs and normal dogs of brachycephalic breeds. Contrast material or gas may accumulate in the pseudopouches, mimicking a pulsion diverticulum. Repeat radiography with the neck in an extended position

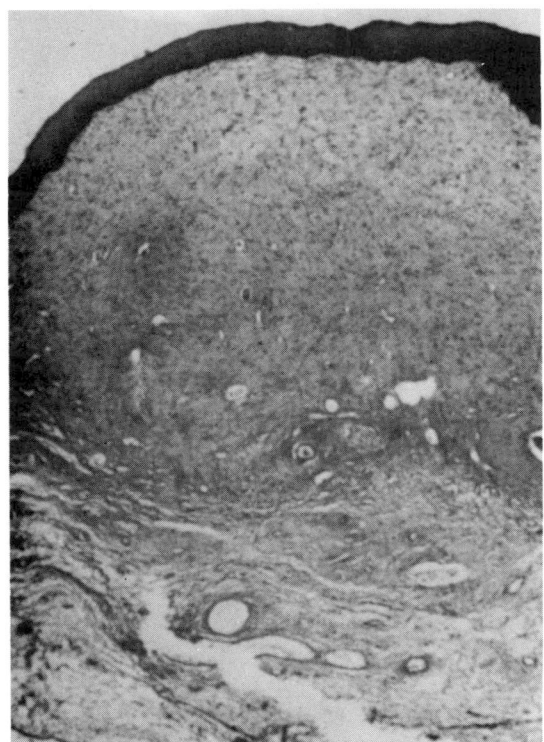

FIGURE 83–17. Photomicrograph of a section from a wall of a true pulsion diverticulum. A normal layer of stratified squamous epithelium, which was well keratinized in the luminal surface, rested on a sheet of connective tissue. The connective tissue on which the stratified squamous epithelium rested was composed of relatively immature collagen fibers. No muscle bundles and no muscle fibers were in any of the tissue. This arrangement contrasts with that of a traction diverticulum, which consists of all layers of the esophagus (adventitia, muscle, submucosa, and stratified squamous mucosa). (From Jones, BD (ed): Canine and Feline Gastroenterology. Philadelphia, WB Saunders, 1986.)

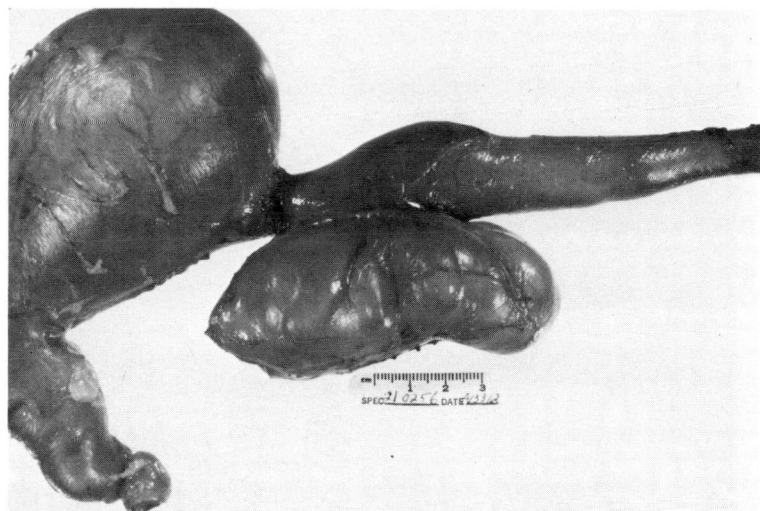

FIGURE 83–18. A large epiphrenic diverticulum is readily visualized in this necropsy specimen. (From Jones, BD (ed): Canine and Feline Gastroenterology. Philadelphia, WB Saunders, 1986.)

removes any esophageal "slack" and results in the disappearance of a false diverticulum. Small diverticula can be incidental findings and may be of little clinical significance. However, once a diverticulum is formed, it has the potential of progressing to esophageal impaction, chronic esophagitis with mucosal ulceration, and rupture of the diverticulum wall with resultant mediastinitis or esophagotracheal fistula formation.

Diverticula that cause clinical signs are usually large and multilobulated and may be inflamed or filled with food, bone, or foreign bodies (Figure 83–18).[98] Typical signs are distress or gasping shortly after eating, postprandial regurgitation, intermittent anorexia, fever, weight loss, thoracic or abdominal pain, and respiratory signs. Diverticula can be identified on survey radiographs as either air- or food-filled masses in the area of the esophagus. Contrast procedures will demonstrate a focal portion of the esophageal lumen that fills partially or completely with contrast material (Figures 83–19 and 83–20). Esophagoscopy is a valuable tool for confirming the diagnosis while identifying associated complications such as ulceration and scarring.

Small diverticula, without other esophageal lesions, may be treated conservatively by using a soft bland diet, feeding the animal in an upright position, and providing ample liquids to discourage food accumulation in the pouch. Large diverticula require surgical excision and reconstruction of the esophageal wall, which warrants a less favorable prognosis. Any underlying cause must be treated appropriately.

Esophageal Neoplasia

Primary malignant neoplasms involving the canine esophagus are rare but include squamous cell carcinoma, osteosarcoma, fibrosarcoma, and undifferentiated carcinomas.[109, 110] Benign tumors are occasionally observed at necropsy and are usually leiomyomas.[110] Feline primary esophageal neoplasms are most frequently carcinomas.[111] Metastatic neoplasms to the esophagus are diagnosed more often than primary tumors but are still uncommon.[27] Reported metastatic tumors include bronchogenic carcinoma, gastric carcinoma, thyroid carcinoma, mammary adenocarcinoma, and squamous cell carcinoma.[110]

The most common primary esophageal neoplasias are sarcomas that arise secondarily to the formation of granulomas caused by the helminth parasite *Spirocerca lupi*.[112, 113] Fibrosarcomas and osteosarcomas are often associated with *Spirocerca* infections and are most commonly located in the thoracic esophagus between the aortic arch and hiatus. The dog family acts as the

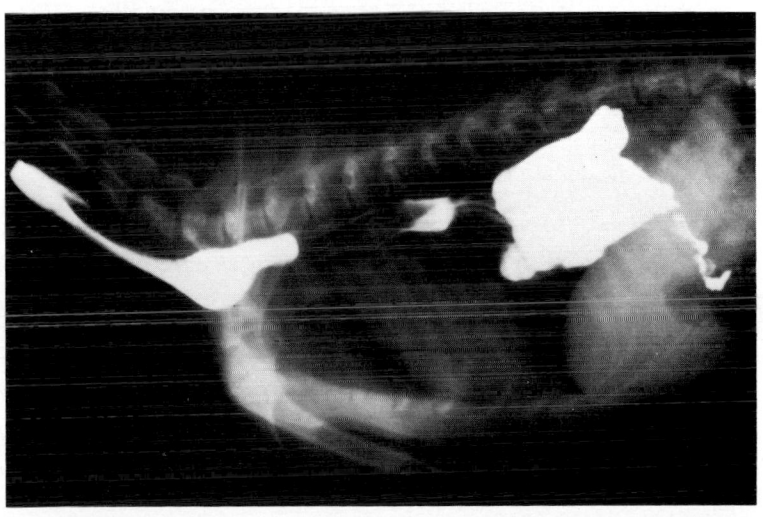

FIGURE 83–19. Lateral view of a positive contrast esophagram demonstrating the large epiphrenic diverticulum shown in Figure 83–18. (From Jones, BD (ed): Canine and Feline Gastroenterology. Philadelphia, WB Saunders, 1986.)

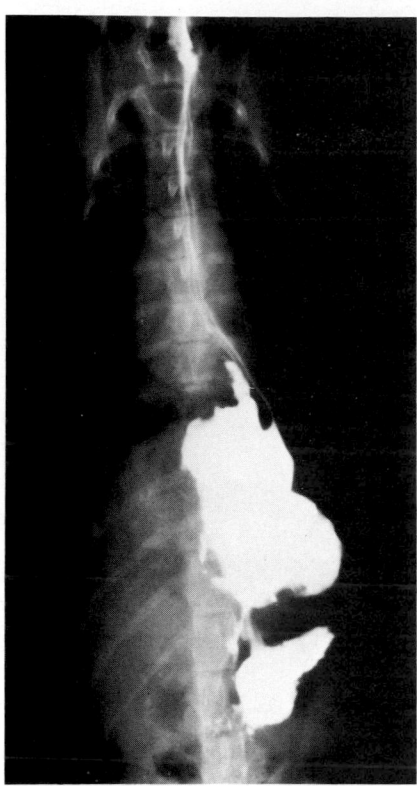

FIGURE 83–20. Ventrodorsal view of a positive contrast esophagram demonstrating a large epiphrenic diverticulum. This should not be confused with a gastric herniation into the thoracic cavity because the stomach is in its normal position. (From Jones, BD (ed): Canine and Feline Gastroenterology. Philadelphia, WB Saunders, 1986.)

definitive host for this parasite, which lives in the wall of the esophagus. Infection is established by ingesting beetles or transport hosts (rodents, birds) that harbor encysted larvae. Following ingestion, the encysted larvae are freed and migrate through the wall of the stomach and the aorta to the esophagus where they mature. Larval migration can cause aortic aneurysms, vertebral spondylitis, esophageal granulomas, as well as neoplasia of the esophagus. Hypertrophic osteopathy has been reported in cases of esophageal fibrosarcoma with and without pulmonary metastasis.[114]

Clinical Signs. The predominant clinical signs in dogs with esophageal neoplasia include slowly progressive regurgitation, dysphagia, drooling, weight loss, and debilitation. Regurgitation may or may not be related to eating. Esophageal tumors usually occur in dogs and cats over six to eight years of age.[27]

Diagnosis. Diagnosis may be aided by radiography; however, esophagoscopy and biopsy are required for a definitive diagnosis. The earliest and most consistent radiographic sign is the retention of intraluminal gas cranial to the tumor as a consequence of disturbed esophageal motility. Other abnormalities observed on survey films include a displacement of periesophageal structures and an increase in soft tissue or mineral density in the mediastinum. Positive contrast radiography is often required to delineate mural infiltration. Endoscopy will allow visualization of the mass and permit biopsy (Figure 83–21).

Treatment. Response to treatment and prognosis are dependent upon the cause for the neoplasia. Malignant tumors carry a poor prognosis with surgical intervention often not practical. Radiation therapy may be palliative for radiosensitive tumors; however, radiation-induced esophagitis is a potential sequela. Treatment for *Spirocerca lupi* infections has included the use of disophenol, diethylcarbamazine, and dithiazine iodide.[31] Fenbendazole and related compounds may be a useful adjunct, since they are effective against spirocerca larvae in extraintestinal tissues.[115]

Disorders of the Esophageal Hiatus

The esophageal hiatus is that diaphragmatic perforation that allows the esophagus to pass from the thoracic cavity into the abdominal cavity. The esophageal wall is secured to this hiatus by a phrenoesophageal membrane, which normally allows only minor cranial movement of the abdominal esophageal segment. Congenital or acquired lesions of the hiatus may allow for a hiatal hernia. a periesophageal hiatal hernia, gastroesophageal intussusception, or a diaphragmatic hernia to occur.[5]

Hiatal hernias allow for herniation of the abdominal esophagus, gastroesophageal junction, and stomach into the thoracic cavity and are uncommonly seen in the dog and cat. Reflux esophagitis is often associated with hiatal hernia. Paraesophageal hiatal hernias are very rare and involve displacement of a portion of the stomach through a diaphragmatic defect adjacent to the esophageal hiatus. Gastroesophageal intussusception describes the invagination of all or parts of the stomach into the thoracic esophagus. In severe cases, the spleen and pancreas may be herniated as well. Idiopathic megaesophagus or incompetency of the LES mechanism may predispose dogs to this disorder.[116, 117] Although uncommon, gastroesophageal intussusception is most often seen in large breed dogs less than three months of age.[118]

Clinical Signs. Clinical signs associated with hiatal disorders include occasional or persistent regurgitation, hematemesis, respiratory distress, and cyanosis. Abdominal pain may be evident on palpation. Dehydration may lead to death in affected puppies. Survey radiographs frequently demonstrate esophageal dilatation with a well-circumscribed area of increased density in the caudal thoracic esophagus. Barium contrast procedures may be necessary for diagnosis. Surgical correction of the hiatal disorder is the recommended mode of therapy.

Esophageal Fistula

Fistula formation between the esophagus and airways may be due to congenital or acquired causes and is rarely reported in small animals. The fistula may be esophagotracheal, esophagobronchial, or esophagopulmonary. The esophagobronchial fistula is the most often reported esophageal fistula in the dog.[119] Congenital occurrence is thought to result from incomplete separation of the esophagus and airways during embryonic development.[98] The pathogenesis of acquired esophageal fistulas is poorly understood but usually includes a history of foreign body obstruction.

Clinical Signs. Clinical signs principally relate to respiratory dysfunction and include coughing, choking,

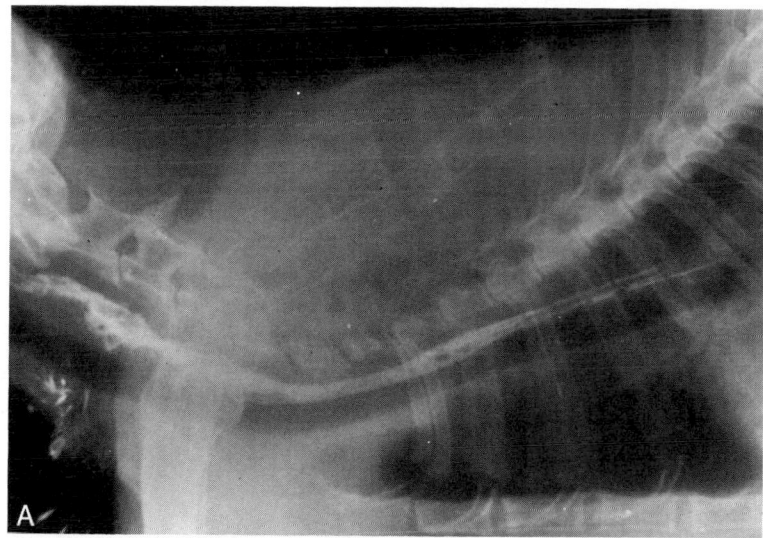

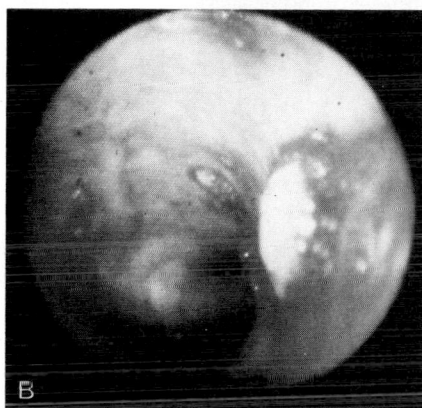
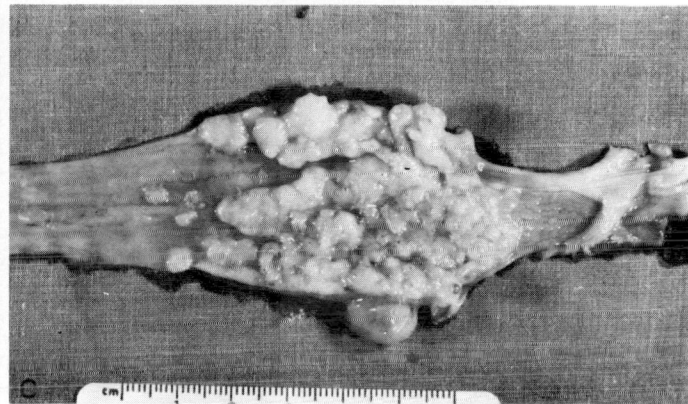

FIGURE 83–21. *A,* A positive contrast esophagram of a 14-year-old neutered male Siamese cat that had a history of dysphagia and regurgitation of three months duration. The cervical esophagus showed an abnormal roughened mucosal pattern with what appeared to be numerous small and large filling defects. *B,* An endoscopic examination revealed numerous nodular growths that were present in the caudal pharynx and diffusely involved the entire proximal third of the esophagus. This is a view through a flexible endoscope of one of the nodules. A biopsy specimen of a nodule was obtained through the endoscope. A histologic diagnosis was squamous cell carcinoma. *C,* The proximal esophagus at necropsy. The final diagnosis was squamous cell carcinoma of the esophagus. (From Jones, BD (ed): Canine and Feline Gastroenterology. Philadelphia, WB Saunders, 1986.)

regurgitation, and dysphagia. Coughing associated with drinking liquids is frequently observed in dogs with esophagobronchial fistulas but may not be present in all cases.[120] Anorexia, lethargy, weight loss, and pyrexia are also observed and are attributable to aspiration pneumonia with systemic infection. Crackles may be auscultated over consolidated lung regions on physical examination.

Diagnosis. Survey thoracic radiographs may demonstrate radiopaque foreign bodies, pulmonary consolidation, and pleural fluid accumulation. Contrast radiography will confirm the presence of esophageal perforation and locate the site of respiratory tract communication. Contrast esophagrams have been shown to be a reliable method for diagnosing esophagobronchial fistulas in dogs.[120] Esophagoscopy and bronchoscopy should be attempted but may prove futile in identifying the origin of the fistulous tract.

Treatment. Clinical management is aimed at surgical correction of the fistulous tract and its associated complications. Esophagotomy to remove foreign bodies and pneumonectomy of consolidated pulmonary tissues may

be indicated. With thoracic cavity infection, appropriate bacteriologic cultures and antibiotic sensitivity testing should be performed. Those cases with limited esophageal trauma and minimal pulmonary pathology carry a favorable prognosis. A poor prognosis should be given to dogs with severe complications such as pneumonia, pulmonary abscesses, and significant pleural effusion.

References

1. Kneller, SK and Lewis, RE: Contrast radiography of the normal cat esophagus. JAAHA 9:50, 1973.
2. Watrous, BJ and Suter, PF: Normal swallowing in the dog: A cineradiographic study. Vet Radiol 20:99, 1979.
3. Levitt, MN, et al.: The cricopharyngeus muscle, an electromyographic study in the dog. Laryngoscope 75:122, 1965.
4. Palmer, ED: Disorders of the cricopharyngeus muscle: A review. Gastroenterology 71:510, 1976.
5. Watrous, BJ: Esophageal disease. *In* Ettinger, SJ (ed): Textbook of Veterinary Internal Medicine, 2nd ed. WB Saunders, Philadelphia, 1983, p 1191.
6. Janssens, J, et al.: Studies on the necessity of a bolus for the progression of secondary peristalsis in the canine esophagus. Gastroenterology 67:245, 1974.

7. Nakayama, S, et al.: Effects of electrical stimulation and local destruction of the medulla oblongata on swallowing movements in dogs. Rendic Gastroenterol 6:6, 1974.

8. Lynch, VP, et al.: Autotransplantation of the canine esophagus. Surg Gynecol Obstet 138:396, 1974.

9. Higgs, B, et al.: The experimental production of esophageal achalasia by electrolytic lesions in the medulla. J Thoracic Cardiovasc Surg 50:613, 1965.

10. Greenwood, RK, et al.: The effect of sympathectomy, vagotomy, and oesophageal interruption on the canine gastroesophageal sphincter. Thorax 17:310. 1962.

11. Ingelfinger, FJ: Esophageal motility. Physiol Rev 38:533, 1958.

12. Strombeck, DR: Pathophysiology of esophageal motility disorders. Vet Clin North Am 8:229, 1978.

13. Shelton, GD: Swallowing disorders in the dog. Comp Cont Ed Pract Vet 4:607, 1982.

14. DeNovo, RC: Therapeutics of gastrointestinal diseases. In Kirk, RW (ed): Current Veterinary Therapy IX. WB Saunders, Philadelphia, 1986.

15. Magne, ML: Esophageal Motility Disorders in the Dog, Proc Fourth Annual Veterinary Medical Forum, 12:9, 1986.

16. Hall, AW, et al.: The effects of premedication drugs on the lower oesophageal high pressure zone and reflux status of Rhesus monkeys and man. Gut 16:347, 1975.

17. Gaynor, F, et al.: Physiologic features of the canine esophagus: Effects of tranquilization on esophageal motility. Am J Vet Res 41:727, 1980.

18. Freiman, JM and Diamant, NE: Upper esophageal sphincter (UES) response to esophageal distention and acid, and its alteration with nerve blockade. Gastroenterology 70:970, 1976.

19. Harvey, CE and O'Brien, JA: Esophageal diseases and disorders. Scientific Presentations of the Annual Meeting AAHA, (2):155, 1975.

20. Aronson, E, et al.: Radiology of the gastrointestinal system. In Jones BD (ed.): Canine and Feline Gastroenterology. Philadelphia, WB Saunders, 1986, p 399.

21. Kealy, JK: Diagnostic Radiology of the Dog and Cat. Philadelphia, WB Saunders, 1979.

22. Hendricks, JC, et al.: Transient esophageal dysfunction mimicking megaesophagus in three dogs. JAVMA 185:90, 1984.

23. Schwartz, A, et al.: Congenital neuromuscular esophageal disease in a litter of Newfoundland puppies. J Am Vet Radiol Soc 17:101, 1976.

24. Jones, BD: The use of fiberoptic endoscopy in veterinary medicine. Proc AAHA 45:241, 1978.

25. O'Brien, JA: Esophagoscopy. Vet Clin North Am 2:99, 1972.

26. Zimmer, JF: Gastrointestinal fiberoptic endoscopy. In Kirk, RW (ed): Current Veterinary Therapy VII. Philadelphia, WB Saunders, 1980, p 954.

27. Roudebush, P, et al.: Medical aspects of esophageal disease. In Jones BD (ed.): Canine and Feline Gastroenterology. Philadelphia, WB Saunders, 1986, p 54.

28. Clifford, DH and Malek, R: Diseases of the canine esophagus due to prenatal influence. American Journal of Digestive Diseases. New Series 14:578, 1969.

29. Knauer, CM, et al.: Alimentary Tract and Liver. In Krupp, MA, et al. (eds): Current Medical Diagnosis and Treatment. Lange Publ, Los Altos, 1985.

30. Harvey, CE, et al.: Megaesophagus in the dog: A clinical survey of 79 cases. JAVMA 165, 443, 1974.

31. Strombeck, DR: Diseases of swallowing. In Small Animal Gastroenterology. Stonegate Publishing, Davis, 1979.

32. Leib, MS: Megaesophagus in the dog. Comp Cont Ed Pract Vet 5:825, 1983.

33. Sharp, NJH and Nash, AS: Feline Dysautonomia. In Kirk, RW (ed): Current Vet Therapy IX. Philadelphia, WB Saunders, 1986, p 802.

34. Diamant, N, et al.: Manometric characteristics of idiopathic megaesophagus in the dog: An unsuitable animal. Gastroenterology 65:216, 1973.

35. Diamant, N, et al.: Idiopathic megaesophagus in the dog: Reasons for spontaneous improvement and a possible method of medical therapy. Can Vet J 15:66, 1974.

36. Strombeck, DR: Pathophysiology of esophageal motility disorders in the dog and cat. Vet Clin North Am 8:229, 1978.

37. Hofmyer, CFB: An evaluation of cardioplasty for achalasia of the oesophagus in the dog. J Sm Anim Pract 7:281, 1966.

38. Clifford, DH, et al.: Comparison of motor nuclei of the vagus nerve in dogs with and without achalasia. Proc Soc Ex Bio Med 142:878, 1973.

39. Gray, GW: Acute experiments on neuroeffector function in canine esophageal achalasia. Am J Vet Res 35:1075, 1974.

40. Leib, MS: Megaesophagus in the Dog. In Kirk, RW (ed.): Current Veterinary Therapy IX. Philadelphia, WB Saunders, 1986, p 848.

41. O'Brien, JA, et al.: The Esophagus. In Anderson, NV (ed): Veterinary Gastroenterology. Lea & Febiger, Philadelphia, 1980, p 372.

42. Strombeck, DR and Troya, L: Evaluation of lower motor neuron function in two dogs with megaesophagus. JAVMA 169:411.

43. Rogers, WA, et al.: Electromyographic and esophagomanometric findings in clinically normal dogs and in dogs with idiopathic megaesophagus. JAVMA 174:181, 1979.

44. Hoffer, RE: Primary Esophageal Neuromuscular Diseases. In Jones, BD (ed.): Canine and Feline Gastroenterology. Philadelphia, WB Saunders, 1986, p 89.

45. Hoffer, RE, et al.: Management of acquired achalasia in dogs. JAVMA 175:814, 1979.

46. Hoffer, RE: Surgical esophageal diseases. In Bojrab, MJ (ed.): Pathophysiology In Small Animal Surgery. Philadelphia, Lea and Febiger, 1981, p 90.

47. Clifford, DH, et al.: Congenital achalasia of the esophagus in four cats of common ancestry. JAVMA 158:1554, 1971.

48. Forbes, DC and Leishman, DE: Megaesophagus in a cat. Can Vet J 26:354, 1985.

49. Crawley, AJ and Gendreau, CL: Esophageal achalasia in a cat. Can Vet J 10:195, 1969.

50. Boudrieau, RJ and Rogers, WA: Megaesophagus in the dog: A review of 50 cases. JAAHA 21:33, 1985.

51. Krum, SH, et al.: Polymyositis and polyarthritis associated with systemic lupus erythematosus in a dog. JAVMA 170:61, 1977.

52. Marsden, PD and Hagstrom, JWC: Experimental Trypanosoma cruzi infection in beagle puppies. Trans Royal Soc Tropical Medicine and Hygiene 62:816, 1968.

52a. Walvoort, HC, et al.: Canine glycogen storage disease type II: A clinical study of four affected Lapland dogs. JAAHA 20:279, 1984.

53. Kornegay, JN, et al.: Polymyositis in dogs. JAVMA 176:431, 1980.

54. Haupt, KH, et al.: Familial canine dermatomyositis: Clinical, electrodiagnostic, and genetic studies. Am J Vet Res 46:1861, 1985.

55. Darke, PGG, et al.: Suspected botulism in foxhounds. Vet Rec 99:98, 1976.

56. Van Nes, JJ: Electrophysiological evidence of peripheral nerve dysfunction in six dogs with botulism type C. Res Vet Sci 40:372, 1986.

57. Mason, KV: A case of myasthenia gravis in a cat. J Sm Anim Pract 17:467, 1976.

58. Miller, LM, et al.: Congenital myasthenia gravis in 13 smooth fox terriers. JAVMA 182:694, 1983.

59. Harris, LD, et al.: Esophageal aperistalsis and achalasia produced in dogs by prolonged cholinesterase inhibition. J Clin Invest 39:1744, 1960.

60. Cummings JF, et al.: Ganglioradiculitis in the dog. Acta Neuropathologica 60:29, 1983.

61. Zook, BC and Gilmore, CE: Thallium poisoning in dogs. JAVMA 151:206, 1967.

62. Duncan, ID and Griffiths, IR: Canine giant axonal neuropathy; some aspects of its clinical, pathological and comparative features. J Sm Anim Pract 22:491, 1981.

63. Shell, LG, et al.: Spinal muscular atrophy in two Rottweiler littermates. JAVMA 190:878, 1987.

64. Zook, BC: The pathologic anatomy of lead poisoning in dogs. Vet Path 9:310, 1972.

65. Van Ee, RT, et al.: Bronchoesophageal fistula and transient megaesophagus in a dog. JAVMA 188:874, 1986.

66. Cassella, RR, et al.: Achalasia of the esophagus: Pathologic and etiologic considerations. Ann Surg 160:474, 1964.

67. Hara, T: Experimental study on the pathogenesis of achalasia. Jpn J Smooth Muscle Res 5:33, 1969.

68. Osborne, CA, et al.: Hereditary esophageal achalasia in dogs. JAVMA 151:572, 1967.

69. Fox, JG, et al.: Familial reflex myoclonus in Labrador retrievers. Am J Vet Res 45:2367, 1984.
70. Pidgeon, G: Unpublished observations, 1987.
71. Chastain, CB and Ganjam, VK: Clinical Endocrinology of Companion Animals. Philadelphia, Lea & Febiger, 1986.
72. Feldman, EC and Tyrrell, JB: Hypoadrenocorticism. Vet Clin N Am 7:555, 1977.
73. Schaer, M, et al.: Autoimmunity and Addison's disease in the dog. JAAHA 22:789, 1986.
74. Ridgeway, RL and Suter, PF: Clinical and radiographic signs in primary and metastatic esophageal neoplasms of the dog. JAVMA 174:700, 1979.
75. Carpenter, JL and Holzworth, J: Thymoma in 11 cats. JAVMA 181:248, 1982.
76. Darke, PGG, et al.: Myasthenia gravis, thymoma and myositis in a dog. Vet Rec 97:392, 1975.
77. Pearson, H, et al.: Pyloric and oesophageal dysfunction in the cat. J Sm Anim Pract 15:487, 1974.
78. Bishop, LM, et al.: Megaloesophagus and associated gastric heterotopia in the cat. Vet Pathol 16:444, 1979.
79. Strating, A and Clifford, DH: Canine achalasia with special reference to hereditary. Southwest Vet 19:135, 1966.
80. Cox, VS, et al.: Hereditary esophageal dysfunction in the miniature schnauzer dog. Am J Vet Res 41:326, 1980.
81. Breshears, DE: Esophageal dilation in six-week-old male German shepherd pups. VM/SAC 60:1034, 1965.
82. Palmer, CS: Achalasia or cardiospasms in Great Dane puppies. VM/SAC 63:574, 1968.
83. Spy, GM: Megaesophagus in a litter of greyhounds. Vet Rec 75:853, 1963.
84. Guilford, WG: Unpublished observations (1986).
85. Sokolovsky, V: Achalasia and paralysis of the canine esophagus. JAVMA 160:943, 1972.
86. Lobis, IF and Fisher, RS: Anticholinergic therapy for achalasia: A controlled trial. Gastroenterology 70:976, 1976.
87. Weiser, HF, et al.: Clinical and experimental studies on the effect of nifedipine on smooth muscle of the oesophagus and LRS. In Duthie, HL (ed): Gastrointestinal Motility in Health and Disease. Lancaster, England, MTP Press, 1978, p 565.
88. Lobis, IF and Fisher, RS: Anticholinergic therapy for achalasia: a controlled trial. Gastroenterology 70:976, 1976.
89. Hoffer, RE, et al.: Physiologic features of the canine esophagus: Effect of modified Heller's esophagomyotomy. Am J Vet Res 41:723, 1980.
90. Guffy, MM: Esophageal Disorders. In Ettinger, SJ, (ed): Textbook of Veterinary Internal Medicine. Philadelphia, WB Saunders, 1975, p 1098.
91. Shires, PK and Liu, W: Persistent right aortic arch in dogs: A long term follow-up after surgical correction. JAAHA 17:773, 1981.
92. Ettinger, SJ and Suter, PF: Diseases of the great vessels. In Ettinger, SJ (ed): Textbook of Veterinary Internal Medicine. WB Saunders, Philadelphia, 1975, p 980.
93. Leipold, HW: Nature and causes of congenital defects of dogs. Vet Clin North Am 8:47, 1977.
94. Patterson, DF: Epidemiologic and genetic studies of congenital heart disease in the dog. Circ Res 23:171, 1968.
95. Patterson, DF: Canine congenital heart disease: Epidemiology and etiological hypotheses. J Sm Anim Pract 12:263, 1971.
96. Adler, PL: Phycomycosis in fifteen dogs and two cats. JAVMA 174:1216, 1979.
97. O'Brien T.R.: Radiographic Diagnosis of Abdominal Disorders in the Dog and Cat. WB Saunders, Philadelphia, 1978.
98. Suter, PF and Lord, PF: Swallowing problems and esophageal abnormalities. In Thoracic Radiography—A Text Atlas of Thoracic Diseases of the Dog and Cat. Peter F. Suter, Wettswil, Switzerland, 1984.
99. Davenport, HW: Physiology of the digestive tract. 3rd ed, Year Book Medical Publishers Inc. Chicago, 1971.
100. Pearson, H, et al.: Reflux esophagitis and stricture formation after anesthesia: A review of seven cases in dogs and cats. J Sm Anim Pract 19:507, 1978.
101. Clifford, DH, et al.: The esophagus. In Bojrab, MJ (ed): Current Techniques in Small Animal Surgery. Lea and Febiger, Philadelphia, 1975, p 104.
102. Pope, CE: Gastroesophageal reflux disease (reflux esophagus). In Sleisenger, MO and Fordtran, JS (eds): Gastrointestinal Disease. Philadelphia, WB Saunders, 1978, p 568.
103. Strombeck, DR: Acute Gastritis in Small Animal Gastroenterology. Davis, CA, Stonegate, 1979, p 98.
104. Ryan, WW and Greene, RW: The conservative management of esophageal foreign bodies and their complications. A review of 66 cases in dogs and cats. JAAHA 11:243, 1975.
105. Lantz, GC, et al.: Pharyngostomy tube induced esophagitis in the dog: An experimental study. JAAHA 19:207, 1983.
106. Clifford, DH, et al.: Stricture and dilatation of the esophagus of the cat. JAVMA 156:1007, 1970.
107. Pearson, H, et al.: Oesophageal diverticulum formation in the dog. J Sm Anim Pract 19:341, 1978.
108. Lantz, GC, et al.: Epiphrenic esophageal diverticulectomy. JAAHA 12:629, 1976.
109. McCaw, D, et al.: Squamous cell carcinoma of the esophagus in a dog. JAAHA 16:561, 1980.
110. Ridgway, RL and Suter, PF: Clinical and radiographic signs in primary and metastatic esophageal neoplasms of the dog. JAVMA 74:700, 1979.
111. Vernon, FF and Roudebush, P: Primary esophageal carcinoma in a cat. JAAHA 16:547, 1980.
112. Ivoghli, B: Esophageal sarcomas associated with canine spirocercosis. VM/SAC 73:47, 1978.
113. Seibold, HR, et al.: Observations on the possible relations of malignant esophageal tumors and Spirocera lupi lesions in the dog. Am J Vet Res 16:5, 1955.
114. Daily, WS: Parasites and cancer—sarcoma in dogs associated with Spirocerca lupi. Ann NY Acad Sci 180:890, 1963.
115. Corwin, RM and Green, SE: Gastrointestinal parasitism in the dog and cat. In Jones, BD (ed): Canine and Feline Gastroenterology. Philadelphia, WB Saunders, 1986, p 487.
116. Pollock, S and Rhodes, WH: Gastroesophageal intussusception in an Afghan hound: A case report. J Am Vet Rad Soc 11:5, 1970.
117. Hoffer, RE: Surgical esophageal diseases. In Bojrab, MJ (ed.): Pathophysiology in Small Animal Surgery. Philadelphia, Lea and Febiger, 1981, p 90.
118. Rowland, MG and Robinson, M: Gastro-oesophageal intussusception in an adult dog. J Sm Anim Pract 19:121, 1978.
119. Caywood, DD and Feeney, DA: Acquired esophagobronchial fistula in a dog. JAAHA 18:590, 1982.
120. Park, RD: Bronchoesophageal fistula in the dog: Literature survey, case presentations, and radiographic manifestations. Comp Cont Ed Pract Vet 6:669, 1984.

DRUG INDEX

Generic	(Trade)	Dosage	Route	Frequency	Description
Cimetidine	Tagamet	2–5 mg/lb	PO, IV, IM	TID	H_2 blocker: Can be used for reflux esophagitis
Ranitidine	Zantac	0.20 mg/lb	PO	BID	H_2 blocker: Can be used for reflux esophagitis
Metoclopramide	Reglan	0.05–0.15 mg/lb 0.005–0.01 mg/lb/hr	PO, IV, SQ IV	QID Continuous	Increases LES pressure; beneficial for reflux esophagitis; may also increase strength of esophageal contractions
Acetylpromazine	Acepromazine	0.02–0.5 mg/lb	IV		Tranquilization in uncooperative patients for esophagraphy

84 GASTRIC DILATATION-VOLVULUS-TORSION SYNDROME

CHARLES L. LIPPINCOTT and ALAN J. SCHULMAN

General Comments and Definitions

The gastric dilatation-volvulus-torsion syndrome (GDVT) is a medical and surgical emergency with high mortality in the dog.[1-8] Early recognition of this entity is of paramount importance to successful treatment of this syndrome. The practitioner must be cognizant of the epizootiology, etiology, pathoanatomy, and pathophysiology in order to provide effective therapeutic and surgical management.

Gastric dilatation refers to distention of the stomach, caused most often by swallowed air. Usually, the dilatation also contains fluid and ingesta mixed with a frothy mucoid substrate. Dilatation implies an innocuous condition that can easily be corrected by passing a stomach tube to relieve the distention. Rarely is a dilatation corrected by the passage of a stomach tube. The patient may be temporarily relieved but often may suffer from a coincidental torsion that should be diagnosed by a barium swallow and radiographic examination. Gastric torsion occurs when the tubular stomach rotates on itself (Figures 84–1 to 84–3).

The common rotation begins with the pylorus and the pyloric antrum passing from the right ventral side of the abdomen and rotating under the stomach and coming to rest dorsally above the cardia on the left side. This torsion may remain as an occult occurrence and may not lead to a GDVT syndrome, or the torsion may continue developing into a volvulus. When and if the volvulus occurs, the ensuing GDVT syndrome is a serious pathophysiologic event.

In the torsion, the stomach outflow may not be totally blocked. Many animals may appear quite normal but still are in a torsed condition. An early diagnosis of the torsion allows the clinician to take steps to prevent a gastric volvulus from developing. Gastric volvulus occurs as the torsion continues to twist about its long axis. This volvulus completely obstructs the gastric flow of fluid, food, and gases. Twisting of the hollow organ precipitates strangulation necrosis of segments of the stomach wall. As the exit of gases is blocked, gastric dilatation ensues.

Disease Incidence and Breed Susceptibility

The gastric dilatation-volvulus-torsion complex occurs primarily in the large, deep-chested canine breeds.[1-7] Several investigators have documented a greater prevalence of GDVT in the Great Dane, the Saint Bernard, and the Borzoi.[8, 9] The German shepherd and the Irish setter also frequently develop GDVT. The syndrome is recognized more often in these breeds because of a greater frequency with which they are seen rather than a greater susceptibility to gastric dilatation.[2, 8–10] Although GDVT is typically a disease of large dogs, it does occur rarely in small breeds.[1, 2] The age of affected dogs varies, but GDVT is most likely to develop between the ages of two and ten years.[8–10] Recent studies have shown no sexual predisposition for the disease.[8]

PATHOPHYSIOLOGY

Stomach Torsion With Volvulus and Increased Gastric Pressures

The torsion rotates around the gastroesophageal junction. Because the gastroesophageal orifice is closed, there can be no vomiting or belching. The torsion is continued along the greater curvature of the stomach to the antrum. The fundus and the pyloric antrum expansion compresses the pyloroduodenal region, blocking gas and fluid from exiting into the duodenum. The gastric Auerbach plexus ganglionic cells may be compromised due to distention, creating further atony of the stomach wall.[11] These patients may initially have a low electric activity of contraction potential present in the gastric wall. This may account for the stomach's inability to expel trapped pressures, allowing GDTV to develop.[12] The trapped gas causing the increased distention of the gastric wall comes mainly from aerophagia.[13] Other hypotheses are that clostridial organisms produce gas, bacterial fermentation of a suitable substrate produces CO_2, diffusion of gases associated with trapped blood in the muscle wall increases CO_2 accumulations and intragastric pressures possibly prevent this gaseous diffusion, and gastric acid and bicarbonate react and form CO_2.[14-16] The source of the bicarbonate may be the pancreatic secretions and the swallowed saliva. For each milliequivalent of bicarbonate, 22.4 cc of CO_2 is released. This may account for the increased gaseous distention after the gastric exits are blocked.[14, 16] Ischemia of the gastric musculature occurs when the gaseous intraluminal pressures exceed the arterial systolic pressure supplying the muscle wall. The twisted and distended stomach pathophysiologically initiates a profound "domino effect" on most of the organ systems of the body. If rapid, aggressive, and specific treatment is not instituted within three hours, the patient will usually die.[13, 14, 22, 29, 38]

Effects on Other Organ Systems

Spleen. The changes seen in neighboring organs are related to the pressure applied by the distended stomach and to anatomic movement of the stomach and related organs. As the greater curvature of the stomach moves into a twisted position, the spleen is also pulled into a new position. The splenic vessels are partially occluded, causing secondary venous congestion and splenomegaly. This splenic rotation can also cause gastric necrosis.[15]

Portal Vein and Caudal Vena Cava. The gastric distention restricts the normal portacaval and caudal vena caval blood flow. This causes shunting of blood through the ventral vertebral sinus and the azygos vein to the cranial vena cava and then to the right heart.[17] Occlusion of the portal vein and caudal vena cava causes marked passive chronic congestion of the abdominal viscera. This anatomic obstruction is a factor in the ensuing hypovolemic shock syndrome.

Abdominal Organs. Since the veins draining the cau-

dal abdomen are compressed, venous stasis occurs in the organs. The organs suffer engorgement, increased blood viscosity, and local acidosis. These factors may initiate disseminated intravascular coagulation (DIC).[18, 19] With the sequestration of blood, oxyhemoglobin desaturation occurs, and the vicious circle continues.[15-17]

Liver. The normal liver receives 85 per cent of its blood supply from the portal vein. As this supply is interrupted, the resultant liver ischemia is another factor contributing to the initiation of the hypovolemic shock. Because of the lack of portal circulation, the reticuloendothelial cells of the liver cannot neutralize the gram-negative bacterial endotoxins.[20] These endotoxins precipitate endotoxic shock, which potentiates the hypovolemic shock and hastens death.

Cardiovascular System. Three main components of the cardiovascular system are vital to continued health of the organism. No matter which of the three components fails—fluid volume (blood), the pump (heart), or the tubular structures (arteries, veins, capillaries)—the results are disastrous. In the GDVT syndrome, the hypovolemia that ensues affects the entire cardiovascular system. In GDVT, rarely is there an acute excessive loss of blood, but merely a redistribution of the blood responding to the catecholamine and adrenergic mediation.

Adrenergic Response. The release of epinephrine and norepinephrine from the adrenal cortex causes vasoconstriction of the metarterioles entering the capillary beds and vasoconstriction of the postcapillary venules leaving the capillary beds. This adrenergic response occurs in the capillary beds of all the body organs, except the heart and brain. This hormonal vasoconstriction slows perfusion of the cell.

Blood Volume Conservation. The GDVT patient tries to reestablish circulating blood volume by redirecting fluid from the lungs, bone, liver, cartilage, and extra-

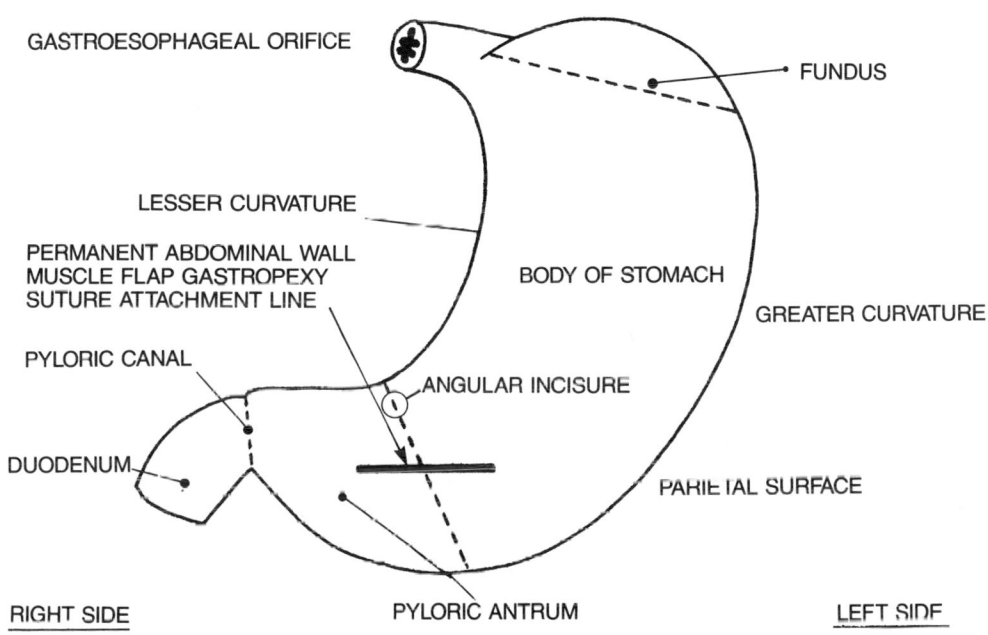

GASTROESOPHAGEAL ORIFICE

FUNDUS

LESSER CURVATURE

PERMANENT ABDOMINAL WALL MUSCLE FLAP GASTROPEXY SUTURE ATTACHMENT LINE

BODY OF STOMACH

GREATER CURVATURE

PYLORIC CANAL

ANGULAR INCISURE

DUODENUM

PARIETAL SURFACE

RIGHT SIDE

PYLORIC ANTRUM

LEFT SIDE

FIGURE 84–1. Normal regional anatomy of the canine stomach.

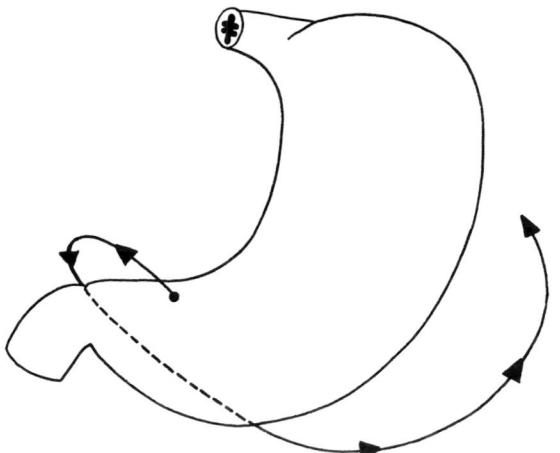

FIGURE 84–2. The normal rotation path of the pylorus creating a torsion. The pylorus moves from its normal right-sided position under the stomach and twists to the left dorsal position.

vascular tissue spaces into the intravascular spaces to compensate for the developing hypovolemia. Hypovolemia may be monitored by measuring the pressure of the volume of blood returning to the right heart (central venous pressure monitoring).

Cardiac Output and Tissue Perfusion. Reduced venous return to the right atrium results in a decreased cardiac output. Early in the GDVT syndrome, the blood pressure can remain normal or be increased. Once shock develops, there is usually a hypotensive state present. The development of shock is not caused by a drop in blood pressure, so vasopressors should not be used in the treatment of GDVT. The stimulation of the gastric sympathetic nerves can also account for added hypotension.

The hypotension, reduced circulating blood flow, low velocity of flow, and adrenergic effect all continue to synergistically reduce tissue perfusion. In summary, the outstanding pathophysiologic feature of GDVT is hypovolemic shock.[2] Gastric dilatation initiates hypovo-

lemic shock by a functional obstruction of blood flow through the caudal vena cava as it passes dorsal to the distended stomach. Increased intragastric pressure also decreases blood flow through the portal vein. Compensatory collateral venous return via the ventral vertebral sinuses to the azygous vein is not great enough to compensate, and sequestration of blood within the dilated splanchnic, renal, and posterior muscle capillary beds occurs.[2, 3, 16]

Many other adverse consequences of hypovolemia and splanchnic congestion occur.[2] Hypotension and vascular stasis result in decreased oxygen delivery to the cells and a shift to anaerobic metabolism, with increased production of organic acids and eventually cell death in many tissues.

Biochemistry of the GDVT Shock Syndrome. With poor tissue perfusion, the cells of the tissues do not receive oxygen and cannot dispose of their CO_2 wastes.[18] Normally the cells use oxygen to convert glucose into pyruvate, pyruvate to acetyl CoA, and acetyl CoA to ATP. When perfusion is low, there is reduced O_2 available to the cell; although anaerobic attempts are made, the end result is that not enough ATP is made. The cells convert pyruvate to lactate, and they develop lactic acidosis. In the untreated metabolic acidotic patient, many cells lose their ability to function and become pyknotic.[18] As this process worsens, cells of many organ systems similarly fail, the organ systems lose their proper function, homeostasis is compromised, and often death follows.

Lungs. The enlarged stomach in the GDVT patient encroaches on the thoracic diaphragm. The abdominal dilatation is extremely painful. The act of breathing deeply is compromised because of a painful decreased compliance resulting in a decrease in the tidal volume of the lungs. As the tidal volume is decreased, the rate of respiration automatically increases to maintain the minute volume needed. Inspiratory and expiratory resistance is increased severely and the lung compliance is decreased. Since the cardiac output is decreased, the

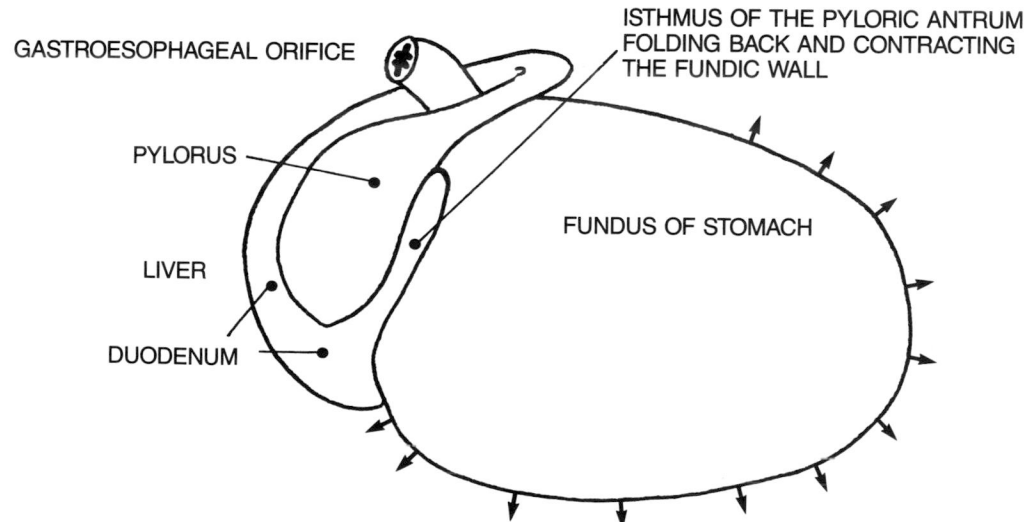

FIGURE 84–3. The relationship of the pylorus, the duodenum, and the gastroesophageal orifice in a GDVT.

lung perfusion is automatically decreased, and since the tidal volume is decreased, the ventilation-perfusion ratio is not maintained adequately. Pulmonary edema, hyperemia, and hemorrhage ensue. This is referred to as "shock lung."[21, 22]

Intestinal Tract. Hypoxia of the intestinal tract may cause a decrease in intestinal motility, and the sequela of paralytic ileus is common.[23] Injury to the gastric wall occurs as the normal gastric mucosa is subject to high transmural pressure that results in congestion, venous stasis, and local anoxia.[22] Subepithelial hemorrhage and edema develop, later followed by hemorrhagic gastritis.[22] Devitalization of the gastric wall may occur, with the most commonly infarcted area being along the greater curvature in the area served by the short gastric vessels.[22]

Myocardial Depressant Factor. Another work cites a vasoactive peptide called myocardial depressant factor (MDF), which is an arrhythmia-inducing compound created in the ischemic pancreas and stored in the spleen. The MDF causes cardiac arrhythmias and reduces cardiac myocardial contractile efficiency, resulting in hypoperfusion of the coronary arteries. Myocardial ischemia and microinfarcts have been demonstrated.[24, 25] It is as yet unclear whether the patients that suffer coronary hypoperfusion and infarcts of the myocardium actually develop ventricular premature beats or other cardiac arrhythmias that complicate the survival of the GDVT patient. On occasion, patients will succumb and never develop cardiac arrhythmias. There is no proven correlation between the lack of cardiac arrhythmias and survival.

CLINICAL SIGNS AND DIAGNOSIS

The clinical symptoms associated with GDVT include acute onset of abdominal distention with tympany, nonproductive retching, sialorrhea and restlessness, respiratory distress, increased heart rate, weak femoral pulses, and poor mucous membrane perfusion.[3, 26] The condition of the patient at the time of presentation should determine the extent of diagnostic testing that is done.[27] If possible, radiography should be utilized. When time is important and stress to the patient must be minimized, the view of choice for the diagnosis of GDVT is the right lateral recumbent view.[23, 27]

A gas-filled pylorus located dorsal and slightly cranial to the gas-filled fundus of the stomach in the right lateral recumbent view is compatible with the diagnosis of GDVT. Passage of a stomach tube does not preclude the presence of torsion, and torsion can remain after successful tube decompression.[7] This makes it essential to radiographically evaluate all dogs that do not have prompt surgical correction following a tube decompression.

Some dogs will have bloating only intermittently despite having gastric torsion. In these cases, a barium sulfate contrast examination will help differentiate simple gastric dilatation from gastric torsion.

EMERGENCY PREOPERATIVE TREATMENT

Medical treatment should include immediate placement of a large-bore intravenous catheter in the cephalic or jugular vein or both. Catheterization of the saphenous vein is to be avoided because caudal vena caval and portal venous obstruction caused by the dilated stomach will interfere with distribution of the administered fluids.[5, 28] Rapid administration of a balanced electrolyte solution at an initial rate of 100 ml/lb of body weight is indicated. Lactated Ringer's solution is generally the crystalloid fluid of choice.[8] The rate is adjusted on the basis of the patient's cardiovascular response and central venous pressure.

Corticosteroid therapy for managing shock consists of IV prednisolone sodium succinate, at a dose of 5 to 10 mg/lb. Broad-spectrum antibiotic therapy is directed against microorganisms absorbed from the gastrointestinal tract and ineffectively removed by the reticuloendothelial system.[7] Ampicillin and gentamicin is an effective bactericidal combination.[8]

Dogs with GDVT are subject to a variety of acid-base and electrolyte abnormalities.[29] Correction of these disorders is ideally based on serum biochemical and blood gas analysis. Metabolic acidosis and hypokalemia are common findings.[29] Sodium bicarbonate, 1 mEq/lb intravenously, and potassium chloride (at a rate not exceeding 0.02 mEq/lb of body weight per hour) are administered with the initial intravenous fluid therapy. If multiple large-bore catheters are used, be careful to avoid hyperkalemia. Sodium bicarbonate and electrolyte therapy should be monitored at frequent intervals and adjusted as needed to satisfy each patient's requirements.[29] Until the blood gas determinations or CO_2 values are obtained from the laboratory, the amount of sodium bicarbonate to administer may be estimated as follows: assuming that a moderate acidosis exists, multiply the weight in pounds by 6. This is the amount of bicarbonate mEq. to be given in 24 hours. Administer 50 per cent of this amount in the first 30 minutes with the initial fluids.[13, 14, 22] Give the balance of the $NaHCO_3$ over the next 12 hours.

The development of GDVT is often complicated by cardiopulmonary deterioration and the occurrence of a variety of cardiac arrhythmias.[30, 31] Electrocardiographic monitoring should be utilized routinely to assess the patient's cardiovascular status at admission and throughout the hospitalization period. Arrhythmias should be treated initially with quinidine gluconate administered by deep intramuscular injection.[30] Antiarrhythmic therapy is maintained by constant infusion of lidocaine throughout the surgical procedure and is continued into the postoperative period.

SURGICAL DECISIONS

One-stage and two-stage surgical techniques are available. Each has its merits and is discussed.[32 35] Gastric decompression must be achieved quickly; decompression immediately improves cardiac output by relieving caudal vena caval and portal venous occlusion.[2, 3, 7, 8] Often, decompression may be accomplished by the passage of a flexible orogastric tube. Factors such as patient cooperation, amount of gastric distention, and degree of gastric torsion determine the ease and feasibility of passing a stomach tube.[3] If the dog resists physical restraint, sedation with oxymorphone may be utilized to allow passage of the orogastric tube. Once positioned, the stomach tube is used to remove as much gastric gas and fluid as possible. Gastric lavage with warm saline aids in the removal of solid gastric contents.[2] The tube must not be forced if resistance is encountered at the gastroesophageal junction, as an iatrogenic esophageal tear may be created. In the event an orogastric tube cannot be passed, immediate temporary gastrostomy under local anesthetic may be performed to achieve gastric decompression.

Two-Stage Surgical Decompression

The surgeon, faced with the need to perform an immediate decompression, may be without adequately trained assistance. Alternatively, the surgeon may not feel confident performing the entire abdominal procedure. A two-stage decompression can often be instituted at an emergency clinic and then the case may be referred back to the regular veterinarian on the following day for the second stage of surgery. This two-stage surgical correction is initiated with a gastrostomy, which is a fistula created over the left abdominal wall, just caudal to the last rib (Figures 84–4 to 84–8). Analgesia, using oxymorphone, 0.20 mg/lb IV, and atropine, 0.02 mg/lb SQ, allows gentle intubation of the patient. An inflated endotracheal cuff permits 10 to 12 intermittent positive pressure respirations per minute. The oxygen drive should be set at 10 cc per pound of weight vaporizing a

concentration of 0.75 per cent isoflurane to produce the needed surgical anesthesia. The area of the greatest distention, just behind the left 13th rib, is clipped and prepared for aseptic surgery. The surgical site is draped and a sterile technique is employed. Incise the skin and muscles and identify the gastric wall. The stomach wall and the skin edges of the original incision are securely sutured together. Once this watertight incision is fashioned, incise the stomach wall, allowing immediate decompression. This simple procedure allows the portal and caudal vena caval circulation to be reestablished. The animal recovers from the hypovolemic state and is a much better surgical risk for the second-stage surgery, usually performed within 24 hours of the gastrostomy. This rapid decompression can be lifesaving in the proper situation. However, there are a few reasons that preclude it from being a primary selection. Two procedures are required, and additional expenses are incurred by the client. The initial gastrostomy must also be closed before the abdominal procedure can be performed, so the patient is ultimately subjected to a longer overall surgical time.

One-Stage Surgical Decompression

The one-stage approach is usually the desirable protocol. It does require the surgeon and staff to be prepared and to have a preestablished plan to allow a quick and efficient response to surgical emergency. The suggested analgesic is intravenous oxymorphone, 0.20 mg/lb. Atropine, 0.02 mg/lb, is administered SQ. This analgesia allows gentle intubation of the patient. An inflated endotracheal cuff allows intermittent positive pressure respirations. This one-stage surgical correction begins with a midline celiotomy. The stomach is visualized and decompressed using a sterile blood collection set, or a large-bore needle is connected to sterile intra-

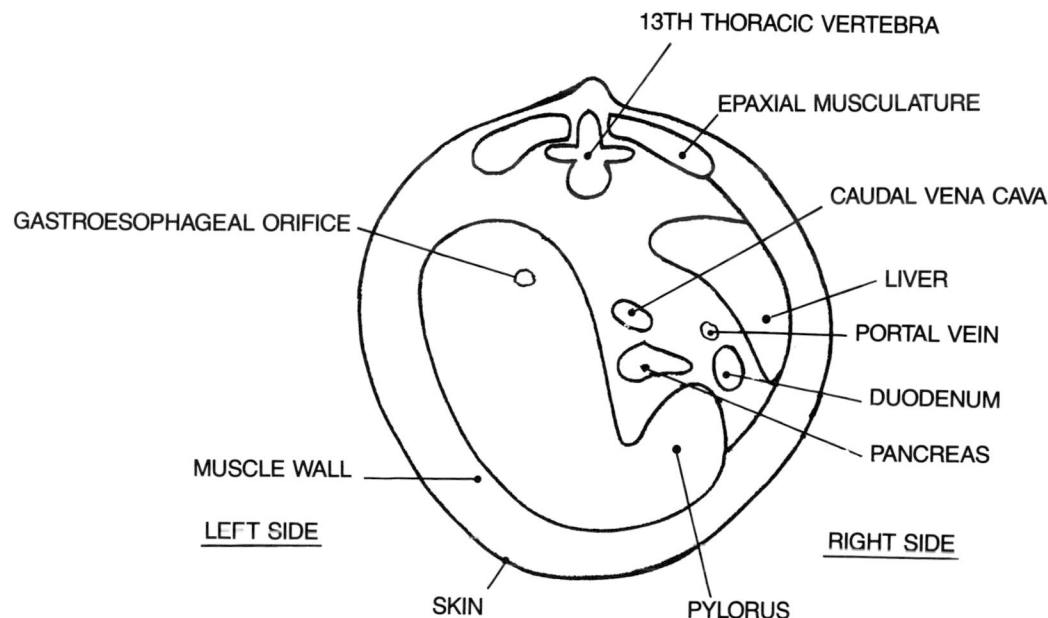

FIGURE 84–4. This is cross-section at the 13th thoracic vertebra showing the normal relationship of the stomach to the adjacent organs.

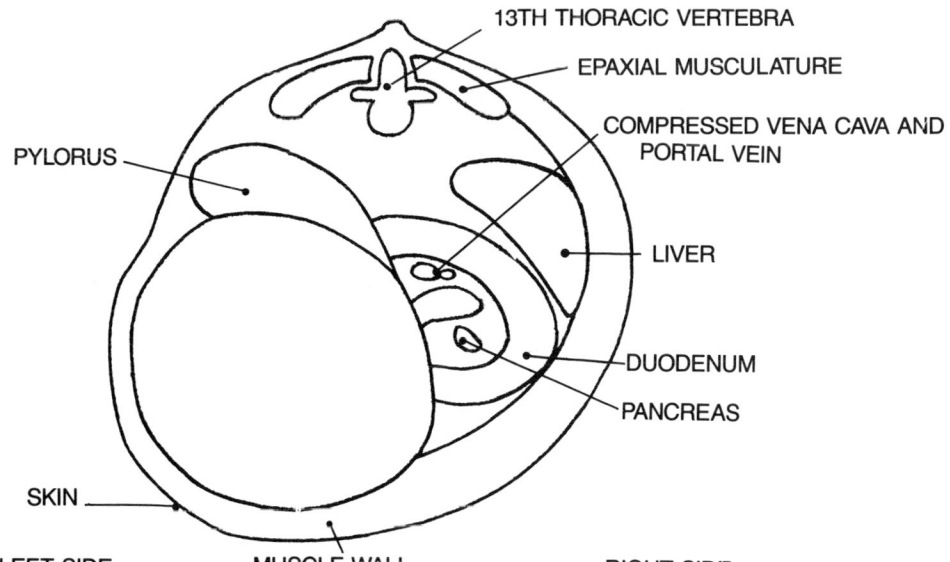

FIGURE 84–5. The same anatomic relationship as in Figure 84–4 but with GDVT.

venous tubing. The tympanic stomach is punctured with a trocar, and the sterile tube hangs pendant over the drapes to allow the trapped gases to escape. The decompressed stomach is untwisted and placed in its normal anatomic position. A large-bore stomach tube is lubricated and is passed into the stomach from the mouth, to further decant gas, fluid, and food. The spleen is examined, and removal may or may not be required. Often a splenic torsion will have occurred and splenectomy is indicated. The splenic venous and arterial blood supply is examined, and if thrombi are present, the spleen is removed. In other cases, the spleen may have

ruptured, necessitating removal. *Worthy of thought is the fact that myocardial-depressant factors are manufactured in the ischemic pancreas and may be stored in the spleen.*[24] Consider removal of the spleen before decompressing the stomach to possibly prevent the showering of the myocardial-depressant factors into the general circulation. The pylorus is then modified to allow rapid and unrestrictive exit of fluid and gas from the stomach.[21, 36]

The abdominal cavity is methodically inspected for abnormalities such as mesenteric suspension irregularities, intestinal serosal tears, hematomas, and ischemic

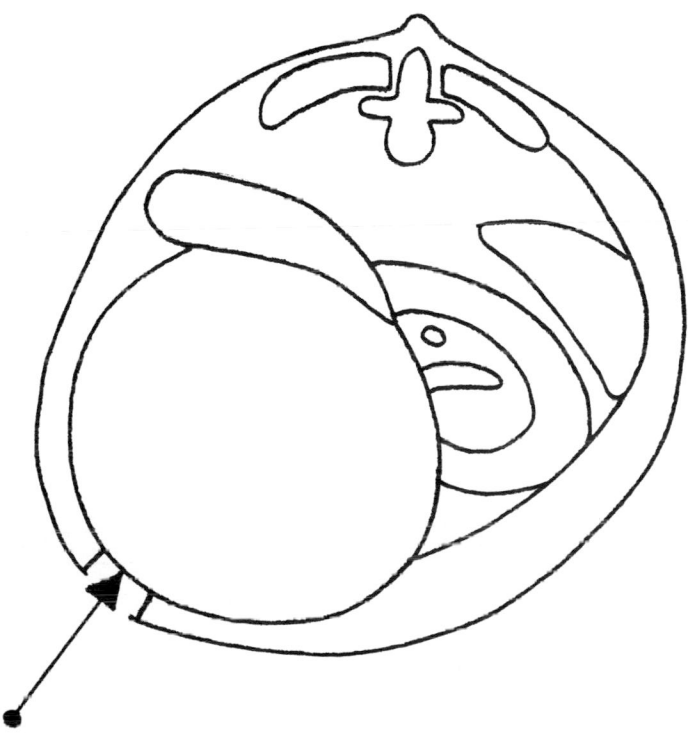

FIGURE 84–6. The first step in the castrostomy procedure. Incise the skin approximately 3 inches vertically. Dissect through the SQ, musculature, and peritoneum. Do not incise the gastric wall at this time.

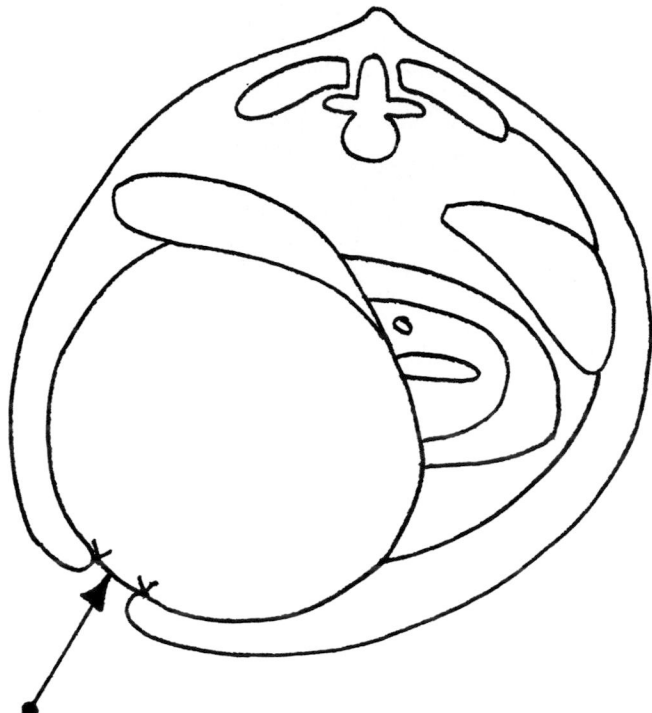

FIGURE 84–7. The second step in the gastrostomy procedure. Using a continuous pattern, suture the skin edge to the seromuscularis gastric wall. A taper point Prolene suture is used to create a watertight seal of the skin to the stomach wall.

areas of the duodenum and stomach wall including the region of the gastroesophageal orifice. The stomach is then permanently affixed to the abdominal wall to prevent recurrence. We employ the permanent abdominal muscular flap gastropexy.[10]

Pyloromyotomy. The muscular valve exiting the stomach is rendered inoperative by either resecting the muscles, as in a pyloromyotomy, or changing the actual orifice relationship, as in a pyloroplasty. Either method offers an enlarged and patent opening exiting the stomach. The risk of peritonitis and death increases as the gastric lumen is invaded. For this reason, we prefer the Fredet-Ramstedt pyloromyotomy over the pyloroplasty. The immediate relief of gastric fluid and entrapped gas is seen as the pylorus is modified. Pyloric surgery affords a rapid exit of fluid, food, and gas and is important in the prevention of recurrence.[21, 36]

Splenectomy. In not every dog is splenectomy necessary. The spleen should be inspected for thrombi and areas of rupture. If in doubt, perform a splenectomy. If there is free hemorrhage in the abdomen, it is vacuumed and discarded; should the PCV drop below 20 per cent, a whole blood transfusion is required. A sterile autotransfusion unit utilizing the free abdominal blood may be recycled and readministered to the patient through a venous catheter.

Decompression. Trocharization is contraindicated due to the risk of organ damage and secondary peritonitis. Probanging a stomach tube past a blocked cardia also must be avoided. Passing plastic tubes and the use of water gavage can also be fatal. However, a rapid, controlled, and effective decompression is mandatory, using either a flexible orogastric tube, a gastrostomy, or a midline celiotomy.

Gastropexy. A number of different gastropexy techniques are effective in preventing recurrence of GDVT. A gastropexy procedure is indicated in all dogs that undergo surgery for GDVT.[10, 28]

Tube gastrostomy, commonly used in the past, is associated with several potential problems. As the gastric lumen is penetrated, postoperative peritonitis may develop and necessitate a second surgical procedure.[42] Refractory peritonitis is a complication that may lead to death. The tube must remain in place for up to ten days to allow time for the formation of adhesions. This aftercare requires additional hospitalization and adequate nursing care to prevent the tube from being prematurely removed by the patient. The Foley catheter's rubber balloon often ruptures due to prolonged

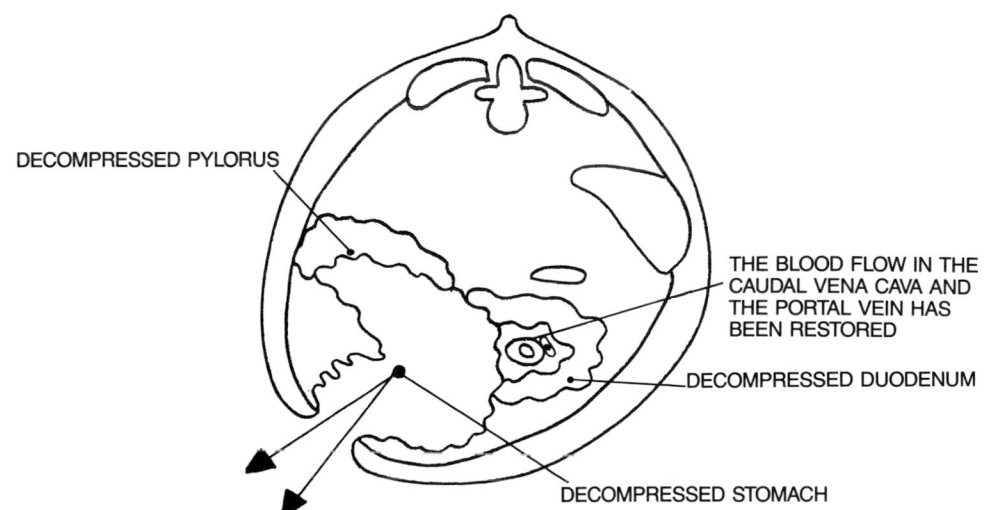

DECOMPRESSED PYLORUS

THE BLOOD FLOW IN THE CAUDAL VENA CAVA AND THE PORTAL VEIN HAS BEEN RESTORED

DECOMPRESSED DUODENUM

DECOMPRESSED STOMACH

FIGURE 84–8. The third step in the gastrostomy procedure. Carefully avoiding the suture line, incise the muscle wall. The stomach is immediately decompressed. The torsion persists. The caudal vena caval and portal circulation is restored.

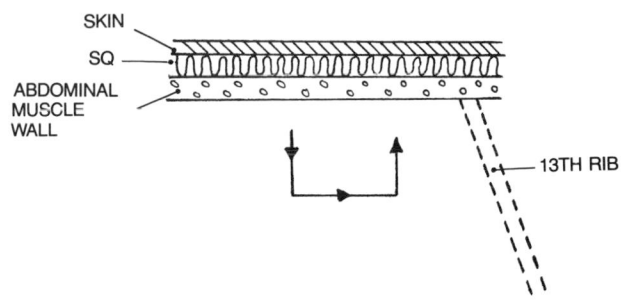

FIGURE 84–9. The first step in the permanent abdominal wall muscular flap gastropexy procedure. Incise the peritoneum and muscle wall in a U-shaped pattern.

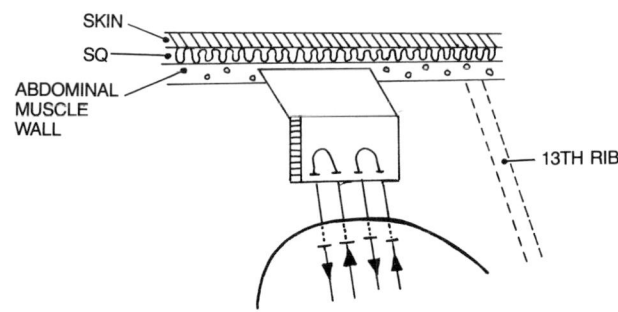

FIGURE 84–11. The third step in the permanent abdominal wall muscular flap gastropexy procedure. Using a taper point 2/0 Prolene suture, place two horizontal mattress sutures through the stomach and abdominal wall. Try not to penetrate the gastric lumen. (See Figure 84–1 for the stomach wall suture placement.)

contact with gastric juices. This allows stomach contents to seep into the abdomen, often causing peritonitis. The circumcostal gastrostomy has resolved most of the potential problems inherent in the tube gastrostomy procedure.[1]

Circumcostal gastropexy does not require penetration of the gastric lumen. Therefore, the risk of iatrogenic peritonitis is reduced markedly. The need for postoperative tube maintenance and extended hospitalization also is alleviated. However, the possibility of iatrogenic pneumothorax due to accidental penetration of the diaphragm does exist. The permanent abdominal wall muscular flap gastropexy technique is an effective means of producing a long-lasting fixation of the pyloric antrum to the body wall (Figures 84–9 to 84–15).[10] This technique, performed easily, does not require penetration of the gastric lumen; therefore, it also reduces the risk of peritonitis and alleviates the need for postoperative tube maintenance and extended hospitalization. Iatrogenic pneumothorax is not a concern when performing a permanent abdominal wall muscular flap gastropexy.

CARDIAC DYSRHYTHMIAS IN GDVT

Cardiac arrhythmias are a frequent finding in dogs with GDVT and contribute significantly to the overall mortality rate observed with the syndrome.[9, 24, 27, 29–31, 37] Electrocardiographic monitoring should be performed on all patients throughout hospitalization. The mechanisms that initiate and maintain these arrhythmias are

varied and include acid-base abnormalities, electrolyte abnormalities, autonomic imbalances, myocardial depressant factors, and myocardial ischemia.[30] Metabolic acidosis and hypokalemia can affect antiarrhythmic therapy.[30] Blood gas determinations allow accurate assessment and determination of proper amounts of bicarbonate supplementation.

To assess potassium levels accurately, immediate laboratory analysis is needed. Hypokalemia should be treated by appropriate intravenous administration of potassium-containing solutions.[14] The use of potassium chloride infusion in the face of hypokalemia reduces the incidence of cardiac arrhythmias and leads to a faster return to oral alimentation for dogs recovering from GDVT surgery.[1] Potassium chloride replacement therapy is indicated during postoperative recovery but must be performed with strict serum potassium electrolyte determinations. The importance of autonomic imbalance in the evolution of cardiac arrhythmias in dogs with GDVT has not been fully ascertained. However, both parasympathetic and sympathetic neural activity can lead to a wide variety of supraventricular and particularly ventricular cardiac arrhythmias frequently observed in dogs with GDVT.[37]

Any explanation advanced for the initiation and maintenance of cardiac arrhythmias associated with GDVT must take into account the predominance of their delayed onset.[37] In humans, myocardial ischemia and infarction trigger rapid arrhythmias. In animals, however,

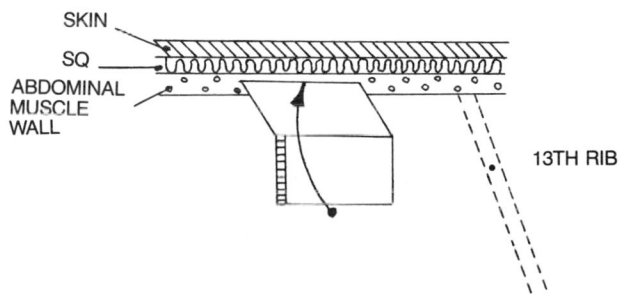

FIGURE 84–10. The second step in the permanent abdominal wall muscular flap gastropexy procedure. Open the peritoneum-muscle flap.

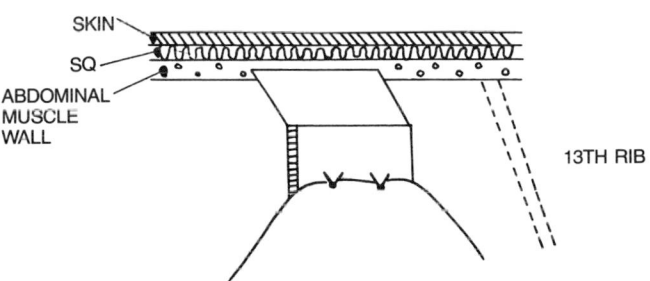

FIGURE 84–12. The fourth step in the permanent abdominal wall muscular flap gastropexy procedure. Tie the mattress sutures. This pattern secures the stomach wall to the edge of the gastrostomy pocket.

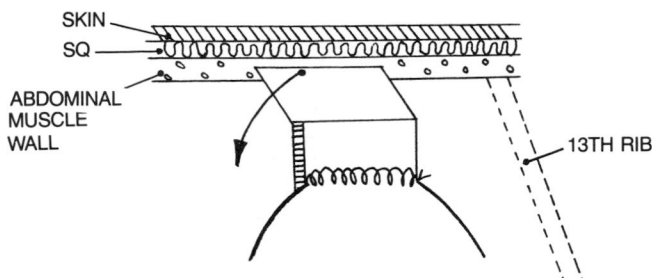

FIGURE 84–13. The fifth step in the permanent abdominal wall muscular flap gastropexy procedure. Using 2/0 Prolene, whip-stitch the gastric wall to the deeper muscle tissue inside the gastrostomy pocket. This pulls the stomach well into the gastrostomy pocket.

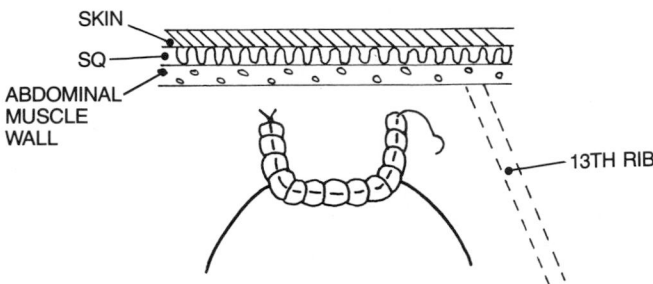

FIGURE 84–15. The seventh step in the permanent abdominal wall muscular flap gastropexy procedure. Using 2/0 Prolene, the flap is closed securely to the stomach wall. This completes the permanent abdominal wall muscular flap gastropexy.

several investigators have indicated that myocardial ischemia and the resulting myocardial cellular damage is followed by a 6- to 12-hour period of normal cardiac rhythm.[38] Thereafter, a 24- to 48-hour period of increased ventricular ectopic activity ensues, during which fatal cardiac dysrhythmias may develop.[38]

As the development of GDVT progresses, mechanical compression of the caudal vena cava and portal vein occurs; this results in reduced venous return, central venous pressure, cardiac output, and arterial blood pressure. These hemodynamic changes could reduce coronary arterial blood flow sufficiently to lead to myocardial ischemia and the development of cardiac arrhythmias. Clinical, experimental, and histologic studies have shown that a direct cause and effect relationship between cardiac arrhythmias and mortality has not been established.[1, 9, 26, 30] It has been shown, however, that cardiac arrhythmias commonly develop in GDVT in dogs, and prompt antiarrhythmic therapy is indicated on the basis of the potentially fatal electric and hemodynamic consequences of these arrhythmias.[9, 10, 30] Most ventricular arrhythmias can be effectively converted with antiarrhythmic therapy consisting of lidocaine, procainamide, and quinidine.[8, 10, 30, 39, 40, 44–47] The antiarrhythmic properties of these drugs are related to their ability to depress membrane responsiveness and excitability, depress cardiac conduction and automaticity, and suppress accelerating ectopic foci.[1, 30]

The usual criteria for initiating antiarrhythmic drug treatment include sustained and nonsustained atrial or ventricular premature contractions, ventricular tachy-

cardia, atrial flutter or fibrillation, and development of an R on T phenomenon.[8, 30, 40]

Although most of the arrhythmias observed in GDVT are life-threatening and require therapy, current literature recommendations suggest that drug therapy administration be delayed until there is electrocardiographic confirmation of these arrhythmias.[38, 44] The rationale behind this approach is the occasional induction of toxic effects (nausea, vomiting, depression, and aggravation of the arrhythmias by the antiarrhythmic agents). The prophylactic utilization of antiarrhythmic agents in dogs with GDVT may be warranted because of the high mortality rate experienced with conservative therapy. The recommended dosages of these drugs must not be exceeded. Ventricular tachycardias associated with GDVT are initially treated with an infusion of lidocaine. Although conversion to normal sinus rhythm in the majority of patients occurs after a single bolus injection of lidocaine, the arrhythmias usually return.[30] For this reason, rapid infusion of lidocaine for a short period followed by constant infusion is indicated. It is essential that constant ECG monitoring occur during this infusion, and if the infusion is continued postoperatively, an ICU nurse must monitor the patient continuously.

When the patient's condition is stable, intravenous antiarrhythmic therapy is replaced with oral administration of procainamide in conjunction with quinidine.[10] Oral administration of procainamide with quinidine is a safer approach to antiarrhythmic therapy, because lower total dosages may be used for each drug and the potential initiation of side effects encountered with therapy is reduced.[39] Oral antiarrhythmic therapy is continued 7 to 14 days postoperatively and then is discontinued. The patient should receive electrocardiographic examinations before the drugs are stopped.

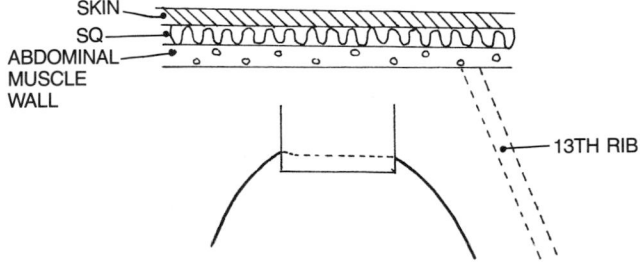

FIGURE 84–14. The sixth step in the permanent abdominal wall muscular flap gastropexy procedure. The peritoneum-muscle flap is closed over the entrapped stomach.

POSTOPERATIVE CARE

Antiarrhythmic Therapy. The immediate postoperative care is extremely important. The surgeon must not relax vigilance postoperatively. As we have emphasized, antiarrhythmic drug therapy must be continued for 7 to 14 days postoperatively, and only then is it stopped if there is no electrocardiographic evidence of arrhythmia.[44]

Feeding. We begin gruel feedings as soon as the patient has recovered. The food is processed in a blender and fed three times daily. Upon discharge, clients are told to divide the regular amount of food into two daily portions. We also advise them to withhold water and strenuous exercise for one hour after feeding.

Fluid Therapy. The intravenous fluids are administered as required but usually are discontinued in 24 hours.

Antibiotics. Cephalexin is dispensed (15 mg/lb PO q12h) for a seven-day period.

RECURRENCE AND PREVENTION

Although no one surgical technique has proven 100 per cent effective in preventing recurrence, decreased recurrence rates have been achieved when multiple procedures were employed.[10] The postsurgical recurrence rates associated with the permanent abdominal wall muscle flap gastropexy and the circumcostal gastropexy techniques compare favorably with recurrence rates reported previously for GDVT.[1, 2, 10, 28, 42–50]

With the etiology of GDVT unresolved, postoperative management often includes a change of dietary regimen.[44] Conventional discharge recommendations include multiple small feedings (twice to three times daily) of moistened softened foodstuffs and restriction of water intake and exercise before and after feeding.

There is no known nonsurgical prevention of GDVT. Many suggestions are given: do not overfeed, do not "roughhouse" immediately after eating, do not allow the pet to consume inordinate amounts of water, do not let the pet jump with a full stomach, and do not allow the pet to consume large amounts of dry meal and then drink water. Most preventions suggested revolve around not allowing the pet to exercise strenuously on a full stomach.

References

1. Lieb, MS and Blass, CE: Gastric dilatation-volvulus in dogs: An update. Comp Cont Ed 11:961, 1984.
2. Todoroff, RJ: Gastric dilatation-volvulus. Comp Cont Ed 2:142, 1979.
3. Matthiesen, DT: The gastric dilatation volvulus complex: Medical and surgical considerations. JAAHA 19:925, 1983.
4. Van Kruiningen, HJ, et al.: Acute gastric dilatation: A review of comparative aspects, by species, and a study in dogs and monkeys. JAAHA 10:294, 1974.
5. Wingfield, WE and Hoffer, RE: Gastric dilatation-torsion complex in the dog. In Bojrab, MJ (ed): Current Techniques in Small Animal Surgery. Philadelphia, Lea and Febiger, 1975, p 112.
6. Greene, RW: Gastric dilatation-torsion (volvulus) complex. Proceedings of the AAHA 43:227, 1976.
7. Strombeck, DR: Acute gastric-dilatation volvulus. In Kirk, RW (ed): Current Veterinary Therapy VII. Philadelphia, WB Saunders, 1980, p 896.
8. Orton, EC: Gastric dilatation-volvulus. In Slatter, DE (ed): Textbook of Veterinary Surgery. Philadelphia, WB Saunders, 1984, p 856.
9. Muir, WW: Gastric dilatation-volvulus in the dog, with emphasis on cardiac arrhythmias. JAVMA 180:739, 1982.
10. Schulman, AJ, Lippincott, CL, et al.: Muscular flap gastropexy: A new surgical technique to prevent recurrences of gastric dilatation-volvulus syndrome. JAAHA 22:339, 1986.
11. Twedt, DC and Wingfield, WE: Diseases of the Stomach. In Ettinger, SJ (ed): Textbook of Veterinary Internal Medicine, 2nd ed. Philadelphia, WB Saunders, 1983, p 1270.
12. Burrows, C: Stomach's electrical activity may cause life-threatening condition in canines. DVM Newsletter, Oct, 1986, p 4.
13. Caywood, D, et al.: Gastric gas analysis in the canine gastric-dilatation-volvulus syndrome. JAAHA 13:459, 1977.
14. Wingfield, WE: In Bojrab, MJ (ed): Pathophysiology in Small Animal Surgery. Philadelphia, Lea and Febiger, 1981, p 107.
15. Baronofsky, I and Wangensteen, OH: Obstruction of splenic vein increases weight of stomach and predisposes to erosion and ulcers. Pro Soc Exp Biol Med 59:234, 1945.
16. Wingfield, WE, et al.: Experimental acute gastric dilatation and torsion in the dog. Venous angiographic alterations seen in gastric dilatation. J Small Anim Pract 16:55, 1975.
17. Merkely, DF, et al.: Experimentally induced acute gastric dilatation in the dog: Cardiopulmonary effects. JAAHA 12:143, 1987.
18. Matheson, NA: Factor in tissue perfusion: The microcirculation in shock. Post Grad Med 45:530, 1969.
19. Lees, GE, et al.: Management of gastric dilatation volvulus and disseminated intravascular coagulation in the dog: A case report. JAAHA 13:463, 1977.
20. Olkay, I, et al.: Reticuloendothelial dysfunction and endotoxemia follow portal vein occlusion. Surgery 75:64, 1974.
21. Bojrab, MJ: Pathophysiology in Small Animal Surgery. Philadelphia, Lea and Febiger, 1981.
22. Wingfield, WE, et al.: Pathophysiology associated with gastric dilatation. JAAHA 12:136, 1976.
23. O'Brien, TR: Radiographic diagnosis of abdominal disorders in dog and cat. Philadelphia, WB Saunders, 1987.
24. Lefer, AM: Role of myocardial depressant factors in shock states. Mod Concepts Cardiac Dis XLII:59, 1973.
25. Matheson, NA: Factors in tissue perfusion. The microcirculation in shock. Postgrad Med Jour 45:530, 1969.
26. Ettinger, SJ: Personal communication, 1988.
27. Hathcock, JT: Radiographic view of choice for the diagnosis of gastric volvulus: The right lateral recumbent view. JAAHA 20:967, 1984.
28. Woolfson, JM and Kostolich, M: Circumcostal gastropexy: Clinical use of the technique in 34 dogs with gastric dilatation-volvulus. JAAHA 22:825, 1086.
29. Muir, WW: Acid-base and electrolyte disturbances in dogs with gastric dilatation-volvulus. JAVMA 181:229, 1982.
30. Muir, WW and Bonagura, JD: Treatment of cardiac arrhythmias in dog with gastric distention-volvulus. JAVMA 184:1366, 1984.
31. Muir, WW and Weisbrode, SE: Myocardial ischemia in dogs with gastric dilatation-volvulus. JAVMA 181:363, 1982.
32. Bojrab, MJ: Pathophysiology in Small Animal Surgery. Philadelphia, Lea and Febiger, 1981.
33. Bojrab, MJ: Current Techniques in Small Animal Surgery. Philadelphia, Lea and Febiger, 1975.
34. Gourley, IM and Vasseur, PB: General Small Animal Surgery. Philadelphia, JB Lippincott, 1985.
35. Slater, DH: Textbook of Small Animal Surgery. Philadelphia, WB Saunders, 1985.
36. Bojrab, MJ (ed): Gastric-dilatation syndrome, pyloromyotomy. Philadelphia, Lea & Febiger, 1975, p 114.
37. Muir, WW: Gastric dilatation-volvulus in the dog, with emphasis on cardiac arrythmias. JAVMA 180:739, 1982.
38. Wingfield, WE, et al.: Pathophysiology of the gastric dilatation complex in ten dogs. J Small Anim Pract 14:735, 1979.
39. Johnson, RG, et al.: Gastric dilatation-volvulus: Recurrence rate following tube gastrostomy. JAAHA 20:33, 1984.
40. Flanders, JA and Harvey, HJ: Results of tube gastrostomy as treatment for gastric volvulus in the dog. JAVMA 12:168, 1976.
41. Fox, SM: Gastric dilatation-volvulus: Results from 31 surgical cases of circumcostal gastropexy vs tube gastrostomy. Calif Vet March/April:8, 1985.
42. MacCoy, DM, et al.: A gastropexy technique for permanent fixation of the pyloric antrum. JAAHA 18:763, 1982.
43. Lieb, MS, et al.: Circumcostal gastropexy for preventing recur-

rence of gastric dilatation-volvulus in the dog: An evaluation of 30 cases. JAVMA 187:245, 1985.

44. Schulman, AJ and Lippincott, CL: Prophylactic treatment of cardiac arrhythmias occuring in dogs with gastric dilatation-volvulus. In press.

45. Lasseter, KC: Treatment of arrhythmias: Basic considerations. Med Clin North Am 55:435, 1971.

46. Ettinger, SJ: Cardiac Arrhythmias. *In* Ettinger, SJ (ed): Textbook of Veterinary Internal Medicine. Philadelphia, WB Saunders, 1983, p 980.

47. Muir, WW and Lipowitz, AJ: Cardiac dysrhythmias associated with gastric dilatation-volvulus in the dog. JAVMA 172:683, 1978.

48. Fallah, AM, et al.: Circumcostal gastropexy in the dog. A preliminary study. Vet Surg 11:9, 1982.

49. Betts, CW, et al.: "Permanent" gastropexy as a measure against gastric volvulus. JAAHA 12:177, 1976.

50. Parks, JL and Greene, RW: Tube gastrostomy for the treatment of gastric volvulus. JAAHA 12:168, 1976.

DRUG INDEX

Generic/Trade	Dosage	Route	Frequency	Description
Sodium bicarbonate	1 mEq/lb	IV	Dosage interval depends on acid-base parameters	Alkalyzing agent
Prednisolone sodium succinate (Solu-Delta-Cortef)	5–10 mg/lb	IV	Dosage interval depends upon response to hypovolemic shock treatment	Corticosteroid
Gentamicin sulfate (Gentacin)	1 mg/lb	IM, SQ	Q12h	Antibiotic
Ampicillin (Polyflex)	5–10 mg/lb	SQ	Q12h	Antibiotic
Cephalexin (Keflex)	15 mg/lb	PO	Q12h	Antibiotic
Lidocaine				
1st bolus	2 mg/lb	IV	Dosage depends upon response to therapy and cardiac status	Antiarrhythmic
2nd bolus	1 mg/lb	IV		
IV infusion		IV		
12–25 μg/lb/min				
Quinidine gluconate	3–10 mg/lb	IM	Once	Antiarrhythmic
Procainamide HCl (Pronestyl)	3–10 mg/lb	PO	Q4–6h	Antiarrhythmic
Procan SR (long-acting)	3–10 mg/lb	PO	Q8h	Antiarrhythmic
Quinidine sulfate	3–10 mg/lb	PO	Q4–6h	Antiarrhythmic
Quinidex (long-acting Quinidine)	3–10 mg/lb	PO	Q8–12h	Antiarrhythmic
Note: If Quinidex is used in combination with Procan, reduce the dosage of each drug to 3 mg/lb				
Potassium chloride	Rate not to exceed 0.02 mEq/lb/hr/IV		Dosage depends upon electrolyte and cardiac status	
Oxymorphone (Numorphan)	0.22 mg/lb	IV to effect	Induction	Analgesic

85 DISEASES OF THE STOMACH

DAVID C. TWEDT and MICHAEL L. MAGNE

ANATOMY

Functional Anatomy

The topographic anatomy of the stomach is divided into five regions: cardia, fundus, body, antrum, and pylorus (Figure 85–1). The *cardia* is the entrance of the intra-abdominal esophagus into the stomach. Left and dorsal to the cardia lies the fundus. When filling with food occurs, the fundus fills first.

The *body* is the second part of the stomach to fill and expand. It is the largest region of the stomach and is most capable of dilatation. Together with the cardia and fundus, the body represents the proximal storage portion of the stomach. This capacity for adaptation, known as receptive relaxation, occurs with little change in intra-gastric pressure. The body also represents an important area for secretion of digestive juices. The concave surface of the lesser curvature forms the gastric angle, referred to as the *incisura angularis*, an anatomic landmark important in endoscopy. A line drawn from the incisura angularis to the greater curvature represents the juncture between the body (proximal) and antrum (distal). This distal segment functions in mechanical digestion and release of the hormone gastrin that, in turn, regulates the release of hydrochloric acid. The antrum will expand with peristaltic contractions and the presence of foodstuffs (chyme).

Located between the antrum and duodenum is an anatomic sphincter, the *pylorus*. This muscular structure functions to limit the size of particles entering the duodenum and prevents gastric reflux of duodenal contents. A layer of circular smooth muscle, several times thicker than the outer longitudinal muscle layer, is present at the pylorus. The pyloric region is actually described as two pyloric loops; a proximal and a distal loop. The antral lumen between the two loops is the pyloric canal. There is some species variation, and in the dog, the proximal pyloric loop is very thin and indistinguishable in the intact stomach; therefore, the last two to three centimeters of the canine antrum is usually designated as the terminal antrum. The muscle bundle of the distal pyloric loop is referred to as the pyloric sphincter.[1]

Proximally, the circular muscle fibers form a weak gastroesophageal sphincter. This sphincter is augmented on the greater curvature by transversely running inner oblique fibers. Movement of the stomach is restricted. The gastroesophageal junction is fixed where it passes through the diaphragm. Pyloric movement is restricted by the gastrohepatic ligament and common bile duct. Additional mesenteric attachments include the greater and lesser omentum.

The principal arterial supply to the stomach is derived from the celiac artery. This artery divides into the hepatic, left gastric, and splenic arteries, with each contributing arterial flow to the stomach. Satellite veins to the arteries of the stomach empty into either the gastroduodenal vein on the right or the splenic vein on the left. Both the splenic and gastroduodenal veins contribute to the portal vein just caudal to the hilus of the liver. Lymphatic drainage from the stomach eventually enters the right or left hepatic lymph node. The left hepatic lymph node receives drainage after passage through the splenic and gastric nodes. The right hepatic node receives drainage from the stomach via the duodenal node.

Parasympathetic innervation of the stomach is supplied by the vagal nerves, which stimulate motility of the stomach as well as secretion of acid, pepsin, and gastrin. Vagal fibers are predominantly afferent.[2] Sym-

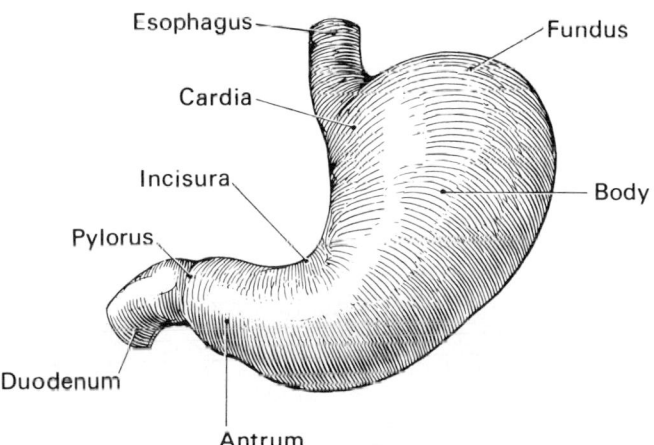

FIGURE 85–1. Diagram of the dog's stomach. The five regions of the stomach are the cardia, fundus, body, antrum, and pylorus. The incisura or gastric angle is an important endoscopic landmark.

pathetic innervation of the stomach is both efferent and afferent and arises from the celiac plexus. In the dog's cardia, sympathetic α-receptors are stimulatory and β-receptors inhibitory, whereas both receptors are inhibitory in other parts of the stomach.[3]

Microscopic Anatomy

The gastric mucosal surface is composed of mucus-secreting columnar epithelial cells. These lining cells extend into numerous invaginations in the mucosal surface, forming gastric pits. At the base of the gastric pits are mitotic foci that renew desquamated surface cells approximately once every one to three days.[4] These cells produce a layer of mucus that lubricates and protects the gastric mucosa. This mucosal cell layer and mucous coat forms the basis of the gastric mucosal barrier that resists hydrochloric acid and digestive enzymes. Three types of glandular regions are found in the stomach: the cardiac, fundic (gastric), and pyloric regions.[5] The gastric glands within each region open into the base of the gastric pits and extend deep into the mucosa (Figure 85–2).

Cardiac Gland Region. Cardiac glands are found in a narrow zone around the cardia, are composed of mucous epithelial cells, and function in secreting mucus for lubrication.

Fundic Gland Region. The fundic gland region comprises the largest area, including the fundus and body of the stomach. These glands function in digestion by producing hydrochloric acid and pepsinogen. The four cell types comprising the fundic glands are chief cells, parietal cells, mucous cells, and argentaffin cells. The chief cells are in highest concentration at the base of the gland and produce pepsinogen. Parietal cells (oxyntic cells) are scattered throughout the midportion of the gland and are responsible for hydrochloric acid secretion. Argentaffin cells are endocrine cells scattered throughout the gastric glands, which contain granules that hold serotonin, a potent vasoconstrictor substance. The exact function of these cells is still unknown. Mucous cells are relatively few in number and are found in the neck region of the glands.

Pyloric Gland Region. The pyloric glands are found in the antral region of the stomach. The major cell type is the mucous cell. In the midgland region are many gastrin-containing cells (G cells), which are pyramidal in shape and extend long processes into the gastric lumen to detect the nature and pH of the gastric contents. Upon stimulation, the hormone gastrin, a potent stimulator for hydrochloric acid secretions, is released. Below the glands lies the lamina propria, the connective tissue portion of the gastric mucosal layer. Scattered throughout both the lamina propria and submucosa are numerous mast cells, which act as one of the mediators of gastric acid secretion.[6]

PHYSIOLOGY

The stomach serves three important functions. First, it provides an adjustable reservoir by adapting quickly

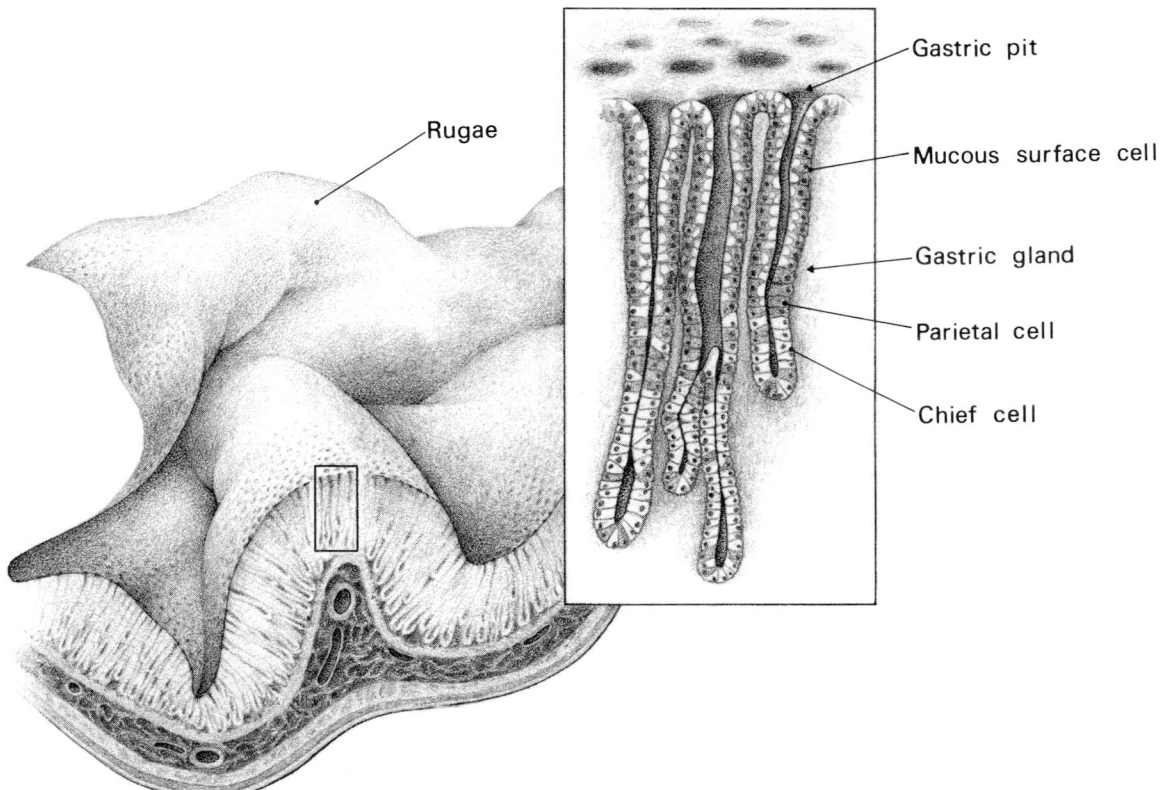

FIGURE 85–2. Cross-sectional anatomy of the dog's stomach, with a microscopic diagram of the gastric glands.

and markedly in volume with the intake of food, without the development of excessive intragastric pressure; second, gastric contents are mixed with gastric secretions; and third, the gastric contents are gradually passed into the intestinal tract for final digestion and absorption.

Gastric Filling

To a certain degree the empty stomach simply unfolds to accommodate a part of the ingested volume. This phenomenon is known as adaptive (receptive) relaxation and is the basis of the storage function of the stomach. In order to maintain constant intragastric pressure, gastric smooth muscle tone changes with varying volumes. This ability to maintain basal intragastric pressure appears to result from two centrally mediated vagal reflexes. The first is receptive relaxation that is initiated when there is inhibition of tonic contraction of the proximal stomach in response to swallowing. The other is gastric accommodation, a local reflex occurring when gastric distention produces activation of vagal relaxatory fibers. The gastric response to activation of the relaxatory fibers consists of a prolonged relaxation, primarily affecting the body and fundic regions. Gastric accommodation may also be regulated by humoral factors.

The capacity of the stomach varies from 0.5 to 8 liters in the dog. Greater ranges in relative size are noted in puppies than in adult dogs.[7] A capacity of 45 to 115 ml/lb (100 to 250 ml/kg) of body weight has been reported by Neumayer and cited by Ellenberger and Baum.[8]

Gastric Secretion

Acid Secretion. The stomach secretes hydrochloric acid, other electrolytes, pepsinogen, gastrin, and mucus into the lumen. These secretions are regulated by neural and hormonal stimulants and inhibitors.

Hydrochloric Acid Production. Parietal cells secrete hydrochloric acid into the gastric lumen. Hydrogen ion concentration in the gastric juice is three million times greater than that in the blood and tissues. Although the electrical and biochemical events that result in hydrochloric acid secretion are not completely understood, the tremendous increase in hydrogen ion concentration represents a large gradient for the ion to be transported against, which concomitantly requires considerable energy. Secretion of one liter of hydrochloric acid at a concentration of 160 mEq/L requires 1500 calories of energy.

For each hydrogen ion secreted, a molecule of CO_2 derived from arterial blood or mucosal metabolism is converted to bicarbonate, which ultimately enters the intestinal fluid. Parietal cells contain a high concentration of the enzyme carbonic anhydrase, which catalyzes this conversion. The amount of bicarbonate entering the blood during acid secretion is directly proportional to the amount of acid secreted, and results in transient alkalosis referred to as the *alkaline tide*. The three major stimulants of gastric-acid secretion are acetylcholine, gastrin, and histamine.[9] It has been debated whether each agent stimulates the parietal cell directly or whether one acts as the final common mediator for the others. A complex interaction between many neural and humoral factors dictates secretion at controlled rates and at the proper time. The mechanisms that control secretion have their effects at three sequential times during digestion: the cephalic phase, gastric phase, and intestinal phase. The *cephalic phase* of gastric secretion is stimulated by the anticipation, sight, taste, smell, and passage of food through the oropharynx. Cortical areas of the brain mediate this phase through efferent vagal fibers, which terminate on gastrin-secreting G cells, parietal cells, and chief cells. Thus, the vagus stimulates release of gastrin, hydrochloric acid, and pepsinogen. The *gastric phase* is the most important determinant of gastric secretion and is initiated via gastric distention and by digested proteins. Distention of either the parietal gland area (fundus and body) or the pyloric gland area results in activity of the G cells and parietal cells, as do the cephalic vagal reflexes.[9]

The introduction of protein foods into the small intestine produces a distinct acid secretory response. In this *intestinal phase*, three components can be discerned: direct stimulation of acid secretion, augmentation of maximal response to histamine and gastrin, and release of antral gastrin.[10]

The role of histamine in gastric secretion is not completely understood. Usually, histamine is not present in body fluids in any significant quantity. In dogs and cats, histamine is contained in eosinophils and mast cells of the gastric mucosa.[11] Some histamine escapes the gastric mucosa and enters the gastric juice. From this observation came the discovery of H_2-receptors and a correlation between histamine output and the output of gastric juice in dogs during psychic and vagal stimulation. Histamine output occurs mainly during the early phases of gastric secretion.[6] The H_2-receptor is visualized to be on the basal membrane of the parietal cells. When occupied by histamine, and in the presence of acetylcholine, gastrin acts to stimulate maximal acid secretion. If all receptor sites are occupied, and then one site is blocked (i.e., by atropine, blocking acetylcholine, or cimetidine, blocking histamine), stimulation of the other receptors will result in less than maximum response (Figure 85–3). Thus, the H_2-receptor on the parietal cell is a major controller of the cell's hydrogen ion production and use of H_2-receptor antagonists makes them effective agents for control of gastric secretion.

Electrolyte Secretion. Chloride, potassium, and sodium are important electrolytes found in significant concentrations in gastric juices. As a result of electrolyte secretion, the mucosal surface of the stomach is electrically negative when compared with the serosal surface. Although the specific cell responsible for generation of this negative potential has not been identified, the potential appears to be generated primarily at the luminal cell border. The active transport of chloride ions from the intracellular space against both concentration and electrical gradients appears to be the principal source of the potential difference. During secretion of acid, proton (hydrogen ion) secretion is coupled with secretion of an equivalent amount of chloride ions; therefore, the potential does not change.

Sodium and hydrogen ion concentration in gastric

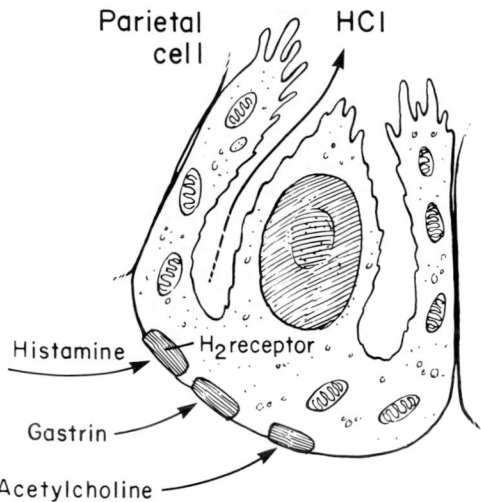

FIGURE 85–3. The factors stimulating hydrochloric acid secretion by the parietal cell. Adjacent mast cells release histamine, stimulating the H₂-receptors. Gastrin and vagal stimulation also mediate receptors for acid production.

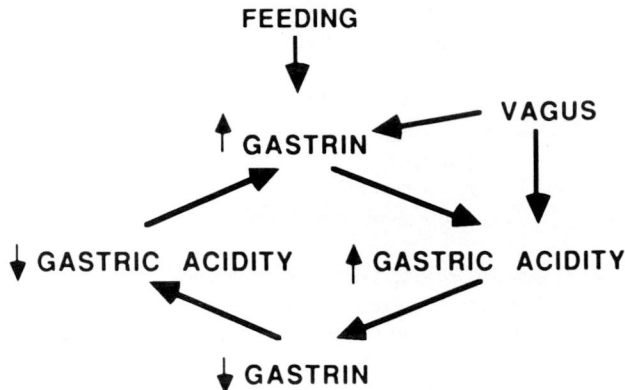

FIGURE 85–4. Regulation of circulating gastrin concentrations resulting from various feedback inhibition loops.

juices varies inversely. The basal membrane of the epithelial cell is highly permeable to chloride and less permeable to sodium. As the intracellular concentrations of sodium and chloride are lower than extracellular fluid, both ions diffuse into the cell. Sodium is then actively pumped out of the cell.

Potassium concentration in gastric secretions is two to four times greater than that in plasma. As gastric secretion rates increase, the potassium in the juices increases, but after a prolonged period the potassium in gastric juices falls, presumably because intracellular potassium is depleted. Most potassium in the gastric juices is derived from intracellular stores. Depletion of these stores is often not reflected in a lowering of plasma potassium.

Pepsin. Pepsinogen is the inactive precursor to pepsin, the principal proteolytic enzyme of gastric juices. The chief cell in the fundic region stores most of the pepsinogens. Pepsinogen is secreted into the gastric lumen, and its secretin is increased by the same stimulants of acid secretion, with the major exception that secretion inhibits acid secretion and stimulates pepsinogen. In the presence of an acid pH, pepsinogens are autocatalytically converted to pepsin by the cleavage of several small peptides. Pepsin is active at an acid pH and irreversibly inactivated at a neutral or slightly alkaline pH. Thus, the proteolytic activity of pepsin ceases when chyme leaves the stomach and enters the more neutral duodenum.

Mucus. Gastric mucosal cells are coated with a gelatinous material called gastric mucus, which is composed of glycoproteins, proteins, and carbohydrates. Stimulation of mucus secretion occurs in response to local mucosal irritation and cholinergic stimulation. In cats, secretin and pentagastrin also stimulate mucus secretion.[12] Mucus is assumed to provide lubrication to gastric contents and protection against physical irritants. Mucus provides little impediment to the movement of water and electrolytes, nor is protection afforded against gastric acid or the proteolytic activity of pepsin. Some components of mucus inhibit pepsin activity, but they

are not effective in the concentrations and pH ranges of the secreting stomach. Mucus has some buffering capacity, which provides some neutralization of acid, but this is negligible during active acid secretion.

Gastrin. G cells synthesize gastrin peptides and release the hormones into the circulation when appropriately stimulated and are numerous in the gastric antrum of the dog. In the canine duodenal bulb there are gastrin-containing cells, but none are found distal to the major duodenal papilla.[13] Distribution of G cells in the cat is similar to that in the dog.

The regulation of circulating gastrin concentrations is best noted in terms of a basic feedback inhibition loop (Figure 85–4). When gastrin concentrations rise, gastric parietal cells are stimulated to secrete acid. When the antral mucosa is bathed in acid, further release of gastrin is inhibited. Feeding is a most important regulator of gastrin release. Partially digested proteins, amino acids, distention of the antrum or fundus, and calcium are known to cause gastrin release in the dog.[14–16] In the dog, serum gastrin levels increase to a peak of about 160 pg/ml after eating. Actions of gastrin that occur at this physiologic level include acid secretion, pepsin secretion, increased mucosal blood flow, and trophic actions. Other actions require much higher levels (Table 85–1).

The kidneys are a major site of metabolism and removal of gastrin from the circulation. Other organs, including the small intestine and liver, also participate in the metabolism of gastrin.

Gastric Motility and Emptying

Motility of the stomach has two functions: mixing and grinding and timely evacuation of gastric contents into the intestine. The stomach can be physiologically divided into proximal and distal motor regions. The proximal

TABLE 85–1. ACTIONS OF GASTRIN ON THE STOMACH

Increases acid, electrolyte, and water secretion
Increases pepsin secretion
Increases smooth muscle contraction of the stomach and lower
　esophageal sphincter
Increases blood flow
Inhibits pyloric sphincter contraction and gastric emptying

stomach consists of the fundus and upper body, which acts as a reservoir as well as regulating emptying of liquids. Motility of the proximal stomach is that of slow, sustained contractions that generate a basal gastric pressure. It is this basal pressure gradient that is responsible for propelling liquids into the duodenum; little contribution is required from the distal stomach.

The distal region of the stomach includes the distal body, the antrum, and pylorus, which together function as a gastric grinder, breaking down solid particles to a size of 2.0 mm or less. Digestible solids are emptied from the stomach only when they have been reduced to an essentially liquefied form. This process is referred to as *trituration* and results from strong distal gastric peristaltic waves that increase in amplitude and velocity as they move distally. Circular rings of contraction propel solids toward the pylorus. Liquids and small particles (<2.0 mm) pass through the open pylorus, while larger solids are ground by the peristaltic wave and then retropelled orally, where this process is repeated.

The electrical and mechanical activities of the distal stomach differ from those of the proximal stomach. Located in smooth muscle cells of the greater curvature is an intrinsic gastric pacemaker that generates the normal distal gastric electric activity. Slow cyclic electrical potential changes referred to as pacesetter potentials arise from this intrinsic pacemaker and are propagated distally as a depolarizing event. These pacesetter potentials occur at a rate of about five per minute in the dog (Figure 85–5).[17] Pacesetter potentials determine the frequency and velocity of gastric contractions and do not initiate them. Muscle contractions result when there is a rapid change in the electric potential, referred to as an *action potential*. The greater the amplitude and duration of the action potentials, the larger the contraction. The pacesetter potentials determine the rate, direction, and velocity of propagation of contractions, while the action potentials determine the strength of contractions. The onset of an action or spike potential is regulated in part by ambient neural and/or hormonal input that favors depolarization of the circular muscle at a particular point in time.

The pylorus has been naively regarded as a muscular sphincter that opens and closes to regulate emptying. The pylorus, in fact, has little sphincter activity, with minimal or no role in regulating gastric emptying of liquids. It is important in preventing large food particles from entering the duodenum as well as reflux of duodenal contents.[18] The pyloric canal is frequently open and only closes simultaneously with contraction of the terminal antrum. The pyloric segment is richly supplied by both excitatory and inhibitory nerves. Excitatory responses lead to only a brief contraction of the pyloric segment. Occasionally, nervous stimulation results in a decrease in basal tension but without complete relaxation.

Emptying of indigestible solids occurs during the fasted state. Strong peristaltic activity, which begins in the stomach and migrates through the small intestine, is called the migrating motor complex (MMC) or interdigestive housekeeper contractions. These cycles occur approximately every two hours and may be mediated by the hormone motilin.[19, 20]

Three main factors control gastric motility and emptying: composition or physiochemical properties of the meal, neural control, and hormonal control. Liquids leave the stomach in a linear fashion that decreases in a manner that is exponential and is proportional to the volume present in the stomach. Solids have a tendency to empty once titrated with liquids in a more direct linear fashion. Emptying is inversely related to the osmolality, acidity, and viscosity of the contents, as well as protein and fat components.[21] The nutritive density (Kcal/ml), and not the initial volume, determines the rate of gastric emptying. The caloric density is also important in that isocaloric amounts of proteins, carbohydrates, and fats all leave the stomach at similar rates.[22]

Neural pathways involve both vagal and sympathetic fibers. Intrinsic control within the stomach may also be related to the effects of various locally released neurotransmitters. Several hormones can influence gastric motility, but only gastrin appears to have a physiologic effect retarding gastric emptying.

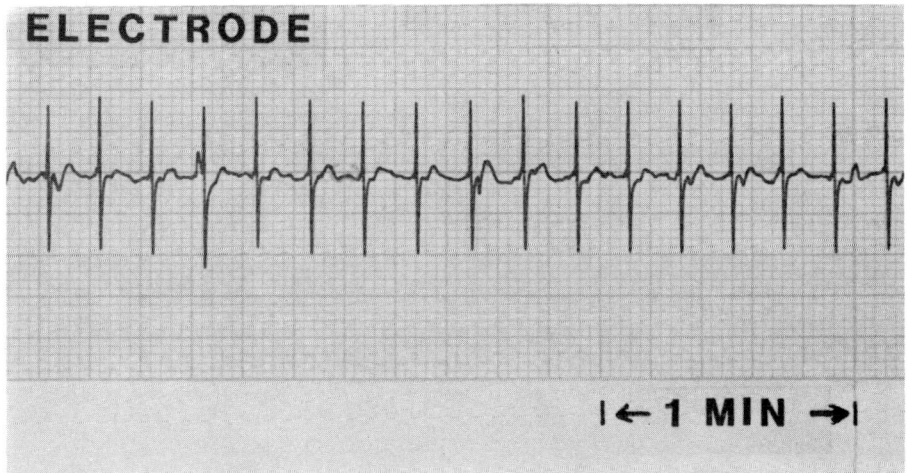

FIGURE 85–5. A representation of simultaneous recordings of gastric myoelectric pacesetter potentials measured by gastric serosal electrodes and gastric mechanical activity measured by gastric serosal strain gauges in a dog. (Courtesy of Dr. Jean Hall, Colorado State University, Fort Collins, CO.)

ELECTRODE

I← 1 MIN →I

CLINICAL EVALUATION

History. The history, taken in a chronological order, helps the clinician localize the disease condition, determine severity of the disease, and decide whether further diagnostic tests or merely symptomatic therapy is required.

Vomiting is the principal clinical sign of gastric disease. It is not, however, synonymous with gastric disease and may be associated with many conditions not involving the stomach. When presented with the complaint of vomiting, it is imperative that the clinician obtain a description of the vomiting episode to adequately differentiate vomiting from regurgitation associated with esophageal disease or coughing and expulsion of phlegm associated with respiratory disease. Vomiting is preceded by a period of nausea, with licking of the lips, salivation, or repeated attempts at swallowing. This is followed by retching or forceful simultaneous diaphragmatic and abdominal contractions, and, with the head lowered, expulsion of the gastric contents. Regurgitation is more passive, lacks retching, and results in the loss of undigested esophageal contents through gravity and increased intrathoracic pressure. Vomiting reported as a forceful or projectile episode, often following shortly after eating, suggests pyloric outflow obstruction. Gastric volvulus or dilatation results in frequent, nonproductive retching, with a rapidly distending abdomen.

In addition to a complete description of the vomiting episodes, it is essential to determine in chronological order the duration and frequency of the episodes as well as any association with feeding or drinking. Acute gastritis often has a sudden onset with numerous vomiting episodes, whereas in chronic gastritis the vomiting may be as infrequent as once every few days.

It is equally important to obtain a complete description of the amount, color, and consistency of the vomitus, and whether it has changed since the onset of vomiting. If the vomitus consists of food, the degree of digestion is noted, thus suggesting the length of time it has remained in the stomach. Vomitus may contain mucus and fluid from gastric and swallowed salivary secretions. Yellow or green-stained vomitus indicates intestinal reflux of bile into the stomach or vomiting of duodenal contents. Fresh blood from gastric bleeding may be present as small red flecks or large blood clots. Blood that has remained in the stomach for some time becomes partially digested and appears to have a brown, "coffee grounds" consistency. The presence of blood in the vomitus signifies serious gastric disease.

Other signs that may occur with gastric disease include nausea, belching, polydipsia, and pica. Melena, or black tarry stools, occurs with upper gastrointestinal bleeding and may imply gastric disease. Coughing may suggest aspiration pneumonia resulting from vomiting. Some owners report increased bowel sounds (borborygmus) or "growling" of the stomach. Animals with gastric pain may assume a position of relief ("praying position"), with the rear legs elevated.[23]

The anamnesis should include environmental factors such as possible exposure to toxins, garbage, or bones, which may precipitate vomiting. Many drugs cause gastric disease, and medication history should be recorded. The chewing and playing nature of young animals makes the possibility of foreign body ingestion a constant concern. Careful questioning for that possibility should always be included in the history.

Physical Examination

The physical examination of an animal with suspected gastric disease should include a complete review of all body systems with careful notation of the animal's hydration, since serious fluid and electrolyte depletion may result in the vomiting animal.

Normally the stomach cannot be palpated, because it lies cradled within the rib cage. Palpation is possible only when the stomach is distended with gas or food and extends past the caudal ribs. The stomach of small dogs and cats is often easier to palpate, and in some cases the fingers can be pushed under the rib cage and the stomach palpated. Palpation of the cranial abdomen may be facilitated by elevating the front legs, allowing the abdominal contents to fall caudally.

Pain on palpation in the region of the stomach is an inconsistent finding with gastric disease. The gas-distended stomach of the gastric dilatation-volvulus syndrome can be balloted and percussed as an air-filled density. Abdominal auscultation may reveal increased bowel sounds that occur from gastrointestinal motility causing movement of gas over fluid. The strongest and loudest bowel sounds generally originate from the stomach. An empty stomach is usually silent but becomes vocal with fluid and gas.[24] Increased bowel sounds may occur in some gastric disease conditions.

Physical examination of the gastrointestinal system is not complete without a rectal examination. The presence of melena suggests high gastrointestinal bleeding, possibly occurring from the stomach.

Laboratory Findings

Few biochemical and hematologic alterations are consistently associated with diseases of the stomach. Gastric lesions can occur secondary to other diseases, and laboratory testing is required to rule out these conditions. Acute gastric disease is usually self-limiting and often requires no laboratory support, while conditions such as pyloric obstruction result in serious fluid, electrolyte, acid base, and biochemical abnormalities in which laboratory support is essential. Indications for laboratory testing are based on history, clinical findings, and past clinical experience. The dehydrated, debilitated, and critical patient or one with a chronic history should have laboratory support.

Minimum laboratory tests include the hematocrit (PCV) and total solids (total protein). These two simple tests reflect the approximate hydration state of the animal. With fluid loss from vomiting and inadequate fluid intake, dehydration occurs and is reflected by a rise in PCV and total solids. A normal PCV in a dehydrated animal with an elevated total solids suggests pre-existing anemia.

A complete blood count (CBC) also provides useful information. Most animals vomiting from gastric disease show a stress leukogram (mature neutrophilia, lymphopenia, eosinopenia). A vomiting animal lacking a stress leukogram and with a lymphocytosis and eosinophilia should suggest the possibility of adrenocortical insufficiency (Addison's disease). Leukopenia might suggest a viral etiology. An increased total eosinophil count may occur with gastrointestinal parasites, eosinophilic gastritis, or allergic conditions. Anemia from blood loss in gastric disease is characterized by regeneration with reticulocytosis, nucleated red blood cells, anisocytosis, and polychromasia. Chronic gastrointestinal blood loss eventually results in iron deficiency anemia with microcytic hypochromic red blood cell indices. Biochemical profiles and urinalysis should be evaluated to exclude systemic causes of gastric disease. Common conditions such as liver disease, uremia, and pancreatitis are easily ruled out on most biochemical profiles.

Vomiting from gastric disease may result in electrolyte depletion and acid-base abnormalities. Substantial losses of water, chloride, sodium, and, to a lesser degree, hydrogen and potassium, result through vomiting. Traditionally, vomiting has been associated with metabolic alkalosis resulting from loss of gastric acid. Clinically, however, the majority of vomiting small animals with acid-base abnormalities have metabolic acidosis. Acidosis occurs from loss of fluid and electrolytes, resulting in extracellular fluid volume contraction with minimal loss of acid. The normal empty stomach has negligible basal acid secretion, and when hydrogen ions are actively secreted, there is a transient extracellular alkalosis. This is normally corrected by equivalent loss of bicarbonate through bile and pancreatic juices. In the vomiting state, an acid deficit does not occur, owing to simultaneous loss of refluxed alkaline-rich duodenal fluid and to reabsorption of hydrogen and chloride ions that pass from the stomach into the intestine. Hypokalemia frequently occurs in vomiting patients and results predominantly from urinary losses and, to a lesser extent, through losses in gastric juices.

Metabolic alkalosis is uncommon but can be precipitated by a net loss in hydrogen ions occurring from frequent and profuse vomiting or pyloric outflow obstruction. Gastric alkalosis is perpetuated through chloride depletion, contraction of the extracellular volume, and hypokalemia.[25]

In the normal animal, most of the sodium and bicarbonate entering the kidney is reabsorbed. When plasma bicarbonate rises and the capacity for renal absorption is exceeded, the excess bicarbonate escapes in the urine, resulting in an increased urine pH. Urinary bicarbonate excretion continues until homeostasis is again achieved. Metabolic alkalosis may, however, be perpetuated when renal bicarbonate absorption occurs concurrently with elevated plasma bicarbonate levels. This can result from contracted extracellular volume and chloride depletion. With loss of salt and water, the effective arterial blood volume contracts, resulting in increased stimulation for proximal nephron reabsorption of sodium. Sodium is reabsorbed with the anion chloride; if chloride levels are reduced, then another anion, bicarbonate, is reabsorbed to maintain electrical neutrality. Thus, extracellular fluid depletion, especially when associated with hypochloremia, results in inadequate urinary bicarbonate excretion, leading to or maintaining a state of metabolic alkalosis.

Potassium deficiency often occurs with metabolic alkalosis. This deficiency may result from etiologic factors that caused hydrogen and chloride losses (e.g., vomiting), from renal loss of potassium, and through increased aldosterone secretion secondary to volume depletion. Loss of cellular potassium also causes a shift of extracellular hydrogen ions (derived from carbonic acid) into cells, producing an increase in extracellular bicarbonate and thus perpetuation of the metabolic alkalosis.

Renal potassium wasting occurs when there is a disparity between the availability of reabsorbable anion (chloride) in the glomerular filtrate and the simultaneous need to conserve body sodium (Figure 85–6).[26] In these conditions, sodium-hydrogen exchange, as well as sodium-potassium exchange in the distal tubule, are accelerated. With severe hypokalemia, sodium reabsorption occurs only by exchange with hydrogen ions. When metabolic alkalosis occurs in conjunction with renal bicarbonate reabsorption and sodium hydrogen exchange, a paradoxical aciduria exists.[27]

The stool should be examined for evidence of gastrointestinal parasites or upper gastrointestinal bleeding. Melena may be the consequence of severe gastric bleeding, while mild gastric hemorrhage is often not evident grossly. The stool can be evaluated for occult blood by using Hematest tablets. Animals eating meat protein diet may show a false-positive occult test and should be put on a meat-free diet several days prior to the test.

Gastric Fluid Analysis. Analysis of gastric contents may offer further information in evaluation of the animal

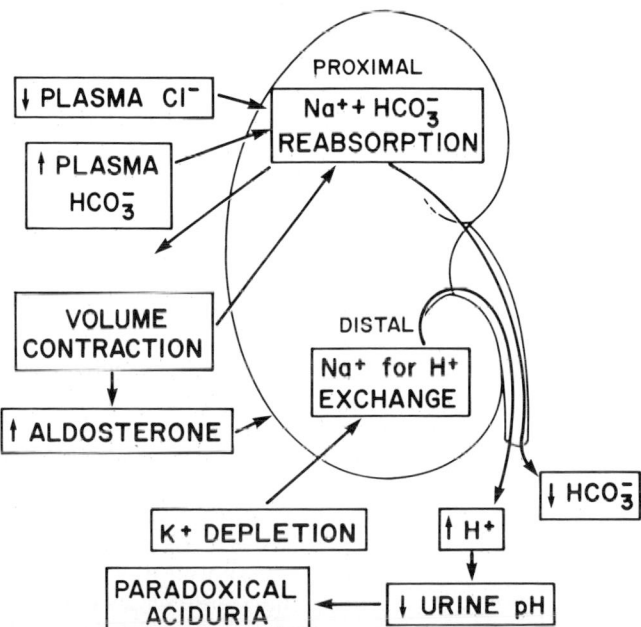

FIGURE 85–6. Renal mechanism for perpetuating a metabolic alkalosis from hypochloremia and hypokalemia of gastric origin. Proximal tubular reabsorption of bicarbonate occurs with sodium when chloride levels are low, and distal tubular sodium reabsorption is exchanged for hydrogen when potassium levels are low. (From Twedt, DC and Grauer, GF: Fluid Therapy for Gastrointestinal, Pancreatic and Hepatic Disorders. Vet Clin North Am 12, 1982.)

with gastric disease. In addition to gross physical examination of the vomitus, certain laboratory tests can be performed; samples of vomitus or fluid collected by aspiration during endoscopy or by placement of a gastric tube are analyzed.

Normal gastric contents of a fasted animal should be clear, with small amounts of mucus and saliva. The pH of gastric fluid in the fasted animal approaches neutrality. With stimulation of gastric acid secretion, the pH of gastric contents may fall to a level of two or less. The pH of vomitus serves as an indication of its origin. With regurgitation from esophageal disease, the pH will usually be alkaline. Duodenal reflux causing bile contamination of gastric juice will also raise the pH of the vomitus.

Microscopic examination of sediment from a centrifuged sample may reveal red blood cells, white blood cells, epithelial cells, bacteria, parasites, foreign material, or food particles. Due to the acidity of gastric juice, only nuclear remnants of cellular elements may remain. In cases of suspected neoplasia, gastric lavage may retrieve neoplastic cells. Normal saline is instilled in the fasted stomach via stomach tube and syringe. The solution is vigorously agitated prior to retrieval. The fluid is collected, centrifuged, and the sediment examined microscopically for neoplastic cells.

The feline gastric nematode *Ollulanus tricuspis* has been associated with chronic vomiting and gastritis.[28] Detection of the parasite is made by examining the gastric fluid followed by either a Baermann technique or straining the contents and examination using a $40\times$ or dissecting microscope.[29] The administration of xylazine (1.0 mg/lb or 2.2 mg/kg IM) to cats stimulates vomiting and is a suggested means of collecting gastric secretions for analysis.

Radiology

Radiology is an important diagnostic tool for evaluating the stomach. Gastric position, shape, intraluminal radiopaque foreign bodies, gastric wall abnormalities, and gastric emptying can be demonstrated radiographically.

When possible, animals should be fasted at least 12 hours before abdominal films are taken. Routine films are taken in two views (ventrodorsal and lateral). A radiograph taken in right lateral recumbency will usually show fluid in the pyloric antrum and gas in the gastric body, while a left lateral radiograph will usually demonstrate gas in the pyloric antrum. In certain instances, other views may be required to demonstrate suspected gastric abnormalities. The normal fasted stomach should be free from ingesta, containing only small amounts of fluid from salivary and gastric secretions and a variable amount of swallowed gas. Radiographic evidence of apparent gastric ingesta in a fasted animal should suggest a foreign body, gastric outflow obstruction, or gastric motility disorder.

Gastric size, shape, and location can usually be evaluated on routine abdominal radiographs. Changes in gastric position and shape are usually due to extragastric masses, organomegaly, or gastric wall lesions. The mu-

cosal surface and character of the rugal folds should be noted; however, these are difficult to assess on routine films. Complete evaluation of luminal surfaces requires contrast and distention of the stomach.

Contrast studies are performed in animals with chronic signs of gastric disease and negative routine films to confirm a suspected gastric lesion or foreign body, to identify gastric position, or to evaluate gastric emptying. Prior to contrast studies, routine films and a laboratory data base should be obtained.

Negative Contrast Study. A negative contrast study of the stomach is performed using either air or carbon dioxide. A stomach tube is passed into the stomach, and gas is introduced until the stomach is moderately distended. This is an inexpensive and easy method of outlining suspected intraluminal foreign bodies or evaluating gastric wall thickness.

Positive Contrast Study. A positive contrast study employs a radiopaque contrast material, usually barium sulfate. Commercially prepared micropulverized contrast agents (30 per cent W/V) give consistent homogeneous gastric filling. The suggested dosage, administered by stomach tube, is 4 to 6 cc/lb (8 to 12 cc/kg) body weight in small dogs and cats and 2 to 3 cc/lb (5 to 7 cc/kg) body weight in large dogs.[30] Barium sulfate powder mixed with water or given in a gelatin capsule does not provide consistent homogeneous gastric filling. Oral liquid organic iodine contrast agents have little use in evaluation of the stomach. These solutions give poor mucosal coating, have very rapid transit, and are used only when gastric perforation is suspected. Due to osmotic draw of fluid into the bowel, these hypertonic contrast agents are contraindicated in dehydrated or debilitated animals.

Positive contrast studies of the stomach are used to demonstrate gastric position, gastric emptying time, foreign bodies, or lesions of the gastric wall. Mucosal and rugal patterns are best evaluated when the stomach is distended for contrast or double contrast studies. Rugal folds are absent in the fundus, longitudinal and parallel in the body, and small and spiral in the antral region. The normal mucosal-contrast interface is smooth and homogeneous. Inflammatory lesions with increased mucus production or gastric wall inflammation and ulceration result in irregular mucosal-contrast interface. Chronic gastritis may sometimes result in rugal fold hypertrophy.

The demonstration of large gastric ulcers or masses involving the gastric wall requires careful radiographic technique and interpretation. These lesions may be obscured by a dense barium mixture and often require other special techniques. Multiple views, including oblique positions, may help bring a lesion into view. When most of the contrast agent has left the stomach, air can be introduced for a double contrast study. Using a simultaneous pneumoperitoneum, gastric wall masses or thickening may be demonstrated.

Contrast studies crudely evaluate gastric motility and emptying. Fluoroscopy is the best means of evaluating gastric wall motility. Without fluoroscopy, multiple radiographs must be taken to observe changes in the gastric wall due to peristaltic contractions. A fixed, rigid, or nondistensible region of the stomach suggests a gastric wall lesion. Delayed gastric emptying results from gastric motility disorders or outflow obstructions. Normally, the duodenum begins to fill in 5 to 15 minutes, and the stomach empties in approximately one to four hours.[31] Total retention of contrast in the stomach for longer than 30 minutes generally indicates a gastric emptying disorder.[32] The rate of gastric emptying can be altered by excitement, nervous inhibition, or various anticholinergic drugs or tranquilizers. If tranquilization is required, acetylpromazine maleate reportedly does not affect gastric transit time.[33]

Liquid barium contrast studies may not demonstrate abnormal gastric emptying. This is due to the fact that the emptying of liquids and solids is controlled by different gastric mechanisms; consequently, the passage of liquid barium may not reveal abnormalities in emptying of solids. In suspected cases, food should be mixed with barium to demonstrate these motility disorders. The average time for the stomach to completely empty is eight to ten hours. This time may, however, be as long as 15 hours in some normal animals.[34] Retention of a barium meal longer than normal suggests gastric stasis or obstruction to pyloric outflow.

Double Contrast Study. Double contrast studies of the stomach involve using both negative and positive contrast agents (Figure 85–7). This technique is useful in outlining gastric foreign bodies, gastric wall contour, and the mucosal surface. This technique is most helpful when foreign bodies absorb or are coated by the positive contrast agent. The technique involves administering approximately 0.5 cc/lb (1 cc/kg) body weight of micropulverized barium sulfate (30 per cent W/V).[35] The

animal is rolled so that contrast material coats the mucosal surface; a stomach tube is then reintroduced, and the stomach distended with gas.

Endoscopy

Endoscopy enables the clinician to visually examine the luminal surface of the stomach. Rigid endoscopes, either hollow tubes or solid optics, offer limited value in examination of the small animal stomach. They have been useful in removal of various gastric foreign bodies.

With the development of flexible fiberoptics, examination of the gastrointestinal system has improved, and the entire stomach can be adequately visualized. Endoscopes used for examination of the stomach consist of a long, flexible insertion tube with a bending distal tip, an eyepiece, and control section. The distal tip of the endoscope is manipulated using either a two- or four-way control knob in the handpiece. In addition to the fiber bundles, two channels are present. One channel permits a variety of endoscopic tools to be passed and fluids to be suctioned. The other channel carries air for insufflation or water for washing away mucus and other material from the viewing port. A separate light source with a pump for instillation of fluid and air and a separate suction apparatus are required. Biopsy forceps, cytology brushes, aspiration tubes, snares, and grasping forceps are available.

Most endoscopes are designed for human use, although less expensive veterinary endoscopes have been developed. Many veterinary endoscopists prefer human

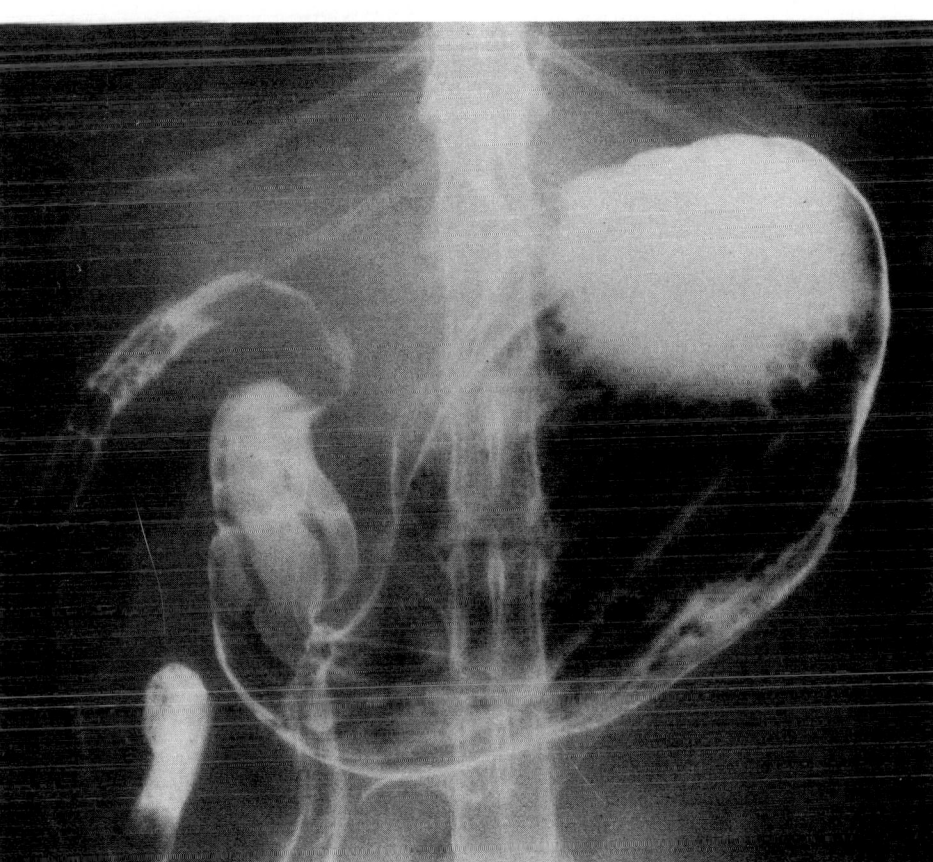

FIGURE 85–7. Double contrast gastrogram showing the gastric luminal surface. This technique is also beneficial for identifying gastric foreign bodies. (From Twedt, DC: Differential Diagnosis and Therapy of Vomiting. Vet Clin North Am 13, 1983.)

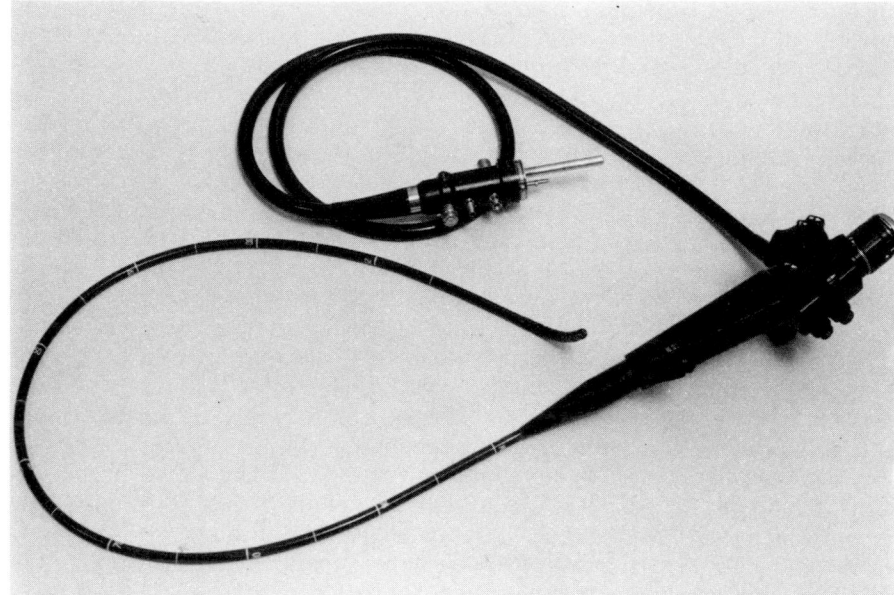

FIGURE 85–8. A gastrointestinal fiberoptic endoscope (Olympus GIF XP10). The insertion tube length of 100 cm with a diameter of 7.9 mm and a four-way control distal end-bending section makes this instrument ideal for evaluating the gastrointestinal system of almost all dogs and cats.

pediatric size endoscopes (Figure 85–8).[36] Most endoscopes have a working length of approximately 110 cm and an outer diameter of 7.9 to 10 mm, making them versatile for small dogs and cats as well as giant breeds.

Indications. Endoscopy has added a new diagnostic modality in gastric disease but has not completely replaced other conventional diagnostic methods. Any animal with signs suggestive of gastric disease (e.g., vomiting, hematemesis, and melena) is a candidate for gastroscopy. The procedure should be preceded by adequate laboratory support and radiology. Endoscopy enables visualization of the luminal surface of the stomach and evaluation for the presence of ulceration, hemorrhage, or tumors. Endoscopy is also used when abnormal radiographic findings need to be confirmed or when radiography fails to demonstrate a lesion. During endoscopy the clinician can obtain guided punch biopsies, brush cytology, or fluid aspiration, or remove certain small foreign bodies.[37]

Technique. Animals are fasted 12 hours before the procedure. General anesthesia with tracheal intubation is recommended; heavy sedation is possible but increases the risk of damage to the endoscope. A mouth gag should always be used to protect the instrument. The animal is placed in left lateral recumbency so that the antrum and pylorus are away from the table and thus less distorted. This position permits good visualization of the stomach and facilitates passage of the instrument into the antrum. As the endoscope is passed into the stomach, air is insufflated to distend the lumen. Distention flattens the mucosal folds and aids in visualization of the mucosal surface. Location of the endoscope tip is known once the prominent incisura, a large fold demarcating the junction of the antrum and lesser curvature, is found. The cardia and fundus are visualized when the endoscope tip is retroflexed. To view the pylorus, the endoscope must be advanced into the antrum. With expertise, the scope can usually be passed through the pyloric sphincter into the proximal duodenum. This procedure may be aided by the use of

intravenous glucagon or metoclopramide, both of which have hypotonic effects on the pyloric sphincter.

The mucosal surface should be evaluated for changes in color or consistency. Submucosal hemorrhage or small mucosal ulcerations can be observed in gastritis. Gastric tumors are often characterized by areas that lack distensibility, such as large protuberances or a large raised ulcer. Small polyps may be observed as incidental findings.

When a lesion is observed, biopsy forceps are passed through the endoscope and directed to the area to be biopsied. A cytology brush is used in a similar manner to obtain tissue. Small four-pronged grasping forceps or snares may be used to remove small gastric foreign bodies.

Complications. Complications of gastroscopy are rare.[38] The major problem occurs with operator inexperience, in both technical aspects and accurate interpretation of findings. Anesthesia and overdistention of the stomach with air are always potential complications.

Gastric Biopsy

Gastric biopsies are obtained with endoscopic biopsy forceps, a biopsy capsule, or during surgery.

Various types of biopsy capsules have been designed with which gastric mucosal biopsies may be obtained perorally. These instruments are relatively simple and noninvasive and can easily be passed into the stomach to obtain random mucosal sections. All instruments employ the basic principle of a capsule attached to a long flexible tube. Suction is created when the operator, using a syringe and vacuum gauge, draws a piece of mucosa into a small hole in the capsule. A knife attached to a cable is pulled and cuts off the piece of tissue. The mucosal biopsy is then retained inside the capsule.

One capsule found suitable for gastric biopsy in small animals is the Quinton multipurpose biopsy instrument (Figure 85–9). Gastric biopsies are best when obtained

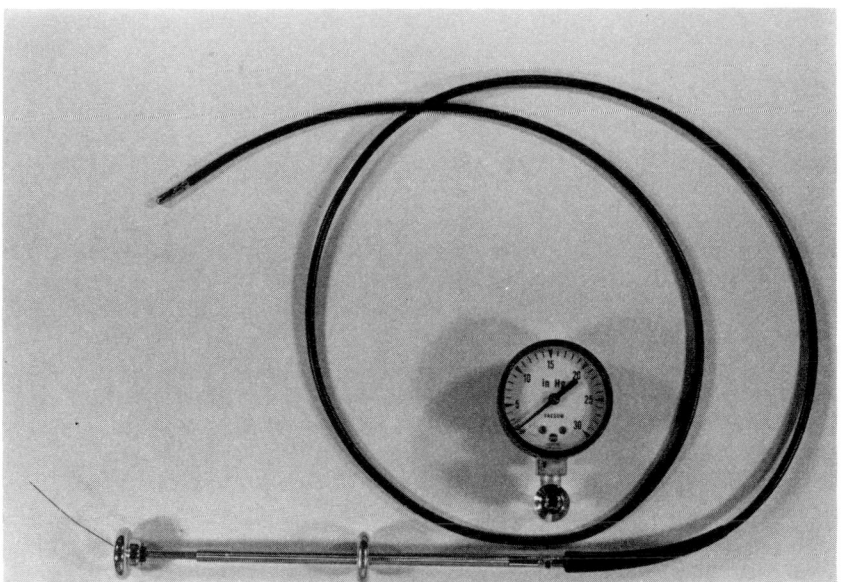

FIGURE 85–9. The Quinton Multipurpose Suction Biopsy Instrument with vacuum gauge. Esophageal, gastric, and colonic mucosal biopsies can be retrieved with this instrument.

using the Quinton colonic capsule with a 2.8 mm or larger capsule hole. It is sometimes possible to obtain an older Wood's gastric biopsy capsule from a human gastrointestinal unit, since these instruments have become outdated by modern endoscopic instruments and hydraulically controlled multiple biopsy probes.[39]

The animal to be biopsied should be held off food for 12 to 24 hours before the procedure. Sedation is usually unnecessary. An oral speculum is used, and the capsule and tube are introduced into the mouth and passed down the esophagus to the stomach. The position of the capsule is not known unless fluoroscopy is used simultaneously to direct the biopsy capsule or it is directed during endoscopy. If the dog is in left lateral recumbency, the greater curvature is usually biopsied, while a right lateral recumbency usually retrieves lesser curvature and antral area. This biopsy technique is most feasible for diffuse mucosal lesions. Focal mucosal lesions or submucosal lesions are often not detected.

Few complications occur.[40] The most serious potential complication is gastric perforation or hemorrhage. The procedure should not be used in any animal with a bleeding disorder.

Exploratory celiotomy provides the best means of establishing a definitive diagnosis of gastric disease. Surgery provides the opportunity to palpate the stomach, examine the luminal surface, obtain a full thickness biopsy of the gastric wall, and remove gastric foreign bodies. Surgery is often required for the removal of gastric ulcers, polyps, or tumors and to correct gastric outflow obstructions. At the time of surgery the animal should be carefully evaluated for other intra-abdominal problems such as pancreatitis, lymphadenopathy, or small, gastrin-secreting pancreatic tumors.

Gastric Secretory Testing

A major function of the stomach is the secretion of hydrochloric acid. Disease states can occur with either an increase or a decrease in gastric acid secretion.

Increased gastric acid secretion potentiates mucosal damage and may result in duodenal or gastric ulcers. A hyperacidic state occurs in the dog due to gastrin-secreting tumors or certain mast cell tumors. Other causes of increased acid production in animals with clinical gastric disease have not been reported and warrant investigation.

The collection of gastric secretions and analysis of the acid content help detect hyperacidic secretory states. Clinical gastric acid collection in the dog is best achieved by temporarily placing a gastric tube into the antral region of the stomach.[41] Basal gastric acid output secretions (BOA) are collected in the fasted dog in 15 minute aliquots. The sample is pH meter titrated to a neutral pH and then expressed in milliequivalents of hydrogen ion per 15 minute period.[42] Basal acid output in the normal fasted dog is usually negligible. The potential acid-secreting ability of the stomach is directly proportional to the parietal cell mass.[43] This maximal acid output (MAO) can be stimulated by various secretagogues such as histamine, betazole, and pentagastrin.

Pentagastrin contains the C-terminal active site of natural gastrins and therefore acts as a physiologic gastric acid stimulator and is preferred for evaluating gastric secretory function. Pentagastrin, given at a dose of 3 μg/lb (6 μg/kg) body weight subcutaneously or intravenously, causes maximal acid secretion within one hour.[44] In the normal dog, a wide range of values are reported, depending on the methods used. Ranges of 3 to 12 mEq of hydrogen ion per 15 minutes are reported using pentagastrin stimulation.[45-47]

GASTRIC MUCOSAL INJURY

Mechanisms of Mucosal Damage

Gastric Mucosal Barrier. The parietal cells of the gastric mucosa produce hydrochloric acid, often generating a luminal secretion with a pH as low as one. The unique ability of the stomach to withstand concentrated acid without cellular damage is referred to as the gastric mucosal barrier.[48] This barrier is resistant to "back-diffusion" of hydrogen ions from the gastric lumen into the mucosa as well as sodium loss into the lumen. The anatomic makeup of the barrier consists of two parts: the mucous layer lining the surface of the epithelial cells and the mucosal cells that compose the epithelial membrane. The true function of the mucous layer is unclear, but it is believed to act predominantly in lubrication. Mucus has only a weak neutralizing and buffering capacity, and acid readily diffuses through it. The gastric epithelial cells seem to be the most important component of the anatomic barrier.[49] The epithelial mucosal cells are held together by strong intracellular tight junctions, and it is these tight junctions or the lipoprotein layer of the plasma membrane that constitutes the barrier.

Local tissue prostaglandins provide a cytoprotective effect against injurious substances. Protection by the gastric mucosal barrier is both morphologic and functional and seems to be mediated by endogenous formation of local prostaglandins. The mechanism by which prostaglandins exert their effect is unknown. In addition to their effect of tightening the gastric mucosal barrier, they also stimulate mucus secretion and the sodium pump, activate cyclic AMP, and increase gastric mucosal circulation.[50]

Back-diffusion of luminal acid into the mucosa is central in the pathogenesis of gastric mucosal damage. Normally there is minimal leakage of secreted acid back into the mucosa. Such leakage occurs at a very slow rate and is rapidly removed by the vascular system.[51] The topical action of many endogenous and exogenous agents can alter this barrier, thereby increasing mucosal permeability to acid. With increased acid entry, a chain of events ensues, beginning with direct damage to the mucosa and followed by destruction of the subepithelium (Figure 85–10). Mast cells in the submucosa and lamina propria degranulate and release histamine upon

contact with acid. Released histamine stimulates parietal cell secretion of hydrochloric acid as well as local inflammation and edema. Acid may also damage blood vessels and stimulate nerves of the stomach wall, leading to increased muscular contractions. When the gastric mucosal barrier is broken, acid enters the gastric wall, and luminal acid concentration decreases if measured by conventional means.

Agents of Mucosal Damage.
Normally, an electrical potential difference of 40 to 60 millivolts exists across the gastric mucosa of the dog.[52] The production of hydrogen ions and the pumping of chloride into and sodium out of the lumen contribute to this potential difference. Only an intact gastric mucosal barrier can maintain such gradients of electrical and chemical activity. With disruption of the barrier and back-diffusion of hydrogen ions, there is a simultaneous decrease in the potential difference. Experimentally, a decrease in potential difference is used as a sensitive indicator of gastric mucosal damage. Various physiochemical agents have been shown to cause such changes, and are classified as exogenous factors, endogenous factors, or conditions that result in mucosal ischemia.

Exogenous Agents.
The ingestion of certain exogenous agents results in direct damage by contact or injury following entry into the mucosal cells. These include drugs, various toxins, infectious agents and corrosive or damaging chemicals. Hypertonic solutions and foreign materials may also stress the gastric mucosal barrier.

Drugs such as aspirin consistently cause gastric lesions in the dog and cat.[53, 54] Aspirin damages the gastric epithelial cells by virtue of its lipid membrane solubility, which allows entry into the cells, causing cellular damage. Aspirin at a dose of 40 mg/lb (100 mg/kg) per day has been shown to consistently cause gastric lesions in the dog,[55] while approximately half that dose is reported to cause gastric lesions in the cat.[56] Buffered aspirin also causes gastric lesions, whereas enteric-coated aspirin produces fewer gastric lesions but has inconsistent drug absorption.[57] Other compounds entering the gastric mucosa by way of lipid solubility include bile acids, short-chain fatty acids, and certain detergents (e.g., digoxin).

Nonsteroidal anti-inflammatory drugs such as flunixin, ibuprofen, phenylbutazone, and indomethacin cause gastric mucosal lesions. These drugs exert their effect via their antiprostaglandin action (blocking cyclo-oxygenase activity), thus altering the gastric cytoprotective activity of prostaglandins. The severity of gastric mucosal ulceration varies with each drug and appears to be dose-related. Indomethacin causes severe gastric ulcers in doses as low as 0.5 mg/lb (1 mg/kg) body weight and therefore should not be used in dogs and cats.[58]

Corticosteroids alone do not alter the permeability of the gastric mucosa but do significantly enhance the effects of aspirin, bile acids, and other mucosal damaging agents. Corticosteroids decrease mucosal cell turnover and mucous production, as well as increasing gastrin levels and gastric acid production.[59]

Alterations in Blood Flow.
A reduction in gastric mucosal perfusion will potentiate the formation of gastric mucosal lesions. Mucosal ischemia alone, without acid or cellular damage, does not break the barrier.[60] There is evidence that ischemia results in profoundly

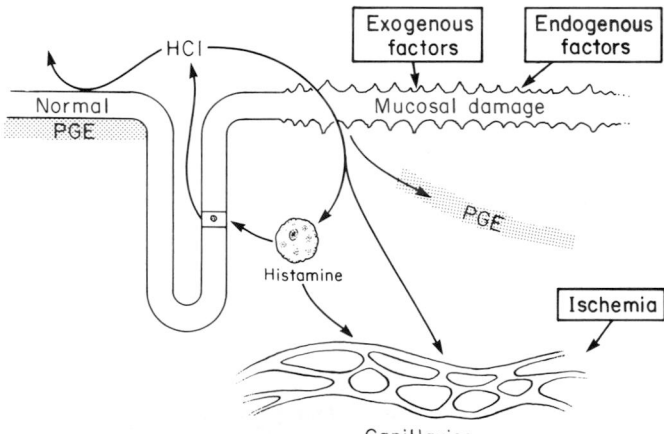

FIGURE 85–10. Disruption of the gastric mucosa occurs from endogenous or exogenous factors or from local ischemia. The mechanism of events resulting from damage to the gastric mucosal barrier includes entry of acid through the damaged mucosa, disruption of local tissue prostaglandins (PGE), and degranulation of mast cells with a release of histamine. All events perpetuate further damage to the gastric wall.

decreased gastric mucosal energy and rapid cellular death.[61] Decreased blood flow to the gastric mucosa may result from a number of causes, including hypotension, shock, and sepsis. Abnormal blood flow may occur with central nervous system lesions and is believed to result from altered equilibrium between sympathetic and parasympathetic pathways. This happens most commonly in spinal cord lesions with a loss of sympathetic inhibitory influences, resulting in paralytic vasodilatation and vagotonia in vessels of the gastric wall. Parasympathetic overdrive also stimulates an increase in gastric acid and enzyme secretion.

Endogenous Factors. Conditions such as excessive gastric hydrochloric acid production will promote mucosal damage. The reflux of bile and pancreatic enzymes causes increased permeability to hydrogen ions and damage to the mucosal barrier. Bile acids alter the barrier by virtue of their lipid solubility. Bile, gastric acid, and ischemia all act synergistically to destroy the gastric mucosal barrier. The importance of bile is emphasized in experimental studies of hemorrhagic shock wherein dogs in which the pylorus had been occluded, preventing duodenal reflux of bile, had a significantly lower incidence of gastric ulcerations.[62] Conditions such as states of excessive gastric hydrochloric acid production will promote mucosal damage.

Stress is associated with gastric lesions by altering the gastric mucosa through a neuroendocrine mechanism. This results from sympathetically mediated vasoconstriction, which promotes vascular stasis, and from endogenous release of corticosteroids, vasoactive catecholamines, and serotonin.[49] (See Gastric Ulceration.)

Gastric lesions may occur secondary to *metabolic diseases.* Renal failure results in the accumulation of uremic toxins that damage the gastric mucosa and vessels of the gastric wall.[63] Serum gastrin levels are also elevated during uremia due to reduced renal clearance.[64, 65] Gastric lesions may occur secondary to liver failure, although the exact mechanism is not completely known. Damage results in part from reduced mucosal blood flow, loss of the mucous barrier, and elevated gastrin levels. Systemic mastocytosis causes gastric ulceration from increased levels of histamine, which stimulate the parietal cells, resulting in increased gastric acid production.[33] Gastric lesions have also been observed in some cases of adrenocortical insufficiency.

ACUTE GASTRITIS

Acute gastritis is a common disease entity in small animals. Strictly defined, acute gastritis is inflammation and mucosal damage that has occurred in response to an insult to the gastric mucosa. Rarely does acute gastritis warrant biopsy and histologic confirmation; therefore, the diagnosis of acute gastritis is given when signs of gastric disease are acute and self-limiting.

Etiology

In most cases of acute gastritis, the etiology is never determined. In contrast to reports of experimentally produced lesions, there is a paucity of published cases of spontaneously occurring acute gastritis. Acute gastritis is associated with a multitude of factors, mainly related to dietary indiscretions of dogs and cats. It is most often associated with ingestion of rancid or spoiled foodstuffs, resulting in what is referred to as "garbage-can" intoxication. The causative agents are derived from fermentation or putrefaction of food products, bacterial enterotoxins, or mycotoxins.[66]

Ingestion of foreign material such as food wrappings of cellophane or aluminum, bones, plastic, rocks, and small toys may damage the gastric mucosa by mechanical means. The incidence of ingested foreign bodies is more common in young animals, possibly owing to their chewing habits and curious nature. Trichobezoars (hairballs) are frequently encountered in the stomachs of some long-haired cats and dogs. Certain drugs (e.g., aspirin, indomethacin, phenylbutazone, corticosteroids) and chemicals reportedly cause gastritis in the dog and cat. Examples of chemical irritants include heavy metals (e.g., lead), cleaning agents, fertilizers, and herbicides.

Many plants and plant toxins can cause acute gastritis, possibly the most common being grass. Ingestion of grass and plants is probably a normal instinctive behavior; however, animals with gastric disease, for some unknown reason, often ingest and vomit plant material. Many common household plants can cause acute gastritis.[67]

Infectious agents may cause acute gastritis. The incidence of bacterial gastritis is low, because the gastric lumen contains few bacteria due to the acid environment. Viruses such as canine distemper, canine hepatitis, coronavirus, and parvovirus may cause gastric lesions as part of a more extensive disease condition. Mycotic infections of the stomach have been reported in the dog.[68–70] Parasites generally do not produce gastric lesions or clinical signs. *Physaloptera* spp. is the most common gastric parasite, although ascarids and tapeworms may infrequently cause gastritis and vomiting. The nematode *Ollulanus tricuspis* has been associated with gastric lesions in cats, and spirochetes have been observed in the gastric mucous layer and parietal cells in some dogs and cats and may be a factor in causing acute or chronic gastritis.[71]

Acute gastritis may result from an allergic reaction to a previously sensitized antigen. Clinical gastritis conditions are often suggested to be simple food allergies. Other disease conditions including uremia, liver disease, neurologic disease, shock, sepsis, or stress may play a role in the etiology of acute gastritis.

Pathophysiology

Acute lesions may be localized or diffuse. Necrosis of surface epithelial cells with extravasation of blood from damaged vessels in the lamina propria produces superficial erosions, edema, and hemorrhage. Variable degrees of polymorphonuclear (PMN) and lymphocytic infiltration occur. Occasionally, inflammation may progress to a purulent gastritis with necrosis and extensive PMN infiltration.

Diagnosis

A tentative diagnosis of acute gastritis is made on the basis of history, clinical signs, and physical examination. Since acute gastritis is far more common than other causes of gastric disease, symptomatic therapy is warranted without extensive diagnostic procedures. Rapid and complete response to therapy confirms the diagnosis. Severely ill animals, or those that fail to respond to symptomatic therapy, require further diagnostic testing (see Clinical Evaluation).

Treatment. Most cases of acute gastritis respond to simple symptomatic therapy within 24 to 48 hours after the onset of signs. Such cases are usually treated on an outpatient basis. Animals displaying severe clinical signs, evidence of dehydration, or failure to respond to previous conservative measures require further medical and laboratory support. Basic principles in therapy of gastric disease include removing the initiating agent, providing proper conditions that promote mucosal repair, correcting secondary complications of gastritis (vomiting, abdominal pain, infection), and correcting fluid, electrolyte, and acid-base abnormalities.

Dietary restriction should be the initial step in therapy of acute gastritis. Ingestion of food or liquids results in gastric distention and increased gastric motility, and is a stimulus for further vomiting. Food results in gastric acid production stimulated through both the cephalic and gastric phases of gastric secretion. This results in greater back-diffusion of hydrogen ions and further mucosal damage. Food may also serve as an exogenous source of bacteria that could potentially invade the damaged gastric mucosa.

The animal with acute gastritis should be given nothing per os (NPO) for a minimum of 12 hours. If no vomiting occurs during that period, the animal is offered frequent, small amounts of water or ice cubes, only enough to keep the mouth moist and to supply modest fluid replacement. Only after a minimum of 24 hours following the onset of signs should feeding be attempted. The animal is fed small amounts of a bland diet, and foods high in fat and protein are avoided. A diet consisting predominantly of carbohydrates is used. Cooked rice or cooked cereals supplemented with cottage cheese, lean boiled ground beef, or baby foods may be recommended. Commercial diets formulated for gastrointestinal disease (e.g., Prescription Diet i/d) may also be prescribed. If a favorable response is obtained with dietary management, the regular diet is gradually reintroduced over several days.

Parenteral fluids are given only when dehydration, electrolyte, or acid-base imbalances occur. The quantity of fluids administered should be enough to supply daily maintenance needs (approximately 20 to 30 ml/lb/day or 40 to 60 ml/kg/day), correct existing dehydration, and replace fluid losses that may occur with continued vomiting. Vomiting in acute gastritis results in volume depletion and losses of sodium, chloride, and potassium with a metabolic acidosis. An isotonic balanced electrolyte solution such as Ringer's lactated solution is usually given. Infrequently, in conditions with profuse vomiting or gastric outflow obstruction, a severe hypochloremia, hypokalemia, and metabolic alkalosis may exist. Normal (0.9 per cent) saline is the fluid of choice for correcting metabolic alkalosis resulting from vomiting. Therapy with chloride corrects the deficit and allows for renal excretion of bicarbonate.[72] In either acidotic or alkalotic states, potassium is usually depleted and necessitates additional supplementation with potassium chloride. The amount of potassium chloride supplemented in parenteral fluids is based on measured serum potassium levels.[73]

Antiemetic drugs are given to control refractory vomiting when pyloric obstruction or gastric foreign body has been ruled out. These drugs inhibit vomiting but do little for primary treatment of the gastritis. Antiemetic drugs act centrally to suppress either the chemoreceptor trigger zone (CTZ), the emetic center, or the vestibular apparatus (see Chapter 7).

Drugs that suppress only the CTZ are generally not useful unless the vomiting is secondary to conditions such as uremia or other toxins that may directly stimulate the CTZ. Phenothiazine tranquilizers (e.g., chlorpromazine) have a broad-spectrum pharmacologic effect. At low doses they block the CTZ and at higher doses they depress the emetic center.[74] Chlorpromazine (Thorazine, 0.20 mg/lb (0.5 mg/kg) IM or SQ, or 0.02 mg/lb (0.05 mg/kg) IV, q6h to q8h) and prochlorperazine (Compazine, 0.2 mg/lb (0.5 mg/kg) IM, SQ or IV, q6h to q8h) are the most widely used and effective antiemetics. These drugs are effective in blocking the visceral input that results from gastritis and should be considered in cases with persistent vomiting. Phenothiazines should not be used in dehydrated or hypotensive animals, owing to their α-adrenergic blocking action, which causes arteriolar vasodilatation. Sedation may also occur because of the tranquilizing properties of these drugs; however, the dose for tranquilization is generally greater than that required for antiemetic activity.

Anticholinergic drugs reduce gastric motility and spasms, which are factors that stimulate vomiting and pain with acute gastritis. In addition to blocking parasympathetic stimulation of smooth muscle of the gastric wall, anticholinergics also block the cephalic and gastric phase stimulation of gastric acid secretion. However, they do not block histamine- or gastrin-stimulated acid secretion. These drugs have the undesirable effect of reducing gastric emptying, which results in gastric distention and further gastric acid secretion. Overuse of these drugs may result in gastric hypotonia and iatrogenic gastric outflow obstruction, which may cause continued vomiting. For this reason they should not be administered for longer than three days. Anticholinergic drugs used in the therapy of gastric disease include atropine, methylscopolamine, isopropamide, and propantheline. Aminopentamide (Centrine, 0.1 to 0.4 mg, q8h to q12h, SQ or IM) is a common anticholinergic for veterinary use. Anticholinergics in combination with the phenothiazine prochlorperazine (Darbazine, prochlorperazine and isopropamide, 0.06 to 0.10 ml/lb (0.14 to 0.22 ml/kg), q12h, SQ) have an increased spectrum of antiemetic activity. Opiates (e.g., camphorated tincture of opium, diphenoxylate) have a similar action in decreasing gastric motility and emptying.

Oral protectants such as kaolin and pectolin compounds and antibiotics are generally not indicated in the treatment of acute gastritis. Protectants may bind certain bacteria or toxins, but they do not coat or protect injured gastric mucosa. Potential benefits are frequently outweighed by difficulty encountered by owners in administration and vomiting that may occur from gastric distention by these compounds. Bismuth subsalicylate (Pepto-Bismol) used as a gastric protectant may be of benefit because of its antiprostaglandin properties. Because of cats' intolerance of salicylates and since the salicylates in bismuth subsalicylates are absorbed systemically, these agents should probably not be used in feline patients. Antibiotics are not indicated unless a bacterial infection is suspected, and in such cases are best given parenterally.

Antacid or H_2-receptor therapies are not usually prescribed for simple cases of acute gastritis but are reserved for refractory cases or those with serious gastric bleeding or ulcers (see Gastric Ulceration). H_2-receptor antagonists (e.g., cimetidine, ranitidine) are effective in reducing gastric acid production in the dog and cat by blocking the histamine receptor of the parietal cells. Indications for these drugs include treatment of duodenal and gastric ulcers, esophagitis from gastroesophageal reflux, prevention and treatment of acute gastric hemorrhage, chronic gastritis, and syndromes resulting in gastric acid hypersecretion.[75] The recommended dosage for cimetidine is 2 to 5 mg/lb (5 to 10 mg/kg) three times a day and for ranitidine is 1 mg/lb (2 mg/kg) three times daily.

Other drugs, such as prostaglandin compounds, have been effective experimentally in reducing gastric acid secretion in the dog and may be clinically available in the future.[76] Corticosteroids are not indicated in treatment of acute gastritis, as they potentiate the formation of gastric lesions; however, corticosteroids given to the dogs in septic shock do protect the gastric mucosa.[77] Severe gastric hemorrhage is treated as an emergency condition, with whole blood and fluids administered to replace losses.

All gastric foreign bodies should be removed. The most common means is via surgical gastrotomy. Surgery also allows examination of the remaining gastrointestinal tract for other foreign bodies or abnormalities. A less invasive procedure is gastroscopy, since some gastric foreign bodies can be successfully removed endoscopically using grasping forceps or snares. Alternative methods include retrieving metallic foreign bodies with magnets or passing grasping forceps under fluoroscopic direction.

With ingestion of small objects (e.g., needles and pins) but without signs of gastric disease, one may elect to attempt natural passage of the foreign object. A high-fiber diet and lubricants are given with the patient under strict observation. Failure of passage in 48 hours generally requires removal of the foreign body. Administration of emetics to cause vomiting of the foreign body should be carried out with great caution and is attempted only when the foreign body is small with smooth surfaces, so that it will not create lacerations, perforations, or esophageal obstruction. The animal should be fed cotton balls to coat the foreign object before initiation of vomiting. Small trichobezoars are treated with Vase-

line or other petroleum products to lubricate passage through the gastrointestinal tract. Owners should not be advised to administer mineral oil, for fear of possible aspiration pneumonitis. Large, indurated trichobezoars require surgical removal.

CHRONIC GASTRITIS

Chronic gastritis describes numerous clinical entities with a vast number of etiologies. The definition of chronic gastritis infers that there are chronic inflammatory changes within the mucosa of the stomach coexisting with clinical signs of gastric disease. There are several subtypes of chronic gastritis that have been observed in both dogs and cats. Often, a diagnosis of chronic gastritis is made clinically but a precise diagnosis requires gastric mucosal biopsy.

Etiology

The etiology of chronic gastritis is seldom determined. Most lesions probably occur as a result of various extrinsic influences, because the gastric mucosa is repeatedly exposed to an infinite number of dietary antigens, chemicals, toxins, and infectious agents. Damage to the mucosa also results in back-diffusion of gastric acid into the gastric wall causing further damage. Mucosal damage may also initiate an allergic or immune-mediated response. Damage causes the release of certain gastric antigens that initiate either a cellular or humoral response, resulting in an immune-mediated mechanism of chronic gastritis.[78]

Many chemicals, drugs, and infectious and physical agents will cause lesions of chronic gastritis. Most of these agents have similarly been incriminated as causes of acute gastritis, but repeated exposure may result in chronic lesions. Chronic ingestion of aspirin is an excellent example of an agent causing chronic gastritis. Gastric foreign bodies, if left in the stomach, result in chronic gastric mucosal irritation and lesions of chronic gastritis. Atrophic gastritis has been produced experimentally in the dog by repeated immunization with gastric juices,[79–81] but naturally occurring immune-mediated gastric disease has not been documented.

Certain infectious agents may also play a role in the pathogenesis of chronic gastritis. The bacterium *Campylobacter pyloridis* has been associated with chronic gastritis in humans but has yet to be identified in affected dogs or cats.[82] The role of spirochetal organisms in the stomach of dogs is unknown. The organism *Spirillium* is considered to be a normal gastric inhabitant and usually innocuous but possibly in large numbers may induce an inflammatory response.[83]

Pathophysiology

Chronic gastritis can be divided into a number of distinct histologic subclassifications. The clinical features, however, cannot be differentiated among the various types.[84] In most cases, the lesions do not result in significant mucosal ulceration and are therefore referred to collectively as nonerosive gastritis. The two major types include chronic superficial gastritis and chronic atrophic gastritis. Other, less frequent, histologic patterns are also reported. *Chronic superficial gastritis* is the most common form of chronic gastritis and is characterized by excessive but variable inflammatory cell infiltrate and fibrosis of the mucosa and submucosa.[85] The inflammatory component consists of lymphocytes, plasma cells, and neutrophils. Mild superficial mucosal erosions, edema, and hemorrhage may also be present but are rare. In this condition there is no obvious change in mucosal thickness.

Chronic atrophic gastritis is a diffuse lesion of the stomach involving particularly the body and fundus. Atrophy is evident by a thinner-than-normal mucosa, with reduction in size and depth of the gastric glands. Chief and parietal cell numbers are reduced and often replaced by mucus-secreting cells. An inflammatory component, as found in chronic superficial gastritis, is almost always present. It is possible that atrophic gastritis is the result of progression from chronic superficial gastritis. The time sequence is unknown but the condition probably takes months to develop, as indicated from experimental studies. Atrophic gastritis that has been experimentally induced appears quite similar to the naturally occurring disease in dogs.

Chronic atrophic gastritis has been reported in dogs in association with achlorhydria.[86] Although not convincingly documented, it is reasonable to assume that hypochlorhydria would result from reduction in parietal cell mass. Further assumptions suggest that serum gastrin levels may be abnormally elevated because of loss of the negative feedback from acid secretion, which inhibits gastrin release. Atrophic gastritis is one predisposing factor for development of gastric ulcers.[87] Acid reduction from achlorhydria may also be associated with secondary intestinal bacterial overgrowth and malabsorption.[88]

There are a number of other less common types of chronic gastritis that have been described in both the dog and cat. These include *granulomatous gastritis*, which is characterized by the presence of tissue granulomas as the predominant histologic finding. This condition may result from allergic, infectious, or possible foreign body migration. Granulomatous gastritis is reported in dogs with gastric phycomycosis and is characterized by a thickened gastric wall.[89, 90] Some cats with the gastric nematode *Ollulanus tricuspis* may develop chronic fibrosing gastritis.[28] There is also a report of chronic histiocytic gastritis in the dog and cat.[91]

Clinical Findings

Signs of chronic gastritis are ill-defined and often obscure, and may occur with periodic exacerbations. Many dogs show symptoms for several months before presentation, while others are asymptomatic. Vomiting is reportedly the most common sign observed in chronic gastritis, although it does not occur in every case.[85] Vomiting is usually infrequent and may or may not be associated with eating. Owners may describe periodic vomiting of bile-tinged or egg white consistency fluid as the only sign. Frequent, severe vomiting occurs with gastric outflow obstructions or in advanced gastritis. With gastric mucosal ulceration, vomitus may contain digested or nondigested blood. Other signs of chronic gastritis may include poor appetite, weight loss, abdominal pain, depression, and polydipsia. Other, less frequent, signs may include chronic belching, pica (such as licking the floors or grass eating), and total anorexia. Usually, animals with chronic gastritis are in good condition and show little evidence of debilitation, weight loss, or diarrhea.

The physical examination is usually unrewarding but should be carefully performed to rule out conditions that may mimic chronic gastric disease.

Diagnosis

Routine laboratory evaluation is generally noncontributory but helps exclude gastritis secondary to other disease conditions. Anemia, electrolyte imbalance, and dehydration are rare but may occur with chronic gastritis and will be reflected in the laboratory tests. Plasma proteins, both albumin and globulin, will be depressed in conditions resulting in protein-losing gastropathy. At present, gastric acid analysis offers limited information, except in confirming suspected states of hypo- or achlorhydria.

The diagnostic value of radiology was described earlier (see Radiology). Very few, if any, radiologic signs are pathognomonic for lesions of chronic gastritis. Contrast studies may demonstrate paucity of rugal folds in atrophic gastritis.

Gastroscopy is a useful tool in the diagnosis of chronic gastritis.[92, 93] In some types of gastritis, the mucosa may appear normal endoscopically, while in severe cases mucosal erosions or hemorrhage may be observed. Atrophic gastritis may allow visualization of submucosal vessels through the thinner-than-normal mucosa. Gastric biopsies are required for a definitive diagnosis of chronic gastritis.

Treatment

The primary aim in the therapy of chronic gastritis is the removal of the etiologic agent. Elimination of chronic drug ingestion or known toxic agents and the removal of gastric foreign bodies is obvious. With elimination of the causative agent, the prognosis is generally good. However, the etiology of most cases is never determined, and therapy must be directed in a logical, but often "trial and error," approach. The prognosis in such cases is quite variable. There have been no reported clinical studies evaluating the effectiveness of therapies for chronic gastritis in the dog and cat.

Dietary control should first be attempted in therapy of chronic gastritis in which the etiologic agent is suspected to have been ingested. Dietary elimination and a positive clinical response confirm those suspicions. Diets high in antigenic proteins or those with many supplements should be avoided. Multiple small feedings of a bland, predominantly carbohydrate diet may be beneficial. Prescription or home diets (such as cottage cheese and rice) developed for (allergic) gastrointestinal disease may also be useful. Generally, canned, meat-based, or semi-moist diets are better tolerated than the dry, high-fiber diets, which cause more distention and mechanical irritation. Dietary trials of two-week intervals should be attempted when eliminating dietary allergies or intolerances.

Corticosteroids are indicated to control chronic gastritis resulting from immune mechanisms in conditions suggestive of an immune response, when biopsy samples show a predominance of lymphocyte and plasma cell infiltration. Corticosteroids stimulate regeneration of gastric parietal cells and may be beneficial in some cases of atrophic gastritis.[94] Corticosteroids do, however, enhance the ulcerogenic potential of mucosal lesions. Initial oral prednisone therapy of 0.5 mg/lb/day (1 mg/kg/day) should be instituted, and the dose tapered over several months. Repeat gastric biopsies are useful in monitoring response to therapy. The immunosuppressant azathioprine (Imuran) prevents experimentally produced immune gastropathy in dogs and may be clinically useful in treating cases with suspected immune-mediated etiologies.[95]

H$_2$-receptor blockers such as cimetidine and ranitidine, which inhibit gastric acid secretion, may play an important role in therapy of chronic gastritis. Some dogs with chronic simple gastritis or mild mucosal atrophy have shown a positive response to this drug. Cimetidine (Tagamet, 2 to 5 mg/lb (5 to 10 mg/kg), q6h to q8h) or ranitidine (Zantac, 1 mg/lb (2 mg/kg) q8h) should be administered for at least two weeks. Longer therapy may be required subject to response. Acid reduction and dietary control often result in resolution of signs of simple chronic superficial gastritis. The use of acid-reducing agents in animals with atrophic gastritis with presumably reduced acid output is somewhat controversial but appears to be clinically beneficial in many patients.

Long-term anticholinergic therapy should be avoided, for it may result in gastric atony and continued vomiting. If signs of vomiting (especially if associated with meals) persist following initial therapy, then a secondary gastric motility disorder should be considered and metoclopramide (Reglan, 0.1 to 0.2 mg/lb (0.2 to 0.4 mg/kg), 30 minutes before meals, q6h to q8h) should be tried. Metoclopramide acts both as a central antiemetic and to promote gastric emptying but has no effect on the primary chronic gastritis.

The prognosis for chronic gastritis is variable. Chronic superficial gastritis generally shows a favorable response to H$_2$-receptor blocker therapy and dietary manipulation. Some cases may require anti-inflammatory therapy as well. Chronic atrophic gastritis is less responsive and less likely to go into complete remission. Granulomatous gastritis generally has a poor prognosis.

EOSINOPHILIC GASTRITIS AND GRANULOMA

Eosinophilic gastritis is a rare condition characterized by diffuse eosinophilic and granulation tissue infiltration involving many or all layers of the stomach wall, or less frequently, as discrete single or multiple granulomatous nodules.[96, 97] Eosinophilic lymphadenitis and vasculitis are also reported in this condition. Hayden and Fleischman[96] describe the gross lesions of diffuse eosinophilic gastritis as a scirrhous thickening of the gastric wall resembling gastric neoplasia.

Pathophysiology

The cause of eosinophilic infiltration in the stomach is unknown but is thought to be immunologically mediated, possibly allergic or parasitic in etiology.[97] In a report of diffuse eosinophilic gastritis in a dog, microfilariae were observed in some histologic sections.[98] Dogs experimentally infected with *Toxocara canis* had focal eosinophilic gastritis, but the lesions rarely contained larvae, and vasculitis was not found.[99] This latter condition may be similar to the syndrome eosinophilic gastroenteritis, in which there is either segmental or diffuse infiltration of eosinophils in the mucosa and submucosa of the stomach and/or intestine. Although the clinical presentation of the two conditions may be similar, they differ significantly in their pathologic features.

Clinical Findings

The clinical features are similar to those of animals with chronic gastritis. Vomiting is the most consistent sign and results from either infiltration within the gastric wall or from a mechanical gastric outflow obstruction. Anorexia and debilitation are frequent. When gastric ulceration occurs, hematemesis or melena may be described. The physical examination usually finds an unthrifty dog with evidence of weight loss. The animal may exhibit pain upon palpation in the region of the stomach. A hard, firm stomach or gastric wall mass may be palpated. Because eosinophilic granulomas may also involve adjacent organs such as regional lymph nodes, spleen, kidneys, and intestines, adjacent organ enlargement may be detected.

Diagnosis

The history and physical findings will suggest a gastric disorder. Leukocytosis with an absolute eosinophilia occurs in most cases of eosinophilic gastritis or granulomas. Consequently, a presumptive diagnosis of eosinophilic gastritis can be made in animals with signs of chronic gastric disease, peripheral eosinophilia, and a positive response to a trial dosage of systemic corticosteroids. Careful examination for heartworms and fecal examination for intestinal parasites should be performed to detect a possible etiology. Other laboratory abnormalities may include anemia, hypoproteinemia, or melena, all from gastric ulceration and blood loss.

Barium contrast studies may demonstrate single or multiple granulomatous nodules as filling defects within the gastric wall, or, with diffuse involvement of the gastric wall, a rigid thickened stomach. Pyloric outflow obstruction may be evident. These radiographic changes frequently appear similar to those of gastric neoplasia.

Endoscopy or surgery will demonstrate the gastric lesions. Biopsy taken by either means generally confirms the diagnosis. Impression smear evaluation of the biopsy sample showing numerous eosinophils supports a preliminary diagnosis.

Treatment

Therapy should include dietary trials, since a dietary allergy may play a role in the etiology. Some dogs with eosinophilic gastritis showed clinical improvement and resolution of circulating eosinophilia when placed on a controlled diet alone.[97] Prescription hypoallergenic diets or homemade diets such as rice with cottage cheese or lamb should be tried. If parasites are identified, appropriate therapy should be instituted.

The basis of medical management in eosinophilic gastritis is corticosteroid therapy. Clinical improvement and reduction in the infiltrative lesions usually result. Prednisone at an initial dose of 0.5 to 1 mg/lb (1 to 2 mg/kg) body weight should be given daily in divided doses for several weeks. The dose is then tapered to a range of 0.05 to 0.2 mg/lb (0.12 to 0.50 mg/kg) every other day. The response to diet and corticosteroids is generally favorable, but prolonged therapy is usually required to maintain remission.

HYPERTROPHIC GASTROPATHIES

Chronic hypertrophic gastropathies include a number of conditions characterized by a thicker-than-normal gastric mucosa. These hypertrophic changes may be either diffuse, regional, or focal in distribution and may be observed radiographically, endoscopically or through gross visual examination. Histopathologically, several forms of hypertrophic gastropathies have been recognized. There may be thickening of the mucosa resulting entirely from proliferation of surface mucosal epithelial cells or from glandular hypertrophy, in which the gastric glands increase in size. There may be an inflammatory infiltrate associated with the changes.

Pathophysiology

Hypertrophic gastropathies vary in their etiology and pathologic characterization. An extensive description of each is hindered by both the lack of a uniform system of classification and a paucity of clinical reports. From the experimental evidence and clinical case reports, there appear to be a number of trophic factors that cause gastric hypertrophy. Chronic irritation to the gastric mucosa can result in hypertrophy and hyperplasia. Mechanical irritation (such as a gastric foreign body), chemical, or inflammatory factors may all be responsible. Focal gastric hypertrophy has been produced by the chronic administration of aspirin.[53] Immune-mediated mechanisms as described in chronic atrophic gastritis may, rather than causing gastric mucosal atrophy, result in gastric mucosal proliferation by stimulating the generative zones in compensation for parietal cell loss or damage.[100] Possibly neuroendocrine factors are trophic to the gastric mucosa. For example, cholecystokinin and acetylcholine are both trophic to the gastric mucosa and could be released in excess due to chronic vagal activity.[97] Excess production of the gastric hormone gastrin will cause gastric glandular hypertrophy. A number of clinical conditions may result in hypergastrinemia. These include chronic gastric distention, chronic renal disease and altered gastrin degradation, gastrin-secreting tumors (gastrinomas), and idiopathic hypertrophy of the G (gastrin-secreting) cells in the antrum. The trophic action of histamine is similar to that of gastrin, and blood levels may be elevated with mastocytomas. Excess histamine levels not only cause mucosal changes but also cause gastric ulceration due to excess gastric acid secretion. Stress-related environmental factors are reported to cause gastric mucosal hyperplasia in mice.[100]

It is believed that stress-related vascular disturbances result in gastric ischemia with parietal cell death initiating an autoimmune proliferative response. This proposed mechanism may be a potential etiology in some canine or feline cases.

The following types of chronic hypertrophic gastropathies have been observed in dogs.

Focal cystic hypertrophic gastropathy is a condition described as well-circumscribed, enlarged, convoluted rugae. Radiographically these focal lesions appear as mucosal filling defects and were observed predominantly in the body or fundic region of the stomach. Prominent features histopathologically are elongated and tortuous mucous glands with frequent mucous cyst formation.[101]

Hypertrophic gastritis of basenji dogs is usually associated with a diffuse, immunoproliferative enteropathy.[102, 103] The gastric lesions are either a diffuse rugal hypertrophy or may be regional in the body of the stomach.[104] There is hypertrophy of the glands and an increase in the mucous, parietal, and chief cells. There is also generally an inflammatory component to the lesion as well as gastric ulceration. The postulated cause of these lesions is thought to be, in part, genetic as well as immunologically mediated. Hypergastrinemia may play a role, since many of these dogs have elevated serum gastrin concentrations.[105]

Hypertrophic glandular gastritis is a condition resulting from trophic hyperplasia of the glandular gastric mucosa. There is an increase in the number of parietal cells and thus a probable corresponding increase in gastric acid secretion. Gastric ulceration is common. These changes have been observed in dogs with systemic mastocytosis (histamine excess) and in dogs with gastrin-secreting tumors (gastrinomas).[106, 107] A hypertrophic glandular gastritis with increased gastric acid secretion and gastric ulceration in conjunction with hypergastrinemia was observed in a bassett hound.[108] Provocative testing found this dog to have gastric antral G-cell hyperplasia. Diffuse gastric rugal hypertrophy has also been described in a Boxer dog, although no etiology was identified.[109]

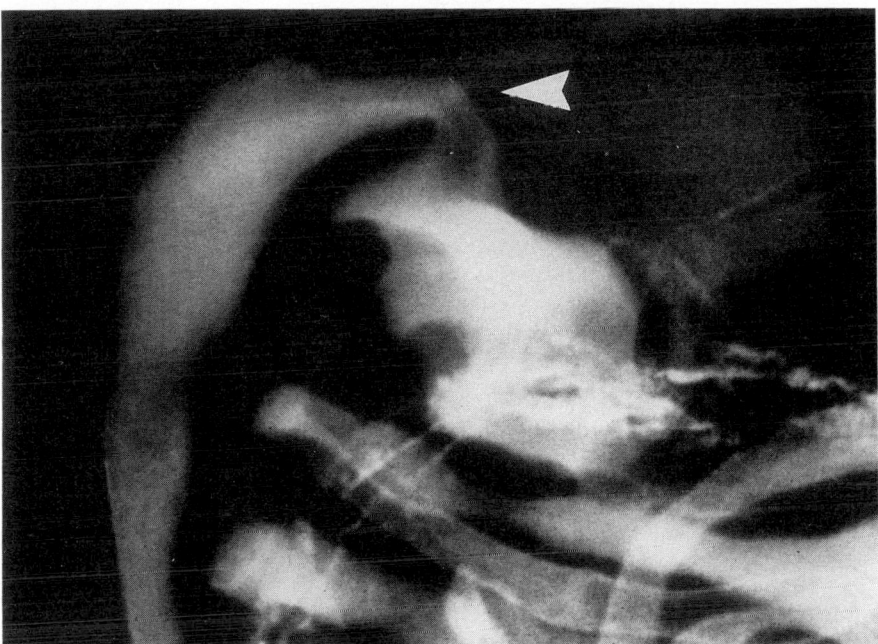

FIGURE 85–11. A liquid barium study demonstrating a partial gastric outflow obstruction in the pyloric-antral region secondary to chronic mucosal hypertrophy. Thickened rugal folds are present just anterior to the pyloric canal (arrowhead). These mucosal lesions were subsequently surgically resected in this case.

Chronic hypertrophic pyloric gastropathy is characterized by antral and pyloric mucosal hypertrophy.[110, 111] The lesions occur as focal or multifocal polypoid thickening or as a regionally generalized rugal enlargement. There are foveolar and glandular hyperplasia, cystic dilatation, and superficial mucosal ulceration and inflammation. These lesions often result in gastric outlet obstruction.[112] The etiology of this condition or group of conditions is unknown. A neuroendocrine or stress-related cause is postulated, since many of the cases are observed in highly excitable and nervous small breed dogs.[111]

Clinical Findings

The clinical signs in dogs with hypertrophic gastropathy are similar to signs of chronic gastritis. Vomiting is the most constant feature. If there is mucosal ulceration, the vomitus may contain blood. If the hypertrophy causes a partial mechanical outflow obstruction, the vomiting may be intermittent, consisting of undigested food, often hours following eating. Other signs include anorexia, belching, abdominal pain, melena, and weight loss. Basenji dogs with hypertrophic gastritis usually have anorexia, diarrhea, and weight loss due to a concurrent immunoproliferative enteropathy. Dogs with hypertrophic pyloric gastropathy are usually described as small breed, middle-aged dogs that have been vomiting intermittently for several months to years.

Diagnosis

The diagnosis of hypertrophic gastropathies is based on a full-thickness gastric biopsy. A suction biopsy or endoscopically directed pinch biopsy is usually not deep enough to adequately demonstrate the hypertrophy. Barium contrast radiographs will demonstrate thickened gastric rugal folds. In some cases, changes will be focal and appear similar to neoplastic filling defects. Lesions that are located in the pyloric-antral portion of the stomach often result in delayed gastric emptying or a narrowed antral region by the filling defects (Figure 85–11). Endoscopic examination may confirm the radiographic findings and will also identify any associated mucosal ulceration. Care should always be taken to adequately insufflate the gastric lumen during endoscopic examination, for in an improperly distended stomach, normal rugae may appear as hypertrophic rugae.[93] Dogs with hypertrophic gastropathies persist in having prominent rugal folds even after complete distention of the stomach. Cases in which there is hypertrophic glandular gastritis with an increase in mucosal, chief, and parietal cells, or hypertrophic gastritis with gastric or duodenal ulceration, should be evaluated for histamine-associated mast cell tumors or conditions associated with elevated serum gastrin levels. Abnormal gastrin elevations are found with gastrinomas (gastrin-secreting tumors), antral G-cell hyperplasia, and compromised renal function.[113] In such conditions, gastric acid production will be abnormal.

Treatment

The therapy for chronic hypertrophic gastropathies is often supportive, especially if an etiology is not determined. Focal or discoid areas of hypertrophy are usually responsive to simple resection. Diffuse hypertrophy, especially associated with hypergastrinemia, hyperchlorhydria, and mucosal ulceration, should be managed with H_2-receptor blockers, or antacids (see Gastric Ulceration). Dietary suggestions for chronic gastritis should also be applied to these disorders.

When the mucosal hypertrophy acts as a mechanical obstruction and pyloric outflow is reduced, surgical intervention is required. Focal mucosal resection, pyloroplasty, or even a pyloric-antral resection may be required.[114] There was apparent higher success rate in dogs with pyloric-antral lesions following a pyloric resection with a gastroduodenostomy.

The prognosis for chronic hypertrophic gastropathy is quite variable based on the etiology, surgical therapy, and secondary complications. Dogs with hypergastrinemic, hypertrophic glandular gastritis have a guarded prognosis. H_2-receptor blocking agents may be beneficial in managing the gastric ulceration. Hypertrophic gastropathy in basenji dogs is only one facet of a complicated disease syndrome and has a very poor prognosis.

GASTRIC ULCERATION

Gastric ulceration refers to grossly detectable mucosal defects. These mucosal defects may occur as multiple, superficial mucosal erosions or as large, circumscribed ulcers that penetrate through the muscularis mucosae. The latter type is less commonly observed in dogs or cats. Erosions and ulcers arise from a number of causes, and the signs may be associated with significant gastric hemorrhage.

Etiology

Gastric ulceration in the dog and cat may result from any of the agents causing acute or chronic gastritis. The basic conditions (exogenous factors, endogenous factors, and altered gastric mucosal blood flow) are responsible for mucosal erosions and ulcerations. Often gastric ulceration is associated with certain clinical situations or drug administration that brings about the mucosal damage. Table 85–2 lists conditions and drugs that have been recognized to be associated with gastric ulceration.

Pathophysiology

The mechanisms of gastric ulcer formation and their description and location vary depending on the etiology.

TABLE 85–2. COMMON FACTORS ASSOCIATED WITH GASTRIC ULCERATION

Drugs
   Aspirin
   Indomethacin
   Phenylbutazone
   Flunixin
   Ibuprofen
   Naproxen
   Corticosteroids
Stress Factors
   Hypotension
   Severe illness
   Environmental stress
Neurologic Disease
Enterogastric Reflux
Metabolic Disorders
   Renal disease
   Liver disease
   Adrenocortical insufficiency
Gastric Hyperacidity
   Systemic mastocytosis
   Gastrinoma

In all conditions the pathophysiologic factors are many, and no one mechanism can be considered solely responsible. *Many drugs* commonly administered to dogs and cats are ulcerogenic to the gastric mucosa; most notable are the nonsteroidal anti-inflammatory agents. Refer to the section on Agents of Mucosal Damage for a description of their action.

Stress ulceration results in multiple erosions in the gastric, duodenal, or colonic mucosa of acutely ill patients. Lesions are usually superficial to the muscularis mucosae and are thus properly termed erosions, but occasionally a penetrating ulcer is noted, surrounded by erosions. Stress ulceration is common, but is infrequently reported in the dog. When present, stress ulcers may have a significant morbidity and mortality.[115–117] Stress conditions such as restraint, severe illness, trauma, shock, and hypotension are associated with stress ulcer formation. It is frequently the intensive care patient that is a high risk for the development of gastric ulcerations.

A multifactorial pathogenesis is suspected in stress ulcer formation. Gastric epithelial cell vitality and renewal are protective against ulcer formation. Gastric mucosal cells have an average four-day lifespan and are constantly undergoing replication. Certain stress conditions impair this epithelial cell renewal.[118] Ischemia to the gastric mucosa is another factor in stress-related ulceration. Shock, hypotension, and sympathetically mediated vasoconstriction promote ischemia. Local ischemia then results in a profound reduction in gastric mucosal aerobic metabolism with subsequent cellular death. Concurrent release of endogenous corticosteroids, vasoactive catecholamines, and serotonin contribute to stress ulceration.[119] Bile acids and pancreatic enzymes, if refluxed into the gastric lumen, promote ulceration.

Neurologic disease is also associated with gastric ulceration.[120, 121] This is most often observed in dogs with severe spinal cord lesions, concurrently receiving glucocorticoid therapy.[122] Severe gastric erosions or deep and possibly perforating ulcers may develop. The pathophysiology of neurologic-related gastric ulceration is thought to include previously described stress-related factors in conjunction with imbalances in sympathetic and parasympathetic innervation to the stomach. Loss in the vascular sympathetic input along with a parasympathetic-mediated vasodilation and stimulation of acid secretion promotes mucosal ischemia and ulceration. The administration of exogenous glucocorticoids in this situation potentiates ulcer formation.

Various diseases and metabolic disturbances frequently result in gastric ulceration as one component of the disease syndrome. Acute or chronic renal failure can lead to mucosal damage. Uremic toxins can directly injure the gastric mucosa and vessels of the gastric wall.[123] Renal failure also results in elevated serum gastrin levels that, in turn, increase gastric acid secretion.[65] It is proposed that abnormal elevations in gastrin are due to decreased renal metabolism of the hormone. Thus, direct mucosal damage, excess acid secretion, and local ischemia all play a role in the formation of uremic ulcerative gastritis.

Gastric ulceration is observed secondary to chronic

liver disease and results from several mechanisms.[124] The catabolic state of the patient and associated hypoalbuminemia result in altered gastric mucus production and reduced epithelial cell turnover. Ulceration is potentiated by reduced gastric blood flow as a result of portal hypertension.[125] In the authors' experience, some but not all dogs with chronic liver disease have elevated serum gastrin levels and increased gastric acid secretion. In experimental studies in dogs with portacaval anastomosis, there is a marked increase in gastric acid secretion.[126] This may be due to elevated circulating bile acid levels that stimulate gastrin release.[127] Another explanation is that histamine, a byproduct of dietary histidine that is normally degraded in passage through the liver, enters the collateral circulation and directly stimulates gastric parietal cells to secrete gastric acid.[128] Gastric lesions have also been observed in some animals with hypoadrenocorticism, in which gastric ulceration is possibly caused by hypotension and abnormal vascular tone.

In *systemic mastocytosis*, histamine produced by mast cells is released in large quantities and causes gastric lesions. Gastric ulcers secondary to mast cell neoplasia in dogs[129, 130] and cats[131] have been reported. In dogs, the concentration of histamine in mast cell tumors varies considerably.[132] Gastric ulceration in the dog is most frequent with mast cell tumors that contain a large tumor mass, but infrequently, small tumors can also cause gastric ulceration.[129]

The mechanism of induction of gastroduodenal lesions with mastocytomas is not completely understood. Interestingly, heparin prevents mucosal ulceration in the stomach.[129, 133] In dogs with mast cell neoplasia there may be pronounced histamine intoxication without concomitant heparinemia. The mast cell contains both compounds in abundance; it therefore follows that in mastocytomas either heparin is not released in significant amounts or it is bound or rapidly metabolized following liberation. In canine mastocytoma, neoplastic cells are often anaplastic and exhibit little cytoplasmic metachromasia, indicating a lack of heparin.[129]

Mucosal lesions in mastocytoma are partially associated with mucosal ischemia and intravascular thrombosis. Small vascular thrombi were observed in the gastric mucosa of dogs with mastocytoma.[129] Serum gastrin levels are low, probably the result of a feedback mechanism from increased acid production.

Clinical Findings

Vomiting is the most frequent clinical sign of gastric ulcers. Vomitus may be either tinged with partially digested blood ("coffee ground" appearance) or with fresh blood and clots in severe ulceration. Melena, variable appetite, and weight loss are often reported. With severe blood loss the patient may show anemia, and with vomiting, dehydration and secondary polydipsia may be noted. Some dogs with gastric ulcers may be asymptomatic, while others are seen following perforation, which rapidly results in death.

Diagnosis

The diagnosis of gastric ulceration should always be considered when clinical circumstances that promote gastric ulceration exist. These include specific drug therapy, stress factors, neurologic disease, and metabolic disorders. Careful investigation should also include examination for cutaneous mast cell tumors. These are usually easily diagnosed by fine needle aspirate.

The presence of blood in the vomitus, either fresh or digested, should signify gastric ulceration unless proven otherwise. Consequently, hematemesis associated with appropriate clinical situations may be all that is required for a presumptive diagnosis of gastric ulceration.

The physical examination is often noncontributory. Abdominal pain may be the most frequently encountered physical examination finding. Although the location of the stomach prevents actual palpation, abdominal splinting should include gastric ulceration as a differential.

There are few hematologic and biochemical alterations specifically associated with gastric ulceration. Regenerative anemia may be associated with gastric ulceration, whereas chronic blood loss may result in iron deficiency anemia. In 16 of 22 cases of peptic ulceration in dogs, liver disease was also noted. The pathologic changes in the liver ranged from severe disease to fatty and degenerative changes.[134] Lead poisoning may also result in gastric ulcers.[135]

Gastric ulcers, mucosal niches, craters, or fissures of varying sizes may be demonstrated by contrast barium radiography. Superficial stress erosions usually cannot be seen by barium contrast examination. For this reason, contrast radiography is a relatively insensitive diagnostic tool for detecting mucosal ulceration, and a negative study does not rule out the diagnosis. If a perforated ulcer is suspected, an iodine contrast agent should be used to avoid barium peritonitis.

Endoscopy provides the best objective evidence of gastric ulcers. With acute ulcers, mucosal lesions may be bleeding, have an inflammatory appearance around the periphery, and usually have no evidence of fibrin in the ulcer craters. Chronic ulcers may show little inflammatory response and have a fibrin-filled crater and wrinkled mucosa peripheral to the ulcer. With stress ulceration, early in the post-stress period, focal areas of pallor and cyanosis are seen. Later, discrete areas of red blood cell extravasation may be observed. Numerous small, well-delineated punctate lesions can be identified along the crests of the rugae within the proximal stomach. These lesions are usually only a few millimeters in size. Fresh or digested blood may be observed within the lumen.

Exploratory gastrotomy can be a useful diagnostic tool in gastric ulceration. Gastric ulceration can occur in association with benign and malignant neoplasms of the stomach, and for this reason, histopathology should always be included in all cases of gastric ulceration.

If the gastric ulceration is suspected to be secondary to hypergastrinemia or conditions associated with hyperchlorhydria, gastric acid analysis or secretory testing may be helpful (refer to section on Gastric Secretory Testing).

Treatment

Therapy for gastric ulceration should begin by correcting the initiating cause. This includes discontinuation of ulcerogenic drugs, adequate fluid expansion, and replacement of major blood loss. Therapy is then directed at decreasing hydrogen ion and peptic activity, or increasing the protective ability of the gastric mucosa to resist the effects of ulceration. Pharmacologic agents that are useful in the management of gastric ulceration include antacids, H_2-receptor antagonists, coating agents, and some newer but still investigational drugs.

Antacids function to reduce the total amount of available hydrogen ions, as well as to irreversibly inactivate pepsin if gastric luminal contents can be brought above pH six. A third effect of antacids is to diminish peptic activity as the pH is raised above the range for optimal proteolysis. Antacids must be administered frequently, as infrequent antacid administration may result in rebound acid hypersecretion. This rebound effect is most frequently noted when antacids are given two to three times a day, rather than being continuously administered. The rate of gastric emptying is a major determinant of antacid effectiveness. Thus, with the exponential emptying characteristic of the stomach, the administration of antacids in large, infrequent doses is less likely to provide sustained buffering. Aluminum-containing antacids delay gastric emptying in some species.[136]

Various preparations are available, but no antacid is free of hazard. Sodium bicarbonate may produce sodium overload and systemic alkalosis. Magnesium preparations may lead to severe diarrhea and are hazardous to renal failure patients. Calcium carbonate may lead to hypercalcemia, renal impairment, and stimulation of gastric acid secretion. Aluminum hydroxide may lead to phosphate depletion, with consequent muscle weakness, bone resorption, and hypercalciuria.[137] Although antacid therapy is effective in the management of gastric ulceration, the frequency and administration difficulty in animals make it less practical. Antacid therapy is generally reserved for the patient with severe gastric ulceration and bleeding.

H_2-receptor antagonists such as cimetidine, ranitidine, and famotidine are effective in reducing gastric acid production by blocking the histamine receptor on the parietal cell.[138] There are few published clinical reports on their effectiveness in the treatment of gastric ulceration in dogs,[139, 140] but clinically they are considered to be efficacious in increasing the healing rate of gastric ulcers and preventing their recurrence.[141] H_2-receptor antagonists are not effective in providing adequate prophylaxis to gastric ulceration. This ineffectiveness results because these agents impair the secretory state of the mucosa, thus decreasing intracellular buffering capacity, and thereby inadequately reducing intraluminal acidity.[142]

H_2-receptor antagonists are clinically indicated in the treatment of gastric ulcerations. A suggested dose of cimetidine (Tagamet) is 2 to 5 mg/lb (5 to 10 mg/kg) q6h IV or PO, and for ranitidine (Zantac), 1 mg/lb (2 mg/kg), q8h IV or PO. Therapy should continue for two weeks. Long-term therapy may be required for the management of gastrinomas, mastocytoma, and uremic gastritis. Both drugs appear to be similarly effective; however, clinical studies are lacking. Ranitidine reportedly has more potent acid inhibition than cimetidine, with a longer duration of action as well as fewer side effects. The antiandrogenic effects of cimetidine observed in humans with prolonged use as well as the potential for altered hepatic biotransformation of concurrently administered drugs may favor the use of ranitidine. Adverse effects of either drug have not been reported in dogs or cats.

Cytoprotective agents such as sucralfate (Carafate), when given orally, bind to proteins in the ulcer site, forming a protective barrier. Other beneficial properties include inhibition of pepsin activity, binding of pancreatic secretions and bile salts, and stimulation of endogenous mucosal cytoprotective prostaglandins.[143]

Sucralfate appears to be as effective as H_2-receptor antagonists for healing gastric or duodenal ulcers. A suggested dose is 1 gm/60 lb (1 gm/30 kg) body weight given orally q6h. Sucralfate is a safe preparation that is not absorbed systemically. It should not be given concurrently with other medications, because of altered gastrointestinal absorption. Since gastric acid is required to break down the tablets, H_2-receptor therapy should follow sucralfate therapy by approximately one hour. Clinical experience has found the combined use of Carafate and H_2-receptor antagonists to be the preferred therapy for gastric and duodenal ulceration.

Another class of cytoprotective agents is the prostaglandins (PGE_2) and their analogs. These agents will soon be available for clinical use. In addition to their cytoprotective capabilities, they also reduce gastric acid secretion and increase mucosal healing rates. The exogenous administration of prostaglandin analogs has been shown to be therapeutically beneficial in various types of gastric mucosal injury.[144, 145]

Emergency therapy is required for severe gastric blood loss from acute ulceration. Whole blood transfusions as well as crystalloid fluids should be administered to replace blood losses. Previous recommendations for the management of life-threatening gastric bleeding included the use of iced gastric lavages, often containing norepinephrine. The rationale was that cooling decreases blood flow and reduces the digestive processes while adrenergic agents further promote local vasoconstriction. Studies in the dog have found that cooling the stomach actually prolongs bleeding times and does not slow hemorrhage.[146, 147] The efficacy of norepinephrine-containing lavages is also unproven. It appears more rational and less stressful to use H_2-receptor antagonists, sucralfate, and possibly frequent oral antacid administration in these patients.

Surgical therapy is occasionally required for gastric ulceration. Partial gastrectomy is generally required for removal of the ulcer. This technique, along with pyloromyotomy and vagotomy, has been successfully used in the dog.[148] With peritonitis secondary to perforation of a gastric ulcer, immediate surgery is indicated.

GASTRIC OUTLET OBSTRUCTIONS

Retention of gastric contents is often associated with pyloric dysfunction, motility disorders of the stomach, or both. The pylorus is an important anatomic structure because of its location at the distal end of the stomach and because it functions to impede gastric emptying of solids and to prevent duodenal reflux. Mechanical obstructions in the gastric antrum or pylorus may result in blockage of the passage of contents into the intestine. Gastric retention, distention, and vomiting are manifestations of these obstructive lesions.

Etiology

Pyloric dysfunction results from intrinsic, extrinsic, or obturative lesions. Intrinsic lesions of the pylorus result either from hypertrophy of the circular muscle fibers (pyloric stenosis) or from intrinsic pyloric neoplasia. Extrinsic pyloric lesions include hepatic and pancreatic abscesses, neoplasia, and inflammatory lesions. Gastric histoplasmosis and phycomycosis may produce intrinsic or extrinsic lesions. Foreign bodies, gastric and/or duodenal ulcers, antral mucosal hypertrophy, and antral polyps (see Hypertrophic Gastropathy section) result in obturative pyloric lesions.

Pyloric stenosis refers to a specific intrinsic lesion associated with hypertrophy of the circular muscle fibers in the pyloric ring that reduces the luminal diameter. The signs are those of a pyloric outflow obstruction. Two clinical syndromes occur with this muscular hypertrophy. The first is a congenital pyloric stenosis that is detected in young dogs and cats shortly following weaning. The second is an acquired form that occurs more commonly in older animals.

Pathophysiology

The net result of clinical and metabolic changes is similar, regardless of the etiology of the pyloric outflow obstruction. The severity of gastric-associated events is, in part, due to the duration and completeness of the pyloric outflow obstruction.

The cause of pyloric stenosis is unknown. It may result from excessive secretion of gastrointestinal hormones. With antral distention, G cells are stimulated to release gastrin, which ultimately leads to a decrease in gastric pH. Gastrin also has potent trophic effects on gastric smooth muscle. Gastrin injections given to pregnant bitches cause 28 per cent of pups to be born with pyloric stenosis. Circular muscle becomes hypertrophied, as in spontaneous disease.[149] This report was recently refuted when it was noted that human-origin gastrin does not cross the canine placenta and also that human maternal and cord-blood gastrin levels may vary independently.[150]

Pyloric stenosis may also be associated with neurogenic dysfunction. The number of myenteric ganglion cells and nerve fiber tracts is reduced in the pyloric region, and the circular muscle of the pylorus is hypertrophied.[151] A nonorganic stenosis accompanied by antral dilatation and muscular hypertrophy can be produced by selective destruction of the intramural ganglia of the pylorus.[152]

Partial obstruction to pyloric outflow in any condition may result in gastric hypersecretion. An obvious consequence of outflow obstruction is gastric distention.

With chronic distention, gastric mucosal hyperplasia occurs as a consequence of increased secretory cell mitosis.[153, 154] From the preceding it can be suggested that gastric retention leads to worsening of outflow obstruction due to the trophic actions of gastrin on smooth muscle and mucosa.

Clinical Findings

Vomiting at fairly regular intervals following ingestion of solid food and accompanied by gastric distention is the primary sign of pyloric outflow obstruction. The vomitus is usually undigested food and is rarely bile-stained. Normally, the stomach should be empty of a meal by eight to ten hours following eating. Vomiting of food greater than eight to ten hours following eating suggests a disorder associated with abnormal gastric retention. Chronic vomiting may be associated with weight loss and dehydration. Animals with gastric neoplasia may have significant debilitation and possibly signs of other organ involvement. Conditions causing a complete outflow obstruction will result in severe and profuse vomiting.

Projectile vomiting has been associated with complete or partial pyloric obstruction and involves the abrupt occurrence of vomiting without the warning signs of increased salivation and retching. In most instances the vomitus is thrown for a considerable distance and readily empties the stomach.

Brachycephalic breeds have a high incidence of congenital pyloric stenosis. It is also reported in Siamese cats.[155] No sex predilection is reported for the dog or cat. Two female kittens with pyloric stenosis have been reported, suggesting a possible heritable basis for the disease.[156] Animals with congenital pyloric stenosis usually begin vomiting following weaning or at an early age. The severity of signs generally progresses with time. These animals often reingest the vomited meal only to vomit again later. The signs of acquired pyloric stenosis are frequently those of chronic intermittent vomiting. The vomiting usually progresses in severity with time.

Diagnosis

There are no specific physical examination findings in animals with pyloric outflow obstructions, and laboratory evaluation will be quite variable depending on the etiology. Laboratory assessment may show hematologic changes of dehydration with an elevation in the PCV and total solids. With a severe and complete gastric outlet obstruction, vomiting will result in metabolic alkalosis. In these patients, there is hypokalemia and hypochloremia and possibly a paradoxical aciduria.[157]

Radiography affords the most definitive method of diagnosing gastric retention. Gastric distention with food and/or air long after ingesta should be in the intestine is diagnostic of gastric retention.[32] In the cat, increased gastric volume, with the fundus and body elongated craniocaudally but remaining on the left side of the midline, and the mucosal folds being stretched and having a smooth appearance, is seen with gastric retention.[155] The pyloric antrum is often enlarged in size and the pyloric canal narrowed and elongated.

Contrast radiography is helpful in assessing the rate of gastric emptying. The term "gastric emptying time" in radiography is usually regarded as the time required for the stomach to begin to empty—but not to empty completely. Less than 30 minutes is reported to be normal gastric emptying time. Normally barium is retained for 5 to 15 minutes. The presence of barium within the stomach for more than 12 to 24 hours is abnormal and should be considered a sign of gastric retention. The stress of chemical[33] or manual restraint may delay gastric emptying.[32]

Contrast barium studies usually identify obturating lesions such as foreign bodies, mucosal hypertrophy, or large ulcers, as well as extrinsic lesions that compromise the pyloric canal. Intrinsic lesions, unless quite prominent, are more difficult to identify. In some cases, fluoroscopy aids in evaluating the pyloric area.[158]

The radiographic features of pyloric stenosis include gastric distention, delayed emptying time, and failure of contrast to fill the pyloric canal. Stenosis from muscular hypertrophy may result in a "beak-sign" when barium appears as a beak-like projection entering the pyloric canal (Figure 85–12). The canal may also appear elongated and narrow, with a string of contrast passing through. Normal findings on a barium contrast do not exclude the possibility of pyloric stenosis, as some animals may have normal emptying.[159] In such cases, the lesion may affect the emptying of food more than liquids, and emptying studies using canned food mixed with barium should be evaluated.

The usefulness of gastroscopy in the canine patient with hypertrophy of the pyloric musculature is not documented. One report suggests that the pyloric orifice is fixed or narrowed and that peristaltic waves result in incomplete closure of the orifice.[160] It is advisable to remember that the pyloric orifice of the dog is usually partially open. With the presence of ulcer, neoplasms, inflammation, or granulomatous changes, biopsies may be taken for diagnosis and prognosis.

Treatment

Pyloric outflow obstructions may result in fluid, electrolyte, or acid-base abnormalities. In such cases, appropriate fluid therapy should be instituted. Metabolic alkalosis resulting from an outflow obstruction must be treated with adequate quantities of potassium and chloride. Ringer's solution or normal saline solution supplemented with additional potassium is indicated. Buffered solutions such as lactated Ringer's should be avoided in animals with metabolic alkalosis. Obstruction to gastric outflow is best managed surgically. Intrinsic hypertrophy of the pylorus may be successfully corrected with pyloromyotomy or pyloroplasty.[156, 161-164] With either technique, the incision must be extended well onto the antrum as well as the duodenum to alleviate the area of hypertrophied muscle. Biopsies should be taken of the hypertrophied muscle to confirm the diagnosis and to rule out neoplasia. Pyloric surgery in normal dogs has little effect on the emptying of solids and causes a slight acceleration in emptying of liquids.[165] Obturative lesions must be carefully assessed. With severe mucosal damage and ulceration it may be necessary to surgically excise the affected area. Occasionally the severity of the lesion necessitates elaborate surgical dismemberment of the pylorus, as in gastroduodenostomy[166] or gastrojejunostomy. Dogs with chronic hypertrophic pyloric gastropathy (either mucosal or muscularis hypertrophy) had a favorable response to pyloric resection followed by a gastroduodenostomy.[114]

MOTILITY DISORDERS

A major function of the stomach is the timely evacuation of gastric contents into the intestine for further

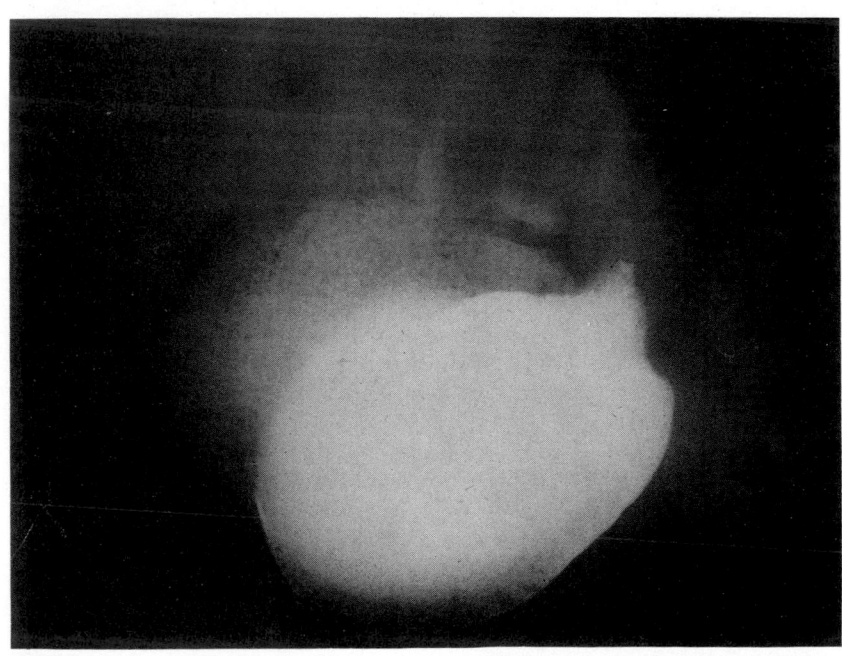

FIGURE 85–12. A liquid barium contrast study demonstrating a narrowed pyloric canal secondary to pyloric muscular hypertrophy in a dog. (Courtesy of Dr. LJ Konde, Las Vegas, NV.)

digestion and absorption. The failure of the stomach to empty its contents in a normal period of time signifies a gastric retention disorder. The previous section (Gastric Outlet Obstructions) dealt with obstructive lesions that possibly comprise most of the clinical causes of gastric retention. In addition to this group of diseases, certain functional motility disorders also cause chronic gastric retention. These motility disorders may result secondary to other conditions or may arise as a primary disease syndrome.

Etiology

There are a number of conditions that are clinically associated with abnormalities in gastric motor function. In order to better understand these conditions and the pathophysiology associated with each, the reader should review the section entitled Gastric Motility and Emptying. There are two basic categories of gastric motility disorders: gastric stasis and disorders of pyloric function.

Gastric Stasis. The failure of normal gastric motility comprises a number of poorly defined conditions that have been observed in the dog and cat. Because there is yet no definitive technique for evaluating normal motor function, the diagnosis of these conditions is often presumptive and made on the basis of appropriate clinical signs and associated clinical situations, and failure to demonstrate an outflow obstructive lesion. Table 85–3 lists conditions that have been associated with delayed gastric emptying due to gastric stasis.

There are many factors that reduce the motility of the stomach and result in retention of gastric contents. *Neurologic inhibition* of gastric motility is mediated through the sympathetic nervous system.[167] Epinephrine has been shown to alter normal gastric electrical and mechanical activity, thereby delaying gastric emptying in the dog.[168] Examples of clinical situations in which nervous inhibition may be a factor include acute stress, trauma, and psychogenic causes. Pain, as with intra-abdominal disorders such as pancreatitis or peritonitis, may also result in gastric stasis from sympathetic stimulation.

TABLE 85–3. CAUSES OF DELAYED GASTRIC MOTILITY

Nervous Inhibition
  Stress
  Trauma
  Pain
  Psychogenic
Metabolic Disorders
  Hypokalemia
  Uremia
  Hepatic encephalopathy
  Hypothyroidism
Drugs
  Anticholinergics
  Narcotic analgesics
Inflammatory Lesions
  Gastritis
  Gastric ulceration
  Parvovirus
Prolonged Gastric Obstruction
Idiopathic

Certain *drugs* cause abnormal gastric motility, and include those with anticholinergic activity and the narcotic analgesic agents. These drugs are often prescribed as therapy for vomiting or diarrhea but have the undesirable side effect of reducing gastric motility. The prolonged administration of these agents may result in severe gastric stasis with signs of retention. These iatrogenic-induced gastric motility disorders resolve with discontinuation of the drug.

A number of *metabolic disturbances* such as electrolyte or acid-base imbalances and certain disease-related changes may be responsible for altered gastric neuromuscular function. Hypokalemia, calcium imbalance, acidosis, uremia, diabetes mellitus, and hepatic encephalopathy have all been associated with abnormal gastric motility.[169] Hypothyroid dogs have been shown to have abnormal gastric myoelectric and mechanical activity.[170] The clinical significance of each is yet to be determined.

Inflammatory lesions of the stomach are often clinically associated with delayed gastric emptying. Ulcerative, inflammatory, or infiltrative lesions alter normal gastric electrical-mechanical activity. It is not unusual for chronic gastritis to be complicated by a secondary gastric stasis. Gastroparesis may also follow viral gastroenteritis.[171] Dogs with parvovirus infections have reduced gastric motility that can be severe enough to cause persistent vomiting for days following otherwise clinical improvement. Chronic gastric outlet obstructions may lead to gastric distention and hypomotility.

There is considerable speculation that the gastric dilatation volvulus complex may, in part, result from abnormal gastric motility.[172] Measurement of gastric myoelectric and mechanical activity is currently being investigated; however, radiographic and isotope studies have failed to demonstrate, as yet, a significant abnormality in emptying times.[173]

Some animals have been identified as having signs and symptoms of gastric stasis without evidence of an underlying primary etiology. These *idiopathic gastric motility disorders* may result from abnormal function of the gastric pacemaker with defective gastric electrical and mechanical activity. Some persons with symptoms of nausea, vomiting and delayed gastric emptying have been found to have abnormal gastric electrical conduction disturbances.[174] Electrical gastric dysrhythmias such as tachygastria, characterized by an ectopic pacemaker firing at a higher rate than normal, or tachyarrhythmias, with irregular electrical cycles, have been recorded in dogs and humans and may account for idiopathic gastric stasis.[17] Chronic trichobezoar formation in cats may be the result of an idiopathic motility abnormality resulting in abnormal migrating motor complexes (interdigestive housekeeper contractions). This consideration arises from the fact that some persons with bezoar formation have been identified with this motility disturbance.[175]

Pyloric Dysfunction. Pylorospasm is a condition described as a functional closure of the pyloric canal resulting in an outflow obstruction. This has been a frequent radiographic diagnosis made when there is a delay in gastric emptying, with a failure of the contrast agent to fill the pyloric canal. True pylorospasm in humans does not exist,[154] but rather is thought to be a function of decreased gastric antral motility.[176]

The pylorus functions to limit the reflux of duodenal contents. Enterogastric reflux occurs when the duodenal pressure exceeds gastric and pyloric pressure. Normal gastric motility prevents prolonged gastric contact with any refluxed material by subsequent peristaltic waves. Bile, pancreatic enzymes, and other constituents of intestinal fluid will produce gastric mucosal damage from persistent reflux. Signs of enterogastric reflux include nausea, vomiting of bile, and gastric pain. This clinical syndrome associated with bilious vomiting is referred to as *reflux gastritis*.

Clinical Findings. Vomiting is the principal clinical sign of gastric or pyloric motility disorders. An undigested meal may be vomited many hours after the stomach should have been empty. The duration and frequency of vomiting may be quite variable. Other signs include nausea, anorexia, belching, and weight loss.

Signs of reflux gastritis consist of vomiting bile-stained gastric fluid, frequently in the early morning when the stomach is empty. Dogs with this condition are generally asymptomatic for the remainder of the day and are, for the most part, in good health.

Diagnosis

A presumptive diagnosis is often made only after excluding other organic-related gastric disease in animals with signs characteristic of a motility abnormality. Vomiting of an undigested meal more than eight to ten hours following eating suggests either a motility disturbance or an outlet obstruction. Failure to identify an obstructive lesion (see Gastric Outlet Obstructions) supports a diagnosis of motility abnormality.

Endoscopic or surgical examination of the stomach is generally unremarkable. Barium radiographic studies may demonstrate delayed emptying but may be normal in some cases. The use of food mixed with liquid barium may better demonstrate delayed emptying in some cases. The retention of a barium meal for longer than ten hours supports the diagnosis.[34]

Additional research-oriented means of evaluating motility disorders include dye-dilution studies,[177] radioisotope studies, real-time ultrasonography, and the measurement of gastric electrical and mechanical activity.[175]

Treatment

Prior to specific therapy for a suspected motility disorder, attempts should be directed at identifying and correcting any underlying etiology. Conditions such as hypokalemia, drug therapies, chronic gastritis, hypothyroidism, and mechanical obstructions, for example, if treated, usually resolve the motility disorder.

The primary therapy of gastric stasis should first begin with dietary modification. A diet based on certain physiologic principles should be formulated that will promote emptying. Liquid diets empty the stomach faster than solids; high caloric density diets of high osmolarity are slower to leave the stomach.[178, 179] A diet should be formulated that is of liquid consistency and low in fiber, fat, and osmolarity. This generally extrapolates to feeding a moderately low fat, canned, meat-based diet that has been blenderized to a semiliquid consistency.[121] Multiple small meals should be fed each day.

Prokinetic gastric drugs should be incorporated if diet therapy is unsuccessful. Metoclopramide (Reglan) is the drug of choice for the management of motility abnormalities in dogs and cats.[176, 180] Metoclopramide is a dopamine antagonist and a cholinergic potentiating agent that acts to increase the tone and amplitude of gastric contractions, relax the pyloric canal, and increase contraction in the proximal small intestine. Metoclopramide also has a central-acting antiemetic effect. A suggested dosage is 0.1 to 0.3 mg/lb (0.2 to 0.5 mg/kg) given three to four times a day, approximately one-half hour before meals. A continuous intravenous infusion of the drug 0.5 to 1 mg/lb/24 hours (1 to 2 mg/kg/24 hours) is suggested for severe emesis, such as that which may occur in dogs with parvovirus.[181] This drug is contraindicated in gastric outflow obstruction, with concurrent phenothiazine or narcotic therapy, and in epilepsy. Side effects of metoclopramide include central nervous system abnormalities (usually hyperexcitability or depression). An agent similar to metoclopramide with antidopaminergic properties is domperidone; however, its clinical use in dogs is limited. A recently developed compound, cisapride, has been shown to stimulate gastric motility by facilitating acetylcholine release at the myenteric plexus. Cisapride is unlike acetylcholine analogues such as bethanechol and cholinesterase inhibitors such as neostigmine in that it has no extragastrointestinal effects nor does it alter gastric secretion.[182] This agent appears to have significant therapeutic potential.

Reflux gastritis syndromes generally respond to a number of therapeutic approaches. The signs generally result from antral gastritis, and consequently antacids, H_2-receptor antagonists, or sucralfate may prove beneficial. Often, multiple feedings are all that is required. If the vomiting is of an early-morning type, the condition may be managed by simply feeding a late bedtime meal. The food may stimulate motility or perhaps acts as a buffer against refluxed duodenal contents. Most animals with this condition will respond to metoclopramide therapy, as will those with primary motility disorders.

Surgery for gastric stasis has not been objectively studied in veterinary patients. Guidelines similar to those used in humans may be useful in assessing veterinary patients with gastric emptying disorders involving decreased motility. Only patients with objective abnormalities in gastric motor function whose symptoms cannot be controlled by medical therapy are considered, and some attempt should be made to verify that other motor disturbances of the digestive tract are absent.[175]

GASTRINOMA

A gastrinoma is characterized by a gastrin-secreting tumor of the pancreas, resulting in hypergastrinemia, gastric acid hypersecretion, and upper gastrointestinal ulceration.[183] This clinical condition observed in humans is referred to as Zollinger-Ellison syndrome. Cases resembling the human Zollinger-Ellison syndrome have also been observed in dogs and in a cat.[184–188]

Etiology

A gastrinoma is a functional, non-β islet cell tumor of the pancreas that produces gastrin. These tumors are believed to arise from δ (D) cells, which normally compose approximately 5 to 10 per cent of the islet cells.

Pathophysiology

Gastrinomas release biologically active gastrin, resulting in a hypergastrinemic state. Elevated serum gastrin levels stimulate parietal cell secretion, which leads to increased hydrochloric acid secretion (hyperchlorhydria). Further, gastrin has a trophic effect on the gastric mucosa, causing mucosal hypertrophy. Increased gastric acid secretion causes gastric mucosal damage, often resulting in large peptic ulcers in the stomach or proximal duodenum (Figure 85–13). Esophagitis may result from the gastric reflux of the highly concentrated acid secretions. Diarrhea may develop with steatorrhea caused by inactivation of pancreatic lipase and precipitation of bile salts in the abnormally acidic upper intestine. The gastric secretions are also irritating to the

intestinal mucosa, causing inflammatory changes, and high plasma levels of gastrin may contribute to diarrhea by altering intestinal absorption of water and electrolytes.[189] Hypocalcemia may be produced by elevated gastrin levels; this in turn stimulates C-cell hyperplasia in the thyroid and elevates calcitonin levels. Elevated secretin levels reported in one dog with a gastrinoma were thought to result from excessive secretion stimulated by an abnormally acidic duodenum.[107]

Clinical Findings

The majority of dogs with gastrin-secreting tumors are middle-aged or older and show signs of chronic vomiting and weight loss. Vomitus often consists of large volumes of gastric secretions and may contain fresh or digested blood. Gastric or duodenal ulcers may result in blood loss and melena, and if an ulcer perforates, the animal will present with signs of peritonitis. Depression, anorexia, polydipsia, and diarrhea have also been reported.

Diagnosis

A gastrinoma should be considered in any animal with persistent vomiting, diarrhea, and upper gastrointestinal ulceration that is only partially responsive or nonresponsive to conservative therapy. Laboratory findings of

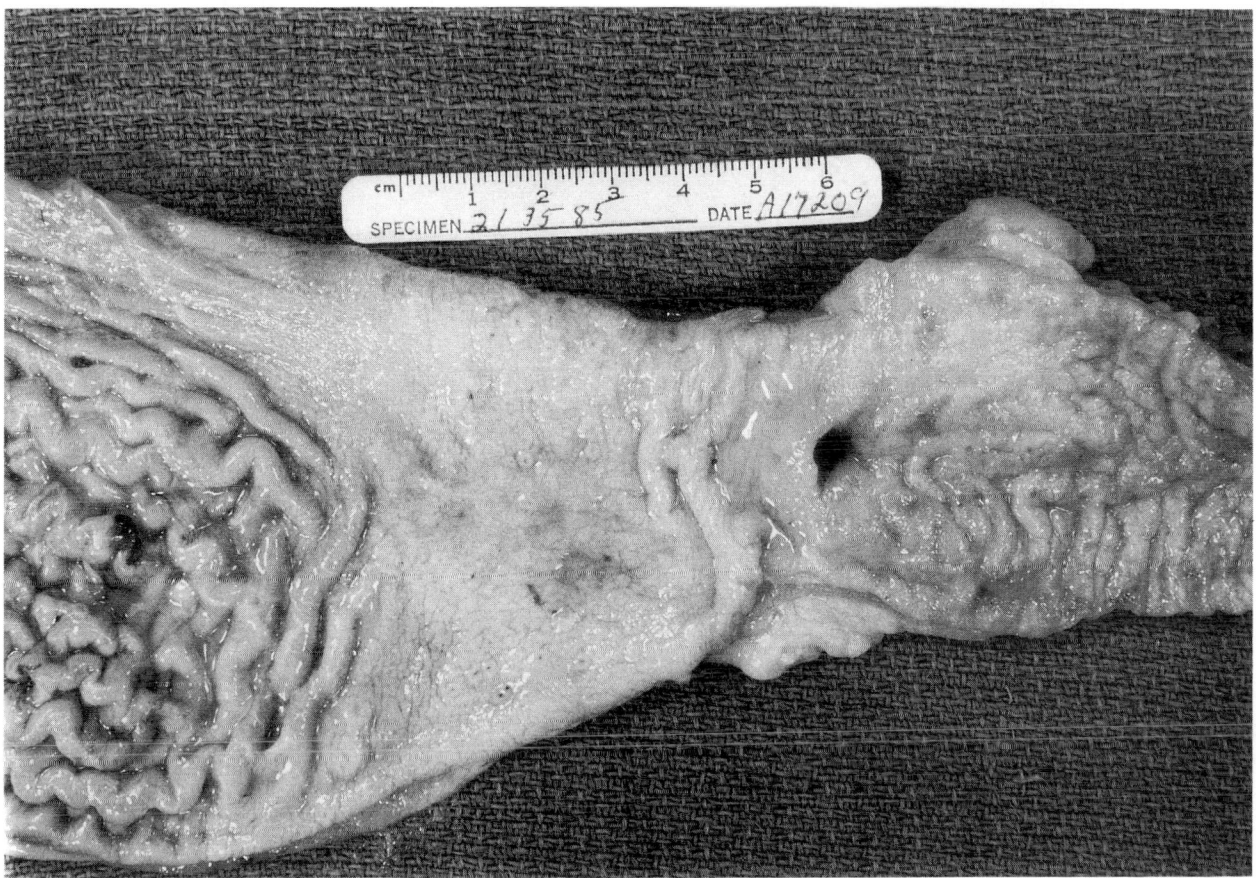

FIGURE 85–13. Perforated ulcer in the proximal duodenum occurring in a dog with a gastrinoma and excessive gastric acid secretion. Also shown is hypertrophy of the gastric mucosa and small gastric erosions.

GASTRIC ACID COLLECTION

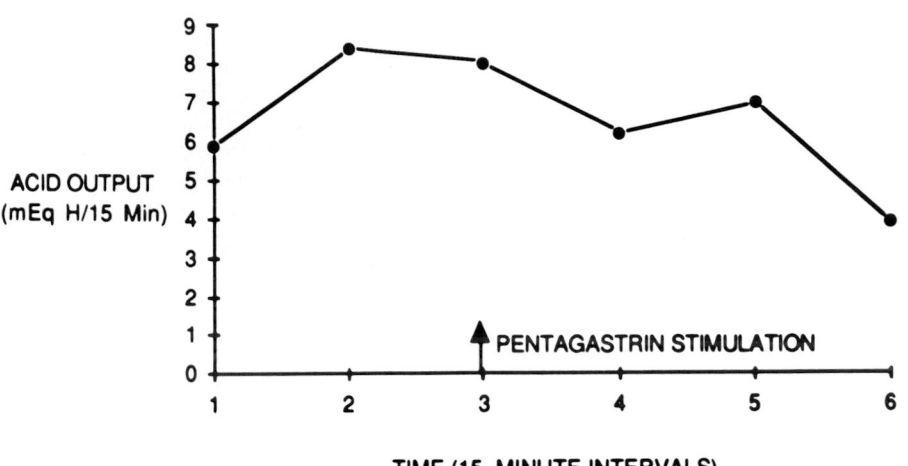

FIGURE 85–14. Gastric acid collection in a dog with a gastrinoma. Basal concentrations are followed by a maximal acid output stimulation by pentagastrin (6 μg/kg subcutaneously). Acid output was collected over 15-minute time periods.

hypochloremia and hypokalemia with a metabolic alkalosis may occur in Zollinger-Ellison syndrome.[185] Abnormal liver-specific enzymes may result from hepatic metastasis, and hypocalcemia occurs from gastrin-stimulated calcitonin secretion. Steatorrhea often develops and is demonstrated with a positive fecal Sudan stain.

Certain contrast radiographic abnormalities may assist in the diagnosis. Gastric rugal folds will be increased and extremely prominent, usually occurring with an ulcer in the stomach or proximal duodenum. The stomach usually contains large amounts of acid-rich fluid, which tends to flocculate the contrast media. There may also be irregularity in the proximal intestinal wall occurring from acid-induced enteritis.

Endoscopy is the best means for evaluating the esophagus, stomach, and proximal duodenum for inflammation and ulceration.[190] Endoscopic examination may reveal inflammation of the distal esophagus due to reflux and vomiting of the acidic gastric contents. The gastric mucosal folds will be prominent, both in number and size. The mucosal surface is often hyperemic, and there may be small superficial ulcerations. The endoscopist may note an increased amount of fluid in the stomach of a fasted animal. There may be a large, one to two cm ulcer in the pyloric antral region or in the proximal duodenum. Biopsies reveal inflammation of the esophageal mucosa, gastric mucosal hypertrophy, and chronic gastritis.

At present, the most reliable means for establishing the diagnosis of a gastrinoma (short of surgery and biopsy) is demonstrating hyperchlorhydria in conjunction with increased serum concentrations of gastrin. Until gastrin levels and secretory testing are evaluated in other clinical gastric diseases in the dog, only a presumptive diagnosis can be made.

Gastric secretory testing is performed as previously described. The normal fasting dog has negligible basal acid output, while fasting levels of 3 to 15 mEq of hydrogen ion per hour have been measured in dogs with gastrinomas.[185, 186] This collection is then followed by measuring maximal acid output. In a dog with a gastrinoma, acid output is already near maximum and therefore, with stimulation, does not show a significant rise as does the acid output of a normal dog (Figure 85–14).

Reported fasting basal plasma gastrin levels in dogs with gastrinomas are approximately 2 to 40 times greater than normal control values. Since gastrin levels may be elevated in other disease conditions, further diagnostic tests are necessary to document a gastrinoma. Because gastrinomas are autonomous in their secretory response, there is generally no stimulated response to a test meal. Both secretin and calcium are known to stimulate the release of gastrin from these tumors and are useful in provocative diagnostic testing. Intravenous infusion of calcium (calcium gluconate, 1 mg/lb or 2 mg/kg body weight) results in a significant rise in serum gastrin levels in gastrinomas, but causes little if any increase in normal animals. An intravenous injection of secretin (2 U/lb or 4 U/kg body weight) lowers serum gastrin levels in normal animals, but with gastrinomas the levels may rise or remain the same (Figure 85–15). Secretin normally inhibits gastrin release; the mechanism resulting in elevated levels in patients with gastrin-secreting tumors is unknown.[191]

Discovery of a gastrin-secreting pancreatic non-β islet cell tumor during exploratory surgery offers the defini-

SECRETIN STIMULATION

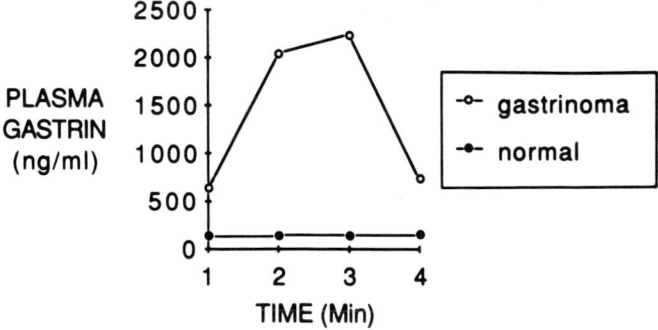

FIGURE 85–15. Gastrin levels following secretin infusion in a normal dog and a dog with a gastrinoma. The normal dog received two clinical units of Secretin-Kabi, and the dog with the gastrinoma was given 4 U/kg of Boots Secretin.

tive diagnosis. Most of these pancreatic tumors are one to a few centimeters in diameter. Regional lymph nodes and the liver should be carefully examined for metastatic lesions, and large gastric or duodenal ulcers should be resected. It must be emphasized that cases involving chronic gastritis or gastric ulcerations in which surgery is performed should include a careful examination of the pancreas for a gastrinoma.

Treatment

The treatment of choice is surgery. Surgery not only offers a definitive diagnosis but also allows removal of the primary pancreatic tumor and evaluation for possible metastasis. Surgery may also be required to remove large peptic ulcers. Medical therapy is frequently unsuccessful because of the high incidence of metastasis. Therefore, patients with this syndrome are often treated with total gastrectomy, which removes the target organ, the stomach.[192]

With the development of H_2-receptor blocking agents (cimetidine and ranitidine), which inhibit gastrin-stimulated gastric acid secretion, beneficial results may be obtained in the medical treatment of canine gastrinomas. Successful medical management of human Zollinger-Ellison syndrome using a combination of cimetidine and an anticholinergic is reported but has yet to be evaluated in the dog.[193]

The prognoses of reported cases of canine Zollinger-Ellison syndrome have been poor, with the major clinical threat being the physiologic effects of elevated gastrin rather than the biologic effects of the tumor. All but one dog had evidence of metastasis, and all the reported dogs and the cat eventually died from complications of the disease. With surgery in conjunction with H_2 blockers and anticholinergic drugs, the prognosis should improve. Other endocrinopathies occur in conjunction with the Zollinger-Ellison syndrome in humans and should be investigated in the dog. Straus[107] reported an ACTH-secreting gastrinoma in a dog showing concurrent signs related to hyperadrenocorticism. Chemotherapy appears to have limited benefit in humans and probably also in animals; however, there are no clinical reports as yet.

GASTRIC NEOPLASIA

The incidence of benign and malignant gastric neoplasia in the dog and cat is low. Adenocarcinoma is the most common neoplasm occurring in the canine stomach, accounting for 1 per cent of all malignant neoplasms and comprising 42 to 72 per cent of all gastric malignancies.[194] The incidence of gastric neoplasia in the cat is unknown, but it occurs far less frequently than in the dog. In reports of gastrointestinal neoplasms in the cat, the stomach was the least commonly affected organ.[195] Lymphosarcoma is the most frequent feline gastric neoplasia.[196]

The clinical signs of gastric neoplasia, regardless of cell type, are the result of either altered gastric motility or gastric outflow blockage. The most common signs include persistent vomiting and weight loss.

Benign Tumors

Benign Adenomatous Polyps. Polyps occur as pedunculated or polypoid nodules of mucosal proliferation that protrude above the mucosal surface. Although there are few reported cases of adenomatous polyps in the dog and cat, the incidence of nonclinical polyps may actually be higher.[197, 198] Most occur as single or multiple solitary nodules ranging from a few millimeters to centimeters in size; however, diffuse, multiple polyps invading the entire gastric mucosa have been reported.[110, 199] Gastric adenomatous polyps are often incidental findings during endoscopy or at necropsy. They generally cause no clinical signs unless they are diffuse or occlude the pyloric antrum and gastric outflow (see Hypertrophic Gastropathies). The etiology is unknown, but it is thought that polyps occur secondary to chronic gastric mucosal damage. It is suggested that adenomatous polyps may be premalignant, although this is not proven in the dog.

Leiomyomas. Leiomyomas are the second most common gastric tumor found in older dogs (average age 15 years).[200] These tumors vary in size and arise from the muscle layers of the gastric wall. Most are found incidentally at necropsy, are distributed randomly, and involve different segments of the muscular layer. Ulceration is infrequent, and the tumor exerts its effect by mass involvement, altering either motility or pyloric outflow.

Malignant Tumors

Adenocarcinoma is the most common malignant tumor in the stomach of the dog; however, it is exceedingly rare in the cat. The average age of dogs diagnosed with gastric adenocarcinoma is eight years,[201] with males more commonly affected than females. Grossly, these gastric tumors appear as raised plaques with a central ulcer, as polypoid lesions projecting into the lumen, or as a very firm, diffusely infiltrating mass invading the stomach wall. This latter type is referred to as scirrhous carcinoma or linitis plastica (leather bottle stomach) because of the rigid nondistensible consistency of the stomach wall (Figure 85–16).[202] Most tumors have superficial mucosal ulcerations, and more than half originate in the pyloric antral area.

Patnaik and Hurvitz[200] describe two main histologic types of adenocarcinoma, diffuse and intestinal, with several subtypes in each group. The most common and most malignant is the diffuse type, lacking a distinct glandular structure. In some unknown way, the neoplastic cells of this type stimulate mesenchymal elements and induce a tremendous fibrous connective tissue component of the tumor.[203] The other histologic group, the intestinal type, has a glandular structure, and often presents as a raised mass in the gastric wall. Regardless of the histologic type, metastasis is frequent, extending to regional lymph nodes, liver, lungs, and adrenals.

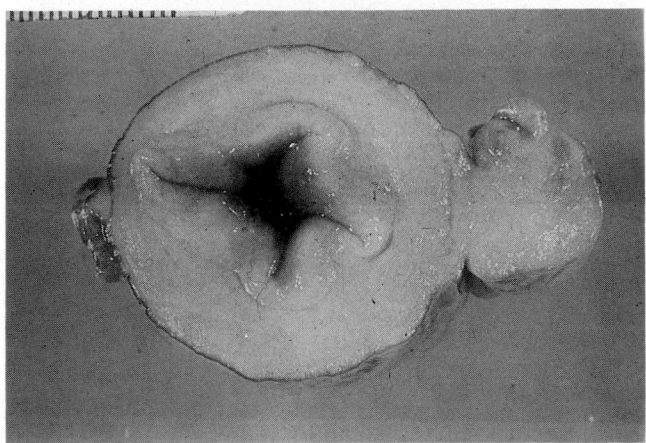

FIGURE 85–16. Cross section of the gastric antrum in a dog with a gastric adenocarcinoma and scirrhous infiltration of the gastric wall, making the stomach thickened and nondistensible.

Primary sarcomas of the stomach occur most frequently as lymphosarcomas and are the most common gastric tumor in the cat. The majority of cats with these β-lymphocyte tumors are FeLV negative. The tumors occur either as raised masses or as diffuse infiltration in the gastric wall, with various sized ulcers in the gastric mucosa. In the dog, gastric lymphosarcoma was more common in males, but there was no breed predisposition.[204, 205]

Other, less frequent, malignant tumors of the stomach include leiomyosarcomas and fibrosarcomas. Rarely, metastatic tumors result from adenocarcinomas (mammary glands, GI tract, liver, pancreas), lymphosarcomas, or hemangiosarcomas.

Clinical Findings

The most consistent sign of gastric neoplasia is vomiting. Vomiting may vary in both frequency and onset after eating, with the severity of signs often related to the amount of gastric wall involvement or pyloric outflow obstruction. With complete pyloric obstruction the vomiting may become projectile. Hematemesis and melena occur with mucosal ulceration and bleeding. Malignant gastric neoplasia often results in anorexia, chronic debilitation, and weight loss. The average duration of clinical signs for most dogs in one report ranges from two weeks to three months.[205, 206]

Diagnosis

Gastric neoplasia should always be suspected in older animals displaying chronic vomiting. Abdominal palpation is generally unrewarding, although occasionally a gastric mass may be palpated. Gastric pain is inconsistent unless perforation of the tumor has resulted in peritonitis. Anemia with melena is a frequent finding with chronic bleeding lesions. Ascites, jaundice, or respiratory distress may result from metastasis to other areas.

In addition to routine laboratory support, radiology is the first step in the diagnosis of gastric neoplasia.

Plain films are usually nondiagnostic, but in extensive involvement may demonstrate a mass or thickened gastric wall. All require contrast studies to definitively demonstrate a gastric lesion (see Gastric Radiology). In many cases a double contrast study best outlines lesions of the gastric wall. Certain characteristic radiographic findings are suggestive of gastric neoplasia. These include thickening and rigidity of the gastric wall as viewed on multiple radiographs, distortion of the gastric lumen and derangement of the rugal folds, filling defects, ulcers, and a marked delay in gastric emptying. Because gastric neoplasia often alters motility and pyloric emptying, fluoroscopy may be beneficial in evaluating some lesions. Lesions invading the gastric wall without a mass effect may not be appreciated without fluoroscopy.

Endoscopy is used to confirm suspected gastric lesions observed with radiology. A skilled endoscopist can often appreciate lesions not demonstrated on gastric contrast studies.[207] Polyps, ulcerations, or raised masses protruding into the luminal surface are easily observed. Gastric neoplasia without mass or mucosal involvement is more difficult to identify. The endoscopist must be aware of areas that have lost distensibility or normal rugal fold patterns. Gastric adenocarcinomas of the linitis plastica type with predominantly submucosal involvement are often missed on endoscopic examination. When lesions are observed, biopsy forceps or cytology brushes can be directed under endoscopic control for obtaining samples. Gastric lavage and cytology may retrieve cells diagnostic of gastric neoplasia; however, there have been no reported cases using this technique in the available veterinary literature.

Surgery offers the best diagnostic method for evaluating gastric neoplasia. The surgeon can palpate the stomach wall for inconsistencies, perform a gastrotomy and evaluate the mucosal surface and pyloric canal diameter, and obtain full-thickness biopsies of the gastric wall. Surgery also allows evaluation of the regional lymph nodes, liver, and adjacent organs for evidence of metastasis.

Treatment

The current treatment of choice for most gastric neoplasia is surgical removal. Partial gastrectomy or segmental resection is usually indicated. Since the majority of gastric neoplasms involve the pyloric antral area, resection of the pylorus may be required. In such cases, surgical anastomosis of the remaining stomach to the intestine (gastroduodenostomy or gastrojejunostomy) is required; however, this procedure is not without complications. Palliative surgery in malignant gastric neoplasia may justifiably increase survival times by several months.[208–210] Chemotherapy is suggested for lymphosarcomas following surgical removal of single or multiple solitary masses and has resulted in a good response in some cases.[211] Therapy for sarcomas involves the use of agents such as vincristine, cyclophosphamide, and prednisone. Sarcomas in which there is diffuse infiltration of the gastric wall and that are not surgical candidates show a poor response to chemotherapy.

Chemotherapy may also be used as an adjunct to surgical removal of other malignant gastric tumor types.[212]

The prognosis for malignant gastric neoplasia is generally poor, owing to the advanced nature of the disease at the time of diagnosis, surgical complications of gastric resection, and frequent metastasis.

References

1. Schulze-Delrieu, K and Anuras S: Chronic esophagitis in two sisters. Dig Dis Sci 28:1101, 1983.
2. Polyak, RI, et al.: Parasympathetic innervation of the stomach. Bull Exp Biol Med 71:373, 1971.
3. Sakamoto, H: A pharmacological study on the autonomic innervation of cardia, corpus and pylorus in the dog stomach. Fukuoka Acta Med 60:561, 1969.
4. Baker, BL: Cell replacement in the stomach. Gastroenterology 46:202, 1964.
5. Banks, WJ: Digestive System. Applied Veterinary Histology. Baltimore, Williams and Wilkins, 1981, p 373.
6. Code, CF: Reflections of histamine, gastric secretion, and the H_2 receptor. N Engl J Med 296:1459, 1975.
7. Evans, HE and Christensen, GC: Anatomy of the Dog. Philadelphia, WB Saunders, 1979.
8. Ellenberger, W and Baum, H: Handbuck der Vergleichender Anatonie der Haustiere. Berlin, Springer-Verlag, 1943.
9. Grossman, MI: The chemicals that activate the "On" switches of the oxyntic cell. Mayo Clin Proc 50:515, 1975.
10. Debas, HT, et al.: Intestinal phase of gastric acid secretion: Augmentation of maximal response of Heidenhaim pouch to gastrin and histamine. Gastroenterology 68:691, 1975a.
11. Aures, D, et al.: Cellular stores of histamine and monoamines in the dog stomach. Life Sci 7.1147, 1968.
12. Vagne, M and Fargier, MC: Effect of pentagastrin and secretin on gastric mucus secretion in conscious cats. Gastroenterology 65:757, 1973.
13. Tobe, T: Distribution of gastrin in canine, cat, and human digestive organs. Am J Surg 132:581, 1976.
14. Debas, HT, et al.: Release of antral gastrin. In Chey, WP and Brooks, SP (eds): Endocrinology of the Gut. Thorofare, Charles B Slack, 1974.
15. Debas, HT, et al.: Proof of a pyloro-oxyntic reflex for stimulation of acid secretion. Gastroenterology 66:526, 1974.
16. Debas, HT, et al.: Evidence for oxynto-pyloric reflex for release of antral gastrin. Gastroenterology 68:687, 1975.
17. You, CH and Chey, WY: Study of electromechanical activity of the stomach in humans and dogs with particular attention to tachygastria. Gastroenterology 86:1460, 1984.
18. Stemper, TJ and Cooke, AR: Effect of a fixed pyloric opening on gastric emptying in the cat and dog. Am J Physiol 230:813, 1976.
19. Debas, HT, et al.: Motilin enhances gastric emptying of liquids in dogs. Gastroenterology 73:777, 1977.
20. Thomas, PA, et al.: Does motilin regulate canine interdigestive gastric motility? Dig Dis Sci 24:577, 1979.
21. Cooke, AR: Control of gastric emptying and motility. Gastroenterology 68:804, 1975.
22. Hunt, JN and Stubbs, DF: The volume and energy content of meals as determinants of gastric emptying. J Physiol 245:209, 1975.
23. Thrall, DE, et al.: Demonstration of a position of relief in dogs with lesions of the stomach or small bowel. JAAHA 14:343, 1978.
24. Politzer, JP, et al.: The genesis of bowel sounds. Influence of viscus and gastrointestinal content. Gastroenterology 71:282, 1976.
25. Dumler, F: Primary metabolic alkalosis. Am Fam Physician 23:193, 1981.
26. Sabatini, S, et al.: Disorders of acid-base balance. Med Clin North Am 62:1223, 1978.
27. Gardham, JRC: Pyloric stenosis. An experimental study of alkalosis and the paradox of acid urine in dogs. Br J Surg 56:628, 1969 (Abst).
28. Hargis, AM, et al.: Chronic fibrosing gastritis associated with *Ollulanus-tricuspis* in a cat. Vet Pathol 3:320, 1982.
29. Tiberio, SR, et al.: A report of *Olluanus tricuspis* and vomiting in cats in Florida. JAAHA 19:887, 1983.
30. Root, CR and Morgan, JP: Contrast radiography of the upper gastrointestinal tract in the dog. J Small Anim Pract 10:279, 1969.
31. Funkquist, B and Garmer, L: Pathogenic and therapeutic aspects of torsion of the canine stomach. J Small Anim Pract 8:523, 1967.
32. Gibbs, C and Pearson, H: The radiological diagnosis of gastrointestinal obstruction in the dog. J Small Anim Pract 14:61, 1973.
33. Zontine, WJ, et al.: Perforated duodenal ulcer associated with mastocytoma in the dog: A case report. J Am Vet Rad Soc 18:162, 1977.
34. Burns, J and Fox, SM: The use of a barium meal to evaluate total gastric emptying time in the dog. Vet Radiol 27:169, 1986.
35. O'Brien, TR: Stomach. In O'Brien, TR (ed): Radiographic Diagnosis of Abdominal Disorders in the Dog and Cat. Philadelphia, WB Saunders, 1978.
36. Johnson, GF and Twedt, DC: Endoscopy and laparoscopy in the diagnosis and management of neoplasia in small animals. Vet Clin North Am 7:77, 1977.
37. Johnson, GF, et al.: Esophagogastric endoscopy in small animal medicine. Gastrointest Endosc 22:226, 1976 (Abst).
38. Johnson, GF: Gastroscopy. In Anderson, NV (ed): Veterinary Gastroenterology. Philadelphia, Lea & Febiger, 1979, p 84.
39. Wood, IJ, et al.: Gastric biopsy: Report on fifty-five biopsies using a new flexible gastric biopsy instrument. Lancet 1:18, 1949.
40. Batt, RM: Technique for single and multiple peroral jejunal biopsy in the dog. J Small Anim Pract 20:259, 1979.
41. Aagaard, P, et al.: Augmented histamine test in dogs. Methods of aspiration technique. Scand J Gastroenterol 7:279, 1972.
42. Isenberg, JI: Gastric secretory testing. In Sleisenger, MH and Fordtran, JS (eds): Gastrointestinal Disease, 2nd ed. Philadelphia, WB Saunders, 1978.
43. Marks, IN, et al.: Maximal secretory response to histamine and its relation to parietal cell mass in the dog. Am J Physiol 199:579, 1960.
44. Baron, JH: Maximal stimuli. In Clinical Tests of Gastric Secretion. New York, Oxford University Press, 1979, p 25.
45. Hirschowitz, BI and Gibson, RG: The effect of cimetidine on stimulated gastric secretion and serum gastrin in the dog. Am J Gastroenterol 70:437, 1978.
46. Grossman, MI and Konturek, SJ: Inhibition of acid secretion in dog by metiamide, a histamine antagonist acting on H_2 receptors. Gastroenterology 66:517, 1974.
47. Bilski, R, et al.: The effect of L-amino acids given intravenously on gastric secretion stimulated by pentagastrin in dogs. Digestion 18:240, 1978.
48. Ivey, KJ: Gastritis. Vet Clin North Am 58:1289, 1974.
49. Skillman, JJ and Slen, W: Gastric mucosal barrier. Surg Annu 4:213, 1972.
50. Robert, A: Cytoprotection by prostaglandins. Gastroenterology 77:761, 1979.
51. Cheung, LH and Chang, N: The role of gastric mucosal blood flow and H^+ back-diffusion in the pathogenesis of acute gastric erosions. J Surg Res 22:357, 1977.
52. Cooke, AR: Gastric damage by drugs and the role of the mucosal barrier. Aust NZ J Med 6:26, 1976.
53. Kuo, YJ and Shanbour, LL: Mechanism of action of aspirin on canine gastric mucosa. Am J Physiol 230:762, 1976.
54. Larsen, EJ: Toxicity of low doses of aspirin in the cat. JAVMA 143:837, 1963.
55. Lev, R, et al.: Effects of salicylates on the canine stomach: a morphological and histochemical study. Gastroenterology 62:970, 1972.
56. Herrgesell, JD: Aspirin poisoning in the cat. JAVMA 151:452, 1967.
57. Lanza, FA, et al.: Endoscopic evaluation of the effects of aspirin, buffered aspirin, and enteric-coated aspirin on gastric and duodenal mucosa. N Engl J Med 303:136, 1980.

58. Ewing, GO: Indomethacin-associated gastrointestinal hemorrhage in a dog. JAVMA 6:1965, 1972.

59. Fenester, LF: The ulcerogenic potential of glucocorticoids and possible prophylactic measures. Med Clin North Am 57:1289, 1973.

60. Davenport, HW and Barr, LL: Failure of ischemia to break the dog's gastric mucosal barrier. Gastroenterology 65:619, 1973.

61. Moody, FG, et al.: Stress and the acute gastric mucosal lesion. Dig Dis Sci 21(2):148, 1976.

62. Guilbert, J, et al.: Role of intestinal chyme in pathogenesis of gastric ulceration following experimental hemorrhagic shock. J Trauma 9:723, 1969.

63. Cheville, NF: Uremic gastropathy in the dog. Vet Pathol 16:292, 1979.

64. Gold, CH, et al.: Gastric acid secretion and serum gastrin levels in patients with chronic renal failure on regular hemodialysis. Nephron 25:92, 1980.

65. Jonas, LD and Twedt, DC: Serum gastrin concentrations in dogs with acute and chronic renal failure. Sci Proc Am Coll Vet Intern Med 1982 (Abst).

66. Harris, WF: Clinical toxicities of dogs. Vet Clin North Am 5:605, 1975.

67. Atkins, CE and Johnson, RK: Clinical toxicities of cats. Vet Clin North Am 5:623, 1975.

68. Osborne, AD and Wilson, MR: Mycotic gastritis in a dog. Vet Rec 85:487, 1969.

69. Howard, EB: Acute mycotic gastritis in a dog. VM/SAC 61:549, 1966.

70. Barsanti, JA, et al.: Phycomycosis in a dog. JAVMA 167:293, 1975.

71. Weber, AF, et al.: Some observations concerning the presence of spirilla in the fundic glands of dogs and cats. Am J Vet Res 19:677, 1958.

72. Finco, DR: Fluid therapy for profuse vomiting. JAAHA 8:200, 1972.

73. Twedt, DC: Jaundice, hepatic trauma, and hepatic encephalopathy. Vet Clin North Am 11:121, 1981.

74. Davis, LE: Clinical pharmacology of the gastrointestinal tract. In Anderson, NV (ed): Veterinary Gastroenterology. Philadelphia, Lea & Febiger, 1980, p 277.

75. Malagelada, JR and Cortot, A: H₂-receptor antagonist in perspective. Mayo Clin Proc 53:184, 1978.

76. Bolton, JP and Cohen, MM: The effect of prostaglandin E2, and metiamide on established canine gastric mucosal barrier damage. Surgery 8:333, 1979.

77. Payne, JG and Bowen, JC: Hypoxia of canine gastric mucosa caused by Escherichia coli sepsis and prevented by methyl prednisolone therapy. Gastroenterology 890:84, 1981.

78. Chisholm, J: Immunology of gastritis. Clin Gastroenterol 5:419, 1976.

79. Hennes, AR, et al.: Atrophic gastritis in dogs. Arch Pathol 73:33, 1962.

80. Krohn, KJE and Finlayson, DC: Interrelations of humoral and cellular immune responses in experimental canine gastritis. Clin Exp Immunol 14:237, 1973.

81. Porteous, JR, et al.: Induction of autoallergic gastritis in dogs. J Pathol 112:138, 1974.

82. Marshall, BT: Campylobacter pyloritis and gastritis. J Infect Dis 153:650, 1986.

83. Henry, GA, et al.: Gastric spirillosis in beagles. Am J Vet Res 48:831, 1987.

84. Twedt, DC and Magne, ML: Chronic gastritis. In Kirk, RW (ed): Current Veterinary Therapy IX. Philadelphia, WB Saunders, 1986.

85. Van Der Gaag, I, et al.: Investigation of the dog stomach. Netherlands Small Anim Vet Assoc Proc 5:60, 1974.

86. Ditchfield, J and Phillipson, MH: Achlorhydria in dogs, with report of a case complicated by avitaminosis C. Can Vet J 1:396, 1960.

87. Sorour, VE: The relationship between atrophic gastritis and gastric ulcer. Suid-Afrikaanse Tydskrif vir Chirurgie 14:47, 1976.

88. Strombeck, DR, et al.: Maldigestion and malabsorption in a dog with chronic gastritis. JAVMA 179:801, 1981.

89. Miller, RI, et al.: Gastrointestinal phycomycosis in a dog. JAVMA 182:1245, 1983.

90. Miller, RI: Gastrointestinal phycomycosis in 63 dogs. JAVMA 186:473, 1985.

91. McLeod, CG, et al.: Ulcerative histiocytic gastritis with amyloidosis in a dog. Vet Pathol 18:117, 1981.

92. Fung, WP, et al.: Endoscopic, histological, and ultrastructural correlations in chronic gastritis. Am J Gastroenterol 71:269, 1979.

93. Sullivan, MF, et al.: Gastrointestinal absorption of metals by rats and swine. Environ Res 35:439, 1984.

94. Jeffries, GH: Gastritis. In Sleisenger, MH and Fordtran, JS (eds): Gastrointestinal Disease, 2nd ed. Philadelphia, WB Saunders, 1978.

95. Davenport, HW: Prevention and suppression by azathioprine of venom-induced protein-losing gastropathy in dogs. Proc Natl Acad Sci USA 73:968, 1976.

96. Hayden, DW and Fleischman, RW: Scirrhous eosinophilic gastritis in dogs with gastric arteritis. Vet Pathol 14:441, 1977.

97. Strombeck, DR: Chronic gastritis, gastric retention and gastric neoplasms. In Small Animal Gastroenterology. Davis, CA, Stonegate Publishing, 1979.

98. Bishop, L, et al.: Eosinophilic gastritis in a dog associated with microfilaria. In press.

99. Hayden, DW and Van Kruiningen, HI: Experimentally induced canine toxocariasis: Laboratory examinations and pathologic changes, with emphasis on the gastrointestinal tract. Am J Vet Res 36:1605, 1975.

100. Greaves, P and Boiziau, JL: Altered patterns of mucin secretion in gastric hyperplasia in mice. Vet Pathol 21:224, 1984.

101. Kipnis, RM: Focal cystic hypertrophic gastropathy in a dog. JAVMA 173:182, 1978.

102. Breitschwerdt, EB, et al.: Clinical and epidemiologic characterization of a diarrheal syndrome in Basenji dogs. JAVMA 180:914, 1982.

103. Breitschwerdt, EB, et al.: Multiple endocrine abnormalities in Basenji dogs with renal tubular dysfunction. JAVMA 182:1348, 1983.

104. Van Kruiningen, HJ: Giant hypertrophic gastritis of Basenji dogs. Vet Pathol 14:19, 1977.

105. Breitschwerdt, EB: Immunoproliferative enteropathy of Basenjis. Proceed 5th Ann Vet Med Forum, 1987, p 683.

106. Willems, G, et al.: Endogenous hypergastrinemia and cell proliferation in the fundic mucosa in dogs. Dig Dis Sci 22:419, 1977.

107. Straus, E and Yalow, RS: Hypersecretinemia associated with marked basal hyperchlorhydria in man and dog. Gastroenterology 72:992, 1977.

108. Twedt, DC: Gastrointestinal peptide hormones. In Small Animal Endocrinology. New York, Churchill Livingstone, 1986.

109. Van Der Gaag, I, et al.: A Boxer dog with chronic hypertrophic gastritis resembling Menetrier's disease in man. Vet Pathol 13:172, 1976.

110. Happe, RP, et al.: Multiple polyps of the gastric mucosa in two dogs. J Small Anim Pract 18:179, 1977.

111. Walter, MC, et al.: Chronic hypertrophic pyloric gastropathy as a cause of pyloric obstruction in the dog. J Am Vet Med Assoc 186:157, 1985.

112. Happe, RP, et al.: Pyloric stenosis caused by hypertrophic gastritis in three dogs. J Small Anim Pract 22:7, 1981.

113. Twedt, D: Chronic Gastritis. Proceedings of the 8th Kal Kan Symposium for the treatment of Small Animal Diseases. Kal Kan Foods Inc, Vernon CA, October 1984, p 87.

114. Matthiesen, DT and Walter, MC: Surgical treatment of chronic hypertrophic pyloric gastropathy in 45 dogs. JAAHA 22:241, 1985.

115. Hoerlein, BF and Spano, JS: Non-neurological complications following decompressive spinal cord surgery. Arch Am Coll Vet Surg IV:11, 1975.

116. Ader, P: Penetrating gastric ulceration in a dog. JAVMA 175:710, 1979.

117. Toombs, JP, et al.: Colonic perforation following neurosurgical procedures and corticosteroid therapy in four dogs. JAVMA 177:68, 1980.

118. Ippoliti, A and Walsh, J: Newer concepts in the pathogenesis of peptic ulcer disease. Surg Clin North Am 56:1479, 1976.

119. Gottleib, JE, et al.: Gastrointestinal complications in critically ill patients: The intensivist's overview. Am J Gastroenterol 81:227, 1986.

120. Halloran, LG, et al.: Prevention of acute gastrointestinal complications after severe head injury; a controlled trial of cimetidine prophylaxis. Am J Surg 139:44, 1980.

121. Twedt, DC: Differential diagnosis and therapy of vomiting. Vet Clin North Am 13:3, 1983.
122. Moore, RW and Withrow, SM: Gastrointestinal hemorrhage and pancreatitis associated with intervertebral disc disease in the dog. JAVMA 180:1443, 1982.
123. Zucherman, GR, et al.: Upper gastrointestinal bleeding in patients with chronic renal failure. Ann Intern Med 102:588, 1985.
124. Twedt, DC: Cirrhosis: A consequence of chronic liver disease. Vet Clin North Am 15:151, 1985.
125. Manabe, T: Changes of gastric blood flow in experimentally induced cirrhosis of the liver. Surg Gynecol Obstet 147:753, 1978.
126. Hein, MF: The effect of portacaval shunting on gastric secretion in cirrhotic dogs. Gastroenterology 44:637, 1983.
127. Hardy, RM: Diseases of the liver. In Ettinger, SJ (ed): Textbook of Veterinary Internal Medicine, 2nd ed. Philadelphia, WB Saunders, 1983.
128. Millward-Sadler, GH and Wright, R: Cirrhosis: An appraisal. In Wright R, et al. (eds): Liver and Biliary Disease. Philadelphia, WB Saunders, 1979.
129. Howard, EB, et al.: Mastocytoma and gastroduodenal ulceration. Pathol Vet 6:146, 1969.
130. Carrig, CB and Seawright, AA: Mastocytosis with gastrointestinal ulceration in a dog. Aust Vet J 44:503, 1968.
131. Seawright, AA and Grono, LR: Malignant mast cell tumor in a cat with perforating duodenal ulcer. J Pathol Bact 87:107, 1964.
132. Howard, EB and Kenyon, AJ: Canine mastocytoma: Altered α-globulin distribution. Am J Vet Res 26:1132, 1965.
133. Watt, J, et al.: The effect of heparin on gastric secretion stimulated by histamine or ametrazole hydrochloride. J Pharm Pharmacol 18:615, 1966.
134. Murray, M, et al.: Peptic ulceration in the dog: A clinicopathological study. Vet Rec 91(19):441, 1972.
135. Sass, B: Perforating gastric ulcer associated with lead poisoning in a dog. JAVMA 157:76, 1970.
136. Hurwitz, A, et al.: Effects of antacids on gastric emptying. Gastroenterology 71:268, 1976.
137. Morrissey, JF and Barreras, RF: Antacid therapy. N Engl J Med 290(10):550, 1974.
138. Daly, MJ, et al.: Inhibition of gastric acid secretion in the dog by the H₂-receptor antagonists, ranitidine, cimetidine, and metramide. Gut 21:408, 1980.
139. Schulman, J: Control of gastric ulcers in a dog using cimetidine. Canine Pract 6(6):42, 1979.
140. Okabe, S, et al.: Effects of cimetidine on healing of chronic gastric and duodenal ulcers in dogs. Dig Dis Sci 23(2):166, 1978.
141. Zimmerman, TW and Schenker, A: A comparative evaluation of cimetidine and ranitidine. Ration Drug Ther 19:1, 1985.
142. Priebe, HJ, et al.: Antacid versus cimetidine in preventing acute gastrointestinal bleeding. N Engl J Med 302:426, 1980.
143. Nagashima, R: Development and characteristics of sucralfate. J Clin Gastroenterol 3:103, 1981.
144. Wilson, EE: The role of prostaglandins in gastrointestinal physiology and digestive diseases. Prostaglandin Digest, November 1985.
145. Van Essen, HA, et al.: Intragastric prostaglandin E2 and the prevention of gastrointestinal hemorrhage in ICU patients. Crit Care Med 13:957, 1985.
146. Waterman, NG and Walker, JL: The effect of gastric cooling on hemostasis. Surg Gynecol Obstet 137:80, 1973.
147. Gilbert, DA and Saunders, DR: Iced saline lavage does not slow bleeding from experimental canine gastric ulcers. Dig Dis Sci 26:1065, 1981.
148. Damiano, S: Chronic follicular hypertrophic gastritis in a dog. Acta Med Vet 13:363, 1967.
149. Dodge, JA: Production of duodenal ulcers and hypertrophic pyloric stenosis by administration of pentagastrin to pregnant and newborn dogs. Nature 225:284, 1970.
150. Janick, JS, et al.: The role of gastrin in congenital hypertrophic pyloric stenosis. J Ped Surg 13:151, 1978.
151. Belding, HH, III and Kernohan, JW: A morphologic study for the myenteric plexus and musculature of the pylorus with special reference to the changes in hypertrophic pyloric stenosis. Surg Gynecol Obstet 97:322, 1953.
152. Okamoto, E, et al.: Selective destruction of the myenteric plexus: Its relation to Hirschsprung's disease, achalasia of the esophagus and hypertrophic pyloric stenosis. J Ped Surg 2:444, 1967.
153. Cream, GP, et al.: Hyperplasia of the gastric mucosa produced by duodenal obstruction. Gastroenterology 56:193, 1969.
154. Kaye, MD, et al.: Manometric studies of the human pylorus. Gastroenterology 70:477, 1976.
155. Pearson, H, et al.: Pyloric and esophageal dysfunction in the cat. J Small Anim Pract 15:487, 1974.
156. Twaddle, AA: Congenital pyloric stenosis in two kittens corrected by pyloroplasty. NZ Vet J 19:26, 1971.
157. Twedt, DC and Grauer, GF: Fluid therapy for gastrointestinal, pancreatic and hepatic disorders. Vet Clin North Am 12, 1982.
158. Douglas, SW: Lesions involving the pyloric region of the canine stomach. J Am Vet Rad Soc 9:89, 1968.
159. Rhodes, WH and Brodey, RS: The differential diagnosis of pyloric obstruction in the dog. J Am Vet Rad Soc 6:65, 1965.
160. Zimmer, JF: Gastrointestinal fiberoptic endoscopy. In Kirk, RW (ed): Current Veterinary Therapy VI. Philadelphia, WB Saunders, 1977.
161. Archibald, RM and Milton, AR: Surgical relief of pyloric stenosis in the dog. Can J Comp Med 18:394, 1954.
162. Archibald, JA, et al.: Surgical technique for correcting pyloric stenosis. Mod Vet Pract 41:28, 1960.
163. Lawther, WA: Pyloric stenosis in a puppy. Aust Vet J 37:317, 1961.
164. Twaddle, AA: Pyloric stenosis in three cats and its correction by pyloroplasty. NZ Vet J 18:15, 1970.
165. Hinder, RA and Bremmer, CG: Relative role of pyloroplasty size, truncal vagotomy, and milk meal volume in canine gastric emptying. Am J Dig Dis 23:210, 1978.
166. Butler, HC: Gastroduodenostomy in the dog. JAVMA 155:1347, 1969.
167. Azpiroz, F and Malagelada, Jr: Pressure activity patterns in the canine proximal stomach: Response to destruction. Am J Physiol 247:265, 1984.
168. Kim, CH, et al.: Characteristics of spontaneous and drug induced gastric dysrhythmias in a chronic canine model. Gastroenterology 90:421, 1986.
169. Minami, H and McCullum, RW: The physiology and pathophysiology of gastric emptying in humans. Gastroenterology 86:1592, 1984.
170. Kowalewski, K and Kolodej, A: Myoelectric and mechanical activity of stomach and intestine in hypothyroid dogs. Dig Dis 22:235, 1977.
171. Mccroff, JC: Abnormal Gastric Motor Function in Viral Gastroenteritis. Ann Int Med 92:370, 1980.
172. Stampley, AR, et al.: Effect of experimental GDV on gastric myoelectrical activity in the dog. Proceedings at the 5th Annual Veterinary Medical Forum (Abst), 1987, p 903.
173. Van Sluijs, FJ: Gastric dilatation volvulus in the dog. Thesis, University of Utrecht, The Netherlands, 1987, p 89.
174. You, CH, et al.: Electrogastrographic study of patients with unexplained nausea, bloating and vomiting. Gastroenterology 79:311, 1980.
175. Malagelada, JR: Physiologic basis and clinical significance of gastric emptying disorders. Dig Dis Sci 24(9):657, 1979.
176. Prove, J and Ehrlein, HF: Motor function of gastric antrum and pylorus for evacuation of low and high viscosity meals in dogs. Gut 23:1250, 1982.
177. Leib, MS, et al.: Gastric emptying of liquids in the dog. I. Serial test meal and modified emptying time techniques. Am J Vet Res 46:1876, 1985.
178. Eeckhout, C, et al.: Different meals produce different digestive motility patterns. Dig Dis Sci 29:219, 1984.
179. Leib, MS, et al.: Gastric emptying of glucose in the dog. Am J Vet Res 47:31, 1986.
180. Tams, TR: Reglan—clinical applications in GI disorders. Proceed of 51st Annual Meeting of AAHA, 1984, p 207.
181. Burrows, CF: Metoclopramide. JAVMA 183:1341, 1983.
182. Van Neuten, JM, et al.: Gastrointestinal motility stimulating properties of cisapride. In Ramon, C (ed): Gastrointestinal Motility. Lancaster, MTP Press, 1984.
183. Zollinger, RM: Islet cell tumors of the pancreas and alimentary tract. Am J Surg 129:102, 1975.
184. Jones, BR, et al.: Peptic ulceration in a dog associated with an islet cell carcinoma of the pancreas and an elevated plasma gastrin level. J Small Anim Pract 17:593, 1976.

185. Straus, E, et al.: Canine Zollinger-Ellison syndrome. Gastroenterology 72:380, 1977.

186. Happe, RP, et al.: Zollinger-Ellison syndrome in three dogs. Vet Pathol 17:177, 1980.

187. Drazner, FH: Canine gastrinoma: A condition analogous to the Zollinger-Ellison syndrome in man. Calif Vet 11:6, 1981.

188. Middleton, DJ and Watson, ADJ: Duodenal ulceration associated with gastrin-secreting pancreatic tumor in a cat. JAVMA 4:461, 1983.

189. McGuigan, JE: The Zollinger-Ellison syndrome. *In* Sleisenger MH and Fordtran JS (eds): Gastrointestinal Disease, 2nd ed. Philadelphia, WB Saunders, 1978.

190. Regan, PT and Malagelada, JR: A reappraisal of clinical, roentgenographic and endoscopic features of the Zollinger-Ellison syndrome. Mayo Clin Proc 53:19, 1978.

191. McGuigan, JE and Wolfe, MW: Secretin injection test in the diagnosis of gastrinoma. Gastroenterology 79:1324, 1980.

192. McCarthy, DM: The place of surgery in the Zollinger-Ellison syndrome. N Engl J Med 302:1344, 1980.

193. Richardson, CT and Walsh, JH: The value of histamine H_2-receptor antagonist in the management of patients with the Zollinger-Ellison syndrome. N Engl J Med 294:133, 1976.

194. Patnaik, AK, et al.: Canine gastric adenocarcinoma. Vet Pathol 15:600, 1978.

195. Brody, RS: Alimentary tract neoplasms in the cat: A clinicopathologic survey of 46 cases. Am J Vet Res 27:74, 1966.

196. Tyler, DE: Gastric neoplasia in the dog and cat. Arch Am Coll Vet Surg 6:47, 1977. (Abst).

197. Murray, M, et al.: Primary gastric neoplasia in the dog: A clinicopathological study. Vet Rec 91474, 1972.

198. Hayden, DW and Nielsen, SW: Canine alimentary neoplasia. Zentralbl Veterinaermed 20:1, 1973.

199. Conroy, JD: Multiple gastric adenomatous polyps in a dog. J Comp Pathol 79:465, 1969.

200. Patnaik, AK and Hurvitz, AI: Neoplasms of the digestive tract in the dog. *In* Kirk, RW (ed): Current Veterinary Therapy VI. Philadelphia, WB Saunders, 1977.

201. Lingeman, CH, et al.: Spontaneous gastric adenocarcinomas of dogs: A review. J Natl Cancer Inst 47:137, 1977.

202. Pollock, S and Wagner, BM: Gastric adenocarcinoma or linitis plastica in a dog. VM/SAC 68:139, 1973.

203. Laurin, P: The two histologic main types of gastric carcinoma: Diffuse and so-called intestinal type carcinoma. An attempt at histo-clinical classification. Acta Pathol Microbiol Scand 64:31, 1965.

204. Priester, WA: The occurrence of tumors in domestic animals. Natl Canc Inst Monograph 54:1980.

205. Couto, CG: Gastrointestinal neoplasia. *In* Van Marthens, E (ed): Proceed 8th Ann Kal Kan Symp. Kal Kan Foods 8:17, 1984.

206. Sautler, JH and Hanlon, GF: Gastric neoplasms in the dog: A report of 20 cases. JAVMA 166:691, 1975.

207. Laufer, MD, et al.: The diagnostic accuracy of barium studies of the stomach and duodenum—correlation with endoscopy. Radiology 115:569, 1972.

208. Douglas, SW, et al.: The surgical relief of gastric lesions in the dog: Report of seven cases. Vet Rec 86:743, 1970.

209. McDonald, AE: Primary gastric carcinoma of the dog: Review and case report. Vet Surg 7:70, 1978.

210. Olivieri, M, et al.: Gastric adenocarcinoma in a dog: Six-and-one-half month survival following partial gastrectomy and gastroduodenostomy. JAAHA 80:78, 1984.

211. MacEwen, EG: Canine lymphosarcoma. *In* Kirk, RW (ed): Current Veterinary Therapy VII. Philadelphia, WB Saunders, 1980.

212. Moertel, CG: Current concepts in cancer: Chemotherapy of gastrointestinal cancer. N Engl J Med 299:1049, 1978.

86 DISEASES OF THE SMALL BOWEL

ROBERT G. SHERDING

STRUCTURE AND FUNCTION OF THE SMALL INTESTINE

Anatomy

The structure of the small intestine provides maximal surface area for optimal performance of the intestinal functions of digestion, absorption, and secretion. The interface between mucosal surface and luminal content, where these functions take place, is increased by (1) the looped and folded, hollow tubular structure of the small bowel; (2) a mucosal lining that is folded and has finger-like mucosal projections called villi; and (3) the covering of the mucosal surface of the villi with a single layer of specialized epithelial cells that possess microvilli on their luminal membrane (brush border).

The small intestine of the dog and cat consists of three parts: the duodenum, the shortest and most proximal portion, which receives the openings of the stomach, common bile duct, and pancreatic ducts and lies largely to the right of midline; the jejunum, the longest portion, which consists of up to eight loops of gut that occupy most of the midabdomen and are covered by the omentum; and the ileum, the short terminal portion, which opens into the ascending colon.

The arterial supply of the small bowel is provided largely via the cranial mesenteric artery, although the duodenum also receives arterial supply via the gastroduodenal artery, which originates from the common hepatic branch of the celiac artery. Venous drainage is into the portal vein via the cranial and caudal mesenteric veins and, for a portion of the duodenum, via the gastroduodenal vein. Intestinal lymphatics generally parallel the intestinal arteries and veins. Intestinal lymph drains via intestinal lymphatics into mesenteric lymph nodes, then into large intestinal lymphatic trunks that converge to become the cisterna chyli (the dilated caudal portion of the thoracic duct); finally, it is transported by the thoracic duct into the venous circulation.[1]

The small intestine is innervated by the autonomic nervous system. Extrinsic parasympathetic and sympathetic supply are via the vagus and splanchnic nerves, respectively. Intrinsic neural control of intestinal function is largely through an intramural network of neurons and nerve fibers called the myenteric and submucosal plexuses.

The layers of the intestinal wall, listed from inside (lumen) to outside (serosa), are the columnar epithelium of the mucosal surface, the basement membrane, the lamina propria, the muscularis mucosae, the submucosa, circular and longitudinal muscle layers, and the serosa. The luminal surface or microvillous border of the epithelium is coated with a glycoprotein substance called the glycocalyx. A one-cell thick layer of epithelium covers the intestinal villi and lines the "valleys" or crypts between the villi. There are four basic types of intestinal epithelial cells: (1) the columnar cell or enterocyte, which is the most populous cell and is specialized for digestion and absorption; (2) the goblet cell, which secretes mucus; (3) the Paneth cell, whose function is unclear but is probably secretory in nature; and (4) the enteroendocrine cell, which secretes hormones in response to chemical stimuli.[2]

Constant turnover of intestinal epithelium is characterized by a balance between cell production in the crypts and cell loss at the villous tips. Only the immature, undifferentiated epithelial cells within the crypts can replicate. These crypt cells proliferate continuously to supply new epithelial cells, which migrate out onto the villi, to be eventually extruded into the gut lumen from the villous tip (Figure 86–1). As the villous epithelial cells migrate, they mature and differentiate, becoming specialized for digestion and absorption. This process of replication, migration, and differentiation of intestinal epithelium is sometimes called epithelial renewal and under normal conditions spans from two to six days. Epithelial renewal time varies with the villous length in different segments of the bowel and varies between species. Epithelial renewal is accelerated by intestinal disease or surgical resection of a portion of the bowel. It is prolonged by factors such as food withdrawal, uremia, radiation, and chemotherapeutic agents that inhibit DNA synthesis.[2, 3] In addition, cell renewal is faster in conventionally reared animals that have a normal microflora than in germ-free animals.[2, 4]

Although the crypt-villus model is somewhat of an oversimplification, it is useful in understanding the morphogenesis of lesions and functional changes in certain diarrheal diseases, especially infections caused by the

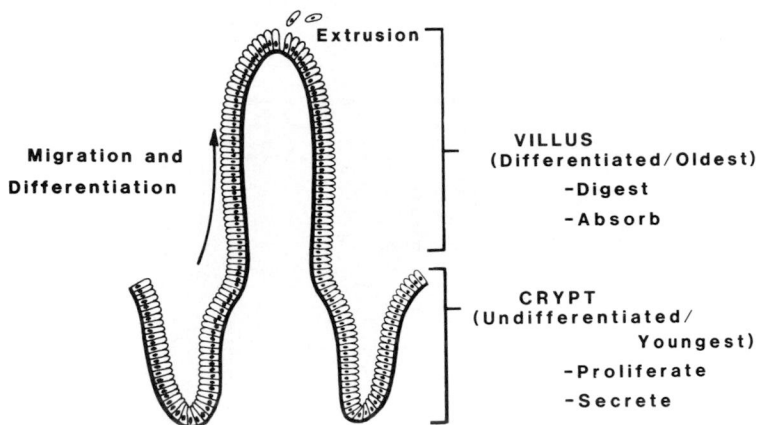

Migration and Differentiation

Extrusion

VILLUS (Differentiated/Oldest)
-Digest
-Absorb

CRYPT (Undifferentiated/ Youngest)
-Proliferate
-Secrete

FIGURE 86–1. The crypt-villus unit of the intestinal mucosa consists of immature proliferative-secretory cells that line the crypts and mature digestive-absorptive cells that populate the villi. The crypt cells proliferate to continuously supply new cells that migrate out onto the villi, where they differentiate into cells specialized for digestion and absorption as they migrate, and are finally extruded into the gut lumen from the villous tip. Villus absorption exceeds crypt secretion, resulting in net absorption by the crypt-villus unit.

epitheliotropic viruses that have a predilection for different parts of the crypt-villus epithelium[5] (Figure 86–2). Normally, absorption by the differentiated digestive-absorptive cells of the intestinal villi exceeds secretion by the immature proliferate-secretory cells of the intestinal crypts, resulting in net absorption by the crypt-villus unit. Enteroviruses that selectively destroy villous epithelium (coronaviruses and rotaviruses) will cause villous atrophy, malabsorption, and crypt hyperplasia, resulting in net secretion by the crypt-villus unit and diarrhea. In general, the severity of the diarrhea will parallel the extent of villous destruction. This contrasts with viruses that selectively destroy crypt epithelium, such as parvoviruses. These virus infections initially destroy the crypts while leaving intact villi; however, without crypt cells to proliferate and replace villous cells as they are lost by normal turnover, complete mucosal collapse eventually occurs. Because of the extensive loss

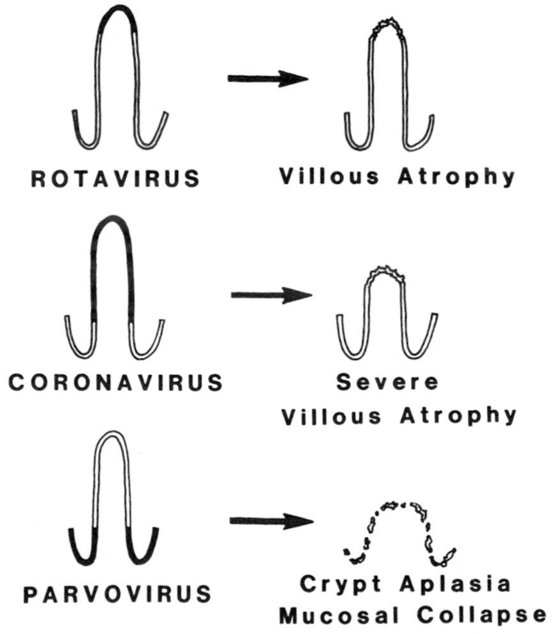

ROTAVIRUS → **Villous Atrophy**

CORONAVIRUS → **Severe Villous Atrophy**

PARVOVIRUS → **Crypt Aplasia Mucosal Collapse**

FIGURE 86–2. Enteric viruses have predilections for different parts of the crypt-villus epithelium. Villus-selective viruses (rotavirus, coronavirus) cause villous atrophy leading to malabsorption and crypt hyperplasia, while crypt-selective viruses (parvovirus) cause crypt aplasia leading to mucosal collapse.

of epithelium, diarrhea is severe and mucosal regeneration is slow.

Another component of the small intestinal microanatomy that deserves special mention is the lymphoid tissue associated with the gut. Immunocompetent cells (lymphocytes and plasma cells) are widely distributed throughout the length of the small bowel. They are located in between mucosal epithelial cells, scattered diffusely throughout the lamina propria beneath the epithelium, located at various sites along the GI tract as structured collections of cells called lymphoid nodules and as unique aggregates of lymphoid nodules called Peyer's patches.[4] These immunocytes participate in the local immune response to antigens that contact the animal via the gastrointestinal mucosal surface largely through the production of immunoglobulin A(IgA), the major Ig in intestinal secretions,[6] but also through the production of other Ig types and through cell-mediated immunity. It is of interest to note that animals reared in a germ-free environment, thereby lacking bacterial colonization of their mucosa, have many fewer lymphocytes and plasma cells in their lamina propria than do conventional animals. Thus, the constant contact of the normal microflora (and their antigens) with the mucosa of the normal animal apparently stimulates a physiologic inflammation.[2] In addition to lymphoid cells, other cells that participate in immune responses are scattered throughout the small intestine, including macrophages, eosinophils, neutrophils, and mast cells.

Digestion and Absorption

The primary function of the small intestine is to provide nutrients, water, and essential ions by the processes of digestion and absorption. Enzymes that are secreted into the gut lumen and associated with the mucosal brush border break down ingested food, and the products of digestion are then transferred from the gut lumen into the blood, where they become available for systemic use as metabolic substances. For the purpose of this discussion, the three major classes of nutrient (fat, carbohydrate, and protein) are discussed in terms of three sequential phases of digestion and absorption: the luminal phase, the mucosal phase, and the delivery phase (Figure 86–3).

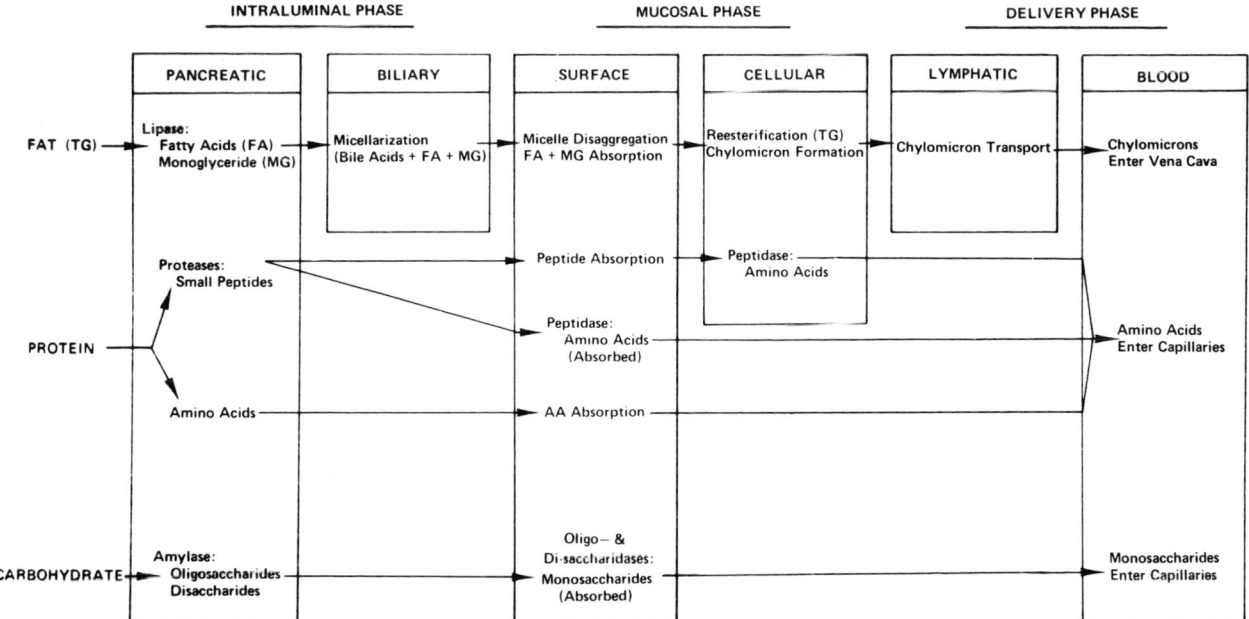

FIGURE 86–3. The phases of digestion and absorption of fat, carbohydrate, and protein. Note the greater complexity of fat assimilation, which includes biliary and lymphatic steps.

FAT

The digestion and absorption of fat is extremely efficient. Under most circumstances, over 95 per cent of ingested fat is absorbed, and fecal fat excretion in the dog remains relatively constant over a wide dietary intake range. A large portion of the fat that is normally found in feces comes from desquamated colonic cells, colonic secretions, and bacterial synthesis, rather than from dietary fat. Long-chain triglycerides made up of three long-chain fatty acids (16 to 18 carbons) on a glycerol backbone are the primary component of dietary fat, although a smaller portion of dietary fat consists of medium-chain triglycerides (fatty acids of 6 to 12 carbons).

The luminal phase of fat digestion includes emulsification, hydrolysis, and micellarization, with participation by pancreatic and lingual lipase and biliary secretions.[7, 8] The stomach does not contribute to the breakdown of fat, but it does perform a reservoir function insofar as gastric emptying, under neurohormonal influence, regulates the rate of fat entry into the duodenum. The first step of intraluminal fat digestion is the release of the hormone cholecystokinin (CCK) from the duodenum. This hormone stimulates enzyme-rich pancreatic secretion, which includes pancreatic lipase. Simultaneously, CCK causes contraction of the gallbladder and relaxation of the sphincter of Oddi, releasing bile into the duodenum. Hence, in a well-orchestrated chain of events, the duodenum is the recipient of fat (ingesta), lipase, and bile acids.

Duodenal triglycerides are insoluble in the intraluminal water, and lipase hydrolyzes lipid mainly at the oil-water interface. The surface area of this interface, and therefore the activity of lipase, is enhanced by intraluminal fat emulsification. Since bile acids promote emulsification because of their detergent properties, they facilitate the action of pancreatic lipase. Lipolysis, how-

ever, can proceed in the absence of bile acids. In the hydrolysis of long-chain triglyceride, lipase preferentially splits off two α-fatty acids, leaving a single β-fatty acid attached to glycerol as a β-monoglyceride.

The free fatty acids and monoglycerides that result from the hydrolysis of fat undergo the final luminal step in fat assimilation, called micellarization. Insoluble fatty acids and monoglycerides are rapidly brought into solution (i.e., "solubilized") by formation of macromolecular aggregates with bile acids, called micelles. Bile acids are amphipathic molecules, containing polar (hydrophilic) and nonpolar (hydrophobic) regions. When a critical concentration of bile acids is attained, they aggregate into a small sphere with the water-soluble (polar) end facing out toward luminal water and the fat-soluble (nonpolar) end toward the center of the sphere. Fatty acids and monoglycerides, as well as fat-soluble vitamins (A, D, E, K) are incorporated into the center of this sphere and are maintained in micellar solution for presentation to the intestinal epithelial cell for absorption.

The first step in the mucosal phase of fat assimilation is disaggregation of the micelle at the mucosal surface. The released fatty acids and monoglycerides passively diffuse into the epithelial cell. The released bile acids remain in the lumen until reaching the terminal ileum, where 95 per cent of the bile acids are then reabsorbed by active transport, recirculated to the liver, and resecreted in bile (enterohepatic circulation). Once inside the cell, free fatty acids and monoglycerides are enzymatically reesterified into triglyceride. To enable transport out of the cell, this newly formed triglyceride is then aggregated with lipoprotein, cholesterol, and phospholipid to form large transport particles called chylomicrons.

Finally, in the delivery phase, these chylomicrons exit from the base of the intestinal epithelial cell into the lamina propria and enter the central lacteal of the villus by a poorly understood mechanism. The pumping action of the villous smooth muscle propels chylomicron-laden lymph into draining lymphatics, which transport the chylomicrons to the thoracic duct and into the venous circulation.

The aforementioned sequence of events occurs in the digestion and absorption of long-chain triglyceride (LCT), the major component of dietary fat. However, triglyceride composed of fatty acids of shorter chain length, i.e., medium-chain triglyceride (MCT), is digested and absorbed differently and more efficiently.[8] The differences are noteworthy, because MCT is commercially available for dietary management of malabsorption syndromes and certain other disorders. Pancreatic lipase is more active against MCT than against LCT, and it is able to split off all three fatty acids, leaving minimal monoglyceride. The resulting medium-chain fatty acids (MCFA) form micelles more readily than LCFA, although micellarization is probably not necessary, since MCFA are more water-soluble. Furthermore, an estimated 30 per cent of an oral MCT dose can be absorbed intact without any prior lipolysis. Once absorbed into the epithelial cell, MCFA are not reesterified or formed into chylomicrons, as LCFA are, but instead leave the cell as fatty acids. Finally, and most importantly, the removal phase of MCFA is by direct entry into the capillary venous system of the villus for transport to the liver via the portal vein, thereby entirely bypassing lymphatic transport.

A thorough knowledge of the physiology of fat digestion and absorption is pertinent to the clinician's understanding of the pathogenesis of steatorrhea, since disruption of the sequence at any step can potentially result in steatorrhea.[7] Of the three classes of nutrient, fat seems to be the most susceptible to deranged assimilation, since its digestion and absorption sequence is the most complex and specialized, requiring the most steps. Fat is the only nutrient that requires micellarization (bile acid-dependent) and lymphatic transport. Also, enterocytes on the apex of the villus tip, the portion of the crypt-villus unit most susceptible to mucosal injury, are the most specialized for absorption of fat.[9] Therefore, fecal fat excretion (quantitated by fecal fat analysis) is an indicator of the functional status of the small bowel, steatorrhea often appearing in maldigestive and malabsorptive states.

CARBOHYDRATE

Dietary carbohydrate consists of disaccharides (sucrose, lactose), which are digested at the brush border surface membrane of intestinal epithelial cells, and polysaccharides (starch, glycogen), which are first hydrolyzed within the lumen by pancreatic amylase to oligosaccharides and then further digested at the brush border surface.[8, 10, 11] In response to the entry of ingesta into the duodenum, the release of CCK stimulates amylase secretion from the pancreas. Intraluminal digestion of starch by pancreatic amylase is extremely rapid (within minutes) and efficient, yielding a mixture of oligosaccharides (maltose, maltotriose, and α-dextrins).

The intestinal epithelial cell functions in the digestion as well as the absorption of carbohydrate. Hydrolytic enzymes called oligosaccharidases (e.g., maltase, isomaltose, sucrase, lactase, amyloglucosidase) are located in the brush border surface membrane of these cells. The oligosaccharide products from the intraluminal digestion of starch, plus the ingested disaccharides sucrose and lactose, are rapidly hydrolyzed to their constituent monosaccharides by these brush border enzymes at the lumen-cell interface. The resulting monosaccharides (glucose, galactose, and fructose) are then absorbed by active transport mechanisms.

Glucose and galactose are actively transported across the brush border into the intestinal epithelial cell by a protein-carrier-mediated process that requires energy and couples their entry with sodium entry. Fructose, the other monosaccharide, is absorbed by facilitated diffusion, involving a specific carrier mechanism that does not require sodium. Once inside the cell, monosaccharides are released from their carriers and exit the cell. They diffuse down a concentration gradient through the lamina propria and into the capillaries of the portal venous system.

In general, the breakdown of carbohydrate into an absorbable form (monosaccharide) is rapid and efficient. It is the active transport of monosaccharide into the cell that is the rate-limiting step for carbohydrate digestion/absorption. Lactose, however, may be an exception. Evidence suggests that the rate-limiting step in the assimilation of lactose is its hydrolysis by brush border lactase, rather than its absorption into the cell. Lactose intolerance may explain the apparent frequency of milk-induced diarrhea.

The clinical settings in which malabsorption of carbohydrate are observed include (1) impaired digestion of starch (amylorrhea) caused by deficiency of amylase, most commonly found in dogs with complete exocrine pancreatic insufficiency and generalized maldigestion (see Chapter 90); (2) generalized carbohydrate malabsorption because of impaired brush border hydrolysis of oligosaccharides together with impaired absorption of monosaccharides, usually resulting from severe diffuse mucosal disease (for example, villous atrophy); and (3) malabsorption of dietary lactose (milk intolerance) resulting from a deficiency of brush border lactase relative to the quantity of milk ingested. Congenital deficiencies of specific brush border enzymes and monosaccharide carrier proteins are rare causes of carbohydrate malabsorption in humans but have not yet been described in dogs or cats.

PROTEIN

Protein digestion is initiated in the stomach by pepsin, but in the absence of pepsin activity protein digestion proceeds normally. Most intraluminal protein digestion occurs in the duodenum and upper jejunum under the influence of pancreatic proteases.[8, 12, 13] These proteases are secreted as inactive proenzymes in response to the CCK that is released when ingesta enters the duodenum and also in response to vagal activity. One of these proenzymes, trypsinogen, is converted to active trypsin by a duodenal brush border enzyme called enterokinase. The active trypsin in turn activates the other proteases and autocatalyzes further trypsinogen activation. The optimal pH for pancreatic protease activity is 7, so the low duodenal pH created by the entry of gastric acid is efficiently buffered by the secretion of the bicarbonate-rich pancreatic juice in response to the hormone secretin.

The intraluminal phase of protein digestion is the result of the sequential action of endo- and exopeptidases, each proteolytic enzyme having optimal activity against specific peptide bonds.[8, 12, 13] Trypsin, elastase, and chymotrypsin are endopeptidases that split internal peptide bonds in the protein molecule, resulting in small peptides. Carboxypeptidase A and B are exopeptidases that act only on terminal peptide bonds to produce small peptides and some amino acids. There is an overabundance of pancreatic proteases secreted normally in response to a meal, such that the intestinal cell phase rather than the intraluminal phase is the rate-limiting step in overall protein assimilation. It has been estimated that pancreatic protease secretion has to decrease to less than ten per cent of normal before noticeable protein maldigestion occurs.

In the mucosal phase of protein digestion and absorption, small peptides resulting from intraluminal digestion are hydrolyzed to amino acids at the brush border surface, and in some cases, within the cell itself.[8, 12, 13] The peptidases involved are found within the brush border membrane of the intestinal epithelial cell as well as inside the cell, and the enzymes found in these two locations appear to be distinctly different. The resulting amino acids are absorbed into and transported across the cell by an active, sodium-dependent, protein-carrier-mediated mechanism. Four different such mechanisms are known, each for a specific group of amino acids. Amino acids then diffuse across the basolateral membranes of the cell and into the capillaries for portal venous delivery.[8, 12, 13]

The aforementioned processes may be impaired in the dog and cat by diseases of the exocrine pancreas or the small intestine. Severe exocrine pancreatic insufficiency, when proteolytic enzyme output drops below ten per cent of normal, may cause protein maldigestion, usually accompanied by fat and starch maldigestion (see Chapter 90). Diseases of the intestinal mucosa may lead to defective protein absorption by causing impaired mucosal digestion of peptides and reduced absorption of amino acids and small peptides. Furthermore, some intestinal diseases are accompanied by excessive loss of endogenous protein (see Protein-Losing Enteropathy).

Intestinal Transport of Water and Solute

Diarrhea, regardless of etiology, is basically the passage of feces containing an excess of water, resulting from abnormal intestinal handling of water and solute. Therefore, to understand the pathophysiology of diarrhea, the concepts of normal intestinal movement of water and solute are important.

In the case of water and ions, the small intestine is both a secretory and absorptive organ. Large volumes of fluid, which are derived largely from endogenous secretions (salivary, gastric, pancreatic, biliary, intestinal) and, to a lesser extent, ingested fluids, enter the lumen of the small bowel to become the absorptive load, but efficient distal recovery (reabsorption) of most of this fluid prevents excessive loss in the feces and rapid depletion of extracellular fluid volume. This has been called the enterosystemic cycle of water.[5, 14] The greatest volume of this fluid is absorbed in the jejunum. By the time the luminal fluid load reaches the colon, it is much reduced in volume. This small residual fluid load is acted on very efficiently by the colon, so that the end result is formed feces rather than diarrhea.

Continuous fluxes of water and ions across the intestinal mucosa occur simultaneously in opposing directions: absorptive fluxes in a lumen-to-blood direction, and secretory fluxes in a blood-to-lumen direction.[5, 15] For the formation of normal feces, absorptive fluxes should exceed secretory fluxes, so that the overall net transmucosal flux is one of net absorption. Even though this net flux is relatively small, it represents the sum of massive, but opposing, fluid shifts. A small percentage change in these large fluid shifts, e.g., slightly increased secretory flux or decreased absorptive flux, is all that is needed to cause massive accumulation of fluid in the intestinal lumen, resulting in diarrhea. Thus, it is not surprising that animals with severe diarrhea may succumb to dehydration, electrolyte imbalance, and shock.

At the cellular level, transepithelial movement of water and solute may occur through transcellular or intercellular pathways and involve active or passive processes.[5, 15, 16] Water transport is passive secondary to osmotic and hydrostatic pressure gradients that are mainly generated by solute transfer. In the transcellular pathway, solute is transported through the epithelial cell itself, usually by active transport mechanisms that involve membrane pumps (basolateral membrane sodium pump) and membrane carriers (brush border carriers). The other major pathway, the intercellular or shunt pathway, involves passive diffusion through aqueous channels or pores in the tight junctions between epithelial cells under the influence of electrochemical, osmotic, and hydrostatic pressure gradients.

Intestinal Motility

Motility of the small intestine consists of mixing and propulsive movements that provide for optimal contact of bowel content (ingesta) with secretions and the absorptive surface.[17, 18] Three basic types of motor activity are recognized in the small intestine: segmentation, peristalsis, and interdigestive motility. Segmentation contractions are localized, circumferential constrictions of the lumen, spaced a few centimeters apart, which divide the content into segments, producing a mixing action. The frequency of these contractions is characteristic of a species, being 18 to 22 per min in the dog and 28 to 30 per min in the cat.[17] Peristalsis, on the other hand, is an advancing wave of contraction that propels bowel content downstream. During the interdigestive state in dogs fasted over 12 hours, there is a unique motility pattern characterized by recurring intense annular contractions that start at the stomach and sweep downstream along the entire length of small bowel. These interdigestive contractions have been called housekeeper contractions since they are thought to cleanse the GI tract in preparation for the next meal.[19]

The major determinants of the patterns of small bowel contractions are the inherent myoelectric properties of smooth muscle and its slow waves of depolarization (basal electrical rhythm). Motor function is modulated, however, by neural factors: the autonomic nervous system regulates motility through intrinsic (intramural) and extrinsic innervation. In general, parasympathetic influence (cholinergic) via the vagus nerve is an excitatory influence and sympathetic influence (adrenergic) via the splanchnic nerves is an inhibitory influence on intestinal smooth muscle. Sensory input is from mechanoreceptors that respond to pressure, movement, and stretch (volume) stimuli, or from chemoreceptors that respond to osmotic stimuli, pH, and digestion products. Gastrointestinal hormones can also affect motility.

Endocrine Function

The gastrointestinal tract contains a variety of endocrine cells, scattered sparsely among the mucosal cells, collectively called APUD cells because of their distinctive biochemical property of *Amine Precursor Uptake and Decarboxylation*. APUD cells are also found in the pancreatic islets. Polypeptide hormone products from alimentary endocrine cells include gastrin, secretin, cholecystokinin (CCK), enteroglucagon, vasoactive intestinal polypeptide (VIP), gastric inhibitory polypeptide (GIP), somatostatin, motilin, and others, all of which have an effect on gastroenteropancreatic function. It is apparent from this list that the alimentary tract should be considered an endocrine organ as well as a digestive organ. Some of these GI peptides may not act as classic circulating hormones but instead are released locally to act on adjacent tissues (paracrine function). Further, the localization of some of these peptides to neural structures within the gut wall suggests a neurotransmitter-like (neurocrine) function. It is beyond the scope of this chapter to discuss the complex functions and interrelationships of each of these hormones; however, numerous reviews on the subject are available.[20]

Immune Function

The small intestine is in the seemingly precarious state of being separated from a potentially hostile external environment by an epithelial barrier that is only one cell thick.[4] Intestinal lymphoid tissue plays a major "watchdog" role in maintaining local immunity of the mucosal surface, as well as contributing to the overall scheme of the body's immune system. Intestinal secretory antibodies, most of which are IgA, originate from plasma cells located in the lamina propria beneath the mucosal surface, and play an essential role in the maintenance of the epithelial surface as a barrier to penetration of harmful microorganisms, enterotoxins, and antigens (allergens) from the lumen.[6, 21] These IgA-secreting plasma cells are first sensitized to intestinal antigens as immunoblasts, then after proliferating and hemolymphatic circulation, they return to the intestinal

mucosa (homing response) to reside in the lamina propria.

Local cell-mediated immunity also plays a role in gut defenses.[22] Other nonimmunologic host defense mechanisms include normal alimentary secretions, peristalsis, and the native microflora that provide a barrier against the colonization of the gut by pathogens.[4, 22] Insufficiency or impairment of intestinal immune function may be important in a number of clinical disorders. On the other hand, an aberrant intestinal immune response has been postulated, but is unproven, for certain inflammatory diseases, e.g., eosinophilic enteritis and lymphocytic-plasmacytic enteritis, in which the lamina propria distends with cells that are known to be primary or secondary participants in immune reactions (lymphocytes, plasma cells, eosinophils).

MECHANISMS OF DIARRHEA

Diarrhea is the most consistent clinical manifestation of intestinal disease in the dog and cat, and is one of the most frequent presenting complaints in small animal practice (see Chapter 8).[23] Diarrhea is defined as the passage of feces that contain an excess amount of water, resulting in an abnormal increase in stool liquidity and weight.[24] The accumulation of water in the intestinal lumen is a passive process. It occurs secondary to derangement of transmucosal solute fluxes associated with abnormal digestion, absorption, secretion, permeability, or motility.

The pathogenesis of diarrhea involves a combination of four mechanisms: (1) decreased solute absorption (osmotic diarrhea), (2) hypersecretion of ions (secretory diarrhea), (3) increased permeability (exudative diarrhea), and (4) abnormal motility.[5, 14, 15, 24] This well-established classification scheme is based on separations that are somewhat artificial and simplistic, insofar as the pathogenesis of diarrhea in most patients is probably a complex integration of several mechanisms.

Osmotic Diarrhea

Osmotic diarrhea occurs when impaired absorption results in an accumulation of unabsorbed exogenous solutes in the gut lumen, where they retain water by their osmotic activity.[5, 14, 15] This excess luminal solute and water causes bowel distention and is then expelled as bulky, fluid diarrhea. These solutes are largely derived from malabsorbed nutrients, especially carbohydrates. Unabsorbed carbohydrates are hydrolyzed by colonic bacteria to small organic acids, adding to the osmotically active molecules that retain water in the lumen, as well as acidifying the colonic content. Malabsorbed fats exert minimal osmotic effect because they are water-insoluble; however, unabsorbed fatty acids are hydroxylated by colonic bacteria to hydroxy fatty acids, which alter water and electrolyte transport in the large intestine to produce secretory diarrhea.[14, 25]

Clinically, osmotic diarrhea is most often the result of maldigestion caused by exocrine pancreatic insufficiency (see Chapter 90) or primary intestinal malabsorption caused by intrinsic intestinal disease, such as diffuse inflammatory, neoplastic, or villous atrophy disorders (Table 86–1).[5] Osmotic diarrhea usually improves or ceases during fasting, and the osmolality of fecal fluid exceeds the sum of fecal electrolyte concentrations (osmol gap), implicating the accumulation of an unabsorbed nonelectrolyte solute.

Another example of the osmotic mechanism is the catharsis produced by laxatives that contain poorly absorbed substances (magnesium sulfate, sodium phosphate, lactulose) that osmotically retain water in the bowel lumen.

Secretory Diarrhea

Secretory diarrhea occurs when there is a net secretory flux of fluid and electrolytes into the intestinal lumen caused by a derangement of the normal intestinal transport processes, independent of changes in mucosal permeability or osmotic gradients generated by exogenous solutes.[5, 24] Normally, the bidirectional mucosal transport of water and ions produces a state of net fluid absorption; however, if hypersecretion overwhelms the absorptive capacity or if absorption is inhibited (usually both occur together), then the net secretion is expelled as watery diarrhea.[16]

The intestinal secretions are usually isotonic and similar to extracellular fluid, although the composition may be altered during transit. Feces contain excess water, electrolytes, and bicarbonate. Therefore, the conse- quences of secretory diarrhea are isotonic dehydration, electrolyte depletion, and acidosis. In pure secretory diarrhea, fecal osmolality is almost entirely accounted for by the concentration of sodium, potassium, and their accompanying anions.

Mediators of intestinal hypersecretion are numerous and diverse, and probably contribute to the pathogenesis of a wide variety of acute and chronic diarrheal diseases. These include bacterial enterotoxins, gastrointestinal neurohumoral peptides (e.g., vasoactive intestinal polypeptide), products of the inflammatory response (e.g., bradykinins and prostaglandins), serotonin, parasympathetic stimulation, dihydroxy bile acids, hydroxylated fatty acids, and certain laxatives.[5, 15, 16] The mechanisms by which many of these secretagogues influence intestinal secretion are poorly understood.

Permeability (Exudative) Diarrhea

The pathogenesis of diarrhea can involve increased mucosal permeability caused by mucosal damage. Because this mechanism becomes most clinically important when permeability is altered enough to allow exudation of plasma proteins, it is often called exudative diarrhea, and it is characterized by the outpouring of plasma proteins, blood, or mucus from sites of inflammation, ulceration, or infiltration of the gut.[5, 14, 24]

The passive transmucosal leakage of fluid, electrolytes, and protein into the lumen is dependent upon not only the disruption of the mucosal membrane, but also on the subepithelial interstitial fluid or hydrostatic pres-

TABLE 86–1. PATHOPHYSIOLOGY OF DISORDERS OF DIGESTION AND ABSORPTION

Stage of Assimilation	Defect	Consequence	Clinical Examples
1. Intraluminal: Pancreatic stage	Deficient enzyme and bicarbonate secretion	Generalized maldigestion (of all nutrients)	Pancreatic acinar atrophy Destructive pancreatitis Impaired function due to protein-calorie malnutrition
2. Intraluminal: Biliary stage	Bile acid deficiency	Fat malabsorption due to defective micellarization	Severe cholestasis (bile duct obstruction) Bacterial overgrowth syndrome Duodenal acidification Ileal disease or resection
3. Intestinal: Mucosal surface stage	Microvillus damage Biochemical brush border disease (altered enzyme levels)	Impaired brush border digestion of oligosaccharides and peptides Impaired lumen-to-cell transport (malabsorption of all nutrients)	Giardiasis Bacterial overgrowth syndrome Exocrine pancreatic insufficiency Lactose intolerance Many other diseases that injure the brush border
4. Intestinal: Cellular stage	Enterocyte damage Villous atrophy	Loss of absorptive surface area (malabsorption of all nutrients)	Infectious agents Gluten-sensitive enteropathy Enteropathy resembling tropical sprue Many other diseases that injure enterocytes
5. Delivery stage	Infiltration of inflammatory or neoplastic cells into lamina propria, distending and distorting core of villi	"Filled villi"—interference with uptake of nutrients into capillaries and lacteals	Chronic inflammatory small bowel diseases (eosinophilic, lymphocytic-plasmacytic, granulomatous)
6. Lymphatic transport stage	Reduced lymph flow due to lymphatic obstruction or elevated lymphatic hydrostatic pressure	Dilatation and rupture of lacteals (steatorrhea, protein-losing enteropathy)	Lymphangiectasia Intestinal lymphosarcoma Abdominal histoplasmosis Right-sided congestive heart failure

From Sherding RG: In Ford RB (ed): Clinical Signs and Diagnosis in Small Animal Practice. New York, Churchill Livingstone, 1988.

sure, which is the driving force for this movement.[15, 26] Any factor that affects mucosal interstitial fluid dynamics, especially factors that increase net transcapillary filtration, may cause the accumulation of mucosal interstitial fluid and elevate mucosal hydrostatic tissue pressure. This increases mucosal permeability and fluid leakage, resulting in permeability diarrhea and, if plasma protein leakage is severe enough, the syndrome of protein-losing enteropathy. Clinical situations in which this occurs are: (1) mucosal inflammation, with increased capillary permeability and arteriolar dilatation; (2) increased portal venous pressure (portal hypertension or right-sided congestive heart failure); (3) circumstances that elevate capillary hydrostatic pressure; (4) obstruction to lymph flow due to intestinal diseases that involve lymphatics (lymphangiectasia, lymphosarcoma, or histoplasmosis); (5) decreased plasma protein oncotic pressure associated with hypoalbuminemic states; and (6) extracellular volume expansion.

Diarrhea Caused by Deranged Motility

Deranged motility by itself rarely plays a primary role in the pathogenesis of diarrhea.[5, 15] Since diarrhea is essentially an abnormality of fluid and ion transport by the intestinal mucosa, derangements of motility mostly occur secondary to the increased volume and fluidity of intestinal contents caused by one of the other previously mentioned mechanisms. Nevertheless, derangements of motility that may be associated with diarrhea include abnormally reduced peristalsis which promotes stasis and bacterial overgrowth in the small intestine, hyper-

motility which accelerates small bowel transit to such a degree that mucosal contact time for digestion and absorption is insufficient, as appears to occur in feline hyperthyroidism, and premature emptying of the colon associated with colonic inflammation or "irritability."[24] Intestinal motility is affected by abdominal surgery, many drugs, numerous hormones, bacterial enterotoxins, and the autonomic nervous system.

DIAGNOSIS

Diarrhea is the most consistent clinical manifestation of small intestinal disease. Therefore, this section will emphasize the clinical diagnostic approach for the animal with diarrhea as a major presenting sign.

The diagnosis of diarrhea can be logically approached in sequential steps that correspond to the temporal (acute versus chronic), anatomic (small bowel versus large bowel), functional (maldigestion versus malabsorption), and etiologic (categorization by histopathologic or other specific criteria) classification schemes for diarrhea found in Table 86–2. As a general rule, common disorders and simple diagnostics should be considered first, then more complex or sophisticated tests and procedures can be chosen based on the most likely diagnostic possibilities. In some cases, it is more important initially to correct dehydration and electrolyte disturbances than to hastily initiate diagnostic procedures.

The first consideration should be to determine whether the diarrhea is acute or chronic (based on history) and to exclude simple or obvious causes such

TABLE 86–2. CLASSIFICATION SCHEMES USED TO CATEGORIZE DIARRHEA AND THE CORRESPONDING SEQUENTIAL STEPS FOR DIAGNOSIS

Classification Schemes Used to Categorize Diarrhea	Sequential Steps for Diagnosis

A. *Mechanistic*
  1. Osmotic diarrhea
  2. Secretory diarrhea
  3. Permeability (exudative) diarrhea
  4. Disordered motility	

B. *Temporal*
  1. Acute diarrhea
  2. Chronic diarrhea
	Step 1
	Historical characterization of the duration of the problem
	  (Many cases of acute diarrhea are self-limiting or resolved in this stage and do not require further evaluation)
	Exclusion of dietary problems, intoxications, parasitism, infectious diseases, or systemic disorders

C. *Anatomic*
  1. Small bowel–type diarrhea (small intestine, pancreas, liver)
  2. Large bowel–type diarrhea (cecum, colon, rectum)
  3. Diarrhea secondary to nonenteric disease
	Step 2
	Anatomic localization of process to small or large bowel using history, physical examination, fecal characteristics, and preliminary laboratory tests

D. *Functional*
  1. Normal assimilation (nonsteatorrheic diarrhea)
  2. Malassimilation (steatorrheic diarrhea)
    a. Maldigestion (pancreatic)
    b. Malabsorption (intestinal)
  3. Diarrhea accompanied by protein-losing enteropathy
	Step 3
	Functional characterization (in chronic small bowel diarrhea) to identify malassimilation and then to differentiate maldigestion from malabsorption

E. *Etiologic*	*Step 4* Definitive etiology or histopathologic diagnosis through an extended data base consisting of more sophisticated laboratory tests, radiographs, biopsies (by endoscopy–small intestine; by colonoscopy–large intestine), and response to therapy

From Sherding RG: In Ford RB (ed): Clinical Signs and Diagnosis in Small Animal Practice. New York, Churchill Livingstone, 1988.

as dietary problems, parasites, infectious diseases, intoxications, or extraintestinal systemic disorders. The clinician frequently applies this temporal categorization in the initial planning of a diagnostic and therapeutic strategy for an animal with diarrhea. Thus, for the purposes of discussion, this chapter will organize intestinal diseases of the dog and cat according to whether they are most likely to present as acute diarrhea or chronic diarrhea.

Acute diarrhea is more common and characterized as diarrhea of abrupt or recent onset and short duration (three weeks or less). Many of the conditions that cause acute diarrhea are self-limiting or easily resolved, typified by simple dietary indiscretion or uncomplicated intestinal parasitism; however, others are fulminant and life-threatening, as typified by parvoviral enteritis or acute hemorrhagic gastroenteritis. Management of acute diarrhea is based on rehydration therapy and dietary restriction. Symptomatic therapy with antidiarrheal agents may also be a consideration. Acute diarrhea often resolves spontaneously in a day or two even without any treatment, suggesting that treatment may not always even be indicated. Diagnostic evaluations in acute diarrhea should not be extensive. In fact, diarrhea in most patients is resolved in the absence of a definitive diagnosis with just the information provided by the history and physical examination. Nevertheless, tests to identify parasites are always justified, and depending on the animal's clinical presentation, tests for infectious agents may be indicated (Table 86–3). Elaborate evaluations of gastrointestinal function, however, are not usually necessary initially in such patients.

In animals with diarrhea that is severe, bloody, or associated with systemic signs such as fever, depression, and dehydration, additional diagnostic considerations might include: virologic testing for enteric viruses, fecal cultures for bacterial enteropathogens such as *Salmonella* or *Campylobacter*, and plain abdominal or even barium contrast upper GI radiography for detection of mechanical or obstructive disorders of the bowel. In situations where maintenance of fluid, electrolyte, and acid-base homeostasis is critically important, frequent comparisons of laboratory parameters such as hematocrit, serum biochemistries, and blood gases with the physical status of the patient can enhance the efficacy of therapy.

Somewhat arbitrarily, diarrhea is categorized as chronic rather than acute if it has not been self-limiting or responsive to symptomatic therapy within three to four weeks.[23] This time frame generally excludes many cases of dietary, parasitic, and infectious diarrhea. Management of chronic diarrhea is based upon diagnosis rather than symptomatic treatment. Once diarrhea achieves chronicity, it is unlikely to resolve on its own or to respond to nonspecific antidiarrheal medications. Specific intervention or treatment is usually necessary, and this requires a specific diagnosis. Furthermore, chronic diarrhea, by its very nature, is a nonspecific sign common to a wide variety of disorders that disrupt normal intestinal function. Thus, there is no justification for a "hit-or-miss" approach to diagnosis and therapy. The veterinarian must be prepared to approach chronic diarrhea in a systematic way using sequential diagnostic tests and procedures such as gut and pancreatic function studies, fecal examinations, radiographic procedures, and endoscopic procedures (Table 86–4). Biopsy of the small or large intestine is also often required to reach a definitive diagnosis. Only with the data obtained from these diagnostic evaluations is there a rational basis on which to institute appropriate, specific therapy. In difficult cases, referral to an internal medicine specialist should be a consideration.

TABLE 86–3. DIAGNOSIS OF INFECTIOUS DISEASES OF THE INTESTINES

Viruses (e.g., parvovirus, coronavirus, rotavirus)
1. Demonstration of virus in feces
   Virus isolation
   Electron microscopy
   Hemagglutination (parvovirus)
2. Serology (paired sera)
3. Demonstration of characteristic lesions
   Villous atrophy (coronavirus, rotavirus)
   Crypt necrosis (parvovirus)
   Fluorescent antibody-positive tissues

Bacteria
1. Fecal microscopy
   Presumptive identification of *Campylobacter*
2. Fecal culture (specialized media)
   Salmonella, Campylobacter, Yersinia
3. Fecal assay for toxin
   Clostridium difficile

Mycoses
1. Fecal culture (Sabouraud's)
2. Cytology–feces or rectal mucosal smears
   Histoplasma, Candida
3. Serology (immunodiffusion, complement fixation)
   Histoplasma
4. Identification of fungi in biopsies
   Histoplasma, Pythium, Aspergillus, Candida

Prototheca
1. Fecal culture (Sabouraud's)
2. Cytology–feces or rectal mucosal smears
3. Identification in biopsies

History

Animals with intestinal disease most often present to the veterinarian because of diarrhea or because of concern over other abnormalities that often accompany or result from diarrhea, such as anorexia, vomiting, inactivity, weakness, or weight loss. In animals that only defecate outside, unobserved by the owner, diarrhea may go entirely undetected and only the vague, nonspecific signs of illness that often accompany diarrhea are noted. Diarrhea does not then become recognized as a prominent part of the animal's illness until it is detected during hospitalization or until the owner is specifically instructed to watch for it at home. In some cases, inconvenience can even be the initial reason for owner concern; examples of client-perceived nuisances include "accidents" in the house or outside the litter box, inability to retain feces throughout the night, more frequent litter changes, haircoat soiled with feces, malodorous feces, or excessive flatus.

Even though diarrhea as a sign is nonspecific, detailed observations made by the veterinarian and elicited from the owner through a careful history are helpful to determining the location, nature, and severity of the

TABLE 86–4. PROCEDURES FOR DIAGNOSIS OF CHRONIC SMALL INTESTINAL DISEASE

Procedure	Interpretation of Abnormal Findings	Comments
Serum trypsin-like immunoreactivity (TLI)	Decreased TLI: exocrine pancreatic insufficiency (EPI)	Easy and reliable; test of choice for confirming EPI
BT-PABA digestion test	Flat PABA curve: exocrine pancreatic insufficiency	Less convenient and more expensive than TLI; fairly reliable
Xylose absorption test	Flat xylose curve: intestinal malabsorption	Relatively insensitive, but provides a basis for recommending biopsy
Quantitative fecal fat analysis	Increased fat excretion: maldigestion/malabsorption	Lacks specificity and convenience; has been replaced by other tests
Serum protein electrophoresis	Panhypoproteinemia: lymphangiectasia or other protein-losing enteropathy	Exception: hyperglobulinemia in basenji enteropathy
Serum folate assay	Decreased folate: malabsorption (jejunal) Increased folate: bacterial overgrowth	Folate/B_{12} assay may be the screening test of choice for bacterial overgrowth
Serum vitamin B_{12} assay	Decreased B_{12}: malabsorption (ileal) or bacterial overgrowth	Nonspecific and somewhat insensitive
Nitrosonaphthol test	Positive: bacterial overgrowth	Screening test only
Duodenal aspirates		
Microscopic examination:	*Giardia* trophozoite identification	Occult giardiasis diagnosed more easily by response to therapy
Quantitative culture:	>10^5 organisms/ml:bacterial overgrowth	Test of choice to confirm bacterial overgrowth but too difficult to procure/process specimens for routine use
Upper GI endoscopy/biopsy	Documents mucosal lesions	Definitive test for many disorders, e.g., inflammatory bowel disease
Upper GI barium radiography	Can delineate sites of infiltration, stenosis, and so on	Low diagnostic yield but may provide basis for recommending surgery/biopsy
Thyroid function tests (T_4, scan)	Hyperactivity: thyrotoxicosis	Run on all cats > 6 yr with diarrhea or weight loss

disease process. This is often the first step in planning the direction of diagnostic evaluations. History is especially helpful for localizing the disease process to small or large bowel. It also may indicate extraintestinal disease (for example, renal failure, hypoadrenocorticism, or hyperthyroidism) as the underlying cause of diarrhea, or identify important predisposing factors, such as breed, diet, environmental stress, exposure to parasites or infectious agents, and drug or toxin exposures. The following historical aspects of the diarrhea may help to determine the nature of the disease process: (1) Mode of onset (abrupt versus gradual), (2) duration (acute versus chronic), (3) clinical course (intermittent versus continuous; progression in severity), (4) correlation with diet (specific intolerances such as milk, gluten, and additives; indiscretions such as ingestion of garbage or abrasives; dietary allergy), (5) correlation with drug exposures (idiosyncrasies), (6) correlation with stressful events (psychogenic, anxiety, or "irritability" factors), (7) response to previous medications (such as prescribed diets, antibiotics, corticosteroids, or anthelmintics), and (8) association with other signs, such as weight loss, vomiting, or dyschezia.

Clinical Differentiation of Small and Large Bowel Diarrhea

The initial step in the diagnosis of intractable diarrhea in the dog and cat is the anatomic localization of the disease process to large or small bowel based on history and fecal characteristics (frequency, volume, consistency, color, odor, and composition) (Table 86–5).[23, 27, 28] This distinction is an important one, because it determines the direction of subsequent diagnostic evaluations. Small bowel diarrhea, which refers broadly to diarrhea caused by diseases of the small intestine or of the accessory digestive glands whose secretions function within the lumen of the small intestine (pancreas–enzymes; liver–bile acids), is then evaluated by function tests that differentiate exocrine pancreatic insufficiency (see Chapter 90) from primary intestinal malabsorption and that identify protein-losing enteropathy. Large bowel diarrhea (see Chapter 87), which refers to diseases of the colon, cecum, and rectum, is then evaluated by endoscopic examination as a relatively easy method for direct visualization of the lumen, sampling of luminal contents, and directed biopsy.[27, 28] Widespread involvement of the intestinal tract in a few diseases, such as diffuse intestinal lymphosarcoma, chronic inflammatory bowel disease, or histoplasmosis, may produce concurrent small and large bowel diarrhea.

Chronic small bowel diarrhea is often associated with maldigestion or malabsorption. Thus, voluminous diarrhea, loss of body weight, failure to gain weight, and decline in body condition (malnutrition) are characteristic. It is important for the clinician to consider fecal volume and frequency separately. Volume (daily amount of feces produced) cannot be estimated from the frequency of defecation. The owner may not differentiate an increase in volume or frequency and may refer to either or both as "diarrhea" or "increased defecation." In small bowel diarrhea, each defecation typically produces a large quantity of malodorous, unformed, watery or mushy feces. Frequency of defecation may be increased, but not usually more than two or three times normal, while urgency and tenesmus are uncommon. The feces in exocrine pancreatic insufficiency can have the appearance of a yellowish, "cowpatty" gruel or even undigested food, whereas the feces of primary small intestinal disease are often more soupy or pudding-like and the consistency is more homogene-

TABLE 86–5. DIFFERENTIATION OF SMALL INTESTINAL FROM LARGE INTESTINAL DIARRHEA

Parameter	Small Intestine	Large Intestine
The Feces		
Volume	Markedly increased	Normal or slightly increased
Mucus	Rarely present	Frequently present
Melena	May be present	Absent
Hematochezia	Absent except in acute hemorrhagic diarrhea	Frequently present
Steatorrhea	Present with maldigestive or malabsorptive disease	Absent
Undigested food	May be present with maldigestion	Absent
Color	Color variations occur (e.g., creamy brown, green, orange or clay color)	Color variations are rare, may be bloody
Defecation		
Urgency	Absent except in acute or very severe disease	Usually but not invariably present
Tenesmus	Absent	Frequent but not invariably present
Frequency	2 to 3 times normal for the patient	Usually greater than 3 times normal
Dyschezia	Absent	Present with distal colonic or rectal disease
Ancillary Signs		
Weight loss	Often present in maldigestive or malabsorptive disease	Rare except with severe colitis, diffuse tumors, or histoplasmosis
Vomiting	May be present in inflammatory diseases	Uncommon but occurs in up to 25 to 30% of dogs with colitis
Flatulence and borborygmus	May be present with maldigestion or malabsorption	Absent
Halitosis in the absence of oral disease	May be present with maldigestion or malabsorption	Absent

From Burrows CF: Chronic diarrhea in the dog. Vet Clin North Am 13:521, 1983.

ous. Small bowel diarrhea is generally free of grossly visible mucus or red blood. Unabsorbed nutrients that are degraded and fermented by intestinal bacteria cause small bowel diarrhea to be rancid and foul-smelling. In addition, increased production of luminal gas by bacteria results in excessive flatulence and borborygmus.

Steatorrhea is often a prominent manifestation of small bowel diarrhea.[27, 29] Consequently, the feces are frequently lighter in color. When steatorrhea is severe, maldigestion due to exocrine pancreatic insufficiency is most likely.[27, 29] In extreme cases of this disease, the feces may contain so much undigested fat that they appear oily or greasy. Hair around the animal's perineum may also have an oily texture from contact with fatty feces, and during hospitalization it may be noticed that in-cage defecations produce grease spots on cage papers. Clay-colored, acholic feces, a rare finding, sig-

nifies complete obstruction of the common bile duct with failure of bile pigments to enter the intestine, and must be differentiated from the light-tan color caused by severe steatorrhea.

By contrast, large bowel diarrhea is characterized by frequent attempts to defecate (usually greater than three times normal frequency), each defecation producing small quantities of feces that often contain excessive mucus and fresh red blood.[28] Since the principal function of the canine and feline colon is the absorption of fluid and electrolytes rather than the absorption of nutrients, there should be no evidence of malabsorption or steatorrhea. Dogs with large bowel diarrhea have been shown to have minimally increased daily fecal output (weight or volume) as opposed to the substantial increase in fecal output of dogs with small bowel diarrhea.[30] At the same time, urgency, resulting from irritability or inflammation of the distal colon, causes premature expulsion of a quantity of feces that would otherwise be insufficient to trigger a defecation reflex.[28] Thus, repeated attempts to defecate, producing only a scant amount of feces or none at all, are observed. Sometimes the frequent attempts to defecate produce small amounts of feces composed almost entirely of mucus, exudate, and blood. In addition, large bowel diarrhea may be associated with excessive straining to defecate (tenesmus) or lapses in house-training ("accidents") caused by urgency and inability to retain the feces. The owner may note that the animal remains in a squatting posture for an extended period of time after defecation or makes repeated attempts to defecate within a few minutes period of time.[23] Vomiting occurs in 30 per cent of dogs with colitis.[23] The reader is referred to Chapter 87 for further discussion of large bowel diarrhea.

Abundant mucus in the feces is a fairly reliable indicator of a large bowel problem.[28] The localizing value of fecal mucus is based on the fact that the colonic mucosa contains a relatively large population of mucus-secreting goblet cells that respond to irritation, inflammation, and ulceration by an outpouring of mucus. Excessive mucus may give the feces a glistening or jelly-like appearance.

Extensive mucosal injury at any location along the digestive tract may result in hemorrhage into the lumen. Because many large bowel diseases are inflammatory in nature, diarrhea of large bowel origin frequently contains fresh red blood (hematochezia).[23, 28] When there is bleeding from a lesion in the proximal gastrointestinal tract, the luminal blood pigment has time to undergo chemical change during small bowel transit (except in instances of very rapid transit), producing dark black discoloration of the feces (melena). Gastrointestinal bleeding generally indicates a parasitic, inflammatory, infectious, or neoplastic disorder.

Comparing food intake to the presence or absence of weight loss can be important in evaluating animals with chronic diarrhea. The typical animal with large bowel diarrhea has a relatively normal appetite and minimal weight loss. Severe protracted small bowel diarrhea is generally associated with obvious weight loss and malnutrition, even when appetite may be normal to increased. Constant hunger is a common sign in long-standing exocrine pancreatic insufficiency and is sometimes accompanied by pica and coprophagia.[27]

Physical Examination

A complete physical examination may reveal important clues about the severity, nature, and cause of intestinal disease (Table 86–6). An effort should be made to identify underlying systemic diseases that are a cause or consequence of diarrhea. Physical examination should be thorough and emphasize the detection of fever, weight loss or malnutrition, dehydration, weakness or depression (which may indicate acid-base or electrolyte imbalances), pallor (bloodloss anemia), and effusions or edema (hypoalbuminemia). The thyroid area should be routinely palpated for thyroid tumors that may be associated with the diarrhea of thyrotoxicosis, especially in aged cats.[31] The liver and other abdominal structures can be examined by palpation. Intestinal loops should be carefully palpated for masses, thickening, distention, aggregation, pain, or associated lymphadenopathy. The rectum is examined by digital palpation for foreign objects, masses, strictures, and abnormalities of rectal wall consistency and architecture. In addition, the fecal material obtained on the gloved finger should be inspected grossly for foreign material (e.g., bone particles), blood and mucus, and microscopically for abnormal constituents (parasites, inflammatory cells, lipid).

TABLE 86–6. CLINICAL SIGNIFICANCE OF ABNORMAL PHYSICAL FINDINGS ASSOCIATED WITH INTESTINAL DISEASE

Physical Finding	Potential Clinical Association
General Physical Examination	
Dehydration	Diarrheal fluid loss
Depression/weakness	Electrolyte imbalance, severe debilitation
Emaciation/malnutrition	Chronic malabsorption, protein-losing enteropathy
Dull unthrifty haircoat	Malabsorption of fatty acids, protein, and vitamins
Fever	Infection, transmural inflammatory bowel disease, lymphosarcoma
Edema, ascites, pleural effusion	Protein-losing enteropathy
Pallor (anemia)	GI blood loss, anemia of chronic illness or inflammation
Intestinal Palpation	
Masses	Foreign body, neoplasia, granuloma
Thickened loops	Infiltration (inflammatory, neoplastic)
"Sausage loop"	Intussusception
Aggregated loops	Linear intestinal foreign body, peritoneal adhesions
Pain	Inflammation, obstruction, ischemia
Gas or fluid distention	Obstruction, ileus
Mesenteric lymphadenopathy	Inflammation, infection, neoplasia
Rectal Palpation	
Masses	Polyp, granuloma, neoplasia
Circumferential narrowing	Stricture, spasm, neoplasia
Coarse mucosal texture	Colitis, neoplasia

From Sherding RG: In Ford RB (ed): Clinical Signs and Diagnosis in Small Animal Practice. New York, Churchill Livingstone, 1988.

TABLE 86–7. HEMATOLOGIC CORRELATES OF CHRONIC INTESTINAL DISEASE

Hematologic Parameter	Abnormality	Clinical Associations
1. Neutrophils (/μL)	Neutrophilia	Widespread or transmural inflammatory bowel disease
	Neutropenia	Parvoviral enteritis
		Endotoxemia or overwhelming sepsis (such as bowel rupture or necrosis)
2. Eosinophils (/μL)	Eosinophilia	Parasitism (e.g., hookworms, whipworms)
		Eosinophilic enterocolitis
		Hypoadrenocorticism
3. Monocytes (/μL)	Monocytosis	Chronic inflammation
		Granulomatous inflammation
		Histoplasmosis
4. Lymphocytes (/μL)	Lymphopenia	Intestinal lymphangiectasia
		Stress
5. Erythrocytes (hematocrit)	Erythrocytosis	Hemoconcentration from enteric fluid loss
		Hemorrhagic gastroenteritis syndrome (HGE)
	Anemia	Enteric blood loss
		Anemia of malnutrition
		Anemia of chronic inflammation
6. Plasma Proteins (gm/dl)	Hypoproteinemia	Intestinal lymphangiectasia
		Other protein-losing enteropathies
		Severe malnutrition
		Enteric blood loss
	Hyperglobulinemia	Basenji enteropathy

From Sherding RG: In Ford RB (ed): Clinical Signs and Diagnosis in Small Animal Practice. New York, Churchill Livingstone, 1988.

Routine Hematology and Blood Chemistry

The initial data base for undiagnosed chronic diarrhea should include a complete hemogram (CBC) (Table 86–7) and routine serum biochemistry determinations. On the CBC, eosinophilia may suggest that diarrhea is associated with endoparasitism, eosinophilic enteritis, mast cell neoplasia, or hypoadrenocorticism. A regenerative neutrophilia may suggest necrosis or a widespread inflammatory process within the bowel wall, likely involving the deeper layers. Degenerative or toxic neutropenia may suggest parvoviral infection, septicemia, endotoxemia, or overwhelming bacterial peritonitis due to bowel necrosis or perforation. Lymphopenia may accompany intestinal lymphangiectasia from persistent loss of lymphocytes into the gut lumen. An increased packed cell volume (PCV) and hemoglobin value are indicative of hemoconcentration from fluid loss. Anemia may result from enteric blood loss and from depressed erythropoiesis due to chronic malnutrition or chronic inflammation. Changes in RBC morphology may provide clues to the nature of the anemia. Microcytic hypochromic RBCs are found in dogs with iron deficiency caused by chronic enteric blood loss, while macrocytic RBCs may be found in some malnutritional anemias. In the cat, macrocytosis is also associated with hyperthyroidism,[31] and feline leukemia virus infection.[32]

A serum biochemical profile and urinalysis should also be considered to exclude metabolic or extraintestinal disorders that could cause or result from diarrhea. For example, underlying systemic disease such as renal failure (increased BUN and creatinine) or hypoadrenocorticism (hyperkalemia and hyponatremia) may be detected. Elevated serum liver enzymes may suggest diarrhea secondary to liver disease. Liver function can then be further evaluated by serum bile acid determination. It should be noted that nonspecific mild elevations of liver enzymes are quite common in many animals with intestinal disease. In cases of diarrhea suspected to be due to thyrotoxicosis (particularly in cats), thyroid function should be evaluated (T_4 assay, thyroid scan).[31]

Total plasma protein is useful for screening for hypoproteinemia associated with protein-losing enteropathy and may be further evaluated by albumin and globulin determinations or serum protein electrophoresis. In most cases of protein-losing enteropathy, serum levels of both albumin and globulin are decreased.[33] The unique exception to this is immunoproliferative enteropathy of the Basenji; in this disorder, hyperglobulinemia usually accompanies hypoalbuminemia.[34] In contrast to most protein-losing enteropathies, hypoproteinemia due to liver disease (impaired hepatic protein synthesis) or kidney disease (protein-losing glomerulonephropathy) usually involves only albumin. In association with hypoproteinemia, a decreased total serum calcium level is often found because of a reduction in the protein-bound fraction.[35]

Fecal Examinations

Fecal examinations that are useful for diagnosis of chronic intestinal disease include gross inspection, parasite examinations, microscopic examinations, quantitative fecal collection, chemical determinations, and cultures (Table 86–8). The diagnostic importance of gross characteristics of feces (volume/weight, consistency, color composition, odor) have been discussed previously in this chapter.

Fecal examinations that should be part of the minimum data base in all animals with intractable diarrhea include fecal flotations and direct smears for parasites; microscopic examinations of stained fecal smears for fat, starch, and leukocytes; and if circumstances suggest infection, fecal culture for specific enteropathogenic bacteria or fungi.

Fecal Examinations for Parasites. The importance of a careful search for parasites through fecal examinations and other procedures cannot be overemphasized (Table 86–9). Endoparasitism can mimic virtually any of the more complex small and large bowel disorders, and in many areas parasites are the most frequent cause of diarrhea. Conventional fecal flotations should be performed to identify metazoan ova. Zinc sulfate centrifugation is used to identify protozoan cysts, such as those of *Giardia*. In warm, humid regions where *Strongyloides stercoralis* infection may be suspected, a direct smear,

sedimentation, or Baermann technique can be utilized to look for larvae in the feces. Motile trophozoites of protozoan parasites, including *Giardia canis*, *Trichomonas* sp., *Entamoeba histolytica*, and *Balantidium coli*, can be identified microscopically in a drop of fresh feces suspended in a few drops of isotonic saline.[36] The distinguishing characteristics of each of these protozoa are discussed in the section on Intestinal Protozoa.

In some cases of chronic small bowel-type diarrhea caused by *Giardia*, the protozoa cannot be found in fecal examinations (occult infection), and the diagnosis

TABLE 86–8. FECAL EXAMINATIONS USED FOR DIAGNOSIS OF INTESTINAL DISEASE

Examination/Procedure	Diagnostic Significance
1. Gross inspection	
Volume (bulk)	Small vs. large bowel diarrhea
Consistency, color, odor	Small vs. large bowel diarrhea
Composition	Blood, mucus, foreign matter
2. Parasite examinations	
Fecal flotation	Parasite ova, cysts
Saline fecal smear	Protozoa
3. Microscopic examinations	
Sudan preparation	Fat (steatorrhea)
Iodine preparation	Starch (amylorrhea)
Cytologic preparation	Leukocytes, infectious agents
4. Quantitative 24-hour fecal collection	
Quantitative fecal fat analysis	Malassimilation
Fecal weight (daily fecal output)	Malassimilation
5. Chemical determinations	
Fat content	Steatorrhea–malassimilation
Water content	Correlated with fecal weight
Nitrogen content	Azotorrhea–malassimilation
Electrolytes	Osmotic vs. secretory diarrhea
Osmolality	Osmotic vs. secretory diarrhea
pH	Carbohydrate malassimilation
Occult blood test	GI bleeding
Proteolytic (trypsin) activity	Pancreatic insufficiency
Alpha$_1$-antitrypsin	Protein-losing enteropthy
Toxin assays	*Clostridium difficile* infection
6. Cultures	
Bacterial	*Salmonella, Campylobacter, Yersinia*, and others
Fungal	Histoplasmosis and others

From Sherding RG: In Ford RB (ed): Clinical Signs and Diagnosis in Small Animal Practice. New York, Churchill Livingstone, 1988.

TABLE 86–9. DIAGNOSIS OF INTESTINAL PARASITES

Examination/Procedure	Diagnostic Findings
Fecal examinations	
Visual inspection	Tapeworm proglottids
Flotation (conventional; e.g., sodium nitrate)	Nematode and cestode ova
Zinc sulfate centrifugation–flotation	*Giardia* and coccidia cysts
Sheather's sugar centrifugation–flotation	*Cryptosporidium* cysts
Saline suspension	*Strongyloides* larvae
Duodenal aspiration	*Giardia* trophozoites
Colonoscopy	Adult whipworms
Therapeutic trial	
Response to fenbendazole	Occult trichuriasis
Response to metronidazole	Occult giardiasis

is made by identification of *Giardia* trophozoites in duodenal aspirates,[37] or by response to a therapeutic trial of metronidazole or atabrine. Similarly, occult infestation of whipworms is a rather frequent cause of chronic large bowel diarrhea. The diagnosis can be established by colonoscopic observation of adult whipworms or by response to a whipcidal drug such as fenbendazole.

Fecal Examinations for Infectious Agents. The diagnosis of infectious diarrhea often depends upon the detection of the offending viral, bacterial, or fungal organisms in the feces. The details of diagnosing these various enteric infections are found in the respective sections of this chapter.

Viral diarrhea is generally acute and confirmed by identification of virus in the feces serologically or electron microscopically. Specific enteropathogenic bacteria such as *Salmonella, Campylobacter,* and *Yersinia* can be isolated from fresh feces using specialized culture media. These invasive enteropathogens should particularly be considered in leukocyte-positive, large bowel diarrhea. Under most circumstances, the special techniques required for isolation of these bacteria will necessitate submission of specimens to a large commercial laboratory, veterinary school laboratory, or human hospital laboratory. *Salmonella* organisms generally survive transport to the lab quite well. *Campylobacter,* on the other hand, is microaerophilic and rather intolerant of conditions outside of the animal. Thus, it is easily destroyed in transit to the laboratory. Specimens for *Campylobacter* should be processed as soon as possible after collection, or held at 4° C and transported in anaerobic transport medium.[38] A presumptive identification of *Campylobacter* organisms can be made from microscopic examination of fresh diarrheic feces by an experienced microbiologist, although positive findings should always then be confirmed by culture. Although special procedures to isolate specific bacterial enteropathogens from feces can be an important aspect of the diagnostic evaluation of a patient with unexplained diarrhea, the clinician must be aware that the submission of feces for conventional aerobic bacterial culture is of practically no value. This is because such cultures will not detect the anaerobic and facultative microorganisms which are of greatest importance as enteropathogens.

Feces can also be cultured for fungal organisms, such as *Histoplasma capsulatum,* using Sabouraud's media; however, isolation attempts often fail.[39] Serodiagnosis of histoplasmosis using immunodiffusion and complement fixation blood tests is usually more rewarding (see Chapter 49). Fungal elements *(Histoplasma, Aspergillus, Pythium, Candida)* may also be identified in cytology preparations (fecal leukocyte examination, rectal mucosal scraping) or biopsy specimens. Prototheca, pathogenic unicellular algae that are a rare cause of necrotizing enterocolitis, may also be identified in feces and biopsies as endosporulated structures (five to ten μ size) or cultured on Sabouraud's media.[40]

Microscopic Examination of Feces. Fecal microscopy includes preparations of direct and indirect Sudan stain, Lugol's iodine stain, and new methylene blue or Wright's stain. Saline smears for protozoa identification are usually done at the same time, and have already been discussed. These basically are simple, in-office qualitative screening tests used to initially identify malabsorbed nutrients or exudative colitis. Since these are only screening tests, they should be performed several times for optimal reliability. Feces for these evaluations should be fresh; either tested within 15 minutes of defecation, or obtained directly from the rectum digitally, or with a loop or swab. In each test, one to two drops of feces and one to two drops of stain are mixed well on a microscope slide, cover slipped, and examined.

The direct Sudan preparation (saturated Sudan III solution in 95 per cent ethyl alcohol) stains excessive undigested (unsplit) fat in the feces as numerous, large, refractile orange droplets, indicating steatorrhea due to exocrine pancreatic insufficiency (Figure 86–4).[41] This preparation is usually strongly positive in dogs with exocrine pancreatic insufficiency that are fed a fat-containing diet, but it does not stain the free fatty acids of intestinal steatorrhea. In the indirect Sudan test (one to two drops each of feces, 36 per cent acetic acid, and Sudan mixed and heated twice to boiling on slide) unabsorbed fatty acids (split fat) stain as well. Thus, numerous large orange lipid droplets on an indirect Sudan preparation in an animal with a negative direct Sudan preparation suggests steatorrhea due to intestinal malabsorption of fatty acids.[41] Occasionally in pancreatic maldigestion, the indirect Sudan test for split fat is more strongly positive than the direct test for unsplit fat. The indirect Sudan preparation must be examined while still warm, or as it cools down the lipid globules form crystalline spicules.[42] Examination of Sudan-stained feces as a method for detecting steatorrhea in humans correlates well with the results of quantitative fecal fat analysis.[41–44]

Lugol's two per cent iodine solution stains excessive undigested starch in the feces (amylorrhea) as dark blue-black granules or identifies light brown, undigested striated muscle fibers in meat-fed animals, either of these findings suggesting maldigestion due to pancreatic insufficiency.[27] This procedure, however, is relatively insensitive and imprecise and depends on the animal's diet. *Giardia* trophozoites and cysts are also stained light brown with iodine.

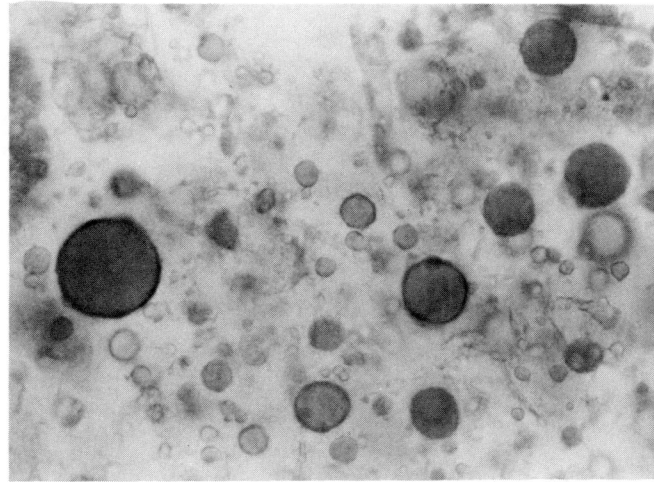

FIGURE 86–4. Refractile orange fat droplets in the Sudan-stained feces of an animal with steatorrhea.

Examination of feces for leukocytes can be useful in patients with colitis. Cytology stains, such as new methylene blue or Wright's, can be used to examine feces for leukocytes, which appear in exudative inflammatory bowel diseases when there is disruption of distal intestinal or colonic mucosa.[45, 46] Similarly, exfoliative cytology of colonic mucosal scrapings or swabbings taken during proctoscopy or directly from the rectum may also reveal colonic mucosal disease. Cytology may, in some cases, provide a definitive diagnosis. For example, in endemic areas, intestinal histoplasmosis may be diagnosed by finding the organisms within macrophages obtained by colonic scraping (Figure 86–5).[28] When lesions are confined to the small intestine, fecal leukocytes are usually absent and colonic scrapings are normal. It is advisable to follow up cases that are positive for fecal leukocytes with colonoscopy and fecal cultures for invasive bacteria such as *Campylobacter* and *Salmonella*.

Fecal Biochemistry Determinations. Chemical analyses that can be performed on feces include occult blood detection, proteolytic (trypsin) activity, fat quantitation, electrolyte concentrations, osmolality, pH, and detection of excess enteric loss of protein. With the exception of chemical tests for fecal occult blood as a means of detecting subtle GI hemorrhage, most of these are too impractical or too unreliable to be of clinical value.

Feces may be chemically tested for the presence of occult blood by a simple, in-office commercial test (Hemoccult test). This is a qualitative test that is sensitive for detecting even very small amounts of gastrointestinal hemorrhage. Because of this sensitivity, it is recommended that the animal's diet not contain meat for at least three days prior to testing for occult blood to avoid false-positive results. The presence of fecal occult blood signifies a bleeding lesion of the GI tract,

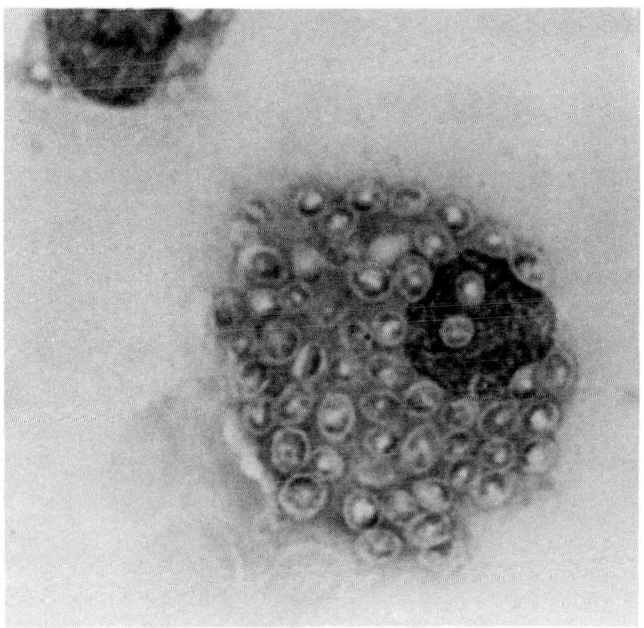

FIGURE 86–5. Numerous *Histoplasma capsulatum* organisms within the cytoplasm of a macrophage obtained by colonic scraping of a dog with chronic diarrhea due to *Histoplasma* enterocolitis (Wright's stain).

thereby suggesting an ulcerative, inflammatory, or neoplastic disorder. The fecal occult blood test is also indicated when GI bleeding is suspected on the basis of hematologic changes (such as chronic blood loss anemia) but cannot be demonstrated by grossly visible fecal hemorrhage (melena).

Quantitative fecal fat analysis can be used as an intestinal function test to confirm steatorrhea, but it is extremely cumbersome and impractical to perform and does not differentiate pancreatic maldigestion from intestinal malabsorption. Feces must be collected for a 24- to 72-hour period while the animal is confined and fed a standard diet. The feces are weighed and sent to a commercial laboratory for analysis. Normally, less than ten per cent of ingested fat is excreted in the feces, or less than 0.3 gm/kg/day in dogs,[29, 47] and less than 0.4 gm/kg/day in cats.[48] If one goes to the trouble of quantitative fecal collection, simply recording the weight of feces produced daily can help to clarify whether the diarrhea is small or large bowel in origin. Daily fecal output (weight) of dogs with pancreatic maldigestion or intestinal malabsorption is three to four times greater than that of normal dogs or dogs with colitis.[30]

In the past, tests for proteolytic activity of feces (such as gel tube and x-ray film digestion tests) were used as indicators of pancreatic secretion of proteases (trypsin) for the diagnosis of exocrine pancreatic insufficiency. These tests are too unreliable to recommend, and they have been replaced with a much more accurate diagnostic test, the serum trypsin-like immunoreactivity assay (see Chapter 90).

Determination of fecal electrolyte concentrations, osmolality, and pH in the supernatant fecal water after centrifugation of diarrheic feces (30 min at 2000 gm) is used in humans to differentiate osmotic and secretory diarrhea.[24] The results of electrolyte and osmolality determinations are meaningful only if the diarrhea is fluid enough that after centrifugation the supernatant water comprises at least a third of the total sample. In osmotic diarrhea, because osmotically active exogenous solutes are retained in the gut lumen and feces, there is an osmol gap such that the calculated osmolality using fecal electrolytes (sum of Na^+ and K^+ concentrations multiplied by two) is much less than the actual osmolality of the fecal fluid measured by freezing point depression. In purely secretory diarrhea, fecal osmolality is almost entirely accounted for by the fecal concentration of Na^+, K^+, and their anions, so that: $[Na^+ + K^+] \times 2$ approximates the actual measured fecal osmolality.[24] The fecal pH in osmotic diarrhea is usually low because carbohydrate malabsorption acidifies colonic content.[24]

Tests to Document GI Protein Loss. For the documentation of protein-losing enteropathy, the gastrointestinal loss of plasma proteins can be measured using the fecal excretion of intravenously administered radiolabeled proteins and macromolecules, such as [51]chromium-labeled albumin.[49, 50] However, these radiolabeled substrates are difficult to obtain and the procedures are too impractical for use in the clinical setting. The fecal concentration and intestinal clearance of α_1-antitrypsin, a natural plasma protein, is in current use as a simple and reliable method for measuring enteric protein loss in human patients without the use of radioisotopes;[51, 52] however, this test has not yet been evaluated in canine protein-losing enteropathy.

Tests of Digestive and Absorptive Function

Once simple dietary, parasitic, and infectious causes for chronic small bowel diarrhea have been excluded, diagnostic efforts should be directed next toward verifying or ruling out exocrine pancreatic insufficiency, and then toward characterization of intestinal malabsorption. This is accomplished by evaluating the function of these organs through tests of digestion and absorption, especially in dogs. The microscopic examination of Sudan-stained feces as a screening test for steatorrhea was described in the previous section. Only a few of the numerous tests of enteropancreatic function that have been used in dogs provide reliable diagnostic information. These include the assay for serum trypsin-like immunoreactivity (TLI test);[53, 54] and the bentiromide (BT-PABA) digestion test,[55–60] both of which evaluate exocrine pancreatic function and are detailed in Chapter 90; and the xylose absorption test,[59, 61, 62] which evaluates intestinal function. In addition, preliminary results suggest that serum concentrations of folate and cobalamin (vitamin B_{12}) are useful indicators of intestinal absorptive function and bacterial overgrowth,[63] while a breath hydrogen excretion test looks promising as an indicator of carbohydrate malabsorption.[64, 65]

In cats, tests of exocrine pancreatic function are rarely necessary since exocrine pancreatic insufficiency is very rare in this species. Older cats with weight loss and diarrhea should routinely be evaluated for hyperthyroidism with at least a baseline serum T_4 test. For evaluating intestinal absorptive function in cats, unfortunately the xylose absorption test is imprecise.[66–68]

There are many other tests of digestive and absorptive function reported in the veterinary literature; however, these are too inaccurate or impractical to be useful. These include fat digestion/absorption tests such as quantitative fecal fat analysis, the plasma turbidity test, vitamin A absorption test, and radiolabeled triolein-oleic acid absorption test; carbohydrate absorption tests such as oral glucose, starch, and lactose tolerance tests; and tests that determine fecal protease (trypsin) activity qualitatively or quantitatively.[29, 47, 48, 62, 69–77]

Xylose Absorption Test. The standard test for evaluating mucosal absorptive function is the xylose absorption test.[61] Xylose is a pentose monosaccharide that is absorbed by both passive and active mechanisms and once absorbed is relatively inert, unaffected by insulin, and excreted mainly by the kidney. After a 12-hour fast, plasma xylose concentration is determined before and at 30, 60, 90, and 120 minutes (60- and 90-minute samples are usually satisfactory for routine diagnostic use) after the oral administration of 0.2 gm D-xylose/lb body weight, given as a five to ten per cent solution (with tap water). In normal dogs, xylose concentration should peak at greater than 60 mg/dl at 60 to 90 minutes, indicative of normal absorption, whereas dogs with severe malabsorption usually have a depressed xylose curve (Figure 86–6). Since some dogs with exocrine pancreatic insufficiency malabsorb xylose, it is important to evaluate pancreatic function (Chapter 90) before interpreting an abnormal xylose test. The test is somewhat insensitive: some animals with significant intestinal disease have a normal xylose absorption test. Therefore, when the test is abnormal it strongly suggests severe diffuse intestinal disease; however, when it is normal, it does not necessarily exclude malabsorption. In normal cats, xylose absorption curves vary widely and peak serum xylose concentrations are lower and less predictable than in normal dogs; thus in cats with diarrhea, the test is difficult to interpret and much less useful than in dogs.[66, 67] In one study, there was no significant difference between xylose absorption in normal cats and cats with diffuse infiltrative intestinal disease.[68]

False results with the xylose test include a factitiously low (or delayed) peak due to delayed gastric emptying, intraluminal bacterial metabolism of xylose in states with bacterial overgrowth, or sequestration of xylose in ascitic fluid, whereas a falsely elevated peak may result

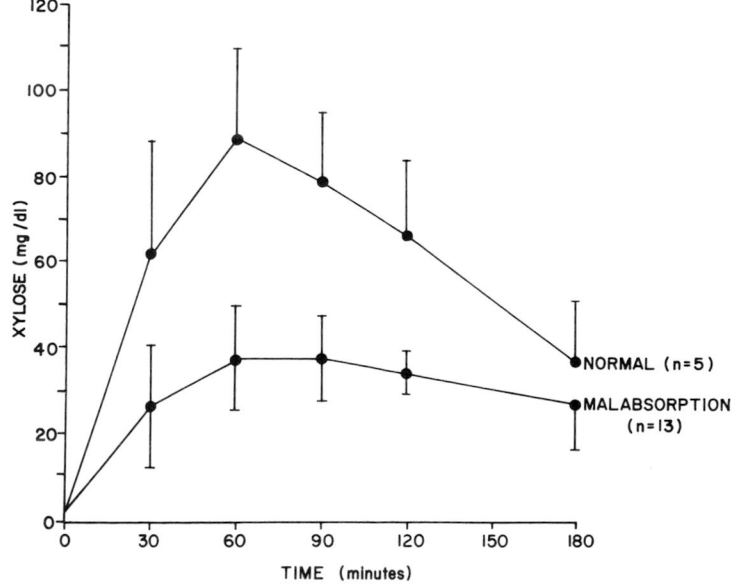

FIGURE 86–6. D-Xylose absorption curve in clinically normal dogs and 13 dogs with malabsorption (brackets = standard deviation).

from decreased urinary xylose excretion because of renal failure. It also has been demonstrated in rats that the absorption of xylose can occur from the stomach as well as the small intestines.[78] As the standard test for intestinal absorptive function, the xylose absorption test can be conveniently combined with a test of pancreatic digestive function, the bentiromide digestion test, for the simultaneous evaluation of pancreatic digestion and intestinal absorption.[59]

Measurement of Serum Folate and Vitamin B_{12}.
Measurement of serum concentrations of folate and vitamin B_{12} (cobalamin) have been helpful in recognizing and characterizing certain chronic malabsorptive diseases of the small intestine in the dog.[63] Serum folate levels depend upon the absorptive function of the proximal small intestine (jejunum), while serum levels of vitamin B_{12} reflect absorption in the distal small intestine (ileum). Accordingly, serum folate concentrations are depressed in enteropathies that affect the proximal small intestine, serum vitamin B_{12} concentrations are reduced in diseases of the ileum, and serum levels of both vitamins are decreased in disorders that cause diffuse intestinal malabsorption.[63] In bacterial overgrowth, serum folate concentrations may actually be elevated due to synthesis of folate by certain bacteria, while serum levels of vitamin B_{12} are decreased because many bacteria can bind vitamin B_{12} making it unavailable for absorption.[63] This same pattern of increased folate and decreased vitamin B_{12} is observed in some dogs with exocrine pancreatic insufficiency. The normal values (12-hour fasted) for one laboratory that accepts serum specimens (2 ml nonhemolyzed serum packed in ice) on a mail-in basis (University of Florida Veterinary Medical Teaching Hospital, Gainesville, FL) are: folate, 3.5 to 11.0 µg/L and vitamin B_{12}, 300 to 700 ng/L.

Diagnosis of Small Intestinal Bacterial Overgrowth

The syndrome of small intestinal bacterial overgrowth is characterized by an excessive number of bacteria in the proximal small bowel leading to malabsorption and diarrhea. Although a naturally occurring enteropathy associated with bacterial overgrowth has been studied in dogs, the importance of the condition in animals is not known because of the difficulty in confirming the diagnosis. The results of intestinal absorption tests generally overlap with other causes of malabsorption, and direct documentation of bacterial overgrowth requires quantitative aerobic and anaerobic culture of intestinal contents obtained by duodenal intubation or aspiration. Thus, specimen procurement, and the laboratory culture procedures as well, are too tedious and expensive to be practical for routine clinical use.

There are also indirect, noninvasive methods of diagnosis that are based on the detection of bacterial metabolites in the blood (serum folate), urine (indican, phenols), or expired air (breath tests).[79, 80] A urine nitrosonaphthol test has been used as a nonspecific screening test for bacterial overgrowth in dogs.[81] This test uses readily available reagents that are mixed with urine to produce a color change indicative of the pres-

ence of parahydroxyphenyl acetic acid and related compounds that are derived from bacterial degradation of dietary tyrosine. As discussed in the section on Measurement of Serum Folate and Vitamin B_{12}, elevated serum folate concentration, presumably due to synthesis of folate by certain bacteria, has been quite reliable as an indirect indicator of bacterial overgrowth in dogs.[63] Decreased serum levels of vitamin B_{12} are usually found concomitantly. The breath tests, which are used widely in humans, have not yet been adapted for clinical use in animals; however, measurement of breath hydrogen excretion appears experimentally in dogs to be a promising tool for indirect assessment of carbohydrate malabsorption and bacterial overgrowth.[64, 65, 82] Patients with suspected small intestinal bacterial overgrowth should respond to a therapeutic trial of antibiotics (e.g., tylosin, tetracycline, metronidazole and chloramphenicol).

Gastrointestinal Radiography and Ultrasonography

An upper gastrointestinal barium series should be considered when other tests fail to determine a cause for chronic diarrhea. Upper GI barium studies have been helpful in detecting intestinal neoplastic, granulomatous, and chronic inflammatory lesions that cause radiographic irregularities of the intestinal mucosal pattern or markedly distort the bowel wall (Figure 86-7).[83] Such findings may in some cases provide the grounds for recommending to the owner that endoscopic or surgical biopsy be performed. In most cases, however, chronic diarrhea involves microscopic or functional changes in the bowel that are not detected by barium radiography. Barium may temporarily interfere with fecal cultures, detection of protozoa, absorption tests, and colonoscopy.

In the animal suspected of having a mechanical or obstructive disorder (foreign body or intussusception), radiography often provides the diagnosis or at least sufficient information to support surgical intervention (Figure 86-8).

Barium enema radiography is helpful in evaluating the cecum and colon for ileocolic intussusceptions, cecal inversions, colonic neoplasms, polyps, strictures, colonic displacement, colonic shortening, and chronic colitis (see Chapter 87).[83] In general, colonoscopy is preferred and performed instead of a barium enema since it is easier and yields more definitive diagnostic information.

In animals with intestinal lymphangiectasia, diagnostic mesenteric lymphangiography can be used to evaluate the intestinal lymphatic system and to delineate sites of obstructed lymph flow within the thoracic duct.[84]

Abdominal ultrasonography can be useful for defining intestinal and other abdominal masses, for evaluating the pancreas for tumors or abscesses, and for detecting evidence of biliary tract disease. This technique is currently available mainly at referral centers.

Gastrointestinal Endoscopy

Duodenoscopy with a flexible fiberoptic endoscope can be used in the anesthetized animal for the visual

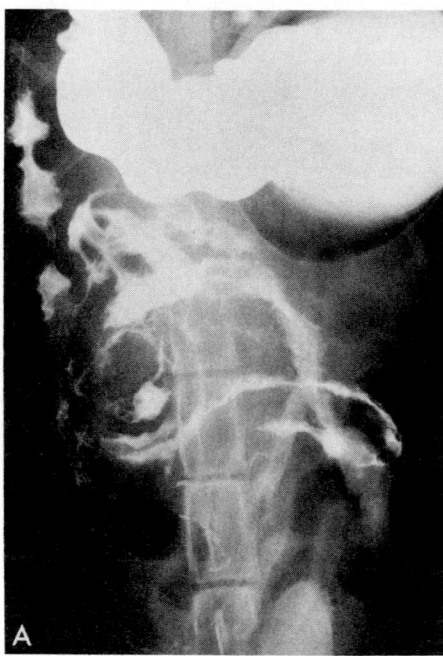
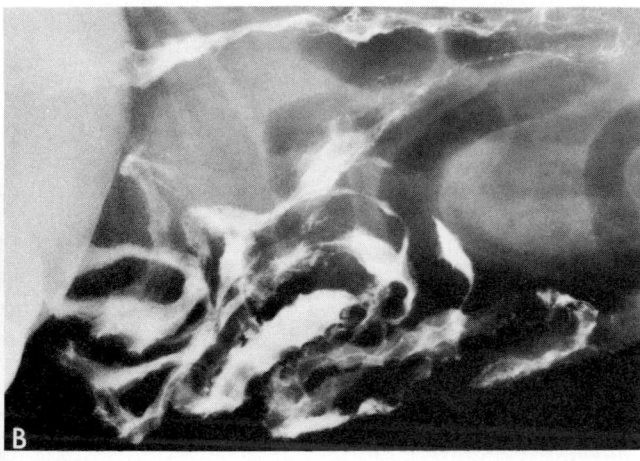

FIGURE 86–7. Ventrodorsal *(A)* and lateral *(B)* radiographs of the abdomen one hour after barium administration in this dog with chronic diarrhea showed diffuse mucosal irregularity and nodular infiltration throughout the duodenum and jejunum. These radiographic abnormalities prompted a small bowel biopsy, which confirmed diffuse intestinal lymphosarcoma.

inspection of the duodenum, duodenal aspiration (for culture, isolation of *Giardia*, and pancreatic response testing), and mucosal biopsy. The equipment required for duodenoscopy is relatively expensive. Accessory instruments that can be used through the endoscope biopsy channel include tubing for aspirations, endoscopic biopsy brush for cytology specimens, and endoscopic biopsy forceps for directed mucosal biopsy. Duodenoscopy has been particularly useful for obtaining mucosal biopsies without the necessity of major abdominal surgery.

Definitive diagnosis of many large bowel diseases, especially colitis, is made by colonoscopy and colon biopsy (see Chapter 87). Colonoscopic biopsy of the

colon may even be useful in the diagnosis of certain generalized enteric diseases, such as chronic inflammatory disease (enterocolitis), prototheocosis, histoplasmosis, and diffuse intestinal lymphosarcoma, any of which can affect both small and large bowel simultaneously. In these diseases, colon biopsy can be diagnostic even though the majority of signs may be of small bowel origin.

Intestinal Biopsy

Definitive diagnosis of the various intestinal malabsorptive diseases is usually best accomplished by exploratory laparotomy with inspection and biopsy of the small intestine and mesenteric lymph nodes. Multiple biopsies should be taken along the length of the gut even if there are no lesions visible by gross inspection, which is often the case. Other abdominal organs, especially the pancreas, liver, and colon, should also be evaluated during laparotomy. Duodenal aspirates or duodenal mucosal impression smears may be examined for *Giardia* or cultured quantitatively for aerobic and anaerobic bacterial overgrowth. In patients in which diffuse mucosal lesions are suspected, mucosal biopsy via duodenoscopy or peroral suction biopsy capsule are less invasive alternatives to full-thickness intestinal biopsy by laparotomy, provided that the necessary equipment is available.

Surgery in those animals with severe hypoproteinemia or emaciation should not be taken lightly—chronic protein depletion and the catabolic state may severely impair healing of biopsy sites. The greatest risk in full-thickness surgical biopsy of the intestines is dehiscence of the enterotomy incision, which leads to subsequent bowel leakage and postoperative peritonitis. Thus, less invasive biopsy methods such as endoscopy or suction biopsy capsule should be used whenever possible in hypoproteinemic or cachexic animals. If these biopsy

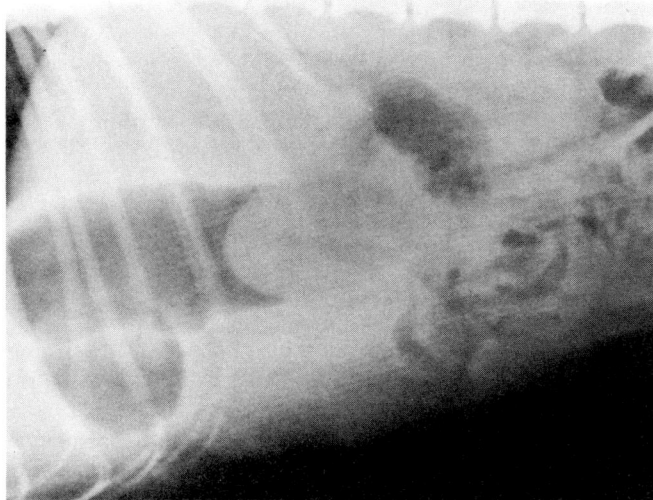

FIGURE 86–8. The radiographic delineation of a gas-distended gut loop associated with an egg-shaped intraluminal object in this vomiting dog suggested intestinal foreign body obstruction and provided the information needed to support surgical intervention. A foam rubber ball was removed from the small bowel.

methods are not available, then the diagnosis of lymphangiectasia (the most common lesion in severe protein-losing enteropathy) may be made from gross appearance and biopsy of serosal and mesenteric lymphatic lesions without risking invasion of the gut for a full-thickness specimen. In severely hypoproteinemic animals, preoperative plasma infusions are also advisable.

A novel approach to the detection of chronic malabsorptive intestinal disease uses biochemical analysis of jejunal mucosal biopsies obtained by a peroral suction biopsy technique.[85, 86] Based on the mucosal enzyme activities, a variety of enteropathies in the dog have been characterized by nonmorphologic criteria, including an enteropathy resembling human tropical sprue,[87] a dietary sensitivity to wheat in the Irish setter,[88–91] and an enteropathy in the German shepherd dog that is associated with bacterial overgrowth in the proximal small bowel.[92–94] Although these procedures are currently only research tools, in the future, biochemical analysis of intestinal biopsies may be as valuable for diagnosis as conventional morphologic evaluation of biopsies.

Diagnosis by Response to Therapy

Response to therapy is a valid means of confirming certain diagnoses when backed up with sufficient supportive evidence. Trial and error test diets, for example, are commonly used to exclude dietary intolerance to certain foods. Response to antibacterial therapy (such as tylosin, tetracycline, or metronidazole) is often a practical method for determining bacterial overgrowth within the small bowel. Occult parasitic diseases, such as occult giardiasis or occult whipworm infestation, may be excluded by response to metronidazole or fenbendazole, respectively.

ACUTE, DIETARY, PARASITIC, AND INFECTIOUS DIARRHEA

Acute diarrhea is usually characterized by a sudden onset of watery or watery-mucoid diarrhea that may be overtly bloody in severe cases. Inappetence, lethargy, and vomiting are concomitant signs in most animals, while fever, abdominal pain, and significant dehydration suggest more serious intestinal disease.

Acute diarrhea in the dog and cat may be caused by dietary indiscretion or intolerance, drugs and toxins, intestinal parasites, infectious agents (viral, bacterial, rickettsial), and a variety of systemic or metabolic disturbances. The diagnosis and treatment of these disorders are tabulated at the end of this chapter. Although there are exceptions, acute diarrhea associated with diet, parasites, and medications generally tends to be mild and self-limiting, whereas acute diarrhea that is severe and life-threatening occurs most frequently in young animals with infectious enteritis (Table 86–10), idiopathic hemorrhagic gastroenteritis, and neonatal ancylostomiasis.

TABLE 86–10. ENTERIC PATHOGENS OF DOGS AND CATS

Viral
  1. Coronavirus
  2. Parvovirus
  3. Rotavirus
  4. Others: Canine distemper, FIP, FeLV, FIV, astrovirus*
Bacterial
  1. Enteropathogenic *E. coli**
  2. *Salmonella* spp.
  3. *Yersinia enterocolitica*
  4. *Campylobacter jejuni*
  5. *Bacillus piliformis* (Tyzzer's disease)
  6. *Clostridium* spp.*
Rickettsial (Salmon Poisoning)
  1. *Neorickettsia helminthoeca*
  2. *Neorickettsia elokomimica*
Mycotic
  1. *Histoplasma capsulatum*
  2. *Aspergillus* spp.
  3. *Candida albicans*
  4. *Pythium* spp.
Other—*Prototheca* spp. (algae)

*Pathogenicity in dogs and cats is likely but not proven.

A presumptive diagnosis of the cause of acute diarrhea can often be determined from information obtained by history and physical examination. The history should include a review of the animal's vaccination status, diet, current medications, and possible exposure to toxins, parasite-infected environments, or infectious disease.

Dietary factors, parasites, and medications are common causes of mild diarrhea that is easily resolved; thus these causes should be initially considered when an animal develops diarrhea acutely but otherwise does not seem very ill. Restriction of food intake for 24 hours or symptomatic therapy (see the Treatment of Intestinal Disease section) in most patients results in rapid resolution of the diarrhea. The inciting cause is seldom determined.

An effort should always be made to identify intestinal parasites by fecal examination (flotations, smears, and sedimentations for ova, larvae, cysts, and trophozoites) and visual inspection of feces for tapeworm proglottids and adult ascarids (see Table 86–9). Treatment with specific parasiticides should result in rapid resolution.

In patients with diarrhea that is severe, bloody, or associated with systemic signs such as fever, depression, and dehydration, additional diagnostic considerations might include virologic testing for parvovirus or other enteric viruses, fecal cultures for bacterial enteropathogens such as *Salmonella* or *Campylobacter*, and plain abdominal or even barium contrast upper GI radiography for detection of mechanical or obstructive disorders of the bowel. In situations in which maintenance of fluid, electrolyte, and acid-base homeostasis is critically important, monitoring of laboratory parameters such as hematocrit, serum biochemistries, and blood gases can facilitate therapy. The symptomatic treatment of acute diarrhea in dogs and cats is discussed at the end of this chapter.

Dietary Diarrhea

Diarrhea as a result of indiscriminate eating and chewing behavior is particularly common in dogs. Die-

TABLE 86-11. ANTHELMINTICS

Drug	Dosage (D = dog, C = cat)	Efficacy (%)					Comments
		Ascarids	Hookworms	Whipworms	Tapeworms	Strongyloides	
Bunamidine HCl (Scolaban)	D/C:25–50 mg/kg, PO	—	—	—	56–90 Dipylidium 100 Taenia 85–100 Echinococcus	—	Do not use with Styquin. May cause idiosyncratic sudden deaths (large dogs).
Butamisole HCl (Styquin)	D:2.4 mg/kg, SC	—	92	99	—	—	Fourfold overdose is fatal. Fatal reactions with Scolaban. Do not use in dogs < 8 wk, debilitated, or heartworm-positive. Pain at injection site.
Dichlorvos (Task)	D:27–33 mg/kg, PO C & pups: 11 mg/kg, PO	95	95	90	—	—	Do not use in debilitated, heartworm-positive, or anticholinesterase-treated animals.
Diethylcarbamazine (many products)	D:6.6 mg/kg/day, PO	80	—	—	—	—	When used as daily heartworm prevention, DEC aids control of ascarids and with additives also aids control of hookworms. Oxibendazole is hepatotoxic in some dogs.
DEC + styrylpyridinium (Styrid-Caricide)		80	80	—	—	—	
DEC + oxibendazole (Filarabits Plus)		80	80	—	—	—	
Disophenol (DNP)	D/C:10 mg/kg SC	—	95	—	—	—	Fourfold overdose is fatal. Do not use in overheated or respiratory-diseased animals. Stains at injection site.
Febantel & Praziquantel (Vercom)	D/C:15 mg/kg Feb. × 3 da, PO 1.5 mg/kg Praz. × 3 da, PO	99	99	100	100 Dipylidium 100 Taenia 100 Echinococcus	—	Very safe and broad-spectrum.

Drug	Dosage				Tapeworm		Comments
Fenbendazole (Panacur)	D/C:50 mg/kg × 3–5 da, PO	99	98	100	0 Dipylidium 88–100 Taenia	100 (5-day Rx)	Safe in cats although not approved. Prenatal and postnatal Rx of bitch can reduce transmission (>90%) of ascarids and hookworms to pups.
Ivermectin	Needs to be determined (PO, SC)	50–98	100	98	—	>90	Appears safe but not yet approved for this use. Inconsistent efficacy for ascarids, especially T. leonina.
Mebendazole (Telmintic)	D:22 mg/kg × 3–5 da, PO	95	95	95	0 Dipylidium 95 Taenia	—	May cause vomiting and occasional acute hepatic necrosis.
Niclosamide (Yomesan)	D/C: 100–157 mg/kg, PO	—	—	—	18–56 Dipylidium 80 Taenia	—	Inconsistent efficacy.
Piperazine (many products)	D/C: 110 mg/kg, PO	85–100	—	—	—	—	Very safe but variable efficacy.
Praziquantel (Droncit)	D/C: consult label	—	—	—	100 Dipylidium 100 Taenia 100 Echinococcus	—	Very safe—drug of choice for tapeworms. For Echino. —10 mg/kg. Pain at injection site.
Pyrantel pamoate (Nemex)	D/C: 5 mg/kg, PO	95	95	95	—	—	Very safe—even nursing pups. Safe in cats although not approved.
Thenium closylate (Canopar) (Thenatol-combo with piperazine)	D: 500 mg (dogs > 5 kg). PO; 125 mg (2.5–5 kg)	—	89	—	—	—	May cause vomiting. Do not use in nursing pups or dogs < 2.5 kg. Occasional fatalities (collies, Airedales).
Thiabendazole (Omnizole)	D: 100–150 mg/kg × 3 da	—	—	—	—	95	May cause vomiting. Not approved for use.
Toluene & Dichlorophene (Vermiplex)	D: size capsule as directed by manufacturer	90	82	—	85 Dipylidium 72 Taenia	—	May cause vomiting. Overdose causes tremors and ataxia.

Adapted from Cornelius LM. Roberson EL: In Kirk RW (ed): Current Veterinary Therapy IX. Philadelphia, WB Saunders Company, 1986, pp 921–924.

tary indiscretions include overeating, ingestion of spoiled garbage or decomposing carrion, and ingestion of abrasive or indigestible foreign material such as bones, stones, hair, plants, wood, cloth, carpeting, foil, and plastic. Animals also may be intolerant of certain foods, such as lactose ingested as milk, fatty foods, spicy foods, and even food additives found in certain commercial diets. True food allergy as a cause of diarrhea in small animals is poorly documented,[95–97] and in most cases these intolerances probably represent idiosyncrasy or the effects of abrupt change in diet. Any change in the composition of the diet should be made in gradual increments over a period of several days to allow for adaptation, especially for a change from a cereal-based diet to a canned meat-based food.

Dietary causes of diarrhea are usually identified by careful history-taking and the response to a restricted diet. The owner should be carefully questioned about all aspects of diet and environment, including recent changes in type and brand of food, all supplemental feeding practices using people foods, patterns of chewing behavior involving nonfood items (including toys and haircoat), likelihood of garbage ingestion, and potential for unobserved indiscretions in free-roaming animals. Dietary diarrhea is self-limiting with feeding of a restricted diet, elimination of identifiable offending substances from the diet, and prevention of indiscriminate eating or chewing behavior.

Drug and Toxin-Induced Diarrhea

Diarrhea is frequently caused by medications and exogenous chemical toxins. Medications that frequently cause diarrhea as a side effect include insecticides used for flea control, nonsteroidal anti-inflammatory agents (aspirin, indomethacin, phenylbutazone, ibuprofen, flunixin meglumine, and numerous others), digitalis and many other cardiac drugs, dithiazanine (Diazan), magnesium-containing compounds, lactulose (used for hepatic encephalopathy), many of the antiparasitic drugs, most anticancer drugs, and many antibacterial drugs (due in part to adverse effects on normal gut flora). Hemorrhagic gastroenteritis, with erosion, ulceration, necrosis, and sometimes fatal colonic perforation, is an important complication in dogs with intervertebral disc disease treated with dexamethasone.[98, 99] Drug-induced diarrhea usually resolves after discontinuation of the offending medication or a reduction in its dosage. The reader is referred to Chapter 57 for a comprehensive discussion of adverse drug reactions in dogs and cats.

Many exogenous toxins cause diarrhea. These may be biologic toxins such as the enterotoxin that causes staphylococcal food poisoning, as well as various diarrheogenic chemical poisons, including heavy metals (lead, arsenic, thallium), insecticides (such as organophosphate dips and flea treatments), lawn and garden products (insecticides, herbicides, fungicides), and some house plants. In addition, a thirsty free-roaming animal may drink from stagnant or run-off water that may be polluted or potentially contaminated with any number of toxic industrial, auto, or farm chemicals. Most poisonings are accompanied by emesis, and sometimes even

dramatic extraintestinal signs; for example, the neurologic manifestations of lead or organophosphate toxicity. The reader is referred to Chapter 55 for a comprehensive discussion of toxicoses in dogs and cats.

Toxin-induced diarrhea is usually suspected on the basis of history of exposure (or opportunity for exposure), clinical signs, and exclusion of other causes of diarrhea. In most patients, the diarrhea resolves with symptomatic antidiarrheal therapy, prevention of further exposure to the toxin, and simply time for elimination of the substance from the body; however, if the exact toxin is known, other sources of information (Chapter 55) should be consulted for additional specific treatments and antidotes.

Parasitic Diarrhea

The common helminths and protozoa that parasitize the intestinal tract of the dog and cat and drugs used in their treatment are listed in Table 86–11. The most consistent clinical features of intestinal parasitism are diarrhea and weight loss, although the overwhelming majority of infections are asymptomatic. Young growing animals are generally more frequently and severely parasitized, but endoparasitism should never be overlooked as a possible cause of acute or chronic diarrhea of either the small or large bowel in dogs and cats of all ages. Other intestinal diseases, such as viral or bacterial enteritis, are often complicated by intestinal parasite infection.

The diagnosis of parasitism depends upon the identification of eggs, cysts, larvae, trophozoites, or proglottids in the feces (Figure 86–9). Methods may include (1) gross inspection of feces for tapeworm proglottids or adult ascarids, (2) conventional saline or sugar fecal flotation for parasite ova and cysts, (3) zinc sulfate centrifugation-flotation for cysts of *Giardia* and other protozoa, (4) fresh saline smears of feces for motile protozoan trophozoites, and (5) Baermann concentration technique for *Strongyloides* larvae. Since the appearance of parasite elements in feces can be intermittent, it is important to perform fecal examinations several times before an animal with diarrhea is regarded as free of intestinal parasites. Sometimes even then, occult infection cannot be ruled out. Parasites that are notorious for evading detection include *Giardia* in dogs and cats with small bowel diarrhea and whipworms in dogs with large bowel diarrhea. In such cases, therapeutic response using metronidazole for *Giardia* or an anthelmintic such as fenbendazole for whipworms may provide an indirect method of diagnosis.

Some basic differences between canine and feline intestinal parasite infections should be mentioned. Helminths are generally less of a clinical problem in the cat than in the dog, largely because the cat's fastidious habit of burying its feces reduces widespread environmental contamination with ova. In addition, prenatal ascarid infection, which is extremely commonplace in the dog, does not occur in the cat.[100] Feline hookworms are not voracious bloodsuckers and thus are not as injurious as canine hookworms.[101] Feline whipworms are rare and almost never cause clinical signs. A large bowel parasite

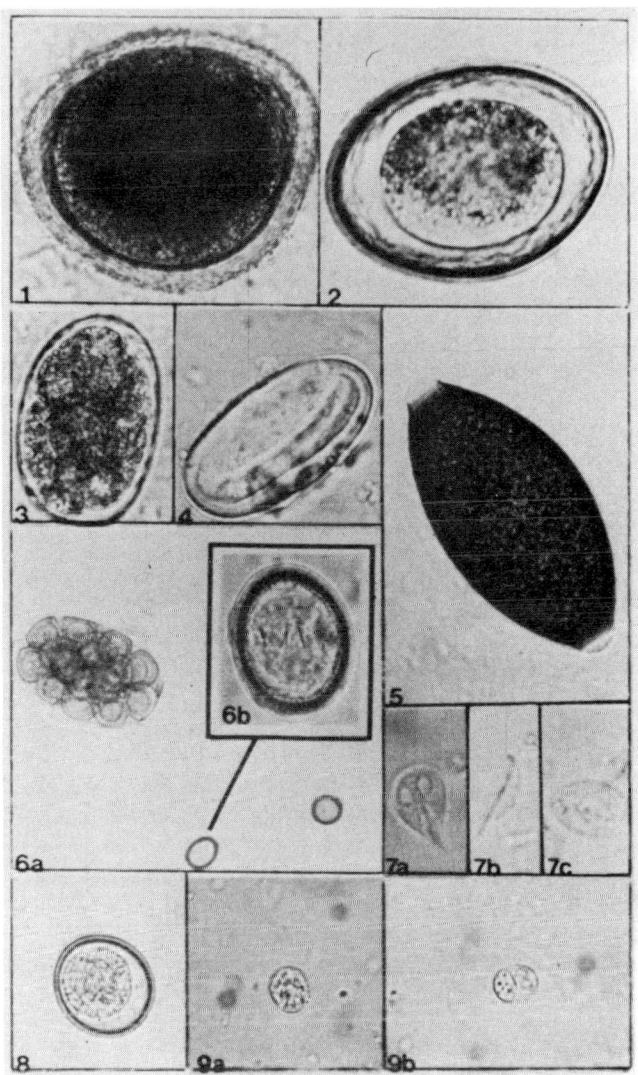

FIGURE 86–9. Composite of common parasite ova and cysts as identified by fecal examinations. Frame 1, egg of *Toxocara* spp. (×540). Frame 2, egg of *Toxascaris leonina* (×450). Frame 3, egg of *Ancylostoma* spp. or *Uncinaria stenocephala* (×560). Frame 4, egg of *Physaloptera* spp. (×610). Frame 5, egg of *Trichuris vulpis* (×480). Frame 6a, egg packet of *Dipylidium caninum* and two eggs of *Taenia* spp. (×160). Frame 6b, egg of *Taenia* spp. enlarged to show hook and striated egg shell (×720). Frame 7a, trophozoite form of *Giardia* spp. dorsal view (×1200). Frame 7b, trophozoite form of *Giardia* spp. lateral view (×1200). Frame 7c, cyst form of *Giardia* spp. (×1200). Frame 8, unsporulated oocyst of *Isospora* spp. from fresh feces (×670). Frame 9a, unsporulated oocyst of *Toxoplasma gondii* from fresh cat feces (×720). Frame 9b, sporulated oocyst of *Toxoplasma gondii* (×720). (From Hendrix CM, Blagburn BL: Common gastrointestinal parasites. Vet Clin North Am 13:627, 1983.)

of the cat, *Strongyloides tumefaciens*, causes chronic diarrhea associated with peculiar tumor-like nodular proliferations in the colonic mucosa.[102, 103] The cat is of tremendous public health concern with regard to the protozoal disease toxoplasmosis, insofar as the cat appears to be the primary host for *Toxoplasma gondii* and the only shedder of oocysts.[104]

ASCARIDS

Ascarid nematodes are the most prevalent parasites of dogs and cats worldwide. The ascarids of the dog are

Toxocara canis and the less common *Toxascaris leonina*, while those in the cat are *Toxocara cati* and *T. leonina*.[105–107]

Clinical signs of ascariasis are most often seen with heavy infections in young puppies and kittens, in which the adult worms in the small intestine may cause abdominal discomfort, whimpering and groaning, potbellied appearance, dull haircoat, unthriftiness, stunted growth, and diarrhea. Worms are frequently passed in vomitus or diarrhea (Figure 86–10). Occasionally, large tangled masses of worms occlude the lumen in young pups and cause death from intestinal obstruction, intussusception, or intestinal perforation (Figure 86–11). In the neonatal pup, the migration of large numbers of *T. canis* larvae through the lungs can cause severe damage and fatal pneumonia. In young animals with light infections and in adults, infection is most commonly asymptomatic, or merely evidenced by loss of body condition.

Ascarid infection occurs by four routes: (1) prenatal infection as a result of transplacental migration, which occurs only with *T. canis;* (2) milk-borne infection as a result of transmammary migration, which occurs with both *T. canis* and *T. cati;* (3) infection by ingestion of infective eggs, which occurs with all three ascarids, *T. canis, T. cati, T. leonina;* and (4) infection by ingestion of a paratenic (transport) host (*T. canis, T. cati*) or intermediate host (*T. leonina*). In addition, there are three types of migration patterns that occur once an animal is infected: liver-lung migration (*T. canis, T. cati*), migration within the wall of the GI tract (all three ascarids), and somatic tissue migration (*T. canis, T. cati*).

Since *T. canis* is the most common intestinal parasite in small animals, and since it may be transmitted by all four routes, its life cycle will be discussed in detail. It appears that the neonatal pup (less than five weeks) and the whelping bitch lack resistance to *T. canis*. In North America, virtually 100 per cent of pups are infected with *T. canis:* most are born infected because of transplacental migration of the bitch's somatic larvae into the fetus (prenatal infection). The prenatally infected pup is born with the third-stage larvae (L3) of *T. canis* within its lungs. These L3 are coughed up, swallowed, and then develop into mature egg-producing adult worms in the small intestine within three weeks after birth. Many pups, therefore, begin passing large numbers of eggs in their feces at about three weeks of age and continue to shed eggs (see Figure 86–9) for most of early puppyhood (four to six months) if untreated. Neonatal puppies may also become infected with L3 contained in the dam's milk for the first month of lactation. These larvae develop to adults in the gut without going through a migrating phase.

Dogs of all ages may be infected by the ingestion of embryonated (infective) eggs from their environment, mainly from the soil. In pups less than five weeks old, this results in liver-lung migration followed by intestinal ascarid infection. In older dogs, however, there is an age-related resistance that causes instead a somatic migration and subsequent arrest of *T. canis* larvae (L3) in somatic tissues such as muscles, kidneys, eyes, and brain. It is these larvae arrested in somatic tissues that are reactivated at about 42 days of gestation in the

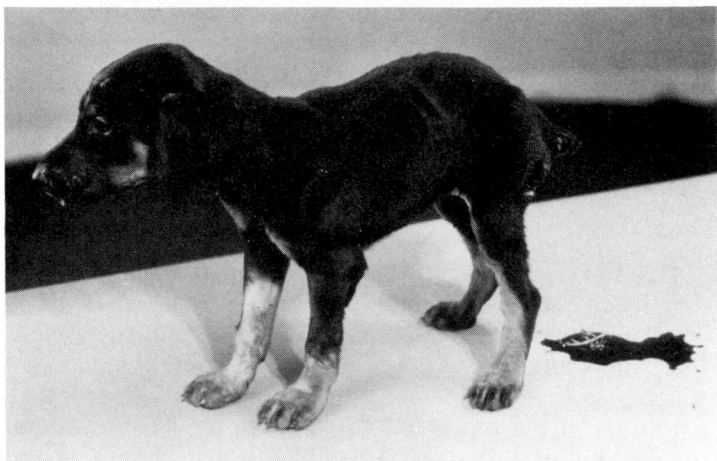

FIGURE 86–10. A parasitized puppy passing ascarids in diarrheic feces.

pregnant bitch; they then migrate to the placenta or mammary gland to produce prenatal or milk-borne infection of the pup.

In contrast to *T. canis* in pups, prenatal infection is not known to occur with *T. cati* in cats. The other routes of infection do occur in the cat, however. The ingestion of paratenic hosts (mice, birds, and insects) is not a very important source of infection of *T. canis* in the dog, although it occurs; in the adult cat, however, this route is a major source of *T. cati* infection. Infection of *T. cati* in the cat is followed by all three forms of migration; liver-lung migration and migration within the wall of the GI tract result in adult worms in the small intestine, while somatic migration, similar to that for *T. canis*, may culminate in milk-borne (but not transplacental) infection of nursing kittens. This is the major source of ascariasis in kittens.

T. leonina infection in dogs and cats is less common than *T. canis* or *T. cati*. Infection occurs by ingestion of embryonated eggs or an intermediate host such as the mouse. Migration is confined to the intestinal wall.

Numerous effective anthelmintics of adult ascarids are available (see Table 86–11). Since most pups are born

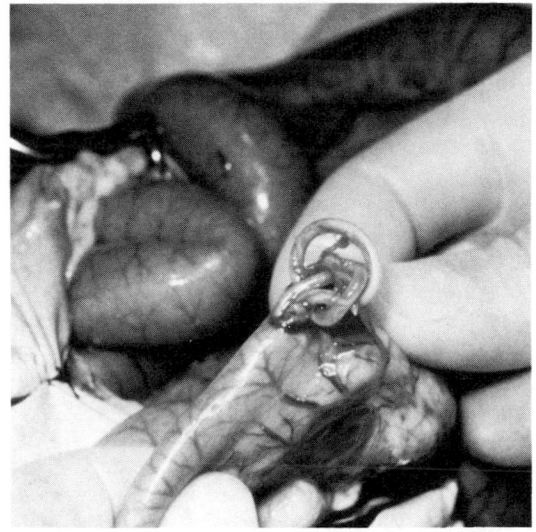

FIGURE 86–11. This tangled mass of ascarids protruding from an enterotomy incision was associated with an intussusception.

infected with *T. canis*, it is recommended that treatment be started at two weeks of age, before eggs are first passed in the feces, and then continued at four, six, and eight weeks to kill all worms derived from prenatal infection, milk-borne infection, and ingestion of infective ova. Pyrantel pamoate has been convenient for this purpose because it is well-tolerated in puppies and also effective in controlling hookworms. Treatment of the nursing bitch should also be part of the roundworm control program.

Because of activation and transplacental or transmammary migration of somatic larvae during gestation, treatment of the pregnant or nursing bitch should be another consideration in the overall roundworm control program. Extended fenbendazole therapy has been used experimentally at 22 mg/lb q12h for 14 days to reduce the number of larvae in somatic tissues.[108] In another study, fenbendazole at 22 mg/lb/day given to bitches from the 40th day of gestation through the 14th day of lactation was highly effective for reducing perinatal roundworm and hookworm burdens in pups.[109] Although these regimens were apparently safe and effective, they are probably too expensive for routine use.

Because of toxocaral visceral larva migrans (VLM), a serious disease of humans (especially children) produced by the invasion of visceral tissues by migrating *T. canis*, *T. canis*–infected pups are considered public health hazards.[106] Human fatalities from VLM have been reported. In addition to the prevalence of prenatal *T. canis* infection in pups, two other features of the parasite increase its potential as a public health problem. First, *T. canis* is a prolific egg layer; each adult female worm may shed 200,000 ova per day. Second, once these eggs embryonate in three to four weeks and become infective for dogs or humans, their resistance to inactivation enables them to remain viable in the soil for months or years.

HOOKWORMS

The most common hookworm in the dog is *Ancylostoma caninum*, a voracious bloodsucker.[101, 107, 110, 111] The common hookworm in the cat, *Ancylostoma tubaeforme*, is more of a tissue feeder than a bloodsucker and is far less pathogenic than *A. caninum* in dogs. Two other less common hookworms, *Ancylostoma braziliense* and *Un-*

cinaria stenocephala, occur in both dogs and cats and are only mildly pathogenic, because they are not as hematophagous. *A. braziliense* is most prevalent in the southern United States and in tropical or subtropical regions, whereas *U. stenocephala* is a "cold weather" hookworm and is most prevalent in Canada.[110]

The pathogenicity of the hookworm is directly related to its bloodsucking activity and capacity for causing intestinal blood loss.[112, 113] Hookworms "graze" along the intestinal mucosa, embedding their mouthparts into the mucosa, sucking blood and tissue fluid, and leaving bleeding ulcers as they go.[114] The most pathogenic hookworm, *A. caninum*, may cause a daily blood loss per adult worm of 0.01 to 0.2 ml; by comparison, daily blood loss from *A. braziliense* (0.001 ml per adult) or *U. stenocephala* (0.0003 ml per adult) is relatively insignificant. The severity of this blood loss peaks at 10 to 15 days after infection as adult worms mature, and hemorrhage may be accentuated by anticoagulant compounds produced by the hookworms.[115] Hence, an important consequence of severe *A. caninum* infection is blood loss anemia.

The clinical signs of ancylostomiasis in the dog include tarry (melena) or bloody diarrhea accompanied by pallor, weakness, emaciation, and dehydration. In heavily infected young pups, severe acute GI hemorrhage and rapidly progressive blood loss anemia may result in death. In others, chronic blood loss from chronic infection eventually causes iron deficiency anemia, and erythrocytes show hypochromasia and microcytosis.[110] One study has shown impaired intestinal absorption of fat, carbohydrate, and amino acids in dogs with severe ancylostomiasis.[116] Infections with the other species of hookworm, and light *A. caninum* infections, especially in partially resistant older dogs, are often asymptomatic.

Hookworm infection can occur by five routes: prenatal, milk-borne, ingestion of infective larvae (L3), skin penetration by infective larvae, and ingestion of paratenic hosts.[110] It is thought that ingestion of larvae and active penetration of the skin by larvae are the most common routes of infection, and in contrast to *T. canis*, *A. caninum* infects neonatal pups more frequently by the milk-borne route than prenatally. Oral ingestion (including milk-borne ingestion) is followed mainly by direct development in the intestine, while larvae penetrating the skin migrate by somatic or circulatory transport to the lung before reaching the intestine. Prenatal or milk-borne infection occurs in pups from bitches that have migrating somatic larvae from past infection. With all routes of infection, eggs are passed in feces after two or three weeks. The strongyloid-type hookworm eggs (see Figure 86–9) rapidly hatch into infectious free-living larvae that survive well for three to four months in warm, moist environments but are killed by drying, direct sunlight, or cold winter conditions. Acute pruritic dermatitis is occasionally associated with the active penetration of skin by hookworm larvae.

Anthelmintics effective against both hookworms and ascarids include pyrantel pamoate (safest in young pups), dichlorvos, mebendazole, and fenbendazole.[107] Thenium, disophenol, and butamisole are hookworm-specific (see Table 86–11).[107] Severely anemic animals should also receive whole blood transfusions, iron supplementation, and supportive therapy. In areas where *A. caninum* is a frequent problem, bitches and puppies should be routinely treated. Because of prenatal and milk-borne infection, treatment of pups can be started at two weeks of age, along with treatment for *T. canis*. Pyrantel pamoate suspension is an excellent choice for nursing pups because it is well tolerated and active against both hookworms and ascarids. Parasite control is aided by good sanitation and impervious flooring in kennels and dog runs. Styrylpyridinium chloride (Styrid-Caricide) or oxibendazole (Filaribits Plus) have been combined with daily heartworm preventative (diethylcarbamazine) to aid control of hookworm infection.

WHIPWORMS

Trichuris vulpis is the whipworm of dogs and *Trichuris campanula* is the whipworm of cats. Infection occurs by ingestion of infective eggs and the life cycle is direct. *Trichuris vulpis* is commonly found attached to the cecum and colon of dogs of all ages and has a distinctive thread-like head end (or "whip"), which firmly embeds deep within the mucosa to feed on blood and tissue fluids.[117, 118] In many animals, there are minimal clinical signs, but whipworms are a frequent cause of colitis and typhlitis characterized by chronic or intermittent mucoid, large bowel-type diarrhea with urgency, tenesmus, and sometimes hematochezia. Therefore, since they are primarily large bowel parasites, whipworms are discussed in Chapter 87. Whipworm infections in cats are considered to be very rare and usually not associated with any clinical signs.[119]

STRONGYLOIDES

Strongyloides stercoralis is a tiny (two mm) rhabditoid nematode that burrows in the mucosa of the proximal small bowel, causing mucosal destruction and hemorrhagic diarrhea.[120, 121] Strongyloidiasis is mainly a problem in puppies in warm, humid tropical regions, and fatalities are common. Infection of dogs with third-stage larvae is by the oral or cutaneous route, and adult worms develop in the small intestine following migration in the circulation and lung. Verminous pneumonia may result from migration. Parthenogenetic female adults produce eggs that hatch within the gut lumen, so that first-stage (rhabdoid) larvae are passed in the feces. These larvae may develop either into infectious third-stage (filariform) larvae or into free-living adults. Another *Strongyloides*, *S. tumefaciens*, sometimes parasitizes the large intestine of cats in the southern United States. It is usually an asymptomatic infection but may cause mucosal and submucosal nodular lesions in the colon with signs of chronic diarrhea and debilitation.[102, 103]

The diagnosis of strongyloidiasis depends on finding motile first-stage larvae, 0.8 to 1.6 mm long and 30 to 80 μ wide, in fresh feces, preferably using a Baermann procedure. *Strongyloides* infection has also been associated with shedding of both larvae and unusually large ova in fresh feces.[122] *S. stercoralis* larvae must be distinguished from larvae of *Filaroides* spp., or in old fecal samples from hookworm larvae that have hatched from ova in the feces.

The treatment for *Strongyloides* spp. is a five-day course of fenbendazole (22 mg/lb/day).

TAPEWORMS

Tapeworms (cestodes) that parasitize the small bowel of dogs and cats are relatively harmless, rarely causing more than a subtle decline in body condition. The most common tapeworm is *Dipylidium caninum*.[107] Fleas and lice are intermediate hosts. The proglottids of *D. caninum* are highly motile and may cause anal pruritus as they crawl on the perineum, and crawling proglottids are often detected in the stool or on the perineum by observant owners. Several species of *Taenia* can be acquired by dogs and cats (most commonly *T. pisiformis* in the dog, *T. taeniaformis* in the cat) from ingestion of cysticerci-infected tissues from intermediate hosts, e.g., rabbits, rodents, sheep, and ungulates. *D. caninum* proglottids are distinguished from *Taenia* by their barrel shape and double genital pore. Also, a proglottid can be squashed in a drop of water between a slide and coverslip to find the characteristic *D. caninum* egg capsules that contain up to 20 eggs (see Figure 86–9). Other cestode infections that rarely occur include *Echinococcus* spp., *Multiceps* spp., *Mesocestoides* spp., and *Spirometra* spp. Praziquantel and bunamidine HCl are the most effective all-round drugs for cestodiasis, although others are available (see Table 86–11). Flea and lice control are important for preventing *D. caninum* reinfection, while control of predation and scavenging help prevent infection with other cestodes.

OTHER METAZOAN PARASITES

Transient hemorrhagic enteritis with bloody diarrhea was observed in a cat with trichinosis.[123] Numerous adult *Trichinella spiralis* nematodes (1.5 to 4.0 mm) were found in the sediment of a centrifuged fecal suspension, and migrating larvae (100 μ) were identified in the blood with a modified Knott's test. The illness was self-limiting without treatment, but eosinophilia persisted for three months. The source of infection was undetermined, but predation of an infected rodent was considered most likely.

Trematodes occasionally parasitize the small intestine but usually without causing clinical signs.[101] The intestinal fluke *Nanophyetus salmincola* is endemic to the Pacific Northwest and acquired from eating raw fish. The fluke itself is unimportant; however, it is the vector of the fatal rickettsial disease of dogs called salmon poisoning. Asymptomatic infection of the jejunum of a dog by the fluke *Alaria arisaemoides* (alariasis) has been reported.[124]

Parasitic schistosomiasis caused by *Heterobilharzia americana* in dogs is characterized by extensive schistosome egg deposition in the intestinal wall and liver, accompanied by granulomatous inflammation.[125, 126] One dog with chronic bloody-mucoid diarrhea, weight loss, and hypercalcemia associated with intestinal *H. americana* infection responded to treatment with praziquantel and fenbendazole.[126]

The intestinal thorny-headed worm *Macracanthorhynchus ingens* was responsible for episodic bloody diarrhea in a kennel of Doberman puppies in New Jersey.[127] Millipedes are the intermediate hosts for this parasite and the usual definitive hosts are wild animals, especially raccoons. Large white adult worms as well as distinctive football-shaped eggs were recovered from the feces of affected dogs over a period of several months, but infection resolved without treatment.[127]

COCCIDIA

Canine and feline intestinal coccidia are protozoan parasites that belong to six genera: *Isospora*, *Besnoitia*, *Hammondia*, *Sarcocystis*, *Toxoplasma*, and *Cryptosporidium*. Most enteric coccidia infections of dogs and cats are commensal and nonpathogenic. Since primary enteric disease in small animals has only been described with *Isospora* and *Cryptosporidium*, the following discussion will be limited to infections caused by these two genera.[128, 129] In addition, *Toxoplasma gondii*, a coccidia that causes multisystemic infection, is discussed in Chapter 46.

Isospora. *Isospora* (also called *Cystoisospora*) species of coccidia that infect dogs are *I. canis*, *I. ohioensis*, *I. burrowsi*, and *I. neorivolta*, while *I. felis* and *I. rivolta* infect cats. Infection can occur either by ingestion of infective (sporulated) oocysts from a contaminated environment or occasionally from ingestion of infective cyst-containing tissues of a paratenic or transport host. Although the direct form of transmission is most common, many mammals can serve as paratenic hosts, including rodents and other prey, and uncooked meat from herbivores.

Many young pups and kittens are asymptomatically infected and diagnosed by the massive shedding of unsporulated oocysts in their feces. When clinical disease occasionally does occur, it is usually related to massive oocyst ingestion in newborn animals and associated with overcrowded, unsanitary, high-stress conditions in settings such as pet shops, kennels, pounds, catteries, and laboratory colonies. Concurrent disease, malnutrition, and immunosuppression are predisposing factors. Thus, coccidia are opportunists. The principal clinical sign of coccidiosis is diarrhea that varies from soft to fluid and is occasionally mucoid or bloody. Other signs include vomiting, lethargy, weight loss, and dehydration. *Isospora* spp. have occasionally been associated with chronic malabsorption,[129] and one isolate of *I. ohioensis* was shown to cause intestinal mucosal lesions of epithelial necrosis and villous atrophy in dogs.[130, 131]

The diagnosis is made by identification of oocysts in fresh feces (see Figure 86–9). Since many normal dogs and cats harbor intestinal coccidia and these protozoa are generally regarded as minimally pathogenic, the clinical significance of finding coccidial oocysts is often questionable, and treatment may be unnecessary. Even in animals with diarrhea, oocysts are usually incidental findings and other causes for the diarrhea should be sought.

Identification of oocysts in a healthy animal with normal feces indicates a self-limiting commensal infection and does not necessarily even warrant treatment, although treatment may help to reduce environmental contamination with oocysts. If clinical signs are attributed to coccidiosis, such as in neonates under six weeks of age with diarrhea, effective coccidiostats should be used for treatment: intestinal sulfas (usually at 22 to 26 mg/lb/day orally for one to three weeks), nitrofurazone 4 to 9 mg/lb/day orally for one week), and amprolium. Amprolium is unapproved for use in dogs but is often recommended for treating kennel animals or other groups of dogs.[101, 129] It is given orally as 20 per cent powder in gelatin capsules at a total dose of 100 mg once daily for small-breed pups or 200 mg daily for larger-breed pups, for 7 to 12 days. Another approach is to mix one-fourth teaspoon 20 per cent powder per four pups with the puppy ration or to add 1.5 to 2 tablespoons of 96 per cent amprolium solution per gallon of free-choice water.

Cryptosporidia. Cryptosporidia are very small coccidia that have occasionally been associated with chronic diarrhea in cats,[132, 133] and acute diarrhea in neonatal puppies.[134–136] Diarrheic calves and lambs are considered the primary reservoir for this parasite, and since cryptosporidia are not very host-specific, they also infect humans, sometimes fatally in the presence of severe immunosuppression.[137] As with the other coccidia, infection is often incidental and subclinical in dogs and cats,[136, 138, 139] although isolates of *Cryptosporidium* differ markedly in their virulence.[140] These coccidia can complicate other infectious diseases that are immunosuppressive, such as feline leukemia virus,[129, 133] and canine distemper.[135]

Profuse watery diarrhea, the most consistent clinical sign of cryptosporidiosis, has been attributed to malabsorption caused by villous atrophy.[140] Mesenteric lymphadenopathy may also be a feature of the disease.[132]

Cryptosporidia oocysts are so small (as little as one-tenth the size of common *Isospora* oocysts) that they can be very difficult to diagnose by fecal examinations. Oocysts can be isolated for identification using Sheather's sugar flotation (with brightfield or phase-contrast microscopy), Kinyouin's carbol fuchsin negative staining, or modified acid fast staining.[140] Careful examination of slides under oil immersion is necessary to visualize the tiny oocysts. Histologic or electron microscopy identification of the organisms in intestinal biopsies is also an appropriate means of diagnosis.[132, 133]

Cryptosporidiosis is self-limiting in immunocompetent hosts, but in the severely immunocompromised animal or human, the infection has a poor prognosis. Spiramycin or quinine and clindamycin have been used to treat humans, but their use in dogs or cats with cryptosporidia infection has not been reported.

GIARDIA

Giardia spp. are pear-shaped, binucleated, flagellated protozoa that infect the proximal small intestine, where they may interfere with mucosal absorption and produce diarrhea.[141–146] *Giardia* has two forms, the trophozoite and the cyst (see Figure 86–9). Motile trophozoites attach to the brush border surface of the mucosal epithelium by means of ventral cup-shaped suction disks or float free within the adjacent mucus layer.[142] They

are mainly found in the duodenum in the dog and in the jejunum and ileum in the cat.[146] Trophozoites can be seen in diarrheic feces but not usually in formed stool. The infective stage, the nonmotile cyst, is usually found in formed feces and is thought to be an encysted trophozoite that has transformed into a cyst during transit through the terminal small bowel and colon.[143] The life of *Giardia* is direct and the usual source of infection is the ingestion of food or water contaminated with cysts.[142, 143] Since wild animals are potential reservoirs, drinking from contaminated streams and ponds may be a source of infection.

Giardia has a worldwide distribution, and although prevalence rates vary widely, in part because of differences in detection methods, the prevalence in most populations has been at least 5 per cent.[142, 143, 146] At the Colorado State University Teaching Hospital, 10.5 per cent of 1785 fecal examinations were positive, and in a sampling of the same population examined by duodenal aspiration, the infection rate was considerably higher.[37] The prevalence may be greatest in young animals and animals confined together in groups. For example, in a cattery experiencing episodic diarrhea problems, 50 per cent of 14 cats were infected with *Giardia*[145] and 68 per cent of 37 clinically normal dogs from an Ohio animal shelter[147] and 86 per cent of 78 dogs in a private kennel[148] were found to be excreting *Giardia*.

The majority of *Giardia* infections are thought to be subclinical, especially in mature animals. This is supported by numerous prevalence surveys that have found that the majority of animals from which *Giardia* are isolated are clinically normal[142, 143, 149] and by the failure of experimental *Giardia* infection in dogs and cats to consistently produce clinical signs.[144, 147] Clinically apparent giardiasis occurs most frequently in young dogs and cats and is characterized by intestinal malabsorption with large volumes of foul-smelling, light-colored, watery or cow patty–like diarrhea, steatorrhea, and weight loss.[37, 141, 146, 150] Diarrhea, the most prominent sign, may be acute or chronic, intermittent or continuous, and self-limiting or persistent. Some animals are presented for a sudden onset of explosive watery diarrhea with depression and anorexia, which may mimic acute enteritides such as viral enteritis. One author has observed an onset of diarrhea that coincides with parturition in bitches that harbor *Giardia*.[37]

The pathogenesis of diarrhea and clinical illness due to *Giardia* probably results from the complex interplay of several mechanisms, which is emphasized by the lack of correlation between the severity of illness, morphologic mucosal damage (if any), and number of protozoa present. Malabsorption induced by trophozoites appears to play an important role, and mechanical, toxic, biochemical, and immunologic mechanisms of mucosal injury may be involved.[142, 143, 146, 151] Impaired absorption of carbohydrate (xylose, lactose), fat, folate, vitamin A, and vitamin B_{12} has been demonstrated in humans.[152] The severity of *Giardia* infection is possibly enhanced by concomitant viral, bacterial, or parasitic infection. Puppies and kittens with giardiasis are frequently coinfected with helminths or other protozoa.[153] Immune deficiency states and malnutrition predispose to giardiasis in humans.[151, 152]

The diagnosis of *Giardia* (see Figure 86–9) depends upon identification of cysts (oval; 8 to 12 μm × 7 to 10 μm) or flagellated trophozoites (pear-shaped; 9 to 21 μm × 5 to 15 μm × 2 to 4 μm) and should be considered in any dog or cat with unexplained diarrhea or malabsorption, especially when several animals confined together are affected.[143, 148] *Giardia* cysts stain well with Lugol's two per cent iodine, and the most reliable method for recovery of cysts from feces is by zinc sulfate centrifugation-flotation.[143, 148] Motile trophozoites can be identified in fresh diarrheic feces suspended in saline, although they are found in feces less consistently than cysts.[148] Since excretion of cysts and trophozoites is intermittent, multiple fecal specimens should be examined, preferably a minimum of three on consecutive or alternate days.[144, 148] The presence of *Giardia* may be temporarily masked for about a week by barium, certain antibiotics, antacids, antidiarrheals, laxatives, and enemas.[143]

Negative fecal examinations do not exclude a diagnosis of giardiasis. Thus, if protozoa cannot be demonstrated by repeated fecal examinations, then another approach is to identify trophozoites in duodenal aspirates, brushings, mucosal impression smears, or biopsies obtained via endoscopy or laparotomy.[37, 150] Duodenal aspirates appear to be significantly more reliable than fecal examinations for the detection of *Giardia* in dogs[37] but, of course, have the disadvantage of being difficult to obtain. In situations in which fecal examinations are negative, endoscopy is not available for procurement of duodenal samples, and laparotomy is not otherwise contemplated, "occult" giardiasis may be diagnosed indirectly by the response to a therapeutic trial of an antigiardial drug.

Three drugs currently available in the United States are considered to be effective in the treatment of *Giardia*—metronidazole (Flagyl), quinacrine HCl (Atabrine), and furazolidone (Furoxone). Metronidazole at 12 to 14 mg/lb orally q12h for 5 to 10 days is usually effective with minimal side effects, although up to one-third of infections may be metronidazole-resistant.[153] Furazolidone at 2 mg/lb orally q12h for five days is both effective and convenient in cats because it is available in a suspension form.[145] Quinacrine at 3 mg/lb q12h orally for five days was highly effective in treating canine giardiasis but was associated with a high incidence of side effects (anorexia, lethargy, vomiting, fever).[153] An experimental drug that is not yet currently available, tinidazole, appears to be highly effective in humans after just a single oral dose but was comparable to metronidazole in one study that compared treatments of giardiasis in dogs.[153] Some dogs and cats require a longer course of therapy than is generally recommended, and others must have treatment repeated when initial treatment fails to eliminate the infection completely. Repeat exposure can cause recurrence of infection, and in groups of animals confined together, giardiasis can be a troublesome enzootic problem.[145, 148, 153]

PENTATRICHOMONAS

Pentatrichomonas hominas are motile, pear-shaped, flagellated protozoa that inhabit the large intestine of dogs and cats, and have been found in both normal and diarrheic feces.[36, 154–159] The pathogenicity of these protozoa in small animals has not been conclusively established, but massive numbers of trichomonads are sometimes found in diarrheic feces of pups and kittens, especially associated with overcrowded, unsanitary housing conditions and coinfections with other parasites.

The diagnosis of trichomoniasis is established by identification in saline fecal smears of motile, pear-shaped flagellated trophozoites with characteristic wavelike motion of an undulating membrane and a constant, erratic turning and rolling motion. Feces for detecting trichomonads should be taken directly from the rectum or examined within minutes of defecation while trophozoites are still motile. Trichomonads lack a cyst stage. Pentatrichomonads can be effectively eliminated with a five day course of metronidazole (12 to 14 mg/lb, q12h) or a three day course of tinidazole (20 mg/lb, q24h).[153] In addition, concurrent infection with other parasites or enteropathogens should be searched for and treated.

OTHER PROTOZOA

Amebiasis, caused by *Entamoeba histolytica*, and balantidiasis, caused by *Balantidium coli*, are characterized by bloody mucoid diarrhea (colitis). Both diseases are diagnosed by identification of the protozoa in fresh saline fecal smears and are treated with metronidazole. Because these are primarily large bowel pathogens, the details are discussed in Chapter 87.

Viral Diarrhea

During the last two decades, numerous viruses have been discovered in canine and feline feces by either virus isolation or electron microscopy.

In the dog, these viruses include the "minute virus" isolated from normal dogs (now known to be a parvovirus that is distinct from the enteritis-producing parvovirus), canine coronavirus, canine parvovirus (cause of parvoviral enteritis), canine rotavirus, astrovirus, paramyxo-like virus, adenovirus, and picornavirus.[160–165] In addition, human ECHO and coxsackieviruses have been isolated from canine feces.[166, 167] Some of these are found with equal frequency in normal feces and feces from animals with diarrhea and as yet have not been established as enteropathogens.[168, 169] Coronavirus, parvovirus, and rotavirus have been established as causes of viral enteritis and diarrhea in the dog. Canine distemper virus can also cause diarrhea.

In the cat, the most clinically important primary enteric virus is the parvovirus, feline panleukopenia virus (FPV). Diarrhea in the cat has also been attributed to enteric coronavirus, rotavirus, and astrovirus.[170–174] In addition to these, other viruses of uncertain importance as enteric pathogens that were found by electron microscopic screening of 185 feline fecal samples includes calicivirus, reovirus Type III, and noncultivable enteric picornaviridae-like virus.[174] Also in the cat, the intestine may be involved as part of generalized viral infection due to feline leukemia virus (FeLV), feline immunodeficiency virus (FIV), or feline infectious peritonitis (FIP)

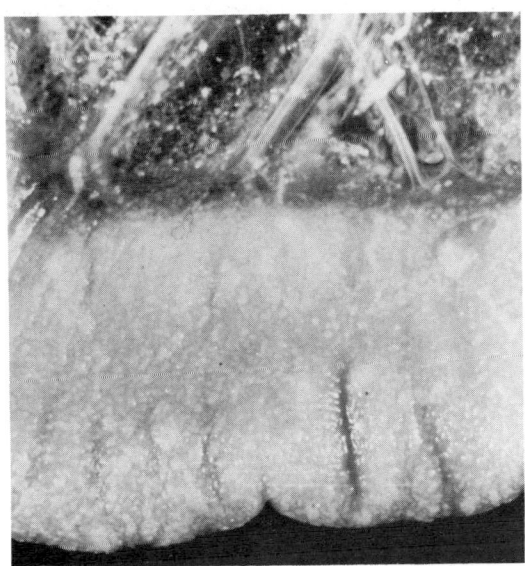

FIGURE 86–12. Pyogranulomatous serositis and enteritis in a kitten with feline infectious peritonitis (FIP). Notice the granular fibrinous deposits on the serosa and mesentery.

coronavirus. A panleukopenia-like syndrome characterized by severe enterocolitis has been associated with FeLV infection.[175] In FIP, pyogranulomatous enteritis or serositis may occur (Figure 86–12). Canine and feline viral diseases are discussed in detail in Chapters 47 and 48; however, pertinent aspects of those with primary intestinal involvement will be briefly described here.

CANINE PARVOVIRUS

Canine parvovirus (CPV) infection is an acute, highly contagious enteritis of dogs that has been prevalent worldwide since the late 1970s.[162, 176] The virus has an affinity for the rapidly dividing cells of the intestine, bone marrow, and lymph tissues, and thus causes intestinal crypt necrosis, severe diarrhea, leukopenia and lymphoid depletion.[162, 165, 176–179] Parvovirus infection occurs by the feco-oral route, and, because the virus can survive for long periods in the environment, fomites and environmental contamination play a major role in transmission. Signs of enteric disease usually occur five days after experimental inoculation of CPV, coincident with localization of virus in the mitotically active zones of intestinal crypt epithelia.[180, 181] The severity of intestinal disease is correlated with the magnitude and duration of viremia.[182]

Dogs of any age can be infected, but the incidence of clinical disease is highest in puppies between 6 and 20 weeks of age.[176] Puppies younger than six weeks are generally protected by passive maternal immunity, while most mature animals have either been immunized or fail to show clinical signs if they become infected. In susceptible populations, most adult animals seroconvert without manifesting signs, indicating that mild or inapparent infection is common, while enteritis may spread rapidly through the younger animals.

Clinical Signs. Clinical signs include anorexia, depression, and vomiting (which are often noticed first); intractable fluid diarrhea that may be profuse and hem-

orrhagic; and rapidly progressive dehydration. Most dogs with CPV are febrile. Hypothermia, icterus, or hemorrhagic diathesis (DIC) may develop terminally in those with endotoxic shock. The severity of clinical illness may be increased by factors such as stress, crowded or unsanitary conditions, secondary bacterial infection, and concurrent diseases such as canine distemper, salmonellosis, campylobacteriosis, and parasitism. Death may occur in severe cases, particularly in very young puppies, and is usually attributable to dehydration, electrolyte imbalances, endotoxic shock, or overwhelming bacterial infection associated with the leukopenia. Mild or inapparent infections that result in seroconversion are probably common.

Diagnosis. Parvovirus infection should be suspected in dogs that have an abrupt onset of vomiting and diarrhea along with supportive clinical findings such as young age (peak incidence at 6 to 20 weeks of age), exposure history, severity of clinical signs (especially extreme depression, intractable vomiting, hematochezia, fever), and hematologic abnormalities.[176] Prior vaccination does not necessarily exclude the possibility of parvoviral infection.

A hemogram is particularly useful and should be routine in any dog with acute gastroenteritis, especially when accompanied by fever or hematochezia. During the first 72 hours of clinical signs, approximately 85 per cent of dogs with parvoviral enteritis develop severe leukopenia due to lymphopenia and granulocytopenia, often with a total of 500 to 2000 WBC/μl, or even less.[183, 184] Depletion of circulating mature neutrophils is caused by extensive loss of neutrophils through the damaged intestinal wall.[180] The severity of the leukopenia may be proportional to the severity of the clinical illness,[180] and a rebound in the WBC is a useful indicator of impending recovery. The hematocrit is usually normal or slightly decreased, which helps to clinically differentiate this disease from hemorrhagic gastroenteritis (HGE), in which profound hemoconcentration usually causes a markedly elevated hematocrit.

In addition to HGE, parvoviral enteritis must be differentiated from other viral enteritides, salmonellosis, and small intestinal obstruction (e.g., GI foreign body, intussusception). Gas and fluid distention of the gut are frequent radiographic findings in parvoviral enteritis and may mimic intestinal obstruction.[185]

Definitive diagnosis of parvoviral enteritis requires either demonstration of active excretion of virus in the feces or specific IgM analysis as serologic evidence of recent infection.[186] Since the results of these often take one or more days to obtain, the diagnosis is usually made retrospectively after nonspecific treatment measures appropriate for acute enteritis of any cause have already been initiated.

Fecal tests for viral excretion are based on the fact that during the acute illness dogs shed massive quantities of virus in their feces.[186] The fecal hemagglutination (HA) test, based on the distinctive hemagglutinating properties of parvovirus, determines the highest dilution (titer) of patient feces that agglutinates monkey or porcine erythrocytes as a measure of the level of virus in the fecal specimen (see Figure 86–13).[186, 187] Fecal specimens (20 to 30 gm) can be refrigerated and sent to

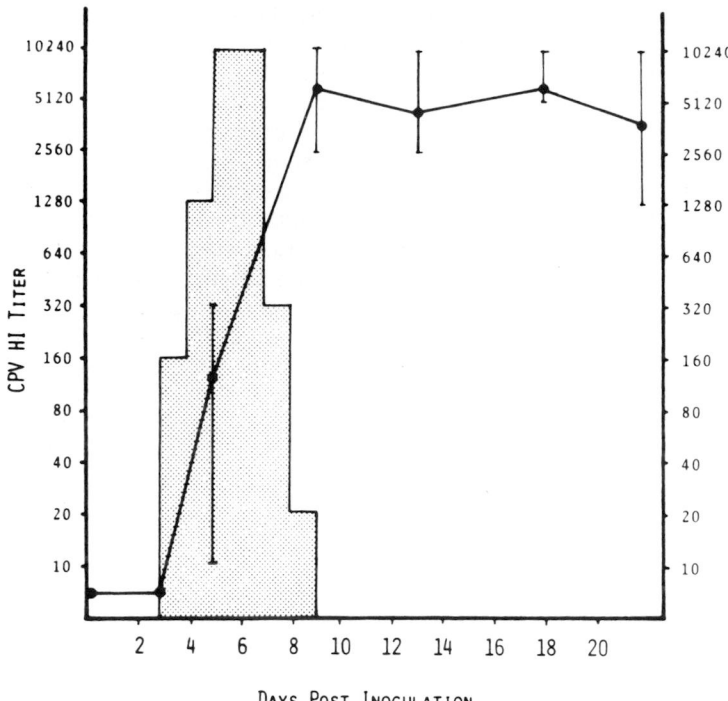

FIGURE 86–13. The CPV HI antibody and fecal HA responses after oral infection with CPV. Shaded portion represents the period of fecal viral shedding as measured by fecal HA test (right axis), while the solid line represents the mean HI antibody titer (left axis). (From Carmichael, LE, et al.: Hemagglutination by canine parvovirus: Serologic studies and diagnostic applications. Am J Vet Res 41:784–791, 1980.)

a commercial diagnostic laboratory for HA analysis. A titer of greater than 1:64 is generally considered diagnostic, although false-positive low titers sometimes occur. Fecal titers can also be determined using ELISA methodology.[188] Electron microscopy and virus isolation to demonstrate fecal excretion of parvovirus are not practical for routine clinical use.

Serologic determination of an anti-CPV antibody titer (by hemagglutination-inhibition, virus neutralization, and other methods) is not sufficient for diagnosis since an estimated 75 to 95 per cent of dogs in the population have seroconverted from prior vaccination or exposure. However, demonstration that an anti-CPV antibody titer consists of predominantly IgM (by indirect immunofluorescent antibody test or a 2-mercaptoethanol procedure) indicates recent infection, because IgM is only found in the first few weeks after infection.[176]

Necropsy diagnosis of parvovirus is based on detection of the characteristic histopathologic lesion of necrosis of the rapidly proliferating intestinal crypt cells with secondary villous collapse and dilatation of the crypts with necrotic debris. Myeloid degeneration and widespread lymphoid depletion are also seen. Parvovirus can be demonstrated in frozen tissue samples by fluorescent antibody methods.[182]

Treatment. Since the treatment of parvovirus is mainly supportive and similar to what would be used in most animals with severe gastroenteritis, therapy should be instituted whether or not definitive tests are done or while the return of results is being awaited.

The cornerstone of treatment is rehydration. In most cases, intravenous fluid and electrolyte replacement is preferred, and lactated Ringer's solution supplemented with potassium according to guidelines in Chapter 53 is suggested. Dextrose may also be added to IV fluids at a 2½ per cent solution to control complicating hypoglycemia of sepsis. The severe leukopenia seen in many

patients should be a consideration in whether fluids are administered subcutaneously, since there is a high incidence of complicating infection, cellulitis, and skin necrosis at administration sites.

Parenteral antibiotics are indicated to control secondary bacterial sepsis. In dogs with severe depression, high fever, marked leukopenia, hypoglycemia, shock, disseminated intravascular coagulation, or hematochezia, a parenteral broad-spectrum antibiotic regimen directed at potentially life-threatening sepsis should be used, such as cephalothin, chloramphenicol, trimethoprim-sulfadiazine, or ampicillin-gentamicin.

Additional measures may include antiemetic therapy for persistent vomiting, oral bismuth subsalicylate for its nonspecific antidiarrheal activity, and plasma infusion or blood transfusion if hypoproteinemia or severe blood loss anemia occurs. Metoclopramide (Reglan) given as a continuous infusion of 0.5 to 1 mg/lb per 24 hours diluted in intravenous fluids is beneficial for control of refractory vomiting associated with delayed gastric emptying that sometimes occurs in parvoviral infection.[189]

Nothing is given per os until vomiting has ceased for at least 24 hours and diarrhea is subsiding and free of gross hemorrhage. This can take three to five days in severe cases. When feeding is resumed, small bland feedings are given until GI function appears to have recovered. The transition back to regular feeding should be gradual.

Dogs with parvovirus shed massive amounts of virus in their feces during illness and are highly infectious for other dogs. Thus, they should be kept isolated from other dogs until at least a week after full recovery. Elimination of the virus from infected premises is difficult since the virus is so resistant; however, disinfection with dilute (1:30) chlorine bleach is suggested.[179]

Prognosis and Complications. Most patients having parvovirus enteritis that are treated appropriately for dehydration recover. Complications during the course of parvovirus infection are common, however, and some animals succumb to sepsis or endotoxemia with disseminated intravascular coagulation, which are attributable to the extreme immunosuppression caused by this virus. In general, the younger the animal the higher the mortality risk. Other complications include hypoglycemia (probably secondary to sepsis), hypoproteinemia, anemia, intussusception, liver disease, CNS signs (likely due to concomitant canine distemper), and numerous potential secondary bacterial infections; for example, endocarditis, thrombophlebitis, pneumonia (caused by aspiration in some dogs), urinary tract infection, injection site abscesses, and intestinal salmonellosis and campylobacteriosis.

Prevention. Vaccination is the only realistic and effective means of prevention and control of this disease. The virus is ubiquitous, and since it is so stable outside of the animal and easily transmitted by fomites, prevention of exposure is almost impossible.[176]

Although widespread vaccination against CPV has markedly reduced the incidence of the disease in North America, parvoviral enteritis continues to be a problem in puppies as they are nearing the end of their maternal antibody protection at 6 to 20 weeks of age. This is despite vaccination because of a phenomenon called the *critical period of susceptibility*.[190] In the first weeks of life, maternal antibody protects the puppy from infection, but at the same time it can also interfere with active immunization. As the level of this maternal antibody gradually declines, there is a period of two to four weeks during which the titer is high enough so that the puppy is refractory to vaccination but at the same time too low to be protective, which leaves the animal susceptible to parvoviral infection if exposed.[190] Almost all apparent "vaccination failures" in puppies probably result from exposure to infection during this critical period of susceptibility. Vaccination strategies for canine parvovirus are described in Chapter 47.

CANINE CORONAVIRUS

Canine coronaviral enteritis (CCV) is an acute contagious disease of dogs caused by an epitheliotropic virus that preferentially invades the enterocytes of the villous tips.[161, 162, 165, 168, 179] The resulting villous destruction, atrophy, and fusion cause diarrhea of variable severity. Clinical signs of canine coronaviral enteritis are the acute onset of anorexia and depression followed by vomiting and diarrhea. The character of the diarrhea varies from yellow-orange and mushy to watery or overtly bloody. Increased fecal mucus may be seen, and the odor is often fetid. Most dogs infected with CCV are afebrile.

Most infections are subclinical, although occasional epizootics of severe enteritis have occurred, mostly associated with kennels and dog shows.[168] Canine coronavirus spreads rapidly through contact with infective feces. The clinical importance of canine coronavirus as a cause of enteritis may be relatively minor—in a survey of 1100 fecal specimens from dogs with suspected viral enteritis, only 3 cases of coronaviral enteritis were identified.[191]

Coronaviral enteritis should be considered in dogs with gastroenteritis of acute onset, especially if other dogs are simultaneously affected. In contrast to parvoviral enteritis, fever, leukopenia, and severe hematochezia are infrequent findings; in an epizootic coronaviral outbreak, the overall severity of illness and mortality rate are generally less than that expected for parvovirus. Definitive diagnosis requires laboratory confirmation, either by demonstration of viral particles in feces by electron microscopy or virus isolation during the acute illness or demonstration of a fourfold or greater rise in serum antibody titer in paired sera (at the time of illness and two to six weeks later). Both false-positives and false-negatives are a problem with electron microscopy, virus isolation is not readily available to the clinician, and serology provides only a retrospective diagnosis.[186] However, since coronaviral enteritis is usually nonfatal and the only treatment is supportive, definitive laboratory confirmation is not needed for effective case management except to document an epizootic outbreak.

The treatment of coronaviral enteritis consists of fluid therapy and symptomatic treatment as described in the section on Treatment of Acute Diarrhea. Most animals recover rapidly, although some dogs have had persistent diarrhea for three to four weeks. Fatalities have been reported, especially in neonates, but are considered to be rare.

A killed (inactivated) canine coronavirus vaccine is commercially available (see Chapter 47); however, its efficacy (completeness and duration of immunity) or the need for parenteral vaccination for this disease remains to be established.[186] In general, immunity to coronaviruses is brief and mediated by local (IgA) immunity rather than the serum antibodies that would result from a parenteral vaccine.

CANINE ROTAVIRUS

Rotaviruses have been recognized as one of the most important causes of neonatal diarrhea in humans and many other species of mammals and birds.[192] Rotaviruses replicate exclusively in the mature enterocytes of the villous tip, causing blunted villi that are populated mainly with immature secretory cells from the crypts.[193, 194] Rotaviruses have been isolated from the feces of puppies with self-limiting diarrhea as well as those with fatal enteritis[163, 195-198] and surveys have shown an incidence of antirotavirus antibodies as high as 79 per cent in dogs, suggesting that many dogs go through mild or subclinical infection.[199, 200] In most species, rotaviruses cause potentially fatal diarrhea and dehydration mostly in neonates but only subclinical infection in adults. Experimental inoculation of neonatal gnotobiotic pups with canine rotavirus results in diarrhea and mild-to-moderate villous atrophy; however, deprivation of colostrum in neonatal puppies predisposes to severe diarrhea following rotaviral inoculation.[194, 201] On the other hand, it has almost been impossible to experimentally produce signs of rotavirus infection in dogs over six months of age.[163]

Clinically, this viral agent has not been shown to be an enteropathogen of major importance in the dog or cat. Clinical signs of acute enteritis attributed to rotavirus are occasionally seen in young puppies. The diarrhea, which may be watery to mucoid, is usually self-limiting and of brief duration, although rare fatalities have been reported.[163] Active rotavirus infection can be established by detection of virus in feces by enzyme immunoassay, electron microscopy, or virus isolation.

Rotaviral enteritis is treated like any other acute diarrhea with emphasis on supportive measures such as fluid therapy and dietary restriction. Most animals recover uneventfully. There is currently no vaccine available for canine rotavirus.

FELINE PANLEUKOPENIA VIRUS

Feline panleukopenia is a severe, highly contagious parvoviral infection of cats. The virus has a predilection for rapidly dividing cells, particularly for the intestinal crypt epithelium (acute enteritis), for hemopoietic tissue (panleukopenia), and for lymphoid tissues (lymphoid depletion).[202] Clinical features are similar to canine parvoviral enteritis: anorexia, depression, high fever, persistent vomiting, diarrhea, and progressive dehydration. Vomitus is usually a bile-stained fluid, and feces may be watery, mucoid, or bloody. The incidence and mortality rate are highest in young kittens.

Infection probably occurs by oropharyngeal contact with the virus, and the extreme resistance of panleukopenia virus to inactivation potentiates fomite transmission. The pathogenesis of panleukopenia infection has been studied extensively.[203-210] Replication of virus in oropharyngeal lymphoid tissues is followed by viremia, and then by hematogenous invasion of the intestinal crypt epithelium, resulting in crypt necrosis. The severity of the crypt lesion appears to depend on the rate of crypt cell proliferation (mitotic activity). The indigenous bacterial microflora provide the conditions for viral-induced injury through their stimulatory effect on mitotic activity of crypt epithelium.[207-209] The virus destroys crypt cells. Without crypt cells available to proliferate and replace villous cells as they migrate and are extruded, the villi shorten and extensive mucosal disruption occurs. Severe damage to intestinal epithelial cells results in diarrhea and dehydration. Colonic lesions similar to those in the small intestine also occur, although they tend to be more focal and less severe.[210]

Feline panleukopenia enteritis is usually diagnosed presumptively on the basis of clinical signs and the profound panleukopenia (nadir often less than 500 WBC/μl) in a susceptible (unvaccinated) cat.[202] The leukopenia is fairly consistent and usually lasts only two to four days. If leukopenia persists for longer or is accompanied by anemia, then the panleukopenia-like syndrome associated with feline leukemia virus infection should be considered (see Chapter 48). Serologic diagnosis (paired neutralizing antibody titers) and virus isolation have been used in research but are rarely necessary in clinical practice. Necropsy diagnosis is based on the lesion of severe crypt necrosis.

The treatment of feline panleukopenia is similar to that discussed for canine parvoviral enteritis; mainly nonspecific supportive treatment such as rehydration, parenteral antibiotics, antiemetics, good nursing care, and restriction of dietary intake. In most cases, a guarded prognosis is justified until impending recovery is indicated by cessation of emesis and diarrhea, return of appetite, return of normal body temperature, and rebound leukocytosis. On the other hand, complications such as hypothermia (endotoxemia), icterus, secondary bacterial and mycotic infection, and disseminated intravascular coagulation, usually indicate a fatal outcome.

Widespread prevention of this disease has been achieved through the availability and use of highly effective vaccines. The reader is referred to Chapter 48 for a discussion of vaccination strategies for prevention of this disease.

FELINE ENTERIC CORONAVIRUS

Feline enteric coronavirus, a virus antigenically related to but distinct from the feline infectious peritonitis (FIP) virus, appears to be ubiquitous in the cat population.[170, 171] The virus is shed in the feces of many normal cats and a high percentage of cats are seropositive, indicating that inapparent infection is extremely prevalent. In young kittens, especially 4 to 12 weeks of age, feline enteric coronavirus causes an acute but mild enteritis that may be subclinical or characterized by vomiting and diarrhea.[170] These signs are usually mild and self-limiting within two to four days; however, fatal peracute hemorrhagic gastroenteritis was reported with coronavirus in one adult cat.[211] Like enteric coronaviruses of other species, the feline enteric coronavirus appears to invade the villous tip epithelium, resulting in villous atrophy.

Serology can identify a convalescent rise in coronaviral antibody titer. This, however, is more important because of the confusion it causes in interpretation of FIP testing than as a diagnostic aid for enteric disease (see Chapter 48). Research facilities can identify coronaviral particles in feces electron microscopically. Treatment is not usually necessary except perhaps rehydration therapy.

FELINE ROTAVIRUS

As in the canine, rotavirus has been isolated from both normal and diarrheic feces of cats, especially kittens, but its enteropathogenic significance is currently unclear.[172, 173, 198] Subclinical infection in mature animals is probably frequent, as indicated by one survey that found antibodies to rotavirus in 26 of 94 clinically healthy cats (28 per cent).[172]

Bacterial, Rickettsial, and Enterotoxigenic Diarrhea

Enteropathogenic bacteria produce intestinal disease either by invading and damaging the epithelium (invasive bacteria) or by remaining attached to the epithelium without penetrating it, where they liberate diarrheogenic enterotoxins (noninvasive or enterotoxigenic bacteria).

Bacteria capable of invading the mucosa include *Salmonella, Campylobacter, Yersinia, Shigella, Bacillus piliformis, Mycobacterium*, and invasive strains of *Escherichia coli*. They primarily invade the colon and distal small bowel, leading to inflammation, exudation, mucous secretion, and bleeding. Thus, invasive bacteria cause enterocolitis characterized by watery-mucoid or bloody-mucoid diarrhea. In severe cases, diarrhea may be leukocyte-positive and accompanied by abdominal pain and fever. These agents are also discussed in Chapter 87. In addition, some invasive organisms can invade the submucosa and enter lymphatics and the bloodstream, producing serious systemic infection (bacteremia) as well as intestinal infection.

Enterotoxigenic bacteria, on the other hand, produce diarrhea without penetration of the mucosal surface. They elaborate enterotoxins that bind to enterocytes and either act as secretagogues that stimulate intestinal epithelial cell secretion or as cytotoxins that directly injure the mucosal epithelium. Secretory enterotoxins cause a voluminous watery, electrolyte-rich diarrhea, mediated through the adenyl cyclase–cyclic AMP and guanyl cyclase–cyclic GMP mechanisms, serotonin, and vasoactive intestinal polypeptide in the upper small intestinal mucosa. The prototypical enteropathogenic bacteria that produce secretory diarrhea in humans are *Vibrio cholera* and enterotoxigenic strains of *E. coli.* Their clinical significance in dogs and cats, however, is unknown. Experimentally, cholera toxin is diarrheogenic in dogs.[212] Cytotoxin-producing enterotoxigenic bacteria, such as *Clostridium difficile*, cause inflammatory large bowel diarrhea that mimics dysentery caused by the invasive enteropathogens. *Staphylococci* produce enterotoxin exogenously while growing in contaminated foods, and the secretory diarrhea associated with staphylococcal food poisoning then develops when this preformed toxin is ingested with the food. Some organisms considered to be primarily invasive, such as *Salmonella*, may also stimulate concomitant hypersecretion through the local release of products of inflammation such as prostaglandins and bradykinins.[213]

Although the clinical importance of the various enteropathogenic bacteria in canine and feline diarrhea has not yet been fully defined, dogs and cats are known to harbor many potential enteropathogens, including *Salmonella, Campylobacter, Yersinia, Shigella,* enteropathogenic *E. coli, Clostridium,* and *Bacillus piliformis.* Since some of these are also human pathogens, particularly *Salmonella, Campylobacter,* and *Yersinia,* pets may be an important reservoir for human infection.

SALMONELLA

Salmonellosis is caused by gram-negative bacilli belonging to the genus *Salmonella* of the family *Enterobacteriaceae. Salmonella* spp. are frequently isolated from the feces of normal dogs and cats, but clinical signs of salmonellosis are uncommon, indicating a prevalent asymptomatic carrier state.[214] The prevalence in the United States canine population has been estimated at 10 per cent, but 15 to 20 per cent or higher has been reported in certain areas with overcrowded or unsanitary conditions.[215] Fecal isolations have generally indicated a somewhat lower prevalence rate in cats, ranging from 0.5 to 13.6 per cent.[216, 217]

Salmonella infection is transmitted by the feco-oral route, mainly through ingestion of contaminated food or water. The organisms can survive in the environment for long periods outside of the host so that fomite transmission may also occur.[214] Infection risk depends on activity of the strain, size of the inoculum, competition from the established flora, age of the host, and host defense factors. Thus *Salmonella* is an opportunistic invader and young animals that are diseased, stressed, immunosuppressed or debilitated and kept in overcrowded or unsanitary kennel conditions are most susceptible. Hospitalized animals are also at risk, especially those with severe illness, those undergoing major surgery, those hospitalized for five or more days, and those receiving glucocorticoids, anticancer chemotherapy, or oral antibiotics that upset the normal flora.[214, 218-221] Infections in hospitalized animals may either be nosocomial or the result of activation of preexisting subclinical infection.[219, 221] One hospital outbreak in cats was associated with a high morbidity (32 per cent) and mortality (61 per cent).[218]

The public health significance of *Salmonella* infection in pets is emphasized by documented reports of animal-to-human transmission.[215, 222, 223]

Clinical Signs. Manifestations of *Salmonella* infection can be categorized into three syndromes: (1) asymptomatic carrier state, (2) gastroenteritis, and (3) gastroenteritis with bacteremia (with or without extraintestinal localization).[221] Clinical salmonellosis is relatively uncommon compared with the prevalence of the subclinical carrier state. When it does occur, salmonellosis in most patients is limited to mucosal invasion and is manifested by typical signs of acute enterocolitis—watery or mucoid diarrhea, containing blood in severe cases, vomiting, tenesmus, fever, anorexia, lethargy, abdominal pain, and progressive dehydration.[214, 218, 221] Also, there is often an associated mesenteric lymphadenitis. These signs usually begin within three to five days after exposure or following stress in a carrier. Most animals with acute *Salmonella* diarrhea recover within three to four weeks, although shedding of organisms continues for up to six weeks. In rare cases of overwhelming *Salmonella* infection, acute enterocolitis may develop into a potentially fatal bacteremia or endotoxemia with signs of systemic illness, endotoxic shock, or disseminated intravascular coagulopathy.[221, 224] *Salmonella* is occasionally associated with chronic or intermittent diarrhea.

Diagnosis. The diagnosis depends upon isolation of *Salmonella* spp. from properly cultured fecal specimens or from blood cultures in bacteremic cases. Salmonellosis should be suspected in any dog or cat with inflammatory diarrhea, especially if probable exposure or any of the aforementioned risk factors can be identified. This includes hospitalized animals that develop signs of acute gastroenteritis.[221] Salmonellosis may mimic other infectious enteritides, including parvovirus infection. The presence of fecal leukocytes may be demonstrable by cytologic examination, suggesting the possibility of an invasive bacterial infection. In severe cases with septicemia and endotoxemia, a neutropenia with a left shift and toxic neutrophils may be seen.[214, 221]

Treatment. The use of antibacterials in the treatment of salmonellosis is controversial. *Salmonella* invasion that is confined locally to the mucosa produces enteritis that is both self-limiting and not likely affected by antibacterial agents. In addition, antibacterial therapy, especially with oral nonabsorbable antibiotics, may actually prolong shedding of the organism and encourage development of a prolonged carrier state.[214, 221] Antibacterials are also unreliable for eliminating chronic asymptomatic carriers of *Salmonella,* which is the most prevalent form of infection found in surveys of dogs and cats. Antibiotics are, however, indicated whenever *Salmonella* invasion becomes severe or complicated by septicemia or endotoxemia, as evidenced by systemic signs such as shock, dehydration, high fever, and extreme depression and laboratory findings such as azotemia, electrolyte imbalances, neutropenia, hypoproteinemia, and coagulopathy. Severe hematochezia may be an indication of impending systemic invasion and should also prompt antibiotic therapy. The choice of an antibiotic should be based on culture and sensitivity, especially since it appears that *Salmonella* are becoming more resistant with time.[221] Trimethoprim, cephalothin, and chloramphenicol are often effective.[221] In addition to antibiotics, fluid and electrolyte replacement and detection and correction of underlying predisposing conditions are important aspects of therapy.

The prognosis for most animals with salmonellosis is good; infection in most patients tends to be self-limiting or antibiotic-responsive. It is difficult, however, to prevent or eliminate the carrier state even with antibiotics. The mortality rate may be higher in outbreaks that occur within extremely susceptible populations, for example, veterinary hospital outbreaks.[218, 221] Also, the prognosis is guarded for those occasional cases complicated by septicemia, endotoxemia, or disseminated intravascular coagulation. Factors in one survey of 58 dogs in a veterinary teaching hospital with clinical salmonellosis that were predictive of a guarded prognosis included peracute onset, high fever (above 104° F), hypothermia, severe bloody diarrhea, degenerative left shift leukogram, and hypoglycemia.[221] The mortality rate in these dogs was 28 per cent,[221] and in an outbreak in hospitalized cats, the mortality rate was 61 per cent.[218]

CAMPYLOBACTER

Campylobacter jejuni are fastidious, microaerophilic, gram-negative, motile, slender curved bacteria that have emerged as important enteric pathogens of animals and humans worldwide. *Campylobacter* is widespread in domestic and wild animals as both an enteropathogen and as an organism shed in the feces of normal animals (Figure 86–14).[38, 225–229] Numerous surveys have indicated that a significant number of normal dogs and cats shed *Campylobacter* in their feces. Although the prevalence of *Campylobacter* shedding is generally less than 1 per cent in pet populations, shedding may occur in as high as 30 per cent of humane shelter animals and in over 40 per cent of commercially reared research dogs.[226, 230, 231] Thus, conditions of close confinement or poor sanitation apparently provide the greatest opportunity for environmental exposure.

In humans, *Campylobacter* is tissue invasive, causing acute enterocolitis and sometimes even bacteremia. Since many of the dogs and cats that shed *Campylobacter* are clinically normal and since it has been difficult to

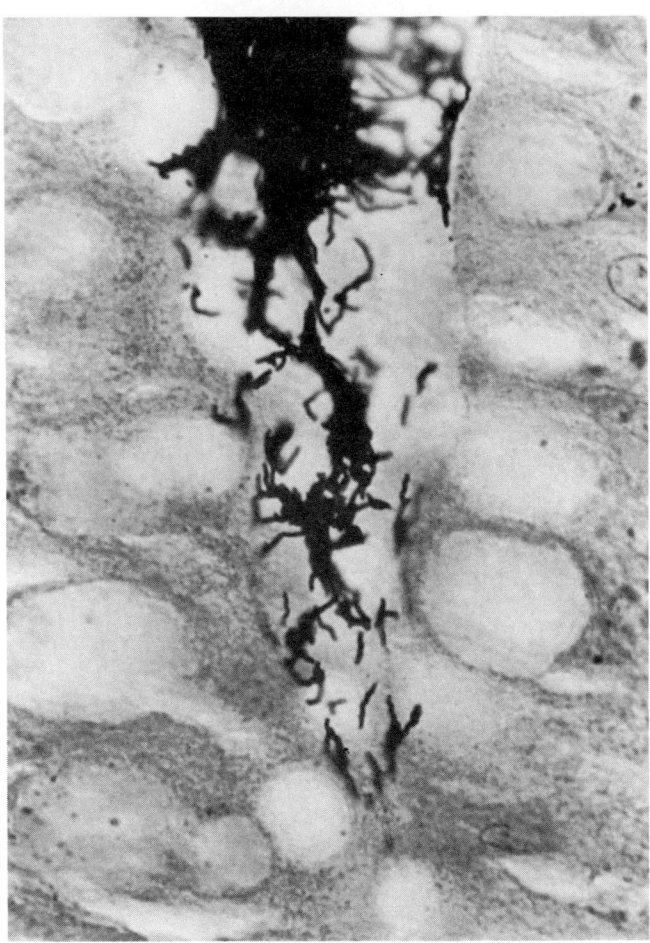

FIGURE 86–14. Histopathologic specimen of canine colon showing numerous *Campylobacter* organisms filling a crypt (Warthin-Starry stain).

produce enteritis with this organism experimentally, the pathogenicity of *Campylobacter* in dogs and cats remains to be fully defined.[228, 229]

Clinical Signs. The full spectrum of clinical manifestations of campylobacteriosis in the dog and cat remains to be determined, although it is clear from the numerous reported surveys that the majority of animals that harbor these organisms are asymptomatic.[228, 229] Since most studies have shown an equal incidence of *Campylobacter* in normal versus diarrheic animals, it has even been debated whether *Campylobacter* by itself causes diarrhea in the dog or cat. Clinical signs associated with *Campylobacter* in dogs and cats have been attributed to superficial erosive enterocolitis and are characterized by a 5- to 15-day course of watery-mucoid diarrhea that occasionally contains blood and may be accompanied by vomiting and tenesmus.[38, 228, 229, 232] Fever is usually mild or absent. *Campylobacter* is occasionally associated with chronic diarrhea.[233] A *Campylobacter* sp. has also been associated with an unusual proliferative enteritis in a litter of pups.[234]

Diagnosis. A presumptive diagnosis of campylobacteriosis may be made by identifying gram-negative, slender curved rods that have a characteristic W-shape in stained fecal smears.[38, 214, 229] The presence of fecal leukocytes may also be noted. In fresh saline smears, the organisms may be seen with dark-field or phase-contrast microscopy as highly motile, darting, spiral or S-shaped bacteria; however, they should not be confused with spirochetes and other motile bacteria that are part of the normal flora.[38, 214]

Confirmation of campylobacteriosis depends upon isolation of the organism from feces utilizing special selective media.[232, 235] Since *Campylobacter* are microaerophilic and difficult to isolate, fecal specimens should be obtained directly from the rectum and processed soon after collection.

Treatment. The antibiotic of choice for human campylobacteriosis is erythromycin, which can be used to treat animals at 5 mg/lb, q8h, orally.[229] Other effective antibiotics include furazolidone, doxycycline, chloramphenicol, and aminoglycosides such as neomycin.[236] The prognosis is considered good. Bacteremia[237] and fatalities in dogs[214] and cats[238] have been reported but are probably rare occurrences.

The duration of fecal shedding of *Campylobacter* in untreated dogs and cats is unknown, but antibiotics are effective in rapidly eliminating excretion of organisms, which thereby reduces the chance of spread of infection to humans or other animals.[228] Since contact with animal feces is a potential source of infection in humans, owners of infected pets should be advised to take appropriate precautions.

YERSINIA

Both *Yersinia pseudotuberculosis* and *Yersinia enterocolitica* are motile gram-negative, rod-shaped bacteria which may occasionally infect the intestinal tract of dogs and cats. Cats acquire *Y. pseudotuberculosis* infection mainly through ingestion of infected rodent and avian prey. Clinical signs include vomiting and diarrhea due to gastroenteritis, icterus due to hepatic invasion, and nonspecific signs of fever, depression, and weight loss.[239–243] Mesenteric lymph nodes, liver, and spleen may be markedly enlarged by pyogranulomatous inflammation. The clinical course ranges from acute (days) to chronic (months), but almost always progresses to death. Although feline pseudotuberculosis is generally a serious, highly fatal disease, *Y. pseudotuberculosis* has also been isolated from healthy cats that are apparently asymptomatic carriers.[244]

Yersinia enterocolitica, a motile gram-negative rod, is recognized worldwide as a cause of acute and chronic enterocolitis in humans,[245] and has been isolated from small numbers of dogs and cats. The carrier prevalence in normal dogs is under one per cent in North America but up to six per cent in Japan and the Scandinavian countries.[244, 246–250] On rare occasions, *Yersinia* has been associated with enterocolitis in young dogs, characterized by bloody-mucoid diarrhea, increased frequency of defecation, tenesmus, and an absence of systemic signs.[250, 251] *Yersinia* infection of dogs may be a public health concern.[252]

Yersinia grows best at colder temperatures and specialized isolation methods are needed to culture the organism from feces. *Yersinia* may also be cultured from blood or infected tissues. The infection is usually susceptible to a trimethoprim-sulfa combination, tetracycline, chloramphenicol, and aminoglycosides; however, culture and antibiotic sensitivity testing is recommended.

BACILLUS PILIFORMIS

Tyzzer's disease, caused by a pleomorphic, gram-negative, spore-forming, obligate intracellular bacillus called *Bacillus piliformis*, is a rare but fatal disease characterized by hemorrhagic-necrotizing enterocolitis and hepatic necrosis.[253–258] Puppies and kittens are most often affected and the disease may complicate parasitism, parvovirus infection, feline leukemia virus infection, and canine distemper. The progression of Tyzzer's disease is rapid, most animals dying within 48 hours after the initial onset of signs of anorexia, depression, and diarrhea. Successful therapy has not been reported.

Diagnosis is difficult since the organism cannot be cultured on artificial media. Instead, mouse inoculation or embryonated egg culture techniques can be used to isolate the organism. Most cases are diagnosed by the histologic identification of typical intracellular filamentous bacilli at the margins of necrotic foci within liver and intestinal lesions using methenamine silver, Giemsa, or PAS staining. Rodents are the principal reservoir of *Bacillus piliformis*.

ESCHERICHIA COLI

Invasive and enterotoxigenic strains of *E. coli* are well-established causes of acute infectious diarrhea in many animals including humans, but the role of *E. coli* as primary enteropathogens in dogs and cats is unclear. Since *E. coli* are normal components of the resident microflora of both the large and small bowel, the mere isolation of *E. coli* from the feces or bowel of the dog or cat is not in itself significant. To establish enteropathogenicity of an *E. coli* isolate, specialized assays that are available only in research laboratories, such as bioassays, tissue culture assays, immunoassays, and genome probes, must be performed to differentiate invasive or enterotoxigenic isolates from nonpathogenic strains.[259–262] Serotyping is also used but is considered less reliable.[263]

Definitive assays such as these to document enteropathogenicity of *E. coli* isolates from dogs and cats with naturally occurring diarrhea are needed. In one study, enterotoxin of *E. coli* isolated from a human patient with secretory diarrhea was shown to stimulate adenyl cyclase activity and fluid secretion by canine jejunum.[264] An atypical slow-acting heat-labile *E. coli* enterotoxin was isolated from two dogs with diarrhea,[265] but earlier surveys for the presence of classic heat-labile enterotoxin in dogs were negative.[266] Enterotoxigenic *E. coli* were isolated from 4 of 148 dogs with diarrhea, and bioassays characterized these isolates as producers of heat-labile and heat-stable enterotoxins.[267] However, since in this study the isolates were so few, the incidence of enterotoxigenic *E. coli* diarrhea in the canine appears to be low.

CLOSTRIDIUM

Clostridium spp. constitute part of the normal intestinal flora of the dog and cat.[268] A severe form of colitis in humans, often described as pseudomembranous, is caused by colonic overgrowth of cytotoxin-producing clostridia, especially *C. difficile*, subsequent to antimicrobial suppression of the normal flora.[269] Toxigenic *C. difficile* have been isolated from normal dogs and cats[270] and from dogs with chronic diarrhea.[271] Since the infections appeared to be transient and generally not associated with enteritis, the role of toxin-producing clostridia in antibiotic-associated diarrheas of small animals remains to be clearly established.

The diagnosis of *C. difficile* is generally based on a positive assay for the cytotoxin in feces. This test is now available in many full-service human hospitals. Infection in humans is usually treated with oral vancomycin, an extremely expensive antibiotic.[272] Metronidazole, bacitracin, or tetracycline may also be effective, and mild cases can be successfully treated with oral nonselective toxin-binding agents such as cholestyramine.

Clostridium perfringens (welchii), a large anaerobic gram-positive bacillus and part of the normal microflora of the dog, has been incriminated as a cause of acute hemorrhagic gastroenteritis (see Canine Hemorrhagic Enteritis).[273-275] A toxigenic *Clostridium perfringens type A* was also isolated from one dog with chronic intermittent watery-mucoid diarrhea.[276]

Although there is only circumstantial evidence that *Clostridium perfringens* or its toxins cause diarrhea in dogs and cats, it is likely that further study will establish clostridia as a cause of bacterial diarrhea of small animals. High doses of metronidazole, penicillin, ampicillin, or chloramphenicol are considered to be effective for treating infections caused by *C. perfringens*.

CANINE HEMORRHAGIC ENTERITIS

Hemorrhagic gastroenteritis (HGE) is a syndrome of unknown etiology characterized by sudden onset of vomition, profuse bloody diarrhea, and marked hemoconcentration.[277-279] Despite its name, HGE does not appear to be primarily an inflammatory disease, but rather a condition of altered intestinal mucosal permeability and perhaps mucosal hypersecretion. Cultures of intestinal contents from dogs with HGE have yielded large numbers of *Clostridium perfringens*, mostly in pure culture, leading to speculation that this organism or its toxins are the primary cause. The clinical signs and explosive onset of HGE have been compared to experimental models of endotoxic shock, anaphylaxis, and immune-mediated bowel disease in dogs;[277, 279] however, there is no direct evidence yet that such mechanisms are involved in HGE.

Clinical Signs. Hemorrhagic gastroenteritis affects dogs of all ages, but especially young adults, two to four years of age. The disease has a predilection for toy and miniature breeds, particularly schnauzers and toy poodles, but any breed can be affected.[279] The first signs are usually sudden onset of vomiting and severe depression, followed within hours by a profuse, bloody fluid diarrhea with fetid odor. Progressive prolongation of capillary refill time and other indicators of circulatory failure are noted as shock develops. If untreated by volume expansion, HGE can cause circulatory failure and death in less than 24 hours. Most dogs experience a single episode, but some (about 10 per cent) have recurrences sporadically throughout their lifetime.[279]

Diagnosis. The diagnosis is suggested by evidence of extreme hemoconcentration without comparable loss of skin turgor in an animal with fetid bloody diarrhea. In most dogs with HGE, the hematocrit is well above 60 per cent, reaching as high as 70 to 80 per cent in some dogs, especially schnauzers. Hemoconcentration is attributable to a combination of rapid shift of fluid out of the effective vascular compartment, rapid secretory and exudative fluid loss into the gut, and splenic contraction. Radiography and other laboratory findings are generally unremarkable, but nevertheless they are useful for excluding other causes of bloody diarrhea. The high hematocrit and lack of fever or leukopenia help to distinguish HGE from parvoviral enteritis, but for greater certainty, a fecal test for parvovirus is necessary.

Treatment. The mortality rate of HGE is low if treated promptly by vigorous fluid volume replacement. A balanced multiple electrolyte solution should be infused rapidly, preferably by indwelling IV catheter, at a rate of 40 ml/lb/hr until return of capillary refill time to normal and hematocrit to below 50 per cent; then, IV fluids are continued over the next 24 hours at a more moderate rate as needed to maintain adequate circulatory function and keep the hematocrit below 50 per cent. Most animals show marked improvement within hours, although diarrhea may not subside for 24 to 48 hours. Occasionally, a dose of corticosteroid may be needed during the initial hours if shock appears to be refractory to IV fluid therapy.

Food and water should be restricted initially until vomiting and bloody or fluid diarrhea have ceased, then small amounts of bland food can be fed. Nonspecific antidiarrheal and antiemetic therapy may be helpful. Antibiotics effective against gram-negative bacteria and *Clostridium perfringens*, such as ampicillin or chloramphenicol, are used empirically because of the possibility that gram-negative endotoxins or clostridial enterotoxins play a role in the disease. Excessive bleeding may occasionally require a fresh whole-blood transfusion.

Failure of the animal to improve dramatically within 24 to 48 hours should prompt a search for other diseases that may mimic HGE; for example, parvovirus, GI foreign body, intussusception, and volvulus.

MYCOBACTERIA

The alimentary form of tuberculosis occurs in cats that ingest unpasteurized milk infected with *Mycobacterium* spp. Since the incidence of feline tuberculosis is closely linked to tuberculosis in dairy cows, the disease is now rare in countries where bovine tuberculosis is controlled.[280] The clinical signs include chronic diarrhea, weight loss, anorexia, and lethargy.[281] The physical findings of palpable intestinal masses (granulomas) in association with mesenteric lymphadenopathy and hepatosplenomegaly make this disease easily confused with alimentary lymphosarcoma.[281] Laboratory and radiographic findings may indicate intestinal malabsorption or obstruction, respectively. The diagnosis of tuberculosis in the cat depends upon identification of characteristic mycobacterial organisms in cytology or biopsy specimens stained with acid-fast stain or Ziehl-Neelsen stain.[280] Intradermal tuberculin testing is unreliable in the cat and cultures for the organism are prohibitively slow to grow. Euthanasia rather than treatment is usually recommended for public health reasons; however, successful remissions (not necessarily cures) have been obtained in cats with isoniazid and streptomycin.[280]

OTHER BACTERIA

Shigella spp., invasive enteropathogenic bacteria that cause bacillary dysentery in humans and other primates, have occasionally been isolated from the feces of clinically normal dogs; however, diarrhea or other indications of enteropathogenicity have not been associated with *Shigella* in small animals.[214, 282] Dogs apparently become transient asymptomatic excretors of this organism following exposure to human feces under conditions of poor sanitation or sewage contamination of water.[214] Natural infection of cats has not been reported.

Staphylococcal food poisoning, a well-known cause of enterotoxigenic diarrhea in humans, has not been well documented in dogs or cats but may be plausible since in one study in Japan, enterotoxigenic staphylococci were isolated from the large bowel of 26 (5.8 per cent) of 451 random-source dogs.[283] Enterotoxigenic *Klebsiella pneumoniae* was isolated from 2 of 148 dogs with diarrhea, but the role of the bacteria in the pathogenesis of diarrhea in these dogs was not determined.[267]

Enteropathogenicity has not been established for the spirochetes often found in feces from dogs and cats. Diarrhea of any cause may dislodge spirochetes that comprise part of the normal canine flora from their normal location within the colonic crypts, resulting in increased numbers in the feces. There is, however, no convincing evidence that spirochetes themselves cause diarrhea.[284, 285] Spirochetes in fecal smears should not be confused with *Campylobacter*.

RICKETTSIAL DIARRHEA (SALMON POISONING DISEASE)

Salmon poisoning is a highly fatal systemic rickettsial infection of dogs in the Pacific Northwest caused by *Neorickettsia helminthoeca* or *Neorickettsia elokominica*, two related rickettsial organisms acquired by ingestion of raw salmon that harbor the disease vector, metacercariae of a fluke called *Nanophyetus salmincola*.[286, 287] Following an incubation of five to seven days after ingestion of infected fish, the fluke matures and attaches to the intestinal mucosa of the host; the rickettsiae cause severe hemorrhagic gastroenteritis and invade the bloodstream, disseminating widely. Signs of infection include high fever, vomiting, diarrhea, anorexia, depression, naso-ocular discharge, dehydration, and peripheral lymphadenopathy. In untreated patients, the mortality rate is 50 to 90 per cent.

The diagnosis should be suspected when these signs are seen in a dog from an endemic area and confirmed by examination of feces for characteristic operculated fluke eggs by direct smear, sugar flotation, or wash-sedimentation methods; or by detection of purple-staining intracytoplasmic rickettsial bodies in macrophages from Giemsa-stained lymph node aspirates.[286, 287] Leukocytosis or leukopenia may be found on routine laboratory studies. Salmon poisoning disease must be differentiated from other causes of febrile hemorrhagic gastroenteritis, especially parvovirus infection.

Tetracycline is the treatment of choice as a specific antirickettsial agent. Vomiting may preclude oral treatment initially, so oxytetracycline, IV at 3 mg/lb q12h, can be used until oral therapy is tolerated.[286] Chloramphenicol, sulfonamides, and penicillin may also be effective.[286] Antibiotics should be continued for two to three weeks. General supportive measures such as parenteral fluid therapy should also be considered and the trematode vector is treated with oral fenbendazole (25 mg/lb/day for 10 to 14 days).[287]

Mycotic Diarrhea

Mycotic infections of the small bowel are uncommon; however, fungi are opportunists that capitalize on predisposing factors such as lowered host resistance, malnutrition, antecedent debilitating illness, or prolonged therapy with antimicrobials or corticosteroids. Fungi may cause acute, dysentery-like diarrhea or chronic diarrhea accompanied by emaciation. Multisystemic involvement is frequent with the systemic mycoses (see Chapter 49). The principal causes of mycotic intestinal disease are *Histoplasma capsulatum*, *Pythium* spp., *Aspergillus* spp., and *Candida albicans*.

INTESTINAL HISTOPLASMOSIS

Histoplasma capsulatum is a chronic systemic fungal infection that usually invades by way of the respiratory tract and affects primarily the lung and macrophage system. Ingestion or widespread dissemination can occur in the dog and cat, leading to an intestinal form of the disease characterized by diffuse granulomatous inflammation of the bowel wall and mesenteric lymph nodes.[39, 288-297] The principal environmental reservoir of infection is the soil throughout the geographic regions bordering the Mississippi River and its tributaries and Texas. For a detailed discussion of histoplasmosis, the reader is referred to Chapter 49.

Intestinal histoplasmosis occurs most often in young dogs and cats, although any age can be affected. Typically, granulomatous inflammation involves all layers of the intestinal wall (Figure 86-15) and associated lymph nodes, which results in severe chronic malabsorption with profuse, intractable watery diarrhea and rapidly progressive weight loss (Figure 86-16).[39, 291, 294, 296] Melena is observed in many cases.[291, 294] Associated protein-losing enteropathy can occur. In addition, when the large bowel is also affected (enterocolitis), signs of tenesmus, hematochezia, and abundant fecal mucus may be observed (see Chapter 87).[39, 290, 291, 294-296] Systemic signs such as fever, pallor, inappetence, depression and weight loss are common.[39, 290, 291, 294, 296]

Emaciation is a consistent feature of intestinal histoplasmosis. Abdominal palpation may reveal diffusely thickened intestinal loops, mesenteric lymphadenopa-

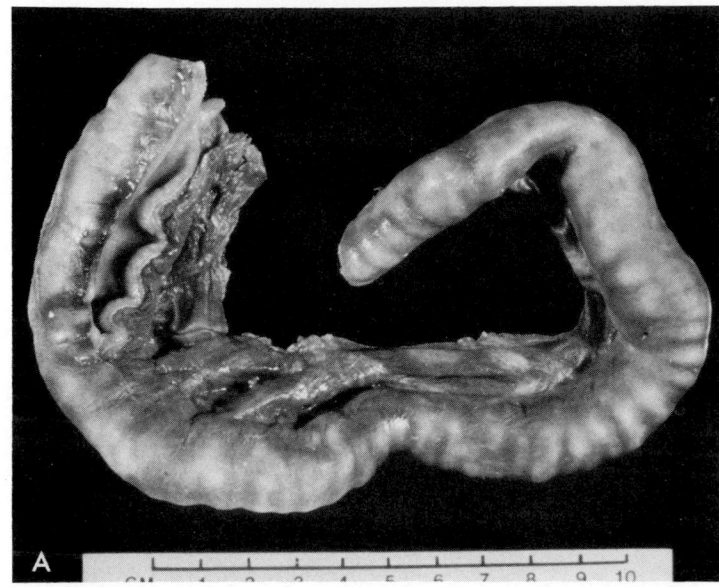

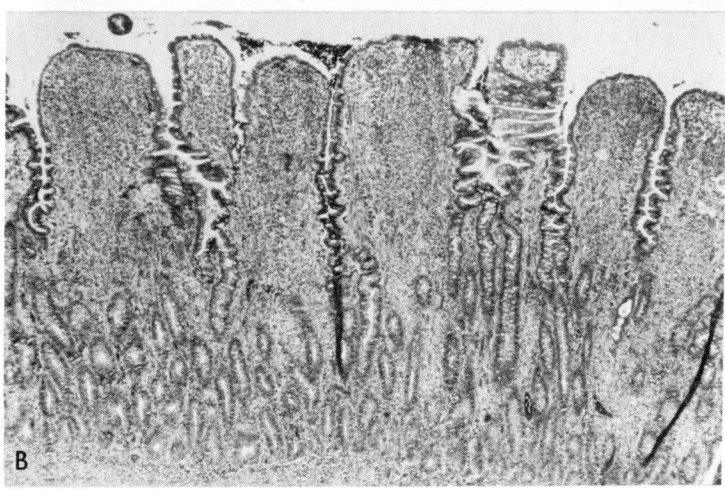

FIGURE 86–15. Thickened corrugated segment of small intestine from a dog with histoplasmosis *(A)*. The lesion was characterized by extensive distortion and thickening of the villi and deeper layers with granulomatous inflammation *(B)*.

thy, mass-like thickenings of the intestine and mesentery or abdominal effusion.[289, 290, 293, 295, 296]

Intestinal histoplasmosis should be considered in any young dog or cat with intractable small or large bowel diarrhea that has lived in an endemic region. The index of suspicion should be increased when the diarrhea is associated with any of the following: extreme emaciation, fever, lymphadenopathy, leukocytosis, evidence of a multisystemic disorder, and a biopsy or cytology finding of granulomatous inflammation. Laboratory find-

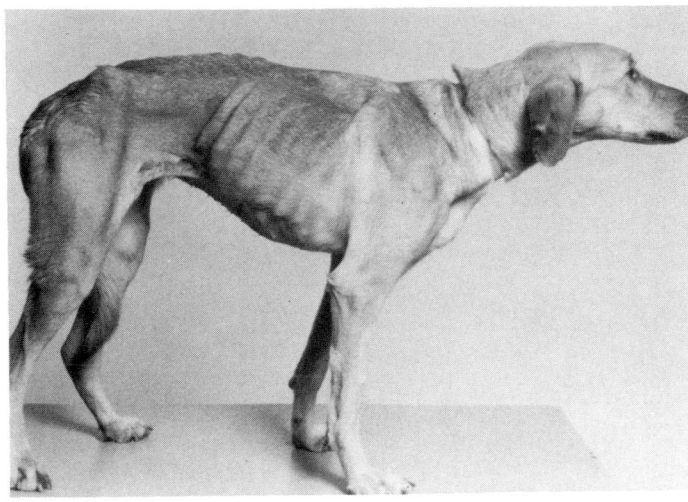

FIGURE 86–16. Intestinal histoplasmosis caused malabsorption, chronic diarrhea, and weight loss in this dog. The bowel lesions are depicted in Figure 86–15.

ings may include steatorrhea, xylose malabsorption, hypoproteinemia, and abnormal liver biochemistries. Barium contrast GI radiography may demonstrate an irregular mucosal pattern indicative of a diffuse infiltrative lesion. Definitive diagnosis depends on identification of *Histoplasma* organisms in cytology preparations (see Figure 86–5), biopsies, or cultures (Sabouraud's medium); although serologic tests (immunodiffusion, complement fixation) are a fairly reliable means of presumptive diagnosis (see Chapter 49 for details).[39]

Intestinal histoplasmosis is usually progressive without treatment. Amphotericin B and ketoconazole, used separately and in combination, have been effective in treating some but not all animals with disseminated histoplasmosis (see Chapter 49). Since treatment failures and relapses are relatively frequent, the prognosis for intestinal histoplasmosis is fair at best.

PHYCOMYCOSIS

The term phycomycosis is a nonspecific designation for infections caused by a variety of poorly septate molds and fungi that primarily invade the digestive tract and include *Pythium* spp. (pythiosis) and members of the Zygomycetes class (zygomycosis), such as Entomophthoraceae (*Basidiobolus* spp., *Conidiobolus* spp.) and Mucoraceae (*Absidia* spp., *Rhizopus* spp., *Rhizomucor* spp., *Mucor* spp., *Mortierella* spp.).[298] Pythium is the most common etiology of canine intestinal phycomycosis, accounting for 60 of 63 cases in a large retrospective survey.[298]

In dogs, phycomycotic organisms can infect any part of the digestive tract, but lesions most commonly involve the stomach, small intestine, mesentery, and mesenteric lymph nodes, resulting in extensive granulomatous tissue reaction and clinical syndromes of chronic diarrhea and/or vomiting.[298, 304] Rare cases of phycomycosis in cats are characterized by ulcerative gastroenteritis.[303, 307]

Phycomycosis most commonly affects young large breed dogs, over 80 per cent being three years of age or less.[298, 303] Cases due to *Pythium* spp. are most prevalent by far and found mainly in the states bordering the Gulf of Mexico, especially Louisiana, whereas cases due to other species of phycomycotic organisms are considerably less common and occur sporadically

throughout the Untied States and Europe.[298] *Pythium* is a waterborne pathogen, and dogs are thought to become infected primarily from ingestion of spore-contaminated water in swampy areas during late summer when the warm water temperature favors growth of the fungi. Subsequently, the lesions within the GI tract and abdominal lymphatics develop slowly and insidiously so that most infected animals then develop overt clinical signs during the period of October through March.[298]

Most animals with intestinal phycomycosis have a chronic clinical course characterized by either intractable diarrhea or vomiting or both, anorexia, depression, and progressive weight loss.[298, 303] Diarrhea may be quite bloody in some cases. The signs are caused by regions of diffuse or multifocal transmural granulomatous inflammation and areas of necrosis within the intestinal wall, often similar lesions in the adjacent mesentery and mesenteric lymph nodes, and variable ulceration of the mucosa (Figure 86–17).[298–304] The extensive granulomatous proliferations may produce palpable enteromesenteric masses.[298] The infection may also disseminate to other abdominal viscera.

Hematologic findings in many cases include mild-to-moderate nonregenerative anemia and mild neutrophilia, with or without a left shift.[303] Routine abdominal radiography frequently demonstrates an abdominal mass, while contrast barium GI study can often delineate a thickened, stenosed segment of bowel.[303]

Intestinal phycomycosis should be considered when chronic intractable small bowel-type diarrhea is associated with an abdominal mass or marked regional thickening of the bowel, especially in any young large breed dog from a state bordering the Gulf of Mexico. Confirmation of the diagnosis depends upon histologic identification of sparsely septate hyphae within biopsies of stomach, intestine, or abdominal lymph nodes. The organisms stain with Gridley's or methenamine silver stains and are found mostly within the necrotic regions of granulomas in the submucosa and muscularis mucosa (Figure 86–18).[298] Intestinal phycomycosis must be differentiated from other granulomatous and neoplastic proliferations of the GI tract including histoplasmosis, lymphosarcoma, and regional (granulomatous) enteritis. The extensive tissue reaction of phycomycosis can easily be mistaken for neoplasia at laparotomy (or necropsy);

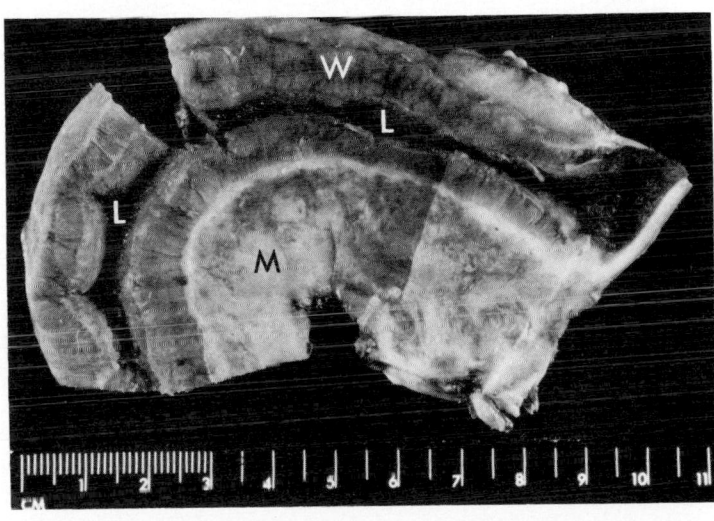

FIGURE 86–17. Longitudinal section of a resected segment of bowel from a dog with chronic diarrhea and weight loss due to phycomycosis. Note the extensive granulomatous thickening of the bowel wall (W), narrowed lumen (L), and extensive involvement of the mesentery (M).

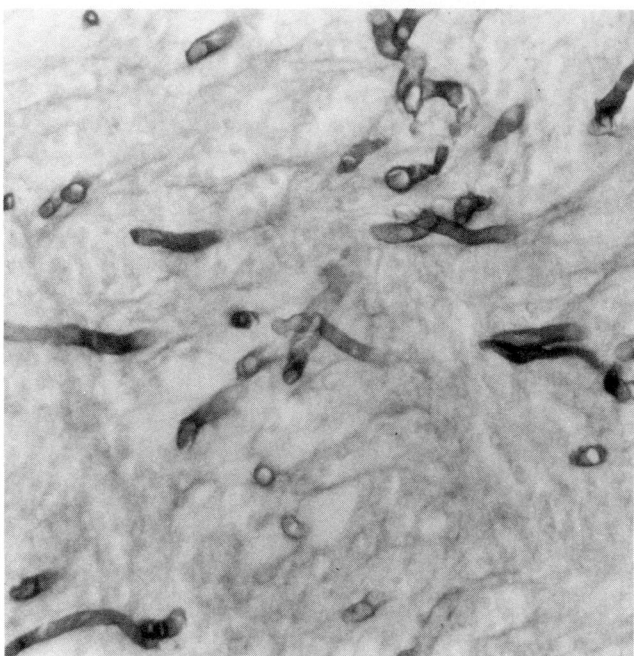

FIGURE 86–18. Histologic section of the lesion in Figure 86–13 showing broad, nonseptate fungal hyphae invading the intestinal submucosa (Silver stain).

therefore, careful histologic evaluation including use of fungal stains is essential for accurate diagnosis.

Successful treatment of phycomycosis has rarely been reported, and thus the prognosis must be considered poor. In the largest reported series of cases, less than 5 per cent of 63 animals were alive 3 months following diagnosis.[298] Amphotericin B and iodide antifungal regimens have not been effective.[298, 303] Surgical excision has been successful in a few cases and thus is the currently recommended treatment, perhaps with long-term follow-up therapy with oral ketoconazole at 5 to 13 mg/lb/day. Unfortunately, euthanasia is appropriate in many cases because tissue damage and infiltration is too extensive by the time a diagnosis is made to allow surgical resection of involved tissues.

OTHER INTESTINAL MYCOSES

In addition to intestinal histoplasmosis and phycomycosis, other mycoses that are rarely associated with enteritis and diarrhea in dogs and cats include *Aspergillus* spp. and *Candida* spp.[307–314] Both *Aspergillus* and *Candida* are considered opportunists since they usually infect young animals already compromised by a preexisting infection or parasitism, or animals that have received prolonged antibiotic corticosteroid therapy. Parvovirus infection in both the dog and cat appears to increase the susceptibility to tissue invasion by opportunistic fungi.[307, 309–312, 314]

Both *Aspergillus* and *Candida* cause chronic diarrhea with mucosal ulceration and necrotizing lesions that extend into the deeper layers of the bowel wall.[307, 308, 311, 312, 314] Pseudomembrane formation and vascular invasion by hyphae have also been observed in cats with aspergillosis.[307, 313] *Aspergillus* may also cause severe pulmonary infection in the cat.[307] The antemortem di-

agnosis of these intestinal mycoses is difficult, usually requiring histologic identification of the fungi in tissue specimens. Fecal cultures for fungi are generally unreliable.

Most reports of intestinal aspergillosis and candidiasis in dogs and cats have been based on necropsy studies. Thus, information on which to base treatment is limited. Localized nasal aspergillosis in dogs sometimes responds to ketoconazole or thiabendazole, but not amphotericin B. Nystatin or ketoconazole can be used to treat candidiasis.

CHRONIC ENTEROPATHIES

Enteropathies that cause chronic small bowel diarrhea as the principal presenting sign in dogs and cats are diverse and sometimes challenging to diagnose; these include chronic inflammatory small bowel diseases, infectious diseases such as giardiasis (see Protozoan Diarrhea section) and histoplasmosis (see Mycotic Diarrhea section), lymphangiectasia, villous atrophy, bacterial overgrowth syndrome, short bowel syndrome, thyroid-related enteropathy, and diffuse intestinal lymphosarcoma (see Neoplasia section). The diagnosis and treatment of these diseases is tabulated at the end of the chapter. Diarrhea caused by these primary intestinal disorders must be differentiated from the diarrhea of exocrine pancreatic insufficiency (see Chapter 90).

Chronic Inflammatory Small Bowel Diseases

The term chronic inflammatory bowel disease refers to a diverse group of disorders characterized by idiopathic infiltration of the intestinal mucosa and sometimes deeper layers of the bowel wall with inflammatory cells. Histopathologic categorization depends upon intestinal biopsy to determine the predominant infiltrating cell: eosinophilic enteritis, lymphocytic-plasmacytic enteritis, or granulomatous enteritis. In some cases, a mixture of inflammatory cells in the lesion makes classification difficult and the infiltrative lesion may involve the stomach and/or colon as well as the small intestine.[315–317] Chronic intractable diarrhea is the hallmark of these diseases. In addition, they may be associated with nutrient malabsorption, protein-losing enteropathy, or both.

The etiology and pathogenesis of these disorders are unknown, but it is plausible that in each type the pathologic infiltrate represents nonspecific, immunologically mediated recruitment of inflammatory cells in response to a variety of inciting causes. Although the cause of these diseases has not been determined, they are often responsive to medical treatment.

LYMPHOCYTIC-PLASMACYTIC ENTERITIS

Diffuse infiltration of an excessive number of lymphocytes and plasma cells into the lamina propria of the small intestine is often found in dogs and cats with chronic diarrhea, with or without vomiting, malabsorption or protein-losing enteropathy.[315-320] Lymphocytes and plasma cells are normal components of the lamina propria, but in lymphocytic-plasmacytic enteritis these cells accumulate in much greater numbers. The etiology is unknown, but since the infiltrating cells are immunocytes, it is probable that immune mechanisms play a central role in the pathogenesis. Instead of being a single disease entity, lymphocytic-plasmacytic enteritis may represent a nonspecific response of the gut to a variety of causative agents and insults that recruit immunocytes.[321] The lesion has been associated with giardiasis, bacterial overgrowth, food allergy,[322, 323] immunoproliferative enteropathy of basenjis,[324] lymphangiectasia,[49] and villous atrophy.[73, 87, 325] Notwithstanding these known associations, lymphocytic-plasmacytic enteritis in many patients is idiopathic.[315-321]

Clinical Signs. Chronic unresponsive small bowel-type diarrhea and weight loss are the usual signs in dogs. In the cat, chronic intermittent vomiting and listless behavior are the most consistent signs and may occur with or without diarrhea.[316] The vomitus usually consists of clear or bilious fluid or foam, and occurs unrelated to eating. Diarrhea may vary from mild to profuse and intermittent to continuous and the consistency from soft to liquid. Occasionally, increased fecal mucus and hematochezia may suggest colonic involvement.[316, 317, 323] In contrast to both eosinophilic and granulomatous enteritis, mucosal ulceration is not a common lesion in lymphocytic-plasmacytic enteritis; therefore, GI bleeding is not a prominent clinical feature. In most animals, physical examination is unremarkable; however, findings may include cachexia, palpable intestinal thickening, and palpable enlargement of mesenteric lymph nodes. Signs of protein-losing enteropathy (ascites, hydrothorax, edema) may be seen in advanced cases.

Diagnosis. Routine hematologic and biochemical parameters are usually normal except for frequent hypoproteinemia in affected dogs, but rarely cats. Most patients have mild to moderate steatorrhea, and normal or decreased xylose absorption.[318] Vitamin K-deficiency and bleeding were associated with malabsorption in two cats with lymphocytic-plasmacytic enteritis.[320] Barium contrast upper GI radiography occasionally reveals diffuse mucosal irregularities (Figure 86–19), a nonspecific finding compatible with an infiltrative lesion, but in most cases radiographic findings are unremarkable.

Intestinal biopsy is the only means of definitive diagnosis. The lesion is characterized by a diffuse infiltrate of well-differentiated lymphocytes and plasma cells in the lamina propria, usually filling the villus core, and sometimes extending into the submucosa.[315-321] Other types of inflammatory cells may also be increased in the lamina propria, but to a lesser extent. The villi may be normal in size or atrophic and fused, and intestinal fibrosis may be seen. Mild dilatation of the central lacteal can also be seen. The intestine containing these lesions may appear grossly normal during endoscopy or laparotomy, emphasizing the importance of procuring biopsies even in the absence of visible lesions.

The differential diagnosis of lymphocytic-plasmacytic enteritis should include dietary hypersensitivity, giardiasis, bacterial overgrowth syndrome, intestinal lymphosarcoma, intestinal lymphangiectasia, and the other types of chronic inflammatory bowel disease.

Treatment. Lymphocytic-plasmacytic enteritis often responds to anti-inflammatory therapy using oral prednisolone (1 to 1.5 mg/lb/day divided q12h).[316, 317] In dogs, a low-fat diet consisting of Prescription Diets i/d, d/d or r/d fed in small amounts at frequent intervals may help to control the diarrhea. In some cats, dietary hypersensitivity may be a cause of lymphocytic-plasmacytic enterocolitis, and thus it may be appropriate before use of corticosteroid therapy to first consider a dietary trial using lamb and rice, horse meat, or Prescription Diets d/d or c/d.[323] Antibiotics such as tylosin are empirically efficacious in some animals,[326] which may suggest a role for bacterial overgrowth or bacterial-derived antigens in the pathogenesis. For dogs, the author recommends ½ to 1 tsp Tylan Plus Vitamins with food, q12h, and ⅛ to ¼ tsp for cats. Alternatively, tetracycline (10 mg/lb, q8h) or metronidazole (5 to 10 mg/lb, q12h) may be used. Because giardiasis may closely mimic this disease, consideration should be given to eliminating the possibility of "occult" *Giardia* infection by initial treatment with an antigiardial dosage of metronidazole (12 to 14 mg/lb, q12h for five days). In glucocorticoid-resistant cases, the addition of azathioprine (Imuran) to the steroid regimen at an oral dosage of 1 mg/lb/day for dogs or 0.14 mg/lb/day for cats may induce a remission of the disease.[316, 317] Laboratory parameters should be monitored for hematologic (leukopenia) and hepatotoxic side effects. In patients that respond to a four- to six-week induction regimen of prednisolone and/or azathioprine, the dosages are gradually tapered to lower maintenance dosages of prednisolone at 0.2 to 0.45 mg/lb once every other day, with or without azathioprine at the dosage above on the alternate days. Therapy may be discontinued on a trial basis after six to eight weeks of remission; however, continuous anti-inflammatory therapy is often required to prevent relapse. Sulfasala-

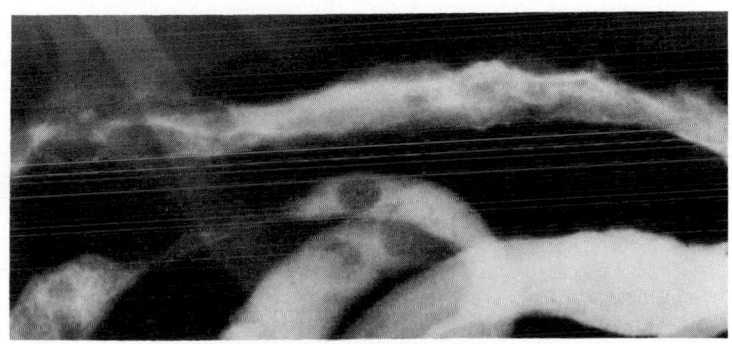

FIGURE 86–19. Barium radiography in this eight-year-old male Alaskan malamute with chronic watery diarrhea and protein-losing enteropathy demonstrated diffuse mucosal irregularity suggestive of an infiltrative bowel disorder. Intestinal biopsy showed diffuse lymphocytic-plasmacytic enteritis.

zine (12 to 18 mg/lb q8h) may be beneficial in patients in which the colon is involved (see Chapter 87).

Some animals with a biopsy diagnosis of lymphocytic-plasmacytic enteritis fail to respond to any treatment initially or later have relapse and rapid deterioration. This subgroup eventually dies (or is euthanatized) and is found at necropsy to have diffuse intestinal lymphosarcoma. Although misinterpretation of initial biopsies is always a possibility, more likely these animals represent progression of what was initially a precancerous lesion. In humans, immunoproliferative small intestinal disease is known to eventually evolve into enteromesenteric lymphoma.[327]

IMMUNOPROLIFERATIVE ENTEROPATHY OF BASENJIS

Immunoproliferative enteropathy is a progressive wasting disease of basenji dogs that is characterized by chronic intractable diarrhea and severe lymphocytic-plasmacytic infiltration of the lamina propria of the small intestine.[34, 324, 328–332] The underlying cause has been postulated to be a genetically determined abnormality of immunoregulation with variable phenotypic expression explained by environmental influences such as stress, diet, and concurrent illnesses.[331] The lesion of lymphocytic-plasmacytic enteritis in these dogs is thought to be the result of a chronic inflammatory reaction to intestinal antigens caused by the altered immunologic responsiveness. Because of extensive inbreeding, there is a high incidence of the disease in North American basenjis.

Clinical Signs. The onset of immunoproliferative enteropathy is insidious and may occur any time from shortly after birth up to several years of age, although most dogs are affected by three years of age.[329] Intermittent signs of anorexia, vomiting, and diarrhea are accompanied by progressive weight loss. Alopecia and dry haircoat are common physical findings, and some dogs have alopecia, pigmentation, and hyperkeratosis of the ear pinnae, occasionally with crusting and ulceration of the margins.[331] Affected dogs may have intestinal malabsorption complicated by functional exocrine pancreatic insufficiency, intestinal bacterial overgrowth, or hypergastrinemia.[34] The clinical course may extend from months to years with signs gradually increasing in frequency and severity. Historically, onset or exacerbation of clinical signs is often associated with stressful events such as boarding, transport, dog shows, surgery, vaccination, estrus, and pregnancy.[329]

A high incidence of associated disorders may contribute to the overall clinical syndrome, including hypothyroidism due to thyroid acinar atrophy, hypertrophic gastritis, membranous glomerulonephritis, and ulcerative dermatitis.[34, 324, 329] Because of extensive inbreeding, it is not uncommon for other genetic diseases of the basenji breed to be seen concurrently with immunoproliferative enteropathy, including pyruvate kinase deficiency anemia, persistent pupillary membranes, and Fanconi's syndrome.[329]

Diagnosis. The diagnosis of immunoproliferative enteropathy should be considered in any basenji with unexplained anorexia, vomiting, diarrhea, or weight loss. A history of chronic diarrhea in a littermate or close relative should increase the index of suspicion. Laboratory tests are generally not helpful until the disease is advanced, and only histologic evaluation of gastrointestinal biopsies provide a definitive diagnosis.

Overall, the most helpful screening test is probably serum protein electrophoresis. Serum albumin concentration is usually decreased and may drop below 1.0 gm/dl, while at the same time serum gamma globulin concentration is often increased.[34, 330] Decreased albumin is due to protein-losing enteropathy in some dogs, but inanition, malabsorption, and reciprocal effect from hypergammaglobulinemia probably also contribute. Mild ascites has been the only recognized consequence of hypoalbuminemia in these animals. Hypergammaglobulinemia may be the result of chronic antigenic stimulation or caused by some underlying defect in immunoregulation. It should be noted that this increased serum globulin concentration is unusual compared with the panhypoproteinemia typical for other canine protein-losing enteropathies (see Lymphangiectasia section). In addition to these protein derangements, mild anemia and mild liver enzyme elevations are found in some cases.[34]

The results of enteropancreatic function tests have been inconsistent. Xylose absorption tests usually demonstrate mild to moderate intestinal malabsorption, although severe impairment is found in some advanced cases.[34] Dogs with immunoproliferative enteropathy often have a depressed PABA curve in response to the bentiromide digestion test, suggesting either incomplete functional exocrine pancreatic insufficiency or PABA malabsorption.[34]

The diagnosis of immunoproliferative enteropathy is established by finding the characteristic lesion of diffuse lymphocytic-plasmacytic infiltration of the intestinal lamina propria in biopsy specimens.[324, 329] The villi are often short, blunt, and fused, and there may be variable lymphangiectasia of lacteals. Gastric mucosal biopsies may identify the associated lesions of hypertrophic or lymphocytic gastritis.[324, 329]

Treatment. Medical treatments that may improve immunoproliferative enteropathy include dietary manipulation, oral antibiotics, corticosteroids, and control of stress.[329, 331] Antibiotics such as tylosin, metronidazole, and trimethoprim-sulfadiazine have been used successfully to control diarrhea in affected animals. This beneficial response has been attributed to control of secondary intestinal bacterial overgrowth. Oral prednisolone at 1 mg/lb/day divided into two doses for five days followed by 0.5 mg/lb/day has produced dramatic improvement in some patients. If a beneficial response occurs, the dose is continued on an alternate-day basis for six months and then an attempt is made to gradually withdraw the animal from steroids.[331] Since exacerbations are often precipitated by stressful events, an effort should be made to minimize stress and changes in the dog's environment. In addition, client education in the area of genetic counseling is advisable.

Most dogs improve initially; some even seem to recover. However, stress-related exacerbations are frequent. The overall clinical course tends to be progressive in spite of treatment, with a survival time after first appearance of signs of generally less than two years, although five-year survival times have been recorded in a few cases.[329] Sequential biopsy studies have shown that the lesion in some dogs progresses from lymphocytic-plasmacytic enteritis to intestinal lymphosarcoma.[329]

CANINE EOSINOPHILIC GASTROENTERITIS

Eosinophilic gastroenteritis is a relatively uncommon and poorly understood disorder that is characterized by diffuse or segmental infiltration of some portion of the GI tract with mature eosinophils, usually accompanied by a peripheral eosinophilia.[315, 333–339] The disease may affect one or more layers of the stomach, small intestine, or colon, resulting in clinical syndromes of chronic vomiting (eosinophilic gastritis, see Chapter 85), chronic small bowel-type diarrhea (eosinophilic enteritis), chronic large bowel-type diarrhea (eosinophilic colitis, see Chapter 87), or any combination of these. Regional lymph nodes may also be enlarged and infiltrated with eosinophils.

The cause of eosinophilic gastroenteritis is unclear, but in humans evidence suggests that allergic or immunologic mechanisms that provoke infiltration of eosinophils into enteric tissues play a role.[340, 341] Some, but not all, human patients fulfill criteria for true food allergy, including positive skin test reactions and high serum IgE antibody concentrations to specific food substances.[340, 341] In animals, elimination diets and intradermal allergy testing have mostly been unsuccessful in implicating allergy to specific antigens. There is evidence in dogs that in at least some cases, the lesions may be associated with the visceral migration of *T. canis* larvae.[337, 342]

Clinical Signs. Eosinophilic gastroenteritis may affect any breed. Signs are usually chronic and determined by both the segment of the digestive tract involved as well as the predominant tissue layer infiltrated. Chronic diarrhea is the most consistent feature of the intestinal form. It may be accompanied by vomiting. Diffuse infiltration of eosinophils into the mucosal layer of the small bowel may cause malabsorption with watery diarrhea and weight loss and sometimes protein-losing enteropathy. Abdominal palpation may reveal diffusely thickened bowel loops. Diarrhea or vomitus may contain blood from mucosal erosions or ulcers. With submucosal or deeper involvement, intramural eosinophilic granulomatous lesions affecting the muscle layers occasionally cause a segmental tumor-like thickening in the gut wall that can partially obstruct the lumen and produce a palpable intestinal mass. When the large bowel is affected, bloody-mucoid diarrhea typical of colitis is the major sign (see Chapter 87).

The clinical course is generally one of chronically recurring diarrhea and progressive weight loss. Because eosinophilic gastroenteritis is usually steroid-responsive, it should be ascertained in the history if any previous use of glucocorticoids produced clinical improvement.

Diagnosis. Eosinophilic gastroenteritis must be differentiated from other malabsorptive and protein-losing enteropathies, and from intestinal parasitism. Once parasites have been ruled out, a diagnosis of eosinophilic gastroenteritis should be considered in any dog with chronic diarrhea and peripheral eosinophilia, although an increase in circulating eosinophils is not found in every patient. Laboratory findings may also include hypoproteinemia. Results of absorptive function tests are inconsistent but may indicate mild steatorrhea and impaired xylose absorption.[315]

In cases of diffuse infiltration of the mucosa, barium radiography may be normal or may indicate nonspecific thickening and mucosal irregularities and filling defects. In other cases with segmental mass-like lesions, barium may delineate sites of intramural thickening and partial luminal obstruction.

The diagnosis of eosinophilic gastroenteritis is established by identifying eosinophilic infiltration in intestinal biopsies. The lamina propria and submucosa often contain the heaviest accumulation of eosinophils, sometimes producing considerable distortion of the villi. Fibrosis and a mixture of other types of inflammatory cells may also be a component of the lesion. Mucosal biopsies taken endoscopically or by suction capsule are usually adequate; however, full-thickness biopsies may be necessary in patients in which infiltration predominates in the deeper layers of the bowel wall. Eosinophilic lesions that cause a localized nodular thickening of the gut wall, particularly within the muscle layer, may also have features of granulomatous inflammation. When these eosinophilic granulomas involve the ileocolic region, they are difficult to distinguish from regional granulomatous enteritis.[343, 344]

Unlike typical eosinophilic gastroenteritis in which the lesions are confined to the GI tract and regional lymph nodes, visceral larva migrans is a multi-visceral disease with widespread involvement of other organs. It probably should be considered a distinct disease in which eosinophilic enteritis and peripheral eosinophilia are components. In eosinophilic gastroenteritis associated with visceral larva migrans in dogs, focal granulomatous lesions are found in liver, spleen, lymph nodes, intestine, kidney, pancreas, lung, heart and diaphragm.[337, 342] These focal lesions are grossly visible as firm white nodules, one to three mm in diameter, randomly distributed on the surface and within the parenchyma of the various organs.

Treatment. Since eosinophilic gastroenteritis may potentially be due to food allergy, a feeding trial using an elimination or hypo-allergenic diet (such as lamb and rice or Prescription Diet d/d) may be considered initially; however, this approach is seldom effective in the author's hands.

The disease in dogs responds well to glucocorticoids and clinical signs improve rapidly, particularly when infiltration is limited mostly to the mucosa. Initially, oral prednisolone is given at 1 to 1.5 mg/lb daily in divided doses until the disease has been controlled for two to four weeks, then the dose is gradually tapered over an additional two to four weeks. In some dogs, the drug can eventually be discontinued, while others require prolonged alternate-day maintenance therapy to control signs. If relapses occur but are infrequent, then control of flare-ups with intermittent therapy is preferred to minimize the side effects of continuous steroid use. Azathioprine may be used to reestablish remission in patients that eventually fail to respond to prednisolone. Obstructing transmural eosinophilic granulomas involving a localized segment of bowel wall may be best managed by surgical excision followed by corticosteroid therapy.

Because visceral larva migrans has been implicated as a cause of eosinophilic gastroenteritis in at least some dogs,[337] there may be a role for the use of drugs such as fenbendazole (22 mg/lb q12h for 14 days),[108] ivermectin, thiabendazole, or Levamisole that potentially could have activity against migrating larvae of *T. canis*.

FELINE HYPEREOSINOPHILIC SYNDROME

Eosinophilic gastroenteritis also occurs as one manifestation of a hypereosinophilic syndrome in the cat that is characterized by widespread infiltration of eosinophils into various organs, including intestine, liver, spleen, lymph nodes, bone marrow, lung, pancreas, adrenals, and skin.[345–349] The extraintestinal involvement, progressive nature and high mortality rate of this syndrome indicate that it should be considered distinct from the more benign eosinophilic gastroenteritis that is confined to the GI tract. The etiopathogenesis is not known, but the feline disorder may be comparable with human hypereosinophilic syndrome.[350]

Vomiting, diarrhea (sometimes bloody), anorexia, and weight loss have been the most consistent clinical signs in cats with hypereosinophilic syndrome.[345, 346, 348, 349] Abdominal palpation may reveal intestinal thickening, hepatosplenomegaly, or mesenteric lymphadenopathy because of the disseminated visceral infiltration of eosinophils.[345, 349] In one cat, a large tumor-like enteropancreatic mass composed of eosinophilic and granulomatous inflammation was detected by palpation.[348] Another cat manifested a generalized pruritic exfoliative dermatitis.[347]

Persistent severe eosinophilia has been a consistent finding in affected cats.[345–349] The eosinophil count usually exceeds 1,500 cells/μl, and may reach as high as 40,000 cells/μl.[349] The diagnosis depends upon histopathologic confirmation of tissue infiltration of eosinophils in biopsies of affected organs. Ulceration and fibrosis may also be components of the intestinal lesion.

In contrast with the favorable prognosis for canine eosinophilic gastroenteritis, feline hypereosinophilic syndrome is often refractory to treatment; even with glucocorticoids, the usual outcome is progressive deterioration and death.[345, 346, 349] Nevertheless, remissions have been obtained using high-dose prednisolone induction (2 to 2.5 mg/lb/day for 2 to 4 weeks), followed by half this dose for 2 to 4 weeks, and then 0.5 to 1.0 mg/lb daily or on alternate days for maintenance.[349] Glucocorticoids must be continued indefinitely to maintain remission. Azathioprine (0.14 mg/lb, q48h) should be added in refractory cases. Surgical excision of intestinal segments that contain obstructing eosinophilic-granulomatous masses may also be beneficial.

GRANULOMATOUS (REGIONAL) ENTERITIS

Regional enteritis is a rare disease characterized by transmural granulomatous inflammation that usually involves the ileum and colon and results in a stenosing, mass-like thickening of a region of the bowel wall.[351–354] Regional lymph nodes and adjacent mesentery may also be involved. The lesion in some animals is heavily infiltrated with eosinophils,[343] making it difficult to distinguish from eosinophilic enterocolitis. Eosinophilic granuloma may be a more appropriate term to use for such cases.

The pathologic lesions in animals with regional granulomatous enteritis are comparable to those of regional enteritis in humans, also known as Crohn's disease.[351–354] The cause of the disease is unknown in either animals or humans; however, factors considered most likely to have a pathogenetic role include infectious agents, aberrant host immune or inflammatory responses, and immune-mediated processes that cause intestinal damage.[355] True regional granulomatous enteritis is idiopathic and must be differentiated from specific infectious or parasitic diseases of small animals that produce granulomatous intestinal lesions, such as histoplasmosis, phycomycosis, prototfecosis, mycobacteriosis, FIP, and whipworm infection.[281, 289, 291, 293, 294, 297, 298, 303, 354, 356–358]

Clinical Signs. Reports of canine regional enteritis have been in young dogs, four years of age or less, and predominantly in males.[343, 351, 353]

The author has seen similar lesions in cats. Chronic diarrhea and weight loss are the major clinical signs, sometimes accompanied by abdominal pain, tenesmus, anorexia, or lethargy.[343, 351, 353] The feces frequently contain fresh blood and may be characteristic of either small or large bowel disease or a combination of the two. The diseased segment of bowel is often palpable as a firm mass in the midabdomen. The adjacent intestinal loops may also be thickened and regional lymph nodes may be enlarged.

Diagnosis. Regional enteritis must be differentiated from other chronic inflammatory and neoplastic diseases of both the large and small intestine. The diagnosis should particularly be considered in any young dog with chronic debilitating hemorrhagic diarrhea and a palpable or radiographically demonstrated intestinal mass. Barium contrast radiography of the distal small intestine and colon may delineate a thickened or stenosed segment of bowel (Figure 86–20). Routine hematologic evaluation frequently reveals an eosinophilia and occasionally neutrophilia or monocytosis.[343, 351, 353] Panhypoproteinemia, presumably from excessive enteric protein loss, may also be a feature of this disorder.[353]

Definitive diagnosis of regional enteritis requires histopathologic examination of biopsies (taken by colonoscopy or laparotomy), along with appropriate special staining of the tissues for fungal and acid-fast organisms to rule out an infectious cause. The key histopathologic feature of regional enteritis is deep granulomatous inflammation involving all layers of the bowel wall.[343, 351, 353] Aggregates of epithelioid cells and giant cells are often found deep in the lesion.[353] In addition to granulomatous foci, other types of inflammatory cells and areas of fibrosis may be diffusely scattered through the layers of the bowel wall. Deep ulceration may also be a feature.

Treatment. Medical treatment of regional enteritis is based on the use of anti-inflammatory and immunosup-

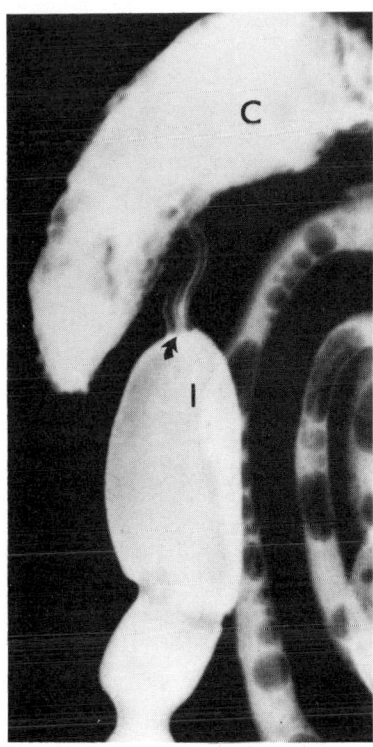
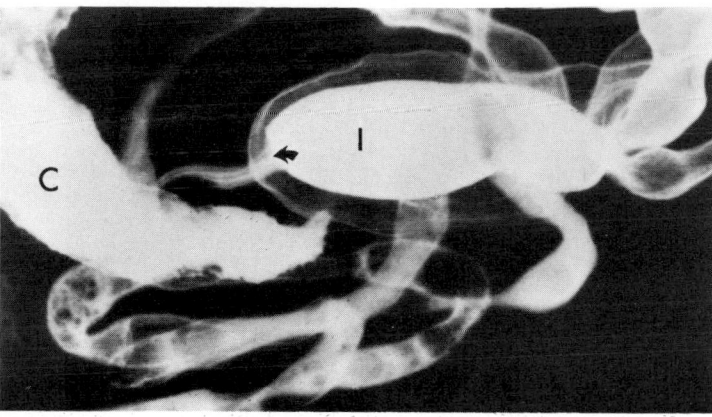

FIGURE 86–20. Ventrodorsal and lateral barium radiographs of this 13-year-old female (spayed) DSH revealed a circumferential constrictive lesion involving the terminal ileum (arrow). Notice the abrupt narrowing of the lumen of the ileum just before it enters the colon *(C)*, and the dilatation of the ileum *(I)* proximal to the stenosis. The tentative diagnosis was neoplasia (adenocarcinoma); however, histopathologic sections of the surgically resected segment revealed granulomatous ileitis. The same lesion was found several months later when surgery was again performed because of recurrence of regional thickening and stenosis of the terminal ileum. After the second surgery, remission was maintained for over a year with alternate-day corticosteroids. (Courtesy of Dr. Kirk Haupt.)

pressive agents, including oral prednisolone, sulfasalazine, azathioprine, and metronidazole.[355] Treatment suppresses the disease process but does not cure it, and response is unpredictable. The results in a limited number of cases of canine regional enteritis have been relatively disappointing. If a remission is obtained, usually treatment must continue indefinitely to maintain it. The regimens for use of these anti-inflammatory and immunosuppressive agents in inflammatory bowel disease are described in the Lymphocytic-Plasmacytic Enteritis section and in Chapter 87.

Surgical excision of the lesion is recommended because the degree of thickening and cicatrization of the affected segment of bowel wall is usually extreme, often producing stenosis and obliteration of the lumen. Surgery should be followed by medical therapy since a high recurrence rate at the surgical site is expected.

Protein-Losing Enteropathy and Intestinal Lymphangiectasia

The term protein-losing enteropathy refers to a variety of intestinal diseases that are associated with hypoproteinemia caused by an excessive loss of plasma proteins into the gut. The syndrome occurs most frequently in association with idiopathic intestinal lymphangiectasia;[49, 315, 359-373] however, other causes include chronic inflammatory small bowel diseases (lymphocytic-plasmacytic enteritis, granulomatous enteritis, eosinophilic enteritis, immunoproliferative enteropathy of basenjis), intestinal histoplasmosis, and intestinal lymphosarcoma.[33] The following discussion will emphasize lymphangiectasia; the other enteropathies are discussed in their respective sections of this chapter.

PATHOGENESIS

Under normal conditions, there is a daily loss of plasma proteins into the intestinal tract, probably resulting from leakage of protein from the lamina propria at sites of epithelial cell extrusion on the villous tips.[50] Once in the lumen, most of these extravasated plasma proteins are digested to their constituent amino acids and then reabsorbed. Gastrointestinal loss accounts for approximately 40 per cent of the normal daily turnover of plasma protein in the dog.[374] This enteric loss of protein is accelerated by disease processes that either disrupt the mucosal barrier or interfere with normal intestinal lymphatic drainage. Thus, protein-losing enteropathies can be classified as lymphogenic or mucosal, depending upon the primary mechanism of increased enteric loss of protein, namely: (1) disturbance of intestinal lymphatic drainage with reflux of protein-rich lymph into the lumen, or (2) disease of the mucosa with protein leakage resulting from exudation, bleeding, or increased permeability.[50] Hypoproteinemia, the hallmark of protein-losing enteropathy, develops when the rate of protein loss exceeds compensatory synthesis.

Lymphangiectasia is a chronic protein-losing enteropathy of the dog that is characterized by insufficiency and marked dilatation of the intestinal lymphatic network (Figure 86–21).[49, 315, 359-373] The intestinal lymphatics transport the products of fat absorption from the intestinal mucosa to the thoracic duct, which in turn channels chyle into the venous circulation.[375] Impaired intestinal drainage, presumably caused by obstruction to the normal lymphaticovenous flow, leads to stasis of chyle within dilated lacteals and lymphatics of the bowel wall and mesentery. Overdistended lacteals then release intestinal lymph into the gut lumen by rupture or extrav-

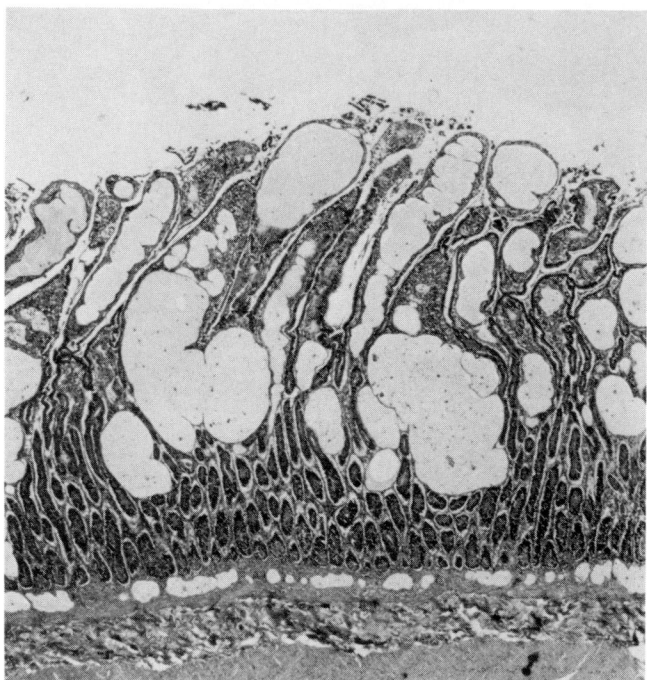

FIGURE 86–21. The hallmark lesion of lymphangiectasia is marked dilatation of lacteals (cystic-appearing areas distorting the villi) and deeper lymphatics, as demonstrated by this mucosal biopsy from a dog with protein-losing enteropathy. (From Fossum TW, et al.: Intestinal lymphangiectasia associated with chylothorax in two dogs. JAVMA 190:61, 1987).

asation, causing loss of the constituents of chyle–plasma proteins, lymphocytes, and lipid (chylomicrons). The protein concentration in chyle is 20 to 40 per cent of that found in plasma with a lymphocyte count of 900 to 7000/μl.[376] The disorder also interrupts lymphatic transport of chylomicrons from intestinal mucosa to venous circulation, which impairs the delivery phase of fat absorption. The functional consequences of lymphangiectasia, therefore, are panhypoproteinemia, lymphocytopenia, hypocholesterolemia, and fat malabsorption (steatorrhea and fat-soluble vitamin deficiency).

Canine intestinal lymphangiectasia is usually idiopathic; however, the potential causes include: (1) congenital malformation of the lymphatic system; (2) infiltration or obstruction of intestinal lymphatics due to an inflammatory, fibrosing, or neoplastic process; (3) obstruction of lymph flow through the thoracic duct; and (4) abnormal drainage and increased production of intestinal lymph resulting from the elevated central venous pressure of congestive heart failure, particularly constrictive pericarditis.[50] Intestinal lymphangiectasia with hypoproteinemia but not diarrhea has been produced experimentally in dogs by complete occlusion of all mesenteric lymphatics for one year.[377] Blockage of the thoracic duct for six months, however, failed to produce the lesion.[378] Pathologic studies of some cases of canine lymphangiectasia have demonstrated lymphangitis and extensive granulomatous inflammation in tissues adjacent to intestinal and mesenteric lymphatics (Figure 86–22),[49, 366–368, 370, 373, 379] observations that would seem to suggest acquired blockage of lymphatics by inflammatory lesions as the cause. However, it remains

to be established whether these lesions are a cause or effect of chyle stasis.[370, 373]

CLINICAL SIGNS

The clinical manifestations of lymphangiectasia are attributable mainly to the secondary effects of enteric loss of lymph constituents, particularly albumin, more so than to any direct impact the disease has on the function of the intestine itself. In fact, hypoproteinemia may be the only apparent manifestation of intestinal disease; affected animals may pass normal-appearing feces and be free of any other signs of intestinal disease.[367, 368]

The excessive enteric loss of plasma proteins in lymphangiectasia leads to hypoalbuminemia and reduced colloidal osmotic pressure of plasma. This in turn allows fluid transudation from capillaries and altered distribution of body fluid, resulting in edema and effusion. Consequently, presenting signs may include dependent pitting edema of subcutis and limbs, fluid distention of the abdomen (ascites), and respiratory distress (hydrothorax).[49, 315, 359–369, 372, 373]

Primary intestinal manifestations may be observed in lymphangiectasia, but they are usually relatively mild. Chronic intermittent or persistent diarrhea of a watery to semisolid consistency and often described as yellowish may be observed, but not all patients have diarrhea. Sporadic vomiting and lethargy have also been reported. Weight loss and progressive emaciation are commonly

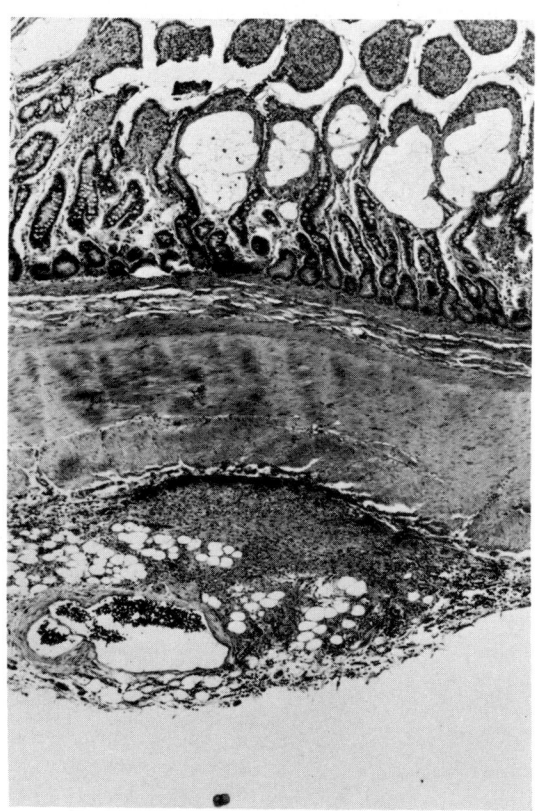

FIGURE 86–22. Full-thickness biopsy from a dog with protein-losing enteropathy, showing villous lesion of lymphangiectasia on the mucosal side, and a lipogranuloma associated with the lymphatics on the serosal (mesenteric) side.

associated with long-standing protein-losing enteropathy.

The signs of intestinal lymphangiectasia are often insidious in onset and tend to fluctuate in intensity, generally producing a clinical course that progresses slowly over a period of several weeks before the typical features of protein-losing enteropathy become apparent.

Lymphangiectasia can affect any breed of dog, but two breeds are reported to be predisposed–the lundehund, a spitz-like Norwegian breed,[362] and the basenji (see the Immunoproliferative Enteropathy of Basenjis section).[34]

DIAGNOSIS

A diagnosis of lymphangiectasia should be considered in animals manifesting hypoproteinemia, with or without edema or effusion, particularly when accompanied by lymphocytopenia, hypocholesterolemia, or hypoglobulinemia. The initial step in diagnosis is to exclude the nonenteric causes of hypoproteinemia, liver failure (impaired hepatic synthesis of albumin), and renal disease (protein-losing glomerulonephropathies), through liver function testing and urine protein determinations. In hypoproteinemia due to liver or kidney disease, it is usually only albumin that is decreased, whereas serum levels of both albumin and globulins are depleted in most patients with lymphangiectasia. Dogs with severe ascites due to intestinal lymphangiectasia may be misinterpreted as having congestive heart failure.

After exclusion of nonenteric causes of hypoproteinemia, intestinal lymphangiectasia must then be distinguished from other protein-losing enteropathies. Compared to the relatively mild or inapparent diarrhea of lymphangiectasia, dogs with protein-losing enteropathy caused by primary mucosal disease generally have persistently severe small intestinal diarrhea that begins before the development of hypoproteinemia. The findings of lymphocytopenia and/or hypocholesterolemia[49, 315, 359, 361–363, 367, 368, 372, 373] are more suggestive of lymphangiectasia than the nonlymphogenic (mucosal) protein-losing enteropathies. Gut function studies such as fecal fat determination and the xylose absorption test may be abnormal in dogs with lymphangiectasia but are not consistently so.[49, 315, 363, 365] Steatorrhea is the predominant abnormality since dilated lacteals leak chylomicron-laden lymph into the lumen and also prevent the normal assimilation of dietary fat.

Hypocalcemia is a frequent finding in lymphangiectasia.[49, 360, 362, 365, 368, 372, 373] A number of factors are probably responsible: decreased protein-bound fraction of calcium associated with hypoalbuminemia, vitamin D malabsorption, and malabsorption of calcium that is complexed in the intestinal lumen with fatty acids and proteins. One hypocalcemic dog with lymphangiectasia was reported to have had calcium-responsive seizures.[49]

Ancillary diagnostic procedures that may be helpful include (1) cardiac evaluation to exclude a cardiac cause of lymphangiectasia; (2) radiography to detect or confirm ascites and pleural effusion; and (3) fluid analysis of body cavity effusions. The effusion associated with lymphangiectasia is usually a transudate. Chylous ascites is sometimes found, apparently due to leakage of chy-

lous lymph fluid from distended or diseased mesenteric and serosal lymphatics.[364] Intestinal lymphangiectasia has also been associated with chylothorax in two dogs.[84] Mesenteric lymphangiography in one of these demonstrated retrograde flow of contrast agent into the intestinal lymphatics and failure of the contrast agent to enter the thoracic duct.[84]

A definitive diagnosis of lymphangiectasia is established by histologic confirmation of the characteristic mucosal lesion in intestinal biopsies. This also is often the best means of differentiating the various other chronic protein-losing and malabsorptive enteropathies. Biopsies may be obtained via laparotomy, or less invasively by endoscopy or peroral suction biopsy capsule. When the animal is severely hypoproteinemic and the less invasive biopsy techniques are unavailable, consideration should be given to obtaining the diagnosis from gross appearance and biopsy of the characteristic serosal and mesenteric lymphatic lesions described below. These lesions, when present, are distinctive and as indicative of the diagnosis as the mucosal and intramural lesions, and this approach avoids the risk of dehiscence that is inherent with a full-thickness enterotomy incision.

Dilated, chyle-filled lacteals and intestinal lymphatics are the hallmarks of lymphangiectasia.[49, 315, 359–373] At surgery a prominent, web-like network of distended, milky-white lymphatic channels are usually seen in the mesentery and on the serosal surface of the gut (Figure 86–23). In many cases, yellow-white nodular masses 1 to 5 mm in size and foamy granular deposits are observed in and around mesenteric and subserosal lymphatics, especially adjacent to the mesenteric attachment (Figures 86–22 and 86–24).[49, 367, 370, 372, 373, 379] These so-called lipogranulomas consist of focal accumulations of large, foamy lipid-laden macrophages (lipophages). The pathogenesis of these lipogranulomatous lesions associated with lymphangiectasia is unknown, but it has been proposed that they are evoked by extravasation of stagnated chyle and fat into perilymphatic tissues.[367, 370, 373]

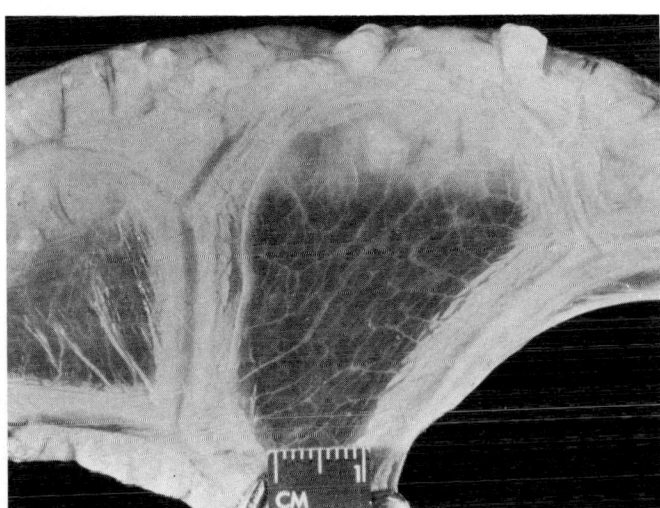

FIGURE 86–23. A web-like network of dilated lymphatic channels is seen in the mesentery of a dog with lymphangiectasia. Also, notice the nodular lesions (lipogranulomas) at the mesenteric border of the intestine.

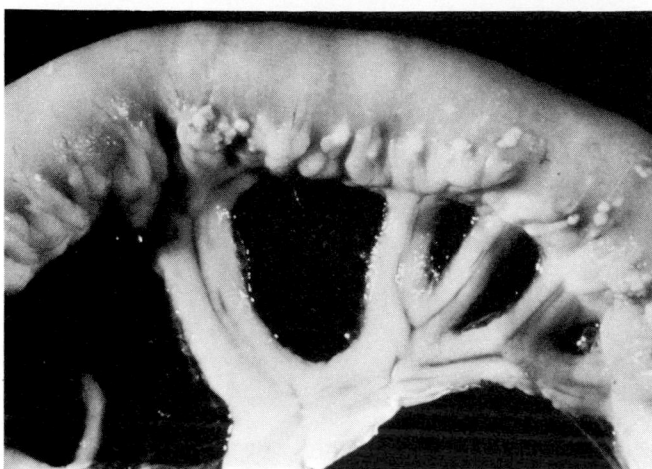

FIGURE 86–24. Lipogranulomas are visible as white nodules along the mesenteric border of the intestine and associated with lymphatics in a dog with lymphangiectasia.

The characteristic histopathologic lesion of the mucosa in intestinal lymphangiectasia is a ballooning distortion of villi caused by markedly dilated lacteals (see Figure 86–21). There also is usually edema and a diffuse or multifocal accumulation of lymphocytes and plasma cells in the lamina propria. Lymphangitis, with or without lipogranulomatous lesions, can involve lymph channels in all layers of the bowel wall and mesentery.[370]

TREATMENT

The major goal in treating intestinal lymphangiectasia is to decrease the enteric loss of plasma proteins so that normal plasma protein levels can be restored and edema and effusions controlled. This is accomplished with dietary manipulation and anti-inflammatory therapy.[33, 372]

The absorption of dietary long-chain triglyceride (LCT) is a major stimulus for intestinal lymph flow. Restriction of dietary intake of LCT reduces the protein loss in lymphangiectasia.[380, 381] This is presumably because reduction of lymph flow and lymphatic hydrostatic pressure decreases the distention and rupture of lacteals. Since LCT incorporated into chylomicrons possibly escapes from diseased lymphatics into surrounding tissues and contributes to the formation of perilymphatic lipogranulomas, restriction of dietary LCT may also have a beneficial effect in reducing these lesions.[367] Fat restriction also ameliorates diarrhea by reducing steatorrhea.

The ideal diet for the dog with lymphangiectasia should contain minimal fat (LCT) and provide an ample quantity of high-biologic quality protein. A special commercial diet that fulfills these requirements is generally adequate and convenient in most cases (Prescription Diet r/d). Because of the fat malabsorption that occurs in lymphangiectasia, diets should be supplemented with fat-soluble vitamins (vitamins A, D, and E by IM injection and vitamin K, orally). Daily food intake should be divided into two or three feedings.

Homemade diets are another alternative; for example, one part low-fat cottage cheese or yogurt as the protein source expanded with three to four parts rice or potatoes as the carbohydrate source. Homemade diets are not balanced, so vitamin-mineral supplements should be added, again with extra fat-soluble vitamins.

Low-fat diets are inherently low in calories; this works against another goal of the therapy, to promote regain of lost weight. Therefore, medium-chain triglyceride (MCT) can be added to the diet to replace the calories lost by removal of conventional fat (LCT) from the diet. MCT is useful as a source of calories in states of fat malabsorption because they are hydrolyzed more rapidly and efficiently than LCT, and then are absorbed directly into the portal venous system, bypassing chylomicron formation and the diseased, nonfunctional lymphatic transport system. Commercially available MCT is derived from coconut oil and can be added to the daily ration as an oil (MCT Oil; 8.3 Kcal/gm; 1 tbsp weighs 14 gm and contains 115 Kcal) at 0.5 to 1 ml/lb body weight, or as a powdered elemental diet mixture (Portagen; 1½ cups added to water to make 1 quart of mixture with 30 Kcal/fluid oz). This latter mixture is hypertonic and may cause vomiting or aggravate diarrhea. With either MCT source, a low dose should be used at first and then gradually increased in daily increments for better patient acceptance and to minimize diarrhea.

The plasma protein loss and diarrhea of lymphangiectasia often benefit from anti-inflammatory doses of corticosteroids (prednisolone, 1.0 to 1.5 mg/lb/day, PO).[33, 372] Once remission has been achieved, this dosage should be adjusted to a lower maintenance level. The beneficial effects of anti-inflammatory therapy may be in reducing the associated inflammatory lesions of intestinal lymphangiectasia: lymphangitis, lipogranulomas, and lymphocytic-plasmacytic lamina propria infiltrate. However, not all cases of lymphangiectasia are steroid-responsive.[367] In addition to dietary management and corticosteroids, antibiotics to control secondary bacterial overgrowth should be considered.

Lymphangiectasia does not respond predictably to therapy. In most patients, the combination of dietary and anti-inflammatory therapy relieves clinical signs, maintains normal plasma protein values, and eliminates effusions (Figure 86–25), but a cure should not be expected. Remissions of several months' duration are not uncommon, and in some patients remissions have been maintained for years.[367, 369, 372] On the other hand, some animals entirely fail to respond. Many of those dogs that do respond eventually relapse and finally succumb to severe protein-calorie depletion, incapacitating effusions, or intractable diarrhea.

Villous Atrophy

Villous atrophy is a lesion characterized by short, blunted mucosal villi that is found in some animals with unexplained intestinal malabsorption and chronic diarrhea.[73, 87–91, 315, 325, 382–384] Dietary, secondary, and idiopathic forms of villous atrophy occur, and they may be categorized as follows: (1) idiopathic canine villous atrophy;[73, 87, 315, 325, 382–384] (2) wheat-sensitive enteropathy in the Irish setter[88–91, 384] and possibly other breeds that resembles gluten enteropathy of humans (celiac disease,

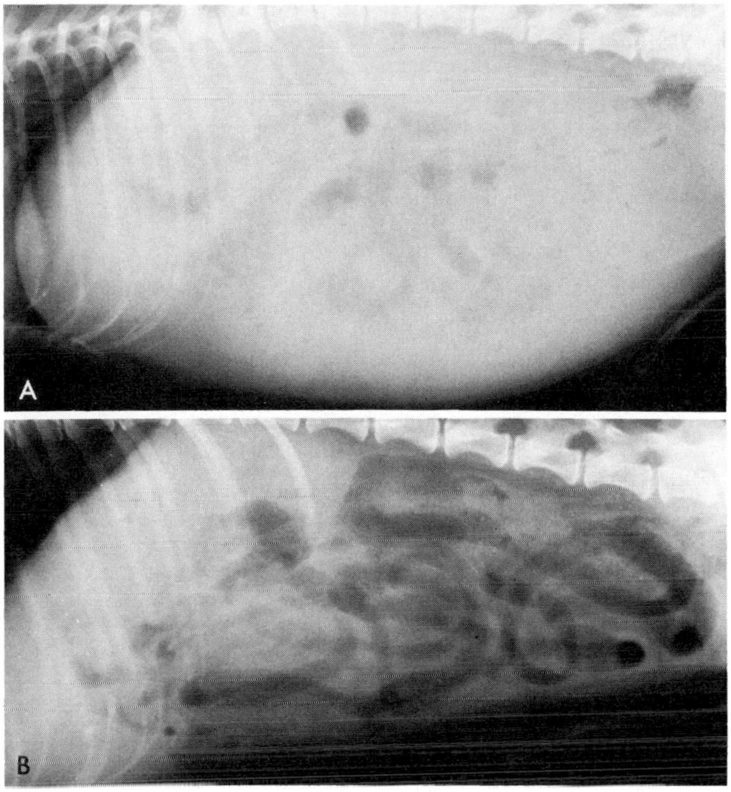

FIGURE 86–25. Although the lesions of lymphangiectasia may be irreversible, medical management based on dietary restriction of long-chain fatty acids can elevate plasma protein levels and control effusions. Abdominal radiographs of a dog with lymphangiectasia and an initial serum albumin of 0.9 mg/dl were taken before *(A)* and during *(B)* treatment to show resolution of abdominal effusion in response to therapy.

nontropical sprue); (3) villous atrophy secondary to infiltrative diseases of the intestinal wall, such as lymphosarcoma[73, 315, 485] or chronic inflammatory bowel disease;[315] and (4) villous atrophy secondary to specific enteric infections, such as from viruses (coronavirus,[188] rotavirus[194]), bacteria (bacterial overgrowth syndrome),[93] or parasites *(Giardia)*.[143]

In addition, findings in infants indicate that mucosal atrophy may also occur as a nonspecific response to severe protein-calorie malnutrition.[368] The discussion that follows focuses on the first two categories listed above in which villous atrophy is apparently the primary disturbance.

Histologic examination is usually adequate for documentation of villous atrophy, but since this is a nonspecific lesion found in a variety of different enteropathies, the diagnosis and characterization of these enteropathies are mainly based on breed predilection, the response to withdrawal of gluten from the diet, tests or procedures to identify enteric infections, and the combination of morphologic and biochemical abnormalities in jejunal biopsies.[384]

IDIOPATHIC VILLOUS ATROPHY

Unexplained villous atrophy is occasionally found in dogs with moderate to severe malabsorption.[73, 315, 325] Although there are similarities between this canine disease and a human enteropathy called tropical sprue,[87, 382, 383] a severe progressive tetracycline-responsive malabsorption syndrome endemic in humans inhabiting tropical regions, there is little evidence that the two diseases share a common cause. Therefore, for now, the disease in dogs should be considered an idiopathic villous atrophy.

Clinical Signs. Idiopathic villous atrophy is associated with severe, chronic small bowel-type diarrhea and weight loss.[73, 87, 315, 325] Overt steatorrhea may[73, 315, 325] or may not[87] be observed. The mechanism of the diarrhea is presumably intestinal malabsorption caused by the loss of mucosal surface area and impairment of microvillus membrane function.[87] There is generally no history of response to dietary manipulations, including withdrawal of gluten from the diet.

Reported cases have been predominantly middle-aged dogs, although a four-month-old German shepherd puppy in one early report was so severely affected that its growth was stunted by approximately 50 per cent compared with an unaffected littermate.[325] Interestingly, the majority of dogs reported with idiopathic villous atrophy have been German shepherds.[73, 87, 325] However, it remains to be determined whether this represents a true breed predilection or whether the villous atrophy is a secondary response to bacterial overgrowth or some other underlying disorder.

Diagnosis. Results of gut function studies in idiopathic villous atrophy reflect impaired mucosal function and include variable steatorrhea;[73, 315, 325] decreased or low-normal xylose absorption;[87, 315] decreased serum concentrations of vitamin A,[325] vitamin B$_{12}$,[87, 384] and folate;[87, 384] normal pancreatic function tests (bentiromide test and serum trypsin-like immunoassay);[87] and sometimes hypoproteinemia.[73, 315] Regarding the vitamin assays, the serum folate value depends upon the absorptive function of the proximal small intestine (jejunum), while the serum value of vitamin B$_{12}$ reflects absorption in the distal small intestine (ileum). Accordingly, serum concentration of both folate and vitamin B$_{12}$ are decreased in enteropathies such as this one that cause diffuse intestinal malabsorption.[63] Biochemical analysis of jejunal biopsies from dogs with idiopathic villous atrophy have indicated reduced activities of many brush border enzymes.[63] Since villous atrophy may be a secondary lesion, underlying causes such as bacterial overgrowth should be considered.

Histopathologic examination of biopsy specimens from dogs with idiopathic villous atrophy generally reveals a severe mucosal lesion that varies from a patchy distribution of short, plump villi with blunt tips interspersed among relatively normal villi,[87] to a more obliterative lesion characterized by complete absence of villi.[73, 315, 325] There are ultrastructural changes in some enterocytes, including damaged microvilli. In addition, mucosal cellularity is usually increased due to an infiltration of lymphocytes and plasma cells, and in some cases there is fibrosis in the lamina propria and submucosa.[87, 315, 325] Because of the dense infiltrate of mononuclear cells in the lamina propria in some patients, it is difficult to determine if the lesion should be categorized as a primary idiopathic villous atrophy or as a chronic inflammatory disease (lymphocytic-plasmacytic enteritis) with secondary villous atrophy (see Lymphocytic-Plasmacytic Enteritis section). Whether or not this distinction is important will depend on future understanding of the etiopathogenesis of these disorders.

Treatment. Dogs with idiopathic villous atrophy are refractory to dietary management (gluten restriction) and are treated with pharmacologic doses of folate and vitamin B_{12}, oxytetracycline, and prednisolone. In this disorder, both folate and vitamin B_{12} are often deficient due to malabsorption, which can lead to further impairment of mucosal integrity.[384] In tropical sprue of humans, treatment with folic acid ameliorates or cures the disease, indicating that folate deficiency may even play a role in perpetuating the intestinal lesion.[387] Therefore, folate is given orally at 5 mg/day and continued indefinitely, and vitamin B_{12} administered IM at 500 µg/month for six months.[384]

In some patients a favorable response is obtained with the use of antibiotics such as oxytetracycline, tylosin, or metronidazole to empirically treat bacterial overgrowth (see Bacterial Overgrowth section). Tetracyclines are highly successful for treatment of tropical sprue in humans. Use of the antibiotic metronidazole may also treat an undiagnosed *Giardia* infection.

Dogs with a diagnosis of idiopathic villous atrophy frequently fail to respond to dietary modification, vitamin supplementation, and antibiotics. In such patients, anti-inflammatory dosages of glucocorticoids may produce clinical improvement.[87] Thus, oral prednisolone (0.5 to 1.5 mg/lb/day) should be initiated when the combination of these other measures does not alleviate signs. The beneficial effect may be due to anti-inflammatory, immunosuppressive, or enterocyte-stimulating[388] actions. If effective, the prednisolone should be continued at this dosage for at least four weeks and then gradually reduced to an alternate-day regimen for an additional six to eight weeks. Oral prednisolone is not helpful in all patients, but those which do benefit may require it indefinitely.

A novel but as yet unsubstantiated approach to stimulate regrowth of the atrophic mucosa is through administration of cimetidine to induce meal-stimulated hyper-gastrinemia, which in turn has a trophic effect on the mucosa. This reportedly was effective in a human patient.[389]

The prognosis for idiopathic villous atrophy is guarded. Approximately half of the animals fail to respond to these treatment measures and either are euthanatized because of intractable diarrhea and debilitation or die of malnutrition.

WHEAT-SENSITIVE ENTEROPATHY

Another distinct enteropathy of dogs is characterized by partial villous atrophy, deficiency or delayed development of specific microvillus enzymes, dietary sensitivity to wheat, and an apparent breed predilection for Irish setters in Great Britain.[88–91, 384] Preliminary studies have demonstrated an early-age onset of this enteropathy in a litter bred from two affected Irish setters, suggesting that it is an inherited disorder.[88–91, 384] When placed on a gluten-free diet (e.g., rice), afflicted animals demonstrate dramatic villous regeneration, restoration of normal biochemical parameters, and resolution of clinical signs, and then when subsequently rechallenged with wheat flour, there is relapse with recurrence of villous atrophy.[91] Because of these observations, this disorder is considered to resemble gluten-sensitive enteropathy (celiac disease, nontropical sprue) of humans.[88–91, 384] This human disorder is characterized by severe villous atrophy and malabsorption from the interaction of gluten, the water-insoluble protein moiety of certain cereal grains (wheat, barley, rye, oats), with the intestinal mucosa in susceptible individuals.[390] The pathogenesis of gluten-induced mucosal damage is not entirely understood; however, proposed mechanisms have included (1) immune hypersensitivity to dietary gluten, (2) receptor-like defect of intestinal cell membrane that allows gluten to bind to the cell surface like a lectin leading to cytotoxicity, and (3) accumulation of cytotoxic, partially digested products of gluten because of an inborn deficiency of an enzyme (missing peptidase) necessary for complete digestion of the protein.[390] As in wheat-sensitive enteropathy of Irish setters, genetic factors are considered important in gluten-induced enteropathy of humans, and additionally, withdrawal of the offending substance, gluten, from the diet results in prompt clinical remission in human patients.

Clinical Signs. The predominant sign of wheat-sensitive enteropathy of Irish setters is weight loss or poor weight gain, with or without mild chronic intermittent diarrhea.[88–91, 384] Afflicted dogs are thin and may have a poor quality haircoat. Appetite varies from periodic inappetence to polyphagia. The age of onset is usually four to seven months, but the disease has been seen in a dog as old as seven years. The mucosal lesion and degree of malabsorption are generally quite mild, and thus diarrhea is not as consistent a feature or as severe as seen in many other chronic enteropathies.

Diagnosis. In wheat-sensitive enteropathy, xylose absorption and serum folate concentration are usually either normal or both mildly depressed, whereas serum concentration of vitamin B_{12}, quantitative bacterial culture of the small intestine, and results of pancreatic function tests are all within normal limits.[88–90, 384] Biochemical analyses reveal decreased activity of selected brush border enzymes; notably, peptidases are reduced while disaccharidases are not, indicating perhaps a greater propensity for malabsorption of protein.[88–91] These findings are compatible with mild or patchy mucosal disease of the proximal small intestine, which is consistent with the morphologic alterations found in affected dogs.[88–91, 384]

The lesion identified in intestinal biopsies from Irish setters with wheat-sensitive enteropathy is partial villous atrophy with a noticeably patchy distribution.[88–91, 384] The villous atrophy in these animals is generally less severe than typically seen in the dogs with idiopathic villous atrophy or in humans with gluten-sensitive enteropathy.[88–91, 384] Rarely, however, these Irish setters can have extreme mucosal flattening. There is also a lymphocytic-plasmacytic infiltration of the lamina propria.[91] By definition, affected dogs should respond to gluten (wheat) withdrawal. Thus, the villous atrophy is completely reversed with elimination of wheat from the diet but then predictably recurs if wheat is reintroduced into the diet.[88–91, 384]

Treatment. The role of gluten in the pathogenesis of this disease needs to be further defined. Nevertheless, in wheat-sensitive Irish setters, and possibly in other breeds, the signs and lesions of villous atrophy resolve with complete elimination of cereal grains from the diet.[91, 384] Thus, since dietary modification may result in rapid clinical improvement with no additional treatment, trial feeding of a gluten-restricted diet should be used initially in all Irish setters with villous atrophy. Most commercial dog foods contain gluten; however, the following gluten-free diets are available: d/d and i/d Prescription Diets; Science Maximum Stress Diet, Canine Growth Diet, Iams Chunks, Plus, and Eukanuba. Alternately, since corn and rice do not contain gluten, homemade diets formulated with these grains and lean meat, low-fat cottage cheese, and potatoes can be used. Other general dietary measures mentioned in the Treatment section also apply.

If the animal responds to dietary modification, then the prognosis is excellent, although gluten restriction must continue for life. Since wheat-sensitive enteropathy appears to be hereditary in Irish setters, breeding of affected animals should be discouraged.

Small Intestinal Bacterial Overgrowth

Bacterial overgrowth syndrome is an overproliferation of microflora within the proximal small intestine that results in malabsorption and diarrhea (also called the contaminated bowel, blind loop, or stagnant loop syndrome).[79, 80, 391–393] In the dog, bacterial overgrowth is defined as a fasting bacterial count in duodenal juice of greater than 10^5 organisms per ml.[92–94, 394–397]

PATHOGENESIS

The normal small intestinal microflora is a sparse but stable population of aerobic and facultative anaerobic bacteria whose growth is regulated and influenced by a combination of host factors, bacterial interactions, and dietary composition. Factors that normally control the growth of bacteria in the small bowel include: (1) the mechanical self-cleansing action of normal intestinal motility and continuous downstream flow of ingesta, (2) the decontamination of ingesta by normal gastric acidity, (3) the inhibitory properties of luminal bile acids and pancreatic juice, (4) the characteristics of the intestinal mucous barrier, (5) the gastrointestinal immune mechanisms, (6) the competitive interactions between bacteria such as mutual competition for nutrients and inhibitory effects of bacterial metabolic by-products on other bacteria, and (7) an ileocolic valve that functions as an antireflux barrier separating the small and large bowel, thereby maintaining an enormous bacterial population gradient across this valve of 10^{11} organisms per ml in the colon versus 10^5 or less in the small bowel.[79, 80, 391–393]

Failure of any one of these normal regulatory mechanisms may produce an environment in the intestinal lumen favorable for bacterial proliferation. Numerous underlying conditions in humans are known to be associated with bacterial overgrowth, especially abnormalities of intestinal structure or motor function that result in stasis of intestinal contents. In dogs, only recently has small intestinal bacterial overgrowth been recognized as a cause of diarrhea.[92–94, 396–401] Since documentation of bacterial overgrowth is difficult, the syndrome may occur more frequently in dogs and cats than is generally recognized. Development of an abnormal small bowel flora should be considered a potential secondary complication of intestinal surgery; stasis-producing mechanical obstructions such as chronic intestinal foreign bodies and stenosing neoplastic or inflammatory (regional enteritis) lesions of the gut; destructive lesions of the ileocecocolonic junction that allow colonoenteric reflux; motility disorders such as idiopathic intestinal pseudo-obstruction; immune deficiency states; conditions associated with hyposecretion of gastric acid; and exocrine pancreatic insufficiency.[402] A demonstrable underlying anatomic or functional predisposition is not identified in most cases of canine bacterial overgrowth. Exocrine pancreatic insufficiency in the dog is frequently complicated by bacterial overgrowth (see Chapter 90).[397] In addition, there may be a breed predilection in German shepherds for an enteropathy associated with bacterial overgrowth,[92–94] possibly related to the relative deficiency of serum IgA found in this breed.[403]

The pathogenesis of malabsorption and diarrhea associated with the bacterial overgrowth syndrome involves complex disturbances of both luminal digestion and mucosal function.[79, 80, 391–393] Absorption of ingested fat, carbohydrate (including xylose), and protein is impaired by mucosal damage combined with the intraluminal degradation of those nutrients as substrates for bacterial metabolism. Mucosal injury is mediated by the toxic effect of bacterial metabolites on epithelial cells and not by bacterial invasion of the mucosa. Mucosal morphology in bacterial overgrowth may be normal or characterized by shortening and broadening of villi with an increased mononuclear cell population within the lamina propria. Even when histologic changes in the mucosa are minimal or absent, distinct biochemical abnormalities suggestive of enterocyte damage and disturbance of the microvillus membranes are demonstrable in animals with bacterial overgrowth syndrome.[93, 94]

Bacterial action on intraluminal bile acids and fatty acids may also play a role in the pathogenesis of diarrhea.[79, 80, 391–393] Bacterial deconjugation of bile acids further impairs fat absorption, contributing substantially to the steatorrhea. Unconjugated bile acids may also stimulate intestinal water and electrolyte secretion and cause mucosal brush border damage. Hydroxylated fatty acids, produced from bacterial metabolism of unabsorbed fatty acids, may also promote diarrhea by stimulating intestinal fluid secretion.

Abnormalities of vitamin metabolism are important clinical consequences of intestinal bacterial overgrowth. Deficiency of vitamin B_{12} together with an increased serum concentration of folate is a relatively unique combination of manifestations that is highly suggestive of bacterial overgrowth.[63] Malabsorption of vitamin B_{12} is attributed to intraluminal retention of the vitamin because of avid binding by bacteria and to direct bacterial metabolism of vitamin B_{12} to inactive derivatives. Consequently, serum concentration of vitamin B_{12} in dogs with bacterial overgrowth is often abnormally low. At the same time, serum folate concentration is usually elevated due to bacterial synthesis of folate within the intestinal tract.[63, 92, 93, 404]

CLINICAL SIGNS

The clinical signs of bacterial overgrowth are variable, depending somewhat on the underlying cause of the abnormal proliferation of flora. The syndrome is most often characterized by chronic, foul-smelling watery diarrhea, steatorrhea, and weight loss.[93, 399, 401] Blood or mucus are not usually present in the feces. Bacterial overgrowth may be responsible for failure of some dogs with exocrine pancreatic insufficiency to respond adequately to enzyme supplementation.[397]

DIAGNOSIS

Small intestinal bacterial overgrowth should be considered in any animal with unexplained small bowel diarrhea and malabsorption, especially if accompanied by any of the following observations which aid in the recognition of bacterial overgrowth syndrome: (1) responsiveness to antibiotics, (2) evidence of delayed intestinal transit of barium radiographically (whether due to anatomic or motility disturbances), (3) absence of definitive morphologic abnormalities in intestinal biopsies, or (4) failure to obtain the expected treatment response in other intestinal disorders known to be conducive to bacterial overgrowth (such as exocrine pancreatic insufficiency). Animals with bacterial overgrowth should be evaluated for underlying disorders or predisposing factors.

Definitive diagnosis of small intestinal bacterial overgrowth can be established only by quantitative aerobic and anaerobic cultures of aspirated duodenal juice obtained by intestinal intubation or laparotomy, either collection method generally requiring general anesthesia. Culture specimens are taken after an 18-hour

fast and must be processed promptly and meticulously. A criterion of greater than 10^5 organisms/ml is used in the dog for diagnosis of bacterial overgrowth.[92–94, 397] The overgrowth is usually composed mostly of various bacteria that make up the normal flora—aerobes, anaerobes, or a combination of both.

There are also indirect, noninvasive methods of diagnosis that are based on the detection of bacterial metabolites in the blood (serum folate), urine (indican, phenols), or expired air (breath tests).[79, 80, 393] Breath tests measure the breath excretion of volatile metabolites produced by the intraluminal action of bacteria on orally administered test substrates. They may use radiolabeled substrates, such as bile acids, amino acids, or xylose, which release radioactive $^{14}CO_2$, or nonlabeled carbohydrates, which release hydrogen. These breath tests are widely used in humans, and investigation of a hydrogen excretion breath test in dogs with malabsorption has shown promise as a clinical diagnostic tool.[64, 65, 82] A urine nitrosonaphthol test has been used as a screening test for bacterial overgrowth in dogs but is relatively nonspecific since various other disorders of the small intestine frequently affect the results.[81]

Since intraluminal bacteria may synthesize folate and bind or compete for vitamin B_{12}, as mentioned previously, a finding of elevated serum folate concentration accompanied by reduced serum level of vitamin B_{12} has been clinically reliable as an indirect indicator of bacterial overgrowth in dogs.[63, 92, 93]

Currently the diagnosis of bacterial overgrowth in most clinical situations is made circumstantially on the basis of signs and results of indirect laboratory tests. Then, diarrhea and abnormal intestinal function tests should resolve with appropriate antibacterial therapy.

Once bacterial overgrowth has been diagnosed, an effort should be made to rule out underlying causes. Bacterial overgrowth has been associated with chronic inflammatory bowel disease,[400] basenji enteropathy,[34] parasitism (Giardia, ascarids),[93] exocrine pancreatic insufficiency,[397] and idiopathic pseudo-obstruction (dilated, hypomotile segment of gut).[398] An effort should be made to identify if these and other associated disorders may be present. Biopsy of the intestine may be useful for differentiating bacterial overgrowth from primary mucosal diseases. Intestinal biopsies from animals with bacterial overgrowth usually have minimal or mild lesions that are patchy in distribution and relatively nonspecific, such as partial villous atrophy and mild lymphocytic-plasmacytic infiltrate.

TREATMENT

The presence of a treatable underlying cause should always be sought and managed appropriately. In cases involving stasis caused by anatomic abnormalities, this may include surgery. Overgrowth of microflora usually responds to antibiotic therapy and dietary modification. The choice of an antibiotic is empiric, since any of several different bacteria with variable antibacterial susceptibilities may be involved. Oral broad-spectrum antimicrobials and those with activity against anaerobes are recommended, such as tetracycline, oxytetracycline, chloramphenicol, ampicillin, metronidazole, tylosin, lincomycin, and erythromycin. Treatment should continue for at least 10 to 14 days, and can be repeated as necessary. Some animals need treatment at frequent intervals or even continuously, while others may remain in remission for months after just one course of antibiotics. The clinical signs and abnormal function tests usually resolve within the first week of therapy, which in itself is good indirect evidence in support of the diagnosis.

In addition to antibacterial therapy, general principles of dietary management for malabsorption should be followed (see Treatment section). Vitamin supplementation should be considered, particularly vitamin B_{12}, which can be given as a 500 μg injection monthly. Treatment with lactobacillus or yogurt culture is generally considered not to be effective for altering the enteric microflora.

Short Bowel Syndrome

Short bowel syndrome refers to a condition of intestinal malabsorption with diarrhea and malnutrition that follows resection of a large portion of the small intestine. It is important clinical syndrome of humans and a relatively uncommon one in animals.[405, 406] The syndrome is manifested by progressive weight loss and chronic persistent watery diarrhea that is foul-smelling without obvious blood or mucus.[405, 406] Weight loss may occur in spite of a ravenous appetite.[406] Signs may be ameliorated by feeding of a low-fat diet.[406]

Some of the more likely underlying disorders that may potentially require extensive bowel resection in dogs and cats include intussusception, intestinal volvulus, bowel infarction (necrosis), and severe intestinal damage associated with certain foreign bodies such as linear ("string") intestinal foreign bodies. The minimum intestinal remnant, i.e., remaining absorptive surface area, that is capable of eventually adapting adequately to prevent gastrointestinal insufficiency following massive bowel resection depends on a number of factors: the site and extent of the resection, the presence or absence of a functioning ileocolonic valve, the functional integrity of the residual gut, and the degree of adaptive change in the remnant.[407–409] The ileum is a superior remnant to the jejunum because of its inherently slower transit time, its role in vitamin B_{12} and bile acid absorption, and its greater capacity for adaptation.[409] In addition, the preservation of the ileocolonic valve in the remnant may influence the outcome of resection because of the role it plays as a barrier to small intestinal bacterial overgrowth.[409]

The functional reserve capacity of the small intestine is impressive. Experimental dogs have functioned well following resection of up to 85 per cent of their small intestine.[405] The function of the remaining gut after resection will progressively improve over a period of several weeks through mucosal adaptation.[407–409]

Short bowel syndrome should be suspected in any animal that develops intractable diarrhea and weight loss following extensive intestinal resection. Parameters of intestinal function may indicate malabsorption. Findings may include subnormal xylose absorption, marked steatorrhea, abnormal bentiromide test, and positive urine nitrosonaphthol test.[406] Dilated intestinal loops may be seen on routine abdominal radiographs, while barium contrast radiography of the upper GI tract usually demonstrates markedly accelerated stomach-to-colon transit time.[405, 406] Mild to moderate nonregenerative normochromic-normocytic anemia may also be found.[405, 406]

The aim of treatment is amelioration of diarrhea and restoration of normal nutritional status. Initially, before there has been substantial bowel adaptation, profuse diarrhea may require parenteral fluid therapy to maintain fluid and electrolyte balance. In humans, the use of total parenteral nutrition has greatly facilitated successful treatment of short bowel patients in the early postoperative phase.[409]

Animals should be returned to oral food intake as early as possible to stimulate adaptive hyperplasia. Frequent small meals should be fed, as many as six to eight per day, consisting of a low-fat diet such as Prescription Diet r/d. Daily vitamin and mineral supplementation is recommended. Eventually, the caloric density of the diet can be increased with supplementation of medium chain triglyceride (MCT oil).

Treatment is also directed at selectively controlling many of the complicating mechanisms of diarrhea: intestinal bacterial overgrowth is controlled with appropriate antibiotics such as tylosin or tetracycline; secondary gastric acid hypersecretion is controlled by use of an oral H_2-receptor blocker such as cimetidine (2.2 mg/lb, q8h); rapid intestinal transit time is controlled with motility-modifying antidiarrheal drugs such as codeine, diphenoxylate, loperamide, or propantheline; and bile acid-mediated diarrhea in cases of ileal resection is treated with oral bile acid-binding agents such as cholestyramine.[407–410] Animals that develop diarrhea following intestinal resection should be given the benefit of the doubt and managed with optimism, using whatever measures are necessary to maintain the animal long enough for adaptation to occur.

Thyroid-Related Diarrhea

Chronic diarrhea is sometimes associated with thyroid disease in the dog and cat. In a dog, medullary thyroid carcinoma was associated with chronic watery diarrhea that resolved within 48 hours after tumor excision.[411] This case resembles the secretory diarrhea syndrome seen in humans with medullary thyroid carcinoma in which diarrheogenic humoral substances such as serotonin and prostaglandins are secreted by the tumor.[412]

Feline hyperthyroidism has been associated with chronic diarrhea in 31 per cent of the patients.[31, 413, 414] In some thyrotoxic cats, along with severe weight loss and polyphagia, feces are soft, voluminous, and steatorrheic. Daily fecal fat excretion in five hyperthyroid cats was 2 to 15 times the upper limit of normal.[31] Proposed mechanisms for the apparent state of relative maldigestion and malabsorption in feline hyperthyroidism include intestinal hypermotility, intestinal overload due to overeating, and depressed pancreatic enzyme secretion, possibly caused by the catecholamine-like effect of

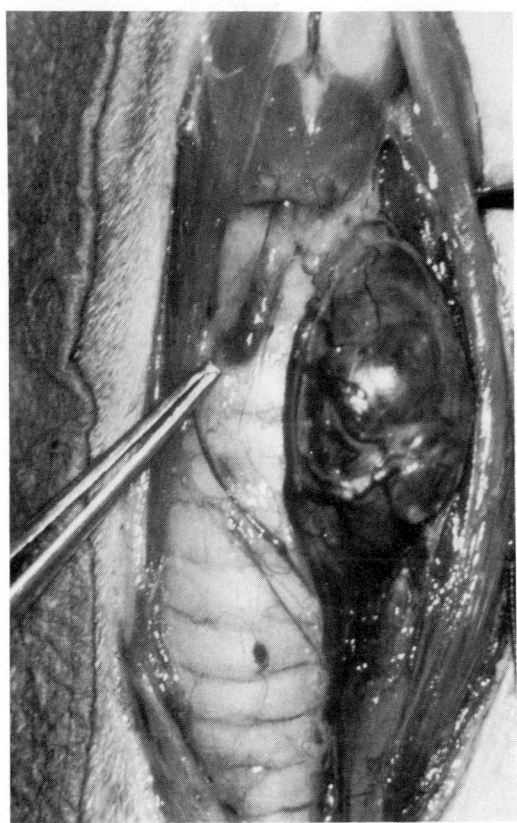

FIGURE 86–26. Thyroid gland adenoma in a cat with chronic diarrhea and weight loss associated with hyperthyroidism (thyrotoxicosis).

thyroxin.[31] The most common cause of feline hyperthyroidism is a functional thyroid adenoma (Figure 86–26), and the diagnosis is based on palpation of a thyroid nodule, measurement of elevated serum thyroxin concentration, or thyroid scan.

The treatment of thyroid-associated diarrhea is excision of the offending thyroid tumor, or alternatively, euthyroidism can be restored in cats with hyperthyroidism by means of radioiodine treatment or antithyroid drugs such as methimazole and propylthiouracil.[414] For a comprehensive discussion of thyroid disorders and their treatment, the reader is referred to Chapter 95.

INTESTINAL NEOPLASIA

Adenocarcinoma and lymphosarcoma are the most common GI tumors of dogs and cats.[415–423] Less frequent neoplasms include leiomyoma, leiomyosarcoma, fibrosarcoma, mastocytoma, and carcinoid tumors.[424] The clinical signs of GI neoplasia are typically vague, and the onset is slow and insidious. The clinical course is usually progressive in parallel with tumor growth. Anorexia and weight loss may be the only early signs, but often diarrhea, vomiting, dehydration, and anemia develop. Abdominal effusion may also occur.

Intestinal Adenocarcinoma

Intestinal adenocarcinomas account for 25 per cent of all GI neoplasia in dogs and 52 per cent in cats.[419] They occur predominantly in older animals with a higher incidence in males and in the Siamese breed of cat.[420] Any region of the GI tract can be affected but, in the cat, adenocarcinomas most commonly occur in the jejunum and ileum,[416, 417, 420, 422, 423] while canine adenocarcinomas occur more frequently in the large intestine and duodenum.[418, 424]

Morphologically, intestinal adenocarcinoma may produce a segmental thickening within the bowel wall with the effect of an expanding mass, or it may grow inward toward the lumen (especially in cats), producing an annular fibrous constricting band with minimal outward enlargement (Figure 86–27).[417, 420, 422, 423] This stenotic type produces partial obstruction and is easily confused with a stricture on barium radiography and even at surgery. Mucosal ulceration is frequent, sometimes resulting in melena and blood loss anemia. Local invasion of the mesentery, omentum, and regional lymph nodes is common. More widespread metastasis may also occur.

The diagnosis of intestinal adenocarcinoma may be suspected from clinical signs and abdominal palpation. Outwardly expanding adenocarcinomas can be palpated as firm, irregular abdominal masses, whereas stricturelike adenocarcinomas may not be palpable at all. Mesenteric lymphadenopathy (metastasis) may be palpable. Radiography, particularly the barium study, is helpful

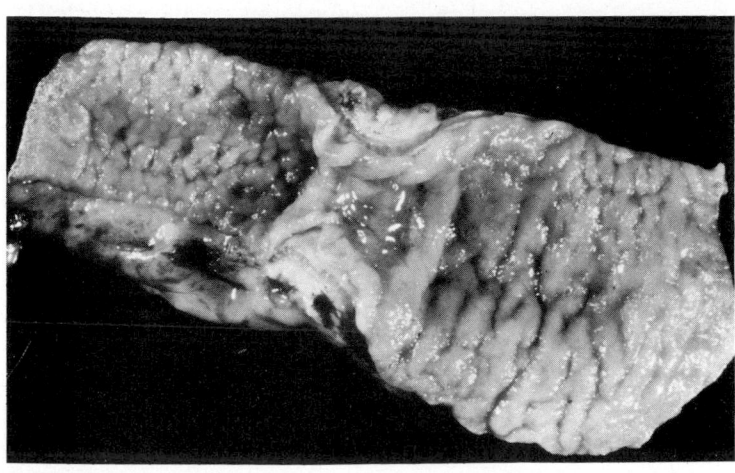

FIGURE 86–27. Opened segment of intestine showing an annular constricting adenocarcinoma that caused intestinal obstruction.

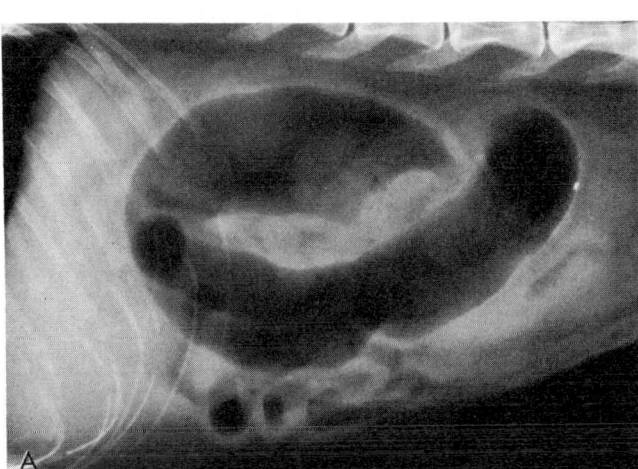
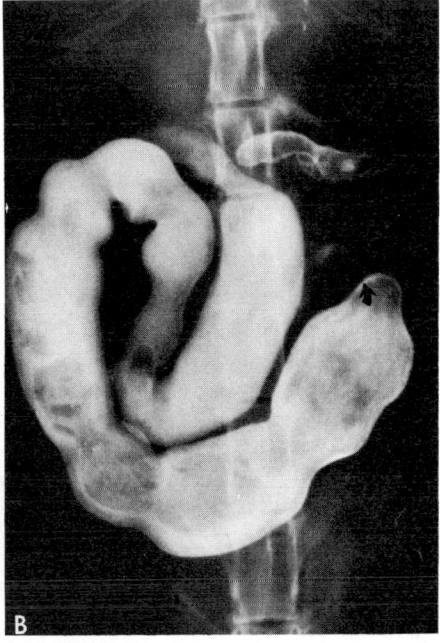

FIGURE 86–28. Lateral radiograph of the abdomen *(A)* of an eight-year-old female Siamese with chronic anorexia and weight loss, showing a gas-distended loop of intestine. A ventrodorsal barium radiograph *(B)* delineates the narrowed lumen at the site of obstruction (arrow) and dilatation proximal to it. Exploratory laparotomy revealed an annular stricture-like lesion in the ileum that was an adenocarcinoma.

in delineating tumor masses, partial obstruction, constrictive lesions, mucosal defects, or wall thickening (Figure 86–28). Definitive diagnosis is usually made by surgical excision or biopsy of the affected segment of bowel. Generally, the prognosis for adenocarcinoma is poor in that the surgical margins, peritoneum, or regional lymph nodes are usually invaded.[420, 423] Mean survival time after surgery is 4 to 6 months; however, survivals of 28 and 54 months after resection of an intestinal adenocarcinoma has been reported in two cats.[420, 425, 426]

Intestinal Lymphosarcoma

Lymphosarcoma (LSA) of the GI tract, usually composed of β-lymphocytes and arising from the "gut-associated lymphoid tissue" (GALT), is the most common extranodal LSA in dogs and cats and is the second most common GI malignancy behind adenocarcinoma, accounting for 10 and 21 per cent of GI malignancies in the dog and cat, respectively.[419, 421] In the cat, LSA is caused by feline leukemia virus (Chapter 48), although as few as one-fourth of cats with alimentary LSA are viremic.[427]

Intestinal LSA may occur at any age, but most affected dogs and cats are middle-aged or older.[349, 421] In the dog, the prevalence is higher in males.[419] Intestinal LSA has two morphologic types, the diffuse type and the nodular type. In diffuse LSA, extensive infiltration of the lamina propria and submucosa with neoplastic lymphocytes may cause malabsorption, steatorrhea, diarrhea, and weight loss (Figure 86–29). In the nodular type, a segmental thickening of the bowel, most often

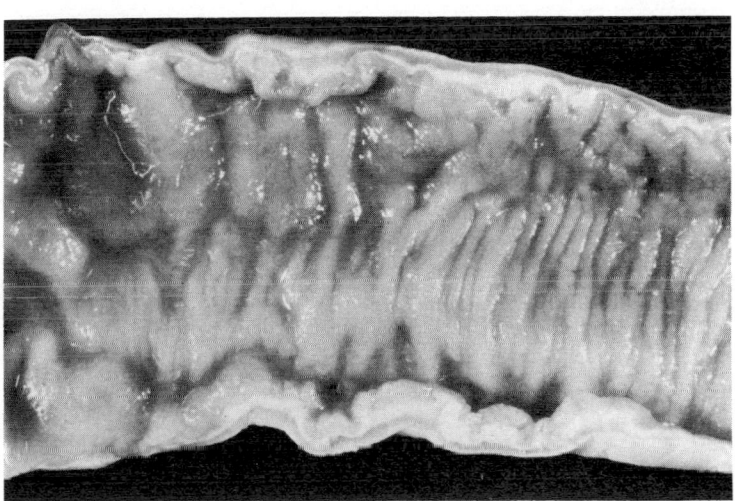

FIGURE 86–29. Opened section of intestine from a dog with diffuse intestinal lymphosarcoma. Notice the thickened gut wall and puffy, infiltrated-appearing mucosal lining.

in the ileocecocolic region, may cause luminal narrowing and partial intestinal obstruction (Figure 86–30). Metastasis to regional lymph nodes in either type is common.

The clinical course usually begins insidiously with vague signs such as anorexia and lethargy, progressing to diarrhea and intermittent vomiting.[349, 421, 428] Weight loss develops and progresses in severity in parallel with tumor growth. Melena, hematemesis, fever, ascites, and icterus may also occur. The diarrhea is usually a small bowel-type diarrhea, attributable to malabsorption caused by severe morphologic changes such as secondary villous atrophy and mucosal ulceration, diffuse infiltration of neoplastic cells into the lamina propria ("filled villi"), bowel wall disfigurement from deeper neoplastic infiltration of the submucosa and muscularis, and obstruction of intestinal lymphatic drainage associated with mesenteric lymphadenopathy.

Multifocal GI LSA may invade the stomach, small intestine, or colon, in any combination, thereby varying the clinical presentation. Furthermore, signs of extraintestinal involvement of organs such as the liver, spleen, or kidney may add to the clinical signs and physical findings.

The diagnosis of intestinal LSA may be suspected from clinical signs and abdominal palpation of intestinal thickening, mesenteric lymphadenopathy, or midabdominal mass. Radiography, particularly barium contrast study, can be helpful for delineating regions of mucosal irregularity, luminal narrowing, and intramural infiltration, thickening, or nodularity (Figure 86–31). Abdominal ultrasound examination may be used to better define abdominal mass lesions.

Laboratory abnormalities in dogs and cats with intestinal LSA may include anemia, neutrophilic leukocytosis with left shift, hypoproteinemia, and elevated serum hepatic enzyme concentrations.[421] In advanced cases, intestinal function studies are likely to show steatorrhea and xylose malabsorption. Definitive diagnosis is usually made by biopsy of the affected segment of bowel, most commonly during exploratory laparotomy. Gastric, duodenal, or colonic lesions are accessible to endoscopic biopsy. Percutaneous fine needle aspiration can be used to make a cytologic diagnosis in selected cases in which the neoplastic intestinal mass or loop can be well-delineated and stabilized by palpation.

In some dogs and cats, an initial biopsy is interpreted as inflammatory bowel disease (lymphocytic-plasmacytic enteritis), but later biopsy (or necropsy) prompted by progression of signs in spite of therapy is read out as neoplastic. It is unclear in such cases whether the initial

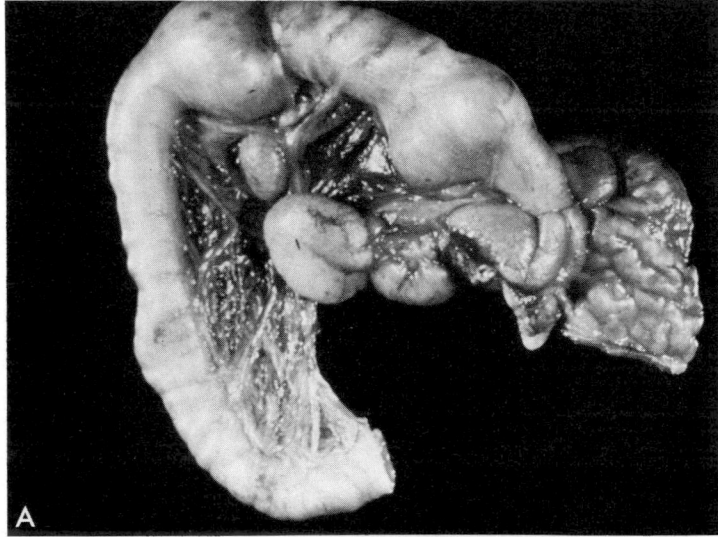
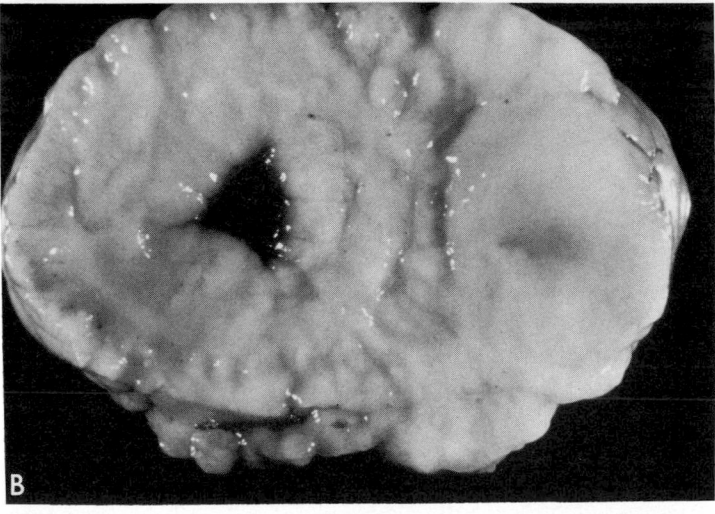

FIGURE 86–30. A typical segmental-nodular type intestinal lymphosarcoma (A) at the ileocecocolic junction and with involvement of the regional lymph nodes. Cross-section of the neoplasm (B) shows narrowing of the lumen, resulting in partial intestinal obstruction.

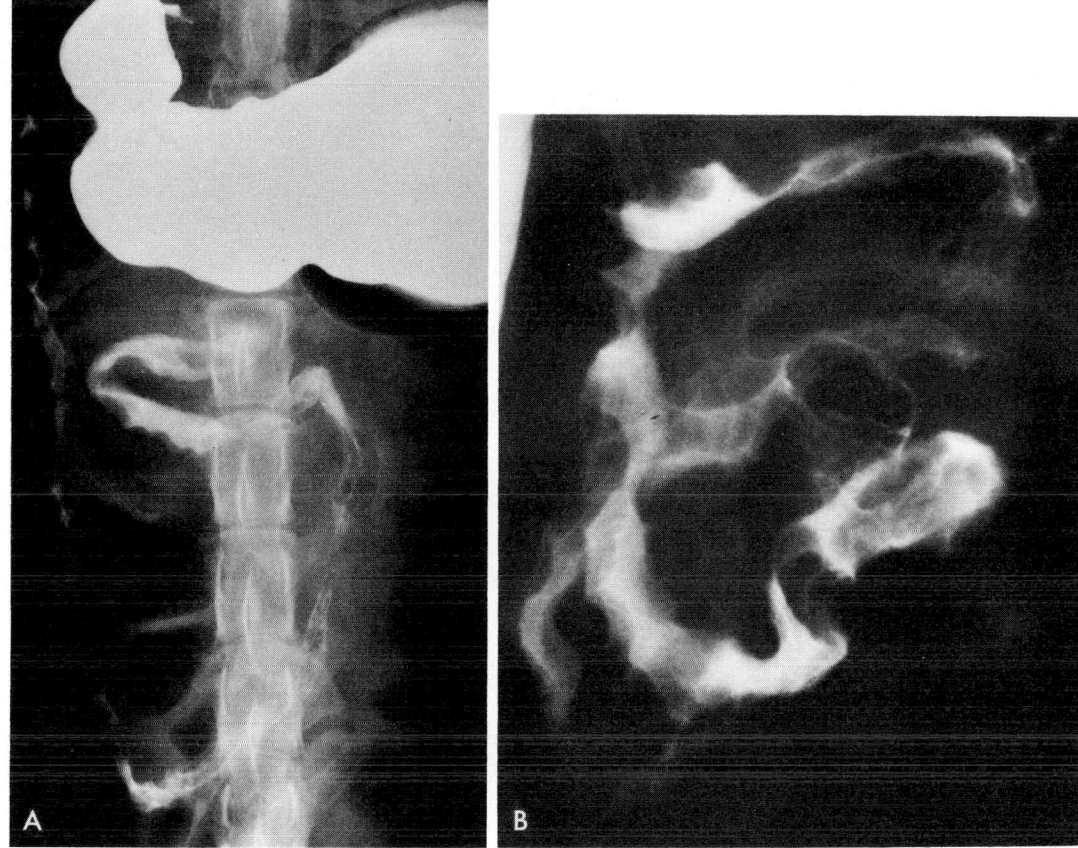

FIGURE 86–31. Ventrodorsal *(A)* and close-up lateral *(B)* barium radiographs of a dog with diffuse intestinal lymphosarcoma. Notice the nodular distortion and infiltration of the gut wall causing luminal filling defects and narrowing.

lesion represented prelymphomatous change or whether it was erroneous because of sampling error or misinterpretation.

Various antineoplastic chemotherapy regimens (see Chapter 59) have been used to treat unresectable GI LSA and as follow-up treatment after resection; however, the number of reports of treatment have been too few to evaluate the response rate. In general, the results of treating GI LSA have been discouraging, especially when advanced to the point of significant malabsorption or protein-losing enteropathy.[421]

The prognosis may be worsened by complications such as severe GI bleeding and anemia, intestinal obstruction, intussusception, and GI perforation leading to fatal septic peritonitis. In addition, involvement of other vital organs, such as the liver or kidneys, may complicate the animal's condition.

If treatment is attempted, consideration should be given to supportive measures such as nutritional management, prevention of sepsis, blood transfusion, and control of small bowel bacterial overgrowth.

Intestinal Mast Cell Tumors

Primary mast cell tumors occur mainly in aged cats as segmental nodular thickenings involving the small bowel. These distinctive tumors resemble carcinoid tumors and are unlike the mast cell tumors that occur in

other body sites in cats.[429] Histochemical and ultrastructural examination may be required to confirm the tumor cells as mast cells which are apparently in a degranulated state.[429] Metastases occur most frequently in mesenteric lymph nodes, liver, and spleen.

DUODENAL ULCERS

Duodenal ulcers occur rarely in dogs and cats. They usually cause signs of vomiting (hematemesis), melena, weight loss, and abdominal pain (Figure 86–32).[430] Blood-loss anemia and perforation are potential complications. Gastroduodenal ulceration is found in dogs and cats with mast cell tumors and disseminated mastocytosis, presumably resulting from chronic stimulation of gastric acid hypersecretion by histamine released from the mast cells.[431, 432] Perforation of these mast cell–associated duodenal ulcers has been reported in both dogs and cats.[433–435] An association between liver disease and peptic ulcer in dogs has been found.[430] Gastroduodenal ulceration in dogs can also result from ulcerogenic drugs such as corticosteroids, aspirin, indomethacin, and other nonsteroidal anti-inflammatory drugs.[436] Finally, duodenal ulceration from gastric hypersecretion has been described in association with gastrin-producing pancreatic islet cell tumors (gastrinoma) in dogs (canine Zollinger-Ellison syndrome),[437–439] and in one cat.[440]

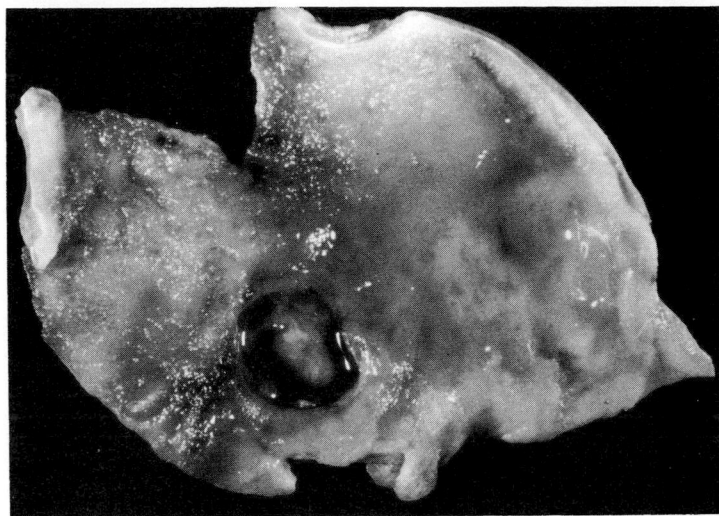

FIGURE 86–32. Duodenal ulcers in dogs are typically well-circumscribed oval lesions, as demonstrated by this ulcer that extended through the mucosa and submucosa down to the circular muscle layer.

Some ulcers are idiopathic. The diagnosis of duodenal ulcer is usually made by endoscopy and occasionally by radiography. The aim of therapy is to promote rapid healing of the ulcer and protect against further mucosal damage using an H_2-receptor antagonist such as cimetidine (Tagamet) to decrease gastric acid secretion and a cytoprotective binding agent such as sucralfate (Carafate). For a more complete discussion of upper GI ulcer disease, including pathogenesis and treatment, the reader is referred to Chapter 85.

INTESTINAL OBSTRUCTION

Intestinal obstruction in dogs and cats may be caused by intraluminal objects, intramural thickening or stenosis, and extramural compression. Specific causes include foreign body, intussusception, volvulus, intestinal torsion, incarceration of bowel in a hernia (includes abdominal hernias of all types, diaphragmatic hernia, and internal herniation of gut loops through a tear in the mesentery), adhesions or stricture (post-trauma or post-surgery), intramural abscess or granuloma, intramural hematoma, congenital malformation (stenosis or atresia), persistent ligamentum pancreaticoduodenale in cats, and intestinal neoplasia.[441–453] The clinical manifestations and consequences of obstruction depend on its location, completeness, and duration, as well as the vascular integrity of the affected bowel segment. Vomiting, anorexia, and depression of acute onset are the most consistent clinical signs. Others include abdominal distention, diarrhea, and abdominal pain, evidenced by restlessness, panting, or abnormal body posture (Figure 86–33).[454]

A syndrome of chronic intestinal pseudo-obstruction has been described in a few dogs in which ineffective propulsive motility and persistent dilatation of the intestine mimics the signs of obstruction, yet the intestinal lumen is patent.[398, 455] The disorder is associated with lesions of intestinal sclerosis characterized by diffuse atrophy, fibrosis, and mononuclear infiltration of the tunica muscularis.[455] Intestinal pseudo-obstruction tends to be progressive and unresponsive to treatment.[398, 455]

Generally, the more proximal and complete the obstruction, the more intense and fulminating the signs will be, and the greater the likelihood of dehydration, electrolyte imbalance, and shock. Proximal duodenal obstructions cause, in effect, gastric outlet occlusion leading to persistent vomiting, loss of gastric secretions (HCl), and metabolic alkalosis (see Chapter 85). Obstructions at more distal sites cause varying degrees of metabolic acidosis. Distal and incomplete obstructions can be insidious, with vague, intermittent signs of chronic anorexia and occasional vomiting that span several days or even weeks, leading to progressive starvation (Figure 86–34).

Intestinal obstructions can also be simple or strangulated. Simple obstructions occlude the lumen without significant loss of vascular integrity, while strangulation involves vascular compromise of the obstructed bowel

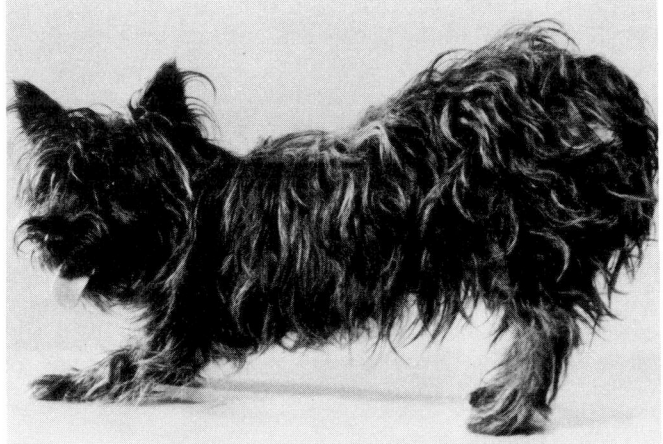

FIGURE 86–33. The abdominal pain of intestinal obstruction is sometimes manifested as a distinctive "praying" posture, also called the "position of relief." This dog was found to have an intussusception.

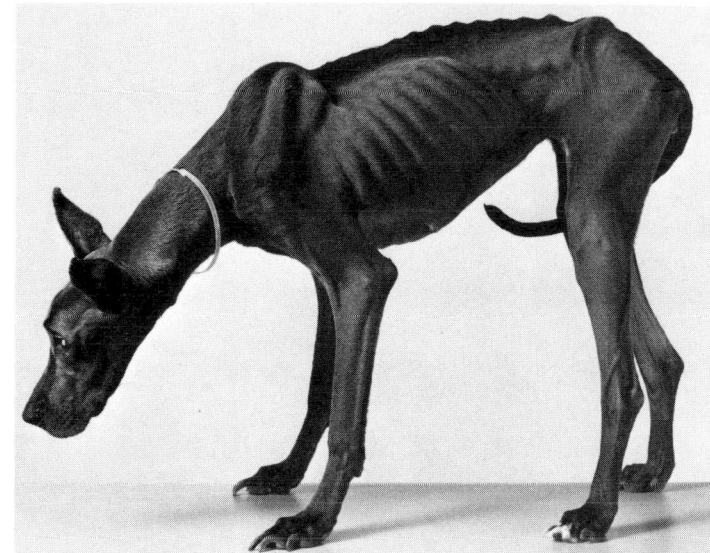

FIGURE 86–34. Incomplete intestinal obstruction may have a chronic course characterized by prolonged anorexia and progressive starvation. This severely emaciated Great Dane had panty hose removed from its small bowel.

segment. This occurs most often with intussusception, volvulus, and incarcerated hernia. The sequence of events following strangulation are edema and engorgement of the affected loop, tissue hypoxia and infarction of the bowel wall, accumulation of gut bacteria and toxins in the peritoneal fluid, and rapidly progressive toxemia and shock, culminating in death.

The diagnosis of obstruction may be established by palpation of a foreign body, intussusception ("sausage loop"), or gas- and fluid-distended loops of bowel proximal to the obstruction. Radiography can usually confirm the presence of obstruction and often delineate the cause, especially when contrast studies are used. Radiographic findings that suggest obstruction include gas or fluid distention (mechanical ileus) of the bowel (Figure 86–35), delayed transit of contrast material, fixation or displacement of gut loops, luminal filling defects (Figure 86–36), or the presence of foreign objects within the lumen (Figure 86–37).[453] Almost any object that the curious or indiscriminant animal takes into its mouth may become a GI foreign body if swallowed; common examples are bones, toys, cloth (Figure 86–38), metallic objects, stones, peach pits, acorns, rubber nipples, or rubber balls. Cats commonly ingest radiolucent linear intestinal foreign bodies (such as thread, string, cloth, fishing line, dental floss, decorative tinsel) that cause aggregation and plication of the bowel and a distinctive radiographic pattern (Figures 86–39 and 86–40).[456]

Intestinal obstructions are treated surgically. Close attention is given to supportive care, especially to maintenance of fluid, electrolyte, and acid-base homeostasis before, during, and after surgery. Although surgical management is appropriate in most cats with linear intestinal foreign bodies, in one study the foreign body passed in 9 of 19 cats diagnosed early and treated conservatively by cutting of sublingually fixed objects along with in-hospital supportive care and observation.[457] For further information regarding the surgical considerations of intestinal obstruction, the reader should consult the standard veterinary surgical text-

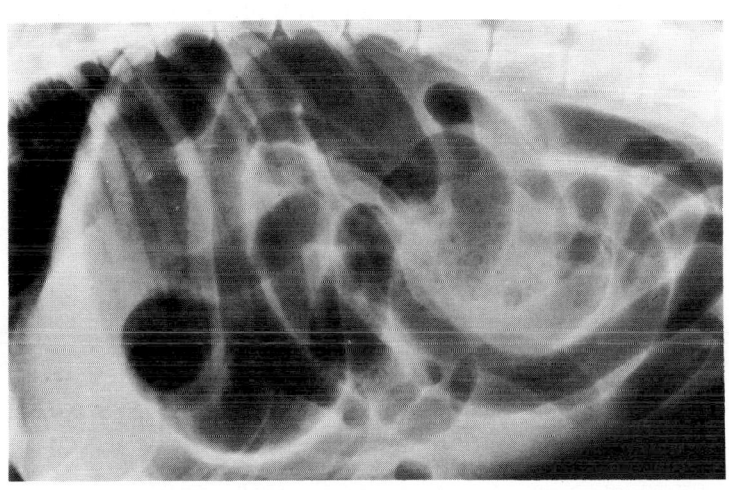

FIGURE 86–35. Lateral radiograph of the abdomen showing gas-distended bowel suggestive of intestinal obstruction. Intestinal volvulus was found by exploratory laparotomy.

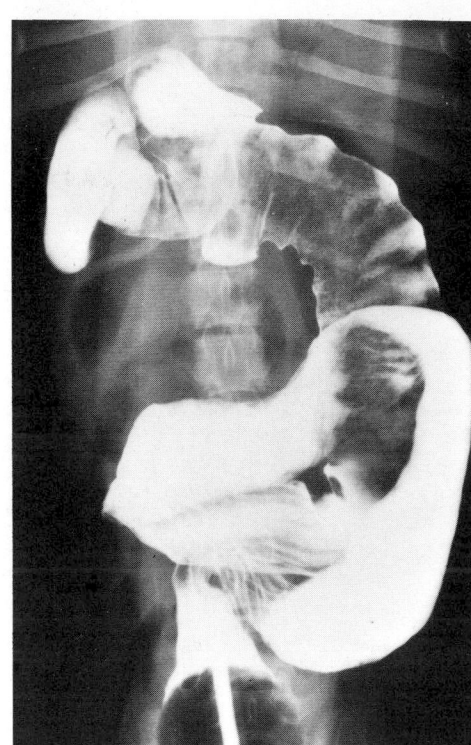

FIGURE 86–36. Barium enema radiography showing a coiled intraluminal filling defect within the colon indicative of ileocolonic intussusception.

FIGURE 86–37. Ventrodorsal *(A)* and lateral *(B)* barium radiographs showing obstructed passage of contrast material by a radiolucent spherical foreign body within the lumen. A rubber ball was removed surgically.

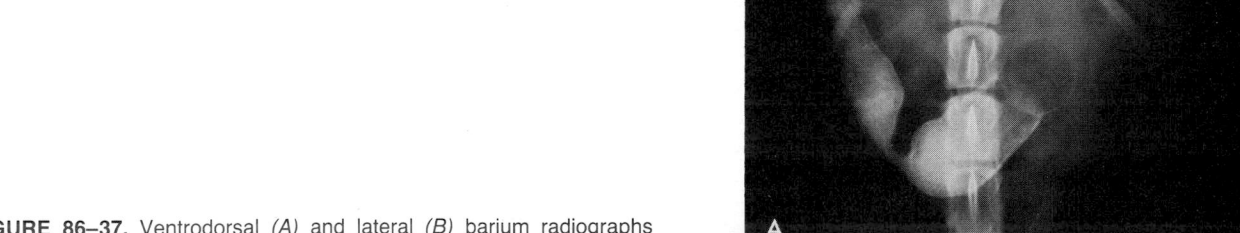

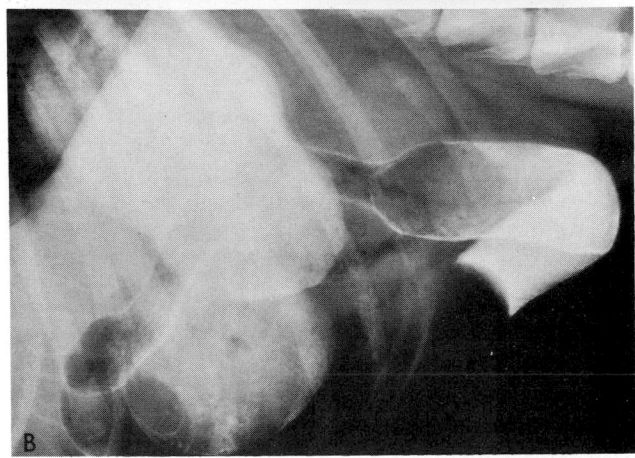

FIGURE 86–38. A cloth intestinal foreign body is removed through an enterotomy incision.

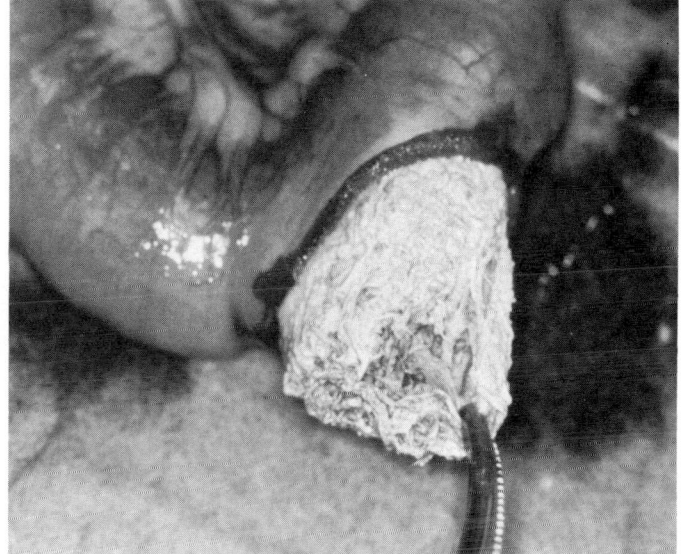

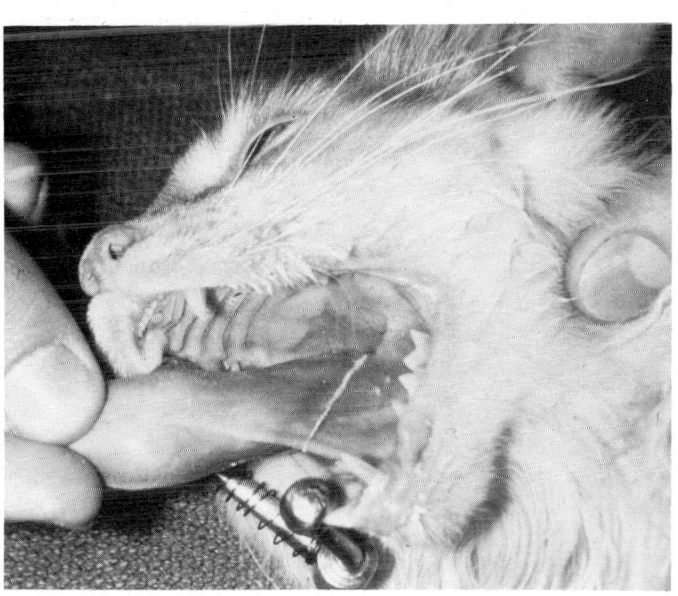

FIGURE 86–39. Linear intestinal foreign bodies such as thread are often looped around the base of the tongue in cats and can be detected by careful examination under the tongue. The free end of the thread is swallowed and passes into the intestine where it causes plication.

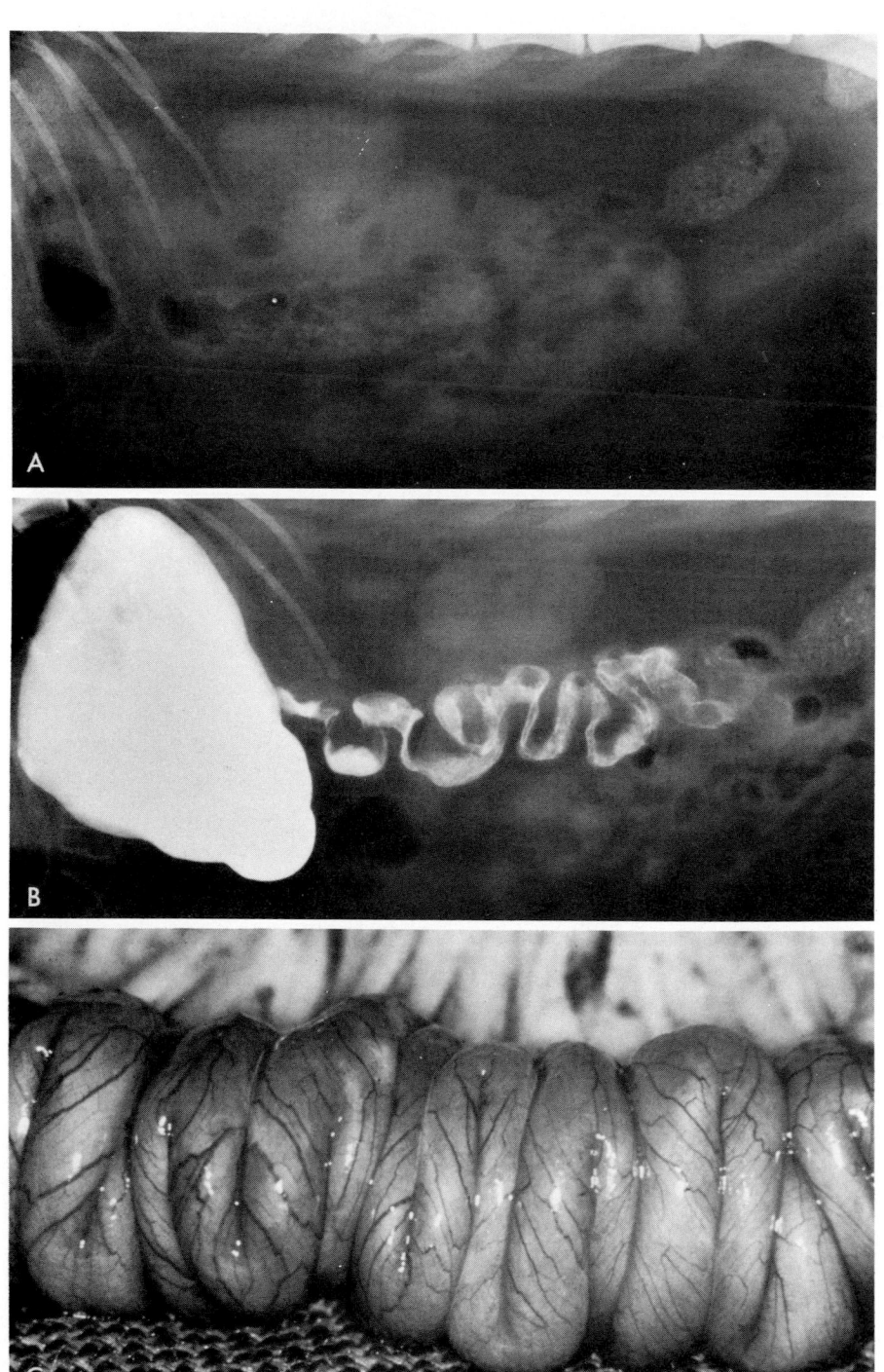

FIGURE 86–40. A lateral abdominal radiograph of a one-year-old male DSH with anorexia, vomiting, and abdominal pain shows aggregation and bunching of gut loops into the midabdomen and eccentrically located gas bubbles in the lumen *(A)*. These findings suggest radiolucent linear foreign body. The diagnosis is confirmed by a barium study showing characteristic intestinal plication *(B)*. The plication caused by the linear foreign body is seen at surgery *(C)*.

books. Complications of intestinal obstruction are necrosis or perforation of the bowel, peritonitis, and endotoxic shock.

TREATMENT OF INTESTINAL DISEASE

Principles of Treatment of Acute Diarrhea

Acute diarrhea in dogs and cats is frequently self-limiting and resolves without treatment. Nevertheless, supportive or symptomatic therapy can be beneficial in many cases, regardless of cause; and in animals with severe diarrhea, rehydration therapy can be life-saving. Supportive therapy includes: (1) dietary restriction; (2) restoration and maintenance of fluid, electrolyte, and acid-base balance; and (3) symptomatic treatment with antidiarrheal drugs that affect intestinal motility or secretion. Along with these nonspecific treatments, additional specific therapies as described in other sections of this chapter for each disease are also used (Table 86–12).

Diet. The initial dietary goal in acute diarrhea is to put the GI tract at rest by restricting food intake for at least 24 hours. When feeding is resumed, bland low-fat foods are fed in small amounts at frequent intervals to maximize digestion and absorption. Examples of appropriate foods include low-fat prescription diets, and homemade diets of boiled rice, tapioca, macaroni, or potatoes combined with cooked lean meat, eggs, cottage cheese, or yogurt. The diet is gradually changed back to the animal's regular food once the diarrhea resolves.

Fluid Therapy. In severe acute diarrhea, dehydration may lead to shock and death. Thus, fluid and electrolyte replacement therapy can be essential. Parenteral fluid therapy is appropriate in most cases of dehydrating diarrhea, but oral glucose solutions have also been used successfully, particularly in humans and calves. Glucose is known to facilitate intestinal absorption of sodium and water. Thus, oral glucose-electrolyte solutions used in secretory diarrhea exploit the intact absorptive capacity of the gut so that enhanced absorption of fluid and electrolytes counterbalances the losses from hypersecretion.[458] In animals, Entrolyte or Pedialyte can be used. Principles of fluid therapy are discussed in detail in Chapter 53.

Antidiarrheal Drugs. Symptomatic antidiarrheal therapy uses drugs that modify motility or secretion or drugs that act locally within the lumen as so-called protectants. The commonly used antidiarrheal agents and their dosages are found in Table 86–13. In most cases, these drugs are reserved for short-term use, usually less than 5 to 7 days. Anticholinergics and narcotic analgesics have traditionally been used as so-called motility modifiers; however, their most beneficial antidiarrheal effects are probably mediated through their influence on mucosal fluid and electrolyte transport (inhibition of intestinal secretions) rather than their effects on smooth muscle. The opiate and opioid narcotic analgesics (e.g., paregoric, diphenoxylate, loperamide, codeine) are probably the most effective antidiarrheal agents. For a long time, the belief had been that these drugs impeded bowel transit by stimulating nonpropulsive contractions (segmentation) while decreasing propulsive motility. Current evidence now indicates that opiates are potent inhibitors of intestinal secretions and they may enhance mucosal absorption.[458, 459] Anticholinergics may not be as useful since they cause generalized suppression of all motility, propulsive and nonpropulsive, and thus may potentiate ileus. Prostaglandin inhibitors, chlorpromazine, and numerous other drugs which are currently under investigation as potential antisecretory agents for diarrhea are reviewed elsewhere.[458]

Oral protectants such as kaolin-pectin, bismuth, magnesium, aluminum compounds, activated charcoal, and barium are purported to act locally within the gut lumen to adsorb injurious bacteria and toxins and to provide a protective coating on inflamed mucosal surfaces; however, efficacy of most of these agents is doubtful. Bismuth subsalicylate, which is the active ingredient of Pepto-Bismol, is an exception. This drug has antienterotoxin, antibacterial, antisecretory, and anti-inflammatory actions that are presumably mediated through the antiprostaglandin effects of its salicylate component. In humans, bismuth subsalicylate has been effective for relieving the symptoms of viral gastroenteritis and enterotoxigenic *E. coli* infections (traveler's diarrhea). There is significant absorption of salicylate from this agent in dogs and cats, which must be taken into consideration, especially in cats because of the long half-life for salicylates in this species.[460] Parenteral antiprostaglandins (Banamine) have also been used empirically for short-term (24 to 48 hours) anti-inflammatory therapy in dogs with parvoviral enteritis, and hemorrhagic gastroenteritis, but extreme caution is advised because of the tendency of these agents to produce GI ulceration.

Antibiotics. Antibiotics have no place in the routine management of acute diarrhea in the dog and cat. Antibiotics are indicated, however, when specific bacterial or rickettsial enteropathogens such as *Salmonella*, *Campylobacter*, or *Neorickettsia* are suspected (see Infectious Diarrhea section). Antibiotics should also be considered in conditions associated with severe mucosal damage and a high risk of secondary sepsis or endotoxemia, such as in parvoviral enteritis or hemorrhagic gastroenteritis. Thus, bloody diarrhea, fever, leukocytosis, leukopenia, fecal leukocytes, and signs of shock are all legitimate indications for antimicrobial therapy in the animal with acute diarrhea. Otherwise, use of antibiotics as empirical therapy in uncomplicated acute diarrhea of undetermined cause is not recommended because of the adverse effects on the normal intestinal flora and its tendency to promote resistant strains of bacteria.

Principles of Treatment of Chronic Diarrhea

Chronic diarrhea does not usually resolve spontaneously or respond to nonspecific antidiarrheal medications. Specific intervention or treatment is desirable and requires a specific diagnosis (Table 86–14). In this chap-

TABLE 86–12. DIAGNOSIS AND TREATMENT OF ACUTE DIARRHEA

Causes	Basis for Diagnosis	Mode of Treatment

Dietary
  1. Abrupt change in diet
  2. Overfeeding
  3. Indiscretion—"garbage" ingestion, ingestion of abrasive or indigestible material
  4. Intolerance—idiosyncrasy, allergy
	History, response to diet modification	Restricted diet

Drug and Toxin Induced
  1. Anti-inflammatory drugs—steroidal, nonsteroidal
  2. Antimicrobials
  3. Parasiticides—anthelmintics, dithiazanine
  4. Antineoplastic agents
  5. Heavy metals—lead, arsenic, thallium
  6. Insecticides—organophosphates, and so on
	History of exposure	Eliminate exposure to the offending drug or toxin

Parasitic
  Helminths
  1. Ascarids
  2. Hookworms
  3. Whipworms
  4. *Strongyloides*
  5. Others—cestodes, trematodes, *Trichinella*
  Protozoa
  1. Coccidia—*Isospora, Cryptosporidia*
  2. *Giardia*
  3. Others—*Pentatrichomonas, Entamoeba, Balantidium*
	Fecal examinations	Specific anthelmintics and antiprotozoal drugs

Viral
  1. Parvovirus
  2. Coronavirus
  3. Rotavirus
  4. Astrovirus
  5. Others—canine distemper, infectious canine hepatitis, FIP, FeLV, FIV
	Clinical signs, demonstration of virus in feces by EM or serologic methods	Supportive (fluid therapy; control of secondary bacterial complications)

Bacterial
  1. *Salmonella*
  2. *Campylobacter*
  3. *Yersinia*
  4. *Bacillus piliformis*
  5. Other—*E. coli,* clostridia, staphylococci, and others
	Specialized fecal cultures	Specific antibiotics

Rickettsial Salmon poisoning disease	Clinical signs, endemic habitat, fecal exam for fluke eggs, lymph node cytology	Tetracycline
Idiopathic—Hemorrhagic gastroenteritis	Clinical signs, hematocrit	Supportive (fluid therapy); antibiotics

Obstructive
  1. Intestinal foreign body
  2. Intussusception
  3. Intestinal volvulus
	Abdominal palpation, barium contrast GI radiography	Surgery

Extraintestinal
  1. Renal failure
  2. Hepatic disease
  3. Hypoadrenocorticism
  4. Acute pancreatitis
	Serum biochemistry determinations and organ function tests	Various treatments to control the underlying extraintestinal disorder

TABLE 86–13. DRUGS USED FOR SYMPTOMATIC TREATMENT OF ACUTE DIARRHEA

Drug	Product (Manufacturer)	Preparations	Dosage	Frequency
*Narcotic Analgesics**				
Diphenoxylate	Lomotil (Searle)	Tab–2.5 mg; Liq–0.5 mg/ml	0.02–0.05 mg/lb	q 6–8h
Loperamide	Imodium (Janssen)			
Codeine	Many	Cap–2 mg; Liq–0.2 mg/ml	0.02–0.05 mg/lb	q 8–12h
		Tab; Cap; Liq	0.11–0.23 mg/lb	q 6–8h
*Narcotic Analgesic Mixtures**				
Paregoric (w/kaolin-pectin)	Parapectolin (Rorer)	Liq	0.11–0.23 ml/lb	q 6–8h
(w/bismuth subsalicylate)	Corrective Mixture (Beecham)	Liq	0.11–0.23 ml/lb	q 6–8h
Opium (w/kaolin-pectin and anticholinergics)	Donnagel-PG (Robins)	Liq	0.11–0.23 ml/lb	q 6–8h
(w/bismuth subsalicylate)	Infantol Pink (Scherer)	Liq	0.11–0.23 ml/lb	q 6–8h
Anticholinergics/Antispasmodics				
Aminopentamide	Centrine (Bristol)	Tab–0.2 mg/Inj–0.5 mg/ml	0.1–0.4 mg total dose	q 8–12h
Dicyclomine	Bentyl (Merrell-Dow)	Tab–20 mg; Cap–10 mg; Liq–2 mg/ml; Inj–10 mg/ml	0.07 mg/lb	q 8–12h
Isopropamide	Darbid (SmithKline Beckman)	Tab–5 mg	0.09–0.05 mg/lb	q 8–12h
Propantheline	Pro-Banthine (Searle)	Tab–15 mg	0.11 mg/lb	q 8–12h
Methscopolamine	Pamine (Upjohn)	Tab–2.5 mg	0.14–0.68 mg/lb	q 8–12h
Hyoscyamine	Levsin (Rorer)	Tab–0.125 mg; Liq–0.025 mg/ml, 0.125 mg/ml	0.001–0.003 mg/lb	q 8–12h
Clidinium	Quarzan (Roche)	Cap–2.5 mg, 5 mg	0.05–0.11 mg/lb	q 8–12h
Anticholinergics Plus CNS Depressant				
Isopropamide plus prochlorperazine	Darbazine (Norden)	Cap #1 / Cap #3 / Inj	< 4.5 lb: #1 capsule / > 4.5 lb: #3 capsule / 0.06–0.10 ml/lb, SC	q 8–12h
Clidinium plus chlordiazeproxide	Librax (Roche)	Cap–2.5 mg clidinium; 5 mg chlordiazeproxide	0.11–0.5 mg/lb (clidinium)	q 8–12h
Hyoscyamine plus phenobarbital	Donnatal (Rorer)	Tab, Cap, Liq	0.001–0.003 mg/lb (hyoscyamine)	q 8–12h
Antisecretory/Protectant				
Bismuth subsalicylate+	Pepto-Bismol (Procter & Gamble)	Liq–9 mg salicylate/ml	0.5 ml/lb	q 4–6h

*Narcotic analgesics not recommended for use in cats and contraindicated in bacterial enteritis or liver disease
+Avoid long-term (> 3 days) use in cats because of low tolerance for salicylates
(Tab = tablets; Cap = capsules; Inj = injectable; Liq = elixir, suspension or drops)
From Sherding RG, Burrows CF: In Anderson NV (ed.): Veterinary Gastroenterology, 2nd ed. Philadelphia, Lea & Febiger, in press.

TABLE 86–14. DIAGNOSIS AND TREATMENT OF DISEASES OF THE SMALL INTESTINE

Disorder	Diagnosis	Treatment
Exocrine pancreatic insufficiency	Fecal stains, serum trypsin assay, BT-PABA test	Enzyme replacement
Chronic inflammatory small bowel disease		
Eosinophilic enteritis	Eosinophilia, biopsy	Prednisolone
Lymphocytic-plasmacytic enteritis	Biopsy	Lamb and rice diet; prednisolone (or also tylosin, metronidazole, azathioprine)
Immunoproliferative enteropathy of basenjis	Serum protein electrophoresis, biopsy	Diet, prednisolone, antibiotics
Granulomatous enteritis	Radiography, biopsy	Prednisolone, surgical resection
Lymphangiectasia	Hypoproteinemia, hypocholesterolemia, lymphopenia, biopsy	Low-fat diet (MCT), prednisolone
Villous atrophy		
Gluten enteropathy	Response to gluten-free diet, biopsy	Gluten-free diet
Idiopathic	Biopsy	Diet, prednisolone, antibiotics (±)
Histoplasmosis	Serology, cytology, biopsy	Amphotericin B, ketoconazole
Phycomycosis	Biopsy	Surgical excision ± ketoconazole
Lymphosarcoma	Biopsy	Chemotherapy (antineoplastic drugs)
Bacterial overgrowth syndrome	Culture intestinal aspirate, serum B_{12}/folate, response to antibiotics	Antibiotics (tetracycline, tylosin, metronidazole, and so on)
Giardiasis	Fecal examination, response to parasiticides	Metronidazole or quinicrine
Lactase deficiency	Response to lactose-free diet	Eliminate milk from diet

From Sherding RG: In Ford RB (ed): Clinical Signs and Diagnosis in Small Animal Practice. New York, Churchill Livingstone, 1988.

ter, specific treatment, when available, is discussed separately with each disease. In addition, chronic diarrhea, regardless of etiology, may benefit from dietary restriction, modification, or supplementation (Table 86–15).[461] This section will emphasize treatment measures applicable to small bowel diarrhea. Diets suitable for large bowel diarrhea are discussed in Chapter 87.

The diet of the animal with chronic small bowel diarrhea or malabsorption should require minimal digestion, provide adequate amounts of high-biologic quality protein derived from one or two known food sources, and contain a minimum of fat, lactose, and additives.[461, 462] In addition, gluten-containing grains such as wheat, barley, rye, and oats should be restricted in animals suspected of gluten-sensitive enteropathy.[91, 384] Daily food intake should be divided into three or four small feedings to avoid overload of intestinal digestive-absorptive functional capacity. In severe malnutrition, digestibility of the diet may be enhanced by the addition of a pancreatic enzyme supplement (Viokase or Pancreazyme). This is because prolonged malabsorption or protein-losing enteropathy may impair pancreatic exocrine function secondary to severe protein-calorie malnutrition.[12]

Adequate quantity and quality of dietary proteins are important for controlling secondary hypoproteinemia, facilitating recovery from intestinal disease, and promoting adaptive mucosal hyperplasia in response to intestinal injury. Restriction of dietary fat (long-chain triglyceride) may produce some amelioration of diarrhea by reducing steatorrhea. Intraluminal hydroxylated fatty acids derived from unabsorbed fat contribute to the pathogenesis of malabsorptive diarrhea, as described previously in the Pathophysiology section. Unfortunately, since the fat content of the diet normally provides a substantial portion of daily caloric intake, fat restriction promotes further weight loss. Therefore, medium-chain triglyceride (MCT) can be used to replace calories lost by removal of conventional fat from the diet. MCTs are useful because they are hydrolyzed more efficiently and rapidly than LCTs, and are absorbed directly into

the portal venous system, bypassing lymphatic transport.[462] Commercially available MCT is derived from coconut oil and can be mixed in with home-prepared and commercial low-fat diets as MCT oil. Because of poor palatability, the addition of MCT to the diet should be started at a low dose and increased gradually up to the maximal tolerated dose, aiming for 0.5 to 1 ml/lb/day. In cats, the value of a fat-restricted diet in the treatment of diarrhea is less clear. Paradoxically, the observation has been made by many that cats with chronic intestinal disease often do best on a high-fat prescription or commercial diet. Even in normal cats, comparison of various diets shows that high-fat/high-calorie diets result in decreased amount of feces and threefold reduction in fecal water excretion.[463]

In the dog with malassimilation, the diet should consist mainly of carbohydrates; however, the source of carbohydrate should be selective. Evidence suggests that dogs digest and absorb starch more completely when it is derived from rice (especially in flour form) rather than wheat or corn.[64, 65, 82] Cats, on the other hand, are observed to have a low tolerance for starch, especially when they have diarrhea, and thus should be fed a diet restricted in starch and based instead on poultry protein.[82]

In both dogs and cats, restriction of lactose content in the diet may be necessary. Brush-border lactase activity may be insufficient for digestion of large amounts of this carbohydrate in animals, which can be compounded by disease of the small intestines. Unabsorbed dietary lactose may contribute osmotically to the pathogenesis of diarrhea. If dairy products are desired as a protein source, cottage cheese or yogurt should be used. One-fourth cup of cottage cheese provides nearly as much protein (7.5 gm) as one cup of whole milk (8.0 gm), but contains considerably less lactose (1.5 gm versus 11.8 gm).[462] Yogurt is an excellent dairy source of protein because it is low in fat, and the lactose in yogurt is absorbed much more efficiently than from milk, apparently due to the intraluminal action of lactase produced by the bacteria in the yogurt.[464]

Diets that are most suitable for dogs with chronic small bowel diarrhea include ready-made low-fat diets such as Prescription Diet r/d or i/d, and low-fat home-prepared diets with a carbohydrate-to-protein ratio of approximately 4:1 consisting of rice or potatoes as the carbohydrate source and low-fat cottage cheese, yogurt, eggs, or boiled lean meat such as chicken or lamb as the protein source.[461] Any of these low-fat diets may be supplemented with MCT oil to enhance the animal's caloric intake to help prevent further weight loss, while all home-prepared diets in particular should also be supplemented daily with a multiple vitamin-mineral product. Although very little is known concerning dietary therapy of feline diarrhea, cats with chronic diarrhea seem to do best on diets such as Prescription Diet c/d or Tender Vittles, which are lower in carbohydrate and higher in fat than most commercial feline diets.[461]

Vitamin and mineral absorption may be impaired in many animals with small bowel diarrhea, and thus supplementation may be indicated. In human patients with malabsorption, subclinical deficiencies of many vitamins and minerals have been documented. The

---

TABLE 86–15. NONSPECIFIC MEDICAL MANAGEMENT OF INTESTINAL MALABSORPTION

1. Frequent small feedings (3–4 per day)
2. Dietary modification
   a. High-protein, fat-restricted diet with minimal lactose (such as r/d, i/d, or rice and uncreamed cottage cheese)
   b. MCT to replace calories lost by removal of fat (LCT) from the diet (1–2 ml/kg/day)
   c. Vitamin-mineral supplements (fat-soluble vitamins—A, D, E, K; folate; B_{12}; calcium)
3. Special nutritional supplementation (in selected cases)
   a. Parenteral (IV) hyperalimentation
   b. Enteral hyperalimentation (liquid elemental diets)
4. Eradicate concomitant parasite infections
5. Antibiotics, e.g., tylosin, metronidazole, tetracycline (When bacterial overgrowth is a cause or complication of malabsorption)
6. Corticosteroids
   (Used in idiopathic chronic inflammatory bowel diseases, lymphangiectasia, and idiopathic villous atrophy)
7. Pancreatic enzyme supplementation
   (Transient exocrine pancreatic insufficiency may potentially occur with severe malabsorption)

deficiencies of greater clinical significance include fat-soluble vitamins (A, D, E, and K), folic acid, vitamin B_{12}, and calcium. Reduced serum concentrations of folate and vitamin B_{12} have been measured in dogs with chronic malabsorptive enteropathies.[63] Deficiency of folate and B_{12} should be prevented since the intestinal mucosa has a rapid turnover of cells and these vitamins are involved in DNA replication.[384] Dosages of 5 mg oral folate per day and 500 µg parenteral B_{12} per month have been used empirically in dogs with chronic enteropathy.[384]

Parenteral (intravenous) and enteral hyperalimentation are two modalities of specialized nutritional support for more intensive treatment or prevention of malnutrition associated with GI disease.[462] Parenteral hyperalimentation is used in humans for temporary in-hospital maintenance of nutrition when there is almost complete inability to use the gut, while awaiting for bowel adaptation to occur.[465, 466] The expense, technical expertise, and intensive monitoring required for parenteral hyperalimentation have limited its usefulness in dogs and cats. Liquid elemental diets can be used for enteral hyperalimentation as an alternative to IV feeding, or in the transition from IV to oral feeding, especially during the recovery or adaptation phase of bowel resection.[467, 468] Commercial elemental diets consist of liquid mixtures of amino acids, dextrins, glucose, electrolytes, small amounts of fat, trace minerals, and vitamins, but no lactose. They are administered by oral instillation, intermittent oronasogastric intubation, or infusion through indwelling pharyngostomy, gastrostomy, or enterostomy tubes.

Other therapies such as antimicrobials and corticosteroids may be considered in certain cases of chronic diarrhea. However, the use of these is best restricted to treatment of specific disorders; for example, antimicrobials are used when there is evidence for a specific bacterial enteropathogen or small intestinal bacterial overgrowth. Corticosteroids, such as oral prednisolone, are frequently used to treat chronic inflammatory bowel disorders. In addition to their immunosuppressive and anti-inflammatory effects, glucocorticoids have also been beneficial in some dogs with villous atrophy, presumably through induction of functional proteins within enterocytes that enhance their digestive-absorptive capacity.[384, 388] Sulfasalazine, a drug with both antimicrobial and anti-inflammatory actions, appears to be efficacious for many dogs with various forms of chronic colitis, as discussed in Chapter 87.

References

1. Anderson, WD and Anderson, BG: Comparative Anatomy. *In* Anderson, NV (ed): Veterinary Gastroenterology. Philadelphia, Lea & Febiger, 1980, p 127.
2. Eastwood, GL: Gastrointestinal epithelial renewal. Gastroenterol 72:962, 1977.
3. Williamson, RCN and Chir, M: Intestinal adaptation (Part 2). Mechanisms of control. N Engl J Med 298.1443, 1978.
4. Hirsh, DW: Microflora, Mucosa, and Immunity. *In* Anderson, NV (ed): Veterinary Gastroenterology. Philadelphia, Lea & Febiger, 1980, p 199.
5. Moon, HW: Mechanisms in the pathogenesis of diarrhea: A review. JAVMA 172:443, 1978.
6. Walker, WA and Isselbacher, KJ: Intestinal antibodies. N Engl J Med 297:767, 1977.
7. Riley, JW and Glickman, RM: Fat malabsorption: Advances in our understanding. Am J Med 67:980, 1979.
8. Gray, GM: Mechanisms of digestion and absorption of food. *In* Sleisenger, MH and Fordtran, JS (eds): Gastrointestinal Disease, 3rd ed. Philadelphia, WB Saunders, 1983, p 844.
9. Shiau, YF, et al.: Apical distribution of fatty acid esterification capacity along the villus-crypt unit of rat jejunum. Gastroenterol 79:47, 1980.
10. Gray, GM: Carbohydrate digestion and absorption. N Engl J Med 292:1225, 1975.
11. Noon, KF, et al.: Detection and definition of canine intestinal carbohydrates, using a standardized method. Am J Vet Res 38:1063, 1977.
12. Freeman, HJ, et al.: Protein digestion and absorption in man: normal mechanisms and protein-energy malnutrition. Am J Med 67:1030, 1979.
13. Sleisenger, MH and Kim, YS: Protein digestion and absorption. N Engl J Med 300:659, 1979.
14. Phillips, SF: Diarrhea: A current view of the pathophysiology. Gastroenterol 63:495, 1972.
15. Argenzio, RA and Whipp, SC: Pathophysiology of diarrhea. *In* Anderson, NV (ed): Veterinary Gastroenterology. Philadelphia, Lea & Febiger, 1980, p 220.
16. Binder, HJ: Absorption and secretion of water and electrolytes by small and large intestine. *In* Sleisenger, MH and Fordtran, JS (eds): Gastrointestinal Disease, 3rd ed. Philadelphia, WB Saunders, 1983, p 811.
17. Davenport, HW: Motility of the small intestine. *In* Physiology of the Digestive Tract, 4th ed. Chicago, Year Book Med., 1977, p 58.
18. Meshkinpour, H: State of the art. Intestinal motility: Current concepts. Am J Gastroenterol 71:101, 1979.
19. Itoh, Z, et al.: Characteristic motor activity of the gastrointestinal tract in fasted conscious dogs measured by implanted force transducers. Am J Dig Dis 23:229, 1978.
20. Walsh, JH: Gastrointestinal peptide hormones. *In* Sleisenger, MH and Fordtran, JS (eds): Gastrointestinal Disease, 3rd ed. Philadelphia, WB Saunders, 1983, p 54.
21. Doe, WF: An overview of intestinal immunity and malabsorption. Am J Med 67:1077, 1979.
22. Welliver, RC and Ogra, PL: Importance of local immunity in enteric infection. JAVMA 173:560, 1978.
23. Burrows, CF: Chronic diarrhea in the dog. Vet Clin North Am 13:521, 1983.
24. Krejs, GJ and Fordtran, JS: Diarrhea. *In* Sleisenger, MH and Fordtran, JS (eds): Gastrointestinal Disease, 3rd ed. Philadelphia, WB Saunders, 1983, p 257.
25. Ammon, HV and Phillips, SF: Inhibition of colonic water and electrolyte absorption by fatty acids in man. Gastroenterol 65:744, 1973.
26. Duffy, PA, et al.: Intestinal secretion induced by volume expansion in the dog. Gastroenterol 75:413, 1978.
27. Sherding, RG: Canine exocrine pancreatic insufficiency. Comp Cont Ed 1:816, 1979.
28. Sherding, RG: Canine large bowel diarrhea. Comp Cont Ed Small Anim Pract 2:279, 1980.
29. Burrows, CF, et al.: Determination of fecal fat and trypsin output in the evaluation of chronic canine diarrhea. JAVMA 174:62, 1979.
30. Burrows, CF: The assessment of canine gastrointestinal function: Recent advances and future needs. *In* Proceedings of the 31st Gaines Veterinary Symposium, 1981.
31. Peterson, ME, et al.: Feline hyperthyroidism: Pretreatment clinical and laboratory evaluation of 131 cases. JAVMA 183:103, 1983.
32. Weiser, MG and Kociba, GJ: Erythrocyte macrocytosis in feline leukemia virus associated anemia. Vet Pathol 20:687, 1983.
33. Tams, TR and Twedt, DC: Canine protein-losing gastroenteropathy syndrome. Comp Cont Ed 3:105, 1981.
34. Breitschwerdt, EB, et al.: Clinical and laboratory characterization of the Basenji dog with immunoproliferative small intestinal disease. Am J Vet Res 45:267, 1984.

35. Meuten, DJ, et al.: Relationship of serum total calcium to albumin and total protein in dogs. JAVMA 180:63, 1982.

36. Greene, JE and Thorson, RE: Canine intestinal protozoa as related to enteritis. 4th Gaines Veterinary Symposium, 1954, p 6.

37. Pitts, RP, et al.: Comparison of duodenal aspiration with fecal flotation for diagnosis of giardiasis in dogs. JAVMA 182:1210, 1983.

38. Dillon, AR and Wilt, GR: Campylobacter species in the dog and cat. A cause for concern? Vet Clin North Am 13:647, 1983.

39. Ford, RB: Canine histoplasmosis. Comp Cont Ed 2:637, 1980.

40. Migaki, G, et al.: Canine protothecosis: Review of the literature and report of an additional case. JAVMA 181:794, 1982.

41. Drummey, GD, et al.: Microscopical examinations of the stool for steatorrhea. N Engl J Med 264:85, 1961.

42. Ghosh, SK, et al.: Stool microscopy in screening for steatorrhoea. J Clin Pathol 30:749, 1977.

43. Masamune, O, et al.: Diagnostic significance of the Sudan III staining for fecal fat. Tohoku J Exp Med 122:397, 1977.

44. Luk, GD and Hendrix, TR: Microscopic examination of stool as a screening test for steatorrhea (abstr). Gastroenterol 74:1134, 1978.

45. Harris, JC, et al.: Fecal leukocytes in diarrheal illness. Ann Intern Med 76:697, 1972.

46. Pickering, LK, et al.: Fecal leukocytes in enteric infections. Am J Clin Pathol 68:562, 1977.

47. Merritt, AM, et al.: Fecal fat and trypsin in dogs fed a meat-base or cereal-base diet. JAVMA 174:59, 1979.

48. Lewis, LD, et al.: Fat excretion and assimilation by the cat. Feline Pract 9:46, 1979.

49. Finco, DR, et al.: Chronic enteric disease and hypoproteinemia in nine dogs. JAVMA 163:262, 1973.

50. Jeffries, GH: Protein-losing gastroenteropathy. In Sleisenger, MH and Fordtran, JS (eds): Gastrointestinal Disease, 3rd ed. Philadelphia, WB Saunders, 1983, p 280.

51. Bernier, JJ, et al.: Diagnosis of protein-losing enteropathy by gastrointestinal clearance of α_1-antitrypsin. Lancet 2:763, 1978.

52. Florent, C, et al.: Intestinal clearance of α_1-antitrypsin. A sensitive method for the detection of protein-losing enteropathy. Gastroenterol 81:777, 1981.

53. Williams, DA and Batt, RM: Diagnosis of canine exocrine pancreatic insufficiency by the assay of serum trypsin-like immunoreactivity. J Small Anim Pract 24:583, 1983.

54. Williams, DA and Batt, RM: Sensitivity and specificity of radioimmunassay of serum trypsin-like immunoreactivity for the diagnosis of canine exocrine pancreatic insufficiency. JAVMA 192:195, 1988.

55. Freudiger, M and Bigler, B: The diagnosis of chronic exocrine pancreatic insufficiency by the PABA test. Kleintier-Praxis (Bern) 22:73, 1977.

56. Strombeck, DR: New method for evaluation of chymotrypsin deficiency in dogs. JAVMA 173:1319, 1978.

57. Stradley, RP, et al.: A method for the simultaneous evaluation of exocrine pancreatic function and intestinal absorptive function in dogs. Am J Vet Res 40:1201, 1979.

58. Batt, RM, et al.: A new test for the diagnosis of exocrine pancreatic insufficiency in the dog. J Small Anim Pract 20:185, 1979.

59. Rogers, WA, et al.: Simultaneous evaluation of pancreatic exocrine function and intestinal absorptive function in dogs with chronic diarrhea. JAVMA 177:1128, 1980.

60. Batt, RM and Mann, LC: Specificity of BT-PABA for diagnosis of exocrine pancreatic insufficiency in the dog. Vet Rec 108:303, 1981.

61. Hill, FWG, et al.: A xylose absorption test for the dog. Vet Rec 87:250, 1970.

62. Hill, FWG: Malabsorption syndrome in the dog: A study of thirty-eight cases. J Small Anim Pract 13:575, 1972.

63. Batt, RM and Morgan, JO: Role of serum folate and vitamin B12 concentrations in the differentiation of small intestinal abnormalities in the dog. Res Vet Sci 32:17, 1982.

64. Washabau, RJ, et al.: Use of pulmonary hydrogen gas excretion to detect carbohydrate malabsorption in dogs. JAVMA 189:674, 1986.

65. Washabau, RJ, et al.: Evaluation of intestinal carbohydrate malabsorption in the dog by pulmonary hydrogen excretion. Am J Vet Res 47:1402, 1986.

66. Sherding, RG, et al.: Bentiromide: Xylose test in healthy cats. Am J Vet Res 43:2272, 1982.

67. Emms, SG, et al.: The rate of D-xylose absorption in normal cats. Aust Vet J 60:30, 1983.

68. Hawkins, EC, et al.: Digestion of bentiromide and absorption of xylose in healthy cats and absorption of xylose in cats with infiltrative intestinal disease. Am J Vet Res 47:567, 1986.

69. Hayden, DW and VanKruiningen, HJ: Control values for evaluating gastrointestinal function in the dog. JAAHA 12:31, 1976.

70. Anderson, NV and Low, DG: Juvenile atrophy of the canine pancreas. Anim Hosp 1:101, 1965.

71. Brobst, DF and Funk, A: Simplified test of fat absorption in dogs. JAVMA 161:1412, 1972.

72. Sateri, H: Investigations on the exocrine pancreatic function in dogs suffering from chronic exocrine pancreatic insufficiency. Acta Vet Scand (Suppl) 53:1, 1975.

73. Kaneko, JJ, et al.: Malabsorption syndrome resembling nontropical sprue in dogs. JAVMA 146:463, 1965.

74. Kallfelz, FA, et al.: Intestinal absorption of oleic acid ^{131}I and triolein ^{131}I in the differential diagnosis of malabsorption syndrome and pancreatic dysfunction in the dog. JAVMA 153:43, 1968.

75. Hill, FWG and Kidder, DE: The oral glucose tolerance test in canine pancreatic malabsorption. Br Vet J 128:207, 1972.

76. Hill, FWG: A starch tolerance test in canine pancreatic malabsorption. Vet Rec 91:169, 1972.

77. Westermarck, E and Sandholm, M: Faecal hydrolase activity as determined by radial enzyme diffusion: A new method for detecting pancreatic dysfunction in the dog. Res Vet Sci 28:341, 1980.

78. Stradley, R, et al.: Gastric absorption of D-xylose in the rat: Its influence on the D-xylose absorption test. J Lab Clin Med 107:10, 1986.

79. King, CE and Toskes, PP: Small intestinal bacterial overgrowth. Gastroenterol 76:1035, 1979.

80. Isaacs, PET and Kim, YS: The contaminated small bowel syndrome. Am J Med 67:1049, 1979.

81. Burrows, CF and Jezyk, PF: Nitrosonaphthol test for screening of small intestinal diarrheal disease in the dog. JAVMA 183:318, 1983.

82. Washabau, RJ, et al.: Evaluation and management of carbohydrate malassimilation. In Kirk, RW (ed): Current Veterinary Therapy IX. Philadelphia, WB Saunders, 1986, p 889.

83. Gomez, JA: The gastrointestinal contrast study—methods and interpretation. Vet Clin North Am 4:805, 1974.

84. Fossum, TW, et al.: Intestinal lymphangectasia associated with chylothorax in two dogs. JAVMA 190:61, 1987.

85. Batt, RM and Peters, TJ: Subcellular fractionation studies on peroral jejunal biopsies from the dog. Res Vet Sci 25:94, 1978.

86. Batt, RM: Techniques for single and multiple peroral jejunal biopsy in the dog. J Small Anim Pract 20:259, 1979.

87. Batt, RM, et al.: Subcellular biochemical studies of a naturally occurring enteropathy in the dog resembling chronic tropical sprue in human beings. Am J Vet Res 44:1492, 1983.

88. Batt, RM, et al.: Morphologic and biochemical studies of a naturally occurring enteropathy in the Irish setter dog: A comparison with coeliac disease in man. Res Vet Sci 37:339, 1984.

89. Batt, RM, et al.: Specific brush border abnormalities associated with a wheat-sensitive enteropathy (WSE) in the Irish Setter dog. Gastroenterol 86:1021, 1984.

90. Batt, RM, et al.: Developmental brush border defect associated with cereal sensitivity in the Irish Setter dog. Clin Sci 66:38, 1984.

91. Batt, RM, et al.: Sequential morphologic and biochemical studies of a naturally occurring wheat-sensitive enteropathy in Irish Setter dogs. Digest Dis Sci 32:184, 1987.

92. Batt, RM, et al.: Bacterial overgrowth associated with a naturally occurring enteropathy in the German Shepherd dog. Res Vet Sci 35:42, 1983.

93. Batt, RM, et al.: Biochemical changes in the jejunal mucosa of dogs with a naturally occurring enteropathy associated with bacterial overgrowth. Gut 25:816, 1984.

94. Batt, RM and McLean, L: Comparison of the biochemical changes in the jejunal mucosa of dogs with aerobic and anaerobic bacterial overgrowth. Gastroenterol 93:986, 1987.

95. Povar, R: Food allergy in dogs (a preliminary report). JAVMA 111:61, 1947.

96. Knowles, JO: Provocative exposure for the diagnosis and treatment of certain canine allergies. JAVMA 149:1303, 1966.

97. Michaux, HR: A mutton and rice diet for treating chronic diarrhea in the dog. JAVMA 149:296, 1966.

98. Toombs, JP, et al.: Colonic perforation following neurosurgical procedures and corticosteroid therapy in four dogs. JAVMA 177:68, 1980.

99. Moore, RW and Withrow, SJ: Gastrointestinal hemorrhage and pancreatitis associated with intervertebral disk disease in the dog. JAVMA 180:1443, 1982.

100. Swerczek, TW, et al.: Transmammary passage of Toxocara cati in the cat. Am J Vet Res 32:89, 1971.

101. Hendrix, CM and Blagburn, BL: Common gastrointestinal parasites. Vet Clin North Am 13:627, 1983.

102. Malone, JB, et al.: Strongyloides tumefaciens in cats. JAVMA 171:278, 1977.

103. Lindsay, DS, et al.: Strongyloides tumefaciens infection in a cat. Comp Anim Pract 1:12, 1987.

104. Dubey, JP: Toxoplasmosis in cats. Feline Pract 16:12, 1986.

105. Glickman, LT, et al.: Canine and human toxocariasis: Review of transmission, pathogenesis, and clinical disease. JAVMA 175:1265, 1979.

106. Schantz, PM and Glickman, LT: Canine and human toxocariasis: The public health problem and the veterinarian's role in prevention. JAVMA 175:1270, 1979.

107. Roberson, EL and Cornelius, LM: Gastrointestinal parasitism. In Kirk, RW (ed): Current Veterinary Therapy VIII. Philadelphia, WB Saunders, 1983, p 797.

108. Dubey, JP: Effect of fenbendazole on Toxocara canis larvae in tissues of infected dogs. Am J Vet Res 40:698, 1979.

109. Burke, T and Roberson, EL: Fenbendazole treatment of pregnant bitches to reduce prenatal and lactogenic infections of Toxocara canis and Ancylostoma caninum in pups. JAVMA 183:987, 1983.

110. Miller, TA: Vaccination against the canine hookworm diseases. Adv Parasitol 9:153, 1971.

111. Migasena, S, et al.: Studies in Ancylostoma caninum infection in dogs. II: Anatomical changes in the gastrointestinal tract. Ann Trop Med Parasitol 66:203, 1972.

112. Miller, TA: Blood loss during hookworm infection, determined by erythrocyte labeling with radioactive ^{51}chromium. I. Infection of dogs with normal and with x-irradiated ancylostoma caninum. J Parasitol 52:844, 1966.

113. Miller, TA: Blood loss during hookworm infection, determined by erythrocyte labeling with radioactive ^{51}chromium. II: Pathogenesis of Ancylostoma braziliense infection in dogs and cats. J Parasitol 52:856, 1966.

114. VanKruiningen, HJ: Comparative Gastroenterology. Springfield, IL, Charles C Thomas, 1982, p 65.

115. Hotez, PJ and Cerami, A: Secretion of a proteolytic anticoagulant by Ancylostoma hookworms. J Exp Med 157:1594, 1983.

116. Migasena, S, et al.: Studies in Ancylostoma caninum infection in dogs. I: Absorption from the small intestine of amino-acids, carbohydrates, and fat. Ann Trop Med Parasitol 66:107, 1972.

117. Rubin, R: Studies on the common whipworm of the dog, Trichuris vulpis. Cornell Vet 44:36, 1954.

118. Burrows, RB and Lillis, WG: The whipworm as a blood sucker. J Parasitol 50:675, 1964.

119. Hass, DK: Feline whipworms do exist. Feline Prac 8:31, 1978.

120. Soulsby, EJL: Helminths, Arthropods, Protozoa of Domesticated Animals, 6th ed. Baltimore, Williams & Wilkins, 1968.

121. Dunn, AM: Veterinary Helminthology. London, Heinemann Medical Books, 1978.

122. Malone, JB, et al.: Strongyloides stercoralis-like infection in a dog. JAVMA 176:130, 1980.

123. Holzworth, J and Georgi, JR: Trichinosis in a cat. JAVMA 165:186, 1974.

124. Hayden, DW: Alariasis in a dog. JAVMA 155:889, 1969.

125. Pierce, KR: Heterobilharzia americana infection in a dog. JAVMA 143:496, 1963.

126. Troy, GC, et al.: Heterobilharzia americana infection and hypercalcemia in a dog. A case report. JAAHA 23:35, 1987.

127. Fahnestock, GR: Macracanthorhynchiasis in dogs. Mod Vet Prac 66:31, 1985.

128. Dubey, JP: A review of Sarcocystis of domestic animals and of other coccidia of cats and dogs. JAVMA 169:1061, 1976.

129. Greene, CR and Prestwood, AK: Coccidial infections. In Greene, CE (ed): Clinical Microbiology and Infectious Diseases of the Dog and Cat. Philadelphia, WB Saunders, 1984, p 824.

130. Dubey, JP, et al.: Canine coccidiosis attributed to an Isospora ohioensis-like organism: a case report. JAVMA 173:185, 1978.

131. Dubey, JP: Pathogenicity of Isospora ohioensis infection in dogs. JAVMA 173:192, 1978.

132. Poonacha, KB and Pippin, C: Intestinal cryptosporidiosis in a cat. Vet Pathol 19:708, 1982.

133. Monticello, TM, et al.: Cryptosporidiosis in a feline leukemia virus-positive cat. JAVMA 191:705, 1987.

134. Wilson, RB, et al.: Cryptosporidiosis in a pup. JAVMA 183:1005, 1983.

135. Fukushima, K and Helman, RG: Cryptosporidiosis in a pup with distemper. Vet Pathol 21:247, 1984.

136. Sisk, DB, et al.: Intestinal cryptosporidiosis in two pups. JAVMA 184:835, 1984.

137. Anderson, BC: Cryptosporidiosis: A review. JAVMA 180:1455, 1982.

138. Iseki, M: Cryptosporidium felis sp. n (Protozoa: Eimeriorina) from the domestic cat. Jpn J Parasitol 28:285, 1979.

139. Current, WL, et al.: Human cryptosporidiosis in immunocompetent and immunodeficient persons. N Engl J Med 308:1252, 1983.

140. Current, WL: Cryptosporidiosis. JAVMA 187:1334, 1985.

141. Brightman, AH and Slonka, GF: A review of five clinical cases of giardiasis in cats. JAAHA 12:492, 1976.

142. Barlough, JE: Canine giardiasis: A review. J Small Anim Pract 20:613, 1979.

143. Kirkpatrick, CE, et al.: Giardiasis. Comp Cont Ed Pract Vet 4:367, 1982.

144. Kirkpatrick, CE and Farrell, JP: Feline giardiasis: observations on natural and induced infections. Am J Vet Res 45:2182, 1984.

145. Kirkpatrick, CE and Laczak, JP: Giardiasis in a cattery. JAVMA 187:161, 1985.

146. Kirkpatrick, CE: Feline giardiasis: a review. J Small Anim Pract 27:69, 1986.

147. Hewlett, EL, et al.: Experimental infection of mongrel dogs with Giardia lamblia cysts and cultured trophozoites. J Infect Dis 145:89, 1982.

148. Zimmer, JF and Burrington, DB: Comparison of four techniques of fecal examination for detecting canine giardiasis. JAAHA 22:161, 1986.

149. Belosevic, M, et al.: Observations on natural and experimental infections with Giardia isolated from cats. Can J Comp Med 48:241, 1984.

150. Roudebush, P and Delivorias, MH: Duodenal aspiration via flexible endoscope for diagnosis of giardiasis in a dog. JAVMA 187:162, 1985.

151. Hartong, WA, et al.: Giardiasis: Clinical spectrum and functional structural abnormalities of the small intestinal mucosa. Gastroenterol 77:61, 1979.

152. Solomons, NW: Giardiasis: nutritional implications. Rev Infect Dis 4:859, 1982.

153. Zimmer, JF and Burrington, DB: Comparison of four protocols for the treatment of canine giardiasis. JAAHA 22:169, 1986.

154. Bruce, KL: Trichomoniasis in a puppy. Vet Med 36:261, 1941.

155. Wenrich, DH: Morphology of the intestinal trichomoniasis flagellates in man and of similar forms in monkeys, cats, dogs, and rats. J Morphol 74:189, 1944.

156. O'Donnell, FA: Intestinal trichomoniasis in a dog. Vet Med 49:390, 1954.

157. Burrows, RB and Lillis, WG: Intestinal protozoan infections in dogs. JAVMA 150:880, 1967.

158. Burrows, RB and Hunt, GR: Intestinal protozoan infections in cats. JAVMA 157:2065, 1970.

159. Narayana, GS: Intestinal trichomoniasis in a dog—a case study. Indian Vet J 53:477, 1976.

160. Binn, LN, et al.: Recovery and characterization of a minute virus of canines. Infect Immun 1:503, 1970.

161. Keenan, KP, et al.: Intestinal infection of neonatal dogs with canine coronavirus I-71: Studies by virologic, histologic, his-

tochemical, and immunofluorescent techniques. Am J Vet Res 37:247, 1976.

162. Appel, MJG, et al.: Status report: Canine viral enteritis. JAVMA 173:1516, 1978.

163. England, JJ and Poston, RP: Electron microscopic identification and subsequent isolation of a rotavirus from a dog with fatal neonatal diarrhea. Am J Vet Res 41:782, 1980.

164. Willimas, FP: Astrovirus-like, coronavirus-like, and parvovirus-like particles detected in the diarrheic stools of Beagle pups. Arch Virol 66:215, 1980.

165. Appel, MJG, et al.: Enteric viral infections of dogs. Gaines 29th Veterinary Symposium 1979, p 3.

166. Pindak, FF and Clapper, WE: Isolation of enteric cytopathogenic human orphan virus type 6 from dogs. Am J Vet Res 25:52, 1964.

167. Lundgren, DL, et al.: Isolation of human enteroviruses from beagle dogs. Proc Soc Exp Biol Med 128:463, 1968.

168. Carmichael, LE and Binn, LN: New enteric viruses in the dog. Adv Vet Sci Comp Med 25:1, 1981.

169. Marshall, JA, et al.: Viruses and virus-like particles in the faeces of dogs with and without diarrhoea. Aust Vet J 61:33, 1984.

170. Pederson, NC, et al.: An enteric coronavirus infection of cats and its relationship to feline infectious peritonitis. Am J Vet Res 42:368, 1981.

171. Pederson, NC: Feline infectious peritonitis and feline enteric coronavirus infections. Feline Pract 13:13, 1983.

172. Snodgrass, DR: A rotavirus from kittens. Vet Rec 104:70, 1979.

173. Chrystie, IL, et al.: Rotavirus infection in a domestic cat. Vet Rec 105:404, 1979.

174. Hoshino, Y, et al.: New insights in gastrointestinal viruses. Cornell Feline Health News 2:2, 1981.

175. Reinacher, M: Feline leukemia virus-associated enteritis-a condition with features of feline panleukopenia. Vet Pathol 24:1, 1987.

176. Pollock, RVH and Zimmer, JF: Canine Viral Enteritis. Proceedings of the 8th Kal Kan Symposium:105, 1984.

177. Appel, MJG, et al.: Isolation and immunization studies of a canine parvo-like virus from dogs with haemorrhagic enteritis. Vet Rec 105:156, 1979.

178. McCandlish, IAP, et al.: Isolation of a parvovirus from dogs in Britain. Vet Rec 105:167, 1979.

179. Pollock, RV and Carmichael, LE: Canine viral enteritis. Recent developments. Mod Vet Pract 60:375, 1979.

180. Macartney, L, et al.: Canine parvovirus enteritis 1: Clinical haematological and pathological features of experimental infection. Vet Rec 115:201, 1984.

181. Macartney, L, et al.: Canine parvovirus enteritis 2: Pathogenesis. Vet Rec 115:453, 1984.

182. Meunier, PC, et al.: Pathogenesis of canine parvovirus enteritis: The importance of viremia. Vet Path 22:60, 1985.

183. Jacobs, RM, et al.: Clinicopathologic features of canine parvoviral enteritis. JAAHA 16:809, 1980.

184. Stann, SE, et al.: Clinical and pathologic features of parvoviral diarrhea in pound-source dogs. JAVMA 185:651, 1984.

185. Farrow, CS: Radiographic appearance of canine parvovirus enteritis. JAVMA 180:43, 1982.

186. Pollock, RVH and Carmichael LE: Canine viral enteritis. Vet Clin North Am 13:551, 1983.

187. Carmichael, LE, et al.: Hemagglutination by canine parvovirus: Serologic studies and diagnostic applications. Am J Vet Res 41:784, 1980.

188. Mathys, A, et al.: Comparison of hemagglutination and competitive enzyme-linked immunosorbent assay procedure for detecting canine parvovirus in feces. Am J Vet Res 44:152, 1983.

189. Burrows, CF: Topics in drug therapy. Metoclopramide. JAVMA 183:1341, 1983.

190. Pollock, RV and Carmichael, LE: Maternally derived immunity to canine parvovirus infection: transfer, decline, and interference with vaccination. JAVMA 180:37, 1982.

191. Hammond, MM and Timoney, PJ: An electron microscopic study of viruses associated with canine gastroenteritis. Cornell Vet 73:82, 1983.

192. Woode, GN and Crouch, CF: Naturally occurring and experimentally induced rotaviral infections of domestic and laboratory animals. JAVMA 173:522, 1978.

193. Middleton, PJ: Pathogenesis of rotaviral infection. JAVMA 173:544, 1978.

194. Johnson, CA, et al.: Gross and light microscopic lesions in neonatal gnotobiotic dogs inoculated with a canine rotavirus. Am J Vet Res 44:1687, 1983.

195. Eugster, AK and Sidwa, T: Rotaviruses in diarrheic feces of a dog. VM/SAC 74:817, 1979.

196. Dagenais, L, et al.: Presence of rotavirus in fecal matter of dogs with diarrhea. Ann Med Vet 124:449, 1980.

197. Fulton, RW, et al.: Isolation of a rotavirus from a newborn dog with diarrhea. Am J Vet Res 42:841, 1981.

198. Schroeder, BA, et al.: The isolation of a rotavirus from calves, foals, dogs and cats in New Zealand. NZ Vet J 31:114, 1983.

199. McNulty, MS, et al.: Antibody to rotavirus in dogs and cats. Vet Rec 102:534, 1978.

200. Dagenais, L, et al.: Incidence of rotavirus antibodies in dog, cat, and horse sera in Belgium. Ann Med Vet 124:422, 1980.

201. Johnson, CA, et al.: Inoculation of neonatal gnotobiotic dogs with a canine rotavirus. Am J Vet Res 44:1682, 1983.

202. Pollock, RVH: The parvoviruses. Part I. Feline panleukopenia virus and mink enteritis virus. Comp Cont Ed 6:227, 1984.

203. Csiza, CK, et al.: Pathogenesis of feline panleukopenia virus in susceptible newborn kittens. I. Clinical signs, hematology, serology and virology. Infect Immun 3:833, 1971.

204. Csiza, CK, et al.: Pathogenesis of feline panleukopenia virus in susceptible newborn kittens. II. Pathology and immunofluorescence. Infect Immun 3:838, 1971.

205. Rohovsky, MW and Fowler, EH: Lesions of experimental feline panleukopenia. JAVMA 158:872, 1971.

206. Larsen, S, et al.: Experimental feline panleucopenia in the conventional cat. Vet Pathol 13:216, 1976.

207. Carlson, JH, et al.: Feline panleukopenia. I. Pathogenesis in germfree and specific pathogen-free cats. Vet Pathol 14:79, 1977.

208. Carlson, JH, et al.: Feline panleukopenia. II. The relationship of intestinal mucosal cell proliferation rates to viral infection and development of lesions. Vet Pathol 14:173, 1977.

209. Kahn, DE: Pathogenesis of feline panleukopenia. JAVMA 173:628, 1978.

210. Shindel, NM, et al.: The colitis of feline panleukopenia. JAVMA 14:738, 1978.

211. McKiernan, AJ, et al.: Isolation of feline coronaviruses from two cats with diverse disease manifestations. Feline Pract 11:16, 1981.

212. Pierce, NF, et al.: Antitoxic immunity to cholera in dogs immunized orally with cholera toxin. Infect Immun 27:632, 1980.

213. Giannella, RA, et al.: Pathogenesis of salmonella-mediated intestinal fluid secretion. Gastroenterol 69:1238, 1975.

214. Greene, CE: Enteric bacterial infections. In Greene, CE (ed): Clinical Microbiology and Infectious Diseases of the Dog and Cat. Philadelphia, WB Saunders, 1984, p 617.

215. Morse, EV and Duncan, MA: Canine salmonellosis: Prevalence, epizootiology, signs, and public health significance. JAVMA 167:817, 1975.

216. Shimi, A and Barin, A: Salmonella in cats. J Comp Pathol 87:315, 1977.

217. Fox, JG: Feline salmonellosis. In Kirk, RW (ed): Current Veterinary Therapy VII. Philadelphia, WB Saunders, 1980, p 1305.

218. Timoney, JF, et al.: Feline salmonellosis: A nosocomial outbreak and experimental studies. Cornell Vet 68:211, 1978.

219. Ketaren, K, et al.: Canine salmonellosis in a small animal hospital. JAVMA 179:1017, 1981.

220. Calvert, CA and Leifer, CE: Salmonellosis in dogs with lymphosarcoma. JAVMA 180:56, 1982.

221. Calvert, CA: Salmonella infections in hospitalized dogs: Epizootiology, diagnosis, and prognosis. JAAHA 21:499, 1985.

222. Kaufmann, AF: Pets and salmonella infection. JAVMA 149:1655, 1966.

223. Morse, EV, et al.: Canine salmonellosis: A review and report of dog to child transmission of Salmonella enteritidis. Am J Public Health 66:82, 1976.

224. Krum, SH, et al.: Salmonella arizonae bacteremia in a cat. JAVMA 170:42, 1977.

225. Blaser, MJ and Reller, BL: Campylobacter enteritis. N Engl J Med 305:1444, 1981.

226. Fox, JG: Campylobacteriosis - a "new" disease in laboratory animals. Lab Anim Sci 32:625, 1982.

227. Fleming, MP: Association of *Campylobacter jejuni* with enteritis in dogs and cats. Vet Rec 113:372, 1983.

228. Fox, JG, et al.: Canine and feline campylobacteriosis: Epizootiology and clinical and public health features. JAVMA 183:1420, 1983.

229. Dillon, AR, et al.: Campylobacter enteritis in dogs and cats. Comp Cont Ed 9:1176, 1987.

230. Blaser, MJ, et al.: Reservoirs for human campylobacteriosis. J Infect Dis 141:665, 1980.

231. Prescott, JF and Munroe, DL: *Campylobacter jejuni* enteritis in man and domestic animals. JAVMA 181:1524, 1982.

232. Fox, JG, et al.: *Campylobacter jejuni*-associated diarrhea in dogs. JAVMA 183:1430, 1983.

233. Fox, JG, et al.: Chronic diarrhea associated with *Campylobacter jejuni* infection in a cat. JAVMA 189:455, 1986.

234. Collins, JE, et al.: Proliferative enteritis in two pups. JAVMA 183:886, 1983.

235. Skirrow, MB: Campylobacter enteritis: A "new" disease. Br Med J 2:9, 1977.

236. Fox, JG, et al.: Antibiotic sensitivity patterns of *Campylobacter jejuni/coli* isolated from laboratory animals and pets. Lab Anim Sci 34:264, 1984.

237. Slee, A: Hemorrhagic gastroenteritis in a dog. Vet Rec 104:14, 1979.

238. Murtaugh, RJ and Lawrence, AE: Feline *Campylobacter jejuni*-associated enteritis. Feline Pract 14:37, 1984.

239. Mollaret, HH: L'infection a bacille de malassez et vignal chez le chat. I: La maladie naturelle. Recl Med Vet 141:1079, 1965.

240. Mair, NS, et al.: *Pasteurella pseudotuberculosis* infection in the cat: two cases. Vet Rec 81:461, 1967.

241. Hubbert, WT: Yersiniosis in mammals and birds in the United States. Am J Trop Med Hyg 21:458, 1972.

242. Allard, AW: *Yersinia pseudotuberculosis* in a cat. JAVMA 174:91, 1979.

243. Spearman, JG, et al.: *Yersinia pseudotuberculosis* infection in a cat. Can Vet J 20:361, 1979.

244. Yanagawa, Y, et al.: Isolation of *Yersinia enterocolitica* and *Yersinia pseudotuberculosis* from apparently healthy dogs and cats. Microbiol Immunol 22:643, 1978.

245. Vantrappen, G, et al.: Yersinia enteritis and enterocolitis: Gastroenterological aspects. Gastroenterol 72:220, 1977.

246. Pederson, KB: Isolation of *Yersinia enterocolitica* from Danish swine and dogs. Acta Pathol Microbiol Scand [B]84:317, 1976.

247. Kaneko, K, et al.: Occurrence of *Yersinia enterocolitica* in dogs. Jpn J Vet Sci 39:407, 1977.

248. Pederson, KB and Winblad, S: Studies on *Yersinia enterocolitica* isolated from swine and dogs. Acta Pathol Microbiol Scand [B]87:137, 1979.

249. Wooley, RE, et al.: Isolation of *Yersinia enterocolitica* from selected animal species. Am J Vet Res 41:1667, 1980.

250. Papageorges, M, et al.: *Yersinia enterocolitica* enteritis in two dogs. JAVMA 182:618, 1983.

251. Farstad, L, et al.: Isolation of *Yersinia enterocolitica* from a dog with chronic enteritis. A case report. Acta Vet Scand 17:261, 1976.

252. Wilson, HD, et al.: *Yersinia enterocolitica* infection in a 4-month-old infant associated with infection in household dogs. J Pediatr 89:767, 1976.

253. Kovatch, RM and Zebarth, G: Naturally occurring Tyzzer's disease in a cat. JAVMA 162:136, 1973.

254. Kubokawa, K: Two cases of feline Tyzzer's disease. Jpn J Exp Med 43:413, 1973.

255. Poonacha, KB and Smith, HL: Naturally occurring Tyzzer's disease as a complication of distemper and mycotic pneumonia in a dog. JAVMA 169:419, 1976.

256. Qureshi, SR, et al.: Tyzzer's disease in a dog. JAVMA 168:602, 1976.

257. Schneck, G: Tyzzer's disease in an adult cat. VM/SAC 70:155, 1975.

258. Bennett, AM: Tyzzer's disease in cats experimentally infected with feline leukemia virus. Vet Microbiol 2:49, 1977.

259. Formal, SB, et al.: Invasive *Escherichia coli*. JAVMA 173:596, 1978.

260. Thorne, GM and Gorback, SL: Enterotoxigenic *Escherichia coli*: Detection and importance in diarrheal disease of children. JAVMA 173:592, 1978.

261. Gyles, CL: Comments on detection and importance of entero-pathogenic *Escherichia coli* in diarrheal disease of human beings. JAVMA 173:598, 1978.

262. Guerrant, MD, et al.: Evaluation and diagnosis of acute infectious diarrhea. Am J Med 78:91, 1985.

263. Echeverria, PD, et al.: Enterotoxigenicity and invasive capacity of "enteropathogenic" serotypes of *Escherichia coli*. J Pediatr 89:8, 1976.

264. Guerrant, RL, et al.: Effect of *Escherichia coli* on fluid transport across canine small bowel. Mechanism and time-course with enterotoxin and whole bacterial cells. J Clin Invest 52:1707, 1973.

265. Olson, P, et al.: *Escherichia coli* infection in two dogs with acute diarrhea. JAVMA 184:982, 1984.

266. Whipp, SC and Donta, ST: Serum antibody to *Escherichia coli* heat-labile enterotoxin in cattle and swine. Am J Vet Res 37:905, 1976.

267. Olson, P, et al.: Enterotoxigenic *Escherichia coli* (ETEC) and *Klebsiella pneumoniae* isolated from dogs with diarrhoea. Vet Microbiol 10:577, 1985.

268. Smith, HW: The development of the flora of the alimentary tract in young animals. J Pathol Bacteriol 90:495, 1965.

269. Bartlett, JG, et al.: Antibiotic-associated pseudomembranous colitis due to toxin-producing clostridia. N Engl J Med 298:531, 1978.

270. Borriello, SP, et al.: Household pets as a potential reservoir for *Clostridium difficile* infection. J Clin Pathol 36:84, 1983.

271. Berry, AP and Levett, PN: Chronic diarrhoea in dogs associated with *Clostridium difficile* infection. Vet Rec 118:102, 1986.

272. George, WL, et al.: Treatment and prevention of antimicrobial agent-induced colitis and diarrhea. Gastroenterol 79:366, 1980.

273. Prescott, JF, et al.: Haemorrhagic gastroenteritis in the dog associated with *Clostridium welchii*. Vet Rec 103:116, 1978.

274. Berg, JN, et al.: Occurrence of anaerobic bacteria in diseases of the dog and cat. Am J Vet Res 40:876, 1979.

275. Tilton, RC, et al.: Toxigenic *Clostridium perfringens* from a parvovirus-infected dog. J Clin Microbiol 14:697, 1981.

276. Carman, RJ and Lewis, JCM: Recurrent diarrhea in a dog associated with *Clostridium perfringens* type A. Vet Rec 112:342, 1983.

277. Hill, FWG: Acute intestinal haemorrhage syndrome in dogs. *In* Grunsell, GSG and Hill, FWG (ed): Vet Annual. England, John Wright, 1973, p 98.

278. Bernstein, M: Hemorrhagic gastroenteritis. *In* Kirk, RW (ed): Current Veterinary Therapy VI. Philadelphia, WB Saunders, 1977, p 951.

279. Burrows, CF: Canine hemorrhagic gastroenteritis. JAVMA 13:451, 1977.

280. Biberstein, EL and Holzworth, J: Bacterial Diseases. *In* Holzworth, J (ed): Diseases of the Cat: Medicine & Surgery. Philadelphia, WB Saunders, 1987, p 279.

281. Orr, CM, et al.: Tuberculosis in cats. A report of two cases. J Small Anim Pract 21:247, 1980.

282. Butler, CW and Herd, BR: Human enteric pathogens in dogs in central Alaska. J Infect Dis 115:233, 1965.

283. Kato, E, et al.: Enterotoxigenic staphylococci of canine origin. Am J Vet Res 39:1771, 1978.

284. Pindak, FF, et al.: Incidence and distribution of spirochetes in the digestive tract of dogs. Am J Vet Res 26:1391, 1965.

285. Turek, JJ and Meyer, RC: Studies on a canine intestinal spirochete: Scanning electron microscopy of canine colonic mucosa. Infect Immun 20:853, 1978.

286. Gorham, JR and Foreyt, WJ: Salmon poisoning disease. *In* Greene, CE (ed): Clinical Microbiology and Infectious Diseases of the Dog and Cat. Philadelphia, WB Saunders, 1984, p 538.

287. Hibler, SC, et al.: Rickettsial infections in dogs. Part III. Salmon disease complex and hemobartonellosis. Comp Cont Ed 8:251, 1986.

288. Menges, RW: Canine histoplasmosis. JAVMA 119:411, 1951.

289. Robinson, VB and McVickar, DL: Pathology of spontaneous histoplasmosis. A study of twenty-one cases. Am J Vet Res 13:214, 1952.

290. Cole, CR, et al.: Histoplasmosis in animals. JAVMA 122:471, 1953.

291. Patnaik, AK, et al.: Canine histoplasmosis. A report of two cases. JAAHA 10:493, 1974.

292. Mahaffey, E, et al.: Disseminated histoplasmosis in three cats. JAAHA 13:46, 1977.

293. Stickle, JE and Hribernik, TN: Clinicopathological observations in disseminated histoplasmosis in dogs. JAAHA 14:105, 1978.

294. Mitchell, M and Stark, DR: Disseminated canine histoplasmosis: a clinical survey of 24 cases in Texas. Can Vet J 21:95, 1980.

295. Stark, DR: Primary gastrointestinal histoplasmosis in a cat. JAAHA 18:154, 1982.

296. Dillon, AR, et al.: Canine abdominal histoplasmosis: A report of four cases. JAAHA 18:498, 1982.

297. Wolf, AM and Belden, MN: Feline histoplasmosis: A literature review and retrospective study of 20 new cases. JAAHA 20:995, 1984.

298. Miller, RI: Gastrointestinal phycomycosis in 63 dogs. JAVMA 186:473, 1985.

299. Gleiser, CA: Mucormycosis in animals. A report of three cases. JAVMA 123:441, 1953.

300. Dawson, C, et al.: Canine phycomycosis: A case report. Vet Rec 84:633, 1969.

301. Heller, RA, et al.: Three cases of phycomycosis in dogs. VM/SAC 66:472, 1971.

302. Lee, CG, et al.: Phycomycosis in the ileum of a dog. Austr Vet J 52:388, 1976.

303. Ader, PL: Phycomycosis in fifteen dogs and two cats. JAVMA 174:1216, 1979.

304. Gaunt, PS: Intestinal phycomycosis in a dog: A case report. Southwest Vet 35:51, 1982.

305. Pavletic, M, et al.: Intestinal infarction associated with canine phycomycosis. JAAHA 19:913, 1983.

306. Miller, RI, et al.: Gastrointestinal phycomycosis in a dog. JAVMA 182:1245, 1983.

307. Fox, JG, et al.: Systemic fungal infections in cats. JAVMA 173:1191, 1978.

308. Smith, JMB: Mycoses of the alimentary tract of animals. New Zealand Vet J 16:89, 1968.

309. Langheinrich, KA and Nielsen, SW: Histopathology of feline panleukopenia: A report of 65 cases. JAVMA 158:863, 1971.

310. Bolton, GR and Brown, TT: Mycotic colitis in a cat. VM/SAC 67:978, 1972.

311. McCausland, IP: Systemic mycoses of 2 cats. New Zealand Vet J 20:10, 1972.

312. Stokes, R: Intestinal mycosis in a cat. Aust Vet J 49:499, 1973.

313. Vogler, GA and Wagner, JE: What's your diagnosis? Lab Anim 5:14, 1975.

314. Anderson, PG and Pidgeon, G: Candidiasis in a dog with parvoviral enteritis. JAAHA 23:27, 1987.

315. Hill, FWG and Kelly, DF: Naturally occurring intestinal malabsorption in the dog. Dig Dis 19:649, 1974.

316. Tams, TR: Chronic feline inflammatory bowel disorders. Part I. Idiopathic inflammatory bowel disease. Comp Cont Ed Pract Vet 8:371, 1986.

317. Tams, TR: Chronic canine lymphocytic plasmacytic enteritis. Comp Cont Ed 9:1184, 1987.

318. Hayden, DW and VanKruiningen, HJ: Lymphocytic-plasmacytic enteritis in German Shepherd dogs. JAAHA 18:89, 1982.

319. Willard, MD, et al.: Lymphocytic-plasmacytic enteritis in a cat. JAVMA 186:181, 1985.

320. Edwards, DF and Russell, RG: Probable vitamin K-deficient bleeding in two cats with malabsorption syndrome secondary to lymphocytic-plasmacytic enteritis. J Vet Intern Med 1:97, 1987.

321. VanKruiningen, HJ and Hayden, DW: Interpreting problem diarrheas of dogs. Vet Clin North Am 2:29, 1972.

322. Walton, GS, et al.: Spontaneous allergic dermatitis and enteritis in a cat. Vet Rec 83:35, 1968.

323. Nelson, RW, et al.: Lymphocytic-plasmacytic colitis in the cat. JAVMA 184:1133, 1984.

324. Ochoa, R, et al.: Immunoproliferative small intestinal disease (IPSID) in Basenji dogs: Morphological observations. Am J Vet Res 45:482, 1984.

325. Vernon, DF, Jr: Idiopathic sprue in a dog. JAVMA 140:1062, 1962.

326. VanKruiningen, HJ: Clinical efficacy of tylosin in canine inflammatory bowel disease. JAAHA 12:498, 1976.

327. Khojasteh, A, et al.: Immunoproliferative small intestinal disease. N Engl J Med 308:1401, 1983.

328. Breitschwerdt, EB, et al.: A hereditary diarrhetic syndrome in the Basenji characterized by malabsorption, protein losing enteropathy, and hypergamma-globulinemia. JAAHA 16:551, 1980.

329. Breitschwerdt, EB, et al.: Clinical and epidemiologic characterization of a diarrheal syndrome in Basenji dogs. JAVMA 180:914, 1982.

330. Breitschwerdt, EB, et al.: Serum proteins in healthy Basenjis and Basenjis with chronic diarrhea. Am J Vet Res 44:326, 1983.

331. Breitschwerdt, EB: Immunoproliferate enteropathy of Basenjis. Proceedings of the 8th Kal Kan Symposium:111, 1984.

332. Barta, O, et al.: Lymphocyte transformation and humoral immune parameters in Basenji dogs with immunoproliferative small intestinal disease. Am J Vet Res 44:1954, 1983.

333. Hall, CL: Three clinical cases of eosinophilic enteritis. Southwest Vet 21:41, 1967.

334. Bartsch, RC and Irvine-Smith, B: Eosinophilic gastroenteritis: Report of a case in a dog. J S Afr Vet Med Assoc 43:263, 1972.

335. Easley, JR: Gastroenteritis and associated eosinophilia in a dog. JAVMA 161:1030, 1972.

336. Legendre, AM and Krehbiel, JD: Eosinophilic enteritis in a Chesapeake Bay Retriever. JAVMA 163:258, 1973.

337. Hayden, DW and VanKruiningen, HJ: Eosinophilic gastroenteritis in German shepherd dogs and its relationship to visceral larva migrans. JAVMA 162:379, 1973.

338. Quigley, PJ and Henry, K: Eosinophilic enteritis in the dog: a case report with a brief review of the literature. J Comp Path 91:387, 1981.

339. Itoh, N, et al.: Eosinophilic enteritis in a dog. Comp Anim Pract 1:29, 1987.

340. Cello, JP: Eosinophilic gastroenteritis—a complex disease entity. Am J Med 67:1097, 1979.

341. Greenberger, N: Allergic disorders of the intestine and eosinophilic gastroenteritis. In Sleisenger, MH and Fordtran, JS (eds): Gastrointestinal Disease, 3rd ed. Philadelphia, WB Saunders, 1983, p 1069.

342. Hayden, DW and VanKruiningen, HJ: Experimentally induced canine toxocariasis: Laboratory examinations and pathologic changes, with emphasis on the gastrointestinal tract. Am J Vet Res 36:1605, 1975.

343. Strande, A, et al.: Regional enterocolitis in Cocker Spaniel dogs. Arch Pathol 57:357, 1954.

344. Tedesco, FJ, et al.: Eosinophilic ileocolitis. Expanding spectrum of eosinophilic gastroenteritis. Dig Dis Sci 26:943, 1981.

345. Hendrick, M: A spectrum of hypereosinophilic syndromes exemplified by six cats with eosinophilic enteritis. Vet Pathol 18:188, 1981.

346. Moore, RP: Feline eosinophilic enteritis. In Kirk, RW (ed): Current Veterinary Therapy VIII. Philadelphia, WB Saunders, 1983, p 791.

347. Scott, DW, et al.: Hypereosinophilic syndrome in a cat. Feline Pract 15:22, 1985.

348. Tolias, SW: Hypereosinophilic syndrome in a cat. Mod Vet Pract 66:1008, 1985.

349. Tams, TR: Chronic feline inflammatory bowel disorders. Part II. Feline eosinophilic enteritis and lymphosarcoma. Comp Cont Ed Pract Vet 8:464, 1986.

350. Hardy, W and Anderson, R: Hypereosinophilic syndromes. Ann Intern Med 68:1220, 1968.

351. VanKruiningen, HJ: Canine colitis comparable to regional enteritis and mucosal colitis of man. Gastroenterology 62:1128, 1972.

352. Rechenberg, R: Regional enteritis in dogs. Monatschr Vet Med 29:352, 1974.

353. DiBartola, SP, et al.: Regional enteritis in two dogs. JAVMA 181:904, 1982.

354. VanKruiningen, HJ, et al.: The classification of feline colitis. J Comp Pathol 93:275, 1983.

355. Donaldson, RM, Jr: Crohn's disease. In Sleisenger, MH and Fordtran, JS (eds): Gastrointestinal Disease, 3rd ed. Philadelphia, WB Saunders, 1983, p 1088.

356. VanKruiningen, HJ: Prothecal enterocolitis in a dog. JAVMA 157:56, 1970.

357. Holscher, MA, et al.: Disseminated canine protothecosis: A case report. JAAHA 12:49, 1976.

358. Widmer, WR and VanKruiningen, HJ: Trichuris-induced trans-

mural ileocolitis in a dog-an entity mimicking regional enteritis. JAAHA 10:581, 1974.

359. Campbell, RSF, et al.: Intestinal lymphangiectasia in a dog. JAVMA 153:1050, 1968.
360. Schwartz-Porsche, DM, et al.: Enteric protein loss syndrome in a dog. Zentbl Vet Med A 17:665, 1970.
361. Mattheeuws, D, et al.: Intestinal lymphangiectasia in a dog. J Sm Anim Pract 15:757, 1974.
362. Flesja, K and Yri, T: Protein-losing enteropathy in the Lundehund. J Small Anim Pract 18:11, 1977.
363. Milstein, M and Sanford, SE: Intestinal lymphangiectasia in a dog. Can Vet J 18:127, 1977.
364. Barton, CL, et al.: The diagnosis and clinicopathological features of canine protein-losing enteropathy. JAAHA 14:85, 1978.
365. Olson, NC and Zimmer, JF: Protein-losing enteropathy secondary to intestinal lymphangiectasia in a dog. JAVMA 173:271, 1978.
366. Hartigan, PJ, et al.: Intestinal lymphangiectasia in a dog. Irish Vet J 33:156, 1979.
367. Burns, MG: Intestinal lymphangiectasia in the dog. A case report and review. JAAHA 18:97, 1982.
368. Griffiths, GL, et al.: Lymphangiectasia in a dog. Aust Vet J 59:187, 1982.
369. Malo, D, et al.: Protein-losing enteropathy secondary to intestinal lymphangiectasia in three dogs. Can Vet J 23:129, 1982.
370. VanKruiningen, HJ, et al.: Lipogranulomatous lymphangitis in canine intestinal lymphangiectasia. Vet Pathol 21:377, 1984.
371. Suter, MM, et al.: Primary intestinal lymphangiectasia in three dogs: A morphological and immunopathological investigation. Vet Pathol 22:123, 1985.
372. Sherding, RG: Intestinal lymphangiectasia. In Kirk, RW (ed): Current Veterinary Therapy IX. Philadelphia, WB Saunders, 1986, p 885.
373. Meschter, CL, et al.: Intestinal lymphangiectasia with lipogranulomatous lymphangitis in a dog. JAVMA 190:427, 1987.
374. Kallfelz, FA and Wallace, RJ: Studies of albumin metabolism in dogs using 51Cr- and 125I- labeled albumin. Digest Dis 20:594, 1975.
375. Freeman, LW: Lymphatic pathways from the intestine in the dog. Anat Rec 82.543, 1942.
376. Frank, BW and Kern, F: Intestinal and liver lymph and lymphatics. Gastroenterol 55:408, 1968.
377. Danese, CA, et al.: Studies of the effects of blockage of intestinal lymphatics. I. Experimental procedure and structural alterations. Am J Gastroenterol 57:541, 1972.
378. Bank, S, et al.: The lymphatics of the intestinal mucosa. A clinical and experimental study. Am J Digest Dis 12:619, 1967.
379. Loppnow, H and Schwartz-Porsche, D: Further study of protein-losing enteropathy in the dog. Vet Pathol 17:105, 1980.
380. Holt, P: Dietary treatment of protein loss in intestinal lymphangiectasia. Pediatrics 34:629, 1964.
381. Jeffries, GH, et al.: Low-fat diet in intestinal lymphangiectasia: Its effect on albumin metabolism. N Engl J Med 270:761, 1964.
382. Batt, RM, et al.: Morphologic and biochemical studies of a naturally occurring enteropathy in the dog resembling chronic tropical sprue in man (abstr). Gastroenterol 76:1096, 1979.
383. Batt, RM, et al.: Naturally occurring enteropathy in the dog resembling chronic tropical sprue in man. Gut 20:A441, 1979.
384. Batt, RM: Chronic small intestinal disease in the dog. Proceedings of the 8th Kal Kan Symposium:93, 1984.
385. Hart, IR and Kidder, DE: The quantitative assessment of mucosa in canine small intestinal malabsorption. Res Vet Sci 25:163, 1978.
386. Brunser, O, et al.: Jejunal mucosa in infant malnutrition. Am J Clin Nutr 21:976, 1968.
387. Klipstein, FA: Tropical sprue. In Sleisenger, MH and Fordtran, JS (eds): Gastrointestinal Disease, 3rd ed. Philadelphia, WB Saunders, 1983, p 1040.
388. Batt, RM and Scott, J: Response of the small intestinal mucosa to oral glucocorticoids. Scand J Gastro 17(suppl):75, 1982.
389. Fisher, SE, et al.: Chronic protracted diarrhea and jejunal atrophy in an infant. Cimetidine-associated stimulation of jejunal mucosal growth. Digest Dis Sci 26:181, 1981.
390. Trier, JS: Celiac sprue. In Sleisenger, MH and Fordtran, JS (eds): Gastrointestinal Disease, 3rd ed. Philadelphia, WB Saunders, 1983, p 1050.

391. Gracey, M: The contaminated small bowel syndrome: pathogenesis, diagnosis, and treatment. Am J Clini Nutrition 32:234, 1979.
392. Banwell, JG, et al.: Small intestinal bacterial overgrowth syndrome. Gastroenterol 80:834, 1981.
393. Toskes, PP and Donaldson, RM, Jr: The blind loop syndrome. In Sleisenger, MH and Fordtran, JS (eds): Gastrointestinal Disease, 3rd ed. Philadelphia, WB Saunders, 1983, p 1023.
394. Bishop, RF: Bacterial flora of the small intestine of dogs and rats with intestinal blind loops. J Path Bact 87:189, 1962.
395. Greenlee, HB, et al.: The influence of gastric surgery on the intestinal flora. Am J Clin Nutrition 30:1826, 1977.
396. Batt, RM, et al.: Subcellular biochemical changes in the jejunal mucosa of dogs with naturally occurring bacterial overgrowth. Clin Sci 63:55, 1982.
397. Williams, DA, et al.: Bacterial overgrowth in the duodenum of dogs with exocrine pancreatic insufficiency. JAVMA 191:201, 1987.
398. Arrick, RH and Kleine, LJ: Intestinal pseudoobstruction in a dog. JAVMA 172:1201, 1978.
399. Hoeing, M: Intestinal malabsorption attributed to bacterial overgrowth in a dog. JAVMA 176:533, 1980.
400. Strombeck, DR, et al.: Maldigestion and malabsorption in a dog with chronic gastritis. JAVMA 179:801, 1981.
401. Simpson, JW: Bacterial overgrowth causing intestinal malabsorption in a dog. Vet Record 110:335, 1982.
402. Drude, RB and Hines, C, Jr: The pathophysiology of intestinal bacterial overgrowth syndromes. Arch Intern Med 140:1349, 1980.
403. Whitbread, TJ, et al.: Relative deficiency of serum IgA in the German Shepherd dog: A breed abnormality. Res Vet Sci 37:350, 1984.
404. Bernstein, LH, et al.: Experimental production of elevated serum folate in dogs with intestinal blind loops: Relationship of serum levels to location of the blind loop. Gastroenterol 63:815, 1972.
405. Joy, CL and Patterson, JM: Short bowel syndrome following surgical correction of a double intussusception in a dog. Can Vet J 19:254, 1978.
406. Williams, DA and Burrows, CF: Short bowel syndrome—a case report in a dog and a discussion of the pathophysiology of bowel resection. J Small Anim Pract 22:263, 1981.
407. Weser, E, et al.: Short bowel syndrome. Gastroenterol 77:572, 1979.
408. Weser, E: Nutritional aspects of malabsorption. Short gut adaption. Am J Med 67:1014, 1979.
409. Tilson, MD: Pathophysiology and treatment of short bowel syndrome. Surg Clin North Am 60:1273, 1980.
410. Greenberger, NJ: The management of the patient with short bowel syndrome. Am J Gastroenterol 70:528, 1978.
411. Leav, I, et al.: Adenomas and carcinomas of the canine and feline thyroid. Am J Pathol 83:61, 1976.
412. Steinfeld, CM, et al.: Diarrhea and medullary carcinoma of the thyroid. Cancer 31:1237, 1973.
413. Holzworth, J, et al.: Hyperthyroidism in the cat: Ten cases. JAVMA 176:345, 1980.
414. Petersen, ME: Feline hyperthyroidism. Vet Clin North Am 14:809, 1984.
415. Brodey, RS: Alimentary tract neoplasms in the cat. A clinicopathological survey of 46 cases. Am J Vet Res 27:74, 1966.
416. Lingeman, CH and Garner, FM: Comparative study of intestinal adenocarcinomas of animals and man. J Natl Cancer Instit 48:325, 1972.
417. Patnaik, AK, et al.: Feline intestinal adenocarcinoma. A clinicopathologic study of 22 cases. Vet Pathol 13:1, 1976.
418. Patnaik, AK, et al.: Canine gastrointestinal neoplasms. Vet Pathol 14:547, 1977.
419. Priester, WA: The occurrence of tumors in domestic animals. Natl Canc Inst Monogr 54.1980.
420. Turk, MAM, et al.: Nonhematopoietic gastrointestinal neoplasia in cats: A retrospective study of 44 cases. Vet Pathol 18:614, 1981.
421. Couto, CG: Gastrointestinal neoplasia. Proceedings of the 8th Kal Kan symposium:17, 1984.
422. Birchard, SJ, et al.: Nonlymphoid intestinal neoplasia in 32 dogs and 14 cats. JAAHA 12:307, 1986.

423. Kosovsky, JE, et al.: Small intestinal adenocarcinoma in cats: 32 cases (1978-1985). JAVMA 192:233, 1988.
424. Patnaik, AK, et al.: Canine intestinal adenocarcinoma and carcinoid. Vet Pathol 17:149, 1980.
425. Patnaik, AK, et al.: Surgical resection of intestinal adenocarcinoma in a cat with survival of 28 months. JAVMA 178:479, 1981.
426. Carpenter, JL, et al.: *In* Holzworth, J (ed): Diseases of the cat. Medicine & Surgery. Philadelphia, WB Saunders, 1987, p 406.
427. Hardy, WD: Hematopoietic tumors of cats. JAAHA 17:921, 1981.
428. Leib, MS and Bradley, RL: Alimentary lymphosarcoma in a dog. Comp Cont Ed 9:809, 1987.
429. Alroy, J, et al.: Distinctive intestinal mast cell neoplasms of domestic cats. Lab Invest 33:159, 1975.
430. Murray, M, et al.: Peptic ulceration in the dog: A clinico-pathological study. Vet Rec 91:441, 1972.
431. Howard, EB, et al.: Mastocytoma and gastroduodenal ulceration. Pathol Vet 6:146, 1969.
432. O'Keefe, DA, et al.: Systemic mastocytosis in 16 dogs. J Vet Int Med 1:75, 1987.
433. Seawright, AA and Grono, LR: Malignant mast cell tumor in a cat with perforating duodenal ulcer. J Pathol Bacteriol 87:107, 1964.
434. Carrig, CB and Seawright, AA: Mastocytosis with gastrointestinal ulceration in a dog. Aust Vet J 44:503, 1968.
435. Zontine, WJ, et al.: Perforated duodenal ulcer associated with mastocytoma in a dog: A case report. J Am Vet Radiol Soc 18:162, 1977.
436. Ewing, GO: Indomethacin-associated gastrointestinal hemorrhage in a dog. JAVMA 161:1665, 1972.
437. Jones, BR, et al.: Peptic ulceration in a dog associated with an islet cell carcinoma of the pancreas and an elevated plasma gastrin level. J Small Anim Pract 17:593, 1976.
438. Straus, E, et al.: Canine Zollinger-Ellison syndrome. Gastroenterol 72:380, 1977.
439. Happe, RP, et al.: Zollinger-Ellison syndrome in three dogs. Vet Pathol 17:177, 1980.
440. Middleton, DJ and Watson, ADJ: Duodenal ulceration associated with gastrin secreting pancreatic tumor in a cat. JAVMA 183:461, 1983.
441. Wilson, GP and Burt, JK: Intussusception in the dog and cat: A review of 45 cases. JAVMA 164:515, 1974.
442. Weaver, AD: Canine intestinal intussusception. Vet Rec 100:524, 1977.
443. Kipnis, RM: A case history of postoperative intussusception in a dog. JAAHA 13:197, 1977.
444. Koike, T, et al.: Clinical cases of intestinal obstruction with foreign bodies and intussusception in dogs. Jpn J Vet Res 29:8, 1981.
445. Runyon, CL, et al.: Intussusception associated with a paracolonic enterocyst in a dog. JAVMA 185:443, 1984.
446. Lewis, DD and Ellison, GW: Intussusception in dogs and cats. Comp Cont Ed 9:523, 1987.
447. Parker, WM and Presnell, KR: Mesenteric torsion in the dog. Canadian Vet J 13:283, 1972.
448. Harvey, HJ and Rendano, VT, Jr: Small bowel volvulus in dogs. Vet Surg 13:91, 1984.
449. Marks, A: Torsion of the colon in a rough Collie. Vet Rec 118:400, 1986.
450. Wolfe, DA and Meyer, CW: Obstructing intestinal abscess in a dog. JAVMA 166:518, 1975.
451. Moore, R and Carpenter, J: Intramural intestinal hematoma causing obstruction in three dogs. JAVMA 184:186, 1984.
452. Ockens, N: Ileus in cats - an unknown cause: Ligamentum pancreaticoduodenale. Proceedings of the 20th World Veterinary Congress, Thessalonica, Greece 2:1822, 1975.
453. Hornbuckle, WD and Kleine, LJ: Obstruction of the small intestine. *In* Kirk, RW (ed): Current Veterinary Therapy VI. Philadelphia, WB Saunders, 1977, p 952.
454. Thrall, DE, et al.: Demonstration of a "position of relief" in dogs with lesions of the stomach or small bowel. JAAHA 14:343, 1978.
455. Moore, R and Carpenter, J: Intestinal sclerosis with pseudoobstruction in three dogs. JAVMA 184:830, 1984.
456. Felts, JF, et al.: Thread and sewing needles as gastrointestinal foreign bodies in the cat. A review of 64 cases. JAVMA 184:56, 1984.
457. Basher, AWP and Fowler, JD: Conservative versus surgical management of gastrointestinal linear foreign bodies in the cat. Vet Surg 16:135, 1987.
458. Willard, MD: Newer concepts in treatment of secretory diarrheas. JAVMA 186:86, 1985.
459. Primi, MP, et al.: Central regulation of intestinal basal and stimulated water and ion transport by endogenous opiates in dogs. Digest Dis Sci 31:172, 1986.
460. Papich, MG, et al.: Absorption of salicylate from an antidiarrheal preparation in dogs and cats. JAVMA 23:221, 1987.
461. Chiapella, AM: Treatment of intestinal disease. Vet Clin North Am 13:567, 1983.
462. Regan, PT and DiMagno, EP: The medical management of malabsorption. Mayo Clin Proc 54:267, 1979.
463. Sauer, LS, et al.: Effect of diet composition on water intake and excretion by the cat. Feline Pract 15:16, 1985.
464. Kolars, JC, et al.: Yogurt - an autodigesting source of lactose. N Engl J Med 310:1, 1984.
465. Fischer, JE: Hyperalimentation. Med Clin North Am 63:973, 1979.
466. Sheldon, GF: Role of parenteral nutrition in patients with short bowel syndrome. Am J Med 67:1021, 1979.
467. Heymsfield, SB, et al.: Enteral hyperalimentation: An alternative to central venous hyperalimentation. Ann Intern Med 90:63, 1979.
468. Koretz, RL and Meyer, JH: Elemental diets: Facts and fantasies. Gastroenterol 78:393, 1980.

87 DISEASES OF THE LARGE BOWEL

KEITH P. RICHTER

NORMAL STRUCTURE[1]

The large intestine and rectum together are approximately 0.2 to 0.6 m in length in the dog, and 0.2 m in the cat (10 to 20 per cent as long as the small intestine). The cecum is 0.08 to 0.3 m long in the dog and 0.02 to 0.04 m long in the cat. The large bowel begins as a short segment termed the *ascending colon*. At the ileal orifice is a distinct anatomic sphincter, the *ileocecal sphincter*. This structure is a true sphincter in that intraluminal pressure is higher than in adjacent areas.[2] The transverse colon is the most cranial portion of the large intestine at the level of the twelfth thoracic vertebra, and connects the ascending to the descending colon. The transverse colon passes cranial to and around the root of the mesentery. The descending colon blends into the rectum at the pelvic inlet. The colon is connected to the ascending duodenum by the duodenocolic fold. The colon is palpable on physical examination, with the exception of the cranial portion in deep-chested dogs.

Normal blood supply to the large intestine is via the cranial and caudal mesenteric vessels. Venous drainage is into the portal vein.

Nervous control is from the autonomic system. The parasympathetic system is most important for normal function. The vagus nerve supplies parasympathetic innervation to the cranial portion of the large intestine, and sacral parasympathetics supply the remainder of the large intestine by way of the pelvic nerves. The sympathetic system plays little role in normal function. It arises in the paravertebral sympathetic trunk and passes to the large intestine via abdominal sympathetic ganglia.

Microscopically, the colonic mucosa is smooth and villi are absent. Tubular glands, containing mucus and epithelial cells, extend from the surface to the muscularis mucosae. These glands are closely packed, leaving a sparse lamina propria. The remainder of the colonic wall is similar to the small intestinal wall.

NORMAL FUNCTION[1, 3]

Motility

The main function of the colon is to act as a reservoir for storage, allowing completion of absorption of fluids and electrolytes. Motor activity in the colon is similar to that in the small bowel, consisting of propulsive movements (peristalsis), and segmental contractions acting to delay transit. The latter allows for mixing so that fluid and electrolytes are presented to the mucosal surface for absorption. The rate of rhythmic segmentation in the colon is less than that of the small intestine, thus allowing for aboral movement of ingesta. This electrical control activity is affected by neurologic stimuli, humoral factors, drugs, and intraluminal contents. Within the colon, there is a reversed gradient of electrical activity, with the highest rate occurring in the colonic pacemaker in the middle part of the colon, decreasing in frequency in the oral direction. This delays movement of contents in the aboral direction, allowing storage in this area until absorption of fluid and electrolytes is complete. There is little gradient of electrical control activity over the caudal half of the colon, except the most caudal ten per cent. Diarrhea from various disease states often develops when multiple pacemakers arise in the cranial large intestine and the reversed gradient is lost.

The colon possesses another type of electrical activity, characterized by prolonged bursts originating in the middle of the colon and progressing in the aboral direction. This activity is responsible for rapid discharge of colonic contents during defecation.

The main stimulus for motility in the large intestine is distention by intraluminal contents, the degree of which is mainly determined by the amount of undigested material entering the colon. This will stimulate segmental contractions, thus limiting transit of intraluminal contents. Distention will also stimulate the mass propulsive activity, thus allowing evacuation of the colon. This explains the paradoxic beneficial effects of bulk agents with both diarrhea and constipation. With diarrhea, adding bulk to stimulate segmental contractions limits transit and allows more complete absorption. With constipation, increasing bulk will stimulate mass propulsive activity necessary for fecal evacuation. These concepts are important to understand proper therapeutic interventions with motility-modifying drugs. Anticholinergic drugs will reduce rhythmic segmentation, allowing minimal propulsive activity to propel contents in the aboral direction through a relatively flaccid tube. In contrast, narcotic analgesics will increase rhythmic segmentation.

Large Intestinal Secretions

The main secretory product of the large intestine is mucus, which is produced by the large number of mucous cells on the mucosal surface. Mucus acts as an important lubricant for easy passage of feces and as a protectant for the wall of the colon. The rate of secretion of mucus is determined by direct tactile stimuli to the mucous cells and by local nervous reflexes. Parasympathetic stimulation via the pelvic nerves also increases mucus secretion, in addition to stimulating motility. Mucus protects the wall from excoriation and from fecal bacterial activity. Mucus also contains a high concentration of bicarbonate, which helps buffer acid end-products of bacterial activity. Whenever a segment of the colon becomes irritated, the mucosa secretes large quantities of mucus, water, and electrolytes, often resulting in diarrhea.

Large Intestinal Absorption

Approximately 10 to 15 per cent of the fluid entering the gastrointestinal tract either from ingestion or secretions ends up entering the large intestine, the remainder being absorbed in the small intestine. Water absorption in the large intestine is passive (osmosis) following the active absorption of sodium and chloride. This is also coupled to a transport mechanism resulting in bicarbonate secretion. Most of the absorption occurs in the proximal half of the colon. Feces are normally about 75 per cent water and 25 per cent solid material. The brown color of feces is from stercobilin and urobilin, pigments derived from bilirubin. Odor is caused by bacterial action resulting in the production of compounds such as indole, scatole, mercaptans, and hydrogen sulfide.

Normal Microflora of the Large Intestine[1, 4]

The highest concentration of bacteria in the normal gastrointestinal tract is in the large intestine, usually 10^{10} to 10^{11} bacteria per gram. Normal microflora are necessary to prevent colonization by pathogens and to maintain normal structure and function of the mucosa. The most common bacteria in the large intestine are anaerobes, especially *Bacteroides* and *Bifidobacterium*. Other bacteria commonly found in large numbers include members of the Enterobacteriaceae family, streptococci, *Clostridium*, and lactobacilli. Several factors are necessary to maintain normal bacterial populations and prevent pathologic changes from bacteria. These include normal colonic motility, the normal mucus layer against the mucosa, and the local immune response (primarily immunoglobulin A). Other factors affecting the colonic flora include diet, interrelationships among the resident microflora, endogenous bile acids, and antimicrobial agents.

EVALUATION OF THE LARGE INTESTINE

History and Clinical Signs

Since the diagnostic and therapeutic approach to large intestinal disease differs from that of small intestinal disease, it is important to localize the problem to the principal site in the intestine in which the abnormality is located. This can usually be accomplished by obtaining a complete history and asking specific questions regarding the stool. The history should be obtained in a chronological order, and include: (1) character of the problem at onset; (2) previous treatment and response; (3) current and previous diet, including responses to dietary changes; (4) parasite control; (5) environment; and (6) aggravating factors. Often, responses to these questions will give clues as to potential etiology, as well as characterize the severity of the problem and aid the clinician in determining how aggressive to be with the diagnostic and therapeutic plan. In addition to a gastrointestinal history, a review of other systems should be obtained. Many systemic diseases involve gastrointestinal signs, including hepatic disease, renal disease, hypoadrenocorticism, hyperthyroidism, and pancreatic disease.

Specific features of the stool will also help localize the problem to the large intestine. Information that should be obtained includes (1) color; (2) consistency; (3) character (blood, mucus, and the like); (4) frequency; (5) quantity; (6) duration; and (7) concurrent problems (weight loss, vomiting). If an animal's bowel movement is never seen, it might be assumed to be normal. Therefore, the client should be questioned as to whether bowel movements are observed.

The most common primary sign of large intestinal disease is diarrhea (defined as a change in frequency, fluidity, or volume of bowel movements), although certain large intestinal diseases cause constipation (infrequent or incomplete bowel movements). Typical signs that aid the clinician to distinguish large intestinal from small intestinal disease are listed in Table 87–1. Characteristic clinical features of large bowel diarrhea include passage of increased amounts of mucus in the stool, with occasional fresh blood, often accompanied by straining and urgency. As the problem progresses, the volume of each bowel movement decreases and the frequency increases. Often earlier bowel movements of the day are more normal, and as the day progresses, the bowel movements become more liquid, with increasing frequency and urgency. Often there is unproductive straining following a bowel movement with frequent squatting episodes and subsequent passage of only mucus or dripping of stool. Well-trained pets will sometimes defecate in the house due to their sense of urgency. Occasionally, the only sign may be increased licking at the anal area or pain during the act of defecation along with just occasional diarrhea. In general, animals with large intestinal disease appear healthy with the exception of their gastrointestinal signs. All of these signs suggest large intestinal disease; work-up and treatment should be directed accordingly.

TABLE 87–1. CLINICAL FEATURES USED TO LOCALIZE ANATOMIC SITE OF PROBLEM

Sign	Small Intestine	Large Intestine
Weight loss	Prominent	Minimal
Appetite	May be ravenous	Usually normal
Vomiting	Occasional	Rare
Belching	Occasional	Rare
Flatulence	Common	Occasional
Bloated abdomen	Common	Rare
Stool quantity	Increased	Normal to small
Stool frequency	Normal or increased	Increased
Tenesmus	Rare	Common
Gross examination of stool:		
Blood	Melena	Fresh
Mucus	Absent	Present
Fat	May be present	Absent
Rectal examination	Normal	Blood, mucus, pain
Anal pruritus	Absent	May be present
Setting	Little importance	Stress and psychological factors may be important

Examination and Laboratory Evaluation of the Large Intestine

GROSS EXAMINATION OF FECES

The feces should be inspected to confirm the owner's interpretation of such features as blood, mucus, and color, which can help localize the source of the problem as just described. The dark-brown color of feces is from bile pigments, mainly stercobilin and urobilin. Lighter color can result from absence of bile pigments as can occur with bile duct obstructions (acholic stools). Since bile pigment metabolism depends on bacterial action, changes in intestinal flora will alter color. Increased transit rate and decreased intestinal bacterial numbers will cause lighter-colored feces due to incomplete metabolism of bile pigments. Antibiotics can have this effect until colonic bacteria repopulate. Diet will also alter fecal color. Compared with conventional diets, diets high in milk proteins such as cottage cheese will typically produce a light-colored or mustard-colored stool, possibly owing to decreased stimulation of bile secretion, or owing to its potential to alter colonic bacteria. Excess bile pigments entering the colon will darken stool color, as occurs with hemolytic disease, upper gastrointestinal bleeding, and liver or meat diets.

ABDOMINAL PALPATION AND DIGITAL RECTAL PALPATION

In most cases of large intestinal disease, abdominal palpation is normal. Occasionally, strictured areas of the large intestine are palpable per abdomen or per rectum. Other conditions that may be palpable include distention of the colon with feces or foreign material, certain neoplasms, and intussusceptions involving the large intestine. The performance of rectal palpation also affords a good opportunity to obtain a fresh fecal sample.

FECAL FLOTATION AND SEDIMENTATION

Many parasites can be identified by variations of these techniques. Some parasites are identified by their ova, such as ascarids, hookworms, and whipworms. Others are identified by their cysts, such as *Giardia* and coccidia. It is important to repeat the fecal flotation several times to detect certain parasites such as whipworms. Although standard flotation solutions using concentrated sucrose or salt solutions are adequate for most parasites, zinc sulfate flotation is necessary for detection of *Giardia* and *Balantidium* cysts.[5, 6] Fluke ova are concentrated by sedimentation.

DIRECT FECAL SMEARS

Direct fecal smears are used to detect motile trophozoites of *Giardia*, *Trichomonas*, *Balantidium*, and *Entamoeba*. In addition, those parasites that are typically found in fecal flotations can also be found on a direct smear if present in large numbers. It is important to obtain the direct smear from a fresh fecal specimen (less than ten minutes) or directly from a rectal glove or swab in order to detect motile trophozoites of protozoa. As the feces cool, the trophozoites encyst and disintegrate, making their detection more difficult. The smear is prepared by mixing a small amount of feces with a drop of saline on a microscope slide. Care must be taken not to make the smear too thick, or detection of parasites will be obscured by fecal debris. Previous administration of bismuth, kaolin, radiographic contrast material, certain antibiotics, and enemas can interfere with parasite detection. Spirochetes are often seen in direct fecal smears from animals with diarrhea, but since they are normal inhabitants of colonic crypts, their presence is of little significance.[1, 4]

FECAL STAINING

Direct staining of fecal smears with standard hematology stains is occasionally useful in identifying white blood cells, which can be increased with inflammatory diseases. Trichrome staining of preserved feces is useful for the detection of *Giardia*.[6a] Bacterial pathogens, mainly *Salmonella*, *Campylobacter*, invasive or enterotoxin-producing *Escherichia coli*, and *Yersinia* cannot be reliably identified in fecal smears. Fecal staining for the presence of maldigestion or malabsorption is discussed in Chapter 86.

COMPLETE BLOOD COUNT, BIOCHEMISTRY PROFILE, AND URINALYSIS

In general, these tests reveal little information specifically regarding the colon. However, they are useful in establishing a complete data base to evaluate other organ systems. This is often necessary when diagnostic procedures requiring sedation or general anesthesia (such as colonoscopy) are being considered. Hemograms will occasionally reflect specific large intestinal disease states, such as an eosinophilia (seen with eosinophilic colitis and parasites) or neutrophilia (seen with invasive bacterial infections).

BACTERIAL CULTURE

In general, bacterial cultures are only useful for enteric pathogens, mainly *Salmonella* and *Campylobacter*. Invasive and enterotoxin-producing strains of *Escherichia coli* cannot be distinguished from nonpathogenic strains by standard culture techniques. Laboratory animal inoculation and specific *in vivo* and *in vitro* tests are required to make this distinction.[7, 8] Since there are numerous bacteria normally present in feces, their identification and quantitation do not allow the clinician to speculate on their relative pathogenicity. Localized or diffuse changes in small or large intestinal flora are seldom reflected in quantitative changes in fecal bacteria.[1] In addition, 99.9 per cent of fecal bacteria are anaerobes, which have not been extensively studied. This makes the value of aerobic fecal cultures even more questionable. Cause and effect relationships in quantitative or qualitative fecal flora changes cannot be established in animals with diarrhea. Therefore, fecal bacterial cultures should be attempted only for the purpose of identifying known bacterial pathogens. Special culture techniques are required for their identification.

FECAL OCCULT BLOOD

Feces may contain blood that is not grossly visible. Chemical tests are employed to identify fecal blood. Certain tests are based on the pseudoperoxidase activity of blood, which oxidizes a color reagent. However, these tests vary in sensitivity and specificity and can be falsely positive if meat or certain drugs are in the diet. Therefore, meat should be withheld from the diet for a minimum of three days.[1, 8a] A fluorometric method for the quantitative assay of fecal hemoglobin has also been evaluated in the dog.[8a] This method can take into account the amount of hemoglobin in the diet when fecal hemoglobin is evaluated.

Endoscopic Examination of the Colon

Endoscopic examination of the colon can be accomplished with either a rigid proctoscope (allowing visualization of the descending colon and rectum), or with a flexible colonoscope (allowing visualization of the entire colon up to the level of the ileum).

PROCTOSCOPY

Indications. The indications for proctoscopy include any suspected disease of large intestinal origin that would produce an abnormal gross or microscopic mucosal appearance of the descending colon or rectum. In general, this is the test of choice for evaluating signs referable to the large intestine. Since most inflammatory diseases of the large intestine in the dog and cat are diffuse, their presence is usually detected in this region. Neoplastic diseases involving the mucosa of this region can also be investigated with a rigid proctoscopic examination. Non-neoplastic strictures can also be visualized directly, although the length of the stricture can be difficult to determine if the scope cannot fit through the lumen; therefore, a barium enema should be performed to evaluate its extent. Many diffuse diseases primarily causing small intestinal dysfunction can be detected via proctoscopy, since the descending colon can be involved to some extent in the same disease process. Examples of such disorders include lymphocytic-plasmacytic enterocolitis, eosinophilic enterocolitis, and intestinal lymphosarcoma. The diagnosis is more readily obtained via proctoscopy because of the relative ease of its use in obtaining biopsy samples, its lack of invasiveness, and availability of its equipment compared with that used in obtaining small intestinal biopsies. Finally, parasitic diseases such as trichuriasis can sometimes be detected via proctoscopy.

Equipment. The rigid proctoscope (sleeve) contains a large central lumen for visualization and obtaining biopsies. Light is usually transmitted via a fiberoptic cable from a remote light source and exits at either the proximal or distal aspect of the scope. The proctoscope also includes an obturator (stylus) and air insufflation bulb to distend the colon (Figure 87–1). Proctoscopes are available in several sizes. The author uses a 30 cm long, 21 mm diameter scope for dogs larger than 5 kg, and a 20 cm long, 12 mm diameter scope for smaller dogs and for cats.

Technique. Patient preparation is extremely important to perform a reliable examination, as residual fecal material can prevent complete visualization of the mu-

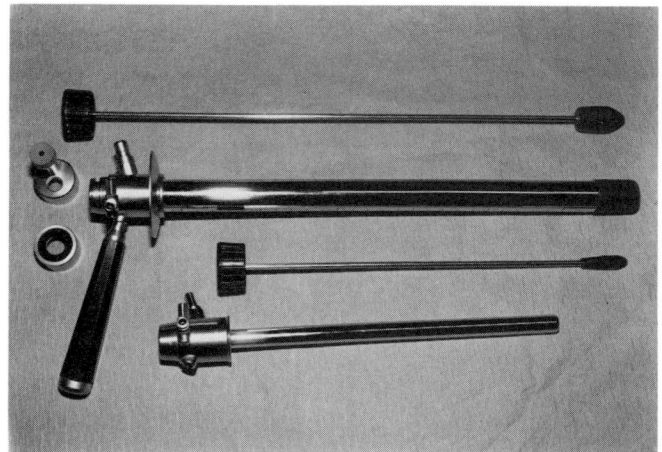

FIGURE 87–1. Rigid adult (top) and pediatric (bottom) proctoscope, with obturators and glass covers (with and without biopsy port). Insufflation bulb and fiberoptic light cable for attachment to light source are not shown.

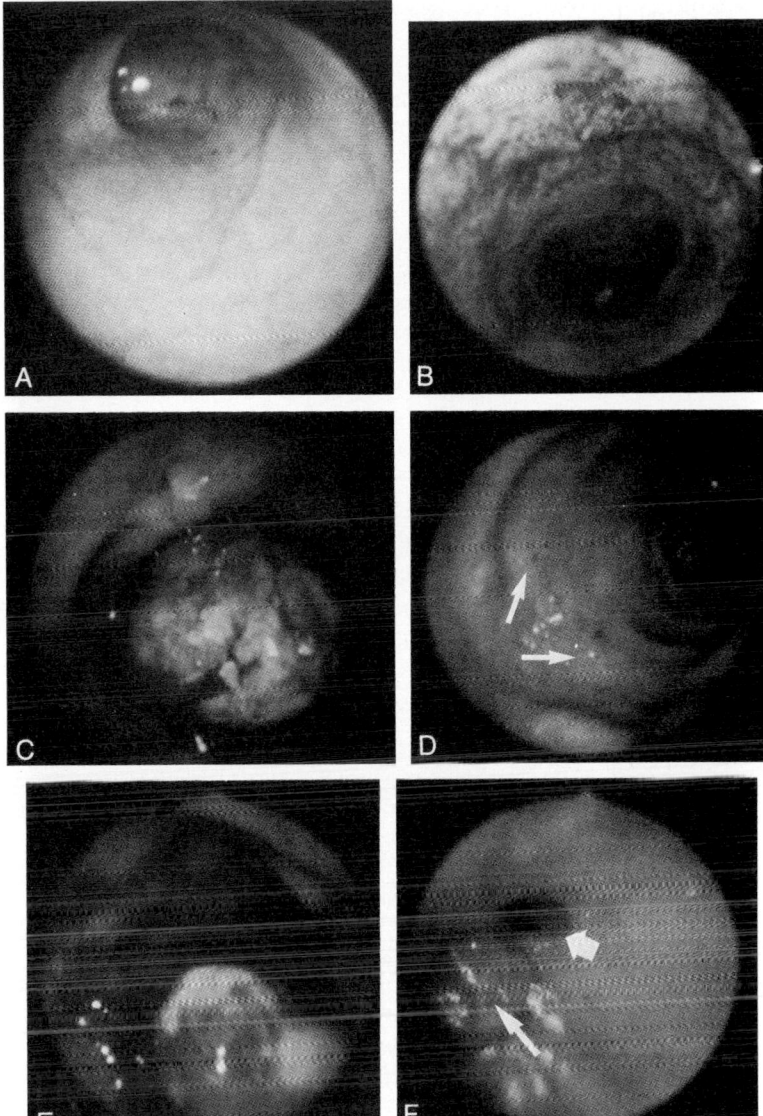

FIGURE 87–2. Colonoscopic findings with *A,* normal colon. *B,* Hyperemic colon in a dog with lymphocytic plasmacytic colitis. *C,* Lymphosarcoma in the colon of a dog, seen as a large, ulcerated mass. *D,* Superficial ulcers (arrows) and thick, nondistensible folds in the colon of a dog with lymphocytic plasmacytic colitis. Submucosal vessels are not visualized. *E,* Carcinoma in situ in the colon of a dog. *F,* The normal ileocecal-colic junction in the dog. The arrow is pointing to the opening to the ileum; the arrowhead is pointing to the opening of the cecum.

cosal surface. Patients should be fasted for 24 to 48 hours prior to the procedure. One method of preparation involves administration of multiple warm-water enemas. Phosphate or soapy enemas are not used because of their potential to cause colonic irritation.[9] The last enema should result in the return of clean fluid without fecal material and should be given at least one to two hours before the procedure to facilitate evacuation and minimize artifactual hyperemia of the mucosa. Phosphate enemas should not be given to cats because of their potential to cause severe alterations in serum calcium and other electrolyte concentrations, which can be fatal.[10, 11] An alternative method of preparation involves the use of an oral gastrointestinal lavage solution, containing polyethylene glycol as the main nonabsorbed solute (Golytely). The principle of this solution is that it results in a severe osmotic diarrhea with virtually no net absorption or secretion of electrolytes, bicarbonate, or water.[12] This method of preparation is contraindicated with confirmed or suspected intestinal strictures. This method has been shown to result in superior colonic preparation compared with multiple enemas when given

at 12 cc/lb (25 cc/kg) via orogastric tube twice, one hour apart, 12 to 18 hours before proctoscopy.[13]

Although proctoscopy can be performed without chemical restraint, the use of sedation or general anesthesia is usually desirable. Patients often have pain and may have a structurally weakened colon wall that makes perforation with the instrument possible if the patient moves suddenly. The patient is placed in right lateral recumbency to pool any residual fluid in the transverse and ascending colon. The instrument is slowly passed into the colon after the sleeve and obturator are lubricated. If resistance is encountered, gentle manipulation and redirection often allows continued passage. The scope is never forced past an area of resistance.

When the scope is completely advanced, the obturator is removed and glass lens placed to allow air insufflation. The entire circumference is examined while the scope is slowly removed. The normal colon wall when distended with air is smooth, glistening, pink, and easily distended (Figure 87–2). The colon wall is examined for texture, color, friability, parasites, erosions, and ulcerations. Lymphoid follicles, seen as small, grey plaques, are normally seen. Multiple biopsies can be obtained as the instrument is slowly withdrawn. It is not recommended to advance the instrument and/or insufflate the colon past previous biopsy sites, especially if the wall is friable. If no gross lesions are visible, multiple biopsies should still be taken, since many diffuse inflammatory diseases and lymphosarcoma (especially in cats) can be grossly normal.

Complications. The main complication of a proctoscopic procedure is perforation of the colon. This can occur upon introduction of the instrument, when the colon is insufflated with air, or when biopsies are taken. If a perforation is known to have occurred, immediate surgical intervention is indicated. If a perforation goes undetected, as can happen following biopsy, the animal will show signs of peritonitis, including fever, abdominal pain, and vomiting. The diagnosis can be confirmed radiographically (noting free gas in the abdomen and an abdominal effusion) or by evaluating a peritoneal tap and/or diagnostic lavage (noting purulent inflammation with phagocytized bacteria).

FLEXIBLE COLONOSCOPY

Flexible colonoscopy is indicated when the transverse colon, ascending colon, or cecum needs to be examined. The suspicion of lesions in these areas can be based on abdominal palpation, contrast radiology, or a negative proctoscopic examination with persistence of large intestinal signs. The equipment needed is any flexible fiberoptic endoscope of sufficient length to reach the cecum (1 m in most dogs). The same instruments used for upper gastrointestinal endoscopy are suitable for colonoscopy. Patient preparation is identical to that described for proctoscopy. Colonoscopy must be performed under general anesthesia. The scope is carefully passed using insufflation to facilitate passage. The lumen should always be visible and the scope should advance easily. If resistance is met, the scope should be withdrawn and the tip gently manipulated to straighten any flexures or redundant folds in the colon. With practice, the cecum can be reached in most animals. The types of lesions seen and complications encountered while flexible colonoscopy is performed are similar to those described for rigid proctoscopy.

LARGE INTESTINAL BIOPSY TECHNIQUES

The large intestine can be biopsied under direct visualization through a rigid proctoscope or flexible colonoscope, or biopsied "blind" using a flexible suction capsule system. When biopsies are obtained through a flexible colonoscope, the size of the biopsy instrument is limited by the diameter of the biopsy channel, usually 2.0 or 2.7 mm (Figure 87–3). However, mucosal biopsies obtained with these instruments, usually including muscularis mucosa, are often diagnostic. The likelihood of perforating the colon with such an instrument is extremely remote, unless there is a severely diseased wall. These instruments can also be used through a rigid proctoscope, or alternatively a large rigid forceps can be used (Figure 87–3). Although the latter can harvest larger biopsy samples, it carries the risk of a greater

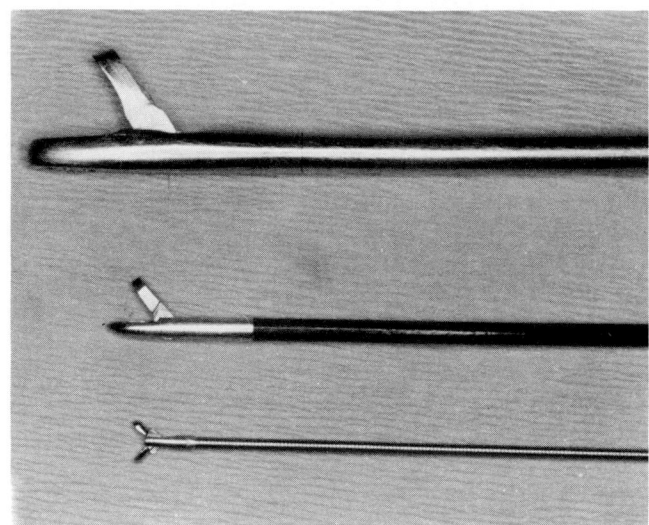

FIGURE 87–3. Rigid colon biopsy instruments (top and middle) and flexible 1.8 mm diameter biopsy instrument (bottom).

likelihood of causing a perforation. Samples are fixed in ten per cent buffered formalin.

Suction capsule systems, such as the Quinton (Seattle, WA) or Microvasive (Milford, MA) systems, employ a flexible tube with a small, blunt metal capsule at the end (Figure 87–4). There is a small hole (2.0 mm) on the side of the capsule through which a small portion of the colonic mucosa enters when suction is applied. A sharp knife controlled by a wire running through the tube is used to cut off this portion of the mucosa, yielding a suitable biopsy within the capsule. Since the tube is passed blindly, no sedation is needed in most cases. This method is extremely safe, with minimal risk of perforation.

Full-thickness colon biopsies can also be obtained via laparotomy. However, the risk of dehiscence from a colonic incision is much greater than in other regions of the bowel. Therefore, this method should only be used when a lesion deep to the mucosa is suspected (such as neoplasia).

Radiographic Examination

SURVEY ABDOMINAL RADIOGRAPHS

Plain abdominal radiographs are generally of little value in assessing large intestinal disorders. Certain diseases that could result in abnormal plain radiographs include megacolon (seen as a large, distended colon filled with feces), certain cases of neoplasia (when the mass itself can be visualized, or sublumbar lymphadenopathy from metastatic spread exists), or compression of the large intestine from extraintestinal structures (such as an enlarged prostate gland, pelvic bones, and so on). Since most other cases of large intestinal disease involve mucosal abnormalities, contrast radiology is necessary to evaluate such problems.

BARIUM ENEMA

Most cases of large intestinal disease can be diagnosed without the aid of a radiographic contrast study. Usually,

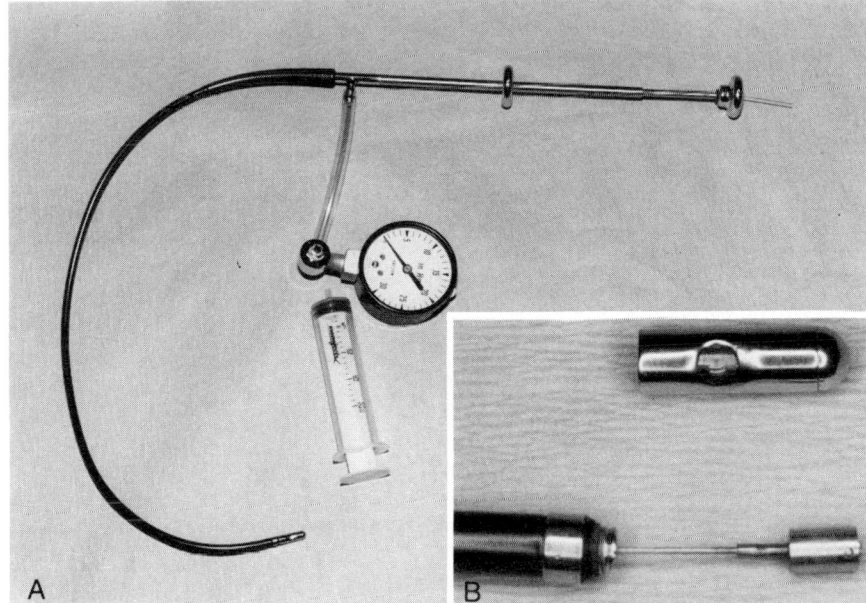

FIGURE 87–4. *A,* Suction capsule biopsy instrument (Quinton Instrument Company, Seattle, Washington), capable of obtaining blind colon biopsies. *B,* Closeup of the capsule with its hole into which mucosal tissue is drawn when suction is applied, and the knife that fits inside the capsule that is drawn by its wire to cut the biopsy sample.

colonoscopy, proctoscopy, or colon biopsy is the most sensitive and accurate way to evaluate the large intestinal mucosa. In clinical practice, the main value of contrast radiology is to evaluate conditions that result in inability to pass a colonoscope, or when such equipment is unavailable. Table 87–2 lists the indications for performing a barium enema. The main contraindication to performing a barium enema is suspected large intestinal perforation (organic iodides may be substituted with caution). An upper gastrointestinal series should not be used to evaluate the large intestine, since lack of distention, incomplete filling, and artifacts from residual fecal material will make interpretation difficult.

As with colonoscopy, proper patient preparation is essential. Patients should be fasted for 24 to 48 hours. Cleansing of the colon is performed in a manner identical to that described for colonoscopy. Either multiple enemas or an oral lavage solution can be used. Survey radiographs are obtained first to ensure adequate patient preparation. General anesthesia is usually required for an adequate examination, since large intestinal distention with barium is necessary, which in an awake animal would otherwise stimulate a normal defecation reflex or reflex contractions of the large intestine, making interpretation difficult. The contrast agent of choice is a 20 per cent weight/volume suspension of barium sulfate.[14] A balloon-tipped catheter is positioned with the balloon inflated just inside the rectum. The barium solution is placed in a disposable enema bag and administered by

TABLE 87–2. INDICATIONS FOR PERFORMING BARIUM ENEMA

Strictures
Neoplasia
Extraintestinal compression
  Prostate enlargement
  Pelvic bones (previous fractures)
  Sublumbar masses
Technical failure to pass colonoscope/proctoscope
Suspected intussusception or cecal inversion

gravity flow at the rate of approximately 6 to 10 ml/lb (13 to 22 ml/kg).[14] This rate will vary with the disease state, which affects the distensibility of the large intestine. Ideally, fluoroscopy is used to observe the flow of barium and to ensure adequate distention and complete filling up to the level of the cecum. Attempts should be made to avoid getting barium in the small intestine because this can overlie the colon and make interpretation more difficult.

Once the colon is filled, radiographs should be taken in multiple views, ideally including left lateral, ventrodorsal, and left and right ventrodorsal-oblique projections.[15] These projections maximize the likelihood of locating profiles of lesions such as filling defects and mucosal irregularities. If desired, a double contrast study can be performed by removing as much barium as possible through the catheter and infusing 10 to 15 ml/lb (22 to 33 ml/kg) of room air.[14] This will result in barium coating the mucosa of the air-filled colon, thus giving excellent mucosal detail. The same views as in the positive contrast study are obtained.

Complications include perforation of the large intestine (usually the result of overdistention by barium of a diseased wall or overinflation of the balloon in the rectum). If the potential for this complication is anticipated, water-soluble iodinated contrast material should be used. Barium can also move retrograde through the entire gastrointestinal tract and be aspirated upon vomiting if too much pressure is used.

Lesions that can be identified from a barium enema include cecocolic or ileocolic intussusception, strictures, neoplasia, or severe inflammatory mucosal disease such as histiocytic ulcerative colitis. The barium enema is sometimes performed in conjunction with or after endoscopy. It can help differentiate mucosal and transmural disease and evaluate the extent of a lesion identified by endoscopy.[15] Ideally, the barium enema should not be performed for three to four days after colon biopsy to prevent extravasation of barium at the biopsy site. However, the author and others[15] have performed a barium enema immediately after obtaining colon biopsies without any complications.

PNEUMOCOLON

The pneumocolon is a safe and easy procedure that can usually be performed without sedation. It is mainly used to evaluate the position of the colon when this cannot be determined from plain radiographs, and to evaluate intraluminal masses or strictures. It is performed by infusing approximately 5 ml/lb (11 ml/kg) of room air directly into the colon.[15] Left lateral and ventrodorsal projections are obtained as soon as possible, before the air is expelled by the patient.

INFLAMMATORY DISEASES OF THE LARGE INTESTINE

Idiopathic Chronic Inflammatory Bowel Disease

Idiopathic chronic inflammatory bowel disease (IBD, chronic colitis) represents the most common category of disease affecting the large intestine. The most common inflammatory diseases of the large intestine seen in the dog and cat are lymphocytic-plasmacytic colitis, eosinophilic colitis, suppurative colitis, and histiocytic ulcerative colitis. Collectively, they are also referred to as chronic inflammatory bowel disease. These diseases are named for the predominant inflammatory cell in the colonic mucosa. Since there are many similarities in etiology, clinical presentation, response to treatment, and prognosis, much of the discussion will concern the common features of IBD with specific differences pointed out where appropriate. Other diseases that result in mucosal inflammation that have a specific etiology, such as bacterial or parasitic infections, will be discussed separately. There are several similarities between IBD in animals and humans, suggesting that animals may be a model for certain aspects of the human disease.[1]

ETIOLOGY OF CHRONIC INFLAMMATORY BOWEL DISEASE

The etiology of IBD is unknown, although there is evidence for several causes.

Bacterial Etiology. Evidence for a bacterial etiology is based primarily on response to antibiotic therapy, mainly sulfasalazine, tylosin, and metronidazole. Bacterial cultures have failed to yield a consistent causative organism.[1] Other pathogens known to be causative agents in colitis, such as *Salmonella, Campylobacter,* and invasive strains of *Escherichia coli,* are rarely isolated in clinical cases. In addition, experimental transmission of bacteria has failed to reproduce the disease.[1]

Although there is clearly a profound therapeutic effect of certain antibiotics, it is doubtful that such success can be attributed to the antibacterial effect alone. Sulfasal-

azine contains a sulfa antibiotic and an anti-inflammatory salicylate. Studies have shown that the sulfa moiety has little effect on the colonic flora.[1, 16] In addition, infusion of the colon via enema solution of each of the components separately has shown the salicylate moiety to be of main therapeutic benefit.[17] Tylosin is another antibiotic reported to be effective in managing IBD.[18] However, its mode of action is unknown, and it is not clear whether therapeutic benefits can be attributed to its antimicrobial activity alone. Metronidazole has also been reported to be effective in managing IBD in dogs[19] and in humans.[16] Although metronidazole is effective against a wide variety of anaerobic bacteria,[20] it also has other properties that may be more significant in explaining its effectiveness, including an antiprotozoan effect and its ability to inhibit cell-mediated immunity.[21] These drugs will be discussed in detail in the treatment section.

Some experimental studies have suggested that bacteria may play a role in the perpetuation of chronic colitis, because antibiotic therapy reduces the severity of induced colonic disease.[22, 23] It is possible that the normal microflora of the large intestine may secondarily affect or mediate changes in a colon predisposed to IBD. In addition, antibiotics can induce colitis, presumably because of their effect on the normal fecal flora, allowing selective bacterial overgrowth.

Immune-Mediated Etiology. Most of the evidence available suggests that immunologic factors play a major role in IBD. Many of the inflammatory cells that are present, including lymphocytes, plasma cells, and eosinophils, are mediators of the immune response. The presence of these inflammatory cells may represent a nonspecific response of the colon to a variety of antigens, including bacterial, dietary, or those contained within the colonic mucosal epithelium. (The latter may be further exposed or released following cellular disruption from the inflammatory process, thus perpetuating the reaction.) The types of immune responses and the character of the antigens determine the nature and severity of the inflammatory disease.[1] Antigens can be processed by all four types of hypersensitivity reactions leading to changes resulting in IBD,[24] with cell-mediated immunity appearing to be the most important reaction.[1] The results of these immune responses include antibody-dependent cell-mediated cytotoxicity, and antibodies directed against colonic tissue, bacteria, and dietary constituents, with subsequent fixation of complement resulting in histamine release, neutrophil infiltration, and kinin-mediated inflammatory changes.[1] The response is seen histologically as an influx of inflammatory cells (usually lymphocytes, plasma cells, and lesser numbers of neutrophils and eosinophils) and changes in the architecture of the colonic mucosa. If antigen stimulation persists, the immune response continues, resulting in continued inflammation and eventually fibrosis. This cycle can be broken by eliminating the offending antigens or by modulating the immune response pharmacologically.[1]

Additional evidence for immune-mediated causes is clinical response to hypoallergenic diets.[1, 25] Such diets minimize the amounts of dietary antigens reaching the colon. Clinical improvement in patients with IBD following treatment with immune-modulating drugs provides additional evidence of an immune-mediated etiology. Such drugs include sulfasalazine, metronidazole, glucocorticoids, and azathioprine. As mentioned previously, most of these drugs have other properties, so the mechanism by which they have therapeutic benefit is unclear.

Despite these observations, there is no direct evidence for an immune-mediated or autoimmune etiology of IBD in animals or humans. However, an abnormal immune response may be triggered by bacteria or dietary antigens in a susceptible host that already has clones of sensitized B and T cells.[24] A hypothesis that suggests a multifactorial etiology and pathogenesis that has been proposed for human IBD probably has merit in animals.[26] In susceptible individuals with abnormal host defenses, external agents (such as bacteria or dietary antigens) or those involving cross-reactivity between lumenal antigens and the colonic mucosa, are involved in many autoimmune features of IBD. Any insult that increases intestinal permeability to these antigens can precipitate colonic inflammation. Although this concept has not been proven, it provides a useful basis to evaluate and treat dogs and cats with IBD.

PATHOPHYSIOLOGY OF INFLAMMATORY BOWEL DISEASE

Changes that occur in the large intestine with IBD result in structural and functional abnormalities causing large bowel diarrhea. Normal colonic motility is necessary for normal fluid absorption. This occurs primarily in the absorptive portion of the colon (i.e., the ascending and transverse colon) where there is normally a reversed gradient of muscular contractions that promotes retention of feces, thus allowing for complete absorption. This gradient is lost in patients with IBD resulting in incomplete absorption. In addition, there is loss of normal rhythmic segmental contractions that would otherwise slow down passage of fecal contents.[1] Therefore, very little peristaltic activity is needed to expel fecal contents. When pathology in the cranial portion of the colon is minimal, normal formation of fecal material can occur. If the caudal portion of the colon is affected in such cases, the function as a storage reservoir is affected. Inflammation causes increased sensitivity to the defecation reflex, resulting in increased frequency of defecation.[1] Also, the normal colonic pacemaker is lost and multiple pacemakers arise, resulting in frequent bowel movements.[1] Often there is an urge to defecate when only a small amount of fecal material is present in the descending colon. Tenesmus is often present, usually as a result of direct stimulation of the defecation reflex from the inflammatory process.

In addition to abnormal colonic motility, there is a decreased absorptive ability in the cranial portion of the colon. With chronic ulcerative colitis in humans, the normal electrical potential across the colonic mucosa is lost. This results in a decreased ability to actively absorb sodium across an electrochemical gradient (and therefore decreased passive water absorption).[19] With large bowel diarrhea, even though the volume of each individual bowel movement is usually decreased, the total fecal volume is usually increased.[27] Irritation of the mucosa also stimulates goblet cells to secrete mucus.[1] Another change occurring with chronic inflammation is increased epithelial turnover. Loss of superficial epithelium can result in hemorrhage and ulceration, seen as fresh blood in the stool.[1]

CLINICAL FINDINGS

Animals with large intestinal IBD have large bowel diarrhea as the most common presenting complaint. Historically, patients will typically have increased frequency of defecation, usually with small volumes at a time. Often, the first bowel movement of the day is more normal, with subsequent movements becoming progressively more liquid and decreasing in volume. Mucus either covering or within the feces is very common. Frank blood in the feces and tenesmus are also frequently seen. Many well-trained dogs will defecate in the house due to an increased sense of urgency. The presence of tenesmus, increased urgency, and mucus in the feces are the most common signs seen with chronic colitis. However, the absence of any of the signs does not rule out IBD. Similar signs also occur in cats, but infrequent owner observance of the cat's pattern of defecation may allow these signs to go unnoticed.

Other signs may occur but are less common. These include vomiting and weight loss, which can be either a result of severe colitis or of involvement of the small intestine or stomach with the same inflammatory process. However, in general, most animals appear healthy with normal appetite and physical appearance. There is seldom a history suggesting involvement of other body systems, usually only single animals in multiple-pet households are affected, and environmental history is usually noncontributory. Stress may be a precipitating factor in some animals, but its relative contribution is difficult to evaluate. In the author's practice, there does not seem to be a breed or sex predisposition. Most affected animals are middle aged, although the disease occasionally occurs in the very young and old.

Physical examination is usually unremarkable except in severe cases when weight loss might be a feature. Occasionally, there is excess discomfort upon rectal palpation, and feces seen on the rectal glove reflect historical information.

LABORATORY FINDINGS

Laboratory findings in patients with chronic colitis are usually unremarkable. However, these tests are run to rule out other causes of chronic diarrhea and to evaluate other body systems. These tests should include fecal flotations, sedimentation, and direct smears to rule out parasites, and fecal cultures to rule out bacterial pathogens. Hemograms are usually normal but may show neutrophilia and monocytosis in severe cases (reflecting chronic, active inflammation) or eosinophilia when this inflammatory cell predominates histologically. Serum chemistry profiles will occasionally show hypoalbuminemia, hyperglobulinemia, and mild-to-moderate liver enzyme elevation. The latter is from absorption of toxins through a damaged mucosal barrier and resultant hepatocellular degeneration.

1406   SECTION IX—The Gastrointestinal System

COLONOSCOPIC FINDINGS

Proctoscopy or colonoscopy is the procedure of choice in evaluating disorders of the large intestine in general, and especially IBD. In most cases, the descending colon is most severely involved or at least concurrently involved. Therefore, rigid proctoscopy usually provides adequate diagnostic information. Gross findings are extremely variable (Figure 87–2). The colon might appear grossly normal (pink, smooth, glistening, easily distended) despite severe histologic abnormalities. In other cases, the mucosa can be extremely hyperemic, with pale patches in areas with more severe cellular infiltrates. Ulcers and erosions are often visible. The mucosa is often friable and bleeds easily following introduction of the scope or bleeds excessively following superficial biopsies. The mucosa can also appear thickened with a cobblestone-like appearance and nondistensible wall. Such cases are usually chronic and severe, with extensive fibrosis seen histologically. An uncommon sequela to chronic ulceration and fibrosis is stricture formation. These strictures can be small enough to prevent passage of even a small-diameter endoscope. The need for taking multiple biopsy samples, even when the mucosa appears normal, should be emphasized, since histologic evaluation is critical to the diagnosis.

RADIOGRAPHIC FINDINGS

Plain abdominal radiographs contribute little in patients with IBD. However, they may be a useful screening procedure to rule out other abdominal disorders. Barium enemas are rarely indicated in IBD. The main indication for this study is failure of proctoscopy to obtain a diagnosis and when flexible colonoscopy is not available. Barium enemas are also useful to define strictures, a rare complication of chronic colitis. Lesions commonly seen on barium enemas in patients with IBD include irregular mucosal borders (seen as "serrations"), thickened mucosal wall and folds, decreased distensibility, shortening of the colon, and mucosal ulcers. However, these changes are not specific, and a definitive diagnosis can only be made histologically.

HISTOLOGIC FINDINGS

The histologic abnormalities in IBD are not unique to this syndrome but can be seen in other specific disease entities, such as parasitic or bacterial colitis. Therefore, the diagnosis depends on a combination of clinical and pathologic features, primarily meant to rule out these specific disease entities. Once this is accomplished, histologic evaluation is necessary for a definitive diagnosis of IBD.

The most consistent feature of IBD is an accumulation of a varied population of inflammatory cells in the lamina propria of the colonic mucosa, usually lymphocytes, plasma cells, and a lesser number of eosinophils and neutrophils. There is also crypt dilatation, loss of the surface epithelial cells, and flattening and vacuolation of epithelial cells.[1] The colonic glands are also dilated and goblet cells are decreased in number.[19] Immaturity of colonic glands indicates mucosal regeneration in many cases of IBD. There is an absence of periodic acid-Schiff (PAS) positive histiocytes, unlike the case in histiocytic colitis. As the disease progresses, fibrosis first appears in the lamina propria. More severe loss of superficial epithelium results in ulceration. Eventually, inflammation and fibrosis can extend into the submucosa.

The types of inflammatory cells vary among patients. Although most cases involve a mixture of inflammatory cells, lymphocytes and plasma cells usually predominate. Some cases with a severe lymphocytic infiltration can be difficult to distinguish from mature, lymphocytic lymphosarcoma. A lymphocytic inflammatory infiltrate may also progress to lymphoma, a phenomenon well documented in humans with immunoproliferative small intestinal disease.[28] Other cases have eosinophils or neutrophils as the predominant cell type. The presence of eosinophils may suggest an allergic or parasitic cause, but such an infiltrate can occur without evidence of these. Other clinical features, including therapeutic response, are similar to that of lymphocytic-plasmacytic colitis. The presence or predominance of neutrophils as an inflammatory infiltrate does not necessarily indicate a bacterial etiology, but may be a response to cellular degeneration or necrosis.[1, 29]

TREATMENT

Diet. Dietary control is critical in managing many cases of chronic colitis. During acute phases, resting the gastrointestinal tract by minimizing oral intake of food is often useful in controlling signs of colitis. This will reduce the amount of dietary antigens reaching the colon. In humans, total parenteral nutrition is sometimes effective in managing severe cases.[30] However, this is not practical for small animals in most clinical settings, and those measures aimed at complete rest of the gastrointestinal tract are not suitable for long-term management.

Since some patients have dietary antigens as a cause of the inflammatory response, a hypoallergenic diet designed to use a single protein and carbohydrate source that is highly digestible is indicated to minimize such antigens.[1] Homemade diets best fulfill these objectives, including cottage cheese or lamb mixed with rice. Cottage cheese is preferred because it is more completely digested and absorbed than is meat.[1] Rice is the preferred carbohydrate source since its starch is more completely assimilated than starches in the flours from other cereal sources.[31] These types of controlled diets have been used successfully as the only form of therapy in clinical cases treated by the author and others.[25, 32]

In cases when a true dietary allergy exists, elimination diets are necessary to determine the nature of the offending allergen. Some animals cannot tolerate meat products and do well when cottage cheese is the main protein source, while others cannot tolerate glutens and do well when grains such as wheat, rye, barley, oats, and buckwheat are eliminated from the diet. Appropriate diet trials will help reduce or eliminate the need for concomitant drug therapy. Other diets containing a different protein source should be tried before dietary therapy is discarded. Seven to ten days of feeding a given diet may be necessary before calling it a failure.

Once remission is achieved (with or without concomitant drug therapy), commercial diets may be gradually introduced. Those containing a limited number of nutrient sources should be used. Although the author has achieved good success with dry nonmeat, gluten-free diets, others have recommended the use of canned all-meat dog food because this may result in lighter, less bulky feces.[19] They also recommend the addition of bulk agents such as bran because of the potential benefit of altering colonic motility.[19] Dietary fiber will also bind bile acids and bacteria, both of which can cause further insult to an already inflamed colon.[1]

The need for client education cannot be overstated. If owners understand that the problem is controllable and not curable, they are more likely to avoid giving offending foods that may precipitate a relapse. Likewise, unnecessary dependence on drug therapy can often be avoided with proper controlled diets.

Antimicrobial Drugs. Most antimicrobial drugs are of little value in the long-term management of patients with IBD. Since a primary bacterial infection is rarely the etiology of the disease, these drugs are rarely indicated.[33] Occasionally, bacterial overgrowth may accompany IBD, or a damaged colonic mucosa might be further damaged by the effects of normal bacterial flora. In these instances, there may be temporary improvement with antibiotic therapy. Broad-spectrum antibiotics given systemically might also be necessary in severe cases when extensive mucosal damage increases the likelihood of systemic infection following absorption of normal colonic flora. However, in most cases the routine use of antibiotics is not justified, and in some cases the condition will be worsened due to their disruptive effect on normal colonic flora.[22, 32, 33] An exception to this rule is the use of sulfasalazine, metronidazole, and tylosin, antibiotics that have been shown to have long-term therapeutic benefit. As will be discussed, these drugs may be helpful for reasons other than their antimicrobial properties.

SULFASALAZINE. Sulfasalazine (salicylazosulfapyridine, Azulfadine) is the drug of choice in most cases of IBD.[1, 19] It is a combination of the sulfa drug sulfapyridine and the antileukotriene and antiprostaglandin 5-aminosalicylate. The two compounds are linked by an azo bond and undergo minimal small intestinal absorption (10 to 15 per cent).[1, 17, 34] Other studies suggest that small intestinal absorption occurs, but most of the drug is returned to the gastrointestinal tract via the biliary system.[35] Cleavage of the azo bond occurs in the colon and is caused by the action of colonic bacteria. The sulfapyridine moiety is almost completely absorbed from the colon, metabolized in the liver, and excreted in the urine.[17, 34] Most of the 5-aminosalicylate moiety remains in the colon, where it is active locally and binds to colonic connective tissue.[35] In humans, about 30 per cent of the 5-aminosalicylate is absorbed.[29] The effectiveness of sulfasalazine is most likely due to the 5-aminosalicylate moiety. Rectal infusion of the separate ingredients has shown 5-aminosalicylate to have the most therapeutic effect in humans with ulcerative colitis.[17] It is doubtful that the antibacterial effect of the sulfapyridine portion is of benefit, since it has minimal effect on colonic flora,[16] and antibiotics in general are only effective in suppressing colonic flora for a few days.[1, 33]

The benefits seen from the 5-aminosalicylate portion have been attributed to its antiprostaglandin effects, but there is now evidence that the benefits are due to its properties to inhibit leukotriene production.[35a-35c] Leukotrienes are inflammatory mediators derived from arachidonic acid metabolism through the lipoxygenase pathway. They are potent chemotactic agents, induce neutrophil aggregation and degranulation, increase vascular permeability, and induce release of lysosomal enzymes.[35a, 35b] Leukotrienes are increased in human colonic mucosa with IBD compared with normal colonic mucosa, and more so than prostaglandins.[35a, 35c] In addition, the concentration of leukotrienes in the rectum of humans with IBD correlates with disease activity before and following treatment with 5-aminosalicylate.[35c] Prostaglandins, products derived from arachidonic acid metabolism through the cyclo-oxygenase pathway, were once thought to be mediators in the inflammatory process and affect mucosal transport, thus contributing to diarrhea.[36] However, other drugs that suppress prostaglandins to a greater extent than sulfasalazine lack therapeutic benefit.[35b, 36] Sulfasalazine changes the abnormal net secretion of sodium and water in the colon to a net absorption.[35] However, the precise mechanism of drug action remains to be explained. Nonetheless, the drug is considered to be effective in dogs and cats.[1, 9, 19, 25, 29, 32]

The usual starting dosage for the dog is 10 to 15 mg/lb (20 to 30 mg/kg) q8h orally. Most dogs respond well to this regimen. When histologic lesions are mild, the drug can usually be stopped after three weeks. However, in severe cases, treatment for six weeks or longer is often necessary. The drug is supplied in 500-mg tablets, 500-mg enteric-coated tablets, and liquid form containing 50 mg/ml. The dosage has not been as well established in the cat, and caution must be used because of the species' sensitivity to salicylates. This author currently uses 10 to 12 mg/lb (20 to 25 mg/kg) q12h to q24h, which is similar to the dosage reported by others.[25, 29] The liquid form allows more accurate administration to smaller cats. Vomiting and partial anorexia will occasionally occur in cats, and can often be successfully managed using the enteric-coated tablets.

Side effects of sulfasalazine are uncommon, and include keratoconjunctivitis sicca (KCS),[37, 38] cholestatic jaundice, allergic dermatitis, and vomiting.[19] Of these, KCS is the most common, and usually requires discontinuation of the drug. The onset of signs averages six to eight months after starting sulfasalazine (but can be sooner), and KCS is usually permanent in these dogs.[37, 38]

METRONIDAZOLE. Metronidazole (Flagyl) is another drug that has been used successfully in managing cases of chronic colitis. This drug has several properties that could explain its effectiveness. In addition to its well-known antiprotozoal effect,[39] metronidazole is effective against a wide variety of anaerobic bacteria,[20] is a potent suppressor of cell-mediated immunity,[21] affects leukocyte chemotaxis, and may have other immunosuppressive effects.[39a–39c] Metronidazole has been shown to be effective in treating humans with IBD,[16] and has been shown to have a protective effect against experimentally induced colitis.[40] It is unlikely that its success is caused by its antiprotozoal effect. Although occult protozoal infections occur, patients with chronic colitis relapse when metronidazole administration is stopped after five days, the usual treatment course for many protozoal infections, suggesting another mechanism requiring long-term administration. Its effectiveness against anaerobic bacteria suggests the possible contribution of anaerobic bacterial antigens to the inflammatory reaction, although it is not clear whether there is significant long-term alteration of colonic microflora after metronidazole therapy.[16] Metronidazole's effects on inhibiting the immune response is another likely mechanism of benefit in chronic colitis. As already mentioned, the contribution of the immune system to the etiology of IBD justifies the use of immune-modulating drugs.

Although there have been no controlled studies on the effectiveness of metronidazole in animals as there have been in humans, it has been used successfully by the author and by others in dogs and cats.[19] Although sulfasalazine seems to be the drug of first choice, metronidazole has been useful in patients that suffer undesirable side effects of sulfasalazine. It is also a useful adjunct when a patient is being treated with corticosteroids, in that it allows a marked reduction in corticosteroid doses. An effective dose of metronidazole is less than that required for protozoan infections. Most animals respond well to 5 to 7 mg/lb (10 to 15 mg/kg) q12h. It appears safe for long-term administration. It is supplied in 250 mg and 500 mg tablets, as a ready to use solution for IV use containing 5 mg/ml, and as a lyophilized powder to be reconstituted for IV use after dilution. Side effects are rare, but the author has seen self-limiting neurologic signs (including seizures) in two dogs inadvertently given overdoses. Neurotoxicity is also a reported side effect in humans[20] and has been described in the dog.[20, 41]

TYLOSIN. Tylosin (Tylan) is a macrolide antibiotic that has been reported to be effective in a variety of long-standing forms of IBD.[18] In this uncontrolled study, 81 per cent of the dogs recovered, although the diagnosis was confirmed by biopsy in only a small percentage of dogs. The mechanism of action of tylosin is unknown. Its effectiveness among cases seems variable, although some patients unresponsive to other forms of therapy have responded to tylosin. Dosage is imprecise, but the agent has been used successfully at 5 to 100 mg/lb (11 to 200 mg/kg)[18] and 10 to 20 mg/lb (20 to 40 mg/kg) q12h.[42] Tylosin is supplied in a powdered form containing 440 mg per teaspoon (along with vitamins). It appears safe for long-term administration, with no side effects.[18]

Corticosteroids. Since IBD most likely has an immunologic basis, the use of immunosuppressive drugs appears justified. Corticosteroids have been used successfully in controlled studies in humans with IBD,[43] and the author and others have had success in treating animals.[1, 9, 19, 32] The benefits seen with corticosteroids are most likely due to their anti-inflammatory, antiprostaglandin, antileukotriene, and immunosuppressive effects, although they also increase salt and water absorption across the normal colonic mucosa and regulate basal colonic electrolyte transport. It appears that this mechanism could be of value in treating large bowel diarrhea.[44]

The main indication for corticosteroid administration appears to be in patients only partially responsive to sulfasalazine or metronidazole. In these animals, prednisone can be used to manage acute exacerbations and to allow a decreased dosage of the other drugs. Corticosteroids do not appear to be suitable as the sole drug used or for long-term management because of detrimental side effects[9] (and in humans their efficacy decreases with prolonged daily treatment).[44] Others have suggested that corticosteroids are the drug of choice for eosinophilic colitis.[1, 9, 19, 41, 42] The initial dose of prednisone for chronic inflammatory bowel disease is 0.5 to 1 mg/lb/day (1 to 2 mg/kg/day) for the dog, and 1 to 2 mg/lb/day (2 to 4 mg/kg/day) for the cat. Once clinical remission is achieved, the dosage is tapered over a three- to five-week period. Corticosteroids can also be given locally by rectal infusion. Steroid absorption from the rectum and colon is about half that after ingestion; thus, systemic side effects can be reduced.[44] However, the effect of a true retention enema is difficult to achieve in animals due to lack of cooperation, and therefore rectal administration is of most value when there is proctitis along with colitis or when systemic side effects become intolerable. They are especially useful for treating acute exacerbations. Several rectal infusion products are available, including hydrocortisone acetate foam, hydrocortisone acetate mixed with an anesthetic foam containing pramoxine, hydrocortisone retention enema, and hydrocortisone acetate suppositories. Side effects with prolonged administration of any corticosteroid are those of iatrogenic Cushing's syndrome and hypothalamic-pituitary-adrenal axis suppression. Additional side effects particular to the gastrointestinal tract include inhibition of the normal cytoprotective action of prostaglandins (thus predisposing to intestinal ulceration and perforation), predisposition to acute pancreatitis, the development of steroid hepatopathy, and predisposition to parasitic, bacterial, and fungal infections.[44]

Other Immunosuppressive Drugs. **AZATHIOPRINE.** Azathioprine (Imuran), an antimetabolite, is a synthetic purine analogue that blocks the incorporation of natural purines into DNA and thereby interferes with cell metabolism. It is apparently a somewhat less toxic imidazolyl derivative and metabolic precursor of the closely related compound 6-mercaptopurine.[45] Azathioprine has been reported to be beneficial in several human patients with ulcerative colitis and Crohn's disease. Although controlled trials have not shown significant improvement compared with sulfasalazine in treating ulcerative colitis, azathioprine has reliable steroid-sparing effects in Crohn's disease.[45] However, there appears to be a subgroup of patients that especially benefit from azathioprine. The author has found a need for azathioprine in only rare instances, but in these few cases it has been helpful. The dose is 50 mg/m² once daily for two weeks, followed by alternate-day administration. It is supplied in 50 mg tablets. The most significant adverse effect is bone marrow suppression and leukopenia. A complete blood count should be obtained periodically during azathioprine therapy.

OTHER CYTOTOXIC AGENTS. Other cytotoxic agents, including chlorambucil (Leukeran), busulfan (Myleran), and nitrogen mustard (mechlorethamine, Mustargen), have not been used much or have not undergone controlled trials in humans or animals. Occasional beneficial results have been reported in humans, but these agents' undesirable side effects and lack of controlled trials prohibit their indication in treating IBD.[45]

CROMOLYN SODIUM. Cromolyn sodium (disodium cromoglycate) is used for inhalation therapy of asthma in humans, acting locally to prevent mast cell degranulation in immediate hypersensitivity reactions.[45, 46] Some benefit has been seen in controlled trials with oral and rectal administration in humans with ulcerative colitis, presumably because of the same mechanism.[46] However, the results have not been dramatic, and since available forms are extremely expensive and inconvenient, its use is likely unjustified at this time.

Motility Modifiers. Motility-modifying drugs offer only temporary symptomatic relief rather than correcting the primary problem in IBD. However, they are occasionally helpful during acute exacerbations. As mentioned previously, motility derangements include primarily a decrease in rhythmic segmental contractions, which normally provide resistance to flow of feces. Since the colon is already hypomotile, there is no indication for the routine use of anticholinergic drugs that further depress rhythmic segmentation, and their use can exacerbate or prolong diarrhea.[1, 19, 32] Narcotic analgesics, on the other hand, act to increase rhythmic segmentation and thus help slow passage of feces and restore normal motility. In addition, these drugs help re-establishment of normal colonic secretion and absorption.[32] Examples of narcotic analgesics with primarily gastrointestinal effects are loperamide (Imodium, supplied in 2 mg capsules, given at 0.05 mg/lb (0.1 mg/kg), or about one capsule per 15 kg of body weight in the dog, q8h to q12h), diphenoxylate (Lomotil, supplied in tablets and liquid containing 2.5 mg diphenoxylate and 0.025 mg atropine per tablet or five ml liquid, given at 0.05 to 0.1 mg/lb (0.1 to 0.2 mg/kg) or about one tablet per 10 to 15 kg of body weight, q8h), and paregoric (usually supplied with intestinal protectants and absorbents, given at 0.03 mg/lb (0.06 mg/kg), q8h to q12h).

On the rare occasion that colonic spasm is contributing to clinical signs, anticholinergic drugs might be helpful, although long-term use is not justified.[19, 32] Anticholinergic drugs with relative specificity to the gastrointestinal tract include propantheline bromide (Pro-Banthine, supplied in 7.5 and 15 mg tablets, given at 0.1 to 0.25 mg/lb (0.25 to 0.5 mg/kg) q8h), and clidinium bromide (Quarzan, Librax, supplied in capsules containing 2.5 mg clidinium with and without five mg of the tranquilizer chlordiazepoxide, given at about one capsule per 50 lb of body weight, q12h). The latter drug may be useful in rare cases where stress and behavior problems contribute to the pathogenesis of the problem.

PROGNOSIS

Although no controlled studies have been performed to assess the outcome in patients with IBD, clinical experience has shown that most patients can be successfully managed. Most therapeutic failures are caused by (1) lack of proper dietary management; (2) reliance on one or two drugs alone; (3) lack of patience when making therapeutic changes; (4) failure to educate clients regarding the nature of the disease and treatment, and the need for strict compliance with dietary and drug treatment; (5) failure to recognize that some animals require long-term or even lifetime management; and (6) inadequate diagnostic workup, with failure to obtain a definitive diagnosis by biopsy, and failure to identify underlying diseases such as parasitic or bacterial pathogens.

When the disease has progressed to gross stricture formation or extensive fibrosis histologically, successful management is less likely. However, aggressive medical treatment is still indicated, with surgical removal of the diseased portion of the colon reserved as a salvage procedure only in cases not responsive to medical management.

Eosinophilic Colitis

Eosinophilic colitis is a variant of inflammatory bowel disease characterized by an infiltration of the lamina propria with eosinophils as the predominant inflammatory cell. The etiology of the disease is unknown, although a food allergy or parasitic reaction may be involved.[1, 19] Since there is no evidence to support this, and because hypoallergenic diet trials alone and broad-spectrum anthelmintic therapy are generally unsuccessful, the disease should probably be regarded as an idiopathic entity similar to that described for inflammatory bowel disease, with an immunologic basis as the most likely etiology. In cats, there appear to be two forms of the disease. One form is similar to that occurring in the dog, with an eosinophilic infiltration limited to the gastrointestinal tract. The other form is one in which the eosinophilic enterocolitis is a component of a hypereosinophilic syndrome with systemic involvement (including eosinophilic infiltration of the spleen, liver, and bone marrow).[47]

Clinical findings in animals with eosinophilic colitis are similar to that described for inflammatory bowel disease (with the exception of the severe systemic involvement in cats with the hypereosinophilic syndrome). In animals that have enterocolitis, small intestinal signs often accompany those of colitis. Abnormal laboratory findings often include an absolute and relative cosinophilia (seen in approximately 50 per cent of affected animals). Other causes of eosinophilia that result in gastrointestinal signs should be ruled out, including intestinal parasites and hypoadrenocorticism. In cats with the hypereosinophilic syndrome, additional findings include signs reflecting systemic involvement. Often the bowel is palpably thickened, there may be hepatosplenomegaly, and the colon is affected in nearly one-half of affected cats.[47] Eosinophil counts can be in excess of $100,000/\mu l$, making the syndrome difficult to distinguish from eosinophilic leukemia.

Diagnosis is established only by obtaining a colon biopsy revealing numerous eosinophils in the colonic mucosa. A rectal cytologic smear showing numerous eosinophils is also highly suggestive. Although a peripheral eosinophilia along with gastrointestinal signs supports the diagnosis, these signs are not diagnostic of eosinophilic colitis alone, and a biopsy is required.

Treatment is similar to that described for chronic inflammatory bowel disease, and the reader is referred to this section. First, attempts are made to rule out dietary and parasitic antigens with a controlled hypoallergenic diet and a broad-spectrum anthelmintic. Many animals do not respond to these attempts and require anti-inflammatory medication. Many authors suggest using corticosteroids initially as the drug of choice.[1, 9, 19, 41, 42] The initial dose is 0.5 to 1 mg/lb/day (1 to 2 mg/kg/day) of prednisone in the dog, and 1 to 2 mg/lb/day (2 to 4 mg/kg/day) in the cat. Once clinical remission is achieved, this dose is maintained for about three weeks, after which it is tapered over an additional three weeks. Some animals will require long-term administration. In these cases, alternate-day therapy is preferred. If side effects become a concern, other drugs such as sulfasalazine, metronidazole, tylosin, or azathioprine can be used. These drugs and other symptomatic treatment measures described in the section on inflammatory bowel disease may be useful in some patients.

Histiocytic Ulcerative Colitis

ETIOLOGY

Histiocytic ulcerative colitis is a relatively uncommon disease characterized by mucosal ulcers and an inflammatory cell infiltrate composed mainly of periodic acid-Schiff (PAS) positive histiocytes. There appears to be a marked breed predisposition in Boxer dogs, but the disease has also been described in the French bulldog[48] and in the cat.[49] Although the etiology of the disease is unknown, many theories have been proposed. The hallmark of the disease is an accumulation of histiocytes engorged with polysaccharides that are PAS-positive. Since these histiocytes develop from macrophages phagocytizing these substances, their accumulation might be caused by a deficiency of lysosomal enzymes necessary for degradation. Another theory is that macrophages are unable to process normal amounts of foreign material absorbed from the colon.[50] Alternatively, the macrophages may be normal but are ingesting some substances that inhibit the degradation process.[50] An infectious etiology has also been proposed on the basis of the finding of coccoid structures resembling *Chlamydia* in ultrastructural studies.[51] However, similar work failed to detect such organisms.[50] Researchers have not been able to produce the disease experimentally by the transmission of any agent.[1] Due to the marked breed predisposition in the Boxer dog, it has also been suggested that there is a genetic predisposition.[52] Ischemia is an unlikely cause of epithelial injury, as vascular studies did not demonstrate reductions in mucosal blood flow, but only nonspecific changes reflecting the stage and severity of inflammation.[53] Since crypt epithelial cells are unable to repair defects at the luminal surface, affected dogs may have a defect in the kinetics of epithelial regeneration, or there may be a defect in the surface barrier allowing nonspecific injury by normal microflora and toxins.[50] However, the etiology remains unclear, and the pathogenic mechanism for epithelial injury remains unknown.

CLINICAL FEATURES

Histiocytic ulcerative colitis is a very uncommon cause of colitis, accounting for less than two per cent of all cases of colitis.[19] The disease affects primarily young boxers, with most cases occurring in dogs less than two years of age.[19, 54, 55] Presenting signs are those features that suggest large bowel diarrhea, including bloody mucoid diarrhea. As the disease progresses, weight loss and general debilitation occur. There are often spontaneous remissions and relapses. Laboratory findings are similar to those described for chronic inflammatory bowel disease.

The diagnosis is based on characteristic changes of the colon seen grossly and histologically. The earliest gross changes are patchy red foci, either punctate or diffuse. These progress in severity and eventually ulcerate.[52] At this point there are thick irregular folds giving a cobblestone appearance, with ulcers varying in size. Areas of granulation tissue are also seen. Microscopic changes begin with focal, acute inflammation, and epithelial cell degeneration, suggesting that the initial lesion is epithelial cell injury.[50] Neutrophils are often present within the epithelium, with occasional microabscess formation. There are numerous PAS-positive histiocytes in the deep lamina propria and submucosa as the lesions progress. Chronic changes also include infiltration of lymphocytes and plasma cells.[52] Eventually, mucosa of reduced thickness progresses to frank ulceration.

TREATMENT AND PROGNOSIS

Treatment is the same as that described for chronic inflammatory bowel disease, with sulfasalazine the drug of choice. When treatment is begun early, the outcome is often favorable, although these dogs often relapse later in life and may require lifelong treatment. The prognosis is poor in dogs that have treatment begun after the disease has progressed. In these dogs, there are often treatment failures or repeated recurrences.

Parasitic Diseases of the Large Intestine

TRICHURIASIS

Whipworm (*Trichuris vulpis*) infection is a very common cause of acute, chronic, or intermittent large intestinal diarrhea in the dog. Although *Trichuris* sp. has been reported in the cat, it is extremely rare and not a significant pathogen in this species.[56–58] The parasite generally lives in the cecum and proximal colon of the dog, where the long thread-like esophageal region of the worm is imbedded in the mucosa, and the stout "handle" portion of the worm is free in the lumen.[56] With heavy infestations, the worms can be seen throughout the entire colon. The presence of the parasite results in extensive mucosal hyperplasia and a chronic inflammatory cell infiltrate.[19] The life cycle of *Trichuris vulpis* is simple and direct. Adults shed eggs in the feces, which develop into infective larvated eggs in two to four weeks. The parasite then undergoes a mucosal migration lasting three months before developing into the adult worm in the cecum and colon.[56]

The severity of the signs depend on the number of parasites and the individual response of the host. Often stress, concurrent disease, or the administration of corticosteroids will cause a previously asymptomatic dog to show clinical signs, which are similar to those of other causes of large bowel diarrhea.

Since the signs cannot be distinguished from other causes, the diagnosis usually depends on identifying the typical bioperculated eggs in a fecal flotation or direct fecal smear. Many dogs will shed the eggs in the feces intermittently, requiring at least three to four negative samples over a three- to four-day period before the presence of whipworms can be ruled out. Occasionally, the diagnosis is made by observing the adult worms in the colon during colonoscopy. The author and others have identified the parasite in this manner when repeated fecal examinations were negative.[19, 58] Other colonoscopic findings depend on the severity of the infection, ranging from grossly normal to severe hyperemia with superficial ulcers. Biopsy changes are nonspecific and cannot readily be distinguished from chronic inflammatory bowel disease.

Treatment consists of an effective anthelmintic, several of which are now available. The author prefers fenbendazole (Panacur) at an oral dose of 22 mg/lb (50 mg/kg) daily for three days. This regimen is reported to be 100 per cent effective for *Trichuris*, with minimal adverse side effects.[58] Other drugs with activity against *Trichuris* include phthalofyne (Whipcide, 90 per cent effective), glycobiarsol (Milibus V, 90 per cent effective), butamisole HCl (Styquin, 99 per cent effective), dichlorvos (Task, 90 per cent effective), mebendazole (Telmintic, 95 per cent effective), and febantel (Vercom, 100 per cent effective).[58, 59, 60] The efficacy of these drugs may vary with the number of adult parasites. Animals should be retreated or have repeated fecal examinations at three month intervals to check for re-establishment of patent infections. Since eggs are very resistant in the environment, it may be necessary to treat the areas the animal frequents to prevent reinfection. Supportive care is generally not necessary, and the prognosis for recovery is good.

GIARDIASIS

Giardia is a flagellate protozoan parasite thought to be primarily a small intestinal parasite, although some dogs will show signs typical of large intestinal involvement.[61-63] Inside the host, *Giardia* exists as a motile trophozoite, while outside the host, *Giardia* exists as a resistant cyst.[5] The life cycle is simple and direct, with trophozoites becoming infective cysts in the large intestine and subsequently being passed in feces. When ingested, they excyst in the duodenum to the trophozoite stage.[5] The pathogenic mechanisms by which *Giardia* causes intestinal disease remain unclear.

Diagnosis of giardiasis is made by identification of the parasite or by response to specific treatment. However, the diagnosis of *Giardia* based on response to treatment with metronidazole should be made with caution because of this drug's effects on anaerobic bacteria and host immune responses, effects that would improve

other diseases (see section on Chronic Inflammatory Bowel Disease). There are several methods by which *Giardia* can be detected. Motile trophozoites can be found in fresh saline smears of feces, a technique that is simple to perform. However, modified zinc sulfate concentration technique was found to be the most sensitive method of diagnosis, detecting the cyst stage of the parasite.[6] In another study, a trichrome stain of preserved feces was found to be the most sensitive method of detection studied.[6a] Since shedding of the organism is often intermittent, repeated examinations may be necessary to identify the parasite. Identification of *Giardia* can also be made from duodenal aspirates obtained during endoscopy or surgery.[61] However, response to treatment may be a less invasive diagnostic alternative.

Treatment of *Giardia* is usually successful with either metronidazole (12 mg/lb (25 mg/kg) q12h for 5 days), or with quinacrine (3 mg/lb (6.6 mg/kg) q12h for 5 days). In one study, metronidazole was 67 per cent effective against *Giardia* and 100 per cent effective against *Pentatrichomonas*, while quinacrine was 100 per cent effective against *Giardia* and zero per cent effective against *Pentatrichomonas*.[39] These authors recommended the use of metronidazole because of its lack of side effects when compared with quinacrine (anorexia, lethargy, fever, vomiting, diarrhea, and abdominal pain), and its superior efficacy for *Pentatrichomonas*. Those animals that do not respond to metronidazole should then be treated with quinacrine. Another drug that has been successful in treating *Giardia* is ipronidazole hydrochloride, a feed or water additive for the treatment of blackhead in turkeys.[64] It is added to the dog's drinking water at a concentration of 126 mg/L of water for seven days.

Although there are many species of *Giardia* depending on the host infected, they are morphologically similar, and species found in animals can be infective for humans.[5, 61] Due to this public health risk, proper treatment for all infected animals is recommended.

TRICHOMONIASIS[5]

Trichomoniasis is caused by the pyriform flagellate *Pentatrichomonas hominis*. The parasite inhabits the large intestine of dogs and cats, as well as other species including humans. Trophozoites have a large single posterior flagellum opposite multiple anterior flagella, an appearance that distinguishes them from *Giardia* (multiple flagella along the same pole). Although *P. hominis* does not form true cysts, pseudocysts may be seen. Transmission occurs when trophozoites in feces, food, or water are ingested.

It is unknown whether *Pentatrichomonas* is pathogenic in dogs and cats. Although the parasite is sometimes found in animals with diarrhea, a cause-and-effect relationship has not been established.[5, 39] While some authors suggest the organism may be an opportunistic pathogen,[5] others suggest it is a clinical entity, especially in the young.[39]

Diagnosis of the infection depends on identification of the motile trophozoites in feces. Smears may be stained with iron hematoxylin, Giemsa, or silver stains to examine morphologic details that distinguish *P. hom-*

inis from *Giardia*. Treatment of trichomoniasis with metronidazole has been shown to be 100 per cent effective at a dose of 12 mg/lb q12h (25 mg/kg).[39]

AMEBIASIS[5]

Amebiasis is caused by infection with the protozoan parasite *Entamoeba histolytica*. Although *E. histolytica* is more common in humans, it can invade the large intestine of dogs and cats. The incidence is more widespread in tropical countries than in the United States. The major source of infection is ingestion of food or water contaminated with human feces.[65] The infection is acquired upon ingestion of the resistant cyst form, which then descend and colonize the large intestine. Animals then excrete primarily the motile trophozoites in the feces. Since this form is extremely fragile and noninfective, animals do not represent a significant reservoir for infection.[65] Humans, however, also excrete infective cysts in addition to trophozoites, and thus represent a source of continued infection. In the large intestine, trophozoites of *E. histolytica* lyse colonic epithelial cells and invade the intestinal wall, producing characteristic flask-shaped ulcers.[65] This results in typical signs of large bowel diarrhea. Some animals may be asymptomatic carriers. With deeper penetration, the parasite can invade blood vessels or lymphatics, and subsequently invade other tissues, such as the liver and skin.[65] Extraintestinal involvement is less common in dogs than in humans.

The diagnosis depends on identification of the motile trophozoites in feces or mucosal colon biopsy. It is important that a saline fecal smear be examined while fresh due to the fragile nature of the trophozoites. Nonpathogenic amebic species are rare in the dog, so that definitive identification of the species is usually not necessary.[5] Trophozoites in tissue sections stain strongly with periodic acid-Schiff stain, allowing easier identification.

The drug of choice for treatment of amebiasis is metronidazole; however, clinical reports of its use in amebiasis are limited.[65] Furazolidone was also used successfully in a dog at a dose of 1.1 mg/lb q8h (2.3 mg/kg) for seven days.[66]

BALANTIDIASIS[5]

Balantidium coli is a ciliated protozoan that resides in the large intestinal mucosa in the trophozoite form. *B. coli* is more common in pigs and humans, with few reports of clinical infection in dogs.[67–69] Both trophozoites and cysts can be found in the feces. The cyst form is the infective stage, and upon ingestion the parasite excysts and the trophozoites invade the large intestinal mucosa. This process results in inflammation and flask-shaped ulcers similar to those produced by *E. histolytica*. Clinical signs range from asymptomatic to severe large bowel diarrhea. Since reported cases of *B. coli* infection involved concurrent *Trichuris* infection, it is unclear what the relative contribution of *B. coli* was in causing signs.[67–69]

Diagnosis of balantidiasis can be made by finding trophozoites or cysts in direct fecal smears, by finding cysts in feces processed by the zinc sulfate flotation technique, or by finding trophozoites in tissue sections from colon biopsies. Metronidazole has been suggested as the proper treatment,[9] although elimination of concurrent *Trichuris* infection alone may be sufficient.[19, 67, 68] Oxytetracycline for ten days and dichlorvos 40 mg/lb (80 mg/kg) have also been suggested as alternative treatments.[9]

Fungal Infections of the Large Intestine

HISTOPLASMA COLITIS

Histoplasma capsulatum is a pathogenic yeast that usually affects the respiratory tract but can involve the intestines through direct ingestion, or secondarily following systemic dissemination. When the intestines are involved, there can be lesions and subsequent clinical signs associated with small intestinal involvement, large intestinal involvement, or both.[19] Histoplasmosis is more common in dogs, although involvement of primarily the large intestine has been described in the cat.[70] The organism colonizes the lamina propria and submucosa of the intestine and elicits a severe granulomatous reaction, resulting in corrugation, thickening, and distortion of the wall.[9] *Histoplasma* organisms are often present intracellularly within macrophages in these lesions. The organisms can be restricted to the intestine when this organ is primarily affected, or they can invade intestinal lymphatics and blood vessels and then undergo systemic dissemination.[19]

Clinical signs and physical examination findings depend on the extent of tissue involvement. When only the large intestine is involved, signs cannot be distinguished from other disorders of the large intestine. More extensive involvement may be accompanied by signs of small intestinal disease, liver disease, or respiratory disease.

The diagnosis of *Histoplasma* can be obtained by several methods. The simplest method is to identify the organism on a rectal mucosal scraping or fecal cytology.[9, 71] The organism is found intracellularly in macrophages or histiocytes. A more reliable method is to identify the organism in tissue section from a colon biopsy.[9, 19, 71] A granulomatous reaction is seen, with the organisms best seen with special stains such as the periodic acid-Schiff or Gomori's silver stain.[71] Colon biopsies represent a noninvasive method to obtain a definitive diagnosis even in cases in which signs of other organ involvement predominate. The diagnosis can also be established with serologic tests, such as the complement-fixation and agar gel precipitin tests. However, these tests can sometimes yield false-positive or false-negative results.[71] The organism can sometimes be cultured from feces or tissue biopsies. However, cultures are frequently negative in cases confirmed histologically.[71]

Treatment can be effective with either ketaconazole or with amphotericin B.[9, 71] The prognosis is guarded when there is evidence of dissemination, as many of these patients have decreased immunocompetence.[19, 71] The infection in animals does not represent a significant human health risk but can indicate the presence of a contaminated environment.

PROTOTHECAL COLITIS

Prototothecosis is caused by an alga of the genus *Prototheca*, with the species *P. zopfii* and *P. wickerhamii* considered the most important pathogens.[72] The organism is ubiquitous in the environment, and the low incidence of infection suggests that *Prototheca* is an opportunistic pathogen in an immunocompromised host.[73] The route of entry of the pathogen is thought to be through the gastrointestinal tract, since nearly all reported cases involve gastrointestinal signs, especially of large bowel origin.[72, 73] In the colon, the organism causes nodular thickening of the mucosa with scattered hemorrhagic ulcers. The nodules consist of masses of *Prototheca* organisms. An inflammatory cell response is usually minimal.[73] Following intestinal infection, dissemination occurs via hematogenous or lymphatic routes to other organs, including the central nervous system and eyes.

The most common presenting sign in dogs with protothecosis is bloody diarrhea, which is often chronic and intermittent.[73] As the disease becomes advanced, weight loss and debilitation occur. Ocular involvement is also common, occurring in about half of the reported cases and suggesting disseminated disease.

Diagnosis is based on identification of the organism on tissue section, most easily obtained from a colon biopsy. Special staining with either paraphenylenediamine, periodic acid-Schiff, or Gomori's silver stain aids in identifying the organism,[72] although it is usually seen on routine hematoxylin and eosin-stained tissue. The organism can also be seen on biopsy of other involved organs or rectal scraping. The organism can also be cultured on Sabouraud's cyclohexamide-free dextrose agar.[72, 73] Samples can be obtained from a vitreous tap or from CSF when these tissues are involved. Species can be identified by a fluorescent antibody technique.[72, 73]

There have been no reports of successful treatment of protothecosis in the dog or cat. The use of ketaconazole has not been thoroughly evaluated. Because of widespread tissue involvement, the prognosis is grave.

Bacterial Infections

Bacterial infections are a relatively uncommon cause of large bowel diarrhea in the dog and cat. There are several defense mechanisms to prevent bacterial overgrowth or colonization by pathogens, including normal motility, gastric acid secretion, the protective mucus layer, the local immune system, and microbial interactions. Microbial interaction is especially important in the colon, and disruption of normal populations, as would occur with antibiotic therapy, can lead to certain bacteria causing disease.[8] This discussion will concern the effects of known pathogens not part of the normal flora.

CAMPYLOBACTER

Campylobacter jejuni, now a recognized pathogen in humans, is a curved, motile, microaerophilic, gram-negative rod. Its pathogenicity in dogs and cats is less clear, mainly because of similar isolation rates in normal and diarrheic animals.[8, 74] The prevalence of *C. jejuni* varies from 0 to 49 per cent in normal animals and from 2.2 to 38 per cent in diarrheic animals.[74] Attempts to induce diarrhea in pups and kittens experimentally have been equivocal.[75, 76] However, chronic diarrhea has resolved in clinical cases when specific antibiotic therapy has been used.[77] Failure to consider *C. jejuni* as a pathogen until recently may also stem from the special environmental and cultural growth requirements of the organism.[75, 78, 79] Different isolation rates may also reflect the environment and age of the animals. There seems to be a higher prevalence of infection in animals that are young, stray, kenneled, stressed, or have concurrent disease.[76, 80] The organism survives poorly in the environment, and food or water contamination is the most likely source of infection.[75] The organism can survive in feces up to four weeks, however, and since the duration of excretion in infected animals can vary from one to four months, this represents another potential source.[76]

The incubation period following ingestion ranges from one to seven days. The organism colonizes the mucosal surface of the terminal small intestine and colon, usually without epithelial invasion.[76] The exact mechanism by which *Campylobacter* causes diarrhea is unknown. Clinical signs are most common in young pups and kittens, often with concurrent diseases. Depression, mucoid or bloody diarrhea, and vomiting are the most common signs, usually lasting from 3 to 15 days.[75, 80] Most animals are afebrile, and bacteremia and fatal cases are rare.[76] Infections in humans are often self-limiting.

Diagnosis is based on a positive fecal culture. Fresh rectal swabs should be placed immediately into transport media. Selective enrichment and isolation media for *Campylobacter* have been described and are commercially available.[78] Cultures are incubated at 42 to 43°C in a microaerophilic, high nitrogen environment.[76, 78–80] Direct microscopic fecal smears can also identify the curved, motile rods, but this method is unreliable. Gross and histopathologic lesions are nonspecific.[76]

Treatment with antibiotics may not be necessary because some cases are self-limiting. However, if clinical signs are prolonged or the animal is debilitated, treatment is indicated. Also, animals that persistently shed the organism should be treated due to the zoonotic potential.

The drug of choice for human *Campylobacter* infections is erythromycin, and it has been suggested that this is the drug of choice in animals.[74, 76, 77, 80] A dose of 15 to 20 mg/lb/day (30 to 40 mg/kg/day) for five days eliminates infection in dogs and cats.[74, 77] An alternative antibiotic is oral tylosin at a dose of 20 mg/lb/day (45 mg/kg/day) for five days.[74, 76] The efficacy of treatment should be confirmed by fecal cultures one and four weeks after treatment. Negative cultures are usually obtained within 48 hours after treatment.[76, 80] Other antibiotics that show *in vitro* effectiveness include tetracycline, aminoglycosides, clindamycin, chloramphenicol, and furazolidone. Variable susceptibility is seen with metronidazole, ampicillin, and trimethoprim-sulfonamide. There is usually resistance to penicillin, cephalosporins, rifampin, trimethoprim, vancomycin, and polymyxin B.[76] Antibiotics do not appear to prolong the carrier state as is thought to occur with *Salmonella* infections.

Campylobacter infection should be considered zoonotic. If both pet and owner were affected simultaneously, they most likely acquired the infection from the same source, usually contaminated food or water.[8] It is estimated that only five per cent of human infections are associated with a canine or feline source, with most infections associated with dogs.[74, 81] When pets are a source of human infections, the animals usually have diarrhea and are often in conditions with poor hygiene.[74] Appropriate hygiene should be stressed to clients.

SALMONELLA[76]

Salmonella infections can be limited to the gastrointestinal tract where they produce an acute or chronic enterocolitis, or the organism can undergo systemic invasion producing signs referable to other organ systems. Salmonellae are motile gram-negative rods in the family Enterobacteriaceae. They are pathogenic to a variety of mammals, birds, and reptiles. The most common isolate causing disease in animals is *S. typhimurium*. The organisms are ubiquitous, with contaminated food, water, or fomites the most likely source of infection. They can also survive long periods outside the host. The incidence of infection in normal dogs varies from 1 to 36 per cent, and in normal cats from 0 to 14 per cent. Young animals and those with concurrent disease, immunodeficiency, or stress are more susceptible to infection and clinical illness. Normal bacterial flora is especially important in minimizing the likelihood of *Salmonella* colonization.[33] *Salmonella* requires a relatively large inoculum to produce colonization compared with *Campylobacter*. Once ingested, *Salmonella* colonizes the ileum and to a lesser extent the colon.[8] The organism is capable of mucosal invasion, although some strains stimulate intestinal secretion by stimulating cAMP.[8] Bacteremia can occur with severe mucosal invasion, allowing the organism to disseminate throughout the body. When localized to the intestine, the infection is usually self-limiting. However, intermittent shedding of the organism can occur for three to six weeks.

Clinical signs depend on the number of organisms, host status, and concomitant disease. Gastrointestinal signs are usually acute and are typical of both small and large bowel diarrhea. When systemic invasion occurs, signs are referable to the organs involved.

Diagnosis is based on a positive fecal culture. Because of subclinical carriers, positive cultures are not diagnostic of illness. Concurrent disease or stress can reactivate shedding in carrier animals. Special enrichment broths (selenite or tetrathionate) and culture media (deoxycholate) are used to inhibit the growth of other organisms and favor the growth of *Salmonella*. A negative culture does not rule out *Salmonella*. Culture of other organs and body fluids can be used to detect systemic disease. Serologic testing has not been shown to be helpful in animals.

The use of antibiotics in salmonellosis remains controversial. In cases in which clinical infection is confined to the intestine, it is doubtful that antibiotic therapy alters the course of illness, but the likelihood of increased shedding, the development of resistant strains, and the prolongation of the carrier state become much greater.[8] Therefore, in the absence of systemic involvement, only supportive care is indicated. In asymptomatic carriers, antibiotic therapy may reactivate clinical illness. With systemic involvement, parenteral antibiotics are indicated on the basis of results of culture and sensitivity testing. In such cases, chloramphenicol, trimethoprim-sulfonamide, and gentamicin are usually effective, although resistance to these may occur.[33] *Salmonella* does have zoonotic potential, so clients must be made aware of the importance of proper hygiene.

YERSINIA

Yersinia enterocolitica is a motile gram-negative coccobacillus capable of causing enterocolitis in humans and animals. However, there are few reports of documented clinical cases in dogs,[82, 83] and no reports in cats. The organism has been cultured in normal dogs, with a prevalence ranging from 0.4 to 6 per cent depending on geographic location. Clinical signs are typical of large intestinal involvement, including increased frequency of defecation, blood and mucus in the feces, and tenesmus.[82] Systemic involvement or fever have not been seen in dogs. The pathogenesis of infection is unknown, although an enterotoxin is suspected,[84, 85] and mucosal invasion may occur.[8, 84]

Diagnosis is based on culture of the organism and subsequent response to an appropriate antibiotic. *Yersinia* selectively replicates in refrigerated temperatures, and cold enrichment with subculture is recommended.[8] Treatment is indicated in animals with persistent diarrhea from whom the organism is isolated. The organism is usually sensitive to chloramphenicol, trimethoprim-sulfonamide, tetracycline, cephalosporins, and gentamicin.[76] In clinical cases reported to respond to treatment, one dog recovered following cephadrine therapy, and the other dog recovered following trimethoprim-sulfamethoxazole therapy.[82] Since humans are susceptible to *Y. enterocolitica*, public health concerns should exist for this organism.

ESCHERICHIA COLI

E. coli is part of the normal gastrointestinal flora, present in highest concentration in the large intestine and terminal small intestine.[4] Although certain strains of *E. coli* are invasive or can produce an enterotoxin resulting in diarrhea in some species, their role in producing illness in dogs and cats is unknown. Since *E. coli* is part of the normal fecal flora, fecal cultures would be expected to grow the organism. Documenting the presence of enterotoxin-producing strains requires specific *in vivo* and *in vitro* tests,[7] and demonstrating invasive strains requires laboratory animal inoculation.[8] Therefore, it is difficult to distinguish pathogenic from nonpathogenic strains. When mucosal invasion occurs, it is difficult to say whether it results from decreased host resistance or from bacterial pathogenicity.[8]

Two dogs with diarrhea were shown to have a heat-labile enterotoxin of *E. coli* origin.[7] However, an etiologic relationship could not be established. It was suggested that this strain of *E. coli* might have thrived as a result of concurrent intestinal disease, or it might have made the intestinal environment suitable for other infectious agents, thus worsening an otherwise mild infection. However, the identification of such strains of *E. coli* should be considered to be involved in the pathogenesis of diarrhea, if isolated. Antibiotics should be used with caution to prevent the development of multiple resistant strains, which readily occurs with *E. coli*.[86] Since most pathogenic strains of *E. coli* are host-specific, the zoonotic potential is low.[8]

PSEUDOMEMBRANOUS COLITIS

Pseudomembranous colitis is a condition seen in humans and attributed to a toxin produced from an overgrowth of *Clostridium difficile*, which occurs after antibiotic suppression of normal flora. Many antibiotics have been associated with the disease, but lincomycin, clindamycin, ampicillin, and cephalosporins are most commonly involved. Gross findings in humans include an erythematous mucosa covered with small, raised plaques. Histologically, there is a pseudomembrane composed of mucin, fibrin, neutrophils, sloughed epithelial cells, and a variety of bacteria.[22] The disease is usually successfully treated with either vancomycin or metronidazole.[87]

There have been very few reports of this condition in animals. Toxigenic *Clostridium difficile* was isolated from three dogs with chronic diarrhea, all of whom responded to metronidazole.[87a] Two dogs had diarrhea associated with *Clostridium welchii*,[88] and another dog was described that was treated with clindamycin and had lesions identical to those seen with pseudomembranous colitis in humans.[19] Another dog had recurrent diarrhea associated with *Clostridium perfringens* type A.[88a] Despite these observations, the evidence linking *Clostridium* species as a causative agent of diarrhea in dogs is only circumstantial. Colitis can also be induced in hamsters with clindamycin administration.[22] However, the lesions induced are not identical to those seen in humans.

MECHANICAL DISORDERS OF THE LARGE INTESTINE

Idiopathic Megacolon

ETIOLOGY

Idiopathic megacolon is a disorder that is manifested by a large, distended, poorly motile colon, with decreased ability to expel its contents. The cause of the disorder is unknown, and it is much more common in cats than dogs. The disorder has mistakenly been referred to as Hirschsprung's disease, but there is no evidence that it is analogous to this condition in humans. Hirschsprung's disease, which occurs in children, is caused by an absence or loss of ganglion cells of the intrinsic plexuses in a narrowed segment of the rectum.[1, 19] This results in a functional obstruction, and fecal material distends the colon proximal to the aganglionic segment. The portion of the colon that was normal at first eventually becomes irreversibly dilated. This form of megacolon is extremely rare in clinical

cases in dogs or cats.[89] More commonly, the colon dilates for no apparent reason and the condition is thus labeled idiopathic. Other forms of acquired megacolon can be secondary to mechanical obstruction caused by neoplasia, strictures, extracolonic masses, or foreign bodies. In addition, functional motility disorders resulting in fecal retention can be caused by spinal cord lesions, chronic inflammation, electrolyte disturbances, and hypothyroidism.[1, 19, 89, 90, 91, 92]

HISTORY

Idiopathic megacolon occurs in cats and dogs usually in middle-age. The disorder is much more common in cats than dogs, and most cases described occurred in male cats.[89] Most affected cats have a chronic history of tenesmus and constipation. When fecal retention is severe, depression and vomiting may result. As the disease progresses, cats are unable to expel any feces despite conservative management with laxatives.

DIAGNOSIS

The presence of severe constipation or obstipation is readily apparent on abdominal palpation. The colon is distended with firm feces. Abdominal radiographs confirm the presence of fecal material and rule out predisposing causes such as a mass compressing the colon. Usually, fecal material provides enough contrast to visualize the entire colon and rectum, but occasionally a pneumocolon or barium enema radiograph is necessary to rule out a rectal stricture. A digital rectal or proctoscopic examination can also be performed to rule this out.

TREATMENT

The treatment depends on the severity of the disease. Animals with complete obstipation must have the feces manually removed. This can be accomplished with warm water enemas in the awake state in a few animals but usually requires general anesthesia. Enemas and sponge forceps are used to evacuate the colon in these patients. Care must be taken to avoid colonic perforation since in some cases the wall is thin. Once the animal is completely evacuated of feces, medical management consists of dietary modifications and laxatives. The author has had the most success with high-fiber diets, including bulk agents such as bran or methylcellulose. This can be combined with laxatives such as docusate sodium (50 to 200 mg q8h). In refractory cases, diarrhea can be induced with the osmotic cathartic lactulose (starting at 0.5 cc/lb (1 cc/kg) q8h). The dose is adjusted to achieve the necessary fecal consistency.

Surgical removal of the colon represents a salvage procedure in animals nonresponsive to medical management. Total or subtotal colectomy has been performed successfully in the author's practice and by others in cats and dogs.[89, 93, 94] Most animals have had few complications and are able to pass normal feces within two weeks postoperatively, although loose feces and tenesmus persist in some cases. Despite these successful outcomes, surgery should be reserved as a salvage procedure, since surgery of the large intestine can be accompanied by numerous complications.

PROGNOSIS

The prognosis is guarded, because most cases are progressive. Clients must be made aware that medical management requires continual dietary and therapeutic measures.

Irritable Bowel Syndrome

The irritable bowel syndrome is thought to be a disorder of colonic muscle dysfunction,[19] or a psychosomatic problem resulting in constipation, diarrhea, or abnormal defecation patterns. However, no colonic muscle dysfunction has been documented in these dogs, and the diagnosis is usually made by ruling out other causes of colonic disease. Often stress and emotional stimuli will precipitate or worsen signs. This effect may be mediated by sympathetic or parasympathetic nervous stimulation. Abnormal motility patterns and physiologic reflexes seen in the disorder in humans have not been documented in the dog.[1] Often signs of inflammatory diseases of the colon will be worsened during stress. This should not be confused with the irritable bowel syndrome.

Clinical signs in dogs are variable and cannot be distinguished from inflammatory diseases of the colon. The diagnosis is based on exclusion of other diseases, requiring a complete evaluation including negative findings on fecal examinations, diet trials, colonoscopy, colon biopsy, and barium enema radiography.

Treatment consists of anticholinergics, tranquilizers, dietary modification, environment modification, or a combination of these. Anticholinergic and antispasmodic drugs include propantheline bromide and clidinium bromide. The latter drug is often combined with the tranquilizer chlordiazepoxide. Occasionally, a narcotic analgesic such as loperamide or diphenoxylate is used to control diarrhea. These drugs were discussed in the section on motility modification in chronic inflammatory bowel disease. Dietary modification consists of adding a bulk agent such as bran or methylcellulose.

The prognosis is guarded, since the cause of the disease is unknown, and the possibility of an undiagnosed organic disease still remains. Symptomatic treatment is often prolonged in the absence of a definitive diagnosis.

Intussusception

Two types of intussusceptions involving the colon include ileocolic and cecocolic. The latter is also termed *cecal inversion*. Both conditions can cause complete or partial obstruction. In one large series, ileocolic intussusception accounted for 50 per cent of all intestinal intussusceptions, while no cases of cecal inversion were seen.[95] The average age of these dogs was less than six months. In another series of 45 cases of intestinal intussusception, ileocolic intussusception was seen in 32

dogs and cecal inversion in two dogs.[96] One reported series of eight dogs as well as multiple single case reports described most cases of cecal inversion in young, large-breed male dogs.[97–100] Cecal inversion has also been described in the cat.[101] Although the cause of intussusception is unknown, it has been suggested that parasitism is a predisposing factor.[97] Intestinal lymphosarcoma has also been described associated with intussusception.[102]

Clinical signs can be acute or chronic. Bloody diarrhea, often intermittent, is the most common sign. Vomiting and weight loss can also occur. Although some intussusceptions are detected on abdominal palpation, many are not palpable.

The diagnosis is usually established with contrast radiography (noting a filling defect in the colon on barium enema, pneumocolon, or when barium is administered by orogastric intubation) or by colonoscopy (noting the inverted tissue as an intraluminal mass within the colon). Treatment is surgical reduction of an ileocolic intussusception (with intestinal resection, if necessary) and amputation of the cecum in cases of cecal inversion.

Injury to the Large Intestine

Injury to the large intestine can result from sharp or blunt trauma, intraluminal trauma, diagnostic procedures (colonoscopy, colon biopsy, barium enema), or from nontraumatic perforation associated with glucocorticoid administration.

TRAUMA TO THE LARGE INTESTINE

Perforation of the colon causes rapidly progressive septic peritonitis. Initial signs include abdominal pain, vomiting, and fever. Pale mucous membranes, slow capillary refill, and rapid pulse are seen as septic shock develops. Deterioration in animals is rapid, making rapid diagnosis important.[103] Because prior glucocorticoid administration may mask early signs of peritonitis, early detection may be difficult.[44]

Radiographic findings may include free air or lack of detail in the peritoneal cavity. Barium enema should not be used in cases of suspected colon rupture, as leakage of barium through the colon is almost always fatal.[103] The diagnosis can be confirmed by evaluating a peritoneal aspirate or diagnostic peritoneal lavage. Degenerate neutrophils and bacteria are seen microscopically, although these can also be seen in animals with localized intestinal devitalization without actual rupture.

Treatment consists of immediate surgical repair of the perforation. Broad-spectrum antibiotics are indicated before and after surgery. In cases of blunt trauma, continual re-evaluation of physical parameters, radiographs, and abdominal lavage are used to determine if surgical exploration is indicated.

NONTRAUMATIC PERFORATION OF THE LARGE INTESTINE

The administration of corticosteroids to dogs with neurologic injury has been associated with colonic rupture in several cases.[104] Most of these animals have undergone a major surgical procedure, and most have received dexamethasone as the corticosteroid. The dosage and duration of dexamethasone given to these dogs varied, ranging from a cumulative dose of 1.3 to 7 mg/lb (2.7 to 15.5 mg/kg) (mean, 3 mg/lb) (mean 6.4 mg/kg) and a duration ranging from one to ten days (mean, 5.1 days). Causes of corticosteroid-induced colonic perforation are unknown but may include the deleterious effect of corticosteroids on normal cytoprotective mechanisms and thus a predisposition to mucosal injury.[44] There might also be an autonomic nervous imbalance associated with neurologic injury and stress.[104] It was suggested that the most common site of perforation, the proximal portion of the descending colon, is the location of a changeover between vagal and sacral sources of parasympathetic innervation and between celiacomesenteric and caudal mesenteric sources of sympathetic innervation. An imbalance of innervation in the transition zone could affect motility and microvascular blood supply, thus increasing the likelihood of ulceration.[104]

Clinical signs, diagnostic findings, and treatment are similar to those described for traumatic perforation. The prognosis for recovery is grave, as almost all cases are fatal despite surgical intervention. Therefore, careful monitoring of animals with neurologic conditions receiving corticosteroids is mandatory. Additional preventive measures include use of corticosteroids other than dexamethasone, limitation of dosage and duration of usage, avoidance of concurrent drugs with ulcerogenic potential, and avoidance of large volume enemas, if possible.[104]

NEOPLASIA OF THE LARGE INTESTINE

Incidence

Neoplasia of the large intestine represents 36 to 60 per cent of all canine and 10 to 15 per cent of feline alimentary tract neoplasia.[105] Most tumors are malignant in both species, with adenocarcinoma the most common malignant tumor in dogs and lymphosarcoma the most common in cats. Other tumors seen include leiomyosarcoma, carcinoid, anaplastic sarcoma, mast cell tumor, extramedullary plasmacytoma, adenomatous polyp, and leiomyoma.[19, 105-113] Most nonhematopoietic intestinal tumors in cats occur in the ileum and jejunum, whereas they occur most commonly in the colon and rectum in the dog.[106-108]

Adenocarcinomas can be variable in appearance and behavior. They can (1) infiltrate the colon wall creating a fibrotic stricture, (2) cause ulceration of the mucosa, (3) proliferate within the lumen of the colon and subsequently ulcerate, or (4) infiltrate the submucosa without causing an obstruction.[105] All types are usually slowly progressive and do not cause signs until they result in a severe stricture, ulceration and frank hemorrhage, or metastasis. Most animals are over eight years of age. There may be an increased incidence in males, and

collies and German shepherds may have a higher incidence than other breeds.[19]

Clinical Findings

Clinical signs vary with the type and location of the neoplasm, and are essentially the same as with inflammatory and obstructive processes. Often the signs are slowly progressive. Most animals are in good physical condition until late in the course, when there is severe mucosal ulceration, almost complete obstruction, or metastasis. Adenocarcinomas usually metastasize to local lymph nodes, liver, and occasionally the lungs. Spread into adjacent blood vessels and lymphatics can occur, resulting in circulatory obstruction and subsequent inguinal and hind leg edema.

Lymphosarcoma can diffusely infiltrate the colonic mucosa. This process can remain confined to this area of the bowel or involve other regions of the intestine and the liver. Clinical signs depend on the extent of involvement, including large bowel signs only, or a mixture of large and small bowel signs. Lymphosarcoma can also appear as a discrete mass infiltrating the colonic wall. This can result in ulceration, and in some cases perforation.

Certain tumors may result in signs associated with the release of certain chemical or hormonal mediators. Carcinoids, which are uncommon in the dog and cat, are derived from intestinal endocrine cells capable of releasing vasoactive amines, such as serotonin and kallikrein.[109] Mast cell tumors are capable of releasing vasoactive substances including histamine, which has the potential to induce gastroduodenal ulceration. However, the intestinal form of mast cell tumors does not seem to result in gastroduodenal ulceration as occurs when this neoplasm is in other sites in either the dog or cat.[110, 114]

Diagnostic findings in cases of large intestinal neoplasia depend on the nature of the tumor. Fecal examination and laboratory tests generally do not contribute to the diagnosis. Survey abdominal radiographs may show a large intraluminal mass if it is contrasted with gas in the colon. Sublumbar lymph node enlargement may also be seen if metastasis has occurred. Demonstration of large intestinal neoplasia is best accomplished with barium enema radiography or colonoscopy. Barium enema can outline filling defects, mucosal ulceration, or identify strictures. These lesions can also be seen during colonoscopy (see Figure 87–2). Definitive diagnosis is made from a biopsy specimen obtained during the procedure. The limitations of biopsies performed in this manner are that lesions not involving the mucosa may be missed, since only superficial samples are obtained. Biopsy instruments capable of taking deeper samples carry an increased risk of perforation.

Treatment

The treatment of most large intestinal neoplasia is surgical removal. The location and extent of the lesion determine which surgical approach is used. In general, large intestinal surgery carries more risk and potential complications than that in other areas of the bowel. Certain neoplasms may be amenable to chemotherapy, such as lymphosarcoma and mast cell tumors. Adenocarcinomas have also been treated successfully with radiation.[115] The prognosis of benign or localized slow-growing malignant tumors is good if surgical removal is successful. Poorly differentiated or advanced malignant tumors have a poor prognosis because local recurrence and/or metastasis usually occurs.

References

1. Strombeck, DR: Small Animal Gastroenterology. Davis, California, Stonegate Publishing, 1979.
2. Conklin, JL and Christensen, J: Local specialization at ileocecal junction of the cat and opossum. Am J Physiol 228:1075, 1975.
3. Guyton, AC: Textbook of Medical Physiology, 7th ed. Philadelphia, WB Saunders, 1986.
4. Greene, CE: Gastrointestinal, intra-abdominal and hepatobiliary infections. In Greene CE (ed): Clinical Microbiology and Infectious Diseases of the Dog and Cat. Philadelphia, WB Saunders, 1984, p 247.
5. Kirkpatrick, CE: Enteric protozoal infections. In Greene, CE (ed): Clinical Microbiology and Infectious Diseases of the Dog and Cat. Philadelphia, WB Saunders, 1984, p 806.
6. Zimmer, JF and Burrington, DB: Comparison of four techniques of fecal examination for detecting canine giardiasis. JAAHA 22:161, 1986.
6a. Baker, DG, et al.: Laboratory diagnosis of Giardia duodenalis infection in dogs. JAVMA 190:53, 1987.
7. Olson, P, et al.: Enterotoxigenic Escherichia coli infection in two dogs with acute diarrhea. JAVMA 184:982, 1984.
8. Dillon, R: Bacterial enteritis. In Kirk, RW (ed): Current Veterinary Therapy IX. Philadelphia, WB Saunders, 1986, p 872.
8a. Boulay, JP, et al.: Evaluation of a fluorometric method for the quantitative assay of fecal hemoglobin in the dog. Am J Vet Res 47:1293, 1986.
9. Sherding, RG: Canine large bowel diarrhea. Comp Cont Ed Pract Vet 2:279, 1980.
10. Jorgensen, LS, et al.: Electrolyte abnormalities induced by hypertonic phosphate enemas in two cats. JAVMA 187:1367, 1985.
11. Schaer, M, et al.: Iatrogenic hyperphosphatemia, hypocalcemia and hypernatremia in a cat. JAAHA 13:39, 1977.
12. Davis, GR, et al.: Development of a lavage solution associated with minimal water and electrolyte absorption or secretion. Gastroenterology 78:991, 1980.
13. Richter, KP and Cleveland, MB: Comparison of an oral gastrointestinal lavage solution with traditional mechanical bowel evacuation as a preparation for proctoscopy in dogs. Proceed Fifth ACVIM Forum, 1987.
14. Burt, JK: Contrast radiology of the gastrointestinal tract. Proceed Eighth Ann Kal Kan Symp for Treatment of Sm Anim Diseases. Oct 1984, p 57.
15. Brawner, WR and Bartels, JE: Contrast radiography of the digestive tract. Indications, techniques and complications. Vet Clin North Am 13:599, 1983.
16. Ursing, B, et al.: A comparative study of metronidazole and sulfasalazine for active Crohn's disease: The cooperative Crohn's disease study in Sweden. II. Result. Gastroenterology 83:550, 1982.
17. Azad Khan, AK, et al.: An experiment to determine the active therapeutic moiety of sulphasalazine. Lancet 2:892, 1977.
18. Van Kruiningen, HJ: Clinical efficacy of tylosin in canine inflammatory bowel disease. JAAHA 12:498, 1976.
19. Burrows, CF: Diseases of the colon, rectum, and anus in the dog and cat. In Anderson, NV (ed): Veterinary Gastroenterology. Philadelphia, Lea and Febiger, 1980, p 553.
20. Roe, FJC: Metronidazole: review of uses and toxicity. J Antimicrob Chemother 3:205, 1977.
21. Grove, DI, et al.: Suppression of cell-mediated immunity by metronidazole. Int Arch Allergy Appl Immunol 54:422, 1977.
22. Onderdonk, AB, et al.: The role of the intestinal microflora in experimental colitis. Am J Clin Nutr 30:1819, 1977.
23. Van Der Waaij, D, et al.: Mitigation of experimental inflammatory bowel disease in guinea pigs by selective elimination of the aerobic gram-negative intestinal microflora. Gastroenterology 67:460, 1974.
24. Kirsner, JB: Chronic inflammatory bowel disease: Overview of etiology and pathogenesis. In Berk, JE (ed): HL Bockus Gastroenterology, 4th ed. Philadelphia, WB Saunders, 1985, p 2093.
25. Nelson, RW, et al.: Lymphocytic-plasmacytic colitis in the cat. JAVMA 184:1133, 1984.
26. Kirsner, JB and Shorter, RG: Recent developments in nonspecific inflammatory bowel disease. N Engl J Med 306:837, 1982.
27. Burrows, CF, et al.: Determination of fecal fat and trypsin output in the evaluation of chronic canine diarrhea. JAVMA 174:62, 1979.
28. Khojasteh, A, et al.: Immunoproliferative small intestinal disease. A "third-world lesion." N Engl J Med 308:1401, 1983.
29. Leib, MS, et al.: Suppurative colitis in a cat. JAVMA 188:739, 1986.
30. Driscoll, RH and Rosenberg, IH: Total parenteral nutrition in inflammatory bowel disease. Med Clin North Am 62:185, 1978.
31. Washabau, RJ, et al.: Evaluation and management of carbohydrate malassimilation. In Kirk, RW (ed): Current Veterinary Therapy IX. Philadelphia, WB Saunders, 1986, p 889.
32. Ridgway, MD: Management of chronic colitis in the dog. JAVMA 185:804, 1984.
33. Dillon, R: Therapeutic strategies involving antimicrobial treatment of the gastrointestinal tract in small animals. JAVMA 185:1169, 1984.
34. Das, KM and Sternlieb, I: Salicylazosulfapyridine in inflammatory bowel disease. Dig Dis 20:971, 1975.
35. Goldman, P and Peppercorn, MA: Sulfasalazine. N Engl J Med 293:20, 1975.
35a. Sharon, P and Stenson, WF: Enhanced synthesis of leukotriene B₄ by colonic mucosa in inflammatory bowel disease. Gastroenterology 86:453, 1984.
35b. Donowitz, M: Arachidonic acid metabolites and their role in inflammatory bowel disease. An update requiring addition of a pathway. Gastroenterology 88:580, 1985.
35c. Lauritsen, K, et al.: Effects of topical 5-aminosalicylic acid and prednisolone on prostaglandin E₂ and leukotriene B₄ levels determined by equilibrium in vivo dialysis of rectum in relapsing ulcerative colitis. Gastroenterology 91:837, 1986.
36. Kirsner, JB and Shorter, RG: Recent developments in "nonspecific" inflammatory bowel disease (first of two parts). N Engl J Med 306:775, 1982.
37. Morgan, RV and Bachrach, A: Keratoconjunctivitis sicca associated with sulfonamide therapy in dogs. JAVMA 180:432, 1982.
38. Sansom, J, et al.: Keratoconjunctivitis sicca in the dog associated with the administration of salicylazosulphapyridine (sulphasalazine). Vet Rec 116:391, 1985.
39. Zimmer, JF and Burrington, DB: Comparison of four protocols for the treatment of canine giardiasis. JAAHA 22:168, 1986.
39a. Gnarpe, H, et al.: Influence of metronidazole and tinidazole on leukocyte chemotaxis in Crohn's disease. Infection 6:S107, 1978.
39b. Kostakis, A and Caine, RY: The immunosuppressive action of metronidazole. IRCS Med Sci 5:142, 1977.
39c. Tanga, MR, et al.: Clinical evaluation of metronidazole as an anti-inflammatory agent. Int Surg 60:75, 1975.
40. Onderdonk, AB, et al.: Protective effect of metronidazole in experimental ulcerative colitis. Gastroenterology 74:521, 1978.
41. Chiapella, A: Diagnosis and management of chronic colitis in the dog and cat. In Kirk, RW (ed): Current Veterinary Therapy IX. Philadelphia, WB Saunders, 1986, p 896.
42. DeNovo, RC: Therapeutics of gastrointestinal diseases. In Kirk RW (ed): Current Veterinary Therapy IX. Philadelphia, WB Saunders, 1986, p 862.
43. Kaplan, HP, et al.: A controlled evaluation of intravenous adrenocorticotropic hormone and hydrocortisone in the treatment of acute colitis. Gastroenterology 69:91, 1975.
44. Scott, J: Physiological, pharmacological and pathological actions of glucocorticoids on the digestive system. Clin Gastroenterol 10:627, 1981.

45. Sachar, DB and Present, DH: Immunotherapy in inflammatory bowel disease. Med Clin North Am 62:173, 1978.
46. Mani, V, et al.: Treatment of ulcerative colitis with oral disodium cromoglycate. Lancet 1:439, 1976.
47. Moore, RP: Feline eosinophilic enteritis. *In* Kirk, RW (ed): Current Veterinary Therapy VIII. Philadelphia, WB Saunders, 1983, p 791.
48. Van der Gaag, I, et al.: Histiocytic ulcerative colitis in a French Bulldog. J Sm Anim Pract 19:283, 1978.
49. Van Kruiningen, HJ and Dobbins III, WO: Feline histiocytic colitis. A case report with electron microscopy. Vet Pathol 16:215, 1979.
50. Gomez, JA, et al.: Canine histiocytic ulcerative colitis. An ultrastructural study of the early mucosal lesion. Dig Dis 22:485, 1977.
51. Van Kruiningen, HJ: The ultrastructure of macrophages in granulomatous colitis of boxer dogs. Vet Pathol 12:446, 1975.
52. Russell, SW, et al.: Canine histiocytic ulcerative colitis. The early lesion and its progression to ulceration. Lab Invest 25:509, 1971.
53. Lawson, TL, et al.: Vascular alterations in canine histiocytic ulcerative colitis. Invest Radiol 10:212, 1975.
54. Ewing, GO and Gomez, JA: Canine ulcerative colitis. JAAHA 9:395, 1973.
55. Kennedy, PC and Cello, RM: Colitis of boxer dogs. Gastroenterology 51:926, 1966.
56. Georgi, JR: Parasitology for Veterinarians. Philadelphia, WB Saunders, 1974.
57. Kelly, JD: Occurrence of *Trichuris serrata* von Linstow, 1879 (Nematoda: Trichuridae) in the domestic cat *(Felis catus)* in Australia. J Parasitol 59:1145, 1973.
58. Roberson, EL and Cornelius, LM: Gastrointestinal parasitism. *In* Kirk, RW (ed): Current Veterinary Therapy VIII. Philadelphia, WB Saunders, 1983, p 797.
59. Cornelius, LM and Roberson, EL: Treatment of gastrointestinal parasitism. *In* Kirk, RW (ed): Current Veterinary Therapy IX. Philadelphia, WB Saunders, 1986, p 921.
60. Corwin, RM, et al.: Effect of febantel against *Ancylostoma caninum* and *Trichuris vulpis* infections in dogs. Am J Vet Res 43:1100, 1982.
61. Pitts, RP: Giardiasis. *In* Kirk, RW (ed): Current Veterinary Therapy VIII. Philadelphia, WB Saunders, 1983, p 796.
62. Ewing, GO and Aldrete, AV: Canine giardiasis presenting as chronic ulcerative colitis: A case report. JAAHA 9:52, 1973.
63. Watson, ADJ: Giardiasis and colitis in a dog. Aust Vet J 56:444, 1980.
64. Abbit, B, et al.: Treatment of giardiasis in adult greyhounds, using ipronidazole-medicated water. JAVMA 188:67, 1986.
65. Wittnich, C: *Entamoeba histolytica* infection in a German shepherd dog. Can Vet J 17:259, 1976.
66. Northway, RB: *Entamoeba histolytica* in a dog. VM/SAC 70:306, 1975.
67. Ewing, SA and Bull, RW: Severe chronic canine diarrhea associated with *Balantidium-Trichuris* infection. JAVMA 149:519, 1966.
68. Hayes, FA and Jordan, HE: Canine helminthiasis complicated with Balantidium species. JAVMA 129:161, 1956.
69. Bailey, WS and Williams, AG: Balantidium infection in the dog. JAVMA 114:238, 1949.
70. Stark, DR: Primary gastrointestinal histoplasmosis in a cat. JAAHA 18:154, 1982.
71. Barsanti, JA: Histoplasmosis. *In* Greene, CE (ed): Clinical Microbiology and Infectious Diseases of the Dog and Cat. Philadelphia, WB Saunders, 1984, p 687.
72. Migaki, G, et al.: Canine protothecosis: Review of the literature and report of an additional case. JAVMA 181:794, 1982.
73. Tyler, DE: Prototheosis. *In* Greene, CE (ed): Clinical Microbiology and Infectious Diseases of the Dog and Cat. Philadelphia, WB Saunders, 1984, p 747.
74. Holt, PE: The role of dogs and cats in the epidemiology of human Campylobacter enterocolitis. J Sm Anim Pract 22:681, 1981.
75. Fox, JG, et al.: Canine and feline campylobacteriosis: Epizootiology and clinical and public health features. JAVMA 183:1420, 1983.
76. Greene, CE: Enteric bacterial infections. *In* Greene, CE (ed): Clinical Microbiology and Infectious Diseases of the Dog and Cat. Philadelphia, WB Saunders, 1984, p 617.
77. Fleming, MP: Association of *Campylobacter jejuni* with enteritis in dogs and cats. Vet Rec 113:372, 1983.
78. Patton, CM, et al.: Comparison of selective media for primary isolation of *Campylobacter fetus* subsp. *jejuni.* J Clin Microbiol 13:326, 1981.
79. Fox, JG: Campylobacteriosis—a "new" disease in laboratory animals. Lab Anim Sci 32:625, 1982.
80. Fox, JG, et. al.: *Campylobacter jejuni*-associated diarrhea in dogs. JAVMA 183:1430, 1983.
81. Skirrow, MB: Campylobacter enteritis in dogs and cats: A "new" zoonosis. Vet Res Commun 5:13, 1981.
82. Papageorges, M, et al.: *Yersinia enterocolitica* enteritis in two dogs. JAVMA 182:618, 1983.
83. Farstad, L, et al.: Isolation of *Yersinia enterocolitica* from a dog with chronic enteritis. Acta Vet Scand 17:261, 1976.
84. Mors, V and Pai, CH: Pathogenic properties of *Yersinia enterocolitica.* Infect Immun 28:292, 1980.
85. Robins-Browne, RM, et al.: Mechanism of action of *Yersinia enterocolitica* enterotoxin. Infect Immun 25:680, 1979.
86. Moss, S and Frost, AJ: The resistance to chemotherapeutic agents of *Escherichia coli* from domestic dogs and cats. Aust Vet J 61:82, 1984.
87. Cherry, RD, et al.: Metronidazole: An alternate therapy for antibiotic-associated colitis. Gastroenterology 82:849, 1982.
87a. Berry, AP and Levett, PN: Chronic diarrhoea in dogs associated with *Clostridium difficile* infection. Vet Rec 118:102, 1986.
88. Prescott, JF, et al.: Haemorrhagic gastroenteritis in the dog associated with *Clostridium welchii.* Vet Rec 103:116, 1978.
88a. Carman, RJ and Lewis, JCM: Recurrent diarrhoea in a dog associated with *Clostridium perfringens* type A. Vet Rec 112:342, 1983.
89. Bright, RM, et al.: Subtotal colectomy for treatment of acquired megacolon in the dog and cat. JAVMA 188:1412, 1986.
90. Belshaw, BE: Thyroid diseases. *In* Ettinger, SJ (ed): Textbook of Veterinary Internal Medicine, 2nd ed. Philadelphia, WB Saunders, 1983, p 1592.
91. Schuster, MM: Megacolon in adults. *In* Sleisenger, MH and Fordtran, JS (eds): Gastrointestinal Disease, 2nd ed. Philadelphia, WB Saunders, 1978, p 1812.
92. Hudson, EB, et al.: Acquired megacolon in a cat. Mod Vet Pract 60:625, 1979.
93. Fellenbaum, S: Partial colectomy in the treatment of recurrent obstipation/megacolon in the cat. VM/SAC 73:737, 1978.
94. Webb, SM: Surgical management of acquired megacolon in the cat. J Sm Anim Pract 26:399, 1985.
95. Weaver, AD: Canine intestinal intussusception. Vet Rec 100:524, 1977.
96. Wilson, GP and Burt, JK: Intussusception in the dog and cat: A review of 45 cases. JAVMA 164:515, 1974.
97. Miller, WW, et al.: Cecal inversion in eight dogs. JAAHA 20:1009, 1984.
98. Guffy, MM, et al.: Inversion of the cecum into the colon of a dog. JAVMA 156:183, 1970.
99. Schlotthauer, CF: Inverted cecum in a dog. JAVMA 125:123, 1954.
100. Edwards, NJ, et al.: Cecocolic invagination in the dog. VM/SAC 72:376, 1977.
101. Kolata, RJ and Wright, JH: Inflammation and inversion of the cecum in a cat. JAVMA 162:958, 1973.
102. Morris, BJ: Intussusception associated with intestinal lymphosarcoma. VM/SAC 78:1384, 1983.
103. Abcarian, H and Lowe, R: Colon and rectal trauma. Surg Clin North Am 58:519, 1978.
104. Toombs, JP, et al.: Colonic perforation in corticosteroid-treated dogs. JAVMA 188:145, 1986.
105. Crow, SE: Tumors of the alimentary tract. Vet Clin North Am 15:577, 1985.
106. Patnaik AK, et al.: Canine intestinal adenocarcinoma and carcinoid. Vet Pathol 17:149, 1980.
107. Turk, MAM, et al.: Nonhematopoietic gastrointestinal neoplasia in cats: A retrospective study of 44 cases. Vet Pathol 18:614, 1981.
108. Lingeman, CH and Garner, FM: Comparative study of intestinal adenocarcinomas of animals and man. J Natl Cancer Inst 48:325, 1972.
109. Sykes, GP and Cooper, BJ: Canine intestinal carcinoids. Vet Pathol 19:120, 1982.

110. Patnaik, AK, et al.: Intestinal mast cell tumour in a dog. J Sm Anim Pract 21:207, 1980.
111. Seiler, RJ: Colorectal polyps of the dog: A clinicopathologic study of 17 cases. JAVMA 174:72, 1979.
112. MacEwen, EG, et al.: Extramedullary plasmacytoma of the gastrointestinal tract in two dogs. JAVMA 184:1396, 1984.
113. Carb, A and Barrett, RB: Leiomyosarcoma of the cecum in the dog. JAAHA 14:631, 1978.
114. August, JR: Gastrointestinal disorders of the cat. Vet Clin North Am 13:585, 1983.
115. Turrel, JM and Theon, AP: Single high-dose irradiation for selected canine rectal carcinomas. Vet Radiol 27:141, 1986.

DRUG INDEX

Generic (Trade)	Dosage	Route	Frequency	Brief Description
Sulfasalazine (Azulfadine)	10–15 mg/lb	PO	q 8 hr (dog)	Anti-inflammatory effects in the colon in
	10–12 mg/lb	PO	q 12–24 hr (cat)	inflammatory bowel disease
Metronidazole (Flagyl)	5–7 mg/lb	PO	q 12 hr	Effective for inflammatory bowel disease
	12 mg/lb	PO	q 12 hr × 5 days	Effective for protozoan parasites
Tylosin (Tylan)	5–90 mg/lb	PO	q 12 hr	Effective for inflammatory bowel disease
	20 mg/lb day	PO	Divided	Effective for *Campylobacter*
Prednisone	0.5–1 mg/lb	PO	q 24 hr	Effective for inflammatory bowel disease
	(dog)	PO	q 24 hr	
	1–2 mg/lb (cat)			
Azathioprine (Imuran)	50 mg/m^2	PO	q 24–48 hr	Effective for inflammatory bowel disease
Loperamide (Imodium)	0.05 mg/lb	PO	q 8–12 hr	Motility modifier
Diphenoxylate (Lomotil)	0.05–0.1 mg/lb	PO	q 8 hr	Motility modifier
Paregoric	0.03 mg/lb	PO	q 8–12 hr	Motility modifier
Propantheline bromide (Pro-Banthine)	0.12–0.25 mg/lb	PO	q 8 hr	Motility modifier
Clidinium (Librax, Quarzan)	0.05 mg/lb	PO	q 12 hr	Motility modifier
Fenbendazole (Panacur)	25 mg/lb	PO	q 24 hr × 3 days	Anthelmintic
Quinacrine (Atabrine)	3 mg/lb	PO	q 12 hr × 5 days	Effective for *Giardia*
Ipronidazole HCl	126 mg/L in drinking water		for 7 days	Effective for *Giardia*
Erythromycin	15–20 mg/lb/day	PO	Divided for 5 days	Effective for *Campylobacter*
Lactulose	0.5 ml/lb	PO	q 8 hr	Osmotic cathartic
Docusate sodium (Colace)	50–200 mg	PO	q 8 hr	Stool softener

88 PATHOPHYSIOLOGY AND LABORATORY DIAGNOSIS OF LIVER DISEASE

S. A. CENTER

The liver plays a central role in the homeostatic balance of many essential biologic processes. Its broad spanning functions encompass the synthesis, regulation, activation, integration and storage of a myriad of substances (Table 88–1). The liver has phenomenal storage capacity, functional reserve, and regenerative capabilities. While these characteristics protect the body from loss of the biologic processes for which the hepatobiliary system is an integral component, they also complicate the clinical recognition of hepatobiliary disease. As a consequence, injury must be severe, occur in strategic anatomic localizations, or be associated with cholestasis before laboratory tests reveal the presence or result of hepatobiliary injury.

LABORATORY DIAGNOSIS OF LIVER DISEASE

The laboratory diagnosis of liver disease is a confusing and continually expanding area with which the clinician must deal on a daily basis. Judicious selection of tests takes into consideration their cost, the desired completeness of study, and their diagnostic efficacy. The efficacy of a test is expressed in its ability to indicate the presence or absence of disease. This can be considered in terms of the test sensitivity, specificity, positive predictive value, and negative predictive value. Sensitivity is the ability of the test to identify patients with liver disease. Specificity is the test's correctness in determining a disease-free individual. The positive predictive value is the accuracy of the test in identifying patients with disease. The negative predictive value is the accuracy of the negative prediction that a patient is free of disease when the test is negative. Some tests are sensitive but nonspecific and have a low positive predictive value, such as alkaline phosphatase in the dog. Others are specific yet not sensitive and therefore have a low

negative predictive value for the detection of disease, as do many of the function tests. To maximize the return from clinical tests, they should be used in conjunction with one another. The goal of the clinician should be to select the best test armamentarium that will include both sensitive and specific screening and diagnostic tests. This is achieved through the collection of a baseline screening

TABLE 88–1. SUMMARY OF MAJOR HEPATOBILIARY FUNCTIONS

Carbohydrate Metabolism
 Glucose homeostasis
 Glycogen metabolism
 Glycogen storage
 Insulin degradation

Lipid Metabolism
 Cholesterol synthesis
 Ketogenesis
 Triglyceride metabolism
 Lipoprotein metabolism
 Phospholipid metabolism
 Fatty acid mobilization

Protein Metabolism
 Albumin turnover
 Amino acid regulation
 Ammonia: synthesis
  detoxification
 Urea synthesis
 Coagulation factor synthesis
 Globulin synthesis

Vitamin Metabolism
 Water-soluble vitamins:
  activation
 Fat-soluble vitamins:
  activation
  storage

Immunologic Functions
 Kupffer cell population
 Complement metabolism
 Immunomodulation (metabolic
  products)

Endocrine Hormone Metabolism
 Polypeptide hormones:
  target organ
  degradation
 Steroid hormone conjugation

Storage Function
 Water-soluble vitamins
 Fat-soluble vitamins
 Glycogen
 Trace metals: iron, copper
 Lipids

Detoxification and Excretion
 Bilirubin
 Steroids
 Ammonia
 Drugs
 Microsomal enzyme induction

Hematologic Functions
 Coagulation system
  homeostasis
 Hematopoietic factors:
  storage
  activation
 Iron homeostasis
 Potential extramedullary
  hematopoiesis

Digestive Functions
 Bile acids:
  synthesis
  regulation
  enterohepatic circulation

profile including a complete history, physical examination, a complete hemogram, serum biochemical profile, urinalysis, and fecal examination. The initial laboratory evaluations are aimed at obtaining objective support for clinically suspected conditions. These lead to further diagnostic efforts such as tests of liver function, radiography, ultrasonography, and hepatic biopsy for definitive diagnosis.

Spontaneous liver disease usually involves several types of histologic lesions simultaneously. Through the experimental induction of liver injury, particular types of hepatocellular lesions have been studied, such as extrahepatic cholestasis, intrahepatic cholestasis, necrosis, lipidosis, portosystemic venous anastomosis, and glucocorticoid hepatopathy. Much of the basic research pertaining to humans in liver disease has been conducted using the dog or cat as an animal model. These references are drawn on in this chapter where appropriate.

PHYSIOANATOMIC FEATURES

Familiarity with the normal anatomy of the hepatobiliary system fosters the clinical ability to select and interpret laboratory tests, to consider a thorough list of differential diagnoses, and to choose the most appropriate treatment.

Blood Supply

The liver has a dual blood supply, which under normal circumstances perfuses it with 25 per cent of the cardiac output.[1] Two-thirds of the hepatic circulation is derived from the portal vein and one-third from the hepatic artery, which supplies 80 per cent of its oxygenation. Blood from the low pressure-low resistance valveless portal system merges with blood from the high pressure-high resistance hepatic artery in the hepatic sinusoids. More than 40 per cent of the hepatic blood is contained in the capacitance vessels (hepatic arteries, portal veins, hepatic veins) with the remainder in the hepatic sinusoids.[2] The liver is dynamic in its ability to store blood and to release it when necessary. Ordinarily, it contains 25 to 30 ml blood per 100 gm tissue accounting for 10 to 15 per cent of the total blood volume.[3] During rapid blood volume expansion in cats, the liver can accommodate up to 20 per cent of the infused fluid.[3] During moderate hemorrhage, it can expel enough blood to compensate for 25 per cent of a lost blood volume. The ability of the liver to serve as a blood reservoir can markedly affect hepatic size. Animals with chronic passive congestion can have substantial hepatomegaly attributable to blood storage as up to 60 ml blood per 100 gm of liver can be stored.[4] Regulation of hepatic blood flow occurs via the hepatic arterioles in response to nervous stimulation, hormones, metabolites, and bile salts.[5] Smooth muscles around the arterioles and precapillary sphincters continually adjust the sinusoidal blood flow. Momentary differences in lobule perfusion may be responsible for the multifocal distribution of some hepatic lesions.

The quality and not the quantity of blood flowing to the liver determines the size of the hepatic mass. The portal venous blood supply is an important determinant of hepatic size because of its delivery of hepatotrophic factors derived from the gastrointestinal tract and pancreas. Hepatotrophic factors consist of nutrients and hormonal substances, and these determine the size of individual hepatocytes. Reduction of portal circulation results in hepatocyte atrophy, loss of glycogen stores, hepatocellular vacuolation, and a marked reduction in liver size.

Following occlusion of the hepatic artery, the portal circulation does not compensatorily increase.[6] Instead, the liver may develop a collateral arterial supply from mesenteric vessels and from an increase in the pericholedochal arterial bed.[6] Extrahepatic portal vein occlusion may result in the development of hepatopetal circulation in which normal portal collaterals interconnecting with the liver enlarge to accommodate a greater blood flow.[5] Intrahepatic portal vein occlusion results in heptofugal blood flow, in which blood follows an extrahepatic route around the portal obstruction.[5] In clinical cases, this develops as a result of severe hepatic fibrosis causing portal hypertension that leads to the portosystemic shunting of blood through mesenteric collaterals.

The portal circulation transports gut-derived microorganisms and endotoxins along with ingested nutrients and hepatotrophic substances. Gram-positive cocci, gram-negative bacilli, and clostridial organisms have been cultured from the liver of normal dogs.[7] Experimental work in the dog has shown that clostridial organisms may become established as resident flora in the liver after the middle of the first year of life. In the mature dog, acute interruption of the hepatic artery can result in lethal hepatic necrosis associated with unabated growth of gut-derived microorganisms, particularly those that are anaerobic.[8]

Anatomy

To improve the morphologic and functional classification of hepatobiliary injury, the structural and functional units of the liver have been separately defined.[9, 10] The basic *structural* unit of the liver is the classic hepatic lobule, shown in Figure 88–1. The hepatic lobule consists of cords of hepatocytes radiating concentrically around the central hepatic vein. The boundaries of the classic lobule are demarcated by regularly distributed portal triads composed of portal venules, hepatic arterioles, bile ductules, lymphatics, and nerves.

The basic *functional* unit of the liver is the hepatic acinus, also shown in Figure 88–1. The liver acinus is composed of irregularly sized and shaped hepatic parenchyma situated around the vascular axis of the acinus, which is centered in the portal triad.[9, 10] The liver acinus is bordered by the terminal hepatic venules or the "central veins" of the hepatic lobule. The concept of the acinus representing a functional unit of the liver evolved from the recognition that hepatocyte perfusion and thus oxygen and nutrient delivery does not correspond with the structural organization of the hepatic lobule. Blood flows from the portal triad into the hepatic

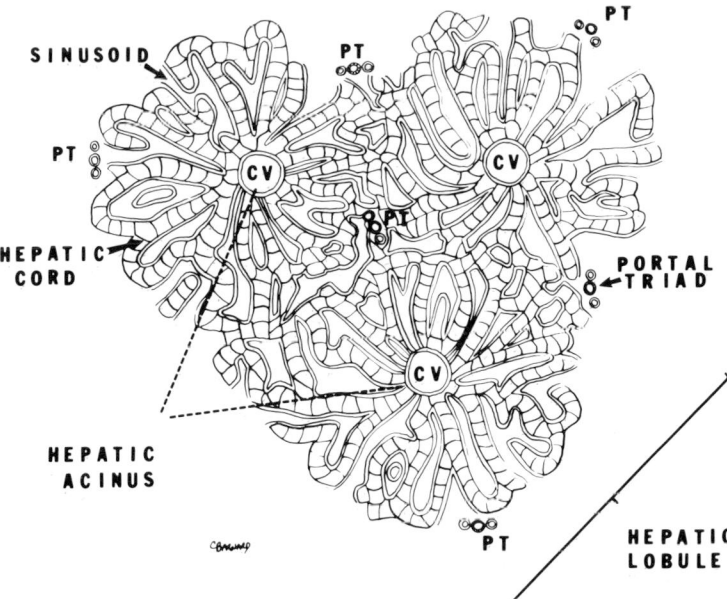

FIGURE 88–1. Schematic illustration of the structural unit of the liver: hepatic lobule, the functional unit of the liver: liver acinus.

sinusoids before exiting through the terminal hepatic venules or "central veins." Subdividing the acinus into circulatory or nutritional zones has proven to be useful in identifying and understanding hepatocyte heterogeneity in terms of function, enzymatic activity, and susceptibility to noxious insults (Figure 88–2). Hepatocyte enzymic activity is largely determined by the microcirculatory environment to which the cells are exposed and is therefore related to their zone localization. This concept helps explain the susceptibility of hepatocytes in specific zones to certain drugs and drug metabolites and to hypoxia. Although marked cellular differences between zones exists, the designated activity of hepatocytes remains flexible.

The hepatic sinusoids comprise a vascular network that converges on the terminal hepatic venule. The major structural components of the sinusoid are endothelial cells, Kupffer cells, and Ito cells.[10, 11] These cells line the vascular channel of the sinusoid and separate it from adjacent hepatocytes by the space of Disse or perisinusoidal space. The vascular channels of the sinusoids are more variable in diameter than most capillaries and the endothelium contains larger fenestrations.[10] The sinusoids serve as a fluid conduit providing hematogenous access to the hepatocytes and serving as the means for the dissemination and excretion of their metabolic products. A protein-rich ultrafiltrate of blood (hepatic lymph) penetrates the endothelial fenestrations and perfuses the perisinusoidal space. This hepatic lymph bathes the surface of the hepatocytes and Kupffer cells. The hepatocytes are arranged into cords of cells that are interconnected by a central bile canaliculus. Each hepatocyte has contact with adjacent hepatocytes, the biliary network and the perisinusoidal space. The bile canaliculi are composed of specially modified portions of the hepatocyte cell membrane. Canaliculi intercommunicate, forming a continuous three-dimensional network surrounding the hepatocytes. These are the initial conduits through which bile flows toward the portal

triad, opposite in direction to the flow of sinusoidal blood.

The *Kupffer cells* are phagocytic, motile, and self-replicating. They can extend cytoplasmic processes through the endothelial fenestrations of the sinusoid to

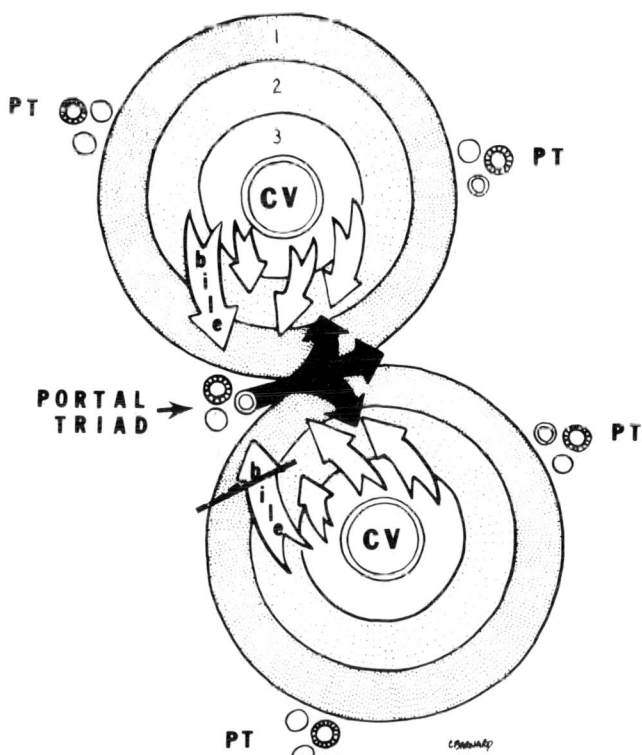

FIGURE 88–2. Schematic illustration of the nutritional or circulatory zones of the liver acinus. Zone 1 hepatocytes receive the best perfusion since they are positioned in the afferent vascular pathways. These cells are most resistant to nutritional or circulatory deprivations. Zone 3 hepatocytes are least resistant to circulatory or nutritional insults being located in the efferent circulatory pathway. Zone 2 hepatocytes are intermediate in their resistance. The black arrows indicate blood flow. CV represents central vein.

reach the hepatocytes.[10] They are derived from a bone marrow precursor and comprise the largest group of fixed macrophages in the body.[12, 13] They function as the important initial component of the monocyte/macrophage reticuloendothelial system in the processing of bilirubin and as scavengers clearing the sinusoidal area of particulate matter, gut origin antigens, endotoxins, bacteria, and senescent erythrocytes.[10] They also play a role in the metabolism of iron, lipids, cholesterol and certain hormones.[14–16] *Ito cells* are believed to be resting fibroblasts with fat storage and vitamin A storage capabilities.[11] Nodular hyperplasia in the dog has been associated with an increase in the Ito cell population.[17.]

The hepatocytes are rich in organelles, as would be expected in light of their immense metabolic responsibilities. Organelles present in abundance include smooth and rough endoplasmic reticulum, mitochondria, Golgi apparatus, primary and secondary lysosomes, cytoplasmic vesicles, microtubules, and microfilaments. Normal cytoplasmic inclusions include triglycerides, lipoproteins, glycogen, and lipofuscin granules.[10] Ceroid pigments may accumulate as an oxidation product of unsaturated lipid.[17] The liver has a large capacity for glycogen storage. In glycogen storage disorders and glucocorticoid hepatopathy in dogs, hepatic glycogen content can become markedly increased to the point of causing hepatomegaly.

The mitochondria of the hepatocytes are large and numerous, and it is here that oxidative phosphorylation and oxidation of fatty acids occur. The endoplasmic reticulum of the hepatocytes is one of its most dynamic organelles. It can hypertrophy causing an increase in size of individual hepatocytes and the liver as a whole and can increase the activity of its constituent enzymes on demand. It contains enzymes essential for gluconeogenesis, the microsomal steps in cholesterol biosynthesis, and the rate-limiting step in synthesis of bile acids from cholesterol. Many enzyme-inducing substances are metabolized in the hepatic microsomes by the mixed function oxidase system, a chain of enzymes that includes NADPH cytochrome C reductase and cytochrome P 450. Cytochrome P 450 is important in drug detoxification, hormone metabolism, and lipid synthesis. Induction of hepatocellular enzymes may follow exposure to inducing agents such as phenobarbital and cortisol. Inhibition may follow exposure to agents such as cimetidine, chloramphenicol, and quinidine.[18, 19] Enzyme induction and inhibition can have diverse metabolic effects depending on the systems involved. Following cessation of exposure to an enzyme-inducing or -suppressing agent, the cellular and enzymatic changes usually resolve over a period of days to a few weeks.

The hepatocellular lysosomes provide digestive enzymes that function in the disposal of exogenous substances, effete organelles, and polypeptide hormones.[10] They also serve as a storage depot for extraneous materials such as copper and in this manner protect the remainder of the cytosol from deleterious effects. The lysosomes are the site of copper accumulation in Bedlington terriers affected with copper storage hepatopathy. Lipofuscin granules are sometimes observed in the livers of dogs and cats. These are considered to be secondary lysosomes or storage residual bodies.[10] Micro-

tubules and microfilaments are present in the bile canalicular membrane. These are thought to be associated with endocytosis, membrane transport and exocytosis associated with movement of lipids into bile or plasma, and the secretion of bile into the canalicular lumen.[20]

The supporting network of the liver is supplied by the vascular and biliary structures and the stroma or connective tissue. Connective tissue follows and interdigitates with the vascular and biliary network and carries the hepatic lymphatics and nerve fibers. The orderly structure of the hepatic cords and plates is supported by the reticulum framework. It is this substructure that promotes the organized regrowth of the lobular structure following injury. If the connective tissue framework is severely damaged, repair is accomplished by unorganized regeneration of hepatic cords. The capsule of the liver is an extension of the supporting stroma. It is supplied with pain receptors that may be stimulated following acute distention. The capsule has limited expansion capabilities. If passive congestion engorges the liver beyond the available expansion space, the increased hydrostatic pressure causes a weeping of protein-rich hepatic lymph from the capsule surface.

Biliary System and Bile Production

The biliary system is composed of canaliculi, bile ductules, bile ducts, cystic duct, gallbladder, and common bile duct. Bile is initially secreted by the hepatocytes into the bile canaliculi. It is then transported through the bile ductules and ducts, which are lined by metabolically active biliary epithelium that actively modifies the electrolyte and fluid content of canalicular bile. Following delivery to the gallbladder, bile is concentrated and stored. At mealtimes, the presence of an acid duodenal pH, or protein or fat within the duodenum, signals the intestinal release of cholecystokinin and pancreozymin, which evoke gallbladder contraction and expulsion of bile into the alimentary canal. Gallbladder contraction also appears to be under the influence of other mediators (such as motilin), and it has been shown that spontaneous contraction occurs in the dog as in man unrelated to meals.[21]

Bile is an isotonic aqueous solution containing bile acids, cholesterol, phospholipids, bilirubin pigments, inorganic electrolytes and small amounts of immunoglobulins (IgA).[22] Bile production relies on three separate mechanisms: (1) a spontaneous basal flow of bile acids from the hepatocytes (the bile acid–dependent fraction), (2) a canalicular flow driven by Na^+, K^+-ATPase mediated by sodium transport (bile acid–independent fraction), and (3) modification of preformed bile by reabsorption and secretion of fluids and electrolytes by the bile ductules and bile ducts. Various pharmacologic and physiologic substances influence the rate and volume of bile production; some of these are presented in Table 88–2.

Hepatic Regeneration

How liver regeneration is initiated and terminated is unknown. The process is regulated by several hormones

TABLE 88–2. SUBSTANCES INFLUENCING THE FLOW OR VOLUME OF BILE

Substance or Condition	Mechanism
Bile salts	Increase flow by osmotic activity
Organic anion dyes	Increase flow by osmotic activity
BSP	
ICB	
rose bengal	
Phenobarbital	Increases bile acid–independent flow
Hyperthyroidism	Increases bile acid–independent flow
Glucagon	Increases bile acid–independent flow
Theophylline	Increases bile acid–independent flow
Prostaglandins	Inhibit duct fluid reabsorption
Salicylates	Increase bile acid–independent flow
Secretin	Increases bile acid–independent flow
Hypothyroidism	Decreases bile acid–independent flow
Estrogen	Decreases bile acid–independent flow

including insulin, glucagon, epidermal growth factor, parathormone, calcitonin, thyroxine, and glucocorticoids, and by the availability of essential and nonessential amino acids.[23] The liver can regenerate to its original mass and function following 70 per cent hepatectomy over a period of six weeks.[24–26] Following massive hepatocellular injury, immediate survival depends on the continuous provision of intravenous glucose. Within 4 to 12 hours, intermittent supplementation with coagulation factors also becomes necessary.[27–30]

The Enterohepatic Circulation

Any substance secreted in bile that is resorbed in the intestine and recirculated in the portal circulation to the liver for re-extraction and elimination in bile is said to undergo an enterohepatic circulation. This recycling process has received most consideration in regard to the normal metabolism of bile acids, bilirubin, and urobilinogen. A number of other endogenous and exogenous substances undergo an enterohepatic circulation, including cholesterol, phospholipids, vitamin B_{12}, folic acid, some of the steroid hormones such as the estrogenic sterols, copper, and many drugs (e.g., chloramphenicol and digitalis glycosides).[31, 32] Interruption of biliary secretion, intestinal absorption, portal circulation, or hepatocellular uptake can impair the regulation of substances having an extensive enterohepatic circulation.[31, 32]

Alterations in Hepatic Size

In health, the liver varies from 1.3 to 6.0 per cent of the body weight. In the neonate, it occupies a large portion of the abdominal cavity. As the animal ages, the ratio of the liver weight to the body weight declines. In young dogs, the ratio may be as great as 40 to 50 gm/kg, while in older dogs the ratio is 20 gm/kg.[33] Microhepatica (small liver) may develop due to acute changes in hepatic perfusion (hypotension), chronic liver disease associated with fibrosis in the dog but not in the cat, hepatocellular atrophy, and deprivation of the normal portal circulation.

Hepatomegaly may develop as a result of acute or chronic disorders impairing outflow from the hepatic veins, extramedullary hematopoiesis, hyperplasia of the reticuloendothelial system, or infiltrative disorders. Differential diagnoses for alterations in hepatic size are given in Table 88–3.

TABLE 88–3. DIFFERENTIAL DIAGNOSIS FOR ALTERATIONS IN HEPATIC SIZE

Microhepatica		Hepatomegaly

Decreased Hepatic Perfusion
Hypotension
  Severe dehydration
  Shock
  Endotoxemia
  Hypoadrenocorticism
Impaired Portal Perfusion
  Congenital portal shunt
  Portal vein atresia
Hepatocellular Atrophy
Congenital
  Portosystemic shunt
Hepatocyte Destruction
Cirrhosis (dog)
  Severe necrosis
	Impaired Venous Outflow
	Cardiac Disease
	  Congestive heart failure
	  Pericardial disease
	  Pericardial tamponade
	  Dirofilariasis
	  Atrial hemangiosarcoma
	  Cardiomyopathy
	  Arrhythmias
	Venous Occlusion
	  Vena caval occlusion
	  Hepatic vein occlusion
	  Vena caval syndrome (Dirofilariasis)
	Reticuloendothelial Hyperplasia
	  Immune-mediated diseases:
	    anemia
	    thrombocytopenia
	    vasculitis (SLE, other)
	  Infectious diseases:
	    bacterial
	    protozoan
	    mycotic
	    rickettsial
	  Septicemia
	Nodular Hyperplasia
	  Idiopathic
	  Hepatic regeneration
		Infiltrative Disorders
		Amyloid (rare)
		Glycogen:
		  hyperadrenocorticism
		  glycogen storage disease
		Lipid:
		  diabetes mellitus
		  idiopathic lipidosis (cat)
		Neoplasia:
		  lymphosarcoma
		  malignant histiocytosis
		  myeloproliferative disease
		  hemangiosarcoma
		  metastatic
		Hemochromatosis (iron)
		Extramedullary hematopoiesis
		Inflammatory Disease
		Hepatitis
		Acute necrosis
		Cholangitis
		Cholangiohepatitis
		Cirrhosis (cat)
		Abscess
		Extrahepatic Bile Duct Occlusion
		Neoplasia
		Pancreatitis
		Cholelithiasis
		Inspissated bile
		Cystic Disease
		Isolated cysts
		Polycystic disease

INTERMEDIARY METABOLISM AND THE LIVER

Hormone Metabolism

Interactions between the hepatobiliary system and endocrine hormones are numerous and include the liver functioning as a major target organ for hormone effect, as an activator of prohormones, as a source of second messenger hormones, and as the site of hormone degradation or excretion.[34, 35] Certain hormones also undergo an enterohepatic circulation. Because of the many ways that the liver interacts with the endocrine system, diminished hepatic function can disrupt normal endocrine physiology (Table 88–4). Patients with hepatobiliary disease may have diminished or altered hormonal effects despite an apparently normal circulating hormone concentration.[34, 35] Documented interactions between the hepatobiliary system and endocrine hormones are outlined in Table 88–5.

Vitamin Metabolism

The liver has an important role in the metabolism, utilization, storage, and degradation of many of the vitamins. Liver function can be altered by deficiencies or excess of certain vitamins.[36] Examples include the inability of the liver to activate the coagulation factors II, VII, IX, and X in the absence of active vitamin K, and the hepatopathy associated with vitamin A toxicity. Most of the water-soluble vitamins act as coenzymes in biochemical pathways operative in the liver and other tissues.[36] Many of these are activated in the liver. Hepatocellular necrosis, functional insufficiency, biliary obstruction, and the nutritional and hormonal dysregulations that develop in liver disease may each play a role in the deprivation of active vitamins. The importance of individual vitamins in metabolic processes inherent to the hepatobiliary system and the role of the liver in vitamin activation and regulation are summarized in Table 88–6.

One of the more important hepatobiliary-vitamin interactions is with vitamin K, one of the fat-soluble vitamins. Vitamin K_2 is acquired from intestinal microorganisms and has 60 per cent of the potency of vitamin K_1, which is acquired from dietary sources.[37] Normally,

TABLE 88–4. MECHANISMS OF ENDOCRINE ABNORMALITIES IN HEPATOBILIARY DISEASE

Decreased hepatic hormone production
Decreased hepatic hormone activation
Decreased hepatic hormone degradation
Decreased hepatic hormone excretion
Increased production of inappropriate hormones
Increased hepatic production of variant hormones (vitamin D)
Impaired feedback mechanisms regulating hormone production
Abnormal hepatic response to hormones
Impairment of hormone production by other organs
Interference in endocrine balance due to nutritional alterations and drugs involved in management of liver disease

TABLE 88–5. SPECIFIC HEPATOBILIARY-HORMONE INTERACTIONS

Hormone	Hepatobiliary Interaction
Estrogens	Biliary excretion
	Enterohepatic circulation
	Metabolized by P 450 oxidases
	Influences bile formation and flow
Progesterone	Hepatic catabolism
Glucocorticoids	Induce hepatic protein synthesis, especially albumin, fibrinogen
	Hepatic clearance
Aldosterone	Hepatic biotransformation for renal excretion
	Increased production in cirrhosis due to decreased albumin and renal blood flow
T_4, T_3	Hepatic storage, metabolism, excretion
	Important site of deiodination ($T_4 \rightarrow T_3$)
	Enterohepatic circulation
	Influence bile formation and flow
Growth hormone	Hepatic clearance
	Increased production in cirrhosis
Somatomedin	Hepatic synthesis
	Decreased synthesis in chronic liver disease
Vitamin D	Enterohepatic circulation
	Hepatic activation
Parathyroid hormone	Hepatic catabolism
Glucagon	Increased synthesis in chronic liver disease
	Catabolism in kidney and liver
Insulin	Catabolism in kidney and liver
	Insufficient hepatic delivery for carbohydrate homeostasis if portosystemic shunting
ADH Calcitonin Oxytocin TSH TRH Angiotensin II Bradykinin	Catabolized by liver and other tissue(s)

vitamin K_1 is rapidly absorbed from the intestines in the presence of bile salts, enters the systemic circulation via intestinal lymph, and is delivered to the liver and other tissues for storage. In the liver, vitamin K is a cofactor in the activation of factors II (prothrombin), VII, IX, and X.[38] During the generation of active factors, vitamin K is converted to its biologically inactive form. Normally this is rapidly reactivated in the liver. The availability of active vitamin K may be critically limited by anticoagulants such as warfarin, hepatic insufficiency, and obstructive jaundice. Anticoagulants such as warfarin competitively inhibit the hepatic reactivation of vitamin K;[39, 40] liver insufficiency may limit vitamin K reactivation as well as factor synthesis; and obstructive biliary tract disease prohibits vitamin K replenishment. In the absence of functional vitamin K, precursor forms of the vitamin K–dependent coagulation factors cannot be activated and a hemorrhagic diathesis ensues. The inactive factors accumulate in plasma and can be quantified as evidence of vitamin K deficiency.[41–43] The reader is referred to the section on coagulation in this chapter for further discussion of vitamin K and liver disease.

TABLE 88–6. METABOLIC INTERACTIONS OF VITAMINS WITH THE HEPATOBILIARY SYSTEM

Vitamin	Metabolic Interactions
Water-Soluble Vitamins	
Vitamin C	Component of NADH hydroxylation system
	Transformation of cholesterol to bile acids
	Maintains copper and iron in reduced state
	Essential for collagen synthesis
Biotin	Cofactor in acetyl coenzyme A
	Component of carboxylation reactions
Cyanocobalamin (Vitamin B_{12})	Hepatic activation
	Enterohepatic circulation
Folic acid	Hepatic storage and activation
	Enterohepatic circulation
Nicotinic acid	Hepatic synthesis and conversion to NAD+ and NADP+
Pantothenic acid	Hepatic metabolism to coenzyme A
Pyridoxine (Vitamin B_6)	Hepatic metabolism to pyridoxal phosphate, an important enzyme system cofactor
Riboflavin (Vitamin B_2)	Hepatic metabolism to FMN/FAD, important enzyme system cofactors
	Hepatic storage
	Enterohepatic circulation
Thiamine	Hepatic activation
	Coenzyme for transketolase, pyruvate dehydrogenase, α-ketoglutarate dehydrogenase
Fat-Soluble Vitamins	
Vitamin A	Hepatic storage
	Minor enterohepatic circulation
Vitamin D	Hepatic metabolism: $D_3 \rightarrow$ 25-hydroxyvitamin D_3
Vitamin E	Located in mitochondrial membranes
	Protects microsomal membranes from peroxidation
Vitamin K	Hepatic storage and activation
	Activates coagulation factors II, VII, IX, and X

HEMATOLOGIC AND HEMOSTATIC FUNCTIONS

The liver plays an important role in hemopoiesis and hemostasis. In the fetus, it serves as an important site of extramedullary hematopoiesis. With maturation, this function ceases but the potential for hematopoiesis remains.[44] The hepatic reticuloendothelial system participates in the removal of senescent or damaged erythrocytes. It is involved in the synthesis and ultimate metabolism and excretion of bilirubin, and as the source of transferrin, the major carrier protein for iron. To a limited extent, the liver acts a storage depot for iron, which is stored in the form of ferritin, a water-soluble protein iron complex, or as hemosiderin, an insoluble compound contained within Kupffer cells.[45, 46] Storage of other hematopoietic and hemostatic substances (B_{12}, folate, and vitamins A and K) is also provided.

HEMATOLOGIC ABNORMALITIES

Hematologic changes observed in patients with liver disease include aberrations in erythrocyte morphology,

platelet numbers or function, the development of anemia, and the presence of lipemic or jaundiced plasma.

Abnormalities in red cells have been recognized in humans and in dogs and cats with liver disease.[47–51] These erythrocytic changes may be induced by circulatory changes in the spleen or by alterations in the concentration and types of circulating lipoproteins.[52] Under normal circumstances, the spleen acts as a mechanical filter that can identify, trap, and destroy erythrocytes with mild defects caused by reduced membrane deformability. Its normal sluggish circulation enhances its efficiency in recognizing and entrapping effete or abnormal erythrocytes.[52] When the hepatic RE function is disabled, subsequent systemic immune stimulation may cause hyperplasia of immunocompetent cells in lymphoreticular tissue. Hyperplasia of the splenic pulp increases its propensity to detain abnormal erythrocytes. This propensity may be furthered by circulatory congestion, which may result from portal hypertension. Together, these changes exaggerate the normally adverse conditions to which red cells are exposed in the spleen and further promote a reduction in erythrocyte life span.

In humans, a mild abnormality in the erythrocyte membrane fluidity seems to be associated with alterations in the types and concentrations of circulating lipoproteins. Excessive amounts of red cell membrane cholesterol, phospholipid, and lecithin have been shown.[52] Unusual acanthocytes such as spur cells and poikilocytes have been described in both humans and animals with hepatobiliary disease.[47–51, 53] Spur cells are mature red cells with multiple, irregularly arranged surface projections. It is believed that the spleen plays a role in the continued modification of spur cells by reduction of cell surface area and consequent exaggeration of their spiculation, which inhibits return to their normal shape.[52] Loss of surface area renders the cell more rigid and less able to conform to the demands of the vascular passages within the spleen, leading to their entrapment and destruction.

Target cells and poikilocytes have been observed in dogs and cats with different forms of liver disease including hepatic lipidosis, cholangiohepatitis, hepatic necrosis, and portal venous anomalies (Figure 88–3). The mechanism of cell deformation has not been proven. Erythrocyte microcytosis is commonly observed in dogs with portosystemic shunts.[54] Affected animals seem to have normal iron-binding capacity, serum iron concentrations, and bone marrow iron stores. The cause of the microcytosis has not been confirmed. Normocytic, normochromic anemia may develop in patients with liver disease owing to inefficient utilization of marrow iron stores (anemia of chronic disease), decreased nutritional intake, decreased nutrient availability from the liver to the bone marrow, inadequate erythropoietin levels, chronic blood loss due to coagulopathies, and decreased red cell survival.[44]

Quantitative as well as qualitative defects in platelets may be associated with hepatobiliary disorders.[44, 55] Quantitative abnormalities result from alterations in platelet distribution or production or from increased destruction. Splenomegaly associated with portal hypertension can cause sequestration of as many as 60 to 90 per cent of the platelets at a given time in humans.[56, 57]

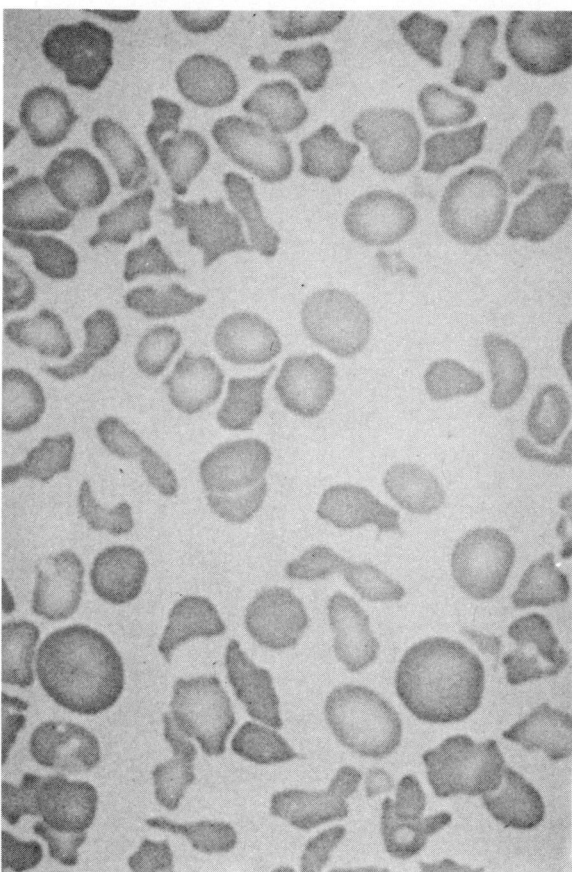

FIGURE 88–3. Photomicrograph of poikilocytes observed in the peripheral blood of a cat with hepatic insufficiency. (Courtesy of Dr. Tracy French, NYS Coll Vet Med, Cornell Univ, Ithaca, New York.) (From Comp Cont Educ 8:886, 1986.)

Fortunately, splenomegaly is relatively rare in dogs and cats with portal hypertension. Qualitative platelet defects may also develop and are considered to result from abnormal responses to extrinsic platelet stimuli, abnormal extrinsic stimuli stemming from deranged hepatic function, and intrinsic platelet defects.[58, 59] Qualitative defects characterized in humans include decreased factor III availability and impaired platelet adhesiveness and aggregation.[55, 58, 59] Ultrastructural platelet defects have been shown in some humans.

HEMOSTASIS

The liver plays a central role in the modulation and interaction of the coagulation, fibrinolytic, and inhibitor systems. It is the origin of all the coagulation factors, with the exceptions of factor VIII and calcium. It synthesizes and/or regulates the activity of plasminogen, the physiologic inhibitors of plasmin (antithrombin III, α_2-antiplasmin, and α_2-macroglobulin), and the plasmin activators.[44, 60–64] Activated coagulation factors, fibrinolytic enzymes, and many breakdown products are cleared from the circulation by the liver. In this way the liver protects against unrestrained clotting, fibrinolysis, and coagulation factor consumption.

Tests evaluating coagulation factors such as prothrom-

bin time (PT), activated coagulation time (ACT), activated partial thromboplastin time (APPT), and thrombin time (TT) reflect the adequacy of hepatic function. The PT evaluates the extrinsic coagulation system, while the ACT and APPT evaluate the intrinsic coagulation system. The TT evaluates the quantitative availability and function of fibrinogen. The PT, ACT, and APTT each reflect abnormalities in the common pathway. During synthetic failure the onset of factor deficiency is determined by factor utilization and factor half-life. The factor half-lives vary from hours to days and their estimated half-lives are shown in Table 88–7.[44, 65] Factor depletion to less than 30 per cent of normal factor activity causes prolonged clotting times and bleeding tendencies.[66] Depletion due solely to hepatic synthetic failure usually is not as severe as that due to congenital factor deficiencies. Bleeding in patients with liver disease is primarily due to provocative local factors such as gastritis, ulcers, surgical procedures, and other medical problems rather than to spontaneous hemorrhage from profound coagulation abnormalities.[64] Only 15 per cent of human patients with severe hepatic dysfunction evidence pathologic bleeding.[60] It is unknown what percentage of dogs or cats with liver disease demonstrate bleeding disorders.

It is important to realize that hemorrhagic tendencies may exist even though laboratory evaluations of coagulation indicate normalcy. A propensity to bleed should be anticipated in any patient with decreased hepatic function or major bile duct occlusion. Prolongation of the prothrombin time seems to be more common than prolongation of the other coagulation tests in humans with liver disease. Comparison of the PT and PTT in dogs with naturally occurring hepatic disease showed that abnormal clotting times (prolongation or shortening) may develop but that neither test is consistently superior.[67] Prolongation of coagulation time was more common than shortening, but abnormalities were not frequent enough to warrant their use as screening or diagnostic indicators of liver disease.[67] The sensitivity of these tests can be improved by using dilutions of the patient's citrated platelet-poor plasma.[67]

Factor deficiency may develop in patients with liver disease from synthetic failure, acquired qualitative factor defects, excessive consumption, and proteolysis. The severity of coagulation abnormalities seems to depend

TABLE 88–7. HALF-LIVES OF COAGULATION PROTEINS

Protein	Site of Synthesis	Half-Life
Factor XIII	Liver	5–12 days
Factor XII	Liver	2–3 days
Factor XI	Liver	2–3 days
Factor X	Liver	32–48 hours
Factor IX	Liver	20–24 hours
Factor VIII:Ag/c	Endothelial cells	12–40 hours
Factor VIII:vWF	Endothelial cells	12–40 hours
Factor VII	Liver	1.2–6 hours
Factor V	Liver	12–24 hours
Prothrombin	Liver	2–3 days
Fibrinogen	Liver	2–3 days
Plasminogen	Liver	2 days
Antithrombin III	Liver	12–40 hours

upon the degree and type of hepatocellular injury.[68] Specific factor deficiencies have been described in dogs with various types of liver disease.[28, 69] In dogs undergoing experimental CCl_4 hepatic injury, dramatic reductions in factors II, VII, and IX developed within 48 hours and resolved within five days.[28] Hepatectomized dogs given intravenous glucose survive for 20 hours and then succumb to hemorrhagic diathesis owing to coagulation factor deficiencies.[30] Blood transfusions can prolong but not ensure survival. In acute severe liver disease or after partial (75 per cent) hepatectomy, factor VII deficiency seems to be the earliest detectable change.[27] In humans with hepatobiliary disease the prognosis seems to correlate with the concentration of factor VII.[70, 71] It is unknown whether this is true in the dog and cat. In a study of naturally occurring hepatic disease in dogs, changes in specific factors were more frequent than abnormalities in the PT or PTT or in serum liver enzyme activities.[69] Unfortunately, although assays for clotting factors seem to have discriminant value in the differential diagnosis of liver disease, such measurements are neither practical nor expediently accomplished in most clinical settings.

The prothrombin coagulant factors II, VII, IX, and X are dependent on vitamin K for activation. These factors comprise a unique class of coagulation proteins that contain a glutamic acid residue that requires activation by a vitamin K–dependent carboxylation reaction that exclusively occurs within the hepatocyte.[68, 77] During factor activation, vitamin K is oxidized to its epoxide form, which then must be regenerated by vitamin K epoxide reductase. This so-called "vitamin K cycle" must be intact if factors II, VII, IX, and X are to be normally activated. In the absence of vitamin K, these factors are present in plasma but lack coagulant activity.[72] The inactive proteins may be measured as evidence of insufficient vitamin K activation and are referred to as proteins induced by vitamin K absence or antagonists (PIVKA).[42, 43] Vitamin K can be derived from preformed dietary sources or can be synthesized within the lower bowel by intestinal microbes. Conditions resulting in vitamin K deficiency include dietary deficiency, intestinal malabsorption, major bile duct obstruction, biliary fistula, intestinal sterilization, and antagonism by warfarin-like compounds. Major bile duct obstruction leads to vitamin K depletion as a result of the absence of intestinal bile salts and the ensuing fat malabsorption. Although the normal liver stores vitamin K, these depots are quickly depleted without continued replenishment.[66] The oral administration of antibiotics to humans on a vitamin K–deficient diet results in vitamin K depletion in 21 to 28 days.[73] It is unknown how long it takes in the dog or cat to deplete vitamin K in this manner. Although the PT and PTT are not practically useful in the differential diagnosis of liver disease, they can assist in differentiation between parenchymal and cholestatic disorders associated with extrahepatic bile duct obstruction. Correction of a PT prolongation by greater than 30 per cent within 12 to 24 hours following the administration of 5 to 15 mg of active vitamin K (K_1, Aquamephyton) corroborates the presence of vitamin K deficiency as a major causative factor.[73, 74] Prolongation of

the PT is the first demonstrable abnormality following vitamin K depletion because of its dependency on the short-lived factor VII. The APTT and ACT are also usually prolonged in clinical patients with liver disease having coagulopathies induced by vitamin K deficiency. Parenteral administration of vitamin K to patients with coagulation defects due primarily to hepatocellular synthetic failure provides no reliable benefit. Occasionally, minor improvements may be observed.[73, 74]

Fibrinogen is exclusively synthesized in hepatocytes. It is an acute phase reactant and therefore may increase due to acute or chronic liver disease or any other major systemic inflammatory, infectious, or necrotic process.[63, 75] The liver apparently has a huge capacity to synthesize fibrinogen, and it is only with acute hepatic failure or decompensated chronic hepatic disease that synthetic failure is realized. Normally, about 75 per cent of the total fibrinogen is located in the intravascular compartment, where it is readily available for coagulation purposes.[68] Excessive catabolism of available fibrinogen may occur when liver disease is associated with disseminated intravascular coagulation (DIC). Once fibrinogen is transformed to fibrin, proteolysis by plasmin releases fibrin monomers and other degradation products that are cleared by the reticuloendothelial systems in the liver and spleen. Fibrin degradation products share common antigenicity with fibrinogen but are not functional in promoting coagulation. They can be detected in plasma using immunologic techniques. Increases in fibrin degradation products (FDPs) occur as a result of accelerated fibrinolysis or because of impaired clearance by the liver. Simple bleeding into body cavities will not cause an increase in the FDPs in the normal dog, but it is unknown if this is so in patients with hepatic failure or with inflammatory conditions complicated by hemorrhage into body cavities.[76]

Dysfibrinogenemia, an acquired qualitative abnormality of the fibrinogen molecule, has been recognized as a cause of hemorrhagic diathesis associated with liver disease in humans.[77] It is potentially reversible if the underlying hepatic disorder is controlled. Dysfibrinogenemia is suspected when a prolonged TT occurs in the absence of other causal factors. Functional coagulation tests, but not the heat method of fibrinogen estimation, will indicate dysfibrinogenemia.[78, 79] At present, it is unknown if this occurs in animals.

Disseminated intravascular coagulation may be a sequela to a variety of hepatic disorders as well as abnormalities that can lead to hepatic disease.[74, 80–84] Pathogenetic mechanisms include release of thromboplastic substances from damaged hepatocytes, decreased hepatic clearance of gut-origin endotoxins that trigger the intrinsic cascade, impaired hepatic clearance of activated coagulation factors, reduced concentration or activity of antithrombin III, and stagnation of blood flow in mesenteric collaterals.[68] The use of heparin in the management of DIC associated with hepatic dysfunction is controversial. These patients are already at substantial risk from impaired coagulation factor synthesis, quantitative or qualitative platelet defects, and local causes of hemorrhage. Heparin acts by binding to antithrombin III (AT III). Antithrombin III is a glycoprotein synthesized in the liver that functions as a protease inhibitor.[85, 86] It can bind to and inhibit all the proteases of the intrinsic coagulation system and factors IX, X, C1, and thrombin.[78] The molecular size of AT III is comparable to that of albumin and therefore it can be lost in severe protein-losing nephropathies and enteropathies.[82] The AT III inactivation of coagulation factors is greatly accelerated by the presence of heparin, and without it, heparin therapy is largely ineffectual.[86] The concentration of AT III is reduced in veterinary patients with DIC and in human patients with hepatic dysfunction.[86-91] Preliminary studies in dogs with liver disease indicate that AT III values decline as hepatic function worsens. In patients with liver disease, low concentrations of AT III, and evidence of DIC, the risks of heparin therapy and the probability that it may be ineffectual argue against its use. If heparin is administered, it should be combined with transfusions of fresh blood or plasma. AT III activity decreased below 50 per cent of normal creates a thrombotic potential. If normal quantities and activities of coagulation factors exist, coumarin derivatives may be used for antithrombotic therapy.[92-94] Unfortunately, this approach is ill advised for patients with hepatic failure because they may already have subnormal quantities of coagulation factors.

The fibrinolytic system normally assists in the overall homeostatic balance of coagulation.[66] This system depends on the production of the serine protease plasmin, which is derived from plasminogen, a protein synthesized in hepatocytes and activated by a complex series of activators. Plasmin is responsible for maintaining vascular patency by digestion of fibrin.[66] About 60 per cent of the plasminogen is present in the intravascular compartment where its activity is controlled by specific antiproteases (α_2-antiplasmin and α_2-macroglobulin), which are also synthesized in hepatocytes.[66, 95] Liver disease may disrupt the fibrinolytic system in a number of ways. There may be increases in plasminogen activators due to impaired hepatic clearance, reduced levels of plasminogen and α_2 antiplasmin due to impaired hepatic synthesis, or accelerated consumption secondary to DIC.[96]

The overall management of the hemostatic disorders recognized in patients with hepatobiliary disease is dependent on the clinical status of the patient. If active hemorrhage is observed, treatment to alleviate the primary cause of the bleeding is the most important objective. Blood transfusions should be reserved for patients having active hemorrhage or that have documented coagulation deficiencies and that must undergo surgical procedures. Only fresh blood should be transfused to ensure delivery of functional platelets and to minimize the infusion of excessive ammonia, which may accumulate in stored blood. Gastrointestinal bleeding should be treated with H_2 receptor blockers and gastric protectants. A routine fecal examination should be done to detect endoparasitism. Invasive diagnostic procedures should be minimized. It is prudent to remember that patients may remain asymptomatic despite obvious coagulation test abnormalities. Aggressive therapeutic intervention should be reserved for crisis situations and when the patient has a reasonable chance for correction of the underlying defect.

Table 88–8 demonstrates specific defects reported in humans and dogs with different types of liver disease.[27-30, 60, 68, 97-99]

TABLE 88–8. HEMOSTATIC DEFECTS IDENTIFIED IN HUMAN AND CANINE* PATIENTS WITH VARIOUS HEPATOBILIARY DISORDERS

Coagulative Factor	Specific Abnormality	Associated Condition
Thrombocytopenia	↓ Platelets	Cirrhosis*
		Neoplasia*
		Congestive splenomegaly
		DIC*
		Hepatectomy*
Thrombocytosis	↑ Platelets	Hepatoma
		Hepatoblastoma
Quantitative platelet defects	↓ Platelet aggregation	Cirrhosis
		Viral hepatitis
Vitamin K–dependent factors (II, VII, IX, X)	↓ Factor activation	Extrahepatic cholestasis*
		Hepatic failure
	↓ Synthesis	Hepatectomy*
		Hepatic failure*
		Hepatic necrosis*
		Cirrhosis*
Factor V	↓ Synthesis	Hepatic failure*
Factor VIII	↑ or normal synthesis	Acute or chronic disease*
		Extrahepatic cholestasis*
		Biliary cirrhosis
		Hepatoma
		Neoplasia*
		Viral hepatitis
Fibrinogen	↑ Synthesis	Acute or chronic disease*
		Extrahepatic cholestasis
		Biliary cirrhosis
		Hepatoma
		Metastatic neoplasia
		Hepatic necrosis*
	↓ Synthesis	Hepatic failure*
		Cirrhosis*
	↑ Consumption	DIC*
		Hemorrhage*
		Loss into ascites
	Dysfibrinogenemia	Viral hepatitis
		Cirrhosis
		Severe necrosis
		Hepatoma
Factors XI, XII, XIII	↓ Synthesis	Cirrhosis*
		Severe hepatitis
		Hepatoma
		Hepatic failure*
Prekallikrein	↓ Synthesis	Cirrhosis
		Viral hepatitis
Plasminogen activator	↓ Clearance	Cirrhosis
Plasminogen	↓ Synthesis or	Hepatic failure
		Hepatic lipidosis
	↑ Consumption	Hepatic necrosis
Antithrombin III	↓ Synthesis or	Viral hepatitis
		Cirrhosis*
	↑ Consumptiom	Hepatoma
		DIC*
		Hepatic necrosis*
	↑ or normal synthesis	Extrahepatic cholestasis
		Primary biliary cirrhosis

CARBOHYDRATE METABOLISM

The liver plays a crucial role in carbohydrate metabolism. Many of the ingested dietary nutrients are directly delivered to the liver where they are converted and conserved in appropriate storage fuels. In conjunction with insulin and glucagon, the normal liver prevents excessive fluctuations in the blood glucose concentration. It has a large reserve capacity for maintaining glucose homeostasis. Fasting hypoglycemia is uncommon in liver disease because euglycemia can be managed with as little as 30 per cent of the normal parenchymal mass and because the kidney is also capable of gluconeogenesis.[100, 101] Suspected causes of hepatogenic hypoglycemia include insufficient parenchymal mass, insufficient enzymes or substrates for gluconeogenesis or glycogenolysis, glucagon resistance, and portosystemic shunting. When hepatogenic hypoglycemia develops, acute fulminant hepatic failure, end-stage chronic liver disease, or severe portosystemic shunting is usually present.

The liver is important as a target for insulin function and for insulin degradation. Studies in dogs have shown that 50 per cent of pancreatic insulin is degraded during first pass through the liver.[102–104] Hyperinsulinemia is common in humans with hepatic insufficiency. Suspected pathogenetic mechanisms include insulin hypersecretion, insulin resistance, and decreased insulin degradation.[105, 106] Insulin degradation may be limited as a result of diminished hepatocyte function or portosystemic shunting of blood away from the liver. Experimental studies of the effects of diverting portal or pancreatic venous blood to the systemic circulation have yielded conflicting results, some showing hyperinsulinemia and others not.[107–111]

Glucose intolerance is more common than hypoglycemia in humans with severe hepatic dysfunction.[106, 117] Carbohydrate intolerance is more consistent with oral as compared with intravenous carbohydrate loading, and this possibly reflects a greater influence on glucose metabolism of portosystemic shunting than of reduced hepatic mass. Hyperglucagonemia has been demonstrated in humans with hepatic insufficiency and is suspected to occur in dogs with cirrhosis and concurrent glucose intolerance or diabetes mellitus.[112–115] The presence of portosystemic shunting of blood appears to be important in the genesis of hyperglucagonemia. Progressive hyperglucagonemia has been observed following experimental portocaval anastomosis in normal dogs.[108, 116] Shunting decreases glucagon delivery to the liver thereby decreasing and delaying glucagon stimulated glycogenolysis and glucagon degradation.

In animals with portosystemic vascular anomalies there appears to be diminished hepatic glucose production, decreased hepatic glycogen stores, and decreased responsiveness to glucagon.[117] Impaired response to glucagon may be due to diminished delivery of glucagon to the liver, decreased hepatic glycogen stores due to inadequate hepatic mass or chronically increased glycogenolysis, or damaged or resistant glucagon receptors. In some dogs with portosystemic vascular anomalies, hypoglycemia has been recognized as a dominant clinical problem. Toy breeds appear to be at increased risk.

Hypoglycemia has also been reported as an uncommon complication of hepatic tumors in dogs. The proposed yet unproven causes of hypoglycemia in these cases include increased glucose utilization by neoplastic tissue, elaboration of insulin-like activity, release of substances that inhibit normal glycogen mobilization (somatostatin-like activity), and insufficient glycogen reserves due to severe parenchymal destruction.[118]

In summary, the blood glucose concentration is an insensitive indicator of hepatobiliary function because of the very large hepatic reserve for maintaining euglycemia. Acute toxic and ischemic insults, infections, portosystemic shunting, and extensive hepatic neoplasia are all capable of disrupting normal glucose regulation.

LIPID METABOLISM

Lipid metabolism is complex and depends in part on normal hepatic function. Some of the basic research in lipid metabolism has been completed in animal models, including the dog. Comparatively little is known about lipid metabolism in the cat. Although the use of lipid moieties as diagnostic indices for liver disease in veterinary medicine is poorly understood, the current knowledge is presented in this section.

Cholesterol, cholesterol esters, phospholipids, and triglycerides comprise the major plasma lipids. These water-insoluble substances are transported in the circulation as lipoprotein complexes. Liver disease may disrupt the normal balance between the major lipid moieties and in the distributions within the lipoprotein classes.

Cholesterol is the precursor sterol nucleus for the synthesis of bile acids, steroid hormones, and vitamin D. It is a structural component in all mammalian cell membranes. Although all mammalian tissues are capable of cholesterol synthesis, up to 50 per cent occurs in the liver.[119] Serum cholesterol concentrations are adjusted by feedback mechanisms according to the balance between ingestion, synthesis, degradation, and excretion.[119, 120] Alimentary sources of cholesterol are derived from dietary ingestion, epithelial exfoliation, and bile. The cholesterol nucleus is not degraded but is lost from the body in balance with ingress from alimentary uptake and de novo synthesis. Although cholesterol undergoes an enterohepatic circulation, excretion largely occurs via the alimentary canal in feces in the form of biliary and dietary cholesterol, bile salts, and metabolites of unabsorbed cholesterol. Minor losses occur through shedding of cellular cholesterol from skin and intestinal epithelia.[119, 121–123] Intestinal absorption of cholesterol occurs by passive diffusion into the enterocytes, where it is esterified and packaged with triglycerides, apoproteins (carrier proteins), and newly synthesized cholesterol into chylomicrons. Being large molecules, the chylomicrons gain access to the systemic circulation through the mesenteric lymphatics.

Total serum cholesterol (nonesterified and esterified cholesterol) is usually measured in dogs and cats on routine screening profiles. In the normal dog, 60 to 80 per cent of the circulating cholesterol is esterified.[124]

Cholesterol esterification is catalyzed by acyl coenzyme A:cholesterol-acyltransferase (ACAT) and lecithin-cholesterol acyltransferase (LCAT).[125] The interaction of LCAT with cholesterol is believed to occur on the surface of certain lipoprotein particles, following activation by specific apoproteins.[126] LCAT has been measured in the serum of dogs with experimentally induced hepatic injury but not as a diagnostic parameter in clinical cases.

Diet seems to be an important determinant of the total serum cholesterol content in dogs. Pet dogs have a higher fasting total serum concentration than do research dogs, the difference purportedly due to their differing nutritional intake.[127, 128] The effect of dietary cholesterol supplementation on the serum cholesterol concentration in dogs has been studied. Feeding 2 raw eggs per kg diet for 15 weeks results in minor changes while feeding 4, 8, or 16 eggs per kg diet results in substantial increases in the total serum cholesterol.[129] Despite increases in serum cholesterol induced by dietary cholesterol, dogs do not develop atherosclerotic lesions unless they have some other metabolic derangement such as hypothyroidism.[127, 130]

Lipoproteins can be differentiated by size and density into chylomicrons, very-low-density lipoproteins (VLDLs), low-density lipoproteins (LDLs), and high-density lipoproteins (HDLs). These can be separated by electrophoresis and quantified by density gradient ultracentrifugation. The protein components of the lipoproteins are called *apoproteins*; several groups have been identified and classified alphabetically. Apoproteins are synthesized in the hepatic microsomes and are linked to lipid in the smooth endoplasmic reticulum, where the enzymes for lipogenesis are located.[131]

Chylomicrons float in stored plasma and remain at the origin on electrophoresis. They are very short lived in the circulation, being cleared within 30 to 60 minutes following intestinal production.[132] While bound to vascular endothelium they are enzymicly degraded to yield free fatty acids, which diffuse into adjacent tissues, and a cholesterol remnant. VLDLs are produced in the intestines and liver.[133] Hepatic VLDL production is increased when carbohydrate or fat is metabolized to triglycerides.[134] VLDLs and chylomicrons are the primary route of triglyceride transport in the systemic circulation. Like chylomicrons, VLDLs are catabolized by lipoprotein lipase. LDLs and HDLs are produced from the catabolism of VLDLs or by direct synthesis in the liver, intestines, or plasma.[133]

The metabolism of lipoproteins is complex and involves the activity of three enzymes: lipoprotein lipase, hepatic lipase, and LCAT. These enzymes implement the transfer of constituent lipids among lipoproteins and promote lipoprotein catabolism.[135] In certain tissues, lipoprotein lipases are bound to capillary endothelia and are activated by a heparin-like substance. Lipoprotein lipase catalyzes the hydrolysis of triglycerides in chylomicrons and VLDL, releasing them for uptake by peripheral tissues. Hormonal modulation of lipoprotein lipase activity has been shown; it is increased by insulin and is decreased by glucagon, ACTH, and TSH.[133] Hepatic lipase is thought to hydrolyze surface phospholipids present on lipoproteins and to promote the inter-

conversion of different classes of HDL and the catabolism of VLDL to LDL.[135] Lipoprotein lipase and hepatic lipase can be activated by the intravenous injection of heparin. In normal dogs, fasting for 12 hours is usually adequate to clear postprandial lipemia. In those in which gross lipemia persists, the intravenous administration of 50 IU/lb (100 IU/kg) sodium heparin and the collection of blood 15 minutes later can be used to clear lipemia.[127]

The physical characteristics of different lipid moieties may allow quick assessment of lipemic samples. Following refrigerated storage, a flocculent surface layer with clearing beneath indicates chylomicronemia. Persistently turbid samples are rich in triglycerides (lipoproteins), which remain distributed throughout plasma.[136]

EFFECT OF LIVER DISEASE ON PLASMA LIPIDS AND LIPOPROTEINS

Reduced LCAT has been shown in dogs with experimental liver injury as in humans with liver disease.[137–143] The decline in enzyme activity is attributed to synthetic failure or hepatocyte necrosis. The net result is reduced plasma cholesterol esterification.

In humans, hypertriglyceridemia may develop in acute and chronic hepatitis and in cholestasis.[137, 144] Obstructive jaundice may lead to hypercholesterolemia and hypertriglyceridemia.[137, 142, 145] Most of the hypertriglyceridemia is associated with LDL particles, which may represent the accumulation of remnant lipoproteins remaining in the circulation because of impaired lipolysis or ineffective hepatic clearance.[135] Cholesterol synthesis is increased in obstructive jaundice. This may be the origin of hypercholesterolemia observed in dogs and cats with major bile duct occlusion.[146, 147] Increased synthesis may result from the lack of feedback inhibition via chylomicron remnants.[132] In addition to increased cholesterol synthesis, regurgitation of biliary lipids into the systemic circulation also occurs. Studies of obstructive jaundice in the dog have shown either no change in cholesterol esterification or a transient (two to six days after obstruction) decrease followed by a gradual rise to normal.[137] Hypercholesterolemia may also be associated with metabolic derangements stemming from other primary disease processes such as hypothyroidism, diabetes mellitus, hyperadrenocorticism, and the nephrotic syndrome.

An unusual lipoprotein may accumulate in patients with reduced LCAT activity and obstructive jaundice. This lipoprotein is an abnormal VLDL (lipoprotein X) and is characterized by reduced cholesterol ester and triglyceride components.[135, 142, 144, 148, 149] The clinical observations associated with lipoprotein X are inconsistent. Not all patients with lipoprotein X have reduced LCAT activity. Although lipoprotein X is common in humans with extrahepatic bile duct occlusion, it can also develop in patients with any cause of severe cholestasis. The most likely explanations for the occurrence of lipoprotein X include the regurgitation of biliary lipids, substrate accumulation secondary to LCAT deficiency, and the fact that lipoprotein X is a poor substrate for LCAT activity.[132] Lipoprotein X has been identified in normal dogs following experimental complete extrahepatic bile duct occlusion.[150] Hypercholesterolemia and hypertriglyceridemia developed as early as day 3 and remained through 17 days of observation. These dogs also developed an increase in the relative percentage of α_1 lipoproteins and a decrease in the α_2 fraction.

Other studies of lipids in animals with hepatic disease are sparse. Experimentally induced hepatic necrosis in dogs (CCl_4) results in reduced serum triglyceride concentrations for two days.[128] Hypocholesterolemia has received more attention than other lipid aberrations, having been reported in animals with congenital portosystemic vascular anomalies, in those with acquired hepatic insufficiency, and in dogs treated with anticonvulsant drugs. After surgical creation of portacaval shunts, dogs develop a 40 to 45 per cent decrease in the total cholesterol concentration.[151] The mechanism remains undetermined but is conjectured to involve decreased synthesis of cholesterol, triglyceride, or lipoproteins or a shift in the localization of cholesterol so that it is no longer distributed in the routinely measured pool.[116, 152-154] In dogs with surgically created shunts, the size of the shunting vessels, the completeness of visceroportal shunting, and the longevity of patient survival seem to correlate with the severity of the ensuing hypocholesterolemia. In patients with congenital portosystemic vascular anomalies, hypocholesterolemia seems to resolve after surgical correction of the aberrant circulation.

A moderate decline in serum cholesterol concentrations develops in normal dogs given oral primidone. Their cholesterol concentrations return to pretreatment levels within two weeks after drug discontinuation.[155] In some dogs receiving anticonvulsants, a progressive hepatopathy may develop. In these animals, marked hypocholesterolemia correlates with severely impaired hepatic function. Both the esterified and the nonesterified cholesterol fractions may decline in hepatic failure. Persistent severe hypocholesterolemia in patients with acquired hepatic insufficiency warrants a grave prognosis if other causes of low cholesterol have been discounted. The hypocholesterolemia in animals with portosystemic vascular anomalies or cirrhosis is associated with markedly increased concentrations of serum bile acids, further documenting hepatic insufficiency. Whether the high serum bile acids are linked to the hypocholesterolemia is controversial. Experimentally, the feeding of bile salts decreases hepatic cholesterol synthesis. Although bile salts may have a direct inhibitory effect on some of the key enzymes essential for cholesterol synthesis, it is unclear if this occurs naturally.[132] There is some evidence that chenodeoxycholate acts to decrease cholesterol synthesis directly.[132]

The ramifications of abnormal lipoprotein metabolism are multisystemic. Abnormal HDLs that develop in certain forms of liver disease may be immunosuppressive.[135] The best recognized effects are those resulting from cell membrane adsorption of abnormal lipids. Membrane changes include deleterious alterations in membrane permeability, surface receptors, transport proteins, enzymes, and reduced concentrations of prostaglandin and thromboxane precursors.[135] Membrane alterations are morphologically conspicuous in erythrocytes and may cause platelet dysfunction, discussed further in the hematology section of this chapter.

The formation of VLDL is an important mechanism by which the liver can extract excess fatty acids from plasma and mobilize it for storage elsewhere. Defects in this mechanism can cause fat accumulation in the liver. Abnormalities in the transport of VLDL from the liver or any imbalance resulting in a greater accumulation than dispersal of triglycerides can result in hepatic lipidosis. This syndrome can lead to hepatic failure and death in the cat. The exact mechanisms responsible for the hepatic lipidosis syndrome in cats are unknown but are considered to be multifactorial. Affected animals have not been shown to be consistently hypertriglyceridemic, hypercholesterolemic, or hyperglycemic.

For the interested reader, further discussion of lipoprotein metabolism is available in Chapters 39 and 40.

PROTEIN SYNTHESIS AND REGULATION

The liver is essential for normal protein homeostasis. It is the exclusive or primary site of synthesis for a majority of the plasma proteins and the site of degradation or regulation for many other proteins and hormones. It processes amino acids derived from ingested protein for its own requirements and for those of the peripheral tissues and receives amino acids from peripheral tissues for gluconeogenesis and transamination reactions. It is also the site for detoxification of the nitrogenous end products of protein metabolism through the Krebs-Henesleit urea cycle and for the conversion of uric acid to allantoin.

Albumin

Hepatic synthesis of constituent and export proteins comprises about 20 per cent of the total body protein turnover.[157] Albumin is the major hepatic export protein. In health it constitutes around 50 to 60 per cent of the total plasma protein and 75 per cent of the plasma oncotic pressure. It is the principal binding and transport protein for many substances in the systemic circulation, including hormones, fatty acids, trace metals, tryptophan, bilirubin, bile acids, other organic anions of both endogenous and exogenous origin, and many drugs.[158] Albumin is exclusively synthesized in hepatocytes, which usually work at one-third their maximal albumin synthesizing potential.[158] The plasma albumin concentration is the net result of synthesis, secretion, distribution, and degradation. Variables including the age of the animal, availability of amino acid precursors, hormonal balance, and the osmotic environment of the hepatocyte influence albumin homeostasis by regulating the rates of albumin production or degradation. The synthesis of albumin is increased by both cortisol and thyroxine, but the most important factors controlling albumin production are the nutritional status of the animal and the oncotic pressure of the interstitial fluids bathing the hepatocytes.[158] In fasted animals and those fed low protein diets, hepatic albumin production declines by 40 to 50 per cent within 24 hours.[158] In comparison to other protein synthesis, however, albumin synthesis is relatively spared.[158, 159] Albumin synthesis is exquisitely sensitive to the availability of amino acids (especially tryptophan) and this is considered to be an important inhibiting influence during starvation.[160] The rate of albumin synthesis seems to correlate best with changes in the oncotic pressure of the perisinusoidal extracellular space rather than those in the plasma. It is thought that small changes in the concentration of osmotically active macromolecules in the interstitial space directly signal the hepatocytes to adjust albumin synthesis.[161, 162] Newly synthesized albumin is released directly into the sinusoidal plasma rather than into the perisinusoidal space. This prohibits immediate negative feedback on the rate of albumin synthesis. Substantial monoclonal or polyclonal increases in the immunoglobulins can inhibit albumin synthesis according to the changes induced in the oncotic pressure.

The normal half-life of albumin in the dog is estimated at 8.5 to 8.7 days, but this can vary because albumin catabolism can be accelerated or decreased depending on the animal's nutritional status and plasma oncotic pressure.[163, 164] The exact mechanism and control of albumin degradation is poorly understood. The rate of albumin degradation seems to be primarily controlled by the total exchangeable albumin mass, although the rate of degradation also declines when albumin synthesis is reduced.[165] In health, degradation of albumin occurs in many tissues but primarily the liver, gut, and muscle.[166]

Since albumin is a major plasma protein and is synthesized entirely by the liver, it can be used as an indicator of hepatic function. It must be remembered, however, that the serum concentration reflects not only the rate of albumin synthesis but also the rate of degradation, pathologic excretion from the body, and its volume of distribution. Any chronically anorectic animal may have minor decreases in the serum albumin concentration as result of malnutrition. Pathologic processes associated with continuous losses of albumin from the body such as protein losing nephropathies or enteropathies may moderately to markedly reduce the plasma albumin concentration. In certain disease states, the volume of distribution for albumin may expand. The serum albumin concentration inconsistently reflects these changes because of concurrent adjustments in the size of the exchangeable pool. In patients with cirrhosis associated with ascites, low albumin may be more a reflection of the increased volume of distribution than of impaired hepatic synthesis.[167] In those with reduced albumin synthesis, a secondary reduction in albumin turnover may conceal the decreased production.[167-169] The salt and water retention that develops in severe liver disease may cause dilutional hypoalbuminemia even if albumin synthesis remains normal or increases.[170, 171] Furthermore, in some patients with ascites, newly synthesized albumin is released directly from hepatic lymphatics or the liver capsule into the ascitic fluid, thereby circumventing the vascular compartment.[161, 172]

From the foregoing discussion, it is obvious that use of the serum albumin concentration as a measure of hepatic function is fraught with many complications. All of the factors and exceptions discussed influence the concentration of albumin in the plasma pool. The serum albumin concentration is therefore not a reliable indicator of albumin synthesizing capacity or the overall functional capacity of the liver.

Serum Globulins

The total serum globulin concentration is composed of a number of different proteins serving a myriad of functions. A partial list is given in Table 88–9. With the exception of the immunoglobulins, the majority of the serum globulins are synthesized and stored in the liver. Seventy-five to 90 per cent of the α-globulins are produced by the liver but only about 50 per cent of the β-globulins.[173] The total serum globulin concentration is not a good measure of liver function because of the large fraction composed of immunoglobulins derived from other sources. The electrophoretic separation of the serum globulins in patients with liver disease has shown a variety of patterns. β1-globulins are increased in neoplastic conditions, β_2-globulins are increased in jaundiced animals, and the τ-globulin fraction is increased nonspecifically in most patients with compromised hepatic function. A bridging of the β- and τ-

TABLE 88–9. PROTEINS SYNTHESIZED IN THE LIVER

Protein	Major Function
Albumin	Regulates plasma oncotic pressure
	Major transport protein in plasma
Globulins:	
α_1-antitrypsin	Major serum protease inhibitor, inhibits: pancreatic trypsin, chymotrypsin, elastase, collagenase, kallikrein, plasmin, renin, urokinase, and thrombin
α_1-fetoprotein	Synthesized by fetal liver
	Elaborated by regenerating hepatocytes
α_2-macroglobulin	Protease inhibitor
	Immunoregulatory
α_2-antiplasmin	Protease inhibitor
Antithrombin III	Protease inhibitor activated by heparin, inhibits: serine proteases of the intrinsic coagulation system and factors IX, X, C_1, thrombin, plasmin, kallikrein, and urokinase
C-reactive protein	Acute-phase protein
	Activates complement
	Enhances phagocytosis of bacteria, RBCs
	Immunomodulator
Ceruloplasmin	Copper and iron transport
Coagulation proteins: Factors II, V, VII, IX, X, XI, XII	Important constituents of the intrinsic, extrinsic, and common pathway of the coagulation cascade
Fibrinogen:	Acute phase protein
	Constituent of the common pathway of the coagulation cascade
Plasminogen:	Major fibrinolytic protease
	Maintains vascular patency
Haptoglobin	Hemoglobin transport
Hemopexin	Binds and transports heme
Thyroid-binding protein	Circulatory transport of thyroid hormone
Transferrin	Binds and transports iron

globulin fractions has been noted in patients with cirrhosis.

Hyperglobulinemia is common in animals with hepatobiliary disease. The magnitude of hyperglobulinemia may be great enough to mask significant hypoalbuminemia if the serum total protein content is the only parameter determined. Because of the strategic anatomic position of the liver between the gastrointestinal tract and the systemic circulation, it modulates the exposure of the body to gut-derived antigens, endotoxins, and microorganisms. The reticuloendothelial system has its largest component in the liver. In health it acts as a filter against exogenous substances transported in the portal circulation, thereby reducing the systemic exposure to antigens. When this system is dysfunctional, systemic antigenic stimulation causes hyperglobulinemia. Increased systemic antibody production in response to diminished hepatic RE function usually occurs in the lymph nodes and spleen and may cause hypertrophy of these tissues.

The macrophages of the hepatic reticuloendothelial (RE) system (Kupffer cells) play a role in the management of antigen and T and B cell interactions and in the repair of damaged hepatic tissue.[174] Following hepatic injury, their normal function may be reduced because of quantitative cell loss, a redesignation of cell function, or abnormalities in liver blood flow and shunting of portal blood around the hepatic sinusoids.[174-176] There is also evidence of disturbed T and B cell function in liver disease, which may contribute to the hyperglobulinemia that develops in some patients. The derangements in the function and regulatory balance between B and T cells may affect the liver directly. An abnormal immunologic response to initial injury may result in perpetuation of hepatic inflammation eventuating in hepatic fibrosis. Autoantibodies have been identified in humans with chronic liver disease. These include antinuclear antibody, anti-DNA antibody, anti-smooth muscle antibody, antimitochondrial antibody, bile canalicular antibody, and liver membrane antibody. Some of these abnormal globulins have been postulated to play a causal role in the perpetuation of certain types of hepatic disease. Their importance in naturally developing liver disease in animals has not been investigated.

AMINO ACID REGULATION

The liver modifies the amino acid composition of the systemic circulation by selective uptake of amino acids from the portal circulation at mealtimes. The aromatic amino acids (AAAs) (phenylalanine, tyrosine, and methionine) are preferentially extracted and metabolized by the liver. The branched-chain amino acids (BCAAs) (valine, leucine, and isoleucine) are routed to the muscles and other tissues and are minimally metabolized by the liver. BCAAs serve as a source of energy for muscle, of carbon skeletons for pyruvate synthesis, and of nitrogen for transamination of pyruvate to alanine and glutamine.[177] In health, the sum of the concentrations of the BCAAs in the systemic circulation exceeds the sum of the AAAs by about 3:1. In patients with hepatic

insufficiency, this ratio is usually reduced to approximately 1.[177-179] Amino acid concentrations have been determined in dogs subjected to experimental liver injury and in those with spontaneous hepatobiliary disorders. Dogs with massive hepatic necrosis develop increases in all of the amino acids except arginine and citrulline.[180-184] Decreased citrulline concentrations are speculated to reflect impaired urea cycle activity and decreased arginine to reflect increased arginase release from injured hepatocytes.[180, 184, 185] Increased serum concentrations of α-amino-N-butyric acid were observed in two dogs with hepatocellular carcinoma.[184] The consistency of this observation has not been further investigated. The amino acid ratio in a group of dogs with portosystemic vascular anomalies was 0.94 and in dogs with acquired hepatic insufficiency was 1.31.[184]

Specific causes for the amino acid derangements in liver disease include (1) increased peripheral uptake and oxidation of BCAAs, (2) increased utilization of BCAAs for ketogenesis, (3) increased utilization of BCAAs for hepatic and renal gluconeogenesis, (4) increased production of AAAs as a result of increased proteolysis, and (5) altered hepatic metabolism of AAAs.[186] The hyperaminoacidemia that develops in acute hepatic necrosis results from compromised hepatic function, lysis of necrotic liver tissue, catabolism of protein in peripheral tissues, and hormonal imbalance (increased catecholamines, cortisol). Most of the plasma amino acid aberrations in patients with chronic liver disease may be explained on the basis of impaired hepatic function, portosystemic shunting of blood, and hyperinsulinemia and hyperglucagonemia that induce extensive muscle catabolism.[186]

The ratio of the BCAA:AAA has been extensively investigated as to its value as a diagnostic and prognostic parameter in humans with liver disease. Although there remains much controversy, an abnormal ratio seems to correlate with the histologic severity of liver disease and abnormalities in other biochemical liver tests.[186] Therapeutic manipulations aimed at normalizing amino acid imbalances have given inconsistent clinical results. Intravenous administration of specially formulated solutions high in branched-chain amino acids has produced remarkable clinical improvement in some patients but no improvement or detrimental effects in others.[187-194]

The administration of keto-analogues of the BCAAs has been suggested as a superior form of nutritional therapy in encephalopathic patients. In theory, keto-analogues of amino acids can be used in the synthesis of essential amino acids and, in the process, will help consume generated ammonia. Response to the use of these solutions in humans has given variable results. The infusion of protein-containing fluids (amino acid solutions or blood transfusions) to patients with impaired hepatic function requires careful consideration of the many potential detrimental effects. Of the commercial amino acid solutions available, none is specifically balanced for canine or feline patients. Their therapeutic use has not been adequately investigated and therefore cannot be recommended. Diets that are low in protein and have favorable BCAA:AAA ratios have been designed for animals having hepatic encephalopathy.[195] Long-term use of these diets in affected dogs has given excellent results. Whether beneficial effects are derived from corrected amino acid imbalances or general protein restriction remains unclear.

LIVER ENZYMES

Liver enzymes customarily included in serum biochemical screening profiles include alanine aminotransferase (ALT, formerly SGPT), aspartate aminotransferase (AST, formerly SGOT), alkaline phosphatase (ALP), and γ-glutamyltransferase (GGT). Increases in the serum activity of these enzymes are common. Unfortunately, although they are considered to be sensitive indicators of hepatobiliary disturbances, they lack specificity as to the nature or severity of the initiating condition. There are four major variables that influence the activity of liver enzymes in the circulation: (1) their intracellular localization, (2) their baseline intracellular activity, (3) their tendency to leak from the cell following changes in membrane permeability, and (4) their serum half-life.[196] Increased enzyme activity may develop in association with reversible or irreversible changes in hepatocyte cell membrane permeability, microsomal enzyme induction, or structural injury resulting from hepatobiliary ischemia, necrosis, neoplasia, or cholestasis. Medications and conditions associated with increased serum enzyme activity in the absence of serious hepatobiliary consequences are frequent in small animal practice; examples are shown in Table 88–10. Liver enzyme induction is common in the dog and is the major reason for confusion in the interpretation of abnormal enzyme activity. Different pathologic processes involv-

TABLE 88–10. CONDITIONS ASSOCIATED WITH INCREASED SERUM ACTIVITY OF LIVER ENZYMES BUT *NOT NECESSARILY* WITH CLINICALLY IMPORTANT HEPATOBILIARY DISEASE

Hypoxia	Gastrointestinal Disorders
pulmonary disease	diarrhea (acute or chronic)
acute anemia	(large or small bowel)
severe chronic anemia	pancreatitis
cardiac failure	severe constipation
Hypotension	Mechanical Injury
cardiac disease	blunt abdominal trauma
arrhythmias	iatrogenic surgical trauma
cardiomyopathy	Drugs
pericardial disorders	glucocorticoids (dog)
severe dehydration	anticonvulsants (dog)
shock	thiacetarsamide
Endocrine Disorders	ketaconazole (dog)
diabetes mellitus	others
hyperadrenocorticism	Systemic Infections
hyperthyroidism (cat)	rickettsial (ehrlichia)
hypothyroidism	viral (parvovirus, others)
hypoadrenocorticism	dirofilariasis
Bone Disorders	abscessation
growth (birth to 7 mo)	pyometra
osteomyelitis	severe dental disease
metabolic bone disease	septicemia
osseous neoplasia	Other
Neoplasia	systemic tissue necrosis
enzyme induction	renal disease
liver origin	following general anesthesia
paraneoplastic	fever

ing the liver can cause proportionately different elevations in serum enzyme activity owing to variation in enzyme localization within the hepatic lobule. Sometimes these variations can be used to differentiate between possible diagnoses.

It is well known that liver enzyme activity is an unreliable indicator of hepatic disease because severe dysfunction (end-stage cirrhosis and portosystemic vascular anomalies) can exist in the absence of serum enzyme abnormalities. Caution must always be exercised in the use of liver enzymes as prognostic indicators. If sequential blood samples are monitored, continuous abnormal enzyme activity may indicate continuing hepatobiliary disease or continued enzyme induction. Diminished enzyme activity may indicate improvement, resolution of an enzyme-inducing process, or a paucity of viable hepatocytes capable of releasing enzyme. Use of single measurements of enzyme activity as the basis for important irrevocable clinical decisions or as prognostic indicators of the severity of liver disease must be avoided.

Alanine Aminotransferase

Alanine aminotransferase (ALT) is a cytosolic enzyme regarded as liver-specific in the dog and cat, although it is also present in the heart and kidneys.[197] The serum half-life of ALT in the dog has been reported as three hours and four days.[198, 199] Immediate increases in serum ALT activity may follow hepatocellular injury or reversible or irreversible changes in cell membrane permeability because of its ready liberation from the hepatocellular cytosol. The magnitude of an ALT increase generally correlates with the number of involved cells, although focal and diffuse hepatic disorders cannot be differentiated. Largest increases develop in association with hepatocellular necrosis and inflammation. A series of gradual and sequential decreases in ALT activity can be a sign of recovery, but also it can indicate a poor prognosis, reflecting a paucity of remaining viable hepatocytes.[200] In acute liver disease, a 50 per cent or more decrease in serum ALT activity over 24 to 48 hours is considered a good prognostic sign.[200]

After acute severe diffuse hepatocellular necrosis, serum ALT activity sharply increases within 24 to 48 hours up to 100 times normal or higher to peak during the first five days after injury.[201–205] If the injurious agent or event is removed, the ALT activity gradually declines to normal over two to three weeks.

Extrahepatic bile duct occlusion is associated with a more gradual ALT increase of lesser initial magnitude than that associated with necrosis. Within three days of major bile duct occlusion, ALT activity may increase 5 to 45 times normal in the cat and 20 to 70 times in the dog.[146, 147, 201–203, 206–208] Within one to two weeks, ALT may peak at increases 20 to 40 times normal and sometimes higher in the dog, and up to 15 to 45 times normal in the cat.[146, 147, 201, 202, 204] Severe cholestasis induces hepatic necrosis and membrane alterations as a result of the noxious influence of bilirubin and bile salts on the hepatocytes and biliary network. After the initial one-to three-week increase in ALT activity, ALT declines but usually does not return to the normal range for several weeks.

Microsomal enzyme induction in dogs generally causes smaller increases in ALT activity than does necrosis or bile duct occlusion. Anticonvulsant medications given in usual therapeutic dosages may be associated with up to four-fold ALT increases. Following high-dose phenobarbital treatment (2 mg/lb or 4.4 mg/kg q8h), ALT has increased over 50 times normal in certain individuals.[209] Whether such large increases are consistently associated with morphologically evident hepatocellular injury is unknown. The administration of glucocorticoids (prednisone 2 mg/lb or 4.4 mg/kg q24h) to dogs may result in ALT activity two to five times normal within one week and up to ten times normal within 14 days.[210, 211] Dogs developing a glucocorticoid hepatopathy may have ALT activity increase up to 40 times normal. After discontinuation of short-acting glucocorticoids, ALT activity may persist for several weeks.

In the dog, marked increases in serum ALT activity may develop in association with primary hepatic neoplasia (hepatocellular carcinoma, hepatoma), secondary neoplasia and nodular hyperplasia.[118, 205, 211–214] Increased serum ALT activity from 3 to 35 times normal has been observed in dogs with hepatocellular carcinoma. Such increases could be caused by tumor-associated necrosis, compression and necrosis of adjacent normal hepatocytes, isoenzyme production, or abnormal membrane permeability in neoplastic cells (paraneoplastic enzyme liberation). Metastatic hepatic neoplasia in dogs and cats may be associated with normal serum ALT activity or with only slight to moderate increases. In exceptional cases, values as high as ten times normal have developed.

The serum activity of ALT in cats may be increased from 2 to 45 times normal in hepatic necrosis, cholangitis, or cholangiohepatitis, two to ten times normal in hepatic lipidosis, and two to five times normal in severe acute anemia, septicemia, and feline leukemia virus-associated disorders (lymphosarcoma, myeloproliferative disease).

Aspartate Aminotransferase

Aspartate aminotransferase (AST) is present in substantial concentrations in a wide variety of tissues. In the dog and cat, highest tissue concentrations are present in the heart, liver, skeletal muscle, kidney, and brain.[198, 203, 215–218] The plasma half-life of AST is reported as five hours in the dog and 77 minutes in the cat.[198, 216] Hepatic AST is located in the cytosol and associated with mitochondrial membranes. In humans, AST from hepatocellular mitochondria and cytosol is immunochemically distinct.[219] While most of the circulating AST is of cytosolic origin, the majority of the hepatocellular enzyme is in the mitochondrial form. In humans, the mitochondrial enzyme has a very short half-life in the systemic circulation; therefore, its presence in serum implies a severe hepatocellular insult involving organelle injury.[219] It is unknown if similar AST isoenzyme identification would be useful in the dog or cat.

Increased serum AST activity can result from altered membrane permeability, necrosis, inflammation, and, in the dog, microsomal enzyme induction. AST activity that is related to liver disease should parallel increases in ALT. In some circumstances, AST activity becomes quiescent before the ALT activity. Increases in the AST activity in the absence of abnormal ALT activity implicate an extrahepatic source of enzyme.

Following acute diffuse severe hepatic necrosis, AST activity increases sharply within the first three days, 10 to 30 times normal in dogs and up to 50 times normal in cats.[146, 203, 220] If the necrosis resolves, AST activity gradually declines over a period of two to three weeks.

Complete extrahepatic bile duct occlusion is associated with a marked rapid increase in AST during the first week, up to 25 times normal in the dog and 20 times normal in the cat. Enzyme activity may continue rising through three weeks or plateau and then gradually decline.[146, 147, 204] In experimentally induced obstructive jaundice, surgical trauma to muscle and viscera may be responsible for increased AST activity during the early postoperative period.

In some cats with liver disease, AST may be a more sensitive indicator of hepatobiliary disease than is ALT. This observation has been made in individual cats with hepatic necrosis, cholangiohepatitis, myeloproliferative disease, lymphosarcoma, and chronic bile duct obstruction.[147, 220, 221] Similar disparity between these two enzymes has been observed in humans with widespread, gross, or severe necrosis; as a result, it has been suggested that an AST:ALT ratio might be useful in projecting a prognosis.[222, 223] A ratio greater than 1.0 is associated with a poor prognosis. The application of this ratio has not been investigated in the dog or cat. A recent study of the diagnostic value of different liver enzymes in dogs with naturally developing hepatic disease indicated that increases in the AST activity were overall more sensitive than ALT.[224] The contribution of AST activity from other tissues, particularly in animals with metastatic cancer and in those with congestive heart failure, was suspected.

Dogs treated with glucocorticoids may have normal or only mild increases in the serum AST activity.[211] The induced enzyme activity resolves one to two weeks after glucocorticoid withdrawal.

Arginase

Arginase is considered a liver specific enzyme because it is present in higher concentrations in the hepatocytes than in any other tissue. It is a major constituent of the urea cycle, with large quantities located in the hepatocyte cytosol associated with mitochondria.[225, 226] A simplified method for analysis has made this test applicable for clinical practice.[227] Simultaneous measurements of serum arginase and transaminase activity may provide prognostic information concerning the nature of the associated hepatic disorder. With acute necrosis, ALT and arginase are immediately released from hepatocytes causing sharp increases in the serum enzyme activity.[228] If both plasma arginase and transaminase activities are continually increased, progressive hepatic necrosis is probable.[225] In dogs and cats, experimentally induced hepatic necrosis with CCl_4 results in a 500- to 1000-fold increase in arginase, which persists for only two to three days. During recovery from necrosis, leakage of transaminases but not arginase continues, ALT and AST activity remaining increased for one week or longer.[225, 228, 229]

Dogs treated with dexamethasone (1.5 mg/lb or 3 mg/kg q24h for 11 days), underwent a transient increase (five- to eight-fold) in arginase activity by day four.[230] With chronicity of treatment, a steady increase in the serum arginase activity was observed. On termination of the study (day 12), the serum arginase activity was ten times normal. It is possible that induction by glucocorticoids or the associated catabolism caused the increase in arginase activity, as has been reported in other species.[226, 230]

Alkaline Phosphatase

Increased serum alkaline phosphatase (ALP) activity is the most common biochemical abnormality observed in screening profiles of the canine patient. In the dog, ALP has high sensitivity but low specificity as a test for liver disease. In the cat it has a lower sensitivity but is more specific. ALP is a membrane bound enzyme present in many tissues.[215, 218, 231, 232] The tissue containing the greatest amount of ALP is the intestinal mucosa with lesser, yet substantial, amounts also present in the kidney cortex, placenta, liver and bone. The ALP extracted from these tissues are distinctly different isoenzymes.[208, 232–235] The four isoenzymes identifiable in canine serum include bone, liver, and glucocorticoid-induced isoenzymes and an isoenzyme of unknown origin and significance.[232] In the dog, the half-life of the placental, renal, and intestinal ALP is very short, less than six minutes.[232, 236] In the cat, the half-life of the intestinal isoenzyme is less than two minutes. Since the structures of the placental and renal isoenzymes in the cat are similar to those of the intestinal isoenzyme, they are also surmised to have a short half-life.[237, 238] The isoenzymes with ultra-short half-lives have not been observed in the serum of dogs or cats with increased ALP activity. The exception is the placental isoenzyme, which has been detected in late-term pregnant cats.[208] The liver isoenzyme is primarily responsible for the serum ALP activity in the normal dog and cat. The half-life of the liver isoenzyme is about six hours in the cat, while the half-lives of the liver and glucocorticoid-induced isoenzymes in the dog are approximately 70 hours.[232, 235, 236] The specific activity of ALP in liver extract from the normal dog has been reported as equal to or two-fold greater than that of the normal cat.[208, 215] Smaller increases in ALP activity are realized in cats with hepatobiliary disorders than in the dog as a result of the differences between serum ALP half-life and possibly because of the smaller inherent liver ALP content in this species. Regardless of the small magnitudes of change, ALP remains an important and useful diagnostic clue for feline hepatobiliary disease.[201, 202, 239]

The use of ALP in the dog is complicated by the accumulation of different isoenzymes in the serum and the ease with which the hepatic and glucocorticoid enzymes are induced. Clinical utility of ALP in the dog is improved through isoenzyme determination. The interpretation of ALP activity is less complicated in the cat than in the dog since there is no glucocorticoid isoenzyme and limited evidence of drug-initiated ALP induction. Since multiple isoenzymes do not accumulate in the serum of cats, isoenzyme determination is not clinically useful in this species.

The ALP bone isoenzyme increases as a result of osteoblast activity. It is present in the serum of young growing animals and may be associated with bone tumors and secondary renal hyperparathyroidism. Increases in ALP due to bone isoenzyme usually do not exceed four to six times normal.[232] Bone tumors may not affect serum ALP activity or they may cause a two- to three-fold increase. In the young cat, the magnitude of serum ALP activity attributable to the bone isoenzyme may simulate enzyme activity associated with hepatobiliary disease.

The liver ALP isoenzyme is thought to be derived from canalicular and hepatocyte cell membranes. This isoenzyme increases in serum as a result of increased de novo hepatic synthesis rather than merely through regurgitation into plasma.[232, 240] While ALT is immediately liberated as a result of acute hepatocellular necrosis, membrane-bound ALP, which is present in lesser amounts within the cytosol, is not immediately released.[232] Rather, it takes several days for induction to gear up and for ALP to spill into the circulation. Largest increases in the serum ALP liver isoenzyme activity (as high as 100 times normal or greater) are associated with diffuse or focal cholestatic disorders, primary hepatic neoplasms (hepatocellular carcinoma and bile duct carcinoma), and, in the dog, with enzyme induction. Marked increases in the serum ALP activity have also been reported in dogs with mammary cancer, but in that report osseous or hepatic metastasis was not clearly ruled out.[241] Circumstantial evidence suggested that the enzyme was liberated from the mammary neoplasia because tumor resection was followed by long-term survival and reduction in the serum ALP activity.

Following acute severe hepatic necrosis, ALP activity in the dog or cat increases two to five times normal, stabilizes, and then gradually declines over a two- to three-week interval.[201, 202, 208] In the cat, serum enzyme increases are less predictable than in the dog after an acute insult, and abnormalities seem to resolve faster.

Extrahepatic bile duct obstruction in the dog results in serum ALP activity that initially increases within eight hours. Values may reach 15 times normal by two to four days and as much as 50 to 100 times normal within one to two weeks. After this, the activity stabilizes and gradually declines, but not into the normal range.[146, 205–207, 242] In the cat, extrahepatic bile duct obstruction results in a two-fold increase within two days, as much as a four-fold increase within one week, and up to a nine-fold increase within two to three weeks. After this, activity stabilizes and gradually declines but never to the normal range.[147, 208, 243] The specific activity of ALP in liver extracts from normal dogs was equivalent to those observed in liver extracts of cats having common bile duct occlusion for 21 days.[208] Cats with partial occlusion of the biliary tree (ligation of major hepatic ducts) showed serum ALP activity approximately half that observed in cats with complete occlusion of the common duct.[208] In contrast, even partial occlusion of the biliary tree in the dog causes huge increases in the serum ALP activity.

Many different extrahepatic and hepatic conditions may promote increased production of the hepatic ALP isoenzyme. Hepatic parenchymal inflammation and systemic inflammation may cause secondary intrahepatic cholestasis.[232, 244] It has been speculated that alterations in the energy-dependent sodium-potassium membrane pump cause isosmotic fluid imbibition within the hepatocyte. This results in hepatocellular swelling and subsequent cholestasis. Any involvement of biliary structures causes increased ALP synthesis and regurgitation of enzyme into blood. Processes associated with increased local accumulations of bile salts may potentiate this regurgitation by alteration of the cell membrane permeability.[245] This facilitates release of newly synthesized ALP. Increases in hepatic isoenzyme owing to secondary hepatic effects are especially common in the dog and may cause ALP activity to increase up to 5 times normal.

The glucocorticord isoenzyme in the dog is produced in the intestine and liver.[232, 246, 247] It can be identified in serum by many different techniques. This isoenzyme develops in animals treated with glucocorticoids, in those with spontaneous or iatrogenic hyperadrenocorticism, and in some dogs with hepatic neoplasia or chronic illness.[233, 246] Dogs with hepatic neoplasia may have increased hepatic and glucocorticoid isoenzymes in the absence of exposure to exogenous corticosteroids. It has not been proved whether this isoenzyme is of tumor origin or is induced by the neoplasm.[233, 248] There is no apparent correlation between the magnitude of increased serum ALP activity due to the glucocorticoid isoenzyme and the presence of a steroid hepatopathy.[211] In the dog, serum ALP activity increases as early as one week after daily administration of prednisolone (1 mg/lb or 2 mg/kg q24h),[249] as early as two days after the daily administration of prednisone (2 mg/lb or 4.4 mg/kg q24h),[210] and as early as three days after daily administration of dexamethasone (1 mg/lb or 2.2 mg/kg q24h).[211] The initial increase in ALP activity is attributed to the liver isoenzyme. Thereafter, the glucocorticoid isoenzyme is present. Different magnitudes of enzyme activity develop depending on the type of glucocorticoid administered, the dosage, and the individual patient response.[210, 232, 250, 251] Increases in serum ALP activity due to the glucocorticoid isoenzyme are often greater than those observed with liver or bone isoenzymes. Following 14 consecutive daily doses of 2 mg/lb or 4.4 mg/kg prednisone after which treatment was discontinued, dogs reached a maximum ALP activity of 64 times normal by day 20. These values decreased gradually to eight-fold normal by day 56.[251] In these dogs, histopathologic evaluation revealed a vacuolar change in hepatocytes by day two, which progressed to maximum severity between days 5 and 14. This study is particularly relevant to clinical practice since commonly prescribed immunosuppressive dosages of prednisone were used. The plasma concentrations of prednisone, prednisolone, and cortisol remained increased for a total of 30 days (14 days of treatment and 16 days after

withdrawal of the aqueous prednisone therapy).[251] The production of the glucocorticoid ALP isoenzyme does not imply that a dog treated with cortisone has iatrogenic hyperadrenocorticism, a suppressed pituitary adrenal axis, or clinically important glucocorticoid hepatopathy. The corticosteroid isoenzyme can also increase in chronically ill dogs, perhaps as a result of endogenous corticosteroid release. Liver biopsy in some chronically ill dogs has shown a glucocorticoid-like hepatopathy (vacuolar hepatopathy) in spite of normal dexamethasone suppression and ACTH response tests and in the absence of historical exposure to glucocorticoids.

The relative insensitivity of the feline liver to glucocorticoids has been demonstrated. Administration of prednisolone (5 mg q12h) to normal cats for 30 days failed to elicit an increase in the activity of ALP in serum or liver tissue.[237] In another study, when cats received 1 mg/lb (2 mg/kg) prednisolone q24h for 16 days, changes in serum ALP activity and morphologic hepatocellular alterations were rare or minor when present.[252]

In the dog, the serum activity of the liver ALP isoenzyme may be increased by administration of the anticonvulsants phenobarbital, primidone, and phenytoin.[209, 253] Induced changes in serum ALP activity usually approximate two- to six-fold increases. During a 30-day study of drug administration to normal dogs, phenytoin (10 mg/lb or 22 mg/kg q8h) produced a uniform, yet small, increase in serum ALP activity. Phenobarbital (2 mg/lb or 4.4 mg/kg q8h) produced peak serum enzyme activity of 30 times normal by 24 days, which then declined. One of two dogs receiving phenobarbital had biochemical evidence of hepatic necrosis, which was speculated to have been drug induced. Primidone (8 mg/lb or 17.6 mg/kg q8h) produced a five-fold increase in serum ALP activity by day 28. Since this preliminary study, in-depth examination of normal dogs and clinical patients receiving chronic anticonvulsant therapy has been completed.[155, 253] Normal dogs receiving combination therapy (primidone and phenytoin) developed ALP increases that ranged from 2 to 12 times normal and some receiving high dose phenobarbital had ALP activity 30 to 40 times normal. Since primidone and phenobarbital are microsomal enzyme inducers, increases in serum ALP activity are not unexpected.

In contrast to the dog, the administration of phenobarbital (0.25 grain q12h) for 30 days in cats failed to elicit an increase in serum or liver ALP activity.[237]

Gamma-Glutamyltransferase

Gamma-glutamyltransferase, also known as γ-glutamyltranspeptidase (GGT), is a glycoprotein important in amino acid membrane transport, foreign compound detoxification, and glutathione metabolism.[254–256] Most body cells contain GGT. Highest tissue GGT concentrations in the dog and cat are present in the kidney and pancreas,[206, 257] with lesser quantities present in the liver, gallbladder, intestines, spleen, heart, lungs, skeletal muscle, and erythrocytes.[210] Renal GGT is located mainly in the microvillus border of the proximal convoluted tubules. The renal enzyme is excreted in the urine and the pancreatic enzyme is excreted with other exocrine pancreatic substances; therefore, neither source of enzyme is thought to be an important source of serum GGT activity.[258–261] It is believed that the major source of serum GGT activity is the liver. There is considerable species variation in the localization of GGT within the liver. Hepatic microsomal localization has been shown in the dog, in which it is associated with the bile ducts and perilobular parenchyma.[257, 262–264] Similar to serum ALP increases, increased GGT activity is the result of increased de novo hepatic synthesis and regurgitation or elution of enzyme from cell membranes rather than of release of free cytosolic enzyme.[265, 266]

Studies of serum GGT activity in dogs and cats undergoing acute severe diffuse necrosis have shown either no change or a mild one- to three-fold increase that resolves over the ensuing ten days. Extrahepatic bile duct obstruction in the dog causes increases of 10- to 50-fold within one to two weeks, after which values may plateau or continue to increase as high as 100-fold.[204, 206] In the cat, serum GGT activity may increase up to two-fold within three days, two- to six-fold within five days, three- to 12-fold within a week, and four- to 16-fold within two weeks.[201, 202] The activity in liver extract from cats with a ligated bile duct had a 1.5-fold increase in tissue GGT activity as compared with that of healthy cats.[202]

Increased serum GGT activity is commonly associated with intrahepatic or extrahepatic cholestasis or pancreatitis. The diagnostic performance of GGT in clinical cases has been examined.[206, 239, 267] In the dog, GGT appears to offer little if any diagnostic advantage over ALP. Glucocorticoids and certain other microsomal enzyme-inducing drugs stimulate GGT production in many tissues similar to their influence on ALP. Administration of dexamethasone (1.5 mg/lb or 3 mg/kg q24h) or prednisone (2 mg/lb or 4.4 mg/kg q24h IM) induced GGT activity within one week from four to seven times normal and up to ten times normal within two weeks.[210, 230, 251] Increased serum GGT activity observed in dogs

given glucocorticoids is thought to be of hepatic origin. Most dogs given anticonvulsants develop only a modest increase in serum GGT activity (up to two- or three-fold) in contrast to the profound induction of ALP.[155]

In the cat, GGT activity in certain hepatobiliary disorders may be more markedly increased than is ALP (Figure 88–4).[239] Differences between individual cats and the hepatic zonal involvement may be influential in causing these variations. Cats with cirrhosis, major bile duct obstruction, or intrahepatic cholestasis usually have a larger magnitude of serum GGT increase as compared to ALP. Cholestasis is thought to enhance the synthesis as well as the release of hepatic GGT. Release may be facilitated by the local accumulation of bile acids.[245] It is unknown whether glucocorticoids or other enzyme inducers influence serum GGT activity in the cat. Clinical experience of the author suggests that this does not occur.

In humans, a unique GGT isoenzyme has been identified in association with hepatocellular carcinoma.[268] It is unknown if this occurs in the dog or cat. Eight- to ten-fold and higher increases in the serum GGT activity have been observed in some dogs with hepatocellular carcinoma and biliary carcinoma.[206, 224] In humans who have ascites associated with liver tumors or active cirrhosis, GGT activity may be detected in the ascitic fluid, and its presence used as a diagnostic test.[269] It is unknown if this is true in the dog or cat. Although GGT is renowned as an indicator of hepatic metastasis in humans, it is not apparently suitable for this purpose in the dog or cat.[270]

Like ALP, GGT lacks specificity in differentiating between parenchymatous hepatic disease and obstructive cholestatic disease. Although it is less sensitive in the dog than is ALP it is more specific in the diagnosis of liver disease.[224] In the cat, it appears that GGT is more sensitive but less specific than ALP. These enzymes are most informative when they are evaluated simultaneously in the cat. The prediction of hepatic lipidosis is possible if the history, physical findings, and

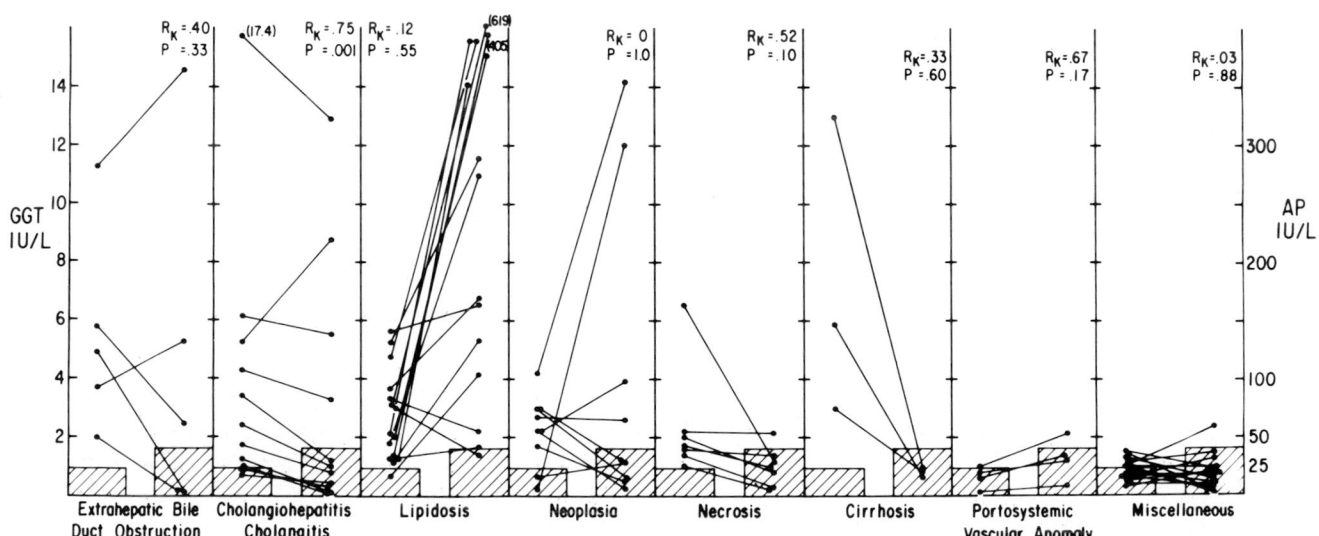

FIGURE 88–4. Comparison of serum activity of gamma-glutamyltransferase (GGT) and alkaline phosphatase (ALP) in cats wtih different hepatobiliary disorders confirmed by histologic examination. Cats with miscellaneous disorders had no morphologic evidence of liver disease. (From Center, SA et al.: JAVMA 188:509, 1986, Fig 1.)

routine biochemical features are considered along with the GGT and ALP activities. In most hepatobiliary disorders in the cat the magnitude of increased serum GGT activity exceeds that of ALP.[239] In hepatic lipidosis, there is usually a marked increase in ALP in contrast to the GGT activity, which may be within the normal range.

MISCELLANEOUS CAUSES OF LIVER ENZYME ABNORMALITIES

One of the most common causes of increased liver enzyme activity in the dog is treatment with glucocorticoids. These drugs are commonly used for their anti-inflammatory and immunosuppressive effects. A glucocorticoid hepatopathy has been well characterized in dogs treated with glucocorticoids or that have spontaneous or iatrogenic hyperadrenocorticism. Glucocorticoid-induced enzyme activity is far more common than the development of a clinically important glucocorticoid hepatopathy. Several investigators have studied the chronologic response of the hepatobiliary system to different glucocorticoids in the dog by documenting the induced changes in serum enzymes, liver function, and morphology. Exposure to daily 2 mg/lb (4.4 mg/kg IM) injections of aqueous prednisone for 14 days resulted in increases in ALP, AST, and GGT activities and no change in leucine aminopeptidase or sulfobromophthalein retention.[210, 251] Histologic findings confirmed the development of hepatocellular changes during the first week of treatment.

Although it is important to recognize biochemical changes induced by glucocorticoids, it must be realized that the enzymic changes depend on individual response, dose of drug, and the particular drug used. Many variables influence the different times of peak serum enzyme activities in relation to the drug administration.[251] Increased enzyme activity may result from enzyme liberation from damaged hepatocytes, altered metabolism and/or elimination rates, altered protein anabolism, or combinations of mechanisms.[251, 271, 272] A demonstrated disparity between the time of maximal morphologic change and peak serum enzyme activity supports the concept of enzyme induction. Continued enzyme induction after drug discontinuation probably depends on the persistence of high glucocorticoid concentrations in the circulation and/or their continued biologic effects after drug elimination.[272, 273] Longer duration of effects is expected with the longer-acting glucocorticoids. Although severe glucocorticoid hepatopathy can cause functional disturbances, most dogs with enzyme induction have not developed hepatic dysfunction. Functional insufficiency seems restricted to dogs with clinical evidence of spontaneous or iatrogenic hyperadrenocorticism, those given inappropriately large glucocorticoid dosages for long periods, or those with some underlying hepatic disorder. There is no proved correlation between the degree of enzyme induction or the presence of a glucocorticoid hepatopathy and the status of the pituitary adrenal axis. A liver biopsy *cannot* be used to confirm the presence of hyperadrenocorticism.

The anticonvulsant drugs primidone, phenytoin, and phenobarbital, administered singly or in combination, cause variable increases in liver enzyme activity in the dog. Some dogs receiving chronic anticonvulsant therapy develop morphologic evidence of liver disease and functional impairment. The majority, however, merely develop increased serum activities of ALP, ± ALT, AST, and GGT. Primidone and phenobarbital seem more consistently to be associated with increased liver enzyme activity than is phenytoin, perhaps owing to the ultra-short half-life of the latter drug in the dog. Combination anticonvulsant therapy with primidone and phenytoin or phenobarbital more consistently induces enzyme activity and to larger magnitudes than does single drug therapy.[155] Increases in ALT and AST activity up to two times baseline may develop with each drug used alone. Combination therapy may induce transaminase activity 3 to 5 times normal. Serum alkaline phosphatase activity appears to be more remarkably and consistently affected by anticonvulsants than are the transaminases. Changes in the serum ALP activity are discussed elsewhere in this chapter. A significant linear association has been shown between the primidone dosage and the magnitude of the serum ALT increase and between dosage of primidone and of phenytoin and the magnitude of serum ALP activity.[155] GGT activity is infrequently altered in dogs receiving phenytoin but values as high as two times baseline may develop with primidone and combination treatment.[155] Delayed BSP (sulfobromophthalein) plasma clearance was common in a group of clinical patients with seizure abnormalities treated long term with anticonvulsants.[253] Histologic examination of hepatic tissue could not be obtained for each patient and therefore the presence of morphologic disease was not determined. It is possible that the pharmacokinetics of BSP were influenced by the anticonvulsants. It seemed that serum fasting bile acids more distinctly differentiated dogs with severe liver disease from those with mere enzyme induction.

On the basis of the cumulative information regarding the idiosyncratic development of liver disease in dogs on extended anticonvulsant therapy, the following recommendations are advised. Re-evaluation should include a thorough history, physical examination, and biochemical assessment, including liver enzymes, cholesterol, albumin, and total bilirubin. This is recommended at 6- to 12-month intervals. In patients with compromised hepatic function, seizure activity is usually well controlled owing to decreased excretion of the anticonvulsant. Severe hypocholesterolemia and hypoalbuminemia may reflect hepatic failure. Marked increases in liver enzymes or decreases in albumin or cholesterol should be followed with quantification of the fasting and two-hour postprandial serum bile acids to assess the adequacy of hepatic function. It is the author's opinion that BSP retention is unreliable as a measure of liver function in this population of dogs.

Hyperthyroidism in the cat is often associated with increases in the serum transaminases and ALP activity; this can distract the clinician from pursuing and treating the underlying endocrinopathy.[274] Careful palpation of the cervical area for a thyroid-associated mass is essential in any aged cat showing nonspecific enzyme activity.

The origin of the ALP in hyperthyroid cats is unknown. In hyperthyroid humans, increased serum ALP activity is the most common biochemical abnormality identified on routine screening tests. The source of enzyme has been identified as bone and liver. In humans, severe thyrotoxicosis is associated with changes in hepatic morphology due to cardiac failure, severe weight loss, or the direct toxic effects of thyroid hormone.[275–277] Similar considerations seem applicable to the cat. In most cases, only modest and nonspecific histologic lesions are found in liver tissue, including centrilobular fatty infiltration and mild necrosis.[276] Evidence of liver dysfunction is uncommon. Despite the increase in cardiac output that occurs in hyperthyroidism, the liver does not realize an increased circulation.[278] At the same time, the splanchnic oxygen consumption increases owing to the increased metabolic rate.[278] Any pre-existent hepatic disease may flourish under these conditions. The liver enzyme abnormalities associated with hyperthyroidism resolve with restitution of a euthyroid status.

Acute and chronic passive congestion of the liver may result in mild to moderate increases in the serum ALP and transaminase activity.[279] Abnormal retention of BSP may occur owing to the circulatory maladjustments. These patients usually have normal serum bile acid concentrations. In humans, evidence of decreased hepatic function may develop in some patients with congestive heart failure, including prolonged coagulation time, hypoalbuminemia, and hyperbilirubinemia.[280] Similar abnormalities are uncommon in the dog and cat.

Increases in liver enzymes, particularly ALP, are common in dogs with hypothyroidism and in dogs and cats with diabetes mellitus and pancreatitis.[281] Disorders associated with endotoxemia, septicemia, anoxia, hyperthermia, thromboembolism, changes in hepatic perfusion caused by hypotension, and microsomal enzyme induction in the dog may also be associated with increased liver enzyme activities. In most instances the magnitudes of increase do not exceed two to three times normal. Some septicemic patients may develop hyperbilirubinemia as a result of intrahepatic cholestasis. The manifestations of the underlying infection usually dominate the clinical signs. Toxic effects of microbial organisms (bacterial products, induced hypotension, organ infiltration) are believed to underlie the intrahepatic cholestasis.[280]

Primary and secondary hepatic neoplasia are commonly associated with biochemical evidence of liver involvement. Increases in the transaminases, ALP, and GGT are variable. The dual blood supply of the liver makes it a frequent site for metastasis. In a study of metastatic liver disease in the dog,[214] AST was the most sensitive indicator of hepatic involvement, and the ALT and ALP together detected liver disease in 70 per cent of 95 dogs. Of these dogs, 25 had lymphosarcoma and 9 had hemangiosarcoma. In another report of 15 dogs with metastatic hepatic neoplasia, abnormalities included increased ALT in 46 per cent, increased ALP in 50 per cent, and hyperbilirubinemia in 46 per cent.[213] Of these, five had lymphosarcoma and two had hemangiosarcoma. Canine tumors that have been associated with increased serum ALP activity include pancreatic adenocarcinoma, intestinal adenocarcinoma, leiomyo-sarcoma, giant cell tumor, adrenal cortical adenocarcinoma, mixed mammary tumor, hemangiosarcoma, lymphosarcoma, and oral carcinoma. Although metastatic hepatic involvement seems likely in most instances, the development of unique isoenzymes cannot be discounted.[214, 281] Laboratory findings reported in 8 dogs with primary hepatocellular carcinoma included increased ALT and ALP activity in 100 per cent, hypoalbuminemia and hyperglobulinemia in 83 per cent, hypoglycemia in 38 per cent, and hyperbilirubinemia in 25 per cent.[213] GGT activity is also markedly increased in dogs with hepatocellular carcinoma.

In addition to glucocorticoids and anticonvulsants, other drugs may cause transient increases in the serum activity of liver enzymes. Idiosyncratic drug reactions resulting in biochemical changes and hepatic pathology are discussed in Chapter 89. Increased transaminases and ALP may follow the administration of thiacetarsamide and ketoconazole.[282–284] In each case, substantial hepatic necrosis has not been proved to occur every time enzyme changes are realized. Dogs with severe heartworm disease may be more susceptible to the toxic effects of thiacetarsamide owing to sluggish hepatic perfusion and underlying anoxia. It is difficult to consistently induce extensive hepatic necrosis in normal dogs given this drug at therapeutic dosages.[282] Biochemical changes during ketoconazole therapy have been observed in dogs and have been extensively studied in humans.[283, 284] In humans, the number of patients with functional impairment and progressive hepatic disease seems small. Since increased hepatic enzymes were common in patients before any treatment it was suggested that hepatotoxic mycotoxins may be responsible for increased serum enzyme activity. In addition, destruction of organisms during treatment may accelerate the release of hepatotoxic fungal products. In many patients, the increased serum enzyme activity normalized despite continued ketaconazole treatment.

Alpha-Fetoprotein

Alpha-fetoprotein (α-fetoprotein) is a glycoprotein synthesized by hepatocytes and released into the systemic circulation. Mammalian liver cells have the capacity to synthesize α-fetoprotein and secrete it into the blood during fetal life. This capability decreases during the perinatal period. In humans, increased serum α-fetoprotein concentrations develop in patients with hepatocellular carcinoma, hepatomas, malignant disease of yolk-sac cell origin (gonadal carcinomas), and a variety of liver diseases including viral hepatitis, chronic active hepatitis, and cirrhosis.[285] Following an 80 per cent hepatectomy, α-fetoprotein does not increase in humans. In contrast, 70 per cent hepatectomy in normal dogs causes an increase in serum α-fetoprotein on postoperative day four, reaching peak activity during days 8 and 12, after which values return to normal by day 24.[286] Alpha-fetoprotein activity is more consistently and chronically increased during hepatic regeneration than are conventional serum enzymes and total bilirubin. Alpha-fetoprotein therefore appears to be a superior marker for normal hepatic regeneration in the dog.[286]

Increases in α-fetoprotein have been reported in dogs with experimentally induced hepatic carcinomas.[287] If present in a patient with neoplasia, α-fetoprotein might serve as a paraneoplastic marker. The clinical application of this test in the dog or cat has not been investigated.

BILIRUBIN METABOLISM

The serum bilirubin concentration reflects the balance between the rate of heme pigment liberation, hepatocellular uptake, storage, and conjugation of bilirubin, and its ultimate biliary disposal. An overview of bilirubin metabolism is given in Figure 88–5.

Bilirubin pigments are derived in part from nonhemoglobin hemoproteins available from myoglobin, cytochromes, and other heme containing enzymes located primarily in the liver.[46, 288, 289] From 60 to 80 per cent of the serum bilirubin is derived from hemoglobin released from senescent erythrocytes and ineffective erythropoiesis. This major source of heme is initially catabolized in phagocytic cells of the monocyte-macrophage or reticuloendothelial (RE) system. Globin is dissociated from heme and is hydrolyzed to its constituent amino acids. Iron is mobilized bound to transferrin to be recycled to erythrogenic progenitors in the bone marrow for hemoglobin synthesis. The heme moiety is converted to biliverdin by microsomal heme oxygenase in RE cells of the bone marrow, spleen and liver, and the parenchymal cells of the liver and kidney.[200, 290] Biliverdin reductase converts biliverdin to unconjugated bilirubin, which is transported into the vascular compartment. There it is avidly bound to albumin. Unconjugated bilirubin is lipid soluble. Avid binding to albumin improves its water solubility while restricting its distribution to within the vascular compartment. As a result, unconjugated bilirubin is not filtered through glomeruli into urine. Dissociation of unconjugated bilirubin and albumin occurs at the surface of the hepatocyte, where a carrier-mediated mechanism transports bilirubin inside the cell.[46, 289, 291] As unconjugated bilirubin enters the hepatocyte, it is taken up and transported by an anionic binding protein, ligandin or Y protein, which is associated with the enzyme glutathione S transferase. A secondary cytoplasmic binding factor, Z protein or fatty acid–binding protein, also assists in the hepatocellular storage and transport of bilirubin.[292–294] Intracellular binding of bilirubin to storage proteins may accelerate its cellular uptake, enhancing its diffusion into and its concentration within the hepatocellular cytosol.[292–294]

Transformation of unconjugated bilirubin to the water-soluble, conjugated form occurs by binding of bilirubin to glucuronide, forming mono- and diglucuronide conjugates. This process is catalyzed by glucuronyl transferase in the endoplasmic reticulum of the hepatocyte associated with the canalicular membranes.[295, 296] Transport of bilirubin conjugates into canaliculi is energy dependent and is the rate-limiting step in the hepatobiliary processing of bilirubin.[288] When bilirubin has decreased entry into bile or when excessive liberation of heme pigments overwhelms the capability of the hepatobiliary system to process or excrete bilirubin, it may regurgitate into the systemic circulation, causing hyperbilirubinemia.[289]

Conjugated bilirubin is less avidly protein bound than is unconjugated bilirubin; therefore, it can be filtered through the glomeruli. Detection of excessive bilirubinuria indicates conjugated hyperbilirubinemia or decreased bilirubin-protein binding that would allow increased glomerular filtration of free bilirubin. Decreased protein binding can result from hypoalbuminemia or the competitive displacement of bilirubin from albumin by a variety of exogenous substances.[297] Urine bilirubin can also be directly produced in the renal tubule cells from hemoglobin or biliverdin.[298–304] Hemoglobinemia severe enough to exceed the haptoglobin-binding capacity allows free hemoglobin to be filtered into urine. Subsequent uptake and metabolism of hemoglobin by renal tubule cells may yield bilirubinuria. In the process, iron is liberated from heme and may be retained as hemosiderin in the renal tubule cells. The detection of iron-positive tubule cells in urine sediment implies recent hemoglobinemia (intravascular hemolysis). In the dog, the kidney, spleen, and intestines can conjugate bilirubin, although the quantitative significance of this alternate route of bilirubin metabolism is small in health.[302] Male dogs seemingly have a greater capacity than females to excrete renally produced bilirubin in urine.[304]

After entering the bile, bilirubin is expelled into the intestines. Conjugated bilirubin is not absorbed by the intestinal mucosa owing to its poor lipid solubility. Rather, it is excreted in the feces or is metabolized by colonic bacteria to other products (urobilinogens, stercobilinogens). The presence of large amounts of bilirubin pigments in feces causes a dark orange-brown to green stool coloration.

Urobilinogen is a colorless product of enteric bacterial degradation of conjugated bilirubin. Only around 20 per cent of the urobilinogens are reabsorbed in the large intestine.[288] Of that reabsorbed, most is efficiently extracted by the liver and is re-excreted in bile, completing an enterohepatic circulation. The remainder is eliminated in urine. The detection of urobilinogenuria provides evidence of an intact enterohepatic circulation of bilirubin pigments. The best clinical application of the test occurs when urobilinogenuria is absent during jaundice. This indicates cessation of bilirubin entry into the intestines, usually as a result of extrahepatic bile duct obstruction. Unfortunately, the test has many shortcomings. While complete extrahepatic bile duct obstruction theoretically should prohibit the enteric production of urobilinogen and therefore the appearance of urobilinogenuria, this is not always so. Bleeding tendencies and ulcerogenic complications of liver disease frequently cause enteric hemorrhage, resulting in an alternate route of bilirubin entry into the bowel. False-negative test results may be produced by alteration of the intestinal flora by chronic antibiotic administration, altered intestinal transit rates, malabsorption syndromes, and improper urine sample management. Urine stored too long or in the presence of light encourages the conversion of urobilinogen to urobilin that is undetected by the routine dipstick test for urobilinogen. The alimentary urobilinogens that are not absorbed (80 per cent) may undergo

BILIRUBIN METABOLISM

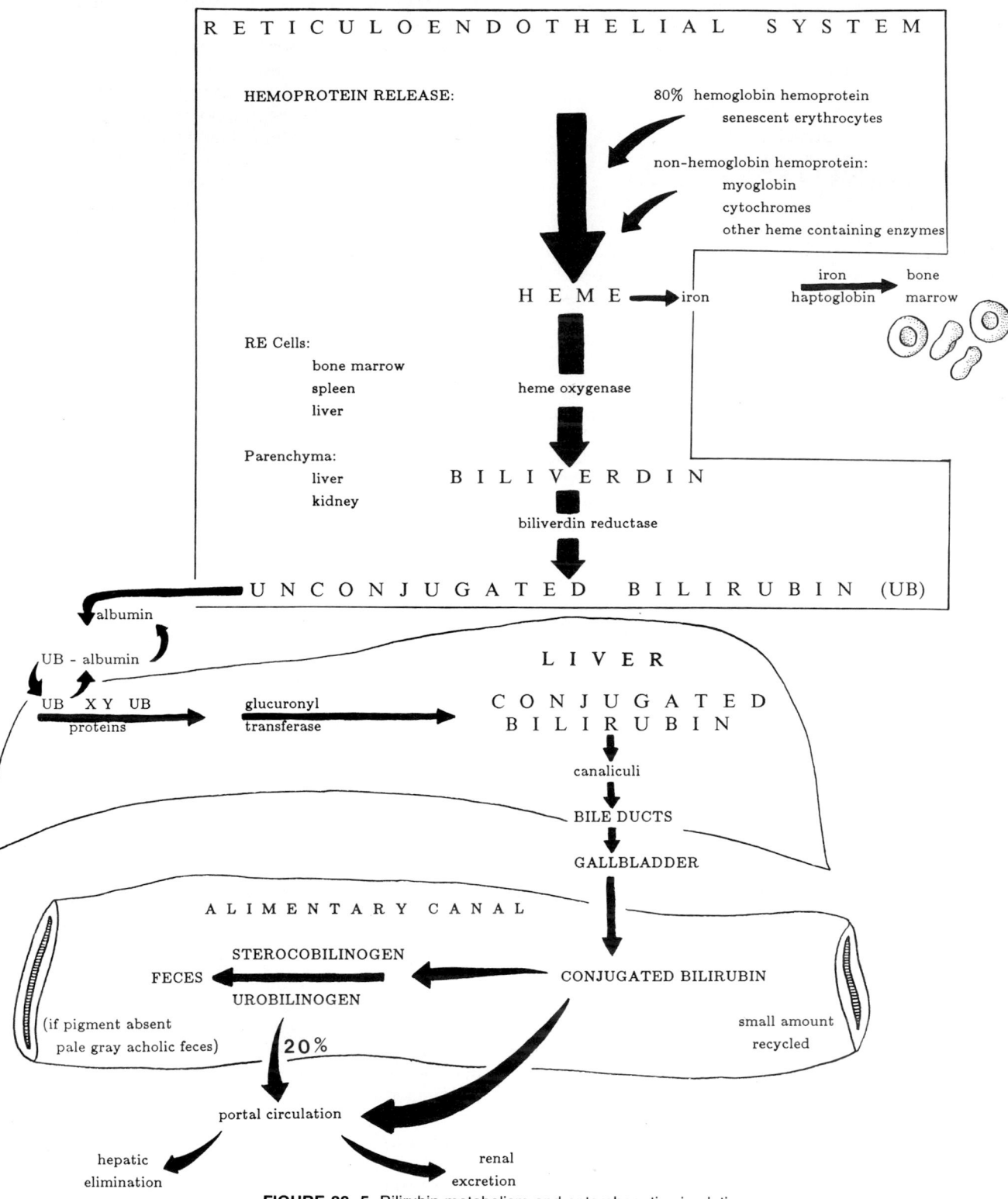

FIGURE 88–5. Bilirubin metabolism and enterohepatic circulation.

oxidation to urobilins and stercobilins. These substances are responsible for the normal brown fecal pigmentation and when absent result in pale-colored or acholic stools that indicate obstructed biliary drainage.

The total serum bilirubin can be fractionated into the unconjugated and conjugated moieties using the van den Bergh reaction. Conjugated bilirubin reacts directly (direct bilirubin) with the van den Bergh reagents, while unconjugated bilirubin does not (indirect bilirubin). Unconjugated bilirubinemia indicates increased heme pigment liberation and/or delayed hepatic bilirubin uptake, storage, or conjugation. Acute hemolytic disorders are principally responsible for unconjugated bilirubinemia in the dog and cat. These conditions are generally associated with serum total bilirubin values less than 10 mg/dl. Unconjugated hyperbilirubinemia exists only transiently without an associated conjugated component. Clinical experience with hemolytic disorders in the dog and cat suggests that the development of predominantly unconjugated hyperbilirubinemia occurs only during the very early stages of hemolysis. Since most animal patients are presented after clinical signs are obvious to their owner, the veterinarian has limited opportunity to evaluate bilirubin concentrations during peracute disease. As more unconjugated bilirubin is produced, an equilibration between the unconjugated and conjugated forms occurs. Minor alterations in hepatocellular function secondary to hypoxia or bilirubin toxicity may be partially responsible for the development of conjugated hyperbilirubinemia associated with hemolysis.

Owing to its water solubility and higher frequency of occurrence, conjugated bilirubinemia is the principal cause of tissue jaundice in the dog and cat. Because of the common occurrence of conjugated bilirubinemia, the "late" owner presentation for hemolytic jaundice, and because of the valuable information gleaned from history, physical examination, and screening blood tests, fractionation of serum bilirubin by the van den Bergh technique is usually unnecessary. This procedure rarely provides information not already apparent from other examinations.

Although less sensitive than the liver enzymes in identifying hepatobiliary disorders, the concentration of total bilirubin is a more specific indicator of hepatic disease. Using bilirubin values adjunctively with the serum enzymes improves the diagnostic performance of each test. Jaundice becomes clinically detectable when bilirubin values exceed 1.5 to 2.0 mg/dl. Conditions associated with jaundice in the dog and cat are listed in Table 88–11. When liver disease is responsible for jaundice, a severe diffuse cholestatic disorder or major bile duct obstruction is suspected. When primary cholestasis is the underlying disorder, jaundice often develops earlier in the course of the disease than with parenchymal disorders. Total bilirubin concentrations documented in dogs and cats with different forms of hepatobiliary disease are shown in Figure 88–6.

In animals with extrahepatic bile duct obstruction, hyperbilirubinemia is evident within several hours and jaundice may be detectable as early as 48 hours. Within three to five days after the obstruction, serum bilirubin concentrations may increase 10 to 20 times normal.[146, 147, 204, 207] With chronic bile duct obstruction exceeding two weeks, serum bilirubin levels may plateau at levels up to 50 to 70 times normal and then gradually decrease, but not to normal concentrations. It has been suggested that the gradual decrease occurs because of development of alternate routes of bilirubin excretion.[302] A compensatory increase in the renal elimination of bilirubin has been shown.[305]

In severe acute diffuse hepatic necrosis, bilirubin may increase two-fold within one to four days but then declines if reparative processes and reserve capacity can re-establish normal liver function. In dogs with 70 per cent hepatectomy, total bilirubin increased two-fold during the first postoperative week and then gradually declined over two to three weeks as regeneration occurred.[24]

Because bilirubinuria is evident before tissue jaundice becomes apparent, it has been acknowledged as a useful screening test for liver disease, although it is not specific. Bilirubin is normally present in the urine of dogs, albeit in small amounts. Detection at any urine specific gravity in the cat is a strong (specific) indication of hepatobiliary or hemolytic disorders.[306, 307] The sensitivity of urine bilirubin for the detection of hyperbilirubinemia and liver disease in cats is unknown. The use of the tablet method (Ictotest) for the detection of bilirubinuria is more sensitive and reliable than the reagent strip method and is therefore the preferred procedure.

The clinician is often faced with differentiating between intrahepatic and extrahepatic causes of jaundice. Accurate differentiation is important because these conditions require profoundly different managements. Extrahepatic jaundice is a mechanical problem that usually requires prompt surgical intervention. Intrahepatic cholestasis requires nonsurgical therapy; this condition may be worsened by the stresses of general anesthesia and surgical exploration.

Differential diagnosis of these conditions should be carefully explored according to the algorithm provided in Chapter 24. A thorough data base should include a complete history, physical examination, complete hemogram, routine serum biochemical profile, urinalysis, and abdominal radiographs. Cholangiography has not proven to be useful as a routine test in dogs or cats. Ultrasonographic examination of the abdomen is a valuable addition to the diagnostic armamentarium and may disclose distention or changes in structure or contents of the gallbladder and bile ducts, changes in the density and size of the liver, or the presence of abdominal fluid or other abdominal abnormalities. If cholestasis is suspected on the basis of the baseline laboratory data and the patient is jaundiced, liver function tests are superfluous. The clinical evaluation (history, physical, and routine laboratory tests) is more useful in the differentiation of extrahepatic from intrahepatic cholestasis than is any one specific test procedure. In two separate studies of the methods used to differentiate intrahepatic from extrahepatic jaundice in humans, the clinical evaluation had a better overall accuracy than did computed tomography, ultrasonography, or radioisotope scanning.[308, 309]

Some of the most challenging cholestatic conditions to differentiate are those associated with pancreatitis. Affected animals may develop intrahepatic or extrahepatic jaundice or have components of each. Some patients will develop occlusion of the extrahepatic bile duct subsequent to focal peritonitis and ascending cholangitis and these may require surgical biliary diversion. Not all such patients require immediate surgical intervention. The provision of conservative medical management may allow the resolution of the biliary obstruction as the pancreatic inflammation resolves. Sequential evaluation of total bilirubin concentration is more useful than measurements of alkaline phosphatase, transaminases, lipase, or amylase in deciding whether surgical

TABLE 88–11. DIFFERENTIAL DIAGNOSIS OF JAUNDICE

Prehepatic or Hemolytic Jaundice	Extrahepatic Jaundice	Hepatic Jaundice	
Hemolytic Anemias	Bile Duct Occlusion	Miscellaneous Disorders	
Erythrocyte parasitemia:	Cholecystitis	Endotoxemia	Hemolytic disease
Babesia	Cholangitis	Shock	Anoxia
Hemobartonella	1° and 2° peribiliary disease	Chronic passive congestion	DIC
Incompatible blood tranfusion	Congenital malformation:		
Neonatal isoerythrolysis	choledochal cysts		
Microangiopathic hemolytic anemia:	Intraluminal bile duct occlusion:		
DIC	inspissated bile (cats)		
vasculitis	cholelithiasis	Intrahepatic Cholestasis	
dirofilariasis	trauma blood clot		
vascular neoplasia (hemangiosarcoma)	Neoplasia:	Infectious:	
Congenital erythrocyte defects:	1° and 2° peribiliary involvement	viral (FIP, ICH, canine	
pyruvate kinase deficiency (basenji, beagle)	Pancreatic disease	parvovirus) bacterial	
phosphofructose kinase deficiency	Parasitic infection (flukes)	(leptospirosis,	
hereditary stomatocytosis (malamute)		septicemia)	
Immune-mediated hemolytic anemia	Ruptured Biliary Tract: (bile ducts	mycotic	
autoimmune hemolytic anemia	or gallbladder)	Neoplasia:	
SLE		mechanical-infiltrative	
infectious disease associated	Trauma		paraneoplastic
idiopathic	Cholelithiasis	Drug-associated:	
drug associated	Cholecystitis	methyltestosterone	
Infectious:	Cholangitis	(anabolics)	mebendazole
FeLV		tribrissen	
Ehrlichia		anticonvulsants	thiacetarsamide
dirofilariasis			acetaminophen
Toxins:		Specific hepatic disorders:	
lead		Cholangitis	
copper		Cholangiohepatitis	
propylene glycol		syndrome (cat)	Breed specific disorders:
Heinz body anemia		Chronic active hepatitis	Bedlington terrier
Toxins/oxidant stress:		Lobular dissecting	Doberman pinscher
acetaminophen		hepatitis	Cocker spaniel
phenazopyridine		Cirrhosis	W. H. white terrier
benzocaine, cetacaine		Hepatic lipidosis:	others?
methylene blue		idiopathic feline disease	
onions		diabetes mellitus	
vitamin K		2° to other disorders	
methionine		Severe steroid	
		hepatopathy (dog)	
		Hepatic necrosis	
Increased Hemoprotein Liberation		Infiltrative disease	
body cavity hemorrhage			
large hematoma formation			
ineffective erythropoiesis		Impaired Hepatobiliary Bilirubin Processing	
congenital porphyria (cats, rare)			
		Congenital Defects:	
		Impaired uptake ± storage:	Gilbert's syndrome (man)
			Mutant Southdown sheep
			Rotor's syndrome (man)
		Impaired conjugation:	Crigler-Najjar syndrome (man)
			Gunn rat
			anorexic cats(?)
		Impaired excretion:	Dubin-Johnson syndrome (man)
			Mutant Corriedale sheep

therapy is indicated. Animals with serum bilirubin concentrations continuously increasing over a course of ten days or more require surgery.

It is well established that bilirubin is toxic. The most common manifestation of bilirubin toxicity and the most written about is kernicterus, the neuropathy associated with severe unconjugated hyperbilirubinemia in human infants. Clinical signs range from subtle developmental and neurologic abnormalities to peracute encephalopathy that may be fatal.[46, 288] Kernicterus is characterized by yellow discoloration and degenerative lesions in the brain. Bilirubin has been shown to be toxic for a variety of enzymes and enzyme systems, and there is evidence that bilirubin may impair membrane function.[308–310] The toxic effects seem aggravated by hypoalbuminemia or decreased albumin binding.[311–312b] Infants are at increased risk for the development of kernicterus as a

result of reduced selectivity of the blood-brain barrier, immature enzyme systems for bilirubin metabolism, and the increased amount of neural lipids having preferential binding for bilirubin.[288] In comparison with humans, bilirubin toxicity is rare as a clinical diagnosis in the dog or cat. Neurologic lesions similar to those observed in infants were demonstrated in a kitten with naturally developing neonatal jaundice and encephalopathic signs.[313] Similar lesions have been induced in neonatal kittens by repeated intravenous injections of a bilirubin-albumin solution.[314] Lesions attributed to hyperbilirubinemia have also been demonstrated in dogs severely jaundiced as a result of choledochocaval anastomoses.[315] Renal changes were characterized by bile casts and pigmented droplets within tubular epithelium and glomerular mesangium. These dogs also developed cholestatic hepatic lesions. The ability of bilirubin to induce

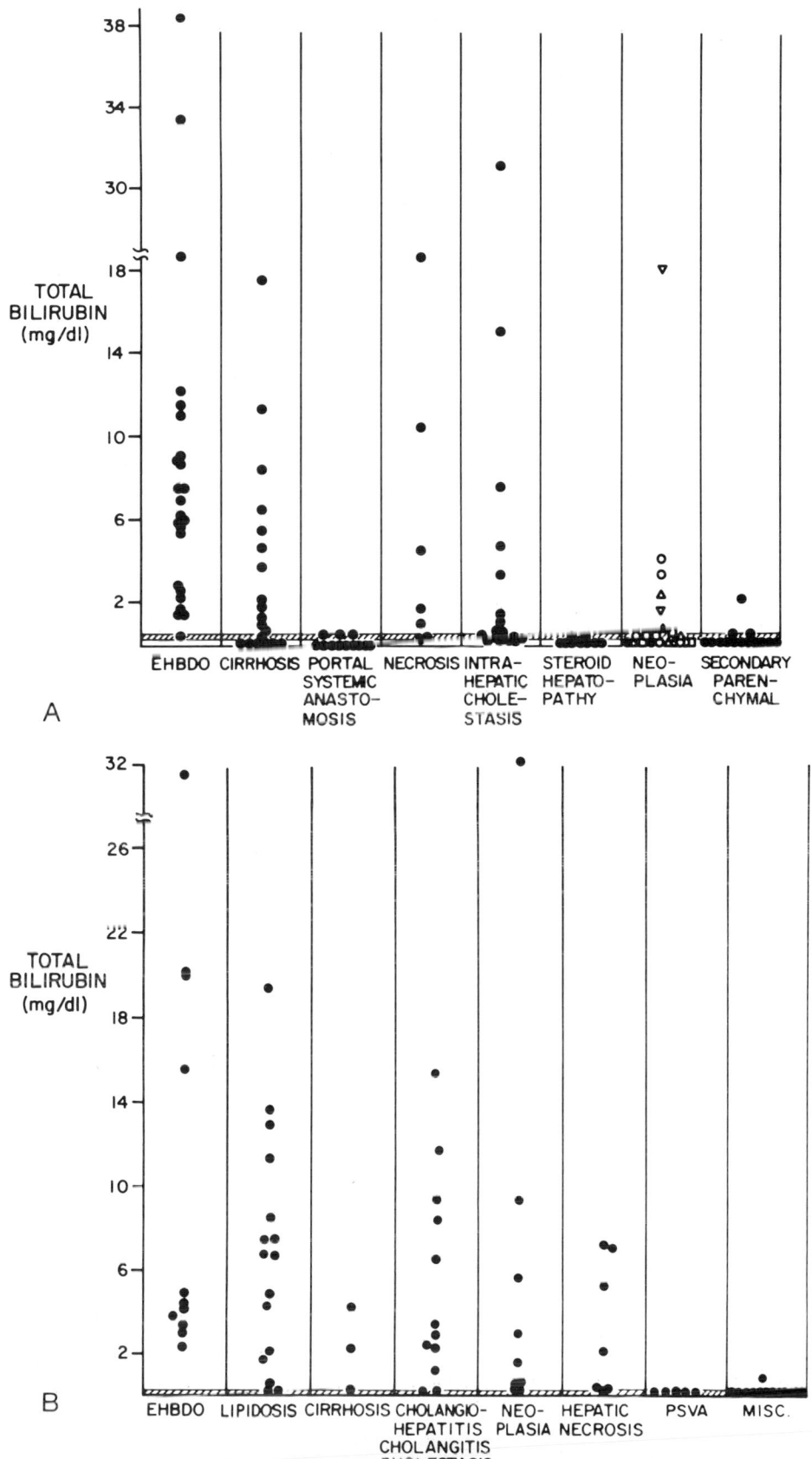

FIGURE 88-6. Serum total bilirubin values in dogs *(A)* and cats *(B)* with different hepatobiliary disorders confirmed by histologic examination. Animals with EHBDO had complete extrahepatic bile duct occlusion. Cats with PSVA had portosystemic vascular anomalies. Dogs with secondary parenchymal disorders and cats with miscellaneous (MISC) had mild or no morphologic lesions on histologic examination. (From Center, SA: JAVMA 187:937, 1985; 189:893, 1986.)

cholestasis has been documented in other studies in which the severity of cholestasis paralleled the magnitude of hyperbilirubinemia.[316, 317] Bilirubin cytotoxicity has been shown in dogs given massive intravenous doses of unconjugated bilirubin in which total bilirubin levels attained 60 and 70 mg/dl 15 minutes following injection and were 20 mg/dl in 3 to 4 hours.[315] Toxic effects were characterized by circulatory collapse, acute diarrhea, and death within 24 hours. Bilirubin and bile salt toxicity may play a role in the hepatocellular injury associated with cholestasis.[318] Bilirubin impairs hepatic mitochondrial function and uncouples oxidative phosphorylation. Bile salts damage hepatic microsomes, impair the function of cytochrome P450 and alter membrane permeability.[318] Morphologic injury to hepatocytes including feathery degeneration, cell necrosis, and subsequent focal reactive inflammation has been described as a sequela to cholestasis.

Heritable defects in bilirubin metabolism have been described in many animal species.[319] These, however, have not been documented in the dog or cat. It has been observed that certain ill and anorectic cats seem to have a tendency to develop unconjugated hyperbilirubinemia, but this remains controversial as it has not been adequately studied.

ORGANIC ANION CHOLEPHILIC DYES

Sulfobromophthalein (BSP) and indocyanine green (ICG) are cholephilic water-soluble dyes that have been used to clinically evaluate hepatic perfusion and hepatobiliary function. ICG is entirely dependent on hepatobiliary excretion, with a 97 per cent recovery in bile, whereas BSP has a bile recovery ranging between 50 and 80 per cent.[320, 321] Following intravenous injection, each dye is instantaneously bound to plasma proteins. The major binding proteins are albumin and an α_1-lipoprotein.[322] Protein binding restricts dye distribution to within the vascular compartment, more so for ICG, which is 90 per cent bound, than for BSP, which is less avidly protein bound. The removal of BSP and ICG from the plasma is closely associated with hepatic blood flow.[320, 323–326] Both dyes are high-extraction substances with clearance primarily determined by the rate of circulatory delivery to the hepatocytes. Hepatobiliary excretion involves a complex series of processes including delivery to the hepatocyte, uptake into the cell, binding to cytosolic carrier proteins, cytosolic storage, biotransformation (BSP conjugation), passage into the canalicular network, and biliary excretion. Abnormalities in any excretory step will alter the plasma dye disappearance. ICG may be a better indicator of hepatic function than is BSP. The avid protein binding allows a more predictable volume of distribution and restricts its extrahepatic removal.[325–327] In addition, unlike BSP, ICG does not undergo an enterohepatic circulation.

Despite the fact that the plasma disappearance of these dyes has long been regarded as a sensitive indicator of abnormalities in hepatic perfusion or function, there are many shortcomings in their use for the assessment of liver function. Although the administered dose of dye is determined on the basis of body weight, it is known that lean body mass is more closely correlated with hepatic mass and plasma volume. Markedly obese patients and those with ascites or edema may be given doses of dye that are too great for their plasma volume and hepatic mass. Dye overdosage will cause a factitious increase in the percentage of retention, because the standard curves used for analysis are based on the dose calculated for lean body weight.[328, 329]

Decreased protein binding caused by hypoalbuminemia or competitive displacement by other substances (drugs) will result in accelerated dye disappearance owing to extravascular dye dispersal and renal excretion. Dye diffusion into edema or ascites may also cause spurious increases in plasma dye clearance. Test results in the presence of hypoalbuminemia warrant careful scrutiny because they will underestimate the extent of hepatobiliary dysfunction.

Any systemic disorder causing sluggish hepatic perfusion such as congestive heart failure, pericardial disease, pericardial tamponade, heartworms, and systemic hypotension may delay plasma dye clearance. The presence of portosystemic venous anastomoses with or without accompanying hepatic lesions increases plasma dye retention. Patients with portosystemic vascular anomalies often but *not always* have increased dye retention. The preferential flow of blood through the anomalous shunting vessel and the degree of hepatic circulatory deprivation and hepatocellular atrophy all contribute to increased dye retention. Patients with acquired portosystemic venous anastomoses associated with hepatic fibrosis and cirrhosis tend to have greater dye retention than patients with portosystemic venous anomalies.

The sensitivity of BSP and ICG as screening tests for the detection of mild to moderate liver disease is poor. These tests are best used as diagnostic tests for the estimation of hepatobiliary function once hepatic disease is suspected. ICG has been shown to be capable of detecting liver dysfunction following 60 per cent but not 40 per cent hepatectomy in the dog.[330] Plasma retention in dogs with 60 per cent hepatectomy was found to correlate well with ammonia intolerance. When the plasma clearance of ICG was sequentially followed in dogs with 70 per cent hepatectomy, normalization of hepatic function correlated with the regeneration of hepatic mass at 6 weeks.[24] The sensitivity for detection and the quantitative estimation of functional liver mass are improved with large dye doses, which saturate the hepatic uptake and storage processes.[200, 326] Doses this large are not advocated for use in clinical diagnostic testing.

In the normal individual, the rate-limiting factor in plasma dye elimination is hepatocyte dye excretion rather than hepatic uptake from the plasma. Dye is stored in the hepatocyte, bound to cytosolic Y and Z proteins, as is bilirubin. Most BSP is conjugated to glutathione before biliary excretion. Many factors have been shown to affect the plasma clearance or hepatobiliary processing of BSP and ICG.[200] Fever has been shown to alter the kinetics of BSP plasma clearance.[331, 332] Drugs may alter the plasma protein binding, reduce hepatic uptake or excretion, reduce binding to intracellular hepatic storage proteins, inhibit the conjugating enzyme for BSP (glutathione-S-transferase), or alter hepatic blood flow thereby influencing the circulatory presentation of dye for hepatic extraction.[200, 333] Diseases interfering with hepatocellular dye uptake, storage, or biliary excretion delay plasma dye disappearance.[321, 326] The hepatocellular uptake of BSP and ICG is carrier-mediated and is competitively inhibited by other organic anions, including bilirubin but not bile acids.[316, 326, 333] The use of BSP or ICG to assess hepatic function in the jaundiced patient is pointless owing to the competitive inhibition of transcellular transport and cytosolic binding by bilirubin.

Congenital abnormalities in the hepatobiliary processing of bilirubin, BSP, or ICG have been well researched in the human, the Gunn rat, and Southdown mutant and Corriedale sheep, but such aberrations are rare in the dog and unreported in the cat.[200, 319] A disorder of hepatic uptake and storage of BSP in the absence of other evidence of hepatobiliary disease has been described in one dog.[334]

The information provided by measuring the plasma dye concentration at a single time is of limited value because it represents the combined effects of hepatic blood flow, uptake, metabolism, and biliary excretion and is subject to many inaccuracies. Monitoring plasma dye disappearance using several sequential measurements is a more sensitive and reliable method for detection of hepatobiliary dysfunction. In humans the initial fractional disappearance rate of BSP provides the best discrimination between normal controls and patients with liver disease.[335] Clearance studies, however, are too cumbersome for routine clinical use because they require multiple venipunctures and carefully timed samples.

The BSP 30-minute retention test has been the preferred test of liver function in the dog. It is completed using a dose of 2.2 mg/lb (5.0 mg/kg) lean body weight given as a 5.0 per cent solution as a rapid intravenous bolus. At precisely 30 minutes following dye injection, a blood sample is collected from a different vein. The percentage of dye remaining in the circulation is calculated from an expected standard initial concentration in the blood. Less is known regarding the use of BSP as a liver function test in the cat. The plasma clearance of BSP and ICG is much faster in the cat than in the dog, and it appears that ICG is the preferable dye for use in the cat.[336, 337] ICG can be used in a manner similar to the BSP 30-minute retention test, given at a dose of 0.7 mg/lb (1.5 mg/kg) in the cat and 0.45 mg/lb (1.0 mg/kg) in the dog. Plasma clearance can be examined using plasma samples obtained before and 5, 10, and 15 minutes following injection. Normal clearance and 30-minute retention values for BSP and ICG in the dog and cat are given in Table 88–12.[336, 337]

Retention of the organic anion dyes cannot differentiate the causes of jaundice in the dog and cat. The major value of these tests is in the detection of abnormalities in hepatic circulation or hepatobiliary function in patients with anicteric or occult liver disease. During the last decade, the availability of BSP has been limited owing to its discontinuation as a test of liver function in humans following reports of lethal anaphylactoid reac-

TABLE 88–12. HEPATIC FUNCTION TESTS: NORMAL VALUES FOR DOGS AND CATS

	Dose	Normal Values
Ammonia tolerance test	0.045 gm/lb NH$_4$Cl PO (not to exceed 3 gm)	30 minute: $\leqq$ 50–70 µM/L
Sulfobromophthalein (BSP)	2.2 mg/kg lb	30 minute % retention: dog $\leqq$ 5.0% cat $\leqq$ 3.0%
Indocyanine Green (ICG)	0.45 mg/lb IV (dog) 0.7 mg/lb IV (cat)	30 minute % retention: dog $\leqq$ 14.7 $\pm$ 5.0 cat $\leqq$ 7.3 $\pm$ 2.9 Clearance ml/min/kg (0–15 minutes): dog 3.7 $\pm$ 0.7 cat 8.6 $\pm$ 4.1
Total serum bile acids	Endogenous test dog p/d* cat c/d*	12-hour fasting µM/L: dog $\leqq$ 5.0 cat $\leqq$ 2.0 2-hour postprandial µM/L: dog $\leqq$ 15.5 cat $\leqq$ 10.0 (values >30 µM/L in dogs and >20 µM/L in cats indicate substantial hepatic dysfunction or cholestasis)

*Hills Pet Products.

tions and of severe perivascular inflammation associated with extravasation of dye during injection.[338, 339] Similar inflammatory reactions to extravasated BSP have been observed in the dog and cat. Anaphylactoid reactions to BSP have been rarely observed in the dog. Compared with BSP, ICG is less convenient for clinical testing. The chemical analysis is more difficult and ICG is supplied in freeze-dried form and must be dissolved only in a specific diluent, immediately before injection. The use of BSP and ICG has been largely replaced by other more convenient and reliable tests of hepatic function, primarily the measurement of serum bile acids.

BILE ACIDS

Bile acids are synthesized in the liver from cholesterol and then conjugated to an amino acid, mainly taurine, in the dog and cat.[340–342] They are then transported into the canalicular network and travel through the biliary system to the gallbladder for storage and concentration in bile. The primary bile acids are cholic acid and chenodeoxycholic acid. These may be modified by intestinal flora to the secondary bile acids (cholate to deoxycholate, chenodeoxycholate to lithocholate) and to the deconjugated and sulfated forms. At mealtime numerous neurohumoral and hormonal factors induce bile secretion and gallbladder contraction, resulting in the passage of bile acids into the intestines. Factors important in initiating gallbladder contraction include fat and protein dietary constituents and acidification of the duodenum by gastric juices.[342] In humans, it is common for gallbladder contraction to occur during the night and for up to half the bile acid pool to be in the circulation before breakfast. Periodic contraction of the gallbladder during fasting has also been reported in the dog.[21, 342] Noncholecystokinin peptides such as motilin are thought to cause gallbladder contraction during the interdigestive phase.[21, 342–345]

Once in the intestines, the detergent action of bile acids facilitates lipid digestion and absorption. Bile acids promote the function of digestive lipases and the formation of micelles, which improve lipid miscibility, increasing the surface area of lipid constituents for digestion and absorption.[343] Most of the conjugated primary bile acids are efficiently reabsorbed by an active transport process in the ileum. Once in the circulation, bile acids are bound to albumin and to lipoproteins. They are efficiently extracted on first pass through the liver. In the normal individual, the enterohepatic bile acid circulation is so efficient that the fecal loss constitutes only two to five per cent of the total circulating pool of bile acids each day.[31] As a result of the system's efficiency, only a very small bile acid pool is necessary for normal physiologic purposes. The total pool recycles between two and five times during each meal, depending on the integrity of the enterohepatic circulation, illustrated in Figure 88–7. Following a 12-hour fast and in the presence of normal portal circulation, hepatobiliary, and gallbladder function, only small amounts of bile acids are present in the systemic circulation. The mean concentration of bile acids in the portal blood is as much as six times greater than in the peripheral blood during a fast and much higher than this at mealtimes.[346, 347] The hepatic extraction of bile acids during first pass ranges from 70 to 90 per cent.[348] The proportion extracted remains fairly constant, with a fixed proportion escaping

into the systemic circulation. This accounts for the two-hour postprandial rise observed in healthy individuals. Normal fasting and two-hour postprandial concentrations of bile acids in the dog and cat are given in Table 88–12. When given intravenously, the clearance of bile acids is limited mainly by hepatic blood flow. In mild to moderate liver disease with normal hepatic blood flow, the extraction efficiency of the functional hepatic mass limits their clearance.

The measurement of serum bile acid concentrations is regarded as a more sensitive test for the detection of liver dysfunction or perfusion abnormalities than is serum bilirubin.[349, 350] They have a greater pool size as compared with bilirubin and undergo a more extensive enterohepatic circulation and storage in the gallbladder. They have a greater flux than that of bilirubin owing to their efficient conservation. As a result of these differences, a slight defect in organic anion excretion (cholestasis) creates a larger relative increase in the serum concentration of bile acids than in bilirubin.

Since bile acids and bilirubin are taken up and excreted by separate mechanisms, bile acids may be used in the differential diagnosis of jaundice, unlike BSP or ICG.[200] Hemolytic causes of hyperbilirubinemia are not associated with increases in the serum bile acid concentration unless hypoxia induces substantial secondary hepatocellular changes.

Although bile acid synthesis depends on hepatic function, hepatic failure does not limit their availability. The liver maintains a tremendous reserve capacity for bile acid synthesis and this reserve is rarely maximally utilized because only very small amounts of bile acids are

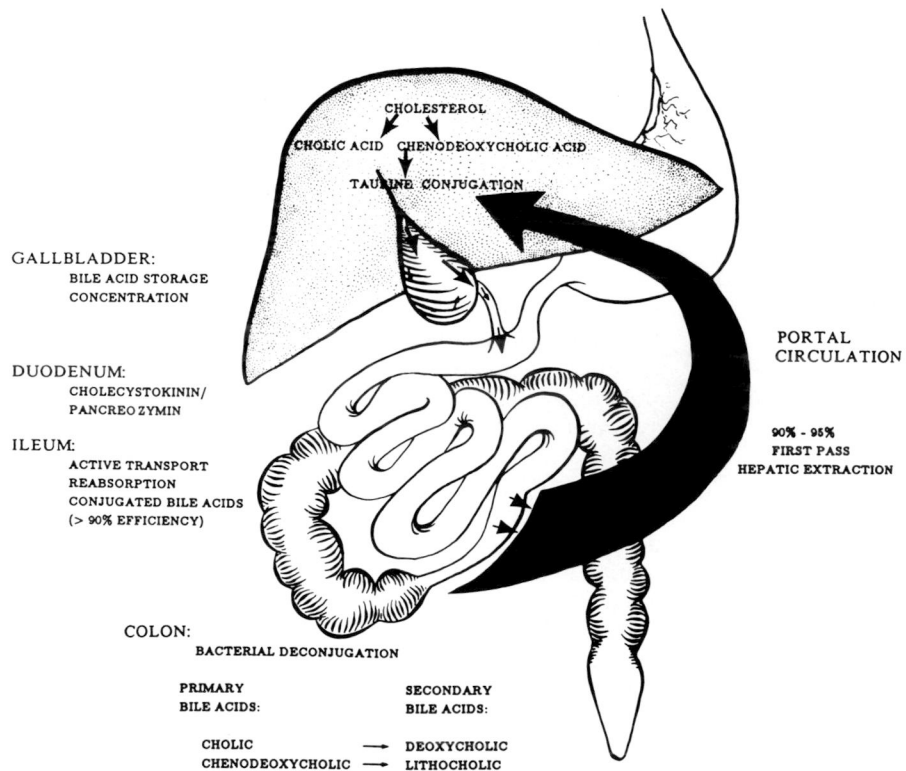

FIGURE 88–7. Enterohepatic circulation of bile acids.

required for normal physiologic purposes. The principal regulators of the serum bile acid concentration are ileal absorption, hepatic perfusion, hepatocellular uptake, storage, and biliary excretion. Impaired ileal absorption may cause a decreased serum bile acid concentration by continual fecal losses in excess of the maximal hepatic synthesizing capacity; such conditions are rare in dogs and cats. Otherwise, abnormalities in hepatic uptake, storage, excretion, or hepatic perfusion delay bile acid extraction from the portal circulation or cause regurgitation into the systemic circulation. Each of these results in increased serum bile acid concentrations.

The diagnostic value of fasting serum bile acid concentrations in the dog and cat have been reported.[350–355] They have been shown to improve the diagnostic performance of routine tests in patients with all types of hepatobiliary diseases. They are more sensitive than BSP and equivalent in sensitivity to the ammonia tolerance test in the diagnosis of portosystemic venous anastomosis.[351–356] Examples of fasting serum bile acid concentrations in various hepatobiliary diseases in the dog and cat are shown in Figure 88–8. Bile acid concentrations are not appropriate for use as screening tests but are best applied as diagnostic tests. They are appropriately used in an adjunctive capacity, with the other routinely used tests for hepatobiliary disease. Because they offer a specific insight into hepatic function and portal circulation, they may be used to determine the seriousness of a clinical disorder, the likelihood of hepatoencephalopathy, and the need for liver biopsy. On the basis of retrospective studies in dogs and cats with liver disease, it is suggested that liver biopsy be sought when fasting or postprandial values exceed 30 μM/L in the dog and 20 μM/L in the cat.

Different approaches have been examined to optimize the use of bile acids in the assessment of hepatobiliary function. In addition to the conventional testing procedures, these have included the oral administration of exogenous bile acids, the intravenous injection of loading and isotope tracer doses of exogenous bile acids, and cholecystokinin-evoked gallbladder contraction. The value of the endogenous challenge that naturally occurs following a meal in humans is controversial. Some investigators have concluded that it offers no advantage over fasting values,[357] while others have found that it markedly improves the test's diagnostic performance.[358–364] Observations in dogs and cats with liver disease indicate that the postprandial values improve the diagnostic capabilities of the fasting values, particularly when portosystemic shunting exists. In addition, the relative pattern of change in serum bile acid concentration between fasting and postprandial samples in an individual occasionally predicts the type of hepatobiliary lesion (Figure 88–9). Following a prolonged fast, serum bile acid values may be normal in animals with substantial portosystemic shunting. This occurs because of the continuous circulation of bile acids to the liver via the hepatic artery and the gradual extraction of bile acids from this circulation. If the fast is prolonged, the liver may eventually be able to extract bile acids from the systemic circulation. In these cases, the challenge of the timed extraction during the postprandial interval demonstrates the inefficiency of the enterohepatic circula-

tion. For this reason the endogenous challenge appears to be an important clinical test. Oral loading or the intravenous administration of bile acids has not proven to be clinically superior to the postprandial endogenous challenge in humans.[357, 365, 366] Preliminary studies using these techniques in dogs and cats have not been encouraging. Challenge testing with intravenously injected bile acids is complicated by their tendency to cause hemolysis and their relative insolubility. In studies of isotope-labeled bile acids conducted in humans with liver disease, fasting serum bile acid values were more sensitive in detecting hepatic dysfunction.[366] Measurement of bile acid concentrations following the injection of cholecystokinin has not demonstrated a superiority to the endogenous meal-invoked gallbladder contraction.

Together, the fasting and two-hour postprandial tests seem to be useful and reliable for the detection of hepatobiliary functional or circulatory abnormalities in the dog and cat. Shortcomings of the postprandial test include delays in gastric emptying and gallbladder contraction, variation in the rate of intestinal transit delaying ileal presentation of bile acids for absorption, and ileal disease causing bile acid malabsorption.[341, 367–370] Fasting values that exceed postprandial values have been observed in individual normal dogs and cats. Although the cause of this phenomenon is unknown, it is suspected that the following factors may be involved: spontaneous gallbladder contraction during the fast and individual variation of gallbladder contraction at mealtime and of intestinal transit rate. In cases in which such variables are believed to influence the test results, sequential blood sampling over four to six hours may improve the diagnostic performance of the test. Standardization of the test meal is important to reduce variations in gastric emptying and meal-invoked gallbladder contraction. Diets that have been used in bile acid studies in normal and diseased animals include commercial canned dog food (P/D, Hills Pet Products) and cat food (C/D, Hills Pet Products). In patients in which encephalopathic effects of protein are anticipated, a low protein food mixed with a small amount of corn oil is recommended to induce gallbladder contraction.

There are several laboratory methods used to quantify serum bile acid concentrations. Measurement of total 3-hydroxylated serum bile acids by an enzymatic method is easy, inexpensive, and reliable.[371, 372] Radioimmunoassays can be used, but these may measure specific bile acid moieties rather than the total concentration. Attention must be given to the specific bile acid moiety measured in a radioimmunoassay to ensure that it is one that is prevalent in the dog and cat and that the assay is validated in these species.[373] Taurine conjugates predominate in the dog and cat; therefore radioimmunoassays quantifying glycine conjugates cannot be recommended.

AMMONIA AND UREA METABOLISM

The liver is of central importance in the regulation of ammonia. Eighty to 90 per cent of ammonia delivered

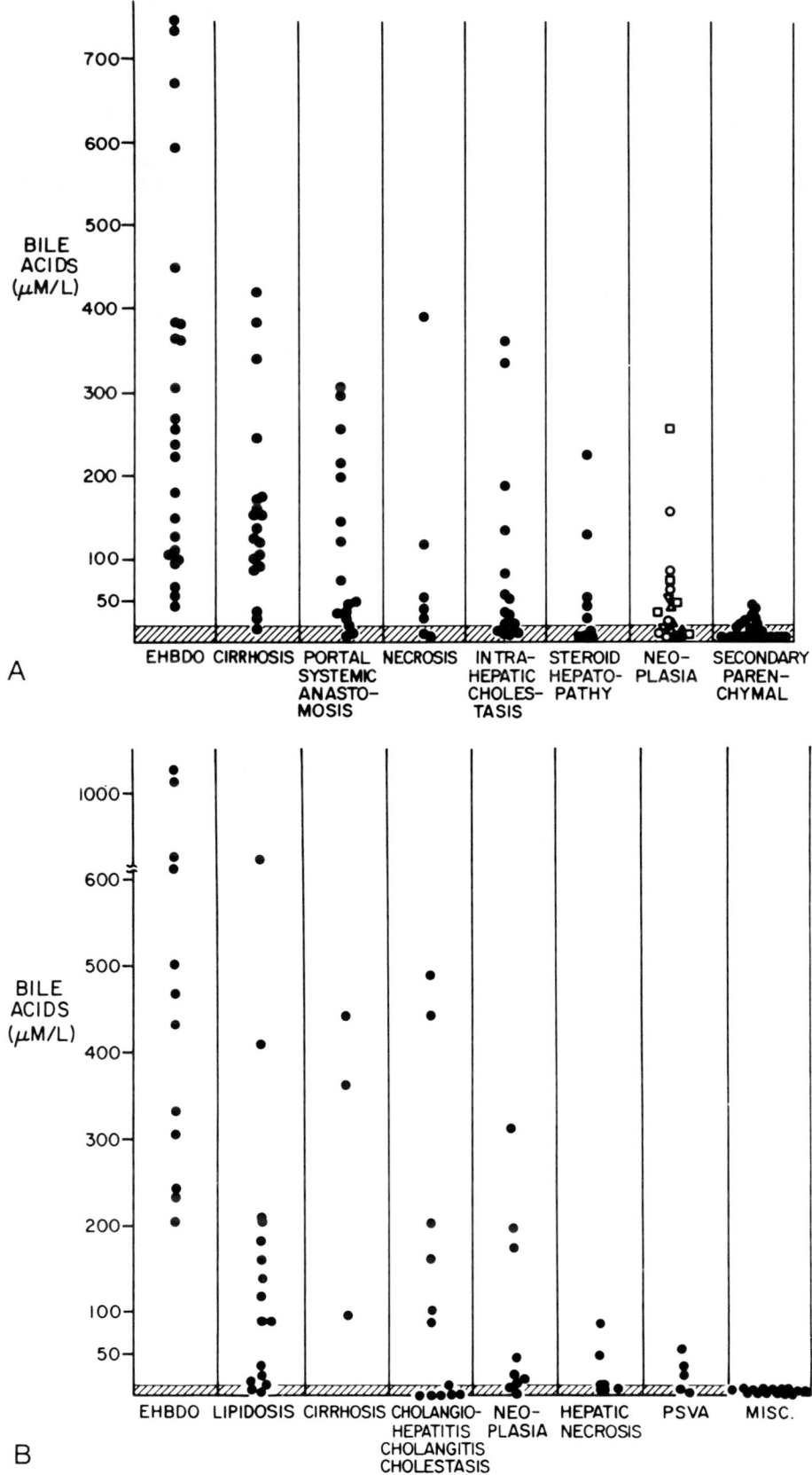

FIGURE 88–8. Fasting total serum bile acids in dogs *(A)* and cats *(B)* with different hepatobiliary disorders confirmed by histologic examination. Animals with EHBDO had complete extrahepatic bile duct occlusion. Cats with PSVA had portosystemic vascular anomalies. Dogs with secondary parenchymal disorders and cats with miscellaneous (MISC) had mild or no morphologic lesions on histologic examination. (From Center, SA: JAVMA 187:937, 1985; 189:893, 1986.)

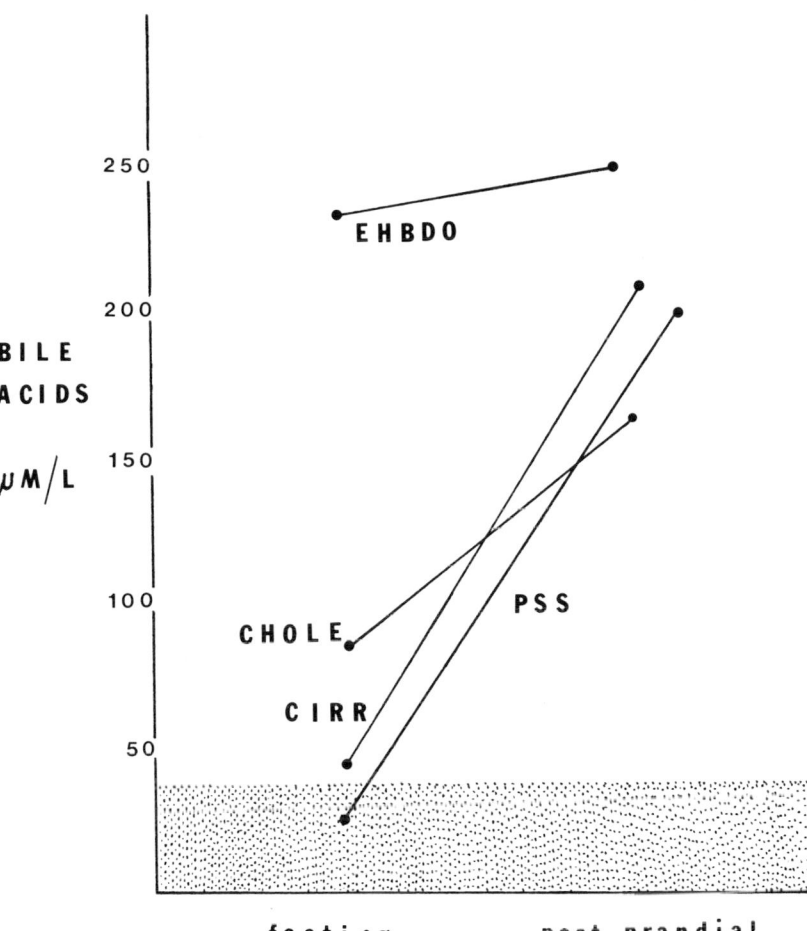

FIGURE 88–9. Serum bile acid concentrations in dogs and cats after a 12-hour fast and two hours following a meal. This diagram depicts patterns commonly observed in patients with extrahepatic bile duct obstruction (EHBDO), intrahepatic cholestasis (CHOLE), cirrhosis (CIRR), and portosystemic shunts (PSS). The normal range is indicated by black stippling. Values are approximated from clinical patients with biopsy confirmed hepatobiliary disease. (NYS Coll Vet Med, 1987.)

to the liver is converted to urea in the urea cycle. The other 10 to 20 per cent exits through the hepatic veins to be distributed in the systemic circulation.[374] Other organs involved with ammonia metabolism include the kidney, heart, brain, skeletal muscle, and gastrointestinal organs.[375]

Ammonia is generated from catabolism of proteins, nucleic acids, and urea. It is consumed in the synthesis of nonessential amino acids, nucleic acids, and other nitrogenous compounds. Specific endogenous sources of ammonia include glutamine, glutamate, other amino acids, adenylate, and urea that diffuses into the gastrointestinal tract. About 25 per cent of the urea produced in the liver diffuses into the alimentary canal, where it undergoes conversion to ammonia and enterohepatic circulation. Exogenous ammonia is derived from the gastrointestinal tract where it is produced by microbial and mucosal enzyme digestion of ingested nitrogenous substances, bacterial debris, and exfoliated epithelial protein.[376] Most of the ammonia (75 per cent) generated in the gastrointestinal tract is produced in the colon, largely through the action of microbial ureases on urea and the degradation of dietary amines (Figure 88–10).[375, 376] Anaerobic microorganisms and coliforms are the major source of colonic ureases.[376, 379] Reduction in the pH of the alimentary lumen reduces the hydrolysis of urea to ammonia, the prevalence of urea-metabolizing organisms, and the intestinal absorption of ammonia. Ammonia is passively absorbed across the bowel wall,

but the rate of absorption depends on the ionization state of the ammonia molecule. The ammonium ion (NH_4^+) diffuses poorly across cellular membranes, and since the ionized form is favored by an acidic pH, ammonia absorption is reduced.[380, 381] This ionization principle also influences the passage of ammonia across other biologic membranes, most importantly, the blood-brain barrier.

In patients with hepatic insufficiency, ammonia is not detoxified and enters the systemic circulation without conversion to urea. Although it is highly neurotoxic, the exact mechanism of its role in hepatic encephalopathy remains controversial. Production of ammonia in the gastrointestinal tract increases following the ingestion of meat or other protein, gastrointestinal hemorrhage, constipation, and the ingestion of ammonium salts.[382] The increase in ammoniagenic substrates in the bowel during hemorrhage can lead to profound hyperammonemia if hepatic function is compromised. Similarly, the transfusion of whole blood can "exogenously" load the urea cycle with unmanageable sources of nitrogen and ammonia. If blood transfusions are necessary, only fresh blood should be used to optimize erythrocyte survival and because stored blood may contain a considerable quantity of preformed ammonia. Patients with encephalopathic tendencies that develop azotemia are in danger of continuous spontaneous hyperammonemia as a result of the enterohepatic circulation of urea as ammonia. Constipation is also detrimental in hepatic insufficiency

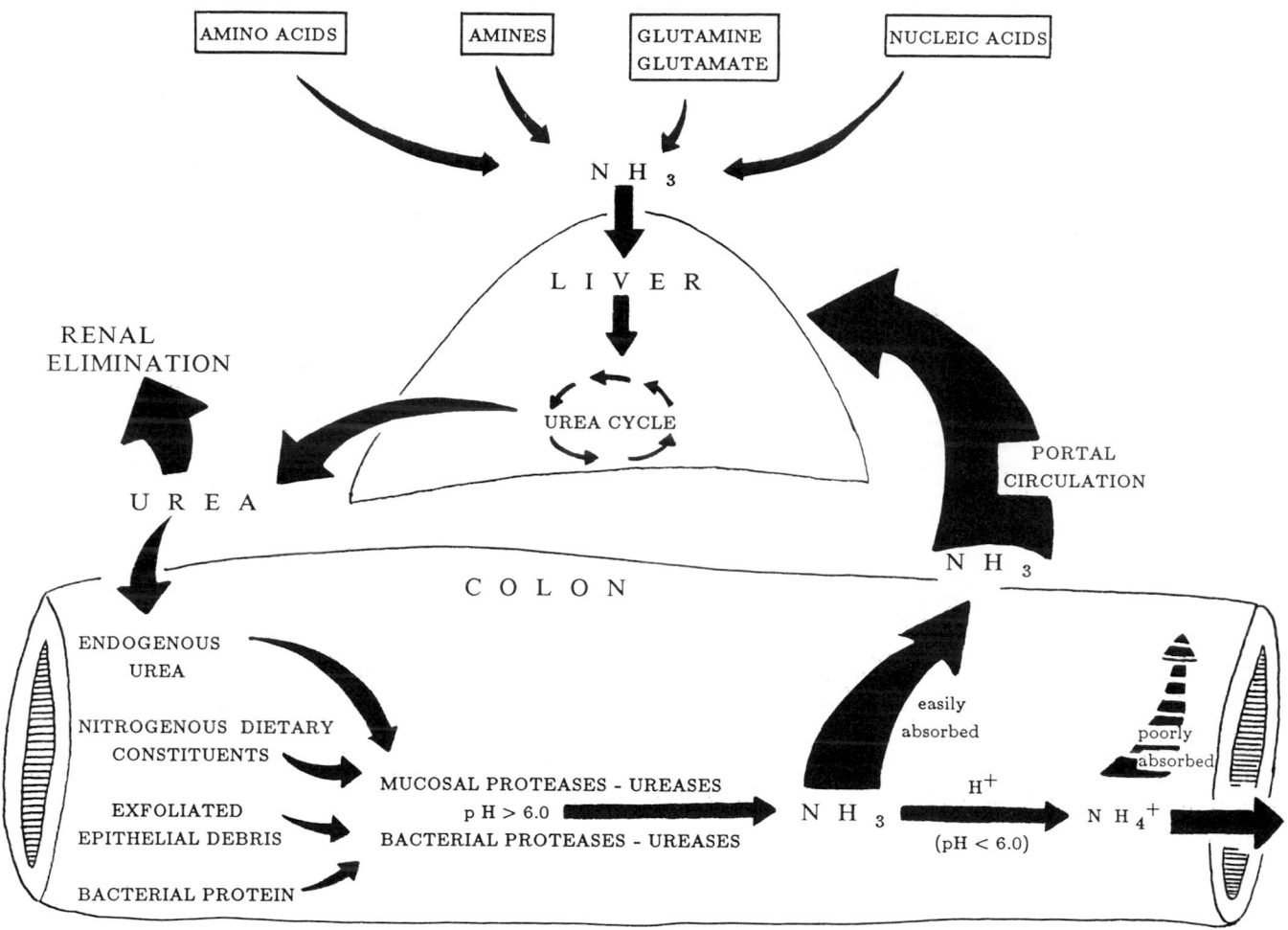

FIGURE 88–10. Schematic representation of ammonia metabolism.

because of the increased risk of ammonia production and absorption from retained *colonic residue.*

Metabolism of glutamate and glutamine deserves attention because the availability of these substances is closely linked to the serum ammonia concentration and to encephalopathic signs.[383] Glutamate is initially produced in larger concentrations than ammonia from protein catabolism and by transamination reactions between α-ketoglutarate and amino acids. Other sources of glutamate include direct hydrolysis of protein and the degradation of proline, histidine, and glutamine.[375, 383] Quantitatively, glutamine is the second major product of hepatic ammonia metabolism. Ammonia can be detoxified as glutamine and in this form can be stored and transported around the body. The discussion of hepatic encephalopathy in this chapter further defines the role of these substances.

Urea is synthesized in the liver as the major metabolic end product of hepatic ammonia detoxification. This is accomplished in the Krebs-Henseleit urea cycle, a cyclical chain of reactions controlled by five major enzymes.[384] Under normal circumstances, the urea cycle is operating at only 60 per cent of its maximum capacity.[177] The activity and amount of the urea cycle enzymes self-adjust according to the intake of dietary protein. Two- to three-fold increases in urea cycle enzymes and urea formation occur with high protein intake or starvation

and a two- to five-fold decrease occurs with protein-free diets.[383, 385–387] Because of the large functional hepatic reserve and tremendous regenerative capabilities, evidence of an insufficient urea cycle is a fairly late development in liver disease. A reduced capacity to degrade ammonia develops when more than 70 per cent of the normal hepatic synthetic capacity has been lost.[388] Urea cycle insufficiency can develop from reduction in hepatic mass, a decline in activity of hepatocellular enzymes, or portosystemic shunting. Experimentally, insufficient ammonia detoxification correlates better with derangements in portal circulation than with loss of functional hepatic mass.[387, 389–391] The activities of urea cycle enzymes have been evaluated in dogs with experimentally created portacaval shunts of three months' duration. Enzyme activity was not significantly different from that in control dogs, although very low concentrations of arginine, which could have been limiting to a key urea cycle enzyme (argininosuccinate synthetase), were found.[392] Investigations in dogs with 40 and 60 per cent hepatectomy demonstrated that ammonia intolerance was only evident in those with 60 per cent hepatectomy.[330] Clinically, abnormalities in the ability to detoxify ammonia are observed most consistently in patients with congenital portosystemic shunts or in those with acquired liver disease associated with intrahepatic or extrahepatic circulatory deviations. Patients with hepatic fibrosis and cirrhosis develop transhepatic shunting due to the intrahepatic architectural changes allowing functional anastomosis between branches of the portal veins and hepatic artery with the hepatic veins. Extrahepatic portosystemic deviations do not always develop.

Reduced concentrations of blood urea nitrogen (BUN) can occur in patients with severely compromised hepatic function. As a test of liver insufficiency, the BUN has low sensitivity and low specificity. There are too many extrahepatic variables influencing the BUN, including the hydration status of the animal, fluid or solute diuresis, protein content of the diet, the presence of gastrointestinal hemorrhage, and renal disease. In addition, individual variation alone can result in a BUN below the standard range. It is not uncommon for patients with acquired liver disease to have aberrations in body fluid homeostasis and concurrent derangements in renal function and urine concentration. These further complicate the use of a subnormal BUN as evidence of hepatic dysfunction. When renal dysfunction coexists with hepatic insufficiency, the serum creatinine must be used to monitor the degree of azotemia.

In exceptional cases, hyperammonemia has developed as a result of disorders not associated with acquired hepatocellular dysfunction or congenitally aberrant portal circulation.[393–398] Hyperammonemia has been reported in two dogs with suspected congenital absence of argininosuccinate synthetase, one of the urea cycle enzymes.[397] These dogs were small in stature, one had chronic recurrent gastrointestinal signs and the other a history of seizures. Normal biochemical profiles, normal BUN, normal BSP percentage retention, normal hepatic histology, and markedly reduced levels of argininosuccinate synthetase as compared with those in one normal dog were described. Contrast venography was not reported for these dogs. Hyperammonemia has been reported in cats fed an experimental diet deficient in arginine.[398, 399] Since arginine is an essential amino acid in the cat, hyperammonemia was thought to have developed from insufficient urea cycle enzyme activity. Obstructive uropathies complicated by infection with urease-producing bacteria have also been reported as a cause of hyperammonemia in humans[395, 396] and in a dog.[396a]

Fasting Blood Ammonia and Ammonia Tolerance Testing

The measurement of blood ammonia has been used as evidence of hepatic encephalopathy because it is one of the few cerebral toxins that can be routinely quantified. This test has high specificity but is limited by its only moderate sensitivity in the diagnosis of liver disease. It is a function test and therefore indicates compromised ammonia tolerance after substantial depletion of hepatic reserves or after the development of portosystemic circulatory diversion. The use of blood ammonia is fraught with many difficulties and inconveniences. The concentration of ammonia in arterial blood seems to be more reliable than that in venous blood because venous samples may reflect regional circulatory changes and local tissue metabolism.[391, 400, 401] Occlusion of a vein for blood collection for too long an interval or vigorous muscular activity can result in increased venous ammonia concentrations.[391, 401]

Although arterial samples seem to be subject to fewer artifactual influences, such samples are technically difficult and injudicious to obtain in patients with a potential for hemorrhage. As a result, venous samples are routinely used to measure blood ammonia concentrations in clinical patients. Samples for ammonia determinations must immediately be stored on ice, centrifuged in a cooled environment, and assayed as soon as possible. Insufficient separation of plasma from erythrocytes can invalidate ammonia measurements since erythrocytes contain two to three times as much ammonia as plasma.[402–407] Ammonia may spontaneously generate in stored plasma, although the exact nature of this process is poorly understood. It may involve hydrolysis of protein or other ammoniagenic substances.[402, 407, 408] A study of the lability of ammonia in feline blood showed that plasma samples can be stored frozen at $-20°$ C for up to 48 hours before assay if promptly separated from erythrocytes.[408] A similar study with canine plasma indicated that storage for any length of time resulted in spurious high or low ammonia values.[409]

In addition to the technical difficulties, hyperammonemia is not consistently demonstrable in patients with hepatic encephalopathy because other toxic substances are involved in the genesis of the syndrome. Ammonia tolerance is not adequately or uniformly assessed by measurement of fasting or postprandial plasma ammonia concentrations. Hyperammonemia is more consistently documented in patients with hepatic insufficiency or portosystemic shunting following a provocative test of hepatic ammonia detoxification.

Ammonia tolerance testing can be accomplished using solutions of ammonium chloride (NH_4Cl) administered orally, per rectum by catheter enema, or by oral administration of a NH_4Cl powder in a gelatin capsule.[400, 410, 411] The gelatin capsule method yields results comparable to solutions administered orally or rectally and is technically simpler to perform.[411] The standard oral tolerance test is conducted following the oral administration of 45 mg/lb (100 mg/kg) body weight of NH_4Cl in a dilute solution (concentration not to exceed 20 mg/ml or a total dose of 3 gm). Heparinized blood samples are obtained before and 30 minutes after administration. Use of concentrated solutions may induce vomiting, which will invalidate the test. The oral test depends on normal gastric emptying and intestinal transit rates for optimal challenge of the subject's ability to extract ammonia from the portal circulation. The rectal tolerance test is conducted after a 12-hour fast and cleansing enema. Ammonium chloride is administered as a 5 per cent solution at a dose of 1 ml/lb (2 ml/kg) body weight by catheter at a depth of 20 to 35 cm in the rectum. Heparinized blood samples are collected before and at 20 and 40 minutes following NH_4Cl administration. Some animals expel the solution immediately. Those with preexistent diarrhea are poor subjects for the rectal tolerance test. Spurious hyperammonemia can result from solution administered too shallow in the colon as a result of absorption through hemorrhoidal veins.

The oral tolerance tests are more commonly used than is the rectal test. Regardless of the type of test performed, a control sample from a fasted, healthy animal should be concurrently evaluated to ensure that proper procedures were used in managing blood samples and that the ammonia assay was correctly performed.

In normal animals, blood ammonia concentrations remain unchanged or increase up to two-fold greater than baseline fasting values at 30 minutes following oral NH$_4$Cl administration (Table 88–12). In animals with compromised hepatic function, fasting ammonia values may be normal or up to ten times normal. Following the administration of NH$_4$Cl, blood ammonia concentrations usually range between three and ten times baseline values (Figure 88–11).

In conclusion, although evaluation of ammonia tolerance is useful in the diagnosis of hepatic insufficiency and hepatic encephalopathy, the technical difficulties associated with the test limit its convenient use in clinical practice. The comparable sensitivity in detecting hepatic insufficiency (Figure 88–12), the increased convenience, and the stability of bile acids during sample transport make the serum bile acid tolerance test more appropriate for routine clinical testing.[353, 355] Each of these tests is more specific than is BSP.

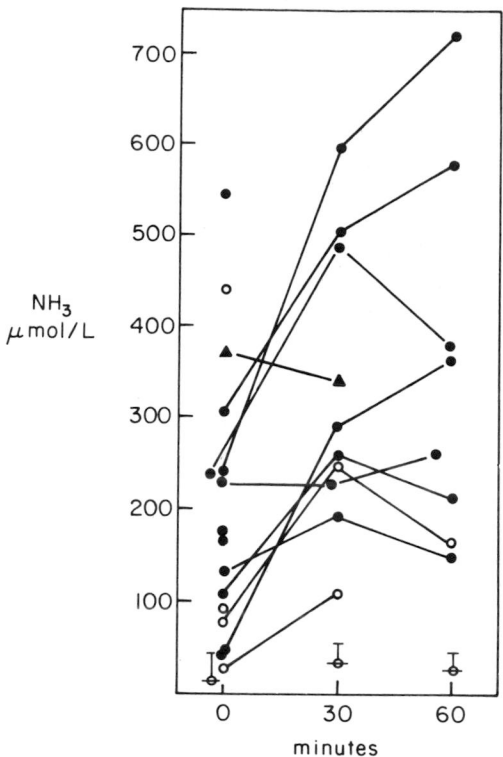

FIGURE 88–11. Blood ammonia concentrations in dogs and cats with portosystemic vascular anomalies. Samples were taken after a 12-hour fast (0 time), and following the oral administration of ammonium chloride (30 and 60 minutes). Normal values are depicted by the ⊖ at each interval. Solid circles and triangle are dogs, open circles are cats. (From Center, SA: JAVMA 186:1092, 1985.)

URIC ACID

Uric acid is a by-product of purine nucleotide catabolism.[412] Most dogs transform uric acid to water-soluble allantoin in the liver via the action of uricase. Some dogs, particularly Dalmatians, have an inborn error of uric acid metabolism whereby they cannot transform uric acid to allantoin. These animals are unable to transport uric acid across membranes but have normal uricase activity.[413, 414] In animals with normal uric acid membrane transport but insufficient hepatic function, serum uric acid may increase owing to the absence of hepatic uricase.[124, 415–417] Hyperuricemia has also been associated with conditions other than liver failure such as diffuse tissue destruction or inflammation causing increased catabolism of purine nucleotides (pyometritis, trauma, hypoxia, and hemorrhagic shock) and glycogen storage disease.[416–418] Early study of uric acid as a diagnostic test for liver disease in the dog showed that it was a relatively insensitive reflection of hepatic function. Since then its clinical use has been largely abandoned.

AMMONIUM URATE CRYSTALLURIA OR CALCULI

Ammonium urate crystals may develop in the urine of dogs and cats with recurrent hyperammonemia. Ammonium biurate crystalluria or calculi, especially in young animals, should inspire a thorough investigation for anomalous portal circulation. Prior to the advent of ultrasonography, ammonium-urate calculi were rarely detected in shunt patients unless clinical symptomatology drew attention to the urinary system and radiographic contrast studies were completed. The routine use of abdominal ultrasonography has shown the presence of renal or cystic calculi to be relatively common in these animals. Once calculi are identified, treatment should be jointly directed to the underlying hepatic disorder and urinary tract signs. When surgical correction of the aberrant hepatic circulation is not elected or is unsuccessful, medical management of hepatic encephalopathy has reduced the recurrence of ammonium urate calculi. The success of allopurinol in these patients has not yet been adequately studied in a significant number of animals.

PORTAL HYPERTENSION

The portal circulatory bed is a low resistance system with a normal venous pressure of around ten cm of water (to convert to mm Hg, divide by 1.36).[419–425] In health, the portal pressure exceeds the pressure in the hepatic veins and caudal vena cava, thereby providing a circulatory gradient across the hepatic sinusoids. Increased portal pressure can develop from increased portal blood flow, increased intrahepatic vascular resistance, or obstruction of a major vessel compromising flow. Any derangement in the flow of portal blood has the potential to affect the entire portal circulation as a result of the paucity of valves in the system. Beyond a certain critical level portal hypertension results in the development of collateral shunting to the systemic cir-

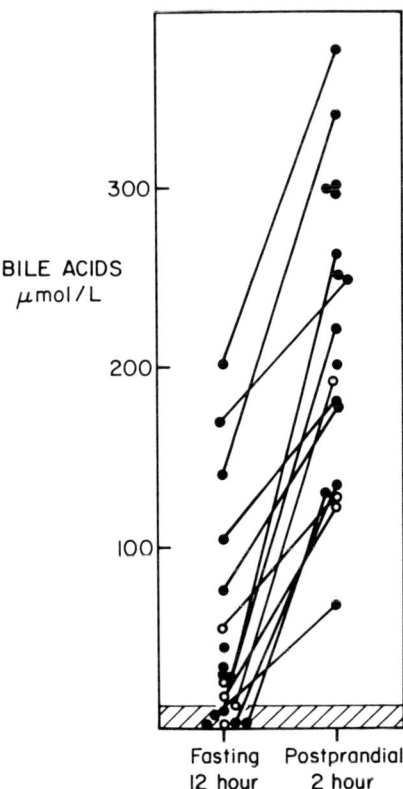

FIGURE 88–12. Total serum bile acid values in the same dogs and cats depicted in Figure 88–11. Samples were taken after a 12-hour fast and 2 hours after a meal. Normal values are depicted by the hatched area.

culation. This compensatory diversion of blood helps partially relieve the increased portal pressure, but it never completely abolishes the hypertension.[422–425] The clinical and pathologic sequelae of obstructed portal flow depend on the location, completeness, and rate of onset of the causal mechanism. If major portosystemic shunting develops, blood deviated from the liver carries increased amounts of bile acids, ammonia, bacteria, endotoxins, and other alimentary-derived substances to the systemic circulation.

Locating the cause of portal venous hypertension allows classification into four major categories: (1) increased portal blood flow, or increased vascular resistance originating in (2) presinusoidal, (3) intrahepatic-

sinusoidal, or (4) postsinusoidal locations (see Table 88–13).[422–425] Ultrasonographic examination of the portal vein before and after arborization within the liver is a noninvasive method for locating the origin of portal hypertension. Alternatively, direct or indirect measurement of portal pressure can be used (Figure 88–13).[422–425] The direct portal pressure may be estimated by catheter placement into a mesenteric portal vein tributary. Pressure is expressed in mm H_2O using a manometer calibrated at the level of the right atrium. Indirect estimates of portal pressure may be accomplished by using splenic pulp pressure, hepatic tissue pressure, or hepatic vein wedged pressure. Splenic pulp pressure is estimated using needle perforation of the body of the spleen; a free flow of blood is obtained and pressure estimated using a water manometer. This technique can also be used with the liver. Wedged hepatic vein pressure may be estimated by threading a catheter through jugular vein and right atria to the caudal vena cava and wedging a catheter tip in a parenchymal hepatic vein. Expected normal values are shown in Figure 88–13.[422–425]

Increased portal blood flow is an uncommon cause of portal hypertension. When portal blood flow increases, portal venous pressure rises secondary to the hepatic vascular resistance to the expanded flow. Arterialization of the liver due to an arteriovenous fistula can cause this type of portal hypertension.[426] Arteriovenous fistulas result from congenital vascular malformations or visceral trauma or are associated with neoplasia. Although rare, reported cases have involved congenital malformations possibly due to failure of the embryologic vascular anlage to differentiate. Animals with congenital arterioportal fistulas demonstrate clinical signs similar to those observed in patients with portal vein anomalies. These patients differ from routine portosystemic vascular anomaly cases in that they have ascites and multiple portosystemic collaterals that are open and shunting mesenteric blood to the systemic circulation. Overall hepatic size may be reduced or individual lobes may be large or small. Diagnosis may be accomplished by selective catheterization of the celiac trunk, nonselective jugular venography, radioisotope methods, or ultrasonography. Arterioportal fistulas are grossly evident during laparotomy as tortuous pulsating vessels on the surface of the affected liver lobe. A palpable thrill may

TABLE 88–13. CAUSES OF PORTAL HYPERTENSION

Increased Portal Blood Flow	Increased Vascular Resistance	
Arterialization of Liver	Intrahepatic	Extrahepatic
Arterioportal fistula	Sinusoidal fibrosis	Postsinusoidal Causes
congenital	Portal fibrosis	Cardiomyopathy
trauma	Collagen in space of Disse	Congestive heart failure
neoplasia	Hepatic vein occlusion	Pericardial disease
Hepatic Fibrosis	Nodular regeneration	Pericardial tamponade
Microvascular arteriovenous	Hepatocyte hypertrophy	Vena caval occlusion
communications	Infiltrative disease	Hepatic vein occlusion
Increased Splenic Blood Flow		Presinusoidal Causes
Chronic liver disease (rare)		Portal vein occlusion
Other causes of splenomegaly		thrombi
		neoplasia
		maldevelopment
		inflammatory disease

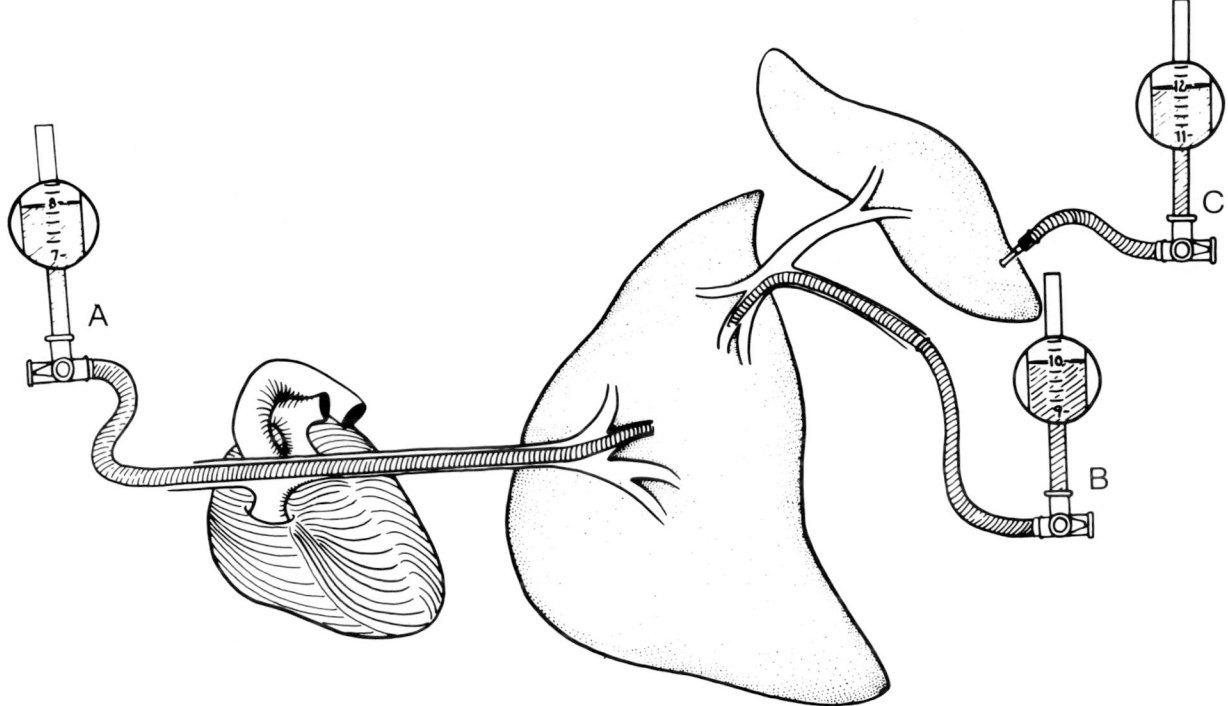

FIGURE 88–13. Estimation of portal pressure by *(A)* hepatic vein "wedged" pressure, *(B)* mesenteric portal tributary catheterization, and *(C)* splenic pulp pressure. Expected normal values are depicted by the manometer readings.

also be obvious. The routine radiographic contrast techniques used for diagnosis of portosystemic vascular anomalies (mesenteric or splenic vein injections) will fail to demonstrate a hepatic arteriovenous fistula. These studies will document the existence of open portosystemic collaterals while missing the primary lesion. Although arterioportal fistulas are difficult to diagnose, once they are identified, surgical ligation or excision can be curative if performed before permanent architectural hepatic changes have developed.

Increased vascular resistance is the most common cause of portal hypertension. Presinusoidal causes include occlusion of the portal vein by thrombi, tumor, congenital maldevelopment, or external compression. The liver is normal in size and ascites is unusual. When ascites is present, it has low protein content, being derived from intestinal lymph. Portosystemic collaterals may develop with chronicity.[424–426]

The most common cause of increased vascular resistance leading to portal hypertension is obstruction to blood flow through the hepatic sinusoids. Any form of chronic progressive hepatic disease promoting fibrogenesis can culminate in sinusoidal portal hypertension.[422–425] In the dog, this form of portal hypertension commonly coexists with cirrhosis, in which sinusoidal circulatory obstruction results from regenerating nodules, fibrosis, and collagenization of the sinusoids.[422–425] Portal pressures ranging from 18 to 39 cm H_2O have been reported in dogs with cirrhosis.[422] Chronic obstruction of the common bile duct in the dog causes intrahepatic portal hypertension after eight weeks.[427–429] In conjunction with the portal hypertension, dogs also develop extensive portosystemic shunts and a hyperdynamic systemic circulation. Histologic and ultrastructural changes include distortion of the normal architec-

ture by fibrosis of the central veins and collagen deposition along the sinusoids. Any sinusoidal cause of portal hypertension may be worsened by the development of intrahepatic arteriovenous anastomoses.[426, 430] Such secondary arteriovenous communications arterialize the hepatic portal circulation and thereby increase the flow of blood through restricted conduits. Infiltrative liver diseases can also cause sinusoidal hypertension if they compromise normal sinusoidal architecture and restrict circulatory pathways.[422–426]

Postsinusoidal causes of portal hypertension include disorders causing passive hepatic circulatory congestion by increasing resistance to blood flow in the major hepatic veins, caudal vena cava, or heart. Examples include right-sided heart failure, cardiac tamponade, restrictive or constrictive pericardial disease, and right atrial or caudal vena caval tumors or thrombi. Increased venous pressure is quantitatively transmitted to the hepatic veins, sinusoids, and portal vein. Hepatomegaly is expected and ascites may develop acutely or with chronicity. This type of portal hypertension should not result in portosystemic shunting because a gradient does not exist between the portal and systemic venous beds.

Ascites

Although portal hypertension is commonly associated with ascites, it is not the only pathophysiologic determinant of ascites formation. The formation of ascites is multifactorial, involving the following mechanisms: hypoalbuminemia, portal hypertension, sodium retention, abnormal water retention, altered renal function, altered rates of intestinal and hepatic lymph formation, altered reabsorption of ascites by peritoneal lymphatics, and the

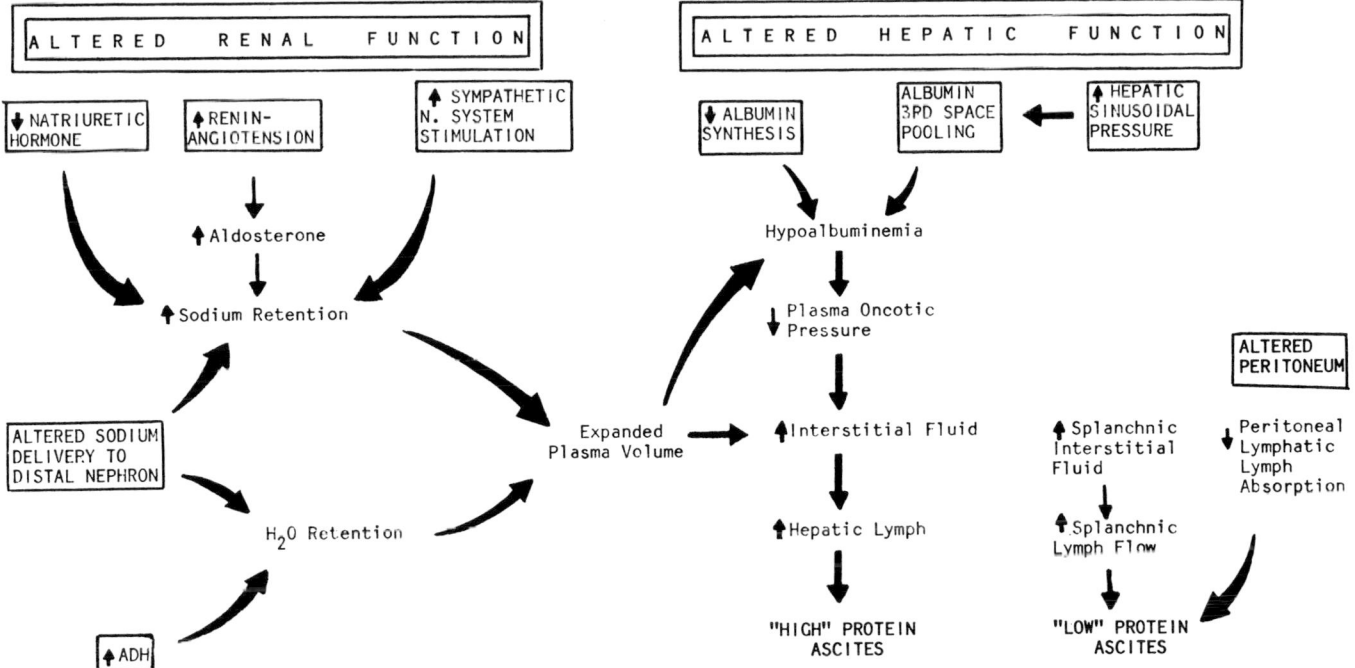

FIGURE 88–14. Pathogenetic mechanisms involved with the generation of ascites in patients with compromised hepatic function.

presence of inflammatory visceral or peritoneal lesions.[431, 432] Ascitic fluid may be largely derived from high protein content hepatic lymph or lower protein content splanchnic lymph. As a result of its diverse origins, the physicochemical attributes of ascitic fluid vary. Figure 88–14 demonstrates numerous variables influencing the formation of ascites in patients with liver disease. For a more detailed discussion, the reader is referred to Chapter 28.

PLASMA ELECTROLYTE, FLUID, AND RENAL DISORDERS

Electrolyte and fluid aberrations are common in humans with liver disease. The frequency of similar disorders in dogs and cats with naturally developing liver disease is unreported. The following discussion highlights the most important complications of electrolyte and fluid balance associated with hepatobiliary disorders.

Potassium depletion in humans with liver insufficiency seems to precipitate hepatic encephalopathy. Hypokalemia increases renal ammonia production and forces a sodium-hydrogen ion exchange in the distal convoluted tubule.[433, 434] The latter effect promotes a metabolic alkalosis that facilitates uptake of ammonia across the blood-brain barrier. Hypokalemia has been shown to promote renal ammonia production in dogs made potassium deficient by hemodialysis and dietary restriction.[133] The pathogenesis of hypokalemia in liver disease may include the following mechanisms: hyperaldosteronism, polydipsia and polyuria in conjunction with anorexia, vomiting or diarrhea, renal tubular acidosis, respiratory alkalosis, magnesium depletion, and admin-

istration of loop diuretics (furosemide) for the management of ascites.[432, 435]

Chronic compensated hepatic insufficiency in humans is associated with decreased sodium and urea excretion and impaired renal concentrating ability.[435, 436] Impaired water diuresis may also develop due to increased concentrations or activity of ADH and decreased delivery of glomerular filtrate to the diluting segments of the nephron.[435] It is unknown if these effects also develop in dogs or cats with spontaneous liver disease. Fluid retention leading to ascites and edema may accompany reduced sodium excretion. Coexistent hypoalbuminemia aggravates fluid retention and its dispersal in extravascular localizations. Hyperaldosteronism develops in approximately one-third of human patients afflicted with hepatic insufficiency–associated ascites.[437] The hyperaldosteronism develops as a result of increased adrenal secretion and decreased hepatic degradation of aldosterone.[437]

Fluid retention in these patients is aggravated by sodium retention. There are many mechanisms responsible for sodium retention besides hyperaldosteronism. These include increased renal prostaglandins, decreased activity of natriuretic factor, alterations in the kallikrein-kinin system, increased estrogens, vasoactive intestinal peptide, or prolactin, increased sympathetic nervous system activity, and alterations in the distribution of intrarenal blood flow.[431, 437] Although sodium retention appears to be common in humans with liver disease, it is unknown how this relates to liver disease in the dog or cat. An important complicating factor of diagnostic importance is that sodium retention or potassium depletion is not always indicated by changes in plasma electrolyte concentrations. Retained sodium is dispersed and "diluted" with retained fluids, and depleted potassium stores can be hidden by the patient's acid-base status that influences ion shifts between the intracellular and extracellular compartments.

Polyuria and polydipsia are common in animals with hepatic insufficiency. These features have been dominant clinical signs in some animals with portosystemic vascular anomalies and occult cirrhosis. Dogs presenting with polydipsia and polyuria may show partial responses to water deprivation in their ability to concentrate urine.[438, 439] The concentration defect may resolve if the hepatic disorder can be corrected, as is seen in patients with congenital portosystemic shunts undergoing successful surgical correction. The pathogenesis of polyuria is multifactorial. Polyuria may develop due to central or primary (psychogenic) neuronal stimulation of the thirst center as an effect of hepatic encephalopathy, alterations in portal vein osmoreceptors, or a renal concentrating defect.[440–446] In health, the osmoreceptors in the portal venous system send stimuli to the CNS via the vagus nerve.[440] In liver disease, these portal osmoreceptors may be dysfunctional and stimulate thirst in the absence of changes in plasma osmolality.[438] The osmostats may be reset to a new critical threshold that triggers thirst and water retention at a lower plasma osmolality than in health. Polyuria and polydipsia may follow the development of renal concentrating defects associated with potassium depletion, increased endogenous corticosteroid concentrations, renal medullary solute washout, or renal disease. Hypokalemia can further impair urine concentration and can also induce a central polydipsia. Morphologic evidence of a hypokalemic nephropathy has not been documented in patients with polyuria and hepatic disease.[446] Increased cortisol concentrations may develop in patients with hepatic insufficiency as a result of decreased hepatic degradation and increased adrenal hormone production. Polydipsia and polyuria may follow increased cortisol concentrations as a result of central stimulation of the thirst center, impaired action of antidiuretic hormone, and a general increase in glomerular filtration.

Renal medullary solute washout develops in patients with chronic polydipsia and polyuria and depletion of the important renal interstitial solutes sodium and urea. Water diuresis induced by primary polydipsia promotes renal medullary solute washout and reduces renal responsivity to ADH. Diminished production of urea due to hepatic insufficiency and anorexia further impairs the maintenance of the medullary solute gradient. There may also be a shift in the distribution of blood flow within the kidney, from the cortical to the juxtaglomerular nephrons. This perfusion change further compromises the development of the renal interstitial concentration gradient. All of the aforementioned factors probably play a role in the reduced ability to concentrate urine in patients with hepatic disease.[431, 435] How many of them are functional in the dog and cat remains unproven.

Treatment of polyuria and polyuria is limited in patients with hepatic disease. The underlying disorders must receive primary attention and, if they improve, the polyuria and polydipsia may resolve. If central polydipsia is suspected, a cautious gradual reduction in water intake may be imposed to re-establish a normal renal medullary concentration gradient. Since polydipsia and

polyuria may be manifestations of hepatic encephalopathy, caution is warranted to avoid volume contraction, induced prerenal azotemia, and acid-base imbalances resulting from excessive water restriction. Each of these iatrogenic complications can promote hepatic encephalopathy. Salt supplementation aimed at re-establishing the medullary concentration gradient is contraindicated in patients with encephalopathy since they also probably have salt-conserving tendencies.

A hepatorenal syndrome has been described in humans with liver disease.[431, 435, 447] It is unknown to what extent a similar abnormality develops in small animal patients. This syndrome is characterized as progressive oliguric renal failure associated with hepatic insufficiency and for which other causes of renal failure cannot be identified. Despite aggressive investigation, the pathogenesis of the syndrome is poorly understood. The renal failure is thought to be functional since the kidneys are morphologically normal and retain their ability to conserve sodium and to concentrate urine. A transient and reversible functional pathogenetic mechanism involving active renal vasoconstriction is suspected. Mediating factors may include abnormal activation of the renin-angiotensin system, increased intrarenal prostaglandin liberation, subnormal activity of the kallikrein-kinin system, endotoxins derived from the incompletely filtered portal circulation, or an increase in sympathetic discharge.[431, 435, 447]

Renal disease may precede, occur simultaneously with, or follow the diagnosis of liver disease. Concurrent renal and hepatic dysfunction complicates the management of each condition. Azotemia aggravates hyperammonemia and the attendant encephalopathic signs. Renal disorders impairing urine concentration promote the tendency for dehydration and the development of prerenal azotemia and hypovolemia, which can worsen metabolic disturbances promoting hepatic encephalopathy. If hypoalbuminemia is a concurrent problem, large volumes of fluid may be redistributed into the extravascular space. Judicious selection and administration of intravenous fluids and albumin transfusions may improve the hemodynamic status of these patients. Fluid therapy to improve renal perfusion is fraught with many complications. Patients with pre-existent ascites or edema may further expand their extravascular fluid and sodium stores as a result of fluid therapy. Fluids low in sodium should be selected for such patients. The use of diuretics to mobilize ascites or to improve urine output may jeopardize a patient in the promotion of dehydration, hypovolemia, hypotension, and azotemia.[448]

The presence of a large volume of ascites may substantially impair renal perfusion. Paracentesis may improve renal hemodynamics by reducing intra-abdominal fluid pressure. If hypoalbuminemia is a concurrent problem, paracentesis should not be performed on the ventral midline. Rather, puncture of the abdomen from a lateral aspect is advisable, being careful to avoid visceral structures. A lateral approach will reduce the gravitational effects promoting the continued leakage of ascitic fluid from the paracentesis site. Paracentesis is not routinely used to therapeutically remove ascites. Acceptable indications for fluid removal by paracentesis include the diagnostic examination of fluid for unexplained pyrexia, encephalopathy, or other constitutional signs, the relief of abdominal discomfort, the relief of dyspnea, the alleviation of detrimental intra-abdominal pressure, the facilitation of physical or radiologic examination, and in preparation for surgery.[438] Paracentesis and removal of ascites can result in punctured viscera, iatrogenic septic peritonitis, and worsening hypoalbuminemia. Too rapid removal of large volumes of fluid can lead to serious complications such as hypovolemia, hepatic encephalopathy, and renal failure, although these sequelae are rare.

Renal enlargement has been observed in animals with portosystemic vascular anomalies. Renal hypertrophy is thought to be associated with increased metabolic activity in the kidneys and the influence of trophic factors deviated from the liver by the aberrant portal circulation. Work-related hypertrophy could also explain the increased renal size developing in response to increased metabolic demands. This may involve gluconeogenesis and ammonia detoxification.

ACID-BASE DISORDERS

Disorders of the acid-base status in patients with liver disease can encompass either acidemia or alkalemia. In human patients with hepatic insufficiency, respiratory and metabolic alkalosis are most common.[432, 449] Hyperventilation is frequent and seems to correlate with the severity of the clinical abnormalities, although the exact pathogenesis remains uncertain.[150] A number of factors can stimulate either the medullary respiratory center or the peripheral respiratory stretch receptors to cause hyperventilation.[450, 451] These include hypoxemia caused by ventilation-perfusion imbalances, hyperammonemia, hyponatremia, potassium depletion, increased concentrations of short-chain fatty acids, acidosis of the respiratory center, and physical stimuli associated with restricted thoracic expansion such as impaired diaphragmatic motion caused by large volumes of ascites.[449-452] Respiratory alkalosis is usually spontaneous in occurrence while metabolic alkalosis develops following overzealous use of diuretics (furosemide), or in conjunction with chronic vomiting, intravascular volume contraction, hyperaldosteronism, or hypokalemia. Excessive renal production and excretion of urinary acid in the form of ammonium are major mechanisms of metabolic alkalosis.[453] They are usually associated with excessive mineralocorticoid activity, potassium deficiency, and adequate sodium delivery to the distal nephron. The enhanced renal absorption of sodium in exchange for potassium and hydrogen ion generates and perpetuates the hypokalemia and alkalosis. Contraction alkalosis caused by reduction in the extracellular fluid volume without proportional reduction of the extracellular bicarbonate may be induced by overwhelming diuresis. Extensive volume contraction leads to increased reabsorption of sodium, chloride, and bicarbonate in the proximal tubule. Mineralocorticoid excess also promotes sodium and bicarbonate reabsorption and hydrogen ion secretion in the distal tubules.[439]

Lactic acidosis can develop in patients with insufficient hepatic function due to the importance of the liver in the metabolism of lactate. Greater than 50 per cent of the lactate produced each day is metabolized by the liver.[454, 455] The occurrence of lactic acidosis is said to be an ominous sign and lends a grave prognosis in consideration of the underlying pathophysiologic mechanisms.[454] Factors known to promote lactate production in liver disease include hypotension, seizures, sepsis, hyperventilation, alkalosis, thiamine deficiency, and renal failure.[449] In some patients, the metabolic acidosis expected with lactate accumulation may be offset by concurrent alkalosis (respiratory and/or metabolic).[453] A primary impairment in the use of lactate in hepatic gluconeogenesis is suspected if lactic acidosis and hypoglycemia develop concomitantly.[454-456]

Mixed acid-base disorders are common in patients with hepatic disease. Combinations of respiratory alkalosis, metabolic alkalosis, and metabolic acidosis may be deduced from examination of the serum electrolytes, bicarbonate, PCO_2, pH, and PO_2, and the clinical status of the patient. Treatment must be individualized on the basis of serum electrolyte concentrations and the acid-base profile. Correction of dehydration, infection, renal dysfunction, and electrolyte aberrations will usually improve the acid-base status. Specific recommendations for correction of acid-base disorders in patients with liver disease have been published.[457] Correction should not be undertaken if the pH is greater than 7.10 or less than 7.55 or if the base deficit is less than 10 mEq/L. If the pH is greater than 7.55 and the patient is asymptomatic, therapy should be directed to the suspected primary cause of the alkalemia, such as diuretic therapy or the liver disorder. If the patient is symptomatic (encephalopathic, cardiac arrhythmias), cautious treatment of the alkalosis is indicated. Fluid therapy should include half-strength saline supplemented to 2.5 per cent glucose and potassium replacement calculated from serum potassium measurements, and use of a standard sliding scale for potassium supplementation. Solutions containing lactate should be avoided if hepatic function is impaired. Fluid administration to patients in which edema, ascites, or hypoalbuminemia is pre-existent requires intensive monitoring to guard against overhydration and sodium loading. If the pH is less than 7.1 and the patient is symptomatic, cautious administration of bicarbonate is recommended over a 24- to 48-hour period while the clinical status is carefully monitored. Repeat acid-base profiles should guide the continued administration of bicarbonate because of the dangers of promoting alkalosis in encephalopathic patients. Bicarbonate therapy may result in excessive sodium administration, and this should be considered in patients with sodium- and fluid-retaining tendencies.

A particularly difficult problem to cope with is the concurrent development of metabolic and respiratory alkalosis. Compensation for the metabolic alkalosis initially depends on the respiratory system, which, in this situation, cannot fulfill the normal physiologic obligation of decreased ventilation. Compensation for the respiratory alkalosis depends on renal excretion of bicarbonate and retention of hydrogen ion, which in this circum stance is improbable. Treatment must be aimed at the underlying or associated problems. In very rare circumstances, severe alkalemia may require the cautious administration of hydrochloric acid as a last-chance or salvage effort.[458]

GASTROINTESTINAL ULCERATION AND HEMORRHAGE

Gastrointestinal ulceration can be a sequela to impaired hepatobiliary function or extrahepatic bile duct occlusion and can result in severe vomiting, hematemesis, and melena. Pre-existent coagulation disorders developing from hepatic insufficiency or vitamin K depletion may worsen hemorrhage from enteric ulcers. Since alimentary bleeding may cause a neurologic crisis in patients with encephalopathic tendencies, it must be efficiently identified and managed. The pathogenesis of gastrointestinal ulceration in liver disease is multifactorial (see Figure 88–15).[422] Reduced turnover of gastric mucosal cells, an altered gastric mucus barrier, and diminished mucosal circulation are promoted by hypoalbuminemia, negative nitrogen balance, and portal hypertension.[422, 459-461] Compromised hepatic function may also promote hypergastrinemia and gastric hydrochloric acid production, which favors the development of gastritis and ulcer formation.[424, 459-461] Increased serum bile acids may have causal importance in stimulating gastrin and hydrochloric acid secretion. The etiologic influence of excessive hydrochloric acid in ulcer formation warrants the use of H_2 blockers in addition to gastric protectants. Further discussion of the manage-

ment of gastrointestinal complications associated with liver disease is provided in Chapters 85 and 89.

HEPATIC ENCEPHALOPATHY

Hepatic encephalopathy is a clinical syndrome of multifactorial cause, characterized by abnormal neurologic status in a patient with severe hepatic insufficiency.[384, 462] The associated clinical signs may include lethargy, dementia, amaurosis, maniacal behavior, aggressiveness, uncontrolled barking, evidence of hallucinations, anorexia or polyphagia, vomiting, diarrhea or constipation, polydipsia, polyuria, ptyalism (especially in cats), ataxia, neuromuscular weakness, seizures, and coma. The onset can be obvious and abrupt or insidious. The patient may appear to be normal between exacerbations. Histologic lesions in the central nervous system have been characterized in patients with chronic recurrent hepatic encephalopathy. The pathogenetic mechanisms and the substances suspected to be causal to the syndrome are summarized in Figure 88–16. Certain factors appear to be synergistic in their toxic effects. The combination of factors responsible for the neurologic signs probably varies among individuals and within individuals at different times.[462] Since many of the putative toxins are derived from foodstuffs or are produced within the alimentary canal, the major therapeutic focus is to prevent toxin formation and to eliminate toxins from the gastrointestinal tract. This is largely accomplished by careful restriction of toxin-promoting dietary constituents and by modification of the intestinal microbial flora and pH. Hepatic encephalopathy should be

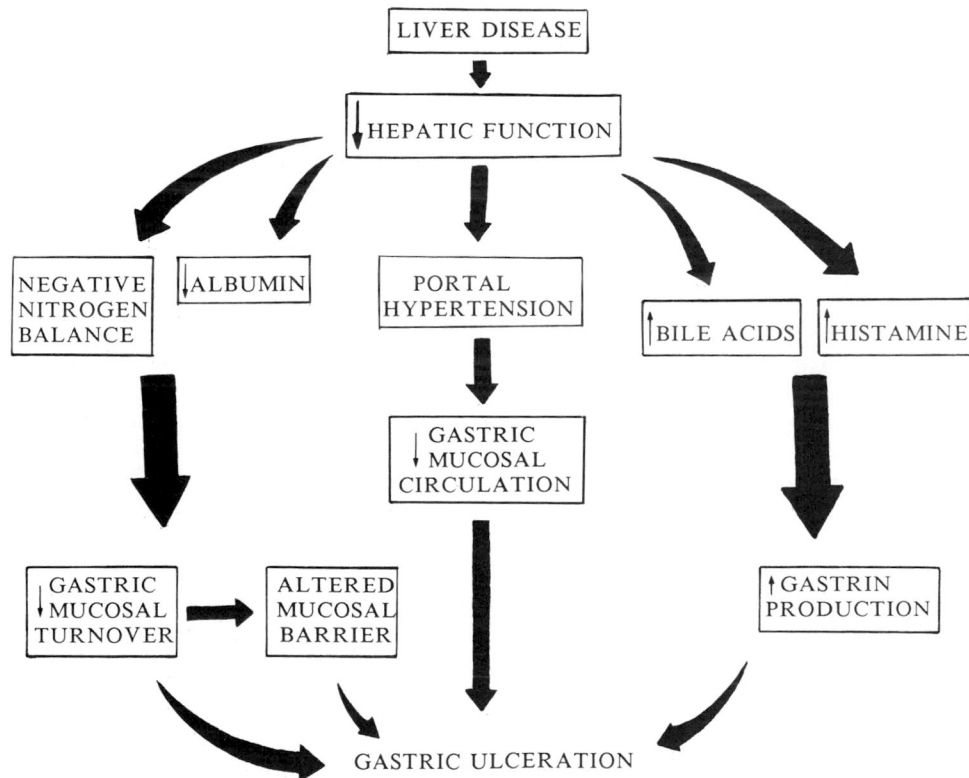

FIGURE 88–15. Pathogenetic mechanisms of gastric ulceration in patients with hepatobiliary disorders. (Modified from DeTwedt, Vet Clin of North Am 15:167, 1985.)

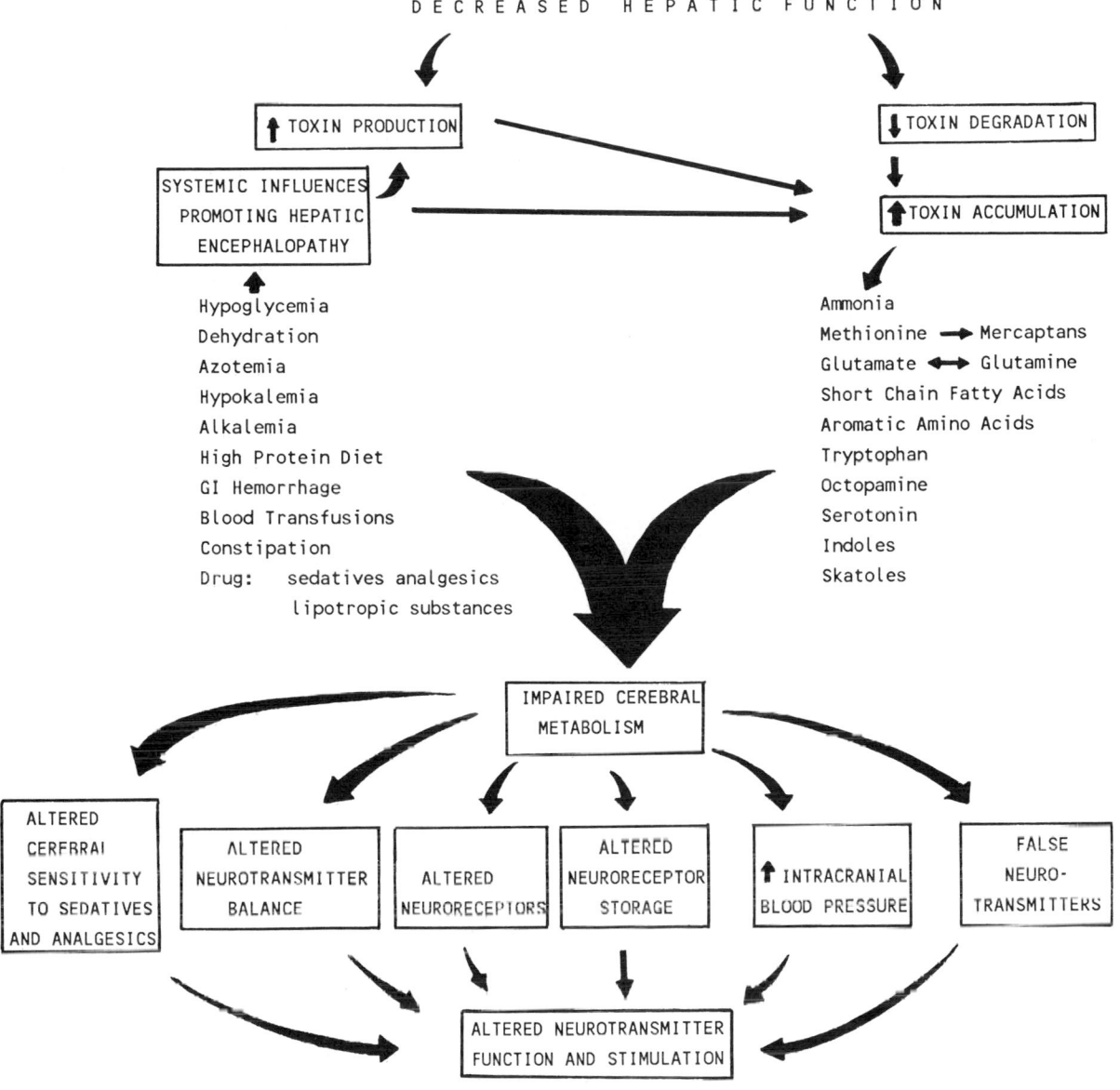

HEPATIC ENCEPHALOPATHY

FIGURE 88–16. Pathogenesis of hepatic encephalopathy.

treated as a medical emergency. Appropriate acute and chronic management is presented in Chapter 89.

Toxins Implicated in the Pathogenesis of Hepatic Encephalopathy

AMMONIA

Since the early investigations of patients with hepatic insufficiency, ammonia has been incriminated as the major pathogenetic mechanism. The neurotoxicity of ammonia has been established from indirect and direct evidence. Hyperammonemic encephalopathy develops in patients with inborn errors of urea cycle enzyme production but otherwise normal hepatic function. In addition, administration of ammonia to normal subjects reproduces many of the clinical signs of hepatic enceph-

alopathy. Nevertheless, although patients with hepatic encephalopathy are commonly hyperammonemic and benefit from measures designed to reduce the blood ammonia concentration, a consistent relationship has not been established. Some patients with unequivocal encephalopathy have normal blood ammonia concentrations while others, showing few or no signs, have remarkable hyperammonemia. There is no correlation between the severity of neurologic signs and the magnitude of the blood ammonia concentration.[384, 462] When ammonia administration has been used to induce encephalopathy in normal animals, blood ammonia concentrations necessary to induce toxic effects have greatly exceeded those documented in natural cases.[384, 462]

Ammonia is known to depress neuronal membrane activity and to interfere with cerebral energy metabolism. Acute hyperammonemia also increases cerebral blood flow and intracranial pressure and diminishes normal autoregulatory tone in cerebral vessels.[463–465] Although many other mechanisms have been proposed to explain the toxic effects of ammonia, the issue of which is most important remains controversial. Ammonia toxicity seems to be responsible, at least in part, for the amino acid imbalances that develop in hepatic insufficiency. Increased blood ammonia stimulates glucagon secretion, which promotes gluconeogenesis from BCAA.[465, 466] Increased protein catabolism, coupled with the decreased functional capacity of the urea cycle, results in perpetuation of systemic hyperammonemia.

Management of hyperammonemia centers on the restriction of ammoniagenic dietary components, control of gastrointestinal hemorrhage, conservative use of blood transfusions, administration of antibiotics and lactulose to curtail ammoniagenesis by gastrointestinal microorganisms, acidification of the lower gastrointestinal tract to promote ammonium ion trapping, osmotic catharsis, prompt treatment of infectious processes that might increase protein catabolism, and careful avoidance of metabolic alkalosis and hypokalemia that potentiate the availability and toxicity of ammonia in the central nervous system.

GLUTAMINE, GLUTAMATE, α-KETOGLUTARATE

The CSF concentrations of α-ketoglutarate and glutamine have shown a more consistent correlation with hepatic encephalopathy than has ammonia, in some investigations.[467–469] In the CNS, ammonia combines with α-ketoglutamate to form glutamic acid, which then combines with more ammonia to form glutamine. The net result is the depletion of α-ketoglutarate and ATP, which are necessary for normal brain metabolism. Glutamine and glutamate promote abnormal plasma and brain amino acid concentrations, which may lead to deranged cerebral neurotransmission.[462] Therapy aimed at reducing the blood ammonia concentration should also alleviate maladjustments in glutamate and glutamine.

AROMATIC AMINO ACIDS

Amino acid dysregulation develops as a consequence of increased gluconeogenesis, protein catabolism and increased insulin, factors that promote the uptake and metabolism of branched-chain amino acids by muscle. Increased concentrations of aromatic amino acids have been consistently observed in patients with hepatic encephalopathy. Certain of the aromatic amino acids are suspected to be neurotoxic. Of particular interest is tryptophan, which is present in abnormal concentrations in the CSF in humans and animals with hepatic insufficiency.[470, 471] The concentration of tryptophan metabolites (octopamine, serotonin, dopamine, skatoles, and indoles) may also be increased in the CNS, and it is thought that these products are the cause of at least some of the neurotoxicity. Some of these metabolites function as false neurotransmitters (octopamine) and inhibitory neurotransmitters (serotonin) and some appear to decrease the synthesis of the normal excitatory neurotransmitters.[472] Unfortunately it is unclear whether aromatic amino acids are primary mediators of hepatic encephalopathy because amino acid imbalances show a more consistent association with severe liver disease than with the onset of encephalopathy.[473]

METHIONINE AND MERCAPTANS

Methionine has also been implicated as a mediator of neurotoxicity in hepatic encephalopathy. Oral administration but not intravenous injection results in toxic effects in experimental animals. It is thought that the toxic factor is a metabolic product formed in the alimentary canal, because oral antibiotics can provide protection against methionine-induced encephalopathy.[474] Mercaptans (methanethiol, methyl mercaptan) are derived from methionine by bacterial metabolism. Methyl mercaptans are further metabolized to dimethyl sulfoxide, which seems to be involved in the production of fetor hepaticus (the abnormal breath odor associated with hepatic failure in humans).[475, 476] Methyl mercaptans are known to be highly neurotoxic and to produce signs of hepatic encephalopathy.[477–479] The toxicity of methyl mercaptan is synergistic with ammonia and free fatty acids, but the mechanism of toxicity remains undetermined.[480] The administration of methionine to dogs with reduced hepatic function can induce hepatic coma.[481] Methionine is a constituent of certain lipotropic veterinary products (drugs purported to mobilize fat). These products are indicated only if a nutritional deficiency of lipotropic substances exists, but this is rare or nonexistent in clinical practice. The prescription of lipotropic drugs is rarely indicated in clinical practice and should especially be avoided if hepatic insufficiency is suspected.

SHORT-CHAIN FATTY ACIDS

Short-chain fatty acids increase in the peripheral circulation and CSF of humans with cirrhosis or surgically created portosystemic shunts. As much as a 10-fold increase in plasma concentration of free fatty acids per gram of serum albumin has been documented.[482] These acids also increase in experimental animals undergoing hepatectomy and in cirrhotic humans fed medium-chain triglycerides.[483, 484] Short-chain fatty acids appear to be derived from the gastrointestinal tract as a result of bacterial digestion of medium-chain triglycerides, from incomplete hepatic metabolism of long-chain fatty acids, and from intestinal microbial digestion of amino acids and carbohydrates.[483] When administered to normal animals, short-chain fatty acids produce unconsciousness and electroencephalographic changes similar to those in humans with hepatic coma.[484, 485] Synergism with ammonia, mercaptan, and methanethiol has been recognized.[486] Short-chain fatty acids may also contribute to the neurotoxicity of tryptophan by reducing its protein binding and hence its availability for diffusion across the blood-brain barrier.[487] The exact toxic mechanism of short-chain fatty acids remains controversial. They appear to inhibit brain cellular respiration and membrane transport mechanisms.[463]

NEUROTRANSMITTERS

Abnormal neurotransmitter availability and function are also important pathogenetic mechanisms of hepatic encephalopathy. Brain neurons become depleted of the normal neurotransmitters, epinephrine and dopamine. Increased CNS concentrations of tryptophan promote the synthesis of brain serotonin, which may displace normal neurotransmitters from storage depots and/or receptors.[488] Both the concentration of serotonin and that of its major metabolite, 5-hydroxyindole acetic acid (5-HIAA), increase in the serum of animals following surgical creation of a portacaval shunt and in the brain and CSF of humans with acute and chronic hepatic encephalopathy. Successful management of hepatic encephalopathy in dogs and primates has rectified abnormal serotonin and 5-HIAA concentrations simultaneous with clinical improvement.[489] Imbalances in plasma amino acids also seem to be associated with increased brain 5-HIAA. Correction of plasma amino acid imbalances by infusion of branched-chain amino acids reduces the brain indole concentration.

FALSE NEUROTRANSMITTERS

The accumulation of false neurotransmitters in the CNS is also considered to be a pathogenetic mechanism of hepatic encephalopathy. False neurotransmitters are molecules that accumulate in synaptic areas and mimic the metabolism and function of natural neurotransmitters.[384] Although they are structurally similar to physiologic neurotransmitters, they are less potent in eliciting a normal response from the target tissue. Substances classified as false neurotransmitters include octopamine (an analog of norepinephrine), tyramine, β-phenylethanolamine, serotonin, histamine, catecholamines, and γ-aminobutyric acid. These substances impose important inhibitory and stimulatory effects on neuronal transmission.[384] Some of them exhibit weak sympathetic activity and can displace norepinephrine and dopamine from nerve terminal storage granules.

Treatment with L-dopa improves the clinical status of human patients with hepatic encephalopathy, presumably because of the competition with and displacement of false neurotransmitters.[490–491] L-dopa also seems to normalize concentrations of serum and CNS ammonia and this effect may underlie its apparent efficacy.[486] Bromocriptine, a dopamine agonist, has also been shown to improve mental status in encephalopathic patients. Abnormal cerebral concentrations of some of the false neurotransmitters precede their accumulation in the systemic circulation. This implicates CNS synthesis or selective brain uptake following peripheral synthesis.[473, 489] Considered independently, the false neurotransmitters cannot be promoted as a major cause of hepatic encephalopathy. Experimental work has shown that concentrations exceeding those usually found in clinical patients must be present to evoke similar clinical signs in normal animals. Furthermore, humans with hepatic failure but without signs of hepatic encephalopathy have concentrations of false neurotransmitters as high as or exceeding those in patients with neurologic signs.

INHIBITORY NEUROTRANSMITTERS

Gamma-aminobutyric acid (GABA) is the most potent inhibitory neurotransmitter implicated in the pathogenesis of hepatic encephalopathy.[492] The increased CNS concentrations of GABA are derived from increased colonic microbial production coupled with decreased hepatic extraction from the portal circulation, permeability changes in the blood-brain barrier, and direct metabolism of glutamic acid in the CNS. The availability of brain glutamate in hepatic encephalopathy would favor the latter mechanism. In humans with fulminant hepatic failure, increased plasma GABA correlates with declining neurologic status. Increased plasma GABA, however, is not closely associated with neurologic signs in dogs with chronic encephalopathy resulting from experimental portacaval shunts.[493]

ALTERATIONS IN THE BLOOD-BRAIN BARRIER

A substantial increase in the passive permeability of the blood-brain barrier and in its transport of amino acids has been shown in experimentally produced hepatic failure.[494] Alterations in the blood-brain barrier would increase the access of many substances to the brain. Experimental models of acute hepatic failure have demonstrated changes in the blood-brain barrier permeability before the onset of overt encephalopathic signs. Increased concentrations of serum bile acids have been implicated in the pathogenesis of these permeability changes.

ALTERATIONS IN NEURORECEPTORS

Recent studies have explored the changes in brain neuroreceptors during hepatic encephalopathy.[495] It is possible that the response to metabolic toxins is intensified by changes in the availability or avidity of receptors in binding neurotoxins. Increased sensitivity to and avidity for inhibitory neurotransmitters and decreased sensitivity to and avidity for excitatory neurotransmitters have been suggested.

ALTERED CEREBRAL SENSITIVITY

Alterations in the neurotransmitters and their receptors seem to increase the cerebral sensitivity to a variety of insults, including sedative and anesthetic drugs, infection, hypoxia, and disturbances of fluid, electrolytes, and pH. Relatively small changes in these variables may promote profound neurologic signs. Caution is warranted in using drugs with known CNS effects or that require hepatic biotransformation or excretion in patients with compromised hepatic function. The effects of drugs such as certain anesthetics, acepromazine, and anticonvulsants may be prolonged.

HYPOGLYCEMIA

Hypoglycemia has been shown to augment the encephalopathic effects of ammonium chloride and to increase the brain ammonia concentration. Synergism has also been observed between hypoglycemia and short-chain fatty acids in the induction of encephalopathic signs. Hypoglycemia must be anticipated and monitored for in patients with impaired hepatic function because the signs of neuroglycopenia simulate those of other encephalopathic toxins. Early prophylaxis with intravenous glucose is warranted because of the possibility of permanent neurologic impairment. Glucose administration also promotes the normalization of blood ammonia concentrations.

RADIOGRAPHY AND ULTRASONOGRAPHY OF THE HEPATOBILIARY SYSTEM

Radiography of the liver is a nonsensitive method of disease detection. Radiographically visible abnormalities are uncommon and nonspecific. Owing to the insensitivity of survey radiography, alternative procedures have been devised to improve its usefulness. Cholangiography, cholecystography, pneumoperitoneography, portovenography, and celiac angiography have each been used clinically with varied success. In exceptional cases, radioisotope scanning of the liver has been used to detail hepatic lesions. Ultrasonography has largely replaced the use of complicated or invasive radiologic procedures for examination of the hepatobiliary system.

Radiography

The liver is situated in the intrathoracic portion of the abdominal cavity. By nature of its anatomic associations, it is influenced by the position and continuity of the diaphragm, the strength and stretch of hepatic-diaphragmatic ligaments, the respiratory phase, conformation of the patient, abnormalities in adjacent organs, and the position of the patient during radiography. Movement of the diaphragm with the respiratory phases may shift the position of the liver in relation to the costal arch by one centimeter. Thoracic distention causing a caudal displacement of the diaphragm may create the appearance of hepatomegaly, while diaphragmatic rupture or congenital peritoneopericardial diaphragmatic hernia may create the illusion of microhepatica. Positioning a patient in right lateral recumbency promotes the caudad movement of the left hepatic mass and the impression of hepatomegaly.[496] An impression of reduced hepatic size may also occur in normal animals as a result of individual variation. There are minor differences in the lobulation of the liver between the dog and cat but these are not apparent on radiographic examination. Survey radiography of the liver reveals only an approximation of its multilobed structure and biliary and vascular components owing to soft tissue superimposition.

The most important features apparent by radiographic assessment of the liver include alterations in hepatic size, position, shape, and variation in density.[496–497] The position of the adjacent viscera provides an approximation of liver size. The angle of the gas pocket in the stomach can be used as an anatomic landmark. In health, the gastric silhouette lies parallel to the inter-costal spaces, following the arch of the ribs at about the tenth intercostal space. With a reduction of hepatic volume, the gastric gas pattern assumes a more upright posture with cranial displacement reducing the distance between the stomach and diaphragm.[496] Positional shift of the right kidney, pyloric antrum, proximal duodenum and transverse colon to a more cranial location also may signify a reduction in hepatic mass. In general, the radiographic impression of microhepatica is unreliable and inexact. Radiographic features of hepatomegaly include a rounding of the liver lobe margins, extension of the hepatic lobes beyond the costal arch (particularly the left lateral lobe on the lateral view), caudal-dorsal leftward displacement of the stomach, caudal displacement of the proximal duodenum and right kidney, and caudal medial displacement of the transverse colon. Assessment for surface irregularities is rewarding only in the caudoventral margins of the liver. This is enhanced by the presence of fat within the falciform ligament. Radiographs made with the patient in left lateral recumbency may result in a merging of the hepatic and splenic shadows, thus obscuring the ordinarily visible margins of the liver. Blunting or rounding of the liver margins suggests diffuse hepatomegaly. Irregular or bumpy liver margins indicate hepatic neoplasia, regenerative nodules, hepatic cysts, or other focal lesions.

The detection of intrahepatic gas in the common bile duct, gallbladder, or hepatic ducts may follow recent surgical intervention involving these structures. This may also indicate infection with gas-producing organisms. Gas has been reported within the portal venous system following severe necrotizing or ulcerative gastroenteritis, paralytic ileus, and gastric torsion, as evidence of discontinuity in the gastrointestinal microcirculatory bed or infection with gas-producing organisms.[496, 497] Gas in the hepatic veins creates a linear, branching pattern similar to an air bronchogram in the lung. Emphysematous cholecystitis, gas accumulation within the wall and lumen of the gallbladder, has been seen in dogs, some of which have been diabetics.[498, 499] Organisms associated with emphysematous cholecystitis in humans include *E. coli*, staphylococci, anaerobic streptococci, and clostridia.[499, 500]

Mineralization or calcifications of intrahepatic structures have been observed in both dogs and cats. Dystrophic calcification may appear as multifocal intrahepatic "lithiasis" and may be associated with postnecrotic scarring, granulomas, hematomas, neoplasia, or parasitic cysts (see Figure 88–17).[496–497] Diffuse cholelithiasis associated with radiodense choleliths lodged in bile ducts may produce a similar radiographic appearance.

Pneumoperitoneography has been used to investigate the hepatic silhouette. This technique is accomplished by injecting air, CO_2, or O_2 into the abdominal cavity. The negative contrast is used to outline different areas of the liver by manipulation of patient position and exposure angles. Further discussion of this technique is available.[501]

Positive contrast studies of the biliary tree have been advocated for differentiation of intrahepatic and extrahepatic causes of jaundice. Cholecystography and cholangiography are completed by use of cholephilic iodi-

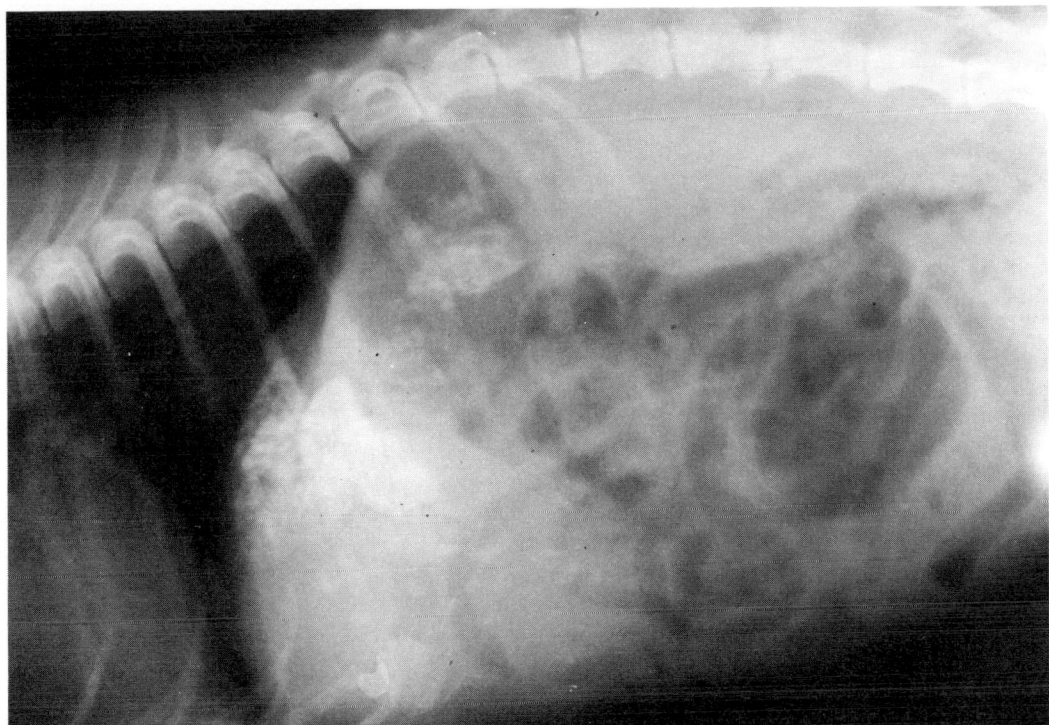

FIGURE 88–17. Radiograph made of a dog with multifocal dystrophic mineralization resulting from hepatic inflammation and necrosis.

nated contrast media that are excreted through the biliary system. Cholecystography following the oral administration of iopanoic acid (Telepaque) and the intravenous administration of iodipamide (Cholografin) has been completed in healthy dogs and cats.[496, 502–504] The intravenous procedures seem preferable to the oral methods.[505] The concentration of contrast in the biliary tree is inconsistent because it represents the cumulative effects of contrast-induced choleresis, contrast excretion, and the patient's basal flow of bile. Contraindications to the procedure include severe hyperbilirubinemia, severe hepatocellular disease, and known adverse responses to iodinated contrast media.[505] In veterinary clinical practice, these procedures are unreliable in the differentiation of cholestatic abnormalities. Test inadequacy may be due to poor intestinal contrast absorption induced by prolonged fasting, vomiting or diarrhea, a low intestinal pH, delayed gastric emptying, ileus associated with inflammatory visceral lesions, disorders of the gallbladder, biliary stasis, rapid biliary tree absorption of the contrast agent, or hepatic dysfunction.[505] Cholangiographic procedures have been largely replaced by ultrasonographic examinations.

Arteriography and venography may be used to assess hepatic and portal vasculature. Arteriography requires selective catheterization of the celiac or anterior mesenteric artery or nonselective catheterization of the jugular vein with radiographs made during arterial perfusion after bolus injection of contrast. Image-intensified fluoroscopy and the equipment for producing rapid serial radiographs are necessary for these studies.[505] Hepatic arteriography may be used to localize focal intrahepatic lesions and intrahepatic arteriovenous fistulas. Examination of the portal venous system is possible by contrast injection into a mesenteric vein, a splenic vein, or the splenic pulp, or by selective catheterization of the anterior mesenteric artery with radiographs made during the portal venous phase of circulation. Portography is used to visualize abnormalities in the portal venous circulation such as those present in congenital or acquired portosystemic shunts. Lateral and dorsoventral views should be obtained for correct vessel identification. This procedure is recommended for localization of congenital portosystemic shunts prior to surgical intervention.

Ultrasonography

Ultrasonography is an important diagnostic modality for evaluation of the hepatobiliary system. It is exceptionally useful in the detection of focal hepatic parenchymal abnormalities or biliary tract disease. This technique allows inspection of the hepatic parenchyma, biliary system, and vascular structures. Detectible abnormalities include changes in tissue density, vascular distention, focal or diffuse changes in hepatic size, the presence of ascites, congenital malformations, neoplasia, cysts, abscesses, cholelithiasis, inflammation of the biliary tree, and extrahepatic bile duct occlusion. The deposition of fat or fibrous tissue in the hepatic parenchyma may produce a diffuse increase in echogenicity.[506–508] Infiltration of the parenchyma with lymphoma or acute inflammation may result in a diffuse decrease in echogenicity.[509] Ultrasonographic features of passive congestion include hepatomegaly, hepatic vein distention, portal vein distention, and ascites. Ultrasonography allows noninvasive localization of the cause of portal hypertension by inspection of the caudal vena cava, hepatic veins, and portal circulatory system.

Focal or multifocal lesions are more easily recognized than diffuse parenchymal disease. Liver masses as small as 1 to 2 cm can be detected. Ultrasonography has been shown to be a sensitive method for detecting metastatic hepatic lesions.[507] Focal abnormalities are described in terms that differentiate them from the surrounding tissues: anechoic (no internal echoes, fluid filled), hypoechoic (reduced internal echoes), hyperechoic (increased internal echoes), and mixed echogenicity (any combination).[506] Since many different pathologic processes may produce similar ultrasonographic patterns, the nonspecific nature of the findings must be considered. Table 88–14 provides a reference to the reported ultrasonographic characteristics associated with focal hepatic lesions.[505–510]

The gallbladder is easily examined by ultrasonography. It normally appears round, is anechoic, and is located to the right of midline between the quadrate and right medial liver lobe.[506, 508] The size of the gallbladder is determined by the interval between meals during which the patient is examined. In the anorectic patient it is often large or distended. The wall of the gallbladder is usually not well defined in the healthy animal. If the wall is thickened by inflammation or edema associated with ascites, hypoproteinemia, or congestive heart failure, a double-rimmed effect may be produced.[506] The detection of biliary sediment seems to

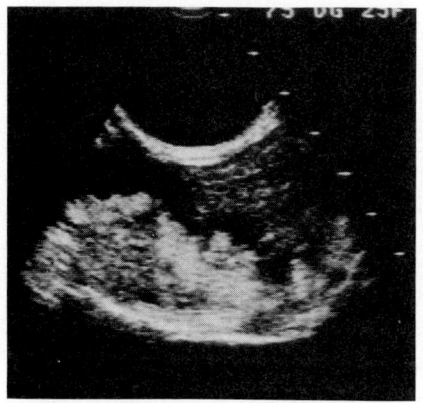

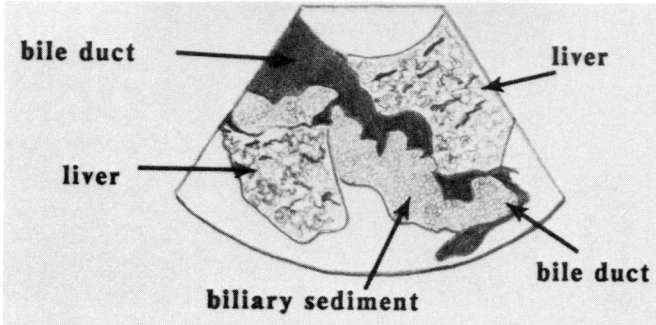

FIGURE 88–18. Two-dimensional ultrasonogram and diagrammatic sketch of the sonogram of a cat with complete occlusion of the common bile duct. The tortuous, dilated, irregular bile duct and biliary sediment indicated a need for surgical biliary diversion. (Courtesy of Dr. Amy Dietze, NYS Coll Vet Med, Ithaca, New York.)

TABLE 88–14. ULTRASONOGRAPHIC FEATURES OF FOCAL HEPATOBILIARY LESIONS

Echogenicity	Lesion
Parenchymal Lesions	
Anechoic Lesions	
Absence of internal echoes Sharply demarcated margins Posterior acoustic enhancement Septations Internal debris	Congenital cysts Acquired cysts
Irregular internal margins Varying degrees acoustic enhancement	Abscesses Hematoma Hepatic necrosis Neoplasia
Hypoechoic Lesions	Hematomas Abscesses Neoplasia Regenerative nodules
Hyperechoic Lesions	Dense fibrosis Hematomas Abscesses Choleliths Mineralization Emphysematous lesions (gas)

Mixed
Lesions solid with fluid
  components or fluid with
  solid debris
	Hepatic necrosis
	Neoplasia
	Hematomas
	Abscess

Gallbladder Masses	Cystic hyperplasia Adenoma Adenocarcinoma Choleliths

be common in small animal patients. The significance of this observation remains to be established. In the clinically icteric patient, ultrasound can be used to ascertain the presence of biliary obstruction. Extrahepatic bile duct occlusion may be differentiated from intrahepatic cholestasis (Figure 88–18). In the normal animal, intrahepatic bile ducts are not easily visualized.[498] If dilated bile ducts are seen and obstructive biliary disease seems probable, surgical intervention should be considered. Experimental work completed in dogs has characterized the temporal development of gallbladder dilatation and sequential retrograde dilatation of the biliary tract after complete extrahepatic bile duct occlusion.[510] Within 48 hours the common bile duct distends, within three days the extrahepatic bile ducts dilate, and within seven days the intrahepatic lobar and interlobar ducts dilate. Enlarged dilated bile ducts differ from the adjacent portal veins in their tortuosity and by the nature of their irregularly branching patterns.[510] It is also known that bile duct dilatation may persist ultrasonographically for some time after extrahepatic bile duct occlusion is alleviated.

Prior to the availability of ultrasonographic techniques, cholelithiasis and choledocholithiasis were infrequently diagnosed in the dog and cat. The diagnosis of these disorders seems more common now that ultrasonography is routinely used at referral centers. Ultrasonography allows detection of biliary calculi regardless of their radiodensity. Calculi and biliary sediment gravitate to dependent portions of the gallbladder with changes in the patient's position and can thus be differentiated

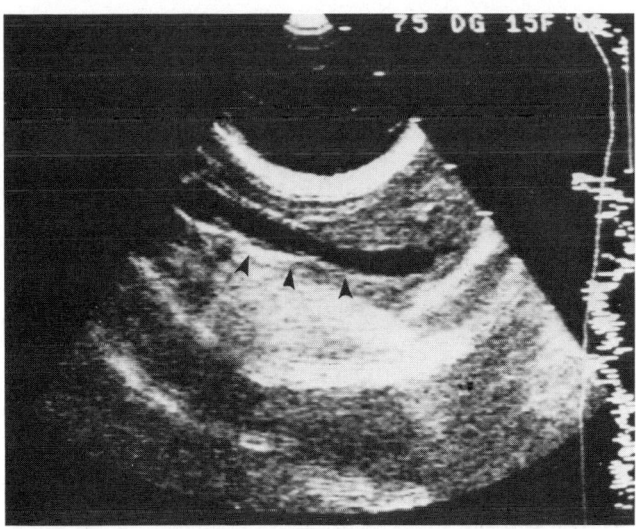

FIGURE 88–19. Two-dimensional ultrasonogram of a cat with a congenital extrahepatic portosystemic shunt. Careful examination of the portal vasculature allowed identification of the anomalous vessel indicated by the black arrows. (Courtesy of Dr. Amy Dietze, NYS Coll Vet Med, Ithaca, New York.) (From Comp Cont Educ 8:896, 1986.)

from fixed structural abnormalities. Intraductal calculi are more difficult to visualize than choleliths situated within the gallbladder.

Ultrasonography can also be used to confirm the presence of intrahepatic or extrahepatic, single or multiple, portosystemic shunts (Figure 88–19). Intrahepatic venous anomalies are the easiest to visualize. The presence of single extrahepatic shunts may also be confirmed, but these necessitate a greater expertise and a more tedious examination than does localization of large intrahepatic shunts. Intrahepatic arteriovenous fistulas have also been identified using ultrasonography.

Although ultrasonographic examination of the hepatobiliary system seems to be more sensitive as a diagnostic test for disease than is radiography, it is critical that an experienced ultrasonographer interpret the findings. Inexperience with this technique can easily lead to a false sense of security and an inaccurate diagnosis.

Hepatic Biopsy

Liver biopsy is indicated on the basis of historical and physical examination and clinicopathologic findings in order to ascertain a correct definitive diagnosis, specific therapy, and accurate prognosis. This is an invasive procedure that must be carefully considered before implementation. Major complications experienced in veterinary and human patients range between 0.015 and 3.5 per cent, varying with the procedure used and the experience of the clinician collecting the sample.[511-513] The indications and contraindications for biopsy must be carefully considered before a biopsy is taken. The major indications for hepatic biopsy are listed in Table 88–15. To gain maximum information from biopsied tissue the clinician should consider the alternatives for biopsy examination. Before fixation in formalin, cytologic imprints should be made and a portion of the tissue aseptically retained for bacterial culture. Special

stains for determining the presence of glycogen, fat, fibrosis, and infectious agents should be requested if deemed appropriate in context of the case. Stains for fat must be applied to tissue that has not been paraffin-embedded for routine histologic examination.

Prior to the biopsy procedure, the coagulation status of the patient must be assessed and a source of compatible blood for transfusion should be located. Hemorrhagic tendencies may exist but fail to be evidenced by *in vitro* assessments of coagulation (see section on coagulation in this chapter). As a result, the clinician must *always* be prepared for and anticipate postbiopsy hemorrhage. If extrahepatic bile duct occlusion is suspected in a jaundiced patient, vitamin K_1 should be given at least 24 hours prior to the scheduled procedure.

Several different techniques may be used for hepatic biopsy, including transabdominal fine needle aspirate, keyhole needle biopsy, transthoracic needle biopsy, ultrasonographic guided needle biopsy, laparoscopy guided needle biopsy, and laparotomy for wedge biopsy. Consideration of the benefits and risks of each procedure, the medical condition of the patient, and the expertise of the clinician in obtaining needle biopsies will guide technique selection. If the liver is enlarged and can be unequivocally localized and a diffuse disorder is suspected, a fine needle aspirate or transthoracic or key hole approach for needle biopsy may be used. Contraindications for blind biopsy procedures include the suspected presence of hepatic abscesses, cysts or vascular tumors, extensive abdominal adhesions, septic peritonitis, obstructive jaundice, severe obesity, and the inability to restrain the patient adequately.[511] In cases in which needle biopsy is used, gallbladder contraction should be stimulated six hours before the procedure by ingestion of a fatty meal. The biopsy should be taken from liver lobes not adjacent to the gallbladder. While occasional needle biopsies may contain too few acinar units for optimal histopathologic assessment, wedge biopsies are more reliable. The presence of hepatic fibrosis should be suspected when repeated needle biopsy attempts yield insufficient tissue. If the patient's condition is stable, a laparotomy is advantageous because it allows direct visual selection of the biopsy site, postbiopsy observation for hemorrhage, and the opportunity for surgical therapy should it be indicated. If extrahepatic bile duct occlusion is suspected, laparotomy would allow treatment by biliary diversion without the risk of lacerating a distended gallbladder during a blind biopsy procedure. If focal hepatic lesions are suspected, laparoscopic techniques, ultrasonographic guided biopsy, or laparotomy is indicated. Animals with severe hypoalbuminemia are best biopsied using a paralumbar

TABLE 88–15. INDICATIONS FOR HEPATIC BIOPSY

1. Fulminant hepatic failure of unknown cause.
2. Abnormal liver enzyme activity exceeding 4 to 8 weeks in the absence of drug related enzyme induction in the dog and hyperthyroidism in the cat.
3. Acute or chronic, unexplained abnormal liver function tests.
4. Unequivocal, unexplained changes in hepatic size.
5. To confirm or stage neoplasia.
6. To sequentially assess disease progression.
7. To sequentially assess response to treatment.

approach, regardless of the technique utilized, since ventral midline approaches are complicated by gravitational pooling of edema fluid. A complete review of the methods and instruments used for hepatic biopsy in the dog and cat is available for the interested reader.[511]

References

1. Bradley, SE, et al.: The estimation of hepatic blood flow in man. J Clin Invest 24:890, 1945.
2. Greenway, CV and Stark, RD: Hepatic vascular bed. Physiol Rev 51:23, 1971.
3. Greenway, CV and Lister, GE: Capacitance effects and blood reservoir function in the splanchnic vascular bed during non-hypotensive haemorrhage and blood volume expansion in anesthetized cats. J Physiol 237:279, 1974.
4. Hanson, KM: Liver. In Johnson, PC (ed): Peripheral Circulation. New York, John Wiley & Sons, 1978, p 285.
5. Campra, JL and Reynolds, RB: The hepatic circulation. In Arias, I, et al. (eds): The Liver: Biology and Pathobiology. New York, Raven Press, 1982, p 627.
6. Ternberg, JL and Butcher, HR, Jr: Blood flow relation between hepatic artery and portal vein. Science 150:1030, 1965.
7. Cobb, LM and McKay, KA: A bacteriological study of the liver of the normal dog. J Comp Pathol 72:92, 1962.
8. Schatten, WE: The role of intestinal bacteria in liver necrosis following experimental excision of the hepatic arterial supply. Surgery 36:256, 1954.
9. Gumucia, JJ and Miller, DL: Liver cell heterogeneity. In Arias, I, et al. (eds): The Liver: Biology and Pathobiology. New York, Raven Press, 1982, p 647.
10. Rappaport, AM: Physioanatomic considerations. In Schiff, L and Schiff, ER (eds): Diseases of the Liver, 5th ed. Philadelphia, JB Lippincott, 1982, p 1.
11. Ito, T and Shibasaki, S: Electron microscopic study on the hepatic sinusoidal wall and the fat-storing cells in the normal human liver. Arch Histol Jpn 29:137, 1968.
12. Gale, RP, et al.: Bone marrow origin of hepatic macrophages (Kupffer cells) in humans. Science 201:937, 1978.
13. Editorial: Bone marrow origin of Kupffer cells. Lancet 1:130, 1980.
14. Rogers, DE: Host mechanisms which act to remove bacteria from the blood stream. Bacteriol Rev 24:50, 1960.
15. Friedman, M, et al.: Observations concerning the production and excretion of cholesterol in mammals. Am J Physiol 177:77, 1954.
16. Berliner, DL, et al.: The role of hepatic and adrenal reticulo-endothelial cells in steroid biotransformation. J Reticuloendothel Soc 1:1, 1964.
17. Bergman, JR: Nodular hyperplasia in the liver of the dog: An association with changes in the Ito cell population. Vet Pathol 22:427, 1985.
18. Jones, AL and Fawcett, DW: Hypertrophy of the agranular endoplasmic reticulum in hamster liver induced by phenobarbital (with a review of the function of this organelle in the liver). J Histochem Cytochem 14:215, 1966.
19. Spring-Mills, E and Hones, AL: Ultrastructural concepts of drug metabolism. II. The hepatocyte: Phenobarbital and microsomal enzyme induction. Am J Drug Alcohol Abuse 1:271, 1974.
20. Phillips, MJ, et al.: Microfilament dysfunction as a possible cause of intrahepatic cholestasis. Gastroenterology 69:48, 1975.
21. Takahashi, I, et al.: Comparison of gallbladder contraction induced by motilin and cholecystokinin in dogs. Gastroenterology 82:419, 1982.
22. Mullock, B, et al.: Sources of protein in rat bile. Biochem Biophys Acta 543:497, 1978.
23. Leffert, HL, et al.: Hormonal control of rat liver regeneration. Gastroenterology 76:1470, 1979.
24. Rikkers, LF and Moody, FG: Estimation of functional reserve of normal and regenerating dog livers. Surgery 75:421, 1974.
25. Wienbreu, K: Regeneration of liver. Gastroenterology 37:657, 1959.
26. Harkness, RD: Regeneration of liver. Br Med Bull 13:87, 1957.
27. Furnival, CM, et al.: The mechanism of impaired coagulation after partial hepatectomy in the dog. Surg Gynecol Obstet 143:81, 1976.
28. Osbaldiston, GW and Hoffman, MW: Coagulation defects in experimental hepatic injury in the dog. Can J Comp Med 35:129, 1971.
29. Mann, FC and Magath, TB: The effect of administration of glucose in the condition following total extirpation of the liver. Arch Intern Med 30:171, 1922.
30. Schenk, WG, et al.: The coagulation defect after hepatectomy. Surgery 42:822, 1957.
31. Dowling, RH: The enterohepatic circulation. Gastroenterology 62:122, 1972.
32. Kuipers, F, et al.: Enterohepatic circulation in the rat. Gastroenterology 88:403, 1985.
33. Nickel, R, et al.: The viscera of the domestic mammals. Berlin, Verlag Paul Parey, 1973.
34. Johnston, DG and Alberti, KGMM: The liver and the endocrine system. In Wright, R, et al. (eds): Liver and Biliary Disease, 2nd ed. Philadelphia, WB Saunders, 1985, p 161.
35. van Thiel, DH: Endocrine function. In Arias, I, et al. (eds): The Liver: Biology and Pathobiology. New York, Raven Press, 1982, p 717.
36. Herman, RH: Metabolism of vitamins by the liver in normal and pathologic conditions. In Zakim, D and Boyer, TD (eds): Hepatology—A Textbook of Liver Disease. Philadelphia, WB Saunders, 1982, p 152.
37. Wagner, AF and Folkers, K: The vitamin K group. In Vitamins and Coenzymes. New York, Interscience Publishers, 1964, p 407.
38. Stenflo, J, et al.: Vitamin K dependent modifications of glutamic acid residues in prothrombin. Proc Natl Acad Sci USA 71:2730, 1974.
39. Bell, RG, et al.: Mechanism of action of warfarin. Warfarin and metabolism of vitamin K_1. Biochemistry 11:1959, 1972.
40. Bell, RG and Matschiner, JT: Warfarin and the inhibition of vitamin K activity by an oxide metabolite. Nature 237:32, 1972.
41. Hemker, HC and Muller, AD: Kinetic aspects of the interaction of blood clotting enzymes: VI. Localization of the site of blood-coagulation inhibition by the protein induced by vitamin K absence (PIVKA). Thromb Diath Haemorrh 20:78, 1968.
42. Gaudernack, G and Prydz, H: Studies on PIVKA-X. Thromb Diath Haemorrh 34:455, 1975.
43. Mount, ME: Proteins induced by Vitamin K absence or antagonists (PIVKA). In Kirk, RW (ed): Current Veterinary Therapy, IX. Philadelphia, WB Saunders, 1986, p 513.
44. Steinberg, SE and Hillman, RS: The liver and hematopoiesis. In Zakim, D and Boyer, TD (eds): Hepatology—A Textbook of Liver Disease. Philadelphia, WB Saunders, 1982, p 537.
45. Robinson, SH: Degradation of hemoglobin. In Williams, WJ, et al. (eds): Hematology, 3rd ed. New York, McGraw-Hill, 1983, p 388.
46. Blanckaert, N and Schmid, R: Physiology and pathophysiology of bilirubin metabolism. In Zakim, D and Boyer, TD (eds): Hepatology—A Textbook of Liver Disease. Philadelphia, WB Saunders, 1982, p 246.
47. Douglass, CC, et al.: The acanthocyte in cirrhosis with hemolytic anemia. Ann Intern Med 68:390, 1968.
48. Smith, JA, et al.: Spur-cell anemia: Hemolytic anemia with red cells resembling acanthocytes in alcoholic cirrhosis. N Engl J Med 271:396, 1964.
49. Grahn, EP, et al.: Burr cells, hemolytic anemia and cirrhosis. Am J Med 45:78, 1968.
50. Silber, R, et al.: Spur-shaped erythrocytes in Laennec's cirrhosis. N Engl J Med 275:639, 1966.
51. Shull, RM, et al.: Spur cell anemia in a dog. JAVMA 173:978, 1978.
52. Cooper, RA and Jandl, JH: Destruction of erythrocytes. In Williams, WJ, et al. (eds): Hematology, 3rd ed. New York, McGraw-Hill, 1983, p 377.
53. Zieve, L: Hemolytic anemia in liver disease. Medicine 45:497, 1966.
54. Griffiths, GL, et al.: Hematologic and biochemical changes in dogs with portosystemic shunts. JAAHA 17:705, 1981.

55. Weiss, HJ: Acquired qualitative platelet disorders. *In* Williams, WJ, et al. (eds): Hematology, 3rd ed. New York, McGraw-Hill, 1983, p 1356.

56. Harker, LA and Finch, CA: Thrombokinetics in man. J Clin Invest 48:963, 1969.

57. Aster, RH: Pooling of platelets in the spleen: Role in the pathogenesis of "hypersplenic" thrombocytopenia. J Clin Invest 45:645, 1966.

58. Thomas, DP, et al.: Platelet aggregation in patients with Laennec's cirrhosis of the liver. N Engl J Med 276:1344, 1967.

59. Thomas, DP: Abnormalities of platelet aggregation in patients with alcoholic cirrhosis. Ann NY Acad Sci 201:243, 1972.

60. Roberts, HR and Cederbaum, AI: The liver and blood coagulation: Physiology and pathology. Gastroenterology 63:297, 1972.

61. Walls, WD and Losowsky, MS: The hemostatic defect of liver disease. Gastroenterology 60:108, 1971.

62. Lechner, K, et al.: Coagulation abnormalities in liver disease. Semin Thromb Hemost 4:40, 1977.

63. Flute, PT: Clotting abnormalities in liver disease. Prog Liver Dis 6:301, 1979.

64. Spector, I and Corn, M: Laboratory tests of hemostasis. The relation to hemorrhage in liver disease. Arch Intern Med 119:577, 1967.

65. Colman, RW and Rubin, RN: Blood coagulation. *In* Arias, I, et al. (eds): The Liver: Biology and Pathobiology. New York, Raven Press, 1982, p 761.

66. Aledort, LM: Blood clotting abnormalities in liver disease. *In* Popper, H and Schaffner, F (eds): Progress in Liver Diseases. New York, Grune & Stratton, 1976, p 352.

67. Badylak, SF and Van Vleet, JF: Alterations of prothrombin time and activated partial thromboplastin time in dogs with hepatic disease. Am J Vet Res 42:2053, 1981.

68. Martinez, J and Palascak, JE: Hemostatic alterations in liver disease. *In* Zakim, D and Boyer, TD (eds): Hepatology—A Textbook of Liver Disease. Philadelphia, WB Saunders, 1982, p 546.

69. Badylak, SF, et al.: Plasma coagulation factor abnormalities in dogs with naturally occurring hepatic disease. Am J Vet Res 44:2336, 1983.

70. Green, G, et al.: Factor VII as a marker of hepatocellular synthetic function in liver disease. J Clin Pathol 29:971, 1976.

71. Dymock, IW, et al.: Coagulation studies as a prognostic index in acute liver failure. Br J Haematol 29:385, 1975.

72. Friedman, PA: Vitamin K-dependent proteins. N Engl J Med 310:1458, 1984.

73. Koller, F: Die blutgerinnung und ihre klinische bedeutung. Dtsch Med Wochenschr 80:516, 1956.

74. Deutsh, E: Blood coagulation changes in liver diseases. *In* Popper, H and Schaffner, F (eds): Progress in Liver Diseases. New York, Grune & Stratton, 1976, p 69.

75. Ham, TH and Curtis, FC: Plasma fibrinogen response in man. Influence of the nutritional state, induced hyperpyrexia, infectious disease and liver damage. Medicine 14:413, 1938.

76. McCaw, DL, et al.: Effect of internal hemorrhage on fibrin(ogen) degradation products in canine blood. Am J Vet Res 47:1620, 1986.

77. Lane, DA, et al.: Acquired dysfibrinogenaemia in acute and chronic liver disease. Br J Haematol 33:301, 1977.

78. Millar, HR, et al.: An evaluation of the heat precipitation method for plasma fibrinogen estimation. J Clin Pathol 24:827, 1971.

79. Kaneko, JJ and Smith, R: The estimation of plasma fibrinogen and its clinical significance in the dog. Calif Vet Aug, 21, 1967.

80. Penwick, GD, et al.: Hemorrhagic states secondary to intravascular clotting. An experimental study of their evolution and prevention. Arch Path 66:708, 1958.

81. Strombeck, DR, et al.: Coagulopathy and encephalopathy in a dog with acute hepatic necrosis. JAVMA 169:813, 1976.

82. Green, RA: Clinical implications of antithrombin III deficiency in animal diseases. Comp Cont Ed 6:537, 1984.

83. Weiss, RC, et al.: Disseminated intravascular coagulation in experimentally induced feline infectious peritonitis. Am J Vet Res 41:663, 1980.

84. Wigton, DH, et al.: Infectious canine hepatitis: Animal model of viral-induced disseminated intravascular coagulation. Blood 47:287, 1976.

85. Moore, DH and Kowlessar, OD: Hepatic synthesis and degradation of plasma proteins. *In* Zakim, D and Boyer, TD (eds): Hepatology—A Textbook of Liver Disease. Philadelphia, WB Saunders, 1982, p 137.

86. Biggs, R, et al.: Antithrombin III, antifactor Xa and heparin. Br J Haematol 19:283, 1970.

87. Rodzynek, JJ, et al.: Diagnostic value of antithrombin III and aminopyrine breath test in liver diseases. Arch Intern Med 146:677, 1986.

88. Feldman, BF, et al.: Disseminated intravascular coagulation: Antithrombin, plasminogen, and coagulation abnormalities in 41 dogs. JAVMA 179:151, 1981.

89. Raymond, SL and Dodds, WJ: Plasma antithrombin activity: A comparative study in normal and diseased animals. Proc Soc Exp Biol Med 161:464, 1979.

90. Mannucci, L, et al.: Value of Normotest and antithrombin III in the assessment of liver function. Scand J Gastroenterol 19:103, 1973.

91. Duekert, F: Behaviour of antithrombin III in liver disease. Scand J Gastroenterol 19:109, 1973.

92. Rake, MO, et al.: Intravascular coagulation in acute hepatic necrosis. Lancet 1:533, 1970.

93. Rake, MO, et al.: Early and intensive therapy of intravascular coagulation in acute liver failure. Lancet 2:1215, 1971.

94. Marciniak, E, et al.: Familial thrombosis due to antithrombin III deficiency. Blood 43:219, 1974.

95. Aoki, M and Yamanaka, T: The α-2-plasmin inhibitor levels in liver diseases. Clin Chim Acta 84:99, 1978.

96. Fletcher, AP, et al.: Abnormal plasminogen-plasmin system activity (fibrinolysis) in patients with hepatic cirrhosis: Its cause and consequences. J Clin Invest 43:681, 1964.

97. Green, RA: Hemostasis and disorders of coagulation. Vet Clin North Am: Sm Anim Pract 11:289, 1981.

98. Furie, B: Disorders of hemostasis-acquired disorders of blood coagulation. *In* Williams, WJ, et al. (eds): Hematology, 3rd ed. New York, McGraw-Hill, 1983, p 1421.

99. Reeve, EB, et al.: Studies with ^{131}I labelled antithrombin III in dogs. Thromb Res 20:375, 1980.

100. Sumols, E and Holdsworth, D: Disturbances in carbohydrate metabolism: Liver disease. *In* Dickins, F, et al. (eds): Carbohydrate Metabolism and Its Disorders. New York, Academic Press, 1968, p 289.

101. Owen, OE, et al.: Gluconeogenesis in normal, cirrhotic and diabetic humans. *In* Hanson, RW and Mehlman, MA (eds): Gluconeogenesis: Its Regulations in Mammalian Species. New York, John Wiley & Sons, 1976, p 533.

102. Camu, F: Hepatic balances of glucose and insulin in response to physiological increases of endogenous insulin during glucose infusions in dogs. Eur J Clin Invest 5:101, 1975.

103. Kanazaawa, Y, et al.: Plasma insulin responses to glucose in femoral, hepatic and pancreatic veins in dogs. Am J Physiol 211:442, 1966.

104. Kaden, M, et al.: Effect of intraduodenal glucose administration on hepatic extraction of insulin in the anesthetized dog. J Clin Invest 52:2016, 1973.

105. Johnston, DG, et al.: Hyperinsulinism of hepatic cirrhosis: diminished degradation or increased secretion. Lancet 1:10, 1977.

106. Johnson, DG and Alberti, KGMM: The liver and the endocrine system. *In* Wright, R, et al. (eds): Liver and Biliary Disease. 2nd ed. Philadelphia, WB Saunders, 1985, p 1.

107. Lickley, HLA, et al.: Effects of portacaval anastomosis on glucose tolerance in the dog: Evidence of an interaction between the gut and the liver in oral glucose disposal. Metabolism 24:1157, 1975.

108. Soeters, P, et al.: Insulin, glucagon, portal systemic shunting and hepatic failure in the dog. J Surg Res 23:183, 1977.

109. Sherwin, R, et al.: Hyperglucagonemia in Laennec's cirrhosis: The role of portal-systemic shunting. N Engl J Med 290:239, 1974.

110. Waddell, WR and Sussman, KE: Plasma insulin after diversion of portal and pancreatic venous blood to vena cava. J Appl Physiol 22:808, 1967.

111. Collin, J, et al.: Carbohydrate tolerance with portal and systemic venous drainage of the pancreas. Br J Surg 64:180, 1977.

112. Megyesi, C, et al.: Glucose tolerance and diabetes in chronic liver disease. Lancet 2:1051, 1967.

113. Marco, J, et al.: Elevated plasma glucagon levels in cirrhosis of the liver. N Engl J Med 289:1107, 1973.

114. Sherwin, RS, et al.: Hyperglucagonemia in cirrhosis: Altered secretion and sensitivity to glucagon. Gastroenterology 74:1224, 1978.

115. Walton, D, et al.: Ulcerative dermatosis associated with diabetes mellitus in the dog: A report of four cases. JAAHA 22:79, 1986.

116. Francavilla, A, et al.: The effect of portacaval shunt upon hepatic cholesterol synthesis and cyclic AMP in dogs and baboons. J Surg Res 28:1, 1980.

117. Magne, ML and Macy, DW: Intravenous glucagon challenge test in the diagnosis and assessment of therapeutic efficacy in dogs with congenital portosystemic shunts. (abstract). ACVIM Scientific Proceedings, 1984, p 36.

118. Magne, ML and Withrow, SJ: Hepatic Neoplasia. Vet Clin North Am 15:243, 1985.

119. Turley, SD and Dietschy, JM: Cholesterol metabolism and excretion. In Arias, I, et al. (eds): The Liver: Biology and Pathobiology. New York, Raven Press, 1982, p 467.

120. Brown, MS: Regulation of plasma cholesterol by lipoprotein receptors. Science 212:628, 1981.

121. Dietschy, JM and Wilson, JD: Regulation of cholesterol metabolism (three parts). N Engl J Med 282:1128, 1970.

122. Bunch, SE: Hypocholesterolemia in dogs. ACVIM Proceedings, 1986, p 13-7.

123. Abell, LL: Cholesterol metabolism in the dog. J Biol Chem 220:527, 1956.

124. Bloom, F: The diagnosis and treatment of liver disease of the dog. North Am Vet 38:17, 1957.

125. Erickson, SK, et al.: Rat liver acyl coenzyme A: cholesterol acyltransferase. Its regulation in vivo and some of its properties in vitro. J Lipid Res 21:930, 1980.

126. Cooper, AD: Hepatic lipoprotein and cholesterol metabolism. In Zakim, D and Boyer, TD (eds): Hepatology—A Textbook of Liver Disease. Philadelphia, WB Saunders, 1982, p 109.

127. Rogers, WA, et al.: Lipids and lipoproteins in normal dogs and in dogs with secondary hyperlipoproteinemia. JAVMA 166:1092, 1975.

128. Bass, VD, et al.: Normal canine lipid profiles and effects of experimentally induced pancreatitis and hepatic necrosis on lipids. Am J Vet Res 37:1355, 1976.

129. Cho, BHS, et al.: Effects of feeding raw eggs on levels of plasma and lipoprotein cholesterol in dogs. Nutrition Reports International 30:163, 1984.

130. Steiner, A and Kendall, FE: Atherosclerosis and arteriosclerosis in dogs following ingestion of cholesterol and thiouracil. Arch Pathol 42:433, 1946.

131. Glickman, RM and Sabesin, SM: Lipoprotein metabolism. In Arias, I, et al. (ed): The Liver: Biology and Pathophysiology. New York, Raven Press, 1982, p 123.

132. Cooper, AJ: Hepatic lipoprotein and cholesterol metabolism. In Zakim, D and Boyer, TD (eds): Hepatology—A Textbook of Liver Disease. Philadelphia, WB Saunders, 1982, p 109.

133. Jones, AL, et al.: Electron microscopic and biochemical study of lipoprotein synthesis in the isolated perfused rat liver. J Lipid Res 8:429, 1967.

134. Redgrave, TC: Formation of cholesterol ester rich particulate lipid during metabolism of chylomicrons. J Clin Invest 49:465, 1970.

135. Harry, DS, et al.: Plasma lipoproteins and the liver. In Wright, R, et al. (eds): Liver and Biliary Disease, 2nd ed. Philadelphia, WB Saunders, 1985, p 65.

136. Fredrickson, DS, et al.: Fat transport in lipoproteins—an integrated approach to mechanisms and disorders. N Engl J Med 276:34, 1967.

137. Simon, JB and Scheig, R: Serum cholesterol esterification in liver disease: Importance of lecithin-cholesterol acyltransferase. N Engl J Med 283:841, 1970.

138. Friedman, M and Byers, SO: Observations concerning the production and excretion of cholesterol in mammals. XVI. The relationship of the liver to the content and control of plasma cholesterol ester. J Clin Invest 34:1369, 1955.

139. Fex, G and Wallinder, L: Liver and plasma cholesteryl ester metabolism after partial hepatectomy in the rat. Biochem Biophys Acta 316:91, 1973.

140. Sugano, M, et al.: Hepatotoxicity and plasma cholesterol esterification by rats. Arch Biochem 129:588, 1969.

141. Calandra, S, et al.: Plasma lecithin: Cholesterol acyltransferase activity in liver disease. Eur J Clin Invest 1:352, 1971.

142. Agorastos, J: Lecithin-cholesterol acyltransferase and the lipoprotein abnormalities of obstructive jaundice. Clin Sci Molec Med 54:369, 1978.

143. Gjone, E and Norum, KR: Plasma lecithin-cholesterol acyltransferase and erythrocyte lipids in liver disease. Acta Med Scand 187:153, 1970.

144. Muller, P, et al.: Hypertriglyceridaemia secondary to liver disease. Eur J Clin Invest 4:419, 1974.

145. Quarfordt, SH: Liquid crystalline lipid in the plasma of humans with biliary obstruction. J Clin Invest 51:1979, 1972.

146. Van Vleet, JF and Alberts, JO: Evaluation of liver function tests and liver biopsy in experimental carbon tetrachloride intoxication and extrahepatic bile duct obstruction in the dog. Am J Vet Res 29:2119, 1968.

147. Center, SA, et al.: Hematologic and biochemical abnormalities associated with induced extrahepatic bile duct obstruction in the cat. Am J Vet Res 44:1822, 1983.

148. Milewski, B and Palynyczko, Z: Evaluation of the usefulness of serum lipoprotein-X (LP-X) detection test for the diagnosis of cholestasis in chronic liver diseases. Pol Arch Med Wewn 53:445, 1975.

149. Ritland, S: Quantitative determination of the abnormal lipoprotein of cholestasis, LP-X, in liver disease. Scand J Gastroenterol 10:5, 1975.

150. Bauer, JE, et al.: Cholestasis induced changes in canine serum lipids and lipoproteins. (abstract). ACVIM Scientific Proceedings, 1986, p 14.

151. Coyle, JJ, et al.: The effect of portacaval shunt on plasma lipids and tissue cholesterol synthesis in the dog. Surgery 80:54, 1976.

152. Guzman, IJ, et al.: Combined hypolipidemia of portacaval transposition and ileal resection in the dog. Surg Gyn Obst 150:475, 1980.

153. Coyle, JJ, et al.: Cholesterol pool sizes and turnover following portacaval shunt in the dog. Surg Gyn Obst 148:723, 1979.

154. Guzman, IJ: The effect of selective visceral caval shunt on plasma lipids and cholesterol dynamics. Surgery 82:42, 1977.

155. Bunch, SE: Effects of anticonvulsant drugs phenytoin and primidone on the canine liver. Thesis, Cornell University, 1983, p 81.

156. Rogers, WA, et al.: Idiopathic hyperlipoproteinemia in dogs. JAVMA 166:1087, 1975.

157. Waterlow, JC and Stephen, JML: The effect of low protein diets on the turnover rates of serum, liver and muscle proteins in the rat measured by continuous infusion of L-(U^{14}C) lysine. Clin Sci 35:287, 1968.

158. Rothschild, MA, et al.: Albumin synthesis (first of two parts). N Engl J Med 286:748, 1972.

159. Wilson, SH, et al.: Physiology of rat-liver polysomes: Protein synthesis by stable polysomes. Biochem J 103:567, 1967.

160. Rothschild, MA, et al.: Amino acid regulation of albumin synthesis. J Nutr 98:395, 1969.

161. Rothschild, MA, et al.: Role of hepatic interstitial albumin in regulating albumin synthesis. Am J Physiol 210:57, 1966.

162. Dich, J, et al.: Effect of albumin concentration and colloid osmotic pressure on albumin synthesis in the perfused rat liver. Acta Physiol Scand 89:353, 1973.

163. Kallfeltz, FA and Wallace, RJ: Studies of albumin metabolism in dogs using 51Cr and ^{125}I labelled albumin. Dig Dis 20:594, 1975.

164. Dixon, FJ: Half-lives of homologous serum albumins in several species. Proc Soc Exp Biol Med 83:287, 1953.

165. Moore, DH and Kowlessar, OD: Hepatic synthesis and degradation of plasma proteins. In Zakim, D and Boyer, TD (eds): Hepatology—A Textbook of Liver Disease. Philadelphia, WB Saunders, 1982, p 137.

166. Yedgar, S, et al.: Tissue sites of catabolism of albumin in rabbits. Am J Physiol 244:E101, 1983.

167. Hasch, E, et al.: Albumin synthesis rate as a measure of liver function in patients with cirrhosis. Acta Med Scand 182:83, 1967.

168. Berson, SA and Yalow, RS: The distribution of I^{131}-labeled

human serum albumin introduced into ascitic fluid: Analysis of the kinetics of a three-compartment quaternary transfer system in man and speculation on possible sites of degradation. J Clin Invest 33:377, 1954.

169. Dykes, PW: The rates of distribution and catabolism of albumin in normal subjects and in patients with cirrhosis of the liver. Clin Sci 34:161, 1968.

170. Sterling, K: Serum albumin turnover in Laennec's cirrhosis as measured by I^{131}-tagged albumin. J Clin Invest 30:1238, 1951.

171. Wilkinson, P and Mendenhall, CL: Serum albumin turnover in normal subjects and patients with cirrhosis measured by I^{131}-labelled human albumin. Clin Sci 25:281, 1963.

172. Zimmon, DS, et al.: Albumin to ascites: demonstration of a direct pathway by passing the systemic circulation. J Clin Invest 48:2074, 1969.

173. Kukral, JC, et al.: Synthesis of α- and β-globulins in normal and liverless dog. Am J Physiol 204:262, 1963.

174. Triger, DR and Wright, R: Immunological aspects of liver disease. *In* Wright, R, et al. (eds): Liver and Biliary Disease, 2nd ed. Philadelphia, WB Saunders, 1985, p 215.

175. Canalese, J, et al.: Reticuloendothelial system and hepatocyte function in fulminant hepatic failure. Gut 23:265, 1982.

176. Rimola, A, et al.: Reticuloendothelial system phagocytic activity in cirrhosis and its relation to bacterial infections and prognosis. Hepatology 4:53, 1984.

177. Tavill, AS: Protein metabolism and the liver. *In* Wright, R, et al. (eds): Liver and Biliary Disease. 2nd ed. Philadelphia, WB Saunders, 1985, p 87.

178. Morgan, MY, et al.: Plasma ratio of valine, leucine and isoleucine to phenylalanine and tyrosine in liver disease. Gut 19:1068, 1978.

179. Morgan, MY, et al.: Plasma amino-acid patterns in liver disease. Gut 23:362, 1982.

180. Strombeck, DR, et al.: Plasma amino acid, glucagon, and insulin concentrations in dogs with nitrosamine induced hepatic disease. Am J Vet Res 44:2028, 1983.

181. McMenamy, RH, et al.: Amino acid and α-keto acid concentrations in plasma and blood of the liverless dog. Am J Physiol 209:1046, 1965.

182. Iob, V, et al.: Alterations in plasma free amino acids in dogs with hepatic insufficiency. Surg Gynecol Obstet 130:794, 1970.

183. Aguirre, A, et al.: Plasma amino acids in dogs with two experimental forms of liver damage. J Surg Res 16:339, 1974.

184. Strombeck, DR and Rogers, Q: Plasma amino acid concentrations in dogs with hepatic disease. JAVMA 173:93, 1978.

185. Rutgers, C, et al.: Plasma amino acid analysis in dogs with experimentally induced hepatocellular and obstructive jaundice. Am J Vet Res 48:696, 1987.

186. McCullough, AJ, et al.: The nature and prognostic significance of serial amino acid determinations in severe chronic active liver disease. Gastroenterology 81:645, 1981.

187. Cerra, FB, et al.: Cirrhosis, encephalopathy, and improved results with metabolic support. Surgery 94:612, 1983.

188. Freund, H, et al.: Infusion of branched-chain enriched amino acid solution in patients with hepatic encephalopathy. Ann Surg 196:209, 1982.

189. Fischer, JE, et al.: The effect of normalization of plasma amino acids on hepatic encephalopathy in man. Surgery 80:77, 1976.

190. Freund, H, et al.: Chronic hepatic encephalopathy: Long-term therapy with a branched-chain amino-acid-enriched elemental diet. JAMA 242:347, 1979.

191. Walser, M, et al.: Synthesis of essential amino acids from their α-keto analogues by perfused rat liver and muscle. J Clin Invest 52:2865, 1973.

192. Millikan, WJ, Jr, et al.: Total parenteral nutrition with F080$_R$ in cirrhotics with subclinical encephalopathy. Ann Surg 197:294, 1983.

193. Sapir, DG and Walser, M: Nitrogen sparing induced early in starvation by infusion of branched-chain ketoacids. Metabolism 26:301, 1977.

194. Herlong, HF, et al.: The use of ornithine salts of branched-chain ketoacids in portal-systemic encephalopathy. Ann Intern Med 93:545, 1980.

195. Strombeck, DR, et al.: Dietary therapy for dogs with chronic hepatic insufficiency. *In* Kirk, RW (ed): Current Veterinary Therapy VIII. Philadelphia, WB Saunders, 1983, p 817.

196. Price, CP and Alberti, KGMM: Biochemical assessment of liver function. *In* Wright, R, et al. (eds): Liver and Biliary Disease, 2nd ed. Philadelphia, WB Saunders, 1985, p 455.

197. Cornelius, CE, et al.: Serum and tissue transaminase activities in domestic animals. Cornell Vet 49:116, 1959.

198. Zinkl, JG, et al.: Comparative studies on plasma and tissue sorbitol, glutamic, lactic, and hydroxybutyric dehydrogenase and transaminase activities in the dog. Res Vet Sci 12:211, 1971.

199. Duncan, JR and Prasse, KW: Liver. *In* Veterinary Laboratory Medicine Clinical Pathology, 2nd ed. Ames, IA, Iowa State University Press, 1986, p 121.

200. Kaplowitz, N, et al.: Biochemical Tests for liver disease. *In* Zakim, D and Boyer, TD (eds): Hepatology—A Textbook of Liver Disease. Philadelphia, WB Saunders, 1982, p 583.

201. Meyer, D: Serum γ-glutamyltransferase as a liver test in cats with toxic and obstructive hepatic disease. JAAHA 19:1023, 1983.

202. Spano, JS, et al.: Serum γ-glutamyl transpeptidase activity in healthy cats and cats with induced hepatic disease. Am J Vet Res 44:2049, 1983.

203. Cornelius, CE and Kaneko, JJ: Serum transaminase activities in cats with hepatic necrosis. JAVMA 137:62, 1960.

204. Noonan, NE and Meyer, DJ: Use of plasma arginase and γ-glutamyl transpeptidase as specific indicators of hepatocellular or hepatobiliary disease in the dog. Am J Vet Res 40:942, 1979.

205. Hoe, CM and Jabara, AG: The use of serum enzymes as diagnostic aids in the dog. J Comp Pathol 77:245, 1967.

206. Shull, RM and Hornbuckle, W: Diagnostic use of serum γ-glutamyltransferase in canine liver disease. Am J Vet Res 40:1321, 1979.

207. Guelfi, JF, et al.: Value of so called cholestasis markers in the dog. Res Vet Sci 33:309, 1982.

208. Everett, RM, et al.: Alkaline phosphatase, leucine aminopeptidase and alanine aminotransferase activities with obstructive and toxic hepatic disease in cats. Am J Vet Res 38:963, 1977.

209. Sturtevant, F, et al.: The effect of three anticonvulsant drugs and ACTH on canine serum alkaline phosphatase. JAAHA 13:754, 1977.

210. Badylak, SF and Van Vleet JF: Tissue γ-glutamyl transpeptidase activity and hepatic ultrastructural alterations in dogs with experimentally induced glucocorticoid hepatopathy. Am J Vet Res 43:649, 1982.

211. Dillon, AR, et al.: Prednisolone induced hematologic, biochemical and histological changes in the dog. JAAHA 16:831, 1980.

212. Trigo, FJ, et al.: The pathology of liver tumors in the dog. J Comp Pathol 92:21, 1982.

213. Strombeck, DR: Clinicopathologic features of primary and metastatic neoplastic disease of the liver in dogs. JAVMA 173:267, 1978.

214. McConnell, MF and Lumsden, JH: Biochemical evaluation of metastatic liver disease in the dog. JAAHA 19:173, 1983.

215. Boyd, JW: The mechanisms relating to increases in plasma enzymes and isoenzymes in diseases of animals. Vet Clin Pathol 12:9, 1983.

216. Nilkumhang, P and Thornton, JR: Plasma and tissue enzyme activities in the cat. J Small Anim Pract 20:169, 1979.

217. Nagode, LA, et al.: Enzyme activities of canine tissues. J Am Vet Res 27:1385, 1966.

218. Keller, P: Enzyme activities in the dog: tissue analyses, plasma values, and intracellular distribution. Am J Vet Res 42:575, 1981.

219. Morino, Y, et al.: Immunochemical distinction between glutamic-oxalacetic transaminases from soluble and mitochondrial fractions of mammalian tissues. J Biol Chem 239:943, 1964.

220. Mia, AS and Koger, HD: Comparative studies on serum arginase and transaminases in hepatic necrosis in various species of domestic animals. Vet Clin Pathol 8:9, 1979.

221. Cornelius, LM and DeNovo, RC: Icterus in cats. *In* Kirk, RW (ed): Current Veterinary Therapy VIII. Philadelphia, WB Saunders, 1983, p 822.

222. Gitlin, N: The serum glutamic oxaloacetic transaminase/serum glutamic pyruvic transaminase ratio as a prognostic index in severe acute viral hepatitis. Am J Gastroenterol 77:2, 1982.

223. Ideo, G, et al.: Serum cytosolic/mitochondrial enzyme ratio: A tool for the estimation of the severity of acute hepatitis. Z Klin Chem Klin Biochem 10:74, 1972.

224. Abdelkader, SV and Hauge, JG: Serum enzyme determination in the study of liver disease in dogs. Acta Vet Scand 27:59, 1986.

225. Cornelius, CE, et al: Comparative studies on plasma arginase and transaminases in hepatic necrosis. Cornell Vet 53:181, 1963.

226. Cargill, CF and Shields, RP: Plasma arginase as a liver function test. J Com Pathol 81:447, 1971.

227. Mia, AS and Koger, HD: Direct colorimetric determination of serum arginase in various domestic animals. Am J Vet Res 173:1381, 1978.

228. Cacciatore, L, et al.: Arginase activity, arginine and ornithine of plasma in experimental liver damage. Enzyme 17:269, 1974.

229. Ugarte, G, et al.: Serum arginase activity in subjects with hepatocellular damage. J Lab Clin Med 55:522, 1960.

230. DeNovo, RC and Prasse, KW: Comparison of serum biochemical and hepatic functional alterations in dogs treated with corticosteroids and hepatic duct ligation. Am J Vet Res 44:1703, 1983.

231. Fishman, WH: Perspectives on alkaline phosphatase isoenzymes. Am J Med 56:617, 1974.

232. Hoffmann, WE: Diagnostic value of canine serum alkaline phosphatase and alkaline phosphatase isoenzymes. JAAHA 13:237, 1977.

233. Hoffmann, WE and Dorner, JL: Separation of isoenzymes of canine alkaline phosphatase by cellulose acetate electrophoresis. JAAHA 11:283, 1975.

234. Saini, PK, et al.: Diagnostic evaluation of canine serum alkaline phosphatase by immunochemical means and interpretation of results. Am J Vet Res 39:1514, 1978.

235. Hoffmann, WE and Dorner, JL: The clearance rates of intravenous injected canine alkaline phosphatase isoenzymes. Am J Vet Res 38:1553, 1977.

236. Bengmark, S and Olsson, R: Elimination of alkaline phosphatases from serum in dog after intravenous injection of canine phosphatases from bone and intestine. Acta Chir Scand 140:1, 1974.

237. Hoffmann, WE, et al.: Alkaline phosphatase and alkaline phosphatase isoenzymes in the cat. Vet Clin Pathol 6:21, 1977.

238. Hoffmann, WE and Dorner, JL: Serum half-life of intravenously injected intestinal and hepatic alkaline phosphatase isoenzymes in the cat. Am J Vet Res 38:1637, 1977.

239. Center, SA, et al.: Diagnostic value of serum γ-glutamyl transferase and alkaline phosphatase activities in hepatobiliary disease in the cat. JAVMA 188:507, 1986.

240. De Broe, ME, et al.: Liver plasma membrane: the source of high molecular weight alkaline phosphatase in human serum. Hepatology 5:118, 1985.

241. Hamilton, JM, et al.: Alkaline phosphatase levels in canine mammary neoplasia. Vet Rec 121, 1973.

242. Aronsen, KF, et al.: Enzyme studies in dogs with extra-hepatic biliary obstruction. Scand J Gastroenterol 3:355, 1968.

243. McLain, DL, et al.: Alkaline phosphatase and its isoenzymes in normal cats and in cats with biliary obstruction. JAAHA 14:94, 1978.

244. LaVia, MF and Hill, RB: Principles of Pathobiology. London, Oxford University Press, 1971, p 27.

245. Righetti, ABB and Kaplan, MM: Disparate responses of serum and hepatic alkaline phosphatase and nucleotidase to bile duct obstruction in the rat. Gastroenterology 62:1034, 1972.

246. Hoffmann, WE and Dorner, JL: A comparison of canine normal hepatic alkaline phosphatase and variant alkaline phosphatase of serum and liver. Clin Chim Acta 62:137, 1975.

247. Saini, PK and Saini, SK: Origin of serum alkaline phosphatase in the dog. Am J Vet Res 39:1510, 1978.

248. Oluju, MP, et al.: Simple quantitative assay for canine steroid-induced alkaline phosphatase. Vet Rec 7:17, 1984.

249. Dorner, JL, et al.: Corticosteroid induction of an isoenzyme of alkaline phosphatase in the dog. Am J Vet Res 35:1457, 1974.

250. Dillon, AR, et al.: Effects of dexamethasone and surgical hypotension on hepatic morphologic features and enzymes of dogs. Am J Vet Res 44:1996, 1983.

251. Badylak, SF and Van Vleet, JF: Sequential morphologic and clinicopathologic alterations in dogs with experimentally induced glucocorticoid hepatopathy. Am J Vet Res 42:1310, 1981.

252. Middleton, DJ, et al.: Suppression of cortisol responses to exogenous adrenocorticotrophic hormone and the occurrence of side effects attributable to glucocorticoid excess in cats during therapy with megestrol acetate and prednisolone. Can J Vet Med 51:60, 1986.

253. Bunch, SE, et al.: Hepatic cirrhosis associated with long-term anticonvulsant drug therapy in dogs. JAVMA 181:357, 1982.

254. Albert, Z, et al.: Histochemical and biochemical investigations of γ glutamyl transpeptidase in tissues of man and laboratory rodents. Acta Histochem 18:78, 1964.

255. Hanes, CS and Hird, FJ: Synthesis of peptides in enzymic reactions involving glutathione. Nature 166:288, 1950.

256. Hagenfeldt, L, et al.: The γ glutamyl cycle and amino acid transport. N Engl J Med 299:587, 1978.

257. Braun, JP, et al.: γ glutamyl transferase in domestic animals. Vet Res Comm 6:77, 1983.

258. Shaw, LM, et al.: Isolation of γ glutamyl transferase from human liver, and comparison with the enzyme from human kidney. Clin Chem 24:905, 1978.

259. Lum, G and Gambino, SR: Serum γ glutamyl transpeptidase activity as an indicator of disease of liver, pancreas or bone. Clin Chem 18:358, 1972.

260. Naftalin, L, et al.: Observations on the site of origin of serum γ-glutamyl transpeptidase. Clin Chim Acta 26:297, 1969.

261. Kokot, F, et al.: Glutamyl transpeptidase (GGTP) in the urine and intestinal contents. Arch Immunol Ther Exp 13:549, 1965.

262. Kokot, F, et al.: Experimental studies on γ-glutamyl transpeptidase. IV. Histoenzymatic and biochemical changes in parenchymatous hepatitis in rabbits and in obstructive jaundice in dogs. Acta Med Pol 6:379, 1975.

263. Aronsen, KF, et al.: Enzyme histochemical studies of the liver remnant following partial hepatectomy in dogs. Acta Chir Scand 136:521, 1970.

264. Aronsen, KF, et al.: Enzyme studies in dogs with extra-hepatic biliary obstruction. Scand J Gastroenterol 3:355, 1968.

265. Moss, DW: Clinical enzymology—a perspective. Enzyme 25:2, 1980.

266. Moss, DW: Contribution of clinical enzymology to the study of hepatobiliary disease—the enzymologist's view. Clin Biochem 12:236, 1979.

267. Krebs, C: γ-glutamyltransferase activity in the cat. Inaugural Dissertation. Munchen, Ludwig-Maximilans Universitat. 1979, p 122.

268. Sawabu, N, et al.: Novel γ-GTP isoenzyme as diagnostic tool for hepatocellular carcinoma. Ann Acad Med 9:206, 1980.

269. Peters, RJ, et al.: γ-glutamyltransferase levels in ascitic fluid and liver tissue from patients with primary hepatoma. Br Med J 1:1576, 1977.

270. Mircea, P, et al.: Value of γ-glutamyltransferase in the diagnosis of liver metastases. Rev Roum Med Med Int 19:339, 1981.

271. Takeda, Y, et al.: The effect of corticosteroids on leakage of enzymes from dispersed rat liver cells. J Biol Chem 239:3590, 1964.

272. Schulster, D, et al.: Molecular Endocrinology of the Steroid Hormones. New York, John Wiley & Sons, 1976, p 148.

273. Spencer, KB, et al.: Adrenal gland function in dogs given methylprednisolone. Am J Vet Res 41:1503, 1980.

274. Peterson, ME, et al.: Feline hyperthyroidism: Pretreatment clinical and laboratory evaluation of 131 cases. JAVMA 183:103, 1983.

275. Gavin, LA and Cavalieri, RR: Interrelationships between the thyroid gland and the liver. In Zakim, D and Boyer, TD (eds): Hepatology—A Textbook of Liver Disease. Philadelphia, WB Saunders, 1982, p 508.

276. Beaver, DC and Pemberton, J: The pathologic anatomy of the liver in exophthalmic goiter. Ann Intern Med 7:687, 1933.

277. Pipher, J and Poulsen, E: Liver biopsy in thyrotoxicosis. Acta Med Scand 127:439, 1947.

278. Meyers, JD, et al.: A correlative study of the cardiac output and the hepatic circulation in hyperthyroidism. J Clin Invest 29:1069, 1950.

279. Hoe, CM and O'Shea, JD: The correlation of biochemistry and histopathology in liver disease in the dog. Vet Rec 77:1164, 1965.

280. Cello, JP and Sleisenger, MH: The liver in systemic conditions. In Arias, I, et al. (eds): The Liver: Biology and Pathobiology. New York, Raven Press, 1982.

281. Schall, WD: Laboratory diagnosis of hepatic disease. Vet Clin North Am 6:679, 1976.

282. Himes, JA and Cornelius, CE: Hepatic excretion and storage of sulfobromophthalein sodium in experimental hepatic necrosis in the dog. Cornell Vet 63:424, 1973.

283. Janssen, PAJ and Symoens, JE: Hepatic reactions during ketoconazole treatment. Am J Med 24:80, 1983.

284. Heiberg, JK and Svejgaard, E: Toxic hepatitis during ketoconazole treatment. Br Med J 283:825, 1981.

285. Ruslahti, E, et al: Serum α-fetoprotein diagnostic significance in liver disease. Br Med J 2:527, 1974.

286. Madsen, AC, et al.: α-fetoprotein as a marker for hepatic regeneration in the dog. J Surg Res 28:71, 1980.

287. Hirao, K, et al.: Primary neoplasms in dog liver induced by diethylnitrosamine. Cancer Res 34:1870, 1974.

288. Gollan, J and Schmid, R: Bilirubin metabolism and hyperbilirubinemia disorders. In Wright, R, et al. (eds): Liver and Biliary Disease, 2nd ed. Philadelphia, WB Saunders, 1985, p 301.

289. Schmid, R: Bilirubin metabolism: State of the art. Gastroenterology 74:1307, 1978.

290. Tenhunen, R, et al.: Enzymatic degradation of heme. Oxygenative cleavage requiring cytochrome p-450. Biochem 11:1716, 1972.

291. Litwach, G, et al.: Ligandin: A hepatic protein which binds steroids, bilirubin, carcinogens and a number of exogenous organic anions. Nature 234:466, 1971.

292. Levi, AJ, et al.: Two hepatic cytoplasmic protein fractions, Y and Z, and their possible role in the hepatic uptake of bilirubin, sulfobromophthalein, and other anions. J Clin Invest 48:2156, 1969.

293. Wolkoff, AW, et al.: Role of ligandin in transfer of bilirubin from plasma into liver. Am J Physiol 236:E638, 1979.

294. Cornelius, CE, et al.: Heterogeneity of bilirubin conjugates in several animal species. Cornell Vet 65:90, 1975.

295. Robinson, SH: Degradation of hemoglobin. In Williams, WJ, et al. (eds): Hematology, 3rd ed. New York, McGraw-Hill, 1983, p 388.

296. Bissell, DM: Formation and elimination of bilirubin. Gastroenterology 69:519, 1975.

297. Yeary, RA and Davis, DR: Protein binding of bilirubin: Comparison of in vitro and in vivo measurements of bilirubin displacement by drugs. Toxicol Appl Pharmacol 28:269, 1974.

298. De Schepper, J: Degradation of haemoglobin to bilirubin in the kidney of the dog. Tijdschr Diergeneeskd 99:699, 1974.

299. De Schepper, J and Van der Stock, J: Increased urinary bilirubin excretion after elevated free plasma haemoglobin levels. II. Variations in the calculated renal clearances of bilirubin in isolated normothermic perfused dog's kidneys. Arch Intern Physiol Biochim 80:339, 1969.

300. Van Der Stock, J and De Schepper, J: The urinary excretion of bilirubin after increased plasma hemoglobin concentration in dogs. Experientia 25:814, 1969.

301. De Schepper, J and Van Der Stock, J: Increased urinary bilirubin excretion after elevated free plasma haemoglobin levels. I. Variations in the calculated renal clearances of bilirubin in whole dogs. Arch Intern Physiol Biochim 80:279, 1972.

302. Royer, M and Noir, BA, et al.: Extrahepatic bilirubin formation and conjugation in the dog. Digestion 10:423, 1974.

303. Fulop, M and Braqeau, P: The renal excretion of bilirubin in dogs with obstructive jaundice. J Clin Invest 43:1192, 1964.

304. De Schepper, J and Van Der Stock, J: Influence of sex on the urinary bilirubin excretion at increased free plasma haemoglobin levels in whole dogs and in isolated normothermic perfused dog kidneys. Experientia 27:1264, 1971.

305. Cameron, JL, et al.: Bilirubin excretion in the dog. J Surg Res 3:39, 1963.

306. Osborne, CA, et al.: Clinical significance of bilirubinuria. Comp Cont Ed Pract Vet 2:897, 1980.

307. Lees, GE, et al.: Clinical implications of feline bilirubinuria. JAAHA 20:765, 1984.

308. Scharschmidt, BF, et al.: Approach to the patient with cholestatic jaundice. N Engl J Med 308:1515, 1983.

309. O'Connor, KW, et al.: A blinded prospective study comparing four current noninvasive approaches in the differential diagnosis of medical versus surgical jaundice. Gastroenterology 84:1498, 1983.

310. Rozdilsky, B: Toxicity of bilirubin in adult animals. Arch Pathol 72:22, 1961.

311. Ernster, L, et al.: Experimental studies on the pathogenesis of kernicterus. Pediatrics 20:647, 1957.

312. Karp, WB: Biochemical alterations in neonatal hyperbilirubinemia and bilirubin encephalopathy: A review. Pediatrics 64:361, 1979.

312a. Schiff, D, et al.: Sephadex G-25 quantitative estimation of free bilirubin potential in jaundiced newborn infants' sera: A guide to the prevention of kernicterus. J Lab Clin Med 80:455, 1972.

312b. Bratlid, D and Rugstad, HE: Effect of albumin binding on bilirubin conjugation and toxicity in cell culture of a clonal strain of rat hepatoma cells. Scand J Clin Lab Invest 29:461, 1972.

313. Tryphonas, L and Rozdilsky, B: Nuclear jaundice (kernicterus) in a newborn kitten. JAVMA 157:1084, 1970.

314. Rozdilsky, B: Kittens as experimental model for study of kernicterus. Am J Dis Child 111:161, 1966.

315. Arhelger, RB, et al.: Experimental cholemia in dogs. Electron microscopy of glomerular lesions. Arch Pathol 89:355, 1970.

316. Witzleben, CL: Bilirubin as a cholestatic agent, physiologic and morphologic observations. Am J Pathol 62:181, 1971.

317. Witzleben, CL and Boyce, WH: Bilirubin as a cholestatic agent III. Prevention of bilirubin related cholestasis by sulfobromophthalein. Arch Pathol 100:492, 1975.

318. Schaffner, F and Popper, H: Classification and mechanism of cholestasis. In Wright, R, et al. (eds): Liver and Biliary Disease, 2nd ed. Philadelphia, WB Saunders, 1985, p 359.

319. Cornelius, CE: Comparative bile pigment metabolism in vertebrates. In Ostrow, JD (ed): Bile Pigments and Jaundice: Molecular, Metabolic and Medical Aspects. New York, Marcel Dekker, 1986, p 601.

320. Cherrick, GR, et al.: Indocyanine green: observations on its physical properties, plasma decay and hepatic extraction. J Clin Invest 39:592, 1960.

321. Jablonski, P and Owen, JA: The clinical chemistry of bromosulfophthalein and other cholephilic dyes. In Bodansky, O and Stewart CP (eds): Advances in Clinical Chemistry. New York, Academic Press, 1969, p 309.

322. Baker, KJ: Binding of sulfobromophthalein (BSP) sodium and indocyanine green (ICG) by plasma α1-lipoproteins. Proc Soc Exp Biol Med 122:957, 1966.

323. Paumgartner, G, et al.: Kinetics of indocyanine green removal from the blood. Ann NY Acad Sci 170:134, 1970.

324. Leevy, CM, et al.: Physiology of dye extraction by the liver: Comparative studies of sulfobromophthalein and indocyanine green. Ann NY Acad Sci 111:161, 1963.

325. Leevy, CM, et al.: Indocyanine green clearance as a test for hepatic function. JAMA 200:236, 1967.

326. Paumgartner, G: The handling of indocyanine green by the liver. Schwiz Med Wochenschr. Suppl 1975, p 1.

327. Wheeler, HO, et al.: Hepatic uptake and biliary excretion of indocyanine green in the dog. Proc Soc Exp Biol Med 99:11, 1958.

328. Frestin, JW and Englert, E: The influence of age and excessive body weight on the distribution and metabolism of bromophthalein. Clin Sci 33:301, 1967.

329. Ingelfinger, FJ, et al.: Studies with bromosulphthalein. Its disappearance from blood after a single intravenous injection. Gastroenterology 11:646, 1948.

330. Prasse, KW, et al.: Indocyanine green clearance and ammonia tolerance in partially hepatectomized and hepatic devascularized anesthetized dogs. Am J Vet Res 44:2320, 1983.

331. Blaschke, TF, et al.: The effect of induced fever on sulfobromophthalein kinetics in man. Ann Intern Med 78:221, 1971.

332. Hicks, MM, et al.: The effect of spontaneous and artificially induced fever on liver function. J Clin Invest 27:580, 1958.

333. Hunton, DB, et al.: The plasma removal of indocyanine green and sulfobromophthalein: Effect of dosage and blocking agents. J Clin Invest 40:1648, 1948.

334. Strombeck, DR and Qualls, C: Hepatic sulfobromophthalein uptake and storage defect in a dog. JAVMA 172:1423, 1978.

335. Hacku, W, et al.: A new look at the plasma disappearance of sulfobromophthalein (BSP): correlation with the BSP transport maximum and the hepatic plasma flow in man. J Lab Clin Med 88:1019, 1976.

336. Center, SA, et al.: Comparison of sulfobromophthalein and indocyanine green clearances in the cat. Am J Vet Res 44:727, 1983.

337. Center, SA, et al.: Comparison of sulfobromophthalein and indocyanine green clearances in the dog. Am J Vet Res 44:722, 1983.

338. Iber, FL: Reactions to sulfobromophthalein sodium injections. Bull Johns Hopkins Hosp 116:132, 1965.

339. Walker, CH and Koszalka, MF: Fatal bromosulphthalein reaction. Ann Intern Med 47:362, 1957.

340. Haselwood, GAD: The biological significance of chemical differences in bile salts. Biol Rev 39:537, 1964.

341. Rabin, B, et al.: Dietary influence on bile acid conjugation in the cat. J Nutr 106:1241, 1976.

341a. Smallwood, RA and Hoffman, NE: Bile acid structure and biliary secretion of cholesterol and phospholipid in the cat. Gastroenterology 71:1064, 1976.

342. Papageorgiou, G and Lynn, JA: The physiology of the extrahepatic biliary tree. *In* Wright, R, et al. (eds): Liver and Biliary Disease, 2nd ed. Philadelphia, WB Saunders, 1985, p 267.

343. Scharschmidt, BF: Bile formation and cholestasis, metabolism and enterohepatic circulation of bile acids, and gallstone formation. *In* Zakim, D and Boyer, TD (eds): Hepatology—A Textbook of Liver Disease. Philadelphia, WB Saunders, 1982, p 297.

344. Svenberg, T, et al.: Interdigestive biliary output in man: Relationship to fluctuations in plasma motilin and effect of atropine. Gut 23:1024, 1982.

345. Cox, UL, et al.: Noncholecystokinin peptides in human serum which cause gallbladder contraction. Life Sci 31:3023, 1982.

346. Angelin, B, et al.: Hepatic uptake of bile acids in man. Fasting and postprandial concentrations of individual bile acids in portal venous and systemic blood serum. J Clin Invest 70:724, 1982.

347. Ahlberg, J, et al: Individual bile acids in portal, venous and systemic blood serum in fasting man. Gastroenterology 73:1377, 1977.

348. Berk, PD and Javitt, NB: Hyperbilirubinemia and cholestasis. Am J Med 64:311, 1978.

349. Skrede, S, et al.: Bile acids measured in serum during fasting as a test for liver disease. Clin Chem 24:1095, 1978.

350. Center, SA, et al.: Bile acid concentrations in the diagnosis of hepatobiliary disease in the dog. JAVMA 187:935, 1985.

351. Johnson, SE, et al.: Determination of serum bile acids in fasting dogs with hepatobiliary disease. Am J Vet Res 46:2048, 1985.

352. Center, SA, et al.: Bile acid concentrations in the diagnosis of hepatobiliary disease in the cat. JAVMA 189:891, 1986.

353. Center, SA, et al.: Evaluation of serum bile acid concentrations for the diagnosis of portosystemic venous anomalies in the dog and cat. JAVMA 186:1090, 1985.

354. Hauge, JG and Abdelkader, SV: Serum bile acids as an indicator of liver diseases in dogs. Acta Vet Scand 25:495, 1984.

355. Meyer, DJ: Liver function tests in dogs with portosystemic shunts: measurement of serum bile acid concentration. JAVMA 188:168, 1986.

356. Festi, D, et al.: Diagnostic effectiveness of serum bile acids in liver diseases as evaluated by multivariate statistical methods. Hepatology 3:707, 1983.

357. Korman, MG, et al.: Development of an intravenous bile acid tolerance test: Plasma disappearance of cholylglycine in health. N Engl J Med 292:1205, 1975.

358. Thjodleifsson, B, et al.: Assessment of the plasma disappearance of cholyl-1^{14}G-glycine as a test of hepatocellular disease. Gut 18:697, 1977.

359. Kaplowitz, N, et al.: Postprandial serum bile acid for the detection of hepatobiliary disease. JAMA 225:292, 1973.

360. Barnes, S, et al.: Diagnostic value of serum bile acid estimations in liver disease. J Clin Pathol 28:506, 1975.

361. Fausa, O: Serum bile acid concentration after a test meal. Scand J Gastroenterol 11:229, 1976.

362. Osuga, T, et al.: Evaluation of fluorimetrically estimated serum bile acid in liver disease. Clin Chim Acta 75:81, 1977.

363. Angelico, M, et al.: Fasting and postprandial serum bile acids as a screening test for hepatocellular disease. Am J Dig Dis 22:941, 1977.

364. Linnet, K and Andersen, J: Differential diagnostic value in hepatobiliary disease of serum conjugated bile acid concentrations and some routine liver tests assessed by discriminant analysis. Clin Chim Acta 127:217, 1983.

365. Gilmore, IT and Thompson, RPH: Plasma clearance of oral and intravenous cholic acid in subjects with and without chronic liver disease. Gut 21:123, 1980.

366. Gilmore, IT and Thompson, RPH: Kinetics of ^{14}C-glycocholic acid clearance in normal man and in patients with liver disease. Gut 19:1110, 1978.

367. Ashkin, JR, et al.: Factors affecting delivery of bile to the duodenum in man. Gastroenterology 74:560, 1978.

368. Ponz de Leon, M, et al.: Physiological factors influencing serum bile acid levels. Gut 19:32, 1978.

369. Duane, WC and Hanson, KC: Role of gallbladder emptying and small bowel transit in regulation of bile acid pool size in man. J Lab Clin Med 92:858, 1978.

370. Low-Beer, RS, et al.: The effect of coeliac disease upon bile salts. Gut 14:204, 1973.

371. Mashige, F, et al.: Direct spectrometry of total bile acids in serum. Clin Chem 27:1352, 1981.

372. Center, SA, et al.: Direct spectrometric determination of serum bile acids in the dog and cat. Am J Vet Res 45:2043, 1984.

373. Bunch, SE, et al.: Radioimmunoassay of conjugated bile acids in canine and feline sera. Am J Vet Res 45:2051, 1984.

374. Aldrete, JS: Quantification of the capacity of the liver to remove ammonia from the circulation of dogs with portacaval transposition. Surg Gynecol Obstet 141:399, 1975.

375. Black, M: Hepatic detoxification of endogenously produced toxins and their importance for the pathogenesis of hepatic encephalopathy. *In* Zakim, D and Boyer, TD (eds): Hepatology—A Textbook of Liver Disease. Philadelphia, WB Saunders, 1982, p 397.

376. Nance, FC, et al.: Role of urea in the hyperammonemia of germ-free Eck's fistula dogs. Gastroenterology 66:106, 1974.

377. Vince, A, et al.: Ammonia production by intestinal bacteria. Gut 14:171, 1973.

378. Dawson, AM: Regulation of blood ammonia. Gut 19:504, 1978.

379. McDermott, WV, Jr: Metabolism and toxicity of ammonia. N Engl J Med 257:1076, 1957.

380. Pirotte, J, et al.: Comparative study of basal arterial ammonemia and of orally-induced hyperammonemia in chronic portal systemic encephalopathy, treated with neomycin, lactulose and an association of neomycin and lactulose. Digestion 10:435, 1974.

381. Carter, CC, et al.: Organ uptake and blood pH and concentration effects of ammonia in dogs determined with ammonia labeled with 10 minutes half lived nitrogen 13. Neurology 23:204, 1973.

382. Hoyumpa, AM, Jr, et al.: Hepatic encephalopathy. Gastroenterology 76:184, 1979.

383. Powers, SG and Meister, A: Urea synthesis and ammonia metabolism. *In* Arias, I, et al. (eds): The Liver: Biology and Pathobiology. New York, Raven Press, 1982, p 251.

384. Fraser, CL and Arieff, AI: Hepatic encephalopathy. N Engl J Med 313:865, 1985.

385. Schimke, RT: Differential effects of fasting and protein free diets on levels of urea cycle enzymes in rat liver. J Biol Chem 237:1921, 1962.

386. Aebi, H: Coordinated changes in enzymes of the ornithine cycle and response to dietary conditions. *In* Grisolia, S, et al. (eds): The Urea Cycle. New York, John Wiley & Sons, 1976, p 275.

387. Schimke, RT: Studies on factors affecting the levels of urea cycle enzymes in rat liver. J Biol Chem 238:1012, 1963.

388. Rudman, D, et al.: Maximal rates of excretion and synthesis of urea in normal and cirrhotic subjects. J Clin Invest 52:2241, 1973.

389. Khatra, BS, et al.: Activities of Krebs-Henseleit enzymes in normal and cirrhotic human liver. J Lab Clin Med 84:709, 1974.

390. Conn, HO: Ammonia tolerance in assessing the potency of portacaval anastomoses. Arch Intern Med 131:221, 1973.

391. Stahl, J: Studies of the blood ammonia in liver disease: Its diagnostic, prognostic, and therapeutic significance. Ann Intern Med 58:1, 1963.

392. Millikan, WJ, et al.: Effects of portacaval shunt on hepatic Krebs-Henseleit enzymes in dogs. Surg Forum 25:248, 1974.

393. Hsia, YE: Inherited hyperammonemic syndromes. Gastroenterology 67:347, 1974.

394. Msall, M, et al.: Neurologic outcome in children with inborn errors of urea synthesis: outcome of urea-cycle enzymopathies. N Engl J Med 310:1500, 1984.

395. Drayna, CJ, et al.: Hyperammonemic encephalopathy caused by infection in a neurogenic bladder. N Engl J Med 304:766, 1981.

396. Ullman, MA, et al.: Hyperammonemic encephalopathy and urinary obstruction. N Engl J Med 304:1546, 1981.

396a. Hall, JA, et al.: Hyperammonemia associated with urethral obstruction in a dog. J Am Vet Med Assoc 191:1116–1118, 1987.

397. Strombeck, DR, et al.: Hyperammonemia due to a urea cycle enzyme deficiency in two dogs. JAVMA 166:1109, 1975.

398. Morris, JG: Nutritional and metabolic responses to arginine deficiency in carnivores. J Nutr 115:524, 1985.

399. Rogers, QR and Visek, WJ: Metabolic role of urea cycle intermediates: Nutritional and clinical aspects. J Nutr 115:505, 1985.

400. Rothuizen, J and Van den Ingh, RSGAM: Rectal ammonia tolerance test in the evaluation of portal circulation in dogs with liver disease. Res Vet Sci 33:22, 1982.

401. Rothuizen, J: Arterial and venous ammonia concentrations in the diagnosis of canine hepato-encephalopathy. Res Vet Sci 33:17, 1982.

402. Prytz, B, et al.: In vitro formation of ammonia in blood of dog and man. Clin Chem 16:277, 1970.

403. Reif, AE: The ammonia content of blood and plasma. Anal Biochem 1:351, 1960.

404. Svensson, G and Anfialt, R: Rapid determination of ammonia in whole blood and plasma using flow injection analysis. Clin Chim Acta 119:7, 1982.

405. Seligson, D and Hirahara, K: The measurement of ammonia in whole blood, erythrocytes and plasma. J Lab Clin Med 49:962, 1957.

406. Davidovich, A, et al.: Effects of storage temperature and mercuric chloride on preservation of blood samples for later determination of ammonia-N. J Anim Sci 46:862, 1977.

407. Reinhold, JG and Chung, C: Formation of artifactual ammonia in blood by action of alkali: Its significance for the measurement of blood ammonia. Clin Chem 7:54, 1961.

408. Ogilvie, GK, et al.: Effects of plasma sample storage on blood ammonia, bilirubin, and urea nitrogen concentrations: Cats and horses. Am J Vet Res 46:2619, 1985.

409. Hitt, ME and Jones, BD: Effects of storage temperature and time on canine plasma ammonia concentrations. Am J Vet Res 47:363, 1986.

410. Meyer, DJ, et al.: Ammonia tolerance test in clinically normal dogs and in dogs with portosystemic shunts. JAVMA 173:377, 1978.

411. Davenport, DJ, et al.: Ammonia tolerance test: Comparison of three methods of ammonia administration. (abstract). ACVIM Scientific Proceedings, 1985, p 130.

412. Briggs, OM and Harley, EH: The fate of administered purines in the dalmatian coach hound. J Comp Pathol 96:267, 1986.

413. Giesecke, D and Tiemcyer, W: Defect of uric acid uptake in Dalmatian dog liver. Experientia 40:1415, 1984.

414. Kuster, G, et al.: Uric acid metabolism in Dalmatian and other dogs. Arch Intern Med 129:492, 1972.

415. Duncan, H, et al.: The effects of intravenous administration of uric acid on its concentration in plasma and urine of Dalmatian and non-Dalmatian dogs. J Lab Clin Med 58:876, 1961.

416. Hoe, CM and Harver, DG: An investigation into liver function tests in dogs: Tests other than transaminase estimation. J Small Anim Pract 2:109, 1961.

417. Wooliscroft, JO, et al.: Hyperuricemia in acute illness: A poor prognostic sign. Am J Med 73:58, 1982.

418. Fox, IH, et al.: Hyperuricemia: A marker for cell energy crises. N Engl J Med 317:111, 1987.

419. Witte, CL, et al.: Relationship of splanchnic blood flow and portal venous resistance to elevated portal pressure in the dog. Gut 17:122, 1976.

420. Strombeck, DR: Small Animal Gastroenterology. Davis, CA, Stonegate Publishing, 1979, p 393.

421. Schmidt, S and Suter, PF: Indirect and direct determination of the portal vein pressure in normal and abnormal dogs and normal cats. Am J Vet Rad Soc 21:246, 1980.

422. Twedt, DC: Cirrhosis: a consequence of chronic liver disease. Vet Clin North Am 15:167, 1985.

423. Crossley, IR, et al.: Portal hypertension. In Wright, R, et al. (eds): Liver and Biliary Disease, 2nd ed. Philadelphia, WB Saunders, 1985, p 1283.

424. Boyer, TD: Portal Hypertension and its complications. In Zakim, D and Boyer, TD (eds): Hepatology—A Textbook of Liver Disease. Philadelphia, WB Saunders, 1982, p 464.

425. Reynolds, TB: Portal hypertension. In Schiff, L and Schiff, ER (eds): Diseases of the Liver, 5th ed. Philadelphia, JB Lippincott, 1982, p 393.

426. Moore, PF and Whiting, PG: Hepatic lesions associated with intrahepatic arterioportal fistulae in dogs. Vet Pathol 23:57, 1986.

427. Bosch, J, et al: Chronic bile duct ligation in the dog: hemodynamic characterization of a portal hypertensive model. Hepatology 3:1002, 1983.

428. Ohlsson, EG, et al.: Changes in portal circulation after biliary obstruction in dogs. Am J Surg 120:16, 1970.

429. Ohlsson, EG, et al.: The effect of biliary obstruction on hepatosplanchnic blood flow in dogs. J Surg Res 10:120, 1970.

430. Suter, PF: Hepatic circulatory anatomy and its role in liver disease. Sci Proc AAHA 43:240, 1976.

431. Epstein, M: Renal functional abnormalities in cirrhosis: Pathophysiology and management. In Zakim, D and Boyer, TD (eds): Hepatology—A Textbook of Liver Disease. Philadelphia, WB Saunders, 1982, p 446.

432. Wilkinson, SP and Williams, R: Ascites, electrolytes and renal. In Wright, R, et al. (eds): Liver and Biliary Disease, 2nd ed. Philadelphia, WB Saunders, 1985, p 1341.

433. Gabuzda, GJ and Hall, PW: Relation of potassium depletion to renal ammonium metabolism and hepatic coma. Medicine 45:481, 1966.

434. Warren, KS, et al.: The effect of alterations in blood pH on the distribution of ammonia from blood to cerebrospinal fluid in patients with hepatic coma. J Lab Clin Med 56:687, 1966.

435. Epstein, M: The kidney in liver disease. In Arias, I, et al. (eds): The Liver: Biology and Pathobiology. New York, Raven Press, 1982, p 745.

436. Vaamonde, CA, et al.: Renal concentrating ability in cirrhosis: I. Changes associated with the clinical status and course of the disease. J Lab Clin Med 70:179, 1967.

437. Saruta, R, et al.: Regulation of aldosterone in cirrhosis of the liver. In Epstein, M (ed): The Kidney in Liver Disease, 2nd ed. New York, Elsevier Biomedical, 1978, p 271.

438. Grauer, GF and Nichols, CER: Ascites, renal abnormalities, electrolyte and acid-base diorders associated with liver disease. Vet Clin North Am 15:197, 1985.

439. Grauer, GF and Pitts, RP: Primary polydipsia in three dogs with portosystemic shunts. JAAHA 23:197, 1987.

440. Haberich, FJ: Osmoreception in the portal circulation. Fed Proc 27:1137, 1968.

441. Chwalbinska-Moneta, J: Role of hepatic portal osmoreception in the control of ADH release. Am J Physiol 236:E603, 1979.

442. Berl, T, et al: On the mechanism of polyuria in potassium depletion: The role of polydipsia. J Clin Invest 60:620, 1977.

443. Kozlowski, S and Drzewiecki, K: The role of osmoreceptors in portal circulation in control of water intake in dogs. Acta Physiol Pol 24:325, 1973.

444. Whang, R and Papper, S: The possible relationship of renal cortical hypoperfusion and diminished renal concentrating ability in Laennec's cirrhosis. J Chron Dis 27:263, 1974.

445. Bennet, CM: Urine concentration and dilution in hypokalemic and hypercalcemic dogs. J Clin Invest 49:1447, 1970.

446. Hollander, W and Blythe, WB: Nephropathy of potassium depletion. In Strauss, MB (ed): Diseases of the Kidney, 2nd ed. Boston, Little, Brown, and Co, 1971, p 933.

447. Papper, S: Renal failure in cirrhosis (the hepatorenal syndrome). In Epstein, M (ed): The Kidney in Liver Disease, 2nd ed. New York, Elsevier Biomedical, 1978, p 91.

448. Conn, HO: Diuresis of ascites: Fraught with or free from hazard. Gastroenterology 73:619, 1977.

449. Oster, JR: Acid-base homeostasis. In Epstein, M (ed): The Kidney in Liver Disease, 2nd ed. New York, Elsevier Biomedical, 1982, p 147.

450. Wichner, J and Kazenii, H: Ammonia and ventilation: Site and mechanism of action. Resp Physiol 20:393, 1974.

451. Wilder, CE, et al.: Relationship between serum sodium and hyperventilation in cirrhosis. Am Rev Resp Dis 96:971, 1967.

452. Wolfe, JD, et al.: Hypoxemia of cirrhosis. Detection of small pulmonary vascular channels by a quantitative radionuclide method. Ann Intern Med 63:746, 1977.

453. Sebastian, A, et al.: Metabolic alkalosis. In Brenner, BM and Stein, JH (eds): Contemporary Issues in Nephrology. Acid-Base and Potassium Homeostasis. New York, Churchill Livingstone, 1978, p 101.

454. Frommer, JP: Lactic acidosis. Med Clin North Am 67:815, 1983.

455. Heinig, RE, et al.: Lactic acidosis and liver disease. Arch Intern Med 139:1229, 1979.

456. Marliss, EB, et al.: Amino acid metabolism in lactic acidosis. Am J Med 52:474, 1972.

457. Magne, ML and Chiapella, AM: Medical management of canine chronic hepatitis. Comp Cont Ed 8:915, 1986.

458. Worthley, LIG: The rational use of I.V. hydrochloric acid in the treatment of metabolic alkalosis. Br J Anaesth 49:811, 1977.

459. Hein, MF: The effect of portacaval shunting on gastric secretion in cirrhotic dogs. Gastroenterology 44:637, 1963.

460. Manabe, R, et al.: Changes of gastric blood flow in experimentally induced cirrhosis of the liver. Surg Gynecol Obstet 147:753, 1978.

461. Millward-Sadler, GH, et al.: Cirrhosis: An appraisal. In Wright, R. et al. (eds): Liver and Biliary Disease, 2nd ed. Philadelphia, WB Saunders, 1985, p 821.

462. Duffy, TE and Plum, F: Hepatic encephalopathy. In Arias, IM, et al. (eds): The Liver: Biology and Pathobiology. New York, Raven Press, 1982, p 693.

463. Raabe, W and Gumnit, RJ: Disinhibition in cat motor cortex by ammonia. J Neurophysiol 38:347, 1975.

464. Andersson, KE, et al.: Cerebrovascular effects of ammonia in vitro. Acta Physiol Scand 113:349, 1981.

465. James, JH, et al.: Hyperammonaemia, plasma amino acid imbalance, and blood brain amino acid transport: A unified theory of portal-systemic encephalopathy. Lancet 2:772, 1979.

466. Sherwin, R, et al.: Hyperglucagonemia in Laennec's cirrhosis: The role of portal systemic shunting. N Engl J Med 290:239, 1974.

467. Hourani, BT, et al.: Cerebrospinal fluid glutamine as a measure of hepatic encephalopathy. Arch Intern Med 127:1033, 1971.

468. Gilon, E, et al.: Glutamine estimation in cerebrospinal fluid in cases of liver cirrhosis and hepatic coma. J Lab Clin Med 53:714, 1959.

469. Vergara, F, et al.: α-Ketoglutarate: Increased concentrations in the cerebrospinal fluid of patients in hepatic coma. Science 183:81, 1974.

470. Hirayama, C: Tryptophan metabolism in liver disease. Clin Chim Acta 32:191, 1971.

471. Ogihara, K, et al.: Tryptophan as cause of hepatic coma. N Engl J Med 275:1255, 1966.

472. Fischer, JE: Portal-systemic encephalopathy. In Wright, R, et al. (eds): The Liver and Biliary Disease, 2nd ed. Philadelphia, WB Saunders, 1985, p 1245.

473. Morgan, MY, et al.: Plasma amino acid patterns in liver disease. Gut 23:362, 1982.

474. Knell, A: Serum methionine in liver failure. Lancet 2:1036, 1980.

475. Cavidson, LSP: Mercaptan in the breath of patients with severe liver disease. Lancet 2:197, 1949.

476. Challenger, F and Walshe, JM: Fetor hepaticus. Lancet 2:1239, 1955.

477. Phear, EA, et al.: Methionine toxicity in liver disease and its prevention by chlortetracycline. Clin Sci 15:93, 1956.

478. Rossi-Fanelli, F, et al.: Induction of coma in normal dogs by infusion of aromatic amino acids and prevention by addition of branched chain amino acids. Gastroenterology 83:664, 1982.

479. Ljunggren, G and Norberg, B: On the effect and toxicity of dimethyl sulfide, dimethyl disulfide and methyl mercaptan. Acta Physiol Scand 5:248, 1943.

480. Zieve, L, et al.: Synergism between mercaptans and ammonia or fatty acids in the production of coma: A possible role for mercaptans in the pathogenesis of hepatic coma. J Lab Clin Med 83:16, 1974.

481. Merino, GE, et al.: Methionine-induced hepatic coma in dogs. Am J Surg 130:41, 1975.

482. Mays, ET: Encephalopathy and fatty acid toxicity. Surg Forum 23:352, 1972.

483. Schenker, S, et al.: Hepatic encephalopathy: Current status. Gastroenterology 66:121, 1974.

484. Walker, CO, et al.: Cerebral energy metabolism in short chain fatty acid induced coma. J Lab Clin Med 76:569, 1970.

485. Walker, CO and Schenker, S: Pathogenesis of hepatic encephalopathy with specific reference to the role of ammonia. Am J Clin Nutr 23:619, 1970.

486. Zieve, FJ, et al.: Synergism between ammonia and fatty acids in the production of coma: Implications for hepatic coma. J Pharmacol Exp Ther 191:10, 1974.

487. Curzon, G, et al.: Plasma and brain tryptophan changes in experimental acute hepatic failure. J Neurochem 21:137, 1973.

488. Baldessarini, RJ and Fisher, JE: Serotonin metabolism in rat brain after surgical diversion of the portal venous circulation. Nature 245:25, 1973.

489. Smith, AR, et al.: Alterations in plasma and CSF amino acids, amines and metabolites in hepatic coma. Ann Surg 187:343, 1978.

490. Lunzer, M, et al.: Treatment of chronic hepatic encephalopathy with levodopa. Gut 15:555, 1974.

491. Zieve, L, et al.: Reversal of ammonia coma in rats by L-dopa: A peripheral effect. Gut 20:28, 1979.

492. Roberts, E: The γ-aminobutyric acid (GABA) system and hepatic encephalopathy. Hepatology 4:342, 1984.

493. Thompson, JS, et al.: γ-aminobutyric acid plasma levels and brain binding in Eck fistula dogs. J Surg Res 38:143, 1985.

494. Goldstein, GW: The role of brain capillaries in the pathogenesis of hepatic encephalopathy. Hepatology 4:565, 1984.

495. Frenci, P, et al.: Changes in the status of neurotransmitter receptors in rabbit model of hepatic encephalopathy. Hepatology 4:186, 1984.

496. Kealy, JK: The abdomen. In Diagnostic Radiology of the Dog and Cat, 2nd ed. Philadelphia, WB Saunders, 1987, p 26.

497. Obrien, TR: Liver, spleen and pancreas. In Radiographic Diagnosis of Abdominal Disorders in the Dog and Cat: Radiographic Interpretation, Clinical Signs, Pathophysiology. Philadelphia, WB Saunders, 1978, p 396.

498. Wrigley, RH: Radiographic and ultrasonographic diagnosis of liver diseases in dogs and cats. Vet Clin North Am 15:21, 1985.

499. Lord, PF and Wilkins, RF: Emphysema of the gall bladder in a diabetic dog. JAVMA 13:49, 1972.

500. Meutzer, RM, et al.: A comparative appraisal of emphysematous cholecystitis. Am J Surg 129:10, 1975.

501. Ticer, JW: Abdomen. In Radiographic Technique in Veterinary Practice, 2nd ed. Philadelphia, WB Saunders, 1984, p 312.

502. Allan, GS and Dixon, RT: Cholecystography in the dog: The choice of contrast media and optimal dose rates. J Am Vet Res 16:98, 1975.

503. Goldberg, HI, et al.: Contractility of the inflamed gall bladder: An experimental study using the technique of cholecystokinin cholecystography. Invest Radiol 7:447, 1972.

504. Buergener, FJA and Gutierrez, OH: Comparison of diatrizoate, iopamidol and ioxaglate for arterial portography. An experimental study in normal dogs and dogs with portal hypertension. Invest Radiol 20:399, 1985.

505. Pechman, RD: The liver and spleen. In Thrall, DE (ed): Textbook of Veterinary Diagnostic Radiology. Philadelphia, WB Saunders, 1986, p 391.

506. Nyland, TG and Hager, DA: Sonography of the liver, gallbladder, and spleen. Vet Clin North Am 15:1123, 1985.

507. Taylor, KJW, et al.: Gray scale ultrasound imaging. Radiology 119:415, 1976.

508. Nyland, TG and Park, RD: Hepatic ultrasonography in the dog. Vet Radiol 24:74, 1983.

509. Nyland, TG: Ultrasonic patterns of canine hepatic lymphosarcoma. Vet Radiol 25:167, 1984.

510. Nyland, TG and Gillett, NA: Sonographic evaluation of experimental bile duct ligation in the dog. Vet Radiol 23:252, 1982.

511. Jones, BD, et al.: Hepatic biopsy. Vet Clin North Am 15:39, 1985.

512. Boyce, HW: Laparoscopy. In Schiff, L and Schiff, E (eds): Diseases of the Liver, 5th ed. Philadelphia, JB Lippincott, 1982, p 333.

513. Lettow, E: Laparoscopic examinations in liver diseases in dogs. Vet Med Rev 2:159, 1972.

89 DISEASES OF THE LIVER AND THEIR TREATMENT

ROBERT M. HARDY

The liver is essential to the maintenance of life and is the largest and one of the most important secreting/excreting organs in the body. It functions in hundreds of diverse metabolic activities that maintain the body's normal homeostatic mechanisms. Because of its key role in many metabolic processes, the liver is subject to injury by a wide variety of infectious, metabolic, and toxic diseases. It has been estimated that hepatic diseases account for three per cent of all diseases seen by veterinarians.[1] With the increased interest in the diagnosis and therapy of hepatic diseases over the past few years, this estimate is likely too low.

The knowledge base concerning hepatic diseases in companion animals has increased dramatically in the past several years. A number of new diseases or syndromes have been described, improved methods of diagnosis have been developed, and advances in therapeutic management have taken place.

HEPATIC DISEASES

Because the liver is intimately involved with so many diverse metabolic functions within the body, any factors that significantly alter normal physiology will often produce hepatic damage. Causes for such injury include numerous inflammatory processes, toxin exposure, metabolic abnormalities, degenerative diseases, and neoplastic infiltration. Hepatic disease may be primary such as with infectious canine hepatitis, toxic injury, and neoplasia or secondary to such diverse metabolic diseases as hyperadrenocorticism, diabetes mellitus, and pancreatitis. Unfortunately, many hepatic diseases are similar clinically and biochemically, yet their prognosis and therapy may differ markedly. As more veterinary clinicians become adept at hepatic biopsy, the ability to accurately diagnose, prognose, and treat these diverse disorders will improve.

The hepatic disease classification that follows is somewhat arbitrary, as is the case for man-made schemes of natural diseases; nevertheless, it should enable the reader to approach logically the diagnosis and therapy of patients with hepatic disease. The ultimate goal is to provide the best patient care possible.

Inflammatory Diseases

Inflammation or necrosis characterizes the majority of hepatic diseases diagnosed in clinical practice. From a biochemical standpoint, inflammation is defined as significant elevation in the enzymes associated with hepatocellular injury–serum alanine aminotransferase (ALT), serum aspartate aminotransferase (AST), and arginase. Serum ALT concentrations are sensitive indicators of hepatic parenchymal injury. Most hepatic diseases associated with significant functional impairment will have increases in ALT concentrations. Notable exceptions are animals with congenital portal systemic shunts and those with cirrhosis.

Inflammatory hepatopathies can be infectious or noninfectious and acute or chronic in nature. Noninfectious inflammatory diseases predominate. Unfortunately, labeling a hepatic disease in a dog or cat as "hepatitis" does little toward establishing the etiology, nor does it help in terms of prognosis or therapy. Nearly all cases of clinically apparent inflammatory hepatic disease warrant biopsy for diagnostic, therapeutic, and prognostic reasons.

INFECTIOUS INFLAMMATORY HEPATIC DISEASES

The liver is prone to infection by a number of primary or secondary infectious agents. An adenovirus causes infectious canine hepatitis and canine herpesvirus infection, which are the only well documented viral hepatic diseases in the dog and are discussed in Chapter 47. Recently, a transmissible hepatitis has been described in dogs from England, which is distinct from canine adenoviral infections and has been termed canine acidophil hepatitis.[2] Affected dogs vary widely in age and have typical signs of hepatic disease (anorexia, depression, lethargy, and occasional vomiting). Intermittent fever spikes are present is some animals, and in late stages of the disease, ascites develops. Affected animals may present as acute severe hepatitis, subacute hepatitis, or end-stage cirrhosis. Diagnostic tests are nonspecific. Typically, increases in transaminases and serum alkaline phosphatase (SAP) occur; hypoalbuminemia is a late complication.

Evidence suggests that dogs may have progressive disease for two years or longer. Histologically, lesions vary from acute hepatitis to chronic active hepatitis to cirrhosis. Hepatocytes develop a characteristic necrobiotic acidophilic appearance. Acidophilic granules develop within the cytoplasm of hepatocytes, which coalesce into larger granules. An infectious etiology was suggested by the occurrence of the disease in several dogs in a household and clusters of cases in certain geographic areas. A similar disease was produced experimentally in normal dogs by inoculating them with serum and hepatocyte suspensions from affected dogs. This disease has not been recognized in North America at this time, but as the international transport of pets is commonplace, it would be expected that this disease would eventually have a worldwide incidence.

Although no primary hepatotropic viruses are known in the cat, the feline coronavirus, responsible for feline infectious peritonitis (FIP), and the feline leukemia virus can produce significant hepatic disease. FIP produces hepatic failure due to granulomatous hepatitis. In the author's experience, this is a very uncommon presentation for this disease. Diagnosis is based on biopsy findings of granulomatous hepatitis, the absence of other definable causes for granulomas (fungi, mycobacteria), and other clinical data supporting FIP. Feline leukemia virus–associated hepatic lymphosarcoma will be discussed later in this chapter.

In addition to viruses, the liver may be invaded by pyogenic and granulomatous bacteria, systemic fungi (blastomycosis, histoplasmosis, and coccidioidomycosis), protozoans (toxoplasmosis), spirochetes (leptospirosis), and parasites. The canine liver harbors a normal, low level resident bacterial population. Most adult dogs have one or more species of anaerobic bacteria within their liver by 10 to 12 months of age, with *Clostridium* spp. predominating.[3, 4] These bacteria are presumed to be of gut origin and enter the liver though the biliary system. Resident hepatic anaerobes become of pathogenic importance only if hepatic arterial blood flow is compromised so that tissue hypoxia develops. In addition to resident hepatic flora causing disease, bacteria may gain entry to the liver later in life via hematogenous, lymphatic, and biliary routes, as well as by direct extension from adjacent organs. However, only under exceptional circumstances is bacterial hepatitis a significant clinical problem in dogs.[5] Recent clinical reports include bacterial hepatitis in a three-week-old dog, with the bacteria presumed to be of umbilical vein origin; bacterial hepatitis diagnosed at surgery in a seven-year-old Samoyed in which *Clostridium perfringens* was cultured (the origin of the bacteria was not determined); and a fatal hepatic abscess induced by trauma which ultimately caused peritonitis.[6–8] Diagnosis of hepatic abscess frequently requires exploratory surgery for confirmation

and allows for culture of hepatic tissue and/or bile. Occasionally, radiographs will indicate the presence of gas pockets within liver parenchyma or within the biliary system (Figure 89–1). Patients are usually febrile, may have abdominal tenderness, and have increased white blood cell counts and elevated levels of serum ALT, AST, SAP, and bilirubin concentrations.

Tuberculosis organisms are rare causes for granulomatous hepatitis. Two recent reports, one in a dog and one in a cat, indicate that veterinarians must still consider tuberculosis in the differential diagnosis for chronic inflammatory hepatitis.[9, 10] The dog's disease was presumed to have originated from an owner's friend known to have tuberculosis. The cat had been receiving glucocorticoids for several years prior to developing its fatal illness, but no known source for the infection was identified.

Cholangitis-Cholangiohepatitis Syndrome in Cats.

The cholangitis-cholangiohepatitis syndrome (CCHS) is an important but poorly understood disease of cats.[11–16] This disease complex is considered one of the three most common biopsy-proven diagnoses for feline liver disease.[12, 15–19] I have chosen to include three pathologic processes in the discussion of CCHS: acute suppurative cholangitis, chronic lymphocytic cholangitis/ cholangiohepatitis, and biliary cirrhosis.[12–15] Cholangitis implies that inflammation is limited to intrahepatic bile ducts, while cholangiohepatitis refers to cases in which inflammation has extended to involve peribiliary hepatocytes. Biliary cirrhosis appears to be the end stage of this chronic progressive disease. Opinions are varied as to whether these three pathologic entities are actually separate diseases or whether they represent progressive stages of the same process.[13]

SUPPURATIVE CHOLANGITIS/CHOLANGIOHEPATITIS. Suppurative cholangitis/cholangiohepatitis is an uncommon disease. It is considered by most investigators to be caused by bacteria of intestinal origin, which ascend the common bile duct, eventually involving smaller intrahepatic bile ducts and periportal hepatocytes in the inflammatory process.[12, 15] Rare infectious agents, other than intestinal coliforms, have been identified as causes for CCHS. These include an organism resembling *Hepatozoon canis*, a coccidia-like organism, *Toxoplasma*, and *Bacillus piriformis*.[15] Although infectious agents appear to be the primary cause, other pathologic processes are seen in a large number of cats with suppurative cholangitis and are thought to predispose these cats to ascending bacterial infections. These abnormalities include chronic pancreatitis, cholecystitis, thickened inspissated bile, cholelithiasis, and duodenitis.[12, 16] Whether these latter processes actually predispose to or are a result of this disease is unresolved. Affected cats are of variable age and no breed predisposition is recognized. Clinical signs usually include weight loss, depression, anorexia, vomiting, fever, polydipsia, hypersalivation, and icterus.[12] Physical examination findings are unremarkable except for mild icterus and dehydration. The liver is usually of normal size on radiographs. Hemograms often indicate the presence of an immature neutrophilia. Biochemical abnormalities include mild to moderate hyperbilirubinemia (mostly conjugated), mild increases in SAP (two to four times),

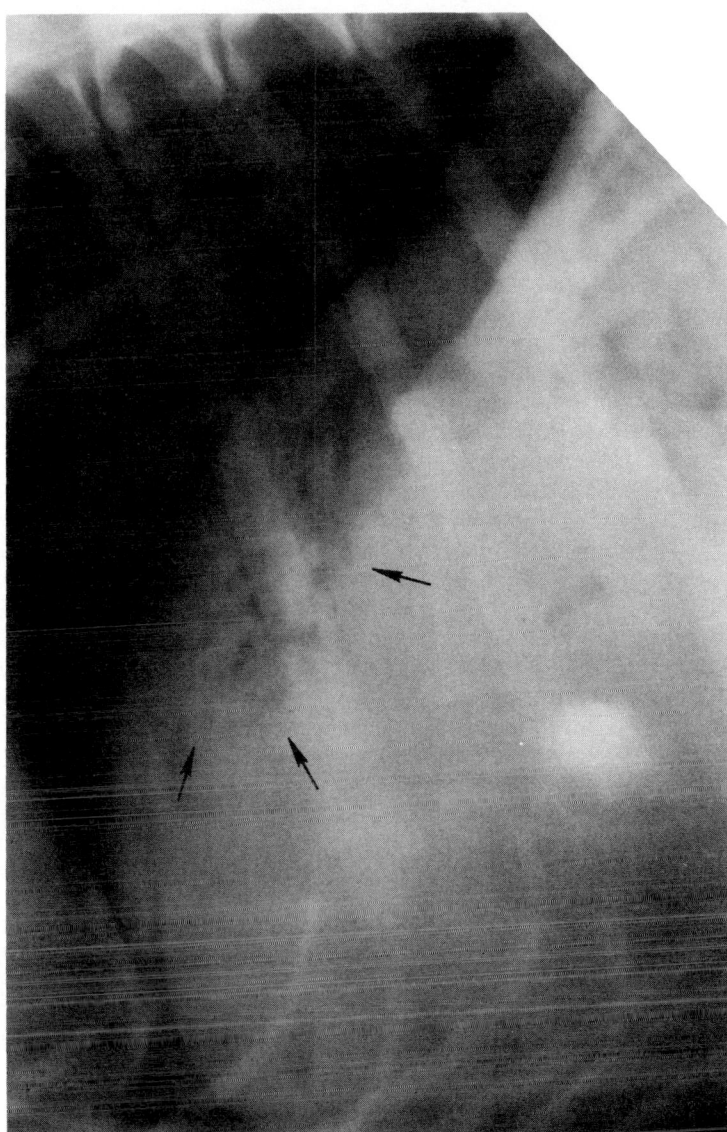

FIGURE 89–1. Abscess is visible within the liver because of gas produced by clostridial organisms (arrows).

and moderate rises in ALT, gamma glutamyl transpeptidase, and serum bile acid concentrations.[11, 12, 15, 20] Hepatic enzymes (ALT, SAP) are normal in some cats. Urinalyses may be positive for bilirubin and urobilinogen. Diagnosis requires hepatic biopsy. Since this disease process is diffuse, biopsies obtained by percutaneous needle techniques, laparoscopy, or laparotomy will be diagnostic. However, biopsy via laparotomy has the advantage of allowing for evaluation of the extrahepatic biliary system and pancreas. If choleliths or inspissated bile exist, they may be mechanically corrected at the time of surgery. Hepatic tissue and/or bile should be cultured both aerobically and anaerobically. Histologic findings include portal hepatic fibrosis, biliary hyperplasia, and suppurative exudate within dilated intrahepatic biliary ducts.[12] The presence of primarily neutrophils within intrahepatic bile ducts is the characteristic feature of this disease and distinguishes it from chronic lymphocytic cholangitis.

Therapy of suppurative CCHS is primarily supportive and symptomatic, and these aspects will be discussed at the end of this chapter. However, this is one hepatic disease in which antibiotics are specifically indicated.

The choice should be made based on culture and sensitivity of tissue or bile taken at biopsy. Drugs such as chloramphenicol, erythromycin, and tetracycline reach high concentrations in bile but have disadvantages for use in this disease. Erythromycin has a poor spectrum of activity for gram-negative bacteria, and causes frequent gastrointestinal upsets and anorexia. Tetracycline frequently causes anorexia in cats, may induce hepatic lipidosis, and is a hepatic enzyme repressor that inhibits protein synthesis. Chloramphenicol may induce anorexia and bone marrow dysplasia and is a potent repressor of hepatic enzyme systems, making it also a poor choice for liver failure. The author currently prefers ampicillin or metronidazole because of their effect on hepatic anaerobes and gastrointestinal coliforms. Aminoglycosides given orally are useful in controlling intestinal flora, which produce many of the toxins associated with hepatic encephalopathy. Aminoglycosides may also be injected parenterally and combined with ampicillin or metronidazole to increase the antibacterial spectrum of activity. Oral antibiotics should be continued for two to four weeks or longer depending on whether fever and neutrophilia persist. There is no evidence that glucocorticoids are beneficial in suppurative CCHS. A number of clinical reports have recommended the use of a hydrocholeretic drug, dehydrocholic acid (Decholin), 5 to 7 mg/lb/os (10 to 15 mg/kg/os) three times daily to aid in improving bile flow.[15] This product has only one use in humans—as an irritant laxative. Data to support its efficacy as a choleretic in cats are totally lacking. Serum bile acids are already increased in most cats with CCHS and would serve as an endogenous choleretic anyway. The author cannot recommend the use of this product. Several other compounds stimulate bile flow by what is termed bile salt-independent mechanisms.[21] Such drugs stimulate flow by increasing ionic transport of water into bile, causing a choleresis. Drugs known to possess this property are furosemide, ethacrynic acid, theophylline, phenobarbital, and hydrocortisone.[21] These would have a more rational basis for use in suppurative CCHS than would dehydrocholic acid.

The short-term prognosis for cats with suppurative CCHS is guarded to fair, but the long-term outlook is highly variable and often poor.[11, 13, 16] Some cats appear to undergo spontaneous remission and have long asymptomatic periods. Others respond to specific and symptomatic care but must remain on medication for their signs to be controlled. Still others respond poorly to therapy and die or are euthanatized. Several reports suggest that the suppurative disease may remain asymptomatic in many cats before it manifests itself as chronic lymphocytic CCHS.[11, 16]

CHRONIC LYMPHOCYTIC CHOLANGITIS/CHOLANGIO-HEPATITIS. Chronic lymphocytic CCHS is the most commonly reported form of feline CCHS.[11, 13, 14] Cats range in age from six months to ten years, with the majority being less than four years old.[13] Persian cats were considered to be at increased risk in one report but not in another.[11, 13] Lymphocytic CCHS differs from suppurative CCHS in several ways. Cats are generally less ill and ascites occurs fairly often, in over 50 per cent of the cats in some studies. Vomiting, depression, and lethargy are uncommon. Icterus was detected clinically in 10 of 21 cats in one series.[13] On physical examinations, significant findings include icterus, ascites, and hepatomegaly. Fever was not present in any of 21 cats from one series, but was present in two of three cats in another report.[13, 14] Hemograms are generally unremarkable, although a mild anemia may exist. White blood cell counts typically remain normal, and little if any left shift is present. Biochemical profiles support the presence of inflammatory, cholestatic liver disease similar to suppurative CCHS. Unique to this syndrome is the presence of hyperglobulinemia and hypoalbuminemia in many cats.[13] The increase in globulins is primarily due to increases in the gamma globulin fraction on electrophoresis.[13] Because of the lymphocytic inflammatory infiltrate that typifies this disease and a possible immune-mediated etiology, tests to detect the presence of antimitochondrial and/or antismooth muscle antibodies have been attempted in a few cases.[13, 14] Results were inconclusive in one study and negative in four cats in another.[13, 14]

A definitive diagnosis requires hepatic biopsy. Needle biopsies are diagnostic but an exploratory allows for examination of the gallbladder, common bile duct, pan-creas, and duodenum. Grossly, the liver will be normal to enlarged. The surface may be smooth or finely nodular depending on the duration and severity of the disease, and it may be quite firm if significant fibrosis is present.

Inspissated bile, formed as a result of dehydration and sludging of biliary secretions, may be present in intrahepatic and extrahepatic bile ducts and the gall bladder. This material must be surgically removed and the entire duct system flushed out to reestablish patency of the biliary system. If patency cannot be reestablished, surgical procedures that will allow bile flow to be normalized must be performed (cholecystoduodenostomy, cholecystojejunostomy). In some cats "white bile" will be present within the biliary system. This material represents fluid secreted by gallbladder and bile duct epithelium without bile pigments being present; some consider this to be a poor prognostic sign.[16]

Histologic findings are characterized by fibrous septa that link portal tracts and form complete or incomplete circumscribed nodules of hepatocytes.[13] A prominent feature is the presence of lymphocytes in the portal tracts which may extend within the fibrous septa. A few plasma cells may also be noted. Destruction of small bile ducts by this inflammatory reaction is often marked, and bile duct proliferation is typical.[13] In some of the cats with ascites, features of biliary cirrhosis become evident.[13] Biopsies should be cultured, as with suppurative CCHS, to determine if specific antibiotic therapy is indicated.

Therapy of chronic lymphocytic CCHS is similar to the suppurative form except that the addition of glucocorticoids appears to improve survival in some cases. The histological features of this disease are similar to an immune-mediated disease of man, chronic nonsuppurative destructive cholangitis (primary biliary cirrhosis), in which steroids improve survival. Because of this histologic similarity, glucocorticoids have been utilized as specific therapy in this feline disease. Limited clinical observations seem to indicate that steroids may help some feline cases as well, although relapses may occur when steroids are withdrawn.[11, 14] Immunosuppressive doses of prednisone, 1 to 2 mg/lb/day (2.2 to 4.4 mg/kg/day) have been used initially with doses tapered off over a 30- to 60-day period. Diuretics are useful in controlling ascites and will be discussed in the section on supportive and symptomatic therapy.

The prognosis for cats with lymphocytic CCHS is guarded to fair. Many animals will fail to adequately respond to supportive care and will die or be euthanatized. Some have an initial response to therapy but are prone to relapses if steroids and/or antibiotics are withdrawn. One cat has been reported to have had multiple relapses but to still be surviving over four and a half years.[14] Others appear normal clinically but have persistent biochemical abnormalities, and still others recover completely from their illness. Cats must be followed both clinically and biochemically until all evidence for persistent disease has ceased. Those cats with illness that continues to progress may develop biliary cirrhosis.

BILIARY CIRRHOSIS. Biliary cirrhosis appears to be the end stage of the chronic cholangitis/cholangiohepatitis complex in some cats.[11, 14, 16] This is the least common of the three disorders comprising this syndrome. These cats are typically icteric, depressed, and very thin, have ascites, and are in functional hepatic failure. Hepatomegaly is usually present (in contrast to cirrhosis in dogs), in which reduced liver mass is expected. In addition to mild to moderate increases in hepatic enzymes, hypoalbuminemia, hyperglobulinemia, and coagulopathies are often present.[16] A definitive diagnosis is dependent upon liver biopsy, but if coagulopathies exist, these cats should receive fresh whole blood transfusions prior to any biopsy procedures. Grossly, these livers will be firm and nodular. Histopathologic findings include severe bridging portal fibrosis, bile duct proliferation and hyperplasia, and nodular hepatic regeneration.[11] Inflammatory cells are minimal in this state of the process, but small numbers of lymphocytes may be present in portal areas. Therapy is supportive and symptomatic, but significant clinical improvement rarely occurs owing to the advanced stage of the disease. Survival is usually a few days to weeks following diagnosis.

Parasitic Infestations of the Liver. Parasitic infestations of the liver occur in both dogs and cats, with the latter species most often affected. Reported cases occur primarily in tropic and subtropic areas of the United States, with cases from Florida and Hawaii predominating. Low grade infestations usually are not associated with clinical disease.[22] Heavy infestations can be associated with chronic biliary disease that may ultimately lead to chronic cholangitis and biliary cirrhosis both in dogs and cats. Species of flukes reported to infect dogs and/or cats include *Opisthorchis felineus*, *Amphimerus pseudofelineus*, *Metorchis conjunctis*, *M. albidis*, *Clonorchis sinensis*, and *Platynosomum concinnum*.[22-24] Cats apparently are more frequently affected because of their ingestion of the intermediate hosts (snails or fish). For *Platynosomum concinnum*, the snail is the first intermediate host, with a reptile (lizard) or amphibian serving as the second and infective intermediate host.[22] Clinical signs include anorexia, depression, weight loss, vomiting, and mucoid diarrhea.[22, 25] Physical examination findings include depression, emaciation, icterus, hepatomegaly, and slight fever. Too little diagnostic information has been published to make conclusions about expected hematologic or biochemical profiles for this disease. It is interesting to note that one seriously affected cat had normal liver enzyme levels.[25] Reported radiographic abnormalities include hepatomegaly and multiple mineralized densities within the liver. Diagnosis is based on whether fluke eggs are found in fecal samples. This may be difficult in some cases, however, because eggs are often passed in low numbers.[22] Concentration techniques using formalin or ether have been recommended to improve diagnostic sensitivity. Liver biopsy can also provide the diagnosis, but if no flukes are identified in the biopsy sections, a diagnosis of idiopathic chronic cholangitis will be made.[25] Although no proven anthelmintic is available, a single dose of praziquantel (Droncit), 91 mg/lb (200 mg/kg), has been reported to markedly decrease the number of eggs passed in an infested cat.[25] An alternative therapeutic choice is nitroscanate catrodifene at 45 mg/lb (100 mg/kg), but reports of efficacy are lacking.[22, 25] Supportive care including antibiotics, fluids, vitamins, dietary management, and possibly glucocorticoids would also be indicated.

Dirofilariasis in dogs is infrequently associated with acute hepatic failure and death, a condition referred to as the vena cava syndrome. It is characterized by sudden weakness, bilirubinuria, hemoglobinuria, azotemia, marked elevation of BSP and serum ALT, and death. Large numbers of adult heartworms are found in both the pre- and postcava, and severe passive congestion of the liver is seen pathologically. Therapy is directed at surgically removing the heartworms in order to return systemic blood flow to normal.

Systemic Mycoses. Systemic mycoses, particularly histoplasmosis, may cause significant hepatic disease. Because these organisms are polysystemic in nature, the liver is usually one of several organ systems involved (pulmonary, skin, gastrointestinal, reticuloendothelial). From a diagnostic standpoint, the liver may assume prominence because confirming the diagnosis of deep mycoses requires identification of the organism in tissue specimens. Hepatic biopsy is much less complicated and generally carries less risk than does a full thickness intestinal biopsy. The liver serves as an easy access to reticuloendothelial tissue in which the organisms are proliferating and allows a diagnosis to be established.

NONINFECTIOUS INFLAMMATORY DISEASES

Noninfectious inflammatory hepatic diseases account for the majority of liver diseases in clinical practice. They include injuries to the liver that are secondary to disease in other organ systems, such as acute pancreatitis, chronic inflammatory colitis, and hyperthyroidism in cats, or that may follow severe trauma. Noninfectious inflammatory liver disease is more commonly caused by one or more of the following primary liver disorders: chronic hepatitis, chronic active hepatitis, copper-associated hepatitis in several breeds, toxic or drug-induced disease, and the end stage of many of these disorders, cirrhosis.

HEPATIC DISEASE SECONDARY TO OTHER DISORDERS

Acute Pancreatitis. Acute pancreatitis in the dog is nearly always associated with some degree of hepatic injury. Abnormalities in biochemical profiles occur owing to local injury to the right lobes of the liver, which lie adjacent to the inflamed pancreas, or are subsequent to absorption of toxic ferments via hepatic lymphatics or portal vein. Biochemically, these dogs have mild to severe increases in both serum ALT and AP concentrations. Serum bilirubin concentrations can be markedly increased in association with toxic cholestasis and/or common bile duct compression by the inflamed pancreas. The severity of hepatic injury correlates with the severity and duration of the pancreatitis. Hepatic lesions observed following experimental pancreatitis in dogs include hemorrhage, necrosis, and fatty infiltration.[26] These abnormalities are generally completely reversible once the pancreatitis is controlled.

Chronic Bowel Disease. Chronic inflammatory bowel disease in humans has a fairly high incidence of associated inflammatory or cholestatic hepatic disease.[27] Increases in SAP are observed most often, and a perichol-

1484   SECTION IX—The Gastrointestinal System

angitis is usually found on biopsy specimens. Therapy for the colitis usually results in resolution of the hepatic biochemical abnormalities. The author has observed a few dogs with chronic large or small bowel disease that have had mild increases in ALT and SAP that resolved with correction of the bowel disorder. It was presumed the bowel disease allowed portal vein absorption of toxic intestinal products, which resulted in injury to the liver.

Shock, Anemia, Congestive Heart Failure. Significant hepatic disease is often detected in animals following an episode of shock, severe anemia, or advanced congestive heart failure. The cause is presumed to be related to decreased hepatic perfusion and hypoxia. Except for the patient with congestive heart failure, resolution of the primary disorder results in complete resolution of the liver abnormalities. Animals with congestive heart failure and chronic passive congestion develop a mild degree of "cardiac cirrhosis." Anoxia and centrilobular necrosis are thought to be responsible for the changes observed. Ascites will develop in advanced cases, but clinical jaundice is rare. Functional failure is not expected with chronic passive congestion. The animal usually succumbs to the primary disease prior to liver failure. Laboratory evaluations usually indicate mild hyperbilirubinemia, slightly increased serum ALT and AP concentrations, and mild BSP retention.[28]

Trauma to the Liver and Bile Ducts. Abdominal trauma may result in significant injury to the liver and biliary system. In most cases in which only hepatic contusions have occurred, and no lacerations of hepatic parenchyma, bile ducts, or gallbladder exist, enzyme activity will be increased for a number of days, but repair and recovery should be complete. Lacerations of hepatic parenchyma can result in severe hemoperitoneum, and immediate surgical intervention is needed to save the patient. The gallbladder or, more commonly, the common bile duct or one of the hepatic ducts may be torn following blunt abdominal trauma and can lead to bile peritonitis.[29, 30] If the bile remains sterile, which is often the case, animals may remain asymptomatic. The presence of ascites and jaundice several days following abdominal trauma may be the first indications that a problem exists. The mean time from initial trauma to diagnosis was 13 days in one series of 29 dogs.[29] Septic bile peritonitis causes rapid deterioration of the animal and should be diagnosed as soon as possible. Clinical signs include ascites, jaundice, abdominal pain, anorexia, weight loss, vomiting, retching, and chalky, pale feces.[30, 31] Biochemically, mild increases in serum ALT, SAP, and bilirubin occur in all cases. Bilirubinuria is consistently present in large quantities. Urine urobilinogen concentrations vary depending upon whether significant quantities of bile are still able to enter the duodenum. Correction of the problem requires surgical intervention, and specifics will be discussed in Chapter 91 of this section.

Feline Hyperthyroidism. Clinical signs seen in hyperthyroid cats are similar to those associated with cats in liver failure, such as vomiting, weight loss, diarrhea, polydipsia, and polyuria. In addition, hyperthyroid cats have significant elevations in hepatic enzymes and bilirubin.[32] Serum alkaline phosphatase concentrations are increased in 72 per cent, AST concentrations in 61 per cent, ALT concentrations in 51 per cent, and serum bilirubin concentrations in 21 per cent of cats with this disease. Because the clinical signs and laboratory data strongly support the presence of primary liver disease, these cats may be misdiagnosed as having primary liver disease unless a serum thyroxine concentration is determined. Histologic findings are nonspecific and include centrilobular fatty infiltration and mild hepatocellular necrosis.[32] Conversely, we have diagnosed several cats in which both hyperthyroidism and primary liver disease coexisted. The presence of hepatomegaly and increases in hepatic serum enzymes and bilirubin above concentrations usually associated with hyperthyroid cats suggest that hyperthyroidism was not likely the sole cause for liver disease in these cats. Liver biopsy was necessary to establish a definitive diagnosis. Once hyperthyroid cats are treated for their disease, hepatic biochemical profiles return to normal.

PRIMARY NONINFECTIOUS INFLAMMATORY HEPATIC DISEASES

Chronic Hepatitis/Chronic Active Hepatitis. Chronic hepatitis is an important clinical syndrome in dogs and has been reported with increasing frequency over the last several years. In addition to an idiopathic group, several other disorders are now recognized that present as chronic hepatitis but do not appear to have an immune-mediated basis (Table 89–1). The most important of these disorders include: chronic hepatitis in Bedlington terriers; copper-associated hepatitis in West Highland white terriers; chronic hepatitis in Doberman pinschers; leptospirosis-associated hepatitis; lobular dissecting hepatitis; idiopathic hepatoportal fibrosis; and chronic hepatitis associated with infectious canine hepatitis virus. Because most of the above chronic inflammatory liver diseases are clinically and biochemically similar, differentiating between them usually requires hepatic biopsy. Further, because prognosis and therapy vary widely within this clinically homogeneous group of diseases, clinicians should make every attempt to be as precise in their diagnostic efforts as possible.

Much of what we know about chronic hepatitis in dogs, particularly what has been called chronic active

TABLE 89–1. DISEASES PRESENTING AS CHRONIC HEPATITIS IN DOGS

Cause Known or Suspected	Cause Unknown
1. Copper-associated hepatitis in Bedlington terriers	1. Idiopathic chronic active hepatitis
2. Copper-associated hepatitis in Doberman pinschers	2. Lobular dissecting hepatitis
3. Copper-associated hepatitis in West Highland white terriers	3. Idiopathic hepatic portal fibrosis
4. Leptospirosis-associated chronic active hepatitis	4. Cirrhosis
5. Infectious canine hepatitis virus–associated chronic active hepatitis	

6. Drug-induced chronic active hepatitis
  a. Anticonvulsants (primidone, phenytoin)
  b. Anthelmintics (oxibendazole)	

7. Primary neoplasms of the liver (hepatocellular carcinoma, cholangiocellular carcinoma)	

hepatitis (CAH), has been extrapolated from findings in humans with chronic liver disease. Whether dogs or cats are truly affected by immune-mediated liver disease remains to be proven. Even more important is whether glucocorticoids and other immunosuppressive drugs should be used indiscriminately in the therapy of so-called idiopathic canine CAH.

Most of what has been written by veterinarians about chronic hepatitis in dogs has been based on data from human CAH cases. Therefore, it is important to have a perspective on what chronic hepatitis, and especially what chronic active hepatitis, mean in the human medical field. Conceptually, chronic hepatitis refers to a group of liver diseases characterized by clinically apparent necroinflammatory processes that differ significantly as to cause, natural history, and therapeutic response.[33] For a disease to receive the designation of chronic, there must be evidence of continuing inflammation for at least six months.[33, 34] Some hepatitis viruses may persist in humans for six months before resolution occurs. Chronic hepatitis has only three recognized forms: chronic persistent hepatitis (CPH), chronic active hepatitis, and chronic lobular hepatitis, which is rare.[33, 35, 36]

Chronic persistent hepatitis is a benign disease that probably is caused by viral infection or drugs.[35] Most patients are asymptomatic, being diagnosed after routine biochemical screening for other problems. The only significant laboratory abnormalities are persistent mild to moderate increases in serum aminotransferases. Because these enzyme abnormalities persist for over six months, patients are biopsied to determine whether they have CPH or CAH. Histologic lesions in CPH are confined primarily to portal tracts and have minimal evidence of hepatocellular necrosis. Lobular architecture is preserved and little or no fibrosis is evident. Piecemeal necrosis is usually absent or, if present, is mild.[33, 35]

Follow-up biopsies at two- to three-month intervals show no progression of disease. Biochemical and histologic evidence of mild disease may persist for years before spontaneous resolution occurs. No specific or supportive care is indicated in this disease. Repeat biopsies are indicated because early lesions of CAH resemble those of CPH and are especially important for those in which long-term glucocorticoid therapy is contemplated. Certain patients with CAH benefit from steroid therapy, while those with CPH should not receive it.

The author is unaware of any published evidence that a disease similar to CPH exists in small animals. A few dogs have been evaluated with mild periportal hepatitis of unknown cause showing biochemical evidence of hepatic inflammation for months to years. These patients remained asymptomatic and had no biochemical evidence for progression of their disease, which may resolve spontaneously.

Chronic active hepatitis refers to an etiologically diverse group of diseases that have widely varying clinical, biochemical, and therapeutic responses and are linked solely by histologic similarities.[36, 37] Chronic active hepatitis is not a final diagnosis; it is a label for a group of diseases that tend to progress to cirrhosis but that require different therapeutic approaches.[38] Patients usu-

ally have obvious clinical illness, and biochemical abnormalities exist for six months or longer. Serum aminotransferases are typically five to ten times normal during this period. Hepatic biopsies are necessary for a definitive diagnosis.[33, 39–41] The lesions of CAH are characterized by portal inflammation that spills over into liver parenchyma, piecemeal necrosis, and periportal fibrosis.[40] Histologic evidence for cirrhosis may or may not be present at the time of initial diagnosis; however, lesions frequently progress to macronodular cirrhosis, hepatic insufficiency, and death.

Etiologic categories for human CAH include at least three subgroups in this classification: (1) viral-induced CAH; (2) drug-induced CAH; and (3) autoimmune, cryptogenic, or idiopathic CAH.[33–35, 39, 40, 42] Several other chronic inflammatory liver diseases that can progress to cirrhosis and have some features in common with CAH include: (1) metabolic disorders such as Wilson's disease (chronic copper toxicity), α-1-antitrypsin deficiency, chronic ethanol ingestion, and hemochromatosis; (2) chronic biliary tract disease, in particular, primary biliary cirrhosis; and (3) gastrointestinal disorders, such as pancreatitis and chronic bowel disease, which may induce a periportal cholangitis and be confused with CAH.[33] Most authors exclude these latter disorders because they can usually be diagnosed via clinical, biochemical, and histologic criteria.[35]

Viruses are responsible for 10 to 30 per cent of all cases of CAH.[35] Viruses incriminated are hepatitis B and non-A, non-B hepatitis virus. Some cases previously considered autoimmune or cryptogenic now appear to have an underlying viral association.[39, 42] Most hepatitis B-associated CAH patients have circulating antibodies to hepatitis B surface antigens (HBsAg-pos). Recently, new diagnostic tests have detected antibodies to a hepatitis B core antigen in many CAH patients previously considered idiopathic, suggesting a relationship between prior viral exposure and development of CAH.[42, 43]

Drugs are known to induce two to five per cent of all cases of human CAH.[41] The most important drugs are oxyphenisatin (once used in many laxatives but no longer available in the United States), α-methyldopa, and isoniazid.[33, 41] Very rare cases have been associated with exposure to halothane, nitrofurantoin, dantrolene, and propylthiouracil.[33, 41] A tenuous etiologic association exists with the drugs aspirin, acetaminophen, sulfonamides, and chlorpromazine.[41] Drug-induced CAH typically develops weeks to months following initiation of drug therapy. Recovery almost always occurs when the incriminated agent is discontinued.[40]

Autoimmune, cryptogenic, or idiopathic causes make up the remainder of cases of CAH not caused by viruses or drugs. These patients are the least well understood etiologically and pathophysiologically but are the most likely to respond to immunosuppressive therapy.[34] These patients have a large number of abnormal immunologic tests that, although not specific for CAH, suggest the presence of altered immune regulation, manifested by hypergammaglobulinemia and excessive quantities of circulating antibodies against nuclear protein (ANA), smooth muscle, and mitochondria. Thirty per cent of patients with CAH have positive LE cell preparations.

Recent immunologic work has detected the presence

of antibodies directed against specific liver cell surface antigens, lending strong support to the concept that immunologic mechanisms play an important part in the cause or perpetuation of CAH. Two diagnostically important liver-specific antigens have so far been identified: liver-specific membrane lipoprotein (LSP) and liver membrane antigen, a poorly characterized hepatocyte membrane component. If lymphocytes from patients with CAH are incubated with normal rabbit or human hepatocytes, an antibody-dependent cell-mediated cytotoxicity to the hepatocytes occurs.[44] High titers of antibodies to LSP are not specific for CAH, being found in several other chronic liver diseases as well.[33] High titers do correlate with disease activity, as patients with high titers receiving steroids are very prone to relapse if steroids are withdrawn.[38] In contrast, high titers of antibodies to liver membrane antigen are more specific for CAH, occurring in 38 per cent of these patients and 61 per cent of those with HBsAg-negative cirrhosis.[33, 42]

Regardless of the cause, the pathogenesis of CAH involves autoimmune reactions against hepatocytes. Genetic predisposition also appears to play a role, as affected patients have consistent patterns of histocompatible antigens,[38] and first and second degree relatives have increased T-cell sensitization to LSP when compared to spouses.[45] Some initiating event occurs that leads to injury to hepatocytes (viruses, drugs, and so forth). Binding of drugs, drug metabolites, or viruses to the cell surface results in antibodies and sensitized lymphocytes being directed against these altered hepatocyte membranes; eventually cellular death occurs. Once hepatocyte-specific antigens are exposed, additional immunologic reactions are initiated, leading to complement-mediated cytotoxic reactions, which eventually become self-perpetuating. Immunologic injury is critical in early phases of the disease but assumes less importance in chronic phases. Vascular alterations and increases in collagen formation are important in the chronic phases of the disease.

A definitive diagnosis of CAH requires several diagnostic criteria to be verified: (1) clinical data supporting the presence of active hepatic disease for six months or longer; (2) the presence of multiple abnormal immunologic findings as described above; and most importantly, (3) biopsy confirmation. Biopsy data not only allows for differentiation of CAH patients from those with other chronic liver disorders but helps to stage the disease process.[33] Biopsies are best evaluated by individuals with knowledge of the histopathological spectrum of this disorder. Diagnostic accuracy is especially important because some, but not all, forms of CAH require immunosuppressive therapy.[34] If needle biopsies are obtained, core samples should be at least two cm in length to reduce the chance of sampling errors.[33, 35] Diagnostic accuracy is poorer when cirrhosis is present.[35]

Histopathologic features typical of CAH include piecemeal necrosis, bridging necrosis, and active cirrhosis.[35] Piecemeal necrosis is a specific pattern of periportal necrosis and inflammation typical of CAH. This lesion is not pathognomonic, however, as it is also seen in some nonprogressive hepatic diseases.[33–35] Inflammation begins in the portal triad and extends outward into hepatic lobular parenchyma. In this process of expansion, the limiting plate (a single-cell thick row of hepatocytes surrounding the portal triad) is obscured or destroyed. The inflammatory cells producing the necrosis are typically lymphocytes and plasma cells, although variable numbers of neutrophils may also be present. Small groups or islands of hepatocytes tend to be isolated and surrounded by inflammatory cells. Additional pathologic changes accompany piecemeal necrosis but are more variable and include bile duct proliferation, bile stasis, fatty metamorphosis, bridging necrosis, lobular collapse, and eventually cirrhosis.[46]

The final pathologic stage of CAH is active cirrhosis.[33–35] Inflammatory cells are replaced by fibrosis in areas of bridging necrosis, regenerative nodules are widespread, and marked architectural distortion is evident. Patients may not be diagnosed until this advanced stage is present, and confirmation that these changes are a result of CAH is difficult. By combining clinical signs, biochemical profiles, immunodiagnostics, and biopsy, a diagnosis of CAH can be established in most cases.

General therapeutic guidelines followed in humans are a useful starting point for consideration in animals. The ultimate goal is to eliminate signs of both liver disease and drug side effects while allowing the patient to reach near normal life expectancy.[40] Determining which patients to treat, how long to treat, and with what drugs remain unresolved. Attempts should be made to identify a causative agent first, such as viruses, drugs, or genetic disorders. All drugs taken by patients have the potential to induce chronic hepatitis, and their administration should be stopped, if possible. Drug-induced chronic liver disease responds well to drug elimination alone in most cases. Other diseases with morphologic similarities to CAH should be ruled out (Wilson's disease, α-1-antitrypsin deficiency, primary biliary cirrhosis, and sclerosing cholangitis).[47] Finally, glucocorticoids should be considered. Available information suggests that steroids are indicated neither in *asymptomatic* patients (regardless of biopsy findings) nor in symptomatic patients with mild histopathologic findings.[36, 41] Glucocorticoid use is contraindicated in viral-induced CAH.[40, 48] Good evidence exists to show that glucocorticoids improve the quality of life, lengthen survival, and decrease progression of early lesions to cirrhosis in patients with *moderate to severe symptomatic autoimmune CAH*.[40, 41] Prednisone is used in immunosuppressive doses (1 mg/lb/day) for 10 to 14 days and then gradually tapered down to maintenance doses over 4 to 6 weeks.[39, 40] Maintenance dosages are generally 0.15 to 0.33 mg/lb/day. Patients are monitored clinically and biochemically during the tapering period for signs of their disease worsening. Biochemical remissions usually occur within three months, while histologic improvement may not occur for months to years.[40, 41] If steroid side effects are severe, or if continued high dosages are required for control of the disease, azathioprine (Imuran) can be combined with low dosage prednisone as an alternative and equally effective form of therapy.[39, 40] White blood cell and platelet counts must be monitored with this combined immunotherapy approach. Follow-up liver biopsies should ideally be taken at six-month intervals during therapy and after drug cessation to determine the histologic state of the disease.

The optimal duration of therapy has not been established, but two to four years or more of daily prednisone may be necessary before remissions are complete. Steroids are tapered off at the end of the maintenance period over four to six weeks.

A limited number of long-term studies have been published comparing prednisone with placebo treatment for CAH.[33, 35, 40, 49, 50] Spontaneous recovery occurs in 20 to 33 per cent of patients on placebo alone.[33, 35, 40] Of those receiving steroids, 20 per cent continue to progress in spite of therapeutic efforts. Sixty per cent of patients receiving steroids improve significantly, but relapses occur in half of these if steroids are withdrawn.[49] Complete cures occur in only 10 to 15 per cent of patients. The mean time for complete remission varies from three to four and a half years.[33, 40] If cirrhosis is present on biopsy, death occurs in 20 per cent of patients.[51]

If steroids and azathioprine are ineffective in controlling the progression of CAH the use of D-penicillamine and polyunsaturated phosphatidylcholine may be considered.[43, 52, 53] D-penicillamine has antifibrotic and immunomodulating properties and may be of some therapeutic use in human CAH. Polyunsaturated phosphatidylcholine is a highly unsaturated phospholipid extracted from soya beans and appears to protect hepatocytes against cytotoxic lymphocytes. When fed at 45 mg/lb/day (100 mg/kg/day) to rabbits, it was hypothesized to become incorporated into hepatocyte plasma membranes and protect them from *in vitro* lymphocytotoxicity.[43]

Chronic Hepatitis in Dogs. The complete spectrum of chronic hepatitis in dogs is just beginning to be realized (Table 89–1). During the past several years a number of newly recognized causative agents for chronic hepatitis have been identified in dogs.[54–57] In addition, several breeds of dogs appear to have a genetic predisposition to develop chronic inflammatory liver disease.[57-59] Lastly, several reports have been published describing an entity in dogs considered similar to idiopathic or autoimmune CAH in humans.[51, 54, 60–65] There is a great deal of overlap between these areas.

IDIOPATHIC CHRONIC ACTIVE HEPATITIS IN DOGS. Chronic active hepatitis appears to be the disease of the 1980s in veterinary hepatology. Unfortunately, this diagnostic designation has been applied indiscriminately to virtually any inflammatory liver disease that persists for a few weeks and has lesions even remotely resembling those seen in human CAH. One veterinary pathologist has questioned whether CAH, as it is defined for humans, even exists in the dog.[46] This lack of diagnostic specificity results from semantic differences between authors, poor definition of diagnostic criteria, unknown specificity of diagnostic tests, lack of available supportive immunodiagnostic tests, and lack of controlled therapeutic trials. A study involving 11 dogs reported by Strombeck and Gribble is probably the best documented report on a canine disease resembling idiopathic CAH in humans.[63] Clinical signs were nonspecific with depression, weakness, and anorexia present in all 11 dogs. Polydipsia and polyuria were observed in eight, jaundice in six, and encephalopathy in one dog. Serum ALT concentrations were generally quite high (mean 15 times normal), serum AP concentrations averaged five times normal, and the total bilirubin was

increased in 9 of 11 (mean = 2.6 mg/dl). The retention of BSP ranged from 6 to 48 per cent (mean = 33 per cent). Hypoalbuminemia and hypergammaglobulinemia were documented in only three animals. Hepatic biopsy information was used as the primary diagnostic test to make the diagnosis of CAH and to determine whether glucocorticoids were utilized.

The designation of a liver disease as chronic is often based on historic information (often unreliable), repetitive biochemical evaluations (often not obtained), or histopathologic findings supporting chronicity (fibrosis), also frequently unavailable. Currently, 12 weeks has been suggested as sufficient time for a chronic designation to be applied to dogs with liver disease.[63] How do we define active liver disease in dogs? Activity means evidence for continuing inflammation or necrosis, which is most easily determined via laboratory evaluations of serum aminotransferases. Serum alanine aminotransferase concentrations have been stated to average 15 times normal in canine CAH, however, several cases of presumed canine CAH have had ALT concentrations within the normal range.[51, 60, 63, 64]

Immunologic criteria to support an immune-mediated basis for this disease in dogs are also lacking. Some cases have been found to have elevated IgG concentrations, a nonspecific finding in many chronic liver diseases. Occasional dogs have titers against nuclear protein (ANA positive) or abnormal LE cell phenomena, but the significance of these findings is unresolved. Measurements of antibodies against mitochondria, smooth muscle, or liver-specific antigens have not been reported.

Biopsy data provide the most specific information for diagnosing CAH; in fact, a definitive diagnosis requires it. Lesions compatible with human CAH have been used by most investigators to substantiate this diagnosis in dogs.[51, 60, 62–65] Unfortunately, biopsy alterations are not pathognomonic for CAH and great care must be taken not to overinterpret histologic findings.

The situation as it stands today regarding idiopathic chronic active hepatitis in dogs is anything but resolved. A group of dogs exists in which there is biochemical evidence for chronic hepatitis; no cause has been identified, and biopsy features resemble CAH.[51, 60–63, 65] What should we call the disease(s), and how should we treat the dogs? Establishing a diagnosis of idiopathic CAH involves several steps. First, it should be confirmed that active liver disease exists. This can be done by using the clinical history and appropriate biochemical tests (ALT, AST). If no identifiable cause can be found and the patient has mild or intermittent disease, it is likely that only supportive care will be necessary (no steroids). If the dog's signs worsen or there is biochemical evidence of a continuing necroinflammatory process or that the disease is chronic, a liver biopsy should be obtained. Biopsies should be reviewed by pathologists knowledgeable of the features of CAH. Veterinarians should send as much pertinent clinical data as are available to assist the pathologist in establishing a diagnosis, since biopsy data are only one piece of the diagnostic puzzle. If the biopsy findings are compatible with idiopathic CAH, immunosuppressive therapy should be considered along with general supportive and symptomatic measures.

The therapy of idiopathic chronic active hepatitis combines supportive and symptomatic care with specific immunosuppressive therapy. General supportive measures are discussed in the therapy section at the end of this chapter; drugs unique to the therapy of CAH will be discussed here. These drugs include glucocorticoids, azathioprine, D-penicillamine, and polyunsaturated phosphatidylcholine. Glucocorticoids are used alone or in combination with azathioprine (Imuran). Only one report of clinical usage of steroids in canine CAH has been published.[63] Five of nine dogs treated with steroids were considered to have improved. However, multiple approaches to therapy were utilized in this group of dogs and no control group was evaluated, making conclusions speculative at best. Until results of well-controlled clinical trials become available, the author has the following recommendations. Dogs should be given 1 mg/lb/day of prednisone for 10 to 14 days. Dosages are decreased by 25 per cent every week thereafter until a maintenance dosage of approximately 0.25 mg/lb/day is achieved (one month), at which time dogs should be reevaluated clinically and biochemically. If improvement is noted, this dosage should be continued for another month and then decreased to alternate day therapy. A recheck at this time should determine whether continued steroid therapy is indicated. If the dog is active, alert, and eating well, and if biochemical profiles are improving, steroid withdrawal should be considered. Because of the profound effect of glucocorticoids on canine hepatic enzymes, it may be difficult to determine whether the dog's disease is improving, unless functional tests are also run, e.g., serum bile acids, albumin concentrations, BSP retention, ammonia tolerance. The dog must be reassessed following steroid withdrawal to determine if the disease is recurring. If relapses occur, reinitiation of steroid therapy is indicated. The optimal duration of such therapy is totally arbitrary, and good clinical judgment is necessary here.

If glucocorticoids are poorly tolerated by the dog, consideration should be given to decreasing the steroid dosage to one that is tolerated and adding azathioprine at 0.45 mg/lb/day (1 mg/kg/day) to the therapy. Hemograms must be monitored at two- to three-month intervals when azathioprine is used. This regimen has been reported to result in clinical remission in dogs with chronic hepatitis.[66]

Therapy using D-penicillamine in the dog for CAH should be considered if steroids and azathioprine are ineffective. No data are available for dogs supporting its efficacy in CAH. It has had limited clinical trials in humans as an antifibrotic drug.[52, 53] Penicillamine inhibits collagen synthesis, causes reductions in IgM and circulating immune complexes, and may inhibit cell-mediated immunity. Steroids have not been effective in reversing or delaying hepatic fibrosis in human CAH, while penicillamine has been shown to have a beneficial effect. The dosage for this drug in dogs is 4.5 to 6.8 mg/lb (10 to 15 mg/kg) given every 12 hours.

The use of polyunsaturated phosphatidylcholine in canine CAH should be considered experimental, but preliminary drug trials in humans have been encouraging.[67] Histologic evidence of significantly decreased disease activity was found in patients who had received this drug in combination with prednisone and azathioprine and who had failed to respond to the latter two drugs. Human recommended dosages are three grams/day. Experimental animals (rabbits) have been given 45 mg/lb/day (100 mg/kg) in experiments to try and define the mechanism through which this drug alters the immune system.

COPPER-ASSOCIATED HEPATITIS IN BEDLINGTON TERRIERS. In 1975, Bedlington terriers were first recognized as having a genetically predisposed chronic liver disease characterized by massive accumulations of copper within their livers.[57] The disease is inherited as an autosomal recessive trait, and owing to extensive inbreeding, its incidence in the breed is quite high.[68] In spite of attempts by a few dedicated Bedlington breeders to reduce its incidence in the breed, many affected dogs are still being bred.

Clinical signs and physical findings associated with Bedlington liver disease are highly variable. Affected dogs may be asymptomatic, present acutely with signs of mild, moderate, or fulminant hepatic failure, or be first diagnosed in the end stages of chronic liver disease. Asymptomatic dogs tend to be younger (one to six years old), and are in the copper accumulating phase of their illness. They are identified after routine biochemical screening is performed and/or a liver biopsy is obtained. This group is the most likely to respond well to prophylactic therapy.

The majority of symptomatic Bedlingtons present as middle-aged, mildly or moderately sick dogs. Varying degrees of vomiting, depression, lethargy, and weight loss are reported. Physical findings, except for the presence of jaundice, are nonspecific. Laboratory evaluations support the presence of mild to moderately severe inflammatory, cholestatic liver disease. Hemograms are usually unremarkable. Serum ALT concentrations generally are from two to ten times normal. Mild hyperbilirubinemia, mostly conjugated, is present. Supportive care is usually associated with recovery in several days. These dogs may have similar acute recurrent attacks throughout their lives or may ultimately develop cirrhosis.

Rarely, a young to middle-aged Bedlington will present in fulminant hepatic failure and have had no previous evidence of liver disease. Signs exhibited by the dog include acute onset of depression, lethargy, vomiting, jaundice, and possibly coma. On physical examination these dogs are icteric and may have prominent hepatomegaly. Serum biochemical profiles support the existence of an acute, severe, inflammatory liver disease. Serum transaminases are in the thousands, total bilirubin concentrations may be 10 to 20 mg/dl, and blood ammonia concentrations are very high. A less common finding is the presence of acute hemolytic anemia. Dogs have a rapid decline in packed cell volume, severe jaundice, hemoglobinemia, and hemoglobinuria.[69] Serum copper concentrations, which are normal in most affected Bedlingtons, may be dramatically elevated in these animals. Mortality tends to be quite high in this group in spite of intensive therapeutic efforts. Death may occur within 48 to 72 hours following the onset of clinical signs. Dogs surviving the acute attack develop chronic progressive hepatitis and cirrhosis if left untreated.

Some affected Bedlingtons are first identified when they are old and have signs of cirrhosis. Usually, no history of prior clinical disease is evident. Their signs are similar to those of the younger affected dogs but are less severe. Ascites may be present, and the dogs' livers are usually small and nonpalpable. These dogs may respond to supportive and symptomatic care for a few weeks to months, but long-term survival is the exception.

The pathogenesis of this disease is incompletely understood. It is known that the cause of hepatocellular injury is directly related to the progressive accumulation of copper within hepatic lysosomes.[70] Copper is known to be hepatotoxic once significant intracellular concentrations exist. It has been determined that absorption of copper from the gastrointestinal tract is normal in affected dogs; the defect appears to be an inability to effectively excrete stored copper into the biliary system leading to a net positive copper balance.[70] Normal canine hepatic copper concentrations are from 91 to 377 μgm/gm (mean = 200 μgm/gm) on a dry weight basis. Hepatic copper concentrations in normal puppies appear to increase until they are four months old and remain fairly stable after that.[71] In affected Bedlingtons, hepatic copper concentrations may be significantly increased as early as four months of age.[72] Six of seven affected puppies in one study had quantitative hepatic copper concentrations greater than 1000 μgm/gm dry weight at six months of age.[73] The seventh dog's hepatic copper concentration was determined to be abnormal at 17 months of age. Hepatic copper concentrations continue to increase until the dogs are five to six years old.[73, 74] Hepatic copper content slowly declines after this peak period but never declines into the normal range. Affected dogs have hepatic copper concentrations of 850 to 12,000 μgm/gm dry weight.[75] The copper that accumulates within hepatic lysosomes gives them a characteristic histologic picture (Figure 89–2). Until hepatic copper concentrations exceed 2000 μgm/gm, little evidence of morphologic injury is evident.[73] Once this occurs, progressive morphologic and functional damage becomes clinically and biochemically apparent. When massive numbers of hepatocytes undergo rapid lysis, large quantities of copper may be released into the circulation and cause acute severe hemolysis. In the majority of dogs, however, serum copper values remain normal.

A definitive diagnosis requires liver biopsy combined with special histochemical stains to detect the presence of copper and/or quantitative copper assays. Although the presence of inflammatory liver disease in a Bedlington terrier strongly suggests that copper toxicosis is present, biopsy is mandatory to assess the severity of the liver lesions and to determine the need for specific therapy, which is expensive, lifelong, and may not be effective in all cases. Biopsies are also indicated for those Bedlingtons that are being considered for use in a breeding program. Generally, biopsies are delayed until the animals are over one year old because occasional affected animals may not accumulate pathologic increases in hepatic copper until this age. Normal biochemical profiles do not rule out this disease, as significant numbers of younger animals will have no increases in serum ALT or other liver parameters while still having significantly increased copper concentrations.[73] Histologically, biopsies will show a wide spectrum of lesions depending on the duration and severity of the illness. The earliest lesions are only evident as numerous brownish eosinophilic granules dispersed throughout hepatocyte cytoplasm primarily in centrilobular regions. Once the cells' tolerance for increased copper is exceeded, focal hepatitis becomes evident. Later, piecemeal necrosis, mononuclear inflammatory cell infiltrates, bridging necrosis, and other features of CAH exist.[73] Eventually macro- and micronodular cirrhosis, the end stage of this disease, develops.

Three special stains can be utilized for histochemical estimations of hepatic copper content—rhodanine, rubeanic acid, and Timm's silver sulfide stains. Timm's silver sulfide is the most sensitive of these stains, but it detects the presence of excess iron as well as copper, so it is less specific.[76] Rhodanine and rubeanic acid are specific for tissue-localized copper and have been used as semiquantitative methods to determine hepatic copper content.[72, 77] Both these stains consistently detect the presence of copper in liver biopsies when its concentration exceeds 400 μgm/gm dry weight. The sensitivity of rhodanine for detecting increased hepatic copper in affected dogs has been reported to be 95 per cent (20 of 21 dogs were positive), while none of 19 normal dogs

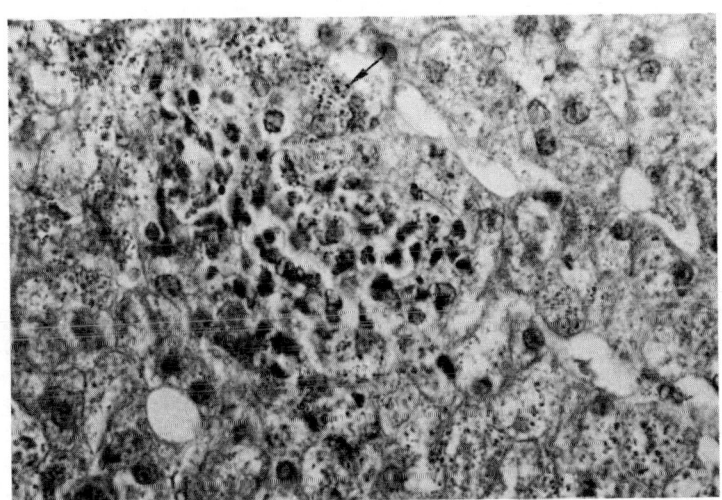

FIGURE 89–2. Foci of neutrophils associated with necrotic hepatocytes in a liver biopsy from a Bedlington terrier with copper storage disease. Large copper-containing lysosomal granules are prominent throughout the specimen (arrow). 320×.

stained positively.[72] It has been determined that hepatic biopsies stored in formalin for extended periods lose their ability to pick up these copper-sensitive stains.[77] Although good staining was maintained on samples preserved for six weeks, samples restained after seven months in formalin were negative for copper. It is important to note that, in contrast to special stains for copper, quantitative copper results from samples stored for prolonged periods were unchanged from results obtained on these same samples when fresh.[78]

Therapy of this disease is both specific and supportive and symptomatic. This is one of the few hepatic diseases for which a specific mode of therapy exists. Two copper chelating agents, D-penicillamine and trientine dihydrochloride, can be utilized to put affected dogs in negative copper balance. The drug for which there is the most information is D-penicillamine. D-Penicillamine is a chelator of divalent cations. It has been used for years to treat Wilson's disease, a copper accumulating hepatic disease in humans. Its beneficial effects are thought to be attributed to its ability to chelate copper within the circulation. The chelated copper is eventually excreted in urine, preventing its accumulation in the liver. The currently recommended dosage for Bedlingtons is 125 mg every 12 hours. The drug should be given 30 minutes before eating. Common side effects are anorexia and vomiting. These reactions can be reduced by giving only 125 mg/day initially and increasing the dosage up to 125 mg twice daily after several days. Another disadvantage of the drug is its slow rate of decoppering, which makes it generally ineffective in severely ill dogs or in those with advanced cirrhosis.

Objective evidence of therapeutic efficacy, e.g., reductions in serum ALT concentrations or reductions in quantitative copper values, often require months or years of continuous therapy. Limited clinical evaluations of this drug have been done in Bedlington terriers. Quantitative hepatic copper concentrations from an affected dog treated 26 months with D-Penicillamine were reduced from 5298 μgm/gm dry weight to 228 μgm/gm dry weight.[74] In another study of two dogs receiving D-penicillamine for one year, no significant change in histopathology was detected on follow-up biopsy in either dog. Quantitative copper results available from one of the dogs was unchanged from pretherapy values.[79] The author has follow-up biopsies and quantitative hepatic copper values in one Bedlington followed over seven months. The hepatic copper content was 8884 μgm/gm dry weight when therapy was initiated and 6785 μgm/gm dry weight seven months later. No significant change in hepatic morphology was noted. One recent report indicates that hepatic copper concentrations in two affected Bedlingtons decreased by 900 μgm/gm/year when D-penicillamine was administered.[80]

Trientine dihydrochloride (Cuprid) has recently been approved for use in the United States as an alternative therapy for humans with Wilson's disease who do not tolerate D-penicillamine. It is no more effective than D-penicillamine as a cupruretic agent but has many fewer adverse side effects. It has been evaluated experimentally in normal dogs as a potential cupruretic agent with encouraging results.[81] A derivative of this compound, 2,3,2,tetramine tetrahydrochloride, has also been tried on an experimental basis in affected Bedlington terriers and has been found to have significantly faster reductions in hepatic copper than was noted with D-penicillamine.[80] When compared with trientine dihydrochloride in normal animals, 2,3,2,tetramine tetrahydrochloride has found to be four to nine times more potent as a cupruretic agent. This latter drug is still experimental at this time and is not commercially available. Since both compounds were effective in normal dogs, without apparent side effects, it would seem that trientine dihydrochloride warrants further investigation in affected Bedlington terriers. A potential starting dose is 250 mg every 12 hours. Adverse reactions reported in humans include iron deficiency and systemic lupus erythematosus. This drug should be given an hour before meals and no other therapeutic agents; including vitamin and mineral supplements, should be given at the same time.

An alternative to the administration of systemically active chelators is the use of zinc sulfate or zinc gluconate. Zinc increases fecal excretion of copper by stimulating production of an intestinal mucosal metallothionein with high affinity for both zinc and copper, which impairs absorption of these metals.[82] Zinc gluconate has been suggested as an alternative to the usually prescribed zinc sulfate because it induces less gastric irritation. According to one author, it is equal in effectiveness and less expensive than D-penicillamine as therapy for copper-associated hepatitis in Bedlington terriers.[83] No data to substantiate this claim were presented. Recommended dosages, based on criteria in humans, are 0.9 to 1.4 mg/lb/day (2 to 3 mg/kg/day) in three divided doses.[82] The drug should be given 30 to 60 minutes before meals.

No objective criteria have been established for determining which affected Bedlingtons should receive therapy with decoppering agents. The author routinely initiates therapy in any dog that has had one attack of liver disease and is not exhibiting any signs of vomiting. Therapy is also indicated in asymptomatic dogs with persistently increased serum ALT concentrations of approximately 300 IU or higher, as an attempt to prevent either an acute crisis or the progression of the disease to cirrhosis. These dogs must be treated for life on the premise that hepatic disease will continue unless therapy is constant. In general, no attempts to limit copper intake are made except to avoid foods high in copper, such as chocolate, nuts, and liver, and to avoid supplementing the diet with vitamin-mineral compounds containing copper.

Owners of Bedlington terriers who plan to breed their dogs should be aware of methods available to limit the genetic perpetuation of this disease. Because this is an autosomal recessive trait, only homozygous recessive dogs will manifest this disease. All dogs being considered for inclusion in a breeding program should have both biochemical profiles and hepatic biopsies obtained. Quantitative copper assays should be performed on liver samples that appear negative for copper by histochemical means. Since both normal mature Bedlingtons and heterozygotes have normal hepatic copper concentrations, it is difficult to identify heterozygotes except through breeding trials and serial biopsies. On the basis of one limited study, it appears that heterozygotes may be detected by obtaining serial hepatic biopsies, one at 5 to 7 months of age and another at 14 to 15 months of age or later.[84] Heterozygote Bedlingtons have moderately increased hepatic copper concentrations at six months of age (over 400 μgm/gm dry weight but less than 1000 μgm/gm dry weight) which generally return to normal levels at approximately one year of age.

Affected Bedlingtons will have progressively increasing hepatic copper concentrations on the two samples. Although it appears that most heterozygotes have hepatic quantitative copper values within the normal range after 14 to 15 months of age, several documented cases have had values that persisted over 400 μgm/gm dry weight, but less than the 850 μgm/gm dry weight concentration considered the lowest value typical of affected animals.[72, 84] These dogs do not develop hepatic disease, and copper concentrations do not appear to increase during the life of the dog.

CHRONIC HEPATITIS IN DOBERMAN PINSCHERS. Doberman pinschers are affected by what is presumed to be an inheritable, copper-associated hepatitis that clinically and histologically resembles idiopathic chronic active hepatitis.[58, 85–87] This disease so closely resembles CAH that in two earlier reports, 6 of 15 dogs considered to have idiopathic CAH were Dobermans.[51, 62] One unique feature of this disease is the high ratio of females to males. Females strongly outnumber males in reported cases (39 females to 2 males). The age range of affected dogs is 1½ to 11 years (mean = 5 years). Clinical signs are typical of liver failure and are present from 1 to 20 weeks prior to examination by veterinarians. Polydipsia, polyuria, weight loss, ascites, icterus, anorexia, depression, vomiting, and diarrhea are the most commonly reported signs. Polydipsia and polyuria are prominent in many affected dogs that have few other signs. The overwhelming majority of dogs so far evaluated have been in advanced stages of liver failure regardless of the severity of clinical signs. Prominent biochemical abnormalities include increases in serum concentrations of alkaline phosphatase (mean = ten times normal), ALT (mean = ten times normal), and bilirubin (mean = 3.9 mg/dl). Hypoalbuminemia is present in 62 per cent, and prothrombin and partial thromboplastin times are prolonged in 55 per cent of affected dogs. Thrombocytopenia and overt bleeding are occasionally seen.[85] Resting concentrations of blood ammonia are nearly always elevated and BSP retention is dramatically prolonged. A few of these dogs have had low resting T_4 concentrations and have been positive for von Willebrand's disease. Significant bacteriuria is present in many of these dogs. Liver size is usually reduced on survey radiographs of the abdomen.

Pathologic findings are most compatible with CAH. The liver is generally small and has an irregular or coarsely nodular surface. Upon microscopic examination, piecemeal necrosis is typical, mononuclear infiltrates predominate in periportal areas, varying degrees of fibrosis are present throughout the lobule, and bridging fibrosis does occur.[58, 85] Hepatic copper and iron concentrations are often increased but not to the levels seen in Bedlington terriers (copper is usually less than 1500 μgm/gm dry weight), and a number of dogs have had high normal values for copper.[58] The role copper

and iron accumulations play in the pathogenesis of this disease is unknown. Copper accumulations were initially considered to be secondary to chronic cholestasis since cholestasis results in decreased elimination of copper in bile.[58] Two young Dobermans have recently been described that had significantly increased hepatic copper concentrations but no biochemical or histological evidence of cholestasis. The copper was hypothesized to be the cause for the liver disease rather than a consequence of it.[87] The importance of copper and iron in this disease remains unresolved.

Therapeutic efforts have been directed at modifying the inflammatory reaction occurring in the liver while continuing to provide supportive and symptomatic care. Both D-penicillamine and prednisone have been used in various combinations in an effort to decrease excess copper and inflammation. D-Penicillamine has been given at 4.5 to 6.8 mg/lb (10 to 15 mg/kg) twice daily. Sequential biopsies performed on an affected Doberman at the University of Minnesota indicated that hepatic copper content normalized within three and a half months following D-Penicillamine therapy (2482 μgm/gm dry weight to 194 μgm/gm dry weight). In spite of copper concentrations returning to the normal level, this dog's clinical, biochemical, and histologic findings worsened. In addition, hepatic iron concentrations increased from 2013 μgm/gm dry weight to 7654 μgm/gm dry weight (normal – <891 μgm/gm dry weight).[88] Prednisone was added to the D-Penicillamine therapy at 1 mg/lb/day. Associated with prednisone administration, hepatic iron declined to 1750 μgm/gm dry weight within 30 days. D-Penicillamine was stopped and prednisone dosages tapered down over several months. Attempts have been made on several occasions to withdraw steroids completely, resulting in worsening of both clinical signs and biochemical parameters within several weeks of drug cessation. The dog has remained stable on five mg prednisone every other day for five years. This dog is normal clinically but not biochemically or histologically. No evidence for progression of disease can be detected.

Another recent report also documents improvement in the clinical and biochemical status of affected Dobermans following prednisone treatment alone.[85] Because of the advanced stage of clinical illness when these dogs are first evaluated, neither duration nor quality of life has been extended beyond a few weeks to a few months, except in rare instances.[58, 85, 86] Early biochemical detection and histologic confirmation of asymptomatic Dobermans is likely the only way to improve our therapeutic success. From a genetic standpoint, no information is available regarding the presumed genetic mode of inheritance of this disease.

COPPER-ASSOCIATED HEPATITIS IN WEST HIGHLAND WHITE TERRIERS. West Highland white terriers also have a tendency to accumulate abnormal concentrations of copper in their livers and to develop chronic hepatitis and cirrhosis.[59, 89] Detailed clinical features of this syndrome have not been published. The initial report on 71 dogs stressed the histopathologic features in either asymptomatic dogs or those that died of cirrhosis.[59] Histologic features vary from normal to multifocal, centrilobular hepatitis to postnecrotic cirrhosis (three dogs). Increased hepatic copper has been detected either histochemically or quantitatively in all clinically ill dogs thus far studied. Many clinically normal West Highland white terriers also have evidence for abnormal accumulations of hepatic copper. Quantitative assays for copper indicate that values may reach 3500 μgm/gm dry weight, although the mean value for 38 dogs was 1261 μgm/gm dry weight.[59] It appears that hepatic copper values do not progressively increase with age as is seen in Bedlington terriers. The disease occurs with equal frequency in males and females. Although definitive genetic studies have not been performed, a recent publication indicated that 24 of 44 affected dogs were closely related.[59] A mating between an affected male and a normal beagle yielded three puppies, all with increased hepatic copper concentrations at five and a half months of age (600 μgm/gm, 700 μgm/gm, and 930 μgm/gm) suggesting a dominant mode of inheritance.

D-Penicillamine has been recommended for therapy, although no data are available to support its efficacy nor is there convincing evidence that these dogs even need treatment. The only way to identify asymptomatic, affected animals is through liver biopsy and the use of special stains that identify copper in tissue sections.[77] Since many of these dogs do not accumulate copper to concentrations that appear to cause hepatic necrosis (greater than 2000 μgm/gm dry weight), it would seem reasonable to recommend therapy only in animals with signs of hepatic necrosis on biopsy, or in those that have quantitative hepatic copper values greater than 2000 μgm/gm dry weight, or in those that are clinically ill from their disease. Therapeutic recommendations are similar to those for Bedlington terriers.

The role copper plays in the development and perpetuation of chronic liver disease in dogs deserves a great deal more attention. At least three breeds, Bedlington terriers, West Highland white terriers, and Doberman pinschers, have chronic hepatic disorders that are apparently familial and are associated with accumulating large concentrations of intrahepatic copper. One author notes that potential problems of copper toxicosis exist in Labrador retrievers, cocker spaniels, German shepherds, Pekinese, English bulldogs, keeshonds, schnauzers, Kerry blue terriers, and occasional crossbreeds.[90, 91] One isolated clinical observation has been reported of several Skye terriers, all related, that developed "chronic cirrhosing hepatitis."[92] No cause was identified. This report came from England; the author is unaware of a similar problem being identified in the United States.

LOBULAR DISSECTING HEPATITIS. An unusual form of chronic hepatitis has recently been described in six dogs, termed lobular dissecting hepatitis.[93] The primary clinical sign was ascites caused by portal hypertension. Biochemical abnormalities included hypoalbuminemia (all six), increased BSP retention (greater than 23 per cent in all six), and increased fasting blood ammonia concentrations (1.5 to 6 times normal in all six). Alanine transaminase and alkaline phosphatase concentrations were normal to moderately increased. Lesions were characterized microscopically by a mild, mixed inflammatory reaction. Cells were mostly neutrophils, lymphocytes, and macrophages. Reticulin and fine collagen fibers dissected lobular parenchyma. Limiting plates were disrupted by this process but portal inflammation was inconsistent and seldom marked. Lesions were described as different from CAH in dogs and other chronic hepatitides in humans. No cause was identified.

LEPTOSPIROSIS-ASSOCIATED CHRONIC HEPATITIS. An outbreak of chronic active hepatitis associated with leptospirosis in five American foxhounds has recently been reported.[54] Biochemical data were taken on only one of the dogs, and mild increases in serum AP, ALT, gamma globulin concentrations, and BSP retention were noted. Spirochetes were identified histologically in four of five dogs using special staining techniques (Warthin-Starry). Other lesions identified in the liver were compatible with idiopathic CAH. Efforts should be made to consistently identify this organism in dogs with chronic inflammatory liver disease in order to determine its possible significance as a causative agent in chronic canine liver diseases.

INFECTIOUS CANINE HEPATITIS–ASSOCIATED CHRONIC HEPATITIS. The adenovirus responsible for infectious canine hepatitis has been associated with the production of chronic hepatitis in experimental dogs.[56] Dogs with partial immunity to infectious canine hepatitis were exposed to virulent virus and developed a chronic hepatitis with lesions resembling CAH. Virus was not identifiable in tissue sections except in the early phase of the disease course. Recently, formalinized tissue sections from 53 dogs diagnosed as having chronic hepatitis of unknown cause were stained with an avidin-biotin immunoperoxidase procedure designed to detect the presence of canine adenoviral antigen.[94] Five of the 53 samples were positive for the presence of viral antigens. It was interesting to note that two of the five dogs were female Dobermans. It was suggested that canine adenovirus may play a role in the cause of chronic hepatitis in dogs. This area of investigation deserves further study.

HEPATOPORTAL FIBROSIS. Three four- to six-month-old purebred dogs have been described that had main presenting complaints of anorexia, weight loss, apathy, and ascites.[95] Biochemically, each dog had mild to severe increases in ALT, AST, and GGT concentrations, decreased serum albumin concentrations, and markedly abnormal ammonia tolerance tests. Severe portal hypertension and collateral venous anastomoses were documented using portal angiographic techniques. Hepatic biopsies indicated the presence of widespread portal fibrosis associated with portal vein atrophy or atresia. No cirrhotic changes were observed, although the livers were small, firm, and irregular. No cause was identified and a comparison to human idiopathic congenital hepatic fibrosis was made. Once again, clinical and biochemical findings could be considered compatible with idiopathic CAH. Hepatic biopsy is critical for correct diagnostic and therapeutic recommendations to be made.

Toxic and Drug-Induced Liver Disease. **TOXIC LIVER INJURY.** The liver is subject to damage by a wide variety of chemical products by virtue of its central role in metabolism and detoxification of the body. Hepatotoxins are agents that cause a predictable pattern of hepatic damage in animals, usually associated with a short latent period.[96] Some of the more common toxins are chemicals and heavy metals, e.g., copper, iron, selenium, arsenic, phosphorus, mercury, chloroform, chlordane, dieldrin, tannic acid, tetrachloroethylene, trinitrotoluene, cinchophen, tetrachlorethane, dimethylnitrosamine, carbon tetrachloride, coal tar pitch, and gossypol. Certain plants, especially those associated with fungal growth and aflatoxin production (moldy corn poisoning) and metabolic or nutritional deficiencies (methionine and choline), also produce toxic hepatitis.[97] In cases of severe, acute, diffuse toxic reactions, the animal only survives a few days, since a majority of hepatocytes are injured. In others, complete recovery may be possible. Certain toxins associated with nutritional deficiencies may develop so slowly that no acute signs are seen, and chronic fibrotic liver disease is the first indication that a toxic process is present. Hepatotoxins may cause necrosis of parenchymal cells and its sequelae, biochemical evidence of disease, or morphologic alterations in the liver, for example, lipidosis or fibrosis.

Multiple factors appear to predispose an animal to toxic liver injury. Individual host susceptibility is related to the animal's sex and nutritional status. Females appear to be more susceptible than males to hepatotoxins, while diets high in fat increase the toxic effect of many poisons, especially lipid soluble ones.[98] Diets deficient in carbohydrate and protein also increase the animal's susceptibility to toxic damage. Diets adequate in quantity and quality of protein, specifically the lipotrophic substances methionine and choline, protect against carbon tetrachloride and chloroform injury. Other factors that determine host response to toxic agents are dose, duration of exposure, and type of agent. The duration of exposure is critical with toxins that have a cumulative effect, and exposure may require weeks for effects to be seen. Once hepatocellular necrosis begins, it is resolved with fibrosis, a process that may be self-perpetuating even if the agent is no longer present. Animals with toxic liver injury present with signs of liver disease similar to diseases already discussed. The spectrum is one that runs from subtle signs to fulminant failure. Laboratory evaluations are nonspecific. Generally, hepatotoxins cause inflammation, necrosis, and cholestasis. A definitive diagnosis is rarely established unless exposure to known hepatotoxins can be verified. Many mild, reversible liver diseases of short duration in animals are ascribed to "toxic" episodes. In most cases this is purely speculative, but it sounds good to clients and fits what we expect toxic liver disease to look like. Therapy for toxic hepatitis involves removal of the toxin from the environment, as well as supportive and symptomatic care. If antidotes exist, they should be used, but for most toxic injuries, no antidotes are available.

DRUG-INDUCED LIVER DISEASE. Drug-induced liver injury is merely part of the spectrum of toxic hepatitis. While we do not commonly associate hepatic injury with the use of therapeutic agents, drug-induced liver disease accounts for 5 per cent of all cases of jaundice and 25 per cent of all cases of acute severe hepatic failure in humans.[99, 100] Similar figures for animals are not available, since no organized system for evaluating such reactions has been established in veterinary medicine.

A list of potentially hepatotoxic drugs is included in Table 89–2.

Two major factors appear to be involved in determining why the liver is so often involved in adverse drug reactions. The first relates to the central role of the liver in drug metabolism. Hepatocytes metabolize stable chemical compounds to potent alkylating, arylating, or acetylating compounds that are toxic to the liver. Second, because the liver is anatomically situated between the venous effluent of the intestinal tract and the systemic circulation, noxious compounds gain access to the liver before the rest of the body is exposed.[100] Patients with acute drug-induced liver disease usually have cytotoxic, cholestatic, or mixed types of injury. Cytotoxic reactions induce either necrosis or lipidosis. In general, cytotoxic injuries carry a more grave prognosis than do cholestatic types. Less commonly, chronic drug use is associated with the development of neoplasms of the liver.

Toxic drug reactions are most often classified as either intrinsic and predictable or idiosyncratic and unpredictable.[101, 102] Intrinsic hepatotoxins typically produce reactions in high numbers of exposed individuals, are dose dependent, and can often be reproduced in experimental animals. These drugs produce damage either directly by inducing injury to hepatocyte membranes (chloroform, carbon tetrachloride, tannic acid) or indirectly by entering the cell and disrupting critical metabolic pathways that lead secondarily to structural changes. Drugs in this latter category include methotrexate, ethanol, tetracycline, paromomycin, L-asparaginase, azaserine, azacytidine, azauridine, acetaminophen, urethane, 6-mercaptopurine, mithramycin, contraceptive steroids, C-17 alkylated steroids, lithocholic acid, flavaspidic acid, cholecystographic dyes, rifampicin, and novobiocin.[99]

Idiosyncratic reactions may occur within one to four weeks of initiation of drug therapy or may require many months of continuous therapy. Idiosyncratic reactions are present in low numbers of individuals (less than one per cent), have little if any dose dependency, and cannot be reproduced in experimental animals.[102, 103] This particular group of hepatotoxins is very difficult to identify and substantiate as responsible for liver disease because they require widespread usage before sufficient numbers of toxic events are recognized. Immunologic mechanisms have for many years been considered responsible for idiosyncratic drug reactions. The presence of fever, rashes, and eosinophilia in humans with idiosyncratic injury has been used to support this premise.[100, 102]

TABLE 89–2. DRUGS THAT MAY CAUSE HEPATIC INJURY IN DOGS AND CATS

Acetaminophen	Methoxyflurane
Acetylsalicylic acid	Oxibendazole
Androgenic anabolic steroids	Phenazopyridine
(methyltestosterone, mibolerone)	Phenobarbital
Antineoplastic drugs	Phenylbutazone
Chloroform	Phenytoin
Chlortetracycline	Primidone
Erythromycin	Thiacetarsemide
Glucocorticoids	Tolbutamide
Halothane	Trimethoprim/sulfa
Ketoconazole	
Mebendazole	

Recent information casts doubt on the concept that allergic reactions actively mediate these types of hepatic reactions.[103, 104]

It is currently believed that most, if not all, idiosyncratic reactions occur so rarely because affected individuals have a unique variation (probably genetically determined) in the way drugs or their metabolites are handled. The drugs are biotransformed to toxic metabolites that exist in higher concentrations or are cleared more slowly in genetically predisposed individuals, resulting in hepatic injury. Environmental factors and exposure to other drugs may increase biotransformation of a drug to its toxic metabolites.[105] Both phenobarbital and phenytoin are potent enzyme inducers and have been shown to increase the hepatotoxicity of certain drugs by accelerating degradation of parent compounds to toxic metabolites.[100] The toxicity of acetaminophen and furosemide occurs only when massive dosages are consumed; an increase in toxic metabolites produces hepatic damage.[100] Cats are known to have a relative deficiency of glucuronic acid, which limits their ability to conjugate many drugs including morphine, chloramphenicol, salicylic acid, indomethacin, dapsone, certain sulfas, metabolites of phenacetin, acetaminophen, phenobarbitone, and codeine.[106] This results in signs of drug toxicity in cats at what would be low dosages or safe dosing intervals for other species.

Establishing a diagnosis of drug-induced liver disease is often a process of exclusion.[103] Clinical signs are usually nonspecific. Clinicians should suspect such reactions in all cases of jaundice or unexplained hepatitis.[85] Exposure to a known hepatotoxic drug, development of a characteristic clinical syndrome, typical histologic findings, and rapid recovery following drug withdrawal are commonly utilized as diagnostic criteria.[102] Recurrence of hyperbilirubinemia following a test dose of the suspect drug is highly supportive of drug-induced injury in cholestatic types of damage; however, only 40 to 60 per cent of patients develop jaundice following a single test dose of a suspected drug.[102] Drug testing of agents known to produce cytotoxic reactions is generally not indicated unless the patient is likely to need the drug again, as serious hepatic reactions can develop upon readministration of such compounds.

Histologic features of drug-induced hepatic diseases are often similar between patients, but some variation is possible.[107] Histology provides support that drugs are likely causative agents for a given liver disease, but lesions are rarely pathognomonic.[105, 107] Absolute histologic criteria for idiosyncratic drug-induced hepatotoxicity have not been established. Histologic features of drug-induced acute hepatitis often resemble viral hepatitis lesions in humans.[103] Hepatic lobules and or portal tracts are often infiltrated by inflammatory cells (neutrophils, lymphocytes, macrophages, and eosinophils).[107] Common observed abnormalities include necrosis, vacuolation, and swelling of hepatocytes. Bile duct epithelial cells may undergo similar changes. Zonal necrosis is commonly observed in association with drug reactions in humans.[108] Most often, damage is localized to the terminal hepatic venule (centrilobular), but midzonal and periportal lesions may also be seen. Factors influencing the regional distribution of lesions include lobular gradients for oxygen tension, drug concentration, rates of drug uptake, intracellular concentration of drug metabolizing enzymes, and the cellular concentration of cytoprotective compounds such as glutathione.[108] Inflammatory lesions caused by drugs often result in bridging necrosis between adjacent lobules and occasionally inducing pathologic changes compatible with chronic active hepatitis.[103] Other less commonly observed lesions include granulomatous reactions, vascular injury, and micro- and macrovesicular hepatic lipidosis.[103]

Reports of confirmed or suspected hepatotoxic drug reactions in companion animals are very infrequent. A number of drugs have been implicated as causes for hepatic injury in dogs and cats that the author considers important. This is because the drug is commonly used, and therefore, practitioners are likely to observe toxic reactions, or because reactions may be particularly severe. Drugs in these two categories are: glucocorticoids, anticonvulsants (primidone, phenytoin, phenobarbital), anthelmintics (mebendazole, oxibendazole), organic arsenicals (caparsolate), and inhalant anesthetics (halothane, methoxyflurane). In addition, a few other compounds have been implicated in rare reports of adverse reactions and will be briefly discussed (tolbutamide, phenazopyridine, acetaminophen, sulfonamides, ketoconazole, and methotrexate).

GLUCOCORTICOID HEPATOPATHY. The canine liver is uniquely sensitive to the development of hepatic disease following exogenous administration or endogenous production of excess glucocorticoids. This condition has been termed steroid hepatopathy.[109] Steroid hepatopathy occurs most often following the administration of exogenous glucocorticoids, while hyperadrenocorticism is the most common naturally occurring disease associated with this condition. Clinical signs relate to the effects of glucocorticoids in dogs, the most prominent are polydipsia, polyuria, polyphagia, and hepatomegaly. They will also develop bilateral symmetrical alopecia if administration of steroids is prolonged or if long-standing hyperadrenocorticism exists.

Other dogs represent diagnostic challenges for practitioners because of the profound effect of steroids on serum biochemical profiles. Glucocorticoids cause major increases in the serum concentrations of alkaline phosphatase, gamma glutamyltransferase, and alanine transaminase. The levels of these enzymes become increased rapidly after exogenous administration of glucocorticoids, making interpretation of biochemical profiles a diagnostic challenge. The cause for rise in serum AP and gamma glutamyltransferase appears due to enzyme induction.[110, 111] For serum AP, there is a unique isoenzyme produced by the liver.[111] At least 86 per cent of dogs with hyperadrenocorticism have increased serum AP concentrations and 53 per cent have elevated serum ALT concentrations.[112] Experimental work in dogs indicates that serum AP can become significantly increased within 48 hours following daily administration of 2 mg/lb of prednisone intramuscularly.[113] The magnitude of rise in serum AP is nearly always greater than that of serum ALT. Serum AP concentrations can be increased to 64 times normal. Even after only two weeks of such therapy, serum AP concentrations remained eight times normal six weeks after the drug was stopped.[113] Serum

ALT concentrations increased within 72 hours after the prednisone was administered and were 10 times normal after 12 days, declining to three times normal six weeks after the drug was stopped. Serum gamma glutamyltransferase concentrations were increased by the sixth day, reached a maximal value of 23 times normal, and also remained persistently increased six weeks after the drug was stopped. Even a single injection of a long-acting glucocorticoid has been shown to significantly elevate serum enzymes for 32 weeks.[114] Other laboratory abnormalities that may develop include prolonged BSP retention (generally less than 10 per cent retention at 30 minutes), and increased serum bile acid concentration.[114, 115] The type of glucocorticoid does not appear to make a major difference in whether serum enzymes become elevated; however, dexamethasone is generally not associated with the magnitude of rise noted with prednisone.[114, 115, 116]

In the absence of obvious clinical signs of hyperadrenocorticism or knowledge of iatrogenic steroid administration, the presence of marked hepatomegaly and major increases in hepatic enzymes would warrant hepatic biopsy for diagnostic purposes. Lesions of steroid hepatopathy develop within two days of steroid administration. Grossly these livers are smooth, swollen, pale, and friable. Microscopic findings are typically those of severe vacuolar change or hydropic degeneration of hepatocytes (Figure 89–3).[110, 113, 117, 118] These changes will occur in some dogs that do not develop serum enzyme abnormalities.[117] The cause of this vacuolar change has variably been ascribed to increases in cellular water, fat, or glycogen. Although glycogen was discounted by earlier investigations, recent work using electron microscopy and special fixation techniques, or using alcohol rather than formalin, supports that glycogen is the primary component of the cytoplasmic vacuoles.[110, 118, 119] These lesions are reversible following cessation of steroid administration or treatment of the hyperadrenocorticism but take weeks or months to resolve.

The importance of this disease as a cause of overt hepatic failure is unknown. The author is aware of three dogs that rapidly developed severe hepatic failure after receiving massive steroid dosages for autoimmune disorders. All three had biopsy lesions compatible only with steroid hepatopathy. The dogs improved dramatically when steroid dosages were decreased. These cases appear to be the exception rather than the rule. Other than having signs of polydipsia, polyuria, and hepatomegaly, dogs generally remain healthy. It is important for clinicians to recognize the profound effect that glucocorticoids have on canine biochemical profiles and not to assume some other disease is present when dogs are receiving these drugs. In addition, once dogs are receiving steroids, the clinician should expect serum profiles to become dramatically altered. In dogs with hyperadrenocorticism but without typical skin or biochemical changes, liver biopsy may prove an efficient means of establishing the probable diagnosis.

ANTICONVULSANT-ASSOCIATED HEPATOPATHY. A series of recent reports has emphasized the importance of anticonvulsants (primidone, phenytoin, phenobarbital) as potential causes of serious liver disease.[120–123] It has been recognized for some time that many dogs receiving anticonvulsants develop increases in hepatic biochemical profiles, but these changes were generally thought to be of little clinical significance.[123] Until recently, only one report of serious hepatic failure associated with the use of primidone and phenytoin had been published.[124] A more recent clinical report of 48 dogs receiving either primidone alone, phenytoin alone, or combinations of these two drugs and phenobarbital for six months or more indicates that significant hepatic disease can develop in from 6 to 15 per cent of treated dogs.[120] Clinical signs are those expected with chronic liver disease, anorexia, depression, and weight loss. Two dogs developed ascites. Consistent increases in serum ALT, AP, and decreased albumin will be noted in the most severe cases. Three dogs were euthanatized because of the severity of their illness, and cirrhosis was present at necropsy. A direct relationship was noted between the magnitude of rise in ALT values and the dose of primidone and between the magnitude or rise in serum AP and the dose of phenytoin. The higher the dosage, the greater the rise in enzyme levels. The mean dose of primidone was 15 mg/lb/day (33 mg/kg/day) and that of phenytoin was 10 mg/lb/day (21 mg/kg/day).

Recent experimental work using these two drugs in dogs has helped to clarify the pathogenesis of anticonvulsant-induced hepatic disease.[121, 123] Primidone and phenytoin, when given at normal therapeutic dosages, caused persistent increases in ALT and AP concentrations in some dogs but not in others. Primidone was most consistently associated with increases in ALT concentrations, while phenytoin most often caused a rise in serum AP concentrations. Enzyme increases can be noted within two weeks of initiating drug therapy. Values return to normal within five weeks of stopping either drug. No significant changes occurred in the serum concentrations of bilirubin, gamma glutamyltransferase, fasting bile acids, or BSP retention when the drugs were given for 82 days.[123] Longer studies (dogs treated for 7.5 months) identified significant increases in serum gamma glutamyltransferase concentrations as well as hypoalbuminemia in some dogs.[121] All dogs remained healthy in spite of significant biochemical disease. Lesions present on liver biopsy included hepatocellular hypertrophy, single cell necrosis, and multifocal lipidosis. When eight dogs received combined therapy, three developed severe, fatal hepatic disease within 15 weeks. Those dogs not developing severe illness had serum AP values less than 300 IU/L and ALT values less than 150 IU/L. Three clinical patients have recently been reported that also developed fatal hepatic disease in association with high dose phenytoin therapy (dosages in excess of 14 mg/lb/day or 30 mg/kg/day), in combination with either phenobarbital or primidone.[122] All three dogs were treated for 15 to 23 months. Biochemical findings were indicative of functional liver failure with evidence for hypoalbuminemia, hypocholesterolemia, hyperbilirubinemia, and increased serum bile acid, gamma glutamyltransferase, ALT, and AP concentrations. Histopathologic findings included hepatomegaly, diffuse hepatocellular swelling, cytoplasmic vacuolation, centrilobular atrophy, multiple intracanalicular bile casts, and multifocal small areas of hepatocellular necrosis.[122] In-

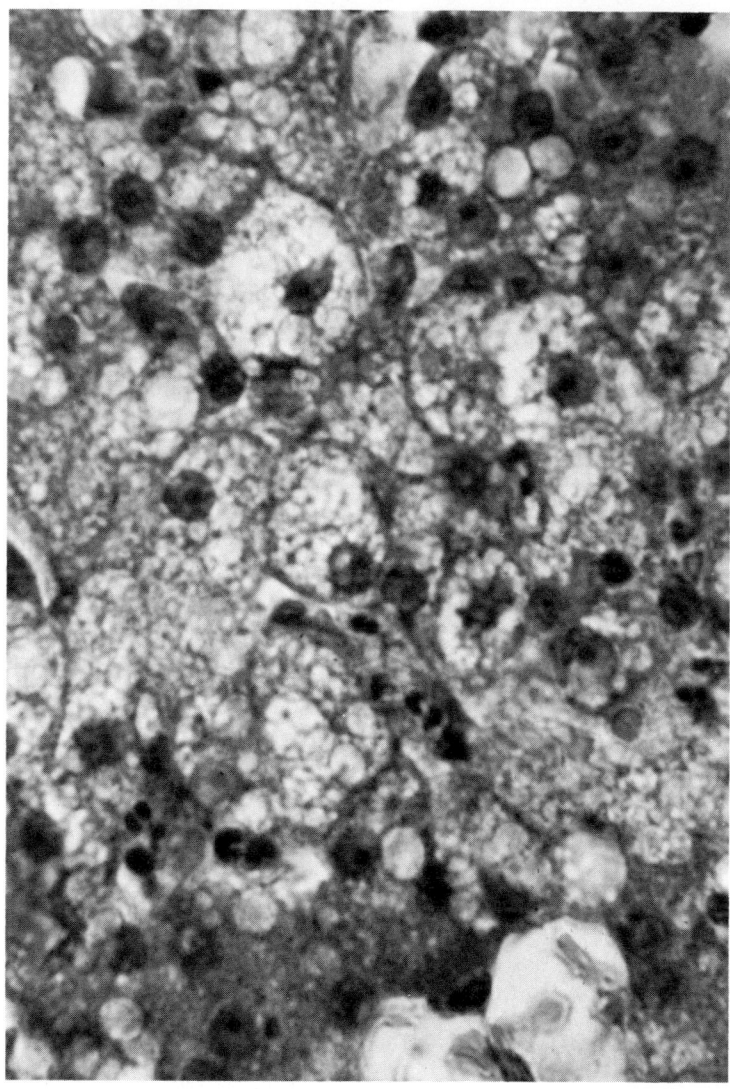

FIGURE 89–3. Diffuse vacuolation of hepatocytes typical for dogs with glucocorticoid-induced hepatopathy (100×).

flammation was remarkably slight considering the severity of failure present. These clinical patients were quite similar to the experimental dogs just discussed.

From the above observations several recommendations can be made regarding the use of anticonvulsants in dogs and the risk of liver failure. High dosages of phenytoin, or phenytoin plus primidone or phenobarbital, appear to carry the greatest risk of inducing serious liver disease and should be avoided, if possible. Since phenytoin is considered by most veterinary neurologists to have minimal efficacy, it is a poor choice anticonvulsant at best. Much data are available to support that primidone has little, if any, advantage over phenobarbital and thus should be avoided as a first choice drug for seizures.[125] Phenobarbital is believed to be the safest and most effective antiepileptic agent available for dogs and should be used as the first choice drug. For patients receiving any of these drugs, periodic monitoring is indicated to determine if hepatic enzymes are increased beyond the ranges indicated as safe.

ANTHELMINTIC-ASSOCIATED HEPATITIS. Two benzimidazole anthelmintics, mebendazole and oxibendazole, have been associated with significant numbers of cases of hepatic disease.[126, 127] Mebendazole is more typically associated with acute fulminant hepatitis with signs of vomiting, depression, anorexia, and jaundice following single or repeated administrations of the drug. At least 45 adverse drug reactions have been reported to the Food and Drug Administration in association with the use of this drug. Mortality has generally been high when reactions occur, since there is no antidote and lesions are very severe in most cases. More recently, oxibendazole was incriminated as a cause of periportal hepatitis in 13 dogs.[127] Dogs received the drug in combination with diethylcarbamazine as a combination heartworm-hookworm preventative. Clinical signs included anorexia, depression, vomiting, and weight loss. Biochemical profiles substantiated the presence of inflammatory and cholestatic liver disease. Hepatic function tests were abnormal in most cases. Histologic findings indicated mild to severe periportal hepatitis and vacuolar hepatopathy. Most dogs improved clinically soon after drug withdrawal; however, two were euthanatized in end-stage liver disease. Drug challenge tests in two dogs suggested that this compound was causing idiosyncratic toxic hepatitis in these dogs.

The organic arsenical, caparsolate, is the only approved drug for use in the treatment of adult heartworms. This drug is a direct, intrinsic hepatotoxin and has a small margin of safety between that dose which is effective as an anthelmintic and that which induces serious hepatic disease. The author has never monitored a dog receiving caparsolate that did not develop significant increases in serum ALT concentrations within 24 to 48 hours following an injection of the drug; and values are often in the high thousands. Unless the animal becomes icteric or shows other signs of being metabolically ill, the author does not routinely stop therapy for the heartworms just because enzymes are increased. There is no specific therapy for arsenical toxicity other than supportive and symptomatic care.

INHALANT ANESTHETIC TOXICITY. Inhalant anesthetics have been associated with fulminant hepatic failure in humans following repeated exposures, particularly to halothane. Similar reports in the veterinary literature are meager and usually circumstantial.[128–130] Halothane was implicated as a cause for acute hepatic necrosis and death in a ten-year-old male dachshund following surgery for prostatic disease.[128] This dog had also received trimethoprim-sulfa and diethylstilbestrol preoperatively and had received banamine and gentamicin in the postoperative period. The dog had been anesthetized two years previously with halothane. Two other case reports of acute hepatic failure following repeated exposures to methoxyflurane have been published.[129, 130] Lesions seen at necropsy were said to be suggestive of those observed in humans with idiosyncratic halothane- or methoxyflurane-associated hepatic failure. These reactions would appear to be quite rare and unpredictable considering the large number of animals anesthetized with these agents every year and the paucity of reports of adverse reactions.

MISCELLANEOUS TOXIC COMPOUNDS. There have been isolated reports of toxicity in clinical cases or experimental work in dogs or cats with a number of other drugs. Ketoconazole, a relatively new imidazole used in the therapy of systemic mycoses, may occasionally be associated with adverse hepatic reactions.[131, 132] These reactions generally occur in dogs receiving doses of over 18 mg/lb/day (40 mg/kg/day). At this dosage, increases in ALT and AP and liver weight occur.[131] At 27 mg/lb/day (60 mg/kg/day) for 20 weeks, marked increases in enzymes take place, and at 36 mg/lb/day (80 mg/kg/day), enzyme increases, severe gastritis, icterus, and death occur by two to four weeks. At the lower dosages, hepatic lesions are reversible following drug withdrawal. Two toxic reactions to trimethoprim-sulfadiazine antibiotics have been reported in dogs.[133, 134] Animals became depressed, anorectic, and jaundiced. Withdrawal of the drug was associated with clinical recovery in both dogs, although biochemical profiles remained abnormal for 18 weeks in one dog. Acetaminophen and phenazopyridine can be hepatotoxic to cats. Acetaminophen induces methemoglobinemia and increased serum ALT concentrations in cats and should not be used as an anti-inflammatory drug.[135] Phenazopyridine, a human urinary tract analgesic, was administered to a cat with feline lower urinary tract disease. The cat developed Heinz body hemolytic anemia and hepatic injuries and died. The hepatic injuries were mild but probably contributed to the cat's death.[136]

Methotrexate was incriminated as a cause for acute severe generalized hepatic necrosis in a nine-year-old dog receiving multiple drugs for chemotherapy of a maxillary neoplasm.[136a] Because this agent has been associated with acute hepatitis in humans, it may have played a role in this dog's disease, but it was unproved.

Therapy of drug-induced hepatic disease is primarily supportive. Major goals involve removing the offending drug, providing supportive care, and waiting for the resolution of a self-limited bout of necrosis.[104] These general principles will be covered later.

Cirrhosis. Cirrhosis should be thought of clinically as end-stage chronic liver disease regardless of its cause. Any process that causes progressive inflammation, necrosis, and fibrosis will ultimately result in cirrhosis, if the process cannot be halted. Potential causes in animals include toxins, drugs (anticonvulsants, oxibendazole), heavy metals (copper, iron), chronic viral infections, chronic bacterial disease (cholangitis/cholangiohepatitis), chronic hypoxia, and probably immune factors. Specific details concerning these causes for chronic hepatitis and potentially cirrhosis have been discussed previously. The incidence of cirrhosis in dogs and cats is unknown. However, at teaching institutions performing many liver biopsies, it varies from 5 per cent (Minnesota) to 15 per cent (Colorado).[137] In a recent World Health Organization publication, hepatic cirrhosis was defined as a diffuse process characterized by fibrosis and a conversion of normal hepatic architecture into structurally abnormal nodules.[138] Most veterinary pathologists characterize cirrhosis as widespread hepatic fibrosis coupled with varying degrees of necrosis and attempts at parenchymal cell regeneration.[98, 139] This process results in a loss of normal hepatic lobular architecture and in development of multiple fine to coarse regenerative nodules separated by connective tissue septa. The pathologic appearance of an end-stage liver gives little clue to the initiating factors responsible for its failure. These livers may be characterized grossly as micronodular or macronodular in appearance, but this serves little purpose, as these findings do not correlate clinically with any specific causes. Generally, macronodular forms predominate in small animals. Liver size is generally decreased in dogs with cirrhosis, but interestingly, in most cats with cirrhosis, the liver is normal to enlarged. In cats, the most often recognized form of cirrhosis is biliary cirrhosis and results from chronic cholangitis/cholangiohepatitis as discussed previously. Cirrhosis tends to be an active, chronic, and progressive disease that ultimately leads to hepatic failure and death in nearly all cases.

The pathogenesis of cirrhosis has recently been reviewed.[137] It is a complex process that involves interactions among dying hepatocytes, the liver's attempt to repair the lesion (inflammation and scarring), and regeneration of new hepatocytes (that develop into nodules); this compromises blood supply, which leads to further necrosis, and so on. Dead and dying hepatocytes stimulate an inflammatory reaction in the liver. It may be neutrophilic early in the disease but progresses to a more mononuclear reaction with chronicity. In the healing process following inflammation, fibrous tissue is deposited in the liver. The production of collagen by both hepatocytes and fibroblasts may be accelerated to ten times normal, while collagenase activity is decreased.[140] This leads to a net gain in fibrous connective tissue within the liver. Regeneration of hepatic tissue is a response to necrosis of hepatocytes and a loss of functional capacity of the liver, and it is the body's attempt to return functional capacity back to normal. Unfortunately, regenerative nodules often are not functionally normal. As they enlarge, they compress adjacent stroma and decrease blood flow to surrounding parenchyma. Compression leads to regional hypoxia, hypoxia causes more necrosis, more inflammation, more fibrosis, more regeneration, and so forth.

Abnormal vascularity of cirrhotic livers is typical.[141] The portal venous supply of regenerative nodules gets pushed to the periphery of the nodule. This leads to increased resistance to portal flow, which leads to portal hypertension. Portal veins may communicate directly with central veins, bypassing sinusoidal flow entirely. Arteriovenous shunts also develop between the hepatic artery and hepatic veins, which further decreases hepatic oxygenation and exacerbates portal hypertension. When hepatic arterial and portal blood bypass hepatic parenchyma, toxins and metabolic wastes are allowed to enter the systemic circulation directly without being processed by the liver. These products are responsible for many of the signs of hepatic encephalopathy. The vomiting and diarrhea seen in cirrhotic animals are associated with gastritis and gastric ulceration in some cases. Animals with cirrhosis have decreased ability to maintain the normal gastric mucosal barrier. In one study of 22 dogs with intestinal ulcers, 16 had severe liver pathology and 4 had cirrhosis.[142] Ulcers are predisposed to by several mechanisms in cirrhosis. Gastric mucosa has decreased capabilities for repair owing to a negative nitrogen balance in cirrhosis. Hypoalbuminemia, which accompanies cirrhosis, has traditionally been associated with decreased production by the liver; however, recent evidence suggests it may be more associated with malnutrition than decreased synthesis in humans.[143] Gastric blood flow is also decreased in cirrhosis in association with portal hypertension. Increased hydrochloric acid secretion may play a role in ulcerogenesis of hepatic failure as well. Experimental dogs with portacaval anastomoses have increased gastric acid secretion, and circulating bile acids also have this effect.[144] Decreased hepatic metabolism of histidine absorbed from the intestines causes increased histamine secretion. Histamine in turn stimulates gastric parietal cells to secrete hydrochloric acid.[145]

The clinical manifestations of cirrhosis are typically associated with impaired liver function, jaundice, and ascites. There is little unique to the clinical presentation of dogs or cats with cirrhosis, except their signs are more typical of chronic than acute hepatic failure. The onset of signs is usually gradual, taking weeks to months for owners to appreciate the presence of serious disease. Evidence for marked weight loss and ascites is often noted. Signs of central nervous system derangements other than depression, anorexia, lethargy, polydipsia, and polyuria are very uncommon. In rare instances, animals will exhibit classic signs of hepatic encephalopathy, such as dementia, circling, pacing, amaurotic blindness, and ultimately coma.

Laboratory evaluations of animals with cirrhosis tend to be fairly typical, but great individual variation is possible. Biochemical evidence of inflammation is nearly always present but occasionally may be mild or even absent. Serum ALT concentrations are mildly to moderately increased (mean = 425 IU/L, 9 times normal).[137] Three out of 20 confirmed cirrhotic dogs had normal ALT concentrations in a recent study.[137] Normal enzymes occur in very advanced disease at which point little inflammatory reaction still exists and a small quantity of functioning hepatocytes is present. Alkaline phosphatase concentrations are also increased (mean = 375 IU/L, four times normal).[137] Five per cent of cirrhotic dogs (1/20) had normal values for SAP in this same study. Hyperbilirubinemia is inconsistent and depends on the location of lesions within the liver. Periportal lesions are associated with more severe hyperbilirubinemia than centrilobular lesions. The mean serum bilirubin concentration in 20 cirrhotic dogs was 3.6 mg/dl (6 times normal); however, 35 per cent were in the normal range. Biochemical assessments of liver function (other than bilirubin) often are dramatically and disproportionately elevated in cirrhosis when compared to enzyme tests. Serum albumin concentrations are frequently depressed, often to less than 2.0 gm/dl. Hypoalbuminemia reflects altered synthesis, malnutrition, and dilution by an expanded plasma volume. Retention of BSP is typically in the 10 to 30 per cent range, correlating with the degree of altered hepatic perfusion. Ammonia tolerance test results are variable in cirrhotic animals, but too few have been evaluated to allow for meaningful conclusions. The author has generally found them to be normal in fasting animals without signs of encephalopathy and unpredictable following ammonia challenge. Serum bile acids have been evaluated in a limited number of cirrhotic dogs and found to be consistently increased.[146] Mean values were 148 μmol/L (normal 1.8 μmol/L). Coagulation parameters, prothrombin time, partial thromboplastin time, and platelets may become abnormal in end stage liver disease. This is typically a late clinical finding and generally associated with a very poor prognosis. The blood urea nitrogen concentration may become subnormal in cirrhosis. A decreased synthesis of urea from ammonia is the usual cause, and thus, blood urea nitrogen concentrations become poor estimates of glomerular function in dogs or cats with cirrhosis. Abdominal radiographs and ultrasound can be helpful in the assessment of cirrhotic patients. Liver size is generally reduced in cirrhotic dogs but not in cats. Microhepatica generally reflects a loss of hepatocytes and their replacement by fibrous tissue. Hepatic ultrasonography is helpful in determining the size of the liver in dogs with ascites, in which abdominal contrast is typically poor. These livers are small and have a generalized mottled increase in echogenicity.

A definitive diagnosis of hepatic cirrhosis requires pathologic confirmation since clinical and laboratory parameters are nonspecific. Hepatic biopsy in cirrhosis may miss the major lesion, particularly if a hepatic regenerative nodule is sampled. Specimen size may also be a problem, especially if needle biopsies are used. The diagnosis of cirrhosis is often made not just on the pathologic findings but often also includes the physical characteristics of the liver, if it is visualized at the time of biopsy.[147] This is only possible if biopsies are obtained via laparoscopy or laparotomy. In one study of the accuracy of percutaneous needle biopsies in human liver diseases, cirrhosis was missed 20 per cent of the time if only one biopsy was obtained. If three biopsy cores were obtained, diagnostic accuracy improved to 100 per cent.[148]

Therapy for cirrhosis generally involves supportive and symptomatic care, since lack of an identifiable cause and the advanced stage of this disease (regardless of the cause) often preclude specific therapy from being beneficial. These approaches to treatment will be discussed later.

Noninflammatory Hepatic Diseases

Noninflammatory hepatic diseases, although seen less frequently than inflammatory ones, form an important group of clinical disorders. They often differ dramatically from inflammatory hepatic diseases in terms of diagnosis, prognosis, and therapy. Disorders to be considered include: (1) congenital portal vascular anomalies; (2) intrahepatic arteriovenous fistulas; (3) lipidosis; (4) congenital hepatic cysts; (5) glycogen storage disease; (6) urea cycle enzyme deficiencies; and (7) amyloidosis.

PORTAL VASCULAR ANOMALIES

Portal systemic shunts (PSS) are a relatively common phenomenon in companion animals and may be either congenital or acquired. Shunts develop as collaterals between the hepatic portal vein and major systemic veins. Blood from the intestinal tract is diverted around hepatic parenchyma and enters the systemic circulation without undergoing hepatic metabolism. Such shunts may involve single large communicating vessels or multiple smaller veins. Multiple shunting vessels are nearly always acquired and develop secondary to diseases that induce portal hypertension (cirrhosis, chronic hepatitis, hepatic neoplasia, arteriovenous fistulas, congestive heart failure, and hepatoportal fibrosis). Acquired shunts accounted for 20 per cent of 120 cases recently reviewed.[149] Normal portal vein pressures are between 6 and 12 mmHg.[149] Processes that cause sustained portal pressures of 12 to 15 mmHg or more lead to development of multiple intra-abdominal portal shunts (Figure 89–4).[149] Breeds commonly identified with these types of acquired shunts are Doberman pinschers and German shepherds, and they usually have ascites as well.[149] Normal values for portal vein pressure are frequently listed in either mmHg or cm water. To convert mmHg to cm water, multiply the value given in mmHg by 1.36.[150]

The most commonly identified shunts are single large intrahepatic or extrahepatic shunts.[149, 151–168] They are likely to be congenital rather than acquired, since they are usually diagnosed in dogs and cats under one year of age. One author has suggested that because of significant geographic differences in the incidence of congenital shunts, some in utero event, such as exposure to an inciting agent, may cause malformation of fetal portal vascular development.[149] To date, five major types of shunt have been recognized: (1) patent ductus venosus, (2) portal vein atresia with development of multiple collateral portal systemic communications (rare), (3) drainage of the portal vein into the caudal vena cava (portal-caval shunt), (4) drainage of the portal vein into the azygous vein (portal-azygous shunt), and (5) drainage of the portal vein and caudal vena cava into the azygous vein with discontinuation of the prerenal segment of the caudal vena cava (Figure 89–5). No breed or sex predisposition has been identified for animals with PSS. There is, however, a significant difference in the types of shunts generally seen in large dogs versus small dogs or cats.[149, 165] Large breeds of dogs (Doberman pinschers, golden retrievers, Labrador retrievers, Irish setters, Samoyeds, Irish wolfhounds) typically have single, large intrahepatic shunts. The shunt is most often a remnant of the fetal ductus venosus that remains patent; however, other large intrahepatic venous communications may also develop. Twenty-eight per cent of 120 PSS cases had this type of anomaly.[149] The ductus venosus is an embryonic venous channel originating from the umbilical vein which traverses the liver and drains into the left hepatic vein and then into the caudal vena cava.[154] Small breeds of dogs (miniature schnauzers, miniature poodles, Yorkshire terriers, dachshunds) and cats generally have single large extrahepatic shunts between the portal vein and post cava (45 per cent) or between the portal vein and azygous vein (5 per cent).[149] Complete absence of portal vein entry into the liver is very rare (1.5 per cent).[149]

Clinical signs seen with PSS are highly variable, but all result from hepatic encephalopathy or progressive functional impairment of the liver. This is one of the few hepatic diseases in small animals that consistently produces signs of hepatic encephalopathy. Diversion of portal blood around the liver leads to progressive hepatic atrophy. The severity of clinical signs depends on the volume of blood shunted and the location of the shunting vessels. Blood draining the gastric, pancreatic, duodenal, and splenic areas is most critical for normal hepatic growth. Insulin plays a particularly important hepatotropic role, although other nonpancreatic factors are also necessary.[169, 170] Thus, clinical signs and hepatic atrophy are most severe in animals with gastroduodenal-pancreatic venous shunting. In many cases the clinical signs have an episodic nature; they are present for a few hours to a day or two, and then the animal returns to "normal." An association between onset of clinical signs following ingestion of meals, particularly high protein meals, is helpful diagnostically. This observation is inconsistent, however, as it is found in approximately 25 per cent of cases.[149]

The great majority of animals with PSS are diagnosed under one year of age, but some dogs will be as old as eight years when first identified. Many animals can be characterized as "chronic poor doers." They are stunted, thin, depressed, and in poor general condition, and have trouble gaining weight. Nearly all dogs have some type of central nervous system sign that may be the best clue for the clinician to determine what might be going on. Particularly bizarre behavioral signs or dementia char-

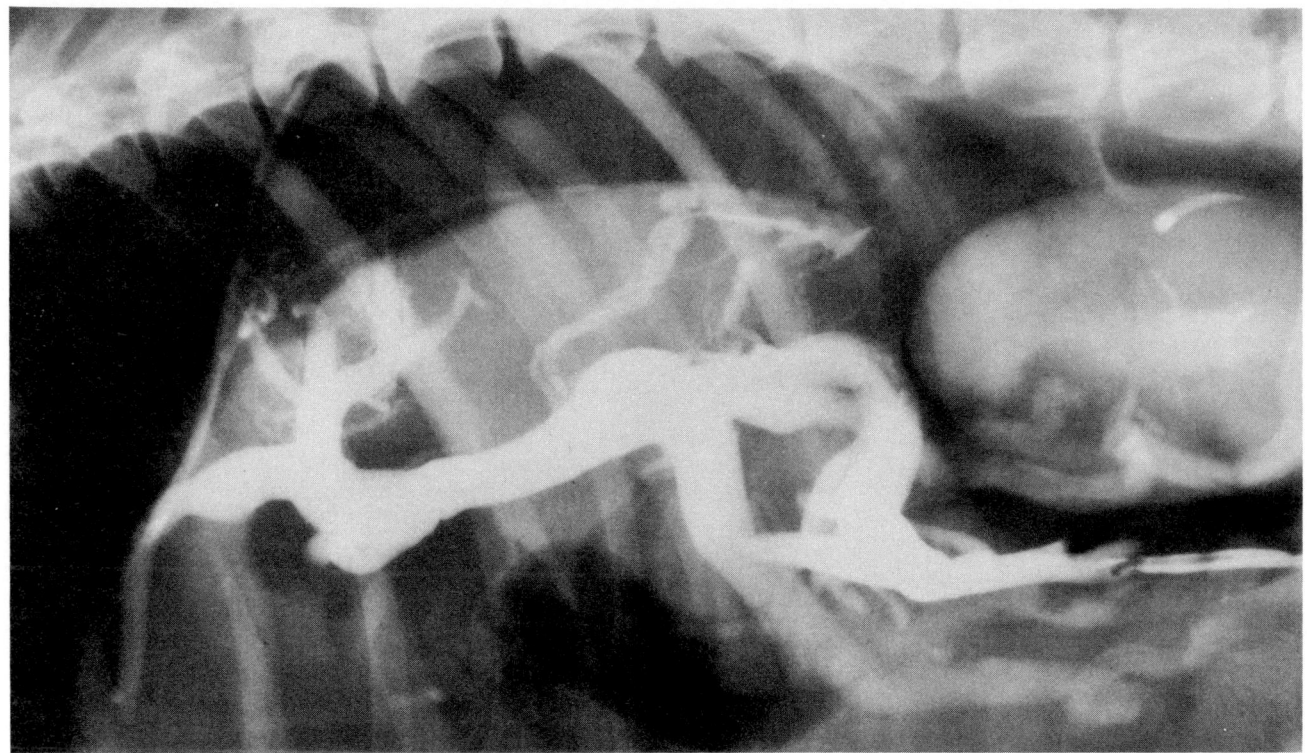

FIGURE 89–4. Operative splenoportogram from a five-year-old female Doberman pinscher with acquired portal systemic shunts caused by portal hypertension. Dilated, tortuous portal veins communicating with the abdominal post cava are evident.

acterized by hysteria, unpredictable bouts of aggression, staggering, pacing, circling, head pressing, amaurotic (cortical) blindness, intermittent deafness, tremors, seizures, and coma may all be seen. Occasional animals will present with signs of upper motor neuron disease and ataxia. Gastrointestinal signs are present in 75 per cent of the animals with PSS.[149] These signs are usually mild and intermittent as well. They include anorexia, vomiting, hypersalivation (which may be prominent), diarrhea, pica, and sometimes polyphagia. Several dogs in our clinic consistently ingested all their cage paper during periods of encephalopathy. We considered this

almost pathognomonic for PSS. Signs of less localizing value include polydipsia and polyuria, rare ascites, and anesthetic or tranquilizer intolerance. Eighteen of 20 dogs that had anesthetic experiences prior to being diagnosed as having a shunt had histories of prolonged anesthetic recovery.[149] Two recent reports stressed the importance of recurrent urinary calculi as another possible presenting complaint for dogs with PSS.[164, 165]

Physical examination findings in these animals are usually nonspecific. The most severely affected animals are stunted and cachectic and may have mild ascites (rare), but these signs are of little localizing value. If a

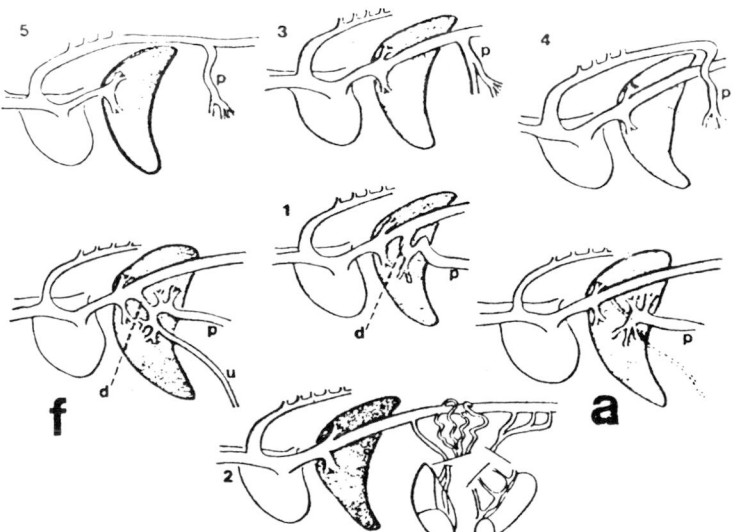

FIGURE 89–5. Illustrations of the five types of congenital portal vein anomalies found in dogs. In addition, the normal fetal (f) and adult (a) portal system is illustrated. In the fetus, the umbilical vein (u) perfuses the liver, but most of its volume is diverted through the ductus venosus (d) to the fetal heart. Soon after birth, the umbilical vein and ductus venosus atrophy. Portal vein blood (p) then perfuses hepatic sinusoids completely, being collected by the hepatic veins. The abnormal portal systemic shunts are (1) Patent ductus venosus (d) with or without a hypoplastic portal system; (2) Portal vein atresia, associated with the development of multiple portopostcaval anastomoses; (3) Major solitary portopostcaval anastomosis; (4) Isolated, major portal azygous shunt; (5) Portal azygous shunt with discontinuation of the prerenal segment of the caudal vena cava. (Reprinted with permission from Suter, PT; Portal vein anomalies in the dog: Their angiographic diagnosis. J Am Vet Radiol Soc 16:84, 1975.)

patient exhibits signs of dementia as described above, however, then a diagnosis of PSS becomes a real probability.

The definitive diagnosis of portal vascular anomalies requires a combination of urinalysis and hematologic, biochemical, and radiographic evaluations. Hematologic abnormalities are nonspecific, but they may lead you to consider liver disease as a cause for an animal's vague clinical signs. Mild nonregenerative anemia is present in one-third of patients. In addition, microcytosis and decreased mean corpuscular volume are present in 72 per cent of shunt cases without either anisocytosis, poikilocytosis, or hypochromia evident on blood smears.[147, 149, 171] The mean corpuscular hemoglobin concentration (MCHC) has also been determined to be normal in spite of the microcytosis.[171] The author has observed marked increases in target cells in dogs with PSS (Figure 89–6). This finding is uncommon in other forms of hepatic disease. A mild, mature neutrophilia is present in one-third of shunt patients. Hypoproteinemia is commonly found if an estimate of total plasma proteins is made with a refractometer (65 per cent of cases).

Biochemical data are most likely to indicate that significant hepatic disease is present in suspected patients. However, hepatic enzymes are not the best screening tests for PSS cases. Serum ALT and AST concentrations are only increased in approximately 50 per cent of affected animals, and increases are generally minimal.[149] Serum AP concentrations may be increased in two-thirds of cases but most likely reflect an increase in circulating bone isoenzyme in young, growing animals, and again, the rise is mild. This should not be too surprising, since the major pathologic change in these livers is atrophy, and there is minimal inflammation in most cases. Total serum bilirubin concentrations remain normal in congenital PSS cases because no impingement on bile flow occurs, and the liver requires very little functional reserve to conjugate the normal daily turnover of free bilirubin.

Other hepatic function tests are nearly always abnormal, however. Diagnostically useful evaluations include serum concentrations of albumin, fasting and postprandial bile acids, uric acid, and cholesterol, fasting and postchallenge blood ammonia concentrations, as well as prolonged retention of BSP.[149, 171, 172] Mild hypokalemia has been documented in 44 per cent of cases.[149] Serum albumin concentrations are subnormal in 41 per cent of

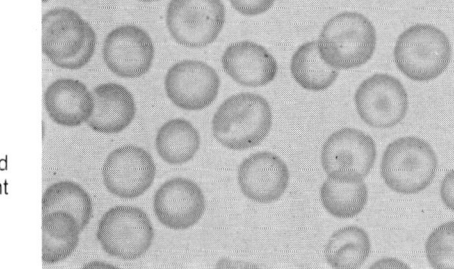

FIGURE 89–6. Multiple target cells (arrows) as seen in a blood smear from a dog with a congenital portal systemic shunt (450×).

PSS patients.[149] This reflects the effects of decreased production and malnutrition. Serum bile acids increase dramatically in PSS patients.[172] In fact, all cases evaluated to date have had significantly increased fasting and/or postprandial serum bile acids. Mean reported fasting serum bile acid concentrations in dogs are 78.9 μmol/L (normal = < 3.4 μmol/L), while comparable values in cats with PSS are 24.4 μmol/L (normal = < 3 μmol/L).[172, 172] Mean two hour postprandial values for dogs are 177 μmol/L and for cats are 120.6 μmol/L (normal = < 12.6 for dogs and < 10 for cats). Serum uric acid concentrations have been increased in a significant number of patients evaluated by the author. Values are usually between 1.2 and 4.0 mg/dl. Increases are presumed due to an inability of the failing liver to convert uric acid to allantoin. Increased serum uric acid concentrations lead to increased urinary excretion of uric acid and likely cause the increased incidence of uric acid or ammonium urate urinary tract calculi seen in dogs and cats with PSS. Serum cholesterol concentrations are below normal in 57 per cent of PSS animals.[149] Since the liver is responsible for endogenous production of cholesterol, decreased concentrations reflect impaired synthesis. Blood urea nitrogen concentrations are subnormal in 70 per cent of cases. This most likely reflects decreased hepatic synthesis from urea, decreased intake, and loss associated with polydipsia and polyuria. Fasting blood ammonia concentrations are abnormal in 93 per cent of cases, while 100 percent of cases have abnormal ammonia tolerance tests. Ammonia challenge tests should be reserved for animals showing no clinical signs of encephalopathy. Adding an ammonia load to an already encephalopathic animal is unnecessary and may be harmful to the patient. Blood ammonia is a very labile substance and unless tests can be run "in house," the likelihood of reliable data being obtained is questionable. A recent study indicated that blood ammonia concentrations run on freshly frozen samples had no correlation to values run immediately after collection.[174] Ammonia concentrations can increase due to storage and decrease following vaporization. Although the sensitivity of blood ammonia as a diagnostic test is equal to that of serum bile acid assays, the ease of collection and stability of bile acids will make them the preferred test.

Prolonged retention of BSP is found in nearly all cases of PSS (93 per cent).[149] However, values may occasionally be normal, (less than 5 per cent) or only marginally increased (e.g., 5 to 10 per cent retention), making interpretation of their significance difficult. Fasting blood glucose concentrations may be below normal in as many as 25 per cent of cases.[159] Although hypoglycemia may be responsible for some of the neurologic signs in this disease, many animals with hypoglycemia were asymptomatic at the time the blood was obtained. The above biochemical abnormalities reflect the severity of portal shunting and the degree of hepatic functional insufficiency in an individual patient. They are not unique to PSS cases and would be expected to occur in any advanced, generalized liver disease in which significant portal systemic shunting exists.

The urinalysis of dogs or cats with PSS may have findings that aid in establishing the diagnosis. Ammonium urate crystalluria is found in roughly half the cases (Figure 89–7).[149, 165, 171] These crystals are infrequently observed in other types of hepatic disease but are common in Dalmatians in which enzyme defects prevent conversion of uric acid to allantoin. Urine specific gravities are low in 44 per cent of cases.[149] Urinary calculi are present in the kidney, bladder, and urethra of many cases.[149, 164, 165] Calculi are usually composed of ammonium urate and/or ammonium magnesium phosphate.[175] Several animals with PSS and urinary tract calculi have been evaluated at the author's hospital to determine their 24-hour urinary excretion of ammonia and uric acid. In all cases studied so far, dramatically increased urinary excretion of both these substances has been measured. Any dog other than a Dalmatian in which a uric acid calculus is identified should be evaluated as a possible PSS case. A recent study confirmed that the hyposthenuria seen in many animals with PSS may be due to primary polydipsia.[161] Three animals with consistent urine specific gravities below 1.008 and with mild serum hypo-osmolality concentrated their urine to greater than 1.035 following water deprivation (1.037, 1.038, and 1.040). Since the dogs failed to concentrate urine maximally, some impairment in renal concentrating ability was present. An additional two animals also failed to respond to water deprivation, implying that severe medullary solute washout had occurred.

Radiography is one of the most important diagnostic procedures for establishing a diagnosis of PSS in dogs and cats and is the only method of confirming the diagnosis short of major surgery. Portal angiographic procedures help determine whether medical or surgical therapy should be considered. Survey abdominal radiographs are valuable initial screening tests since most affected animals have significant reductions in liver size. This will be particularly evident on lateral projections. Renomegaly has also been detected in a number of animals.[165] Because abdominal contrast is generally poor in these thin animals, administering a small quantity of positive or negative contrast material into the stomach will allow a better appreciation of hepatic size. In addition to reductions in liver size, radiopaque calculi may be visualized in the kidneys, bladder, or urethra of many animals. These are usually ammonium urate calculi, and their radiographic density is much less than struvite calculi, so they are easily overlooked. Small liver size coupled with bizarre neurologic signs in a young dog or cat is strong supportive evidence that a shunt exists, and that further diagnostic tests are indicated.

Several contrast radiographic procedures have been evaluated for use in dogs to delineate the portal vein and to determine if it is normal or abnormal. Four techniques provide useful information: cranial mesenteric arteriography, transabdominal splenoportography, operative mesenteric portography, and celiac arteriography.[176] Cranial mesenteric arteriography or splenoportography provides the most diagnostic information.[159] The author has used percutaneous and operative splenoportography in most cases and believes this technique is easily performed in clinical practice. It does not require special injection equipment or rapid speed cassette changers for diagnostic films to be obtained. Ap-

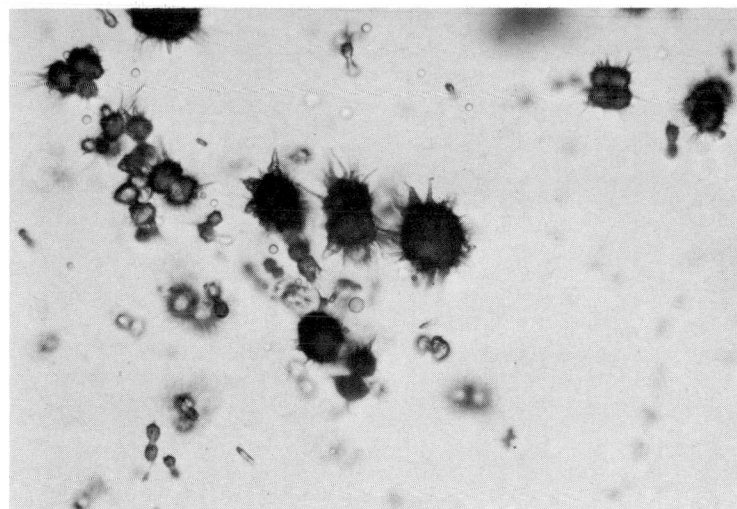

FIGURE 89–7. Ammonium urate (biurate) crystals from the urine sediment of a dog with a portal vascular anomaly (450×).

proximately 0.5 ml/lb body weight of intravenous contrast agent (iothalamate, Conray-400) is administered rapidly, either directly into the splenic pulp or into a cannulated splenic vein. Films should be exposed as soon as the injection is completed. In general, lateral radiographs provide the best diagnostic films; however, ventrodorsal radiographs following a second injection of contrast material may add useful information. A needle biopsy of the liver may also be obtained at this time to assess the severity of hepatic atrophy. Angiography should provide evidence for one of the acquired shunts illustrated in Figure 89–5. We generally do not attempt corrective surgery the same day as the angiography is performed even when an operable PSS is diagnosed (Figure 89–8). These animals are quite fragile metabolically, and we usually close the abdomen and treat the animal medically for a few days prior to attempting shunt ligation. It is important to appreciate that in most cases no evidence for a normal appearing portal vein entering and perfusing the liver will be identified. This is particularly true with single large extrahepatic shunts. There is nearly always a hypoplastic portal vein. No contrast material is visualized in the hypoplastic vessels because the pressure to drive blood through this rudimentary vessel is much greater than that necessary to perfuse the shunt. Portal blood will take the route of least resistance. Only after surgical attenuation or ligation of the shunt will these vessels become evident.

Two other radiographic techniques may be used to diagnose PSS, hepatic ultrasonography, and quantitative hepatic scintigraphy.[177–180] Ultrasonographic findings include reduced liver size, little or no evidence for hepatic veins or intrahepatic branches of the portal vein, and evidence for large intrahepatic vascular communications from the portal vein area to the caudal vena cava.[178] Only *intra*hepatic shunts are consistently diagnosed using this technique. Additional success can be had by applying positive pressure ventilation during the procedure. This displaces the liver caudally and distends the portal vascular system, allowing for better ultrasonographic visualization of the liver. Extrahepatic shunts are not usually identifiable using ultrasonography. Hepatic quantitative scintigraphy is a research tool that allows for noninvasive measures of relative arterial and

venous portal blood flow to the liver using the radioisotope technetium 99m sulfur colloid. Dogs with shunts have decreased hepatic uptake and increased splenic and pulmonary uptake of the radiocolloid.

Histologic findings in animals with PSS are those associated with diffuse hepatic atrophy, but in mild cases the changes are very subtle.[149, 165, 166] There are prominent lobular collapse, indistinct or absent portal veins in the portal triad area, close proximity of adjacent portal triads, compressed hepatic cords, and mild centrilobular or diffuse fatty infiltration. Peripheral liver cells may be hypertrophied, while centrilobular hepatocytes are atrophied.

An organized approach to the diagnosis of PSS should involve the following sequence of events. If the history, clinical signs, and biochemical changes are strongly supportive of hepatic disease in young dogs and cats, PSS should be ruled out. If radiographs indicate the liver is small and the kidneys are enlarged or that slightly radiopaque urinary calculi are present, portal angiography should be performed. Portal angiography will assist in determining whether the animal is a good surgical candidate.

Therapy for congenital shunts may be surgical and/or medical. Medical therapy is used primarily to improve the health status of the animal prior to attempting surgical correction or to help prolong the functional life of PSS animals if owners will not consider surgery. Hepatic functional failure tends to progress in most animals that are diagnosed prior to one year of age, even though medical therapy keeps them relatively asymptomatic. They eventually become refractory to medical management and succumb to their disease.[181] Thus, surgical attenuation or ligation of the shunting vessel will most likely lead to complete reversal of signs and long duration quality survival. The objective of surgery is to redirect shunting blood back into the liver, providing hepatic parenchyma with hepatotropic factors necessary for its normal growth and metabolism. Numerous reports of surgical correction of portal venous anomalies have been published.[154, 182–184] As indicated previously, large breeds of dogs generally have large intrahepatic shunts, and smaller breeds of dogs usually have single, large extrahepatic shunts. The goal of

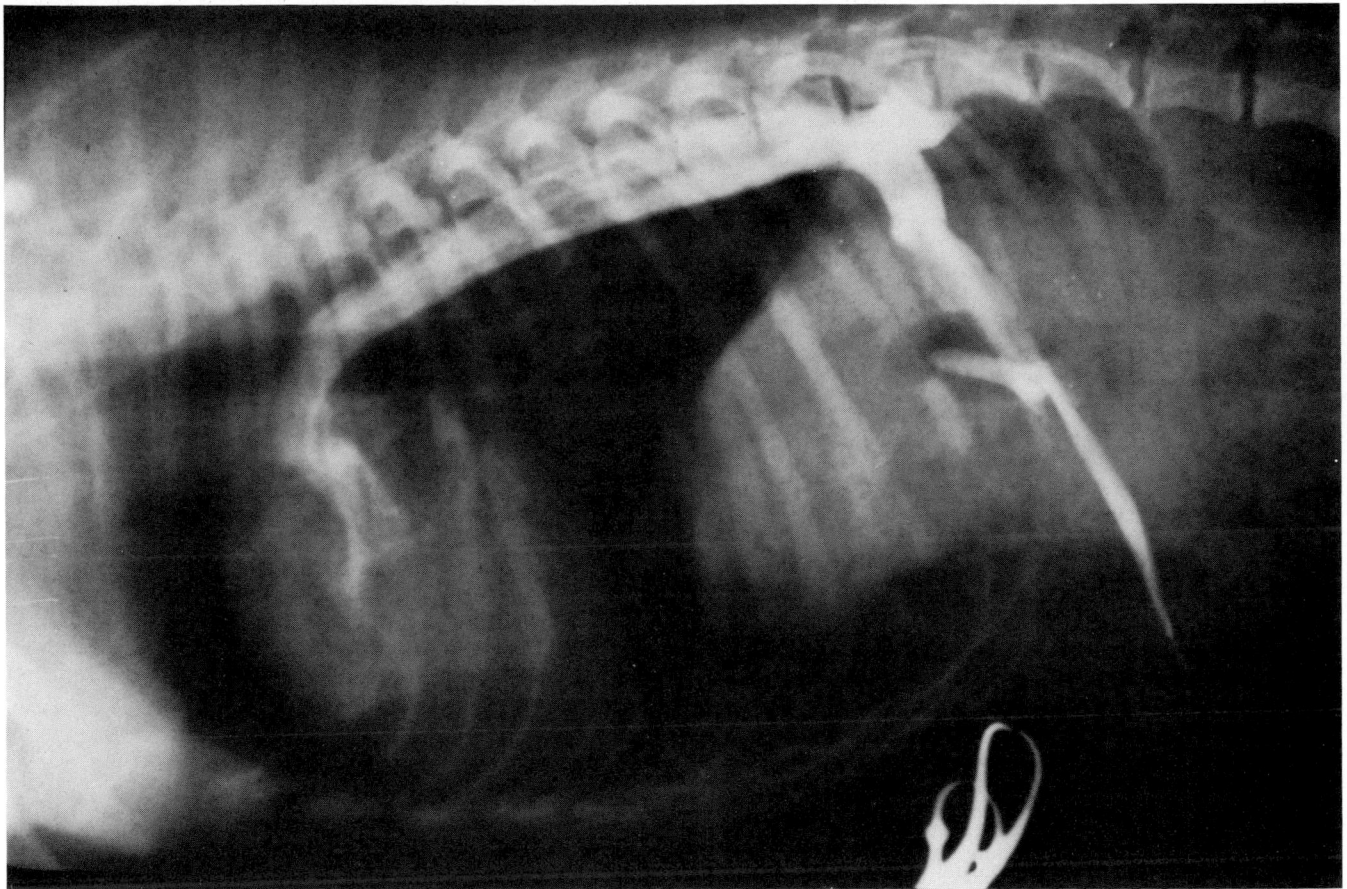

FIGURE 89–8. Operative splenoportogram from a two-year-old female miniature schnauzer with a single large extrahepatic portal systemic shunt (portal-azygous).

surgery is to isolate the shunting vessel and to attenuate or ligate the vessel. Reducing or eliminating shunt flow causes significant volumes of portal blood to be redirected so that it perfuses the liver through the hypoplastic intrahepatic portal system.

Several surgical approaches are available to attempt to correct intrahepatic shunts.[149, 154] These techniques are much more difficult than those utilized for extrahepatic single shunts and are well described in the literature.[149, 154] In the author's practice, surgical success with intrahepatic shunts has been much less rewarding than for extrahepatic ones. Correction of portocaval and portal-azygous shunts is less technically demanding and has a higher rate of success and fewer postoperative complications. Once the location of the shunt has been identified through angiography, the patient should be scheduled for an exploratory laparotomy. The extrahepatic shunt is isolated and temporarily occluded while portal vein pressure is simultaneously measured. A heparinized catheter is placed in the remnant portal vein or an intestinal branch of the portal drainage to measure portal pressure. The catheter is hooked up to a heparinized central venous pressure manometer with the base of the manometer at the level of the right atrium (usually located in the right inguinal region). Portal pressures should not exceed 20 to 23 cm of water following shunt ligation. If this occurs, the ligature must be loosened until portal pressures approach 20 cm of water. Pressures above this are associated with venous stagnation of the

bowel, shock, and death. It has also been suggested that postligation portal vein pressure should not be greater than 10 cm of water over preligation values, even if this value is less than 24 cm of water (18 mmHg).[185] Other parameters that should be monitored include heart rate, central venous pressure, systemic blood pressure, and color of the viscera, especially of the pancreas. Observation of intestinal color as an indication of congestion is a poor substitute for direct portal pressure measurements. Deaths will occur 12 to 24 hours later if postligation splanchnic pressures are too high.

Many of the cases operated on at the University of Minnesota had major drops in blood pressure when shunt manipulations began. Careful monitoring of blood pressure and instituting appropriate measures to correct hypotension (fluids, blood or plasma, alpha-adrenergic agents) must be utilized rapidly for consistent surgical success. If portal hypertension does not develop following temporary shunt occlusion, the shunt may be permanently ligated. If pressures are too high, the ligature is slowly loosened until portal pressures drop to 20 cm of water or less and the ligature is tied at that point. Incomplete shunt occlusion allows a safety valve to reduce the chance for serious postoperative complications associated with acute portal hypertension. If shock is avoided, serious postoperative complications are uncommon. One dog operated on at the author's hospital developed complete thrombosis of its shunt vessel 24 hours postoperatively. The thrombus produced total occlusion of the dog's pancreatic drainage and caused hemorrhagic pancreatitis. Another case of postoperative portal vein thrombosis has also been reported.[149] For this reason, it has been suggested that a single intravenous dose of heparin, 45 units/lb (100 u/kg), given immediately postsurgically, may be beneficial in cases where extensive manipulations of the portal vein occur.[149]

Ascites is a minor and transient complication in some cases. This occurs when portal pressures are increased in animals with depressed albumin concentrations. Ascites does not exist presurgically because portal pressures are normal. Ascites can generally be managed quite easily with diuretics. In most cases it resolves within a few days and does not require long-term management. Dogs generally have dramatic clinical and biochemical improvement following shunt correction. They are usually clinically improved within 24 to 48 hours. Follow-up function studies return to normal within a few weeks to a few months. Some animals will have persistently abnormal, but improved, ammonia tolerance tests or slightly prolonged retention of BSP but will remain clinically asymptomatic and require no special therapy. A number of postoperative portal angiograms have been reported and all show improved portal circulation of the liver, but the perfusion pattern is aberrant (Figure 89–9).[182] It is not necessary to reoperate to completely ligate previously attenuated shunts. The dog's improved functional status appears to remain stable for years.[149] The overall prognosis for dogs with single extrahepatic shunts appears to be excellent if they survive the surgery and immediate postoperative period. For intrahepatic shunts the outlook is more guarded, but numerous successful surgeries have been performed by surgeons knowledgeable in the intricacies of this procedure.

If urinary calculi cannot be removed during the surgery to correct the shunt, they may be either removed at a later date or managed medically. The author has observed spontaneous dissolution of several renal calculi (presumed to be ammonium urate) following shunt correction. Calculi present in the bladder may also be successfully dissolved using a combination of a reduced purine diet (Prescription Diet u/d) combined with allopurinol, 4.5 mg/lb every 8 hours (10 mg/kg), and sufficient sodium bicarbonate to alkalinize the urine. Calculi will generally disappear in 4 to 12 weeks with this therapy. Recurrences of calculi should not be a problem once the shunt is corrected, as metabolic abnormalities causing increased urinary ammonia and uric acid excretion should cease.

Medical therapy for nonsurgical cases involves measures used to control the signs of hepatic encephalopathy and maximize remaining hepatic function. These measures are covered in detail in the section on hepatic therapy which follows. Although medical therapy may provide dramatic short-term improvement, hepatic atrophy continues to progress in most cases. Rare animals appear to plateau at some survivable level of hepatic function, and their disease does not progress. They will require medical management for life.

Portal systemic shunts in cats appear to be much less common than in dogs. The first two cases to be reported were in 1981.[168] Since then, an additional 21 cases have been described.[153, 160, 162, 165, 166, 168, 186, 187] Although clinical signs and diagnostic approaches to cats with PSS are similar to dogs, some significant differences exist. No breed or gender predisposition is known. The mean age of onset of clinical signs documented in 16 of 23 reported cases was 5 months. Thirteen of 16 affected cats were 6 months of age or younger when they first started showing clinical signs. However, these cats remained symptomatic for long periods of time before a definitive diagnosis was made. The mean age at the time of diagnosis for the 23 cats was 14.8 months old (range = 3 to 36 months). Half of the cats were under one year old when diagnosed.

Central nervous system signs predominate in cats as in dogs. Some of the signs of feline hepatic encephalopathy are rather unique, however. Ptyalism was a major clinical sign in 17 of 23 animals. Several cats had been treated for recurrent upper respiratory tract infections because of the similarity of signs between these two diseases. Interestingly, cats usually have temporary improvement when given antibiotics due to the beneficial effect of oral antibiotics on intestinal ammonia production. Another dramatic sign was that of grand mal seizures. They occurred in roughly 33 per cent of the cats and may have been the primary reason for seeking veterinary care. Seizures were often a late sign in the progressive history of these cats. Since idiopathic epilepsy is so uncommon in cats, any cat with an onset of seizures between three months and three years of age should be evaluated as a possible PSS animal unless another obvious cause for the seizures exists.

Other central nervous system abnormalities are somewhat similar to those seen in dogs. Generally they reflect diffuse symmetrical abnormalities of the cerebral cortex. Abnormalities of behavior predominate. Signs recognized include depression, agitation or aggression, staring blankly into space, blindness with dilated but responsive pupils, head pressing, circling or aimless running, quadriataxia, generalized tremors, stupor, and coma. For the most part, these signs are intermittent, occurring at intervals of once a month to several times per week. Most of the animals are thin or stunted and have histories of anorexia, occasional vomiting or gagging, and intolerance to protein. Several cats had consistent hypersalivation associated with eating. Physical examinations are usually non-localizing, although occasional cats are examined when in hepatic coma. Three of seven cats in one study had significant cardiac murmurs, although this abnormality was not reported by others.[166]

Laboratory evaluations of these cats show a consistent pattern. The only significant finding in the hemogram is significant poikilocytosis in the absence of anemia. White blood cell counts are usually normal. Biochemical abnormalities are typically those that support a functional problem rather than an inflammatory one. Serum ALT and AP concentrations are increased in less than 30 per cent of cases and, when elevated, are generally less than three times normal. Fasting blood ammonia concentrations were elevated in 11 of 17 animals that were tested. Ammonia tolerance tests were performed in three animals, and all three were abnormal. Normal fasting blood ammonia concentrations in cats have been

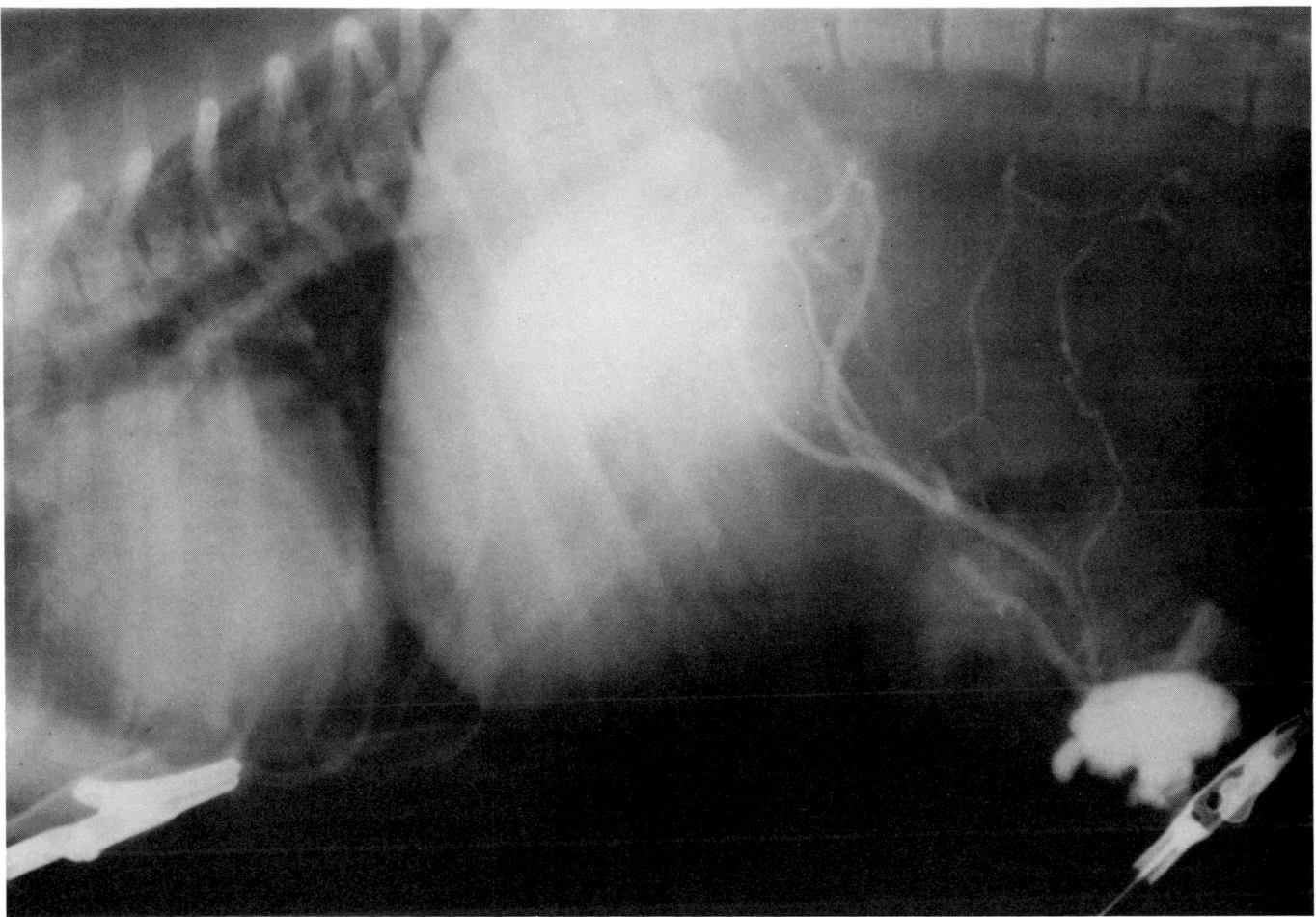

FIGURE 89–9. Operative splenoportogram four months after surgical attenuation of a portal-azygous shunt (presurgical angiography, Figure 89–8). Several new smaller shunting vessels are now evident and radiocontrast material can still be seen in the azygous vein. Much improved intrahepatic portal blood flow is evident.

reported to be from 100 to 350 μgm/dl by one author and from 80 to 120 μgm/dl by another.[168, 188] Normal values for ammonia challenge testing are reported to be from 260 to 530 μgm/dl.[168] Retention of BSP is less sensitive in cats than dogs; just over 50 per cent of affected cats had significantly prolonged retention of BSP. Serum bile acids have not been evaluated in large numbers of cats with PSS, but postprandial bile acids were dramatically increased in all cats tested so far. Fasting bile acids are also frequently increased, but in animals that have been anorectic for some time, these levels may be normal. Hypoalbuminemia is *not* a common finding. It was present in only one of 21 cats. The blood urea nitrogen concentrations were below normal in half of the reported cases. Since normal cats rarely have low urea nitrogen concentrations, this is a useful indicator of impaired urea formation. Ammonium urate crystalluria has only been documented in two cats and cystic calculi in one.

Survey radiographs of the abdomen often indicate the liver is reduced in size (8 of 13 cases). Angiography to confirm the presence of the shunt typically identifies a single, extrahepatic shunt (20 of 22 cases). The most common shunt is a communication between the left gastric vein and the caudal vena cava. Only two cases

of intrahepatic shunts have been identified; both had a ductus venosus.[153]

Therapy involves ligation or attenuation of the shunting vessel as with dogs. Nine of ten cats that had surgical closure of their shunts had successful outcomes. Most were able to be ligated completely without inducing significant portal hypertension. Several cats maintained for short periods of time on a reduced protein diet combined with lactulose and neomycin had decreased frequency and severity of their encephalopathy but were not asymptomatic. Signs rapidly returned if medical therapy was discontinued. At this time, it appears that surgery is the best therapeutic option for cats with PSS.

Now that clinicians have become more aware of the many possible signs associated with hepatic encephalopathy, PSS patients are being correctly diagnosed much more commonly. This disease should not be considered one of academic curiosity, never to be seen in the "real world." Portal vascular anomalies are one of the most common causes for CNS signs in young dogs and cats.

ARTERIOVENOUS FISTULAS

Arteriovenous fistulas (AVF) occasionally develop between a branch of the hepatic artery and the portal vein.[189, 190] This leads to great disparity in pressures between the two systems with resultant retrograde flow of blood in the portal vein, development of multiple extrahepatic portocaval shunts, and ascites. These fistulas may be congenital or acquired. Acquired AVF develop secondary to hepatic trauma, rupture of hepatic artery aneurysms, or following surgery on the liver. Seven cases that were surgically managed have been reported.[190] Dogs ranged in age from 4 to 13 months (mean = 6 months). Clinical signs are of acute onset and reflect a combination of those caused by hepatic encephalopathy and those caused by portal hypertension. Signs exhibited were depression, lethargy, stupor or coma, weight loss, bizarre behavior, ptyalism, painful abdomen, vomiting and diarrhea (7 of 7), ascites (7 of 7), fever and sepsis (3 of 7), cardiac murmur (3 of 7), and an auscultable murmur in the cranial abdomen (5 of 7).

Important laboratory abnormalities include increased retention of BSP, increases in fasting and post-ammonia tolerance, blood ammonia concentrations, and hypoalbuminemia. A diagnosis is usually established by exploratory surgery. Portal venous angiography will only indicate that multiple extrahepatic portal postcaval communications exist, and will not identify the cause. At surgery, arteriovenous fistulas will be easily recognized by the presence of multiple large, tortuous vessels coursing through the involved liver lobe(s). Multiple extrahepatic portocaval venous communications will also be easily visualized. Temporary occlusion of the hepatic artery leads to a decrease or elimination of the fremitus associated with the fistula. Correction involves excision of the involved liver lobe. If a resection cannot be performed, selective dearterialization of the affected tissue can be tried.[119] Four of seven dogs undergoing lobectomies had successful surgical outcomes. These animals still had problems with signs of encephalopathy owing to the continued presence of acquired portocaval shunts. All four required a second surgery to redirect portal flow into the liver. In the second surgery, the caudal vena cava was banded to increase the pressure gradient between the vena cava and the portal vein, favoring flow toward the liver. All four dogs were doing well five months to three years postoperatively.[190]

HEPATIC LIPIDOSIS

Hepatic lipidosis is the most frequent cause for severe liver failure in cats seen at the University of Minnesota Veterinary Teaching Hospital and is also the most common primary hepatobiliary disease seen in cats at the Animal Medical Center in New York.[16] Although lipidosis occurs in dogs, it is a relatively mild phenomenon and is not often associated with clinical signs. The normal liver contains approximately 5 per cent lipid, which may exist as triglycerides, fatty acids, phospholipids, cholesterol, and cholesterol esters.[191] However, when significant fat accumulates in the liver, it is nearly always triglyceride and may be 40 to 50 per cent of the total liver weight.[191] Normal hepatic lipid arises from multiple sources (the most important is the diet), from mobilization of fatty acids out of peripheral fat stores, and from endogenous fatty acid synthesis in the liver.

Circulating fatty acids are carried in the bloodstream bound to albumin. Upon reaching the liver, they are removed and incorporated into triglycerides, if they are not oxidized for energy. Triglycerides are complexed with specific proteins (apoproteins) forming lipoprotein particles (very low density lipoprotein, VLDL), which are secreted back into the circulation. If the rate at which fatty acids are brought to the liver exceeds the liver's ability to metabolize or resecrete them back into the circulation as VLDL, storage of fatty acids as triglycerides (lipidosis) occurs.[191] The normal liver is capable of extracting fatty acids from blood at rates that exceed the liver's capacity either for synthesis or secretion of VLDL.[192] Thus, excess triglyceride accumulation in the liver is easily accomplished.

Processes that lead to lipidosis are associated with one or more of the following: increased delivery of fatty acids to the liver, either from the diet or in association with peripheral lipolysis; decreased hepatic fatty acid oxidation; or decreased ability to secrete VLDL back into the circulation.[191] In the process of VLDL formation, adequate dietary intermediates such as choline, methionine, cysteine, betaine, or casein are necessary for phospholipid formation. Thus, fatty livers that respond to lipotropic agents such as choline are physiologic fatty livers and are due to dietary deficiencies of these compounds. In most clinical diseases associated with lipidosis, deficiencies of these substances do not exist; supplementation with lipotropic agents, especially methionine, has no beneficial effect and may be harmful (see Therapy section).

The most important causes for lipidosis in dogs and cats are starvation, diabetes mellitus, obesity, drug injury, and toxicities. Of these, the severe lipidosis seen in obese cats associated with prolonged anorexia is the most clinically significant and may account for as much as 62 per cent of all cases.[192] Although lipidosis may develop in cats in association with any of the above mentioned mechanisms, in the overwhelming majority of cases with severe, clinically apparent liver failure, the cause, other than the association with starvation, is unknown. This syndrome has been called idiopathic feline lipidosis to distinguish it from cases induced by other recognizable causes, such as diabetes mellitus, drugs, and so forth.[11, 16, 192–196] Starvation in other species is generally associated with mild degrees of fatty liver and subtle clinical disease. In cats, however, severe idiopathic lipidosis often has a fatal outcome. Why anorexia is associated with such a severe disease in cats is currently unknown. With starvation, a lack of availability of dietary glucose causes increased growth hormone secretion and sympathetic activity and decreased insulin release. These processes lead to accelerated peripheral lipolysis and massive free fatty acid release into the circulation.[191] Fatty acids are taken up by the liver and converted to triglycerides. In states of protein-calorie malnutrition, it appears that accumulated triglycerides are not efficiently converted to VLDL due to failure of lipoprotein synthesis and secretion.[191]

Several hypotheses have been proposed as to why some cats, particularly obese cats, develop such severe lipidosis in association with anorexia.[15, 194, 195, 197] Cats of normal size are apparently able to tolerate long periods of starvation without developing this severe complication. A relative deficiency of arginine may be important as a cause for idiopathic feline lipidosis. Arginine is an essential amino acid for cats, and during periods of starvation, it is supplied by muscle catabolism. Arginine is an important intermediate in the urea cycle, and deficiencies lead to rapid development of hyperammonemia and encephalopathy in cats.[198] If a relative deficiency of this amino acid exists, it would lead to encephalopathy, which would lead to anorexia and perpetuate the disease.

A deficiency of arginine can also result in reduced quantities of ornithine, another intermediate in the urea cycle. Lack of sufficient ornithine causes concentrations of carbamoyl phosphate to increase within hepatocytes. Carbamoyl phosphate is metabolized to orotic acid. Orotic acid is known to induce severe lipidosis by interfering with lipoprotein secretion from the liver, which can be reversed by adenine.[191] Cats require a minimum of 1.1 per cent of arginine in the diet, and when arginine is deficient, urinary orotic acid concentrations increase proportionately.[198] Serum concentrations of orotic acid and arginine have not been evaluated in these cats.

Carnitine deficiency has also been proposed as a possible mechanism for idiopathic feline lipidosis.[15] This is based on information from humans in which rare cases of severe lipidosis are due to a deficiency of carnitine.[199] Carnitine is necessary for oxidation of hepatic triglycerides, and in its absence, patients develop severe lipidosis, hepatomegaly, and hypoglycemia. Concentrations of carnitine are decreased in plasma, muscle, and liver tissue. The feline disease bears minimal resemblance to the human syndrome.

Endocrine abnormalities, particularly a relative or absolute insulin deficiency, has been proposed to play a role in feline lipidosis.[16] A few cats have had impaired glucose tolerance and mild intermittent hyperglycemia. Such cats are often obese, and obesity can cause insulin resistance. Insulin resistance or decreased insulin secretion results in accelerated lipolysis and increased circulating fatty acids. The role that subclinical diabetes may play in this disease is unknown. A recent study of 150 cats found that fasting blood glucose values were higher in cats with mild to moderate lipidosis than in those with the most severe disease.[192]

Cats with lipidosis have no age, sex, or breed predispositions, although most cats are over two years of age.[192] Nearly all cats have been partially or completely anorectic for some period of time (median two to three weeks). The more complete the anorexia and the longer the duration, the more severe is the disease. The cause for anorexia may be associated with some stress in the cat's life, such as moving, kenneling, addition of new pets, or a minor clinical disease. Some cases are caused by attempts to change the cat's diet. Cats that have marked dietary preferences will starve rather than eat a new type of food and may develop severe lipidosis. Many cats were obese prior to the onset of the disease and have had significant weight loss, up to 50 per cent of their body weight. Cats are typically depressed and lethargic and may vomit occasionally, hypersalivate, and show other signs of hepatic encephalopathy. Upon phys-

ical examination, these cats are usually thin, and have pronounced muscle wasting but still maintain intraabdominal fat stores. Hepatomegaly is considered uncommon by some but has been frequent in cases evaluated by the author.[194, 195] Jaundice is present in many animals.

Laboratory evaluations on cats with lipidosis support the severity of the hepatic failure. Mild to moderate nonregenerative anemias and mild neutrophilia are present in a few cases. Biochemical profiles usually indicate marked increases in serum concentrations of AP, ALT, and AST. Bilirubin, gamma glutamyltransferase, and serum bile acid concentrations are also mildly to markedly increased. Blood glucose, serum cholesterol, and triglyceride concentrations are infrequently increased, and hypoalbuminemia is uncommon. Blood ammonia concentrations may be increased. The most consistent abnormality in the urinalysis is the presence of bilirubin. A definitive diagnosis requires biopsy. This is a diffuse disease, and percutaneous needle biopsies are an efficient, rapid method of obtaining a diagnosis. In fact, the diagnosis can sometimes be made from cytologic evaluations of fine needle aspirations alone. An estimate of clotting status is important prior to obtaining a liver biopsy in cats with lipidosis. Mild to marked coagulopathies are sometimes present. Fresh whole blood should be given to cats with coagulopathies prior to attempting a liver biopsy. Grossly, these livers are swollen, yellow, and friable. They have a prominent reticulated pattern to their surface. The biopsy specimen will float when placed in formalin. A rapid tentative diagnosis can be made cytologically from a touch imprint of the specimen. Hepatocytes are diffusely swollen with numerous palestaining, large, fat droplets that displace the majority of the cytoplasm to the periphery of the cell (Figure 89–10).

Two forms of vacuolation may be observed histologically: macrovesicular and microvesicular.[98, 192] The macrovesicular form is characterized by one to several very large vacuoles within the hepatocyte that displace the nucleus and cytoplasm to the periphery of the cell. The microvesicular pattern has multiple small fat vacuoles distributed throughout the hepatocyte cytoplasm, and the nucleus is centrally located. In humans, the macrovesicular pattern is most often seen with alcoholism, starvation, and malnutrition, while the microvesicular pattern is typical of Reye's syndrome and acute fatty liver of pregnancy associated with tetracycline use. Although this difference has been thought to represent a different pathogenesis, it more likely reflects a difference in the severity and duration of fat accumulation.[191] With chronic, progressive lipidosis, there is aggregation of smaller triglyceride droplets into large aggregates. For fat to be definitively identified on tissue sections, specimens must be stained with oil red-O on fresh frozen samples or formalinized tissue. Fat is normally lost in the processing of most tissue sections. Inflammatory reactions are usually minimal in these biopsies. Prominent cholestasis will be seen in many specimens and be evident as bile plugged canaliculi.

The therapy of lipidosis should be directed at the cause, if known, combined with aggressive supportive and symptomatic care. Most published reports of idio-

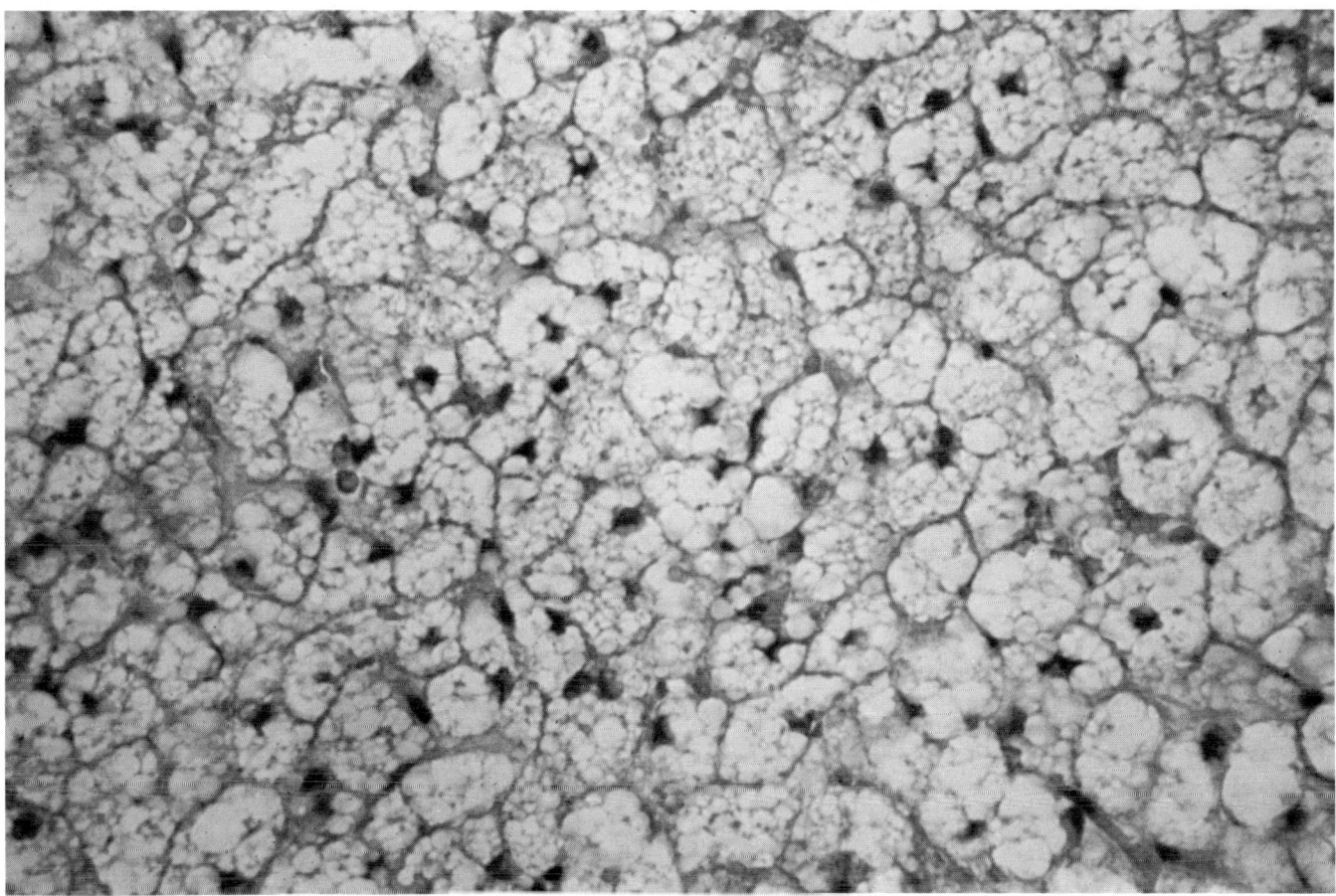

FIGURE 89–10. Photomicrograph of a liver biopsy taken from a cat with idiopathic lipidosis. All hepatocytes are pale and swollen with lipid (250×).

pathic feline lipidosis indicate the disease is nearly always uniformly fatal.[194] Until the past two to three years, this has been the author's experience as well. However, once we began utilizing aggressive nutritional support in these cats, our success rate has improved dramatically. We have increased the survival rate from 5 to 10 per cent to 50 to 60 per cent. The only significant change has been more aggressive oral alimentation and persistence. In addition to standard supportive and symptomatic therapy for animals in hepatic failure (fluids, oral neomycin and/or lactulose, vitamin supplementation), we combine force-feeding of a reduced protein diet (feline k/d) either as meatballs or as a gruel if the animal will tolerate that method.

If we have to fight the cat to force-feed it, or if it is too depressed for that method to be effective, we feed it with a 3 or 5 French diameter soft rubber nasoesophageal catheter. The distal end of the catheter is sutured to the cat's forehead and an Elizabethan collar is put on the cat to keep it from removing the catheter. Commercial canned cat foods cannot be blenderized sufficiently to get them to pass through these small catheters. A nutritionally complete liquid diet for use in humans (Ensure-HN) has worked well as nutritional support in many of these cats. This diet must be mixed 50:50 with water to get it to flow easily through the catheter. The catheter must be flushed with water after each feeding to keep it from plugging. We attempt to administer the total daily caloric requirement by this means. The cat will have to be fed small quantities multiple times per day. If large volumes are administered, vomiting often results. We start with 2 to 3 ml/lb/feeding initially and gradually increase this volume until 5 to 7 ml/lb can be given at one time. Some cats will not tolerate intermittent boluses, and we have used a continuous feeding pump to slowly infuse the required food throughout the day. Not only can the caloric requirements of the cat be met this way, but fluids, electrolytes, lactulose, and neomycin can also be given by this route. Although pharyngostomy tubes allow feeding tubes of larger diameter to be used, they require general anesthesia for placement and are not well-tolerated by many cats for long-term use. Once the patient is stabilized in the hospital, it can be sent home with the tube in place, allowing the owner to provide the necessary nursing care. We also use benzodiazepines to stimulate appetite in cats that are still willing to voluntarily consume food. These agents will be covered in the therapy section to follow.

Recovery in moribund cats is not a rapid process. We have maintained several cats on forced alimentation for eight weeks or longer, until they began to show an interest in eating. Such cats will look unhealthy for quite some time before they start to make any obvious clinical improvement. Once they start eating on their own, the prognosis is good. The author firmly believes many more cats can be saved with persistent effort. Several survivors looked as though they were not going to improve after three or four weeks of effort, but through perseverance, these cats are now totally normal. They serve as a reminder not to quit too early in the treatment of this disease.

Biochemical recovery is also slow to become evident. A number of animals returned to eating on their own, yet chemistry profiles were not significantly different from those obtained at the height of their illness. Idiopathic feline lipidosis is potentially completely reversible.

Diabetes is the only other major cause for lipidosis that occurs with any frequency in dogs and cats. In dogs, the disease is primarily a biochemical problem; rarely is it associated with clinical illness. This is generally true in diabetic cats as well. However, some diabetic cats with severe lipidosis do not reverse rapidly once the diabetes is regulated and will need to be managed as described above for the idiopathic disease. In diabetic dogs, serum ALT concentrations are increased mildly in approximately 50 per cent of cases. In contrast, serum AP concentrations are nearly always increased. The magnitude of rise is variable, but three- to five-fold increases are common. Retention of BSP may be in the 6 to 12 per cent range.[200] Hyperbilirubinemia is uncommon and, when present, is mild.

An important drug-induced cause for lipidosis in dogs is the use of tetracycline. Oral tetracyclines are associated with mild lipidosis in dogs, which is reversible upon withdrawal of the drug. The milder forms of tetracycline-induced lipidosis are thought to result from impaired hepatic lipoprotein formation.

Toxic injury is another potentially important cause for lipidosis. Many toxins can induce hepatic lipidosis if they interfere with hepatic protein synthesis. Bacterial endotoxins absorbed from the gut are well established causes for mild lipidosis. Treatment with oral antibiotics significantly reduces the severity of these lesions by suppressing colonic bacterial toxin production.

CONGENITAL HEPATIC CYSTS

Single or multiple hepatic cysts may occasionally be found in both dogs and cats.[201, 202] Animals are often asymptomatic, but the cysts may become large enough to cause abdominal distention or be easily palpated. Biochemical profiles are unremarkable. Diagnosis is usually established by exploration for an ill-defined abdominal mass. Although surgical correction is not always necessary, solitary large cysts may be removed by lobectomy. Frequently, multiple cysts of the liver and kidney are identified. Large cysts can be opened and drained, but they may recur several times during the life of the animal.[201] These cysts generally arise as congenital abnormalities of the intra- and extrahepatic biliary system and are lined by a secretory epithelium. The fluid present is usually a transudate.

UREA CYCLE ENZYME DEFICIENCIES

Two dogs have been described with signs of hepatic encephalopathy that were determined to have deficiencies of hepatic urea cycle enzymes.[203] One dog was a stunted four-month-old golden retriever with neurologic signs compatible with hepatic coma. The other dog was a stunted four-year-old beagle with a history of seizures since it was nine months old. The only abnormalities detected during a medical workup were hypoalbuminemia and increased blood ammonia concentrations. Hepatic biopsy material was quantitatively analyzed for enzymes important in the conversion of ammonia to urea. Both dogs had significant reductions in the urea cycle enzyme, arginosuccinate synthetase. A deficiency in this enzyme would lead to inability to handle endogenous ammonia and to signs of encephalopathy. Portal angiographic studies were normal in these dogs. Dietary and antibiotic therapy designed to minimize intestinal ammonia production resulted in significant amelioration of clinical signs in both dogs.

Sodium benzoate might be considered as an alternative drug to decrease blood ammonia concentrations in such cases.[204, 205] This drug has been very effective in lowering the blood ammonia in children with inborn errors of urea synthesis and in a limited number of patients with cirrhosis. Sodium benzoate results in increased conjugation of nitrogenous compounds with glycine or glutamine and facilitates their excretion in urine as hippuric acid.[204]

These cases might not be as rare as first supposed. They were only diagnosed on the basis of fasting blood ammonia concentrations. Since this test is not routinely available, it is possible that other dogs with seizures or behavioral signs could manifest signs of hepatic encephalopathy and not be diagnosed because other hepatic biochemical tests remain normal. Obviously, a definitive diagnosis requires very sophisticated assay techniques to quantitate intracellular hepatic enzymes.

AMYLOIDOSIS

Amyloidosis refers to the accumulation of abnormal types of hyaline-like deposits primarily within the liver, spleen, kidneys, and adrenal glands. Primary amyloidosis is very uncommon and occurs principally in the islet cells of the feline pancreas. Secondary amyloidosis occurs most often in the dog, and its presence is associated with a number of chronic diseases that stimulate antigen-antibody reactions. Amyloidosis most often occurs in chronic infections such as osteomyelitis, tuberculosis, and neoplastic conditions. Amyloid fibrils have an amino acid sequence identical to that of light chain immunoglobulins. On this basis, amyloid is thought to be an abnormal degradation product of the antibody molecule which remains as an extracellular accumulation in various target organs.

Hepatic amyloid accumulates within Disse's spaces, adjacent to the cords of hepatocytes lining the liver sinusoids. As this material accumulates, sinusoidal blood supply is reduced, and anoxia and necrosis develop. The liver becomes quite enlarged with palpably rounded edges. Liver failure may be the cause of death from amyloidosis. Only one case of hepatic failure secondary to amyloidosis has been reported.[206] This case occurred in a dog and was secondary to coccidioidomycosis. A definitive diagnosis requires biopsy and special staining techniques to detect the presence of amyloid. Amyloidosis is a progressive and fatal disorder. There is no specific therapy. Therapeutic efforts are aimed at identifying and eliminating the primary stimulus for amyloid production. Therapeutic success is not expected.

GLYCOGEN STORAGE DISEASES

A number of hereditary deficiencies of enzymes necessary for the breakdown of hepatic glycogen have been identified in humans. Only one form has been well documented in dogs, that of a deficiency of the debranching amyloclastic enzyme amylo-1,6-glucosidase (Cori's disease).[207, 208] Hepatic glycogen is necessary for the maintenance of normal fasting blood glucose levels, and an inability to mobilize hepatic glycogen results in hypoglycemic attacks. Because no defect in hepatic synthesis of glycogen exists in these diseases, the continued accumulation of glycogen without removal leads to severe hepatomegaly. This disease was diagnosed in four female German shepherds of similar genetic background. The most obvious clinical sign was massive hepatomegaly. Other signs included poor weight gain and muscle weakness. Signs began as early as two months of age and progressed slowly. Significant pathologic findings included massive increases in the glycogen content of the liver, cardiac and skeletal muscles, and the brain. A reduction in the hepatic concentration of the glycogen debranching enzyme amylo-1,6-glucosidase was confirmed. Hepatic concentrations were zero to 7 per cent of normal in these dogs. In nonfasted animals, a normal glucagon response is seen, but in the fasted state, no elevation in blood glucose occurs in response to glucagon administration. It is possible that some of the intermittent hypoglycemic attacks observed in hunting dogs after exercise are due to such a defect.

Hepatic Neoplasia

PRIMARY HEPATIC TUMORS

Primary hepatic tumors are uncommon in both dogs and cats. They are estimated to comprise between 0.6 and 1.3 per cent of all tumors.[208] Data taken from recent necropsy surveys indicate that primary hepatic tumors are found in 0.63 to 2.6 per cent of all necropsies performed.[208-210] These tumors may arise from either epithelial or mesenchymal tissue (Table 89–3). The two

TABLE 89–3. HEPATIC NEOPLASMS IN DOGS AND CATS

Primary Neoplasms

Epithelial Origin	Mesenchymal Origin
Benign	Malignant
Hepatocellular adenoma	Hemangiosarcoma
Cholangiocellular adenoma	Fibrosarcoma
	Extraskeletal osteosarcoma
	Leiomyosarcoma
Malignant	
Hepatocellular carcinoma	
Cholangiocellular carcinoma	
Hepatic carcinoids	

Metastatic Neoplasms

Hematopoietic origin (lymphosarcoma)
Epithelial origin (pancreatic adenocarcinoma)
Mesenchymal origin (hemangiosarcoma)

most common tumors are hepatocellular carcinoma and cholangiocellular carcinoma. These tumors most often develop in aged dogs and cats. The mean age of occurrence is between 10 and 11 years of age, but animals as young as 4 years old have been reported.[208, 209] It appears that hepatocellular carcinomas and some sarcomas of hepatic origin occur slightly more frequently in male dogs, while cholangiocellular carcinomas are slightly more common in females.[208]

The cause for these tumors in dogs and cats is unknown, but a number of factors have been associated with the development of primary hepatic tumors in humans and laboratory animals.[211] Incriminated factors include: (1) chemicals such as azo-compounds, nitrosamines, aflatoxins, methylcholanthrene, acetylaminofluorene, senecio alkaloids, chlorinated hydrocarbons, cycasin, and vinyl chloride; (2) Thorotrast, a radiographic contrast agent; (3) anabolic steroids; (4) malnutrition; (5) cirrhosis; (6) hepatitis B virus; and (7) parasites (schistosomiasis, clonorchiasis). The best documented carcinogens of this list are aflatoxins, polycyclic hydrocarbons, cycasin, and dimethylnitrosamine. The association of hepatic neoplasia with cirrhosis in dogs and cats is rare, while it is much more important in humans. Only 6 animals of 110 with primary liver tumors had any evidence of coexisting cirrhosis.[208] The rate of metastasis present at the time of diagnosis is high with these tumors. Hepatic carcinoids are metastatic 93 per cent of the time, while for hepatocellular carcinomas this figure is 61 per cent.[208] Metastasis occurs through direct extension to adjacent organs, and through both the blood and lymph to distant sites. Tumors of epithelial origin most often metastasize to regional lymph nodes and the lungs. Sarcomas of hepatic origin most often metastasize to the spleen. These tumors may also spread to the brain, kidneys, omentum, peritoneum, adrenals, pancreas, gastrointestinal tract, spine, and pituitary gland.[208, 211]

Hepatocellular Carcinomas. Hepatocellular carcinomas are the most common primary hepatic neoplasms. They accounted for 76 of 159 (47.7 per cent) of hepatic tumors identified in two extensive necropsy studies.[210, 212] Clinical signs are nonspecific but generally are those associated with hepatic failure. Lethargy, weakness, anorexia, weight loss, vomiting, and a pendulous abdomen are often present. Other less commonly observed signs include ascites, diarrhea, jaundice, and dyspnea. A large palpable cranial abdominal mass can be identified in 80 per cent of these cases.[210]

The definitive diagnosis of this tumor requires a biopsy; however, hematologic and biochemical changes are useful for localizing the patient's disease to the liver. Significant abnormalities in the hemogram include the presence of anemia in approximately 50 per cent of patients and neutrophilia in 66 per cent of patients.[212] Hepatic biochemical profiles are typically abnormal.[209, 210, 212] Hepatic enzyme profiles resemble those of nonneoplastic, inflammatory liver diseases. Moderate to marked increases in serum concentrations of ALT and AST occur in over half the cases. Serum alkaline phosphatase concentrations are increased in 82 per cent of the patients.[209] Hepatic functional indicators are more often normal than abnormal. Serum bilirubin concentrations are mildly increased in 26 per cent of the cases, while hypoalbuminemia is rare (16 per cent). Hypoglycemia may occur, but it was identified in only 4 of 65 cases. However, it may be so severe that it is the primary reason for the patient being evaluated.[213]

Additional diagnostic tests utilized in the evaluation of these patients include radiographs (survey and ultrasonograms), cytology of ascitic fluid, and biopsy. Radiographs serve primarily as a localizing tool, since most of these tumors are identified upon physical examination. The presence of ascites may limit the diagnostic usefulness of survey radiographs. Hepatic ultrasonography has been a useful presurgical tool to identify the site of origin of abdominal masses, to determine if they are solitary and likely primary, or whether they are multifocal and most likely metastatic lesions (Figure 89–11).[214] Hepatic ultrasonograms may detect lesions as small as 0.5 to 1.0 cm in diameter. Cytologic evaluation of peritoneal fluid from cases of hepatocellular carcinoma is usually unrewarding. These tumors rarely exfoliate into the fluid; a modified transudate is most often found. Biopsy of these masses is the diagnostic method of choice. Samples may be obtained by fine needle aspiration, needle core, or incisional and excisional techniques. Needle aspirations or core biopsies are generally rapid, safe, and technically uncomplicated approaches to the diagnosis of neoplasia. However, establishing a diagnosis of hepatocellular carcinoma from small biopsy samples is often difficult. Hepatocellular carcinoma cells often retain a normal appearance, mitoses are rare, and reasonably normal architecture is usually maintained.[215]

Exploratory surgery is the diagnostic method of choice. This technique allows for a visually guided biopsy, and surgical excision may be performed at the same time if no metastases are seen. Hepatocellular carcinomas do not fulfill the usual criteria for malignancy.[215] They are most often found as large, solitary masses with a predisposition for the left lateral lobe of the liver.[208] They tend to be well encapsulated and grow primarily by expansion and compression of adjacent tissue. When metastases are absent, their malignant potential is often based on their size and degree of local invasion. However, metastases will be identified at the time of diagnosis in 61 per cent of cases.[212] Thoracic radiographs should always be taken preoperatively since these cancers often metastasize to the lungs.

Surgical excision is the treatment of choice for solitary hepatocellular carcinomas. Unfortunately, the debilitated state, age, and degree of hepatic and other organ dysfunction in these animals makes major surgery a high risk choice. As an alternative to lobectomy, ligation of either the portal vein or the hepatic artery supplying the involved lobe has been attempted in humans. Significant improvement has been noted in human patients with surgically inoperable or metastatic hepatocellular carcinomas following segmental ligation of the portal vein.[216] Tumor vascularity significantly affects whether venous or arterial ligation is chosen. Hypovascular neoplasms respond best to segmental portal venous ligation, while hypervascular tumors regress more if the regional hepatic artery is ligated. The vascularity of the tumor is determined by presurgical nuclear scans of the liver. A study has been performed in normal dogs to determine if they will tolerate segmental hepatic artery ligation.[216a] All nine dogs survived the procedure well, suggesting this may be an alternative in clinical patients with unresectable tumors. Chemotherapy of hepatocellular carcinomas in humans primarily involves the use of systemic or intra-arterial 5-fluorouracil, Adriamycin, or methotrexate.[211, 217] No controlled clinical trials in dogs or cats using these agents has been performed. One ten-year-old Scottish terrier received 5-fluorouracil at a dosage of 200 mg/m²/week for six months after a solitary hepatocellular carcinoma was surgically removed.[218] The dog died acutely following rupture of the tumor, which had reoccurred at the previous surgical site. Metastases to the lung were identified at necropsy.

The prognosis for patients with hepatocellular carcinoma is usually poor. Their high rate of metastasis, coupled with the size and degree of local invasion of these tumors, and the physical status of the patient often preclude corrective surgery. Even resectable tumors

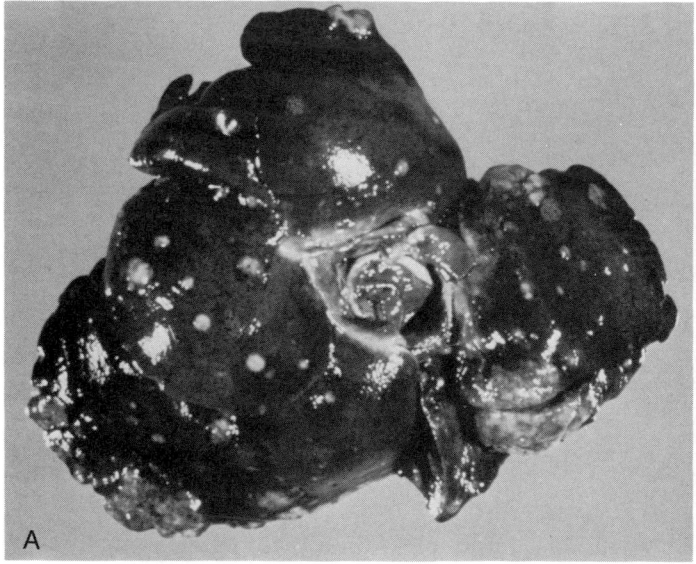
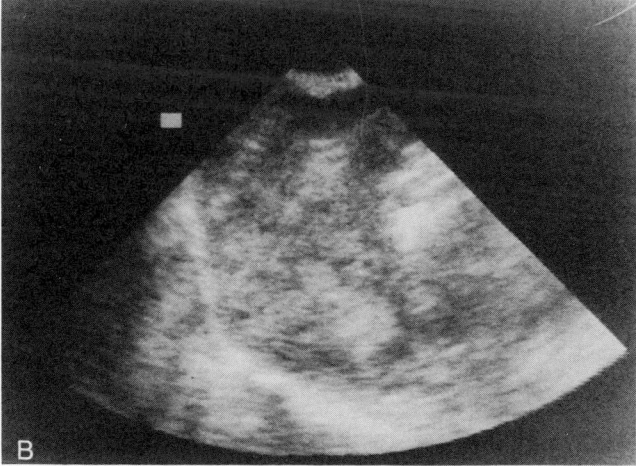

FIGURE 89–11. *A* and *B*. Gross liver specimen (A), and hepatic ultrasonogram (B) from a dog with multiple intrahepatic metastases from a pancreatic adenocarcinoma.

with no evidence of metastases had mean survival times of less than 80 days in one study.[219] Earlier detection and innovative chemotherapeutic approaches will, it is hoped, improve this situation in the future.

Cholangiocellular Carcinoma (Bile Duct Carcinoma). Cholangiocellular carcinomas account for 27 per cent of primary hepatic neoplasms.[208, 210] They almost always arise from intrahepatic bile duct epithelium, but a rare case may arise from the extrahepatic bile ducts or gallbladder. These tumors are known to be induced by the presence of the Chinese liver fluke, *Clonorchis sinensis,* or by exposure to *o*-aminoazotoluene, and the organic sulfite insecticide, aramite.[215]

Clinical signs and laboratory data are similar to those described for hepatocellular carcinomas and will not differentiate these two primary hepatocellular neoplasms.[210, 220] The diagnosis is made following biopsy of the tumor. Exploratory celiotomy is the diagnostic and therapeutic approach of choice. Cholangiocellular carcinomas are often of the massive type and, like hepatocellular carcinomas, most often involve the left lateral hepatic lobe. Metastases are more frequent with bile duct carcinomas occurring in 87 per cent of cases.[220] Metastases occur most often in the regional lymph nodes, lung, and peritoneum, and widespread metastases are common. Cure is not to be expected, both because of dissemination of the tumor prior to diagnosis and the tumor's tendency to massively infiltrate the liver, making surgery impossible.

Hepatic Carcinoids. Hepatic carcinoids have only been mentioned in two reports in dogs and one in the cat.[208, 221, 222] These tumors originate from neuroectodermal tissue scattered throughout the liver. These cells are classified as enterochromaffin or APUD cells. APUD is an acronym for a biochemical characteristic of this group of cells, i.e., they are capable of *A*mine *P*recursor *U*ptake and *D*ecarboxylation. Fifteen of 110 primary hepatic tumors in dogs were of this type.[208] Hepatic carcinoids occur at a slightly younger mean age (8 years) than the other primary hepatic tumors (10 years). Except for the absence of hepatomegaly, clinical signs, diagnostic criteria, and prognosis for carcinoids are similar to the other two primary hepatic neoplasms. All 15 of the identified tumors were metastatic throughout the liver at necropsy and 14 of 15 had extrahepatic metastases present.

Nonepithelial (Mesenchymal) Hepatic Neoplasms. Benign and malignant tumors of mesenchymal origin occur within the livers of dogs and cats. They are much less common than those of epithelial origin discussed previously. Tumor types recognized include hemangiosarcoma, fibrosarcoma, leiomyosarcoma, hepatic mixed sarcoma, hepatic mesenchymoma, and extraskeletal osteosarcoma.[208, 210, 215, 222, 222a] Clinical features of hepatic sarcomas are similar to other primary tumors; therefore, biopsy is the sole method of differentiating them. No effective therapy, short of early surgical excision, is available. The prognosis is universally poor.

Hepatocellular Adenoma/Nodular Hyperplasia. Nodular hyperplasia is a common finding, reportedly occurring in 15 to 60 per cent of aged dogs.[223] Differentiating nodular hyperplasia from hepatocellular adenomas appears to be difficult.[208, 224] Nodular hyperplasia occurs most often in dogs over 11 years of age and is not thought to be a "precancerous" lesion.[224] Hyperplastic nodules range from 0.1 to 5 cm in diameter and may be single or multiple. They are not associated with clinical signs. They are most often identified during exploratory surgery or at necropsy, and it is important to histologically distinguish them from hepatocellular carcinomas.

METASTATIC LIVER DISEASE (SECONDARY TUMOR)

The liver is a major site for metastasis of malignancies. Through its portal circulation, the liver serves as a filter between other major abdominal organs and the systemic circulation. Thus, it is vulnerable to metastatic cells arising from other gastrointestinal organs. In a series of 1867 necropsies, 129 cases of metastasis to the liver were identified (6.9 per cent), which was 2.6 times the frequency at which primary hepatic tumors were identified.[210] Malignancies of nonhepatic origin had a tendency to metastasize to the liver in 30.6 per cent of cases, which exceeded that for the lung (24.2 per cent). The mean age of animals with metastatic cancer was 7.8 years compared to 10 years for primary hepatic neoplasms.

Clinical signs associated with metastatic hepatic malignancies are highly variable. Most often signs relate to the type and location of the primary tumor, not to its liver involvement. The degree of involvement of the liver must be great before signs of impaired function develop. Hepatomegaly is uncommon with metastatic disease.[209, 210] Biochemical abnormalities are unpredictable. In general, metastatic disease of the liver induces much less dramatic changes in biochemical profiles than those induced by primary hepatic tumors. Mild to moderate increases in serum concentrations of ALT occur in 46 to 70 per cent of cases.[209, 210] Serum concentrations of alkaline phosphatase may be mildly to markedly increased in roughly half the cases, which usually reflects the degree of bile duct occlusion induced by the tumor. Hyperbilirubinemia occurs in 30 to 46 per cent of cases.[209, 210]

Tumors metastatic to the liver arise from three major tissues—hematopoietic, epithelial, and mesenchymal.[225] Hematopoietic neoplasms, in particular lymphosarcoma, accounted for 63 per cent of the metastatic tumors in one survey.[210] Epithelial tumors account for 27 per cent of metastatic hepatic neoplasms. One-third of these are pancreatic adenocarcinomas. Mesenchymal tumors cause only 16 per cent of hepatic metastatic disease. Hemangiosarcomas make up 75 per cent of this group, and over 90 per cent of these originated in the spleen. Therapy for metastatic hepatic neoplasia is directed at the primary cancer if possible. Since signs and laboratory abnormalities indicative of hepatic disease may dominate the clinical picture, a diagnosis of disseminated cancer may not be made until a liver biopsy is obtained.

Hepatic Therapy

General objectives for therapy of hepatic failure revolve around attempts to eliminate causative agents, if known, to suppress or eliminate mechanisms that potentiate the illness, to provide optimal conditions for hepatocellular regeneration, and to control manifestations of complications that develop. Clinical manifestations are often similar in acute and chronic hepatic failure, differing primarily in the severity and number of complications that develop. Little controlled work has been done on therapy of spontaneous hepatic diseases in the dog or cat. Most therapeutic recommendations are based on conclusions obtained from trials in experimental animals or in humans.

SPECIFIC THERAPY FOR HEPATIC FAILURE

Therapy for hepatic diseases may be either specific (directed at a causative agent) or supportive and symptomatic (directed at the signs of failure regardless of the cause). At present, there is little specific therapy available for the majority of known hepatic diseases. This is because the cause for many is not identified or known. If the cause is known, it has no specific treatment (viruses), or it is no longer present when the disease is diagnosed (cirrhosis). Clinicians are compelled to treat the manifestations of hepatic failure symptomatically in an attempt to prolong the patient's life until there is sufficient repair and regeneration to sustain life. Even if complete recovery is not possible, as is often the case, by utilizing appropriate therapeutic manipulations, many animals can remain asymptomatic for months or years. Specific therapies were covered in the previous discussion of known hepatic diseases.

SUPPORTIVE AND SYMPTOMATIC THERAPY

Regardless of the cause for hepatic failure in dogs and cats, most cases will receive supportive and symptomatic therapy in addition to any specific drugs that may be indicated. Such care is designed to reduce or eliminate the severity of clinical signs while providing optimal conditions for hepatic regeneration. Even if cures are not possible, improvement in the patient's quality and quantity of life can be attained in many instances. In addition to rest and dietary modifications, a number of drugs may be given to patients in hepatic failure to reduce major complications that develop.

Rest and Confinement. Rest and confinement are beneficial for animals with liver failure because liver regeneration is facilitated by the increased blood flow and the reduction in workload. Decreased activity reduces pain and tenderness associated with stretching of the liver capsule in acute inflammatory diseases. The subjective signs of illness reported by humans (malaise, nausea, and anorexia) are reduced if activity is curtailed, and presumably this may be true for animals as well. Once biochemical evidence of improvement in hepatic function occurs, exercise restriction is unnecessary. Most dogs and cats in liver failure usually voluntarily curtail their activity because they are so depressed.

Dietary Modifications. Dietary therapy is the single most important means of modifying the clinical course of most spontaneous liver diseases in dogs and cats. Dietary modifications are likely to be most effective in animals with subacute or chronic diseases because these patients will often be willing to voluntarily consume sufficient quantities of nutrients and calories to meet their body's maintenance needs as well as those necessary for hepatic repair and regeneration. Animals with acute severe liver disease usually are unwilling to consume any food at all and must be force-fed or given parenteral hyperalimentation to meet their caloric needs.

Dietary therapy involves adjusting the diet so that optimal quantities and types of nutrients are provided to the animal. The intake of the animal must be balanced with its ability to metabolize these foodstuffs using a failing liver. Protein restriction and modification are of major importance. The goal is to minimize the alterations in nitrogen metabolism induced by hepatic failure. Appropriate adjustments in the type and quantity of protein ingested by the patient will lead to a reduction in blood ammonia and a return to normal ratios of circulating branched-chain to aromatic amino acids. The type and quantity of protein, as well as the frequency of feeding, are all important in reducing clinical signs of hepatic failure.[63, 226]

Cottage cheese is a high quality protein source for animals in hepatic failure. Dogs usually find this food more palatable than do cats. Cottage cheese contains no additives, is easily and completely digested, and has a good ratio of branched-chain to aromatic amino acids. The beneficial effects of cottage cheese are related to the fact that it undergoes less putrefaction and ammonia production by intestinal bacteria during digestion, and that there is a reduction in urease-positive bacteria within the colon when it is fed.[227] Cottage cheese is superior to intravenous casein hydrolysates in terms of both nitrogen retention and stabilization of plasma amino acid ratios.[228] The lack of food additives in cottage cheese is important, as many commercial pet foods contain additives that are metabolized by intestinal bacteria to potent hepatotoxins.[226] The efficient digestion of cottage cheese within the small bowel results in little residue available for colonic bacteria to metabolize. Decreasing intestinal residues reduces both the numbers of colonic bacteria and the toxic waste products of their metabolism. Low residue diets also decrease intestinal ammonia production by reducing desquamation of intestinal epithelium. Reduced intestinal cell turnover also results in less protein loss through intestinal lymphatics. Food should be provided to patients with hepatic failure three to four times per day. Hepatic failure patients have reduced ability to handle normal quantities of dietary substrate. By dividing the total daily nutrient intake into several smaller meals, these patients will maintain their appetite and intake, which will speed their recovery.

Dogs with hepatic failure should receive approximately 1 gm/lb/day (2 gm/kg/day) of high biologic value protein. This amount should be adequate for maintenance needs as well as that needed for repair and regeneration of the liver, without leading to signs of encephalopathy. Cats have significantly higher protein needs and should receive sufficient good quality protein to provide 30 per cent of their caloric needs as protein.[229] In estimating the protein requirements of patients it is important to know the serum albumin concentration.

Severe protein restriction in hypoalbuminemic patients may further deplete serum albumin concentrations and lead to ascites or edema. If clinical signs improve on reduced protein diets but serum albumin concentrations do not, the protein content of the diet should be supplemented. The author recommends increasing the protein available by 0.25 gm/lb/day (0.5 gm/kg/day) at weekly intervals until either protein anabolism is evident or signs of encephalopathy develop. It is not necessary to increase the protein beyond 2.5 gm/lb/day (5 gm/kg/day). A commercially available reduced protein diet that works well in many dogs and cats with hepatic failure is canine or feline k/d. If animals will eat enough to meet their caloric needs, this diet will provide sufficient protein for their metabolic demands. In some animals, even this reduced protein diet cannot be tolerated and an ultra-low protein prescription diet, u/d, must be utilized. Although this diet may not totally meet the protein needs of the liver failure patient, it may allow them to survive longer and more comfortably than with other available foods.

An easily digested carbohydrate source should form the bulk of the required daily calories for animals with hepatic failure. The carbohydrate source should be easily digested so that minimal residues remain in the colon where intestinal flora may convert them to volatile fatty acids. An inexpensive and useful carbohydrate source that meets these needs is boiled white rice. A high carbohydrate diet provides an easily assimilated source of nonprotein calories, which spares body tissues from catabolizing muscle protein for energy and reduces the catabolism of dietary nitrogen for energy.

Fats should be given so that they comprise 6 per cent of the dietary calories on a dry weight basis. This will be accomplished by supplying 0.51 gm/lb/day (1.32 gm/kg/day) of fat in the diet. Fats are necessary to supply essential fatty acids and fat soluble vitamins (A, D, E, K) and to improve palatability. Excessive fat supplementation may worsen signs of encephalopathy if the fat source contains large quantities of short chain fatty acids, e.g., coconut oil. However, short chain fatty acids are primarily derived from dietary carbohydrates and to some extent amino acids, not from ingested fats.[230] In general, milk fat and seed oils are not sources of short chain fatty acids. Another reason for moderate fat restriction is that patients with hepatic failure may have reduced intestinal bile salts, which are important for normal fat assimilation. If excessive fats are fed, the animal may develop fat malassimilation and steatorrhea.

Vitamin and mineral supplementation can be important, especially when diets are formulated at home.[231] Hypovitaminosis is common in liver failure and is caused by multiple factors. Decreased intake associated with anorexia is of major importance. In addition, increased physiologic demands, accelerated intestinal losses, malutilization, and impaired storage capacity all combine to increase dietary needs for vitamins.[232, 233] Vitamins most often deficient in humans with hepatic failure include folic acid, B_6, B_{12}, thiamine, A, E, riboflavin, nicotinic acid, and pantothenic acid. In addition, the minerals zinc and cobalt are often deficient. Vitamins B_6 and B_{12} are particularly important for normal cell regeneration. Cats normally have two to eight times the needs of dogs

for B-complex vitamins.[229] It is recommended that daily B-complex vitamin requirements for dogs and cats be doubled. Vitamin C has recently been shown to be reduced in the blood of dogs with experimental hepatic insufficiency, and it should be supplemented at 12 mg/lb/day (25 mg/kg/day).[231]

Zinc acetate has been supplemented in cirrhotic humans with chronic hepatic encephalopathy, and in short-term studies, patients receiving zinc supplementation had significantly improved neurologic status.[234] Blood urea nitrogen concentrations returned to normal following zinc supplementation, implying that zinc deficiency impaired the efficiency of the urea cycle. The recommended dosage for zinc in dogs and cats is 22 mg/lb/day (50 mg/kg/day).[235] Vitamin and mineral supplements that contain copper should be avoided. This is particularly important for dogs that have copper storage defects or in animals with chronic cholestasis. Of the fat soluble vitamins, K and D are the most important. If hemorrhagic tendencies develop in association with prolonged cholestasis, parenteral vitamin K_1, 0.5 to 1.5 mg/lb/day (1 to 3 mg/kg/day), IM may help to return clotting parameters to normal in a few days. If coagulopathies are a result of chronic hepatocellular failure, parenteral vitamins will not be utilized by the failing liver. Fresh whole blood is necessary to stabilize clotting abnormalities in this situation.

The routine use of lipotropic agents containing methionine in dogs and cats in hepatic failure should not continue. Metabolites of oral methionine can induce signs of hepatic encephalopathy quite easily in experimental dogs. It also acts synergistically with short chain fatty acids and ammonia to induce coma. Recently, it has been shown that methionine can also induce a severe Heinz body hemolytic anemia in cats at dosages of 0.25 to 0.5 mg/lb/day (0.5 to 1 gm/kg/day).[236] Lipotropic drugs are of proven value only in cases in which confirmed deficiencies exist. Animals receiving a nutritious diet with adequate quantities of protein have no need for methionine supplementation, which may actually worsen signs of disease.[237]

For animals that are totally anorectic, nutritional support may be supplied by force-feeding one of several nutritionally complete liquid diets formulated for use in humans. They can be force-fed by syringe or administered through a nasoesophageal catheter or pharyngostomy tube. Isocal has been used as the sole source of nutrition in experimental dogs that had portocaval shunts surgically constructed (Eck fistula dogs).[238] The dogs maintained normal weight and serum albumin concentrations and had no central nervous signs, while those eating standard dog food continued to deteriorate. Although the liver of Isocal-treated dogs continued to atrophy, the dogs appeared clinically normal. This diet has a relatively high ratio of carbohydrate per gram of protein, which has a protein-sparing effect on the body. The author has experience with a similar diet, Ensure-HN, which is used commonly in anorectic cats with idiopathic lipidosis. These formulations provide one calorie per milliliter of diet and are an efficient and useful method of providing oral alimentation to patients in liver failure which will not eat on their own.

Several benzodiazepine derivatives may be tried as

appetite stimulants for anorectic cats.[234] These drugs are not as effective in dogs. Benzodiazepine compounds stimulate the hunger center in the brain and can cause voracious feeding in normal cats. Of the available compounds, oxazepam is the most potent, followed by lorazepam, and then diazepam. Dosages as low as 0.05 mg/lb (0.1 mg/kg) increased food intake by 50 per cent, while 0.12 mg/lb (0.3 mg/kg) caused a 72 per cent increase in food intake in normal cats. This effect occurred even when the drug was given 12 hours prior to feeding. Dosages of 4.5 mg/lb (10 mg/kg) resulted in sleepiness and ataxia. Diazepam was not as effective, but dosages of 0.12 mg/lb (0.3 mg/kg) caused a 39 per cent increase in food intake, and 0.45 mg/lb (1.0 mg/kg) caused an 82 per cent increase in feeding. In the author's experience, diazepam stimulates a very transient interest in eating in cats with hepatic failure and usually makes them sleepy, even at 1.5 to 3 mg total dose. Oxazepam deserves more clinical evaluation in anorectic cats with liver failure to see if it will shorten the time necessary for forced feeding.

Drugs in Hepatic Failure. The liver is quantitatively the most important organ involved with drug metabolism, although the kidney, brain and other organs make significant contributions. For many drugs metabolized in the liver, their duration and intensity of action may be increased in the presence of liver disease. However, not all enzyme systems are equally affected by hepatic failure. A number of therapeutic agents cause nonspecific induction of hepatic drug metabolizing enzymes, and their metabolism may actually be increased, even in the presence of liver failure. There is no test of liver function that can be run to determine if a given drug will be metabolized normally in a patient with liver failure.[240] As a general rule, most commonly used drugs are well tolerated by patients with hepatic failure and can be prescribed, as long as animals are monitored for signs of toxicity.

ANTIBIOTICS. Adequate hepatic function does not seem to be a critical factor in the patient's capability to handle most antibiotics. They are generally given at standard recommended dosages and dosage intervals.[241] Antibiotics are indicated as specific treatment for primary bacterial hepatitis, hepatic abscesses, bacterial cholangitis, and cholecystitis and are of great value in the suppression of intestinal bacteria, which are responsible for many of the signs of hepatic encephalopathy (see Complications of Hepatic Failure).

The selection of antibiotics to be used for the treatment of nonhepatic infections should be made with caution. It is best to avoid drugs that require hepatic inactivation or excretion, since they may reach toxic levels if the failing liver is unable to effectively remove them from the circulation. Conversely, for treating specific infections of the liver, drugs that are metabolized and eliminated by the liver are ideal since very high tissue concentrations will develop.[242]

All tetracyclines are concentrated in the liver and excreted in bile. Biliary concentration may reach 5 to 32 times the serum concentration. Parenteral preparations are known to be toxic in high dosages in humans. A reversible lipidosis occurs in dogs given chlortetracycline, which is the most hepatotoxic of the group.

Tetracyclines also suppress hepatic protein synthesis and thus impair albumin synthesis and enzyme activity in the liver. Prolonged use of these drugs has been associated with decreased vitamin K absorption in humans. Because they generally cause anorexia in dogs and cats and have toxic side effects, they are poor choices for animals with hepatic failure.

Penicillins and their newer derivatives, ampicillin and amoxicillin, reach high tissue concentrations in the liver. They are primarily excreted renally and are quite safe to use in animals in hepatic failure. Hetacillin requires conversion to ampicillin by the liver, so this would not be a good choice for animals with liver failure.[243] Cephalosporins also do not require hepatic metabolism for biologic activity and are useful for treating systemic infections in patients with liver failure.

Chloramphenicol is conjugated by the liver and then excreted by the kidney. Concentrated hepatic tissue and biliary levels are attained. Disadvantages associated with chloramphenicol outweigh the potential benefits. The drug is a potent inhibitor of hepatic microsomal enzyme systems and thus inhibits the clearance of many other drugs and waste products produced endogenously. Its half-life is often prolonged in chronic liver disease and may augment its toxic potential. It also produces anorexia and reversible erythroid hypoplasia both in dogs and cats and thus cannot be recommended for use.

Lincomycin, clindamycin, and erythromycin estolate are all cleared by the liver or known to be hepatotoxic and should be avoided in patients with liver disease because it may potentiate their toxicity.[240]

SEDATIVES, ANTICONVULSANTS, ANESTHETICS, AND ANALGESICS. Sedatives should be avoided in hepatic failure, since their use is commonly associated with the development of hepatic coma. Phenobarbital is primarily excreted by the kidney and is the safest hypnotic. Convulsive states are best controlled using short-acting compounds like diazepam (Valium) or chlordiazepoxide (Librium) at reduced dosages. The potential toxicity associated with the use of phenytoin and primidone has already been discussed. They should not be used to control seizures in animals with evidence of pre-existing liver disease.

Avoid analgesics, anesthetics, and barbiturates in patients with hepatic failure. If analgesia is required, meperidine, codeine, butorphenol, oxymorphone, or combinations of diazepam and ketamine are tolerated better than morphine. Start with smaller dosages than you would normally use and give more if necessary, rather than give a relative overdose to start with. Of all the inhalant anesthetics, halothane has been frequently incriminated in cases of fulminant hepatic failure in humans following repeated exposures. Similar experiences in dogs or cats are extremely rare. Halothane in combination with hypoxia and metabolic acidosis may be hepatotoxic.[244] Because of its relative safety compared to other anesthetics, the author has no concern about using halothane for anesthetizing metabolically fragile patients in hepatic failure.

ANABOLIC ANDROGENIC STEROIDS. Several reports have attributed beneficial effects to the use of androgenic anabolic steroids in the treatment of chronic liver disease in humans.[245-248] Drugs evaluated include testosterone propionate, methandrostenolone, testosterone, methenolone enanthate, and norethandrolone.[246] Administration of these drugs generally was continued for many months. The bulk of clinical studies indicates a trend in favor of a positive effect for anabolic steroids in the course and prognosis of patients with cirrhosis and possibly other liver diseases. Anabolic steroids appear to stimulate both hepatic RNA and protein synthesis in the regenerating liver and to protect against the induction of fatty liver.[246] One interesting report concerns the use of norethandrolone at 120 mg once daily for severe alcoholic fatty liver in humans. The lipidosis was dramatically reversed in two weeks of this treatment. This effect was not observed when 25 mg of daily testosterone was used. These compounds warrant clinical evaluations in cirrhosis and idiopathic lipidosis. Regardless of the drug used, for anabolic steroids to be effective, sufficient nonprotein calories must be taken in to meet metabolic demands, or no anabolic effects will be seen. Methyltestosterone has been shown to have a mild toxic effect on the dog liver and should be avoided.[249]

GLUCOCORTICOIDS. The use of glucocorticoids in hepatic failure remains a controversial subject. They have proven efficacy only in human chronic active hepatitis and primary biliary cirrhosis. Their potential for use in canine CAH and feline cholangitis/cholangiohepatitis has already been discussed. The potential benefits to steroid use include increased appetite, reductions in serum bilirubin concentrations, reductions in transaminases, lessened BSP retention, and increased serum albumin concentrations.[250] Glucocorticoids also have a mild choleretic effect and might be useful in diseases associated with cholestasis. In spite of these many potential benefits, they are known to have many disadvantages. Glucocorticoids fail to prevent the progression of most acute liver diseases to chronic phases; they may increase the chance of intercurrent infections developing; they generally do not increase life expectancy; they fail to alter the histology of most liver diseases; and they can aggravate the management of ascites by promoting sodium retention.[250, 251] Previously stable cirrhotic dogs may deteriorate rapidly following the administration of steroids.[137] Recent information indicates they also increase the incidence of peptic ulceration in cirrhotic men.[252] In general, patients in which steroids may have a beneficial effect are those with prolonged anorexia and weight loss, those that would benefit by an increased food intake, and those with suspected immune-mediated hepatobiliary diseases.

The dosage and type of glucocorticoid used may be more important in patients with hepatic failure than with other steroid responsive diseases. Short-acting steroids should be chosen; prednisone or prednisolone are the drugs of choice. Prednisone must be converted to its active form, prednisolone, by the liver. This should make prednisolone the best choice for animals in liver failure, but most pharmacologic studies of this problem have concluded the benefits of one drug over the other are minimal.[253, 254] Another important factor to consider in the use of steroids is that the drug's half-life is often prolonged in animals with liver failure. Unless the dosage is reduced or the dosage interval is increased

from those usually considered, signs of iatrogenic hyperadrenocorticism may develop. Maintenance dosages in dogs may be as low as 0.1 mg/lb/day.

DRUGS TO CONTROL HEPATIC FIBROSIS. One of the most significant pathologic changes in chronic liver diseases is the development of fibrosis. Both increased synthesis and decreased degradation of collagen occur in cirrhosis.[140] If causative agents can be identified early in the course of chronic diseases, fibrosis may be completely reversible. However, at some point in the progression of chronic liver diseases, fibrosis becomes self-perpetuating, even if the causative agent is removed. Immunologic factors appear to play a role in the development and progression of fibrosis in many chronic liver diseases.

COLCHICINE. Of all the experimental antifibrotic drugs available, colchicine appears to have the most potential benefit. Colchicine is an alkaloid, antimitotic agent. This drug has unique anti-inflammatory properties but is only licensed for use in gouty arthritis.[255] It binds to microtubule protein and interferes with the function of mitotic spindles, which can arrest cell division.[255] Colchicine prevents transcellular movement of collagen in fibroblasts and stimulates a two- to ten-fold increase in collagenase activity.[256] Preliminary clinical trials in human cirrhotics indicate that histologic progression was halted and mortality was decreased by 25 per cent over a 53-month period of study.[256] In addition, serum albumin concentrations were consistently increased in cirrhotic humans receiving colchicine.[257] Therapeutic trials in primary biliary cirrhosis also show benefit. Serum albumin concentrations again increased, while those of bilirubin, cholesterol, and ALT decreased, and mortality was reduced by 50 per cent after four years.[258] Only one clinical report of its use in dogs has been published.[259] A four-year-old cirrhotic dog was treated for seven months (0.014 mg/lb/day or 0.03 mg/kg/day orally). The dog had deteriorated with the administration of steroids but improved clinically after colchicine was started. No toxicity was observed. Reported signs of acute toxicity in humans include nausea, vomiting, diarrhea, and abdominal pain. These signs may be reduced by administering the drug intravenously. Chronic toxicity includes agranulocytosis, aplastic anemia, myopathy, and alopecia. The author has evaluated colchicine in several dogs with severe chronic liver disease. The dogs showed no clinical improvement, but periods of evaluation were less than one month.

D-PENICILLAMINE. D-Penicillamine is another drug that may be used to modify hepatic fibrosis. Large dosages given to cirrhotic rats (140 mg/lb/day or 300 mg/kg/day) induced significant reductions in hepatic fibrosis. This dose is much higher than currently recommended for the dog (5 to 7 mg/lb/day or 10 to 15 mg/kg/day) and would not likely be tolerated.

THERAPY FOR COMPLICATIONS OF HEPATIC FAILURE

A number of potentially serious complications of hepatic failure may develop in any given patient. It is often one or more of these complicating factors that causes the death of the patient. It is important for clinicians to recognize these complications early in their course and manage them vigorously if any degree of success is to be obtained.

Hepatic Coma. Hepatic coma is a serious complication of hepatic failure. It is seen most often in young dogs and cats with congenital portal systemic shunts. Occasionally, an older dog or cat with chronic liver failure will manifest encephalopathic signs as well. In adult animals, signs of encephalopathy are much less dramatic and often are those of depression, lethargy, vomiting, and diarrhea. The goal of therapy is to control the pathophysiologic mechanisms responsible for inducing the encephalopathy while the liver attempts to regenerate sufficient tissue to maintain life. This is accomplished by reducing the entry, production, and absorption of gastrointestinal "toxins" and by administering systemic drugs that counteract the effects of the absorbed toxins.

The mainstays of therapy for encephalopathy involve reduction of protein intake, suppression or elimination of urease-containing intestinal bacteria, and catharsis. In addition, steps must be taken to recognize and eliminate any precipitating factors that may have induced the encephalopathy (Table 89–4). For animals exhibiting signs of encephalopathy, all oral intake of food should cease until CNS signs abate. This is particularly important for protein. Cessation of food intake eliminates dietary sources of ammonia, toxic amines, aromatic amino acids, and short-chain fatty acids which induce encephalopathy. Next, complete catharsis of the colon should be undertaken. Emptying the colon rapidly decreases numbers of colonic bacteria and removes potentially toxic by-products of bacterial metabolism. Although warm water enemas are most often used, a more effective method combines substances that impair ammonia production or absorption in the enema solution. Using a 10 per cent povidone iodine solution as the enema fluid or adding liquid neomycin sulfate (10

mg/lb) to the enema fluid results in more efficient, rapid suppression of colonic bacteria, which generate the majority of the blood ammonia. Enemas should be repeated until no fecal material in evident in the evacuated fluid.

Another drug that is highly effective in lowering blood ammonia concentrations when added to enema fluid is lactulose (1-4-β-galactosidofructose) (Cephulac). Lactulose is a semisynthetic disaccharide that is not metabolized by mammalian intestinal disaccharidases.[260] When this undigested sugar reaches the colon, intestinal bacteria hydrolyze it to lactic, acetic, and formic acids, which dramatically lower colon pH.[261] In addition to the pH effect, when large quantities of unabsorbed solutes are produced in the colon an osmotic diarrhea results.[260] Blood ammonia concentrations are lowered because of several unique attributes of lactulose. By-products of lactulose fermentation produce what is termed ionic trapping of ammonia within the colon.[261] In an acid environment, ammonia (NH_3) accepts a proton to form ammonium (NH_{4+}). Ammonium is much less diffusible than ammonia. Thus, ammonium ions remain within the colon and are excreted rather than being absorbed. This effect occurs when the colon pH is 6.2 or lower and is most noticeable if the colon pH is 5.0 or lower.[261, 262]

In addition to ionic trapping, lactulose apparently inhibits ammonia generation by colonic bacteria through a process known as catabolite repression.[262] By providing a carbohydrate source to intestinal bacteria, less proteolysis, peptide degradation, and deamination of bacterial proteins occurs. This results in significantly less generation of ammonia by colonic bacteria than would be produced under other circumstances, and this effect is independent of the pH effect. Lactulose enemas are much more effective than warm water enemas in reducing blood ammonia concentrations and improving clinical signs.[263] Lactulose is diluted with warm water (30 per cent lactulose, 70 per cent water) and given as a

TABLE 89–4. COMMON PRECIPITATING CAUSES OF HEPATIC COMA

Cause	Proposed Mechanism Producing Coma
Increased dietary protein	Source for NH_3, false neurotransmitters, SCFA
Gastrointestinal hemorrhage	Provides substrate for increased ammonia (100 ml blood yields 15 to 20 gm of protein)
	Hypovolemia may compromise hepatic, cerebral, and renal function; decreased renal perfusion leads to urea retention and increased ammonia production
	Transfusions: Storage of blood for 1 day = 170 μg/100 ml, 4 days = 330 μg/100 ml, 21 days = 900 μg/100 ml
	Role of shock and/or hypoxia
Diuretics	Induced hypokalemic alkalosis, increased renal vein ammonia, enhanced ammonia transfer across blood brain barrier
	Overzealous diuresis (+ paracentesis) may lead to hypovolemia and prerenal uremia
	Separate role of acetazolamide and hypokalemia on cerebral function
Sedatives and anesthetics	Direct depressive effect on brain; hypoxia
Uremia	Increased enterohepatic circulation of urea nitrogen and thus ammonia production
	Direct cerebral effect of uremia
Infection	Increased tissue catabolism leading to increased endogenous urea nitrogen load and increased ammonia
	Dehydration and diminished renal function
	Hypoxia and hyperthermia may potentiate ammonia toxicity
Constipation	Increased production and absorption of ammonia and other nitrogenous derivatives

retention enema. Approximately 10 to 15 ml/lb is infused and retained in the colon for 20 to 30 minutes before evacuation. The pH of the evacuated fluid is measured, and if greater than 6.0, another lactulose enema should be administered. Improvement in neurologic status can occur in two hours in humans.

As soon as patients are able to tolerate oral liquids, attempts should be made to "sterilize" the gut. Nonabsorbable intestinal antibiotics are used to suppress potent urea-splitting intestinal flora, which contribute significantly to blood ammonia concentrations. The antibiotic used most commonly for this purpose is neomycin sulfate, although kanamycin, vancomycin, and paromomycin may be used interchangeably. The recommended dose for use in dogs and cats is ten mg/lb three to four times daily. Other beneficial effects of the use of oral antibiotics are to decrease bacterial deamination of amino acids and reduce the production of aromatic amino acids, circulating false neurotransmitters, and short chain fatty acids by gut bacteria.[261, 266] Occasional rare complications to the chronic use of neomycin are oto- and nephrotoxicity, severe diarrhea, and intestinal malabsorption.[267] A number of other systemically absorbed antibiotics may be used in animals with hepatic failure as alternatives to aminoglycosides. One that has received a great deal of interest is metronidazole (Flagyl). Metronidazole is active against many of the urease-positive, gram-negative anaerobes, which are potent generators of ammonia in the intestinal tract.[268, 269] Most clinical studies have indicated that metronidazole is equal in effectiveness to neomycin in controlling blood ammonia concentrations.[269] The recommended dose is nine mg/lb given every eight hours. Toxicity to metronidazole has not been reported in dogs and cats, but in humans, nausea, ataxia, dizziness, and paresthesias occur.[270] Many animals will also respond to other antibiotics, such as ampicillin, which are effective against intestinal anaerobes. These animals improve clinically while receiving antibiotics but develop signs of illness when antibiotics are stopped. This likely corresponds to the effect the drug has on GI flora, an effect that stops soon after the drug is discontinued.

Oral lactulose may be used as an alternative to, or in conjunction with, intestinal antibiotics in the management of hepatic coma. Most surveys indicate that lactulose alone or neomycin alone provides clinical improvement in 80 per cent of humans with chronic encephalopathy.[260, 271–273] An additional group of patients will benefit from the combination of neomycin and lactulose since these are sometimes synergistic. Because these two drugs control intestinal ammonia formation by different mechanisms, this should not be surprising. It is interesting that neomycin does not impair the effectiveness of lactulose in most patients. Since lactulose requires metabolism by intestinal bacteria and neomycin kills bacteria, one would think that oral antibiotics would be contraindicated for maximal effectiveness of lactulose. This is not the case. Neomycin inhibits bacterial degradation of lactulose in less than one-third of patients.[274–276] Lactulose is degraded by lactulosophilic bacteria of which *Bacteroides* spp. predominate. *Bacteroides* spp. are fairly resistant to the effects of neomycin. To determine whether lactulose degradation is occurring

in animals receiving both drugs, stool pH should be measured after 7 to 14 days of combined therapy. If the stool pH is lower than 6.0, then the lactulose is being metabolized and neomycin is not impairing its effectiveness. If the stool pH remains around 7.0, lactulose will be ineffective and should be discontinued. Lactulose is dosed so that a decrease in fecal pH is produced, but diarrhea is avoided. Usually cats require 2.5 to 5 ml three times daily and dogs require 2.5 to 25 ml three times daily. If watery diarrhea develops, the dosage should be reduced.

Alternative methods of controlling hepatic encephalopathy may be tried but are not likely to be as effective as lactulose and neomycin. Attempts may be made to repopulate the colon with lactose-fermenting, non-urease-containing bacteria such as lactobacilli. Unfortunately, supplementing the diet with lactobacillus-containing drugs or yogurt in quantities sufficient to maintain desirable flora in adequate numbers has not had much clinical success.[277]

Specifically formulated intravenous solutions containing primarily branched chain amino acids as the nitrogen source have been marketed for use in the therapy of acute hepatic encephalopathy (Hepatamine). These solutions are designed to help normalize plasma amino acid patterns by decreasing muscle catabolism. Decreasing muscle breakdown reduces the concentration of circulating aromatic amino acids, which are considered to be important in the genesis of hepatic encephalopathy. Experimental work in encephalopathic dogs indicates that use of these preparations results in marked improvement in neurologic status.[149, 278] However, the majority of the published results in humans with chronic encephalopathy does not support any significant benefit over other well balanced amino acid solutions.[197, 279–281] Clinicians must be extremely cautious when using inexpensive intravenous protein hydrolysates in animals in hepatic coma. Such solutions have extremely high ammonia concentrations, 1500 to 1900 μgm/dl, and may rapidly worsen the clinical status of the patient.[282] Stored blood may also be dangerous in this regard.

Another drug that may be considered for use in encephalopathic dogs or cats that fail to respond to traditional therapy is levodopa (Larodopa, Roche). Levodopa is a precursor to norepinephrine and dopamine, and when given orally, it raises cerebral dopamine concentrations.[283] It has been used with some success in humans with acute hepatic coma. Patients usually respond by regaining full consciousness in 6 to 12 hours. Unfortunately, responses may be transient even though therapy is continued. The recommended dosage, based on those used in humans, would be an initial dose of 15 mg/lb followed by 3 mg/lb every six hours. No information regarding the safety or efficacy of levodopa in animals is available.

Oral cation exchange resins such as cholestyramine have been used in humans and experimental animals to decrease the absorption of endotoxins from the intestines.[284, 285] Reticuloendothelial function of the liver is known to be impaired in cirrhosis and predisposes patients to bacterial infections.[286] Cholestyramine binds bacterial endotoxin and prevents it from being absorbed systemically. No dosage is available for dogs and cats.

Additional supportive measures may be necessary in the management of animals with hepatic encephalopathy. Parenteral fluid therapy is often required for several days in patients with hepatic failure, and the fluid you choose can be an important therapeutic decision. Animals with chronic liver failure are often hypokalemic, alkalotic, and prone to sodium retention.[137] The ideal fluid should be supplemented with potassium, low in sodium, and nonalkalinizing. Sodium bicarbonate is given only if metabolic acidosis develops and is severe (pH is less than 7.1). Fluids containing lactate may be ineffective as alkalinizing agents, since the liver is the site of conversion for lactate to bicarbonate and glucose. Either half-strength saline (0.45 per cent) or half-strength saline plus 2.5 per cent dextrose is a good choice for fluid needs in the liver failure animal. These fluids should be supplemented with approximately 20 mEq/L of potassium chloride. Glucose supplementation is beneficial in preventing hypoglycemia, in decreasing peripheral catabolic processes, and in decreasing brain ammonia concentrations.

Ascites and Edema. Ascites is a fairly common complication of chronic hepatic failure, while peripheral edema is very infrequent. Ascites, although varying in severity, is not necessarily harmful. Moderate amounts have minimal physiologic importance. When ascites is severe (marked by the presence of respiratory distress or hypotension), therapy should be directed at reducing the volume pharmacologically or mechanically and also toward measures that will improve hepatic function. Patients with advanced hepatic failure and ascites may not have significant diuresis until there is improvement in hepatic function.

Low sodium diets and diuretics are the most commonly used means of controlling ascites formation. If these methods fail, mechanical measures such as peritoneovenous or portocaval shunting procedures may be tried. Low sodium diets and diuretics form the basis for management of most cases. Salt restriction must be severe in cirrhotic animals in order to effectively manage ascites and may require reductions in sodium intake that are much below those used in congestive heart failure.[287] Commercially available low sodium diets (k/d, h/d) may be tried initially, but if a poor response is noted, home-formulated diets should be tried.[231] Ultralow sodium intake is on the order of 7 mg/lb/day (15 mg/kg/day) in dogs.

Active sodium reabsorption by the kidney plays a major role in the development and perpetuation of cirrhotic ascites. Potent "loop" diuretics are useful in many cases in preventing this reabsorption and inducing a diuresis. Either furosemide (0.5 to 1 mg/lb every 8 to 12 hours) or ethacrynic acid may be used. If a significant diuresis does not develop in 4 to 7 days, the initial dose is doubled. If there is no response to this increased dose, an aldosterone antagonist should be added to the therapy. A number of complications can develop following furosemide administration in cirrhotic patients, nearly all of which are dose related.[288] The most important are electrolyte disturbances (hypokalemia, hypochloremia, and hyponatremia), hypovolemia, and hepatic coma. Periodic serum electrolyte profiles need to be evaluated in animals receiving potent diuretics for

any period of time. In addition, animals must be monitored carefully to avoid inducing dehydration.

Some animals fail to respond to furosemide. This probably reflects the fact that serum aldosterone levels are very high in many cirrhotics.[289] Hyperaldosteronism causes significant reabsorption of sodium in the distal tubules. Since furosemide promotes sodium excretion primarily from the loop of Henle, much of the sodium that reaches the distal tubules is reabsorbed under the influence of aldosterone, negating furosemide's diuretic effect. Aldosterone antagonists should be used in animals whose ascites is refractory to furosemide. Ascitic human cirrhotics who are refractory to furosemide usually respond when spironolactone (Aldactone or Aldactone-A) or triamterene is added to the diuretic regime.[289] Spironolactone should be administered at 0.5 to 1 mg/lb twice daily. Response may take several days to be noted. If neither a diuresis nor a decrease in ascites is noted, the dosage of spironolactone should be doubled. In humans, dosages of spironolactone may be 6 to 20 times the usual recommended dose before an appropriate diuresis is produced.[290] In humans, it is possible to predict those who are likely to need large doses of spironolactone by measuring the U_{Na}/U_K ratio.[290] Patients likely to respond poorly to low dosages of aldosterone antagonists have U_{Na}/U_K ratios of less than 1.0, while those with good initial responses have ratios greater than 1.0. Potassium supplements should *not* be given to patients receiving aldosterone antagonists, as this may lead to hyperkalemia.

Do not attempt to remove ascites too vigorously through pharmacologic means. Ascitic fluid has a maximal rate of mobilization of 700 to 900 ml/day in humans. Any net fluid loss beyond this is at the expense of plasma water. Patients are not normally allowed more than 200 to 300 ml of net water loss per day (0.2 to 0.3 kg/day weight loss).[291] Diuretics should be stopped once ascites is no longer clinically evident. If it reoccurs after drug withdrawal, the lowest dosage necessary to control ascites build-up should be continued indefinitely. If serum albumin concentrations can be raised, ascites will often spontaneously regress.

If two weeks of salt restriction and appropriate diuretic use do not result in significant reductions in the degree of ascites present, more heroic measures should be considered. Such measures include intermittent paracentesis, surgical implantation of some type of peritoneovenous shunt, and creating a surgical portocaval shunt. Paracentesis for removal of ascites should generally be avoided except as a temporary measure to provide immediate relief for a dyspneic or painful patient or for patients in which aggressive medical therapy has been unsuccessful. Small quantities may be removed for diagnostic purposes. Complications associated with paracentesis of patients in hepatic failure include albumin depletion, peritonitis, hypovolemia, hepatic coma, and oliguria.[292]

Two surgical procedures have been used clinically in humans and experimentally in dogs to control chronic, diuretic, resistant ascites. The first is the LaVeen shunt, initially developed in 1972. The LaVeen shunt is a one-way pressure-actuated valve. The valve is inserted into the peritoneal cavity and connected by subcutaneous tubing to the jugular vein. Ascitic fluid is propelled into the venous system by the pumping action of the diaphragm.[293] Such surgical drainage systems have been well tolerated by experimental dogs.[294] These shunts are often successful in controlling ascites in humans; however, their use is associated with many major complications.[290, 295] Shunt failure due to clogging of the valve occurs in 10 per cent of cases. An alternative surgical procedure for ascites management is the creation of a portal-systemic venous shunt. Such shunts decompress the portal system and relieve portal hypertension. If portal hypertension can be alleviated, ascites may disappear. Unfortunately, this procedure is associated with high surgical mortality, and patients are prone to develop hepatic coma. The trade-off lies in whether the ascites is a worse problem than managing the encephalopathy.

Intercurrent Infections. Intercurrent infections are one of the most frequent complications of hepatic cirrhosis. Gram-negative septicemias often develop in humans, with the bowel being the presumed source of the infection. Because many cases of chronic active liver disease are associated with a nonspecific fever, an infection tends to be overlooked and must be guarded against. The normal dog liver harbors anaerobic gram-positive organisms that may proliferate if hypoxic conditions develop within the liver. The addition of prophylactic antibiotics to the therapeutic regimen of animals with acute hepatic failure is justified in such cases.

Malabsorption. Clinically significant malabsorption associated with chronic hepatic and biliary tract diseases is uncommon in animals. Steatorrhea owing to reduced bile salt excretion probably occurs in many cholestatic liver diseases but its magnitude has not been assessed. Several products may help alleviate or reduce the severity of the problem. Oral bile salts may increase the emulsification of triglycerides and aid in the digestion and absorption of intestinal fats (Decholin). These products contain unconjugated fractions that are irritating to the bowel and may cause diarrhea. Neutral fats may be added to the diet in the form of water soluble medium chain triglycerides (Portagen), which do not require the action of lipase or bile salts for absorption. This preparation may increase caloric intake and promote weight gain, but it has the risk of aggravating hepatic encephalopathy because it contains significant quantities of short chain fatty acids. Lastly, occasional cases of biliary tract disease with steatorrhea may benefit from the addition of pancreatic enzymes to the diet.

Hemorrhage and Anemia. Coagulopathies associated with hepatic disease are common, but clinical bleeding associated with the coagulopathy is rare, except in acute fulminant hepatic failure or chronic end-stage liver disease. Abnormalities associated with prothrombin deficiencies are frequent. Prothrombin synthesis is impaired in any hepatic disease that compromises the ability of the liver to synthesize prothrombin from dietary precursors. Chronic cholestatic diseases or prolonged bile duct obstruction can induce vitamin K deficiencies owing to impaired absorption of fat soluble vitamins. If overt hemorrhage occurs secondary to a coagulopathy, fresh whole blood is necessary to provide clotting factors and red blood cells. Injections of parenteral vitamin K_1 0.5

mg/lb/day will reverse hypoprothrombinemia associated with bile duct obstruction but are of no benefit when hemorrhage is secondary to hepatic functional failure. Disseminated intravascular coagulation (DIC) can occur with severe hepatic failure and is very difficult to manage successfully. If evidence for DIC exists, the patient should be transfused and heparin therapy instituted (50 units/lb sq, three times daily). Frequent monitoring of coagulation parameters must be done when heparin is given. Bleeding into the gastrointestinal tract is particularly devastating to patients in hepatic failure. Blood is a highly effective protein source for inducing hepatic coma. If bleeding is secondary to gastric or duodenal ulcers, the patient should be given cimetidine (Tagamet) at 2.5 mg/lb every 8 hours or ranitidine (Zantac) at 0.25 mg/lb every 12 hours. In addition, ulcer protective agents such as sucralfate (Carafate) can be given at 1 gm/60 lbs every 6 hours. Anemia of liver failure is multifactorial. Blood loss, lack of production secondary to malnutrition, and sequestration and destruction of red blood cells all may play a role. If bleeding tendencies can be controlled and the liver disease stabilized or reversed, these anemias will resolve. In most animals, the degree of anemia is not severe and the patient will not need transfusions.

Fulminant Hepatic Failure. Fulminant hepatic failure (FHF) is a syndrome associated with acute, massive necrosis of parenchymal cells and with sudden severe impairment of hepatic function. This syndrome is uncommon in small animals. The causes are variable, but most cases are associated with viral infections (rare) or with exposure to drugs or toxins. The author has observed a number of cases in Bedlington terriers with copper toxicosis. Occasional cases occur following severe abdominal trauma or prolonged hypotension. Before beginning intensive therapy, it is important to be sure that the situation is acute and that the patient is not in end-stage chronic liver failure. This is because acute severe failure is potentially completely reversible, while the outcome of animals with chronic failure is invariably death. The primary goals of therapy are supportive and symptomatic. The animal is supported long enough for sufficient repair and regeneration to occur to allow for survival.

Fulminant hepatic failure is associated with multiple organ system abnormalities that may need to be aggressively managed (Table 89–5). The majority of humans that die in fulminant failure do not succumb from the loss of hepatic parenchyma, rather, they most often die from cerebral edema, hemorrhage, or sepsis.[296–298] Central nervous signs in FHF are due to both hepatic

TABLE 89–5. SYSTEM ABNORMALITIES SEEN IN FULMINANT HEPATIC FAILURE

Major Organ Failure	Metabolic Derangements
Hepatic coma	Jaundice
Cerebral edema	Hypoalbuminemia
Circulatory failure	Coagulopathies
Respiratory failure	GI bleeding (ulcers)
Renal failure	Hypoglycemia
Pancreatitis	Hypothermia
	Electrolyte abnormalities
	Acid-base disorders (alkalosis)
	Sepsis

encephalopathy and cerebral edema. Cerebral edema is not seen in chronic hepatic failure. Cerebral edema of FHF is thought to be primarily of vasogenic origin.[296] Permeability of the blood-brain barrier is altered, allowing circulating toxins and plasma proteins to egress from intracerebral capillaries into the extracellular space. The permeability of the blood-brain barrier is increased by ammonia, short-chain fatty acids, and mercaptans, which are known to be increased in the circulation in FHF. If patients are hypoproteinemic, fluid transudation out of capillaries is also promoted. Determining whether cerebral edema is present and causing some of the CNS signs in these patients is difficult. If the neurologic status of the patient continues to deteriorate in spite of aggressive management of hepatic encephalopathy, it is better to treat for cerebral edema for 12 to 24 hours than do nothing.

Steroids are ineffective in controlling cerebral edema in FHF.[297, 298] Mannitol (20 per cent solution) is given at 0.45 gm/lb/IV (1 gm/kg/IV) over a 30-minute period and is repeated every four hours if the patient does not improve neurologically. Furosemide is also given at 0.5 to 1 mg/lb/IV (1 to 2 mg/kg/IV) every eight hours for two or three doses. If patients are hypoproteinemic, plasma transfusions should be given, if available. Hypoglycemia can be severe in FHF and contribute to the CNS signs. Anorexia, depleted glycogen reserves, and reduced hepatic insulin degradation all contribute to this effect. Intravenous glucose may have to be given as 10 or 20 per cent solutions in order to maintain blood glucose concentrations in the normal range. Frequent blood glucose monitoring is essential.

Sepsis is responsible for the death of 10 to 15 per cent of humans with FHF. It is extremely important to take great care maintaining asepsis in catheter placement and to rapidly control any infections that develop. Broad spectrum antibiotics should be routinely administered.

Hemorrhage occurs early and often in FHF. Bleeding may be evident from any location in the body. Hemorrhage is usually secondary to decreases in prothrombin-dependent clotting factors. Increasing gastric pH to greater than 4.0 with intravenous cimetidine or ranitidine significantly reduces gastrointestinal bleeding.[297] Hemorrhagic tendencies are managed as indicated previously. The use of injectable vitamin K_1 is indicated because it may be rapidly incorporated into prothrombin by newly regenerating hepatocytes.

Renal failure occurs in up to 40 per cent of patients with FHF and is termed hepatorenal syndrome. When present, the prognosis is usually very poor. This appears to be a result of intense renal vasoconstriction, which may cause acute tubular nephrosis. Therapeutic measures are often ineffective in reversing this problem. Prerenal components must be reversed rapidly. Hemodialysis is often necessary in humans to support patients with hepatorenal syndrome.[296]

Glucocorticoids have been used for years in patients with FHF. Recent clinical trials in humans with viral-induced FHF indicate they have no benefit and may be harmful.[254] However, when methylprednisolone was given to rabbits with galactosamine-induced FHF, significantly improved survival was noted when compared

to control animals.[299] Most cases of FHF in humans are viral-induced and it was suggested that steroids may have benefit in nonviral FHF.

References

1. Candlin, FT: Diseases of the liver, pancreas and peritoneum. *In* Catcott, EJ (ed): Canine Medicine, 1st ed. Wheaton, American Veterinary Publications, Inc, 1968.
2. Jarrett, WHF and O'Neil, BW: A new transmissible agent causing acute hepatitis, chronic hepatitis and cirrhosis in dogs. Vet Rec 116:629, 1985.
3. Cobb, LM and McKay, KA: A bacteriological study of the liver of the normal dog. J Comp Pathol 72:92, 1962.
4. Lykkegaard, NM, et al.: Anaerobic bacteriological study of the human liver, with a critical review of the literature. Scand J Gastroenterol 9:671, 1974.
5. Speaman, JG, et al.: Yersinia (Pasturella) pseudotuberculosis infection in a cat. Can Vet J 20:361, 1979.
6. Valentine, BA and Porter, WP: Multiple hepatic abscesses and peritonitis caused by eugonic fermenter-4-bacilli in a pup. JAVMA 183:1324, 1983.
7. Smith, LT: Hepatitis due to *Clostridium perfringens* in a dog. Vet Med Small Anim Clin 75:1380, 1980.
8. Lord, PF, et al.: Emphysematous hepatic abscess associated with trauma, necrotic nodular hyperplasia and adenoma in a dog: A case history report. Vet Radiol 23:46, 1982.
9. Ferber, JA, et al.: Tuberculosis in a dog. JAVMA 183:117, 1983.
10. Grossman, A: Mycobacterial hepatitis associated with long-term steroid therapy. Fel Pract 13:37, 1983.
11. Center, SA: Feline liver disorders and their management. Comp Cont Ed Small Anim Pract 8:889, 1986.
12. Hirsh, VM and Doige, CE: Suppurative cholangitis in cats. JAVMA 182:1223, 1983.
13. Lucke, VM and Davies, JD: Progressive lymphocytic cholangitis in the cat. J Small Anim Pract 25:249, 1984.
14. Prasse, KW, et al.: Chronic lymphocytic cholangitis in three cats. Vet Pathol 19:99, 1982.
15. Rogers, KS, and Cornelius, LM: Feline icterus. Comp Cont Ed Small Anim Pract 7:391, 1985.
16. Zawie, DA and Garvey, MS: Feline hepatic disease. Vet Clin North Am 14:1201, 1984.
17. Center, SA, et al.: Bile acid concentrations in the diagnosis of hepatobiliary diseases in the cat. JAVMA 189:891, 1986.
18. Cornelius, LM and DeNovo, RC: Icterus in cats. *In* Kirk, RW (ed): Current Veterinary Therapy VIII. Philadelphia, WB Saunders, 1983, pp 822–829.
19. Hitt, ME, et al.: The feline liver: Identifying and treating its diseases. Vet Med Small Anim Clin 82:139, 1987.
20. Center, SA, et al.: Diagnostic value of serum gamma glutamyl-transferase and alkaline phosphatase activities in hepatobiliary diseases in the cat. JAVMA 188:507, 1986.
21. Papich, MG and Davis LE: Drugs and the liver. Vet Clin North Am 15:17, 1985.
22. Bielsa, LM and Greiner, EC: Liver flukes (*Platynosomum concinnum*) in cats. JAAHA 21:269, 1985.
23. Levine, ND, et al.: Hepatitis due to *Amphimerus pseudofelineus* in a cat. Ill Vet 1:47, 1958.
24. Rothenbacker, H and Lindquist, WD: Liver cirrhosis and pancreatitis in a cat infected with *Amphimerus pseudofelineus*. JAVMA 143:1099, 1963.
25. Barriga, OO, et al.: Liver flukes (*Platynosomum concinnum*) in an Ohio cat. JAVMA 179:901, 1981.
26. Tuzhilin, SA, et al.: Hepatic lesions in pancreatitis: clinicoexperimental data. Am J Gastroenterol 64:108, 1975.
27. Dew, MJ, et al.: The spectrum of hepatic dysfunction in inflammatory bowel disease. J Med 48:113, 1979.
28. Ettinger, SE and Suter PF: Canine Cardiology. Philadelphia, WB Saunders, 1970.
29. Hunt, CA and Gofton, N: Primary repair of a transected bile duct. JAAHA 20:57, 1984.

30. Watkins, PE, et al.: Traumatic rupture of the bile duct in the dog: a report of seven cases. J Small Anim Pract 24:731, 1983.

31. Harari, J, et al.: Extrahepatic bile duct obstruction due to cholecystitis and cholelithiasis: A case report. JAAHA 18:347, 1982.

32. Peterson, ME: Feline hyperthyroidism. Vet Clin North Am 14:809, 1984.

33. Mackay, JR: Immunologic disorders in liver disease. In Schiff, L and Schiff, ER (eds): Diseases of the Liver, 5th ed. Philadelphia, JB Lippincott, 1982.

34. Kaplan, MM: The spectrum of chronic active liver disease. Hosp Pract 18:67, 1983.

35. Seefe, LB and Koff, RS: Therapy for chronic active hepatitis. Adv Intern Med 29:109, 1984.

36. Zakim, D and Boyer, TD (eds): Hepatology: A Textbook of Liver Disease. Philadelphia, WB Saunders, 1982.

37. Whitcomb, FF: Chronic active liver disease. Definition, diagnosis and management. Med Clin North Am 63:413, 1979.

38. Gitlin, N: Corticosteroid therapy for chronic active hepatitis. Am J Gastroenterol 79:573, 1984.

39. Eddleston, AL: Immunology of chronic active hepatitis. J Med 55:191, 1985.

40. Fitzgerald, JF: Chronic hepatitis. Semin Liver Dis 2:282, 1982.

41. Schalm, SW: Treatment of chronic active hepatitis. Liver 2:69, 1982.

42. Mackay, JR: Immunologic aspects of chronic active hepatitis. Hepatology 3:724, 1983.

43. Neuberg, J, et al.: Effect of polyunsaturated phosphatidylcholine immune mediated hepatocyte damage. Gut 24:751, 1983.

44. Stefannini, GF, et al.: Relationship between lymphocytotoxicity to rabbit hepatocytes and circulating antibodies against hepatocyte membrane antigens in chronic active hepatitis. Gastroenterol Clin Biol 6:971, 1982.

45. O'Brien, CJ, et al.: Cell mediated immunity and suppressor T-cell defects to liver-derived antigens in families of patients with autoimmune chronic active hepatitis. Lancet 1:350, 1986.

46. Thornburg, LP: Chronic active hepatitis. What is it, and does it occur in dogs. JAAHA 18:21, 1982.

47. Popper, H: Changing concepts of the evolution of clinical hepatitis and the role of piecemeal necrosis. Hepatology 3:758, 1983.

48. Wu PC, et al.: Prednisolone in HBsAg-positive chronic active hepatitis: Histologic evaluation in a controlled prospective study. Hepatology 2:777, 1982.

49. Czaja, AJ, et al.: Autoimmune features as determinants of prognosis in steroid treated chronic active hepatitis of uncertain etiology. Gastroenterology 85:713, 1983.

50. Muting D, et al.: Is chronic active hepatitis curable? Lancet 17:905, 1982.

51. Doige, CE and Lester, S: Chronic active hepatitis in dogs: A review of fourteen cases. JAAHA 17:725, 1981.

52. Chen, TS, et al.: Studies of nucleic acid and collagen synthesis: Current status in assessing liver repair. Med Clin North Am 63:583, 1979.

53. Popper, H and Schaffner, F: Chronic hepatitis: Taxonomic, etiologic and therapeutic problems. In Popper, H and Schaffner, F (eds): Progress in Liver Diseases, Vol 5. New York, Grune & Stratton, 1976.

54. Bishop, L, et al.: Chronic active hepatitis in dogs associated with leptospires. Am J Vet Res 40:839, 1979.

55. Bunch, SE, et al.: Compromised hepatic function in dogs treated with anticonvulsant drugs. JAVMA 184:444, 1984.

56. Gocke, DJ, et al.: Experimental viral hepatitis in the dog: Production of persistent disease in partially immune animals. J Clin Invest 46:1506, 1967.

57. Hardy, RM, et al.: Chronic progressive hepatitis in Bedlington terriers associated with elevated liver copper concentrations. Minn Vet 15:13, 1975.

58. Johnson, GF, et al.: Chronic active hepatitis in doberman pinschers. JAVMA 180:1438, 1982.

59. Thornburg, LP, et al.: Hereditary copper toxicosis in west highland white terriers. Vet Pathol 23:166, 1986.

60. Barton, C: Chronic active hepatic disease with cirrhosis in a dog. Missouri Vet 28:17, 1977.

61. Meyer, DJ and Burrows, CF: The liver, part II. Biochemical diagnosis of hepatobiliary disorders in the dog. Comp Cont Ed Pract Vet 4:706, 1982.

62. Meyer, DJ, et al.: Obstructive jaundice associated with chronic active hepatitis. JAVMA 176:41, 1980.

63. Strombeck, DR and Gribble, DG: Chronic active hepatitis in the dog. JAVMA 173:380, 1978.

64. Strombeck, DR, et al.: Chronic active hepatic disease in a dog. JAVMA 169:802, 1976.

65. Thornburg, LP, et al.: An unusual case of chronic active hepatitis in a kerry blue terrier. Vet Med Small Anim Clin 76:363, 1981.

66. Magne, ML and Chiapella, AM: Medical management of canine chronic active hepatitis. Comp Cont Ed Small Anim Pract 8:915, 1986.

67. Jenkins, PJ, et al.: Use of polyunsaturated phosphatidyl choline in HBsAG negative chronic active hepatitis: Results of a prospective double-blind controlled trial. Liver 2:77, 1982.

68. Johnson, GF, et al.: Inheritance of copper toxicosis in Bedlington terriers. Am J Vet Res 41:1865, 1980.

69. Watson, ADJ, et al.: Copper storage disease with intravascular haemolysis in a Bedlington terrier. Aust Vet J 60:305, 1983.

70. Su, LC, et al.: A defect of biliary excretion of copper in copper-laden Bedlington terriers. Am J Physiol 243:231, 1982.

71. Keen, CL, et al.: Age related variations in hepatic iron, copper, zinc, and selenium concentrations in beagles. Am J Vet Res 42:1884, 1981.

72. Johnson, GF, et al.: Cytochemical detection of inherited copper toxicosis of Bedlington terriers. Vet Pathol 21:57, 1984.

73. Twedt, DC, et al.: Clinical, morphologic and chemical studies on copper toxicosis of Bedlington terriers. JAVMA 175:269, 1979.

74. Ludwig, J, et al.: The liver in the inherited copper disease of Bedlington terriers. Lab Invest 43:82, 1980.

75. Su, LC, et al.: A comparison of copper-loading disease in Bedlington terriers and Wilson's disease in humans. Am J Physiol 243:6226, 1982.

76. Hultgren, BD, et al.: Inherited chronic progressive hepatic degeneration in Bedlington terriers with increased liver copper concentrations: Clinical pathologic observations and comparison with other copper associated liver diseases. Am J Vet Res 47:365, 1986.

77. Thornburg, LP, et al.: Histochemical demonstration of copper and copper associated protein in the canine liver. Vet Pathol 22:327, 1985.

78. Thornburg, LP and Rottinghaus, G: What is the significance of hepatic copper in dogs with cirrhosis? Vet Med 80:50, 1985.

79. Robertson, HM, et al.: Inherited copper toxicosis in Bedlington terriers. Aust Vet J 60:235, 1983.

80. Hunsaker, HA, et al.: 2-3-2-tetramine as a hepatic copper chelator in treatment of copper hepatotoxicity in Bedlington terrier dogs. JAVMA (accepted for publication).

81. Allen, KGD, et al.: Tetramine cupruretic agents: A comparison in dogs. Am J Vet Res 48:28, 1987.

82. Brewer, GJ, et al.: Oral zinc therapy for Wilson's disease. Ann Intern Med 99:314, 1983.

83. Hoogenraad, TU and Rothuizen, J: Compliance in Wilson's disease and in copper toxicosis of Bedlington terriers. Lancet 2:170, 1986.

84. Owen, CA and McCall, JT: Identification of the carrier of the Bedlington terrier copper disease. Am J Vet Res 44:694, 1983.

85. Crawford, MA, et al.: Chronic active hepatitis in 26 doberman pinschers. JAVMA 187:1343, 1985.

86. Crawford, MA, et al.: Hepatopathy in 24 doberman pinscher dogs. Proceedings of the 2nd Annual Forum and 12th Annual Coll Prog ACVIM:34, 1984.

87. Thornburg, LP, et al.: High liver copper levels in two doberman pinschers with subacute hepatitis. JAAHA 20:1003, 1984.

88. Feldman, BF, et al.: Anemia of inflammatory disease in the dog: Measurement of hepatic superoxide dismutase, hepatic non-heme iron, copper, zinc, and ceruloplasm, and serum iron, copper and zinc. Am J Vet Res 42:1114, 1981.

89. Thornburg, LP and Crawford, SJ: Hereditary copper associated liver diseases in West Highland White Terriers. Vet Rec (in press).

90. Thornburg, LP, et al.: The diagnosis and treatment of copper toxicosis in dogs. Canine Pract 11:36, 1984.

91. Thornburg, LP, et al.: Copper toxicosis in dogs, part 3: Diagnosis and treatment. Canine Pract 13:10, 1986.

92. Christian, MK: Liver disease in Skye terriers. Vet Rec 114:127, 1984.

93. Bennett, AM, et al.: Lobular dissecting hepatitis in the dog. Vet Pathol 20:179, 1983.

94. Thornburg, LP, et al.: Hereditary copper toxicosis in west highland white terriers. Vet Pathol 23:148, 1986.

95. Van den Ingh, TS and Rothuizen, J: Hepatoportal fibrosis in three young dogs. Vet Rec 110:575, 1982.

96. Jeffries, GH: Diseases of the liver. *In* Beeson, PB and Mc-Dermott, W (eds): Cecil and Loeb Textbook of Medicine. 13th ed. Philadelphia, WB Saunders, 1971.

97. Smith, AR, et al.: Sulfur containing amino acids in experimental hepatic coma in the dog and monkey. Surgery 85:677, 1979.

98. Jubb, KVF and Kennedy, PC: The liver and biliary systems. *In* Jubb, KVF and Kennedy, PC (eds): Pathology of Domestic Animals, 2nd ed. New York, Academic Press, 1970.

99. Zimmerman, HJ: Drug-induced liver disease. Drugs 16:25, 1978.

100. Mitchell, JR and Potter, WZ: Drug metabolism in the production of liver disease. Med Clin North Am 59:877, 1975.

101. Schaffner, F and Popper, H: Adverse drug reactions involving the liver: Probable mechanisms. Mt Sinai J Med 44:813, 1977.

102. Zimmerman, HJ: Liver disease caused by medicinal agents. Med Clin North Am 59:897, 1975.

103. Maddrey, WC: Drug and chemical induced hepatic injury. *In* Berk, JE (ed): Bockus Gastroenterology. 4th ed. Philadelphia, WB Saunders, 1985.

104. Black, M: Hepatotoxicity: Pathogenesis and therapeutic intervention. Clin Gastroenterol 8:89, 1979.

105. Kaplowitz, N, et al.: Drug induced hepatotoxicity. Ann Intern Med 104:826, 1986.

106. Wilcke, JR: Idiosyncrasies of drug metabolism in cats. Vet Clin North Am Small Anim Pract 14:1345, 1984.

107. Scheuer, PJ and Bianchi, L: Guidelines for diagnosis of therapeutic drug induced liver injury in liver biopsies. Lancet 1:854, 1974.

108. Koets, BE and Langfitt, M: Drugs and the liver. Comp Ther 10:55, 1984.

109. Rogers, WA and Ruebner, BH: A retrospective study of probable glucocorticoid induced hepatopathy in dogs. JAVMA 170:603, 1977.

110. Badylak, SF and VanFleet, JF: Tissue gamma glutamyl transpeptidase activity and hepatic ultrastructural alterations in dogs with experimentally induced glucocorticoid hepatopathy. Am J Vet Res 43:649, 1982.

111. Wellman, ML, et al.: Immunoassay for the steroid induced isoenzyme of alkaline phosphatase in the dog. Am J Vet Res 43:1200, 1982.

112. Peterson, ME: Hyperadrenocorticism. Vet Clin North Am Small Anim Pract 14:731, 1984.

113. Badylak, SF and VanFleet, JF: Sequential morphologic and clinicopathologic alterations in dogs with experimentally induced glucocorticoid hepatopathy. Am J Vet Res 42:1310, 1981.

114. Meyer, DJ: Prolonged liver test abnormalities and adrenocortical suppression in a dog following a single intramuscular glucocorticoid dose. JAAHA 18:725, 1982.

115. DeNovo, RC and Prasse, KW: Comparison of serum biochemical and hepatic functional alterations in dogs treated with corticosteroids and hepatic duct ligation. Am J Vet Res 44:1703, 1983.

116. Dillon, AR, et al.: Effects of dexamethazone and surgical hypotension on hepatic morphologic features and enzymes of dogs. Am J Vet Res 44:1996, 1983.

117. Dillon, AR, et al.: Prednisolone induced hematologic, biochemical and histologic changes in the dog. JAAHA 16:831, 1980.

118. Fittschen, C and Bellany, JEC: Prednisone induced morphologic and chemical changes in the liver of dogs. Vet Pathol 21:399, 1984.

119. Thompson, SW, et al.: Vacuoles in the hepatocytes of cortisone treated dogs. Am J Pathol 63:135, 1971.

120. Bunch, SE, et al.: Compromised hepatic function in dogs treated with anticonvulsant drugs. JAVMA 184:444, 1984.

121. Bunch, SE, et al.: Effects of long-term primidone and phenytoin administration on canine hepatic function and morphology. Am J Vet Res 46:105, 1985.

122. Bunch, SE, et al.: Toxic hepatopathy and intrahepatic cholestasis associated with phenytoin administration in combination with other anticonvulsant drugs in three dogs. JAVMA 190:194, 1987.

123. Meyer, DJ and Noonan, NE: Liver tests in dogs receiving anticonvulsant drugs (diphenylhydantoin and primidone). JAAHA 17:261, 1981.

124. Nash, AJ: Phenytoin toxicity: A fatal case in the dog with hepatitis and jaundice. Vet Rec 1:280, 1977.

125. Farnbach, GC: Efficacy of primidone in dogs with seizures unresponsive to phenobarbital. JAVMA 185:867, 1984.

126. Polzin, DJ, et al.: Acute hepatic necrosis associated with the administration of mebendazole. JAMVA 179:1013, 1981.

127. Hardy, RM, et al.: Periportal hepatitis associated with the use of a heartworm-hookworm preventative (diethylcarbamazine oxibendazole) in thirteen dogs. JAAHA (accepted for publication).

128. Gaunt, PS, et al.: Hepatic necrosis associated with the use of halothane in a dog. JAVMA 184:478, 1984.

129. Nidirtu, CG and Weigel, J: Hepatorenal injury in a dog associated with methoxyflurane (a case report). Vet Med Small Anim Clin 72:545, 1977.

130. Thornburg, LP amd Rottinghaus, GB: Drug induced hepatic necrosis in a dog. JAVMA 183:327, 1983.

131. Moriello, KA: Ketoconazole: Clinical pharmacology and therapeutic recommendations. JAVMA 188:303, 1986.

132. Sherding, RG: Acute hepatic failure. Vet Clin North Am 15:119, 1985.

133. Anderson, WI, et al.: Hepatitis in a dog given sulfadiazine-trimethoprim and cyclophosphamide. Modern Vet Pract 65:115, 1984.

134. Toth, DM and Derulis, SK: Drug induced hepatitis in a dog: A case report. Vet Med Small Anim Clin 75:421, 1980.

135. Stomar, VD and McKnight, ED: Acetylcysteine for treatment of acetaminophen toxicosis in the cat. JAVMA 176:911, 1980.

136. Harvey, JW and Kornick, HP: Phenazopyridine toxicosis in the cat. JAVMA 169:327, 1976.

136a. Pond, EC and Morrow, D: Hepatotoxicity associated with methotrexate in a dog. J Small Anim Pract 23:659,1982.

137. Twedt, DC: Cirrhosis: A consequence of chronic liver disease. Vet Clin North Am 15:151, 1985.

138. Anthony, PP, et al.: The morphology of cirrhosis: Definition, nomenclature, and classification. Bull WHO 55:521, 1977.

139. Smith, HA, et al.: Veterinary Pathology, Philadelphia, Lea & Febiger, 1972.

140. Rojkind, M and Kershenobich, D: Hepatic Fibrosis. *In* Popper, H and Schaffner, F (eds): Progress in Liver Diseases, Vol 5. New York, Grune & Stratton, 1976.

141. Silk, DBA and Williams, R: Portal Hypertension. *In* Wright, R, Alberti, KGM and Karran, S (eds): Liver and Biliary Disease. Philadelphia, WB Saunders, 1979.

142. Ng, BK and Noor, F: Hepatic cirrhosis with duodenal ulcers in a dog. Aust Vet Pract 11:14, 1981.

143. O'Keefe, SJ: Protein turnover in acute and chronic liver disease. Acta Chir Scand Suppl 507:91, 1981.

144. Hein, MF: The effect of portacaval shunting on gastric acid secretion in cirrhotic dogs. Gastroenterology 44:637, 1963.

145. Millward-Sadler, GH and Wright, R: Cirrhosis: An Appraisal. *In* Wright, R, Alberti, KGM and Karran, S (eds): Liver and Biliary Diseases. Philadelphia, WB Saunders, 1979.

146. Johnson, SE, et al.: Determination of serum bile acids in fasting dogs with hepatobiliary disease. Am J Vet Res 46:2048, 1985.

147. Pagliaro, L, et al.: Percutaneous blind biopsy versus laparoscopy with guided biopsy in diagnosis of cirrhosis. A prospective randomized trial. Dig Dis Sci 28:39, 1983.

148. Wondwosen, A, et al.: Sampling variability on percutaneous liver biopsy. Arch Intern Med 139:667, 1979.

149. Breznock, EM and Whiting, PG: Portacaval shunts and anomalies. *In* Slatter, DH (ed): Textbook of Small Animal Surgery. Philadelphia, WB Saunders, 1985, pp 1156-1173.

150. Johnson, SE: Portal hypertension, part II: Clinical assessment and treatment. Comp Cont Ed Small Anim Pract 9:917, 1987.

151. Audell, I, et al.: Congenital portal caval shunts in the dog. A description of three cases. Zentralbl Veterinarmed 21:797, 1974.

152. Barrett, RE: Four cases of congenital portacaval shunt in the dog. J Small Anim Pract 17:71, 1976.

153. Berger B, et al.: Congenital feline portosystemic shunts. JAVMA 188:517, 1986.

154. Breznock, EM, et al.: Surgical manipulation of intrahepatic portocaval shunts in dogs. JAVMA 182:798, 1983.

155. Birchard, SJ: Surgical management of porto-systemic shunts in dogs and cats. Comp Cont Ed Small Anim Pract 6:795, 1984.

156. Carr, SH and Thornburg, LP: Congenital portacaval shunt in two kittens. Fel Pract 14:43, 1984.

157. Center, SA, et al.: Congenital portosystemic shunts in cats. *In* Kirk, RW (ed): Current Veterinary Therapy, Vol IX. Philadelphia, WB Saunders, 1986, pp 825-830.

158. Cornelius, LM, et al.: Anomalous portosystemic anastomoses associated with chronic hepatic insufficiency in six young dogs. JAVMA 167:220, 1975.

159. Ewing, GO, et al.: Hepatic insufficiency associated with congenital anomalies of the portal vein in dogs. JAAHA 10:463, 1974.

160. Gondolfi, RC: Hepatoencephalopathy associated with patent ductus venosus in a cat. JAVMA 185:301, 1984.

161. Grauer, GE and Pitts, RP: Primary polydipsia in three dogs with portosystemic shunts. JAAHA 23:197, 1987.

162. Howe, RS and Mullen, HS: An unusual portacaval anomaly as a cause of hepatic encephalopathy in a cat. JAAHA 20:987, 1984.

163. Lohse, CL, et al.: Hepatoencephalopathy associated with situs inversus of abdominal organs and vascular anomalies in a dog. JAVMA 168:687, 1976.

164. Maretta, SM, et al.: Urinary calculi associated with portosystemic shunts in six dogs. JAVMA 178:133, 1981.

165. Rothuizen, J, et al.: Congenital porto-systemic shunts in sixteen dogs and three cats. J Small Anim Pract 23:67, 1982.

166. Scavelli, TD, et al.: Portosystemic shunts in cats: Seven cases. JAVMA 189:317, 1986.

167. Simpson, ST and Hribernik, TN: Portosystemic shunts in the dog. Two case reports. J Small Anim Pract 17:163, 1976.

168. Vulgamott, JC, et al.: Congenital portacaval anomalies in the cat. Two case reports. JAAHA 16:915, 1981.

169. Starzyl, TE, et al.: Intraportal insulin protects from the liver injury of portacaval shunt in dogs. Lancet 2:1741, 1975

170. Starzyl, TE and Tciblanche, J: Hepatotrophic Substances. *In* Popper, H and Schaffner, F (eds): Progress in Liver Diseases, Vol 6. New York, Grune & Stratton, 1979.

171. Griffiths, GL, et al.: Hematologic and biochemical changes in dogs with portosystemic shunts. JAAHA 17:705, 1981.

172. Meyer, DJ: Liver function tests in dogs with portosystemic shunts: Measurement of serum bile acid concentrations. JAVMA 188:168, 1986.

173. Center, SA, et al.: Evaluation of serum bile acid concentrations for the diagnosis of portosystemic venous anomalies in the dog and cat. JAVMA 186:1090, 1985.

174. Hitt, ME and Jones, BD: Effects of storage temperature and time on canine plasma ammonia concentrations. Am J Vet Res 47:363, 1986.

175. Hardy, RM and Klausner, JK: Urate calculi associated with portal vascular anomalies. *In* Kirk, RW (ed): Current Veterinary Therapy, Vol IX. Philadelphia, WB Saunders, 1983, pp 1073–1076.

176. Suter, PF: Portal vein anomalies in the dog: Their angiographic diagnosis. J Am Vet Radiol Soc 16:84, 1975.

177. Wrigley, RH, et al.: Ligation of ductus venosus in a dog using ultrasonographic guidance. JAVMA 183:1461, 1983.

178. Wrigley, RH, et al.: Ultrasonographic diagnosis of portocaval shunts in young dogs. JAVMA 191:421, 1987.

179. Hornoff, WJ, et al.: Radiocolloid scintigraphy as an aid to the diagnosis of congenital portacaval anomalies in the dog. JAVMA 182:44, 1983.

180. Koblik, PD, et al.: Use of quantitative hepatic scintigraphy to evaluate spontaneous portosystemic shunts in twelve dogs. Vet Radiol 24:232, 1983.

181. Maddison, JE: Portosystemic encephalopathy in two young dogs: Some additional diagnostic and therapeutic considerations. J Small Anim Pract 22:731, 1981.

182. Breznock, EM: Surgical manipulation of portosystemic shunts in dogs. JAVMA 174:819, 1979.

183. Gofton, N: Surgical ligation of congenital portosystemic shunts in the dog: A report of three cases. JAAHA 14:728, 1978.

184. Strombeck, DR, et al.: Surgical treatment for portosystemic shunts in two dogs. JAVMA 170:1317, 1977.

185. Martin, RA, et al.: Left hepatic vein attenuation for treatment of patent ductus venosus in a dog. JAVMA 189:1465, 1986.

186. Levesque, DC, et al.: Congenital portacaval shunts in two cats: Diagnosis and surgical correction. JAVMA 181:143, 1982.

187. Ware, W, et al.: Atypical portosystemic shunt in a cat. JAVMA 188:187, 1986.

188. Ogilvie, GK, et al.: Effects of plasma sample storage on blood ammonia, bilirubin and urea nitrogen concentrations: Cats and horses. Am J Vet Res 46:2619, 1985.

189. Moore, PF and Whiting, PG: Hepatic lesions associated with intrahepatic arterioportal fistulae in dogs. Vet Pathol 23:57, 1986.

190. Whiting, PG, et al.: Partial hepatectomy with temporary hepatic vascular occlusion in dogs with hepatic arteriovenous fistulas. Vet Surg 15:171, 1986.

191. Alpers, DH and Sabesis, SM: Fatty Liver: Biochemical and Clinical Aspects. *In* Schiff, L (ed): Diseases of the Liver. Philadelphia, WB Saunders, 1982, pp 813-845.

192. Center, SA: Hepatic lipidosis in the cat. Proceedings of the 4th Annual Veterinary Medicine Forum, Vol 2, 13:71, 1986.

193. Barsanti, JA, et al.: Prolonged anorexia associated with hepatic lipidosis in three cats. Feline Pract 7:52, 1977.

194. Burrows, CF, et al.: Idiopathic feline lipidosis: A syndrome and speculation on its pathogenesis. Florida Vet J 10:18, 1981.

195. Cornelius, LM and Rogers, KS: Idiopathic lipidosis in cats. Modern Vet Pract 66:377, 1985.

196. Thornburg, LP, et al.: Fatty liver syndrome in cats. JAAHA 18:397, 1982.

197. Millikan, WJ, et al.: Total parenteral nutrition with F080 in cirrhotics with subclinical encephalopathy. Ann Surg 197:294, 1983.

198. Rogers, QR, et al.: Amino acid nutrition and metabolism in the cat. Kal Kan Symposium, 1977.

199. Chapoy, PR, et al.: Systemic carnitine deficiency—a treatable inherited lipid storage disease presenting as Reye's syndrome. N Engl J Med 303:1389, 1980.

200. Ling, GV, et al.: Diabetes mellitus in dogs: A review of initial evaluation, immediate and long-term management and outcome. JAVMA 170:521, 1977.

201. Black, AP: A solitary congenital hepatic cyst in a cat. Aust Vet Pract 13:166, 1983.

202. Ingh, TSGAM and Rothuizen, J: Congenital cystic disease of the liver in seven dogs. J Comp Pathol 95:405, 1985.

203. Strombeck, DR, et al.: Hyperammonemia due to a urea cycle enzyme deficiency in two dogs. JAVMA 166:1109, 1975.

204. Batshaw, MI and Brusilow, SW: Treatment of hyperammonemic coma caused by inborn errors of urea synthesis. J Pediatr 97:893, 1980.

205. Mendenhall, CL, et al.: A new therapy for portal systemic encephalopathy. Am J Gastroenterol 81:540, 1986.

206. Thornburg, LP and Moody, GM: Hepatic amyloidosis in a dog. JAAHA 17:721, 1981.

207. Ceh, L, et al.: Glycogenosis type III in the dog. Acta Vet Scand 17:210, 1976.

207a. Rafiquazzaman, M, et al.: Glycogenosis in the dog. Acta Vet Scand 17:196, 1976.

208. Patnaik, AK, et al.: Canine hepatic neoplasms: A clinicopathologic study. Vet Pathol 17:553, 1980.

209. Strombeck, DR: Clinicopathologic features of primary and metastatic neoplastic disease of the liver in dogs. JAVMA 173:267, 1978.

210. Trigo, FJ, et al.: The pathology of liver tumors in the dog. J Comp Pathol 92:21, 1982.

211. Theilen, GH and Madewell, BR: Tumors of the digestive tract. *In* Theilen, GH and Madewell, BR (eds): Veterinary Cancer Medicine. Philadelphia, Lea & Febiger, 1979.

212. Patnaik, AK, et al.: Canine hepatocellular carcinoma. Vet Pathol 18:427, 1981.

213. Strombeck, DR, et al.: Hypoglycemia and hypoinsulinemia associated with hepatoma in a dog. JAVMA 169:811, 1976.

214. Feeney, DA, et al.: Two dimensional, gray scale ultrasonography for assessment of hepatic and splenic neoplasia in the dog and cat. JAVMA 184:68, 1984.

215. Moulton, JE: Tumors of the pancreas, liver, gall bladder and mesothelium. Berkeley, University of California Press, 1978.

216. Honjo, I, et al.: Ligation of a branch of the portal vein for carcinoma of the liver. Am J Surg 30:296, 1975.

216a. Gunn, C, et al.: Hepatic dearterialization in the dog. Am J Vet Res 47:170, 1986.

217. Sciarrino, E, et al.: Adriamycin treatment for hepatocellular carcinoma. Experience with 109 patients. Cancer 56:2751, 1985.

218. Harcum, DB: Hepatic carcinoma in a dog. Canine Pract 10:21, 1983.

219. Magne, ML: Primary epithelial hepatic tumors in the dog. Comp Cont Ed 6:506, 1984.

220. Patnaik, AK, et al.: Canine bile duct carcinoma. Vet Pathol 18:439, 1981.

221. Patnaik, AK, et al.: Canine hepatic carcinoids. Vet Pathol 18:445, 1981.

222. Alexander, RW and Kock, RA: Primary hepatic carcinoid (APUD cell carcinoma) in a cat. J Small Anim Pract 23:767, 1982.

222a. Jeraj, K, et al.: Primary hepatic osteosarcoma in a dog. JAVMA 179:1000,1981.

223. Mulligan, RM: Neoplasms of the Dog. Baltimore, Williams & Wilkins, 1949.

224. Fabry, A, et al.: Nodular hyperplasia of the liver in the Beagle dog. Vet Pathol 19:109, 1982.

225. Analyan, WG: Carcinoid tumors and the carcinoid syndrome. In Sabiston, DC (ed): Textbook of Surgery. Philadelphia, WB Saunders, 1977, pp 1045–1049.

226. Strombeck, DR: Management of chronic active hepatitis. In Kirk, RW (ed): Current Veterinary Therapy, vol 7. Philadelphia, WB Saunders, 1980.

227. Fenton, JCB, et al.: Milk and cheese diet in portal systemic encephalopathy. Lancet 1:164, 1966.

228. Patel, D, et al.: Amino acid adequacy of parenteral casein hydrolysate and oral cottage cheese in patients with gastrointestinal disease as measured by nitrogen balance and blood aminogram. Gastroenterology 65:427, 1973.

229. Kronfeld, DS: Feeding cats and feline nutrition. Comp Cont Ed Pract Vet 5:419, 1983.

230. Bauer, JE: Nutrition and liver function: Nutrient metabolism in health and disease. Comp Cont Ed Small Anim Pract 8:923, 1986.

231. Strombeck, DR, et al.: Dietary therapy for dogs with chronic hepatic insufficiency. In Kirk, RW (ed): Current Veterinary Therapy, vol 8. Philadelphia, WB Saunders, 1983, pp 817–822.

232. Russell, RM: Vitamin and mineral supplements in the management of liver disease. Med Clin North Am 63:537, 1979.

233. Twedt, DC: Jaundice, hepatic trauma, and hepatic encephalopathy. Vet Clin North Am 11:121, 1981.

234. Reding, P, et al.: Oral zinc supplementation improves hepatic encephalopathy: Results of a randomized controlled trial. Lancet 1:493, 1984.

235. Lewis, LD, et al.: Small Animal Clinical Nutrition. 3rd ed. Topeka, Mark Morris Associates, 1987.

236. Maede, Y, et al.: Methionine toxicosis in cats. Am J Vet Res 48:289, 1987.

237. Branam, JE: Suspected methionine toxicosis associated with a portacaval shunt in a dog. JAVMA 181:929, 1982.

238. Thompson, JS, et al.: The dietary prevention of hepatic coma in ECK fistula dogs: Ammonia and the carbohydrate to protein ratio. Surg Gynecol Obstet 162:1265, 1986.

239. Fratta, W, et al.: Benzodiazepine induced voraciousness in cats and inhibition of amphetamine anorexia. Life Sci 18:1157, 1976.

240. Riviere, JE: Calculation of dosage regimens of antimicrobial drugs in animals with renal and hepatic dysfunction. JAVMA 185:1094, 1984.

241. Rosenoer, VM and Gualberto, G: Management of patients with chronic obstructive jaundice. Med Clin North Am 56:759, 1972.

242. Jacobs, I: Antibiotics and liver disease. Calif Med 111:382, 1969.

243. Tams, TR: Hepatic encephalopathy. Vet Clin North Am 15:177, 1985.

244. Hoenig, V: Management of acute liver damage in man. In Popper, H and Schaffner, F (eds): Progress in Liver Diseases vol 3. New York, Grune & Stratton, 1970.

245. Figueroa, RB: Mesterolone in steatosis and cirrhosis of the liver. Acta Hepato-Gastroenterol 20:282, 1973.

246. Gluid, C: Anabolic-androgenic steroid treatment of liver diseases. Liver 4:159, 1984.

247. Islam, N and Islam, A: Testosterone propionate in cirrhosis of the liver. Br J Clin Pract 27:125, 1973.

248. Pulliyel, MM, et al.: Testosterone in the management of cirrhosis of the liver—a controlled study. Aust NZ J Med 7:596, 1977.

249. Heywood, R, et al.: Toxicity of methyl testosterone in the beagle dog. Toxicology 7:357, 1977.

250. Schiff, L: The use of steroids in liver disease. Medicine 45:565, 1966.

251. Rogers, AE: Therapeutic considerations in selected forms of acute and chronic liver disease. Med Clin North Am 55:373, 1971.

252. Christensen, E, et al.: Aspects of the natural history of gastrointestinal bleeding in cirrhosis and the effect of prednisone. Gastroenterology 81:944, 1981.

253. Madsbad, S, et al.: Impaired conversion of prednisone to prednisolone in patients with liver cirrhosis. Gut 21:52, 1980.

254. Tanner, AR and Powell, LW: Corticosteroids in liver disease: Possible mechanisms of action, pharmacology and rational use. Gut 20:1109, 1979.

255. Flowers, RF, et al.: Analgesics, antipyretics and antiinflammatory agents: Drugs used in the therapy of gout. In Goodman, LS and Gilman, A (eds): The Pharmacological Basis of Therapeutics. 6th ed. New York, Macmillan Publishing Co, 1980, pp 718–722.

256. Rojkind, M, et al.: Antiinflammatory and antifibrogenic activities of colchicine: Treatment of liver cirrhosis. Prog Clin Biol Res 154:475, 1984.

257. Kershenobich, D, et al.: Treatment of cirrhosis with colchicine: A double-blind randomized trial. Gastroenterology 77:532, 1979.

258. Kaplan, MM, et al.: A prospective trial of colchicine for primary biliary cirrhosis. N Engl J Med 315:1448, 1986.

259. Boer, HH, et al.: Colchicine therapy for hepatic fibrosis in a dog. JAVMA 185:303, 1984.

260. Fingl, E: Laxatives and cathartics. In Goodman, A and Gilman, LS (eds): The Pharmacological Basis of Therapeutics. 6th ed. New York, Macmillan Publishing Co, 1980, pp 1009–1010.

261. Editorial: Lactulose. Can Med Assoc J 112:203, 1975.

262. Vince, AJ, et al.: Ammonia production by intestinal bacteria: The effects of lactose, lactulose and glucose. J Med Microbiol 13:177, 1980.

263. Van Waes, L: Emergency treatment of portal-systemic encephalopathy with lactulose enemas: A controlled study. Acta Clin Belg 34:122, 1979.

264. Breen, KJ and Schenker, S: Hepatic coma: Present concepts of pathogenesis and therapy. In Popper, H and Schaffner, F (eds): Progress in Liver Diseases, vol 4. New York, Grune & Stratton, 1972.

265. Fischer, JE, et al.: An alternative mechanism for beneficial effects of intestinal sterilization in hepatic encephalopathy. Surg Forum 25:369, 1974.

266. Schenker, S, et al.: Hepatic encephalopathy: Current status. Gastroenterology 66:121, 1974.

267. Maddrey, WC and Weber, FL: Chronic hepatic encephalopathy. Med Clin North Am 39:937, 1975.

268. Grossley, IR and Williams, R: Progress in the treatment of chronic portasystemic encephalopathy. Gut 25:85, 1984.

269. Morgan, MH, et al.: Treatment of hepatic encephalopathy with metronidazole. Gut 23:1, 1982.

270. Farrell, G, et al.: Impaired elimination of metronidazole in decompensated chronic liver disease. Br Med J 287:1845, 1983.

271. Atterbury, CE, et al.: Neomycin-sorbitol and lactulose in the treatment of acute portal systemic encephalopathy. Dig Dis Sci 23:398, 1978.

272. Bircher, J, et al.: Treatment of chronic portal-systemic encephalopathy with lactulose. Am J Med 51:148, 1971.

273. Conn, HO, et al.: Comparison of lactulose and neomycin in the treatment of chronic portal systemic encephalopathy. Gastroenterology 72:573, 1977.

274. Conn, HO and Lieberthal, MM: Lactulose and neomycin: Combined therapy. In Conn, HO and Lieberthal, MM (eds): The Hepatic Coma Syndromes and Lactulose. Baltimore, Williams & Wilkins, 1979, pp 340–345.

275. Orlandi, F, et al.: Comparison between neomycin and lactulose in 173 patients with hepatic encephalopathy. A randomized clinical study. Dig Dis Sci 265:498, 1981.

276. Weber, FL, et al.: Effects of lactulose and neomycin on urea metabolism in cirrhotic subjects. Gastroenterology 82:213, 1982.

277. Fischer, JE and Baldessarini, RJ: Pathogenesis and therapy of hepatic coma. In Popper, H and Schaffner, F (eds): Progress in Liver Diseases, vol 5. New York, Grune & Stratton, 1976.

278. Fruend, H, et al.: Chronic hepatic encephalopathy. Long-term therapy with a branched-chain amino acid enriched diet. J Am Med Assoc 24:347, 1979.

279. McGhee, A, et al.: Comparison of the effects of Hepatic-Aid and a casein modular diet on encephalopathy, plasma amino acids, and nitrogen balance in cirrhotic patients. Ann Surg 197:288, 1983.

280. Michel, H, et al.: Treatment of acute hepatic encephalopathy in cirrhotics with a branched chain amino acid enriched vs a conventional amino acid mixture. A controlled study of 70 patients. Liver 5:282, 1985.

281. Wahren, J, et al.: Is intravenous administration of branched chain amino acids effective in the treatment of hepatic encephalopathy? A multi-center study. Hepatology 3:475, 1983.

282. Strombeck, DR, et al.: Hyperammonemia and hepatic encephalopathy in the dog. JAVMA 166:1105, 1975.

283. Szczerban, J and Rozya, J: Treatment of acute and chronic portal encephalopathy with the precursors of dopamine. Acta Med Pol 20:249, 1979.

284. Nolan, JP and Ali, MV: Effect of cholestyramine on endotoxin toxicity and absorption. Am J Dig Dis 17:161, 1972.

285. Nolan, JP: The role of endotoxin in liver injury. Gastroenterology 69:1346, 1975.

286. Rimola, A, et al.: Reticuloendothelial system phagocyte activity in cirrhosis and its relation to bacterial infections and prognosis. Hepatology 4:53, 1984.

287. Arroyo, V and Rodes, J: Treatment of ascites—a rational approach to the treatment of ascites. Post Grad Med J 51:558, 1975.

288. Nararyo, CA, et al.: Furosemide induced adverse reactions in cirrhosis of the liver. Clin Pharmacol Ther 25:154, 1979.

289. Perez-Ayuso, RM, et al.: Randomized comparative study of efficacy of furosemide versus spironolactone in nonazotemic cirrhosis with ascites. Gastroenterology 85:961, 1983.

290. Rocco, VK and Ware, J: Cirrhotic ascites. Ann Intern Med 105:573, 1986.

291. Boyer, TD and Goldman, TS: Treatment of cirrhotic ascites. Adv Intern Med 31:359, 1986.

292. Zeegen, R and Dawson, AM: The neuro-psychiatric disturbances of liver disease. Br J Clin Pract 22:170, 1968.

293. Wyllie, R, et al.: Ascites: Pathophysiology and management. J Pediatr 97:167, 1980.

294. Levy, M, et al.: Sodium retention in dogs with experimental cirrhosis following removal of ascites by continuous peritoneovenous shunting. J Lab Clin Med 94:933, 1979.

295. Kinney, MJ, et al.: The "hepatorenal" syndrome and refractory ascites. Successful therapy with the LaVeen-type peritoneal-venous shunt and valve. Nephron 23:228, 1979.

296. Corall, I and Williams, R: Management of liver failure. Br J Anaesth 58:234, 1986.

297. Hetzel, DJ: Fulminant hepatic failure. Anesth Intensive Care 13:272, 1985.

298. Payne, JA: Fulminant hepatic failure. Med Clin North Am 70:1067, 1986.

299. Minuk, GY, et al.: A comparative study of the effects of insulin/glucagon infusions, parenteral amino acids and high dose corticosteroids on survival in a rabbit model of fulminant hepatitis. Hepatology 6:73, 1986.

90 EXOCRINE PANCREATIC DISEASE

DAVID A. WILLIAMS

The major function of the exocrine pancreas is to secrete digestive enzymes.[1] The exocrine pancreas also fulfills several other functions (Table 90–1). Pancreatic juice contains substances that play a role in the absorption of cobalamin (vitamin B_{12}),[2-5] zinc,[6] and perhaps other nutrients, as well the coenzyme colipase, a protein that facilitates the action of pancreatic lipase.[7] Bicarbonate in pancreatic juice contributes to the neutralization of gastric acid,[8] and antibacterial factors inhibit bacterial proliferation in the proximal small intestine.[9] Pancreatic secretions also influence the function of the small intestine by contributing to the normal degradation of exposed brush border enzymes[10, 11] and, together with biliary secretions, by exerting a trophic effect on the mucosa.[12, 13] Finally, the pancreas protects itself against autodigestion by several mechanisms, including the synthesis of a specific enzyme inhibitor that is stored and secreted together with the digestive enzymes.[14, 15]

ANATOMY

The pancreas of dogs and cats consists primarily of right and left lobes and a small central body where the lobes join together (Figure 90–1).[16, 17] It develops from ventral and dorsal bud-like primordia that arise from the embryonic small intestine and therefore represents an extension of the glandular mucosa of the duodenum, to which it remains connected by secretory ducts.[17] Since either the dorsal or ventral primordium or their associated ducts may involute during development, there is

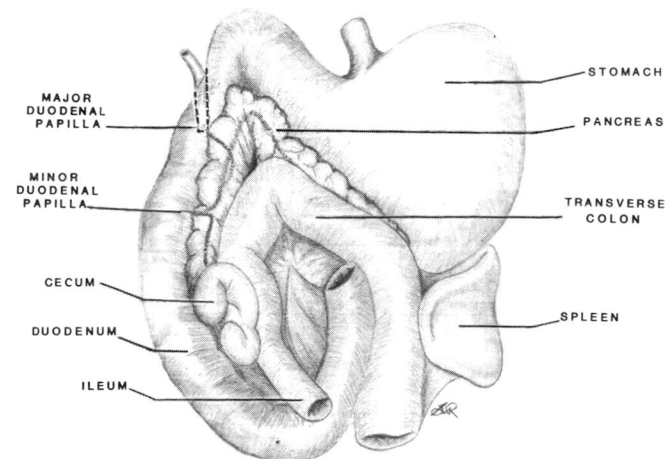

FIGURE 90–1. Anatomic associations of the canine pancreas.

marked species, and to a lesser extent individual, variation in the origin of the gland and the pattern of its duct system.[16, 17] While the areas of pancreas derived from the two primordia resemble one another histologically, that tissue derived from the ventral pancreatic bud, which contributes primarily to the right lobe, contains most of the pancreatic polypeptide-producing cells. In contrast, glucagon-secreting cells predominate in the tissue that develops from the dorsal bud, which contributes primarily to the left lobe.[18]

In the dog both primordia usually persist and fuse, and the two original ducts are retained. The duct of the ventral primordium is the pancreatic duct (Wirsung's duct) and opens adjacent to bile duct on the major duodenal papilla. The duct of the dorsal primordium is the accessory pancreatic duct (Santorini's duct) and opens on the minor duodenal papilla a few centimeters distal to the major duodenal papilla. These two duct systems usually intercommunicate within the gland.[16] In some dogs only the accessory pancreatic duct (the larger of the two) is present, and all pancreatic juice enters the duodenum through the minor duodenal papilla.[16, 17] In the cat only the duct of the ventral primordium, the pancreatic duct, generally persists, and it fuses with the

TABLE 90–1. FUNCTIONS OF THE EXOCRINE PANCREAS

Secretion of digestive enzymes
Secretion of colipase
Secretion of bicarbonate
Facilitation of cobalamin and zinc absorption
Secretion of antibacterial factors
Modulation of intestinal mucosal function
Protection against autodigestion

bile duct before opening on the major duodenal papilla.[17, 19] However, in approximately 20 per cent of cats, the accessory pancreatic duct is also present.[17]

The color of the pancreas varies from pale pink to dark red depending on the amount of blood it contains; it is particularly dark in color following a meal.[1, 17] Anatomically, the pancreas is closely associated with the stomach, liver, and duodenum (Figure 90–1). The body lies in the bend of the cranial part of the duodenum where it is crossed dorsally by the portal vein on its way to the liver.[17] The right lobe lies in the mesoduodenum and accompanies the descending duodenum, in some cases extending to the cecum. The left lobe lies in the deep wall of the greater omentum and accompanies the pyloric part of the stomach to the left where it also makes contact with the liver, transverse colon, and sometimes the left kidney and spleen. Additional accessory pancreatic tissue may be present sporadically in some individuals.[16, 17]

Each microscopic pancreatic lobule is composed mainly of cells that synthesize the digestive enzymes and store them in zymogen granules (acinar cells) and of a smaller number of cells that make up the branching duct system (intralobular, interlobular, and main pancreatic ducts).[16, 17] The cells comprising the initial part of the intralobular, or intercalated, ducts are termed centroacinar cells, and they line the tubular segments of the gland into which acinar cells secrete.[20] These centroacinar cells are the major site of pancreatic bicarbonate and fluid secretion. The pancreas also contains endocrine tissue, the islets of Langerhans, but this accounts for only one to two per cent of the gland, whereas the exocrine tissue together with associated vessels and nerves account for more than 98 per cent of pancreatic mass.

The pancreas is well supplied with blood by branches of the celiac and cranial mesenteric arteries.[16] The main vessels to the right lobe are the cranial and caudal pancreaticoduodenal arteries that anastomose within the gland and arise from the celiac and cranial mesenteric arteries respectively. The left lobe is supplied predominantly by the pancreatic branch of the splenic artery arising from the celiac artery. Small branches from the common hepatic and gastroduodenal arteries as well as direct branches from the celiac artery may also supply portions of the gland. Satellite veins corresponding to the caudal and cranial pancreaticoduodenal arteries, and other veins terminating in the splenic vein drain the right and left lobes respectively and enter the portal vein leading to the liver.[16]

Recent morphologic studies have demonstrated that in many species, including dogs and cats, an islet-acinar portal system communicates between the endocrine islet tissue and the exocrine acinar tissue.[18] Pancreatic intralobular arteries give branches that divide to form capillary glomeruli within the islets. Numerous efferent vessels (insuloacinar portal vessels) emerge from the glomeruli and enter the surrounding exocrine tissue capillary beds, from which vessels emerge and coalesce into venules. It is believed that essentially all of the blood leaving the islets goes into acinar capillaries before leaving the pancreas and that the acinar cells, particularly those surrounding the islets, are therefore exposed

to high concentrations of islet hormones. This is thought to be an important mechanism by which insulin, and perhaps other peptides, may exert a regulatory role on the exocrine pancreas.[18]

While the pancreas is not supplied by well-defined extrinsic nerves, it is richly supplied with myelinated and unmyelinated nerve fibers, and nerve trunks and intrapancreatic ganglia are found scattered throughout the tissue.[21] These neurons are either derived from the vagus and splanchnic nerves and reach the organ by following branches of the celiac and cranial mesenteric arteries, or are intrinsic to the gland. In addition to the traditional cholinergic (parasympathetic) and adrenergic (sympathetic) transmitters, it is now apparent that serotonin, dopamine, and a variety of regulatory peptides including vasoactive intestinal polypeptide (VIP), gastrin-releasing peptide (GRP), substance P, neuropeptide Y, and enkephalin-related peptides are also present in these nerve fibers and play a role in the regulation of pancreatic function.[21]

BIOCHEMISTRY AND PHYSIOLOGY

Digestive Enzymes

The acinar cells secrete a fluid rich in enzymes that degrade proteins, lipids, and polysaccharides (Table 90–2).[22] Trypsins, chymotrypsins, and elastases are endopeptidases that cleave peptide bonds at specific sites within polypeptide chains, while the carboxypeptidases are exopeptidases that cleave specific carboxyl-terminal residues.[22] Alpha-amylase hydrolyzes 4-glycosidic bonds in starches, phospholipase A_2 hydrolyzes fatty acid esters at the two-position of some membrane phospholipids, and lipase, in the presence of the coenzyme colipase, hydrolyzes ester bonds in the one and three positions of triglycerides.[22]

This protein-rich secretion is diluted and carried along the duct system by the profuse, watery, bicarbonate-rich secretion of the centroacinar and duct cells.[23] While this bicarbonate contributes to the neutralization of gastric acid emptied into the duodenum, it is probably not indispensable for the maintenance of a neutral pH. Secretion of bicarbonate and absorption of hydrogen ions by the intestinal mucosa itself provide the duo-

TABLE 90–2. MAJOR SECRETORY PROTEINS OF THE EXOCRINE PANCREAS OF THE DOG

Enzymes secreted as inactive zymogens	
Trypsinogens (1 (anionic), 2 and 3 (cationic))	trypsins
Chymotrypsinogens (1, 2, and 3)	chymotrypsins
Proelastases (1 and 2)	elastases
Procarboxypeptidases (A_1, A_2, A_3, and B)	carboxypeptidases
Prophospholipase A_2	phospholipase A_2
Coenzyme	
Procolipase	colipase
Enzymes	
α-Amylase	
Lipase	
Inhibitor	
Pancreatic secretory trypsin inhibitor	

denum with a tremendous capacity to dispose of acid to which it is exposed, even in the absence of alkaline biliary and pancreatic secretions.[8]

Defenses Against Autodigestion

Several mechanisms exist that discourage autodigestion of the pancreas by the enzymes that it secretes.[22] Firstly, proteolytic and phospholipolytic enzymes are synthesized, stored, and secreted by the pancreas in the form of catalytically inactive zymogens (indicated by the addition of the prefix "pro-" or the suffix "-ogen" to the enzyme name) (Table 90–2). These zymogens are activated by enzymatic cleavage of a small peptide, the activation peptide, from the amino-terminal of the polypeptide chain (Figure 90–2).[22] Enzymes from several sources, including some lysosomal proteases, are capable of activating pancreatic zymogens, but ordinarily activation of zymogens does not occur until they are secreted into the small intestine. The enzyme enteropeptidase (enterokinase), which is synthesized by the enterocytes lining the duodenal mucosa, is particularly effective at cleaving the activation peptides from trypsinogens to form trypsins. Active trypsins subsequently cleave the activation peptides from other digestive zymogens (Figure 90–3). Enteropeptidase therefore plays a crucial role in the activation of digestive enzymes.[22]

Secondly, from the moment that synthesis of digestive enzymes begins, they are segregated, along with potentially damaging lysosomal enzymes, into the lumen of the rough endoplasmic reticulum.[24] This is part of the cisternal space of the acinar cell, a compartment separate from the cell cytosol, which contains other enzymes with the potential to activate the zymogens. Biochemical studies have demonstrated that this segregation is due to the presence of a transient peptide extension on the amino terminal of the enzymes as they are translated from mRNA on the ribosomes. This extension, the signal sequence or signal peptide, serves only to route the protein being synthesized into the cisternal space, and its presence is indicated by the addition of the prefix "pre-" to the name of the enzyme or zymogen (e.g., preamylase, preproelastase, pretrypsinogen).[24] The signal peptide is removed by the action of a signal peptidase located on the inside surface of lumen of the rough

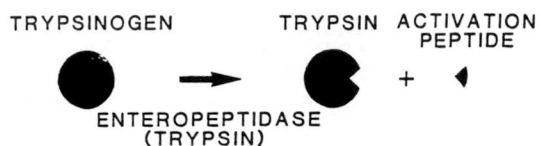

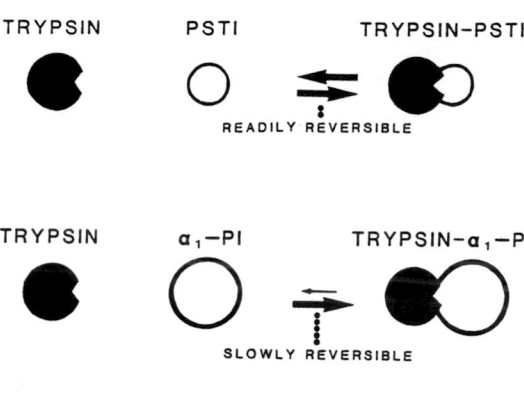

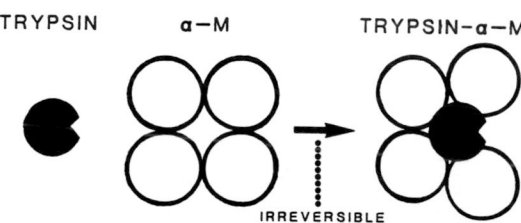

FIGURE 90–2. Diagrammatic representations of zymogen activation (trypsinogen) and the binding of proteases (trypsin) by major inhibitors.

endoplasmic reticulum while the remainder of the peptide is being synthesized, so complete polypeptide chains representing the enzyme or zymogen with its signal peptide extension, such as preamylase, never actually exist in vivo.[24] Segregation of enzymes in the cisternal space is continued as they are processed through the Golgi apparatus, where lysosomal enzymes are selectively routed to lysosomes. The digestive enzymes are incorporated into condensing vacuoles and ultimately zymogen granules, in which they are stored prior to secretion (Figure 90–4).[25]

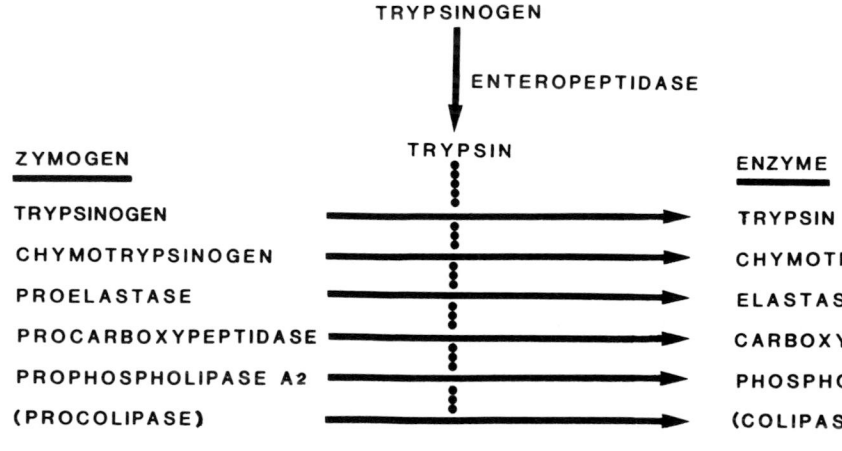

FIGURE 90–3. Activation of pancreatic proteases and phospholipase.

TABLE 90–3. MAJOR PROTEASE INHIBITORS IN CANINE PANCREAS AND PLASMA

Inhibitor	Pancreatic Secretory Trypsin Inhibitor (PSTI)	α_1-Protease Inhibitor (α_1-Antitrypsin) (α_1-PI)	α-Macroglobulins (α-M$_1$ and α-M$_2$)
Principal locations	Pancreas, pancreatic juice	Plasma, intercellular space	Plasma
Approximate mol. wt.	6000	55,000	750,000
Specificity	Trypsin only	Broad-spectrum (serine proteases)	Broad-spectrum (serine and other proteases)
Inhibition	Temporary (slowly degraded by trypsin)	Transient (transfers enzyme to α-M)	Irreversible (permanent trap for captured enzyme)
Function	Inhibits intrapancreatic autoactivation of trypsin	Readily diffusible inhibitor present in the intercellular space	Traps proteases prior to removal by reticuloendothelial system

Finally, the acinar cells contain a specific trypsin inhibitor that is synthesized, segregated, stored, and secreted along with the digestive enzymes.[14, 15, 22] This low molecular weight pancreatic secretory trypsin inhibitor (PSTI) is distinct from the much larger plasma protease inhibitors (Table 90–3). It is believed that PSTI immediately inhibits any trypsin activity produced should there be activation of trace amounts of trypsinogen within the acinar cell or duct system and therefore blocks further intrapancreatic activation of the digestive enzymes (Figure 90–2).[22]

Regulation of Pancreatic Secretion

The exocrine pancreas secretes juice into the duodenum both in the absence of food (basal or interdigestive secretion) and in response to a meal. The basal rate of secretion in dogs is about 10 per cent of the maximal secretory rate in response to a meal. The response following feeding is biphasic; an initial phase that peaks at about two hours and is rich in enzymes, and a second more voluminous phase that peaks at about eleven hours and is rich in bicarbonate.[26]

Pancreatic secretion related to feeding occurs as a response to cephalic stimulation, such as the anticipation and smell of food, as well as to gastric and intestinal stimulation due to the presence of food in the stomach and small intestine.[27] The response to these stimuli is mediated by a complex interplay of excitatory and inhibitory nervous and hormonal mechanisms; in dogs and cats the endocrine mechanisms are probably of particular importance.[27] Secretin and cholecystokinin, released into the blood from the proximal small intestine when acid and partly digested food are emptied from the stomach into the duodenum, stimulate the secretion of bicarbonate-rich and enzyme-rich components of pancreatic juice, respectively.[27, 28]

Pancreatic Enzymes in the Blood

It has long been known that amylase and lipase are present in the plasma of normal healthy animals, and it has recently been shown that the zymogens of pancreatic proteases are also normal constituents of blood.[29–31] These pancreatic enzymes and their zymogens are believed to leak directly from the gland into the bloodstream, from which they are cleared by glomerular filtration, with subsequent degradation by renal tubular epithelial cells.[29–31] Detectable amounts of intact pancreatic digestive enzymes are not absorbed from the intestinal lumen, and reports of a significant "enteropancreatic" circulation of these enzymes are now discounted.[32, 33] If there were such a circulation, then pancreatic proteases would be present in blood in active forms, whereas only inactive zymogens are detectable in serum from normal mammals.[29–33]

DISEASES OF THE EXOCRINE PANCREAS

Pancreatitis

Inflammatory disease of the human pancreas is usually divided into acute and chronic types based on a combi-

TABLE 90–4. CLASSIFICATION OF PANCREATITIS

Acute
Etiology–Various
Severity–Mild
    No multisystem failure
    Uncomplicated recovery
–Severe
    Multisystem failure
    Complication (e.g., pseudocyst, abscess)
Chronic
Etiology–Various
Severity–Mild
    Minimal morphologic change
    Subclinical loss of exocrine or endocrine function
–Severe
    Severe morphologic damage
    Clinical exocrine pancreatic insufficiency or diabetes mellitus

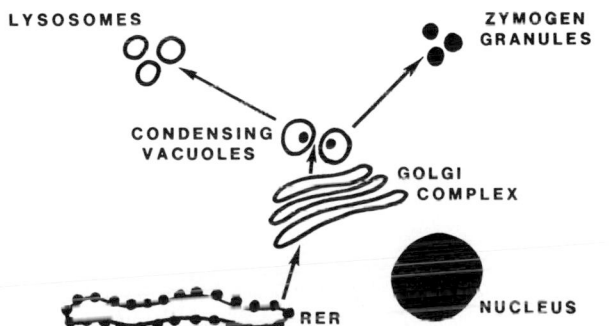

FIGURE 90–4. Normal intracellular routing of digestive and lysosomal enzymes by the pancreatic acinar cell.

nation of diagnostic criteria that may be loosely applied to cats and dogs (Table 90–4).[34] Acute pancreatitis may be defined as inflammation of the pancreas with a sudden onset. Recurrent acute disease refers to repeated bouts of inflammation with little or no permanent pathologic changes. Chronic pancreatitis is a continuing inflammatory disease characterized by irreversible morphologic change and possible permanent impairment of function. Both acute and chronic pancreatitis may be further subdivided based on the etiology, if known, and the degree of severity. Diagnostic limitations often preclude the strict application of these criteria in veterinary medicine, and the true prevalence of each is not known, but acute and recurrent acute disease are more commonly diagnosed than chronic pancreatitis.

Acquisition of knowledge about naturally occurring pancreatitis in dogs and cats has been hindered by the lack of specific laboratory tests, the inaccessibility of the gland, and the reluctance to biopsy pancreatic tissue. When examined at exploratory laparotomy or necropsy, affected pancreas is edematous and soft, or swollen and firm with fibrinous adhesions to adjacent organs.[19] Severely affected areas of pancreas may be liquefied, secondary infection with enteric organisms may produce abscesses, and sterile pseudocysts may form.[19, 35] Hemorrhages may be present in the omentum and in the pancreas, and there are often chalky areas of fat necrosis both adjacent to the pancreas and also in fat as far away as the anterior mediastinum. The peritoneal cavity may contain a small amount of blood-stained fluid containing fat droplets. Histologically, there is extensive multifocal infiltration by neutrophils, and varying degrees of hemorrhage, necrosis, edema, and vessel thrombosis.[19]

If an initial acute episode is not fatal, there may be complete resolution, or alternatively the inflammatory process may smolder continuously and asymptomatically. Extensive destruction of pancreatic tissue may reduce the gland to a few distorted lobules adjacent to where the ducts enter the duodenum.[19]

Chronic mild interstitial pancreatitis characterized by inflammation of interstitial tissue apparently spreading from the ducts is the type of pancreatic inflammation most commonly reported in cats.[19, 36, 37] This type of pancreatitis is often accompanied by cholangiohepatitis, and sometimes by interstitial nephritis, either of which may be of greater clinical significance than the pancreatitis.[19, 36, 37]

PATHOPHYSIOLOGY

Numerous experimental procedures lead to the development of pancreatitis models (Table 90–5), but the relevance of many of these models, which often cause extremely severe and rapidly fatal pancreatitis, to the spontaneous disease is questionable.[38] Recently, however, models have been developed based on hyperstimulation of the pancreas or dietary manipulation, which induce a mild to moderate inflammation that probably more closely mimics the natural disease.[38]

TABLE 90–5. EXPERIMENTAL MODELS OF PANCREATITIS

Pancreatic duct obstruction
Intraductal bile injection
Intraductal enzyme injection
Intraductal fatty acid injection
Duodenal reflux (closed duodenal loop)
Pancreatic ischemia
Diet-induced (ethionine supplemented, choline deficient)
Hyperstimulation-induced (caerulein, carbamylcholine, scorpion venom)

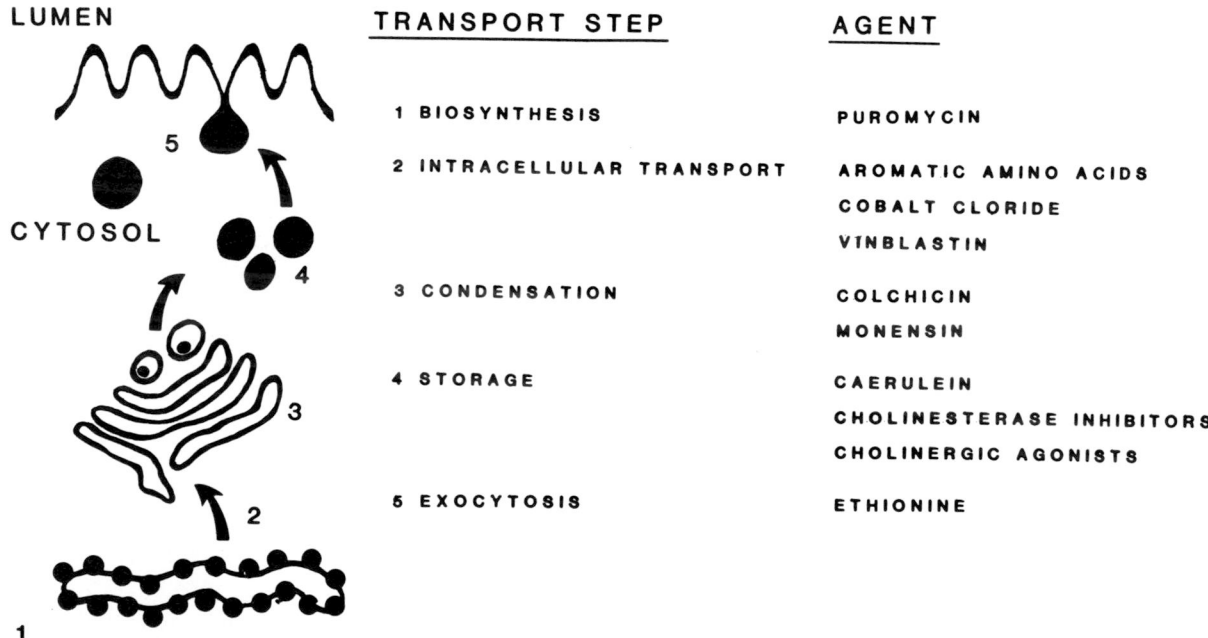

LUMEN	TRANSPORT STEP	AGENT
	1 BIOSYNTHESIS	PUROMYCIN
	2 INTRACELLULAR TRANSPORT	AROMATIC AMINO ACIDS
		COBALT CLORIDE
		VINBLASTIN
	3 CONDENSATION	COLCHICIN
		MONENSIN
	4 STORAGE	CAERULEIN
		CHOLINESTERASE INHIBITORS
		CHOLINERGIC AGONISTS
	5 EXOCYTOSIS	ETHIONINE

FIGURE 90–5. Experimental disruption of protein transport in acinar cells. Abnormal accumulation of secretory proteins within the cisternal compartment stimulates lysosomal degradative pathways (autophagy, crinophagy) with resultant mixing of zymogens and lysosomal proteases. (Modified from Adler, G, et al.: Experimental models and concepts in acute pancreatitis. *In* Go, VLW, et al. (eds): The Exocrine Pancreas: Biology, Pathology and Diseases. New York, Raven Press, 1986, p 407.)

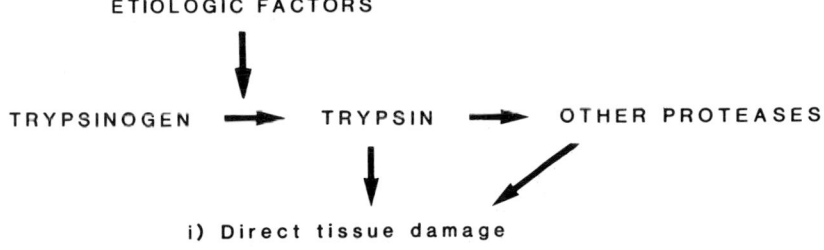

ETIOLOGIC FACTORS

TRYPSINOGEN → TRYPSIN → OTHER PROTEASES

i) Direct tissue damage

ii) Cascade initiation:

Coagulation

Fibrinolysis

Complement

Kallikrein–kinin

FIGURE 90–6. Local and systemic effects of trypsin in pancreatitis.

It is generally believed that pancreatitis develops when there is activation of digestive enzymes within the gland with resultant pancreatic autodigestion. The site of initiation of enzyme activation has been assumed to be the intercellular space or duct system, but recent studies of both diet-induced and hyperstimulation-induced pancreatitis have indicated a common intracellular basis for abnormal zymogen activation.[38] Using these models it has been shown that prior to the development of overt pancreatitis abnormal fusion of lysosomes and zymogen granules occurs, probably due to failure of normal intracellular transport, storage, or exocytosis of zymogen granule contents (Figure 90–5).[38] It is known that lysosomal proteases, such as cathepsin B, are capable of activating trypsinogen,[38, 39] and that the trypsin inhibitor present in zymogen granules is ineffective at the acid pH present in lysosomes.[40] Failure of the normal subcellular mechanism for effective segregation of zymogens and lysosomal proteases (Figure 90–4) may well explain spontaneous and experimental pancreatitis due to a variety of otherwise dissimilar causes (Figure 90–5).[22, 38–40]

Whatever the underlying cause or mechanism by which enzyme activation is initiated, recent evidence has suggested that oxygen-derived free radicals may be important in the progression of pancreatitis.[41] These radicals can damage cell membranes directly by peroxidation of lipids within the membrane. Under normal circumstances, the small amounts of free radical which form are detoxified by scavenger enzymes such as superoxide dismutase and catalase, but under some pathologic conditions, the capacity of the defense mechanisms is exceeded and tissue injury ensues. An important aspect of this injury is thought to be increased capillary permeability due to endothelial cell membrane damage, with resultant pancreatic edema.[42] Perfusion of the pancreas with free-radical scavengers ameliorated the severity of pancreatitis induced by experimental ischemia, duct obstruction, and free fatty acid infusion in a canine model.[41]

Once intracellular and intraductal activation of trypsinogens to trypsins takes place, further activation of all enzymes, particularly proelastase and prophospholipase,

will amplify pancreatic damage. Experimental and clinical studies indicate that activation of progressively larger amounts of protease and phospholipase within the gland is associated with transformation of mild edematous pancreatic inflammation to hemorrhagic or necrotic pancreatitis with multisystem involvement and consumption of plasma protease inhibitors (see Figure 90–6 and Table 90–6).[43–59]

Plasma protease inhibitors (see Table 90–3 and Figure 90–2) are vital in protecting against the otherwise fatal effects of proteolytic enzymes in the vascular space.[15, 48, 55–58] Alpha-macroglobulins are particularly important in this regard. Dogs tolerate intravenous injection of trypsin or chymotrypsin without showing adverse effects providing that free α-macroglobulins are available to bind the active proteases. Once α-macroglobulins are no longer available, however, dogs die rapidly from acute disseminated intravascular coagulation and shock, as the free proteases activate the kinin, coagulation,

TABLE 90–6. THE ROLE OF ENZYMES IN THE PATHOPHYSIOLOGY OF PANCREATITIS

Enzyme	Pathophysiologic Action
Trypsin	Activation of other proteases
	Coagulation and fibrinolysis (disseminated intravascular coagulation)
Phospholipase A₂	Hydrolysis of cell membrane phospholipids
	Pulmonary surfactant degradation
	Demyelination (cell necrosis and liberation of toxic substances such as myocardial depressant factor; respiratory distress; neurologic signs–pancreatic encephalopathy)
Elastase	Degradation of elastin in blood vessel walls (hemorrhage, edema, respiratory distress)
Chymotrypsin	Activation of xanthine oxidase and subsequent generation of oxygen-derived free radicals (membrane damage)
Kallikrein	Kinin generation from kininogens
Kinins	Vasodilation, pancreatic edema (hypotension, shock)
Complement	Cell membrane damage, aggregation of leukocytes (local inflammation)
Lipase	Fat hydrolysis (local fat necrosis, hypocalcemia)[43–56, 59]

fibrinolytic, and complement cascade systems (Figure 90–6).[48, 55, 56]

Binding of proteases by α-macroglobulins results in a change in conformation which allows the complex to be recognized and rapidly cleared from the plasma by the reticuloendothelial system.[55] This removal is important since α-macroglobulin–bound proteases retain catalytic activity, particularly against low molecular weight substrates (see Figure 90–2);[55] normal functioning of the reticuloendothelial system is an important factor determining survival in experimental pancreatitis.[60, 61]

Eighty per cent of plasma α$_1$-protease inhibitor is still available to bind proteases when α-macroglobulins are saturated with trypsin, but the available α$_1$-protease inhibitor is not life-saving.[48] While pancreatic proteases bound to α$_1$-protease inhibitor are effectively inhibited, the binding is reversible (Figure 90–2).[48] Alpha$_1$-protease inhibitor probably functions largely as a transient inhibitor and an intermediary in the transport of protease to the protective α-macroglobulins, particularly in the extravascular spaces into which the large α-macroglobulin molecules cannot permeate.[55]

ETIOLOGY

The inciting cause of spontaneous canine and feline pancreatitis is usually unknown, but based on causes documented in human patients and experimental studies, the following potential factors should be considered.[62]

Nutrition. The exocrine pancreas is highly responsive to changes in nutritional substrates present in the diet, and it has been reported that pancreatitis is more prevalent in obese animals.[63–66] Malnutrition has also been reported to cause pancreatic inflammation and atrophy in human patients, and pancreatitis has been observed after refeeding following a prolonged fast, particularly in extremely malnourished individuals.[67]

Hyperlipoproteinemia. Hyperlipoproteinemia, often grossly apparent, is common in dogs with acute pancreatitis and may develop secondary to pancreatitis as a result of abdominal fat necrosis, or may be a cause of the disease.[68] Some familial hyperlipoproteinemias of humans are associated with frequent episodes of pancreatitis that respond to control of serum triglyceride levels.[69, 70] There is anecdotal evidence that pancreatitis in dogs often develops following a fatty meal and may be particularly prevalent in miniature schnauzers with idiopathic hyperlipoproteinemia.[68, 71] It is not known why hyperlipidemia might cause pancreatitis, but it has been suggested that toxic fatty acids are generated within the pancreas by the action of lipase on abnormally high concentrations of triglycerides in pancreatic capillaries.[69, 70]

Drugs. A number of drugs may cause pancreatitis, although absolute proof of a causal relationship is often unavailable. Suspect drugs commonly used in veterinary medicine include thiazide diuretics, furosemide, azathioprine, L-asparaginase, sulfonamides, and tetracycline.[72, 73] Considerable controversy exists as to whether or not corticosteroids may induce pancreatitis, a particular problem since they may be of value in the treatment of pancreatitis.[72]

Infection. Viral and parasitic infections may be associated with pancreatitis, although this is usually recognized as part of a more generalized disease.[69, 74–76] It is not known if infection plays a role in the development of isolated pancreatitis in some instances, but it has been reported that bacterial infection may increase the severity of experimental pancreatitis, and it may act similarly in spontaneous disease.[77]

Duct Obstruction. Experimental obstruction of the pancreatic ducts produces inflammation, particularly when the gland is stimulated to secrete. The pathology in this model is characterized by pancreatic edema, chronic inflammation, atrophy, and fibrosis rather than fulminating acute pancreatitis.[69] Clinical conditions that may lead to partial or complete obstruction of the pancreatic ducts include biliary calculi, sphincter spasm, edema of the duct or duodenal wall, tumor, parasites, and surgical interference.[69] Biliary calculi are a major cause of pancreatitis in humans, but this has not been reported in dogs and cats presumably because of the low incidence of gallstones in these species, and in dogs, the separation of the pancreatic and bile ducts. Coexistent chronic interstitial pancreatitis and cholangiohepatitis have been observed in cats, and although the relationship between the changes in the two organs is not clear, the convergence of the feline biliary and pancreatic ducts may be a factor.[19, 36, 37, 78]

Duodenal Reflux. Reflux of duodenal juice into the pancreatic ducts secondary to surgical creation of a closed duodenal loop causes severe acute pancreatitis.[62] Enteropeptidase, activated pancreatic enzymes, bacteria, and bile present in the duodenal juice may all contribute to development of pancreatitis.[62] Under normal circumstances such reflux is unlikely to occur, since the duct opening is surrounded by a specialized compact, smooth mucosa over the duodenal papilla and is equipped with an independent sphincter muscle.[79] This anti-reflux mechanism may sometimes fail in the face of abnormally high duodenal pressure, however, such as may occur with vomiting.[62]

Hypercalcemia. Pancreatitis has been considered a complication of hypercalcemia due to hyperparathyroidism and other causes in human patients,[80] but the validity of this association has been questioned.[69] Pancreatitis has been reported in a dog with primary hyperparathyroidism and also in a dog following induction of iatrogenic hypercalcemia.[81, 82]

Trauma. Surgical manipulation, automobile accidents, and falling from high buildings are potential causes of pancreatic trauma, but reports of pancreatitis following such insults are rare, and in most cases of abdominal trauma, injury to the pancreas is probably mild or unrecognized.[69, 83] Pancreatitis is a rare complication of pancreatic biopsy using either wedge or needle techniques and is also uncommon following resection of pancreatic neoplasms.[84–87]

Uremia. Morphologic changes in the pancreas have been associated with renal failure in a number of species.[88] Uremic pancreatitis may contribute to clinical signs of depression and anorexia in end-stage renal disease, although severe acute pancreatitis is clearly not a common complication of renal failure in dogs and cats.[88] It is likely that renal failure secondary to acute pancreatitis is encountered more frequently.[89]

Ischemia. Experimental and clinical reports have indicated ischemia to be important in the pathogenesis of acute pancreatitis, either as a primary cause or as an exacerbating influence.[90] Pancreatic ischemia may develop during shock and secondary to hypotension during general anesthesia and may explain some instances of postoperative pancreatitis in which areas remote from the pancreas are operated upon.[69, 90]

Hereditary. Hereditary factors are important in some forms of pancreatitis recognized in human patients, such as those associated with familial hyperlipoproteinemia and developmental abnormalities of the duct system.[69, 70, 80, 91] Similar mechanisms may explain the anecdotal high prevalence of pancreatitis in some animal breeds such as miniature schnauzers.

Miscellaneous. Scorpion stings are frequent causes of pancreatitis in human beings in Trinidad, and experimental administration of scorpion venom to dogs also elicits pancreatitis via a hyperstimulation-type mechanism.[69, 80] Administration of cholinesterase-inhibitor insecticides and cholinergic agonists has similarly been associated with the development of pancreatitis, probably also due to hyperstimulation of the gland.[80, 92] Pancreatitis and gastrointestinal hemorrhage have been reported in association with intervertebral disk disease in dogs, although it is not known if this arises as a direct consequence of spinal cord trauma, corticosteroid therapy, or a combination of these factors.[93]

DIAGNOSIS

History and Clinical Signs. Animals with acute pancreatitis are usually presented because of depression, anorexia, vomiting and, in some cases, diarrhea. Severe acute disease may be associated with shock and collapse, while other cases may have a history of less dramatic signs extending over several weeks. Some dogs demonstrate abdominal pain by assuming a "prayer" position with the forelimbs outstretched, the sternum on the floor, and the hindlimbs raised. Signs of pain are usually elicited on abdominal palpation, although some animals do not react even though they have severe acute pancreatitis. An anterior abdominal mass is palpable in some cases, and occasionally there is mild ascites. Most affected animals are mildly to moderately dehydrated and febrile. Uncommon systemic complications of pancreatitis that may be apparent on physical examination include jaundice, respiratory distress, bleeding disorders, and cardiac arrhythmias.[35, 81, 94–97] Although dogs of any age may develop pancreatitis, affected animals are usually middle-aged or older, sometimes obese, and the onset of signs may have followed ingestion of a large amount of fatty food.[63, 68, 81, 94–98] The clinical signs of chronic pancreatitis are poorly documented but are probably extremely variable and nonspecific, if the disease is clinically apparent at all.

Radiographic Signs. History and clinical signs associated with pancreatitis are nonspecific and common to numerous gastrointestinal and metabolic disorders. Abdominal radiographs may provide evidence leading to one of these alternative diagnoses or support a tentative diagnosis of pancreatitis. Radiographic signs reported with pancreatitis include increased density, diminished contrast, and granularity in the right cranial abdomen, displacement of the stomach to the left, widening of the angle between the pyloric antrum and the proximal duodenum, displacement of the descending duodenum to the right, presence of a mass medial to the descending duodenum, static gas pattern in or thickened walls of the descending duodenum, static gas pattern in or caudal displacement of the transverse colon, gastric distension suggestive of gastric outlet obstruction, and delayed passage of barium through the stomach and duodenum with corrugation of the duodenal wall indicating abnormal peristalsis.[83, 95, 96, 99–101] Unfortunately, definitive radiographic evidence supporting a diagnosis of pancreatitis is usually not present, the most common finding being a somewhat subjective loss of visceral detail ("ground glass appearance") in the anterior abdomen.

Ultrasonic imaging is a promising new approach to visualization of the diseased pancreas. Nonhomogeneous masses and loss of echodensity have been noted in dogs with experimental pancreatitis, while ultrasonography confirmed the presence of a complex cystic mass in the anterior abdomen of a dog that had a pancreatic pseudocyst associated with acute pancreatitis.[35, 102, 103]

Laboratory Aids to Diagnosis. Leukocytosis is a common hematologic finding in acute pancreatitis. The packed cell volume may be increased as a result of dehydration, although in some cases anemia is observed.[81, 104–107] The mechanism for development of anemia is not known.

Azotemia is frequently present and usually reflects dehydration, but sometimes there may be acute renal failure secondary to hypovolemia or to other mechanisms, such as circulating vasotoxic agents and plugging of the renal microvasculature by either fat deposits or microthrombi from the sites of disseminated intravascular coagulation.[81, 89, 104–108]

Liver enzyme activities are often increased, reflecting hepatocellular injury as a result of either hepatic ischemia or exposure of the liver to high concentrations of toxic products delivered from the pancreas in portal blood.[81, 109, 110] In some cases, there is marked hyperbilirubinemia with clinically apparent icterus, which may indicate severe hepatocellular damage and/or intrahepatic and extrahepatic obstruction to bile flow.

Hyperglycemia is also common, probably as a result of hyperglucagonemia and stress-related increases in the concentrations of catecholamines and cortisol. Some affected animals are diabetic following recovery from acute episodes of pancreatitis.[63, 82, 94, 98]

Hypocalcemia has often been reported but is usually mild to moderate and is not associated with clinical signs of tetany.[81, 94, 104–107] The mechanism leading to development of hypocalcemia is not clear, but deposition of calcium as soaps following excessive breakdown of fat by released pancreatic lipase is one potential explanation.[59, 81, 95]

Hypercholesterolemia and hypertriglyceridemia are very common, and hyperlipemia is often grossly apparent even though food has not been ingested for many hours.[59, 81, 95] Extreme hyperlipemia may prevent accurate determination of other serum biochemical values.

Assays of pancreatic enzymes and zymogens in serum provide more specific tests for pancreatitis.[104–107, 111–114]

Numerous different assay methods exist, including conventional catalytic assays and newer highly specific immunoassays (Figure 90–7) and it is important that an appropriate method for each species be utilized. Canine amylase can be reliably assayed by amyloclastic methods, but saccharogenic methods will give falsely high values because of the presence of maltase and glucoamylase in canine serum.[115-116] Immunoassays are generally only applicable to the species for which they were developed. Clinical and experimental observations have involved primarily amylase and lipase, but recently phospholipase A_2 and serum trypsin-like immunoreactivity have been investigated.[45, 46, 104-107, 111-114]

While experimental studies in general indicate parallel changes in results of different enzyme determinations during the course of canine pancreatitis, clinical observations do not always indicate this to be the case. Marked elevations of one enzyme may be accompanied by minimal elevations of another. Furthermore, normal enzyme activities may be present in dogs with spontaneous disease.[81, 114, 117] It is possible that by the time some clinical cases are investigated, the inflamed pancreas is depleted of stored enzyme, and release into the bloodstream is therefore no longer increased. Similar reasoning may explain the lack of correlation between the magnitude of the increases in enzyme activities and the clinically perceived severity of disease and eventual outcome.

Increased concentrations of circulating pancreatic enzymes may also arise secondary to reduced clearance from the plasma, as happens in renal failure.[88, 118] Because azotemia is common in acute pancreatitis, it is sometimes difficult to determine whether increased levels of pancreatic enzymes are due to pancreatic inflammation or renal disease. It is generally believed that increases of more than two to three times above the upper limit of normal are unlikely to result from renal dysfunction alone, although there are exceptions.[88, 113]

Amylase and lipase also originate from extrapancreatic sources, including gastric and small intestinal mucosa, and activities of both enzymes may be increased in dogs with hepatic, renal or neoplastic disease in the absence of pancreatitis.[117-121] Lipase activity has been reported to be a more reliable marker for the diagnosis of pancreatitis than that of amylase.[117] However, dexamethasone administration has been shown to increase canine serum lipase activity up to five-fold without histologic evidence of pancreatitis, although parallel increases in amylase activity do not occur.[122] Moderate elevations of serum lipase in dogs receiving dexamethasone should therefore not be taken as strong evidence for pancreatitis unless amylase is also increased.

Attempts to identify a pancreas-specific isoenzyme of canine amylase, as has been possible in humans, have produced contradictory findings.[120, 121, 123-125] While a pancreas-specific isoenzyme has not yet been conclusively demonstrated, a proportionately greater increase in a distinct amylase fraction, which appears to originate predominantly from the pancreas, has been identified.[124] This test is promising and may prove to have greater specificity than simple determination of total amylase.

The presence of trypsin complexed with the plasma protease inhibitor α_1-antiprotease is reported to be a specific marker for pancreatitis, since in the absence of pancreatitis only trypsinogen is present in the plasma.[31, 43-47, 55-58, 80] Furthermore, there is evidence that the concentration of this inhibited trypsin complex may correlate with the severity and clinical course of the disease.[44-47, 55-58] However, the value of this test in naturally occurring canine pancreatitis has not been determined, and technical complexities may limit its usefulness.

Methemalbumin is formed in humans with hemorrhagic pancreatitis as pancreatic enzymes degrade hemoglobin, with subsequent binding of oxidized heme (hemin) to albumin.[118] Hemin does not bind to canine albumin, however, but rather to a variety of different serum proteins, so true methemalbuminemia cannot exist in dogs.[125a] While these protein-bound forms of hemin may also be formed in other conditions, such as hemolytic dyscrasias and intestinal infarctions, their presence in patients with other evidence of pancreatitis is highly suggestive of the hemorrhagic form of the disease, and their concentration may be of prognostic value.[104, 118]

Reports of acute pancreatitis in cats are few, but elevations of serum amylase and lipase are less than in dogs, as are normal activities of these enzymes.[37, 68, 81, 83, 98, 107, 126] An experimental study demonstrated that while serum lipase increased significantly in cats following induction of pancreatitis, amylase activity was never increased above normal but rather decreased significantly during the course of the disease.[107]

Clearly there is no widely available ideal test or combination of tests for the diagnosis of acute pancreatitis, and in the absence of direct examination of pancreatic tissue, the diagnosis can only be tentative. Nonetheless, careful evaluation of the entire clinical picture will in many instances give a high degree of confidence in the presumptive diagnosis. If gross or histopathologic confirmation of the diagnosis is required, or the possibility of other abdominal disease is to be eliminated, it is important that attention be given to stabilization of fluid and electrolyte status prior to general anesthesia and surgical exploration of the abdomen.

IMMUNOLOGIC ASSAY   CATALYTIC ASSAY

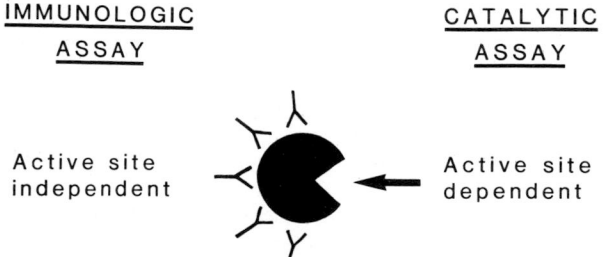

Active site independent   Active site dependent

FIGURE 90–7. Assay of pancreatic enzymes and zymogens in serum. Catalytic assays detect degradation of specific substrates exposed to the active site of the molecule, and therefore measure enzyme activity. Immunoassays detect antigenic sites over the surface of the molecule and therefore measure enzyme or zymogen concentration.

TREATMENT

The basis for therapy of acute pancreatitis is maintenance of fluid and electrolyte balance while the pancreas is "rested" by withholding food and thereby allowed to recover from the inflammatory episode.[127, 128] If drug-induced pancreatitis is suspected, then any incriminated agents should be withdrawn and replaced by an unrelated alternative drug if necessary. Sufficient IV balanced electrolyte solution should be given to replace fluid deficits and provide maintenance requirements while all oral intake is suspended for three or four days. Mild cases of pancreatitis are probably self-limiting and may spontaneously improve after one or two days. Other patients require aggressive fluid therapy over several days to treat severe dehydration and ongoing fluid and electrolyte loss due to vomiting and diarrhea. Many animals become hypokalemic during such therapy, and serum potassium should be monitored and supplemented as needed by addition of potassium chloride to the IV fluids (see Chapter 53). Serum creatinine or BUN should also be followed to document resolution of azotemia. While metabolic acidosis is probably common in acute pancreatitis, this may not always be the case, and vomiting patients may be alkalotic.[81, 128] Blind correction of suspected acid base abnormalities should therefore not be attempted unless documented by appropriate tests.[128] Excessive bicarbonate administration may precipitate signs of hypocalcemia in individuals with subclinical hypocalcemia. It is common practice to give antibiotics during this supportive period, particularly when toxic changes are evident in the hemogram or when the patient is febrile.[127, 128]

If abdominal pain is severe, then analgesic therapy (meperidine hydrochloride) should be given to provide relief. Hyperglycemia is often mild and transient, but in some cases, frank diabetes mellitus may develop and require treatment with insulin. Respiratory distress, neurologic problems, cardiac abnormalities, bleeding disorders, and acute renal failure are all poor prognostic signs. Attempts should be made to manage these complications by appropriate supportive measures, but recovery is unlikely unless the underlying pancreatitis resolves.

Some affected animals do not improve or continue to deteriorate in spite of supportive care. Recent observations have indicated that in severe pancreatitis there is marked consumption of plasma protease inhibitors as activated pancreatic proteases are cleared from the circulation, and that saturation of available α-macroglobulins is rapidly followed by acute disseminated intravascular coagulation, shock, and death.[45–48, 55–58, 129–131] Transfusion of plasma or whole blood to replace α-macroglobulins may be life-saving in these circumstances and has the additional benefit of maintaining plasma albumin concentrations.[131, 132] Albumin is probably beneficial in pancreatitis because of its oncotic properties that not only help maintain blood volume and prevent pancreatic ischemia but also limit pancreatic edema formation.[12, 42] Low molecular weight dextrans have also been used to expand plasma volume, but they may aggravate bleeding tendencies, contain no protease inhibitor, and provide no major advantages over plasma administration.[127, 128]

The use of corticosteroids in pancreatitis has been recommended because they stabilize lysosomal membranes, reduce inflammation, and alleviate shock, but they have not been shown to be of value in experimental acute studies.[133] They should be given only on a short-term basis to animals in shock associated with fulminating pancreatitis, and then in concert with fluids and plasma as described above.[128] Longer periods of administration may impair removal of α-macroglobulin–bound proteases from the plasma by the reticuloendothelial system, with resultant complications due to systemic effects of circulating uninhibited enzymes.[60, 61]

The use of peritoneal lavage to remove toxic material accumulated in the peritoneal cavity is experimentally beneficial, and is thought by many to be useful in human patients.[127] While impractical in most veterinary hospitals, peritoneal lavage may be of value in some cases. Certainly in those patients in which acute pancreatitis is confirmed at exploratory laparotomy, removal of as much free fluid as possible by abdominal lavage is advisable. In some cases pancreatitis may be localized to one lobe of the gland or a pancreatic abscess may be present, and surgical resection and drainage of the affected area may be followed by complete recovery.[134, 134a] Surgical intervention may also benefit those dogs with common bile duct obstruction secondary to chronic fibrosing pancreatitis: cholecystoduodenostomy was followed by resolution of clinical signs in a group of six such cases.[134b]

Indirect approaches to inhibition of pancreatic secretion which have been employed, in addition to withholding food, include nasogastric suctioning of gastric secretions and inhibition of gastric secretion by use of antacids or cimetidine.[127] None of these methods has been consistently shown to be effective, and their use is not recommended.[127] Attempts to rest the pancreas by use of direct inhibitors of secretion, such as atropine, acetazolamide, glucagon, calcitonin, and somatostatin or its analogs, have also not yet been proved to be effective.[127, 133] Pancreatic gamma irradiation is an effective if impractical method that reduces pancreatic secretion and lessens the severity of experimental pancreatitis.[135] Administration of a variety of naturally occurring and synthetic enzyme inhibitors with selective actions against individual pancreatic digestive enzymes has shown promise in experimental studies, but their value remains to be demonstrated in clinical trials.[127, 136–138] Future clinical and experimental trials will probably be directed at the use of agents to modify intracellular events that are currently believed to be important in the pathobiology of pancreatitis, including free radical scavengers, inhibitors of enzyme synthesis or transport, and factors that may stabilize lysosomal and other membranes.[138–140]

As soon as there has been no vomiting for one to two days, small amounts of water should be offered, and if there is no recurrence of clinical signs food may be gradually reintroduced. The diet should have a high carbohydrate content (rice, pasta, potatoes), since protein and fat are more potent stimulants of pancreatic secretion and are perhaps more likely to promote a relapse. If there is continued improvement, gradual introduction of a low fat maintenance diet should be attempted. Another period of food deprivation should be instituted if signs of pancreatitis recur.[96, 128]

In many patients a single episode of pancreatitis occurs, and all that is necessary in the way of long-term therapy is to avoid feeding meals with an excessively high fat content. In other patients repeated bouts of pancreatitis occur, and it may be beneficial to feed a moderately or severely fat restricted diet permanently. In spite of this, some animals experience recurrent disease.[96]

Oral pancreatic enzyme supplements have been shown to decrease the pain that accompanies chronic pancreatitis in humans, probably by feedback inhibition of endogenous pancreatic enzyme secretion.[141] It is not known if they are of similar value in dogs or cats, but in individuals with chronic or recurrent signs attributed to pancreatitis, a trial period of enzyme therapy may be warranted.

PROGNOSIS

Pancreatitis is an unpredictable disease of widely varying severity, and it is difficult to give a prognosis even when a diagnosis is definitively established. Life-threatening signs accompanying acute fulminating pancreatitis are usually followed by death in spite of supportive measures, but some dogs recover fully following an isolated severe episode. In other cases, relatively mild or moderate chronic or recurrent pancreatitis persists despite all therapy, and the patient either dies in an acute severe exacerbation of the disease or is euthanatized because of failure to recover and because of the expense of long- term supportive care. Most patients with uncomplicated pancreatitis probably recover spontaneously after a single episode and do well as long as high fat diets are avoided.

Exocrine Pancreatic Insufficiency

Progressive loss of exocrine pancreatic acinar cells ultimately leads to failure of absorption due to inadequate production of digestive enzymes. The functional reserve of the pancreas is considerable, however, and signs of exocrine pancreatic insufficiency (EPI) do not occur until a large proportion of the gland has been destroyed. Steatorrhea and azotorrhea do not develop in humans until more than 90 per cent of the secretory capacity of the pancreas has been lost.[142] Similarly in dogs with naturally occurring EPI, both the amylase secretory capacity[143] and the serum concentration of trypsin-like immunoreactivity[144] are reduced to less than 15 per cent of normal. The most common cause of such severe loss of exocrine tissue in the dog is pancreatic acinar atrophy (PAA). Pancreatic insufficiency is caused less commonly by chronic pancreatitis and rarely by pancreatic neoplasia.[63, 94, 145–150] While not yet documented, it is likely that congenital abnormalities of canine pancreatic exocrine function such as pancreatic hypoplasia, and isolated deficiencies of individual pancreatic enzymes, and deficiency of enteropeptidase also occur.[19, 151]

Although pancreatic enzymes perform essential digestive functions, alternative pathways of digestion do exist. Following experimental exclusion of pancreatic secretion from the intestine, dogs can still absorb up to 63 per cent of ingested protein and 84 per cent of ingested fat.[152–155] This residual enzyme activity probably originates from lingual and/or gastric lipases and gastric pepsins and also from intestinal mucosal esterases and peptidases.[119, 156–158] Nonetheless, when exocrine pancreatic function is severely impaired, these alternative routes of digestion are inadequate, and clinical signs of malabsorption occur.

ETIOLOGY

Pancreatic Acinar Atrophy (PAA). Atrophy of the pancreatic acinar cells in the absence of a pronounced inflammatory response may occur in a variety of experimental circumstances. Spontaneous development of severe PAA in previously healthy adult animals appears to be uniquely common in the dog, although reports indicate that similar conditions occur sporadically in other species.[159–162]

The underlying cause of canine PAA is unknown, but numerous nutritional deficiencies, such as amino acid imbalance and copper deficiency in the rat and protein-calorie malnutrition in humans, cause atrophy of exocrine tissue.[80, 163–166] Whether canine PAA is caused by a nutritional imbalance is unknown, but such an imbalance, acquired perhaps as a consequence of an underlying small intestinal mucosal abnormality, is an attractive explanation for the development of pancreatic atrophy in dogs with previously normal exocrine pancreatic function. Although preexisting small intestinal disease in dogs with PAA has not been documented, it has been observed that affected dogs sometimes have a history of gastrointestinal disturbances long before the development of severe weight loss.[167, 168] Alternative explanations for development of PAA include: (1) pancreatic duct obstruction, (2) a primary congenital abnormality in the pancreas itself, (3) toxicosis, (4) ischemia, (5) viral infection, (6) immune-mediated disease, and (7) defective secretory and/or trophic stimuli, although there is little evidence to support the role of any of these etiologies in naturally occurring canine PAA.[167] While PAA may occur at any age in a wide variety of breeds, a high prevalence in young German shepherds is recognized.[143, 167–171] Investigations of family histories have suggested that predisposition to development of the disease is inherited in an autosomal recessive fashion in this breed.[170, 171]

The pancreatic atrophy of CBA/J mice is the only naturally occurring disorder that resembles canine PAA.[159] Morphologic study of pancreata from affected mice has implicated destabilization of zymogen granules as one of the earliest ultrastructural abnormalities, while biochemical studies indicate that premature activation of trypsinogen and chymotrypsinogen occurs within the zymogen granules.[159, 172] Inflammatory cell infiltration occurs relatively late in the course of the disease.[159, 172] Whether similar changes occur in canine PAA is unknown, but the CBA/J mouse model illustrates that the variable inflammatory response observed in affected dogs may arise secondary to an earlier and more subtle underlying abnormality in the acinar cells themselves.[143, 148, 149, 168]

Chronic Pancreatitis. While chronic pancreatitis resulting in progressive destruction of pancreatic tissue is

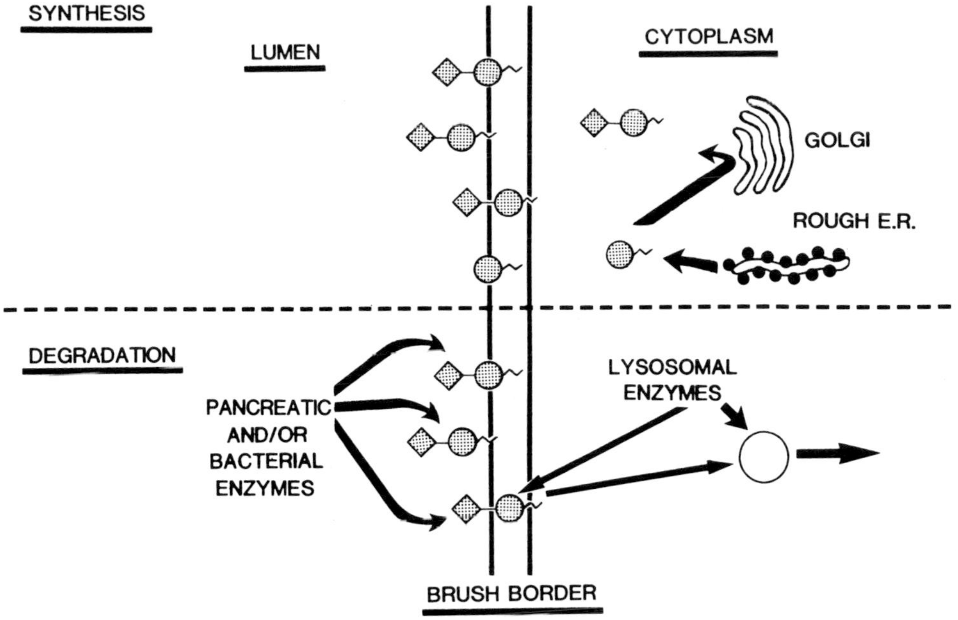

FIGURE 90–8. Factors influencing activities of jejunal brush border enzymes. The importance of degradation by intraluminal proteases depends at least in part on the location of the enzyme in the membrane, and hence its susceptibility to proteolytic attack. (Modified from Alpers, DH and Seetharam, B: Pathophysiology of diseases involving intestinal brush-border proteins. N Engl J Med 296: 1047, 1977.)

a common cause of EPI in adult humans, gross and histologic examination rarely reveals end-stage pancreatitis as the underlying cause of EPI in dogs.[63, 94, 143, 146–149, 168, 169] There are no well-documented reports of dogs with either chronic relapsing pancreatitis or severe acute pancreatitis that resulted in EPI, but those animals with EPI and coexistent diabetes mellitus probably fall into this category. A similar combination of clinical signs is seen in association with chronic pancreatitis in humans, reflecting damage to both exocrine and endocrine tissue as occurs in pancreatitis, in contrast to PAA in which islet tissue is spared.[173, 174] Exocrine pancreatic insufficiency is seldom diagnosed in cats and is apparently uncommon. Chronic pancreatitis has been the underlying cause in the majority of the few cases reported.[68, 145, 175, 176]

Hereditary, Congenital and Miscellaneous Causes of EPI. Cystic fibrosis and congenital hypoplasia (Shwachman syndrome) are common causes of EPI in children, but these disorders differ from canine EPI in that there are also abnormalities of organs other than the pancreas.[177] Other extremely rare causes of EPI in children include congenital deficiencies of individual pancreatic digestive enzymes or of intestinal enteropeptidase, but these have not been described in dogs or cats.[151] Occasionally young dogs are seen that have signs of EPI and diabetes mellitus from a very early age, and congenital pancreatic hypoplasia or aplasia may be the underlying causes.[19]

Finally, EPI has been reported as a complication of proximal duodenal resection and cholecystoduodenostomy in cats, a finding that probably reflects the absence of dual pancreatic ducts in this species, such that damage to the major duodenal papilla blocks pancreatic secretion.[178]

PATHOPHYSIOLOGY

Nutrient malabsorption in canine EPI probably does not arise simply as a consequence of failure of intraluminal digestion. Morphologic changes (villous atrophy, inflammatory cell infiltrates) in the small intestine of dogs with EPI have occasionally been reported, and studies of naturally occurring and experimental EPI in several species have revealed abnormal activities of mucosal enzymes and impaired function as indicated by abnormal transport of sugars, amino acids, and fatty acids.[143, 147, 179–190] The cause of this mucosal pathology is unknown, but the absence of the trophic influence of pancreatic secretions, bacterial overgrowth in the small intestine, and endocrine and nutritional factors may all be contributory.[12, 13, 191–196]

Small Intestinal Mucosa. Exocrine pancreatic insufficiency in humans and dogs is associated with increased activities of jejunal brush border maltase and sucrase.[197, 198] Similar increases in disaccharidase activities have been reported in hamsters with ligated pancreatic ducts, in rats after subtotal pancreatectomy, and in the CBA/J mouse with PAA.[10, 11, 180] These increased activities have been attributed to reduced degradation of exposed brush border proteins as a consequence of decreased pancreatic protease activity within the gut lumen (Figure 90–8).[197] This explanation is supported by the normalization of jejunal maltase and sucrase activities in both murine and canine EPI in response to treatment with pancreatic enzymes.[11, 199, 200] The abnormal accumulation of these enzymes and perhaps other proteins on the surface of the brush border membrane may interfere with normal absorption.

In contrast to the increased activities of maltase and sucrase, the activity of brush border peptidase (leucyl-2-naphthylamidase) is unchanged, while that of alkaline phosphatase is decreased in dogs with EPI.[198–200] These proteins are relatively resistant to degradation by intraluminal proteases.[201–206]

Protein synthesis by jejunal mucosa is decreased in dogs with EPI, but returns to normal following treatment.[199, 207] Jejunal alkaline phosphatase activity also normalizes following treatment suggesting that the activity of this enzyme is particularly dependent on the rate of protein synthesis (Figure 90–8). The mechanism for the defect in protein synthesis is not known, but contributory factors may include malnutrition and intraluminal or humoral factors. Intraluminal pancreatic secretions and the products of digestion exert a trophic effect on the small intestine,[12, 13] and both are deficient in untreated dogs. Hormones and other regulatory peptides including gastrin, enteroglucagon, glucagon, insulin, and epidermal growth factor may mediate these trophic effects.[195, 196]

Disturbances of glucose homeostasis are common in dogs with EPI, and in these dogs, insulinopenia may be an additional factor affecting intestinal mucosal function. Insulin receptors are present both on basolateral and brush border membranes of enterocytes, and insulin has a stimulatory effect on DNA synthesis in the gastrointestinal tract.[195, 196, 208–213]

Small Intestinal Microflora.
Bacterial overgrowth ($> 1 \times 10^5$ organisms/ml duodenal juice) is common in dogs with EPI.[191] Changes in the intestinal microflora may arise secondary to loss of the antibacterial properties of pancreatic juice[9] or as a consequence of as yet undefined abnormalities of intestinal immunity or motility. Achlorhydria, a factor predisposing to development of bacterial overgrowth, has been reported to be common in human patients with chronic disease of the exocrine pancreas but has not been documented in canine EPI.[192, 214, 215]

The pathologic changes associated with bacterial overgrowth depend on the type of bacteria involved. In those dogs with increases in aerobic and facultative anaerobic bacteria, changes are similar to those observed in dogs with EPI that do not have bacterial overgrowth.[191] In these dogs, activities of brush border enzymes other than alkaline phosphatase are either normal or increased (see above). In contrast, when the overgrowth includes obligate anaerobic bacteria, there is often an associated decrease in many enzyme activities, and in some cases, partial villous atrophy.[191] These findings are consistent with the known ability of some strains of obligate anaerobic bacteria to produce enzymes that release or destroy exposed brush border enzymes.[105, 216, 217] Even when bacterial overgrowth does not include large numbers of obligate anaerobes, the abnormal microflora may be of clinical significance, since bacteria may indirectly impair absorption by competing for nutrients and by changing intraluminal factors such as the concentration of conjugated bile salts.[192]

Pancreatic Regulatory Peptides.
Histopathologic examination of pancreata from dogs with PAA reveals almost total atrophy of acinar tissue but plentiful, disorganized islet tissue, accompanied by numerous ganglia and patent exocrine ducts.[143, 148] Immunohistochemical staining of PAA pancreas shows many insulin-, glucagon-, somatostatin-, and pancreatic polypeptide-immunoreactive cells scattered haphazardly throughout residual islet tissue. This differs from the more organized arrangement of cells in healthy canine pancreas, in which a central core of insulin- and scattered somatostatin-immunoreactive cells is surrounded by a halo of glucagon- (left lobe) or pancreatic polypeptide- (right lobe) immunoreactive cells.[218, 219] In addition, enkephalin- and vasoactive intestinal polypeptide (VIP)-immunoreactive

nerve fibers are extremely profuse in PAA islet tissue, accompanied by numerous enkephalin- and VIP-immunoreactive nerve cell bodies; whereas in normal pancreas, enkephalin-immunoreactive fibers are very rare, while VIP-immunoreactive innervation is moderate in acinar tissue but rarely present in islets.[218] Enkephalin-like immunoreactivity in PAA pancreas is probably due to a precursor immunochemically related to proenkephalin.[220]

Disturbance of the morphologic relationships among cells in islet pancreatic tissue may impair intra-islet and/or entero-islet homeostatic mechanisms and might account for subnormal basal plasma insulin concentrations in dogs with PAA. The neuronal regulatory peptide abnormalities may represent a primary defect in canine PAA, or they may occur secondary to the atrophy of acinar tissue, perhaps arising as a result of neuronal overgrowth in response to loss of target tissue.

Glucose Intolerance.
In dogs with EPI secondary to pancreatitis, there may be frank diabetes mellitus secondary to islet cell destruction. Oral and intravenous glucose tolerance is also abnormal in untreated dogs with PAA, although diabetes mellitus has not been reported in these dogs.[221–223]

The "incretin" effect is reduced in dogs with experimental pancreatic atrophy.[224] Incretin refers to insulinotropic factors released from the gut which are responsible for the augmentation of insulin secretion in response to orally administered glucose compared with that stimulated by the same dosage of intravenously administered glucose.[225] Gastric inhibitory polypeptide (GIP) is probably an important factor contributing to incretin activity, and feeding does not stimulate GIP release from the small bowel of dogs with PAA unless pancreatic enzymes are added to the food.[225, 226] Similar observations have been made in children with cystic fibrosis, and the failure of GIP secretion appears to arise because products of digestion (glucose, amino acids, fatty acids) are the stimuli for GIP release rather than the act of feeding or the undigested constituents of food itself.[226] The relationship of plasma GIP responses to oral glucose intolerance in canine PAA and whether oral glucose tolerance returns to normal following treatment have not been reported.

Intravenous glucose tolerance in untreated dogs with PAA is associated with subnormal resting and stimulated insulin concentrations,[200, 223] abnormalities that are presumably independent of incretin. Similar abnormalities have been reported in dogs with experimental pancreatic atrophy.[224, 227] Treatment of PAA is followed by normalization of intravenous glucose tolerance, although basal plasma insulin concentrations remain subnormal.[200, 223]

It is probable that the abnormalities in glucose homeostasis are related at least in part to metabolic changes associated with the catabolic state of many untreated dogs with EPI. Withholding food from dogs for a period of two weeks produces a decrease in circulating insulin concentrations.[228] This probably represents an adaptation to reduced food intake, since lower insulin levels facilitate enhanced lipolysis, leading to increased concentrations of plasma free fatty acids that are available as an energy source.[228]

Nutritional Status. Many dogs with EPI suffer from malabsorption for a considerable period of time before a diagnosis is made. Thus, the clinical and pathophysiologic features associated with EPI may in some instances be due to malnutrition rather than EPI per se. For example, malnutrition may have direct effects on the gastrointestinal mucosa as well as produce systemic endocrine and immunologic changes, which may in turn have an effect on gastrointestinal function.[229–232]

PROTEIN-CALORIE MALNUTRITION. In many cases, dogs with EPI are cachectic secondary to long-term protein-calorie malnutrition, and in such malnourished individuals, alterations in circulating concentrations of insulin and other hormones may contribute to changes in glucose homeostasis and intestinal mucosal function.[12, 13, 195, 208, 209, 218] Changes in small intestinal mucosal enzyme activities have been observed in severely malnourished children and may be a direct effect of nutrient deficiency impairing protein synthesis.[12, 13, 193, 230] Severe protein-calorie malnutrition may also affect the normal immune response, and this in turn may contribute to development of changes in the intestinal microflora.[192, 229] Furthermore, malnutrition in rats impairs the capacity to maintain protective mucosal mucin content and accelerates the development of brush border enzyme deficiency in intraluminal bacterial overgrowth.[231, 232] Finally, protein-calorie malnutrition per se may contribute to EPI, perhaps through impairment of pancreatic protein synthesis, and this may worsen already impaired exocrine pancreatic function.[163]

TRACE ELEMENTS. Absorption of trace elements in EPI may be promoted or inhibited secondary to either loss of specific factors affecting absorption or to a change in intraluminal pH.[6, 233–235] Preliminary investigations have not revealed any trace element deficiencies in dogs with EPI, though only serum copper and zinc levels have been assessed.[200]

VITAMINS. Malabsorption of cobalamin (vitamin B_{12}) is well-documented in association with EPI in humans, and mildly to severely subnormal serum cobalamin levels have been observed in dogs with EPI.[200, 236, 237] The mechanism for malabsorption of cobalamin in canine EPI is not known, but overgrowth of cobalamin-binding bacteria in the proximal small bowel may be responsible.[191, 192] In addition, deficiency of pancreatic proteases may prevent the normal release of cobalamin from salivary and/or gastric R proteins.[5] These proteins bind ingested cobalamin in the stomach, where the low pH prevents binding to gastric intrinsic factor.[5] Cobalamin is absorbed in the ileum only when it is coupled with intrinsic factor, and degradation of proteins in the proximal small bowel by pancreatic proteases is an important factor in the successful transfer of cobalamin from R proteins to intrinsic factor.[5, 238] A deficiency of an intrinsic factor–like protein in canine pancreatic juice may also directly contribute to malabsorption of cobalamin.[2–4] Because serum concentrations do not necessarily normalize following otherwise effective treatment, cobalamin malabsorption is probably not solely due to lack of pancreatic enzymes in the gut lumen.[200] Cobalamin is essential for DNA synthesis, and severely subnormal serum cobalamin concentrations may adversely affect the normal proliferation of crypt cells in the intestinal mucosa, hence the specific activities of jejunal mucosal enzymes.[239, 240] It is therefore possible that persistent cobalamin deficiency may be a contributory factor in those cases in which response to treatment is suboptimal.

Serum folate concentrations may be increased, normal, or decreased in dogs with EPI, both before and after treatment.[200, 237] High serum folate levels may reflect overgrowth of bacteria in the small intestine.[191, 195, 241] Intraluminal bacteria commonly synthesize and release folate, and overgrowth of such bacteria in the proximal small intestine, the site for folate absorption in the dog, may elevate serum concentrations of this vitamin.[241] Alternatively, folate absorption may be promoted due to decreased duodenal pH secondary to reduced pancreatic bicarbonate secretion;[242] however, this is perhaps a less likely explanation since pancreatic bicarbonate secretion is relatively well preserved in canine PAA, and the duodenum itself has significant ability to neutralize acid.[8, 143] The elevations of serum folate associated with canine EPI are probably of little functional significance except that they may help protect against the development of cobalamin deficiency–associated anemia, which does not seem to be a feature of EPI even when serum cobalamin concentrations are severely subnormal.

Serum tocopherol (vitamin E) concentrations are often severely subnormal in canine EPI,[200] which is not surprising given the severe fat malabsorption that occurs. Overgrowth of bacteria may contribute to deficiencies of fat-soluble vitamins by exacerbating fat malabsorption.[192, 243] Serum tocopherol concentrations do not increase in response to treatment,[200] perhaps because treatment does not return fat absorption to normal even though clinical signs of EPI resolve,[244] or because intraluminal bacterial overgrowth persists.

Tocopherol deficiency decreases the proliferative response of canine lymphocytes to mitogenic stimulants,[245] and if this reflects an *in vivo* defect in immune function, tocopherol deficiency may be an additional factor predisposing to overgrowth of intestinal bacteria in dogs with EPI. Tocopherol deficiency may cause pathologic change in smooth muscle, central nervous system, skeletal muscle, and retina,[246–250] and although not yet reported, similar changes may accompany chronic untreated tocopherol deficiency in dogs with EPI.

Subnormal serum concentrations of vitamin A have also been observed in dogs with EPI, but no associated signs of deficiency were reported.[63] The author is aware of one dog with EPI which had a vitamin K–responsive coagulopathy, characterized by prolonged prothrombin and activated partial thromboplastin times but normal platelet count and fibrin degradation product concentration, and in which there was no evidence of anticoagulant toxicosis.[251] The potential for selective chronic nutrient deficiencies in EPI deserves further investigation.

DIAGNOSIS

History. Animals with EPI usually have a history of weight loss in the face of a normal or increased appetite. Polyphagia is often severe, and owners may complain that dogs ravenously devour all food offered to them as well as scavenge from waste bins and so forth. This is by no means always the case, however, and some dogs may even have periods of inappetence. Coprophagia and pica are also common, probably as manifestations of polyphagia but also perhaps as a consequence of specific nutritional deficiencies. Water intake may also increase in some dogs, and in chronic pancreatitis, there may be polyuria and polydipsia due to diabetes mellitus.[63, 68, 94, 145–147, 149, 167, 169]

Diarrhea often accompanies EPI, but this can be very variable in character. Most owners report frequent passage of large volumes of semiformed feces, although some dogs have intermittent or continuous explosive watery diarrhea, while in other instances diarrhea is infrequent and is not considered a problem. Diarrhea generally improves or resolves in response to fasting. Introduction of a low-fat diet may also decrease or eliminate diarrhea. There may be a history of vomiting, and commonly there is marked borborygmus and flatulence. Owners sometimes consider the dog to be suffering from episodes of abdominal discomfort.[63, 68, 94, 143, 145–149, 167–169, 252]

In some dogs there has been a protracted history of gastrointestinal disturbances prior to the final diagnosis of EPI, the significance of which is not clear but which may merely represent initial failure to diagnose EPI.[147, 167] Unless signs of vomiting, diarrhea, borborygmus, or flatulence are severe, many owners may not seek veterinary advice until weight loss is marked, and even when animals are presented early, the diagnosis may be missed because the "classic" signs have not yet appeared. Appropriate testing in such early cases will allow the diagnosis of EPI to be made before the animal's body condition severely deteriorates.

Pancreatic acinar atrophy is very prevalent in young German shepherds, thus EPI is often initially suspected because of the age and breed of the affected dog. It must be emphasized, however, that even in young German shepherds, small intestinal disease is more prevalent than EPI, and that PAA may occur in a wide variety of breeds at any age. Chronic pancreatitis is probably more common in older dogs, but the true prevalence of EPI due to chronic pancreatitis is not known. Whatever the underlying pathology, results based on radioimmunoassay of serum trypsin-like immunoreactivity indicate that in the United States numerous breeds are affected and that only approximately fifty per cent are German shepherds.[253]

Clinical Signs. Mild to marked weight loss is usually seen in association with EPI. Some dogs are very emaciated at presentation, with severe muscle wasting and no palpable body fat, and in extreme cases, dogs may be physically weak owing to loss of muscle mass. The hair coat is often in poor condition, and some animals may give off a foul odor because of soiling of the coat with fatty fecal material and passage of excessive flatus.[63, 68, 94, 143, 145–149, 167–169, 252]

Laboratory Aids to Diagnosis. The history and clinical signs of EPI are nonspecific, vary in severity, and do not distinguish the condition from other causes of malabsorption. While replacement therapy with oral pancreatic enzymes is generally successful, response to treatment is not a reliable diagnostic approach. Not all dogs with EPI respond to treatment, and dogs with self-limiting small intestinal disease may improve spontaneously, giving the false impression of a response to enzyme supplementation. Furthermore, veterinarians often advise a change in diet when treating dogs with EPI, and this in itself can lead to clinical improvement in some dogs with small intestinal diseases. It is also possible that pancreatic enzymes might have a favorable effect in the treatment of malabsorption due to causes other than EPI.[188]

In dogs with PAA, extreme atrophy of the pancreas is readily observed on gross inspection at either exploratory laparotomy or laparoscopy,[84] although in dogs with chronic pancreatitis, it may be impossible to gauge accurately the amount of residual exocrine pancreatic tissue because of severe adhesions and fibrosis. These procedures involve unnecessary anesthetic and surgical risks and therefore cannot be recommended as diagnostic procedures given the availability of reliable noninvasive tests.

Many laboratory tests for the diagnosis of EPI have been described, but their sensitivities and specificities[254] are often highly questionable. The most reliable tests currently available include assay of serum trypsin-like immunoreactivity (TLI), assay of fecal proteolytic activity using a casein-based substrate, and the bentiromide (N-benzoyl-L-tyrosyl-p-aminobenzoic acid or BT-PABA) absorption test.

DIRECT MEASUREMENT OF PANCREATIC ENZYME ACTIVITY. Pancreatic juice secreted into the gut lumen can be collected following peroral intubation of the canine duodenum, and the enzyme activity of this intestinal juice can then be assayed in vitro.[143] This technique has been used to investigate secretion of pancreatic amylase and bicarbonate by dogs with EPI in response to stimulation with exogenous secretin and cholecystokinin, but the value of this test as a diagnostic aid has not been assessed.[143] Moreover, this procedure is technically difficult, and therefore has limited clinical application.

SERUM TESTS. SERUM TRYPSIN-LIKE IMMUNOREACTIVITY (TLI). Trypsinogen is synthesized exclusively by the pancreas, and measurement of the serum concentration of this zymogen by radioimmunoassay* provides a good indirect index of canine pancreatic function.[255] This immunoassay detects both trypsinogen and trypsin (see Figure 90–7), hence the use of the term trypsin-like immunoreactivity (TLI) to describe the total concentration of these two immunoreactive species. Measurement of serum TLI is much simpler than most of the other tests in that analysis of just a single serum sample obtained after food has been withheld for several hours is all that is required. Serum TLI is quite stable under normal conditions, and samples can therefore be mailed to an appropriate laboratory. Administration of oral pancreatic extracts does not affect serum TLI concentrations in either normal dogs or dogs with EPI, so withdrawal from enzyme supplementation prior to testing of dogs that are already receiving treatment is unnecessary.

---

*Diagnostic Products Corporation, 5700 West 96th St., Los Angeles, CA 90045.

Measurement of serum TLI has been shown to be a highly sensitive and specific test for the diagnosis of canine EPI. Serum TLI concentrations are dramatically reduced in dogs with EPI, whereas TLI concentrations in dogs with small intestinal disease are not significantly different from normal (Figure 90–9).[255, 256]

While not yet documented, it can be predicted that serum TLI concentrations will be normal in those rare dogs with EPI due to tumors obstructing the pancreatic ducts or due to congenital deficiencies of enzymes other than trypsinogen. A very small proportion of samples submitted to the author's laboratory for analysis have subnormal serum TLI concentrations (<5.0 µg/l) that are greater than those observed in dogs with EPI (<2.5 µg/l). These dogs have not been available for additional clinical investigation, but on retesting, serum TLI concentrations have usually been either clearly consistent with EPI or normal. Failure to withhold food prior to taking the blood sample, recovery of pancreatic function following an episode of pancreatitis, or exposure of the sample to excessive heat during shipping may explain these "gray zone" results. A few dogs have consistently had serum TLI concentrations in the gray zone on retesting, but none of these individuals has thus far required enzyme therapy. It is likely that they have some reduction of pancreatic secretory capacity that is not sufficient to cause clinical signs.

Radioimmunoassays for trypsin are usually species-specific, and assays for human TLI do not detect canine TLI. The canine TLI radioimmunoassay developed by the author is not suitable for use in the cat.

BENTIROMIDE (*N*-BENZOYL-L-TYROSYL-*P*-AMINO-BENZOIC ACID OR BT-PABA) ABSORPTION TEST. Chymotrypsin activity in the proximal small intestine may be assayed *in vivo* by the oral administration of the synthetic substrate bentiromide.[155] Free PABA is released from this substrate by chymotrypsin, absorbed from the gut lumen, and subsequently excreted in the urine. Absorption may be assessed by measuring PABA either in plasma or in urine (Figure 90–10). The relatively high cost of the substrate, the requirement for either multiple blood sampling or collection of urine in a metabolism cage, and the technical expertise required for the PABA assay have largely restricted its use to referral practices and institutions. Moreover, results of this test are equivocal in some cases, since there is overlap between results from dogs with EPI and those with small intestinal disease (Figure 90–11).[155, 188, 189, 255–260]

In some dogs with small intestinal disease, free PABA is not adequately absorbed or a "functional" pancreatic insufficiency may occur, possibly due to impaired release of pancreatic secretagogues from diseased intestinal mucosa.[188, 189, 255] The results of the BT-PABA test are more confidently interpreted if combined with a simultaneous xylose absorption test, since normal xylose absorption indicates that gastric contents have passed into the small intestine.[188, 189] Furthermore, small intestinal disease severe enough to cause malabsorption of free PABA is likely to be associated with obvious xylose malabsorption. Markedly subnormal PABA absorption accompanied by normal xylose absorption is therefore clearly diagnostic for EPI. Since xylose malabsorption is common in dogs with EPI, however, exocrine pancreatic function cannot be reliably assessed in those dogs with both abnormal xylose and PABA absorption on the basis of these tests alone.[188–190]

The explanation for the appreciable PABA absorption seen in some dogs with EPI is not known. Bacterial degradation could significantly increase BT-PABA hydrolysis in those individuals with bacterial overgrowth.[261] Alternatively there may be compensatory synthesis of increased amounts of an intestinal peptidase with chymotrypsin-like substrate specificity.[262]

An advantage of the bentiromide absorption test over serum TLI assay is that it should detect EPI caused by obstruction to the flow of pancreatic juice; in such animals release of trypsinogen into the blood, and hence the concentration of TLI, may not be abnormal.[150]

Combined bentiromide/xylose absorption test results in healthy cats vary considerably and differ from those seen in dogs.[263, 264] Results from cats with malabsorption due to EPI have not been reported, but the diagnostic usefulness of the bentiromide/xylose test is probably limited in this species because of the wide variation seen in normal cats.[263, 264]

PLASMA TURBIDITY TEST. Lipemia (plasma turbidity) develops in normal dogs following the oral administration of fat, but this response is absent or diminished in

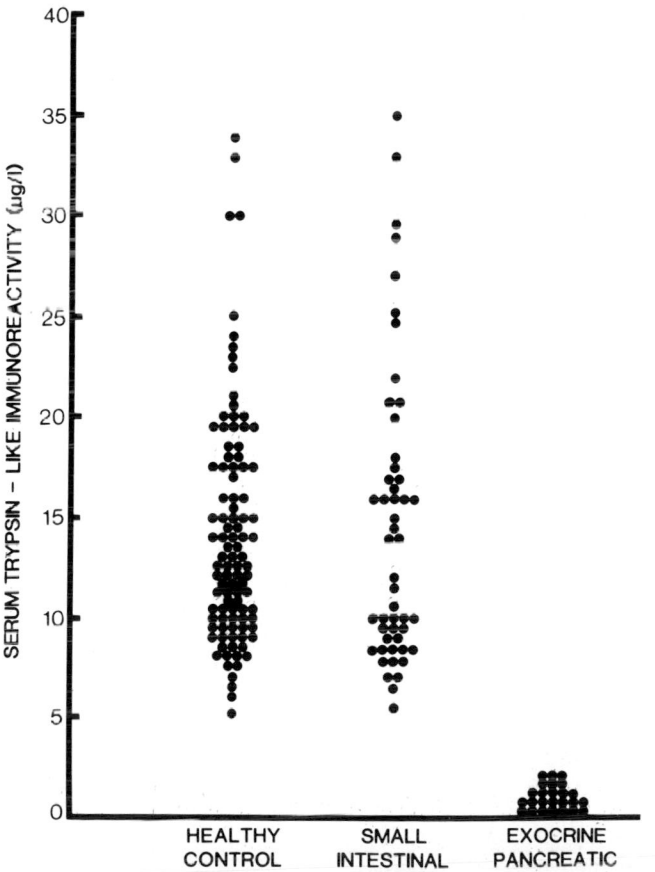

FIGURE 90–9. Serum trypsin-like immunoreactivity in 100 healthy dogs, 50 dogs with small intestinal disease, and 25 dogs with exocrine pancreatic insufficiency. (Reproduced from Williams, DA and Batt, RM: Sensitivity and specificity of assay of serum trypsin-like immunoreactivity for the diagnosis of canine exocrine pancreatic insufficiency. J Am Vet Med Assoc 192:195, 1988.)

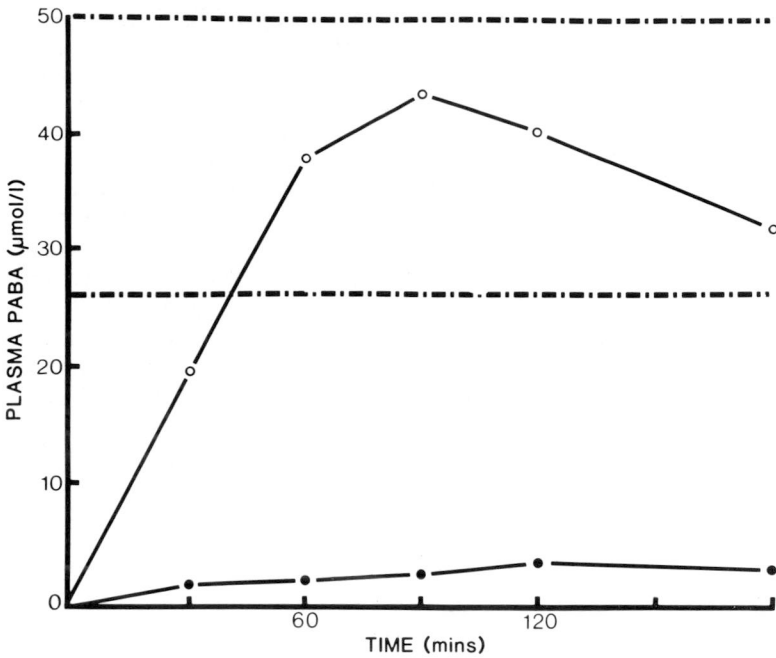

FIGURE 90–10. Bentiromide (BT-PABA) test results from a dog with exocrine pancreatic insufficiency (closed circles) and from a dog with normal exocrine pancreatic function (open circles). The horizontal lines indicate the limits of peak plasma *p*-aminobenzoic acid (PABA) levels in healthy control dogs. (Reproduced from Williams, DA: The diagnosis of canine exocrine pancreatic insufficiency. Vet Ann 25:330, 1985.)

dogs with fat malabsorption.[265] It has been suggested that EPI can be distinguished from other causes of fat malabsorption by repeating the test after addition of pancreatic extract to the fat meal. Plasma turbidity should then develop in dogs with EPI but not in dogs with other causes of fat malabsorption. This test is relatively simple to perform since biochemical analysis of serum samples is not required; however, its sensitivity is questionable since even in severe EPI 80 per cent or more of ingested fat may be absorbed.[147, 152–155, 189, 266] It is unlikely that such a subtle reduction in the normal variable post-prandial lipemia can be accurately assessed

by visual inspection of serum or plasma. Moreover, there is considerable normal variation in both the degree of lipemia and the time it takes for lipemia to develop due to factors such as variation in clearance of plasma lipids and gastric emptying times. There is also evidence that absorption of free fatty acids after oral administration of hydrolyzed fat is decreased in canine EPI; thus development of lipemia may be impaired even when affected dogs are given fat with pancreatic enzymes.[143, 186, 187] Such a failure to develop lipemia was reported in one of eight dogs with EPI tested in a recent study.[267] Biochemical quantitation of serum triglyceride levels

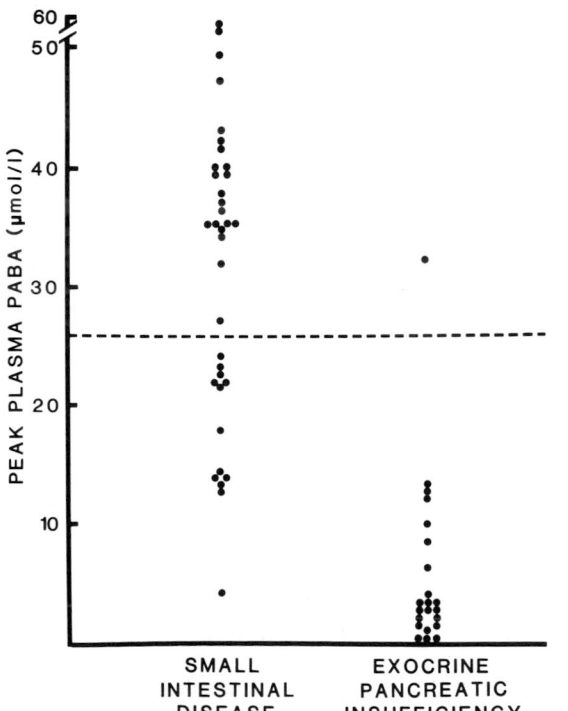

FIGURE 90–11. Peak plasma *p*-aminobenzoic acid (PABA) concentration after combined bentiromide/xylose absorption testing of 35 dogs with small intestinal disease and 22 dogs with exocrine pancreatic insufficiency. The dashed line indicates the lower limit of the range of peak plasma PABA values in healthy dogs. (Reproduced from Williams, DA and Batt, RM: Sensitivity and specificity of assay of serum trypsin-like immunoreactivity for the diagnosis of canine exocrine pancreatic insufficiency. J Am Vet Med Assoc 192:195, 1988.)

after oral fat administration barely distinguishes dogs with EPI from healthy dogs,[268] and the results of such testing in dogs with small intestinal disease have not been reported.

STARCH TOLERANCE TEST. Oral administration of starch is followed by a small increase in blood glucose in normal dogs, but due to carbohydrate malabsorption, the magnitude of this response is reduced in dogs with EPI.[147, 190] The poor specificity of this test is predictable, since the degradation of starch and subsequent absorption of glucose involve brush border as well as pancreatic enzymes, and this has been confirmed by the finding of abnormal starch tolerance in dogs with small intestinal disease.[147] The sensitivity of this test is also questionable in view of the evidence for amylase activity of intestinal origin in the dog.[120, 121]

GLUCOSE TOLERANCE TEST. Oral and intravenous glucose tolerance is often abnormal in dogs with EPI but may occur as a result of malnutrition rather than EPI per se.[221, 222] Since glucose intolerance is not seen in all cases[148] and may occur in some dogs with small intestinal disease,[147] this test is of limited diagnostic value.

OTHER SERUM TESTS. Routine laboratory test results are generally not helpful in establishing the diagnosis of EPI. Serum alanine aminotransferase levels are mildly to moderately increased and may reflect hepatocyte damage secondary to increased uptake of hepatotoxic substances through an abnormally permeable small intestinal mucosa.[143, 147, 269] Other routine serum biochemical tests results are unremarkable, except that total lipid, cholesterol, and polyunsaturated fatty acid concentrations are often reduced.[143, 147, 252] Dogs with EPI display a remarkable ability to maintain normal serum protein concentrations even when severely malnourished. Mild lymphopenia and eosinophilia are occasionally seen in dogs with EPI, but complete blood count results are usually within normal limits, and major abnormalities should be pursued as evidence of additional or alternative underlying disorders.[167, 252]

Serum amylase, lipase, and phospholipase A_2 activities are generally normal or only slightly reduced in EPI, and these tests are not useful in the identification of affected dogs.[143, 252, 270] Nonpancreatic sources of these enzymes are clearly present in dogs, and although their activities may increase in inflammatory disease of the pancreas, they do not decrease proportionately as the mass of functional exocrine pancreatic tissue declines. For example, even though amylase secreted into the gut lumen in response to stimulation with cholecystokinin and secretin is reduced to less than 10 per cent of the normal value in dogs with EPI, serum amylase activity is decreased only to approximately 66 per cent of normal.[120, 143] Quantitation of putative pancreas-specific iso-amylase using either electrophoresis or selective inhibition has not yet proved to be reliable in the identification of dogs with EPI.[120, 123]

FECAL ANALYSIS. EXAMINATION FOR UNDIGESTED FOOD PARTICLES. Microscopic examination of feces for evidence of undigested food (starch grains, muscle fibers) has long been used as a test for canine EPI; however, such assessment is subjective and therefore not very precise. Interpretation of results is further complicated by the variation in fecal characteristics, which occurs with different diets and with changes in intestinal transit time.[271] Moreover, the presence or absence of undigested food particles in feces does not consistently distinguish malabsorption due to EPI from that due to primary intestinal disease.[266, 267]

EXAMINATION FOR STEATORRHEA. Exocrine pancreatic insufficiency is often associated with severe steatorrhea. Steatorrhea may be assessed qualitatively by microscopic examination of fecal samples stained with Sudan III dye, but this is a subjective and inaccurate technique.[266] Using this technique, it has been reported that the observation of "heavy" fecal fat, when present, is almost always associated with EPI, but this identifies less than 50 per cent of affected dogs.[266] The majority of dogs with EPI have only trace, mild, or moderate fecal fat content. Quantitative assessment of fecal fat output is necessary to document steatorrhea but does not differentiate EPI from other causes of fat malabsorption (Figure 90–12).[266, 272] Microscopic evaluation of canine feces for the presence of "split" (i.e., digested) and "neutral" (i.e., undigested) fat, while theoretically attractive, does not appear to be useful in differentiating pancreatic from nonpancreatic steatorrhea.[267]

FECAL PROTEOLYTIC ACTIVITY. Fecal proteolytic activity has been used as an index of pancreatic enzyme activity for many years, but the reliability of the test varies widely depending on the method employed. The widely used x-ray film digestion test is certainly unreliable as performed in many laboratories. Gelatin digestion is difficult to evaluate with precision, and the test gives many false-negative and false-positive results. This may to some extent reflect poor standardization of

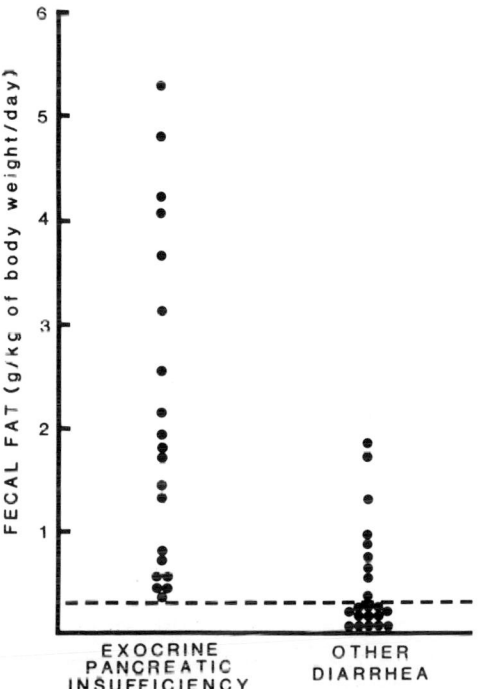

FIGURE 90–12. Fecal fat output in dogs with exocrine pancreatic insufficiency and dogs with chronic diarrhea due to other causes. The dashed line indicates the upper limit of normal in healthy dogs. (Modified from Burrows, CF, et al.: Determination of fecal fat and trypsin output in the evaluation of chronic canine diarrhea. J Am Vet Med Assoc 174:62, 1979.)

technique (perhaps the use of nongelatin-coated film),[258, 266, 273, 274] but might also be due to the presence of bacterial proteases that can digest gelatin.[261] Proteolytic activity can be measured more precisely using dyed protein substrates such as azocasein.[147, 271] Fecal proteolytic activity as assessed by this method is consistently low in most dogs with EPI, but because dogs with normal pancreatic function occasionally pass feces with low proteolytic activity, repeated determinations must be made (Figure 90–13).[147, 271] Some dogs with EPI have normal fecal proteolytic activity as assessed by this assay, but this is rare.[255, 256] Limited evidence suggests that this type of substrate is suitable for use in the cat, but it is likely that similar caution should be exercised in the interpretation of results, since healthy cats may also pass feces with negligible proteolytic activity.[175] A new assay for fecal proteolytic activity, which uses radial enzyme diffusion into agar gel containing a calcium paracaseinate substrate, has recently been developed.[274] Using this method, it has been shown that dogs with low fecal proteolytic activity not associated with EPI can be stimulated to pass feces with normal proteolytic activity by feeding crude soybean meal, which contains a trypsin inhibitor, for two days prior to testing.[274] While this modification increases the specificity of the test, it is not clear if this occurs at the expense of decreased sensitivity.

Synthetic substrates degraded only by enzymes with trypsin- or chymotrypsin-like specificities have been used to investigate the value of assay of true fecal trypsin or chymotrypsin activities in the identification of dogs with EPI.[252, 266] These assays require expensive laboratory equipment and appear to offer no advantages over simple assays of general proteolytic activity based on casein.

SUMMARY. The measurement of serum TLI appears to be the most sensitive and specific test for the identification of dogs with EPI. A combined bentiromide/xylose absorption test and/or measurement of fecal proteolytic activity in several samples using an azocasein or calcium paracaseinate substrate will also identify most affected dogs, although these tests will also give subnormal results in a proportion of dogs with small intestinal disease. Unlike assay of serum TLI, however, these latter tests should identify those rare dogs with EPI due to obstruction of the pancreatic ducts. Microscopic examination of the feces for undigested food, assessment of fecal proteolytic activity using x-ray film gelatin digestion, starch tolerance, plasma turbidity, and glucose tolerance are all unreliable and have limited value given the availability of more sensitive and specific tests. Assay of proteolytic activity in multiple fecal samples using a casein substrate is probably the most reliable test for EPI in the cat, preferably combined with quantitation of fecal fat output in order to document steatorrhea.

TREATMENT

Enzyme Replacement. Most dogs with EPI can be successfully managed by supplementing each meal with pancreatic enzymes from ox or pig pancreas. This can be accomplished using commercially available dried pancreatic extracts.[275] Numerous formulations of these extracts are available (tablets, capsules, powders, granules), some of which are enteric-coated, and their enzyme content and bioavailability vary widely.[275–277] Addition of two teaspoons of powdered nonenteric-coated preparation with each meal per 45 lb (20 kg) of body weight is generally an effective starting dose. This can be mixed with a maintenance dog food immediately prior to feeding. Two meals a day are usually sufficient to promote weight gain. Dogs will generally gain 1 to 2 lb (0.5 to 1.0 kg) per week, and diarrhea will resolve within four to five days. In some cases, the reduction in frequency of defecation is dramatic, and other signs such as coprophagia and polyphagia often disappear within a few days. As soon as clinical improvement is apparent, owners can determine a minimum effective dose of enzyme supplement to prevent return of clinical signs. This varies slightly between batches of extract, and also from dog to dog. Most affected animals require at least one teaspoonful of enzyme supplement per meal. One meal per day is sufficient in some dogs, while others continue to require two. Commercial dried pancreatic extracts are expensive, and when available, substitution of three to four ounces per 45 lb (20 kg) of body weight of chopped raw ox or pig pancreas obtained from animals certified as healthy following appropriate postmortem inspection is a more economical alternative. Pancreas can be stored frozen at −20°C for at least three months, and enzyme activity will be adequately maintained.

MEASURES TO INCREASE THE EFFECTIVENESS OF EN-

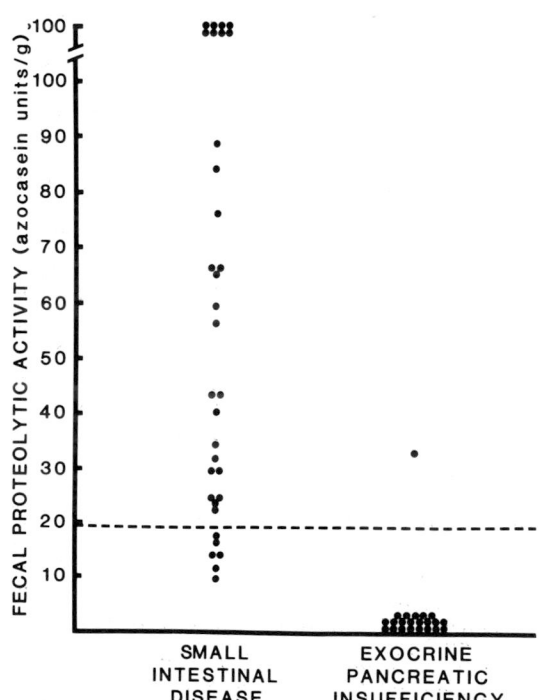

FIGURE 90–13. Fecal proteolytic activity determined by azocasein assay of three-day collections from 34 dogs with small intestinal disease and 22 dogs with exocrine pancreatic insufficiency. The dashed line indicates the lower limit of the range of values in healthy dogs. (Reproduced from Williams, DA and Batt, RM: Sensitivity and specificity of assay of serum trypsin-like immunoreactivity for the diagnosis of canine exocrine pancreatic insufficiency. J Am Vet Med Assoc 192:195, 1988.)

ZYME SUPPLEMENTATION. While administration of pancreatic enzymes with food as described above is generally successful, only a small proportion of the oral dose of each enzyme is delivered functionally intact to the small intestine, and fat absorption does not return to normal.[244, 275–279] Pancreatic lipase is rapidly inactivated at the acid pH encountered in the stomach, while trypsin and other pancreatic proteases, although relatively acid resistant, are susceptible to degradation by gastric pepsins.[278] In humans with EPI, as much as 90 per cent of ingested lipase and 80 per cent of ingested trypsin is inactivated prior to delivery to the jejunum.[275] In view of the expense of pancreatic enzyme preparations, attempts have been made to increase the effectiveness of enzyme supplementation.[244, 279] These include preincubation of enzymes with food prior to feeding, supplementation with bile salts, neutralization or inhibition of secretion of gastric acid, and use of enteric-coated preparations.

Preincubation of food with enzyme powder for 30 minutes prior to feeding does not improve the effectiveness of oral enzyme treatment in promoting fat absorption in dogs with ligated pancreatic ducts.[244] This is not surprising, since optimal activity will not be achieved unless lipase is in solution at the appropriate pH and temperature and is in the presence of appropriate concentrations of colipase and bile acids, conditions that are unlikely to be encountered in the feeding bowl.

There is no evidence that bile release is deficient in naturally occurring EPI in humans or dogs, and addition of bile salts to enzyme supplement does not improve fat absorption over that obtained when enzymes alone are given with food to dogs with ligated pancreatic ducts.[244] It is possible that bile salts may be precipitated in individuals with abnormally low small intestinal intraluminal pH, and while this may contribute to development of steatorrhea due to a functional bile salt deficiency, supplementation with oral bile salts will not rectify such a situation.[280] Drastic reductions in intraluminal pH in canine EPI are unlikely, so functional bile salt deficiency is probably not of importance.

Gastric acid secretion may be reduced by administration of the histamine type 2 receptor antagonist cimetidine. When given at a dosage of 300 mg/45 lb (300 mg/20 kg) body weight with oral pancreatic enzymes to dogs with ligated pancreatic ducts, this drug does improve fat absorption but does not decrease fecal wet or dry weight.[244] The routine use of cimetidine in the treatment of EPI is not recommended given the expense of the drug and the fact that so many dogs respond well to enzymes alone. The use of oral antacids (sodium bicarbonate, aluminum and magnesium hydroxide) to decrease intragastric lipase destruction does not increase the effectiveness of enzyme therapy in experimental EPI.[244] Indeed, it is possible that antacids may be detrimental.[156, 281] While antacids may increase the quantity of orally administered pancreatic lipase reaching the small intestine, lingual and/or gastric lipase activity, which probably accounts for the considerable residual fat absorption in dogs with EPI, may be inhibited since an acid pH is optimal for intragastric lipolysis.[156]

Enteric-coated preparations have been formulated in an attempt to protect orally administered enzymes from gastric acid. In studies in humans, these preparations have generally proved to be no more effective than non-enteric coated extracts.[275, 278, 279] In the author's experience, enteric-coated preparations have been either ineffective or less effective than powdered pancreatic extract in treating dogs with EPI. This may reflect selective retention of enteric-coated particles in the stomach or perhaps rapid intestinal transit such that adequate enzyme release does not occur.[279] Similar mechanisms may explain the ineffectiveness of an uncrushed tablet formulation of pancreatic enzymes in treating EPI in pancreatic duct–ligated dogs, while in contrast the same formulation was effective when crushed prior to feeding.[244] In those dogs with suboptimal weight gain in response to pancreatic enzymes alone, the author has found no advantage either in increasing the dose of enzymes above two teaspoonfuls per meal or giving cimetidine, suggesting that factors other than enzyme delivery to the small intestine are involved.

Dietary Modification. Clinical studies in humans and experimental studies in dogs show that fat absorption does not return to normal despite appropriate enzyme therapy.[244, 279] Dogs appear to compensate by eating slightly more than usual, and as with any individual dog, it is necessary to regulate the amount of food given in order to maintain ideal body weight.[281]

While therapy with regular maintenance dog food and appropriate enzyme replacement is usually effective, feeding of a highly digestible, low-fiber diet has been advocated.[282] Results of experimental studies have been contradictory, however, and definitive conclusions about the value of special diets in EPI cannot be made.[244, 281, 283] Dietary fiber does impair pancreatic enzyme activity, and high-fiber diets probably should be avoided.[284] Highly digestible diets may be of particular value in promoting caloric uptake in those dogs with EPI that do not regain normal body weight when fed regular food with enzyme replacement. These patients may also benefit from addition of medium-chain triglycerides to the food. Some medium-chain triglyceride is absorbed intact, and its hydrolysis by lipase proceeds much faster than that of long-chain triglycerides, so that fat absorption is facilitated.[278] Highly digestible diets may also be beneficial in dogs in which enzyme replacement does not cause complete resolution of diarrhea.

Vitamin Supplementation. Dogs with EPI may have severely subnormal concentrations of serum cobalamin and tocopherol, which do not necessarily increase in response to treatment with oral pancreatic enzymes, even in cases in which the clinical response in terms of weight gain and resolution of diarrhea is excellent.[200] Clinical signs associated with naturally occurring deficiencies of these vitamins in the dog have not been documented, but both may contribute to intestinal mucosal changes and perhaps cause systemic signs of deficiency, including either myopathy or myelopathy and other abnormalities of nervous tissue as reported in other species. It therefore seems prudent to supplement with these vitamins if serum concentrations are subnormal. In the author's experience, supplementation with large oral doses of tocopherol (400 to 500 IU given once daily with food for one month) is effective in returning serum concentrations to normal. In contrast, cobalamin must be given parenterally (250 μg by intramuscular or subcutaneous injection once a week for several weeks) to normalize serum concentrations.

Potential deficiencies of other vitamins in canine EPI have not been investigated in detail. Malabsorption of fat-soluble vitamins is to be expected both before and after treatment in view of the failure of pancreatic replacement therapy to return fat absorption to normal, but malabsorption of vitamins A, D, and K may not be as marked as with tocopherol, since tocopherol appears to be particularly sensitive to abnormalities in the intestinal lumen.[243] It should be noted that doses of individual vitamins in multivitamin preparations may be insufficient to normalize serum concentrations and that parenteral or very high oral doses may be required for adequate supplementation.

Antibiotic Therapy. Dogs with PAA commonly have overgrowth of bacteria in the small intestine, but in most cases this is a subclinical abnormality and affected individuals respond very well to treatment with oral enzyme replacement alone.[191] Bacterial overgrowth can cause malabsorption and diarrhea, however,[192] and in those individuals that do not respond to oral enzymes alone, antibiotic therapy may be of value. Oral oxytetracycline, metronidazole, or tylosin may be effective in improving the clinical response in some of these dogs.[191] Long-lasting untreated bacterial overgrowth may cause mucosal damage that is only partially reversible following even prolonged antibiotic therapy,[285] and this may explain why some dogs fail to return to normal body weight. Whether overgrowth persists following treatment with enzymes alone is not known, nor is it known if a predisposition to recurrent development of overgrowth exists following antibiotic therapy.

Glucocorticoid Therapy. In those few dogs that respond poorly to the above treatments, oral prednisolone (or prednisone) at an initial dose of ½ to 1 mg/lb (1 to 2 mg/kg) q12h for seven to 14 days may be beneficial. Inflammatory bowel disease, for example lymphocytic-plasmacytic enteritis, coexists with EPI in some of these dogs. Long-term glucocorticoid administration is generally unnecessary, and the dose can be reduced over four to six weeks.

PROGNOSIS

The underlying pathologic process leading to EPI is generally irreversible, and lifelong treatment is required. It has been suggested that enzyme therapy may be withdrawn without return of clinical signs in some affected dogs,[167] although this must be very rare judging by the infrequency with which such claims are made. Nonetheless, given the expense of treatment, it is reasonable to withdraw enzyme supplement for a trial period every six months or so and observe the dog for recurrence of polyphagia and diarrhea. Pancreatic acinar tissue does have some capacity to regenerate, and it is not inconceivable that following either pancreatitis or PAA, residual acinar tissue might regenerate sufficiently to prevent clinical signs of EPI. In most cases treatment will be required for life, but providing owners are willing to accept the cost of enzyme replacement, the prognosis

is generally good. Some dogs may fail to regain normal body weight, but these animals usually have total resolution of diarrhea and polyphagia and are quite acceptable as pets.

Treatment of dogs with diabetes mellitus and EPI due to chronic pancreatitis is likely to be more troublesome and expensive. Diabetes mellitus may be particularly difficult to regulate in view of probable coexistent derangement in the secretion of glucagon and somatostatin. Inflammation in residual pancreatic tissue may cause anorexia, vomiting, or other signs of pancreatitis, and this may further complicate treatment of diabetes mellitus.

Neoplasia of the Exocrine Pancreas

Pancreatic adenocarcinomas may be acinar or duct cell in origin, but both are uncommon and they are particularly rare in cats. In both species they are seen in older animals. Pancreatic carcinoma may be more common in Airedale terriers than in other breeds.[19, 286–288]

Adenocarcinomas are usually highly malignant tumors and have often metastasized to the liver and local lymph nodes, or less commonly to the lungs, at the time of presentation. Clinical signs are usually nonspecific: weight loss, anorexia, depression, and vomiting. Affected animals are often icteric due to associated obstruction of the bile ducts or widespread hepatic metastasis. Occasionally, dogs will present with characteristic signs of diabetes mellitus or EPI due to obstruction of the pancreatic ducts or β cell destruction.[118, 150, 286]

There are usually no specific findings on physical examination, but there may be abdominal tenderness due to associated pancreatitis, and occasionally an anterior abdominal mass is palpable. Abdominal radiographs may suggest pancreatitis or indicate the presence of an anterior mass, while thoracic radiographs may reveal pulmonary metastasis. Ultrasonographic examination may help further define pancreatic abnormalities, and cytologic examination of abdominal fluid or of material aspirated from suspect areas may reveal neoplastic cells.

There are no specific laboratory tests for pancreatic carcinoma, and results of routine tests may be misleading. Elevated activities of amylase and lipase are seen in some dogs with pancreatic carcinoma. Hepatic involvement is usually indicated by marked elevations of alkaline phosphatase and bilirubin, with lesser increases in alanine aminotransferase, suggesting an obstructive hepatopathy.[118, 286] In most cases, definitive diagnosis requires exploratory laparotomy. It is important to biopsy abnormal pancreatic tissue since chronic pancreatitis may grossly resemble pancreatic carcinoma.

Given the frequency of metastasis at the time of diagnosis, the prognosis for animals with carcinomas of the exocrine pancreas is extremely poor. There are no reports of curative therapy, but surgical excision of localized lesions, perhaps in combination with chemotherapy, may be palliative. Therapy with insulin and pancreatic enzymes may be required to treat associated diabetes mellitus and EPI.[150, 286]

Pancreatic Flukes in Cats

There are several reports of infection with the pancreatic fluke, *Eurytrema procyonis*, in domestic cats.[289-291] Associated pathology generally includes pancreatic atrophy and fibrosis that in some cases, together with duct obstruction, may severely decrease exocrine pancreatic secretory capacity.[289] In spite of marked loss of exocrine tissue, however, weight loss and diarrhea have not been reported, and the infection is usually subclinical.[289]

Infection is often an incidental finding based on observation of characteristic eggs in the feces.[290] However, one report described an infected cat that had marked inflammatory infiltrates in association with the parasites, and a two-year history of weight loss and intermittent vomiting, consistent with pancreatitis perhaps progressing to clinical EPI.[291] Treatment with fenbendazole has been reported to be effective.[290]

References

1. Bernard, C: Memoir on the pancreas and on the role of pancreatic juice in digestive processes. Particularly in the digestion of neutral fat. Translated by Henderson, J. Monographs of the Physiological Society No. 42, New York, Academic Press, 1985.
2. Abels, J and Muckerheide, MM: Absorption of vitamin B_{12} in dogs. Clin Res 18:530, 1970.
3. Abels, J, et al.: A dual role for the dog pancreas in the absorption of vitamin B_{12}. Program, 17th Mtg Am Soc Hematology, Atlanta, 1974.
4. Horadagoda, NU, et al.: Identification and characterization of a pancreatic intrinsic factor in the dog. Gastroenterology 90.1464, 1986.
5. Herzlich, B and Herbert, V: The role of the pancreas in cobalamin (vitamin B_{12}) absorption. Am J Gastroenterol 79:489, 1984.
6. Evans, GW, et al.: A proposed mechanism for zinc absorption in the rat. Am J Physiol 228:501, 1975.
7. Borgstrom, B: Relative colipase deficiency as a cause of fat malabsorption in humans and the importance of the law of mass action for clinical medicine. Gastroenterology 86:194, 1984.
8. Dorricott, NJ, et al.: Mechanisms of acid disposal in canine duodenum. Am J Physiol 228:269, 1975.
9. Rubinstein, E, et al.: Antibacterial activity of the pancreatic fluid. Gastroenterology 88:927, 1985.
10. Alpers, DH and Tedesco, FJ: The possible role of pancreatic proteases in the turnover of intestinal brush border proteins. Biochim Biophys Acta 401:28, 1975.
11. Kwong, WKL, et al.: Effect of exocrine pancreatic insufficiency on small intestine in the mouse. Gastroenterology 74:1277, 1978.
12. Williamson, RCN: Intestinal adaptation: Structural, functional and cytokinetic changes. N Engl J Med 298:1393, 1978.
13. Williamson, RCN: Intestinal adaptation: Mechanisms of control. N Engl J Med 298:1444, 1978.
14. Eddeland, A and Ohlsson, K: Purification of canine pancreatic secretory trypsin inhibitor and interaction in vitro with complexes of trypsin-macroglobulin. Scand J Clin Lab Invest 36:815, 1976.
15. Laskowski, M and Kato, I: Protein inhibitors of proteinases. Annu Rev Biochem 49:493, 1980.
16. Evans, HE and Christensen, GC: The digestive apparatus and abdomen. *In* Evans, HE and Christensen, GC (eds): Miller's Anatomy of the Dog. Philadelphia, WB Saunders, 1985.
17. Schummer, A, et al.: The alimentary canal, general and comparative. *In* Nickel, R, et al. (eds): The Viscera of the Domestic Mammals. New York, Springer-Verlag, 1979, p 99.
18. Williams, JA and Goldfine, ID: The insulin-acinar relationship.
19. Jubb, KV, et al.: The pancreas. *In* Jubb, KV (ed): Pathology of Domestic Animals. New York, Academic Press, 1985, p 313.
20. Bockman, DE: Anastomosing tubular arrangement of dog exocrine pancreas. Cell Tissue Res 189:497, 1978.
21. Holst, JJ: Neural regulation of pancreatic exocrine function. *In* Go, VLW, et al. (eds): The Exocrine Pancreas: Biology, Pathology and Diseases. New York, Raven Press, 1986.
22. Rinderknecht, H: Pancreatic secretory enzymes. *In* Go, VLW, et al. (eds): The Exocrine Pancreas: Biology, Pathology and Diseases. New York, Raven Press, 1986.
23. Case, RM and Argent, BE: Bicarbonate secretion by pancreatic duct cells: Mechanisms and control. *In* Go, VLW, et al (eds): The Exocrine Pancreas: Biology, Pathology and Diseases. New York, Raven Press, 1986.
24. Scheele, GA: Biosynthesis, segregation and secretion of exportable proteins by the exocrine pancreas. Am J Physiol 238:G467, 1980.
25. Scheele, G: Cellular processing of proteins in the exocrine pancreas. *In* Go, VLW, et al. (eds): The Exocrine Pancreas: Biology, Pathology and Diseases. New York, Raven Press, 1986, p 69.
26. Itoh, Z, et al.: Biphasic secretory response of exocrine pancreas to feeding. Am J Physiol 238:G332, 1980.
27. Singer, MV: Neurohormonal control of pancreatic enzyme secretion in animals. *In* Go, VLW, et al. (eds): The Exocrine Pancreas: Biology, Pathology and Diseases. New York, Raven Press, 1986, p 315.
28. Williams, JA and Hootman, SR: Stimulus-secretion coupling in pancreatic acinar cells. *In* Go, VLW, et al. (eds): The Exocrine Pancreas: Biology, Pathology and Diseases. New York, Raven Press, 1986, p 123.
29. Geokas, MC, et al.: Molecular forms of immunoreactive pancreatic elastase in canine pancreatic and peripheral blood. Am J Physiol 238:G238, 1980.
30. Borgstrom, A: The fate of intravenously injected trypsinogens in dogs. Scand J Gastroenterol 16:281, 1981.
31. Geokas, MC, et al.: Plasma pancreatic trypsinogens in chronic renal failure and after nephrectomy. Am J Physiol 242:177, 1982.
32. Levitt, MD, et al.: Study of the possible enteropancreatic circulation of pancreatic amylase in the dog. Am J Physiol 241:G54, 1981.
33. Florholmen, J, et al.: The "endocrine" enzyme secretion from the pancreas. Scand J Gastroenterol 21:513, 1986.
34. Sarner, M: Pancreatitis: Definitions and classification. *In* Go, VLW, et al. (eds): The Exocrine Pancreas: Biology, Pathology and Diseases. New York, Raven Press, 1986.
35. Rutgers, C, et al.: Pancreatic pseudocyst associated with acute pancreatitis in a dog: Ultrasonographic diagnosis. JAAHA 21:411, 1985.
36. Kelly, DF, et al.: Jaundice in the cat associated with inflammation of the biliary tract and pancreas. J Small Anim Pract 16:163, 1975.
37. Duffel, SJ: Some aspects of pancreatic disease in the cat. J Small Anim Pract 16:365, 1975.
38. Steer, ML and Meldolesi, J: The cell biology of experimental pancreatitis. N Engl J Med 316:144, 1987.
39. Rinderknecht, H: Activation of pancreatic zymogens. Normal activation, premature intrapancreatic activation, protective mechanisms against inappropriate activation. Dig Dis Sci 31:314, 1986.
40. Steer, ML, et al.: Pancreatitis, the role of lysosomes. Dig Dis Sci 29:934, 1984.
41. Sanfey, H, et al.: The role of oxygen-derived free radicals in the pathogenesis of acute pancreatitis. Am Surg 200:405, 1984.
42. Sanfey, H and Cameron, JL: Increased capillary permeability—an early lesion in acute pancreatitis. Surgery 96:485, 1984.
43. Brodrick, JW, et al.: Molecular forms of immunoreactive pancreatic cationic trypsin in pancreatitis patient sera. Am J Physiol 237:E474, 1979.
44. Borgstrom, A and Lasson, A: Trypsin-α_1-protease inhibitor complexes in serum and clinical course of acute pancreatitis. Scand J Gastroenterol 19:1119, 1984.
45. Borgstrom, A and Ohlsson, K: Immunoreactive trypsins in sera from dogs before and after induction of experimental pancreatitis. Hoppe Seyler's Z Physiol Chem 361:625, 1980.

46. Geokas, MC, et al.: Immunoreactive forms of cationic trypsin in plasma and ascitic fluid of dogs with experimental pancreatitis. Am J Pathol 105:31, 1981.

47. Durie, PR, et al.: Serial alterations in the forms of immunoreactive pancreatic cationic trypsin in plasma from patients with acute pancreatitis. J Pediatr Gastroenterol Nutr 4:199, 1984.

48. Ohlsson, K, et al.: In vivo interaction between typsin and some plasma proteins in relation to tolerance to intravenous infusion of trypsin in dogs. Acta Chir Scand 137:113, 1971.

49. Kwaan, HC, et al.: A study of pancreatic enzymes as a factor in the pathogenesis of disseminated intravascular coagulation during acute pancreatitis. Surgery 69:663, 1970.

50. Izquierdo, R, et al.: Comparative study of protease inhibitors on coagulation abnormalities in canine pancreatitis. J Surg Res 36:606, 1984.

51. Nevalainen, TJ: The role of phospholipase A in acute pancreatitis. Scand J Gastroenterol 15:641, 1980.

52. Geokas, MC, et al.: The role of elastase in acute hemorrhagic pancreatitis in man. Lab Invest 19:235, 1968.

53. Lungarella, G, et al.: Pulmonary vascular injury in pancreatitis: Evidence for a major role played by pancreatic elastase. Exp Mol Pathol 42:44, 1985.

54. Sanfey, H, et al.: The pathogenesis of acute pancreatitis: The source and role of oxygen-derived free radicals in three different experimental models. Ann Surg 201:633, 1985.

55. Lasson, A: Acute pancreatitis in man. A clinical and biochemical study of pathophysiology and treatment. Scand J Gastroenterol (Suppl) 99:1, 1984.

56. Lasson, A and Ohlsson, K: Acute pancreatitis: The correlation between clinical course, protease inhibitors, and complement and kinin activation. Scand J Gastroenterol 19:707, 1984.

57. Lasson, A and Ohlsson, K: Protease inhibitors in acute human pancreatitis: The correlation between biochemical changes and clinical course. Scand J Gastroenterol 19:779, 1984.

58. Largman, C, et al.: Correlation of trypsin-plasma inhibitor complexes with mortality in experimental pancreatitis in rats. Dig Dis Sci 31:961, 1986.

59. Kornegay, JN: Hypocalcemia in dogs. Comp Cont Ed Pract Vet 4:103, 1982.

60. Adham, NF, et al.: Relationship between the functional status of the reticuloendothelial system and the outcome of experimentally induced pancreatitis in young mice. Gastroenterology 84:461, 1983.

61. Adham, NF, et al.: The effect of reticuloendothelial system (RES) stimulation on the outcome of bile-induced pancreatitis in dogs. Gastroenterology 84:1088, 1983.

62. Adler, G, et al.: Experimental models and concepts in acute pancreatitis. In Go, VLW, et al. (eds): The Exocrine Pancreas: Biology, Pathology and Diseases. New York, Raven Press, 1986, p 407.

63. Coffin, DL and Thoradal-Christensen, A: The clinical and some pathological aspects of pancreatic disease in dogs. Vet Med 48:193, 1953.

64. Haig, TH: Cellular membranes in the etiology of acute pancreatitis. Surg Forum 20:380, 1969.

65. Haig, TH: Pancreatic digestive enzymes: Influence of a diet that augments pancreatitis. J Surg Res 10:601, 1970.

66. Goodhead, B: Importance of nutrition in the pathogenesis of experimental pancreatitis in the dog. Arch Surg 103:724, 1971.

67. Pitchumoni, CS, et al.: Effects of nutrition on the exocrine pancreas. In Go, VLW, et al. (eds): The Exocrine Pancreas: Biology, Pathology and Diseases. New York, Raven Press, 1986, p 69.

68. Anderson, NV and Strafuss, AC: Pancreatic disease in dogs and cats. JAVMA 159:885, 1971.

69. Steer, ML: Etiology and pathophysiology of acute pancreatitis. In Go, VLW, et al. (eds): The Exocrine Pancreas: Biology, Pathology and Diseases. New York, Raven Press, 1986.

70. Guzman, S, et al.: Impaired lipid clearance in patients with previous acute pancreatitis. Gut 26:888, 1985.

71. Rogers, WA, et al.: Idiopathic hyperlipoproteinemia in dogs. JAVMA 166:1087, 1975.

72. Mallory, A and Kern, F: Drug-induced pancreatitis: A critical review. Gastroenterology 78:813, 1980.

73. Hansen, JF and Carpenter, RH: Fatal acute systemic anaphylaxis and hemorrhagic pancreatitis following asparaginase treatment in a dog. JAAHA 19:977, 1983.

74. Smart, ME, et al.: Toxoplasmosis in a cat associated with cholangitis and progressive pancreatitis. Can Vet J 14:313, 1973.

75. Sherding, RG: Feline infectious peritonitis. Comp Cont Ed 1:95, 1979.

76. Rothenbacher, H and Lindquist, WD: Liver cirrhosis and pancreatitis in a cat infected with Amphimerces pseudofelineus. JAVMA 143:1099, 1963.

77. Keynes, MW: A nonpancreatic source of the proteolytic-enzyme amidase and bacteriology in experimental acute pancreatitis. Ann Surg 191:187, 1980.

78. Hirsch, VM and Doige, CE: Suppurative cholangitis in cats. JAVMA 182:1223, 1983.

79. Keane, FB, et al.: Interdigestive canine pancreatic juice composition and pancreatic reflux and pancreatic sphincter anatomy. Dig Dis Sci 26:577, 1981.

80. Geokas, MC, et al.: Acute pancreatitis. Ann Intern Med 103:86, 1985.

81. Schaer, M: A clinicopathologic survey of acute pancreatitis in 30 dogs and 5 cats. JAAHA 15:681, 1979.

82. Neuman, NB: Acute hemorrhagic pancreatitis associated with iatrogenic hypercalcemia in a dog. JAVMA 166:381, 1975.

83. Suter, PF and Olsson, SE: Traumatic hemorrhagic pancreatitis in the cat. A report with emphasis on the radiological diagnosis. J Am Vet Radiol Soc 10:4, 1969.

84. Dalton, JRF and Hill, FWG: A procedure for the examination of the liver and pancreas in dogs. J Small Anim Pract 13:527, 1972.

85. Lightwood, R, et al.: The risk and accuracy of pancreatic biopsy. Am J Surg 132:189, 1976.

86. Moossa, AR and Altorki, N: Pancreatic biopsy. Surg Clin North Am 63:1205, 1983.

87. Wilson, JW and Caywood, DD: Functional tumors of the pancreatic beta cells. Comp Cont Ed Pract Vet 3:458, 1981.

88. Polzin, DJ, et al.: Serum amylase and lipase activities in dogs with chronic primary renal failure. Am J Vet Res 44:404, 1983.

89. Goldstein, DA, et al.: Acute renal failure in patients with acute pancreatitis. Arch Intern Med 136:1363, 1976.

90. Sanfey, H, et al.: Experimental ischemic pancreatitis: Treatment with albumin. Am J Surg 150:297, 1985.

91. Gross, JB: Hereditary pancreatitis. In Go, VLW, et al. (eds): The Exocrine Pancreas: Biology, Pathology and Diseases. New York, Raven Press, 1986, p 829.

92. Dressel, TD, et al.: Pancreatitis as a complication of anticholinesterase insecticide intoxication. Ann Surg 189:199, 1979.

93. Moore, RW and Withrow, SJ: Gastrointestinal hemorrhage and pancreatitis associated with intervertebral disk disease in the dog. JAVMA 180:1443, 1982.

94. Holroyd, JB: Canine exocrine pancreatic disease. J Small Anim Pract 9:269, 1968.

95. Anderson, NV: Pancreatitis in dogs. Vet Clin North Am 2:79, 1972.

96. Pidgeon, G: Exocrine pancreatic disease in the dog and cat. Part I: Acute pancreatitis. Comp Anim Pract 1:67, 1987.

97. Lees, GE, et al.: Pulmonary edema in a dog with acute pancreatitis and cardiac disease. JAVMA 172:690, 1978.

98. Garvey, MS and Zawie, DA: Feline pancreatic disease. Vet Clin North Am 14:1231, 1984.

99. Kleine, LJ and Hornbuckle, WE: Acute pancreatitis: The radiographic findings in 182 dogs. J Am Vet Radiol Soc 19:102, 1978.

100. Kleine, LJ: Clinical and radiographic aspects of acute pancreatitis in the dog. Comp Cont Ed Pract Vet 2:295, 1980.

101. Gibbs, C, et al.: Radiological features of inflammatory conditions of the canine pancreas. J Small Anim Pract 13:531, 1972.

102. Nyland, TG, et al.: Ultrasonic features of experimentally induced acute pancreatitis in the dog. Vet Radiol 24:260, 1983.

103. Murtaugh, RJ, et al.: Pancreatic ultrasonography in dogs with experimentally induced acute pancreatitis. Vet Radiol 26:27, 1985.

104. Feldman, BF, et al.: Biochemical and coagulation changes in a canine model of acute rectalizing pancreatitis. Am J Vet Res 42:805, 1981.

105. Mulvany, MH, et al.: Clinical characterization of acute necrotizing pancreatitis. Comp Cont Ed Pract Vet 4:394, 1982.

106. Jacobs, RM, et al.: Review of the clinicopathological findings of

acute pancreatitis in the dog: Use of an experimental model. JAAHA 21:795, 1985.

107. Kitchell, BE, et al.: Clinical and pathologic changes in experimentally induced acute pancreatitis in cats. Am J Vet Res 47:1170, 1986.

108. Wells, AD and Schenk, WG: Effectiveness of normal saline solution, dextran 40 and dextran 75, and aprotinin (Trasylol) on renal blood flow preservation during acute canine pancreatitis. Am J Surg 148:624, 1984.

109. Tuzhilin, SA, et al.: Hepatic lesions in pancreatitis. Clinicoexperimental data. Am J Gastroenterol 64:108, 1975.

110. Andrzejewska, A, et al.: The ultrastructure of the liver in acute experimental pancreatitis in dogs. Exp Pathol 18:167, 1985.

111. Mia, AS, et al.: Serum values of amylase and pancreatic lipase in healthy mature dogs and dogs with experimental pancreatitis. Am J Vet Res 39:965, 1978.

112. Stickle, JE, et al.: Isoamylases in clinically normal dogs. Am J Vet Res 41:506, 1980.

113. Wagner, AE and Macy, DW: Nephelometric determination of serum amylase and lipase in naturally occurring azotemia in the dog. Am J Vet Res 43:697, 1982.

114. Westermarck, E and Rimaila-Parnanen, E: Serum phospholipase A_2 in canine acute pancreatitis. Acta Vet Scand 24:477, 1983.

115. Rapp, JP: Normal values for serum amylase and maltase in dogs and the effect of maltase on the saccharogenic method of determining amylase in serum. Am J Vet Res 23:343, 1962.

116. O'Donnell, MD and McGeeney, GF: Amylase and glucoamylase activities in canine serum. Comp Biochem Physiol 50B:269, 1975.

117. Strombeck, DR, et al.: Serum amylase and lipase activities in the diagnosis of pancreatitis in dogs. Am J Vet Res 42:1966, 1981.

118. Cornelius, LM: Laboratory diagnosis of acute pancreatitis and pancreatic adenocarcinoma. Vet Clin North Am 6:671, 1976.

119. Blum, AL and Linscheer, WG: Lipase in canine gastric juice. Proc Soc Exp Biol Med 135:565, 1970.

120. Jacobs, RM, et al.: Isoamylases in clinically normal and diseased dogs. Vet Clin Pathol 11:26, 1982.

121. Stickle, JE, et al.: Isoamylases in clinically normal dogs. Am J Vet Res 41:506, 1980.

122. Parent, J: Effects of dexamethasone on pancreatic tissue and on serum amylase and lipase activities in dogs. JAVMA 180:743, 1982.

123. Simpson, JW, et al.: Serum isoamylase values in normal dogs and dogs with exocrine pancreatic insufficiency. Vet Res Commun 8:303, 1984.

124. Murtaugh, RJ and Jacobs, RM: Serum amylase and isoamylases and their origins in healthy dogs and dogs with experimentally induced acute pancreatitis. Am J Vet Res 46:742, 1985.

125. Williams, DA, et al.: Comments on isoamylases (letters). Am J Vet Res 46:1598, 1985.

125a. George, JW: Methemalbumin: Reality and myth. Vet Clin Path 17:43, 1988.

126. Owens, JM, et al.: Pancreatic disease in the cat. JAAHA 11:83, 1975.

127. Lankisch, PG: Acute and chronic pancreatitis. An update on management. Drugs 28:554, 1984.

128. Drazner, FM: Diseases of the pancreas. In Jones, BD and Liska, WD (eds): Canine and Feline Gastroenterology. Philadelphia, WB Saunders, 1986, p 295.

129. Murtaugh, RJ and Jacobs, RM: Serum antiprotease concentrations in dogs with spontaneous and experimentally induced acute pancreatitis. Am J Vet Res 46:80, 1985.

130. McMahon, MJ, et al.: Relation of α_2-macroglobulin and other antiproteases to the clinical features of acute pancreatitis. Am J Surg 147:164, 1984.

131. Wendt, P, et al.: Proteinases and inhibitors in plasma and peritoneal exudate in acute pancreatitis. Hepatogastroenterology 31:277, 1984.

132. Cuschieri, A, et al.: Treatment of acute pancreatitis with fresh frozen plasma. Br J Surg 70:710, 1983.

133. Attix, E, et al.: Effects of an anticholinergic and a corticosteroid on acute pancreatitis in experimental dogs. Am J Vet Res 42:1668, 1981.

134. Denny, HR and Lucke, JN: A case of acute pancreatic necrosis in the dog. J Small Anim Pract 13:545, 1972.

134a. Salisbury, SK, et al.: Pancreatic abscess in dogs: Six cases (1978–1986). JAVMA 193:1104, 1988.

134b. Matthiesen, DT and Rosin, E: Common bile duct obstruction secondary to chronic fibrosing pancreatitis: Treatment by use of cholecystoduodenostomy in the dog. JAVMA 189:1443, 1986.

135. Musa, BE, et al.: Evaluation of gamma radiation therapy in experimentally induced hemorrhagic pancreatitis in dogs. Am J Vet Res 40:927, 1979.

136. Balldin, G and Ohlsson, K: Trasylol prevents trypsin-induced shock in dogs. Hoppe-Seyler's Z Physiol Chem 360:651, 1979.

137. Balldin, G, et al.: Aprotinin turn-over studies in dog and in man with severe acute pancreatitis. Hoppe-Seyler's Z Physiol Chem 365:1417, 1984.

138. Hermon-Taylor, J and Heywood, GC: A rational approach to the specific chemotherapy of pancreatitis. Scand J Gastroenterol (Suppl) 117:39, 1985.

139. Gabryelewicz, A, et al.: Prostacyclin: Effect on pancreatic lysosomes in acute experimental pancreatitis in dogs. Mt Sinai J Med 50:218, 1983.

140. Triebling, AT, et al.: The renal lysosomes in acute experimental pancreatitis in dogs treated with prostacyclin (PGI_2). Pathol Res Pract 178:280, 1984.

141. Slaff, J, et al.: Protease-specific suppression of pancreatic exocrine secretion. Gastroenterology 87:44, 1984.

142. Dimagno, EP, et al.: Relations between pancreatic enzyme outputs and malabsorption in severe pancreatic insufficiency. N Engl J Med 288:813, 1973.

143. Sateri, H: Investigations on the exocrine pancreatic function in dogs suffering from chronic exocrine pancreatic insufficiency. Acta Vet Scand (Suppl) 53:1, 1975.

144. Williams, DA and Batt, RM: Diagnosis of canine exocrine pancreatic insufficiency by the assay of serum trypsin-like immunoreactivity. J Small Anim Pract 24:583, 1983.

145. Holzworth, J and Coffin, DL: Pancreatic insufficiency and diabetes mellitus in a cat. Cornell Vet 43:502, 1953.

146. Anderson, NV and Low, DG: Diseases of the canine pancreas: A comparative summary of 103 cases. Anim Hosp 1:189, 1965.

147. Hill, FWG: Malabsorption syndrome in the dog: A study of 38 cases. J Small Anim Pract 13:575, 1972.

148. Pfister, K, et al.: Morphological studies in dogs with chronic pancreatic insufficiency. Virchows Arch [A] 386:91, 1980.

149. Rimaila-Parnanen, E and Westermarck, E: Pancreatic degenerative atrophy and chronic pancreatitis in dogs. A comparative study of 60 cases. Acta Vet Scand 23:400, 1982.

150. Bright, JM: Pancreatic adenocarcinoma in a dog with maldigestion syndrome. JAVMA 187:420, 1985.

151. Lerner, J, et al.: Hereditary abnormalities of pancreatic function. In Go, VLW, et al. (eds): The Exocrine Pancreas: Biology, Pathology and Diseases. New York, Raven Press, 1986.

152. Vermeulen, C, et al.: The effect of pancreatectomy on fat absorption from the intestines. Am J Physiol 138:792, 1943.

153. Pessoa, VC, et al.: Fat absorption in the absence of bile and pancreatic juice. Am J Physiol 174:209, 1953.

154. Douglas, GJ, et al.: The effect on digestion and absorption of excluding the pancreatic juice from the intestine. Gastroenterology 23:452, 1953.

155. Imondi, AR, et al.: Synthetic peptides in the diagnosis of exocrine pancreatic insufficiency in animals. Gut 13:726, 1972.

156. Abrams, CK, et al.: Lingual lipase in cystic fibrosis. Quantitation of enzyme activity in the upper small intestine of patients with exocrine pancreatic insufficiency. J Clin Invest 73:374, 1984.

157. Curtis, KJ, et al.: Protein digestion and absorption in rats with pancreatic duct occlusion. Gastroenterology 74:1271, 1978.

158. Meyer, JH: Pancreatic physiology. In Sleisenger, MH and Fordtran, JS (eds): Gastrointestinal Disease, 3rd ed. Philadelphia, WB Saunders, 1983.

159. Eppig, JJ and Leiter, EM: Exocrine pancreatic insufficiency syndrome in CBA/J mice. Ultrastructural study. Am J Pathol 86:17, 1977.

160. Balk, MW, et al.: Exocrine pancreatic dysfunction in guinea pigs with diabetes mellitus. Lab Invest 32:28, 1975.

161. Port, CD, et al.: Chronic exocrine pancreatic insufficiency in two Indian lions (Panthera leo persica). J Comp Pathol 91:483, 1981.

162. Hasholt, J: Atrophy of the pancreas in budgerigars. Nord Vet 25:436, 1972.

163. Barbezat, GO and Hansen, JDL: The exocrine pancreas and protein-calorie malnutrition. Pediatrics 42:77, 1968.

164. Levenson, SM, et al.: Strange hemolytic anemia and pancreatic acinar atrophy and fibrosis. Fed Proc 30:1785, 1971.

165. Fell, BF, et al.: Pancreatic atrophy in copper-deficient rats: Histochemical and ultrastructural evidence of a selective effect on acinar cells. Histochem J 14:665, 1982.

166. Mizunuma, T, et al.: Effects of injecting excess arginine on rat pancreas. J Nutr 114:467, 1984.

167. Van Kruiningen, HJ: Pancreatic atrophy. In Van Kruiningen, HJ (ed): Comparative Gastroenterology. Springfield, IL, Charles C Thomas, 1982, p 42.

168. Hill, FWG, et al.: Pancreatic degenerative atrophy in dogs. J Comp Pathol 81:321, 1971.

169. Anderson, NV and Low, DG: Juvenile atrophy of the canine pancreas. Anim Hosp 1:101, 1965.

170. Weber, von W and Freudiger, U: Erbanalytische untersuchungen uber die chronische. Exokrine pankreasinsuffizienz beim deutschen schaferhund. Schweiz Arch Tierheilk 119:257, 1977.

171. Westermarck, E: The hereditary nature of canine pancreatic degenerative atrophy in the German Shepherd dog. Acta Vet Scand 21:389, 1980.

172. Leiter, EH, et al.: Exocrine pancreatic insufficiency syndrome in CBA/J mice. Biochemical studies. Am J Pathol 86:31, 1977.

173. Andriulli, A, et al.: Circulating trypsin-like immunoreactivity in chronic pancreatitis. Dig Dis Sci 26:532, 1981.

174. Grendell, JH and Cello, JP: Chronic pancreatitis. In Sleisenger, MM and Fordtran, JS (eds): Gastrointestinal Disease, 3rd ed. Philadelphia, WB Saunders, 1983.

175. Watson, ADJ, et al.: Weight loss in cats which eat well. J Small Anim Pract 22:473, 1981.

176. Hoskins, JD, et al.: Feline pancreatic insufficiency. VM/SAC 77:1745, 1982.

177. Grand, RJ, et al.: Pancreatic disorders in childhood. In Sleisenger, MM and Fordtran, JS (eds): Gastrointestinal Disease, 3rd ed. Philadelphia, WB Saunders, 1983.

178. Tangner, CH, et al.: Complications associated with proximal duodenal resection and cholecystoduodenostomy in two cats. Vet Surg 11:60, 1982.

179. Balas, D, et al.: Effects of pancreatic duct ligation on the hamster intestinal mucosa. Digestion 20:157, 1980.

180. Senegas-Balas, F, et al.: Effect of pancreatic duct ligation on the hamster intestinal mucosa. Digestion 21:83, 1981.

181. Senegas-Balas, F, et al.: Histological variations of the duodenal mucosa in chronic human pancreatitis. Dig Dis Sci 27:917, 1982.

182. Kotler, DP, et al.: Effects of luminal contents on jejunal fatty acid esterification in the fat. Am J Physiol 238:G414, 1980.

183. Shiau, YF, et al.: Can normal small bowel morphology be equated with normal function? Gastroenterology 76:1246, 1979.

184. Milla, PJ, et al.: Small intestinal absorption of amino acids and a dipeptide in pancreatic insufficiency. Gut 24:818, 1983.

185. Morin, CL, et al.: Small bowel mucosal dysfunction in patients with cystic fibrosis. J Pediatr 88:213, 1976.

186. Clark, CH: Pancreatic atrophy and absorption failure in a boxer. JAVMA 136:174, 1960.

187. Kallfelz, FA, et al.: Intestinal absorption of oleic acid I and triolein I in the differential diagnosis of malabsorption syndrome and pancreatic dysfunction in the dog. JAVMA 153:43, 1968.

188. Rogers, WA, et al.: Simultaneous evaluation of pancreatic exocrine function and intestinal absorptive function in dogs with chronic diarrhea. JAVMA 177:1128, 1980.

189. Batt, RM and Mann, LC: Specificity of the BT-PABA test for the diagnosis of exocrine pancreatic insufficiency in the dog. Vet Rec 108:303, 1981.

190. Washabau, RJ, et al.: Use of pulmonary hydrogen gas excretion to detect carbohydrate malabsorption in dogs. JAVMA 189:674, 1986.

191. Williams, DA, et al.: Bacterial overgrowth in the duodenum of dogs with exocrine pancreatic insufficiency. JAVMA 191:201, 1987.

192. King, CE and Toskes, PP: Small intestine bacterial overgrowth. Gastroenterology 76:1035, 1979.

193. Romer, H, et al.: Moderate and severe energy malnutrition in childhood: Effects of jejunal mucosal orophology and disaccharidase activities. J Pediatr Gastroenrol Nutr 2:459, 1983.

194. Sherman, P, et al.: Sequential disaccharidase loss in rat intestinal blind loops: Impact of malnutrition. Am J Physiol 248:626, 1985.

195. Scheving, LA, et al.: Circadian stage-dependent effects of insulin and glucagon on incorporation of ^{3}H-thymidine into deoxyribonucleic acid in the esophagus, stomach, duodenum, jejunum, ileum, caecum, colon, rectum and spleen of the adult female mouse. Endocrinology 111:308, 1982.

196. Gallo-Payet, N and Hugon, JS: Insulin receptors in isolated adult mouse intestinal cells: Studies in vivo and in agar culture. Endocrinology 114:1885, 1984.

197. Arvanitakis, C and Olsen, WA: Intestinal mucosal disaccharidases in chronic pancreatitis. Am J Dig Dis 19:417, 1974.

198. Batt, RM, et al.: Biochemical changes in the jejunal mucosa of dogs with naturally occurring exocrine pancreatic insufficiency. Gut 20:709, 1979.

199. Williams, DA, et al.: Reversible impairment of protein synthesis may contribute to jejunal abnormalities in exocrine pancreatic insufficiency. Clin Sci 68:37P, 1985.

200. Williams, DA: Studies on the diagnosis and pathophysiology of canine exocrine pancreatic insufficiency. PhD Thesis, University of Liverpool, Liverpool, England.

201. Eicholz, A: Studies on the acquisition of the brush border in intestinal epithelial cells. V. Subfractionation of enzymatic activities of the microvillus membrane. Biochim Biophys Acta 163:101, 1968.

202. Critchley, DR, et al.: Solubilization of brush borders of hamster small intestine and fractionation of some of the components. Biochim Biophys Acta 394:361, 1975.

203. Louvard, D, et al.: Topological studies on the hydrolases bound to the intestinal brush border membrane. I. Solubilization by papain and Triton X-100. Biochim Biophys Acta 375:236, 1975.

204. Louvard, D, et al.: The brush-border intestinal aminopeptidase, a transmembrane protein as probed by macromolecular photolabelling. J Molec Biol 106:1023. 1976.

205. Jonas, A, et al.: Pathogenesis of mucosal injury in the blind loop syndrome. Brush horder enzyme activity and glycoprotein degradation. J Clin Invest 60:1321, 1977.

206. Kenny, JA and Maroux, S: Topology of microvillar membrane hydrolases of kidney and intestine. Physiol Rev 62:91, 1982.

207. Williams, DA, et al.: Reductions in both protein synthesis and degradation may contribute to jejunal abnormalities in canine exocrine pancreatic insufficiency. Proceedings of the Third Annual Medical Forum of the ACVIM, San Diego, 1985.

208. Malo, C and Menard, D: Synergistic effects of insulin and thyroxine on the differentiation and proliferation of epithelial cells of suckling mouse small intestine. Biol Neonate 44:177, 1983.

209. Olsen, WA and Korsmo, H: The intestinal brush border membrane in diabetes. J Clin Invest 60:181, 1977.

210. Helman, CA, et al.: Jejunal monosaccharide, water, and electrolyte transport in patients with chronic pancreatitis. Gut 19:46, 1978.

211. Mahmood, A, et al.: Effect of chronic alloxan diabetes and insulin administration on intestinal brush border enzymes. Experientia 34:741, 1978.

212. Pothier, P and Hugon, JS: Immediate and localized response of intestinal mucosal enzyme activities in streptozotocin-diabetic mice. Comp Biochem Physiol 72A:505, 1982.

213. Gourley, GR, et al.: Intestinal mucosa in diabetic rats: Studies of microvillus membrane composition and microviscosity. Metabolism 30:1053, 1983.

214. MacLaren, IF, et al.: Achlorhydria associated with chronic disease of the exocrine pancreas. Surgery 59:676, 1966.

215. Williams, DA, et al.: Duodenal bacterial overgrowth may occur in canine exocrine pancreatic insufficiency but is not due to achlorhydria. Scientific Proceedings of the ACVIM, Washington, DC, 1984.

216. Riepe, SP, et al.: Effect of secreted Bacteroides proteases on human intestinal brush border hydrolases. J Clin Invest 66:314, 1980.

217. Jonas, A, et al.: Pathogenesis of mucosal injury in the blind loop syndrome. Release of disaccharidases from brush border membranes by extracts of bacteria obtained from intestinal blind loops in rats. Gastroenterology 75:791, 1978.

218. Vaillant, C, et al.: Regulatory peptide abnormalities in dogs with pancreatic acinar atrophy. Regul Pept 7:304, 1983.

219. Orci, L: Patterns of cellular and subcellular organization in the endocrine pancreas. J Endocrinol 102:3, 1984.

220. Vaillant, C, et al.: Pancreatic enkephalin immunoreactivity in canine pancreatic acinar atrophy. Dig Dis Sci 29:92S, 1984.

221. Hill, FWG and Kidder, DE: The oral glucose tolerance test in canine pancreatic malabsorption. Br Vet J 128:207, 1972.

222. Greve, T and Anderson, NV: The high-dose, intravenous glucose tolerance test (H-IVGTT) in dogs. Nord Vet Med 25:436, 1973.

223. Williams, DA and Batt, RM: Reversible intravenous glucose intolerance in canine exocrine pancreatic insufficiency. In Proceedings of the Fourth Annual Medical Forum of the ACVIM, Washington, DC, 1986.

224. Schwille, PO, et al.: Long-term pancreatic duct occlusion impairs the entero-insular axis in the dog—failure of plasma VIP to respond as "incretin." Peptides 4:445, 1984.

225. Creutzfeldt, W: The incretin concept today. Diabetologia 16:75, 1979.

226. Rogers, WA, et al.: Postprandial release of gastric inhibitory polypeptide (GIP) and pancreatic polypeptide in dogs with pancreatic acinar atrophy. Dig Dis Sci 28:345, 1983.

227. Bewick, M, et al.: Canine pancreatic endocrine function after interruption of pancreatic exocrine drainage. Transplantation 36:246, 1983.

228. de Bruijne, JJ, et al.: Fat mobilization and plasma hormone levels in fasted dogs. Metabolism 30:190, 1981.

229. Dowd, PS and Heatley, RV: The influence of undernutrition on immunity. Clin Sci 66:241, 1984.

230. Salazar de Sousa, J: Malnutrition and small intestinal mucosa. J Pediatr Gastroentcrol Nutr 3:321, 1984.

231. Sherman, P, et al.: Mucin depletion in the intestine of malnourished rats. Am J Physiol 248:G418, 1985.

232. Sherman, P, et al.: Sequential disaccharidase loss in rat intestinal blind loops: Impact of malnutrition. Am J Physiol 248:G626, 1985.

233. Jamison, MH, et al.: The influence of pancreatic juice on ^{64}Cu absorption in the rat. Br J Nutr 50:113, 1983.

234. Jacob, RA, et al.: Zinc status and vitamin A transport in cystic fibrosis. Am J Clin Nutr 31:638, 1978.

235. Seal, CJ and Heaton, FW: Chemical factors affecting the intestinal absorption of zinc in vitro and in vivo. Br J Nutr 50:317, 1983.

236. Brugge, WR, et al.: Development of a dual label Schilling test for pancreatic exocrine function based on the differential absorption of cobalamin bound to intrinsic factor and R protein. Gastroenterology 78:937, 1980.

237. Batt, RM and Morgan, JO: Role of serum folate and vitamin B$_{12}$ concentrations in the differentiation of small intestinal abnormalities in the dog. Res Vet Sci 32:17, 1982.

238. Marcoullis, G and Rothenberg, SP: Intrinsic factor-mediated intestinal absorption of cobalamin in the dog. Am J Physiol 241:G294, 1981.

239. Dowling, RH and Gleeson, MH: Cell turnover following small bowel resection and by-pass. Digestion 8:176, 1973.

240. Arvanitakis, C: Functional and morphological abnormalities of the small intestinal mucosa in pernicious anemia—a prospective study. Acta Hepatogastroenterol 25:313, 1978.

241. Bernstein, LM, et al.: Experimental production of elevated serum folate in dogs with intestinal blind loops: Relationship of serum levels to location of the blind loop. Gastroenterology 63:815, 1972.

242. Russell, RM, et al.: Influence of intraluminal pH on folate absorption: Studies in control subjects and in patients with pancreatic insufficiency. J Lab Clin Med 93:428, 1979.

243. Sokol, RJ, et al.: Comparison of vitamin E and 25-hydroxyvitamin D absorption during childhood cholestasis. J Pediatr 103:712, 1983.

244. Pidgeon, G and Strombeck, DR: Evaluation of treatment for pancreatic exocrine insufficiency in dogs with ligated pancreatic ducts. Am J Vet Res 43:461, 1982.

245. Langweiler, M, et al.: Effect of vitamin E deficiency on the proliferative response of canine lymphocytes. Am J Vet Res 42:1681, 1981.

246. Desai, ID, et al.: A time sequence study of the relationship of peroxidation, lysosomal enzymes, and nutritional muscular dystrophy. Arch Biochem Biophys 108:60, 1964.

247. Machlin, LJ, et al.: Effects of a prolonged vitamin E deficiency in the rat. J Nutr 107:1200, 1977.

248. Cordes, DO and Mosher, AH: Brown pigmentation (lipofuscinosis) of canine intestinal muscularis. J Pathol Bact 92:197, 1966.

249. Hayes, KC, et al.: Plasma tocopherol concentrations and vitamin E deficiency in dogs. JAVMA 157:64, 1970.

250. Nelson, JS, et al.: Progressive neuropathologic lesions in vitamin E-deficient rhesus monkeys. J Neuropathol Exp Neurol 40:166, 1981.

251. Lee-Parritz, D and Williams, DA: Unpublished observations, 1985.

252. Freudiger, U: Die diagnose der chronischen exokrinen pankreasinsuffizienz. Schweiz Arch Tierheilk 114:476, 1972.

253. Williams, DA: Unpublished observations, 1988.

254. Boyd, JW: The interpretation of serum biochemistry test results in domestic animals. Vet Clin Pathol 13(2):7, 1984.

255. Williams, DA and Batt, RM: Sensitivity and specificity of assay of serum trypsin-like immunoreactivity for the diagnosis of canine exocrine pancreatic insufficiency. JAVMA 192:195, 1988.

256. Williams, DA and Batt, RM: Exocrine pancreatic insufficiency diagnosed by radioimmunoassay of serum trypsin-like immunoreactivity in a dog with a normal BT-PABA test result. JAAHA 22:671, 1986.

257. Freudiger, U and Bigler, B: The diagnosis of chronic exocrine pancreatic insufficiency by the PABA test. Kleintier-Prax 22:73, 1977.

258. Strombeck, DR: New method for evaluation of chymotrypsin deficiency in dogs. JAVMA 173:1319, 1978.

259. Batt, RM, et al.: A new test for the diagnosis of exocrine pancreatic insufficiency in the dog. J Small Anim Pract 20:185, 1979.

260. Strombeck, DR and Harrold, D: Evaluation of 60-minute blood p-amino-benzoic acid concentration in pancreatic function testing of dogs. JAVMA 180:419, 1982.

261. Gyr, K, et al.: Chymotrypsin-like activity of some intestinal bacteria. Am J Dig Dis 23:413, 1978.

262. Sterchi, EE, et al.: Nonpancreatic hydrolysis of N-benzoyl-L-tyrosyl-p-aminobenzoic acid (PABA peptide) in the rat small intestine. J Pediatr Gastroenterol Nutr 2:539, 1983.

263. Sherding, RG, et al.: Bentiromide:xylose test in healthy cats. Am J Vet Res 43:2272, 1982.

264. Hawkins, EC, et al.: Digestion of bentiromide and absorption of xylose in healthy cats and absorption of xylose in cats with infiltrative intestinal disease. Am J Vet Res 47:567, 1986.

265. Brobst, DF: Pancreatic Function. In Kaneko, JJ (ed): Clinical Biochemistry of Domestic Animals. New York, Academic Press, 1980.

266. Burrows, CF, et al.: Determination of fecal fat and trypsin output in the evaluation of chronic canine diarrhea. JAVMA 174:62, 1979.

267. Zimmer, JF and Todd, SE: Further evaluation of bentiromide in the diagnosis of canine exocrine pancreatic insufficiency. Cornell Vet 75:426, 1985.

268. Simpson, JW and Doxey, DL: Quantitative assessment of fat absorption and its diagnostic value in exocrine pancreatic insufficiency. Res Vet Sci 35:249, 1983.

269. Walker, WA and Isselbacher, KJ: Uptake and transport of macro-molecules by the intestine—Possible role in clinical disorders. Gastroenterology 67:531, 1974.

270. Westermarck, E, et al.: Quantitation of serum phospholipase A$_2$ by enzyme-diffusion in lecithin agar gels. A comparative study in man and animals. Acta Vet Scand 25:229, 1984.

271. Canfield, PJ, et al.: Effect of various diets on fecal analysis in normal dogs. Res Vet Sci 34:24, 1983.

272. Lewis, LD and Boulay, JP: Fat excretion and assimilation by the cat. Feline Pract 9:46, 1979.

273. Westermarck, E: The diagnosis of pancreatic degenerative atrophy in dogs—a practical method. Acta Vet Scand 23:197, 1982.

274. Westermarck, E and Sandholm, M: Faecal hydrolase activity as determined by radial enzyme diffusion: A new method for detecting pancreatic dysfunction in the dog. Res Vet Sci 28:341, 1980.

275. Dimagno, EP: Medical treatment of pancreatic insufficiency. Mayo Clin Proc 54:435, 1979.

276. Graham, DY: Enzyme replacement therapy of exocrine pancreatic insufficiency in man. N Engl J Med 296:1314, 1977.

277. Niessen, KH, et al.: Studies on the quality of pancreatic prepa-

rations: Enzyme content, prospective bioavailability, bile acid pattern, and contamination with purines. Eur J Pediatr 141:23, 1983.

278. Grendell, JH: Nutrition and absorption in diseases of the pancreas. Clin Gastroenterol 12:551, 1983.
279. Dutta, SK, et al.: Comparative evaluation of the therapeutic efficacy of a pH-sensitive enteric coated pancreatic enzyme preparation with conventional pancreatic enzyme therapy in the treatment of exocrine pancreatic insufficiency. Gastroenterology 84:476, 1983.
280. Zentler-Munro, PL, et al.: Effect of intrajejunal acidity on aqueous phase bile acid and lipid concentrations in pancreatic steatorrhoea due to cystic fibrosis. Gut 25:500, 1984.
281. Pidgeon, G: Exocrine pancreatic disease in the dog and cat. Part 2: Exocrine pancreatic insufficiency. Canine Pract 14:31, 1987.
282. Lewis, LD, et al.: Gastrointestinal, pancreatic and hepatic diseases. In Small Animal Clinical Nutrition, 3rd ed. Topeka, KS, Mark Morris Assoc, 1987.
283. Pidgeon, G: Effect of diet on exocrine pancreatic insufficiency in dogs. JAVMA 181:232, 1982.
284. Dutta, SK and Hlasko, J: Dietary fiber in pancreatic disease:

Effect of high fiber diet on fat malabsorption in pancreatic insufficiency and in vitro study of the interaction of dietary fibres with pancreatic enzymes. Am J Clin Nutr 41:517, 1985.
285. King, CE and Toskes, PP: Protein-losing enteropathy in the human and experimental rat blind-loop syndrome. Gastroenterology 80:504, 1981.
286. Anderson, NV and Johnson, KH: Pancreatic carcinoma in the dog. JAVMA 150:286, 1967.
287. Banner, BF, et al.: Acinar cell carcinoma of the pancreas in a cat. Vet Pathol 16:543, 1979.
288. Priester, WA: Data from eleven United States and Canadian colleges of veterinary medicine on pancreatic carcinoma in domestic animals. Cancer Res 34:1372, 1974.
289. Fox, JN, et al.: Pancreatic function in domestic cats with pancreatic fluke infection. JAVMA 178:58, 1981.
290. Roudebush, P and Schmidt, DA: Fenbendazole for treatment of pancreatic fluke infection in a cat. JAVMA 180:545, 1982.
291. Anderson, WI, et al.: Pancreatic atrophy and fibrosis associated with *Eurytrema procynosis* in a domestic cat. Vet Rec 120:235, 1987.

DRUG INDEX

Generic	(Trade)	Dosage	Route	Frequency	Brief Description
Pancreatin	Gastrizyme Pancrezyme Viokase-V	½–2 teaspoon	Oral	With each meal	Pancreatic digestive enzymes
Oxytetracycline		5 mg/lb (10 mg/kg)	Oral	q 12 h for 7–28 days	Antibiotic to treat bacterial overgrowth in small intestine
Metronidazole	Flagyl	5–10 mg/lb (10–20 mg/kg)	Oral	q 12–24 h for 7 days	Antibiotic to treat bacterial overgrowth in small intestine
Tylosin	Tylan Plus Vitamins	¼–1 teaspoon	Oral	With each meal as needed	Antibiotic to treat bacterial overgrowth in small intestine
Prednisolone or prednisone		½–1 mg/lb (1–2 mg/kg) initially	Oral	q 12 h for 7–14 days	Glucocorticoid to treat idiopathic inflammatory bowel disease or villous atrophy
Cimetidine	Tagamet	5 mg/lb (10 mg/kg)	Oral	With or 30 min before each meal	Histamine type 2 receptor antagonist; inhibits gastric acid secretion
Medium-chain triglyceride oil	MCT Oil	¼–4 teaspoons per day with food	Oral	Divided dose with meals	Readily absorbed caloric supplement (excess may cause diarrhea)
Meperidine hydrochloride	Demerol	1–2.5 mg/lb (2–5 mg/kg)	SQ	q 6 h	Narcotic analgesic
Fenbendazole	Panacur	15 mg/lb (30 mg/kg)	Oral	q 24 h for 6 days	Anthelmintic

91 DISEASES OF THE GALLBLADDER AND THE EXTRAHEPATIC BILIARY SYSTEM

DAVID A. HAGER

Over the past several years our ability to diagnose and treat gallbladder and biliary tract diseases has greatly improved. This has largely come about through new developments in biochemical testing, biliary imaging, and refined surgical techniques. The diagnosis of biliary disease even with these advancements remains difficult. Although the classic clinical feature of biliary disease is icterus, affected animals may also present with vague nonspecific clinical signs that include anorexia, depression, vomiting, lethargy, and abdominal pain or distention.[1] The goal of the diagnostic work-up is to localize the disease process to the gallbladder and to differentiate the medically treated diseases from surgically managed extrahepatic biliary obstruction and biliary tract rupture.

DIAGNOSTIC APPROACH

The diagnosis of diseases of the gallbladder and extrahepatic biliary tract relies heavily on evaluation of historic and clinical information, biochemical testing, and biliary imaging. Abdominal palpation is generally not helpful, since the gallbladder is located within the cranial abdomen surrounded by liver. Plain film radiographs help only if there is gas or mineral density associated with the gallbladder. Biochemical analysis of the biliary system (liver enzymes, bilirubin levels, and liver function tests) supplies the needed information in the icteric animal in determining the presence of biliary obstruction and its intrahepatic (hepatocellular) or extrahepatic origin (see Chapter 24). Biochemical analysis is also helpful in detecting a nonobstructing inflammatory process in the biliary tract. When biochemical values are equivocal or additional information is needed, noninvasive or invasive biliary imaging techniques are required.

The noninvasive imaging techniques currently being used include oral and intravenous cholecystography, diagnostic ultrasound, and biliary scintigraphy.[2-6] Ultrasound has become the preferred method because it is rapid and safe, and easily demonstrates the gallbladder while providing important information about surrounding organs. Oral and intravenous cholecystography will frequently not delineate the gallbladder in the icteric animal; however, ultrasound is not limited by jaundice. Biliary scintigraphy requires large expensive equipment and radioactive pharmaceuticals to image the gallbladder, and because of this, it is available only at a few teaching institutions.

One important advantage of ultrasound is its ability to help differentiate extrahepatic obstruction from intrahepatic disease. On examination of a normal liver with ultrasound, the intrahepatic and extrahepatic biliary tree and common bile duct are not detectable (Figure 91–1). With a distal extrahepatic biliary obstruction, there is rapid dilation of the gallbladder, followed within 48 hours by common bile duct enlargement. Dilation of the extrahepatic biliary structures occurs by three days

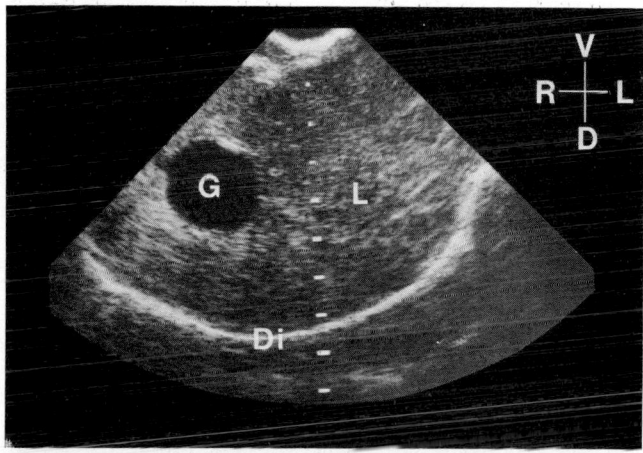

FIGURE 91–1. Transverse ultrasound scan of a normal liver. The liver has a homogenous tissue texture, and the gallbladder lumen is free of debris. G = gallbladder, L = liver, Di = diaphragm, D = dorsal, V = ventral, R = right, L = left.

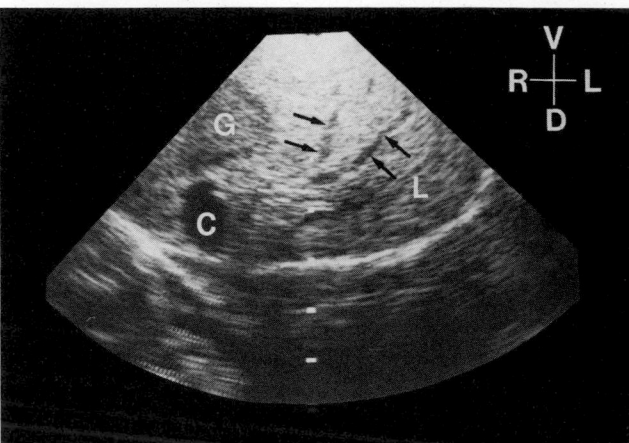

FIGURE 91–2. Transverse ultrasound scan of a liver with extrahepatic biliary obstruction. The gallbladder is filled with debris, the common bile duct is distended, and there is dilation of intrahepatic bile ducts (arrows). Intrahepatic bile ducts may be distinguished from hepatic vessels by their tortuous appearance and irregular branching pattern. G = gallbladder, L = liver, C = common bile duct.

and dilation of the intrahepatic ducts by seven days post obstruction (Figure 91–2). Intrahepatic bile ducts may be distinguished from hepatic vessels by their tortuous appearance and irregular branching pattern. Gallbladder distention also commonly occurs in fasted and anorectic animals. To rule out early obstructive disease in these animals, induction of gallbladder contraction (i.e., fatty meal) and sequential ultrasound exams may be required.[7]

Percutaneous cholecystography is an invasive method of diagnosing biliary disease. With fluoroscopic guidance, a small-gauge needle is placed into the gallbladder and radiopaque contrast is injected, delineating the gallbladder and the common bile duct.[8] This procedure gives excellent definition of the biliary system for the diagnosis of a variety of biliary disorders, although biliary tract leakage is a potential complication.

CLASSIFICATION AND TREATMENT OF GALLBLADDER DISEASE

Nonobstructive Diseases

There are a variety of extrahepatic biliary tract and gallbladder diseases that may not cause obstruction. These diseases are frequently incidental findings and can be difficult to diagnose. They are classified as to their location in the gallbladder and extrahepatic biliary tract (intraluminal and mural) (Table 91–1).

INTRALUMINAL: CHOLELITHIASIS/ GALLBLADDER SEDIMENT

Calculi in the gallbladder (cholelithiasis) are considered rare in the dog (incidence of less than one per cent of dogs with liver disease)[9] and cat and are frequently an incidental finding.[10] In veterinary medicine, little is known about the pathogenesis of stone formation, but they are thought to result from bacterial infection,

TABLE 91–1. CLASSIFICATION OF GALLBLADDER AND EXTRAHEPATIC BILIARY TRACT DISEASES

Nonobstructive Diseases
Intraluminal
Cholelithiasis/gallbladder sediment
Parasitic *(Platynosomum concinnum)*
Mural
Cholecystitis
Acute or chronic cholecystitis
Emphysematous cholecystitis
Cystic mucinous hypertrophy
Obstructive Diseases (Extrahepatic)
Intraluminal
Cholelithiasis
Parasitic *(Platynosomum concinnum)*
Foreign body
Mural
Cholecystitis and cholangitis
Biliary tract neoplasia
Extramural
Inflammation, infection, or neoplasia of the pancreas, duodenum, or cranial abdominal lymph nodes
Biliary Tract Rupture

biliary stasis, a change in bile composition, or a combination of these factors.[9, 10] Detailed information on the quantitative analysis of the biliary tract stones is lacking but most stones are composed of cholesterol, bilirubin, calcium, magnesium, and oxalates.[9] The diagnosis of gallstones in the past has been based mainly on identification of radiopaque stones on plain films. Unfortunately, not all biliary stones contain sufficient mineral to be radiopaque. In humans only 10 to 15 per cent of cholesterol and mixed stones and approximately 50 per cent of pigmented stones are apparent on plain films.[11] No such studies are available in small animals. Ultrasound allows easy diagnosis of both radiolucent and radiopaque biliary calculi (Figure 91–3), but more importantly it can be used to differentiate hepatic calcification from biliary tract calculi. When biliary calculi are discovered, the animal should be carefully examined for signs (symptoms) of biliary disease, and consideration should be given to stone removal. If the stones are removed, a cholecystotomy rather than a cholecystectomy is the preferred surgical technique. To determine an etiology for the stone formation and to aid in future

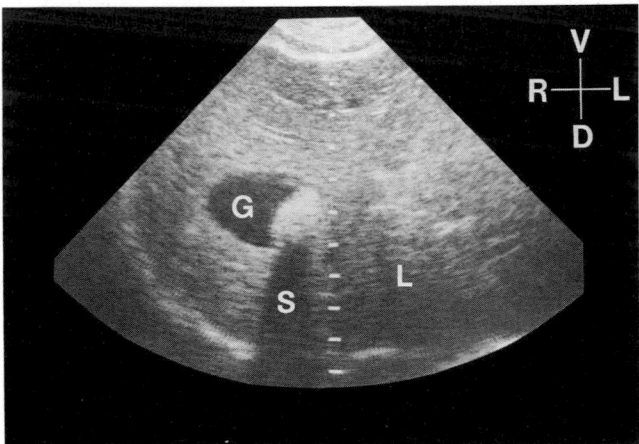

FIGURE 91–3. Transverse ultrasound scan of the liver. Within the lumen of the gallbladder is a cholelith. The stone creates an ultrasound artifact called acoustic shadowing. G = gallbladder, L = liver, S = acoustic shadowing.

medical management of the patient, a culture of the gallbladder bile, biopsy of the gallbladder mucosa, and analysis of the calculi are recommended. Appropriate medical therapy may include antibiotics for the management of cholecystitis, combined with a high protein and low cholesterol diet to slow calculi formation.[1]

Sediment is frequently seen within the gallbladder lumen with ultrasound. The significance of this gallbladder debris is unknown, but it may be secondary to biliary stasis.[4]

INTRALUMINAL: PARASITIC GALLBLADDER DISEASE (PLATYNOSOMUM CONCINNUM)

Platynosomum concinnum is a fluke that inhabits the gallbladder, bile ducts, and rarely the small intestines of cats. It has been reported primarily in Florida and Hawaii, with sporatic cases seen in other states.[12] This trematode causes fibrosis of the bile duct walls, which can progress and cause extrahepatic biliary obstruction.[13] Secondary cirrhosis and hepatic lipidosis may also occur. The lifecycle of the fluke includes a first intermediate host of a land snail followed by a second intermediate reptile or amphibian host, such as a lizard or a toad, which the cat ingests. The clinical signs depend upon the amount of liver damage and biliary obstruction but may range from normal signs to icterus, vomiting, mucoid diarrhea, anorexia, emaciation, depression, and death. The diagnosis is made upon fecal examination using fecal sedimentation or formalin ether methods. Routine sugar and zinc sulfate floatation are not consistent in detecting the fluke eggs. Eggs may not be shed into the gastrointestinal tract if there is complete biliary obstruction. Treatment remains controversial (Table 91–2), although a single dose of praziquantel (9 mg/lb or 20 mg/kg) and nitroscanate (45 mg/lb or 100 mg/kg) has been shown to decrease the number of eggs passed in infected cats.[14] Drug and dosage protocols need to be established and evaluated for the treatment of these flukes. The prognosis for animals with extensive liver disease is guarded.

MURAL: CHOLECYSTITIS

Acute and chronic forms of cholecystitis are poorly documented, rarely reported diseases in small animals. They are thought to occur from reflux of intestinal bacteria into the gallbladder or from blood-borne bacteria from the hepatic circulation.[10] Acute cholecystitis in humans is nearly always the result of obstruction of the cystic duct by a gallstone.[11] There may or may not be associated cholelithiasis in small animals.[15]

Emphysematous cholecystitis is an inflammatory condition of the gallbladder with formation of gas within the wall and/or lumen of the gallbladder. This occurs secondary to a proliferation of gas-forming organisms such as *Escherichia coli* and *Clostridium welchii (C. perfringens)*. It has been reported in dogs associated with diabetes mellitus[16] but is also seen in nondiabetic animals.[17]

The clinical signs of cholecystitis are frequently vague. Animals may display cranial abdominal pain, pyrexia, anorexia, and vomiting. Depending upon the cause of cholecystitis, there may be partial or complete outflow obstruction of the gallbladder. Treatment of acute, chronic, and emphysematous cholecystitis should be aimed at the underlying disease.

MURAL: CYSTIC MUCINOUS HYPERTROPHY

Cystic hypertrophy of the mucus-producing glands of the gallbladder is a condition identified at necropsy in dogs and may not cause clinical signs. It is generally found in dogs older than six years of age with no breed or sex predilection.[18] On ultrasound these lesions may appear as sessile or polypoid masses.[4]

Obstructive Biliary Diseases (Extrahepatic)

Complete or partial biliary obstruction can occur in the major hepatic ducts, the cystic duct, or the common bile duct. Obstruction can be classified as intraluminal, mural, or extramural (Table 91–1). The most common clinical features of biliary obstruction are icterus and vomiting; however, anorexia, weight loss, abdominal pain, emaciation, depression, dehydration, diarrhea, and acholic feces may be noted.[19] Biochemically, there is a marked increase in serum alkaline phosphatase (ALP) and only a slight to moderate increase in serum alanine aminotransferase (SALT). The total serum bilirubin is generally very high, composed of primarily the conjugated form.

INTRALUMINAL

The most common intraluminal cause of biliary obstruction is cholelithiasis. Although stones within the gallbladder may be incidental findings, stones within the lobar, hepatic,[20] and common bile duct (choledocholithiasis) generally cause biliary obstruction.[15, 21, 22] Other causes for intraluminal biliary obstruction include biliary flukes and common bile duct foreign bodies.

MURAL: INFLAMMATION/BILIARY NEOPLASIA

Both severe inflammation changes of the extrahepatic biliary tree and neoplasia can cause extrahepatic biliary obstruction. Biliary neoplasms such as adenomas, adenocarcinomas, and bile duct carcinomas are very rare.[23]

TABLE 91–2. DRUGS USED FOR TREATING *PLATYNOSOMUM CONCINNUM*

Generic	Trade	Dosage	Route	Frequency	Description
Praziquantel	(Droncit)	9 mg/lb (20 mg/kg)	PO	Once	Anthelmintic
Nitrosanate	(Lopatol)	45 mg/lb (100 mg/kg)	PO	Once	Anthelmintic

EXTRAMURAL

Inflammation, infection, and neoplasia of the pancreas, duodenum, and cranial abdominal lymph nodes can all lead to extrahepatic biliary obstruction.[4] The pancreas is a common cause of extrahepatic biliary obstruction. In one study of 11 animals with extrahepatic biliary obstruction, seven had acute or chronic pancreatitis.[19] When obstruction is diagnosed, surgical exploration is indicated. The goal of surgery for obstructive disease is to identify the obstruction and to reestablish patency of the biliary tract or to redirect bile flow. In diseases with severe damage to the extrahepatic biliary tract, bile flow may be redirected by anastomosing the gallbladder to the duodenum (cholecystoduodenostomy) or jejunum (cholecystojejunostomy).[24]

When dealing with extrahepatic biliary obstruction secondary to pancreatitis, the obstruction may be relieved without surgical intervention if the inflammatory process can be controlled.

Biliary Tract Rupture

There are several causes for gallbladder or biliary tract rupture including blunt trauma, penetrating wound, pathologic rupture secondary to inflammation or neoplasia, and following percutaneous liver biopsies or abdominal exploratory surgery.[24] Traumatic ruptures are usually associated with other disorders such as shock, hemorrhage, liver fracture, skeletal trauma, or pneumothorax,[25] which may mask the clinical manifestations of the rupture.

The clinical course of biliary rupture is generally protracted due to a failure to recognize the problem and to a lack of specific clinical signs. These animals generally experience abdominal pain for the first 48 hours. This is followed by anorexia, depression, fever, abdominal distention, and icterus.[24] Diagnosis of gallbladder or biliary tract rupture is based primarily on obtaining a bile stained modified transudate on abdominocentesis. Other supporting data would include appropriate historic and clinical findings, an elevated total serum bilirubin, and elevated liver enzymes (SAP, SALT). Radiographs usually show peritoneal fluid. Biliary tract imaging is often nonrewarding. Ultrasound rarely demonstrates the site of leakage, and to confuse the diagnosis, the gallbladder may remain distended. Oral and intravenous contrast studies are not helpful. Percutaneous cholecystography holds the most promise of defining rupture sites but may be difficult to interpret with peritoneal contrast leakage that commonly occurs with the procedure.

Exploratory surgery is indicated when biliary tract rupture is suspected. The technique of surgical repair depends on the site and extent of damage. Complete removal of the gallbladder and cystic duct (cholecystectomy) is recommended when there is extensive damage to these structures. Surgical repair of the common bile duct is a little more difficult due to its small size and its tendency for stricture. Techniques for repair of partial tears of the common bile duct utilize straight, T- or Y-shaped polyethylene tubes implanted temporarily within the lumen of the common bile duct to prevent stricture formation. Avulsion of the common bile duct or a complete tear should be repaired by reimplantation of the common bile duct into the duodenum or by a biliary enteric anastomosis. Ruptures or tears of the hepatic ducts may be ligated, since the flow of bile will be redirected through other hepatic ducts.[24]

References

1. Strombeck, DR: Diseases of the gallbladder. *In* Small Animal Gastroenterology. Davis, CA, Stonegate Publishing, 1979, p 485.
2. Allan, GS and Dixon, RT: Cholecystography in the dog: The choice of contrast media and optimum dose rate. J Am Vet Rad Soc 16:98, 1975.
3. Carlisle, CH: A comparison of techniques for cholecystography in the cat. Vet Rad 18:173, 1977.
4. Nyland, TG and Park, RD: Hepatic ultrasonography in the dog. Vet Rad 24:74, 1983.
5. Nyland, TG and Hager, DA: Sonography of the liver, gallbladder and spleen. Vet Clin North Am 15:1123, 1985.
6. Kerr, LY and Hornoff, WJ: Quantitative hepatobiliary scintigraphy using 99M TC-DISIDA in the dog. Vet Rad 27:173, 1986.
7. Nyland, TG and Gillett, NA: Sonographic evaluation of experimental bile duct ligation in the dog. Vet Rad 23:252, 1982.
8. Wrigley, RH and Reuter, RE: Percutaneous cholecystography in normal dogs. Vet Rad 23:239, 1982.
9. Schall, WD, et al.: Cholelithiasis in dogs. JAVMA 163:459, 1973.
10. Schall, WD and Griener, TP: Diseases of the gallbladder. *In* Ettinger, SJ (ed): Textbook of Internal Medicine. Philadelphia, WB Saunders, 1975, p 1270.
11. McPhee, MS and Greenberger, NJ: Diseases of the gallbladder and bile ducts. *In* Braunwald, E, et al. (eds): Harrison's Principles of Internal Medicine. New York, McGraw-Hill, 1986, p 1358.
12. Bielsa, LM and Greiner, EC: Liver flukes (*Platynosomum concinnum*) in cats. JAAHA 21:269, 1985.
13. Jenkins, CC, et al.: Extrahepatic biliary obstruction associated with *Platynosomum concinnum* in a cat. Comp Cont Ed 10:628, 1988.
14. Evans, JW and Green, PE: Preliminary evaluation of four anthelmintics against the cat liver fluke, *Platynosomum concinnum*. Aust Vet J 54:454, 1978.
15. Matthiesen, DT and Lammerding, J: Gallbladder rupture and bile peritonitis secondary to cholelithiasis and cholecystitis in a dog. JAVMA 184:1282, 1984.
16. Lord, P and Wilkin, RJ: Emphysema of the gallbladder in a diabetic dog. Vet Rad 13:49, 1972.
17. Burk, R and Johnson, G: Emphysematous cholecystitis in the nondiabetic dog: Three case histories. Vet Rad 21:242, 1980.
18. Kovatch, RM, et al.: Cystic mucinous hypertrophy of the mucosa of the gallbladder in the dog. Pathol Vet 2:574, 1965.
19. Martin, RA, et al.: Surgical management of extrahepatic biliary tract disease: A report of eleven cases. JAAHA 22:301, 1986.
20. Cantwell, HD, et al.: Radiopaque hepatic and lobar duct choleliths in a dog. JAAHA 19:373, 1983.
21. Harari, J, et al.: Extrahepatic bile duct obstruction due to cholecystitis and choledocholithiasis: Case report. JAAHA 18:347, 1982.
22. Wolf, AM: Obstructive jaundice in a cat resulting from choledocholithiasis. JAVMA 185:85, 1984.
23. Moulton, JE: Tumors of the pancreas, liver, gallbladder, and mesothelium. *In* Tumors in Domestic Animals. Los Angeles, University of California Press, 1978, p 273.
24. Blass, CE: Surgery of the extrahepatic biliary tract. Comp Cont Ed 5:801, 1983.
25. Suter, PF and Olson, SE: The diagnosis of injuries to the intestines, gallbladder and bile ducts in the dog. J Small Anim Pract 11:575, 1970.

92 RECTO-ANAL DISEASE

COLIN F. BURROWS and GARY V. ELLISON

Diseases of the anus and rectum are fairly common in the dog and cat; they are more prevalent in the dog than in the cat but have similar signs in both species, with tenesmus, dyschezia, and hematochezia the predominating signs. Since the rectum functions as a fecal reservoir and plays an important role in defecation and the anus functions to maintain fecal continence, it is not surprising that diseases of these areas usually involve complaints of abnormal defecation or appearance of the feces.

Parts of the body relevant to signs of recto-anal disease include the rectum, the anal canal, the internal and external anal sphincter, the pelvic diaphragm, and the integument immediately circumferential to the anus.

ANATOMY

The rectum is that portion of the large intestine which begins at the pelvic inlet and lies within the pelvic canal.[1] It lies mainly caudal to the peritoneal reflexion and forms a straight tube, about five cm long and three cm in diameter in a medium-sized dog and slightly smaller in the cat (Figure 92–1). The rectal mucosa is thrown up into a number of longitudinal folds and is comprised of columnar epithelial cells rich in mucus-secreting cells. The mucus secreted by the rectum serves to lubricate fecal material in its final passage from the alimentary tract. Another prominent feature of the rectal mucosa in dogs and cats is the presence of approximately 100 solitary lymph nodes. In dogs, the free surface of each nodule forms a crater or rectal pit, which is visible as a small indentation about one mm in diameter in the rectal mucosa.

The anal canal is about one cm long in both dogs and cats,[1, 2] and is surrounded by both the smooth and striated muscle sphincters. The mucosa of the anal canal represents the transition from columnar to stratified squamous epithelium and is characterized by two prominent zones. The inner columnar zone is about seven cm wide in both medium-sized dogs and cats and is thrown up into short anal columns that terminate in blind anal sinuses. A narrow one mm wide intermediate zone, also called the anocutaneous line, separates the columnar zone from the cutaneous zone. The cutaneous zone is divided into an inner and an outer zone. The inner cutaneous zone is only a few mm wide and is the area in which the ducts of the anal sacs open.

The anal sacs are round invaginations of the inner cutaneous zone, sandwiched between the internal and external anal sphincters at the four and eight o'clock positions. They vary from 7 to 15 mm in diameter in dogs and are pea-sized in cats. The walls of the sacs are lined with keratinized epithelium supported by connective tissue stroma intermingled with large coiled apocrine tubules and occasional sebaceous glands. Anal sac fluid is composed of glandular secretions, desquamated epithelium, and bacteria. Each excretory duct is approximately two mm in diameter and five mm in length in a medium-sized dog.

The outer cutaneous zone is distinguished by its hairless stratified squamous keratinized epithelium and constitutes the nonhaired portion of the anus. The anus varies greatly in width particularly in adult male dogs because of the varied development of the underlying circumanal (perianal) glands. These modified sebaceous glands are located in a subcutaneous zone around the anus for a radius of four cm and a thickness of eight mm in dogs. Since these perianal glands continue to develop throughout life in unaltered males, perianal adenomas are common in older male dogs. Circumanal glands are also present in cats but are of little clinical significance.

The internal anal sphincter is the caudal thickened part of the circular smooth muscle coat of the anal canal. The role that this involuntary muscle plays in fecal continence is poorly defined in the dog and cat. The external anal sphincter is a large circular band of striated voluntary muscles which varies from 1 to 2 cm in width and from 0.5 to 1.5 cm in thickness in dogs and is important in the maintenance of fecal continence. Dorsally, fibers of the external anal sphincter blend with those of the rectococcygeal muscle which attach to the fifth and sixth coccygeal vertebrae (Figure 92–2). This attachment of the rectococcygeal muscles to the tail serves to anchor the rectum and anal canal. Movement of the tail during the act of defecation also moves the anal canal and rectum caudally and helps promote evacuation of feces. The retroperitoneal part of the rectum and anal canal is supported by fatty connective tissue and the pelvic diaphragm. The pelvic diaphragm (Figure 92–2) is composed of the levator ani muscle

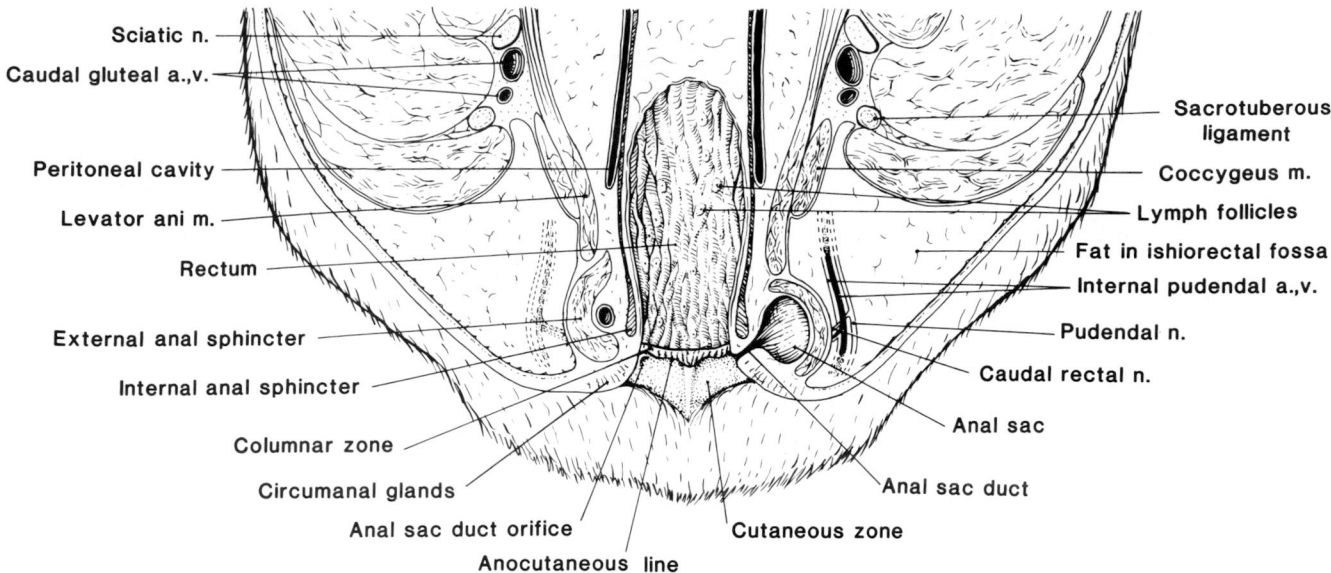

Sciatic n.

Caudal gluteal a.,v.

Peritoneal cavity

Levator ani m.

Rectum

External anal sphincter

Internal anal sphincter

Columnar zone

Circumanal glands

Anal sac duct orifice

Anocutaneous line

Cutaneous zone

Sacrotuberous ligament

Coccygeus m.

Lymph follicles

Fat in ishiorectal fossa

Internal pudendal a.,v.

Pudendal n.

Caudal rectal n.

Anal sac

Anal sac duct

FIGURE 92–1. Horizontal cross sectional diagram of the normal anus and rectum showing the interrelationships of clinically relevant structures. The right side is cut at a slightly lower level to show the duct of the anal sac.

medially and the coccygeal muscle laterally. These muscles course obliquely from their ischial attachment to their insertion on the coccygeal vertebra.

Vascular supply to the intra-abdominal rectum is via the cranial rectal artery that arises from the caudal mesenteric artery, whereas the retroperitoneal rectum, anus, and perianal area are supplied by the caudal rectal and internal pudendal arteries, respectively. Autonomic innervation to the smooth muscle of the rectum and internal anal sphincter is provided by the parasympathetic pelvic nerve plexus, which originates from the first and second sacral nerve segments and the sympathetic hypogastric nerves, which arise from the caudal

mediastinal plexus. The external anal sphincter receives its motor innervation from the caudal rectal branch of the pudendal nerve. The perineal branch of the pudendal nerve is sensory to the anus and perineal area. The pudendal nerve can be destroyed unilaterally without fecal incontinence occurring, but bilateral destruction results in a flaccid anus.

PHYSIOLOGY OF DEFECATION

The anus and anal canal are normally devoid of fecal material and are in a collapsed state with the walls in apposition. Defecation commences when the rectum is

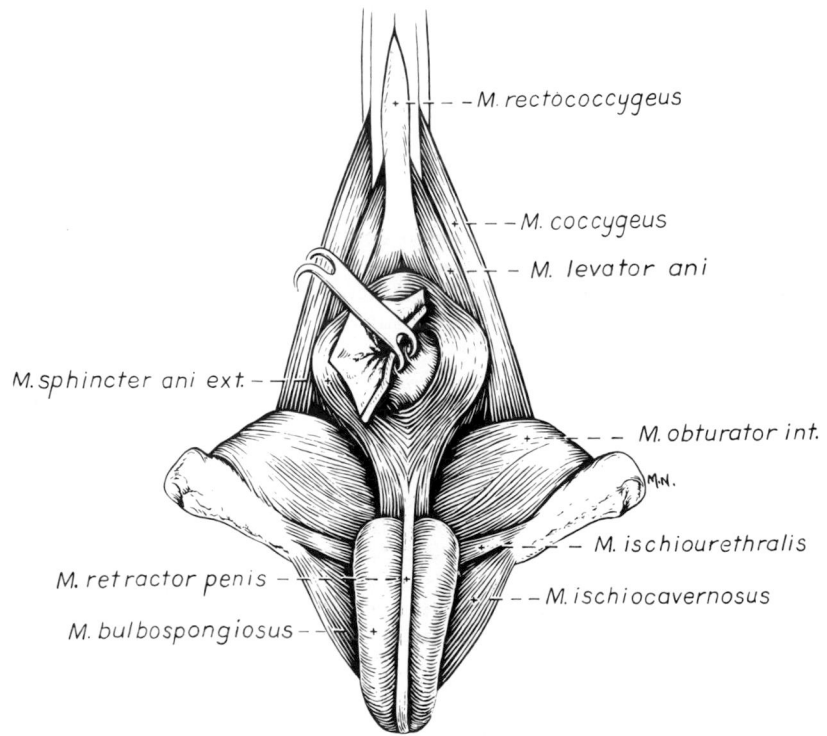

M. rectococcygeus

M. coccygeus

M. levator ani

M. sphincter ani ext.

M. obturator int.

M. retractor penis

M. ischiourethralis

M. bulbospongiosus

M. ischiocavernosus

FIGURE 92–2. Diagrammatic representation of the pelvic diaphragm, showing how the anal sphincter and rectum are supported dorsally by the rectococcygeal muscle, laterally by the coccygeal muscle, and ventrally by the internal obturator muscle. (Reproduced from Miller, W (ed): Anatomy of the Dog. 2nd Ed. WB Saunders Company, 1979.)

distended by fecal material. This causes the internal anal sphincter to relax and stimulates stretch receptors in the distal anal canal and medial coccygeal muscles. Initially, rectal distention causes the external anal sphincter and the medial coccygeal muscles to undergo a reflex contraction which forms a high pressure zone to counter the force of peristaltic movement, and prevents spontaneous expulsion of feces from the anal canal. The desire or stimulus to defecate is thus temporarily suppressed and continence is maintained, a process that in the normal animal can be repeated until the rectum is maximally distended. Constipation can ensue, however, if such stimuli are continually suppressed. The opposite situation occurs when the rectal stimulus is augmented by colonic or rectal inflammatory disease to cause urgent defecation with tenesmus.

An intact nerve supply to the external anal sphincter is essential for normal defecation. Spinal cord disease, peripheral nerve transection, or sphincter division may lead to a loss of continence and of the ability to defecate normally.

Controlled defecation can occur at any time when a stimulus from the rectum reaches the animal's consciousness. During defecation the animal assumes a squatting position; abdominal pressure is increased by closure of the glottis, the diaphragm fixates, the abdominal wall contracts, and the external anal sphincter relaxes. Intense "migrating contractions" in the colon push the feces distally and defecation ensues.[3] Contraction of the medial coccygeal and other intrapelvic muscles enhances the increased abdominal pressure and enables the rectum to push the last part of the fecal bolus to result in expulsion. Following defecation, the muscles of the pelvis relax and return to their normal position with concomitant obliteration of the now empty lumen.

HISTORY AND PHYSICAL EXAMINATION IN RECTO-ANAL DISEASE

The primary complaint in animals with rectal or anal disease almost invariably involves abnormal defecation. The client may complain of constipation, feces of small diameter, reduced fecal volume, tenesmus, dyschezia, and blood or mucus in the feces. Diarrhea is uncommon. Other complaints may include perineal swelling or a vague complaint of malodor from the area.

Physical examination should include both a careful visual inspection of the perineum and careful rectal examination. If rectal examination is too painful at the time of initial examination, it can be postponed until the animal is anesthetized, allowing the examination to be carried out in conjunction with and as a prelude to colonoscopy.

SPECIAL EXAMINATION IN RECTO-ANAL DISEASE

Specific diagnosis of rectal disease frequently necessitates colonoscopy and biopsy. If the lesion is in the anal canal or in the distal rectum, then colonoscopy and biopsy may be performed without prior preparation with enemas or colonic lavage; indeed, this is frequently preferable, as passage of the enema tube may be painful,

may disrupt underlying lesions, and may cause unnecessary bleeding.

Diseases of the Rectum

PERINEAL HERNIA

Perineal hernia is a well recognized entity in the dog and is thought to result from a weakness of the pelvic diaphragm, which is composed of the muscles that form the caudal limit to the pelvic canal. Perineal hernia has been defined as herniation of a rectal diverticulum or abdominal or pelvic contents through an opening bordered by the external anal sphincter medially, the coccygeal muscle laterally, and the internal obturator muscle ventrolaterally, or more simply, as a failure of the pelvic organs.[4]

Incidence and Etiology. Perineal hernia is a condition seen primarily in intact male dogs with a mean age of about eight years. The disease is rarely seen in the female dog and has been reported in only five cats.[5, 6, 7] Boston terriers, Boxers, collies, Welsh corgies, and Pekingese are apparently at increased risk.[8, 9] Hernias may occur unilaterally or bilaterally, but curiously, up to 80 per cent of unilateral hernias are located on the right side.[8, 10, 11] Most hernias have the external anal sphincter as their medial boundary, the levator ani and coccygeal muscle as their lateral boundary, with the internal obturator muscle located ventrally.[4] Occasionally, the hernia will develop between the levator ani and coccygeal muscles.

The exact etiology and pathogenesis of perineal hernia remains obscure but several possible causes have been proposed. A predisposition in brachycephalic breeds suggests that inherent conformational deficiencies may contribute to the disease in these breeds.[12] Hormonal imbalance is suggested as a cause and is supported by several interesting studies. Absolute or relative increases in androgens might be involved, since a relatively high incidence of hernias was reported with interstitial cell tumors (15 per cent), seminomas (19 per cent), or mixed-type tumors (11 per cent), whereas dogs with estrogen-secreting Sertoli cell tumors had a low incidence of herniation (2 per cent).[13] Prostatic enlargement is commonly associated with perineal hernia, and castration may have a sparing effect on the recurrence of the disease.[9] However, the sparing effect may be due entirely to resolution of the prostatic disease and associated tenesmus rather than to removal of any hormonal influence. This is supported by the observation that perineal hernias may occur secondary to other medical conditions that cause tenesmus.

Regardless of the cause, fascial weakening and separation of the external anal sphincter from the pelvic diaphragm ensue, and muscle atrophy and degeneration occur. Muscular changes may be due to stretching or to neurogenic atrophy.[14] Three types of rectal pathology may ensue: (1) rectal deviation, (2) rectal diverticulum, and (3) rectal sacculation.[15, 16] These are not separate entities from perineal hernia but are merely extensions of the same disease process. Once the pelvic diaphragm is destroyed, the rectum can divide laterally and impair fecal passage. With rectal diverticulum, a defect develops in the muscularis, allowing the mucosa and submucosa to prolapse, while in sacculation the muscularis remains intact and the whole rectum dilates and expands to fill the space formed by the weakened pelvic diaphragm.[15, 17] The rectal muscle is intact in most dogs with perineal hernia, and thus rectal sacculation is more common than rectal diverticulum.

History and Presenting Signs. Most dogs with perineal hernia are presented because of difficult defecation and an obvious swelling lateral to the anus. Tenesmus, constipation, and dyschezia are common complaints, and fecal incontinence occurs in about 10 per cent of afflicted dogs. Occasionally, the bladder or prostate retroflexes into the hernia creating acute urethral obstruction, uremia, hyperkalemia, and the potential for strangulation of the bladder (Figure 92–3). If this occurs, the urethra should be catheterized in an attempt to empty the bladder. However, this is seldom possible, and cystocentesis must be performed to decompress the bladder sufficiently to pass a urinary catheter (Figure 92–4). An indwelling urethral catheter allows time for correction of azotemia and hyperkalemia, but surgery must ultimately be performed in all patients with perineal hernia and retroflexed bladder.

Diagnosis. The hernial defect can sometimes be palpated externally, immediately lateral to the external anal sphincter, but definitive diagnosis comes from rectal palpation, identification of a dilated rectum, and a flaccid pelvic diaphragm. Digital rectal examination reveals a right- or left-sided rectal diverticulum or sacculation that is almost invariably filled with inspissated feces. The rectum feels lax and loosely anchored, and there may be varying degrees of rectal deviation. If the finger is moved laterally, it may be observed to move the skin medial to the ischial tuberosity. The flaccid dilated rectal wall tends to prevent easy evacuation of feces, suggesting a reason for difficulty in defecation. Some dogs may present with complaints of dyschezia and tenesmus but have only a rectal dilatation and no obvious perineal swelling, although close examination

of the perineum in short-haired dogs may reveal a slight bulge in the perineum. However, these animals also have perineal hernia, since the rectum can dilate only if the muscles of the pelvic diaphragm (mainly the levator ani) are weakened.

Treatment. The conventional approach to treatment is surgical repair of the hernia. Medical treatment may be attempted in uncomplicated cases, since about 20 per cent of dogs can be maintained free of signs by the use of fecal softeners and occasional enemas. Owners should be told that the hernia may enlarge with time and should be advised of the dangers of bladder retroflexion. If dyschezia persists and the problem is still apparent with medical treatment, a perineal herniorrhaphy should be performed. The conventional technique has been described in detail and consists of approximation of the external anal sphincter to the coccygeal muscle dorsally and laterally, the sacrotuberous ligament laterally, and the internal obturator muscle ventrally.[4] Plication of the redundant rectal wall to reduce the sacculation or diverticulum is also commonly performed concurrently. Long-term recurrence is common, even for experienced surgeons, and ranges from 37 to 46 per cent over a follow-up period of five years.[8, 14] Although early success rates are good, most breakdowns occur more than 12 months after the initial repair, and clients should be advised of this before surgery, as well as of potential surgical complications, such as wound infection, sciatic nerve paralysis, fecal incontinence, and rectal prolapse.

Transplanting the superficial gluteal muscle has been described as an alternative technique.[16] However, the 12-month follow-up success rate, judged by remission of signs and lack of recurrence, was higher in the conventional technique (81 per cent) than in gluteal transplantation (64 per cent). So this technique seems to have little place in modern surgical therapy.[18]

Transplantation of the internal obturator muscle is a new surgical technique that appears to have a higher success rate.[19] In this, the origin of the internal obturator muscle is elevated off the ischial plateau, and the tendinous insertion is cut, allowing the muscle to be rotated

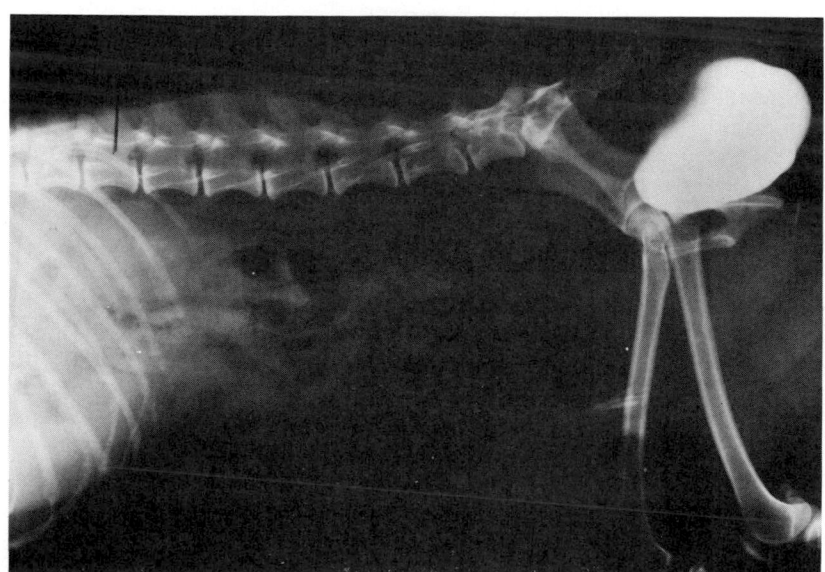

FIGURE 92–3. Radiograph of an eight-year-old male poodle cross dog that was presented with a history of dysuria, anorexia, lethargy, vomiting, and a perineal swelling. Rectal examination revealed rectal diverticulum and diverticulum compatible with perineal hernia. Contrast cystography revealed retroflexion of the bladder into the pelvic canal.

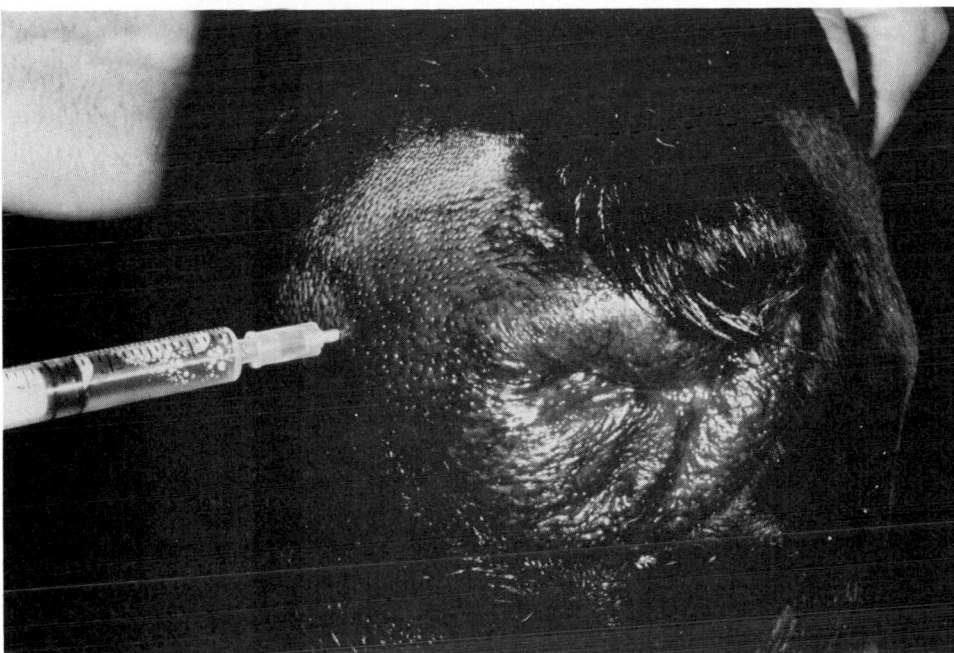

FIGURE 92–4. Obvious perineal swelling in a four-year-old Boston terrier with a history of anuria. Perineal centesis obtained urine from a bladder that had retroflexed into the hernial sac.

up and sutured to the external anal sphincter medially and to the sacrotuberous ligament laterally. Short-term success rates are encouraging, with 25 patients operated on successfully over a two-year period without recurrence. However, long-term objective data are not presently available.

In large or recurrent hernias, polyester mesh has been used to successfully repair the defect in four of five dogs,[20] with the single recurrence documented at 19 months. However, the risk of wound infection and postoperative draining tracts is high with this technique.

A technique using porcine dermal collagen for repair has been described with results equal or slightly better than conventional techniques.[21] The author also suggests that the technique may be useful in closing defects that cannot be repaired by conventional means. With all perineal herniorrhaphy techniques it is essential that fecal softeners (following section) be continued after surgery, since dyschezia may persist in animals with a dilated or deviated rectum.

Anal splitting is an alternative surgical treatment to perineal herniorrhaphy in dogs with excessive tenesmus, large rectal sacculation, and little other tissue in the hernia.[10, 22] In this procedure, two fingers are placed through the anus into the rectum and an incision is made from the anal opening through the skin, external anal sphincter muscle, and rectal wall. This lays open the rectum, the edge of which is then sutured to the skin edge. The incision must be carefully placed to avoid the pudendal nerve and anal sac. The technique is judged to be not too successful because of postoperative fecal incontinence.[18]

Regardless of the technique used, the benefit of castration, both in the prophylaxis of perineal hernia as well as in the prevention of recurrence after surgical repair, is still unclear. There are conflicting reports of statistical studies of the effects of castration. Two studies failed to demonstrate any beneficial effect,[8, 14] while another two studies of much larger populations dem-

onstrated a significant sparing effect of castration on recurrence.[9, 23] When the sum of the literature was tabulated, 43 per cent of 102 uncastrated dogs had recurrent hernias compared with 23 per cent of 633 castrated dogs. Castration has also been shown to be useful in the treatment of perianal gland neoplasms,[24] as well as in the prophylaxis of testicular tumors. Both are common diseases of the older male dog. Castration is now an accepted and integral part of the treatment of perineal hernia.

Prognosis. The prognosis must be guarded in view of the tendency for breakdown of the surgical repair, the need for persistent treatment, and the postsurgical complications. In one survey only 42 per cent of clients were completely satisfied with the results of surgery.[8]

RECTAL PROLAPSE

Rectal prolapse is a disorder characterized by the protrusion of one or more layers of the rectum through the anus. It may be either partial or complete depending upon the structures involved. In partial prolapse, also called rectal eversion, only the rectal mucosa protrudes. Complete rectal prolapse is a double layer evagination of the rectum, sometimes including the anorectal junction through the anal canal.

History and Resulting Signs. The disorder can occur whenever there is persistent and severe tenesmus from intestinal, anorectal, or urogenital disease. Rectal prolapse occurs in dogs and cats of any age, breed, or sex, but is seen most frequently in young animals with severe diarrhea and tenesmus. Rectal foreign bodies can also cause severe straining and prolapse. Other predisposing factors include tumors of the distal colon, rectum, or anus, dystocia, cystitis, urethral obstruction, prostatitis, prostatic hypertrophy, colitis, and proctitis. Defects in the pelvic musculature, such as occur in perineal hernia, also predispose to prolapse, as does mechanical interference with the external anal sphincter.[25]

Physical Findings. Diagnosis is made by the presence of a tube-like mass of varying length which protrudes from the anus. It is important to distinguish a true rectal prolapse from a prolapsed ileocolic intussusception. A well-lubricated thermometer or finger is gently passed between the anus and the prolapsed mass. With a rectal prolapse, the fornix is located within a centimeter of the anus, whereas with a prolapsed intussusception, a probe or finger can be easily passed for a distance of five to six cm past the mass (Figure 92–5).

Treatment. Treatment is based on identification and correction of the underlying cause and reduction of the prolapse. The various techniques for treatment of rectal prolapse have been described in detail and range from simple reduction to resection.[26] Partial prolapse usually responds well to medical treatment. The mucosa is gently replaced through the anus, and antibiotic-steroid ointments such as Panalog are applied topically for at least one week. If prolapse recurs, 0.05 mg/lb (0.1 mg/kg) q8h of loperamide (Imodium), increases anal sphincter tone and reduces tenesmus, thereby helping to prevent reappearance. A purse-string suture can be placed around the anus. Concomitant treatment of the underlying cause is mandatory.

Management of complete rectal prolapse depends upon (1) the degree of tissue viability and (2) the number of recurrences. If the rectal mucosa is viable as determined by a warm temperature and the appearance of red oxygenated blood oozing from its surface and it is the animal's first occurrence, treatment by simple reduction and an anal purse-string suture should be the initial approach. Under general anesthesia or epidural analgesia, the edematous mucosa should be lubricated with KY jelly and gently massaged to reduce swelling. Cold hypertonic solutions such as 50 per cent dextrose have been advocated to reduce edema by vascular constriction and osmosis; however, warm isotonic solutions may serve to dilate the blood vessels and better allow interstitial edema to be removed by gentle manipulation.[26] After reduction of the prolapse, a purse-string suture of 2-0 nylon is preplaced at the anocutaneous line immediately cranial to the anal sac duct orifices. A well-lubricated small lavender top blood collection tube is then placed into the rectum, and the purse-string is tied tight enough to gently appose the rectal mucosa against the tube. The tube is then removed, leaving a purse-string that is tight enough to prevent recurrence but loose enough to allow defecation of soft feces. The suture can usually be left in for a week or more without major problems.

If the rectal prolapse is viable but cannot be reduced digitally, or if there is a history of multiple recurrences, then a colopexy procedure is recommended. Colopexy has been an especially effective prophylactic treatment in cats in which purse-string management is often ineffective and the risks of suture line dehiscence or rectal stricture after amputation are high. The colopexy is performed to the left abdominal wall with the colon in slight traction. A five mm × one cm elliptical section of peritoneum is removed from the abdominal wall two cm lateral to the midline and a corresponding area is then removed from the adjacent colonic serosa. The raw bleeding surfaces are then apposed with five or six simple interrupted sutures of 3-0 nylon or polypropylene, taking

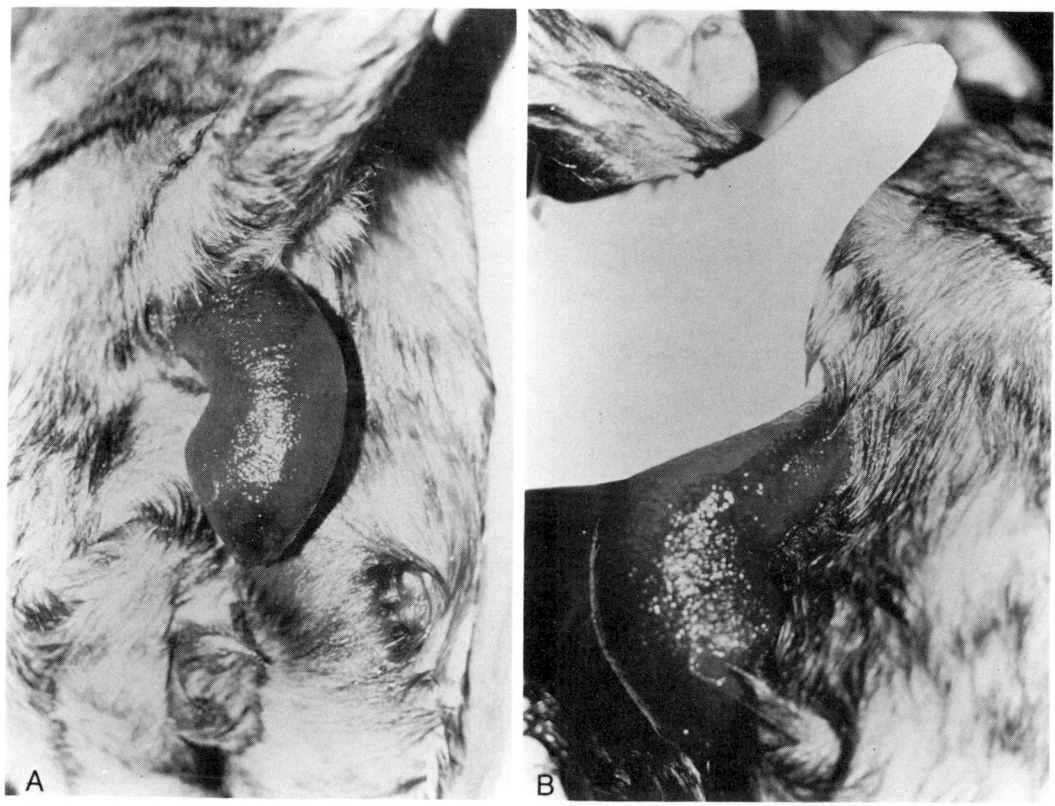

FIGURE 92–5. *A,* An 18-month-old greyhound with chronic whipworm infection, diarrhea, and tenesmus and an apparent rectal prolapse. *B,* Insertion of a gloved index finger for a distance of five cm revealed that this was in fact a prolapsed ileocolic intussusception.

care not to penetrate into the lumen of the colon. It is usual to create three or four colopexy sites along the length of the colon.

When the prolapsed segment is devitalized, amputation and rectal anastomosis should be performed.[27] A devitalized prolapse is usually dark purple or black in appearance and exudes dark cyanotic blood from its often ulcerated surface. Potential complications after amputation and anastomosis of rectal prolapse include dehiscence and stricture formation. Suture line dehiscence may be fatal unless detected early. Postoperative strictures are initially managed by dilating the constricting ring with a rectal or vaginal speculum under general anesthesia followed by two weeks of corticosteroid therapy. If the stricture recurs, excision of the fibrous ring must be attempted surgically.

Postoperative Care. Elimination of postoperative tenesmus is often essential for a successful outcome. Local anesthetic ointments instilled rectally or epidural analgesia may achieve this over the short term. Fecal softeners such as dioctyl sodium sulfosuccinate or Metamucil are useful supplements to kibbled food, which is higher in fiber than canned meat-based diets and produces softer feces. Symptomatic treatment in the form of nonabsorbable antibiotics, intestinal protectants, or anticholinergics is advisable if diarrhea is present. Identification and treatment of the primary cause is mandatory.

Prognosis. The prognosis depends upon degree, duration, and underlying cause. It is usually good provided the underlying cause can be identified and corrected.

COLONIC AND RECTAL TUMORS

Tumors of the colon and rectum represent 36 to 60 per cent of all canine and 10 to 15 per cent of all feline alimentary tract neoplasms.[28, 29] The benign adenomatous polyp is the most common tumor in the dog, accounting for about 50 per cent of all large bowel tumors in this species.[30] Lymphosarcoma and adenocarcinoma are the most frequently diagnosed malignant tumors, but carcinomas, leiomyosarcomas, carcinoid tumors, and anaplastic sarcomas have also been reported.[30–34] The most common large intestinal tumor in the cat is lymphoma. The location of the tumor varies in different species. In the cat most tumors occur in the ileocecal area,[34] while in the dog the majority are found in the rectum.[30, 33, 35]

Based on their gross characteristics, adenocarcinomas have been classified into three main types: (1) infiltrative, (2) ulcerative, and (3) proliferative.[36] The infiltrating tumor spreads within the rectal or colonic wall to cause fibrosis and strictures of varying length. The ulcerative type produces a typical malignant ulcer with a hard base and raised edge, while the proliferative type has a wart-like appearance. All three types are slow-growing and may be present for months and occasionally even years before diagnosis. The tumor eventually spreads through the rectal wall, penetrates the lymphatics, and metastasizes to the local lymph nodes, lungs, and liver. Adenocarcinomas occur predominantly in dogs older than nine years,[37] more frequently in males than females, and have a particularly high incidence in collies and German shepherds.[30, 33]

Colonic and rectal lymphosarcomas are uncommon in the dog but are the most common large bowel tumor of the cat.[34, 38] They occur either as a discrete mass or as a diffuse infiltrate in the colonic and rectal mucosa. This tumor occurs in older cats and in dogs younger than four years.

Carcinoid tumors, though rare, occur in both the small and large intestine.[33, 39] The tumor is associated with diarrhea and gastrointestinal hemorrhage and, as a result of its secretion of serotonin, with systemic vasomotor effects.

Adenomatous polyps are the most common benign neoplasms of the colon and rectum with most being found in the rectum.[31, 32] There appears to be a breed predilection in collies and the West Highland white terrier.[30, 32] Carcinomas may arise within adenomatous polyps in the canine rectum.[32, 40]

History and Physical Findings. Dogs and cats with large intestinal tumors usually have a history of dyschezia, hematochezia, tenesmus, and mucoid diarrhea (Figure 92–6). Intermittent anal eversion is not uncommon. As with most malignant tumors, afflicted animals appear chronically ill and debilitated. Specific signs depend upon tumor location and type. All three types of adenocarcinoma cause tenesmus with the frequent passage of small amounts of mucoid and often bloody feces. Tenesmus worsens as the lesion develops, especially in the proliferative or obstructive type which can obliterate the lumen to completely obstruct fecal passage, and causes secondary colonic impaction (Figure 92–7). If the tumor does not cause an obstruction, its presence may change the character of the feces. A thin ribbon of feces is not uncommon with infiltrating adenocarcinomas, and hematochezia is a frequent complaint in the ulcerating type. Rectal irritation also causes a mucoid diarrhea or mucus-covered feces passed with excessive tenesmus and rectal eversion. Digital rectal examination typically reveals a painful ring-like mass or stenotic area, the so-called "napkin-ring lesion," anterior to which a hard fecal mass may be palpated. Abdominal palpation may reveal a large painful colon full of hard noncompressible fecal material.

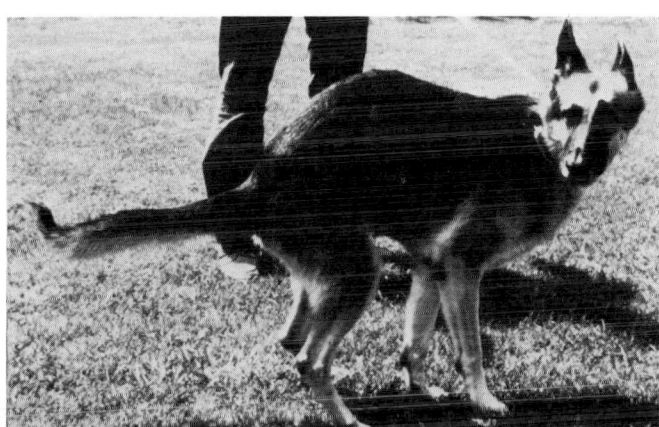

FIGURE 92–6. A 10-year-old German shepherd with rectal carcinoma. The animal was presented with a history of diarrhea and tenesmus. When walked, the dog continually adopted the semisquatting position shown in the picture. This is compatible with a severe rectal lesion; note the abnormal tail carriage. Rectal examination revealed almost total obliteration of the lumen.

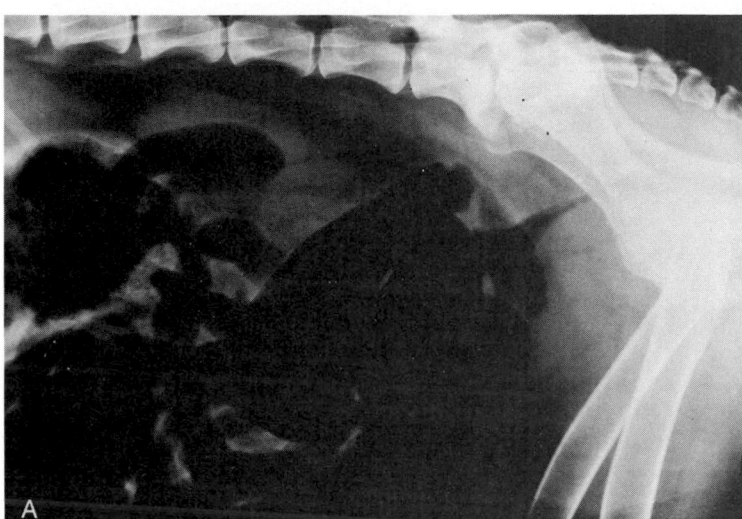
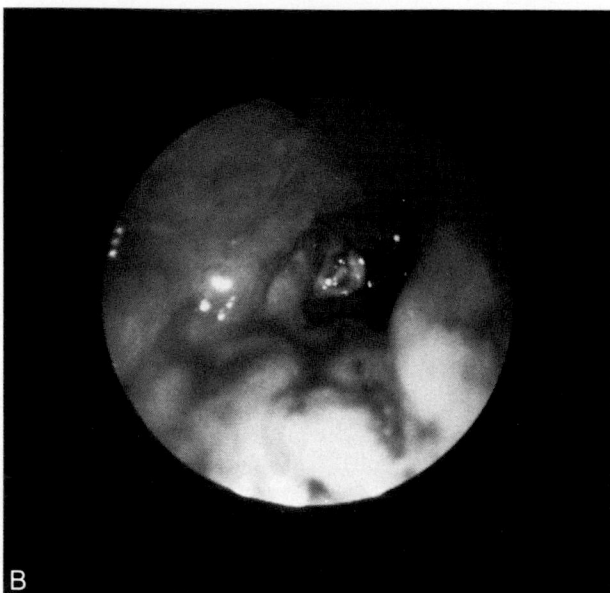

FIGURE 92–7. *A,* Lateral abdominal radiograph of the dog shown in Figure 92–6. There is a megacolon with marked fecal retention and widespread ileus. The colon can be seen to narrow at the pelvic inlet consistent with a mural stricture. Enlarged iliac lymph nodes are also present suggesting metastasis. *B,* Endoscopic view of the stricture. The lumen is almost totally obliterated and bled readily when touched with the tip of the endoscope.

If diffusely infiltrated through the colon wall, lymphosarcomas of the large intestine cause a chronic unresponsive diarrhea similar to that seen in chronic histoplasmosis or severe idiopathic colitis. Occasionally, a single focus of lymphosarcoma may be identified, in which case the signs resemble those of an adenocarcinoma.

Dogs with colonic or rectal polyps do not appear as debilitated as dogs with malignant tumors. With this disorder, the predominant signs are tenesmus following defecation and a chronic unresponsive bloody or mucoid diarrhea. Animals are sometimes presented with the tumor prolapsed from the rectum if tenesmus is particularly severe.

Diagnosis. Digital rectal examination is sufficient to confirm the presence of a rectal mass, and proctoscopy with biopsy or cytologic examination of an impression smear is usually diagnostic. In some patients a superficial biopsy may reveal only inflammatory cells, and a second deeper biopsy is required to confirm the diagnosis. The presence of a colonic tumor can also be confirmed by colonoscopy or contrast radiography. Since lymphosarcoma seldom involves the mucosa, superficial mucosal biopsy may be negative, even though a mass is palpated. Pararectal aspiration cytology can help to identify such lesions.

Polyps appear either as dome-shaped, lobulated friable masses with a cobbled surface or as a mass of finger-like projections of soft, dark red or pink tissue (Figure 92–8); palpation or slight trauma from the colonoscope usually causes bleeding. Distinct pedicles such as occur in humans are rare. Colonoscopy may be difficult or impossible when the tumor causes rectal stenosis.

Treatment. Surgical resection of carcinomas and adenocarcinomas can be attempted but is usually unrewarding, since metastasis has usually occurred before presentation.[41] In addition, morbidity and mortality is high in patients with rectal resection and anastomosis. Anastomotic leakage occurs about 30 per cent of the time, and fecal incontinence occurs when over 6 cm of the rectum is removed.[42]

About 75 per cent of polyps are accessible through the anus and can be easily exposed if the rectal mucosa is everted by gentle traction. Polyps can be removed either by surgical excision or by electrocautery. Polyps located more proximally can be removed with an electrocautery snare passed through the colonoscope or via a colotomy. The prognosis is good, even if biopsy shows submucosal invasion;[30] however, new polyps may occur and there is always a risk of postoperative rectal stricture.

RECTAL AND ANAL STRICTURES

Strictures of the rectum and anus are uncommon in the dog and cat. They usually occur as a complication of an inflammatory disease, such as perianal fistula, chronic anal sac disease, or anorectal trauma, or as a

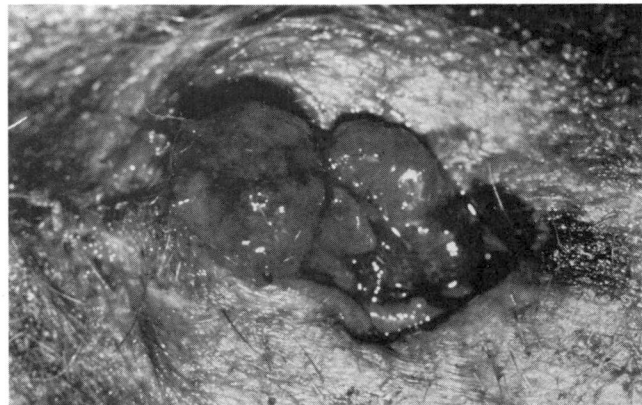

FIGURE 92–8. Rectal polyp in a four-year-old male Doberman with a history of hematochezia. Rectal examination revealed a lobulated friable mass that could easily be exteriorized. Submucosal resection was performed with total resolution of the problem.

47. Christie, TF: Perianal fistula in the dog. Vet Clin North Am 5:353, 1975.
48. Liska, WD, et al.: Cryosurgery in the treatment of perianal fistulae. Vet Clin North Am 5:449, 1975.
49. Lane, JG and Burch, DGS: The cryosurgical treatment of canine anal furunculosis. J Small Anim Pract 16:387, 1975.
50. Van Ee, RT and Palminteri, A: Tail amputation for treatment of perianal fistulas in dogs. JAAHA 23:95, 1987.
51. Vasseur, P.B.: Perianal fistulae in dogs: a retrospective analysis of surgical techniques. JAAHA 17:177, 1981.
52. Vasseur, PB: Results of surgical excision of perianal fistulas in dogs. JAVMA 186:60, 1984.
53. Goring, RL, et al.: Perianal fistulas in the dog: Retrospective evaluation of surgical treatment by deroofing and fulguration. Vet Surg 15:293, 1986.
54. Rawlings, CA and Capps, WF: Rectovaginal fistula and imperforate anus in a dog. JAVMA 159:320, 1971.
55. Harvey, CE: Incidence and distribution of anal sac disease in the dog. JAAHA 10:573, 1974.
56. Halnan, CRE: The frequency of occurrence of anal sacculitis in the dog. J Small Anim Pract 17:537, 1976a.
57. Halnan, CRE: The experimental reproduction of anal sacculitis. J Small Anim Pract 17:693, 1976b.
58. Halnan, CRE: The anal sacs of the dog. FRCVS Thesis. London, Royal College of Veterinary Surgeons, 1973.
59. Halnan, CRE: The diagnosis of anal sacculitis in the dog. J Small Anim Pract 17:527, 1976c.
60. Halnan, CRE: Therapy of anal sacculitis in the dog. J Small Anim Pract 17:685, 1976d.
61. Halnan, CRE: Canine anal sac disease. In Grunsell, CS and Hill, FWD (eds): Veterinary Annual No 18. Bristol, England, Scientechnica, 1978, p 225.
62. Bostock, D: Neoplasms of the skin and subcutaneous tissues in dogs and cats. Brit Vet J 142:1, 1986.
63. Hayes, HM and Wilson, GP: Cancer Res 37:2068, 1977.
64. Gillette, EL: Veterinary radiotherapy. JAVMA 157:1707, 1970.
65. Liska, WD and Withrow, SJ: Cryosurgical treatment of perianal gland adenomas in the dog. JAAHA 14:457, 1978.
66. Rijnberk, A, et al.: Pseudohyperparathyroidism associated with perirectal adenocarcinoma in elderly female dogs. Tijdschr Diergeneeskd 103:1069, 1978.
67. Meuten, DJ, et al.: Hypercalcemia associated with an adenocarcinoma derived from the apocrine glands of the anal sac. Vet Pathol 18:454, 1981.
68. Rubinard, S., and Slivaprasad, H.L.: Hypercalcemia associated with an anal sac adenocarcinoma in a castrated male dog. Comp Vet Cont Ed 7:348, 1985.
69. Leeds, EB and Renegar, WR: A modified fascial sling for the treatment of fecal incontinence—surgical technique. JAAHA 17:663, 1981.

DRUG INDEX

Motility Modifier
Loperamide (Imodium–Janssen) 0.05 mg/lb (0.1 mg/kg)
Antibiotic for Gastrointestinal Disease
Sulfasalazine (Azulfidine–Pharmacia) 12–18 mg/lb (25–40 mg/kg) q8h
Bulk-forming Laxative
Psyllium (Metamucil–Searle) 1–3 tsp mixed with food SID or BID

THE ENDOCRINE SYSTEM

93 PITUITARY-HYPOTHALAMIC DISEASES

J. E. EIGENMANN

HISTORIC BACKGROUND

The view that the pituitary gland is a phlegm gland (Latin "Pituita," phlegm) appears to have begun with Galen in approximately 130–200 A.D. Yet, Vesalius first recognized the hypophysis cerebri (attachment underneath the brain) not necessarily as a separate entity but as an identifiable part. He believed the pituitary secreted mucus into the nose and named the pituitary the glandula pituitaria cerebri excipiens, "the little phlegm corndrawn out of the brain." Several investigators in the 17th century ascribed an exocrine function to the pituitary. Sylvius, Vieussens, and Willis believed that the pituitary produced the cerebrospinal fluid. Diseases of humans now known to be of pituitary origin may have been recognized for centuries. An old English medical record (1738) shows the facial characteristics of acromegaly. However, the connection between the pituitary and acromegaly was not made until 1886 when Pierre Marie, a French physician, recognized the latter relationship and named the disease "acromegalie" because of the hypertrophy of the distal body parts. Fourteen years later, another investigator ascribed the syndrome to an adenoma of pituitary eosinophil cells.

In the late 19th century, the suspicion of a relation between pituitary destruction and certain clinical states began to emerge. Lorain pointed to the association of a destroyed pituitary gland and dwarfism. In 1914, Morris Simmonds' famous report on an emaciated woman who had destruction of the anterior pituitary appeared. In the early 20th century, clinicians started to relate tumors of the pituitary gland with the syndrome of what is now known as pituitary insufficiency. In 1901, Fröhlich reported on the successful removal of a cystic tumor of the pituitary, probably a craniopharyngioma, from a boy with failed vision but without acromegaly. This was the beginning of what is now known as Fröhlich's syndrome, later named adiposogenital dystrophy. Such tumors are known to be derived from the pharyngeal derivative of the Rathke's pouch, the embryologic "anlage" of the anterior hypophysis.

The second development of major significance was the finding that the anterior lobe not only has the cytologic characteristics of most other secreting glands but also undergoes changes during altered physiologic and pathologic states. It was observed that the pituitary undergoes enlargement in the human male and female following gonadectomy.

A brief historic synopsis of the major advances in pituitary physiology and disease is given below.[1]

Growth Hormone (GH) and Prolactin

Hypophysectomies on dogs and cats were done as early as 1907. However, because of inappropriate techniques, no valid conclusions could be drawn from these experiments. Yet, as early as 1909, proof for the importance of the pituitary as a growth-promoting organ was obtained. Dogs hypophysectomized by Aschner failed to grow. From then on, knowledge about pituitary physiology has increased rapidly and continues to expand. In 1921, gigantism was produced in rats by administering pituitary extracts. The breakthrough in pituitary physiology was the discovery that implants of fresh anterior lobe tissue induced an immediate and remarkable growth and maturation of the ovaries. In 1928 prolactin was identified and later purified and analyzed.

Adrenocorticotropic Hormone (ACTH)

Some of the pioneers in research on pituitary factors and their influence on the adrenals include: Smith, who demonstrated that hypophysectomy leads to adrenal atrophy in 1926; Cushing, who showed the syndrome of hyperfunction of the pituitary-adrenal system in 1932; Li and Schwyzer, who isolated ACTH in 1942; Hofmann, Li, and Schwyzer, who synthesized ACTH in 1962; and Schwyzer and Sieber, who synthesized β-corticotropin in 1966.

Thyroid-Stimulating Hormone (TSH)

In 1927, the existence of TSH was shown and by 1969, the hormone was purified for the first time.[2, 3]

History of the Neurohypophysis

The physiology and pharmacology of active principles of the neurohypophysis date from experiments performed by Sir Edward Ackert Sharpey-Schafer. It led to the discovery of the pressor effect exerted by pituitary extracts, and evidence was presented that the activity resided in the posterior part of the mammalian hypophysis. The blood-pressure–raising action of pituitary extracts was confirmed by many other investigators.

In 1898, Howell made an important advance by showing that the pressor principle of pituitary extracts resided in the posterior lobe, or as he preferred to call it, the infundibular body. Until shortly before he undertook his experiments, the posterior lobe was, on morphologic grounds, commonly regarded as a rudimentary organ without physiologic function.

The antidiuretic effect of posterior pituitary extracts was made by Fanici and von der Velden. Historically, the most important paper on the mechanisms of the antidiuretic effect was probably that of Starling and Verney who observed in 1924 that there is an antidiuretic effect of posterior pituitary extracts on the isolated kidney.

Sir Henry Dale described his discovery in 1906 as follows: "When I injected an appropriate dose of the pituitary extract, I observed that it had not only retained its normal pressor action, in contrast to the reversed depressor action of adrenaline, but that it also produced a powerful, contractile response of the uterus, not hitherto described."[4] This was the discovery of oxytocin.

The History of Clinical Pituitary Diseases in Small Animals

Although descriptions of pituitary tumors in the dog appeared as early as 1935, it was not until 1939 that the first description of hyperadrenocorticism (Cushing's disease) in the dog was given.[5] Clinical, biochemical, and pathologic studies are milestones in the history of a now frequently recognized and treatable disease.[6–8]

Acromegalic features in a dog suffering from an eosinophilic adenoma were reported as early as 1923.[9] Acromegaly was again tentatively diagnosed in 1963 in a female dog with a pituitary adenoma.[10] It was conclusively diagnosed as iatrogenic acromegaly in a dog,[11] and iatrogenic or spontaneous acromegaly in 1981.[12]

Dwarfism in German shepherds was tentatively diagnosed to be of pituitary origin as early as 1953. It was not until recently that dwarfism in German shepherds could be unequivocally addressed as dwarfism of pituitary origin (growth hormone deficiency).[13, 14] With the advancement of hormone assays and the growing interest of owners in the treatment of their pets' diseases, knowledge about pituitary disease continues to increase.

INTRODUCTION (CONCEPTS)

Feedback

One of the axioms of physiology has been Claude Bernard's concept of the constancy of the organism's internal environment ("milieu interne"); however, it has become clear that the milieu interne is subjected to changing environmental stimuli as well as to the presence of circadian variation. Despite such variation, it is still true that there is a relatively constant internal milieu and that this requires the interaction of numerous body processes involving complex physiologic control mechanisms. The neuroendocrine system forms the major regulatory area in this regard. Both long- and short-loop systems are operative. The long-loop systems are those from the target gland to the anterior pituitary, hypothalamus, and other areas of the central nervous system. Tissue metabolites, such as glucose and free fatty acids, may also function in such a long-loop system. Most of the feedback processes are considered to be inhibitory (negative feedback); however, occasionally there may be a positive feedback. In case of a negative feedback, the product of the pituitary hormone's target gland, e.g., T_4 or cortisol, depresses the pituitary hormone secretion at either the pituitary or hypothalamic level. An example of a positive feedback is low estrogen levels. They can stimulate the release of luteinizing hormone-releasing hormone (LHRH), while higher estrogen levels usually inhibit LHRH release. Another example is adrenocorticotropin (ACTH) secretion. The cell regulating ACTH secretion is programmed to stop secreting ACTH above a certain level, while below a certain corticosteroid level it will initiate ACTH secretion. In certain situations such as neuroendocrine disease or stress, the setpoint may be changed. For instance, a change in the setpoint of gonadal steroid inhibition has been invoked as an explanation for the onset of puberty. Short-loop feedback systems involving the effect of anterior pituitary hormones on releasing hormone concentrations have not been as thoroughly investigated. Most such feedback systems are inhibitory in nature allowing self-regulation and avoiding overshoot in the production of any secretory product.[15]

HYPOPHYSIOTROPIC CONCEPT

It is generally accepted that the central nervous system regulation of anterior pituitary function is mediated by hypophysiotropic hormones (factors). Although these hypothalamic hormones are called releasing hormones, there is evidence that they also stimulate pituitary hormone synthesis. Hypophysiotropic hormones are believed to be products of specialized neurosecretory cells, which are concentrated within the hypothalamus.

The role of the hypothalamus was emphasized in early studies in which fragments of anterior pituitary lobe tissue were transplanted into different parts of the hypothalamus of hypophysectomized rats. Pituitary function was preserved only when the pituitary implants were placed in direct contact with the hypothalamus. It is clear from such studies and from anatomic studies, which demonstrated essential lack of innervation of the anterior pituitary, that neural regulation of pituitary function must be accomplished by humoral substances that would normally reach the pituitary gland via its portal vascular system supply.[15]

ANATOMY

Developmental Anatomy

At an early developmental stage, contact between the oral and neural ectoderm occurs. A small portion of oral ectoderm evaginates and contacts the ventral surface of the neural tube. This portion ultimately is freed entirely from the remaining ectoderm. With continued differentiation, a small evagination of the neural tube develops at the point of adhesion with the oral ectoderm. This structure becomes surrounded by the collapsing vesicle of oral ectoderm. The surrounding mesenchyme provides the stroma and vascularization of the pituitary.

A portion of the neuroectoderm forms the neurohypophysis consisting of the pars proximalis and pars distalis. The oral ectoderm surrounds the neurohypophysis. The surface of the oral ectoderm vesicle contacting the neurohypophysis develops into the pars intermedia. The remaining part of the vesicle, not being in direct contact with the neurohypophysis, evolves into the pars proximalis and the pars distalis of the adenohypophysis. Pituitary size varies among breeds of dogs, and variation occurs even in the same breed. In the 22 lb (10 kg) dog, the weight of the pituitary ranges from less than 100 mg to about 300 mg. The larger the dog, the bigger the pituitary. This merely represents an increase in absolute weight; the relative pituitary weight in a large dog is less than in a small dog.

Macroscopic Anatomy

The main part of the pituitary is embedded in a recess in the sphenoid bone. The recess is shallow in the dog but not in humans. The cranial and caudal margins of the fossa are formed by the tuberculum sellae. Dorsally, the pituitary is confined by the dorsum sellae. Although the external or endosteal layer of the dura mater extends into the pituitary fossa and thereby lines the fossa, the inner meningeal part does not enter and forms the diaphragma sellae (dorsum sellae). In the dog, in contrast to humans, a large foramen ovale is present in the center of the diaphragm, thus allowing for dorsal expansion in case of tumor growth. On both sides of the pituitary, large cavernous sinuses can be found. In the dog, they are connected by a smaller caudal transverse sinus. Within each of the cavernous sinuses lies the rostral portion of the middle meningeal artery and the anasto-motic ramus of the external ophthalmic artery. In addition, the internal carotid artery courses through each of the sinuses. In the proximity of the hypophysis pass the oculomotor, trochlear, and abducent nerves and the ophthalmic branch of the trigeminal nerve.[16–18]

Parts of the Pituitary

PROXIMAL PART OF THE PITUITARY

The proximal part consists of the infundibular portions of the neuro- and adenohypophysis. Together, they form a funnel-like structure enclosing the infundibular recess and the pituitary stalk. This structure, therefore, consists of a neural and an epithelial component. The epithelial cells are of a cuboidal, undifferentiated nature. The infundibular part of the adenohypophysis contains the long portal vessels and some of the capillary network draining into the portal vessels. The neural tissue consists mainly of unmyelinated nerve fibers from the hypothalamus, blood vessels, and pituicytes. The neural tissue is composed of distinct internal and external zones. The internal zone contains fibers extending from the supraoptic and paraventricular nuclei of the hypothalamus into the pituitary. It is assumed that the external zone is the site of termination of the tuberoinfundibular fiber system. The fiber system is likely to originate from the parvocellular nuclei located in the region called the hypophysiotropic area (Figure 93–1).

DISTAL PART OF THE PITUITARY

This part consists of the pars distalis and pars intermedia of the adenohypophysis and the infundibular process of the neuro-hypophysis. The pars distalis of the adenohypophysis is composed of cuboidal epithelial cells and contains a network of sinusoids. The cells can be characterized according to content of granules, staining properties, and size as acidophils, basophils, and chromophobes. Sophisticated staining techniques have revealed that both basophils and acidophils consist of distinct classes of cell types. Among acidophils, GH-secreting cells and prolactin-secreting cells are recognized. The latter can be differentiated from GH-producing cells by light microscopy. Basophils secrete thyroid-stimulating hormone (TSH), gonadotropins (luteinizing hormone, follicle-stimulating hormone), and ACTH. Some of the anterior pituitary cells, depending on the staining technology used, are 15 to 40 per cent chromophobic by light microscopy. Depending on the stain, these cells will resemble either basophils or acidophils and have been named amphophils. Although in the normal pituitary no hormone secretory role for these cells has been identified, it is possible that they are actively secreting or resting degranulated cells. Moreover, in pituitary tumors, these cells have been associated with hormone oversecretion. Cells of a given type tend to be clustered together in certain regions of the pars distalis.

PARS INTERMEDIA

The pars intermedia varies considerably in extent and demarcation in various animal species. While in the pituitary of adult humans there is no distinct pars intermedia, the pars intermedia in the canine consists of a broad band of epithelial cells. Although the cat has a pars intermedia, the zone is not as prominent as in the dog. The band is intimately attached to the infundibular

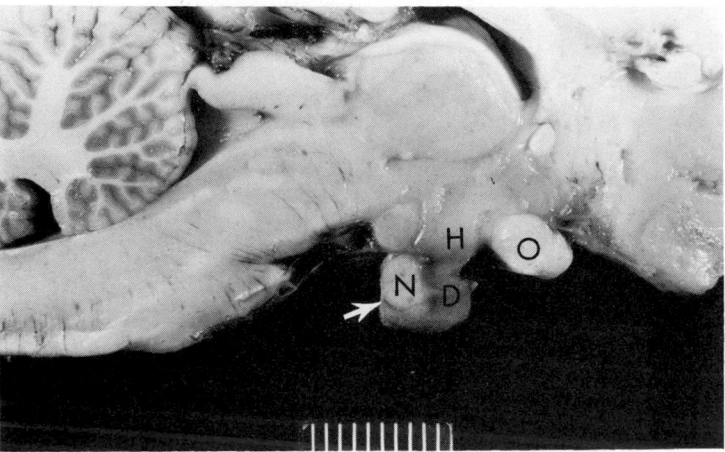

FIGURE 93–1. The pituitary region from a dog illustrates the close relationship to the optic chiasm (O), hypothalamus (H), and overlying brain. The pars distalis (D) forms a major part of the adenohypophysis and completely surrounds the pars nervosa (N). The residual lumen of Rathke's pouch (white arrow) separates the pars distalis and pars nervosa and is lined by the pars intermedia. Scale at bottom = 1 cm.

process but partly separated from the pars distalis by the Rathke's cleft (the residual lumen of the Rathke's pouch). There are two cell types in the pars intermedia, A and B cells. These epithelial cells are either large and rounded or smaller and more angular. Together, these cells secrete melanotropin, ACTH, and β-lipoprotein. While the A cells secrete all of these hormones, the B cells secrete only ACTH and lipotropin.[19] There are few blood vessels and only occasional nerve fibers in the pars intermedia.

THE INFUNDIBULAR PROCESS

The infundibular process comprises the distal part of the neural component of the pituitary gland. Here, the majority of nerve fibers of the supraoptic-paraventriculo-hypophyseal tract terminate. Ramification of these fibers extends into the posterior lobe. There is stainable neurosecretory material containing vasopressin, oxytocin, and their carrier proteins, particularly present around the blood vessels.

VASCULARIZATION OF THE PITUITARY

The major arterial supply is provided by the internal carotid arteries and the caudal communicating arteries. Several branches provide blood supply directly to the pituitary stem from the rostal and caudal intercarotid arteries and the caudal communicating arteries. Four to ten branches leading to the proximal part of the neurohypophysis stem from the rostral intercarotid artery. Another extensive group of vessels arises from the rostral communicating arteries. All of these vessels pass toward the proximal part of the neurohypophysis. Here, through anastomosis, they form the mantle plexus. On the cranial and lateral surfaces of the median eminence, major vessels arise from the mantle plexus or as direct branches of the intercarotid vessels, named the rostral hypophyseal arteries. Several of these provide capillaries to the median eminence and the proximal part of the neurohypophysis. The capillaries receive neurohumoral substances (releasing factors) subsequently carried from the hypothalamus via the portal system to the pituitary. The capillaries of the adenohypophysis form the secondary blood capillary network. The veins that connect the secondary with the primary (situated in the infundibu-lum) plexus are the portal vessels of the pituitary (Figure 93–2).[17]

HYPOTHALAMIC-HYPOPHYSEAL CONNECTIONS

Between the hypothalamus and the pituitary gland are located both the neural and neurovascular connections. Unmyelinated axons arise from the supraoptic and paraventricular nuclei and pass through the infundibulum as the supraoptic-paraventricular-hypophyseal tract. This tract conveys vasopressin, oxytocin, and their neurophysins (carrier proteins). This system is referred to as the magnocellular neurosecretory system (Figure 93–3).

The parvocellular system is represented by the tubero-infundibular tract. This tract originates from the periventricular and infundibular nuclei and terminates on the portal vessels of the tuberal area of the infundibulum. This system is believed to transport corticotropin-releasing factor (CRF).

The portal system consists of a primary capillary plexus in the infundibulum which is continuous with both the vascular bed of the hypothalamus and the secondary capillary plexus situated within the pituitary. Connection is provided by the long portal vessels. A second, primary capillary plexus supplied by the inferior hypophyseal arteries is situated in the infundibular process. This plexus is connected with the adenohypophyseal plexus by short portal vessels. Thus, all blood ultimately reaching the pituitary passes through one of the two primary plexuses.[20–24]

HYPOTHALAMUS

The hypothalamus lies at the base of the diencephalon on either side of the midline and is bounded externally by the rostral perforated substance, the pyriform lobe, and the crura cerebri. The hypothalamus is divided into a rostral hypothalamic region, an intermediate or tuberal hypothalamic region, and a caudal hypothalamic region. Each of these regions is subdivided into a number of subsidiary nuclei.[15]

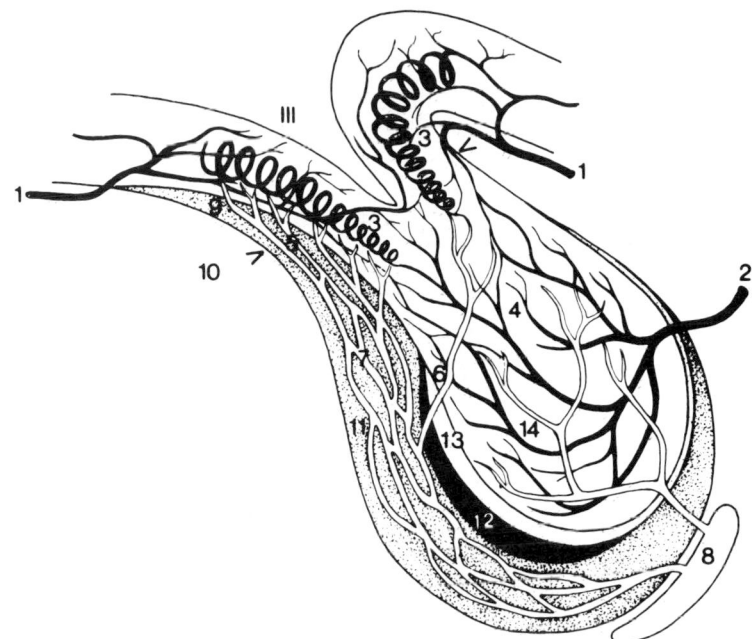

FIGURE 93–2. Diagrammatic representation of the pituitary gland and its vascular supply. 1. Superior hypophyseal artery. 2. Inferior hypophyseal artery. 3. Primary plexus of the infundibular stem. 4. Primary plexus of the infundibular process. 5. Long portal vessels. 6. Short portal vessels. 7. Secondary plexus in the adenohypophysis. 8. Collecting vein. 9. Pars tuberalis (infundibularis of the adenohypophysis.) 10. Pituitary stalk. 11. Pars distalis. 12. Residual hypophyseal lumen (intraglandular cleft). 13. Pars intermedia. 14. Infundibular process of the neurohypophysis. III. Infundibular recess of the third ventricle. (From Meijer, JC: An investigation of the pathogenesis of pituitary-dependent hyperadrenocorticism in the dog. Utrecht, Elinkwijk, 1980.)

NEUROTRANSMITTER REGULATION OF HYPOPHYSIOTROPIC CELLS

There are no anatomically or histologically demonstrable central nervous system areas involved in the regulation of a specific hypophysiotropic hormone. Rather, there seems to be neurotransmitter coding for such hormones.

The neurosecretory cell can be described as having receptors for several neurotransmitters, each arriving via different anatomic pathways and activated by different stimuli. Neurotransmitters can be either excitatory or inhibitory. Virtually all the postulated neurotransmitters (catecholamines, indolamines, acetylcholine, histamine, and γ-aminobutyric acid [GABA]) have been identified in the hypothalamus and specifically within the median eminence. There is incomplete agreement as to the specific effects of a given neurotransmitter on a specific hypophysiotropic hormone.[15]

HYPOPHYSIOTROPIC HORMONES

Several factors have been isolated and definitively characterized.

Thyrotropin-releasing Hormone (TRH). Thyrotropin-releasing hormone, a tripeptide, was the first of the hypophysiotropic hormones to be identified. TRH has been synthesized and is widely available for clinical as well as experimental use. The mechanism of TRH action on the pituitary is believed to involve activation of the adenyl cyclase-cAMP system. This effect is blocked by thyroid hormone through a mechanism involving synthesis of an inhibitory protein blocking the action of TRH. In patients with pituitary tumors, acromegaly, or Cushing's disease, TRH has been shown to increase the release of growth hormone and of ACTH, respectively. TRH may have a direct effect on CNS function. TRH

may be effective behaviorally, not only through an action on neural cells but also by altering brain neurotransmitter turnover.[15, 25, 26]

Gonadotropin-releasing Hormone (GnRH). Gonadotropin-releasing hormone, a decapeptide, has been demonstrated to be contained almost solely in the median eminence. The effects of GnRH on luteinizing hormone (LH) release are mediated via the adenyl cyclase-cAMP system. Behavioral effects consist of the induction of estrus behavior.[15, 25, 26] Corticotropin-releasing factor (CRF) obtained from ovine, rat, and human hypothalamic tissue has potent stimulatory effects on ACTH and β-endorphin secretion from the pituitary *in vivo* and *in vitro*.[27–29]

Growth Hormone-releasing Hormone (GH-RH). GH-RH, a peptide containing either 40 or 44 amino acids, was first isolated from a human pancreatic islet tumor. Later, the peptide was isolated from ovine, caprine, rat, porcine, bovine, and human hypothalami. It is likely that α-adrenergic substances or α-adrenergic impulses stemming from the CNS act to increase GH secretion by increasing hypothalamic growth hormone-releasing factor (GRF) secretion. In some patients suffering from isolated GH deficiency as diagnosed by a failure of GH to increase in response to classic stimuli (hypoglycemia, clonidine), GHRH can cause release of GH.[30–33]

Prolactin (Inhibitor, Releasing Factor). Although the control of secretion of prolactin by the hypothalamus is predominantly inhibitory, some evidence exists to indicate the presence of a stimulating hypothalamic prolactin-releasing factor. Available evidence indicates that much of the prolactin inhibitory-like activity of hypothalamic extracts may be accounted for by dopamine. There is evidence that there are different forms of prolactin-releasing factor.[34, 35]

Somatostatin. Somatostatin is a tetradecapeptide that has been identified in several body fluids. Somatostatin not only blocks GH release but also blocks the release of many other hormones including insulin, glucagon, secretin, gastrin, and renin secretion.[15, 36, 37]

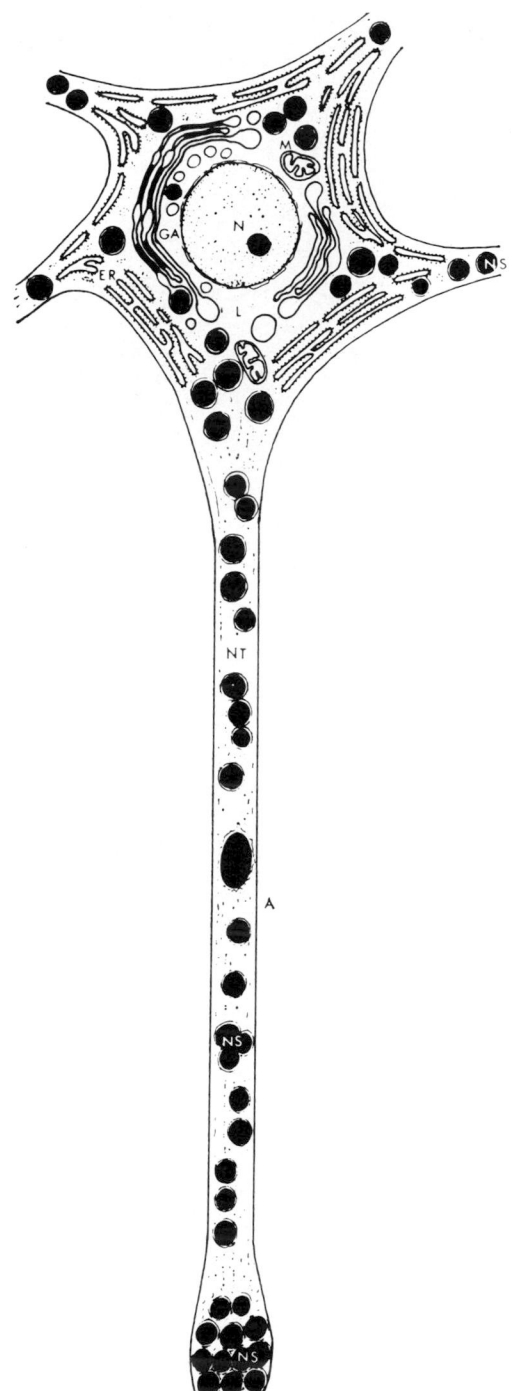

FIGURE 93–3. Structural characteristics of a neurosecretory neurone in the hypothalamus. The nerve cell body (M, nucleus) has dendritic and axonal (A) processes with arrays of rough endoplasmic reticulum, a prominent Golgi apparatus, and neurotubules (NT). Hormone-containing membrane-limited neurosecretory granules (NS) are formed in the Golgi apparatus and are transported along the axon to the site of release at the termination on capillaries. Neurosecretory neurones synthesize the releasing and release-inhibiting hormones of the adenohypophysis (oxytocin, ADH).

ENDOCRINE RHYTHMS AND NEUROENDOCRINE FUNCTION

The major classifications are daily, seasonal, or annual rhythms. Rhythms with an approximate 24-hour period are called circadian. Ultradian rhythms are those with periods shorter than 24 hours, and infradian rhythms are those with periods longer than 24 hours. Some endogenous rhythms may be synchronized by a periodic environmental influence, such as with light changes or the phases of the moon. In the dog there is evidence for episodic but not circadian activity in plasma concentrations of adrenocorticotropin, cortisol, and thyroxine. Equally, GH secretion is episodic, but there is a close association of GH secretion with sleep.[15, 38, 39]

Pituitary Hormones

Growth hormone (GH) is a single-chain polypeptide of pituitary origin. In most species, including the dog, it has a molecular weight of approximately 22,000 daltons.[40] By employing analytic and preparative techniques, it was found that growth hormone as usually extracted from the pituitary is not a single substance but a mixture of variants differing in amino acids.[41] In contrast to other pituitary hormones, the action of GH is not confined to one single target and the hormone displays diametrically opposed intrinsic anabolic and catabolic activities. Its catabolic activity (enhanced lipolysis and restricted glucose transport as a result of insulin resistance) is directly caused by the peptide. It is now widely held that the anabolic effects of GH are mediated by insulin-like growth factors or somatomedins (Figure 93–4).[42]

In normal animals, an increase in plasma insulin concentration acutely leads to an increase in glucose transport by adipose tissue. In hypophysectomized GH-deficient animals, however, basal glucose transport oc-

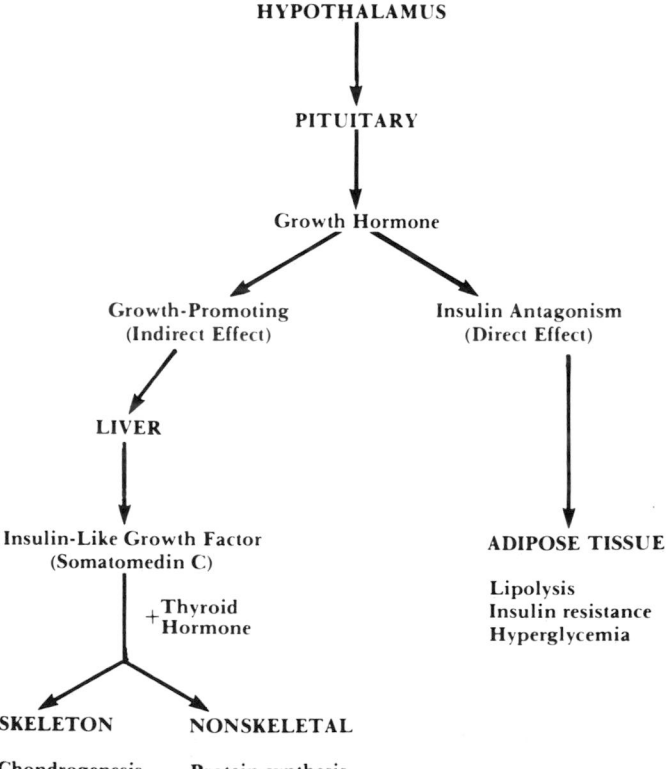

FIGURE 93–4. The main actions of growth hormone (GH) are outlined.

curs at a maximal rate, and adipose tissue glucose transport in such animals is insensitive to the action of insulin. GH administration in this animal model reduces glucose transport back to normal. Thus, GH normally restricts glucose transport, and this transport can be acutely modulated by insulin. Hence, insulin appears to inhibit a GH-controlled "glucose transport limiting factor." The glucose transport limiting factor may be the high-affinity CA^{2+}-ATPase found in fat cell membranes. Insulin decreases and GH increases the CA^{2+}-ATPase activity. Additionally, it has been suggested that the high affinity CA^{2+}-ATPase of isolated fat cells may be involved in early metabolic steps influenced by insulin, which regulates intracellular CA^{2+} levels. The above concept is in keeping with the finding that excessive GH produces insulin resistance at a site distal to the insulin binding site by modifying one or several intracellular processes involved in insulin action.[43–49]

The regulation of GH secretion is complex. The hypothalamus acts predominantly in a stimulatory fashion on GH secretion, while destruction of the hypothalamus in humans leads to GH deficiency. When measuring GH levels throughout the day and night, there is a variation in plasma GH concentrations in humans and dogs. The profile of the secretion bursts of GH and their nonsuppressibility by potential metabolic regulators of growth hormone secretion suggest that the diurnal variation results from primary activation of GH secretion by neural mechanisms.

GH secretion is governed by a dual system of hypothalamic hypophysiotropic hormones, one inhibitory and the second stimulatory. The fact that many pharmacologic stimuli affect GH secretion in humans led to extensive investigations of the role of monoamines, in particular, norepinephrine, dopamine, and serotonin. Substances or situations leading to GH secretion include hypoglycemia, amino acids, peptides, monoamines (levodopa, dopamine agonists), α-adrenergic substances such as epinephrine and clonidine, serotonin precursors, and melatonin. The situation is slightly different in the dog. Hypoglycemia and amino acids are very weak and undependable stimuli of GH secretion in the dog, while dopamine or α-adrenergic substances such as clonidine are potent stimulators of GH secretion.[37, 38, 49–52] An appreciable amount of attention has been given to a long-suspected hypothalamic GH-releasing factor (GRF). Recently, a peptide with a potent intrinsic GH-releasing activity was isolated from pancreatic tumors of two patients suffering from acromegaly. These patients did not suffer from primary GH overproduction but from primary GRF overproduction. This peptide thus is called hp (human pancreatic)-GRF. In both reports the GH-releasing effects of hp-GFR were highly specific both *in vivo* and *in vitro*.[30, 32] It is highly likely that α-adrenergic substances or α-adrenergic impulses stemming from the CNS act to increase GH secretion by increasing hypothalamic GRF-secretion. These drugs do not act directly on the pituitary. Additionally, in some patients suffering from isolated GH deficiency, as diagnosed by a failure of GH to increase in response to classic stimuli (hypoglycemia, clonidine), hp-GRF can cause release of GH.[33]

In the dog, hp-GRF given intravenously at doses similar to those employed in humans leads to a dramatic increase in GH levels. The hypothalamic system inhibiting pituitary GH release is represented by somatostatin variably called GIF (GH-inhibiting factor) or SRIF (somatotropin release-inhibiting factor). In the dog, SRIF inhibits the GH surge normally provoked by L-dopa administration.[37]

Insulin-like Growth Factors

Separate lines of research, initially perceived as unrelated, have converged to form the present field of the insulin-like growth factors or somatomedins. In one series of studies, it was demonstrated that GH exerts *in vivo* growth-promoting activity but fails to do so when incubated *in vitro* with cartilage. In the presence of serum, however, cartilage was found to be highly responsive to a GH-dependent serum factor (sulfation factor) that was eventually named somatomedin.[42] A second major line of research on this subject was derived from the investigation of a serum fraction whose insulin-like activity, as assessed by glucose uptake in adipose tissue, could not be abolished by anti-insulin antibodies.[54] Five factors or groups of factors meeting the criteria of insulin-like growth factors have been found thus far: insulin-like growth factors I and II (IGF I and II), somatomedin A, somatomedin C, and multiplication-stimulating activity (MSA).[55–58] IGFs were the first to be purified and amino acid sequenced, and recently, it has been shown that somatomedin C (SM-C) is identical to IGF I.[55, 59, 60]

IGF II is probably similar to or contained in somatomedin A.[61] The principal properties of insulin-like growth factors/somatomedins include: (1) single chain, acid-soluble polypeptides of molecular weight 5000 to 10,000, (2) weak *in vitro* insulin-like activity in adipose tissue, (3) stimulation of sulfate uptake by cartilage *in vitro*, (4) stimulation of nucleic acid, protein, and glycogen synthesis in calvaria cells, (5) preferential enhancement of myoblast differentiation in chicken embryonic cells, and (6) interaction with cell surface receptors specific for somatomedins and some interaction with insulin receptors. Additionally, in contrast to other peptide hormones, IGF, like steroid, thyroid, and vitamin D hormones, is bound to a serum carrier protein. IGF I thus exhibits an unusually high plasma half-life of approximately four hours in the rat.[62–64] The primary structures of IGF I and II show striking similarity to proinsulin, suggesting that IGF I and II and proinsulin all have evolved from a common ancestral molecule (Figure 93–5).[55, 59, 65] Both IGF I and II appear to be GH-dependent. IGF I levels are high in human acromegalics and low in patients affected by hypopituitarism. The GH dependency of IGF II becomes apparent only when GH secretion falls below normal.[60, 61] The reason for this divergent regulation is not entirely clear. IGF II may well play a role in fetal life, while in adult life IGF I appears to be more important.[67]

IGF I regulation appears to be governed by multifactorial processes. For instance, both insulin and prolactin may contribute to the regulation of IGFs.[67, 70] Recent studies have shown that the peptides are synthesized

PROINSULIN / INSULIN

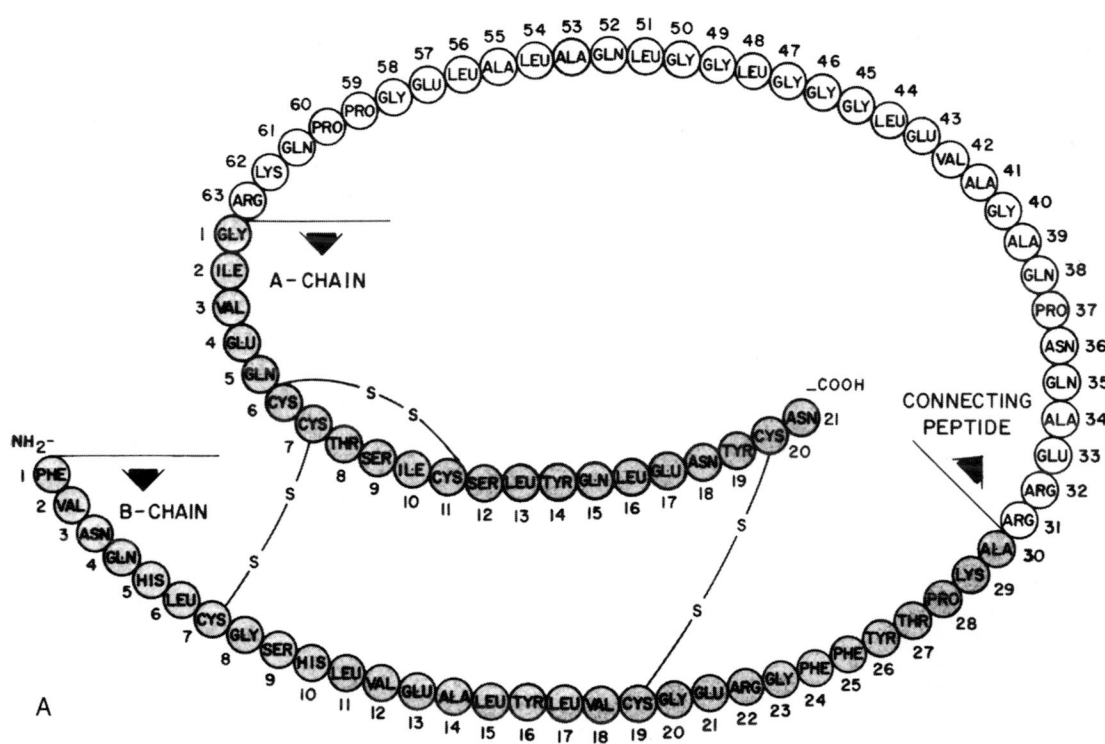

INSULIN - LIKE GROWTH
FACTOR I

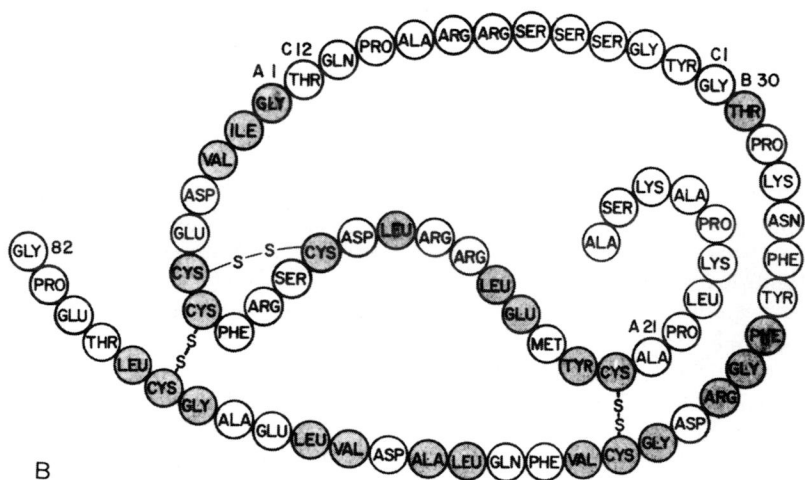

FIGURE 93–5. Bovine proinsulin/insulin *(A)* and human insulin-like growth factor *(B)*. Filled circles in *B* denote amino acid identity with insulin. Note: Both molecules exhibit three disulfide bridges.

and promptly released from the liver into the circulation under the influence of GH.[71] In conclusion, the finding that IGFs share structural homology with proinsulin and that these levels are low in some catabolic and high in some anabolic *in vivo* situations suggests an important growth-promoting role for these factors. Yet, almost all evidence gathered so far is indirect. The question as to whether GH, IGF I, or both are primarily responsible for body growth remains unclear. Although small size in GH-deficient patients is associated with low IGF I levels, no conclusion can be drawn, since both GH and IGF I are lowered. Similarly, in acromegaly both GH and IGF I levels are elevated. Some light has been shed on this problem recently; IGF I given to hypophysectomized rats by constant infusion provokes body growth similar to that obtained by GH administration.[72]

Prolactin

Prolactin is closely related to growth hormone. When the amino acid sequence of human GH is compared with that of ovine prolactin, three homologous segments comprising approximately 50 per cent of each peptide chain have been found. Therefore, it is assumed that both GH and prolactin have evolved from a common ancestral molecule by gene duplication. Also, for prolactin there is extensive interspecies similarity. The primary site of prolactin action is the breast where, in conjunction with other hormones, mammary tissue development and lactation are stimulated. Prolactin is somehow involved in normal breast development in many species, although an essential role is yet to be demonstrated.

During pregnancy, the increase in prolactin in conjunction with sex steroid hormones and in the presence of insulin results in additional breast development, leading eventually to milk formation. Prolactin specifically stimulates the synthesis of milk proteins. Continued prolactin secretion is required to maintain lactation once it has begun. Metabolic actions of prolactin in hypophysectomized animals resemble those of growth hormone, including stimulation of protein synthesis and chondroitin sulfate formation in cartilage. Stimulatory and inhibitory effects are almost entirely the same as for the regulation of GH. Additional stimuli include pregnancy, nursing, and nipple stimulation.[73–75]

Thyroid-Stimulating Hormone

Thyroid-stimulating hormone (TSH) is a glycoprotein with a molecular weight of approximately 28,500 daltons. TSH is composed of subunits termed A and B, as are the other pituitary glyco-protein hormones (LH and FSH). Within a single species, including humans, the β subunits of LH, FSH, and TSH are identical. The B subunit varies among species, providing the biologic specificity to each hormone.

The effects of TSH on the thyroid glands are largely the same as those of ACTH on the adrenal glands. TSH promotes thyroid hormone synthesis and, probably in conjunction with other serum factors, controls thyroid size. In the thyroid, TSH stimulates mRNA and protein synthesis. Chronic overstimulation by TSH leads to an increase in thyroid size (goiter).

TSH secretion is governed by two main factors, the feedback effect of thyroid hormones and central nervous system stimuli and TSH-releasing hormone. Both T_4 and T_3 are potent feedback-regulating hormones at the level of the pituitary. Thus, in the presence of low T_3 but normal T_4 concentrations, e.g., in chronic illness, TSH levels remain within normal range. T_4 appears to be efficiently and preferentially deiodinated to T_3 within the pituitary, providing evidence that T_3 is the major hormone exerting feedback inhibition on TSH secretion. The influence of TRH on TSH secretion is of modulatory nature. TSH is further influenced by glucocorticoids that suppress TSH secretion.[76–81]

Follicle-Stimulating and Luteinizing Hormone

Follicle-stimulating hormone (FSH) stimulates ovarian follicular and testicular growth and spermatogenesis. Luteinizing hormone (LH) acts to promote ovulation and luteinization of the ovarian follicle, as well as to stimulate testicular interstitial (Leydig) cell function and enhance steroid production (progesterone, testosterone) in both the ovaries and the testes. The control of secretion is complex, involving the gonadal and hypothalamic system, and there are differences between species. For detailed information, the reader is referred to textbooks of reproductive endocrinology.[82, 83]

Adrenocorticotropic Hormone

Adrenocorticotropic hormone (ACTH) is a single chain, 39 amino acid peptide. The N-terminal end, 1-24 amino acids are identical in all species thus far studied. The first 18 amino acids are required for full biologic activity. A number of related peptides share a portion of the ACTH molecule. Two of these are fragments of ACTH, α-melanocyte-stimulating hormone (α-MSH; identical to $ACTH_{1-13}$) and corticotropin-like intermediate lobe peptide (CLIP, identical to $ACTH_{18-39}$). Further, β-lipotropin (β-LPH), a 91 amino acid peptide, contains a heptapeptide that is identical to $ACTH_{4-10}$. α-MSH and CLIP are primarily found in species with a more fully developed intermediate lobe, such as sheep and dogs. β-LPH contains the structures of α-MSH and β-endorphin. It is now accepted that ACTH and other peptides are cleavage products from a common precursor glycoprotein molecule. This molecule has been variously named pro-ACTH/endorphin, procorticomelanotropin, proopiomelanocortin, and procorticolipotropin.

The primary effects of ACTH are on the adrenal cortex where the hormone stimulates the secretion of glucocorticoids, mineralocorticoids, and androgenic steroids. The effect of ACTH on mineralocorticoid synthesis is only transient. ACTH stimulates protein synthesis; a persistent ACTH oversecretion results in adrenal hypertrophy and hyperplasia.

Three major control systems contribute to ACTH

secretion: a feedback system responsive to cortisol, an inherent diurnal rhythm (humans), and a neurally mediated stimulus, commonly referred to as "stress." ACTH is secreted in a pulsatile manner and, hence, a diurnal rhythm is observed for both ACTH and cortisol secretion (humans). Cortisol exhibits a negative feedback effect at the level of the central nervous system and the pituitary. Moreover, evidence exists that cortisol exerts a negative feedback effect on corticotropin-releasing factor (CRF) via both the hypothalamus and extrahypothalamic sites.[84–89]

Measurement of Pituitary Hormones in the Dog

Plasma concentrations of most pituitary hormones can be reliably assessed by radioimmunoassay (RIA) techniques. Hormones that can be measured include GH, ACTH, FSH, LH, and prolactin. An RIA for canine TSH has recently been reported.[52, 90–93]

Hypopituitarism

Primary hypopituitarism is referred to as a condition in which the disease process that gives rise to hypopituitarism is located in the pituitary (congenital defects, tumors, inflammatory processes) (Table 93–1). Secondary hypopituitarism results from either hypothalamic deficiency or from drugs (T_4, glucocorticoids). Hypopituitarism is characterized by a failure of a single (monotropic failure), several (multitropic failure), or all pituitary hormones. The latter is also referred to as panhypopituitarism or, in adult humans, Simmond's disease.[94] Pituitary failure leads to an impaired production of target gland hormones such as T_4, T_3, corticosteroids, and sex steroids. As a result, the same signs may appear as those observed in primary target gland deficiency (Table 93–2). In adult humans, panhypopituitarism is associated with clinical signs and symptoms such as changes in menstruation, loss of libido, inability to lactate, loss of pubic hair growth, hypoglycemia, intolerance to cold, adynamia, oliguria, and somnolence. Diabetes insipidus may occur temporarily. Hypopituitarism is encountered in adulthood or childhood; in the latter instance, it causes dwarfism. In humans, the incidence of panhypopituitarism in adulthood is very low (1 in 10,000).

TABLE 93–1. CAUSES OF HYPOPITUITARISM

Hypothalamic/Pituitary Causes
  Congenital
  Traumatic
  Degenerative
  Inflammatory
  Vascular
  Neoplastic
Functional Causes
  Systemic disease
  Thyroid/adrenal disorders
  Administration of thyroid hormones, glucocorticoids
  Neuropharmacological medication
Extrasellar structural causes
  Space-occupying lesions

TABLE 93–2. CLINICAL SIGNS OF HYPOPITUITARISM

Hormone Deficiency	Manifestations During Puppyhood	Manifestations During Adulthood
GH	Short stature, hair loss	Hair loss
TSH	Signs of hypothyroidism	Signs of hypothyroidism
ACTH	Adrenal atrophy: Signs of glucocorticoid withdrawal (e.g., weakness, hypotension)	
Gonadotropins	Failure of sexual maturation	Loss of libido, testicular atrophy, absence of estrus
Prolactin	None	Failure of lactation possible

Pituitary failure may be due to processes directly impairing the hypothalamic-pituitary system (that is, congenital, traumatic, functional inflammatory, vascular, degenerative and neoplastic factors, functional impairment by drugs, and excessive autonomous secretion of peripheral hormones [T_4/T_3] and corticosteroids) or to structural diseases that are anatomically separate from the hypothalamic-pituitary region (that is, space occupying lesions, aneurysms, and meningiomas).[95]

Hypopituitarism in German Shepherds

Dwarfism is a condition characterized by short stature. Short stature may have a hereditary cause, as occurs in some dog breeds or in certain human families, or may be caused during intrauterine or postnatal life by pathologic processes that prevent the full development of the genetically determined growth potential. Only the latter condition is called dwarfism. Besides short stature, other striking clinical signs of pituitary dwarfism in German shepherds include hyperpigmentation and fragility of the skin, deficiency of primary (guard) hairs, retention of puppy-hair coat, and partial or total alopecia. Alopecia, if not present at the time of presentation, is likely to develop and to eventually affect the entire body except the head.

The growth rate usually diminishes a few weeks after birth. Growth plates may be open or closed. The dogs appear alert and playful. Owners seem more concerned about the skin condition than about the dog's size (Figure 93–6).

Pedigree analysis in dogs suggests that the disease has a genetic background. It appears that the condition is inherited through an autosomal recessive trait.

GH deficiency is a primary endocrine abnormality. There is no GH secretion in response to either clonidine or xylazine administration (Table 93–3). Equally, the mean insulin-like growth factor I (IGF I) concentration is very low (280 ± 23 ng/ml in normals and 11 ± 2 ng/ml in dwarfs). In affected animals, T_4 levels are only slightly subnormal, and there is an increase in these levels in response to TSH administration. The mean plasma cortisol concentration is normal, and there is a distinct increase in cortisol after ACTH administration.

In most of the dwarfs reported in the literature, a colloid-filled cyst has been found in the pituitary region

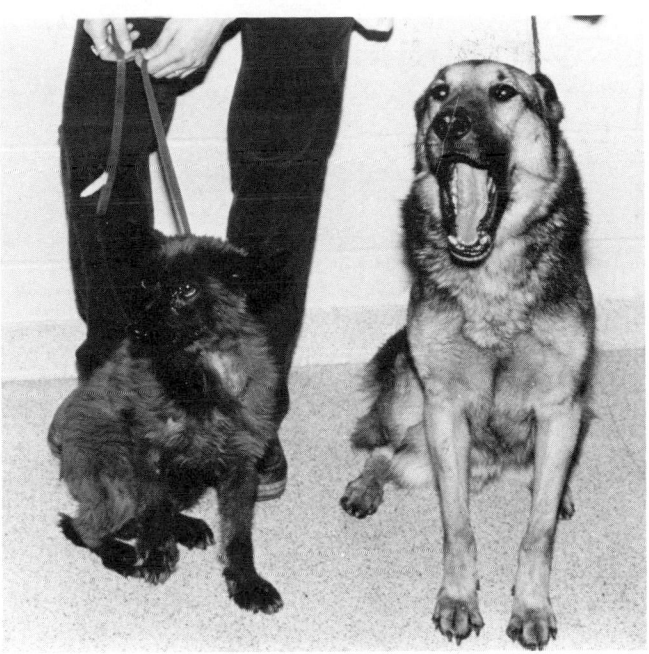

FIGURE 93–6. German shepherd with pituitary dwarfism and normal German shepherd. (From Eigenmann, JE, et al.: Growth hormone and insulin-like growth factor in German shepherd dwarf dogs. Acta Endocrinol 105:289, 1984.)

(Figure 93–7). Most authors suggest that the fluid-filled cyst induces pituitary hypofunction by exerting pressure on the surrounding tissues. Although attractive, this hypothesis is questionable because many normal adult dogs have pituitary cysts (up to 7 per cent in mongrels). Because of the continued secretion of colloid, these cysts may enlarge progressively. An attractive hypothesis would be that cells of the anterior hypophysis fail to differentiate into normal tropic hormone-secreting cells. These cells may secrete osmotically active proteinaceous material into the cleft. Analysis of cystic fluid obtained from rats has shown that the osmotically active protein-aceous material could attract water and thereby contribute to the growth of the cyst.

Capen has presented evidence that dwarfism in German shepherds is usually associated with a failure of the oropharyngeal ectoderm of Rathke's pouch to differentiate into tropic hormone-secreting cells of the pars distalis.[7] This may result in progressively enlarging, multiloculated cysts in the sella turcica and an absence of the adenohypophysis. The cysts are lined by pseudostratified, often ciliated, columnar epithelium with interspersed mucin-secreting goblet cells. The mucin-filled cysts eventually occupy the entire pituitary area in the sella turcica and severely compress the pars nervosa

and infundibular stalk. Permanent dentition is delayed or completely absent. Closure of epiphysis may be appreciably delayed. There are few trabeculae in the primary and secondary spongiosa of the metaphysis of long bones, and osteoblasts are decreased in dwarf pups, as compared with normal littermates. Cutaneous lesions include hyperkeratosis, follicular keratosis, hyperpigmentation, a loss of elastin fibers, and the loose network of collagen fibers in the dermis. Hair shafts are absent, and hair follicles are primarily in the telogen (resting) phase of the growth cycle.

Dwarfism also occurs in the Carelian bear dog. However, no endocrine studies are available characterizing the condition.[96–103]

Growth Hormone Deficiency in the Mature Dog

Congenital GH deficiency may be idiopathic (sporadic, familial) or caused by malformation of the central nervous system. Acquired GH deficiency may be idiopathic or caused by tumors, trauma, irradiation, or medication. In adult humans, GH deficiency occurs as a result of insults including postpartum pituitary necrosis (Sheehan's syndrome), pituitary tumors, irradiation, infiltrative diseases, infectious diseases, or as a result of underlying metabolic disorders (chronic renal failure, diabetes mellitus). However, adult onset disorders in general are characterized by failure of several pituitary hormones. It has been proposed that GH failure is the most common adult endocrine pituitary disorder, secondary to chromophobe adenoma. GH deficiency may result from either a primary hypothalamic or a primary pituitary defect. Pituitary GH deficiency is either isolated or occurs in conjunction with failure of other pituitary hormones.

Dogs affected by the disorder are presented with the complaint of moderate to severe skin changes. Depending upon the severity of the disorder, the skin is marked by sparse or absent hair of thin diameter and by hyperpigmentation. Hair loss and hyperpigmentation are most pronounced over the trunk. Skin changes do not involve the head and affect the legs to a lesser extent than the trunk (Figure 93–8). In one study, the mean age of presentation was five years. However, hair loss and other skin changes appear to start at an earlier age. There is no sex predilection for the disease. Routine laboratory examination is unremarkable in all cases.

Routine endocrine studies are normal including basal T_4 or T_4 in response to TSH administration and basal plasma cortisol in response to dexamethasone or ACTH

TABLE 93–3. PLASMA GH (NG/ML) BEFORE AND IN RESPONSE TO CLONIDINE ADMINISTRATION IN GERMAN SHEPHERDS

	Minutes After Clonidine Administration					
	0	*15*	*30*	*45*	*60*	*90*
Dwarfs (n = 9) Mean ± SEM	0.48 ± 0.09	0.46 ± 0.05	0.56 ± 0.09	0.47 ± 0.05	0.49 ± 0.07	0.56 ± 0.09
Normal dogs	1.5 ± 9.6	29.6 ± 9.6	44.4 ± 13.9	16.5 ± 4.9	10.3 ± 2.9	6.0 ± 2.7

From Eigenmann, JE and Eigenmann, RY: Influence of medroxyprogesterone acetate (Provera) and plasma growth hormone levels and on carbohydrate metabolism. II. Studies in the ovariohysterectomized, oestradiol-primed bitch. Acta Endocrinol (Copenh) 98:603, 1981.

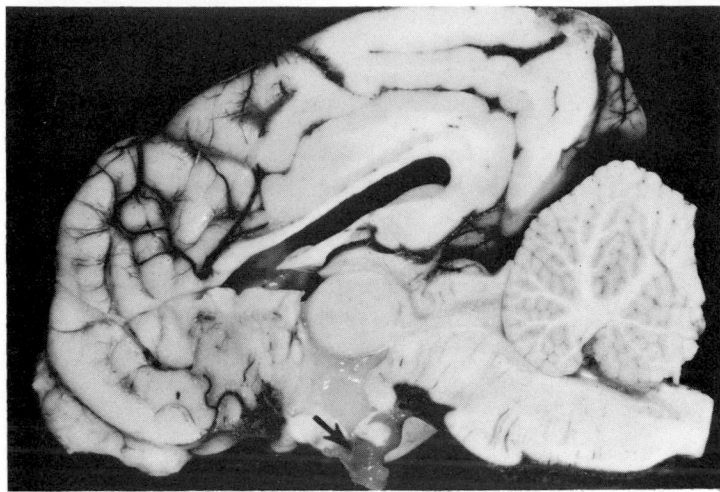

FIGURE 93–7. Panhypopituitarism in a dog associated with failure of the embryonic oropharyngeal epithelium of Rathke's pouch to differentiate into secretory cells of the adenohypophysis. Longitudinal section of the pituitary region and brain to illustrate the large multiloculated cyst. The pars nervosa was formed normally but was compressed by the mucin-filled cyst.

administration, indicating normal thyroid and normal pituitary/adrenal function.

Growth hormone secretory capacity, assessed by plasma GH measurements during clonidine or xylazine stimulation, are subnormal. In some animals, GH cannot be detected at all. In some animals there is a slight increase in plasma GH after stimulation; in others, the increase is more pronounced (Figure 93–9). The latter finding as well as the fact that the animals are not short in stature indicate that GH deficiency developed during adulthood.

Routine histologic examination of skin biopsies reveals a decreased number of elastin fibers. The condition occurs in breeds such as the Pomeranian, poodle, terrier, Lhasa apso, chow chow, and keeshond. Other breeds may be involved in the disorder. The underlying defect resulting in GH deficiency remains unknown.

Necropsy studies are not available. It remains unknown whether GH deficiency is of primary pituitary or primary hypothalamic origin. Moreover, it is unknown whether the condition has a familial background.[104–110]

Hypopituitarism Caused by Pituitary Tumors

Hypopituitarism in adult dogs caused by pituitary tumors and documented by hormonal studies has been

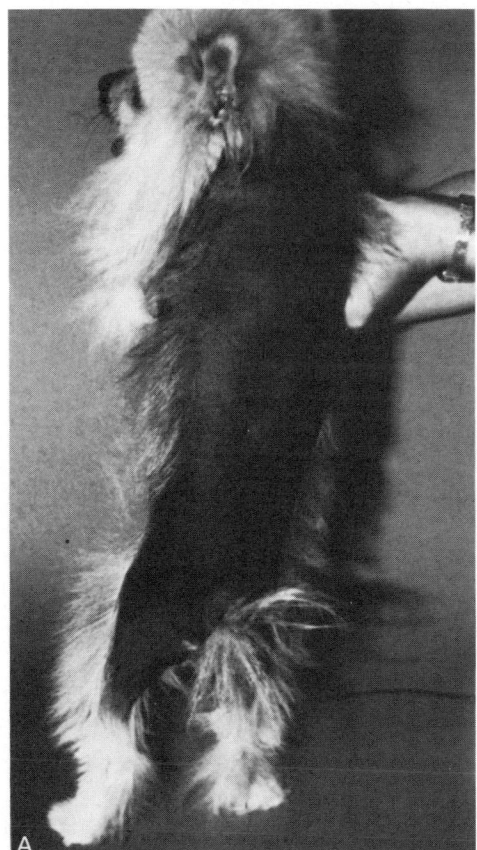

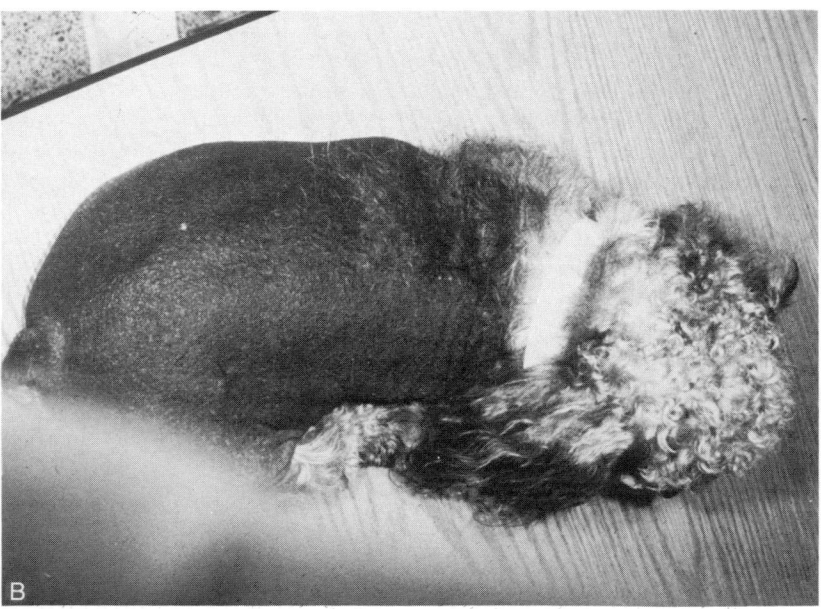

FIGURE 93–8. Growth hormone deficiency in two mature dogs. Note alopecia and hyperpigmentation. (From Eigenmann, JE and Patterson, DF: Growth hormone deficiency in the mature dog. JAAHA 20:741, 1984.)

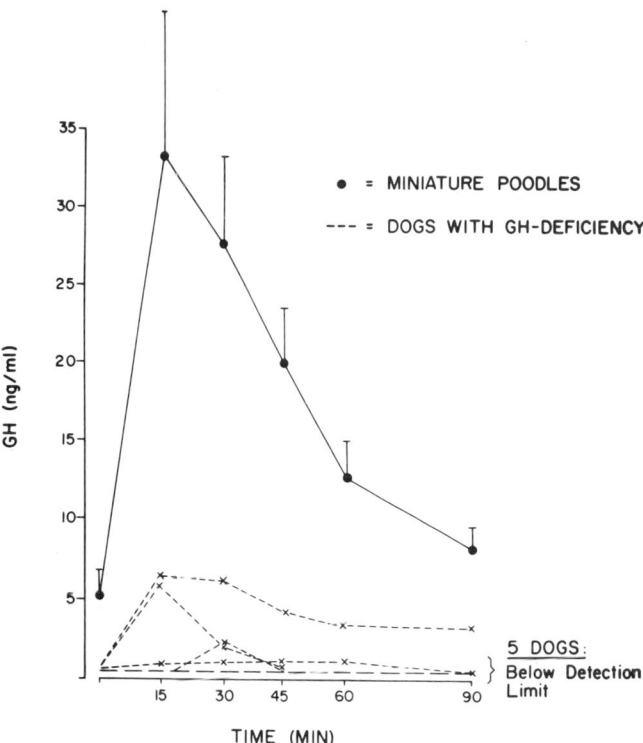

FIGURE 93–9. Growth hormone secretory capacity in miniature poodles and dogs with growth hormone deficiency.

reported infrequently. Most of the diagnoses are based on clinical and pathologic findings.

Endocrinologically Inactive Chromophobe Adenoma Arising in the Pars Distalis

Nonfunctional pituitary tumors occur frequently in dogs, cats, and horses but are uncommon in other species. There is no apparent breed or sex predisposition. Chromophobe adenomas by virtue of their space-occupying nature may lead to significant pituitary impairment. Dogs may be presented with neurologic signs or signs of hypopituitarism.

In long-standing cases there may be evidence of blindness, with dilated and fixed pupils owing to compression and disruption of optic nerves by extension of the tumor. Affected dogs also may have progressive weight loss. The gonads may become atrophied. Polyuria and polydipsia may eventually develop. Disturbance of water balance is the result of interference with the synthesis of antidiuretic hormone in the supraoptic nucleus or release of the hormone into capillaries of the pars nervosa. The posterior lobe, infundibular stalk, and hypothalamus are compressed or disrupted by neoplastic cells.

Pituitary adenomas usually reach considerable size before they cause obvious signs or kill the animal. There is usually no evidence of erosion of the sphenoid bone, and because of an incomplete diaphragma sellae, there is dorsal expansion (Figure 93–10). The cells comprising nonfunctional pituitary adenomas are cuboidal to polyhedral and are either arranged in diffuse sheets or subdivided into small packets by fine connective tissue septa.

The histogenesis of nonfunctional chromophobe adenomas in dogs is uncertain, but the adenomas appear to be derived from pituitary cells.[7, 111]

Functional Corticotropic Adenoma of the Adenohypophysis Associated with Hypercortisolism

Depending upon the author, pituitary Cushing's disease is reported to be associated with a pituitary tumor in as few as 20 per cent or in as many as 84 per cent of the cases. This rather striking difference in the frequency of pituitary tumors remains unexplained. It is possible that the high frequency observed in one of the studies is the result of more refined sectioning techniques and a more conscientious search for tumors. The pituitary tumors of animals suffering from Cushing's disease may stem from the pars distalis or, in contrast to many other species, from the pars intermedia. It appears that dogs have an unusual number of pars intermedia cells capable of producing ACTH, thereby explaining why canine Cushing's disease can be caused by tumors of the pars intermedia (up to 20 per cent). Most commonly, the tumors are microadenomas. They are rarely malignant. Some pituitary tumors are basophilic but most are chromophobic (Figure 93–11).

Although pituitary ACTH-producing tumors (at least initially) do not lead to hypopituitarism, eventually they may. Nelson's syndrome, that is, hypopituitarism caused by mechanical and/or functional impairment of remaining pituitary tissue by an ACTH-producing tumor, is also observed in the dog. Such tumors may actually develop preferentially in individuals treated for Cushing's disease (as a result of the administration of Lysodren or from adrenalectomy). Patients treated for Cushing's disease lack endogenous glucocorticoids.[7, 8, 19, 112–114]

In a survey on the functional morphology of spontaneous hyperplastic and neoplastic lesions in the canine pituitary gland, a frequent occurrence of chromophobe or basophil cell adenomas staining for ACTH was ob-

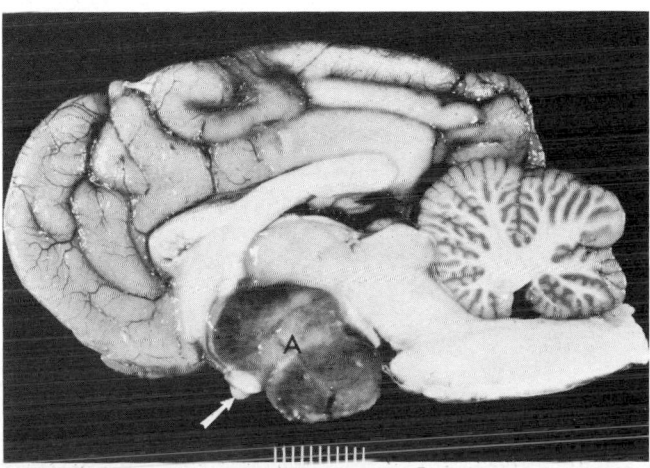

FIGURE 93–10. Large pituitary adenoma (A) in a dog extending dorsally out of the sella turcica into the overlying brain. The optic chiasm (white arrow) is severely compressed by the large adenoma. The adenohypophysis, neurohypophysis, and hypothalamus are incorporated and destroyed by the neoplasm, resulting in clinical disturbances of panhypopituitarism and diabetes insipidus.

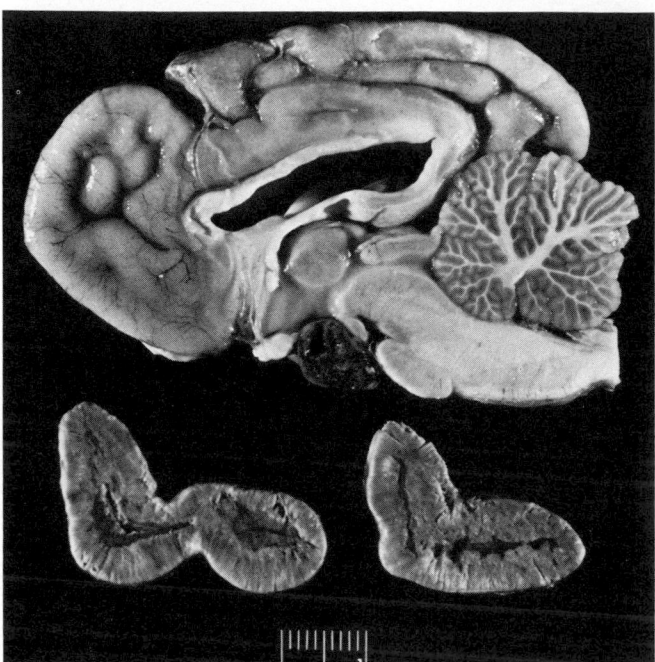

FIGURE 93–11. ACTH-secreting chromophobe adenoma in the pituitary gland from a dog with bilateral adrenal hyperplasia. Scale = 1 cm.

served, while neoplasms from granulated acidophils were not seen.[115, 116] Other pathology reports highlight the fact that ACTH-producing tumors are indeed the most frequent pituitary tumors in the canine.[7, 117] This high frequency of ACTH-producing tumors is striking, but perhaps it is in agreement with the frequency by which spontaneous Cushing's disease is observed in the dog. While in humans the frequency is about 1/1000 (hospital population), the frequency in the dog is about 1/100. This striking difference between humans and dogs remains unexplained.

Craniopharyngioma

Fröhlich's syndrome (dystrophia adiposogenitalis) has been reported in a number of dogs. This syndrome is caused by a craniopharyngioma, which alters pituitary function primarily by mechanical/functional impairment of the hypothalamus and by failure of hypophysiotropic hormones. Equally, obesity associated with Fröhlich's syndrome is a result of hypothalamic impairment. Diabetes insipidus is commonly found. Common endocrine changes in humans include failure of growth hormone and gonadotropin secretion. TSH and ACTH failures occur less often. In the dog with a craniopharyngioma, clinical and pathologic findings similar to those in humans are seen. Endocrine function studies are uncommonly reported.

Panhypopituitarism (growth hormone failure, secondary hypothyroidism/hypoadrenocorticism) associated with diabetes insipidus was described in an adult dog (Figure 93–12). This dog had a pure suprasellar tumor, possibly a craniopharyngioma (Figures 93–13 and 93–14).

Secondary hypoadrenocorticism generally does not lead to clinical signs. Electrolyte disturbances, such as

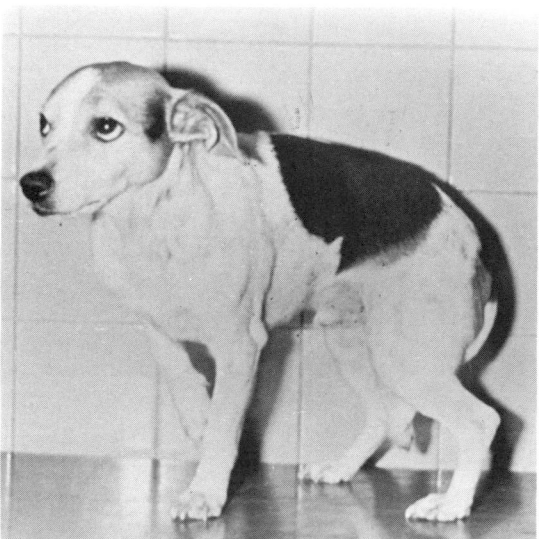

FIGURE 93–12. Dog with a suprasellar tumor (craniopharyngioma). Note weight loss. (From Eigenmann, JE, et al.: Panhypopituitarism caused by a supracellar tumor in a dog. JAAHA 19:377, 1983.)

changes in serum sodium concentration, may actually be caused by hypothalamic derangement. Physiologically, the thirst center, located in the hypothalamus, is controlled by osmoreceptor cells located in the anterior (cranial) hypothalamus.

Alterations in structural and/or functional integrity of osmoreceptors may give rise to adipsia or exaggerated drinking behavior.

This may or may not be associated with impaired antidiuretic hormone (ADH) secretion. At any rate, appreciable changes in hydration status may induce hypernatremia, as in ADH deficiency and/or adipsia, or hyponatremia as in the case of overdrinking.[118–120]

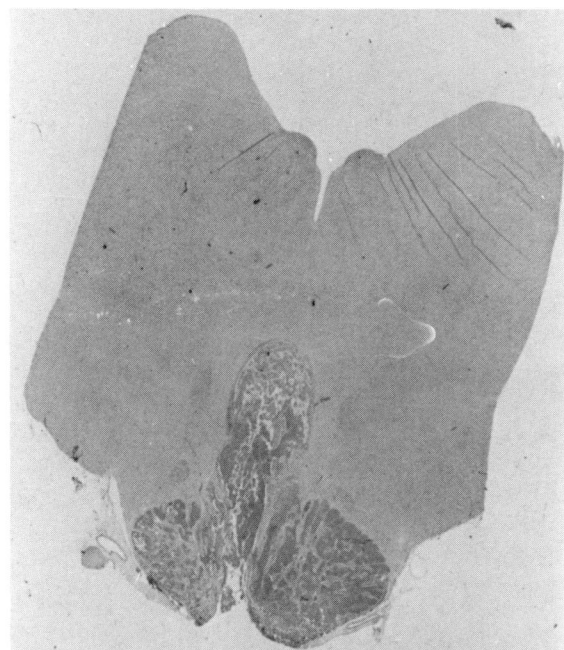

FIGURE 93–13. Photomicrograph, sagittal section through hypothalamic area (5 ×). Note symmetric tumor, invasion of surrounding brain tissue, invasion of third ventricle, no visible pituitary gland. (From Eigenmann, JE, et al.: Panhypopituitarism caused by a supracellar tumor in a dog. JAAHA 19:377, 1983.)

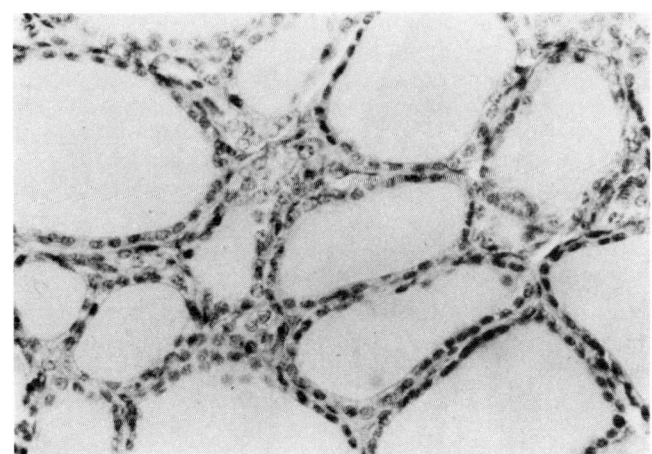

FIGURE 93–14. Section through thyroid of the same dog as in Figure 93–13. Note flat epithelium.

Pars Intermedia Adenoma

Adenomas derived from the pars intermedia of the posterior lobe of the pituitary occur in nonbrachycephalic breeds of dogs and are not often functionally active. If, in the case of a large pituitary neoplasm, diabetes insipidus occurs, then this is the result of expansion up into the third ventricle and a result of lesions of the supraoptico-hypophyseal system. Ultrastructural studies in such dogs demonstrate compression of neurons within the supraoptic nucleus by slow expansion of the neoplasm (Figure 93–15).[98]

DIAGNOSIS OF HYPOPITUITARISM

The diagnosis of hypopituitarism must be based on the measurement of pituitary hormones, for example, GH. In normal individuals, resting plasma GH may be low or even below the assay's limit of detection. A conclusive diagnosis must be based on plasma GH measurements during a provocation test. Clonidine (14 μg/lb IV or 30 μg/kg IV), an effective antihypertensive drug with intrinsic α-adrenergic activity, has been found to be a reliable stimulus for this purpose. Xylazine (Rompun) can be used as well (45 μg/lb IV or 100 μg/kg IV).[52] There are other means for the direct assessment of pituitary integrity. Measurements of canine plasma

prolactin, FSH, LH, or GH are performed in very few laboratories.

Indirect assessment can be performed by stimulation of pituitary hormone secretion and by subsequent estimation of plasma concentration of target gland hormones such as T₄ and cortisol. Indirect tests should be preceded by tests with pituitary hormones such as ACTH and TSH to assess the responsiveness of target glands.[119]

Secondary hypothyroidism is characterized by subnormal T_4 levels, but in contrast to primary hypothyroidism, T_4 increases in response to TSH administration. Multiple TSH administration may be necessary.

Assessment of adrenal function is performed by ACTH testing. In secondary hypoadrenocorticism, basal cortisol levels are usually low, but there is a distinct increase in cortisol levels in response to ACTH. Indirect testing of pituitary ACTH secretory capacity can be performed by administering lysine-vasopressin (LVP), a drug with intrinsic ACTH-releasing activity. Cortisol is measured before LVP injection and at multiple intervals after LVP injection.[119] Absent or subnormal response supports the possibility of impaired ACTH secretion. ADH secretory capacity is best evaluated by the modified water deprivation test.

Computed tomography is becoming more readily available and is invaluable in the diagnosis of pituitary tumors.

PITUITARY IMPAIRMENT BY DRUGS

Certain drugs may induce hypopituitarism. For instance, administration of glucocorticoids or thyroid hormones will cause suppression of ACTH and TSH secretion, respectively. Other commonly used drugs will suppress secretion of other pituitary hormones.

In humans, glucocorticoids are known to suppress GH and TSH levels. GH suppression in canine Cushing's disease has recently been documented. It is not unusual for thyroid hormone concentrations to be low in dogs with iatrogenic or spontaneous Cushing's disease. It is conceivable that in dogs, glucocorticoids, in addition to having other effects, actually suppress TSH levels. In humans suffering from excessive glucocorticoids, TSH levels may be suppressed. Megestrol acetate (Ovaban),

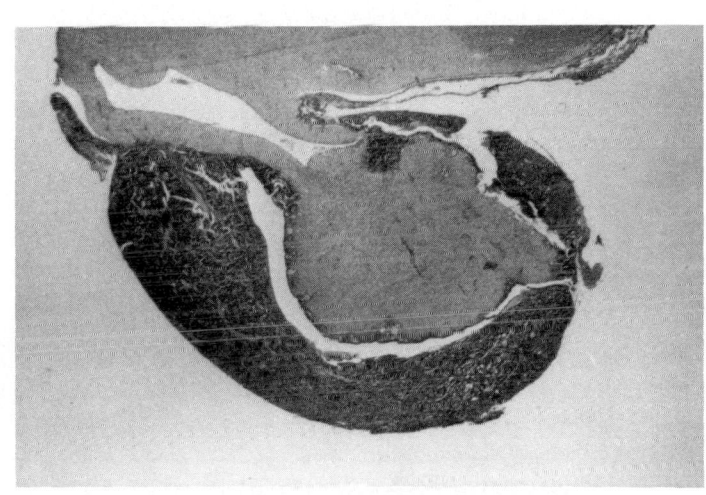

FIGURE 93–15. Pars intermedia adenoma. Note compression of pars distalis.

which is commonly used in feline practice, suppresses pituitary adrenal function probably by virtue of intrinsic glucocorticoid activity.[122-128]

Limited information is available concerning the treatment of GH deficiency in dogs. GH is difficult to obtain and is expensive. Although GH of nonprimate origin is biologically inactive in humans, human GH appears to be active in phylogenetically lower animals such as dogs. Growth hormones of nonprimate origin (e.g., canine, porcine, ovine, bovine) are immunologically interrelated and all appear to be effective for treatment.

The recommended dose of GH is 0.05 U/lb (0.1 U/kg) administered subcutaneously three times a week. Treatment should be continued for up to five weeks, at which time hair regrowth should be evident. If alopecia develops again, the GH treatment can be repeated. Some dogs may become nonresponsive or refractory to treatment, possibly because of the development of antibodies against GH, which decrease its biologic activity. In German shepherd dwarf dogs, thyroxine (10 μg/lb/day or 20 μg/kg/day) should also be given if concurrent hypothyroidism is present.

Synthetic human GH, manufactured by recombinant DNA techniques, is currently available to a limited extent. Although synthetic human GH appears to be effective for treatment of human GH-deficient disorders, long-term results are not yet available. A possible future treatment includes the use of GH-releasing factor in dogs with primary hypothalamic disease resulting in GH deficiency (Figures 93–16 and 93–17).

GROWTH HORMONE-INDUCED DIABETES MELLITUS

Diabetes mellitus (DM) is the metabolic disorder characterized by disturbances of carbohydrate, lipid, and protein metabolism. Diabetes mellitus may be either overt (frank, persistent hyperglycemia) or chemical in nature (normal or slightly elevated blood glucose concentrations accompanied by abnormal glucose tolerance). The hyperglycemia of DM results from either an absolute or a relative lack of insulin or as a defect in insulin action at the target tissues. In the latter situation,

in which there is a diminished responsiveness of tissues to the action of insulin, circulating insulin concentrations may be subnormal, normal, or even elevated. Therefore, hyperglycemia associated with diabetes mellitus is not always the result of a lack of insulin. Hyperglycemia with high levels of insulin (characteristic of an insulin-resistant state) may develop in association with other endocrine disorders (such as GH excess) and may be reversible if the underlying cause of the insulin resistance is detected and treated.

In humans, primary or idiopathic diabetes can be divided into two main types. Type I (insulin-dependent, ketosis-prone) diabetes mellitus usually occurs in young people, whereas Type II (noninsulin-dependent, non-ketosis-prone) DM occurs primarily in mature individuals and is usually associated with obesity. DM may also develop secondary to pancreatic disease or hypersecretion of hormones with actions antagonistic to those of insulin. Compared with idiopathic (Types I and II) forms of DM, however, secondary diabetes is a less common cause of human diabetes mellitus.[129]

In dogs, DM is a relatively frequent disease, but because of a lack of comprehensive endocrinologic, pathologic, immunologic, and genetic studies, data on canine DM are less complete than on humans. In an epizootiologic study of diabetes in dogs, its prevalence was estimated to range from 1:100 to 1:500 dogs presented to veterinary hospitals. The risk was found to be lowest in young dogs, with about two to three per cent of affected animals being one year of age or younger. In young animals, the risk is approximately equal for males and females, but in older dogs, females are at greater risk.[130]

Although DM similar to juvenile-onset Type I does occur, the majority of cases of DM develop in mature dogs. As opposed to mature-onset (Type II, noninsulin-dependent) diabetes of humans, however, most adult diabetic dogs require insulin therapy to survive. In addition, insulin levels (a prerequisite for categorizing cases into Type I or II diabetes) have been measured infrequently in diabetic dogs, and conflicting results have been obtained. In one study, investigators demonstrated that diabetic dogs brought to a veterinary clinic had very

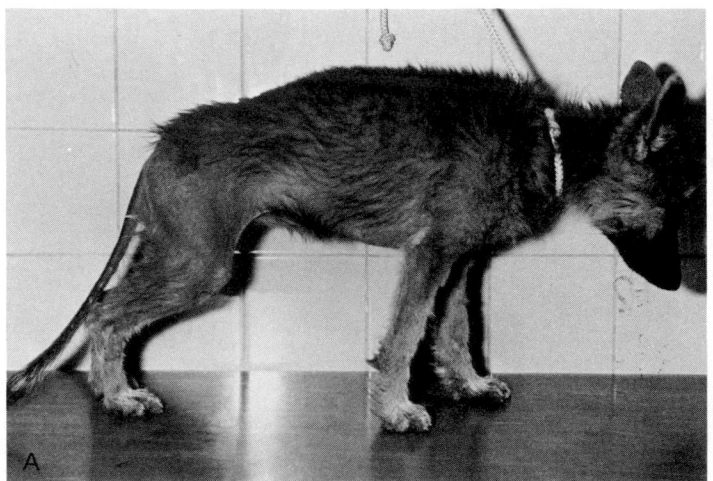
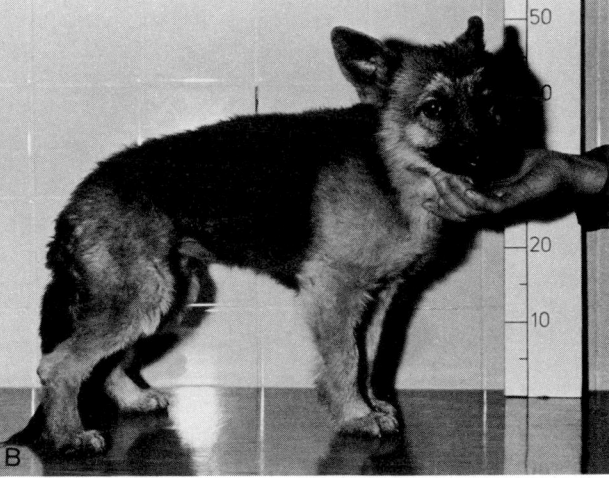

FIGURE 93–16. German shepherd before and after GH treatment. (From Eigenmann, JE, et al.: Growth hormone and insulin-like growth factor in German shepherd dwarf dogs. Acta Endocrinol 105:289, 1984.)

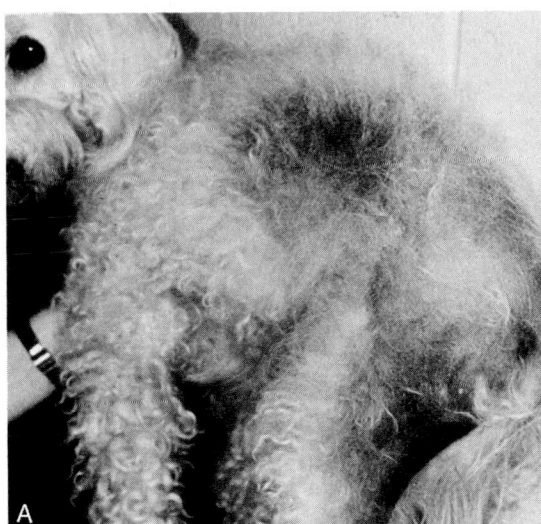
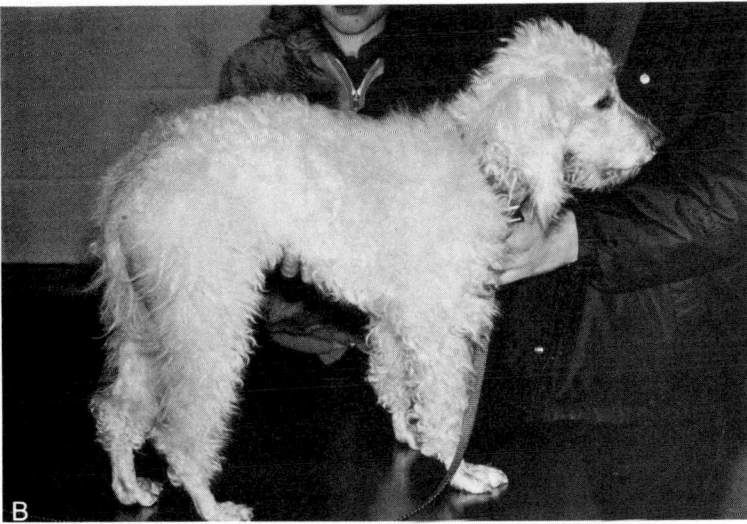

FIGURE 93-17. GH deficiency (A) in a dog and its treatment (B). (From Eigenmann, JE, et al.: Growth hormone and insulin-like growth factor in German shepherd dwarf dogs. Acta Endocrinol 105:289, 1984.)

low circulating insulin levels, suggesting that canine DM generally is associated with hypoinsulinemia, similar to human Type I DM. In another study, dogs with diabetes were classified into several groups by measuring the insulin response to a glucose load. These investigators showed that insulin levels in diabetic dogs may be low, normal, or elevated. They also attempted to compare dogs having undetectable insulin levels with humans affected by Type I diabetes, and dogs having normal or elevated insulin levels with humans affected by Type II diabetes. However, a classification based solely on plasma insulin levels seems questionable, because it provides no clues as to the pathogenesis or origin of the disorder. Moreover, regardless of the diabetes-inducing principle, insulin levels may be high, normal, or undetectable depending on the stage of the disease. For instance, if normal dogs are rendered diabetic by GH treatment, DM can be transient or permanent, depending on the duration of treatment. Insulin levels in such dogs are initially high and later become normal and eventually subnormal. If the administration of GH is stopped after a few days, the disease reverses. However, if GH therapy is continued for several days and then stopped, the disease persists and insulin levels decline steadily, despite cessation of the treatment. This process occurs over a period of several months, and affected dogs survive for months even if no insulin is given.[129]

There are few known causes of DM in mature dogs. However, it is known that several underlying disturbances can be associated with canine DM, and it is possible that secondary DM may be the most common form of the disease in mature dogs. Although it is well recognized that severe pancreatic disease can produce secondary diabetes in dogs, pancreatitis appears to be an uncommon cause of DM in this species. A more important cause of secondary diabetes in dogs, however, appears to be endogenous GH excess.

When factors precipitating DM in dogs are evaluated carefully, it becomes clear that the disease occurs frequently in aged females and is manifested during the corpus luteum phase (diestrus) of the estrous cycle, when the synthesis of progesterone is maximal.[131] This

is in keeping with the findings from epizootiologic studies that indicate that intact female dogs are at higher risk than males.[130] Thus, it appears that progesterone may induce diabetes mellitus in some dogs. However, progesterone cannot be solely responsible for the precipitation of the disease because only a minor fraction of intact females develop DM. Thus, progesterone in conjunction with a genetically determined predisposition or another progesterone-controlled diabetogenic factor must be responsible for the induction of the disease.

Despite the known relationship between the development of diabetes and the period following estrus (progesterone phase), the pathogenesis involved in the disorder has remained obscure. Recent studies of mammary tumor induction by progestagens revealed that progestagens, in addition to their tumor induction potency in some dogs, induced DM and soft tissue changes reminiscent of human acromegaly.[131] From the latter observations, the hypothesis was derived that both conditions (i.e., diabetes and acromegalic changes) could have been caused by progestagen-induced GH overproduction. This could explain why some intact female dogs develop diabetes during their progesterone phase.

GH exerts a powerful diabetogenic action, especially in carnivores (dogs, cats).[133] There is ample evidence that the diabetogenic action of GH is mainly brought about by induction of insulin resistance on insulin targets such as adipose tissue. GH appears to induce insulin resistance at a site on the insulin receptor distal to the insulin-binding site (i.e., transduction) or at one or more of the intracellular reactions important in insulin action.[134] It has been shown that GH-induced diabetes in dogs may be reversible or permanent, depending on the dose of GH administered, the duration of GH treatment, and an animal's individual response to GH. At any rate, during the early stage of treatment, circulating insulin levels increase approximately 20 fold, whereas a 90 per cent decrease in pancreatic insulin content occurs. This striking shift of pancreatic insulin toward peripheral insulin is likely to be the result of the appreciable insulin resistance GH can induce. Yet, the rate of secretion of insulin is elevated over the rate of formation of insulin,

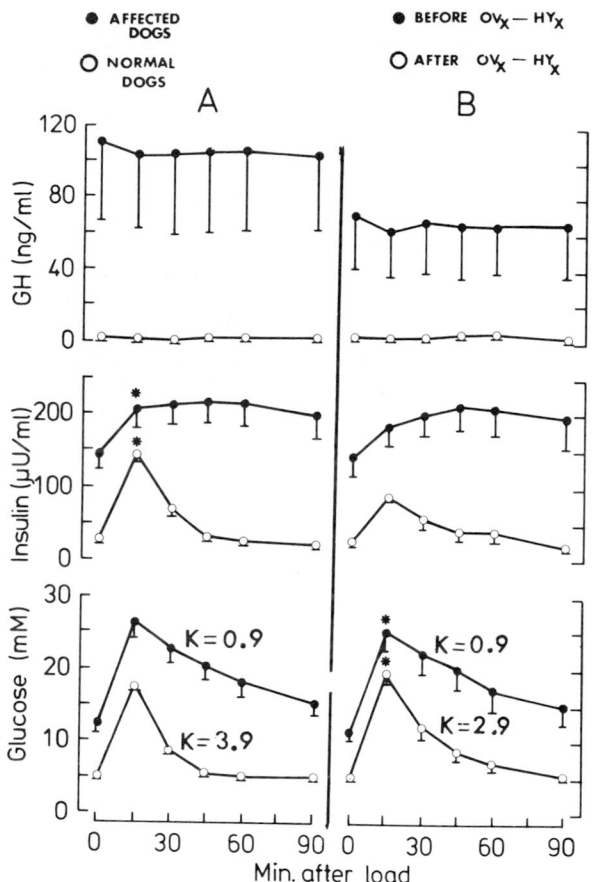

FIGURE 93–18. *Left,* Glucose, GH, and insulin levels during IVGTT in normal dogs and in affected dogs. *Right,* the same parameters before and after ovariohysterectomy. (From Eigenmann, JE and Peterson, ME: Diabetes mellitus associated with other endocrine disorders. Vet Clin North Am 14:837, 1984.)

thus explaining the final exhaustion of pancreatic B cells taking place in GH diabetes.

HISTORIC SIGNS AND LABORATORY FINDINGS IN DOGS WITH GH EXCESS

Female dogs with either glucose intolerance or frank DM were investigated to determine the relationship of progesterone or progestagen excess. Some dogs developed glucose intolerance or DM during diestrus, whereas others were affected after treatment with medroxyprogesterone acetate (MPA), an estrus-repressing agent. More than half of the dogs also showed signs of acromegaly, at least to some degree.

Laboratory findings revealed that about half of the dogs studied had frank hyperglycemia (plasma glucose concentration greater than 10 mM, or greater than 180 mg/dl), whereas the remainder had fasting basal glucose levels that ranged from 5.4 to 7.7 mM (95–140 mg/dl). In addition, despite extreme elevation of basal insulin levels, these dogs exhibited glucose intolerance during intravenous glucose tolerance testing, as well as drastic elevation of GH levels when compared with results obtained in normal dogs. Thus, as expected from the initial hypothesis, GH levels are high, and diabetes in such animals is characterized by hyperinsulinemia rather than hypoinsulinemia; this is consistent with insulin

resistance. If such animals are subjected to progestagen withdrawal and ovariohysterectomy, GH levels drop and, despite appreciably lowered insulin levels, glucose tolerance improves (Figures 93–18 and 93–19). However, DM may not disappear in some animals. The trend for development of associated acromegalic changes appears to be higher in animals with only moderate glucose intolerance, whereas dogs with frank DM do develop acromegaly less frequently.

Dogs exhibiting signs of glucose intolerance (with or without acromegaly) during a natural progesterone phase (diestrus) have progesterone levels within the normal range but have elevated GH levels. In animals developing signs during diestrus, ovariohysterectomy or a spontaneous reduction in progesterone levels is followed by a slight but inevitable drop in GH levels (Figure 93–19). In animals that develop signs after MPA administration, plasma levels of the compound at the time of presentation are usually low. GH levels in pregnant dogs that are invariably under the influence of progesterone are only occasionally elevated.

PATHOGENESIS OF GH-INDUCED GLUCOSE INTOLERANCE

The findings of hyperinsulinemia in dogs with GH excess point to insulin resistance as the factor responsible for the hyperglycemia or glucose intolerance. This is further supported by the fact that, despite elevated endogenous insulin levels, the insulin requirement of diabetic dogs with GH elevation is appreciably higher than the insulin requirement of diabetic dogs not having GH elevations. These findings are compatible with GH-induced diabetes. GH causes glucose intolerance mainly by inducing insulin resistance. In contrast to other species such as the rat, carnivores are particularly sensitive to the diabetogenic actions of GH. Administration of GH to dogs can produce a diabetic state within a matter of days which initially was characterized by hyperinsulinemia. If exposure to high GH levels persists, exhaustion of pancreatic B cells and hypoinsulinemia ensue. It is important to note that in affected dogs there is generally no correlation between the degree of GH elevation and the degree of hyperglycemia. The fact that GH is elevated in animals exhibiting diabetes during progestagen exposure but not in dogs developing diabetes independently of such exposure precludes the possibility that GH elevation may be caused by hyperglycemia or the diabetic state as such.

The fact that GH levels drop after ovariohysterectomy and progestagen withdrawal is evidence for a progestagen-GH interrelationship. Compared with dogs having high GH concentrations, most pregnant dogs have normal GH levels. This suggests that GH production in some dogs is paradoxically controlled by natural levels of progesterone.

The mechanism by which the GH axis becomes responsive to progesterone remains unknown. The disorder may be present at birth or may develop later in life. The fact that GH levels in some diabetic dogs were already elevated to an extent certainly sufficient to induce diabetes earlier in life suggests that the condition, for some unknown reason, only develops in older age.

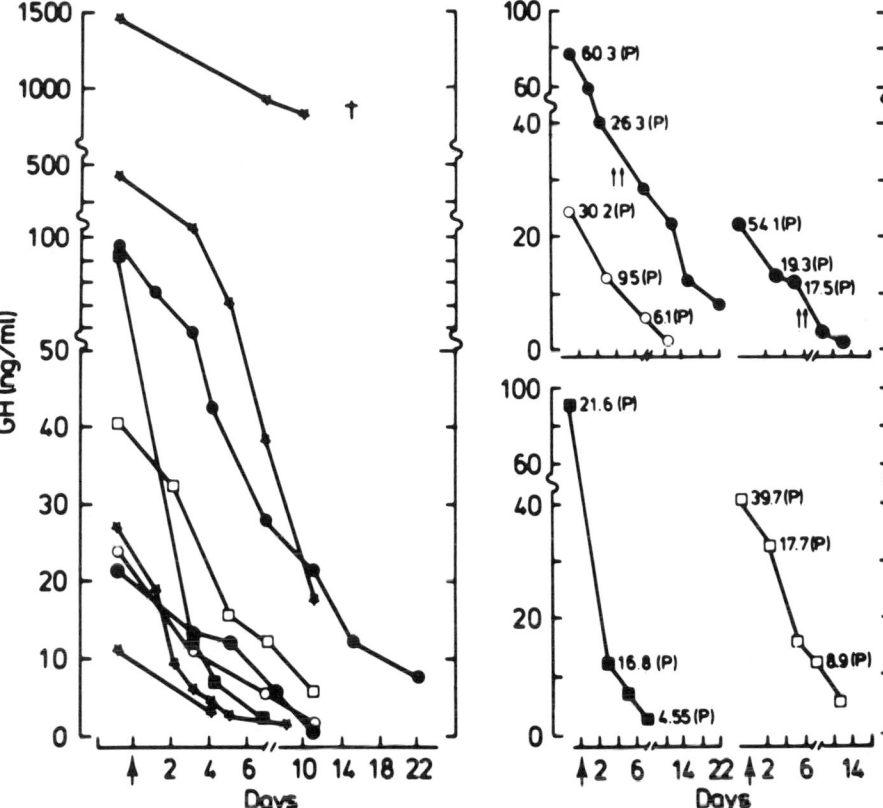

FIGURE 93–19. GH levels before and after ovariohysterectomy (left). Decline in progesterone levels (P) and simultaneous decrease in GH levels.

In this context, it is important to realize that dogs, in contrast to other species, exhibit almost identically high postestrus progesterone concentrations whether pregnant or not. Additionally, a dog's reproductive cycle does not cease in old age. Whether such lifelong exposure to "pregnancy progesterone levels" contributes to or provides the necessary environment for the development of the disorder is unknown but remains an interesting possibility.

TREATMENT

In dogs with glucose intolerance resulting from GH excess, the following diagnostic and therapeutic points are emphasized: (1) prompt recognition of hyperglycemia or impaired glucose intolerance, (2) prompt correction of hyperglycemia, and (3) performance of ovariohysterectomy or cessation of progestagen treatment or both in order to lower plasma GH levels and insulin output and preserve most of the remaining B-cell activity.

RECOGNITION OF HYPERGLYCEMIA OR GLUCOSE INTOLERANCE

In any intact female dog presenting with signs of acromegaly or diabetes (such as respiratory stridor, increased number of skin folds, increased abdominal size, fatigue, polyuria, polydipsia) either during progestagen treatment or during a natural progesterone phase, the plasma glucose level should be evaluated immediately. Testing only the urine for glucose is insufficient for the diagnosis, since a number of animals affected by the disorder may have mild elevations of fasting plasma glucose. However, because of their glucose intolerance, these animals may readily spill some glucose into the urine after food ingestion. If the fasting plasma glucose is only moderately elevated (less than 150 mg/dl), the most appropriate means of diagnosing glucose intolerance is with an intravenous glucose tolerance test. Although normal animals generally have glucose assimilation coefficient (k) values greater than three, affected animals have glucose intolerance manifested by k values of less than two. In normal dogs, plasma glucose levels should return to a preload concentration within 60 minutes of the glucose load.

OVARIOHYSTERECTOMY

It has proven practical to ovariohysterectomize affected intact females as soon as possible regardless of whether the animal has developed the disease when treated with progestagens or during a luteal phase. Even in dogs in which the chance for recovery from diabetes is minimal, ovariohysterectomy is recommended. Intact female dogs that have developed diabetes because of progesterone-induced GH excess will invariably have an increased insulin demand during the following progesterone phase. Progesterone at that time will again lead to high GH levels; the resulting resistance to insulin may develop abruptly and be extreme. It is impossible to predict the degree of insulin resistance, and the owners of such dogs are often unable to cope with the changes in insulin requirement. It is also possible that such dogs, because of insufficient insulin administration, may develop ketoacidosis. Treatment at that time may be frustrating, especially if the animal is also affected by pyometra or renal failure. The recommendation to ovariohysterectomize dogs as soon as possible, provided the animal is not ketotic, appears to be advantageous. Early ovariohysterectomy in dogs that still suffer from appreciable GH elevation leads to a rapid decrease in plasma GH elevation, which leads to a rapid decrease in plasma GH levels and thus to an amelioration of the insulin resistance. Moreover, if ovariohysterectomy is performed early, the time course for the decrease in insulin requirement becomes more predictable.

Finally, it must be emphasized that suppression of estrus (chemical ovariohysterectomy) in such animals is contraindicated. Some veterinarians believe that estrus and diestrus are somehow involved in the pathogenesis of diabetes in intact females and attempt to eliminate cycles by administering estrus-suppressing agents such as MPA. By doing this, they directly provoke the hormonal situation (e.g., progestagen-induced GH excess) that is responsible for the development and dysregulation of diabetes in such animals. The safety of testosterone derivatives such as mibolerone remains unknown. Although testosterone derivatives are C^{19} steroids, it is conceivable that by cross-reacting with progesterone receptors they may have progestagen-like activities.

INSULIN TREATMENT

A crucial question is at what blood glucose level to start insulin replacement. The question is complex and, in a clinical setting, has no straightforward answer. In general, the clinician does not have data concerning the dog's actual plasma insulin, GH, and progesterone concentrations. Even if these determinations were available, they do not always indicate the actual pancreatic insulin reserve or the degree of insulin resistance. Plasma insulin concentrations, however, should be measured whenever possible. The finding of a high plasma insulin concentration indicates that the dog has a fair chance of recovery from the diabetic state if adequately treated; in contrast, a subnormal plasma insulin level indicates that the chance of recovery is minimal. In a dog that has a fair chance for recovery, strict control of the blood glucose concentration is warranted because of its positive influence on recovery from the diabetic state.

In general, a longer duration of clinical signs lessens the chance for recovery. By questioning owners carefully, one can often learn that the dog has had similar signs during earlier progesterone phases. The frequency of episodes is likely to provide an additional negative influence on the chance of recovery from the diabetic state.

It is important to know whether the dog has developed diabetes following estrus or during progestagen medication. In dogs treated with progestagens, plasma GH concentrations can remain elevated for prolonged periods of time, thus decreasing the chance of recovery. Progestagens, probably because of their depot effect, appear to influence GH secretion more profoundly. As a rule, one should initiate insulin therapy if the fasting plasma glucose concentration is greater than 150 mg/dl in the progestagen-treated dog and when the plasma glucose level is greater than 200 mg/dl in dogs that develop diabetes during the progesterone phase.

Both GH-induced insulin resistance and the functional recovery of the residual pancreatic β cells play significant roles in determining the dog's initial and subsequent insulin requirements. Plasma GH concentrations usually normalize within a matter of days after ovariohysterectomy. However, recovery of residual β-cell function may take days to weeks. After ovariohysterectomy, it is recommended to keep such dogs in the hospital for a few days and to adjust their daily insulin requirement

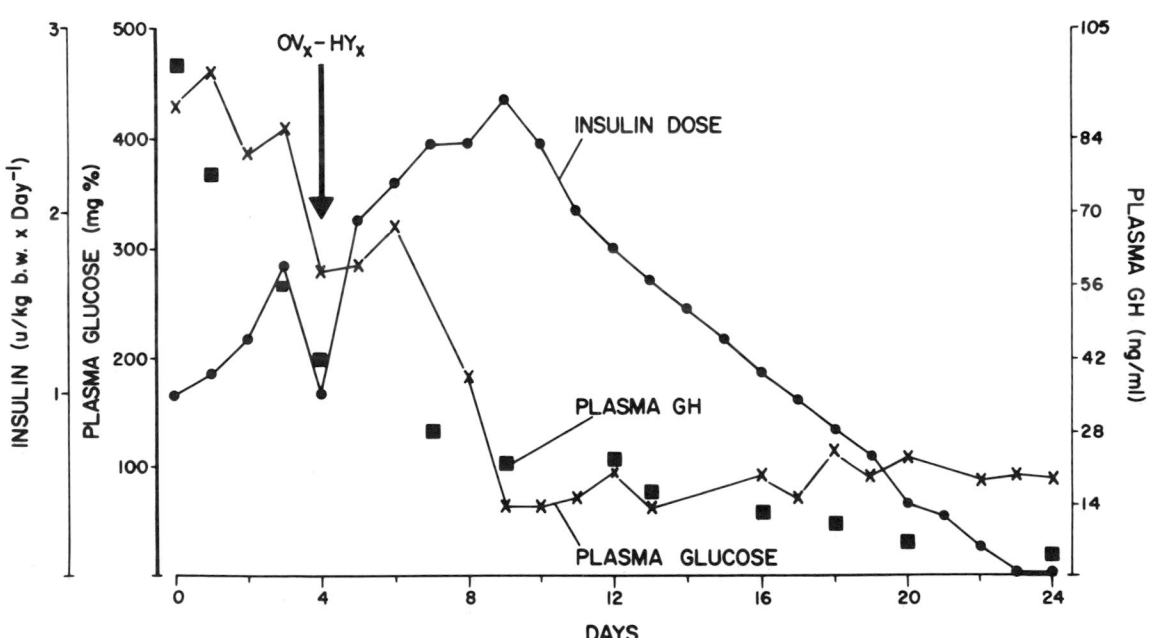

FIGURE 93–20. Plasma glucose levels, insulin dose, and plasma GH levels in a dog with spontaneous GH-diabetes. (From Eigenmann, JE and Peterson, ME: Diabetes mellitus associated with other endocrine disorders. Vet Clin North Am 14:837, 1984.)

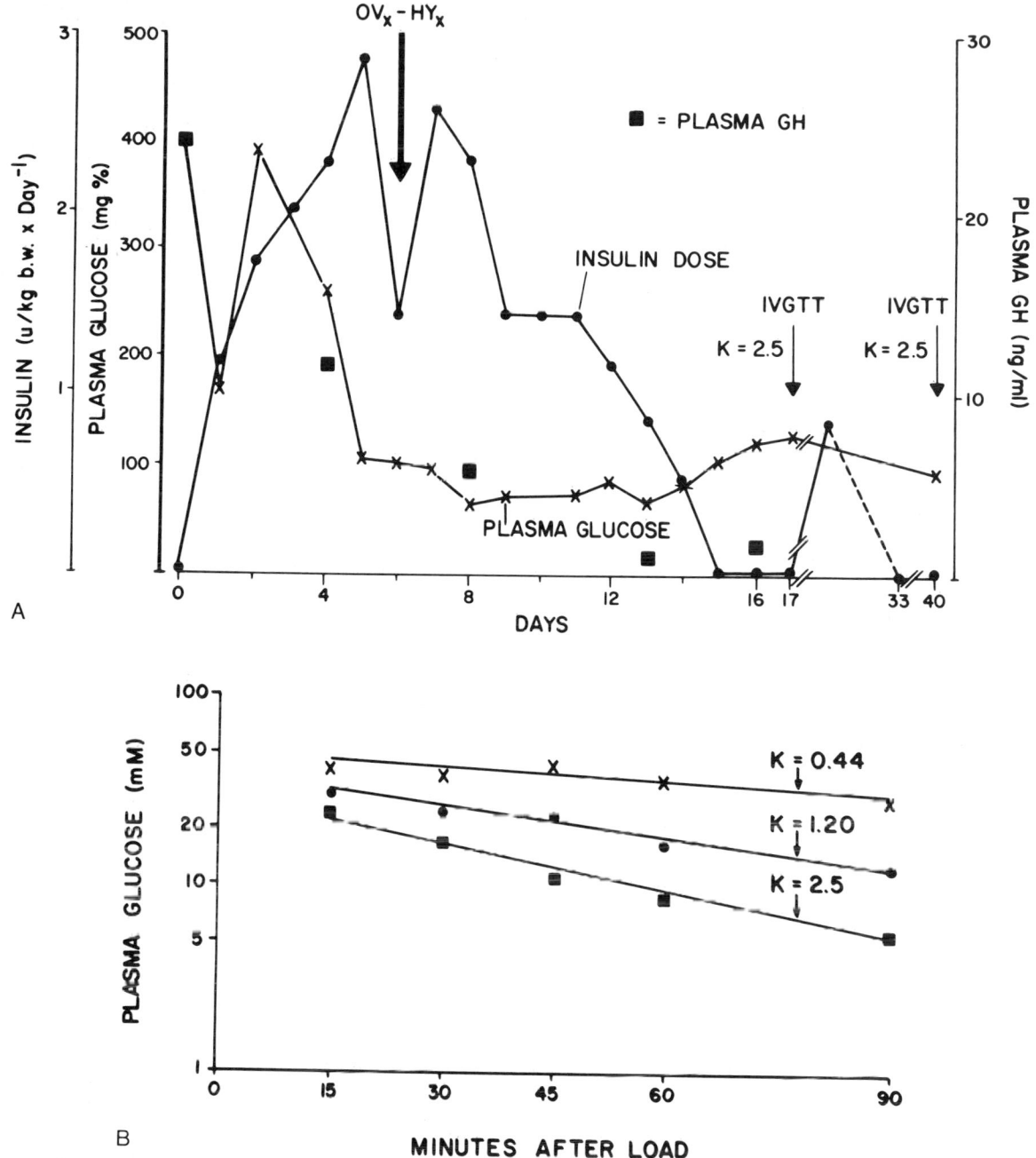

FIGURE 93-21. *A.* Plasma glucose levels, insulin dose, and plasma GH levels in a dog with spontaneous GH diabetes Note: Initial increase in insulin requirement and drop after ovariohysterectomy; drop of elevated GH levels; resting plasma glucose levels increased again after insulin withdrawal and after the dog is glucose intolerant (K = 1.2); glucose tolerance improved after the animal had been given insulin again for two weeks. *B.* Plasma glucose disappearance curves and glucose assimilation coefficient (K) in the dog shown in part A. X _____ X before treatment; O _____ O after ovariohysterectomy and insulin withdrawal when afternoon blood glucose levels had normalized; ■ _____ ■ seven days after the dog had been given insulin again for two weeks. Note: Diabetic glucose tolerance (K = 1.2) despite only slightly elevated resting blood glucose levels and negative urine glucose readings and improvement of the glucose tolerance after the dog had been given insulin again for two weeks.

by monitoring serial blood glucose concentrations. As soon as the blood glucose concentrations begin to decrease, the daily insulin dose should be decreased accordingly. In some dogs, the insulin requirement may drop to zero during the initial postoperative period. In other dogs, the daily insulin requirement may initially decrease, then plateau, and finally continue to gradually decrease over a longer period of time. Figure 93-20 illustrates the insulin adjustments before and after ovar-

iohysterectomy in a dog that developed diabetes mellitus during the progesterone phase.

If a dog does not recover from the diabetic state during its hospital stay, it is discharged and the insulin requirement is adjusted at home. Diabetic monitoring is slightly more complicated at home because blood glucose measurements cannot be easily performed. During this time, blood glucose concentrations should be evaluated at least once a week and the daily insulin dose

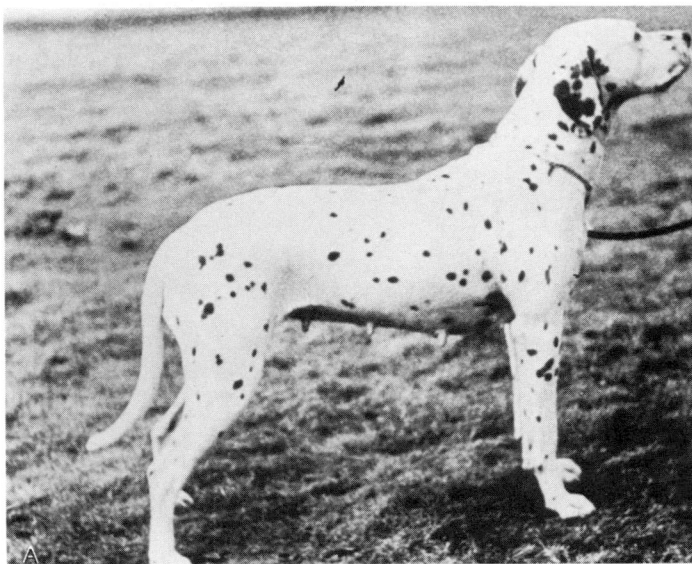
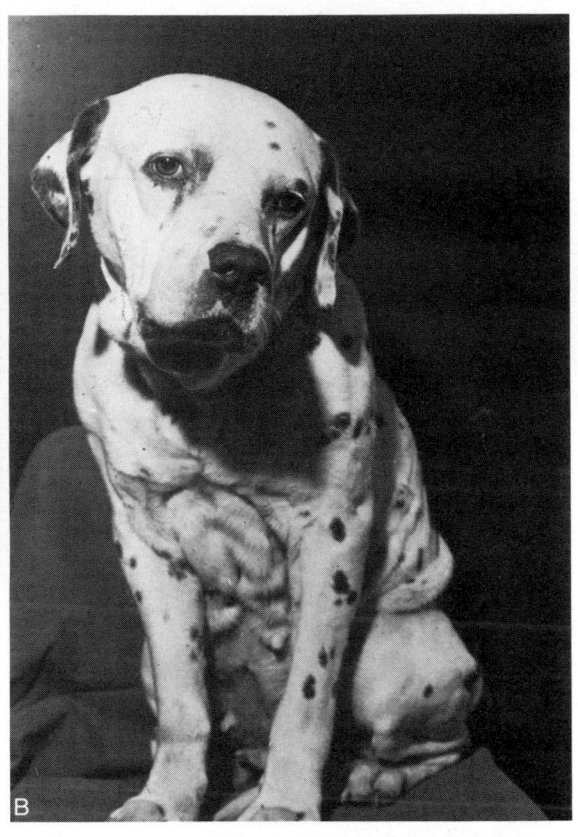

FIGURE 93–22. *A,* Dalmatian while still normal. *B,* Same dog with severe spontaneous acromegaly. (From Eigenmann, JE and Venker van Haagen, A.: Progestagen-induced and spontaneous canine acromegaly due to reversible growth hormone overproduction: clinical picture and pathogenesis. JAAHA 17:813, 1981.)

lowered if necessary. In a number of dogs, however, weekly blood glucose monitoring is insufficient, and the insulin dose has to be lowered according to clinical signs of mild hypoglycemia. Although hypoglycemia is undesirable, it is still the best biologic indicator of improving β-cell function. The owners should be advised to observe the dog closely and to take action as soon as mild signs of hypoglycemia develop. At that time, the dog must be given carbohydrates orally, and several smaller meals should be offered subsequently throughout the day. The daily insulin dosage should also be lowered the following morning. Tapering of the insulin dose should be continued until it reaches another plateau or drops to zero.

It is recommended that insulin therapy not be withdrawn simply on the basis of negative morning urine glucose concentrations. Although complete insulin withdrawal may be appropriate in some cases, there is no way to predict this possibility, since urine glucose measurements are an insensitive way of assessing glucose tolerance. Even basal plasma glucose measurements may be insensitive. After appropriate insulin treatment and ovariohysterectomy in a dog with GH-induced diabetes, the insulin dose was lowered according to afternoon blood glucose readings until it was totally discontinued. Over a period of two days off insulin treatment, the afternoon glucose started to rise again. An intravenous glucose tolerance test performed at that time revealed that the dog was still diabetic. Over the next two weeks, the dog was treated again with decreasing amounts of insulin. Another glucose tolerance test performed seven days later showed greatly improved glucose tolerance, and insulin therapy was permanently discontinued (Figure 93–21). This is compatible with the known fact that recovery of the β cells may take time

and that strict control of blood glucose levels is important if total recovery is to occur.[129, 135–137]

Acromegaly

In humans, acromegaly is a chronic endocrine disorder characterized by overgrowth of soft tissues and bony structures in adulthood. The disorder is caused by excessive GH secretion, usually resulting from a pituitary tumor or hyperplasia of pituitary acidophils. Patients suffering from the disorder exhibit profound soft tissue increases of their face, hands, and feet. Fatigue, headache, amenorrhea, loss of libido, and diabetes mellitus may also occur. There is no sex predilection in human patients.

In dogs, spontaneous acromegaly was first confirmed in 1980, although an intact female dog with clinical signs suggestive of acromegaly had previously been reported.[11] Recently, the results of high-dose, long-term toxicity studies with progestagens such as MPA have also been reported in dogs. Although these studies were primarily aimed at the elucidation of mammary gland tumor induction by these compounds, they showed that some dogs treated with progestagens developed signs of acromegaly or diabetes. Therefore, it appeared that acromegaly might occur spontaneously in female dogs during the progesterone phase (diestrus) or in dogs treated with progestagens.

HISTORIC FINDINGS AND CLINICAL SIGNS ENCOUNTERED IN CANINE ACROMEGALY

All dogs thus far diagnosed as having acromegaly have been intact females. Some of the dogs develop

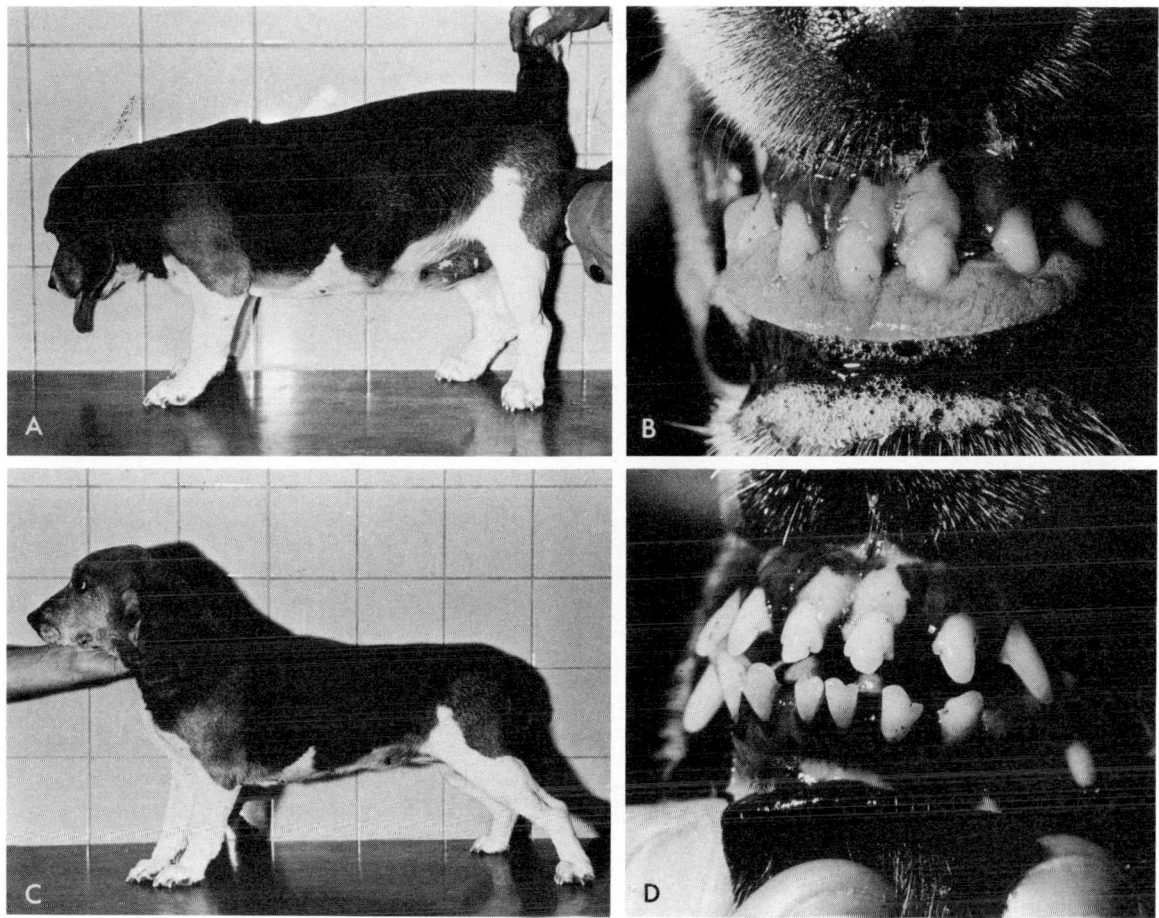

FIGURE 93–23. Severe spontaneous acromegaly (A, B). Reduction of soft tissue after treatment (C, D). (From Eigenmann, JE, et al.: Progesterone-controlled growth hormone overproduction and naturally occurring canine diabetes and acromegaly. Acta Endocrinol 104:167, 1983.)

acromegaly during MPA treatment for estrus suppression. In other dogs, acromegaly develops during diestrus (progesterone phase). In one study of 22 acromegalic dogs, clinical signs included inspiratory stridor, polydipsia and polyuria, fatigue, increased abdominal size, prominent skin folds, and mammary gland tumors (Figures 93–22 and 93–23). Respiratory stridor, a prominent sign in these dogs, occurs because of excessive soft tissue proliferation in the orolingual, pharyngeal, and laryngeal regions. On physical examination, increased interdental spaces may also be observed. Frequent abnormalities in laboratory data include elevated serum alkaline phosphatase, hyperglycemia, and a slightly lowered packed cell volume. In some dogs, the increase in soft tissue of the head, neck, and trunk is dramatic, but only subtle changes may be observed in other dogs.

Diagnosis of Acromegaly. A tentative diagnosis of acromegaly can be made based on the dog's history, clinical signs, and laboratory findings. Radiographs of the head and neck can be helpful in establishing the diagnosis. In most dogs with acromegaly, there is diffuse proliferation of the soft tissues of the orolingual, oropharyngeal, and laryngeal regions (Figure 93–24). In a dog with inspiratory stridor, it must be determined whether the respiratory distress (particularly in brachycephalic, intact female dogs) is caused by acromegaly or simply by an elongated soft palate. The comparison of

photographs taken of the dog early in life and again during the disease state has also proven particularly helpful in recognizing changes typical of acromegaly.

A conclusive diagnosis of acromegaly requires the demonstration of persistent elevations of plasma GH concentrations. Basal GH levels in acromegalic dogs vary greatly, and there is no correlation between the degree of GH elevation and the extent of acromegaly. In addition, basal GH concentrations may be elevated in conditions other than acromegaly. Therefore, to definitively diagnose acromegaly, one must demonstrate that plasma GH concentrations remain elevated during a suppression test, such as the intravenous glucose tolerance test (0.45 gm of glucose/lb body weight) (Figure 93–25). Finally, measurement of insulin-like growth factors or somatomedins may also be helpful in diagnosing canine acromegaly. Since these peptides are GH-dependent, acromegalic dogs have elevated plasma levels compared with normal animals.

Treatment. Canine acromegaly may be diagnosed in dogs under MPA treatment and in dogs under the influence of progesterone during diestrus. Since the GH elevations in acromegalic dogs are induced by progestagen exposure, treatment should include withdrawal of the progestagen and/or ovariohysterectomy. After treatment (progestagen withdrawal), circulating GH concentrations normalize and soft tissue abnormalities re-

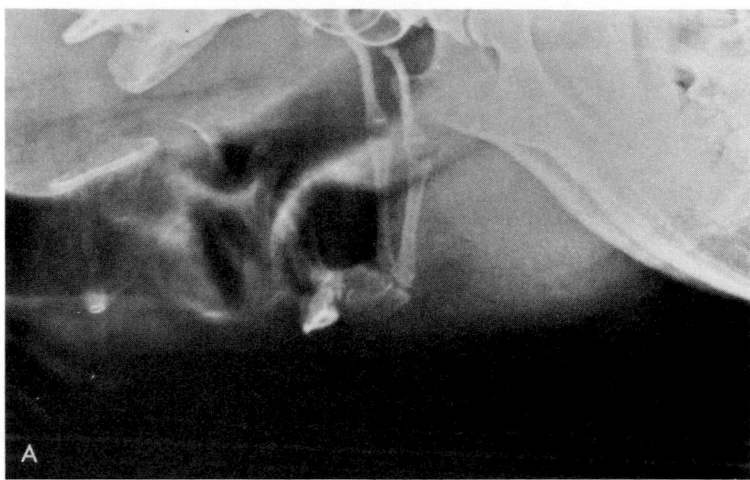

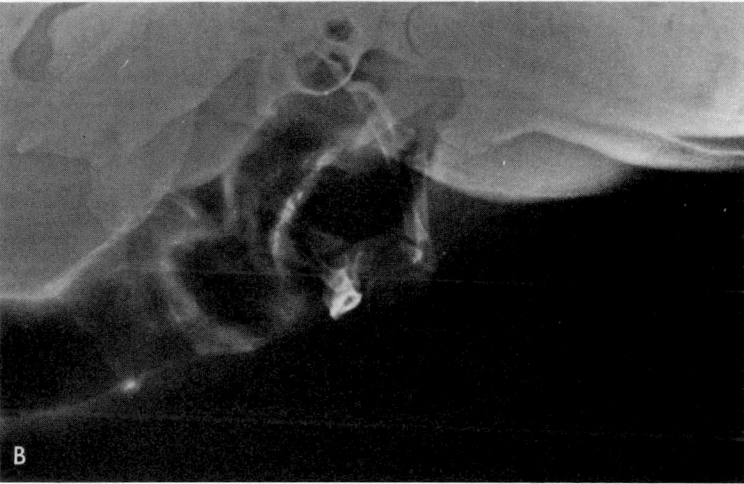

FIGURE 93–24. Lateral radiographs taken from a dog during active acromegaly (A) and after treatment (B). (From Eigenmann, JE and Venker van Haagen, A.: Progestagen-induced and spontaneous canine acromegaly due to reversible growth hormone overproduction: clinical picture and pathogenesis. JAAHA 17:813, 1981.)

solve.[12, 52, 135, 137, 138] Increased levels of growth hormone can also be induced by medroxyprogesterone acetate administration (Figure 93–26).[139, 140]

GROWTH HORMONE EXCESS IN THE FELINE

We recently studied an old, castrated, male domestic short-haired cat with insulin-resistant diabetes mellitus.

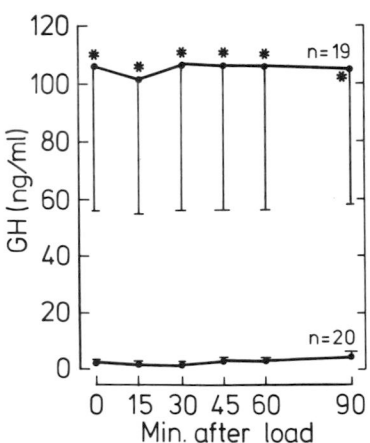

FIGURE 93–25. Plasma GH levels during an IVGTT in normal dogs (lower curve) and in acromegalic dogs (upper curve). (From Eigenmann, JE and Venker van Haagen, A.: Progestagen-induced and spontaneous canine acromegaly due to reversible growth hormone overproduction: clinical picture and pathogenesis. JAAHA 17:813, 1981.)

Despite extremely elevated levels of endogenous insulin, the cat exhibited hyperglycemia. In order to adequately control the animal's hyperglycemia, insulin (lente) doses as high as 70 U/day had to be administered. GH levels were approximately 100 times normal. In multiple samples obtained over a period of one year, GH concentration was persistently elevated. Lesions in the endocrine pancreas were compatible with GH-induced diabetes. In addition to diabetes, the cat exhibited signs of acromegaly (enlarged abdomen, prognathia inferior) (Figure 93–27). A mass in the pituitary region was diagnosed by computerized axial tomography and gamma camera imaging (Figure 93–28). A pituitary tumor was confirmed at necropsy.[141, 142]

Besides this cat, we have seen similar extreme plasma GH elevations in a few other diabetic cats with high insulin requirements. Furthermore, pathology reports support the view that GH may be involved in the development of the disease in cats. An adenoma of pituitary acidophil cells in two diabetic cats has been described.[143]

Insulin-like Growth Factor I (IGF I) in Pituitary-Hypothalamic Disease

As in humans, IGF I appears to be growth hormone (GH)-dependent in the dog.[99] IGF I decreases signifi-

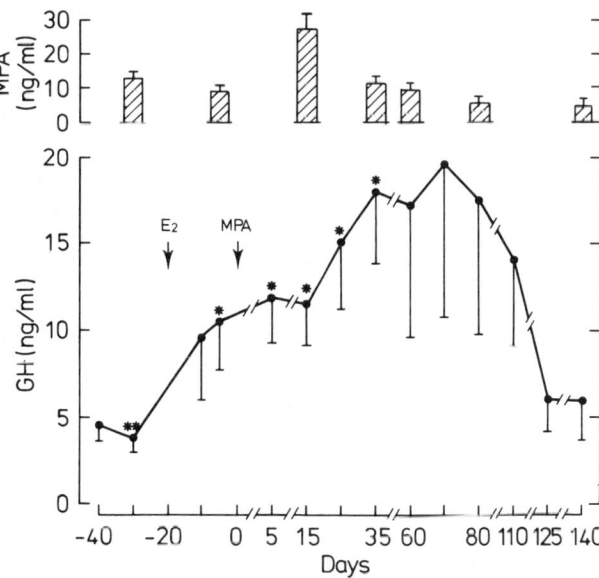

FIGURE 93–26. Plasma GH levels in experimental dogs during medroxyprogesterone acetate (MPA) exposure, when estradiol was given, and again when MPA was given. (From Eigenmann, JE and Eigenmann, RY: Influence of medroxyprogesterone acetate (Provera) on plasma growth hormone levels and on carbohydrate metabolism. II. Acta Endocrinol 98:603, 1981.)

cantly after hypophysectomy.[144] German shepherd dwarf dogs that invariably lack GH show exceedingly low levels of IGF I (Figure 93–29). In dogs with GH elevation (dogs with acromegaly or those with GH-diabetes), there is a striking elevation of IGF I levels. These elevated IGF I levels drop significantly in response to a drop in GH levels (Figure 93–30). However, there is no correlation between GH and IGF I concentration. A similar lack of correlation exists in human patients suffering from GH elevation.[145] In the dog with GH elevation, measurement of IGF I could be helpful in assessing the quality of treatment; improvement of the diabetic or acromegalic condition is associated with a drop in IGF levels.

In dogs of breeds that differ in body size, there is a parallel relationship between body size and plasma IGF I levels.[145] In smaller breeds, the IGF I levels decrease progressively with decreasing body size. IGF I levels in German shepherds are similar to those found in adult humans.

Another example is found in poodles; standard poodles exhibit six times the mean plasma IGF I concentration found in toy poodles (Figure 93–31). There is a

highly significant linear correlation between circulating IGF I levels and body size.[146] Theoretically, the measurement of IGF I levels should be diagnostically helpful in isolated GH deficiency (German shepherds, adult-onset GH deficiency). GH deficiency thus should be associated with low IGF I levels. However, adult-onset GH deficiency often occurs in small dogs that have already normally low IGF I levels. Thus, especially in this condition, IGF I measurement is not helpful.

Hypernatremia

Hyponatremia reflects a low concentration of total solutes in the extracellular compartment. Sodium solutes are the most abundant solutes in the extracellular fluid, and hence, sodium is the major factor determining plasma osmolality. Because water (H_2O) freely moves across cell membranes in response to osmotic pressure gradients, hyponatremia means that solutes are diluted throughout the body. However, the same concept in reverse holds true for hypernatremia.

Hypernatremia is a state of relative H_2O deficit and, therefore, is a state of excessive concentration of solutes in all body fluids. The latter condition represents a hyperosmolar, hypertonic situation. Hyperosmolar conditions without hypertonicity exist equally. An example of this is hyperosmolality, but not hypertonicity, induced by alcohol (alcohol diffuses into cells, while Na does not).

Body fluid tonicity and serum sodium concentrations are usually maintained in a narrow range by regulatory mechanisms of water homeostasis. Hypertonicity induces both release of anti-diuretic hormone (ADH) and thirst. Hence, ADH-induced urinary concentration comes into play. By minimizing the volume of water lost during solute excretion, a maximum of water is retained by the body. The most crucial defense against hypertonicity is thirst that is followed by water intake. As long as enough water is ingested, hypertonicity should never be more than transient.

The syndrome thus occurs most frequently in the

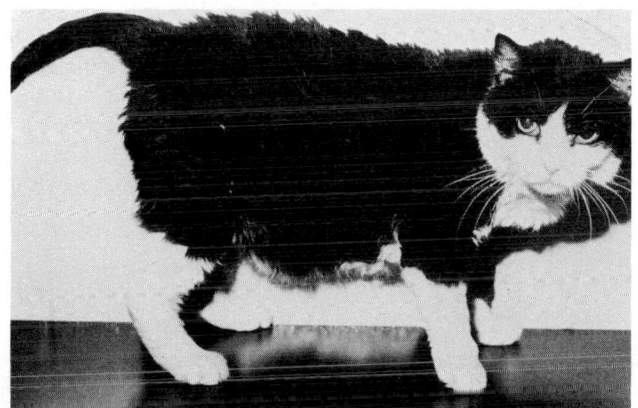

FIGURE 93–27. Cat with diabetes and acromegaly. Note heavy appearance. (From Eigenmann, JE, et al.: Elevated growth hormone levels and diabetes mellitus in a cat with acromegalic features. JAAHA 20:747, 1984.)

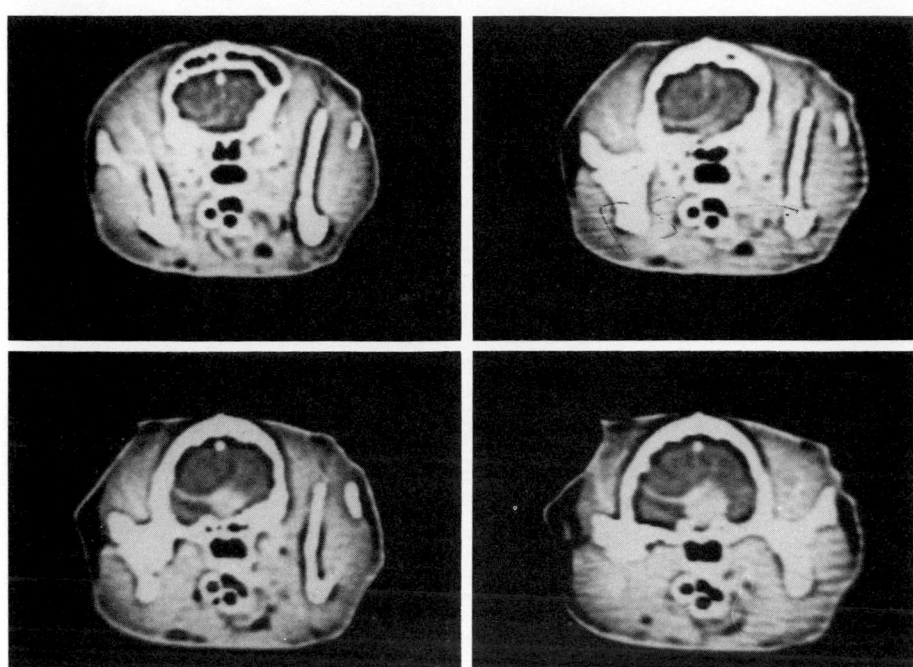

FIGURE 93–28. Computer-assisted tomogram from the same cat. Note mass in the pituitary region. (From Eigenmann, JE, et al.: Elevated growth hormone levels and diabetes mellitus in a cat with acromegalic features. JAAHA 20:747, 1984.)

individual with diminished water intake caused by an inability to take in and/or retain H_2O (e.g., unavailability, weakness, and vomiting).

Because of primary loss through the kidneys (e.g., diabetes insipidus), hypernatremia should not occur as long as enough water is ingested. Hypernatremia caused primarily by an absence of thirst occurs but is extremely rare.

A common denominator to all hypertonic syndromes is cellular dehydration (= volume contraction of the intracellular fluid compartment). This cellular dehydration, as far as osmoreceptors are concerned, is thought to be the mechanism leading to thirst and ADH release.

Principally, hypernatremic states can be subdivided into two entities: (1) water loss (pure or hypotonic) and (2) salt gain. Salt gain could supervene as a result of high salt intake or infusion of hypertonic salt solutions. Water loss in its most pure form is found in patients

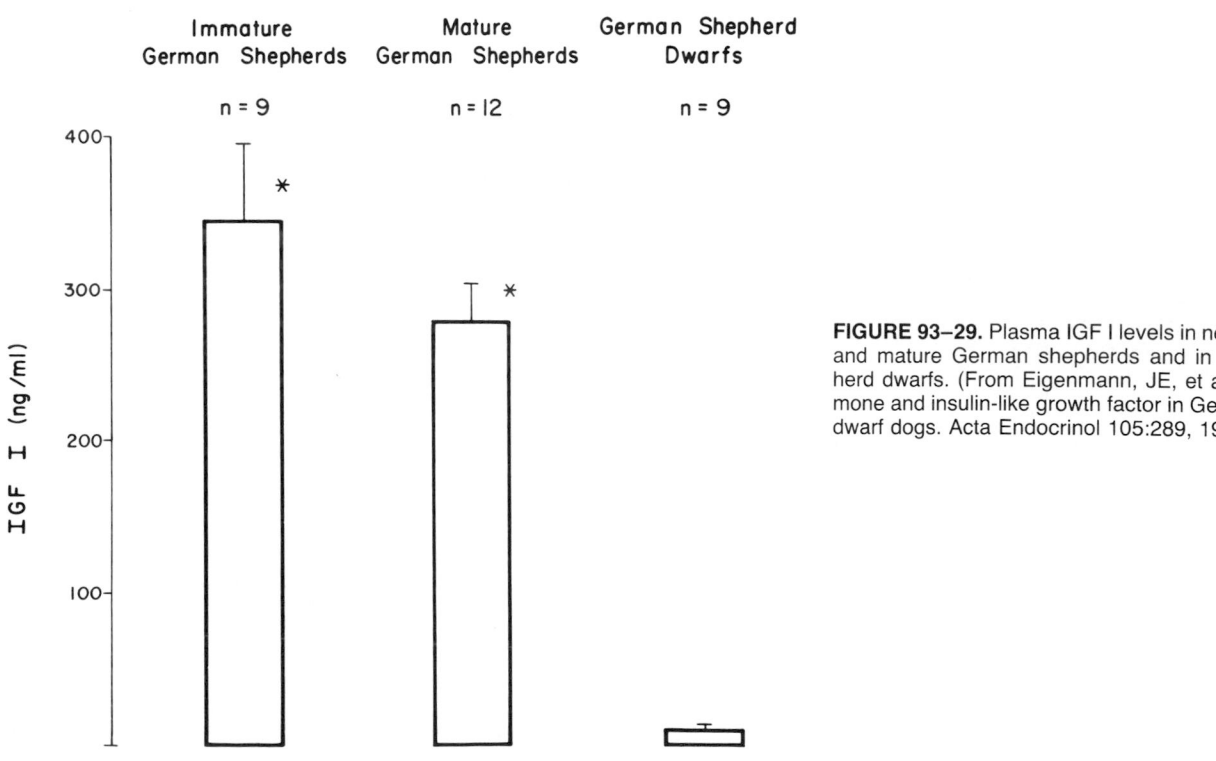

FIGURE 93–29. Plasma IGF I levels in normal immature and mature German shepherds and in German shepherd dwarfs. (From Eigenmann, JE, et al.: Growth hormone and insulin-like growth factor in German shepherd dwarf dogs. Acta Endocrinol 105:289, 1984.)

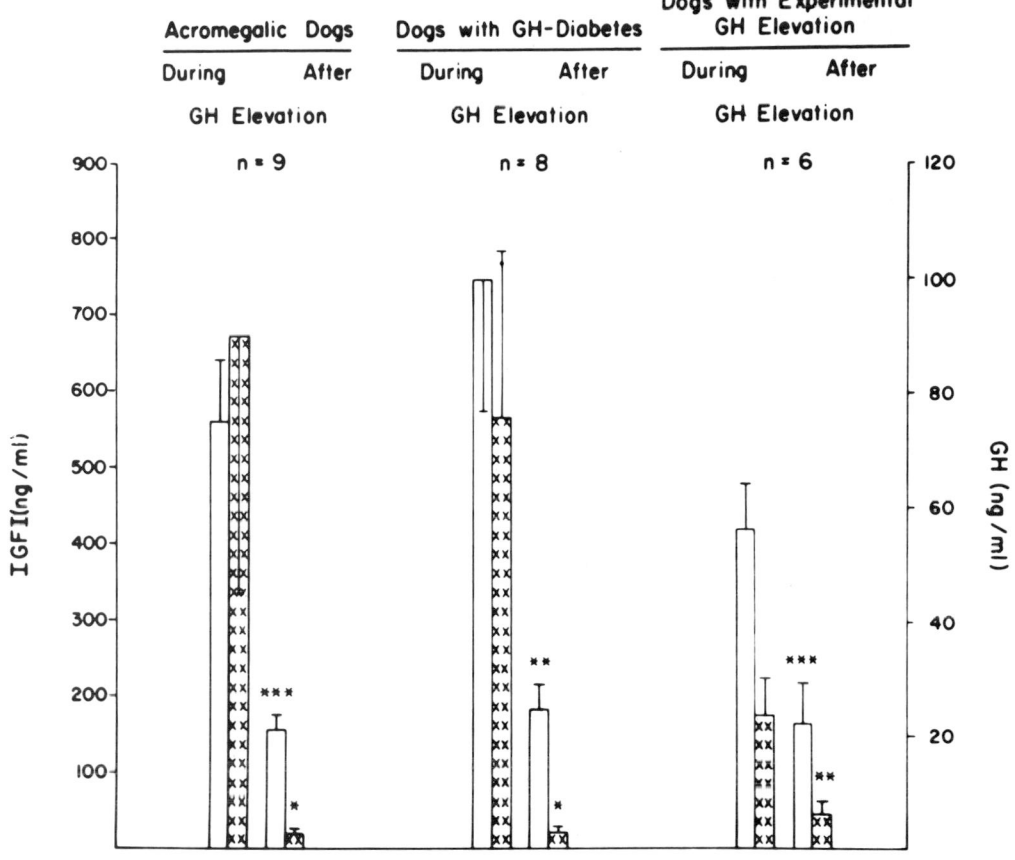

FIGURE 93–30. Plasma GH and IGF levels in acromegalic dogs, dogs with GH diabetes, and dogs with experimentally induced GH elevation during and after a stage of GH elevation. Open bars = IGF; filled bars = GH. (From Eigenmann JE, et al.: Insulin-like growth factor I in the dog: a study in different dog breeds and in dogs with growth hormone elevation. Acta Endocrinol 105:294, 1984.)

with diabetes insipidus. Hypotonic fluid loss (water loss that contains some solutes but less than plasma) most commonly occurs as a result of gastroenteritis.

SIGNS AND SYMPTOMS OF HYPERNATREMIA

The most prominent manifestations of hypernatremic (hyperosmolar) disorders are neurologic in nature, primarily as a result of dehydration. Irritability, restlessness, lethargy, muscle twitching, hyperreflexia, and spasticity can occur and end in coma, seizures, and death.

TREATMENT

The primary goal is restoration of serum tonicity. The euvolemic, hypernatremic patient with pure water loss requires water orally or parenterally as five per cent dextrose. Water deficit in this situation can be calculated on the basis of serum Na concentration and on the assumption that 60 per cent of the total body weight is water. Most authorities recommend lowering plasma osmolality by not more than 2 mOSM/hour. Thus, rehydration in the above case should occur over at least 14 hours.[147, 150]

Pituitary Diabetes Insipidus

Failure to synthesize or secrete vasopressin normally limits maximal urinary concentration ability and, de-

pending on the severity of the disease, causes varying degrees of polyuria and polydipsia.

In humans, in approximately half the patients with pituitary diabetes insipidus, no underlying pathologic condition is found. In others, head trauma, hypophysectomy, and neoplasms, either primary or metastatic, are the cause of diabetes insipidus. Others include encephalitis, sarcoidosis, and eosinophilic granuloma.

There is also a familial form of the disease. The onset of the disorder is frequently abrupt and occurs with equal frequency in both sexes.[150]

In the dog with pituitary diabetes insipidus, laboratory examination is normal and usually no specific historic or clinical findings are present. The suspicion of pituitary diabetes insipidus (= central diabetic insipidus) arises when all other possible causes for polyuria and polydipsia (e.g., diabetes mellitus, chronic renal failure, hyperthyroidism, Cushing's disease, hypercalcemia, and the like) have been ruled out. The diagnosis is usually established by employing the so-called water deprivation test. The water deprivation test may be followed by administration of vasopressin. Vasopressin (ADH) function is assessed by measuring urinary concentration and its changes. The animals are dehydrated up to five per cent and their plasma osmolality and/or urine osmolality (specific gravity) is recorded.

In the dog with total central or total renal diabetes insipidus essentially no changes in urinary specific grav-

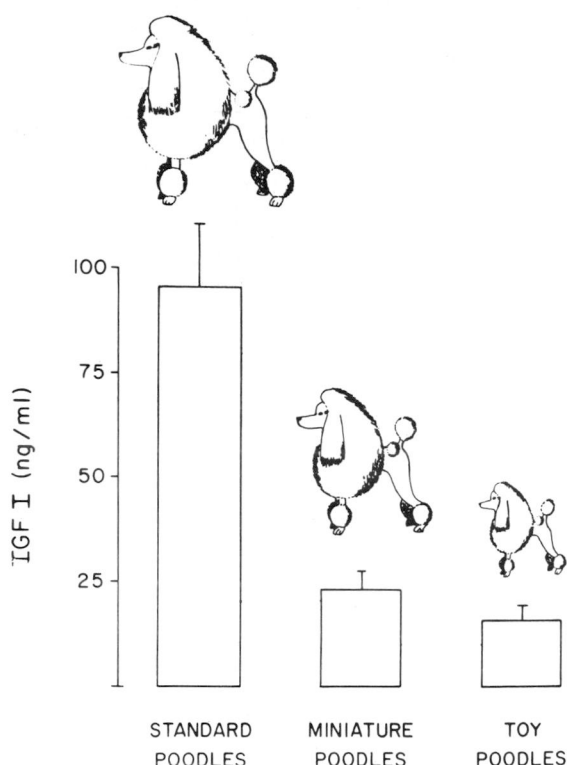

FIGURE 93–31. Mean plasma concentrations of insulin-like growth factor I (IGF I) (bars) in 10 standard, 10 miniature, and 10 toy poodles. (From Eigenmann JE, et al.: Body size parallels insulin-like growth factor I levels but not growth hormone secretory capacity. Acta Endocrinol 106:448, 1984.)

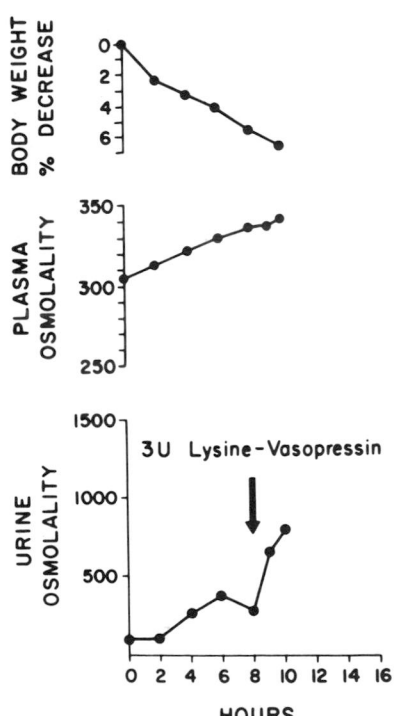

FIGURE 93–32. Body weight, plasma osmolality, and urine osmolality in a dog with central diabetes insipidus. Note virtually no change in urine osmolality during dehydration; increase in urine osmolality after LVP administration.

ity occur. During ADH administration, urinary specific gravity increases in the case of central diabetes insipidus (Figure 93–32), while there are no changes observed in the case of renal diabetes insipidus.

In humans, it has become clear that several conditions and partial forms of diabetes insipidus are difficult to distinguish from one another, and direct measurements of AVP are needed. Recently, Biwenga et al. have tried to correlate the results of the modified water deprivation test and direct AVP measurements.[156] A misdiagnosis was especially apparent in animals that had been suspected of having primary polydipsia on the basis of the water deprivation test.

In most patients initially diagnosed as having neph-rogenic diabetes insipidus, a disturbance in vasopressin secretions was found. It is likely that the latter condition was caused by medullary sodium washout known to lead to ADH resistance. The problem may be avoided if after water deprivation, NaCl (1 gm per 60 lb body weight q12h) is given for five days while water intake is decreased, and then the water deprivation test is repeated.

A comparison of plasma vasopressin measurements with a standard indirect test in the differential diagnosis of polyuria in humans has shown similar results. Severe neurogenic diabetes insipidus diagnosed by the indirect test was confirmed by the vasopressin assay.[151–157]

TREATMENT OF CENTRAL DIABETES INSIPIDUS

Two and a half units of Pitressin tannate is given at intervals of two to three days. Instead of Pitressin tannate, 1-deamino-8-D-arginine vasopressin (DDAVP) can be given. One drop of DDAVP is given two to three times into the conjunctival sac.

References

1. Christy, N: Harvey Cushing as clinical investigator and laboratory worker. Am J Med Sci 281:79, 1981.
2. Labhart, A: The adenohypophysis. *In* Labhart, A (ed): Clinical Endocrinology. New York, Springer-Verlag, 1984, p 77.
3. Greep, RO: History of research on anterior hypophyseal hormones. *In* Greep, RO and Astwood, EB (eds): Handbook of Physiology, Vol IV. Washington, DC, American Physiological Society, 1974, p 1.
4. Heller, H: History of neurohypophyseal research. *In* Greep, RO and Astwood, EB (eds): Handbook of Physiology, Vol IV. Washington, DC, American Physiological Society, 1974, p 103.
5. Verstraet, A and Thoonen, J: Twee nieuwe gevallen van hypo-physarte Stoornissen bij den hond. Vlaams Diergeneesk Tijdschr 8:304, 1939.
6. Coffin, DL and Munson, TD: Endocrine disease of the dog associated with hair loss. JAVMA 123:402, 1953.
7. Capen, CC, et al.: Neoplasms in the adenohypophysis of dogs. Pathol Vet 4:301, 1967.
8. Rijnberk, A, et al.: Spontaneous hyperadrenocorticism in the dog. J Endocrinol 41:397, 1968.
9. Luksch, F: Ueber Hypophysentumoren beim Hunde. Tierarztl Arch 3:1, 1923.
10. Groen, JJ, et al.: Observations on a case of spontaneous diabetes mellitus in a dog. Diabetes 13:492, 1969.
11. Rijnberk, A, et al.: Acromegaly associated with transient over-

production of growth hormone in a dog. JAVMA 177:534, 1980.

12. Eigenmann, JE and Venker van Haagen, A: Progestagen-induced and spontaneous canine acromegaly due to reversible growth hormone overproduction: clinical picture and pathogenesis. JAAHA 17:813, 1981.

13. Scott, DW, et al.: Clinicopathological findings in a German shepherd with pituitary dwarfism. JAAHA 14:183, 1978.

14. Eigenmann, JE: Diagnosis and treatment of dwarfism in a German shepherd dog. JAAHA 17:798, 1981.

15. Krieger, DT: Neuroendocrine physiology. In Felig, P, et al. (eds): Endocrinology and Metabolism. New York, McGraw-Hill, 1981, p 125.

16. Goldberg, RD and Chaikoff, IL: On the occurrence of six cell types in the dog anterior pituitary. Anat Rec 112:265, 1952.

17. Hullinger, RL: The endocrine system. In Evans, HI and Christensen, GC (eds): Miller's Anatomy of the Dog, 2nd ed. Philadelphia, WB Saunders, 1979, p 602.

18. Meijer, JC, et al.: Adrenocortical function tests in dogs with hyperfunctioning adrenocortical tumors. J Endocrinol 80:315, 1979.

19. Halmi, NS, et al.: Pituitary intermediate lobe in the dog: two cell types and high bioactive adrenocorticotropin content. Science 211:72, 1981.

20. Daniel, PM and Prichard, MML: Studies of the hypothalamus and the pituitary gland. Acta Endocrinol (Kbh) 80:1, 1975.

21. Etreby, FL, et al.: Effect of 17-β-estradiol on cells of the pars distalis of the adenohypophysis in the beagle bitch. An immunocytochemical and morphometric study. Endokrinologie 19:202, 1977.

22. Krieger, DT and Liotta, AS: Pituitary hormones in brain: Where, how and why. Science 205:366, 1979.

23. Palkovits, M: Neural pathways involved in ACTH regulation. Ann NY Acad Sci 297:455, 1977.

24. Spaulding, SW and Utiger, RD: The thyroid: physiology, hyperthyroidism, hypothyroidism and the painful thyroid. In Felig, P, et al. (eds): Endocrinology and Metabolism. New York, McGraw-Hill, 1981, p 281.

25. Sandow, J and Konig, W: Chemistry of the hypothalamic hormones. In Jeffcoate, SL and Hutchinson, JSM (eds): The Endocrine Hypothalamus. New York, Academic Press, 1978, p 149.

26. Meites, J and Sonntag, WE: Hypothalamic, hypophysiotropic hormones and neurotransmitter regulation: current views. Am Rev Pharmacol Toxicol 21:295, 1981.

27. Vale, W, et al.: Characterization of a 41 residue ovine hypothalamic peptide that stimulates secretion of corticotropin and endorphin. Science 213:1394, 1981.

28. Rivier, J, et al.: Characterization of rat hypothalamic corticotropin-releasing factor. Proc Natl Acad Sci USA 80:4851, 1983.

29. Shibahara, S, et al.: Isolation and sequence analysis of the human corticotropin-releasing factor precursor gene. EMBO J 2:775, 1983.

30. Rivier, J, et al.: Characterization of a growth hormone releasing factor from a human pancreatic islet tumor. Nature 300:276, 1982.

31. Brazeau, P, et al.: Growth hormone-releasing factor from ovine and caprine hypothalamus: Isolation sequence analysis and total synthesis. BBRC 135:606, 1984.

32. Guillemin, R, et al.: Growth hormone-releasing factor from a human pancreatic tumor that caused acromegaly. Science 218:585, 1982.

33. Borges, JL, et al.: Effect of human pancreatic tumor growth hormone-releasing factor on growth hormone and somatomedin C levels in patients with idiopathic growth hormone deficiency. Lancet 16:119, 1983.

34. Boyd, AE, et al.: Prolactin-releasing factor (PRF) in porcine hypothalamic extract distinct from TRH. Endocrinology 99:861, 1976.

35. Yasuda, N: Heterogencity of activity of the prolactin-releasing factor in the bovine hypothalamo-neurohypophyseal complex. J Endocrinol 103:243, 1984.

36. Richardson, S and Twente, S: Inhibition of rat hypothalamic somatostatin release by somatostatin: Evidence for somatostatin ultrashort loop feedback. Endocrinol 118:2076, 1986.

37. Lovinger, RL: Effect of synthetic somatotropin release inhibiting factor on the increase in plasma growth hormone elicited by L-Dopa in the dog. Endocrinol 95:943, 1974.

38. Takahashi, Y, et al.: A model of human sleep-related growth hormone secretion in dogs: effects of 3, 6 and 12 hours of forced wakefulness on plasma growth hormone, cortisol and sleep states. Endocrinology 109:262, 1977.

39. Kemppainen, RJ and Sartin, JL: Evidence for episodic but not circadian activity in plasma concentrations of adenocorticotropin, cortisol and thyroxine in dogs. J Endocrinol 103:219, 1984.

40. Wilhelmi, AE: Canine growth hormone. Yale J Biol Med 41:199, 1968.

41. Lewis, UJ, et al.: Human growth hormone: complex of proteins. Recent Prog Horm Res 36:477, 1980.

42. Daughaday, WH, et al.: Somatomedin: proposed designation for sulphation factor. Nature 235:107, 1972.

43. Rosenfeld, RG, et al.: Both human pituitary growth hormone and recombinant DNA-derived human growth hormone cause insulin resistance at a postreceptor site. J Clin Endocrinol Metab 54:1033, 1982.

44. Schoenle, E, et al.: Effect of insulin on glucose metabolism and glucose transport in fat cells of hormone-treated hypophysectomized rats: evidence that growth hormone restricts glucose transport. Endocrinology 105:1237, 1979.

45. Schoenle, E and Froesch, ER: In vivo control of the insulin-suppressible high-affinity Ca^{2+} ATPase of fat cell membranes by growth hormone and its possible involvement in the regulation of glucose transport. FEBS Lett 123:219, 1981.

46. Schoenle, E, et al.: In vivo control of insulin-sensitive phosphodiesterase in rat adipocytes by growth hormone and its parallelism to glucose transport. Endocrinology 109:561, 1981.

47. Schoenle, E, et al.: Glucose transport in adipocytes and its control by growth hormone in vivo. Am J Physiol 242:E368, 1982.

48. Zapf, J, et al.: Effect of insulin on glucose transport and metabolism in adipose tissue and skeletal muscle of hypophysectomized rats. FEBS Lett 135:199, 1981.

49. Reichlin, S: Regulation of somatotrophic hormone secretion. In Greep, RO and Astwood, EB (eds): Handbook of Physiology, Vol IV. Washington, DC, American Physiological Society, 1974, p 405.

50. Weiner, RI and Ganong, WF: The role of brain monoamines and histamine in the regulation of anterior pituitary secretion. Physiol Rev 58:905, 1978.

51. Martin, JB: Neural regulation of growth hormone secretion. Med Clin North Am 62:327, 1978.

52. Eigenmann, JE and Eigenmann, RY: Radioimmunoassay of canine growth hormone. Acta Endocrinol (Copenh) 98:514, 1981.

53. Zimmerman, H, et al.: Evidence that the effects of 5-hydroxytryptophan on the secretion of ACTH and growth hormone in dogs are not mediated by central release of serotonin. Neuroendocrinology 34:27, 1982.

54. Froesch, ER, et al.: Antibody suppressible and nonsuppressible insulin-like activities in human serum and their physiologic significance. An insulin assay with adipose tissue of increased precision and specificity. J Clin Invest 42:1816, 1963.

55. Rinderknecht, E and Humbel, RE: The amino acid sequence of human insulin-like growth factor I and its structural homology with proinsulin. J Biol Chem 253:2769, 1978.

56. Marquardt, H, et al.: Purification and primary structure of a polypeptide with multiplication-stimulating activity from rat liver cell cultures. J Biol Chem 256:6859, 1981.

57. Van Wyk, JJ, et al.: The somatomedins. A family of insulin like hormones under growth hormone control. Recent Prog Horm Res 30:259, 1974.

58. Pierson, RW and Temin, HM: The partial purification from calf serum of a fraction with multiplication-stimulating activity for chicken fibroblasts in the cell culture and with nonsuppressible insulin-like activity. J Cell Physiol 79:319, 1972.

59. Rinderknecht, E and Humbel, RE: Primary structure of human insulin-like growth factor II. FEBS Lett 89:283, 1978.

60. Klapper, DG, et al.: Sequence analysis of somatomedin C: confirmation of identity with insulin-like growth factor I. Endocrinology 112:2215, 1983.

61. Zapf, J, et al.: Radioimmunological determination of insulin-like growth factors I and II in normal subjects and in patients with growth disorders and extrapancreatic tumor hypoglycemia. J Clin Invest 68:1321, 1981.

62. Froesch, ER: From NSILA to IGF: A look back on the major advance and breakthrough. *In* Spencer, EM (ed): Insulin-like growth factors/somatomedins. Basic chemistry, biology, clinical importance. New York, W de Gruyter, 1983, p 13.

63. Schmid, CH, et al.: Preferential enhancement of myoblast differentiation by insulin-like growth factors (IGF I and II) in primary cultures of chicken embryonic cells. FEBS Lett 61:117, 1983.

64. Schmid, C, et al.: Insulin-like growth factors stimulate synthesis of nucleic acids and glycogen in cultured calvaria cells. Calcif Tissue Int 35:578, 1983.

65. Blundell, TL, et al.: Insulin-like growth factors: a model for tertiary structure accounting for immunoreactivity and receptor binding. Proc Natl Acad Sci USA 75:180, 1978.

66. Merimee, TJ, et al.: Dwarfism in the pygmy: An isolated deficiency of insulin-like growth factor I. N Engl J Med 305:965, 1981.

67. Adams, SO, et al.: Developmental patterns of insulin-like growth factors I and II synthesis and regulation in rat fibroblasts. Nature 302:150, 1983.

68. Clemmons, DR, et al.: Hyperprolactinemia is associated with increased immunoreactive somatomedin C in hypopituitarism. J Clin Endocrinol Metab 52:731, 1981.

69. Daughaday, WH, et al.: The effects of insulin and growth hormone on the release of somatomedin by the isolated rat liver. Endocrinology 98:1214, 1976.

70. Phillips, LS and Young, HS: Nutrition and somatomedin. II Serum somatomedin activity and cartilage growth activity in streptozotocin-diabetic rats. Diabetes 25:516, 1976.

71. Schwander, J, et al.: Synthesis and secretion of insulin-like growth factor and its binding protein by the perfused rat liver: Dependence on growth hormone status. Endocrinology 113:297, 1983.

72. Schoenle, EJ, et al.: Insulin-like growth factor I stimulates growth in hypophysectomized rats. Nature 296:252, 1982.

73. Li, CH: Chemistry of ovine prolactin. *In* Greep, RO and Astwood, EB (eds): Handbook of Physiology, Vol IV. Washington, DC, American Physiological Society, 1974, p 103.

74. Neill, JD: Prolactin: Its secretion and control. *In* Greep, RO and Astwood, EB (eds): Handbook of Physiology, Vol IV. Washington, DC, American Physiological Society, 1974, p 469.

75. Nicoll, CS: Physiological actions of prolactin. *In* Greep, RO and Astwood, EB (eds): Handbook of Physiology, Vol IV. Washington, DC, American Physiological Society, 1974, p 253.

76. Connors, JM and Hedge, GA: Feedback regulation of thyrotropin by thyroxine under physiological conditions. Am J Physiol 240:E308, 1981.

77. Florsheim, WM: Control of thyrotropine secretion. *In* Greep, RO and Astwood, EB (eds): Handbook of Physiology, Vol IV. Washington, DC, American Physiological Society, 1974, p 449.

78. Pierce, JG: Chemistry of thyroid-stimulating hormone. *In* Greep, RO and Astwood, EB (eds): Handbook of Physiology, Vol IV. Washington, DC, American Physiological Society, 1974, p 79.

79. Scanlo, MF, et al.: The neuroregulation of human thyrotropin section. *In* Martini, C and Ganong, WF (eds): Frontiers in Neuroendocrinology, Vol 6. New York, Raven Press, 1980, p 333.

80. Spaulding, SW and Utiger, RD: The thyroid: Physiology, hyperthyroidism, hypothyroidism and the painful thyroid. *In* Felig, P, et al. (eds): Endocrinology and Metabolism. New York, McGraw-Hill, 1981, p 281.

81. Wartofsky, C and Burman, KD: Alterations in thyroid function in patients with systemic illness: the euthyroid sick syndrome. Endocr Rev 3:164, 1982.

82. Greenwald, GS: Role of follicle-stimulating hormone and luteinizing hormone in follicular development and ovulation. *In* Greep, RO and Astwood, EB (eds): Handbook of Physiology, Vol IV, Section 7. Washington, DC, American Physiological Society, 1974, p 293.

83. Sairam, MR and Papkoff, H: Chemistry of pituitary gonadotrophins. *In* Greep, RO and Astwood, EB (eds): Handbook of Physiology, Vol IV. Washington, DC, American Physiological Society, 1974, p 111.

84. Chretien, M, et al.: From B-lipotropin to B-endorphin and "pro-opiomelanocortin." Can J Biochem 57:1111, 1979.

85. Johnston, SD and Mather, EC: Feline plasma cortisol (hydrocortisone) measured by radioimmunoassay. Am J Vet Res 40:190, 1979.

86. Krieger, DT, et al.: Abolition of circadian periodicity of plasma M-OHCS levels in the cat. Am J Physiol 215:959, 1968.

87. Muller, J and Baumann, K: Multifactorial regulation of the final steps of aldosterone biosynthesis in the rat. J Steroid Biochem 5:795, 1974.

88. Rijnberk, A, et al.: Investigations on the adrenocortical function of normal dogs. J Endocrinol 41:387, 1968.

89. Sayers, G and Portanova, R: Regulation of the secretory activity of the adrenal cortex: Cortisol and corticosterone. *In* Greep, RO and Astwood, EB (eds): Handbook of Physiology, Vol IV. Washington, DC, American Physiological Society, 1974, p 41.

90. Boyns, AR, et al.: Development of a radioimmunoassay for canine luteinizing hormone. J Endocrinol 55:279, 1972.

91. Graf, KJ, et al.: Homologous radioimmunoassay for canine prolactin and its application in various physiological states. J Endocrinol 75:93, 1977.

92. Reimers, TJ, et al.: Radioimmunologic measurement of follicle stimulating hormone and prolactin in the dog. Biol Reprod 19:673, 1978.

93. Quinlan, WJ and Michaelson, S: Homologous radioimmunoassay for canine thyrotropin: response of normal and x-irradiated dogs to propylthiouracil. Endocrinology 108:937, 1981.

94. Simmond, H: Ueber Hypophysischwund mit toedlichem Ausgang. Dtsch Med Wochenschr 40:322, 1914.

95. Abboud, CF and Laws, ER, Jr: Clinical endocrinological approach to hypothalamic-pituitary disease. J Neurosurg 51:271, 1979.

96. Andresen, E and Willeberg, P: Pituitary dwarfism in German shepherds: additional evidence of simple autosomal recessive inheritance. Nord Vet Med 28:481, 1976.

97. Eigenmann, JE: Diagnosis and treatment of pituitary dwarfism in dogs. *In* van Martens, E (ed): Sixth Annual Kal-Kan Symposium, p 107, 1983.

98. Capen, CC and Martin, SL: Diseases of the pituitary gland. *In* Ettinger, SJ (ed): Textbook of Internal Medicine. Philadelphia, WB Saunders, 1983, p 1542.

99. Eigenmann, JE, et al.: Growth hormone and insulin-like growth factor I in German shepherd dwarf dogs. Acta Endocrinol (Copenh) 105:289, 1984.

100. Andresen, E and Willeberg, P: Pituitary dwarfism in Carelian bear dogs: evidence for simple, autosomal recessive inheritance. Hereditas 83:232, 1976.

101. Andresen, E, et al.: Pituitary dwarfism in German shepherd dogs: genetic investigations. Nord Vet Med 16:692, 1974.

102. Rao, RR and Bhat, NG: Incidence of cysts in pars distalis of mongrel dogs. Indian Vet J 48:128, 1971.

103. Benjamin, M: Review: cysts (large follicles) and colloid in pituitary glands. Gen Comp Endocrinol 45:425, 1981.

104. McGillivray, MH and Voorhees, ML: Disorders of growth and development. *In* Felig, P (ed): Endocrinology and Metabolism. New York, McGraw-Hill, 1981, p 1385.

105. Sheehan, HL: Postpartum necrosis of the anterior pituitary. J Pathol Bacteriol 45:189, 1937.

106. Siegel, ET: Hypofunction of the anterior pituitary gland. *In* Siegel, ET (ed): Endocrine Diseases of the Dog. Philadelphia, Lea & Febiger, 1977, p 23.

107. Parker, WM and Scott, DW: Growth hormone responsive alopecia in the mature dog: a discussion of 13 cases. JAAHA 16:824, 1981.

108. Phillips, JA, et al.: Molecular basis for familial isolated growth hormone deficiency. Proc Natl Acad Sci USA 78:6312, 1981.

109. Eigenmann, JE and Patterson, DF: Growth hormone deficiency in the mature dog. JAAHA 20:741, 1984.

110. Eigenmann, JE: Growth hormone-deficient disorders associated with alopecia in the dog. *In* Kirk, RW (ed): Current Veterinary Therapy IX. Philadelphia, WB Saunders, 1986.

111. Capen, CC: Tumours of the endocrine glands. *In* Moulton, JE (ed): Tumors in Domestic Animals. Berkeley, University of California Press, 1978, p 377.

112. Peterson, ME, et al.: Immunocytochemical study of the hypophysis in 25 dogs with pituitary-dependent hyperadrenocorticism. Acta Endocrinol (Copenh) 101:15, 1982.

113. Nelson, DM, et al.: ACTH-producing pituitary tumors following

adrenalectomy for Cushing's syndrome. Ann Int Med 52:560, 1960.
114. Lubberink, AAME: Diagnosis and treatment of canine Cushing's syndrome. Ph.D. Thesis, University of Utrecht, Drukkerij Elinkwijk, 1977.
115. Attia, MA: Cytological study on pituitary adenomas in senile untreated beagle bitches. Arch Toxicol 46:287, 1980.
116. El Etreby, MF, et al.: Functional morphology of spontaneous hyperplastic and neoplastic lesions in the canine pituitary gland. Vet Pathol 17:109, 1980.
117. Dammrich, K: Die morphologische und funktionelle Pathologie der Geschwulste der Adenohypophyse bei Hunden. Zentralbl Vetinarmed 14:137, 1967.
118. Saunders, LZ: Craniopharyngioma in a dog with apparent adiposogenital syndrome and diabetes insipidus. Cornell Vet 42:490, 1952.
119. Eigenmann, JE, et al.: Panhypopituitarism caused by a suprasellar tumor in a dog. JAAHA 19:377, 1983.
120. Neer, MT and Reavis, DU: Craniopharyngioma and associated central diabetes insipidus and hypothyroidism in a dog. JAVMA 182:519, 1983.
121. Hampshire, J and Altszuler, N: Clonidine or xylazine as provocative tests for growth hormone secretion in the dog. Am J Vet Res 42:1073, 1981.
122. Belshaw, BE and Rijnberk, A: Hypothyroidism. In Kirk, RW (ed): Current Veterinary Therapy VII. Philadelphia, WB Saunders, 1980, p 994.
123. Chastain, CB, et al.: Adrenocortical suppression in cats given megestrol acetate. Am J Vet Res 42:2029, 1981.
124. Duick, DS and Wahner, MW: Thyroid axis in patients with Cushing's syndrome. Arch Intern Med 139:767, 1979.
125. Feldman, EC: Effect of functional adrenocortical tumors on plasma cortisol and corticotropin concentrations in dogs. JAVMA 178:823, 1981.
126. Kemppainen, RJ, et al.: Adrenocortical suppression in the dog after a single dose of methylprednisolone acetate. Am J Vet Res 42:822, 1981.
127. Pamenter, RW and Hedge, GA: Inhibition of thyrotropin secretion by physiological levels of corticosterone. Endocrinology 106:162, 1980.
128. Peterson, ME and Altszuler, N: Suppression of growth hormone secretion in spontaneous canine hyperadrenocorticism and its reversal after treatment. Am J Vet Res 42:1881, 1981.
129. Eigenmann, JE and Peterson, ME: Diabetes mellitus associated with other endocrine disorders. Vet Clin North Am 14:837, 1984.
130. Marmor, M, et al.: Epizootiologic patterns of diabetes mellitus in dogs. Am J Vet Res 43:465, 1982.
131. Wilkinson, JC: Spontaneous diabetes mellitus. Vet Rec 72:548, 1960.
132. Sloan, JM and Oliver, EM: Progestagen-induced diabetes in the dog. Diabetes 24:337, 1975.
133. Young, FG: Growth hormone and diabetes. Recent Prog Horm Res 8:471, 1953.
134. Rosenfeld, RG, et al.: Both human pituitary growth hormone and recombinant DNA-derived human growth hormone cause insulin resistance at a postreceptor site. J Clin Endocrinol Metab 54:1033, 1982.
135. Eigenmann, JE, et al.: Progesterone-controlled growth hormone overproduction and naturally occurring canine diabetes and acromegaly. Acta Endocrinol (Copenh) 104:167, 1983.
136. Eigenmann, JE: Diabetes mellitus in elderly female dogs: Recent findings on pathogenesis and clinical implications. JAAHA 17:805, 1981.
137. Eigenmann, JE: Disorders associated with growth hormone oversecretion: Diabetes mellitus and acromegaly. In Kirk, RW (ed): Current Veterinary Therapy. Philadelphia, WB Saunders, 1985, p 1006.
138. Eigenmann, JE: Acromegaly in the dog. Vet Clin North Am 14:827, 1984.
139. Eigenmann, JE and Rijnberk, A: Influence of medroxyprogesterone acetate (Provera) on plasma growth hormone levels and on carbohydrate metabolism. I. Studies in the ovariohysterectomized bitch. Acta Endocrinol (Copenh) 98:599, 1981.
140. Eigenman, JE and Eigenmann, RY: Influence of medroxyprogesterone acetate (Provera) on plasma growth hormone levels and on carbohydrate metabolism. II. Studies in the ovariohysterectomized, oestradiol-primed bitch. Acta Endocrinol (Copenh) 98:603, 1981.
141. Eigenman, JE, et al.: Elevated growth hormone levels and diabetes mellitus in a cat with acromegalic features. JAAHA 20:747, 1984.
142. Lichtensteiger, CA, et al.: Functional pituitary acidophil adenoma in a cat with diabetes mellitus and acromegalic features. Vet Pathol 23:518, 1986.
143. Gembhardt, C and Loppnow, H: Zur Pathogenese des spontanen Diabetes mellitus der Katze. II. Mitteilung: Azidophile Adenome des Hypophysenvorderlappens und Diabetes mellitus in zwei Fallen. Tierarztl Wochenschr 89:336, 1976.
144. Eigenmann, JE, et al.: The influence of hypophysectomy on NSILAs-concentrations in the dog. Evidence for partially pituitary independent regulation. Acta Endocrinol (Copenh) 86:498, 1977.
145. Eigenmann, JE, et al.: Insulin-like growth factor I in the dog: a study in different dog breeds and in dogs with growth hormone elevation. Acta Endocrinol (Copenh) 105:294, 1984.
146. Eigenmann, JE, et al.: Body size parallels insulin-like growth factor I levels but not growth hormone secretory capacity. Acta Endocrinol (Copenh) 106:448, 1984.
147. Crawford, MA, et al.: Hypernatremia and adipsia in a dog. JAVMA 184:818, 1984.
148. Feig, PU: Hypernatremia and hypertonic syndromes. Med Clin North Am 65:271, 1981.
149. Hall, EJ: Hypernatremia and adipsia in a dog. (Letter). JAVMA 185:4, 1984.
150. Schrier, RW and Berl, T: Disorders of water metabolism. In Schrier, RW (ed): Renal and Electrolyte Disorders. Boston, Little, Brown, 1980, p 1.
151. Trasher, TN: Osmoreceptor mediation of thirst and vasopressin secretion in the dog. Fed Proc 41:2528, 1982.
152. Wade, CE, et al.: Osmotic control of plasma vasopressin in the dog. Am J Physiol 243:E287, 1982.
153. Ruggles, BT, et al.: The vasopressin-sensitive adenylate cyclase in collecting tubules and in thick ascending limb of Henle's Loop of human and canine kidney. J Clin Endocrinol Metab 60:914, 1985.
154. Hardy, RH and Osborne, CA: Water deprivation test in the dog: maximal normal values. JAVMA 74:479, 1979.
155. Mulnix, JA, et al.: Evaluation of a modified water deprivation test for diagnosis of polyuric disorders in dogs. JAVMA 169:1327, 1976.
156. Biewenga, AWE, et al.: Vasopressin in polyuric syndromes in the dog. In Rijnberk, A and Wimersma Greidanus, TJB (eds): Comparative Pathophysiology of Regulatory Peptides. Basel, Karger (in press).
157. Zerbe, RL and Robertson, GL: A comparison of plasma vasopressin measurements with a standard indirect test in the differential diagnosis of polyuria. N Engl J Med 305:1539 1981.

94 PARATHYROID DISEASE AND CALCIUM METABOLISM

DONALD J. MEUTEN and P. JANE ARMSTRONG

With some systems it is the physical abnormalities and/or signs an animal exhibits that lead a veterinarian to suspect that disease x or y may be present. Laboratory data are used to help distinguish which of these diseases is most probable. With diseases of the parathyroid glands, however, a laboratory abnormality (hypercalcemia or hypocalcemia) is generally detected first. The exceptions to this may include a lactating female in tetany, a history of polyuria and polydipsia, or an animal with marked enlargement of the facial bones. Because diseases of the parathyroid glands are usually considered after an abnormal concentration of serum calcium is detected, it seems appropriate to discuss hypercalcemia and hypocalcemia, which include diseases that affect the parathyroid glands directly or indirectly. Previous editions of this text contain excellent reviews of the physiology, pathology, and anatomy of the parathyroid glands.

HYPERCALCEMIA

General Considerations

Hypercalcemia exists when the serum concentration of calcium exceeds the reference range on more than one determination. A single high value of calcium must always be confirmed with a second sample. Many times the second and subsequent samples have calcium concentrations within the established reference range.[1] These spurious and generally unexplained increases in serum calcium are relatively common and have been reported as one of the most frequent causes of an increased serum concentration of total calcium. Young animals frequently have mild hypercalcemia (less than 13 mg/dl) that is best interpreted as physiologic and need not be investigated.[2, 3] Pups will also have mild hyperphosphatemia and increased serum concentrations of alkaline phosphatase and vitamin D, probably related to the positive calcium balance and rapid skeletal remodeling that occur during growth. Comparable changes in serum calcium and phosphorus have not been reported in cats.

Hemoconcentration can produce mild hypercalcemia (less than 13 mg/dl), and correction formulas for dogs can help to identify if all or part of an increased serum calcium concentration is due to an increase in albumin (dehydration) or total serum protein (Figure 94-1). Lipemia and/or hemolysis can falsely increase serum total calcium determined with autoanalyzers that use alizarin red, methythymol blue, or O-cresolphthalein complexone. Samples that are grossly lipemic and/or hemolyzed can have values of calcium greater than 20 mg/dl. Lipemic and hemolyzed samples may also have false increases in other substances, such as albumin, bilirubin, and some of the hepatic enzymes. Therefore, a sample should not be interpreted as hypercalcemic if there is evidence of lipemia or hemolysis. Ethylenediaminetetraacetic acid (EDTA) will complex with calcium and falsely lower the calcium concentration when determined with an autoanalyzer. If the concentration of calcium is determined by atomic absorption spectrophotometry, however, EDTA may falsely increase the concentration of calcium. Before pursuing a differential diagnosis for hypercalcemia be sure none of the possibilities above exist. It is important to eliminate these problems, since the practical list of differential diagnoses for hypercalcemia is short (Table 94-1) and a final diagnosis should be relatively easy. After hypercalcemia of malignancy, other causes of hypercalcemia are uncommon.

Malignancy

Hypercalcemia associated with malignancy is the most common cause of symptomatic hypercalcemia in both

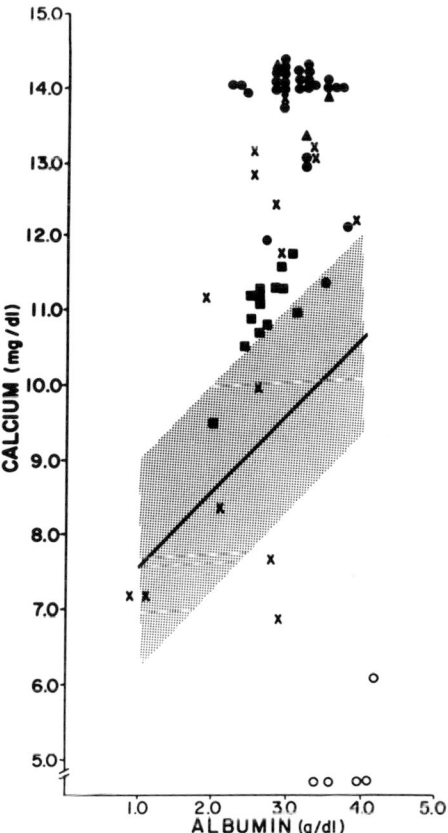

FIGURE 94–1. Relation of serum total calcium to serum albumin concentration in 209 dogs. The shaded area represents the 95 per cent confidence limits for the population, and the solid line, the least square regression line. As the concentration of albumin increases or decreases there is a concurrent increase or decrease in serum total calcium. One third of the variability in calcium was attributable to the change in the concentration of albumin (R^2 = .33). Approximately 90 per cent of dogs with disorders of calcium metabolism and 85 per cent of young dogs were outside the 95 per cent confidence limits for serum albumin. ● = hypercalcemia of malignancy; ■ = young dogs; X = renal failure; 0 = hypoparathyroidism; ▲ = primary hyperparathyroidism.

human and canine patients. Production of bone-resorbing compounds that stimulate the resorption of bone adjacent to the tumor (local osteolysis) or distant from the tumor (humoral osteolysis) is one of the major mechanisms by which a neoplasm can induce hypercalcemia.[4–6] Increased absorption of calcium from the gastrointestinal tract and renal tubules also contributes to the hypercalcemia in some human and animal patients with this paraneoplastic syndrome.[4, 7, 8] Bone-resorbing factors or other calcemic factors purportedly produced by tumor cells are parathyroid hormone (PTH), parathyroid hormone–related protein (PTH-rP) factors, transforming growth factors, 1,25-dihydroxyvitamin D, prostaglandin E_2 (PGE_2), cytokines such as osteoclast activating factor, interleukin-1, interleukin-2, gamma interferon, lymphotoxin, colony-stimulating factor and other partially characterized compounds.[9–19] These factors may act on bone, gut, or renal cells individually or synergistically to induce hypercalcemia. Clearly the mechanisms responsible for the hypercalcemia associated with malignancies are heterogeneous.

The term pseudohyperparathyroidism was initially used to characterize the syndrome of hypercalcemia of malignancy because of the similarity to primary hyperparathyroidism. Both syndromes are associated with hypercalcemia, hypophosphatemia, hyperphosphaturia, and an absence of bone metastases. It was concluded that ectopic production of PTH was probably the cause of pseudohyperparathyroidism. More recent work indicates that true PTH seldom causes the hypercalcemia associated with malignancy. Although some tumors produce a factor that mimics some of the actions of PTH, it is different from true PTH in that (1) it is larger than PTH, (2) it is not detected by probes for PTH messenger RNA,[20] (3) it does not cross-react with multiple antisera for PTH,[5] (4) it does not consistently increase nephrogenous cAMP[21] nor increase serum 1,25-dihydroxyvitamin D,[5] (5) it does not increase the serum concentration of osteocalcin,[22] and (6) it does not consistently interact with PTH receptors in bone.[23] Recently, a protein has been isolated from tumors in man and animals that has an amino terminus which is very similar to true PTH.[23a] This protein (PTH-rP) contains 141 amino acids, and 8 of the first 13 amino acids are identical to those of human PTH.[23a, 23b] Since the amino terminus of the PTH molecule is responsible for the biologic action of PTH, it is easy to understand why PTH-rP, by binding with receptors for PTH, mimics the biologic action of PTH. The mid- and carboxy regions of PTH and PTH-rP are different, which explains why PTH-rP is not detected by present immunoassays for true PTH. It has also been shown that the gene for PTH-rP is located on chromosome 12, whereas the gene for PTH is on chromosome 11.[23c] The role PTH-rP plays in normal calcium homeostasis in the adult and fetus needs to be determined.[23d]

Despite spontaneous, transplantable, and chemically induced models for hypercalcemia associated with malignancy the pathogenesis of the hypercalcemia is still not clear.[24–28] It is apparent that different factors may produce this syndrome, and that these factors may act as primary or secondary messengers to stimulate hypercalcemia. Furthermore, whether these factors act on

**TABLE 94–1. DIFFERENTIAL DIAGNOSIS
FOR HYPERCALCEMIA***

Practical
1. Malignancy
    Lymphosarcoma
    Adenocarcinoma—apocrine glands of anal sac
    Other (multiple myeloma, carcinomas)
Uncommon
2. Hypoadrenocorticism
3. Renal failure
4. Primary hyperparathyroidism
5. Bone lesion
    Metastases
    Septic (bacterial/mycotic osteomyelitis)
    Disuse osteoporosis
6. Blastomycosis
7. Hypervitaminosis D
8. Others
    Young age
    Laboratory error, artifact—hemolysis, lipemia
    Severe hypothermia
    Hyperproteinemia
    Unclassified

*The eight general headings are arranged in order of probable occurrence.

bone, gut, or renal cells alone or in concert with other factors is an area of research that needs clarification.

LYMPHOSARCOMA

The most common cause of symptomatic hypercalcemia in dogs is cancer; it is probably the most common cause of hypercalcemia in cats as well. The combination of *hypercalcemia and hypophosphatemia* limits the differential diagnoses to hypercalcemia of malignancy and primary hyperparathyroidism. Finding a large nonparathyroid tumor is usually the easiest way to differentiate these two diagnoses. In both dogs and cats the tumor most frequently associated with hypercalcemia is lymphosarcoma.

The association of hypercalcemia with lymphosarcoma in dogs has been documented in numerous reports.[29–31] Approximately one third of dogs with lymphosarcoma have hypercalcemia. In fact the presence of hypercalcemia is often a clue that a careful evaluation for lymphosarcoma is needed. Greater than 90 per cent of dogs with lymphosarcoma and hypercalcemia have clinically detectable lymphadenomegaly. Most reports conclude that the majority of dogs with lymphosarcoma and hypercalcemia also have a mass in the anterior mediastinum. Some of the other characteristics of dogs with hypercalcemia and lymphosarcoma include weight loss, lethargy, lymphopenia, polyuria, polydipsia, and tumor in bone marrow, liver, spleen, and tonsil.[31]

A dog with marked lymphadenomegaly, a mass in the anterior thoracic cavity, and persistent hypercalcemia (serum calcium greater than 12.5 mg/dl on more than one determination) is not a diagnostic challenge. The problem arises when persistent hypercalcemia is detected but the tumor(s) is not obvious. In dogs a careful search for occult lymphosarcoma or a tumor of the apocrine glands of the anal sac (CA) must be made, since these two tumors are the most common causes of symptomatic hypercalcemia. A thorough rectal examination and palpation and/or radiographs of the sublumbar region may reveal a mass, in which case a CA is probably the cause of the hypercalcemia. If no mass can be found with these techniques and no other mass is detectable, then the dog may have occult lymphosarcoma. When lymphosarcoma is strongly suspected but enlarged lymph nodes are not detected, several procedures may be helpful: (1) cytologically evaluate the bone marrow from several bones for lymphosarcoma, (2) radiograph the thorax and evaluate the cranial mediastinum for a neoplasm (if a mass is found, then aspirational cytology may confirm the diagnosis of lymphosarcoma), (3) cytologically evaluate one or more peripheral lymph nodes even if they are not enlarged, and (4) administer prednisone or prednisolone, 1 mg/lb (2 mg/kg) q12h for 2 days, and determine serum calcium daily. If the concentration of serum calcium returns to the reference range within 12 to 48 hours of steroid administration, then occult lymphosarcoma, especially in bones, should be suspected (Figure 94–2). Aspirational cytology of lymph nodes or bone marrow at this time may be useless because of the lympholytic effect of the corticosteroids. When hypercalcemia recurs there probably is also recurrence of lymphosarcoma, and at this time the cytologic evaluation of multiple lymph nodes and bone marrow from several bones may confirm the diagnosis. The mechanisms by which corticosteroids decrease the serum concentration of calcium in hypercalcemic dogs with lymphosarcoma include the following: (1) lympholytic effect of steroids destroys the tumor and the source of calcemic factors, (2) high doses of corticosteroids inhibit the production of osteoclast activating factor, (3) steroids inhibit the action of osteoclast activating factor on bone, (4) corticosteroids are potent inhibitors of osteoclastic bone resorption stimulated by prostaglandins and vitamin D, (5) steroids block the synthesis of prostaglandins, and PGE_2 is necessary for the release of osteoclast activating factor, (6) steroids have a hypercalciuric effect, and (7) steroids decrease the absorption of calcium from the intestine.[32–35] The lympholytic effect of corticosteroids is probably the most important factor in the rapid decrease of serum calcium in dogs with lymphosarcoma. Because steroid therapy may exacerbate other diseases that cause hypercalcemia, such as blastomycosis and osteomyelitis, these diseases should be ruled out or deemed unlikely before a prednisone trial is initiated.

Although hypercalcemia is associated with feline lymphosarcoma and/or feline leukemia virus infection, it is an uncommon complication of both problems.[36–38] Some of these cats had generalized lymphosarcoma, including a large cranial mediastinal mass. There is one report of a hypercalcemic cat that was infected with the feline leukemia virus and that also had proliferative and myelosclerotic bone lesions, but without solid tissue neoplasia.[38] As in dogs, the destruction of the tumor in cats results in remission of hypercalcemia. The pathogenesis of the hypercalcemia in these cats is unknown; however, it seems reasonable that the mechanism of the hypercalcemia is similar to that for dogs and other species.

A major contribution to the hypercalcemia in animals with lymphosarcoma is increased bone resorption.[31, 39] Dogs with lymphosarcoma and hypercalcemia have decreased trabecular bone volume and markedly increased osteoclastic osteolysis.[31, 39] However, the identity of the factor that stimulates this bone resorption and the importance of tumor in bone are not clear.[39, 40] Dogs with lymphosarcoma and hypercalcemia can have increased bone resorption in bones with or *without* lymphosarcoma in the marrow ("humoral hypercalcemia").[39, 40] Separate investigations concluded that the factor(s) produced by canine lymphosarcoma was not PGE_2, 1,25-dihydroxyvitamin D_3, or an immunoreactive form of parathyroid hormone (iPTH).[30, 31] Furthermore, extracts of tumors from hypercalcemic dogs with lymphosarcoma did not contain detectable iPTH[31] or messenger RNA for parathyroid hormone.[20] Although PGE_2 was not increased in the plasma of hypercalcemic dogs with lymphosarcoma, its metabolite was increased approximately twofold.[31] This small increase in the metabolite may indicate there was local PGE_2 production in bone, stimulated by humoral factors produced elsewhere, or the PGE_2 metabolite may be important to stimulate the release of other bone-resorbing compounds, such as osteoclast activating factor. Tumor tissue from hypercalcemic and normocalcemic dogs with lymphosarcoma has been shown to produce a bone-resorbing factor(s) *in vitro*.[30]

FIGURE 94–2. Longitudinal section through the lumbar vertebrae of a hypercalcemic dog with lymphosarcoma. There is marked osteolysis of bone and tumor replacement of bone marrow in the body (ventral) and arch (dorsal) of multiple vertebrae. This dog had marked hypercalcemia and moderate hypophosphatemia that could not be diagnosed from the usual ancillary tests or physical examination techniques. She was a candidate for exploratory neck surgery; however, the serum total calcium returned to reference ranges within 24 hours of prednisolone administration. Occult lymphosarcoma was suspected. When hypercalcemia returned, aspirational cytology was performed on several normal-sized peripheral lymph nodes and several bones, but no abnormalities were detected. Prednisolone administration again produced normocalcemia within 24 hours of its administration. This pattern was repeated several times over the next 18 months. At necropsy lymphosarcoma was present in lumbar and thoracic vertebrae, several other bones, and a few internal lymph nodes on both sides of the diaphragm. This case emphasizes the use of prednisolone as a diagnostic tool and how lymphosarcoma can occasionally be difficult to diagnose.

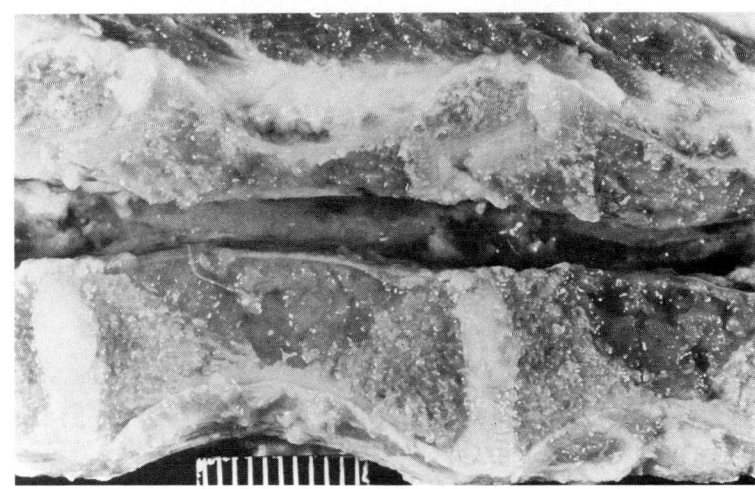

Recent investigations indicate that lymphosarcoma tissue from hypercalcemic, but not normocalcemic, dogs contains an adenylate cyclase-stimulating protein that interacts with a PTH receptor.[40] If this substance can be shown to stimulate bone resorption, it may be one of the factors responsible for hypercalcemia associated with lymphosarcoma in dogs. Messenger RNA for PTH-rP has been identified in tumor tissue from a hypercalcemic dog with lymphosarcoma but not in tissue from a normocalcemic dog with lymphosarcoma.[40a] Comparable mRNA has been identified in a variety of animal and human tumors associated with humoral hypercalcemia of malignancy.[40a] Other factors implicated in the pathogenesis of the hypercalcemia associated with hematopoietic tumors include the lymphokine osteoclast activating factor, colony-stimulating factor, interleukins, gamma interferon, PTH-rP, and 1,25-hydroxyvitamin D.[9, 13, 14, 16, 17, 24] Although these factors may work individually, it seems more likely that they work synergistically to induce the resorption of calcium from bone and from soft tissues such as the gut or kidneys.

ADENOCARCINOMA FROM THE APOCRINE GLANDS OF THE ANAL SAC

The perineum of dogs contains circumanal glands, which are modified sebaceous glands; anal glands, which are merocrine glands and are located in the submucosa of the anus; apocrine glands, which surround the anal sac; and both sebaceous and apocrine sweat glands associated with hair follicles. Dogs develop a unique adenocarcinoma derived from the apocrine glands of the anal sac (CA).[41] This tumor is distinct from the relatively common circumanal (perianal) gland tumor both clinically and pathologically (Table 94–2). Circumanal gland tumors are benign, occur most commonly in males, regress with castration, and are not associated with hypercalcemia. In contrast, CA are malignant tumors that occur most commonly in females, are difficult to ablate surgically or chemically, and are frequently associated with hypercalcemia.[42] The clinical syndrome produced by this tumor is distinct (Table 94–3). Dogs with CA are usually older females, and they present with problems such as polyuria and polydipsia that may

be referable to the hypercalcemia, or with problems related to the tumor in the perineum (mass, pruritus, tenesmus). The primary tumor is generally covered by haired skin, may be small, and often is not found unless thorough rectal and perirectal examinations are done (Figure 94–3).[42–44]

In a survey of more than 7000 tumors it was found that CA is the most common malignant tumor in the perineum of female dogs.[42] Approximately 90 per cent of dogs with CA are hypercalcemic. Whenever a tumor is detected in the perineum of an older female dog a CA is the most likely diagnosis. Serum should be col-

TABLE 94–2. DIFFERENTIATION OF PERIANAL (CIRCUMANAL) ADENOMA AND CA*

Feature	Apocrine Adenocarcinoma	Circumanal Adenoma
Sex	Female	Male
Gross tumor	Often occult	Usually visible
Histology	Acini, columnar cells, solid areas	Solid "hepatoid"
Behavior	Malignant	Benign
Prognosis	Poor	Good
Serum calcium	Increased	Normal

*Adenocarcinoma derived from apocrine glands of anal sac.

TABLE 94–3. CLINICAL CHARACTERISTICS IN 58 DOGS WITH CA*

Characteristic	Number of Dogs
Sex	
Female	52
Male	6
Age	
Range (yr)	7–16
Mean (yr)	10
Breeds	Varied
Clinical signs frequently reported by owner	
Perirectal mass	34
Polyuria and polydipsia	21
Anorexia	14
Lethargy and weakness	12
Metastases to regional lymph nodes evaluated	34/44 evaluated
Hypercalcemia	29/31 evaluated

*Adenocarcinoma derived from apocrine glands of anal sac; this information is summarized from references 41 through 43.

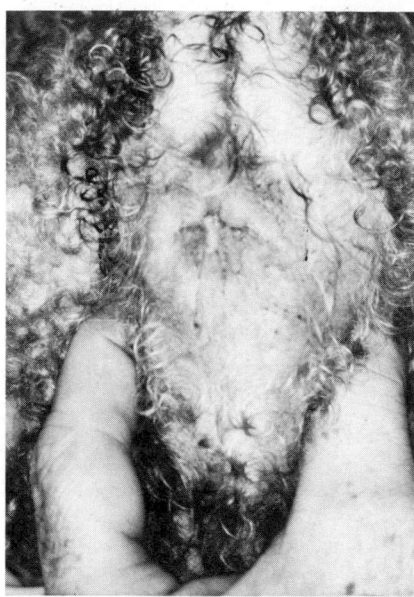

FIGURE 94–3. Perineum of an older female dog with hypercalcemia and hypophosphatemia. The perineum is fully haired and a protruding mass was not seen. On perirectal and rectal examination a large mass was palpated ventrally and laterally to the anus. The final diagnosis was an apocrine gland adenocarcinoma emerging from one anal sac.

lected, both preoperatively and postoperatively, from any female dog with a mass in the perineum. Calcium can be determined immediately or after a histopathologic diagnosis is obtained. Histopathology does not always confirm the diagnosis, since many times the tumor is misinterpreted as a circumanal (perianal) gland neoplasm, a rectal neoplasm, or an epithelial tumor of undetermined origin. If serum samples are submitted after a histopathologic diagnosis, there are several points relevant to the management of the dog: (1) if hypercalcemia was present preoperatively and is absent postoperatively, then it essentially confirms the diagnosis of CA and suggests that most of the tumor has been removed, (2) furthermore, the recurrence of hypercalcemia in a dog with CA can be used as an indicator of tumor recurrence, and (3) if hypercalcemia is present preoperatively and postoperatively, then a careful examination of the perineum, pelvic cavity, sublumbar region, and thoracic cavity should be completed in an attempt to find more tumor. After removal of a CA the serum calcium will return to the normal reference range within 12 to 48 hours. Postoperative hypocalcemia is not a problem, despite inactive to atrophic parathyroid glands.[44] The endogenous secretion of PTH in response to the decreasing serum calcium concentrations postoperatively is sufficient to prevent hypocalcemia.[44] Although postoperative hypocalcemia is a frequent complication after the removal of a functional parathyroid tumor, this is not the case when a tumor associated with hypercalcemia of malignancy is destroyed or removed.

Tumors from the anal sac apocrine glands are invariably malignant, and unfortunately the majority will have metastasized by the time they are recognized (Figure 94–4).[42] The opposite biologic behavior is expected with circumanal gland neoplasms. Recurrence of hypercalcemia in a dog with CA is a good indicator that the tumor has regrown. The most likely areas for regrowth are the primary site, within the pelvic cavity, and in lymph nodes in the sublumbar region. Distant metastases to the lungs and liver are less common. Despite vigorous treatments with chemotherapy, radiation therapy, and/or surgical excision, these tumors recur and/or metastasize. The average survival of dogs with CA was nine months (range 2 to 21 months) in one study.[42] It is important to accurately recognize these tumors as adenocarcinoma derived from the apocrine glands of the anal sac because of their *poor prognosis.*

The pattern of serum calcium decreasing and phosphorus increasing after surgical removal of the tumor and then the return of hypercalcemia and hypophosphatemia with recurrence or metastases suggests that CA produces a hypercalcemic factor(s).[42] This factor or factors results in hypercalcemia, hypophosphatemia, and increased osteoclastic bone resorption distant from the tumor.[27, 44] Tumor extracts and a tumor line (CAC-8) stimulate *in vitro* bone resorption, and this bone resorption can be *partially* inhibited by a PTH receptor antagonist.[44a] Messenger RNA for PTH-rP has been identified in tumor tissue from a dog with CA.[40a] The PTH-rP is approximately 16,000 daltons and resembles human PTH-rP. Earlier studies have indicated that the factor produced by this tumor is not iPTH or PGE_2.[44] Serum concentration of vitamin D is not suppressed in hypercalcemic dogs with spontaneous CA or in hypercalcemic nude mice with transplanted CA.[27, 44] Transplantation of CA to nude mice produces a syndrome similar to that seen naturally in dogs.[27] This adaptation of the canine tumor to mice should facilitate studies that try to identify the factor or factors that cause the hypercalcemia.

OTHER TUMORS

Multiple myeloma has been associated with hypercalcemia in dogs. In one study 10 of 60 dogs (16.6 per cent) with multiple myeloma had hypercalcemia.[45] Fifty per cent of the dogs also had radiographic evidence of bony lysis or diffuse osteoporosis. Hypercalcemia contributed to the development of renal failure in these dogs. Hypercalcemia, along with light-chain proteinuria and extensive bony lesions, was associated with a worse prognosis.[45] Although myeloma cells produce osteoclast activating factor, there is actually a relatively poor correlation between the production of osteoclast activating factor and hypercalcemia.[16] There is only a weak correlation between hypercalcemia and the presence of bony lesions in both animals and human beings with multiple myeloma. This implies that factors other than the production of a bone-resorbing factor contribute to the hypercalcemia associated with multiple myeloma. As in most cases of hypercalcemia associated with malignancy, probably several factors work individually or in concert to produce hypercalcemia. Although the concentration of total serum protein is often markedly increased in animals and people with multiple myeloma, the hypercalcemia is seldom caused by increased binding of calcium by abnormal serum proteins.[46]

Several other carcinomas and sarcomas have been associated with hypercalcemia in dogs. These are singular observations, and none represent a series on a particular tumor type associated with hypercalcemia.[47–49]

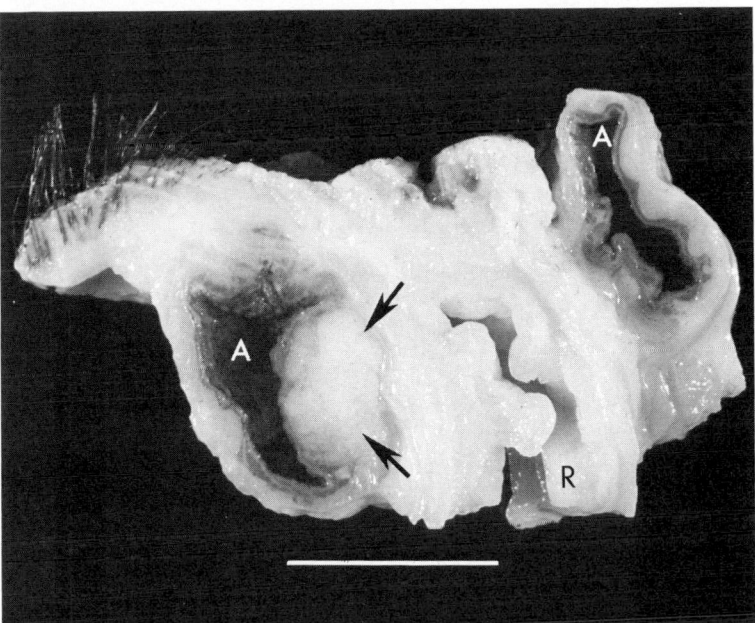

FIGURE 94–4. Transverse section of rectum (R) and anal sacs (A) from an eight-year-old female dog with hypercalcemia (16 mg/dl) and hypophosphatemia (2.6 mg/dl). Adenocarcinoma (arrows) arises from the apocrine glands in the wall of the left anal sac. Despite the small size of the primary tumor it had already spread through the pelvic canal and metastasized into regional lymph nodes. The apocrine glands are visible as a dark band surrounding the lumen of each anal sac. (Bar = 1 cm)

Literally any tumor could produce this syndrome. Several of the reports that identified carcinomas of undetermined origin associated with hypercalcemia may have been describing CA.[47, 49] Lymphosarcoma, multiple myeloma, and adenocarcinoma derived from the apocrine glands of the anal sac probably account for greater than 98 per cent of dogs with hypercalcemia and malignancy.

Hypoadrenocorticism

Hypercalcemia is present in approximately 33 per cent of dogs with hypoadrenocorticism (Addison's disease).[50, 51] Hypercalcemia has been reported in a cat with primary adrenal cortical failure.[52] In dogs the degree of hypercalcemia correlates roughly with the severity of the hypoadrenocorticism, but usually the hypercalcemia is mild, often less than 13.5 mg/dl. Clinical problems resulting from hypoaldosteronism generally overshadow any problem that could be attributed to hypercalcemia. The pathogenesis of the hypercalcemia associated with hypoadrenocorticism is not entirely known, but is probably associated with the following factors[35, 51]: (1) increased concentration of calcium citrate, which complexes with calcium, (2) hemoconcentration results in increased albumin and total serum protein, which contributes to an increase in protein-bound calcium, thereby increasing total serum calcium, (3) increased renal tubular reabsorption of calcium, and (4) increased affinity of serum proteins for calcium, which may be partly due to hyponatremia. Although the total serum concentration of calcium is increased in adrenalectomized dogs, the concentration of ionized calcium in the serum remains within reference ranges.[35]

The presence of hypercalcemia associated with hypoadrenocorticism can usually be determined by clinical laboratory tests. In one report all hypercalcemic dogs with hypoadrenocorticism were azotemic, and most were hyperkalemic (88 per cent) and hyperphosphatemic (75 per cent); many dogs were also hyponatremic and had increased concentrations of serum albumin.[50] A combination of laboratory data that includes mild hypercalcemia, hyponatremia, hyperkalemia, hyperphosphatemia, and azotemia strongly suggests hypoadrenocorticism. Renal insufficiency is the only other problem that could have this combination of electrolyte abnormalities and azotemia. Some dogs with hypoadrenocorticism, hypercalcemia, and/or medullary washout from inadequate reabsorption of sodium can produce dilute urine. In this case dehydrated dogs with hypoadrenocorticism may not have concentrated urine, which will further complicate the clinical distinction between hypercalcemia caused by hypoadrenocorticism and hypercalcemia caused by renal insufficiency. If the laboratory and physical abnormalities can be rapidly corrected by fluid therapy alone, then hypoadrenocorticism is the more likely diagnosis. This diagnosis should be confirmed by determining the serum concentration of cortisol pre-stimulation and post-stimulation with adrenocorticotropic hormone (ACTH). Specific therapy for the hypercalcemia should not be necessary in dogs with hypoadrenocorticism because steroid treatment of the primary problem will correct the abnormalities in calcium metabolism. A complete discussion of the diagnosis and treatment of hypoadrenocorticism is covered in Chapter 97 of this text.

Renal Disease

Primary renal disease is usually associated with normocalcemia or mild hypocalcemia. Occasionally, however, dogs and cats with renal failure will be hypercalcemic.[1, 53, 54] In the dog this is most often seen in such breeds as Shih Tzu, Lhasa apso, and Doberman pinscher, in which familial renal disease occurs. Affected dogs of these breeds will be presented for evaluation when they are quite young, often at less than one year of age. The owners' complaints may involve signs specifically related to chronic renal failure or hypercalcemia, such as stunted growth, vomiting, and polyuria and polydipsia. Although most reports involve young dogs, hypercalcemia can develop as a consequence of renal failure in dogs of any age or breed. A recent report indicated that hypercalcemia was present in 7 of 61 cats (11.5 per cent) with renal failure.[54] The group was not subdivided by age. The increase in serum calcium concentration in these cats was small, the highest value being 12.7 mg/dl.

Patients with primary renal failure and hypercalcemia will be azotemic and markedly hyperphosphatemic, and will generally have isosthenuric urine. It is challenging to determine whether hypercalcemia is due to renal disease or is the cause of it. Polyuria and hyposthenuria are common early signs of hypercalcemia of any cause. These reversible effects of hypercalcemia are due to a reduced concentration of cAMP in cells that normally respond to antidiuretic hormone (nephrogenic diabetes insipidus).[55] Hypercalcemia can also result in nephrocalcinosis, which may be mild and easily reversible, or severe and progressive. Mineralization occurs most commonly in tubular basement membranes, compromising the regenerative ability of damaged tubular epithelial cells, and in tubular epithelial mitochondria, which can result in cell death. The outflow of urine may be obstructed as mineralized necrotic cell debris is sloughed into tubular lumina.[56] Hypercalcemia can also markedly alter renal hemodynamics.[57] In dogs with induced hypercalcemia pronounced vasoconstriction of glomerular afferent arterioles occurred when serum calcium exceeded 20 mg/dl and was less consistent when the serum calcium was between 15 and 20 mg/dl.[58] Because of these renal functional and structural changes induced by hypercalcemia, the temporal relation between renal failure and hypercalcemia is often difficult to determine. This differentiation can be facilitated by a careful search for other causes of hypercalcemia, determination of the presence of hyperphosphatemia, evaluation of kidney size, and examination of urine samples for abnormalities associated with primary renal disease. If hypercalcemia is associated with normophosphatemia, or especially hypophosphatemia, then the serum calcium abnormality is *not* caused by primary renal failure.

The pathogenesis of hypercalcemia associated with acute or chronic renal failure in any species is not fully understood. It has been demonstrated that the development of hypercalcemia in experimentally nephrectomized dogs depends on the presence of the thyroparathyroid complex.[59] Hyperplasia of the parathyroid glands is a characteristic lesion in chronic renal failure, and thyroparathyroidectomy will decrease the serum concentration of calcium and PTH in dogs with hypercalcemia and renal failure.[53] A large fraction of the increased concentration of PTH in the serum of patients with chronic renal failure is the inactive carboxy terminal fragment of PTH. However, it appears that the presence of parathyroid glands and increased serum concentrations of iPTH are important in the pathogenesis of hypercalcemia associated with renal failure. Other factors that contribute to the hypercalcemia are decreased renal excretion of calcium; increased responsiveness to

vitamin D; an increased concentration of citric acid, which complexes with calcium; and autonomous parathyroid gland secretion. During the oliguric phase of acute renal failure there may be deposition of mineral in soft tissues. With treatment and improved renal function the calcium phosphate may be mobilized, resulting in hypercalcemia and hyperphosphatemia during the diuretic phase.[60–62]

Primary Hyperparathyroidism

Primary hyperparathyroidism is infrequently diagnosed in animals.[63–65a] The most common lesion that produces primary hyperparathyroidism in dogs is an adenoma of one parathyroid gland.[65] Carcinomas of the parathyroid gland in the cervical region and cranial mediastinum have also been reported.[66] Familial hyperparathyroidism has been described in two young German shepherd siblings.[67] With either primary parathyroid hyperplasia or parathyroid neoplasia there are excessive amounts of PTH in the serum. Despite marked hypercalcemia the parathyroid glands continue to secrete PTH, and this secretion is not suppressed by the usual concentrations of calcium. The excessive amounts of PTH act on renal tubular epithelium to potentiate calcium and chloride reabsorption and phosphorus and bicarbonate excretion. PTH will also stimulate increased bone resorption and may stimulate both osteoid and fibrous tissue production in bone. Receptors for PTH are located on osteoblasts,[68] and apparently a second messenger from the osteoblast communicates with the osteoclast to stimulate the increased resorption of bone.[69] The net result of these effects should be hypercalcemia, hypophosphatemia, hyperchloremic metabolic acidosis, and dilute urine. Although increased bone resorption is expected in dogs with primary hyperparathyroidism and is present histologically, it is often not detectable antemortem.

The clinical signs seen in dogs with primary hyperparathyroidism are caused by hypercalcemia. These signs include polyuria and polydipsia, listlessness, weakness, seizures, and anorexia. A palpable enlargement in the thyroparathyroid region should not be expected. Primary hyperparathyroidism is seen in aged dogs ($\geq$ 6 years) and there may be a breed predilection for this disorder in keeshonden.[65, 70] A diagnosis of primary hyperparathyroidism should be suspected when the other, more common causes of hypercalcemia have been eliminated and when the laboratory data are more suggestive of hyperparathyroidism than other causes of hypercalcemia. Dogs with primary hyperparathyroidism are hypercalcemic and usually normophosphatemic or hypophosphatemic, even if mildly azotemic. The combination of *hypercalcemia* and *hypophosphatemia* is seen *only* with primary hyperparathyroidism and the hypercalcemia of malignancy. Primary hyperparathyroidism has not been reported in cats.

Most dogs with primary hyperparathyroidism also have dilute urine (specific gravity less than 1.020), and some may have increased serum concentrations of alkaline phosphatase. These animals will also have increased serum concentrations of PTH and vitamin D and increased urine concentration of cAMP.[44, 70, 71] Although these latter determinations will generally confirm primary hyperparathyroidism, they are expensive, not routinely available, and are used infrequently in veterinary medicine. They can be measured in dogs, however, and may provide a definitive diagnosis without exploratory surgery of the neck region. Submit samples to a laboratory that gives specific instructions on how to collect samples for these determinations and that will help with the interpretation of the results. For instance, a concentration of PTH within reference range in a *nonazotemic* patient with hypercalcemia and hypophosphatemia is still indicative of primary hyperparathyroidism even though the serum concentration of PTH does not exceed the reference range. A diagnosis of hyperparathyroidism should be suspected when hypercalcemia and hypophosphatemia or normophosphatemia are identified in an older dog and no underlying malignancy can be found. In addition, combinations of the following data further support the diagnosis of primary hyperparathyroidism: hypophosphatemia or normophosphatemia in the presence of azotemia,[65] a serum chloride–phosphorus ratio greater than 33,[72, 73] absence of anemia (anemia is more likely in an animal with an underlying malignancy than it is in one with hyperparathyroidism), marked phosphaturia, and radiographic evidence of bone loss in the lamina dura of teeth and subperiosteally in multiple bones. Other than in multiple myeloma, radiographic evidence of bone loss is extremely rare in hypercalcemia of malignancy. Administration of corticosteroids will return the serum calcium concentration to reference range if the cause is lymphosarcoma, but not if the cause is hyperparathyroidism.

As an alternative to measuring the serum concentration of PTH to confirm the diagnosis of primary hyperparathyroidism, the thyroparathyroid complex can be explored surgically. An attempt should be made to identify all four parathyroid glands before one is excised. If an enlarged gland is cystic, it probably is not the neoplasm, but rather a cyst of the duct that connected the parathyroid gland with the thymus during embryonic development (Kürsteiner's cyst). The thymus and the internal parathyroid glands develop from pharyngeal pouch III. These cysts are common microscopically in dogs and occasionally are visible grossly (Figure 94–5). If a cystic mass is found in the region of the parathyroid during exploratory surgery of a dog with suspected primary hyperparathyroidism, then exploration should be continued. In primary hyperparathyroidism the lesion that should be sought is a solid adenoma of one gland. There will probably be atrophy of the nonneoplastic parathyroid glands, making their identification difficult. Intravenous infusion of methylene blue (6.6 mg/lb or 3 mg/kg) has been described to aid surgical identification of parathyroid tumors.[73a] At our institution, use of this dose of methylene blue was associated with severe hemolysis precipitating fatal acute renal failure in a dachshund with primary hyperparathyroidism. The best approach to the parathyroid glands is ventral, splitting the sternohyoid and sternothyroid muscles longitudinally to expose the trachea. The thyroid glands will be located on, or lateral to, the first four tracheal rings, and the parathyroids are located just cranial to (external gland)

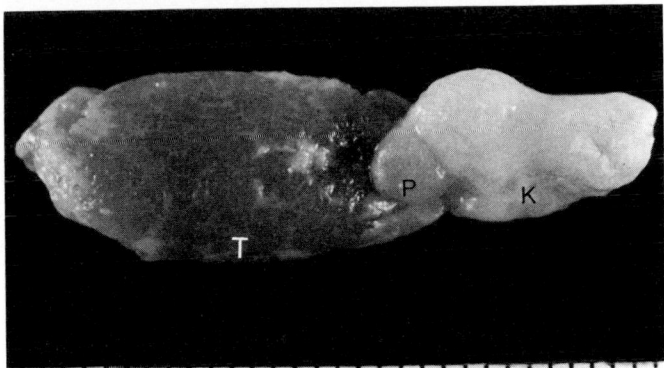

FIGURE 94–5. Thyroid gland (T), parathyroid (P), and Kürsteiner's cyst (K). Laboratory results from this dog included PCV 30 per cent, total plasma protein 9.1 gm/dl, urine s. g. 1.018, UN 234 mg/dl, Ca 9.3 mg/dl, and P 19.7 mg/dl. Kürsteiner's cysts are derived from an embryonic duct that connected the parathyroid gland (III) and the thymus. They are common microscopically and, as evident in this dog, can occasionally be large enough to be seen grossly. These cysts should not be misinterpreted as parathyroid adenomas, which are solid nodules located in the same region. The parathyroid gland is enlarged because of renal secondary hyperparathyroidism.

and on the medial aspect of (internal gland) the thyroid lobes (Figure 94–6). The external parathyroid is normally larger, approximately three to four times the size of the internal parathyroid. The external parathyroid gland is most frequently located one to ten mm cranial to the thyroid in the fascia. The internal parathyroid glands are subcapsular, and are usually located on the medial aspect of the lobes of the thyroid glands. There may be multiple (up to seven) parathyroids per thyroid, but this is the exception. The external parathyroid gland receives blood from a branch of the cranial thyroid artery, and the internal parathyroid gland from multiple small vessels that supply the thyroid. Special attention is required to protect the blood supply to these tissues and not to damage the recurrent laryngeal nerve.

The identification and removal of a parathyroid adenoma may be relatively easy compared with the postoperative care required by these patients. Most dogs with a parathyroid adenoma will become hypocalcemic

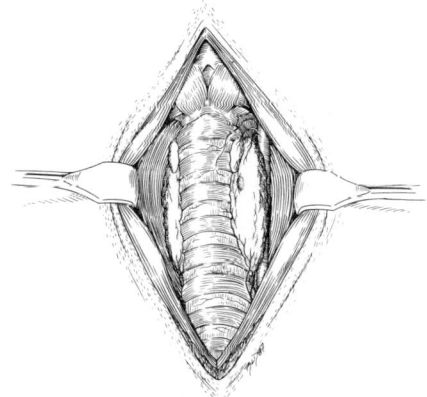

FIGURE 94–6. Ventral approach to the thyroid and parathyroid glands in the cat. The external parathyroid is outside the capsule on the cranial aspect of the thyroid gland. The subcapsular location of the internal parathyroid is indicated by the shaded dot on the left thyroid gland. The internal parathyroid glands are difficult to visualize and will be excised during bilateral thyroidectomy. Care must be taken to preserve the external parathyroids and their blood supply from the cranial thyroid artery.

within 96 hours of tumor removal.[65] Hypocalcemic dogs may exhibit nervousness, excitement, muscle tremors, muscle cramping, stiff gait, tetany, and/or convulsions. If clinical signs are present and hypocalcemia is confirmed, then intravenous treatment with a calcium preparation and/or subcutaneous calcium should be started. If clinical signs are not present, these dogs can be treated orally with vitamin D and/or calcium. Treatment will be needed until the remaining parathyroid tissues start to function properly and can maintain the serum calcium within reference ranges (see Puerperal Tetany below).

Familial hyperparathyroidism has been described in two German shepherd pups. These puppies had hypercalcemia, hypophosphatemia, increased fractional excretion of phosphorus, autonomous secretion of iPTH, and hyperplasia of all four parathyroid glands.[67] The infusion of intravenous calcium to one of the pups would not suppress iPTH. Neither pup was azotemic at the time of initial diagnosis. At necropsy there was diffuse hyperplasia of parathyroid chief cells in all parathyroid glands, nodular hyperplasia of thyroid C cells, fibrous osteodystrophy, hypercalcemic nephropathy, and extensive mineralization of the pulmonary and gastric tissues. The sire and dam were half siblings, and one pup from an earlier litter had clinical problems and radiographic lesions comparable with those found in these two pups. Although primary parathyroid hyperplasia is a rare cause of hypercalcemia, if it were diagnosed, subtotal parathyroidectomy of three of the four parathyroid glands would be recommended. The best gland to leave would be the one in which the blood supply to the gland was clearly identified and was left undisturbed.

Perhaps the most difficult cause of hypercalcemia to diagnose would be that of an ectopic parathyroid adenoma.[66] These tumors occasionally arise from nests of parathyroid tissue located in the cranial mediastinum. The clinical and laboratory findings mimic those of other causes of primary hyperparathyroidism. However, at exploratory surgery of the neck, an enlarged parathyroid gland would not be found. If all the clinical and laboratory evidence still suggests primary hyperparathyroidism, it will be essential to establish that diagnosis before exploring the thoracic cavity for a mass on or near the cranial portion of the pericardium. The best way to confirm this diagnosis would be to determine that the serum concentration of PTH is increased *or* inappropriately high (perhaps even within reference range) for the serum concentration of calcium. The concentration of iPTH should also be determined after removal of the mass and the tumor evaluated microscopically and perhaps with immunohistochemistry to determine if it contains iPTH. The diagnosis of primary hyperparathyroidism owing to an ectopic parathyroid neoplasm would be confirmed if (1) the serum calcium returns to the reference range or below after the tumor is excised, (2) a postoperative decrease in iPTH occurs, and (3) iPTH can be identified in the tumor.

If the diagnosis and treatment of primary hyperparathyroidism are carried out early in the course of the disease, then the prognosis for patients with this problem may be much better than previously thought. In a recent study of 21 dogs with hypercalcemia and primary hyperparathyroidism, 19 had the tumor surgically removed.[65]

Three of these dogs died within two weeks of surgery; however, 16 dogs lived for an extended postoperative period. Eight of these 16 dogs lived 9 to 37 months after removal of the parathyroid tumor and died of causes unrelated to the tumor. The remaining dogs were still alive at the time of publication.

Bone Disease

The increased resorption of bone secondary to septic osteomyelitis, primary and secondary tumors of bone, and disuse osteoporosis is an uncommon cause of hypercalcemia in animals. The mild hypercalcemia associated with disuse osteoporosis is associated with increased bone resorption and urinary hydroxyproline excretion, decreased bone production, hypercalciuria, and osteopenia.[74, 75] Decreased bone formation has been reported in the extremities of dogs and ponies immobilized with plaster casts as well as in laboratory rodents held in a weightless environment.[76] Bacterial and mycotic infections of bone can produce hypercalcemia in dogs and cats. The inflammation associated with septic lesions apparently causes sufficient destruction of bone to mobilize an excess amount of calcium, exceeding the renal compensatory mechanisms. Bone-resorbing factors such as prostaglandins and osteoclast-activating factor are produced by monocytes and activated lymphocytes, and are important mediators of bone resorption associated with chronic inflammatory lesions.[77, 78] Endotoxin can stimulate osteolytic activity of viable macrophages.[79] Furthermore, if the lesions associated with these septic problems are granulomatous, then it is possible that the hypercalcemia may be due to a mechanism comparable with that seen in sarcoidosis and other granulomatous diseases of humans.[80, 81] In sarcoidosis, increased production of 1,25-dihydroxyvitamin D by the granulomas and increased sensitivity of the body to vitamin D result in hypercalcemia.[80]

Several reports indicate that tumors metastatic to bone are more common in the dog and cat than previously suspected.[82, 83] These reports did not include clinical laboratory data; therefore, the percentage of dogs and cats with bone metastases that have increased serum concentrations of calcium, phosphorus, and/or alkaline phosphatase is unknown. It would seem, however, that hypercalcemia is uncommonly associated with secondary bone tumors in animals. The opposite is true in human medicine, in which bone metastases from breast carcinoma are one of the most common causes of hypercalcemia.[84, 85] Presumably animals with hypercalcemia secondary to bone metastases would also be hyperphosphatemic and possibly would have an increased alkaline phosphatase owing to increased bone turnover.

Epithelial tumors are the neoplasms most likely to spread to bone in dogs and cats. Mammary gland, liver, lung, and prostate carcinomas are the most common secondary bone tumors identified in dogs. The most likely sites for tumor metastases in dogs are the proximal ends of long bones and the vertebrae.[82] In one study all dogs that had bone metastases also had concurrent metastases in soft tissues. In cats the local invasion of bone by a tumor was more common than distant metastases.[83] Squamous cell carcinoma that invaded the bones of the skull was the most common secondary tumor of bone in cats. Cats with secondary or primary bone tumors rarely have metastases in soft tissues.

Blastomycosis

Hypercalcemia associated with blastomycosis has been described in several dogs.[86, 87] It was concluded that the hypercalcemia was due to the blastomycosis infection and the granulomatous inflammation.[86] Although all dogs had some degree of azotemia, it was suggested that renal disease was a consequence of the persistent hypercalcemia rather than a cause of it. In the dogs evaluated and with the methods used, parathyroid hyperplasia or extensive bone lesions were not detected. The serum concentration of calcium returned to the reference range in two dogs after successful treatment of the blastomycosis.[86] It was further suggested that increased production of 1,25-dihydroxyvitamin D by mononuclear cells in the granulomas may have been the mechanism of hypercalcemia in these dogs with extensive granulomatous disease.[86] A comparable pathogenesis has been speculated for hypercalcemia associated with sarcoidosis, tuberculosis, a variety of other granulomatous diseases, as well as several neoplasms in humans.[13, 14, 24, 80, 81, 88, 89] It is important to determine if hypercalcemia and/or azotemia is present in dogs with blastomycosis before initiating treatment with nephrotoxic drugs. Although not reported, we have also seen hypercalcemia associated with histoplasmosis and coccidioidomycosis[90] in dogs. Because the disease caused by blastomycosis or the other mycotic organisms is usually so severe, recognition of hypercalcemia is often a fortuitous finding. Treatment of the mycotic disease should also remedy the hypercalcemia. It is important to rule out a systemic mycotic infection before using corticosteroids as a diagnostic test for hypercalcemia associated with occult lymphosarcoma. This can usually be accomplished by critical evaluation of pulmonary radiographs, aspirational cytology of enlarged lymph nodes, and cytologic examination of impression films from any ulcerated skin lesion.

Hypervitaminosis D

The excessive intake of vitamin D can cause hypercalcemia and hyperphosphatemia in dogs and cats. The most common source of vitamin D in veterinary medicine is the administration of vitamin D to patients with spontaneous hypoparathyroidism or in the postoperative treatment of primary hyperparathyroidism. Overzealous supplementation of diets with vitamin D and ingestion of plants containing glycosides of vitamin D will also cause hypercalcemia. Iatrogenic intoxication with vitamin D is accomplished relatively easily because of the cumulative effect of vitamin D and its continued action even after therapy is stopped. The ingestion of toxic plants containing glycosides of vitamin D is best documented in horses and cattle.[91] Plants containing glycosides of vitamin D include *Cestrum diurnum* (day jes-

samine), *Solanum malacoxylon*, and *Trisetum flavescens*. The use of the common name "day jessamine" instead of the botanical name *Cestrum diurnum* could lead to some confusion, in that the common houseplant jasmine could be incorrectly implicated. The active ingredient in the rodenticide Quintox is cholecalciferol, and the lethal effects of this poison are due to hypercalcemia and hypervitaminosis D. Hypercalcemia associated with the ingestion of Quintox has been recognized in at least one dog.[91a] Increased resorption of bone coupled with increased gastrointestinal absorption of calcium and phosphorus causes hypercalcemia and may cause hyperphosphatemia. Although vitamin D is a potent stimulator of bone resorption *in vitro* and *in vivo,* it also stimulates the production of bone. Increased osteoid deposition (hyperosteoidosis), but without mineralization of this osteoid, is one of the lesions reported with vitamin D toxicity.[92]

Hypercalcemia and hyperphosphatemia are the expected electrolyte abnormalities in animals with vitamin D intoxication; however, there may be periods in which the serum concentration of phosphorus and/or calcium is normal.[91] A diagnosis of vitamin D intoxication depends on an accurate history. Mineralization of soft tissues may be detected radiographically in animals with vitamin D toxicity, since in these animals soft tissue mineralization is the most severe of any of the causes of hypercalcemia.

Evaluation of the Patient with Hypercalcemia

Although the list of differential diagnoses for hypercalcemia can be quite long for dogs and cats, the practical list is relatively short (Table 94–1). The first step in diagnosis is to be sure that the hypercalcemia cannot be attributed to the young age of the patient or to sample errors such as lipemia and/or hemolysis, and that the serum concentrations of albumin and total protein cannot account for the entire increase in serum calcium. Second, confirm that hypercalcemia is present on two or more determinations (Table 94–4). The results of a complete history, physical examination, chemistry panel, and hemogram and determination of electrolyte levels will establish the cause of the hypercalcemia in the majority of cases. Concurrent hypercalcemia and hypophosphatemia are rare in small animals, and only *two* possibilities are practical: hyperparathyroidism and hypercalcemia of malignancy. Because hypercalcemia associated with malignancy is much more common than primary hyperparathyroidism the first procedures used should attempt to identify the tumor. In most animals with hypercalcemia of malignancy the tumor is obvious clinically. The tumor most commonly associated with this paraneoplastic syndrome is lymphosarcoma. This diagnosis can be confirmed in the majority of dogs by the cytologic examination of an enlarged lymph node. If lymphadenomegaly or hepatosplenomegaly is not detected, thoracic radiographs should be made to look for a cranial mediastinal mass. If occult lymphosarcoma is still suspected, a trial dose(s) of corticosteroids may be helpful, but this should be done only after infectious causes of hypercalcemia have been deemed unlikely.

TABLE 94–4. EVALUATION OF A HYPERCALCEMIC PATIENT

1. Consider age of patient and influence of albumin and total protein
2. Repeat serum calcium determination
3. Hypercalcemia of malignancy (number one cause of persistent hypercalcemia in dogs and cats)
   Lymphosarcoma (most common tumor associated with hypercalcemia in dogs)
      Evaluation of lymph nodes, anterior mediastinum, bone marrow
      Determination of presence of hepatosplenomegaly
      Response to corticosteroids (after eliminating other causes)
   Adenocarcinoma from apocrine glands of anal sac (second most common tumor associated with hypercalcemia in dogs)
      Female
      Thorough rectal–perirectal examination
      Sublumbar metastases usually present
   Myeloma
      Markedly increased total protein
      Radiographic bone lesions
   Other tumors
      Mammary, pulmonary, and others
4. Hypoadrenocorticism
   Hyponatremia, hyperkalemia
   Na:K less than 25:1
   Azotemia, hyperphosphatemia
   ACTH stimulation test
5. Renal disease
   Usually young
   Azotemia and marked hyperphosphatemia
   Urinalyses
   Evaluate renal size
6. Primary hyperparathyroidism
   Hypophosphatemia or normophosphatemia; *hyperphosphaturia*
   Ratio of Cl to P greater than 33
   Radiographic evaluation (lamina dura, subperiosteum)
   Parathyroid hormone determination
   Exploratory surgery of cervical region
7. Bone lesions
   Lame, painful
   Radiographic evaluation of bones and lungs
   Osteomyelitis: bacterial, mycotic
      Aspirational cytology and culture of lesions
   Secondary bone tumors
      Dogs—epithelial tumors metastasize to metaphyseal region of humerus, vertebrae, femur; soft tissue metastases will be present
      Cats—epithelial tumors invade adjacent bones of skull

The easiest procedure to identify adenocarcinoma derived from the apocrine glands of the anal sac is a thorough rectal and perirectal examination. Radiographic evaluation of the sublumbar region may also be helpful. Animals with multiple myeloma and hypercalcemia will have multiple foci of radiolucencies in bones and a markedly increased concentration of total serum protein, characterized as a monoclonal gammopathy.

Hypoadrenocorticism is the next diagnosis to consider. Mild azotemia and hyperphosphatemia coupled with a serum sodium-potassium ratio less than 25 suggest that the hypercalcemia is due to hypoadrenocorticism. Hypoadrenocorticism should be confirmed by performing an ACTH response test. Marked hyperphosphatemia, azotemia, nonregenerative anemia, and abnormal urinalyses (e.g., urine not concentrated, sediment abnormalities) indicate that primary renal disease is a probable cause of hypercalcemia. Hypercalcemia with normophosphatemia, or especially with hypophosphatemia, even in an azotemic patient, suggests that a nonrenal problem is causing the hypercalcemia.

Primary hyperparathyroidism is a probable cause of hypercalcemia if there is concurrent hypophosphatemia or normophosphatemia, a chloride-phosphorus ratio greater than 33, and marked phosphaturia and a neoplasm cannot be found. Increased serum concentration of PTH in an animal with normal renal function and the problems stated above would confirm a diagnosis of hyperparathyroidism. If these assays are not readily available and the physical and laboratory data are compatible with primary hyperparathyroidism, then exploratory surgery of the cervical region can help to establish a diagnosis and provide definitive treatment. Return of the serum calcium concentration to reference range after removal of the suspected parathyroid tumor, coupled with histologic diagnosis of parathyroid neoplasia, confirms the diagnosis in the absence of measuring serum PTH. Other causes of hypercalcemia are extremely unlikely in dogs and cats. Because vitamin D intoxication requires an exogenous source, historical information will usually establish this diagnosis. Physical and radiographic examinations and radiolabeled bone scans are often the best procedures to identify bacterial or mycotic osteomyelitis or bone neoplasms as causes of hypercalcemia.

Treatment of Hypercalcemia

Although often listed as a medical emergency, hypercalcemia rarely requires emergency therapy. Animals with hypercalcemia may have had this abnormality for weeks or months before it is first recognized. Often the clinical problems are mild and may be due to the primary disease. The animals that do require vigorous therapy are those that are already azotemic, hyperphosphatemic, or dehydrated, or those in which it is known that the hypercalcemia is acute (hours to days). When the calcium x phosphorus product is greater than 70, soft tissue mineralization is probable. Hyperphosphatemia is more important for the development of mineralization than is hypercalcemia. A serum total calcium of 17 mg/dl and a phosphorus of 1.9 mg/dl yields a calcium x phosphorus of 32, whereas a serum total calcium of 14 mg/dl and a phosphorus of 9 mg/dl have a product of 126. The combination of hyperphosphatemia and azotemia will probably result in mineralization of soft tissues. Patients with these laboratory abnormalities should be treated vigorously to avoid mineralization of heart, kidneys, lungs, and stomach. Although some mineralization of soft tissues can eventually be reversed, serious consequences and permanent damage in the heart and kidneys may result. Overzealous treatment of the hypercalcemia before a cause is established may actually interfere with identification of the primary disease. *Before* any therapy is initiated, serum should be collected for routine clinical biochemistry evaluation and a serum sample saved for specific diagnostic tests. Collection of a urine sample *before* therapy is also helpful. Because hypercalcemia is always a manifestation of some other primary problem, recognition and treatment of the primary disease are necessary and will correct the hypercalcemia.

The best symptomatic treatment of hypercalcemia and the one that would be least likely to interfere with establishing a primary diagnosis is volume expansion and diuresis with 0.9 per cent sodium chloride (NaCl). A large portion of filtered calcium is reabsorbed independent of PTH in the proximal tubule and loops of Henle, following gradients established by NaCl and water reabsorption. Owing to the passive nature of this process, calcium transport will be affected by changes in net NaCl transport. The first principle of treatment, therefore, is to administer normal saline solution intravenously to increase urinary calcium excretion by maximizing glomerular filtration rate and urinary sodium excretion. Hypercalcemic patients may become dehydrated owing to vomiting, decreased oral intake of fluids, and hypercalcemia-induced defects in concentrating ability. Dehydration is particularly detrimental to a hypercalcemic patient, as the resultant drop in glomerular filtration rate will stimulate proximal tubular reabsorption of sodium and, consequently, calcium. Dehydration may also potentiate the structural nephrotoxic effects of hypercalcemia. Although fluid therapy will decrease the serum calcium concentration, it often will not return calcium to reference ranges without additional therapy directed against the primary disease. Corticosteroids may reduce the serum calcium concentration through a variety of mechanisms, as mentioned earlier. Their administration should be delayed, if possible, until attempts to establish a primary diagnosis have been initiated, since it could significantly interfere with the diagnosis of lymphosarcoma or hypoadrenocorticism and could be detrimental to the patient if the cause of hypercalcemia is an infectious agent.

Loop diuretics such as furosemide will increase calcium excretion in direct proportion to sodium excretion in normal dogs.[92a, 92b] High doses of furosemide appear to be required, however, to reduce serum calcium concentration in hypercalcemic dogs.[93] In one study a 2.2 mg/lb (5 mg/kg) intravenous bolus of furosemide followed by a 2.2 mg/lb/hr (5 mg/kg/hr) infusion effectively reduced serum calcium concentration, whereas twice-daily intramuscular injections (1.0–7.0 mg/lb or 2.5–15 mg/kg) did not.[93] At these high dosages there is a great risk of causing or potentiating dehydration. A dosage of 1–2 mg/lb (2–4 mg/kg) intravenously every 12 hours has been used if the use of furosemide is required because of a poor response to saline diuresis. It is critical to prevent volume contraction and electrolyte abnormalities by careful monitoring and volume replacement therapy.[94] Thiazide diuretics should be *avoided* because they decrease the urinary excretion of calcium and may contribute to or cause hypercalcemia.

A variety of other therapies have been suggested for hypercalcemia.[73, 95] However, their use is usually precluded by toxicity, lack of information on dosages for the dog and cat, and lack of availability. Fortunately symptomatic treatment is generally not necessary once the primary problem has been identified and treated.

HYPOCALCEMIA

General Considerations

Hypocalcemia is a common laboratory abnormality in dogs and cats. In one survey of nearly 2000 samples of canine serum, hypocalcemia was detected in 13.5 per cent of the samples.[1] Seventy per cent of 262 hypocalcemic samples were due to hypoalbuminemia (50 per cent) and causes that could not be classified (20 per cent).[1] The list of differential diagnoses for hypocalcemia is considerably longer than that for hypercalcemia; however, the practical list, or the list of diseases that are clinically important, is relatively short (Table 94–5). The two most common causes for *symptomatic hypocalcemia* (e.g., tetany) are hypoparathyroidism and puerperal tetany. Most other causes of hypocalcemia do not have clinical signs referable to the low serum calcium concentration.

Hypoalbuminemia is the single most common cause of hypocalcemia and accounted for approximately 50 per cent of hypocalcemic dogs in one study.[1] Hypocalcemia resulting from hypoalbuminemia or low total serum protein is not associated with clinical signs referable to hypocalcemia. Hypocalcemia resulting from decreased serum proteins is usually mild, in the range of 7.0 to 8.5 mg/dl. A total serum calcium concentration less than 6.5 mg/dl is more likely to be caused by a calcium metabolic disorder than by changes in the serum concentration of albumin or total protein. Serum total calcium consists of protein-bound, complexed (citrate, carbonate, phosphate), and ionized fractions. Most of the decrease in serum total calcium associated with low serum proteins is due to a decrease in the calcium fraction bound to proteins (see Figure 94–1). However, if the concentration of serum ionized calcium is measured in hypocalcemic dogs with hypoalbuminemia, it also is often decreased, although only mildly so as compared with the decrease in serum total calcium. Correction formulas have been derived for *dogs* to compensate for the decrease in total serum calcium associated with hypoalbuminemia and hypoproteinemia.[3] These formulas may not be applicable to other species. The correction formula using albumin is easier to work with:

Adjusted calcium (mg/dl) = 3.5 − albumin (g/dl) + measured calcium (mg/dl).

TABLE 94–5. DIFFERENTIAL DIAGNOSIS OF HYPOCALCEMIA

Practical
*1. Hypoalbuminemia
 2. Primary renal disease
   Acute
   Chronic
   Ethylene glycol intoxication
 3. Hypoparathyroidism
   Primary
   Secondary
 4. Puerperal tetany/eclampsia
*5. Unclassified (cause not defined)
Complete
 6. Pancreatitis
 7. Malabsorption syndrome
 8. Iatrogenic chelators
   EDTA, citrates, phosphate, oxalate, ethylene glycol, massive blood transfusion with citrate
   Phosphate enema
 9. Canine distemper virus
10. Rhabdomyolysis–soft tissue trauma
11. Laboratory error, artifact

*Hypoalbuminemia (50 per cent) and unclassified (20 per cent) accounted for 70 per cent of 262 hypocalcemic dogs in one study.[1]

The correction formula for calcium based on the concentration of total serum protein in dogs is as follows:

Adjusted calcium (mg/dl) = measured calcium (mg/dl) − 0.4 [total serum protein (g/dl)] + 3.3.

Application of these formulas to correct for hypoalbuminemia and hypoproteinemia often results in a corrected calcium concentration that is within the reference range. This is just a crude estimate of the corrected calcium value, and depending on the underlying disease, there are probably different correction formulas for different diseases. For instance, some of the highest correlation coefficients of albumin to calcium have been found in human patients with hepatic disease.[96] With different underlying diseases it seems logical that there may be different binding kinetics of calcium not only to albumin and serum proteins but also to other substances that complex calcium, such as citrates and phosphates. To devise correction formulas for each disease would be tedious and would negate the usefulness of a correction formula that can be used when first interpreting an abnormal calcium value.

The purpose of the correction formulas is to determine if a significant abnormality in calcium is present before a primary diagnosis is established. One report indicated that when the concentration of serum total calcium was less than or equal to 6.5 mg/dl, or greater than or equal to 12 mg/dl, these animals had calcium metabolic disorders that could not be attributed to changes in the concentration of albumin or total protein.[3] Young dogs and dogs with disorders of calcium metabolism had concentrations of calcium that were outside the 95 per cent confidence intervals for albumin and total serum protein (see Figure 94–1). Dogs with these conditions had serum calcium concentrations that remained outside the reference ranges after correction formulas were applied.

In several species alkalemia is associated with a decrease in the serum concentration of ionized calcium, supposedly with little or no change in the serum concentration of total calcium. The converse is characteristic for acidemia. Induction of alkalemia or acidemia in awake dogs produces these expected changes in serum ionized calcium; however, changes in serum total calcium were also produced, and these paralleled the changes in ionized calcium.[97] The correlation coefficients for serum ionized calcium and serum pH were considerably higher (r = −.96, R^2 = .91) than for serum total calcium (r = −.71, R^2 = .50). Comparable observations have been made in the cat. The practical use of this information may be that determinations of serum total calcium during periods of alkalemia or acidemia do in fact reflect changes induced by the perturbation in acid-base status.

Primary Renal Disease

Chronic or acute renal failure may cause hypocalcemia in dogs and cats. It is apparent that dogs and cats with primary renal failure may be normocalcemic, hypocalcemic, or, infrequently, hypercalcemic. Regardless of the serum calcium concentration, animals with reduced glomerular filtration rates will also be hyperphosphatemic and azotemic. These laboratory abnormalities, coupled with urinalyses, will usually establish the diagnosis of primary renal disease. Several mechanisms may work synergistically to result in hypocalcemia in animals with renal disease. These factors are: (1) decreased renal tubular cells to reabsorb calcium, (2) decreased functioning renal mass and/or hyperphosphatemia, resulting in decreased formation of 1,25-dihydroxycholecalciferol, (3) hyperphosphatemia, promoting deposition of calcium and phosphorus in soft tissues, (4) hypoalbuminemia, and (5) chelation of calcium with oxalate, which may occur if the cause of renal failure was intoxication with ethylene glycol.

The parathyroid glands respond to the decreasing serum calcium concentration by hypertrophy and hyperplasia. If the response is sufficient, then normocalcemia will be maintained, although periods of hypocalcemia may recur. Animals with chronic renal failure and compensatory parathyroid hyperplasia may have lesions in bones owing to the increased concentration of PTH. This increased concentration causes increased bone resorption and will often stimulate the excessive deposition of soft tissue, either fibrous or osteoid (unmineralized), in bones. These lesions result in loose teeth, loss of the lamina dura around teeth (Figure 94–7), marked enlargement of the facial or maxillary bones (Figures 94–8A and B), and possibly soft malleable bones, referred to as rubber jaw (Figure 94–8C). The physical problems in bones may be the reason some of these animals present clinically.

In renal secondary hyperparathyroidism the parathyroid glands are responding to changes in the serum concentration of calcium, and are not the primary problem. If the response is adequate, the serum concentration of calcium generally remains within reference ranges. The parathyroid gland may fluctuate its production and secretion of PTH in response to changes in the serum concentration of calcium that remain within reference ranges. For example, the calcium may decrease from 10 to 9 mg/dl and stimulate the secretion of PTH. A fluctuation in the concentration of calcium of 0.25 mg/dl may affect the secretion of PTH. It is this close regulation between serum calcium and PTH that generally keeps the serum calcium within reference ranges.

Hypocalcemia associated with renal failure is usually mild and not accompanied by clinical signs attributable to the hypocalcemia. However, in ethylene glycol intoxication[98] the hypocalcemia may be so severe that some clinical signs are due to the low serum calcium. In addition, animals in renal failure are often acidotic, which favors an increased proportion of calcium in the biologically active ionized compartment. If intravenous therapy to correct the acidosis associated with severe renal failure is so vigorous as to produce a rapid shift in acid-base balance toward alkalosis, ionized calcium will decrease. This may have detrimental consequences if the serum total calcium concentration was already low. Monitoring serum calcium and acid-base status during fluid therapy may prevent further aggravation of the hypocalcemic condition. Hypocalcemia may accompany the marked hyperphosphatemia, hyperkalemia, and azotemia seen in cats with urethral obstruction. In one study approximately 15 per cent of cats with chronic renal failure had mild hypocalcemia (6.7 to 8.3 mg/dl).[54]

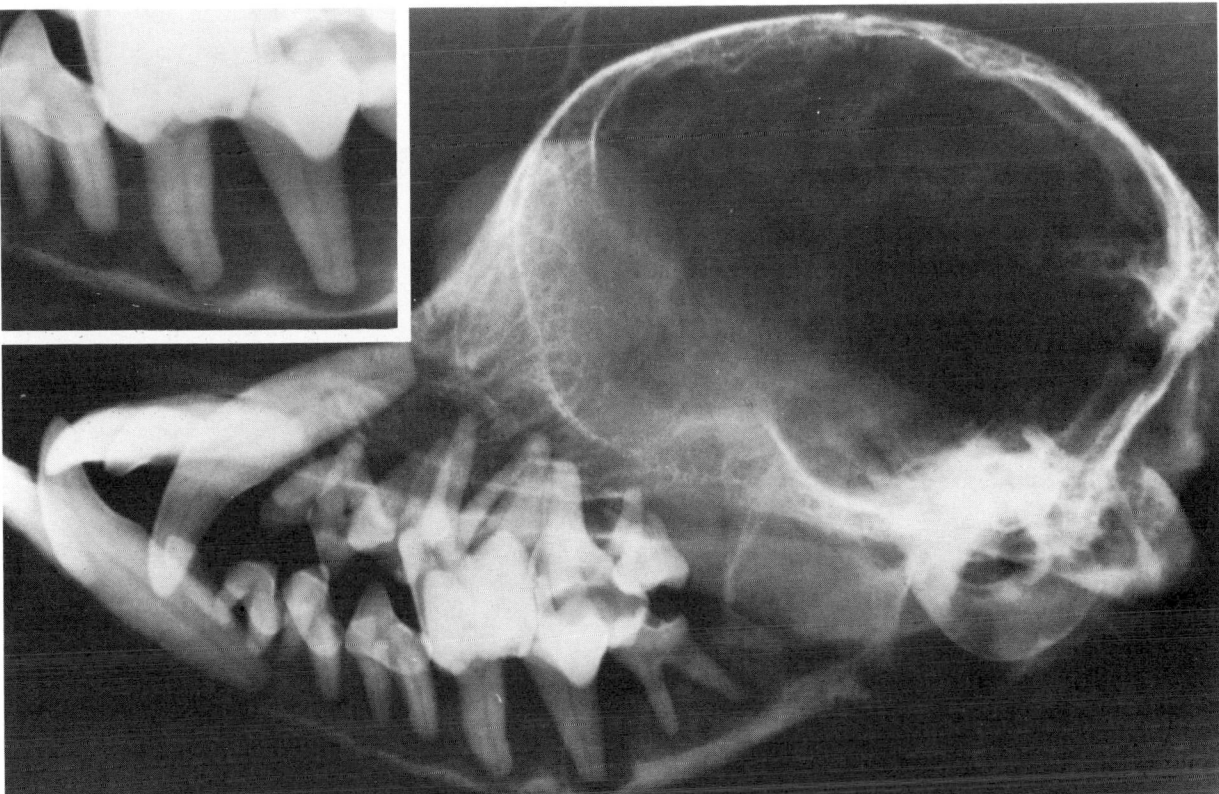

FIGURE 94–7. Marked resorption of bone around teeth and in the calvarium of a dog with chronic renal failure. Laboratory abnormalities included total serum calcium 12.3 mg/dl, phosphorus 11.4 mg/dl, serum urea nitrogen 143 mg/dl, and plasma iPTH >13,000 pg/ml.

Hypoparathyroidism

Hypoparathyroidism is always listed as a differential diagnosis for hypocalcemia, but as a spontaneous condition, it is relatively uncommon in dogs and has not been reported in cats. Hypoparathyroidism is the result of insufficient production of PTH to maintain a total serum calcium concentration and/or ionized serum calcium concentration within reference ranges. This can be caused by the removal of the parathyroid glands during thyroidectomy, destruction of the parathyroid glands by a lymphocytic inflammatory reaction, infarction of a parathyroid adenoma, agenesis of the parathyroid glands, or severe atrophy of the parathyroid glands from prolonged hypercalcemia and hyperparathyroidism.[65, 99, 100] In cats the most common cause of hypoparathyroidism is the inadvertent removal of and/or damage to the parathyroid glands associated with thyroidectomy[99] for hyperthyroidism (secondary hypoparathyroidism) (see Figure 94–6). In dogs the most common known cause of primary hypoparathyroidism is lymphocytic infiltration and destruction of the parathyroid glands (Figure 94–9).[100] Approximately 30 dogs with hypoparathyroidism have been described, and certainly many more cases have been diagnosed and treated but never reported.[73, 100–102] Dogs with hypoparathyroidism are often middle-aged females, but any age or breed could be affected. A consistent finding is that all of the dogs reported with hypoparathyroidism have had clinical signs referable to hypocalcemia.[100–102] These problems include muscle tremors, tetany, seizures, changes in behavior, and an ataxic or stiff gait. These signs occur

periodically. Some of the dogs developed cataracts, which has been described with hypocalcemia and hypoparathyroidism in other species as well. Characteristic laboratory findings are marked hypocalcemia (<6.5 mg/dl) and mild hyperphosphatemia. Hypocalcemia is present in all dogs with hypoparathyroidism, but hyperphosphatemia is not always present. The only other disease that tends to produce hypocalcemia and hyperphosphatemia is renal disease. The distinction between renal disease and hypoparathyroidism is usually straightforward, based on physical and laboratory findings. Furthermore, the hypocalcemia associated with renal disease is not accompanied by detectable neuromuscular disturbances, and the hyperphosphatemia is usually severe.

In dogs with hypoparathyroidism the serum concentration iPTH is undetectable or within reference ranges and is interpreted as inappropriately low for the serum concentration of calcium.[44, 100] In fact the substances being detected in these patients by assays for iPTH may not be measuring true PTH, but rather substances that nonspecifically dissociate the PTH antibody from the radioactively labeled PTH antigen. Comparable results are seen in other species. Therefore, the presence of marked hypocalcemia with low concentrations of iPTH is consistent with hypoparathyroidism. If the serum concentration of iPTH is measured, then the sample should be collected *before* therapy with vitamin D or calcium and when the patient is hypocalcemic.

If the parathyroid glands from these dogs can be found and are examined histologically, the most common lesion is lymphocytic parathyroiditis.[100, 102] The majority of the gland is destroyed and replaced by lymphocytes. Scattered through the infiltrate are small

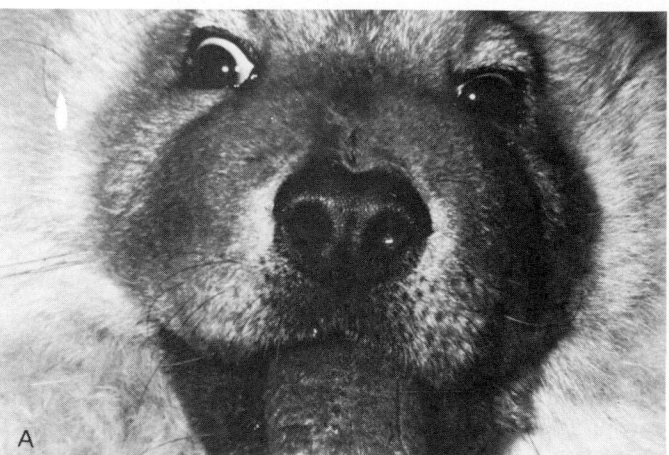
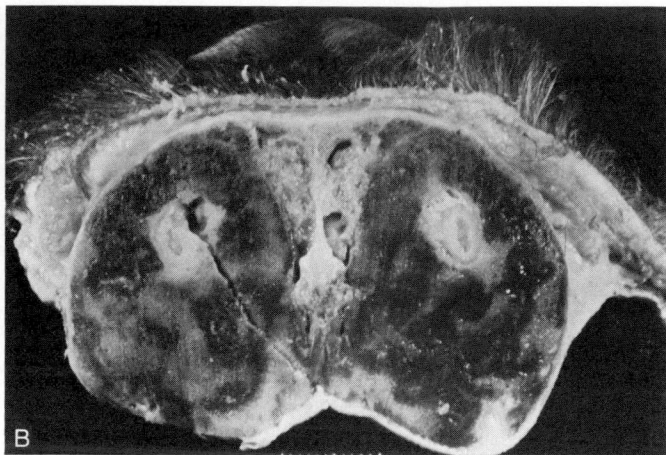
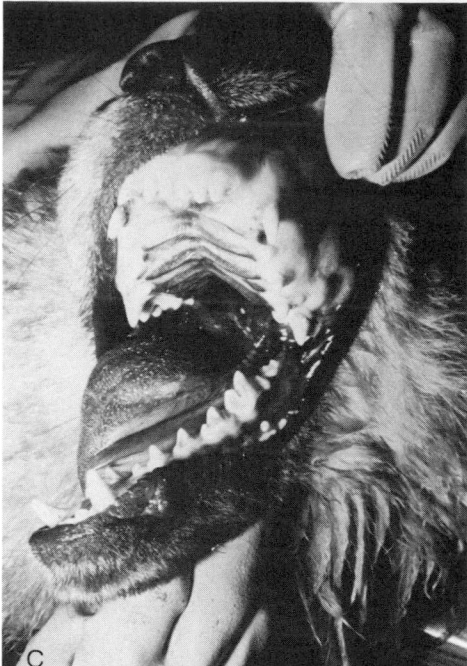

FIGURE 94–8. Chow chow with markedly enlarged maxillae due to renal secondary hyperparathyroidism (A). Transverse sections through the maxillae (B) demonstrate the marked loss of bone and replacement by fibrous tissue interpreted as fibrous osteodystrophy. The fibrous tissue proliferation is so extensive that airways have been obstructed. The dog was presented for dyspnea. The marked loss of bone, coupled with the soft tissue proliferation, results in malleable bones that can be twisted post-mortem (C).

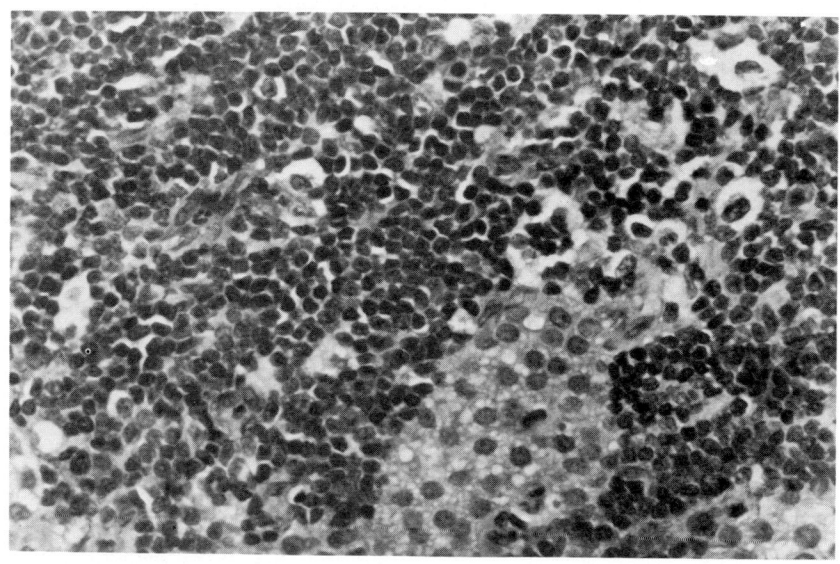

FIGURE 94–9. Parathyroid gland from a dog with hypocalcemia (3.9 mg/dl) and hyperphosphatemia (7.2 mg/dl). Most of the gland has been replaced by a lymphocytic infiltrate. There are a few islands of viable and hypertrophic chief cells. The dog had hypoparathyroidism caused by lymphocytic parathyroiditis.

islands of hypertrophic chief cells (Figure 94–9). It has been suggested that this may be an immune-mediated lesion, and a comparable lesion can be produced by the injection of homologous parathyroid tissue into dogs.[103] The important observation is that the parathyroid glands are physically destroyed and regeneration is *not* expected. Therefore, these animals will require treatment for the rest of their lives. Treatment of hypocalcemia and parathyroiditis is covered at the end of this section.

Secondary hypoparathyroidism is seen in dogs after the removal of a parathyroid tumor that produced iPTH and caused hypercalcemia.[65] In these situations the hypoparathyroidism is due to atrophy of the parathyroid glands induced by the prolonged hypercalcemia and increased concentrations of PTH. Secondary hypoparathyroidism is a temporary problem, and once the glands regenerate, hypocalcemia should not occur. The goal in these cases is to judiciously supplement the animals postoperatively with vitamin D and calcium so that hypocalcemia is prevented yet iatrogenic hypercalcemia is not produced. If this goal is accomplished, the parathyroid glands will return to a normal functioning state so they can appropriately respond to increases and decreases in the concentration of serum calcium. Of interest is that secondary hypoparathyroidism is not seen in dogs with hypercalcemia associated with malignancy after the tumor is destroyed.[29, 44] Although destruction of the tumor by physical removal and/or chemical destruction will result in a fall in serum calcium to reference ranges within 12 to 48 hours after tumor ablation, hypocalcemia is *not* a problem. Perhaps the combination of hypercalcemia and increased serum PTH in dogs with primary hyperparathyroidism results in a greater suppression of parathyroid chief cells than does the hypercalcemia caused by malignancy.

An extremely rare cause of hypoparathyroidism in dogs is infarction of a parathyroid adenoma.[103a] Presumably there is concurrent atrophy of the remaining nonneoplastic parathyroid glands. If the tumor becomes infarcted, there is inadequate parathyroid tissue to produce PTH. The consequence of this is hypocalcemia and tetany. Agenesis of the parathyroid glands, pseudohypoparathyroidism, and production of biologically inactive PTH are listed as other causes of hypoparathyroidism but have not been reported in dogs or cats. These diagnoses at least deserve some consideration when other causes for hypocalcemia cannot be established.

Spontaneous hypoparathyroidism has not been reported in cats. The most common cause of hypoparathyroidism in cats is inadvertent removal of and/or trauma to the parathyroid glands during bilateral thyroidectomy[99] for hyperthyroidism (secondary hypoparathyroidism). Despite attempts to leave untraumatized parathyroid tissue in the cervical region and to leave the blood supply intact to this tissue, hypocalcemia occurs in 10 to 15 per cent of thyroidectomized cats. Not all of these cats will need vitamin D and calcium postoperatively, and some may need these compounds only temporarily. If viable parathyroid tissue is left in the cervical region and/or accessory parathyroid tissue exists in the animal, then, given time, these tissues will begin producing PTH and can maintain adequate serum calcium concentrations. If vitamin D and calcium are needed, the goal is the same as stated previously: to prevent hypocalcemia without suppressing the remaining parathyroid tissue. Vitamin D and calcium independently inhibit the production and secretion of PTH. See Tables 94–6 through 94–8 for recommended doses of calcium and vitamin D.

Surgical removal of the parathyroid glands for experimental purposes in dogs results in hypocalcemia and decreased concentrations of serum PTH. However, these dogs generally do well clinically and do not exhibit signs referable to hypocalcemia even though their total serum calcium may be decreased to 7 mg/dl or less. The concentration of ionized calcium will also be decreased in these dogs and can be below 3.5 mg/dl. Neuromuscular problems may not be detected until some other factor further stresses the animal. This also correlates fairly well with the observation that signs are only present intermittently in animals with naturally occurring hypoparathyroidism despite the constant presence of hypocalcemia.[100–103] It seems that some other factors, such as stress and alkalosis, are needed to precipitate the clinical problems. (Editor's Note: The editor has observed several dogs with primary hypoparathyroidism that developed clinical signs after receiving cortisone injections for skin problems.) One dog with surgical parathyroidectomy had serum total calcium concentrations less than 6 mg/dl, and serum ionized calcium concentrations less than 2.5 mg/dl, was asymptomatic, and maintained a pregnancy until full term. Only during whelping did the dog become tetanic and require immediate calcium therapy. With oral calcium and oral vitamin D she successfully reared four puppies.

Eclampsia (Puerperal Tetany)

Puerperal tetany is a hypocalcemic syndrome seen in dogs and cats and is probably comparable to the condition seen in cows and horses. Along with hypoparathyroidism, it is one of the few causes of hypocalcemia that have clinical signs caused by the low concentration of serum calcium.[104] Eclampsia, or puerperal tetany, is most often seen in small bitches with large litters, approximately two to four weeks post-whelping. However, the condition can occur in a variety of dogs and cats and may occur prepartum. Presumably the hypocalcemia is due to an imbalance in calcium metabolism, such that the influx of calcium entering the serum pool is insufficient to maintain the efflux of calcium exiting through the mammary gland. There is no evidence to suggest that inadequate production of PTH during the hypocalcemic crisis is responsible for eclampsia. In fact dairy cows with a similar condition have adequate production of PTH in response to postparturient hypocalcemia but have an inadequate pool of osteoclasts for PTH to stimulate.[105] The decreased osteoclast pool is due to maintenance of nonlactating animals on relatively high intake of dietary calcium, which suppresses parathyroid gland secretion and stimulates C cell secretion of calcitonin. The defective osteoclast pool is ultimately responsible for the hypocalcemia, and not inadequate production of PTH during hypocalcemia. The paresis seen in cattle rather than the tetany seen in dogs is

TABLE 94–6. CALCIUM PREPARATIONS FOR PARENTERAL ADMINISTRATION

Calcium Salt	Calcium Content (%)	Form	Elemental Calcium Content (mg/ml)	Elemental Calcium Content (mEq/L)	Route	Osmolality (mOsm/L)
Calcium gluconate	10	10-ml vials, 10% solution	9.3	465	IV*	680
Calcium chloride	27	10-ml vials	27.2	1360	IV (only)	2040
Calcium gluceptate	8.2	5-ml vials, 22% solution	18.0	900	IV, IM	900

*Calcium gluconate can be administered subcutaneously if diluted 1:1 with 0.9 per cent NaCl.

Dosage for hypocalcemia: 2–7 mg of elemental calcium per pound per hour (0.25–0.75 mEq/kg/hr) (i.e., calcium gluconate, 0.2–0.75 ml/lb/hr IV; calcium chloride, 0.1–0.3 ml/lb/hr IV). It is critical to calculate the dosage of calcium based on the *elemental* calcium available in each product.

probably due to a combination of the mild hypermagnesemia; failure to release acetylcholine at neuromuscular junctions; increased volatile fatty acids, which are inhibitory to neuromuscular synapses; and the higher threshold for firing of neuromuscular junctions in the cow.[106]

The clinical diagnosis of puerperal tetany is made from the history, clinical signs, and response to treatment. Intravenous therapy with calcium is often started before a serum calcium concentration is determined. Intravenous ten per cent calcium gluconate *to effect* (0.2 to 0.7 ml/lb or 0.5 to 1.5 ml/kg) usually results in rapid clinical improvement and correction of all clinical signs within 15 minutes. A dose of 2 to 7 mg/lb/hr (5 to 15 mg/kg/hr) of elemental (available) calcium intravenously is recommended. For ten per cent calcium gluconate this converts to approximately 0.2 to 0.7 ml/lb/hr (0.5 to 1.5 ml/kg/hr). If possible, do not let the pups or kittens suckle for 24 hours, and if the tetany recurs in the same lactation, the litter should be weaned. Approximately 12 to 22 mg/lb/day (25 to 50 mg/kg/day) of elemental calcium per day per os with or without dihydrotachysterol can be used for the remainder of the lactation. If vitamin D is used, monitor the concentration of serum calcium once a week. Although corticosteroids are also used to treat eclampsia, they have multiple effects by which they should lower serum calcium, and are contraindicated. A successful response

TABLE 94–7. VITAMIN D PREPARATIONS

Preparation	Commercial Name	Dosage Form	Dosage	Time for Maximal Effect	Time for Toxicity to Be Abated
Dihydrotachysterol	DHT (Roxane)	*Tablets* 0.125 mg 0.2 mg 0.4 mg *Oral solution* 0.04 mg/ml	Initial: 0.01–0.02 mg/lb/day for 3 days. 0.005–0.013 mg/lb/day for next 7 days.	1–7 days	1–2 wks
	Hytakerol (Winthrop)	*Capsules* 0.125 mg *Oral solution* 0.25 mg/ml	Maintenance: 0.005–0.01 mg/lb/day or every other day.		
1,25-Dihydroxyvitamin D_3 (calcitriol)	Rocaltrol (Roche)	*Capsules* 0.25 µgm 0.5 µgm	0.013–0.03 µgm/lb/day.	1–4 days	1–7 days
Vitamin D_2 (ergocalciferol)	Calciferol (Kremers–Urban) Drisdol (Winthrop) Deltalin (Lilly) Drisdol (Winthrop)	*Capsules/tablets* 25,000 U 50,000 U *Oral solution* 8,000 U/ml	Initial: 2,000–3,000 U/lb/day. Maintenance: 500–100 U/lb every 3 days.	5–20 days	1–18 wks
	Calciferol (Kremers–Urban)	*Injectable, IM* 500,000 U/ml			
25-Hydroxycholecalciferol (calcifediol) 25-$(OH)D_3$	Calderol (Organon)	*Capsules* 20 µgm 50 µgm	0.1–0.45 µgm/lb/day	5–14 days	1–4 wks
Cholecalciferol D_3	Vitamin D_3 (Freeda)	*Tablets* 1000 U			
	Delta D (Freeda)	*Tablets* 400 U			

TABLE 94–8. CALCIUM PREPARATIONS FOR ORAL ADMINISTRATION

Calcium Salt	Calcium Content (%)	Dosage Forms	Dosages	Elemental Calcium Content (mg)
Calcium carbonate	40.0	Suspension	1.0–1.25 gm/5 ml*	400–500 mg/5 ml*
		Tablets	650–1500 mg/tab	260–600 mg/tab
		Tablets, chewable	350–850 mg/tab	140–340 mg/tab
Calcium gluconate	10.0	Tablets	500–1000 mg/tab	45–93 mg/tab
Calcium chloride	27.2	Powder		0.27 mg/mg powder
Calcium lactate	13.0	Tablets	325 and 650 mg	42 and 85 mg/tab
Calcium glubionate	6.4	Solution	1.8 gm/5 ml	120 mg/5 ml
Calcium phosphate tribasic	40.0	Tablets	1604 mg/tab	600 mg/tab

Food	Amount	Elemental Calcium Content (mg)[113]
Cottage cheese	1 tbsp	25
Cheddar cheese	¾-inch cube	110
Swiss cheese	1 oz	260
Yogurt	1 cup	280
Milk	8 oz	300
Macaroni and cheese	1 cup	400

Dosage for hypoparathyroidism: 12–22 mg of elemental calcium per pound per day in two to four divided doses. It is critical to calculate the dosage of calcium based on the *elemental* calcium in each product (i.e., calcium chloride, 12–22 mg/lb/day ÷ 44–80 mg of powder/lb/ day ÷ 4 doses [derivation: 12 mg ÷ 0.272 = 44 mg; 22 mg ÷ 0.272 = 80 mg]; calcium gluconate, 120–220 mg of tablet/lb/day ÷ 4 doses [derivation: 12 mg ÷ 0.10 = 250 mg; 22 mg ÷ 0.10 = 500 mg]).

*Ranges of preparation and calcium content indicate that there are a variety of dosage forms within the ranges indicated.

to treatment despite the use of corticosteroids probably attests to the body's ability of compensating for our tendency to overtreat.

Pancreatitis

In one series of cases of acute pancreatitis, hypocalcemia (mean 8.2 mg/dl) was present in about one half of the dogs.[107] None of the patients exhibited hypocalcemic tetany. A slight reduction in serum calcium concentration occurs in experimentally induced pancreatitis in the dog and cat but is clinically innocuous.[108, 109] The lowest values occurred at 48 hours (dogs) and 96 hours (cats) after induction of pancreatitis; however, even at these times the serum calcium concentrations were *not* in the hypocalcemic ranges.

The pathogenesis of the hypocalcemia associated with pancreatitis is unknown but has been attributed to the deposition of calcium during the saponification of mesenteric fat, decreased concentrations of PTH, and inability to respond to adequate concentrations of PTH. In experimentally acute pancreatitis of dogs, the serum concentration of PTH increased six hours after the onset and then decreased, but with wide variations in the concentration of PTH.[110]

Further complicating the association of pancreatitis and calcium are the reports of acute pancreatitis secondary to hypercalcemia.[110a] This has been described with several spontaneous diseases that cause hypercalcemia in humans. In cats, experimentally induced acute hypercalcemia but not chronic hypercalcemia increases the permeability of the pancreatic duct to large molecules and increases enzyme secretion in response to cholecystokinin.[110a]

Other Causes

Table 94–5 identifies other causes associated with hypocalcemia in dogs and cats.[110b] Most of these conditions do not have clinical signs referable to the hypocalcemia. Malabsorption syndromes may be associated with hypocalcemia, not only because of the hypoalbuminemia, but also because of the failure to absorb sufficient quantities of calcium. If severe steatorrhea is present, then the loss of fat-soluble vitamin D and intestinal calcium in the steatorrhea may further compound the hypocalcemia. The intravenous administration of chelators such as EDTA and citrate will complex calcium, resulting in hypocalcemia, but this is not a diagnostic dilemma. The administration of enemas rich in phosphates may produce hypernatremia (160–170 mEq/L), severe hyperphosphatemia (12–45 mg/dl), hypocalcemia (<6.0 mg/dl), and tetany.[111] Apparently there is sufficient absorption of the phosphates through the colonic mucosa to produce severe hyperphosphatemia and subsequent hypocalcemia. Massive blood transfusions have produced hypocalcemia in humans as a result of the excess citrate in the anticoagulants. Hypocalcemia has also been associated with the experimental infection of pups with canine distemper virus.[112] These pups had viral particles in the parathyroid chief cells and had ultrastructural evidence of parathyroid gland inactivity. The concentration of serum proteins or phosphorus was not reported in these pups, and a cause and effect relationship between the presence of virus and hypocalcemia was not established. Rhabdomyolysis is a cause of hypocalcemia in humans and may be partially responsible for hypocalcemia seen in a number of trauma cases in dogs. The hypocalcemia is attributed to the deposition of calcium and phosphate in the damaged muscle. If there is concurrent oliguric renal failure (hyperphosphatemia), this may enhance the deposition of minerals in soft tissue because of the increased calcium x phosphorus product. Furthermore, during the diuretic phase of renal failure this mineral may be mobilized and hypercalcemia produced. Collection of blood in tubes that prevent clot formation by chelating calcium, such as EDTA, citrate, or oxalate, will result in *in vitro* hypocalcemia. Serum samples are preferred for the determination of calcium; however, heparinized plasma is acceptable.

Treatment of Hypocalcemia

Hypoparathyroidism and puerperal tetany are the most common causes of symptomatic hypocalcemia and require specific therapy to increase the serum concentration of calcium. The hypocalcemia associated with other causes of decreased calcium rarely requires treatment. Two criteria can help to determine whether the hypocalcemia should be treated: (1) if the total serum calcium is less than 6.5 mg/dl, then treatment may be necessary and (2) if a hypocalcemic animal has signs associated with decreased serum calcium, such as muscle tremors, muscle weakness, tetany, or seizures, then treatment is needed. Animals with hypocalcemia caused by hypoalbuminemia do not need to receive treatment for the hypocalcemia. When the primary disease is corrected the hypocalcemia will abate.

PARENTERAL CALCIUM THERAPY

Puerperal tetany and hypoparathyroidism can be treated with the same dosages of calcium, 2 to 7 mg/lb/hr (5 to 15 mg/kg/hr) of elemental (available) calcium. The higher dosage range should be infused slowly during the initial emergency therapy (4.5 to 7 mg/lb/hr or 10 to 15 mg/kg/hr). Once life-threatening problems of hypocalcemia are controlled, the lower dose range is appropriate ($\leq$ 2 mg/lb/hr or $\leq$ 5 mg/kg/hr). If bradycardia or a shortening of the Q-T interval is detected, the rate of calcium infusion should be decreased. Monitor the serum concentration of calcium as frequently as feasible. Table 94–6 indicates the amount of elemental calcium available in several commercial products. For ten per cent calcium gluconate a dose of 2 to 7 mg/lb/hr (5 to 15 mg/kg/hr) would convert to approximately 0.2 to 0.7 ml/lb/hr (0.5 to 1.5 ml/kg/hr). This is often administered by slow intravenous infusion over 10 to 30 minutes. Lactating bitches often respond to one or two doses of intravenous calcium. Additional therapy for eclampsia was discussed previously. Hypoparathyroid patients may require continued intravenous therapy with calcium until oral vitamin D and calcium take effect. Even then, periods of hypocalcemia, if accompanied by clinical signs, may necessitate repeated intravenous administration of calcium.

Once clinical signs of hypocalcemia have been controlled, calcium can be added to the intravenous fluids (5 per cent dextrose) and infused at a rate of approximately 1 to 2 mg of elemental calcium per pound per hour. Calcium gluconate (9 mg of elemental calcium per pound two to three times per day) can be administered by the subcutaneous route if the tonicity of the solution is reduced by dilution with normal saline solution one to one (see Table 94–6). Calcium chloride cannot be administered subcutaneously. If the underlying cause of hypocalcemia has not been corrected, oral therapy with calcium and vitamin D should be started as soon as oral medication can be tolerated, as the effects of parenteral calcium administration are short-lived.

ORAL THERAPY WITH VITAMIN D AND CALCIUM

General. Although the same drugs are used to treat primary and secondary hypoparathyroidism, the goal of therapy is different for each. For primary hypoparathyroidism (lymphocytic parathyroiditis), therapy will continue for the life of the animal, but with secondary hypoparathyroidism (i.e., removal of a parathyroid neoplasia, atrophy of remaining glands, or damage to parathyroid glands during thyroidectomy) the goal is to eventually stop all medication. It is a difficult task to juggle vitamin D and calcium therapy so that hypocalcemia is prevented yet hypercalcemia is not produced, causing continued suppression of the parathyroid glands. Vitamin D and calcium are both inhibitory to the parathyroid glands and will decrease the secretion of PTH. Many dogs, perhaps the majority, become hypercalcemic with therapy. This is due to the difficulty in regulating the dosages of vitamin D and calcium and the tendency to overtreat. Iatrogenic hypercalcemia is usually mild and asymptomatic. Simply reducing the dose of vitamin D and/or calcium will usually correct the hypercalcemia, but this may take several days, owing to the continued function and body stores of vitamin D. Hypercalcemia is not a desirable effect, especially in treating secondary hypoparathyroidism, since it will continue to suppress the parathyroid glands, preventing their return to normal function.

There are several vitamin D compounds that can be administered (see Table 94–7); however, dihydrotachysterol is often the drug of choice in veterinary medicine. It is administered orally, the cost is reasonable, and the delay in onset of action, as well as the continued toxicity, is intermediate in duration compared with the other vitamin D compounds. This synthetic analog of vitamin D requires hydroxylation in the liver but does not require hydroxylation in the kidney mitochondria, which is the rate-limiting step in the production of 1,25-dihydroxyvitamin D_3 (the most active form of vitamin D). A recommended maintenance dose of dihydrotachysterol is approximately 0.002 to 0.01 mg/lb (0.005 to 0.02 mg/kg) every 24 hours. The drug is administered orally, and during the first few days the dose may be increased to get a loading effect and then be reduced to maintenance levels. Patience must be used before increasing the dose of dihydrotachysterol. Hypocalcemia is not rapidly reversed by therapy with vitamin D because of the delay in onset of action of dihydrotachysterol for several days (vitamin D stimulates the production of calcium binding and translocating proteins in gastrointestinal epithelium). If the patient is mildly hypocalcemic and asymptomatic, then do not increase the dose of vitamin D. Just as there was a delayed onset of action of the dihydrotachysterol, there is also a delayed response (one to two weeks) after the dose of vitamin D is decreased. Hence iatrogenic hypercalcemia can be expected to remain for 7 to 14 days after vitamin D therapy is ceased.

If vitamin D compounds other than dihydrotachysterol are selected, consult Table 94–7 for recommended doses, time required for onset of action, and time required for toxicity to cease. Ergocalciferol (vitamin D) products require hydroxylation in the liver and kidney; they are the least expensive and least potent, and have the longest delay before onset of action as well as the longest continued action (toxicity) after administration of the drug is stopped. Calcitriol [1,25-

TABLE 94–9. INTERCONVERSION FACTORS FOR CALCIUM

Ion	Atomic Weight	To mg/dl from:		From mg/dl to:	
		mM/L	mEq/L	mM/L	mEq/L
Calcium++	40.08	4	2	0.25	0.5

To convert mgCa++ to mEqCa++, multiply by 0.05; to convert mEqCa++ to mgCa++, multiply by 20.

(OH)$_2$D$_3$] requires no further hydroxylation; it is the most expensive and most potent, and has the shortest time required for activity and the shortest time for its effect to stop after administration of the drug ceases. If one of these compounds is selected, then dosages need to be adjusted to compensate for their biologic behavior.

Calcium should be administered orally concurrent with vitamin D therapy (Tables 94–6 and 94–7). It is important to calculate the dosage of calcium based on the *elemental* calcium content of the product selected; to get 1 gm of elemental calcium may require the administration of 10 gm of certain calcium products.

Secondary Hypoparathyroidism. The goal of therapy in secondary hypoparathyroidism is to prevent serious hypocalcemia and give the remaining parathyroid tissue a chance to rejuvenate. If therapy is too aggressive and hypercalcemia is produced, the parathyroid glands will remain suppressed.

Serum concentration of calcium should be monitored once or twice daily during the initial loading period with vitamin D and calcium. This usually takes five to ten days. If hypocalcemia and clinical signs are observed, then intravenous calcium should be given. After the serum calcium is stabilized, calcium should be checked weekly. The dosage of vitamin D and oral calcium should be gradually decreased over two to three weeks, or as needed. A loading dose of dihydrotachysterol is 0.01 to 0.022 mg/lb/day (0.02 to 0.05 mg/kg/day) for two to three days and then 0.005 to 0.013 mg/lb/day (0.01 to 0.03 mg/kg/day) for one week; vitamin D is administered once per day. Once a low normal serum calcium concentration has been achieved, a dose of 0.005 mg/lb/day (0.01 mg/kg/day) can be administered every other day and then every third day and so on, until it is finally stopped. The exact doses chosen will depend on the serum concentration of calcium and must be individualized for each animal. The effect of every dose of dihydrotachysterol will persist for approximately 7 to 14 days. During the loading period with vitamin D, calcium should be given orally two to four times per day at a dose of 12 to 22 mg/lb/day (25 to 50 mg/kg/day) of elemental calcium. After one week decrease the oral calcium to 7 to 12 mg/lb/day (15 to 25 mg/kg/day) and continue a gradual reduction concurrent with the decrease in vitamin D. The goal is to maintain the serum calcium between 7.5 and 9.5 mg/dl, or in the low range of normal. This will permit the remaining parathyroid tissue to establish a normal feedback mechanism with the serum calcium concentration and PTH secretion. Hypercalcemia is a common complication; therefore, do not overtreat. Owners should be instructed as to some of the signs of hypercalcemia: polyuria, polydipsia, anorexia, weakness, listlessness, and vomiting. Cats with hypoparathyroidism secondary to thyroidectomy may require therapy with vitamin D and calcium for several months. The dosages of these compounds for cats is

empirical but should be approximately the same as those used for dogs.

Primary Hypoparathyroidism. Treatment of primary hypoparathyroidism will continue for the animal's life. The goals of treatment are to attain a serum calcium that prevents tetany, not to produce hypercalcemia, and to use as little vitamin D and calcium therapy as possible. The loading dose of vitamin D and calcium is the same as for secondary hypoparathyroidism. After this, dihydrotachysterol can be given at 0.005 mg/lb/day (0.01 mg/kg/day) and then, if the serum calcium permits, at 0.005 mg/lb (0.01 mg/kg) every other day. Oral calcium should gradually be decreased to as low a dosage as possible. Rather than maintain the dog on oral calcium supplements, it may be preferable to administer dairy foods that have a high concentration of calcium (see Table 94–8). After the loading period with vitamin D and stabilization of the serum concentration of calcium, serum calcium should be checked once or twice a month and the dosages of vitamin D and oral calcium adjusted with changes of approximately 25 per cent. Eventually serum calcium may only need to be checked several times a year.

If hypercalcemia should develop, stop all therapy with vitamin D and calcium. If hypercalcemia is accompanied by clinical signs and/or hyperphosphatemia, then 0.9 per cent NaCl should be given and furosemide and/or corticosteroids considered. The hypercalcemia may persist for two to four weeks because of the body stores of vitamin D. When hypercalcemia is corrected vitamin D and calcium therapy can be started but at appropriately lower-adjusted dosages.

Thiazide diuretics may be useful in the treatment of hypoparathyroidism, since they promote the reabsorption of calcium from renal tubules. This has a dual benefit of helping to maintain the serum calcium concentration and decreasing the urinary excretion of calcium, possibly avoiding hypercalciuria and nephrocalcinosis. There is increased urine loss of calcium in hypoparathyroidism because of the low concentrations of PTH. If thiazide diuretics are used, then the dosages of vitamin D and oral calcium may need to be decreased.

References

1. Chew, DJ and Meuten, DJ: Disorders of calcium and phosphorus metabolism. Vet Clin North Am 12:411, 1982.
2. Fletch, SM and Smart, ME: Blood chemistry of the giant breeds: Bone profile. Bull Am Soc Vet Clin Pathol 2:30, 1973.
3. Meuten, DJ, et al.: Relationship of calcium to albumin and total proteins in dogs. JAVMA 180:63, 1982.
4. Mundy, GR: Hypercalcemia of malignancy revisited. J Clin Invest 82:1, 1988.
5. Stewart, AF, et al.: Quantitative bone histomorphometry in humoral hypercalcemia of malignancy: Uncoupling of bone cell activity. J Clin Endocrinol Metab 55:219, 1982.

6. McDonnell, GD, et al.: Quantitative bone histology in the hypercalcemia of malignant disease. J Clin Endocrinol Metab 55:1066, 1982.
7. Doppelt, SH, et al.: Gut-mediated hypercalcemia in rabbits bearing VX_2 carcinoma: New mechanism for tumor-induced hypercalcemia. Proc Natl Acad Sci 79:640, 1982.
8. Ralston, SH, et al.: Hypercalcemia of malignancy: Evidence for a nonparathyroid humoral agent with an effect on renal tubular handling of calcium. Clin Sci 66:187, 1984.
9. Greenberg, PB, et al.: Synthesis and release of parathyroid-hormone by a renal carcinoma in cell culture. Clin Sci 45:183, 1973.
10. Stewart, AF, et al.: Biochemical evaluation of patients with cancer-associated hypercalcemia. N Engl J Med 303:1377, 1980.
11. Rodan, SB, et al.: Factors associated with humoral hypercalcemia of malignancy stimulate adenylate cyclase in osteoblastic cells. J Clin Invest 72:1511, 1983.
12. Ibbotson, KJ, et al.: Tumor-derived growth factor increases bone resorption in a tumor associated with humoral hypercalcemia of malignancy. Science 221:1291, 1983.
13. Breslau, NA, et al.: Hypercalcemia associated with increased serum calcitriol levels in three patients with lymphoma. Ann Int Med 100:1, 1984.
14. Shigeno, C, et al.: Identification of 1,24(R)-dihydroxyvitamin D_3-like bone-resorbing lipid in a patient with cancer associated hypercalcemia. J Clin Endocrinol Metab 61:761, 1985.
15. Tashjian, AH, Jr.: Role of prostaglandins in the production of hypercalcemia by tumors. Cancer Res 38:4138, 1978.
16. Mundy, GR, et al.: Bone-resorbing activity in supernatants from lymphoid cell lines. N Engl J Med 290:869, 1974.
17. Dodd, RC, et al.: Lymphokine-induced monocytic differentiation as a possible mechanism for hypercalcemia associated with adult T-cell lymphoma. Cancer Res 45:2501, 1985.
18. Kondo, Y, et al.: Association of hypercalcemia with tumors producing colony-stimulating factor(s). Cancer Res 43:2368, 1983.
19. Bringhurst, FR, et al.: Humoral hypercalcemia of malignancy. J Clin Invest 77:456, 1986.
20. Simpson, EL, et al.: Absence of parathyroid hormone messenger RNA in nonparathyroid tumors associated with hypercalcemia. N Engl J Med 309:325, 1983.
21. Rude, RK, et al.: Urinary and nephrogenous adenosine 3',5'-monophosphate in the hypercalcemia of malignancy. J Clin Endocrinol Metab 52:765, 1981.
22. Delmas, PD, et al.: Serum bone γ carboxyglutamic acid-containing protein in primary hyperparathyroidism and in malignant hypercalcemia. J Clin Invest 77:985, 1986.
23. D'Souza, SM, et al.: Failure of parathyroid hormone antagonists to inhibit in vitro bone resorbing activity produced by two animal models of the humoral hypercalcemia of malignancy. J Clin Invest 74:1104, 1984.
23a. Suva, LT, et al.: A parathyroid hormone-related protein implicated in malignant hypercalcemia: cloning and expression. Science 237:893, 1987.
23b. Thompson, DD, et al.: Direct action of the parathyroid hormone-like human hypercalcemic factor on bone. Proc Natl Acad Sci USA 85:5673, 1988.
23c. Mangin, M., et al.: Identification of a cDNA encoding a parathyroid hormone-like peptide from a human tumor associated with humoral hypercalcemia of malignancy. Proc Natl Acad Sci USA 85:597, 1988.
23d. Rodda, CP: Evidence for a novel parathyroid hormone-related protein in fetal lamb parathyroid glands and sheep placenta: comparisons with a similar protein implicated in humoral hypercalcemia of malignancy. J Endocrinol 117:261, 1988.
24. Ralston, SH, et al.: Circulating vitamin D metabolites and hypercalcemia of malignancy. Acta Endocrinol 106:556, 1984.
25. Insogna, KL, et al.: Biochemical and histomorphometric characterization of a rat model for humoral hypercalcemia of malignancy. Endocrinology 114:888, 1984.
26. Carlson, HE, et al.: Hypercalcemia in rats bearing growth hormone and prolactin secreting transplantable pituitary tumors. Endocrinology 117:1602, 1985.
27. Rosol, TJ, et al.: Humoral hypercalcemia of malignancy in nude mouse model of a canine adenocarcinoma derived from apocrine glands of the anal sac. Lab Invest 54:679, 1986.

28. Gkonos, PJ, et al.: Squamous carcinoma model of humoral hypercalcemia of malignancy. Endocrinology 115:2384, 1984.
29. Weller, RE, et al.: Chemotherapeutic responses in dogs with lymphosarcoma and hypercalcemia. JAVMA 181:891, 1982.
30. Heath, H, III, et al.: Canine lymphosarcoma: A model for study of the hypercalcemia of cancer. Calcif Tissue Int 30:127, 1980.
31. Meuten, DJ, et al.: Hypercalcemia in dogs with lymphosarcoma: Biochemical, ultrastructural and histomorphometric investigations. Lab Invest 49:553, 1983.
32. Strumpf, M, et al.: Effects of glucocorticoids on osteoclast-activating factor. J Lab Clin Med 92:772, 1978.
33. Raisz, LG, et al.: Effect of glucocorticoids on bone resorptions in tissue culture. Endocrinology 90:961, 1972.
34. Yoneda, T and Mundy, RG: Release of the lymphokine osteoclast activating factor requires cyclic AMP accumulation. Calcif Tissue Int 34:204, 1982.
35. Walser, M, et al.: The hypercalcemia of adrenal insufficiency. J Clin Invest 42:456, 1963.
36. Chew, DJ, et al.: Pseudohyperparathyroidism in a cat. JAAHA 11:46, 1975.
37. Engleman, RW, et al.: Hypercalcemia in cats with feline-leukemia-virus-associated leukemia-lymphoma. Cancer 56:777, 1985.
38. Zenoble, RD and Rowland, GN: Hypercalcemia and proliferative, myelosclerotic bone reaction associated with feline leukovirus infection in a cat. JAVMA 175:591, 1979.
39. Norrdin, RW and Powers, BE: Bone changes in hypercalcemia malignancy in dogs. JAVMA 183(4):441, 1983.
40. Weir, EC, et al.: Humoral hypercalcemia of malignancy in canine lymphosarcoma. Endocrinology 122:602, 1988.
40a. Ikeda, K, et al.: Identification of transcripts encoding a parathyroid hormone-like peptide in messenger RNAs from a variety of human and animal tumors associated with humoral hypercalcemia of malignancy. J Clin Invest 81:2010, 1988.
41. Rijnberk, et al.: Pseudohyperparathyroidism associated with perirectal adenocarcinomas in elderly female dogs. Tijdschr Diergneeskd 103:1069, 1978.
42. Meuten, DJ, et al.: Hypercalcemia associated with an adenocarcinoma derived from the apocrine glands of the anal sac. Vet Pathol 18:454, 1981.
43. Goldschmidt, MH and Zoltowski, C: Anal sac gland adenocarcinoma in the dog: 14 cases. J Small Anim Pract 22:119, 1981.
44. Meuten, DJ, et al.: Hypercalcemia in dogs with adenocarcinoma derived from apocrine glands of the anal sac. Lab Invest 48:428, 1983.
44a. Rosol, TJ, et al.: Inhibition of in vitro bone resorption by a parathyroid hormone receptor antagonist in the canine adenocarcinoma model of humoral hypercalcemia of malignancy. Endocrinology 122:2098, 1988.
45. Matus, RE, et al.: Prognostic factors for multiple myeloma in the dog. JAVMA 188:1288, 1986.
46. Annesley, TM, et al.: Artifactual hypercalcemia in multiple myeloma. Mayo Clin Proc 57:572, 1982.
47. Zenoble, RD, et al.: Adenocarcinoma and hypercalcemia in a dog. Vet Pathol 16:122, 1979.
48. Wilson, RB and Bronstad, DC: Hypercalcemia associated with nasal adenocarcinoma in a dog. JAVMA 182:1246, 1983.
49. Weller, RE, et al.: Paraneoplasia and hypercalcemia. Calif Vet 34:25, 1980.
50. Peterson, ME and Feinman, JM: Hypercalcemia associated with hypoadrenocorticism in sixteen dogs. JAVMA 181:802, 1982.
51. Willard, MD, et al.: Canine hypoadrenocorticism: Report of 37 cases and review of 39 previously reported cases. JAVMA 180:59, 1982.
52. Johnessee, JS, et al.: Primary hypoadrenocorticism in a cat. JAVMA 183:881, 1982.
53. Finco, PR and Rowland, GN: Hypercalcemia secondary to chronic renal failure in the dog: A report of four cases. JAVMA 173:900, 1978.
54. DiBartola, SP, et al.: Clinicopathologic findings associated with chronic renal disease in cats: 74 cases (1973-1984). JAVMA 190:1196, 1987.
55. Jamison, RL and Maffly, RH: The urinary concentrating mechanism. N Engl J Med 295:1059, 1976.
56. Duffy, JL, et al.: Acute calcium nephropathy. Arch Pathol 91:340, 1971.
57. Benabe, JE and Maktinez-Maldonado, M: Hypercalcemic nephropathy. Arch Intern Med 138:777, 1978.

58. Liu, LE: Renal function in hypercalcemic dogs during hydropenia and during saline infusion. Acta Physiol Scand 106:177, 1979.
59. Tuna, SN and Mallette, LE: Hypercalcemia after nephrectomy in the dog: role of the kidneys and parathyroid glands. J Lab Med 102(2):213, 1983.
60. Fuss, M, et al.: Parathyroid hormone and calcium blood levels in acute renal failure. Nephron 20:196, 1978.
61. Llach, F, et al.: The pathophysiology of altered calcium metabolism in rhabdomyolysis-induced acute renal failure. N Engl J Med 305:117, 1981.
62. Segal, AJ, et al.: Hypercalcemia during the diuretic phase of acute renal failure. Ann Intern Med 68:1066, 1968.
63. Carrillo, JM, et al.: Primary hyperparathyroidism in a dog. JAVMA 174:67, 1979.
64. Wilson, JW, et al.: Primary hyperparathyroidism in a dog. JAVMA 164:942, 1974.
65. Berger, B and Feldman, EC: Primary hyperparathyroidism in dogs: 21 cases (1976–1986). JAVMA 191:350, 1987.
65a. Ihle, SL, et al.: Seizures as a manifestation of primary hyperparathyroidism in a dog. JAVMA 192:71, 1988.
66. Patnaik, AK, et al.: Mediastinal parathyroid adenocarcinoma in a dog. Vet Pathol 15:55, 1978.
67. Thompson KG, et al.: Primary hyperparathyroidism in German shepherd dogs. Vet Pathol 21:370, 1984.
68. Rouleau, MF, et al.: Parathyroid hormone binding in vivo to renal, hepatic and skeletal tissues of the rat using a radioautographic approach. Endocrinology 118:919, 1986.
69. Chambers, TJ, et al.: Osteoclastic bone resorption is induced by contact with bone mineral. Calcif Tissue Int 36:455 (abstr), 1984.
70. Weir, EC, et al.: Primary hyperparathyroidism in a dog: biochemical bone histomorphometric and pathologic findings. JAVMA 189:1471, 1986.
71. Fox, J and Heath, H, III: Parathyroid hormone does not increase nephrogenous cyclic AMP excretion by the dog. Endocrinology 107:2124, 1980.
72. Reeves, CD, et al.: The differential diagnosis of hypercalcemia by the chloride phosphate ratio. Am J Surg 130:166, 1975.
73. Feldman, EC and Nelson, RW: Canine and feline endocrinology and reproduction. Philadelphia, WB Saunders, 1987, p 328.
73a. Fingeroth, JM, et al.: Intravenous methylene blue infusion for intraoperative identification of parathyroid gland and pancreatic islet-cell tumors in dogs, Part 1: Experimental determinations of dose-related staining efficacy and toxicity. JAAHA 24:166, 1988.
74. Meythaler, JM, et al.: Immobilization hypercalcemia associated with Landry-Guillain-Barré syndrome. Arch Intern Med 146:1567, 1986.
75. Evans, RA, et al.: Immobilization hypercalcemia. Miner Electrolyte Metab 10:244, 1984.
76. Eagle, MT, et al.: Mineral metabolism and immobilization osteopenia in ponies treated with 25-hydroxychole-calciferol. Cornell Vet 73:372, 1982.
77. Robinson, DR, et al.: Prostaglandin-stimulated bone resorption by rheumatoid synovia. J Clin Invest 56:1181, 1975.
78. Torbinejad, M, et al.: A cat model for the evaluation of mechanisms of bone resorption: induction of bone loss by stimulated immune complexes and inhibition by indomethacin. Calcif Tissue Int 29:207, 1979.
79. McArthur, W, et al.: Bone solubilization by mononuclear cells. Lab Invest 42(4):450, 1980.
80. Koide, Y, et al.: Increased 1,25-dihydroxycholecalciferol as a cause of abnormal calcium metabolism in sarcoidosis. J Clin Endocrinol Metab 52:494, 1981.
81. Felsenfeld, AJ, et al.: Hypercalcemia and elevated calcitriol in a maintenance dialysis patient with tuberculosis. Arch Intern Med 146:1941, 1986.
82. Geodegebuure, SA: Secondary bone tumors in the dog. Vet Pathol 16:520, 1979.
83. Quigley, PJ and Leedale, AH: Tumors involving bone in domestic cats: A review of fifty-eight cases. Vet Pathol 20:670, 1983.
84. Eilon, G and Mundy, GR: Direct resorption of bone by human breast cancer cells in vitro. Nature 276:726, 1978.
85. Galasko, CSB: Mechanisms of bone destruction in the development of skeletal metastases. Nature 263:507, 1976.
86. Dow, SW, et al.: Hypercalcemia associated with blastomycosis in dogs. JAVMA 188:706, 1986.
87. Legendre, Am, et al.: Canine blastomycosis: A review of 47 clinical cases. JAVMA 178:1163, 1981.
88. Lemann, J and Gray, RW: Calcitriol, calcium, and granulomatous disease. N Engl J Med 311:1115, 1984.
89. Kozeny, GA, et al.: Hypercalcemia associated with silicone-induced granulomas. N Engl J Med 311:1103, 1984.
90. Lee, JG, et al.: Hypercalcemia in disseminated coccidioidomycosis. N Engl J Med 297:431, 1977.
91. Harrington, DD and Page, EH: Acute vitamin D_3 toxicosis in horses: case reports and experimental studies of the comparative toxicity of vitamins D_2 and D_3. JAVMA 182:1358, 1983.
91a. Gunther, R, et al.: Toxicity of a vitamin D_3 rodenticide to dogs. JAVMA 193:211, 1988.
92. Boyce, RA and Weisbrode, SE: Effect of dietary calcium on the response of bone to $1,25(OH)_2D_3$. Lab Invest 48:683, 1983.
92a. Eknoya, G, et al.: Effect of diuretics on urinary excretion of phosphate, calcium, and magnesium in thyroparathyroidectomized dogs. J Lab Clin Med 76:257, 1970.
92b. Walser, M: Calcium clearance as a function of sodium clearance in the dog. Am J Physiol 200:1099, 1961.
93. Ong, SC, et al.: Effect of furosemide on experimental hypercalcemia in dogs. Proc Soc Exp Biol Med 145:227, 1974.
94. Suki, WN, et al.: Acute treatment of hypercalcemia with furosemide. N Engl J Med 283:836, 1970.
95. Mundy, GR, et al.: The hypercalcemia of cancer: clinical implications and pathogenic mechanisms. N Engl J Med 310:1718, 1984.
96. Payne, RB, et al.: Interpretation of serum calcium in patients with abnormal serum proteins. Br Med J 4:643, 1973.
97. Meuten, DJ: Hypercalcemia. Vet Clin North Am 14:891, 1984.
98. Thrall, MA, et al.: Clinicopathologic findings in dogs and cats with ethylene glycol intoxication. JAVMA 184:37, 1984.
99. Birchard, SJ, et al.: Surgical treatment of feline hyperthyroidism: result of 85 cases. JAAHA 20:705, 1984.
100. Sherding, RG, et al.: Primary hypoparathyroidism in the dog. JAVMA 176:439, 1980.
101. Kornegay, JN, et al.: Idiopathic hypocalcemia in four dogs. JAAHA 16:723, 1980.
102. Jones, BR and Alley, MR: Primary idiopathic hypoparathyroidism in St. Bernard dogs. NZ Vet J 33:94, 1985.
103. Lupulescu, A, et al.: Experimental investigations on immunology of the parathyroid gland. Immunology 14:475, 1968.
103a. Rosol, TJ, et al.: Acute hypocalcemia associated with infarction of parathyroid gland adenomas in two dogs. JAVMA 192:212, 1988.
104. Capen, CC and Martin, SC: Calcium metabolism and disorders of parathyroid glands. Vet Clin North Am 7:513, 1977.
105. Black, HE, et al.: Ultrastructure of parathyroid glands and plasma immunoreactive parathyroid hormone in pregnant cows fed normal and high calcium diets. Lab Invest 29:173, 1973.
106. Bowen, JM, et al.: Neuromuscular transmission and hypocalcemic paresis in the cow. Am J Vet Res 31:831, 1970.
107. Schaer, M: A clinicopathologic survey of acute pancreatitis in 30 dogs and 5 cats. JAAHA 15:681, 1979.
108. Feldman, BF, et al.: Biochemical and coagulation studies in a canine model of acute necrotizing pancreatitis. Am J Vet Res 42:805, 1981.
109. Kitchell, BE, et al.: Clinical and pathologic changes in experimentally induced acute pancreatitis in cats. Am J Vet Res 47:1170, 1986.
110. Palmieri, BMA, et al.: Plasma parathyroid hormone in acute pancreatitis. Calcif Tissue Int 36:506 (abstr), 1984.
110a. Cates, MC, et al.: Acute hypercalcemia, pancreatic duct permeability, and pancreatitis in cats. Surgery 104:137, 1988.
110b. Abrams, KL: Hypocalcemia associated with administration of sodium bicarbonate for salicylate intoxication in a cat. JAVMA 191:235, 1987.
111. Jorgensen, LS, et al.: Electrolyte abnormalities by hypertonic phosphate enemas in two cats. JAVMA 187:1367, 1985.
112. Weisbrode, SE and Krakowka, S: Canine distemper virus-associated hypocalcemia. Am J Vet Res 40:147, 1979.
113. Peterson, ME: Hypoparathyroidism. In Kirk, RW (ed): Current Veterinary Therapy IX. Philadelphia, WB Saunders, 1987, p 1040.

95 THYROID DISEASES

MARK E. PETERSON and DUNCAN C. FERGUSON

The role and physiologic and cultural significance of the thyroid gland has been under discussion for centuries.[1] In the mid-1600s, Wharton suggested that the purpose of the thyroid gland (most importantly in women) was to enhance the roundness and beauty of the neck.[2] Vercelloni, on the other hand, advanced the idea of a somewhat less pristine role for the thyroid with his argument that "the thyroid is a bag of worms;" his theory was that these worms and their eggs were capable of invading the esophagus to aid in digestion.[3] Parry and Meuli believed the thyroid gland served as a vascular shunt to guard against sudden increases in blood flow to the brain.[4, 5]

However, early in the 19th Century, scientists were beginning to see a correlation between the thyroid gland and various physiologic functions. As early as 1827, experimental thyroidectomies were found to cause death.[6] Of course, the deaths associated with these experiments were largely due to removal of the parathyroids, glands which were not recognized until 1891.[7] A breakthrough came in 1896 when Vassale and Generali separated the entities of myxedema and hypocalcemic tetany following surgical thyroidectomy.[8]

Sporadic cretinism was first reported by Fagge in 1871;[9] this paved the way for Gull's report of the disease in the adult three years later.[10] It was not until 20 years later, however, that researchers reported the successful treatment of myxedema by injection of a glycerine extract of sheep thyroid.[11] In 1893 the British Journal of Medicine published reports of the treatment of myxedema by feeding with lightly cooked sheep thyroids.[12]

The history of hypothyroidism in dogs parallels that of hypothyroidism in humans. In his 1907 paper on the occurrence and nature of thyroid hyperplasia associated with iodine deficiency in the dog and sheep, Marine implied that "cretinism" was already a common and well-recognized entity in the dog.[13] In that report, the author described clinical signs seemingly consistent with thyrotoxicosis, following the feeding of thyroid glands to cretin dogs with goiter. It was not until the 1950s, however, that cases of canine hypothyroidism not induced by iodine deficiency (thyroid atrophy) were well documented.[14]

Thyroid disease in cats, on the other hand, is a recent arrival on the veterinary scene. Whether hyperthyroidism has existed in cats all along is debatable, but the disease was not characterized in the scientific literature until 1979, 144 years after Graves described hyperthyroidism in humans.[15, 16]

ANATOMY AND PHYSIOLOGY

ANATOMY

Canine Thyroid Gland. The canine thyroid gland consists of two separate lobes that lie adjacent to the lateral surface of the trachea (i.e., first five or six tracheal rings). Unlike the human thyroid gland, the connecting isthmus between the two thyroid lobes is usually indistinct in the adult dog, except occasionally in large or brachycephalic breeds.[17] The two normal thyroid lobes of the dog, being deep to the sternocephalicus muscle, are not palpable and have a combined mass of 0.04 to 0.4 gm/kg body weight in iodine-sufficient areas. They are proportionately larger in brachycephalic breeds and in puppies. The size of each thyroid lobe is variable, with the mass of one occasionally exceeding the other by as much as 50 per cent. The thyroid gland is extremely vascular with its major blood supply arising from two vessels, the cranial and caudal thyroid arteries. The cranial thyroid artery arises as a branch of the common carotid artery, whereas the caudal thyroid artery usually arises from the brachycephalic artery and runs along the lateral surface of the trachea to join with the respective cranial thyroid artery. Venous flow from the thyroid gland is primarily from the cranial and caudal thyroid veins, which exit from the respective poles of each thyroid lobe.[17]

Two parathyroid glands are associated with each thyroid lobe, each measuring 2 to 5 mm in diameter and 0.5 to 1 mm in width.[17] The external parathyroid gland most commonly lies on the cranial, dorsolateral surface of the thyroid lobe, superficial to the thyroid capsule. However, the positional relationship between each thyroid lobe and external parathyroid gland varies. In most dogs, the internal parathyroid glands are embedded within the thyroid parenchyma at a variable depth, usually in the caudal portion of the thyroid lobe.[17] Careful thyroidectomy techniques allow the maintenance of the external, but generally must sacrifice the internal, parathyroid glands.

Ectopic or extracervical thyroid tissue is common in dogs and more than 50 per cent of dogs have accessory thyroid tissue near the hyoid bone, along the cervical portion of the trachea, or at the base of the aorta. These sites of thyroid tissue are developmentally related to the primordial aortic sac.[18, 19] Ectopic thyroid tissue is significant in that surgical thyroidectomy will not remove this tissue, resulting in its hyperplasia and, eventually, recrudescence of thyroid function.[20] In addition, ectopic thyroid tissue is occasionally the site of thyroid neoplasia.[21]

Feline Thyroid Gland. In the cat, the thyroid gland consists of two separate lobes that normally lie adjacent to the first five or six tracheal rings.[22] The normal thyroid lobes in the cat are approximately 2 cm long, 0.5 cm thick, and 0.3 cm wide; the combined weight of the two normal lobes ranges from about 0.1 to 0.3 gm.[23, 24] Dorsally, the lobes are in close proximity to the carotid sheath and the vagosympathetic trunk. Fibers of the right recurrent laryngeal nerve pass dorsally in close association with the right thyroid lobe. The principal blood supply to each lobe of the thyroid is the cranial thyroid artery, which arises from the common carotid artery.[22] Unlike the dog, no caudal thyroid artery is present in most cats.[25] The principal venous return from the thyroid gland is by the cranial and caudal thyroid veins, which leave the cranial and caudal poles of each lobe, respectively.

Two parathyroid glands are usually associated with each thyroid lobe. The external parathyroid gland most commonly lies in the fascia at the cranial pole of the thyroid lobe, whereas the internal parathyroid gland is usually embedded in the thyroid parenchyma and varies in location.[25] The external parathyroid glands range in length from 2 mm to 7 mm and can usually be distinguished from the thyroid tissue by their lighter color and spherical shape. The blood supply to the parathyroid glands consists of minute vessels that arise from the cranial thyroid artery.[25]

Accessory thyroid tissue is also very common in the cat and may be found in the neck and thorax.[23] This fact has clinical significance since adenomatous hyperplasia and occasionally carcinoma may arise from thyroid tissue in the ventral cervical or anterior mediastinal region.[24] Such accessory thyroid tissue may explain, at least in part, why most cats are eventually able to maintain normal circulating thyroid hormone concentrations without the need for replacement therapy after bilateral thyroidectomy.

Microstructure of the Normal Thyroid Gland. In both the dog and cat, each thyroid lobe is composed of numerous follicles that are lined by cuboidal or columnar epithelium and contain colloid, a proteinaceous material composed of thyroglobulin.[26] The follicular cell plasma membrane facing the colloid (apical surface of the follicular cell) is characterized by microvilli similar to renal and intestinal brush border membranes. This surface of the cell is the site of thyroidal colloid protein synthesis, hormone organification, and colloid resorption. The basolateral surface of the follicular cell contacts the blood vessels from which circulating iodide is transported and to which thyroid hormones are secreted (Figure 95–1).

THYROID PHYSIOLOGY

Iodine Metabolism. Thyroid hormones are the only iodinated organic compounds in the body. Therefore, the only function of ingested iodine is for thyroid hormone synthesis. The daily maintenance iodine require-

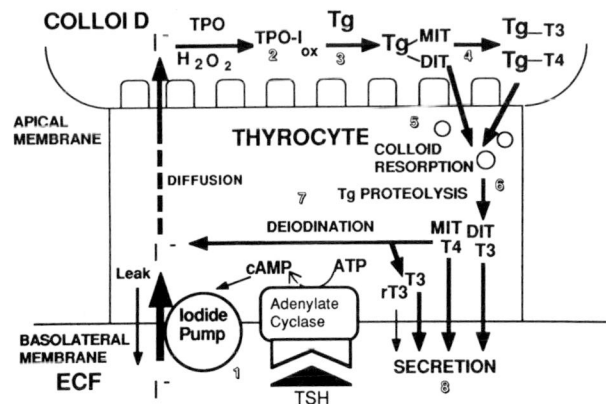

FIGURE 95–1. Iodide uptake, organification, and secretion by the thyroid cell. Step 1—Iodide uptake. Inorganic iodide (I^-) is actively translocated into the thyrocyte from the extracellular fluid (ECF) to the cytosol of the follicular cell. The maintenance of the sodium gradient via the $Na^+K^+ATPase$ appears to be important for this process. This step is stimulated by thyrotropin (TSH) interaction with a plasma TSH receptor and activation of adenylate cyclase. Steps 2 and 3—Oxidation and organification. After diffusion to the apical plasma membrane, the iodide is oxidized by the thyroid peroxidase enzyme (TPO) (Step 2) and organified onto tyrosine residues of preformed thyroglobulin (Tg) (Step 3) to form monoiodotyrosine (MIT) and diiodotyrosine (DIT). Step 4—Coupling. The MIT and DIT residues on Tg couple to form T_3 and two DIT residues couple to form T_4. Step 5—Colloid resorption. Under the stimulus of TSH, follicular colloid containing Tg is resorbed into the thyrocyte. Step 6—Thyroglobulin proteolysis. Thyroid hormones, MIT, and DIT are released from Tg under the stimulus of TSH. Step 7—Deiodination. Also stimulated by TSH at the time of secretion, deiodinase enzymes convert T_4 to T_3 and rT_3 and iodotyrosines are deiodinated to allow recycling of iodide. Step 8—Secretion. T_4, T_3, and rT_3 are released into the bloodstream

ment is about 140 μg for the 20 to 35 lb (10 to 15 kg) dog and 100 μg for the cat. Most commercial dog and cat foods include at least three to five times this minimum requirement for iodine when fed in recommended amounts.[27] As a result, iodine deficiency has become a rare condition in the dog and cat.

Ingested iodine is converted to iodide in the gastrointestinal tract and absorbed into the circulation. The dog has plasma iodide concentrations of 5 to 10 μg/dl, which are ten to twenty times the levels in human plasma.[26, 28] Preliminary data indicate that the normal cat ingesting approximately 250 μg of iodine per day has plasma iodide concentrations that are similar to or even slightly higher than those found in dogs. This nonhormonal iodide bound to plasma protein constitutes about one-half to one-third of the total protein bound iodine (PBI) in the dog, and is the principal reason why PBI determinations are an unsatisfactory index of thyroid hormone levels in dogs.[26, 28, 29]

In the thyroid gland, iodide is concentrated or trapped by active transport mechanisms of the basolateral plasma membrane of the follicular cell, resulting in intracellular iodide concentrations that are 10 to 200 times that of serum. This process is stimulated by the interaction of thyrotropin (TSH) with follicular cell surface receptors, leading to the stimulation of cyclic AMP (Figure 95–1). Although not commonly recognized, tissues other than the thyroid gland can take up iodide in a TSH independent fashion. These tissues, which include the salivary glands, gastric mucosal cells, renal proximal tubule cells, placenta, ciliary body, choroid plexus, and mammary glands, generally do not concentrate iodide to any great extent. However, it has recently been reported that gastric recycling of iodine may be an important factor in iodine metabolism, at least in the normal cat.[30]

Either radioactive iodide or pertechnetate (TcO_4), which, unlike iodine, cannot be organified, can be used diagnostically to assess anion transport function (uptake) by the thyroid gland. Conversely, perchlorate inhibits iodide uptake and promotes efflux of iodide from the thyroid gland.[31] On this basis, oral administration of perchlorate following the administration of a tracer dose of radioiodine can be used to diagnose congenital defects in the thyroidal organification of iodide (perchlorate discharge test).[31, 32]

Thyroid Hormone Synthesis and Secretion. Thyroglobulin, an iodinated glycoprotein with a molecular weight of 660,000 daltons, serves to store thyroid hormone and its precursors.[31] After synthesis within the endoplasmic reticulum of the thyroid follicular cell, membrane vesicles containing noniodinated thyroglobulin fuse with the apical membrane and are released (by exocytosis) into the follicular lumen, where thyroglobulin is stored as colloid.

Once inside the thyroid cell, iodide diffuses down a concentration gradient to the brush border or apical surface of the cell, where it is oxidized to iodine (Figure 95–1). Iodine then diffuses from the cell into the colloid, where it is incorporated into tyrosine residues of thyroglobulin in a process called organification, forming monoiodotyrosine (MIT) and diiodotyrosine (DIT). Thyroxine (T_4) is then formed by coupling two DIT molecules, and 3,5,3'triiodothyronine (T_3) is formed by coupling one MIT molecule with one DIT molecule (Figure 95–1).[31] The thyroid organification and coupling steps are sensitive to inhibition by the antithyroid thiourylene drugs (propylthiouracil and methimazole), which act to block thyroid hormone secretion (Figure 95–1, Steps 3 and 4).[31]

When iodine intake is adequate, production of T_4 is favored. However, in iodine-deficient states and impending thyroid failure, the intrathyroidal synthesis of T_3 is preferred over that of T_4. By this autoregulation, the thyroid gland produces the most active thyroid hormone (T_3 is three to five times more potent than T_4) while using less iodide. Conversely, chronic iodine excess may lead to excessive storage of thyroidal hormone.[31]

An intrathyroidal regulatory mechanism, the Wolff-Chaikoff effect, is key to understanding the potential acute antithyroid effect of large amounts of iodine (see Treatment of Hyperthyroidism). Believed to be mediated via inhibition of thyroid peroxidase, the administration of iodine as potassium iodide to hyperthyroid humans or animals decreases both the percentage of the administered iodide incorporated and the absolute rate of organic iodine formation.[31, 33] In humans, this effect is transient and escape is seen within several weeks. The Wolff-Chaikoff effect may be an intrathyroidal mechanism that protects the animal from massive thyroid hormone release following a large dietary iodine load.

Thyroid hormone secretion is initiated as the follicular cells take up thyroglobulin colloid droplets by a process called pinocytosis. Simultaneously, lysosomes (containing proteases and hydrolytic enzymes) migrate from the basal region of the cell and fuse with the colloid droplets (Figure 95–1). Degradation of thyroglobulin by the lysosomal proteolytic enzymes produces both the iodotyrosines (MIT and DIT) and iodothyronines (T_4 and T_3). Little of the released MIT and DIT enters the circulation because the iodine is removed from these molecules by a specific dehalogenase enzyme (Figure 95–1, Step 7). Some of this iodine is recycled internally for iodination of new tyrosine residues in thyroglobulin, but in the dog (and presumably in the cat) much of the iodine is released into the circulation.[26] This inefficient thyroidal reuse of iodine helps explain the high daily iodine requirements of the dog and cat compared with those of humans.

Proteolysis of thyroglobulin, as described above, liberates relatively large amounts of T_4 but only small quantities of T_3 into the cytosol. Enzymes present within the thyroid gland, however, can deiodinate T_4 to either T_3 or 3,3',5'-T_3 (reverse T_3, rT_3).[34-36] As a result, although the ratio of T_4 and T_3 stored in the canine thyroid gland is 12:1, the ratio of secreted products is 4:1. Production rates of the thyroid hormones in the dog have been estimated to be 1.0 to 1.5 μg/lb/day (2.5 to 3.2 μg/kg/day) for T_4 and 0.4 to 0.7 μg/lb/day (0.8 to 1.5 μg/kg/day) for T_3.[37] Similarly, a recent study of six normal cats found mean ($\pm$SD) secretion rates of 2.5 $\pm$ 0.6 μg/lb/day (5.6 $\pm$ 1.2 μg/kg/day) and 0.2 $\pm$ 0.05 μg/lb/day (0.4 $\pm$ 0.1 μg/kg/day) for T_4 and T_3, respectively.[30] These production rates are more than twice that seen in humans.[38]

Thyrotropin (thyroid stimulating hormone, TSH), a glycoprotein produced in the thyrotrophs of the pituitary pars distalis, has profound stimulatory effects on thyroid hormone synthesis and secretion.[31] In addition, TSH acts to stimulate thyroid growth, probably in conjunction with actions of the insulin-like growth factors (IGF I and II). Thyrotropin has a molecular weight of about 30,000, consisting of an α subunit (identical to the α subunit of the other glycoprotein pituitary hormones LH and FSH) and a β subunit that is specific to the TSH molecule. Thyrotropin binds to a specific receptor on the thyroid follicular cell membrane and stimulates adenylate cyclase, the production of cyclic AMP, and the active uptake of inorganic iodide (Figure 95–1). It also stimulates the synthesis of thyroglobulin, its release into the colloid, and its iodination by thyroid peroxidase (organification). As a final step in the delivery of hormone into plasma, TSH stimulates thyroglobulin resorption and proteolysis to release T_3 and T_4. The thyroidal enzymes deiodinating T_4 to T_3 and rT_3 are also stimulated by TSH.[36]

Metabolism of Thyroid Hormone. The metabolically active thyroid hormones are the iodothyronines T_4 and T_3. Thyroxine is the main secretory product of the normal thyroid gland. However, T_3, which is about three to five times more potent than T_4, as well as smaller amounts of rT_3 (a thyromimetically inactive product) and other deiodinated metabolites is also secreted by the canine (and presumably feline) thyroid gland (Figure 95–1).[34, 35]

Although all T_4 is secreted by the thyroid, a considerable amount (40 to 60 per cent in the dog)[37] of T_3 is derived from extrathyroidal enzymatic 5'-deiodination of T_4. Therefore, although it also has intrinsic metabolic activity, T_4 has been called a "prohormone;" and its activation to the more potent T_3 is a step regulated individually by peripheral tissues (Figure 95–2). The vast majority (approximately 90 per cent) of rT_3 is derived from extrathyroidal sources in the dog.[39] The identification of two distinct types of 5'deiodinase enzymes (Type I in most peripheral tissues, Type II in brain, pituitary, and brown adipose tissue) has underscored the importance of T_3 produced locally from T_4. For example, hypothyroidism dramatically reduces the activity of the Type I 5'-deiodinase while increasing the activity of the Type II enzyme (Figure 95–3).[40] Through this type of regulation, the brain may continue to obtain adequate cellular T_3 levels necessary to prevent or delay neurologic dysfunction resulting from T_4 deficiency, while the liver reduces its production of T_3, leading to decreased systemic metabolism. Although most tissues are able to deiodinate T_4 to T_3, the liver and kidney appear to be the most active.[40, 41] Muscle and skin, although they have low enzyme activity, may produce a significant amount (approximately 60 per cent in the rat) of the body's T_3 solely because of their large mass.[40]

After the formation of active T_3 and inactive rT_3, the process of deiodination continues until the thyroid hormone nucleus is stripped of its remaining iodine molecules, allowing iodine to recycle for hormone resynthesis (Figure 95–2). These further deiodinated metabolic products do not have thyromimetic activity. A number of nonthyroidal illnesses and drugs may affect the local tissue regulation of thyroid hormone deiodination (see Extrathyroidal Factors Altering Thyroid Hormone Me-

tabolism and Circulating Thyroid Hormone Concentrations).[42] Other pathways of thyroid hormone metabolism include conjugation to form soluble glucuronides and sulfates for biliary or urinary excretion, as well as cleavage of the ether linkage between the tyrosine nuclei (Figure 95–2).

In the dog, over 50 per cent of the T_4 and about 30 per cent of the T_3 produced each day are lost into the feces.[43] The authors' preliminary results in the cat indicate that fecal excretion may account for as much as 50 per cent of the daily turnover of T_4 and T_3. In both the normal dog and cat, the extrathyroidal body stores of T_4 are eliminated (metabolized or excreted) and replaced in about one day, whereas stores of T_3 are lost and replaced twice daily.[26] As in human patients with hyperthyroidism, the overall rate of thyroid hormone turnover in hyperthyroid cats is even higher, approximately 50 per cent greater than in normal cats.[30] Both the per cent hormone lost in the feces and overall rates of thyroid hormone turnover are much higher in the dog and cat than in humans. Such fecal wastage is responsible, in part, for the higher daily replacement doses of thyroid hormone required on a per lb basis in hypothyroid dogs and cats.

With oral administration of thyroid hormone preparations, the first-pass effect must be considered. The first-pass consists of that proportion of administered hormone that is absorbed from the gastrointestinal tract into the hepatoportal system, metabolized by the liver, and excreted into the bile before ever reaching the systemic circulation.

Plasma Hormone Binding of Thyroid Hormone. Thyroid hormones are water-insoluble lipophilic com-

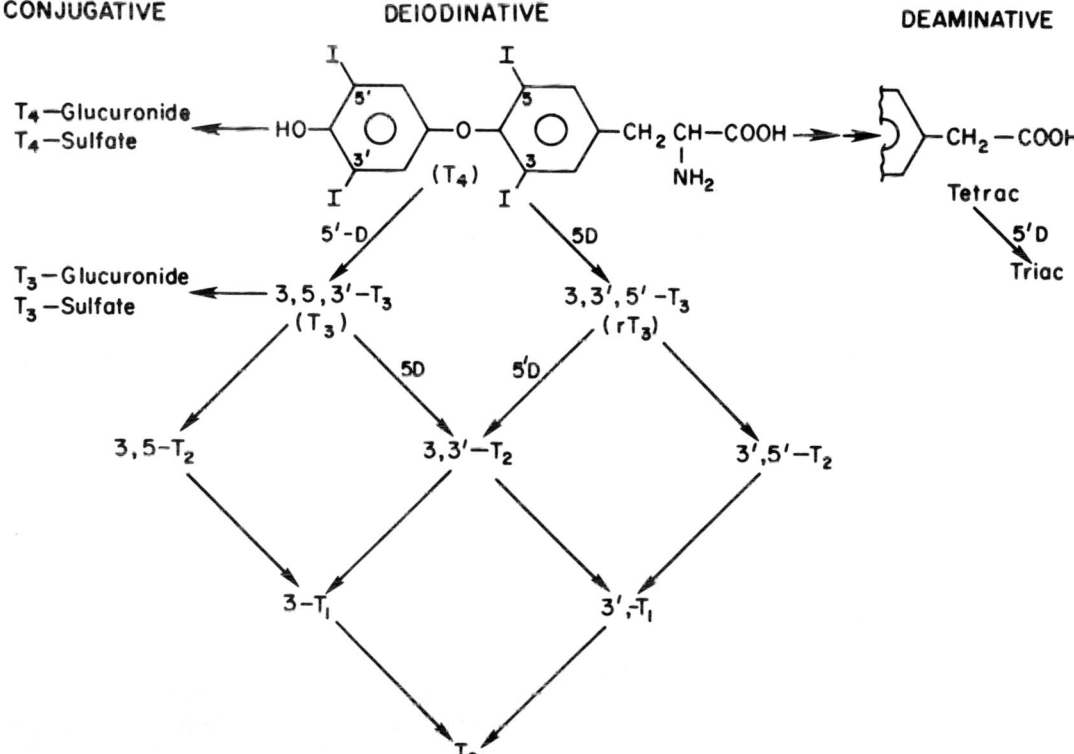

FIGURE 95–2. Pathways of metabolism of thyroid hormones. 5'-D = 5'-deiodinase; 5-D = 5-deiodinase. (From Ferguson, DC: Thyroid function tests in the dog: Recent concepts. Vet Clin North Am 14:570, 1984.)

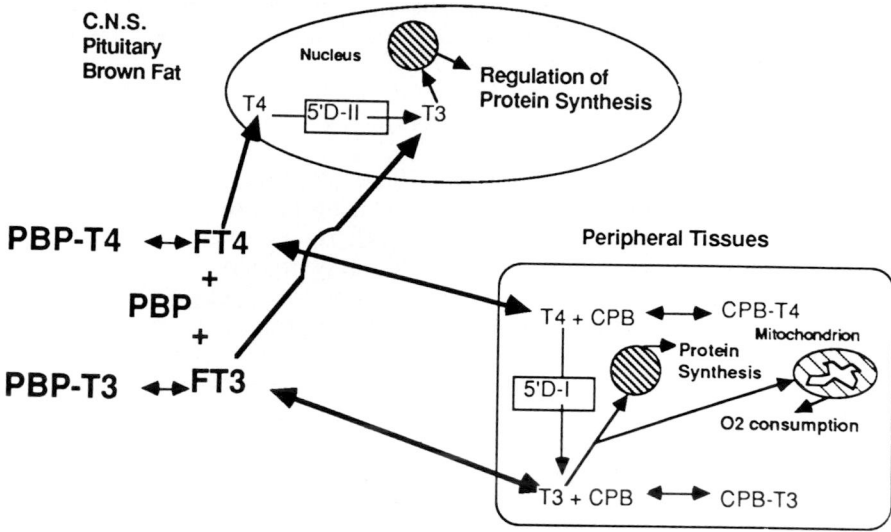

FIGURE 95–3. Peripheral action of thyroid hormone. Thyroxine and T_3, in amounts proportional to their free forms (FT_4 and FT_3) in plasma at equilibrium with plasma binding proteins (PBP), are taken up by peripheral tissues such as liver and kidney, which have the Type I 5'-deiodinase enzyme (5'-D-I). Triiodothyronine from the plasma (or that derived from T_4) interacts wtih mitochondrial receptors to rapidly increase oxygen consumption and with nuclear receptors to initiate protein synthesis. Cytosolic binding proteins (CPB) buffer the effects of intracellular hormones and provide a relatively unsaturable hormone reservoir. In the brain, pituitary and brown fat, another isoenzyme of the 5'-deiodinase (5'-D-II), converts T_4 to T_3 in these tissues. This enzyme is regulated very differently from the Type I enzyme.

pounds. Their ability to circulate in plasma depends on binding by specific binding proteins, thyroxine-binding protein (TBG) and thyroxine-binding prealbumin (TBPA; transthyretin), as well as by albumin itself. The major function of the thyroid hormone binding proteins is probably to provide a hormone reservoir in the plasma and to buffer hormone delivery into tissue (Figure 95–3). Recent evidence suggests that TBPA, and possibly albumin, also may serve as intermediary carriers for specific uptake of the hormone by tissues.[44]

The dog does have a high affinity thyroid hormone binding protein comparable to TBG in humans, but plasma concentrations of TBG in the dog are only 25 per cent of those in humans.[45] In addition to TBG, TBPA, and albumin, circulating T_4 in canine plasma appears to bind to certain plasma lipoproteins. These include a high density lipoprotein (HDL_2) that migrates in the α_1 region on the electrophoretic pattern and a very low density lipoprotein (VLDL) that migrates in the β region.[45] At normal serum T_4 concentrations in the dog, about 60 per cent of T_4 is bound to TBG, 17 per cent to TBPA, 12 per cent to albumin, and 11 per cent to the HDL_2. Thyroxine-binding globulin in the dog is not saturated until the total T_4 concentration is about 12 μg/dl, about six times the normal serum T_4 value, while the other serum proteins are virtually unsaturable.[45] The cat does not appear to have a high affinity thyroid binding protein (such as TBG) but has only TBPA and albumin as plasma thyroid hormone binding proteins.[45, 46] The overall affinity of the thyroid hormone binding proteins for T_4 is lower in the dog and cat than in humans. Partly as a result of this weaker protein binding, total T_4 concentrations are lower, the unbound or free fraction of circulating T_4 is higher, and hormone metabolism is more rapid in the dog and cat than in humans.

In the healthy euthyroid dog or cat, about 0.1 per cent of total concentration of serum T_4 is free (not bound to thyroid hormone binding proteins), whereas about one per cent of circulating T_3 is free.[47] Clinically, it is important to recognize that circulating thyroid hormones normally are highly bound to thyroid hor-

mone binding proteins because the proportion of free versus bound hormone may change in response to drug administration or illness. For example, in uremia, plasma compounds (possibly free fatty acids) compete for hormone binding, resulting in a transient increase in serum free T_4 (FT_4) and serum free T_3 (FT_3) concentrations but decreased total hormone values.[48] However, such alterations in hormone binding by the thyroid hormone binding proteins generally do not affect the thyroid status, since the absolute level of the free hormone concentrations tends to return to within the normal range or remain relatively constant.[48]

Most evidence suggests that the fractions of circulating FT_4 and FT_3 determine the amount of hormone that is available for uptake by tissues. Although routine thyroid hormone determinations are limited to the plasma compartment, approximately 50 to 60 per cent of the body's T_4 and 90 to 95 per cent of the body's T_3 is located in the intracellular compartment.[38] Certain organs, particularly the liver and kidney, can concentrate thyroid hormones and exchange hormone rapidly with the plasma. In humans, about 60 per cent of the intracellular T_4 is in these rapidly equilibrating tissues (liver and kidney), whereas only six per cent of the intracellular T_3 is in these tissues.[38] About 80 per cent of all extrathyroidal T_3 is located in the slowly equilibrating tissues (e.g., muscle, skin), while only 20 per cent of intracellular T_4 is in this compartment.[38] As a result, most T_4 is located in plasma, interstitial fluid, liver, and kidney. The majority of the body's extrathyroidal T_3 is in the cells of the muscle and skin. Therefore, because T_3 is primarily an intracellular hormone and a considerable amount is derived from extrathyroidal sources, the isolated measurement of its serum concentration is a less meaningful estimate of thyroid function than is the determination of serum total T_4 concentration.

The free fraction of circulating thyroid hormone is also a primary determinant of the rate of fractional metabolic and excretory turnover. As discussed above, humans have higher concentrations of TBG than the dog or cat, resulting in stronger protein binding and much lower fractions of circulating FT_4 and FT_3. As a result of these differences in hormone binding, the plasma half-life of T_4 in the dog has been estimated to be between 10 and 16 hours, compared with a plasma half-life of about 7 days in humans.[29, 38, 43, 49] Similarly, the plasma half-life of T_3 in the dog has been estimated to be 5 to 6 hours,[50] compared with 24 to 36 hours in humans. Preliminary studies in the normal cat indicate that the plasma half-lives of T_4 and T_3 are similar to that of the dog, whereas the thyroid hormones disappear from the circulation at a faster rate in cats with hyperthyroidism. It should be emphasized that these figures reflect plasma disappearance rates and do not necessarily indicate extent or duration of biological action.

Regulation of Thyroid Hormone Secretion (Hypothalamic-Pituitary-Thyroid-Extrathyroid Axis).

A detailed study of the canine and feline hypothalamic-pituitary-thyroid-extrathyroid axis (Figure 95–4) has not been possible without the availability of a valid canine or feline TSH radioimmunoassay (RIA). Results of one study, however, in which serum TSH concentrations increased in response to a lowering of circulating thyroid hormone values produced by administration of antithyroid drugs or thyroid x-irradiation,[51] as well as indirect evidence for a TSH rise (based on an increase in serum T_4 and T_3 concentrations) following thyrotropin releasing hormone (TRH) administration,[52-55] suggest that the hypothalamic-pituitary regulation in the dog is similar to that in rats and humans.

The tripeptide TRH is produced in the paraventricular nucleus of the hypothalamus and transported to the pituitary pars distalis by the hypophyseal portal system in the pituitary stalk. In the pituitary gland, TRH binds to specific receptors on the thyrotroph cell and stimulates TSH secretion (Figure 95–4). In the dog as in other species, TRH also stimulates the secretion of prolactin.[54] The hypothalamic hormone somatostatin acts to inhibit TSH secretion and may function as a thyrotropin inhibitory factor.

Current evidence suggests that under normal physiologic conditions, the negative feedback effect of thyroid hormones (in the free or unbound form) is the principal mechanism regulating TSH secretion and that tonic stimulation by TRH is permissive to its secretion (Figure 95–4).[40] The pituitary thyrotroph cell rapidly and completely deiodinates T_4 (derived from the plasma) to T_3, which subsequently acts via pituitary nuclear receptors to inhibit TSH synthesis and secretion (Figure 95–3). This negative feedback effect involves the generation of an inhibitory protein that blocks TSH release. The end result may be a decrease in the number of TRH receptors on the thyrotroph.[56] Thus, although T_3 acts as the active hormone intracellularly to suppress TSH release, circulating T_4 taken up by the pituitary (rather than plasma T_3 itself) is the preferred source of T_3 in the pituitary, at least in the rat.[40] In human patients with hypothyroidism, however, there is some evidence that the plasma T_3 concentration may be more important than T_4 as a determinant of TSH secretion T_4.[57] There is now some evidence that thyroid hormones may have a direct negative feedback effect on the hypothalamus, inhibiting the release of TRH (Figure 95–4). Also, TSH and TRH may have "short-loop" and "ultrashort-loop" negative feedback effects, respectively, on the hypothalamus to inhibit TRH release.[58] Pulses of TSH secretion and an evening rise in serum TSH concentrations (possibly resulting from a fall in circadian circulating cortisol concentrations) have been described in humans and may contribute to this direct negative-feedback effect on TRH secretion.[59] Although similar investigations of TSH secretion have not yet been performed in the dog and cat because of the lack of a valid assay for canine or feline TSH, studies have failed to demonstrate a circadian rhythm in circulating thyroid hormone concentrations in either the dog or cat.[60]

EXTRATHYROIDAL FACTORS ALTERING THYROID HORMONE METABOLISM AND CIRCULATING THYROID HORMONE CONCENTRATIONS

Effect of Illness and Malnutrition in Humans.

In humans, a wide range of clinical conditions such as chronic starvation or malnutrition, surgery, diabetes mellitus, hepatic and renal disease, and other chronic systemic illnesses may result in decreased serum T_3 concentrations together with elevated serum rT_3 values.[42] This situation (which has been called the "low T_3" or "euthyroid sick" syndrome) results from inhibition of 5'-deiodinase, the enzyme necessary for conversion of T_4 to T_3 and the conversion of rT_3 to $3,3'$-T_2. Since the conversion of circulating T_4 to rT_3 is not affected, T_4 continues to be deiodinated along this pathway and rT_3 accumulates in the peripheral circulation.[42]

The reduction in the production of T_3, the most potent thyroid hormone, appears to be a beneficial adaptive

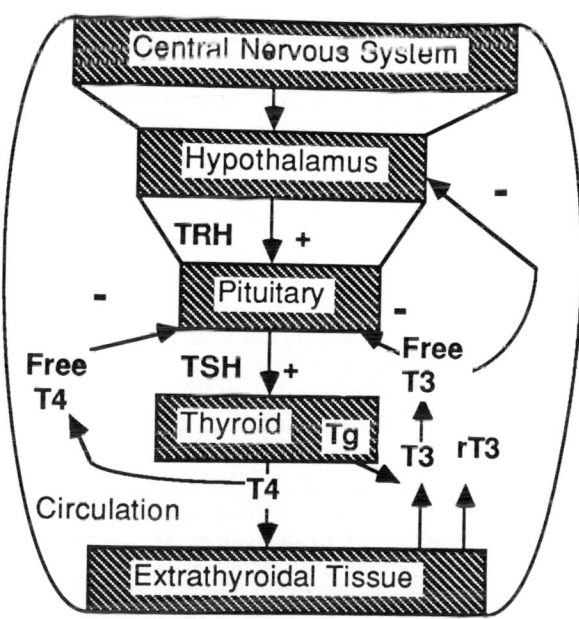

FIGURE 95–4. Hypothalamic-pituitary-thyroid-extrathyroid axis. TRH = thyrotropin releasing hormone; TSH = thyrotropin; Tg = thyroglobulin. TRH has a stimulatory effect on pituitary TSH synthesis and release. TSH stimulates thyroidal hormone synthesis and secretion. The free forms of T_4 and T_3 have a negative feedback effect on the pituitary and the hypothalamus, decreasing TSH and TRH secretion, respectively. Extrathyroidal tissue takes up T_4, the main secretory product of the thyroid, and produces T_3, a more active hormone, or rT_3, a thyromimetically inactive compound.

mechanism by which the body limits the loss of protein and perhaps blunts the metabolic rate during illness.[61] Maintenance of serum T_3 concentrations (with triiodothyronine replacement) in euthyroid fasting humans leads to excessive nitrogen excretion and blunting of the pituitary's TSH response to TRH, as if a state of hyperthyroidism had supervened.[62] Current evidence does not support the contention that lowering of serum T_3 during malnutrition and illness is associated with tissue hypothyroidism.[61, 63] It remains unknown whether a chronic block in T_4 to T_3 conversion might result in adverse effects associated with thyroid hormone deficiency.[38, 42, 64]

Particularly in acute and severe illnesses in humans, both serum T_4 and T_3 concentrations may fall precipitously.[42, 63–66] Several pathophysiologic mechanisms may contribute to this low T_4 state of medical illness. Impaired serum protein binding of T_4 caused by an endogenous inhibitor of binding (such as free fatty acids) or a reduction in binding protein concentrations results in reduced total serum T_4 concentrations and an increased fraction of FT_4. In most cases, however, the absolute FT_4 concentrations remain normal.[48, 63] A fall in serum TSH concentrations may also contribute to the subnormal serum T_4 concentrations, especially in patients treated with dopamine or glucocorticoids, drugs that inhibit TSH release.[63] Some workers have raised the question whether this syndrome causes a state of transient secondary hypothyroidism, based on the finding of low serum thyroid hormone concentrations in combination with normal or slightly reduced serum TSH concentrations.[64] However, studies of critically ill patients with low serum T_4 and T_3 concentrations have revealed that thyroxine therapy is not beneficial and fails to improve survival.[67] Upon recovery from the severe nonthyroidal illness, the depressed serum thyroid hormone concentrations return to normal.[42]

Serum T_4 concentrations have been reported to provide an objective means for quantifying the severity and predicting the clinical outcome of humans with severe nonthyroidal illness.[65, 66] A persistent decrease in serum T_4 concentration is a poor prognostic sign, and in one study, correctly predicted mortality in 70 per cent of cases.[49]

The Canine "Euthyroid Sick" Syndrome. In a study of the effects of prolonged fasting in the dog, serum T_3 concentrations fell significantly after two days and reached one-third of baseline values after two weeks.[68] No significant fall in the mean serum T_4 level was observed in the nine dogs studied, and, in contrast to humans, serum rT_3 concentrations did not rise. In that study, it was postulated that the absence of an increase in rT_3 was somehow related to the dog's resistance to the development of ketosis during fasting.[68] Another study of the effects of a short-term (4 days) fast on serum thyroid hormone values in 12 dogs again found a significant decrease in mean serum T_3 concentrations, but also found a transient fall in serum rT_3 concentrations 24 hours after the start of a fast and a slight fall in mean serum T_4 concentrations after 4 days.[69] Overall, the results of the two studies indicate that, although low serum T_3 concentrations do develop in the fasted dog, the concomitant high serum rT_3 concentrations found in humans do not occur in the dog.

The effects of nonthyroidal illness on thyroid hormone metabolism in the dog are less well characterized than in humans. In the dog, depressed serum T_4 concentrations have been reported in various nonthyroidal illnesses such as hyperadrenocorticism, diabetes mellitus, hypoadrenocorticism, chronic renal failure, hepatic disease, as well as a variety of other critical medical illnesses requiring intensive care.[70–72] In addition, the subnormal serum T_4 concentrations are usually, but not always, accompanied by a fall in total serum T_3 concentrations. The reverse situation (low serum T_3 with normal T_4) as occurs in the low T_3 syndrome of humans does not appear to be a frequent phenomenon in the dog.

The suppressive effects of spontaneous hyperadrenocorticism on serum thyroid hormone concentrations in the dog are well recognized. In a study of 102 dogs with spontaneous hyperadrenocorticism, basal serum T_4 and/or T_3 concentrations were decreased in 57 per cent and 52 per cent of the dogs, respectively.[70] In a follow-up study on the mechanism of these alterations in circulating thyroid hormone concentrations, the authors determined FT_4 and total T_4, T_3, and rT_3 concentrations in an additional 45 dogs with Cushing's syndrome.[47] In that study, the fractional FT_4 (determined by equilibrium dialysis) was elevated in about 25 per cent of the dogs, consistent with diminished serum protein binding. In most of the dogs with reduced total T_4 concentrations, however, the absolute FT_4 values (total T_4 concentration $\times$ fractional FT_4) were also below the normal range. Low serum rT_3 concentrations were found in most of these dogs, supporting the contention that the FT_4 (from which virtually all rT_3 is derived) was decreased.

These low absolute FT_4 concentrations found in some dogs with hyperadrenocorticism suggest that reduced thyroid hormone secretion, probably mediated via inhibition of pituitary TSH release, plays an important role in the pathogenesis of low serum thyroid hormone concentrations in this syndrome. It has also been reported that dogs with hyperadrenocorticism lack a normal response to exogenous TRH, consistent with pituitary TSH suppression.[73] In addition, impaired serum protein binding (as described above) and alterations in peripheral thyroid hormone metabolism may contribute to the low hormone values.[70] In contrast to the situation in dogs given acute doses of glucocorticoids, inhibition of 5′-deiodinase appears to play a less important role in the development of subnormal serum T_3 concentrations in canine hyperadrenocorticism because the serum rT_3 values remain normal or fall.[47] It is not yet clear whether a true state of secondary hypothyroidism exists in these dogs with low FT_4 concentrations. However, it is known that correction of the hypercortisolism alone (with either o,p,′-DDD or adrenalectomy) will result in normalization of resting serum thyroid hormone concentrations.[70] There is little evidence that thyroid hormone supplementation in a dog with hyperadrenocorticism is clinically beneficial, and its use could enhance the catabolic state of chronic cortisol excess.

The effect of diabetes mellitus on serum thyroid hormone concentrations has been examined in several studies. One report of six dogs with spontaneous diabetes mellitus demonstrated normal basal T_4 and T_3

concentrations; however, a slightly blunted serum T_4 response to TSH was observed.[71] Another study of 22 untreated diabetic dogs found normal concentrations of serum T_4 but elevated serum concentrations of T_3, rT_3, and thyroxine-binding prealbumin (TBPA).[72] The elevated serum T_3 concentrations are not consistent with observations in untreated human diabetics, where low serum T_3 concentrations are usually found.[42] However, the authors have observed subnormal serum concentrations of both T_4 and T_3 in dogs with uncontrolled diabetic ketoacidosis. Therefore, the severity of the diabetic state, the adequacy of treatment, and presence of concurrent illness all may contribute to the alterations in serum thyroid hormone concentrations reported in canine diabetes mellitus. In accord with this, it has been shown in human patients that the degree of diabetic control affects basal thyroid hormone values.[74] Interpretation of the effects of the diabetic state on thyroid function is complicated by the association between the development of diabetes mellitus and overt hypothyroidism in the dog, as well as the high incidence (38 per cent) of circulating anti-thyroglobulin antibodies in spontaneously diabetic dogs (compared with 59 per cent incidence in spontaneous canine hypothyroidism).[75, 76] Therefore, in at least some dogs, diabetes mellitus and primary hypothyroidism may coexist as manifestations of polyglandular autoimmune endocrinopathies.

Chronic renal failure has a profound effect on serum thyroid hormone concentrations. In 16 dogs with chronic renal disease associated with severe azotemia, 14 had subnormal serum T_4 concentrations, and four of these had undetectable T_4 concentrations (unpublished observations). Most of these dogs also had subnormal serum T_3 values but elevated serum rT_3 concentrations, a pattern confirmed by other workers.[72] The serum concentrations of TBPA tend to be subnormal in dogs with chronic renal failure, possibly resulting from loss of the protein through the glomeruli. The lowered circulating concentrations of TBPA could contribute to the subnormal serum T_4 concentrations commonly found in dogs with renal disease.[72]

Effect of Drugs on Thyroid Function in the Dog. A variety of drugs may impair plasma or tissue binding of the thyroid hormones or alter thyroid hormone metabolism.[77] Drugs used in veterinary medicine that are most likely to alter circulating thyroid hormone concentrations include the glucocorticoids, anticonvulsants, quinidine, salicylates, phenylbutazone, and radiographic contrast agents. The mechanisms by which these drugs exert their effects vary. Glucocorticoids, quinidine, and other membrane-stabilizing drugs may inhibit 5'-deiodinase, salicylates may directly displace thyroid hormone from plasma binding sites, phenylbutazone appears to have a direct antithyroid effect, and radiographic contrast agents (e.g, diatrizoate, iopanoic acid, ipodate, tyropanoate, and metrizamide) may act by preventing the uptake of T_4 by tissue, by directly inhibiting 5'-deiodinase, or by releasing the iodine they contain to exert an antithyroid effect on the thyroid gland.

Exogenous glucocorticoids have also been shown to have a profound effect on thyroid function tests in the dog. A single dose of 1.0 mg/lb (2.2 mg/kg) of prednisone intramuscularly had no effect on serum T_4 concen-

trations but lowered serum T_3 concentrations when retested 8 and 24 hours after administration.[78] In another study, a single injection of dexamethasone using a relatively high dosage (0.25 mg/lb or 0.6 mg/kg) had no effect on serum T_4 concentrations but produced a significant decrease in mean serum T_3 concentration (to about one-half of the control value) at 24 hours posttreatment.[69] Dexamethasone also increased serum rT_3 concentrations by two-thirds, an effect observed at 24 and 48 hours.[69] Therefore, the acute effect of a single high dose of glucocorticoids appears to be mainly inhibition of 5'deiodination.

Most dogs on chronic, high dose, daily glucocorticoid therapy have very low or undetectable serum T_4 concentrations, as well as subnormal serum T_3 values. Administration of prednisone (1.0 mg/lb IM or 2.2 mg/kg, IM) on alternate days for a total of six doses produced significant decreases in the serum concentrations of both T_4 and T_3 (to values below the normal range).[78] Based upon electron microscopic examination of thyroid tissue, it was postulated that glucocorticoids may interfere with thyroid hormone secretion by inhibiting lysosomal hydrolysis of colloid in the follicular cell.[78, 79] Because the thyroid retains its responsiveness to TSH during chronic glucocorticoid excess,[70, 79] suppression of pituitary TSH secretion is probably the primary and most important mechanism by which serum T_4 concentrations are suppressed. In accord with this, glucocorticoids have been shown to decrease the secretion of TSH in humans.[80] Serum T_3 concentrations may be decreased because of glucocorticoid inhibition of 5'-deiodinase or simply because of a reduced availability of plasma T_4, the substrate for the enzyme. Other possible mechanisms by which glucocorticoids may alter thyroid hormone metabolism include a direct or indirect reduction in serum hormone binding (as suggested by the observations in spontaneous hyperadrenocorticism), decreased tissue binding of hormone, and increased nondeiodinative degradation and clearance of T_4 and T_3.

A variety of other drugs alter thyroid hormone metabolism or serum or tissue binding of the thyroid hormones in the dog. The anticonvulsants phenytoin and phenobarbital, which are mixed function oxidase inducers, consistently decrease serum T_4 concentrations to subnormal values, possibly by enhancing the rate of deiodinative metabolism and biliary excretion.[26, 81] Ipodate, a radiographic contrast agent, significantly increased mean serum T_4 concentrations, decreased mean T_3 values, but had no effect on serum rT_3 concentrations when given in one large dose to dogs.[69] The antithyroid drug propylthiouracil, administered to dogs in high doses (600 mg, twice daily) for three days, reduced serum T_3 and rT_3 concentrations while having no effect on serum T_4 concentrations.[69]

In humans, estrogens increase the synthesis of TBG and increase total serum T_4 concentrations.[77] In one study of dogs, however, administration of one dose of estradiol benzoate failed to alter serum T_4 or T_3 concentrations.[82] Similarly, normal serum T_4 or T_3 concentrations were found in dogs with hyperestrogenism secondary to Sertoli cell testicular tumor.[71] Pregnancy, on the other hand, has been reported to increase circulating protein-bound iodine concentrations (consisting primarily of T_4) in the dog, presumably as the result of increased circulating progesterone levels.[83]

Effect of Obesity on Thyroid Function in the Dog.
An increase in serum T_3 and T_4 concentrations (into the high-normal or slightly high range) has been reported in obese euthyroid dogs.[71] In agreement with the results of that study, the authors have observed slightly high basal concentrations of T_4 or T_3 (or both) in dogs suspected of having hypothyroidism primarily because of moderate to severe obesity. Excessive caloric intake, rather than the resultant obesity, is believed to result in increased production of the thyroid hormones.[42]

Effect of Age on Thyroid Function in the Dog.
Thyroid hormone concentrations vary with age, most notably early in life. Total serum T_4 concentrations are elevated from two to five times the adult level during the first three months of a puppy's life.[84] Total serum T_4 concentrations peak at one month of age in the dog, probably as a result of a transient increase in serum binding proteins.[84] In the human infant and in the foal, serum T_3 values rise and rT_3 concentrations fall shortly after birth.[42, 84, 85] This increase in T_3 production is probably an adaptation to the decreased environmental temperature and is designed to increase shivering thermogenesis upon leaving the warmth of the uterus. These acute perinatal changes have not been examined in the puppy or kitten.

One study of 91 beagles from 1 to 13 years of age showed that basal serum T_4 and post-TSH T_4 were highly inversely correlated with age.[86] In another cross-sectional study of 5 groups of 10 beagles (average ages of 2, 5, 8, 11, and 15 years), basal and TSH-stimulated responses of serum T_4, T_3, and rT_3 were examined (unpublished observations). These studies showed a decline in the mean serum T_4 concentration from 2.1 μg/dl in the youngest group to 1.6 μg/dl and 1.4 μg/dl in the oldest groups. The most striking change was in the increment of the T_4 concentration six hours after TSH administration. In the youngest group, the mean T_4 concentration increased by almost 4 μg/dl, whereas in the oldest group mean T_4 increased only about 2 μg/dl. Although the youngest group of dogs had the highest mean basal serum T_3 concentration, a progressive age-related decline in serum T_3 concentrations was not apparent. The most age-sensitive parameter appeared to be the T_3 increment above baseline 6 hours post-TSH (which averaged about 80 ng/dl in the youngest group and only about 40 ng/dl in the two oldest groups). Although these trends were seen, individual variation was considerable. Basal rT_3 concentrations showed no consistent pattern of change with aging; however, post-TSH increments showed qualitatively the same patterns as for T_4 and T_3. Despite these changes in laboratory colony dogs, the authors did not observe a significant correlation of basal serum total or FT_4 with age in a group of 28 normal pet dogs.[47] The reason for the discrepancy between the effect of aging and of serum thyroid hormones in beagle laboratory dogs and a variety of breeds of pet dogs is not yet clear. However, the progressive development of subclinical thyroid insufficiency in the beagles must be ruled out, as this breed has a high incidence of autoimmune thyroiditis.[75]

Effect of Surgery and Anesthesia on Thyroid Function in the Dog.
In an experimental study of normal dogs subjected to anesthesia alone (with a combination of thiopental and methoxyflurane) or anesthesia together with an abdominal laparotomy, notable effects on serum thyroid hormone concentrations were observed (unpublished observations). Anesthesia, alone or combined with the surgical procedure, resulted in significant fall in mean serum concentrations of T_4, T_3, and rT_3 for a period of 30 hours. However, the ratios of T_3 to T_4 and rT_3 to T_4 increased, suggesting inhibition of hormone secretion and possibly stimulation in the deiodinative metabolism of T_4. In other species, thiobarbiturates are known to inhibit hormone organification and deiodination.[87, 88] In contrast, methoxyflurane has little to no effect on serum concentrations of T_4 and T_3, at least in humans.[87] Some of the other inhalant agents, such as halothane and isoflurane, may increase serum thyroid hormone concentrations by displacing T_4 from peripheral tissue storage pools, most notably the liver.[87]

MECHANISMS OF THYROID HORMONE ACTION

No single reaction or metabolic event can be equated with the action of thyroid hormone. It acts on many different cellular processes via specific ligand-receptor interactions with the nucleus, the mitochondria, and the plasma membrane (Figure 95–3).[89] Thyroid hormones affect most body tissues. Although both L-T_4 and L-T_3 have intrinsic metabolic activity, L-T_3 is three to five times more potent in binding to the nuclear receptors and similarly more potent in stimulating oxygen consumption.

The effects of thyroid hormone can generally be divided into those that are rapid and evident within minutes to hours of administration, such as stimulation of amino acid transport and mitochondrial oxygen consumption and those that require protein synthesis and a longer period of time (usually no sooner than six hours) to become manifest (Figure 95–3). About one-half of the increment in oxygen consumption produced by thyroid hormone has been related to activation of the plasma membrane–bound $Na^+K^+ATPase$. This effect, at least in the kidney and liver, is secondary to increases in passive K^+ fluxes.[89] Thyroid hormone also directly stimulates mitochondrial oxygen consumption. These changes have been linked directly to the calorigenic effect of thyroid hormone. The rapid hormone effects can be observed clinically in the hypothyroid patient starting on thyroid replacement therapy, by signs such as increased physical and mental activity. Of course, the clinical manifestations may require weeks to months to be clearly appreciated.

More chronic effects of thyroid hormone invariably are related to the cellular actions of the hormone, requiring interaction with nuclear T_3 receptors followed by an increase in protein synthesis crucial to physiological processes such as growth, differentiation, proliferation, and maturation (Figure 95–3).[89] A common clinical presentation of thyroid insufficiency is bilaterally symmetrical alopecia, the result of diminished turnover of shafts of hair within the hair follicle, resulting in greater amounts of telogen hairs. Such changes are slow in onset and, upon treatment, slow to resolve.

Thyroid hormones, in physiological quantities, are anabolic. Working in conjunction with growth hormone and insulin, protein synthesis is stimulated and nitrogen excretion is reduced. However, in excess (hyperthyroidism), thyroid hormones can be catabolic, with increased gluconeogenesis, protein breakdown, and nitrogen wasting.

CANINE HYPOTHYROIDISM

Causes of Hypothyroidism

Hypothyroidism results from impaired production and secretion of thyroid hormone. Although dysfunction anywhere in the hypothalamic-pituitary-thyroidal axis may result in thyroid hormone deficiency, more than 95 per cent of clinical cases of hypothyroidism appear to result from destruction of the thyroid gland itself (primary hypothyroidism).

THYROIDAL (PRIMARY) HYPOTHYROIDISM

The two most common causes of canine adult-onset primary hypothyroidism are lymphocytic thyroiditis and idiopathic atrophy of the thyroid gland.[90, 91] These appear to occur with equal frequency. Other rare forms of canine hypothyroidism include iatrogenic conditions, neoplastic destruction thyroid tissue, and congenital (or juvenile-onset) hypothyroidism.

Lymphocytic Thyroiditis. Lymphocytic thyroiditis is characterized histologically by a diffuse infiltration of the gland by lymphocytes, plasma cells, and macrophages, resulting in progressive destruction of follicles and secondary fibrosis.[26, 90, 91] Clinical signs of hypothyroidism develop when more than 75 per cent of the gland is destroyed. Lymphocytic thyroiditis is probably an immune-mediated disease, as suggested by the morphology of the thyroid lesions (including electron microscopic evidence of antigen-antibody complexes in the follicular cell basement membrane) and the frequent occurrence of circulating thyroglobulin autoantibodies.[71, 76, 90] Antibody binding to follicular cell, colloid, or thyroglobulin antigens may activate the complement cascade or antibody-dependent cell-mediated cytotoxicity, causing follicular cell destruction.

Idiopathic Atrophy of the Thyroid. Idiopathic atrophy of the thyroid gland is the second major histologic form of canine primary hypothyroidism.[26, 90, 91] Histologically, there is loss of thyroid parenchyma, with replacement by adipose tissue. The cause of idiopathic thyroid atrophy is unknown. Although this follicular atrophy may represent the end-stage form of lymphocytic thyroiditis, this is unlikely because of the lack of an inflammatory cell infiltrate in this form of hypothyroidism. Idiopathic follicular atrophy is most probably a primary degenerative disorder of the thyroid gland affecting individual follicular cells.[90]

Congenital or Juvenile-onset Hypothyroidism. Congenital hypothyroidism in human infants is a relatively rare but well-recognized syndrome, occurring about once in every 4000 births. In humans, 80 to 90 per cent of congenital thyroid defects are caused by various forms of thyroid dysgenesis such as athyreosis (no demonstrable thyroid tissue, hypoplasia), small thyroid remnant demonstrable in the normal anatomic region, and thyroid ectasia (small amount of thyroid tissue only in an ectopic location).[92] The second most common cause of congenital hypothyroidism in human infants is dyshormonogenesis, most commonly resulting from an inherited inability to organify iodide. Other forms of dyshormonogenesis, although rare, include circulating thyroid hormone transport abnormalities and metabolic defects (e.g., induced by severe iodine deficiency or ingestion of goitrogens). When hypothyroidism first develops later in childhood, it is most often caused by chronic autoimmune thyroiditis.[92]

The incidence of congenital or juvenile-onset primary hypothyroidism in the dog is not known but appears to be extremely rare, with only six reported cases.[29, 32, 93–96] It is likely that congenital hypothyroidism usually results in undiagnosed puppy death. In two reported cases, the exact cause of the hypothyroid state was not determined.[93, 96] The cause of the congenital or juvenile-onset primary hypothyroidism in the remaining four dogs included deficient dietary iodine intake, dyshormonogenesis (iodine organification defect), and thyroid dysgenesis.[29, 32, 94, 95]

Neoplastic Destruction of the Thyroid Gland. Clinical and laboratory features of hypothyroidism occasionally may develop following destruction of more than 75 per cent of normal thyroid tissue by a nonfunctional thyroid tumor.[97] These thyroid tumors are usually primary thyroid carcinoma but rarely may be secondary tumors (metastases from other organs).

Iatrogenic Hypothyroidism. Since naturally occurring hyperthyroidism is rare in the dog, the development of iatrogenic hypothyroidism following treatment with radioiodine (^{131}I), surgical thyroidectomy, or use of an antithyroid drug is also extremely rare in dog. However, this has become the most common cause of hypothyroidism in the cat.

PITUITARY (SECONDARY) HYPOTHYROIDISM

Hypothyroidism may result from an impaired ability of the pituitary gland to secrete thyrotropin (TSH), resulting in secondary follicular atrophy. In the dog, secondary hypothyroidism accounts for less than five per cent of clinical cases of hypothyroidism.[26] Potential etiologies include large pituitary tumors, congenital malformation of the pituitary gland, and isolated TSH deficiency, as well as surgical or irradiation treatment of pituitary tumors.

Pituitary Tumors. The most common cause of secondary hypothyroidism is destruction of pituitary thyrotrophs by an expanding, space-occupying pituitary tumor.[26, 98] Because of the nonselective nature of the resulting compressive atrophy and replacement of pars distalis tissue by such large pituitary tumors, deficiencies of one or more other pituitary hormones also usually occur. Secondary hypothyroidism may also develop following surgical or irradiation treatment of pituitary tumors.[97]

Pituitary Malformation. Congenital secondary hypothyroidism has been documented only in German shepherd dogs with pituitary dwarfism associated with a cystic Rathke's pouch.[99, 100] The degree of TSH deficiency in these dogs is variable, however, and clinical signs are usually caused primarily by growth hormone (rather than thyroid hormone) deficiency.

Isolated TSH Deficiency. While TSH deficiency usually occurs in association with deficiency of other pituitary hormones, rare cases of isolated familial deficiency have been described in humans with hypothyroidism.[92] Such an isolated deficiency of TSH has yet to be documented in the dog.

HYPOTHALAMIC (TERTIARY) HYPOTHYROIDISM

Although a poorly defined disorder in the dog, deficient production or release of TRH also has been reported to cause hypothyroidism.[26] In humans, this type of hypothyroidism can result from traumatic, destructive, or infiltrative diseases of the hypothalamus or biochemical defects in TRH production.[92] Humans with documented hypothalamic hypothyroidism have subnormal serum TSH concentrations but show normal increases in circulating TSH after administration of TRH. Until a valid TSH assay is available in the dog, it may be difficult to differentiate pituitary (secondary) hypothyroidism from hypothalamic hypothyroidism with certainty.

DEFECTS IN PERIPHERAL CONVERSION OF T$_4$ TO T$_3$ (POOR CONVERTERS)

An inability to convert T$_4$ to T$_3$ by peripheral tissues (caused by a selective absence or reduction of 5'-deiodinase activity), although considered by some to be a possible cause of canine hypothyroidism, has yet to be documented to produce a hypothyroid state in any species. The finding of low serum T$_3$ concentrations in conjunction with normal serum T$_4$ concentrations is most likely the result of concurrent illness, drug therapy, or anti-T$_3$ antibodies.

Clinical Signs in Adult-Onset Canine Hypothyroidism

Although the onset of clinical signs is variable, hypothyroidism most commonly develops in middle-aged dogs (four to ten years of age).[26, 97, 101, 102] The disorder usually affects mid- to large-size breeds of dogs, while hypothyroidism is rare in toy and miniature breeds of dogs. Breeds reported to be predisposed to developing hypothyroidism include the golden retriever, Doberman pinscher, Irish setter, miniature schnauzer, dachshund, cocker spaniel, and Airedale terrier.[101] German shepherds and mongrels have a lower than expected risk for developing the disease. There does not appear to be a sex predilection, but spayed female dogs appear to be at greater risk of developing hypothyroidism than intact females.[101]

General Signs Associated with Decreased Metabolic Rate. Thyroid hormone is needed for the normal cellular metabolic functions throughout the body.[89] A deficiency in circulating thyroid hormone affects the metabolic function of all organ systems. As a result, clinical signs are diffuse, variable, often nonspecific, and rarely pathognomonic for hypothyroidism. Therefore, one must maintain a high index of suspicion for the disorder. Overdiagnosis, however, should also be avoided; many diseases, especially those of the skin, can easily be misdiagnosed as being the result of thyroid deficiency.

The common clinical signs associated with canine hypothyroidism are listed in Table 95–1. Many of the clinical signs are directly related to the slowing of cellular metabolism. This results in the development of mental dullness, lethargy, unwillingness to exercise, intolerance of exercise, and weight gain without a corresponding increase in appetite. Mild to marked obesity develops in some dogs. The reduced metabolic rate may result in difficulty in maintaining body temperature, leading to frank hypothermia in some dogs. As a result, the "classic" hypothyroid dog is a heat-seeker because of intolerance to cold.

Skin and Hair Coat. Alterations in the skin and hair coat are common in dogs with hypothyroidism. Dryness of the hair coat, excessive shedding, and retarded regrowth of hair are usually the earliest dermatologic changes observed in dogs with hypothyroidism. Nonpruritic hair thinning or alopecia (usually bilaterally symmetric in distribution), which may involve the ventral and lateral trunk, the caudal surfaces of the thighs, dorsum of the tail, ventral neck, and the dorsum of the nose, occurs in about two-thirds of dogs with hypothyroidism (Table 95–1). Such hair thinning or alopecia, sometimes associated with hyperpigmentation, often initially starts over points of wear. Occasionally, secondary pyoderma (which may produce pruritus) is observed.

In moderate to severe cases of hypothyroidism, thickening of the skin secondary to accumulation of glycos-

TABLE 95–1. FREQUENCY OF COMMON CLINICAL SIGNS AND ROUTINE LABORATORY FINDINGS IN CANINE HYPOTHYROIDISM

	Percentage of Dogs
Clinical signs	
Lethargy/mental dullness	70
Alopecia/hair loss	65
Weight gain/obesity	60
Dry hair coat/excessive shedding	60
Anestrus (15 intact females)	40
Hyperpigmentation	25
Cold intolerance/hypothermia	15
Bradycardia	10
Laboratory findings	
Hypercholesterolemia	80
Normocytic, normochromic anemia	50

Compiled from 30 dogs diagnosed at The Animal Medical Center and 26 cases reported in references 102, 115–118, 126, and 127. Hypothyroidism was confirmed in all cases on the basis of the results of either TSH stimulation testing or thyroid biopsy.

aminoglycans (mostly hyaluronic acid) in the dermis is observed.[26, 92, 103] In such cases, myxedema is most commonly recognized on the dog's forehead and face, resulting in a puffy appearance and thickened skin folds above the eyes. This puffiness, together with slight drooping of the upper eyelid, gives some dogs the appearance of a "tragic" facial expression. These changes may not be localized only to the skin, since analogous accumulations of interstitial mucoid material have been described in the intestinal tract, heart, and skeletal muscles.[103]

Cardiovascular System. Cardiovascular signs associated with severe canine hypothyroidism include bradycardia (Table 95–1), a weak apex beat, and decreased QRS amplitudes.[104] In humans with hypothyroidism, a reversible type of cardiomyopathy has been documented; however, cardiac failure is a rare consequence of hypothyroidism in the absence of underlying cardiac disease.[105] Similarly, impaired myocardial contractility has clearly been demonstrated in dogs with experimentally induced hypothyroidism.[106, 107] Echocardiographic studies of dogs with induced hypothyroidism have revealed evidence of impaired myocardial function, as shown by thinning of the left ventricular posterior wall and interventricular septum, decreased shortening fraction, and decreased left ventricular posterior wall excursion.[108] Despite the impairment in myocardial function associated with severe canine hypothyroidism, hemodynamic, echocardiographic, or pathologic signs suggestive of congestive heart failure have not been found.

Although hypothyroidism has been suspected of inducing dilated cardiomyopathy in some dogs, the relationship between hypothyroidism and overt congestive heart failure has yet to be convincingly documented. In a recent study of thyroid function in dogs with congestive cardiomyopathy, resting serum thyroid hormone concentrations were subnormal in 5 of the 13 dogs evaluated, but only one dog had concurrent hypothyroidism based on the results of TSH response testing.[109] Care must be taken not to misdiagnose hypothyroidism in dogs with heart failure, since any severe illness can falsely lower basal thyroid hormone levels when thyroid function is actually normal.

Nervous System and Muscle. Clinical signs of peripheral nervous dysfunction that only very rarely develop in hypothyroid dogs include dragging of the front feet, lateral head tilt (vestibular nerve paralysis), and inability to close the eyelid or retract the lip (facial nerve paralysis).[26] The cause of the ineffective lifting of the front feet is unclear but may result from a peripheral neuropathy, analogous to the carpal tunnel syndrome (compression of the median nerve at the wrist) commonly seen in humans with myxedema.[92] Likewise, the exact pathogenesis of the vestibular and facial nerve paralysis that can develop is not known, but such neuropathies are likely to result from compression by mucinous deposits in and around the affected nerves as they pass through the internal acoustic meatus of the temporal bone.[26] If the peripheral neuropathies are not of long duration, the changes are usually reversible after thyroid hormone replacement therapy. An association between hypothyroidism and laryngeal paralysis also has been suggested but remains to be proven.[110] Although

extremely rare, CNS signs of seizures, disorientation, and circling also have been reported in dogs with cerebrovascular atherosclerosis caused by the hyperlipidemia associated hypothyroidism.[111] Clinical signs suggestive of musculoskeletal dysfunction in the hypothyroid dog may include weakness, exercise intolerance, muscle cramps, and stiffness. Although the cause of such musculoskeletal signs in canine hypothyroidism is unclear, it is possible that distention of muscle tissue with glycosaminoglycans is a contributing factor.[92] Type II muscle fiber atrophy has also been described in dogs with hypothyroidism.[112] Although a hypothyroid state has been reported to induce megaesophagus,[113] such an association is extremely uncommon and a cause and effect relationship between the two disorders has yet to be documented.

Reproductive System. In the sexually intact dog, hypothyroidism may cause a variety of reproductive disturbances. When breeding bitches are affected, the primary complaints associated with the hypothyroid state are failure to cycle (anestrus) or sporadic cycling, infertility, abortion, or poor litter survival.[97, 114] In addition, inappropriate galactorrhea is a rare sign of hypothyroidism that develops in some intact female dogs whose mammae have been primed for lactation.[115] Hyperprolactinemia, resulting from the excessive stimulation of prolactin-secreting pituitary cells by TRH, appears to be the cause of such galactorrhea in susceptible bitches and may be at least partially responsible for the infertility associated with canine hypothyroidism. Lack of libido, testicular atrophy, hypospermia, or infertility can be seen in the male. The incidence of reproductive abnormalities associated with hypothyroidism in dogs used for breeding purposes has not been reported.

Gastrointestinal Signs. Dogs with hypothyroidism usually have normal bowel movements but a few have somewhat dry feces and prolonged intestinal transient times.[26] Studies in hypothyroid dogs have demonstrated a decrease in the electrical and motor activity of the stomach, intestine, and colon.[116] Occasionally, however, mild diarrhea may develop; the cause is unknown.

Eyes. Although rarely observed, a multitude of ocular abnormalities may develop in dogs with hypothyroidism. These include corneal lipid deposits (arcus lipoides), chronic uveitis, lipid effusion into the aqueous humor, secondary glaucoma, and keratoconjunctivitis sicca.[117, 118] All of these abnormalities appear to develop as a result of severe hyperlipidemia associated with the hypothyroid state.

Coagulation System (Bleeding Disorders). It has been suggested that a cause and effect relationship exists between canine hypothyroidism and the development of an acquired coagulation defect (von Willebrand's disease).[119, 120] While an association between hypothyroidism and a bleeding tendency (e.g., easy bruising) is recognized in human patients, clinically significant bleeding is extremely rare.[121–123] In many of these human patients, the precise nature of the hemostatic defect is unclear, but in some cases the laboratory features do resemble those of von Willebrand's disease.[123]

It is widely recognized that a relationship between factor VIII and factor VIII-related antigen and the thyroid hormones exists. Both hyperthyroidism and the administration of thyroxine to euthyroid human subjects consistently increase factor VIII coagulant activity and related antigen.[124, 125] Similarly, in dogs with von Willebrand's disease treated with thyroid hormone, a rise in factor VIII antigen may occur within 24 hours despite the fact that results of TSH testing are not always consistent with hypothyroidism. The mechanism of action of thyroxine in these circumstances is uncertain, but may reflect the nonspecific action of thyroid hormone on protein synthesis (especially with large doses of thyroid hormone).

Since von Willebrand's disease is most prevalent in many of the same breeds that are predisposed to developing hypothyroidism (e.g., Doberman pinscher, golden retriever, miniature schnauzer),[101, 119] it is likely that the von Willebrand's disease is primary in nature and is not directly caused by the hypothyroid state, at least in most of these dogs. However, in a dog with mild or subclinical von Willebrand's disease, the development of hypothyroidism (together with a further decrease in factor VIII activity) would predispose to the development of overt bleeding.

Endocrine System. The hypothyroid state also can affect the secretion of nonthyroidal hormones from other endocrine glands, especially many of the pituitary hormones (e.g., growth hormone, gonadotropins, and prolactin). Deficient growth hormone secretion secondary to the hypothyroid state is clinically the most important alteration because two of the common differential diagnoses for a dog with "endocrine" alopecia include hypothyroidism and GH deficiency (GH responsive alopecia in the mature dog).[100] Therefore, the finding of a suppressed circulating GH response to provocative stimuli (e.g., xylazine or clonidine) is not diagnostic for primary GH deficiency unless the diagnosis of hypothyroidism has been excluded. In dogs with secondary GH deficiency associated with hypothyroidism, the impaired GH secretory capacity will normalize following thyroid hormone replacement therapy.[96, 100]

Myxedema Coma. Myxedema coma is a rare syndrome representing the extreme expression of severe hypothyroidism.[92] Although well characterized in human hypothyroid patients, there have been only a few reports of the condition in the dog.[126, 127] The course, which can develop rapidly, is one of lethargy progressing to stupor and then coma. The common signs of hypothyroidism (e.g., hair loss) are usually present but other signs of hypoventilation, hypotension, bradycardia, and profound hypothermia are usually observed as well. Laboratory findings may include hypercarbia (CO_2 retention), hypoxia, hyponatremia, and hypoglycemia.[92, 126, 127]

Because of the extremely high mortality associated with untreated myxedema coma, it is essential that treatment be instituted promptly and vigorously as soon as the diagnosis is made. Treatment should include intravenous doses of L-T_4 (2.2 µg/lb or 5 µg/kg twice daily), slow, passive rewarming (wrapping in blankets), and mechanical respiratory support as needed. Therapy for hypotension and shock should include fluid and electrolyte replacement, as well as glucocorticoid supplementation, if needed.

Clinical Signs in Adult-Onset Secondary Canine Hypothyroidism

Since the majority of dogs with adult-onset pituitary hypothyroidism have pituitary tumors, clinical signs associated with other hormonal disturbances (e.g., hyperadrenocorticism, hypoadrenocorticism, diabetes insipidus, hypogonadism) are common. In addition, progressive neurological abnormalities commonly develop in these dogs.[98]

Clinical Signs in Congenital or Juvenile-Onset Canine Hypothyroidism

During the fetal period and in the first few months of postnatal life, thyroid hormones are crucial for growth and development of the skeleton and CNS. Therefore, in addition to the well-recognized signs of adult-onset hypothyroidism, disproportionate dwarfism and impaired mental development (cretinism) are prominent signs of congenital and juvenile-onset hypothyroidism.[29, 32, 93–96] With primary congenital hypothyroidism, enlargement of the thyroid gland (goiter) also may be detected, depending on the cause of the hypothyroid state.[32] Radiographic signs of epiphyseal dysgenesis (underdeveloped epiphyses throughout the long bones), shortened vertebral bodies, and delayed epiphyseal closure are common.[32, 93–96]

In dogs with congenital hypopituitarism (pituitary dwarfism), there may be variable degrees of thyroidal, adrenocortical, and gonadal deficiency, but clinical signs are primarily related to growth hormone deficiency. Clinical signs that develop in these dogs include proportionate dwarfism (rather than the disproportionate form of dwarfism characteristic of congenital hypothyroidism), loss of primary guard hairs with retention of the puppy coat, hyperpigmentation of the skin, and bilateral, symmetric alopecia of the trunk.[99, 100]

Screening Laboratory Tests

There are well-recognized clinical pathologic abnormalities associated with hypothyroidism, the severity of which usually correlates with the severity and chronicity of the hypothyroid state. It is important to remember that these alterations are nonspecific and may be associated with many other diseases in the dog. Their presence, however, adds supportive evidence for a diagnosis of hypothyroidism in a dog with appropriate clinical signs.

Complete Blood Count. The classic hematologic finding associated with hypothyroidism is a normocytic, normochromic, nonregenerative anemia (Table 95–1). Decreased erythropoietin production, decreased peripheral demands for oxygen, and a direct effect of thyroid hormone deficiency on bone marrow may all contribute to the anemia associated with hypothyroidism.[128, 129]

Serum Biochemical Tests. The classic serum biochemical abnormality is hypercholesterolemia, which occurs in most dogs with hypothyroidism (Table 95–1).

Serum triglyceride concentrations are less consistently increased. Lipoprotein electrophoresis may reveal increases in the pre-β, β, and α_2 regions.[130, 131] Both hypercholesterolemia and hypertriglyceridemia result from decreased metabolism and clearance of these substances from the blood. Less commonly, an elevated concentration of serum creatine phosphokinase is detected, which is also a result of decreased turnover of the enzyme.[132]

Thyroid Function Tests

Most of the serum thyroid hormone (and thyroid-related protein) measurements are based upon radioimmunoassay (RIA) techniques. Although thyroid hormone molecules are not species specific, all assays used to measure them must be validated for the species of interest because the nonspecific effects of serum binding proteins vary among species. It is recommended that test results be compared only to the normal range for a species established by the laboratory performing the test.[133] In general, thyroid hormone concentrations are relatively stable in serum or plasma through freezing and thawing and do not vary despite storage at room temperature for as long as eight days.[134] The various thyroid function tests discussed here are listed in approximate order of their availability and utility.

Serum Total T_4 Concentration. The determination of basal serum total T_4 concentration by RIA may provide important information to rule out a diagnosis of hypothyroidism. Since T_4 is produced only from the thyroid gland, dogs with hypothyroidism can, in most cases, be distinguished from normal dogs on the basis of a low resting serum T_4 concentration.[81] However, as previously discussed, many nonthyroidal illnesses and certain drugs may also falsely lower baseline serum T_4 concentrations in the dog.[69–72, 78, 79] Even when historical and physical findings do not suggest the presence of other factors that would lower serum T_4, it is wise to confirm the diagnosis of hypothyroidism with a dynamic thyroid function test (e.g., TSH or TRH stimulation test).

Serum Total T_3 Concentration. Because T_3 is the most potent thyroid hormone at the cellular level, it would seem logical to measure its concentration for diagnostic purposes. Indeed, it has been reported that the serum T_3 concentration is about as useful in distinguishing normal from hypothyroid dogs as is the serum T_4 concentration.[81] However, many other investigators have reported low, normal, or occasionally high serum T_3 concentrations in dogs with subnormal serum T_4 concentrations documented to have hypothyroidism.[71, 72, 135] Overall, it is clear that determination of resting serum T_3 (or T_4) concentrations alone cannot always separate dogs with hypothyroidism from normal dogs or dogs with falsely low resting values secondary to nonthyroidal illness. The diagnostic value of a serum T_3 determination appears particularly weak during early thyroid failure because the failing thyroid has the tendency to increase the relative synthesis and secretion of T_3 over T_4.[136] There is also evidence in humans that peripheral tissues may autoregulate 5'-deiodination in hypothyroidism in order to preserve the circulating T_3 concentration as

long as possible.[137] In the hypothyroid dog in which high values for serum T_3 are found, anti-T_3 antibodies, which produce spurious results in most T_3 RIAs,[135] should be suspected (see section on Circulating Autoantibodies to T_3 and T_4).

Thyrotropin (TSH) Stimulation Test. The administration of exogenous bovine TSH followed by the measurement of serum T_4 provides important information in the diagnosis of hypothyroidism because it tests thyroid secretory reserve. At present, the TSH stimulation test is the most definitive noninvasive test for the diagnosis of primary hypothyroidism.

Protocols for this test vary widely.[138] Because the TSH dose and serum sampling times used are often dictated by practical and economic considerations, it seems logical that the TSH stimulation test should use the lowest TSH dose required to give a maximal thyroidal T_4 response, and that the post-TSH blood sample be obtained at the time of the peak T_4 response. Because the response of serum T_3 concentration to TSH stimulation tends to be less consistent than the T_4 response, determination of post-TSH serum T_3 values is not routinely recommended. For the dog, the authors suggest collecting a baseline blood sample for serum T_4 determination, administering TSH at the dosage of 0.05 U/lb (0.1 U/kg), IV (up to a maximum dose of 5 units), and collecting the post-TSH serum sample for T_4 determination six hours after injection. Although the manufacturer states that the shelf life of reconstituted TSH is only 48 hours, a recent study found that reconstituted TSH can be stored at 4°C for at least three weeks without loss of biologic activity.[139] Accordingly, multiple TSH stimulation tests could potentially be performed following the reconstitution of one vial of TSH, thereby helping to minimize the cost of the test. The TSH stimulation test may be performed concurrently with the adrenocorticotropin (ACTH) stimulation test for hypo- or hyperadrenocorticism without significant effects on the results of either test.[140] Although rare, anaphylaxis may develop in dogs after repeated IV injections of bovine TSH. Therefore, retesting with TSH (at least using the IV route of administration) should be performed under close supervision, if at all.

Figure 95–5 summarizes the various possibilities for results of TSH stimulation tests (and TRH stimulation tests, see next section). In primary hypothyroidism, the post-TSH serum T_4 concentration remains below the normal range for basal T_4 (usually less than 1.0 μg/dl) and rarely increases by more than 0.2 μg/dl above the baseline value.[81] With TSH stimulation testing, primary hypothyroidism can be distinguished from other causes of depression of basal serum T_4 concentrations (e.g., drugs and nonthyroidal illness), in which the serum T_4 response may be suppressed but the slope of the increase is similar to that of normal dogs. However, the test can not always differentiate the effects of illness and drug therapy from secondary (and tertiary) hypothyroidism or from early stages of primary hypothyroidism where the thyroid gland may remain somewhat responsive to TSH.[81, 98] Cases of long-standing pituitary or hypothalamic hypothyroidism with subsequent thyroid atrophy, on the other hand, usually fail to show a serum T_4 response after a single dose of TSH (e.g., dogs with

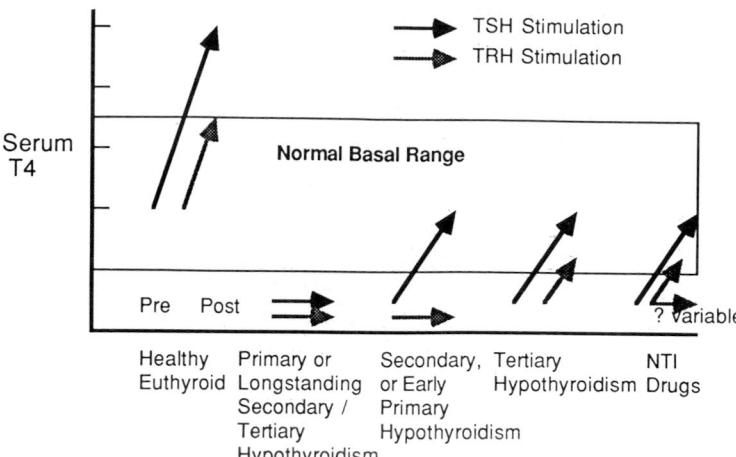

FIGURE 95–5. Serum T_4 responses to TSH and TRH in various conditions. The arrows represent in a stylized fashion the classical response of serum T_4 concentrations to optimal doses of TSH and TRH.

primary hypothyroidism) and may require two or three consecutive daily doses of TSH to eventually demonstrate thyroid responsiveness.[26, 28]

Some investigators have advocated that adequate thyroidal response to TSH be considered a doubling of the baseline serum T_4 concentration. In one study of normal dogs sampled at various times after administration of TSH (5 U, IV), a doubling of the basal serum T_4 concentration was not achieved by four hours in 80 per cent of the dogs but was achieved in all cases by six hours after TSH administration.[141] While such a "doubling" standard recognizes the importance of demonstrating thyroid secretory reserve, this empirical criterion is unreasonable to apply when the pre-TSH and post-TSH serum T_4 concentrations are both low (e.g., basal serum T_4, 0.4 µg/dl; post-TSH T_4, 0.8 µg/dl) and when the pre-TSH value is normal but the post-TSH value is not double (e.g., basal serum T_4, 3 µg/dl; post-TSH T_4, 5 µg/dl). Furthermore, as previously discussed, interpretation of results of TSH testing must take into consideration the fact that the maximal serum T_4 response following TSH injection tends to decrease with age.

In general, when evaluating the results of a TSH stimulation test, calculation of the difference between the basal serum T_4 concentration and the post-TSH T_4 value is more discriminative in the diagnosis of hypothyroidism than is the ratio between the two values. According to the results of one study, the increase in serum T_4 concentration should be at least 18 nmol/l (approximately 1.5 µg/dl) 4 hours after IV administration of 10 units of TSH in normal dogs.[72] However, not all hypothyroid dogs could be detected using this criterion. An increase in diagnostic precision was achieved, however, when the evaluation was performed by combining the TSH response with the basal T_4 value, as described in the following equation (calculated by discriminant analysis): $k = 0.5 \times$ basal T_4 concentration (nmol/l) + difference between post-TSH and pre-TSH T_4 concentration (nmol/l) or $k = 6.4 \times$ basal T_4 concentration (µg/dl) + 12.9 $\times$ T_4 increment following TSH (µg/dl).[72] In that study, all dogs with a k value less than 15 were hypothyroid, whereas dogs with a value greater than 30 were considered euthyroid. In dogs with a k value between 15 and 30, other diagnostic tests (e.g., thyroid biopsy, thyroid imaging) were required.

The value of a diagnostic test for hypothyroidism cannot be judged unless the results of the test are compared to a histological diagnosis (e.g., lymphocytic thyroiditis, thyroidal atrophy) or are based upon the success in predicting a response to replacement therapy. Based on these criteria, the post-TSH T_4 concentration should generally either increase by at least 2.0 µg/dl over the basal serum T_4 value or exceed the normal range of basal T_4 concentrations (approximately 4 µg/dl in most laboratories) by six hours after injection of TSH (0.22 U/lb or 0.1 U/kg, IV) to rule out a diagnosis of hypothyroidism. Dogs that fail to meet these criteria can be considered to have hypothyroidism and their response to thyroid hormone replacement therapy should be evaluated. Although the discriminant functions (k values), as described above, may further aid in the diagnosis of canine hypothyroidism, similar equations ideally should be established in each laboratory to enhance diagnostic interpretation.

Thyrotropin-Releasing Hormone (TRH) Stimulation Test. The TRH stimulation test, as used in the diagnosis of human pituitary-thyroid disease, is designed to evaluate the pituitary's responsiveness to TRH as manifested by the change in serum TSH concentration. The serum TSH response to TRH is increased in primary thyroid gland failure and decreased in secondary hypothyroidism states (as well as in hyperthyroidism). Since a valid homologous canine TSH assay is not yet widely available, application of the TRH stimulation test requires the measurement of serum T_4 concentrations. In theory, the administration of TRH should lead to an increase in T_4 only if the pituitary-thyroid axis is intact (Figures 95–4 and 95–5). Therefore, responsiveness to TRH should only be observed in normal dogs and dogs with the hypothalamic form of thyroid insufficiency, a rare finding.

Several studies have examined a range of TRH doses for use in the dog.[52–55] In one study, no difference in the peak T_4 response to TRH was noted, using intravenous dosages ranging from 0.001 to 5 mg/lb (0.002 to 10 mg/kg).[52] However, increasing the TRH dose increased the duration of the serum T_4 response. Side effects were more common at dosages greater than 0.05 mg/lb (0.1 mg/kg) and included salivation, urination, defecation, vomiting, miosis, tachycardia, and tachypnea. The recommended protocol for the TRH stimulation test is to collect blood samples for T_4 determination before and six hours after administration of TRH, using a dosage of 0.05 mg/lb (0.1 mg/kg) IV. Using this protocol in normal dogs, resting serum T_4 concentrations increased by at least 50 per cent in 28 of 31 dogs and increased by at least 0.5 μg/dl in all dogs.[52]

The TRH stimulation test has been touted by some investigators as a replacement for the TSH stimulation test in the diagnosis of hypothyroidism.[52, 55] Because the TRH tripeptide is not species-specific, it is not antigenic (as is bovine TSH), a theoretical advantage if repeated testing is required. Like TSH, pharmaceutical preparations of TRH can be expensive (using recommended dosages). Most important, however, is the fact that the rise in the serum T_4 concentration following TRH in euthyroid dogs may be small compared to that observed after TSH (minimum response is 0.5 μg/dl for TRH and 2.0 μg/dl for TSH).[52] Therefore, the successful application of the TRH stimulation test requires the use of an assay with extremely good internal reproducibility. For example, the serum T_4 result may vary as much as 20 per cent in many "acceptable" T_4 RIAs (two standard deviations if the coefficient of variation is 10 per cent) when a sample containing a low T_4 concentration is run repeatedly in one assay. Finally, the TRH stimulation test cannot be recommended for diagnosis of hypothyroidism until the effects of drugs or nonthyroidal illness on test results have been investigated. For example, it has been reported that approximately half of dogs with spontaneous hyperadrenocorticism lack a normal response to TRH, consistent with pituitary TSH suppression (secondary hypothyroidism).[73] After correction of the hypercortisolism, however, the subnormal serum T_4 and T_3 concentrations return to normal and treatment of the reversible hypothyroid state does not appear to be necessary.[70]

Serum Total Reverse T_3 (rT_3) Concentration. Reverse T_3, the inactive product of T_4 5-monodeiodination, also may be measured by specific RIA. The major usefulness of serum rT_3 determinations is to aid in differentiating hypothyroidism from the nonthyroidal causes of low serum total T_4 and T_3 concentrations.[42] Since virtually all circulating rT_3 is derived from T_4 secreted from the thyroid gland, the finding of low serum rT_3 concentrations provides confirmatory evidence for low amounts of available (free) T_4 and therefore is generally consistent with a hypothyroid state. When the serum concentration of rT_3 is high, on the other hand, it suggests that the free T_4 (FT_4) concentration is normal and 5'-deiodination has been inhibited, as occurs in certain nonthyroidal illnesses.

One nonthyroidal illness that appears to be a notable exception is canine hyperadrenocorticism. In one study, suppression of serum T_4 or T_3 concentrations (or both) into the subnormal range was seen in over half of the dogs, while serum rT_3 concentrations remained normal or were decreased.[47] The absence of an increase in serum rT_3 values in canine hyperadrenocorticism is probably related to the reduction in serum FT_4 concentrations, observed in about 25 per cent of the cases.[47] As discussed above, it appears that at least some dogs with hyperadrenocorticism have a secondary form of hypo-

thyroidism that is reversible after correction of the cortisol excess.

Serum Free T_4 Concentration. Because the free concentration of T_4 reflects the hormone available for entry into cells, free T_4 determinations provide a more consistent assessment of thyroid status at the tissue level than does measurement of total T_4. Furthermore, the FT_4 concentration is not as likely as total T_4 determinations to be affected by nonthyroidal illness or drug therapy. The fraction of FT_4 by equilibrium dialysis is about 0.1 per cent of the total T_4 concentration in the healthy euthyroid dog.[47] This free fraction may rise in certain nonthyroidal illnesses (e.g., chronic renal failure) or after administration of certain drugs (e.g., aspirin, phenylbutazone, phenytoin), as a consequence of impaired serum protein binding of thyroid hormones or decreased concentrations of the thyroid binding proteins.[38, 48, 77]

Two general methods are available for the determination of the FT_4 concentration. The standard method involves the determination of the FT_4 fraction (%FT_4) by equilibrium dialysis and the total T_4 (TT_4) concentration by RIA. The absolute FT_4 concentration (AFT_4) is then calculated as follows: AFT_4 (ng/dl) = %FT_4 × TT_4 (μg/dl) × 10. The absolute concentrations of FT_4 are very similar among species (0.7 to 3.3 ng/dl for dog).[47] The main disadvantage for routine use of equilibrium dialysis is that the procedure is time-consuming and technically difficult.[142] In addition, a relatively large volume of serum (1–2 ml) is required, because canine serum cannot be diluted before equilibrium dialysis or artificially low results will be obtained (unpublished observations).

Use of commercial RIA kits is the second method for determination of the FT_4 concentrations. These kits, which theoretically measure the FT_4 concentrations directly (but in reality do not), are being used with increasing frequency by some veterinary diagnostic laboratories. Such kits (which generally employ either a labeled thyroxine analogue method or use a microcapsule dialysis membrane technique)[142, 143] are more rapid and, at least seemingly, more practical than equilibrium dialysis. In humans, however, the reliability and validity of results obtained with these FT_4 kits has recently been seriously questioned.[63, 143–145] Use of these kits has been reported to underestimate or provide inaccurate values, especially in situations when the serum protein binding of thyroid hormones is impaired (e.g., nonthyroidal illness and after treatment with certain drugs). Until proven reliable in states of thyroid dysfunction as well as in nonthyroidal illness, these RIA methods for FT_4 determination in the dog and cat should be interpreted with caution. Ultimately, to be valid, the results should compare closely to those obtained by equilibrium dialysis.

Serum Free T_3 Concentration. All of the considerations for the measurement of the FT_4 concentrations, as discussed, also hold for free T_3 (FT_3) determinations. Although serum FT_3 concentrations should reflect the cellular availability of the most active thyroid hormone, the nonthyroidal factors that alter the total serum T_3 concentrations will also affect FT_3 concentrations, reducing their value as a single discriminator of the thyroid status.

Triiodothyronine Resin Uptake (Thyroid Hormone Binding Ratio). The T_3 resin uptake (or T_3 uptake) test is an indirect method for estimating changes in thyroid hormone binding by plasma proteins.[92] Because the term "T_3 uptake" has been confused with total serum T_3 measurements, the American Thyroid Association recently recommended changing the name of the test to the "Thyroid Hormone Binding Ratio (THBR)."[145] In humans, the results of the T_3 resin uptake (THBR) test correlate well with FT_4 concentrations determined by equilibrium dialysis. The product of the T_3 uptake result and total T_4 concentration is called the free thyroxine index and is commonly used as a reliable estimate of the serum FT_4 concentration in humans.[92] However, it may be inaccurate when marked increases or decreases in TBG concentrations are present.

Unfortunately, because of the relative lack of high affinity serum thyroid hormone binding proteins (e.g., TBG), the T_3 uptake test is very insensitive to changes in canine (and feline) thyroid function and cannot be used to reliably estimate the FT_4 concentration.[49, 146] Likewise, since the value for free thyroxine index is derived from the T_3 resin uptake (THBR) test result, the free thyroxine index is also an unreliable indicator of the serum FT_4 concentration in the dog and cat.

Circulating Thyroid Hormone Autoantibodies. Autoantibody binding of thyroid hormone is widely documented in humans with autoimmune thyroid disease (including lymphocytic thyroiditis), although some of these individuals remain clinically euthyroid.[147–149] The exact mechanism for induction of thyroid hormone autoantibodies has not been clarified but may be related to the T_4 and T_3 binding capacity of anti-thyroglobulin antibodies.[149] The effect of the abnormal antibody binding of thyroid hormone in euthyroid subjects (or in hypothyroid patients given thyroid hormone replacement therapy) is to elevate total serum thyroid hormone concentrations. While these autoantibodies alter plasma binding, free concentrations of T_4 or T_3 remain normal. The main importance of thyroid hormone autoantibodies is that they present serious practical and interpretative problems when the serum concentrations of T_4 and T_3 are measured by RIA.[147–149] The type of interference that thyroid hormone autoantibodies produce in RIAs depends on the separation method employed in the assay. Nonspecific separation methods (e.g., charcoal extraction) result in spuriously low or undetectable thyroid hormone concentrations, while specific separation systems (e.g., double-antibody or solid phase techniques) produce spuriously high values for T_4 or T_3.[147–149] Accurate total hormone concentrations may be determined in these patients only by special extraction techniques or by removing the endogenous immunoglobulin prior to assay.[147–149] Because the autoantibodies also interfere with the RIA determination of FT_4 and FT_3, equilibrium dialysis is the only reliable method to determine the free hormone fraction.[148]

In a large series of canine serum samples submitted to a veterinary diagnostic laboratory for thyroid hormone determinations, approximately 0.2 per cent had apparent T_3 concentrations (determined by a solid phase RIA method) greater than 500 ng/dl, a finding that was virtually pathognomonic of anti-T_3 antibodies.[135] Unfor-

tunately, neither the clinical history nor results of thyroid biopsy were available in the dogs with T_3 autoantibodies of that report. Although no dogs with elevated total T_4 values were reported in that study, the authors have observed low, normal, and elevated serum T_4 concentrations in hypothyroid dogs with apparent high T_3 concentrations (both measured by solid phase RIA technique). In addition, using electrophoretic techniques to study tracer thyroid hormone binding to TBG, TBPA, and gamma globulin,[147] the authors have documented the presence of anti-T_4 antibodies, as well as T_3 autoantibodies, in eight dogs with hypothyroidism caused by lymphocytic thyroiditis. As in humans, the presence of T_3 or T_4 autoantibodies appears to be of no clinical significance to the dog, since the binding capacity of the antibody is easily exceeded by administration of standard dosages of L-thyroxine. Evaluation during thyroid hormone replacement therapy depends primarily on the presence or lack of clinical improvement. Therapeutic monitoring of serum thyroid hormone concentrations ("post-pill testing") is not routinely recommended in these dogs since the autoantibodies will continue to produce spurious RIA results.[147] Because thyroid hormone autoantibodies may develop in clinically euthyroid dogs as well as in dogs with lymphocytic thyroiditis, confirmation of the hypothyroid state in these dogs is best obtained by thyroid biopsy.

Circulating Antibodies to Thyroglobulin. Antibodies to thyroglobulin are often generated early in the course of thyroidal destruction associated with lymphocytic thyroiditis. A recent study found antithyroglobulin antibodies by ELISA methods in 59 per cent of 34 hypothyroid dogs. The incidence of antibodies to thyroglobulin in 1057 normal dogs evaluated was 13 per cent.[76] Another study of 25 dogs with hypothyroidism showed circulating antibody titers against thyroglobulin and thyroid microsomal antigens in 48 per cent and 4 per cent, respectively, using the chromic chloride passive hemagglutination test.[71] Although only reported as a research tool, determination of antithyroglobulin antibodies potentially could provide a method for the early diagnosis of lymphocytic thyroiditis.

Serum Thyroxine Binding Prealbumin. A recent study of dogs with liver or kidney disease found that mean serum concentrations of TBPA (measured by a immunoelectrophoresis method) were significantly decreased in both groups, as compared to normal dogs.[72] In addition, there was a direct correlation between serum T_4 values and TBPA concentrations in these two groups of "sick" dogs. These findings suggest that the low serum T_4 concentrations seen in these nonthyroidal illnesses may be attributed, at least in part, to depressed TBPA levels resulting from decreased hepatic production or increased renal excretion of the serum binding protein.[72] However, since TBPA concentrations may be normal or elevated when serum T_4 concentrations are subnormal, especially in disorders such as canine diabetes mellitus and hyperadrenocorticism,[72] changes in TBPA (and TBG) binding affinity or other factors unrelated to TBPA must also be important in determining the total T_4 concentration in nonthyroidal illness. Although clearly only a research tool at the present time, determination of serum TBPA concentrations may someday aid in distinguishing between hypothyroidism and low serum T_4 concentrations secondary to canine nonthyroidal illnesses.

Endogenous Serum TSH Concentrations. The measurement of basal and TRH-stimulated endogenous serum TSH concentrations has proven to be extremely important for the early diagnosis of thyroid disorders in humans.[92] Basal and TRH-stimulated serum TSH concentrations are invariably elevated in humans with primary hypothyroidism. In contrast, humans with pituitary (secondary) hypothyroidism generally have low basal serum TSH concentrations that fail to increase after the administration of TRH. Because TSH is a species-specific glycoprotein, attempts to use commercially available anti-human TSH RIA kits in the dog have generally failed to aid in the diagnosis of hypothyroidism.[54, 150, 151]

Although results of one validated canine TSH RIA have been reported (apparently satisfactory for use in canine research studies),[51] the reagents for this assay have not been made available for commercial distribution. Recently, a commercial homologous canine TSH assay kit was introduced but the widespread consensus has been that the results from this assay do not allow the discrimination of hypothyroid from normal dogs. Once a valid TSH assay is made available for widespread use in dogs and cats, it is certain to greatly contribute to the diagnosis and management of thyroid disorders.

Thyroid Radionuclide Uptake and Imaging. The radioiodine uptake determination, one of the oldest thyroid function tests, involves administration of a tracer dose of radioiodine followed by measurement (using external γ counting) of the proportion of the dose present in the thyroid gland at a particular time.[152] The fraction of the radioiodine that is taken up by the thyroid gland depends on a number of factors, including the functional capacity of the thyroid, the endogenous secretion of TSH, and the dietary iodine intake.[152] In normal dogs, peak uptake of radioiodine (which occurs between 48 and 72 hours after administration) is about 15 per cent of the administered dose, whereas the per cent thyroid uptake value is usually less than five per cent of the dose in dogs with primary hypothyroidism.[26, 28, 37] Because values vary inversely with the intake of stable iodine, however, thyroid uptake determinations also may be depressed in normal dogs receiving a relatively high iodine diet.[28] Even in the absence of dietary factors, thyroid radioiodine uptake measurement can be a relatively insensitive diagnostic test for hypothyroidism and is impractical for routine clinical use. Therefore, thyroid uptake determinations are no longer used as a general screening test for canine hypothyroidism but are reserved as an aid in characterizing congenital defects of thyroid hormone synthesis.[32, 152, 153]

Although not widely available, thyroid imaging is a useful technique to evaluate the functional status of the thyroid gland and to aid in the differentiation between hypothyroidism, euthyroidism, and the sick euthyroid syndrome.[26] Although radioiodine (^{131}I, ^{123}I) can be used,[29] γ camera imaging of the canine thyroid gland can be most easily performed using pertechnetate ($^{99m}TcO_4{}^-$) as the radionuclide. The imaging procedure can begin only 20 minutes after the administration of $^{99m}TcO_4{}^-$ (approximately 1 to 2 mCi, IV), with a scanning time of about one to two minutes.[26] With thyroid imaging, the normal canine thyroid lobes appear as two uniform, symmetric densities in the cervical region (Figure 95-6). A one-to-one ratio usually exists between the size and intensity of the parotid salivary glands, also visualized with $^{99m}TcO_4$ scanning, and the normal thyroid lobes. In dogs with nonthyroidal illness or drug-induced lowering of the basal serum thyroid hormone concentrations, the thyroid concentrates $^{99m}TcO_4$ normally, thereby excluding hypothyroidism. In both thyroidal (primary) and pituitary (secondary) hypothyroidism, the thyroid image is markedly reduced or virtually absent, especially compared to the radionuclide uptake into the salivary glands (Figure 95–6). Stimulation of atrophied thyroid tissue for three days with exogenous TSH causes little or no change in the reduced thyroid image in dogs with thyroidal hypothyroidism but does result in a normal thyroid image in dogs with pituitary or hypothalamic hypothyroidism.[26, 29]

Thyroid Biopsy. The histologic examination of a biopsy of the thyroid gland is an extremely useful and reliable means of diagnosing hypothyroidism and differentiating the primary and secondary forms of hypothyroidism. In primary hypothyroidism, there is loss of thyroid follicles, resulting from either lymphocytic thyroiditis or thyroidal atrophy (see Causes of Hypothyroidism). In dogs in which the hypothyroid state is secondary to TSH deficiency, the thyroid follicles become distended with colloid and the lining epithelial cells become flattened. The colloid is uniformly dense with complete or nearly complete absence of resorption vacuoles at the periphery of the colloid. Grossly, the thyroid gland appears normal to slightly enlarged, because of the accumulation of colloid.[26]

Treatment

The goal of hormone administration in an endocrine deficiency state is the reversal of the pathophysiologic effects of deficiency in a manner that mimics the natural pattern of secretion and metabolism of that hormone. Before therapy, care should be taken in establishing the diagnosis of hypothyroidism because, with very few exceptions, therapy will be necessary for the remainder of the animal's life. This discussion emphasizes the physiological bases for choice of appropriate thyroid hormone products and replacement regimes.

DETERMINANTS OF BIOAVAILABILITY AND CLINICAL EFFICACY OF THYROID HORMONE PREPARATIONS

The ultimate determinants of bioavailability and efficacy of administered thyroid hormone preparations include the following: route of administration, gastrointestinal absorption, peripheral metabolism, persistence of cellular stores, and persistence of biological effects. All of these factors bear on the clinician's design of a rational thyroid replacement regime.

Although the daily thyroidal secretion of T_4 has been estimated to be approximately 2.5 μg/kg/day in the

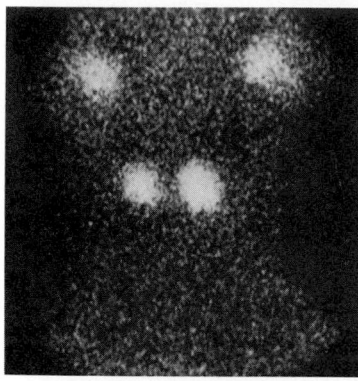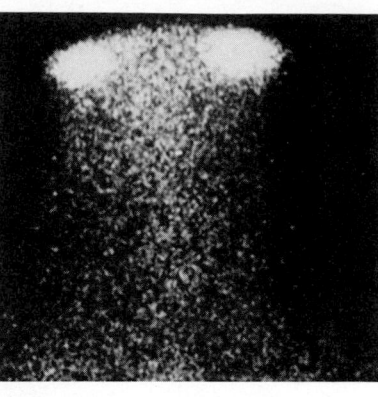

FIGURE 95–6. *Left,* Thyroid scan of a normal dog obtained with $^{99m}TcO_4$. Note that a one-to-one ratio exists between the size and intensity of the parotid salivary glands, also visualized with $^{99m}TcO_4$ scanning, and the two normal thyroid lobes. *Right,* Thyroid scan of a dog with hypothyroidism. With either thyroidal (primary) or pituitary (secondary) hypothyroidism, the thyroid image is markedly reduced or virtually absent, especially compared to the radionuclide uptake into the salivary glands.

dog,[37] the administration of this dose once or divided twice daily subcutaneously or intravenously to surgically thyroidectomized dogs did not normalize serum T_4 concentrations. Serum T_4 concentrations were not normalized until a divided intravenous daily dose of 4.5 μg/lb (10 μg/kg) was given.[154] Thus, if normalization of serum T_4 is the therapeutic goal, then parenterally administered doses of thyroid hormone must exceed the amounts secreted physiologically. With the standard use of oral thyroid hormone products in clinical practice, the additional variability of gastrointestinal absorption is introduced. Although systematic studies have not been performed in the dog, comparison of oral T_4 doses necessary to normalize serum T_4 concentrations (10 to 20 μg/lb day or 20 to 40 μg/kg/day) to parenteral doses (1.2 to 5 μg/lb/day or 2.5 to 10 μg/kg/day) suggests that net gastrointestinal absorption is probably in the range of 10 to 50 per cent. Similarly, in the normal cat, the oral L-T_4 dosage must be approximately five- to tenfold higher than the parenteral dosage required to normalize serum T_4 concentrations. This is in contrast to the situation in humans, where absorption of T_4 preparations is higher (50 to 80 per cent)[155] and explains, in part, why the thyroid hormone replacement dose in the dog and cat is so much higher than in humans. Intraluminal contents, including plasma protein, dietary factors, and intestinal flora, may bind T_4 and make it less available for diffusion.[155] Therefore, it is recommended that dose administration be made at a consistent time relative to meals. Additionally, the administered dose of thyroid hormone should always be tailored to the clinical and/ or biochemical response, as gastrointestinal absorption of orally administered products is variable and unpredictable.

THYROID HORMONE PREPARATIONS

Thyroid hormone preparations can be classified into the following groups: (1) crude hormones prepared from animal thyroid gland, (2) synthetic L-thyroxine (L-T_4), (3) synthetic L-triiodothyronine (L-T_3), and (4) synthetic combinations of L-T_4 and LT$_3$. An extensive list of the available commercial preparations has been published.[97, 156, 157]

Crude Thyroid Products. Thyroid hormone products derived from thyroid tissue from hogs, sheep, or cattle are available in the form of desiccated thyroid. There appear to be no good reasons to continue to use these

products for replacement therapy. Problems, which include a highly variable content of T_4 and T_3, unphysiologically low ratios of T_4/T_3 (2:1 to 4:1), and short shelf-life, outweigh the lower cost of these products.[155] The newer standards set by the U.S. Pharmacopoeia for control of hormone content may improve the reproducibility of these products but are unlikely to eliminate the other disadvantages.

Synthetic L-Thyroxine. Thyroxine (L-T_4) is the thyroid hormone replacement compound of choice in the dog. It is generally formulated and used as levothyroxine sodium for oral administration. Injectable forms are also available (for treatment of myxedema coma). Thyroxine is recommended for the following reasons: (1) L-T_4 is the main secretory product of the thyroid gland. (2) L-T_4 is the physiological prohormone; administration of L-T_4 does not bypass the cellular regulatory processes controlling the production of the more potent T_3 from T_4 (5'-deiodination) (Figure 95–7, bottom). (3) In humans, therapy is often tailored to normalize the serum TSH concentration. In humans with untreated hypothyroidism, serum TSH concentrations correlate inversely with serum T_4 concentrations, but to a lesser extent with serum T_3 concentrations.[158] A more recent study of humans treated with L-T_4 revealed that suppression of serum TSH concentrations into the normal range usually requires high-normal to slightly high circulating T_4 concentrations, while serum T_3 concentrations are usually normal.[57] In that study, suppression of pituitary secretion was more closely related to the serum concentration of T_4 than to T_3.[57] (4) Despite these apparent discrepancies in humans, there is no debate that the therapeutic goal should be to normalize both tissue and serum T_4 and T_3 concentrations, and this is only accomplished in all tissues with exogenous T_4 administration. The central nervous system and pituitary derive a large proportion of their intracellular T_3 from local 5'-deiodination of T_4 (Figure 95–7). (5) With administration of T_3, the serum T_3 concentrations must be higher than normal to normalize serum TSH. Although the same is true for serum T_4 in humans, the adequacy of T_4 replacement can more accurately be monitored by post-pill hormone measurements. (6) In general, variability in bioavailability of synthetic T_4 preparations is less than that of the crude products. (7) L-T_4 is less expensive than other synthetic preparations.

In 1982, the U.S. Pharmacopoeia (USP) adopted a new method for the assay of hormone content in thyroid

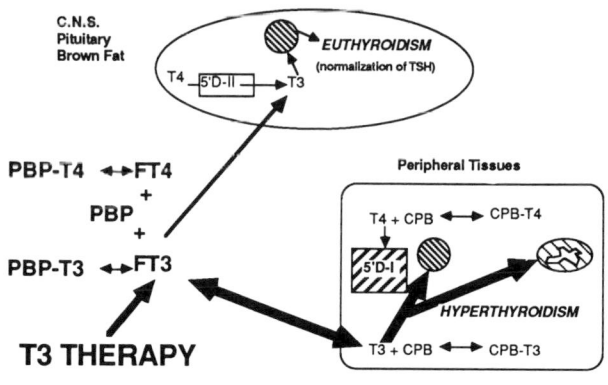

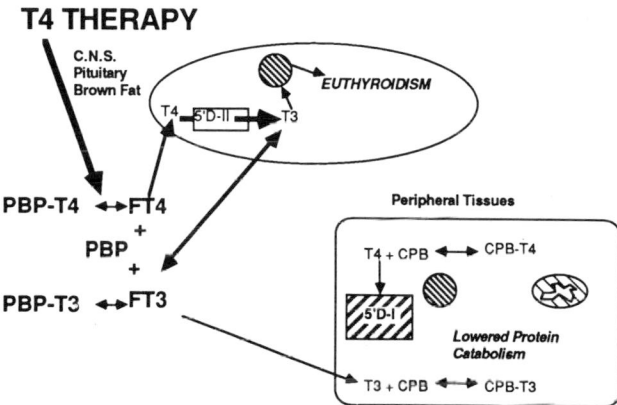

FIGURE 95–7. Thyroid replacement therapy of hypothyroidism with L-T_3 (top) or L-T_4 in supervening nonthyroidal illness. *Top*, L-T_3 therapy during nonthyroidal illness bypasses the individual tissue regulation of the 5'-deiodinase enzymes. Shown is the scenario when the amount of T_3 administered is sufficient to recreate euthyroidism in the pituitary, brown fat, or CNS. In the pituitary, TSH secretion would be reduced to normal. This amount of T_3 would be excessive for tissues such as the liver and kidney, which are trying to limit protein catabolism during illness. A state of tissue hyperthyroidism results. *Bottom*, In contrast to therapy with L-T_3, L-T_4 therapy allows individual tissues to regulate T_3 production. Therefore, the brain, pituitary, and brown fat continue to produce adequate amounts of T_3 derived from plasma T_4, but the liver, kidney, and other tissues reduce local T_3 production, allowing a lowering of protein catabolism in illness.

hormone preparations. The old, less accurate determinations based upon iodine content were replaced by high pressure liquid chromatographic (HPLC) determination. Recent studies of brand-name and generic L-thyroxine preparations showed that the hormonal content of some generic tablets may be as little as 30 per cent of the amount stated on the label.[159] Therefore, when starting an animal on a thyroid replacement product, it is recommended to start with a brand-name product (or proven generic product) with which broad experience has been obtained and use this product until a distinct clinical response is observed. If no response is seen at a reasonable dose after a period of at least four to six weeks, and normal serum T_4 concentrations are achieved after administration, then the diagnosis should be reevaluated. Except for financial reasons, the concern about mild over-replacement is minimal in most cases, since dogs (as well as cats) are very resistant to the development of thyrotoxic signs, requiring 10 to 20 times the replacement dose chronically in order to demonstrate signs. This is likely the result of the capacity of

the dog and cat to efficiently clear thyroid hormone via biliary and fecal excretion.

With very few exceptions, thyroid hormone replacement therapy will be necessary for the remainder of the animal's life. Therefore, careful initial diagnosis and tailoring of treatment are essential. A variety of dosage regimens for T_4 therapy have been recommended. This probably reflects the variation among animals in hormone absorption and metabolism, the variable degree of remaining endogenous hormone secretion by the failing thyroid, the possible effect of circulating anti-T_4 antibodies in a subgroup of animals, the resistance to the development of thyrotoxicosis with overdoses in the dog, and the vague and variable criteria by which clinical improvement is judged.

In general, reported replacement doses for T_4 in the dog range from a total dose of 0.01 mg/lb (0.02 mg/kg) to 0.02 mg/lb (0.04 mg/kg) daily. It has also been proposed that dosage be calculated according to body surface area (0.5 mg/M²), which is proportional to the metabolic rate.[160] When L-T_4 dosage is determined on a body weight basis, large breed dogs have a greater tendency to develop thyrotoxicosis or at least elevated serum T_4 concentrations. For example, according to body surface area, an 11 lb (5 kg) (0.29 M² BSA) dog would start on a dose of 0.15 mg L-T_4 daily, or 0.015 mg/lb (0.03 mg/kg). A 110 lb (50 kg) dog (1.36 M² BSA) would start on 0.70 mg/day, or less than half the dose according to body weight, 0.07 mg/lb (0.014 mg/kg). There are no published experimental studies, however, to confirm the validity of this dosing method.

As thyroid replacement therapy is initiated, a common practice is to divide the total daily dosage into two separate doses given at 12 hour intervals. Because of the significant intracellular capacity for storage of T_4, particularly in rapidly exchanging pools like the liver and kidney, the initial oral doses of thyroid hormone may be substantially distributed into tissue stores. As previously outlined, hypothyroidism reduces the deiodinative and conjugative rate of thyroid hormone metabolism. Division of the daily dose reduces the metabolic effect of a bolus of thyroid hormone on hypothyroid tissues and decreases the first-pass effect (hepatic metabolism and excretion of a portion of a bolus dose of hormone before it ever reaches the systemic circulation). During the initial days to weeks of replacement therapy in a hypothyroid animal, the hormone stores of the liver and kidney are repleted to euthyroid levels, and then can serve to buffer serum concentrations when the circulating hormone store bound to binding proteins begins to be depleted. The result is that many hypothyroid animals can be maintained on once-daily T_4 therapy despite the fact that the serum half-life for T_4 in normal dogs is 10 to 16 hours. In humans, it seems that clinical improvement and suppression of serum TSH can be maintained by any replacement regimen which, over the course of a day, leads to a normal average serum concentration without leading to the acute toxic effects of thyroid hormone. Although the serum T_4 concentration may be high at one time of the day and low at another, the tissue response "integrates" the serum concentration throughout the day, thereby reflecting the average concentration. Once-daily administration also leads to greater compliance by owners. In an animal that has responded to twice-daily therapy, the reappearance of clinical signs of hypothyroidism on a once-daily regimen should be a signal to return to the successful twice-daily regimen.

Gradual introduction of hormone is ideal, particularly in animals with decreased ability to metabolize T_4 and increased risk of developing thyrotoxicosis, such as hypoadrenal, aged, cardiac, or diabetic patients. In these dogs, it is recommended to use divided dose protocols, gradually increasing the daily dose in 20 to 25 per cent increments (over a period of four to eight weeks) until the desired level is reached. Glucocorticoid replacement should begin prior to thyroid replacement therapy in patients with concomitant hypoadrenocorticism (e.g., hypopituitarism), since correction of hypothyroidism increases metabolism and, hence, the demand for endogenous steroids. In all cases, because the metabolism of thyroid hormone changes with correction of hypothyroidism, dosage regimens should be reassessed by clinical and laboratory criteria after at least four weeks of initial therapy.

Synthetic L-Triiodothyronine. Although T_3 is the active intracellular hormone, there are few valid reasons to use this product for replacement therapy and some good reasons not to use it. Triiodothyronine replacement is not physiological, and bypasses the final cellular regulatory step of $5'$-deiodination of T_4 (Figure 95–7). Thyroxine does have intrinsic thyromimetic activity. Its role is particularly important in the central nervous system and pituitary, tissues in which normalization of the intracellular T_3 concentration depends on the normalization of both serum T_4 and T_3. Treatment with T_3 alone may provide amounts sufficient for organs like the liver, kidney, and heart, which derive a high proportion of T_3 from plasma. However, the brain and pituitary, which derive a majority of their T_3 from T_4 intracellularly, may be deficient in thyroid hormone. Conversely, T_3 therapy adequate for the brain and pituitary may be excessive for the liver, kidney, and heart (Figure 95–7, top).

At present, it cannot be recommended that T_3 therapy be instituted in the "low T_3 syndrome" associated with nonthyroidal illness. Because of its higher oral bioavailability, it may be used to improve the clinical response in a dog with demonstrated or suspected poor T_4 absorption in which post-therapy serum T_4 and T_3 concentrations remain low despite increases in the oral daily T_4 dose. Triiodothyronine therapy may be indicated when thyroid replacement is necessary with the simultaneous administration of drugs that inhibit the conversion of T_4 to T_3, an important example being pharmacological doses of glucocorticoids.

Anecdotal reports suggest that a small fraction of hypothyroid dogs convert T_4 to T_3 poorly in the absence of obvious nonthyroidal illness and, therefore, do not respond to L-T_4 therapy. Triiodothyronine therapy has been recommended in these cases as an adjunct to T_4 or as sole therapy. The response to T_3 in these purported "poor converters" following the failure of T_4 therapy does not constitute sufficient evidence for a selective $5'$-deiodinase defect. The most likely cause of apparently low serum T_3 concentrations and normal or high T_4

concentrations following T_4 therapy is the presence of anti-T_3 antibodies which, in certain T_3 RIAs, results in extremely low reading for the T_3 concentration. As previously discussed, this observation is an in vitro artifact that has no relevance to the choice of replacement therapy products. It is recommended that usual dosages of L-T_4 be given to these dogs and the dose increased (if needed) until a clinical response is seen. The post-treatment serum T_3 concentration should be ignored in these dogs with T_3 autoantibodies. Other possible causes of low serum T_3 concentrations during L-T_4 therapy for hypothyroidism or the rare observation of a response to T_3 after failure of T_4 treatment include concomitant nonthyroidal illness, greater oral bioavailability of T_3 than of T_4, or increased serum T_4 binding, possibly due to T_4 antibodies that may impair T_4 uptake into tissue.

A divided dose regimen of 2 to 3 μg/lb (4 to 6 μg/kg) three times or possibly twice daily appears necessary to maintain adequate serum T_3 concentrations without high peaks which appear to be associated with signs of thyrotoxicosis.

Synthetic Combinations of L-T_4 and L-T_3. The use of commercial combinations of synthetic L-T_4 and L-T_3 has little rational basis in human or veterinary medicine. These preparations, containing a 4:1 mixture of T_4 and T_3, were designed to mimic the ratio of T_4:T_3 in thyroidal secretion (approximately 6:1 in the dog) and tablets were designed to provide the equivalent of one grain (65 mg) of desiccated thyroid (50 to 60 μg T_4:12.5 to 15 μg T_3). A variety of dosage schemes have been proposed, but the most common suggests dosing according to the T_4 content and division of the dose to account for the shorter serum half-life of T_3. Administration of these preparations commonly leads to a low-normal to normal serum T_4. Because of the high T_3 content of these products, increasing the dose to normalize serum T_4 can result in high serum T_3 concentrations and can produce thyrotoxicosis. Compared with L-T_4, these preparations share the disadvantages of the T_3 preparations, including increased cost, increased complexity of dosing regimens, and a higher incidence of thyrotoxic signs.

POTENTIAL FACTORS AFFECTING DOSE

Clinically adequate doses of thyroid hormone can be quite variable from animal to animal. In addition to the effects of concomitant drug therapy on thyroid hormone metabolism, increased doses of T_4 appear to be necessary in hypothyroid humans during the colder months of winter. While similar studies have not been performed in animals, it is possible that an animal housed outdoors might require a higher dose of T_4 than an animal predominantly in the house, particularly during the colder months. In the dog, as in humans, basal serum concentrations of T_4 decrease with age. It has been observed in humans that older hypothyroid patients require lower doses of T_4 for adequate replacement and are more apt to develop the adverse effects of slight thyroid hormone overdoses.

SIGNS OF OVERDOSE (THYROTOXICOSIS)

Animals on replacement therapy, particularly with a T_3 or T_3-containing product, can develop signs of thyrotoxicosis. However, the incidence at recommended doses is rare. Signs suggesting an overdose include polyuria, polydipsia, nervousness, weight loss, increased appetite, panting, and fever.[29] Diagnosis is confirmed by elevated serum T_4 and/or T_3 concentrations and the amelioration of signs by temporary discontinuation of therapy.

THERAPEUTIC TRIAL FOR DIAGNOSIS OF HYPOTHYROIDISM

Thyroid replacement therapy, without confirmatory laboratory evidence of hypothyroidism, has been suggested as a valid diagnostic step in a dog suspected to be hypothyroid. Although the major factor cited in defense of this practice is the cost of the diagnostic testing for the owner, it should be emphasized to an owner that replacement therapy is generally necessary for the remainder of the animal's life. Therefore, an incorrect diagnosis (and unnecessary long-term thyroid hormone treatment) can also be quite expensive. Furthermore, a delayed diagnosis of another disease could be detrimental, and diagnostic procedures following a therapeutic trial with equivocal results can be quite difficult to interpret because secretion of the normal thyroid gland is inhibited by usual replacement doses of thyroid hormone. In one study of normal dogs given L-T_4 at the dosage of 0.5 mg/m² twice daily, the mean serum T_4 response to exogenous TSH had been suppressed to 56 per cent and 46 per cent of the pretreatment value when retested at four and eight weeks on treatment, respectively. Four weeks after cessation of L-T_4 therapy, the serum T_4 response to TSH was still slightly suppressed.[161] Therefore, if TSH stimulation testing is used to confirm the diagnosis of hypothyroidism in a dog that has recently been receiving thyroid hormone, TSH testing should not be performed for at least four weeks following discontinuation of thyroid hormone replacement therapy.

MONITORING THERAPY

The most important indicator of the success of thyroid replacement therapy is clinical improvement. Before therapy is begun, the clinician and owner should have a clear idea of the goals of therapy and the time frame in which these goals can reasonably be achieved. The reversal of changes in haircoat and body weight should be assessed only after one to two months of therapy. In cases in which clinical improvement is marginal or signs of thyrotoxicosis are seen, the clinical observations can be supported by therapeutic monitoring of serum thyroid hormone concentrations (post-pill testing). Clearly, the documentation of distinctly elevated serum T_4 concentrations following T_4 administration and elevated serum T_3 concentrations following T_3 administration, concomitant with signs of thyrotoxicosis, confirm an overdose. The interpretation of post-pill serum thyroid hormone concentrations in cases of suspected underdosing can be more complicated because the timing of sampling may be critical to the proper interpretation. Ideally, therapeutic monitoring should not be attempted until steady-state conditions are reached, minimally one month after

the initiation of therapy. With once daily T_4 administration, the peak serum concentrations of T_4 generally should be in the high-normal to slightly high range four to eight hours after dosing and should be low normal to normal 24 hours after dosing. Given the dog's resistance to signs of thyrotoxicosis, it may be reasonable and adequate to check the serum T_4 concentration 24 hours after the previous day's dose, expecting it to still be in the normal range. Animals on twice daily administration probably can be checked at any time, but peak concentrations can be expected at the middle of the dosing interval (four to eight hours) and the nadir just prior to the next dose. When the dog's dose is stabilized, once or twice yearly checks of serum T_4 (with or without T_3) concentrations are recommended.

If serum T_3 concentrations are to be measured following T_4 administration, something not routinely recommended, they should be interpreted carefully together with the serum T_4 results and, most importantly, the clinical response. Low serum T_3 and T_4 concentrations, together with a poor clinical response, suggest an underdose or inadequate bioavailability (absorption). With T_3 administration, serum concentrations are reported to peak two to three hours after administration.[50] Serum T_4 concentrations are routinely low or undetectable in dogs receiving T_3 therapy. Any remaining endogenous thyroidal T_4 secretion is inhibited because of the suppression of pituitary TSH secretion by T_3.

THERAPEUTIC FAILURE

If clinical signs of hypothyroidism remain despite the use of reasonable doses of thyroid hormone, the following possibilities must be considered: (1) the dose or frequency of administration is improper, (2) the owner is not complying with instructions or is not successfully administrating the product, (3) the animal may not be absorbing the product well, or is metabolizing and/or excreting it too rapidly, (4) the product is outdated, or (5) the diagnosis is incorrect. A syndrome of tissue resistance to thyroid hormone, while described in humans,[162] has not yet been described in the dog or cat.

FELINE HYPOTHYROIDISM

Causes of Hypothyroidism

Naturally occurring hypothyroidism is an extremely rare clinical disorder in the cat. Although surveys of the histologic evaluation of the feline thyroid gland have revealed several pathologic abnormalities consistent with the development of hypothyroidism (thyroid atrophy, lymphocytic thyroiditis, and goiter),[24, 163, 164] spontaneous acquired primary (thyroidal) hypothyroidism has yet to be convincingly documented in the adult cat. Despite the apparent lack of adult-onset feline hypothyroidism, congenital or juvenile-onset hypothyroidism appears to develop with some frequency in the cat. One kitten with congenital hypothyroidism associated with thyroid gland enlargement (goiter) resulting from a suspected defect in thyroid hormone biosynthesis (defective peroxidase activity resulting in an iodine organification defect) has been reported.[165] In addition, five other cats with congenital hypothyroidism have recently been identified. One of these cats also had a goiter associated with an iodine organification defect (which was documented on the basis of a thyroid scan, radioiodine uptake studies, and a perchlorate discharge test), whereas the other four cats had thyroid dysgenesis confirmed by thyroid biopsy. As in hypothyroid puppies, it is likely that congenital hypothyroidism results in early death in most affected kittens and therefore goes undiagnosed. Neither secondary (pituitary) or tertiary (hypothalamic) hypothyroidism has been described in either the juvenile or mature cat.

The most common cause for the development of feline hypothyroidism is iatrogenic destruction or removal of the thyroid gland (following radioiodine or surgery) for treatment of hyperthyroidism.[166, 167] Although antithyroid drug overdosage could also produce hypothyroidism, this appears to be uncommon. As discussed in the section on antithyroid drug treatment for hyperthyroidism, cats treated with methimazole that develop subnormal T_4 concentrations usually maintain normal circulating T_3 concentrations and thus fail to demonstrate any clinical signs of hypothyroidism.[168]

Clinical Signs

The clinical signs associated with iatrogenic primary hypothyroidism in the adult cat usually include lethargy and nonpruritic seborrhea sicca. Matting of hair over the back (because of failure to groom) and hair loss over the lateral and medial distal halves of both pinnae may also develop. Bilateral, symmetric alopecia, with the exception of the pinnae involvement, does not appear to develop. In addition, hair removed by clipping usually regrows. Obesity, although it may develop, is not a consistent sign.[169]

Cats with congenital hypothyroidism typically have signs of disproportionate dwarfism, with an enlarged broad head but a short neck and limbs. Severe lethargy, mental dullness, constipation, hypothermia, and bradycardia have been observed in most cats. Hair is usually present all over the body but consists mainly of undercoat, with primary hairs scattered throughout. Obesity is generally not present. Radiographic examination has revealed almost complete absence of ossification centers in long bones.[165]

Diagnosis

Diagnosis of iatrogenic hypothyroidism can be difficult because of the vague clinical signs that these cats usually display. The tentative diagnosis in these cats should be based on the clinical signs described previously, together with a history of surgical thyroidectomy or treatment with radioiodine for hyperthyroidism. Congenital or juvenile-onset hypothyroidism should be suspected in any young cat with stunted growth and other clinical signs characteristic of cretinism (mental dullness).[165] Because of the multiple factors that can falsely lower baseline serum thyroid hormone values in cats with diseases other than hypothyroidism, the definitive diagnosis of iatrogenic or spontaneous feline hypothyroidism should be confirmed by the finding of a subnormal resting serum T_4 concentration that fails to rise adequately six hours after administration of bovine TSH (0.5 IU/lb or 1.0 IU/kg, IV).[170] Alternately, the TSH can be administered intramuscularly using a dosage of 2.5 units per cat and the post-TSH T_4 sample collected at 8 to 12 hours post-injection.[171] Using either protocol, a normal response is a post-TSH T_4 concentration that either is 2.0 to 3.0 μg/dl higher than the basal serum T_4 value or exceeds the normal range of basal T_4 concentrations (approximately 4 μg/dl in most laboratories). In kittens with documented hypothyroidism, other procedures (e.g., thyroid scanning, radioiodine uptake studies, perchlorate discharge testing, thyroid biopsy, biochemical analysis of thyroid tissue) should be considered to help better classify the underlying causes of the congenital feline hypothyroidism.[153]

Treatment

As in the dog, the recommended treatment for feline hypothyroidism is daily administration of L-T_4, using an initial dose of 5 to 10 μg/lb/day (10 to 20 μg/kg/day). This dosage should subsequently be adjusted on the basis of the cat's clinical response and post-pill serum T_4 evaluation (as described for the dog). Complete resolution of clinical signs can usually be expected in cats with adult-onset iatrogenic hypothyroidism. Thyroid hormone is crucial for normal growth and development of the central nervous system and skeleton. Consequently, the dwarfism and mental dullness that develops in kittens with hypothyroidism usually persists because of the delayed period of time from onset to diagnosis in these cats.

FELINE HYPERTHYROIDISM

Hyperthyroidism (thyrotoxicosis) is a multisystemic disorder resulting from excessive circulating concentrations of the two thyroid hormones, thyroxine (T_4) and triiodothyronine (T_3). Although first documented within the last decade,[15, 172] hyperthyroidism has become the most common endocrine disorder of middle-aged to old cats and is one of the most frequently diagnosed disorders in small animal practice.

Causes of Feline Hyperthyroidism

Functional thyroid adenomatous hyperplasia (or adenoma) involving one or both thyroid lobes is the most common pathologic abnormality associated with feline hyperthyroidism.[24, 172, 174] In about 70 per cent of hyperthyroid cats, both thyroid lobes are enlarged, whereas in the remaining cats, only one lobe is involved.[175–177] On histologic examination, such enlarged thyroid lobes contain one or more easily discernible foci of hyperplastic tissue, sometimes forming nodules ranging in diameter from less than 1 mm to 3 cm.[24, 172-174] Thyroid carcinoma, the primary cause of canine hyperthyroidism, only very rarely causes hyperthyroidism in the cat, with a prevalence of approximately one to two per cent.[178]

Although the thyroid pathologic abnormalities associated with feline hyperthyroidism have now been well characterized, the pathogenesis of the adenomatous hyperplastic changes associated with the disorder remains unclear. Until very recently, few references to pathologic abnormalities of the feline thyroid gland had been reported. In the authors' review of approximately 7,000 cats that had necropsies performed at The Animal Medical Center during the 14-year period from 1970 to 1984, an average of only 1.9 cats per year were found to have gross evidence of thyroid enlargement (caused by adenomatous hyperplasia, adenoma or carcinoma) in the period before 1977 when the first cat with hyperthyroidism was diagnosed at that institution. Since 1977, both the prevalence of thyroid pathologic abnormalities and the associated clinical state of hyperthyroidism have been detected at a markedly increasing frequency. At the present time, hyperthyroidism is being diagnosed at a rate of approximately 1:300 cats examined at The Animal Medical Center. Although a greater awareness of this disease has undoubtedly contributed to diagnosis of larger numbers of cases, it does appear that the incidence of feline hyperthyroidism has also increased. It also is possible that hyperthyroidism is really a "new" disorder of the cat. Further studies of this disorder are needed in order to better define the pathogenesis of feline hyperthyroidism.

Feline hyperthyroidism most resembles toxic nodular goiter in humans, which is also caused by one or more hyperfunctioning adenomatous thyroid nodules. Diffuse hyperplasia of the thyroid (Graves' disease), the most common type of hyperthyroidism in humans, is an autoimmune disorder in which circulating antibodies that act like thyroid stimulating hormone (TSH) bind to TSH receptors and stimulate thyroid hormone secretion.[92] Cats do not appear to develop a Graves-like disease. The authors and others have been unable to detect circulating thyroid stimulating immunoglobulins (TSIs) in serum collected from cats with hyperthyroidism.[179, 180] In accord with these findings, when adenomatous thyroid tissue removed from cats with hyperthyroidism is transplanted into nude mice, the thyroid tissue retains a histological appearance identical to that of the donor tissue.[174] This transplanted adenomatous tissue also continues to demonstrate hyperfunction (based on the ability to accumulate an increased fraction of radioiodine) and continues to grow (based on the demonstration of ^{3}H-thymidine incorporation into the adenomatous thyroid tissue).[174] These findings are similar to the situation observed with thyroid tissue from humans with toxic nodular goiter. In contrast, since circulating TSIs are responsible for the hyperthyroid state in human Graves' disease patients, the associated hyperplastic thyroid changes normalize after transplantation into the nude mouse (an environment without abnormal circulating thyroid stimulating autoantibodies).[181]

Although it is clear that circulating TSIs are not responsible for feline hyperthyroidism, increased titers of serum thyroid growth-stimulating immunoglobulins (TGIs) have been measured in cats with hyperthyroidism.[180] These autoantibodies, which act to promote thyroid growth but not to stimulate thyroid hormone secretion, also have been reported in humans with toxic nodular goiter, as well as in patients with Graves' disease, Hashimoto's thyroiditis, and euthyroid goiter.[182] Based on the authors' results of transplantation of feline adenomatous tissue into nude mice, however, it is clear that the growth of this thyroid tissue does not depend on humoral extrathyroidal stimulators such as TSIs.[174] The role, if any, of TGIs in the pathogenesis of hyperthyroidism remains unknown.

Clinical Manifestations of Feline Hyperthyroidism

Feline hyperthyroidism occurs in middle-aged to old cats, with a reported range of 4 to 22 years (mean age, approximately 12 to 13 years). There is no breed or sex predilection.[168, 173, 175, 177]

General Considerations. Table 95–2 lists the most common historical and clinical signs recorded in cats with hyperthyroidism. Since the actions of the thyroid hormones are generally stimulatory, the clinical signs of hyperthyroidism are usually manifested by evidence of increased thyroid hormone effects on one or more organ systems. Thyroid hormones regulate metabolic processes from heat production to carbohydrate, protein, and lipid metabolism in virtually all body systems; increased energy metabolism and heat production cause the increased appetite, weight loss, muscle wasting, weakness, heat intolerance, and slightly elevated body temperature characteristic of hyperthyroidism. Thyroid hormones also appear to interact with the central nervous system; increased overall sympathetic drive causes the hyperexcitability or nervousness, behavioral changes, tremor, and tachycardia characteristic of hyperthyroidism.

The clinical manifestations of feline hyperthyroidism may be mild to severe and are modified by the duration

TABLE 95–2. FREQUENCY OF HISTORICAL AND CLINICAL SIGNS IN FELINE HYPERTHYROIDISM

Clinical Finding	Percentage of Cats
Weight loss	95–98
Hyperactivity/difficult to examine	68–81
Polyphagia	65–75
Tachycardia	57–65
Polyuria/polydipsia	45–55
Cardiac murmur	10–54
Vomiting	33–50
Diarrhea	30–45
Increased fecal volume	13–28
Decreased appetite	19–28
Lethargy	15–25
Polypnea (panting)	13–28
Muscle weakness	15–20
Muscle tremors	15–30
Congestive heart failure	10–15
Dyspnea	10–15

Compiled from data reported in references 166, 175, and 177.

of hyperthyroidism, presence of concomitant abnormalities in various organ systems, and the inability of a body system to meet the demands imposed by thyroid hormone excess. Because of the multisystemic effects of hyperthyroidism, most cats have clinical signs that reflect dysfunction of many organ systems. In some, however, clinical signs of one body system predominate and may obscure other features of hyperthyroidism. Since clinical signs of feline hyperthyroidism are so variable, the presence or absence of one sign can neither diagnose nor exclude hyperthyroidism. In addition, cats might be misdiagnosed because of the resemblance of hyperthyroidism to many other diseases of the cat.

In most cats, the hyperthyroid state is slowly progressive. In addition, the fact that most cats maintain a good to excellent appetite and are active (or hyperactive) for their age usually makes the owner feel that the cat is in good health until obvious weight loss or other troublesome signs develop. As hyperthyroidism has become more commonly recognized, veterinarians are diagnosing more and more cats with the disease at an early stage of the disease, even before most owners realize that their cats are ill.

General Appearance and Behavior. Most cats with hyperthyroidism show evidence of weight loss. About half have an unkempt haircoat, with excessive shedding and matting of hair. Cats with hyperthyroidism are usually restless, can show a frantic, anxious expression, and can be difficult to handle and become aggressive during the restraint of a physical examination.[166, 175, 177]

Cats with hyperthyroidism tend to have impaired tolerance for stressful situations. In some cats, the stress of a car ride to the veterinary hospital together with the restraint of a physical examination may result in marked respiratory distress and weakness, with the development of cardiac arrhythmias (and even cardiac arrest) in a few cases. This decreased ability to cope with stress must be considered when planning diagnostic or therapeutic procedures.

Thyroid Gland. On physical examination, enlargement of one or both thyroid lobes can be detected in over 90 per cent of cats with hyperthyroidism.[166, 175] The thyroid gland is not usually palpable in the normal cat. However, the finding of enlargement of one or both thyroid lobes on physical examination cannot always be equated with an associated hyperthyroid state, since thyroid enlargement occasionally can be detected in cats without clinical and laboratory evidence of hyperthyroidism. Although some of these cats may remain euthyroid (at least for prolonged periods of time), many of these cats with enlargement of one or both lobes of the thyroid gland eventually develop clinical and biochemical signs of hyperthyroidism as the thyroid nodules continue to grow and begin to oversecrete thyroid hormone.

To palpate an enlarged thyroid gland, the cat's neck should be slightly extended with the head tilted backward. Using the thumb and index finger, one should gently pass the fingers over both sides of the trachea, starting at the laryngeal area and moving ventrally toward the thoracic inlet. Since the thyroid lobes of the cat are loosely attached to the trachea, the enlarged lobe(s) frequently descends ventrally from its normal location adjacent to the larynx. In hyperthyroid cats in which thyroid gland enlargement is not palpable, the possibility that the affected lobes have descended into the thoracic cavity should always be considered.

Nervous System and Muscle. Increased circulating concentrations of thyroid hormone, presumably through a direct effect upon the nervous system, cause hyperactivity, restlessness, pacing, or irritability in many cats with hyperthyroidism.[166, 175, 177] Even with careful questioning, however, such abnormal nervous behavior may not be apparent to many cat owners. During physical examination, the hyperactivity and restlessness characteristic of feline hyperthyroidism quickly become obvious to the veterinarian. Many of these cats cannot remain still for even the time it takes to complete a physical examination, and become aggressive if restraint is attempted.

Weakness and fatigability, common complaints in humans with hyperthyroidism, are reported less frequently in cats with hyperthyroidism. Although the biochemical basis for the weakness remains unclear, the generalized muscle wasting that accompanies severe weight loss is likely to contribute.

Gastrointestinal System. Increased appetite and food intake are common signs of feline hyperthyroidism and occur in response to increased calorie use. In most cats, however, compensation is inadequate, and mild to severe weight loss also develops.[166, 175, 177] Although the cause is unclear, about 20 per cent of hyperthyroid cats also have periods of decreased appetite that usually alternate with periods of normal to increased appetite (see Apathetic Hyperthyroidism).

Other gastrointestinal signs that occur in feline hyperthyroidism include vomiting, diarrhea, increased frequency of defecation, and increased volume of feces (Table 95–2). Rapid overeating, common in the hyperthyroid cat, appears to contribute to vomiting since it usually occurs shortly after eating. Intestinal hypermotility appears to be responsible for the increased frequency of defecation and diarrhea. Malabsorption with increased fecal fat excretion also develops in some cats with hyperthyroidism.[175] Although the exact mechanism for steatorrhea is unknown, a reversible reduction in pancreatic exocrine secretion has been documented in humans with hyperthyroidism.[183] In addition, it is likely that excessive fat intake resulting from polyphagia contributes to the increased fecal fat excretion that develops in some cats.[175]

Renal System. Renal blood flow, glomerular filtration rate, and tubular reabsorptive and secretory capacities are increased in humans with hyperthyroidism and in animals given large doses of thyroid hormone.[184] Clinically, there is no specific renal pathology associated with hyperthyroidism, and renal azotemia, although a relatively common finding in the middle-aged to old cats that develop hyperthyroidism, does not appear to be caused by the hyperthyroid state. In contrast, the increased renal hemodynamics associated with untreated hyperthyroidism may be beneficial in maintaining sustainable renal function (and delaying the clinical and biochemical consequences of severe renal failure) in some cats with chronic renal failure. Deterioration of renal function, with marked rises in both the BUN and serum creatinine concentrations, as well as clinical signs of renal failure (e.g., anorexia, vomiting, depression), occurs after correction of the hyperthyroid state in some cats in which normal (or only slightly increased) values for serum creatinine and BUN were measured prior to treatment of the hyperthyroidism.

Thyroid hormones also have a diuretic action, an effect that was reported in cats approximately 50 years ago.[185] In accord with those experimental findings, polydipsia and polyuria are frequent clinical signs in feline hyperthyroidism (Table 95–2). Although concurrent primary renal disease contributes to polyuria and polydipsia in some cats with hyperthyroidism, these signs also occur in many cats without evidence of renal dysfunction, in which resolution of polyuria and polydipsia usually occurs after treatment of hyperthyroidism. The exact cause of these signs in hyperthyroidism is unknown. The hyperthyroid state may, however, impair urine concentrating ability by increasing total renal blood flow and thereby decreasing renal medullary solute concentration; such medullary washout may cause polyuria with secondary polydipsia. Alternately, in cats with normal renal concentrating ability, a hypothalamic disturbance caused by thyrotoxicosis may produce compulsive polydipsia with secondary polyuria.[166]

Respiratory System. Some cats with hyperthyroidism exhibit dyspnea, panting, or hyperventilation at rest.[166, 175, 177] Such respiratory signs develop most commonly after the stress of travel to the veterinary hospital and the restraint of a physical examination, but are occasionally observed by the owner at home.

The hyperthyroid state can produce multiple alterations in respiratory function, including a decreased vital capacity, decreased pulmonary compliance, and an increased minute respiration.[166] These abnormalities in respiratory function probably result from a combination of respiratory muscle weakness and increased CO_2 production. In some cats, thyrotoxic congestive heart failure also contributes to dyspnea and hyperventilation.

Cardiovascular System. On physical examination, cardiovascular abnormalities, including tachycardia, systolic murmurs, gallop rhythm, arrhythmias, and signs of congestive heart failure (e.g., dyspnea, muffled heart sounds, ascites), are fairly common in cats with hyperthyroidism.[166, 175, 186] Table 95–3 shows the frequency of cardiac abnormalities in cats with hyperthyroidism, as detected by thoracic radiography, electrocardiography, and echocardiography. Radiographic findings may include mild to severe cardiomegaly, pleural effusion, and pulmonary edema.[175, 186] Electrocardiographic abnormalities may include tachycardia, increased R-wave amplitude in lead II, various atrial and ventricular arrhythmias, and intraventricular conduction disturbances.[175, 177, 187] Echocardiographic abnormalities frequently found in cats with hyperthyroidism include left ventricular hypertrophy, thickening of the interventricular septum, left atrial and ventricular dilatation, and myocardial hypercontractility (manifested by increased shortening fraction and velocity of circumferential fiber shortening).[188] Postmortem examination has confirmed the presence of symmetrical hypertrophy of the left ventricular free wall and interventricular septum in most cats with either experimentally induced or naturally occurring hyperthyroidism.[189, 190] Less commonly, echocardio-

TABLE 95–3. APPROXIMATE FREQUENCY OF CARDIAC ABNORMALITIES IN FELINE HYPERTHYROIDISM DETECTED WITH THORACIC RADIOGRAPHY, ELECTROCARDIOGRAPHY, AND ECHOCARDIOGRAPHY

	Percentage of Cats
Thoracic radiographs	
Cardiomegaly	50
Pulmonary edema/pleural effusion	10
Electrocardiography	
Sinus tachycardia	70
Increased R wave amplitude in lead II	30
Intraventricular conduction defects	10
Atrial premature contractions/fibrillation	10
Ventricular premature contractions	2
Echocardiography	
Left ventricular hypertrophy	70
Hypertrophy of the intraventricular septum	40
Left atrial dilatation	70
Left ventricular dilatation	45
Hyperdynamic wall motion (hypercontractility)	20

Compiled from data reported in references 175, 187, and 188.

graphic evidence of a dilatative type of cardiomyopathy is observed, as evidenced by subnormal myocardial contractility and marked ventricular dilatation; these cats also usually have clinical and radiographic findings consistent with severe congestive heart failure.[186, 188]

These studies confirm that hyperthyroidism can induce a secondary form of cardiomyopathy in the cat, either a hypertrophic form of cardiomyopathy or, less commonly, a dilatative type of cardiomyopathy. Either form of cardiomyopathy may result in congestive heart failure, but severe cardiac failure develops much more frequently in hyperthyroid cats with dilated cardiomyopathy. In cats that develop signs of congestive heart failure, treatment with furosemide (with or without vasodilator and digitalis therapy) may be required.[191] Propranolol should be used with caution in these cats, however, and should never be administered until the congestive heart failure has stabilized.

After correction of the hyperthyroid state, the hypertrophic form of thyrotoxic cardiomyopathy is usually reversible.[187, 188] In contrast, the dilated form of cardiomyopathy is usually not reversible despite correction of the hyperthyroid state.[188] In those cats in which cardiomyopathy persists or worsens despite treatment, it is possible that the presence of excess thyroid hormone may cause irreversible cardiac structural damage, or underlying primary cardiomyopathy may be present.

Although the exact pathogenesis of cardiac abnormalities associated with hyperthyroidism is unclear, cardiac changes that compensate for altered peripheral tissue function caused by thyrotoxicosis appear to play an important role. Hyperthyroidism results in a high-output cardiac state in which vascular resistance is low and cardiac output is high because of increased tissue metabolism and oxygen requirements. A volume overload is created by low peripheral vascular resistance and by reflex renal mechanisms that conserve fluid. The principal cardiac compensatory mechanisms in high-output states such as hyperthyroidism are dilatation (in response to volume overload) and hypertrophy (in response to dilatation). In addition, the direct action of thyroid hormones on heart muscle and interactions of

T_4 and T_3 with the sympathetic nervous system also appear to be factors that influence cardiac function in hyperthyroidism.

Apathetic Hyperthyroidism. Apathetic or masked hyperthyroidism is a clinical form of thyrotoxicosis that develops in about 10 per cent of cats with hyperthyroidism.[175] In these cats, hyperexcitability or restlessness is replaced by depression and weakness as the dominant clinical features. Weight loss remains a common clinical sign but is usually accompanied by anorexia rather than increased appetite. These cats also frequently have cardiac abnormalities, including arrhythmias and congestive heart failure. Ventroflexion of the neck, which usually responds to supportive fluid and thiamine supplementation and therefore may be the result of thiamine deficiency, is also observed in a few of these cats.[175, 177]

Screening Laboratory Tests

Screening laboratory tests (complete blood count, serum biochemical profile, urinalysis) should always be performed in a cat suspected of having hyperthyroidism. Results of these tests may show alterations that aid in the diagnosis of hyperthyroidism. Even more importantly, however, results of such routine screening tests may reveal the presence of a concurrent disorder not directly related to the hyperthyroid state, a situation that should not be surprising considering the old age of most cats with hyperthyroidism. Finally, chest and abdominal radiographs, electrocardiogram, echocardiogram, or other studies may also be warranted, especially if signs of congestive heart failure are present.

Complete Blood Count. Mature leukocytosis and eosinopenia are common hematologic findings in feline hyperthyroidism and appear to reflect a stress response to thyroid hormone excess.[166, 175] The red blood cell count (RBC), packed cell volume (PCV), and hemoglobin concentrations are usually in the high-normal to slightly high range in these cats. Although such erythrocytosis is generally mild to moderate in severity, an elevated value for the PCV is found in approximately half of cats with hyperthyroidism. The erythrocytosis of hyperthyroidism appears to result from both a direct effect of thyroid hormones on erythroid marrow and an increased production of erythropoietin.[166]

Serum Biochemical Tests. The most common serum biochemical abnormalities (which occur in approximately 50 to 75 per cent of cats with hyperthyroidism) include elevation in concentrations of alanine aminotransferase (ALT), aspartate aminotransferase (AST), alkaline phosphatase (SAP), and lactic dehydrogenase (LDH).[166, 175, 177] Histologic examination of liver usually reveals only modest and nonspecific changes, including centrilobular fatty infiltration and mild hepatic necrosis or degeneration. The causes of hepatic damage and elevation in liver enzymes in thyrotoxicosis are unknown. Malnutrition, congestive heart failure, infection, hepatic hypoxia, and direct toxic effects of thyroid hormone on the liver may all contribute. Since only ALT is specific for hepatic necrosis in the cat, it is likely that other organs may also contribute to the elevations of SAP, AST, and LDH concentrations. Whatever the cause, elevated concentrations of ALT, AST, SAP, and LDH normalize with treatment of hyperthyroidism.[166, 177]

Evidence of concurrent renal dysfunction in untreated cats with hyperthyroidism is also fairly common, with mild to moderate elevations in serum creatinine and BUN concentrations being reported in 20 to 40 per cent of cases.[175, 177] Careful consideration should be given to the method of treatment selected for the hyperthyroid state in these cats with concomitant azotemia since deterioration of renal function with development of clinical signs of renal failure develops in at least some of these cats after correction of the hyperthyroid state. In general, medical therapy with methimazole is usually favored as initial therapy of the hyperthyroid state in cats with concurrent azotemia. If no significant deterioration of renal function develops after medical control of the hyperthyroid state for at least two to four weeks, surgical thyroidectomy or radioiodine treatment for hyperthyroidism can then be considered.

Mild hyperphosphatemia develops in 20 to 50 per cent of cats with hyperthyroidism.[175, 177] Although azotemia contributes to the elevated serum phosphate concentrations in some cats, approximately 50 per cent of cats with hyperphosphatemia do not have elevations in serum creatinine or BUN concentrations. Increased renal tubular absorption of phosphate and increased phosphate loads from exaggerated bone resorption and muscle catabolism appear to be responsible for the hyperphosphatemia of hyperthyroidism, at least in cats without detectable renal impairment.[166, 177]

Thyroid Function Tests

Resting Serum Thyroid Hormone Concentrations. Increased basal serum thyroid hormone concentrations are the biochemical hallmark of hyperthyroidism. Resting serum concentrations of both T_4 and T_3 are above the normal range in the vast majority of cats with hyperthyroidism.[166, 177] Approximately five to ten per cent of hyperthyroid cats maintain normal serum concentrations of T_3, however, despite clearly elevated T_4 concentrations. Although the cause is unclear, most hyperthyroid cats with normal serum T_3 concentrations have only mild clinical signs of hyperthyroidism; therefore, it is likely that the normal T_3 levels found in these cats will eventually increase into the thyrotoxic range if the disorder is allowed to progress untreated.[166] Nevertheless, a serum T_4 determination is usually of greater diagnostic value than determination of serum T_3.[175, 177]

Thyroid hormone concentrations in cats with hyperthyroidism are subject to a considerable degree of fluctuation over time.[192] In cats with thyroid hormone values well above the normal range, this fluctuation does not appear to be of great clinical or diagnostic significance (Figure 95-8). However, in cats with mild hyperthyroidism, the degree of serum T_4 and T_3 fluctuation that can occur (into the normal range in some cats) (Figure 95-9) suggests that a diagnosis of hyperthyroidism cannot be excluded on the basis of the finding of a single normal to high-normal serum T_4 (and T_3) result alone. In cats with clinical signs consistent with hyperthyroidism (and especially in cats with palpable goiters), it is possible

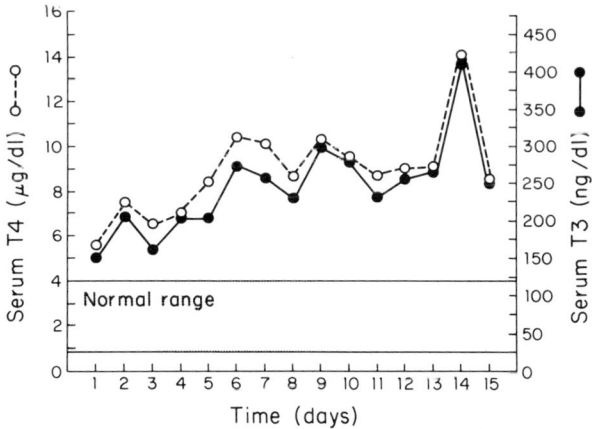

FIGURE 95–8. Serum T_4 and T_3 concentrations determined daily over a 15-day period in a cat with hyperthyroidism. (From Peterson, ME, et al.: Serum thyroid hormone concentrations fluctuate in cats with hyperthyroidism. J Vet Intern Med 1:142, 1987.)

that more than one serum T_4 determination could be required to confirm a diagnosis. In addition, the finding of a more pronounced thyroid hormone fluctuation over a period of days compared to a period of hours within the same day suggests that multiple blood samples for thyroid hormone determinations, if needed, should be collected on separate days (one to three weeks apart) rather than at different times during the same day.[192]

In hyperthyroid cats with severe concurrent nonthyroidal illness (renal disease, diabetes mellitus, primary hepatic disease, and other chronic illnesses), high-normal or only slightly elevated serum thyroid hormone concentrations may be found at time of initial evaluation. Despite the normal total serum T_4 concentrations, one would expect levels of FT_4 to be elevated in these situations. Since severe nonthyroidal illness is expected to decrease serum thyroid hormone concentrations into the subnormal range, concomitant hyperthyroidism

should be suspected in any middle-aged to old cat with severe nonthyroidal illness and high-normal serum T_4 and T_3 concentrations, especially if signs of hyperthyroidism are also present. Upon stabilization of, or recovery from, the concurrent nonthyroidal disorder, serum thyroid hormone concentrations increase into the "diagnostic" thyrotoxic range in these cats with hyperthyroidism.

Thyroid Hormone (Triiodothyronine) Suppression Test. Inhibition of TSH secretion by exogenous thyroid hormone is a characteristic feature of normal pituitary-thyroid interaction. This decrease in TSH secretion results in a decreased secretion of endogenous thyroid hormone. In contrast, when thyroid hormone secretion is autonomous and independent of endogenous TSH regulation, exogenous thyroid hormone has little to no effect on endogenous thyroid hormone secretion (since TSH secretion has already been inhibited under these circumstances). In cats in which hyperthyroidism is suspected but high-normal serum concentrations of T_4 and T_3 are found, use of the triiodothyronine (T_3) suppression test should be considered.[92]

In the cat, the T_3 suppression test can be performed by determining basal serum concentrations of T_4, administering exogenous T_3 at the dosage of 25 μg every eight hours for two days, and giving the last (seventh) dose on the morning of the third day. Approximately four hours after the last dose of T_3 is administered, serum for determination of T_4 is again collected. In the normal cat, suppression of the serum T_4 concentration to approximately 50 per cent or greater of the pretreatment value (with a decrease in the absolute serum T_4 concentration to less than 1.5 μg/dl in the authors' laboratory) occurs after administration of T_3 at this dosage. In contrast, little to no decrease in serum T_4 concentration is found in cats with mild hyperthyroidism.

Thyroid Stimulating Hormone (TSH) Response Test.

FIGURE 95–9. Serum T_4 and T_3 concentrations determined daily over a 15-day period in a cat with hyperthyroidism. Note the fluctuation in and out of the normal range for both serum T_4 and T_3 values. (From Peterson, ME, et al.: Serum thyroid hormone concentrations fluctuate in cats with hyperthyroidism. J Vet Intern Med 1:142, 1987.)

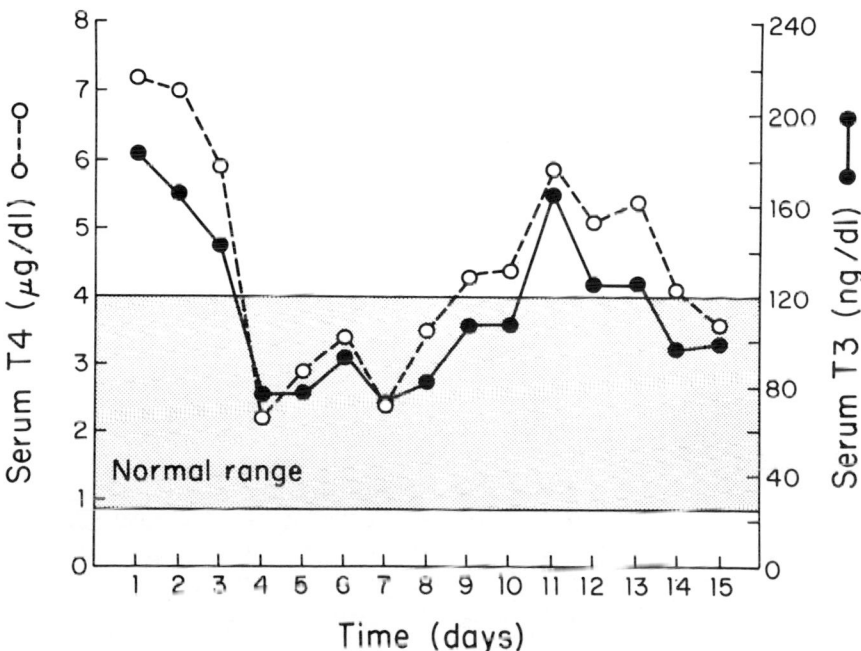

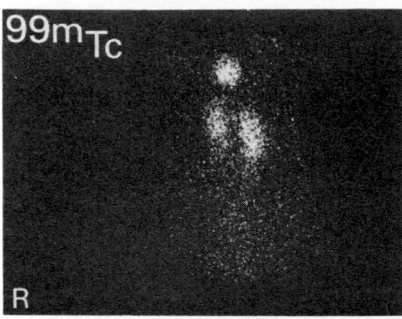
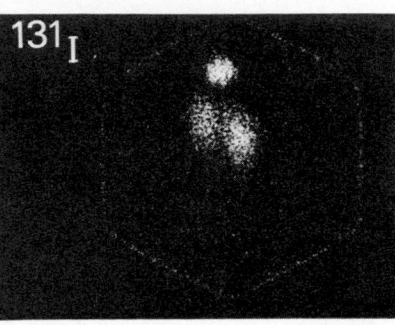

FIGURE 95-10. Thyroid scans of a normal cat obtained with $^{99m}TcO_4$ and ^{131}I. With either isotope, the thyroid lobes are symmetric in both position and size, with uniform distribution of radioactivity throughout the gland. A 2-cm^2 marker placed over the larynx is visible at the top of the scan. (From Peterson, ME and Becker, DV: Radionuclide thyroid imaging in 135 cats with hyperthyroidism. Vet Radiol 25:23, 1984.)

In cats with hyperthyroidism, little to no increase in resting serum T_4 concentrations (less than a twofold increase) generally occurs four to six hours after the administration of exogenous TSH (using doses of 0.5 U/lb, IV (1.0 U/kg IV).[175] In contrast, the serum T_4 concentration usually will increase by at least twofold (and by at least 2.5 µg/dl) over resting values in the normal cat.[170, 171] Therefore, in cats in which hyperthyroidism is suspected but serum concentrations of T_4 and T_3 are found to be in the high-normal range, use of a TSH stimulation test can also be considered. As with the T_3 suppression test, TSH stimulation testing of cats in which mild hyperthyroidism is suspected should only be considered when resting serum thyroid hormone concentrations are borderline or only slightly increased. Because of the variability in response to TSH that may occur among both normal and hyperthyroid cats, as well as the considerable cost of the TSH preparation needed for the TSH response test, use of the T_3 suppression test is generally preferred over the TSH stimulation test as an aid in diagnosis of mild feline hyperthyroidism.

Thyroid Radionuclide Uptake and Imaging. A characteristic feature of hyperthyroidism is an increased thyroidal uptake of radioiodine, after administration of a small tracer dose of a radionuclide.[166] Because values vary inversely with the intake of stable iodine, however, thyroid uptake determinations may be low or normal in hyperthyroid patients that have been on a high iodine diet or have recently received iodine-containing drugs or radiographic contrast agents.[92] Even in the absence of such factors, thyroid radioiodine uptake measurement can be a relatively insensitive diagnostic test for hyperthyroidism and its use is generally reserved for determining various parameters of thyroid kinetics used in calculation of the therapeutic ^{131}I dose (see Radioactive Iodine Treatment).

Thyroid imaging (scanning) is useful in the evaluation of hyperthyroidism because it delineates functioning thyroid tissue. Although thyroid scanning with either radioiodine (^{131}I, ^{123}I) or pertechnetate (^{99m}Tc) produces similar thyroid images in both normal cats and cats with hyperthyroidism (Figures 95-10, 95-11, and 95-12),[176] there are several advantages to using ^{99m}Tc rather than radioiodine. Because of the rapid uptake of ^{99m}Tc, the imaging procedure can begin only 20 minutes after administration, as opposed to 4 and 24 hours for ^{123}I and ^{131}I, respectively. In addition, because higher doses of ^{99m}Tc can be safely administered without delivering a high radiation dose, thyroid scanning with ^{99m}Tc can be completed more rapidly than with radioiodine. Finally, the quality of ^{99m}Tc thyroid scans is consistently equal or superior to that of radioiodine.[176]

Thyroid imaging can be an useful adjunct in diagnosing feline hyperthyroidism. With pertechnetate (^{99m}Tc) thyroid scanning, a one-to-one ratio usually exists between the size and intensity of the salivary glands and the two thyroid lobes. In contrast, most cats with hyperthyroidism have obvious enlargement of one or both thyroid lobes, together with an increased uptake of pertechnetate into the abnormal thyroid tissue, as compared to the salivary glands.[193]

The major usefulness of thyroid imaging, however, is in determining the extent of thyroid gland involvement and in detecting possible metastasis. In about 70 per cent of hyperthyroid cats, thyroid imaging reveals enlargement of both lobes and increased radionuclide accumulation in both lobes (Figure 95-11), whereas involvement of only one lobe is seen in the remaining cats (Figure 95-12).[175, 176] With unilateral thyroid lobe involvement, the normal contralateral lobe is completely suppressed and cannot be visualized. Thyroid imaging is also helpful in the hyperthyroid cat in which no enlargement of the thyroid gland can be palpated; in many of these cats, thyroid imaging demonstrates that an affected lobe has descended into the thoracic cavity. Finally, scanning is of value in detecting regional or

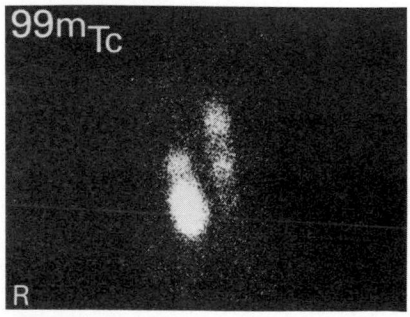
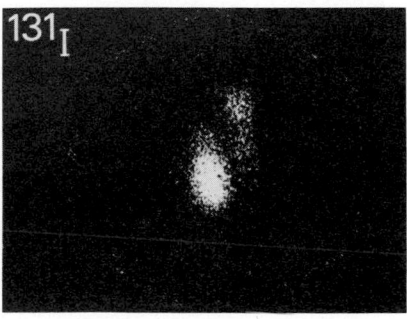

FIGURE 95-11. $^{99m}TcO_4$ and ^{131}I thyroid scans of a hyperthyroid cat with adenomatous hyperplasia of both thyroid lobes. Note that with both radionuclides, the distribution of activity is heterogeneous, with defects in tracer uptake into the enlarged gland. (From Peterson, ME and Becker, DV: Radionuclide thyroid imaging in 135 cats with hyperthyroidism. Vet Radiol 25:23, 1984.)

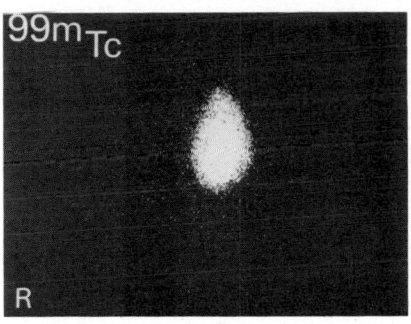 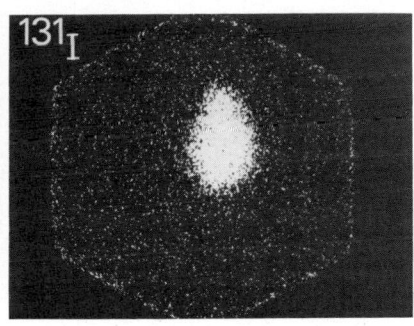

FIGURE 95–12. $^{99m}TcO_4$ and ^{131}I thyroid scans of a hyperthyroid cat with an adenoma (adenomatous hyperplasia) of one thyroid lobe. The left lobe is enlarged and has descended ventrally toward the thoracic inlet. Note that the uninvolved lobe cannot be visualized on either scan. (From Peterson, ME and Becker, DV: Radionuclide thyroid imaging in 135 cats with hyperthyroidism. Vet Radidol 25:23, 1984.)

distant metastasis of functional thyroid carcinoma causing feline hyperthyroidism (Figure 95–13).[175, 176]

Treatment

The underlying etiology of the thyroid adenomatous hyperplasia that causes feline hyperthyroidism is not known. Since spontaneous remission of the disorder does not occur, the aim of treatment is to control the excessive secretion of thyroid hormone from the adenomatous thyroid gland. Feline hyperthyroidism can be treated in three ways: surgical thyroidectomy, radioactive iodine (^{131}I), or chronic administration of an antithyroid drug. Antithyroid drug therapy is also extremely useful as short-term treatment (three to six weeks) in the preparation of the hyperthyroid cat prior to thyroidectomy. The advantages and disadvantages of each form of treatment are summarized in Table 95–4 and should always be considered when selecting the most appropriate treatment

The treatment of choice for an individual cat depends

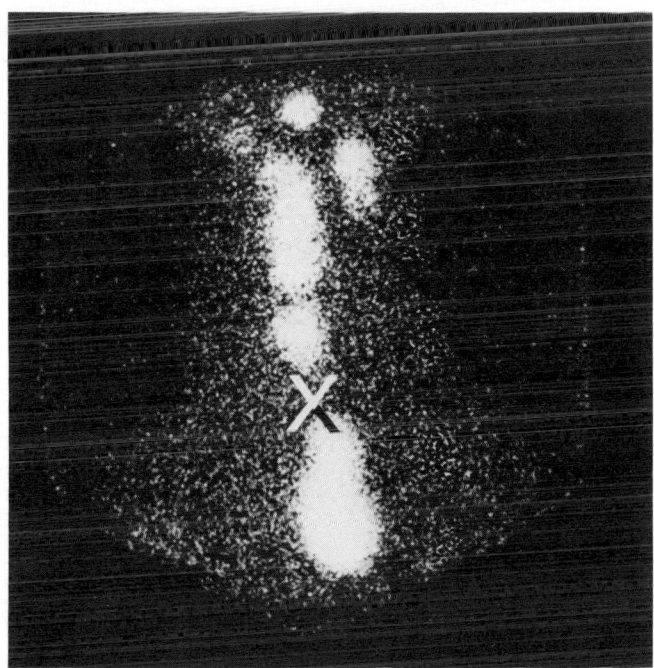

FIGURE 95–13. Thyroid scan from a hyperthyroid cat with thyroid adenocarcinoma. Note the multiple thyroid nodules that accumulate radioactivity and extension of the tumor into the thoracic cavity. X = thoracic inlet. (From Peterson, ME and Becker, DV: Radionuclide thyroid imaging in 135 cats wtih hyperthyroidism. Vet Radiol 25:23, 1984.)

on several factors, including the age of the cat, presence of associated cardiovascular diseases or other major medical problems (e.g., renal disease), availability of a skilled surgeon or nuclear medicine department, and owner's willingness to accept the form of treatment advised. Of the three forms of treatment available, it must be emphasized that only surgery and radioactive iodine remove and destroy the adenomatous thyroid tissue, respectively, and thereby "cure" the hyperthyroid state. Use of an antithyroid drug (e.g., methimazole) blocks thyroid hormone synthesis; however, since antithyroid drugs do not destroy adenomatous thyroid tissue, relapse of hyperthyroidism invariably occurs within 24 to 72 hours after the medication is discontinued.[168, 194]

ANTITHYROID DRUGS

Methimazole (Tapazole) and propylthiouracil (PTU) are the two thiourylene antithyroid drugs available for use in the United States. After administration, these drugs are actively concentrated by the thyroid gland, where they act to inhibit the synthesis of thyroid hormones through the following mechanisms: (1) by blocking the incorporation of iodine into the tyrosyl groups in thyroglobulin (Figure 95–1, Steps 2 and 3), (2) by preventing the coupling of iodotyrosyl groups (mono- and diiodotyrosines) into T_4 and T_3 (see Figure 95-1, Step 4), and (3) through direct interactions with the thyroglobulin molecule. Antithyroid drugs do not interfere with the thyroid gland's ability to concentrate or trap inorganic iodine, nor do they block the release of stored thyroid hormone into the circulation.

Advantages of long-term antithyroid drug treatment over other available treatment modalities (surgery and radioactive iodine) include absence of certain complications, such as permanent hypothyroidism and postsurgical hypoparathyroidism (Table 95–4). In addition, unlike surgery or radioiodine, use of antithyroid drugs requires no advanced skills, training, or special licensing, and is a practical treatment choice for most practitioners.

Although both PTU and methimazole are effective in decreasing serum thyroid hormone concentrations into the normal or low range, PTU produces a high incidence of mild to serious adverse effects, which include anorexia, vomiting, lethargy, immune-mediated hemolytic anemia, thrombocytopenia, and the development of serum antinuclear antibodies in both normal and hyperthyroid cats.[194-196] Because of the prevalence of severe hematologic complications, use of PTU for control of feline hyperthyroidism can no longer be recommended.

TABLE 95–4. ADVANTAGES AND DISADVANTAGES OF TREATMENT MODALITIES FOR FELINE HYPERTHYROIDISM

	Methimazole	Surgery	Radioiodine
Persistent hyperthyroidism	Low (dose-related)	Rare	Low (dose-related)
Complications			
Hypoparathyroidism	Never	Common	Never
Permanent hypothyroidism	Never	Intermediate	Rare (dose-related)
Anorexia, vomiting	Common	Rare	Never
Hematologic effects	Rare (thrombocytopenia, agranulocytosis, serum ANA)	Never	Rare (only with very high doses)
Neurologic damage	Never	Rare (vocal cord paralysis, Horner's syndrome)	Never
Hospitalization time required	None	1–3 days	1–4 wk
Time until euthyroid	1–3 wk	1–2 days	1–12 wk
Relapse/recurrence	High	Intermediate	Low
Ease of treatment	Simple	Most difficult	Intermediate (but not readily available)

The authors recently reported the results of a three-year evaluation of the efficacy and safety of methimazole in 262 cats with hyperthyroidism.[168] Overall, the studies show that methimazole is better tolerated and safer than PTU in the cat and can be considered the antithyroid drug of choice for both the preoperative and long-term medical management of feline hyperthyroidism.

Initial Treatment. Initially, methimazole should be administered at a dose of 10 to 15 mg per day, depending on the severity of the hyperthyroid state. This methimazole dosage ensures that serum T_4 concentrations will decrease to normal or low values within two to three weeks of treatment in most cats (Figure 95–14). During the first three months of therapy (time period when the most serious side effects associated with methimazole therapy develop), the cat should be examined every two to three weeks in order to make necessary dose adjustments and to monitor for adverse effects. At each of these rechecks, serum T_4 concentrations and complete blood and platelet counts should be determined. If little to no decrease in serum T_4 concentration occurs during this initial treatment period, the daily methimazole dosage should be gradually increased (in 5 mg increments), after poor compliance by owners or difficulty in giving the medication has been excluded as the cause of persistent hyperthyroidism. Although a few cats appear to be resistant to the effects of the drug, euthyroidism can be restored in virtually all cats if a high enough dosage of methimazole (25 to 30 mg/day in a few cases) is reliably administered on a daily basis.

If methimazole is given as preoperative preparation, surgical thyroidectomy can be performed once serum T_4 concentrations decrease to normal or low values (usually within two to four weeks). Surgical risks in cats with subnormal circulating T_4 concentrations do not appear to be increased, probably because normal serum T_3 concentrations are maintained in these cats. The last dose of methimazole should be administered on the morning of surgery.

Long-Term Treatment. In cats in which long-term methimazole treatment is planned, the goal of treatment is to maintain serum T_4 values within the low-normal range with the lowest possible daily dosage, since some side effects (at least serum ANA development) appear to develop less frequently with lower doses of methimazole. Therefore, if serum T_4 concentrations fall to low or low-normal values during methimazole treatment in these cats, the daily drug dosage should be decreased by 2.5 to 5 mg increments and further testing continued at two- to three-week intervals until the lowest daily dose is found that effectively maintains serum T_4 concentrations within the low-normal range. Although a few cases of feline hyperthyroidism can be effectively controlled on a long-term basis with a daily dosage as low as 2.5 to 5 mg, the great majority require a dose of 7.5 to 10 mg/day. Other cats may continue to require dosages of 15 to 20 mg/day to maintain serum T_4 concentrations within normal range.

Although subnormal serum T_4 concentrations commonly develop during both short- and long-term treatment with methimazole (Figures 95–14 and 95–15), serum T_3 values usually remain within the normal range and clinical signs suggestive of hypothyroidism have not been observed. Unlike PTU, methimazole does not

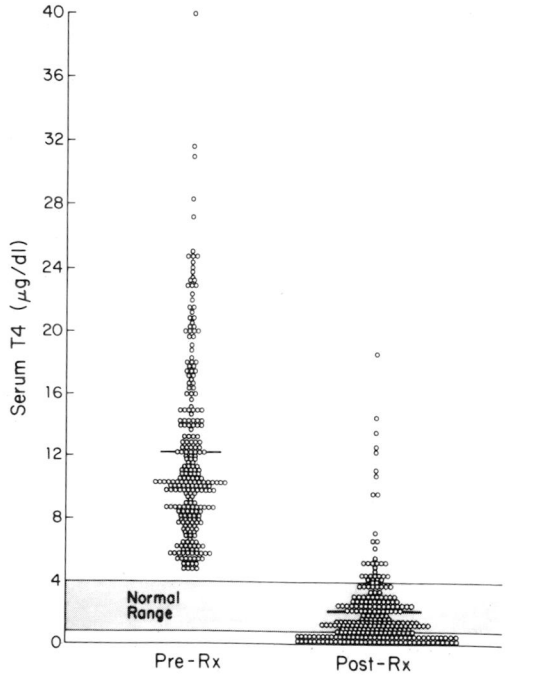

FIGURE 95–14. Serum T_4 concentrations in 262 cats with hyperthyroidism before and two to three weeks after treatment with methimazole (10 to 15 mg/day). Horizontal lines indicate mean values. (From Peterson, ME, et al.: Methimazole treatment of 262 cats with hyperthyroidism. J Vet Intern Med 2:150, 1988.)

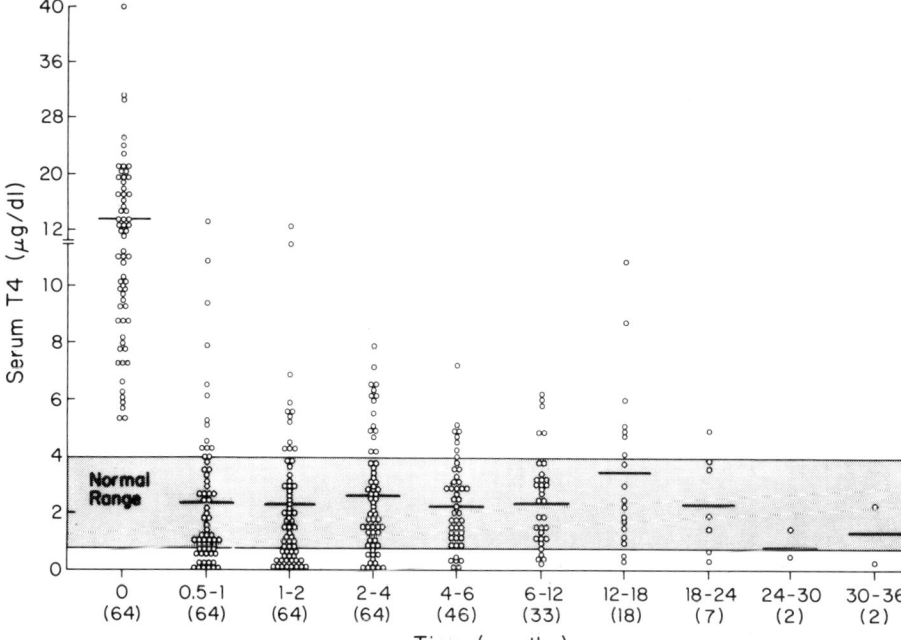

FIGURE 95–15. Serum T$_4$ concentrations in 64 cats with hyperthyroidism before and during long-term treatment with methimazole. Horizontal lines indicate mean values. Numbers in parentheses indicate number of cats treated during each time period. (From Peterson, ME, et al.: Methimazole treatment of 262 cats with hyperthyroidism. J Vet Intern Med 2:150, 1988.)

appear to inhibit the 5′-deiodination of T$_4$ to T$_3$. Since T$_3$ appears to be the most metabolically active thyroid hormone, normal circulating T$_3$ concentrations explain the absence of clinical signs of hypothyroidism.

While divided doses of methimazole (given every 8 or 12 hours) tend to be most effective in controlling the hyperthyroid state, euthyroidism can often be maintained when the necessary dose is given only once daily. Despite a serum half-life for methimazole of only 4 to 6 hours, studies in human hyperthyroid patients have shown that the drug has an intrathyroidal residence time of approximately 20 hours.[197] Since antithyroid drugs act to inhibit thyroid hormone synthesis only after they are concentrated within the thyroid gland, serum half-life of these drugs is of less importance than the intrathyroidal drug concentration for adequate control of the hyperthyroid state. In addition, many cat owners, especially those using methimazole on a long-term basis, may find a treatment regimen of once-daily medication easier to maintain than having to give medication two or three times daily. However, methimazole must be given at least once daily or serum thyroid hormone concentrations will again rise into the thyrotoxic range. Consequently, elevated circulating T$_4$ concentrations will develop in many cats treated with methimazole on a long-term basis because of a decrease in compliance by the owners or increased difficulty in giving daily medication (Figure 95–15).

Adverse Effects Associated with Methimazole Treatment. Mild clinical side-effects associated with methimazole treatment are relatively common (approximately 15 per cent of cats) and include anorexia, vomiting, and lethargy (Table 95–5).[168] In most cats, these adverse signs are transient and resolve despite continued administration of the drug. Severe gastrointestinal signs persist in some cats, however, necessitating discontinuation of the drug. Self-induced excoriations of the face and neck also may develop in a few cats within the first six weeks of therapy (Table 95–5). Although these cutaneous lesions tend to be partially responsive to treatment with systemic glucocorticoids, cessation of methimazole administration is usually required for complete resolution of these excoriations. Finally, hepatic toxicity is an uncommon but serious reaction that can develop during drug treatment.[168] Methimazole-induced hepatopathy is characterized by the development of marked increases in serum concentrations of ALT, AST, SAP, and total bilirubin. Clinical improvement, with resolution of anorexia, vomiting, and lethargy, usually occurs within a few days after cessation of methimazole, but jaundice and abnormal serum biochemical tests indicative of liver disease may not resolve for several weeks. Rechallenge with the drug will again induce clinical signs and serum biochemical abnormalities indicative of hepatic disease within a few days.[168]

TABLE 95–5. CLINICAL SIDE EFFECTS AND HEMATOLOGIC AND IMMUNOLOGIC ABNORMALITIES ASSOCIATED WITH METHIMAZOLE TREATMENT IN 262 CATS WITH HYPERTHYROIDISM

Sign	No. of Cats (%)	Time When Signs Developed (days)	
		Range	Median
Anorexia	29 (11.1)	1–78	18.0
Vomiting	28 (10.7)	7–60	15.0
Lethargy	23 (8.8)	1–60	21.0
Excoriations	6 (2.3)	6–40	19.0
Bleeding	6 (2.3)	15–50	22.5
Hepatopathy	4 (1.5)	15–60	41.0
Thrombocytopenia	7 (2.7)	14–90	24.0
Agranulocytosis	4 (1.5)	26–95	62.5
Leukopenia	12 (4.7)	10–41	23.0
Eosinophilia	30 (11.3)	12–490	21.0
Lymphocytosis	19 (7.2)	14–90	18.5
Antinuclear antibodies*	52 (21.8)	10–870	46.0
Positive Coombs' test*	3 (1.9)	45–60	50.0

*Antinuclear antibodies determined in 239 cats and direct antiglobulin (Coombs') tests performed in 160 cats

(Modified from data in Peterson, ME, et al.: J Vet Intern Med 2:150, 1988.)

A variety of hematologic abnormalities may develop in cats during treatment with methimazole (Table 95–5). Those abnormalities that do not appear to be associated with any adverse effects include eosinophilia, lymphocytosis, and transient leukopenia with a normal differential count.[168] As with PTU treatment,[194–196] more serious hematologic reactions that develop in a few cats treated with methimazole include severe thrombocytopenia (platelet count less than 75,000 cells/mm^3) and agranulocytosis (severe leukopenia with a total granulocyte count less than 250 cells/mm^3).[168, 196] Immune-mediated hemolytic anemia, a major side effect associated with PTU treatment,[195, 196] has not been observed with methimazole therapy. Most cats that develop severe thrombocytopenia also show concomitant overt bleeding (epistaxis, oral hemorrhage). Development of agranulocytosis during methimazole treatment predisposes to severe bacterial infections, systemic toxicity, and fever. If serious hematologic reactions develop during methimazole therapy, the drug should be stopped and supportive care given; these adverse reactions should resolve within five days after the methimazole is withdrawn.[168] Since most life-threatening side-effects (e.g., hepatopathy, thrombocytopenia, agranulocytosis) caused by methimazole treatment usually again develop quickly after rechallenge with the drug, alternative therapy with either surgery or radioiodine should be considered in these cases.

During methimazole therapy, serum antinuclear antibodies (ANA) develop in a high percentage of cats after treatment with methimazole.[168] The risk of developing ANA appears to increase with the duration of methimazole treatment, with ANA developing in approximately half of cats treated for more than six months in the author's study (Figure 95–16). The risk of developing serum ANA also appears to be greater for cats treated with higher daily methimazole doses, since most cats that develop ANA are receiving doses greater than or equal to 15 mg/day and ANA disappears in most cats after the dosage is decreased. Despite the high prevalence of ANA development during long-term treatment with methimazole, clinical signs associated with a lupus-like syndrome (dermatitis, polyarthritis, glomerulonephritis, hemolytic anemia, or fever) have not been observed in any of these cats. However, the potential for lupus development in cats with methimazole-induced ANA still exists. The daily drug dosage should therefore be decreased to as low as possible (while still maintaining serum T$_4$ values within the low-normal range), since ANA tests will become negative in many cats when the methimazole dosage is decreased.

Although the most serious adverse effects of methimazole treatment usually develop during the first few weeks of drug administration, side effects can potentially occur at any time during treatment. After the first three months of methimazole therapy, one should continue to measure serum T$_4$ concentrations at three- to six-month intervals in order to monitor dosage requirements and response to treatment. Although it does not appear to be necessary to continue to monitor complete blood and platelet counts during these rechecks, the cell counts should be performed if agranulocytosis or thrombocytopenia is suspected. In addition, although methimazole-

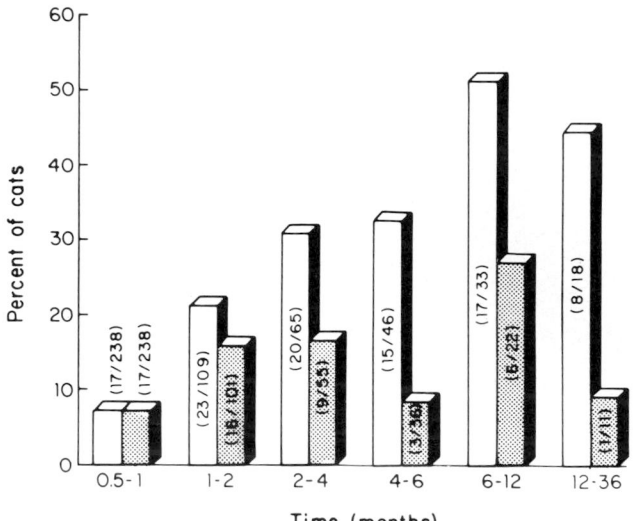

FIGURE 95–16. Percentage of cats developing serum antinuclear antibodies (ANA) during treatment with methimazole. Shaded bars represent the percentage of cats that first developed ANA during each time period. Unshaded bars represent total percentage of cats with ANA during each time period. For example, of the 55 cats that did not have ANA at the beginning of the two- to four-month treatment interval, nine cats developed ANA during this period (shaded bar). Of the 65 total cats treated during the same interval, 20 had ANA, 11 of which had developed ANA before the two- to four-month interval (unshaded bar). (From Peterson, ME, et al.: Methimazole treatment of 262 cats with hyperthyroidism. J Vet Intern Med 2:150, 1988.)

induced lupus has not been detected in cats that develop ANA during treatment, periodic monitoring of serum biochemical screening values and urinalysis, as well as serum ANA determinations, is also recommended if signs consistent with a lupus-like syndrome develop.

SURGERY

Surgical thyroidectomy is a highly effective treatment for feline hyperthyroidism. While thyroidectomy is most often successful, it can be associated with significant morbidity and mortality. Hyperthyroidism is a systemic illness that affects all body systems; although thyroidectomy in itself is a relatively simple procedure, cardiovascular, hepatic, and gastrointestinal dysfunctions associated with hyperthyroidism greatly increase anesthetic and surgical risks.[87, 88, 198] All hyperthyroid cats should therefore be prepared for surgery by administration of an antithyroid drug, propranolol, or iodide to decrease the metabolic and cardiac complications associated with hyperthyroidism.

Preoperative Preparation. Use of the antithyroid drug methimazole, as described previously, is the method of choice for the preoperative preparation of a hyperthyroid cat. After methimazole treatment has maintained euthyroidism for one to three weeks, most systemic complications associated with hyperthyroidism will have improved or resolved, and the anesthetic and surgical complications will be greatly minimized. The last dose of methimazole should be administered on the morning of surgery.

In hyperthyroid cats that cannot tolerate antithyroid drug treatment, alternate preoperative preparation with propranolol or stable iodine, alone or in combination, should be used. Although propranolol, a β-adrenergic blocker, does not lower elevated serum thyroid hormone concentrations, this drug blocks many of the cardiovascular and neuromuscular effects of excess thyroid hormone and controls the tachycardia and hyperexcitability associated with feline hyperthyroidism. In addition, treatment with a β-adrenergic blocker helps prevent arrhythmias that commonly develop during the anesthetic period in untreated cats with hyperthyroidism.[87] Propranolol should be administered for 7 to 14 days before surgery at the dosage of 2.5 to 5.0 mg (every eight hours), as required to decrease resting heart rate to within the normal range and to control hyperexcitability.[167] In cats with congestive heart failure secondary to chronic thyroid hormone excess, propranolol should not be initiated until cardiac failure has been stabilized with diuretics (and digitalis when indicated).[191] In these cases, propranolol should be used with caution, since the drug depresses myocardial function.

Large doses of stable iodine block T_4 and T_3 release from the thyroid gland and lower serum thyroid hormone concentrations.[31] In addition, iodine treatment causes a reduction in the size and vascularity of the adenomatous thyroid gland. Iodine has major limitations as antithyroid therapy, however, since serum T_4 and T_3 concentrations may not ever completely normalize during iodine treatment, and the drug often loses its antithyroid effect within a few weeks.[31] Therefore, iodine should not be used as sole therapy in preparation for thyroidectomy, but can be given in conjunction with propranolol or an antithyroid drug. Iodine should be administered as either oral potassium iodide (saturated solution of potassium iodide—SSKI), Lugol's solution, or intravenous sodium iodide at a dosage of 50 to 100 mg per day for 7 to 14 days prior to surgery.[167] Common side effects of oral potassium iodide treatment include excessive salivation and decreased appetite; such adverse signs appear to result from the unpleasant taste of iodine. To prevent this adverse effect, the dose of SSKI can be placed within a small gelatin capsule and immediately administered.

Anesthesia. Anesthetic management of the hyperthyroid cat should include the judicious use of agents that have minimal cardiac arrhythmic effects. A variety of anesthetic agents and techniques can be used and none has advantages that exclude use of all others, especially if the hyperthyroid state has been controlled with methimazole prior to surgery.[88, 198]

Premedication with acetylpromazine is useful because this drug reduces autonomic manifestations of hyperthyroidism and may prevent arrhythmias induced by thiobarbiturates and inhalation agents.[87, 88] Use of xylazine (Rompun) is contraindicated because it potentiates the development of cardiac arrhythmias induced by inhalation or barbiturate anesthesia. Atropine should also be omitted because it stimulates adrenergic activity and may induce tachycardia and arrhythmias.[87, 88, 198] If an anticholinergic agent is used, glycopyrrolate (Robinul-V) is the drug of choice because it has minimal effects on cardiac rate and rhythm. Because hyperthyroid cats are particularly sensitive to catecholamine-induced arrhythmias, anesthetic agents that stimulate sympathoadrenal activity, such as ketamine, should be avoided.[87, 88]

Thiobarbiturates are acceptable induction agents because they possess antithyroid activity and do not stimulate catecholamine secretion. Many inhalation agents are acceptable for maintaining anesthesia in cats with hyperthyroidism. If available, enflurane or isoflurane is preferred over methoxyflurane and halothane because the latter inhalation agents sensitize the heart to catecholamine-induced arrhythmias to a lesser extent.[87, 88]

During the anesthetic period, continuous monitoring of the anesthetic level and electrocardiogram is essential. Ventricular arrhythmias are common, especially in cats not rendered euthyroid prior to surgery. If arrhythmias develop, the anesthetic concentration should be lowered and the cat ventilated with a higher concentration of oxygen. If the arrhythmias persist, small doses (0.1 mg) of intravenous propranolol usually restore normal sinus rhythm.[88, 198]

Surgical Considerations. About 30 per cent of hyperthyroid cats have disease in only one thyroid lobe, whereas the remaining 70 per cent have bilateral thyroid lobe involvement.[175, 176] In cats with unilateral thyroid tumors, the contralateral lobe is normal in position and either normal or small in size when inspected at surgery. Hemithyroidectomy corrects the hyperthyroid state in these cats, and relapse resulting from the development of adenomatous changes in the remaining "normal" thyroid lobe is extremely rare and takes years to develop. In cats with bilateral thyroid adenomas (adenomatous hyperplasia), removal of both lobes with preservation of parathyroid function is necessary to control hyperthyroidism and avoid postoperative hypocalcemia. With bilateral thyroid tumors, enlargement of both lobes can easily be identified at surgery in most cats; about 15 per cent of cats with bilateral lobe involvement, however, have one lobe, which is only slightly enlarged and may be mistaken as normal. Preoperative thyroid imaging is helpful in defining the extent of thyroid lobe involvement in these cases.[175, 176] If thyroid imaging is not feasible, the authors recommend removal of the obviously enlarged lobe with preservation of the associated external parathyroid gland in all cats with suspected unilateral lobe involvement. If bilateral lobe involvement was initially present, relapse of hyperthyroidism usually occurs within nine months of surgery. Preservation of the external parathyroid gland during hemithyroidectomy minimizes the risk of hypoparathyroidism, should removal of the contralateral lobe be required.

Techniques for unilateral and bilateral thyroidectomy have been reported for cats with hyperthyroidism.[198–200] Both intracapsular and extracapsular methods designed for removal of thyroid tissue while preserving parathyroid function have been described.[198, 201] With the intracapsular technique for thyroidectomy, however, it can be difficult to remove the entire thyroid capsule (and therefore all abnormal thyroid tissue) while concurrently preserving parathyroid function. Small remnants of thyroid tissue that remain attached to the capsule may regenerate and produce recurrent hyperthyroidism.[200, 201] The main advantage of the extracapsular, as compared to the intracapsular, technique is that the incidence of relapse is much less because using this method, the entire thyroid capsule is removed together with the thyroid lobe.

Postoperative Complications. There are many potential complications associated with thyroidectomy, including hypoparathyroidism, Horner's syndrome, and laryngeal paralysis (most commonly voice change).[198–201] The most serious complication is hypocalcemia, which develops after the parathyroid glands are injured, devascularized, or inadvertently removed in the course of bilateral thyroidectomy. Since only one parathyroid gland is required for maintenance of normocalcemia, hypoparathyroidism develops only in cats treated with bilateral thyroidectomy. After bilateral thyroidectomy, the serum calcium concentration should be monitored on a daily basis until it has stabilized within the normal range. In most cats with iatrogenic hypoparathyroidism, clinical signs associated with hypocalcemia develop within one to three days of surgery.[202, 203] Although mild hypocalcemia (6.5 to 7.5 mg/dl) is a common finding during this immediate postoperative period, laboratory evidence of hypocalcemia alone does not require treatment. However, if accompanying signs of muscle tremors, tetany, or convulsions develop, therapy with vitamin D and calcium is indicated (see Chapter 94).[202, 203] Although hypoparathyroidism may be permanent in some cats, spontaneous recovery of parathyroid function may occur weeks to months after surgery. In most cases, such transient hypocalcemia probably results from reversible parathyroid damage and ischemia incurred during surgery. Alternatively, accessory parathyroid tissue may compensate for the damaged parathyroid glands and maintain normocalcemia.[24]

Long-Term Management. Serum thyroid hormone concentrations fall to subnormal levels for two to three months after hemithyroidectomy for unilateral thyroid lobe involvement. However, thyroxine supplementation is rarely required during this period. If bilateral thyroidectomy has been performed, thyroxine (0.1 to 0.2 mg/day) should be started 24 to 48 hours after surgery. Although thyroxine supplementation at this dosage can be safely continued indefinitely, the low serum concentrations of T_4 and T_3 that develop 24 to 48 hours after bilateral thyroidectomy may spontaneously increase to within normal range weeks to months postoperatively. Thyroxine administration can then be discontinued. Because of the potential for recurrence of hyperthyroidism, all cats treated by surgical thyroidectomy should have serum thyroid hormone concentration monitored once or twice a year. In cases of recurrent thyrotoxicosis after bilateral thyroidectomy, treatment with either methimazole or radioiodine is favored over a second operation, since the incidence of surgical complications (especially permanent hypoparathyroidism) is considerably higher in subsequent operations than in the initial procedure.[200]

RADIOACTIVE IODINE

Radioactive iodine provides a simple, effective, and safe treatment for cats with hyperthyroidism. The basic principle behind treatment of hyperthyroidism with radioiodine is that thyroid cells do not differentiate between stable and radioactive iodine; therefore, radioiodine, like stable iodine, is concentrated by the thyroid gland after administration. In cats with hyperthyroidism, radioiodine is concentrated primarily in the hyperplastic or neoplastic thyroid cells, where it irradiates and destroys the hyperfunctioning tissue. Normal thyroid tissue, however, tends to be protected from the effects of radioiodine, since the uninvolved thyroid tissue is suppressed and receives only a small dose of radiation (unless very large doses are administered).

The radioisotope most frequently used to treat hyperthyroidism is radioiodine-131 (^{131}I). Iodine-131 has a half-life of eight days and emits both β particles and γ radiation.[166] The β particles, which cause 80 per cent of the tissue damage, travel a maximum of 2 mm in tissue and have an average path length of 400 microns. Therefore, β particles are locally destructive but spare adjacent hypoplastic thyroid tissue, parathyroid glands, and other cervical structures.

The ideal goal of ^{131}I therapy is to restore euthyroidism with a single dose of radiation without producing hypothyroidism. Three major methods have been used to estimate the activity of ^{131}I required to destroy the hyperfunctioning thyroid tissue in cats with hyperthyroidism.

With the first method of ^{131}I dose determination, various parameters of thyroid kinetics are determined with a small "tracer" dose of radioiodine.[167, 204, 205] Using an estimated desired radiation dose of 15,000 to 20,000 rad per gram of thyroid tissue, the therapeutic dose of ^{131}I is calculated from the following parameters: (1) the effective half-life of ^{131}I (which accounts for both the physical half-life and duration of radioiodine retention by the thyroid), (2) the fraction of ^{131}I deposited in the thyroid gland (the per cent thyroid uptake), and (3) estimated thyroid gland weight. Using this method, the calculated ^{131}I dose may range from 1 to 10 mCi, which can be administered either orally or as a single subcutaneous or intravenous injection. With this ^{131}I dose method, approximately 80 per cent of hyperthyroid cats become euthyroid within three months (most within two weeks) after a single dose of radioiodine, while the remaining cats require a second ^{131}I treatment for complete resolution of the hyperthyroid state.[204–206] Very few cats develop hypothyroidism from ^{131}I overdosage and require thyroid hormone supplementation with this regimen. The major disadvantage of this method of dose determination is that the procedures used may necessitate sedating the cat on one or more occasions.

The second method of dose determination is to select a relatively low dose of ^{131}I without determining thyroid gland kinetics. Administration of 2 to 6 mCi of ^{131}I (based on the size of the thyroid nodule and the T_4 value) produces euthyroidism in the majority of cats with hyperthyroidism. However, use of this approach also results in under- or overtreatment of a number of cats, resulting in persistent hyperthyroidism or hypothyroidism, respectively. The advantage of this method is that nuclear medicine equipment is not needed, the time required to determine thyroid kinetics is eliminated, and sedation of the cat is not required.

The third method of radioiodine therapy is to administer extremely large doses of radioiodine (10 to 30 mCi). These doses of ^{131}I almost always totally destroy the adenomatous thyroid tissue as well as normal thyroid tissue. Thus, this method is effective in curing the hyperthyroidism in almost all cats but also has the disadvantage of inducing hypothyroidism in the majority of cases. In general, the authors recommend use of such large does of ^{131}I only in cats with hyperfunctioning thyroid adenocarcinoma to ensure complete destruction of the malignant tissue.[167]

Regardless of the method of dose determination selected, there are certain radiation safety restrictions and procedures that must be followed. The cats should be confined to restricted areas of the hospital that have minimal traffic and be housed in metabolic cages so that urine and feces can be collected safely. All personnel handling the cats, cages, food dishes, and excreta should wear long laboratory coats, disposable plastic gloves, and film badges. All material removed from the cage must be handled as radioactive waste and be disposed of accordingly. The cats are discharged from the hospital when the radiation dose rate has decreased to a safe level that has been determined by the state radiation control office (usually after a one- to three-week period). The owners are advised prior to radioiodine therapy that their cat will be radioactive when discharged and are given instructions to minimize their risk.

Overall, use of radioiodine may be the optimal treatment for feline hyperthyroidism when nuclear medicine facilities are available. Radioactive iodine treatment involves a single, nonstressful procedure that is without associated morbidity or mortality. Untoward systemic effects have not been observed. Unlike surgery, anesthesia is not required. A single ^{131}I treatment restores euthyroidism in most cats with hyperthyroidism, whereas cats that remain persistently hyperthyroid can be successfully retreated with radioiodine and those that become hypothyroid can be supplemented readily with thyroxine. At present, the major disadvantage of radioiodine therapy is the unavailability of facilities that can safely handle ^{131}I and accurately determine the ideal dose to administer.

CANINE THYROID NEOPLASIA AND HYPERTHYROIDISM

In the dog, thyroid tumors represent approximately one to two per cent of all canine neoplasms and account for 10 to 15 per cent of all primary tumors in the head and neck region.[707] As opposed to the relatively small, noninvasive thyroid tumors (i.e., adenomatous hyperplasia) associated with feline hyperthyroidism, most canine tumors are large, invasive carcinomas that are not hyperfunctional (i.e., do not produce hyperthyroidism). Because many of these tumors are malignant and have reached an advanced state at the time of diagnosis, the prognosis is often poor.

Pathology of Canine Thyroid Tumors

About 90 per cent of canine thyroid tumors detected clinically (in the living dog) are malignant (thyroid carcinomas).[26, 177, 208–211] Most adenomas are small (less

than 2 cm in maximal diameter) and are detected only at necropsy. Thyroid carcinomas are usually much larger than adenomas and are characterized by rapid growth, extensive vascularization, and necrosis. Local invasion and extension of the malignant thyroid tumor into adjacent structures (e.g., esophagus, trachea, cervical musculature, nerves, and thyroid vessels) occurs frequently. In addition, distant metastasis is also common, with a 60 to 80 per cent rate of metastasis reported in most surveys.[208, 212] Because malignant thyroid tumors have a propensity for invading veins within the tumor mass, metastasis to the lungs occurs more frequently and earlier than to the regional lymph nodes.[208] In approximately one third of dogs with adenocarcinoma, pulmonary metastasis is already evident at the time the dog is examined (Table 95–6). If lymphatic extension does occur, the retropharyngeal lymph nodes are most likely to be involved, since the major lymphatic drainage is from the anterior rather than the posterior pole of each thyroid lobe.[213] In general, the probability of metastasis increases in proportion to the size and duration of the tumor.

Thyroid carcinomas may arise from follicular epithelium or parafollicular cells (C cells). Tumors of follicular cell origin can be further classified as follicular, solid (compact cellular), mixed solid-follicular, papillary, or anaplastic, depending on their pattern of growth. The majority of canine adenocarcinomas contain both follicular and solid cellular patterns (solid-follicular tumor type), while pure follicular cell tumors are less common.[208, 212] Papillary carcinoma, the most common thyroid tumor type in humans, is rare in the dog. Parafollicular cell tumors (medullary carcinomas) are rare and account for less than five per cent of all canine thyroid tumors.[212] Histologically, medullary carcinomas are difficult to distinguish from the solid cellular type of follicular cell tumor.[214, 215]

In humans, it is very helpful to classify thyroid tumors into follicular versus papillary types because the prognosis for cancers containing papillary elements is gen-

TABLE 95–6. INCIDENCE OF CLINICAL SIGNS IN DOGS WITH THYROID TUMOR

Sign	Percentage of Cases
Nontoxic (euthyroid or hypothyroid) thyroid tumor (N = 168)	
Goiter	100
Respiratory distress/cough	28
Metastases to lung or lymph nodes	35
Vomiting	11
Dysphagia	10
Anorexia	9
Weight loss	7
Hyperfunctional (hyperthyroid) thyroid tumor (N = 18)	
Goiter	100
Polydipsia and polyuria	94
Weight loss	78
Weakness and fatigue	72
Polyphagia	67
Heat intolerance	56
Nervousness	50
Hyperdefecation/diarrhea	28
Tremors	22

Compiled from data reported in references 29, 177, 211, 216, 217, 220–223, 228, and 231.

erally much better than that of pure follicular carcinoma. Such classification schemes may also have prognostic value in the dog, since some investigators found that follicular carcinomas grow more rapidly than the majority of mixed solid-follicular tumors.[26, 212] This suggestion, however, has not been supported by other recent studies.[207, 216] Overall, much more than the type of carcinoma must be considered in predicting the prognosis: the size of the primary tumor, the presence or absence of direct extension and invasion of tumor into the juxtathyroidal tissues, and the presence or absence of foci of metastatic tumor.

Clinical Features

Signalment. As with thyroid tumors of the cat, thyroid tumors in the dog usually occur in dogs of middle to old age (reported range, 7 to 15 years).[208, 210, 211] There does not appear to be a sex predilection in the dog. However, the risk of thyroid carcinoma rose in older, neutered bitches as compared with older males in one study, suggesting that ovarian hormones may protect against the development of thyroid malignancy.[209] Breeds reported to be at increased risk for developing thyroid tumors include the boxer, beagle, and golden retriever.[208, 209, 212]

Clinical Signs. Most dogs with thyroid tumors are presented because the owner has noticed an enlargement of the neck (Table 95–6).[207, 208, 210–212, 216–218] Less commonly, the tumor may be an incidental finding on physical examination. Unlike the relatively small, freely movable thyroid tumors of the cat, most of the tumors in dogs are very large and easily palpable, and are fixed to the soft tissues of the neck. The tumors are usually unilateral (approximately two thirds of cases), firm, asymmetrical, and irregular in shape. In general, most dogs remain fairly healthy, with only a few being obviously cachectic or depressed. Other clinical signs that may be reported, however, especially in dogs with nonfunctional thyroid tumors, include dyspnea, cough, hoarseness, dysphagia, vomiting, anorexia, weight loss, voice change, and facial edema (Table 95–6).[207, 208, 210–212, 216–218] Respiratory signs in dogs with thyroid carcinoma may be caused by tracheal obstruction or pulmonary metastasis. Rarely, metastasis to the cervical vertebrae produces lysis of vertebral bodies and laminae, with resultant neurological signs (e.g., neck pain, ataxia, tetraparesis).[219]

Some canine thyroid tumors develop autonomous hyperfunction, leading to signs of hyperthyroidism, and in these dogs the hyperthyroid state is usually the major reason for examination.[29, 212, 218, 220, 221] Although one group of investigators reported hyperthyroidism in 20 percent of dogs with thyroid tumor,[29, 212, 218] others have found the prevalence of thyrotoxicosis to be much less (e.g., only six per cent in one study).[177] Histologically, these tumors are almost always carcinomas of the follicular or compact-follicular cellular type. In general, hyperfunctional tumors producing hyperthyroidism are usually smaller (2 to 5 cm in diameter) than the nontoxic tumors and therefore display less of a compressive effect on adjacent structures.[29, 212] Polydipsia and polyuria are

usually the earliest and most predominant signs associated with canine hyperthyroidism. Weight loss, despite an increase in appetite, is also common. Compared with most cats with hyperthyroidism, however, the degree of weight loss is usually much less severe. Other signs that may develop in dogs with hyperthyroidism (usually in proportion to the severity and duration of the hyperthyroid state) include weakness and fatigue, heat intolerance, nervousness or restless behavior, and more frequent defecation with semiformed feces (Table 95–6).[29, 212, 218, 220, 221] Cardiac signs may include a more forceful apex beat and arterial pulse, and the electrocardiogram may show high voltage in all leads.

In dogs with the rare thyroid tumors that arise from the parafollicular cells (medullary carcinoma), the most striking clinical feature that may be observed is diarrhea, as well as a visible mass or swelling in the neck.[212, 214, 215] The cause of the diarrhea is unclear, but may be due to the elaboration of a substance (such as serotonin or prostaglandins) by the thyroid tumor.[212, 224] Medullary carcinomas also are widely known to hypersecrete calcitonin in both humans and dogs.[224, 225] Although calcitonin decreases serum calcium concentration when administered acutely, serum calcium values almost always remain normal in humans and dogs with medullary carcinoma. Of the few clinical reports of canine medullary carcinoma, only one dog has had profound hypocalcemia (resulting in signs of seizures and tetany).[215]

Diagnosis

Thyroid neoplasia should be suspected in any dog with an enlarging mass in the ventral cervical region. The differential diagnosis for a mass in the ventral cervical region should include inflammatory conditions (e.g., abscess, granuloma) and nonthyroid neoplasia (e.g., regional soft tissue sarcomas, lymphosarcoma, metastatic oral tumors), as well as thyroid tumors. Fine needle aspiration cytology (using a 21- to 23-gauge needle) may be very helpful in differentiating a thyroid tumor from an abscess, salivary mucocele, or enlarged lymph node.[226] In addition, cytological examination of fine needle aspirates can be a useful aid in the preoperative differential diagnosis of benign or malignant thyroid disease. Because of the vascular nature of the thyroid neoplasm, however, fine needle aspiration cytology may be unrewarding because of blood contamination. A definitive diagnosis usually requires an excisional biopsy and histopathology.

Screening laboratory tests (e.g., complete blood count, serum biochemical profile, urinalysis) should always be performed in a dog with suspected thyroid neoplasia. Results of such pretreatment screening tests may reveal the presence of a concurrent disorder not directly related to the thyroid tumor that may influence subsequent surgical and anesthetic management or use of chemotherapy. Chest radiographs should always be reviewed, since about a third of these dogs will have pulmonary metastasis at time of diagnosis. It is important to realize, however, that metastatic nodules smaller than 5 mm in diameter may not be visible radiographically. In addition, electrocardiography, echocardiography, or other studies may also be warranted in dogs with hyperfunctional thyroid tumors, especially if signs of thyrotoxic congestive heart failure are present.

Most dogs with thyroid tumors remain euthyroid. Therefore, unless clinical signs suggestive of hypo- or hyperthyroidism are present, determination of basal serum thyroid hormone (T_4 and T_3) concentrations is usually unnecessary. Although some investigators have reported hypothyroidism in 40 per cent of cases (secondary to destruction of normal thyroid tissue of both lobes by the expanding, nonfunctioning tumor),[177] the majority of other reports suggest that the development of overt hypothyroidism is relatively uncommon. Hyperthyroidism has been reported to occur in up to 20 per cent of cases by some investigators,[29, 218] but most reports indicate a much lower prevalence.[177, 211, 216] In general, the severity of the hyperthyroid state (based on both the degree of elevation in serum thyroid hormone concentrations and severity of clinical signs) is usually milder in dogs than in most hyperthyroid cats. As in cats with mild hyperthyroidism, the serum T_4 concentration may be increased but the T_3 value may remain within the normal range in some dogs.[26] Once the thyroid tumor is recognized, diagnostic studies for the hyperthyroid state are largely academic because the fundamental (and more life-threatening) problem is the malignant tumor. However, the management of dogs with hyperthyroidism may differ from those with hypothyroidism since ^{131}I would be expected to be more effective in hyperfunctional thyroid tumors (because of the higher uptake of the radioactivity into the tumor). In addition, the persistence or recurrence of either clinical or laboratory signs of hyperthyroidism after attempted excision of the tumor may signify recurrence or metastasis of the carcinoma.

Imaging of canine thyroid tumors is valuable both for diagnosis and localization of the tumor. Thyroid imaging may also detect regional and distant thyroid metastasis, as well as identify the presence of any ectopic thyroid tumor tissue. Although thyroid imaging with either radioiodine or $^{99m}TcO_4$ is likely to produce similar results, use of radioiodine is generally preferred for imaging of canine thyroid tumors because a thyroid uptake determination can be performed at the time of imaging with ^{123}I or [131]I. Thyroid uptake determinations are very useful in assessing thyroid function and may aid in the calculation of a therapeutic ^{131}I dose (see Treatment, below).

Based on thyroid imaging, most dogs with thyroid tumors show varying degrees of radionuclide uptake into the tumor. Tumors without any radionuclide accumulation are usually of the anaplastic type or are medullary (C cell) carcinomas, whereas the predominant solid and mixed solid-follicular cellular types usually have rather extensive areas of uptake of the radioisotope. Those dogs that show extensive radionuclide uptake into the tumor (and have normal to high values for thyroidal uptake of radioiodine) may show a better response to treatment with radioiodine, whereas ^{131}I would be of limited value in dogs without any radioiodine accumulation by the tumor (since ^{131}I would not be concentrated by the cells that need to be destroyed).

Treatment

Surgery. For most dogs with thyroid tumors, the initial treatment of choice is attempted surgical resection. Small, well-encapsulated thyroid tumors (generally up to 3 cm in diameter) are relatively easy to remove, whereas complete excision of large invasive carcinomas is usually difficult and may be impossible. However, even in the latter cases, debulking of the tumor mass may be beneficial in preparation for other treatment, as well as in making the dog more comfortable (relief of dyspnea, dysphagia). Dogs with distant metastasis should not be treated with surgery alone, but debulking of the primary thyroid mass may improve the effectiveness of adjunct chemotherapy or radiotherapy. Although debulking of the tumor can be very helpful in treatment of thyroid cancer, aggressive attempts to completely remove all malignant thyroid tissue can do more harm than good for the dog, since recurrent laryngeal nerves, parathyroid glands, and major blood vessels may be seriously damaged in the process of surgical removal. Even if complete excision of the thyroid carcinoma is not possible, attempted thyroidectomy allows for the excisional biopsy (and subsequent histopathologic examination) of the tumor needed to confirm the diagnosis.

The major complication associated with excision of thyroid carcinoma during the intraoperative period is extensive blood loss. Because highly vascular thyroid carcinomas often infiltrate local blood vessels, massive (sometimes uncontrollable) hemorrhage develops during attempted thyroidectomy in some dogs. In addition, after resection of large thyroid tumors, acceptable wound closure may be difficult as the result of the large dead space.[207]

Postoperatively, unilateral removal of thyroid and parathyroid tissue does not require replacement therapy, since the contralateral thyroid lobe and associated parathyroid glands compensate for the loss. When dogs with bilateral thyroid tumor are treated with surgery, it is usually very difficult to recognize and preserve the parathyroid glands. In addition to full thyroid replacement, treatment of hypoparathyroidism is therefore necessary[202, 203] (also see Chapter 94). In an attempt to prevent rapid progression of inoperable thyroid tumor, one may administer L-T_4 at the dosage of 10 to 20 µg/lb/day (20 to 40 µg/kg/day). The resulting suppression of TSH secretion is believed to decrease the rate of progression of thyroid tumor growth, at least in humans.[227]

Chemotherapy. Although surgery cures thyroid adenoma, total removal of all malignant thyroid tissue is not common, especially in dogs with large, invasive carcinomas. Therefore, chemotherapy becomes an important adjunctive mode of therapy when complete surgical removal was not successful, when distant metastatic lesions are identified, or when the size of the primary tumor is so large (more than 4 cm in diameter) that metastasis is likely even though it cannot be identified with thoracic radiographs or other routine diagnostic tests. In addition, preoperative reduction in tumor volume with chemotherapy may reduce the morbidity of surgical thyroidectomy and improve the chance for a more complete resection in dogs with massive local disease.[207]

Doxorubicin has thus far been the most effective chemotherapeutic agent for canine thyroid carcinoma.[228, 229] Doxorubicin should be administered at a dose of 30 mg/m^2 body surface area (BSA), IV, every three weeks for a total of five treatments (cumulative dose 150 mg/m^2 BSA). Doxorubicin causes a severe slough if extravasated and may produce immediate hypersensitivity reactions if given too rapidly. Therefore, the drug should be diluted in normal saline and administered as a continuous infusion over a 15- to 30-minute period. Acute adverse reactions associated with doxorubicin therapy include generalized anaphylaxis, facial swelling and urticaria, gastrointestinal dysfunction (vomiting, diarrhea), hypotension, and cardiac arrhythmias.[229] Pretreatment administration of diphenhydramine hydrochloride (e.g., Benadryl), using a dosage of 0.2 to 0.5 mg/lb (0.5 to 1.0 mg/kg) helps to prevent the development of these acute reactions associated with doxorubicin. The most limiting chronic toxicosis associated with doxorubicin therapy is congestive cardiomyopathy. Doxorubicin-induced cardiomyopathy is an irreversible condition and may develop weeks to months after the last treatment was administered. The risk of drug-induced cardiomyopathy increases in proportion to the cumulative doses administered, especially at doses greater than 150 mg/m^2 BSA. At this time, there is no reliable method to predict which dogs will develop this doxorubicin-induced cardiomyopathy. Other chronic adverse reactions associated with doxorubicin therapy, which are usually self-limiting, include weight loss, diarrhea, anorexia, bone marrow hypoplasia, focal or generalized alopecia, and testicular atrophy.[229]

Although the response to doxorubicin treatment is variable and only rarely produces complete remission of the tumor, approximately half of dogs treated with this regimen will demonstrate at least a 50 per cent decrease in tumor volume. Combination chemotherapy with cyclophosphamide (Cytoxan) appears to enhance the effectiveness of doxorubicin. With this regimen, oral cyclophosphamide is administered using a dosage of 50 mg/m^2 BSA for four consecutive days, starting two days after each doxorubicin treatment (cumulative dose 1000 mg/m^2 BSA). In addition to antineoplastic agents, thyroid hormone therapy (10 to 20 μg/lb/day or 20 to 40 μg/kg/day of L-T_4), as described previously, may be of value in suppressing thyroid growth after tumor excision or debulking procedures have been performed.[227]

External Beam Irradiation. External beam (cobalt) irradiation is commonly used as adjunct therapy for thyroid carcinoma in humans,[227] but a controlled study of the efficacy of this treatment for canine thyroid tumors has not been reported. A dose of 4800 to 5200 cGy fractionated into 30 doses and given five times a week over a six-week period has been successful in reducing tumor volume in a few dogs with large, unresectable thyroid tumors. With that regimen, side effects (e.g., skin changes, esophagitis, pharyngitis, laryngitis) are uncommon. As in humans, a combination of surgical debulking followed by external beam irradiation would probably be very effective in destroying residual tumor tissue in the dogs. Alternately, a combination of chemotherapy (e.g., doxorubicin) and external radiation, as has been described in humans with unresectable thyroid carcinoma,[230] may work in other dogs.

Radioiodine. Most canine thyroid carcinomas retain the ability to concentrate radioiodine. Therefore, a favorable response to treatment of these tumors with large doses of ^{131}I might be expected, especially in dogs that have a high degree of radioiodine uptake by the tumor. The results of ^{131}I treatment for treatment of functioning thyroid carcinoma has only been reported in a few dogs. Rijnberk described four hyperthyroid dogs in which ^{131}I doses of 10 to 35 mCi resulted in improvement in the thyrotoxic state and a decrease in tumor volume.[29, 221, 231] However, in another hyperthyroid dog with functioning lung metastasis reported by Rijnberk, administration of 100 mCi ^{131}I resolved the signs of hyperthyroidism but failed to control the metastatic growth.[29]

As in humans, it appears that radioiodine treatment alone can result in palliation of clinical signs in dogs that have large unresectable primary tumors or massive thyroid metastasis. However, very large, repetitive ^{131}I doses may be required for an adequate response. The authors have treated one dog with hyperthyroidism resulting from a large, nonresectable thyroid carcinoma with three doses of ^{131}I of 60 to 75 mCi each, given at six-month intervals.[232] The dog became euthyroid following each treatment and the size of the tumor decreased, resolving the dyspnea, but both the hyperthyroidism and breathing difficulty recurred each time within a few months. The dog was euthanatized shortly after the last ^{131}I treatment because of progressive tracheal compression and pulmonary metastasis. Although radioiodine therapy definitely prolonged survival time in this dog, this therapy is prohibitively expensive for most cases.

Although the authors have only limited clinical experience in treating these cases with combination therapy, it appears that a combination of surgical debulking with chemotherapy, external radiotherapy, or radioiodine may offer the best chance for cure.

Prognosis

The prognosis for thyroid adenomas is excellent with surgical excision alone. The prognosis for thyroid carcinomas is related to the size of the tumor, resectability, and presence of metastasis. As might be expected, there appears to be a correlation between the size of the thyroid carcinoma and presence of metastasis. One study demonstrated that when tumor volume was less than 21 cm^3, only 14 per cent of dogs had metastasis. In dogs with a tumor volume between 21 and 100 cm^3, on the other hand, metastasis was present in 74 per cent, and all dogs with tumor volumes greater than 100 cm^3 had metastasis.[212] In general, dogs with well-encapsulated thyroid carcinomas that are easily resected have a relatively good prognosis with surgical treatment alone (median survival times of two to three years). In contrast, survival times of only 8 to 12 months can be expected in dogs with large, unresectable carcinomas treated with chemotherapy alone. Thus, smaller tumors carry a better prognosis, and aggressive therapy (combination of surgery with chemotherapy or radiation therapy, or both) is warranted in dogs with moderate to large invasive thyroid carcinomas.

References

1. Werner, SC: Historical resume. *In* Ingbar, SH and Braverman, LE (eds): The Thyroid, 5th ed. Philadelphia, JB Lippincott, 1986, p 3.
2. Wharton, T: Adeniographia: Sive glandularum tolius corporis descripto, Cap XVIII De glandulis thyroidaeis. Londonis, Typis JG Impensis Authoris, 1656:118.
3. Vercelloni, J: De glandulus oesophagi conglomeratis humore vero digestivo et vermibus dissertatio. Typ JB de Zagrandis, 1711.
4. Parry, CH: Collections from the unpublished papers of the late Caleb Hilliel Parry. (Lond) 2:111, 1825.
5. Meuli, J: Zur Funktion der Schilddruse. Eine experimentellphysiologische Studie. Pfluegers Arch 33:378, 1884.
6. Cooper, AP: Notes on the structure of the thyroid gland. Guys Hosp Rep 1:448, 1836.
7. Gley, E: Sur les fonctions du corps thyroïde. CR Soc Biol (Paris) 43:841, 1891.
8. Vassale, G and Generali, F: Sur les effets de l'extirpation des glandes parathyreoïdiennes. Arch Ital Biol 26:61, 1896-97.
9. Fagge, CH: On sporadic cretinism occurring in England. Br Med J 1:279, 1871.
10. Gull, WW: On a cretinoid state supervening in adult life in women. Trans Clin Soc (Lond) 7:180, 1974.
11. Murray, GR: Note on the treatment of myxoedema by hypodermic injections of an extract of the thyroid gland of a sheep. Br Med J 2:796, 1891.
12. Howitz, F: The treatment of myxoedema by feeding with thyroid glands. Br Med J 1:266, 1893.
13. Marine, D: On the occurrence and physiological nature of glandular hyperplasia of the thyroid (dog and sheep) together with remarks on the important clinical (human) problems. Johns Hopkins Hosp Bull, September 1907.
14. Govings, LS: Clinical diagnosis and therapy of hypothyroidism in dogs. JAVMA 141:341, 1962.
15. Peterson, ME, et al.: Spontaneous hyperthyroidism in the cat. Scientific Proc ACVIM 1979, p 108.
16. Graves, RJ: Clinical lectures. Lond Med Surg J 7:516, 1835.
17. Hullinger, RL: The endocrine system. *In* Evans, HE and Christensen, GC (eds): Miller's Anatomy of the Dog, 2nd ed. Philadelphia, WB Saunders, 1979, p 602.
18. Godwin, MC: The early development of the thyroid gland in the dog with special reference to the origin and position of accessory thyroid tissue within the thoracic cavity. Anat Rec 66:233, 1936.
19. Kameda, Y: The accessory thyroid gland of the dog around the intrapericardial aorta. Arch Histol Jpn 34:375, 1972.
20. Ganjam, VK, et al.: Recrudescence of extra-thyroidal tissue, T₄ and T₃ kinetics following thyroidectomy, and effects of replacement therapy in the canine. Fed Proceed 39:947 (#3572), 1980.
21. Thake, DC, et al.: Ectopic thyroid adenomas at the base of the heart of the dog. Vet Pathol 8:421, 1971.
22. Crouch, JE: Text Atlas of Cat Anatomy. Philadelphia, Lea and Febiger, 1969.
23. Carlson, AJ: On the cause of congenital goiter (thyroid hyperplasia) in dogs and cats. Am J Physiol 33:143, 1914.
24. Carpenter, JM, et al.: Tumors and tumor-like lesions. *In* Holzworth, J (ed): Diseases of the Cat. Philadelphia, WB Saunders, 1987, p 406.
25. Nicholas, JS and Swingle, WW: An experimental and morphological study of the parathyroid glands of the cat. Am J Anat 34:469, 1933.
26. Belshaw, BE: Thyroid diseases. *In* Ettinger, SE (ed): Textbook of Veterinary Internal Medicine, 2nd ed. Philadelphia, WB Saunders, 1983, p 1592.
27. Mumma, RO, et al.: Toxic and protective constituents in pet foods. Am J Vet Res 47:1633, 1986.
28. Belshaw, BE, et al.: The iodine requirement and influences of iodine intake on iodine metabolism and thyroid function in the adult beagle. Endocrinology 96:1280, 1975.
29. Rijnberk, A: Iodine metabolism and thyroid disease in the dog. PhD thesis. University of Utrecht, Drukkerij, Elinkwijk, 1971.
30. Broome, MR, et al.: Peripheral metabolism of thyroid hormones and iodide in healthy and hyperthyroid cats. Am J Vet Res 48:1286, 1987.
31. Taurog, A: Hormone synthesis: Thyroid iodine metabolism. *In* Ingbar, SH and Braverman, LE (eds): The Thyroid, 5th ed. Philadelphia, JB Lippincott, 1986, p 53.
32. Chastain, CB, et al.: Congenital hypothyroidism in a dog due to an iodine organification defect. Am J Vet Res 44:1257, 1983.
33. Nagataki, S and Ingbar, SH: Autoregulation: effects of iodine. *In* Ingbar, SH and Braverman, LE (eds): The Thyroid, 5th ed. Philadelphia, JB Lippincott, 1986, p 319.
34. Laurberg, P: Iodothyronine release from the perfused canine thyroid. Acta Endocrinol (Suppl) 236:1, 1980.
35. Laurberg, P: Iodothyronine deiodination in the canine thyroid. Dom Anim Endocrinol 1:1, 1984.
36. Wu, S: Thyrotropin-mediated induction of thyroidal iodothyronine monodeiodinases in the dog. Endocrinology 112:417, 1983.
37. Belshaw, BE, et al.: A model of iodine kinetics in the dog. Endocrinology 95:1078, 1974.
38. Nicoloff, JT: Physiologic and pathophysiologic implications of hormone binding. *In* Ingbar, SH and Braverman, LE (eds): The Thyroid, 5th ed. Philadelphia, JB Lippincott, 1986, p 128.
39. Laurberg, P: Non-parallel variations in the preferential secretion of 3,5,3′ triiodothyronine (T₃) and 3,3′,5′-triiodothyronine (rT₃) from dog thyroid. Endocrinology 102:757, 1978.
40. Larsen, PR, et al.: Relationships between circulating and intracellular thyroid hormones: Physiological and clinical implications. Endocr Rev 2:87, 1981.
41. Yoshida, K, et al.: Monodeiodination of thyroxine to 3,5,3′-triiodothyronine and to 3,3′,5′-triiodothyronine in isolated dog renal cortical tubuli. Endocrinol Jpn 30:211, 1983.
42. Wartofsky, L and Burman, KD: Alterations in thyroid function in patients with systemic illness: The "euthyroid sick syndrome." Endocr Rev 3:164, 1982.
43. Furth, ED, et al.: Thyroxine metabolism in the dog. Endocrinology 82:976, 1968.
44. Schussler, GC and Divino, CM: Transthyretin (TTR, prealbumin) stimulates the uptake and 5′deiodination of T₄ by hepatocytes (HEP G2) in vitro. Proc 69th Annu Mtg Endocrine Society, (abstr 375), 1987, p 115.
45. Larsson, M, et al.: Thyroid hormone binding in serum of 15 vertebrate species. Isolation of thyroxine-binding globulin and prealbumin analogs. Gen Comp Endocrinol 58:360, 1985.
46. Bigler, B: Thyroxine-binding serum proteins in the cat: A comparison with dog and man. Schweiz Archiv Tierheilkd 118:559, 1976.
47. Ferguson, DC and Peterson, ME: Serum free thyroxine concentrations in spontaneous canine hyperadrenocorticism. Proc Fourth Annu Vet Med Forum. ACVIM sec 14, 1986, p 39.
48. Woeber, KA and Maddux, BA: Thyroid hormone binding in nonthyroidal illness. Metabolism 30:412, 1981.
49. Kallfelz, FA and Erali, RP: Thyroid function tests in domestic animals: Free thyroxine index. Am J Vet Res 34:1449, 1973.
50. Fox, LE and Nachreiner RF: The pharmacokinetics of T₃ and T₄ in the dog. Proceed 62nd Conference of Research Workers in Animal Disease, 1981, p 13.
51. Quinlan, WJ and Michaelson, S: Homologous radioimmunoassay for canine thyrotropin: Response of normal and x-irradiated dogs to propylthiouracil. Endocrinology 108:937, 1981.
52. Lothrop, CD, et al.: Canine and feline thyroid function assessment with the thyrotropin-releasing hormone response test. Am J Vet Res 45:2310, 1984.
53. Evinger, JV, et al.: Thyrotropin-releasing hormone stimulation testing in healthy dogs. Am J Vet Res 46:132, 1985.
54. Kaufman, J, et al.: Serum concentrations of thyroxine, 3,5,3′-triiodothyronine, thyrotropin, and prolactin in dogs before and after thyrotropin-releasing hormone administration. Am J Vet Res 46:486, 1985.
55. Li, WI, et al.: Effects of thyrotropin-releasing hormone on serum concentrations of thyroxine and triiodothyronine in healthy, thyroidectomized, thyroxine-treated, and propylthiouracil treated dogs. Am J Vet Res 47:163, 1986.

56. Hinkle, PM, et al.: Mechanism of thyroid hormone inhibition of thyrotropin-releasing hormone action. Endocrinology 108:199, 1981.

57. Fish LH, et al.: Replacement dose, metabolism, and bioavailability of levothyroxine in the treatment of hypothyroidism: Role of triiodothyronine in pituitary feedback in humans. N Engl J Med 316:764, 1987.

58. Reichlin, S: Neuroendocrine control of thyrotropin secretion. In Ingbar, SH and Braverman, LE (eds): The Thyroid, 5th ed. Philadelphia, JB Lippincott, 1986, p 241.

59. Parker, DC, et al.: Effect of normal and reversed sleep cycles upon nycterohemeral rhythmicity of plasma thyrotropin: Evidence suggestive of an inhibitory influence in sleep. J Clin Endocrinol Metabol 43:318, 1976.

60. Kemppainen, RJ and Sartin, JL: Evidence for episodic but not circadian activity in plasma concentrations of adrenocorticotropin, cortisol, and thyroxine in dogs. J Endocrinol 103:219, 1984.

61. Utiger, RD: Decreased extrathyroidal triiodothyronine production in nonthyroidal illness: Benefit or harm? Am J Med 69:807, 1980.

62. Gardner, DF, et al.: Effect of triiodothyronine replacement on the metabolic and pituitary responses to starvation. N Engl J Med 300:579, 1979.

63. Faber, J, et al.: Pituitary-thyroid axis in critical illness. J Clin Endocrinol Metabol 65:315, 1987.

64. Heinen, E, et al.: Secondary hypothyroidism in severe nonthyroidal illness? Horm Metabol Res 13:284, 1981.

65. Slag, MF, et al.: Hypothyroxinemia in critically ill patients as a predictor of high mortality. JAMA 245:43, 1981.

66. Kaptein, EM, et al.: Relationship of altered thyroid hormone indices to survival in nonthyroidal illnesses. Clin Endocrinol 16:565, 1982.

67. Brent, GA and Hershman, JM: Thyroxine therapy in patients with severe nonthyroidal illnesses and low serum thyroxine concentration. J Clin Endocrinol Metabol 63:1, 1986.

68. de Bruijne, JJ, et al.: Fat mobilization and plasma hormone levels in fasted dogs. Metabolism 30:190, 1981.

69. Laurberg, P and Boye, N: Propylthiouracil, ipodate, dexamethasone, and periods of fasting induce different variations in serum rT$_3$ in dogs. Metabolism 33:323, 1984.

70. Peterson, ME, et al.: Effects of spontaneous hyperadrenocorticism on serum thyroid hormone concentrations in the dog. Am J Vet Res 45:2034, 1984.

71. Gosselin, SJ, et al.: Biochemical and immunological investigation on hypothyroidism in dogs. Can J Comp Med 44:158, 1980.

72. Larrson, M: Diagnostic methods in canine hypothyroidism and influence of non-thyroidal illness on thyroid hormones and thyroxine-binding proteins. PhD thesis, Uppsala, Sweden, 1987.

73. Lothrop, CD and Nolan, HL: Pituitary-thyroid function in canine Cushing's syndrome. Proc Third Annu Vet Med Forum. ACVIM 1985, p 147.

74. Alexander, CM, et al.: Pattern of recovery of thyroid hormone indices associated with treatment of diabetes mellitus. J Clin Endocrinol Metabol 54:362, 1982.

75. Hargis, AM, et al.: Relationship of hypothyroidism to diabetes mellitus, renal amyloidosis, and thrombosis in pure-bred beagles. Am J Vet Res 45:1077, 1981.

76. Haines, DM, et al.: Survey of thyroglobulin autoantibodies in dogs. Am J Vet Res 45:1493, 1983.

77. Wenzel, KW: Pharmacological interference with in vitro tests of thyroid function. Metabolism 30:717, 1981.

78. Woltz, HH, et al.: Effect of prednisone on thyroid gland: Morphology and plasma thyroxine and triiodothyronine concentrations in the dog. Am J Vet Res 44:2000, 1983.

79. Kemppainen, RJ, et al.: Effects of prednisone on thyroid and gonadal endocrine function in dogs. J Endocrinol 96:293, 1983.

80. Wilber, JF and Utiger, RD: The effect of glucocorticoids on thyrotropin secretion. J Clin Invest 48:2096, 1969.

81. Belshaw, BE and Rijnberk, A: Radioimmunoassay of plasma T$_4$ and T$_3$ in the diagnosis of primary hypothyroidism in dogs. JAAHA 15:17, 1979.

82. Afifi, A and Kraft, W: Influence of dexamethasone, triamcinolone-acetonide and estradiol benzoate on thyroid function in the dog. Zbl Vet Med [A] 24:856, 1977.

83. Monty, DE, et al.: Thyroid studies in pregnant and newborn beagles using [125]I. Am J Vet Res 40:1249, 1979.

84. Book, SA: Age related changes in serum thyroxine and ^{125}I-triiodothyronine resin sponge uptake in the young dog. Lab Anim Sci 27:646, 1977.

85. Dudan, FE, et al.: Circulating serum thyroxine (T$_4$), triiodothyronine (T$_3$), and reverse tri-iodothyronine (rT$_3$) in neonatal term and preterm foals. Proc Fifth Annu Vet Med Forum. ACVIM 1987, p 881.

86. Weller, RE, et al.: Basal serum thyroxine concentration in euthyroid, hypothyroid, and aged dogs. Proc 12th Sci Mtg. ACVIM 1984, p 31.

87. Murkin, JM: Anesthesia and hypothyroidism: A review of thyroxine physiology, pharmacology, and anaesthetic implications. Anesth Analg 61:371, 1982.

88. Peterson, ME: Considerations and complications in anesthesia with pathophysiologic changes in the endocrine system. In Short, CE (ed): Principles and Practice of Veterinary Anesthesia. Baltimore, Williams and Wilkins, 1987, p 251.

89. Sterling, K: Thyroid hormone action at the cellular level. In Ingbar, SH and Braverman, LE (eds.): The Thyroid, 5th ed. Philadelphia, JB Lippincott, 1986, p 219.

90. Gosselin, SJ, et al.: Histologic and ultrastructural evaluation of thyroid lesions associated with hypothyroidism in dogs. Vet Pathol 18:299, 1981.

91. Lucke, VM, et al.: Thyroid pathology in canine hypothyroidism. J Comp Pathol 93:415, 1983.

92. Spaulding, SW and Utiger, RD: The thyroid: Physiology, hyperthyroidism, hypothyroidism, and the painful thyroid. In Felig, P, et al. (eds): Endocrinology and Metabolism. New York, McGraw Hill, 1981, p 281.

93. Brouwers, J: Goitre et hérédité chez le chien. Ann Med Vet 94:173, 1950.

94. Schwalder, VP: Zwergwuchs beim Hund. Kleintier-Praxis 23:3, 1978.

95. Greco, DS, et al.: Juvenile-onset hypothyroidism in a dog. JAVMA 187:948, 1985.

96. Medleau, L, et al.: Congenital hypothyroidism in a dog. JAAHA 21:341, 1985.

97. Feldman, EC and Nelson, RW: Hypothyroidism. In Canine and Feline Endocrinology and Reproduction. Philadelphia, WB Saunders, 1987, p 55.

98. Chastain, CB, et al.: Secondary hypothyroidism in a dog. Canine Pract 6(5):59, 1979.

99. Eigenmann, JE: Diagnosis and treatment of dwarfism in the German shepherd dog. JAAHA 17:798, 1981.

100. Eigenmann, JE: Growth hormone-deficient disorders associated with alopecia in the dog. In Kirk, RW (ed): Current Veterinary Therapy IX. Philadelphia, WB Saunders, 1986, p 1015.

101. Milne, KL and Haynes, HM: Epidemiologic features of canine hypothyroidism. Cornell Vet 71:3, 1981.

102. Kaelin, S, et al.: Hypothyroidism in the dog: A retrospective study of sixteen cases. J Sm Anim Pract 27:533, 1986.

103. Goldberg, RC and Chaikoff, IL: Myxedema in the radiothyroidectomized dog. Endocrinology 50:115, 1952.

104. Nijhuis, AH, et al.: ECG changes in dogs with hypothyroidism. Tijdschr Diergeneeskd 103:736, 1978.

105. Santos, AD, et al.: Echocardiographic characterization of the reversible cardiomyopathy of hypothyroidism. Am J Med 68:675, 1980.

106. Taylor, RR, et al.: Influence of the thyroid state on left ventricular tension-velocity relations in the intact, sedated dog. J Clin Invest 48:775, 1969.

107. Skelton, CL and Sonnenblick, EH: The cardiovascular system. In Ingbar, SH and Braverman, LE (eds): The Thyroid, 5th ed. Philadelphia, JB Lippincott, 1986, p 1140.

108. Miller, CW, et al.: Echocardiographic assessment of cardiac function in beagles with experimentally produced hypothyroidism. J Ultrasound Med (Suppl) 3:157, 1984.

109. Calvert, CA, et al.: Congestive cardiomyopathy in Doberman pinscher dogs. JAVMA 181:598, 1982.

110. Harvey, HJ: Laryngeal paralysis in hypothyroid dogs. In Kirk, RW (ed): Current Veterinary Therapy VIII. Philadelphia, WB Saunders, 1983, p 694.

111. Patterson, JS, et al.: Neurologic manifestations of cerebrovascular atherosclerosis associated with primary hypothyroidism in a dog. JAVMA 186:499, 1985.

112. Braund, KG, et al.: Hypothyroid myopathy in two dogs. Vet Pathol 18:589, 1981.

113. Wastrous, B: Esophageal disease. *In* Ettinger, SE (ed): Textbook of Veterinary Internal Medicine, 2nd ed. Philadelphia, WB Saunders, 1983, p 1191.

114. Johnston, SD: Diagnostic and therapeutic approach to infertility in the bitch. JAVMA 176:1335, 1980.

115. Chastain, CB and Schmidt, B: Galactorrhea associated with hypothyroidism in intact bitches. JAAHA 16:851, 1980.

116. Kowalewski, K and Kolodej, A: Myoelectrical and mechanical activity of stomach and intestine in hypothyroid dogs. Am J Digest Dis 22:235, 1977.

117. Crispin, SM and Barnett, KC: Arcus lipoides corneae secondary to hypothyroidism in the Alsatian. J Sm Anim Pract 19:127, 1978.

118. Kern, TJ and Riis, RC: Ocular manifestations of secondary hyperlipidemia associated with hypothyroidism and uveitis in a dog. JAAHA 16:907, 1980.

119. Dodds, WJ: Canine von Willebrand's disease. Veterinary Reference Laboratory Newsletter 7(4), 1983.

120. Romatowski, J: Intercurrent hypothyroidism, autoimmune anemia, and a coagulation deficiency (von Willebrand's disease) in a dog. JAVMA 185:309, 1984.

121. Egeberg, O: Influence of thyroid function on the blood clotting system. Scand J Clin Lab Invest 15:1, 1963.

122. Edson, JR, et al.: Low platelet adhesiveness and other hemostatic abnormalities in hypothyroidism. Ann Intern Med 82:342, 1975.

123. Dalton, RG, et al.: Hypothyroidism as a cause of acquired von Willebrand's disease. Lancet 1:1007, 1987.

124. Rogers, JS, et al.: Factor VIII activity and thyroid function. Ann Intern Med 97:713, 1982.

125. Rogers, RS and Shane, SR: Factor VIII activity in normal volunteers receiving oral thyroid hormone. J Lab Clin Med 102:444, 1983.

126. Chastain, CB, et al.: Myxedema coma in two dogs. Canine Pract 9(4):20, 1982.

127. Kelly, MJ and Hill, JR: Canine myxedema coma and stupor. Comp Cont Ed Pract Vet 6:1049, 1984.

128. Cline, MJ and Berlin, NI: Erythropoiesis and red cell survival in the hypothyroid dog. Am J Physiol 204:415, 1963.

129. Hollander, CS, et al.: Repair of the anemia and hyperlipidemia of the hypothyroid dog. Endocrinology 81:1007, 1967.

130. Rogers, WA, et al.: Lipids and lipoproteins in normal dogs and dogs with secondary hyperlipoproteinemia. JAVMA 166:1092, 1975.

131. Zerbe, CA: Canine hyperlipidemias. *In* Kirk, RW (ed): Current Veterinary Therapy IX. Philadelphia, WB Saunders, 1986, p 1045.

132. Karlsberg, RP and Roberts, R: Effect of altered thyroid function on plasma creatine kinase clearance in the dog. Am J Physiol 235:E614, 1978.

133. Reimers, TJ: Radioimmunoassays and diagnostic tests for thyroid and adrenal disorders. Comp Cont Ed Pract Vet 4(1):65, 1982.

134. Reimers, TJ, et al.: Effects of storage, hemolysis, and freezing and thawing on concentrations of thyroxine, cortisol, and insulin in blood samples. Proc Soc Exp Biol Med 170:509, 1982.

135. Young, DW, et al.: Abnormal canine triiodothyronine-binding factor characterized as a possible triiodothyronine autoantibody. Am J Vet Res 46:1346, 1985.

136. Larsen, PR: Thyroid hormone concentrations. *In* Ingbar, SH and Braverman, LE (eds): The Thyroid, 5th ed. Philadelphia, JB Lippincott, 1986, p 479.

137. Lum, SMC, et al.: Peripheral tissue mechanism for maintenance of serum triiodothyronine values in a thyroxine-deficient state in man. J Clin Invest 73:570, 1984.

138. Ferguson, DC: Thyroid function tests in the dog: Recent concepts. Vet Clin North Am 14:783, 1984.

139. Bruyette, DS, et al.: Effect of thyrotropin storage on thyroid-stimulating hormone response testing in normal dogs. J Vet Intern Med 1:91, 1987.

140. Reimers, TJ, et al.: Changes in serum thyroxine and cortisol in dogs after simultaneous injection of TSH and ACTH. JAAHA 18:923, 1982.

141. Wheeler, SL, et al.: Serum concentrations of thyroxine and 3,5,3'-triiodothyronine before and after intravenous or intramuscular thyrotropin administration in dogs. Am J Vet Res 46:2605, 1985.

142. Elkins, RP: Principles of measuring free thyroid hormone concentrations in serum. Nucl Compact 16:305, 1985.

143. Kaptein, EM, et al.: Free thyroxine estimates in nonthyroidal illness: Comparison of eight methods. J Clin Endocrinol Metab 52:1073, 1981.

144. Elkins, RP, et al.: Euthyroid sick syndrome and free thyroxine assay. Lancet 2:402,1983.

145. Larsen, PR, et al.: Letter to the Editor: Revised nomenclature for tests of thyroid hormones and thyroid-related proteins in serum. J Clin Endocrinol Metabol 64:1089, 1987.

146. Kallfelz, FA: The triiodothyronine-131I resin sponge uptake test as an indicator of thyroid function in dogs. JAVMA 152:1647, 1968.

147. Premachandra, BN and Walfish, PG: Effects and clinical significance of exogenous thyroxine therapy in patients with circulating thyroid hormone autoantibodies. Am J Clin Pathol 78:63, 1982.

148. Beck-Peccoz, P, et al.: Evaluation of free thyroxine methods in the presence of iodothyronine-binding autoantibodies. J Clin Endocrinol Metabol 58:736, 1984.

149. Sakata, S, et al.: Autoantibodies against thyroid hormones or iodothyronine. Ann Intern Med 103:579, 1985.

150. Chastain, CB: Human thyroid stimulating hormone radioimmunoassay in the dog. JAAHA 14:368, 1978.

151. Larsson, M: Evaluation of a human TSH radioimmunoassay as a diagnostic test for canine primary hypothyroidism. Acta Vet Scand 22:589, 1981.

152. Cavalieri, RR: Isotopic tests: Quantitative in vivo tests. *In* Ingbar, SH and Braverman, LE (eds): The Thyroid, 5th ed. Philadelphia, JB Lippincott, 1986, p 445.

153. Stanbury, JB: Inherited metabolic disorders of the thyroid system. *In* Ingbar, SH and Braverman, LE (eds): The Thyroid, 5th ed. Philadelphia, JB Lippincott, 1986, p 687.

154. Hulter, HN, et al.: Thyroid replacement in thyroparathyroidectomized dogs. Miner Electrolyte Metab 10:228, 1984.

155. Brennan, MD: Thyroid hormones. Mayo Clin Proc 55:33, 1980.

156. Rosychuk, RAW: Thyroid hormones and antithyroid drugs. Vet Clin North Am 12:111, 1982.

157. Ferguson, DC: Thyroid hormone replacement therapy. *In* Kirk, RW (ed): Current Veterinary Therapy IX. Philadelphia, WB Saunders, 1986, p 1018.

158. Utiger, RD: Thyrotropin. Assay and secretory physiology. *In* Ingbar, SH and Braverman, LE (eds): The Thyroid, 5th ed. Philadelphia, JB Lippincott, 1986, p 304.

159. Sawin, CT, et al.: Oral thyroxine: Variation in biological action and tablet content. Ann Intern Med 100:641, 1984.

160. Chastain, CB: Canine hypothyroidism. JAVMA 181:349, 1982.

161. Panciera, DL, et al.: Tests of the pituitary-thyroid axis in euthyroid dogs treated with L-thyroxine. Proc Fourth Annu Vet Med Forum. ACVIM 1987:880.

162. Refetoff, S: Thyroid hormone resistance syndromes. *In* Ingbar, SH and Braverman, LE (eds): The Thyroid, 5th ed. Philadelphia, JB Lippincott, 1986, p 1292.

163. Clark, ST and Meier, H: A clinicopathological study of thyroid disease in the dog and cat. Zbl Vet Med (A)5:17, 1958.

164. Lucke, VM: A histologic study of thyroid abnormalities in the domestic cat. J Sm Anim Prac 5:351, 1964.

165. Arnold, U, et al.: Goitrous hypothyroidism and dwarfism in a kitten. JAAHA 20:753, 1984.

166. Peterson, ME: Feline hyperthyroidism. Vet Clin North Am 14:809, 1984.

167. Peterson, ME and Turrel, JM: Feline hyperthyroidism. *In* Kirk, RW (ed): Current Veterinary Therapy IX. Philadelphia, WB Saunders, 1986, p 1026.

168. Peterson, ME, et al.: Methimazole treatment of 262 cats with hyperthyroidism. J Vet Intern Med 2:150, 1988.

169. Thoday, KL: Differential diagnosis of symmetric alopecia in the cat. *In* Kirk, RW (ed): Current Veterinary Therapy IX. Philadelphia, WB Saunders, 1986, p 545.

170. Hoenig, M and Ferguson, DC: Assessment of thyroid functional reserve in the cat by the thyrotropin-stimulation test. Am J Vet Res 44:1229,1983.

171. Kemppainen, RJ, et al.: Endocrine responses of normal cats to TSH and synthetic ACTH administration. JAAHA 20:737, 1984.

172. Holzworth, J, et al.: Hyperthyroidism in the cat: Ten cases. JAVMA 176:345, 1981.

173. Hoenig, M, et al.: Toxic nodular goiter in the cat. J Sm Anim Pract 23:1, 1982.

174. Peter, HJ, et al.: Autonomy of growth and of iodine metabolism in hyperthyroid feline goiters transplanted onto nude mice. J Clin Invest 80:491, 1987.

175. Peterson, ME, et al.: Feline hyperthyroidism: Pretreatment clinical and laboratory evaluation of 131 cases. JAVMA 183:103, 1983.

176. Peterson, ME and Becker, DV: Radionuclide thyroid imaging in 135 cats with hyperthyroidism. Vet Radiol 25:23, 1984.

177. Feldman, EC and Nelson, RW: Hyperthyroidism and thyroid tumors. In Feldman, EC and Nelson, RW (ed): Canine and Feline Endocrinology and Reproduction. Philadelphia, WB Saunders, 1987, p 91.

178. Turrel, JM, et al.: Thyroid carcinoma causing hyperthyroidism in cats: 14 cases (1981-1986): JAVMA 193:359, 1988.

179. Peterson, ME, et al.: Lack of thyroid stimulating immunoglobulins in cats with hyperthyroidism. Vet Immunol Immunopathol 16:277, 1987.

180. Brown, RS, et al.: Increased serum thyroid growth immunoglobulins in feline hyperthyroidism. Proc 69th Annu Meeting Endocrine Society, 1987:115.

181. Peter, HJ, et al.: Pathogenesis of heterogeneity in human multinodular goiter: A study on growth and function of thyroid tissue transplanted onto nude mice. J Clin Invest 76:1992, 1985.

182. Valente, WA, et al.: Antibodies that promote thyroid growth: A distinct population of thyroid-stimulating autoantibodies. N Engl J Med 309:1028, 1983.

183. Wiley, ZD, et al.: The effect of hyperthyroidism on gastric emptying rates and pancreatic exocrine and biliary secretion in man. Digest Dis 23: 1003, 1978.

184. Vaamonde, CA and Michael, UF: The kidney in thyroid dysfunction. In Suki, WN and Eknoyan, G (eds.): The Kidney in Systemic Disease, 2nd ed. New York, John Wiley and Sons, 1981, p 361.

185. Radcliffe, CE: Observations on the relationship of the thyroid to the polyuria of experimental diabetes insipidus. Endocrinology 32:415, 1943.

186. Jacobs, G, et al.: Congestive heart failure associated with hyperthyroidism in cats. JAVMA 188:52, 1986.

187. Peterson, ME, et al.: Electrocardiographic findings in 45 cats with hyperthyroidism. JAVMA 180:934, 1982.

188. Bond, BR, et al.: Echocardiographic findings in 103 cats with hyperthyroidism. JAVMA (in press).

189. Liu, SK, et al.: Hypertrophic cardiomyopathy and hyperthyroidism in the cat. JAVMA 185:52, 1984.

190. Skelton, CL and Soonblick, EH: Heterogeneity of contractile function in cardiac hypertrophy. Circ Res [Suppl II] 1974(34 & 35):83.

191. Bond, BR: Hyperthyroid heart disease in cats. In Kirk, RW (ed): Current Veterinary Therapy IX. Philadelphia, WB Saunders, 1986, p 399.

192. Peterson, ME, et al.: Serum thyroid hormone concentrations fluctuate in cats with hyperthyroidism. J Vet Intern Med 1:142,1987.

193. Beck, KA, et al.: The normal feline thyroid: Technetium pertechnetate imaging and determination of thyroid to salivary gland ratios in 10 normal cats. Vet Radiol 26:35, 1985.

194. Peterson, ME: Propylthiouracil treatment of feline hyperthyroidism. JAVMA 179:485, 1981.

195. Peterson, ME, et al.: Propylthiouracil-associated hemolytic anemia, thrombocytopenia, and antinuclear antibodies in cats with hyperthyroidism. JAVMA 184:806, 1984.

196. Aucoin, DP, et al.: Propylthiouracil-induced immune-mediated disease in cats. J Pharmacol Exp Ther 234:13, 1985.

197. Jansson, R, et al.: Intrathyroidal concentrations of methimazole in patients with Graves' disease. J Clin Endocrinol Metabol 57:129, 1983.

198. Peterson, ME, et al.: Anesthetic and surgical management of endocrine disorders. Vet Clin North Am 14:911, 1984.

199. Black, AP and Peterson, ME: Thyroid biopsy and thyroidectomy. In Bojrab, MJ (ed): Current Techniques in Small Animal Surgery. Philadelphia, Lea and Febiger, 1983, p 388.

200. Birchard, SJ, et al.: Surgical treatment of feline hyperthyroidism: Results of 85 cases. JAAHA 20:705, 1984.

201. Peterson, ME and Randolph, JR: Endocrine disorders. In Sherding, RG (ed): Diseases of the Cat: Diagnosis and Management. Philadelphia, Lea and Febiger (in press).

202. Peterson, ME: Treatment of canine and feline hypoparathyroidism. JAVMA 181:1434, 1982.

203. Peterson, ME: Hypoparathyroidism. In Kirk, RW (ed): Current Veterinary Therapy IX. Philadelphia, WB Saunders, 1986, p 1039.

204. Becker, DV and Peterson, ME: Radioactive iodine treatment of feline hyperthyroidism. Proc First Annu Vet Med Forum. ACVIM 1983, p 40.

205. Turrel, JM, et al.: Radioactive iodine therapy in cats with hyperthyroidism. JAVMA 184:554, 1984.

206. Meric, S, et al.: Serum thyroxine concentrations after radioactive iodine therapy in cats with hyperthyroidism. JAVMA 188:1038, 1986.

207. Loar, AS: Canine thyroid tumors. In Kirk, RW (ed): Current Veterinary Therapy IX. Philadelphia, WB Saunders, 1986, p 1033.

208. Brodey, RS and Kelly, DF: Thyroid neoplasms in the dog: A clinicopathological study of 57 cases. Cancer 22:406, 1968.

209. Hayes, HM, Jr and Fraumeni, JF, Jr: Canine thyroid neoplasms: Epidemiologic features. J Natl Cancer Inst 55(4):931, 1975.

210. Mitchell, M, et al.: Canine thyroid carcinomas: Clinical occurrence, staging by means of scintiscans, and therapy in 15 cases. Vet Surg 8:112, 1979.

211. Birchard, SJ and Roessel, OF: Neoplasia of the thyroid gland in the dog: A retrospective study of 16 cases. JAAHA 17:369, 1981.

212. Leav, I, et al.: Adenomas and carcinomas of the canine and feline thyroid. Am J Pathol 83:61, 1976.

213. Sterns, EE and Doris, P: Thyroid lymphography of the dog. Cancer 21:468, 1968.

214. Zarrin, K: Naturally occurring parafollicular cell carcinoma of the thyroid in dogs: A histological and ultrastructural study. Vet Pathol 14:556, 1977.

215. Patnaik, AK, et al.: Canine medullary carcinoma of the thyroid. Vet Pathol 15:590, 1978.

216. Harari, J, et al.: Clinical and pathologic features of thyroid tumors in 26 dogs. JAVMA 188:1160, 1986.

217. Weller, RE, et al.: Thyroid carcinoma in two dogs. Mod Vet Prac 67: 116, 1986.

218. Rijnberk, A and Leav, I: Thyroid tumors. In Kirk, RW (ed): Current Veterinary Therapy VI. Philadelphia, WB Saunders, 1977, p 1020.

219. Gilmore, DR: Neoplasia of the cervical spinal cord and vertebrae in the dog. JAAHA 19:1009, 1983.

220. Reid, CF, et al.: Functional adenocarcinoma of the thyroid gland in a dog with mitral insufficiency. J Am Vet Rad Soc 4:36, 1963.

221. Rijnberk, A and van der Horst, CJG: Investigations on iodine metabolism of normal and goitrous dogs. Zbl Vet Med [A]16:495, 1969.

222. Chastain, CB, et al.: Excess triiodothyronine production by a thyroid carcinoma in a dog. JAVMA 177:172, 1980.

223. Ackerman, LJ, et al.: Thyroid adenocarcinoma in a dog. Mod Vet Prac 65:303, 1984.

224. Long, GG, et al.: Metastatic canine medullary carcinoma. Vet Pathol 17:323, 1980.

225. Peterson, ME, et al.: Multiple endocrine neoplasia in a dog. JAVMA 180:1476, 1982.

226. Thompson, EJ, et al.: Fine-needle aspiration cytology in the diagnosis of canine thyroid carcinoma. Can Vet J 21:186, 1980.

227. Blahd, WH: Treatment of malignant thyroid disease. Semin Nucl Med 9:95, 1979.

228. Jeglum, KA and Whereat, A: Chemotherapy of canine thyroid carcinoma. Comp Cont Ed Pract Vet 5:96, 1983.

229. Susaneck, SJ: Doxorubicin therapy in the dog. JAVMA 182:70, 1983.

230. Kim, JH and Leeper, RD: Treatment of anaplastic giant cell and spindle cell carcinoma of the thyroid with combination adriamycin and radiation therapy: A new approach. Cancer 52:954, 1983.

231. Rijnberk, A: Hyperthyroidism in the dog and its treatment with radioactive iodide. Tijdschr Diergenesk 91:789, 1966.

232. Peterson, ME, et al.: Use of radioactive iodine for treatment of hyperthyroidism resulting from thyroid carcinoma in a dog. J Vet Intern Med (in press).

DRUG INDEX

Generic	Trade	Dosage	Route	Frequency	Description
L-Thyroxine	(Synthroid, Soloxine, Levothroid, Noroxine, Thyro-Tab)	0.01–0.02 mg/lb 0.02–0.04 mg/kg	Orally	q24h or divided q12h	Thyroid repl. (dog or cat)
Methimazole	(Tapazole)	5 mg (initial) 5–20 mg (maint.)	Orally Orally	q8h–q12h q24h or divided	Antithyroid drug
Propranolol	(Inderal)	2.5–5.0 mg	Orally	q8h	β-blocker (preop. prep. of hyperthyroidism)
		0.1 mg	IV	As needed	Intraop. treatment hyperthyroid-induced arrhythmias
Potassium Iodine (Lugol's)		50 mg	Orally	q12h–q24h	Preop prep. of hyperthyroidism
Doxorubicin	(Adriamycin)	30 mg/m^2	IV	Every 3 weeks for 5 treatments	Chemotherapeutic drugs for canine thyroid carcinoma
Cyclophosphamide	(Cytoxan)	50 mg/m^2	Orally	Every 3 weeks for 4 days following doxorubicin injection	

96 DISORDERS OF THE ENDOCRINE PANCREAS

RICHARD W. NELSON

The endocrine pancreas is composed of the islets of Langerhans, which are surrounded by the exocrine secreting acinar cells of the pancreas. Four cell types have been identified in the pancreatic islets on the basis of staining properties and morphology: α cells, which secrete glucagon; β cells, which secrete insulin; Δ cells, which secrete somatostatin; and F cells, which secrete pancreatic polypeptide.[1, 2] Other cell types (e.g., C and E cells) have been identified but their function is unknown.

Dysfunction involving any of these cell lines ultimately results in either an excess or a deficiency of the respective hormone in the circulation. In dogs and cats the primary disorders associated with the endocrine pancreas involve a deficiency of insulin (i.e., diabetes mellitus), an excess of insulin (i.e., insulin-secreting islet cell tumor), or an excess of gastrin (i.e., gastrinoma). The cell of origin of the pancreatic gastrinoma is believed to be the Δ cell, which normally secretes gastrin during fetal development and somatostatin during adult life.[3, 4] Gastrinomas are discussed elsewhere in this text. Dysfunction involving other cell lines (e.g., glucagonoma, somatostatinoma) have been well documented in humans but have not yet been described in dogs and cats.[5]

DIABETES MELLITUS

Etiology and Pathogenesis

On the basis of fasting plasma glucose and insulin concentrations, plus β cell secretory responses to glucose tolerance testing, dogs and cats with diabetes mellitus can be categorized into insulin-dependent (IDDM) and non-insulin-dependent (NIDDM) types, similar to what is described in humans.[6–8] Of these, the most common clinically recognized form appears to be IDDM, which is characterized by hypoinsulinemia, impaired insulin secretion after a glucose challenge, a necessity for insulin injections, and a tendency to develop ketoacidosis (Fig-

ure 96–1).[9, 10] The etiology has been poorly characterized in dogs and cats but is undoubtedly multifactorial. Genetic predispositions have been suggested by familial associations in dogs and by pedigree analysis of keeshonden.[11–13] β cell absence in inherited diabetes mellitus of keeshonden and in four dogs with canine juvenile diabetes mellitus, reported by Atkins and colleagues,[14] suggests that in some dogs an extreme form of inheritance occurs, represented by lack of development of β cells. Less severe, genetic-based changes in β cells may predispose an animal to the development of diabetes mellitus after exposure to environmental factors, such as viral infections, toxic chemicals, and chronic stressful situations, or prolonged exposure to insulin antagonists. The necessity for some predisposing factor in the development of diabetes mellitus gains credence in reviewing the findings of a recent epidemiologic study. A number of common dog breeds, including cocker spaniels, German shepherds, collies, Pekingese, and Boxers, appear

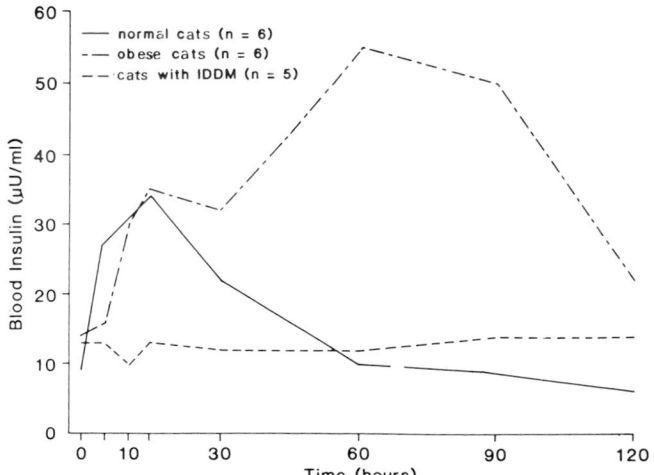

FIGURE 96–1. Mean blood insulin concentrations following the intravenous injection of 0.5 g glucose/Kg body weight in normal cats (———), extremely obese cats (– – –), and cats with insulin dependent diabetes mellitus (–·–·–). The insulin secretory pattern in the obese cats is similar to humans with noninsulin dependent diabetes mellitus.

to be at relatively low risk. This indicates a possible genetic resistance of these breeds to diabetes or precursor illnesses. Pulik, Cairn terriers, and miniature pinschers are breeds at higher risk than explained by breed popularity, which reflects a definite probability of genetic predisposition.[15]

Immune-mediated destruction of the islets is considered an important factor in the development of IDDM in humans. Anti-islet cell antibodies of the IgG class are present in more than 50 per cent of humans with IDDM at the time of initial diagnosis.[16] Similar anti-islet cell antibodies have been found in some dogs with IDDM.[17] Although the humoral immune system plays a role, the cell-mediated immune system is believed to be the major determinant of β cell destruction.[18]

The development of IDDM has been conceptually divided into six stages, beginning with genetic susceptibility.[19] Stage 2 involves a triggering event that leads to β cell autoimmunity. Environmental factors that trigger the development of β cell immunity are poorly defined but probably include drugs and infectious agents. Stage 3 is the period of active autoimmunity, but normal insulin secretion is maintained. During stage 4, immunologic abnormalities persist, but glucose-stimulated insulin secretion is progressively lost, despite the maintenance of euglycemia. Overt diabetes develops in stage 5, although some residual insulin secretion remains. Stage 6 is characterized by complete β cell destruction.

Clinically, pancreatitis is often seen in dogs with diabetes mellitus and has been suggested as a cause of diabetes after destruction of the islets. A 40 per cent to 70 per cent incidence of preexisting or concurrent inflammation of the pancreas has been reported.[20, 21] In contrast, histologic changes consistent with pancreatitis were absent in a majority of diabetic dogs evaluated in another study.[22] Although destruction of β cells secondary to pancreatitis is an obvious explanation for the development of hypoinsulinemic diabetes mellitus, other, perhaps more complex factors are involved in the development of diabetes mellitus in dogs without obvious pancreatic lesions.

A strong association exists between insular amyloid deposits and diabetes mellitus in the cat. Insular amyloid deposits occur in about 45 per cent of nondiabetic cats five years of age and older, and in 65 per cent of adult diabetic cats.[23, 24] Diabetic cats have significantly greater numbers of pancreatic islets with amyloid deposits and more extensive deposition of amyloid within islets than nondiabetic cats, suggesting that diabetes mellitus and insular amyloid are causally related. It has been hypothesized that insular amyloid may be a product of some alteration in the biosynthesis or degradation of insulin.[25, 26] Disease or environmental stress factors may produce elevated blood glucose levels in cats, which, in turn, may promote the secretion of quantitatively or qualitatively altered insulin. These altered insulin products may be assembled into amyloid fibrils and accumulate in the islets. In essence, the presence of amyloid in pancreatic islets would represent a morphologic marker of a primary β cell abnormality.

Clinical recognition of NIDDM is less common than IDDM. A juvenile form of canine diabetes mellitus that closely resembles human maturity-onset diabetes of the young, a subclassification of NIDDM, has been described.[14, 27] Insulin kinetics for juvenile canine NIDDM is usually characterized by normal to increased basal insulin concentrations and a sluggish initial insulin response to intravenous (IV) glucose tolerance tests, with an exaggerated response in the second hour of testing, resulting in a normal total insulin secretion.[28] Unfortunately clinical characteristics of juvenile canine NIDDM resemble IDDM, in that insulin therapy is usually required to manage hyperglycemia and these dogs are prone to ketosis and other complications frequently associated with IDDM.[27]

Insulin secretory patterns comparable to those described in juvenile canine NIDDM have been observed in obese dogs and cats after a glucose challenge (Figure 96–1).[29, 30] Obesity is an important predisposing factor in the development of NIDDM in humans. Obesity results in peripheral insulin antagonism and initial hyperinsulinemia. The causes of insulin antagonism in obesity are heterogeneous. The plasma insulin concentration appears to inversely regulate the concentration of cellular insulin receptors. The hyperinsulinism induced by overeating results in decreased insulin receptor sites on peripheral cells and may interfere with insulin binding to these sites.[31, 32] With progressively worsening hyperinsulinemia, a postreceptor defect also develops that involves the activity of the plasma membrane glucose transport carrier.[33, 34] These defects appear to be reversible once the hyperinsulinism is corrected.

The influence of obesity on insulin kinetics may play a role in the transient nature of diabetes in some cats. Most cats with apparent transient diabetes are obese animals that may have NIDDM. Because β cells still have the ability to secrete insulin in NIDDM, albeit the secretion is abnormal, cats with NIDDM could exist for prolonged periods of time in the unstressed home environment in a compensated state without clinical signs. If insulin action is impaired as a result of such factors as concurrent illness, administration of certain pharmaceuticals, and severe stress, blood glucose concentrations could increase above the renal tubular threshold for glucose, resulting in clinical signs of diabetes mellitus. At the time of presentation to the veterinarian, overt diabetes mellitus, frequently requiring insulin therapy, is correctly diagnosed. However, these cats often are not difficult to manage on a day-to-day basis. With resolution of the insulin antagonist state (e.g., stress, illness), these cats may spontaneously recover from their insulin dependence and revert to a mild form of NIDDM that no longer requires insulin therapy. Unfortunately identifying this reversion from insulin-requiring to non-insulin-requiring NIDDM may be difficult and insulin injections may be continued, predisposing the cat to hypoglycemia.

Measurement of basal blood insulin concentrations during periods of hyperglycemia may allow differentiation between IDDM and NIDDM in both dogs and cats. Normal basal plasma insulin concentrations in the dog and cat range from 5 to 20 μU/ml, although this range may vary, depending on the laboratory in which the insulin concentration is evaluated. Dogs and cats with hypoinsulinemic diabetes mellitus that require life-long insulin therapy have basal insulin concentrations within or frequently below the normal range, which, for our radioimmunoassay, is less than 5 μU/ml.[6, 29] Insulin concentrations below normal are inappropriately low when hyperglycemia is present, and imply severe β cell failure with an inability to secrete insulin. Insulin concentrations that are normal in the presence of hyperglycemia, especially severe hyperglycemia, implies β cell degeneration or loss of beta cell function, and may be consistent with either IDDM or NIDDM. This may also be an end stage development from a persistent peripheral insulin antagonistic state (e.g., hyperadrenocorticism), or a primary disorder of the β cells.

Hyperglycemic dogs and cats with functioning β cells have high normal or increased plasma insulin concentrations, often exceeding 50 μU/ml.[6, 29] Hyperinsulinemia implies the existence of a functioning pool of β cells that are secreting large quantities of insulin in an attempt to correct the hyperglycemic state. These conditions suggest the existence of insulin antagonism and are not an absolute indication of NIDDM. Hormonally induced diabetes mellitus can resemble NIDDM. Increased plasma concentrations of any of the diabetogenic hormones (i.e., glucocorticoids, epinephrine, glucagon, or growth hormone) owing to excessive secretion, impaired degradation, or exogenous administration will result in insulin antagonism in peripheral tissues and/or enhanced hepatic gluconeogenesis and glycogenolysis, hyperinsulinemia, and impaired glucose tolerance.[35–37] Progesterone may result in insulin antagonism owing to stimulation of growth hormone secretion.[38]

In dogs and cats with hyperinsulinemia, the presence of clinical signs depends on the degree of insulin antagonism and the compensatory insulin response by the β cells. If insulin antagonism can be identified and the cause corrected while the β cells are still functioning, permanent diabetes mellitus requiring insulin therapy may not develop. Therefore, the identification of hyperinsulinemia in the diabetic dog or cat is an indication to pursue potential causes of insulin antagonism before arbitrarily diagnosing NIDDM and attempting therapy with diet and oral hypoglycemic agents.

Pathophysiology

Nonketotic Diabetes Mellitus. A relative or absolute deficiency in insulin results in decreased utilization of glucose, amino acids, and fatty acids by peripheral tissues, including the liver, muscle, and fat cells. Glucose obtained from the diet or from hepatic gluconeogenesis, which occurs at a modest rate with hypoinsulinemia, accumulates in the circulation, causing hyperglycemia. As the plasma glucose concentration increases, the ability of the renal tubular cells to resorb glucose from the glomerular ultrafiltrate is exceeded, resulting in glycosuria. This occurs when the plasma glucose concentration exceeds 180 to 220 mg/dl in the dog. Diabetic cats subjectively appear to have a renal threshold for glucose of approximately 200 mg/dl, whereas the reported mean threshold for normal cats is 290 mg/dl.[39] Glycosuria creates an osmotic diuresis, causing polyuria. Compensatory polydipsia prevents dehydration. Glycosuria also represents a caloric loss and, in conjunction with dimin-

ished peripheral tissue metabolism of ingested glucose, results in weight loss.

The satiety center in the ventromedial region of the hypothalamus is responsible for controlling the amount of food ingested. The amount of plasma glucose entering the cells in this region of the brain directly affects the feeling of hunger; the more glucose that enters these cells, the less the feeling of hunger and the more the satiety center is inhibited. The ability of glucose to enter these cells is under the influence of insulin. In diabetes mellitus with a relative or absolute lack of insulin, glucose does not enter these cells, the satiety center is not inhibited, and the individual becomes polyphagic despite the presence of hyperglycemia.[40] Therefore, the four classic signs of diabetes mellitus are polyuria, polydipsia, polyphagia, and weight loss. As these signs become obvious to the owner, the pet is brought to the veterinarian for care.

Ketoacidosis. Unfortunately, some cats and dogs are not identified by their owners as having signs of disease, and these untreated diabetics may ultimately develop diabetic ketoacidosis (DKA). Four major alterations are believed to be responsible for the increase in ketogenesis and gluconeogenesis: an insulin deficiency, diabetogenic hormone excess, fasting, and dehydration.[41] Virtually all dogs and cats with DKA have a relative or absolute insulin deficiency. Some dogs and cats have plasma insulin concentrations similar to those observed in normal, fasted nondiabetics (i.e., 5 to 20 μU/ml). However, this insulin concentration is inappropriately low for the severity of hyperglycemia encountered. Diabetic ketoacidosis may also develop in dogs and cats that receive inappropriately low insulin dosages. Impaired insulin action and/or insulin resistance also plays a major contributory role in the development of ketosis.[42]

Insulin deficiency is essential in initiating lipolysis. The nonesterified fatty acids released from adipose tissue are used extrahepatically as oxidative fuels and are also assimilated by the liver at a rate dependent on their plasma concentration. With insulin present, fatty acids are incorporated into triglycerides in the liver. With insulin deficiency, these fatty acids are converted into the coenzyme A (CoA)-derivative acyl-CoA, which is oxidized to acetyl-CoA.[43] In severe diabetes acetyl-CoA is diverted almost entirely to the formation of acetoacetyl-CoA, and hence to acetoacetic acid. Acetoacetic acid is further metabolized to β-hydroxybutyric acid. Acetone is formed by spontaneous decarboxylation of acetoacetate (Figure 96–2). These ketone bodies—acetoacetic acid, β-hydroxybutyric acid, and acetone—cause the ketosis and acidosis of ketoacidosis.

In a short-term situation the conversion of free fatty acids to ketone bodies is a safety measure. Diabetes mellitus is interpreted physiologically as a state of starvation. With glucose deficiency, ketone bodies can be utilized as an energy source by many tissues. The rate of ketogenesis is linked to the rate of gluconeogenesis and lipolysis; the more rapid the latter factors, the more rapidly ketone production proceeds.[44] Linking of the two processes may explain why ketogenesis is more active in uncontrolled diabetes than in starvation, since gluconeogenesis proceeds at an accelerated rate in a state of insulin deficiency. Insulin deficiency also impairs

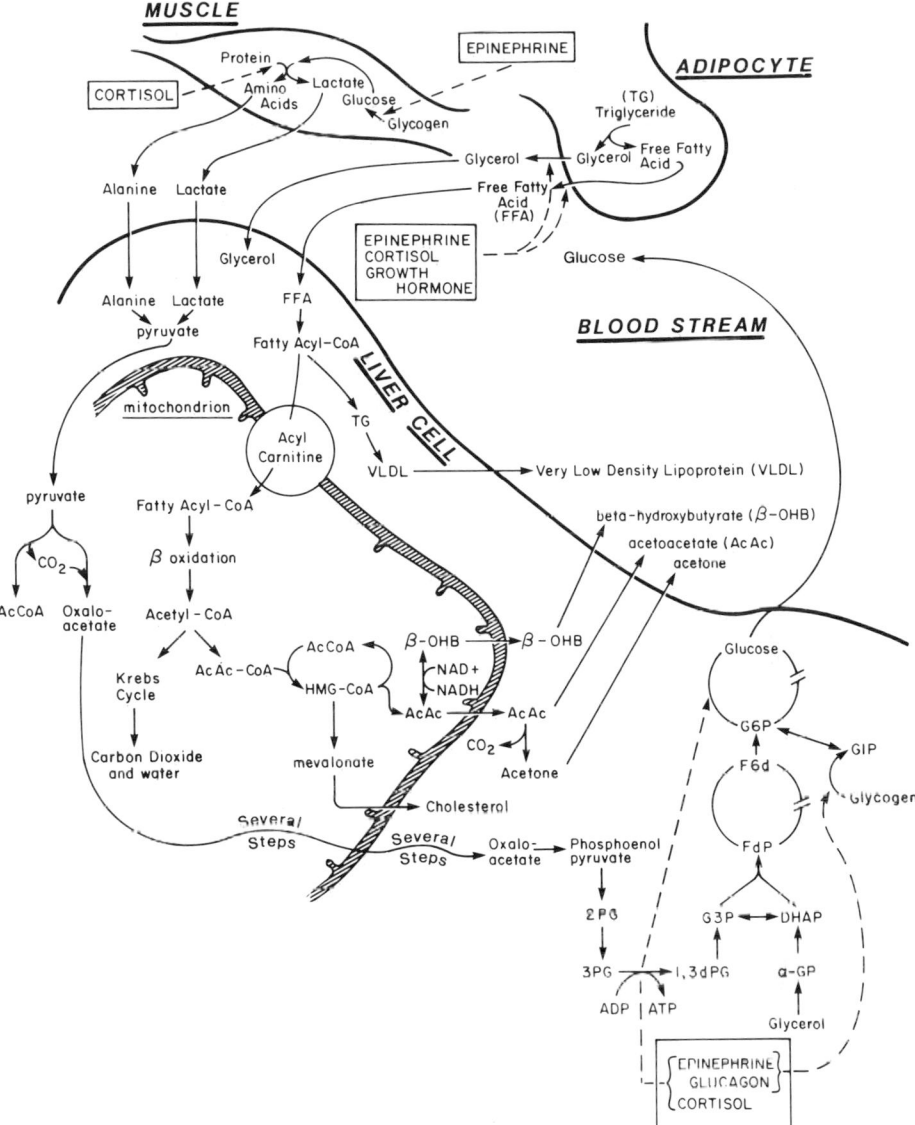

FIGURE 96–2. In response to a wide variety of stress situations, the body increases its production of the gluco-regulatory hormones—insulin, glucagon, epinephrine, cortisol, and growth hormone. In diabetes, the lack of insulin allows the gluconeogenic effects of the stress hormones to be unopposed in liver, muscle, and adipose tissue. This results in excess ketone formation, fat and muscle breakdown, and a classic catabolic state. (From Feldman, EC and Nelson, RW: Canine and Feline Endocrinology and Reproduction. Philadelphia, WB Saunders, 1987, p 276).

the utilization of ketones by peripheral tissues.[45] This, in conjunction with their increased production, results in accumulation of ketones in the blood. Excessive serum ketones can overwhelm the body's buffering system, causing an increase in arterial hydrogen ion concentration and a decrease in serum bicarbonate. As ketones accumulate in the extracellular space, they eventually surpass the renal tubular threshold of complete reabsorption and spill into the urine, contributing to the osmotic diuresis. In the short term the production of ketones can be life-preserving, but in the long term the severe metabolic consequences of uninhibited excessive ketone production, which include severe acidosis, osmotic diuresis, dehydration, vomiting, and obtundation, can be terminal.

The development of DKA in the diabetic patient appears to involve more than a relative or absolute deficiency in insulin. Evidence to negate insulin deficiency as the sole factor in the development of DKA includes: (1) normal plasma insulin concentrations in most human ketoacidotic patients initially seen at the hospital, (2) delayed onset of DKA after insulin withdrawal from diabetic patients, and (3) lack of hypolipolytic and hypoketonemic effects after insulin administration without prior stimulation of adipocytes and hepatocytes by diabetogenic hormones.[46–48]

Evidence that diabetogenic hormones (glucagon, catecholamines, cortisol, and growth hormone [GH]) contribute to the metabolic alterations of DKA materialized when measurement of these hormones in plasma became feasible, after 1960. Their concentrations were increased in every case of DKA in which these hormones were measured (Figure 96–3).[46] The only exception to this generalization was the concentration of plasma GH. It is now suggested that the diabetogenic effects of GH may be expressed at a time when the plasma concentration has returned to normal.[49]

Additional evidence that diabetogenic hormones play a role in the pathogenesis of DKA includes: (1) pharmacologic blockade of each of these hormones (e.g., somatostatin injections to suppress glucagon) reduces the rate and/or frequency of metabolic decompensa-

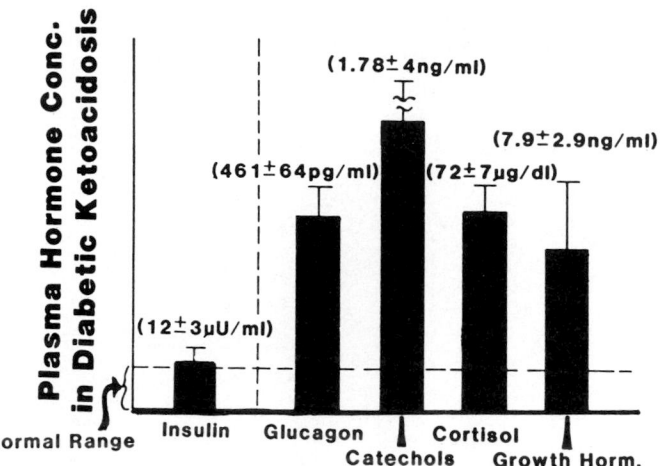

FIGURE 96–3. Plasma insulin and counterregulatory hormone concentrations in DKA (mean ± SEM). (From Schade, DS, et al.: Diabetic ketoacidosis: Pathogenesis, prevention, and therapy, diabetic coma. Albuquerque, The University of New Mexico Press, 1981, p 84).

tion,[50, 51] (2) removal of the pituitary and/or the adrenal glands prevents the development of DKA after insulin withdrawal in diabetic animals, and (3) administration of each of these hormones under appropriate conditions induces metabolic decompensation in diabetics despite "normal" circulating concentrations of plasma insulin.[46]

The body increases its production of the diabetogenic hormones in response to a wide variety of stress situations (physical or mental). This response is usually positive. In the stress of DKA, however, the activity of these hormones as insulin antagonists usually worsens the developing hyperglycemia and ketonemia, provoking acidosis, fluid depletion, and hypotension. These factors act as further stresses in a self-perpetuating spiral of metabolic decompensation (Figure 96–4). It is rare for the dog or cat with DKA not to have some coexisting disorder, such as pancreatitis, infection, gastroenteritis, or congestive heart failure. These disorders have the potential for increasing diabetogenic hormone secretion. The recognition and treatment of disorders that coexist with DKA represent good general patient care and specific management of the DKA as well (Figure 96–5).

It is common for hyperketonemia and associated problems to induce a state of nausea that results in diminished food intake and enhanced mobilization of endogenous lipid stores for fuel. This may be helpful in some situations but can be catastrophic in the diabetic pet, since the metabolic conversion from carbohydrate to fat metabolism augments ketone body production. Thus the inappetence that accompanies hyperketonemia accentuates ketone body production and worsens anorexia.

In diabetic pets, fasting, intentional or owing to illness, may also induce DKA by increasing plasma diabetogenic hormone concentrations. The owners of diabetic pets are often mistakenly taught to withhold insulin injections if the animal does not eat. This combination of hormone fluxes augments gluconeogenesis and ketogenesis. The omission of insulin plus excess plasma stress hormones results in a progressive domino effect in the development of DKA (Figure 96–4).

Nonhormonal factors may also contribute to the en-

hanced ketogenesis. Fasting may cause a decline in available alanine, pyruvate, and lactate. These substrates are important inhibitors of ketogenesis in the perfused rat liver.[52] Fasting also results in decreased peripheral utilization of ketone bodies.[53] This can be reversed only with insulin therapy. Thus the augmented hepatic ketogenesis, in conjunction with the decreased utilization of ketone bodies, results in the potential for development of severe hyperketonemia and metabolic acidosis in fasting diabetics.

The increasing serum concentrations of both glucose and ketones in the diabetic patient eventually result in their spillage into the urine, creating an osmotic diuresis. Daily urinary losses of glucose add a solute load of about 6 mOsm and each gram of ketone, about 20 mOsm.[42] In addition, the anionic nature of ketones, even at maximally acid urine pH, obligates the excretion of positively charged ions, such as sodium and potassium. The total urinary osmolar load from glucose and ketones alone can amount to two to four times normal daily urinary osmolar losses. The accompanying loss of fluid and salt is a major contributor to the development of dehydration. Severe dehydration results from a lack of fluid intake because of the nausea, abdominal pain, confusion, or obtundation associated with hyperosmolarity, hyperglycemia, and DKA. Vomiting, diarrhea, and hyperventilation are later contributing factors. Loss of fluids and the resultant dehydration cause contraction of the intravascular fluid space, leading to prerenal azotemia and a decline in the glomerular filtration rate. Hyperglycemic patients with reduced glomerular filtration rates lose the ability to excrete glucose and, to a lesser degree, hydrogen ions. Glucose and ketones then accumulate in the vascular space at a more rapid rate. The result is increasing hyperglycemia and ketonemia, predisposing the diabetic patient to worsening DKA (Figure 96–4).

Hyperosmolar Nonketotic Diabetes Mellitus. The hyperglycemia and associated osmotic diuresis and prerenal uremia that occur in some diabetic dogs, and probably cats, have the potential to cause severe hyperosmolarity of the extracellular fluid and the development of the hyperosmolar nonketotic syndrome (DHNS). This syndrome is characterized by: (1) severe hyperglycemia (blood glucose concentration > 600 mg/dl), (2) hyperosmolarity (> 350 mOsm/kg), (3) severe clinical dehydration, (4) lack of urine or serum ketone bodies, (5) lack of or moderate metabolic acidosis, and (6) some central nervous system (CNS) depression, at least to the point of lethargy.[54–56] As with DKA, a precipitating condition such as renal insufficiency, pneumonia, or other severe stress is associated with DHNS. Certain drugs, such as anticonvulsants, glucocorticoids, and thiazide diuretics, may also precipitate or contribute to the progression of this syndrome.

The pathogenesis of DHNS is poorly understood but is believed to involve impaired CNS function or interference with fluid intake induced by increasing osmolality, azotemia, and nausea. As the extracellular space becomes contracted, tissue perfusion diminishes, resulting in a decreased glomerular filtration rate that, in turn, causes or aggravates the azotemia. It also causes worsening hyperglycemia due to glucose retention. An

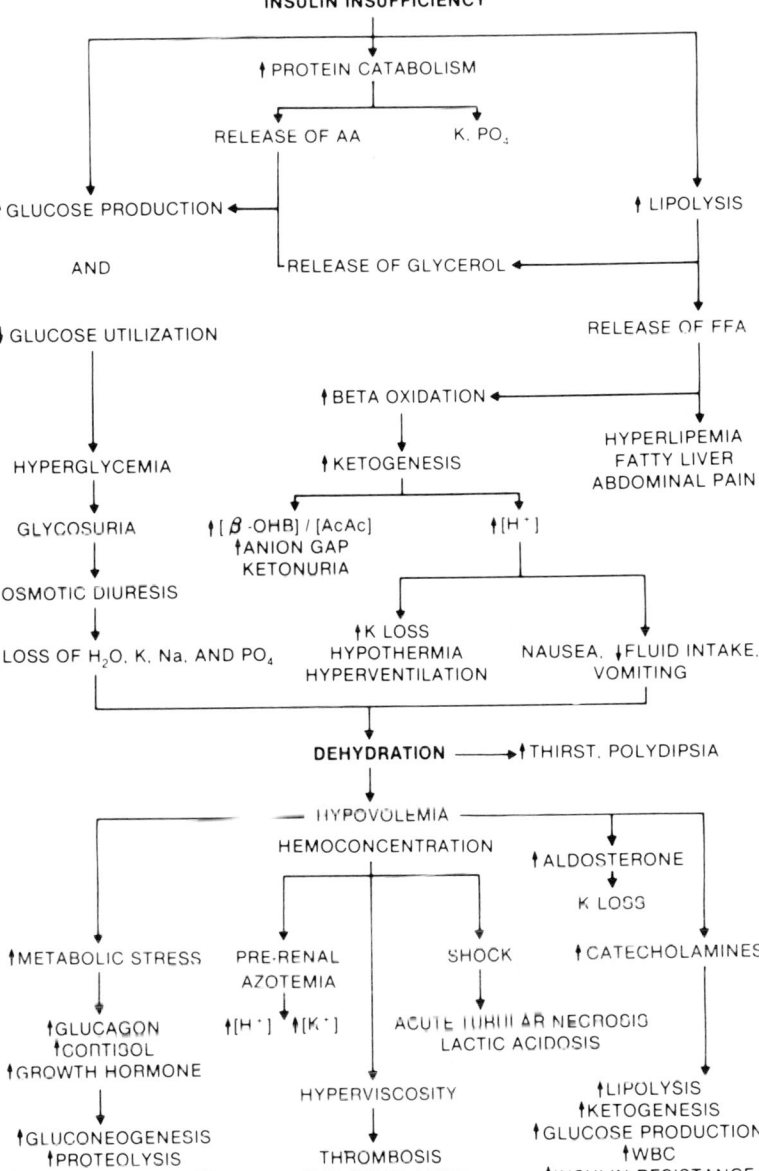

FIGURE 96–4. The interrelationship of the pathophysiologic mechanisms that result in DKA. AA = amino acids, FFA = free fatty acids, K = potassium, AcAc = acetoacetic acid, B-OHB = β-hydroxybutyric acid. (From Feldman, EC and Nelson, RW: Canine and Feline Endocrinology and Reproduction. Philadelphia, WB Saunders, 1987, p 275).

uric or oliguric renal failure interferes with and limits renal glucose excretion. This, in turn, contributes markedly to the rise in serum glucose concentration and osmolality. Hyperosmolality causes mental confusion, further contributing to reduced or absent fluid intake and thus adding to the overall complexity of the problem.

The absence of ketosis is not well understood. In humans with NIDDM, endogenous insulin secretion is present and should be antiketogenic. Furthermore, the stimulus for lipolysis is reduced in these patients because of low plasma concentrations of GH, cortisol, and glucagon, as compared with that in ketoacidotic patients. The plasma free fatty acid levels are lower in DHNS than in DKA.[57] In contrast with the short time course of developing ketoacidosis, DHNS may be gradual and prolonged.[50]

Some dogs and cats with DHNS are acidotic but have

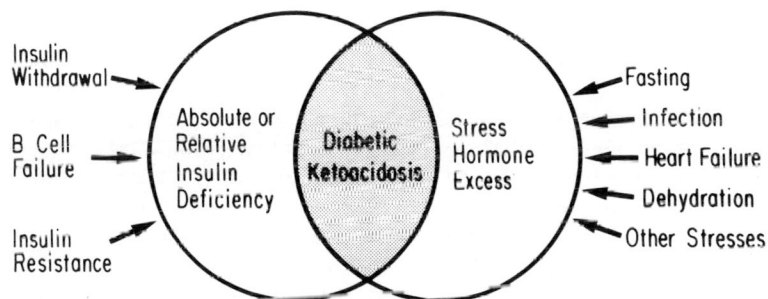

FIGURE 96–5. The hormonal pathogenesis of DKA, illustrating the interaction of insulin deficiency and stress hormone excess necessary in the development of the ketoacidotic state. (From Feldman, EC and Nelson, RW: Canine and Feline Endocrinology and Reproduction. Philadelphia, WB Saunders, 1987, p 280).

low or undetectable concentrations of ketoacids in the plasma or urine. One reason for this disparity in expected versus real results is that β-hydroxybutyrate is not recognized by the commonly used urine and plasma reagent strips or tablets. Unrecognized DKA appears to be an uncommon entity in dogs and cats. Another cause for acidosis in nonketotic diabetics is lactic acidosis. Lactic acid is the end product of anaerobic metabolism of glucose. The principal sources of this acid are erythrocytes (which lack the enzymes for aerobic oxidation), skeletal muscle, skin, and brain. Removal of lactic acid is by way of hepatic and, to some degree, renal uptake with conversion first to pyruvate and eventually back to glucose, a process that requires oxygen. Lactic acidosis occurs when excess lactic acid accumulates in the blood. This can be the result of overproduction (tissue hypoxia), deficient removal (hepatic failure), or both (circulatory collapse). Dogs and cats with lactic acidosis are usually severely ill, with problems such as sepsis, hemorrhage, anemia, pulmonary disease, liver disease, and renal failure.

Signalment

The age and sex distributions of dogs with diabetes mellitus in several series reveal that most affected dogs are 4 to 14 years old, with a peak incidence at 7 to 9 years of age.[15] Females are affected about twice as frequently as males. Controversy exists regarding a sex predilection for juvenile-onset diabetes in puppies. A female predilection was reported whereas others found six of nine dogs with juvenile-onset diabetes mellitus to be male.[14, 27, 58]

Genetic predispositions to the development of diabetes have been suggested by familial associations in dogs and by pedigree analysis of keeshonden.[11-13] Pulik, Cairn terriers, and miniature pinschers are breeds at higher risk than explained by breed popularity, which reflects a definite probability of genetic predisposition.[15] Certainly, the author's experience with diabetic poodles, dachshunds, miniature schnauzers, and beagles allows their inclusion into a list of frequently affected breeds. A number of common dog breeds, including cocker spaniels, German shepherds, collies, Pekingese, and Boxers, appear to be at relatively low risk. This indicates a possible genetic resistance of these breeds to diabetes or precursor illnesses.

Diabetes mellitus may be diagnosed in cats of any age or breed. Most diabetic cats are six years of age or older, and the disease appears to be more common in males.

Anamnesis

The history in virtually all diabetics includes the classic alterations of polydipsia, polyuria, polyphagia, and weight loss. Owners will often bring a previously housebroken pet to the veterinarian because they notice the dog or cat urinating in the home. The other signs are established by further questioning the owner. A complete anamnesis is extremely important even in the so-called "obvious diabetic" because the clinician must be aware of any complicating or concurrent problem in the patient. Because these dogs and cats are usually older animals, all the potential disorders of any geriatric animal must be evaluated. The clinician also must ask, "Why has the patient shown symptoms now?" In many instances these patients may be borderline or latent diabetics that develop overt diabetes secondary to drug therapy, pancreatitis, congestive heart failure, estrus, urinary tract infections, or a myriad of other potential causes.

Occasionally an owner will present a dog because of sudden blindness caused by cataract formation. The classic signs of diabetes mellitus may have gone unnoticed or been considered insignificant by the owner. Cataract formation is the most common complication in the diabetic dog but appears to be rare in the diabetic cat.

If the clinical signs associated with uncomplicated diabetes are not observed by the owner and cataracts do not develop, a diabetic dog or cat is at risk for developing systemic signs of illness as progressive ketonemia and metabolic acidosis develop. It is perhaps not surprising that the time sequence for initiation of severe decompensation is so unpredictable. We have seen diagnosed diabetic dogs and cats continue rather normal existences for 6 to 24 months without any therapy. Once ketoacidosis develops, however, the duration of severe illness before presentation to the veterinarian is usually one to seven days.

Physical Examination

The physical examination remains an extremely important tool in evaluating diabetics, despite the lack of pathognomonic abnormalities. A simple diagnosis of diabetes mellitus falls short of revealing the entire picture in any animal. The incidence of infection (especially urinary tract infections), pancreatitis, endocrine-appearing alopecia, pyoderma, congestive heart failure, prostatitis, testicular tumors, pyometra, and other disorders is so common that it is imperative that a thorough physical examination be performed on any suspected or known diabetic before treatment or hospital admission.

The findings on physical examination of the diabetic dog and cat will depend on the presence and severity of DKA. In the nonketotic diabetic there are no classic physical findings. Many diabetic dogs and cats are obese but are otherwise in good physical condition. Dogs and cats with prolonged untreated diabetes may have lost weight but are rarely thin. Secondary to mobilization of fats is the development of hepatic lipidosis and therefore hepatomegaly. Cataracts are another common clinical finding in canine diabetics. Diabetic cats may develop a plantigrade posture (i.e., the hocks touch the ground when the cat walks) (Figure 96–6). This posture, possibly caused by diabetic neuropathy, is not common, and such a gait and/or stance has also been observed in cats with chronic polyarthritis.

In the ketoacidotic diabetic dog or cat, physical findings include dehydration, depression, weakness, tachypnea, vomiting, and sometimes a strong odor of acetone

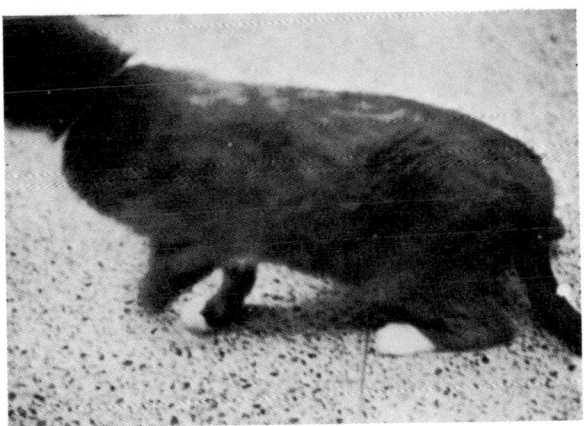

FIGURE 96–6. Plantigrade posture in a diabetic cat. (From Feldman, EC and Nelson, RW: Canine and Feline Endocrinology and Reproduction. Philadelphia, WB Saunders, 1987).

on the breath. With severe metabolic acidosis slow, deep breathing (i.e., Kussmaul respiration) may be observed. Gastrointestinal signs of vomiting, abdominal pain, and distention are common in DKA and must be differentiated from similar signs associated with pancreatitis, peritonitis, or other intra-abdominal disorders. The vomiting and abdominal pain that accompany DKA are usually acute in onset, beginning after the diabetes mellitus is well established. Conversely, a history of intermittent abdominal pain or vomiting occurring over a period of days or weeks before presentation should enhance suspicion of a separate abdominal problem, especially chronic pancreatitis. It is critical not to overlook a potentially treatable abdominal crisis.

The owners of pets that develop DIINS usually observe the classic signs of diabetes mellitus (i.e., polydipsia, polyuria, polyphagia, and weight loss). These signs precede the progressive weakness, anorexia, vomiting, and lethargy that the pet may develop. Physical examination will often reveal profound dehydration. These pets are typically lethargic, extremely depressed, or actually comatose. Hypothermia and slow capillary refill time are common.

Establishing a Diagnosis

Cardinal features of diabetes mellitus include persistent fasting hyperglycemia and glycosuria. In-hospital measurement of blood glucose and urine glycosuria with appropriate blood (Chemstrip bG) and urine (Keto-Diastix) reagent test strips allows rapid confirmation of diabetes mellitus in both dogs and cats. The concurrent documentation of ketonuria establishes diabetic DKA. In the ill dog or cat with hyperglycemia, glycosuria, and ketonuria, treatment should be initiated while confirmatory blood glucose and acid-base studies are performed. If ketonuria is not present, but DKA is suspected, the serum can be tested with Acetest tablets. The color reaction after a drop of either serum or plasma is placed on a crushed tablet determines whether ketones are present. If they are present, the concentrations of plasma ketones may not have reached the renal threshold that would result in ketonuria. The serum tablets

and urine reagent strips do not detect one of the most important ketoacids, β-hydroxybutyric acid. It is rare for DKA to develop without an excess of this anion.

A diagnostic dilemma arises when the plasma glucose concentration is between 120 and 200 mg/dl. Most of the blood panels from pets are randomly obtained. Therefore, a mild postprandial elevation in plasma glucose concentration is the most common explanation, especially if the diet consists of semimoist foods that are rich in sugar. Postprandial hyperglycemia is not common in normal dogs fed high-protein (canned food) and/or low-sugar (kibbled food) diets (Figure 96–7).[59] If postprandial hyperglycemia is present in a dog that is on a canned or kibbled diet, impaired insulin secretion or function should be suspected.

Mild hyperglycemia, with plasma glucose concentrations below the renal threshold, may be stress-induced or associated with excessive endogenous secretion or exogenous administration of the diabetogenic hormones, most commonly glucocorticoids and progestogens. Such hormones commonly cause mild hyperglycemia as a result of peripheral antagonism to the effects of insulin. Diabetes-induced polyuria and polydipsia do not develop until glycosuria and the resultant osmotic diuresis occur. In the normal dog this does not happen until the plasma glucose concentration exceeds 180 to 220 mg/dl, and in the cat, until a level of 200 to 300 mg/dl is achieved. Another diagnosis, especially disorders associated with insulin antagonism, should be sought in pets with polyuria, polydipsia, mild hyperglycemia (120–175 mg/dl), and no glycosuria. Insulin therapy is not indicated in these animals, since overt diabetes mellitus per se is not responsible for the clinical signs.

In cats the diagnosis of insulin-requiring diabetes mellitus is reserved for hyperglycemic, glycosuric cats that are observed by their owners to have at least three of the four major signs seen in this disturbance (i.e., polydipsia, polyuria, polyphagia, and weight loss). Hyperglycemic cats that are receiving megestrol acetate and those that are ketoacidotic are also assumed to have diabetes mellitus. A diagnosis of diabetes is questionable in all other hyperglycemic cats that do not have typical signs. A transient elevation in blood glucose concentration may not consistently result in measurable glycosuria. Hyperglycemia, reaching levels in the range of 300 to 400 mg/dl, may be seen in stressed cats. Unfortunately "stress" is a subjective term that cannot be measured, is not always easily recognized, and may evoke inconsistent responses among cats. Hyperglycemia in ill or frightened cats is usually stress-induced. Stress-induced hyperglycemia is thought to be the result of sudden secretion of epinephrine, causing both a release of glucose and a simultaneous inhibition of insulin action at the level of the cell membrane.[60] Epinephrine is a potent cause of hyperglycemia, making the diagnosis of feline diabetes mellitus anything but routine. The owner and veterinarian should be aware of the hyperglycemia, and extra care should be taken in observing the animal for onset of the classic signs. Admitting a hyperglycemic cat to the hospital overnight for adjustment to a frightening environment, followed by a repeated blood glucose determination the next day, will often separate stress-induced hyperglycemia from

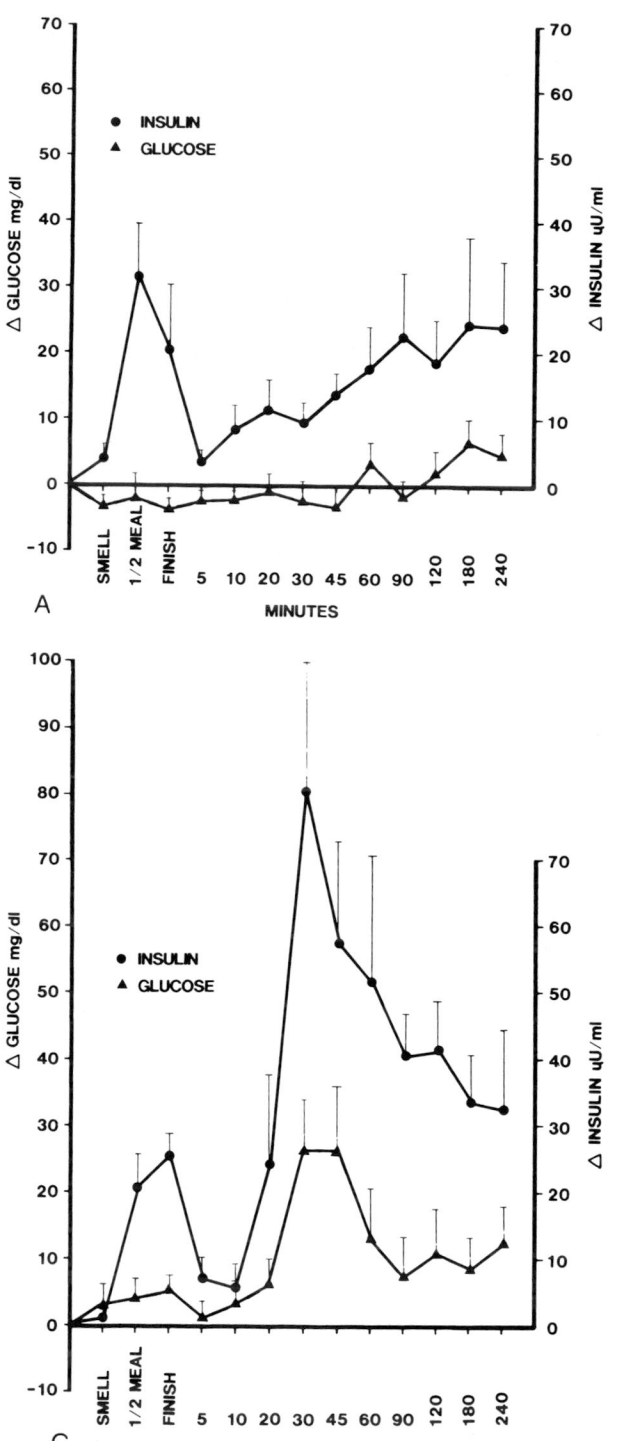

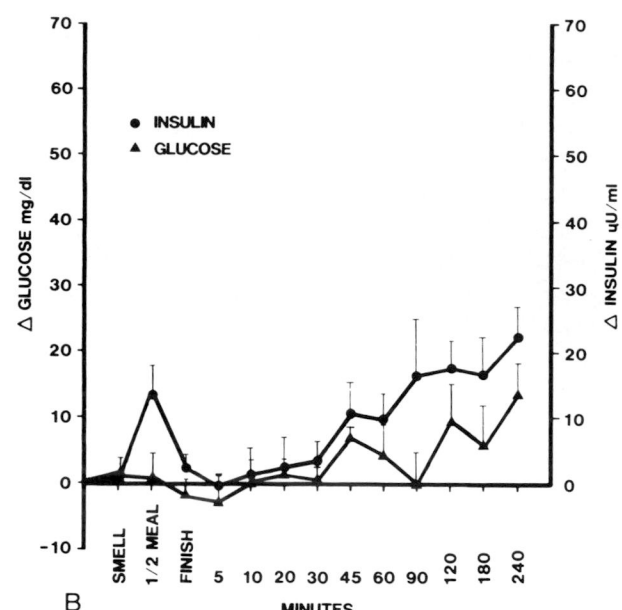

FIGURE 96–7. The effect of feeding on blood glucose and insulin concentrations in ten normal dogs. Each dog was given 30 Kcal of food/lb body weight. Bars represent SEM. *A*, Canned food. *B*, Dry kibble food. *C*, Semimoist food. (From Feldman, EC and Nelson, RW: Canine and Feline Endocrinology and Reproduction. Philadelphia, WB Saunders, 1987, p 236).

diabetic hyperglycemia. One could also recheck the urine for persistence of the glycosuria either in the hospital or at home. Another, more aggressive option would be to place an IV catheter into a jugular vein 12 to 24 hours before rechecking the blood in order to avoid the stress of venipuncture.

Primary renal glycosuria is a renal tubular defect that involves the reabsorption of glucose, resulting in persistent glycosuria with euglycemia.[61, 62] The syndrome has been reported in many breeds but appears to be most common in the basenji and Norwegian elkhound.

This syndrome may be mistaken for diabetes mellitus if only a urinalysis is evaluated. Therefore, a definitive diagnosis should not rely solely on the presence of glycosuria.

Patient Evaluation

Non-Ketotic Diabetic. A thorough laboratory evaluation is recommended for any suspected or known diabetic dog or cat. The clinician must be aware of any disease that might be causing or contributing to the carbohydrate intolerance, such as hyperadrenocorticism, infection, pancreatitis, congestive heart failure, or liver or kidney disease. Finally, the practitioner should be searching for abnormalities that are a result of the diabetic state, such as prerenal uremia and urinary tract infection.

The minimum laboratory evaluation in any healthy nonketotic diabetic should include a complete blood count, biochemical panel, serum lipase, and urinalysis with bacterial culture. Additional tests may be warranted after obtaining the anamnesis and performing the physical examination. Long-acting insulin therapy may be initiated while awaiting the laboratory results.

Ketoacidotic Diabetic. The laboratory evaluation of apparently healthy dogs and cats with both glucose and ketones present in the urinalysis is similar to the nonketotic diabetic. The healthy ketotic diabetic can usually be managed conservatively, without fluid therapy or intensive care. In contrast, ketoacidotic diabetic dogs and cats that present with lethargy, inappetence, vomiting, diarrhea, and dehydration are critical metabolic emergencies that require a much more aggressive therapeutic plan.

To aid in the formulation of a treatment protocol, a group of critically important studies must be performed. Without this evaluation, a clinician cannot adequately assess a patient's biochemical status, and therefore cannot be expected to have sufficient knowledge of the specific abnormalities that require correction. The minimum required tests include urinalysis, hematocrit, blood glucose, venous total carbon dioxide or arterial acid-base evaluation, blood urea nitrogen (BUN) or serum creatinine, serum electrolytes, and an electrocardiogram.

These studies are needed for the immediate assessment and intensive care of the patient. Knowing the results of the tests allows for proper choice of fluid therapy as well as for corrections that must be made with respect to electrolyte alterations, acidosis, and renal function. Other data, such as radiographs or further clinical pathologic studies, may be needed for the complete medical assessment of the animal. However, the "ketoacidosis profile" provides the information necessary to begin proper emergency therapy.

Clinical Pathologic Abnormalities

Hemogram. The hemogram is usually normal in the uncomplicated diabetic pet. A mild, apparent polycythemia may be present if the animal is dehydrated. An elevation of the white blood cell count may be caused by either an infectious process or a severe inflammation, especially if an underlying pancreatitis is present. The presence of toxic or degenerative neutrophils or a significant left shift toward immaturity of the cells would support the presence of an infectious process as the cause of the leukocytosis.

Biochemical Panel. Serum alanine aminotransferase and, in dogs, alkaline phosphatase concentrations are commonly increased. Ten to 20 per cent of diabetic cats also have elevated total bilirubin concentrations. The

bromsulphalein retention time may also be prolonged in some diabetic dogs. Abnormalities in the liver enzymes and liver function tests are primarily a result of hepatic lipidosis that accompanies the peripheral mobilization of fats common in most diabetics. Concurrent pancreatitis and obstruction of the biliary ducts may also be involved. Because liver function tests are frequently abnormal, the diagnosis of concurrent liver disease in the animal with diabetes mellitus is difficult, and the veterinarian should rely on histologic evaluation of a liver biopsy specimen.

The BUN and serum creatinine concentrations are usually normal in the uncomplicated diabetic. An elevation in these parameters may be due to either primary renal failure or prerenal uremia secondary to dehydration. Primary renal failure as a result of glomerulosclerosis, damage specifically related to hyperglycemia, is a well-recognized complication in humans. This has only rarely been reported in dogs and has tended to be a subclinical problem.[63-65] This complication is characterized by progressive azotemia with gradually worsening oliguria and the eventual development of anuric renal failure. Evaluation of urine specific gravity should help to differentiate primary renal failure from prerenal uremia.

Obvious lipemia is frequently encountered in many endocrinopathies of small animals, including the untreated diabetic (Table 96–1). In uncontrolled diabetes there is an increase in the plasma concentration of triglycerides, cholesterol, lipoproteins, chylomicrons, and free fatty acids. These factors contribute to the development of lipemic plasma. The rise in these constituents is mainly due to decreased movement of plasma triglycerides into fat depots. The enzyme lipoprotein lipase aids in the metabolism of very low density lipoproteins and chylomicrons. Without insulin, lipoprotein lipase fails to be activated, and lipemia is produced. With insulin therapy the triglyceride-rich low-density lipoproteins and chylomicrons are metabolized and triglyceride concentrations are reduced. Low-density lipoprotein, which is high in cholesterol, is a by-product of chylomicron metabolism. Therefore, the treated diabetic may be seen to have reduced serum triglyceride concentrations and elevated serum cholesterol concentrations.

Increased plasma cholesterol concentrations may play a role in the accelerated development of arteriosclerotic vascular disease, which is a major long-term complication of diabetes in humans. There is evidence that in severe diabetes, cholesterol synthesis is decreased. Part

TABLE 96–1. CLINICAL SYNDROMES ASSOCIATED WITH LIPEMIA IN THE DOG AND CAT

Postprandial
Hyperadrenocorticism
Hypothyroidism
Diabetes mellitus
Hepatopathy
Pancreatitis
Nephrotic syndrome
Protein-losing enteropathy
Starvation
Hyperchylomicronemia syndrome
Familial hypertriglyceridemia
Primary hypercholesterolemia

of the rise in plasma cholesterol is due to an increase in the cholesterol-containing very low-density and low-density lipoproteins secondary to an increase in circulating triglycerides. Another factor may be a decline in hepatic degradation of cholesterol.[40]

Alterations in serum electrolytes and acid-base parameters are common in pets with DKA and are discussed in the section dealing with therapy for the severe ketoacidotic diabetic.

Pancreatic Enzymes. Chronic and acute pancreatitis is associated with diabetes mellitus in both the dog and cat. Animals with concomitant pancreatitis should have hyperlipasemia and hyperamylasemia. Unfortunately lipase and amylase concentrations do not always correlate accurately with the presence or absence of pancreatitis. Chronic inflammation and renal failure are two of the nonpancreatic conditions that may increase serum pancreatic enzyme concentrations. In both prerenal azotemia and primary renal failure, hyperlipasemia or hyperamylasemia may develop as a result of reduced renal excretion or reduced renal degradation of these pancreatic enzymes without concomitant pancreatitis being present.[66, 67] We also have experience with dogs that have histologically confirmed pancreatitis and normal pancreatic enzyme concentrations. In animals with normal serum lipase and amylase concentrations, a suspicion of pancreatitis must rely on the presence of appropriate clinical signs, biochemical alterations other than hyperlipasemia and hyperamylasemia, and radiographic or ultrasound abnormalities consistent with pancreatitis. The concomitant presence of pancreatitis may necessitate the instigation of intensive fluid therapy and a controlled diet, which would otherwise not have been done.

Urinalysis. Abnormalities identified in the urinalysis that are consistent with diabetes mellitus include glycosuria, ketonuria, proteinuria, and bacteriuria with or without associated pyuria and hematuria. The patient with uncomplicated diabetes usually has glycosuria without ketonuria. However, a relatively healthy diabetic may also have trace to small amounts of ketones in the urine. If large amounts of ketones are present in the urine, especially in an animal with systemic signs of illness (e.g., lethargy, vomiting, diarrhea, or dehydration), a diagnosis of DKA should be made and the animal treated appropriately.

Proteinuria may be the result of urinary tract infection or glomerular damage secondary to disruption of the basement membrane.[68] Because of the high incidence of infection, the urine sediment should be carefully inspected for changes consistent with infection, including white blood cells, red blood cells, protein, and bacteria.[20] Whenever possible, urine obtained by antepubic cystocentesis using aseptic techniques should be submitted for bacterial culture and sensitivity testing, even if pyuria and hematuria are not present.

Therapy: III Diabetic Ketoacidotic

The goals in the treatment of the severely ill ketoacidotic diabetic pet are (a) to provide adequate amounts of insulin to normalize intermediary metabolism, (b) to

restore water and electrolyte losses, (c) to correct acidosis, (d) to identify precipitating factors, and (e) to provide a carbohydrate substrate when required by the insulin treatment. Proper therapy does not imply forcing as rapid a return to normal as possible. Because osmotic and biochemical problems can be created by overly aggressive therapy as well as by the disease process itself, rapid changes in various vital parameters can be as harmful as, or more harmful than, no change. If all abnormal parameters can be slowly returned toward normal (i.e., over a period of 36 to 48 hours), there is better likelihood of success in therapy.

Fluid Therapy

Replacement and maintenance of normal fluid balance are important to ensure adequate cardiac output, blood pressure, and blood flow to all tissues. Improvement of renal blood flow is especially critical. In addition to the general beneficial aspects of fluid therapy in any dehydrated patient, fluid therapy can lower the plasma glucose concentration in the patient with DKA, even in the absence of insulin administration (Figure 96–8).[69, 70] Fluids enhance glucose excretion by increasing glomerular filtration and urine flow, and they decrease secretion of the diabetogenic hormones that stimulate hyperglycemia. Concentrations of acetoacetate and β-hydroxybutyrate, in contrast to the glucose concentrations, do not fall when fluids are given without insulin.[71]

Fluid Composition and Rate. The type of fluids initially used will depend on the animal's electrolyte status, blood glucose concentration, and osmolality. With rare exceptions, all dogs and cats with DKA have significant deficits in total body sodium, regardless of the measured serum concentration. Excessive urinary sodium loss is

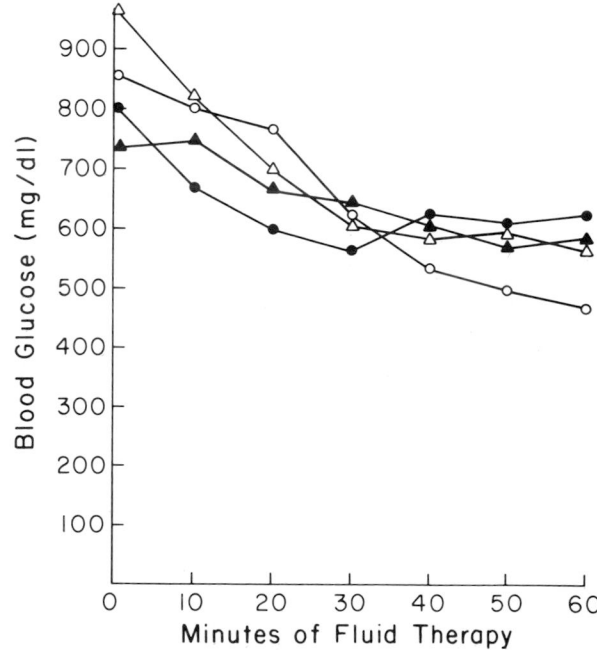

FIGURE 96–8. The effect of fluid therapy on four severely diabetic ketoacidotic dogs over a period of one hour, without insulin administration.

thought to result from the osmotic diuresis induced by glycosuria and ketonuria, and from the insulin deficiency per se. Insulin enhances renal sodium reabsorption in the distal portion of the nephron, and its absence results in sodium wasting. Hyperglucagonemia, vomiting, and diarrhea also contribute to the sodium loss in DKA.[71]

The dog or cat with severe DKA usually is sodium-depleted and, therefore, not suffering from dramatic hyperosmolality despite potentially remarkable elevations in both the plasma glucose concentration and the BUN. Direct measurements of serum osmolality are rarely performed in the clinical veterinary setting, but can be estimated from the following formula:

$$\frac{\text{Osmolality}}{\text{(mOsm/kg)}} = \frac{2\ (\text{Na} + \text{K})}{\text{(mEq/L)}} + \frac{0.05\ (\text{glucose})}{\text{(mg/dl)}} + \frac{0.33\ (\text{BUN})}{\text{(mg/dl)}}$$

The initial IV fluid of choice is 0.9 per cent sodium chloride, unless severe hyperosmolality (> 350 mOsm/kg) is present. In the mildly hypertonic patient (310 to 350 mOsm/kg), this solution (tonicity of 308 mOsm/L) will be hypotonic to the patient's plasma osmolality. If the dog or cat is not hypertonic, normal saline remains the IV fluid of choice. Only if the osmolality is greater than 350 mOsm/kg should hypotonic fluids (i.e., 0.45 per cent saline) be considered. Patients rarely die of hypertonicity, but they may die from the effects of volume contraction caused by infusion of too much free water (i.e., hypotonic fluids). In humans, contraction of the vascular space is associated with myocardial infarction, stroke, and irreversible shock.[42] Overzealous administration of water in the form of hypotonic fluids may also cause cerebral edema.

The initial volume and rate of fluid administration are determined by assessing the degree of shock, the dehydration deficit, and the patient's maintenance require-ments. The patient's size and the presence or absence of cardiac disease are also important factors. The typical dog or cat with DKA is 6 per cent to 12 per cent dehydrated. Fluid administration should be directed at gradually replacing all deficits over a period of 24 to 48 hours. Rapid replacement of fluids is rarely indicated except if the dog or cat is in shock. Once out of this critical phase, fluid replacement should be decreased in an effort to correct the fluid imbalance in a slow but steady manner. Once fluid deficits are corrected, a maintenance fluid rate (20 to 30 ml/lb/day or 40 to 60 ml/kg/day) should be initiated. Frequent reevaluation of fluid requirements should be completed and adjustments made as changes in urine output and the severity and frequency of vomiting and diarrhea are noted.

Potassium Supplementation. During the development of DKA the serum potassium concentration changes little because the renal losses are replenished from the intracellular compartment, primarily from muscle. The metabolic acidosis, lack of insulin, and serum hypertonicity combine to cause a shift of potassium into the serum from the cells (Figure 96–9). Because 98 per cent of the total body potassium is located in the intracellular compartment, large quantities of potassium are available for shifting into the vascular space. Most dogs with DKA initially have either normal or decreased serum potassium concentrations (Table 96–2). Individual patients may have low, normal, or elevated potassium concentrations, depending on the duration of illness, renal function, and previous nutrition. Knowing the serum potassium concentration is critical. Insulin and bicarbonate therapy will cause a shift of plasma potassium into the intracellular compartment. Dogs and cats with DKA and hypokalemia require aggressive potassium replacement therapy to replace deficits and

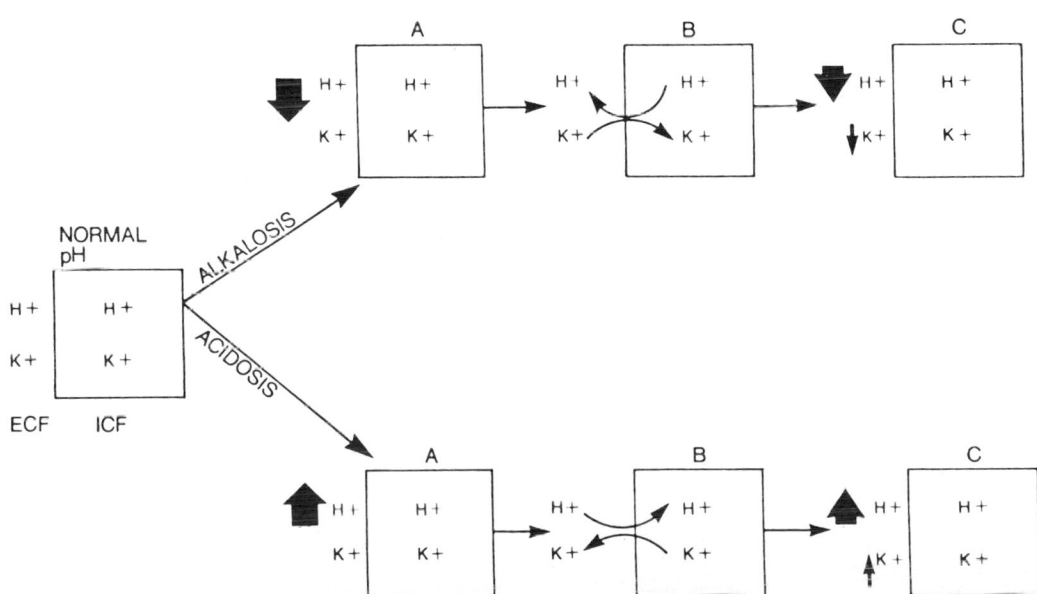

FIGURE 96–9. Redistribution of extracellular fluid (ECF) and intracellular fluid (ICF) potassium and hydrogen ions in response to changes in ECF pH. Alkalosis: A, H+ concentration decreases. B, H+ then moves out of cells and K+ moves into cells to maintain electrical neutrality. C, Hypokalemia develops. Acidosis: A, H+ concentration increases. B, H+ then moves into cells and K+ moves out of cells to maintain electrical neutrality. C, Hyperkalemia develops. The size of the arrow represents the amount of change from normal. (From Gabow, P: *In* Schrier, RW (ed): Renal and Electrolyte Disorders. Boston, Little, Brown and Company, 1976.)

TABLE 96–2. INITIAL CHEMISTRY VALUES IN 49 DOGS WITH SEVERE DKA

	Venous or Arterial Bicarbonate (mEq/L)	Blood Glucose (mg/dl)	Serum Sodium (mEq/L)	Serum Potassium (mEq/L)	Serum Chloride (mEq/L)	Blood Urea Nitrogen (mg/dl)	Osmolality (mOsm/kg)
Mean	5.8	535	130	3.6	85	87	310
Range	2–11	320–1075	116–145	1.7–5.1	54–112	41–213	272–426
Normal values	18–27	80–110	141–192	3.5–5.1	105–144	11–22	290–300

to prevent worsening hypokalemia after initiation of insulin therapy. Those dogs and cats with normal serum potassium concentrations also require immediate potassium replacement therapy in the IV infusion solution, but at initially lower doses (Table 96–3). Severe acidosis and/or renal failure can result in hyperkalemia. Potassium supplementation should initially be withheld in these dogs and cats until glomerular filtration is restored and the hyperkalemia is resolving.

Normal saline does not contain potassium, so supplementation of these fluids is required, especially with initially low or normal plasma potassium concentrations. During therapy for DKA the serum potassium concentration will fall in virtually all patients because of rehydration (dilution), correction of acidemia (shift of hydrogen out of cells in exchange for potassium), insulin-mediated cellular uptake of potassium, and continued urinary losses. Therefore, if an accurate measurement of plasma potassium is not available, it is recommended that 10 mEq of potassium initially be added to each 250 ml (40 mEq/L) of IV fluids.

Because abnormalities in serum potassium are common both before and during therapy, an electrocardiogram (ECG) is recommended as part of the initial evaluation of these animals. If an ECG and a serum potassium determination are obtained prior to therapy, the ECG becomes an important tool for monitoring potassium levels as therapy continues. Ideally, serum potassium levels should be monitored every two to four hours. However, laboratory facilities for these tests are often not available, especially in the evening. When such facilities are available, continual monitoring of serum electrolyte levels can be extremely expensive. For these reasons, monitoring the ECG can be a safe, inexpensive, and relatively reliable technique for detecting worrisome changes in the serum potassium concentration.

Phosphate Supplementation. Attention has recently been directed to phosphorus concentrations in human patients with DKA. Like potassium, phosphorus also

TABLE 96–3. A GENERAL GUIDELINE FOR POTASSIUM SUPPLEMENTATION IN IV FLUIDS

Serum K+ (mEq/L)	K+ Supplement/250 ml of Fluids
>3.5	5
3.0–3.5	7
2.5–3.0	10
2.0–2.5	15
<2.0	20

The amount of supplementation is based on evaluation of the serum potassium concentration and is added to 250 ml of IV fluids. Regardless of the amount of supplementation, total hourly potassium administration should not exceed 0.5 mEq/lb (1 mEq/kg) body weight.

shifts from tissues (including bone) to the extracellular compartment during DKA. Consequently patients rarely develop hypophosphatemia even though they have severe total body phosphorus deficiency because of excessive renal losses. Phosphorus concentrations in patients with untreated DKA are typically normal or elevated. Almost invariably, however, the serum phosphorus concentration falls progressively during therapy, potentially dropping to extremely low levels within 12 to 24 hours.[72]

The clinical effects of hypophosphatemia are not completely defined but appear to affect almost every organ system (e.g., confusion and seizures, decreased myocardial contractility with congestive heart failure, respiratory failure, and red blood cell lysis). Phosphorus depletion may also impair the migration and phagocytic capability of white blood cells, increase resorption of skeletal calcium, and cause muscle weakness and/or paralysis.

Despite the frightening aspects of induced hypophosphatemia, the phosphate depletion in ketoacidosis is usually clinically silent and shows up only in chemical measurements.[71] Two studies in humans have indicated that phosphate infusion has no effect on the hospital course of patients with DKA and does not diminish the morbidity, mortality, rate at which acidosis resolves, or enhancement of oxygen delivery to the tissue.[73, 74] Nevertheless, various treatment protocols, including phosphate replacement, have been proposed and may be indicated if clinical signs referable to hypophosphatemia develop.[42, 71, 72]

The recommended dosage for phosphate supplementation in the dog is 0.005 to 0.015 mMol of phosphate per lb (0.01 to 0.03 mMol of phosphate per kg) of body weight per hour for three to six hours, at which time the blood phosphorus concentration should be rechecked.[75] Phosphate is usually supplemented by administering a potassium phosphate solution, preferably in a calcium-free solution (e.g., physiologic saline). The commonly available potassium phosphate solution for parenteral administration contains 224 mg of KH_2PO_4 and 236 mg of K_2HPO_4 per milliliter, which provides 4.4 mEq of potassium and 3.0 mMol of phosphate per milliliter.[75] Adverse effects from overzealous phosphate administration include iatrogenic hypocalcemia and its associated neuromuscular signs, hypernatremia, hypotension, and metastatic calcification.[76] Phosphorus supplementation is not indicated in dogs with hypercalcemia, hyperphosphatemia, oliguria, or suspected tissue necrosis.

Glucose Supplementation. The initial blood glucose concentration will dictate, in part, when glucose-containing fluids are required. The clinician should not allow the blood glucose concentration to decline below

200 mg/dl during the initial 24 to 48 hours of therapy. Mild hyperglycemia will maintain an osmotic diuresis that aids in the correction of azotemia and DKA. If the initial blood glucose concentration is near 300 mg/dl, a glucose-containing fluid will be needed fairly soon after initiation of fluid and insulin therapy. However, if the initial blood glucose level is above 700 mg/dl, glucose-containing fluids should not be required for a few hours. Hourly blood glucose evaluations are important in all patients with extremely increased blood glucose concentrations to ensure that a slow but steady decline in the blood glucose concentration is occurring. Too rapid a decline in the blood glucose level can result in cerebral edema and hypoglycemia.

Rapidly falling blood glucose concentrations seen during the initial stages of therapy can be attributed, in part, to the IV infusion of fluids. Intravenous fluids lead to an increase in the glomerular filtration rate, an increased glucose excretion rate, and a decline in blood glucose concentrations, independent of the administration of insulin. A rapid decline in the blood glucose concentration in these animals may require the initiation of glucose-containing fluids earlier than anticipated.

Patient Monitoring. The rate of fluid administration and its effects on the patient must be monitored. Overzealous fluid therapy can lead to fluid overload, pulmonary edema, and potentially serious consequences. Inadequate fluid administration can result in prolonged tissue underperfusion, hypoxia, continuing pancreatitis (if present), persistent prerenal azotemia, and the potential for development of primary renal failure. Evaluation of fluid therapy should include subjective and objective assessments. Subjectively, the clinician should monitor the patient's alertness, heart rate, mucous membrane moisture, capillary refill time, pulse pressure, and skin turgor. Objectively, serial evaluation of central venous pressure (CVP), urine output, and body weight should ideally be done. Central venous pressure should remain below 10 cm H_2O. Although pulmonary and cardiac auscultation should be performed, this procedure is an ineffective way to monitor fluid therapy. If pulmonary rales are heard on auscultation, fluid therapy has been excessive and the dog or cat has already reached a point one must try to avoid. The fasted dog or cat should also lose approximately 0.5 per cent to 1.0 per cent of its body weight daily.

Accurate assessment of urine output is extremely important in the ill ketoacidotic dog or cat. Diabetes-induced glomerular microangiopathy and/or the hemodynamic effects of DKA, concurrent necrotizing pancreatitis, or prolonged severe dehydration can lead to oliguric or anuric renal failure. Failure to produce urine within several hours of initiating fluid therapy is an alarming sign, one that demands rapid recognition and an aggressive course of action. Because this is a relatively common complication, all severely ill patients with DKA should have a urinary catheter secured in the bladder. The catheter should be attached to a closed collection system. Frequent, accurate monitoring of urine production is imperative. A minimum of 0.5 to 1.0 ml of urine/lb (1.0 to 2.0 ml of urine/kg) of body weight per hour should be produced after the initial phase of fluid therapy.

If urine is not being produced or the rate of flow is minimal, one must first be certain that the catheter is in the bladder. The next question to be answered is whether the amount of IV fluid administered was sufficient to restore adequate blood pressure needed for renal perfusion. This is best assessed by measuring arterial blood pressure with a Doppler monitor or by obtaining a CVP measurement. Several readings over a short period are usually required for the CVP. If the patient is hypotensive, the CVP is very low (< 1 to 2 cm H_2O), or questions concerning fluid volume remain, the rate of fluid administration should be increased for an additional one to two hours. Urine output, CVP, blood pressure, and signs of overzealous fluid administration should be carefully monitored during this time.

If the fluid volume administered is deemed adequate and anuria or severe oliguria persists, one can attempt to induce or increase the volume of urine produced with diuretics (e.g., furosemide, 1 to 2 mg/lb or 2 to 4 mg/kg IV) or dopamine (1 to 3 μgm/lb/min or 2 to 5 μgm/kg/min IV). Dopamine is useful as a renal vasodilator and may work synergistically with furosemide. It needs to be diluted in saline or Ringer's solution and cannot be added to solutions containing sodium bicarbonate. The dopamine solution is best administered by means of a pediatric minidrip that can be either infused into the patient directly or piggy-backed into the primary IV fluid lines. The dose can be increased if urine production does not increase within two to three hours. The development of tachycardia or arrhythmias indicates that the dose administered is excessive and should be reduced. If significant diuresis develops, the dopamine infusion should be slowly decreased over 6 to 12 hours, until urine production is maintained with fluid therapy alone. If this therapy fails, peritoneal dialysis or hemodialysis is the only alternative.

Urinary tract infections are a definite reality with indwelling urinary catheters. The vast majority of iatrogenically induced infections can be successfully managed with appropriate antibiotic therapy after removal of the catheter. Palpation of the bladder is not an accurate method for assessing urine output, especially in obese dogs, dogs with painful abdomens, or small dogs that may normally pass small volumes of urine.

An important aid in fluid therapy is the frequent assessment (i.e., every four to six hours) of serum sodium and potassium concentrations and total venous carbon dioxide or arterial blood gases. Electrolyte balance is an integral part of fluid therapy. After the initial four to six hours of therapy, if the serum sodium concentration is between 140 and 155 mEq/L, the IV fluid should be changed to Ringer's solution, which has less sodium than normal saline. If the serum sodium concentration is still less than 140 mEq/L, the patient should be maintained on normal saline. If the serum sodium concentration is greater than 155 mEq/L, then 0.45 per cent sodium chloride (one-half strength) should be given. The IV infusion may need to be changed several times during the initial 24 hours of therapy.

Insulin Therapy

Large doses of insulin are not required in the management of DKA. Any regimen that provides stable high physiologic insulin concentrations would seem appropriate. Early rehydration and meticulous clinical care are equally as important as the insulin protocol utilized.[77] The amount of insulin needed by an individual animal is difficult to predict. Therefore, one needs to use an insulin that has a rapid onset of action and a brief duration of effect. If these criteria are met, the effectiveness of one to two insulin doses can be assessed and adjustments in dose made accordingly. Rapid-acting regular insulin meets the criteria and is the only insulin to be used in DKA.

Intermittent Intramuscular Insulin Regimen. Arguments abound regarding the most appropriate route for insulin administration. The choices are few, and when applying available information to veterinary practice, the intermittent intramuscular (IM) regimen used in humans appears to be best suited to veterinary practice. Insulin administered IM has a half-life of approximately two hours. The intermittent IM protocol is simple, reliable, and consistent, and avoids the inherent difficulties of IV or subcutaneous (SQ) regimens. Successful management of spontaneous DKA in dogs, using low insulin doses, has been reported.[78] Presently, the author recommends giving dogs and cats with severe DKA an initial regular insulin loading dose of 0.1 U/lb IM (0.2 U/kg), followed by 0.05 U/lb IM (0.1 U/kg), every hour. The insulin should be administered into the muscles of the rear legs to ensure that the injections are IM and not going into fat or subcutaneous tissue.

The dose of insulin used in low-dose regimens in small dogs and cats can seem minuscule. Diluting regular insulin with special diluting agents or saline is beneficial for managing these animals. The insulin is usually diluted 1:10 for convenience, and half-strength (i.e., 0.5 ml) insulin syringes are used. These syringes, when filled, contain 5 units of insulin.

Once the initial hourly insulin therapy brings the blood glucose concentration below 250 mg/dl (usually within 6 to 12 hours), begin to administer regular insulin every four to six hours IM or, if the hydration status is good, every six to eight hours SQ. The dose used is usually 0.05 to 0.2 U/lb (0.1 to 0.4 U/kg). The blood glucose concentration should still be monitored every one to two hours with Chemstrip bG reagent strips. Longer-acting insulins, such as isophane (NPH) insulin or protamine zinc insulin (PZI), are not administered until the dog or cat is stable, eating, not vomiting, maintaining fluid balance without any IV infusions, and no longer acidotic, azotemic, or electrolyte-deficient.

The goal of insulin therapy is to slowly lower the blood glucose concentration to the range of 200 to 250 mg/dl. Ideally, this should take approximately eight hours. However, lowering of the blood glucose concentration is not easy to control because the rate of decline depends on many factors, including the initial degree of hyperglycemia, aggressiveness of fluid therapy, acidemia, diabetogenic hormone concentrations, and body temperature.

Because of the numerous factors that influence both insulin therapy and the rate of blood glucose decline, one cannot reliably predict the course of treatment. Therefore, it is recommended that the blood glucose concentration be monitored hourly. In most veterinary hospitals this can be accomplished using Chemstrip bG reagent strips and an automated test strip analyzer. Ideally, the blood glucose concentration should decrease by 50 to 100 mg/dl/hr; this provides a steady and moderate decline while avoiding large osmolality shifts. Whenever the blood glucose concentration reaches 250 to 300 mg/dl, the IV infusion solution should have enough 50 per cent dextrose added to create a 5 per cent dextrose solution (100 ml of 50 per cent dextrose added to each liter of fluids). The blood glucose concentration should be maintained between 150 and 250 mg/dl until the patient is stable and eating. Usually a 5 per cent dextrose solution is adequate in maintaining the desired blood glucose concentration. If the blood glucose concentration dips below 150 mg/dl or rises above 250 mg/dl, the IM insulin dose can be lowered or raised accordingly. The total dose being used is usually quite small, and changes of 10 per cent in the hourly dose are sufficient for initial corrections.

One may want to monitor urine ketone concentrations in addition to the other parameters previously discussed. Although it is a good sign to see ketone concentrations decline, this is one constituent that remains of little value in monitoring the initial treatment of DKA. Inhibition of lipolysis is much more sensitive to insulin than is stimulation of glucose uptake. Therefore, if the plasma glucose concentration is falling, one can be certain that lipolysis, and the supply of free fatty acids for ketone production, has been effectively turned off. Glucose concentrations, however, fall much more rapidly than do ketone levels. In general, hyperglycemia is corrected in 4 to 8 hours, but ketosis takes 10 to 30 hours to resolve.[42]

Alternative Approaches for Insulin Therapy. Although IV and SQ routes of insulin administration are also effective in initially managing the DKA patient, these methods have potential drawbacks not found with the intermittent IM regimen. Insulin given as an IV bolus has a plasma half-life of approximately 6 minutes and a biologic half-life of about 20 minutes in tissues.[79] Therefore, IV insulin therapy should be given as a continuous infusion, rather than by intermittent bolus injections. The continuous infusion system is based on doses of 0.02 to 0.5 U/lb/hr (0.05 to 0.1 U/kg/hr).[80, 81] Insulin can absorb to glassware and plastic.[82] However, an insulin-electrolyte infusion mixture can be expected to deliver approximately 100 per cent of the insulin in solution if the first 50 ml of mixture is discarded after running it through the plastic tubing.[83] By using this wash-through procedure, no extra protein additives are necessary. IV infusion by pump is favored, although these pumps require careful attention, and the insulin solution must be given separate from the primary fluid therapy used to correct dehydration deficits, electrolyte imbalances, and acidosis. This is necessary because the rate of administration of the primary fluids is in a constant state of flux as the fluid demands of the patient change from hour to hour. In the average veterinary practice, two IV infusion lines, or a piggyback pediatric infusion system, can become cumbersome and time-consuming.

Subcutaneous administration of insulin also has major drawbacks. In the dehydrated patient or in the patient in shock, subcutaneous blood flow, and hence insulin absorption, is likely to be decreased. In addition, insulin depots are more likely to accumulate after SQ administration, complicating later management.[77] Subcutaneously injected regular insulin has a half-life of approximately four hours, which suggests that the initial rise in concentration will be too slow for effective early management of DKA. The therapeutic response has been slower in those studies using the SQ route.[84] Nevertheless, for many years the author has successfully used initial IM followed by intermittent SQ insulin given every six to eight hours in the management of DKA.

Bicarbonate Therapy

A tremendous amount of controversy exists concerning therapy specifically directed at the acidosis component of DKA. Objections to bicarbonate therapy include (a) therapy with alkali may result in metabolic alkalosis, which is as potentially serious as metabolic acidosis, (b) any alkalization can cause a shift to the left of the oxygen dissociation curve, thereby limiting tissue oxygen delivery, (c) a rapid elevation in arterial pH may be accompanied by an exaggerated fall in the cerebrospinal fluid (CSF) pH with resultant worsening of CNS function,[85] and (d) alkalization leads to a greater incidence of hypokalemia.[86] In addition, recent reports from two different centers on bicarbonate therapy in humans with DKA found no difference in the rates of recovery between patients who received bicarbonate therapy (regardless of the regimen used) and those who did not receive such therapy.[87]

Some investigators believe that the paradoxical fall in CSF pH after bicarbonate therapy is of real concern, while others do not.[42, 87, 88] If it occurs, the reason for the paradoxical fall in CSF pH is that carbon dioxide rapidly diffuses across the blood-brain barrier, whereas hydrogen ions and bicarbonate move slowly across this barrier. If the metabolic acidosis is corrected rapidly with bicarbonate therapy, the serum carbon dioxide concentration increases. Most of this carbon dioxide can be "blown off" through the lungs, but significant amounts will also diffuse across the blood-brain barrier. This will, by virtue of the following equation, increase the CSF hydrogen ion concentration and decrease the pH within the CNS, resulting in worsening CNS acidosis. The equation is:

$$H_2O + CO_2 \leftrightarrow H_2CO_3 \leftrightarrow H^+ + HCO_3^-$$

The severity of CNS depression caused by metabolic acidosis primarily depends on the pH of the CSF, and not on that of the peripheral circulation. An alert dog or cat that is brought to the hospital with a severely depressed peripheral pH probably has a normal or near-normal pH in the CSF. However, an acidotic patient that is brought to the hospital with severe depression may have severe CNS acidosis. These are difficult patients to treat, and the only safe therapy is to correct the metabolic acidosis slowly in the peripheral circulation, thereby avoiding major alterations in the pH of the CSF.[89]

Despite these arguments, the deleterious effects of severe uncorrected acidemia far outweigh the negative aspects of bicarbonate therapy. When the blood pH falls below 7.2, and particularly below 7.1, serious consequences ensue, including lack of insulin binding to receptors; significant depression of cardiac output; constriction of the pulmonary arterial bed, arrhythmias, antagonism of endogenous pressor activity with the potential for peripheral vascular collapse; significant dilation of the cerebrovascular bed, leading to increased CSF pressure and coma; renal and mesenteric vascular constriction, which predisposes the patient to acute renal tubular necrosis and ischemic bowel disease; and decreased buffer reserve.[90-93] The last factor is a major concern in the severely acidotic dog or cat with DKA because small changes in either PCO_2 or serum bicarbonate concentration can produce life-threatening changes in the blood pH. A low buffer reserve in a patient with unrecognized and untreated DKA or lactic acidosis can lead to severe acidemia and irreversible cardiovascular collapse.[42]

Acetoacetic acid and β-hydroxybutyric acid are usable anions, and 1 mEq of bicarbonate is generated from each 1 mEq of ketoacid metabolized. In addition, insulin therapy dramatically diminishes production of ketoacids, causing the serum bicarbonate concentration to return toward normal without using alkali-containing solutions. For these reasons the author recommends that animals with a serum bicarbonate concentration (or total venous carbon dioxide concentration) of 12 mEq/L or greater not be treated with bicarbonate.

When the plasma bicarbonate concentration is 11 mEq/L or less (the total venous carbon dioxide is below 12), bicarbonate should be given IV during the first six hours of treatment. The bicarbonate deficit (i.e., the milliequivalent of bicarbonate initially needed to correct acidosis to the critical level of 12 mEq/L over six hours) is calculated as mEq bicarbonate = body weight (kg) × 0.4 × (12—patient's bicarbonate) × 0.5.

The difference between the patient's serum bicarbonate concentration and the critical value of 12 mEq/L represents the treatable base deficit in DKA. The factor 0.4 corrects for the extracellular fluid space in which bicarbonate is distributed (40 per cent of body weight). The factor 0.5 provides one half of the required dose of bicarbonate in the IV infusion. In this manner a conservative dose is given over six hours. Bicarbonate should never be given by bolus infusion.[94] After six hours of therapy the acid-base status should be reevaluated and the calculations repeated. Once the plasma bicarbonate level is greater than 12 mEq/L, further bicarbonate supplementation is not needed.

Therapy: Healthy Diabetic Ketoacidotic

If the dog or cat appears healthy but mild ketonuria persists, or if the ketoacidotic animal initially presents "healthy," short-acting regular insulin can be administered three or four times daily until the ketonuria resolves. The insulin dose should be based solely on blood glucose concentrations. To minimize hypoglycemia, the dog or cat should be fed one-third or one-fourth of its daily caloric intake at the time of each insulin injection. The blood glucose and urine ketone concentrations, as well as the patient's clinical status, should be monitored. If the blood glucose concentration is well controlled, the ketone concentrations will fall, although this may take a few days. Prolonged ketonuria is suggestive of a (significant) concurrent illness. Once the ketoacidotic state has resolved and the dog or cat is stable, eating, and drinking, insulin regulation may be initiated using the long-acting insulin preparations.

Therapy: Nonketotic Diabetic

Oral Hypoglycemic Agents. Oral hypoglycemic agents have been used in humans with NIDDM, but they are not often used in veterinary practice. The two major groups of oral hypoglycemic drugs are the sulfonylureas and the biguanides. The sulfonylureas have several antidiabetic actions, including the acute stimulation of insulin secretion by β cells, the chronic antidiabetic actions of insulin on muscle and adipose tissue carbohydrate transport, a direct action on the liver to decrease hepatic glucose output, and the potentiation of insulin action on the liver.[95] The biguanides delay gastrointestinal absorption of ingested nutrients and promote the peripheral utilization of blood glucose.

Church recommends the use of two sulfonylureas: glipizide (Glucotrol, 0.12 to 0.25 mg/lb or 0.24 to 0.5 mg/kg q12h; maximum, 5 mg/day) or glibenclamide (Diabeta, 0.1 mg/lb daily or 0.2 mg/kg) for diabetic dogs that have a measurable insulin response to a glucose challenge.[80] However, chronic treatment with some of the sulfonylureas, including glibenclamide, has resulted in decreased insulin content in β cells and decreased nutrient-stimulated insulin secretion in normal animals.[95] Therefore, caution must be used in the long-term treatment of canine and feline diabetes with these oral hypoglycemic agents. In addition, diabetic dogs and cats with high normal or increased blood insulin concentrations should be evaluated for the presence of treatable underlying problems. Some diabetic dogs and cats with measurable blood insulin levels have concurrent disorders that cause insulin antagonism (e.g., hyperadrenocorticism, diestrus). Identification of these potentially treatable disorders should be attempted before arbitrarily initiating hypoglycemic drugs.

The author has successfully managed several diabetic dogs with oral hypoglycemic drugs; however, there has been a poor response with these agents in diabetic cats. The blood glucose concentration is routinely evaluated before oral hypoglycemic drugs are initiated and weekly for one month post therapy. If there has been no response to therapy (i.e., no decrease in blood glucose concentrations) or if clinical signs of DKA develop, oral hypoglycemics are discontinued and insulin therapy initiated. If the blood glucose concentration has decreased, the dosage of the oral hypoglycemic is adjusted to maintain blood glucose concentrations between 80 and 170 mg/dl. Appropriate dietary therapy is also initiated to help control blood glucose concentrations. Once glycemic control has been obtained, the blood glucose should be rechecked every two to three months and

appropriate adjustments made in the dosage of the oral hypoglycemic agent.

Insulin Therapy. Commercial insulin is categorized by promptness, duration, and intensity of action after SQ administration (Table 96–4). The solubility of insulin is determined by the size of the insulin crystals, the zinc content, and the nature of the buffer in which it is suspended. Commonly used insulins for the long-term management of diabetics include NPH insulin, Lente insulin, and PZI. NPH insulin is perhaps the most commonly used insulin preparation for canine and feline diabetics. Unfortunately the duration of effect of NPH insulin often is only 12 to 18 hours in the dog and 4 to 10 hours in the cat.[96] In the dog, NPH insulin frequently needs to be administered twice daily if good glycemic control is to be achieved. Some dogs, however, do obtain good glycemic control with once-daily NPH insulin injections. Because of this, NPH insulin is the initial insulin of choice for regulation of the diabetic dog, until serial glucose determinations dictate otherwise. In the diabetic cat, even when administered twice a day, NPH insulin often causes wide fluctuations in the blood glucose concentration from hour to hour (Figure 96–10, top panel). Thus this insulin is not usually satisfactory in gaining good glycemic control in diabetic cats, and its use is not recommended.

Longer-acting insulins (e.g., PZI) appear to be best suited for the cat and are the initial insulins of choice for glycemic regulation. PZI begins to lower blood glucose concentrations in 1 to 3 hours, peaks in 4 to 10 hours, and has a duration of 12 to 24 hours (Table 96–4). There is significant individual variation (Figure 96–10, middle, lower panels). Approximately half of the diabetic cats receive PZI once daily and the remaining cats receive this insulin twice daily. Most cats would be best treated with twice-daily injections, but owner/cat willingness may not allow frequent administration.

Long-acting insulin therapy is begun using NPH insulin in the dog and PZI in the cat as a single morning injection. Small dogs (< 15 kg) receive approximately 0.5 U/lb (1.0 U/kg) of body weight, and large dogs (> 25 kg) receive 0.22 U/lb (0.5 U/kg). Diabetic cats can usually be controlled with insulin doses of 0.1 to 0.5 U/lb (0.2 to 1.0 U/kg) of body weight. The average cat is started on 1 to 3 units of PZI per cat. Insulin is better dosed on a square meter basis than on a simple body weight basis. Thus the larger the animal, the smaller the typical dose needed per kilogram or pound.

An animal will usually require two to four days to equilibrate to changes in insulin dosage or preparation. Therefore dogs and cats that initially receive insulin are not closely monitored for the first two or three days. Blood glucose concentrations are determined once or twice in the afternoon during this time to identify insulin overdosage and potential hypoglycemia. One could teach the owner to administer the insulin and send the animal home for this equilibration period. However, the author prefers and recommends hospitalization during this period for a previously untreated diabetic dog or cat. A thorough evaluation of the dog or cat can be completed during the two- to four-day equilibration period, thus simultaneously accomplishing the medical assessment of the patient and the initial therapy.

TABLE 96–4. PROPERTIES OF BEEF-PORK INSULIN PREPARATIONS USED IN DOGS AND CATS

| Type of Insulin | Route of Administration | Onset of Effect | Time of Maximum Effect | | Duration of Effect | |
			Dog	Cat	Dog	Cat
Regular crystalline	IV	Immediate	½–2 hr		1–4 hr	
	IM	10–30 min	1–4 hr		3–8 hr	
	SQ	10–30 min	1–5 hr		4–10 hr	
NPH (isophane)	SQ	½–3 hr	2–10 hr	2–8 hr	8–24 hr	6–12 hr
PZI	SQ	1–4 hr	5–20 hr	3–12 hr	8–30 hr	12–24 hr
Lente	SQ	Immediate	2–10 hr	?	8–24 hr	?
IZS-P	SQ	Immediate	2–10 hr	?	8–20 hr	?

Purified-pork regular insulin, NPH insulin, and PZI appear to be more potent, act faster, and have a shorter duration of action than beef-pork insulins.

Dietary Therapy. Dietary management should be initiated at the same time as long-acting insulin therapy. The presence of concurrent disease (e.g., pancreatitis) may dictate the type of diet consumed by the diabetic dog or cat. Successful diets for diabetic patients with concurrent pancreatitis have included low-fat cottage cheese mixed 1:2 with cooked white rice or a 1:1 mixture of cooked white rice and kibbled dog food. Regardless of the presence or absence of pancreatitis, semimoist foods should be avoided. Their high simple sugar content is rapidly assimilated, causing dramatic excursions in postprandial blood glucose levels and greater difficulty in maintaining glycemic control.[59] Most canned and dry foods contain complex carbohydrates that require intestinal digestion, and thereby prolong their assimilation. Rapid fluctuations in postprandial blood glucose concentrations are less likely with these diets.

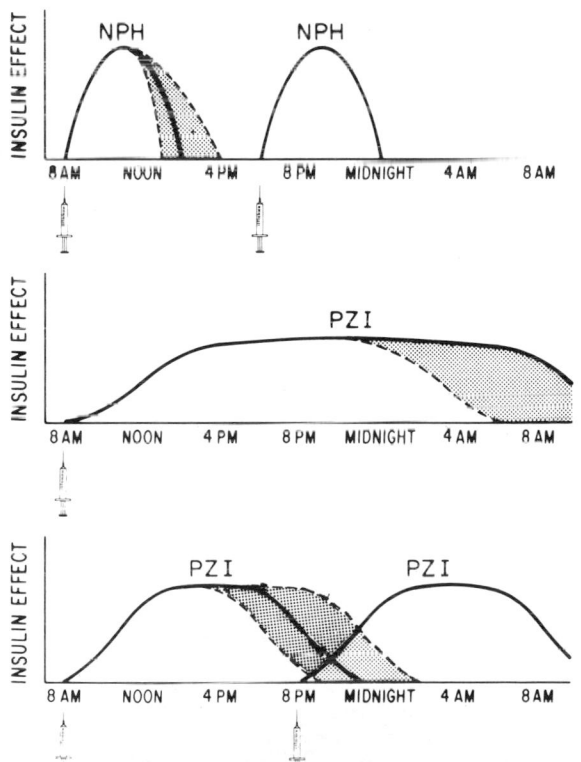

FIGURE 96–10. The effects of NPH and PZI insulins in diabetic cats. Note the variability in effect seen with each type of insulin, requiring serial glucose monitoring to assess response to insulin therapy in each cat. (From Feldman, EC and Nelson, RW: Canine and Feline Endocrinology and Reproduction. Philadelphia, WB Saunders, 1987, p 268).

A feeding program should be initiated that minimizes postprandial hyperglycemia, while preventing or correcting obesity. Studies in both the dog and cat have documented the deleterious influence obesity has on insulin function and glucose tolerance. Daily caloric intake (20–30 kcal/lb or 40–60 kcal/kg in the geriatric pet) should be based on ideal body weight, which must be estimated in the obese animal. Intuitively, food should be absorbed with glucose in the blood ready to be utilized when the injected insulin has its maximum effect. Feeding multiple (i.e., 3 to 4) small meals throughout the day, beginning at the time of insulin administration, is the best way to minimize an increase in the postprandial blood glucose. Feeding one half of the total daily caloric intake at the time of the insulin injection and the remainder approximately six to ten hours later is also an acceptable protocol. Feeding one large meal often results in hyperglycemia, especially when given in the morning or early evening and should therefore be avoided (Figure 96–11).

Several short-term studies have emerged during the past decade that evaluate the influence of dietary fiber supplementation on improving glycemic control in both IDDM and NIDDM in humans. Although controversial, soluble fiber (e.g., guar, pectin), rather than insoluble fiber (e.g., cellulose, lignin), is better at improving glycemic control.[97] By increasing daily soluble fiber consumption from levels of 3 to 10 gm/day to greater than 30 gm/day, an improvement in glycemic control is observed in both IDDM and NIDDM patients, including a decrease in fasting and postprandial blood glucose concentrations, urine glucose excretion, glycosylated hemoglobin concentrations, daily insulin requirements, and adverse insulin reactions.[98, 99] Soluble fibers are believed to exert their effects on glycemic control by altering gastrointestinal transit time, carbohydrate absorption, the secretion of gastrointestinal hormones, and tissue sensitivity to insulin.[97, 100–102] Carbohydrates have a synergistic influence on fiber supplementation.[99, 100] For fiber supplementation to be effective, daily carbohydrate intake must exceed 40 per cent of the diet and must be intimately mixed with the fiber before ingestion.[100]

Soluble fiber supplementation also affects lipid metabolism in human diabetics. Total blood cholesterol concentrations and the LDL cholesterol fraction decrease, while the HDL cholesterol fraction increases with high-soluble fiber diets.[103, 104] Although somewhat controversial, soluble fiber supplements also seem to lower plasma triglyceride concentrations, especially in patients with hypertriglyceridemia.[103, 105] The beneficial effects on

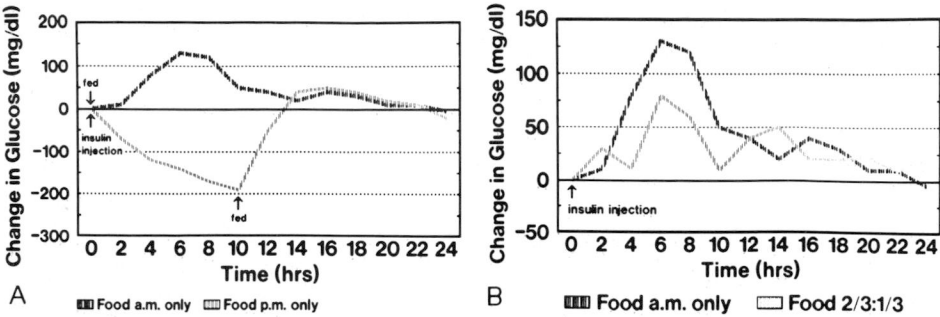

FIGURE 96–11. Mean change in blood glucose concentrations in eight dogs with IDDM fed 30 kcal of canned dog food/lb body weight. A fixed amount of NPH insulin was administered to each dog at 8 AM. *A*, all the food was given in one meal at either 8 AM or 6 PM. *B*, all the food was given in one meal at 8 AM or in two meals at 8 AM ($\frac{2}{3}$ of the food) and 6 PM ($\frac{1}{3}$ of the food). Note the reduction in the mean blood glucose excursion in *B*, merely by feeding multiple meals rather than one meal daily.

plasma triglyceride concentrations are more apparent on postprandial rather than fasting concentrations.[106] High-fiber diets also reduce the total lipid and triglyceride content of the liver in laboratory animals.[107] These alterations in lipid metabolism have antiatherogenic implications and are beneficial in diabetes mellitus, in which derangements in cholesterol metabolism and hypercholesterolemia are frequently found.

The influence of soluble and insoluble fiber on glycemic control in IDDM dogs is currently under investigation. Preliminary results would suggest comparable improvement in glycemic control in the diabetic dog as has been reported in humans. Beneficial effects, however, have been documented with both soluble and insoluble fiber supplementation. Subjectively, prescription R/D and W/D diets, which are high in insoluble fiber, have been beneficial in improving glycemic control in a few poorly regulated diabetic dogs. Until studies dictate otherwise, the use of these high fiber diets is indicated in diabetic dogs and cats that are difficult to manage with conventional diets and insulin therapy.

Dietary therapy may be the only therapy required to manage the obese cat with mild NIDDM. If the diabetic cat is stable, a conservative therapeutic approach relying solely on dietary therapy may be tried initially. Daily caloric intake should correct and prevent obesity. In addition, a high-fiber diet (e.g., Prescription diet feline R/D) should be fed to take advantage of the beneficial effects of dietary fiber on improving glycemic control. A fasting and 2- to 3-hour postprandial blood glucose concentration should be determined weekly during the initial month. If the blood glucose concentrations decline to less than 200 mg/dl during this month, urine becomes negative for glucose, and clinical signs improve, insulin therapy is not indicated and the cat should be managed with dietary therapy. Conversely, if hyperglycemia, glycosuria, and clinical signs persist during the first month of conservative therapy, insulin therapy should be initiated.

In-Hospital Adjustments of Insulin and Dietary Therapy. After the first few equilibration days, close monitoring of the blood glucose response to the insulin and dietary therapy is imperative. The remarkable variation in onset, peak, and duration of effect of NPH insulin and PZI necessitates the evaluation of serial blood glucose measurements every one to two hours through-

out the day. This will allow the clinician to determine the time of peak insulin effect, the duration of effect, and the degree of fluctuation in blood glucose concentrations obtained in that particular dog or cat. Obtaining only one or two blood glucose concentrations has not been reliable for evaluating the effect of a given insulin dose (Figure 96–12). The dosage of insulin, type of insulin, frequency of administration, and time of feeding may be altered, depending on the results of the blood glucose measurements. An ideal graph of the serial

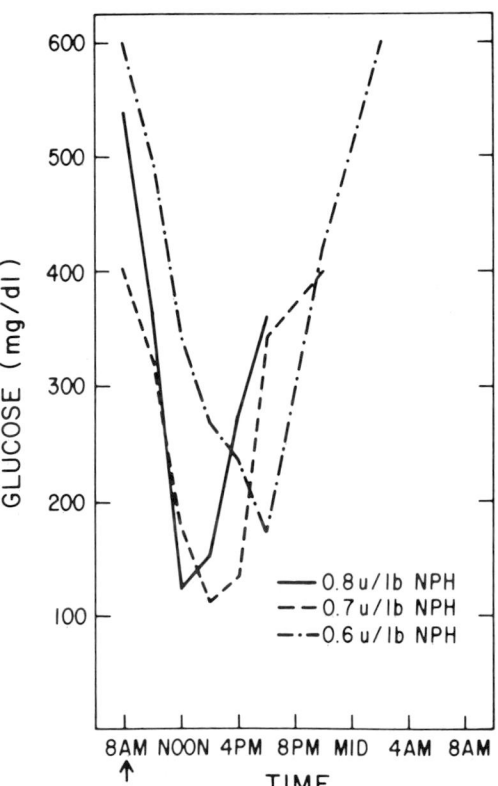

FIGURE 96–12. Blood glucose curves from three dogs receiving similar doses of NPH insulin, demonstrating the remarkable individual variation seen in response to exogenous insulins. Rapid insulin metabolism is present in all three dogs. If a blood glucose was only determined at 4 PM, good control would have been assumed in one dog and hyperglycemia found in the other two dogs. However, in one of these hyperglycemic dogs the insulin effect is wearing off, while in the other it has not yet reached maximum. (From Nelson, RW and Feldman, EC: JAVMA 182:1321, 1983.)

glucose concentrations has the lowest blood glucose concentration of 80 to 120 mg/dl occurring 10 to 12 hours after insulin administration. The duration of insulin effect should be 22 to 24 hours, with the highest blood glucose concentration of 180 to 200 mg/dl 24 hours after the insulin injection (Figure 96–13).

Knowing exact plasma glucose concentrations is not necessary. Therefore, laboratory glucose measurements that require 2 to 3 ml of sodium fluoride–treated blood for each sample may be expensive and are not mandatory. The author routinely uses Chemstrip bG reagent strips, which only require one drop of whole blood. These strips are perfect for the in-hospital management of diabetics. As currently marketed, these reagent strips can be cut into halves or thirds and be that much more cost-effective. Use of these strips allows the veterinarian a chance to offer a relatively inexpensive, safe, nonpainful (use a 25-gauge needle to obtain blood), scientifically sound approach to diabetes management.

The nadir in the blood glucose concentration should be above 80 mg/dl. This is important because the chances of actually taking a blood sample at the moment the blood glucose concentration reaches its lowest point are nil. Therefore, if the lowest measured blood glucose concentration is 80 mg/dl, the lowest real blood glucose concentration is presumably at a safe level, assuming that the concentrations are being checked hourly.

Adjusting the insulin dosage will usually affect the lowest blood glucose concentration obtained without altering the duration of effect of insulin. In the dog, if the duration of effect of NPH insulin is between 14 and 20 hours, a longer-acting insulin (i.e., Lente, PZI) given once a day should be tried. As a general rule, longer-

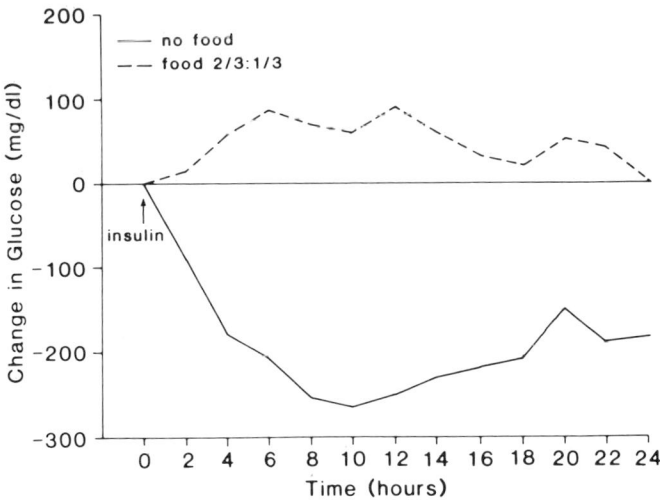

FIGURE 96–14. Mean change in blood glucose concentrations in eight dogs with IDDM given a fixed amount of NPH insulin at 8 AM and either not fed (———) or fed 30 kcal of canned dog food/lb body weight in two meals at 8 AM (2/3 of the food; time 0) and 6 PM (1/3 of the food; time 10 hr) (– – – –).

acting insulins increase the duration of action by no more than six to eight hours. Therefore, if the duration of effect of NPH insulin is 10 to 14 hours, NPH insulin administered twice daily may be necessary to achieve better glycemic control. If the duration of effect of NPH insulin is eight hours or less, Lente insulin or PZI administered twice daily should be considered. In the cat, if the duration of PZI is less than 14 hours, PZI administered twice a day may be needed.

When generating the initial blood glucose curve in the hospital, the dog or cat should be fed as outlined under the section on dietary therapy, with the main meal given six to ten hours after the insulin injection. Generating a curve without feeding the animal will allow evaluation of the peak time of insulin action but will not allow evaluation of dosage or duration of action because of the effects eating has on blood glucose (Figure 96–14). By feeding the ideal caloric requirements at the time of the blood sampling, the clinician will be able to assess all of the important variables previously discussed.

Determining the time of peak insulin effect will help to establish a feeding schedule. If the lowest blood glucose concentration occurs before the dog or cat receives its evening meal, the time interval between the insulin injection and the evening feeding should be shortened accordingly, or a longer-acting insulin used. If the effects of the insulin are wearing off at the time of the evening feeding, a dramatic increase in the blood glucose concentration will be seen in the samples obtained after feeding the dog (Figure 96–15). This is an indication of rapid metabolism of the insulin, and either a switch to PZI or administration of insulin twice a day should be considered. With twice-daily insulin administration, the owner's schedule must be considered and the treatment protocol altered to comply with what is feasible. Most clients who are giving insulin twice daily feed their pets two equal meals, one meal immediately after each insulin injection.

Fine control of the blood glucose concentration and

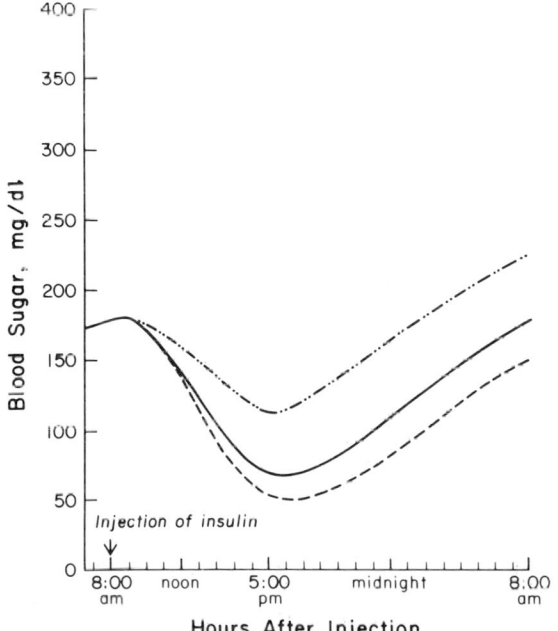

FIGURE 96–13. Ideal blood glucose concentrations over a 24-hour period after a single injection of insulin (———). Also illustrated is the ideal response to a high dose of insulin (– – – –) as well as an insufficient dose of insulin (–··–··–). In reality, these ideal responses are virtually never seen, forcing the veterinarian to rely on serial blood glucose concentrations to monitor diabetic dogs and cats. (From Feldman, EC: In Ettinger, SJ (ed): Textbook of Veterinary Internal Medicine, 2nd ed., Philadelphia, WB Saunders, 1983, p 1628)

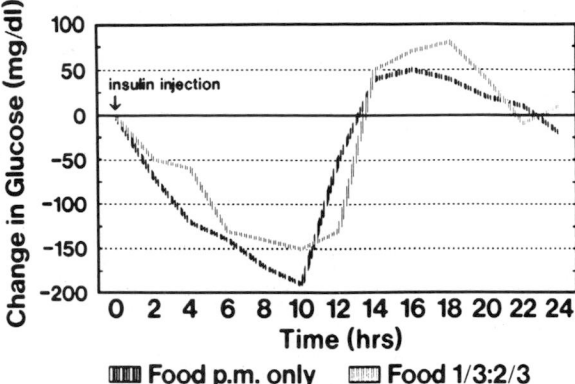

FIGURE 96–15. Mean change in blood glucose concentrations in 8 dogs with IDDM and rapid insulin metabolism. A fixed amount of NPH insulin was given at 8 AM (time 0) and 30 kcal of canned dog food/lb body weight was given as a single meal at 6 PM or in two meals at 8 AM (1/3 of the food; time 0) and 6 PM (2/3 of the food; time 10 hr). Note the marked reduction in the change in glucose excursion (i.e., recurrence of hyperglycemia) in these dogs shortly after the evening meal, which is frequently seen with rapid metabolism of insulin.

determination of the "exact" insulin dose should not be the objectives of hospital regulation. Diet and exercise are two important variables that affect blood glucose and thus insulin requirements; these variables will change in the home environment. The main objectives of hospital regulation are to determine a "ballpark" insulin dose, as well as to determine the type of insulin, frequency of administration, and approximate feeding schedule to maintain optimum glycemic control. The basic objective of insulin therapy is to eliminate the symptoms of diabetes mellitus. This is accomplished if the majority of each day's blood glucose concentrations are below 180 mg/dl. By doing this, many of the long-term complications of diabetes mellitus can be delayed or avoided completely (Table 96–5).

Home Management. Once the type of insulin, frequency of administration, approximate dosage, and feeding schedule have been determined in the hospital, the diabetic dog or cat can be sent home. Insulin requirements will often change at home because of differences in caloric intake and exercise. The goal of home therapy is to maintain the plasma glucose concentration as close to euglycemia as possible, thereby preventing both the recurrence of clinical signs and the long-term complications associated with poorly controlled diabetes mellitus.

It is recommended that, initially, the diabetic pet be reevaluated once every 7 to 14 days until satisfactory glycemic control is achieved. On the day of reevaluation, the owner should administer insulin and feed the pet as usual that morning. The animal should then be seen at the veterinary hospital as soon after the injection as possible, and blood glucose concentrations should be checked hourly throughout the day (at least) or for 24 hours (ideally). Adjustments in therapy are made based on the results of the study. These blood glucose concentrations not only check the animal's response to insulin, but also assess the owner's ability to administer insulin. Once the pet is reasonably controlled, similar rechecks are recommended every two to four months.

Daily urine monitoring is an integral facet in the care of the diabetic dog. Historically, daily insulin adjustments have been based on morning urine glucose concentrations and were designed to compensate for day-to-day variations in food consumption and exercise. By measuring morning urine glucose concentrations and adjusting the insulin dose accordingly, fluctuations in blood glucose concentration were theoretically minimized and complications of insulin therapy more rapidly recognized. Daily adjustments in insulin dose, based on the urine checks, should be done with caution and an understanding of potential pitfalls. Although this approach to the home management of the diabetic dog works in some, the vast majority of dogs have developed complications as a result of owners being misled by urine glucose concentrations. Potentially serious problems may arise when attempting to adjust the insulin dosage based on morning urine glucose concentrations.

It is difficult to interpret persistently elevated morning glycosuria. As detailed later in the "complications" section, persistent morning glycosuria may suggest an underdosage but will also occur with a problem with the insulin administration technique, a problem in the insulin potency, rapid metabolism of insulin, insulin-induced hyperglycemia (overdose), or insulin antagonism. Thus, morning glycosuria is correct in suggesting underdosage in only a minority of cases. The appropriate therapy to reestablish blood glucose control is different for each of these situations. In addition, persistent negative urine glucoses are suggestive of a well-controlled diabetic animal more often than of an insulin overdosage. Therefore, if this method of home monitoring is adopted, it should be discontinued at the slightest indication of a problem.

The author currently relies on owner observation for recurrence of signs and the monitoring of afternoon urine glucose levels. Most important is the owner's subjective opinion of water intake and urine output. If these factors are normal, the animal is usually well controlled. It should have a good (not ravenous) appetite. Diabetic pets that are well controlled should not have problems with vomiting, diarrhea, anorexia, weight gain, weight loss, or persistent ketonuria. The author also has the owners check the urine daily for glucose and ketones before the evening meal and not in the morning. The urine should be negative for glucose before feeding if the animal is properly responding to the injections. Owners are also encouraged to check the urine as many times during the day as possible. All urine test results should be recorded in a daily diary. As would be expected, the well-controlled diabetic pet will have urine that is free of glucose for most of each 24-hour period. This animal should be rechecked with

TABLE 96–5. COMPLICATIONS ASSOCIATED WITH DIABETES MELLITUS IN THE DOG AND CAT

Common	Uncommon (Often Subclinical)
Cataracts-blindness	Retinopathy
Hepatic lipidosis	Neuropathy
Bacterial infections	Glomerulosclerosis
Ketoacidosis	Gastric paresis
Chronic pancreatitis	Diabetic diarrhea
Iatrogenic hypoglycemia	

blood glucose concentrations once every two to four months. Persistent glycosuria suggests a problem that would require evaluation by means of in-hospital blood glucose determinations at the owner's earliest convenience, regardless of the dog's condition.

A similar approach is taken to the home management of the diabetic cat. Attempts are not made to adjust the insulin dosage based on morning urine glucose concentrations. Rather, a fixed dosage of insulin is administered, based on results of in-hospital serial blood glucose testing. Once glycemic control is established, the insulin dosage is reevaluated every two to four months by serial evaluations of blood glucose concentrations in the hospital. These evaluations are performed earlier if clinical signs of diabetes recur or other complications (e.g., hypoglycemic reactions) develop. Urine monitoring is not mandatory; however, it can be used to identify problems with insulin therapy. As in the dog, persistent glycosuria suggests a problem that would require evaluation by means of in-hospital blood glucose determinations.

Glycosylated Hemoglobin

During the lifespan of the circulating erythrocyte, a small portion of the hemoglobin becomes irreversibly bound to glucose in a nonenzymatic reaction. The extent of glycosylation of hemoglobin is directly related to the plasma glucose concentration. Because red blood cells are insulin-independent, hyperglycemia for long periods causes increased production of this glycosylated hemoglobin (HbA_1). Therefore, measurement of this hemoglobin should aid in determining the success of any particular insulin regimen, since good diabetic control should result in normal or near-normal HbA_1 concentrations.

There are two major fractions of glycosylated hemoglobin: a minor fraction (HbA_{1a+b}) that does not bind to glucose and a major fraction (HbA_{1c}) that binds to glucose at the NH_2-terminal valine of the β chains of the hemoglobin molecule.[108, 109] Two forms of HbA_{1c} have also been identified: one form is stable and is present in similar concentrations before and after dialysis, while the second form is cleaved by the dialysis step of the assay.[110] Acute hyperglycemia will cause an increase in the concentration of HbA_{1c} in undialyzed hemolysates, with almost no effect on the HbA_{1c} concentration of dialyzed hemolysates. In the original technique the red cell hemolysates were dialyzed before chromatographic separation was performed, whereas the newer kit techniques omit the dialysis step. Therefore, interpretation of the glycosylated hemoglobin concentration should take into consideration the technique used to determine HbA_{1c}. Depending on the methodology used, acute hyperglycemia could elevate the concentration of HbA_1.[110, 111]

Glycosylated hemoglobin concentrations have been infrequently reported in dogs. Wood and Smith found the mean HbA_{1c} concentration in seven normal dogs to be three per cent, while it was between three per cent and seven per cent in seven diabetic dogs.[112] Similarly, Mahaffey and Cornelius found mean HbA_{1c} concentra-

tion for 16 clinically normal dogs to be 6.4 per cent while it was 9.6 per cent in 16 diabetic dogs.[113] Periodic evaluations of HbA_1, beginning with the initial regulation of the dog, should provide the clinician with some indication of the success of the insulin and dietary regimen used in that animal. However, this test does not identify the underlying problem if HbA_1 concentrations should be increased. Therefore, periodic determination of serial blood glucose concentrations is as valuable as, if not more so than, measurement of HbA_{1c} in the continuing management of diabetic pets.

Complications of Insulin Therapy

Veterinary reevaluation should take place before the planned visit if any one of several situations develops. Dogs or cats with symptoms of hypoglycemia, persistent glycosuria, anorexia, ravenous appetite, polydipsia, polyuria, weight loss, persistent ketonuria, or any illness are easier to understand and properly manage with one veterinary evaluation than with repeated changes in treatment over the phone. These symptoms indicate a problem with the insulin therapy, and an investigation should be undertaken to determine its cause.

An effort to eliminate the simple or obvious causes for poor diabetic control should be done before expensive, sophisticated, or time-consuming studies are performed. A thorough review of the owner's injection method is extremely important. Lack of a satisfactory response to insulin may involve improper insulin storage, or inaccurate or outdated urine glucose test strips. The veterinarian should also compare the syringes used with the type of insulin administered (i.e., U-100 insulin requires the use of U-100 syringes). The author routinely asks owners to bring their syringes and insulin along with their dogs or cats and then ask them to administer insulin (or saline) so that owner technique can be observed and evaluated. The method of mixing is checked and storage habits are reviewed. Once these obvious potential problems are demonstrated not to be responsible for poor diabetes control, the dog or cat should be hospitalized for further evaluation.

The author's approach to the problem diabetic dog or cat is to determine the effects of the current insulin dose and feeding schedule on blood glucose levels before recommending alterations in therapy. Beginning at the owner's normal time for insulin injection, the owner's insulin and current dose should be administered and the daily feeding schedule followed. Blood glucose concentrations (usually using Chemstrip bG reagent strips) are determined every 1 to 2 hours for 14 to 24 hours, beginning with the injection of insulin. A graph of the serial blood glucose determinations will then help to define the problem. An ideal graph of the serial blood glucose concentrations has the lowest blood glucose concentration at 80 to 120 mg/dl. The duration of once- or twice-daily insulin effect should be 22 to 24 hours, with the highest blood glucose concentration not exceeding 180 to 200 mg/dl.

The duration of insulin action, peak insulin activity as measured by the lowest blood glucose concentration, and time of peak insulin effect are extremely variable from animal to animal. These factors must be evaluated in the diabetic dog or cat that is having problems before a logical adjustment in therapy can be recommended. The following are the common disturbances that have been identified using serial blood glucose determinations.

Insulin-induced Hyperglycemia (Somogyi Overswing). Administering an overdosage of insulin to a patient, causing usually subclinical but severe hypoglycemia followed by significant hyperglycemia, has been recognized in human diabetics virtually since the discovery and use of insulin.[114, 115] Insulin increases glucose utilization by tissues and decreases glucose production by the liver. When the glucose concentration decreases below approximately 60 mg/dl, several physiologic mechanisms begin to raise it back toward normal. Hypoglycemia directly increases glucose production in the liver by increasing glycogenolysis, a reaction that is not hormone-mediated.[116, 117] Hypoglycemia also stimulates glucoreceptors in the hypothalamus, resulting in stimulation of the sympathoadrenal pathway, with subsequent release of catecholamines, specifically epinephrine.[118, 119]

Release of epinephrine stimulates hepatic glycogenolysis and diminishes tissue utilization of blood glucose. Epinephrine is also a potent stimulus for glucagon release from the α cells of the pancreatic islets.[120, 121] Glucagon, in turn, stimulates hepatic glycogenolysis and gluconeogenesis. Glucagon, epinephrine, and the direct hepatic effects of hypoglycemia are believed to be responsible for the acute increase in glucose production, which often prevents the clinical signs of hypoglycemia.[120, 122]

Hypoglycemia and increased catecholamine secretion augment the release of cortisol, by way of adrenocorticotropin (ACTH), and growth hormone (GH).[120, 123] Increased concentrations of these hormones are not detectable for 30 to 60 minutes after the initial rise in epinephrine, glucagon, and blood glucose concentrations.[124] Growth hormone and cortisol are not believed to be involved in the acute response to hypoglycemia, but are responsible for the persistent hyperglycemia and ensuing glucose intolerance in diabetics with insulin-induced hyperglycemia.[125] A high GH concentration is associated with decreased utilization of glucose.[126]

Secretion of these diabetogenic hormones results in increased hepatic gluconeogenesis and glycogenolysis and in decreased peripheral utilization of blood glucose, partly because of insulin antagonism at the cell receptor sites. Insulin overdosage and its attendant hypoglycemia are thus seen to result in a rapid response by epinephrine, glucagon, cortisol, and GH.

As a result of the response to hypoglycemia, blood glucose concentrations begin to increase, usually preventing a hypoglycemic convulsion. However, because these dogs are diabetic, sufficient endogenous insulin cannot be secreted to dampen the continuing rise in the blood glucose concentration (Figure 96–16). By the next morning the blood glucose concentration can be extremely elevated (400 to 800 mg/dl), and the morning urine glucose concentration is consistently 1 to 2 gm/dl, as measured with urine glucose test strips. If the owners are adjusting the daily insulin dose based on morning urine glucose concentrations, they interpret these read-

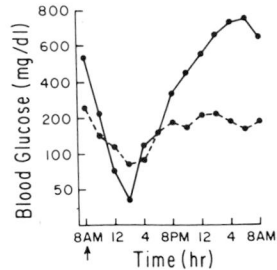

FIGURE 96–16. Blood glucose concentrations in a 6.1 kg Cairn terrier after receiving NPH insulin at 8 AM. The dog was fed at 8 AM and 6 PM. Solid line, 20 units; broken line, four units; ↑, insulin injection. (From Feldman, EC, Nelson, RW: JAVMA 180:1432, 1982).

ings as indicating that the dogs received insufficient amounts of insulin, especially if hypoglycemic signs (i.e., weakness, ataxia, bizarre behavior, or convulsions) are not observed. Therefore, owners will increase the insulin dose the next morning, and a continuous cycle of worsening insulin-induced hyperglycemia occurs.

The confusion surrounding this complex disorder may be compounded if the veterinarian elects to obtain only one late afternoon blood glucose concentration. In most dogs and cats with insulin-induced hyperglycemia, secretion of the diabetogenic hormones has commenced before 2 to 3 PM. The resultant hyperglycemia may suggest an inadequate dose of insulin or insulin antagonism when only one late afternoon blood glucose is evaluated, further supporting an incorrect diagnosis.

Insulin-induced hyperglycemia is a common problem when daily insulin adjustments are based on morning urine glucose concentrations, but it can also occur in the diabetic dog or cat that receives a fixed insulin dosage. The dosage of insulin that will induce posthypoglycemic hyperglycemia is variable. Although insulin-induced hyperglycemia can occur at any dose of insulin, it most commonly occurs at high doses (> 1 U/lb or > 2.2 U/kg). Insulin-induced hyperglycemia should be suspected when there is persistent morning glycosuria (> 1 gm/dl on urine glucose test strips), continued polyuria and polydipsia, symptoms of hypoglycemia, weight loss, or insulin dosages approaching 1 U/lb (2.2 U/kg).

Diagnosis of insulin-induced hyperglycemia requires demonstration of hypoglycemia (< 65 mg/dl) followed by hyperglycemia (> 300 mg/dl) within one 24-hour period after insulin administration. Therapy involves reducing the insulin dose by 25 per cent to 50 per cent, allowing three or more days for the dog or cat to equilibrate to this new dose, and then reassessing the dog's or cat's blood glucose concentrations. Further adjustments in the insulin dose should be made after reviewing these results. Unrecognized rapid insulin metabolism is a common cause for the induction of the Somogyi phenomenon (Figure 96–17). Therefore, reevaluation of serial glucose determinations after the insulin dosage is reduced is extremely important. Insulin dosage adjustments based on the morning concentration of glucose in the urine should be discontinued, and a fixed insulin dosage with afternoon urine checks should be initiated instead.

Rapid Metabolism of Insulin. In some diabetic dogs

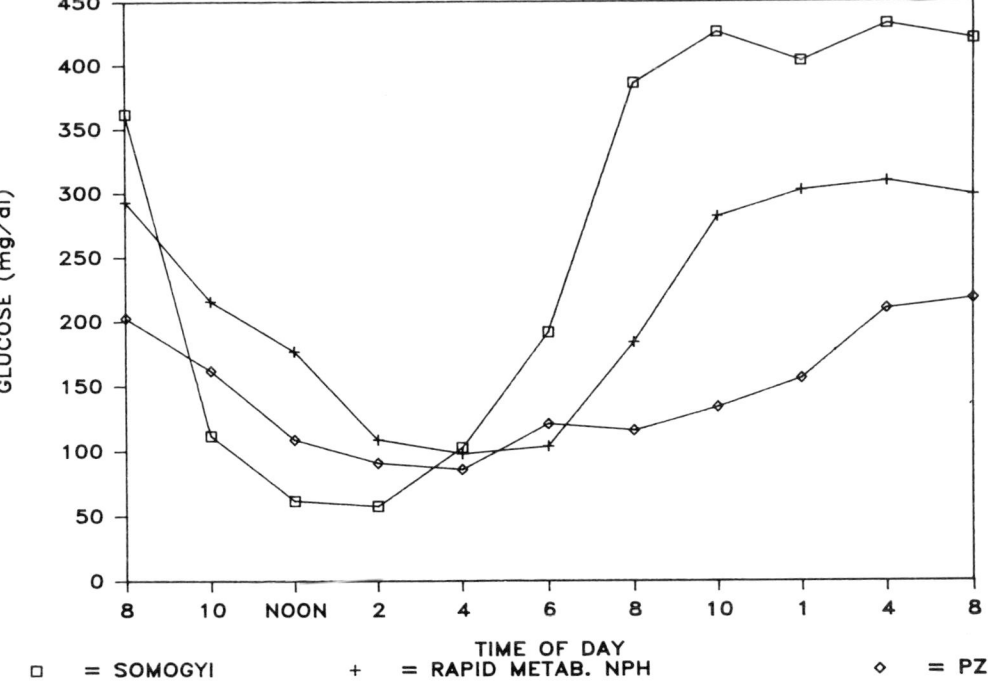

FIGURE 96–17. A 22-pound miniature poodle with insulin-induced hyperglycemia. On initial presentation, the owner was administering 28 units of NPH insulin once daily (squares). Following identification of the problem, the insulin was reduced to eight units of NPH insulin once daily (crosses), which revealed rapid insulin metabolism. The insulin was switched to PZI insulin once daily and finally fixed at 13 units once daily (diamonds). Insulin was given at 8 AM in each case. The dog was fed at 8 AM and 6 PM.

□ = SOMOGYI   + = RAPID METAB. NPH   ◇ = PZI

and cats the duration of effect of NPH insulin or PZI is considerably less than 24 hours. As a result, significant hyperglycemia (> 200 mg/dl) occurs for prolonged periods each day. This hyperglycemia may begin as early as eight hours after insulin administration. Diabetic dogs and cats that rapidly metabolize insulin will have persistent morning glycosuria (> 1 gm/dl on urine glucose test strips). Owners of these pets usually mention continuing problems with evening polyuria and polydipsia.

A diagnosis of rapid insulin metabolism is made by demonstrating significant hyperglycemia (> 200 mg/dl) within 18 hours or less of the insulin injection, while the lowest blood glucose concentration is maintained above 80 mg/dl. If owners are adjusting the daily insulin dosage based on the morning urine glucose concentration, they may increase the insulin dosage and cause insulin-induced hyperglycemia. Veterinarians who obtain single afternoon blood glucose determinations may find normal glucose concentrations or mild or severe hyperglycemia. Such findings may not be consistent with the worries of the owner, and thus become confusing to both owner and veterinarian. Therefore, diabetic dogs and cats that may not have an ideal duration of insulin action can be diagnosed only by determining serial blood glucose concentrations.

For the diabetic dog, if the duration of NPH insulin is between 16 and 20 hours, a switch to Lente insulin or PZI should be considered (Figure 96–17). In the author's experience, Lente is similar to NPH insulin, whereas PZI theoretically has a longer duration of action (i.e., 4 to 8 hours longer) when compared with NPH insulin. Many diabetic dogs, however, will also metabolize PZI in a similar manner to NPH insulin (Figure 96–18). As a general rule, the dose of PZI is approximately 25 per cent greater than that of NPH to achieve the same degree of effect. Therefore, the correct dosage should

be based on serial blood glucose determinations. The duration of effect and time of peak effect can thus be determined, and the insulin dosage and feeding schedule adjusted accordingly.

If the effect of NPH insulin lasts for 10 to 14 hours, then NPH insulin given twice a day should be considered. If the effect of NPH insulin lasts for less than ten hours, twice-daily administration of Lente insulin or PZI should be considered. Similar rules of thumb hold for the diabetic cat. However, the author initially gives most cats PZI, so the decision is usually whether to give PZI once or twice a day.

If insulin is administered twice each day, similar doses given at 12-hour intervals initially are recommended. Ideally, the dog or cat should be fed four meals—one at the time of each insulin administration and one two hours before each peak effect of the insulin. Each meal should be one fourth of the total daily caloric requirement. However, the owner's schedule must be considered and the treatment protocol altered to comply with what is feasible. Most owners who administer insulin twice daily feed two equal-sized meals, one immediately after each injection.

For the diabetic dog, twice-daily insulin injections can be crudely monitored by checking urine glucose concentrations before each insulin injection. The well-controlled diabetic dog that is treated with this regimen may have persistent negative tests for urine glucose. If the dog is clinically well and not symptomatic for hypoglycemia, the author recommends serial blood glucose determinations every two to four months. Dogs with persistent 1 or 2 per cent glycosuria may be overdosed or underdosed and should be brought to the veterinarian. Those with 1/10 per cent, 1/4 per cent or 1/2 per cent glycosuria are considered "adequately" controlled if they are not polyphagic, polyuric, and polydipsic.

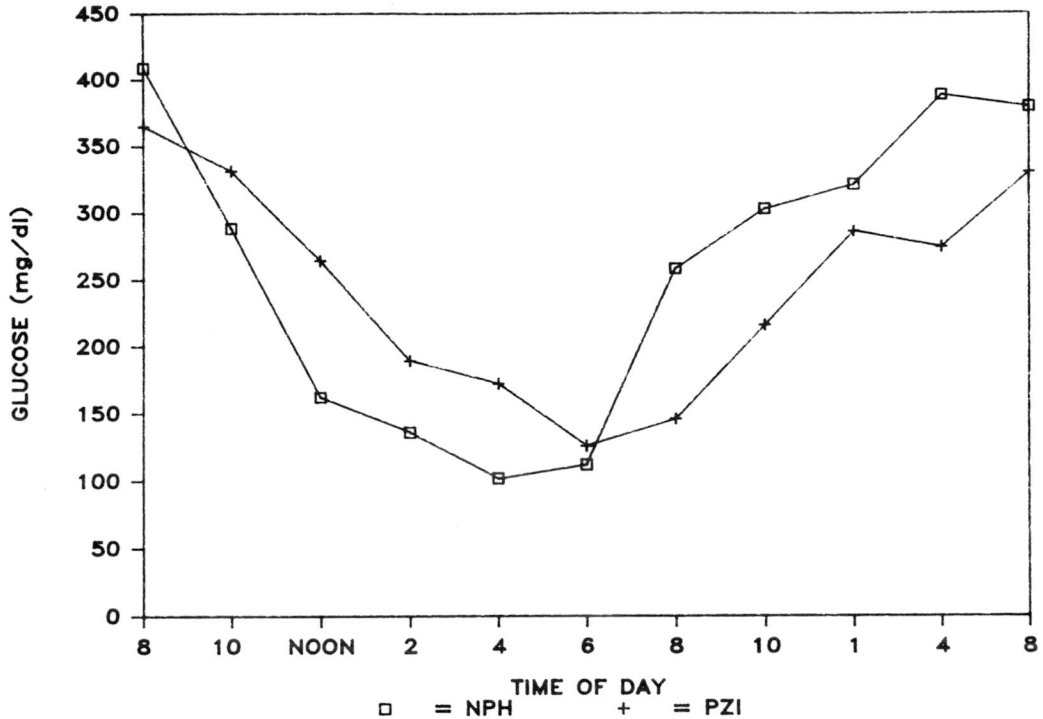

FIGURE 96–18. A 29-pound beagle with rapid insulin metabolism of both NPH and PZI insulin. 18 units of insulin was administered once daily at 8 AM in both instances. The dog was fed at 8 AM and 6 PM.

These dogs can be monitored with serial blood glucose determinations at the scheduled recheck. However, if the owners of such dogs do not believe that their dogs are well controlled, an earlier recheck is always advisable. Reevaluation of most cats on twice-daily insulin involves periodic serial glucose determinations in the hospital, although some owners will measure urine glucose concentrations.

Insulin Antagonism/Resistance. Insulin resistance implies peripheral antagonism to the effects of insulin. As a result, there is persistent hyperglycemia (> 300 mg/dl) and glycosuria, as well as continued polyuria, polydipsia, polyphagia, and weight loss, despite insulin therapy. Increasing the insulin dosage is ineffective in controlling these signs. Diabetic dogs and cats with this problem will often be receiving more than 1 unit of insulin per pound (2.2 units of insulin per kg) body weight. Recognized causes of insulin resistance in the dog and cat are listed in Table 96–6.

A diagnosis of insulin resistance is made by demonstrating either persistent hyperglycemia (> 300 mg/dl) on serial blood glucose studies with continuing inability to decrease the blood glucose concentration despite increasing the insulin dosage above 1 U/lb (2.2 U/kg) (Figure 96–19), or unusually high dosage requirements to obtain desired blood glucose concentrations. Endogenous hyperinsulinemia, rather than hypoinsulinemia, may be found, depending on the underlying cause. If insulin resistance and hyperinsulinemia are both present, and the cause for the insulin resistance can be corrected, permanent insulin-requiring diabetes mellitus may not develop.

Problems with the handling of insulin and with owner administration can result in serial blood glucose concen-

trations that resemble insulin resistance. The same is true if the animal is simply markedly underdosed. These causes should be adequately investigated before embarking on a diagnostic evaluation for insulin resistance. If an adequate dose of new insulin administered by the veterinarian, rather than the old insulin given by the owner, is still ineffective in decreasing the blood glucose concentration, a diagnostic evaluation for a cause for insulin resistance is justified.

Progesterone. If insulin resistance is diagnosed in an intact diabetic bitch, estrus or diestrus (with or without pregnancy) should be suspected. The serum progester-

TABLE 96–6. DIFFERENTIAL DIAGNOSIS FOR PERSISTENT HYPERGLYCEMIA DESPITE INSULIN THERAPY IN THE DIABETIC DOG AND CAT

Improper insulin administration
Inactive, outdated insulin
Rapid insulin metabolism
Insulin-induced hyperglycemia
Hyperadrenocorticism
   Spontaneous
   Iatrogenic
Elevation in progesterone
   Spontaneous (diestrus)
   Iatrogenic
Acromegaly
Pheochromocytoma
Improper feeding schedule
Improper food
Stress
   Infection
   Recurring pancreatitis
   Renal failure
   Cancer
Anti-insulin antibodies
Subcutaneous insulin degradation

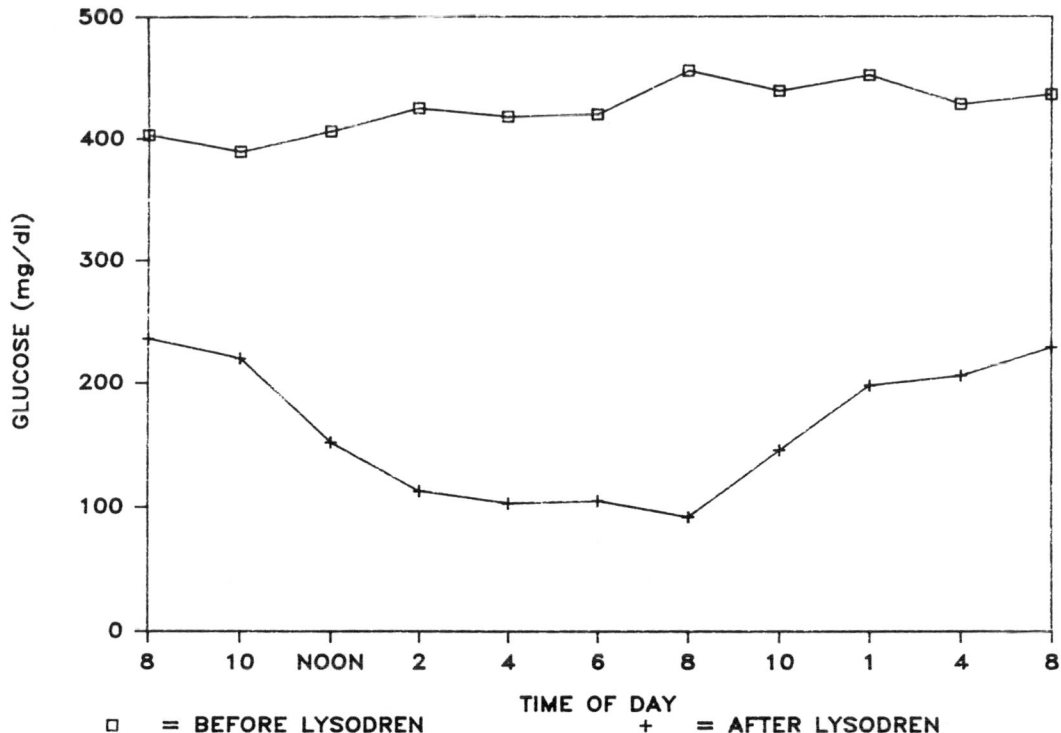

□ = BEFORE LYSODREN   + = AFTER LYSODREN

FIGURE 96–19. An 18-pound diabetic miniature schnauzer with pituitary-dependent hyperadrenocorticism and insulin resistance. On initial presentation, the owner was administering 25 units NPH insulin once daily (squares). Following the diagnosis and treatment of the hyperadrenocorticism with o,p′DDD, the insulin resistance resolved and the dog was eventually stabilized on 7 units NPH insulin once daily (crosses). Insulin was administered at 8 AM and the dog was fed at 8 AM and 6 PM.

one concentration will be increased above anestrus levels for two to three months after standing heat. This is believed to stimulate the secretion of GH, an insulin antagonist.[38, 127] Increased circulating GH concentrations appear to decrease the number of insulin receptors in cell membranes, alter the affinity of cell receptors for insulin, and possibly alter or inhibit postreceptor cellular reactions normally stimulated by insulin.[40, 128, 129] The resultant insulin antagonism may lead to poor control of a previously well-controlled diabetic dog or result in the appearance of signs of diabetes mellitus in a previously undiagnosed diabetic bitch. Several reviews of canine diabetes have revealed that if the intact bitch is prone to develop diabetes mellitus, she is likely to first show symptoms during estrus or diestrus.[130–132] Exogenous administration of progestogens, such as medroxyprogesterone acetate, also stimulates secretion of GH in dogs.[133] Diabetes mellitus in cats is also associated with megestrol acetate therapy, although the mechanism for inducing diabetes remains unclear.[134, 135]

If the owners are not certain of recent estrus activity, a serum progesterone determination will identify the presence of functioning corpora lutea. Ovariohysterectomy will result in a rapid decline in the serum progesterone and GH concentrations with subsequent loss of insulin resistance. An occasional diabetic bitch may no longer require insulin therapy either after being spayed or at the end of diestrus.

Glucocorticoids. Glucocorticoids promote hepatic gluconeogenesis, decrease peripheral tissue utilization of glucose, inhibit cellular receptor affinity for insulin, and exert a postreceptor influence that inhibits insulin action.[40, 129, 136] The resultant insulin resistance can occur with spontaneous hyperadrenocorticism or exogenous steroid administration (Figure 96–19).[36, 137] Careful questioning of the owner for recent glucocorticoid administration or recent "unknown" shots given by another veterinarian may explain the difficulties in diabetic control.

Unfortunately polyuria, polydipsia, and polyphagia are common owner complaints for both diabetes mellitus and hyperadrenocorticism. Some dogs and cats with both diseases will not initially have other clinical signs consistent with hyperadrenocorticism (e.g., truncal alopecia, abdominal distention). Therefore, a high index of suspicion for hyperadrenocorticism should be maintained in a diabetic dog or cat that requires large doses of insulin (> 1 U/lb/day or > 2.2 U/kg/day). An ACTH stimulation test and a low-dose dexamethasone screening test should be performed to diagnose spontaneous or iatrogenic hyperadrenocorticism.

With appropriate medical or surgical therapy, as well as discontinuation of exogenous glucocorticoid administration, plasma glucocorticoid concentrations will decline, insulin antagonism will resolve, and the daily insulin dosage will decrease (Figure 96–19). Diabetic dogs with hyperadrenocorticism that are treated with o,p′-DDD, may be prone to the development of hypoglycemia as a result of loss of peripheral insulin antagonism, decreased hepatic gluconeogenesis, and inappropriately high insulin dosages. A more gradual decline in plasma glucocorticoid concentrations may be obtained by decreasing the initial induction dosage of o,p'-DDD from 23 mg/lb to 12 to 16 mg/lb (50 mg/kg to 25 to 35 mg/kg), thereby minimizing the chances of hypoglycemia. In addition, afternoon urine glucose concentrations should be measured daily to help the owner identify when the insulin antagonism is resolving. As long as the afternoon urine glucose concentrations remain at 1 or 2 per cent, insulin antagonism can be assumed to be present. A negative urine glucose is an indication for immediate reduction in the insulin dose. Once the hyperadrenocorticism is controlled, regulation of the diabetic dog or cat should be done, based on serial glucose determinations.

Growth Hormone. As previously discussed, GH is believed to mediate the insulin antagonistic actions of progesterone. Excessive GH secretion (i.e., acromegaly) can also result from a functional tumor of the pituitary somatotrophs, a syndrome that has been described in several aged diabetic cats with insulin antagonism.[138, 139] A diagnosis should rely on evaluation of a basal GH concentration and the demonstration of a pituitary mass by means of computerized tomography (Figure 96–20). If the excessive GH concentrations can be controlled, the insulin antagonism will resolve (Figure 96–21).

Glucagon. Glucagon stimulates gluconeogenesis, glycogenolysis, and ketogenesis and decreases the affinity of cell receptors for insulin.[40] Hyperglucagonemia may be associated with bacterial infections, trauma, congestive heart failure, azotemia, and functioning tumors of the α cells of the islets of the pancreas or gastrointestinal tract (i.e., glucagonoma).[140, 141] Glucagonomas are rare tumors in humans and have not been reported in dogs or cats. In humans glucagon-secreting tumors are characterized by anemia, a rash referred to as necrolytic migratory erythema, glucose intolerance, and/or diabetes mellitus.[142] A definitive diagnosis requires documentation of hyperglucagonemia. With correction of the underlying problem, plasma glucagon concentrations should decline and the insulin antagonism resolve.

Renal Failure and/or Acidosis. Severe renal insufficiency may result in insulin antagonism and carbohydrate intolerance owing to hyperglucagonemia, decreased concentrations of insulin receptors, defective transport of glucose into cells, and metabolic acidosis.[141, 143, 144] Acidosis may decrease the affinity of insulin receptors for insulin and result in deranged intracellular glycolysis.[145, 146]

Catecholamines. Epinephrine/norepinephrine stimulates hepatic glycogenolysis, inhibits insulin secretion, and stimulates glucagon secretion.[120, 121, 147] Excessive secretion of epinephrine/norepinephrine is most commonly associated with pheochromocytoma. Clinical signs develop either as a result of the space-occupying nature of the tumor and its metastases, or as a result of excessive secretion of catecholamines. Most of the signs related to catecholamine excess are believed to result after the development of systemic hypertension. Common clinical signs observed in 31 dogs with pheochromocytoma included weakness, anorexia, vomiting, weight loss, and panting.[5] The diagnosis of pheochromocytoma can be tentatively established by biochemical or pharmacologic tests that demonstrate excessive production of catecholamines or their metabolites (i.e.,

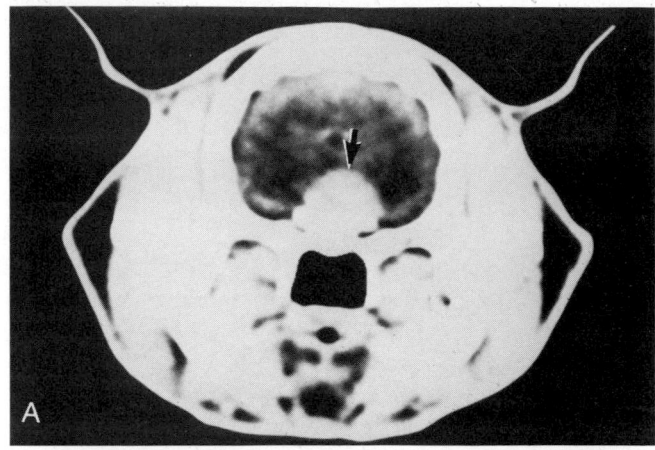

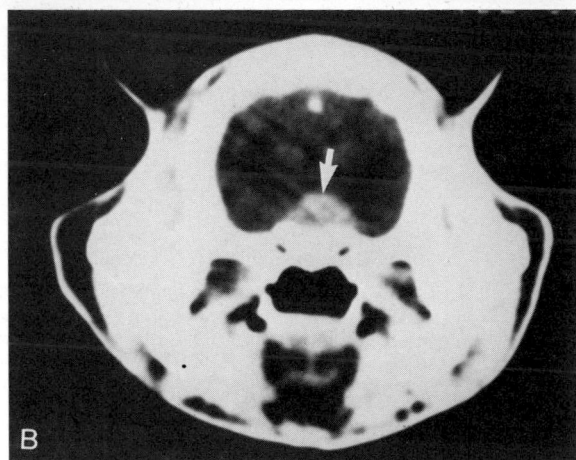

FIGURE 96–20. *A*, CT scan of the pituitary region of a 13-year-old male castrated cat with diabetes mellitus and acromegaly. A basal GH concentration was 54 ng/ml (normal, < 5 ng/ml). A mass is evident in the pituitary region following the intravenous administration of a positive contrast agent (arrow). *B*, CT scan of the same cat pictured in *A* two months after completion of cobalt radiation therapy. A basal GH concentration at this time was 7 ng/ml. Although pooling of the contrast agent is still evident (arrow), the mass has decreased in size by more than 50 per cent. (From Feldman, EC and Nelson, RW: Canine and Feline Endocrinology and Reproduction. Philadelphia, WB Saunders, 1987, p 44).

metanephrine, normetanephrine, vanillylmandelic acid), by radiographic, ultrasonographic, or computer tomographic demonstration of an adrenal mass, or by means of exploratory surgery.

Excessive catecholamine secretion may also play a role in creating an insulin antagonistic glucose curve in the extremely fractious or hyperexcitable dog or cat in which insulin is actually effective in the home environment. For these animals, the author relies on owner observation for signs of poor regulation and the measurement of urine glucose concentrations at home. If clinical signs of diabetes are not evident, the urine glucose is negative in the home environment, but an insulin antagonism glucose curve is generated in the hospital, excessive catecholamine secretion induced by the hospital environment should be suspected.

Anti-insulin Antibodies. Because insulin is a protein, prolonged administration may result in anti-insulin antibody production and insulin resistance. Therapy with conventional insulin has been associated with the formation of insulin antibodies in human diabetics.[148] How-

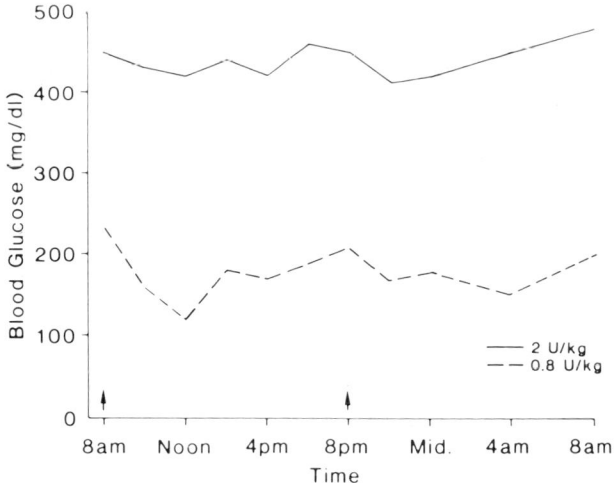

FIGURE 96–21. A 13-pound diabetic cat with acromegaly and insulin resistance (see Figure 96–20). On initial presentation, the owner was administering 12 units PZI insulin twice daily (———). Following the diagnosis and treatment of the pituitary mass with cobalt radiation, the insulin resistance resolved and the cat was stabilized on five units PZI insulin twice daily (– –). Insulin was administered at 8 AM and 8 PM.

ever, the development of insulin resistance as a result of insulin antibody formation is relatively uncommon.[149] The most common commercially available insulin preparations are a combination of beef and pork insulins. The amino acid sequence of pork and canine insulins is identical; however, the amino acids at positions 8 and 10 of the A chain are different in the cow versus the dog.[40] The immunogenic sites on the insulin molecule are amino acids 8 to 11 on the A chain and 3 and 30 on the B chain.[150] Therefore, beef insulin injected into the dog is potentially antigenic and could result in antibody production and the development of insulin resistance.

Anti-insulin antibody production was consistently documented in a group of dogs with IDDM that were receiving beef-pork insulin, however, the amount of antigenicity associated with beef-pork insulin was not significant enough to cause problems.[151] Anti-insulin antibodies were not detected in dogs with IDDM that were receiving pork insulin. Subjectively and objectively, however, pure pork insulin tended to be quicker in onset but briefer in duration of action than beef-pork insulin. On a clinical basis, the beef-pork insulins are easier to use and, as a general rule, are preferred for the treatment of diabetes mellitus. Only if other potential causes of insulin antagonism have been ruled out should a switch to pure pork insulin be done.

Synthetic insulin (Humilin) with a structure identical to human insulin is now commercially available. It is produced either by chemical synthesis, exchanging the terminal alanine at position B30 of pork insulin for the threonine found in that position in human insulin, or by recombinant DNA techniques. The biologic effects of pork insulin and synthetic human insulins are essentially identical.[152] Theoretically the human hormone should be less antigenic, but this has not proved of clinical importance.[153] Although studies that involve the dog and cat have yet to be reported, there is probably little advantage in using the synthetic insulins over purified pork

insulin in dogs and cats with undetermined insulin antagonism.

Antibodies directed against the insulin receptor on the cell membrane are a rare cause of insulin resistance in diabetic humans and have not been reported in the dog or cat.[154, 155] In humans, this form of insulin resistance is usually associated with other, concomitant immunologic abnormalities, such as systemic lupus erythematosus and acanthosis nigricans.

Subcutaneous Degradation. Insensitivity to subcutaneously deposited insulin but normal sensitivity after IV administration is a rare cause of insulin antagonism in humans.[156, 157] This syndrome is thought to be related to excessive protease activity in the subcutaneous tissue, resulting in excessive degradation of insulin at the site of injection.[158, 159] Insulin degradation at the site of injection would decrease the amount of insulin available for absorption, thereby lowering plasma insulin concentrations. Measurement of blood insulin concentrations in conjunction with blood glucose concentrations after SQ insulin administration will allow a differentiation between impaired insulin absorption and insulin receptor/postreceptor abnormalities (Figure 96–22). Therapy for this form of insulin antagonism has involved the use of alternative routes of insulin delivery, additives (e.g., aprotinin) to prevent the enzymatic degradation of insulin, and medications to increase circulation in subcutaneous tissues.[160]

Hypoglycemia. One of the most common complications associated with insulin therapy is hypoglycemia. If the diabetic dog or cat receives too much insulin or exercises too strenuously, severe hypoglycemia may occur before the diabetogenic hormones (i.e., glucagon, cortisol, epinephrine, and GH) are able to compensate for and reverse the low sugar level. Signs of hypoglycemia include weakness, lethargy, shaking, head tilting, ataxia, convulsions, and coma. Occurrence of clinical signs is thought to depend on the rate of decline of plasma glucose as well as on the degree of hypoglycemia. As plasma glucose decreases, areas of the brain with the highest metabolic rate (i.e., the cerebral cortex) are affected first, while areas with the lowest metabolic rate (i.e., brain stem nuclei) are affected last. Therefore, the initial clinical signs are cortical in origin and include disorientation, weakness, and hunger. With progressive hypoglycemia, convulsions and coma occur. If hypoglycemia is prolonged, death may occur from depression of the respiratory centers.

If mild signs of hypoglycemia occur, the animal should be fed its normal food. If severe signs are present, or if convulsions occur, IV dextrose or oral sugar water (e.g., Karo syrup) rubbed on the buccal mucosa should be given until the convulsions stop. Fluid should not be forced down the mouth of a convulsing animal, nor should fingers be placed inside the mouth. Once the animal is conscious and sternal, food should be offered. Whenever signs of hypoglycemia occur, the insulin dose needs to be decreased. Serial blood glucose determinations should be used to make appropriate insulin dosage adjustments.

White recently reported a series of nine human diabetic patients who were having problems with severe hypoglycemia in whom deficient secretion of the coun-

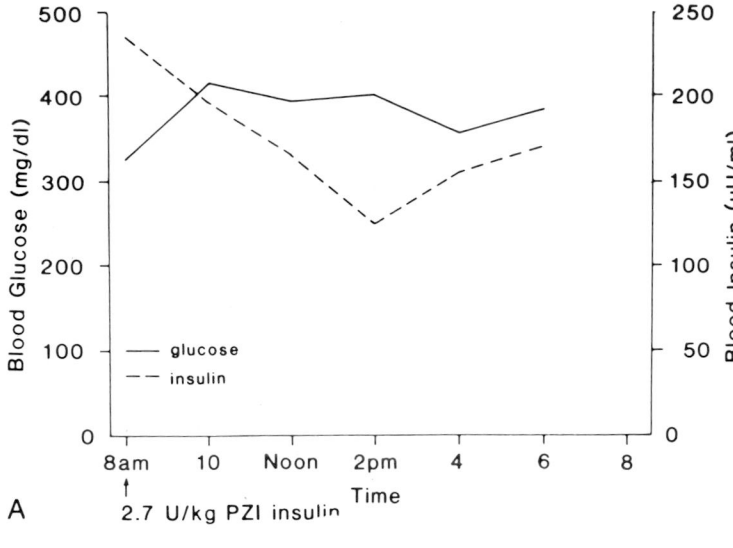

A

2.7 U/kg PZI insulin

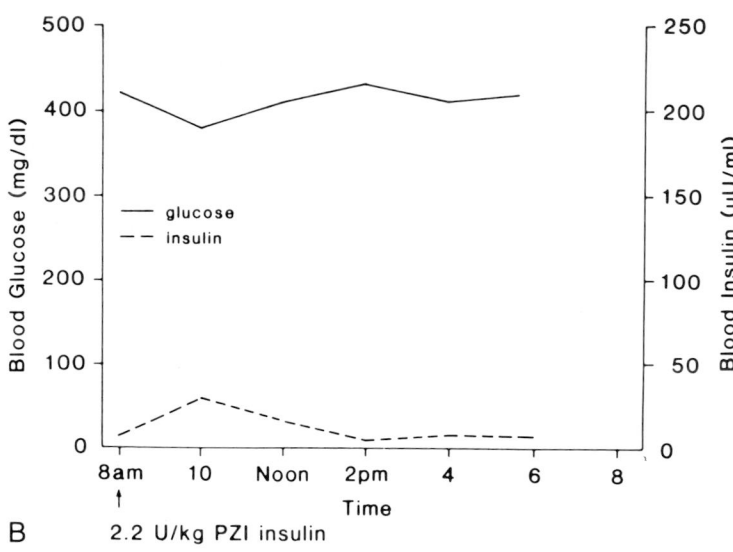

B

2.2 U/kg PZI insulin

FIGURE 96–22. Blood glucose and insulin concentrations following insulin administration in two dogs with diabetes mellitus and apparent insulin antagonism. For both dogs, insulin was given SC at 8 AM and they were fed at 8 AM and 6 PM. *A,* A 20 pound mixed-breed dog given 25 units PZI. The increased blood insulin concentrations with no apparent effect on blood glucose would imply a receptor/postreceptor problem. *B,* A 32 pound mixed-breed dog given 32 units PZI. The low blood insulin concentrations would imply problems with absorption or rapid degradation of the insulin.

terregulatory hormones was present.[161] As a result, when the blood glucose concentration approached 60 mg/dl, there was no compensatory response by the body to attempt to increase the blood sugar, and prolonged hypoglycemia ensued. A similar problem should be considered in a dog or cat with IDDM that is exquisitely sensitive to small doses of insulin.

Diabetic Complications

Cataracts. Cataract formation is the most common and one of the most important long-term complications associated with diabetes mellitus in the dog but is rare in the cat. The rate of onset of diabetic cataracts in rats has been demonstrated to be directly related to the degree of hyperglycemia.[162] The incidence of cataracts in diabetic dogs is quite high because many of these patients have significant hyperglycemia despite insulin therapy. Indeed, the majority of canine patients are maintained on insulin doses that result in mild hyperglycemia and glycosuria. Occasionally the initial presenta-

tion of the dog is not for the systemic manifestations of diabetes mellitus, but for sudden development of cataracts and blindness.

The pathogenesis of diabetic cataract formation is thought to be related to altered osmotic relations in the lens. The lens of the eye is freely permeable to glucose, which enters the lens from the aqueous humor by facilitated transport. In the normal lens the glucose concentration is approximately 10 per cent of the blood glucose level and is converted to lactic acid by way of the anaerobic glycolytic pathway. In the presence of elevated glucose concentrations, the glycolytic enzymes become saturated. Glucose is then metabolized through the sorbitol pathway, with the production of sorbitol occurring by the action of the enzyme aldose reductase. Sorbitol is then converted to fructose by the enzyme sorbitol dehydrogenase.[163] Although glucose is freely permeable to the cell membrane, sorbitol and fructose are not. As a result, they act as potent hydrophilic agents, causing an influx of water into the lens, which leads to swelling and rupture of the lens fibers and the development of cataracts.

Cataract formation is an irreversible process once it begins, and the development of cataracts can occur quite rapidly. Clinically, dogs may progress from having normal vision to being blind over a period of days to months. The owner of a diabetic pet should be made aware of the high probability of cataract formation. Good glycemic control decreases the likelihood of cataracts, whereas blindness caused by cataracts reduces the need for stringent blood glucose control. The blindness may be corrected by removing the abnormal lens, assuming the retina is functioning normally.[164] Experimental work with aldose reductase inhibitors, primarily sorbinil, shows promise for the future prevention of cataract formation by inhibiting the production of sorbitol within the lens.[165]

Retinopathy. Diabetic retinopathy is an uncommon complication in the dog and cat, presumably because of their relatively short lifespan after the development of diabetes mellitus. In human diabetics less than 10 per cent develop retinal changes during the first 10 years of the disease, whereas 95 per cent develop retinopathies within 25 years of the initial development of the disease.[166] The onset of the retinal changes appears to be related to the severity and duration of the diabetes. Engerman and associates found a reduced incidence of retinal disease in diabetic dogs with good glycemic control versus diabetic dogs with poor regulation.[167] Microaneurysms, hemorrhages, and varicose and shunt capillaries may be observed with an ophthalmoscope.[168] Histologic changes include an increased thickness of the capillary basement membrane, loss of pericytes, capillary shunts, and microaneurysms. The histologic changes are believed to be a response to retinal ischemia. Increased red blood cell and platelet aggregation causes sluggish blood flow, decreased oxygen delivery, and microinfarction.[169] Unfortunately the rapid development of cataracts often inhibits the ability to evaluate the retina in the dog with diabetes mellitus. Because of the high incidence of cataract formation, the retinas should always be evaluated in the newly diagnosed diabetic pet to ensure normal function and lack of grossly visible disease, if cataract formation and subsequent lens removal should become necessary in the future. Lens removal would be unwarranted in a diabetic dog with retinal changes sufficiently severe to result in blindness itself. An electroretinogram can also be used to evaluate the function of the retina before cataract surgery.

Pancreatitis. Destruction of pancreatic islet cells by inflammatory disease of the exocrine pancreas is one cause of diabetes mellitus.[170] In addition, the hyperlipemia and poor diet associated with some dogs with diabetes mellitus may induce pancreatitis.[171] Unfortunately pancreatitis is often a chronic, smoldering disease, which periodically results in clinical signs, such as abdominal pain, vomiting, and anorexia. It is not unusual for dogs with diabetes mellitus to suffer from periodic bouts of pancreatitis, sometimes severe, requiring intensive fluid therapy and a controlled diet. In fact, the author has several diabetic dogs that must remain on a controlled low-fat diet (low-fat cottage cheese and rice or kibbled dog food and rice) to prevent clinical recurrence of pancreatitis. Some diabetic dogs die or are eventually euthanized because of intractable pancreatitis.

Hepatic Lipidosis. Hepatic lipidosis is commonly encountered in the unregulated or poorly regulated diabetic dog or cat. It is a direct consequence of insulin deficiency and resultant expansion of hepatic triglyceride stores. Hypoinsulinemia results in increased release of free fatty acids from adipose tissue, thus providing increased substrate for hepatic triglyceride synthesis.[172] Insulin deficiency also decreases triglyceride secretion by the liver, allowing further accumulation of lipids in the liver.[173] Hepatomegaly is a frequent finding on physical examination. Hepatic lipidosis is partially reversible with good glycemic control of the diabetes mellitus. Additional management should include prevention of excessive caloric intake and the feeding of adequate protein to maintain adequate lipoprotein synthesis for transporting lipids from the liver. The diabetic has not lost the ability to synthesize lipoproteins for mobilization of fats from the liver;[174] therefore, providing the necessary protein to ensure lipoprotein synthesis should help to mobilize the hepatic triglycerides. The use of lipotrophic agents, such as choline and methionine, is of little, if any, value in humans with well-regulated diabetes,[175] and is probably not indicated in the management of canine or feline hepatic lipidosis resulting from diabetes mellitus.

Ketoacidosis. Insulin-requiring diabetic dogs and cats are prone to the development of DKA and its associated systemic manifestations. Ketoacidosis may develop in a previously well-controlled diabetic dog or cat during periods of illness, chronic stress, or estrus. Secretion of the diabetogenic hormones results in insulin antagonism, ineffective insulin actions, and the eventual development of ketonemia. Inappropriate insulin administration or the use of inactivated insulin may also result in the development of DKA. Frequent owner checking of the urine with reagent strips for the presence of ketones is an effective way to identify the presence of ketonuria and thus ketonemia. The occasional presence of small amounts of ketones in the urine should not cause concern as long as the dog or cat is not systemically ill. However, persistent ketonuria is an indication that the injected insulin is not providing adequate control. If persistent ketonuria is present, the dog or cat should be evaluated by the veterinarian to determine the underlying cause. If ketonuria and ketonemia go unrecognized, systemic signs of illness will eventually develop, requiring the immediate attention of a veterinarian.

Bacterial Infections. Concurrent bacterial infections are common with the initial presentation of a diabetic dog or cat to the veterinarian. Diabetics also are prone to the development of infections in the future, especially if the blood glucose concentration is poorly controlled. Bacterial infections may induce ketoacidosis as a result of stimulation of secretion of glucagon, an insulin antagonist.[140] Soler and colleagues found that 28 per cent of cases of recent-onset ketoacidosis in human diabetics were due to bacterial infections,[176] whereas Muller and coworkers found 77 per cent of cases to be due to infections.[177] Bacterial infections should be suspected in any diabetic dog or cat that suddenly develops DKA. In the author's experience, the most common sites of infection in the diabetic dog and cat are the urinary tract, pulmonary system, and skin. The author routinely performs a complete blood count, urinalysis, and bacterial culture of urine obtained by cystocentesis in any diabetic dog or cat with ketonemia.

There are many proposed mechanisms for the increased susceptibility to infections in diabetics. These mechanisms include: (1) decreased blood supply secondary to the associated microangiopathy and atherosclerosis, resulting in decreased delivery of oxygen, phagocytes, and antibodies to the site of infection, (2) impaired humoral immunity, resulting in decreased antibody production, (3) abnormal chemotaxis of neutrophils, (4) defects in the phagocytosis and intracellular killing of organisms and (5) impaired cell-mediated immunity.[178-184] Many of these host defense abnormalities improve, at least partially, with better glycemic control.

Diabetic Neuropathy. Although diabetic neuropathies are the most common complication in humans with diabetes mellitus, they are rarely reported in the dog and cat.[185-187] Subclinical neuropathy is probably more common than severe neuropathy resulting in clinical signs.[188] Clinical signs supportive of a coexistent neuropathy in the diabetic dog or cat include weakness, knuckling, muscle atrophy, depressed limb reflexes, and deficits in postural reaction testing.[186, 187] In the dog it is primarily a distal polyneuropathy, characterized by segmental demyelination/remyelination and axonal degeneration/regeneration.[189] Electrophysiologic testing may reveal fibrillation potentials and positive sharp waves, suggesting denervated muscle, and occasionally fasciculation potentials and bizarre high-frequency discharges.[188] There also is a decrease in motor and sensory nerve conduction velocities.

The etiopathogenesis of diabetic neuropathy is poorly understood. In humans, mononeuropathies are believed to result from vascular dysfunction, whereas symmetrical polyneuropathies and autonomic neuropathies, such as diabetic diarrhea and gastric paresis, are believed to be due to metabolic derangements.[185] Polyneuropathies appear to be the most common neuropathy in the canine diabetic. The primary abnormality appears to be an axonal degeneration, resulting in a "dying back" neuropathy, with distal portions of the neuron most severely involved. The metabolic derangement may be related to excessive sorbitol accumulation within the Schwann cells, resulting in impaired nerve conduction. This would explain the improved nerve conduction velocity in a group of diabetic humans with polyneuropathy treated with the aldose reductase inhibitor sorbinil.[190] There is currently no specific therapy for the neuropathic signs other than to maintain good glycemic control, although the future use of aldose reductase inhibitors may hold promise.[191] The reversibility of the neuropathy is variable and spontaneous; it does not appear to be under the influence of metabolic control of the diabetes mellitus per se.[185, 192]

Diabetic Nephropathy. Although diabetic nephropathy has occasionally been reported in the dog,[63-65, 193] its incidence appears to be relatively low. This may be due, in part, to the presence of concurrent oliguric or anuric renal failure in addition to diabetes mellitus and DKA, resulting in death of the animal before therapy can be instituted. The author has seen several diabetic ketoacidotic animals develop or present with concurrent oliguric renal failure and die within one to two days after presentation. In many of these animals glomerulosclerosis was found on histologic examination of the kidneys.

Histopathologic findings in diabetic nephropathy depend on the duration of the disease before evaluation of the dog or cat and on the degree of glycemic control. Histologic findings consistent with diabetic nephropathy include membranous glomerulonephropathy with fusion of the foot processes, glomerular and tubular basement membrane thickening, an increase in the mesangial matrix material, the presence of subendothelial deposits, and glomerular fibrosis.[63, 65, 193, 195]

Clinical signs depend on the severity of the glomerulosclerosis and the functional ability of the kidney to excrete metabolic wastes. Diabetic nephropathy is initially manifested as severe proteinuria, primarily albuminuria, as a result of the glomerular dysfunction.[65, 195] As the glomerular changes progress, glomerular filtration becomes progressively impaired, resulting in the development of azotemia and, eventually, uremia. With severe fibrosis of the glomeruli, oliguric and then anuric renal failure develop.

The development of renal insufficiency secondary to the glomerular pathology may result in prolonged insulin action owing to impaired insulin degradation.[196] Severe renal insufficiency may also result in insulin antagonism.[143] The progression of the glomerulosclerosis is related to the degree of glycemic control. There appears to be a definite decrease in the incidence of the glomerular microvascular changes with improved glycemic control.[197, 198]

Islet Cell Transplantation

Although the life expectancy of humans with IDDM has considerably improved since the introduction of exogenous insulin, SQ administered insulin exhibits nonphysiologic pharmacokinetics and fails to reproduce the stimulus-coupled pulsatile secretory responses of normal β cells. The consequence is an altered state of metabolism that contributes to the complications associated with the disease. During the last decade, remarkable advances have been made in islet cell transplantation. Increasing experimental evidence has shown that transplantation of the endocrine pancreas can normalize blood glucose levels and result in physiologic insulin secretion.[199] The problem of rejection remains the biggest obstacle to successful transplantation. Current research efforts are centered around the prevention of rejection by immunomodulation of the graft and the recipient or by isolation of allografted islets from the host immune system, and therapeutic strategies to prevent recurrence of the autoimmune process in the transplanted islet tissue.

If an attempt is not made to alter islet immunogenicity or the host immune response, islet allografts will normally be rejected in five to ten days in all animal species, depending to some degree on the site of transplantation and the histocompatibility barrier.[200] Islet immunogenicity may be diminished by deleting resident immunostimulatory nonendocrine cells without destroying the endocrine secretory cells. This can be accomplished through short-term tissue-culturing techniques, treatment of islets with monoclonal antibody and complement directed against the immunostimulatory cells, or use of ultraviolet radiation alone or in conjunction with cyclosporine.[201-204]

Cyclosporine A, a relatively new immunosuppressive drug, has been used to alter the host immune response to the transplant. Cyclosporine A interferes with the initial T-cell activation process by inhibiting the synthesis of interleukin-2, but spares the generation of antigen-specific suppressor cells, allowing the development of an active mechanism of suppression.[205, 206] Short-term cyclosporine A therapy has been shown to prolong survival of highly purified islet allografts and induce a state of immune unresponsiveness to islet alloantigens in dogs with experimental diabetes.[207]

Even with alteration of the immunogenicity of islets and the immune responsiveness of the recipient sufficiently to prevent rejection, transplanted islets may still be destroyed by the ongoing autoimmune process (i.e., isletitis) in humans (and possibly dogs) with IDDM.[208, 209] To circumvent islet-directed alloimmunity and autoimmunity, procedures are being developed to immuno-isolate islets in microcapsules that present a physical barrier between the islet graft and the host's immune system.[210, 211] The artificial biomembranes must be biocompatible with the recipient, have permeability characteristics that facilitate the movement of nutrients and hormones across the membrane, and be a barrier to the passage of mediators of immune destruction. The success of this approach would undoubtedly also facilitate the use of xenografts as a source of donor islets.

Much of this experimental work is being done in dogs, which is of obvious interest to us as veterinarians. Although long-term (i.e., years) success has been documented in dogs, especially with autograft techniques,[212] islet transplantation currently remains an investigational technique.

INSULIN-SECRETING ISLET CELL NEOPLASIA

Etiology

Functional tumors of the β cells of the pancreatic islets secrete insulin or proinsulin independent of the suppressive effects typically associated with hypoglycemia. β cell tumors, however, are not completely autonomous, and respond to provocative stimuli (e.g., glucagon) by secreting insulin, often in excessive amounts. Immunohistochemical analysis of β cell tumors has revealed a high incidence of multihormonal production, including pancreatic polypeptide, somatostatin, glucagon, serotonin, and gastrin.[213] Insulin, however, has been the most common product demonstrated within the neoplastic cells, and clinical signs are primarily a result of the effects of hyperinsulinemia.

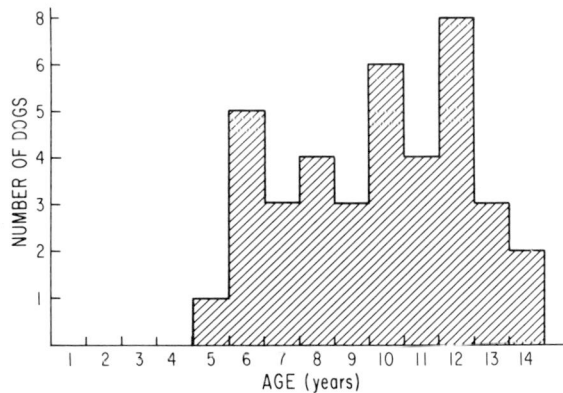

FIGURE 96–23. Age of 36 dogs at the time of initial diagnosis of an insulin-secreting islet-cell tumor.

Signalment

Insulin-secreting tumors typically occur in the middle-aged or older dog, with an age range of 6 to 14 years (Figure 96–23). There is no apparent sex predilection.[214, 215] Various breeds are suggested to have a higher incidence of insulin-secreting tumors than would be predicted simply by breed popularity. These include the standard poodle, Boxer, fox terrier, German shepherd, and Irish setter.[214-217] Because of the wide variety of breeds in which this diagnosis has been confirmed (Table 96-7), a diagnosis of an insulin-secreting tumor should not be excluded because of breed alone.

A Siamese cat with an insulin-secreting tumor has been described; however, this remains a rare diagnosis in cats. Insulin-secreting tumors have also been documented in ferrets.[218-221]

Pathophysiology

The β cells of the pancreatic islets are primarily responsible for monitoring and controlling the blood glucose concentration. Unlike most other cells, entrance of glucose into β cells is independent of insulin. When blood glucose concentrations exceed approximately 110 mg/dl, insulin is secreted and the blood glucose concen-

TABLE 96–7. BREED DISTRIBUTION OF 25 DOGS WITH ISLET CELL TUMORS

Breed	No. of Dogs	(%)
German shepherd	5	(20)
German shepherd-X	2	(8)
Irish setter	4	(16)
Collie	2	(8)
Collie-X	1	(4)
Golden retriever	2	(8)
Poodle	2	(8)
Samoyed	2	(8)
West Highland white terrier	1	(4)
Wire-haired pointing griffon	1	(4)
Weimaraner	1	(4)
Labrador retriever	1	(4)
Boxer	1	(4)

From Kruth, SA, et al.: Insulin-secreting islet cell tumors: Establishing a diagnosis and the clinical course of 25 dogs. JAVMA 181:54, 1982.

X, mixed-breed dog

tration declines into the normal physiologic range. When blood glucose concentrations decrease below 60 mg/dl, insulin secretion is normally depressed, thus limiting continued tissue utilization of glucose and increasing the blood glucose concentration back into the normal physiologic range.[222]

Insulin-secreting tumors and the associated hyperinsulinemia interfere with glucose homeostasis by decreasing the rate of glucose release from the liver and by increasing the uptake of glucose by insulin-sensitive tissues. Insulin interferes with mechanisms that promote hepatic glucose output by limiting circulating concentrations of substrates needed for gluconeogenesis. This effect is accomplished by inhibiting enzymes necessary for mobilizing amino acids from muscle and glycerol from adipose tissue. In addition, insulin decreases the activity of hepatic enzymes utilized in gluconeogenesis and glycogenolysis.[223] Insulin also lowers blood glucose concentrations by stimulating glucose uptake and utilization in liver, muscle, and adipose tissue. Thus insulin increases tissue utilization of glucose present within the extracellular space, while interfering with hepatic production of glucose. The net effect is promotion of hypoglycemia and a reduction of fuel available to the CNS.

Glucose is the primary fuel utilized by the CNS. Carbohydrate reserves in neural tissue are quite limited, and normal function by these cells depends on a continuous supply of glucose from sources outside the CNS. If the blood glucose concentration drops below a critical level, nervous system dysfunction occurs. In mammals the cerebral cortex is the first area to be affected by a critical shortage of glucose. The metabolically slower vegetative centers in the brain stem have less demand for blood glucose and are affected after the cerebral cortex.

Glucose entrance into the neurons of the CNS primarily occurs by diffusion and is not insulin-dependent. Therefore, blood insulin concentrations do not affect neuronal glucose utilization. However, if hyperinsulinemia results in an inadequate glucose supply for intracellular oxidative processes within neurons, there is a resultant decline in energy-rich phosphorylated compounds (adenosine triphosphate) within the cell. This, in turn, results in cellular changes typical of hypoxia, with increased vascular permeability, vasospasm, vascular dilatation, and edema. Neuron death from anoxia follows. In acute hypoglycemia histologic alterations are most marked in the cerebral cortex, basal ganglia, hippocampus, and vasomotor centers.[224] Although most of the damage from hypoglycemia occurs in the brain, peripheral nerve degeneration and demyelination are sometimes encountered.[40, 225] Other major organ systems, such as the heart, kidneys, and liver, also depend on glucose. However, an acute decrease in blood glucose concentration will result in clinical signs that involve the CNS before signs of any other major organ system dysfunction become apparent.[40]

Prolonged, severe hypoglycemia may result in irreversible brain damage; however, it is rare for a dog to die during a hypoglycemic episode. Hypoglycemia is a potent stimulus for the release of the diabetogenic hormones that function to antagonize the effects of

insulin and stimulate an increase in blood glucose concentrations. The temporal relation between the elevations in these hormones and the reversal of the effects of insulin on glucose kinetics suggest that catecholamines and glucagon exert the major counterregulatory influence.[117, 226, 227] A normal glucose rebound after insulin-induced hypoglycemia has been observed in adrenalectomized patients and in those animals with cervical cord transection or thoracolumbar sympathectomy, emphasizing the importance of other mechanisms, especially glucagon, in the counterregulatory response.[226, 228] Overall, the data suggest that under normal circumstances, both adrenal medullary secretion and sympathetic nervous system activity are stimulated and are responsible, in part, for the reversal of acute hypoglycemia.[229]

The clinical manifestations of hypoglycemia are believed to result from both a lack of glucose supply to the brain (neuroglycopenia) and stimulation of the sympathoadrenal system. The neuroglycopenic signs common to dogs include lethargy, weakness, ataxia, bizarre behavior, convulsions, and coma (Table 96–8). The signs resulting from stimulation of the sympathoadrenal system consist of muscle tremors, nervousness, restlessness, and hunger. In humans, the symptoms related to an elevation in circulating catecholamines often precede those of neuroglycopenia and act as an early warning sign of an impending hypoglycemic attack. This illustrates the rapid response of catecholamine secretion to hypoglycemia and, in part, explains why canine patients with insulin-secreting tumors do not always progress to generalized seizure activity during a fast.[223, 229]

Clinical manifestations depend on the duration, as well as the severity, of hypoglycemia. Animals with chronic and/or recurring fasting hypoglycemia appear to tolerate low blood glucose levels (i.e., 20 to 30 mg/dl) for prolonged periods without symptoms, and only small additional changes in the blood glucose level are then required to produce symptomatic episodes.[230] The mechanism whereby some humans and animals adapt to exceedingly low blood glucose concentrations without showing symptoms is not well understood.

TABLE 96–8. CLINICAL SIGNS ASSOCIATED WITH INSULIN-SECRETING TUMORS IN 82 DOGS

Clinical Sign	No. of Dogs	(%)
Seizures	52	(63)
Posterior paresis	30	(37)
Weakness	28	(34)
Collapse	28	(34)
Muscle fasciculations	18	(22)
Bizarre behavior	17	(21)
Depression, lethargy	16	(20)
Ataxia	15	(19)
Polyphagia	12	(15)
Exercise intolerance	11	(13)
Polyuria, polydipsia	8	(10)
Weight gain	6	(7)
Diarrhea	4	(5)
Syncope	3	(4)
Nervousness	2	(3)
Head tilt	2	(3)
Blindness	1	(1)

From Feldman, EC and Nelson, RW: Canine and Feline Endocrinology and Reproduction. Philadelphia, WB Saunders, 1987; and Leifer, CE, et al.: JAVMA 188:60, 1986.

Anamnesis

Clinical signs of an insulin-secreting tumor may be present for as long as three years or as briefly as one day before veterinary care is sought. Most dogs, however, are symptomatic for one to six months before presentation to the veterinarian.[215]

The signs associated with an insulin-secreting tumor typically are related to neuroglycopenia (hypoglycemia) and an elevation in circulating catecholamine concentrations (Table 96–8). One characteristic of hypoglycemic signs, regardless of the cause, is their episodic nature. Signs are generally observed for only a few seconds to minutes because of the compensatory counterregulatory mechanisms that are designed to increase the blood glucose concentration when hypoglycemia develops. If these mechanisms are inadequate, syncope, seizures, or coma may occur as the blood glucose concentration continues to fall. Seizure activity is more common than syncope or coma (Table 96–8), and appears to be self-limiting, typically lasting from 30 seconds to 5 minutes. The seizure may stimulate further catecholamine secretion and other counterregulatory mechanisms that increase the blood glucose level above critical concentrations.

There is a strong association between the development of clinical signs of hypoglycemia, and fasting, excitement, exercise, and eating. Exercise results in an increased demand for glucose production. In the normal exercising dog, stimulation of the sympathetic nervous system inhibits insulin secretion and enhances hepatic release of glucose. Thus the increased glucose utilization is balanced by increased hepatic production. Exercising muscles continue to utilize glucose despite a decrease or lack of insulin secretion, owing to a "pooling" or "trapping" of previously secreted insulin in this tissue. The balance between glucose utilization and production maintains the circulating blood glucose concentration, allowing the brain to continue to function.[231]

The exercising dog with an insulin-secreting tumor has increased glucose utilization not just by muscle, but by all tissues, owing to the abnormal availability of insulin.[231] In addition, hepatic release of glucose is impaired. The potential for hypoglycemia is great, and this fact is supported by the number of owners who associate symptoms in their pets with jogging, play, or long walks. A similar pathophysiology is thought to explain the development of symptoms during periods of excitement.

Insulin-secreting tumors are usually responsive to increases in the blood glucose concentration. Food consumption stimulates insulin secretion, which is often excessive and results in postprandial hypoglycemia two to six hours after a meal.

Physical Examination

The physical examination of dogs with insulin-secreting tumors is surprisingly unremarkable. These dogs are usually free of visible or palpable abnormalities. Weight gain is evident in some dogs and is probably a result of the potent anabolic effects of insulin.

Peripheral neuropathies have been reported in dogs with insulin-secreting tumors,[225, 232] which may produce detectable alterations on physical examination, including proprioception deficits, depressed reflexes, and muscle atrophy. The pathogenesis of the polyneuropathy is not known. Proposed theories include metabolic derangements of the nerves induced by the hyperinsulinemia, a paraneoplastic effect of the tumor, and an immune-mediated reaction as a result of shared antigens between tumor and nerves.[233, 234]

Differential Diagnosis

In virtually all dogs with an insulin-secreting neoplasm, the veterinary clinician is usually attempting to make diagnostic and therapeutic decisions about a pet with a vague history of repeated seizures, weakness, ataxia, posterior paresis, muscle fasciculations, bizarre behavior, and/or lethargy. In the broadest sense, most of these animals have the common history of episodic weakness or seizures, which encompasses a wide variety of organic disorders (see Table 96–9). The minimum diagnostic evaluation for these dogs should include screening blood and urine tests. Therapy other than that required for an emergency situation should be withheld until a diagnosis is made.

Once fasting hypoglycemia has been confirmed, reviewing the possible causes in conjunction with the anamnesis and physical examination should enable the practitioner to develop a priority ranking of likely diagnoses (Table 96–10). With the priority ranking constructed, one can proceed with confirmatory tests to achieve a definitive diagnosis.

TABLE 96–9. A PARTIAL LISTING OF THE NUMEROUS DISORDERS THAT MAY RESULT IN EPISODIC WEAKNESS (INCLUDES SEIZURES)

Neuromuscular disorders
Infectious: viral encephalitis (canine distemper), cryptococcosis, toxoplasmosis
Congenital: hydrocephalus
Trauma
Acquired: myasthenia gravis, tetanus, discospondylitis, idiopathic polyradiculoneuritis (coon hound paralysis), polymyositis, polyarthritis
Neoplasia
Toxin: lead poisoning
Idiopathic epilepsy
Idiopathic polyneuropathy
Cardiovascular disorders
Congenital: anatomic defects
Acquired: tachyarrhythmias or bradyarrhythmias, heartworm, bacterial endocarditis
Neoplasm: hemangiosarcoma
Coagulopathy (warfarin-induced)
Metabolic disorders
Hepatic encephalopathy
Hypocalcemia
Polycythemia
Hypoadrenocorticism
Hyperviscosity syndrome
Pheochromocytoma
Hypoglycemia
Hypokalemia
Anemia

TABLE 96–10. CLASSIFICATION OF FASTING HYPOGLYCEMIA

I. Endocrine
  A. Excess insulin or insulin-like factors
    1. Insulin-producing islet cell tumors
    2. Extrapancreatic tumors producing and secreting insulin-like substances
    3. Iatrogenic-insulin overdose
  B. Growth hormone deficiency
    1. Hypopituitarism affecting several tropic hormones (i.e., ACTH, GH)
    2. Monotropic growth hormone deficiency
  C. Cortisol deficiency
    1. Hypopituitarism
    2. Isolated ACTH deficiency
    3. Hypoadrenocorticism
II. Hepatic
  A. Congenital
    1. Vascular shunts
    2. Glycogen storage diseases
  B. Acquired
    1. Vascular shunts
    2. Chronic fibrosis (cirrhosis)
    3. Hepatic necrosis: toxins, infectious agents
III. Substrate
  A. Extrapancreatic tumors that utilize large quantities of glucose
  B. Fasting hypoglycemia of pregnancy
  C. Puppy hypoglycemia ± ketonemia (alanine deficiency?)
  D. Uremia
  E. Severe malnutrition
  F. Severe polycythemia
IV. Miscellaneous
  A. Artifact
  B. Iatrogenic-insulin overdose

Clinical Pathologic Abnormalities

Virtually all dogs with insulin-secreting tumors remain undiagnosed and often unsuspected of having such tumors after completion of the anamnesis and physical examination. A complete data base, including a hemogram, biochemical panel, and urinalysis, should be performed in an effort to identify evidence supportive of one of the disorders outlined in Table 96–9.

Results of the hemogram and urinalysis from dogs with an insulin-secreting tumor are usually normal. Results of the biochemical panel, aside from the blood glucose, are also usually normal. Hypoalbuminemia, hypophosphatemia, hypokalemia, and an increase in alkaline phosphatase and alanine aminotransferase have been reported,[68, 235] but these findings are considered nonspecific and not helpful in achieving a definitive diagnosis. A correlation has not been found between liver enzyme elevations and obvious metastasis of the pancreatic tumor to the liver.

The only consistent abnormality found in the biochemistry panel is hypoglycemia. The mean initial blood glucose concentration in 31 dogs with an insulin-secreting tumor was 50 mg/dl, with a range of 18 to 77 mg/dl, in one report[5] and in another study of 46 dogs was 46 mg/dl, with a range of 7 to 77 mg/dl.[235] Dogs with insulin-secreting tumors may occasionally have a normal blood glucose concentration on random testing. Such a finding does not eliminate hypoglycemia as a cause of episodic weakness or seizure activity. Fasting with hourly evaluations of the blood glucose should be done in these dogs. A fast of eight or fewer hours was successful in demonstrating hypoglycemia in 33 of 35

trials in 31 dogs with insulin-secreting tumors.[5] Longer fasts have been reported to be needed in some dogs;[236] however, it is rare that fasts beyond 12 hours would fail to produce hypoglycemia in dogs with insulin-secreting tumors.

Radiography/Ultrasonography

Insulin-secreting tumors are usually quite small. Thus it is not surprising that abdominal radiographs are routinely interpreted as normal and are usually of limited value in this disorder. Displacement of viscera or a visible mass in the right cranial quadrant of the abdominal cavity is considered extremely rare. Thoracic radiographs are also of limited help in documenting metastatic disease.[237] Ultrasonic evaluation of the cranial abdomen, however, has been useful in detecting mass lesions in the region of the pancreas and within the hepatic parenchyma, thus establishing the existence of metastatic disease in several dogs.

Confirmation of an Insulin-secreting Tumor

In 1935 the report that established insulin-secreting tumors of the pancreas as a clinical entity included a discussion of the three criteria to be used in confirming the diagnosis.[238] These standards, now referred to as Whipple's triad, are as follows: (1) the patient's symptoms occur after fasting or exercise, (2) at the time of symptoms, the serum glucose concentration is less than 50 mg/dl, and (3) the symptoms are relieved by the administration of glucose. Unfortunately this triad can result from numerous causes of hypoglycemia and, as such, is nonspecific. More sophisticated diagnostic tests should be used to distinguish patients with insulin-secreting tumors from those with other potential causes of fasting hypoglycemia.

Basal Insulin and Glucose Determinations. The easiest and perhaps best way to establish a diagnosis of an insulin-secreting tumor is to evaluate the blood insulin concentration at a time when hypoglycemia is present. Hypoglycemia suppresses insulin secretion in normal animals, the degree of suppression being directly related to the severity of the hypoglycemia. Hypoglycemia would fail to have this same suppressive effect on insulin secretion if the insulin arose from autonomous neoplastic cells. Tumor cells that produce and secrete insulin are less responsive to hypoglycemia than normal β cells. Invariably the dog with an insulin-secreting tumor will have an insulin concentration greater than that needed for a particular blood glucose concentration. The relative excess of insulin becomes easier to recognize when the blood glucose concentration is low. If the blood glucose concentration is below normal and the insulin concentration is within a normal range or increased, the animal has a relative or absolute excess of insulin that can be explained if an insulin-secreting tumor, insensitive to hypoglycemia, is present.

The diagnostic approach to a dog with fasting hypoglycemia suspected of having an insulin-secreting tumor of the pancreas is straightforward (Table 96–11). The

TABLE 96–11. PROTOCOL FOR DOCUMENTING INAPPROPRIATE INSULIN SECRETION IN THE DOG WITH HYPOGLYCEMIA

8:00 AM	Blood glucose concentration is checked with Chemstrip bG.
Every 30 minutes	Check blood glucose concentration with Chemstrip until blood glucose level is approximately 40 mg/dl (any concentration ≤ 60 mg/dl is ideal).
When 40 mg/dl is attained:	Obtain blood for a laboratory blood glucose determination. Obtain blood for an insulin determination by radioimmunoassay. Feed dog several small meals over next few hours.

dog is fed a normal meal early in the day (8:00 AM). For the remainder of the study the animal should be kept as quiet as possible and fasted in its cage or run. A drop of blood is obtained every hour and the glucose concentration evaluated with Chemstrip bG test strips. When the "strip" glucose concentration is approximately 40 mg/dl, a blood sample should be assayed for both glucose and insulin by standard laboratory methods. The patient is then fed several small meals over the next one to three hours to avoid postprandial reactive hypoglycemia. When stable, the dog should be returned to the owners and fed every six hours until a diagnosis is confirmed and definitive therapy instituted.

The protocol discussed above is not necessary if serum or plasma from the blood obtained for the initial screening tests has been stored frozen and if those tests reveal a blood glucose less than 60 mg/dl. In this instance an insulin concentration can be determined from the frozen serum or plasma.

Most dogs with insulin-secreting tumors develop hypoglycemia on this protocol within four to ten hours of the morning meal.[215, 237] If the blood glucose concentration should fail to decline below 60 mg/dl during the ten-hour fast, a longer period of withholding food may be attempted. If this becomes necessary, the dog should be fed at 5:00 PM, 8:30 PM, and midnight. Food should not be given after midnight and blood glucose concentrations should be monitored beginning at 8:00 AM the next morning. If necessary, monitoring and fasting should continue until 5:00 PM. It is not recommended to continue a fast beyond 5:00 PM unless the patient is monitored by veterinary personnel.

If the blood glucose concentration is less than 60 mg/dl and the blood insulin concentration is above normal, the presence of an insulin-secreting neoplasm is likely. If the blood insulin is in the normal range, the presence of an insulin-secreting tumor remains possible. In one report, 31 dogs with an insulin-secreting tumor had a mean blood glucose concentration of 50 mg/dl and a mean blood insulin concentration of 32 μU/ml (N: 5 to 22 μU/ml), with an insulin range of 6 to 95 μU/ml.[5] In another report of 46 dogs, the mean blood glucose concentration was 46 mg/dl and the mean blood insulin concentration was 90 μU/ml (N: 4 to 26 μU/ml), with an insulin range of 6 to 571 μU/ml.[235] In the author's experience, no dog with fasting hypoglycemia caused by an insulin-secreting tumor has had a plasma insulin concentration below the normal range. Any plasma insulin concentration that is below the normal range is

consistent with insulinopenia and is inconsistent for an insulin-secreting tumor.

Eight of 82 blood samples from 77 dogs with insulin-secreting tumors had plasma insulin concentrations in the low normal range (i.e., less than 10 μU/ml).[5, 235] Insulin values in the low normal range may be found with hypoglycemia associated with nonislet cell tumors, as well as insulin-secreting tumors. In one report, eight dogs with a nonislet cell tumor and hypoglycemia had plasma insulin concentrations between four and 10 μU/ml.[239] Therefore, insulin values in the low normal range in a dog with hypoglycemia are an indication for further diagnostics, including repeating the blood glucose and insulin determinations, to determine the underlying cause.

Insulin-Glucose Ratios. A diagnosis of an insulin-secreting tumor can usually be made based on the anamnesis, physical examination, and results of the initial data base and blood glucose/insulin concentrations. Rarely, this information fails to establish a diagnosis (i.e., hypoglycemia is marginal and insulin concentrations remain in the normal range). Several insulin-glucose ratios, including the insulin:glucose ratio, the glucose:insulin ratio, and the amended insulin:glucose ratio, have been recommended in these instances to evaluate the interrelationship between blood glucose and insulin concentrations and to help establish the diagnosis.[215, 237, 240] Of these ratios, the amended insulin:glucose ratio is believed to be the most reliable.[215]

The diagnostic approach is as described above. Once the "strip" glucose concentration is approximately 40 mg/dl, a blood insulin and glucose concentration should be determined from the same blood sample and the values plugged into the formula for the amended insulin:glucose ratio:

$$\frac{plasma\ insulin\ (\mu U/ml) \times 100}{plasma\ glucose\ (mg/dl) - 30}$$

The use of −30 in the formula is based on the theory that in normal humans, plasma insulin concentrations are virtually undetectable when the plasma glucose concentration is 30 mg/dl or less. Whenever the glucose is less than 30 mg/dl, the number 1 is used as the divisor. Extrapolating from the human literature, most authors have suggested that an amended insulin:glucose ratio greater than 30 is diagnostic of an insulin-secreting tumor.[215, 240, 241] However, this test is not specific, that is, some dogs with other causes of hypoglycemia may have abnormal amended ratios.[235]

Provocative Testing. Several tests have been described that use agents that stimulate insulin secretion by normal and neoplastic β cells, including the glucagon tolerance test, the oral and IV glucose tolerance test, the tolbutamide tolerance test, and the epinephrine stimulation test.[5] By evaluating the response of blood glucose and insulin concentrations for a period of time after the administration of these agents, a differentiation between normal and neoplastic β cells can potentially be made. Fortunately these tests are rarely, if ever, needed to establish the diagnosis of an insulin-secreting tumor.

The glucagon tolerance test is the best known and most widely used of these provocative tests. The administration of glucagon causes a rapid elevation in the blood glucose concentration, and stimulates the secretion of insulin by pancreatic β cells. Stimulation of insulin secretion is either the result of a direct effect of glucagon on β cells (normal or neoplastic) or an indirect effect caused by the rise in the blood glucose concentration.[40] Because glucagon administration results in insulin release from neoplastic insulin-secreting cells, the summation of glucagon effects in a dog with an insulin-secreting tumor could include: (1) a rise in the blood glucose concentration less than the expected levels, (2) the blood glucose concentration quickly decreasing to subnormal concentrations owing to secretion of excess insulin, and (3) insulin concentrations that rapidly rise to levels that exceed normal glucagon-induced concentrations.

This test ideally should commence after a fast sufficient to lower the blood glucose concentration below 70 mg/dl but may be initiated with higher blood glucose levels. Glucagon (USP) is injected IV at a dose of 0.014 mg/lb (0.03 mg/kg). Sodium fluoride-treated or EDTA-treated anticoagulated blood should be obtained before the glucagon injection and at 1, 3, 5, 15, 30, 45, 60, 90, and 120 minutes after administration. Glucose concentrations can be assessed with Chemstrip bG test strips before any sample is submitted. Each blood sample should be assayed for both glucose and insulin concentrations. Because this number of glucose and insulin analyses can become extremely expensive, the veterinarian may elect to request only blood glucose concentrations initially. Another alternative would be to obtain blood only at 1, 15, 60, and 120 minutes after glucagon administration. An IV catheter should be in place during the test and 50 per cent glucose available for immediate administration in case a hypoglycemic crisis occurs during or after the test as a result of excessive insulin secretion.

Five major criteria have been suggested for establishing the diagnosis of an insulin-secreting tumor, using the glucagon tolerance test: (1) the peak blood glucose concentration at any time during the test should be less than 135 mg/dl, (2) hypoglycemia (glucose concentration below 70 mg/dl) should be documented within 60 to 120 minutes after glucagon administration, (3) the plasma insulin concentration should be greater than 50 μU/ml one minute after glucagon infusion, (4) the blood glucose concentration should decrease one to two minutes after glucagon injection, and (5) an insulin:glucose ratio should be greater than 0.75 one minute into the test.[236] Although the glucagon tolerance test is relatively simple to perform and is not time-consuming, it is expensive, potentially dangerous to the animal (i.e., glucagon-induced hypoglycemia 90 to 150 minutes after glucagon administration), and only moderately effective as a diagnostic tool.[215] The test is not reliable and certainly less consistent than evaluation of fasting blood glucose and insulin concentrations.

Surgical Therapy

Surgery as a therapeutic approach for insulin-secreting tumors in the dog remains controversial because of the high incidence of metastatic disease at the time of diagnosis, the age of many of these dogs, and an inability to document improvement in the long-term prognosis after surgery. Nevertheless, surgical exploration is the best diagnostic, therapeutic, and prognostic tool for insulin-secreting tumors. Surgery offers a chance to "cure" dogs with benign tumors. With nonresectable tumors or those with obvious metastasis, removal or debulking of as much abnormal tissue as possible has frequently resulted in remission of, or at least reduction in, clinical signs and improved response to medical therapy. Regardless of the findings at surgery, the author does not recommend euthanasia. Many dogs with metastatic disease can be managed medically with minimal complications for several months to more than a year.

Until surgery is performed, the dog with an insulin-secreting tumor must be protected from episodes of severe hypoglycemia. This can usually be accomplished with frequent small meals and glucocorticoid therapy. A continuous IV infusion of a five per cent dextrose solution before, during, and immediately after surgery is helpful in preventing hypoglycemia. The blood glucose concentration should be monitored once or twice during surgery to help identify hypoglycemia. Alterations can then be made in the rate of administration of the dextrose-containing fluids to prevent severe hypoglycemia.

Adequate fluid therapy just before, during, and immediately after surgery is also helpful in minimizing the development of pancreatitis after digital and surgical manipulation of the pancreas. Providing adequate fluid therapy before and during the surgery ensures good circulation through the microvasculature of the pancreas. The author routinely gives fluids at two times the maintenance rate during and for 24 to 48 hours after surgery.

A complete inspection of the abdominal contents is imperative to identify unsuspected abnormalities as well as sites of metastasis. The most common sites of tumor spread include the lymphatics and lymph nodes (duodenal, mesenteric, hepatic, splenic), liver, mesentery, and omentum. As much of the pancreas as possible should be visually examined. A complete, gentle digital inspection of this organ should then be undertaken. The necessity for gentle handling of the pancreas cannot be overemphasized. Failure to do so may result in severe, potentially life-threatening pancreatitis. Most dogs with insulin-secreting tumors have masses that are visible to the surgeon inspecting the pancreas (Figure 96–24). In a smaller group of dogs the tumor may not be visible, but is palpable during a gentle but thorough digital examination of the pancreas.

There is no predisposition of tumor location within the pancreas. In one series of 31 dogs with an insulin-secreting tumor, the tumor was located in the right (duodenal) lobe of the pancreas in 13 dogs and in the left (splenic) lobe in 16 dogs.[5] Two dogs had the mass removed from the central area of the pancreas. If the surgeon fails to recognize a mass and the diagnosis has been confirmed by glucose/insulin measurements, the surgeon should attempt to remove at least one half of the pancreas in the hope of removing the portion that contains the tumor. In 2 of 25 cases in one study, a

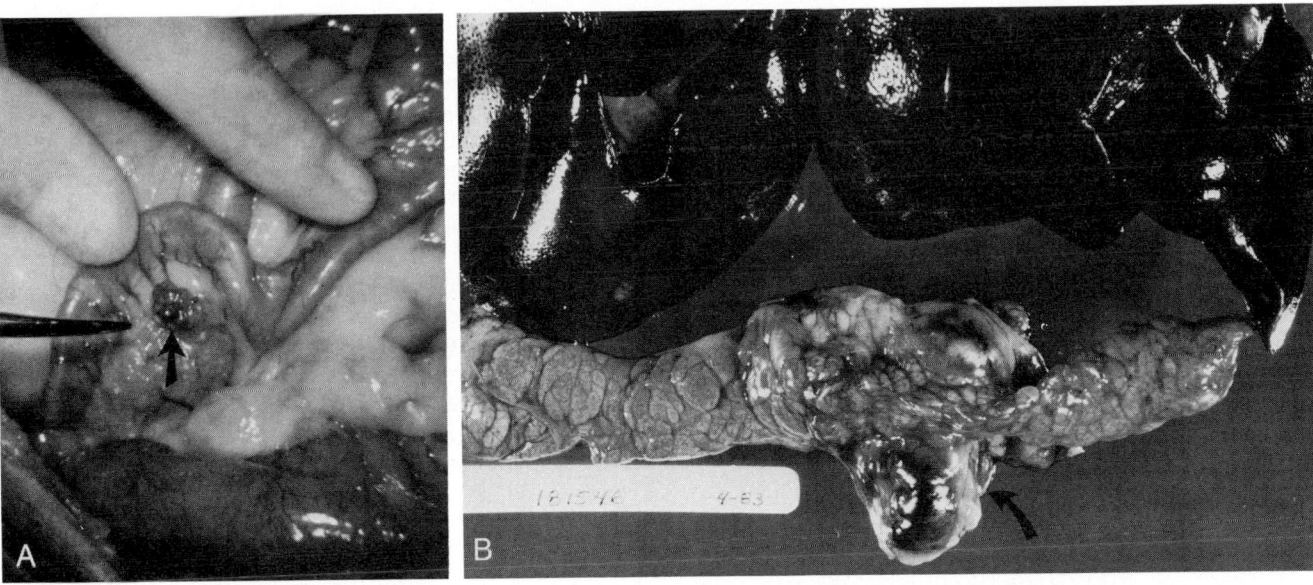

FIGURE 96–24. *A* and *B*, Photographs of pancreatic insulin-secreting islet-cell tumors (arrows).

diffuse microscopic islet cell carcinoma was recognized histologically in the resected portion of the pancreas despite an inability to visualize or palpate abnormal tissue.[215]

Regardless of the findings at surgery, each dog should be treated for pancreatitis during the initial 36 to 48 hours after surgery. Nothing should be given to the patient orally during this time. An IV balanced electrolyte and glucose infusion is provided at 1.5 to 2 times maintenance requirements. The blood glucose concentration should be determined twice daily and blood electrolytes once daily during the initial 48 hours after surgery. Adjustments in the electrolyte or dextrose composition of the fluids should be made accordingly. If there are no problems, water is offered on day three. If the water is consumed and no vomiting is seen on day three, bland food is offered on day four. Circulating pancreatic enzyme concentrations (e.g., lipase and amylase) are rarely determined after surgery because the test results offer little additional information for managing the dog. Treating each dog for pancreatitis without determining serum pancreatic enzyme concentrations beforehand has provided excellent results.

Occasionally dogs develop diabetes mellitus after surgery for an insulin-secreting tumor.[237] Diabetes mellitus is believed to result from inadequate insulin secretion by atrophied normal β cells. Removal of all, or a majority, of the neoplastic cells acutely deprives the animal of insulin. Until the atrophied normal cells regain their secretory capabilities, the animal will be hypoinsulinemic and may require exogenous insulin injections to maintain euglycemia. It was once thought that postsurgical hyperglycemia and glycosuria were excellent prognostic signs indicating total removal of insulin-secreting neoplastic cells. However, in the author's experience, some dogs that require exogenous insulin after surgery ultimately require medical management for an exacerbation of an insulin-secreting tumor several months after discontinuing insulin injections.

Postsurgical insulin therapy is initiated only when hyperglycemia and glycosuria persist for longer than two or three days after all dextrose-containing IV fluid therapy has been discontinued. Diabetes mellitus is usually transient, lasting from two days to six months. These dogs still may have metastases of neoplastic β cells that will cause hypoglycemic symptoms at a later date. Evaluation of urine glucose in the home environment is helpful in identifying when insulin therapy is no longer needed. Persistent negative urine glucose results, especially with low daily insulin requirements, is an indication to discontinue insulin therapy. If hyperglycemia and glycosuria recur, insulin therapy can be reinstituted.

If the dog is still hypoglycemic despite surgical removal or debulking of the tumor, medical therapy should be initiated, beginning with feeding small meals frequently (see discussion below). Three or four small meals daily are recommended. If the frequent feedings should succeed in keeping the dog in clinical remission, the various medical approaches to therapy can be set aside for potential future use. If a dog becomes symptomatic despite the frequent feedings, medical therapy should be attempted before recommending euthanasia.

Medical Therapy for an Acute Hypoglycemic Crisis

The dog or cat with suspected hypoglycemia should have a blood sample obtained for a glucose determination and then glucose should be administered IV slowly until all symptoms have been reversed and the animal is no longer in distress. Two to 15 ml of 50 per cent dextrose is usually required to alleviate the symptoms. Dogs and cats with hypoglycemia should respond to the administration of glucose within 30 to 120 seconds. Any dog or cat with CNS symptoms that responds to exogenous glucose satisfies a portion of Whipple's triad and should be thoroughly investigated for disorders known to cause hypoglycemia.

If an owner contacts a veterinarian by telephone and reports that the pet is having a hypoglycemic seizure, the author does not recommend transporting the dog to a veterinary hospital. Rather, the owner is instructed to pour a sugar solution (e.g., Karo syrup) over the fingers and rub the syrup on the pet's buccal mucosa. Hypoglycemic dogs and cats usually respond in 30 to 120 seconds. Never have an owner place a hand or object into an animal's mouth during a seizure because the person is likely to be bitten. Never recommend pouring a sugar solution directly into the animal's mouth because the owner is likely to be bitten and the animal may aspirate the liquid.

If a dog or cat responds to glucose administration, it should be fed a small, high-protein meal and should be kept as quiet as possible. The dog or cat should be fed three to six small meals each day and veterinary attention should be sought.

Rarely, a hypoglycemic dog or cat with CNS signs fails to respond to glucose administration. These signs could be the result of a disorder unrelated to hypoglycemia. However, irreversible cerebral lesions may result from long-term, severe hypoglycemia and the resultant cerebral hypoxia. Cerebral hypoxia predisposes the nervous tissue to edema, causing increased CSF pressure and cell death. These animals have a guarded to grave prognosis. Therapy is directed at providing a continuous supply of glucose as a 5 per cent solution IV. Simultaneously, seizure activity is controlled with diazepam or stronger anticonvulsant medication. Lastly, if cerebral edema is suspected, it may be treated with mannitol and glucocorticoids.

Medical Therapy for Chronic Hypoglycemia

Medical management for chronic hypoglycemia should be initiated when an exploratory celiotomy is not performed or when a metastatic or an inoperable tumor results in recurrence of clinical signs. The goals of chronic therapy are to reduce the frequency and severity of clinical signs and to avoid an acute hypoglycemic crisis. Medical management includes nonspecific antihormonal therapy and specific chemotherapy directed against the neoplastic β cells.

Antihormonal Therapy. Antihormonal therapy is palliative and designed to minimize hypoglycemia by increasing absorption of glucose from the intestinal tract, increasing hepatic gluconeogenesis and glycogenolysis, or inhibiting the synthesis, secretion, or peripheral cellular actions of insulin. Each therapeutic method should be continued until signs of hypoglycemia recur. At that time, another treatment should be initiated without discontinuing prior therapy. Using this technique, many dogs can be successfully managed for more than a year after the diagnosis of hyperinsulinism. Antihormonal therapy primarily consists of frequent feedings, and glucocorticoid and diazoxide therapy.

FREQUENT FEEDINGS. Dogs with insulin-secreting tumors have a persistent absolute or relative excess of circulating insulin. If a constant source of calories is provided as a substrate for this insulin, hypoglycemic episodes can be reduced in frequency or avoided. Diets that are high in proteins, fats, and complex carbohydrates are recommended. If dog food is used, a combi-

nation of canned and dry food, fed in three to six small meals daily, is recommended. Exercise should be limited to short walks on a leash. Simple sugars (including semi-moist dog foods) may stimulate insulin secretion by neoplastic β cells and should be avoided. Any signs of hypoglycemia should prompt the owner to feed the pet immediately. As long as the dog can eat, honey, maple syrup, corn syrup, and other sugar solutions should be avoided because they may delay one hypoglycemic episode but predispose the animal to another episode within 30 to 120 minutes.

GLUCOCORTICOID THERAPY. Glucocorticoids should be initiated when dietary manipulations are no longer effective in preventing signs of hypoglycemia. Glucocorticoids antagonize the effects of insulin at the cellular level, which results in decreased tissue utilization of glucose and an indirect increase in the blood glucose. Glucocorticoids also increase blood glucose concentrations directly by stimulating hepatic glycogenolysis, and indirectly by providing the necessary substrates for hepatic gluconeogenesis.[242]

Prednisone is the glucocorticoid most often used. The initial dose is 0.22 mg/lb/day (0.5 mg/kg/day) given in divided doses. If this controls the signs of hypoglycemia, the medication is continued without adjusting the dose. If signs are still not controlled, the dose should be gradually increased until signs of hypoglycemia abate or the daily prednisone dose is 2 to 3 mg/lb/day (4 to 6 mg/kg/day). If the latter occurs, other medications will be needed to control hypoglycemic signs.

Hypoglycemic signs commonly recur within months of instituting glucocorticoid therapy, presumably owing to tumor growth. When this happens, the dose of prednisone can gradually be increased in a stepwise manner, not to exceed 2 to 3 mg/lb/day (4 to 6 mg/kg/day). Signs of iatrogenic hypercortisolism may develop as the amount of prednisone administered increases. These signs include polydipsia, polyuria, polyphagia, infections, obesity, weakness, and bilaterally symmetrical alopecia. With evidence of hypercortisolism, the dose of prednisone should be reduced and diazoxide therapy initiated.

DIAZOXIDE THERAPY. Diazoxide (Proglycem) is a benzothiadiazide diuretic. It inhibits the secretion of insulin by decreasing the intracellular release of ionized calcium, thereby blocking emiocytosis of insulin granules.[243] However, it neither inhibits insulin synthesis nor has antineoplastic effects. Diazoxide also stimulates hepatic gluconeogenesis and glycogenolysis by stimulating the adrenergic nervous system and the secretion of epinephrine, respectively.[244] Finally, diazoxide inhibits tissue use of glucose by directly inhibiting cellular uptake of glucose and by stimulating epinephrine secretion.[245] The net effect is the development of hyperglycemia.

Unfortunately, the availability of diazoxide is extremely limited at this time. If available, the initial dosage of diazoxide is 5 mg/lb (10 mg/kg), divided into two doses daily. The dose may gradually be increased as needed to control signs of hypoglycemia but should not exceed 27 mg/lb (60 mg/kg). Thiazide diuretics, which may potentiate the effects of diazoxide, can be administered in conjunction with diazoxide to enhance the hyperglycemic effect if diazoxide alone is not effective. The dose of hydrochlorothiazide is 1 to 2 mg/lb/day (2 to 4 mg/kg/day).

The goal of diazoxide therapy is to establish a dosage in which hypoglycemia and its clinical signs are reduced or absent, while avoiding hyperglycemia (greater than 180 mg/dl) and its associated clinical signs. Cataracts, one complication associated with diazoxide therapy, are believed to be due to diazoxide overdosage and resultant hyperglycemia.[246] Other potential complications related to diazoxide usage include anorexia, vomiting, diarrhea, tachycardia, bone marrow suppression, aplastic anemia, thrombocytopenia, diabetes mellitus, and sodium and fluid retention.[243]

Reports of diazoxide usage have appeared in the veterinary literature only sporadically.[235, 237, 247] Eleven of 13 dogs with an insulin-secreting tumor in the author's series have had good clinical responses lasting from 6 weeks to 17 months. In another report, 9 of 14 dogs had a good response to diazoxide therapy.[235] The most common adverse reactions in these dogs were anorexia and vomiting. Administering diazoxide with a meal or decreasing the dosage, at least temporarily, is usually effective in controlling adverse gastrointestinal signs. Diazoxide is metabolized in the liver, and the metabolites are excreted primarily by way of the kidneys and biliary system.[248] Adverse reactions or complications may develop more rapidly or at a lower dosage of diazoxide in a dog with concurrent hepatic dysfunction.

Miscellaneous Drugs. Several other drugs have been used for the antihormonal management of chronic hypoglycemia in humans, including phenytoin, propranolol, and L-asparaginase.[244] The efficacy and therapeutic protocol for these drugs have not been adequately evaluated in the dog. In addition, potentially serious adverse reactions are possible, especially with L-asparaginase. Therefore, until properly evaluated, these drugs should not be used except as a last resort in the management of canine insulin-secreting tumors.

Chemotherapy. Chemotherapeutic drugs directed against neoplastic β cells have not been adequately evaluated in the dog. Streptozotocin and alloxan have been used for the treatment of human insulin-secreting tumors, but such use has appeared only sporadically in the veterinary literature.[243, 249–251] Acute renal failure is a potentially serious complication for both of these drugs. Until further studies have been completed, they should be used only as a last attempt to treat dogs with insulin-secreting tumors.

STREPTOZOTOCIN. Steptozotocin is a naturally occurring nitrosourea isolated from the fermentation cultures of *Streptomyces achromogenes*.[252] This drug selectively destroys pancreatic β cells by depressing the pyridine nucleotides NAD (nicotinamide-adenine dinucleotide) and NADH, the reduced form of NAD.[253] In humans a dose of 500 mg/m² daily for five consecutive days has been beneficial.[244] Only two dogs with confirmed insulin-secreting tumors that were treated with this agent have been reported.[250, 251] Unfortunately an acute nephropathy developed after two doses of streptozotocin (500 mg/m² body surface area) administered seven days apart. If used at all, the dose of streptozotocin should be less than 500 mg/m² once every seven days for two to four treatments. The dog should be carefully monitored for

signs of renal damage (i.e., proteinuria, casts in the urine, elevation in urea nitrogen or creatinine). If renal damage occurs, further therapy with streptozotocin should be discontinued.

ALLOXAN. Alloxan is an unstable uric acid derivative that has a direct cytotoxic effect on the pancreatic β cells, primarily by altering β cell membrane permeability.[254] The toxic effect of alloxan on β cells appears to be dose-related.[255] Alloxan also enhances hepatic gluconeogenesis, possibly by enhancing glucagon secretion from pancreatic α cells.[254]

Alloxan, which theoretically would be an ideal drug, has not been helpful in the management of insulin-secreting tumors in humans.[229] Its use for canine insulin-secreting tumors is yet to be critically evaluated, although it was effective in producing hyperglycemia for three months in one of three dogs with metastatic insulin-secreting tumors at the author's clinic. The primary toxicity associated with alloxan therapy is renal tubular necrosis and resultant acute renal failure. This toxicity is dose-dependent and potentially reversible with appropriate fluid therapy and supportive care.[256]

Prognosis

Owing to the extremely high likelihood of malignancy in any dog with an insulin-secreting tumor, the long-term prognosis, at best, is guarded to poor. The author has been able to follow 33 dogs with hyperinsulinism until they died or received at least six months of therapy. One dog died during surgery from cardiac arrest, and four dogs were euthanized at the time of surgery owing to the finding of tumor metastasis. Three dogs died within seven days of surgery, with the cause of death potentially the result of severe hypoglycemic episodes.

Fourteen dogs were euthanized owing to recurrent hypoglycemic seizure activity after the hospitalization when surgery was performed. Of these dogs, the mean survival time was 15.9 months, with a range of 2 to 38 months. At the time of euthanasia one dog was being treated with frequent feedings, six dogs were being given frequent meals and prednisone, and seven dogs were receiving frequent feedings, prednisone, and diazoxide. These owners, for the most part, worked diligently at helping their pets. Time and expense for the owners were important considerations in electing euthanasia. These dogs were usually re-checked every three to four months with at least a history, physical examination, and blood glucose determination. Other studies were performed as dictated by signs and findings on the physical examination. The owners of these animals were generally pleased with the additional time their pets were given to live. In addition, these people did not feel that their dogs had suffered with their illness.

Eleven dogs are still alive. These include dogs living 6 to 60 months beyond the initial diagnostic surgical procedure. These pets are in various stages of treatment, and 9 of the 11 dogs have confirmed malignancy. One dog is currently treated only with frequent meals, six are given frequent meals and prednisone, and four receive frequent meals, prednisone, and diazoxide. The dogs are comfortable and appear not to be suffering.

The major problem these dogs face is progressive obesity. The author encourages owners to take these animals for short slow walks but to limit vigorous exercise. Again, the cost of treating these dogs is not prohibitive, and owners are pleased with the longer lives their pets are able to have. The mean survival time of these dogs is 19.4 months postsurgically, surprisingly long in the face of malignancy.

References

1. Bloom, WF and Fawcett, D: A Textbook of Histology, 10th ed. Philadelphia, WB Saunders, 1975.
2. Munger, GL: Morphological characterization of islet cell diversity. *In* Cooperstein, SJ and Watkins, D (eds): The Islets of Langerhans: Biochemistry, Physiology, and Pathology. New York, Academic Press, 1981, p 3.
3. Like, AA and Orci, L: Embryogenesis of the human pancreatic islets. Diabetes 21:511, 1972.
4. Larsson, LI, et al.: Pancreatic gastrin in foetal and neonatal rats. Nature 262:609, 1976.
5. Feldman, EC and Nelson, RW: Canine and Feline Endocrinology and Reproduction. Philadelphia, WB Saunders, 1987.
6. Kaneko, JJ, et al.: Glucose tolerance and insulin response in diabetes mellitus of dogs. J Small Anim Pract 118:85, 1978.
7. Manns, JG and Martin, CL: Plasma insulin, glucagon, and nonesterified fatty acids in dogs with diabetes mellitus. Am J Vet Res 33:981, 1972.
8. Hendricks, HJ, et al.: Studies on glucose and insulin levels in the blood of normal and diabetic dogs. Zentralbl Veterinarmed 23:206, 1976.
9. Bennett, P: Classification of diabetes. *In* Ellenberg, M and Rifkin, H (eds): Diabetes Mellitus: Theory and Practice, 3rd ed. New York, Medical Examination Publishing, 1983, p 409.
10. Eigenmann, JE: Diabetes mellitus in dogs and cats. Proceed Sixth Ann Kal Kan Symp, Columbus, OH, 1982, p 51.
11. Williams, M, et al.: Characterization of naturally occurring diabetes in a colony of golden retrievers. Fed Proc 40:740, 1981.
12. Gershwin, LJ: Familial canine diabetes mellitus. JAVMA 167:479, 1975.
13. Kramer, JW, et al.: Inherited, early-onset, insulin-requiring diabetes mellitus of keeshond dogs. Diabetes 29:558, 1980.
14. Atkins CE, et al.: Diabetes mellitus in the juvenile dog: A report of four cases. JAVMA 175:362, 1979.
15. Marmor, M, et al.: Epidemiologic patterns of diabetes mellitus in dogs. Am J Vet Res 43:465, 1982.
16. Srikanta, S, et al.: Assay for islet cell antibodies: Protein A-monoclonal antibody method. Diabetes 34:300, 1985.
17. Alejandro, R: Personal communication, 1987.
18. Koevary, S, et al.: Passive transfer of diabetes in the BB/W rat. Science 220:727, 1983.
19. Eisenbarth, GS: Type I diabetes mellitus: A chronic autoimmune disease. N Engl J Med 314:1360, 1986.
20. Ling, GV, et al.: Diabetes mellitus in dogs: An overview of initial evaluation, immediate and long-term management, and outcome. JAVMA 170:521, 1977.
21. Anderson, NV and Low, DG: Disease of the canine pancreas: A comparative summary of 103 cases. Anim Hosp 1:189, 1965.
22. Gepts, W and Toussaint, D: Spontaneous diabetes in dogs and cats. A pathological study. Diabetologia 3:249, 1967.
23. Yano, BL, et al.: Feline insular amyloid: Incidence in adult cats with no clinicopathologic evidence of overt diabetes mellitus. Vet Pathol 18:310, 1981.
24. Yano, BL, et al.: Feline insular amyloid: Association with diabetes mellitus. Vet Pathol 18:621, 1981.
25. Westermark, P and Wilander, E: Islet amyloid in Type II (non-insulin dependent) diabetes is related to insulin. Diabetologia 24:342, 1983.
26. O'Brien, TD, et al.: High dose intravenous glucose tolerance test and serum insulin and glucagon levels in diabetic and non-diabetic cats: Relationships to insular amyloidosis. Vet Pathol 22:250, 1985.
27. Atkins, CE: Disorders of glucose homeostasis in neonatal and juvenile dogs: Hyperglycemia. Comp Cont Ed 5:851, 1983.
28. Atkins, CE and Chin, H: Insulin kinetics in juvenile canine diabetics after glucose loading. Am J Vet Res 44:596, 1983.
29. Mattheeuws, C, et al.: Diabetes mellitus in dogs: Relationship of obesity to glucose tolerance and insulin response. Am J Vet Res 45:98, 1984.
30. Nelson, RW, et al.: Unpublished data, 1987.
31. Flier, JS, et al.: Receptors, antireceptor antibodies, and mechanisms of insulin resistance. N Engl J Med 300:413, 1979.
32. Olefsky, JM, et al.: Insulin action and resistance in obesity and noninsulin-dependent type II diabetes mellitus. Am J Physiol 243:E15, 1982.
33. Kolterman, OG, et al.: Mechanisms of insulin resistance in human obesity—evidence for receptor and post-receptor defects. J Clin Invest 65:1273, 1980.
34. Cushman, SW and Wardzala, LJ: Potential mechanisms of insulin action on glucose transport in the isolated rat adipose cell. Apparent translocation of intracellular transport system to the plasma membrane. J Biol Chem 255:4752, 1980.
35. Sloan, JM and Oliver, FM: Progestagen-induced diabetes in the dog. Diabetes 24:337, 1975.
36. Peterson, ME, et al.: Diagnosis and management of concurrent diabetes mellitus and hyperadrenocorticism in thirty dogs. JAVMA 178:66, 1981b.
37. Feldman, EC and Tyrrell, JB: Plasma testosterone, plasma glucose, and plasma insulin concentration in spontaneous canine Cushing's syndrome. ACVIM Scientific Proceedings, Salt Lake City, 1982, p 81.
38. Eigenmann, JR: Diabetes mellitus in elderly female dogs: Recent findings on pathogenesis and clinical implications. JAAHA 17:805, 1981.
39. Kruth, SA and Cowgill, LD: Renal glucose transport in the cat. ACVIM Scientific Proceedings, Salt Lake City, 1982, p 78.
40. Ganong, WF: Review of Medical Physiology, 10th ed. Los Altos, CA, Lange Medical Publications, 1981.
41. Schade, DS and Eaton, RP: Diabetic ketoacidosis—pathogenesis, prevention and therapy. Clin Endocrinol Metab 12:321, 1983.
42. Barrett, EJ and DeFronzo, RA: Diabetic ketoacidosis: Diagnosis and treatment. Hosp Pract 19:89, 1984.
43. Alberti, KGMM and Hockaday, TDR: Diabetic coma. Clin Endocrinol Metab 6:421, 1977.
44. Blackshear, PB, et al.: The effects of inhibition of gluconeogenesis on ketogenesis in starved and diabetic rats. Biochem J 148:353, 1975.
45. Balasse, EO and Neef, MA: Isotopic studies in the ketosis of fasting and diabetes in man. Diabetologia 11:331, 1975.
46. Schade, DS and Eaton, RP: Pathogenesis of diabetic ketoacidosis: A reappraisal. Diabetes Care 2:296, 1979.
47. Muller, WA, et al.: Hyperglucagonemia in diabetic ketoacidosis—its prevalence and significance. Am J Med 54:52, 1973.
48. Mahler, R, et al.: The effect of insulin on lipolysis. Diabetes 13:297, 1964.
49. Schade, DS, et al.: The regulation of plasma ketone body concentrations by counterregulatory hormones in man. II. Effects of growth hormone in diabetic man. Diabetes 27:916, 1978.
50. Gerich, JE: Metabolic effects of long-term somatostatin infusion in man. Metabolism 25:1505, 1976.
51. Dobbs, R, et al.: Somatostatin analogs as glucagon suppressants in diabetes. Diabetes 26:360, 1977.
52. McGarry, JD and Foster, DW: The regulation of ketogenesis from oleic acid and the influence of antiketogenic agents. J Biol Chem 246:6247, 1971.
53. Owen, OE, et al.: Rapid intravenous sodium acetoacetate infusion in man. Metabolic and kinetic responses. J Clin Invest 52:2606, 1973.
54. Podolsky, S: Hyperosmolar nonketotic coma in the elderly diabetic. Med Clin North Am 62:815, 1978.
55. Schaer, M, et al.: Hyperosmolar syndrome in the non-ketoacidotic diabetic dog. JAAHA 10:357, 1974.
56. Schaer, M: Diabetic hyperosmolar nonketotic syndrome in a cat. JAAHA 11:42, 1975.
57. Gerich, JE, et al.: Clinical and metabolic characteristics of hyperosmolar nonketotic coma. Diabetes 20:228, 1971.

58. Kramer, JW and Evermann, JF: Early-onset genetic and familial diabetes mellitus in dogs. Proceed Sixth Ann Kal Kan Symp, Columbus, OH, 1982, p 59.

59. Holste, LC, et al.: Effect of a dry, soft moist, and canned dog food on postprandial blood glucose and insulin concentrations in healthy dogs. Am J Vet Res 1989 (in press).

60. Hamburg, S, et al.: Influence of small increments of epinephrine on glucose tolerance in normal humans. Ann Intern Med 93:566, 1980.

61. Finco, DR, et al.: Familial renal disease in Norwegian elkhound dogs. JAVMA 156:747, 1970.

62. Easley, JR and Breitschwerdt, EB: Glucosuria associated with renal tubular dysfunction in three Basenji dogs. JAVMA 168:939, 1976.

63. Bloodworth, JBM: Experimental diabetic glomerulosclerosis. The dog. Arch Pathol 79:113, 1965.

64. Bloodworth, JBM, et al.: Experimental and diabetic microangiopathy. Basement status in the dog. Diabetes 18:455, 1969.

65. Janle-Swain, E, et al.: Improvement in kidney function with continuous intraperitoneal insulin infusion (CPI) in severe diabetic glomerulopathy. Diabetic Nephropathy 2:16, 1983.

66. Wagner, AE and Macy, DW: Nephelometric determination of serum amylase and lipase in naturally occurring azotemia in the dog. Am J Vet Res 43:697, 1982.

67. Polzin, DJ, et al.: Serum amylase and lipase activities in dogs with chronic primary renal failure. Am J Vet Res 44:404, 1983.

68. Feldman, BF and Feldman, EC: Routine laboratory diagnosis of endocrine disease. Vet Clin North Am 7:443, 1977.

69. Waldhausl, W, et al.: Severe hyperglycemia: Effects of rehydration on endocrine derangements and blood glucose concentration. Diabetes 28:577, 1979.

70. Owen, OE, et al.: Renal function and effects of partial rehydration during diabetic ketoacidosis. Diabetes 30:510, 1981.

71. Foster, DW and McGarry, JD: The metabolic derangements and treatment of diabetic ketoacidosis. N Engl J Med 309:159, 1983.

72. Willard, MD, et al.: Severe hypophosphatemia associated with diabetes mellitus in six dogs and one cat. JAVMA 190:1007, 1987.

73. Keller, U and Berger, W: Prevention of hypophosphatemia by phosphate infusion during treatment of diabetic ketoacidosis and hyperosmolar coma. Diabetes 29:87, 1980.

74. Wilson, HK, et al.: Phosphate therapy in diabetic ketoacidosis. Arch Intern Med 142:517, 1982.

75. Willard, MD: Severe hypophosphatemia: Significance and treatment. Proceed ACVIM, San Diego, 1987, p 141.

76. Stoff, JS: Phosphate homeostasis and hypophosphatemia. Am J Med 72:489, 1982.

77. Alberti, KGMM: Insulin therapy in diabetic ketoacidosis and surgery. In Skyler, JH (ed): Insulin Update: 1982. Princeton, NJ, Excerpta Medica, 1982, p 160.

78. Chastain, CB and Nichols, CS: Low-dose intramuscular insulin therapy for diabetic ketoacidosis in dogs. JAVMA 178:561, 1981.

79. Turner, RC, et al.: Measurement of the insulin delivery rate in man. J Clin Endocrinol Metab 33:279, 1971.

80. Church, DB: Diabetes mellitus. In Kirk, RW (ed): Current Veterinary Therapy VIII. Philadelphia, WB Saunders, 1983, p 838.

81. Schall, WD and Cornelius, LM: Diabetic ketoacidosis. In Kirk, RW (ed): Current Veterinary Therapy VII. Philadelphia, WB Saunders, 1980, p 1016.

82. Perry, C and Cunningham, NL: Insulin adsorption by glass infusion bottles, polyvinylchloride infusion container and intravenous tubing. Anesthesiology 40:400, 1974.

83. Peterson, L, et al.: Insulin adsorbance to polyvinylchloride surfaces with implication for constant-infusion therapy. Diabetes 25:72, 1976.

84. Ionescu-Tirgoviste, C and Mincu, I: Our experience in the insulin treatment of diabetic ketoacidosis. Rev Roum Med Ser Med Int 15:281, 1977.

85. Kaye, R: Diabetic ketoacidosis—the bicarbonate controversy. J Pediatr 87:156, 1975.

86. Schade, DS and Eaton, RP: Dose response to insulin in man: Differential effects on glucose and ketone body regulation. J Clin Endocrinol Metab 44:1038, 1977.

87. Lever, N and Jaspan, J: Sodium bicarbonate therapy in severe diabetic ketoacidosis. Am J Med 75:263, 1983.

88. Felig, P: Diabetic ketoacidosis. N Engl J Med 290:1360, 1974.

89. Posner, JB and Plum, F: Spinal-fluid pH and neurologic symptoms in systemic acidosis. N Engl J Med 277:605, 1967.

90. Phear, DH: Conference on diabetes, effects of acidosis. Br Med J 2:1581, 1963.

91. Wang, H and Katz, RL: Effects of changes in coronary blood pH on the heart. Circ Res 17:114, 1965.

92. Gerst, PH, et al.: A quantitative evaluation of the effects of acidosis and alkalosis upon ventricular fibrillation threshold. Surgery 59:1050, 1966.

93. Zimmet, PZ, et al.: Acid production in diabetic acidosis; a more rational approach to alkali replacement. Br Med J 3:610, 1970.

94. Ryder, RE: Lactic acidosis: High-dose or low-dose bicarbonate therapy. Diabetes Care 7:99, 1984.

95. Lebovitz, HE and Feinglos, MN: The oral hypoglycemic agents. In Ellenberg, M and Rifkin, H (eds): Diabetes Mellitus: Theory and Practice, 3rd ed. New York, Medical Examination Publishing, 1983, p 591.

96. Moise, NS and Reimers, TJ: Insulin therapy in cats with diabetes mellitus. JAVMA 182:158, 1983.

97. Anderson, JW, et al.: Fiber and diabetes. Diabetes Care 2:369, 1979.

98. Anderson, JW and Ward, K: High carbohydrate, high fiber diets for insulin-treated men with diabetes mellitus. Am J Clin Nutr 32:2312, 1979.

99. Anderson, JW: Dietary fiber and diabetes. In Spiller, GA and Kay, RM (eds): Medical Aspects of Dietary Fiber. New York, Plenum, 1980, p 193.

100. Jenkins, DJ: Dietary fiber and carbohydrate metabolism. In Spiller, GA and Kay, RM (eds): Medical Aspects of Dietary Fiber. New York, Plenum, 1980, p 175.

101. Morgan, LM, et al.: The effect of unabsorbable carbohydrate on gut hormones: Modification of postprandial GIP secretion by guar. Diabetologia 17:85, 1979.

102. Hjollund, E, et al.: Increased insulin binding to adipocytes and monocytes and increased insulin sensitivity of glucose transport and metabolism in adipocytes from noninsulin-dependent diabetics after low-fat/high-starch/high-fiber diets. Metabolism 32:1067, 1983.

103. Gatti, E, et al.: Effects of guar-enriched pasta in the treatment of diabetes and hyperlipidemia. Ann Nutr Metab 28:1, 1984.

104. Riccardi, G, et al.: Separate influence on dietary carbohydrate and fiber on the metabolic control in diabetes. Diabetologia 26:116, 1984.

105. Anderson, JW: High-fiber diets for diabetic and hypertriglyceridemic patients. Can Med Assoc J 123:975, 1980.

106. Anderson, JW and Chen, WC: Plant fiber. Carbohydrate and lipid metabolism. Am J Clin Nutr 32:346, 1979.

107. Chang, MW and Johnson, MA: Influence of fat level and type of carbohydrate on the capacity of pectin in lowering serum and liver lipids of young rats. J Nutr 106:1562, 1976.

108. Trivelli, LA, et al.: Hemoglobin components in patients with diabetes mellitus. N Engl J Med 284:353, 1976.

109. Bookchin, RM and Gallop, PM: Structure of hemoglobin A_{1c}: Nature of the N-terminal B chain blocking group. Biochem Biophys Res Commun 32:86, 1968.

110. Widness, JA, et al.: Rapid fluctuations in glycohemoglobin (hemoglobin A1c) related to acute changes in glucose. J Lab Clin Med 95:386, 1980.

111. Goldstein, DE, et al.: Effects of acute changes in blood glucose on HbA_{1c}. Diabetes 29:623, 1980.

112. Wood, PA and Smith, JE: Glycosylated hemoglobin and canine diabetes mellitus. JAVMA 176:1267, 1980.

113. Mahaffey, EA and Cornelius, LM: Glycosylated hemoglobin in diabetic and nondiabetic dogs. JAVMA 180:635, 1982.

114. Somogyi, M, et al.: Symposium on the management of unstable, severe, diabetic patients. Wkly Bull St Louis Med Soc 32:498, 1938.

115. Somogyi, M: Exacerbation of diabetes by excess insulin action. Am J Med 26:169, 1959.

116. Bergman, R: Integrated control of hepatic glucose metabolism. Fed Proc 265, 1977.

117. Sacca, L, et al.: Blood glucose regulates the effects of insulin and counterregulatory hormones on glucose production in vivo. Diabetes 28:533, 1979.

118. Goldfein, A, et al.: The effect of hypoglycemia on the adrenal secretion of epinephrine and norepinephrine in the dog. Endocrinology 62:749, 1958.

119. Wallace, J and Harlan, W: Significance of epinephrine in insulin hypoglycemia in man. Am J Med 38:531, 1965.

120. Garber, A, et al.: The role of adrenergic mechanisms in the substrate and hormonal response to insulin-induced hypoglycemia in man. J Clin Invest 58:7, 1976.

121. Gerich, J, et al.: Stimulation of glucagon secretion by epinephrine in man. J Clin Endocrinol Metab 37:479, 1973.

122. Endinli, E and Sokal, J: Comparison of glucagon and epinephrine in the dog. Endocrinology 78:47, 1966.

123. Bruck, E and MacGillivray, M: Interaction of endogenous growth hormone, cortisol, and catecholamines with blood glucose in children with brittle diabetes mellitus. Pediatr Res 9:535, 1975.

124. Mintz, D, et al.: Hormonal genesis of glucose intolerance following hypoglycemia. Am J Med 45:187, 1968.

125. Feldman, J, et al.: The role of cortisol and growth hormone in the counter-regulation of insulin-induced hypoglycemia. Horm Metab Res 7:378, 1975.

126. Fineberg, S and Merimee, T: Acute metabolic effects of human growth hormone. Diabetes 23:499, 1974.

127. P, CE and Chin, H: Insulin kinetics in juvenile canine diabetics after glucose loading. Am J Vet Res 44:596, 1983.

128. Muggeo, M, et al.: The insulin resistance of acromegaly: Evidence for two alterations in the insulin receptor on circulating monocytes. J Clin Endocrinol Metab 48:17, 1979.

129. Kahn, C, et al.: Alterations in insulin binding induced by changes in vivo in the levels of glucocorticoids and growth hormone. J Endocrinol 103:1054, 1978.

130. Joshua, JO: Some clinical aspects of diabetes mellitus in the dog and cat. J Sm Anim Pract 4:275, 1963.

131. Wilkinson, JS: Spontaneous diabetes mellitus. Vet Res 72:548, 1960.

132. Foster, SJ: Diabetes mellitus—a study of the disease in the dog and cat in Kent. J Small Anim Pract 16:295, 1975.

133. Eigenmann, JE and Venker-van Haagen, AJ: Progestagen-induced and spontaneous canine acromegaly due to reversible growth hormone overproduction: Clinical picture and pathogenesis. JAAHA 17:813, 1981.

134. Peterson, ME, et al.: Insulin resistant diabetes mellitus associated with elevated growth hormone concentrations following megestrol acetate treatment in a cat. ACVIM Scientific Proceedings, Salt Lake City, July 1981a, p 63.

135. Pukay, BP: A hyperglycemia—glucosuria syndrome in cats following megestrol acetate therapy. Can Vet J 20:117, 1979.

136. Greenfield, C, et al.: Glucocorticoid—induced insulin resistance in vitro: Evidence for both receptor and postreceptor defects. Endocrinology 109:1723, 1981.

137. Nelson, RW, et al.: Spontaneous hyperadrenocorticism in cats: 6 cases (1978–1986). JAVMA, 1987.

138. Eigenmann, JE, et al.: Elevated growth hormone levels and diabetes mellitus in a cat with acromegalic features. JAAHA 20:747, 1984.

139. Peterson, ME, et al.: Spontaneous acromegaly in the cat. ACVIM Scientific Proceedings, Washington, DC, 1986, p 14.

140. Rocha, DM, et al.: Abnormal pancreatic α-cell function in bacterial infections. N Engl J Med 284:621, 1971.

141. Bilbrey, GL, et al.: Hyperglucagonemia of renal failure. J Clin Invest 53:841, 1974.

142. Mallinson, CN, et al.: A glucagonoma syndrome. Lancet 2:1, 1974.

143. Mondon, CE, et al.: The site of insulin resistance in acute uremia. Diabetes 27:571, 1978.

144. DeFronzo, RA: Pathogenesis of glucose intolerance in uremia. Metabolism 27:1866, 1978.

145. Cuthbert, C and Alberti, KGMM: Acidemia and insulin resistance in the diabetic ketoacidotic rat. Metabolism 27:1903, 1978.

146. Misbin, RI: Insulin resistance in ketoacidosis (letter). N Engl J Med 297:893, 1977.

147. Melmon, KL: Catecholamines and the adrenal medulla. In Williams, RH (ed): Textbook of Endocrinology. Philadelphia, WB Saunders, 1974, p 283.

148. Berson, SA, et al.: Insulin I-131 metabolism in human subjects: Demonstration of insulin binding globulin in the circulation of insulin treated subjects. J Clin Invest 35:170, 1956.

149. Kurtz, AB and Nabarro, JDN: Circulating insulin-binding antibodies. Diabetologia 19:329, 1980.

150. Fineberg, SE: Personal communication, 1984.

151. Feldman, EC, et al.: Reduced immunogenicity of pork insulin in dogs with spontaneous insulin-dependent diabetes mellitus (abstr). Diabetes 32 (suppl 1):153A, 1983.

152. Home, PD, et al.: A comparison of the activity and disposal of semi-synthetic human insulin and porcine insulin in normal man by the glucose clamp technique. Diabetologia 22:41, 1982.

153. Skyler, JS, et al.: Biosynthetic human insulin: Progress and prospects. Diabetes Care 4:140, 1981.

154. Flier, JS, et al.: Characterization of antibodies to the insulin receptor: A cause of insulin resistant diabetes in man. J Clin Invest 58:1442, 1976.

155. Pedersen, 0, et al.: Diabetes mellitus caused by insulin-receptor blockade and impaired sensitivity to insulin. N Engl J Med 304:1085, 1981.

156. Paulsen, ET, et al.: Insulin resistance caused by massive degradation of subcutaneous insulin. Diabetes 28:640, 1979.

157. Henry, DA: Defective absorption of injected insulin. 1978. Lancet 2:741,

158. Freidenberg, GR, et al.: Diabetes responsive to intravenous but not subcutaneous insulin: Effectiveness of aprotinin. N Engl J Med 305:363, 1981.

159. Chandler, ML and Varandanmi, PT: Insulin degradation. The widespread distribution of glutathione-insulin-transhydrogenase in the tissues of the rat. Biochem Biophys Acta 286:136, 1971.

160. Schade, DS and Duckworth, WC: In search of the subcutaneous insulin resistance syndrome. N Engl J Med 315:147, 1986.

161. White, NH, et al.: Identification of type I diabetic patients at increased risk for hypoglycemia during intensive therapy. N Engl J Med 308:485, 1983.

162. Bellows, JC: Cataract and Abnormalities of the Lens. New York, Grune & Stratton, 1975, p 97.

163. Wood, PA: Metabolic complications of diabetes mellitus. Comp Cont Educ 3:218, 1981.

164. Peiffer, RL, et al.: Diabetic cataracts in the dog. Canine Pract 14:18, 1977.

165. Gonzalez, A, et al.: The effect of an aldose reductase inhibitor (sorbinil) on the level of metabolites in lenses of diabetic rats. Diabetes 32:482, 1983.

166. Caird, FI, et al.: Diabetes and the Eye. London, Blackwell Scientific, 1968, p 75.

167. Engerman, R, et al.: Relationship of microvascular disease in diabetes to metabolic control. Diabetes 26:760, 1977.

168. Barrie, KP, et al.: Diseases of the canine posterior segment. In Gelatt, KN (ed): Textbook of Veterinary Ophthalmology. Philadelphia, Lea & Febiger, 1981, p 474.

169. L'Esperance, FA and James, WA: The eye and diabetes mellitus. In Ellenberg, M and Rifkin, H (eds): Diabetes Mellitus: Theory and Practice, 3rd ed. New York, Medical Examination Publishing Co, 1983, p 591.

170. Coffin, DL and Thordal-Christensen, A: The clinical and some pathological aspects of pancreatic disease in dogs. Vet Med 48:193, 1953.

171. Strombeck, DR: The pancreas. In Strombeck, DR (ed): Small Animal Gastroenterology. Davis, CA, Stonegate Publishing, 1979, p 301.

172. Woodside, WE and Heimberg, M: The metabolism of oleic acid by the perfused rat liver in experimental diabetes induced by anti-insulin serum. Metabolism 27:1763, 1978.

173. Basso, LV and Havel, RJ: Hepatic metabolism of free fatty acids in normal and diabetic dogs. J Clin Invest 40:537, 1970.

174. Strombeck, DR: Hepatic lipidosis and steroid-induced hepatopathy. In Strombeck, DR (ed): Small Animal Gastroenterology. Davis, CA, Stonegate Publishing, 1979, p 468.

175. Creutzfeldt, W, et al.: Liver disease and diabetes mellitus. In Popper, H and Schaffner, F (eds): Progress in Liver Diseases, Vol. 3. New York, Grune & Stratton, 1970, p 371.

176. Soler, NG, et al.: Intensive care in the management of diabetic ketoacidosis. Lancet 1:951, 1973.

177. Muller, WA, et al.: Hyperglucagonemia in diabetic ketoacidosis: Its prevalence and significance. Am J Med 54:52, 1973.

178. Brayton, RG, et al.: Effect of alcohol and various diseases on leukocyte mobilization, phagocytosis, and intracellular bacterial killing. N Engl J Med 282:123, 1970.

179. Ludwig, H, et al.: Humoral immunodeficiency to bacterial antigens in patients with juvenile onset diabetes mellitus. Diabetologia 12:259, 1976.
180. Mowat, AG and Baum, J: Chemotaxis of polymorphonuclear leukocytes from patients with diabetes mellitus. N Engl J Med 284:621, 1971.
181. Molenaar, DM, et al: Leukocyte chemotaxis in diabetic patients and their nondiabetic first-degree relatives. Diabetes 25:880, 1976.
182. Nolan, CM, et al.: Further characterization of the impaired bactericidal function of granulocytes in patients with poorly controlled diabetes. Diabetes 27:889, 1978.
183. Tan, JS, et al.: Neutrophil dysfunction in diabetes mellitus. J Lab Clin Med 85:26, 1975.
184. MacCuish, AC, et al.: Phytohemagglutinin transformation and circulating lymphocyte subpopulations in insulin-dependent diabetic patients. Diabetes 23:708, 1974.
185. Ellenberg, M: Diabetic neuropathy. In Ellenberg, M and Rifkin, H (eds): Diabetes Mellitus: Theory and Practice, 3rd ed. New York, Medical Examination Publishing Co, 1983, p 777.
186. Chrisman, CL: Diseases of peripheral nerves and muscles. In Ettinger, SJ (ed): Textbook of Veterinary Internal Medicine. Philadelphia, WB Saunders, 1975, p 459.
187. Katherman, AE and Braund, KG: Polyneuropathy associated with diabetes mellitus in a dog. JAVMA 182:522, 1983.
188. Steiss, JE, et al.: Electrodiagnostic analysis of a peripheral neuropathy in dogs with diabetes mellitus. Am J Vet Res 42:2061, 1982.
189. Braund, KG and Steiss, JE: Distal neuropathy in spontaneous diabetes mellitus in the dog. Acta Neuropathol 57:263, 1982.
190. Judzewitsch, RG, et al.: Aldose reductase inhibition improves nerve conduction velocity in diabetic patients. N Engl J Med 308:119, 1983.
191. Greene, DA and Lattimer, SA: Recent advances in the therapy of diabetic peripheral neuropathy by means of an aldose reductase inhibitor. Am J Med 79:13, 1985.
192. Service, FJ, et al.: Effect of blood glucose control on peripheral nerve function in diabetic patients. Mayo Clin Proc 58:283, 1983.
193. Patz, A, et al.: Studies on diabetic retinopathy. II. Retinopathy and nephropathy in spontaneous canine diabetes. Diabetes 14:700, 1965.
194. Steffes, MW, et al.: Diabetic nephropathy in the uninephrectomized dog: Microscopic lesions after one year. Kidney Int 21:721, 1982.
195. Friedman, EA: Diabetic renal disease. In Ellenberg, M and Rifkin, H (eds): Diabetes Mellitus, Theory and Practice, 3rd ed. New York, Medical Examination Publishing Co, 1983, p 759.
196. Larner, J: Insulin and oral hypoglycemic drugs; glucagon. In Goodman, LS and Gilman, A (eds): The Pharmacologic Basis of Therapeutics, 6th ed. New York, Macmillan, 1980, p 1497.
197. Nyberg, G, et al.: Impact of metabolic control in progression of clinical diabetic nephropathy. Diabetologia 30:82, 1987.
198. Wiseman, MJ, et al.: Effect of blood glucose control on increased glomerular filtration rate and kidney size in insulin-dependent diabetes. N Engl J Med 312:617, 1985.
199. Sutherland, DER, et al.: One hundred pancreas transplants at a single institution. Ann Surg 200:414, 1984.
200. Alejandro, R: Pancreatic transplantation update: Advances in islet cell transplantation, Department of Medicine, Grand Rounds, University of Miami, October 22, 1986.
201. Rabinovitch, A, et al.: Tissue culture reduces Ia antigen-bearing cells in rat islets and prolongs islet allograft survival. Diabetes 31 (Suppl.4):48, 1982.
202. Faustman, DL, et al.: Prevention of rejection of murine islet allografts by pretreatment with anti-dendritic cell antibody. Proc Natl Acad Sci USA 81:3864, 1984.
203. Lau, H, et al.: Prolongation of rat islet allograft survival by direct ultraviolet irradiation of the graft. Science 223:607, 1984.
204. Lau, H, et al.: The use of indirect ultraviolet irradiation and cyclosporine in facilitating indefinite pancreatic islet allograft acceptance. Transplantation 38:566, 1984.
205. Elliott, JF, et al.: Induction of interleukin 2 messenger RNA inhibited by cyclosporin A. Science 226:1439, 1984.
206. Kupiec-Weglinski, JW, et al.: Sparing of suppressor cells: A critical action of cyclosporine. Transplantation 38:97, 1984

207. Alejandro, R, et al.: Successful long-term survival of pancreatic islet allografts in spontaneous or pancreatectomy-induced diabetes in dogs: Cyclosporine-induced immune unresponsiveness. Diabetes 34:825, 1986.
208. Sutherland, DER, et al.: Twin-to-twin pancreas transplantation: Reversal and reenactment of the pathogenesis of type I diabetes. Trans Assoc Am Phys 97:80, 1984.
209. Sibley, RK, et al.: Recurrent diabetes mellitus in the pancreas iso- and allograft: A light and electron microscopic and immunohistochemical analysis of four cases. Lab Invest 53:132, 1985.
210. Sun, AM, et al.: Optimization of microencapsulation parameters: Semipermeable microcapsules as a bioartificial pancreas. Biotech Bioeng 27:146, 1985.
211. O'Shea, GM and Sun, AM: Encapsulation of rat islets of Langerhans prolongs xenograft survival in diabetic mice. Diabetes 35:943, 1985.
212. Cutfield, RG, et al: Long-term follow-up of canine segmental pancreatic autografts. Diabetes 34:174, 1985.
213. Moore, FM, et al.: Pancreatic endocrine tumors in dogs: An immunohistochemical analysis. Lab Invest 52:44, 1985 (abstr).
214. Hill, FWG, et al.: Functional islet cell turnover in the dog. J Small Anim Pract 15:119, 1974.
215. Kruth, SA, et al.: Insulin-secreting islet cell tumors: Establishing a diagnosis and the clinical course of 25 dogs. JAVMA 181:54, 1982.
216. Priester, WA: Pancreatic islet cell tumors in domestic animals. Data from 11 colleges of veterinary medicine in the United States and Canada. J Nat Cancer Institute 53:227, 1974.
217. Caywood, DD and Wilson, JW: Functional pancreatic islet cell adenocarcinoma in the dog. In Kirk, RW (ed): Current Veterinary Therapy VII. Philadelphia, WB Saunders, 1980, p 1020.
218. MacMillan, F: Insulinoma in a cat, ACVIM Scientific Proceedings, New York, 1983, p 51 (abstr).
219. Quesenberry, KE, et al.: Pancreatic insulin-secreting tumor in the ferret. Proceedings of the ACVIM, San Diego, 1987, p 879 (abstr).
220. Kaufman, J, et al.: Pancreatic β cell tumor in a ferret. JAVMA 185:998, 1984.
221. Luttgen, PJ, et al.: Insulinoma in a ferret. JAVMA 189:920, 1986.
222. Marliss, EB: Normalization of glycemia in diabetics during meals with insulin and glucagon delivery by the artificial pancreas. Diabetes 26:663, 1977.
223. Fajans, SS and Floyd, JC: Fasting hypoglycemia in adults. N Engl J Med 294:766, 1976.
224. Krook, L and Kenny, RM: Central nervous system lesions in dogs with metastasizing islet cell carcinoma. Cornell Vet 52:385, 1962.
225. Braund, KG, et al.: Insulinoma and subclinical peripheral neuropathy in two dogs. J Vet Intern Med 1:86, 1987.
226. Bradows, RG, et al.: Mechanism of plasma cyclic AMP response to hypoglycemia in man. Metabolism 25:659, 1976.
227. Cryer, PE and Gerich, JE: Glucose counterregulation, hypoglycemia, and intensive insulin therapy in diabetes mellitus. N Engl J Med 313:232, 1985.
228. Palmer, JP, et al.: Glucagon response to hypoglycemia in sympathectomized man. J Clin Invest 57:522, 1976.
229. Sherwin, RS and Felig, P: Hypoglycemia. In Felig, P, et al. (eds): Endocrinology and Metabolism. New York, McGraw-Hill, 1981, p 869.
230. Scully, RE, et al.: Case records of the Massachusetts General Hospital. N Engl J Med 308:30, 1983.
231. Vranic, M and Kawamori, R: Essential roles of insulin and glucagon in regulating glucose fluxes during exercise in dogs. Diabetes 28 (suppl 1):45, 1979.
232. Shahar, R, et al.: Peripheral polyneuropathy in a dog with functional isle B-cell tumor and widespread metastasis. JAVMA 187:175, 1985.
233. Jaspan, JB: Hypoglycemic peripheral neuropathy in association with insulinoma: Implications of glucopenia rather than hyperinsulinism. Medicine 61:33, 1982.
234. Kudo, M and Noguchi, T: Immunoreactive myelin basic protein in tumor cells associated with carcinomatous neuropathy. Am J Clin Pathol 84:741, 1985.
235. Leifer, CE, et al.: Insulin-secreting tumor: Diagnosis and medical and surgical management in 55 dogs. JAVMA 188:60, 1986.

236. Johnson, RK: Insulinoma in the dog. Vet Clin North Am 7:629, 1977.
237. Feldman, EC, et al.: Insulin-secreting islet cell tumors: Establishing a diagnosis and the clinical course of 29 dogs. Kal Kan Symposium, Columbus, Ohio, 1983, p 101.
238. Whipple, AO and Grantz, VK: Adenoma of islet cells with hyperinsulinism. A review. Ann Surg 101:1299, 1935.
239. Leifer, CE, et al.: Hypoglycemia associated with nonislet cell tumor in 13 dogs. JAVMA 186:53, 1985.
240. Caywood, DD, et al.: Pancreatic islet cell adenocarcinoma: Clinical and diagnostic features of six cases. JAVMA 174:714, 1979.
241. Mattheeuws, D, et al.: Hyperinsulinism in the dog due to pancreatic islet cell tumor: A report on three cases. J Small Anim Pract 7:313, 1976.
242. Baxter, JD and Forsham, PH: Tissue effects of glucocorticoids. Am J Med 53:573, 1972.
243. Haemers, S and Rottiers, R: Medical treatment of insulinoma. Acta Clinica Belgica 36:199, 1981.
244. Schein, PS, et al.: Islet cell tumors: Current concepts and management. Ann Intern Med 79:239, 1973.
245. Altszuler, N, et al.: On the mechanism of diazoxide-induced hyperglycemia. Diabetes 26:931, 1977.
246. Schiavo, DM, et al.: Cataracts in beagle dogs given diazoxide. Diabetes 24:1041, 1975.
247. Parker, AJ, et al.: Diazoxide treatment of metastatic insulinoma in the dog. JAAHA 18:315, 1982.
248. Pruitt, AW, et al.: Metabolism of diazoxide in man and experimental animals. J Pharmacol Exp Ther 188:248, 1974.
249. Smith, CK, et al.: Treatment of malignant insulinoma with streptozotocin. Diabetologia 7:118, 1971.
250. Meyer, DJ: A pancreatic islet cell carcinoma in a dog treated with streptozotocin. Am J Vet Res 37:1221, 1976.
251. Meyer, DJ: Temporary remission of hypoglycemia in a dog with an insulinoma after treatment with streptozotocin. Am J Vet Res 38:1201, 1977.
252. Herr, RR, et al.: Structure of streptozotocin. J Am Chem Soc 89:4808, 1967.
253. Schein, PS, et al.: The use of nicotinamide to modify the toxicity of streptozotocin diabetes without loss of antitumor activity. Cancer Res 27:2324, 1967.
254. Dublin, WE, et al.: Experimental and spontaneous diabetes in animals. *In* Ellenberg, M and Rifkin, H (eds): Diabetes Mellitus, Theory and Practice, 3rd ed. New York, Medical Examination Publishing, 1983, p 361.
255. Rossini, AA, et al.: Studies of alloxan toxicity on the β cell. Diabetes 24:516, 1975.
256. Rerup, CC: Drugs producing diabetes through damage of the insulin-secreting cells. Pharmacol Rev 22:485, 1970.

DRUG INDEX

Generic	Trade	Dosage	Route	Frequency	Indication
Regular insulin	—	0.1 U/lb	IM	Once hourly	Initial treatment of DKA until blood glucose is <250 mg/dl
		0.05 U/lb	IM		
		0.05–0.2 U/lb	IM,SQ	t.i.d.–q.i.d.	Mild DKA or when blood glucose is <250 mg/dl in severe DKA
NPH insulin	—	0.25–0.5 U/lb	SQ	s.i.d.	Initial treatment of healthy diabetic dog
Protamine zinc insulin	—	1–3 units/cat	SQ	s.i.d.	Initial treatment of healthy diabetic cat
Furosemide	(Lasix)	1–2 mg/lb	IV	t.i.d.–q.i.d.	DKA with concurrent oliguric renal failure
Dopamine	(Intropin)	1–3 µgm/lb/min	IV	Continuous drip	DKA with concurrent oliguric renal failure
Glipizide	(Glucotrol)	0.1–0.25 mg/lb (max. 5 mg/day)	PO	b.i.d.	Oral hypoglycemic agent
Glyburide	(Diabeta)	0.1 mg/lb	PO	s.i.d.	Oral hypoglycemic agent
Prednisone	—	0.12 mg/lb	PO	b.i.d.	Initial dosage for treatment of insulin-secreting tumor
Diazoxide	(Proglycem)	2.5 mg/lb	PO	b.i.d	Initial dosage for treatment of insulin-secreting tumor

97 ADRENAL GLAND DISEASE

EDWARD C. FELDMAN

HYPERADRENOCORTICISM— CANINE CUSHING'S SYNDROME (CCS)

In 1932 Dr. Harvey Cushing described 12 humans with a disorder that he suggested was the result of "pituitary basophilism." A careful study of these and later cases in humans suggests multiple causes of this syndrome. The eponym Cushing's syndrome is an inclusive term used to refer to the constellation of clinical and chemical abnormalities resulting from chronic exposure to excess glucocorticoids. The eponym Cushing's disease is applied to those cases of Cushing's syndrome in which hypercortisolism is secondary to inappropriate secretion of adrenocorticotropin (ACTH) by the pituitary (i.e., pituitary-dependent hyperadrenocorticism, PDH). Canine Cushing's syndrome (CCS) also has various pathophysiologic origins, but all have one common denominator: increased concentrations of circulating cortisol.

A pathophysiologic classification of the causes of CCS would include adrenocortical hyperplasia due to a pituitary tumor that produces excess ACTH or excess ACTH resulting from a hypothalamic disorder, primary adrenal disease due to adrenocortical carcinoma or adenoma, and iatrogenic causes such as excessive ACTH administration (rare) or excessive glucocorticoid medication (common). A tumor outside the hypothalamus or pituitary that produces excessive quantities of ACTH has been described in humans, but not in dogs or cats.

REGULATION OF GLUCOCORTICOID SECRETION

Corticotrophin-Releasing Hormone

Since the early descriptions of portal circulation connecting the hypothalamus and the pituitary, it has been recognized that the hypothalamus exerts control over secretion of ACTH by the anterior pituitary. The factor responsible for this control was identified, initially, as corticotrophin-releasing factor. This "factor" has now been identified as a polypeptide that contains 41 amino acid residues and is referred to as corticotrophin-releasing "hormone" (CRH). The CRH-secreting neurons are located in the anterior portion of the paraventricular nuclei within the hypothalamus. Their axons terminate in all parts of the external layer of the median eminence. CRH stimulates the secretion of beta-lipotropin (β-LPH) as well as ACTH.[1] These pituitary hormones are formed from a large precursor molecule called pro-opiomelanocortin and are released in equimolar amounts by exocytosis. There is good evidence that CRH controls ACTH release but does not increase synthesis of the hormone. There is probably feedback control by ACTH on CRH secretion. This internal or "short-loop" feedback system is directly controlled by the blood level of ACTH at the hypothalamic level.[2]

There is a question as to the role that vasopressin (ADH) plays in the control of ACTH secretion. It is likely that ADH is released during certain stresses and that it potentiates the action of CRH.[3] In addition, angiotensin II acts directly on the pituitary to stimulate ACTH secretion, but its physiologic role in the regulation of ACTH secretion is not known.[1]

ACTH and Related Peptides

BIOSYNTHESIS

ACTH and its related peptides, the lipotropins and endorphins, are secreted by basophil-staining cells that are embryologically of intermediate lobe origin. These cells are located in both the intermediate and anterior lobes of the adult canine pituitary. ACTH is a 39-amino acid peptide hormone (MW, 4500). Within the corticotroph, a single mRNA directs the synthesis of the large precursor, which is then processed into smaller biologically active fragments. The function and importance of these related peptides (β-LPH, α-MSH, β-MSH, β-endorphin, and N-terminal fragment) are an evolving area of endocrine research. Most of these peptides are glycosylated to some extent, causing differences in the reporting of their molecular weights. It is these carbohydrate moieties that are responsible for the basophilic staining of corticotrophs. Previous names for portions of the pro-opiomelanocortin precursor, such as "big ACTH," "pro-ACTH," and "pre-pro-ACTH," were based on nonspecific techniques.[4]

Two major peptide fragments are contained within the structure of ACTH: α-MSH is identical to $ACTH_{1-13}$ and corticotropin-like intermediate lobe peptide (CLIP) represents $ACTH_{18-39}$. These fragments are found in species with developed intermediate lobes (e.g., the rat). β-Lipotropin, a fragment with 91 amino acids (1–91), is secreted by the corticotroph in equimolar quantities with ACTH. Within the β-LPH molecule exists the amino acid sequence for β-MSH (41–58), α-LPH (1–58), and β-endorphin (61–91). β-Endorphin appears to have importance in normal endocrine physiology and in disease. Despite the presence of the amino acid sequence for methionine-enkephalin (61–65) within β-LPH and β-endorphin, there is no evidence that it is secreted separately by the pituitary.[4]

The N-terminal fragment (131 amino acids) of pro-opiomelanocortin has been isolated and sequenced; it appears in vitro to have aldosterone-stimulating activity and may be found to have clinical importance.[4]

FUNCTION OF ACTH AND RELATED PEPTIDES

ACTH. The primary effect of ACTH is to stimulate the synthesis and secretion of glucocorticoids, mineralocorticoids, and androgenic steroids from the adrenal cortex. The amino-terminal end (residues 1–18) is responsible for this biologic activity. ACTH binds to receptors on the adrenal cortex and provokes steroidogenesis, through the mediation of cyclic 3′,5′-adenosine monophosphate (cyclic AMP, cAMP). The increases in cAMP stimulate the rate-limiting step of cholesterol metabolism. ACTH has a number of other effects, including increased free cholesterol formation, increased lipoprotein uptake by the adrenal cortex, and increased binding of cholesterol to the cleavage enzyme in mitochondria. Plasma concentrations of cortisol rise within minutes after ACTH administration. Chronic stimulation increases protein, RNA, and DNA synthesis, leading to adrenocortical hyperplasia and hypertrophy. Conversely, ACTH deficiency results in decreased steroidogenesis and is accompanied by adrenocortical atrophy, decreased gland weight, and decreased protein and nucleic acid content.[4]

β-LPH and Associated Peptides. The physiologic function of β-LPH and its family of peptide hormones, including β-endorphin, is not well understood. However, it is known that both β-LPH and β-endorphin have the same secretory dynamics as ACTH: they increase in response to stress and hypoglycemia and are suppressible with glucocorticoids. These hormones also parallel ACTH in disease states; for example, they are elevated in Addison's disease, Cushing's disease, and Nelson's syndrome (growing pituitary tumor after removal of the adrenals). Furthermore, there is evidence that β-endorphin acts as an "endogenous opiate," suggesting a role in pain appreciation. It may affect the endocrine regulation of other pituitary hormones and be a causative factor in disease states.

NEUROENDOCRINE CONTROL

Physiologic Factors. Physiologic factors that influence the secretion of ACTH can conveniently be divided into three main groups: those that are under control of the diurnal mechanism, those resulting from stress, and feedback inhibition by cortisol of ACTH secretion. Although there is no evidence proving that there are different corticotropin-releasing hormones, or different pathways by which CRH acts, this division is a convenient one and is corroborated by much experimental data.[5]

Diurnal Variation. The diurnal variation in glucocorticoid secretion is characterized by high levels of circulating cortisol in the early morning hours (at approximately sunrise) and low levels in the late evening. This daily rhythm is superimposed on episodic secretion in humans. It is the result of central nervous system events that regulate both the number and magnitude of CRH and ACTH secretory episodes. Major secretory bursts occur with rapid frequency in the early morning hours. About half of the total daily cortisol output is secreted during this period. Cortisol secretion then gradually declines during the day, with fewer secretory episodes of decreased magnitude; however, there is increased cortisol secretion in response to eating. Thus, in interpreting plasma corticosteroid determinations in clinical situations, a single determination may be misleading. Diurnal variation in plasma cortisol has been difficult to confirm in the dog.[6] If cortisol concentration levels reflect "bursts" of ACTH secretion, the plasma cortisol value depends on the moment of venous sampling relative to the timing of both the pituitary burst of ACTH and the adrenocortical response.

The circadian rhythm in plasma ACTH and cortisol is usually absent in human patients with hyperadrenocorticism. However, the normal rhythm in ACTH concentrations is present in hypoadrenocorticism, although, owing to the lack of the normal corticosteroid feedback to the pituitary gland, all concentrations are elevated. Thus the periodicity of the circadian rhythm is independent of the negative feedback effects of corticosteroids. The absence of a rhythm in hyperadrenocorticism is assumed to be an associated dysfunction at either the adrenal, pituitary, or hypothalamic level.[3]

There is a circadian rhythm in the ability of natural and synthetic exogenous corticosteroids to suppress ACTH secretion. In humans and rats the maximum inhibitory effect is exerted when these substances are administered four to eight hours before the circadian peak.[7] There is, therefore, a good argument for restricting corticosteroid administration in veterinary patients to the morning only (when possible), thereby limiting the dangers of pituitary suppression.[3]

Although secretion patterns are consistent, there is considerable intra-individual and inter-individual variability, and the circadian rhythm may be altered by changes in sleep pattern, light/dark exposure, and feeding times. The rhythm is also changed by (1) physical stresses such as major illness, surgery, trauma, or starvation; (2) psychologic stress; (3) central nervous system and pituitary disorders; (4) Cushing's syndrome; (5) liver disease and other conditions that alter cortisol metabolism; and (6) chronic renal failure. Cyproheptadine (see section on Therapy) inhibits the circadian rhythm, possibly by its antiserotoninergic effects, whereas other drugs usually have no effect.

Stress. Under normal circumstances, mammals respond to a variety of stressful situations, both physical and psychologic, by increased secretion of ACTH. Studies have demonstrated the importance of the nervous system in the mediation of these responses,[8] illustrated by the marked increase in ACTH secretion after severe trauma to a limb. Denervation of the involved limb decreases the response because the stimulus travels by way of peripheral nerves to central locations in the median eminence of the hypothalamus, where it stimulates secretion of CRH. The hypothalamic transmitter is carried by the hypophyseal portal circulation to the anterior pituitary, where it stimulates production of ACTH. CRH produced in this response cannot easily be suppressed. The corticosteroids do not immediately suppress further ACTH production, which would block the additional surge of corticosteroids needed to combat the stressful situation. In severe and prolonged stress, corticosteroid levels rise and continue at high concentrations over extended periods.[9]

ACTH secretion in response to stress is also episodic. The secretory spike frequency increases under stress, since average spike frequency in the morning and in the evening is statistically lower under non-stressed conditions than during stress.[5]

Feedback Inhibition (Feedback Loops). The third major regulator of ACTH and cortisol secretion is that of glucocorticoid feedback inhibition of CRH, ACTH, and cortisol secretion. In the resting state, ACTH and cortisol bear a reciprocal control relationship to each another. ACTH release produces a rise in the plasma cortisol concentration, which in turn acts on receptors in the hypothalamus to decrease CRH secretion and thus reduce ACTH release. As the effective level of glucocorticoid diminishes, CRH secretion increases and the cycle is completed.

PATHOPHYSIOLOGY

Pituitary-Dependent Hyperadrenocorticism (PDH)

In PDH, ACTH secretion is random, episodic, and persistent. Excessive ACTH secretion results in adrenocortical hyperplasia and excess cortisol secretion with absence of the normal circadian rhythm. Feedback inhibition of ACTH (secreted from hyperplastic cells or a pituitary adenoma) by physiologic levels of glucocorticoids is absent (Figure 97–1). Thus, ACTH secretion persists despite elevations in cortisol secretion. This unbridled release of hormone results in chronic glucocorticoid excess. The episodic secretion of ACTH and cortisol results in fluctuating plasma concentrations that may at times be within the normal range. Studies of cortisol production, such as urine cortisol excretion over 24 hours, confirm the existence of excessive cortisol secretion. This excessive secretion and the absence of diurnal variation (if it exists) in glucocorticoid secretion cause the clinical manifestations of Cushing's syndrome. In addition to the systemic effects of glucocorticoid excess, this disorder also results in inhibition of normal pituitary and hypothalamic function. affecting thyrotropin (TSH), growth hormone (GH), and gonadotropin (luteinizing hormone and follicle-stimulating hormone, FSH) release.

Eighty to 85 per cent of dogs with spontaneous Cushing's syndrome have PDH, that is, excessive secretion of ACTH by the pituitary, causing bilateral adrenal hyperplasia and excessive secretion of glucocorticoids.[10–12] The reported incidence of pituitary tumors in dogs with PDH varies tremendously but is probably dependent, for the most part, on the competence, microdissection capabilities, and staining capacities of the laboratory performing the histology. In one study in which immunocytochemical staining of the pituitary was used, tumors of the pars distalis and pars intermedia, as well as combinations of these abnormalities, were recognized.[13] Despite these new and exciting findings, the primary cause for PDH remains obscure. Both a primary pituitary abnormality (ACTH-secreting adenoma) and a central nervous system derangement with excessive stimulation of pituitary corticotrophs by CRH or other hypothalamic factors have been proposed.[14] Adenomas of the pars distalis are the most common histologic finding in canine PDH, suggesting a primary pituitary cause for the disorder. However, a small number of dogs have pituitary hyperplasia, which suggests a hypothalamic disorder that causes excessive stimulation of pituitary corticotrophs. It is conceivable that adenomas could also arise secondary to prolonged central nervous system stimulation of corticotrophs. It would be difficult for one hypothalamic disorder to account for tumors arising in both the pars distalis and pars intermedia, since regulation of the two lobes is so different. The pars distalis is devoid of a nerve supply and is controlled by hypothalamic CRH that reaches it through the hypophyseal portal vessels, whereas the avascular pars intermedia is innervated by dopaminergic and serotoninergic fibers from the brain.[13, 15] Further confusion is seen in response to treatment. Cyproheptadine, which has antiserotoninergic actions, was reported to have been therapeutically effective in only 3 of 15 cases of canine PDH.[16] It is safe to propose that PDH may result from several physiopathogenic mechanisms that may be further defined in the near future.[17]

Adrenal Tumors

Primary adrenal tumors, both adenomas and carcinomas, arise spontaneously, and autonomously secrete excessive quantities of cortisol. Circulating plasma ACTH levels are suppressed, resulting in cortical atrophy of the uninvolved adrenal and of all normal cells in the involved adrenal (see Figure 97–1). Cortisol secretion by these tumors is independent of hypothalamic-pituitary control. Secretion is randomly episodic. Adrenal tumors are typically unresponsive to manipulation of the hypothalamic-pituitary axis with pharmacologic agents such as dexamethasone. In dogs there have been no recognized features other than tumor size that aid in distinguishing patients with adrenal adenomas from those with adrenal carcinomas (may be large), as has been recognized in humans.[4]

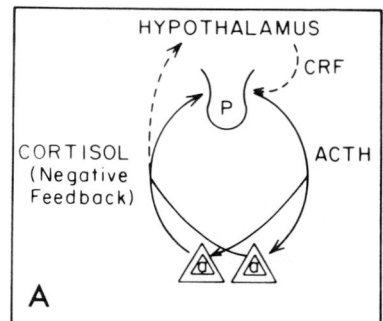 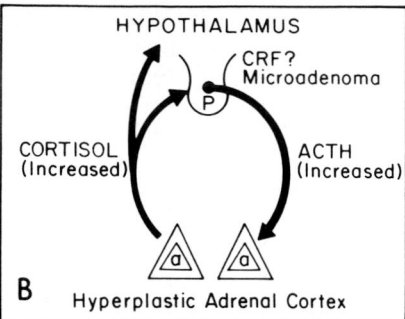 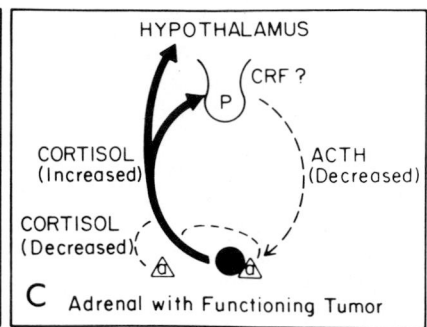

FIGURE 97–1. The pituitary-adrenal axis in normal dogs *(A)*, dogs with pituitary-dependent hyperadrenocorticism *(B)*, and dogs with a functioning adrenocortical tumor *(C)*. a, adrenal; P, pituitary; CRF, corticotropin-releasing factor. (From Feldman, EC: *In* Ettinger, SJ (ed): Textbook of Veterinary Internal Medicine, 2nd ed. Philadelphia, WB Saunders, 1983, p 1673.)

Ectopic ACTH Syndrome

This syndrome has not yet been diagnosed in the dog. In humans it comprises a varying group of tumors that are capable of synthesizing and secreting ACTH, and ultimately cause adrenal hyperplasia with hypercortisolism. Tumors with the potential for causing the ectopic ACTH syndrome in humans include oat cell carcinomas of the lung, thymoma, pancreatic islet cell tumors, carcinoid tumors (lung, gut, pancreas, ovary), medullary carcinoma of the thyroid, and pheochromocytoma.[4] When these tumors synthesize and secrete excessive quantities of biologically active ACTH, the related peptides β-LPH and β-endorphin are also synthesized and secreted, as are inactive ACTH fragments. CRH-like activity has also been demonstrated in ectopic tumors that secrete ACTH; however, secretion of CRH into plasma has not been demonstrated and the role of this tumor-derived CRH is unclear.[4]

PATHOLOGY

The Pituitary

Microadenomas. Eighty to 85 per cent of the dogs with spontaneous Cushing's syndrome have pituitary-dependent disease. The reported incidence of histologically recognized pituitary tumors varies between 20 and 100 per cent.[18, 19] In one study using immunocytochemical staining of the pituitary, pituitary adenomas reactive to ACTH or related peptides (β-LPH, β-endorphin, α-melanocyte-stimulating hormone, α-MSH) were found in 21 of 25 dogs with PDH.[13] In that series, there were also three dogs in which corticotropic hyperplasia was present: one without any associated adenoma, one with hyperplasia of both the pars distalis and the pars intermedia in association with a pars distalis adenoma, and one with hyperplasia of the pars distalis in association with a pars intermedia tumor.[20] It is fair to say that recognition of these pituitary tumors requires careful microdissection, experience, special stains, and a great deal of patience. Because these criteria are not often met, pituitary abnormalities are frequently not appreciated. Most ACTH-secreting

pituitary tumors are usually defined as microadenomas (< 1 cm in diameter). They are not encapsulated, but may be surrounded by a rim of compressed normal pituitary cells. With routine histologic stains, such tumors are seen to be composed of compact sheets of well-granulated basophilic cells in a sinusoidal arrangement. ACTH-secreting adenomas typically show Crooke's changes (a zone of perinuclear hyalinization that results from chronic exposure of corticotroph cells to hypercortisolism). Electron microscopy demonstrates secretory granules that vary in size from 200 to 700 mm. The number of granules varies in individual cells.

Macroadenomas. A significant percentage of dogs with PDH (perhaps 20 to 30 per cent) have large pituitary tumors. A macroadenoma is defined as being visible on gross examination of the pituitary, or > 1 cm in diameter. These tumors have the potential of becoming invasive, leading to their extension out of the sella turcica. The masses usually extend dorsally into the hypothalamus, and may result in depression, anorexia, listlessness, dull behavior, or, rarely, aggressive behavior. It is possible for some dogs to have no clinical signs despite the presence of a large pituitary mass. Large pituitary tumors may appear chromophobic on routine histologic study, but they typically contain ACTH and its related peptides. Malignant pituitary tumors occur rarely.[17]

Hyperplasia. Diffuse hyperplasia of corticotroph cells has been reported in three dogs with PDH (see previous discussion on microadenomas). These cases may be the consequence of excessive stimulation of the anterior pituitary by CRH.

Adrenocortical Hyperplasia

Simple Bilateral Hyperplasia. This disorder is usually secondary to PDH. Combined adrenal weight is typically modestly increased. On histologic study, there is equal hyperplasia of the compact cells of the zona reticularis and the clear cells of the zona fasciculata; consequently, the width of the cortex is increased. Electron microscopy reveals normal ultrastructural features.

Bilateral Nodular Hyperplasia. This occurs in less than five per cent of dogs with CCS. It is not clear whether these animals have PDH or some other disorder. Most cases have been demonstrated to occur secondary to excess secretion of ACTH. Autonomous nodular adrenal hyperplasia has not been reported in the dog. In humans with this disorder, the adrenals are enlarged, sometimes markedly. Grossly, there are multiple nodules within the adrenal cortices, with widening of the intervening cortex. The nodules are typically yellow, and on histologic examination resemble the clear cells of the normal zona fasciculata. The remainder of the adrenal cortices show the histologic features of simple adrenocortical hyperplasia.

Adrenal Tumors

Adenomas. Adrenal adenomas are encapsulated and grossly visible, and range in size from 1 to 6 cm. Microscopically, clear cells of the zona fasciculata type predominate, although cells typical of the zona reticularis may also be seen. Approximately 50 per cent of adrenocortical adenomas are partially calcified.[21]

Carcinomas. Adrenal carcinomas can become quite large. Several carcinomas in our series were two to three times larger than the dog's kidney. Grossly, they are encapsulated and highly vascular; necrosis, hemorrhage, and cystic degeneration are common. Tumor calcification is present in 50 per cent of these dogs. The histologic appearance of these carcinomas varies considerably; they may appear to be benign or may exhibit considerable pleomorphism. Vascular or capsular invasion is predictive of malignant behavior, as is local extension. These carcinomas invade local structures (kidney, liver, vena cava, aorta, and retroperitoneum) and metastasize hematogenously to liver and lung.

Uninvolved Adrenal Cortex. The cortex contiguous to the tumor and that of the contralateral gland are atrophic in the presence of functioning adrenal adenomas and carcinomas. The cortex is markedly thinned, whereas the capsule is thickened. Histologically, the zona reticularis is virtually absent; the remaining cortex is composed of clear zona fasciculata cells. The architecture of the zona glomerulosa is usually normal.

SIGNALMENT

The age at the time of diagnosis of hyperadrenocorticism varies between 2 and 16 years.[22] The author has seen four dogs with PDH less than one year of age at the time of diagnosis (Figure 97–2). It is generally agreed, however, that PDH is usually a disease of middle-aged and older dogs, usually six years of age and older, with a median age of seven to nine years.[23]

Dogs with hyperadrenocorticism caused by functioning adrenocortical tumors have a median age, at the time of diagnosis, of 10 to 11 years.[18] In a review of 47 dogs with adrenocortical tumors in our series, the average age was 11.3 years, ranging between 6 and 16 years.[25]

Dogs with hyperadrenocorticism did not have a significant sex distribution,[22] nor was one sex believed to be more at risk in the PDH group reviewed. Females,

however, were found to have adrenal tumors three times more frequently than males.[18] In our series of 47 dogs with functioning adrenocortical tumors, 32 were female (67 per cent).

No breed preference was seen in dogs with adrenal tumors in one study.[18] In our series, however, German shepherd dogs, toy poodles, dachshunds, and terriers were most common. Poodles, dachshunds, and beagles were found to be at increased risk of developing PDH when compared with the general population of canine patients in our series. The Boston terrier and boxer have also been mentioned to be at increased risk.[25] Both adrenocortical tumors and PDH have been diagnosed in numerous breeds.

HISTORY

General Review. As a result of the chronic relative or absolute elevations in plasma glucocorticoids, affected dogs usually develop a classic combination of dramatic clinical signs and lesions. These are the sequelae of the combined gluconeogenic, lipolytic, protein catabolic, anti-inflammatory, and immunosuppressive effects of glucocorticoid hormones on various organ systems.

The course of the disease is insidious and slowly progressive. The owner typically reports the presence of some alterations typical of hyperadrenocorticism in the pet for one to six years before the diagnosis is made (Table 97–1). A similar time period elapses before the owner seeks veterinary attention for the animal, since changes are quite gradual in onset and are often believed by the client to be simple "aging." It is only when the signs become intolerable to the client or after alterations are specifically pointed out by people who have seen the pet infrequently (therefore noting obvious changes that have developed so slowly the owner does not observe them) that professional opinions are sought. The most common reasons owners give for finally seeking veterinary help for their dogs are usually polydipsia and polyuria, polyphagia, lethargy, panting, and/or hair coat changes.

In a minority of dogs, clinical signs may initially be intermittent, with periods of remission and relapse.[26] Dogs with rapidly growing adrenocortical tumors and some with PDH are occasionally reported by their owners to have a rapid onset and progression of illness. The duration of clinical signs or the signs noticed have not consistently aided in distinguishing PDH from adrenal tumor.[17]

Polydipsia and Polyuria. Polydipsia and polyuria are extremely common signs of CCS, and represent perhaps the major reason for bringing a pet to the veterinarian. Previously housebroken animals are no longer able to endure the night without urinating. The pet pesters the owner to be let outside or urinates indoors, and the situation quickly becomes intolerable for the client. Polydipsia and polyuria are seen in 85 to 97 per cent of dogs with CCS.[18, 22, 23, 27]

The polydipsia occurs secondary to polyuria and the tremendous fluid losses that may occur. Using a normal water intake for the average dog of approximately 20 to

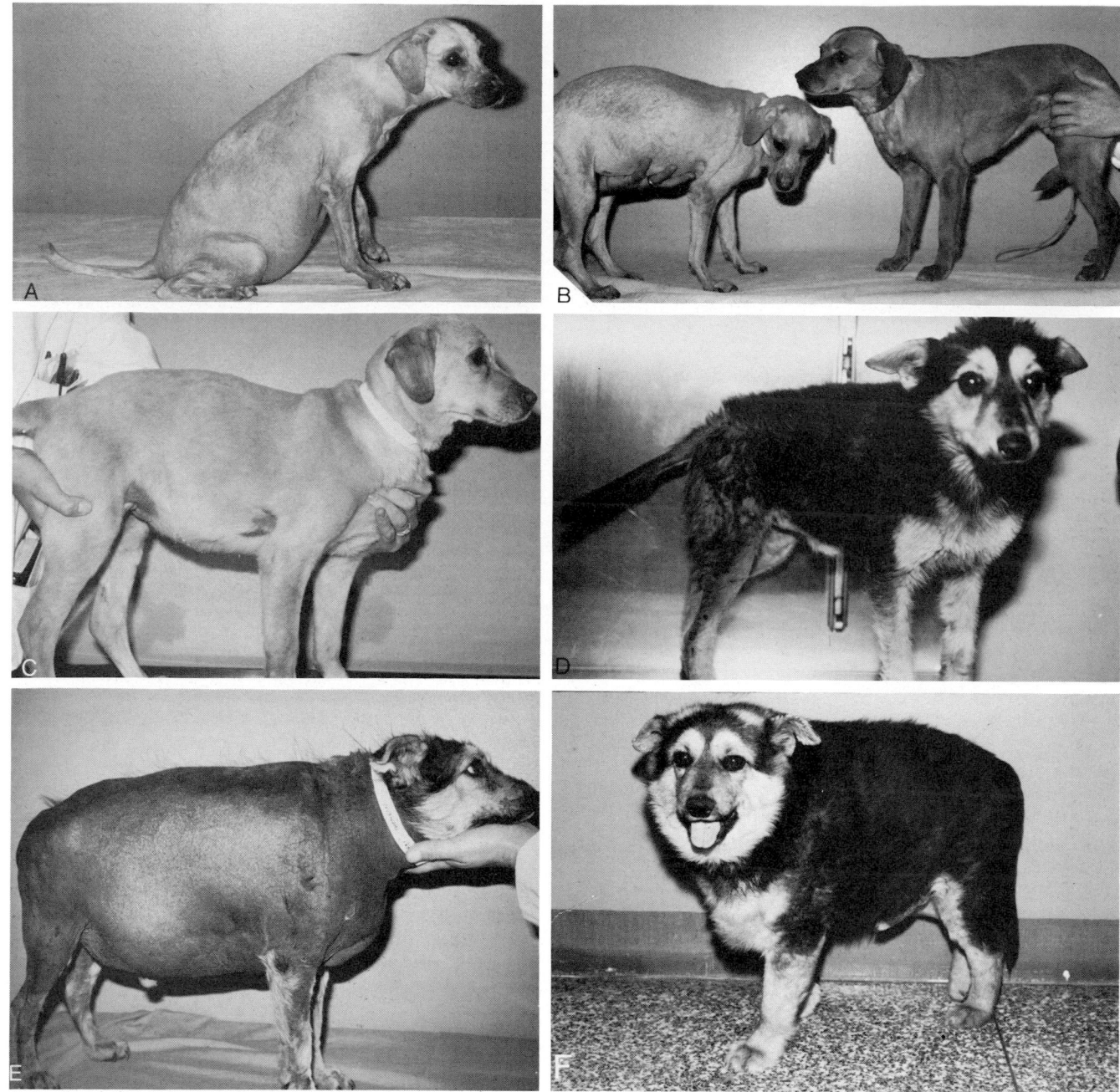

FIGURE 97–2. *A,* Mixed-breed 18-month-old dog with hyperadrenocorticism. *B,* Same dog *(left)* and a normal litter mate. *C,* Five months after initiation of o,p'-DDD therapy. *D,* A six-month-old German shepherd dog with hyperadrenocorticism. *E,* Same dog as in *D,* after four years without therapy. *F,* Same dog as in *D* and *E* four months after initiating therapy with o,p'-DDD.

30 ml per pound of body weight per day,[28] owners will usually report the water intake in polydipsic hyperadrenal dogs to vary between two and ten times normal. The cause of the polyuria remains obscure. Some investigators believe that the polyuria is the result of interference by cortisol with the action of antidiuretic hormone at the level of the renal collecting tubules.[18] It has also been proposed that cortisol may increase the glomerular filtration rate, thus initiating a diuresis.[27] In humans, however, cortisol raises the responsive threshold of osmoreceptors.[29] A direct depression of renal tubular permeability to water has also been noted in normal dogs,[30] and large doses of glucocorticoids may

prevent increased release of vasopressin from the pituitary in adrenalectomized dogs under certain acute stressful conditions.[31] It seems unlikely that direct compression of the posterior pituitary gland by an anterior pituitary tumor or compression of the hypothalamus or hypothalamic stalk would cause the polyuria in most cases of CCS, since these patients usually have quite small microtumors. In addition, the polydipsia and polyuria usually resolve with treatment.[17]

Polyphagia. Increased appetite may be troublesome to some owners because the dog with CCS may resort to stealing food, eating garbage, begging continuously, and, occasionally, aggressively attacking or protecting

TABLE 97–1. INITIAL HISTORY OF DOGS WITH HYPERADRENOCORTICISM

Polydipsia/polyuria
Polyphagia
Abdominal enlargement
Decreased exercise tolerance (muscle weakness)
Increased panting
Lethargy
Obesity
Alopecia
Calcinosis cutis
Anestrus
Testicular atrophy
Heat intolerance
Acne (skin infection, comedones)
Cutaneous hyperpigmentation
Exophthalmos

food. In most instances, however, it is the dog's continued excellent appetite in the face of other abnormalities that convinces the owner that the pet is healthy and does not require veterinary attention. Increased appetite is assumed to be a direct effect of glucocorticoids, but this has not been proved. It is possible that the glucocorticoid-induced anti-insulin effect produces a subclinical (sometimes overtly clinical) case of diabetes mellitus. This could result in an increased appetite, as the patient attempts to compensate for "starvation." Polyphagia is present in 77 to 87 per cent of patients with CCS.[18, 23, 27]

Abdominal Enlargement. The potbellied appearance in hyperadrenocorticism is a classic symptom in humans and is present in 93 to 95 per cent of affected dogs.[18, 23, 27] This pendulous abdomen is believed to be the result of hepatomegaly and the redistribution of fat from various storage areas to the abdomen. The mechanism responsible for this redistribution of fat is not understood,[32] but accounts for a significant increase in the weight of abdominal contents. When this is coupled with the second factor, muscle wasting, a pendulous abdomen results. Protein catabolism accounts for muscle wasting and, therefore, muscle weakness.[32] The abdominal muscles, weakened by glucocorticoid effects, simply cannot prevent the bulging shown in Figure 97–3.[17]

Muscle Weakness and Lethargy. These signs are rarely a major owner concern. Patients with CCS are usually quite capable of rising from a prone position and of going for short walks. Muscle weakness in small dogs is usually reflected as an inability to climb stairs, although these dogs can often come down stairs without hesitation. Owners may also note an inability to jump onto furniture or into an automobile. Infrequently, muscle weakness is more profound. Exercise tolerance is often reduced. Although dogs with CCS can walk without problem, normal running may cause undue fatigue. As with abdominal distention, muscle weakness is the result of muscle wasting caused by protein catabolism. It has been noted in 74 to 82 per cent of patients with CCS.[18, 23, 27]

Lethargy is probably an expression of muscle weakness and muscle wasting. Hyperadrenal dogs are usually alert, but they are often not active. As mentioned, this vague sign is certainly one that most clients attribute to simple aging.

Less common signs of muscle weakness include unilateral or bilateral facial nerve paralysis.[20] Chronic CCS can result in an exaggeration of common problems such as anterior cruciate ligament rupture and patellar luxation lameness. One of our young dogs with Cushing's syndrome suffered a stress fracture across a tibial crest epiphysis, which had failed to close at the typical age. Decubital ulcers are common in large dogs with CCS, owing to their predisposition to remain recumbent.

Alopecia, Skin Atrophy, Thin Skin, and Acne. Endocrine alopecia may be caused by thyroid, ovarian, testicular, and GH disturbances, as well as by hypercortisolism. These are typically bilaterally symmetrical alopecias, which may be severe (Figure 97–4), mild, or involve a poor and abnormal hair coat. Bilaterally symmetrical alopecia has also been noted in cats with hyperadrenocorticism.

The hair loss associated with CCS is one of the most common and major concerns of an owner. This is a slow and progressive problem that begins with hair loss at points of wear (such as bony prominences) and eventually involves the flanks, perineum, and abdomen. The end result (Figure 97–4A) is severe alopecia, with only the head and distal extremities retaining a coat. The pinna and the base of the ears can be alopecic, especially in the dachshund. Endocrine alopecia has been recognized in 55 to 90 per cent of the cases reported.[18, 23, 27]

The thin skin, poor healing, and susceptibility to infection typical of hypercortisolism may cause additional problems. Many of the larger-breed dogs with muscle weakness spend much of their time lying down, and tend to develop decubital ulcers due to prolonged pressure on these areas. These sores are often infected and heal quite slowly. Management of these lesions requires diligent cleaning plus provision of soft bedding to minimize further trauma.

The fragility seen in the thin skin is also present in the blood vessels. Excessive bruising can follow venipuncture (Figure 97–5) or other minor trauma. We have had a number of dogs that underwent ovariohysterectomy years before developing Cushing's syndrome only to have the metal sutures begin to cause bruising after development of CCS. These abnormalities are worsened by decreased subcutaneous tissue secondary to the hypercortisolism. Wounds that do heal do so tenuously,

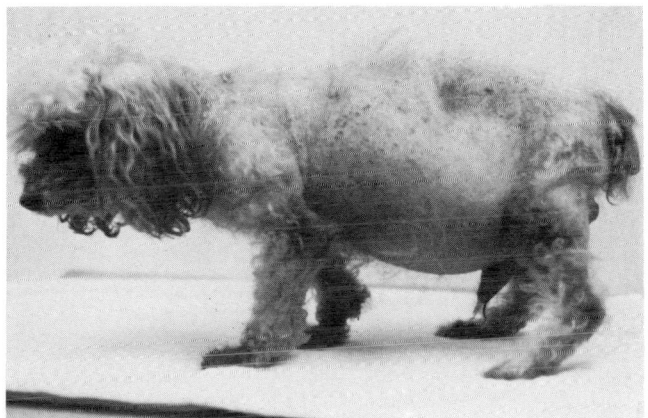

FIGURE 97–3. Poodle with pituitary-dependent hyperadrenocorticism, illustrating the potbellied appearance frequently seen.

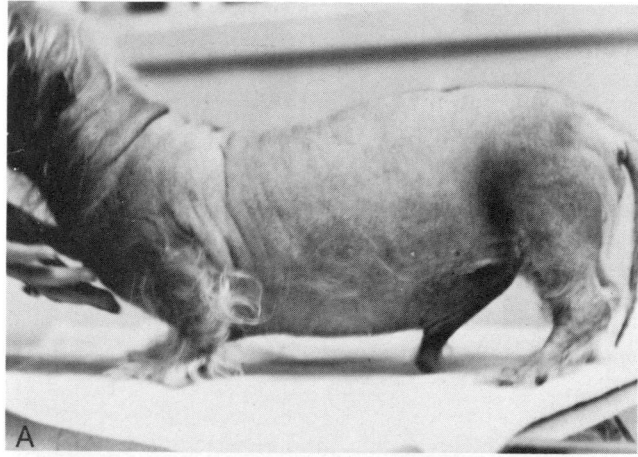

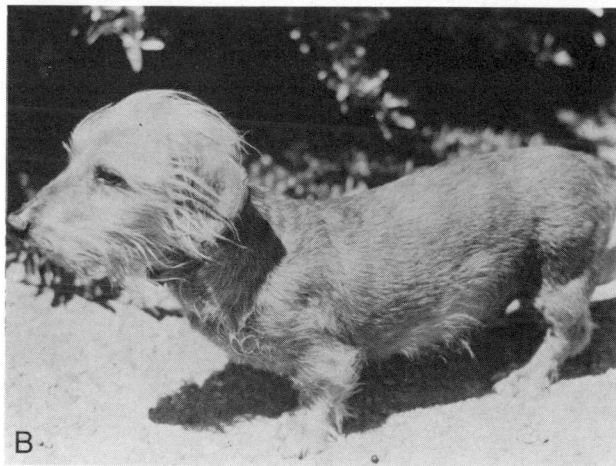

FIGURE 97–4. *A,* Dachshund with pituitary-dependent hyperadrenocorticism (PDH) illustrating severe bilaterally symmetrical alopecia. *B,* Same dog as in *A* two months after therapy with o,p'-DDD. (From Feldman, EC: *In* Ettinger, SJ (ed.): Textbook of Veterinary Internal Medicine, 2nd ed. Philadelphia, WB Saunders, 1983, p 1677.)

with fragile, thin scar tissue equivalent to the striae seen in humans. Healing skin lesions often undergo dehiscence because of the limited amount of fibrous tissue present.

The skin of animals with hyperadrenocorticism is thin and easily wrinkled. Often one can view subcutaneous blood vessels with ease. In addition, keratin-plugged follicles are often found around the nipples and along the dorsal midline, although they may be present anywhere on the trunk.

Prolonged exposure to elevated glucocorticoids may result in atrophy of the skin. Also noted is atrophy of hair follicles and the pilosebaceous apparatus, with keratin accumulation within the atrophic hair follicle being common. This atrophy disrupts the attachment of the hair shaft to the follicle, causing hair loss and lack of hair regrowth. If the hair is shaved, regrowth is poor or nonexistent. New hair is often brittle, sparse, and fine.[27] The abnormal hair follicles and thin skin are quite susceptible to infection, and localized or diffuse pyoderma is common. Skin infection is especially common along the dorsal midline and trunk. At times it may be severe and may be worse in areas of hyperpigmentation. The suppressed immune system associated with hyperadrenocorticism exaggerates the problem.[17]

Obesity. Owners usually notice an apparent weight gain in their pets. In fact, dogs with hyperadrenocorticism do not gain a large amount of weight; rather, they have fat redistribution, as previously mentioned, and a potbellied appearance, which appears to exaggerate the true weight. Truncal obesity is a classic symptom in humans with Cushing's syndrome. In dogs and humans this truncal obesity appears to occur at the expense of muscle and fat wasting from the extremities; true obesity is present in less than half the dogs.[17]

Increased Panting. Dogs with CCS are often noted to be short of breath or to have a rapid respiratory rate while at rest. These animals have increased fat deposition over the thorax, muscle wasting, weakness of the muscles involved in respiration, and increased pressure placed on the diaphragm after fat accumulation in the abdomen and hepatomegaly. All of these factors might be expected to disturb ventilatory mechanics. Nocturnal cough is not a common owner complaint. The signs of mild respiratory distress are believed to be exaggerated by a marked reduction in expiratory reserve volume and decreased chest wall compliance, which increase the work of breathing. If such a dog also has a collapsing trachea, the combination of expiratory distress associ-

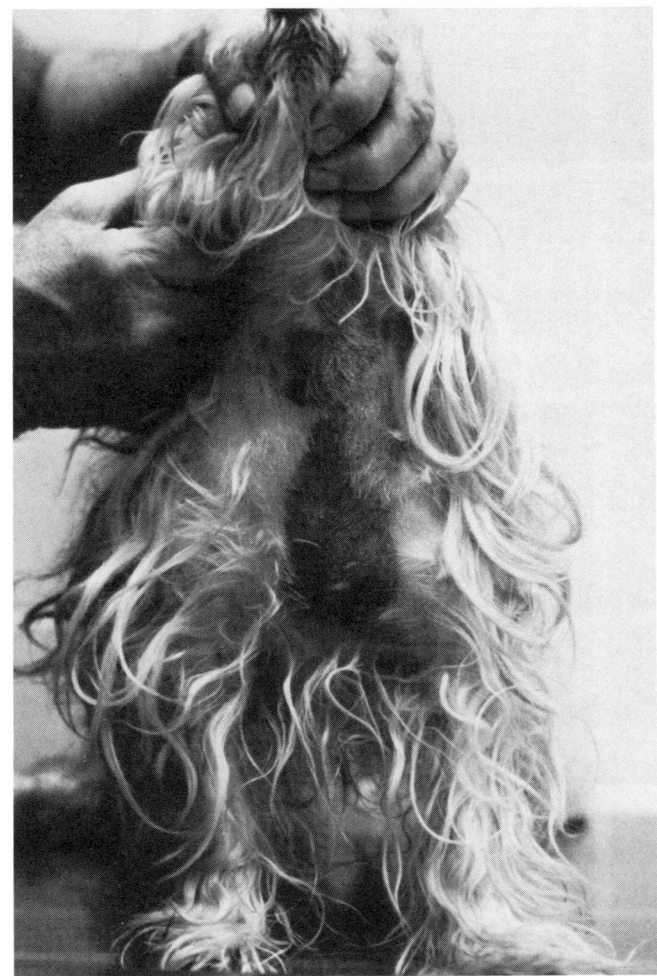

FIGURE 97–5. This dog with hyperadrenocorticism had two blood samples obtained from the jugular vein. The bruising was obvious two hours later. (From Feldman, EC: *In* Ettinger, SJ (ed.): Textbook of Veterinary Internal Medicine, 2nd ed. Philadelphia, WB Saunders, 1983, p 1679.)

ated with the tracheal problem and the changes seen with hyperadrenocorticism obesity can cause marked signs. Similar problems can easily be appreciated if such a dog also has chronic mitral and/or tricuspid valvular fibrosis. Signs become further exaggerated with the stress of excitement, exercise, and trauma.

Thromboembolism is a recognized problem in humans with Cushing's syndrome.[33, 34] Pulmonary thromboembolism occurs in CCS.[35] Dogs with pulmonary thromboembolism can develop acute severe respiratory distress. The pathogenesis and treatment are described in a following section.

Testicular Atrophy or Failure to Cycle. Male dogs with CCS usually have bilaterally symmetrical, small, soft, spongy testes. This is rarely a problem recognized by an owner and has not been a cause for seeking veterinary attention. The female dog with CCS commonly ceases estrous cycle activity. Often the length of anestrus reflects the duration of subclinical or clinical hypercortisolism. Again, this would be an extremely unusual owner concern. Both of these problems are discussed in greater detail in the next section (Physical Examination).

Myotonia (Pseudomyotonia). Rarely, dogs with hyperadrenocorticism develop a distinct myopathy, characterized by persistent active muscle contraction after cessation of voluntary effort (this was noted in 2 of our 303 dogs with Cushing's syndrome). Historically, these dogs have had a stiff gait (especially in the pelvic limbs) that was present from the time the other signs of hyperadrenocorticism developed. Pelvic limb muscle stiffness and proximal appendicular muscle enlargement are obvious on physical examination. Myotonic, bizarre high frequency discharges are noted on electromyography.[36, 37] Histologic, electron microscopic, and histochemical findings in the musculature of five dogs with Cushing's syndrome and this muscular disorder were characteristic of noninflammatory degenerative myopathy.[38] Clinical signs may improve after successful therapy for hyperadrenocorticism. The cause for this unusual phenomenon in hyperadrenocorticism in not known.

Neurologic Problems. See section on Central Nervous System Signs.

PHYSICAL EXAMINATION

General Review. On physical examination of the dog with hyperadrenocorticism, the veterinarian will often note many of the signs seen by owners. These include abdominal enlargement, increased panting, truncal obesity, bilaterally symmetrical alopecia, skin infections, and comedones (hair follicles filled with keratin and debris, usually black and easily expressed). In addition, hyperpigmentation, ectopic calcification, testicular atrophy, clitoral hypertrophy, hepatomegaly, and easy bruisability are common (Table 97–2).

There is, however, a remarkable variation in the number and severity of these signs. These dogs may have a single predominant sign or ten signs. Understanding this inconsistency in signs among animals afflicted

TABLE 97–2. PHYSICAL EXAMINATION FINDINGS IN DOGS WITH HYPERADRENOCORTICISM

Thin skin
Bilaterally symmetrical alopecia
Acne (skin infection, comedones)
Cutaneous hyperpigmentation
Calcinosis cutis
Abdominal enlargement
Muscle wasting of extremities
Hepatomegaly
Panting
Bruising
Exophthalmos
Testicular atrophy
Clitoral hypertrophy

with one underlying problem is an area of continuing study.

Hyperpigmentation. Hyperpigmentation may be diffuse or focal (Figure 97–4*A*). Histologically, there are increased numbers of melanocytes in the stratum corneum, basal epidermis, and dermal tissues.[25] It appears that hyperpigmentation is more common in humans (and dogs) with PDH than in patients with adrenal tumors.[5] Hyperpigmentation, however, is seen with either pituitary or adrenal Cushing's syndrome. Thus the likelihood of α-MSH being the sole cause of the hyperpigmentation in PDH is not strongly supported.[4] As a by-product of ACTH metabolism, however, α-MSH may have some role in the hyperpigmentation.

Hepatomegaly. The enlarged liver seen in CCS contributes to the abdominal enlargement previously discussed. The liver is typically swollen, large, pale, and friable. It is usually easy to palpate, owing to the flaccid and weak abdominal muscles.

Liver biopsy samples from animals with hypercortisolism usually reveal centrilobular hepatocytic vacuolation with few, often single, large vacuoles displacing the nucleus to the periphery of the cell. Hepatocellular glycogen accumulation is concentrated in periportal hepatocytes. Lipid deposits are not demonstrable with Sudan III stains, and hepatocellular necrosis, although present, is not an important feature.[39] Ultrastructural studies of the livers from dogs with glucocorticoid hepatopathy indicated that the principal alterations were abundant glycogen accumulations and few mitochondria in hepatocytes.[40]

The histologic alterations seen in the livers of dogs with spontaneous or iatrogenic excesses in glucocorticoids are quite consistent. When present, there appear to be few differential diagnoses for the group of alterations consistent with steroid excess. However, vacuolization alone can be caused by a variety of problems. "Steroid hepatopathy" does imply chronic elevations in circulating glucocorticoids. For unknown reasons, not all dogs with Cushing's syndrome have steroid hepatopathy, but liver biopsy does have a potential role as a diagnostic test.[17] Liver biopsy, however, is not recommended routinely because of the poor wound healing and potential of infection in dogs with hyperadrenocorticism.

Testicular Atrophy, Anestrus, Clitoral Hypertrophy. The negative feedback effects of hypercortisolism in CCS result in decreased pituitary gonadotropin secretion. This explains the testicular atrophy, decreased libido, and depressed plasma testosterone concentrations typically seen in male dogs with CCS. Testicular androgen secretion is reduced, whereas adrenal androgen secretion is increased. However, conversion of adrenal androstenedione to testosterone accounts for less than 5 per cent of the production rate of this hormone. Thus, the physiologic effect of adrenal androgens is negligible in males, and the male becomes feminized. In one study, the plasma testosterone concentration averaged 4.7 ng/ml in normal males versus the much lower 1.2 ng/ml in male dogs with CCS.[41]

In females, the negative feedback effects of hypercortisolism depress pituitary secretion of gonadotropins, as in the male. This results in prolonged anestrus, one of the common features of CCS in the bitch. In the normal state, ovarian androgen production is low and the adrenal gland substantially contributes to total androgen production. Abnormal adrenal function, as seen in CCS, results in excessive secretion of adrenal androgens, and their peripheral conversion results in clinical androgen excess (virilization). This is reflected in clitoral hypertrophy, frequently noticed in female dogs with CCS. Hormone studies support this finding. The average plasma testosterone concentration in normal female dogs was 20 pg/ml, whereas in females with CCS it was 30 pg/ml, a substantial difference.[41]

The abnormalities in circulating testosterone concentrations in dogs of either sex with CCS do return to or toward normal with successful management of the disorder.[41]

Ectopic Calcification. Calcium deposition in the dermis and subcutis is a common sign of CCS. On examination these areas feel like firm plaques in or under the skin. The common locations of this calcium deposition, called calcinosis cutis, include the temporal area of the head and the dorsal midline, neck, ventral abdominal, and inguinal areas (Figure 97–6A). Ectopic calcification is also seen involving the tracheal rings and bronchial walls, the kidneys, and, rarely, major arteries and veins. This calcification may only be noted histologically in some dogs but occasionally will be visible radiographically if it was not noted on physical examination. The exact pathogenesis is not known.

Bruisability. Easy bruisability is common after venipuncture in the dog with CCS (see Figure 97–5). An unusually bad bruise may result from any trauma. This reflects the poor wound healing associated with suppressed tissue granulation secondary to glucocorticoid excess (see section on Alopecia, Skin Atrophy, Thin Skin, and Acne).

IN-HOSPITAL EVALUATION

General Approach. Any dog or cat suspected of having hyperadrenocorticism should be thoroughly evaluated before specific diagnostic procedures are undertaken. The initial tests should include clinicopathologic studies (complete blood count (CBC), urinalysis, and chemistry profile, including renal function tests, liver enzymes, calcium, phosphorus, cholesterol, blood glu-

cose, total plasma protein, plasma albumin, and total bilirubin levels). Finding a large percentage of abnormalities on initial screening tests that are consistent with hyperadrenocorticism allows the veterinarian to establish a presumptive diagnosis of CCS (Table 97–3). The more expensive and sophisticated studies needed to confirm a diagnosis and localize the cause of the syndrome can then be offered to the client. The initial results not only ensure that the veterinarian is pursuing the correct diagnosis, but also alert the clinician to any concomitant medical problems in the patient. These problems may be common in CCS or unexpected but in either case should not be ignored. Seemingly minor disturbances (e.g., urinary tract infection, pyoderma, and heart murmur) may be of major medical importance in the hyperadrenal dog.[17]

CBC. Excessive production of cortisol results in neutrophilia and monocytosis owing to steroid-produced capillary demargination of these cells and to the subsequent prevention of normal egress of the cells from the vascular system. Lymphopenia is most likely the result of steroid lympholysis, and eosinopenia results from bone marrow sequestration of eosinophils.[42] The red blood cell count is usually normal, although mild polycythemia may occasionally be noted, especially in females.

Blood Glucose and Plasma Insulin. CCS frequently results in elevated fasting plasma glucose concentrations and less commonly in overt diabetes mellitus.[43, 44] Fifty-seven per cent of patients with CCS had an elevated plasma glucose value in one study.[22] Presumably, glucocorticoids increase gluconeogenesis and decrease peripheral utilization of glucose by antagonizing the effects of insulin. Glycosuria may be manifested if the renal threshold for plasma glucose (180 to 220 mg/dl) is exceeded.[45] A suspicion of CCS should be raised in any diabetic dog that requires large amounts of insulin.

A study that compared normal dogs with nondiabetic Cushing's syndrome dogs was recently completed. After an 18-hour fast the average morning plasma insulin concentration in the control dogs was 12 μU/ml, while it was 38 μU/ml in 44 dogs with spontaneous hyperadrenocorticism. Simultaneous plasma glucose concentrations averaged 85 mg/dl in the control dogs and 111 mg/dl in the hyperadrenal dogs.[41] These results perhaps reflect the antagonistic effects that glucocorticoids have on insulin action. Owing to this antagonism, more insulin is required to maintain carbohydrate tolerance. In most dogs with CCS, the increased secretion of insulin partially controls carbohydrate tolerance but is not adequate to normalize glucose parameters. These abnormalities usually dissipate with successful therapy for Cushing's syndrome.[17]

Abnormal elevations in plasma insulin concentration are not consistent, limiting the usefulness of this assay as a diagnostic aid. Using fasting insulin concentrations to assess 30 patients with CCS, we have found abnormally elevated concentrations in less than half the patients.[41] Administration of prednisolone to healthy dogs for three weeks did not cause peripheral insulin resistance, suggesting a need for longer duration of steroid excess before carbohydrate intolerance develops.[46]

Blood Urea Nitrogen (BUN). With the diuresis stimu-

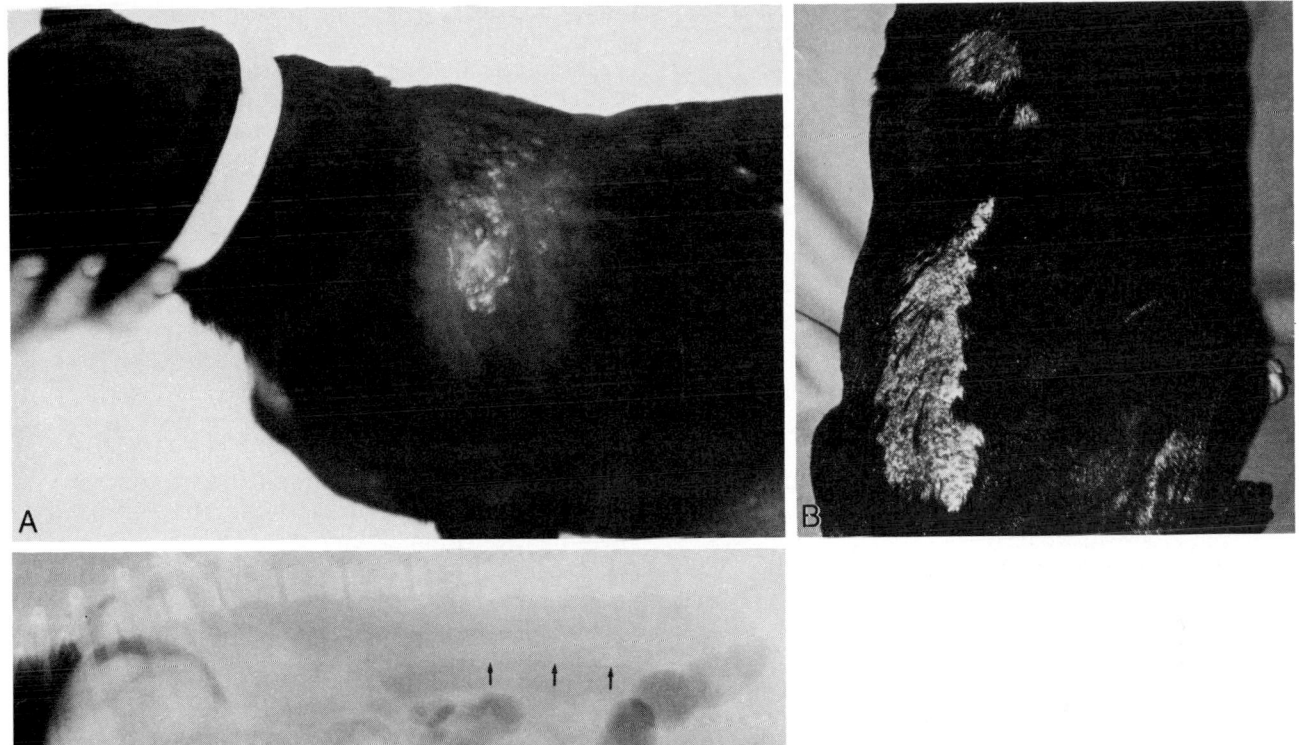

FIGURE 97–6. *A* and *B*, An area of skin altered dramatically by calcinosis cutis *C*, Radiograph showing calcified vena cava (arrows).

lated by glucocorticoids there is a continual urinary loss of urea nitrogen. This diuresis is secondary to several mechanisms described herein. The BUN was below normal in 56 per cent of dogs tested in one review,[23] and a mean BUN concentration half that of normal dogs was noted in another review.[42] The serum creatinine concentrations also tend to be normal or low.

Alanine Aminotransferase (ALT; SGPT). The ALT is commonly elevated in CCS. This is usually a mild elevation believed to occur secondary to liver damage caused by swollen hepatocytes, glycogen accumulation, or some other factor. Hepatocellular necrosis, a minor but important feature of "steroid hepatopathy," was seen with enough frequency to account for the mild elevation in the ALT.[39]

Alkaline Phosphatase. The alkaline phosphatases are a group of enzymes that catalyze the hydrolysis of phosphate esters. The main sources of serum alkaline phosphatase are liver, kidney, bone, and, in some cases, intestine. As a result of hepatic glycogen deposition and vacuolization impinging on the biliary tract in CCS, the alkaline phosphatase production rate increases. This partially accounts for the elevated concentrations of the enzyme in the serum. However, the majority of the increase follows glucocorticoid induction of a specific hepatic isoenzyme of alkaline phosphatase. This isoenzyme is distinct from that seen in normal dogs or in most of those with non-steroid-related illness.[47] An elevated serum alkaline phosphatase is perhaps one of the alterations on a biochemical panel from a dog with hyperadrenocorticism. However, alkaline phosphatase isoenzyme analysis is not recommended as a screening test for this disorder, even though this elevation is commonly 5 to 40 times above the normal mean.

Dogs with spontaneous hyperadrenocorticism do not have pathognomonic findings on serum alkaline phosphatase isoenzyme studies. Dogs with spontaneous hyperadrenocorticism have results that were similar to those of dogs with diabetes mellitus, degenerative hepatic disease, or nonspecific neoplasias and of dogs treated with glucocorticoids, estrogen preparations, or primidone.

Cholesterol and Lipid Levels. Concomitant with glucocorticoid stimulation of lipolysis are increased blood lipid and cholesterol concentrations. Ninety per cent of 71 dogs with CCS were noted to have elevated plasma cholesterol concentrations.[22] Lipemia is at least as frequent, and it may interfere with the accurate assessment

TABLE 97–3. HEMATOLOGIC, SERUM BIOCHEMICAL, URINE, AND RADIOGRAPHIC ABNORMALITIES TYPICAL OF HYPERADRENOCORTICISM*

Test	Abnormality
CBC:	Mature leukocytosis
	Neutrophilia
	Lymphopenia
	Eosinopenia
	Erythrocytosis (females)
Chemistries:	Increased alkaline phosphatase (sometimes extremely elevated)
	Increased ALT (SGPT)
	Increased cholesterol
	Increased fasting blood glucose
	Increased or normal insulin
	Increased BSP retention
	Decreased BUN
	Lipemia
Urinalysis:	Urine specific gravity <1.015, often <1.008
	Urinary tract infection
	Glycosuria (<10% of cases)
Radiographs:	Hepatomegaly
	Excellent abdominal contrast
	Potbelly
	Distended bladder
	Osteoporosis
	Calcinosis cutis/dystrophic calcification
	Adrenal calcification (usually adrenal tumor)
	Congestive heart failure (rare)
	Pulmonary thromboembolism (rare)
	Calcified trachea and main stem bronchi
	Pulmonary metastasis of adrenal carcinoma
Miscellaneous:	Low T_4/T_3 concentrations
	Response to TSH that parallels normal but both "pre" and "post" T_4 concentrations are below normal "pre" and "post" values
	Hypertension

*It would be unusual for an individual animal to have all these abnormalities.
CBC = complete blood count.

of several clinicopathologic test results. Parameters that can be altered by lipemia include red blood cell counts, hemoglobin, red cell indices, total plasma proteins, albumin, total bilirubin, alkaline phosphatase, calcium, phosphorus, amylase, lipase, sodium, and sulfobromophthalein (BSP) retention studies.[42]

Serum Phosphate. Hypophosphatemia had been reported to occur in approximately one third of dogs with hyperadrenocorticism.[20] This had been explained as resulting from a glucocorticoid-induced increase in the urinary excretion of phosphate.

BSP. The BSP retention test is frequently used by veterinarians who are attempting to assess the degree of liver damage in the dog. It has been frequently abnormal in CCS, owing to vascular disease or liver damage caused by glycogen accumulation. These abnormalities may be mild to quite severe and are reversible with successful treatment of the syndrome. The BSP test, however, would not aid in separating dogs with primary liver disorders from those with hyperadrenocorticism.

Serum Electrolytes. Mild abnormalities in the serum sodium (elevation) and potassium (depression) concentrations are seen in approximately half the dogs with CCS. Serum electrolyte concentrations become extremely important if a dog with CCS develops anorexia, vomiting, or diarrhea because exaggeration of these abnormal electrolyte concentrations may become life-threatening.

Urinalysis. The urinalysis is one of the most important initial studies. It is strongly recommended that owners obtain a urine sample by clean-catch before bringing the pet to the hospital or that a urine sample be collected at the time of initial examination. The most frequent abnormality is the finding of dilute urine (specific gravity <1.015), which occurs in 85 per cent of our cases. Other investigators have found dilute urine less frequently because samples were obtained after the dogs had been hospitalized for hours or even days. Hyperadrenal dogs may not consume large quantities of water in a foreign environment. Some animals consume much less water, with the specific gravity reflecting this reduction in intake. It is therefore unreliable to measure water intake in the hospital.[17] The urine-concentrating ability of water-deprived hyperadrenal dogs has been well documented. Such animals can concentrate their urine to an osmolality well above plasma osmolality, although usually this concentrating ability remains less than normal.[48]

In addition to determining specific gravity, the veterinarian can assess a urine sample for the presence of glycosuria. Such a finding has been noted in 10 per cent of one series of cases[18] and indicates that overt diabetes mellitus is probably present. The finding of hyperglycemia and glycosuria is diagnostic of diabetes mellitus, which should be treated, whether or not it is secondary to CCS.

Because urinary tract infection is a common sequela to CCS,[22] the urine obtained should be analyzed for infection. Whenever hyperadrenocorticism is suspected, cystocentesis with culture and sensitivity testing is strongly recommended.

Blood Pressure. Blood pressure is often elevated in humans with Cushing's syndrome. The elevation is moderate and sustained and is caused by expansion of the vascular volume.[5] This hypervolemia is most likely a consequence of enhanced renal tubular sodium reabsorption and secondary fluid retention.[32] Eleven hyperadrenal dogs had blood pressure determinations before therapy. In nine of these dogs both systolic and diastolic pressures were elevated.[23] In another study 8 of 14 dogs with Cushing's syndrome were hypertensive. Normal dogs had systolic, diastolic, and mean blood pressures of 148, 87, and 102 mmHg, respectively. The dogs with CCS had systolic, diastolic, and mean blood pressures of 176, 121, and 142 mmHg, respectively.[49] Hypertension resolves after successful management of the hyperadrenocorticism.

Radiography

General Approach. Radiographs of the abdomen should be obtained in dogs with suspected or proved hyperadrenocorticism. In addition to the possible changes consistent with the diagnosis of CCS, the veterinarian should remember that most dogs with CCS are older animals. Such patients may have serious concurrent (perhaps subclinical) diseases that may be revealed radiographically. Radiographs of the skull are not recommended, as they are usually normal and

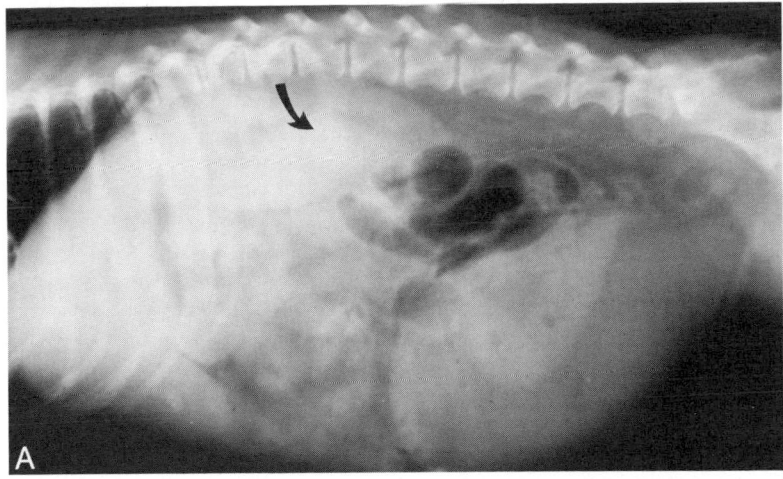
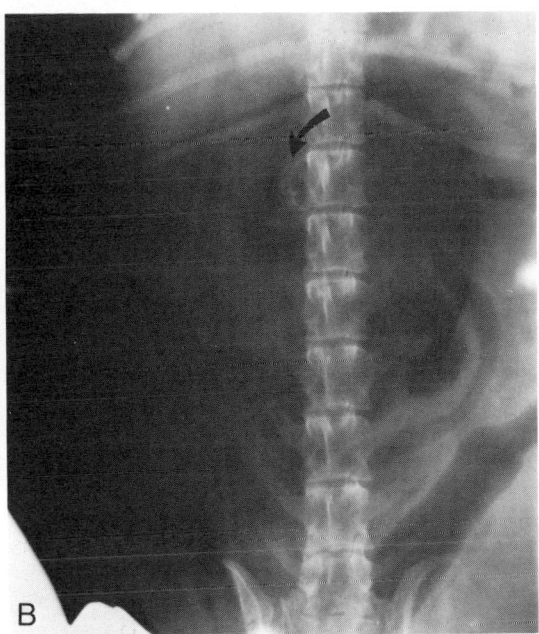

FIGURE 97–7. Lateral *(A)* and ventrodorsal *(B)* abdominal radiographs of a dog with a functioning adrenal tumor causing hyperadrenocorticism. Note the calcified adrenal tumor (arrows), hepatomegaly, distended (atonic) bladder, and excellent contrast owing to fat mobilization. (From Feldman, EC: *In* Ettinger, SJ (ed.): Textbook of Veterinary Internal Medicine, 2nd ed. Philadelphia, WB Saunders, 1983, p 1683.)

require an anesthetized patient. Changes such as the bony erosion seen in the human sella turcica caused by an expanding pituitary tumor[5] are not expected to be seen in the dog, which has an anatomically more open and shallow sella turcica.[27]

ABDOMINAL RADIOGRAPHS

Abdominal Contrast and Hepatomegaly. Radiographs of the abdomen can be a useful aid in establishing a presumptive diagnosis of CCS as well as occasionally helping to define the cause. Good radiographic contrast should allow easy identification of abdominal contents because of the large amounts of fat distributed into the abdomen. The potbellied appearance and hepatomegaly are usually obvious. Thirty-six of 48 dogs with CCS showed evidence of hepatomegaly in a recent report, the degree being classified as mild in 14 dogs, moderate in 12, and severe in 10. There was no obvious association between the duration of illness and the degree of hepatomegaly.[50]

Osteoporosis. Occasionally radiographs may give the impression that osteoporosis involving the lumbar spine is present. Objective radiographic evaluation of skeletal demineralization is notoriously difficult. A distinct reduction in the radiographic density of the lumbar vertebral bodies, relative to vertebral end plates, was detected in 8 of 48 dogs with Cushing's syndrome.[50] Lameness and pathologic fractures were not detected in those animals. However, failure of the epiphyses to close and epiphyseal fractures may occur when young dogs are afflicted with Cushing's syndrome. It is probable that the catabolic effects of corticosteroids are exerted on bone matrix. Furthermore, cortisol increases urinary calcium excretion as well as inhibiting gastrointestinal absorption of calcium by interfering with the action of vitamin D. Thus the depletion of matrix accompanied by loss of mineral may be the cause of osteoporosis.[37]

Calcinosis Cutis and Dystrophic Calcification. Cal-

cinosis cutis and subcutaneous calcification are occasionally observed and are usually focal in appearance (see Figure 97–6). In 48 dogs with Cushing's syndrome, 9 had radiographic signs of calcinosis cutis. In addition, radiographic dystrophic calcification was seen involving the renal pelvis in five dogs, the liver in one, the gastric mucosa in one, and the branches of the abdominal aorta in one.[50]

The Urinary Bladder. A grossly distended urinary bladder may be seen radiographically. Because dogs with CCS are house pets, they are usually housebroken. These animals probably attempt to avoid urinating indoors, and it is our subjective opinion that many such dogs develop secondary mild to moderate atonic bladders. These dogs may not be capable of totally emptying their bladders. If these animals were allowed to urinate on their own before obtaining abdominal radiographs, one may still see a large, partially filled bladder (Figure 97–7*A*).

Enlarged Adrenals. Perhaps the most important finding on abdominal radiographs would be unilateral or bilateral calcification in the area of an adrenal gland (Figure 97–7). Such a finding would be strongly suggestive of an adrenal tumor, although this is not always true in people.[51] Large masses are suggestive of adrenal carcinomas (Figure 97–8). In a review of 23 dogs with CCS caused by an adrenal tumor, 13 had tumor calcification. Six of ten adrenocortical adenomas and seven of 13 carcinomas had radiographically visible calcification.[21] It is possible that an adrenal tumor may be large enough to displace the kidneys or other abdominal organs, as in Figure 97–8.

THORACIC RADIOGRAPHS

Several changes may be observed in the thoracic radiographs of dogs with Cushing's syndrome. Ectopic calcification is frequently seen radiographically, involving the tracheal rings and main stem bronchi. Calcification of these structures, however, can be seen in nor-

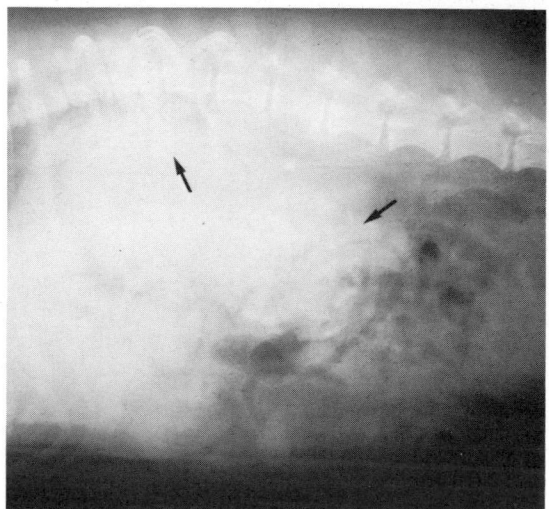

FIGURE 97–8. Lateral abdominal radiograph from a dog with a large calcified functioning adrenocortical carcinoma (arrows).

mally aging dogs and is not considered highly important.[27, 52] Osteoporosis may be suspected from the appearance of the thoracic vertebrae. Any evidence of metastasis of a malignant adrenal tumor must be investigated when examining the lung fields. Three of 17 dogs with adrenal carcinomas in our series have had radiographically visible lung metastases. In evaluation of any dog that has an adrenal tumor, thoracic radiographs are warranted. Another major concern is pulmonary thromboembolism (see section on Pulmonary Thromboembolism).

Thyroid Function Tests

A study of 102 dogs with spontaneous hyperadrenocorticism revealed that 68 per cent had decreases in basal serum T_4 and/or T_3 concentrations. Of those dogs, 61 per cent had low T_4 and T_3 concentrations, 23 per cent had decreases only in T_4 concentrations, while 16 per cent had decreases only in the T_3. TSH stimulation increased serum T_4 concentrations in the dogs with Cushing's syndrome in a manner parallel to increases in normal dogs but usually not to normal concentrations (Figure 97–9).[15, 53] Chronic hypercortisolism may depress pituitary secretion of TSH, leading to secondary hypothyroidism. Hypercortisolism may also change thyroid hormone binding to plasma proteins and enhance the metabolism of thyroid hormone. Glucocorticoids decrease peripheral deiodination of T_4 to T_3.

The abnormalities seen in thyroid function testing of dogs with hyperadrenocorticism are important because of the overlap in some clinical signs between these two disorders (i.e., listlessness, bilateral symmetrical nonpruritic alopecia, apparent weight gain, hypercholesterolemia). This overlap in signs can be a source of confusion to the veterinarian. Treatment of a hyperadrenal dog with thyroid replacement medication does not usually have a deleterious effect. In fact, many such dogs become slightly more active. Because the primary disease is not being treated, however, signs will continue to develop, which should alert the veterinarian that

hypothyroidism is not the total explanation of a dog's problems. Many of the clinical and biochemical features of CCS would not likely be found in hypothyroidism.[17]

GH Secretion

Occasionally the veterinary clinician may have a dog or cat with signs or laboratory data suggestive of acromegaly (GH-secreting tumor) or hyperadrenocorticism (Table 97–4). Dogs with CCS, however, have suppressed plasma GH concentrations, while those with acromegaly have elevated growth hormone concentrations. Interestingly, in four dogs with hyperadrenocorticism, no significant increase in plasma GH concentration occurred after the administration of xylazine, whereas increases were observed in three of those four dogs following successful therapy for the CCS.[54]

The endocrine alopecia and hyperpigmentation found in dogs with adult-onset GH deficiency may mimic the dermatologic signs of hyperadrenocorticism. Evaluation of the history, a thorough physical examination, and an initial data base will usually allow the clinician to differentiate between these two syndromes. However, we have seen a few dogs with CCS that mimicked adult-onset GH deficiency. Because of the suppressive effects of CCS on GH secretion, evaluation of basal GH concentrations and GH response to provocative testing with clonidine or xylazine may not reliably differentiate

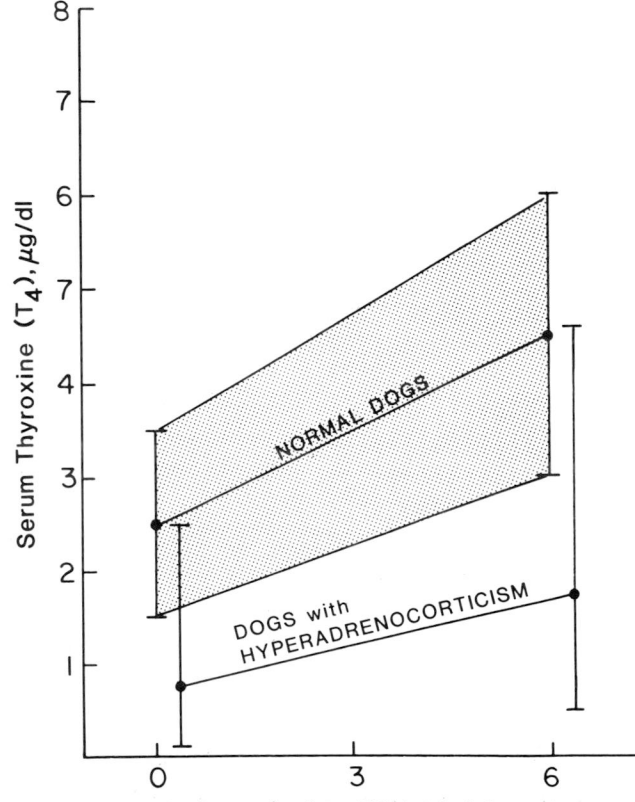

FIGURE 97–9. T_4 concentrations before and after TSH administration in normal dogs and those with hyperadrenocorticism. The Cushing's syndrome dogs may have normal or below but parallel to normal increases in serum T_4 concentrations.

TABLE 97–4. DIFFERENTIAL DIAGNOSES FOR CANINE CUSHING'S SYNDROME (CCS) WITH MAJOR AREAS OF OVERLAP

Differential Diagnosis	Overlap with CCS
Diabetes mellitus	PD/PU/polyphagia
	↑ SAP, ↓ ALT, ↑ FBG, ↑ Chol
	Hepatomegaly
	Urinary tract infection
Renal disease	PD/PU
Liver disease	Hepatomegaly
	↑ SAP, ↑ ALT, ↑ BSP
Hypothyroidism	Bilaterally symmetrical alopecia
	Apparent weight gain
	↑ Chol
Sertoli cell tumor	Bilaterally symmetrical alopecia
Pyelonephritis	Chronic recurring urinary tract infection
Hypercalcemia	PD/PU
Diabetes insipidus	
(Nephrogenic)	PD/PU
(Central)	PD/PU
Primary (psychogenic) polydipsia	PD/PU/polyphagia
	Poor hair coat
	↑ SAP, ↑ ALT
Acromegaly	PD/PU, ↑ SAP
	Enlarged abdomen
	Muscle weakness
	Inspiratory stridor
	↑ FBG
	Hepatomegaly
Ascites	Enlarged abdomen (may be difficult to palpate)
Anticonvulsant therapy	PD/PU; lethargy; polyphagia
	↑ SAP; ↑ ALT; abnormal plasma cortisol concentrations

Abbreviations: PD = polydipsia; PU = polyuria; SAP = serum alkaline phosphatase; ALT (SGPT) = alanine aminotransferase; BSP = sulfobromophthalein sodium; FBG = fasting blood glucose; Chol = cholesterol.

between these two syndromes.[54] Differentiation must rely initially on the evaluation of the pituitary-adrenal axis. If this axis is normal, then provocative testing to evaluate somatotroph function will be more reliable.

COMPLICATIONS

Several life-threatening problems may occur in dogs with CCS. Although most hyperadrenal dogs are surprisingly healthy and vital, the long-term effects of elevated glucocorticoids can be catastrophic in certain circumstances.

Pyelonephritis. As discussed earlier, urinary tract infections are common in dogs with CCS, and such infections can ascend to the kidneys. The result is severe and chronic infection plus, in some cases, renal failure. Suspicion of pyelonephritis should be raised if a urinary tract infection cannot be cleared, even after proper antibiotic therapy chosen in light of the results of culture and sensitivity on a urine sample obtained by cystocentesis. Pyelonephritis is best diagnosed by contrast dye studies of the kidneys, by renal biopsy, or by ultrasonography.

Congestive Heart Failure. One of the sequelae of excess glucocorticoids is hypertension secondary to hypervolemia. This increases the workload of the myocardium and results in myocardial hypertrophy. Congestive heart failure may occur as hypertension and fluid retention become severe. In addition, CCS frequently affects middle-aged and older dogs of breeds commonly known to have acquired chronic mitral and tricuspid valvular fibrosis. The combined effect of valvular insufficiency and CCS is a definite strain on the myocardium. Overt congestive heart failure, however, is not common among dogs with hyperadrenocorticism. Radiographs of the thorax often reveal cardiomegaly associated with a prominent left ventricle and, occasionally, pulmonary edema. Electrocardiographically, left ventricular hypertrophy is a frequent finding. Dogs with CCS and congestive heart failure respond poorly to therapy consisting of digitalization and sodium restriction. In dogs with CCS that are polydipsic and polyuric, diuretic therapy should be used with caution, since it can easily lead to hypokalemia and/or alkalosis. Treatment of the congestive heart failure and hypertension is best accomplished by using drugs that lower blood pressure as well as focusing on the underlying cause of these disorders. With the appropriate diagnosis and treatment, dogs with CCS may be rendered normotensive, leading to control of the cardiovascular complications of this disease.[55]

Pulmonary Thromboembolism. Pulmonary thromboembolism is a potential complication of hyperadrenocorticism as well as of several other disorders (e.g., amyloidosis, renal failure, and pancreatitis). A majority of the hyperadrenal dogs that have developed this serious complication had been undergoing treatment for Cushing's syndrome when the embolic episode began. These dogs usually have acute respiratory distress, orthopnea, and, less commonly, a jugular pulse.[35, 56] The panting may occur secondary to hypoxia and/or pleuritic pain. Radiographs of the thorax are an important part of the diagnostic evaluation of these patients. The radiographs may reveal no abnormalities. Usually, however, they have revealed pleural effusion, increased diameter and blunting of the pulmonary arteries, lack of perfusion of the obstructed pulmonary vasculature, and overperfusion of the unobstructed pulmonary vasculature. Arterial blood gas analysis reveals a decrease in the PCO_2 to the mid 50s or mid 60s (normal, 80 to 100 mmHg) and a decrease in the PO_2 to the range of 17 to 30 (normal, 35 to 45 mmHg). Initially there may be a respiratory alkalosis, but the effects of hypoxia and the complicated physiology of this syndrome usually results in lactic acidosis and a mild metabolic acidosis with mild depression in the arterial pH. Thrombosis may be confirmed with angiography of the lungs or with a radionuclear lung scan. Therapy consists of general support, oxygen, anticoagulants (heparin and/or coumarin), and watchful waiting. The prognosis for this condition is guarded to grave.

Thromboembolic events are thought to occur with increased frequency in Cushing's syndrome, owing to obesity, hypertension, a raised hematocrit, and the presence of a "hypercoagulable state."[34] Additional predisposing factors include prolonged recumbency, surgery, and pancreatitis. Dogs with Cushing's syndrome may be in a hypercoagulable state with elevations of clotting factors V, IX, and X, fibrinogen, antithrombin III (AT III), and plasminogen concentrations. However, factors IX and VIII:C remain in the reference range. The low factor VIII:C and elevated AT III concentrations are not consistent with a hypercoagulable state.[57, 58]

Central Nervous System Signs. Although uncommon, occasionally CCS results from a functioning large pituitary tumor. Such a mass, with dorsal expansion, may compress the optic chiasm and hypothalamus; invaginate the pituitary "stalk," which connects the hypothalamus with the pituitary; and dilate the infundibular recess and third ventricle.[25] The most common clinical signs resulting from this process are extreme "dullness," anorexia, and listlessness. Other described signs include seizures, somnolence, aimless wandering, head pressing, ataxia, blindness, anisocoria, dramatic fluctuations in body temperature, and Horner's syndrome. The author has had experience with one dog that had unpredictable episodes of aggressive and vicious behavior. As will be described, dogs and cats with these large tumors are now being diagnosed using computed tomography (CT) and/or magnetic resonance imaging scans and are being treated with cobalt irradiation.[17]

Several dogs with CCS were initially evaluated for signs related to a large pituitary tumor. Most often, however, the central nervous system signs begin after therapy for PDH using the adrenocorticolytic agent mitotane (see Chemotherapy Using op'-DDD). This sequence of events may be purely coincidental, but another explanation involves the removal of glucocorticoid-negative feedback. Without negative feedback, some pituitary tumors may rapidly enlarge.[59, 60]

DIFFERENTIAL DIAGNOSIS

The combination of clinical signs seen in most dogs with hyperadrenocorticism is strongly suggestive of the final diagnosis. With most dogs the veterinarian gains a suspicion of CCS after completing the history and physical examination. As seen in Table 97–4, however, several diseases do have signs, with or without laboratory data, that may overlap with those of hyperadrenocorticism. The more obvious differential diagnoses are diabetes mellitus, acromegaly, diabetes insipidus, renal disease, liver disease, pyelonephritis, hypothyroidism, hyperthyroidism (in cats), Sertoli cell tumors, and hypercalcemia.

SPECIFIC EVALUATION OF THE PITUITARY-ADRENOCORTICAL AXIS

General Approach

After establishing a presumptive diagnosis of canine or feline hyperadrenocorticism from the signs, physical examination, laboratory data base, and/or radiographs, one must proceed to confirm the diagnosis and, if possible, to determine the cause of the disorder. The mainstay of these diagnostic procedures is the measurement of plasma cortisol concentrations. Assays for these hormone values include fluorometric, competitive protein-binding, radioimmunoassay (RIA), enzyme-linked immunosorbent assay (ELISA), and high-performance liquid chromatography (HPLC) assays. All of these assay systems are reliable. RIA methods are the most commonly used. Urine cortisol assays are similar to those used for plasma.

Screening Tests—Tests to Diagnose Hyperadrenocorticism

URINARY CORTICOSTEROIDS

Several methods are available to measure urinary cortisol and its metabolites. Usually the methods involve 24-hour urine collections, which provide an integrated assessment of the amount of cortisol produced over a 24-hour period. Problems of episodic release of cortisol, present with plasma assays, can be avoided. This study is an excellent diagnostic test that remains one of the recommended initial studies in the diagnostic evaluation of humans suspected of having Cushing's syndrome. Urine free cortisol is the recommended assay because it is rapid and suitable for clinical use, and has advantages over measurement of urine 17-hydroxycorticosteroids or 17-ketogenic steroids. The 24-hour urine specimen is collected in a suitable preservative and is then stable when refrigerated.[61] Despite the advantages of seeing the reflection of the total cortisol production over a 24-hour period, the cumbersome nature of collecting urine for this test has made it rarely used in dogs and cats.

A single cortisol-creatinine ratio from a randomly obtained morning urine sample was evaluated. This simple, inexpensive study was found to be extremely reliable in distinguishing between dogs afflicted and those not afflicted with hyperadrenocorticism. Although not widely used, this screening test will probably gain popularity in the near future. In Europe, one recommended method of evaluating a dog suspected of having hyperadrenocorticism is to have the owner collect voided urine on three consecutive mornings. The mean cortisol: creatinine ratio of the first two samples is used as a screening test. Following the second collection, owners are instructed to administer 0.1 mg/kg of dexamethasone at eight-hour intervals with the third urine sample replacing the high-dose suppression test (decribed later).[62]

RESTING PLASMA CORTISOL CONCENTRATIONS

Basal morning plasma cortisol determination is, by itself, of little diagnostic value when one is attempting to distinguish normal dogs from those with CCS. The mean resting plasma cortisol concentration in a group of dogs with CCS is significantly higher than that of normal dogs, i.e., 3.5 µg/dl. However, most dogs with hyperadrenocorticism have resting plasma cortisol concentrations within the normal range, i.e., 0.5 to 6.0 µg/dl. Several reports disagree with the number of resting plasma cortisol concentrations that are abnormal in a series of dogs with CCS. Our experience indicates that only approximately ten per cent of hyperadrenal dogs have an elevated plasma cortisol concentration on random morning sampling.

Why would an animal with a normal plasma cortisol concentration ever develop clinical features of hyperadrenocorticism? In humans with Cushing's syndrome, this apparent discrepancy is explained by noting a failure of normal circadian rhythm in cortisol concentrations. The morning cortisol values should be the day's highest, with much lower concentrations found at night. Chronic failure in the circadian rhythm will result in signs of hyperadrenocorticism, based on the knowledge that most humans with Cushing's syndrome have morning plasma cortisol concentrations that are normal and that throughout the day these values fail to decrease. Rather, they constantly remain at the morning concentration. When such a lack of rhythm occurs over months to years, the person becomes "cushingoid."[5] This may explain the insidious, progressive development of the syndrome.

Investigators have had difficulty demonstrating diurnal variation in plasma cortisol concentrations in dogs. As noted in one such study, "the stresses of handling, venipuncture, and disruption of both light-dark and sleep-wake cycles during sampling" affect cortisol secretion.[62] With or without circadian rhythms it is known that both ACTH and cortisol are secreted episodically. These bursts of secretion occur throughout the day, creating peaks and valleys in plasma cortisol concentrations. These fluctuations account for the wide normal range for plasma cortisol concentration in the resting dog (usually 0.5 to 6.0 μg/dl with RIA and ELISA). We believe that dogs with hyperadrenocorticism have a greater frequency of cortisol bursts as well as increased amplitude in these secretion patterns. For the most part, these bursts result in cortisol concentrations in the plasma that overlap with normal. During any 24 hour period, however, this hormonal profile creates an overall excess in the amount of cortisol secreted and, during the course of months or years, the clinical syndrome of hyperadrenocorticism.

ACTH STIMULATION TEST

The ACTH stimulation test has been the most commonly used study for diagnosing hyperadrenocorticism during the past two decades.[63–66] The test is safe, simple, relatively inexpensive, not time-consuming, and reliable. During the past few years, the ACTH stimulation test has undergone a few critical studies that have revealed some of its weaknesses and strengths.

Theory. Dogs and cats with PDH have adrenal hyperplasia secondary to chronic excessive stimulation by ACTH. Therefore, it is assumed that these hyperplastic adrenals have abnormally large cortisol reserves as well as excessive tissue capable of synthesizing cortisol. Functioning adrenocortical tumors (adenomas and carcinomas) are similar. Therefore, animals with PDH or adrenocortical tumors have the potential for hyper-responding to a maximal ACTH stimulation. If this is true, and if the adrenals in both disorders maintain ACTH responsiveness, the hyper-responding dogs or cats with Cushing's syndrome can be distinguished from animals without pituitary and/or adrenal disease.

Protocol. Numerous protocols for the ACTH stimulation test have been published. Testing begins between 8 and 10 AM, after a 12-hour fast and a night in the hospital. This approach eliminates some of the "patient" variables that may alter test results. Reliable results are obtained when using porcine aqueous gelatin ACTH at a dose of 1.0 IU/lb (2.2 IU/kg) of body weight. Before and two hours after an IM injection of the drug, plasma samples should be obtained for cortisol assay. Alternatively, one can use synthetic ACTH. This drug is administered at a dose of 0.25 mg/dog (1 vial) IM, regardless of body weight. In cats, 0.125 mg (one-half vial) is administered IM. The 0.25 mg dose causes vomiting in some cats.[67] Plasma is obtained for cortisol assay before and one hour after ACTH administration in dogs and one-half hour after ACTH administration in cats.

Both gelatin and synthetic ACTH cause maximal stimulation of adrenocortical reserve. These two products and their respective protocols can be interchanged without altering test results or reducing one's confidence in the diagnosis.[57] Maximal adrenocortical stimulation is an important criterion that must be met by any stimulation test method. The exogenous ACTH must be more potent than the effects of traveling, hospital environment, handling, and venipuncture. With maximal exogenous stimulation, these important variables are eliminated.

The advantage of using porcine ACTH is its cost (it is less expensive), whereas synthetic ACTH is recommended because of its ease of use, shorter stimulation period, purity, and reduced potential for causing immunogenic reactions.[37, 68] Over the past ten years we have consistently used the synthetic ACTH with confidence.

Results. NORMAL DOGS. Normal values must be established by the individual laboratory. However, most laboratories have reasonably similar results for plasma cortisol concentrations because most laboratories use assays and testing protocols that are similar. In our laboratory the normal baseline morning cortisol concentration is between 0.5 and 6.0 μg/dl, and the normal post-stimulation cortisol concentration is between 6 and 17 μg/dl (Figure 97–10). Post-stimulation values between 17 and 20 μg/dl are considered borderline, and those ≥ 20 μg/dl are consistent with a diagnosis of hyperadrenocorticism. It is important to emphasize that ratios or percentage of change is not a valid criterion.[17]

PDH. In a recent study, the ACTH stimulation test results were abnormal in 86 per cent of dogs with PDH.[11] Thus, this test was a useful diagnostic aid but was not absolutely reliable. It also must be noted that the test results of dogs with PDH were not distinguishable from those of dogs ultimately shown to have functioning adrenocortical tumors.

FUNCTIONING ADRENOCORTICAL TUMORS. The ACTH response test is a valuable screening test in the diagnostic evaluation of adrenal tumor hyperadrenocorticism (ATH). Production and secretion of ACTH are suppressed by the excessive secretion of cortisol from functioning adrenal tumors; low to undetectable concentrations of plasma ACTH are well recognized in dogs with hyperadrenocorticism caused by adrenal tumors (see Figure 97–1).[11, 25] The suppressed endogenous

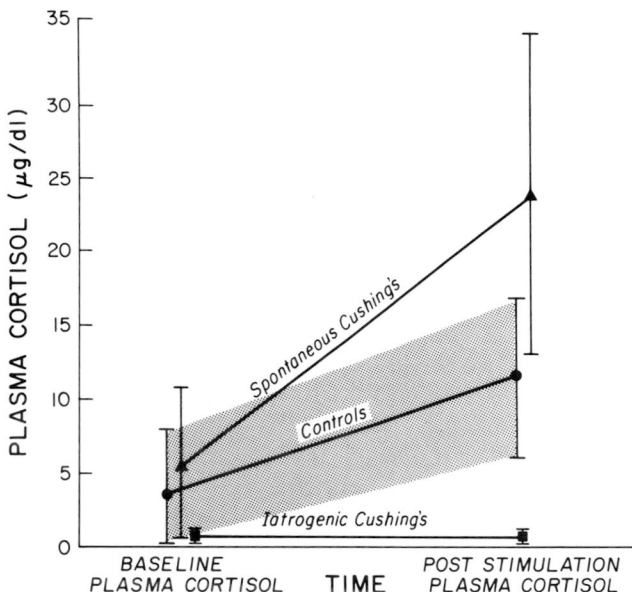

FIGURE 97–10. Mean RIA plasma cortisol concentrations (± 2 SD) determined before and one hour after administration of synthetic ACTH in control dogs, dogs with spontaneous hyperadrenocorticism, and those with iatrogenic hyperadrenocorticism.

ACTH results in atrophy of all normal adrenocortical tissue. Despite the autonomous nature of these tumors, they retain the ability to increase plasma cortisol concentrations by means of synthesis and secretion after administration of exogenous ACTH. The neoplastic cells retain surface ACTH receptors and the intracellular pathways integral to a response caused by ACTH.

In one study four of seven dogs with adrenal tumors had abnormal ACTH stimulation test results.[10] In additional studies 6 of 10 ACTH stimulation test results from 5 dogs with functioning adrenocortical tumors were abnormal (Figure 97–11),[25] and 13 of 22 similar dogs were also shown to have abnormal test results.[26] The ACTH response test remains a good screening test. Dogs with adrenal tumors can be diagnosed as having Cushing's syndrome with this test. However, as in PDH, the test results may occasionally be normal. The test does not distinguish between PDH and ATH.

IATROGENIC CUSHING'S SYNDROME. One of the major advantages of using the ACTH stimulation test as a screening test for dogs with suspected Cushing's syndrome is its ability to readily identify animals with iatrogenic Cushing's syndrome. An animal that is chronically receiving glucocorticoid therapy can develop all the clinical features of spontaneous hyperadrenocorticism. This has been seen with injectable, oral, topical, and even ophthalmic glucocorticoid preparations.[69] Occasionally, owners fail to report or do not realize the importance of all their pets' medications. A dog with clinical signs and routine laboratory test features of Cushing's syndrome with a low-normal baseline cortisol concentration and little or no response to exogenous ACTH is quite likely a patient with iatrogenic Cushing's syndrome (see Figure 97–10). All other test results are identical to those of dogs with spontaneous hypoadrenocorticism. No other screening test differentiates spontaneous hyperadrenocorticism from iatrogenic Cushing's syndrome as well as ACTH stimulation.[17]

Misleading Results. As previously described, not all dogs with spontaneous hyperadrenocorticism have diagnostic ACTH stimulation test results (i.e., the test is diagnostic of hyperadrenocorticism in 80 to 85 per cent of cases). However, not all "diagnostic" tests are found solely in dogs with hyperadrenocorticism. A single test result could always be spurious. Perhaps one of the most confusing clinical situations is dogs with signs of hyperadrenocorticism that are receiving anticonvulsant medication. Such medication (primidone, phenytoin, and even phenobarbital) can cause polydipsia, polyuria, polyphagia, lethargy, increased serum liver enzyme values, and abnormal or bizarre plasma cortisol concentrations. One must be cautious when establishing a diagnosis in dogs receiving these medications (see Table 97–4).

It is also possible for an individual test result to be incorrect, owing to human error in handling or processing the plasma or assay. Animals with clinical evidence of hyperadrenocorticism, supported by abnormalities in the routine in-hospital evaluation, are likely to have hyperadrenocorticism. In this situation the ACTH stimulation test is a reliable screening study.

DEXAMETHASONE SCREENING TEST (LOW-DOSE DEXAMETHASONE TEST)

Theory. Pituitary ACTH, under hypothalamic control, stimulates adrenocortical synthesis and secretion of glucocorticoids. The rising plasma concentrations of glucocorticoids, by way of negative feedback, suppress continued secretion of ACTH (see Figure 97–1). The communication between the pituitary and adrenal cortex is a constantly functioning system of positive and negative stimulation. The result is maintenance of plasma cortisol concentrations in the physiologic range necessary for normal metabolic homeostasis.

In hyperadrenocorticism, disturbances in the pituitary-adrenal axis are encountered. Dogs with functioning adrenocortical tumors autonomously secrete cortisol. This endogenous cortisol suppresses endogenous ACTH secretion; therefore, these tumors function independently of ACTH control.

PDH occurs secondary to the presence of ACTH-secreting pituitary microadenomas, macroadenomas, and/or pituitary hyperplasia. It is a syndrome resulting from cortisol excess because excess ACTH causes adrenocortical hyperplasia and oversecretion. Therefore, the abnormal pituitary is somewhat resistant to the negative feedback action of cortisol. If this were not true, the excess cortisol would suppress ACTH secretion, and hyperadrenocorticism would never develop. This resistance to negative feedback to PDH or independence from ACTH control in dogs with adrenal tumors provides the basis for dexamethasone screening tests.

Secretion of endogenous ACTH can be suppressed with dexamethasone in normal dogs. Plasma cortisol concentrations rapidly decline and remain suppressed for 24 to 48 hours.[70] Distinguishing between normal dogs that have received dexamethasone, which causes declining plasma cortisol concentrations, and dogs with Cushing's syndrome (pituitary-dependent or adrenocortical tumor), which do not exhibit declining cortisol concen-

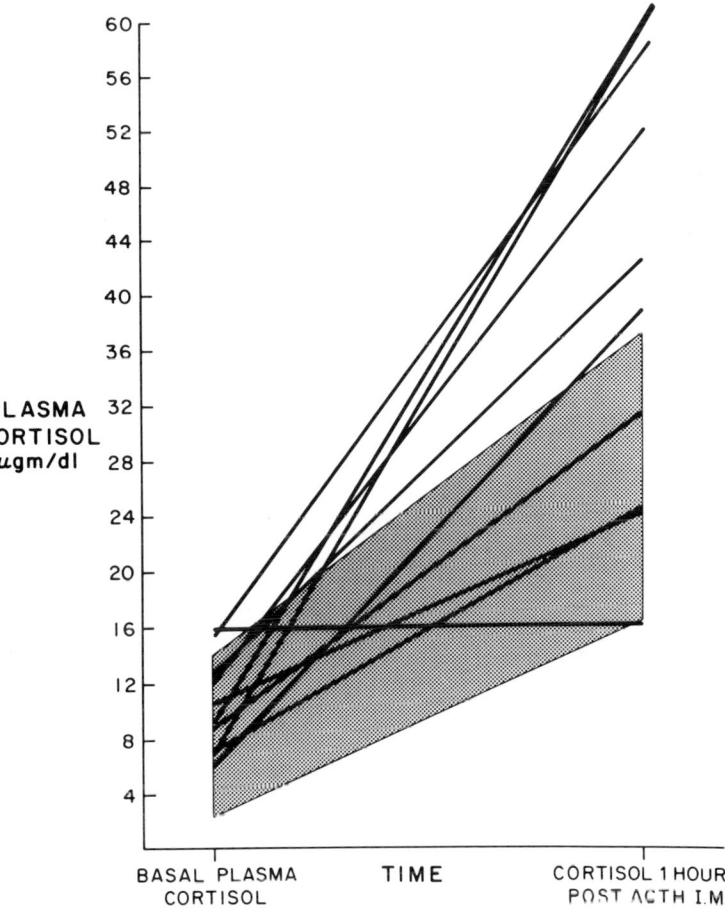

FIGURE 97–11. Plasma cortisol concentrations determined (fluorometric assay) before and one hour after administration of synthetic ACTH from five dogs with functioning adrenocortical tumors. This figure shows the variability in test results seen with functioning adrenal tumors. Shaded area represents results from control dogs.

trations, should be straightforward (Figure 97–12). In addition, it has recently been shown that 75 per cent of dogs with Cushing's syndrome clear dexamethasone from their plasma within a three-hour period. Plasma dexamethasone concentrations in healthy dogs persist for more than eight hours. Thus dexamethasone clear-

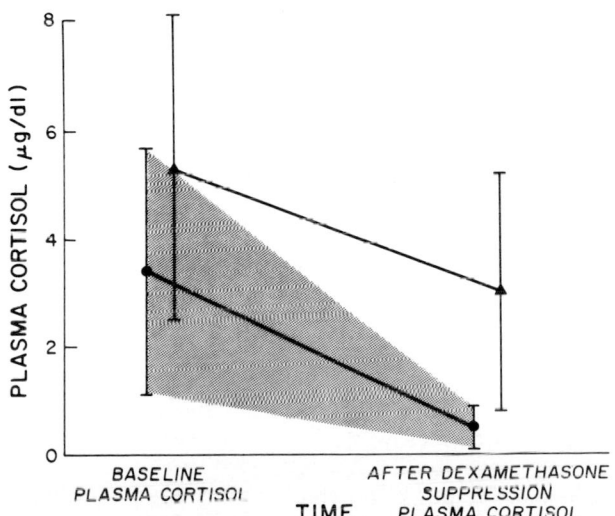

FIGURE 97–12. Mean plasma cortisol concentrations (± 2 SD) determined before and eight hours after administration of a low dexamethasone dose (0.01 mg/kg IV) in control dogs and in dogs with hyperadrenocorticism.

ance rates were altered in dogs with Cushing's syndrome.[71] If the dexamethasone is rapidly cleared, it cannot be present to cause persistent suppression of cortisol.[17]

Protocol. The recommended protocol is to obtain a morning baseline plasma sample for cortisol determination and then administer 0.005 mg of dexamethasone sodium phosphate/lb of body weight (0.01 mg of dexamethasone sodium phosphate/kg of body weight), IV. Samples should be taken eight hours later for cortisol determination.[10]

Other investigators have recommended different protocols, such as administration of 0.007 mg/lb (0.015 mg/kg) of dexamethasone in propylene glycol IM. Only the eight-hour cortisol sample is necessary for a diagnosis of hyperadrenocorticism. However, a three- to five-hour sample may be informative, as explained in the section on discrimination testing. If suppression is not seen at eight hours but is documented at three to five hours, it is likely that the dog has PDH rather than ATH. Dogs with ATH and some with PDH would not suppress at three to five hours (Figure 97–13).

Test Results. NORMAL DOGS. Normal dogs in our laboratory have a plasma cortisol concentration < 1.4 µg/dl eight hours after dexamethasone administration. For convenience, a level of 1.0 µg/dl is used as the criterion for diagnosis. Dexamethasone consistently suppresses plasma cortisol concentration in the normal dogs for the entire eight-hour test period. When comparing

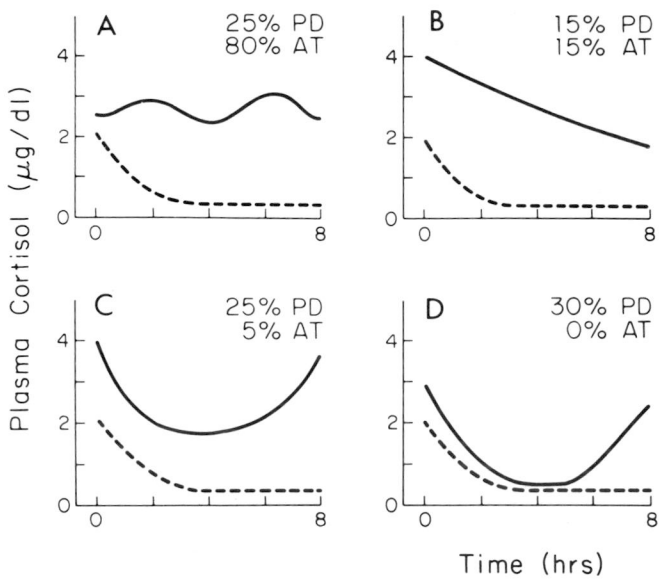

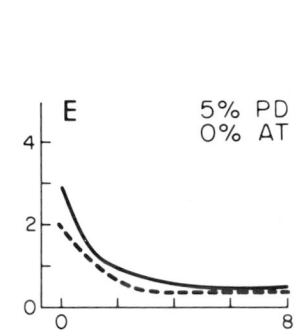

FIGURE 97–13. Pattern of plasma cortisol responses during low-dose dexamethasone screening in normal dogs and dogs with hyperadrenocorticism. *A,* No suppression; *B,* gradual and progressive suppression; *C,* rapid onset of mild suppression but transient effect; *D,* rapid onset of complete suppression but transient effect; *E,* normal complete suppression. PD, Pituitary-dependent hyperadrenocorticism; AT, adrenal tumor. (From Peterson, ME: Vet Clin North Am 14:731, 1984.)

the baseline cortisol concentration with that at eight hours, an obvious suppression is noted in the control dogs (see Figures 97–11 and 97–13).

DOGS WITH CCS. The dexamethasone screening test (low-dose dexamethasone test) has been extremely reliable in differentiating normal dogs from those with hyperadrenocorticism. In compiling the data from three recent reports,[10, 72, 73] the screening test was shown to correctly identify 96 of 102 dogs with hyperadrenocorticism (94 per cent).

Various responses to the low dose of dexamethasone (using Azium 0.007 mg/kg) are seen in dogs with hyperadrenocorticism (Figure 97–13). Dogs with PDH and those with adrenal tumors are resistant to suppression of cortisol with this dose, with five patterns of cortisol response seen in dogs with hyperadrenocorticism. No cortisol suppression occurs in most dogs with adrenal tumors and in 25 per cent of those with PDH (Figure 97–13A). In other dogs with either adrenal tumors or PDH, < 50 per cent suppression of baseline cortisol concentrations occurs during the testing period, and all cortisol values remain > 1.0 μg/dl (Figure 97–13B and C). In about one third of dogs with PDH, cortisol is suppressed to normal concentrations two and five hours after injection, but "escape" from suppression occurs at the sixth to eighth hour, with cortisol rising to presuppression levels (Figure 97–13D). This "escape" may be due to the rapid clearance of dexamethasone and can be used to distinguish between PDH and ATH. Finally, in a minority of dogs with early, mild PDH, normal cortisol suppression is observed (Figure 97–13E); these dogs usually develop abnormal test results when retested 2 to 12 months later. Noting suppression in dogs with an adrenal tumor is unusual. Because plasma cortisol concentrations do fluctuate spontaneously from minute to minute, one may by chance obtain a low cortisol concentration after dexamethasone administration in a dog ultimately shown to have an adrenal tumor. This finding would be interpreted as spurious,[74] rather than as suggesting a response to dexamethasone. Most dogs with CCS that had suppressed

cortisol concentrations on the screening test (4 of 85) were those with PDH. Despite these few unexpected results, the test remains an excellent and reliable screening test for distinguishing between normal dogs and those with Cushing's syndrome.[17]

Misleading Results. As with the ACTH stimulation test, dexamethasone screening test results can be misleading. Anticonvulsant medications can cause dogs to have unusual plasma cortisol concentrations, which may fail to suppress normally. The stress of bathing, hospitalization, illness, and numerous other factors may interfere with the suppressive effects of dexamethasone. Iatrogenic steroids may remain in the blood for long periods, causing an apparent failure to respond to dexamethasone because cortisol assays measure endogenous and iatrogenic glucocorticoids (not dexamethasone). Whenever iatrogenic disease is suspected, the ACTH stimulation test should be performed (see Figure 97–10). The dexamethasone screening test is affected by more variables than is the ACTH stimulation test. When interpreting either test, one must realize that neither is foolproof. It must be remembered that ACTH stimulation and low-dose dexamethasone screening tests are used for confirming a clinical suspicion. The most important initial screening tests are the history and physical examination.

Miscellaneous Screening Tests

GLUCAGON TOLERANCE TEST

The glucagon tolerance test was recently evaluated and advocated as a reliable screening test for the diagnosis of CCS.[75] However, the glucagon tolerance test has major drawbacks: (1) it cannot distinguish between overt diabetic dogs and those with both overt diabetes mellitus and CCS; (2) it cannot distinguish between dogs with mild type III diabetes mellitus and dogs with mild diabetes secondary to CCS; (3) it cannot distinguish between iatrogenic Cushing's syndrome and spontaneous Cushing's syndrome; and (4) it fails to account for dogs with CCS that do not have significant insulin antagonism. Therefore, the recommendation that this is an acceptable screening test remains to be proved with a critical review of the data.

HIGH-PERFORMANCE LIQUID CHROMATOGRAPHY PLASMA GLUCOCORTICOID ASSAYS

The HPLC assay allows quantification of multiple endogenous steroid hormones and synthetic analogues. Each hormone and analogue can be specifically analyzed. In a study of dogs with CCS, measurement of plasma cortisone, corticosterone, and cortisol concentrations provided some additional criteria for the laboratory confirmation of a clinical diagnosis.[71] However, HPLC assay systems are not widely available, the assay procedure is time-consuming, and only a limited number of samples can be analyzed daily. Because HPLC glucocorticoid measurements have their limitations,[71] one must await further studies and test availability before recommending this test for clinical cases.

COMBINED DEXAMETHASONE SUPPRESSION/ ACTH STIMULATION TEST (CDS/AST)

The CDS/AST has been recommended as the initial endocrine study to be performed in dogs suspected of having hyperadrenocorticism. This combined test was devised to provide information concerning pituitary gland and adrenal gland activity in a single, brief, relatively inexpensive trial.[76-78]

As an isolated study, neither ACTH stimulation nor dexamethasone suppression is invariably correct. Therefore, it is not surprising to find a test combining two imperfect studies to be critically lacking as a diagnostic tool. The authors of this test now recommend that it be used solely as a screening test to distinguish dogs with hyperadrenocorticism from those free of the disease. However, the test remains difficult to interpret, and its use is not recommended.[72, 73]

LIVER BIOPSY

Elevations in liver enzymes and abnormal liver function tests are common in CCS. For this reason, patients with vague clinical features of hyperadrenocorticism may be thought to be suffering from primary liver disease. With the increasing use of liver biopsies, this procedure may be performed on hyperadrenal dogs. Dogs with spontaneous hyperadrenocorticism or those given exogenous glucocorticoids usually have histologic evidence of glucocorticoid-induced hepatopathy. This hepatopathy is histologically characterized by centrilobular vacuolization, perivacuolar glycogen accumulation within hepatocytes, and focal centrilobular necrosis.[79] Any dog with these findings on liver biopsy should be evaluated for CCS.

Vacuolar hepatopathy can result from a variety of disorders. Currently there appear to be few differential causes for steroid-induced hepatopathy. Therefore, liver biopsy can be used as a screening test to identify CCS.

This study cannot distinguish between spontaneous and iatrogenic steroid excess. Other disadvantages to the routine use of liver biopsy as a screening test include the complications of infection or inadequate healing after the procedure, due to the systemic effects of hyperadrenocorticism. However, this test remains potentially helpful in patients with vague evidence of CCS. The hepatomegaly typical of hyperadrenocorticism makes most percutaneous biopsy procedures straightforward.[17]

Discrimination Tests to Differentiate Dogs with Pituitary-Dependent CCS from Dogs with Functioning Adrenal Tumors

ENDOGENOUS ACTH CONCENTRATIONS

Theory. In reviewing the underlying causes that lead to development of hyperadrenocorticism (see Figure 97–1), one gains an impression that measurement of the patient's plasma endogenous ACTH concentration would be a helpful discriminating test. Adrenocortical tumors should suppress ACTH secretion, and pituitary-dependent CCS is the result of excessive ACTH secretion. In both humans and dogs, assays for ACTH concentration are not used to diagnose hyperadrenocorticism because a large number of the test results fall into the normal range and because iatrogenic glucocorticoid administration can suppress ACTH concentrations. The plasma endogenous ACTH level remains a valuable aid in distinguishing patients with adrenocortical tumors from those with pituitary-dependent disease.[17]

Protocol. Pituitary secretion of ACTH occurs episodically (i.e., it is released in bursts). Therefore, plasma concentrations fluctuate from minute to minute. Overlying these alterations in plasma levels are potential diurnal variations, with more frequent bursts of a higher magnitude occurring in the early morning hours versus the decreased frequency and magnitude in secretion seen at night.[74] In order to diminish the variables of stress and time of day, dogs spend at least one night in the hospital before plasma is obtained for determination of endogenous ACTH concentration, and the blood is taken only between 8 AM and 9 AM.

Cold, heparinized plastic syringes are used. Blood is obtained, and the filled syringe is placed on ice. The blood is then transferred to cold plastic tubes and cold-centrifuged. Plasma is placed into plastic tubes and frozen at -40 °C. The entire procedure should take less than ten minutes.

Results. The baseline plasma ACTH concentration in healthy dogs averages 46 pg/ml, and the reference range is 20 to 100 pg/ml. Endogenous ACTH concentrations < 20 pg/ml in a dog or cat with spontaneous hyperadrenocorticism are strongly suggestive of a functioning adrenocortical tumor (Figure 97–14). If a dog with iatrogenic hyperadrenocorticism is studied, its plasma endogenous ACTH concentration would also be < 20 pg/ml, but the ACTH stimulation test should reveal the underlying disorder (see Figure 97–10).

Endogenous plasma ACTH concentrations are ex-

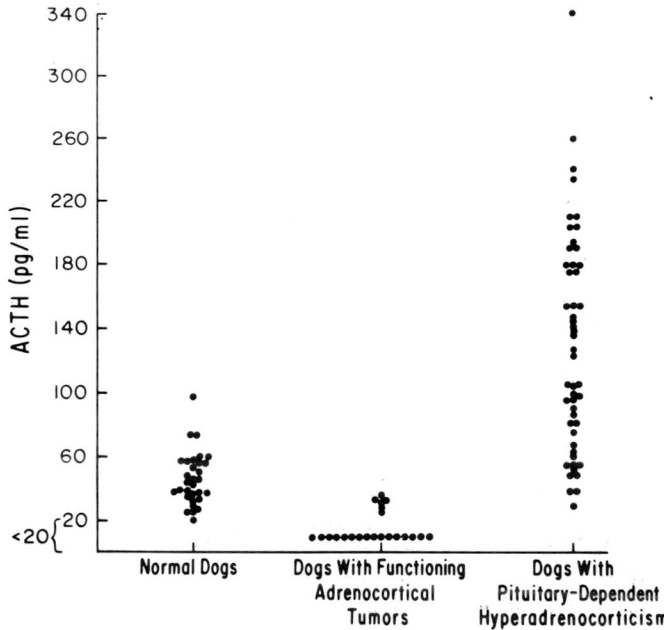

FIGURE 97–14. Endogenous plasma ACTH concentrations from clinically normal dogs, dogs with functioning adrenocortical carcinomas or adenomas, and dogs with pituitary-dependent hyperadrenocorticism.

tremely useful in determining the cause of canine hyperadrenocorticism. Plasma ACTH concentrations are normal to elevated in dogs with PDH and are low in dogs with adrenocortical tumors (Figure 97–14). Difficulty in obtaining plasma ACTH assays may offset their usefulness. Plasma ACTH assays are technically difficult to perform, and many commercial laboratories may be unable to give consistently reliable results.

DEXAMETHASONE SUPPRESSION TEST (HIGH-DOSE DEXAMETHASONE TEST)

Theory. In dogs with functioning adrenal tumors, dexamethasone at any dosage will not suppress cortisol levels because these tumors function independent of ACTH control. In PDH the threshold for glucocorticoid negative feedback of ACTH is higher than normal; ACTH secretion is relatively resistant to glucocorticoid suppression, but high doses of dexamethasone can suppress ACTH secretion in most dogs with PDH, resulting in a decline in circulating cortisol levels.

Protocol. The dexamethasone suppression protocol that was found to be most reliable in several studies was to collect heparinized blood samples before and 8 hours after administration of 0.05 mg/lb (0.1 mg/kg) IV dexamethasone sodium phosphate.[11, 72] Suppression is defined as an 8-hour post-dexamethasone plasma cortisol concentration < 50 per cent of the baseline concentration. Other investigators utilize higher doses of 0.5 mg/lb (1.0 mg/kg) and have defined suppression as a reduction in plasma cortisol concentration below an absolute plasma cortisol value. Attempts at using a specific cut-off figure, however, were not as reliable as utilization of the percentage of change.[11] In addition, percentage of change removes the confusion created by individual laboratory variability in reported cortisol values.

Results. **ADRENOCORTICAL TUMORS.** As has been previously described, adrenocortical tumors function autonomously (i.e., they are independent of ACTH control). As expected, administration of a high dose of dexamethasone does not result in cortisol suppression (Figure 97–15).[11, 72] Suppression is defined as an 8-hour plasma cortisol concentration < 50 per cent of the baseline level. However, in any animal, plasma cortisol concentrations do fluctuate, and one could occasionally see a "suppressed" plasma cortisol concentration by chance. This would be an extremely unusual phenomenon in a dog with an adrenocortical tumor. Dogs with CCS that do have suppressed cortisol concentrations on a high-dose dexamethasone test can be assumed to have pituitary-dependent disease.

PDH. The dexamethasone suppression test (high-dose test) should result in suppression of ACTH secretion from functioning adenomatous or hyperplastic pituitary cells. The test has not been totally reliable. Approximately 75 to 80 per cent of dogs with PDH do have plasma cortisol concentrations < 50 per cent of baseline (Figure 97–15). The percentage remained at that level in dogs tested with the 0.5 mg/lb (1.0 mg/kg) dose of dexamethasone. Almost 100 per cent of the dogs with CCS that demonstrated suppression on the 0.5 mg/lb (1.0 mg/kg) dose of dexamethasone had PDH; however, among the dogs with CCS that failed to demonstrate suppression were some with PDH and others with adrenocortical tumors.[11, 72]

It is not known why some dogs with PDH are extremely resistant to dexamethasone suppression.[60] Meijer reported that lack of cortisol suppression after high-

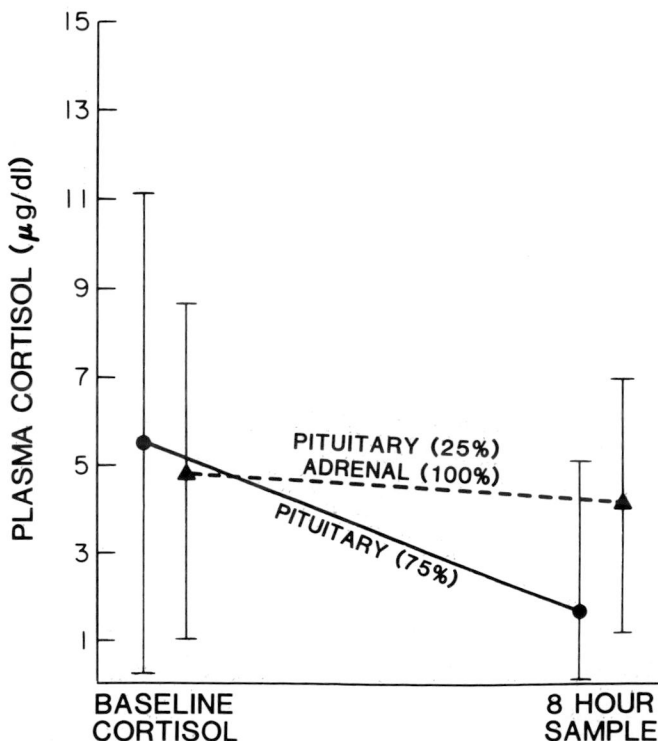

FIGURE 97–15. Pattern of plasma cortisol responses during high-dose dexamethasone suppression in dogs with pituitary-dependent or adrenal tumor hyperadrenocorticism. Note that suppression is diagnostic of pituitary dependency; lack of suppression included all adrenal tumor cases and 25 per cent of the pituitary-dependent cases.

dose dexamethasone testing in cases of PDH is usually associated with a large (macroadenoma) pituitary tumor.[18] In our experience, however, there is no correlation between the size of a pituitary tumor and plasma cortisol response to dexamethasone. In human patients with PDH, a similar finding of occasional resistance to dexamethasone has been reported.[80] Pituitary tumors in some of these patients arise from pars intermedia tissue, accounting for a lesser degree of dexamethasone suppressibility, because this area of the pituitary gland is under neural control versus hormonal control of the pars distalis.[81]

Summary. The dexamethasone suppression test (high-dose test), in contrast to endogenous plasma ACTH determination, is available to veterinarians. Any dog with hyperadrenocorticism that demonstrates cortisol suppressibility can be assumed to have PDH. Failure of dexamethasone to suppress plasma cortisol concentrations < 50 per cent of the baseline level eight hours after administration must be viewed as an inconclusive test result. Failure of suppression is typical of patients with adrenocortical tumors and of some patients with pituitary-dependent CCS.

Four patterns of cortisol responses are seen with the 0.5 mg/kg high-dose dexamethasone suppression test in dogs with hyperadrenocorticism (Figure 97–16).[20] In most dogs with PDH, cortisol concentrations are suppressed diagnostically (Figure 97–16A); in these dogs, the six-hour and eight-hour samples are most important for the interpretation of the test because suppression is greatest at these times. In a few dogs with PDH, cortisol is suppressed at two and five hours after injection but rises to presuppression levels by the eighth hour (Figure 97–16B), making the test difficult to interpret or simply inconclusive. Suppression does not occur in approximately 15 per cent of dogs with PDH (Figure 97–16C and D). Only a few of these dogs will exhibit adequate

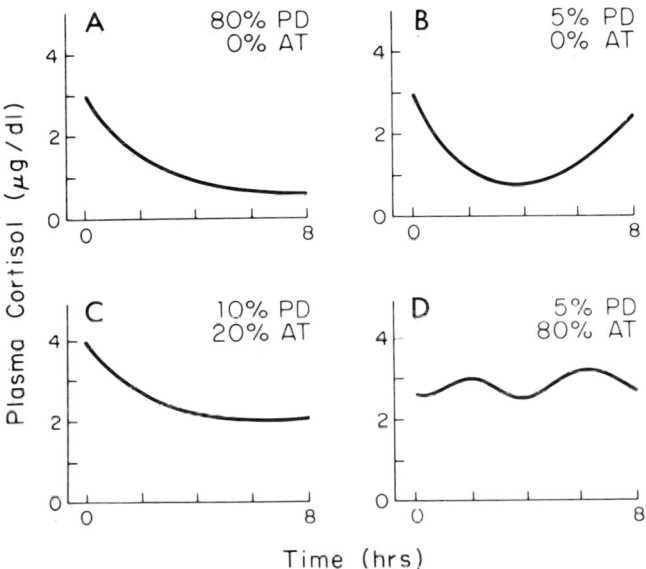

FIGURE 97–16. Pattern of plasma cortisol responses during high dose dexamethasone suppression testing in dogs with hyperadrenocorticism. *A,* Rapid onset and persistent suppression; *B,* rapid onset of suppression but transient effect; *C,* only mild suppression seen; *D,* no suppression. PD, Pituitary-dependent hyperadrenocorticism; AT, adrenal tumor. (From Peterson, ME: Vet Clin North Am 14:731, 1984.)

cortisol suppression with a higher dose of dexamethasone, but in some dogs suppression may not occur even with dexamethasone doses as high as 1 mg/lb (2 mg/kg). In most dogs with adrenal tumors, no cortisol suppression occurs throughout the eight-hour testing period (Figure 97–16D).

Radiography

See previous section.

Ultrasonography

Ultrasound evaluation of dogs with CCS has been moderately helpful as a test in separating dogs with PDH from dogs with adrenocortical tumors.[82] The adrenals of normal dogs cannot be visualized on ultrasound. It is also rare for the adrenals of a dog with bilateral hyperplasia to be visualized. However, approximately 50 per cent of adrenal tumors are large enough to be seen on abdominal ultrasonography (Figure 97–17).

Computed Tomography

Computed tomography is an expensive and sophisticated tool primarily available at veterinary schools and through a small number of veterinary specialists. The CT scan is a noninvasive method of visualizing the anatomy of almost any area of the body. It has been quite successful in distinguishing dogs and cats with one large adrenal from those with two large adrenals from those with normal adrenals. This tool has also been extremely accurate for visualizing large pituitary tumors or cerebral ventricular dilation secondary to a pituitary-hypothalamic mass. Unfortunately, in addition to the expense of such equipment, CT scans require veterinarians with expertise to interpret results and manage the facilities. CT scans require 30 minutes to 2 hours of anesthesia. In addition, many dogs with PDH do not have visible abnormalities in the pituitary region because they have microadenomas.

CRH Stimulation Test

CRH has recently been isolated and made available for scientific study.[83] The effect of exogenous ovine CRH on plasma concentrations of ACTH and cortisol in CCS was recently assessed.[84] The report revealed that a single IV dose of CRH produced increases in plasma ACTH and cortisol concentrations in normal dogs and those with PDH, whereas no significant rise in plasma ACTH or cortisol concentrations was seen in dogs with adrenocortical tumors. Therefore, the CRH test may have value as a discriminating study in CCS. The availability of CRH is quite limited at present.

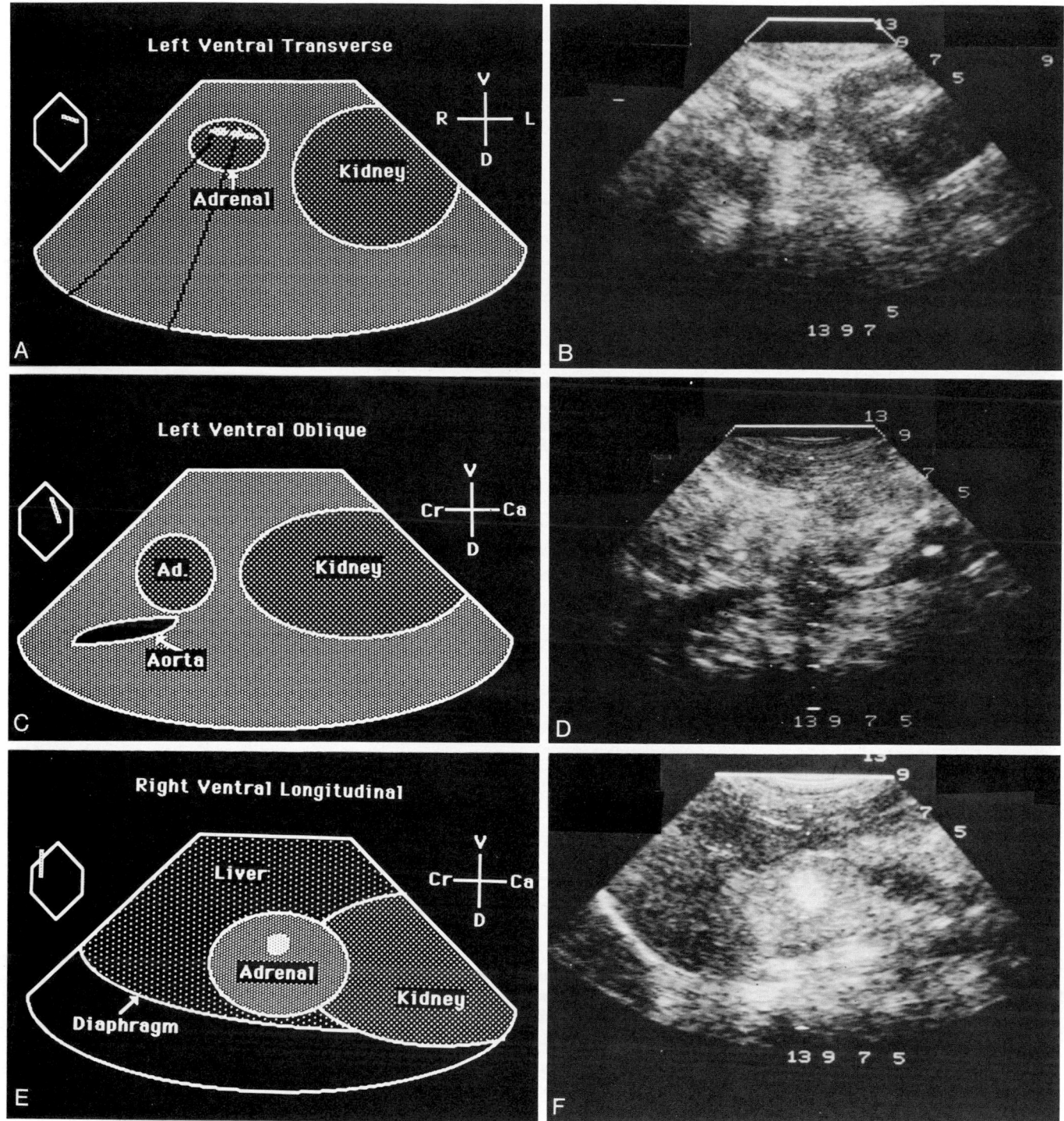

FIGURE 97–17. *A,* A diagrammatic illustration of the ultrasound image shown in *B,* showing the appearance of a calcified adrenal carcinoma in a dog with hyperadrenocorticism. *C,* A diagrammatic illustration of the ultrasound image shown in *D,* illustrating a hyperplastic adrenal gland in a dog with pituitary-dependent hyperadrenocorticism. *E,* A diagrammatic illustration of the ultrasound image shown in *F,* showing the opposite hyperplastic adrenal in the same dog with bilateral adrenal hyperplasia. V, Ventral; D, dorsal; Cr, cranial; Ca, caudal; the symbol in the upper left corner of *A, C,* and *E* is the location and orientation of the transducer in the ventral abdomen. (*A, C,* and *E* courtesy of Dr. Brett Kantrowitz; *B, D,* and *F* from Kantrowitz, BM, et al.: Vet Radiol 27:15, 1986.)

Radioisotope Imaging of the Adrenals

Gamma camera imaging of the adrenal glands has been reported in normal dogs and in dogs with CCS. Dogs were given iodine-131-19-iodocholesterol IV. In normal dogs both adrenal glands could be visualized separately, and there was no difficulty in distinguishing between the images of normal glands, hyperplastic glands, and functioning adrenal tumors.[85]

Metyrapone Testing

Metyrapone is an enzyme blocker that inhibits the action of 11-β-hydroxylase in steroid synthesis. Thus, in normal dogs, plasma cortisol concentrations decline, while 11-desoxycortisol accumulates, owing to continued ACTH stimulation. The suggested dose of metyrapone is 12 mg/lb (25 mg/kg) orally, every six hours for four treatments, with plasma collected before the test and six hours after the final dose. Samples are assayed for both cortisol and 11-desoxycortisol. If metyrapone results in a decrease in the plasma cortisol concentration and a concomitant increase in plasma 11-desoxycortisol level, a diagnosis of PDH can be made. If plasma cortisol and 11-desoxycortisol concentrations both decline after the four metyrapone doses, an adrenal tumor is the probable cause of the hyperadrenocorticism.[86]

TREATMENT

As discussed previously, approximately 80 to 85 per cent of dogs with CCS have PDH, whereas the remainder suffer from functioning adrenal tumors. Therapy depends on the cause of CCS as well as on the veterinarian's surgical experience. Several therapeutic options are available.

Therapy Without Defining the Underlying Cause

A veterinarian may suspect a patient of having CCS and complete the in-hospital evaluation, including data base and screening tests. Many veterinarians cannot or do not proceed diagnostically beyond confirming the diagnosis of CCS. This may occur because of unfamiliarity with tests that distinguish pituitary-dependent from adrenal tumor CCS, owner financial constraints, lack of facilities to perform some tests, or because some test results are not conclusive. One alternative is to refer the patient to a colleague or institution with the capabilities for the required tests. A second alternative is to realize that most dogs with hyperadrenocorticism have pituitary-dependent disease with bilateral adrenal hyperplasia, which is usually responsive to therapy with o,p'-DDD. Such therapy, therefore, is still associated with a good chance of achieving control of the disorder.

Adrenal Tumor Hyperadrenocorticism

SURGERY

Preoperative Evaluation. Dogs diagnosed as having adrenal tumor hyperadrenocorticism carry the best prognosis if the tumor can be surgically removed. Once the diagnosis of Cushing's syndrome and the presence of an adrenal tumor are confirmed, one should attempt to localize the tumor and rule out metastasis. Abdominal radiographs will localize approximately 50 per cent of tumors by means of calcification (see Figures 97–7 and 97–8). Other methods of tumor localization include ultrasound, CT scans, and gamma camera imaging. Each of these procedures does require facilities not found in most veterinary hospitals.

Adrenal tumors that metastasize will usually spread to the liver and/or lungs. Therefore, radiographs of the thorax are mandatory. Ultrasound evaluation of the liver has been quite valuable in detecting metastasis. If metastasis is suspected, an ultrasound-guided biopsy of the liver can be performed to confirm this suspicion.

Screening tests, such as radiographs, ultrasound, and CT scans, may also provide valuable information regarding the size of the tumor present. Small tumors (Figure 97–18) are much more likely to be benign and successfully removed than massive tumors (Figure 97–19). The preoperative evaluation should also be directed at recognizing any concurrent problems that may need to be treated before considering surgery.

Surgical Approach. The recommended surgical approach is by way of a paracostal laparotomy. A ventral midline celiotomy may give excellent exposure of both adrenal glands. However, problems are associated with wound healing in tissues that have been exposed to high concentrations of corticosteroids. Therefore, a ventral weight-bearing incision should be avoided.[87] In addition, the large amount of abdominal fat found in patients with Cushing's syndrome, coupled with the location of the adrenals dorsal and medial to the kidneys, makes the ventral midline approach more difficult. If the ventral midline approach is used, the liver should be thoroughly inspected and a specimen of tissue from any

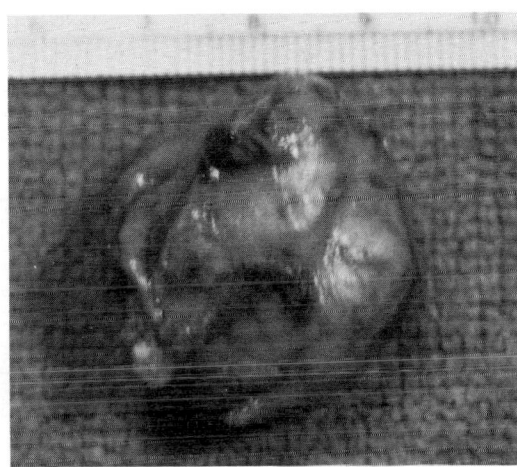

FIGURE 97–18. Photograph of a small, functioning adrenocortical adenoma.

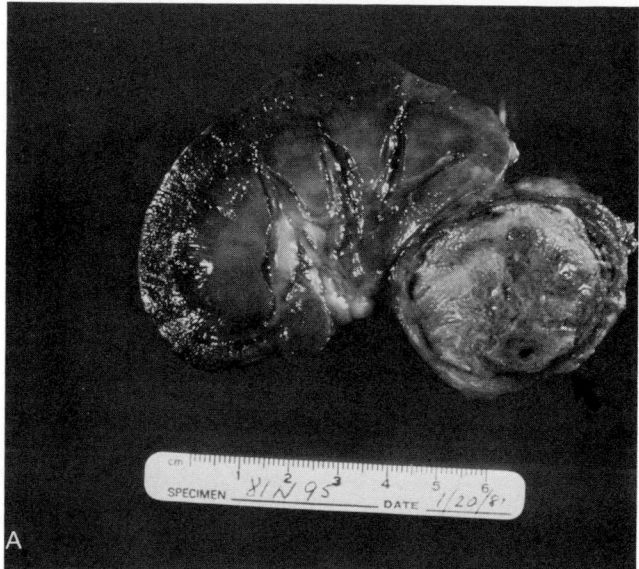

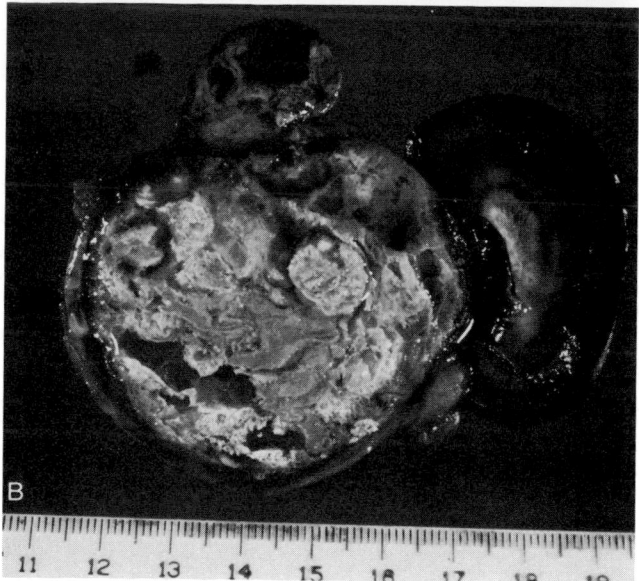

FIGURE 97–19. Photographs of a moderate-sized *(A)* and large *(B)* adrenocortical carcinomas (arrows), closely adhered to the associated kidney.

abnormal areas should be excised for histologic examination.

The paracostal retroperitoneal approach to adrenalectomy gives adequate exposure to the adrenal gland on that side of the abdomen. This approach avoids the wound-healing problems of a ventral midline incision, as well as the difficulties of traversing an abdomen filled with fat. Also, the adrenals, which are dorsolateral to the vena cava and aorta, are much more accessible via the paracostal approach. Several marked disadvantages of the paracostal approach include (1) only being able to explore one adrenal bed (exploration of the opposite side requires closure of the first incision and a second surgical procedure) and (2) inability to evaluate the liver for metastasis.[17]

If the adrenal tumor is not calcified and no other study is used to identify the tumor location, usually one must guess which side to approach first. If the tumor is not on the side chosen, the dog will require a second surgical procedure over the opposite flank to find and remove the tumor.

The actual surgery is well described by Johnston.[87, 88] When an adrenal tumor is recognized, one hopes it will be totally excised. However, the surgeon may encounter a large mass or one that has invaded surrounding tissues and cannot be excised. As much tumor should be removed as possible, since the tissue provides histologic confirmation of the diagnosis and debulking may improve the endocrine status of the dog or cat.

Patient Management During Surgery. Although some investigators have recommended treating surgical patients with corticosteroids for one or two days before the procedure, it is unnecessary and actually potentially harmful. The iatrogenic steroids predispose the patient to overhydration and an increased risk of thromboembolic episodes.

At the time of anesthesia, IV fluids (saline or lactated Ringer's solution) should be administered at a maintenance rate. When the adrenal tumor is recognized by the surgeon, dexamethasone is placed in the IV infusion bottle at a dose of 0.01 to 0.02 mg/lb (0.02 to 0.04 mg/kg) of body weight. This dose is to be given over a six-hour period and will be repeated four times a day for two days before changing to oral prednisone therapy. When the tumor is excised, fludrocortisone (mineralocorticoid) may be administered at a dose of 0.005 to 0.01 mg/lb (0.01 to 0.02 mg/kg) of body weight orally. The blood pressure and BUN, serum electrolyte, and blood glucose concentrations should be closely monitored. It must be remembered that adrenal tumors cause decreased secretion of pituitary ACTH, and this causes atrophy of all normal adrenocortical tissue. When an adrenal tumor is excised, acute hypoadrenocorticism has been created.

After successful recovery from anesthesia, dogs are continued on dexamethasone and mineralocorticoid medications, using the treatment protocol described for hypoadrenocorticism. Parenteral medication is continued for 48 to 72 hours. Dexamethasone is administered at the suggested dose (0.01 to 0.02 mg/lb or 0.02 to 0.04 mg/kg) in IV fluids two to four times a day. Parenteral dexamethasone should be continued daily until the dog is eating and drinking normally, not receiving IV fluids, and considered stable. The mineralocorticoids can be discontinued after a few doses, to be given again only if hyperkalemia or hyponatremia is recognized.

Once the dog is eating and drinking on its own, it is placed on 0.5 mg/lb (1.0 mg/kg) of prednisone orally, twice a day for 2 days. The dosage is then reduced to 0.2 mg/lb (0.5 mg/kg) twice a day for two weeks, 0.12 mg/lb (0.25 mg/kg) twice a day for three weeks, 0.2 mg/lb (0.5 mg/kg) every other day for one month, and finally 0.25 mg/kg every other day for 1 month; the medication is then stopped. Fludrocortisone acetate Florinef (mineralocorticoid) is used at a dosage of 0.01 mg/lb/day (0.02 mg/kg/day) if the serum electrolyte concentrations indicate that it is needed (40 per cent of the dogs have needed this medication). Serum sodium concentrations < 138 mEq/L and serum potassium concentrations > 5.5 mEq/L do indicate a need for mineralocorticoid therapy. Its dosage is then tapered similar to that of the glucocorticoid. Glucocorticoid and mineralocorticoid medication must meet individual requirements; "cookbook" approaches must be avoided.

Ideally, dogs should be on alternate-day therapy within four to eight weeks of surgery and off all medication by three to six months. This time period and tapering of medication should allow sufficient time for return of normal pituitary-adrenal function. ACTH stimulation tests can be used as an adjunct to therapy in determining when to discontinue medication. Any time a patient becomes listless, anorectic, or ill during the tapering process, the glucocorticoid dose may need to be raised and serum electrolytes monitored.

Inoperable Mass, Poor Anesthetic Risk, or Obvious Metastasis.
Surgery cannot be considered for some hyperadrenal dogs with adrenocortical tumors. The reasons for avoiding surgery include finding a large, obviously inoperable mass on radiographs, ultrasound, or CT scan; finding metastatic lesions in the lungs or liver; a patient that is so debilitated that surgery would probably be terminal; and, finally, an owner who refuses surgery.

All these conditions are difficult to manage because little or moderate success has been achieved with o,p'-DDD therapy, following the protocol for dogs with PDH. Many of the dogs with adrenal tumors receive huge quantities of this drug with poor response. However, a few dogs have shown an excellent response. We have recently begun using ketoconazole (see section on Chemotherapy with Ketoconazole) for adrenocortical tumors. Therapy with ketoconazole has been successful in alleviating the signs of hyperadrenocorticism.

Unilateral Versus Bilateral Adrenocortical Tumors.
Although an extremely rare phenomenon, it is possible for a dog to have bilateral adrenocortical tumors. Of 47 dogs with functioning adrenocortical tumors in our series, 4 have had bilateral adrenal adenomas.

Simultaneous Pituitary Tumor and Adrenal Cushing's Syndrome.
One of 47 dogs with a functioning adrenocortical tumor (carcinoma) was also found to have a pituitary microadenoma. This dog had both an adrenal tumor and bilateral adrenocortical hyperplasia. The endocrine evaluation was diagnostic for hyperadrenocorticism. The plasma cortisol concentrations did not suppress when the dog was given a high dose of dexamethasone, but the endogenous plasma ACTH concentration was suggestive of pituitary-dependent disease. The dog was treated first with adrenal tumor excision and then with o,p'-DDD for the remaining adrenal hyperplasia.

A ten-year-old Boxer has also been reported to have both primary adrenal and pituitary-dependent Cushing's syndrome.[89]

Pituitary-Dependent Hyperadrenocorticism

Hypophysectomy.
Surgery to remove the pituitary gland, and thus the source of ACTH in PDH, has been successfully performed in the dog. The procedure has been described;[90] it should be performed by surgeons with considerable experience. Brachycephalic dogs are not good candidates for this surgery. If the procedure is successful, the dog will lose all the features of CCS.

However, these patients also lose all ability to secrete ACTH and will therefore require glucocorticoid therapy for life. These animals may also develop transient or permanent diabetes insipidus as well as hypothyroidism. With an experienced surgeon, hypophysectomy is the ideal treatment. These animals will not suffer from the growth of pituitary tumors, nor will they face the risks associated with chemotherapy or adrenalectomy.

Adrenalectomy.
PDH results in bilateral adrenocortical hyperplasia. Removal of both adrenals will result in a disappearance of the signs caused by CCS. This surgery involves the risk of putting an ill animal, with a compromised immune system and poor wound healing, through a difficult surgical procedure. As with hypophysectomy, in experienced hands (using the flank approach), the risks can be minimized.[88] However, such dogs must be treated for hypoadrenocorticism for the rest of their lives, and they always have the potential for developing a hypoadrenal crisis.

Initial Chemotherapy Using o,p'-DDD

Pretreatment Assessments.
Since the treatment protocol first suggested by Schechter and associates,[66] chemotherapy has been the most common therapeutic approach in CCS.

After in-hospital diagnostic studies are finished, polydipsic animals with hyperadrenocorticism are returned to the owners for water intake monitoring. If an owner has more than one pet, the water intake of the pets at home can be determined while the suspect patient is in the hospital. In this manner the dog with CCS can be returned to its normal environment for water intake monitoring, and the owner will know how much to subtract from the total water consumed to determine the patient's water intake. Water intake is determined for 24 consecutive hours over a minimum of five days to eliminate errors in measuring and to achieve a reliable average figure from which therapy can begin.

Approximately 20 per cent of dogs with PDH are not polydipsic. Like the polydipsic dogs, they can and should be treated by their owners at home. Absence of polydipsia simply eliminates one of the factors that can be monitored during the initial phases of therapy.

o,p'-DDD.
The systemic effects of the insecticide o,p'-DDD were first reported in 1949.[91] The agent was administered to dogs and found to be a potent adrenocorticolytic drug. The drug caused severe, progressive necrosis of the zona fasciculata and zona reticularis. In a subsequent study, partial or complete necrosis was also recognized in the zona glomerulosa.[92] The only other significant pathologic processes involved the liver, including moderate to severe fatty degeneration, moderate centrolobular atrophy, and congestion. No other pathology in the liver or any other organ was considered significant.[91]

It is interesting to note that the normal dogs given o,p'-DDD appear clinically quite resistant to the adrenocorticolytic effects of the drug. In the initial study, four dogs received 22 mg/lb (50 mg/kg), five days per week. Two of the four died after 20 and 21 months of therapy, respectively. The third dog was euthanatized after 21 months of therapy, and the fourth dog was alive after 38 months on the drug.[91] In a subsequent study, ten dogs were treated at a dosage of 22 mg/lb/day (50 mg/kg/day). One dog died after 124 consecutive days of treatment and a second died after 147 days. The remaining eight dogs were clinically healthy at the time of euthanasia, after 36 to 150 consecutive days of drug therapy.[92] In another report, dogs showed decreased adrenocortical reserve and evidence of adrenocortical destruction after three to ten days of therapy, although clinically appearing to be in good health.[93] This final report should remind all veterinarians of the rapid onset of o,p'-DDD effects. The drug must not be used indiscriminately.

The implication from the research on o,p'-DDD is clear. The normal canine adrenal cortex is quickly damaged by o,p'-DDD, but normal animals survive long periods with minimal adrenal support. Dogs with adrenal hyperplasia must be much more sensitive to the destructive effects of o,p'-DDD because they usually respond within 5 to 14 days and often become ill (hypoadrenal) if medication is continued. Any dog diagnosed as having PDH, requiring more than 21 consecutive days of o,p'-DDD therapy, must be carefully reevaluated. One possibility is that the diagnosis is incorrect. A few dogs with PDH have required as much as 60 days of therapy, but these dogs are quite unusual (see Failure to Respond to o,p'-DDD).

Initiating Therapy. Therapy is begun at home with the owner administering o,p'-DDD (Lysodren) at a dosage of 22 mg/lb/day (50 mg/kg/day), divided twice a day (Figure 97–20). Glucocorticoids are not given, but the owner should have a small supply of prednisolone tablets. The owner should receive thorough instructions on the actions of o,p'-DDD and should also have specific instructions on when the drug should be discontinued. Lysodren administration should be stopped when (1) the polydipsic dog consumes less than 30 ml/lb/day (60 ml/kg/day) of water, (2) the dog with an excellent appetite takes 10 to 30 minutes or longer to consume a meal that would be consumed in a shorter time before Lysodren therapy, and (3) the dog vomits, has diarrhea, or is unusually listless. The first two indications for stopping the medication are strongly emphasized. The occurrence of any of these signs strongly indicates that the end point in therapy has been achieved.[17]

Because of the potency of o,p'-DDD, the veterinarian is encouraged not to rely solely on the instructions given to an owner. This drug is highly successful in eliminating the signs of hyperadrenocorticism when its use is coupled with close communication between owner and veterinarian. Either the veterinarian or a technician should call the owner every day, beginning with the third day of therapy. In this way, the owner will be impressed with the veterinarian's concern and will closely observe the animal. It is wise for the owner to feed the dog two small meals each day. The dog's appetite should be observed before each administration of Lysodren. If food is rapidly consumed (± polydipsia), medication is warranted. If food is consumed either slowly or not at all, medication should be discontinued until the veterinarian is consulted. Usually the initial loading dose phase is complete when a reduction in appetite is observed or after water intake approaches or falls below 30 ml/lb/day (60 ml/kg/day).

If before therapy the dog with CCS is neither polydipsic nor polyphagic, the diagnosis must be absolutely positive and the dog closely monitored by the owner. The most important monitoring guide in these dogs is their appetite. Reduction in appetite in any dog receiving o,p'-DDD is an indication that overdosage is imminent.

The water intake in polydipsic dogs may fall to the normal range in as few as 2 days or in as long as 35 days (average is 5 to 16 days). Owners must continue to monitor the water intake daily until it falls below 60 ml/kg/day.

A small percentage of dogs will demonstrate mild gastric irritation from the drug three to four days after medication has been started. If this occurs, the medication should be discontinued until the veterinarian can evaluate the dog. If the gastric upset occurs because of drug sensitivity and not because the treatment is complete, dividing the dose further may be helpful; discontinuing the medication for a few days may be necessary. Also, some dogs develop profound weakness, lethargy, and anorexia within three to four days of beginning this therapy. In our experience this is quite uncommon, but it is recommended that daily treatment be initiated on a Saturday so that if illness develops after three days, the veterinarian will be available during a regular work week, rather than on a weekend.[17]

Veterinary Monitoring. In addition to making daily phone calls, the veterinarian should see the dog eight to nine days after beginning therapy. At this time a thorough history and physical examination should be performed and a recheck of the ACTH response test obtained. A recheck of the BUN, serum sodium, and potassium concentrations may be warranted. Dogs that have responded clinically to the medication (or if the owner is not certain about response) should have therapy withheld until the ACTH response test results can be evaluated. Dogs that have not responded should have an ACTH response test performed but should also remain on daily therapy (see Figure 97–20).

Goal of Therapy. The goal of therapy with Lysodren is to achieve an ACTH response test result that is suggestive of hypoadrenocorticism. In our laboratory successful response to Lysodren is indicated by a pre-ACTH plasma cortisol concentration < 5 μg/dl and a post-ACTH plasma cortisol concentration that is also < 5 μg/dl (Figures 97–10 and 97–20).

Continuing Lysodren Therapy. If the dog with CCS has a normal or exaggerated response to ACTH after the initial eight to nine days of Lysodren therapy, the clinical signs are usually present and medication should be continued. Usually it is continued for three to seven additional consecutive days, the shorter time period being used for dogs that have shown some significant (albeit inadequate) response. Repeat ACTH response tests are continued every seven to ten days until a low post-ACTH plasma cortisol response is achieved. Numerous repeat tests are not usually necessary because most dogs have responded during the initial seven to ten days of medication, and almost all have responded by the 16th day of therapy.

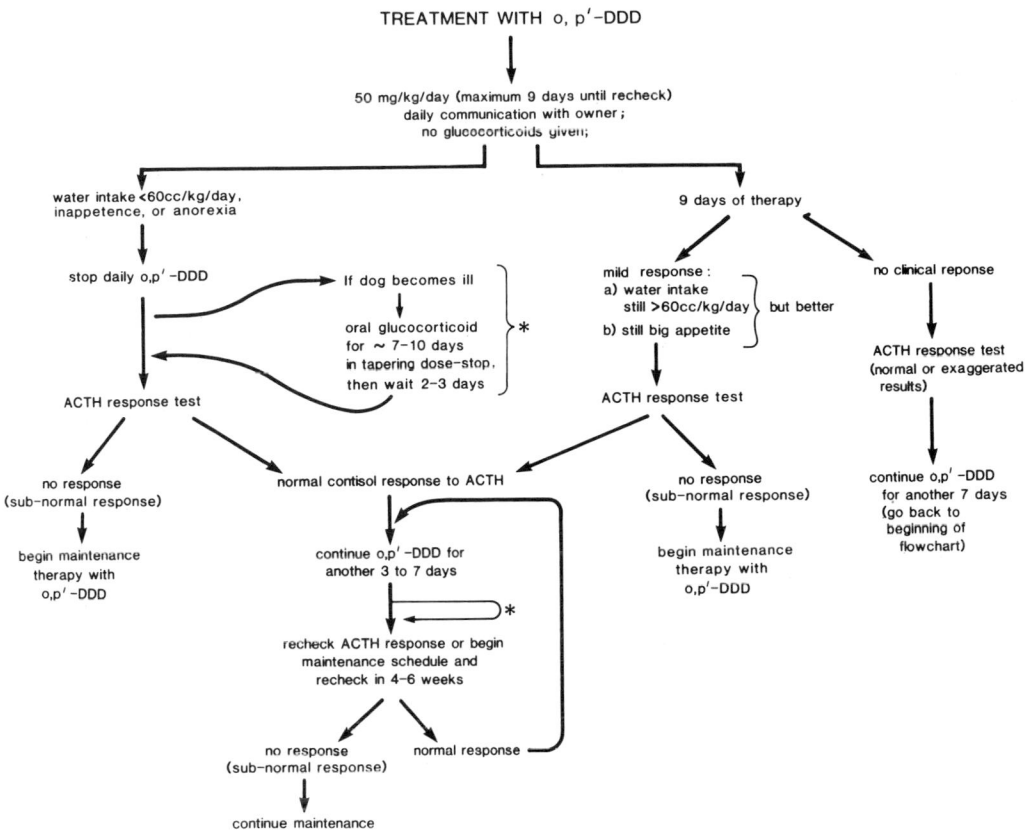

FIGURE 97-20. Flow chart for the management of hyperadrenocorticism using o,p'-DDD. Asterisks indicate similar treatment protocols. (From Feldman, EC, Nelson, RW: Canine and Feline Endocrinology and Reproduction. Philadelphia, WB Saunders, 1987.)

Average Length of Daily Lysodren Therapy. Most dogs with PDH respond to Lysodren within 5 to 16 days. Some dogs respond as quickly as 2 or 3 days, and a few have required more than 60 consecutive days of therapy. The average time for response, however, is 7.7 days. More than 85 per cent of our patients respond in the 5- to 16-day period. It is important to emphasize that each dog must be treated as an individual. There appears to be no reliable method of predicting the length of time a dog will need to respond or the amount of Lysodren necessary to destroy enough of the adrenal cortex for response to be seen.[17]

Concomitant Glucocorticoid Therapy. Some authors have recommended administering glucocorticoids and o,p'-DDD together during the initial phase of therapy.[20, 90] This approach is not recommended here for several reasons. Close communication between veterinarian and client, plus an understanding of when to discontinue medication, has been quite successful. If a dog receives glucocorticoids, it is impossible to know clinically if and when one has administered an adequate amount of o,p'-DDD. Because the end point cannot be seen clinically, one must rely on the ACTH stimulation test. However, in order to perform this test, all glucocorticoid therapy must be withdrawn for two or three days.[20] If glucocorticoids are needed because of Lysodren overdosage, a crisis may develop after their withdrawal. It seems easier to determine if glucocorticoid therapy is needed during treatment. This need has occurred in only five per cent of our patients. If so, one

can be certain that the end point in therapy has been achieved. An ACTH response test may be performed immediately and the dog then placed on glucocorticoids. However, dramatic improvement in an ill dog given glucocorticoid medication would also be diagnostic of surpassing the desired end point of therapy.[17]

If anorexia, vomiting, diarrhea, or listlessness develops, glucocorticoid therapy is warranted. This is true during the initial phase of therapy as well as during the maintenance phase. The same is true if the well-controlled dog undergoes any major stress (e.g., illness, trauma, or elective surgery). Prednisone is administered at 1.0 mg/lb/day (2.2 mg/kg/day) for two days. If signs have developed as a result of o,p'-DDD overdosage, the dog will usually show clinical improvement within one or two hours of initiating prednisone therapy. If oral therapy is not possible because of vomiting, parenteral fluids and glucocorticoids are warranted.

After two days of oral therapy at the high dosage, the prednisone dosage is lowered to 0.5 mg/lb/day (1.0 mg/kg/day) for two days, then to 0.22 mg/lb/day (0.5 mg/kg/day) for three days, and finally to 0.22 mg/lb/day (0.5 mg/kg/day) every other day for one week; the medication is then stopped. Recurrence of signs demands reinstitution of therapy or raising the dosage.

Need for Both Glucocorticoids and Mineralocorticoids. Although o,p'-DDD is reported to spare the zona glomerulosa,[91] and therefore mineralocorticoid secretion, cases of complete adrenocortical failure have rarely developed. Dogs that develop weakness, anorexia, and/or vomiting without electrolyte imbalance require immediate glucocorticoid therapy. Electrolyte disturbances suggestive of deficient mineralocorticoids (elevated serum potassium and/or decreased sodium levels) have been produced iatrogenically with o,p'-DDD; these dogs require both glucocorticoid and mineralocorticoid therapy. However, this finding is extremely rare (seen in one of our closely monitored 256 dogs treated with o,p'-DDD).

Time Sequence for Improvement in Signs. Dogs with PDH treated with o,p'-DDD usually respond within 5 to 16 days. The most obvious and rapid response is the reduction in water intake, urine output, appetite, and activity. These signs usually improve within the initial 5- to 16-day period. Other signs take longer to dissipate. Muscle strength improves within one to two months, as does a reduction in the potbellied appearance.

Alopecia, thin skin, acne, bruisability, calcinosis cutis, and panting often take three to six months before significant improvement is noted. Dogs with hair coat abnormalities may go through a phase of severe seborrhea associated with a terrible hair coat or worsening alopecia and pruritus, which may last for one or two months, before the hair coat shows significant improvement. Some dogs go through a phase of "puppy hair coat" before the normal adult coat returns (Figure 97–21). A few dogs have dramatic changes in coat color after successful therapy (Figure 97–22).

The external appearance of a dog with Cushing's syndrome improves with therapy before internal changes are noted. The liver enzymes and cholesterol may take 6 to 18 months to improve. Similar time periods are needed for return of normal blood pressure. Urinary tract infections clear within weeks to months, and females may begin an estrous cycle within one or two months of beginning successful treatment.

Failure to Respond to o,p'-DDD. It is uncommon for o,p'-DDD to fail to help a dog with PDH. The drug is quite potent, and its effect on destroying the zona fasciculata and zona reticularis is consistent. There are several reasons for apparent treatment failures: (1) adrenocortical tumors (adenomas or carcinomas) are relatively resistant to the cytotoxic effects of o,p'-DDD, (2) the drug itself may not be potent, and replacing the owner's tablets with o,p'-DDD obtained from a new or different bottle may solve an apparent treatment failure, (3) dogs may fail to absorb the drug from the intestines, (4) one often begins to worry about a treatment failure after 14 to 21 days without response, but a small percentage of dogs do require 30 to 60 consecutive days of therapy or they require 45 to 70 mg/lb/day (100 to 150 mg/kg/day) rather than the usual initial dosage of 22 mg/lb/day (50 mg/kg/day), (5) dogs that are diagnosed incorrectly will fail to respond: incorrect diagnoses include dogs with any illness that may mimic hyperadrenocorticism (see Table 97–4), and (6) the dog may have iatrogenic Cushing's syndrome.

The various causes of an apparent treatment failure must be considered before abandoning the use of o,p'-DDD. However, if treatment failure has occurred, either ketoconazole therapy or bilateral adrenalectomy should be considered. Various other medical therapies can be used. Each is described later in this section.

Concurrent Diabetes Mellitus and PDH. Approximately ten per cent of dogs with CCS also have diabetes mellitus (i.e., persistent fasting hyperglycemia and glycosuria). It has been suggested that these dogs be treated with a lower dose of o,p'-DDD (12 to 17 mg/lb/day or 25 to 35 mg/kg/day) and oral glucocorticoids.[43] We have used this method of therapy and not found it to be satisfactory. Our dogs with both diabetes mellitus and PDH are treated in the same manner as the other dogs with PDH (o,p'-DDD at 22 mg/lb/day or 50 mg/kg/day and no glucocorticoids). However, it is recognized that the hyperadrenocorticism does result in insulin antagonism in many dogs. Therefore, successful reduction in the circulating cortisol concentrations should reduce the dog's insulin requirement. Failure to recognize this alteration could result in hypoglycemic reactions.

The treatment of the diabetic dog with CCS does require more work by the owner. These dogs are often receiving more than 1 unit of insulin/lb/day (2.2 units of insulin/kg/day). The complicated nature of the disease and its therapy are explained to the owner. In addition, owners are asked to obtain a urine sample from their pet at least three times daily. Each sample is checked for glucose. Any sample found to be negative for glucose requires that the owner reduce subsequent insulin dose by 10 to 20 per cent. The hyperadrenocorticism in most of these dogs is controlled in the expected 5 to 16 days. The ACTH stimulation test is rechecked after each five days of therapy to avoid unnecessary treatment or dangerous overdosage. On average most dogs respond to one or two five-day cycles of daily treatment. Approximately one third of the dogs in our series require no insulin after successful therapy. An additional one third require significantly less insulin and have better control of the diabetes mellitus after o,p'-DDD therapy. The insulin requirement in the remaining dogs is minimally reduced by control of the PDH.

If a dog is found to have diabetes mellitus and thought to have hyperadrenocorticism, one must treat both disorders. While completing the diagnostic evaluation for hyperadrenocorticism and awaiting test results, insulin therapy should be initiated. Most of these dogs require large doses of insulin. An attempt is not made to achieve perfect control: rather, a dosage of insulin adequate to prevent ketoacidosis is advised (0.22 U/lb [0.5 U/kg] of NPH insulin q12h is a conservative initial dosage). Attempts at extremely good control of the diabetes are less important than is treatment of the hyperadrenocorticism.[17]

Maintenance Therapy

o,p'-DDD. Once the initial daily protocol with o,p'-DDD completes adequate destruction of the adrenal cortex, as determined by clinical signs, reduced water intake, and/or ACTH stimulation test results, maintenance therapy should begin. In dogs with PDH, o,p'-DDD has not affected the abnormal pituitary. Therefore, excessive ACTH secretion continues or becomes exaggerated.[94] Failure to continue o,p'-DDD therapy will result in regrowth of the adrenal cortices and return

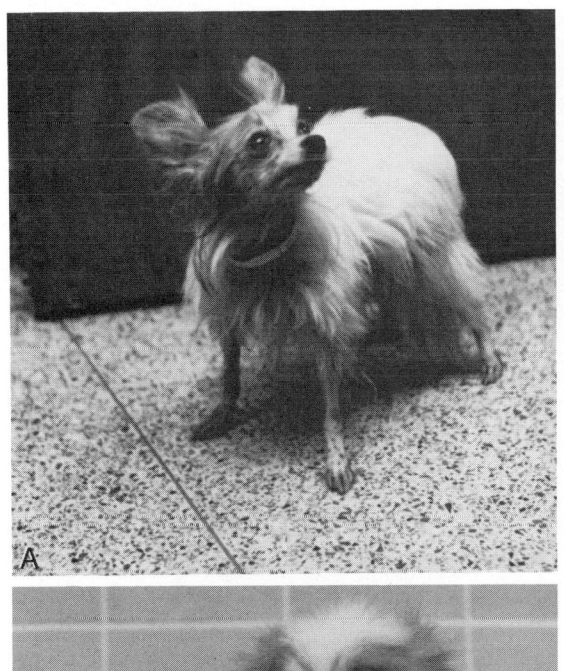
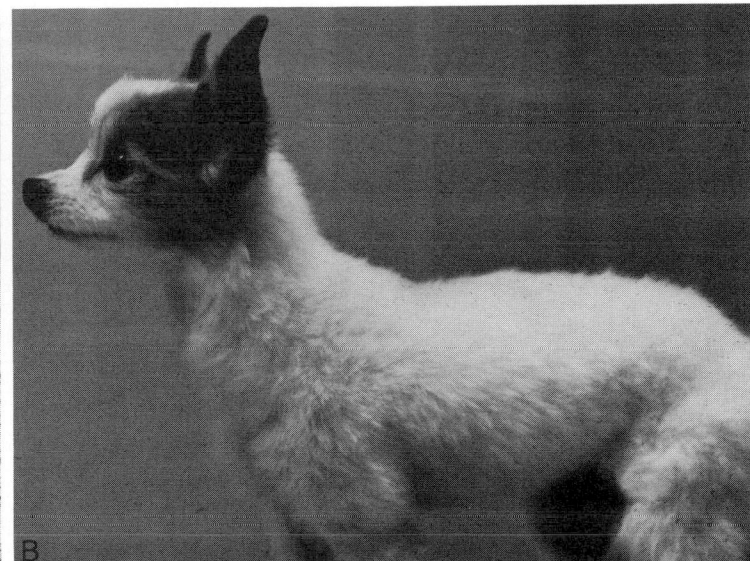
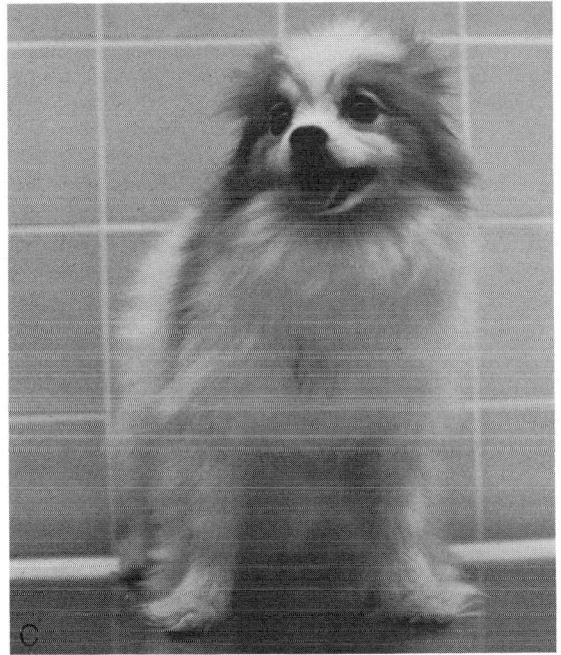

FIGURE 97-21. Photographs of a Papillon with pituitary-dependent hyperadrenocorticism before therapy (A); six weeks after initial o,p'-DDD therapy, which resulted in appearance of a new, puppy-like hair coat (B); and ten weeks later, with a good adult coat (C).

of clinical signs. This exacerbation of the disease usually occurs within 6 to 24 months of stopping therapy.

Maintenance therapy involves choosing a regimen and altering that regimen as required by the patient. Dogs that respond to daily o,p'-DDD therapy within ten days are classified as "sensitive" and begin a maintenance schedule of 12 mg/lb (25 mg/kg) of o,p'-DDD every seven days. Those that initially require more than ten days of therapy are classified as "resistant" and receive 22 mg/lb (50 mg/kg) every seven days. An ACTH response test is performed one and three months after beginning the maintenance therapy. If the plasma cortisol concentration begins to rise after ACTH administration, the o,p'-DDD dosage is increased. Some dogs remain stable for months or years on conservative dosages, whereas others receive o,p'-DDD every two or three days. Return of clinical signs suggestive of hyperadrenocorticism should be managed by performing an

ACTH stimulation test to confirm disease exacerbation, followed by raising the dose of o,p'-DDD. Obvious recurrence of hyperadrenocorticism should be treated with daily o,p'-DDD therapy as initially suggested, whereas any dog with returning signs should also at least be assessed for other diseases, such as renal disease and diabetes mellitus (see Table 97–4).

Overdosage. If the dog becomes weak, anorectic, or lethargic or develops vomiting and/or diarrhea, it may have been overdosed. The easiest method of confirming the diagnosis is to give the dog 5 to 10 mg of prednisone. Clinical improvement in one to three hours confirms that an overdosage of o,p'-DDD has occurred. As long as the dog needs prednisone (usually only one to four weeks), o,p'-DDD is withheld. When prednisone is discontinued, o,p'-DDD should again be given, but at a lower dosage.

Central Nervous System Signs. Rarely, the dog

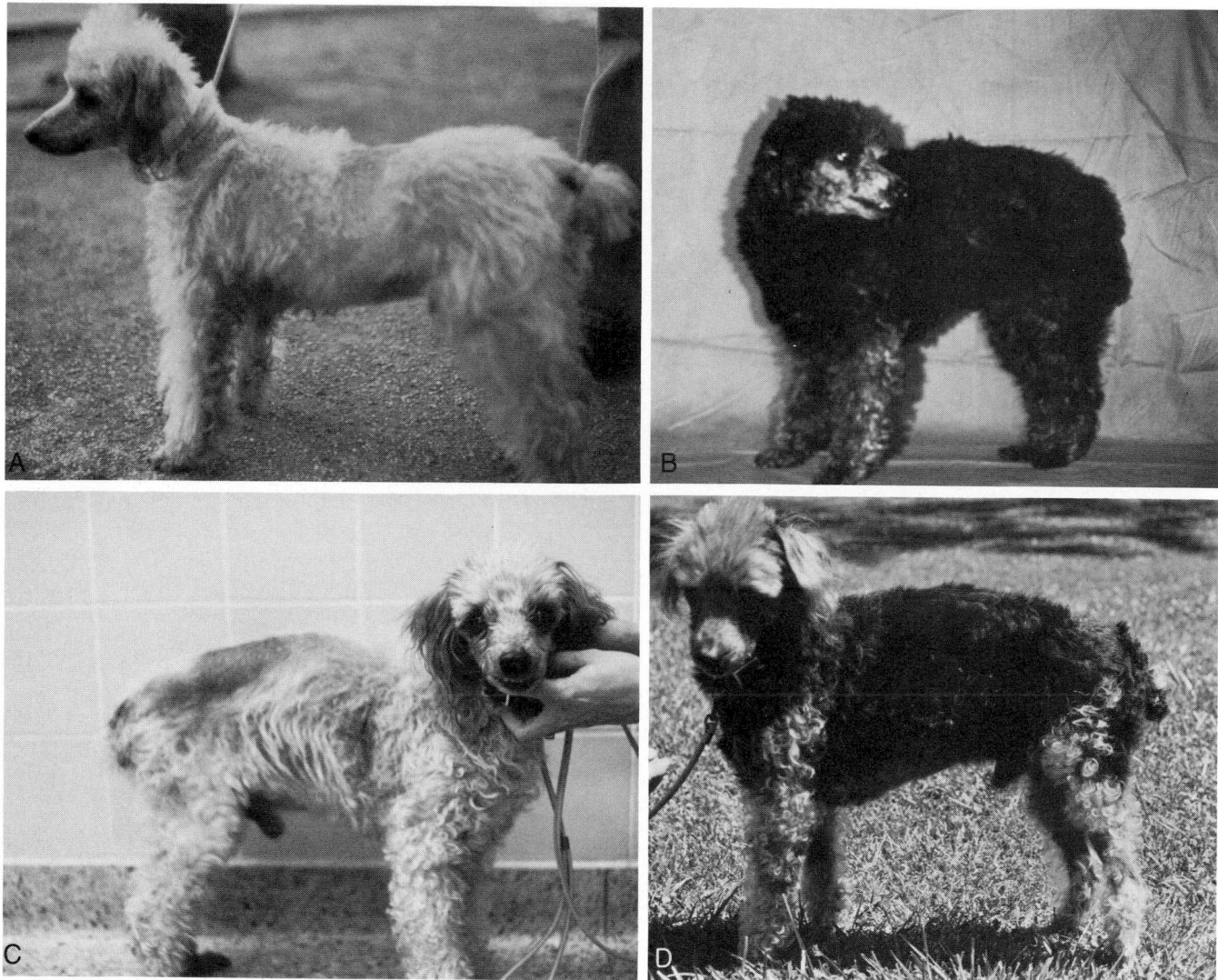

FIGURE 97–22. Photographs of a poodle with pituitary-dependent hyperadrenocorticism before therapy *(A);* two months after o,p′-DDD therapy, showing dramatic hair coat color change *(B);* after a relapse four years later *(C);* and after reinstitution of o,p′-DDD therapy *(D).*

treated with o,p′-DDD develops central nervous system signs induced by the drug. These signs include apparent blindness, ataxia, dull appearance, unawareness of surroundings, circling, walking aimlessly, and head pressing. Another cause for these signs is the presence of a growing pituitary tumor. The drug-induced syndrome is transient, lasting for 12 to 48 hours after each drug administration, versus the more persistent signs associated with a mass lesion. The drug-induced signs occur after 3 to 24 months of therapy and are treated by lowering the dosage or by distributing the dosage in smaller increments given more frequently.

Recommended Rechecks. Many dogs treated with o,p′-DDD remain quite stable on maintenance treatment. It is recommended that these dogs be rechecked with an examination and an ACTH response test every three or four months. Test results allow the veterinarian to adjust maintenance dosages if subclinical problems are occurring. Whenever the post-ACTH plasma cortisol concentration exceeds 5 μg/dl, the dose of o,p′-DDD

should be increased. Whenever listlessness and anorexia are associated with low plasma cortisol results, the o,p′-DDD dose should be reduced.

Stress. Dogs receiving o,p′-DDD that are undergoing any stress (illness, trauma, elective surgery) should be treated with glucocorticoids. Adequately treated dogs with PDH have sufficient adrenal reserve for day-to-day living, but not enough to handle major stresses.

Prognosis. PDH is a serious disorder. We have been able to closely monitor 256 treated dogs. Of the dogs that have died, the life expectancy averaged 23.4 months. These included dogs that lived only 18 days and several that lived longer than seven years. It appears that good owner observation improves the prognosis.

RELAPSES. Relapses were common. Forty-two per cent of the dogs had at least one period in which signs of hyperadrenocorticism recurred, requiring a brief repeat of daily o,p′-DDD therapy or an increase in the maintenance dosage. Forty-five per cent of the dogs that died had a problem that could have been or was related to the hyperadrenocorticism (e.g., thromboembolism, congestive heart failure, infection, pancreatitis, diabetic ketoacidosis, or growing pituitary tumor).

o,p'-DDD OVERDOSAGE. Episodes of o,p'-DDD overdosage were also common. Five per cent of the dogs were mildly overdosed during the induction phase of therapy. A total of 31 per cent were overdosed at some time during therapy. Death from overdosage was seen in 3 per cent of the dogs.

As can be surmised, hyperadrenocorticism is a serious illness that requires conscientious owners and careful veterinary control if a good response to treatment is desired.[17]

ALTERNATIVE CHEMOTHERAPIES

Alternative drugs used in chemotherapy include cyproheptadine, bromocriptine, trilostane, aminoglutethimide, metyrapone, and ketoconazole.

Cyproheptadine. Increased CNS serotonin concentrations are associated with pituitary-adrenal secretory activity. Therefore, the antiserotoninergic agent cyproheptadine may block the stimulatory effects of serotonin or directly inhibit ACTH secretion. It has been used in treating humans and dogs with PDH.[95] Success has been variable.[96]

Ten dogs with PDH were given 0.14 to 1.4 mg/lb (0.3 to 3.0 mg/kg) of cyproheptadine daily for 4 to 27 weeks. All the dogs became polyphagic, indicating a biologic effect caused by the drug. Eight of the ten dogs failed to improve or became worse clinically and biochemically. One dog demonstrated partial improvement, and one had a complete remission.[97] This low rate of success has discouraged most veterinarians from pursuing the use of cyproheptadine for the treatment of PDH. It is likely that a small percentage of the dogs with PDH have a serotonin-mediated disease, and cyproheptadine represents one reasonable mode of therapy. Currently, however, it is not possible to distinguish this population of dogs from the larger group.

Bromocriptine. Bromocriptine, a dopamine agonist, lowers plasma ACTH concentrations and produces remissions in some humans with pituitary-dependent Cushing's disease.[98] Dopamine is a precursor for norepinephrine, a neurotransmitter that indirectly inhibits ACTH secretion. Bromocriptine may enhance the norepinephrine inhibition of ACTH secretion; alternatively, the drug may directly affect the pituitary to decrease ACTH secretion.

The effect of bromocriptine treatment was studied in seven dogs with pituitary-dependent Cushing's disease. The drug was given orally in slowly increasing amounts up to 0.05 mg/lb/day (0.1 mg/kg/day) in divided doses. Side effects were common and included vomiting, anorexia, depression, and behavior changes; treatment was discontinued after one to two weeks in three of these dogs because of severe side effects. The remaining four dogs were treated from two to seven months. Three of these dogs failed to improve clinically, and dexamethasone suppression tests remained abnormal. One dog had a clinical remission after nine weeks of bromocriptine

therapy, and cortisol concentrations were suppressed normally with low-dose dexamethasone.[99]

Bromocriptine appears to have limited usefulness in the management of canine pituitary-dependent Cushing's disease. The drug can induce remission in some of the dogs, but the need for daily administration to maintain remission, frequent relapses, and infrequent successes are problems associated with use of this drug.[16]

Trilostane. Trilostane, a nonproprietary drug, is nonestrogenic, nonprogestational, nonandrogenic, and devoid of glucocorticoid and mineralocorticoid activity. The drug is proposed to act specifically by inhibiting the 3-β-hydroxysteroid dehydrogenase enzyme system. It is reported to reduce elevated corticosteroid levels without producing adrenal insufficiency.[100, 101] The action of trilostane is reversible upon withdrawing medication. In blocking the conversion of pregnenolone to progesterone, trilostane's reduction in corticosteroid output is associated with an increase in biologically inactive pregnenolones.

Early clinical studies of tolerance and efficacy in humans revealed side effects that were largely minor and completely reversible. These side effects included lacrimation, headache, nausea, vomiting, diarrhea, and abdominal cramps. These adverse effects occurred only when initial dosages of 250 mg four times a day or greater were used. They did not occur when therapy was initiated with lower dosages and gradually increased. The reactions were all quickly and spontaneously reversible on withdrawal of trilostane therapy, and no other medication was required. More importantly, a recent report[102] describes the responses of seven humans with Cushing's syndrome (five patients with PDH, two with ATH) to trilostane. There was no consistent fall in serum cortisol levels. In addition, there was no rise in the levels of precursors immediately preceding the proposed site of action of trilostane. These results suggest that trilostane does not effectively block the enzyme 3-β hydroxysteroid dehydrogenase delta-4, delta-5 isomerase in patients with Cushing's syndrome. The report stated that trilostane should no longer be recommended for the treatment of these patients.

This drug has not yet been used in dogs with hyperadrenocorticism.

Aminoglutethimide. Aminoglutethimide was first released in the United States in 1960 as an anticonvulsant but was withdrawn from the market because it caused adrenal insufficiency and hypothyroidism. The drug is now being marketed again, this time for treatment of human patients with Cushing's syndrome.

Aminoglutethimide blocks conversion of cholesterol to δ-5-pregnenolone in the adrenal cortex, inhibiting the synthesis of glucocorticoids, mineralocorticoids, and other steroids. It also blocks the peripheral conversion of androstenedione to estrone.[103]

Aminoglutethimide has been used in a limited number of human patients with Cushing's syndrome, sometimes only to suppress adrenal function preoperatively, but also as medical therapy, either alone or as an adjunct to surgery or irradiation. A retrospective survey of 66 patients with Cushing's syndrome treated with aminoglutethimide suggests that it has been most helpful when given after pituitary irradiation.[104] Only a few patients have been treated with the drug for longer than two years.[105]

This drug has not been used in the dog, and therefore cannot be recommended.

Metyrapone. Metyrapone reduces cortisol production by inhibition of adrenal 11-β-hydroxylase. Although approved only for use in diagnostic testing of pituitary responsiveness to lowering plasma cortisol concentrations in humans, this drug has also been used effectively for long-term control of Cushing's syndrome.[106]

This drug has not been used in treating dogs and its use cannot be recommended (see discrimination test section of this chapter).

Ketoconazole. Ketoconazole (Nizoral), an imidazole derivative, is an orally active antifungal agent. Its antifungal activity is linked to the inhibition of ergosterol synthesis and to interference with other membrane lipids. Ketoconazole has shown efficacy in the treatment of deep mycotic infections in humans and animals and in managing systemic candidal infections and superficial dermatophytosis in humans. In addition to its antifungal activity, ketoconazole has been shown to interfere with gonadal and adrenal[107] steroid synthesis both in vitro and in vivo. This information has led to the suggestion that ketoconazole administration might be of value in the treatment of conditions such as Cushing's syndrome.[17]

The effects of a single daily oral dose of ketoconazole (4.5 to 6 mg/lb or 9.7 to 13.4 mg/kg) were demonstrated in four male beagle dogs. Plasma testosterone concentrations fell markedly within three to four hours and then progressively returned to normal by ten hours. Cortisol levels were not significantly affected. In another study four male dogs were given 4.5 mg/lb (10 mg/kg) of ketoconazole three times a day for five consecutive days. After the five days of treatment, there was a lowering of serum testosterone and cortisol concentrations and cortisol response to exogenous ACTH. Progesterone and 17-hydroxyprogesterone concentrations dramatically increased. No effect on aldosterone concentration was detected. All values returned to normal when rechecked three weeks after stopping therapy.[108] These same investigators reported similar results in dogs given 14 mg/lb (30 mg/kg) of ketoconazole once daily for 64 consecutive days.[109]

We have evaluated the use of this drug in 15 dogs with spontaneous hyperadrenocorticism, including 11 dogs with pituitary-dependent disease as well as four dogs with adrenocortical tumors. They have undergone treatment with ketoconazole at 14 mg/lb (30 mg/kg) once daily or divided into two daily doses. All animals have shown a rapid reduction in serum cortisol concentration and cortisol responsiveness to ACTH. Plasma testosterone concentrations fell markedly with variable changes in plasma concentrations of estrogen and progesterone. In the animals treated for more than two months, there has been significant improvement in their clinical condition as evidenced by a reduction in water intake, urine production, appetite, and weight. Regrowth of hair is occurring and no signs of toxicity have developed.

Ketoconazole, with its low incidence of toxicity, reversible inhibition of adrenal steroidogenesis, and negligible effects on mineralocorticoid production, promises to be an attractive (albeit expensive) alternative in the management of canine hyperadrenocorticism. Ketoconazole may also be useful in two other circumstances: first, in the medical management of those dogs with malignant adrenal tumors for which surgical intervention is not an option, but palliative therapy is desired; and second, in the preoperative stabilization of the surgical patient by providing a rapid decline in the hypercortisolemic state.[17]

TREATMENT OF LARGE PITUITARY TUMORS

As previously described, approximately five to ten per cent of dogs with PDH have clinical signs caused by a growing pituitary tumor that expands dorsally into the hypothalamus. A small number of dogs are initially evaluated because these are the initial signs noted by the owner. In our series most of the dogs with these problems have already been diagnosed and treated for PDH.

The most common signs associated with large pituitary tumors include mental dullness, inappetence, lethargy, and apparent disorientation. Owners have also reported that their pets pace aimlessly, appear blind, are ataxic, head press, circle, are "trapped" in the corner of a room, develop Horner's syndrome, urinate or defecate in the home, or convulse. The least common signs include aggressive, nasty behavior and loss of thermoregulatory capability with wide fluctuations in body temperature, or coma.[17]

The diagnosis is difficult to confirm and is initially made by ruling out other causes for CNS disturbances. The diagnosis can be confirmed with the CT scan.

Limited Modes of Therapy. Some success has been obtained with the use of cobalt irradiation. Cobalt irradiation has successfully reduced tumor size and caused a reduction in or elimination of the CNS signs in several of our dogs and in those in a recent report.[110] However, reduction of the secretory nature of the pituitary tumors is variable, and secretion may even increase despite a confirmed reduction in tumor size. The primary differential diagnosis for the presence of a large pituitary tumor includes the drug-induced neurologic signs occasionally caused by o,p'-DDD therapy (see section on Maintenance Therapy).

Spontaneous Remission of Cushing's Syndrome

Spontaneous remission of Cushing's syndrome is a documented phenomenon in humans.[111] It is possible for CCS to undergo spontaneous remission as well. We have had two dogs with a history and physical examination consistent with CCS. In both cases the owner believed that the pet might be improving after 14 and 24 months of signs, respectively. The in-hospital evaluation was diagnostic of PDH in each dog, but therapy was withheld, owing to the owners' impressions. Reevaluations of each dog over a three-month period revealed a progressive return to normal in all parameters. Both dogs are alive and well. It has been hypothesized that these dogs embolized their pituitary microadenomas, resulting in return of a normal endocrine state.

FELINE CUSHING'S SYNDROME

Feline Cushing's syndrome resembles the canine disorder in many respects.[112-115] Therefore, a complete description of the endocrinopathy will not be presented here. The nine cats with hyperadrenocorticism we have seen over the past seven years are reviewed. In this same time span we have evaluated more than 300 dogs with Cushing's syndrome, illustrating the relative frequency of diagnoses in the two species.[17]

Signalment

Cats with Cushing's syndrome were middle-aged or older (average, 10.4 years). Five of the nine cats were female, five were of the domestic short-hair breed, and eight had concurrent diabetes mellitus.

History and Physical Examination

The significant problems cited by the owners are tabulated in Table 97–5. Eight of the nine cats were polydipsic, polyuric, and polyphagic; four had apparent weight gain and/or alopecia; and three were depressed. On physical examination eight of nine cats had an enlarged abdomen, six had an unkempt and abnormal hair coat, four had muscle wasting and/or hepatomegaly, and three had alopecia. All of these clinical signs are typical of hyperadrenocorticism in the dog, and many of these findings are also consistent with several of the differential diagnoses cited in Table 97–4.

TABLE 97–5. HISTORY AND PHYSICAL EXAMINATION FINDINGS IN 9 CATS WITH HYPERADRENOCORTICISM

	Number of Cats
History	
Polydipsia/polyuria	8
Polyphagia	8
Alopecia	4
Weight gain	4
Depression	3
Poor hair coat	2
Respiratory infection	1
Skin infection	1
Weight loss	1
Diarrhea	1
Physical Examination	
Potbellied appearance	8
Unkempt (rough) hair coat	6
Muscle wasting	4
Hepatomegaly	4
Alopecia	3
Easy bruisability	3
Skin abscess	2
Pruritus	1

In-Hospital Evaluation

CBC, Urinalysis, Chemistry Profile. The CBC from cats with hyperadrenocorticism was not contributory to the final diagnosis. The red and white blood cell counts were consistently within normal limits. Four of the eight cats tested had circulating eosinophils, and six of eight had normal lymphocyte counts.

The urinalysis was not always consistent with the clinical history of polyuria. Six of the eight cats with Cushing's syndrome had urine specific gravities greater than 1.020 in randomly obtained specimens. However, seven of the cats had diabetes mellitus, and six of those had glycosuria. The urine specific gravity in most dogs with hyperadrenocorticism is below 1.020, and in many is below 1.010 on random testing. Only 10 per cent of dogs with Cushing's syndrome have glycosuria.

The only consistent abnormalities on the serum chemistry profile were elevations in the blood glucose concentration and serum cholesterol. The typical low BUN, dramatic elevation in alkaline phosphatase, and mild increase in ALT (SGPT) seen in the dog were not found in hyperadrenal cats.

Radiography. Radiographically, six of seven cats had hepatomegaly and three were felt to have a pendulous abdomen. No other radiographic abnormalities were common.

Serial Blood Glucose Studies. Five cats had multiple blood glucose concentrations evaluated throughout a time period after insulin administration. Three cats had elevated blood glucose concentrations throughout the testing period. These results were suggestive of insulin resistance. Two of these three cats were receiving large doses of insulin. Two cats became hypoglycemic after receiving a large dose (one cat) or low dose (one cat) of insulin. It would appear that significant insulin antagonism occurs in some diabetic cats with hyperadrenocorticism, but not all.

ACTH Stimulation Test. All pre-ACTH administration plasma cortisol samples were obtained between 8 AM and 10 AM. Each cat then received one-half vial (0.125 mg) of synthetic ACTH IM, and the plasma cortisol was assessed 15, 30, and 60 minutes later. The mean baseline plasma cortisol concentration in 19 healthy control cats was 1.8 µg/dl, varying between 0.5 and 4.4 µg/dl. The mean post-ACTH plasma cortisol concentration was 10.1 µg/dl at 30 minutes. Plasma cortisol concentrations had declined by 60 minutes.[116] The results in stable diabetic cats were similar (average baseline concentration, 1.8 µg/dl; average post-stimulation concentration, 10.6 µg/dl) at 30 minutes. Using our plasma cortisol assay, a post-cortisol level ≥ 15.0 µg/dl was suggestive of hyperadrenocorticism, and one between 13 and 15 µg/dl was borderline.[116]

Eight hyperadrenal cats had undergone at least one ACTH response test, and six of eight cats had at least one abnormal test, suggesting hyperadrenocorticism. Eight of the 14 total test results were consistent with Cushing's syndrome, 3 were borderline, and 3 were normal. This test is of diagnostic value as a screening test for hyperadrenocorticism in cats as well as in dogs. The one cat with an adrenocortical tumor had an abnormal test result that was not significantly different from the cats with PDH.

Dexamethasone Screening Test. The dexamethasone screening test (0.005 mg/lb or 0.01 mg/kg, IV dexamethasone; determination of plasma cortisol concentration before and eight hours after administration) was obtained in four cats with PDH. Using the normal values established on cats in one study[116] (post-dexamethasone plasma cortisol concentration ≤ 1.0 μg/dl), three of four cats had an abnormal result.

Endogenous Plasma ACTH. This test is used in the dog as a discriminatory tool. The endogenous ACTH test should aid in separating animals with PDH from those with functioning adrenocortical tumors. Using canine and human values, a result > 40 pg/ml is consistent with PDH, and one < 20 pg/ml is consistent with an adrenocortical tumor (normal, 20 to 100 pg/ml). In the five cats treated, the results were correct for the final diagnosis. The cat with an adrenal tumor had a low endogenous plasma ACTH concentration, and the four cats with PDH had ACTH values of 66, 90, 361, and 487 pg/ml, respectively. However, several normal cats have had endogenous ACTH concentrations < 20 pg/ml.[116]

Therapy

Adrenal Tumor. One cat with an adrenocortical tumor was not treated and was diagnosed at necropsy. A celiotomy was performed on another. An adrenocortical adenoma was successfully removed, and the cat lived approximately 14 months. The cat was in excellent condition after surgery. Within two months its problems were resolving. It no longer required insulin, and the various signs attributed to hyperadrenocorticism had progressively dissipated. The cat died at 12 years of age after being hit by a car.

PDH. NO TREATMENT. Three of the seven cats with PDH were not treated. These three cats were necropsied and the diagnosis was confirmed in each.

O,P'-DDD. Only one cat was treated with this adrenocorticolytic agent. It was treated for 14 consecutive days at a dosage of 12 mg/lb/day (25 mg/kg/day) and an additional 45 consecutive days at 22 mg/lb/day (50 mg/kg/day). The drug appeared to have absolutely no effect on the cat. The cat's physical condition and clinical signs became more consistent with PDH during the treatment period. The ACTH response test was monitored at ten-day intervals, without any change noted.

METYRAPONE. One cat was treated with this agent. Metyrapone is an enzyme inhibitor that blocks adrenal synthesis of glucocorticoids. The cat was treated with 65 mg three times a day orally for six months. The drug was tolerated and the cat reportedly improved slightly. Unfortunately, this cat was then lost to follow-up.

KETACONAZOLE. From initial studies with this drug, cats may be resistant, in contrast to the sensitive nature of dogs to ketaconazole.[109] Two cats with Cushing's disease have been treated. One had an excellent response for six months and the other developed thrombocytopenia and died seven days after beginning medication. The dose used in both cats was 5 mg/lb (10 mg/kg) twice daily.

BILATERAL ADRENALECTOMY. Bilateral adrenalec-tomy was performed on two cats. Both cats had adrenocortical hyperplasia. The cats survived the surgery. One was steadily improving for two months when acute signs of circling, wandering aimlessly, and apparent blindness were observed. The cat was euthanatized but necropsy was not allowed by the owner. An expanding pituitary tumor was suspected. The other steadily improved post-surgically, and it lived for 30 months. It remained a diabetic but was controlled on approximately 1 unit of PZI per day. The cat died of an unrelated problem.

Cobalt Irradiation. The cat that had been treated with o,p'-DDD without response underwent a CT scan. This scan revealed a large pituitary tumor. Cobalt irradiation of the pituitary region, in 12 doses over 4 weeks, was performed. The cat steadily deteriorated, and the cat was euthanatized one month after completion of the irradiation. At that time no clinical improvement had been seen by the owners and no change in the ACTH response test results was noted.

HYPOADRENOCORTISM

The presence of the "superadrenal glands" was well known to early anatomists. However, their importance was not apparent until Thomas Addison (1855) described a clinical syndrome in humans that he associated with dysfunction of these glands. Included in his description were "anemia, general languor, debility, remarkable feebleness of the heart's action and irritability of the stomach." Autopsies revealed either tuberculous destruction or atrophy of the adrenal glands.[5] At that time no therapy was known and patients who developed the disease died. At about the same time that Thomas Addison described the clinical picture of adrenal sufficiency, Brown-Séquard demonstrated that adrenalectomy resulted in death of laboratory animals, thus documenting the necessity of the adrenal glands for maintenance of life.

Seventy-five years later crude lipid extracts from the adrenal cortex were demonstrated to contain substances that maintained the lives of adrenalectomized cats.[117] These extracts were immediately used in humans for the treatment of adrenocortical insufficiency. Unfortunately the extracts were of little help because they were short-acting and contained little cortisol.[5]

The next step in understanding hypoadrenocorticism was documenting both the sodium deficiency of this disease and the beneficial effects of oral or rectal saline solutions as therapy.[118] Synthetic desoxycorticosterone acetate (DOCA) was then shown to be of benefit in the chronic maintenance of patients with adrenal insufficiency.[119] The beneficial effects of salt and desoxycorticosterone administration were related to correction of the electrolyte disturbances and the associated dehydration; although they improved the condition of patients with partial adrenal insufficiency, they were not able to protect hypoadrenal patients from severe stress.

A major advance in the understanding of adrenal insufficiency was the isolation of cortisol and corticosterone from beef and porcine adrenal glands. The isolations were time consuming and expensive, but they demonstrated the importance of these substances in carbohydrate metabolism and maintenance of life, which had not been demonstrated with desoxycorticosterone.[120] Eventually the laboratory synthesis and availability of cortisone and cortisol revolutionized the therapy of hypoadrenocorticism. These substances not only maintained the lives of patients who had undergone adrenalectomy and those with spontaneous adrenal insufficiency, but, in large enough doses, also protected them against stressful situations. Soon, cortisol was isolated from blood and demonstrated to be one of the major secretory products of the adrenal cortex in dogs and humans.[121, 122]

Knowledge of cortisol's structure led quickly to the development of methods to assay concentrations of corticosteroids in blood and urine. Isolation of androgenic substances from adrenal venous blood confirmed that these substances are secreted directly by the adrenal gland.[123] Understanding of adrenal cortical secretions were further advanced with the recognition of a salt-retaining hormone.[124] The three major types of hormones produced by the adrenal cortex were then classified: glucocorticoids—cortisol; mineralocorticoids—aldosterone; and the androgens.

Adrenocortical insufficiency in the dog was initially reported as a clinical entity in 1953.[125] Since then numerous brief accounts have appeared in the veterinary literature, and several small series have also been published.[68, 126–128]

ETIOLOGY

Hypoadrenocorticism is a syndrome that usually results from a deficiency of both glucocorticoid and mineralocorticoid secretion from the adrenal cortices (primary adrenocortical failure). In addition, disease within the hypothalamic-pituitary axis, resulting in reduced secretion of the major tropic hormone, ACTH, can cause atrophy of the adrenal cortices and impaired secretion of glucocorticoids (secondary adrenocortical failure). Isolated hypoaldosteronism is well recognized in humans and is usually due to inadequate secretion of renin by the kidney. Hypoaldosteronism has not yet been described in the dog or cat.

Primary Adrenocortical Failure

Idiopathic adrenal insufficiency is a common diagnosis for patients with adrenal failure because there is no obvious evidence for the cause of the disease and most patients survive, delaying histopathologic evaluation of the glands. A large group of human patients formerly considered to have idiopathic adrenal insufficiency are now known to have had immune-mediated destruction of the glands.[129, 130] With immune-mediated destruction, the glands are usually infiltrated with lymphocytes and plasma cells, and replaced by fibrous tissue. Idiopathic or immune-mediated atrophy of all the layers of the adrenal cortex is the most frequently observed histo-

pathologic lesion in dogs.[25] The pituitary gland is normal in primary immune-mediated adrenocortical atrophy.

Immune-mediated destruction of the adrenal glands in humans is occasionally associated with additional endocrine and related disorders. Since the 1920s hypoadrenocorticism has been found to be associated with thyroid disorders, diabetes mellitus, hypoparathyroidism, primary gonadal failure, pernicious anemia, and vitiligo.[5] The common link has now been shown to be the presence of circulating antibodies directed against these various tissues. In our series of 45 dogs with primary adrenocortical insufficiency, 6 have at least one additional endocrinopathy. Four of these dogs have idiopathic hypothyroidism, one has diabetes mellitus, and one male has partial gonadal failure as evidenced by azoospermia.[17]

Less common causes of canine adrenocortical insufficiency include destruction of the adrenal cortices by granulomatous diseases such as histoplasmosis, blastomycosis, or tuberculosis: hemorrhagic infarctions; metastases of cancer to the adrenal glands; and amyloidosis of the adrenals.[25] Our series includes two dogs with coccidioidomycosis and one with adrenal failure occurring one week after warfarin intoxication. The adrenocorticolytic drug o,p′-DDD inhibits steroid biosynthesis in the dog by destroying the adrenal cortex,[91–93] and thus has the potential for causing primary adrenocortical failure.

Secondary Adrenocortical Failure

Spontaneous. In addition to disease processes that affect the adrenal gland itself, reduced secretion of ACTH by the pituitary gland will result in decreased synthesis and secretion of adrenocortical hormones, especially glucocorticoids.[131, 132] Reduced secretion of CRH by the hypothalamus may also result in secondary adrenocortical failure. Destructive lesions in the pituitary or hypothalamus are usually associated with neoplasia, inflammation, or trauma.

Secondary-Iatrogenic. Adrenal insufficiency secondary to exogenous corticosteroid administration is commonly seen in small animal veterinary practice, although it only rarely results in clinical signs. There is potential for secondary adrenal atrophy in any pet chronically receiving quantities of corticosteroids sufficient to suppress pituitary ACTH secretion. Adrenal atrophy may follow administration of injectable, oral, or topical applications of corticosteroids.[133] Adrenal suppression can occur within a few days of the administration of ACTH-inhibiting doses of corticosteroids. Adrenal function will usually return shortly after discontinuing the hormone, unless long-acting depot forms of glucocorticoids are used.

A wide variety of glucocorticoids are used in veterinary practice. Although estimates of the relative biologic effectiveness of the clinical analogues vary, studies have shown dexamethasone to be 50 to 150 times more potent in suppressing ACTH secretion than is cortisol.[134] Thus very small quantities of dexamethasone may be sufficient to produce adrenal atrophy. The long-acting "depot" injectable corticosteroids, however, are the most potent drugs used in small animal practice for suppressing both the pituitary-adrenal axis and the immune system. One injection of such long-acting agents has been shown to suppress the adrenal glands of dogs for as long as five weeks.[135, 136]

PATHOPHYSIOLOGY

Mineralocorticoids

Mineralocorticoids, primarily aldosterone, are synthesized and secreted from the zona glomerulosa of the adrenal cortex. Mineralocorticoids function to control sodium, potassium, and water homeostasis. They promote sodium, chloride, and water reabsorption as well as potassium excretion in many epithelial tissues, including the intestinal mucosa, salivary glands, sweat glands, and kidneys. Aldosterone's main site of action is the renal tubule, where it promotes proximal convoluted renal tubular absorption of sodium and chloride and distal convoluted renal tubular absorption of sodium by exchange with potassium.[5]

Secretion of aldosterone is primarily influenced by the renin-angiotensin system and by plasma potassium concentrations. The renin-angiotensin system is governed, in part, by the renal juxtaglomerular apparatus. Volume depletion caused by such events as hemorrhage, diuretic administration, or salt restriction is perceived by the juxtaglomerular cells as a decreased "stretch." These cells then release an increased quantity of renin. Renin, in turn, acts on a plasma α_2-globulin produced by the liver, releasing the decapeptide angiotensin I. Converting enzyme in the lung splits off two amino acids from angiotensin I, producing angiotensin II, which is a potent vasoconstrictor and a primary stimulant for aldosterone secretion. The increased plasma aldosterone concentration will cause increased sodium retention, expansion of the extracellular fluid volume, increased renal perfusion, and damping of the initiating signal for renin release (Figure 97–23).[1, 137]

Aldosterone secretion can be regulated independent of the renin-angiotensin system as a function of plasma potassium concentrations. When a solution of potassium ions is injected into adrenal arteries, there is an immediate increase in adrenal venous aldosterone concentration.[138] Potassium appears to have a direct stimulatory effect on the adrenocortical production of aldosterone, presumably through a transmembrane effect.[139] This potassium-mediated aldosterone control system operates in parallel with the renin-angiotensin system and can be of comparable potency.

ACTH can stimulate the release of aldosterone but is not the dominant driving force in secretion by the zona glomerulosa. Apparently ACTH is not an important control mechanism in most physiologic conditions, but exerts a "permissive" influence over aldosterone secretion.[137]

With adrenocortical insufficiency, lack of aldosterone secretion results in impaired ability to conserve sodium and excrete potassium, leading to hyponatremia and

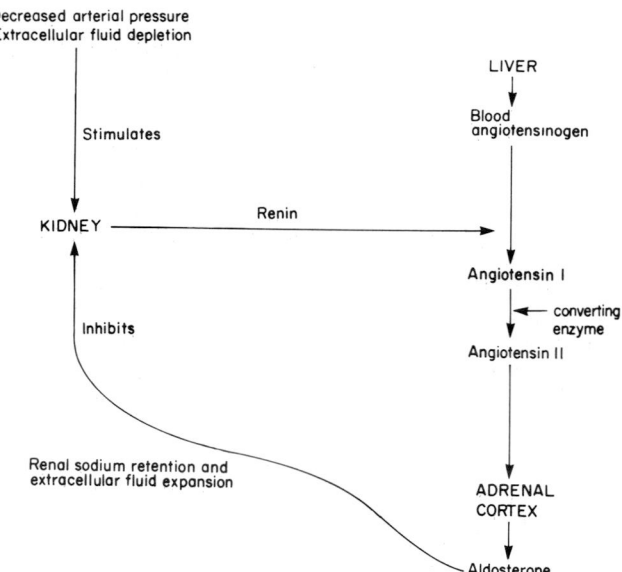

FIGURE 97–23. The renin-angiotensin-aldosterone system.

hyperkalemia. With adequate sodium intake, a mild deficiency of aldosterone may have few, if any, consequences. However, if sodium intake diminishes owing to anorexia or change in diet, or if sodium loss increases because of vomiting and/or diarrhea, the animal's health may quickly deteriorate. Continued loss of sodium through the gastrointestinal tract and kidneys leads to severe depletion of total body sodium stores and the progressive development of hypovolemia, hypotension, reduced cardiac output, and decreased perfusion of the kidneys and other tissues. The decreased glomerular filtration rate causes prerenal azotemia, increased renin production, and mild metabolic acidosis. Weight loss, weakness, microcardia, and depression are common.

Progressively worsening hyperkalemia develops as a result of diminished glomerular filtration and diminished cation exchange by the distal convoluted renal tubules. The most prominent manifestations of hyperkalemia are seen in the heart, where it causes a decrease in myocardial excitability, an increase in the refractory period of the myocardium, and a slowing of conduction. Hypoxia, as a result of hypovolemia and poor tissue perfusion, also contributes to increased myocardial irritability. Ventricular fibrillation or cardiac standstill may eventually occur as the plasma potassium concentration exceeds 10 mEq/L. Mild acidosis develops as a result of impaired ability to reabsorb bicarbonate and chloride ions in the renal tubules, as well as failure to excrete metabolic waste products and hydrogen ions by the poorly perfused kidneys.[140]

Glucocorticoids

Glucocorticoids are synthesized and secreted primarily by the zona fasciculata of the adrenal cortex. Glucocorticoids affect almost every tissue in the body; these effects include stimulation of gluconeogenesis and glycogenesis by the liver and muscle, suppression of peripheral cellular uptake and utilization of plasma glu-

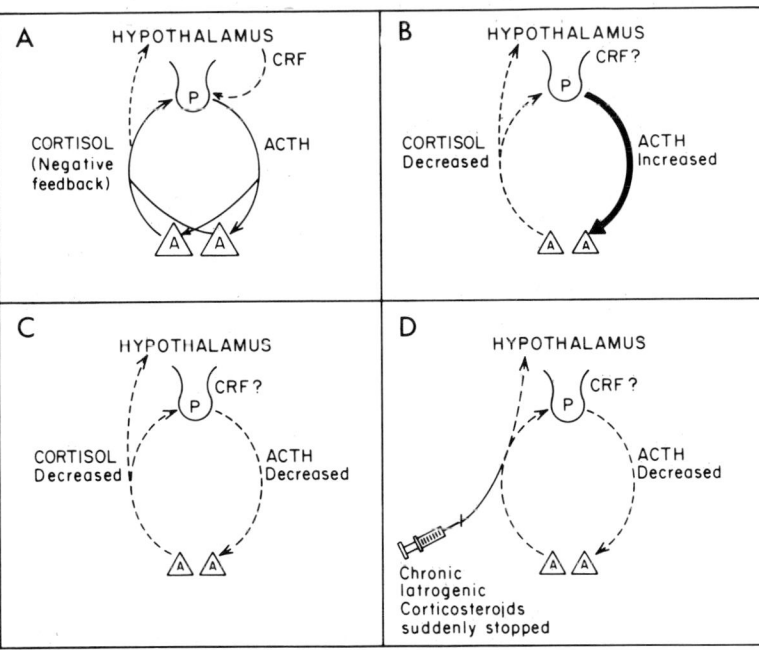

FIGURE 97-24. The pituitary-adrenal axis in normal dogs *(A)*; in dogs with loss of adrenocortical function and excess ACTH secretion owing to a lack of negative feedback (the most common form of hypoadrenocorticism) *(B)*; in dogs with failure to secrete ACTH and secondary atrophy of the adrenal cortex, specifically the zona fasciculata and reticularis *(C)*; and in dogs that are chronically overtreated with exogenous glucocorticoids, causing insufficiency in pituitary ACTH secretion and secondary atrophy of the adrenal cortex *(D)*. A, Adrenal; P, pituitary; CRF, cortico-tropin-releasing factor (hormone). (From Feldman, EC: *In* Ettinger, SJ (ed): Textbook of Veterinary Internal Medicine, 2nd ed. Philadelphia, WB Saunders, 1983, p 1667.)

cose, enhancement of protein and fat catabolism, stimulation of erythrocytosis, suppression of inflammatory responses and lymphoid tissue, maintenance of normal blood pressure, and counteraction of the effects of stress.[1] Secretion of glucocorticoids is controlled, in part, by the hypothalamic-pituitary axis by way of a simple negative-feedback loop (Figure 97-24).

Inadequate glucocorticoid secretion may result from destruction of the adrenal cortex or from dysfunction of the hypothalamus or pituitary gland with insufficient secretion of CRH or ACTH, respectively. Regardless of the underlying cause, lack of cortisol secretion may result in gastrointestinal signs, including anorexia, vomiting, abdominal pain, and weight loss. Mental changes such as diminished vigor and lethargy are also noted. Energy metabolism is diminished owing to impaired gluconeogenesis, impaired fat metabolism and utilization, and depletion of liver glycogen stores. As a result, fasting hypoglycemia may occur. Impaired ability to excrete water free of sodium may result in hyponatremia. With primary adrenal insufficiency, there is an unrestrained secretion of ACTH from the pituitary. One of the hallmark signs of hypocortisolism is impaired tolerance to stress, and clinical signs often become more pronounced when the animal is placed in stressful situations.

In adrenal insufficiency secondary to pituitary or hypothalamic disease, the renin-angiotensin-aldosterone system is preserved; therefore, plasma electrolyte homeostasis is maintained. The same is true in dogs chronically treated with corticosteroids after meditation is acutely discontinued. The exogenously administered corticosteroids inhibit ACTH secretion through negative feedback, resulting in secondary adrenocortical atrophy that spares the zona glomerulosa.[133]

Hypoadrenocorticism produced iatrogenically with the adrenocorticolytic drug o,p'-DDD could produce physiologic changes similar to the natural disease in dogs.

Sex Hormones

The zona reticularis of the adrenal cortex synthesizes and secretes androgens, estrogen-like compounds, and glucocorticoids. The physiologic importance of the sex hormones secreted by the adrenal gland is not clear. Clinical manifestations as a result of impaired secretion of androgens and estrogens are not readily apparent in animals with primary adrenal insufficiency.

Degree of Glandular Destruction

Development of adrenocortical insufficiency is believed to require destruction of at least 90 per cent of the adrenal cortex in people.[141] In most instances destruction of the glands is a gradual process, first leading to a partial deficiency syndrome characterized by inadequate adrenal reserve, with symptoms manifested only during times of stress. Stress may be associated with surgery, trauma, infection, or even psychologic distress, such as when dogs are placed in boarding kennels. However, basal hormone secretion in the unstressed state may be adequate to maintain near-normal plasma electrolyte concentrations and minimal clinical signs. For these dogs the diagnosis can be confirmed only with tests that assess adrenocortical reserve. As destruction of the adrenal glands progresses, hormone secretion becomes inadequate even under nonstressful conditions, and a true metabolic crisis without any obvious inciting event results.

SIGNALMENT

Hypoadrenocorticism is an uncommon endocrine disorder in the dog and is extremely rare in the cat.[25, 45, 130] Data have been accumulated from our initial 47 dogs with spontaneous hypoadrenocorticism and from an additional 76 dogs from one review.[128] Seventy-nine (76 per cent) of these 123 dogs were female. Sex predilection for the female is typical for immune-mediated disorders in the dog[142] and may provide crude but further evidence for an immune-mediated pathogenesis for hypoadrenocorticism. This disorder also appears to be a disease of the young and middle-aged dog. The age range for our series of 39 hypoadrenal dogs was 2 months to 9 years, with a mean of 4.5 years. In a recent review 84 per cent of a series of 37 dogs and 90 per cent of a series of 39 dogs were less than seven years old at the time of diagnosis.[128] No breed predilection has been described, and canine hypoadrenocorticism appears to affect dogs regardless of body size.[17]

HISTORY

Historical owner complaints for dogs with hypoadrenocorticism commonly include anorexia, vomiting, lethargy, depression, and/or weakness (Table 97–6). The signs associated with hypoadrenocorticism are vague and are often suggestive of more common small animal disorders, especially renal, gastrointestinal, and infectious diseases. There are no pathognomonic signs, and each sign can vary in severity from dog to dog. Correlating the signalment, history, and physical examination findings with a suspicion of adrenal insufficiency will allow most practitioners the opportunity to diagnose this condition.

Each of the signs in Table 97–6 can be directly related to a deficiency in glucocorticoid and/or mineralocorticoid secretion. Anorexia, vomiting, lethargy, weakness, loose stools, and abdominal pain can be the result of glucocorticoid deficiency alone. These signs, however, are exaggerated if alterations in the plasma sodium and potassium concentration occur. Weight loss is a sequela of the problems described, and the waxing-waning course is a reflection of the progressive but not absolute deficiency of adrenocortical hormones. Polyuria may be the result of excessive sodium loss into the urine with subsequent renal medullary solute washout. The cause of shivering or shaking in dogs with hypoadrenocorticism is currently believed to be one expression of muscle weakness resulting from depletion of plasma sodium.

One clue in the history of a dog with hypoadrenocor-

TABLE 97–6. CLINICAL SIGNS SEEN IN DOGS WITH HYPERADRENOCORTICISM AND AN ENLARGING PITUITARY TUMOR

Dull behavior, listlessness
Unaware of surroundings
Abandonment of trained behavior
Inappetence
Walking aimlessly
Circling
Ataxia
Apparent or real blindness
Head pressing
Seizures
Aggressive (vicious behavior)
Widely fluctuating body temperature

ticism is the description of a waxing-waning or "episodic" nature of the illness. However, this "classic" alteration was observed in only ten per cent of the dogs described. Thus a waxing-waning course of illness is not obvious to the majority of owners of affected dogs. The period of time that owners observe signs, whether progressive or episodic, is often two weeks or longer. Most dogs that are initially brought to a veterinarian in an acute adrenal crisis have had progressive untreated chronic adrenal or pituitary disease in which mild signs were either not observed or not of concern to the owner. The history from owners whose dogs were brought to the hospital in acute crisis is similar to that provided when the dog is mildly ill. The only difference is in the degree of depression, weakness, or other signs described. Some dogs are so weak that they have to be carried.[17]

PHYSICAL EXAMINATION

Depression was the primary abnormality found on the physical examination of 36 dogs with hypoadrenocorticism. Weakness, dehydration, bradycardia, and weak femoral pulses were present but seen in a surprisingly small number of dogs. Abdominal pain, hypothermia, and emaciation have been mentioned in the veterinary literature but are only rarely seen. A thorough physical examination is of paramount importance in evaluating any animal. In this disorder, as in others, one can assess the severity of an animal's illness on physical examination, but the clinician will often not understand its cause without additional information. Obtaining and evaluating a good medical history as well as carefully choosing one's diagnostic tests are imperative for a definitive diagnosis.[17]

CLINICAL PATHOLOGY

Erythrocyte Parameters. In adrenal insufficiency, a normocytic normochromic anemia secondary to bone marrow suppression from hypocortisolism is common.[1, 126] However, if an animal becomes hemoconcentrated secondary to dehydration, the underlying anemia may not be obvious on a CBC. Once rehydrated, these dogs will exhibit the typical mild anemia of hypoadrenocorticism.[42]

Leukocyte Parameters. In one review, total white blood cell counts in addisonian dogs varied between 7,400 and 28,700 cells/μl.[143] No consistent white blood cell differential count was obvious. An elevated white blood cell count may reflect a granulocytic response to a concurrent bacterial infection.

The presence of an absolute eosinophilia in hypoadrenal dogs is in dispute in the veterinary literature. Eosinophils were absent on admission CBCs in 4 of 36 dogs seen by us, whereas 3 dogs had an absolute eosinophilia. The remaining 29 dogs had eosinophil counts that were within the normal range, both on relative and absolute tabulations. Similar findings were reported in a review involving 62 hypoadrenal dogs.[128] However, the presence of a normal absolute eosinophil count in an ill dog may be significant, because a stress pattern with no or few eosinophils is expected in ill dogs with normal adrenocortical function. It should be remembered that a relative or absolute eosinophilia may also occur with many other diseases. Ten of 62 hypoadrenal dogs had lymphocytosis in the study by Willard and colleagues in 1982.[128] Normal or increased lymphocyte counts in an ill dog with normal adrenocortical function are unusual because enhanced glucocorticoid secretion should result in lymphopenia. Hypoadrenocorticism should be suspected when normal or elevated lymphocyte counts are present in an ill dog.[17]

Blood Urea Nitrogen (BUN) and Urinalysis. Prerenal azotemia in hypoadrenal dogs occurs secondary to reduced renal perfusion and an associated decrease in the glomerular filtration rate. Reduced renal perfusion results from hypovolemia, reduced cardiac output, and hypotension, which in turn result from chronic fluid loss through the kidneys, acute fluid loss through vomiting and/or diarrhea, and lack of adequate fluid intake. The BUN in hypoadrenal dogs is highly variable, with values in excess of 200 mg/dl possible.[143] Thirty-five of 39 hypoadrenal dogs were azotemic when first examined (Tables 97–7 and 97–8). With rehydration and return of an adequate blood volume, the BUN should rapidly return to normal. Occasionally, however, this may not occur, suggesting inadequate fluid therapy or primary renal dysfunction secondary to prolonged impaired renal perfusion and subsequent renal ischemia.

Serum creatinine concentrations were found not to correlate well with the BUN. Serum creatinine concentrations usually are only mildly abnormal while the BUN can be extremely abnormal in dogs with hypoadrenocorticism. An elevated BUN in a dog described by the owner as having clinical signs consistent with either hypoadrenocorticism or renal failure can be misleading to the veterinary practitioner. Confusion may be exacerbated when the practitioner suspects hypoadrenocorticism but the BUN fails to fall rapidly with appropriate fluid therapy.

The urine specific gravity in an animal with prerenal uremia should be elevated (> 1.030), whereas that in an animal with primary renal failure is often isosthenuric or reveals only mild concentration (1.008 to 1.025). Unfortunately many hypoadrenal dogs have an impaired ability to concentrate urine because of chronic sodium loss, depletion of renal medullary sodium, loss of the normal medullary concentration gradient, and impaired water reabsorption by the renal collecting tubules. As a result, some of these dogs with prerenal azotemia will have urine specific gravities that reveal no or only mild increases in concentration (Table 97–7). Twenty-two of 25 dogs with hypoadrenocorticism had pretreatment urine specific gravities < 1.030, including dogs that were severely azotemic (Table 97–7). Ultimately, hormone assay is required to confirm the presence or absence of adrenal disease because of the similarity in screening test results between dogs with renal failure and those with adrenal failure.

Failure of the hypoadrenal dog to increase urine output after aggressive fluid therapy is rare and should be of concern. Most of these dogs are actually polyuric. In the unusual circumstance of oliguria or anuria, concomitant renal or cardiac disease may have been masked by the adrenal-related signs. In some dogs, however, diuresis may be delayed until normal blood pressure is attained with fluid therapy. The measurement of central venous pressure or arterial blood pressure will aid in understanding the cause for anuria or oliguria. Oliguria in conjunction with a low central venous pressure or hypotension suggests inadequate fluid therapy and continued poor renal perfusion. However, oliguria in conjunction with an elevated central venous pressure or hypertension suggests overzealous fluid administration. In these animals primary renal or cardiac dysfunction should be suspected.[17]

Serum Glucose. Glucocorticoids increase hepatic glycogen and glucose production (gluconeogenesis) and decrease glucose uptake and utilization in peripheral tissues.[61] In glucocorticoid deficiency there are decreased glucose production by the liver and increased peripheral cell receptor sensitivity to insulin, which may result in hypoglycemia.[111] Both feeding and a relative decrease in insulin secretion due to the lower blood sugar tend to blunt the tendency for development of hypoglycemia. Ten of 27 (37 per cent) hypoadrenal dogs that we examined had blood glucose concentrations < 70 mg/dl when initially evaluated (Tables 97–7 and 97–8). In a recent review, however, only 4 of 53 (8 per cent) dogs were found to be hypoglycemic.[128] This discrepancy is difficult to understand. Nevertheless, the potential for hypoglycemia should remain a concern of the veterinarian. If a dog with known or suspected adrenal hypofunction is examined, the blood glucose concentration should be measured at least once, realizing that glucose administered IV may be beneficial in managing weakness and is seldom harmful.

TABLE 97–7. SELECTED LABORATORY VALUES IN DOGS WITH PRIMARY HYPOADRENOCORTICISM

Factor	Normal Value	Number Tested	Mean	Number Decreased (%)	Number Increased (%)	Range
Serum sodium	136–150 mEq/L	36	129	22(60)	0(0)	106–146
Serum potassium	3.5–5.0 mEq/L	36	7.2	0(0)	33(92)	4.7–10.8
Sodium:potassium ratio	≥27:1	36	19	35(97)	0(0)	11.2–29.1
BUN (pre-Rx)	9–25 mg/dl	36	84	0(0)	33(92)	12–223
BUN (after 24 hr Rx)	9–25 mg/dl	9	25	0(0)	4(44)	11–47
Serum calcium	8.8–11.0 mg/dl	13	11.5	0(0)	8(62)	9.3–14.4
Serum glucose	70–110 mg/dl	24	81.5	8(33)	4(17)	20–130
Serum bicarbonate	18–24 mM/L	16	14	13(81)	0(0)	9–19
Urine specific gravity	—	25	1.024	—	—	1.008–1.062

TABLE 97–8. SELECTED LABORATORY VALUES IN DOGS WITH PITUITARY FAILURE TO SECRETE ACTH AND SECONDARY ADRENOCORTICAL INSUFFICIENCY

Factor	Normal Value	Number Tested	Mean	Number Decreased (%)	Number Increased (%)	Range
Serum sodium	136–150 mEq/L	3	142	0	0	136–146
Serum potassium	3.5–5.0 mEq/L	3	4.3	0	0	4.0–4.5
Sodium:potassium ratio	≥27:1	3	29	0	0	28–31
BUN	9–25 mg/dl	3	30.5	0	2(66)	25–35
Serum glucose	70–110 mg/dl	3	68	2(67)	0	41–105
Urine specific gravity	—	3	1.044	—	—	1.028–1.052

Serum Calcium. Serum calcium concentrations are occasionally elevated in dogs with adrenal insufficiency. As seen in Table 97–7, 8 of 13 dogs were hypercalcemic when initially evaluated. Sixteen of 62 dogs with adrenal insufficiency were recently reported to be hypercalcemic. Hypercalcemia develops most frequently in extremely ill hypoadrenal dogs. In addition, the severity of the hypercalcemia is usually in direct proportion to the severity of dehydration or the electrolyte abnormalities. However, hypercalcemia is not present in all dogs in hypoadrenal crisis.

Acid-Base Status. Mild to moderate metabolic acidosis is a frequent complication in the ill hypoadrenal dog. Thirteen of 16 dogs that we evaluated had serum bicarbonate concentrations < 18 mM/L (see Table 97–7). Ten dogs had concentrations > 12 and < 18, and three had levels < 12 mM/L. Hypoaldosteronism impairs renal tubular hydrogen ion secretion, which largely accounts for the acidosis.[5] The use of either venous total carbon dioxide or the more expensive arterial blood gas analysis is an adequate method of determining a patient's acid-base status. The mild or moderate acidosis of hypoadrenocorticism rarely requires bicarbonate therapy, since adequate fluid and mineralocorticoid replacement therapy should restore renal perfusion and increase hydrogen ion excretion.

Serum Electrolytes. SODIUM AND POTASSIUM. The classic electrolyte alterations in hypoadrenocorticism include hyponatremia, hypochloremia, and hyperkalemia. These electrolyte abnormalities are primarily due to a deficiency of aldosterone and the associated failure of the kidneys to conserve sodium or excrete potassium. Serum sodium concentrations have varied from normal to as low as 106 mEq/L (see Table 97–7). Because the sodium excreted by the kidney is accompanied by considerable quantities of fluid, the hyponatremic patient often becomes severely dehydrated if fluid intake does not compensate for urinary losses. To some extent this dehydration masks the sodium depletion (mild or severe) that may be present.

Serum potassium concentrations have varied from normal to elevations that induce clinically obvious cardiac rhythm disturbances (see Table 97–7). Hyperkalemia results from both a shift of the ion from the intracellular to the extracellular compartment and a decrease in its renal excretion. The former results from a loss of the effects of cortisol on the sodium-potassium pump, which normally maintains a gradient across the cellular membrane.[5] Hypoaldosteronism and acidosis enhance the extracellular shift of potassium. The deficiency in adrenocortical hormones also allows greater concentrations of sodium to pass into the intracellular compartment as intracellular potassium concentrations decrease. Decreased potassium exchange for sodium in the distal renal tubule leads to decreased potassium excretion and increased sodium excretion in the urine. The shift in electrolytes between body compartments is corrected by the administration of cortisol, but aldosterone or other mineralocorticoids are necessary to prevent renal sodium loss.[5]

THE USE OF RATIOS. The sodium-potassium ratio has frequently been used as a diagnostic tool to identify adrenal insufficiency. The normal ratio varies between 27:1 and 40:1. Values are often below 27 and may be below 20 in primary hypoadrenocorticism. Determination of serum electrolyte concentrations from dogs suspected of having adrenal insufficiency is of paramount importance. The finding of hyperkalemia with or without alterations in serum sodium or chloride concentrations should prompt immediate therapy. The assumption that one is treating hypoadrenocorticism is well warranted and may be lifesaving. If this provisional diagnosis is incorrect, emergency therapy usually will not harm the dog ultimately shown to have renal or gastrointestinal disease. However, the limitations of serum electrolyte determinations must be realized. Reliance on electrolytes as the sole criterion for diagnosing adrenal insufficiency can be misleading if three factors are not kept in mind: first, and most important, is the slow, progressive nature of the development of primary adrenal insufficiency; second, dogs with pituitary failure can secrete aldosterone; and third, hyperkalemia and hyponatremia are not pathognomonic of adrenal insufficiency.[17]

ELECTROLYTE MEASUREMENTS ARE NOT ALWAYS DEFINITIVE. Adrenal insufficiency is usually insidious in onset and gradually progressive, although an acute adrenal crisis may be precipitated by concurrent stress. The results of any diagnostic studies will depend on the severity of clinical signs at the time tests are evaluated. If a dog is severely ill, serum electrolyte determinations may support the diagnosis. However, the same dog may have normal electrolyte concentrations if evaluated when clinical signs are minimal or not present. Three dogs with primary adrenocortical failure had normal serum electrolyte concentrations at the time of diagnosis (see Table 97–7). This uncommon finding has also been seen by other investigators.[145] The diagnosis in these patients must be confirmed by tests that measure adrenocortical reserve.

Electrolyte alterations are attributed, for the most part, to inadequate mineralocorticoids. Therefore, an animal that has pituitary deficiency of ACTH may have a clinical syndrome that reflects only glucocorticoid deficiency. Because aldosterone is only minimally affected by ACTH, such an animal will usually maintain normal electrolyte concentrations. The gastrointestinal, mental, and metabolic changes typical of hypocortisolemia may become obvious to the owner and veterinarian, while those changes ascribed to hypoaldosteronism are absent (see Table 97–8). Electrolyte alterations in such a patient may never be seen. ACTH deficiency may occur as a result of a primary pituitary problem (trauma, infection, cancer) or secondary to long-term corticosteroid medication that is acutely discontinued. Clinically, these dogs may be indistinguishable from those with primary adrenal insufficiency or with renal or gastrointestinal problems. Only a thorough medical history will alert the veterinarian to the possibility of secondary adrenal insufficiency. In addition, hyperadrenal dogs that have been overdosed with o,p'-DDD may develop hypocortisolemia. Clinical signs include depression, anorexia, vomiting, and diarrhea, while serum electrolyte concentrations remain within the normal range.

CAUSES OF HYPERKALEMIA. Dogs with nonadrenal causes of hyperkalemia must be distinguished from those with hypoadrenocorticism. Although the acute management of hyperkalemia is similar regardless of its cause, one must be certain of a diagnosis before pursuing lifelong therapy. The most common nonadrenal cause of hyperkalemia is acute renal failure. Hyperkalemia is uncommon in chronic renal failure unless the patient is terminally anuric or oliguric. Severe hyperkalemia is commonly associated with rupture of the urinary bladder and urine leakage into the peritoneal cavity. In addition, urethral obstruction can cause severe hyperkalemia. Gastrointestinal disorders may also result in serum electrolyte abnormalities suggestive of hypoadrenocorticism. These electrolyte disturbances were reported in dogs with intestinal parasitism (trichuriasis, salmonellosis, ancylostomiasis), perforated duodenal ulcers, and gastric torsion.[146] Similar test results have been seen in some dogs with parvovirus infection, canine distemper, and severe malabsorption syndrome.[17]

Rapid cellular release of potassium and resultant hyperkalemia may occur as a result of severe acidosis or increased tissue destruction after surgery, crush injury, extensive infection, or massive hemolysis. These conditions may also be associated with impaired renal excretion of potassium. Exogenous potassium intake is an uncommon cause of hyperkalemia except in patients with renal insufficiency. The use of potassium-sparing diuretics has the potential of causing mild hyperkalemia.

Artifactual increases in the serum potassium concentration in humans may be associated with significant elevations in the platelet count or may occur when the blood sample is hemolyzed or refrigerated, or if separation of red blood cells from the plasma is delayed. The Akita breed appears to have elevated red blood cell potassium concentrations. Six of eight Akitas had high erythrocyte potassium levels, and plasma from affected dogs displayed hyperkalemia after being refrigerated in contact with red cells for longer than four hours. The rise in plasma potassium concentration (pseudohyperkalemia) was progressive with prolonged red cell contact and was accompanied by a fall in plasma sodium (Table 97–9).[147]

CAUSES OF HYPONATREMIA. Any cause of hyponatremia can alter the serum sodium-potassium ratio. Other than hypoadrenocorticism, conditions associated with hyponatremia include renal tubular diseases, diuretic-induced sodium loss, and urinary sodium loss from osmotic diuresis, such as diabetes mellitus. In addition, hyperglycemia may exacerbate hyponatremia as water shifts from the intracellular to the extracellular fluid compartment.[42] Hyponatremia may also result from inadequate sodium intake, vomiting, diarrhea, or primary polydipsic disorders. Lipemia will cause a false depression in sodium concentration. Lipemia displaces a significant amount of the aqueous phase of plasma in which sodium ions are found. When lipemic plasma is sampled, a less aqueous phase will be obtained, resulting in an erroneous depression in sodium concentration. If the sodium concentration is expressed as plasma water rather than as whole plasma, it will often be normal.

SUMMARY. Electrolyte panels in dogs suspected of having hypoadrenocorticism are extremely valuable. They can be used to support a tentative diagnosis and are tremendously useful in modifying therapy. However, they do not provide a definitive diagnosis, which can only be obtained by evaluating hormone concentrations and adrenocortical reserve. The differential diagnosis for hyperkalemia and hyponatremia is outlined in Table 97–10 (also see Chapter 11).

RADIOLOGY

Hypoadrenal dogs with severe hypovolemia often have microcardia, a flattened and decreased diameter of the descending aortic arch, and a narrow posterior vena cava, as seen in lateral projections of the thorax.[148] Similar radiographic appearances may be seen in some dogs with more insidious signs, such as depression, lethargy, and weakness. These findings support the tentative diagnosis of adrenal insufficiency and are a crude means of evaluating the degree of hypovolemia. However, it should be remembered that microcardia is a nonspecific sign of hypovolemia or shock.

Caution is needed in interpreting lateral thoracic radiographs of dogs with a deep thorax, such as the Irish wolfhound and the borzoi. In these breeds, the heart is frequently not long enough to make contact with the sternum.

Interestingly, two of our hypoadrenal dogs had radiographic and fluoroscopic evidence of an aperistaltic esophageal dilatation. This abnormality disappeared with treatment of the hypoadrenocorticism and may have been a reflection of generalized muscle weakness.

ELECTROCARDIOGRAM (ECG)

Physiology of Hyperkalemia and the Heart. With modest hyperkalemia (K^+ concentration, 5.5 to 6.5

TABLE 97–9. ELECTROLYTE VALUES OF RED CELLS, PLASMA, AND STORED PLASMA*

Dog No.	Breed	Age	Sex	RBC (K⁺) (mEq/L)	Plasma (Na⁺/K⁺) Storage (0 hr) (mEq/L)	Storage (24 hr) (mEq/L)
2	Akita	2½ yr	M	69	161/3.9	148/16.4
3	Akita	4 yr	M	71	160/4.1	142/23.8
4	Akita	5 yr	F	65	159/4.5	145/17.2
5	Akita	2 yr	M	6.0	166/4.0	164/5.6
6	Akita	2 yr	F	4.0	158/3.9	159/4.9
7	Akita	5 yr	F	76	152/3.4	131/21.0
8	Akita	5 yr	M	68	154/4.4	147/14.2
9	Akita	6 yr	F/S	70	151/5.1	146/17.0
10	Japanese tosa	2 yr	F	5.0	154/4.0	152/4.2
11	German shepherd X	7 yr	M/C	3.5	156/4.6	152/5.2
12	Springer spaniel	9 yr	F/S	3.5	151/3.9	152/4.4
13	English bulldog	9 yr	M	4.5	152/4.0	152/5.3
14	Labrador retriever X	9 yr	F/S	5.0	152/4.7	149/5.5
15	Keeshond	3 mo	F	5.5	145/4.4	147/5.6

*Courtesy of Lisa Degen, DVM.
Abbreviations: X = mixed-breed dog; F/S = spayed female; M/C = castrated male.

mEq/L), a transient and minor acceleration of cardiac conduction can be demonstrated. As the serum potassium concentration rises above this level, depression of conduction occurs. Examination of the electrocardiogram (ECG) reveals "peaking" of T waves during modest elevations of the serum potassium concentration in some dogs. As the serum potassium concentration rises, the P-R interval prolongs and the P wave ultimately disappears; the QRS complex widens and R-R intervals become irregular. "Sinoventricular" conduction may be observed at this stage. Later sequential

TABLE 97–10. THE DIFFERENTIAL DIAGNOSIS FOR SIGNIFICANT HYPERKALEMIA AND/OR HYPONATREMIA IN DOGS AND CATS*

I. Hypoadrenocorticism
II. Renal and urinary tract disease
  A. Primary acute renal failure
  B. Chronic severe oliguric or anuric renal failure
  C. Urethral obstruction longer than 24-hour duration
  D. Osmotic- or diuretic-induced diuresis
  E. Urine leakage into the peritoneal cavity
III. Severe liver failure
  A. Cirrhosis
  B. Neoplasia
IV. Severe gastrointestinal disease, including:
  A. Parasitic infestation
    1. Whipworms
    2. Ascarid overload
    3. Salmonellosis
  B. Viral enteritis (parvovirus)
  C. Gastric torsion
  D. Duodenal perforation
V. Severe metabolic or respiratory acidosis, including:
  A. Diabetic ketoacidosis
  B. Pancreatitis
VI. Congestive heart failure
  A. Advanced
  B. Acute
VII. Massive tissue destruction
  A. Crush injury
  B. Extensive infection
  C. Hemolysis
VIII. Primary polydipsia
IX. Pseudohyperkalemia in the Akita breed (see text and Table 97–9)

*Most of these diagnoses are not often associated with these electrolyte alterations, but such changes have been seen.

changes include atrioventricular junctional delay, followed by acceleration of junctional pacemakers, conduction delays in the His-Purkinje system, and delays in ventricular muscle contraction. As potassium concentrations continue to increase, asystole results in cardiac arrest. His bundle and bundle branch recordings indicate that asystole typically results from a block within a distal conducting system. The resultant peripheral ECG shows regular or irregular rhythm with widened QRS complexes. Although the morphology of the QRS complex may suggest that the arrhythmias are of ventricular origin, these rhythms have been shown to be junctional or sinus rhythms. Because hyperkalemia seldom is seen as an isolated finding, one must remember that other electrolyte disturbances, especially in sodium and calcium concentrations, modify pure potassium-mediated alterations.[149]

For those practitioners with ECG machines, hyperkalemia becomes a rapidly recognizable aberration (see Figure 97–25). The most prominent manifestations of hyperkalemia are found on the ECG, which is a vital tool for estimating the severity of hyperkalemia. The veterinarian must always keep in mind that hypoadrenocorticism is only one of several potential causes of hyperkalemia. Once hyperkalemia is diagnosed, however, potentially lifesaving measures can be initiated. No in-hospital screening test is as simple and rapid as an ECG, and none is as easily used in monitoring a patient during treatment.[17]

MILD HYPERKALEMIA. The earliest visible ECG alteration is peaking of the T wave, which occurs when the serum potassium concentration exceeds 5.5 mEq/L. This change is frequently associated with shortening of the Q-T interval. The characteristic tall and narrow T wave occurs before the ECG shows any measurable alteration of the QRS complex. T wave changes are not seen in all cases of mild hyperkalemia. As the serum potassium concentration rises above 7 mEq/L, the T wave may lose its classic peaked shape, if present, because abnormalities that take place secondary to intraventricular conduction disturbances obscure the primary T wave changes.

MODERATE HYPERKALEMIA. Slowing of the intraven-

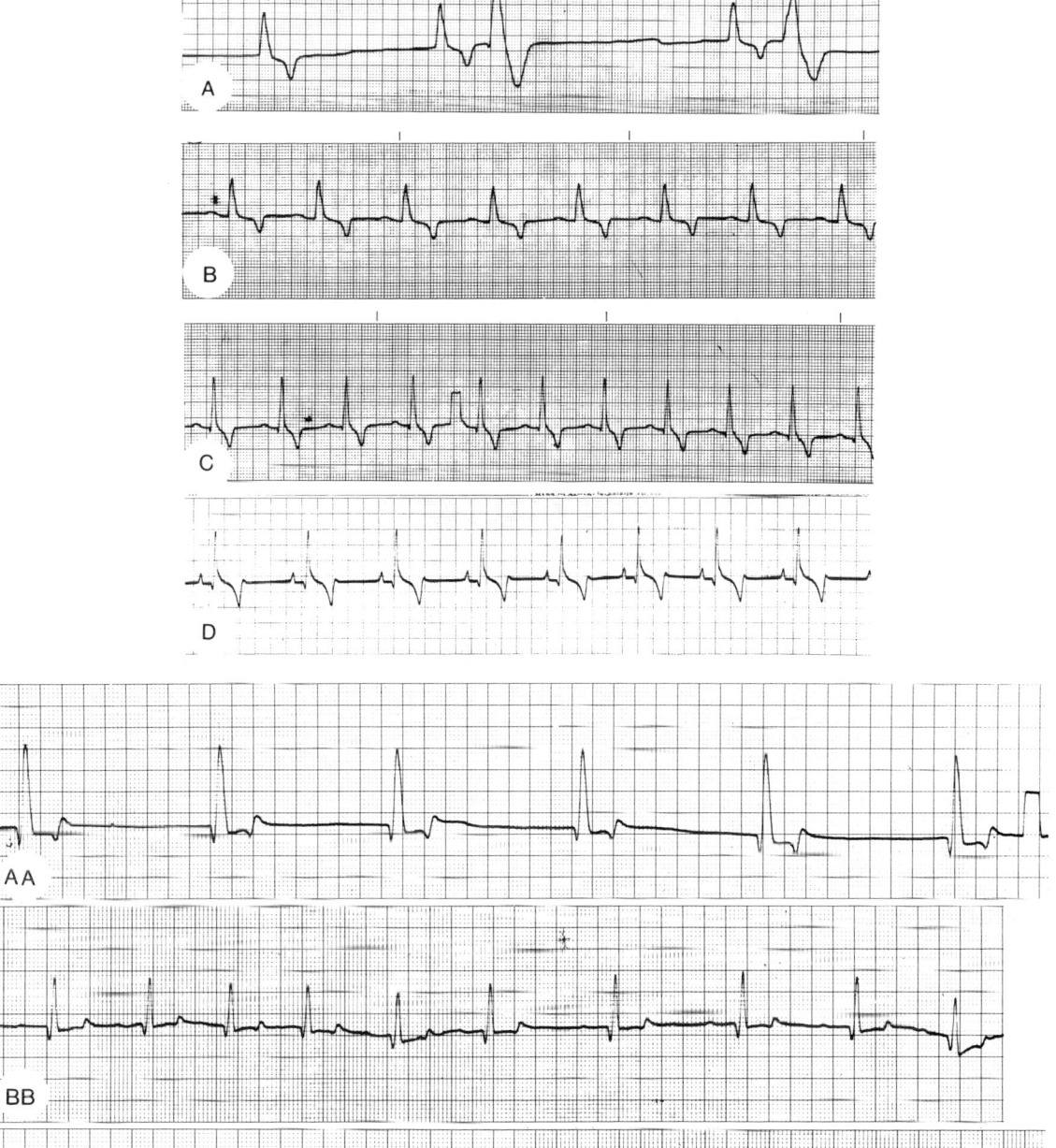

FIGURE 97–25. Serial ECG segments obtained from two dogs wtih hypoadrenocorticism and hyperkalemia. *A* and *AA* both show the effect of severe hyperkalemia, with the former dog having a serum potassium of 8.6 mEq/L and the latter, 9.4 mEq/L. Note the lack of visible P waves, the short and wide QRS complexes, and the T waves, which are not of excessive amplitude. ECG A also reveals a bizarre-looking QRS complex following a more normal-appearing QRS complex. This bizarre wave represents a ventricular escape beat that could be the result of hypoxia and/or hyperkalemia. *B* and *BB* are ECGs from the same dogs as in *A* and *AA*, respectively. They were each obtained approximately one hour after institution of IV normal saline as the only treatment. The serum potassium concentrations had decreased to 7.6 mEq/L and 7.9 mEq/L, respectively. Two important factors to note: First is the improvement seen in each case with return of P waves, a more rapid heart rate, and disappearance of ventricular escape beats. Second, note the abnormalities still present. Most obvious are the prolonged P-R intervals (first degree heart block). This alone suggests hyperkalemia, especially when associated with a widened QRS complex and a short Q-T interval. There are numerous other causes of P-R interval prolongation. In *C* and *CC*, the serum potassium concentrations are considerably lower, 6.2 mEq/L and 5.9 mEq/L, respectively. The P-R interval and P, QRS, and T waves are of shorter duration and the R waves are taller. *D*, ECG from the dog with ECG *A*, when the serum potassium concentration is 5.6 mEq/L and a more "spiked" T wave is seen. (*A-D* From Feldman, EC: *In* Ettinger, SJ (ed): Textbook of Veterinary Internal Medicine, 2nd ed. Philadelphia, WB Saunders, 1983, p 1664.)

tricular impulse conduction is responsible for the QRS complex alterations that occur as the serum potassium concentration exceeds 6.5 mEq/L. At this juncture the T wave abnormalities and the uniformly widened QRS complex allow the presumptive diagnosis of hyperkalemia to be made. With increasing serum potassium concentrations, the QRS duration increases progressively. Thus, a rough correlation between duration of the QRS complex and the degree of hyperkalemia can be made.

MODERATE TO SEVERE HYPERKALEMIA. As the serum potassium concentration rises above 7 mEq/L, the P wave amplitude decreases and its duration becomes prolonged secondary to slowed impulse conduction through the atria. The P-R interval also increases in duration as a result of slower atrioventricular transmission. When serum potassium concentrations exceed 8.5 mEq/L, the P wave frequently becomes invisible. When P waves are absent, an erroneous diagnosis of atrial fibrillation may be made, particularly when the ventricular rate is irregular.

SEVERE HYPERKALEMIA. Continued elevation of the serum potassium concentration can be associated with deviation from the baseline of the S-T segment. When potassium concentrations reach the magnitude of 11 to 14 mEq/L, the electrocardiographer may see ventricular asystole or ventricular fibrillation.

The early diagnosis of hyperkalemia provided in many cases with the ECG allows rapid institution of therapy without waiting for the laboratory report on serum electrolyte concentrations. Regardless of its cause, marked hyperkalemia is an emergency situation that demands a quick therapeutic response from the practitioner.

HORMONE STUDIES—CONFIRMING THE DIAGNOSIS

Cortisol Concentrations

Basal Plasma Cortisol Concentrations. Corticosteroid concentrations in plasma are generally decreased in hypoadrenocorticism. Because partial degrees of adrenal insufficiency occur, and since normal plasma cortisol concentrations can be quite low, reliance on basal concentrations of plasma corticosteroids is unreliable. Tests that measure adrenocortical reserve are necessary to establish the diagnosis.

Urinary Steroids. Urinary 7-hydroxycorticosteroid determinations are accurate in confirming a diagnosis of hypoadrenocorticism, but obtaining the necessary 24-hour urine samples from housebroken pets in metabolism cages can be awkward, if not impossible, for veterinarians.[64, 151, 152] In addition, these determinations do not assess adrenocortical reserve. It remains to be demonstrated whether the amount of cortisol secreted in a 24-hour period (as assessed by urine cortisol assay) or the functional adrenal reserve (as assessed by means of ACTH stimulation) proves to be more reliable in the diagnosis of hypoadrenocorticism.

ACTH Stimulation and Plasma Cortisol Measurement

Protocol. See earlier section under Hyperadrenocorticism. In a patient suspected to be in a hypoadrenal crisis, the ACTH stimulation test is performed on admission to the hospital, regardless of the time of day. Practitioners are urged to follow instructions provided by their laboratory concerning the amount of plasma needed and its handling. Cortisol degradation is minimal in serum or plasma stored at room temperature for up to five days; beyond this time degradation may be significant, especially with initially high cortisol concentrations.[153]

Results. One major criterion is used in confirming the diagnosis of adrenocortical insufficiency: the post-ACTH plasma cortisol concentration using an appropriate, reliable stimulation protocol. A normal plasma cortisol concentration after ACTH administration makes the diagnosis of adrenal insufficiency quite unlikely. An abnormally low or poor response to this provocative test (plasma cortisol concentration < 2 SD below the normal mean) confirms the diagnosis. The ACTH stimulation test will not distinguish dogs with primary adrenal disease from those with secondary insufficiency due to pituitary failure or chronic iatrogenic corticosteroid administration. Primary adrenocortical disease implies cellular destruction of the adrenal cortex, leading to abnormal test results. Secondary adrenal insufficiency, severe enough to result in clinical signs, is associated with significant atrophy of the adrenal cortex (see Figure 97–24). The atrophied cells do not have the capacity to respond to one injection of ACTH; however, they would eventually respond to repeated injections or a chronic infusion of ACTH. Adrenocortical atrophy of cells also follows chronic administration of glucocorticoids.

Dogs with primary or secondary adrenal failure had resting plasma cortisol concentrations that were either normal or below normal. The post-stimulation plasma cortisol concentrations were consistently below normal, and in some of the dogs the plasma cortisol concentration 60 minutes after ACTH administration was actually less than the baseline value. The difference between normal and hypoadrenal animals is shown in Figure 97–25. These studies have also revealed the failure of cortisol response to ACTH administration in dogs having pituitary failure of ACTH secretion and secondary hypoadrenocorticism.[17]

Plasma Endogenous ACTH

Endogenous plasma ACTH concentrations provide the practitioner with academic evidence that confirms the presence or absence of hypoadrenocorticism and can also provide information regarding the site of failure within the pituitary-adrenal axis. As seen in Figure 97–24, a dog with primary adrenocortical failure has little negative feedback to the pituitary, which should result in elevated plasma ACTH concentrations. The same is true of dogs treated with the adrenocorticolytic drug o,p'-DDD. However, a dog with secondary adrenal insufficiency caused by pituitary disease should have insufficient ACTH secretion, resulting in adrenocortical atrophy. This would also be true of a patient that is chronically overtreated with corticosteroids (see Figure 97–24). The endogenous plasma ACTH concentrations in dogs with primary adrenal disease are extremely elevated when compared with the normal range. This lends credence to the supposition that the canine adrenal cortex is controlled by pituitary ACTH and that these dogs had extremely high ACTH concentrations because of primary adrenocortical disease, failure of negative feedback to the pituitary, and an unrestrained secretion of pituitary ACTH (Figures 97–24 and 97–27). However, a few dogs with hypoadrenocorticism had endogenous plasma ACTH concentrations below normal (Figure 97–27). Because these dogs had never received corticosteroid medication before testing, and had normal serum electrolyte concentrations, it can be assumed that they were suffering from pituitary failure to release ACTH (Table 97–8).

TREATMENT

Rapid institution of therapy is vital in dogs known to be or suspected of being in a hypoadrenal crisis. If the serum electrolyte concentrations, ECG, history, or physical examination is strongly suggestive of hyperkalemia and/or hypoadrenocorticism, treatment should be directed toward adrenal disease until this diagnosis is refuted. Treatment in acute adrenal insufficiency is directed toward: (1) correcting hypotension and hypovolemia, (2) improving vascular integrity and providing an immediate source of glucocorticoid, (3) correcting electrolyte imbalances, and (4) correcting acidosis (Table 97–11).

Hypovolemia

Normal saline is the IV fluid of choice because it will aid in correcting hypovolemia, hyponatremia, and hypochloremia. Hyperkalemia is reduced by simple dilution (since saline contains no potassium) and by improved renal perfusion and glomerular filtration. Potassium-containing fluids are a relative contraindication but should be used in lieu of not giving IV fluids. Ringer's and lactated Ringer's solutions contain 4 mEq/L of potassium. Their use in hyperkalemic patients should lower the plasma potassium concentration, albeit at a slower rate, through dilutional effects and enhanced renal perfusion. If the dog is anuric, diuretics such as furosemide (Lasix) would be indicated once sufficient fluids have been administered to restore normal blood pressure (see section on Blood Urea Nitrogen and Urinalysis).

If hypoglycemia is suspected or known to be present, glucose should be added to the IV fluid to produce a 5 per cent dextrose solution. The addition of dextrose to isotonic solutions will produce a hypertonic solution, which should be administered through a jugular vein rather than through the smaller cephalic vein. The ability to measure central venous pressure also makes the use

of a jugular catheter preferable to that of a cephalic or saphenous catheter. It must be emphasized that normal saline alone, given IV, is the most important portion of the therapeutic regimen.

Because death from hyperadrenocorticism is often attributed to vascular collapse and shock, rapid correction of hypovolemia is the first priority. An indwelling IV catheter is placed in the jugular or cephalic vein. In an attempt to both treat the patient and ultimately obtain a diagnosis, a blood sample is taken for serum electrolytes as well as plasma cortisol concentrations once the catheter is in place. ACTH (0.25 mg of Cortrosyn IM) is then given IM, and 0.9 per cent normal saline is administered IV at an initial rate of 10 to 40 ml/pound of body weight. Total fluid replacement is determined from an estimate of the degree of dehydration, urinary output, and insensible fluid loss. The urinary bladder should be catheterized and emptied initially after completion of the ACTH stimulation test, and hourly thereafter, to evaluate urine production and assure that anuric renal failure is not present. Once the post-stimulation plasma cortisol sample is obtained, additional hormone therapy (i.e., mineralocorticoids and glucocorticoids) can be administered.[17]

Glucocorticoids. In order to provide glucocorticoids to the hypoadrenal animal, prednisolone sodium succinate should be administered IV over two to four minutes. It is recommended that the ACTH response test be completed before administration of glucocorticoids. Infusion of IV saline is sufficient therapy during the first hour (while ACTH response is completed). The dosage of prednisolone sodium succinate is 2 to 10 mg/lb (4 to 20 mg/kg) body weight, and this may be repeated in two to six hours. Rather than repeat the administration of this rapid-acting, water-soluble, expensive glucocorticoid, one may elect to add dexamethasone (0.02 to 0.05 mg/lb or 0.05 to 0.1 mg/kg q12h) to the IV infusion. This should provide an adequate and continuous source of glucocorticoid for the dog until oral medication can be safely given (Table 97–11). However, prednisolone sodium succinate has mineralocorticoid action; this is important because no other injectable mineralocorticoid is available.

Electrolyte Imbalance

Recognition of the Problem. The most rapid method of determining the presence of hyperkalemia (the most worrisome electrolyte alteration) is with the ECG, as discussed previously. If P waves are not seen and the heart rate is slow, severe hyperkalemia should be suspected. Invariably the serum potassium concentration with these ECG alterations is > 7.5 mEq/L. The major consideration in the differential diagnosis is atrial fibrillation, which is usually associated with tachycardia and not with vomiting or diarrhea. Adrenal insufficiency or atrial fibrillation will cause weakness, lethargy, anorexia, and weight loss.

Saline. Therapy need not be overzealous when potassium concentrations are < 6.5 mEq/L, whereas intensive therapy must be instituted in animals with serum potassium concentrations > 7.5 mEq/L. With marked hyper-

TABLE 97–11. TREATMENT OF ACUTE ADRENAL INSUFFICIENCY (HYPOADRENOCORTICISM)

Initial Therapy
1. Fluids: sodium chloride injection, USP (normal saline)
2. Baseline cortisol and post-ACTH stimulation cortisol
3. Glucocorticoid and mineralocorticoid
   a. Prednisolone sodium succinate, 4 to 20 mg/kg IV
   b. Dexamethasone, 0.05 to 0.1 mg/kg, into infusion bottle
4. Consider IV glucose and insulin to rapidly lower serum potassium concentration (if serum K is above 9.5 mEq/L; rarely needed)
5. Acidosis: bicarbonate, 25% of calculated dose IV during first 6 hr of therapy if bicarbonate concentration of serum is <12 mEq/L

Guidelines
1. Repeat serum electrolyte and CO_2 levels at 6 to 8 hr intervals
2. Monitor urine production
3. Monitor ECG, if possible
4. Observe central venous pressure, if possible

Subsequent Therapy
1. Fluids: maintain until oral alimentation is possible
2. Glucocorticoids: injectable dexamethasone should be used until oral prednisone (usually low-dose) can be initiated
3. Mineralocorticoid: oral fludrocortisone should be utilized once every 12 hr
4. Bicarbonate: adjust dosage depending on subsequent blood CO_2 levels

---

kalemia, rapid institution of treatment may be lifesaving. IV normal saline is a reliable treatment when one is attempting to lower the serum potassium concentration rapidly. Virtually every dog in hypoadrenocortical crisis we have treated received only rapid administration of 0.9 per cent normal saline during the first hour of treatment. A few dogs also received glucose. This approach alone has resulted in dramatic clinical, biochemical, and electrocardiographic improvement. IV normal saline will, as previously discussed, correct all the life-threatening complications of hypoadrenocorticism in the short term.[17]

Glucose and Insulin. In the unusual circumstance that IV normal saline is not successful, and death from hyperkalemia is believed to be imminent, lowering of the serum potassium concentration can be further aided by the IV infusion of a 10 per cent glucose solution. In the first 30 to 60 minutes, 2 to 5 ml/lb (4 to 10 ml/kg) should be given and may be added to the saline infusion. Glucose uptake by the cells is accompanied by potassium uptake from the vascular compartment. Subcutaneous or IV infusions of regular insulin at a dose of 0.03 to 0.06 U/lb (0.06 to 0.125 U/kg) will enhance the cellular uptake of glucose. For each unit of regular insulin, one should administer at least 20 ml of 10 per cent glucose to avoid precipitating hypoglycemia. Although this therapy would lower serum potassium concentrations, IV saline has negated its need.

Calcium. An IV 10 per cent calcium gluconate infusion has also been recommended in acute hyperkalemia. A dose of 0.2 to 0.5 mg/lb (0.5 to 1.0 mg/kg) IV, given slowly over a period of 10 to 20 minutes, appears to function by "protecting" the myocardium from the deleterious effects of hyperkalemia. This protection provides time for the other modes of therapy to lower the serum potassium. During a calcium infusion the ECG must be continuously monitored and the treatment stopped if any new arrhythmia is observed.

Sodium Bicarbonate. Sodium bicarbonate, as mentioned below, can also be used to decrease elevated serum potassium concentrations. Normal saline, sodium bicarbonate, and IV glucose are the immediate methods of treatment recommended for severe hyperkalemia in hypoadrenocorticism.

DOCA and Hydrocortisone. In addition to these various immediate (rapid-acting) treatment options, mineralocorticoids must be given to the dog to maintain improved electrolyte balance. Mineralocorticoids are administered immediately after completing the ACTH response test. Desoxycorticosterone acetate (DOCA) in oil was the mineralocorticoid of choice at a dosage of 0.1 to 0.2 mg/lb (0.2 to 0.4 mg/kg) by IM injection once daily; however, this form of the drug is no longer available from the manufacturer.

Injectable cortisol (hydrocortisone hemisuccinate or hydrocortisone phosphate) is the drug of choice in managing a hypoadrenocortical crisis. Cortisol has obvious glucocorticoid action and has sufficient sodium-retaining potency to replace mineralocorticoid insufficiency.[11] We have used hydrocortisone hemisuccinate in several hypoadrenal dogs for both its glucocorticoid and mineralocorticoid actions. The recommendation is to administer 0.6 mg/lb (1.25 mg/kg) IV initially, followed by 0.2 to 0.5 mg/lb (0.5 to 1.0 mg/kg) IV every six hours. On the second day the dosage is further tapered, ultimately reaching 0.05 to 0.12 mg/lb (0.1 to 0.25 mg/kg) administered four times a day and then 0.05 to 0.12 mg/lb (0.1 to 0.25 mg/kg) in two oral doses of hydrocortisone per day with mineralocorticoid as needed (see section, Maintenance Therapy).

Acidosis

Dogs with hypoadrenocorticism usually have mild metabolic acidosis, which does not require therapy. Acidosis, when present, is corrected with an infusion of sodium bicarbonate. In a severely ill patient, a base deficit of 10 mEq/L can be assumed to be present, while awaiting laboratory results. When arterial blood gas analysis is not available, total venous carbon dioxide can be used to estimate base deficit by subtracting the patient's venous carbon dioxide concentration from the normal venous carbon dioxide concentration (approximately 22 mEq/L). The number of milliequivalents of bicarbonate needed to correct the acidosis is then determined from the following equation: Deficit in mEq = (body weight in kg)(0.5)(base deficit in mEq).

Patients seldom require the complete bicarbonate replacement dosage. Therefore, it is recommended that 25 per cent of the calculated dose be administered in the IV fluids during the initial six to eight hours of therapy. At the end of this time the acid-base status of the animal should be reassessed. Rarely a dog may require additional parenteral sodium bicarbonate. We do not recommend the indiscriminate use of sodium bicarbonate. If the total venous carbon dioxide or the serum bicarbonate concentration is > 12 mEq/L, sodium bicarbonate therapy is not necessary. If the concentration is < 12 mEq/L, conservative bicarbonate therapy would be helpful.

IV sodium bicarbonate does have more than one favorable effect when used to treat hypoadrenocorticism. It not only aids in correcting metabolic acidosis, but also decreases the serum potassium concentration. Sodium bicarbonate buffers hydrogen ions, decreases the intracellular hydrogen ion concentration, increases the intracellular potassium concentration, and thereby decreases the serum (extracellular) potassium concentration.

General Response After the Initial Crisis

The Acute Phase. Virtually every hypoadrenal dog treated initially with IV saline (first hour) and subsequently with saline, glucocorticoids, and mineralocorticoids has shown rapid improvement. Within one or two hours of rapid and aggressive fluid therapy these dogs are able to stand and walk, when they were initially extremely weak. They have an interest in their owners, food, water, and their environment. Typically, the ECG and serum electrolyte and BUN concentrations correlate with improvement in these parameters toward or to normal. The response to fluid therapy alone is highly suggestive of adrenocortical insufficiency, since dogs with most other illnesses will not have as dramatic a reversal of signs and laboratory abnormalities.[17]

Beyond the Crisis. Each dog should be maintained on IV fluids without oral food or water for at least 24 hours, regardless of the pet's clinical appearance. After this initial 24-hour treatment period, the rate of fluid administration should be reduced by 50 per cent while water is offered in small amounts every one to two hours. If water is consumed and vomiting not seen for 12 additional hours, food may be offered in small amounts. Typically, we offer a 50:50 or 25:75 mixture of cottage cheese (low fat) and cooked white rice. If vomiting is not seen after 12 to 24 hours, the IV fluid administration may be discontinued. Daily injections of hydrocortisone hemisuccinate are continued for 24 hours beyond the time of consuming food and water without vomiting. Then oral fludrocortisone acetate can be initiated (see section on Maintenance Therapy). Each dog should be observed for an additional 24 to 48 hours in the hospital on oral therapies before being returned to the owner. The dog should then be rechecked 7 and 14 days later. These rechecks should include a thorough history, complete physical examination, ECG, and blood tests of the BUN, sodium, potassium, and glucose concentration. If the dog is well and the test results are normal, a recheck every three to four months is strongly encouraged.

Concurrent Problems. If the above test results are normal, yet the dog does not appear to the owner to be in satisfactory condition, two possibilities must be considered. The dog with hypoadrenocorticism that is treated only with mineralocorticoids may not respond completely. Common blood tests may not identify the cause of this incomplete response to treatment (inappetence, lethargy, depression). A trial period (two to four weeks) of low-dose prednisone therapy in addition to the mineralocorticoids may result in the animal's improvement. As mentioned earlier in this chapter, concurrent disease must also be considered. The most common disorder is hypothyroidism, but other endocri-

nopathies should be considered. If the serum electrolyte concentrations are abnormal, an increased dose of mineralocorticoid should be administered. Overdosage of mineralocorticoid is possible but not common.

Maintenance Therapy

DOGS WITH PRIMARY HYPOADRENOCORTICISM

Maintenance therapy can be initiated once the dog is stable with parenteral medication (Tables 97–11 and 97–12). The dog should have a good appetite, and vomiting, diarrhea, weakness, and depression should no longer be problems. In addition, serum electrolyte concentrations should be within the normal range. The veterinary practitioner has several alternatives when choosing long-term mineralocorticoid medications, including subcutaneous implants, intramuscular injections, and oral therapy.

Implants. Pellets of DOCA (125 mg each) have been successfully used in the treatment of adrenocortical insufficiency.[127] These pellets must be surgically placed under the skin, with strict attention given to asepsis to avoid wound contamination. One DOCA pellet should be used for each 0.5 mg of daily DOCA injection required to maintain normal serum electrolyte concentrations. It has been suggested that each pellet releases mineralocorticoid for at least ten months;[154] however, pellets do not always function this long. Therefore, periodic evaluation of serum electrolyte concentrations should be performed to assure adequate function of the pellets. Every ten months the remaining pellet material should be removed and new material implanted. Overdosage, with the development of hypokalemia, has been reported with the use of pellets.[155]

We think that implants are the least reliable and most expensive mode of therapy. Tremendous individual variability has been seen with pellets, both in day-to-day control of the disease and in length of action. Pellets are not recommended because they are not amenable to simple correction of dosage should patient control become inadequate.

TABLE 97–12. LONG-TERM TREATMENT OF PRIMARY ADRENOCORTICAL INSUFFICIENCY

Mineralocorticoid:	Approximately 0.1 mg fludrocortisone/5 kg body weight (divided BID)
Glucocorticoid:	Prednisone as needed, 2.5–10 mg daily or every other day
	OR
Hydrocortisone:	Approximately 0.125 mg/kg body weight daily, divided ¾–⅔ AM; remainder PM
Fludrocortisone:	As needed, approximately 0.05 mg/5 kg body weight (divided BID)

(Divide mineralocorticoid to protect dog against vomiting entire dose should a gastrointestinal problem arise)

Clinical follow-up:	(Re-check every 3–6 months) Maintain normal weight and activity Electrolytes and BUN should be normal
Salt:	No special addition if dog food diet
Times of stress:	Increase glucocorticoid therapy
	Owner education is imperative

IM Injections. Desoxycorticosterone (mineralocorticoid) was available in a pivalate form (DOCP) that slowly released the hormone at a rate of 1 mg/day/25 mg suspension. However, this drug is no longer available from the manufacturer.

Oral Therapy. Fludrocortisone acetate is commonly used in the treatment of humans with hypoadrenocorticism[5] and is recommended for the treatment of canine hypoadrenocorticism.[143] Each tablet contains 0.1 mg of mineralocorticoid. The average 45-lb (20-kg) dog requires two to four tablets daily. The dosage varies, depending on body size, between one-half and nine tablets daily (usually divided twice a day).

The major advantage of tablet administration is the ease of diagnosing and correcting an incorrect dosage (i.e., daily administration is easily altered). Daily therapy also serves as a constant reminder to the dog owner that the animal is afflicted with a serious, life-threatening disease and that it is dependent on the owner for survival. It appears that less reliable owners are best told to administer daily oral medication, since failure to give one or two oral doses is usually not serious, whereas failure to remember a monthly injection or a 6-, 8-, or 10-month implant can have major deleterious consequences. Oral therapy with fludrocortisone acetate is the least expensive approach to management, although all three forms of therapy are relatively expensive.

Monitoring and Drawbacks. Initially the serum electrolyte concentrations should be monitored every one to two weeks until the patient is known to be stable. Rechecks, consisting of physical examination, progress report, and serum analysis of sodium, potassium, and BUN (used for a crude evaluation of blood volume and tissue perfusion), are recommended every three months. Using oral therapy, it has been our experience that the dosage of fludrocortisone acetate must be increased during the first 6 to 18 months of therapy. This may reflect continuing destruction of the adrenal glands. After this period, the required dosage usually remains relatively stable. Similar experience has been noted with monthly injections. This dosage increase constitutes another drawback to the use of subcutaneous implants.

The major drawbacks to oral therapy have been the development of polydipsia and polyuria in some dogs, as well as the extremely high dosages needed in others. Dogs with increased urine output had been satisfactorily treated with monthly injections of DOCP and discontinuation of oral medication. Use of oral hydrocortisone may decrease the polydipsia and polyuria yet control the disease. Dogs that need unusually high doses of oral mineralocorticoids may respond to oral salt and fewer tablets of fludrocortisone.

The use of hydrocortisone alone has been successful in a few of our dogs as a replacement for both insufficient mineralocorticoids and glucocorticoids. We have used approximately 15 mg in the morning and 5 mg in the evening as average doses for a 40-pound dog. In several dogs 0.05 to 0.2 mg of fludrocortisone was also needed.

Glucocorticoids. Approximately 50 per cent of our patients that receive only fludrocortisone do not require glucocorticoid medication. However, a dog may be reported not to be in perfect health yet have normal serum electrolyte concentrations. In this situation, a moderate dosage of prednisone or prednisolone (2.5 to 10.0 mg daily) often improves the dog's well being. Owners quickly note improvement, medication is inexpensive, and adverse reactions are minimal at these low dosages.

Salt Supplementation. Salt tablets or salting of food is only seldom needed to aid in controlling hyponatremia. The use of salt supplementation is reported to be beneficial by other investigators.[155, 156] Salt supplementation may be used to reduce unusually high doses of fludrocortisone. Hydrocortisone therapy in addition to mineralocorticoids is an alternative to salting the food.

DOGS WITH SECONDARY HYPOADRENOCORTICISM

Animals with secondary hypoadrenocorticism do not typically have mineralocorticoid deficiency. Therefore, daily doses of glucocorticoids, as described previously, are usually sufficient to control the signs associated with this disease. However, the veterinarian must periodically monitor serum electrolyte concentrations, since some animals that are believed to be pituitary-deficient ultimately are found to have primary adrenal insufficiency.[145]

Dogs that have developed signs after o,p'-DDD therapy usually can be controlled with glucocorticoids only. However, mineralocorticoid deficiency has been reported and must be ruled out, using serum electrolyte concentrations.[143]

Iatrogenic hypocortisolism caused by the overuse of glucocorticoids must be treated conservatively. Usually such animals are treated by slowly tapering the dose of prednisone. Initially one must attempt to achieve an alternate-day dosage schedule and ultimately wean dogs off all medication.[133]

PROGNOSIS

The prognosis in dogs with hypoadrenocorticism has been excellent when oral therapy has been used. Such

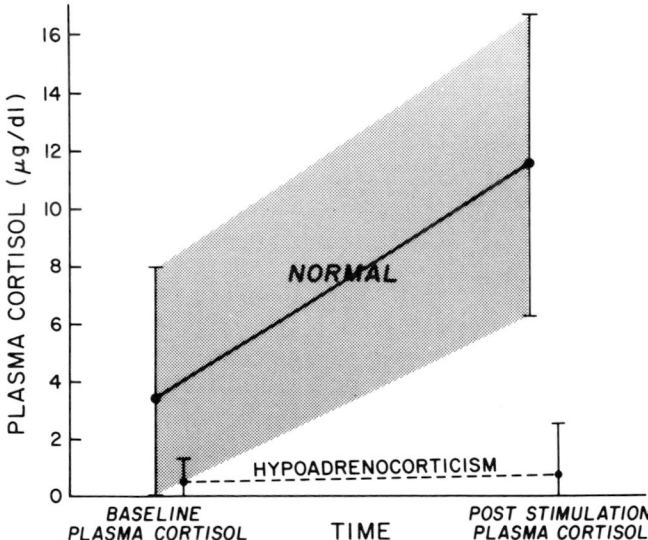

FIGURE 97–26. Radioimmunoassay plasma cortisol concentrations before and after exogenous ACTH stimulation. The ranges are means ± 2 SD.

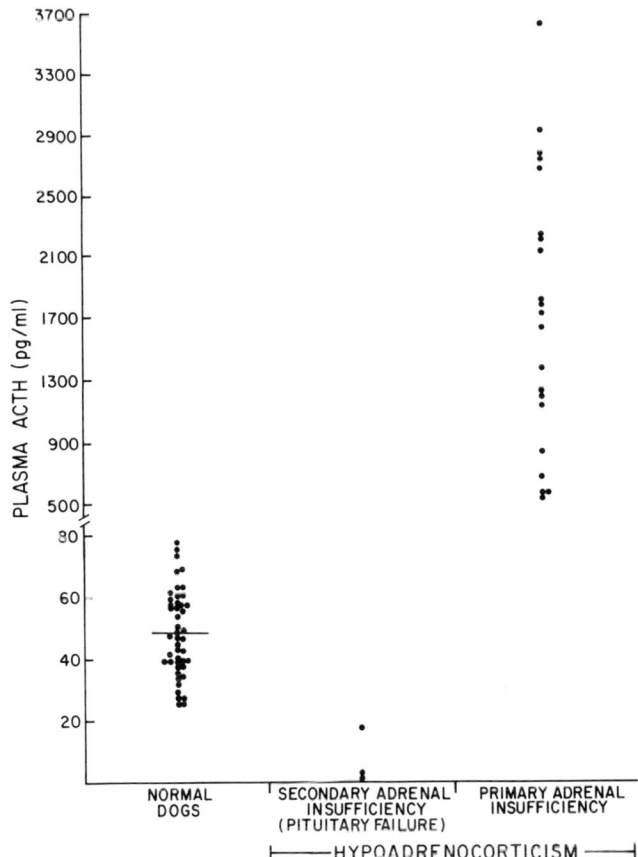

FIGURE 97–27. Plasma endogenous ACTH concentrations in normal dogs, dogs with adrenocortical failure causing lack of negative feedback to the pituitary, and dogs with pituitary failure to secrete ACTH, causing adrenocortical atrophy. (From Feldman, EC: *In* Ettinger, SJ (ed.): Textbook of Veterinary Internal Medicine, 2nd ed. Philadelphia, WB Saunders, 1983, p 1668.)

dogs have led normal lives, with few, if any, restrictions. The most important factor in long-term response to therapy is owner education. This disease must be carefully described and owners warned of the consequences of apparent mild illnesses. All owners should have glucocorticoids available to administer to their dogs in times of stress. Some owners have learned how to give injections and keep parenteral glucocorticoids on hand. Veterinarians should be aware of the increased glucocorticoid requirements of hypoadrenal dogs that undergo surgery or during times of illness with a non-adrenal-related disease.

HYPOADRENOCORTICISM IN THE CAT

Only eight documented cases of spontaneous hypoadrenocorticism have been described in cats.[157, 158] The eight cats were one to nine years of age, with no breed predisposition. Clinical signs observed in these cats included lethargy (eight cats), anorexia (eight cats), dehydration (six cats), weakness (six cats), prolonged capillary refill time (five cats), weak pulse (four cats), microcardia (four cats), vomiting (two cats), polydipsia/polyuria (two cats), bradycardia (one cat), and weight

loss (one cat). Pretreatment hematologic and serum biochemical findings included lymphocytosis (three cats), eosinophilia (one cat), mild anemia (two cats), azotemia (eight cats), hyperphosphatemia (seven cats), and hypercalcemia (one cat). Despite moderate to severe azotemia and dehydration, the urine specific gravity was below 1.030 in four of five cats tested, consistent with the impaired urine-concentrating capability seen in hypoadrenocorticoid dogs (see section on BUN and Urinalysis). All eight cats had serum electrolyte imbalances characteristic of primary hypoadrenocorticism: hyperkalemia, hyponatremia, and hypochloremia. The diagnosis was further supported in each cat by demonstrating lack of adrenocortical reserve on ACTH stimulation (as depicted in the dogs in Figure 97–26). In five cats tested, plasma endogenous ACTH concentrations were extremely elevated (as depicted in the dogs with primary hypoadrenocorticism in Figure 97–27). Four cats at necropsy had severe adrenocortical atrophy. Treated cats are being maintained with daily oral fludrocortisone or monthly injectable desoxycorticosterone pivalate. It would appear that some cats have a slower initial response to therapy than is typical of dogs with hypoadrenocorticism.

Iatrogenic feline hypoadrenocorticism has been reported in association with the use of megestrol acetate. This occurs in cats that receive proper dosages. The adrenocortical suppression occurs as early as two weeks after initiating the medication.[159] Clinical signs suggestive of hypoadrenocorticism have been seen. Withdrawal of medication does result in rapid improvement.

References

1. Ganong, WF: Review of Medical Physiology, 11th ed. Los Altos, Calif, Lange Medical Publications, 1983.
2. Upton, GV, et al.: Evidence for the internal feedback phenomenon in human subjects: Effects of ACTH on plasma CRF. Acta Endocrinol 73:437, 1973.
3. Jones, MT: Control of adrenocortical hormone secretion. *In* James, VHT (ed): The adrenal gland. New York, Raven Press, 1979, p 93.
4. Tyrrell, JB and Forsham, PH: Glucocorticoids and adrenal androgens. *In* Greenspan, FS and Forsham, PH (eds): Basic and clinical endocrinology. Los Altos, Calif, Lange Med Publications, 1983.
5. Nelson, DH: The adrenal cortex. Philadelphia, WB Saunders, 1980, p 240.
6. Kemppainen, RJ and Sartin, JL: Evidence for episodic but not circadian activity in plasma concentrations of adrenocorticotropin, cortisol and thyroxine in dogs. J Endocrinol 103:219, 1984.
7. Retiene, K, et al.: A correlative study of endocrine rhythms in rats. Acta Endocrinol 57:615, 1968.
8. Mangli, G, et al.: Control of adrenocorticotropic hormone secretion. *In* Martini, L and Ganong, WF (eds): Neuroendocrinology. New York, Academic Press, 1966, p 298.
9. Hume, DM, et al.: Blood and urinary 17-hydroxy corticosteroids in patients with severe burns. Ann Surg 143:316, 1956.
10. Feldman, EC: Comparison of ACTH response and dexamethasone suppression as screening tests in canine hyperadrenocorticism. JAVMA 182:505, 1983.
11. Feldman, EC: Distinguishing dogs with functioning adrenocortical tumors from dogs with pituitary-dependent hyperadrenocorticism. JAVMA 183:195, 1983.
12. Feldman, EC: The adrenal cortex. *In* Ettinger, SJ (ed): Textbook

of Veterinary Internal Medicine, 2nd ed. Philadelphia, WB Saunders, 1983, p 1650.

13. Peterson, ME, et al.: Immunocytochemical study of the hypophysis in 25 dogs with pituitary-dependent hyperadrenocorticism. Acta Endocrinol 101:15, 1982.

14. Krieger, DT: Physiopathology of Cushing's disease. Endocrinol Rev 4:22, 1983.

15. Peterson, ME, et al.: Effects of spontaneous hyperadrenocorticism on serum thyroid hormone concentrations in the dog. Am J Vet Res 45:2034, 1984.

16. Peterson, ME and Drucker, WD: Advances in the diagnosis and treatment of canine Cushing's syndrome. In Proceed. Gaines Vet. Symp., Baton Rouge, LA, 1981, p 17.

17. Feldman, EC and Nelson, RN: Canine and Feline Endocrinology and Reproduction. Philadelphia, WB Saunders, 1987.

18. Meijer, JC: Canine hyperadrenocorticism. In Kirk, RW (ed): Current Veterinary Therapy VII. Philadelphia, WB Saunders, 1980, p 975.

19. Capen, CC and Koestner, A: Functional chromophobe adenomas of the canine adenohypophysis: An ultrastructural evaluation of a neoplasm of pituitary corticotrophs. Pathol Vet 4:326, 1967.

20. Peterson, ME: Hyperadrenocorticism. Vet Clin North Am 14:731, 1984.

21. Pennick, DG, et al.: Radiographic features of canine hyperadrenocorticism caused by functioning adrenocortical tumors: 23 cases (1978–1986). JAVMA 192:1604, 1608, 1988.

22. Ling, GV, et al.: Canine hyperadrenocorticism: Pretreatment clinical and laboratory evaluation of 117 cases. JAVMA 174:1211, 1979.

23. Lubberink, AAME: Diagnosis and treatment of canine Cushing's syndrome. PhD Thesis, University of Utrecht, Utrecht, The Netherlands, 1977.

24. Feldman, EC: The effect of functional adrenocortical tumors on plasma cortisol and corticotropin concentrations in dogs. JAVMA 178:823, 1981.

25. Capen, CC, et al.: Endocrine diseases. In Ettinger, SJ (ed): Textbook of Veterinary Internal Medicine. Philadelphia, WB Saunders, 1975, p 1395.

26. Peterson, ME, et al.: Plasma cortisol response to exogenous ACTH in 22 dogs with hyperadrenocorticism caused by an adrenocortical neoplasia. JAVMA 180:542, 1982.

27. Owens, JM and Drucker, WD: Hyperadrenocorticism in the dog: Canine Cushing's syndrome. Vet Clin North Am 7:583, 1977.

28. Osborne, CA, et al.: Canine and feline urology. Philadelphia, WB Saunders, 1972.

29. Aubry, RH, et al.: Measurement of the osmotic threshold for vasopressin release in human subjects, and its modification by cortisol. J Clin Endocrinol Metab 25:1481, 1965.

30. Sadowski, J, et al.: Reduced urine concentration in dogs exposed to cold: Relation to plasma ADH and 17-OHCS. Am J Physiol 222:607, 1972.

31. Share, L and Travis, RH: Interrelations between the adrenal cortex and the posterior pituitary. Fed Proc 30:1378, 1971.

32. Walton, J and Ney, RL: Current concepts of corticosteroids, uses and abuses. Disease-a-Month 3, June, 1975.

33. Sjoberg, HE, et al.: Thromboembolic complications, heparin treatment and increased coagulation factors in Cushing's syndrome. Acta Med Scand 199:95, 1976.

34. Small, M, et al.: Thromboembolic complications in Cushing's syndrome. Clin Endocrinol 19:503, 1983.

35. Burns, MG, et al.: Pulmonary artery thrombosis in three dogs with hyperadrenocorticism. JAVMA 178:388, 1981.

36. Duncan, ID, et al.: Myotonia in canine Cushing's disease. Vet Rec 100:30, 1977.

37. Griffiths, IR and Duncan, ID: Myotonia in the dog: A report of four cases. Vet Rec 93:184, 1973.

38. Greene, CE, et al.: Myopathy associated with hyperadrenocorticism in the dog. JAVMA 174:1310, 1979.

39. Badylak, SF and Van Vleet, JF: Sequential morphologic and clinicopathologic alterations in dogs with experimentally induced glucocorticoid hepatopathy. Am J Vet Res 42:1310, 1981.

40. Badylak, SF and Van Vleet, JF: Tissue gamma-glutamyl transpeptidase activity and hepatic ultrastructural alterations in dogs with experimentally induced glucocorticoid hepatopathy. Am J Vet Res 43:649, 1982.

41. Feldman, EC and Tyrrell, JB: Plasma testosterone, plasma glucose, and plasma insulin concentrations in spontaneous canine Cushing's syndrome. Salt Lake City, The Endocrine Society, 1982, p 343.

42. Feldman, BF and Feldman, EC: Routine laboratory abnormalities in endocrine disease. Vet Clin North Am 7:443, 1977.

43. Peterson, ME, et al.: Diagnosis and management of concurrent diabetes mellitus and hyperadrenocorticism in thirty dogs. JAVMA 178:66, 1981.

44. Katherman, KA, et al.: Hyperadrenalcorticism and diabetes in the dog. JAAHA 16:705, 1980.

45. Feldman, EC: Diabetes mellitus. In Kirk, RW (ed): Current Veterinary Therapy VI. Philadelphia, WB Saunders, 1977, p 1001.

46. Wolfsheimer, KJ, et al.: Effects of prednisolone on glucose tolerance and insulin secretion in the dog. Am J Vet Res 47:1011, 1986.

47. Dorner, JL, et al.: Corticosteroid indication of an isoenzyme of alkaline phosphatase in the dog. Am J Vet Res 35:1457, 1974.

48. Joles, JA and Mulnix, JA: Polyuria and polydipsia. In Kirk, RW (ed): Current Veterinary Therapy VI. Philadelphia, WB Saunders, 1977, p 1050.

49. Kallet, A and Cowgill, LD: Hypertensive states in the dog. In Proceed ACVIM, Salt Lake City, 1982, p 79.

50. Huntley, K, et al.: The radiological features of canine Cushing's syndrome: A review of forty-eight cases. J Small Anim Pract 23:369, 1982.

51. Hoeldtke, RD, et al.: Functional significance of idiopathic adrenal calcification in the adult. Clin Endocrinol 12:319, 1980.

52. Ticer, JW: Roentgen signs of endocrine disease. Vet Clin North Am 7:465, 1977.

53. Ferguson, DC: Thyroid function tests in the dog: Recent concepts. Vet Clin North Am 14:783, 1984.

54. Peterson, ME and Altszuler, N: Suppression of growth hormone secretion in spontaneous canine hyperadrenocorticism and its reversal after treatment. Am J Vet Res 42:1881, 1981.

55. Feldman, EC: Influence of non-cardiac disease on the heart. In Kirk, RW (ed): Current Veterinary Therapy VII. Philadelphia, WB Saunders, 1980, p 340.

56. King, RR, et al.: Pulmonary function studies in a dog with pulmonary thromboembolism associated with Cushing's disease. JAAHA 21:555, 1985.

57. Feldman, EC, et al.: Comparison of aqueous porcine ACTH with synthetic ACTH in adrenal stimulation tests of the female dog. Am J Vet Res 43:522, 1982.

58. Feldman, BF, et al.: Hemostatic abnormalities in canine Cushing's syndrome. Res Vet Sci (in press).

59. Kasperlik-Zaluska, AA, et al.: Nelson's syndrome: Incidence and prognosis. Clin Endocrinol 19:693, 1983.

60. Kemppainen, RJ and Zenoble, RD: Non-dexamethasone-suppressible, pituitary-dependent hyperadrenocorticism in a dog. JAVMA 187:276, 1985.

61. Baxter, JD and Tyrrell, JB: The adrenal cortex. In Felig, P, et al. (eds): Endocrinology and Metabolism. New York, McGraw-Hill, 1981, p 385.

62. Johnston, SD and Mather, EC: Canine plasma cortisol measured by radioimmunoassay: Clinical absence of diurnal variation and results of ACTH stimulation and dexamethasone suppression tests. Am J Vet Res 39:1766, 1978.

63. Rijnberk, A, et al.: Canine Cushing's syndrome. Zentralbl Veterinaermed 16:13, 1969.

64. Siegel, ET, et al.: Cushing's syndrome in the dog. JAVMA 157:2081, 1970.

65. Halliwell, REW, et al.: The value of plasma corticosteroid assays in the diagnosis of Cushing's disease in the dog. J Small Anim Pract 12:453, 1971.

66. Schechter, RD, et al.: Treatment of Cushing's syndrome in the dog with an adrenocorticolytic agent (o,p'-DDD). JAVMA 162:629, 1973.

67. Smith, MC and Feldman, EC: Serum cortisol responses to synthetic ACTH and dexamethasone sodium phosphate in normal felines. Washington, DC, ACVIM Scient Proceed, 1986.

68. Feldman, EC and Tyrrell, JB: Adrenocorticotropic effects of a synthetic polypeptide α1-24 corticotropin in normal dogs. JAAHA 13:494, 1977.

69. Roberts, SM, et al.: Effect of ophthalmic prednisolone acetate

on the canine adrenal gland and hepatic function. Am J Vet Res 45:1711, 1984.

70. Lothrop, CD and Oliver, JW: Diagnosis of canine Cushing's syndrome based on multiple steroid analysis and dexamethasone turnover kinetics. Am J Vet Res 45:2304, 1984.

71. Toutain, PL, et al.: Pharmacokinetics of dexamethasone and its effect on adrenal gland function in the dog. Am J Vet Res 44:212, 1983.

72. Feldman, EC: Evaluation of a combined dexamethasone suppression/ACTH stimulation test in dogs with hyperadrenocorticism. JAVMA 187:49, 1985.

73. Feldman, EC: Evaluation of a six-hour combined dexamethasone suppression/ACTH stimulation test in dogs with hyperadrenocorticism. JAVMA 189:1562, 1986.

74. Van Cauter, E and Refetoff, S: Evidence for two subtypes of Cushing's disease based on the analysis of episodic cortisol secretion. N Engl J Med 312:1343, 1985.

75. Kaufman, J and Macy, DW: The glucagon tolerance test as a screening method for canine hyperadrenocorticism. ACVIM Scient Proc, 1984, p 30.

76. Eiler, H and Oliver, J: Combined dexamethasone suppression and cosyntropin (synthetic ACTH) stimulation test in the dog: New approach to testing of adrenal gland function. Am J Vet Res 41:1243, 1980.

77. Reimers, TJ: Radioimmunoassays and diagnostic tests for thyroid and adrenal disorders. Comp Cont Ed Pract Vet 4:65, 1982.

78. Eiler, H, et al.: AM: Stages of hyperadrenocorticism: Response of hyperadrenocorticoid dogs to the combined dexamethasone suppression–ACTH stimulation test. JAVMA 185:289, 1984.

79. Rogers, WA and Ruebner, BH: A retrospective study of probable glucocorticoid-induced hepatopathy in dogs. JAVMA 170:603, 1977.

80. Aron, DC, et al.: Cushing's syndrome: Problems in diagnosis. Medicine 60:25, 1981.

81. Lamberts, S, et al.: Adrenocorticotropin-secreting pituitary adenomas originate from the anterior or the intermediate lobe in Cushing's disease: Differences in the regulation of hormone secretion. J Clin Endocrinol Metab 54:286, 1982.

82. Kantrowitz, BM, et al.: Adrenal ultrasonography in the dog. Vet Radiol 27:15, 1986.

83. Vale, W and Greer, M: Corticotropin-releasing factor. Fed Proc 44:145, 1985.

84. Peterson, ME and Orth, DN: Corticotropin releasing hormone stimulation test: An aid in the differential diagnosis of canine Cushing's syndrome. Proceed ACVIM, San Diego, 1985, p 151.

85. Mulnix, JA, et al.: Gamma camera imaging of bilateral adrenocortical tumors in the dog. Am J Vet Res 37:1467, 1976.

86. Zerbe, CA, et al.: Use of metyrapone for differentiation of spontaneous hyperadrenocorticism in the dog. Washington, DC, ACVIM Scient Proc, 1986.

87. Johnston, DE: Adrenalectomy in the dog. In Bojrab, MJ, (ed): Current techniques in small animal surgery. Philadelphia, Lea & Febiger, 1983, p 386.

88. Johnston, DE: Adrenalectomy via retroperitoneal approach in dogs. JAVMA 170:1092, 1977.

89. Cohen, SJ and Kneiser, M: Hyperadrenocorticism in a dog with adrenal and pituitary neoplasia. JAAHA 16:259, 1980.

90. Lubberink, AAME: Therapy for spontaneous hyperadrenocorticism. In Kirk, RW (ed): Current Veterinary Therapy VII. Philadelphia, WB Saunders, 1980, p 979.

91. Nelson, AA and Woodard, G: Severe adrenal cortical atrophy (cytotoxic) and hepatic damage produced in dogs by feeding 2,2-bis (parachlorophenyl)-1, 1-trichloroethane (DDD or TDE). Arch Pathol 47:387, 1949.

92. Kirk, GR and Jensen, HE: Toxic effects of o,p'-DDD in the normal dog. JAAHA 11:765, 1975.

93. Kirk, GR, et al.: Effects of o,p'-DDD on plasma cortisol levels and histology of the adrenal gland in normal dogs. JAAHA 10:179, 1974.

94. Nelson, RW, et al.: Effect of o,p'-DDD therapy on endogenous ACTH concentrations in dogs with hypophysis-dependent hyperadrenocorticism. Am J Vet Res 46:1534, 1985.

95. Krieger, DT and Luria, M: Effectiveness of cyproheptadine in decreasing plasma ACTH concentrations in Nelson's syndrome. J Clin Endocrinol Metab 43:1179, 1976.

96. Krieger, DT, et al.: Cyproheptadine-induced remission of Cushing's disease. N Engl J Med 293:898, 1975.

97. Peterson, ME and Drucker, WD: Cyproheptadine treatment of spontaneous pituitary ACTH-dependent canine Cushing's disease. Clin Res 26:703, 1978.

98. Kennedy, AL, et al.: ACTH and cortisol response to bromocriptine and results of long-term therapy in Cushing's disease. Acta Endocrinol 89:461, 1978.

99. Drucker, WD and Peterson, ME: Pharmacologic treatment of pituitary-dependent canine Cushing's disease. Program 62nd Ann Mtg Endocrine Soc, San Francisco, 1980, p 89.

100. Potts, GO, et al.: Selective inhibitor of adrenal 3-β-hydroxysteroid dehydrogenase: Delta^5-isomerase. Endocrinology 96:58, 1975.

101. Potts, GO, et al.: Trilostane, an orally active inhibitor of steroid biosynthesis. Steroids 32:257, 1978.

102. Dewis, P, et al.: Experience with trilostane in the treatment of Cushing's syndrome. Clin Endocrinol 18:533, 1983.

103. Santen, RJ, et al.: Mechanism of action of aminoglutethimide in breast cancer. Lancet 1:44, 1979.

104. Misbin, RI, et al.: Aminoglutethimide in the treatment of Cushing's syndrome. J Clin Pharm 16:645, 1976.

105. Marek, J, et al.: Long-term treatment of Cushing's syndrome with aminoglutethimide. Endokrinologie 58:234, 1971.

106. Jeffcoate, WJ, et al.: Metyrapone in long-term management of Cushing's disease. Br Med J 2:215, 1977.

107. Pont, A, et al.: Ketoconazole blocks adrenal steroid synthesis. Ann Intern Med 97:370, 1982.

108. Willard, MD, et al.: Ketoconazole-induced changes in canine steroidogenesis. San Diego, ACVIM Scient Proc, 1985.

109. Willard, MD, et al.: Hormonal and clinical pathologic changes with long-term ketoconazole therapy in the dog and cat. Washington, DC, ACVIM Scient Proc, 1986.

110. Dow, SW, et al.: Results following radiation therapy of functional pituitary neoplasms in dogs. ACVIM Scient Proc, Washington, DC, 1986.

111. Scott, RS, et al.: Intermittent Cushing's disease with spontaneous remission. Clin Endocrinol 11:561, 1979.

112. Meijer, JC, et al.: Cushing's syndrome due to adrenocortical adenoma in a cat. Tijdschr Diergeneeskd 103:1048, 1978.

113. Fox, JG and Beatty, JO. A case report of complicated diabetes mellitus in a cat. JAAHA 11:129, 1975.

114. Swift, GA and Brown, RH: Surgical treatment of Cushing's syndrome in the cat. Vet Rec 99:374, 1976.

115. Nelson, RW, et al.: Hyperadrenocorticism in cats: Seven cases (1978–1987). JAVMA 193:245, 1988.

116. Smith, MC and Feldman, EC: Plasma endogenous ACTH concentrations and plasma cortisol responses to synthetic ACTH and dexamethasone sodium phosphate in healthy cats. AJVR 48:1719, 1987.

117. Swingle, WW and Pfiffner, JJ: An aqueous extract of the suprarenal cortex which maintains the life of bilaterally adrenalectomized cats. Science 71:321, 1930.

118. Loeb, RF: Effect of sodium chloride in the treatment of a patient with Addison's disease. Proc Soc Exp Bio Med 30:808, 1933.

119. Thorn, GW, et al.: Addison's disease; evaluation of synthetic desoxycorticosterone acetate therapy in 158 patients. Ann Intern Med 16:1053, 1942.

120. Kendall, EC: A chemical and physiological investigation of the supra-renal cortex. Cold Spring Harbor Symp Quant Biol 5:299, 1937.

121. Nelson, DH, et al.: Isolation of a steroid hormone from the adrenal vein blood of dogs. Science 111:578, 1950.

122. Nelson, DH and Samuels, LT: A method for the determination of 17-hydroxycorticosteroids in blood; 17-hydroxycorticosterone in the peripheral circulation. Clin Endocrinol Metab 12:519, 1952.

123. Gassner, FX, et al.: Isolation of an androgenic compound from the adrenal venous blood of cows. Proc Soc Exp Biol Med 77:829, 1951.

124. Simpson, SA, et al.: Secretion of a salt-retaining hormone by the mammalian adrenal cortex. Lancet 2:226, 1952.

125. Hadlow, WJ: Adrenal cortical atrophy in the dog. Report of three cases. Am J Pathol 29:353, 1953.

126. Keeton, KS, et al.: Adrenocortical insufficiency in dogs. Mod Vet Pract 53:25, 1972.

127. Mulnix, JA: Hypoadrenocorticism in the dog. JAAHA 7:220, 1971.

128. Willard, MD, et al.: Canine hypoadrenocorticism: Report of 37

cases and review of 39 previously reported cases. JAVMA 180:59, 1982.

129. Irvine, WJ, et al.: A clinical and immunological study of adrenal cortical insufficiency (Addison's disease). Clin Exp Immunol 2:31, 1967.

130. Irvine, WJ and Barnes, EW: Adrenocortical insufficiency. Clin Endocrinol Metab 1:549, 1972.

131. Bethune, JE: The adrenal cortex. Kalamazoo, MI, The Upjohn Co, Scope Monograph, 1974.

132. Cryer, PE: The adrenal cortex. *In* Cryer, PE (ed): Diagnostic Endocrinology. New York, Oxford University Press, 1976, p 61.

133. Scott, DW and Greene, CE: Iatrogenic secondary adrenocortical insufficiency in dogs. JAAHA 10:555, 1974.

134. Meikle, AW and Tyler, FH: Potency and duration of action of glucocorticoids. Effects of hydrocortisone, prednisone, and dexamethasone on human pituitary-adrenal function. Am J Med 63:200, 1977.

135. Kemppainen, RJ, et al.: Adrenocortical suppression in the dog after a single dose of methylprednisolone acetate. Am J Vet Res 42:822, 1981.

136. Kemppainen, RJ, et al.: Adrenocortical suppression in the dog given a single intramuscular dose of prednisone or triamcinolone acetonide. Am J Vet Res 43:204, 1982.

137. Liddle, GW: The physiology of adrenal cortical function. *In* Thorn, GW: Clinician I, The Adrenal Gland. New York, Medcom, 1971, p 1.

138. Fundor, JW, et al.: Effect of K+ on the secretion of aldosterone. Endocrinology 85:381, 1969.

139. Boyd, JE, et al.: Importance of potassium in the regulation of aldosterone production. Circ Res 32:1, 1973.

140. Liddle, GW and Melmon, KL: The adrenals. *In* Williams, RH, (ed): Textbook of Endocrinology. Philadelphia, WB Saunders, 1974, p 232.

141. Tyrrell, JB and Forsham, PH: Chronic adrenal cortical insufficiency. *In* Conn, HF and Conn, RB, Jr (eds): Current Diagnosis. Philadelphia, WB Saunders, 1974, p 742.

142. Werner, L: Immunological diseases affecting internal organ systems. *In* Ettinger, SJ (ed): Textbook of Veterinary Internal Medicine, 2nd ed. Philadelphia, WB Saunders, 1983, p 2158.

143. Feldman, EC and Tyrrell, JB: Hypoadrenocorticism. Vet Clin North Am 7:555, 1977.

144. Exton, JH: Regulation of gluconeogenesis by glucocorticoids. *In* Baxter, JD and Rousseau, GG (eds): Glucocorticoid hormone action. New York, Springer-Verlag, 1979, p 535.

145. Rogers, W, et al.: Atypical hypoadrenocorticism in three dogs. JAVMA 179:155, 1981.

146. DiBartola, SP, et al.: Clinicopathologic findings resembling hypoadrenocorticism in dogs with primary gastrointestinal disease. JAVMA 187:60, 1985.

147. Rich, LJ, et al.: Elevated serum potassium associated with delayed separation of serum from clotted blood in dogs of the Akita breed. Vet Clin Pathol 15:12, 1986.

148. Rendano, VT and Alexander, JE: Heart size changes in experimentally induced adrenal insufficiency in the dog: A radiographic study. J Am Vet Radiol Soc 17:57, 1976.

149. Ettinger, PO, et al.: Hyperkalemia, cardiac conduction, and the electrocardiogram: A review. Am Heart J 88:360, 1974.

150. Cohen, HC, et al.: The nature and type of arrhythmias in acute experimental hyperkalemia in the intact dog. Am Heart J 82:777, 1971.

151. Rijnberk, A, et al.: Investigation on the adrenocortical function of normal dogs. J Endocrinol 41:387, 1968.

152. Wilson, RB, et al.: Response of dogs to corticotropin measured by 17-hydroxycorticosteroid excretion. Am J Vet Res 28:313, 1967.

153. Olson, PN, et al.: Effects of storage on concentration of hydrocortisone (cortisol) in canine serum and plasma. Am J Vet Res 42:1618, 1981.

154. Mulnix, JA and Smith, KW: Hyperadrenocorticism in a dog: A case report. J Small Anim Pract 16:193, 1975.

155. Schaer, M: Hypoadrenocorticism. *In* Kirk, RW (ed): Current Veterinary Therapy VII. Philadelphia, WB Saunders, 1980, p 983.

156. Lorenz, MD: Canine hyperadrenocorticism: Diagnosis and treatment. Comp Cont Educ 1:315, 1979.

157. Peterson, ME and Feinman, JM: Hypercalcemia associated with hypoadrenocorticism in 16 dogs. JAVMA 181:802, 1982.

158. Peterson, ME and Greco, DS: Primary hypoadrenocorticism in the cat. ACVIM Scient Proc, Washington, DC, May 1986.

159. Chastain, CB, et al.: Adrenocortical suppression in cats administered megestrol acetate. ACVIM Scient Proc, Salt Lake City, 1982, p 54.

THE REPRODUCTIVE SYSTEM

98 REPRODUCTIVE PHYSIOLOGY AND ENDOCRINOLOGY OF THE FEMALE AND MALE

VICTOR M. SHILLE

The major functions of the reproductive system include production of gametes by the male and female, the transport of gametes of both sexes to the fertilization site, the nurturing of the resulting conceptus during its differentiation and growth, and the delivery of the conceptus into independent life. The structures involved in these functions are the gonads, which produce the gametes, the tubular tracts that transport the gametes, and the conceptus.

In this chapter are reviewed the events that constitute healthy functioning of the reproductive system in the domestic carnivores, the dog and the cat. The material presented focuses on clinically significant processes as they are currently understood.

THE CANINE AND FELINE FEMALE

Structural Peculiarities

The vestibule in the bitch is entered through the vulvar labial cleft (Figure 98–1). Immediately cranial to the ventral labial commissure is the well-developed clitoral fossa, containing the clitoris. The vestibule, located dorsocranially, is oriented 60 degrees to the horizontal and terminates at the vestibulovaginal junction, just cranial to the urethral meatus. The junction lies over the ischiatic arch of the pelvis and is formed by the cingulum, an annular, narrow band that slightly constricts the vestibule. Hymen remnants found at the cingulum may interfere with entry into the vagina. The vagina is oriented horizontally in the standing bitch, measuring from the urethral meatus to the dorsal median postcervical fold approximately from 5 cm in a Pomeranian to 14 cm in a beagle or 25 cm in a Great Dane.

There are three anatomic regions distinguishable in the vagina (Figure 98–2). The plicate area that occupies the caudal three fifths with permanent longitudinal folds, the rugose area cranial to the plicate with a smooth, even mucosa, and the pseudocervix, located ventrally to the postcervical fold and caudally to the cervix. The tubular cervix protrudes into the cranial vagina. The cervical os faces caudoventrally at 45 degrees to the horizontal, into a cup shaped depression, the anterior vaginal fossa (Figure 98–3).

When passing instruments into the vagina of the bitch, care should be taken to enter at a dorsocranial angle to avoid the clitoral fossa passing through the vestibule and to reach the vagina proper. A vaginoscope of adequate length is needed to inspect the vagina up to the postcervical fold. Visualization of the cervix is difficult or impossible with currently available instruments.

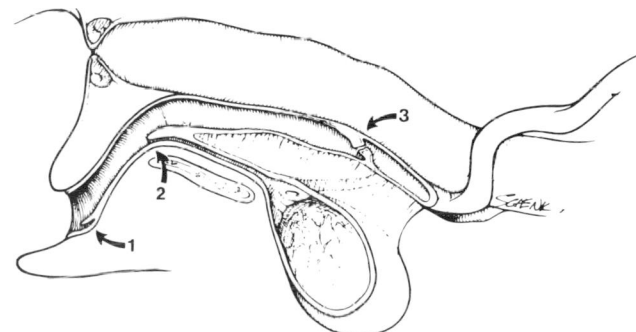

FIGURE 98–1. Midsagittal section of extra-abdominal reproductive organs in the bitch. The clitoral fossa and clitoris (1) are at the caudal border, and the urethral meatus (2) is at the cranial border of the inclined vestibule. The horizontal vagina extends to the dorsal median postcervical fold (3), which overlies the pseudocervix. In the living animal the vaginal lumen is collapsed unless dilated by a speculum or by the penis during coitus. The cervical os faces ventrally on a cup-shaped vaginal fossa,

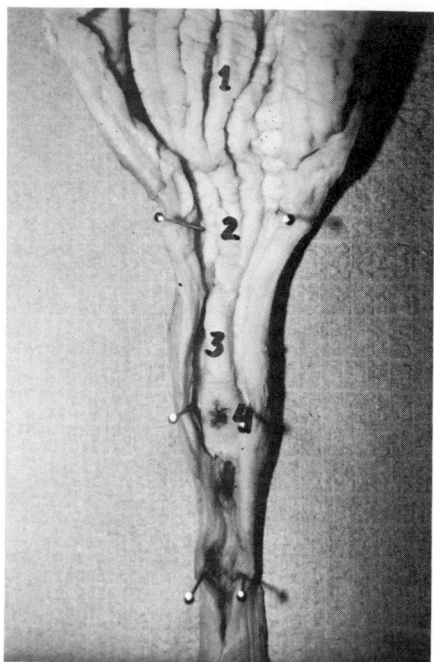

FIGURE 98–2. The anatomic regions in the vagina are the plicate area (1), with permanent longitudinal folds, the rugose area (2), cranial to the plicate, characterized by smooth mucosa during anestrus and diestrus; and the pseudocervix (3), which terminates at the cervix (4).

In the queen, the vulval labiae are less prominent than in the bitch, and the vestibule, vagina, and cervix lie in a straight, horizontal line. The vestibulovaginal junction and cingulum of the queen are narrow and nonelastic when she is not in estrus and, therefore, difficult to enter, even when she is under general anesthesia.

In the bitch and the queen the uterus is a tubular, Y-shaped organ oriented horizontally and situated just ventral to the descending colon. Each horn terminates in a tortuous uterine tube (oviduct) that curves around within the mesovarium. The mesovarium forms a bursa that completely enfolds the ovary and makes viewing the ovary difficult, particularly if there is fat in the bursal tissue. Incising the bursa to inspect the ovary may result in injury to the uterine tube. The ovaries are caudal to the kidneys. The right ovary is more cranial than the left and is dorsal to the descending colon. The left ovary is between the abdominal wall and the left colon. The microstructure of the canine and feline ovary is similar to that described in other mammals.

Hormonally Induced Changes in the Vagina

The vaginal epithelium in many mammals is affected by estrogen. The response is predictable and dose-dependent, forming the basis of a bioassay developed in the rat (Allen-Doisy test) that was used to measure the biologic potency of estrogenic compounds. A similar response is seen in the bitch and queen. Increasing amounts of estradiol-17β produced by the maturing graafian follicles cause multiplication of the epithelial cells that line the basement membrane of the vaginal mucosa. As the cells increase in number they become stacked on one another and the mucosal epithelium thickens from 3 to 5 layers found during anestrus to 20 or more layers found at the end of proestrus. As cells are moved further away from the life-sustaining capillaries in the submucosa, they die (cornify) and form the layers of cornified epithelium characteristic of the estrogen-stimulated vagina. Changes that reflect the progressive cornification of the epithelium may be seen by microscopic and vaginoscopic examination.

Exfoliated cells are collected for microscopic examination by passing a cotton-tipped swab moistened in sterile saline solution into the posterior vagina, rolling the swab on a microscope slide, and staining the preparation with one of several commercial cell stains. Care must be taken not to collect cells from the vestibule or the clitoral fossa; these cells are frequently keratinized and will give a confusing impression of the female's reproductive status. It is possible to microscopically differentiate four distinct types of epithelial cells in the bitch and queen (Figure 98–4).[1, 2]

1. The parabasal cells lie close to the basement membrane and are the smallest, roundest epithelial cells seen in a vaginal smear. These cells have large nuclei, and thus have the largest nucleus-cytoplasm ratio of the

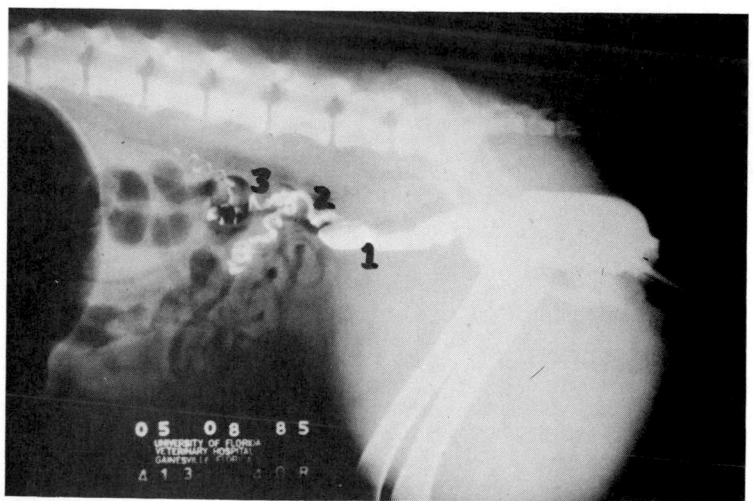

FIGURE 98–3. A lateral contrast vaginogram of a bitch in estrus. Radiographic contrast material (20 ml) was infused into the vagina of a 15-kg bitch through a retention catheter. The cranial vaginal fossa is outlined, cupping the cervix ventrally (1). Contrast material has entered the cervix and is filling the uterine body (2) and horns (3). (Courtesy J. Gossett, 1985.)

epithelial cells. The nuclear membrane is well defined, and the chromatin takes up the stain clearly, giving the nucleus a mottled appearance.

2. The intermediate cells vary in size and shape but are usually twice the size of parabasal cells and may be round, oval, or rectangular. Their nuclei are similar in size and appearance to those in the parabasal cells.

There is some disagreement about the terminology used for the cells in the next stage of cornification. Olson[3] and Concannon[4] separate them into a class by themselves, calling them intermediate-superficial or large intermediate cells, because they are larger than the intermediate cells and have a more angular, folded cytoplasm. The author prefers to classify them with the intermediate cells, since their nuclei have the same size and appearance.

3. Superficial cells are recognized by the diminished nucleus with a nongranular, uniformly dense appearance. These cells have a large, angular, and occasionally wrinkled cytoplasm. They are the largest epithelial cell found in the vaginal smear of the bitch. In the queen there occurs an additional cell, with all the characteristics of a superficial cell, except that it is much smaller than the superficial cell found in estrus. The small superficial cell occurs randomly throughout all stages of the cycle.

4. The anuclear cells, also called anuclear squames, represent the final stage of cornification or cell death. The nuclei are incapable of taking up stain and become virtually invisible. The cytoplasmic borders are indistinct or sharply defined and creased. Anuclear cells may be grouped with superficial cells[3, 4] when doing differential counts, but it is incorrect to refer to superficial cells, which contain visible nuclei, as cornified cells, since that term is reserved for the anuclear squames. In the queen, there is clearly a predominance of anuclear cells during the period of greatest cornification; this appears not to be the case in the bitch.

An alternate method for judging the response of the vaginal epithelium to follicular estrogen is direct observation of the thickening and resultant folding of the mucosa with a vaginoscope.[5] This method is easily used in all but the most nervous bitch but is not practical in the queen. The viewing instrument must be long enough to reach the postcervical fold in the bitch, allowing visualization of the rugose area. In the unstimulated bitch the rugose area is relatively featureless, but after exposure to estrogen, multiple transverse and oblique rugae develop and become sharply angular and "peaked" coincidentally with onset of sexual receptivity.

Microscopic evaluation of the vaginal epithelium and vaginoscopy of the mucosa are methods that serve to semiquantitatively estimate the amount of estradiol-17β in serum, and thus judge the maturity of graafian follicles and the interval remaining to ovulation.

Breeding Season and Puberty

Studies of whelping registrations in England and the United States have shown that when breed is disregarded, dogs cycle with equal frequency throughout the year. Dogs of the sled-dog breeds and the basenji do show a tendency to cycle annually in the spring.[6, 7] Occurrence of anestrus in the bitch thus appears to be unaffected by seasons. In other nonseasonal mammals folliculogenesis begins anew as soon as the luteal phase progesterone declines. In the bitch it is not clear how folliculogenesis is prevented at the end of the luteal phase, only to be restarted after an interval that varies from 3 to 12 months.

Size at maturity has a significant effect on age at onset of puberty in the bitch. Bitches will generally have their first estrus a few months after achieving adult height and body weight, so that a Pomeranian will reach puberty several months earlier than a Great Dane (6 months as opposed to 14 months on the average). This rule of thumb may be compounded by early or late maturation of an individual bitch, particularly in the midsize breeds. Onset of puberty is not affected by season.

The cat is an obligatory seasonal animal, with anestrus being induced by decreasing hours of daylight.[8] There are, however, individual and breed variations in response to light, long-haired breeds being less governed by day length than short-haired breeds.[9] In nature, free-roaming cats will show estrous behavior during spring and summer, from about six weeks after the winter solstice to six weeks after the summer solstice. Cats may be kept sexually active during the short-day season by exposure to artificial illumination adjusted to give 12 hours of light.[2, 8] Cats kept in facilities that do not afford adequate lighting may be sexually suppressed. Estrous behavior may be expected to start within five to six weeks after the inadequate light regimen has been adjusted.

In the cat the age at onset of puberty ranges from four to ten months and depends not only on adequate physical maturation, but also on season. In the northern hemisphere, kittens born in March may attain the mature weight of about 5.25 lbs (2.4 kg) by September; however, they may be affected by shortening day length and may not have their first estrus until January or February of the following year, at 10 or 11 months of age. Conversely, kittens born late in the season (e.g., in October) may reach their mature weight and show first estrus early in March, at five months of age (Figure 98–5).

The Ovarian Cycle

Sexual activity in the bitch and queen is governed, as in other mammals, by effects of the ovarian hormones on various target organs. Ovarian function is generally divided into the follicular, luteal, and quiescent phases. The dominant hormone during the follicular phase is estradiol-17β, produced at an increasing rate by granulosa cells in the growing graafian follicles. After the mature follicle is luteinized and ovulation is stimulated by the surge of luteinizing hormone from the anterior pituitary, the follicular granulosa and theca interna cells change their steroidogenic end point and begin to produce progesterone. The follicle is now a corpus luteum, and this period of the ovarian cycle, dominated by

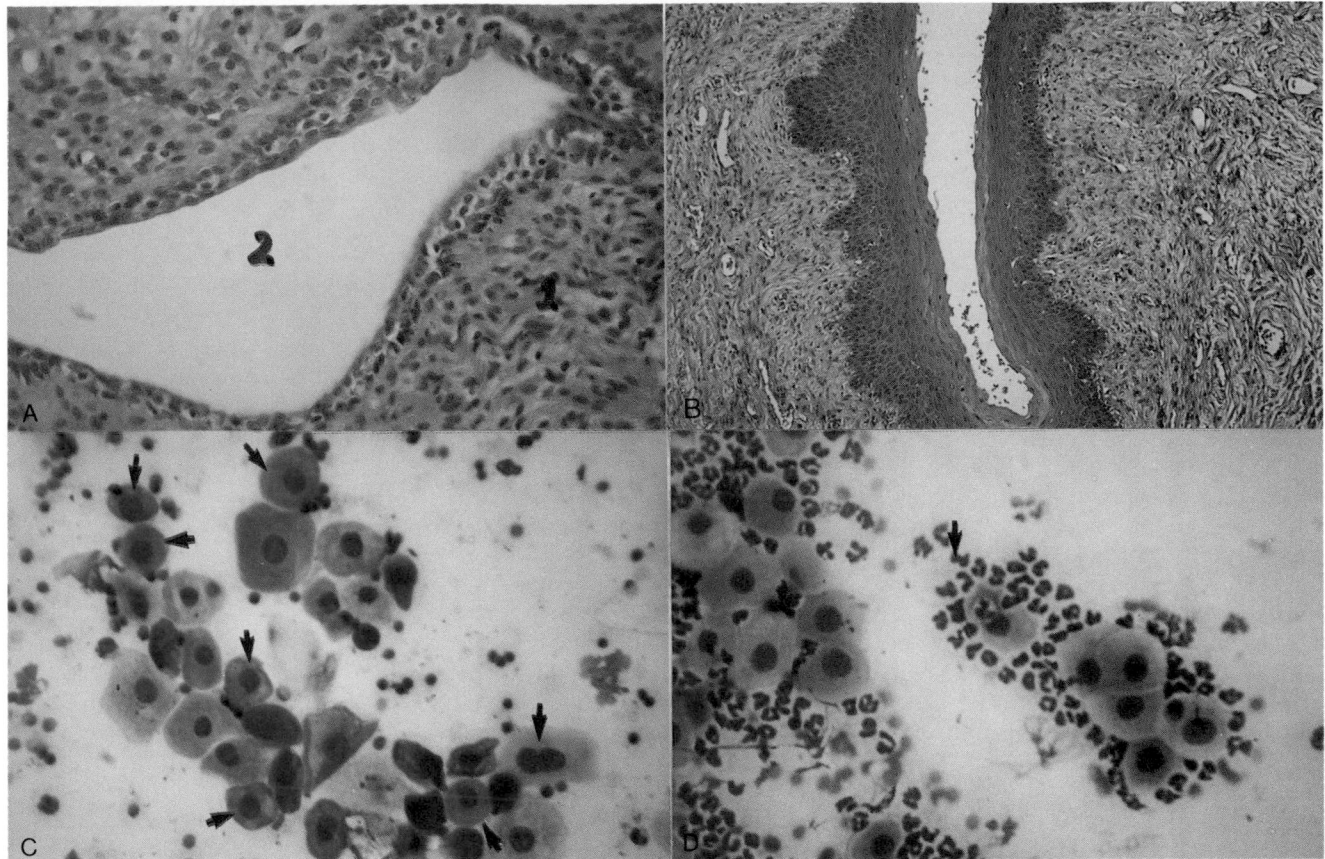

FIGURE 98–4. *A,* Cross-section of a vaginal wall (submucosa, 1; lumen, 2) from a bitch in anestrus. The parabasal and intermediate cells lining the basement membrane are only a few layers thick.

B, Cross-section of a vaginal wall from an estrogen-stimulated bitch. The cells have multiplied and stacked, increasing the number of layers above the basement membrane. Only superficial cells are found in the adluminal layers.

C, Parabasal cells (arrows) (100×). A distinct cytoplasmic membrane encloses the round, small cells. The nuclei are large, with mildly eosinophilic, clearly stained chromatin granules. The mucus strands and droplets surrounding the cells are frequently present during late diestrus and throughout anestrus.

D, Intermediate cells (100×). In comparison to the parabasal cells, intermediate cells are larger, with an oval rather than rounded cytoplasmic outline. The nuclei are like those seen in the parabasal cells. Intermediate cells usually accompany parabasal cells in diestrus and anestrus. Neutrophils (arrows) appear in early diestrus.

progesterone, is the luteal phase. The quiescent phase is seasonally affected by duration of daylight in the cat (seasonal anestrus). In the bitch, anestrus occurs at intervals characteristic for the individual and generally is not affected by seasons. The three phases (follicular, luteal, quiescent) succeed one another in a cyclic manner. The resulting changes in behavior, in the appearance of the external genitalia, and in the structure of the vagina, uterus, and ovaries are collectively called the estrous cycle.

In the bitch, luteinization and progesterone production in follicles occurs before ovulation, concomitantly with the onset of the preovulatory surge of luteinizing hormone (LH). The LH surge occurs spontaneously (it is not affected by coitus) and is mediated by the decline of estradiol from the peak concentrations that occur at the end of proestrus.[10] In an elegant study, Concannon[11] showed that the preovulatory release of progesterone is essential for receptive behavior in the bitch. Ovariectomized bitches were given estradiol alone or estradiol followed by progesterone; onset of estrous behavior occurred only after estradiol was stopped; behavior onset was more synchronous when progesterone was given after withdrawal of estradiol. The luteal phase (serum progesterone > 2.5 ng/ml) is slightly longer in the nonpregnant (75 days) than in the pregnant (63 days) and similar to the hysterectomized (68 days) bitch.[12] Therefore, it is unlikely that the corpus luteum lifespan is modulated by the uterus or by the conceptus.[12, 13]

An outstanding feature of the feline ovarian cycle is that LH surge is induced by coitus, or a comparable stimulus (Figure 98–6). Effective stimuli, other than coitus, are mechanical stimulation of the cervix or administration of LH-containing gonadotrophins or gonadotrophin-releasing hormone.[14] In absence of the LH release, corpora lutea are not formed, and thus there is no luteal phase; successive groups of follicles grow and degenerate, resulting in intermittent estrous periods separated by a period of sexual inactivity. If coitus (or a comparable stimulus) is followed by LH release but fertilization does not occur, corpora lutea are formed

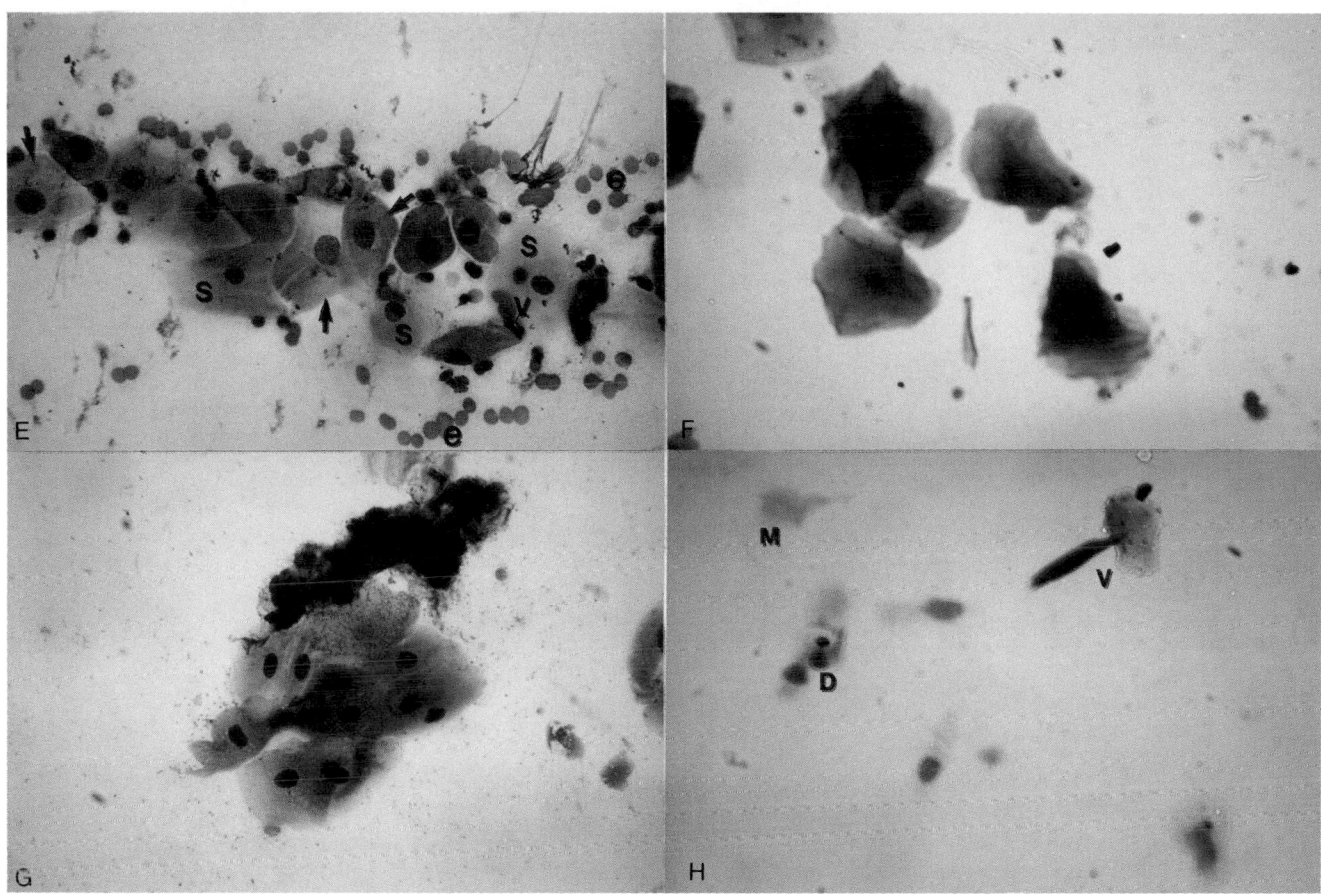

Figure 98–4 *Continued E,* Intermediate-superficial cells (arrows), also known as large intermediate cells, or intermediate cells (100×). Progressing cornification has caused loss of cytoplasmic membrane integrity, resulting in enlargement, folding, and an angular appearance. The nuclei are functional, with clearly indicated chromatin granules. The cells are associated with superficial cells (S) and erythrocytes (e) in proestrus.

F, Superficial and anuclear cells (100×). Large cells with an indistinct cytoplasmic border, showing pyknosis or karyorrhexis. The nuclei are densely stained, usually basophilic, and contain no visible structures. Nuclei also may not stain and become invisible (anuclear cells). Commonly seen in late proestrus and throughout estrus. Bacteria may be seen adhering to or surrounding the cells.

G, Small superficial cells (cat only) (100×). The cells are found in the cat vaginal smear during anestrous, diestrous, and interestrous phases of the cycle. They are replaced by the large superficial cells during proestrus and estrus. The cornified appearance of these cells may be the result of normal epithelial aging, unrelated to fluctuating estrogen levels.

H, Vestibular cells (V), mucus (M), and cellular debris (D) (100×). Artifacts caused by obtaining the sample from the vestibule instead of the vagina, particularly during anestrus, when vaginal mucus has a low water content and tends to precipitate on the slide and take up stain.

but degenerate after about six weeks. A sequence of coitus, LH release, ovulation, formation of corpora lutea, and fertilization may result in pregnancy, during which the serum progesterone remains elevated for over 60 days (Figure 98–7). The source of progesterone before 40 to 45 days of gestation is the corpus luteum; after that it may be the placenta, since the ovaries may be removed without disturbing the pregnancy.

Molecular interactions and the mechanisms that govern folliculogenesis, luteinization, ovulation, and continuing function of the corpus luteum have been studied in detail only in the rat. Because it is still unclear whether the same principles apply to the bitch and queen, the subject will not be discussed here, and the interested reader is directed to read the extensive review on the rat by Richards.[15] Some peculiarities of the endocrine

events in the bitch and cat will be mentioned during the discussion of the estrous cycle.

The estrous cycle is divided into four stages, using a combination of anatomic and behavioral criteria. The stages and their corresponding functional phases are proestrus (follicular phase), estrus and diestrus (luteal phase), and anestrus (quiescent phase). In the queen there is a fifth stage, the interfollicular (interestrous) stage, which is a quiescent phase that occurs between two successive estrous periods if the queen did not ovulate. The occurrence of estrus (sexual receptivity) during the luteal phase is unique in the bitch. It occurs because she ovulates at the onset of sexual receptivity, and thus has freshly formed corpora lutea instead of follicles during estrus. The queen ovulates in response to coital stimulus; thus, if coitus occurs in the beginning

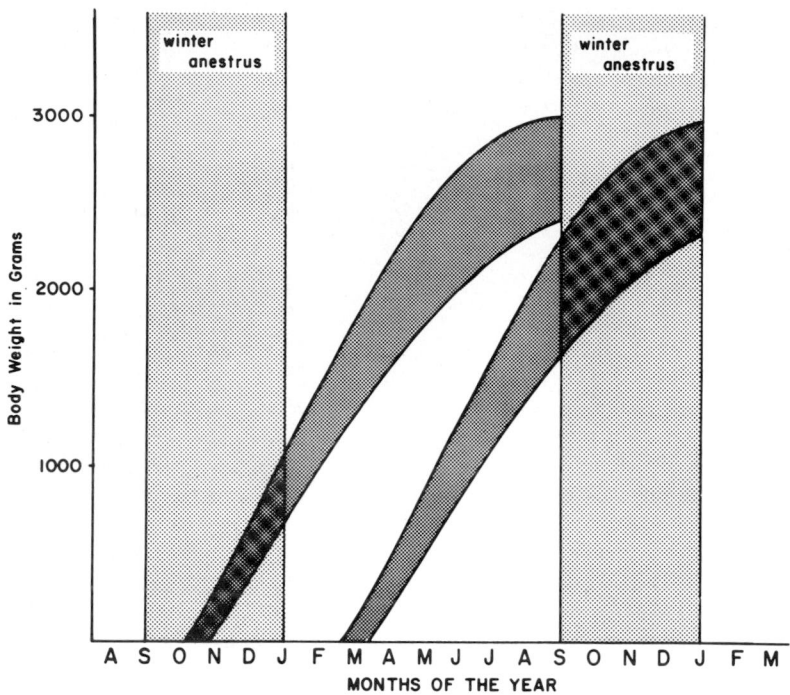

FIGURE 98–5. Effect of season on attainment of puberty in kittens. Weight gain curves depict attainment of mature weight at 2 to 3 kg. Kittens born in October to mothers that were bred late in the summer tend to attain their adult body weight during the reproductive season and may show first estrus in February or March, at four to five months of age. If kittens are born early in the year, they may reach their mature weight at the onset of the seasonal anestrus in September; their pubertal estrus will be postponed until the next spring, at the age of 10 or 11 months.

of estrus, the queen will also have active corpora lutea while continuing to mate.

Clinical Features of the Canine Estrous Cycle

Proestrus and estrus are stages of obvious sexual activity. In the language of the dog breeder, the two stages are combined under the term "heat" or "season," with the first day of heat being the first day of proestrus, the last day of heat being the last day of estrus, while ovulation usually occurs about the 11th day of heat, or day 2 of estrus. A horse or cow breeder would use the term "heat" to mean only the period of sexual receptivity or estrus. The major structural and endocrine features of the cycle are summarized (Figure 98–8).

Anestrus (65 to 281 days, mean 150.3 days). Traditionally known as the quiescent period of the reproductive cycle, anestrus is behaviorally characterized by sexual inactivity. The vaginal mucous membrane in the plicate area shows low-profile, longitudinal, unbranched folds of a translucent, diffuse red-pink. The rugose area is featureless and pale pink. The exfoliated epithelium

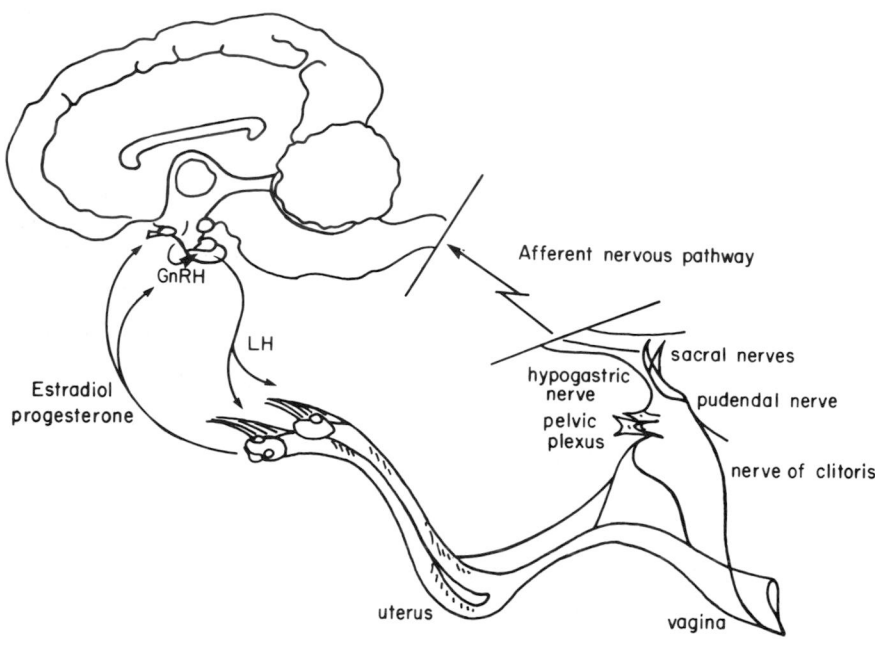

FIGURE 98–6. Schematic of the neuroendocrine signal for induction of ovulation in the cat. Stimulation of the neural pathway occurs at the vagina by coitus or mechanical means. The signal is transmitted to the hypothalamus, where it triggers the gonadotrophin-releasing hormone (GnRH), which in turn releases the preovulatory surge of luteinizing hormone (LH). Ovulation follows, if the ovarian follicles are sufficiently mature. Estradiol produced by the follicles sensitizes the pituitary to GnRH stimulation, facilitating LH release. Progesterone from the corpora lutea hinders GnRH release, preventing follicle maturation and ovulation.

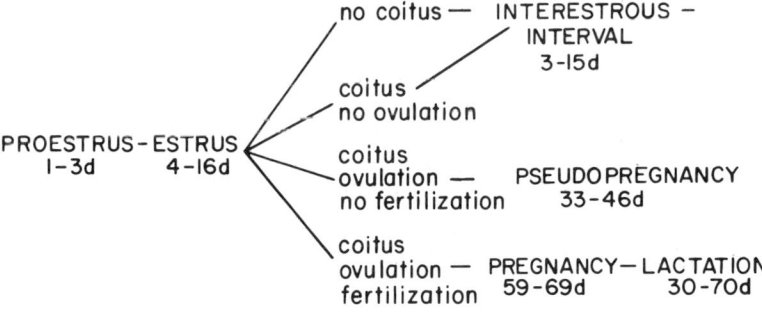

FIGURE 98–7. The occurrence of ovulation (and fertilization) determines the options for subsequent reproductive events in the cat. The interval to return to estrus is short in absence of ovulation (interestrus), longer when a corpus luteum delays folliculogenesis (pseudopregnancy), and longest when pregnancy ensues.

contains a variable mixture of parabasal and intermediate cells, with an occasional superficial cell appearing owing to the natural aging of the mucosa. There is often a paucity of cells, the dominant features on the microscope slide being basophilic mucus strands, eosinophilic mucus droplets, and cell debris. The slide is said to have a "dirty" or "cluttered" appearance.

Patterns of serum hormones have not been studied extensively in anestrus. Serum progesterone and testosterone appear to be at base line concentrations throughout the period. Estradiol concentrations were reported to be elevated in late anestrus and decreasing as proestrus approaches;[16] in early and middle anestrus, estradiol appeared to be at base line concentrations.[17] Concentrations of follicle-stimulating hormone (FSH) begin low in early and middle anestrus[17] and rise in late anestrus to levels comparable to those found during the preovulatory FSH surge.[6, 17] Episodic surges of serum LH may be detected throughout anestrus. The peak concentrations achieved and the frequency of the surges are lower in early anestrus as compared with middle and late anestrus, becoming most intense just before onset of proestrus about 15 days before the preovulatory LH surge.[16, 17]

Proestrus (6 to 11 days, mean 9.1 days). Proestrus is defined as the period when the bitch is sexually attractive while rejecting the male's advances. However, early behavioral clues are indistinct, and it is common to use the appearance of a serosanguineous vaginal discharge to mark the first day of proestrus.

A bitch may be attractive to a male before any vulval swelling or vaginal discharge is seen. She will remain attractive throughout proestrus and estrus, although some experienced males will show little interest in a bitch before she is receptive. During the initial four to five days of proestrus the bitch's response to the male's courtship is usually aggressively negative. Later, a few days before onset of estrus, it will moderate to playful avoidance or passive tolerance.

Throughout proestrus the bitch has a serosanguineous vaginal discharge that varies in volume and intensity of redness. The source of the vaginal discharge is endometrial hemorrhage, arising from erythrocyte diapedesis and subepithelial capillary rupture. Soon after, or coincidental with onset of the discharge, the vulva gradually enlarges, the labia becoming most edematous and firm by the last third of proestrus. A relatively rapid softening of the vulval labia is seen with onset of estrus, as the estradiol-induced edema subsides. The vaginal discharge

and vulval swelling are variable and may be easily missed in long-haired bitches that keep themselves clean. The signs of proestrus and estrus are often indistinct in peripubertal bitches.

The appearance of the vaginal mucosa and of the exfoliated epithelial cells from a bitch in proestrus will vary daily as the follicles mature and serum estradiol rises. Endoscopically, an early proliferative/edematous stage with balloon-like, soft, bulging folds is succeeded by increasing cornification, which gives a shrinking appearance to the growing folds of mucosa. The folds become more convoluted, adding transverse and diagonal branches to the longitudinal ones, but still maintaining a soft, rounded outline of the crests.

The progression of estrogen-induced changes is mirrored in the appearance of the vaginal epithelium (see Figure 98–4). In early proestrus (approximately days 1 to 3), there is a predominance of intermediate cells with a few (10 to 30 per cent) superficial cells. Later, in mid-proestrus (approximately days 4 to 6), superficial and anuclear cells are more frequently found and make up about 50 per cent of the total epithelial cells. As serum estradiol concentrations rise before the LH surge, superficial and anuclear cells predominate, reaching 85 per cent or more of the total cells. Peak cornification is thus reached about one to two days before the actual serum estradiol peak.[18] Erythrocytes are numerous throughout proestrus, appearing rounded and clear as if on a peripheral blood smear in early proestrus, and becoming progressively more crenated and shrunken later. Neutrophils are occasionally seen in the early days but disappear from the slide as cornification progresses and it becomes more difficult for them to migrate into the vaginal lumen. The vaginal and cervical mucus flows more copiously and is diluted with sanguineous uterine fluid; precipitation of mucus on the microscope slide diminishes, and the slide appears "clean" or "uncluttered."

The major hormonal event during proestrus is the continuous rise in serum estradiol levels, culminating in late proestrus with a surge that lasts for one to two days and precedes the serum LH peak by the same interval (Figure 98–8). Serum testosterone also rises, and at onset of estrus it may reach levels comparable to those seen in episodic peaks of the male dog. Progesterone is at base line levels but may start to increase on the last few days, as the LH levels begin to surge. LH is low in early proestrus, but episodic releases begin to increase in amplitude and frequency, the peaks overlapping and

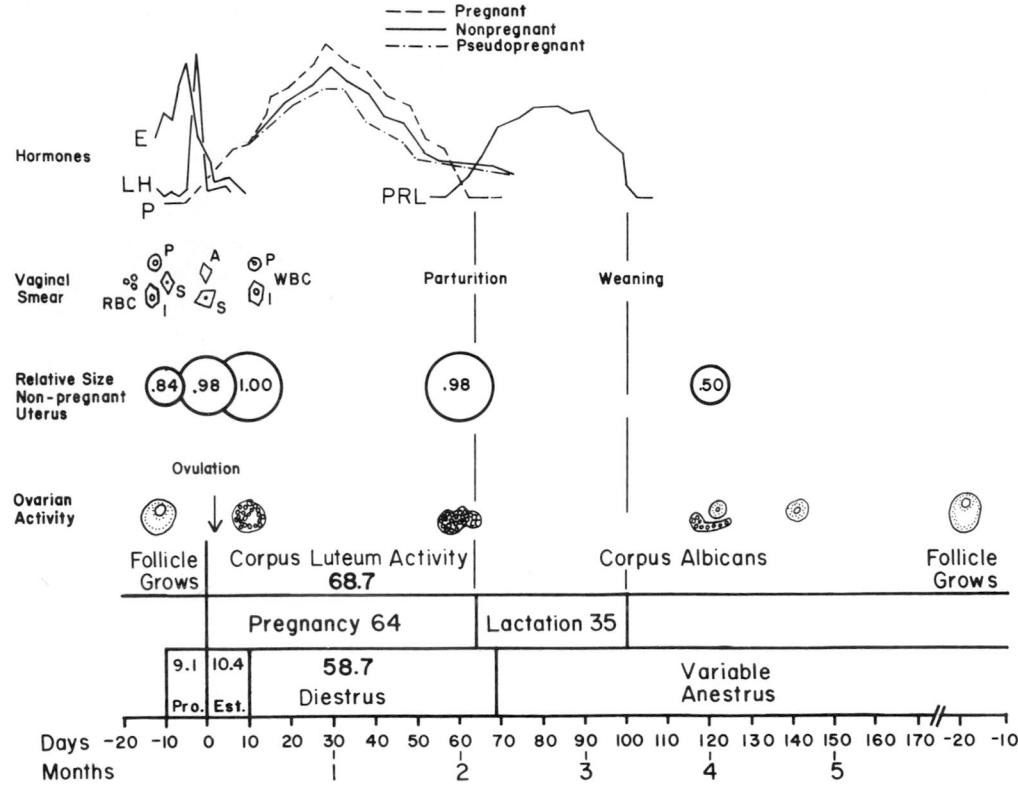

FIGURE 98–8. Schematic representation of events in the estrous cycle of the bitch. The luteinizing hormone (LH) surge (day 0) is assumed to occur at onset of estrus; other events are aligned to day 0. Ovulation occurs on day 2, with corpus luteum activity shown to begin earlier, on day 0. Diestrus follows estrus, starting on day 10. The largest relative uterine size (diameter × length of uterine horns, expressed as a percentage) was found on day 10; the uterus remains the same size through diestrus and does not diminish to 50 per cent until day 120. The estradiol-17β (E) surge occurs on day −2, while serum progesterone (P) levels begin to rise together with the LH on day −1. Progesterone levels in pregnant and nonpregnant bitches as well as in bitches showing signs of clinical pseudopregnancy were similar. Serum prolactin (PRL) is elevated as progesterone declines and prolactin remains high during lactation.

building toward the preovulatory surge. FSH concentrations decline to the lowest level during proestrus.[16]

Estrus (7 to 9 days, mean 10.4 days). Estrus begins when the bitch allows the male to mount and stands with the tail cocked to the side ("flags") when he attempts intromission. Estrus ends with refusal of the male's advances by the bitch. Duration of estrus is quite variable when it is thus defined by the receptive behavior of the bitch (2 to 20 days). The variability in behavior is related to the general attitude and level of sexual experience of the bitch. Direct interference with animal interactions by well-meaning experts, indirect psychological effects of human-animal bonding (presence of the "alpha person" in the bitch's mental hierarchy), and environmental disturbances make unprejudiced behavioral observations difficult. Thus poorly expressed estrous behavior may occur in individuals that have normally functioning ovaries. It is therefore contraindicated to administer gonadotrophins or gonadal steroids without first defining ovarian competence by changes in the vaginal epithelium to estimate estradiol production and assay of serum for progesterone concentrations. In the final analysis it is more important to define the time of ovulation than of estrus. One indirect method is to detect the preovulatory peak of serum estradiol by means of its biologic effect on the vaginal epithelium.

The effects are most intensely expressed four to six days before ovulation,[18] and although not precise, they do provide an acceptable estimate of the most fertile period in the bitch.

Through the endoscope the shrunken and acutely angular appearance of the multiple, branched folds in the plicate and rugose area becomes progressively more obvious as estradiol rises during proestrus. Shortly before the serum estradiol peak there appear sharply defined angular furrows on the postcervical fold. The mucosal appearance then does not change substantially during the ensuing days of estrus. The end of estrus is coincident with rather weakly defined changes, characterized by a gradual loss of definition and a rounding of the mucosal folds.

Cytologically, the early response of the epithelium is defined less precisely than when viewed through the endoscope. There is a gradual increase in cornification until, without a sharply defined end point, only superficial cells are seen on the vaginal smear. On the average the appearance of more than 80 per cent superficial cells precedes the onset of estrous behavior and the LH surge by two to four days. Throughout estrus intermediate cells may be found in small numbers (less than 10 per cent), and the appearance of the vaginal swab remains essentially static, dominated by the superficial cells. The lack of progressive changes in the mucosa during this period makes it impossible to differentiate early estrus from late estrus on the basis of vaginal endoscopy or cytologic examination. Erythrocytes and large numbers of bacteria may be found throughout the period. The bacteria do not elicit a leukocytic response. A clearly defined cytologic end point characterizes the end of estrus and the start of diestrus.

Endocrine patterns are very dramatic at onset of estrus, and their analysis is helpful in timing the events and estimating the effectiveness of pituitary-ovarian function. The precipitous decline of serum estradiol is swiftly followed by a surge in LH that remains elevated for 24 to 96 hours. Progesterone values begin to climb coincidentally with LH, before ovulation has occurred. Progesterone remains elevated throughout estrus. A surge of FSH occurs concomitantly with or immediately after the LH surge. The clearly defined changes in serum progesterone concentrations, which occur just before ovulation, may be measured by any clinical laboratory that does steroid hormone assays. It is advisable to validate the results in canine serum by including samples with known amounts of progesterone with each submitted unknown. Progesterone measurements are useful in confirming the timing and occurrence of ovulation and in estimating the competence of the corpora lutea. Concentrations in the range of 0.1 to 1.0 ng/ml are commonly seen during the follicular phase. Levels above 2.5 ng/ml are required to maintain pregnancy.

Ovulation may occur up to 96 hours after the LH peak, but usually is observed within 24 to 72 hours. The temporal relationships between the first and last ovulation, and the LH peak or first progesterone rise have not been defined more precisely. Because the bitch ovulates a primary oocyte, the first meiotic division is completed in the oviduct within three days after ovulation.

Diestrus (56 to 58 days pregnant, 60 to 75 days nonpregnant). Onset of diestrus may be defined rather precisely by daily examination of microscopic changes in the vaginal epithelium. Somewhat less clearly, it is defined by the first refusal of the male by the female, a behavior that is usually coincident with loss of her attractiveness to males. Subsequently, behavior in diestrus is indistinguishable from that seen in anestrus. The only quantifiable criterion for defining the end of diestrus is the decline of serum progesterone concentration below 1 ng/ml.

The vaginal mucosa, as seen through the endoscope, initially has a rapid rounding out of the dorsal median fold and a disappearance of the folds in the vestibular and rugose areas. Patchy or banded hyperemia is seen throughout the vagina and persists during most of diestrus. There is a noticeable amount of clear to slightly cloudy mucus, which may be colored by reddish uterine fluid in the early days, before the cervix closes.

During the changeover from estrus to diestrus, in an interval of only 24 to 36 hours, at least 30 per cent of the superficial cells on the vaginal swab are replaced by intermediate and parabasal cells. The first day of diestrus may be used to estimate the day of the LH surge (-8 days), ovulation (-6 days), blastocyst attachment (12 days), palpable gestational vesicles (20 to 28 days), and

parturition (56 to 58 days).[18] Note that the cytologic appearance during this stage is similar to that seen during early to mid proestrus, so that it may be impossible to differentiate proestrus from the first or second day of diestrus on the basis of one slide.

Diestrus is completely dominated by progesterone, whereas other hormones are essentially at base line levels. Starting already well above base line at the end of estrus, progesterone continues to rise until about day 15 of diestrus. A gradual decline follows for several weeks until base line levels are reached about six weeks later. Although progesterone concentrations are, on the whole, similar in pregnant, nonmated, and hysterectomized bitches, they decline more abruptly in pregnancy and are at base line at parturition (days 56 to 58 of diestrus).

Events During Pregnancy in the Bitch

Using onset of diestrus as a starting point, the events in pregnancy may be estimated rather accurately. In the following discussion, intervals in days will be given with day 1 equal to first day of diestrus, unless otherwise stated. Measured from the first day of diestrus, gestation length is remarkably consistent, with 85 per cent of the bitches delivering on diestrus days 56 to 58. If a single mating is used to estimate the onset of parturition, the interval may vary from 58 to 69 days, with an average of 63 days; the length of gestation depends, in this case, on whether the interval is measured from a mating that occurred early or late in estrus. Multiple matings usually make the gestation period estimate even less predictable, although the extremes of the range are seldom exceeded. If a problem pregnancy (or parturition) is anticipated, it is advisable to take the trouble to establish the onset of diestrus by daily examination of vaginal smears in the second half of estrus. This will improve the timing of fetal development and onset of parturition.

Fertilization is completed and development proceeds to the morula stage within the oviducts. The morulae enter the uterus between diestrus days 4 and 10 and become blastocysts, which begin attachment and placenta formation by day 12.[18] Before attachment the embryos are mobile and become evenly spaced within both uterine horns. The canine placenta is endotheliochorial (i.e., maternal (endometrial) endothelium is in contact with the chorion) and zonary (i.e., the chorioallantoic tissue where attachment to the endometrium occurs is arranged in a belt-like circumferential loop). Individual enlargements of the uterus (loculi), containing the embryo within the fluid-filled placental vesicle, may be palpated through the abdomen between days 19 and 28. After that the loculi become confluent, and the uniformly enlarged sausage-like uterus may be difficult to recognize as containing fetuses. Embryonal differentiation is completed by day 28, and subsequently the fetus is less vulnerable to teratogenic influences. Loculi become recognizable by ultrasonography as oval, nonechogenic (black) structures appearing in pairs after day 19. Thereafter the developing embryo and growing fetus may be visualized and its viability assessed throughout the pregnancy (Figure 98–9). Enlarged, fluid-filled uter-

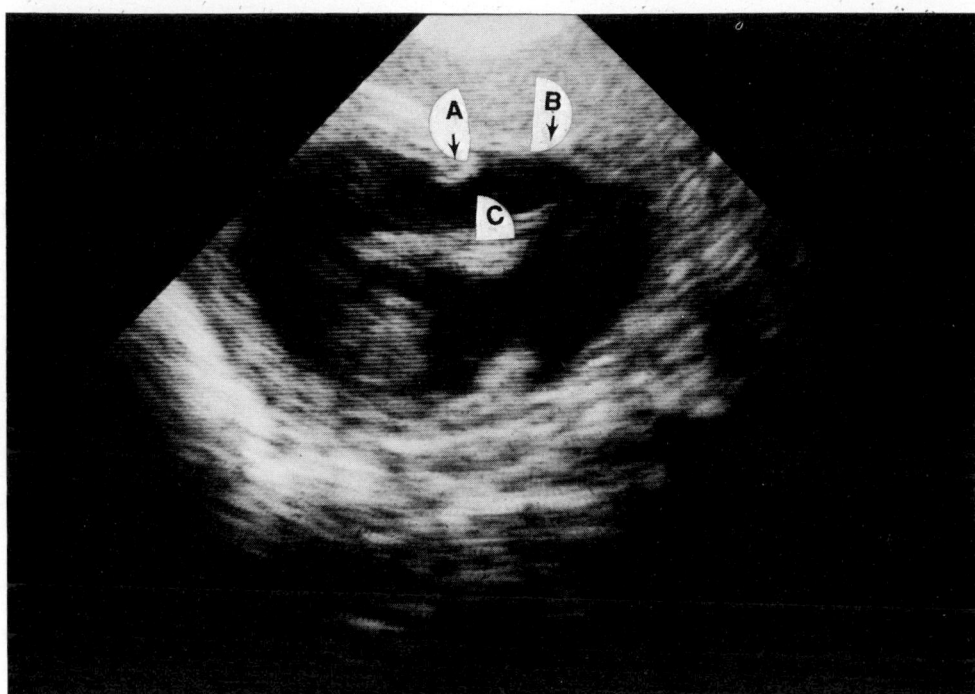

FIGURE 98–9. Sonogram of a canine fetus at day 21 of diestrus. The thickened zonary attachment area of the chorioallantois *(A)* is distinguishable from the thinner, free portion *(B)*. The dense echogenic fetus *(C)* is suspended in the nonechogenic allantoic and amniotic fluid. (Courtesy D. Hager, 1986.)

ine horns may be seen radiographically after day 19, and fetal skeletal elements are unequivocally recognizable after days 38 to 40 of diestrus.

Vaginal walls and the epithelial lining present an appearance similar to that seen in nonpregnant diestrus. In the last seven to ten days of gestation small amounts of clear mucus may be seen passing from the vulva, which will be soft and slightly pendulous. There is gradual mammary gland development after days 38 to 40, and milk usually appears in the last week. Total body weight of the bitch increases by 20 to 55 per cent (average 36 per cent) during the course of gestation. The packed cell volume (40 per cent by day 35 and < 35 per cent at term) and hemoglobin values decline, while the total leukocyte counts rise (17,000 to 26,000) during pregnancy. Pregnancy may aggravate a preexisting subclinical diabetic state and increases the requirement for dietary carbohydrate.

Functional corpora lutea, capable of producing serum progesterone concentrations above 2.0 ng/ml throughout gestation, are essential for maintenance of pregnancy. After the preovulatory surge, estrogen and LH concentrations decline and remain at base line levels during pregnancy. About ten days before parturition estrogen levels show a gradual increase, which is paralleled, to some extent, by a rise in FSH levels. It is likely that LH and prolactin are necessary to support luteal function, particularly in the latter half of gestation, since administration of an anti-LH serum or a prolactin inhibitor (bromoergocryptin) causes luteolysis and abortion.[19]

Parturition

Clinically, the onset of parturition is heralded by two to three days of restlessness, a desire for seclusion, and relative anorexia. The behavior is intensified during the last 12 to 24 hours, when there is panting, nesting, and increased restlessness. Uterine contractions and cervical dilation have begun at this stage (stage I of labor) but are not accompanied by abdominal contractions, and there is no propulsion of the fetuses. Stage I, lasting for 12 to 24 hours, is generally thought to begin with the first decline of rectal temperature to about 99°F (37°C) and to end with the rupture of the chorioallantois as the first pup is pushed through the cervix. The ensuing stretching of the cervix and vagina stimulates involuntary abdominal contraction and intensifies the uterine contractions, all designed to propel the pup through the vaginal canal. This is stage II, the propulsive stage; it occurs with the delivery of each pup and lasts each time no longer than two hours. Prolongation of stage II labor indicates possible obstructive dystocia. The amnion does not rupture during delivery, and the amniotic membranes must be promptly removed by the bitch (or human helper) to prevent suffocation of the neonate. Stage III labor occurs after each pup is delivered. The chorioallantois is expelled and the uterus empties the small amount of lochia from the individual delivery. At this time the bitch may rest for a few minutes up to two to three hours before starting stage II labor with the next pup.

The signals that start parturition have not been elucidated in the bitch, but the known endocrine events suggest that the mechanism is probably similar to that proposed for other species. Maturation of the fetal pituitary-adrenal axis results in an increase of fetal cortisol, which acts at the level of the uterus to release luteolytic doses of prostaglandin $F_{2\alpha}$. Elevated prostaglandin metabolite concentrations have been found on the day of parturition.[20, 21] The subsequent decline of serum progesterone is associated with the prepartum decline of rectal temperature. The progesterone drop occurs while estrogen levels remain slightly elevated, resulting in an increase of the estrogen-progesterone ratio. The ratio change is probably the major cause of placental dissociation, cervical dilation, and increase of myometrial sensitivity to oxytocin. Similar to the sow, the bitch may suffer delayed onset of parturition when a single fetus is apparently incapable of triggering the parturition cascade. A rise in serum prolactin occurs concurrently with the progesterone decline; it continues to be elevated throughout the nursing period and is likely to be associated with lactation and maternal behavior.

Uterine involution is aided by the oxytocin released during nursing. Uterine tone is restored, and new endometrial epithelium grows over the denuded attachment sites. The reepithelialization is slow, with otherwise healthy, fertile bitches showing microscopic evidence of endometrial lesions and a sanguineous vaginal discharge as long as nine weeks postpartum.[22] The postpartum period is characterized by rapidly declining prostaglandin levels and base line concentrations of gonadal steroids and pituitary gonadotrophins.[20]

Clinical Features of the Feline Estrous Cycle

Free-roaming cats usually have one litter in spring, but under domestic or cattery conditions cats will produce two litters per year. If the seasonal anestrus is overcome by ensuring 12 to 14 hours of light, five litters may be reared in two years, each breeding cycle occupying 4.5 months.

Anestrus (about 90 days during short daylight season). The queen is not attractive to the tom during anestrus, and if approached, the free-living, mature queen may be quite vicious in refusing the tom's attentions. A young, shy cat used to the proximity of other cats in a domestic or cattery environment may allow herself to be examined, groomed, and even mounted by a tom, showing her lack of sexual receptivity only by curling her body and tucking her tail firmly over the perineum. The exfoliated vaginal epithelium is dominated by clumped, strongly basophilic parabasal and small superficial cells. The background of the slide visible with the microscope is littered by mucus strands and noncellular debris, which frequently obscure the epithelial cells. Occasional neutrophils may be seen. Estrogen and progesterone are known to remain at base line concentrations during anestrus; serum gonadotrophin concentrations have not been measured.

Proestrus (1 to 2 days in some queens). Proestrus behavior was shown consistently by only 6 of 35 queens in a cattery.[2] The queens attracted the tom by loud "calling" and rolling or rubbing on the ground. Generally the tom would not approach too closely, for he would be immediately rebuffed with hissing, growling, and paw strikes. The major feature seen on the vaginal smear was a clearing of the debris and mucus, so that the well-separated (not clumped), small superficial and intermediate cells became clearly visible. Onset of follicular activity was indicated by a rise of serum estradiol-17β.

Estrus (1 to 21 days, mean 7 days). Most cats progress from sexual inactivity to raucous receptivity in a period that may be as short as six hours. When a male approaches, or when the male's vocal response is heard, the queen will assume a stereotypic posture that incorporates flexion of the forelimbs at the elbow, lordosis, deflection of the tail, and rapid mincing steps with the hindlimbs. She readily accepts the mounting male and allows intromission. At the moment of intromission (which lasts usually under a minute and in the male is immediately followed by ejaculation), the queen emits a bellowing cry and attempts to dislodge the male. When he releases her, she does an elaborate postcoital display, rolling and frantically grooming her vulva and perineum. An approach by the tom (or anyone else) during this time is viciously rejected. Receptive behavior and mating are usually resumed in 20 to 60 minutes. Estrus ends, in most cases, just as abruptly as it began, with the queen suddenly refusing the male's courtship. In a cattery, socially inferior, inexperienced, young, and shy cats may not show any estrous behavior. Because of their lack of posturing they may be ignored by the male or may make coitus impossible. Removal from the influence of the dominant queen and maturation will solve most of these behavioral problems.

Moderate to scant amounts of cloudy and occasionally pink-tinged, watery mucus are seen on swabs taken at estrus from the vagina. Frank bleeding as in the bitch is not seen in the cat. Epithelial cells in the vaginal smear change rapidly; typically, when differential cell counts are done on samples taken 24 hours apart, there will be a drop of parabasal, small superficial, and intermediate cells from more than 60 per cent to 15 to 20 per cent and a concomitant rise in large superficial and anuclear cells from 10 to 15 per cent to more than 80 per cent. Despite the rapid cornification, behavioral signs often precede changes in the vaginal epithelium, making the vaginal smear of little value as a predictive tool in breeding management. The smear, however, is a reliable means of confirming the occurrence of follicular function when behavior is unclear. During estrus no neutrophils are seen and, in contrast to the bitch, few, if any, erythrocytes. Cornified epithelial cells disappear rapidly from the vaginal smear after the decline of serum estradiol-17β. Estrous behavior may continue for a few days after the cells in the vaginal smear are predominantly noncornified.

Follicular activity is defined by a rise in serum estradiol-17β which occurs so rapidly that base line concentrations are doubled or tripled daily (Figure 98–10). In absence of coitus or other ovulatory stimulus, the ovarian follicles eventually become atretic and stop producing estrogen, and the estradiol concentrations decline as rapidly as they rose (interfollicular phase). Mechanisms that govern the duration of follicular activity (3 to 16 days, mean 7.4 days) are unknown at this time. Coitus does not shorten the follicular phase (or estrus): it was shown in 167 estrous cycles that cats that mated and ovulated, those that mated and did not ovulate, and those that were not allowed to mate had mean follicular phases of 7.0, 7.2, and 7.7 days, respectively.[23] Progesterone remains at basal levels during anovulatory cycles, since no corpora lutea are formed.

CAT 9

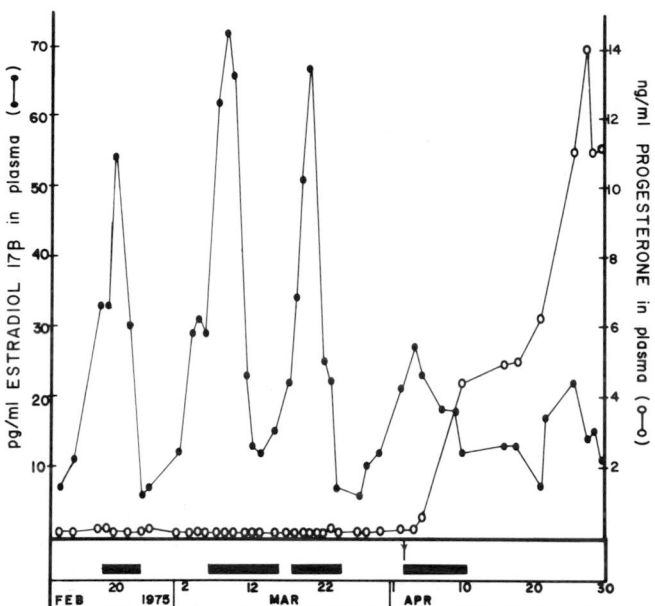

FIGURE 98–10. Endocrine events during estrous cycles in a cat. Repeated estrous behavior (▬) occurred during February and March in absence of coitus. Periods of estrus are correlated with follicle growth, as indicated by elevations of serum estradiol-17β (●——●). Interestrous periods are correlated with low estradiol levels. Progesterone (○——○) remained low until the cat was mated in April (arrow). After that, estradiol remained at or near base line, while onset of luteal activity was reflected in rising progesterone concentrations.

If ovulation occurs, corpora lutea are formed and serum progesterone levels rise above 1 ng/ml 24 to 36 hours later; the cat enters the luteal phase of the cycle. Duration of the progesterone elevation depends on whether ovulation is followed by fertilization (pregnancy) or not (metestrus, pseudopregnancy) (see Figure 98–7).

Interfollicular Stage (2 to 19 days, mean 7 days). Because ovulation is dependent on coital stimulation, unmated queens do not form corpora lutea and the recurrent follicular phases are separated by an interfollicular stage. Thus this is a brief period of sexual inactivity that occurs between successive episodes of estrus in an unmated cat. During this stage, also called interestrus, the cat shows no behavioral, anatomic, physiologic, or endocrine reproductive activity.

Metestrus (nonpregnant, ovulated; 35 to 70 days, mean 45 days). Luteal activity in the cat that ovulated but failed to become pregnant lasts for about 35 to 37 days; an additional variable period (0 to 35 days) is needed for the cat to return to estrus. The period from the end of the luteal phase to the onset of the subsequent follicular phase appears behaviorally and physiologically much like the interfollicular phase. The luteal phase in a nonpregnant cat is also referred to as pseudopregnancy, although it is rarely associated with signs of maternal behavior and lactation as seen in the bitch.

No sexual behavior is shown by the cat during metestrus. Vaginal epithelial cells are predominantly parabasal, intermediate, and small superficial. The back-

ground of the vaginal smear is again cluttered with precipitated mucus and cellular debris. Neutrophils reappear but in fewer numbers and not as dramatically as in the bitch. Because ovulation may be timed rather accurately by observing coitus, onset of metestrus in the cat is not as important clinically as is onset of diestrus in the bitch.

Serum progesterone levels increase within 48 hours after a successful ovulatory stimulus (or 24 hours after ovulation), reach peak concentrations (> 20 ng/ml) in 14 to 18 days, and decline gradually, reaching base line values 30 to 46 days after stimulation. Estradiol remains at base line concentrations except for minor elevations, usually seen between two and three weeks after mating.[23]

Pregnancy (56 to 71 days, mean 63 days). Gestation length, estimated as the interval from coitus to parturition, may vary with breed or family strain, but consistent differences have not been documented. After multiple matings during a long estrus it is advisable to estimate that parturition may occur any time within a period from 63 days after the first mating to 63 days after the last mating. Littermates may have different male parents (superfecundation) if the female is allowed to mate with more than one male.

After coitus, eggs remain in the oviduct for five to six days[24] and are fertilized. Free-floating blastocysts distribute themselves evenly throughout both uterine horns and begin to attach to the endometrium 12 to 15 days postcoitum. Placentation and the sequences of embryonal and fetal growth are the same as in the bitch. Discrete loculi may be palpated after day 17 and will become confluent by day 35. Ultrasonographic imaging of fetuses is successful as early as day 14 or 15, and heartbeats can be seen after day 24.[25] Fetal skeletons may be reliably recognized on radiographs after day 43. No serum or urine tests are available for pregnancy detection in the cat.

The vaginal smear appears the same as that seen during the nonpregnant luteal phase (metestrus). Mammary development occurs in the second half of gestation, and milk is usually produced in the last week.

During the first half of gestation the endocrine patterns are similar to those seen during metestrus. Progesterone levels remain elevated after day 40 until parturition in the pregnant cat, but the ovaries (and corpora lutea) may be removed after day 49 without terminating the pregnancy. It may be assumed that the progesterone in late pregnancy is of placental origin. Concomitant with the progesterone decline in the last two weeks of gestation is a rise in prolactin; the latter continues to be elevated during lactation.[26]

The return to estrus is postponed by pregnancy and lactation. If a female aborts, or loses her nursing kittens, she will return to estrus within two to three weeks.[26]

THE CANINE AND FELINE MALE

Structural Peculiarities

The scrotum is a membranous pouch of pigmented skin, sparsely covered with hair. It contains the paired testes with the attached epididymides. In the dog it is located two-thirds of the distance between the preputial opening and the anus and lies between the thighs. The left scrotal cavity (and testis) is usually more caudal and dorsal than the right, allowing more space for the testes between the thighs. Total scrotal width is measured during breeding soundness examination by gently forcing the testes down into the scrotum and holding them parallel with the thumb and middle finger. Hinged calipers are then applied snug to the scrotal skin at the widest point. Three to five measurements are done and averaged; the scrotum should be released and the testes repositioned between each measurement.[27]

In the cat the scrotum is located immediately below the anus, caudad and dorsal to the thighs. The relation of scrotal width to fertility has not been studied in the cat.

The penis in the dog is directed cranially and ventrally and lies cranial to the hindlegs, along the inguinal region of the abdomen. It is completely enclosed within the prepuce. The os penis is well developed, and it is essential that it occupy the entire length of the glans penis to allow successful intromission of the semierect penis. The glans penis is a bipartite structure, with the pars longa glandis making up the distal three-fourths of the penis and the bulbus glandis surrounding the proximal penis. Both portions enlarge dramatically in circumference and length during erection.

In the cat the penis is immediately ventral to the scrotum and projects caudally so that the dorsum of the penis is ventral and cranial. The penis is enclosed in the prepuce when not erect; an os penis (baculum), when present, is usually rudimentary. The glans forms the cone-shaped tip of the penis and has a variable number of erectile papillae. The structures are testosterone-dependent and usually diminish in size after orchiectomy. During erection there is moderate penile enlargement in length and little in circumference.

The testes are ovoid in the dog and more spherical in the cat. In the dog the testes are oriented at an angle of about 45 degrees to the vertical, with the head of the epididymis pointing dorsocranially. In the cat the testes are more horizontal, and the head of the epididymis points almost directly cranially. In both species the body of the epididymis lies on the dorsolateral aspect of each testis, while the vas deferens returns along the medial border of the epididymis. The epididymis is closely applied to the testis so that its border is difficult to discern. A clearly palpable epididymal border is associated with abnormal changes in the size of either the testis or the epididymis. The testis and epididymis are smooth and of an elastic consistency reminiscent of an unripe grape. Microscopically, the dog testis is similar to that of other domestic mammals; in the cat the interstitial cells are more abundant and practically fill the intertubular spaces.

The prostate gland is the only accessory gland in the dog, whereas the cat has both a prostate gland and bulbourethral glands.

Testicular Function and Its Control

The testes are divided into three functional compartments. The interstitial compartment surrounds the seminiferous tubules and contains the interstitial cells (Leydig cells), which are the primary producers of testosterone (and estradiol). The basal compartment within the seminiferous tubules lies between the basement membrane and the junctional complexes formed by the Sertoli cells. It contains the basal portion of the Sertoli cells and the spermatogonia, which form a pool of cells that proliferate by mitosis (A_1 spermatogonia) and a pool of nonproliferating, reserve cells (A_0 spermatogonia). The central portion of each seminiferous tubule is the adluminal compartment. Macromolecules in the general circulation are kept out of the adluminal compartment by the intercellular junctional complexes between the Sertoli cells. The adluminal compartment contains the inner cytoplasmic processes of the Sertoli cells within which proceed meiosis of the spermatocytes (spermatocytogenesis) and development of spermatids (spermateliosis).

Testosterone of Leydig cell origin is the major gonadal steroid in the male and is essential for all phases of spermatogenesis. Estradiol is produced in minor quantities by aromatization of testosterone in the Leydig cells and in Sertoli cells. Additional estradiol may be produced by aromatization of testosterone in extratesticular tissues such as the brain. Production of testosterone (and estradiol) in the Leydig cells is stimulated by LH; FSH appears to increase spermatogenesis directly by way of the Sertoli cells and does not seem to cause changes in gonadal steroid concentrations. The positive signal for release of LH and FSH consists of pulses of hypothalamic gonadotrophin-releasing hormone (GnRH). Testosterone and estradiol make up the major negative steroid feedback system that governs the release of LH and FSH from the pituitary. In addition to the overall reduction of gonadotrophin release by testosterone, the ratio of testosterone to estradiol contacting the gonadotrophic cells may determine the LH-FSH ratio released by the pituitary.[28]

The basal compartment of the seminiferous tubules is continuously exposed to tissue fluid known to contain testosterone in concentrations that are much higher (50:1) than those measured in serum.[29] Administration of exogenous testosterone, or of anabolic androgens that suppress release of GnRH and thus of pituitary LH, will result in interruption of testosterone synthesis by the Leydig cells. Consequently the cells undergoing spermatogenesis will be deprived of essential testosterone, while the extratesticular serum testosterone concentrations are high. Sterility may result. Suppression of LH release may also result from stress, hyperadrenocorticism, or administration of exogenous glucocorticoids.[30]

The episodic and rather random release of hypothalamic GnRH results in irregular pulses of LH and FSH. LH is metabolized more rapidly than FSH, and thus is characterized by rapidly fluctuating serum concentrations, 5 to 20 excursions within 24 hours ranging in dogs from < 15 to > 90 ng/ml.[27] Serum testosterone values are generally closely correlated with LH, episodic elevations from < 1 to > 6 ng/ml occurring within one hour of the LH surges.[27] In dogs there is no apparent diurnal variation of LH and testosterone, but two to three times higher concentrations were reported in the fall (August and September) for testosterone, but not for LH.[31] With these considerations in mind it becomes clear that a single blood sample taken for measurement of LH, FSH, or testosterone would not be informative. It is recommended that at least three samples be taken, equally spaced over a period of two hours on any given day, to accurately reflect the hormonal status.

Functional Capacity of the Male

A breeding soundness examination should be required before purchase of a breeding male and in cases where breeding failure is suspected. In the evaluation of the male the following factors must be considered: aggressiveness of sexual behavior (libido), general health, soundness of the rear quarters, and spermatogenic capacity.

The obvious critical factor in judging the functional capacity of a male is his ability to deliver potentially fertile spermatozoa into the female on a day-to-day basis. The daily spermatozoal production in the dog is highly correlated with testicular weight (15 to 19 x 10^6 cells/gm of parenchyma; r = .92), and the latter is highly correlated with total scrotal width (r = .72) as measured in the living animal.[32] Thus measurement of total scrotal width is a reliable estimate of the dog's ability to produce and ejaculate spermatozoa.[32] Total scrotal width is influenced by size (weight) of the dog. Dogs ranging from 4.5 to 15.4, 15.9 to 17.7, and 27.3 to 38.2 kg had total scrotal widths of 36 ± 2, 50 ± 1, and 56 ± 1 mm, respectively.[27] Total spermatozoa in any one ejaculate should not be lower than 200 x 10^6. Frequency of ejaculation does not affect daily sperm production, but it depletes sperm reserves in the cauda epididymis and the ductus deferens. Daily or six to eight times per week ejaculation reduces the extragonadal sperm reserve by 26 per cent in one week. In situations in which high sperm concentrations are desired, such as in an aging dog with low total concentrations, or when semen is being collected for cryopreservation, the number of spermatozoa per ejaculate may be maximized by having the dog ejaculate at four- to five-day intervals.[32] Daily spermatozoal production may be estimated by collecting a series of ejaculates once daily for five to seven days. After this interval the total spermatozoa per ejaculate reflect daily spermatogenic capacity. All aspects of the collections should be standardized, since presence or absence of a teaser bitch, interval from the preceding ejaculation, and the degree of sexual arousal before collection will affect the results.[27]

Testicular Descent

The time of testicular descent in the dog and cat has not been established beyond reasonable doubt due to the small size of the neonates, the softness of the immature testes, and the tendency of the cremaster muscle to hold immature gonads in the inguinal region.[33] Final scrotal position in beagles and mixed breed pups was found to occur at seven weeks. In German short-haired pointers a positive correlation was reported between the time of passage of the testes through the inguinal canal and completion of deciduous dentition, with both events occurring at 30 to 35 days of age.[34] It may be assumed that if one or both testes remain within the abdomen after closure of the inguinal canal, a cryptorchid condition will result. Testes are thought to be descended into the scrotum at birth in the cat.

References

1. Schutte, AP: Canine vaginal cytology. Technique and cytological morphology. J Sm Anim Pract 8:301, 1967.
2. Shille, VM, et al.: Follicular function in the domestic cat as determined by estradiol-17β concentrations in plasma: relation to estrous behavior and cornification of vaginal epithelium. Biol Reprod 21:953, 1979.
3. Olson, PN, et al.: Vaginal cytology. A useful tool for staging the canine estrous cycle. Comp Cont Ed 6:288, 1984.
4. Concannon, PW: Clinical and endocrine correlates of canine ovarian cycles and pregnancy. In Kirk, RW (ed): Current Veterinary Therapy IX. Philadelphia, WB Saunders, 1986, p 1214.
5. Lindsay, FEF: The normal endoscopic appearance of the caudal reproductive tract of the cyclic and non-cyclic bitch: post-uterine endoscopy. J Sm Anim Pract 24:1, 1983.
6. Christie, DW and Bell, ET: Some observations on the seasonal incidence and frequency of oestrus in breeding bitches in Britain. J Sm Anim Pract 12:159, 1971.
7. Tedor, JB, and Reif, JS: Natal patterns among registered dogs in the United States. JAVMA 172:1179, 1978.
8. Dawson, AB: Early estrus in the cat following increased illumination. Endocrinology 28:907, 1941.
9. Prescott, CW: Reproduction patterns in the domestic cat. Aust Vet J 49:126, 1973.
10. Concannon, PW, et al.: LH release in ovariectomized dogs in response to estrogen withdrawal and its facilitation by progesterone. Biol Reprod 20:523, 1979.
11. Concannon, PW, et al.: Changes in LH, progesterone and sexual behavior associated with preovulatory luteinization in the bitch. Biol Reprod 17:604, 1972.
12. Olson, PN, et al.: Concentrations of progesterone and LH in serum of diestrous bitches before and after hysterectomy. Am J Vet Res 45:149, 1984.
13. Okkens, AC, et al.: Evidence for the non-involvement of the uterus in the lifespan of the corpus luteum in the cyclic dog. Vet Quart 7:169, 1985.
14. Shille, VM, et al.: Ovarian and endocrine responses in the cat after coitus. J Reprod Fertil 68:29, 1983.
15. Richards, JS: Modulation of folliculogenesis in the rat. Physiol Rev 60:68, 1980.
16. Olson, PN, et al.: Concentrations of canine hormones in canine serum throughout late anestrus, proestrus and estrus. Biol Reprod 27:1196, 1982.
17. Shille, VM, et al.: Concentrations of LH and FSH during selected periods of anestrus in the bitch. Biol Reprod Suppl 36:184, 1987.
18. Holst, PA and Phemister, RD: Onset of diestrus in the beagle bitch: Definitions and significance. Am J Vet Res 35:401, 1974.
19. Concannon, PW, et al.: Suppression of luteal function in dogs by luteinizing hormone antiserum and by bromocriptine. J Reprod Fertil 81:175, 1987.
20. Shille, VM and Thatcher, MJ: Unpublished observations, 1987.
21. Concannon, PW: Personal communication, 1987.
22. Al-Bassam, MA, et al.: Normal postpartum involution of the uterus in the dog. Can J Comp Med 45:217, 1981.
23. Shille, VM: PhD dissertation, University of California at Davis, 1979.
24. Herron, MA and Sis, RF: Ovum transport in the cat and the effect of estrogen administration. Am J Vet Res 35:1277, 1974.
25. Feldman, EC and Nelson, RW: Canine and feline endocrinology and reproduction. Philadelphia, WB Saunders, 1987, p 533.
26. Banks, DR, et al.: Prolactin in the cat: pseudopregnancy, pregnancy and lactation. Biol Reprod 28:923, 1983.

27. Amann, RP: Reproductive physiology and endocrinology of the dog. *In* Morrow, DW (ed.): Current therapy in theriogenology. Philadelphia, WB Saunders, 1986, p 532.
28. Winter, M, et al.: Steroidal control of gonadotropin secretion in the orchidectomized dog. J Reprod Fertil 64:449, 1982.
29. Olson, PN: Clinical approach to infertility in the stud dog. Proc Soc Theriogen 1984, p 33.
30. Feldmann, EC and Tyrell, JB: Plasma testosterone, plasma glucose and plasma insulin concentrations in spontaneous canine Cushing's syndrome. Proc ACVIM, 1982, p 81.
31. Falvo, RE, et al.: Annual variations in plasma levels of testosterone and luteinizing hormone in the laboratory male mongrel dog. J Endocrinol 86:425, 1980.
32. Olar, TT, et al.: Relationships among testicular size, daily production and output of spermatozoa and extragonadal spermatozoal reserves of the dog. Biol Reprod 29:1114, 1983.
33. Ashdown, RR: The diagnosis of cryptorchidism in the young dog: A review of the problem. J Sm Anim Pract 4:216, 1963.
34. Meyer, P: Palpatorische Befunde zum Descenzus Testis beim deutschen Kurzhaar. Dtsch Tierärztl Wchschr 79:590, 1972.

99 PERSISTENT ESTRUS IN THE BITCH

PATRICIA N. OLSON, ROBERT H. WRIGLEY,
PAUL W. HUSTED, RICHARD A. BOWEN, and
TERRY M. NETT

The average length of estrus for normal mature bitches is nine days, but some fertile bitches may be receptive to mating for up to three weeks. Persistent estrus occurs when, for a period of longer than 21 days, a bitch is receptive to mating or greater than 90 per cent of the epithelial cells in a vaginal smear are of the superficial type. If estrus (behavioral or cytologic) exceeds 21 days, the bitch should be evaluated for potential causes of persistent estrus.

OVARIAN CYSTS

An ovarian cyst is a fluid-filled structure, which may be normal or abnormal, in or around the ovary. Normal ovarian cysts in the dog include vesicular follicles and the central cavities in developing corpora lutea.[1-3] Cystic follicles and luteinized cystic follicles are abnormal cysts that may synthesize and secrete varying amounts of sex steroids, depending partly on the degree of luteinization present (Figure 99–1). Normal developing follicles

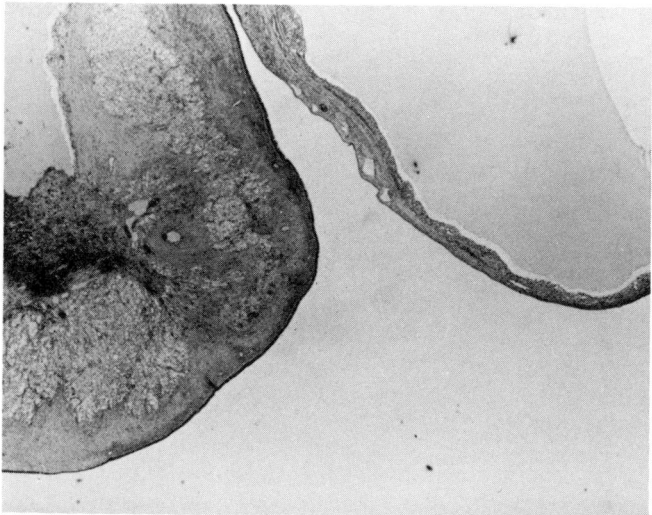

FIGURE 99–1. Histologic appearance of two ovarian cysts within a single ovary. Note differing amounts of luteal tissue among the cysts.

undergo preovulatory luteinization in the bitch;[4-5] however, luteinized cystic follicles do not subsequently ovulate. Abnormal cysts not associated with production of hormones include cysts of the rete ovarii, subsurface epithelial structure (SES) cysts, and cysts within ovarian tumors.

The following discussion will concentrate on abnormal cysts that secrete hormones (e.g., cystic follicles and luteinized cystic follicles), since these cysts are more likely to be associated with persistent estrus in the bitch.

Dow examined 63 bitches with cystic follicles and found that cysts may be solitary or multiple.[2] Solitary cysts were identified in 41 bitches between 2 and 15 years of age, 29 of which were nulliparous. Corpora lutea at various stages of growth and regression were present in the affected and normal ovaries of 31 bitches. Multiple cysts were identified in the other 22 bitches, all of whom were over five years of age, with 18 of the bitches being nulliparous.

Dow identified cysts lined with luteal tissue (luteinized cystic follicles) in another 9 bitches between 2 and 13 years of age, with 6 of the bitches being nulliparous.[2] In each case the luteinized cystic follicle was solitary. Interestingly, of the 72 bitches with cystic follicles, or luteinized cystic follicles, none had histologic evidence of estrogenic stimulation of the vagina. Cystic endometrial hyperplasia was noted in 16 of the bitches. A wide range of signs (persistent estrus to persistent anestrus) may be present in animals with abnormal ovarian cysts. Reportedly, 62 to 85 per cent of cows with cystic follicles are anestrus. Persistent estrus or nymphomania occurs much less frequently.[6]

Thirteen bitches in persistent estrus were evaluated at the Colorado State University Veterinary Teaching Hospital from 1982 to 1986. Abnormal ovarian cysts were diagnosed by ultrasonography, increased concentrations of various sex steroids in the serum, visualizing the cyst(s) at surgery, or response to treatment (Table 99–1). Because 9 of 11 bitches treated medically initially responded to treatment, histologic evaluation is lacking for these cases. Nine bitches were under three years of age, one bitch had recently been aborted with estrogens after a mismating, and two bitches subsequently devel-

TABLE 99–1. CHARACTERISTICS OF BITCHES IN PERSISTENT ESTRUS WITH OVARIAN CYSTS

Animal No. and Breed	Age	Pertinent History	Treatment*	Results	Concentrations of Hormones in Serum			Concentrations of Hormones in Follicular Fluid			Cyst(s) Observed with Ultrasonography
					Estradiol (pg/ml)	Progesterone (ng/ml)	Testosterone (ng/ml)	Estradiol (pg/ml)	Progesterone (ng/ml)	Testosterone (ng/ml)	
1. Malamute	7 mo	In estrus 7 wk	GnRH × 2	Did not resolve	6	1.0	0.8	48,830	2	12	Yes
			GnRH × 3 + surgical drainage	Resolved							
2. Husky X	1.5 yr	In estrus 8 wk	GnRH × 1	Resolved but recurred next cycle, then spayed	24	1.9	0.13	1379	1133	1.9	Yes
3. Malamute	10 mo	In estrus 4 mo	hCG × 1	Did not resolve	38	1.0	0.01	—	—	—	Yes
			GnRH × 2	Resolved							
4. Golden retriever	15 mo	In estrus 4 mo	hCG × 3	Did not resolve	16	6.0	2.8	—	—	—	Yes
			GnRH × 1	Resolved							
5. Yorkshire terrier	3.5 yr	In estrus 3 mo	GnRII × 2	Did not resolve	9	0.8	0.39	—	—	—	Yes
			hCG × 1	Did not resolve							
			GnRH × 3	Resolved but pyometra occurred and bitch was spayed							
6. Chesapeake retriever	16 mo	In estrus 4 wk, out 1 wk, back in estrus	hCG × 1	Resolved	9	1.0	—	—	—	—	—
7. Golden retriever	2.5 yr	In and out of estrus for 2 mo after estrogen treatment for terminating pregnancy	hCG × 2	Resolved; was bred and delivered a single pup	3	2.0	—	—	—	—	ND
8. Greyhound	9.5 yr	Estrous vaginal smear for 2 mo	hCG × 3	Resolved but recurred	143	0.04	0.07	—	—	—	Yes
			GnRH × 3 surgically drained	Did not resolve	19	0.88	ND	138,000	193	35	Yes
			Tamoxifen citrate	Resolved but recurred							
9. Golden retriever	8 mo	In estrus for 8 wk	GnRH × 2	Resolved	26	4.8	0.13	—	—	—	ND
10. Malamute	9 mo	In and out of estrus for 3 mo	PGF$_{2\alpha}$	Did not resolve	ND	1.9	0.06	—	—	—	Yes
			GnRH × 1	Resolved							
11. Scottish terrier	1 yr	In estrus 8 wk	Spayed	Resolved	—	0.39	0.10	—	233	50	—
12. Malamute	3 yr	In estrus 6 wk	Spayed	Resolved	—	0.6	ND	92,000	7392	2.6	—
13. St. Bernard	4 yr	In estrus 4 wk	GnRH × 2	Did not resolve; developed pyometra	24	0.03	0.19	—	—	—	Yes

GnRH, gonadotrophin-releasing hormone; hCG, human chorionic gonadotrophin; ND, not detectable; —, not determined; X, mixed-breed dog.
*Multiple treatments (two or three) were usually separated by 24 to 48 hours.

oped overt pyometra after medical therapy. Concentrations of hormones in follicular fluid varied greatly among five bitches sampled. Data are insufficient to speculate on a breed incidence, although 7 of the 13 bitches with persistent estrus were malamutes or golden retrievers (Table 99–1).

Diagnosis

Abnormal ovarian cysts that secrete hormones should be considered when a bitch has been in behavioral or cytologic estrus for longer than 21 days. A history of incomplete ovariohysterectomy (e.g., a bitch that cycles

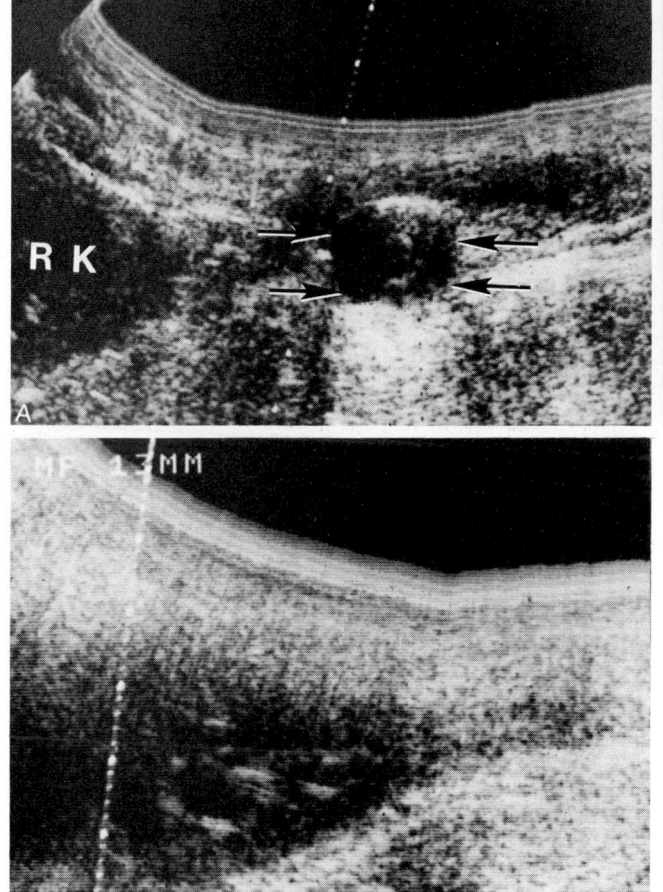

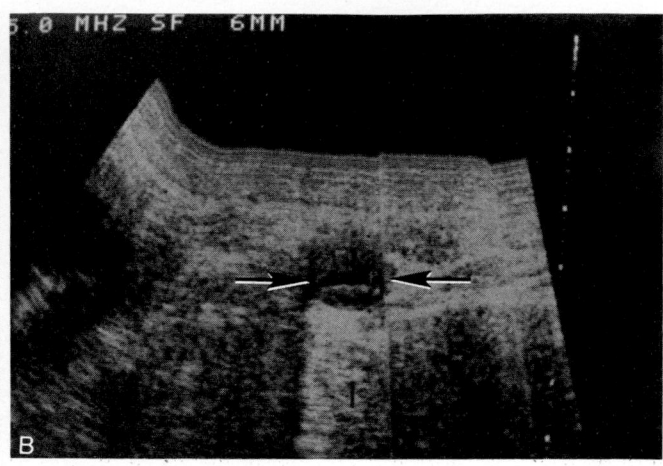

FIGURE 99–2. *A,* Ultrasonogram of the region caudal to the right kidney (RK) revealed a 2-cm fluid-filled ovarian cyst (arrows). *B,* Recheck ultrasonogram six weeks later revealed partial regression of the right ovarian cyst (arrows). *C,* Recheck ultrasonogram nine weeks later revealed further regression of the right ovarian cyst.

after being spayed) or hormone therapy may add support to the diagnosis.[7–9] Concentrations of sex steroids may be measured in the bitch's serum but are not always consistently elevated (Table 99–1). Vaginal smears should be evaluated to verify stimulation of the vaginal epithelium by hormones elaborated from the cyst(s). Ultrasonography may aid in the diagnosis but must be used in conjunction with history and physical examination findings, since antra can be present in normal corpora lutea for two to three weeks after ovulation.[1] Abnormal ovarian cysts vary greatly in size, ranging from < 0.5 to > 19.0 cm in diameter.[1, 2, 10] Normal vesicular follicles before ovulation are reportedly less than 0.5 cm in diameter in beagle bitches.[3]

Treatment

Surgical removal of the abnormal ovaries should be curative. A complete blood count, including a platelet count, should be performed before surgery, since persistent elevation of estrogens in the blood could potentially result in leukopenia, thrombocytopenia, or anemia.[11–13] Medical therapy can be attempted in cases in which the owners desire to breed the bitch at some future time. Although various medical regimens have not been adequately evaluated, abnormal cysts occa-

sionally complete luteinization (Figure 99–2*A* through 2*C*) after the administration of human chorionic gonadotrophin (HCG, 10 units/lb given intramuscularly) or gonadotrophin-releasing hormone (GnRH, 50 to 100 μg/bitch given intramuscularly). In a study using Labrador bitches, 50 μg of GnRH stimulated secretion of luteinizing hormone (LH) similar to that observed during a preovulatory surge.[14] Therefore, ≥ 50 μg of GnRH should be adequate to release preovulatory levels of LH. Whether multiple injections of HCG or GnRH are necessary or beneficial is unknown. Owners should be cautioned that medical therapy might not result in resolution of the problem (Table 99–1). Therefore, bitches should be reevaluated two to three weeks after therapy to determine if estrus has ceased. Vaginal smears should no longer look like estrus smears if treatment was successful. If luteinization of cystic follicles or further luteinization of luteinized cystic follicles follows therapy, concentrations of serum progesterone should be elevated above pretreatment levels. Dow[2] identified corpora lutea at various stages of growth and regression in affected and normal ovaries of 31 of 41 bitches with solitary cystic follicles. Therefore, it seems likely that some bitches with cystic follicles may have concentrations of serum progesterone comparable to those of normal diestrous bitches. Dow also reported that none of the bitches examined had estrogenic stim-

TABLE 99–2. CHARACTERISTICS OF BITCHES IN PERSISTENT ESTRUS WITH OVARIAN TUMORS

Animal No. and Breed	Age	Pertinent History	Treatment	Results	Concentrations of Hormones in Serum			Concentrations of Hormones in Follicular Fluid			Tumor(s) Observed with Ultrasonography
					Estradiol (pg/ml)	Progesterone (ng/ml)	Testosterone (ng/ml)	Estradiol (pg/ml)	Progesterone (ng/ml)	Testosterone (ng/ml)	
1. Golden retriever	11 yr	In estrus >6 wk; was spayed 10 yr ago	Removed ovarian tissue (granulosa cell tumor) and uterine stump (granulation tissue)	Resolved	—	0.43	ND	—	—	—	—
2. Silky terrier	15 yr	In estrus 3 mo	hCG Removed ovaries (bilateral granulosa cell tumors) and uterus (CEH) and mammary growth (papillary adenoma)	Did not resolve Resolved	34	0.49	0.70	—	—	—	ND
3. Malamute	4 yr	In and out of estrus for 8 mo	Removed R ovary (granulosa cell tumor) and R cranial uterine horn (CEH)	Resolved and subsequently whelped puppies	111	0.60	0.97	Four fluid-filled structures on R. ovary evaluated ND / ND / 0.9 ND / 4.2 / 4.8 43 / 107.5 / 28.6 341 / 12.9 / 13.9			Yes
4. Pekingese X	16 yr	In estrus 2.5 mo	Removed ovaries (cystadenocarcinoma) and uterus	Resolved	25	1.32	0.16	—	—	—	—
5. Lhasa apso	17 yr	In estrus 6 wk	Removed ovaries (bilateral granulosa cell tumors) and uterus (edema)		—	0.25	0.05	—	—	—	Yes

ND, not detectable; —, not determined; hCG, human chorionic gonadotrophin; CEH, cystic endometrial hyperplasia; X, mixed-breed dog.

ulation of the vaginal epithelium. All 13 bitches with persistent estrus evaluated at the Colorado State University Veterinary Teaching Hospital had estrogenic stimulation of the vaginal epithelium. Serum concentrations of progesterone in all bitches sampled with ovarian cysts were less than 10 ng/ml before treatment (Table 99–1). Therefore, concentrations of serum progesterone should increase in bitches treated medically for persistent estrus if luteinization of follicles occurs and the bitch enters diestrus.

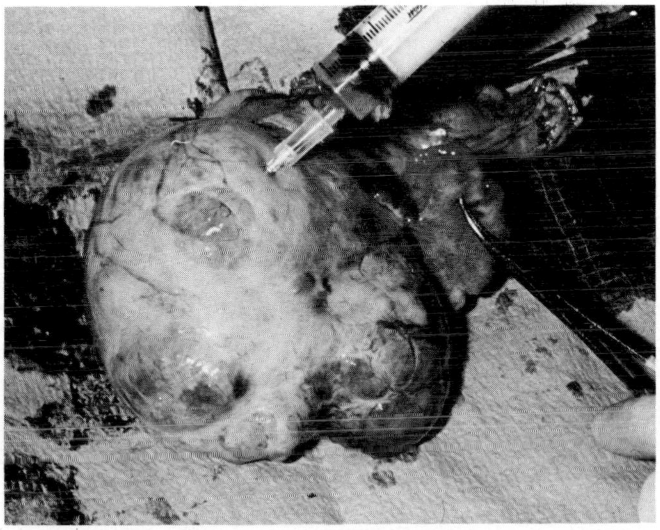

Owners should also be made aware that the problem can recur after apparent resolution. Even when the problem does not recur, subsequent fertility may be reduced, since the incidence of uterine disease appears to be high following "successful" therapy (Table 99–1); further stimulation of the endometrium will occur as ovarian cysts luteinize and serum concentrations of progesterone increase.

OVARIAN TUMORS

Persistent estrus may also occur in bitches with functional ovarian tumors. Although ovarian tumors generally occur in older bitches (mean age of eight years), such tumors occasionally occur in young bitches or bitches with ovarian tissue remaining after incomplete ovariectomy (Table 99–2).[15] Like abnormal ovarian cysts, ovarian tumors can produce a variety of hormones. Functional ovarian tumors frequently originate from sex cord stroma, with 10 to 25 per cent of such tumors being malignant.[15] In the dog the most common hormone-producing ovarian tumor is the granulosa cell tumor. Granulosa cell tumors may be bilateral or unilateral and vary in size from 4 to 16 cm.[13] Although granulosa cell tumors were found in 13 of 115 bitches with ovarian lesions, only in 9 were the ovaries consid-

FIGURE 99–3. Granulosa cell tumor removed from a four-year-old malamute. The bitch later whelped a litter of puppies

ered abnormal at the time of gross autopsy.[2] Hence size and consistency of these tumors can vary considerably (Figure 99–3). Functional ovarian tumors should be considered when persistent estrus is diagnosed in an older bitch. Ovarian tumors are unlikely to respond to medical therapy and should be surgically excised. A thorough examination of the abdominal cavity should be performed when the ovarian tissue is removed to evaluate for possible metastasis.

ESTROGEN THERAPY

A complete drug history should be obtained from the owner when a bitch is presented with signs of persistent estrus. Estrus is frequently lengthened when bitches receive estrogens to terminate unwanted pregnancies. If a bitch remains in estrus for longer than three weeks after a single estrogen treatment, the bitch should be evaluated for abnormal ovarian cysts. Because pyometra, abnormal ovarian cysts, and bone marrow suppression all are associated with estrogen therapy, aborting unwanted pregnancies with estrogens is extremely dangerous. Owners of mismated bitches must be cautioned that terminating pregnancy with estrogens can result in reproductive disease or possibly even death.

LIVER DISEASE

Because the liver is involved in metabolizing many reproductive hormones, bitches in persistent estrus should always be screened for liver disease. Rarely, a bitch with a portosystemic shunt may present for persistent estrus. Because the reserve capacity of the liver is great, abnormal estrous cycles would be anticipated only with severe liver disease.

SPLIT ESTROUS PERIODS

Split estrous periods may be seen occasionally in pubertal bitches and rarely in mature bitches. Although persistent estrus is not a feature of split estrous periods, the owner may consider the bitch in persistent estrus owing to the short interestrus interval. Bitches with split estrous periods exhibit signs of target tissue stimulation by estrogens (vulvar swelling, serosanguineous discharge) for a few days as follicles develop. The bitch may or may not be receptive to mating. This is followed by a regression of vulvar size and cessation of the serosanguineous discharge for a few weeks until the bitch enters a "true" season and ovulates. If the bitch is mated appropriately during the second part of a "split" estrus, fertility should be normal.

References

1. Bloom, F: Ovarian cysts. *In* Pathology of the Dog and Cat. Evanston, IL, American Veterinary Publications, 1954, p 390.
2. Dow, C: Ovarian abnormalities in the bitch. J Comp Pathol 70:59, 1960.
3. Andersen, AC and Simpson, ME: The ovary and reproductive cycle of the dog (beagle). Los Altos, CA, Geron-x, 1973, p 128.
4. Concannon, PN, et al.: Changes in LH, progesterone and sexual behavior associated with preovulatory luteinization in the bitch. Biol Reprod 17:604, 1977.
5. Phemister, RD, et al.: Time of ovulation in the beagle bitch. Biol Reprod 8:74, 1973.
6. Kesler, DJ and Garverick, HA: Ovarian cysts in dairy cattle: A review. J Anim Sci 55:1147, 1982.
7. Miller DM, et al.: Polycystic ovarian tissue in a spayed bitch. Mod Vet Prac 64:749, 1983.
8. Jubb, KVF and Kennedy, PC: Pathology of domestic animals. New York, Academic Press, 1970, p 502.
9. Bowen, RA, et al.: Efficacy and toxicity of tamoxifen citrate in terminating canine pregnancies. Am J Vet Res, 1987.
10. Rowley, J: Cystic ovary in a dog: a case report. VM/SAC, December, 1980, p 1888.
11. Sherding, RG, et al.: Bone marrow hypoplasia in eight dogs with sertoli-cell tumor. JAVMA 178:5, 1981.
12. Chin, T: Studies on estrogen induced proliferative disorders of hemopoietic tissues in dogs. Thesis, University of Minnesota, 1974.
13. Schalm, DW: Exogenous estrogen toxicity in the dog. Canine Prac 5:57, 1978.
14. Chakraborty, PK and Fletcher, WS: Responsiveness of anestrus Labrador bitches to GnRH (39618). Proc Soc Exp Biol Med 154:125, 1977.
15. Withrow, SJ and Susaneck, SJ: Tumors of the canine reproductive tract. *In* Morrow, DA (ed): Current Therapy in Theriogenology, 2nd ed. Philadelphia, WB Saunders, 1986, p 521.

100 UTERINE DISEASES

CHERI A. JOHNSON

ANATOMY AND PHYSIOLOGY

Normal development of the reproductive tract is determined by the chromosomal and gonadal constitution of the individual. During early embryogenesis the müllerian and wolffian ducts develop from the mesonephric kidney. Both duct systems are present in the embryo until sexual differentiation begins, regardless of chromosomal or gonadal sex.[1] In the female the müllerian ducts persist and give rise to the oviducts, uterus, and cranial vagina.[1, 2] The muscular portion of the uterus is derived from the mesenchyme surrounding the müllerian ducts. The urogenital mesentery develops into the broad ligament.[1] Unlike its male counterpart, the müllerian duct never becomes contiguous with the gonad. The wolffian duct is the precursor of the ureteral bud, which ultimately develops into the renal collecting tubules, the ureter, and a part of the urinary bladder in both sexes. Normal müllerian duct development requires the presence of wolffian ducts and the absence of fetal testes.[1, 2] It is unknown how the normal milieu of hormones (steroidal and nonsteroidal) influences female phenotypic development.[1] It appears that in the absence of specific determinants for male development, phenotypic sex will be female.[2]

The uterus is subject to cyclic hormonal stimulation, most importantly from the ovarian hormones (see Chapter 98). The effects of hormonal stimulation are evident macroscopically and microscopically; therefore, the stage of the estrous cycle must always be taken into account when interpreting the appearance of the reproductive tract. During proestrus and estrus, estradiol is the principal hormone produced by ovarian follicles. Estradiol causes the endometrial glands to elongate. The epithelial cells of the glands assume a short columnar shape. Metabolic activity is evidenced by the formation of electron-dense secretory granules.[3] An estrogen-dependent protein has been identified in the lumen of endometrial glands and in the uterine lumen of cats. This protein may play a role in sperm capacitation, sperm or blastocyst viability, and/or implantation.[4] Estradiol also induces the formation of endometrial estrogen and progesterone receptors in both the bitch and queen.[3, 5, 6] In this regard, estradiol has a regulatory effect in the target tissues' responsiveness to continued or subsequent hormonal stimulation.

Following ovulation the ovarian follicles become lu-

teinized and produce progesterone. This luteal phase of the cycle is also known as diestrus or metestrus (see Chapter 98). Progesterone causes hyperplasia and hypertrophy of the endometrial glands.[3] In its presence the estrogen-induced secretory granules are depleted and the glandular epithelial cells begin to synthesize and store glycogen.[3, 4] These progestational effects occur with or without estrogen priming; however, they are delayed in the absence of estrogen.[3] Progesterone decreases the number of endometrial progesterone receptors, thereby regulating its own effects.[5]

Grossly, the uterus has a relatively uniform diameter along its length throughout the nonpregnant estrous cycle. During proestrus and estrus the uterus, especially the endometrium, has an edematous appearance.[7, 8] The endometrial glands are tortuous. They have an increased diameter and thickened epithelial cells, which are columnar and cuboidal. The uterine mucosa is lined by cuboidal cells. There is extravasation of red blood cells into the uterus. There is an increased number of cellular elements in the lamina propria and numerous mitotic figures.[8, 9]

During the luteal phase the uterus develops a corrugated, "corkscrew" appearance grossly.[8] Histologically, there is marked endometrial gland hypertrophy and hyperplasia. Late in the luteal phase there is also cystic dilation of the endometrial glands. The lamina propria and myometrial cells are smaller than during the follicular phase, and there is no edema. Early in the luteal phase the uterine mucosa is composed of small, low cuboidal cells. Late in the luteal phase the mucosal cells become large cuboidal and columnar cells with foamy cytoplasm. At this time there is an increase in the number of leukocytes in the mucosa. The uterine lumen contains necrotic glandular elements and amorphous material.[8, 9]

By the end of the nonpregnant luteal phase, uterine size has decreased to approximately that of proestrus. The uteri of the anestrous bitch, prepuberal bitch, and oophorectomized bitch are similar except for size; after one cycle, the uterus in these animals remains larger than the uterus of an immature or castrated bitch.[8] Histologically, the endometrial glands are short, the epithelial cells are cuboidal, and there is no evidence of secretory activity in either the bitch or queen.[3, 8]

The postpartum uterus is markedly different from the anestrual uterus. During the first postpartum week the uterine horns are grossly dilated and edematous. The

1798   SECTION XI—The Reproductive System

placental sites are covered with mucus and blood clots and are 1.5 to 3 cm wide in the bitch. Histologically, the placental sites are covered with a necrotic mass. There are few intact epithelial cells. Decidual cells are scattered throughout the lamina propria of the placental sites.[10] By the fourth week post partum the placental sites are thick and nodular. They are grayish tan and covered with a few blood clots. Histologically, the placental sites are covered with a mass of collagen fibers.[10] The endometrial glands are greatly dilated, degenerative, and filled with amorphous material. There is a marked mononuclear cell infiltrate in the lamina propria, phagocytized hemosiderin, and increased connective tissue.[8, 10]

During the seventh week post partum the uterine horns are greatly contracted. The placental sites are narrow with few nodules and are light in color. Histologically, large masses of collagen are detached from the luminal surface. The endometrial glands are normal.[10] By the ninth week the uterine horns are uniformly contracted with a narrow lumen and uterine weight approaches that of anestrus.[8, 10] The placental sites are narrow, brown bands. Histologically, the surface sloughing is complete, but replacement of the endometrial lining continues until the 12th week.[10] By 17 weeks post partum the histologic appearance is similar to that of anestrus, except for the presence of hemosiderin deposits. The mucosa is lined with small cuboidal cells.[8]

Like the endometrium, the myometrium responds to many chemicals, the effects of which often vary according to the stage of the estrous cycle. Estrogen, progesterone, oxytocin, prostaglandins, ergonovine, and general anesthetics can all alter uterine motility.[11, 12] The uterus also produces a variety of chemicals, such as histamine and prostaglandins. These are thought to play roles in implantation. The anti-prostaglandin indomethacin and the H_2-receptor antagonist cimetidine have deleterious effects on placentation and fetal viability in some species.[13] In species other than the bitch a uterine luteolytic factor apparently exists because corpora luteal (CL) life is prolonged after hysterectomy.[14] In the bitch the uterus, pregnant or not, has no apparent luteolytic or luteotrophic properties.[14] Unlike in the bitch, certain pregnancy-specific hormones, such as relaxin, have been identified in the queen. It is thought that these are produced by the placenta directly or that some placental substance stimulates ovarian production.[15]

DISORDERS OF THE UTERUS

Cystic Endometrial Hyperplasia—Pyometra

Cystic endometrial hyperplasia (CEH) induced by progesterone is the first lesion in the development of pyometra. The normal physiologic response of the endometrium to progesterone is exaggerated. Endometrial glands become cystic and fluid-filled, and fluid accumulates in the uterine lumen. Although accumulation of sterile fluid (hydrometra/mucometra), causing uterine enlargement and abdominal distention, has been reported in the bitch and queen, this is uncommon.[16]

Secondary bacterial infection occurs in most animals. The fluid accumulation in the uterine lumen and the endometrial glands and decreased myometrial contractility caused by progesterone are thought to favor bacterial invasion.[17] Also, binding of *Escherichia coli* to the brush border of the endometrium and to the myometrium has been shown *in vitro* to be most pronounced during the early luteal phase. *In vitro* binding of *E. coli* is decreased during anestrus.[18] *E. coli* is the most commonly isolated organism. *Streptococcus, Staphylococcus, Pseudomonas, Proteus, Klebsiella, Salmonella,* and mixed bacterial infections also occur.[19–22] Most of the morbidity and mortality associated with CEH-pyometra can be attributed to secondary bacterial infection of the abnormal uterus.[18, 20]

The role of progesterone in the pathophysiology of CEH-pyometra has been investigated.[19, 23–26] When progesterone is administered to oophorectomized bitches, the lesions of CEH and all the typical signs of pyometra are produced. No such lesions are produced when estrogens alone are administered. The occurrence of CEH and pyometra after exogenous progesterone administration are dose- and duration-dependent in both the bitch and queen. Similar uterine pathology has been described after administration of the progestational compounds progesterone, melengestrol acetate, megestrol acetate, medroxyprogesterone acetate, 17-α-acetoxyprogesterone, and chlormadinone acetate to bitches. CEH and pyometra after megestrol acetate and medroxyprogesterone administration to intact, and partially hysterectomized, queens has been reported frequently.[23, 27–29] In addition to CEH, exogenous progestins cause adrenocortical suppression in bitches and queens.[24, 25]

Although exogenous estrogen alone does not cause CEH or pyometra, it does potentiate the effects of progesterone.[19, 20, 30] Pyometra occurred in 25 per cent of bitches given estradiol cypionate (ECP) on the second day of diestrus,[31] a time when endogenous progesterone is rapidly increasing (see Chapter 98). The study simulated the dosages and times of administration of ECP that might be used to prevent pregnancy after accidental mating (mismating). Several (12.5 per cent) of the bitches treated with ECP during diestrus became pregnant. Diethylstilbestrol (DES) was evaluated in the same study. Although none of the bitches developed pyometra, 75 per cent of DES-treated bitches did conceive. Because of the risks of pyometra and the poor efficacy in preventing pregnancy, the authors concluded that estrogens should not be used for pregnancy prevention in the bitch. Others have also recommended that when vaginal cytology is consistent with diestrus, estrogens should never be used as abortifacients in bitches.[32] The mechanism by which estrogen enhances progesterone-induced CEH is unknown. Possibly the estrogenic induction and maintenance of endometrial progesterone receptors[3, 5] play a role.

Dow described four clinical and histologic types of CEH-pyometra in the bitch[19] and queen[22] (Table 100–1). Animals with type I CEH had no signs of illness except for a bloody vaginal discharge in some cats and a mucoid vaginal discharge in some bitches. Grossly and histologically, there was CEH without inflammation. Some cysts were up to 6 cm long, projecting into the

TABLE 100–1. SUMMARY OF DOW'S CLASSIFICATION OF CYSTIC ENDOMETRIAL HYPERPLASIA–PYOMETRA

Type I	Cystic endometrial hyperplasia
	No inflammation
	No clinical signs except ± vaginal discharge
Type II	Cystic endometrial hyperplasia
	With plasma cell infiltrate (bitch)
	With PMN infiltrate (queen)
	± Clinical illness
Type III	Cystic endometrial hyperplasia
	Abscesses around endometrial glands
	Clinically ill
	PMN infiltration of endometrium ± myometrium (bitch)
	Mononuclear infiltration (queen)
Type IV	Open cervix: cystic endometrial hyperplasia, fibrosis, myometrial hypertrophy
	Closed cervix: extreme uterine distention, thin uterine wall, endometrial atrophy
	Clinically ill

uterine lumen in cats. Cysts up to 1 cm in diameter were found in bitches. Type II CEH-pyometra in bitches was characterized clinically by the presence of a vaginal discharge and a slight leukocytosis. Uterine horns were usually less than 2 cm in diameter. CEH was accompanied by plasma cell infiltration in the endometrium. Queens with type II CEH had polymorphonuclear (PMN) cell infiltration in the endometrium and some had such infiltration in the myometrium as well. These queens were clinically ill and may or may not have had a vaginal discharge.

Animals with types III and IV CEH were clinically ill, and the uterine exudate was rarely sterile. A leukocytosis with a left shift was usually present. Uterine size varied inversely with cervical patency. Occasionally only one uterine horn was abnormal. Some animals had annular constrictions along the uterine horns, giving the external appearance of pregnancy. The histopathologic appearance of type III CEH in the bitch was characterized by PMN infiltration of the endometrium and often of the myometrium. There were local abscesses around endometrial glands in both bitches and queens. Plasma cells and other mononuclear cells were the predominant cellular infiltrates found in type III CEH-pyometra in queens. The histologic appearance of type IV CEH-pyometra varied with cervical patency in both the bitch and queen. When the cervix was "open" the uterine horns were usually less than 3 cm in diameter. There was CEH, fibrosis, and myometrial hypertrophy. When the cervix was closed there was extreme uterine distention, a thin uterine wall, and endometrial atrophy.

Although bitches and queens under the influence of endogenous (luteal phase) or exogenous progesterone, and luteal-phase bitches given exogenous estrogens, are obviously at greatest risk for CEH, the reason(s) only certain females are affected is unknown. There are no apparent differences in the concentrations of progesterone or unconjugated estrogens in the blood of bitches with pyometra, bitches with false pregnancy, or normal bitches in the luteal phase of the estrous cycle.[33] There is no evidence that estrus irregularities, pseudopregnancy, or lack of previous pregnancy is in any way associated with the occurrence of pyometra in the bitch.[20, 34] In a survey of 245 bitches, a previous history

of pseudopregnancy was actually more common in bitches without pyometra than in bitches with pyometra.[34] Although hyperplastic changes in the endometrium of bitches with false pregnancy have been described, progesterone was suggested by the author as the causative agent for both conditions.[35] Finally, physical abnormalities that prevent drainage of the uterus may favor the development of pyometra.[36, 37]

Because the bitch normally has a long luteal phase (see Chapter 98) and since the queen experiences a luteal phase only when induced to ovulate, pyometra should be more common in bitches than in queens. Dow reported that pyometra occurred three times as often in bitches as in queens.[22] The clinical findings with CEH-pyometra are essentially the same for both species. The signs of pyometra become evident during the luteal phase, usually four to ten weeks after estrus,[20, 21, 38] or after exogenous progestin administration, as described earlier. The signs include depression, anorexia, vomiting, diarrhea, polydipsia, and polyuria. These otherwise nonspecific signs with a history of progestin exposure are suggestive of pyometra. A purulent vaginal discharge is present in 75 per cent of bitches with pyometra.[20]

Variable severity of depression and dehydration are found on physical examination. A purulent vaginal discharge, often containing blood, may or may not be present. The vaginal discharge may be intermittent or constant, scanty or copious in amount.[19–22] Vaginal cytology, even in the absence of visibly detectable exudate, consists of masses of neutrophils and bacteria.[19, 20] Endometrial cells, mucus, and red blood cells may be observed. The uterus is usually large and palpable; however, its character depends on the volume of fluid within it. Rectal temperature is usually normal. Animals with septicemia or endotoxemia may be hypothermic. These animals are often recumbent and in shock. A leukocytosis with a left shift, monocytosis, and signs of neutrophil toxicity are usually found. However, the white blood cell (WBC) count and differential are extremely variable. There may be a leukopenia and degenerative left shift, or, alternatively, the total WBC count may approach 200,000/μl.[19–22] Anemia, hyperglobulinemia, and/or hyperfibrinogenemia may be detected. Azotemia is common. Isosthenuria and proteinuria were each found in 30 per cent of bitches with pyometra.[20]

The renal lesions associated with pyometra have been investigated. There is reduced ability to concentrate urine associated with bacterial infection of the uterus, but not with hormonal manipulations in the absence of bacterial infection. The tubules are unresponsive to antidiuretic hormone but often can still dilute urine.[39] Tubular lesions have been found by light microscopy.[18, 20] Intact bacteria, attached to tubular epithelium, have also been described.[18] Impaired tubular concentrating ability contributes to polyuria, with compensatory polydipsia. Glomerular lesions characteristic of immune-complex deposition have been identified by electron microscopy and immunofluorescent studies of renal biopsies from bitches with pyometra.[18, 20, 39] *In vitro* studies using *E. coli* recovered from bitches with naturally occurring pyometra have demonstrated *E. coli* binding affinity for the epithelium of the urinary bladder, the parietal and visceral epithelium of Bowman's capsule, and the renal tubular epithelium.[18] The renal lesions associated with pyometra are potentially reversible after removal of the bacterial antigen by ovariohysterectomy.[20]

The essential information for the diagnosis and treatment of pyometra includes a history of the stage of the estrous cycle and/or hormonal therapy and a thorough physical examination. A complete blood count, urinalysis, and biochemical profile are necessary to detect metabolic abnormalities associated with septicemia and/or toxemia, and for the evaluation of renal function. Vaginal cytology will identify the character of the vaginal discharge. Culture and sensitivity of the uterine exudate will direct antibiotic therapy. Abdominal radiography and/or ultrasonography will confirm the presence of a large uterus. The normal, nongravid uterus cannot be distinguished from bowel loops by radiography or ultrasonography.[20, 40]

The most important differential diagnosis for pyometra is pregnancy. Both conditions occur during the luteal phase of the estrous cycle. A leukocytosis in the range of 20,000 WBCs/μl may be detected in normal pregnancy (see Chapter 98); however, there should be no left shift or signs of toxicity. A differential WBC count must be performed on animals suspected of having pyometra. The presence of a purulent vaginal discharge does not negate the possibility of pregnancy. Infection does occasionally occur during pregnancy, and the litter is not necessarily lost in all cases.[41] Finally, vaginal discharge is common during abortion. Sometimes only part of the litter is aborted.[41] The radiographic appearance of the pregnant uterus before fetal calcification (about 42 days) is indistinguishable from that of pyometra. Both have a homogeneous fluid density. Ultrasonography is very helpful in differentiating pyometra from pregnancy. Before day 28, pregnancy diagnosis with ultrasonography is not always accurate,[42] but differentiating pyometra from pregnancy should still be possible. CEH has been identified by ultrasonography.[40] Ascitic fluid such as is seen when uterine contents exude into the abdomen by way of the oviducts may be identified by ultrasonography before it is detectable with radiography. Knowledge that the uterine contents have already contaminated the abdominal cavity might alter the therapeutic plans.

The treatment of choice for CEH-pyometra is ovariohysterectomy. Dehydration should be corrected with aggressive fluid therapy before surgery. Fluid therapy should be continued throughout surgery to ensure that adequate tissue perfusion is maintained. Septicemia and/or endotoxemia can develop at any time. Glucocorticoid therapy may be indicated. Broad-spectrum bactericidal antibiotics should be administered promptly. The antibiotic can be changed, if necessary, when the results of the culture and sensitivity are known. Complications of ovariohysterectomy are peritonitis from leakage of uterine contents into the abdominal cavity, and granuloma formation at the uterine stump.[20]

Ovariohysterectomy may be unacceptable to some owners of purebred animals. The goal of medical management of pyometra is twofold: first, to resolve the clinical illness in the affected females, and second, to preserve their reproductive capability. Prostaglandin $F_{2\alpha}$

($PGF_{2\alpha}$) has been used to treat pyometra in both the bitch[21, 38] and queen.[43] It is administered subcutaneously, once daily, for three to five days. The duration of treatment is determined by uterine evacuation. The uterine discharge usually changes from purulent to serosanguineous and then ceases. The diameter of the uterus decreases. Some animals may need to be treated for longer than five days, but this may indicate a worse prognosis. The dosages reported have been 0.1 mg/kg, 0.25 mg/kg, and 0.5 mg/kg. Untoward effects of $PGF_{2\alpha}$ are dose-dependent and are severest 90 to 120 minutes after administration. They include restlessness, myometrial contraction, salivation, vomiting, defecation, panting, and pupillary dilation and constriction.[21, 44, 45] The LD_{50} for $PGF_{2\alpha}$ in dogs is 5.13 mg/kg.[44] At this high dosage, ataxia and cardiovascular collapse are followed by death. Cats given 5 mg/kg became seriously ill, with signs of ataxia, respiratory distress, muscle tremors, and frequent loose stools, but none died.[45] The dosages of $PGF_{2\alpha}$ used in the treatment of pyometra do not cause luteolysis in either the bitch[44, 46] or queen.[45] The beneficial effects of prostaglandin in the treatment of pyometra are apparently due solely to myometrial contraction and uterine evacuation.

Antibiotics, chosen on the basis of culture and sensitivity, should be administered for two to four weeks.[21, 38, 43] Dehydration is corrected with fluid therapy. Successful resolution of the clinical signs of open-cervix pyometra after the medical management described above varies from 82[21] to 100 per cent.[38] Several bitches required two courses of $PGF_{2\alpha}$ administration within a six-week period. Subsequent pregnancy occurred in 40[38] to 82 per cent[21] of treated bitches. Only one of four bitches with closed-cervix pyometra was treated successfully.[21] There are no reports of successful treatment of closed-cervix pyometra in the queen.

Meyers-Wallen and associates[38] found that histopathologic evidence of periglandular fibrosis was associated with the poorest prognosis for subsequent fertility, although one such bitch did conceive. They also reported a 77 per cent recurrence of pyometra in 27 months after prostaglandin treatment. Pyometra recurred after successful pregnancy in two bitches and during pregnancy in two others. Recurrence of pyometra after the next estrous cycle has also been observed.[21] These observations prompted the suggestion that prostaglandins reduce CEH-pyometra to a subclinical level and/or delay the progression of disease.[38] CEH was still evident histologically after prostaglandin treatment.[38] Therefore, bitches and queens should be bred as soon as possible after medical treatment for pyometra because their reproductive potential will be limited by recurrence of disease.[21, 43]

There are several complications of prostaglandin $F_{2\alpha}$ therapy for pyometra. The most important are the systemic effects of prostaglandins described earlier. These effects (panting, vomiting, etc.) are predictable, and at least some of them will occur at the recommended doses. These effects may limit or preclude treatment with prostaglandin. The uterus may rupture after administration of $PGF_{2\alpha}$[21, 47] especially when the cervix is closed. If the animal is actually pregnant, rather than affected with pyometra, prostaglandin therapy may induce abortion. Medical management of pyometra does not always resolve the clinical signs of pyometra. Also, prostaglandin therapy itself causes some morbidity and therefore cannot be continued indefinitely. Placement, by means of laparotomy, of catheters into the uterine horns reportedly enhanced uterine drainage in bitches treated unsuccessfully with $PGF_{2\alpha}$ for seven to nine days. The catheters were left in place for 9 to 13 days. One of three bitches treated in this manner subsequently became pregnant.[48] The effects of prostaglandin on the interestral interval and/or on estrus itself are not yet known.[45, 49] Two final points must be emphasized. First, the preceding discussion refers only to prostaglandin $F_{2\alpha}$. The more potent prostaglandin analogs, such as fluprostenol and cloprostenol, have not been investigated for the treatment of pyometra in small animals. Finally, prostaglandins do not currently have Food and Drug Administration approval for use in dogs or cats. Therefore, appropriate discrimination should be used in case selection.

Metritis

Metritis is an acute, ascending bacterial infection of the uterus. It is almost always a postpartum disorder.[12, 17, 21, 32] Dystocia, obstetric manipulations, retained fetuses, and retained placentas predispose the development of metritis.[12, 17] Metritis may rarely develop after natural or artificial insemination, or follow abortion.[17] A hematogenous route of infection is unusual. Gram-negative infection, especially with *E. coli*, is most common. Streptococcal and staphylococcal infection also occur.[12, 17]

The clinical signs of metritis are typical for bacterial infection: fever, dehydration, depression, anorexia, and tachycardia. Affected females usually have poor milk production and neglect the neonates.[12, 17] There is a foul-smelling vaginal discharge. Vaginal cytology has degenerate PMNs, intracellular and extracellular bacteria, mucus, cellular debris, and endometrial cells. Muscle fibers from decomposing fetuses may be observed on rare occasions.[12, 32] The uterus is usually large, with a "doughy" consistency. Retained fetuses may or may not be palpable. There is usually a leukocytosis with a left shift. Septic animals may have a leukopenia with a degenerative left shift. There is often prerenal azotemia. Isosthenuria may occur because of endotoxin's interference with antidiuretic hormone.[12]

The diagnosis of acute metritis is based on the typical historical and physical abnormalities. Abdominal radiographs and/or ultrasonography should be done to evaluate the uterine size and uterine contents. Vaginal cytology will differentiate a purulent or septic uterine exudate from normal lochia. Cultures from the cranial vagina should be obtained.

Treatment should be prompt and aggressive because rapid deterioration is common with septicemia and toxemia.[12, 17] Therapy consists of intravenous fluid administration, antibiotics, and evacuation of uterine contents. The latter may be accomplished by ovariohysterectomy. Alternatively, various ecbolic agents may be used. Oxytocin has been the standard medical therapy, at dosages of 0.25 to 0.5 U/lb (0.5 to 1 U/kg), not to exceed 20 units, given once or twice at one- to two-hour intervals. Prostaglandin $F_{2\alpha}$, 0.1 to 0.5 mg/kg subcutaneously once daily for three to five days,[21] and ergonovine, 0.2 mg/35 lb (0.2 mg/15 kg), intramuscularly once,[17] have also been used. Uterine contractions induced by these ecbolic agents are intense and may cause uterine rupture. Occasionally the postpartum cervix can be cannulated. If so, the uterus can be flushed with sterile saline or 2 per cent povidone-iodine (Betadine) solution.[12] Infusion of antibiotics is of questionable value. Nitrofurazone infusion has been shown to reduce subsequent fertility in cattle.[12] Finally, hysterotomy to remove retained placentas, retained fetuses, and other debris, and to flush the uterus, has been performed.[12] The uterus may be friable, and there is danger of uterine rupture with both mechanical and pharmacologic manipulation. Metritis may become chronic and cause infertility.[17]

Congenital Anomalies

Most congenital anomalies of the uterus have been incidental findings at the time of elective ovariohysterectomy. Some are identified during the investigation of infertility. Uterus unicornis,[50] segmental aplasia of the uterine horn,[51] and bifurcation of the cervix[52] have been described. These have not been associated with clinical signs except for infertility. Several animals have had multiple anomalies.[50, 52] The extrauterine anomalies have occasionally caused clinical signs.

Uterine Torsion

Torsion of one or both uterine horns is uncommon in the bitch and queen. When it occurs it is usually with the gravid uterus, near term.[53] Torsion of the nongravid uterus has been described in the bitch.[53, 54] Clinical signs are related to uterine and abdominal distention and abdominal pain. Dystocia will occur in the gravid female with uterine torsion. A sanguineous vaginal discharge may or may not be present. Vaginal cytology is consistent with hemorrhage: red blood cells, debris, and few white blood cells. Abdominal radiographs show a large, fluid-filled uterus in nongravid animals, making pyometra the primary rule-out. The nongravid uterus contains blood (hematometra).[53, 54] Fetuses will be visible radiographically in gravid females; the fetuses may or may not be viable. Treatment of the torsion is surgical. Because torsions of 180 to 1440 degrees occur,[53] ovariohysterectomy is usually necessary. In one pregnant queen the uterine torsion was associated with apparent avulsion of the uterus from the vagina.[55]

Uterine Prolapse

Uterine prolapse is an uncommon complication of parturition. It occurs in primiparous as well as multiparous bitches and queens of any age.[56–59] There may or may not be a history of dystocia. The prolapse usually occurs immediately after delivery of the last neonate.

The diagnosis is established by physical examination of the tubular organ protruding from the vulva. Treatments include manual reduction, reduction by means of laparotomy, and amputation. Ovariohysterectomy is usually performed. Subsequent fertility after reduction of the prolapsed uterus in small animals has not been investigated.

Primary Uterine Inertia

Primary uterine inertia is the failure of the uterus to respond to appropriate signals to begin labor. The cause is unknown, but affected bitches are usually normocalcemic[60] and euglycemic.[61] The condition may or may not recur on subsequent pregnancies.[60] The diagnosis of primary uterine inertia is based on gestation length, a precipitous drop in rectal temperature, and no evidence of labor. Gestation length is usually determined by breeding dates. Because ovulation time is not well correlated with breeding days, and because sperm remain viable in the estrous tract for at least six days, normal gestation length, as determined by breeding dates, is extremely variable: 58 to 71 days in the bitch.[62] When it is determined by the first cytologic day of diestrus, gestation length varies from 57 to 59 days in the bitch.[63] This method of determining gestation length is less likely to result in either premature or delayed intervention. Unfortunately, one cannot determine the onset of diestrus retrospectively. The prospective determination of the first day of diestrus is helpful for managing bitches with histories of problem pregnancies.

Progesterone decreases sharply 36 to 48 hours before parturition in the bitch. Parturition will not occur if progesterone concentrations are greater than 2 ng/ml.[64] Progesterone is thermogenic, and there is a substantial decline in rectal temperature 10 to 14 hours after the fall in progesterone. Thus rectal temperature drops below 100°F, usually to less than 99°F, approximately 24 hours before parturition.[64] This is a very useful clinical tool. Owners should monitor the pregnant bitch's rectal temperature twice daily, beginning a week before the expected due date. If there is no evidence of labor by 24 hours after the drop in rectal temperature, the bitch should be examined.

Physical examination will usually be normal. There is no evidence of labor. No contractions or abdominal press is stimulated by vaginal manipulation. There may be a greenish vaginal discharge. If appropriate endoscopic equipment is available, cervical dilation may be detectable (see Chapter 101). Fetal viability should be assessed with ultrasonography if possible. Therapy for primary uterine inertia is cesarean section since the uterus does not respond to oxytocin or calcium.[60]

Subinvoluted Placental Sites

Subinvolution of placental sites (SIPS) causes persistent postpartum hemorrhage lasting for 7 to 12 weeks. The condition occurs almost exclusively in bitches younger than three years of age. Affected bitches are physically normal, except for the presence of a bloody vaginal discharge. The blood loss from SIPS is rarely severe. Packed cell volume can be monitored if there is concern, keeping in mind that term bitches are normally mildly anemic (see Chapter 98). Vaginal cytology is helpful in differentiating SIPS from metritis and from normal lochia. Red blood cells are the predominant cell type, since the cytologic appearance is that of hemorrhage.[32] Grossly, the placental sites are twice the normal size for the same time post partum. The uterine lumen contains serosanguineous fluid.[65] The diagnosis of SIPS is made on the basis of historical, physical, and cytologic findings. The diagnosis could be confirmed by histopathologic examination of the uterus. Three criteria have been suggested.[65] The presence of large masses of collagen, hemorrhage, and dilated endometrial glands after the seventh postpartum week or no evidence of a massive slough of collagen by 12 weeks post partum is considered abnormal. Finally, trophoblast-like cells invading the myometrium is abnormal at any time post partum. The interplacental endometrium is normal.[65]

The cause of SIPS is not known. The trophoblastic cells do not regress or degenerate normally. Instead, they continue to invade deep into the glandular layer or even into the myometrium, preventing normal involution. Also, evidence of thrombosis of endometrial vessels is often lacking. This results in continued hemorrhage. The reasons for these failures are not known. Both normally involuted and subinvoluted placental sites can be found in the same uterus, suggesting that infectious or hormonal causes are unlikely. Progesterone concentrations were normal in some bitches.[65]

SIPS rarely requires treatment. Recovery is spontaneous and fertility is unaffected.[66] Ovariohysterectomy is curative. Ergonovine could be administered, although it has not been widely investigated for this use in small animals. Transfusions could be administered if hemorrhage is severe, but that is so unlikely that the diagnosis of SIPS should be questioned.

Uterine Rupture

Most tears or ruptures of the uterus are iatrogenic. They occur because of physical or pharmacologic manipulations of the uterus. As mentioned earlier, uterine rupture is a complication during ovariohysterectomy for the treatment of pyometra and metritis. Tears can occur when prostaglandin[21, 47] or oxytocin[67] is administered for treatment of pyometra, metritis, or dystocia. On rare occasions uterine tears occur spontaneously as a result of dystocia or apparently normal parturition.[61] Purulent fluid is occasionally found in the abdominal cavity of bitches with pyometra while no macroscopic tear can be found in the uterus. Whether this represents another instance of spontaneous uterine rupture or whether pus exudes out the oviduct is uncertain.

The clinical signs of uterine rupture are peracute and typical of peritonitis. Abdominal pain and distention and rapid deterioration of the animal's clinical condition are seen. The signs of uterine rupture may be masked by the predisposing pathology such as pyometra or dystocia. Uterine rupture should be considered as a possible but uncommon cause of illness in the postpartum bitch.

The radiographic or ultrasonographic appearance of ascitic fluid would be consistent with, although not specific for, rupture of the uterus. If the ascitic fluid and the uterine discharge recovered from the vagina have the same cytologic appearance, ruptured uterus is likely. The diagnosis is confirmed by exploratory celiotomy. Ovariohysterectomy is the usual treatment. Appropriate fluid therapy, antibiotic therapy, and/or therapy for peritonitis is indicated.

Uterine Neoplasia

Uterine neoplasia is an uncommon condition of older queens and bitches. Leiomyoma, fibroma, lipoma, fibrosarcoma, leiomyosarcoma, and endometrial adenocarcinoma have been reported.[68, 69] Most uterine tumors cause no clinical signs. When signs are present they are usually related to mechanical interference with adjacent viscera. There may be abdominal and/or uterine distention. A sanguineous vaginal discharge may be present.[68, 69] The diagnosis is based on palpation of a large uterus or abdominal mass. Radiography and/or ultrasonography will help to confirm the location of the mass within the uterus. Neoplastic cells are not usually found by cytologic examination of the uterine discharge because the most common tumor, leiomyoma, does not readily exfoliate. Vaginal cytologic examination usually demonstrates blood. The diagnosis of uterine neoplasia is confirmed by excisional biopsy. Details of the biologic behavior and treatment of uterine neoplasia can be found in Chapter 102.

Abortion

Abortion is discussed in Chapter 104. Certain infectious causes of abortion are briefly mentioned here because they are associated with placental lesions. *Brucella canis* infection is the most serious cause of abortion in bitches because there is no effective treatment and no vaccine. Therefore, the entire kennel is at risk of being lost. Abortion is often the only sign of *B. canis* infection, yet infected, asymptomatic animals are an important source of transmission.[70] The only method of eradication of *B. canis* infection from a kennel is colony-wide testing and culling of infected animals.[71] Because the prognosis for eliminating infection from the individual animal as well as from the entire colony is so poor, accurate diagnosis of *B. canis* is paramount.

Despite improved serologic testing, isolation of the *B. canis* organism remains the only certain method of diagnosis.[72] The organism is fastidious and slow-growing. Large numbers of organisms are shed in the postabortion vaginal discharge. This opportunity to establish the definitive diagnosis should not be lost. Recovery of *B. canis* from semen, blood cultures, milk, or vaginal discharge (except after abortion) is unpredictable because shedding of the organism is intermittent and varies according to chronicity of infection. Abacteremic dogs

may still be infectious.[70] Dogs can remain persistently infected for as long as 5.5 years.[72]

Serologic tests have the advantage of being faster and less tedious than microbiologic identification of the organism itself. Cell wall antigens of *Brucella ovis* or *B. canis* are used in the rapid-slide agglutination test (RSAT) and the tube agglutination test (TAT), and in some agar gel immunodiffusion (AGID) tests. These cell wall antigens are common to *B. ovis*, *B. canis*, rough *Brucella abortus*, mucoid *Pseudomonas aeruginosa*, and mucoid *Staphylococcus* species.[72] Therefore, false-positive reactions are possible. In fact, false-positive reactions are very common with the RSAT because it is so sensitive. The cause of most false-positive reactions to cell wall antigens is unidentified.[72] Cytoplasmic antigens, rather than cell wall antigens, are used in some agar gel immunodiffusion tests for *B. canis*. These will cross-react only with certain other brucellae: *B. canis*, *B. ovis*, and both rough and smooth *B. abortus*.[72]

Of course, there is a delay from the time of infection until antibody titers are detectable. Blood cultures are the only reliable method of diagnosis for the first eight to ten weeks of *B. canis* infection.[72] After that, serologic tests using cell wall antigens (RSAT, TAT with or without 2-mercaptoethanol, and AGID) become positive. Most dogs do not have detectable titers to cytoplasmic antigens, using AGID, until the 12th week of infection.[72] All serologic and blood culture tests were positive from 3 months until 40 months after experimental infection in 52 dogs, except for one dog that became abacteremic at month 27.[72] With chronic infection, blood cultures become negative, titers to cell wall antigens become equivocal (1:25 to 1:50), and AGID tests using cell wall antigens become equivocal. AGID using cytoplasmic antigen remains positive for as long as 12 months after the other tests are no longer diagnostic.[72]

Carmichael and colleagues[72] offered the following observations regarding the diagnosis of *B. canis* infection. Culturing the blood for *B. canis* is the most sensitive diagnostic test during the first two months of infection. Bacteremia may subside as early as six months after infection, but it usually persists for more than one year. From the onset of bacteremia until six or more months after the bacteremia becomes intermittent or subsides, serologic tests remain positive. Once bacteremia does subside, serologic tests using cell wall antigen become progressively less certain, with lower titers. Interpretation of the test results must be cautious. Finally, AGID using cytoplasmic antigens becomes positive shortly after the onset of bacteremia and remains positive for at least 12 months after abacteremia, when other serologic tests are equivocal.

Abortion of part or all of the litter occurs with other bacterial infection as well. *E. coli* is the organism most often recovered. *Pasteurella* has also been reported. Antibiotic therapy has enabled some affected bitches to successfully carry part of the litter to term. Possibly *E. coli* endotoxin causes hemorrhage into decidua and separation of the placenta.[41] *Toxoplasma gondii* is known to infect the placenta of sheep and thereby cause abortion.[73] Placental necrosis and abortion occur after experimental intravenous inoculation of feline rhinotracheitis virus in pregnant queens. Intranasal inoculation also results in abortion but not in placental or fetal lesions.[74]

Miscellaneous

Ectopic pregnancy has been reported in cats.[36, 75] It can occur when fertilized ova escape from the oviduct and attach to the mesentery, or after rupture of the gravid uterus, where the developing fetus is lost into the abdominal cavity. Ectopic pregnancy may be an incidental finding with no clinical signs. Signs may be associated with mechanical interference with adjacent viscera or with necrosis of ectopic tissue. Treatment is surgical removal, with or without ovariohysterectomy. If only the ectopic tissue is removed, subsequent normal pregnancy is possible.[36]

Herniation of the gravid uterus through the diaphragm,[76] through the abdominal wall, and through the inguinal canal[61] can occur in the bitch and queen. Treatment is surgical. Although the dam is likely to survive if treatment is prompt, the litter usually does not.

Foreign material, consisting of surgical swabs, has been found in the uterus of a bitch.[77] This foreign material did not cause clinical signs, nor did it prevent pregnancy.

References

1. Wilson, JD: Sexual differentiation. Ann Rev Physiol 40:279, 1978.
2. Johnson, CA: The role of the fetal testicle in sexual differentiation. Comp Cont Ed 5:129, 1983.
3. Boomsma, RA, et al.: The uterine progestational response in cats: changes in morphology and progesterone receptors during chronic administration of progesterone to estradiol-primed and nonprimed animals. Biol Reprod 26:511, 1982.
4. Murray, MK and Verhage, HG: The immunocytochemical localization of a cat uterine protein that is estrogen dependent (CUPED). Biol Reprod 32:1229, 1985.
5. Verhage, HG, et al.: Progesterone effects in cat oviduct and uterus. Anat Rec 208:521, 1984.
6. Johnston, SD, et al.: Cytoplasmic estrogen and progesterone receptors in canine endometrium during the estrous cycle. Am J Vet Res 46:1653, 1985.
7. Christie, DW and Bell, ET: Changes in the dimensions of the uterus of the beagle bitch during the oestrus cycle. J Sm Anim Pract 13:97, 1972.
8. Sokolowski, JH, et al.: Canine reproduction: reproductive organs and related structures of the nonparous, parous and postpartum bitch. Am J Vet Res 34:1001, 1973.
9. Mulligan, RM: Histological studies of the canine female genital tract. J Morphol 71:431, 1942.
10. Al-Bassam, MA, et al.: Normal post-partum involution of the uterus in the dog. Can J Comp Med 45:217, 1981.
11. Wheaton, LG, et al.: Recording uterine motility in the nonanesthetized bitch. Am J Vet Res 47:2205, 1986.
12. Magne, ML: Acute metritis in the bitch. In Morrow, DH, (ed): Current Therapy in Theriogenology, 2nd ed. Philadelphia, WB Saunders, 1986, p 505.
13. Hoos, PC and Hoffman, LH: Effect of histamine receptor antagonists and indomethacin on implantation in the rabbit. Biol Reprod 29:833, 1983.
14. Olson, PN, et al.: Concentrations of progesterone and luteinizing hormone in the serum of diestrous bitches before and after hysterectomy. Am J Vet Res 45:146, 1984.
15. Stewart, DR and Stabenfeldt, GH: Relaxin activity in the pregnant cat. Biol Reprod 32:848, 1985.
16. Johnson, ME: Hydrometra in the dog: A case report. JAAHA 20:243, 1980.
17. Phemister, RD: Nonneurogenic reproductive failure in the bitch. Vet Clin North Amer 4:573, 1974.
18. Sandholm, M, et al.: Pathogenesis of canine pyometra. JAVMA 167:1006, 1975.
19. Dow, C: The cystic hyperplasia-pyometra complex in the bitch. Vet Rec 69:1409, 1957.
20. Hardy, RM and Osborne, CA: Canine pyometra: pathophysiology diagnosis and treatment of uterine and extrauterine lesions. JAAHA 10:245, 1974.
21. Nelson, RW, et al.: Treatment of canine pyometra and endometritis with prostaglandin $F_{2\alpha}$. JAVMA 181:899, 1982.
22. Dow, C: The cystic hyperplasia-pyometra complex in the cat. Vet Rec 74:141, 1962.
23. Austin, AR and Evans, JM: Letter: Pyometritis in spayed cats. Vet Rec 91:77, 1972.
24. Chastain, CB, et al.: Adrenocortical suppression in cats given megestrol acetate. Am J Vet Res 42:2029, 1981.
25. Goyings, LS, et al.: Clinical morphologic and clinico-pathologic findings in beagles treated for 2 years with melengestrol acetate. Am J Vet Res 38:1923, 1977.
26. Sokolowski, JH and Zimbelman, RG: Canine reproduction: Effects of a single injection of medroxyprogesterone acetate on the reproductive organs of the bitch. Am J Vet Res 34:1493, 1973.
27. Wilkins, DB: Letter: Pyometritis in a spayed cat. Vet Rec 91:24, 1972.
28. Long, RD: Letter: Pyometritis in spayed cats. Vet Rec 91:105, 1972.
29. Thornton, DAK and Kear, M: Uterine cystic hyperplasia in a Siamese cat following treatment with medroxyprogesterone. Vet Rec 80:380, 1967.
30. Sokolowski, JH and Zimbelman, RG: Canine reproduction: effects of a single injection of medroxyprogesterone acetate on the reproductive organs of intact and ovariectomized bitches. Am J Vet Res 34:1501, 1973.
31. Bowen, RA, et al.: Efficacy and toxicity of estrogens commonly used to terminate canine pregnancy. JAVMA 186:183, 1985.
32. Olson, PN, et al.: Vaginal cytology. II. Its use in diagnosing canine reproduction disorders. Comp Cont Ed 6:385, 1984.
33. Hadley, JC: Unconjugated oestrogen and progesterone concentrations in the blood of bitches with false pregnancy and pyometra. Vet Rec 96:545, 1975.
34. Fidler, IJ, et al.: Relationship of estrous irregularity, pseudopregnancy and pregnancy to canine pyometra. JAVMA 149:1043, 1966.
35. Whitney, JC: The pathology of the canine genital tract in false pregnancy. J Sm Anim Pract 8:247, 1967.
36. Vasseur, PB and Feldman, EC: Pyometra associated with extrauterine pregnancy in a cat. JAAHA 18:872, 1982.
37. Wildt, DE and Lawler, DF: Laparoscopic sterilization of the bitch and queen by uterine horn occlusions. Am J Vet Res 46:864, 1985.
38. Meyers-Wallen, VN, et al.: Prostaglandin $F_{2\alpha}$ treatment of canine pyometra. JAVMA 189:1557, 1986.
39. Asheim, A: Pathogenesis of renal damage and polydipsia in dogs with pyometra. JAVMA 147:736, 1965.
40. Poffenbarger, EM and Feeney, DA: Use of gray-scale ultrasonography in the diagnosis of reproductive disease in the bitch: 18 cases (1981–1984). JAVMA 189:90, 1986.
41. Linde, C: Partial abortion associated with genital Escherichia coli infection in a bitch. Vet Rec 112:454, 1983.
42. Shille, VM and Gontarek, J: The use of ultrasonography for pregnancy diagnosis in the bitch. JAVMA 187:1021, 1985.
43. Johnson, CA and Wasserfall, JL: Prostaglandin therapy in feline pyometra. JAVMA 20:247, 1982.
44. Sokolowski, JH and Geng, S: Effect of prostaglandin $F_{2\alpha}$-THAM in the bitch. JAVMA 170:536, 1977.
45. Wildt, DI, et al.: Effect of prostaglandin $F_{2\alpha}$ on endocrine-ovarian function in the domestic cat. Prostaglandins 18:883, 1979.
46. Baker, BA, et al.: Luteal function in the hysterectomized bitch following treatment with prostaglandin $F_{2\alpha}$. Therio 14:195, 1980.
47. Jackson, PG: Treatment of canine pyometra with dinoprost. Vet Rec 105:131, 1979.
48. Lagerstedt, AS, et al.: Uterine drainage in the bitch for treatment of pyometra refractory to prostaglandin $F_{2\alpha}$. J Sm Anim Pract 28:215, 1987.

49. Oettle, EE, et al.: Preliminary report on the effect of $PGF_{2\alpha}$ on the duration of the oestrus interval in beagle bitches. Therio 2:409, 1985.
50. Robinson, GW: Uterus unicornis and unilateral renal agenesis in a cat. JAVMA 147:516, 1965.
51. Marcella, KL, et al.: Segmental aplasia of the uterine horn in a cat. JAVMA 186:179, 1985.
52. Ladkin, A: Urethral ectopia and anomalous cervix in a dog. Vet Rec 104:555, 1979.
53. Shull, RM, et al.: Bilateral torsion of uterine horns in a nongravid bitch. JAVMA 172:601, 1978.
54. Homer, BL, et al.: Left horn uterine torsion in a nongravid, multiparous bitch. JAVMA 176:633, 1980.
55. Appleyard, WT and Shelly, J: An unusual uterine anomaly in the cat. Vet Rec 97:182, 1975.
56. Luckhurst, J: Letter: Prolapse of the uterus in the cat. Vet Rec 73:728, 1961.
57. Davies, JE: Letter: Prolapsed uterus in the cat. Vet Rec 103:567, 1978.
58. Newman, MH: Letter: Prolapse of the uterus in the bitch and the cat. Vet Rec 73:680, 1961.
59. Arnall, L: Letter: Prolapse of the uterus in the cat. Vet Rec 73:750, 1961.
60. Johnston, SD: Parturition and dystocia in the bitch. In Morrow, DA (ed): Current Therapy in Theriogenology, 2nd ed. Philadelphia, WB Saunders, 1986, p 500.
61. Johnson, CA: Personal communication, 1988.
62. Johnston, SD, et al.: Prenatal indicators of puppy viability at term. Comp Cont Ed 12:1013, 1983.
63. Holst, PA and Phemister, RD: Onset of diestrus in the beagle bitch: definition and significance. Am J Vet Res 35:401, 1974.
64. Concannon, PW, et al.: Pregnancy and parturition in the bitch. Biol Reprod 16:517, 1977.
65. Al-Bassam, MA, et al.: Involution abnormalities in the postpartum uterus of the bitch. Vet Pathol 18:208, 1981.
66. Schall, WD, et al.: Spontaneous recovery after subinvolution of placental sites in a bitch. JAVMA 159:1780, 1971.
67. Bomzon, L: Rupture of the uterus following Caesarean section in a bitch. Vet Rec 101:38, 1977.
68. Stein, BS: Tumors of the feline genital tract. JAAHA 17:1022, 1981.
69. Herron, MA: Tumors of the canine genital system. JAAHA 19:981, 1983.
70. Zoha, SJ and Carmichael, LE: Serological responses of dogs to cell wall and internal antigens of Brucella canis. Vet Microbiol 7:35, 1982.
71. Pickerill, PA and Carmichael, LE: Canine brucellosis: control programs in commercial kennels and effect on reproduction. JAVMA 160:1607, 1972.
72. Carmichael, LE, et al.: Problems in the serodiagnosis of canine brucellosis: dog response to cell wall and internal antigens of Brucella canis. Develop Biol Standard 56:371, 1984.
73. Dubey, DP, et al.: Placental transfer of specific antibodies during ovine congenital toxoplasmosis. Am J Vet Res 48:474, 1987.
74. Hoover, EA and Griesemer, RA: Comments: Pathogenicity of feline viral rhinotrachcitis virus and effect on germ-free cats, growing bone and the gravid uterus. JAVMA 158:929, 1971.
75. Chivers, AW: Letter: An unusual finding in a cat. Vet Rec 88:560, 1971.
76. Sullivan, JL, et al.: What's your diagnosis. JAVMA 155:941, 1969.
77. Walker, CE: Letter: Foreign body in pekingese uterus. Vet Rec 103:567, 1978.

DRUG INDEX

Drug	Dose	Route	Purpose
Prostaglandin $F_{2\alpha}$ (Prostin; Lutylase)	0.1–0.5 mg/kg q24h	SQ	Uterine evacuation
Oxytocin	0.22–0.5 U/lb once (0.5–1 U/kg once) (20 U max)	IM	Uterine evacuation
Ergonovine	0.2 mg/35 lb once (0.2 mg/15 kg once)	IM	Uterine evacuation

101 VAGINAL DISORDERS

CHERI A. JOHNSON

ANATOMY AND PHYSIOLOGY

The vagina extends from the cervix to the vestibule just cranial to the urethral orifice. In beagle-sized bitches (about 25 pounds body weight) the vagina is 10 to 14 cm in length and 1.5 cm in diameter.[1] The vestibulovaginal junction is demarcated by a mucosal ridge that encircles the vagina. This cingulum is the location of the hymen, which embryologically forms between the vaginal lumen and the external layer of the urogenital sinus.[2] No definite hymen is found in the normal bitch. The embryogenesis of the vagina is unclear, but interaction between the caudal ends of the müllerian ducts and the urogenital sinus is essential for complete vaginal development.[2] The cranial vagina is formed by fusion of the müllerian ducts. The urogenital sinus gives rise to the urinary bladder, urethra, and external genitalia.[2]

Cyclic hormonal stimulation causes changes in the microscopic and macroscopic appearance of the vagina. Estrogen causes proliferation of the vaginal epithelium and diapedesis of red blood cells.[3, 4] During proestrus and estrus there is edema, hypertrophy, and slight to moderate rete pegging of the epithelium. There is a progressive increase in the stratification and cornification of the epithelial cells as estrus approaches. Initially the basal and parabasal layers are three to four cells deep. By estrus the superficial layers predominate and are eight to ten squamous cells thick. Edema is present in the lamina propria. There are no white blood cell infiltrates.

After ovulation the corpus luteum produces progesterone. During the early luteal phase there is a polymorphonuclear cell (PMN) infiltrate in the lamina propria of the vagina. There are no rete pegs and the epithelium is no longer cornified. By the midluteal phase, the epithelium is composed of only two cell layers.[3, 4] Mucin is present in the outer layers during pregnancy.[4] The histologic appearance of the vagina during anestrus is similar to that of the luteal phase except there is no longer a leukocytic infiltrate. The cells of the basal layer are cuboidal, with scanty cytoplasm and dark, oval nuclei.[4] The vagina of the prepuberal and oophorectomized bitch is like that of the intact bitch during anestrus. The cervix has cyclic changes that are similar to those of the vagina.[3]

These changes that occur during the estrous cycle can easily be monitored by vaginal cytology. Vaginal cytology can be used to identify the stage of the cycle, to determine appropriate breeding dates to maximize conception and litter size, to more closely predict whelping dates, to identify "silent heat," and to differentiate normal from abnormal vaginal discharges.[5] Vaginal cytology may also help to determine if a bitch has recently been bred, since sperm heads were detected in vaginal smears from 68 per cent of bitches bred 24 hours earlier, and from 50 per cent of bitches bred 48 hours earlier. Intact sperm were not found.[5a] Vaginal cytology must always be interpreted in light of the stage of the estrous cycle.

Samples are collected with a saline-moistened, cotton-tipped swab inserted into the vagina, or by flushing saline into and aspirating it from the vagina with a pipette.[5–7] Care should be taken to avoid the clitoris, the clitoral fossa, and the skin because those areas normally contain keratinized cells, which could confuse the interpretation.[5, 6] Swabs are gently rolled onto slides. Drops of the saline aspirate are placed on slides. Slides are then stained as desired. Wright's stain, new methylene blue, trichrome stain, and modified Wright's-Giemsa (Diff-Quik) are commonly used, but many other stains are equally acceptable.[5, 6]

The cell types exfoliated from the vaginal epithelium have been described.[5, 6] From the lamina propria to the epithelial surface, in order of increasing maturity, they are basal, parabasal, intermediate, superficial-intermediate, and superficial cells. The basal cells described earlier are on the basement membrane and are not exfoliated. Parabasal cells are small and round with a large nuclear-cytoplasmic ratio. Intermediate cells are round, about twice the size of parabasal cells, with a similar nucleus. Superficial-intermediate cells are larger still, with angular borders. They often are folded. The nucleus is still large but beginning to show karyolysis. The superficial cells are angular and folded. The nucleus is pyknotic, or it takes up no stain[5, 6] (see Figure 101–2).

Estrogen causes proliferation and maturation (cornification) of the vaginal epithelium. During proestrus, parabasal, intermediate, and some superficial cells are exfoliated. Red blood cells (RBCs), white blood cells (WBCs), and bacteria are present. As estrus approaches there is a gradual increase in the maturity of the epithelial cells and a decrease in WBCs. During estrus, superficial cells are the predominant cell type, eventually accounting for more than 90 per cent of the exfoliated epithelial cells. RBCs are often present during estrus. Bacteria may be present. WBCs are absent during estrus unless there is concurrent inflammation.

Diestrus (luteal phase) is marked by an abrupt change in the distribution of epithelial cells. The less mature parabasal and intermediate cells outnumber the superficial cells. Often there are sheets of epithelial cells on the day before diestrus. WBCs almost always return at this time. RBCs and bacteria are often present. Thus it is impossible to differentiate proestrus from diestrus based on a single vaginal smear.[5] RBCs are often present in both. Fewer cells are exfoliated during anestrus. Parabasal and intermediate epithelial cells, with or without a few WBCs and bacteria, are present. Similar changes in vaginal cytology occur during the feline estrous cycle except that RBCs and WBCs are uncommon.[8, 9] Diestrus occurs only if ovulation is induced in the queen.[9]

The macroscopic appearance of the vagina also changes during the estrous cycle. These changes are easily monitored by endoscopy. Thorough knowledge of the normal appearance of the vagina at the various stages of the estrous cycle is essential for recognition and interpretation of abnormal findings. Vaginoscopy is used to evaluate the source of vaginal discharges, to identify the nature and extent of vaginal abnormalities, to obtain specimens for biopsy and/or culture, and to assess cervical patency. Because of the length of the canine vagina, endoscopy equipment should be at least 10 cm long. The diameter of the endoscope will be dictated by the individual bitch. Proctoscopes or anoscopes made for use in children or adults work well for vaginoscopy. The anoscopes are usually too short for viewing the cranial vagina, even in small bitches. Flexible fiberoptic equipment can be passed through a speculum if additional length and/or a smaller diameter is needed. Insufflation of the vagina with air is helpful for thorough inspection.

Vaginoscopy is performed in the awake, standing bitch. Sedation is rarely necessary unless a biopsy is planned.[10, 11] The perineum is inspected and cleansed. The endoscope is lubricated with warm saline solution or a sterile water-soluble lubricant. The clitoris and clitoral fossa must be avoided. Therefore, the speculum is passed through the dorsal commissure of the vulva, in a dorsal direction. There is normally slight resistance at the vestibulovaginal junction. This is especially true for prepuberal and oophorectomized bitches, in which the diameter of that area is sometimes surprisingly narrow. The angle of the speculum is adjusted to a more horizontal direction after the speculum passes through the vestibulovaginal junction.

The normal appearance of the vagina of the bitch has been described.[10] During proestrus the longitudinal folds of the vagina are edematous, round, and smooth. New folds develop, and often the entire vaginal lumen is filled with folds. There is bright red, clear fluid in the vaginal lumen, often in large amounts. As estrus approaches, the vaginal folds become lower and wrinkled. During estrus the vaginal folds have a sharp, angular, crinkled appearance. The mucosa is pale. The vaginal lumen is wide. There is a lesser amount of luminal fluid than during proestrus. This fluid is clear and usually straw-colored; however, it may continue to be bright red throughout estrus.

During the luteal phase of the cycle (diestrus) the vaginal folds are low, round, and soft. The folds in the cranial vagina have a characteristic rosette appearance and may be mistaken for the cervix.[10] Vaginal mucus, which is clear or opalescent, is present in the lumen. The mucous membranes have streaks of hyperemia. During anestrus and in oophorectomized bitches the vaginal folds are low and round and do not fill the vaginal lumen. There is a scant, thin mucous coating, giving the mucous membranes a translucent, pink-red appearance. The mucous membranes are thin and easily traumatized. Submucosal hemorrhages occur from seemingly gentle contact with the endoscope. There is usually some resistance to the passage of the endoscope, especially in neutered animals, so the instrument must be well lubricated.

The appearance of the cranial vagina of the bitch deserves mention because sometimes it is confusing. One of the vaginal folds, known as the dorsal median postcervical fold,[11] is often mistaken for the cervix. This fold extends from the caudal edge of the vaginal portion of the cervix, along the dorsal midline, and eventually blends into lesser folds of the vagina. It is composed of longitudinal and oblique smooth muscle bundles and irregularly arranged collagen. Unlike other folds of the vagina, the dorsal median postcervical fold has no elastic fibers. In beagle-sized bitches this fold is 15 to 42 mm long and 2 to 10 mm wide, compared with the average vaginal length in the same group of bitches of 158 ± 30 mm.[11] Because of its length, location, and inelastic nature, the dorsal median postcervical fold prevents visualization and catheterization of the canine cervix, except on rare occasions.

The vaginal portion of the cervix is tubular. Small furrows radiate from the os, giving it the appearance of a star.[10] The cervical os is not obviously patent, even when uterine fluid is seen flowing from it, except during the puerperium.[10] The vaginal lumen around the cervix and cranial aspect of the dorsal median postcervical fold is quite narrow, and instruments of small diameter (for example, 4.7 mm OD[10]) are necessary to visualize the cervix. The narrow paracervical vaginal lumen, the dorsal median postcervical fold, and/or the rosette appearance of the cranial vagina during diestrus is often confused with the cervix.[10]

Vaginal Anomalies

A variety of congenital and acquired vaginal anomalies have been described in the bitch. Many cause no clinical signs and are incidental findings. Some are discovered during investigation of infertility. Others cause abnormal vaginal discharge, urine pooling, urinary incontinence, or dyspareunia. Congenital abnormalities of the external genitalia are caused by faulty embryogenesis of the urogenital sinus. The posterior vagina may be affected. The cranial vagina, uterus, and the urinary system proximal to the urethra are often normal, since these are derived from the müllerian and wolffian ducts.[2] Congenital rectovaginal fistulas cause abnormal defecation. The diagnosis is established by physical examination. Treatment is surgical reconstruction of the vagina and rectum. One bitch was able to breed and whelp successfully after surgical repair of a congenital rectovaginal fistula.[12] Another bitch had urinary and fecal incontinence after surgery.[13]

Dysgenesis of the perineum such that the vulva and vestibule were not present has been described in bitches.[14, 15] Abnormalities of the uterus, vagina, and/or urethra were also found in these bitches. Abnormal communication between the vulva, vagina, and perineum may be congenital or acquired.[16, 17] Perineal laceration owing to dystocia is rare in the bitch and has not been reported in the queen. Treatment is surgical reconstruction of the vagina and vulva. The anomalies of the external and internal genitalia associated with the intersex condition are discussed in Chapter 104.

More often than not, the external genitalia and vestibule are normal in bitches with vaginal anomalies because of the different embryogenesis of those structures. The most common location of congenital vaginal abnormalities is immediately cranial to the external urethral orifice.[18] This area is easily accessible for digital palpation, even in large bitches. Digital examination is the most sensitive diagnostic procedure for the presence of vaginal anomalies because the endoscope may bypass the lesion.[18] Endoscopy and/or vaginography are useful to determine the cranial extent of the lesion. The following vaginal anomalies have been described in the bitch: vertical septa at the vestibulovaginal junction (Figure 101–1); incomplete fusion of the müllerian ducts, resulting in a partition of the vagina along its length; outpouching of the vagina; and caudal vaginal agenesis.[18–20] Hypoplasia, stenosis, and fibrous annular stricture of the vestibulovaginal junction also occur.[18]

If vaginal anomalies cause no clinical signs in animals not intended for breeding, treatment is unnecessary. If the anomaly causes clinical signs, or if the animal is going to be bred, the abnormality should be surgically corrected by means of episiotomy. Surgery is curative for animals with vertical bands or bifurcation of the vagina.[18] Subsequent fertility is unaffected. The hereditary aspects of vertical septa of the vagina in bitches are not known; however, they are heritable in mice.[18] Pouches from the vagina are usually filled with blood and debris from previous cycles. This material may become infected. Treatment is surgical excision. If the lesion is extensive, most of the vagina may be excised, in which case ovariohysterectomy is also indicated.[19]

Annular vaginal anomalies should be evaluated during estrus because estrogen may cause substantial relaxation of the area.[18] Conversely, vaginal hyperplasia during estrus may accentuate the problem.[18] Annular lesions may relax at parturition, so artificial insemination, without surgical correction of the lesion, might be considered.[18] Dystocia is an obvious possibility if vaginal anomalies are not corrected before pregnancy occurs. The surgical exposure of annular lesions is more difficult than that of vertical ones. Postoperative bouginage for as long as two months may be necessary to prevent adhesions.[18] Clinical signs may persist after attempted surgical correction of annular vaginal lesions.

Acquired ectopic ureter may rarely occur in the bitch or queen after ovariohysterectomy or cesarean section.[21, 22] The clinical sign is the onset of urinary incontinence, with or without a vaginal discharge, after surgery. The diagnosis is best made by excretory urography or, alternatively, by vaginoscopy or exploratory celiotomy. The most likely cause is ureteral incorporation in inflammatory adhesions around the vagina or vaginal stump, with eventual erosion of the ureter. The other possibility is that the ureter is accidentally included with a ligature, and thereby involved in an inflammatory process. Treatment of acquired ectopic ureter is ureteral

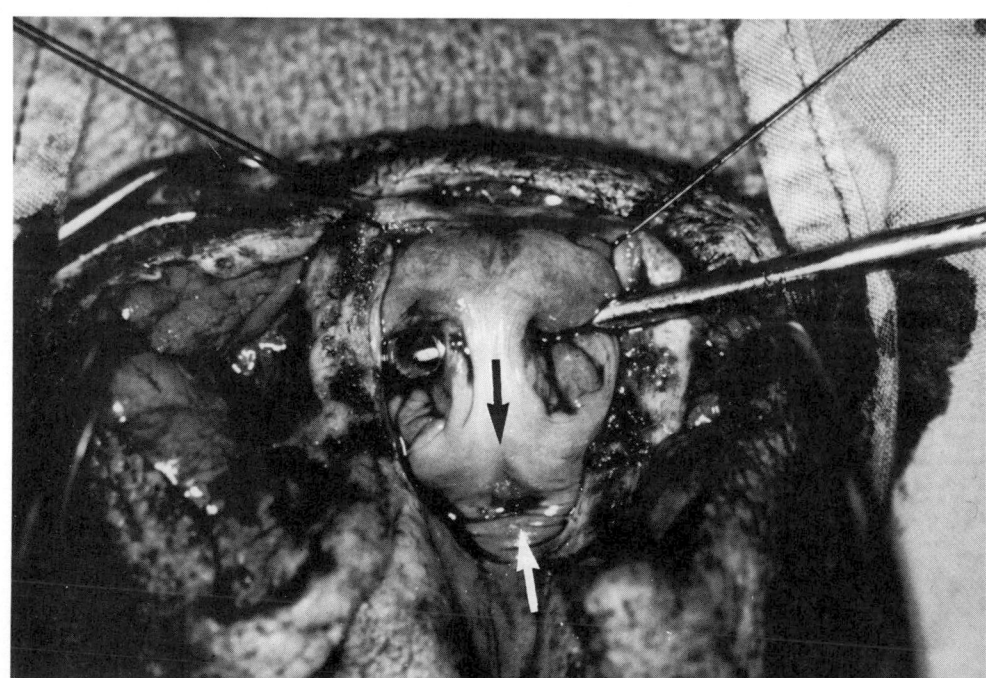

FIGURE 101–1. A vertical vaginal septum is easily identified by means of episiotomy and immobilized by the probe. The urethral orifice is indicated by the arrow.

transplantation or unilateral nephrectomy. Urinary incontinence after ovariohysterectomy should not be automatically attributed to withdrawal of ovarian hormones.

Vaginitis

Inflammation and infection of the vagina are common in bitches and rare in queens. The clinical signs of vaginitis are licking of the vulva and discomfort when the vagina is examined. There may or may not be a vaginal discharge.[23] Male dogs are often attracted to bitches with vaginitis, causing some owners and veterinarians to erroneously assume that the bitch is in season. Physical examination is normal except for the vagina. There may be a vaginal discharge and the vulvar hair may be discolored. Because of the discomfort, sedation may be required to examine the vagina and to obtain samples for cytology and culture.

The severity of the vaginal lesions can be assessed by vaginoscopy. The mucous membranes are hyperemic, and exudate is present on the epithelial surface and/or within the vaginal lumen. Vesicles, ulcers, and lymphoid follicle hyperplasia may be evident. Vaginoscopy also is helpful to identify predisposing causes for vaginitis, such as anatomical abnormalities or pooling of urine in the vagina.

Vaginal cytology consists of PMNs in various stages of degeneration, and bacteria (Figure 101–2). Bacteria may be phagocytized.[23, 24] Macrophages and lymphocytes may be found with chronic vaginitis. Vaginal cytology must be interpreted in light of the stage of the estrous cycle. Large numbers of PMNs are normally present in early diestrus, but unlike in vaginitis, PMNs decrease dramatically as the luteal phase progresses.[7] The anterior vagina should be cultured so that therapy can be as specific as possible. Because urinary tract infection is a common sequela to vaginitis, urinalysis is indicated.

The results of vaginal culture must be interpreted cautiously. The normal bacterial flora of the canine vagina are staphylococci, streptococci (α- and β-hemolytic, and nonhemolytic), *Escherichia coli*, *Pasteurella*, *Proteus*, *Corynebacterium*, *Pseudomonas*, *Klebsiella*, *Moraxella*, *Haemophilus*, and many others.[25–27] There are no qualitative differences in the types of bacteria isolated from normal prepuberal, oophorectomized, or intact mature bitches, nor between the anterior and posterior vagina, nor among the various stages of the estrous cycle.[25–27] There are quantitative differences, however. Coagulase-positive staphylococci are more common in prepuberal bitches than in mature bitches.[25] Also, more organisms are isolated from the posterior vagina (2.4 organisms/bitch) than from the anterior vagina (1.0 organisms/bitch, n = 81).[25]

Mycoplasma and *Ureaplasma* are also normal inhabitants of the canine vagina.[26, 28, 29] They were present in 88 per cent and 50 per cent, respectively, of vaginal cultures from 75 bitches.[28] *Ureaplasma* was always associated with *Mycoplasma*, but not vice versa.[28] Although many of the organisms mentioned are potential pathogens, there are no differences in the types of microbes isolated from normal or infertile bitches or

from vaginal exudates from bitches.[25, 28] *Brucella canis* may be the only bacterial isolate from the vagina that is always considered a pathogen.

Herpesvirus causes vaginal lesions after experimental intravenous and intravaginal inoculation in bitches and queens. The lesions are characterized by hyperemia and edema of the vaginal mucous membranes and petechial, submucosal hemorrhages. In bitches, lymphoid follicle hyperplasia is a prominent feature.[30–32] The gross appearance of the hyperplastic lymphoid nodules may cause them to be mistaken for vesicles.[30] After experimental inoculation, herpesvirus can be recovered from the vagina for several days in both species. Natural infection with herpesvirus is characterized by respiratory disease in adult animals, acute neonatal death in puppies, and, occasionally, in kittens, and abortion in bitches and queens.[32, 33] Vesicular lesions in the vagina and vestibule of bitches have been attributed to naturally occurring canine herpesvirus infection,[34] yet attempts to isolate canine herpesvirus from bitches with lymphofollicular hyperplasia have been unsuccessful.[35] The clinical importance of herpesvirus infection as a cause of vaginal lesions in small animals deserves further investigation. There is no doubt of its clinical importance in other areas of the body, and no doubt of its importance as a cause of venereal disease in other species.[36, 37] Confirmation of herpesvirus vaginitis would include histopathologic evaluation of the vesicular lesions and virus isolation.

Treatment of vaginitis in prepuberal bitches is conservative. The vulva should be kept clean so that dermatitis does not compound the clinical signs. Prepuberal vaginitis resolves spontaneously after the first estrous cycle in the majority of bitches.[23] Therefore, affected animals should be allowed to cycle before being neutered. Treatment of vaginitis in mature bitches is less rewarding.[23] Predisposing causes, such as anatomic abnormalities, urine pooling, vaginal neoplasia, granuloma formation at the vaginal stump after hysterectomy, and foreign material, should be investigated and corrected if discovered. Metabolic diseases in which infection is a common sequela, such as diabetes mellitus and hyperadrenocorticism, might be considered. Often a predisposing cause is not found. Systemic antibiotics, chosen on the basis of culture and sensitivity, are instituted. The efficacy of antibiotic infusion or medicated douche is not known. Because of the anatomy of the canine genital tract and the discomfort caused by vaginitis, owners may not be able to infuse medication without causing additional trauma.

Vaginal Neoplasia

Tumors of the vagina are occasionally found in older bitches and queens. The most common clinical signs associated with vaginal tumors are the presence of a mass protruding from the vulva and a vaginal discharge.[38–40] Less commonly, the mass may cause mechanical interference with surrounding structures, resulting in stranguria, tenesmus, or perineal swelling. The diagnosis is based on the historical and physical findings. Vaginoscopy will help to delineate the extent of the

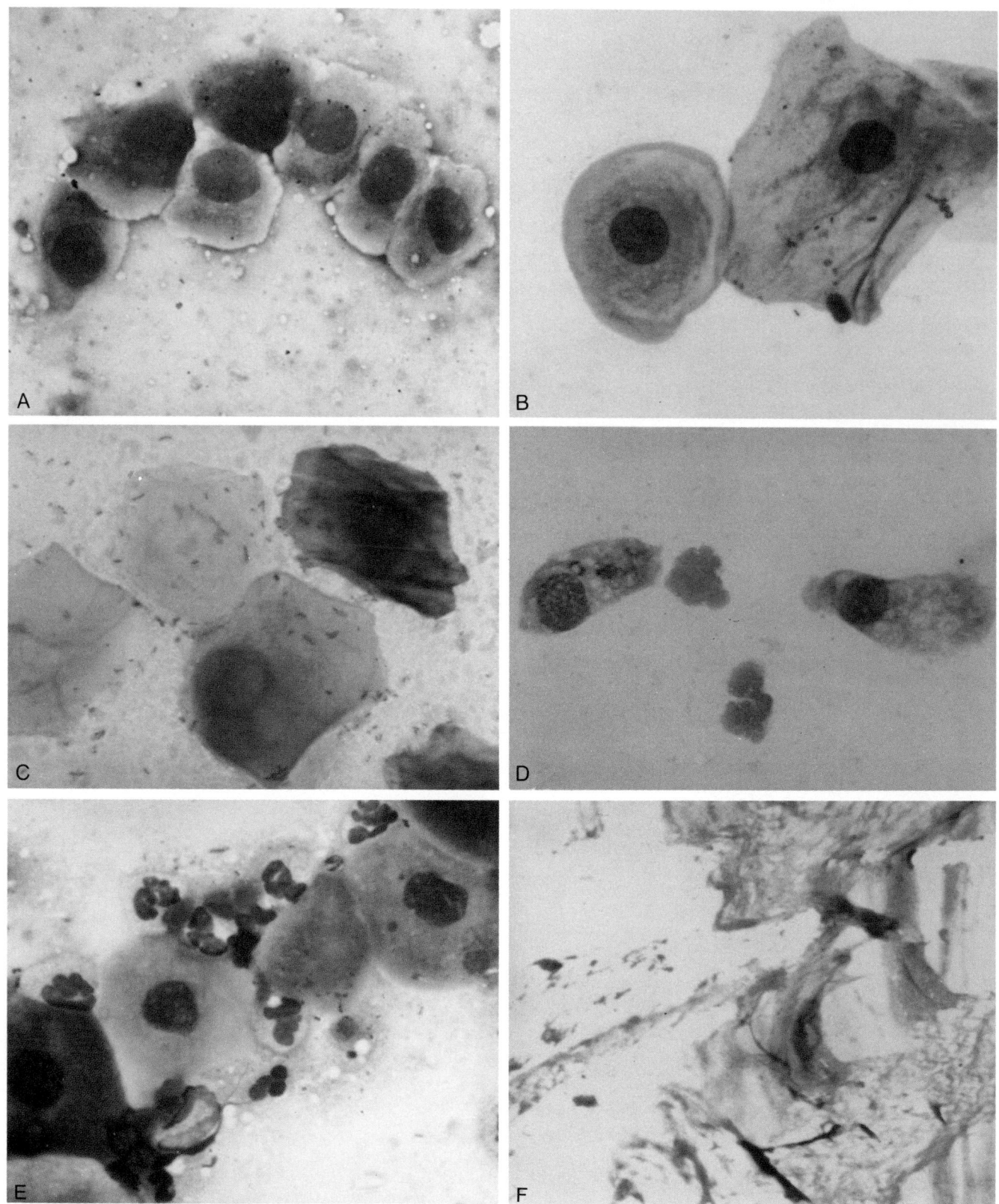

FIGURE 101–2. Vaginal cytology. *A,* parabasal cells; *B,* intermediate and superficial-intermediate cells, bacteria; *C,* superficial cells with bacteria; *D,* columnar endometrial cells; *E,* degenerate PMNs, bacteria, and intermediate cells typical of septic inflammation; and *F,* mucus. (Modified Wright's stain, photographed through a 63-power oil-emersion objective.)

lesion. Biopsy specimens may be obtained through the endoscope.

Leiomyomas and fibromas are the most common vaginal tumors in dogs and cats.[38, 40] Because they arise from smooth muscle and are usually covered by intact vaginal epithelium, neoplastic cells are often not exfoliated. Vaginal cytology is most helpful for the diagnosis of transmissible venereal tumors or transitional cell carcinomas, which tend to exfoliate more readily. The definitive diagnosis of vaginal neoplasia is established by excisional or incisional biopsy and histopathologic examination of the tissues. Treatment of benign vaginal tumors is surgical excision, with or without ovariohysterectomy. Transmissible venereal tumors and malignant vaginal tumors are less common than benign tumors. The details of their biologic behavior and therapeutic options are discussed in Chapter 102.

Vaginal Hyperplasia

The normal physiologic response of the vagina to estrogen is exaggerated in some bitches. The vaginal folds become so edematous and hyperplastic that they protrude from the vulva (Figure 101–3). These abnormal folds arise just cranial to the urethral orifice, from the ventral aspect of the vagina.[41] Rarely, the entire circumference of the vagina is involved but only immediately cranial to the urethra. The remainder of the vagina and vestibule are normal; therefore, this condition is distinct from vaginal prolapse.

Because the inciting cause is estrogen, vaginal hyperplasia is seen during proestrus and estrus in young bitches. It tends to recur with each cycle in affected animals and will rarely recur at parturition.[41] Vaginal hyperplasia resolves spontaneously as soon as estrogen disappears. The diagnosis of vaginal hyperplasia is based on the history of the stage of the estrous cycle and physical examination of the tissue protruding from the vulva. Vaginal hyperplasia must be differentiated from vaginal neoplasia and vaginal prolapse.

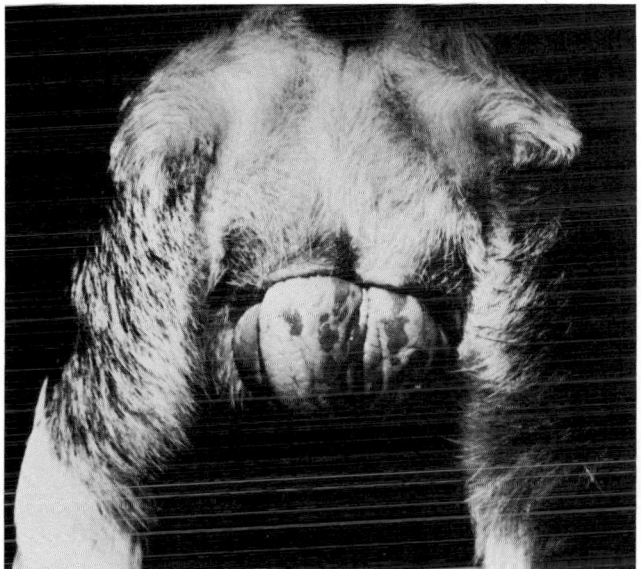

FIGURE 101–3. Vaginal hyperplasia in an estrual bitch.

Treatment of vaginal hyperplasia is both symptomatic and specific. Symptomatic therapy is aimed at protection of the exposed mucous membranes until spontaneous regression occurs during the luteal phase of the cycle. The exposed mucous membranes are easily traumatized. They should be kept clean and moist. Wrapping the tail may be helpful in some cases. Topical antibiotics may be indicated. Usually the hyperplastic tissue prevents natural breeding, so artificial insemination can be considered. The urethra is not incorporated by the hyperplastic tissue. It can be found under, or ventral to, the hyperplastic tissue if urethral catheterization is necessary. If tissue trauma is severe, the hyperplastic tissue can be resected surgically. Resection will not prevent recurrence of vaginal hyperplasia during subsequent cycles in some bitches.[41]

Specific therapy for vaginal hyperplasia is aimed at eliminating the estrogenic stimulation. This is most easily accomplished by ovariohysterectomy. The response is measurable within days of oophorectomy, and the hyperplastic tissue is usually small enough to be covered by the vulvar labia within seven to ten days. Ovariohysterectomy is curative. Because of its anti-estrogenic effects, megestrol acetate has been administered in an attempt to prevent vaginal hyperplasia.[41] Because megestrol also prevents ovulation, it would be contrain-dicated if the bitch was to be bred during that cycle. The possibility of inducing cystic endometrial hyperplasia with megestrol acetate should be considered (Chapter 100). Gonadotrophin-releasing hormone (GnRH) has also been used to treat vaginal hyperplasia.[41] Depending on the degree of follicular maturation, GnRH could cause premature luteinization of immature follicles and a shift in ovarian steroidogenesis from estrogen to progesterone. Ovarian cysts could also occur.[41] If luteinization was already present, GnRH should enhance progesterone production. The relative merits and/or risks of GnRH for the treatment of vaginal hyperplasia deserve further study.

Certain breeds of dogs are reportedly affected with vaginal hyperplasia more often than others.[41] Although this experience is not universal, one should consider the possibility of a hereditary cause. Affected bitches are often difficult to maintain in the breeding program because of the extra care required for the hyperplastic tissue and the extra effort of insemination. Medical therapy may interfere with conception, and surgical resection does not prevent recurrence. Therefore, ovariohysterectomy is currently the treatment of choice for vaginal hyperplasia.

Vaginal Prolapse

The prevalence of vaginal prolapse in bitches and queens is unknown because the terms vaginal prolapse and vaginal hyperplasia have been used interchangeably.[47] True prolapse of the vagina is apparently quite rare (Figure 101–4). It may occur in association with uterine prolapse after dystocia, because of tenesmus, or because of forced separation during coitus.[41] Treatment should include debridement of devitalized tissue and

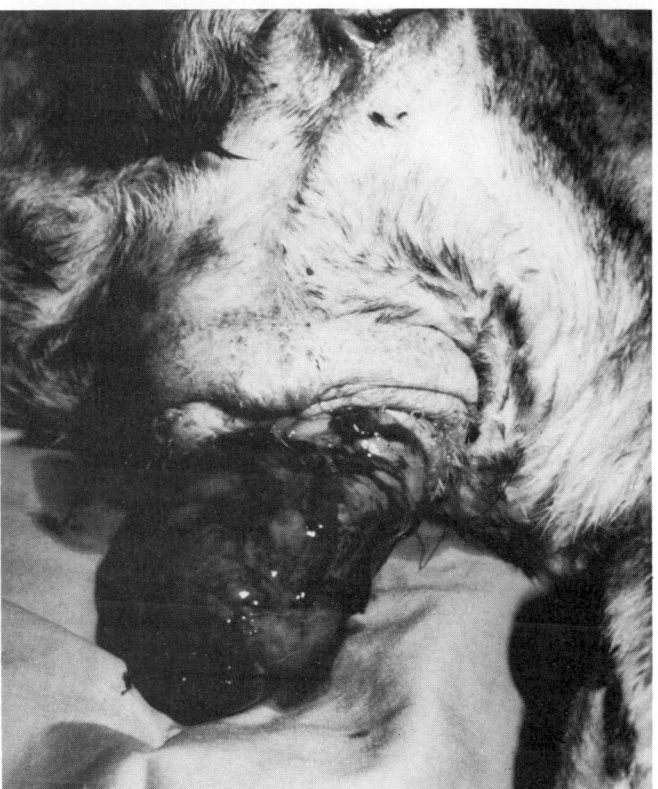

FIGURE 101–4. Vaginal prolapse in a bitch with dystocia.

reduction of the prolapse, with or without ovariohyste-rectomy.

Vaginal Lacerations

Vaginal lacerations are uncommon in the bitch. They are usually a result of obstetric procedures, vaginoscopy, or sodomy. Rarely they are due to breeding trauma or dystocia in bitches.[17] The history is of an acute onset of vaginal hemorrhage after some vaginal manipulation. The diagnosis is confirmed by vaginoscopy. Vaginal tears are most likely to involve the relatively inelastic clitoral folds, the cingulum of the vestibulovaginal junction, or the cranial vagina near the cervix. The location of the tear also depends on the inciting cause. Treatment is surgical repair of the defect by means of episiotomy and/or celiotomy, depending on the location and extent of the lesion.

Summary

Most vaginal abnormalities are associated with some vaginal discharge, which is often the owner's primary concern. The clinician must identify the nature and source of the discharge in order to formulate reasonable therapeutic plans. This is done by obtaining an accurate history of the estrous cycle and the current problem, and by physical examination, vaginal cytology (Figure 101–2), and vaginoscopy. A hemorrhagic (RBC) vaginal discharge is expected with subinvolution of placental sites, vaginal and uterine neoplasia, and vaginal lacera-tions.[23, 24] RBCs with mature or cornified vaginal epithe-lial cells are normal findings during proestrus, estrus, and early diestrus.[5, 23] A similar cytologic appearance can be seen as a result of exogenous estrogen. Occasionally the vagina is the only site of bleeding in animals with coagulopathies.[43]

Septic or purulent (WBCs with or without bacteria) vaginal discharge is present in animals with vaginitis, metritis, or pyometra.[23, 24] Endometrial cells may also be found in vaginal smears from animals with pyometra. Decomposing fetal structures may occasionally be found in animals with metritis. An important differential di-agnosis for the presence of large numbers of PMNs is early diestrus, in which this is an expected finding.[5] Mucus is a normal finding during late pregnancy and in lochia. Lochia also contains abundant cellular debris, RBCs, neutrophils, endometrial cells, and uter-overdin.[6, 24]

References

1. Christensen, GC: The urogenital apparatus. *In* Evans and Chris-tensen (eds): Miller's Anatomy of the Dog. Philadelphia, WB Saunders, 1979, p 590.
2. Wilson, JD: Sexual differentiation. Ann Rev Physiol 40:279, 1978.
3. Sokolowski, JH, et al.: Canine reproductive organs and related structures of the nonparous, parous and postpartum bitch. Am J Vet Res 34:1001, 1973.
4. Mulligan, RM: Histological studies of the canine female genital tract. J Morphol 71:431, 1942.
5. Olson, PN, et al.: Vaginal Cytology. I. A useful tool for staging the canine estrous cycle. Comp Cont Ed 6:288, 1984.
5a. Bowen, KA, et al.: Efficacy and toxicity of estrogens commonly used to terminate canine pregnancy. JAVMA 186:783, 1985.
6. Roszel, JF: Normal canine vaginal cytology. Vet Clin North Am 7:667, 1977.
7. Herron, MA: Feline reproduction. Vet Clin North Am 7:715, 1977.
8. Shille, VM, et al.: Follicular function in the domestic cat as determined by estradiol 17 concentrations in plasma: relation to estrus behavior and cornification of exfoliated vaginal epithe-lium. Biol Reprod 21:953, 1979.
9. Herron, MA: Feline vaginal cytologic examination. Fel Prac 36, 1977.
10. Lindsay, FEF: The normal endoscopic appearance of the caudal reproductive tract of the cyclic and non-cyclic bitch: post-uterine endoscopy. J Sm Anim Pract 24:1, 1983.
11. Pineda, MH, et al.: Dorsal median postcervical fold in the canine vagina. Am J Vet Res 34:1487, 1973.
12. Wilson, CE and Clifford, DH: Perineoplasty for anovaginal cleft in a dog. JAVMA 159:871, 1971.
13. Rawlings, CA and Capps, WF: Rectovaginal fistula and imperfor-ate anus in a dog. JAVMA 159:320, 1971.
14. Capel-Edwards, K: Double vagina with perineal agenesis in a bitch. Vet Rec 101:57, 1977.
15. Schwartz, A, et al.: Urinary incontinence due to multiple urogen-ital anomalies in a mature dog. JAVMA 164:1021, 1974.
16. Burke, TJ and Smith, CW: Vulvo-vaginal cleft in a dog. JAAHA 11:774, 1975.
17. Kock, MD: An unusual sequel to dystocia in a bitch. Vet Rec 101:384, 1977.
18. Wykes, PM and Soderberg, SF: Congenital abnormalities of the canine vagina and vulva. JAAHA 19:995, 1983.
19. Budsberg, SC, et al.: Pyovagina in the dog: A case report. JAAHA 23:108, 1987.
20. Hawe, RS and Loeb, WF: Caudal vaginal agenesis and progressive renal disease in a Shih Tzu. JAAHA 20:123, 1984.
21. Allen, WE and Webbon, PM: Two cases of urinary incontinence in cats associated with acquired vagino-ureteral fistula. J Sm Anim Pract 21:367, 1980.

22. DeBaerdemaecker, GC: Post spaying vaginal discharge in a bitch caused by acquired vagino-urcteral fistula. Vet Rec 115:62, 1984.
23. Barton, CL: Canine vaginitis. 7:711, 1977.
24. Olson, PN, et al.: Vaginal Cytology. Its use in diagnosing canine reproduction disorders. Comp Cont Ed 6:385, 1984.
25. Olson, PN and Mather, EC: Canine vaginal and uterine bacterial flora. JAVMA 172:708, 1978.
26. Ling, GV and Ruby, AL: Aerobic bacterial flora of the prepuce, urethra and vagina of normal adult dogs. Am J Vet Res 39:695, 1978.
27. Osbaldiston, GW: Vaginitis in a bitch associated with *Haemophilus* spp. Am J Vet Res 32:2067, 1971.
28. Doig, PA, et al.: The genital *Mycoplasma* and *Ureaplasma* flora of healthy and diseased dogs. Can J Comp Med 45:233, 1981.
29. Holzmann, A, et al.: Experimentally induced mycoplasmal infection in the genital tract of the female dog. Theriogenology 12:355, 1979.
30. Hill, H and Mare, CJ: Genital disease in dogs caused by canine herpesvirus. Am J Vet Res 35:669, 1974.
31. Bittle, JL and Peckham, JC: Comments: Genital infection induced by feline rhinotracheitis virus and effects on newborn kittens. JAVMA 158:927, 1971.
32. Hoover, EA and Griesemer, RA: Comments: Pathogenicity of feline viral rhinotracheitis virus and effect on germ-free cats, growing bone and gravid uterus. JAVMA 158:929, 1971.
33. Hashimoto, A and Hirai, K: Canine herpesvirus infection. *In* Morrow, DA (ed): Current Therapy in Theriogenology, 2nd ed. Philadelphia, WB Saunders, 1986, p 516.
34. Poste, G and King, N: Isolation of a herpesvirus from the canine genital tract: association with infertility, abortion and stillbirths. Vet Rec 229, 1971.
35. Jackson, JA and Corstvet, RE: Transmission and attempted isolation of the etiologic agent associated with lymphofollicular hyperplasia of the canine species. Am J Vet Res 36:1207, 1975.
36. Kahrs, KF: Effects of infectious bovine rhinotracheitis on reproduction. *In* Morrow, DA (ed): Current Therapy in Theriogenology, 2nd ed. Philadelphia, WB Saunders, 1986, p 250.
37. Lerne, AM: Infections with herpes simplex virus. *In* Petersdorf, et al. (eds): Harrison's Principles of Internal Medicine, 10th ed. New York, McGraw-Hill, 1983, p 1165.
38. Thacker, C and Bradley, RL: Vulvar and vaginal tumors in the dog: a retrospective study. JAVMA 183:690, 1983.
39. Herron, MA: Tumors of the canine genital system. JAAHA 19:981, 1983.
40. Stein, BS: Tumors of the feline genital tract. JAAHA 17:1022, 1981.
41. Wykes, PM: Diseases of the vagina and vulva in the bitch. *In* Morrow, DA (ed): Current Therapy in Theriogenology, 2nd ed. Philadelphia, WB Saunders, 1986, p 476.
42. Rushmore, RA: Vaginal hyperplasia and uterine prolapse. *In* Kirk, RW (ed): Current Veterinary Therapy VII. Philadelphia, WB Saunders, 1980, p 1222.
43. Wheeler, SL, et al.: Persistent uterine and vaginal hemorrhage in a beagle with factor VII deficiency. JAVMA 185:447, 1984.

102 TUMORS OF THE GENITAL SYSTEM AND MAMMARY GLANDS

ANDREW S. LOAR

TUMORS OF THE MALE GENITAL TRACT

Neoplasms of the male reproductive tract include those of the testis, prostate gland, penis, prepuce, and scrotum. In the dog the most common of these are testicular tumors, the vast majority of which are benign. Tumors of the prostate gland are generally malignant, although they are a diagnostic dilemma when benign prostatic hyperplasia is also a differential diagnosis. With the exception of transmissible venereal tumors, the bulk of the neoplasms involving scrotum, penis, and prepuce are similar with regard to behavior and prognosis to those found in other cutaneous sites. Male reproductive tract tumors in the cat are rare, even in nonneutered animals, and are not discussed here.

Testicular Tumors

Tumors of the canine testis are the second most common neoplasm affecting the male dog. These tumors are distinguished by their histologic appearance and are classified as (a) germ cell tumors, which include seminomas, embryonal carcinomas, and teratomas; (b) sex cord–stromal tumors, which include Sertoli (sustentacular) cell and Leydig (interstitial) cell tumors; (c) mesotheliomas; (d) stromal and vascular tumors; and (e) unclassified tumors.[1] Seminomas and Sertoli cell and Leydig cell tumors are by far the most common testicular tumors, and are diagnosed with nearly equal frequency.[2] Testicular neoplasms represent 5 to 15 per cent of tumors recorded in male dogs; they are exceedingly rare in male cats. Breeds known to be at high risk for the development of testicular neoplasms include the Chihuahua, Pomeranian, miniature and standard poodle, miniature schnauzer, Shetland sheepdog, Siberian husky, and Yorkshire terrier; the beagle, Labrador retriever, and mixed breed dogs appeared to be at low risk.[3] For the three major tumor types, the mean age at diagnosis is between 10 and 11 years.[1] Most affected dogs are over age six.

Dogs with undescended testes are approximately 13 times more likely to develop testicular tumors, specifically Sertoli cell tumors and seminomas, than are normal dogs.[2, 4] In cryptorchid testes, Sertoli cell tumors occur in approximately 60 per cent of the cases, whereas seminomas occur in 40 per cent. In addition, cryptorchid dogs appear to develop testicular neoplasms at an earlier age. It has also been reported that the incidence rates for seminomas and Sertoli cell tumors are twice as high in dogs whose retained testis is in the inguinal region versus the abdominal cavity.[5]

In tumors of descended testes, approximately 40 per cent are of Leydig cell origin, 40 per cent are seminomas, and approximately 20 per cent are Sertoli cell tumors. Leydig cell tumors generally do not cause testicular enlargement; therefore, an obvious intrascrotal tumor is twice as likely to be a seminoma as it is to be a Sertoli cell tumor. For each of these tumor types, the right testis is likely to be affected approximately 80 per cent more often than the left; this is identical to the relative frequency of right versus left cryptorchidism.[1] In approximately ten per cent of dogs that develop multiple tumors of the testes, a seminoma or Sertoli cell tumor is generally found to occur concurrently with a Leydig cell tumor. Dogs with inguinal hernias appear to be at a significantly increased risk for the development of testicular neoplasms.[2]

CLINICAL FEATURES

The diagnosis of testicular neoplasm is generally made on physical examination and palpation of the testes. This should be routinely performed on all middle-aged or older intact males. Seminomas or Sertoli cell tumors may result in either diffuse testicular enlargement or a discrete nodule within the testes. Generally the animals are asymptomatic for these changes, although tenderness is occasionally noted. A large mass in the inguinal region ipsilateral to an undescended scrotal testis is suggestive of tumor development.

Leydig (Interstitial) Cell Tumor. Leydig cell tumors in dogs are of little clinical significance. Often this small tumor is not detected unless the involved testis is dissected at castration. It is usually a well-circumscribed nodule less than 1 cm in diameter, yellow or brown, and occurs within normal testicular tissue.[1] This tumor is extremely unlikely to exhibit malignant behavior. In addition, it is generally not associated with other hormonally related clinical syndromes, although one report has suggested such a relationship.[4]

Sertoli Cell Tumors. Generally this neoplasm is relatively slow growing, noninvasive, and varies from 1 mm to 5 cm in diameter. Rarely, a retained testis that develops a Sertoli cell tumor becomes much larger. This tumor has a distinct white capsule, and the cut surface may reveal a spongy network of tissue, brown to white, and is fibrous with interspersed soft lobes within. Occasionally cysts may be noted throughout the tumor tissue.[6] Very large Sertoli cell tumors may cause necrosis and hemorrhage within the tissue. Between 10 and 20 per cent metastasize, most frequently to the regional lymph nodes draining the inguinal and retroperitoneal area. Extension into the ipsilateral kidney or other adjacent sites within the abdomen has been noted from Sertoli cell tumors in abdominally cryptorchid dogs.

The most dramatic and much more common result of Sertoli cell tumors is the clinical syndrome of feminization. As many as 59 per cent of dogs affected with Sertoli cell tumor exhibit this syndrome. Dogs with this tumor in a nonscrotal area are more likely to manifest feminization than those with scrotal tumors.[4, 7] Feminization is associated with significant dermatologic and, occasionally, behavioral changes. Less frequently bone marrow suppression may be noted. Cutaneous manifestation of feminization associated with testicular tumors is similar to that secondary to other more common endocrine diseases. Symptoms include a bilaterally symmetrical, nonpruritic alopecia; hyperpigmentation, often involving the inguinal region and flanks; and gynecomastia.[8, 9] The cause of this syndrome has not been determined in all reported cases; however, it is suggested that the production of estrogenic steroids by the tumor tissue produces these clinical signs. Evidence for this includes (a) recovery of high concentrations of these compounds from the tumor tissues, urine, and spermatic venous blood of affected animals; (b) decreased estrogen levels in urine after tumor removal; (c) positive results of histochemical staining of tumor tissues for steroid receptors; and (d) synthesis of estrogen-like compounds demonstrated in cell cultures of Sertoli cell tumors.[9]

Feminization from testicular tumors, as well as other causes of elevations in circulating estrogen levels, may result in prostatic enlargement owing to squamous metaplasia within the gland. This may or may not result in clinical problems. The differential diagnosis for prostatomegaly is discussed in Chapter 105. A more spectacular problem secondary to feminization is that up to 25 per cent of affected animals will attract other male

dogs in the same manner as estral bitches. Evidence of bone marrow toxicosis secondary to Sertoli cell tumor has also been reported.[7, 9] Typically, the initial response to these substances results in decreased erythropoiesis and thrombopoiesis with a profound myeloid hyperplasia. In the untreated animal, bone marrow aplasia and pancytopenia may ultimately occur.

Seminoma. A seminoma has a homogenous yellow to creamy appearance on cut surface and commonly occupies one pole of the involved testis.[6] Five to ten per cent of seminomas will metastasize, spreading to regional lymphatic sites or to the abdominal viscera. The clinical syndrome of feminization has generally been reported to occur infrequently in dogs with seminomas; however, at least one large study of these tumors has noted the concurrent development of other clinical problems that may be hormonally mediated, such as prostatic disease, alopecia, perineal hernia, perianal gland adenoma, and pendulous penile sheath.[4]

Other Testicular Tumors. Rarely, other primary tumors have been reported to occur in the canine testis. These include hemangioma, granulosa cell tumor, embryonal carcinoma, and sarcoma.[1, 3]

TREATMENT AND PROGNOSIS

Orchiectomy. Surgical removal of the involved testes should be curative, except in the unusual case of a malignant or metastatic neoplasm. Malignant tumors that have not visibly spread from the involved testes have low potential for subsequent recurrence. Nevertheless, animals at increased risk for tumor relapse would include those whose original testicular tumor was of nonscrotal origin. Animals that show visible metastatic disease at the time of inguinal or abdominal exploratory examination may benefit from surgical excision of these lesions, when feasible. Extremely aggressive testicular tumors that manifest widespread regional or distant metastases may show a histologically undifferentiated appearance so that the specific cell type of origin may not be determined. For an animal that shows clinical signs of feminization associated with testicular tumors, castration is generally curative. The clinician must consider other endocrine causes for many of the typical signs of feminization, including hypothyroidism, adrenocortical hyperplasia, and selected pituitary diseases. Although less than 15 per cent of animals that show feminization will manifest signs suggestive of myelosuppression, castration may not reverse the hematologic abnormalities when these changes are advanced.[10]

Palliation for Advanced Disease. In the unusual case in which a malignant seminoma or Sertoli cell tumor has metastasized to regional or more distant sites, certain cytotoxic chemotherapy protocols have been suggested. Most of these treatments are similar to those used in men for advanced testicular cancer. Standard doses and schedules of vinblastine, cyclophosphamide, and methotrexate given in a cyclic (weekly) manner has resulted in greater than 50 per cent tumor reduction in dogs treated at the University of California–Davis.[10] The use of platinum-based chemotherapy protocols at other oncology centers has yielded similarly favorable results. Chemotherapy protocols cannot be expected to eliminate advanced disease in the dog; however, those animals that respond to treatment with a significant reduction in tumor volume should be expected to have at least several months of improved quality of life. The use of radiation or hormonal therapy against advanced testicular cancer in the dog has not yet been studied and reported.

Prostatic Adenocarcinoma

Gross abnormalities of the canine prostate gland include benign prostatic hyperplasia, squamous metaplasia, prostatic adenoma, and prostatic adenocarcinoma. Discussion of these conditions, including their clinical features, diagnosis, and treatment, can be found in Chapter 105. However, a brief review of therapy for prostatic adenocarcinoma is appropriately offered here.

Management of Prostatic Adenocarcinoma. Complete surgical excision of adenocarcinoma of the canine prostate is seldom possible. Partial prostatectomy will probably improve the quality of life of affected animals if significant tumor volume can be resected. Total prostatectomy is more effective in tumor control but is likely to create postoperative urinary incontinence.[11] The reduction of cyst formation and concurrent abscessation may also be a short-term benefit of a surgical approach to prostatic carcinoma. In men, castration is a widely accepted method of antitumor management, presumably by decreased prostatic stimulation due to lowering of testicular androgen levels. Likewise, in the dog, castration at an early age has been alleged to have a sparing effect on the risk of developing prostatic carcinoma. However, a recent report of a large group of dogs with histologically confirmed prostatic carcinoma found that 44 per cent had been neutered at least three years before detectable prostatic disease, and more than one-third of these dogs had been neutered at less than one year of age.[12] This supports the likelihood that nontesticular androgenic steroids may exert a significant influence on the development of canine prostatic carcinoma; it also suggests that castration may be of minimal value in the management of this cancer in dogs.

No studies have been reported concerning nonsurgical management of prostatic carcinoma in the dog; however, cytotoxic chemotherapy has been offered at veterinary oncology centers in the United States. Platinum-based protocols similar to those used in humans have shown significant benefit in fewer than 25 per cent of treated dogs suffering from advanced prostatic carcinoma. Other agents of possible benefit in this disease include hydroxyurea and ketoconazole. The antifungal agent ketoconazole has recently been shown to benefit men with advanced prostatic cancer, presumably by means of its anti-androgen effects.[13] The use of this drug against canine prostatic carcinoma would be best suited in those animals that show massive prostatic enlargement and/or bulky metastatic disease.

Deep-beam radiation therapy may also be helpful in the palliation of prostatic cancer in the dog. Candidates for this therapy would primarily include those animals that show clinical symptoms secondary to large tumor volume in the retroperitoneal areas (see Chapter 59).

Animals that show minimal improvement with the therapies described above can eventually be expected to show signs of tumor involvement in the retroperitoneal and lumbar regions. These signs would include tenesmus, lumbar or posterior abdominal pain, and difficulties with hind limb ambulation. Progression of these problems and subsequent debilitation would be expected prior to significant clinical signs indicating more distant metastatic lesions.

Penile Tumors

Tumors of the penis of the dog and cat are rarely reported. The most common of these in the dog, in certain endemic areas, is the transmissible venereal tumor. Squamous cell carcinoma has also been reported. Other, less common tumors include papilloma, fibroma, hemangioma, fibrosarcoma, hemangiosarcoma, and lymphoma. The most common clinical signs for the more aggressive cell types include ulcers and hemorrhage. Bleeding from the prepuce may be mistaken for hematuria unless a complete examination of the mucosal surface of the penis and prepuce is performed. An impression smear of suspicious lesions may suggest the underlying cell type. Ultimately the diagnosis can be confirmed only by means of incisional or excisional biopsy.

THERAPY

With the exception of transmissible venereal tumors, surgery can be considered the most effective therapy for penile neoplasms. Small tumors may be removed by wide excision, provided normal penile function can be maintained. If the neoplasm is extensive, penile amputation may be the more appropriate therapy. A prepubic or perineal urethrostomy is generally performed before radical penile resection. Epithelial tumors, such as papillomas and squamous cell carcinomas, and some solitary tumors of mesenchymal origin may be best treated using radiotherapy.

Canine Transmissible Venereal Tumor

A contagious round cell tumor of mesenchymal origin, the transmissible venereal tumor (TVT), was the first neoplasm described whose chromosomal structure varies from that of normal canine cells.[10] It was the first and remains the most common tumor known to be transmissible between members of the same species. Spread of this tumor generally occurs by sexual contact, but it has also been spread by licking and contact with nongenital mucosal surfaces. The disease has been reported from many countries all over the world, and it is endemic where dogs are free-roaming.

CLINICAL FEATURES

The transmissible venereal tumor is generally found on the genitals of sexually intact male and female dogs. In the male the external surface of the penis is most often involved, although the tumor may also occur on the inner epithelial surface (visceral or parietal layer) of the prepuce. The base of the penis is commonly involved such that the entire shaft must be extruded to visualize the tumor and obtain a cytologic diagnosis. On the genitals, lesions initially appear as small, raised hyperemic areas that may enlarge to become lobulated cauliflower-like, and may achieve a diameter of 5 cm or more. The tumor is often friable, and a hemorrhagic discharge may accumulate at its surface. Small pieces of the tumor may fracture off the primary mass during manipulation.

Although such tumors have regressed spontaneously, a modest percentage do metastasize. Metastasis may occur early in the course of the disease, but generally it is noted in animals in whom the tumor persists for longer than several months. Metastatic sites include regional lymph nodes and, occasionally, the scrotum or the perineal area. Rarely, more distant areas may become involved, including the orbit, abdominal viscera, lungs, and central nervous system.[10, 14] Primary lesions that appear on the mucous membranes of the face and rectum conceivably result from contact with the genitals of other tumor-bearing dogs.

DIAGNOSIS

The history of the dog, as well as the gross appearance of lesions, should suggest TVT. Differential diagnosis made from the gross appearance of the lesion could include mast cell tumor, histiocytoma, and lymphoma, as well as other nonneoplastic granulomatous lesions. The impression smear or aspiration cytology reveals a homogeneous population of round to ovoid cells that measure 15 to 30 mm in diameter. Mitotic figures may be numerous, and the ratio of nucleus to cytoplasm is low. The cytoplasm is pale with a fine granular appearance. The nuclei are round and should contain coarse chromatin aggregates.[15]

Histologically, the neoplasm resembles other round cell tumors, including histiocytomas, lymphomas, and poorly granulated mast cell tumors. The human histopathologist may not be familiar with this lesion.

THERAPY

Surgical excision may result in long-term control of the tumor, although the experiences of several oncology centers have found relapse rates to approach 50 per cent. Electrosurgical methods of treatment appear to have a more favorable prognosis.[16]

The most effective therapy for TVT is cytotoxic chemotherapy.[17] Although a variety of protocols have been described, the simplest is that reviewed by Calvert and his colleagues. Vincristine is administered weekly at standard cytotoxic doses (see Chapter 59). Therapy should be continued for two treatments past the point where there is no visible evidence of disease. The course of therapy is generally three to four weeks, and visible tumor regression would be expected shortly after the first or second treatment. More than 90 per cent of animals treated with this protocol can be expected to respond; virtually all will remain free of disease. If the

tumor relapses, it may do so locally and be sensitive to subsequent reinitiation of chemotherapy. If this therapy fails, or the animal shows a relapse after a second remission, the author and others have successfully used doxorubicin at standard anticancer doses and schedules. If chemotherapy cannot be administered, TVTs are extremely sensitive to radiation therapy, using multiple fractions or massive solitary doses.

Prepuce and Scrotal Tumors

Tumors arising from the skin of the prepuce and scrotum are generally similar in behavior to those that occur in cutaneous or adnexal structures of other sites (see Chapter 58). The most frequently found tumors of the scrotum and prepuce include mast cell tumors, melanomas, and squamous cell carcinomas. As with skin tumors, the diagnosis can be suggested by the examination of cytologic preparations and, ultimately, confirmed with biopsy. Before radical excision the extent of disease should be evaluated by palpation of the local lymph nodes and by abdominal and thoracic radiographs. In the absence of regional or distant metastatic disease, radical surgical excision is the most effective method of therapy. Depending on the site of the tumor, surgery may include orchiectomy as well as scrotal ablation or amputation of the penis and preputial sheath. Incomplete excision or postoperative relapse would indicate adjunctive therapy dependent on the tumor type. In the author's experience, melanomas of the scrotum have a more aggressive course than those in other cutaneous sites and are more likely to recur postoperatively.

TUMORS OF THE FEMALE GENITAL TRACT

Tumors of the female reproductive tract include those of the ovaries, uterus, cervix, vulva, and vagina. In part because many of the female dogs and cats presented to the veterinary clinician are neutered at a young age, these tumors account for less than one to two per cent of all neoplasms reported. Of these, the most frequently seen are those that occur in the vagina and vulva. By contrast, neoplasia of the canine and feline mammary glands is extremely common. In the female dog, mammary gland tumors are the most common tumor type reported and are most often benign; incidence rates of mammary tumors are second only to neoplasms of the skin. Mammary gland tumors in the female cat are reported less frequently, although most of these tumors have an aggressive natural behavior and ultimately result in the animal's death. It should be noted that mammary gland tissue is not anatomically or histologically considered to be within the reproductive system, and in fact would be more appropriately included in a discussion of dermatologic diseases. However, tradition allows for its inclusion in this chapter.

Tumors of the Ovary

Ovarian tumors are relatively uncommon in the dog and cat, consisting of less than one per cent of all total tumor types reported. Ovarian tumors are distinguished by specific cell types based on their embryologic origin, specifically, epithelial tumors, sex cord–stromal tumors, and germ cell tumors. Epithelial tumors are the most commonly reported in dogs and include papillary adenoma and adenocarcinoma, cystadenoma, cystadenocarcinoma, and undifferentiated carcinoma. Sex cord–stromal tumors arise from endocrine elements of the ovary and include granulosa cell tumors, theca cell tumors, and luteomas. Germ cell tumors are the least common category and include dysgerminomas and teratomas. Benign tumors of epithelial origin (adenomas) are the most common of all canine ovarian neoplasms, accounting for as many as 80 per cent of those studied.[10] They generally result in no clinical signs, and most are noted at routine ovariectomy. Grossly they appear as solitary masses and may be either smooth or roughly granulated and cauliflower-like. Many of these are found bilaterally.

Sex cord–stromal tumors, and particularly granulosa cell tumors, are the most common ovarian tumor of cats, and most of these exhibit malignant behavior. In the dog, granulosa cell tumors account for up to one-third of ovarian tumors reported, although most of these are benign. Grossly, it is difficult to distinguish sex cord–stromal tumors from other ovarian neoplasms.[18, 19] Animals that present with granulosa cell tumors have occasionally manifested clinical signs similar to those of hyperestrogenism, including abnormal estrus cycles, pyometra, and hyperplasia of uterine, vulvar, and vaginal epithelium. However, these features have also appeared in association with other ovarian neoplasms. Presumably this is due to excessive estrogenic steroid production by tumor tissues. The growth and metastatic behavior of feline malignant granulosa cell tumors are similar to those described below for ovarian adenocarcinoma.

Adenocarcinoma is the most common malignant ovarian tumor type reported in the dog and the second most common malignant variety in the cat. It occurs in animals with an average age of eight years; however, dogs as young as one year have been affected. Not infrequently the tumor may be diagnosed as an incidental finding at the time of ovariohysterectomy in the middle aged to older bitch. The potential for ultimate relapse or metastatic spread in these animals is certainly lower than in dogs initially presented with signs secondary to more advanced ovarian cancers. Grossly, the tumor may be difficult to distinguish from other ovarian masses. Unfortunately, histologic examination may not always differentiate between benign and malignant disease. As the neoplasm becomes more advanced it may metastasize to regional lymphatic structures, the adjacent kidney, or other abdominal viscera. Other sites of metastases include the lungs, pleural cavity, and the central nervous system. Lymphatic obstruction secondary to tumor invasion may cause fluid accumulation. In such cases the fluid would probably contain a variable number of carcinoma cells. Tumor cells exfoliated into abdominal fluid may thus implant on other peritoneal surfaces, where larger metastatic lesions may develop. Ovarian carcinomas should thus be among the differential diagnoses in intact female animals presented with abdominal fluid of unknown origin. Abdominal radiographs of these animals may not show evidence of organ enlargement or other abdominal masses. The incidence, behavior, and management of ovarian tumors in the cat are similar to those in the dog.

Differential Diagnosis. Possible causes of ovarian nodules noted as an incidental finding at abdominal surgery should include all of the tumors described as well as nonneoplastic cystic disease. In intact female animals presented with a modified transudate of unknown origin, causes would include nonneoplastic inflammatory disorders resulting in peritoneal lymphatic obstruction, and other neoplastic diseases, including cancers of the liver, pancreas, intestine, kidney, and adrenal gland. On cytologic examination of abdominal fluid, the clinician may not always find suspicious cells, even on centrifuged samples.

THERAPY

Initial Surgical Therapy. Irrespective of embryologic origin, benign ovarian tumors removed with ovariectomy should not recur. Likewise, clinical signs caused by excessive hormonal production should also resolve postoperatively. Virtually no large published studies exist concerning predictable response to therapy of animals with adenocarcinoma or other malignant forms of ovarian tumor; however, the stage of disease at the time of diagnosis is considered to be prognostically important. Lesions that are less than 2 cm in diameter that have not ruptured through the visceral surface of the ovarian tissue are far less likely to relapse postoperatively than larger, ulcerated masses. In the experience of the author and that of clinicians at other veterinary oncology centers, at least 50 per cent of animals presented with small, grossly intact ovarian carcinomas will show no relapse post ovariohysterectomy. In animals presented with evidence of extension beyond the ovary, the likelihood is high for subsequent progression of disease. In these animals surgical resection of large solitary metastatic lesions may be of value in the short-term control of ascites and other effects of the tumors. The surgeon must exercise care during manipulation of the tumor because of its profound tendency for implantation on visceral surfaces; hand and fingerprint lesions on abdominal tissues have been observed postoperatively. In instances in which all gross evidence of disease cannot be removed by surgery, tumor progression and subsequent debilitation can be expected within weeks to months postoperatively.

Adjuvant Therapy. Animals affected with advanced, unresectable ovarian carcinoma may be managed palliatively with a variety of cytotoxic therapy protocols. Doxorubicin-based therapies are indicated in women and have been used with partial success in dogs. Platinum-based treatment programs have yielded a decrease in fluid accumulation and a profoundly better quality of life. Protocols for these drugs can be found in Chapter 59. Solitary lesions may be successfully palliated with deep-beam radiation therapy, if this is available to the clinician. Short-term improvement in overall quality of life may be achieved using various diuretics, analgesics, and other anti-inflammatory treatments, where indicated. The poor short-term prognosis in animals with advanced ovarian carcinoma generally results in euthanasia.

Tumors of the Uterus and Cervix

Uterine tumors of the bitch and queen are uncommon and probably account for less than 0.5 per cent of all tumors reported in either species.[20, 21] In both species, the most common benign tumor type reported is the leiomyoma, which includes 85 to 90 per cent of all tumor types reported in this organ. In the dog, the most common malignant tumor is the leiomyosarcoma and in the cat, endometrial adenocarcinoma. Other rarely reported tumors in both species include adenomas, fibromas, and lymphosarcomas. Uterine tumors generally occur in older animals with an average age of approximately ten years. The benign tumors normally result in few or modest clinical signs and may be reported as incidental findings at surgery or necropsy.

The behavior of virtually all benign tumors of the uterus is characterized by slow growth, generally as an intraluminal mass. Uncommonly, the neoplasm may enlarge and compress adjacent abdominal structures; inflammatory changes leading to vaginal discharge may also result. Accumulation of inflammatory fluid to the degree that a pyometra develops is very rare. In all cases of benign uterine tumors, complete ovariohysterectomy should be curative.

Leiomyosarcoma of the canine uterus involves the growth of an intraluminal or extraluminal mass. Metastases to regional lymphatic or visceral sites are generally late findings. If metastatic lesions are noted at the time of surgery, adjuvant chemotherapy using doxorubicin-based protocols may benefit the animal by delaying progression or shrinking visible disease. However, results of such therapy protocols against leiomyosarcomas have not been published.

Endometrial adenocarcinoma of the feline uterus has a more aggressive behavior than that of leiomyosarcoma.[22] Development of metastatic lesions may occur when the primary tumor is small, and generally involves the regional lymph nodes, abdominal viscera, lungs, and central nervous system. Palliative postoperative chemotherapy for the disease has not been reported, although the clinician may consider the use of cyclophosphamide or doxorubicin-based protocols (see Chapter 59). Radiation therapy to affected sites may aid in delaying progression of the disease postovariohysterectomy.

Tumors of the cervix of the dog and cat are extremely rare and reports have been anecdotal. Behavior and therapy would be similar to those described for uterine tumors.

Tumors of the Vagina and Vulva

Neoplasms found in the vulva and vagina of the dog and cat are by far the most commonly reported tumors in the female genital tract. Most of these, with the exception of animals presented with transmissible venereal tumors, occur in older, sexually intact animals, with an average age of approximately ten years.[20, 23] The majority of vulvar/vaginal tumors are benign, and include tumors of smooth muscle or fibrous tissue origin (i.e., leiomyoma, fibroma, lipoma) as well as polyps. Leiomyosarcoma and squamous cell carcinoma are the two most common malignancies in this site and account for more than 80 per cent of the cancers. Rare miscellaneous tumors reported include hemangiosarcoma, osteosarcoma, mast cell tumors, and adenocarcinomas of adnexal gland origin. Transmissible venereal tumors are a special class of vulvar/vaginal neoplasms that are apt to recur postsurgically, but they metastasize in less than five per cent of the cases reported. Several authors have noted the possibility for hormonal influence on tumor development and postsurgical relapse, particularly with the benign tumor types.

CLINICAL FEATURES

Similar to tumors in the uterus, vaginal/vulvar tumors may be intraluminal or extraluminal. Small benign tumors at these sites are typically intraluminal and may result in a serosanguineous or purulent discharge. Benign tumors tend to be pedunculated and are often noted protruding from the vulvar lips. Visualization of these tumors frequently is possible when the animal strains because of irritation at the time of urination or defecation. Digital examination of the vaginal vault will reveal the size and extent of the mass.

Extraluminal vaginal tumors are less common but may grow to a much larger size before clinical presentation. Deformity and swelling of the perineal region may not be obvious until the tumor becomes more than 3 cm in diameter. Other growth characteristics of malignant vulvar/vaginal tumors include metastases to regional lymphatic tissues, in particular sublumbar lymph nodes. The clinical behavior of squamous cell carcinoma and leiomyosarcoma is similar. Distant metastases are very rare. Generally, malignant vulvar/vaginal tumors progress by way of local invasion and expansion rather than by metastasis. The vulva and vagina are the most common sites of transmissible venereal tumors in the dog. These neoplasms have an appearance similar to that as described in the male, and frequently result in a serosanguineous discharge. As the tumor grows to more than two cm in diameter, it may appear cauliflower-like and friable. Metastasis to regional or more distant sites occurs in less than five per cent of cases. Diagnosis and therapy for this neoplasm in the bitch are identical to those described earlier in the male dog.

THERAPY

Surgical Therapy. The diagnostic management for most of these tumors consists of excisional biopsy. For the benign intraluminal tumor this requires the removal of the pedunculated stalk and adjacent attachments, and is rarely followed by local recurrence if resection has been complete. For neoplasms with wide bases, tumors involving a large portion of the vulva, or those invading extraluminal sites, more aggressive surgical resection, including episiotomy, vulvectomy, or significant perineal dissection, may be required. Occasionally an abdominal approach may be necessary to expose the neoplasm. If malignancy is suspected, surgery should be preceded by abdominal and thoracic radiographs.

In at least one study a hormonal influence on tumor development has been suggested.[23] Estrus cycle abnormalities, recent estrus, pyometra, pseudocyesis, excessive estral discharge, and mammary gland tumors have been reported in many animals presented for vaginal/vulvar tumors. In addition, a small percentage of unspayed animals showed tumor recurrence months to years after initial resection. Although other studies have not confirmed a direct association between the neuter status of affected animals and the development or regrowth of these tumors, it seems reasonable to perform an ovariohysterectomy at the time of tumor resection. No hormonal influences have been noted in animals with malignant tumors at these sites.

The potential for postoperative tumor recurrence depends on the initial size and invasiveness of the cancer. Malignant neoplasms that recur will generally do so within 12 to 24 months of the initial surgery. Unusual cancers of these areas, such as hemangiosarcomas, osteosarcomas, mast cell tumors, and adenocarcinomas of adnexal origin, are generally difficult to resect surgically and may recur rapidly.[20, 23]

Adjuvant Therapy. Adjuvant therapy for malignant tumors should be reserved for those that were incompletely resected. Sarcomas may respond to doxorubicin-based protocols. Carcinomas and mast cell tumors may be controlled with the use of radiation therapy. No studies have been performed to determine the value of these treatments, however.

CANINE MAMMARY GLAND TUMORS

The most common tumor in the female dog is of mammary gland origin. Likewise in this species, malignant mammary tumors are by far the leading form of cancer. In dogs of both sexes only the skin shows a higher reported occurrence rate of neoplastic disease. Despite their high occurrence rate, mammary neoplasms present a therapeutic challenge to the clinician because they exhibit considerable variety in their historical, clinical, and histologic appearance. Prediction of both tumor behavior and response to therapy is extremely difficult and often subjective. Nonetheless, an accurate prognosis is valuable to the clinician in selecting the most appropriate treatment. Certain characteristics of canine mammary gland tumors are of proved, or suspected, prognostic significance and are discussed herein. Surgical and adjunctive therapies are described and are recommended based on the prognosis.

The approximate median age of dogs with mammary tumors is 10 to 11 years. The reported ages range from 2 to 20 years; however, mammary neoplasia in bitches less than 5 years old is extremely uncommon. Cocker spaniels, poodles, and fox and Boston terriers have a higher risk for the development of mammary tumors than other purebred or crossbred dogs; chihuahuas and Boxers are at a decreased risk. Some oncologists have observed that mammary cancer in the German shepherd shows a more malignant behavior than in other breeds. These tumors are very rare in male dogs, accounting for about one per cent of all reported mammary neoplasms. As in humans, the majority of canine mammary tumors in the male are aggressive cancers.

Biologic Behavior and Clinical Features

The tumor characteristics that are most important to the clinician are those associated with an unfavorable prognosis. Certain histologic features are commonly associated with aggressive malignant behavior and correlate with a poor long-term prognosis; however, other clinical factors also have significant impact on the disease outcome. These include the mode and rate of growth of the tumor, the total volume of tumor at the time of presentation, and the involvement of regional or distant lymph nodes.

The rate of tumor growth and duration of clinical signs frequently can be determined by a careful history. Animals with mammary cancer are often presented with a complaint of rapid increase in tumor size. The duration of disease before surgical removal is generally longer for benign tumors than for carcinomas.[24] Rapid growth or regrowth usually indicates an aggressive malignancy and is considered a negative prognostic finding. However, biopsies of small, slow-growing nodules may reveal foci of malignant cells. These observations emphasize two principles in the management of mammary tumors. First, surgical excision of a tumor should not be postponed based on the clinical appearance or history of the mass. Second, to provide the most accurate prognosis, all tumors should be submitted for histologic examination.

The mode of growth of a neoplasm is often an indicator of its relative invasiveness. Well-circumscribed, expansive lesions are more readily excised, and thus have a better prognosis than those with less distinct borders. Gross infiltration of the skin, with or without ulceration, or of tissues deep to the mammary glands suggests an aggressive tumor and a high postoperative recurrence rate. Often, however, assessment for degree of invasiveness is most reliable when based on microscopic examination of biopsy sections (see section on Histopathology).

Enlargement of regional lymph nodes secondary to neoplastic infiltration implies a high metastatic potential for the tumor. In fact, Gilbertson and his colleagues showed that microscopic evidence of tumor invasion into lymph nodes or vessels correlated with a 95 per cent recurrence rate.[25] It is therefore important to examine enlarged lymph nodes microscopically to determine the extent of regional metastases as well as to rule out benign causes of lymphadenopathy.

In general, the clinical characteristics that show the highest influence on disease outcome include the total volume of the primary tumor, the number and extent of regional lymph node involvement, and the presence of distant metastatic disease. Clinical features that have not been shown to be of consistent prognostic significance for dogs with mammary gland neoplasia include the location of the primary tumor burden within the mammary chain, whether tumors are located in single versus multiple mammary glands, right-sided versus left-sided mammary chain involvement, and the type of surgical resection.

The World Health Organization (WHO) has used these important features to develop a clinical staging system for common neoplasms. This tumor-node-metastasis (TNM) system generally classifies four stages of mammary cancer as follows: stage I includes small, localized tumors; stage II involves larger, although discreet, tumors with limited, if any, regional metastases; stage III describes invasion of tumor into surrounding structures or extensive regional metastases; stage IV indicates distant metastases (see Table 102–1 for specific criteria). The author has retrospectively evaluated 204 dogs presented to the Animal Medical Center in New York for treatment of stage I through stage III mammary tumors. For all malignancies, irrespective of the histologic type, animals presented with stage III tumors (primary tumors larger than 3 cm in diameter and/or lymph node infiltration and fixation) showed a significantly higher risk of disease recurrence within two years of surgical excision versus dogs with stage I or stage II tumors (see Figure 102–1).[26]

An uncommon clinical presentation of mammary neoplasia is the inflammatory carcinoma, which has been described in the dog.[27] Animals with inflammatory carcinoma typically show multiple, often bilateral gland involvement with warm, painful tumors. Edema in the mammary glands, overlying skin, and the nearest limb is often present. Nearly all dogs with this aggressive malignancy have systemic metastatic disease at the time of presentation. Surgical resection is seldom complete, and frequently is followed by rapid recurrence. Adjuvant therapy, discussed later in this section, is unlikely to control tumor progression.

Histopathology

Because of the heterogeneous morphology of canine mammary tumors, the development of histopathologic classification systems and the examination of their prognostic significance are among the most controversial topics in veterinary oncology. In 1974 the WHO published a scheme that allows the classification and diagnosis of more than 19 tumor types and is used in some form by many veterinary pathologists. The morphologic basis of this scheme is complex, and is reviewed elsewhere.[28] Table 102–2 summarizes the various tumor types.

Generally clinicians evaluating a surgical pathology report of a mammary tumor have found it difficult to correlate the WHO histologic diagnosis with a specific prognosis. Several published studies have attempted to make such a correlation; however, their results are controversial and have not been reproducible.[29–32]

Many of the histologic classifications created by the WHO have not been of prognostic significance; how-

TABLE 102–1. CLINICAL STAGING SYSTEM FOR CANINE MAMMARY TUMORS

Stage Grouping	T	N	M
I	T_1	N_0 (−) or any N a(−)	M_0
II	T_0	N_1 (+)	M_0
	T_1	N_1 (+)	M_0
	T_2	N_0 (+) or N_1 a(+)	M_0
III	T_3	Any N	M_0
	Any T	Any N b	M_0
IV	Any T	Any N	M_1

Modified from Owen, L. N., ed.: The TNM Classification of Tumours in Domestic Animals. Geneva: World Health Organization, 1980.

KEY: T (Primary Tumor): T_0 = no evidence of tumor; T_1 = tumor less than 1 cm maximum diameter; T_2 = tumor 1 to 3 cm maximum diameter; T_3 = tumor more than 3 cm maximum diameter; T_4 = tumor any size, inflammatory carcinoma; N (Regional Lymph Nodes [RLN]); N_0 = no RLN involved; N_1 = ipsilateral RLN involved; N_2 = bilateral RLN involved; a = not fixed; b = fixed; − = histologically negative; + = histologically positive; M (Distant Metastasis); M_0 = no evidence of distant metastasis; M_1 = distant metastasis.

ever, some distinctions seem to be of importance. The most basic is distinguishing between benign and malignant disease. Dogs with any of the benign mammary neoplasms listed in Table 102–2 are at minimal risk for tumor recurrence, although a second primary tumor may develop in remaining mammary tissue. At least one large retrospective study revealed that a number of neoplasms previously considered malignant by a WHO-based system could be classified as nonmalignant by a newer system.[25] In support of this, a review of more than 5000 dogs whose mammary tumors were removed and submitted for biopsy showed that slightly less than 50 per cent were given a (WHO) histologic diagnosis of cancer.[28] Traditionally, about 50 per cent of dogs with biopsy-proved malignant mammary tumors suffer recurrence or metastasis regardless of the type of surgical excision. Thus, although about one half of all canine mammary tumors show a malignant (WHO) histologic

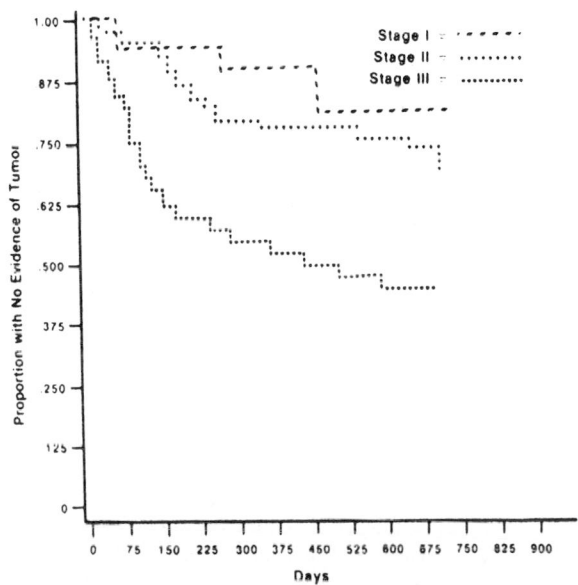

FIGURE 102–1. Disease-free interval by clinical staging—WHO classification (all cancers—WHO histopathologic classification). (From Loar, AS: The management of canine mammary tumors. *In:* Kirk, RW (ed.). Current Veterinary Therapy IX. Philadelphia, WB Saunders, 1986, p 480.)

TABLE 102–2. DIFFERENT MORPHOLOGIC FORMS OF CANINE MAMMARY TUMORS

Benign Mammary Tumors
Benign mixed tumor
Complex adenoma
Fibroadenoma
   Intracanalicular type
   Pericanalicular type
Duct papilloma
Simple adenoma
Malignant Mammary Tumors
Tubular adenocarcinoma
   Simple and complex types
Papillary adenocarcinoma
   Simple and complex types
Papillary cystic adenocarcinoma
   Simple and complex types
Solid carcinoma
   Simple and complex types
Anaplastic carcinoma
Other carcinomas
   Mucinous, squamous cell, spindle cell
Sarcomas
   Osteosarcoma, fibrosarcoma, and combined forms
Malignant mixed tumor (carcinosarcoma)

Based on the International Histological Classification of Tumors of Domestic Animals published by the World Health Organization, 1974. Modified from Theilen and Madewell: Veterinary Cancer Medicine. Philadelphia, Lea & Febiger, 1979, pp 192–203.

appearance, only about one quarter of the total behave in a malignant manner subsequent to tumor removal. To the clinical oncologist, the usefulness of a histologic diagnosis lies in its ability to predict a tumor's biologic behavior. A surgical cure in at least one half of all dogs with a biopsy showing "mammary adenocarcinoma" suggests that the diagnosis of malignancy is offered too liberally. If neither the histologic criteria nor the diagnosis can be shown to have a good correlation with prognosis, then the classification system that contains them should be abandoned.

Histologic malignancy is generally determined by the following poor prognostic features: evidence of microscopic invasion into tissues past the boundaries of tumor stroma; tumor invasion into lymph nodes, lymph vessels, and blood vessels; features indicative of mammary sarcoma; and features indicative of cellular anaplasia.

In a mammary neoplasm with cellular morphology suggestive of a carcinoma, tumor extension into normal adjacent tissue distinguishes an invasive cancer from a well-circumscribed tumor referred to as carcinoma in situ. Demonstration of invasion is more likely when at least two to three sections from the tumor are examined, because many dogs with evidence of invasive cancer also have foci of in situ carcinoma elsewhere in the mastectomy specimen.[25] In addition, not infrequently a pathologist may interpret carcinoma cells infiltrating into surrounding areas of less malignant appearing neoplastic tissue as evidence of invasion; in fact, this finding represents carcinoma in situ. Clinically, well-circumscribed mammary cancers generally appear as distinct nodules within normal glandular tissue. If the histologic diagnosis is discordant with the clinical impression, the author recommends discussion between clinician and pathologist.

Invasive, also called infiltrative, carcinoma is associated with a significantly higher rate of local recurrence or metastases (more than 70 per cent within two years) than noninvasive carcinoma.[25, 30–32] Histologically well-circumscribed carcinomas have generally been associated with less than a 25 per cent rate of tumor death or recurrence after two years. Many authors consider these so-called preinvasive malignant mammary proliferations to be precursor lesions of invasive mammary cancer and, therefore, recommend early mastectomy for the treatment of discrete nodular lesions.

Histologic evidence of tumor invasion into lymph nodes or lymphatic or blood vessels is discussed earlier and appears to represent a poor prognosis. Submission of adequate tissue specimens and the examination of at least several sections are necessary to evaluate these features.

Cellular anaplasia is also generally agreed to be a poor prognostic factor; however, because anaplastic tumors are almost always highly invasive, it is difficult to quantitate the independent significance of this feature in determining prognosis. Overall, the two-year death rate for anaplastic carcinoma is 76 per cent.[31]

Sarcomas of the canine mammary gland are unusual, probably accounting for less than 10 per cent of all mammary tumors. Osteosarcoma, compound osteochondrosarcoma (osteochondrosarcoma), and fibrosarcoma are the most commonly reported cell types, although frequently the tumor cells are too poorly differentiated for the tissue origin to be determined. As opposed to carcinomas, mammary sarcomas rarely metastasize to regional or distant sites. Local tumor regrowth is very likely, however, with a recurrence rate approaching 100 per cent, leading to severe local problems, such as ulceration, infection, and difficulty with locomotion. Most animals with recurrent mammary sarcomas will die as a result of their disease within one to two years of initial therapy. The presence of nonmalignant proliferative mesenchymal elements, such as bone, cartilage, and hyperplastic myoepithelial cells, in biopsy specimens is usually not associated with an unfavorable prognosis.

As many as 65 per cent of dogs presented for mammary neoplasia show evidence of multiple gland involvement. Examination of all excised tumors frequently reveals both malignant and benign lesions, and several histologic types may be noted. The likelihood of disease recurrence in dogs with multiple gland involvement is related to the most aggressive lesion found. Additional less malignant tumors in adjacent tissues do not appear to worsen the prognosis.

Surgical Therapy

Surgical excision of the neoplasm provides the biopsy specimens necessary for a reliable diagnosis and is the single best method for elimination of all visible disease. For most dogs presented with mammary neoplasia the therapeutic objective is to remove all gross evidence of tumor by means of surgical resection. Exceptions to this include those animals that have inflammatory carcinoma or distant metastatic (i.e., stage IV) disease. Among dogs with mammary cancer, the high recurrence rate indicates failure to remove all foci of malignant cells.

Thorough evaluation, including thoracic radiographs, careful palpation of all mammary glands, peripheral lymph nodes, and adjacent soft tissue and bony structures, as well as appropriate laboratory analyses, is a necessary prerequisite to surgical treatment.

If only local disease is detected, the surgeon has a choice of four procedures: *nodulectomy* (lumpectomy), the isolated removal of the tumor(s) from within the gland; *simple mastectomy*, the removal of the affected gland(s); *en bloc mastectomy* (modified radical mastectomy), the removal of a group of glands dependent on their lymphatic drainage; and *complete unilateral mastectomy* (radical mastectomy), the removal of all mammary glands ipsilateral to the tumor(s), intervening tissues, and regional lymph nodes. The clinical stage and site of involvement, as well as the general condition of the dog, should dictate which procedure is used.

Nodulectomy has the advantage of being a rapid, low-cost technique for the excision of small, well-circumscribed nodules, such as in dogs with stage I disease. However, because little of the normal surrounding tissue is removed, it is not possible to evaluate these specimens for histologic evidence of invasiveness or lymph node involvement. If the biopsy subsequently reveals malignancy, then a more aggressive resection, such as a simple or en bloc mastectomy, is indicated.

The primary disadvantage of simple mastectomy is that because most canine mammary glands are intimately associated with their fellow ipsilateral glands, isolated removal of a single gland is often more difficult than an en bloc resection. Also, unless tumor involves the most posterior (fifth) or the most anterior (first) gland, access to the nearest lymph node is not possible without removal of more than one gland. Review of the regional lymphatics thus reveals the usefulness of the en bloc mastectomy.

The lymphatic drainage of mammary tumors suggests that metastatic cells from glands one, two, and three generally traverse cranially to the axillary lymph node, whereas cells from glands four, five, and, occasionally, three usually drain caudally to the inguinal node.[24] Thus, the recommended surgical treatment of the majority of canine mammary tumors is the en bloc mastectomy technique based on these drainage routes. Tumors in glands one and/or two are removed by resection of the three most cranial ipsilateral glands and interposing tissue; the axillary node should also be taken if tumor infiltration is suspected. Tumors in glands four and/or five are removed by resection of the three most caudal ipsilateral glands and intervening tissue; the inguinal lymph node generally adheres to the resected specimen and should also be removed. Tumors associated with gland three can be resected by complete unilateral mastectomy or by simple mastectomy if a less aggressive method is desired; axillary and inguinal lymph nodes should be left intact or removed as described above.

Many clinicians recommend the en bloc mastectomy versus complete unilateral mastectomy for most mammary tumors.[33] Certainly, the former technique should be associated with less overall morbidity and expense. Furthermore, one prospective study by MacEwen and colleagues found no significant differences in the rate of tumor-related death or recurrence in dogs presented for mammary carcinoma that were treated with either type of surgery.

Monitoring after initial surgical therapy depends on the initial clinical stage and histologic diagnosis. Dogs with an increased likelihood for tumor recurrence should be rechecked at least every one to three months, with thoracic radiographs obtained at every other examination visit. In animals with in situ carcinoma, rechecks may be scheduled at three- to six-month intervals, with radiographic evaluation of the chest every six months. Benign tumors suggest less aggressive postoperative monitoring, although new primary tumors may still develop.

Adjuvant Therapy

The indication for postoperative (adjuvant) therapy is histologic evidence that suggests a high risk of tumor recurrence or tumor-related morbidity (e.g., invasive cancer). Forms of adjunctive therapy that may be helpful include the administration of cytotoxic drugs, radiotherapy, and the use of biologic response modifiers (immunotherapy). Adjuvant therapy offers the most benefit when tumor volume is minimal. Candidates for adjuvant therapy include dogs with any of the following: (a) clinical stage III cancers, prior to surgery, including histologically well-circumscribed malignancies; (b) any sized tumor showing histologic evidence of invasion into adjacent normal tissues, lymphatic structures, or blood vessels; and (c) animals with recurrent or inoperable local cancer, or those with distant metastatic (i.e., stage IV) disease. To date, reports regarding the responses to nonsurgical treatment of canine mammary cancer have been anecdotal and poorly controlled. However, some treatments may show promise to clinicians and owners facing the probability of advancing, fatal disease.

CYTOTOXIC DRUG THERAPY

Several protocols for cytotoxic treatment of mammary carcinoma have been recommended in the veterinary literature; however, significant antitumor effects from these therapies have not been reported.[33, 34] In women with advanced mammary carcinoma, the use of doxorubicin as a single agent or in combination with other cytotoxic drugs has resulted in antitumor response rates superior to those reported using other forms of chemotherapy.[35] In a limited number of dogs with metastatic mammary cancer treated with doxorubicin, the author and others have noted objective antitumor responses (see Chapter 59 for protocols and schedules). Controlled studies should ultimately determine the effectiveness of this protocol.

Not infrequently, owners of pets with advanced mammary cancer request treatments to improve their pet's quality of life. When irradiation and cytotoxic agents have failed or are not acceptable, the clinician may still achieve short term palliation with basic supportive therapy. Palliative management for metastatic disease is primarily symptomatic and would include the use of antibiotics, corticosteroids, nutritional support, physical therapy, and other forms of nursing care as needed.

RADIATION THERAPY

In women with breast cancer, radiotherapy is commonly offered as postoperative adjuvant therapy, and is also used for patients with bulky, nonresectable local disease, those with inflammatory carcinoma, and those with painful bony metastases. The intent of this form of therapy in dogs is not to provide a cure or long-term control, but merely to palliate the animal that suffers from advanced disease. The duration of benefit in the limited number of cases reported has been brief, generally less than two to four months. However, despite a grave short-term prognosis, a few pet owners will tolerate the time, expense, and referral required for these treatments. Although no studies have been performed for this purpose, radiotherapy should be expected to delay relapse in animals presented after resection of histologically aggressive lesions.

IMMUNOTHERAPY AND HORMONAL MANIPULATION

The rationale for immunotherapy is that several types of canine mammary tumors generate cellular responses presumed to represent host versus tumor reactivity.[25, 32] Stimulation of the immune system, particularly after tumor removal, may augment these responses and possibly delay recurrence or progression of the tumor.

Immunostimulants. The most frequently suggested therapeutic agents are classified as nonspecific immunostimulants and include levamasole, *Corynebacterium parvum*, and bacillus Calmette-Guérin (BCG). Levamasole and *C. parvum* have been used in several trials by MacEwen and colleagues and have offered no significant benefits.[36] In another study, intravenous therapy with BCG resulted in a significantly lower tumor-associated death rate in dogs that had undergone surgical resection of mammary carcinoma.[28] It remains the most positive study regarding the effectiveness of immunotherapy in animals.

Plasmapheresis. Circulating free tumor antigens, antitumor antibodies, and complexes composed of these antigens and antibodies are all thought to inhibit the host's immune response to its tumor. Researchers have proposed that removal of the immune complexes by either plasmapheresis or selective immunoabsorption may improve the immune reaction and possibly result in tumor regression.[37] Responses to these forms of treatment have been impressive but have not been widely reported and confirmed.

Hormonal Manipulation. In women, hormonal therapy is widely accepted in the adjuvant treatment of mammary cancer. The primary indication for this therapy is the presence of estrogen receptors (ER) on the surface of tumor cells, since animals that are ER positive are more likely to respond favorably to anti-estrogen therapy. However, if patients are ER negative or the ER status cannot be determined, no hormonal manipulations are recommended. ER determinations in a limited number of canine mammary tumors have revealed that about 60 per cent express the receptors, although the most histologically aggressive carcinomas are generally ER negative.[38] Obviously, most clinicians are not routinely able to assay tumors for ER. If future studies confirm that tumors with the poorest prognosis also are usually ER negative, then the various anti-estrogen therapies will rarely be indicated.

Ovariectomy performed before the first estrus virtually eliminates the risk of mammary tumor development in dogs. As ovariectomy is delayed past the first heat, however, the risk of mammary tumor development increases until it plateaus at age two and one-half years. In addition, no improvement has been shown in the rate of tumor recurrence or tumor-associated death in dogs neutered at the time of mammary tumor removal.

MAMMARY TUMORS IN THE CAT

In the cat, the mammary glands are the third most common site of cancer, after tumors of hematopoietic tissues and skin.[39] Similar to the dog, the median age for tumor development is 10 to 12 years. Siamese cat breeds show an increased risk of mammary tumor development in general, but also seem to develop tumors at an earlier age than other cat breeds.[40] No study has shown a difference in tumor development rates for cats spayed before or after their first heat.

The morphology and distribution of feline mammary neoplasms are far less variable than those of the canine. Eighty to 90 per cent of these tumors are malignant, and most are adenocarcinomas.[41] Most feline mammary cancers show local invasion or lymphatic infiltration.[42] Cats with mammary carcinoma will most likely develop tumor recurrence and die within one year after surgery, unless the original tumor was diagnosed as carcinoma in situ.[42, 43] Prognostically, the volume of the tumor and the type of surgical therapy performed appear to be significant factors in determining survival time.[43] Cats with small primary adenocarcinomas (1 to 8 cm in diameter) have longer disease-free intervals and survival times than those with larger cancers.

Surgical therapy techniques for feline mammary tumors are identical to those used in the dog. MacEwen has shown that in the cat, the radical mastectomy technique leads to a longer disease-free interval than the simple mastectomy, but long-term survival times for the two procedures are not significantly different.[43] The en bloc technique is again considered the best method of surgical therapy for the reasons outlined in the canine surgical therapy section.

Cats diagnosed with adenocarcinoma may develop relapses adjacent to the original surgical sites rather than distant metastases. These relapses may best be managed by repeat surgical resections; this may control the disease for up to several years in some cats before the development of distant metastases.

Adjuvant therapy is recommended for any cat with mammary cancer, regardless of other factors. Cats with advanced adenocarcinoma respond impressively to cytotoxic therapy protocols of doxorubicin and cyclophosphamide.[44] Radiation and immunotherapy techniques have yet to be shown beneficial in the cat.

PREVENTION OF REPRODUCTIVE NEOPLASIA

It is rarely possible for texts to specify a method that will protect patients from certain disorders in an entire body system. With the notable exceptions of canine prostatic adenocarcinoma and feline mammary cancer, neutering pets at an appropriately early age will prevent virtually all other tumor types of reproductive tissues. Protecting animals from benign and malignant tumors that as a group account for 15 to 20 per cent of all reported tumor types, including two of the most common neoplasms of the dog as well as an assortment of non-neoplastic conditions of the genital tract, is an uncommon and welcome option.

References

1. Nielson, SW and Leren, DH: Tumors of the testes. WHO 3168:71, 1974.
2. Hayes, HN and Pendergrass, TW: Canine testicular tumors: Pathologic features of 410 dogs. Int J Cancer 18:482, 1976.
3. Pendergrass, TW and Hayes, HM, Jr.: Cryptorchidism and related defects in dogs: epidemiologic comparisons with man. Teratology 12.51, 1975.
4. Lipowitz, AJ, et al.: Testicular neoplasms and concomitant clinical changes in the dog. JAVMA 163:1364, 1973.
5. Reif, AS, et al.: A cohort study of canine testicular neoplasia. JAVMA 175:179, 1979.
6. Cotchin, E.: Testicular neoplasms in dogs. J Comp Pathol 70:232, 1960.
7. Morgan, RV: Blood dyscrasias associated with testicular tumors in the dog. JAAHA 18:970, 1982.
8. Brodey, RS and Martin, JE: Sertoli cell neoplasms in the dog: the clinical pathological findings in 37 dogs. JAVMA 133:249, 1958.
9. Pulley, LT: Sertoli cell tumor. Vet Clin North Am 9:145, 1979.
10. Madewell, BR and Theilen, GH: Tumors of the urogenital tract. In Theilen, GH and Madewell, BR (eds.): Veterinary Cancer Medicine, 2nd ed. Philadelphia, Lea & Febiger, 1987, p 583.
11. Hardie, M, et al.: Complications of prostatic surgery. JAAHA 20:50, 1984.
12. Obradovich, MD, et al.: The influence of castration on the development of prostatic carcinoma in the dog: 43 cases (1978–1985). J Vet Intern Med, in press.
13. Trachtenberg, J: Ketoconazole therapy for advanced prostate cancer. Lancet 2:435, 1984.
14. Higgins, DA: Observations on the canine transmissible venereal tumor as seen in the Bahamas. Vet Rec 79:67, 1966.
15. Duncan, J and Prasse, KW: Cytology of canine cutaneous round cell tumors. Mast cell tumor, histiocytoma, lymphosarcoma, and transmissible venereal tumor. Vet Pathol 16:673, 1979.
16. Idowu, AL: A retrospective evaluation of four surgical methods of treating canine transmissible venereal tumor. J Sm Anim Pract 25:193, 1984.
17. Calvert, C, et al.: Vincristine for treatment of transmissible venereal tumor in the dog. JAVMA 181:163, 1982.
18. Hayes, HM and Young, JL: Epidemiologic features of canine ovarian neoplasms. Gynecol Oncol 6:348, 1978.
19. Nielson, SW, et al.: Tumours of the ovary. Bull WHO 53:203, 1976.
20. Brodey, RF and Roszel, JR: Neoplasms of the canine uterus, vagina, and vulva: A clinical, pathologic study of 96 cases. JAVMA 151:1294, 1967.
21. Stein, BS: Tumors of the feline genital tract. JAAHA 17:1022, 1981.
22. O'Rourke, MD and Geib, LW: Endometrial adenocarcinoma in a cat. Cornell Vet 60:598, 1970.
23. Thatcher, C and Bradley, RL: Vulvar and vaginal tumors in the dog: A retrospective study. 183:690, 1983.
24. Fidler, IJ and Brodey RS: A necropsy study of canine malignant mammary neoplasms. JAVMA 151:710, 1967.
25. Gilbertson, SR, et al.: Canine mammary epithelial neoplasms: biologic implications of morphologic characteristics assessed in 232 dogs. Vet Pathol 20:127, 1983.
26. Loar, AS: The management of canine mammary tumors. In Kirk, RW (ed.): Current Veterinary Therapy IX. Philadelphia, WB Saunders, 1986, p 480.
27. Susaneck, SJ, et al.: Inflammatory mammary carcinoma in the dog. JAAHA 19:971, 1983.
28. Brodey, RS, et al.: Canine mammary gland neoplasms. JAAHA 19:61, 1983.
29. Misdorp, W and Hart, AAM: Prognostic factors in canine mammary cancer. J Nat Cancer Inst 56.779, 1976.
30. Fowler, EH, et al.: Biologic behavior of canine mammary neoplasms based on a histogenetic classification. Vet Pathol 11:212, 1974.
31. Bostock, DE: The prognosis following the surgical excision of canine mammary neoplasms. Eur J Cancer 11:389, 1975.
32. Else, RW and Hannant, D: Some epidemiological aspects of mammary neoplasia in the bitch. Vet Rec 104:396, 1979.
33. Theilen, G and Madewell, BR: Tumors of the mammary gland. In Theilen, G and Madewell, BR (eds.): Veterinary Cancer Medicine, 2nd ed. Philadelphia, Lea & Febiger, 1987, p 327.
34. Harvey, HJ and Gilbertson, SR: Canine mammary gland tumors. Vet Clin North Am 7:213, 1977.
35. Forbes, JF: Advanced breast cancer (and quality of life). Clin Oncol I, 917, 1982.
36. MacEwen, EG, et al.: Evaluation of effects of levamasole and surgery on canine mammary cancer. J Biol Resp Mod 4:428, 1985.
37. Matus, RE: Intensive therapeutic plasmapheresis in veterinary medicine. In Kirk, RW (ed): Current Veterinary Therapy VIII. Philadelphia, WB Saunders, 1983, p 442.
38. MacEwen, EG, et al.: Estrogen receptors in canine mammary cancer. Cancer Res 42:2255, 1982.
39. Dorn, DR, et al.: Survey of animal neoplasms in Alameda and Contra Costa Counties. Cancer morbidity in dogs and cats in Alameda County. J Natl Cancer Inst 40:307, 1968.
40. Hayes, HB, et al.: Feline mammary carcinoma. Vet Rec 108:476, 1981.
41. Hayes, AA and Mooney, S: Feline mammary tumors. Vet Clin North Am 15:513, 1985.
42. Weijer, K, et al.: Malignant mammary tumors. I. Morphology and biology: some comparisons with human and canine mammary carcinomas. J Natl Cancer Inst 49:1697, 1972.
43. MacEwen, EG, et al.: Prognostic factors for feline mammary tumors. JAVMA 185:201, 1984.
44. Jeglum, KA, et al.: Chemotherapy of advanced mammary adenocarcinoma in 14 cats. JAVMA 187:157, 1985.

103 PARTURIENT AND POST-PARTURIENT DISEASES

J. E. MOSIER

Problems arising in association with parturition and the post parturient period primarily focus on the birthing process, the uterus, the mammary glands, metabolism, and behavior. Generally the events and problems that occur in this period are similar in the dog and cat.

In both species prevention of the most common problems depends on the selection of healthy breeding animals of prime breeding age, free of parasites and adequately nourished. Most bitches and queens should gain weight during gestation, with the majority of the weight gain occurring in the latter half of the gestational period. As a guideline, post-whelping weights should not exceed normal pregestational body weight by more than five to ten per cent.[1]

Failure to gain weight during gestation supports a prediction that the puppies and kittens will be small at birth and the lactation will be less than satisfactory.

Obesity may complicate the birthing process owing to clumsiness, early fatigue, and poor muscle tone. Obese animals should undergo weight reduction before breeding. Significant weight reduction during gestation is likely to result in low-birth-weight newborn and inadequate lactation. Moving the dam to the birthing area seven to ten days before parturition will forestall the effect of stress of unfamiliar surroundings on parturition.

NORMAL PARTURITION

Knowledge of normal parturition is essential before recognition of the abnormal is possible.[2]

Normal parturition is the delivery by the bitch or queen of full-term healthy newborn without outside assistance.[2] The length of gestation in the dog and cat averages 63 days, with a usual range of 59 to 67 days. Some maintain that the more accurate estimate for cats would be 65 days with a shorter gestation in cases with large litters.[3, 4] "Normal" birth has been encountered up to 7 days before or after the average 63 days. The greater the deviation from the 63-day average, the greater the probability of abnormal parturition. The common practice of multiple matings and variable ovulation times make determination of the precise length of the gestational period difficult. Beagle females in which the preovulatory luteinizing hormone (LH) peak was determined whelped 64 to 66 days after the LH peak.[5] The date of parturition is usually estimated from the date of the first service.[6] The birthing date is likely to be 56 to 58 days after the first day of diestrus as determined from vaginal cytology.[6]

The exact mechanism for initiation of parturition is not known in the dog and cat. Cortisol and relative estrogen levels increase while progesterone decreases. Stress produced by a decreasingly adequate nutritional supply by the placenta to the fetus stimulates the fetal hypothalamic-pituitary-adrenal axis, resulting in the release of adrenocorticosteroid hormone.[7] The fetal glucocorticoids increase synthesis of estrogen by the placenta through induction of placental aromatizing enzymes.[8] The increased levels of glucocorticoids and estrogen result in the release of prostaglandins from the placenta.[9] Effects attributed to prostaglandins are regression of corpus luteum, inhibition of the production of progesterone, release of oxytocin by the maternal neurohypophysis, and enhancement of uterine contractility. Estrogen sensitizes the myometrium to oxytocin, which in turn initiates strong contractions in the progesterone-free uterus.

Approaching parturition is characterized by anxiety, restlessness, and intermittent nest-making activity. A decrease in the bitch's activity and appetite may occur up to seven days before whelping. Most queens become more vocal and seek a darkened secluded area where they can remain relatively undisturbed. Others will seek out human companionship. The rectal temperature is usually slightly depressed (.5° to 1° F; .2° to .5° C) during the final week of pregnancy. Milk may appear in the mammary glands two to three days before the first stage of parturition in the primiparous dam. In the multiparous bitch it is not uncommon for milk to appear up to seven days before delivery of the first puppy.

Stage I

The nest-building activity of the dam becomes more intense within a few hours of onset of labor, possibly in response to elevated levels of prolactin. The bitch may shiver, pant, refuse food, and sometimes vomit. The queen will become restless and anxious and make frequent trips to her box, where she may indulge in nesting behavior. A drop of 1° to 2° F (.5° to 1° C) in the rectal temperature usually occurs 10 to 24 hours before parturition.[10] Because the drop is transient, the body temperature needs to be taken at least twice daily in order to assure detection.[11] The prepartum hypothermia is thought to represent a transient failure in the temperature compensatory mechanisms during the rapid withdrawal of the hyperthermic effects of progesterone.[5] Sometimes a light green mucoid discharge is noted 24 to 48 hours before onset of labor.[6] Dilation of the cervix and vaginal relaxation occur during stage I. Relaxin, a hormone produced by either the placenta or the ovary, causes relaxation of the pelvic ligaments and the genital tract.[9] The first stage may last from 1 to 36 hours, averaging 6 to 12 hours. Intermittent uterine contractions at approximately 15-minute intervals occur without visible abdominal muscle contraction.[2] The dam may glance occasionally at her flank area. The queen may lick the mammary and perineal areas with particular vigor. Both the bitch and queen generally appear uncomfortable. Active contractions of the uterine muscle become more intense and occur with increasing frequency. Near the end of the first stage the fetus rotates on the long axis.[12] The head, neck, and limbs are extended one to two hours before stage II. The allantochorionic membrane appears in the vagina near the end of stage I. Rupture of the membrane results in some fluid discharge. Shortly after the rupture of the allantochorionic membrane the amniotic sac passes through the vagina and protrudes as a water bag between the lips of the vulva. The engagement of the fetus within the birth canal initiates stage II of parturition.[6]

Stage II

The second stage of parturition is the period of propulsive labor. The length of the second stage depends on the number of young and on the health and vigor of the dam. Generally the dam will lie on her side, although it is commonplace for her to either squat or intermittently stand and strain. Both the bitch and queen will occasionally deliver in the standing position. It is during stage II that the abdominal muscles are brought into play. Most dams will deliver the first pup or kitten within 10 to 30 minutes of onset of the second stage of parturition.[8]

Sensory receptors within the cervix and vagina are stimulated by the pressure from fluid-filled fetal membranes and fetus. Distention of the cervix and vagina leads to a feedback stimulus of the hypothalamus and subsequent release of oxytocin. Afferent stimulation by way of a spinal arc results in stimulation of abdominal muscle contractions.[11] Two to five vigorous straining efforts will propel the fetus through the pelvis in an average parturition.[2] In primiparous dams the lips of the vulva may be insufficiently relaxed to permit unencumbered passage of the first newborn. There may be a sharp cry of pain as the head of the puppy or kitten is forced through the lips of the vulva.[2] The sensation of pain can temporarily inhibit straining. An episiotomy should be performed if simple manipulation proves ineffective.

The delivered pup or kitten may be enclosed within the amniotic membrane. Normally the dam will first remove the membrane and then proceed to thoroughly cleanse the newborn, herself, and the birthing area. It is not uncommon for a queen to cleanse herself before attending to the newborn kitten. Licking appears to stimulate both the circulation and respiration of the newborn. The umbilical cord is usually severed by the dam, and one or more placentas may be ingested. Some bitches will continue to nibble at the umbilical cord until it is quite short and may inadvertently cause accidental evisceration. Puppies are normally suckling within a few minutes of their birth. Most kittens will begin to suckle within an hour or two after delivery of the last fetus,[13] although suckling activity has been noted between deliveries, especially if the parturition time is extended. Suckling should be encouraged as a stimulus for the release of oxytocin, and thus may assist in further deliveries.

Stage III

The third stage of parturition consists of delivery of the placenta, a variable period of uterine rest, and partial segmental involution of the uterus after delivery of a neonate. The placenta may accompany the newborn or be passed within a few minutes of the birth. Sometimes two placentas will be expelled simultaneously after delivery of two puppies or kittens. Kittens may have entangled umbilical cords that must be severed to free the kittens from one another.[14] In any event, the placenta normally will have passed within 45 minutes after the birth of a newborn.

The number of cycles of second and third stages depends on the number of puppies or kittens in the uterus. The length of parturition varies, depending on the breed, the individual animal, and the environment. Time frames are useful guides but must be tempered by careful observation. Examination is recommended for any dam that has initiated and maintained intermittent labor contractions (Stage II) for more than two hours without delivery of a fetus, a dam undergoing concentrated persistent labor for 30 minutes without expulsion of a puppy or kitten, or any dam that has had marginal nonproductive straining for one to one and a half hours after delivery of a prior fetus or the appearance of a water bag. Parturient dams who are resting comfortably, caring for those of the litter already born, are not in trouble but are in a resting phase. The rest period may vary from 10 minutes to 24 hours. In most circumstances a lag of more than four hours is worrisome.[8] Small amounts of warm water or milk should be offered during the resting phase when the parturition period is extended. Gathering the newborn in front of the dam during actual labor will permit greater freedom for the dam in positioning herself for delivery and care of the newest born. Although parturition is usually completed within six hours, delivery of the entire litter can extend to 24 hours without complication.[5]

ABNORMAL PARTURITION

The term abnormal parturition applies to parturition that occurs outside the normal time frame for delivery, a gestational period that is either too long or too short, or a parturition that increases the probability of death of either the newborn or the dam.

Signs that suggest abnormal parturition are dysmaturity of the newborn; abundant green to black, bloody, or abnormal quantities of discharge; unusual odor; ineffective labor; disruption of labor; early or delayed onset of labor; depression and/or fatigue; excessive pain; and stillbirth.

A complete physical examination should be performed. The size and tone of the uterus, the relative number of fetuses, and fetal viability and location may be assessed by abdominal palpation, and the pelvic canal explored by rectal examination.

The perineum should be clipped and washed with antiseptic soap before proceeding with a vaginal examination. Sterile surgical gloves should be worn during vaginal exploration and manipulation.

Radiography will reveal the number, size, location, and viability of the fetuses. Fetal death is confirmed if (1) there is evidence of spinal collapse and maceration, (2) there are intrafetal gas patterns, or (3) overlapping or misalignment of the bones of the skull is noted.[7]

The cause of a specific abnormal parturition may be multifaceted, and the astute clinician will consider the various possibilities before initiating therapy.

Early Onset of Labor. Although the average gestational period is considered to be 63 days from the first breeding, many dogs and cats will have their young before the 63rd day. Parturition at or soon after 56 days of gestation may be normal for an individual female with a particular mating; however, the newborn are likely to be of low birth weight and physiologically immature. In the event of early parturition inquiry should be made relative to previous gestations of the bitch as well as the length of gestations of the dam's mother. Certain males seem to be associated with early parturition. Bitches who experience two or more instances of early onset of labor should be carefully scrutinized for special attributes before further breeding. Parturition before 56 days is definitely abnormal and should be considered abortions.

Delayed Parturition (Prolonged Gestation). Although parturition as late as the 70th day of gestation has resulted in normal delivery of the young, it is appropriate to consider any gestation that extends beyond 67 days from the first breeding or more than 60 days from the beginning of diestrus as abnormal. When the dam is normal insofar as can be determined by clinical examination, her behavior consistent with late gestation, and the owner a careful observer, there is no harm to the puppies from the delay in parturition. Repeated breedings and the inability to determine precise ovulation time make determination of the day of conception difficult; thus most late deliveries may not be delayed as long as the owner might have calculated. Delayed parturition can be associated with dams bred in late middle age or older, with one or two fetuses in a dam that would normally have a litter of four or more, or with in utero death of the fetuses. There is evidence that bitches can actively postpone the delivery of pups for as long as 24 hours when stressed.[5] Other factors that have been incriminated are the injection of exogenous progestogen, hypothyroidism, and delayed involution of the corpora lutea. Rats fed low-zinc diets during pregnancy experienced both delayed and prolonged parturition.[14] Fetuses with defective or abnormal heads may contribute to a prolonged gestational period.[11] Slow initiation of labor owing to subclinical hypocalcemia may be interpreted as delayed parturition. Subclinical hypocalcemia is suspect when the cervix is dilated and stimulation of the Ferguson reflex results in a weak straining action. Immediate response to intravenous calcium would confirm a tentative diagnosis of hypocalcemia.

Prolonged Parturition. The length of the parturition period depends on a variety of factors, including age of dam, number of young, muscle tone, and metabolic rate. Prolonged parturition has been associated with zinc-deficient diets in humans and rats.[14] Personal observation would suggest that an abnormal calcium-zinc ratio (i.e., high calcium, low zinc) has a similar effect in bitches. Obesity may contribute to prolonged parturition because of early fatigue and poor muscle tone. Subclinical hypoglycemia may also significantly prolong parturition.

Live offspring have been delivered 36 hours after earlier delivery. Survival of the fetus in utero depends on the intact placental attachment and adequate oxygen supply. Generally if the dam has delivered one or more newborns and then fails to deliver others present in the uterus within the next one to two hours, she should be examined by the attending veterinarian.[15] From a management view, one might recommend a short walk on the leash for bitches, offering warm milk to the bitch or queen, allowing those already born to nurse for five to ten minutes and then removing them, feathering the vagina, or the administration of calcium and oxytocin. Some dams become very anxious if separated from their owners, whereas others will not settle down in the presence of their owners. Nervous dams may require tranquilization. A promazine-derivative tranquilizer may remove neurogenic inhibition of stage II labor without harming the fetuses.[1, 7, 9] In certain queens a physiologic interruption of the parturition may, for unknown reasons, occur after the birth of the first kitten and can last for 10 to 24 hours. Labor ceases, and the queen rests, lactates, and acts as if the parturition were complete.[16] Completion of parturition may take up to 24 hours in the cat.[17] Bitches exposed to prolonged disturbances cease to labor and appear variously aggressive, agitated, and apprehensive.[10] Parturition resumes 15 minutes to one hour after disturbances are discontinued.[10] Single disturbances result in a delay in the next expected episode of labor or an episode of ineffective labor.[10] Repeated disturbances cause delays of up to six hours. Prolonged vigorous grooming of puppies may be associated with strong but ineffective labor.[10]

Newborns removed from the dam during parturition should be returned to the dam for a suckling period every two hours.

Dystocia

Dystocia is defined as difficult birth or the inability to expel the conceptus from the uterus through the birth canal.[8] Dystocia may be broadly classified as fetal or maternal.[7] Fetal dystocia is due to the shape, size, viability, or position of the fetus. Maternal dystocia can be subdivided into anatomic, endocrine, and psychologic (behavioral) causes.[1] A practical anatomic categorization of dystocia associates dystocia with the uterus, pelvis, fetus, or vaginal vault.[8] Dystocia in the cat is usually associated with uterine inertia secondary to obesity, poor muscle tone, or old age.[18]

The diagnosis of dystocia is based on history, results of a physical examination, and direct observation of the dam in labor. The history should include information relative to previous whelpings; breeding dates; behavior during gestation, with particular focus on the 24 hours immediately preceding the examination; time of onset of labor; the frequency and intensity of labor; the condition and progress of newborn previously delivered in this parturition; and the time intervals between deliveries.

Diagnoses to be ruled out must include uterine inertia, hypoglycemia, and hypocalcemia. Palpation of the abdomen will permit assessment of the uterine tone, relative distention of the abdomen, and location and movement of the fetus(es), especially the most caudal fetus, and may yield information as to the presentation and position. Vaginal examination must be an aseptic procedure. The hair of the perineum should be clipped in long-haired dogs, which should be followed by thorough disinfection of the perineum and vulva. A distended bladder should be emptied and feces removed from the rectum by enema. The degree of relaxation of the vulva and pelvic ligaments should be assessed. The vulva in the primiparous dam may be small, resulting in some physical restriction. Digital examination of the vagina of the bitch may reveal a persistent müllerian duct, contracture of the vagina, or abnormalities of the pelvis resulting from previous injury or a congenital deformity. The diameter of the pelvis of some dogs may be flattened dorsoventrally (e.g., Scottish terriers and Sealyhams).[1] English bulldogs seem more prone to dystocia owing to slackness of the abdominal wall and the angle of the approach to the pelvic inlet.

Maternal dystocia can result from anatomic obstructions, such as failure of the vulva to adequately dilate, flattened or narrow pelvic inlet, incomplete dilation of the cervix, or functional failure (e.g., uterine inertia, uterine torsion, or entrapment). Fibrosis of the cervix has been reported to prevent adequate cervical dilatation. Maternal dystocia may occur in any breed but is more common in breeds with large heads and wide shoulders (e.g., Scottish terriers, Boston terriers, English bulldogs, Sealyham terriers, and Pekingese).[1] Uterine torsion is uncommon but has been reported in both dogs and cats. Usually only one horn of the uterus is involved, and it may be twisted 90 to 360 degrees on its long axis.[11, 19] Hernias, such as inguinal hernias, may entrap a fetus or an entire uterine horn.[8]

When the cervix is dilated and the fetus presented at the pelvic inlet, digital examination may determine the presence of fetal oversize, fetal abnormality, or malpresentation. Fetal oversize is most common in association with small litters, the firstborn of a given litter, or prolonged gestation.[1] Relative fetal oversize may occur when there is a smaller than normal birth canal. Clinical assessment will establish the need for cesarean delivery or the probable risk to the newborn delivered with assistance.

Dystocia of fetal origin may occur as a result of fetal abnormalities (e.g., fetal edema, deformity, hydrocephalus, chondrodystrophy, oversize, or abnormal presentation, position, or posture).[2] Relative oversize of the head is common in brachycephalic breeds.[20] Fetal death can cause maternal dystocia owing to secondary influence on uterine contractions. Inadequate fetal fluid associated with a dead fetus makes passage through the birth canal difficult.[7] The orientation of a fetus as it enters the pelvic canal can be described in terms of the presentation, position, and posture.[7] Presentation reflects the relation of the longitudinal axis of the fetus to that of the mother, and may be cranial (anterior), caudal (posterior), or transverse.[6, 21, 71] Basically the cranial presentation is considered normal; however, caudal presentation occurs in approximately 40 per cent of deliveries and should be considered a normal variant.[6, 7] Position refers to the surface of the uterus to which the fetal vertebral column is applied (i.e., dorsal, ventral, right lateral, left lateral, or oblique). Posture involves the relation between the puppy's extremities and head and its body. Both flexed and extended postures have been described as normal.[7] The presentation, position, and posture of the fetus may be determined by abdominal palpation, digital palpation by way of the vagina, or ultrasonic imagery, or radiographically.

A variety of postures in ventral or lateral position are encountered in dystocia. Breech birth involves a caudal presentation with a coxofemoral flexed posture. The most common fetal position and posture that cause dystocia are the cranial presentation/ventral position and the breast-head posture.[2] Lateral deviation of the head is considered an abnormal posture.[6, 17, 20] Methods used to correct malposition or abnormal posture include repulsion, digital manipulation, and use of instruments.

Uterine inertia is discussed in Chapter 100.

Occasionally caudal presentation of the first fetus may delay dilatation of the cervix and be confused with inertia. The wedge effect of the nose and head is thought to assist in cervical dilatation. Death of the fetuses may result in failure of the sequence of events of parturition, and thus be perceived as dystocia.

Fatigue of the uterine muscle may result in segmental contraction or retraction rings (Bandl's rings).[21] The muscular rings lightly contract around or caudal to the fetus, and thus impede movement of the fetus toward the birth canal.

Oxytocin, calcium, and glucose may be used to convert the weak, irregular contractions of the uterus to regular and forceful contractions. The administration of meperidine hydrochloride, intravenous calcium, and glucose 30 minutes before the administration of oxytocin may be beneficial when Bandl's rings are suspect.

Failure of drugs to produce desired results or when the results of the examination preclude their use forces reliance on either surgery or manipulation to solve the existing dystocia.

Retention of one or more placentas may occur in association with mild uterine inertia, especially in the bitch. When the inertia is due to exhaustion the membranes usually pass within the next 12 hours.[2, 22] The presence of a black or dark green copious discharge is indicative of retained placentas. Retained placenta is seldom a problem in the cat.

The management of dystocia depends on the physical condition of the dam, the number of fetuses involved, the cause of the dystocia, available facilities and/or personnel, the owner's desires, and the judgment of the attending veterinarian.[23]

The options range from the use of oxytocin to delivery by cesarean section. Each option may be exercised with variable success, depending, to some extent, on the experience and judgment of the clinician.

Oxytocin is the traditional initial drug of choice in stimulating uterine contractions.[8] Before the administration of oxytocin the clinician should ascertain (1) position and presentation of the most caudal fetus, (2) the lack of pelvic, vaginal, and vulvar abnormalities, (3) the degree of cervical dilatation, and (4) fetal size relative to the pelvic dimensions. Oxytocin is useful in reinforcing weak uterine contractions, provided the cervix is open and the uterine muscle is not under tension.[24]

Weak, ineffective labor and primary uterine inertia may respond to the administration of oxytocin, provided contraindications are not detected on physical examination. Obstructive dystocia, mouth breathing on the part of the dam, evidence of prolonged uterine muscle fatigue, or a vigorous, actively contracting uterus all preclude the use of oxytocin. The uterine tone and vigor of contraction should be checked by abdominal palpation, noting the length and frequency of the contraction episodes. Intravenous injections of calcium and/or glucose may be helpful in the event of abbreviated or infrequent episodes of labor or of ineffectual contractions in the absence of mechanical obstruction.

Problems associated with the use of oxytocin result from excessive dose, too-frequent administration, and administration in conjunction with an already vigorously contracting uterine muscle. Oxytocin under these circumstances may produce contraction of the cervix, uterine tetany, and prolonged compression of the placental vasculature, and may result in death.

The dose of oxytocin ranges from 5 to 20 units for the dog and 3 to 5 units for the cat. It is given subcutaneously or intramuscularly. The effect of a single dose will last for approximately 15 minutes. When indicated, the dose may be repeated at 20- to 30-minute intervals. If no response is seen to the initial dose and a second dose is contemplated, intravenous calcium gluconate or lactate should precede the second dose.

Oxytocin should not be used for the sole purpose of accelerating the labor process.[25] Oxytocin is particularly recommended in cases of weak labor or uterine bleeding, or after correction of a uterine prolapse and cesarean section.

Feathering of the vagina is especially useful after correction of the position or posture of the presenting fetus. The feathering process consists of using the forefinger to stretch the vaginal wall in a dorsolateral direction. Receptors (Ferguson's reflex) are activated that result in an episode of labor of variable intensity, depending on the degree of maternal fatigue.

On occasion manipulation of the caudal fetus can be achieved through the abdominal wall, especially in small breeds or thin animals. Success of such manipulation is more likely when the fetus is in anterior presentation. The clinician, positioned behind the patient, should place one hand on either side of the abdomen and with the fingers engage the posterior aspect of the occiput of the fetus. The nose and head may be directed into the birth canal and delivery thus assisted. The application of a sling to the abdominal wall may be helpful when inappropriate slackness of the abdominal wall is noted.

Manipulation by way of the vagina should be preceded by adequate preparation of the perineum. Usually the long hair would be removed in anticipation of the whelping. If it is not, it should be removed with clippers or scissors to prevent entanglement and contamination. The perineum and vulva are thoroughly cleansed, and sterile gloves and adequate lubrication are used. The bitch is best restrained on the table in a standing position.[26] Manipulation of the fetus by way of the vagina is most rewarding when an abnormal posture and/or position of the fetus can be successfully righted, or when the finger can be used as a hook and the delivery assisted by traction on the fetus. It is helpful to place the other hand on the dam's abdomen and to stabilize the fetus' position by external abdominal pressure.

Sometimes assistance to delivery of a fetus stalled in the birth canal can be achieved by grasping the puppy's or kitten's feet. This is especially true with caudal presentation and when the feet are at the vulvar opening. Covering the feet with thin gauze will help to avoid slipping of the grasp. In the event of an anterior presentation, traction of the head must be applied with caution. Traction should be applied in concert with straining on the part of the dam, to reduce the possibility of excessive traction causing injury to the neck of the fetus with subsequent hemorrhage, disarticulation, and death.

Sometimes traction can be applied by placing the fingers on the skin overlaying the vaginal wall and grasping the head or pelvis of the fetus through the wall of the vagina. Occasionally mild digital pressure through the rectum may be helpful.

A variety of forceps and obstetric hooks can be used to assist delivery. The relative small size of the queen restricts their probable utilization in cat dystocia.

The need for forceps in delivery of more than one fetus of the litter should cause consideration of the advantages of a cesarean section to the survival and benefit of the bitch and the remainder of the litter. Forceps delivery is particularly indicated when the presenting fetus is dead or slightly oversize and unassisted delivery of the remainder of the litter is anticipated if the presenting fetus is removed, or when the fetus is the last member of the immediate parturition. Forceps can be used with greater vigor when survival of the fetus is not a high priority.

The types of forceps most commonly used are clam shell and sponge forceps. Rampley sponge-holding forceps are especially useful because the sharp angle just distal to the rachet decreases the width of the instrument along its shank when in an open position. Forceps should not be used if the fetus is beyond reach of the fingertip because of the danger of lacerating the uterine wall or the birth canal. Gentle application is essential if the fetus is to survive.

The forceps are inserted in a closed position until contact is made with the fetus. At that point the forceps are sufficiently opened to grasp the head or pelvis, and advanced alongside the fetal head/pelvis until the desired depth of penetration is achieved. Gentle pressure is then applied, and the index finger is inserted along the forceps to determine that neither the uterine nor vaginal wall has been included in the forceps grip. A twisting motion will help to determine whether or not the forceps have engaged the vaginal or uterine wall.

The fetus is lifted or pulled into the birth canal by traction. The forceps may then be used to draw the fetus through the birth canal, provided there is adequate space to maintain the forceps' grasp without harmful pressure on the fetus. Traction should be gently shifted from right to left, or the fetus slightly rotated to facilitate passage through the birth canal. When the head/pelvis is through the vulva, delivery can be completed by use of the fingers. It is important to apply traction in a horizontal plane until the head or buttocks are delivered and then to direct traction ventrally at a 45-degree angle until delivery is complete.[1] Traction should be applied in concert with active contractions on the part of the bitch.

A hook with a short sharp point is useful in some deliveries. It is especially useful when the nose or lower jaw catches on the brim of the pelvis. The hook may be inserted into the intermandibular space of the fetus and judicious tension applied as the dam labors. Blunt hooks are useful to move the fetus to a more favorable position for delivery or to manipulate retained legs or deviated heads. An ovariectomy hook fixed into the soft area between the mandibles, forming, with a finger in the mouth of the fetus, pincers on the mandibular symphysis, may be used to apply traction.

Sterile lubricating gel is essential in most dystocias. Lack of lubrication results in excessive trauma to the birth canal with subsequent swelling and reduction in diameter of the canal. Loss of fetal fluids may result in a dry vagina and friction between the vaginal wall and the fetal hair. The gel should be forced around the body of a fetus before proceeding with traction.

Occasionally the vulva fails to sufficiently relax to permit passage of the first fetus. In such instances an episiotomy will greatly facilitate delivery. Episiotomy should be preceded by attempts to manage the problem without surgery. Management techniques include the liberal use of lubricant, tranquilization, and digital ma-

nipulation to lift the vulvar lips over the protruding head of the presenting fetus. The decision to proceed with a cesarean delivery is based on the judgment of the attending clinician and the acquiescence of the owner. Cesarean deliveries may be preplanned for bitches with a previous dystocia, those prone to dystocia, or those with pelvic abnormalities.

Throughout dystocia the dam should be constantly evaluated for shock, toxicity, and/or fatigue. Parenteral fluids, analgesics, gentle handling of the tissues and of the whole animal, cleanliness, and judicious use of oral feeding are useful in maintaining the expectant but troubled dam in a strong vital state.

DISEASES THAT INVOLVE THE UTERUS

Refer to Chapter 100 on Uterine Diseases.

METABOLIC PROBLEMS

Puerperal Tetany

Puerperal tetany is essentially a hypocalcemic tetany associated with pregnancy in the bitch or queen.[27] The condition may occur as early as 20 days prepartum and as late as 45 postpartum, but is most commonly associated with lactation in bitches or queens one to four weeks after parturition.[8, 28, 29] Small, hyperexcitable breeds of dogs and cats with large litters appear to have the highest frequency.[29] Puerperal tetany rarely occurs in the bitch or queen that is fed a nutritious, well-balanced diet. Serum calcium levels of affected animals generally range from 6 to 7 mg/dl. In one study, 17 of 19 dogs with eclampsia were found to be hypocalcemic (averaging 6.16 mg/dl).[28] The severity of the clinical signs is related to the degree of hypocalcemia. Signs of tetany occur if the serum calcium drops below 8 mg/dl, and at 6 to 7 mg/dl the signs become more severe.[30]

Depletion of serum calcium and often hypophosphatemia develop near the peak of lactation, probably because of an imbalance between inflow and outflow of calcium in the extracellular pool.[31] The available calcium reserve depends on dietary intake, the influence of vitamin D in storage of calcium, and mobilization of calcium by parathyroid hormone to meet emergency needs.[32] Hypoglycemia, acetonemia, and hypercholesterolemia have been noted in puerperal tetany.[27] Blood glucose is usually in the low-normal range or below normal as a result of the intense muscle activity associated with tetany and lack of food intake. Factors that contribute to the development of puerperal tetany include improperly balanced diets, inappropriate dietary supplementation, calcium loss associated with lactation, calcium needs for developing fetal skeletons, reduced appetite, poor calcium utilization, and the stress of lactation. An increase in protein-bound calcium and a decrease in the level of ionized calcium may result from systemic alkalosis secondary to hyperventilation associated with dystocia.[8] Early signs include rapid breathing, nervousness, anxiety, restlessness, and whimpering.[27] The interval between these initial signs and advanced tetany ranges from 15 minutes to 12 hours.[27] As the condition progresses the affected animal begins to show a staggering unsteady gait, stiffness of the legs, and hyperthermia. The inability to stand is accompanied by hyperpnea, a hard and rapid pulse, congested mucous membranes, and excessive salivation. The patient may fall forward or to one side. Affected muscles exhibit fine fibrillary twitching or contractions. Tremors followed by short intervals of relaxation become progressively more severe, leading to convulsive seizures of short duration. Paresis or paralysis is a consequence of the hypocalcemia-induced alteration of cell membrane potentials. Spontaneous repetitive firing of motor nerve fibers induces tonic or tonoclonic contractions of skeletal muscles. Nerve membranes become more permeable to ions as a result of the loss of stabilizing membrane-bound calcium and require a stimulus of lesser magnitude to depolarize. Rectal temperatures up to 108° F (42° C) are associated with the increased muscle activity. Both myosis and mydriasis have been reported.[8, 33] Before death the animal appears to be in shock, the mucosae are pale and dry, the pupils are dilated, and the temperature is subnormal.[33] Death may result from severe respiratory depression, hyperthermia, and associated cerebral edema.[8] The diagnosis of puerperal tetany is based on history, clinical signs, laboratory findings, and response to therapy.[31]

Treatment is generally instituted by the intravenous administration of 10 per cent calcium gluconate (2 to 15 ml). The injection should be given slowly, since emesis is likely to occur following rapid injection. During injection the heart should be monitored for ventricular fibrillation and potential cardiac arrest. If cardiac irregularities occur, calcium administration should be stopped until the heart rate and rhythm return to normal. Intravenous sodium pentobarbital or diazepam should be considered when the administration of calcium and glucose fail to control the neurologic signs.[6] Hyperthermia will normally disappear as the tetany is controlled. Response to treatment is usually rapid and complete. Occasionally bitches with severe hyperthermia will be helped with an ice or alcohol bath.[8] Many veterinarians advise a subcutaneous or intramuscular injection of calcium or calcium orally following up the initial recovery. The dose ranges from one-fourth to one-half of the initial intravenous dose. Hypoglycemia and alkalosis are occasional complicating metabolic problems. Animals that fail to respond well to calcium may have coexisting hypoglycemia. An intravenous dose of approximately 10 ml of 20 per cent solution of dextrose should result in immediate improvement. Alkalosis is most likely to develop during the late stages of lactational tetany, after the animal has been hyperventilating for some time.[33] The respiratory alkalosis, associated with hyperventilation, may result in a blood pH of 7.45 or above, alkaline urine, and a decrease in ionized calcium in the blood. Treatment consists of slow intravenous administration of physiological saline.[33]

Calcium supplementation should be prescribed after initial therapy. Calcium carbonate or calcium gluconate, 500 mg/20 pounds three times a day, or dicalcium phosphate, 500 mg/7 pounds three times a day, should be combined with a review of the diet to assure appropriate mineral balance. The review should focus on the levels of calcium, phosphorus, protein, and fat plus the feed ingredients.

Supplemental dietary calcium and vitamin D plus corticosteroids in certain cases have been useful in preventing relapses in lactating bitches with puerperal tetany.[27, 29] The recommended dose of prednisolone is 0.1 mg/lb of body weight daily for the remainder of the lactation period. The beneficial effect of prednisolone may lie with its effect on release of calcium from bone, preventing deposition of calcium in bone, or its effect on stress of lactation.[34] Prednisolone would be particularly indicated when hypoglycemia, hypercholesterolemia, hypoadrenalemia, or ketonemia is associated with eclampsia.[35] The character of the vaginal discharge and general well-being of the bitch should be carefully monitored to avoid overlooking metritis and/or toxemia. The effect of corticosteroids on calcium metabolism in dogs with puerperal tetany has not been adequately studied.[27] (Editor's Note: Since prednisolone can reduce serum calcium levels in some situations, careful clinical observation is recommended.)

The decision to allow continued suckling depends on the age of the puppies or kittens, the feasibility of the owner caring for the litter, and the initial response of the bitch to therapy. When puerperal tetany is recognized early and treated effectively, the young can be allowed to suckle a few minutes at a time but should not be left with the dam. The suckling time can then be gradually extended.[33] Supplemental feeding of the puppies or kittens along with periodic suckling will reduce the drain on the mother. Usually three to five days are allowed to pass before the young can be left with their mother uninterrupted.[33] When the response to therapy appears delayed or the bitch or queen is in poor condition, it is appropriate to recommend hand-raising the puppies or kittens.

A history of puerperal tetany in a previous litter should command careful scrutiny of the nutritional program and dietary management. Some bitches and queens show a tendency toward hypocalcemia after all pregnancies, and although it might be due to persistent mismanagement, it is debatable whether such animals should be retained in the breeding program.[6] Three of five dogs with previous eclampsia were reported to have recurrence of the condition on subsequent parturition and lactation.[29] Adequate calcium, vitamin D, trace minerals, and a balanced diet are recommended. Bitches or queens with a history of puerperal tetany should be given supplemental calcium throughout lactation. Avoiding excessive amounts of calcium during gestation may help to prepare the calcium homeostatic mechanism to meet the markedly increased demands for calcium and phosphorus imposed by lactation.[31]

Hypoglycemia

The requirement for available carbohydrates in the diet is enhanced in pregnancy in the canine. Bitches maintained on carbohydrate-deficient diets during pregnancy became hypoglycemic during the last two weeks of gestation and had a sevenfold increase in dead puppies at birth and an abnormally high incidence of mortality among puppies during the first three days postpartum.[36]

Hypoglycemia accompanied by ketonemia and ketonuria has been reported but is seldom observed.[37] The condition occurs during the advanced stages of pregnancy. Decreased activity and reduced food intake are followed by vomiting, rapid respirations, abdominal straining, and prostration. Acetone odor on the breath, along with ketonuria and serum glucose levels as low as 7 mg/dl, is diagnostic.[37] Response to intravenous glucose in normal saline solution and subsequent frequent feeding is rapid.[8] Parturition or cesarean delivery alleviates the problem.

Sometimes hypoglycemia exists concurrently with hypocalcemia, and may contribute to uterine inertia and failure of puerperal tetany to respond to calcium therapy. The similarity of presenting signs of a patient with hypoglycemia to those of one with hypocalcemia may lead to misdiagnosis.[38] It has been hypothesized that hypoglycemia may result from the intense muscle activity associated with tetany and lack of food intake.[6]

Prevention depends on adequate nutrition. The most likely cause is failure to eat. Carbohydrate-deficient diets should be avoided, especially in the last two or three weeks of gestation. Exercise is recommended; however, its true value is unknown.

PROBLEMS OF LACTATION

The preparation for lactation begins before breeding. Both milk quality and quantity can be enhanced by genetic selection. The overall health and body condition must be considered in concert with a well-managed breeding program. Energy intake, protein quality, and vitamin B complex are important contributors to the secretion of adequate milk.

A high-protein, high-calorie diet is recommended during the lactation period. Caloric intake should increase slowly, starting with the fifth or sixth week of gestation and reaching a 20 to 40 per cent increase in food intake over prebreeding maintenance levels at the end of gestation. After parturition and a litter of four to five offspring the caloric intake will increase about 25 per cent per week until the peak of lactation is reached three to four weeks after birthing. The percentage of increase will vary, depending on litter size and the activity of the lactating female.

A low caloric density in the food adversely affects milk production, puppy and kitten health, and the maintenance of optimum condition of the bitch or queen.

Among the more common problems of lactation that adversely affect the bitch are agalactia, inadequate milk, mammary congestion, and mastitis.

Agalactia

Agalactia, or lack of milk after parturition, may be due to a failure of milk let-down or milk production.[21] True agalactia, failure of milk production, is uncommon. A lack of mammary development before whelping is the first indication of agalactia. The cause may be complex, involving environmental factors, hormone deficiencies, or defective secretory tissue in the mammary glands.

Suckling stimulates sensory nerve endings in the teat and serves as a stimulus to milk let-down and milk production. Anesthetics and tranquilizers may alter this response and result in temporary agalactia.

Treatment is generally ineffective when mammary gland development is lacking. Certain bitches and queens are extremely nervous and refuse to settle down sufficiently to care for the puppies or kittens. The oral administration of acepromazine has a quieting effect, and subsequent suckling by the puppies or kittens will enhance milk flow. A daily dose of 2 IU of prolactin is sufficient for maintenance of lactation in the bitch.[39]

Failure of milk let-down is more likely to respond to treatment. The mammary glands are usually swollen and firm, but milk is absent in the teat canal. The bitch or queen appears unresponsive to the needs of her young. Failure of milk let-down may occur as a consequence of excessive secretion of epinephrine, resulting from fright or pain.[21] The effect of epinephrine has been variously attributed to blocking of the release of oxytocin from the pituitary gland or to vasoconstriction and reduced supply of blood and oxytocin in the mammary tissue.[24] The administration of oxytocin causes the myoepithelial cells to contract and forces milk from the alveoli and small alveolar ducts into the milk cistern and teat canal.[40] Oxytocin may be administered intramuscularly, intravenously, subcutaneously, or in the form of a nasal spray.[33] Repeated injection or application may be necessary during the first one or two days. The nasal spray is particularly useful when prescribing for use by the owner in follow-up treatment.[41] Once milk flow has been established, administration of oxytocin can be stopped. Other causes of agalactia are premature parturition, physical exhaustion, shock, mastitis, metritis, systemic infection, and endocrine imbalance.[41] Treatment of the underlying condition and continued suckling will result in increased milk flow.

Inadequate Lactation

Inadequate lactation relates to the quality as well as quantity of milk. The quality of milk is markedly influenced by genetics, the presence or absence of vigorous good health, the level of nutrition, and the environment.

The most common scenario involves a poorly nourished bitch, stressed by gestation and compromised by infection. Environmentally excessive heat or cold, noise, commotion, poor sanitation, rough handling, and fear all create levels of stress that adversely affect milk production.

Overcoming the problem of inadequate lactation involves immediate treatment as well as recommendations for prevention.

A thorough physical examination and nutritional review will identify problems (e.g., heart disease, kidney disease, systemic infection, parasitism, malnutrition, metritis, mastitis, enterotoxemia, fever, diarrhea) that may be involved as basic causes.

In most instances the recommendation to feed a highly digestible, high-caloric-density balanced diet will enhance both the quantity and quality of the milk. Administration of B complex vitamins, along with provision of warm, dry, clean, quiet surroundings and gentle handling, is conducive to normal lactation and mothering.

Mammary Congestion (Galactostasis)

Edema and engorgement of the mammary glands and adjacent tissues have been noted before and up to three days after parturition. The enlarged and edematous glands cause pain, discomfort, failure to let down milk, and, rarely, necrosis of the skin. The roles of prolactin, differentials in intravascular pressures, and high caloric intake have not been examined in the dog or cat. In other species, engorgement appears to be a circulatory phenomenon caused by a greater blood supply to the glands than can be accommodated by the venous system.[21]

Milk stasis is most common in heavy milking bitches on a high level of nutrition. Affected animals are uncomfortable and sometimes anorectic. Physical examination reveals grossly enlarged and firm mammary glands and teats that are sometimes difficult to grasp. When teat inversion has occurred, gentle massage of the nipple may be corrective. The glandular tissue appears engorged, the mammae are warm to the touch, and milk may drip from the involved glands.

Treatment consists of withholding food for 24 hours followed by limited feeding for three days and the administration of diuretics. Milking the glands, which are grossly distended, will give temporary relief. The judicious application of cold packs can be combined with massage to reduce the more severe congestion. Careful monitoring is indicated to avoid delayed detection of infection. Bromergocryptine, a dopamine agonist, reduces prolactin secretion in dogs.[5] Its use should be restricted to bitches who have lost their puppies, when the need for lactation no longer exists.

Mastitis

Mastitis may be either acute or chronic, depending on the history and condition of the mammae at the time of examination. Acute mastitis is most frequently noted in hot, humid weather in bitches or queens housed in questionable sanitary surroundings that have recently given birth and have significant congestion of the mammary glands.[42] Acute mastitis in queens may also develop one to two weeks after parturition, due to injury from the sharp nails of the kittens. Usually the source of infection is not found.[5]

A variety of organisms have been incriminated, with the most common being staphylococci, streptococci, and *Escherichia coli*.[43] The contributions of trauma and mammary congestion are a matter of conjecture, but they are generally thought to be involved. Metritis may be a source or a coincidental infection. Early signs include swelling and erythema of the affected gland. The gland feels warm, becomes painful, and is sometimes discolored in association with gangrene and abscessation. Anorexia, listlessness, elevated temperature, and considerable discomfort are usually noted. Dams with septic mastitis may lose interest in their puppies or kittens. Neonates are restless, cry frequently, and may appear bloated.

Affected milk shows increased viscosity and color changes of yellow, pink, or brown, depending on the amount of blood and the degree of purulent exudate present. Cytologic examination of the milk secretion shows bacteria, leukocytes, and red blood cells. A Gram stain is useful in selecting the antibiotic for initial treatment. Aseptically collected milk samples or aspirated material from the affected gland should be cultured, and antibiotic sensitivity tests performed.

Therapy using a broad-spectrum antibiotic should be instituted immediately. More specific antibiotic therapy must await the results of culture and sensitivity testing. If the infection becomes localized, the resulting abscess should be lanced and drainage established. When necrosis is evident, surgical debridement is indicated. Local infiltration of the mammary gland with penicillin or penicillin and streptomycin is sometimes useful in preventing abscess formation. Suckling of abscessed glands should be prevented by use of bandage and tape. When the milk is not frankly purulent, suckling should be encouraged in order to assure constant drainage.[8] If several glands are affected and the condition is severe, it may be appropriate to move the offspring to an incubator and treat them as orphans. Affected glands should be periodically milked out during the day if suckling is not allowed. Chloramphenicol, ampicillin, amoxicillin, penicillin/streptomycin, or kanamycin for at least five days is usually effective.

Cold packs are useful in early stages of congestion and infection, and hot packs are generally indicated once the inflammation is well established. Hot packs hasten localization and drainage and relieve swelling and pain.

There is currently no evidence to indicate that mastitis occurs with greater frequency in previously affected animals.[44] Increased incidence in individual families, within a given breed, suggests a hereditary tendency toward the disease.

Sanitation, early treatment of mammary congestion, and frequent trimming of the nails of the kittens and puppies will help to prevent mastitis.

ABNORMAL MATERNAL BEHAVIOR

Most bitches and queens have strong maternal instincts. Dams in both species are especially protective of their young for several days after birthing and leave them only briefly to defecate or urinate.[6] Maternal behavior patterns depend, to a large extent, on hormonal balance of the mother; the role of the cerebral cortex appears largely confined to assimilating and decoding information supplied by various sense organs.[44] Maternal behaviors involving nest building, nursing, and retrieving depend on genetic makeup, endocrine balance, good health, and environmental factors. Endocrine factors that affect prepartum and postpartum behavior of the bitch or queen have not been adequately determined, but they probably involve elevations in prolactin and oxytocin.[5] Prolactin appears to be responsible for much of the mother's behavior toward her young, especially as serum progesterone levels fall sharply after parturition.[45] The dam's emotional attachment to its owner may distract attention from the newborn to such an extent that even the strongest instinctive urges are overridden.[46] Dams that spend little time with their litter for at least the first two weeks of life are not good mothers.[6]

The underlying cause may be genetic, psychological, or environmental. Poor mothering behavior may be a heritable factor, and some breeds have a high percentage of bad mothering.[6] Most dams that exhibit deficient mothering have the normal instincts, which have been modified by sublimation, close attachment to a human being, or faulty management. A highly nervous human-oriented bitch may, on delivery of the puppy, "manifest blind panic amounting in some cases to actual hysteria and appears to regard her offspring with horror and disgust."[2] The condition may right itself with cessation of uterine pain or if the bitch is controlled while the puppies first suckle. The puppies should not be left unsupervised with the bitch until normal behavior of licking, retrieving, and nursing are apparent. Failure of the maternal instinct may occur in the unusually sensitive, possibly neurotic pet bitch.

Certain dams resent human intervention to such a degree that assisted-birthing and cesarean-delivered newborn are not accepted and on occasion are killed by the dam. Major disturbances during or after parturition may cause killing of newborn.[47] In the bitch, mutilation and cannibalizing activity have been ascribed to mental instability, voiceless newborn, maternal deafness, and malalignment of the teeth. Circumstances in cats that increase the probability are a litter larger than normal, second pregnancy of the season, and an abnormal newborn.[48]

The use of disinfectants with strong odors to sanitize areas for breeding or birthing can have adverse results by blocking perception of pheromones. This can lead to unnatural aggressive behavior and cannibalism of newborn. Females identify their offspring by smell as they clean them after delivery, and they may be inhibited from performing this natural function by strong odors.[46]

Excessively warm birthing areas will cause the dam to move away from the litter. Too little time in close contact with her litter is deleterious not only to the dam, but also, by means of the learning component of behavior, to the subsequent behavior of breeding animals from litters so raised.[6] Some bitches and queens fail to remove the amniotic sac, leaving their young to die of asphyxiation. Such behavior is most likely to occur in the primiparous dam. In others the pain of the first delivery may override instinctive care of the firstborn but allow normal behavior to the remainder of the litter.

Repeated episodes in certain bitches suggest a genetic fault. In other instances the bitch removes the sacs in subsequent litters, suggesting a learned behavior, lack of contributing cause, or maturity.

Quiet, familiar surroundings and the presence of a calm, empathetic, caring owner promote normal maternal behavior. Some bitches and queens prefer isolation and seclusion in a chosen birthing area protected from extraneous noise and distraction. Certainly the sequence of parturition in stage I can be altered by environment. Changing from familiar to unfamiliar or from chosen area to one selected by the owner, or exposure to environmental disturbances, results in a considerable delay in parturition.[7] The presence of strangers and even the owner may disrupt parturient and maternal behavior. Rising prolactin levels in concert with the fall in progesterone may direct the mother's behavior toward her young.[45] Maternal behavior is particularly vulnerable during the first 48 hours postpartum.

Probably the greatest stimulant to maternal behavior is the presence of young. Normal behavior in some queens depends on close contact with their neonate for the first few hours after parturition.[45]

Suckling stimulates nerve endings in the teat and mammary gland that reflexly stimulate the hypothalamus and pituitary gland.[45]

Good health strongly supports normal mothering behavior. Adequate nutrition, freedom from abnormalities arising during or immediately after whelping (e.g., metritis, toxemia, pain, abnormal lactation), clean and dry surroundings, acceptance of the birthing area, and avoidance of environmental disturbances that cause the dam to become overly anxious are all essential to quality mothering.

References

1. Donovan, EF: Dystocia. In Kirk, RW (ed): Current Therapy II. Philadelphia, WB Saunders, 1980, p 1212.
2. Freak, MJ: The whelping bitch. Vet Rec 60:295, 1948.
3. Wilkinson, GT: Diseases of the Reproductive System. Refresher Course on Cats. Proceedings No. 53–55, University of Sydney, 1980, p 39.
4. Nelson, ND and Cooper, J: The growing conceptus of the domestic cat. Growth 39:435, 1975.
5. Concannon, PW: Canine Physiology of Reproduction. In Burke, T (ed): Small animal reproduction and infertility. Philadelphia, Lea & Febiger, 1986, p 23.
6. Jones, DE and Joshua, JO: Reproductive Clinical Problems in the Dog. Boston, Wright & Sons, 1982, p 61.
7. Gaudet, DA and Kitchell, BE: Canine dystocia. Comp Cont Ed 7:406, 1985.
8. Feldman, EC and Nelson, RW: Handbook of canine and feline endocrinology and reproduction. Philadelphia, WB Saunders, 1987, p 444.
9. Bennett, D: Normal and abnormal parturition. In Morrow, DA, (ed): Current Therapy in Theriogenology. Philadelphia, WB Saunders, 1980, p 595.
10. Bleicher, N: Behavior of the bitch during parturition. JAVMA 140:1076, 1962.
11. Bennett, D: Canine dystocia—a review of the literature. J Sm Anim Pract 15:101, 1974.
12. Freak, MJ: Practitioners'-breeders' approach to canine parturition. Vet Rec 96:303, 1975.
13. Hart, BL: Feline behavior—a practitioner's monogram. Collected

from Feline Practice Journal. Santa Barbara, Calif, Veterinary Practice Publishing, 1978, p 18.

14. Bunce, GC, et al.: Efficiency of progesterone withdrawal as a factor in low zinc-induced dystocia. Proc Nutr Soc 41:18A, 1982.

15. Buckner, RG: The genital system. *In* Catcott, ED (ed): Canine Medicine, 4th ed. Santa Barbara, Calif, American Veterinary Publications, 1979, p 501.

16. Joshua, JO: Abnormal behavior in cats. *In* Fox, MW, (ed): Abnormal Behavior in Animals. Philadelphia, WB Saunders, 1968, pp 450–463.

17. Johnston, SD: Personal communication, 1984.

18. Stein, BS: Obstetrics, surgical procedures and anesthesia. *In* Morrow, DA (ed): Current Therapy in Theriogenology. Philadelphia, WB Saunders, 1980, p 865.

19. McIntire, JW and Waugh, SL: Uterine torsion in a cat. Fel Prac 11:41, 1981.

20. Arthur, GH: Wright Veterinary Obstetrics, 3rd ed. Baltimore, Williams and Wilkins, 1964, p 161.

21. Roberts, SJ: Veterinary Obstetrics and Genital Diseases. Ithaca, Author, 1971, p 231.

22. Whitehead, JE: The urogenital system. *In* Catcott, EJ (ed): Feline Medicine and Surgery. Santa Barbara, Calif, American Veterinary Publications, 1964, p 227.

23. Mosier, JE: Normal and abnormal parturition. *In* Burke, T (ed): Small Animal Reproduction and Infertility. Philadelphia, Lea & Febiger, 1986, p 335.

24. McDonald, LE: Veterinary Pharmacology and Therapeutics, 3rd ed. Ames, Iowa State University Press, 1968.

25. Ebert, J: Treatment of reproductive disorders and dystocia in female farm animals with oxytocin. A review. Deutsche Tier Wochen 83:74, 1976.

26. Schille, VM: Diagnosis and management of dystocia in the bitch and queen. *In* Bojrab, MJ (ed): Current Techniques in Small Animal Surgery. Philadelphia, Lea & Febiger, 1983, p 338.

27. Toivola, BE and Mather, GW: Puerperal tetany of the bitch. Norden News, Winter issue, 1968, p 16.

28. Austad, R and Bjerhas, E: Eclampsia in the bitch. J Sm Anim Pract 17:793, 1976.

29. Martin, SL and Capen, CC: The Endocrine System in Canine Medicine, 4th ed. Santa Barbara, American Veterinary Publication, 1979, p 1170.

30. Blakely, CL: Eclampsia or puerperal tetany in the bitch. North Am Vet 19:60, 1938.

31. Martin, SL and Capen, CC: Puerperal tetany. *In* Kirk, RW (ed): Current Veterinary Therapy VII. Philadelphia, WB Saunders, 1980, p 1027.

32. Bourne, RF: The physiology of disease. The tetanies: puerperal tetany of bitches. North Am Vet 33:167, 1952.

33. Colby, ED: Pre and post natal care of female cats. *In* Burke, T (ed): Small Animal Reproduction and Infertility. Philadelphia, Lea & Febiger, 1986, p 317.

34. Kallfelz, FA: Puerperal tetany. *In* Kirk, RW (ed): Current Veterinary Therapy III. Philadelphia, WB Saunders, 1968, p 64.

35. Donovan, EF and Martin, SL: Corticosteroid therapy. *In* Kirk, RW (ed): Current Veterinary Therapy III. Philadelphia, WB Saunders, 1968, p 51.

36. Romsos, D, et al.: Influence of a low carbohydrate diet on performance of pregnant and lactating dogs. J Nutr 111:678, 1981.

37. Jackson, RF, et al.: Hypoglycemia-ketonemia in a pregnant bitch. JAVMA 177:1123, 1980.

38. Irvine, CHG: Hypoglycemia in the bitch. NZ Vet J 12:140, 1964.

39. Christiansen, LBJ: Reproduction in the dog and cat. Bailliere Tindall 154, 1984.

40. Jacobson, NL: The mammary gland and lactation. *In* Swensen, M (ed): Dukes Physiology of Domestic Animals. Ithaca, NY, Cornell University Press, 1970, p 1365.

41. Hosek, JJ: Syntocinon: A treatment for agalactia in the dog. VM/SAC, April, 1972, p 405.

42. Mosier, JE: Pre and postnatal care of female dogs. *In* Burke, T (ed): Small Animal Reproduction and Infertility. Philadelphia, Lea & Febiger, 1986, p 327.

43. Trainor, E: Mastitis. *In* Kirk, RW (ed): Current Veterinary Therapy VIII. Philadelphia, WB Saunders, 1980, p 1214.

44. Johnson, SD and Hayden, DW: Nonneoplastic disorders of the mammary gland. *In* Kirk, RW (ed): Current Veterinary Therapy VIII. Philadelphia, WB Saunders, 1980, pp 1224–1226.

45. Howard, B: Mechanisms in maternal behavior. Proc Soc Vet Ethol 1:5, 1967.

46. Sojka, NJ: Breeding history. *In* Burke, T (ed): Small Animal Reproduction and Infertility. Philadelphia, Lea & Febiger, 1986, p 79.

47. Freak, MJ: Parturient behavior in the bitch. Proc Soc Vet Ethol 1:11–12, 1967.

48. Hart, BF and Hart, LA: Maternal behavior problems in cats. *In* Hart, BF (ed): Canine and Feline Behavioral Therapy. Philadelphia, Lea & Febiger, 1980, p 180.

DRUG INDEX

Generic	Trade	Dose	Route	Frequency	Brief Description
Furosemide	Lasix	0.5–2 mg/lb	Oral, SQ, IM, IV	SID–TID	Diuretic
Oxytocin	Pitocin	C 2–5u D 5–20u	IV, IM SQ	PRN	Ecbolic
Oxytocin	Syntocin	0.2–1 IU	Intranasal	TID–QID	Intranasal nebulization
Prolactin hormone		2 IU		SID	Lactogenic
Acetyl promazine	Acepromazine	0.25–1 mg/lb	Oral, IV, SQ, IM	SID–BID	Tranquilizer
Meperidine	Demerol	D 5 mg/lb C 1.5 mg/lb	IM IM	BID	Analgesia Sedative
Glucose	Dextrose 5%	5–10 ml/lb	IV	PRN	Nutrient
Lubricating gel	K-Y Jelly	NA	Topical	PRN	Lubricant
Diazepam	Valium	D 0.4 mg/lb C 0.5 mg/lb	IV Oral	SID	Sedative
Sodium pentobarbital	Nembutal	4–12 mg/lb	IV	PRN	Sedative anesthetic
Calcium carbonate	Tums	50 mg/lb	Oral	SID	Nutritional supplement
Calcium phosphorus	Calphosan	5–10 ml/lb	IV	SID	
Calcium gluconate (10%)		D 5–30 ml C 5–15 ml	IV IV	SID	Muscle stimulant
Ampicillin	Polyflex	5–20 mg/lb	Oral, IM, SQ	TID	Antibacterial
Amoxicillin	Amoxitabs	5 mg/lb	Oral	BID	Antibacterial
Chloramphenicol	Mychel-Vet	25 mg/lb	Oral	TID	Antibacterial
Bromergocryptine	Parlodel	10 mcg/lb	Oral	BID	Dopamine agonist; inhibits prolactin
Dicalcium phosphate		0.5 gm/7 lb	Oral	Divided dose BID	Nutritional supplement
Prednisolone		0.5 mg/5 lb	Oral	SID	
Procaine G penicillin		1–2 ml	Intramammary	One dose	Antibacterial

104 INFERTILITY

EDWARD C. FELDMAN

INFERTILITY IN THE BITCH

Developing the Problem List

HISTORY (ANAMNESIS)

Infertility or apparent infertility problems in the bitch are common. Veterinary advice will often be sought after a bitch fails to conceive, if she fails to exhibit normal breeding behavior, when her cycles appear to be unusual, or for one of many other disturbances. Infertility, therefore, is a huge category comprising a long list of anatomic, physiologic, and behavioral problems as well as a number of apparent husbandry misconceptions.

Before the bitch is examined by the veterinarian the various potential causes for infertility must be reduced to a workable number. In other words, the differential diagnosis for most infertility disorders is established by obtaining a thorough history from the owner. In order to avoid the time-consuming chore of asking all the questions that aid in establishing a problem list, differential diagnosis, and diagnostic plan, it is recommended that clients be given a list of questions to answer (Table 104–1). This list does not necessarily provide a complete background on every bitch, but it does ask the basic questions that need answers in establishing a foundation from which to work. Items can always be forgotten in reviewing a case history during a busy workday and the question sheet helps to avoid this dilemma.

Small dogs reach sexual maturity at a younger age than large dogs. Virtually all dogs, however, begin estrous cycling before 24 to 30 months of age. In addition, the first and second cycles may be irregular, unusual, short, or long. Therefore, infertility evaluations are delayed in most dogs until they are 24 to 30 months of age. Thus just knowing the age and breed helps one to decide how aggressive to be diagnostically. The small poodle may deserve evaluation earlier in life than the bull mastiff. Each breed does have distinctive average interestrous intervals. These do vary, however, and almost all breeds cycle once every 4.5 to 8 months. The African breeds cycle once yearly. The remainder of the critical factors in an infertility evaluation are described later.

PHYSICAL EXAMINATION

When evaluating a specific organ system, that area of concern should be the last to be examined. This approach assures that each bitch will receive a complete physical examination before evaluation of the reproductive tract. Examination of the reproductive tract usually begins with an external inspection of the vulva, checking the size, conformation, and presence of any discharge. The small, immature vulva or one that is recessed under a fold of tissue because of body type or obesity may present impediments to normal breeding. The obese bitch is prone to perivulvar dermatitis. A swollen, turgid vulva is suggestive of proestrus, and one that is swollen and flaccid can be consistent with standing heat or approaching parturition.

The bitch in anestrus or diestrus usually has no vaginal discharge. A bloody discharge is most suggestive of proestrus, estrus, separation of placental sites, or severe vaginitis. Greenish black or dark bloody discharges are associated with placental separation as well as postpartum lochia. Red-brown, yellowish, greyish, thick, creamy, malodorous vaginal discharges are often seen in open-cervix pyometra and, less commonly, with severe vaginitis. Straw-colored vaginal discharges are sometimes seen in estrus (standing heat). Clear mucus can precede parturition but is otherwise not worrisome.

Mammary glands should be palpated. The primary concern would be the presence of mammary tumors. The glands can also be checked for evidence of lactation, mastitis, inverted teats, or benign nodules.

A digital examination of the vaginal vault should be routinely performed. If a specimen is needed for culture or cytology, it should be obtained before the digital examination. The gloved and lubricated index finger should pass easily into the vaginal vault of a normal bitch. Digital examination allows assessment of clitoral size and shape, vaginal masses, foreign bodies, strictures, or abnormal tissue bands. If the digital examination is abnormal but inconclusive, vaginoscopy provides a more thorough evaluation. Use of an otoscope or a vaginal speculum provides an extremely limited view of the vaginal vault and is of little use in most clinical situations. A pediatric proctoscope is easy to use for vaginoscopy (Figure 104–1), is relatively inexpensive, and can be used in all but the smallest or miniature breeds. In the small breeds an otoscope may be the only method available for examining the vaginal vault.

TABLE 104–1. DATA SHEET—THE INFERTILE BITCH

A. Age _____ Breed _____

B. General Medical History (not including reproduction problems)
    1. Vaccinations current?

    2. Previous significant illnesses requiring hospitalization? If so, please summarize:
        a.

        b.

    3. Does your dog:
        a. have a vomiting problem?   yes _____ no _____
        b. have diarrhea?   yes _____ no _____
        c. drink excessively?   yes _____ no _____
        d. urinate excessively?   yes _____ no _____
        e. have normal ability to play and exercise?   yes _____ no _____
        f. appear to be of normal weight and height?   yes _____ no _____
        g. have a hair coat problem?   yes _____ no _____
        h. any other problem?   yes _____ no _____
            (If yes, please describe)
    4. Has your dog ever had thyroid tests?   yes _____ no _____
    5. Has your dog received thyroid hormone?
        a. in the past?   no _____ yes _____ dose _____
        b. now?   no _____ yes _____ dose _____
    6. Is your dog receiving *any* medication of any type?
        no _____ yes _____ drug and dose _____
    7. Has or is your dog now receiving medicine for fleas or scratching?
        no _____ yes _____ drug and dose _____
    8. Please list all foods and supplements currently being given to your dog:

C. Cycle History
    1. Is the animal cycling?   yes _____ no _____
    2. Time interval between cycles:
    3. Total number of cycles in her life?
    4. For how many days is a bloody discharge present (average in last 2 or 3 cycles)?
    5. How many days does she stand for the male (average in last 2–3 cycles)?
    6. Has a vaginal smear been checked by a veterinarian during a heat?
    7. Has a series of vaginal smears (several during 1 heat) ever been checked?
    8. Have any hormone assays been done?   no _____ yes _____
        Please describe:
    9. Has your dog received any drug to cause a cycle? (no _____ yes _____) or increase fertility? (no _____ yes _____) Please explain:

D. Breeding History
    1. Does your bitch allow the male to mount and breed?
        no _____ yes _____
    2. How often is your dog bred in a cycle?
    3. How are breeding dates chosen?
    4. Has bitch been bred to a male that has successfully sired litters within the past 6 months?
        no _____ yes _____
        1–2 years? no _____ yes _____
    5. Have you observed any ties?   no _____ yes _____
    6. Duration of ties (average)?
    7. Inside tie _____ ? Outside tie _____ ?
    8. Has the bitch been tranquilized before breeding or shipping?
        no _____ yes _____
    9. Is the bitch bred locally, or is she shipped for breeding?

Table continued on following page

TABLE 104–1. DATA SHEET—THE INFERTILE BITCH *Continued*

E. Pregnancy History
  1. Has she had any liters?
    dates: a.   litter size: a.
          b.   b.
          c.   c.
          d.   d.
  2. Any abortions?   no _____ yes _____
    If so, how do you know she aborted?
  3. Any resorption of puppies?   no _____ yes _____
    a) If so, how do you know she resorbed puppies?
    b) How was pregnancy proved?
    c) Was pregnancy examination at:
      1. 7 days _____   4. 28 days _____
      2. 14 days _____   5. 35 days _____
      3. 21 days _____   6. 45 days _____
  4. Ever treated for mismating?
  5. Has she had a *Brucella* titer?
    Date of most recent check _____
  6. Has she ever had:
    pyometra?   yes _____   no _____
    vaginitis?   yes _____   no _____
  7. Has she ever had medication to prevent or delay a heat?
    no _____   yes _____
  8. Does she now have or has she had an abnormal vaginal discharge?
F. Kennel History
  Do any other bitches in your kennel have reproductive disorders? no _____ yes _____
G. Pedigree
  Do any other bitches in this dog's lineage have reproductive disorders?
  no _____   yes _____

A rectal examination ensures that the pelvic canal has been assessed for previous fractures. Compression of the pelvic canal is a potential cause for dystocia. One can also palpate the vagina ventrally.

Brucella-Negative Bitch with Normal Cycles, with Normal Interestrous Intervals, Allowing Breeding

THE MALE

Before embarking on an investigation into the potential causes for infertility in a bitch, the male should be assessed (Figure 104–2). The primary reason for evaluating the male before the female is that the male is much easier to study. The normal male is continuously fertile (i.e., continuously producing spermatozoa). The female is usually fertile only one to three weeks a year.

The easiest and usually most reliable method of establishing male fertility is to review his previous breeding history. Any male that has sired a litter or litters within the preceding three to six months is usually assumed to be fertile. It is also helpful to know if the male specifically sired any litters at the time the bitch in question was in heat and bred.

All active stud dogs should be tested for brucellosis every six months. A less active stud should be checked yearly. A male that has not sired a litter, or that has sired litters in the past but not in the preceding 6 to 12 months, must be viewed with suspicion. Whenever a male has the potential for being infertile, the owner of the bitch has three main alternatives: (1) have a semen analysis and *Brucella* titer performed on the male, (2) use an alternate, proven sire on the next heat, or (3) evaluate the bitch, realizing that she may not be at fault.

Semen analysis is typically simple, safe, and inexpensive. A normal semen analysis is important evidence that the male is not at fault. Abnormal semen, or inability to obtain an ejaculate, leaves some suspicion directed at the male. Any normal male may have one or two abnormal semen studies, but with each abnormal study from one male, the likelihood for his infertility increases. It is also possible for a male to have sperm that appear to be morphologically normal but that may be incapable of fertilization. Sophisticated studies on sperm function are not yet widely available in small animal reproductive medical practice.

OWNER MANAGEMENT PRACTICES

Inaccurate management practices are the cause for a large majority of apparent infertility problems. A bitch that is bred at the incorrect time may be totally normal but fails to conceive as a result of being brought to the male when she is not fertile. Two major errors in breeding management are common. First, many breeders allow only one breeding per cycle. Although a single breeding was associated with excellent conception rates in beagles,[1] breeding several times per cycle does help to eliminate the chances of a poorly timed or mistimed breeding. Second, many dog owners allow breeding only on certain predetermined days of the cycle, that is, days 11 and 13 (first day of vaginal bleeding is day 1), days 10 and 12, day 12 only, or only after the bloody vaginal discharge of proestrus becomes clear or straw-colored. These protocols may work in some or even a majority of bitches, but some normal bitches fail to conceive or refuse to breed if such schedules are followed.

Because the *average* proestrus lasts for nine days and estrus for seven to nine days, predetermined management plans do succeed in the average bitch. The average

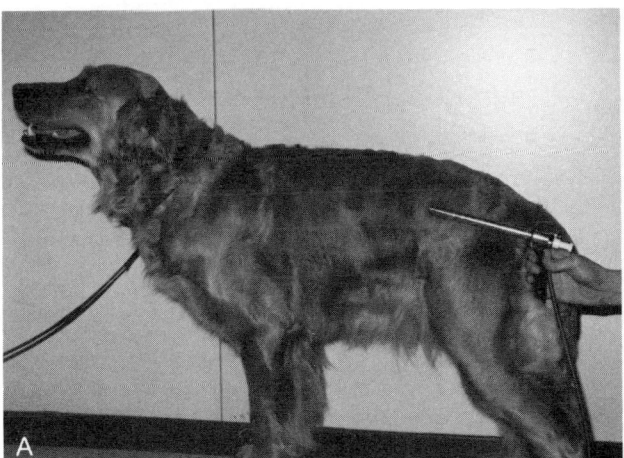
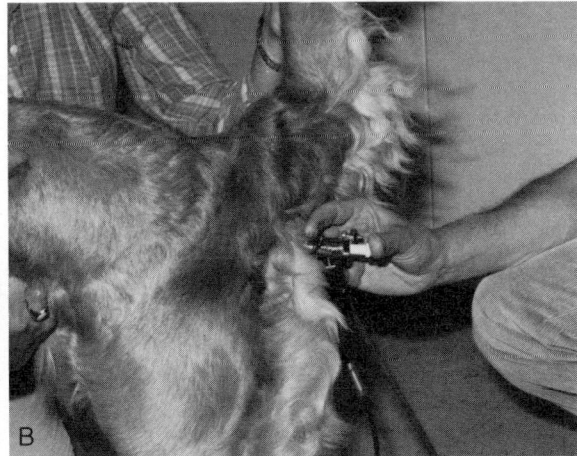

FIGURE 104–1. *A* and *B,* Vaginoscopy can be performed with a pediatric proctoscope. The instrument is easily passed into the vaginal vault for thorough inspection. The pediatric proctoscope does not always allow visualization of the cervix despite its length, illustrating the limited value of using an otoscope for this procedure. (From Feldman, EC and Nelson, RW: Canine and Feline Endocrinology and Reproduction. Philadelphia, WB Saunders, 1987, p 468.)

bitch also has a clear, straw-colored vaginal discharge when in standing heat. However, if a traditional breeding protocol is used in a bitch that fails to conceive, a new approach to management may be more successful.

The initial approach to an apparently normal bitch that fails to conceive is to recommend that the owner adopt a more reliable breeding schedule and simultaneously study follicular function and determine the approximate time of ovulation. The proposed breeding schedule is aimed at better understanding the bitch in question, realizing that in the normal bitch, proestrus can last for 1 or 2 days or as long as 25 days. Estrus (standing heat) can have a duration of 2 to 20 days. The recommendations, therefore, are to bring the bitch to a dominant male for evaluation of behavior beginning on the third or fourth day of proestrus and continue to do so every other day until *diestrus* is demonstrated by behavior or vaginal cytology. It is wise to have one person hold the male and another person attend to the bitch. The dogs are allowed to interact for 5 to 15 minutes in order to assess the response of the bitch to the stud. One is looking for evidence of standing heat. If the male is not the stud to be used in the actual breeding, the handlers must prevent mating. The handlers are also present to prevent fighting, which occasionally does occur. Once the bitch displays standing heat she should be bred on that day and every two to four days thereafter until she refuses to breed. Breeding is continued on this schedule regardless of the duration of standing heat or the interpretation of a vaginal cytology smear. This program assures that viable sperm will be present when eggs become available for fertilization. Bitches with prolonged standing heat should be bred every four days until cytologic or behavioral diestrus is confirmed.

If a bitch is bred only between days 10 and 12 of her cycle, several potential loopholes exist. If proestrus lasts for four days and estrus for six days, she will be bred in diestrus when she is likely to be no longer receptive or, if she is receptive, no longer fertile. If a bitch is in proestrus for 14 days and estrus for 10 days, ovulation is likely on day 18 and fertilization on days 20 through

24. If she was bred on days 10 and 12, few sperm would be alive when fertilization would take place (Figure 104–3). These are simple examples of the problems associated with arbitrary, predetermined breeding dates.

In addition to behavior observation, follicular function can be easily and inexpensively monitored. The owner should be taught how to obtain vaginal smears. The owner is then instructed to obtain vaginal smears beginning with day one of proestrus and continuing, on a daily basis, through to five days into behavioral or cytologic diestrus. Vaginal cytology reflects peripheral estrogen concentrations, which in turn reflects follicular function. Vaginal smears identify the approximate days of estrus and definitively identify the beginning of diestrus. One can count back six days from day one of diestrus to the most likely day of ovulation and/or count back one through four days for the time of fertilization.[1] Taking into account the approximate six-day survival time of viable sperm within the uterus after breeding, the veterinarian can determine if the breeding dates were optimal for fertilization. If they were not, the bitch needs to be managed differently to better coordinate breeding with fertilization. If the breeding dates were optimal, management problems can be excluded from the list of causes for infertility.

The question regarding ovulation needs to be answered. Does the bitch ovulate and, if so, when? Vaginal cytology, by identifying the first day of diestrus, offers an indirect method for determining an approximate ovulation date, as previously described. One can be quite precise, however, by obtaining plasma progesterone concentrations daily or on alternate days. Ovulation occurs two or three days after progesterone rises above 0.5 ng/ml. Obtaining multiple progesterone levels can become prohibitively expensive. A more reasonable approach is the daily vaginal cytology smears to identify day 1 of diestrus (Figure 104–4), coupled with a plasma progesterone concentration obtained between the 10th and 20th days of diestrus. During the initial few weeks of diestrus, the plasma progesterone should be > 3 ng/ml and usually is 10 to 50 ng/ml. Elevation into the ranges mentioned could be attained only through pro-

Clinical Approach to Infertility in

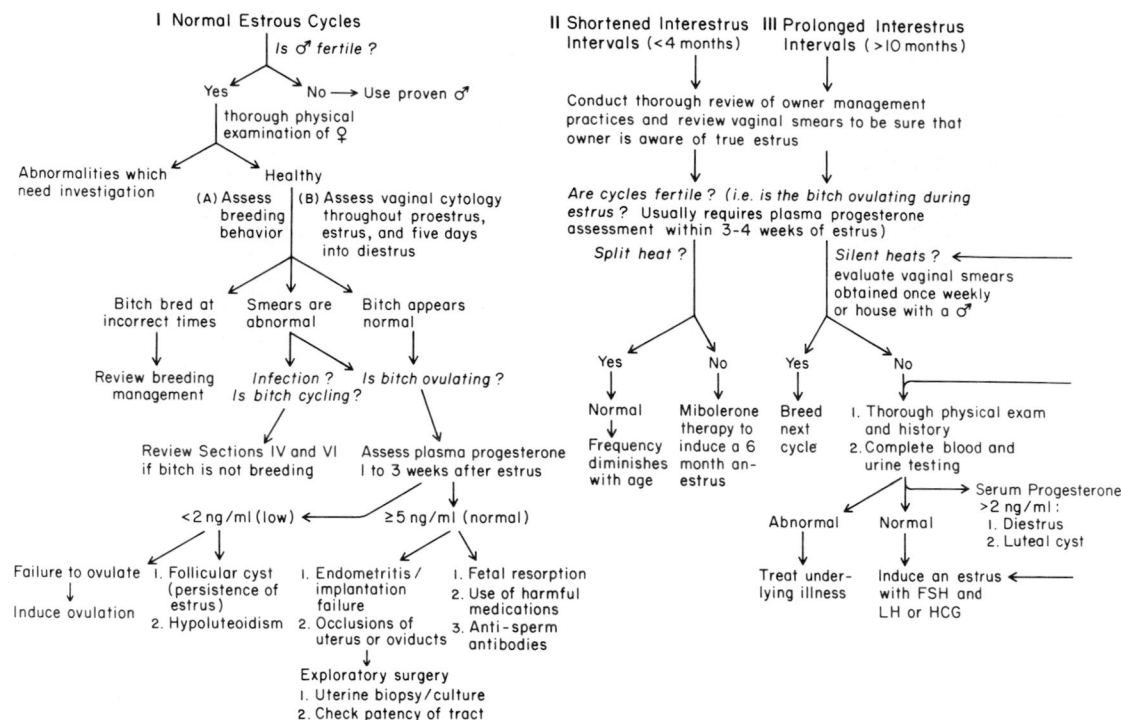

FIGURE 104–2. Step-by-step clinical approach to the diagnosis and treatment of infertility disorders in the bitch. (From Feldman, EC and Nelson, RW: Canine and Feline Endocrinology and Reproduction. Philadelphia, WB Saunders, 1987, p 458.)

gesterone secretion from functioning corpora lutea (excluding exogenous sources), which exist as a result of previous ovulation. Therefore, normal diestrual progesterone concentrations are consistent with successful ovulation and proper luteal function.

Breeding practices need to be reviewed as potential problem areas. For example, it is not known whether tranquilization or the stress of shipping has an undesirable effect on ovulation or early pregnancy. These factors may relate to acquired infertility and are worth avoiding during one cycle to see if the infertility problem is solved. If the owner never observes a breeding, secondhand information is used. Therefore, the owner should witness breedings to assure that normal breeding does occur. If "outside ties" persistently occur, an anatomic problem within the vaginal vault may prevent penetration by the male. Again, careful owner observation is helpful.

All previously or currently used medications should be noted. Previous use of gonadotrophins may have long-term deleterious effects on pituitary function. Previous progesterone or estrogen administration may result in subclinical cystic endometrial hyperplasia, with infertility being the only outward effect that would be seen by the owner or veterinarian.

In summary, management problems are the most common cause of *apparent infertility* in the bitch with a normal cycle. The entire question regarding proper management for an individual bitch can be answered through the relatively inexpensive approach of obtaining a thorough history with corrections made as needed in past practices, behavior observation, vaginal cytology

review, and monitoring the diestrual plasma progesterone concentrations. This approach answers the following questions: (1) how is this owner managing this bitch? (2) when does standing heat begin? (3) how long does standing heat persist? (4) what is the first day of true diestrus? (5) when is the bitch truly fertile? (6) what are her ideal breeding dates? (7) does she ovulate? (8) when does she ovulate? (9) does she have the luteal function necessary to support pregnancy?

GENERAL HEALTH OF THE BITCH

In the clinical evaluation of the infertile bitch, one underlying question is her overall health status. Complete blood counts (CBCs), chemistry panels, urinalyses, and thyroid and adrenocortical function studies have been recommended as an initial step in evaluating the potentially infertile bitch. The bitch that is healthy to an owner, appears healthy on physical examination, and has normal estrus cycles is not likely to have thyroid failure or adrenocortical disease, and rarely has other significant organ disease. Therefore, a CBC, a urinalysis, and blood urea nitrogen (BUN) level are a sufficient data base. If abnormalities on history or physical examination suggest specific or additional problems, appropriate testing can then be chosen.

BRUCELLA

Brucella canis can cause abortion late in gestation. In addition, potential exists for the *Brucella*-infected bitch to be infertile or for the organism to cause resorption

the *Brucella* Negative Bitch

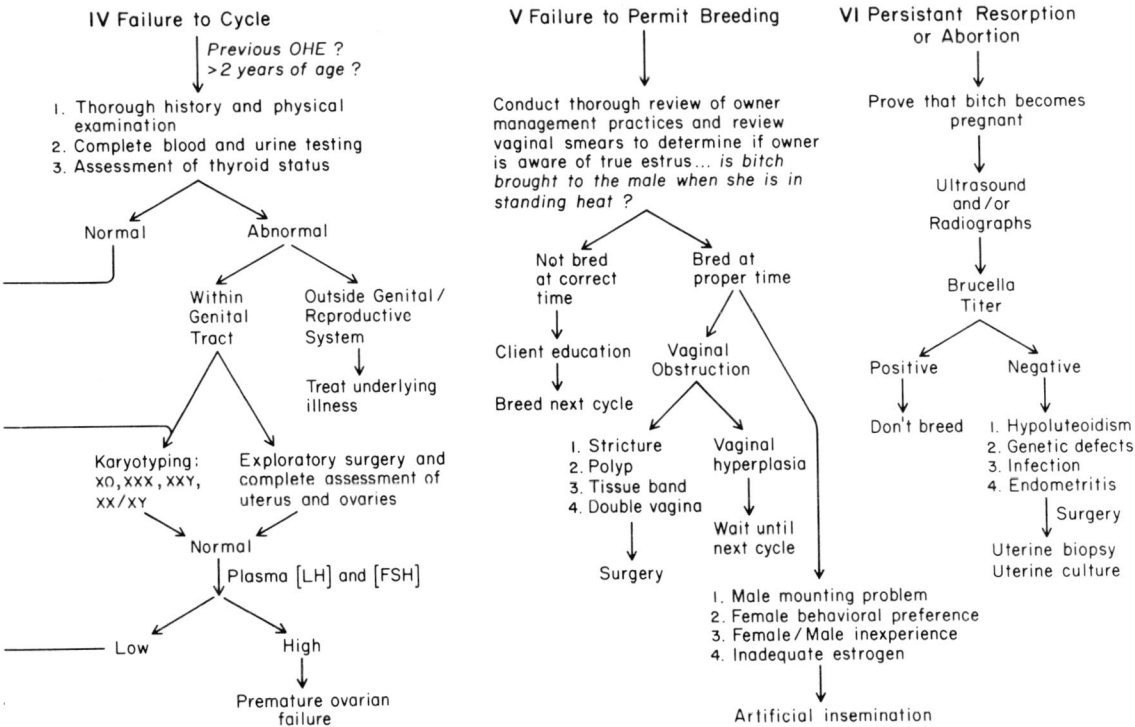

IV Failure to Cycle

Previous OHE ?
>2 years of age ?

1. Thorough history and physical examination
2. Complete blood and urine testing
3. Assessment of thyroid status

Normal   Abnormal

Within Genital Tract   Outside Genital / Reproductive System

Treat underlying illness

Karyotyping: XO, XXX, XXY, XX/XY   Exploratory surgery and complete assessment of uterus and ovaries

Normal

Plasma [LH] and [FSH]

Low   High

Premature ovarian failure

V Failure to Permit Breeding

Conduct thorough review of owner management practices and review vaginal smears to determine if owner is aware of true estrus... *is bitch brought to the male when she is in standing heat ?*

Not bred at correct time   Bred at proper time

Client education

Breed next cycle   Vaginal Obstruction

1. Stricture
2. Polyp
3. Tissue band
4. Double vagina

Surgery

Vaginal hyperplasia

Wait until next cycle

1. Male mounting problem
2. Female behavioral preference
3. Female / Male inexperience
4. Inadequate estrogen

Artificial insemination

VI Persistant Resorption or Abortion

Prove that bitch becomes pregnant

Ultrasound and/or Radiographs

Brucella Titer

Positive   Negative

Don't breed

1. Hypoluteoidism
2. Genetic defects
3. Infection
4. Endometritis

Surgery

Uterine biopsy
Uterine culture

FIGURE 104–2 *Continued*

of fetuses early in gestation, or stillborn or ill puppies.[2] All bitches in active breeding programs, especially those with an infertility problem, should be evaluated for canine brucellosis. The rapid slide agglutination test is an excellent screening test. False-negative tests are unlikely, and a negative result can be trusted. Bitches that are seropositive should be retested using the tube agglutination method because false-positive results do occur.[3]

OTHER INFECTIONS

Bacterial infections have been implicated as a cause for infertility in the bitch.[3, 4] These infections are thought to be subclinical in the infertile bitch, only occasionally resulting in obvious vaginitis, metritis, pyometra, or systemic infection. The recommendation has been made to culture the anterior vagina of infertile bitches with a

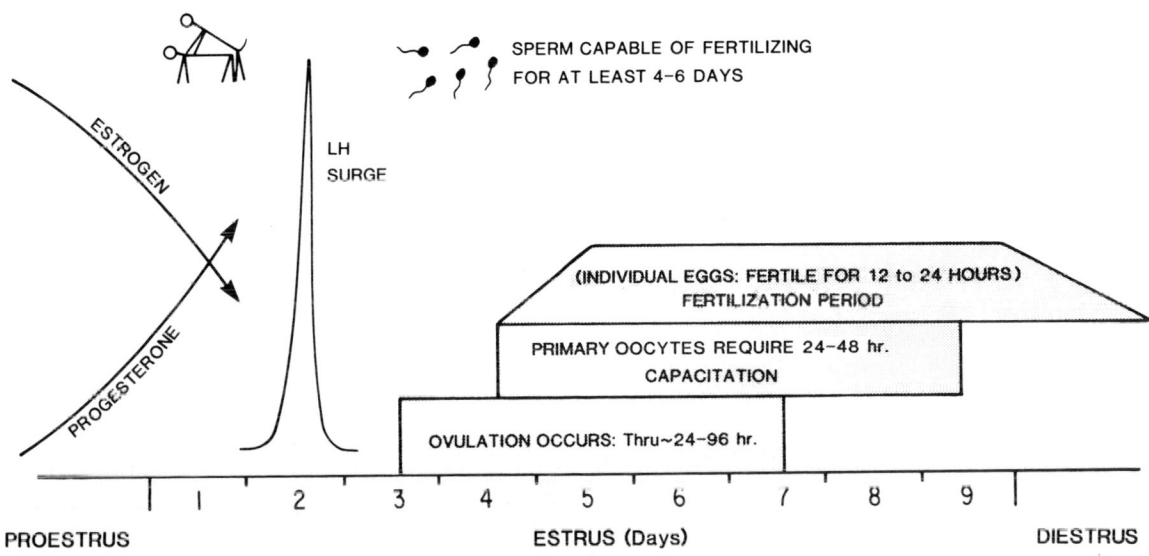

SPERM CAPABLE OF FERTILIZING FOR AT LEAST 4–6 DAYS

ESTROGEN

PROGESTERONE

LH SURGE

(INDIVIDUAL EGGS: FERTILE FOR 12 to 24 HOURS) FERTILIZATION PERIOD

PRIMARY OOCYTES REQUIRE 24–48 hr. CAPACITATION

OVULATION OCCURS: Thru~24–96 hr.

1   2   3   4   5   6   7   8   9

PROESTRUS   ESTRUS (Days)   DIESTRUS

FIGURE 104–3. An illustration of the hormonal changes and sequence of events concerning the timing of ovulation and fertilization of ova in the normal subject. (From Feldman, EC and Nelson, RW: Canine and Feline Endocrinology and Reproduction. Philadelphia, WB Saunders, 1987, p 408.)

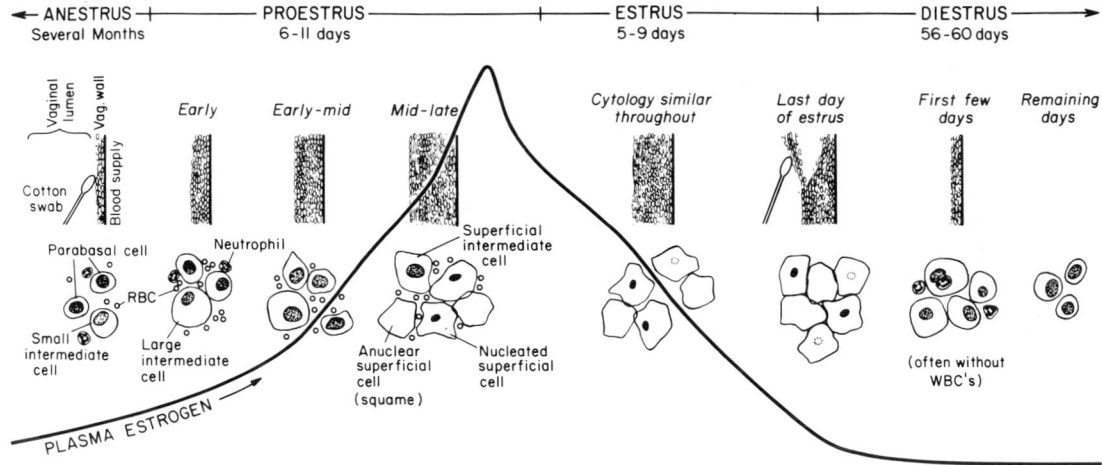

FIGURE 104–4. Changes in vaginal wall thickness, vaginal cytology, and relative plasma estrogen concentrations in a normal subject experiencing an estrous cycle. Note that near the last day of estrus rafts of vaginal cells that are sloughed at that time are present. (From Feldman, EC and Nelson, RW: Canine and Feline Endocrinology and Reproduction. Philadelphia, WB Saunders, 1987, p 402.)

guarded swab. Bacterial isolation, identification, and antimicrobial sensitivity have been suggested in order to place the bitch on appropriate antibiotics for four weeks.[3] However, it is difficult to establish the role of bacterial infections in canine infertility. Most normal bitches have bacterial flora present in the anterior vagina,[5] and similar types of aerobic bacteria are present in the vaginal vaults of infertile bitches.[6]

Approximately 60 per cent of normal bitches harbor aerobic bacteria in the cranial vagina and 90 per cent harbor similar organisms in the caudal vagina (Table 104–2).[2, 5] Merely isolating bacteria from the vagina does not constitute the basis for a diagnosis of disease. Some organisms, such as *B. canis*, may be difficult to isolate. Thus a negative culture does not ensure that a bitch is free of an infectious disease.

The types of bacteria may vary with the age of the bitch; a higher percentage of prepuberal bitches have coagulase-positive staphylococci than do postpuberal bitches. The types of bacteria isolated did not alter with progression through the stages of an estrous cycle, but increased numbers were present in proestrus and estrus.[7, 8] The composition of the gram-positive and gram-negative organisms was found to be unique among individual dogs. Normal flora is usually recovered in mixed cultures of light to moderate growth. If an organism has potential to become a significant pathogen, it usually results in clinical signs, is recovered in large

numbers, and is present in a nearly pure culture because it has gained an advantage and overgrown the normal mixed flora.[2]

Some owners of stud dogs require a "negative" vaginal culture from the bitch to be used in breeding. Most male dogs, however, harbor microorganisms in the prepuce and urethra that are similar to those identified as normal vaginal flora. It is unjustified to refuse to breed a bitch to a stud dog because bacteria have been isolated from the vagina.[2]

Mycoplasma and *Ureaplasma* organisms are commonly cultured from the vaginal tract of the normal bitch. However, a syndrome of poor conception, early embryonic death, embryonal or fetal resorption, abortion, stillborn pups, weak newborns, and neonatal death has been suggested to be caused by these smallest of free-living microorganisms.[9] Current evidence regarding the pathogenesis of these disorders is circumstantial. As with bacterial culture results, if large numbers of these organisms are identified in pure or nearly pure growth from the vaginal vault of a breeding bitch with an infertility problem, the microorganisms may be at fault. Management includes isolation of the animal and tetracycline or chloramphenicol therapy for 10 to 14 days.[9]

Canine herpesvirus (CHV) infection in neonatal pups is a fatal acute infectious disease characterized by generalized focal necrosis and hemorrhage. This disease is one of the best defined neonatal disorders in dogs. The disease in adult dogs is usually subclinical or mild, for example, conjunctivitis, serous or mucopurulent ocular and/or nasal discharges, and vaginal/vestibular/vulvar lesions that are vesicular early in the course of the disease and later become circular and pock-like. Genital lesions usually disappear shortly after infection, but they may reappear with the onset of proestrus. CHV infection can result in infertility, fetal resorption, fetal mummification, small litter size, abortion, or premature birth. A bitch may have dead or mummified fetuses in the same litter as unaffected live pups. Abortion has occurred between 44 and 51 days of gestation after infection on day 30. The fetal placentae from a bitch with CHV

TABLE 104–2. BACTERIAL ISOLATES FROM CLINICALLY NORMAL CANINE VAGINA

A.	B.
Escherichia coli	*Actinomyces* spp.
Streptococcus spp.	*Corynebacterium* spp.
Staphylococcus spp.	*E. coli*
Pasteurella spp.	*Micrococcus* spp.
Proteus spp.	*Mycoplasma* spp.
Corynebacterium spp.	*Pasteurella* spp.
Bacillus spp.	*Propionibacterium* spp.
Others	*Staphylococcus* spp.
	Streptococcus spp.

A. From Olson, P and Mather, E: Canine vaginal and uterine bacterial flora. JAVMA 172:708, 1978.
B. From Kwawer, J: Master's thesis, University of California, Davis, 1986.

infection are typically underdeveloped and congested. Several grey-white foci, ranging in size from miliary to rice grain, can be observed in the placental labyrinth. Sometimes the lesions form zonal structures 2 to 3 mm wide. Typical changes are also seen histologically.

Transmission of herpesvirus can occur venereally, transplacentally, through contact by the neonate during birth, or through respiratory routes of infection. Diagnosis depends on viral isolation. Viral isolation requires fastidious sampling and culture techniques. A negative culture for this virus might be due to inadequate methodology. Separation of infected animals from noninfected animals is advisable. Because there is no vaccine for prevention, one can only recommend careful physical examination and review of the history from dogs to be used in a breeding program.[10, 11]

It is unjustified to associate all positive vaginal cultures with infertility, and it has not been proved that systemic antibiotics alter the bacterial flora of the vagina. However, heavy growth of one bacteria may be abnormal, and treatment with vaginal douches for two to three weeks, with or without systemic antibiotics, may be beneficial, especially if the bacteria are spermicidal. The canine uterus may contain small number of bacteria, yet be normal.[8] A laparotomy must be performed to obtain a uterine culture. The cervix "relaxes" in proestrus and estrus, suggesting that anterior vaginal cultures reflect uterine bacterial growth. Without obvious vaginitis or pyometra, vaginal cultures are not believed to be of major benefit in managing the infertile bitch.

CHRONIC ENDOMETRITIS

The bitch with chronic endometrial disease is likely to be infertile. Such an animal could experience normal estrous cycles, ovulate, have fertilized eggs, but fail to support pregnancy owing to an abnormal uterine environment that prevents implantation or results in fetal resorption. After evaluating the stud and the management practices of an owner, one should be able to assess the likelihood of an ovarian problem. If the stud is normal, the ovaries are normal, the dog is free of brucellosis, and the timing of breeding is correct, an underlying endometrial problem is possible.

Chronic endometritis or cystic endometrial hyperplasia (sterile or infected) can be extremely difficult to confirm. The diagnosis is suspected if the nonpregnant uterus is thickened or abnormally large in anestrus or diestrus. Although a thickened uterine wall is potentially palpable, it is difficult to be certain that it is uterus.

Radiographically, the nonpregnant uterus is seldom visible. If the uterus is visible in a bitch with an infertility problem, endometrial disease is possible. Similarly, visualization of the nonpregnant uterus, using ultrasonography, is a potential method for estimating thickening of the endometrium or the presence of intraluminal fluid. Uterine biopsy, a procedure that usually requires laparotomy, is the only method of confirming a diagnosis of endometrial disease. No definitive treatment has been established for this disorder. Because the diagnosis of chronic endometritis necessitates laparotomy, each bitch that is surgically explored should also be cultured for

bacteria and evaluated for patency of the uterus and oviducts.

EARLY FETAL RESORPTION

Early fetal resorption usually appears to both owner and veterinarian as primary infertility because early pregnancy is so difficult to confirm. It is not possible to diagnose pregnancy on blood or urine tests. Palpably, pregnancy cannot be recognized until after at least 21 days of gestation, and then the diagnosis is subjective. Radiographically, pregnancy cannot be confirmed until 42 to 45 days of gestation. The earliest that pregnancy can be confirmed is approximately 16 days after first breeding, using ultrasonography. This tool has been helpful in recognizing early fetal resorption. Ultrasound abnormalities may be suggestive of an endometrial disorder or evidence of fetal resorption (infection or cystic endometrial hyperplasia), failure of corpora lutea to support pregnancy (hypoluteoidism), infectious disease such as *B. canis*, fetal defects, or some less common disorder.

HYPOLUTEOIDISM

Progesterone concentrations begin to rise in the plasma before the onset of standing heat and decline to basal levels immediately before parturition. The first six to seven weeks of diestrus are usually associated with progesterone concentrations of 10 to 50 ng/ml. Any bitch diagnosed as having an infertility problem should be evaluated with a plasma progesterone concentration 10 to 20 days after standing heat. If the progesterone is below 1.0 ng/ml, either the bitch never ovulated or the corpora lutea have failed to synthesize or secrete progesterone. If the progesterone concentration is 1 to 5 ng/ml, insufficient progesterone (hypoluteoidism) may have resulted in fetal abortion or resorption. Levels of 5 to 10 ng/ml are probably sufficient to maintain pregnancy.

A bitch diagnosed as having hypoluteoidism can be treated, after standing heat, with repositol progesterone. One can use repositol progesterone in polypropylene glycol, 1 mg/lb of body weight, twice weekly until day 50 of diestrus. Another protocol includes 12 to 35 mg of progesterone/dog, giving two injections three days apart and then megestrol acetate (2.5 to 5.0 mg/dog) orally every 24 to 48 hours through day 55 to 60 of gestation. Hypoluteoidism has not been well documented in the bitch. However, the author has successfully managed three bitches with the protocol above after demonstrating suboptimal (< 5 ng/ml) progesterone concentrations and fetal resorption on previous cycles. Progesterone therapy can potentiate the development of pyometra, so the owners must be warned of this serious possible side effect.

To complicate matters, decreased progesterone concentrations in diestrus are not always a primary problem. Fetal factors, placentitis, and exogenous glucocorticoid therapy represent a few of the many potential causes for premature luteal regression. In some situations progesterone administration may be contraindicated, but these conditions are not completely understood. Progesterone therapy is recommended only with great caution.

OCCLUSIONS OF THE UTERUS OR OVIDUCTS

It is impossible to evaluate patency of the uterus and oviducts on a physical examination simply because these structures are too small. Bilateral segmental aplasia or other causes of obstruction of the uterine horns, or occlusion of both oviducts, could result in a bitch that has normal estrus cycles, ovulates, breeds normally, but fails to conceive.[6] Bilateral occlusion prevents the sperm from ever reaching the egg. Diagnosing this rare, but possible, anatomic defect is extremely difficult. The problem of diagnosis lies in the location of these tubular structures and in the physiology governing their accessibility.

Theoretically, one should be able to pass radiopaque dye from the vagina through the cervix and uterus into both oviducts. Radiographs of the abdomen will then allow visualization of the patency of this tract. However, even under a good deal of pressure, dye cannot easily be passed through the cervix except during proestrus and estrus, when cervical dilatation is most pronounced. The uterotabular junction, however, is tight (closed) under the influence of estrogen (i.e., proestrus and perhaps early estrus). Therefore, this dye study (hysterosalpingography) is most likely to be successful only during estrus. Hysterosalpingography is an excellent theoretical tool but is difficult to use on a practical basis.

An alternative to radiographic dye studies would be direct visualization. Laparoscopy is not a good tool because the oviducts cannot be visualized. Laparotomy is the only remaining tool that is realistic. The uterus can be closely studied, and the oviduct patency is assessed by injecting saline solution into the uterus, occluding the uterus at the body, and watching the solution leak out of the oviducts. Others have recommended using dye for the procedure,[12] but its use has not been necessary in our patients. Surgery also allows specimens of the uterus to be collected for biopsy and culture.

There is little that can be done if a bitch is diagnosed as having bilateral uterine or oviductal occlusion. Unilateral occlusion would not result in infertility. Opening an occluded uterine horn or oviduct has not been described. Such bitches are permanently infertile.

MISCELLANEOUS CAUSES OF INFERTILITY

Among the recognized causes of infertility in species other than the dog, when the female has normal cycles and the male is fertile, are anti-sperm antibodies produced by the female or spermicidal substances within secretions of the cervix.[13–18] Anti-sperm antibodies have been recognized in male dogs with *B. canis*.[19] Anti-sperm antibodies have also been induced in dogs.[20] Studies on both systemic antibodies and cervical mucus may soon be part of an evaluation of the infertile bitch. However, such findings remain speculative. Additionally, anti-egg zona pellucida antibodies have been developed in bitches through immunization procedures.[21] Such antibodies do result in infertility. Spontaneous

production of such antibodies may occur but have not yet been recognized.

The Bitch with Shortened Interestrous Intervals

PHYSIOPATHOLOGY

The normal bitch enters the proestrous phase of her cycle every five to nine months (Figure 104–2). In some animals, fertile cycles, culminating in a term pregnancy, are seen every 4 to 4.5 months. The uterus after the phase of progesterone dominance, in which it is in a "pregnant" state, undergoes a period of breakdown and repair in preparation for the next cycle. This recovery period is thought to last for three months.[22] Thus the 2- to 2.5-month duration of diestrus, plus the 0.5 to 1 month needed for both proestrus and estrus, and the 2- to 3-month uterine recovery phase account for the duration of a complete cycle. Clinically, the uterine repair phase is called anestrus. A bitch that enters proestrus before completion of the uterine repair may experience apparent infertility. This infertility could result from an implantation failure caused by an endometrium that has not recovered from the previous effects of progesterone.

Confirmation of these physiopathologic events is difficult. The presumptive diagnosis can be made, however, from a careful review of the history.

OWNER MANAGEMENT PROBLEMS

Before making a diagnosis or instituting therapy, a complete history on the bitch and her estrous cycles must be obtained and reviewed. The goals are to be certain that both veterinarian and client are using the same terminology in describing a cycle and to rule out many of the more obvious causes of infertility. If there is any question regarding management practices, or if the bitch has not been previously evaluated, it is prudent to study the bitch as she progresses through a cycle. In this manner the dates of each cycle and its phases can be confirmed, vaginal cytology performed, progesterone data obtained, and breedings identified. The bitch that cycles at less than four-month intervals is typically normal in all respects and is infertile only as a result of incomplete uterine involution.

Changes in cycle length may be recognized as a bitch matures. Young bitches frequently have irregular, frequent, or silent estrus periods. These can be confusing to an owner who is attempting to predict when an upcoming cycle will begin. By the age of two to three years, however, cycles should become regular, and predicting approximate dates for the next cycle is possible. A segment of the population, however, has cycles that occur every three months at two years of age, but the interestrous intervals progressively increase as the bitch ages, so that the intervals may be four months by three years of age and five months at four years.

Thus it is recommended not to treat any bitch for frequent cycles until she is at least three years of age. In addition, a veterinarian should be allowed to observe and test the bitch through one cycle. Using physical examination, vaginal cytology, and at least one diestrual plasma progesterone level (as described in the previous section) the nature of a cycle can be better understood. Most important, the presence of "split heats" must be ruled out.

SPLIT HEATS

Split heats occur most frequently in young, puberal bitches but can occur at any time in life. The initial phase of a split heat is associated with normal ovarian follicular development and the secretion of estrogen. Adequate estrogen is secreted to cause typical signs of proestrus: vulvar swelling, vaginal bleeding, attraction of males, some behavior changes, and, rarely, breeding. The coordination of endocrine events fails, however, and neither ovulation nor formation of corpora lutea takes place. The follicles regress and all signs of proestrus/estrus dissipate. Two to 12 weeks later a new wave of follicles develop, secreting enough estrogen for signs of proestrus to reappear If the bitch proceeds through proestrus and ovulates, and the cycle continues normally, she has undergone a typical split heat; that is, follicular development is followed by signs of proestrus, which is followed by follicular regression, and then several weeks pass, followed by a return of follicular development and a normal cycle. The final, or "true," heat is typically fertile. Breeding in the true cycle usually results in production of a normal litter.

This entire progression of events can be interpreted as two distinct cycles, and a bitch may be thought to have shortened interestrous intervals. She also may simply be considered to have abnormal cycles. Alternatively, the proestrual bleeding caused by the second follicular wave may be interpreted as the bleeding seen with abortion or resorption of fetuses. Split heats can therefore be confusing. Vaginal cytology can aid in confirming a diagnosis of split heat, since each follicular wave is associated with estrogen secretion and typical estrogen-induced proestrous changes (Figure 104–4).

Greater confusion can be seen in split heats if several follicular waves occur before a successful ovulation(s). In this situation, a bitch may be thought to be cycling every two or three months rather than having incomplete cycles. Two, three, or four independent follicular waves, with external signs of estrogen secretion, can take place before a complete estrous cycle occurs.

Split heats are not considered worrisome. Usually they are seen in young bitches, not in adults. There is no association between split heats and infertility later in life, nor with ovarian or uterine disorders. Recognition of split heats does require close supervision of the bitch and good communication between owner and veterinarian. The possibility of split heats is one reason for not treating any bitch for shortened interestrous intervals until she is at least three years of age.

TREATMENT

Treatment for the bitch that cycles too frequently is to medically induce a normal anestrous period. This can usually be accomplished by treating the bitch with mi-

bolerone drops for six months. Medication is started six to eight weeks after the end of the previous standing heat. A dosage schedule is provided with the medication by the manufacturer, and a separate schedule is used for German shepherd dogs. The veterinarian must be certain that the bitch is not pregnant before beginning mibolerone therapy, since this potent synthetic androgen may cause urogenital defects in female fetuses.[3] The bitch also may undergo some virilization, but these signs are reversible and the drug is not thought to alter future reproductive performance. The bitch should be bred during the first estrus after therapy. This estrus can begin immediately or as long as six to nine months after discontinuation of therapy.

The Bitch with Prolonged Interestrous Intervals

OWNER MANAGEMENT PRACTICES

As with other reproductive problems, a careful review of the history will aid in avoiding unnecessary testing. As a bitch grows older, her interestrous interval lengthens (Figure 104–2). An interval of 10 to 12 months for a bitch older than eight years would not be worrisome. However, such prolonged intervals are not typical of the 2 to 6 year old bitch. Knowing how an owner detects a heat and how closely owners watch their dogs is important. In some instances, estrus may simply be missed by the owner because the bitch may have silent heats. If no males are present and the owner does not specifically examine the vulva once or twice each week, heat cycles can be missed. If the veterinarian and owner are convinced that a bitch is cycling infrequently and that these are infertile cycles, further evaluation is warranted.

IN-HOSPITAL EVALUATION

Prolongation of the interval between the onset of each estrous cycle can occur secondary to underlying illness. Any major medical disorder will usually delay the onset of the estrous cycle. This is an uncommon problem in the apparently healthy bitch, but a general screening panel to establish a data base (CBC, chemistry panel, urinalysis) is recommended. Any abnormality can then be pursued. The disorder most often associated with long interestrous periods is hypothyroidism. Hypothyroid dogs are usually slow, lethargic, inappetent, and dull, and have poor hair coats or endocrine alopecia and blood testing usually reveals a normocytic normochromic anemia and hypercholesterolemia. Appropriate treatment with replacement hormone will usually result in the onset of a cycle within six months. Initiation of normal cycles may follow successful management of any significant underlying disorder.

If all test results are normal one must then be certain that silent heats are not occurring. The owner can then house the infertile bitch with one that is normally cycling, which may induce an earlier cycle. Alternatively, the bitch may be housed with a male to detect silent heats or the owner may wish to obtain weekly vaginal smears, which can be checked for evidence of follicular function. The infrequent cycle can be closely monitored to be certain that proper breeding dates are being chosen. Lastly, an estrous cycle can be medically induced.

Failure to Cycle

Rarely, veterinary advice is sought regarding a bitch that fails to cycle. As with all reproductive disorders, the dog's age, breed, and past history should be assessed before any major tests are undertaken. Some large-breed dogs experience the puberal (first) estrus after they reach two years of age, whereas small breeds of dogs may have several silent heat cycles before exhibiting an obvious cycle. Failure to cycle, therefore, is usually not pursued until the bitch is beyond two to three years of age.

If the past history of a bitch is not known, one cause for failure to cycle is previous oophorohysterectomy. Examination of the ventral midline for an incision scar is suggestive of an earlier spay. One may need to clip hair away from this area to be certain. If one wanted to confirm this finding, plasma can be submitted for a luteinizing hormone (LH) determination. The ovario-hysterectomized female has persistent elevation in LH concentrations. Anestrous bitches may also have higher serum estrogen concentrations than do spayed females.

SILENT HEAT

A silent heat (one that is simply not associated with bleeding) can be difficult to detect. An owner may try bringing the bitch into contact with a male once weekly to help recognize estrus. Close visual examination of the vulva, once or twice weekly, is an excellent method for detecting silent heat. Close observation allows the owner to develop some experience with the anestrous appearance of the vulva. Mild enlargement of the vulva or a slightly bloody discharge will be easier to recognize, and the owner will be more comfortable identifying these signs of early proestrus.

UNDERLYING DISEASE

Any severe illness can delay the onset of an estrous cycle in the bitch. Hypothyroidism is a potential cause for this problem, but those dogs have typical signs of hypothyroidism, such as lethargy, poor appetite, poor hair coats, and bilaterally symmetric alopecia. The alert, active, vibrant bitch is not hypothyroid. When silent heats, previous oophorohysterectomy, and owner error are considered unlikely explanations for apparent failure to cycle, blood and urine testing is advisable. It is recommended that a CBC, chemistry panel, urinalysis, and T_4 ± TSH stimulation test be obtained and reviewed. Hypothyroid dogs should rapidly respond to thyroid replacement by becoming more alert, active, and responsive, as well as having an improved appetite and hair coat. These dogs typically begin to cycle within one to six months of initiating therapy.

GLUCOCORTICOID EXCESS

Glucocorticoids are used in the treatment of numerous small animal problems. Glucocorticoids do have negative feedback effects on pituitary adrenocorticotropin (ACTH) secretion and similar effects on suppressing secretion of both follicle-stimulating hormone (FSH) and LH. A bitch receiving glucocorticoid therapy will usually not have estrous cycles unless dosages are kept to a minimum or administration is discontinued. Specific doses capable of inhibiting estrous cycles are not known. However, any bitch that has a blunted cortisol response to exogenous ACTH is likely to have sufficient negative feedback from its steroid therapy to interfere with ovarian activity.

Spontaneous hyperadrenocorticism (Cushing's syndrome) is not usually a major consideration in the noncycling female because most bitches with Cushing's are older than eight years of age. Therefore, their failure to cycle is not recognized as a problem by the owner, whereas the other major signs of Cushing's are more obvious, dramatic, and worrisome.

DISORDERS OF SEXUAL DEVELOPMENT

Some disorders in embryonic sex development result in a failure to cycle. There are numerous disorders, some of which are briefly outlined here.

Sex Determination. The sex chromosome constitution of the sperm determines the sex of most individual mammals at fertilization. The embryo develops as a male if the fertilizing sperm has a Y chromosome. If the sperm contains an X chromosome, the embryo develops as a female. The genital system of early developing embryos is neither male nor female. Eventually the embryo without a Y chromosome develops an ovary from the undifferentiated gonad and the müllerian system persists as the fallopian tubes, uterus, and cranial vagina. The urogenital sinus and external genitalia develop in a female pattern. In the presence of a Y chromosome the indifferent gonad develops into a testis, which produces both testosterone and müllerian duct inhibiting factor.[23] This factor, secreted by Sertoli cells, causes regression of the müllerian duct system. Testosterone, secreted by Leydig cells, stimulates formation of the epididymis and vas deferens from the wolffian duct system as well as the penis and scrotum.

Dogs have a total chromosome number of 78. These 78 chromosomes include 38 pairs of nonsex chromosomes and 2 sex chromosomes. The sex chromosome constitution of females is XX and that of males is XY.

The XXY Syndrome. During the process of meiosis, which results in gametes (sperm or eggs), abnormalities may occur. Among the abnormalities seen in development of eggs is a condition called nondisjunction, in which one egg contains two X chromosomes and the other contains no sex chromosomes. The two-X chromosome egg, fertilized by a Y chromosome sperm, develops into an XXY individual. The XXY condition has been described in the human, mouse, horse, cow, sheep, cat, and dog.[24] The XXY condition results in a phenotypic male (an individual with male external genitalia), but one having testicular hypoplasia and lack of spermatogenesis.

The XO Syndrome. As described earlier, an egg or sperm may contain no sex chromosome. When fertilized by an X-containing gamete (egg or sperm) the result is an XO zygote. In humans, XO individuals develop as phenotypic females of short stature with other developmental anomalies. The gonads develop as ovaries during fetal life, but they usually degenerate into fibrous streaks lacking germ cells. This condition should be considered in the differential diagnosis of bitches that fail to cycle within their first two to four years. Females that are XO are also sex chromatin–negative. The laboratories of several veterinary schools perform karyotyping (study of the chromosomes), including the University of Minnesota and the University of California, Davis.

Intersexuality. Intersex conditions include individuals with congenital malformations of the genital system such that their sex is ambiguous. Intersex is a general term that includes numerous disorders. True hermaphrodites are individuals with both testicular and ovarian tissue, either combined in one gonad (ovotestis) or existing as separate gonads. Pseudohermaphrodites have the gonads of one sex but reproductive organs that have characteristics of the opposite sex. Male pseudohermaphrodites have testes but have some female features, such as the presence of a uterus, or external genitalia that are primarily female. Female pseudohermaphrodites have ovaries but are masculinized to some degree.[24]

There are several other terms to be defined. The phenotype is the external appearance; a phenotypic female is one that appears to be female. The genotype refers to the genetic makeup of an individual. In terms of sex, the genotype or chromosomal sex refers to XX, XY, XXY, XO, and so on. Gonadal sex type refers to the presence of ovaries or testes.

SURGICAL DIAGNOSIS

Whenever faced with an adult bitch that has apparently never experienced an ovarian cycle, one alternative in the diagnostic evaluation is exploratory laparotomy. In this manner the abdominal organs can be visualized. Although this approach is direct, one may not always be able to distinguish normal from abnormal tissues externally. This approach, therefore, is tempered with the knowledge that a definite diagnosis cannot always be made, even after seeing the organs in question.

PRIMARY VERSUS SECONDARY FAILURE TO CYCLE

Primary failure to exhibit estrous activity involves dogs that have never cycled, and secondary failure to cycle occurs in bitches that have previously had one or more estrous periods. Secondary persistent anestrus can occur after the onset of thyroid or non-endocrine disease. Such patients should be thoroughly evaluated after waiting for at least 16 to 20 months from the previous cycle, in case a heat cycle or two were silent and, therefore, missed. The dog should be closely monitored during this time by the owner.

PREMATURE OVARIAN FAILURE

The functional longevity of the ovaries of bitches is not known. They are believed to gradually decline in function after the bitch is ten years of age on average. Bitches are not usually used in breeding programs beyond eight years of age. The ovaries, however, may cease functioning earlier. This would result in a permanent anestrous state, which could be seen as prolonged anestrous by the owner. This diagnosis is suspected when all other differentials are excluded from the list of potential diagnoses and attempts to induce estrus fail. It is difficult, however, to confirm. One method of confirming such a diagnosis would be random evaluation of plasma FSH and LH concentrations. If these concentrations are extremely increased, premature ovarian failure is likely.

INDUCTION OF ESTRUS

One therapeutic/diagnostic approach to the bitch with prolonged interestrous intervals, primary anestrus, or secondary anestrus is to attempt the medical induction of estrus. Most studies on induction of estrus in the bitch have been performed on healthy females, and success has been variable. When similar protocols are used on a bitch with potential disorders in the pituitary or ovaries, one should not expect great results.

Pregnant mare serum (PMS) was administered to mature anestrous bitches for ten consecutive days at SQ doses of 500 IU/day, 250 IU/day, or 9 IU/lb/day. This was followed by an SQ injection of 500 IU of human chorionic gonadotropin (HCG) on day 10. Fourteen of 25 bitches exhibited behavioral estrus and ovulated.[25] This was one of the most successful induction procedures encountered in the literature. In a more recent study, 8 of 15 bitches ovulated after nine consecutive days of IM or SQ PMS, injected at 20 IU/lb/day, followed by 500 IU of HCG IM on day 10.[26] The responding animals exhibited behavioral estrus 10 to 15 days after treatment was initiated, but only half of those dogs ovulated. Several protocols using FSH, with and without LH, were not promising.[27]

Pretreatment with estrogens, either estrone or estradiol, was useful in inducing estrus in bitches that were in diestrus. Pretreatment with 100 to 300 gm of estrone per day for five or six days was followed by 200 to 400 IU of PMS and 1000 IU HCG IM on the day that vaginal bleeding was first noted and again on the first day of standing heat. This protocol resulted in six of seven bitches becoming pregnant after natural or artificial insemination.[28] Again, the bitches used in that study were normal.

Various other protocols for inducing proestrus and estrus are available (Table 104–3). The author cannot strongly recommend one method because the results have been quite poor when working with bitches that have potential problems. It has been suggested that PMS is more effective in stimulating follicular activity than FSH.[29] However, FSH appears to be readily available commercially and PMS is not.

Investigations are now proceeding to study gonadotrophin-releasing hormone (GnRH). Estrus has been

TABLE 104–3. TREATMENT PROTOCOL FOR INDUCTION OF PROESTRUS AND ESTRUS IN THE BITCH

Method Number	Follicle Development	Ovulation	Source
1	250–500 IU PMS*/day, SQ × 10 days	500 IU HCG,† SQ–day 10	Thun et al., 1977
2	9 IU PMS/lb/day, SQ × 10 days	500 IU HCG, SQ–day 10	Thun et al., 1977
3	20 IU PMS/lb/day SQ × 9 days	500 IU HCG, IM–day 10	Archibald et al., 1980
4	100–300 μgm estrone, SQ × 5 days	200–400 IU PMS and 1000 IU HCG, IM, on day 1 of vaginal bleeding, again on day 1 of standing heat	Takeishi et al., 1976
5	9–23 IU PMS/lb/day, IM × 9 days	500–1000 IU HCG, IM, on days 1 and 2 of standing heat	Chakraborty et al., 1982
6	500–1000 IU PMS, IM, days 1 and 7	50 μgm GnRH‡ IM 2 injections q6h apart on day 1 of standing heat	Chakraborty et al., 1982
7	2 mg FSH§/day, SQ, 5–10 days (until > 80% superficial vaginal cells) (pretreatment with DES, 1 mg/33 lb × 4 days)	1000 IU HCG, IM day after FSH is complete	Olson, 1984
8	1–2 mg FSH/day, IM or SQ, days 1, 3, 6, 9	23 IU HCG/lb, IV–day 9	Burke, 1980
9	0.7 mg FSH/lb/day, SQ × 10 days	5 mg LH,** IV–day 10	
10	1, 2, 4, 8, 16 mg FSH, IM, given on days 1 and 2, 2 and 4, 5 and 6, 7 and 8, 9 and 10		Shille, 1984

*PMS-Sigma Chemical Co., St. Louis, MO.
†HCG Gonamone Fort Dodge Laboratories, Fort Dodge, IA 50501.
‡GnRH Cystorelin-Abbott Laboratories, North Chicago, IL.
§FSH FSH-P Armour-Baldwin Laboratories, Omaha, NE; Burns-Biotec, Oakland, CA.
**FSH FSH-P Armour-Baldwin Laboratories, same as above.

successfully induced with an IV pump that forces a small dose of GnRH into the system (IV or SQ) every 90 minutes for seven to ten days. Induction of proestrus, estrus, ovulation, and pregnancy have been quite successful in normal bitches.

Regardless of the method chosen for estrus induction, the owner must be warned that the protocol may fail. Two of the author's dogs developed severe autoimmune hemolytic anemia during or immediately following induction with FSH and HCG. This may be coincidence, or a side effect of hormone therapy. Once induction is begun, vaginal cytology should be obtained on an alternate-day basis. It is recommended that natural breeding or artificial insemination begin when superficial cells represent ≥ 60 per cent of the exfoliated vaginal epithelial cells. Insemination should continue on an alternate-day basis until diestrus is confirmed.

Failure to Permit Breeding

MISMANAGEMENT

The most common cause for bitches to refuse attempts at mounting by a male is an owner's choosing incorrect breeding dates. For example, if it is predetermined that a bitch is to be bred on days 11 and 13 from the first day of proestrual vaginal bleeding, and if proestrus lasted for 5 days, while estrus lasted for 4 days, breeding will be attempted in diestrus and she will refuse. Simi-

larly, if proestrus was 14 days in duration, again she would not breed because attempts were being made during proestrus. Therefore, bitches that fail to permit breeding are not always at fault. Having an owner better understand the reproductive cycle of the bitch usually results in better management and increased success.

BEHAVIOR

Bitches may be correctly managed but still consistently refuse to breed with a particular male. Mate preference appears to be one potential cause for this problem. Therefore, if no other cause is evident, the owner should attempt breeding the bitch to another, more dominant male before investigating unusual problems.

CONGENITAL ABNORMALITIES OF THE VAGINA AND VULVA

In the normal bitch, the vestibule of the vagina, the urethra, and the urinary bladder are all derived from the embryonic urogenital sinus. The pair of müllerian ducts and anterior vagina are joined to the vestibule of the vagina with two epithelial linings sandwiching a thin layer of mesoderm. In the bitch, this hymen-like structure usually disappears as a recognizable or palpable tissue before the bitch matures. However, abnormalities involving the lumen of the vaginal vault and vestibule remain among the most common types of genital abnormalities of the bitch and can result in failure to permit breeding (see Chapter 101). Bitches with vaginal or vulvar defects are usually brought to veterinarians for one of several owner concerns: difficulty breeding, chronic recurring vaginitis, chronic vulvar licking, attracting male dogs, and the presence of a vaginal discharge.

INFERTILITY IN THE MALE

The diagnostic and therapeutic management of the infertile dog is perhaps one of the most difficult and least rewarding areas of dealing with canine reproduction. Nevertheless, some disorders, if corrected, carry a good prognosis regarding return of fertility.

A thorough, systematic diagnostic approach to the infertile stud offers the best chance of identifying the problem. Therapy should be initiated only after a definitive diagnosis has been established. A definitive diagnosis enables the clinician to formulate a rational therapeutic plan and prognosis. The indiscriminate use of fertility drugs, androgens, or other hormones is usually ineffective, potentially dangerous, and frequently confusing to the owner and veterinarian.

Classification

The historical classification of infertility is based on the dog's previous breeding history and is the easiest to use in practice. The most common history is a proven stud dog that subsequently becomes infertile. These dogs have acquired infertility, of which there are many potential causes (Table 104–4). A dog that has never sired a litter despite numerous matings should be considered congenitally infertile until proven otherwise. Acquired infertility is possible in these dogs if the insult occurred before the onset of sexual use. In addition to acquired causes, the clinician must also consider congenital defects that would not be considered in the

TABLE 104–4. CLASSIFICATION FOR MALE INFERTILITY BASED ON HISTORICAL ABILITY TO SIRE A LITTER

Congenital Infertility	Acquired Infertility
Hormonal	Hormonal
Hypopituitarism	Pituitary neoplasia
Hypothyroidism	Hypothyroidism
Chromosomal aberration	Hyperadrenocorticism
Developmental	Metabolic
Cryptorchidism	Uremia
Penis, prepuce, os penis	Hepatic
anomaly	Neoplasia
Testicular hypoplasia, aplasia	Compression
Duct aplasia	Hormonal secretion
Motility	Stress
Kartagener's syndrome	Infection
Retrograde ejaculation	Fever
	Duct obstruction
	Immune-mediated orchitis
	Drugs, exogenous hormones
	Retrograde ejaculation
	Overuse?
	Psychologic?

previously fertile stud dog with acquired infertility (Table 104–4).

The presence or absence of normal libido will also allow the clinician to categorize an infertile dog and reduce the number of possible causes. Normal libido in an infertile male dog would imply that he has normal Leydig cell function and plasma testosterone concentrations, but an abnormality elsewhere in the testes, epididymides, or prostate gland. Conversely, decreased libido in an infertile dog may result from destruction of the Leydig cells within the testes and from numerous other potential defects.

History

A thorough history is extremely important in the evaluation of the infertile dog. An owner questionnaire (Table 104–5) should be designed to obtain both a complete reproductive history as well as a complete review of the dog's general health. Special attention should be paid to the age of the animal, frequency of sexual use, breeding practices of the kennel, the presence or absence of previous reproductive problems, and the previous or current use of any hormones or medications.

Physical Examination

Abnormalities involving various organ systems can interfere with spermatogenesis; therefore, a complete physical examination is extremely important. Special attention should be given to the size, shape, and location of the os penis in relation to the tip of the glans penis; the preputial opening and the ability to extrude the penis; the size, shape, and consistency of the testes; the size and conformation of the epididymis and spermatic cord; and the size, symmetry, and consistency of the prostate gland. A physical examination should be completed before examination of the external genitalia.

Diagnostic Evaluation

Occasionally the history or physical examination will reveal an abnormality that identifies the cause of infertility. Usually, the history is uneventful and the physical examination is normal or reveals soft testes, which are suggestive of degeneration. The diagnostic evaluation of both groups begins with *B. canis* testing (using the rapid slide or tube agglutination test). A complete semen evaluation, including culture of the ejaculate, also should be performed in a dog with normal libido. An ejaculate may be difficult to obtain in a dog with decreased libido, although it should be attempted. For these dogs evaluation of thyroid gland and Leydig cell function becomes an important initial diagnostic step. Testicular biopsy, epididymal aspiration, or measurement of plasma FSH, LH, and testosterone concentrations may be necessary before a diagnosis can be made and a therapeutic plan formulated (Figure 104–5).

TABLE 104–5. OWNER QUESTIONNAIRE—THE INFERTILE MALE

A. Reproductive History
   1. Is your dog a proven stud?
      no _____   yes _____
      If yes, date of last litter sired? _____
   2. Does your dog show strong sexual desires in the presence of a female in estrus?
      yes _____   no _____

	yes	no
If no, did he in the past?	_____	_____

      If so, when? _____
   3. Can your dog achieve:

	yes	no
a. an erection	_____	_____
b. intromission	_____	_____
c. a tie	_____	_____

      (if yes, duration of tie? _____)

	yes	no
4. Does your dog ejaculate?	_____	_____
If yes, does it occur before intromission?	_____	_____
5. Have you observed the semen?	_____	_____

      If yes, what color is it?
   6. How frequently is your dog used for breeding?

   7. When was your dog last used for breeding?

   8. How do you determine when to mate your dog with a bitch?

   9. How many times do you let your dog mate with a bitch?

	yes	no
10. Has your dog had a *Brucella* titer?	_____	_____

      Date of most recent check _____

	yes	no
11. Has your dog had a semen evaluation?	_____	_____

      If yes, date of most recent evaluation _____
      Results of evaluation:

	yes	no
12. Has your dog ever had a preputial discharge?	_____	_____

      If so, briefly describe what it was, when it occurred, and how it was treated:

   13. Has your dog ever had scrotal

	yes	no
a. swelling	_____	_____
b. pain	_____	_____
c. redness	_____	_____
d. dermatitis	_____	_____
14. Have you noticed any change in the size or consistency of your dog's testes?	_____	_____

      If so, briefly describe:

B. Kennel History

	yes	no
Do any other bitches or dogs in your kennel have reproductive disorders?	_____	_____

   If yes, briefly describe:

C. Pedigree

	yes	no
Do any other bitches or dogs that are related to this dog have reproductive disorders?	_____	_____

   If yes, briefly describe:

SEMEN EVALUATION

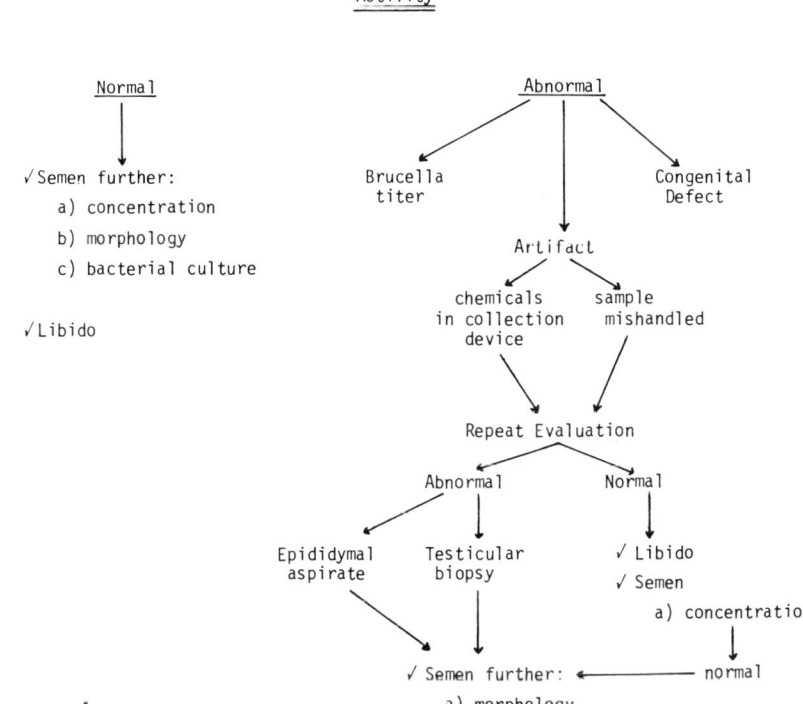

FIGURE 104–5. A diagnostic approach to infertility in the male based on results of the history, physical examination, and semen evaluation. (From Feldman, EC and Nelson, RW: Canine and Feline Endocrinology and Reproduction. Philadelphia, WB Saunders, 1987, p 515.)

Illustration continued on following page

A

Infertility can result from loss of libido or impaired spermatogenesis. Testicular failure may result from primary abnormalities involving the seminiferous tubules, Leydig cells, or hormonal regulation from the pituitary gland.

Treatment

Specific therapy depends on the underlying cause. Fifty-five to 70 days are required for spermatozoa to develop from spermatogonia and subsequently appear in the ejaculate. Any therapy that is expected to increase the sperm count must be given for at least three months before its effectiveness can be critically evaluated. Sexual rest also becomes an important adjunct therapy for many infertility problems and may be all that is required after transient insults to the seminiferous tubules. Stress, sexual overuse, thermal damage, and some drugs are potentially reversible problems, given enough time. Oligospermic and azoospermic dogs should always be re-evaluated three to six months after initial examination before declaring a spermatogenesis problem as being potentially permanent (Table 104–6).

PRIMARY TESTICULAR FAILURE

Dogs with primary testicular failure have loss of function of both the seminiferous tubules and the Leydig cells. Tubular cell degeneration is present with minimal inflammation, and Leydig cells are usually sparse. The pituitary gland is normal. Because of loss of the sup-

pressive effects of inhibin and testosterone, pituitary secretion of FSH and LH is increased. Administration of gonadotrophic hormones is ineffective because the spermatogonia Leydig cell target tissues are absent or nonresponsive. The administration of androgens is also ineffective in promoting spermatogenesis. Dogs with this problem do not respond to any known therapy. Sexual rest and reevaluation should be recommended to be sure a transient insult to the testes was not overlooked. The prognosis for return of fertility in these animals is poor.

PRIMARY FAILURE OF SPERMATOGENESIS

Damage only to the spermatogonia results in infertility and the maintenance of normal libido. Tubular cell degeneration is progressive, and minimal inflammation is present. The associated progressive loss of plasma inhibin results in increasing secretion of pituitary FSH. Leydig cells are present and functional, maintaining normal plasma LH and testosterone concentrations. As with primary testicular failure, there is no known effective therapy if plasma FSH concentrations are increased. Androgens are not indicated, and FSH or pregnant mare serum gonadotrophin (PMSG), which has FSH properties, is ineffective. The prognosis for return of fertility for these dogs is poor. Sexual rest and reevaluation should be recommended.

Some oligospermic dogs will have normal plasma FSH concentrations. This may represent an early stage of primary failure of spermatogenesis or a faulty feedback system between plasma inhibin and pituitary gonadotro-

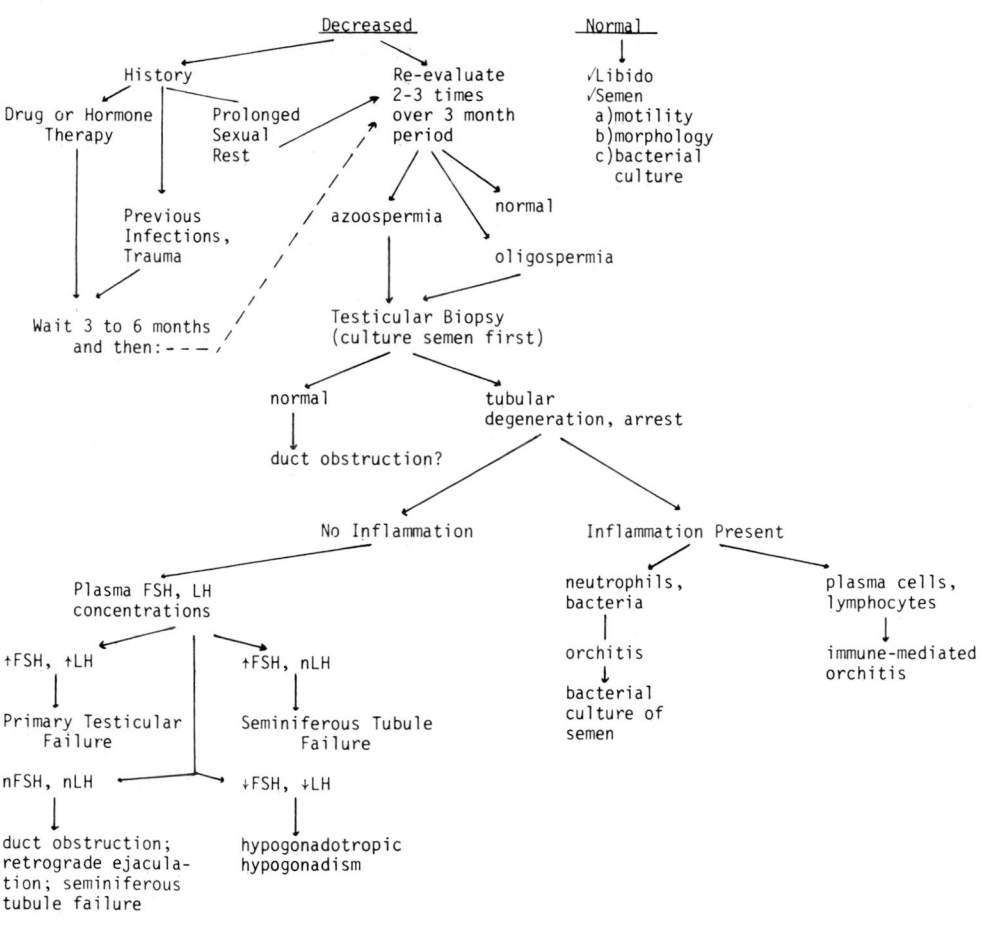

B

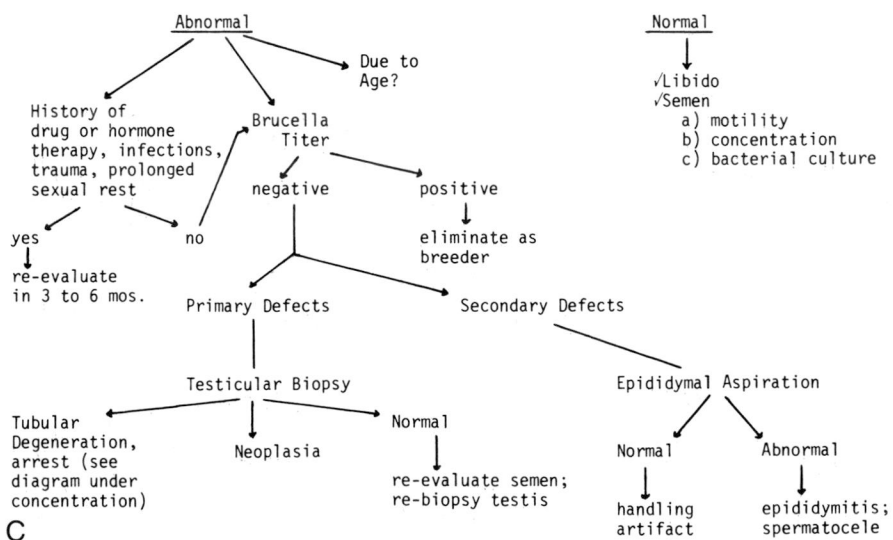

C

FIGURE 104–5 *Continued*

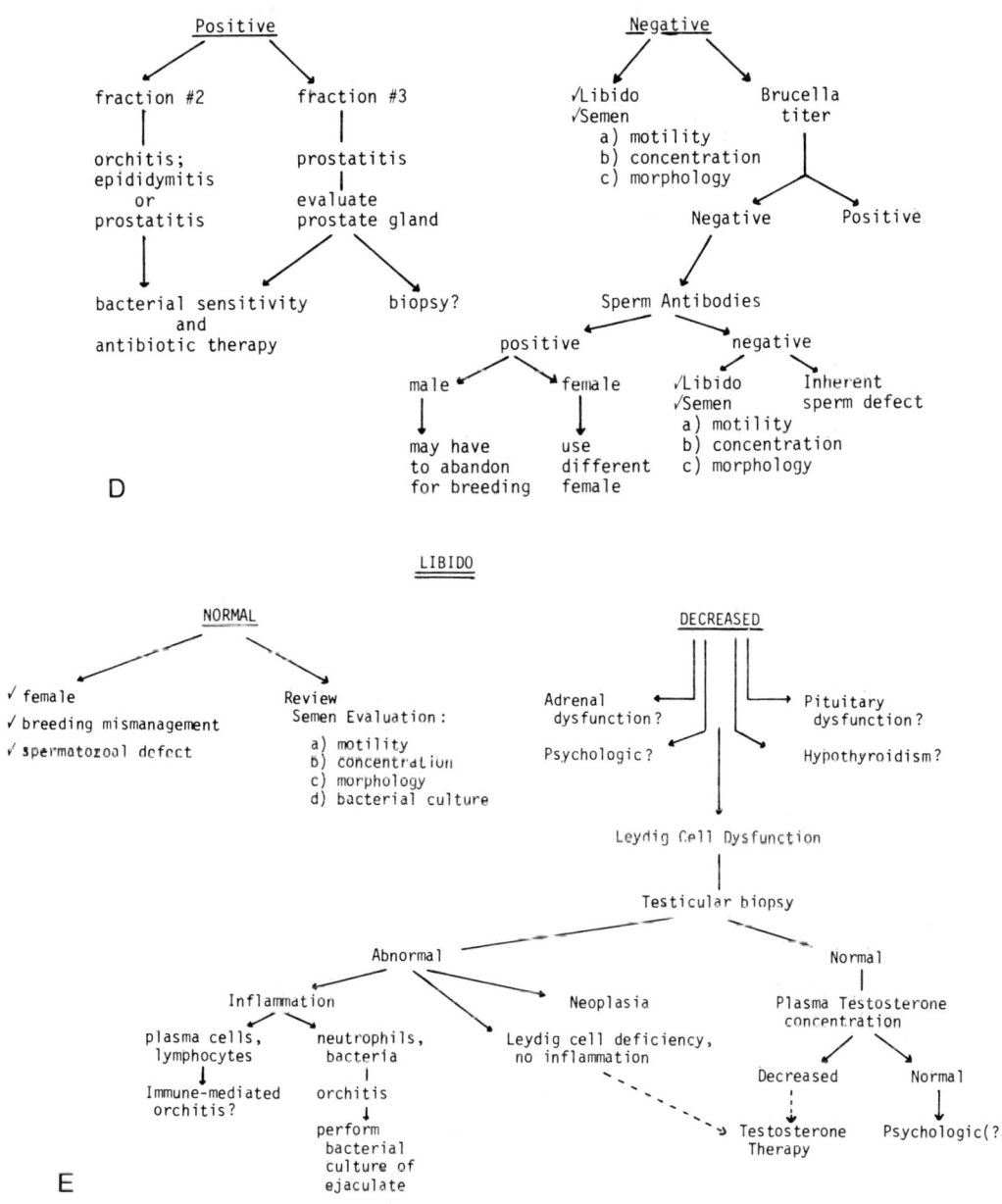

SEMEN EVALUATION

Bacterial Culture

D

LIBIDO

E

FIGURE 104–5 *Continued*

phin secretion. These dogs may respond to clomiphene citrate or tamoxifen therapy.

Clomiphene citrate is a synthetic, nonsteroidal estrogen analog that stimulates pituitary gonadotrophin secretion by excluding estradiol from specific hypothalamic receptor sites, thereby stimulating the secretion of GnRH.[30, 31] It has been used successfully in the management of oligospermia in humans; similar studies in the dog are lacking.[32, 33] One recommended treatment regimen is 25 mg daily in 25-day cycles with 5 days of rest between cycles. This regimen produced an increase in sperm concentration and motility during the first three

months of therapy in 68 per cent of 22 oligospermic humans.[32] Unfortunately a dosage in the dog has not been determined, which is critical in the use of clomiphene citrate. Its effect on the germinal cell epithelium appears to be dose-dependent; the stimulatory response is seen with lower dosages, while higher dosages suppress the gonad, potentially resulting in azoospermia.[34] Long-term therapy, in excess of six months, is also required before the effectiveness of clomiphene citrate can be evaluated. Adverse reactions reported in humans include nausea, vertigo, and weight gain.

The anti-estrogen tamoxifen works in a similar man-

TABLE 104–6. DIAGNOSTIC RESULTS AND THERAPEUTIC RECOMMENDATIONS FOR VARIOUS FORMS OF TESTICULAR FAILURE, OLIGOSPERMIA/AZOOSPERMIA, AND INFERTILITY IN THE DOG

	Libido	Semen Evaluation	Testicular Biopsy	Plasma FSH	LH	Testosterone	Potential Treatments
Primary testicular failure	N/↓	Oligospermia/azoospermia Primary morphologic defects	Tubular degeneration Leydig cells normal or decreased	↑	↑	N/↓	None
Seminiferous tubule failure							
Partial	N	Oligospermia Primary morphologic defects	Tubular degeneration Leydig cells present	N/↑	N	N	Clomiphene citrate Tamoxifen
Complete	N	Azoospermia Primary morphologic defects	Germinal cells absent Leydig cells present	↑	N	N	None
Leydig cell failure	↓	± oligospermia	Leydig cells decreased/ absent Tubules normal ± tubular arrest	N	↑	↓/N	Testosterone Mesterolone Fluoxymesterone
Hypogonadotrophic hypogonadism	↓	Oligospermia/azoospermia	Tubular arrest Leydig cells present	↓	↓	↓	hCG + FSH or PMSG*
Retrograde ejaculation	N	Azoospermia	Normal	N	N	N	Sympathomimetics
Duct obstruction	N	Azoospermia	Normal ± tubular degeneration	N	N	N	Surgery?

*Pregnant mare serum gonadotrophin.

ner as clomiphene citrate but has no undesirable side effects. The recommended dosage in the dog is 10 mg twice a day orally for at least six months.[35]

LEYDIG CELL FAILURE

Functional loss of the Leydig cells will result in loss of libido and variable degrees of impaired spermatogenesis. Results of a testicular biopsy may reveal decreased numbers of Leydig cells. Plasma testosterone concentrations should be decreased. However, because of the greater concentration of testosterone in the testes than in plasma (50:1), plasma concentrations may be normal and not reflect decreased intratesticular concentrations.[36] Pituitary secretion of LH should be increased. The seminiferous tubules should appear normal, with variable degrees of inactivity. Plasma FSH concentrations should be normal.

It is theoretically possible for Leydig cell function to be normal but target cells to be nonresponsive to testosterone. Although the clinical picture would resemble that seen with loss of the Leydig cells, plasma testosterone concentrations would be normal or elevated, plasma LH concentrations increased, and plasma FSH levels normal.

Therapy involves the administration of androgens to promote libido and spermatogenesis. To obtain desired testicular concentrations, large doses of testosterone must be given. Although administration of testosterone may promote libido, it is relatively ineffective in promoting spermatogenesis and may in fact cause oligospermia secondary to its suppressive influence on GnRH and FSH secretion.[37] Use of excessive dosages to promote spermatogenesis may result in aggressive behavior as well as suppression of the hypothalamic-pituitary axis. Nevertheless, androgen therapy may be attempted using oral methyltestosterone, 0.05 mg/lb daily, for three months and then reevaluating a semen sample. Results have been disappointing in the author's experience.

Synthetic androgens that are capable of stimulating seminiferous tissue function without inhibiting the hypothalamic-pituitary axis have been used in human males with oligospermia, androgen deficiency, and infertility.[38] Mesterolone lacks the hepatotoxic side effects that are commonly associated with other orally active androgens. An increase in sperm motility and concentration has been seen in approximately 30 per cent of patients with oligospermia after administration of this androgen.[39] In humans the dose is 25 to 75 mg orally daily. Fluoxymesterone has also been successful in improving semen volume and sperm motility in a small percentage of oligospermic males. There are currently no reports in the literature dealing with the use of these synthetic androgens in dogs.

HYPOGONADOTROPHIC HYPOGONADISM

Pituitary dysfunction with impaired secretion of FSH and LH results in decreased libido and impaired spermatogenesis. Results of a testicular biopsy should reveal Leydig cells, inactive seminiferous tubules, and minimal to no inflammation. Plasma FSH, LH, and testosterone concentrations should be decreased. Depending on the age of the dog, a developmental defect, trauma, or neoplasia involving the pituitary gland may be suspected. A complete diagnostic evaluation of the pituitary gland is warranted to determine the cause and formulate a therapeutic plan. The prognosis for the dog depends on the underlying cause.

If an irreversible but non–life-threatening primary disorder is present, gonadotrophin therapy may be initiated for the infertility problem. Therapy must be designed to stimulate both libido and spermatogenesis. HCG, 500 IU biweekly SQ, may be given to stimulate Leydig cell function. Oral androgens may be used to stimulate libido, but they may be ineffective in enhancing spermatogenesis for reasons previously discussed. Exogenous FSH injections at a dosage of 25 mg SQ once weekly,[40] or 0.5 mg/lb IM every other day,[41] have been recommended to promote spermatogenesis. PMSG has FSH properties and has also been recommended for stimulation of spermatogenesis. The recommended dosage is 10 IU/lb SQ three times weekly. Use of GnRH injections should not be effective in stimulating endogenous FSH and LH secretion in a dog with hypogonadotrophic hypogonadism unless the dysfunction is in the hypothalamus instead of the pituitary gland. Therapy must be continued for at least three months before an assessment of the effectiveness of these injections can be made. The prognosis for return of fertility in these dogs is guarded.

IMMUNE-MEDIATED ORCHITIS

Disruption of the blood-testis barrier may result in exposure of the dog's immune system to spermatozoal antigens, which are not recognized as self antigens. If the damage to the barrier is severe or exposure to these antigens prolonged, an immune-mediated orchitis may develop. It is characterized by an influx of plasma cells and lymphocytes into the testicular parenchyma, seminiferous tubule destruction, and loss of Leydig cells. Clinically, oligospermia to azoospermia with variable loss of libido develops. The involved testis is often small and soft on palpation. Biopsy demonstrates an immunocyte infiltration into the testicular parenchyma. Because of the progressive nature of this condition, the prognosis for return of fertility is poor. Therapy may be attempted using immunosuppressive dosages of glucocorticoids 1 to 1.5 mg/lb/day divided q12h initially) to control the immune reaction. Unfortunately prolonged or excessive dosages of glucocorticoids, which are frequently required for the management of this disorder, will also adversely affect spermatogenesis and lead to infertility. Therefore, the clinician must attempt to control the immune reaction, using the least amount of glucocorticoid given as infrequently as possible to minimize the adverse effects of the therapy. This is seldom possible because controlling the immune-mediated orchitis has usually required large dosages. The effectiveness of other immunosuppressive agents such as azathioprine that do not adversely affect the reproductive tract has yet to be evaluated.

RETROGRADE EJACULATION

Failure of the internal urethral sphincter to contract fully during erection/ejaculation may allow the ejaculated spermatozoa to enter the bladder instead of exiting the penis. The result is azoospermia in a dog with normal libido and mating behavior, which can be a congenital or acquired condition. A diagnosis requires demonstrating the presence of spermatozoa in the urinary bladder of an azoospermic dog after ejaculation. Histologic evaluation of a testicular biopsy is normal, as are plasma gonadotrophin concentrations. The major differential is bilateral duct obstruction and resultant azoospermia. In the latter condition, sperm are not present in the urinary bladder, and results of a testicular biopsy may reveal seminiferous tubule degeneration. Therapy for retrograde ejaculation involves the administration of sympathomimetic agents, such as ephedrine and phenylpropanolamine, that will contract the internal urethral sphincter and force antegrade ejaculation. If this can be accomplished, the prognosis for return of fertility is good.

References

1. Holst, PA and Phemister, RD: Onset of diestrus in the beagle bitch. Definition and significance. J Vet Res 35:401, 1974.
2. Olson, PN, et al.: The use and misuse of vaginal cultures in diagnosing reproductive diseases in the bitch. In Morrow, DA (ed): Current Therapy in Theriogenology II. Philadelphia, WB Saunders, 1986, p 469.
3. Johnston, SD: Diagnostic and therapeutic approach to infertility in the bitch. JAVMA 176:1335, 1980.
4. Lein, DH: Examination of the bitch for breeding soundness. In Kirk, RW (ed): Current Veterinary Therapy VIII. Philadelphia, WB Saunders, 1983, p 909.
5. Olson, PN and Mather, EC: Canine vaginal and uterine bacterial flora. JAVMA 172:708, 1978.
6. Olson, PN, et al.: Infertility in the bitch. In Kirk, RW (ed): Current Veterinary Therapy VIII. Philadelphia, WB Saunders, 1983, p 925.
7. Allen, WE and Dagnall, GJR: Some observations on the aerobic bacterial flora of the genital tract of the dog and bitch. J Sm Anim Pract 23:325, 1982.
8. Baba, E, et al.: Vaginal and uterine microflora of adult dogs. Am J Vet Res 44:606, 1983.
9. Lein, DH: Canine mycoplasma, ureaplasma and bacterial infertility In Kirk, RW (ed): Current Veterinary Therapy IX. Philadelphia, WB Saunders, 1986, p 1240.
10. Hashimoto, A, and Hirai, K: Canine herpesvirus infection. In Morrow, DA (ed): Current Therapy in Theriogenology II. Philadelphia, WB Saunders, 1986, p 516.
11. Poste, G and King, N: Isolation of a herpesvirus from the canine genital tract: association with infertility, abortion, and stillbirths. Vet Rec 88:229, 1971.
12. Senior, DF: Infertility in the cycling bitch. Comp Cont Ed 1:17, 1979.
13. Johnson, MH: Characterization of a natural antibody in normal guinea pig serum reacting with homologous spermatozoa. J Reprod Fertil 16:503, 1968.
14. Nagano, T and Okumura, K: Fine structural changes of allergic aspermatogenesis in the guinea pig. Virchows Arch (Cell Pathol) 14:233, 1973.
15. Bigazzi, PE, et al.: Sperm autoantibodies in vasectomized rats of different inbred strains. Science 197:1282, 1977.
16. Alexander, NJ, et al.: Vasectomy: immunologic effects in monkeys and man. Fertil Steril 25:149, 1974.
17. Bhatt, GN, et al.: Studies on immunoinfertility in repeat breeder cows. Indian Vet J 56:184, 1979.
18. Deo, S and Roy, DJ: Investigations in repeat breeding cows and buffaloes: immunological agglutination of spermatozoa in the cervical mucus. Indian Vet J 48:572, 1971.
19. George, L and Carmichael, L: Antisperm responses in male dogs with chronic Brucella canis infections. Am J Vet Res 45:274, 1984.
20. Rosenthal, RC, et al.: Detection of canine antisperm antibodies by indirect immunofluorescence and gelatin agglutination. Am J Vet Res 45:370, 1984.
21. Mahi-Brown, CA, et al.: Infertility in bitches induced by active immunization with procine zonae pellucidae. J Exp Zoo 222:89, 1982.
22. Al-Bassam, MA, et al.: Normal postpartum involution of the uterus in the dog. Can J Comp Med 45:217, 1981.
23. Wachtel, S: H-Y antigen and the genetics of sex determination. Science 198:797, 1977.
24. Patterson, DF: Disorders of sexual development. AAHA Scientific Proceedings, San Antonio, TX, 1983, p 453.
25. Thun, R, et al.: Induction of estrus and ovulation in the bitch, using exogenous gonadotropins. Am J Vet Res 38:483, 1977.
26. Archibald, LF, et al.: A surgical method for collecting canine embryos after induction of estrus and ovulation with exogenous gonadotrophins. VM/SAC, February, 1980, p 228.

27. Shille, VM, et al.: Induction of abortion in the bitch with a synthetic prostaglandin analog. Am J Vet Res 45:1295, 1984.
28. Takeishi, M, et al: Studies on reproduction in the dog. Induction of estrus by hormonal treatment and results of the following insemination. Jpn J Anim Reprod 22:71, 1976.
29. Chakraborty, PK, et al.: Induction of estrus and evaluation in the cat and dog. Vet Clin North Am 12:85, 1982.
30. Kato, J, et al.: Effect of clomiphene in the uptake of estradiol by the active hypothalamus and hypophysis. Endocrinology 82:1049, 1968.
31. Roy, S, et al.: Effect of clomiphene on the physiology of reproduction in the rat. Acta Endocrinol (Copenh) 47:669, 1964.
32. Paulson, DF, et al: Hypofertility and clomiphene citrate therapy. Fertil Steril 26:982, 1975.
33. Reyes, FL and Faiman, C: Long-term therapy with low-dose cisclomiphene in male infertility: effects on semen, serum FSH, LH, testosterone and estradiol, and carbohydrate tolerance. Int J Fertil 19:49, 1974.
34. Heller, CG, et al.: Clomiphene citrate: a correlation of its effect on sperm concentration and morphology, total gonadotropins, ICSH, estrogen and testosterone excretion, and testicular cytology in normal men. J Clin Endocrinol 29:638, 1969.
35. Feldman, EC and Nelson, RW: Canine and feline endocrinology and reproduction. Philadelphia, WB Saunders, 1987.
36. Olson, PN: Clinical approach to infertility in the stud dog. Proceedings, Society for Theriogenology, Sept. 1984, Denver, p 33.
37. Ganong, WF: The gonads: Development and function of the reproductive system. In Ganong, WF (ed): Review of Medical Physiology, 10th ed. Los Altos, CA, Lange Medical Publications, 1981, p 331.
38. Urry, RL and Cockett, TK: Treating the subfertile male patient: improvement in semen characteristics after low-dose androgen therapy. J Urol 116:54, 1976.
39. Larsen, RE: Testicular biopsy in the dog. Vet Clin North Am 7:747, 1977.
40. Larsen, RE and Johnston, SD: Management of canine infertility. In Kirk, RW (ed): Current Veterinary Therapy VII. Philadelphia, WB Saunders, 1980, p 1226.
41. Burke, TJ: Reproductive disorders. In Ettinger, SJ (ed): Textbook of Veterinary Internal Medicine, 2nd ed. Philadelphia, WB Saunders, 1983, p 1711.

105 CANINE PROSTATIC DISEASES

JEANNE A. BARSANTI and DELMAR R. FINCO

The prostate gland, the only accessory sex gland in the male dog, is a bilobed organ with a median septum on the dorsal surface.[1] It is located predominantly in the retroperitoneal space, just caudal to the bladder in the area of the bladder neck and proximal urethra (Figure 105–1). Only the craniodorsal side is covered by peritoneum. The prostate encircles the proximal urethra at the neck of the bladder, and its ducts enter the urethra throughout its circumference.[2] The position of the prostate in the caudal abdomen depends on age, bladder distention, and disease state.[3] In neonates the prostate is abdominal. After loss of the urachal remnant (at less than two months of age) the prostate resides within the pelvic inlet.[4] With increasing age the prostate again tends to become abdominal in location, so that in intact male dogs over five years of age, most of the prostate gland is abdominal.[3]

Histologically, the prostate gland is composed of glandular acini supported by a stroma of connective tissue and smooth muscle, enclosed by a thick fibromuscular capsule. Columnar glandular epithelium changes to transitional in the excretory ducts opening into the urethra. The cells within the prostate gland are of two types, stromal and epithelial.[5] The epithelial cells are of two types, tall columnar secretory epithelium and basal epithelium located sporadically along the basement membrane. The role of the basal epithelial cells is unknown, but they may be precursors of the secretory epithelium.[5, 6] The stroma consists of fibroblastic and smooth muscle cells enmeshed in collagen with blood vessels and nerves. The fibromuscular stroma is predominant before sexual maturity, at six months to one year of age.[7, 8] After this time the epithelium is predominant.

The purpose of the prostate gland is to produce prostatic fluid as a transport and support medium for sperm during ejaculation. Under parasympathetic stimulation during erection the prostate increases the rate of fluid production, and under sympathetic stimulation it ejects the fluid during ejaculation.[9, 10] Basal secretion of small amounts of prostatic fluid constantly enters the prostatic excretory ducts and prostatic urethra.[11] When neither micturition nor ejaculation is occurring, urethral pressure moves this basally secreted fluid cranially into the bladder (prostatic fluid reflux). During micturition, urine enters the prostate gland in humans (intraprostatic urinary reflux).[12]

With aging the prostate gland increases in weight.[8, 13, 14] Between 4 and 16 months of age (beagles) the prostate grows with a constant doubling time of 0.64 years.[15] This corresponds to the time when serum testosterone is rising to its normal adult level.[15] Once the prostate reaches its normal adult size (12 to 14 gm in beagles), growth stops until prostatic hyperplasia develops. If a dog is castrated before sexual maturity, then normal prostatic growth is completely inhibited.[15] If the dog is castrated as an adult, the prostate will involute to 20 per cent of its normal adult size.[16] Prostatic secretory function, as measured by ejaculate volume, reaches a peak at four years of age in beagles and then begins to decline.[8] There is apparently increased sensitivity of the growth of the prostate gland to testosterone with aging, since testosterone secretion and prostatic testosterone and dihydrotestosterone concentrations decrease with aging.[8] The increase in weight with age is associated with benign prostatic hyperplasia (BPH). BPH has been identified in 40 per cent of beagles by 2.5 years of age, in more than 80 per cent of beagles older than 6 years,[8, 17, 18] and in more than 95 per cent of beagles older than 9 years of age.[18] Thus, with aging, the prostate gland increases in size up to a relative plateau at six years of age, but secretory function begins to decrease after four years of age.[8] In a few older dogs (older than eight years in beagles), another phase of BPH occurs in which the prostate again rapidly increases in size.[18] The reason for this is unknown.

Prostatic diseases are common in the older male dog. With aging, the prostate gradually enlarges because of hyperplasia. Because of the prostate's glandular nature, intraparenchymal prostatic fluid cysts may develop in association with hyperplasia. The prostate is subject to infection from bacteria ascending the urethra. Hematogenous spread of bacteria from the kidneys and bladder by way of urine, or from the testis and epididymis by way of semen is also possible. Bacterial prostatic infections can be acute or chronic and insidious, leading to abscessation. Decreased secretory function in the aging prostate may increase its susceptibility to infection. The aging prostate gland is also subject to neoplastic transformation, most commonly adenocarcinoma. In the presence of excess estrogens, either endogenous or exogenous, the prostatic epithelium will undergo squamous metaplasia.[19, 20] Paraprostatic cysts, which may or

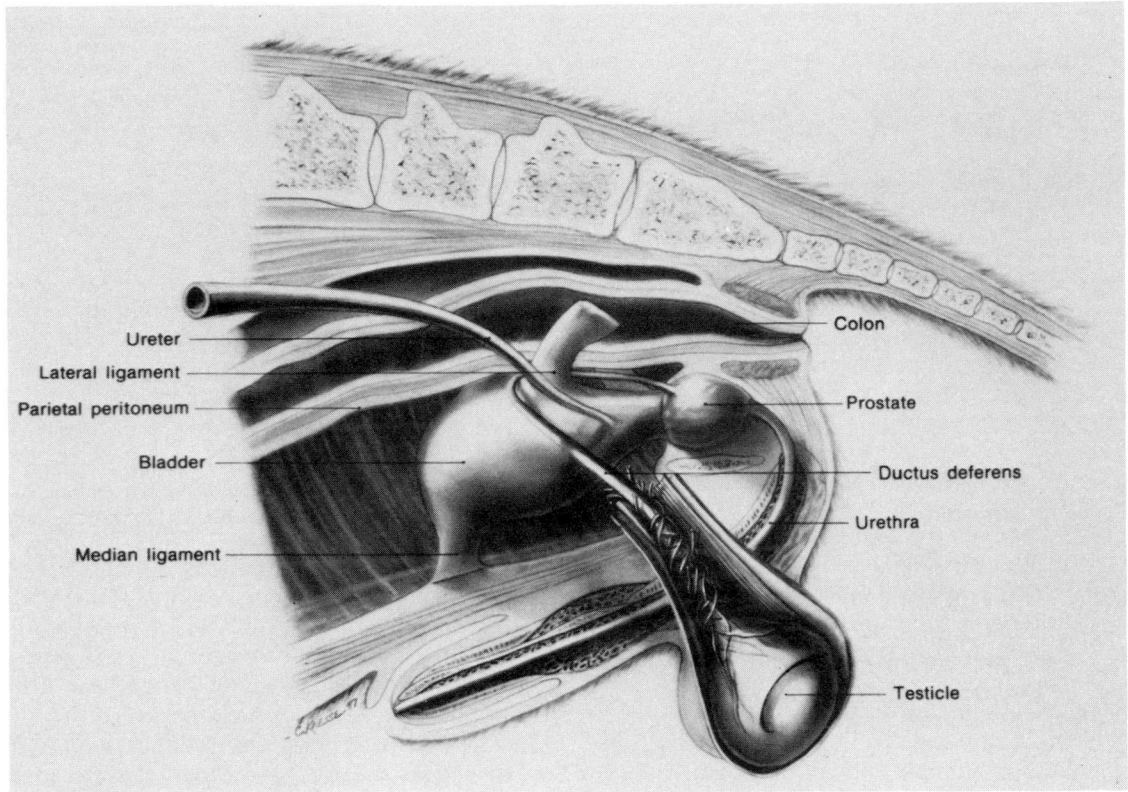

FIGURE 105–1. The relationship of the prostate gland to other structures in the caudal abdomen of the male dog.

may not be of prostatic origin, are usually associated with the prostate and cause the same signs as those associated with prostatomegaly.

Calculi may also be found in canine prostate glands. They are usually small and smoothly marginated.[21] These have been considered incidental findings, unassociated with clinical disease. In recent years in human medicine, prostatic calculi have been identified as the source of chronic infection.[22–24] Human prostatic calculi are largely composed of urinary, not prostatic, constituents.[12, 22] Thus, reflux of urine into the prostate occurs, as well as reflux of prostatic fluid into the bladder.[12, 25] This emphasizes the close association between the two organs. Because no reports of adverse effects of prostatic calculi exist in the veterinary literature, they will not be discussed further.

Other prostatic diseases that are well documented in humans include nonbacterial prostatitis (prostatosis) and prostatodynia.[22, 26] Prostatosis is characterized by the presence of purulent prostatic fluid that is negative for bacteria by routine culture procedures. It may be more common than bacterial prostatitis in humans.[26, 27] The major clinical signs are pain and dysuria without a urethral discharge. The cause is unknown. Some have suggested reflux of urine.[12, 26] Infections with *Mycoplasma* and *Chlamydia* have been implicated by some[28, 29] and discounted by others as causative agents.[22] A similar condition has not been described in dogs. Problems with diagnosis are that experimental infections in dogs indicate that cases of prostatic infection occur in which single samples of prostatic fluid may culture negative and in which prostatic tissue may contain low numbers of organisms, requiring extensive culturing efforts.[30] In

humans as well, the diagnosis must be based on *repeated* inability to culture bacteria and absence of any urinary tract infection.[31] Because little more is known about this condition in dogs at this point, it will not be discussed further.

Prostatodynia refers to prostatic pain with no evidence of inflammation.[22, 26] The cause is unknown, but psychiatric disturbances or micturition disorders such as urethral spasm due to overactivity of pelvic sympathetics have been theorized.[22] Because this type of prostatic disease is currently not recognized in dogs, no further discussion is included.

The purpose of this chapter is to review canine prostatic diseases. In order to do this, the signs associated with prostatic diseases are reviewed, relating the diseases that should be considered to signs. Diagnostic techniques are presented. Signs, diagnosis, and treatment of each disease are reviewed.

CLINICAL SIGNS

Clinical signs vary with the type and severity of prostatic disease (Table 105–1). Any prostatic disease except acute prostatitis can be present without any abnormal signs being evident to the owner. Probable avoidance of some prostatitic diseases is one reason for advocating the neutering of young male dogs. Earlier detection of these diseases may be possible by performing a yearly rectal examination on all mature male dogs.

Tenesmus may be caused by an enlarged prostate gland from any cause encroaching on the rectum in the

TABLE 105–1. CLINICAL SIGNS ASSOCIATED WITH PROSTATIC DISEASES

Fecal Tenesmus	Dysuria	Urethral Discharge	Systemic Signs*	Urinary Tract Infection
Hyperplasia	Cyst	Cyst	Acute bacterial prostatitis	Bacterial prostatitis
Cyst	Abscess	Bacterial prostatitis	Abscess	
Abscess	Neoplasia	Abscess	Neoplasia	
Neoplasia		Neoplasia		

*Fever, depression, pain.
From Barsanti, JA and Finco, DR: Canine prostatic diseases. *In* Morrow, DA (ed.): Current Therapy in Theriogenology II. Philadelphia, WB Saunders, 1986.

pelvic canal. Fecal tenesmus is the only abnormal sign associated with uncomplicated prostatic hyperplasia. Prostatic enlargement also occurs with prostatic abscessation and neoplasia. Detectable prostatic enlargement is uncommon with bacterial prostatitis alone.

If prostatic enlargement is marked, dysuria from urethral obstruction may result. This is an uncommon sign in dogs in contrast to humans, since dogs have much less prostatic tissue lining the urethra. The dog's prostate tends to enlarge outward with hyperplasia, away from the urethra. Partial urethral obstruction is usually noted only in dogs with abscesses, cysts, or neoplasia. However, the authors have encountered one case in which partial urethral obstruction occurred due to chronic prostatic inflammation and hyperplasia with minimal prostatic enlargement (Figure 105–2). If the partial obstruction continues, the bladder detrusor muscle and/or the external bladder sphincter may be damaged, resulting in urinary incontinence. Urodynamic (cystometric and urethral pressure profile) abnormalities are common in dogs with significant prostatic disease, even if there is no history of incontinence.[32] The same is true in humans.[33]

A urethral discharge is a classic sign of prostatic disease. This probably results from increased prostatic fluid production, hemorrhage, and/or exudation of pus from the prostatic acini through the prostatic ducts into the urethra in sufficient quantities not only to reflux into the bladder, but also to drain out the urethral orifice. One must always consider a preputial lesion as a cause for blood or pus from the prepuce. Urethritis is a potential cause of blood or pus dripping from the urethral orifice, but urethritis unassociated with primary

inflammation of the bladder or prostate or urolithiasis is currently considered rare in the dog. Any disease that causes prostatic inflammation or hemorrhage can result in a urethral discharge. Such diseases include cystic hyperplasia, bacterial infection, abscessation, and neoplasia.

Systemic signs of prostatic disease include fever, depression, pain in the caudal abdomen, a stiff gait in the hindlimbs, and leukocytosis. These signs are usually associated with acute bacterial prostatitis, prostatic abscessation (particularly if a localized or diffuse peritonitis has resulted), or prostatic adenocarcinoma. The systemic signs associated with carcinoma may be due to the necrosis and inflammation associated with tumor growth outstripping blood supply. Signs also may be due to metastasis, particularly to vertebral bodies. Another systemic sign seen with suppurative prostatitis or prostatic abscessation is evidence of liver disease (icterus, elevated liver enzymes) and liver dysfunction (prolonged Bromsulphalein retention). This hepatopathy may be due to endotoxemia from prostatic infection with *Escherichia coli*.

Abdominal distention may be noted with very large paraprostatic cysts. Such large cysts may calcify. A firm mass may also be noted in the perineal area if the cyst extends caudally, especially if it is collagenous.

Recurrent lower urinary tract infection in male dogs is often due to chronic bacterial prostatitis and may be the only abnormal sign associated with chronic prostatitis. If the underlying cause of the urinary infection is not suspected, routine antibiotic therapy will result in elimination of bacteriuria. However, the prostatic infection will persist, reinfecting the bladder when antibiotics are discontinued.

DIAGNOSTIC TECHNIQUES FOR PROSTATIC DISEASE

The main diagnostic techniques for prostatic disease are history, prostatic palpation, cytologic examination of any urethral discharge, cytologic and microbiologic examination of prostatic fluid collected by ejaculation or after prostatic massage, radiography, ultrasonography, prostatic aspiration, and prostatic biopsy.

History

A complete history should be obtained, including both the chief complaint and a review of the dog's overall health status. The nature, severity, duration, and pro-

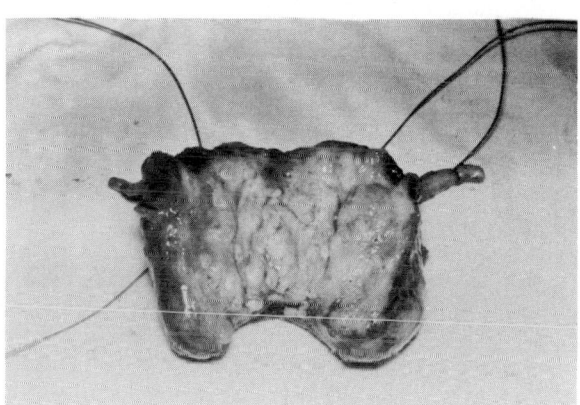

FIGURE 105–2. Prostatectomy specimen opened along the urethra. This tissue was removed from a dog presented for dysuria caused by partial urethral obstruction. The nodular tissue impinging on the urethra was secondary to chronic prostatic inflammation and hyperplasia. (Courtesy of Dr. M. Lappin, University of Georgia.)

gression of the abnormal presenting sign should be determined. It should be established whether urination and defecation are normal or not. Any abnormality should be characterized. The occurrence of any systemic signs of illness (nonlocalized pain, depression, anorexia, vomiting, diarrhea), any lameness, or any changes in water intake or urine output may be important clues to the nature of the disease.

Prostatic Palpation

The prostate is best examined by concomitant rectal and abdominal palpation. The hand palpating the caudal abdomen can both evaluate the cranial aspects of the gland and push the prostate into or near the pelvic canal for better palpation per rectum. The dorsal median groove, the division between the two lobes, is palpable per rectum. The prostate should be evaluated for size, symmetry, surface contour, consistency, movability, and pain. The normal prostate should be symmetric, smooth, movable, and nonpainful. The size in a two- to five-year-old, 25-pound dog was found to vary from ovoid, 1.7 cm in length by 2.6 cm transverse by 0.8 cm dorsoventral, to spheroid, 2 cm in diameter.[34] Size varies, however, with age, body size, and breed, so that judging whether size is normal is subjective. If an increase in size is suspected, estimated measurements should be recorded so that progression can be followed. During the physical examination, the rest of the urinary and reproductive tracts should also be carefully examined.

Urethral Discharge

If a urethral discharge is present, it should be examined microscopically. If sufficient urethral discharge is present, or if the discharge increases with prostatic palpation, the penis can be extruded from the prepuce and cleaned. The discharge can then be collected in a sterile container for culture after extending the penis and cleaning its surface. Quantitative bacterial culture should always be performed because of the presence of normal urethral flora.[35] Any organism isolated by culture should be considered significant only if it is present in large numbers (> 100,000/ml) and if it is also isolated from urine collected by cystocentesis.

Semen Evaluation

An ejaculate is valuable in assessing prostatic disease, since prostatic fluid is the largest component of semen volume (greater than 95 per cent in dogs).[36, 37] The prostatic fluid is the last fraction of the ejaculate, following the sperm-rich fraction. To evaluate a dog for prostatic disease using an ejaculate, the authors first remove any preputial discharge from the penis with gentle, minimal cleansing using gauze sponges and warm water. If any soap is used, it must be thoroughly rinsed off and the penis dried. Contamination of the sample with detergents can invalidate the quantitative bacterial

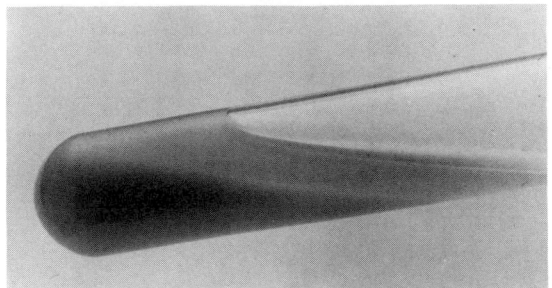

FIGURE 105–3. Ejaculate from a dog with chronic bacterial prostatitis. The sediment contained a large number of neutrophils.

culture.[31] The ejaculate is collected using a sterile funnel and test tube, a sterile large plastic syringe case, or a sterile urine cup. If the dog will not ejaculate by manual stimulation alone, a teaser is used. The bitch may be one in estrus or an anestrous bitch with the dog pheromone methyl-*p*-hydroxybenzoate applied to the vulva.[38] Part of the ejaculate is used for microscopic examination and part for quantitative bacterial culture (Figure 105–3). Quantitative culture is essential, since the distal urethra has a normal bacterial flora.[35]

Both ejaculate cytology and culture must be assessed for accurate interpretation. Normal dogs have occasional white blood cells (WBCs) and positive bacterial cultures.[39] Bacteria are present in less than 100,000/ml and are usually gram-positive. High numbers (> 100,000/ml) of gram-negative organisms with large numbers of WBC indicate infection. High numbers of gram-positive organisms with large numbers of WBC probably also indicate infection if preputial contamination did not occur. Lower numbers of gram-negative or -positive organisms must be correlated with clinical signs, results of urinalysis and urine culture, and ejaculate cytology to determine significance.[30] Dogs with experimental chronic bacterial prostatitis usually had > 1000 organisms/ml.[30] Blood may be found in ejaculates in dogs with bacterial infection, prostatic cysts, prostatic neoplasia, and hyperplasia.

An abnormality in the ejaculate does not localize the problem to the prostate, since the testes, epididymis, deferent ducts, and urethra also contribute to or transport the ejaculate. Collecting and comparing the early fraction of the ejaculate, which is of testicular origin, with a late fraction of prostatic origin may help to localize an abnormal finding.

Use of a urethral swab has been advocated to rule out urethral contamination as a cause of a positive ejaculate culture (Figure 105–4).[37] With this technique, the sterile swab is advanced several centimeters into the distal urethra after cleansing and drying the penis. The swab is placed in 3 ml of sterile saline and agitated. The saline is then cultured quantitatively. Larger numbers of organisms in the ejaculate than from the urethral swab by a factor of 10^2 is reported to be diagnostic of prostatic infection. However, in dogs with experimental prostatitis, some dogs without prostatic infection had higher numbers of gram-positive organisms in the ejaculate than in the urethral swab, and some dogs with urinary tract infection and prostatic infection had high numbers of the same organism in the urethral swab

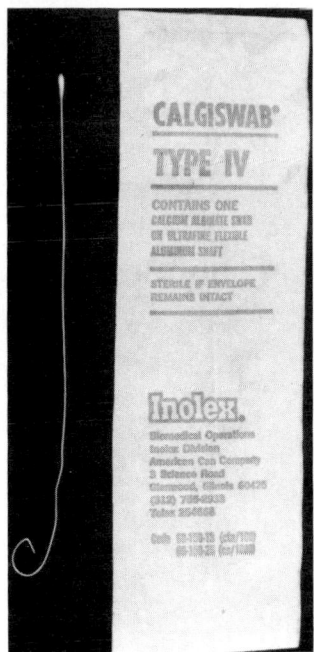

FIGURE 105–4. Swab that can be used to determine the bacterial flora of the distal urethra.

sample. In men as well, contamination with urethral organisms may be greater in the prostatic fluid than in the urethral specimen.[40] Both these problems indicate that results from urethral swabs may be misleading in some cases. The authors use the swabs primarily in dogs without urinary tract infection and with questionable numbers of organisms in the ejaculate, to determine what the distal urethral flora of that particular dog is for comparison with the suspected infecting agent.

Prostatic Massage

Because of the dog's pain, inexperience, or temperament, it is not possible to collect semen in all cases of prostatic disease. An alternative technique to collect prostatic fluid is prostatic massage.[39] The dog is allowed to urinate first to empty the bladder. A urinary catheter is then passed to the bladder, using aseptic technique. The bladder is emptied and flushed several times with sterile saline solution to ensure that it is empty. The last flush of 5 to 10 ml is saved as the preprostatic massage sample. The catheter is then retracted distal to the prostate as determined by rectal palpation. The prostate is massaged rectally, per abdomen, or both for one to two minutes. Sterile physiologic saline is injected slowly through the catheter with the urethral orifice occluded around the catheter to prevent reflux of the fluid out the urethral orifice. The catheter is slowly advanced to the bladder with repeated aspiration, especially from the area of the prostate as determined by rectal palpation. The majority of the fluid will be aspirated from the bladder. Both the premassage and postmassage samples are examined microscopically and by quantitative culture. The authors consider it important to compare the postmassage sample with the premassage sample to be sure any abnormality was due to prostatic fluid

and did not pre-exist in the bladder or urethra (Figure 105–5). Prostatic massage in normal dogs produces only a few red blood and transitional epithelial cells.[39]

Disadvantages of prostatic massage include the inability of knowing whether prostatic fluid has been obtained without comparison with a presample, and the difficulty in detecting increases in bacterial numbers in prostatic fluid if urine is infected.[30, 31] In these cases the authors have administered antibiotics that enter the urine well but do not enter prostatic fluid (e.g., ampicillin) for one day before massage.[30, 31, 41–43] The samples obtained must be cultured immediately so that the antibiotic in the urine does not kill any bacteria in the prostatic fluid after collection.[31] In experimental infection, this method identified three of six cases, but in two of six dogs all cultures became negative despite continuing prostatic infection.[30] When antibiotics are being given, even low counts of bacteria may be significant.[31] Cytologic evidence of inflammation was highly correlated with prostatic infection[30] and is often helpful in determining whether inflammatory prostatic disease exists. Normal prostatic epithelial cells are cuboid and uniform with central round to oval nuclei and moderate, lightly basophilic cytoplasm.[44] A few large transitional cells are often seen that may be binucleate.

In cases in which involvement of the prostatic urethra is suspected (in the presence of dysuria or suggestive radiographic findings), a urinary catheter biopsy technique[43] can be combined with prostatic massage. This can be especially useful in cases of neoplasia of either prostatic or transitional epithelial cell origin.[46] This technique involves placing the catheter in the prostatic urethra by rectal palpation, attaching a syringe containing a small amount of sterile saline solution to the catheter, applying negative pressure, and then rapidly moving the catheter back and forth. Negative pressure is maintained and the catheter quickly withdrawn. Slides for cytology are prepared from the material collected.

Radiography

The size, location, and contour of the prostate may be determined by radiography of the caudal abdomen.[47]

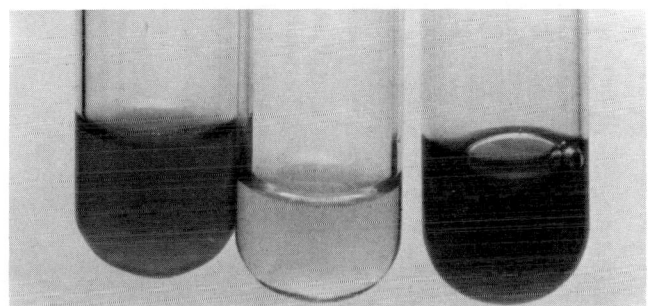

FIGURE 105–5. Samples collected during prostatic massage in a dog with hematuria of unknown origin. Samples from left to right are urine, the preprostatic massage sample, and the postprostatic massage sample. Blood was most predominant in the postmassage sample, suggesting prostatic disease as the origin of the hematuria. Cystic hyperplasia was identified by prostatic biopsy.

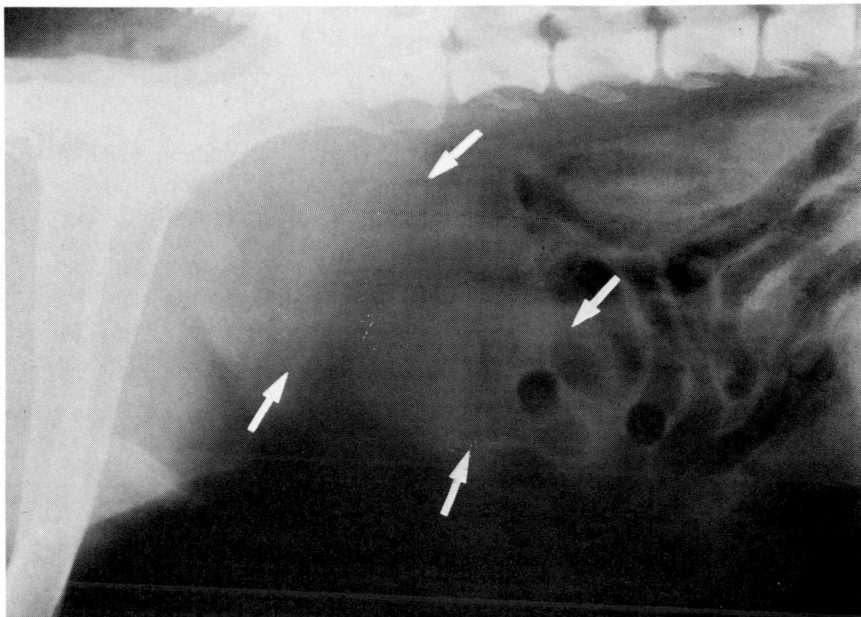

FIGURE 105–6. Lateral radiograph of the caudal abdomen of a dog with marked prostatomegaly (bladder, cranial arrows; prostate, caudal arrows).

The prostate is often distinguishable on lateral and dorsoventral survey views (Figure 105–6). In some cases, contrast cystography may be necessary to delineate the position of the bladder as a landmark for locating the prostate (Figure 105–7). The normal gland is symmetric with a smooth contour and is located near the cranial rim of the pelvic floor. As discussed, the size varies with the age, body size, and breed of dog. However, a normal-sized prostate does not displace the colon or the bladder from their normal positions. On a lateral radiograph there is often a well-defined triangle between the cranioventral aspect of the prostate and the bladder, due to a fat pad.[48]

Survey radiography is often of limited benefit in diagnosis of specific prostatic diseases.[49] In many cases the prostate can be palpated more accurately than it can be visualized on survey radiographs. Poor contrast of

caudal abdominal structures may exist with abscessation, carcinoma, and paraprostatic cysts. Asymmetric shape is also noted with abscess, neoplasia, and cysts.[50] Granular mineralization can be seen with inflammation or neoplasia.[51] Marked prostatic enlargement is most often associated with abscess, cysts, and neoplasia.[50, 51]

Changes in urethral size and presence of reflux of contrast material into the prostate on retrograde urethrography were initially associated with specific diseases. However, more recent surveys have found variable results with different diseases and in normal dogs.[21, 50, 52–56] Characteristics of the prostatic urethra vary with degree of bladder distention.[57, 58] Narrowing of the prostatic urethra can be found normally.[58] In order to avoid variations in technique, distention retrograde urethrocystography has been recommended as the contrast study of choice.[21, 52, 53] With this method the urinary

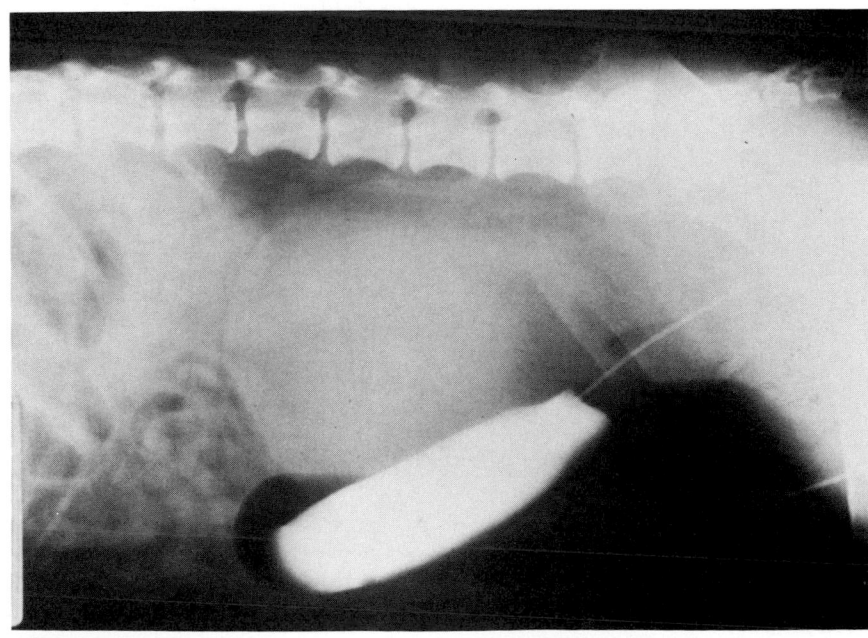

FIGURE 105–7. Positive contrast cystogram. The large structure dorsal to the bladder is a large paraprostatic cyst.

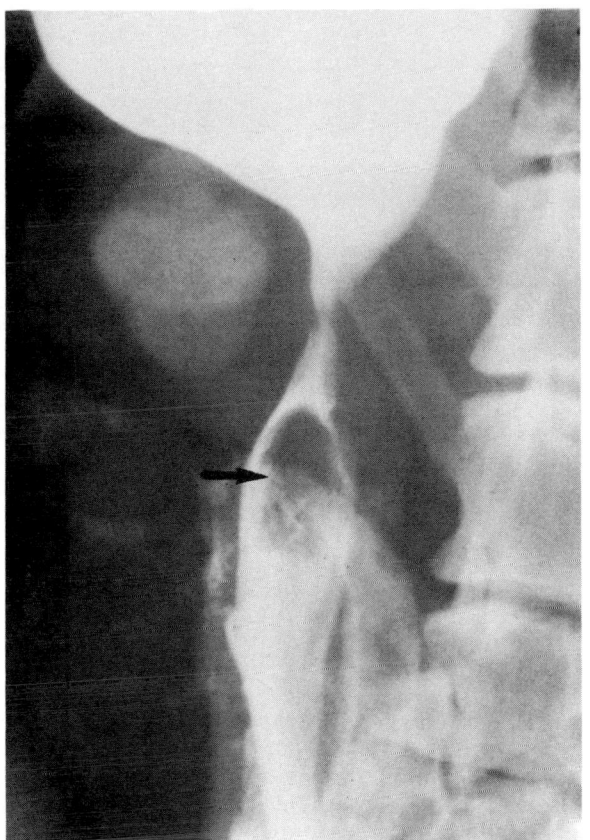

FIGURE 105–8. Retrograde urethrogram in a dog with prostatomegaly, cryptorchidism, and gynecomastia. A large nipple is evident, as is urethroprostatic reflux, and the colliculus seminalis (arrow). A Sertoli-cell tumor of the testis and squamous metaplasia of the prostate were identified in tissue specimens removed surgically.

bladder is palpably distended prior, and then retrograde infusion of the contrast media is performed using end-hole balloon catheters. The normal diameter of the prostatic urethra is 1.0 to 2.7 times the diameter of the midpelvic membranous urethra. The prostate should be symmetric around the urethra. The colliculus seminalis (urethral crest) may be visualized on distention urethrocystography in normal dogs (Figure 105–8).[21] Mild

urethroprostatic reflux is normal.[56] This normal reflux usually does not extend more than one prostatic urethral diameter into the prostatic parenchyma. Marked increases in size are most commonly associated with abscessation, neoplasia, and paraprostatic cysts.[51] A narrowed prostatic urethra can be noted with neoplasia, abscessation, large parenchymal cysts, and, rarely, hyperplasia.[59] If the prostatic urethra is markedly irregular, neoplasia is most likely. If the prostate is markedly asymmetric in relation to the urethra, abscessation, parenchymal cyst, or neoplasia is most likely.[51] Although retrograde urethrography with bladder distention may allow better assessment of the prostatic urethra and prostate gland, the technique has potential complications. These include hematuria and induction of urinary tract infection along with the possibility of bladder rupture if significant bladder wall disease or injury is present.[60–62]

Voiding urethrography has also been used to evaluate the prostatic urethra in normal dogs.[58] With this technique the prostatic urethra may dilate and urethral contractions occur just distal to the prostate gland. The technique has not been systematically evaluated in dogs with prostatic disease.

If the prostate is markedly enlarged, excretory urography is often necessary to determine whether ureteral obstruction is occurring. This is especially important in cases with clinical evidence of reduced renal function, such as reduced concentrating ability or azotemia.

If prostatic neoplasia is a likely possibility, thoracic and abdominal radiographs should be examined for evidence of metastasis (Figure 105–9). The main metastatic route for prostatic adenocarcinoma is by way of pelvic lymphatics to the sublumbar lymph nodes, to the vertebral bodies, and to the lungs.

Ultrasonography

Prostatic consistency can be evaluated better with ultrasound than with radiography.[59, 63, 64] The prostate gland can often be visualized by ultrasound, since it is

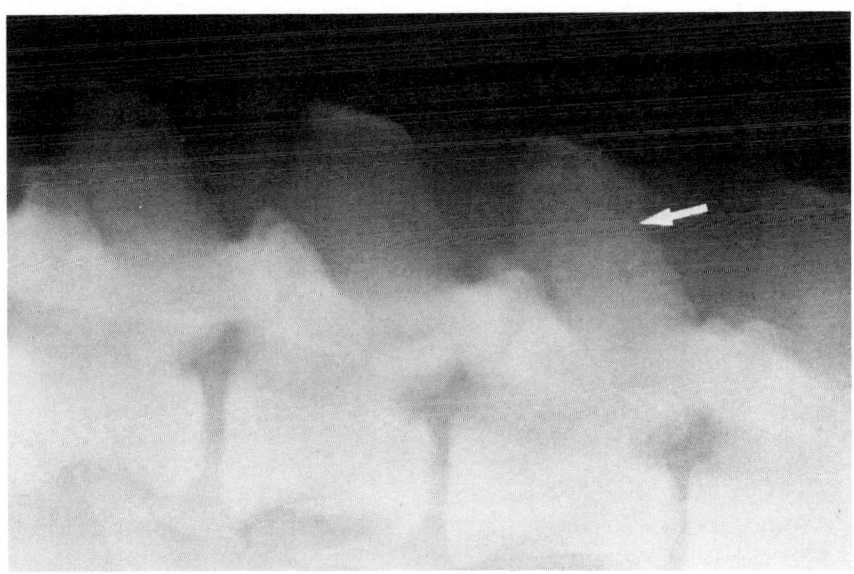

FIGURE 105–9. Metastasis to the dorsal spine of a lumbar vertebra (solid arrow) in a dog with prostatic adenocarcinoma. The dog is the same as shown in Figure 105–6.

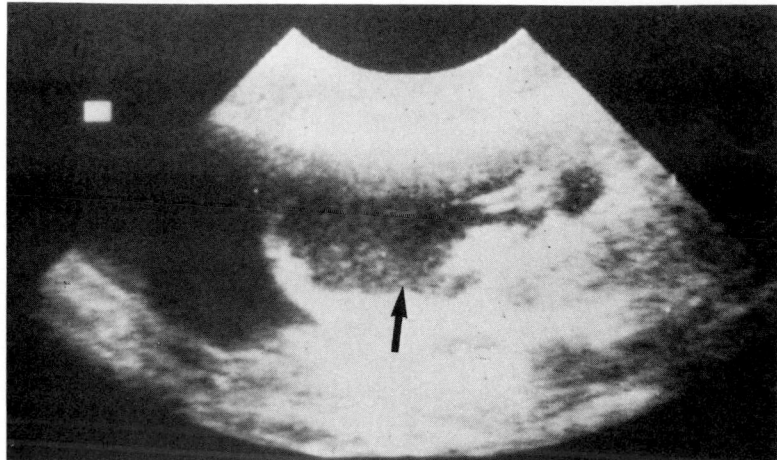

FIGURE 105–10. Ultrasonogram of a dog with a prostatic abscess (bladder, cranial, black area; prostate gland with anechoic area, solid arrow).

usually abdominal in position when enlarged, since there are few other structures between the skin and it, and since the urinary bladder can be used as a landmark. Dogs can usually be examined in dorsal recumbency without sedation. Ultrasound can be useful even in the presence of abdominal fluid or loss of intra-abdominal fat.

Increased general parenchymal echogenicity can be observed with any prostatic disease. Diseases such as inflammation and neoplasia may have focal to multifocal areas of increased echogenicity, whereas cavitating diseases, such as intraparenchymal cysts or abscesses, appear focally hypoechoic to anechoic (Figure 105–10).[59] Ultrasonography can also differentiate paraprostatic cysts from other caudal abdominal masses.[21, 59, 65] Combining retrograde urethrocystography with ultrasonography may be of value, since bladder distention can help

in identification of the prostate gland. Ultrasonography can also provide guidance for aspiration and biopsy.[66, 67]

Prostatic Aspiration

Diagnosis of prostatic disease can be aided by needle aspiration or biopsy. Needle aspiration is most easily done in the dog by the perirectal or transabdominal routes, depending on the location of the prostate. The procedure is done aseptically using a long needle with a stylet, such as a spinal needle. In the perirectal approach the needle is guided by rectal palpation (Figure 105–11). In the transabdominal approach the needle can be guided by palpation or ultrasound.[66] The procedure can be performed in most dogs with mild tranquilization. Needle aspiration is probably best avoided in dogs with

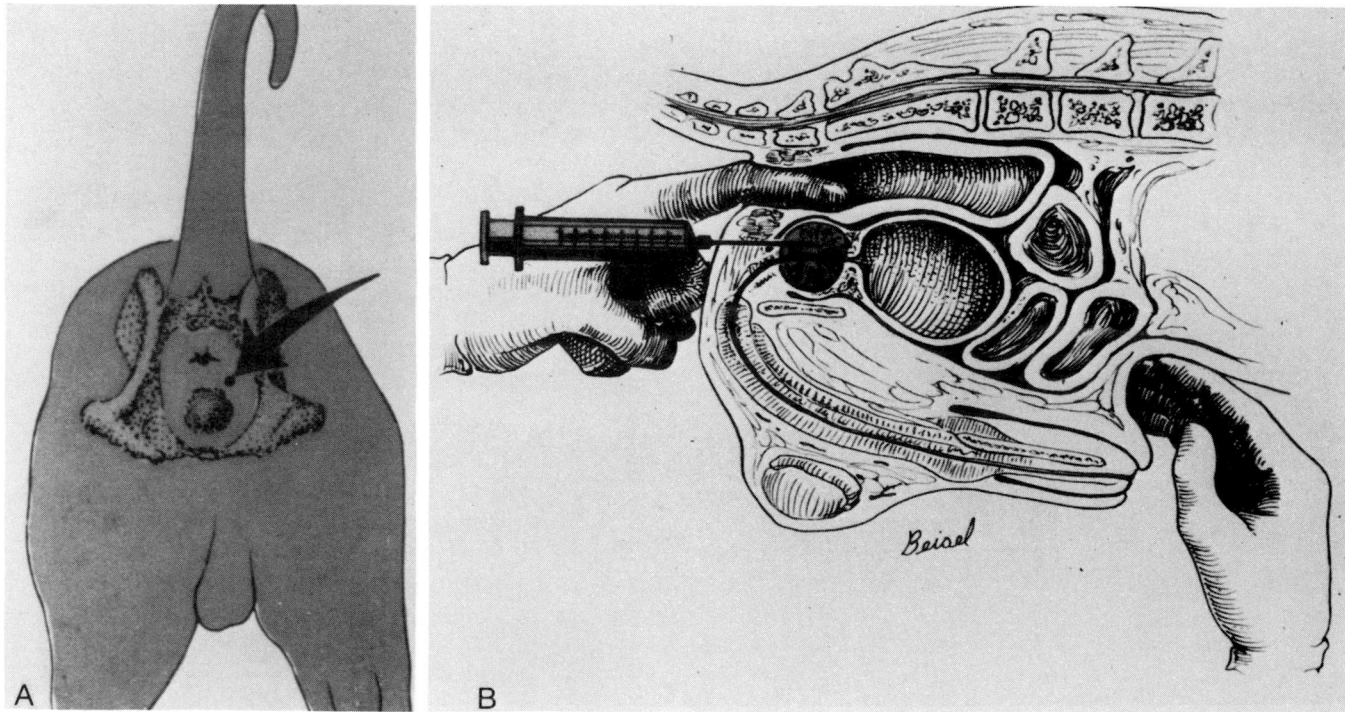

A

B

FIGURE 105–11. *A* and *B,* Perirectal aspiration of the prostate gland. (From Barsanti, JA and Finco, DR: Canine bacterial prostatitis. Vet Clin North Am 9:686, 1979.)

abscessation, since large numbers of bacteria may be seeded along the needle tract. The authors do not perform aspiration in dogs with fever or leukocytosis, or before examining prostatic fluid obtained by ejaculation or massage. Despite these precautions the authors have inadvertently diagnosed abscessation in at least seven dogs by aspiration. All dogs were immediately placed on oral antimicrobial therapy. No complications were noted in four dogs; however, two underwent surgery within 24 hours. In three dogs evidence of a localized peritonitis characterized by fever, pain, and vomiting developed, requiring intravenous antibiotics and fluid therapy. Because of the possibility of an occult abscess, aspiration should always be performed before a closed biopsy. Ultrasonography before or during aspiration is advisable if available. If an abscess is aspirated, antimicrobial therapy should be begun, pending culture results, and the patient should be carefully observed for at least 48 hours.

Prostatic Biopsy

Percutaneous (closed) prostatic biopsy can be performed perirectally (Figure 105–11) or transabdominally, or it can be done directly after the gland is exposed surgically (Figure 105–12).[39, 68, 69] Closed biopsy can be performed with tranquilization and local anesthesia.[69] The biopsy needle can be guided by palpation, as in aspiration, or ultrasound.[66] The authors usually use a Tru-Cut needle. If prostatic abscessation is being considered in the differential diagnosis, aspiration should always precede a blind biopsy technique. Parenchymal cystic lesions, identifiable by ultrasound, should be aspirated rather than biopsied. Acute, septic inflammation is also considered a contraindication to biopsy. With these precautions, the most common complication reported from biopsy in dogs is mild hematuria,[39, 70] although significant hemorrhage is possible, as with any biopsy procedure. Orchitis and scrotal edema were reported in one dog.[68] Dogs should be closely observed for several hours after biopsy. Biopsy samples can be used for bacterial culture as well as for histologic examination.

We often advise prostatic biopsy if castration is recommended as adjunctive therapy. A caudal abdominal incision with traction on the bladder will allow visualization of the prostate for biopsy. An accurate diagnosis can be made and surgical therapy instituted if necessary.

PROSTATIC DISEASES

Benign Hyperplasia

Pathophysiology. Benign prostatic hyperplasia (BPH) is an aging change that occurs in only two species, man and dog.[15, 33, 71] In dogs hyperplasia is primarily uniform and epithelial in contrast to humans, in which the hyperplasia is primarily stromal and nodular.[1, 15, 72–74] However, the natural course of hyperplasia is remarkably similar in both species.[71, 75] It is associated with an altered androgen-estrogen ratio, and requires the presence of the testes.[13, 76–79] In order to produce BPH in young castrated dogs, both androgens and estrogens must be administered.[15, 20] Dihydrotestosterone within the gland probably serves as one hormonal mediator for hyperplasia,[71, 76, 80–83] although some disagree.[84] Dihydrotestosterone accumulates because of changes in catabolism and enhanced binding.[80, 85] Inhibitors of the final enzyme (5-α-reductase) in the synthetic pathway for dihydrotestosterone may hold promise for treatment of BPH.[72] The hyperplastic process is facilitated by estrogens, which may enhance androgen receptors.[80, 86–89] Thus, even in the face of declining androgen production with age, with the presence of increasing estrogen production (estrone and estradiol),[76] hyperplasia develops.[13, 80] Although size increases with hyperplasia, prostatic secretory function decreases (decreased seminal volume).[13, 16, 90]

BPH in the dog begins as glandular hyperplasia.[17] This begins as early as 2.5 years of age in some dogs.[17, 18, 91] After four years of age the tendency to cystic hyperplasia begins,[17, 18] appearing like a honeycomb on cross section. Thus intraprostatic cystic hyperplasia is an extension of glandular hyperplasia.[7, 16, 91, 92] Intraparenchymal cysts often communicate with the urethra and may be largest at the periphery of the gland.[16] The vascularity of the prostate is increased in hyperplasia, and the gland has a tendency to bleed.[16] Evidence of mild chronic inflammation is also common.[13, 14, 93] The cysts vary in size and contour, and contain a thin clear to amber fluid.[7] In an individual dog, BPH seems to develop rapidly (within one year).[18]

Because hyperplasia is an aging change, it occurs concomitantly with the other prostatic diseases to be discussed.

Clinical Signs. Prostatic hyperplasia can be present without abnormal signs. In other dogs, tenesmus associated with defecation may be present because of encroachment on the pelvic canal by the enlarged prostate. In one study of 30 dogs with hyperplasia, the average size of the prostate was 5.5 by 5.1 by 3.1 cm and weight was 34.3 gm, or 1.34 gm/kg.[7]

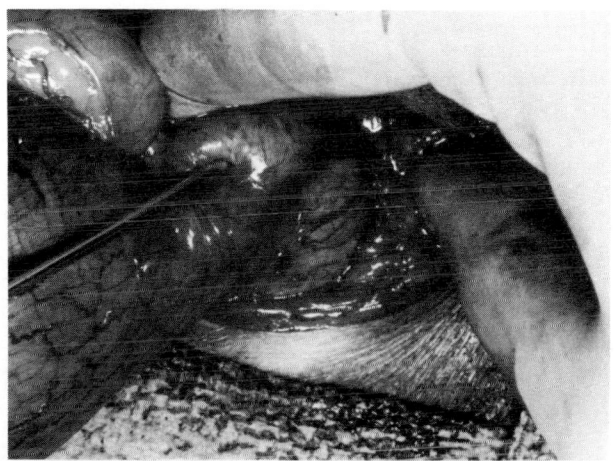

FIGURE 105–12. Tru-Cut needle biopsy of the prostate gland by way of caudal celiotomy. The prostate gland appears normal. (From Barsanti, JA and Finco, DR: Canine prostatic diseases. *In* Morrow, DA (ed): Current Therapy in Theriogenology II. Philadelphia, WB Saunders, 1986.)

An intermittent hemorrhagic or clear light-yellow urethral discharge or intermittent or persistent hematuria occurs in some dogs in which biopsy findings were limited to cystic hyperplasia. Hyperplasia is not associated with any systemic signs of illness. The affected dog is alert, active, and afebrile. Occasional dogs with a hemorrhagic urethral discharge have been found to have von Willebrand's disease. The relation of this finding to the hemorrhagic discharge is unknown.

Diagnosis. On physical examination, the prostate is nonpainful and symmetrically enlarged with normal consistency. Hematologic findings are normal. Urinalysis may be normal or contain blood. Abdominal radiographs confirm mild to moderate prostatic enlargement with dorsal displacement of the colon and cranial displacement of the bladder. Otherwise, the prostate appears normal.[50] On distention retrograde urethrocystography, the prostatic urethra may be normal or it may appear narrowed and undulant without distortion or destruction.[51] Urethroprostatic reflux may be greater than normal. On ultrasonography, the prostate is often normal, but it may also be diffusely hyperechoic with parenchymal cavities if intraparenchymal cysts have developed. If a urethral discharge is present, the discharge is hemorrhagic or clear but not purulent.[94] Semen and postprostatic massage samples may be normal or hemorrhagic (Figure 105–5).[94] Prostatic epithelial cells, when seen, appear normal.[44] Definitive diagnosis is possible only by biopsy. A presumptive diagnosis can be made by history and physical examination with support from hematology, urinalysis, and prostatic fluid analysis, depending on the severity of the presenting complaint. The authors usually do not recommend biopsy for confirmation of the diagnosis if the clinical signs are typical. Response to castration can be used to help confirm the diagnosis.

Treatment. Treatment is required only if related abnormal signs are present. The most effective treatment is castration, which will result in a 70 per cent decrease in prostate size.[16, 79, 95] The prostate gland will begin to involute within days, and a palpable decrease in prostatic size is expected within seven to ten days.[96] Prostatic secretion will become minimal at 7 to 16 days after castration.[16, 36] In both young and old dogs prostatic weight declines most rapidly within the first month after castration.[97] In dogs older than six years, prostatic weight continues to decline for three to four months.[16, 97] With cystic hyperplasia, small irregular spaces may remain postcastration.[16]

If castration is not feasible, low doses of estrogens can be used. Estrogens depress gonadotrophin secretion by the pituitary gland, which reduces the level of androgen secreted by the testes and results in prostatic atrophy. Diethylstilbestrol (DES) administered orally at 0.2 to 0.1 mg/day for five days or every few days for three weeks has been recommended.[98] Low doses of estrogens primarily act to decrease prostatic size. There may be no effect on intraparenchymal cysts.[16] Effective doses of estrogens have not been determined. In one study, 0.1 mg of injectable DES per day for five days markedly reduced prostatic secretory capability for two months.[19] Oral doses of 5 mg/day of DES resulted in death within two months, but doses of 1 mg/day were given for nine

months without development of anemia.[99] The potential side effects of these drugs must be weighed against their clinical benefit in each case before a decision is made to administer them. Initial leukocytosis with a left shift is followed by severe bone marrow depression with resultant anemia, thrombocytopenia, and leukopenia. These effects have been noticed with overdosage, with repeated administration, and at the recommended dose as an idiosyncratic reaction.[100, 101] Although low doses of estrogens decrease prostatic size, repeated administration and overdosage can also cause growth of the fibromuscular stroma of the prostate, metaplasia of prostatic glandular epithelium, and secretory stasis.[16, 102] These changes can result in further prostatic enlargement and a predisposition to cyst formation, bacterial infection, and abscessation.

An experimental drug that avoids the side effects of estrogens is the anti-androgen flutamide. When this drug was administered to research dogs at 2.2 mg/lb (5 mg/kg) per day orally, prostatic size decreased with no change in libido or sperm production.[103] Unfortunately the drug is not commercially available. Megestrol acetate also has anti-androgenic properties.[104–106] In men, megestrol reduces serum testosterone concentrations and competitively inhibits binding of dihydrotestosterone to intracellular receptors and inhibits 5-α-reductase.[104, 105] However, concentrations of plasma testosterone tend to rise again with continued therapy.[105] The efficacy of megestrol for therapy of BPH in dogs has not been studied. The antifungal drug ketoconazole and luteinizing hormone releasing factors are also anti-androgenic.[106–109]

Squamous Metaplasia

Pathophysiology. Squamous metaplasia of prostatic columnar epithelium is secondary to exogenous or endogenous hyperestrogenism.[7, 16, 19, 20, 77, 78, 102, 110] The major endogenous cause is a functional Sertoli-cell tumor. Estrogens also cause secretory stasis. The epithelial change plus secretory stasis predispose to cyst formation, infection, and abscessation.[91, 98]

Clinical Signs. The prostate is usually mildly to moderately enlarged. The testes may be palpably abnormal or one or both testes may be cryptorchid. The opposite testis is usually atrophied. Other clinical signs of hyperestrogenism, including alopecia, hyperpigmentation, gynecomastia, pendulous prepuce, nonregenerative anemia, thrombocytopenia, granulocytosis, or granulocytopenia, may be present (Figure 105–8).[110]

Diagnosis. Increased numbers of squamous epithelial cells may be noted in prostatic fluid or tissue.[9, 44] There may also be evidence of inflammation.[9, 44]

Presumptive diagnosis is based on history, clinical signs, and, in cases of Sertoli-cell tumors, histologic evaluation of the testes. Definitive diagnosis requires prostatic biopsy.

Treatment. Treatment requires removal of the source of estrogens, usually by castration in cases of endogenous hyperestrogenism and by discontinuation of medication in cases of exogenous hyperestrogenism. Squamous metaplasia of the epithelium is reversible.[16]

Paraprostatic Cysts

Pathophysiology. Occasionally a large cyst is found adjacent to the prostate and associated with it by way of a stalk or adhesions.[98, 111] The cyst may also be closely associated with the dorsal wall of the bladder.[4, 111] These large cysts may be remnants of the uterus masculinus or markedly enlarged prostatic cysts (prostatic retention cysts).[9, 111, 112] With a cyst arising from the uterus masculinus, the origin should be on the dorsal midline of the prostate gland.[98] The prostate gland itself should be normal for the age of the dog (e.g., hyperplasia may be present). Proven cases of uterus masculinus are rare.[113] With a prostatic retention cyst, the rest of the prostate gland is abnormal. The origin of most large cysts is obscure.[114] They may be in the abdomen craniolateral to the prostate gland or in the pelvis caudal to the prostate, even extending to the perineum lateral to the anus. Some are in both sites. They can have a thin or thick wall, with a smooth lining or masses of calcified material.[98, 114]

Clinical Signs. With large cysts, clinical signs may be related to their size, with encroachment on the urethra or colon, resulting in dysuria or fecal tenesmus, respectively.[111] If the cyst is sufficiently large, abdominal distention may be seen. Alternatively, the cyst may extend into the perineal region and be palpated there.[111] These cysts may calcify so that they may feel firm.[98, 114] A history of hematuria or intermittent hemorrhagic, serosanguineous, or yellow urethral discharge may be noted.[114]

Diagnosis. Hematologic findings are usually normal, but a neutrophilic leukocytosis has been noted in about 30 per cent of cases in one series.[111] Urinalysis is usually normal, although hematuria is possible if hemorrhage occurs into the cyst and the cyst communicates with the urethra. If a urethral discharge is present, it should be examined cytologically to differentiate a urethral discharge from urine; a fluid analysis can be performed on both and compared in regard to pH, specific gravity, and dipstick analysis. Cyst fluid usually has had more protein than urine from the same patient.[111] Prostatic fluid collected by ejaculation or postprostatic massage should be examined. Prostatic cyst fluid is usually yellow to serosanguineous, has low numbers of WBCs, and is sterile (Figure 105–13).[98] Whether cyst fluid will be obtained by ejaculation or prostatic massage depends on whether the cyst communicates with the urethra.

On survey radiographs there may be poor contrast in the caudal abdomen with asymmetric or irregular prostatic shape.[6] With very large cysts, two "bladders" may be evident. Cystography may be necessary to determine which structure is the bladder (Figure 105–7). Paraprostatic cysts may mineralize, appearing with a density similar to that of egg shells (Figure 105–14).[4, 21, 111, 112, 114] On distention retrograde urethrocystography, the prostate may appear asymmetric around the urethra and the prostatic urethral lumen may be narrowed.[51] Urethroprostatic reflux may be greater than normal. However, contrast material often does not reflux into the large cyst itself.[111] Ultrasound can confirm that the mass is cystic by its being hypoechoic to anechoic with smooth

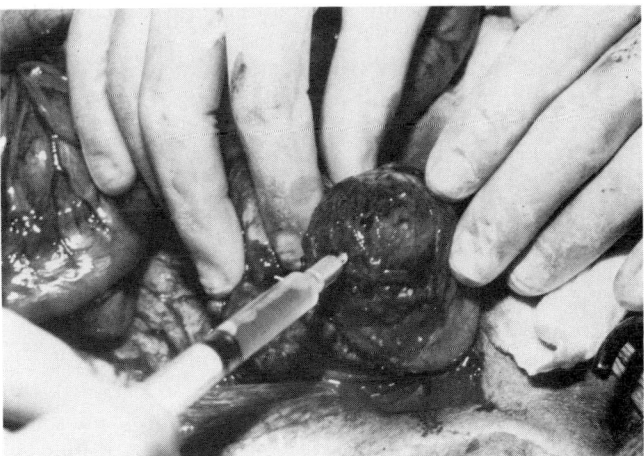

FIGURE 105–13. Aspiration of fluid from a paraprostatic cyst at surgery.

internal margins.[59] Ultrasound can be used to direct fine needle aspiration.

Treatment. The recommended treatment for paraprostatic cysts is surgical drainage with excision or marsupialization if excision is not possible.[98, 111, 115–117] Castration is also recommended. One potential complication of marsupialization is chronic infection.[118]

Bacterial Prostatitis

Pathophysiology. Bacterial prostatitis affects sexually mature male dogs. *E. coli* is the organism most frequently isolated, but infection with other gram-negative and gram positive organisms and with *B. canis* is possible.[119] Infection usually results from ascent of bacteria up the urethra, but it may also result from hematogenous infection, infection of bladder urine, and infection of semen. Signs of infection with *B. canis* are more often

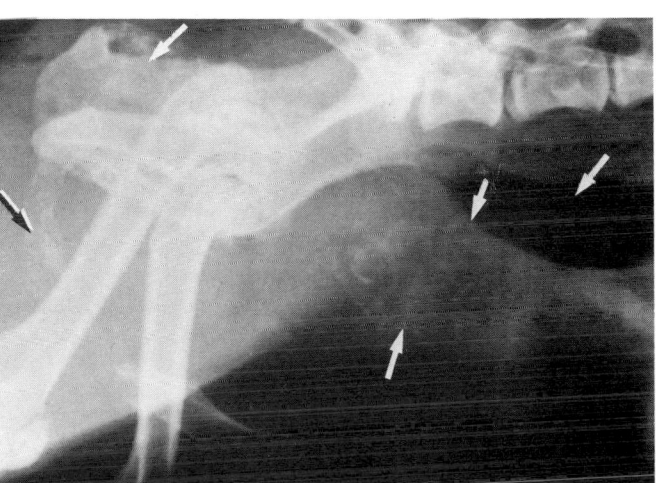

FIGURE 105–14. Survey radiograph of the caudal abdomen, showing a mineralized prostatic cyst (solid arrows). Note that the cyst extends from the caudal abdomen through the pelvic canal and into the perineal area. The colon is visible as the air-filled viscus dorsal to the cyst (black-and-white arrow), and the bladder is visible cranial to the cyst (white arrow, top left).

related to orchitis and scrotal dermatitis than to the prostate gland per se.[119]

The prostate glands of normal male dogs and men produce an antibacterial substance,[11] referred to as prostatic antibacterial factor (PAF).[120] The PAF has been found to be a heat-stable, water-soluble, low-molecular-weight zinc-complexed polypeptide with wide antibacterial efficacy, especially against gram-negative enteric organisms.[22] The antibacterial activity of PAF is due to its zinc content.[120] Men with chronic bacterial prostatitis have decreased prostatic fluid zinc concentrations, but it is unknown whether this is a cause or an effect.[22, 121–125] Dietary supplementation with zinc has no effect on prostatic fluid zinc concentrations.[22, 123] Dogs with chronic prostatitis have normal concentrations of zinc in their prostatic fluid and tissue.[126–128]

Men with prostatic infections have increased prostatic fluid concentrations of IgA antibodies against the specific bacteria involved.[129–131] This has been used as a diagnostic test in men with equivocal culture results.[22] It has been postulated that increased IgA concentrations are a response to a relative lack of PAF in men with chronic bacterial prostatitis, but this remains unproved.[22]

Acute Bacterial Prostatitis

Clinical Signs. Clinical signs include signs of systemic illness, such as anorexia, depression, and fever. Vomiting is possible due to an associated localized peritonitis. Caudal abdominal pain may be present that can be localized to the prostate gland by palpation. A low percentage of affected dogs have a stiff, stilted gait. A constant or intermittent urethral discharge may be present.

Diagnosis. Prostatic palpation often elicits pain. The size, symmetry, and contour of the prostate gland are often normal to mildly enlarged. The enlargement is often due to hyperplasia in the older dog, rather than a direct result of infection. A neutrophilic leukocytosis, with or without a left shift, often exists. Urine usually has blood, WBC, and bacteria present. If the urinalysis indicates urinary tract infection (UTI), a quantitative urine culture and sensitivity testing should be performed on a sample collected by cystocentesis or catheterization. A presumptive diagnosis is based on history, physical examination, hematology, urinalysis, and urine culture. Acute prostatitis often causes too much pain to allow ejaculation. Prostatic massage is contraindicated in human medicine for fear of inducing septicemia.[22, 132] The authors have not induced bacteremia with massage in dogs with experimental infections. However, the results of prostatic massage in dogs with UTI are difficult or impossible to interpret (refer to the section on diagnostic techniques). The prostate on ultrasonography may be diffusely to focally hyperechoic.

Treatment. An antibiotic should be administered for 21 to 28 days. The choice of the antibiotic can be based on urine culture and antibiotic sensitivity testing. The blood–prostatic fluid barrier is usually not intact in acute inflammation, allowing a wide initial antibiotic choice.[133, 134] If the presenting signs are severe, the antibiotic and fluids should initially be given intrave-

nously. Oral antimicrobials can be used once the dog's condition improves. An oral antimicrobial with prostatic penetrance is preferred for the remainder of therapy (refer to section on chronic bacterial prostatitis).[132]

Because acute infections may become chronic, the dog should be reevaluated three to seven days after antibiotic therapy is completed. This reevaluation should include a physical examination, urinalysis, urine culture, and examination of prostatic fluid by cytology and culture.

Chronic Bacterial Prostatitis

Pathophysiology. Chronic prostatic infection may be a sequela to an acute infection, or may develop insidiously without a prior bout of a clinically evident acute infection. It may be secondary to urinary tract infection or urolithiasis, or due to changes in prostatic architecture that interfere with prostatic fluid secretion, such as cysts, neoplasia, or squamous metaplasia. Chronic prostatitis is the most common cause of recurrent bladder infections in men.[43, 135, 136] In dogs, lower urinary tract infections and prostatic infections are almost inseparable. Experimentally, it is difficult to infect the bladder without infecting the prostate and vice versa.[137] Any male dog with a urinary tract infection should be considered to have a prostatic infection until proved otherwise, even if clinical signs are absent. The incidence of chronic prostatic infections in dogs is unknown. However, 6 to 10 per cent of male dogs have UTI,[138] and an accompanying prostatic infection would be expected. This would be similar to the incidence of five per cent reported in human medicine.[22] In humans incidence increases with age, with an incidence of 16 per cent in men over age 80.[22]

Most cases of chronic bacterial prostatitis are due to infections with common bacteria. Granulomatous chronic prostatitis is much less common, but has been noted in association with blastomycosis[139, 140] and cryptomycosis.[141] In humans, besides being caused by a fungal infection or tuberculosis, granulomatous prostatitis is recognized as being a stage in the resolution of acute prostatitis.[22] It is postulated that if prostatic ducts become obstructed secondary to infection, bacterial products or prostatic acinar constituents may leak into the interstitium, thereby gaining exposure to the immune system and causing a hypersensitivity reaction. This in turn may lead to granuloma formation.[22]

Clinical Signs. Chronic bacterial prostatitis can be present without causing any signs referable to the prostate gland. Instead, the dog may be presented for recurrent episodes of cystitis, or a UTI may be found on a routine urinalysis. Chronic bacterial prostatitis is the most common cause of recurrent UTI in men,[132] and the same may be true in the dog. Other dogs may be presented for a constant or intermittent urethral discharge. Some investigators have reported an association of chronic prostatitis with infertility in men.[142] No effects on sperm parameters were found in one study of chronic bacterial prostatitis experimentally produced in dogs.[143]

Diagnosis. The prostate is not painful when palpated, and size is variable, depending on the degree of hyper-

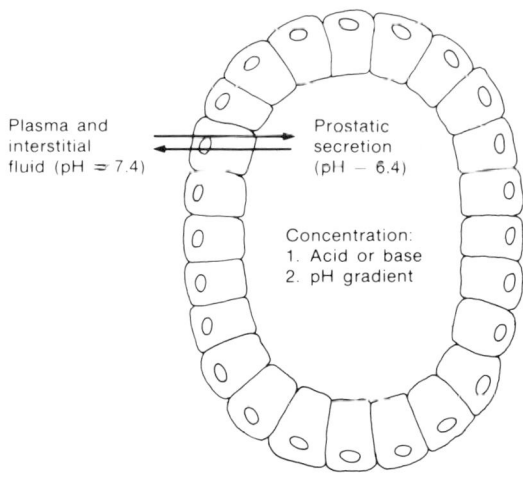

FIGURE 105–15. Factors that determine diffusion and concentration of antimicrobial drugs across epithelium of the prostatic acinus. (From Stamey, TA: Pathogenesis and treatment of urinary tract infections. Baltimore, Williams & Wilkins, 1980.)

plasia and fibrosis. Chronic infection by itself causes no increase in prostatic size. The prostate gland may vary in symmetry and consistency due to formation of fibrous tissue secondary to chronic inflammation. Areas of fibrous tissue are more firm than areas of normal prostatic tissue. The areas of infection may be focal, multifocal, or diffuse.

WBC count is usually normal unless abscessation is present.[30, 94] Pyuria, hematuria, and bacteriuria often are present.[30] Assessment of prostatic fluid is essential in diagnosis of chronic prostatitis, but interpretation of results can be difficult.[144] (Please review the section on diagnostic techniques.) Prostatic fluid collected by ejaculation or after prostatic massage contains inflammatory cells, and quantitative bacterial cultures are usually positive for one species of bacteria.[30] The usual causative organism is *E. coli*. Dogs with experimental chronic bacterial prostatitis had > 1000 organisms/ml.[30] The finding of macrophages in ejaculates correlated with prostatic infection and inflammation.[30] As discussed under diagnostic techniques, results of prostatic massage

are difficult to interpret in the presence of urinary tract infection.[30] In order to use this technique, urinary tract infection must first be controlled.

There are no specific radiographic findings that suggest chronic bacterial prostatitis. Granular parenchymal mineralization has been noted with chronic inflammation. The prostatic size and contour are not affected unless abscessation develops. Distention retrograde urethrocystography is usually normal except for greater than normal urethroprostatic reflux in some dogs.[51] By ultrasound, the prostate gland may be diffusely to focally hyperechoic.[59]

Presumptive diagnosis is by history, physical examination, hematology, urinalysis, and prostatic fluid cytology and quantitative culture. In most cases, if these techniques are carefully done and correctly assessed, a correct diagnosis can be made. Definitive diagnosis is by prostatic tissue culture and histopathology.

Treatment. Chronic bacterial prostatitis is very difficult to treat effectively because the blood–prostatic fluid barrier is intact (Figure 105–15).[129, 132, 134] The blood–prostatic fluid barrier is based partly on the pH difference among the blood, prostatic interstitium, and prostatic fluid; partly on the characteristics of the prostatic acinar epithelium; and partly on the protein-binding characteristics of antibiotics (Table 105–2).[41, 42, 145] Much of the experimental work on antibiotic diffusion into the prostate has used the dog as a model.[3, 41, 42, 146-153] However, the dog model used involves collection of prostatic fluid after pilocarpine stimulation. Pilocarpine-stimulated prostatic fluid is different from basally secreted prostatic fluid, at least in electrolyte content.[154, 155] Therefore, the validity of this model for evaluating antibiotic concentrations in prostatic fluid is unknown. Interestingly, one study that measured drug concentrations of the ejaculum in normal men had markedly different results than those produced by the canine model.[156]

The pH of blood and prostatic interstitium is 7.4. The pH of normal canine prostatic fluid is approximately 6.4.[11, 30, 41, 92, 126, 157-159] The presence of a pH gradient of at least 1.0 pH unit between compartments allows the phenomenon of ion trapping to occur (Figure 105–16). The charged fraction of a drug is greater on one side of

TABLE 105–2. EXPECTED LABORATORY FINDINGS IN PROSTATIC DISEASES

Prostatic Disease	Laboratory Findings						
	Leukocytosis	Hematuria	Pyuria	Bacteriuria	Hemorrhagic Prostatic Fluid	Purulent Prostatic Fluid	Bacteria in Prostatic Fluid
Cystic hyperplasia	No	Yes[h]	No	No	Yes[h]	No	No
Paraprostatic cysts	No[i]	No[i]	No	No	No[i]	No	No
Acute prostatitis	Yes	Yes	Yes	Yes	NA	NA	NA
Chronic prostatitis	No	Yes[c]	Yes[d]	Yes[e]	No[f]	Yes[g]	Yes
Prostatic abscessation	Yes[a]	Yes	Yes	Yes	No[f]	Yes	Yes
Prostatic neoplasia	No[b]	Yes	Yes	No	Yes	Yes	No

a. 60% of cases in one survey had a neutrophilic leukocytosis.[94]
b. Only 20% of dogs with prostatic neoplasia had leukocytosis in one survey.[94]
c. 60% of cases in one survey had hematuria.[94]
d. 72% of cases in one survey had pyuria.[94]
e. 80% of cases in one survey had positive urine cultures.[94]
f. 33% of cases in one survey had hemorrhagic prostatic fluid.[94]
g. 75% of cases in one survey had purulent prostatic fluid.[94]
h. 75% of cases in one survey had bleeding.[94]
i. Leukocytosis and hematuria occasionally reported.

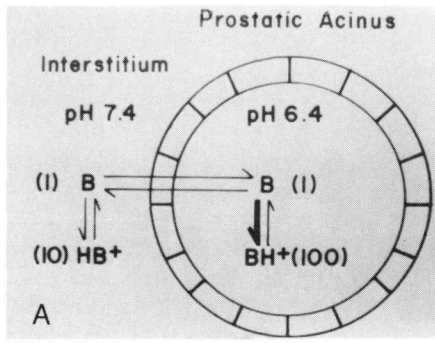

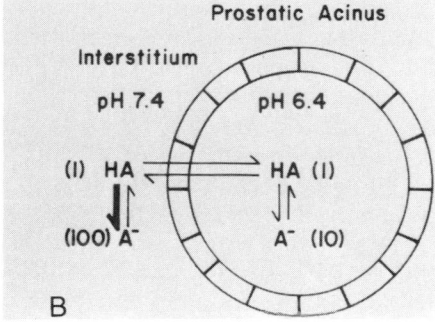

FIGURE 105–16. Ion trapping of basic antibiotics owing to the pH differences between prostatic interstitium and prostatic fluid. Basic antibiotics are trapped within the prostatic acinus (A) while acidic antibiotics are largely excluded from prostatic fluid (B). (From Barsanti, JA and Finco, DR: Canine bacterial prostatitis. Vet Clin North Am 9:679, 1979.)

the system, depending on the pH. Because the uncharged fraction of a lipid-soluble drug equilibrates, there is more total drug (charged plus uncharged) on the side of greater ionization. In contrast to men, in whom prostatic fluid becomes alkaline with infection,[125, 153, 160–163] most dogs with prostatic infection continue to have acidic prostatic fluid.[30, 126, 128, 164, 165] With acidic prostatic fluid, basic antibiotics with high pKa values, such as erythromycin, oleandomycin, clindamycin, and trimethoprim, ionize to a greater extent in prostatic fluid than in plasma (Figure 105–16). In fact, prostatic fluid concentration of trimethoprim can exceed plasma concentrations by two to ten times.[150, 151, 165, 166] The sulfa components of trimethoprim/sulfa (sulfadiazine, sulfamethoxazole) do not concentrate in normal dog prostatic fluid.[3] However, sulfamethoxazole has been reported to

reach therapeutic concentrations in prostatic fluid in men.[167] If infected prostatic fluid is alkaline, acidic antibiotics such as carbenicillin would be more effective. Distribution of nonionizable drugs such as chloramphenicol are not affected by pH differences (see Tables 105–3 and 105–4).

Lipid solubility is also an important factor in determining drug movement across prostatic epithelium. Drugs with low lipid solubility cannot cross into the prostatic acini. Many antibiotics are lipid-insoluble, including penicillin, ampicillin, cephalosporins, oxytetracycline, and the aminoglycosides. Chloramphenicol, the macrolide antibiotics, trimethoprim, the quinolones, and carbenicillin are examples of lipid-soluble drugs that can potentially enter prostatic fluid.

Protein binding in plasma also determines the amount of drug available to enter prostatic fluid. Because protein binding prevents diffusion, only that fraction that is not bound to plasma proteins can diffuse across the membrane. The more protein-bound the drug is, the less drug is available to cross the prostatic epithelium. This factor is probably less important than lipid solubility or pKa, since biologic systems seldom reach equilibrium. Examples of drugs with significant protein binding are clindamycin, chloramphenicol, and nalidixic acid.

In general, diffusion of tetracyclines into canine prostatic fluid is limited. Oxytetracycline does not enter prostatic fluid, whereas tetracycline may, if given intravenously.[149] In clinical studies in men with the newer tetracyclines, some recommend and demonstrate efficacy of minocycline[134, 168, 169] and doxycycline.[29, 170] However, penetration of these drugs into prostatic fluid of normal dogs was minimal.[124, 132, 171, 172] These drugs may diffuse better into alkaline prostatic fluid,[124] and this might explain the differences between the human and canine studies.

Newer quinolone antibiotics have been developed that seem to concentrate in human prostatic fluid.[22] Nalidixic acid is the prototype of this class, but it is highly protein-bound[22] and relatively toxic in dogs.[173–175] Norfloxacin is a lipid-soluble, weak base with a high pKa and low protein binding that is concentrated in human prostate glands.[176] Rosoxacin is also a weak acid with a high pKa, but it is highly protein-bound.[152] In dogs rosoxacin and cinoxacin reached levels in prostatic fluid that were only 10 per cent of plasma levels.[152, 153] Clinical use of these

TABLE 105–3. PHYSIOCHEMICAL CHARACTERISTICS THAT DETERMINE DIFFUSION GRADIENTS BETWEEN PLASMA AND PROSTATIC FLUID OF SELECTED ANTIBIOTICS IN THE DOG[136,172]

Drug	Plasma Conc (μgm/ml)	Prostatic Fluid Conc (μgm/ml)	Acid or Base	Lipid Soluble	pKa	Percentage Unchanged in Plasma
Penicillin G	62.0	0.2	Acid	No	2.7	<0.01
Ampicillin	54.0	0.2	Acid	No	2.5	<0.01
Cephalothin	63.0	0.4	Acid	No	2.5	<0.01
Tetracycline	19.0	4.0	Both	Partial	3.3, 7.7, 9.7	—
Erythromycin	16.0	38.0	Base	Yes	8.8	4.0
Trimethoprim	4.0	7.0	Base	Yes	7.3	56.0
Norfloxacin	—	—	Base	Yes	8.0	—
Carbenicillin	—	—	Acid	Yes	—	100.0
Chloramphenicol	22.5	13.0	NA	Yes	—	—
Clindamycin	9.5	77.0	Base	Yes	7.6	—

Adapted by permission from Stamey, TA: Pathogenesis and Treatment of Urinary Tract Infections. Baltimore, Williams & Wilkins, 1980.

TABLE 105–4. ANTIBIOTICS CURRENTLY THOUGHT TO DIFFUSE INTO PROSTATIC FLUID IN THERAPEUTIC CONCENTRATIONS

Trimethoprim/Sulfa
Chloramphenicol
Carbenicillin
Erythromycin
Clindamycin
Oleandomycin
Norfloxacin

drugs in men has just begun; the drugs are not approved for use in dogs, and toxicity in clinical cases in dogs is unknown.

Most of the penicillins and cephalosporins do not diffuse into prostatic fluid, since they are lipid-insoluble and weak acids.[134, 168, 171, 177, 178] Exceptions are hetacillin (which is lipid-soluble and cleaved to ampicillin within the prostatic acini)[177] and carbenicillin indanyl sodium.[148] In esterified form, carbenicillin is lipid-soluble and uncharged, and reaches prostatic fluid concentrations that are approximately 70 per cent of plasma concentrations.[179] In human studies carbenicillin administered for four to eight weeks resulted in about a 70 per cent cure rate, whereas the use of trimethoprim/sulfamethoxazole for eight weeks resulted in a 40 per cent cure rate.[178, 180] Twelve-week trials of trimethoprim have been variably reported to be 50 to 70 per cent effective.[43, 169, 181, 182] However, prostatic fluid of men with chronic prostatitis is alkaline, and thus an acidic antibiotic, such as carbenicillin, should be more successful than an alkaline antibiotic, such as trimethoprim.[125, 133, 148, 160–162] The opposite may be the case in dogs with acidic prostatic fluid.

Current recommendations depend on whether a gram-positive or gram-negative organism is the infective agent. If the causative organism is gram-positive, erythromycin, clindamycin, oleandomycin, chloramphenicol, or trimethoprim/sulfonamide can be chosen, based on bacterial sensitivity.[172] If the organism is gram-negative, chloramphenicol, trimethoprim/sulfonamide, or carbenicillin would be best. Measurement of prostatic fluid pH could help to determine a potentially effective drug.

Antibiotics should be continued for at least six weeks. Urine and prostatic fluid should be recultured three to seven days and one month after discontinuing antibiotics to be sure the infection has been eliminated, not merely suppressed. The prognosis for cure, based on human medicine, is only fair. Part of the difficulty in curing the infection is that there may be host abnormalities in defense against infection as well as the blood–prostatic fluid barrier.[183] If initial therapy fails, a three-month course of therapy should be instituted, bearing in mind any potential adverse effects of the drug chosen. For such long-term therapy trimethoprim/sulfa or carbenicillin is the best current choice. However, trimethoprim/sulfa can result in keratoconjunctivitis sicca, or mild anemia due to folate deficiency. The authors administer folic acid when using trimethoprim for longer than six weeks at full dosage.

Castration has been recommended as adjunctive therapy to reduce the quantity of prostatic tissue. In experimental chronic prostatitis in dogs, castration performed two weeks after induction of infection hastened spon-

taneous resolution of infection.[127] This research suggests that castration may be beneficial in resolving prostatic infection in clinical cases, but this remains to be proved, since time of castration after initiation of infection may be important.

If oral antibiotics plus castration fail to cure the prostatic infection, only two options remain: low-dose antibiotic therapy or prostatectomy. Low-dose antibiotic therapy can be instituted to suppress the infection so that the infection will be asymptomatic. Trimethoprim at 50 per cent of the usual daily dose each night is useful for this purpose. Other drugs that have been used at one nightly dose include nitrofurantoin and cephalosporins.

Prostatectomy will eliminate infected prostatic tissue and can be used in cases that are refractory to antibiotic therapy and castration. However, the surgical procedure is difficult, and urinary incontinence is a frequent sequela in advanced cases of prostatic disease.[118] Urodynamic evaluation (cystometry and urethral pressure profilometry) should always be done before prostatectomy, to determine preexisting abnormalities.[32] If significant presurgical abnormalities are present, incontinence is very likely. Because of the severity of complications of radical prostatectomy in men, suppressive antibiotic therapy is currently preferred in human medicine.[22]

Another option in human medicine is to inject an antibiotic directly into the prostate gland.[163] This method has not been accepted in the United States.[22, 184]

Prostatic Abscessation

Pathophysiology. Prostatic abscessation is a severe form of chronic bacterial prostatitis in which pockets of septic, purulent exudate develop within the parenchyma of the prostate gland. Aerobic organisms similar to those that cause bacterial prostatitis are most commonly isolated in dogs; however, in human medicine anaerobes have been found in association with aerobes in prostatic abscesses.[185]

Clinical Signs. The dog may be presented for varying signs related to either prostatic enlargement or infection. Prostatic abscesses vary in size and number with each case. If the abscess or abscesses become very large, the dog may be presented with fecal tenesmus from incursion on the colon or rectum, or with dysuria from incursion on the urethra. Incursion on the urethra can lead to partial urethral obstruction, causing a chronically distended bladder, eventual detrusor dysfunction, and overflow urinary incontinence.

Clinical signs related to infection include a constant or intermittent urethral discharge that may be hemorrhagic or purulent. If the abscess ruptures on the outer surface of the prostate, a localized peritonitis results, with fever, pain, and possibly vomiting. Icterus, caused by reactive hepatopathy, may also be present.[118] Reactive hepatopathy refers to abnormal tests of liver function or abnormal liver enzymes, resulting not from primary liver disease, but from the liver's reaction to disease outside of the hepatobiliary system.[186] Reactive hepatopathy is usually noted in association with sepsis or endotoxemia, fever, dehydration, and/or hypoxia.

Diagnosis. On palpation, the prostate gland may or

may not be enlarged, depending on the size and location of the abscess pockets. Occasionally, a fluctuant area may be palpated. The inability to palpate such an area does not rule out abscessation because the abscess may be deeper within the gland or have a firm fibrous capsule. Pain on palpation is more often related to a localized peritonitis than to the abscess itself. Absence of pain does not rule out abscessation. The prostate gland is often asymmetric and may feel of varying consistency (a cobblestone contour with intermixed firmer and softer areas).

A neutrophilic leukocytosis, with or without a left shift, is common with abscessation, but the WBC count may also be normal. A neutrophilic leukocytosis with a left shift and toxic change is common with a localized peritonitis secondary to prostatic abscessation. A urinary tract infection is often present. Prostatic fluid collected by ejaculation or postprostatic massage is usually purulent and septic and may also be hemorrhagic. (Refer to the section on diagnostic techniques for discussion of the difficulty of accurately assessing the results of prostatic massage when urinary tract infection is present.) Quantitative culture of urine and prostatic fluid should have significant numbers of the same organisms. Either aerobic or anaerobic bacteria may be involved in prostatic abscesses. Serum bilirubin and liver enzyme concentrations (especially alkaline phosphatase) may be elevated, and the results of liver function tests, such as Bromsulphalein (BSP) retention, may be abnormal.[118, 187] The pattern of abnormalities usually suggests cholestasis.[186] Liver biopsies are minimally abnormal.[118, 186]

Prostatic enlargement, which can be asymmetric or irregular in outline, may be evident on survey radiographs. There may be poor radiographic contrast of the caudal abdomen. Reflux into the prostate gland may be noted on retrograde urethrography if the abscess communicates with the urethra. The sublumbar lymph nodes may be enlarged. With ultrasound, the prostate gland may be normal to diffusely hyperechoic with parenchymal cavities and irregular outline and asymmetric shape (Figure 105–10).[59] Periurethral asymmetry and narrowing of the prostatic urethra are observed with distention retrograde urethrocystography.[51] The prostatic urethral lumen may appear undulant but is usually not distorted or destroyed.[51]

Presumptive diagnosis is based on history, physical examination, hematology, urinalysis, and prostatic fluid cytology and culture. The diagnosis should be confirmed by aspiration or exploratory celiotomy, since the current treatment of choice is surgical drainage. At surgery the abscess contents should be collected for aerobic and anaerobic culture, and a tissue section should be obtained for microscopic examination and bacterial culture.

Treatment. Surgical drainage is currently the treatment of choice.[98, 116–118] There are many methods to accomplish this, including needle aspiration, tube or Penrose drains, and marsupialization.[118] Alternatively, the prostate may be removed. Complications are common with all methods. Drainage through the abdomen often results in oliguria and septic shock immediately after surgery because of absorption of bacteria and their toxins.[118, 187] Intensive care is often required for several days after surgery.[187] If placed over the prostate, drains may sever the urethra, leading to a urine fistula.[118] Ascending infection with antibiotic-resistant bacteria is possible. Marsupialization leaves a chronic draining stoma in some dogs. If the stoma closes too early, the abscess may reform. Prostatectomy often results in incontinence in dogs with such severe underlying prostatic disease.[118]

If the prostatic enlargement has resulted in partial urethral obstruction, bladder and urethral function should be carefully assessed. It is especially important to assess bladder and urethral function before prostatectomy, since abnormalities before surgery increase the likelihood of incontinence postoperatively.[32] Prolonged bladder distention may have resulted in bladder atony, so the dog may have overflow incontinence.[118] An indwelling urinary catheter may be necessary to let the detrusor muscle recover. If the bladder wall has been chronically distended and infected, it may be irreversibly damaged.

Polyuria and polydipsia, similar to those expected with nephrogenic diabetes insipidus, have been noted in a few dogs after surgical treatment for prostatic abscessation.[118] The polyuria, polydipsia, and preoperative evidence of hepatic dysfunction resolved within one month of initiating treatment.

Castration is recommended along with antibiotic and surgical therapy. Castration without abscess drainage leads to reduction of prostatic tissue but continuation of the abscess pocket(s).

Regardless of which surgical procedure is elected, affected dogs must receive antibiotic therapy. If the dog is systemically ill, intravenous antimicrobials should be used initially. Based on prostatic penetration, chloramphenicol, trimethoprim, and carbenicillin are the drugs of choice. However, the choice should be based on knowledge of the causative organism, its antibiotic sensitivity, and the presence or absence of bacteremia. After improvement of clinical signs, the dog should be managed in the same way as a dog with chronic bacterial prostatitis. If the dog's condition stabilizes and the owner declines surgery, the dog can be managed with long-term suppressive antibiotic therapy as long as the owner realizes that the abscess will persist and potentially result in life-threatening infection. The authors have had two such cases, one with cardiomyopathy and one with chronic renal failure. One was asymptomatic as long as once-a-day antimicrobial therapy was used. This dog lived for two years and died of the underlying disease. The abscess was still present at death. The other dog had recurrent UTI that became increasingly antibiotic-resistant. He then became incontinent as a result of the prostatic disease.

Prostatic abscesses are difficult and expensive to treat.[187] In one survey, survival was approximately 50 per cent after one year.[118] These facts underscore the importance of aggressive treatment of chronic prostatitis to try to halt progression to abscessation.

Prostatic Neoplasia

The most common primary prostatic neoplasm in dogs and in humans is adenocarcinoma.[188] The incidence appears to be low in dogs, with about five per cent of all dogs with prostatic disease having neoplasia.[118, 189, 190] The second most common neoplasm that affects the prostate gland is transitional cell carcinoma.[188] Squamous cell carcinoma has been found in the prostate[191] as well as neoplasms that metastasized from another site. Leiomyosarcomas have been reported but are apparently quite rare.[7] Note that all the above are considered malignant. Benign tumors of the prostate are not reported (other than hyperplasia, which some in human medicine refer to as a form of neoplasia).

PROSTATIC ADENOCARCINOMA

Prostatic adenocarcinoma tends to metastasize through the external and internal iliac lymph nodes to vertebral bodies as well as to the lungs.[48, 192, 193] The tumor may grow into the neck of the bladder and obstruct the ureters.[192] The colon and pelvic musculature may be invaded by way of direct extension through the prostatic capsule.[192] The urethra may also become obstructed from neoplastic extension.[189] Cysts, abscesses, and areas of hemorrhage can be found in association with neoplasia, making diagnosis difficult in some dogs.[188, 189, 194]

Clinical Signs. Prostatic adenocarcinoma arises in old dogs, with a mean age of nine to ten years.[189, 192, 195] Medium to large breeds seem to be more commonly affected.[189, 192, 195] This neoplasm can develop in both intact and neutered males.[48, 195-198] In fact, prostatic neoplasia should be highest on the list of differential diagnoses in an old dog that was neutered when young and that is presented with signs referable to prostatic disease or prostatic enlargement (Figure 105–17).

The presenting complaints by the owner are often related to increased prostatic size, such as fecal tenesmus and dysuria.[189, 192-194, 196, 199] A hemorrhagic urethral discharge may be noted.[192] Hindlimb weakness, or stiffness and pain in the hindquarters are common signs, present in 40 to 50 per cent of affected dogs.[192, 193, 196] The pain may be related to necrosis and inflammation as the tumor outgrows its blood supply, or it may be due to lumbar vertebral metastasis.[193] Chronic weight loss may also be present.[189, 192-194] Hypertrophic osteopathy affecting all four limbs has been reported in one case that had no evidence of lung metastasis.[199] If prostate glands are carefully palpated routinely in older male dogs, a firm neoplastic nodule may be palpated before marked prostatic enlargement and before clinical signs appear.

Diagnosis. On prostatic palpation one or more firm irregular nodules may be detected in early cases. In the majority of cases presented with clinical signs, the prostate gland will be markedly enlarged and asymmetric with increased firmness.[189, 197] It may be painful on palpation and is often nonmovable.[192] The iliac lymph nodes should be palpated rectally and may be enlarged.[192, 199]

WBC counts are usually normal, but a neutrophilic leukocytosis may be present if sufficient necrosis and inflammation are associated with tumor growth.[94, 192] One case has been reported in which neoplastic cells were seen in the blood.[190] If the tumor obstructs both ureters, hydronephrosis and azotemia may result. If the tumor causes partial urethral obstruction, loss of bladder function and azotemia may be present. Hypercalcemia has been noted, although rarely, in association with prostatic carcinoma in men.[200] Plasma acid phosphatase, which is a useful tumor marker in men, was not increased in dogs in one survey[189] and has been reported not to be present in species other than humans.[201] Hematuria is the predominant abnormality on urinalysis, but pyuria may also be present due to prostatic necrosis and inflammation secondary to tumor growth.[94, 192] Semen samples are difficult to collect from dogs with advanced neoplasia, but abnormal epithelial cells may be detected after prostatic massage.[94, 202] These cells are usually large, often in groups, displaying anisocytosis and anisokaryosis. There may be irregular and variably sized nucleoli and, occasionally, abnormal mitotic figures. Because epithelial cells in urine can normally be variable in appearance, identification of such cells should be used as supportive, but not definitive, evidence for neoplasia.[44]

Asymmetric or irregular prostatic enlargement, which may be marked, may be evident on survey abdominal radiography (Figure 105–18).[50] Some prostatic carcinomas are associated with multifocal or granular poorly defined mineral densities.[21] The lumbar vertebral bodies and the pelvic bones should always be carefully examined for areas of lysis or proliferative bone changes suggestive of metastasis (Figure 105–9).[4, 48, 189, 192, 203] Metastasis may also occur to long bones, scapula, ribs, and digits.[192, 193] The degree of enlargement of the iliac lymph nodes should also be determined (Figure 105–

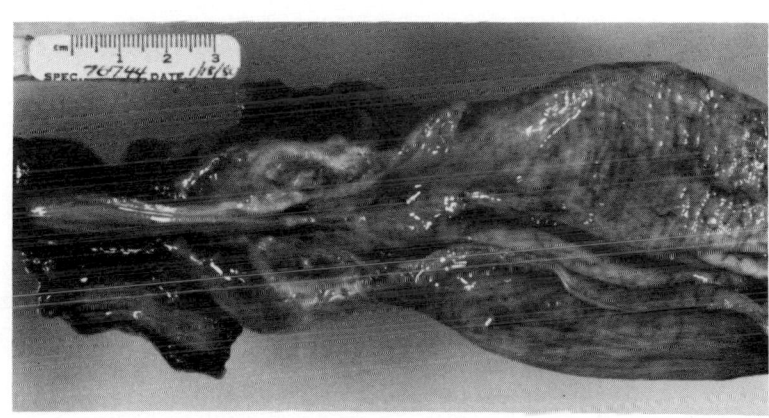

FIGURE 105–17. Necropsy specimens of bladder and urethra opened on the midline from a castrated dog presented for overflow incontinence. Note the flaccid appearance of the bladder. The cause of the incontinence was urethral obstruction caused by prostatic adenocarcinoma. Note that the prostate is not grossly enlarged, but is larger than expected for a dog neutered as a puppy.

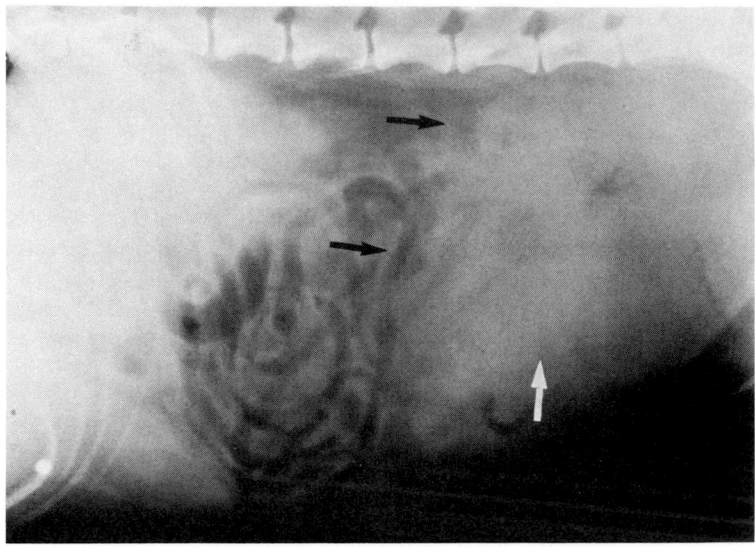

FIGURE 105–18. Marked irregular prostatomegaly (caudal black arrow and white arrow) on a lateral abdominal radiograph. The iliac lymph nodes are also enlarged (dorsal black arrow). Clear differentiation of bladder and prostate is not possible.

18). Thoracic radiographs are indicated to check for metastasis to the lungs. Nuclear scanning techniques can also be used to determine whether metastasis to bone has occurred. The bone scan is a more sensitive indicator of bone pathology than routine radiography. With distention retrograde urethrocystography, periurethral asymmetry and narrowing, distortion, or destruction of the prostatic urethra may be detected.[51] Urethroprostatic reflux that is greater than normal is also common.[51] Spread of the neoplasm into the bladder is possible (Figure 105–19). Ultrasound usually shows focal or multifocal hyperechoic parenchyma with asymmetry and irregular prostatic outline.[59]

A presumptive diagnosis is based on history, physical examination, hematology, urinalysis, cytology of prostatic fluid, radiography, and ultrasonography. Unless metastatic disease is evident radiographically, the diagnosis should always be confirmed by aspiration or biopsy, since the prognosis is poor. If a surgical biopsy is obtained, a biopsy specimen should also be taken from the iliac lymph nodes.

Treatment. Before therapy a thorough search for metastasis should be undertaken to allow a more accurate prognosis. Such a search should include at least thoracic radiographs and contrast radiographs of the lower urinary tract. A bone scan would also be advisable where available.

Radiation therapy is the treatment of choice if metastatic disease is not evident.[204] Intraoperative orthovoltage therapy has recently been recommended.[204] Prostatectomy is alternative therapy, but the owner must be willing to accept the probable postsurgical development of urinary incontinence.[98, 118, 205] The longest reported postoperative survival has been nine months.[118, 206] The one dog that survived nine months had only small foci of neoplasia at the time of initial diagnosis.[118] Median and mean survival times for ten dogs with radiotherapy[204] were 114 and 196 days, respectively. Three dogs with no evidence of metastatic disease appeared to be cured. However, with both therapies, the usual goal is temporary control of the tumor and amelioration of clinical signs. Cure is unlikely, since metastasis is likely to have occurred, even if it is not clinically detectable.[204] In

advanced, metastatic cases euthanasia may be the most humane course because of lack of effective therapy at this time. Palliative therapy includes castration, estrogen therapy, and chemotherapeutic regimens designed for men. Veterinary experience with these treatments is limited, but hormonal therapy does not seem to be effective.[7, 188, 189, 198, 203] Prostatic adenocarcinoma has been reported in a dog with hyperestrogenism and in castrated dogs.[48, 191, 195–197, 202] Lack of decrease in prostatic size after castration may help to differentiate neoplasia from other prostatic diseases. (Refer to Chapter 102 for further discussion.)

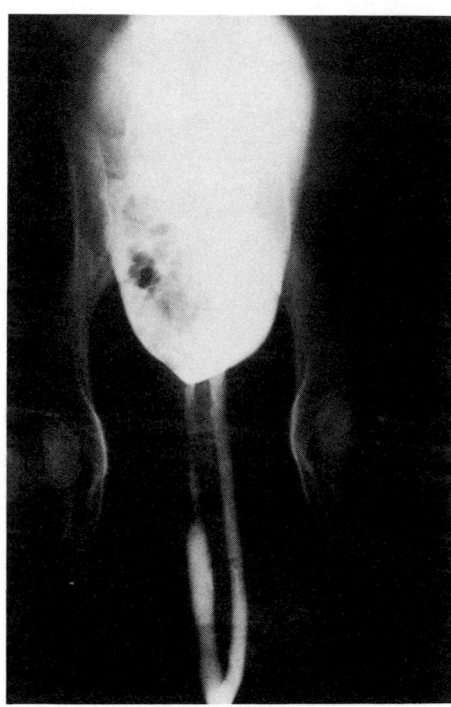

FIGURE 105–19. Retrograde urethrogram and cystogram on the same dog as shown in Figure 105–18. A space-occupying mass is evident in the bladder. Postprostatic massage samples suggested carcinoma. Because the owner refused biopsy or necropsy, the origin of the neoplasm (bladder or prostate) could not be determined.

TRANSITIONAL CELL CARCINOMA

Transitional cell carcinoma of the prostate can occur by way of direct extension from a bladder or urethral lesion or from neoplastic changes in the periurethral prostatic ductal cells themselves (Figure 105–19).[207] Clinical signs are often related to partial urethral obstruction. Radiographic and ultrasonographic findings are similar to those for adenocarcinoma.[51, 59] Only a biopsy may enable differentiation from prostatic adenocarcinoma. Urethral biopsy techniques may be useful.[45, 46] (Refer to Chapter 112 for further discussion.)

METASTATIC NEOPLASIA

Any type of neoplasm may metastasize to the prostate gland. Such neoplastic foci are often subclinical. However, the authors have encountered a few cases of lymphosarcoma in dogs presented primarily for clinical signs related to prostatomegaly. Prostatic lymphosarcoma was also noted in one dog in an early series of cases.[78] However, in this dog, the prostate was reported to be atrophied. Aspiration of the prostate gland has been diagnostic in these cases.

Multiple Diseases

A prostate gland may contain several disease processes. For example, it may be hyperplastic, abscessed, and neoplastic.[111, 188, 194] The occurrence of multiple diseases is a limitation of all diagnostic tests. For markedly abnormal prostate glands, multiple biopsies may be indicated. Clinicians should keep an open mind if the disease course does not fit the disease diagnosed, even when a biopsy has been obtained.

References

1. Neumann, F, et al.: Male accessory sex glands: experimental basis and animal models in prostatic tumour research. In Serio, M and Marteni, L (eds): Animal Models in Human Reproduction. New York, Raven Press, 1980, p 249.
2. Evans, HE and Christensen, GE: Miller's anatomy of the dog, 2nd ed. Philadelphia, WB Saunders, 1979, p 565.
3. Gordon, N: Position of the canine prostate gland. Am J Vet Res 22:142, 1961.
4. Stead, AC and Borthwich, R: The canine urinary bladder and prostate. J Sm Anim Pract 17:629, 1976.
5. Isaacs, WB: Structural and functional components in normal and hyperplastic canine prostates. Prog Clin Biol Res 145:307, 1984.
6. Merk, FB, et al.: Ultrastructural and biochemical expressions of divergent differentiation in prostates of castrated dogs treated with estrogen and androgen. Lab Invest 47:437, 1982.
7. Leav, I and Cavazos, LF: Some morphologic features of normal and pathologic canine prostate. In Goland, M (ed): Normal and Abnormal Growth of the Prostate. Springfield, IL, Charles C Thomas, 1975, p 69.
8. Berry, SJ: Effects of aging on prostate growth in beagles. Am J Physiol 250:R1039, 1986.
9. Rogers, KS, et al.: Diagnostic evaluation of the canine prostate. Comp Cont Ed Pract Vet 8:799, 1986.
10. Bruschini, H, et al.: Neurologic control of prostatic secretion in the dog. Invest Urol 15:288, 1978.
11. Farrell, JI: The newer physiology of the prostate gland. J Urol 39:171, 1938.
12. Kirby, RS, et al.: Intra-prostatic urinary reflux: an aetiological factor in abacterial prostatitis. Br J Urol 54:729, 1982.
13. Brendler, CB, et al.: Spontaneous benign prostatic hyperplasia in the beagle. J Clin Invest 71:1114, 1983.
14. James, RW and Heywood, R: Age-related variations in the testes and prostate of beagle dogs. Toxicology 12:273, 1979.
15. Isaacs, JT: Common characteristics of human and canine benign prostatic hyperplasia. Prog Clin Biol Res 145:217, 1984.
16. Huggins, C and Clark, PG: Quantitative studies of prostatic secretion II. The effect of castration and of estrogen injection on the normal and on the hyperplastic prostate glands of dogs. J Exp Med 72:747, 1940.
17. Ewing, LL, et al.: Testicular androgen and estrogen secretion and benign hyperplasia in the beagle. Endocrinology 114:1308, 1984.
18. Berry, SJ, et al.: Development of canine benign prostatic hyperplasia with age. Prostate 9:363, 1986.
19. Mulligan, RM: Feminization in male dogs: a syndrome associated with carcinoma of the testes and mimicked by the administration of estrogen. Am J Pathol 20:865, 1944.
20. Barrach, ER and Berry, SJ: DNA synthesis in the canine prostate: effects of androgen and estrogen treatment. Prostate 10:45, 1987.
21. Feeney, DA and Johnston, GR: Urogenital imaging: A practical update. Semin Vet Med Surg 1:144, 1986.
22. Orland, SM, et al.: Prostatitis, prostatosis, and prostatodynia. Urology 25:439, 1985.
23. Meares, EM: Infection stones of prostate gland: laboratory diagnosis and clinical management. Urology 4:560, 1974.
24. Eykyn, S, et al.: Prostatic calculi as a source of recurrent bacteriuria in the male. Br J Urol 46:527, 1974.
25. Sutor, DJ and Wooley, SE: The crystalline composition of prostatic calculi. Br J Urol 46:533, 1974.
26. Meares, EM: Etiology of prostatitis. Urology 24:S4, 1984.
27. Greenberg, RN, et al.: Chronic prostatitis: comments on infectious etiologies and antimicrobial treatment. Prostate 6:445, 1985.
28. Peeters, MF, et al.: Role of mycoplasmas in chronic prostatitis. Yale J Biol Med 56:551, 1983.
29. Ristuccia, AM and Cunha, BA: Current concepts in antimicrobial therapy of prostatitis. Urology 20:338, 1982.
30. Barsanti, JA, et al.: Evaluation of various techniques for diagnosis of chronic bacterial prostatitis in the dog. JAVMA 183:219, 1983.
31. Fair, WR: Diagnosing prostatitis. Urology 24:S6, 1984.
32. Basinger, RR, et al.: Mechanism of urinary incontinence in dogs with prostatic disease and surgery. Abstract ACVS, 1987.
33. Andersen, JT and Bradley, WF: Detrusor and urethral dysfunction in prostatic hypertrophy. Br J Urol 48:493, 1976.
34. Roberts, SJ: Veterinary obstetrics and genital diseases. Ithaca, NY, SJ Roberts, 1971, p 607.
35. Ling, GV and Ruby, AC: Aerobic bacterial flora of the prepuce, urethra and vagina of normal adult dogs. Am J Vet Res 39:695, 1978.
36. Huggins, C, et al.: Quantitative studies of prostatic secretion. J Exp Med 70:543, 1939.
37. Ling, GV, et al.: Canine prostatic fluid: techniques of collection, quantitative bacterial culture, and interpretation of results. JAVMA 183:201, 1983.
38. Goodwin, M, et al.: Sex pheromone in the dog. Science 203:559, 1979.
39. Barsanti, JA, et al.: Evaluation of diagnostic techniques for canine prostatic diseases. JAVMA 177:160, 1980.
40. Fowler, JE and Mariano, M: Difficulties in quantitating the contribution of urethral bacteria to prostatic fluid and seminal fluid cultures. J Urol 132:471, 1984.
41. Winningham, DG, et al.: Diffusion of antibiotics from plasma into prostatic fluid. Nature 219:139, 1968.
42. Stamey, TA, et al.: Chronic bacterial prostatitis and the diffusion of drugs into prostatic fluid. J Urol 103:187, 1970.
43. Smith, JW: Recurrent urinary tract infections in men: characteristics and response to therapy. Ann Intern Med 91:544, 1979.
44. Thrall, MA, et al.: Cytologic diagnosis of canine prostatic disease. JAAHA 21:95, 1985.

45. Melhoff, T and Osborne, CA: Catheter biopsy of the urethra, urinary bladder and prostate gland. *In* Kirk, RW (ed): Current Veterinary Therapy VI. Philadelphia, WB Saunders, 1977, p 1173.

46. Holt, PE, et al.: Evaluation of a catheter biopsy technique as a diagnostic aid in lower urinary tract disease. Vet Rec 118:681, 1986.

47. Archibald, J and Bishop, EJ: Radiographic visualization of the canine prostate gland. JAVMA 128:337, 1956.

48. Zontine, WJ: The prostate gland. Mod Vet Pract 56:341, 1975.

49. Douglas, SW and Williamson, HD: Veterinary radiological interpretation. Philadelphia, Lea & Febiger, p 269, 1970.

50. Stone, EA, et al.: Radiographic interpretation of prostatic disease in the dog. JAAHA 14:115, 1978.

51. Feeney, DA, et al.: Canine prostatic disease-comparison of radiographic appearance with morphologic and microbiologic findings: 30 cases (1981–1985). JAVMA 190:1018, 1987.

52. Feeney, DA, et al.: Dimensions of the prostatic and membranous urethra in normal male dogs during maximum distention retrograde urethrocystography. Vet Radiol 25:249, 1984.

53. Johnston, GR, et al.: Effect of intravesical hydrostatic pressure and volume on the distensibility of the canine prostatic portion of the urethra. Am J Vet Res 46:748, 1985.

54. Ackerman, N: Prostatic reflux during positive contrast retrograde urethrography in the dog. Vet Radiol 24:251, 1983.

55. Ackerman, N: Urography—interpretation of the study. Cal Vet 33:29, 1979.

56. Feeney, DA, et al.: Maximum-distention retrograde urethrocystography in healthy male dogs: occurrence and radiographic appearance of urethroprostatic reflux. Am J Vet Res 45:948, 1984.

57. Johnston, GR, et al.: Retrograde contrast urethrography. *In* Kirk, RW (ed): Current Veterinary Therapy VI. Philadelphia, WB Saunders, 1977, p 1189.

58. Poogird, W and Wood, AKW: Radiologic study of the canine urethra. Am J Vet Res 47:2491, 1986.

59. Feeney, DA, et al.: Canine prostatic disease—comparison of ultrasonographic appearance with morphologic and microbiologic findings: 30 cases (1981–1985). JAVMA 190:1027, 1987.

60. Barsanti, JA, et al.: Complications of bladder distension during retrograde urethrography. Am J Vet Res 42:819, 1981.

61. Johnston, GR, et al.: Complications of retrograde contrast urography in dogs and cats. Am J Vet Res 44:1248, 1983.

62. Mehrotra, RML: An experimental study of the vesical circulation during distension and in cystitis. J Pathol Bacteriol 66:79, 1953.

63. Cartee, RE and Rowles, T: Transabdominal sonographic evaluation of the canine prostate. Vet Radiol 24:156, 1983.

64. Cartee, RE: Diagnostic ultrasonography. Mod Vet Pract 61:744, 1980.

65. Feeney, DA, et al.: Gray-scale ultrasonography of the canine prostate gland. Vet Clin North Am 15:1159, 1985.

66. Smith, S: Ultrasound-guided biopsy. Vet Clin North Am 15:1249, 1985.

67. Liddell, HT, et al.: Ultrasound versus digitally directed prostatic needle biopsy. J Urol 135:716, 1986.

68. Weaver, AD: Transperineal punch biopsy of the canine prostate gland. J Sm Anim Pract 18:573, 1977.

69. Finco, DR: Prostate gland biopsy. Vet Clin North Am 4:367, 1974.

70. Leeds, EB and Leav, I: Perineal punch biopsy of the canine prostate gland. JAVMA 154(8):925, 1969.

71. Gloyna, RE, et al.: Dihydrotestosterone in prostatic hypertrophy. J Clin Invest 49:1746, 1970.

72. Hieble, JP and Caine, M: Etiology of benign prostatic hyperplasia and approaches to its pharmacological management. Fed Proc 45:2601, 1986.

73. Mariotti, A, et al.: Collagen and cellular proliferation in spontaneous canine prostatic hypertrophy. J Urol 127:795, 1982.

74. Bartsch, G and Rohr, HP: Comparative light and electron microscopic study of the human, dog, and rat prostate. Urol Int 35:91, 1980.

75. Berry, SJ, et al.: The development of human benign prostatic hyperplasia with age. J Urol 132:474, 1984.

76. Lloyd, JW, et al.: Androgens and estrogens in the plasma and prostatic tissue of normal dogs and dogs with benign prostatic hypertrophy. Invest Urol 13:220, 1975.

77. Zuckerman, S and McKeoun, T: The canine prostate in relation to normal and abnormal testicular changes. J Pathol Bacteriol 46:7, 1938.

78. O'Shea, JP: Studies on the canine prostate gland. Factors influencing its size and weight. J Comp Pathol 72:321, 1962.

79. Schlotthauer, CF: Observations on the prostate gland of the dog. JAVMA 81:645, 1932.

80. Wilson, JD: The pathogenesis of benign hyperplasia. Am J Med 68:745, 1986.

81. Moore, RJ, et al.: Concentration of dihydrotestosterone and 3 α-androstanediol in naturally occurring and androgen-induced prostatic hyperplasia in the dog. J Clin Invest 64:1003, 1979.

82. Isaacs, JT and Coffey, DS: Changes in dihydrotestosterone metabolism associated with the development of canine benign prostatic hyperplasia. Endocrinology 108:445, 1981.

83. Isaacs, JT: Changes in dihydrotestosterone metabolism and the development of benign prostatic hyperplasia in the aging beagle. J Steroid Biochem 18:749, 1983.

84. Ewing, LL, et al.: Dihydrotestosterone concentration of beagle prostatic tissue: effect of age and hyperplasia. Endocrinology 113:2004, 1983.

85. Morimoto, I, et al.: Alteration in the metabolism of dihydrotestosterone in elderly men with prostate hyperplasia. J Clin Invest 66:612, 1980.

86. Rohr, HP, et al.: The dog prostate under defined hormonal influences: an approach to experimentally induced prostatic growth. Path Res Pract 166:347, 1960.

87. Walsh, PC and Wilson, JD: The induction of prostatic hypertrophy in the dog with androstanediol. J Clin Invest 57(4):1093, 1976.

88. Ehrlichman, RJ, et al.: Differences in the effects of estradiol on dihydrotestosterone induced prostatic growth of the castrate dog and rat. Invest Urol 18:466, 1981.

89. Trachtenberg, J, et al.: Androgen and estrogen receptor content in spontaneous and experimentally induced canine prostatic hyperplasia. J Clin Invest 65:1051, 1980.

90. Wheaton, LG, et al.: Relationship of seminal volume to size and disease of the prostate in the beagle. Am J Vet Res 40:1325, 1979.

91. DeKlerk, DP, et al.: Comparison of spontaneous and experimentally induced canine prostatic hyperplasia. J Clin Invest 64:842, 1979.

92. Huggins, C: The physiology of the prostate gland. Physiological Rev 25:281, 1945.

93. Kohnen, PW and Drach, GW: Patterns of inflammation in prostatic hyperplasia: a histologic and bacteriologic study. J Urol 121:755, 1979.

94. Barsanti, JA and Finco, DR: Evaluation of techniques for diagnosis of canine prostatic diseases. JAVMA 185:198, 1984.

95. Huggins, C: The etiology of benign prostatic hypertrophy. Bull NY Acad Med 23:696, 1947.

96. Borthwich, R and Mackenzie, CP: Signs and results of treatment of prostatic disease in dogs. Vet Rec 89:374, 1971.

97. Berry, SJ, et al.: Effect of age, castration and testosterone replacement on the development and restoration of canine benign hyperplasia. Prostate 9:295, 1986.

98. Johnston, DI: The prostate. *In* Slatter, DH (ed): Textbook of Small Animal Surgery. Philadelphia, WB Saunders, 1985, p 1635.

99. Tyslowitz, R and Dingemanse, E: Effect of large doses of estrogens on the blood picture of dogs. Endocrinology 29:817, 1941.

100. Mills, JN and Slatter, DH: Stilbestrol toxicity in a dog. Aust Vet J 57:39, 1981.

101. Pyle, RL, et al.: Estrogen toxicity in a dog. Canine Pract, August, 1976, p 39.

102. Berg, OA: Effect of stilbestrol on the prostate gland in normal puppies and adult dogs. Acta Endocrinol 27:155, 1958.

103. Neri, RO and Monahan, M: Effects of a novel nonsteroidal antiandrogen on canine prostatic hyperplasia. Invest Urol 10:123, 1972.

104. Geller, J, et al.: Effect of megestrol acetate on steroid metabolism and steroid-protein binding in the human prostate. J Clin Endocrinol Metab 43:1000, 1976.

105. Soloway, MS: Treatment of prostatic cancer. Postgrad Med 80:249, 1986.

106. Liu, J, et al.: Effects of androgen blockade with ketoconazole

and megestrol acetate on human prostatic protein patterns. Prostate 9:199, 1986.

107. Trachtenberg, J: Effects of ketoconazole on testosterone production and normal and malignant androgen dependent tissues of the adult rat. J Urol 132:599, 1984.

108. Trachtenberg, J: Ketoconazole therapy in advanced prostatic cancer. J Urol 132:61, 1984.

109. Dube, JY, et al.: Involution of spontaneous benign prostatic hyperplasia in the dog under the influence of chronic treatment with a LHRH agonist. Prostate 5:417, 1984.

110. Sherding, RG, et al.: Bone marrow hypoplasia in 8 dogs with Sertoli cell tumor. JAVMA 178:497, 1981.

111. Weaver, AD: Discrete prostatic (paraprostatitic) cysts in the dog. Vet Rec 102:435, 1978.

112. Akpavie, SO and Sullivan, M: Constipation associated with calcified cystic enlargement of the prostate in a dog. Vet Rec 118:694, 1986.

113. Pinegger, H: Kleintierpraxis 20:231, 1975.

114. Sisson, DD and Hoffer, RE: Osteocollagenous prostatic retention cyst: report of a canine case. JAAHA 13:61, 1977.

115. Smith, CW: Marsupialization of the prostate gland. In Bojrab, MJ (ed): Current Techniques in Small Animal Surgery. Philadelphia, Lea & Febiger, 1975, p 261.

116. Greiner, TP and Betts, CW: Diseases of the prostate gland. In Ettinger, SJ (ed): Textbook of Veterinary Internal Medicine. Philadelphia, WB Saunders, 1975, p 1274.

117. Knecht, CD: Diseases of the canine prostate gland. Surgical techniques. Comp Cont Ed Pract Vet 1:426, 1979.

118. Hardie, EM, et al.: Complications of prostatic surgery. JAAHA 20:50, 1984.

119. Greene, CE and George, LW: Canine brucellosis. In Green, CE (ed): Clinical Microbiology and Infectious Diseases of the Dog and Cat. Philadelphia, WB Saunders, 1984, p 646.

120. Fair, WR and Parrish, RF: Antibacterial substances in prostatic fluid. Prog Clin Biol Res 75:247, 1981.

121. Kavanagh, JP, et al.: The response of seven prostatic fluid components to prostatic disease. Int J Androl 5:487, 1982.

122. Kavanagh, JP, et al.: Zinc in post prostatic massage (VB3) urine samples: a marker of prostatic secretory function and indicator of bacterial infection. Urol Res 11:167, 1983.

123. Fair, WR, et al.: Prostatic antibacterial factor: identity and significance. Urology 7:169, 1976.

124. Meares, EM: Prostatitis. Kidney Int 20(2):289, 1981.

125. Anderson, RU and Fair, WR: Physical and chemical determinations of prostatic secretion in benign hyperplasia, prostatic and adenocarcinoma. Invest Urol 14:137, 1976.

126. Branam, JE, et al.: Selected physical and chemical characteristics of prostatic fluid collected by ejaculation from healthy dogs and from dogs with bacterial prostatitis. Am J Vet Res 45:825, 1984.

127. Cowan, LA, et al.: Effect of castration of experimentally induced chronic prostatic infection in dogs. ACVIM Proc, 1987, p 897.

128. Baumueller, A and Madsen, PO: Experimental bacterial prostatitis in dogs. Urol Res 5:211, 1977.

129. Madsen, PO, et al.: Chronic bacterial prostatitis: theoretical and experimental. Urol Res 11:1, 1983.

130. Fowler, JE and Mariano, M: Immunologic response of the prostate to bacteriuria and bacterial prostatitis. J Urol 128:165, 1982.

131. Fowler, JE, et al.: Immunologic response of the prostate to bacteriuria and bacterial prostatitis. J Urol 128:158, 1982.

132. Meares, EM: Prostatitis syndromes: new perspectives about old woes. J Urol 123:141, 1980.

133. Goldfarb, M: Clinical efficacy of antibiotics in treatment of prostatitis. Urology 24:S12, 1984.

134. Paulson, DF, et al.: Treatment of bacterial prostatitis: comparison of cephalexin and minocycline. Urology 27:379, 1986.

135. Meares, EM: Prostatitis. Annu Rev Med 30:279, 1979.

136. Stamey, TA: Pathogenesis and treatment of urinary tract infections. Baltimore, Williams & Wilkins, 1980.

137. Ling, GV, et al.: Chronic urinary tract infection in dogs: induction by inoculation with bacteria via percutaneous nephropyelostomy. Am J Vet Res 48:794, 1987.

138. Kivisto, AK, et al.: Canine bacteriuria. J Sm Anim Pract 18:707, 1977.

139. Shull, RM, et al.: Urogenital blastomycosis in a dog. JAVMA 171:730, 1977.

140. Barsanti, JA: Blastomycosis. In Green, CE (ed): Clinical Microbiology and Infectious Diseases of the Dog and Cat. Philadelphia, WB Saunders, 1984, p 675.

141. Walde, I and Burtscher, H: Retinal detachment as a result of cryptococcosis in a dog. Kleintierpraxis 25:251, 1980.

142. Giamarellou, H, et al.: Infertility and chronic prostatitis. Andrologia 16:417, 1984.

143. Barsanti, JA, et al.: Effect of induced prostatic infection on semen quality in the dog. Am J Vet Res 47:709, 1986.

144. Drach, GW: Problems in diagnosis of bacterial prostatitis: gram-negative, gram-positive and mixed infections. J Urol 111:630, 1974.

145. Haveland, H: Trimethoprim sulphamethoxazole in bacterial infections. In Bernsteen, LS and Salter, AJ (eds): Prostatic pharmacokinetics. London, Churchill Livingstone, 1973, p 73.

146. Madsen, PO, et al.: Experimental models for determination of antimicrobials in prostatic fluid, interstitial fluid and secretion. Scand J Infect Dis 14:145, 1978.

147. Winningham, DG and Stamey, TA: Diffusion of sulfonamides from plasma into prostatic fluid. J Urol 104:559, 1970.

148. Schaeffer, AJ: Pharmacokinetics of antibiotics used in treatment of prostatitis. Urology 24:8, 1984.

149. Hessl, JM and Stamey, TA: The passage of tetracycline across epithelial membranes with special reference to prostatic epithelium. J Urol 106:253, 1971.

150. Granato, JJ, et al.: Trimethoprim diffusion into prostatic and salivary secretions of the dog. Invest Urol 11:205, 1973.

151. Stamey, TA, et al.: The concentration of trimethoprim in prostatic fluid: nonionic diffusion or active transport? J Infect Dis 128:S686, 1973.

152. Maigaard, S, et al.: Rosoxacin and cinoxacin distribution in prostate, vagina, and female urethra in dogs. Invest Urol 17:149, 1979.

153. Maigaard, S, et al.: Rosoxacin distribution in kidney and prostate: experimental studies in dogs. Urol Res 8:113, 1980.

154. Smith, ER: The secretion of electrolytes by the pilocarpine-stimulated canine prostate gland. Proc Soc Exp Biol Med 132:223, 1969.

155. Smith, ER and Lievski, LV: Secretion of bromide by the canine prostate. Prostate 6:155, 1985.

156. Armstrong, JR, et al.: Concentration of antibiotic and chemotherapeutic agent in the ejaculum. J Urol 100:72, 1968.

157. Nyland, TG, et al.: Gray-scale ultrasonography of the canine abdomen. Vet Radiol 22:220, 1981.

158. Rosenkrantz, H, et al.: The chemical analysis of normal canine prostatic fluid. Am J Vet Res 22:1057, 1961.

159. Bartlett, DJ: Studies in dog semen. I. Biochemical characteristics. J Reprod Fertil 3:190, 1962.

160. Pfau, A, et al.: The pH of the prostatic fluid in health and diseases: implications of treatment in chronic bacterial prostatitis. J Urol 119:384, 1978.

161. Fair, WR and Cordonnier, JJ: The pH of prostatic fluid: a reappraisal and therapeutic implications. J Urol 120:695, 1978.

162. Fair, WR, et al.: A re-appraisal of treatment in chronic bacterial prostatitis. J Urol 121:437, 1979.

163. Plomp, TA, et al.: Treatment of recurrent chronic bacterial prostatitis by local injection of thiamphenicol into the prostate. Urology 15:542, 1980.

164. Baumueller, A, et al.: Prostatic tissue and secretion concentration of rosamicin and erythromycin: experimental studies in the dog. Invest Urol 15:158, 1977.

165. Meares, EM: Observations on activity of trimethoprim-sulfamethoxazole in the prostate. J Infect Dis 128:S679, 1973.

166. Reeves, DS and Ghilchik, M: Secretion of the antibacterial substance trimethoprim in the prostatic fluid of dogs. Br J Urol 42:66, 1970.

167. Dabhoiwala, NF, et al.: A study of concentrations of trimethoprim-sulphamethoxazole in the human prostate gland. Br J Urol 48:77, 1976.

168. Paulsen, DF, et al.: Treatment of bacterial prostatitis. Urology 27:379, 1986.

169. Paulson, DF and White, RD: Trimethoprim-sulfamethoxazole and minocycline hydrochloride in the treatment of culture-proved bacterial prostatitis. J Urol 120:184, 1978.

170. Garnes, HA: Doxycycline levels in serum and prostatic tissue in man. Urology 1:205, 1973.

171. Baumueller, A and Madsen, PO: Secretion of various antimicro-

bial substances in dogs with experimental bacterial prostatitis. Urol Res 5:215, 1977.

172. Reeves, DS, et al.: Twenty-three further studies on the secretion of antibiotics in the prostatic fluid of the dog. Proc, 2nd Int Symp Urinary Tract Infection, London, 1972, p 197.

173. Solleveld, HA, et al.: Nalidixic acid intoxication in two pregnant bitches. Tijdschr voor Diergeneesk 103:899, 1978.

174. Harvey, F and Edelson, J: Species differences in hepatic microsomal oxidation of nalidixic acid. Arch Int Pharmacodyn Ther 229:192, 1977.

175. Duffell, SJ: Unexpected reaction to nalidixic acid. Vet Rec 96:188, 1975.

176. Bologna, M, et al.: Bactericidal intraprostatic concentrations of norfloxacin. Lancet 2:280, 1983.

177. Kjaer, T and Madsen, PO: Prostatic fluid and tissue concentrations of ampicillin after administration of hetacillin ester. Invest Urol 14:57, 1976.

178. Oliveri, RA, et al.: Clinical experience with geocillin in the treatment of bacterial prostatitis. Curr Ther Res 25:415, 1979.

179. Nielsen, OS, et al.: Penicillamic acid derivatives in the canine prostate. Prostate 1:79, 1980.

180. Mobley, DF: Bacterial prostatitis: treatment with carbenicillin idanyl sodium. Invest Urol 19:31, 1981.

181. McGuire, EJ and Lytton, B: Bacterial prostatitis. Treatment with trimethoprim-sulfamethoxazole. Urology 7:499, 1976.

182. Meares, EM: Long-term therapy of chronic bacterial prostatitis with trimethoprim-sulfamethoxazole. Can Med Assoc J 112:22, 1975.

183. McGuire, EJ: Theoretical basis for treatment of prostatitis. Urology 24:S10, 1984.

184. Fair, WA: Roundtable discussion of prostatitis. Urology 24:S16, 1984.

185. Bartlett, JG, et al.: Prostatic abscesses involving anaerobic bacteria. Arch Intern Med 138:1369, 1978.

186. Fenster, LF: Reactive hepatopathy. Postgrad Med 76:62, 1984.

187. Bauer, MS: Prostatic abscess rupture in three dogs. JAVMA 188:735, 1986.

188. O'Shea, JD: Studies on the canine prostate gland. J Comp Pathol 73:244, 1963.

189. Weaver, AD: Fifteen cases of prostatic carcinoma in the dog. Vet Rec 109:71, 1981.

190. Alsaker, RD and Stevens, JB: Neoplastic cells in the blood of a dog with prostatic adenocarcinoma. JAAHA 13:486, 1977.

191. Leib, MS, et al.: Squamous cell carcinoma of the prostate gland in a dog. JAAHA 22:509, 1986.

192. Leav, I and Ling, GV: Adenocarcinoma of the canine prostate. Cancer 22:1329, 1968.

193. Durham, SK and Dietze, AE: Prostatic adenocarcinoma with and without metastasis to bone in dogs. JAVMA 188:1432, 1986.

194. Taylor, PA: Prostatic adenocarcinoma in a dog and a summary of 10 cases. Can Vet J 14:162, 1973.

195. Hargis, AM and Miller, LM: Prostatic carcinoma in dogs. Comp Cont Ed Pract Vet 5:647, 1983.

196. Hornbuckle, WE, et al.: Prostatic disease in the dog. Cornell Vet 68:284, 1978.

197. Evans, JE: Prostatic adenocarcinoma in a castrated dog. JAVMA 186:78, 1985.

198. Dube, JY, et al.: Single case report of prostate adenocarcinoma in a dog castrated 3 months previously. Morphological, biochemical and endocrine determinations. Prostate 5:495, 1984.

199. Rendano, VT and Slauson, DO: Hypertrophic osteopathy in a dog with prostatic adenocarcinoma and without thoracic metastasis. JAAHA 18:905, 1982.

200. Mahadevia, PS, et al.: Hypercalcemia in prostatic carcinoma. Arch Int Med 143:1339, 1983.

201. Frenette, G, et al.: Radioimmunoassay in blood plasma of arginine esterase: the major secretory product of dog prostate. Prostate 10:145, 1987.

202. Gill, CW: Prostatic adenocarcinoma with concurrent Sertoli cell tumor in a dog. Can Vet J 22:230, 1981.

203. Zontine, WJ: Prostatic disease. Mod Vet Pract 56:485, 1975.

204. Turrel, JM: Intraoperative radiotherapy of carcinoma of the prostate gland in 10 dogs. JAVMA 190:48, 1987.

205. Howard, DR: The prostate gland. *In* Bojrab, MJ (ed): Current Techniques in Small Animal Surgery. Philadelphia, Lea & Febiger, 1975, p 255.

206. Pettit, GD: A clinical evaluation of prostatectomy in the dog. JAVMA 136:486, 1960.

207. Sawczuk, I, et al.: Primary transitional cell carcinoma of prostatic periurethral ducts. Urology 25:339, 1985.

106 DISORDERS OF THE EXTERNAL GENITALIA OF THE MALE

SHIRLEY D. JOHNSTON

DEVELOPMENTAL ANATOMY AND PHYSIOLOGY OF THE NORMAL PENIS

Penile Anatomy and Embryology

The penis is embryologically derived from a ventral median thickening of the margin of the urogenital membrane, which becomes the genital (phallic) tubercle.[1,2] Urogenital folds or ridges develop on each side of the opening to the urogenital sinus that elongate and fuse ventrally, starting at the base of the phallus and moving forward until the entire ventral penis closes around the penile urethra. The genital tubercle forms the glans penis, and the urogenital folds form the shaft of the penis.[1,2] Mesenchyme inside the glans in the dog and in some cats ossifies to form an os penis.[1,3]

The penis of the adult dog is composed of the (proximal) continuous roots and body, and the distal glans penis, which includes the bulbus glandis and pars longa glandis.[4] Average length of the penis in 150 male dogs was 17.9 cm, with a range of 6.5 to 24 cm.[4] The bulbus glandis, described as a cavernous expansion of the corpus cavernosum urethrae, surrounds the proximal portion of the os penis in the dog; when engorged during erection it becomes a bulb-like region of greatest diameter, and the most proximal region of the penis to be held within the vagina during copulation.

The penis of the cat is also composed of the roots, body, and glans. In contrast to the dog, the glans, which is an 8 to 10 mm long conical structure, is directed caudally. The glans of the adult intact male contains a band of 120 to 150 penile spines in 6 to 8 circular rows (Figure 106-1).[5] These spines are 0.1 to 0.7 mm in length; they are androgen-dependent, and decrease in size after castration. Their function is unknown; they are proposed to increase cervical stimulation of the female, favoring successful induction of ovulation; to impede withdrawal of the penis from the vagina (as they are directed away from the base of the penis); or to provide sexual stimulation for the male or female.[5]

Normal Bacterial Flora of the Prepuce and Penile Urethra

The prepuce and distal penile urethra of the male dog and cat contain normal aerobic resident bacteria similar to those present in the canine and feline vagina; these bacteria are listed in Table 106-1.[6-11]

Multiple species of bacteria may be present on the preputial mucosa at the same time; 3 to 4 isolates were recovered from 14 of 29 preputial culture samples in one study of 6 fertile cats.[10] The presence of these organisms alone, in the absence of compromise of host defense mechanisms, and in the absence of an inflammatory host response, does not indicate that disease is present.

In the dog, mycoplasmas were recovered from the prepuces of 7 of 11 (64 per cent) clinically normal males and from 8 of 11 (73 per cent) fertile males; mycoplasmas also were cultured from the prepuces of 24 of 26 (92 per cent) infertile males and from the prepuces of 12 of 13 (92 per cent) males with balanoposthitis.[8] The number of positive cultures was higher (P < 0.10) in the infertile/balanoposthitis dogs than in the fertile/clinically normal dogs, but the high number of positive cultures in all groups suggested that a single positive culture cannot be used to classify a dog as infertile, or to suggest that mycoplasmas cause infertility. Ureaplasmas were recovered from the prepuces of 18 of 26 (69 per cent) infertile male dogs, from 1 of 13 (8 per cent) males with balanoposthitis, and from 1 of 11 (9 per cent) clinically normal males: ureaplasmas were not isolated from preputial cultures of 11 fertile male dogs.[8] Culture of the feline prepuce for mycoplasmas and ureaplasmas has not been reported.

Physiology of Erection and Ejaculation

Erection and ejaculation are complex physiologic processes that involve integration of endocrine, neuromuscular, and vascular processes. Erection, which can be elicited by the sensory input of presence of an estrous

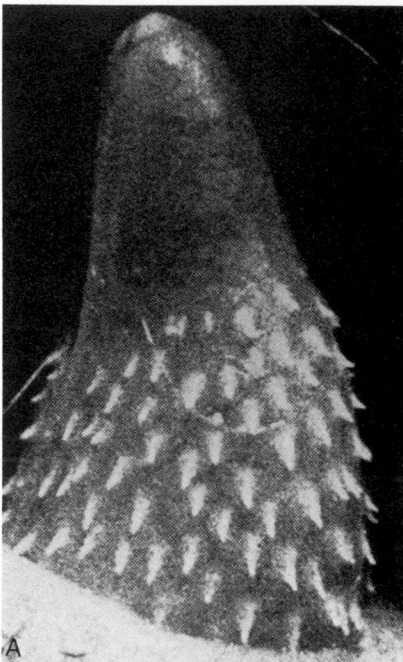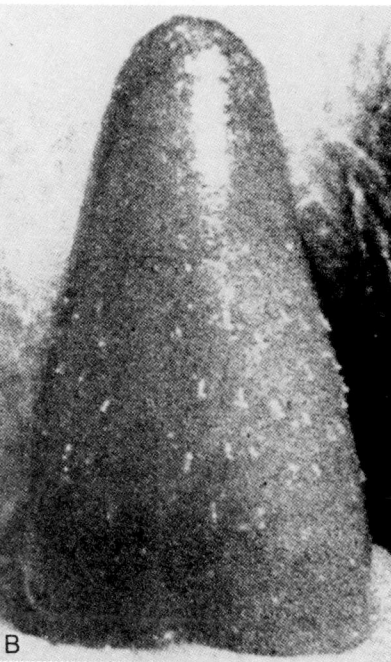

FIGURE 106–1. *A,* Glans penis of an adult intact male cat, and *B,* of an adult male cat six weeks after postpuberal castration. Penile spines after castration are small, thin, and fewer in number. (Aronson, LR, Cooper, ML: Penile spines of the domestic cat: Their endocrine-behavior relations. Anat Rec 157:71, 1967.)

bitch or by pelvic nerve (parasympathetic) stimulation via spinal injury or rectal probe electrical impulse, may be divided into two stages.[12] These are first, filling of the corpus cavernosum urethrae, causing slight penile rigidity, which along with the presence of the os penis enables intromission; and second, stimulation of penile sensory nerve endings, causing complete engorgement of the pars longa glandis and bulbus glandis, leading to entrapment of the penis within the vagina. During this second phase, semen is emitted into the prostatic urethra under α-adrenergic sympathetic stimulation from the T12-L3 region of the sympathetic trunk by way of the hypogastric nerve, the bladder neck closes (also under sympathetic stimulation), and semen is propelled through the pelvic urethra and out the external urethral orifice (ejaculation) by contraction of the striated ischiocavernosus and bulbocavernosus muscles (innervated by the somatic fibers of the pudendal nerve).[13]

TABLE 106–1. BACTERIAL FLORA OF THE NORMAL PREPUCE

Canine	Feline
Acinetobacter sp.	*Bacillus* sp.
Bacillus sp.	*Enterococcus* sp.
Corynebacterium sp.	*Escherichia coli*
Escherichia coli	*Klebsiella oxytoca*
Flavobacterium sp.	*Proteus mirabilis*
Haemophilus sp.	*Pseudomonas aeruginosa*
Klebsiella pneumoniae	*Serratia odorifera*
Moraxella sp.	*Staphylococcus* sp.
Mycoplasma sp.	*Streptococcus* sp.
Proteus mirabilis	*Yersinia intermedia*
Pseudomonas aeruginosa	
Staphylococcus aureus	
Staphylococcus epidermidis	
Streptococcus canis	
Streptococcus equisimilis	
Viridans streptococci	

After emission, and during or after ejaculation of the first, sperm-rich portion of semen, the dog dismounts from the bitch and, with the erect penis still entrapped within the vagina, lifts a hind leg over her back and turns to face away from her in the copulatory lock (Figure 106–2).[14] This results in a 180 degree horizontal flexure of the penile body at a point midway between the distal insertion of the ischiocavernosus muscle and the os penis.[14] During the copulatory lock, which typically lasts 10 to 30 minutes, prostatic fluid is ejaculated. After ejaculation, the extrinsic penile muscles (the ischiocavernosus and bulbocavernosus muscles) relax, arterial blood pressure drops, and venous pressure declines as erectile bodies shrink.[4]

Feline erection, emission, and propulsion of semen through the penile urethra also are mediated by parasympathetic, sympathetic, and somatic nerve fibers.[15, 16] Parasympathetic stimulation of the second sacral nerve roots produces erection, and subsequent sympathetic stimulation at L1-2 or of the hypogastric nerve causes emission; stimulation of the internal pudendal nerve results in propulsion of semen through and out the penile urethra.[15, 16] These events can be elicited by application of electrical impulses by means of rectal probe at electroejaculation. Mechanism of bladder neck closure at emission, or even whether bladder neck closure occurs, is unknown; the cat is known to ejaculate semen into the bladder as well as through the penis at natural copulation.[17]

Influence of Castration on Penile Anatomy and Physiology

Castration does not significantly affect penile anatomy unless performed before time of separation of the common layer of stratified squamous epithelium joining the prepuce to the penis, resulting in penile/preputial adhe-

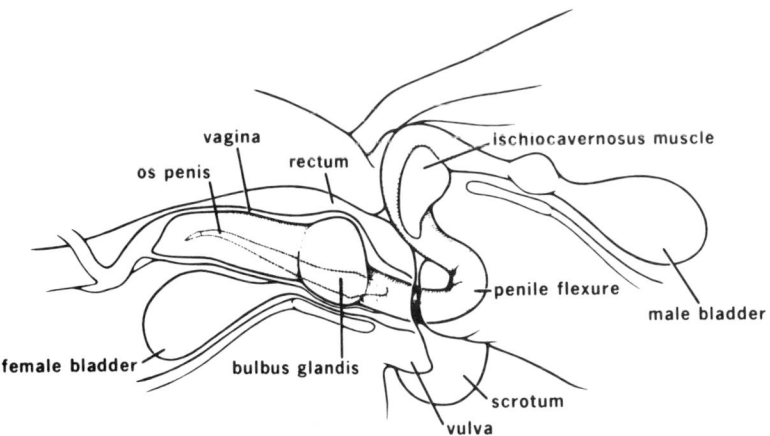

FIGURE 106–2. Diagram of the relationship between the male and female genitalia during second stage coitus. (Adapted from Grandage, J: The erect dog penis: A paradox of flexible rigidity. Vet Rec 91:141, 1972.)

sion. Four of ten male kittens castrated at five months of age showed variable adhesions of the prepuce to the penis, whereas ten kittens left intact and ten kittens castrated at five months of age and given replacement therapy with testosterone did not show such adhesions.[18] Time of complete penile-preputial separation in the dog is unknown. Prepuberal castration does not affect urethral diameter in the cat.[19]

Castration usually results in decrease or elimination of sexual behavior, erection, and ejaculation in the dog and cat.[20] Some males that have been sexually active before castration may, however, continue to copulate after castration.

Congenital Morphologic Disorders of the Penis

Congenital defects of the penis and prepuce were present in 14 of 4074 dogs and in 0 of 242 cats with congenital defects seen at 10 North American veterinary college clinics.[21] Incidence by type of defect or by size of the entire population has not been reported.

Penile Hypoplasia

Penile hypoplasia, a rare disorder, has been reported in the cocker spaniel, collie, Doberman pinscher, Great Dane, and domestic shorthair cat.[22–27]

Two animals with infantile penis have been reported that were karyotyped, and that had an abnormal sex chromosome complement. These were a 2n=78,XX phenotypic male American cocker spaniel with aberrant H-Y antigen transmission, and a 2n=38,XX/3n= 57,XXY chimeric phenotypic male calico cat.[23, 27] Penile hypoplasia was an incidental finding in these patients, both of which otherwise appeared normal except for absence of spermatogenesis in their testes. Penile hypoplasia also has been observed in an 11-month-old Doberman pinscher with a hypoplastic preputial opening, causing urine pooling, chronic urine scald inside the prepuce, and continual dripping of urine from the prepuce.[25, 26] Surgical enlargement of the preputial opening and shortening of the preputial length by excision of a rectangular block of tissue resulted in bringing the tip

of the penis to within 5 mm of the preputial opening, with resolution of the urine pooling signs.

Penile hypoplasia in humans has been associated with numerical abnormality of the sex chromosomes, hypopituitarism, and androgen deficiency states, for which affected dogs and cats should be examined. Therapy is indicated only in those patients in which enlargement of the preputial orifice may facilitate urination.

Hypospadias and/or Preputial Defects

Hypospadias is a congenital defect of urethral closure resulting in abnormal location of the external urethral orifice (Figure 106–3). Types of hypospadias in the male, based on site of the urethral opening, are depicted in Figure 106–4.[28] Glandular, penile, scrotal, and perineal hypospadias have been reported in the beagle, Boston terrier, German shepherd, mixed breed, Shih Tzu, and

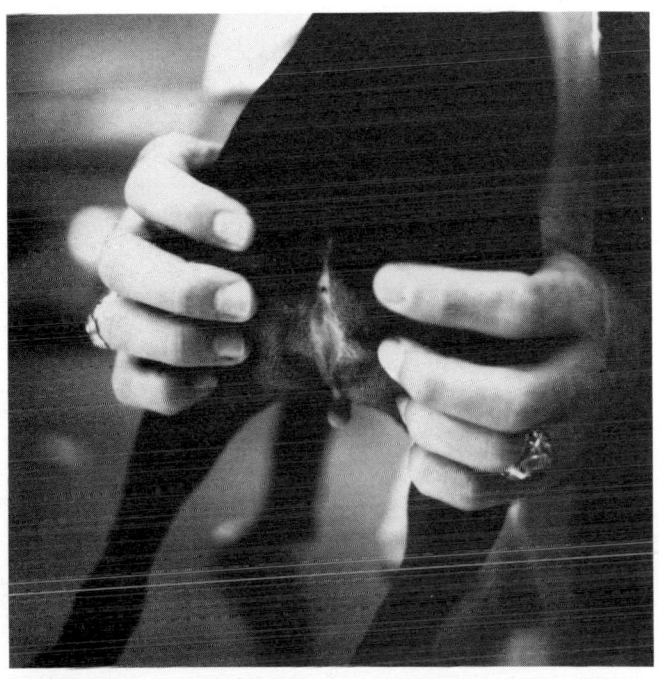

FIGURE 106–3. Scrotal hypospadias in a Boston terrier. The dog urinated through a defect.

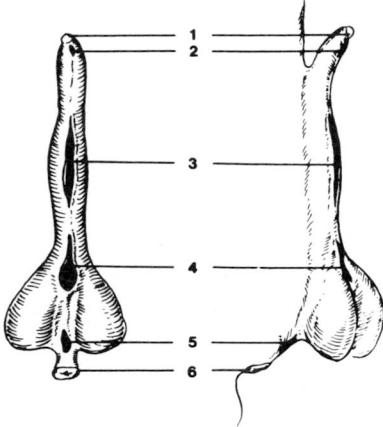

FIGURE 106–4. Types of hypospadias. 1. Normal urethral meatus. 2. Glandular hypospadias. 3. Penile hypospadias. 4. Scrotal hypospadias. 5. Perineal hypospadias. 6. Anal hypospadias. (Ader, PL, Hobson, HP: Hypospadias: A review of the veterinary literature and a report of three cases in the dog. JAAHA 14:721, 1978.)

toy poodle.[28–34] Incontinence was present in two of the affected dogs (one glandular and one perineal), one dog was cryptorchid, one had agenesis of the left kidney, and several had incomplete preputial closure with exposure of the glans penis, necessitating surgical correction.[28] Patients with hypospadias should be observed for evidence of urinary incontinence, and should be evaluated by urinalysis and intravenous urography for evidence of urinary tract infection and other urologic anomalies in addition to the hypospadias. Preputial defects may be present with or without hypospadias, and should be corrected surgically with the objectives of covering the penile mucosa and providing an adequate preputial orifice for penile protrusion.[28, 34]

Persistent Penile Frenulum

Normal separation of the glans penis from the overlying layer of preputial epithelial cells is a testosterone-dependent phenomenon that occurs before birth in some species and days to months after birth in others. Persistence of a sheer, connective tissue penile frenulum in the dog (Figure 106–5) represents partial failure of this normal separation. Persistent penile frenulum in the dog usually occurs on the ventral midline of the penis, and has been reported in the cocker spaniel, miniature poodle, mixed-breed dog, and Pekingese.[35–41] Clinical signs may be absent, or may include unsuccessful breeding attempts, lack of libido, repeated licking of the penis, and urine scald of the rear legs owing to abnormal direction of the urine stream at urination. The fibrous connective tissue bands vary in appearance from 2 mm wide thin bands to wide, flat sheets of tissue; these may cause ventral or lateral deviation of the penis. Diagnosis is by inspection. Treatment is surgical incision of the tissue under local anesthesia or sedation; hemorrhage from the sheer frenuli usually is light. Although heritability of persistent penile frenulum is unknown, one author reports correcting this defect in 16 cocker spaniel puppies from the same kennel, suggesting a heritable basis of the trait.[38]

Herron reported that castration of male kittens at five months of age was associated with adhesions of the prepuce to the penis in four of ten animals.[18] These adhesions were not associated with abnormal clinical signs in the animals examined, but could perhaps predispose to infection of the pockets formed in the adjacent balanopreputial fold. When early castration is considered, therefore, the cat should be examined in order to determine that penile-preputial separation is complete.

Congenital Preputial Stenosis with Phimosis

Congenital preputial stenosis leading to phimosis, or entrapment of the penis inside the prepuce, has been reported in both the dog and cat. It may vary from complete occlusion of the preputial orifice, resulting in obstruction to urinary outflow and early death (Figure 106–6), to asymptomatic narrowing of the urethral orifice, preventing protrusion of the penis. The condition has been reported in the Bouvier des Flandres, German shepherd, Labrador retriever, golden retriever, mixed-breed dog, and domestic shorthair cat.[42–47] Presenting signs include dribbling of urine from the preputial orifice if preputial urine pooling has occurred, dysuria, and/or inability to copulate normally. Diagnosis is by inspection, and treatment is surgical enlargement of the preputial orifice under general anesthesia. Congenital preputial stenosis has been observed in a litter of mixed breed dogs and in multiple related golden retriever litters, suggesting that this condition may be heritable.

Duplication of the Penis (Diphallia)

Penile duplication (Figure 106–7) is an extremely rare congenital anomaly that has been reported in approximately 100 human patients, where incidence is estimated at 1 in 5 million births, and in two dogs.[48, 49] The affected dogs were a five-month-old pointer with concurrent hydronephrosis of the left kidney, and a six-month-old poodle-cross with duplication of the urinary bladder,

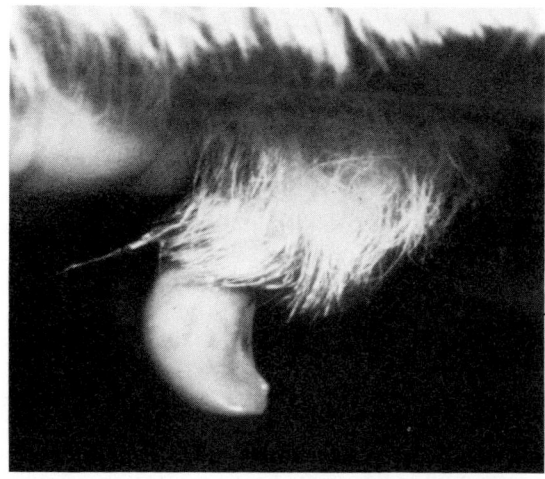

FIGURE 106–5. Persistent penile frenulum in an adult male Shih Tzu, with penis deflected ventrally.

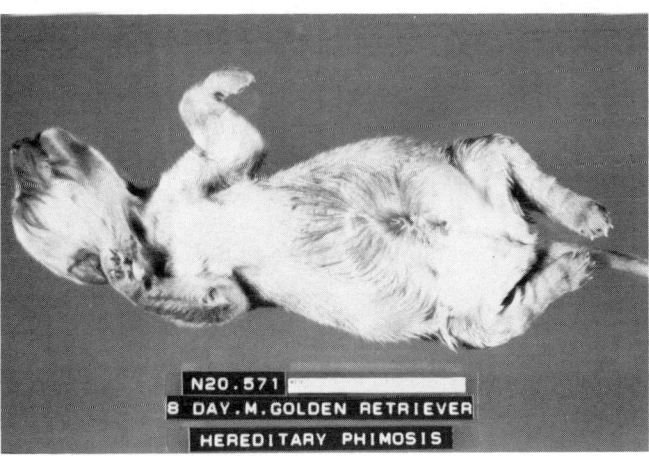

FIGURE 106–6. Eight-day-old golden retriever puppy with phimosis and outflow obstruction to urination.

right renal hypoplasia, bifurcation of the descending colon, and bilateral cryptorchidism. Diphallia may result from anomalous longitudinal duplication of the cloacal membrane, followed by ventral migration of primitive streak mesoderm around two cloacal membranes to form two genital tubercles; more extensive midline duplication may result in duplication or anomaly of other structures of the caudal abdomen, for which affected animals should be carefully examined.

ACQUIRED MORPHOLOGIC DISORDERS OF THE PENIS

Urethral Prolapse

Prolapse of the male urethra through the external urethral orifice at the tip of the penis has been reported in the English bulldog and the Boston terrier (Figure

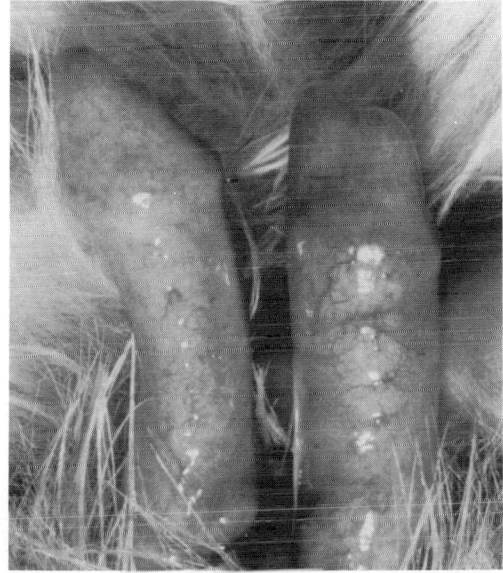

FIGURE 106–7. Diphallia in a six-month-old poodle-cross dog. (Johnston, SD, et al.: Diphallia in a mixed-breed dog with multiple anomalies. Theriogenology, 1987.)

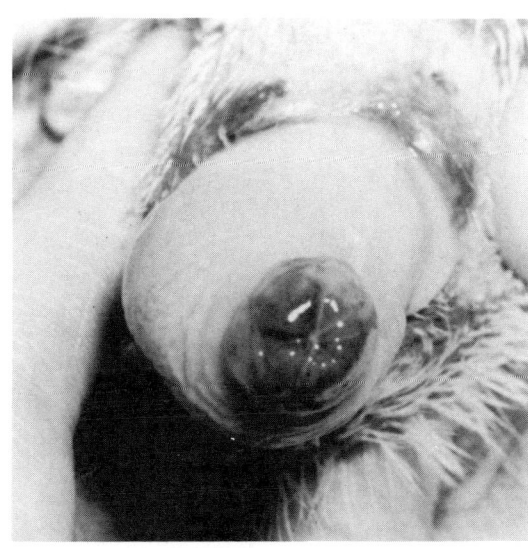

FIGURE 106–8. Urethral prolapse in a one and one-half year old English bulldog.

106–8).[50–52] At time of presentation, affected animals have ranged in age from nine months to three years. Magnitude of eversion may range from 1 to 2 mm in thickness to a pea-sized globe of tissue (8 to 10 mm thick) at the external urethral orifice. Because this condition has been described only in intact males, and because a few affected males appeared to worsen on exposure to an estrous bitch, the condition has been attributed to excessive sexual excitement.[52] Clinical signs may be absent, or bleeding from the tip of the penis (5 to 30 ml per day, randomly or at ejaculation) may occur. Bleeding appears to increase in the presence of an estrous bitch. One author reported success in manually reducing the prolapse and placing a nonabsorbable pursestring suture in the adjacent tissue of the glans penis.[51] Others have reported successful amputation of the prolapsed mass and subsequent normal copulations.[50, 52] The condition has not been reported in neutered males. Hereditary predisposition, if any, is unknown but is suggested by the small number of affected breeds.

Penile Contusion/Injury

Penile trauma may occur in the dog and cat from fights with other animals, from failing to clear fences or other barriers that the animal jumps, from being hit by cars, from mating (secondary to vaginovestibular strictures in the bitch, penile hair rings in the tom), or from the dog being pulled away from the female during the copulatory lock.[47, 53–55] Penile trauma or strangulation may result in formation of a hematoma, with possible subsequent necrosis, and, occasionally, gangrene.[55, 56] Penile trauma usually is very painful, although cats with penile hair rings may be asymptomatic except for prolonged thrusting and breeding attempts.[57, 58]

Urethral integrity and possibility of os penis fracture should be assessed immediately after major penile trauma occurs, using survey radiography, urethral catheterization, and retrograde urethrography. Superficial penile lacerations should be thoroughly cleansed, and antibiotic cream should be liberally applied to prevent adhesion of the healing penis to the prepuce. Deeper wounds should be cleaned, flushed, debrided, if necessary, and sutured with absorbable suture, using meticulous hemostasis and electrocautery. The penis should be protruded twice daily for two weeks for examination and application of antibiotic cream.

Affected animals should have no contact with estrous females or other excitatory circumstances in order to prevent erection and excessive hemorrhage during penile healing. Elizabethan collars should be used if there is licking or chewing at the healing area. Hemorrhage frequently persists for two to three weeks after penile trauma or penile surgery. Penile hair rings in cats can be easily snipped off, and healing of the penis usually is rapid.[57, 58]

Fracture of the Os Penis

Fracture of the os penis has been described in the dog, but not in the cat.[47, 59–64] Such fractures usually are caused by external trauma, and usually are associated with local pain, urethral tear, urine outflow obstruction, and obstructive bony callus formation after healing. Three of four dogs with fractured os penes in one report were originally presented with distended urinary bladders and advanced signs of uremia; seven dogs in other case reports also had these signs.[47, 59–64] All dogs with penile trauma should have survey radiographic examination of the os penis, urethral catheterization, and retrograde urethrography to confirm and localize the area of urethral tear, if present. Cystocentesis can be used to empty the distended urinary bladder before diagnostic evaluation. Treatment depends on the amount of displacement of the bony fragments and on the degree and cause of urethral obstruction. If any urethral compromise is present, urethral catheters and antibiotic therapy should be used for 14 days. Simple fractures with no displacement may not require immobilization, as the os penis is surrounded by fibrous connective tissue.[56] Other fractures have responded well to wiring or plating the os penis fragments together. Urethral tears should be sutured if necessary; a urethrostomy may be performed as a temporary measure during urethral healing or as a permanent measure if adequate urine outflow cannot be maintained. Periodic retrograde urethrography is advised for six to eight months after the fracture to monitor the effect of bony callus formation of the os penis on the urethral lumen. Occasionally perineal urethrostomy and penile amputation are indicated secondary to a fractured os penis and massive urethral trauma.

Balanoposthitis

Infections of the penis and prepuce constituted 20 per cent of 198 cases of canine penile and preputial lesions, and 36 per cent of the 112 cases that excluded tumors.[47] Most cases of balanoposthitis in dogs occur in young intact males with copious yellow or sanguineous purulent preputial discharge.[47] The preputial and penile mucosa of affected dogs is usually erythematous and sometimes ulcerated, and may contain multiple vesicular lesions. Aerobic bacteria cultured from preputial discharge of dogs with balanoposthitis are those of normal preputial mucosa: *Escherichia coli*, *Proteus vulgaris*, *Staphylococcus* sp., hemolytic streptococci, *Pseudomonas aeruginosa*, and *Mycoplasma* sp.[8, 47] Foreign-body or fungal balanoposthitis may occasionally occur in the dog. Balanoposthitis has not been reported in the cat.

Significance of multiple vesicular lesions at the base of the canine penis is unknown. These may be observed in normal, fertile male dogs and in males with clinical signs of balanoposthitis (purulent discharge with inflamed mucosa). Joshua reported finding these vesicles in 62 of 100 dogs ranging in age from 11 weeks to 14 years; the majority of these dogs were asymptomatic.[65, 66] Although no cause was determined, Joshua proposed that the vesicles may be caused by the canine herpesvirus, although no viral inclusions were observed in the vesicular lesions examined, which appeared, histologically, to be lymphoid aggregates.[67]

The diagnostic approach to dogs with balanoposthitis includes careful inspection of the inside of the preputial sheath for foreign bodies or tumors and to confirm presence of mucosal irritation (Figure 106–9); cytologic demonstration of a purulent or granulomatous discharge, bacterial/fungal culture of the discharge as an indicator of antimicrobial therapy; and mucosal biopsy of unusual lesions. Treatment includes a three to four week course of specific parenteral antimicrobial therapy and daily irrigation of the preputial sheath with saline solution and hydrogen peroxide followed by infusion of a broad-spectrum antibiotic ointment (such as bovine mastitis preparations).

Paraphimosis

Paraphimosis refers to failure of the glans penis to be retracted normally into the prepuce. Such failure may occur with an erect or nonerect penis, and may be due to the presence of an abnormally small preputial orifice, presence of a prepuce of inadequate length, or presence of ineffective preputial muscles. Paraphimosis is most typically seen in male dogs after copulation, when the erect glans penis may become strangulated at the preputial orifice; in small excitable breeds that show repeated penile erection not related to copulation; and in pseudohermaphrodite animals that have an abnormally small or short prepuce.[68–74]

Paraphimosis has been reported in one cat, an adult domestic shorthair male, with dysuria, hematuria, and anorexia; an abnormal preputial ring was detected and excised when the cat was examined under anesthesia, and the paraphimosis was resolved.[46]

Paraphimosis is diagnosed by inspection, and determination should be made whether the preputial orifice is abnormally small or abnormally short, and whether the prepuce can be drawn forward over the glans penis (suggesting ineffective preputial muscles). The penis should then be cleaned, well lubricated, and replaced in the prepuce after appropriate surgical correction of the defect. Surgical shortening of the preputial muscles (thin

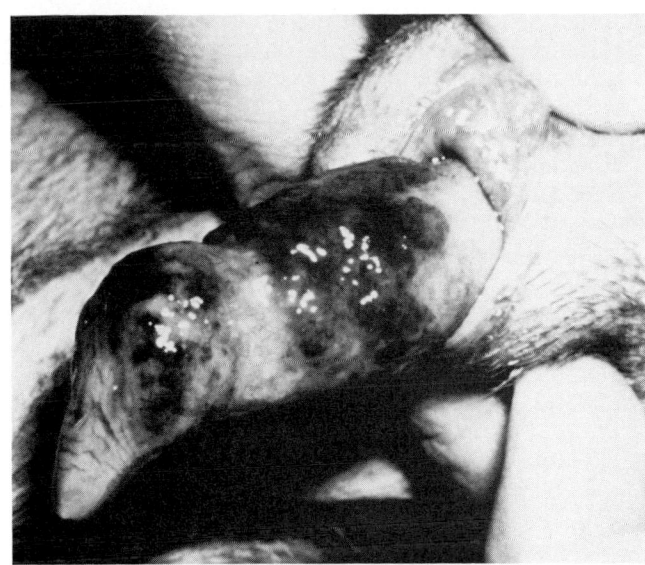

FIGURE 106–9. Ulcerative pyogranulomatous balanoposthitis, which responded to parenteral trimethoprim-sulfa therapy.

ribbons of the cutaneous trunci muscle) has been described, using a through-and-through suture pattern through an S-shaped overlap created in each muscle cranial to the prepuce.[68] Endocrine therapy and castration usually are unsuccessful in resolving true paraphimosis, unless it occurs secondary to persistent erection. Paraphimosis frequently results in gangrene of the glans penis, which necessitates amputation of the penis.

Penile Neoplasia

Tumors of the penis include epithelial tumors (papilloma, squamous cell carcinoma), fibromas, transmissible venereal tumors (TVT), and other mesenchymal tumors (fibrosarcomas, lymphosarcomas, hemangiosarcomas, mast cell carcinomas).[75–79] With the exception of the TVT, which is often acquired by young dogs at coitus, penile tumors occur in older dogs (10 to 11 years of age). Penile neoplasms have not been reported in the cat.

Diagnosis is based on inspection of the penis followed by excisional biopsy (wide surgical excision using electrocautery) and histopathology; the pattern of metastasis and prognosis depends on tumor type. The TVT is a transmissible tumor that grows, invades, and metastasizes most widely in immune-compromised animals. The single TVT should be treated with wide surgical excision. Recurrent or metastatic TVT should be treated weekly with vincristine (0.012 mg/lb or 0.025 mg/kg IV, not to exceed 1 mg) in the absence of leukopenia until the tumor is gone.[76] Doxorubicin and orthovoltage radiotherapy have also been used successfully with the TVT.[78]

FUNCTIONAL DISORDERS OF THE PENIS

Failure to Achieve Erection

Male dogs may fail to achieve normal erection because of inadequate excitatory stimulus of the bitch (bitch not in heat, not periovulatory, mild signs of heat because of ovarian dysfunction), pain (hip dysplasia, vertebral osteoarthritis at mounting the bitch, which normally precedes complete erection), prostate pain secondary to acute prostatitis, parasympathetic (pelvic nerve) deficit, fear/anxiety about the bitch or environment, or androgen deficiency states, such as abnormalities of sexual differentiation (79,XXY, 78,XX, 78,XX/78,XY karyotypes), castration, or anti-androgen therapy (ketaconazole). Erection failure in other species also has occurred secondary to intrapenile vascular shunts preventing normal engorgement with blood.

Diagnostic approach to erection failure is to perform a complete physical examination (to include palpation of the testes and hip joints and rectal palpation of the prostrate), with radiographs of the hips and lower spine in dogs with suspected arthritis. If androgen deficiency is suspected (young dog, small testes, infantile or ambiguous genitalia, congenital infertility), blood should be submitted to a veterinary cytogenetics laboratory for karyotype. As a general rule, serum concentrations of testosterone do not correlate well with libido, but resting serum testosterone (0.5 to 5.0 ng/ml, canine; ND to 3.0 ng/ml, feline) and serum testosterone one hour after IM administration of 1 µg/lb (dog) or 25 µg (cat) of gonadotrophin-releasing hormone (GnRH) IM (3.7 to 6.2 ng/ml, canine; 5.0 to 12.0 ng/ml, feline) can be measured to determine whether the animal can maximally secrete testosterone.[80]

Prognosis usually is grave in the presence of abnormal karyotype, low serum testosterone, or infantile soft testes. If karyotype, serum testosterone, and testicular size are normal, collection of semen, using an artificial vagina, should be attempted in the presence of a docile, periovulatory (usually about 12 days after proestrus onset) bitch. Some authors have reported inducing sexual arousal in male dogs by exposing them to methyl-p-hydrobenzoate, reported to be the major canine sex pheromone.[81]

Failure to Achieve Antegrade Ejaculation

Antegrade ejaculation occurs when semen is emitted into the prostatic urethra (under the influence of α-adrenergic innervation of the cauda epididymides, vasa deferentia, ampullae, and prostate), the smooth muscle of the bladder neck contracts (also under α-adrenergic stimulation), and contraction of the striated bulbocavernosus and ischiocavernosus muscles (by means of pudendal nerve enervation) propels semen through the penile urethra. Retrograde ejaculation of semen into the urinary bladder has been reported in an Alsatian dog.[82] Male cats ejaculate some semen antegrade and some retrograde during normal electroejaculation.[17]

Retrograde ejaculation is diagnosed by detecting semen in the urinary bladder after ejaculation; sperm cells (50 to 150 × 10⁶/ml in semen) and alkaline phosphatase (5,000 to 40,000 μ/L in semen) of appropriate concentration in urine confirm the diagnosis.

Treatment of retrograde ejaculation in the dog has not been reported. Treatment with a sympathomimetic agent (such as phenylpropanolamine, 1.4 mg/lb (3 mg/kg) PO q12h, or pseudoephedrine, 2 to 3.5 mg/lb (5 to 7 mg/kg) PO q12h) would be indicated around time of ejaculation. One patient, a young adult Yorkshire terrier, with small semen volume (one drop of sperm-rich semen present at the urethral orifice, with low sperm numbers and alkaline phosphatase in the urinary bladder after ejaculation) was infertile before and fertile after (with normal semen volume) initiation of pseudoephedrine therapy given one and three hours before copulation.

Persistent Erection (Priapism)

Persistent erection in the absence of sexual stimulus is seen occasionally in dogs with spinal lesions, and rarely in dogs with thromboembolism of penile vasculature. This condition differs from the frequent erections seen in young, excitable small breed dogs, which respond to behavioral modification, castration, and/or progestogen therapy. Dogs with persistent erections should be treated with topical cleansing of the penis, antibiotic creams for penile lubrication, and identification and treatment of spinal lesions. The erection usually subsides with resolution of the spinal lesion. Thromboembolism is diagnosed histologically after amputation of the penis.

References

1. Latshaw, WK: Veterinary Developmental Anatomy. Philadelphia, BC Decker, 1987.
2. Wensing, CJG and Fentener van Vlissingen, JM: Development of the male genital tract in the dog. Tijdschr Diergeneeskd 111:17S, 1986.
3. Jackson, CM: On the structure of the corpora cavernosa in the domestic cat. Am J Anat 2:73, 1902.
4. Miller, ME, et al.: Anatomy of the Dog. Philadelphia, WB Saunders, 1967.
5. Aronson, LR and Cooper, ML: Penile spines of the domestic cat: Their endocrine—behavior relations. Anat Rec 157:71, 1967.
6. Allen, WE and Dagnall, GJR: Some observations on the aerobic bacterial flora of the genital tract of the dog and bitch. J Sm Anim Pract 23:325, 1982.
7. Cox, HU, et al.: Distribution of staphylococcal species on clinically healthy cats. Am J Vet Res 46:1824, 1985.
8. Doig, PA, et al.: The genital mycoplasma and ureaplasma flora of healthy and diseased dogs. Can J Comp Med 45:233, 1981.
9. Figueiredo, C: Contribution to the study of prepuce of dogs: histological aspects; aerobial flora and cytology of the secretion. Arq da Esc Vet Univ Fed Minas Gervais 22:217, 1970.
10. Johnston, SD: Bacterial culture of the reproductive tract: methods and interpretation. Proc 54th Ann Mtg, AAHA, Phoenix, March, 1987, p 185.
11. Ling, GV and Ruby, AL: Aerobic bacterial flora of the prepuce, urethra, and vagina of normal adult dogs. Am J Vet Res 39:695, 1978.
12. Christensen, GC: Angioarchitecture of the canine penis and the process of erection. Am J Anat 95:227, 1954.
13. Arver, S and Sjostrand, NO: Functions of adrenergic and cholinergic nerves in canine effectors of seminal emission. Acta Physiol Scand 115:67, 1982.
14. Grandage, J: The erect dog penis: a paradox of flexible rigidity. Vet Rec 91:141, 1972.
15. Root, WS and Bard, P: The mediation of feline erection through sympathetic pathways with some remarks on sexual behavior after deafferentation of the genitalia. Am J Physiol 151:80, 1947.
16. Semans, JH and Langworthy, OR: Observations on the neurophysiology of sexual function in the male cat. J Urol 40:836, 1938.
17. Dooley, MP, et al.: Retrograde flow of semen caused by electroejaculation in the domestic cat. Proc 10th Intl Congr Anim Reprod Art Insem, Urbana IL, 1984, p 363.
18. Herron, MA: A potential consequence of prepuberal feline castration. Fel Pract 1:17, 1971.
19. Herron, MA: The effect of prepubertal castration on the penile urethra of the cat. JAVMA 160:208, 1972.
20. Rosenblatt, JS and Aronson, LR: The decline of sexual behavior in male cats after castration with special reference to the role of prior sexual experience. Behavior 13:285, 1958.
21. Priester, WA, et al.: Congenital defects in domesticated animals. Am J Vet Res 31:1871, 1970.
22. Bloom, F: Pathology of the dog and cat: The genitourinary system. Evanston, IL, American Veterinary Publications, 1954.
23. Gregson, NM and Ishmael, J: Diploid-triploid chimerism in 3 tortoiseshell cats. Res Vet Sci 12:275, 1971.
24. Hakala, JE: Reproductive tract anomalies in two male cats. Mod Vet Pract 65:629, 1984.
25. Proescholdt, T and DeYoung, D: Infantile penis in the canine. Iowa Vet 2:59, 1977.
26. Proescholdt, TA, et al.: Preputial reconstruction for phimosis and infantile penis. JAAHA 13:725, 1977.
27. Seldon, JR, et al.: Genetic basis of XX male syndrome and XX true hermaphroditism: evidence in the dog. Science 201:644, 1978.
28. Ader, PL and Hobson, HP: Hypospadias: a review of the veterinary literature and a report of three cases in the dog. JAAHA 14:721, 1978.
29. Croshaw, JE and Brodey, RS: Failure of preputial closure in a dog. JAVMA 136:450, 1960.
30. Kipnis, RM: Membranous penile urethra and preputial abnormality in a dog. VM/SAC 69:750, 1974.
31. Larrosa, ET: Hypospadias caninas. Veterinaria (Spain) 38:591, 1973.
32. McFarland, LZ and Deniz, E: Unilateral renal agenesis with ipsilateral cryptorchidism and perineal hypospadias in a dog. JAVMA 139:1099, 1961.
33. Osborne, CA, et al.: Canine and feline urology. Philadelphia, WB Saunders, 1972.
34. Pope, ER and Swaim, SF: Surgical reconstruction of a hypoplastic prepuce. JAAHA 22:73, 1986.
35. Balke, J: Persistent penile frenulum in a cocker spaniel. VM/SAC 76:988, 1981.
36. Belkin, PB: Persistence of penile frenulum in a dog. Mod Vet Prac 50:80, 1969.
37. Biondini, J, et al.: Persistencia do "frenulum preputti" no cao. Arq da Esc Vet Univ Fed Minas Gervais 27:87, 1975.
38. Hutchison, JA: Persistence of the penile frenulum in dogs. Can Vet J 14:71, 1973.

39. Joshua, JO: Persistence of the penile frenulum in a dog. Vet Rec 74:1550, 1962.
40. Pugh, DG, et al.: A persistent penile frenulum in a dog. Canine Prac 14:38, 1987.
41. Ryer, KA: Persistent penile frenulum in a cocker spaniel. VM/SAC 74:688, 1979.
42. Biewenga, WJ: False urinary incontinence in a pup. Tijdschr Diergeneesk 99:841, 1974.
43. Elam, CW and Randle, PO: Peculiar preputial condition in a five-week-old puppy. Vet Rec 64:98, 1952.
44. Elkins, AD: Surgical correction of congenital stricture of the preputial orifice in the cat. Fel Pract 13:20, 1983.
45. Jacobs, D and Baughman, GL: Preputial defect in a puppy. Mod Vet Pract 58:522, 1977.
46. Kirk, H: Phimosis and paraphimosis in the cat. Vet Rec 11:832, 1931.
47. Ndiritu, CG: Lesions of the canine penis and prepuce. Mod Vet Pract 60:712, 1979.
48. Potena, A, et al.: Su di una rarissima difallia in un cane. Acta Med Vet 20:125, 1974.
49. Johnston, SD, et al.: Diphallia in a mixed-breed dog with multiple anomalies. Theriogenology, 1987.
50. Copland, MD: Prolapse of the penile urethra in a dog. NZ Vet J 23:180, 1975.
51. Firestone, WM: Prolapse of the male urethra. JAVMA 99:135, 1941.
52. Hobson, HP and Heller, RA: Surgical correction of prolapse of the male urethra. VM/SAC 66:1177, 1971.
53. Rickards, DA, et al.: Partial phallectomy in a dog. JAVMA 161:290, 1972.
54. Stein, BS: The genital system. In Catcott, EJ (ed): Feline Medicine and Surgery, 2nd ed. Santa Barbara, CA, American Veterinary Publications, 1975, p 303.
55. Coulton, J: Traumatic rupture of the penis in a dog. Rec Med Vet 126:591, 1975.
56. Johnston, DE: Repairing lesions of the canine penis and prepuce. Mod Vet Pract 47:39, 1965.
57. Wooldridge, GH: Retention of urine in a cat, due to spontaneous ligature of the penis with fur. Br Vet J 15:305, 1908.
58. Hart, BL and Peterson, DM: Penile hair rings in male cats may prevent mating. Lab Anim Sci 21:422, 1971.
59. Bradley, RL: Complete urethral obstruction secondary to fracture of the os penis. Comp Cont Ed 9:759, 1985.
60. Denholm, TC: Fracture of the os penis. Vet Rec 69:15, 1957.
61. Jeffery, KL: Fracture of the os penis in a dog. JAAHA 10:41, 1974.
62. Luke, D and Bell, FR: Fracture of the os penis in an Alsatian dog. Vet Rec 54:498, 1942.
63. Stead, AC: Fracture of the os penis in the dog—two case reports. J Sm Anim Pract 13:19, 1972.
64. Woimant, X and Chaffaux, S: Etude d'un cas de fracture de l'os pénien chez le chien. Rec Med Vet 152:235, 1976.
65. Builder, PL, et al.: An eruptive condition affecting mucous surfaces in dogs. Vet Rec 62:796, 1950.
66. Joshua, JO: "Dog pox": some clinical aspects of an eruptive condition of certain mucous surfaces in dogs. Vet Rec 96:300, 1975.
67. Poste, G and King, N: Isolation of a herpesvirus from the canine genital tract: Association with infertility, abortion and still-births. Vet Rec 88:229, 1981.
68. Chaffee, VW and Knecht, CD: Canine paraphimosis: Sequel to inefficient preputial muscles. VM/SAC 70:1418, 1975.
69. Elkins, AD: Canine paraphimosis of unknown etiology: a case report. VM/SAC 79:638, 1984.
70. Flukiger, U and Gonin, P: Welche diagnose stellen sie? - Welche therapeutischen massnahmen schlagen sievor? Schweiz Arch Tierheilkiunde 127:45, 1985.
71. Kogovsek, J and Jazbec, I: Amputation of a gangrene affected penis in a dog. Veterinarski Glasnik 30:1047, 1976.
72. Lee, J: Paraphimosis in a pseudohermaphrodite dog. VM/SAC 71:1076, 1976.
73. Leighton, R: A simple surgical correction for chronic penile protrusion. JAAHA 12:667, 1976.
74. Singh, M, et al.: Surgical management of paraphymosis in a cryptorchid dog. Indian J Vet Surg 2:36, 1981.
75. Ball, V and Rosi, P: Cancer of the prepuce and glans. Vet J 84:530, 1928.
76. Calvert, CA, et al.: Vincristine for treatment of transmissible venereal tumor in the dog. JAVMA 181:163, 1982.
77. Hall, WC, et al.: Tumors of the prostate and penis. Bull WHO 53:247, 1976.
78. Thrall, DE: Orthovoltage radiotherapy of canine transmissible venerable tumors. Vet Radiol 23:217, 1982.
79. Wasman, SC: Cancer of the penis. Vet Med 50:31, 1955.
80. Johnston, SD: Reproductive disorders: diagnostic endocrinology. Proc 54th Ann Mtg, AAHA, Phoenix, AZ, March, 1987, p 182.
81. Goodwin, M, et al.: Sex pheromone in the dog. Science 203:559, 1979.
82. Meinecke, VB: Retrograde ejakulation beim ruden. Zuchthyg 11:122, 1976.

SECTION XII

THE URINARY SYSTEM

107 DIAGNOSIS AND PATHOPHYSIOLOGY OF RENAL DISEASE

D. J. CHEW and S. P. DIBARTOLA

> Superficially it might be said that the function of the kidneys is to make urine; but in a more considered view one may say that the kidneys make the stuff of philosophy itself.
>
> (Homer W. Smith)

INTRODUCTION AND DEFINITION OF TERMS

The clinical methods used in the diagnosis of renal disease are discussed in the first half of this chapter; the second half covers the pathophysiology of uremia and some common syndromes of renal disease (chronic renal failure, acute renal failure, glomerulopathies, and upper urinary tract infection). The reader is referred to Chapter 108 for further information on the diagnosis and treatment of specific diseases.

In veterinary literature, terminology describing the level of renal function, severity of renal lesions, and cause of reduced renal function is confusing. For purposes of this chapter, the following definitions will be used: The term *renal disease* refers to the presence of morphologic or functional lesions in one or both kidneys, regardless of extent. *Renal failure* refers to retention of nonprotein nitrogenous waste products in the body, regardless of the cause. *Azotemia* is defined as the laboratory finding of an increased concentration of nonprotein nitrogenous waste products in blood, typically measured as blood urea nitrogen (BUN) or serum creatinine (S_{cr}), which can result from reduced renal excretion. Inadequate renal excretion of nonprotein nitrogenous waste products can result from primary renal (parenchymal, intrinsic, or intrarenal), prerenal, or postrenal processes. *Uremia* refers to the constellation of clinical signs and biochemical abnormalities associated with a critical loss of functional nephrons and typically includes extrarenal manifestations of disease. Although uremia usually occurs as a consequence of primary renal disease, it may also occur with prerenal and postrenal azotemia. Not all animals with azotemia have clinical signs, and hence are not uremic.

Prerenal azotemia results from disease processes that reduce renal perfusion, such as in hypovolemic shock, severe dehydration, hypoadrenocorticism, heart failure, or any other condition that reduces effective circulating blood volume. Initially, the kidneys are morphologically normal in prerenal azotemia, and are capable of resuming normal function when adequate perfusion is restored. Autoregulation is the ability of the normal kidney to maintain nearly normal glomerular filtration rate (GFR) and renal blood flow (RBF) despite a wide range in systemic blood pressure. In animals with intact renal autoregulation, mean systemic blood pressure must fall below 80 mmHg before GFR decreases. Some diseases impair autoregulation, however, so that azotemia occurs at blood pressures above 80 mmHg. Even when autoregulation is intact, azotemia can result from passive reabsorption of urea from tubular fluid during states of low tubular flow rate, such as dehydration. Sustained renal hypoperfusion can result in the development of primary renal lesions.

In *postrenal* azotemia, elimination of urine from the body is impaired. Either obstruction to urine flow or traumatic rupture of the excretory pathway results in urine accumulation in the body and may cause postrenal azotemia. Early in these processes the kidneys are morphologically normal and can excrete the retained nonprotein nitrogenous waste products after relief of obstruction or repair of urinary tract discontinuity. Long-standing partial obstruction may result in primary renal lesions such as hydronephrosis.

Extensive morphologic or functional lesions in the kidneys themselves result in primary renal (intrinsic, parenchymal, or intrarenal) azotemia when 75 per cent or more nephrons are not filtering. The kidney itself is incriminated in the retention of nonprotein nitrogenous waste products, and correction of dehydration or obstruction does not result in resolution of azotemia. The term *renal insufficiency* has been used to describe a state of reduced renal function resulting from intrarenal lesions that has not yet resulted in retention of nonprotein nitrogenous waste products.

The proper diagnosis of renal disease and evaluation of renal function necessitate answers to the following questions: (1) Is primary renal disease present? (2) Is the renal disease predominantly glomerular, tubular, interstitial, or some combination of these? (3) What is the extent or severity of the renal disease? (4) Is the renal disease acute or chronic, reversible or irreversible, progressive or non-progressive? (5) What is the current level of renal function (glomerular and tubular)? and (6) If azotemia is present, is it prerenal, primary renal, postrenal, nonrenal, or a combination of these? The remainder of the diagnostic portion of this chapter addresses the clinical methods used in answering these questions.

CLINICAL EVALUATION OF RENAL FUNCTION

The diagnosis of renal disease begins with an evaluation of the signalment, a careful history, and a complete physical examination. Pertinent laboratory and radiographic studies to evaluate glomerular and tubular function complete the initial workup.

SIGNALMENT

Consideration of the signalment is important because some renal diseases are more common in certain segments of the animal population. Renal disease in dogs and cats occurs at any age and in either sex, but certain disorders occur more often in dogs than in cats, in older animals than in young, in specific breeds, or in one sex more than in the other. Awareness of these predilections for specific diseases will facilitate an accurate diagnosis.

HISTORY

The patient's history may provide information that suggests the presence of renal disease, and may aid in determining whether it is the primary problem or part of a systemic disease. Often, however, the history is nonspecific, and renal disease may not be suspected. Consideration of the history may allow determination of whether the disease is acute or chronic, and progressive or nonprogressive. The apparent acute onset of clinical signs does not exclude the possibility of chronic underlying renal disease because earlier, more subtle signs may not have been noticed by the owner.

Previous drug therapy, opportunities for exposure to toxins, and previous trauma should be evaluated. A response to previous therapy with corticosteroids or antibiotics may provide insight as to the nature of an underlying immune, neoplastic, or infectious disease. In a review of previous medications, the clinician should pay particular attention to the use of aminoglycosides, cephaloridine, amphotericin B, thiacetarsamide, and nonsteroidal anti-inflammatory agents because of their potential for nephrotoxicity. Exposure to ethylene glycol should be specifically sought during the time of year and in geographical areas in which antifreeze is used.

Specific history related to the urinary system includes questions about the animal's urinations, such as whether there have been any changes in frequency, volume, or color and whether or not dysuria (difficulty in urination) is present. Polyuria (increased urine volume) and polydipsia (increased water intake) occur frequently in progressive renal disease in both dogs and cats. Of these, polydipsia is more readily observed and reported by the owner. Nocturia (voiding during the night) may be the first indication that an animal is polyuric, but it also may be caused by disorders not associated with increased urine volume. The amount of water consumed and urine voided should be determined. Water consumption should be estimated (e.g., number of bowls, cups, or quarts) by the owner and compared with previous intake. Normal water consumption should be less than 100 ml/kg/day for both the dog and cat. The magnitude of polyuria is more difficult for owners to estimate, but increased time to empty the bladder without discomfort may be an indication. Normal urine volume is approximately 25 to 40 ml/kg/day for dogs (12 to 20 ml/lb/day) and 20 to 30 ml/kg/day for cats (10 to 15 ml/lb/day). Polyuria must be clearly distinguished from pollakiuria (increased frequency of urinations), which usually implies pain or inflammation associated with the lower urinary tract. Furthermore, the clinician should be careful to distinguish polyuria from urinary incontinence (involuntary passage of urine). Occasionally the complaint of the owner is incontinence when in reality the animal is actually polyuric but unable to gain frequent enough access to the outdoors. Owners of cats may notice that the litter is more urine-soaked and the litter pan heavier than before. Occasionally an owner may note that the color of the animal's urine has changed from yellow to nearly colorless during polyuria, from dilution of normal urinary pigment. Darker urine can be noted when urine is very concentrated or when abnormal pigments such as bilirubin, hemoglobin, or myoglobin are present.

Dogs and cats with chronic uremia usually are presented for polyuria, polydipsia, anorexia, weight loss, lethargy, or vomiting, but polyuria, polydipsia, and vomiting are reported less frequently in cats.[1] Diarrhea is reported less frequently. Similar signs are seen in acute uremia with the exception of polydipsia, polyuria, and weight loss.

Macroscopic hematuria may occur in animals with renal disease (e.g., nephrolithiasis, renal tumors) but more often occurs in disorders of the lower urinary tract. The time of urinary bleeding in relation to initiation of urination may provide a clue to the origin of hemorrhage. Hematuria at the beginning of urination is more often the result of a urethral or genital lesion, whereas bleeding throughout urination may result from lesions of the kidney, ureter, or bladder. The appearance of blood only at the end of urination suggests lesions of the bladder, urethra, or prostate, whereas dripping of blood unassociated with urination can result from lesions in the urethra, prostate, prepuce, penis, or vagina.

Owners may report reluctance of their animal to move or assumption of a hunched-up posture when the kidneys or bladder is painfully distended or inflamed. Animals with glomerular disease and nephrotic syndrome may present for evaluation of subcutaneous swelling and abdominal distention, or dyspnea, tachypnea, and cyanosis related to acute thromboembolism. Dogs and cats with severe hypertension may be presented for acute blindness due to retinal detachments.[2-5]

PHYSICAL EXAMINATION

Physical examination of animals with renal disease or renal failure often produces nonspecific findings. A complete general physical examination with emphasis on abdominal palpation, however, can suggest disease within the urinary tract.

General observation of the animal may reveal loss of lean body tissues from weight loss, weakness, lethargy, and a poor hair coat. Occasionally an animal with nephrotic syndrome may present with subcutaneous edema and abdominal distention (ascites) (see section on Glomerular Disease). Fibrous osteodystrophy usually is observed in young, growing dogs with renal failure caused by familial renal disease, and is indicated by the presence of a maxilla and mandible that are easily deformed by manipulation (so-called "rubber jaw"). Clinical signs of osteodystrophy are rare in older dogs with chronic renal failure.

The mucous membranes of the oral cavity and eye should be examined for pallor suggestive of anemia and for vascular injection that can occur in advanced uremia. Halitosis specific to uremia (uremic breath) may be detected by some clinicians. Uremic stomatitis and ulcers can occur along the tongue, buccal mucosa, and gingiva, but ulcers are often most prominent in buccal mucosa adjacent to teeth (Figure 107–1A). Oral lesions are more common in dogs than in cats with uremia, and tongue-tip necrosis is a lesion that is apparently unique to uremic dogs (Figure 107–1B). Oral lesions are observed more frequently in animals with long-standing uremia caused by primary renal failure but occasionally are observed in prerenal and postrenal azotemia.

Assessment for dehydration is important for subsequent interpretation of laboratory data. Degree of dehydration should be assessed after evaluation of skin turgor by skin pinch and by moistness of oral mucous membranes. The presence of a large amount of urine in the urinary bladder in a dehydrated animal suggests abnormal renal function and polyuria as the cause for dehydration.

Thoracic auscultation is usually normal, but advanced uremia can result in cardiac arrhythmias and pulmonary crackles. Sinus tachycardia can also occur in animals with dehydration or pain.

Abdominal palpation should include attempts to identify the kidneys, bladder, and urethra; the ureters are not palpable. The kidneys should be palpated near the dorsal costovertebral angle and evaluated for abnormal size (smaller or larger than normal), contour (smooth or irregular), texture (hard or soft), and the presence of pain. At least the caudal portion of the left kidney usually can be palpated in dogs, whereas the right kidney is nonpalpable. Both kidneys are readily palpable in cats. Small, firm, irregular kidneys suggest the presence of chronic renal disease, and there may be asymmetry in their size. Some chronic renal diseases, especially in cats, may be associated with increased renal size (e.g., renal lymphosarcoma, renal FIP, polycystic renal disease).[1] Enlarged, painful kidneys suggest the presence of acute renal disease or obstructive nephropathy.

Palpation of the caudal abdomen, perineum, and rectum is necessary to evaluate the bladder, urethra, and prostate. Intraluminal or intramural masses of the bladder often can be detected by simultaneous rectal and abdominal palpation. An estimate of urine volume residing in the bladder should be made and the presence

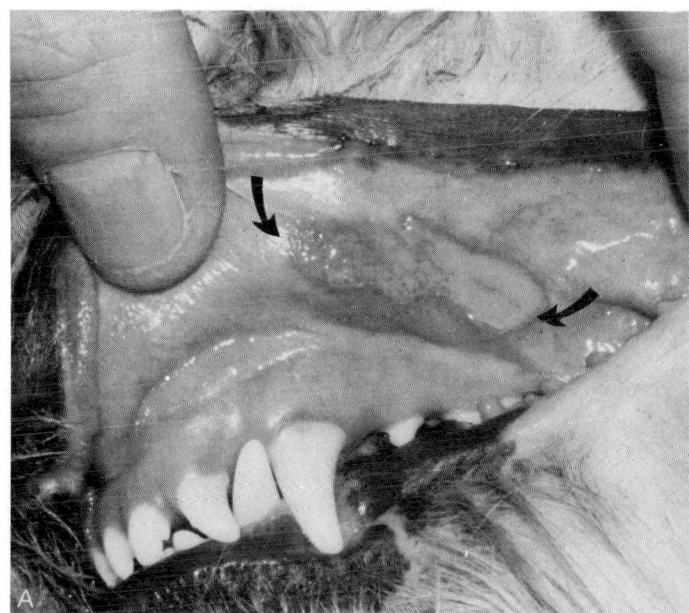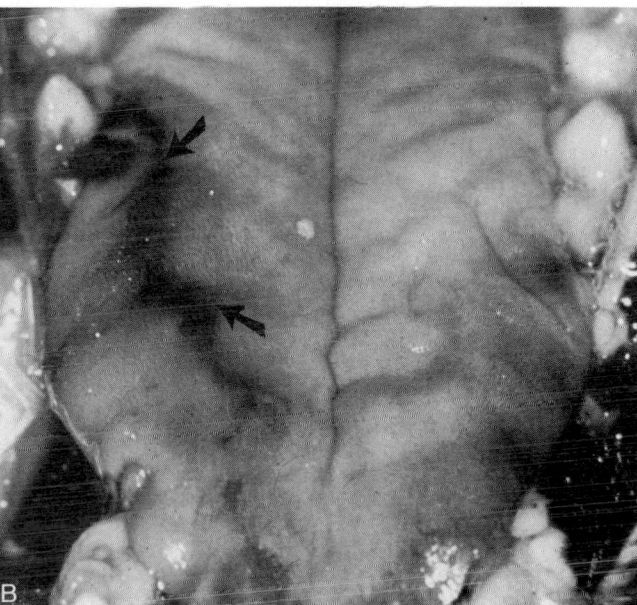

FIGURE 107–1. Uremic oral ulceration. *A,* Buccal ulcer. Uremic ulcers often are found in tissue overlying teeth (arrows). Prerenal, intrinsic renal, or postrenal azotemia may result in oral ulceration, but it is most common in intrinsic renal azotemia. The depicted ulcer is from a dog with parvoviral infection and prerenal azotemia. *B,* Tongue tip necrosis. Arrows denote the area of devitalized tissue which eventually sloughed. This lesion can occur in acute or chronic azotemia in dogs.

of pain noted during bladder palpation. Rectal palpation affords an opportunity to palpate the trigone region of the bladder, the prostate, and the pelvic urethra. The prostate of male dogs should be evaluated for enlargement, asymmetry, or pain.

Systemic blood pressure evaluation is not routinely available for small animal patients but can be helpful, since hypertension is frequent in animals with chronic renal failure, particularly when associated with glomerular disease. Documentation of hypertension is best made with techniques using direct arterial puncture and pressure recording. Ophthalmic funduscopic examination may provide indirect evidence for systemic hypertension (e.g., vascular tortuosity, retinal edema, retinal hemorrhage, and retinal detachments) in visual and nonvisual animals.

CLINICAL EVALUATION OF GLOMERULAR FUNCTION

Evaluation of glomerular function is an essential part of the diagnostic approach to patients with suspected renal disease because GFR is directly related to functional renal mass. BUN and S_{cr} concentrations are commonly used screening tests, while creatinine clearance and sodium sulfanilate half-life are useful in patients with suspected renal disease that have normal BUN and S_{cr} concentrations. Clearance of radioisotopes and nuclear imaging are sophisticated techniques that may be used to determine GFR and effective renal plasma flow (ERPF) but do not require urine collection. Tests of glomerular function are summarized in Table 107–1.

BLOOD UREA NITROGEN

Urea is synthesized in the liver by way of the ornithine cycle, using ammonia derived from amino acid catabolism. The amino acids used in the production of urea result from the catabolism of exogenous (dietary) and endogenous proteins. Urea is freely permeable and is distributed throughout intracellular and extracellular water.

The renal excretion of urea is accomplished by glomerular filtration, and BUN concentrations are inversely proportional to the GFR. Urea is subject to passive reabsorption in the tubules, however, and this occurs to a greater extent at slower tubular flow rates, such as may occur during dehydration and volume depletion. Even at maximal tubular flow rates, up to 40 per cent of filtered urea may be passively reabsorbed.[6] Thus urea clearance is not a reliable estimate of GFR, and in the face of volume depletion, decreased urea clearance may occur without a decrease in GFR.

The production and excretion of urea do not proceed at a constant rate. For example, urea production and excretion will increase after ingestion of a high protein meal. In dogs a mild increase in BUN concentration occurs within eight hours of feeding and is greatest after feeding canned food.[7, 8] A 12-hour fast is recommended

TABLE 107–1. TESTS OF GLOMERULAR FUNCTION

Test	Dog	Cat
Endogenous creatinine clearance (ml/min/kg)	2.98 ± 0.96 (16)* 3.7 ± 0.77 (17) 2.97 ± 0.42 (18)	2.70 ± 1.2 (15)
Exogenous creatinine clearance (ml/min/kg)	4.08 ± 0.5 (18)	2.94 ± 0.32 (20)
Inulin clearance (ml/min/kg)	3.96 ± 0.58 (18) 4.19 ± 1.82; 4.72 ± 1.82 (25) 3.55 ± 0.14 (23)	3.51 ± 0.14 (20) 3.83 ± 0.83 (15) 3.24 ± 0.14 (23)
PAH clearance (ml/min/kg)	12.23 ± 1.65; 10.55 ± 1.5 (25)	10.61 ± 1.71 (20) 15.1 ± 3.48 (15)
Iothalamate clearance (ml/min/kg)	5.6 ± 0.77 (25)	5.12 ± 1.49 (24)
Iodohippurate clearance (ml/min/kg)	16.17 ± 2.99 (25)	14.13 ± 5.74 (24)
^{3}H-TEA clearance (ml/min/kg)	10.51 ± 0.72 (23)	8.14 ± 0.53 (23)
Sodium sulfanilate T½ (minutes)	58 ± 13 (22) 66.1 ± 10.8 (21)	44.4 ± 5.7 (20)
Filtration fraction	0.34 ± 0.02 (23) 0.35 (25)	0.21 (15) 0.39 ± 0.02 (23) 0.33 (20) 0.36 (24)

*Numbers in parentheses are reference articles from which data are taken.

before measuring BUN concentrations to avoid the effect of feeding on urea production. Gastrointestinal bleeding can increase BUN concentrations because blood represents an endogenous protein load. Clinical conditions characterized by increased catabolism such as starvation, infection, fever, or burns also can increase BUN concentrations.[6] Several drugs can increase BUN concentrations by increasing tissue catabolism (glucocorticoids, azathioprine) or decreasing protein synthesis (tetracyclines).[6, 9] BUN concentrations can be decreased by low protein diets, anabolic steroids, severe hepatic insufficiency, or portosystemic shunting.[6] These nonrenal variables limit the usefulness of the BUN concentration as an indicator of glomerular function.

Although urea nitrogen concentrations are the same in blood, plasma, or serum, the term blood urea nitrogen is frequently used. Plasma urea concentration, however, is not synonymous with plasma urea nitrogen because only 47 per cent of urea is nitrogen. BUN is often measured by a diacetylmonoxamine method, and normal values are 8 to 25 mg/dl in the dog and 15 to 35 mg/dl in the cat.

SERUM CREATININE

Creatinine is a spontaneous, nonenzymatic breakdown product of phosphocreatine in muscle, and the daily production of creatinine in the body is largely determined by the muscle mass of the individual. Although one study demonstrated a mild increase after ingestion of cooked meat,[7] it is unlikely that S_{cr} concentration is appreciably altered by diet.[8] Its concentration is more affected by the age, sex, and muscle mass of the individual.[10] Young animals have lower concentrations, whereas males and well-muscled individuals have higher concentrations. Animals with normal renal function that have lost lean body mass may have lower S_{cr} concentrations.

Creatinine does not undergo appreciable metabolism and is excreted by the kidneys almost entirely by glomerular filtration. Its rate of excretion is relatively constant in the steady state, and S_{cr} concentration varies inversely with GFR. Thus determination of creatinine clearance provides a good estimate of GFR. Tubular secretion of creatinine does, however, occur to some extent, and its secretion is increased with reduction in renal mass, making creatinine clearance a less reliable estimate of GFR as renal disease advances.[11]

In the laboratory, creatinine is measured by the alkaline picrate reaction, which is not entirely specific for creatinine and measures another group of substances collectively known as noncreatinine chromagens. These substances are found in plasma, where they may constitute up to 50 per cent of the measured creatinine at normal serum concentrations, but do not appear in urine.[6] As S_{cr} concentration increases due to progression of renal disease and declining GFR, the amount of noncreatinine chromagens is unchanged and contributes progressively less to the total measured S_{cr} concentration. Normal S_{cr} concentrations in the dog and cat are 0.3 to 1.3 mg/dl and 0.8 to 1.8 mg/dl, respectively.

Nonrenal variables that may transiently affect S_{cr} creatinine concentration include massive muscle necrosis or prolonged strenuous exercise. Also, some drugs (cimetidine, trimethoprim) may compete with creatinine for tubular secretion and result in mild increases in S_{cr} concentration.[12, 13] Acetoacetate, present in diabetic ketoacidosis, is measured as a noncreatinine chromagen and can contribute to increased serum S_{cr} concentration in diabetic patients, regardless of renal function.[14]

INTERPRETATION OF BLOOD UREA NITROGEN AND SERUM CREATININE

The relation of BUN or S_{cr} to GFR is a rectangular hyperbola (Figure 107–2). It is important to appreciate the shape of this curve. The slope is small when GFR is mildly or moderately decreased and is large when GFR is severely reduced. Thus, large changes in GFR early in the course of renal disease cause small increases in BUN or S_{cr} that may be difficult to appreciate clinically, whereas small changes in GFR in advanced renal disease cause large changes in BUN or S_{cr}. It must be emphasized that the inverse relation between S_{cr} concentration and GFR is valid only when GFR is relatively constant, and rapid changes in GFR may not be immediately reflected by the S_{cr}.

When nonrenal variables have been eliminated from consideration, an increase in BUN or S_{cr} above normal implies that at least 75 per cent of the nephrons are not functioning (Figure 107–2). Neither the cause nor the reversibility of this malfunction can be predicted from the magnitude of BUN or S_{cr}. The magnitude of the BUN or S_{cr} concentration cannot be used to predict whether azotemia is prerenal, primary renal, or postrenal in origin and cannot be used to differentiate acute versus chronic, reversible versus irreversible, or progressive versus nonprogressive processes.[6] The BUN/creatinine ratio in early prerenal and postrenal azotemia may be increased because of increased tubular reabsorption of urea at lower tubular flow rates or preferential

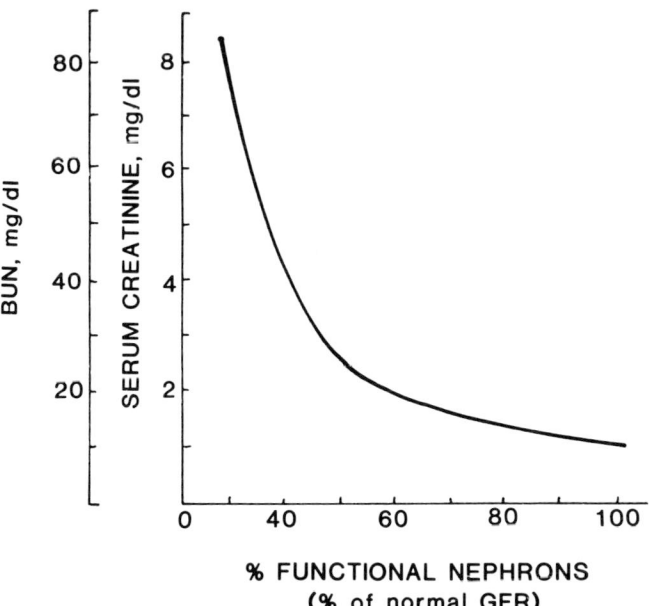

FIGURE 107–2. Relationship of BUN or serum creatinine to percentage of functional nephrons. (From Chew DJ and DiBartola SP: Manual of Small Animal Nephrology and Urology. New York, Churchill Livingstone, 1986.)

absorption of urea across peritoneal membranes in animals with uroabdomen. A decrease in the BUN/creatinine ratio often follows fluid therapy and reflects decreased tubular reabsorption of urea rather than increased GFR.

CONCEPT OF RENAL CLEARANCE

The renal clearance of a substance is that volume of plasma that would have to be filtered by the glomeruli each minute to account for the amount of that substance appearing in the urine each minute. The renal clearance of a substance that is neither reabsorbed nor secreted by the tubules is equal to GFR. For such a substance in a steady state, the amount filtered equals the amount excreted. Thus GFR $\times$ P_x = U_x $\times$ V. Dividing both sides of the equation by P_x gives the standard clearance formula $(U_x V/P_x)$, which in this case is equal to the GFR. Where P_x = plasma concentration of substance x, U_x = urinary concentration of substance x, and V = ml/min of urine formation.

The ideal substance for measurement of GFR should be nontoxic, not bound to plasma proteins, excreted only by the kidneys, and not metabolized elsewhere in the body. It should be freely filtered by the glomeruli and should not undergo tubular secretion or reabsorption. Inulin, a polymer of fructose, meets these criteria but is technically difficult to measure in blood and urine, is not normally present in the body, and must be constantly infused during clearance studies. For these reasons it has not been widely used as a clinical indicator of glomerular function.

CREATININE CLEARANCE

Creatinine is endogenously produced and excreted by the body largely by glomerular filtration and its clearance can thus be used to estimate GFR in the steady state. Tubular secretion of creatinine can lead to up to 25 per cent overestimation of GFR in male dogs with reduced renal mass.[11] In calculation of endogenous creatinine clearance ($U_{Cr}V/P_{Cr}$), the effect of tubular secretion on U_{Cr} is offset by the effect of noncreatinine chromogens on P_{Cr}, making this parameter a reasonable estimate of GFR.[10] Numerous studies in the dog and cat have shown that endogenous creatinine clearance in these species is about 2 to 5 ml/min/kg.[15-18] Published values for glomerular function tests in the dog and cat are presented in Table 107–1.

The main indication for determination of endogenous creatinine clearance is the clinical suspicion of renal disease in a patient with normal BUN and S_{cr}. The only requirements for determination of endogenous creatinine clearance are an accurately timed collection of urine (usually 24 hours), determination of the patient's body weight, and S_{cr} and U_{cr} concentrations. Failure to collect all urine produced will erroneously reduce the calculated clearance value.

To eliminate the inaccuracy caused by noncreatinine chromogens, some investigators have advocated the use of exogenous creatinine clearance.[18, 19] In this procedure creatinine is administered subcutaneously to increase S_{cr} and reduce the relative effect of noncreatinine chromogens. Exogenous creatinine clearance values exceed endogenous creatinine clearance values and closely approximate inulin clearance in the dog.[18] The procedure is somewhat cumbersome, however, and has not replaced endogenous creatinine clearance clinically. In cats exogenous creatinine clearance is slightly lower than inulin clearance, for reasons that are unknown.[20]

SODIUM SULFANILATE HALF-LIFE

Sodium sulfanilate is excreted by glomerular filtration alone, and measurement of its plasma half-life has been used as an indicator of glomerular function. It is administered intravenously at a dosage of 9 mg/lb (20 mg/kg) in the dog and 5 mg/lb (11 mg/kg) in the cat, and heparinized blood samples are collected at 30, 60, and 90 minutes. Normal values in dogs were 50 to 80 minutes in one study[21] and 42 to 82 minutes in another.[22] In cats, normal sodium sulfanilate plasma half-life is 37 to 57 minutes.[20] The test should not be performed if the animal has received sulfonamide medications, as they may cross-react with sulfanilate. The advantage of this procedure is that urine samples are not required, but its disadvantage is that a numerical value for GFR is not obtained.

RADIOISOTOPE STUDIES

Radioisotopes also have been used to determine GFR, effective renal plasma flow (ERPF), and filtration fraction (FF) in dogs and cats. The advantages of these procedures are that they do not require collection of urine and are not time-consuming. The major disadvantages are the use of radioactive compounds and the need for special equipment and expertise. Published values for these radioisotope clearances are presented in Table 107–1. Values obtained using ^{125}I-iothalamate

to measure GFR and ^{131}I-iodohippurate to measure ERPF are slightly higher than values obtained using ^{14}C-inulin and ^{3}H-tetraethylammonium.[23-25] Also, ERPF values for cats are lower than those observed in dogs, and may represent actual species differences in renal blood flow. Thus FF values in cats were 0.39 and 0.34 in dogs.[23] ^{51}Cr-ethylenediaminepentaacetic acid also has been used to assess GFR in dogs, and GFR was estimated to be approximately 3 ml/min/kg for dogs weighing 12 to 40 kg.[26, 27] Nuclear imaging using ^{99m}Tc-diethylenetriaminepentaacetic acid has been used to determine GFR in the dog, and has the advantage of allowing GFR for individual kidneys to be determined.[28]

CLINICAL EVALUATION OF TUBULAR FUNCTION

The kidney has evolved as an organ of water conservation. Depending on the needs of the organism, the kidney is able to produce urine that is highly concentrated or very dilute. Normal urinary concentrating ability depends on the ability of the hypothalamic osmoreceptors to respond to changes in plasma osmolality, release of antidiuretic hormone (ADH) from the neurohypophysis, and the response of the distal nephron to ADH. In addition, medullary hypertonicity must be generated and maintained by the countercurrent multiplier and exchanger systems of the kidney, and there must be an adequate number of functional nephrons to generate the appropriate response to ADH. Tests of tubular function are summarized in Table 107–2.

URINE SPECIFIC GRAVITY AND URINE OSMOLALITY

Total urine solute concentration is measured either by urine specific gravity (USG) or urine osmolality. The latter is preferable because it depends only on the number of osmotically active particles, regardless of their size. USG is defined as the weight of a solution compared with an equal volume of distilled water. It depends on both the number and the molecular weight of the solute particles but has the advantage of requiring only simple, inexpensive equipment for measurement.

TABLE 107–2. TESTS OF TUBULAR FUNCTION

Test	Dog	Cat
Random USG	1.001–1.070	1.001–1.080
USG after 5% dehydration	1.050–1.076	1.047–1.087
U_{OSM} after 5% dehydration (mOsm/kg)	1.787–2.791	1.581–2.984
U_{OSM}/P_{OSM} after 5% dehydration	5.7–8.9	NA*
PSP $T_{1/2}$ (minutes)	21–27	18–31
Fractional clearance of electrolytes (%)		
Sodium	0–0.7%	0.24–0.96%
Potassium	0–20%	6.7–23.9%
Chloride	0–0.8%	0.41–1.33%
Calcium	0–0.4%	NA
Phosphorus	3–39%	17–73%

Data from references 20, 33, 40, and 41.
NA = not available.

Urine normally is composed of solutes of relatively low molecular weight (urea, electrolytes), and there is a roughly linear relation between urine osmolality and specific gravity.[29] Based on this linear relation, the last two digits of the USG may be multiplied by 36 to obtain a rough estimate of urine osmolality in dogs.[30] The range of urine osmolality corresponding to a given USG value, however, may be relatively wide.[31] If the urine contains appreciable amounts of larger molecular-weight solutes, such as glucose, mannitol, or radiographic contrast agents, these substances will have a proportionally greater effect on specific gravity than on osmolality.[29, 32]

The term *isosthenuria* (1.007–1.015 USG, 300 mOsm/kg) refers to urine of the same total solute concentration as unaltered glomerular filtrate. The term *hyposthenuria* refers to urine of lower total solute concentration than glomerular filtrate (< 1.007 USG, < 300 mOsm/kg); *hypersthenuria* (baruria) refers to urine of higher total solute concentration than glomerular filtrate (> 1.015 USG, > 300 mOsm/kg).

The normal range of total urine solute concentration for dogs and cats is wide (USG, 1.001 to 1.080), but despite this wide range, most normal dogs and cats excrete urine that is moderately concentrated. In one study, dogs with access to water produced urine with total solute concentrations of 976 to 2546 mOsm/kg or USG 1.023 to 1.064.[33] The occurrence of dilute urine should be documented on repeated urine samples because low USG on a single sample can be normal.

WATER DEPRIVATION TEST

The water deprivation test is one of the most useful tests of tubular function. It is indicated in the evaluation of animals with polydipsia and polyuria of undetermined cause in which BUN and S_{cr} concentrations are normal. An animal that is dehydrated but has dilute urine has already failed the test and should not be subjected to water deprivation. In such an animal, failure to concentrate urine is due either to structural or functional renal dysfunction (intrinsic renal disease, nephrogenic diabetes insipidus, medullary washout, *Escherichia coli* endotoxin, hypercalcemia, hypokalemia) or to administration of drugs that have interfered with urinary concentrating ability (glucocorticoids, diuretics).

At the beginning of the water deprivation test, the bladder must be emptied and base line data collected (body weight, hematocrit, total plasma proteins, skin turgor, serum osmolality, urine osmolality, and USG). Water is then withheld and these parameters are monitored every six to eight hours. The test is concluded when the patient either demonstrates adequate concentrating ability or becomes dehydrated as evidenced by loss of 5 per cent or more of its body weight. It is important when weighing the animal to use the same scale each time and to allow the animal to empty the bladder at each evaluation.

In normal dogs, dehydration becomes evident after a mean of 42 hours but may not occur until after 96 hours.[33] By the time dehydration is evident, normal dogs develop USG values of 1.050 to 1.076, urine osmolalities of 1787 to 2791 mOsm/kg, and urine/plasma osmolality ratios of 5.7 to 8.9.[33] Normal cats develop USG values

of 1.047 to 1.087 and urine osmolalities of 1581 to 2984 mOsm/kg after water deprivation sufficient to induce 5 per cent loss of body weight.[20] Failure to achieve maximal urinary solute concentration does not localize the level of the malfunction, but a structural or functional defect may be present anywhere along the hypothalamic-pituitary-renal axis.

A modified water deprivation test has been described for the diagnosis of polyuric disorders in dogs.[34] Water is removed from the animal's cage and the urinary bladder emptied, after which urine osmolality or specific gravity is measured and the bladder emptied on an hourly basis. Maximal urine solute concentration is defined as occurring whenever less than five per cent increase in urine osmolality occurs on sequential determinations. This occurred at a mean urine osmolality of 1414 mOsm/kg in normal dogs. At this time, two to three units of aqueous vasopressin are administered subcutaneously and the urine osmolality determined one to two hours later. Further increase in urine osmolality after administration of vasopressin should not exceed 10 per cent in normal dogs. This procedure was found to be valuable in the evaluation of dogs with hyperadrenocorticism and partial pituitary diabetes insipidus.

Gradual water deprivation or the Hickey-Hare test may be considered in animals that fail to concentrate their urine after abrupt water deprivation. Gradual water deprivation over three to five days allows some reestablishment of medullary hypertonicity and partial restoration of urinary concentrating ability. ADH, released in response to plasma hyperosmolality, increases the permeability of the collecting ducts to urea, which constitutes about 50 per cent of the solute composition of the renal papilla.

HICKEY-HARE TEST

In the Hickey-Hare test,[35] water (9 ml/lb or 20 ml/kg) is administered by stomach tube, an indwelling urinary catheter placed, and urine flow (ml/min) determined. Hypertonic saline solution (2.5 per cent) is administered intravenously at a rate of 0.10 ml/min/lb (0.25 ml/min/kg) for 45 minutes. Urine volume is recorded every 15 minutes during the infusion and for 45 minutes afterward. The normal response to this procedure is a decrease in the rate of urine production due to stimulation of ADH release by plasma hypertonicity. It is useful in the differentiation of psychogenic polydipsia with medullary washout from nephrogenic diabetes insipidus after negative water deprivation and exogenous ADH test results. In nephrogenic diabetes insipidus there should be no change or an actual increase in urine flow, whereas in psychogenic polydipsia with medullary washout, repletion of solute (NaCl) should have occurred and the response to hypertonic saline solution should be normal (decreased urine volume).

EXOGENOUS VASOPRESSIN TEST

The exogenous vasopressin test may be used in debilitated patients in which water deprivation is considered hazardous, or to further characterize a concentrating defect detected by the water deprivation test. In the *aqueous vasopressin test*, an intravenous infusion of 5 mU of ADH/lb (11 mU ADH/kg) is given over 60 minutes. The bladder is emptied at the start of the study and parameters of urine solute concentration are measured before and at 30-minute intervals for three hours after beginning the infusion. The bladder is further emptied at each measurement. Maximal response to aqueous vasopressin in water-loaded dogs occurred at 60 minutes and consisted of USG values of 1.009 to 1.033, urine osmolalities of 429 to 1437 mOsm/kg, and urine/plasma osmolality ratios of 1.5 to 5.1.[36]

In the *repositol vasopressin* test, 3 to 5 units of vasopressin tannate in oil are given intramuscularly and the bladder is emptied within six hours of injection. Parameters of urine solute concentration are measured before and at six-hour intervals for 24 hours after injection. Oral water loading should be avoided because of the danger of water intoxication. Maximal response to repositol vasopressin occurred 8 to 12 hours after injection and consisted of USG values of 1.024 to 1.060, urine osmolalities of 1033 to 2001 mOsm/kg, and urine/plasma osmolality ratios of 3.8 to 7.4.[37]

The standard water deprivation test is the preferred initial test of urinary concentrating ability because mean maximal values are usually higher with this test and results are usually easier to interpret. Why higher values for parameters of urinary concentrating ability are achieved with this test as compared with the exogenous vasopressin tests is unknown. Possible explanations include the actions of antidiuretic substances other than ADH that might be present in hydropenic individuals, the effect of slower renal blood flow in dehydrated patients, and intensification of the medullary interstitial gradient in dehydrated individuals.[33]

PHENOLSULFONPHTHALEIN HALF-LIFE

The renal excretion of phenolsulfonphthalein (PSP) may be used as a test of tubular function. Approximately 80 per cent of the administered dose is bound to plasma proteins and the remaining 20 per cent is available for excretion by the kidneys. Only 5 per cent of the administered dose is handled by glomerular filtration, the remainder being handled by tubular secretion. The renal excretion of PSP is thus dependent on renal plasma flow, proximal tubular function, and patency of the urinary collecting system. The test is used in patients suspected of renal disease when BUN and S_{cr} values are normal or when proximal tubular dysfunction is suspected.

The dosage of PSP administered and time allowed for renal excretion may be important factors in the results obtained. Even in the presence of renal disease, the kidneys may excrete most of the dye if a low dosage is used and sufficient time is allowed. In one study, however, approximately 40 per cent of the injected dose was recovered in the urine in the first 20 minutes after injection, regardless of whether a dose of 6 mg or a dosage of 1.4 mg/lb (3 mg/kg) was used.[16] In another study the plasma concentration of PSP 60 minutes after injection of 0.45 mg/lb (1 mg/kg) was determined, and values above 120 μg/dl were considered abnormal.[38]

Tests in which the plasma half-life of PSP is determined may be preferable. PSP half-life is determined by administering 2.3 mg/lb (5 mg/kg) of PSP intravenously and collecting heparinized blood samples at 15, 25, and 35 minutes. The normal value in dogs is 20 minutes and in cats 18 to 31 minutes.[20, 39] Falsely high half-life values may result from poor renal perfusion (dehydration, congestive heart failure) or if there is obstruction of the collecting system. A falsely low half-life may be obtained in the presence of hypoalbuminemia caused by decreased protein binding and increased amount of PSP available for tubular secretion. In cats PSP plasma half-life was poorly correlated with GFR and ERPF.[20]

FRACTIONAL CLEARANCES (CLEARANCE RATIOS)

The extent to which electrolytes appear in the urine is the net result of tubular reabsorption and secretion. The fractional clearance of electrolytes can be used to evaluate tubular function and is defined as the ratio of the clearance of the electrolyte in question to that of creatinine.

$FC_x = (U_xV/P_x)/(U_{Cr}V/P_{Cr}) = (U_xP_{Cr})/(U_{Cr}P_x)$, where FC_x = fractional clearance, U_x = urinary concentration of x, P_x = plasma concentration of x, V = ml/min urine formation, P_{Cr} = plasma creatinine concentration. The advantage of this measurement is that a timed urine collection is not necessary. In normal animals the fractional clearances of all electrolytes are much less than 1.0, implying net conservation, but values are higher for potassium and phosphorus than for sodium and chloride, as might be expected from an understanding of the normal extracellular fluid composition. The fractional clearance of sodium is particularly useful in the differentiation of prerenal and primary renal azotemia. In animals with prerenal azotemia and volume depletion, sodium conservation should be avid and the fractional clearance of sodium very low. On the other hand, in animals with azotemia due to primary parenchymal renal disease, the fractional clearance of sodium will be higher than normal. Values for fractional electrolyte clearances have been reported for dogs and cats and are summarized in Table 107–2.[40, 41]

AMMONIA CHALLENGE TEST

The ammonia challenge test is used to assess urinary acidifying ability and may be useful in the evaluation of renal tubular disorders, specifically renal tubular acidosis. After a 12-hour fast, 0.045 gm of NH_4Cl/lb (0.1 gm NH_4Cl/kg) is given orally, and hourly urine specimens are collected beginning two hours after administration of NH_4Cl. The test is discontinued if urine pH (as measured by pH meter) falls below 6.0. In normal dogs, this should occur between two and eight hours after administration of NH_4Cl.[42]

URINALYSIS

Urine that is properly collected, analyzed, and interpreted can provide meaningful information about the occurrence of lower or upper urinary tract disease and the level of renal function. Abnormalities in the urinalysis can precede serum biochemical changes. The urinalysis is essential for the proper evaluation of dogs and cats with azotemia, polyuria and polydipsia, dysuria, hematuria, or urinary incontinence, and should be included in the minimum data base of any systemically ill animal. The value of the urinalysis is greater when urine is obtained before therapy with drugs or parenteral fluids.

COLLECTION OF URINE

The method by which urine is collected may influence the results that are obtained. Urine can be obtained by voiding, manual compression of the bladder, catheterization, or cystocentesis. A voided sample should be obtained initially in animals with hematuria because other methods of urine collection may add red cells to the sample as a result of trauma. Abnormal urine samples, however, are most easily interpreted when collected by cystocentesis. Ideally, samples should be obtained in the morning, when a concentrated specimen is more likely.

Voided urine should be collected in a clean container that is free of disinfectants that may alter the results of chemical analysis (see below). Styrofoam cups or other inert containers are suitable and should be covered immediately after urine collection. A midstream sample (urine collected after voiding has started) will minimize contamination by the urethra and genital tract. Occasionally it will be useful to collect a sample at the initiation of urination to evaluate animals with suspected urethral or genital disease. Rarely an endstream sample is evaluated for cells that settle out in the bladder and may not be present in midstream samples. Sometimes it is helpful to compare results from initial, midstream, and endstream voided urine samples to anatomically localize the source of red or white blood cells in the urine sediment. Obtaining a voided specimen from cats is more difficult, but sometimes can be accomplished by placing cellophane over the litter, using nonabsorbent litter (NoSorb), or using a freshly washed and dried empty litter pan. Voided urine samples can be collected by owners, require no special equipment, and carry no risk of trauma or infection for the animal. They have the disadvantage that cells, bacteria, and protein can enter the sample as contaminants from the distal urethra, genital tract, skin, and environment and make interpretation of the results difficult.

When a voided specimen cannot be obtained, bladder pressure can be increased by transabdominal compression so that resting urethral pressure is overcome and urine expelled. Furthermore, some animals will void after unsuccessful attempts to express urine. Care must be taken not to rupture the bladder. In one study as many as 50 per cent of dogs and 40 per cent of cats experienced vesicoureteral reflux during manual compression of the bladder.[43] Such an occurrence would be of some clinical concern when bladder urine is infected. Trauma from efforts to express urine can result in microscopic hematuria, which can be misleading.

Urethral catheterization can be performed when urine samples cannot be collected by voiding or cystocentesis, when bacterial cultures are needed, or when a previous voided sample demonstrated cells or bacteria that could have been the result of contamination from the distal urethra or genital tract. Although sterile technique must be followed in all instances, it is impossible to sterilize the distal urethra. Iatrogenic urinary tract infection after urethral catheterization using cleansing and aseptic technique occurred in 20 per cent of female dogs as compared with none of the males.[44] In another study of male dogs urinary infections developed in two of nine dogs after catheterization without cleansing and aseptic techniques, using clean but unsterile catheters.[45] Many types and sizes of urethral catheter are available for use in dogs and cats. Some trauma to the urinary tract during catheterization is common, and may result in mildly increased numbers of red blood cells, transitional epithelial cells, and protein in the sample. Excessive attempts to aspirate urine into a syringe attached to the catheter should be avoided because rafts of transitional epithelium and increased numbers of red blood cells may enter the urine sample. Urethral catheterization for urine collection is difficult in an awake male cat and should be avoided in male cats because of the possibility of creating urethral inflammation and obstruction.

Cystocentesis is well tolerated by both dogs and cats, and urine samples collected by this technique are usually sterile in normal dogs and cats,[46, 47] because contamination by bacteria from the distal urethra and genital tract is avoided. The risk of introducing urinary infection is negligible. Collection of urine by cystocentesis ensures that cells and protein in the specimen did not originate from the distal urethra or genital tract. Cystocentesis can be performed safely in dogs and cats, using a 22 gauge or smaller needle.[48] Cystocentesis should be avoided in the presence of severe caudal abdominal trauma or recent abdominal surgery, including cystotomy. Using cystocentesis, samples can be obtained despite the presence of urethral obstruction or bladder atony, but leakage of urine into the peritoneal cavity could occur in this setting. Accidental puncture of other abdominal viscera may occur but has not been reported to be associated with adverse effects, despite extensive clinical use of this procedure.

PERFORMANCE AND INTERPRETATION OF THE URINALYSIS

A complete urinalysis includes evaluation of the physical and chemical properties of the sample and microscopic examination of the urinary sediment. All three components must be evaluated together, as each evaluates a different aspect of the urinary tract. Urinalysis should be performed as soon as possible after sample collection, preferably within 15 to 30 minutes. Long delays at room temperature may result in dissolution of casts, changes in pH, growth of contaminating microorganisms, and loss of cellular detail. Refrigeration of the specimen is recommended if prompt examination is not possible.[49]

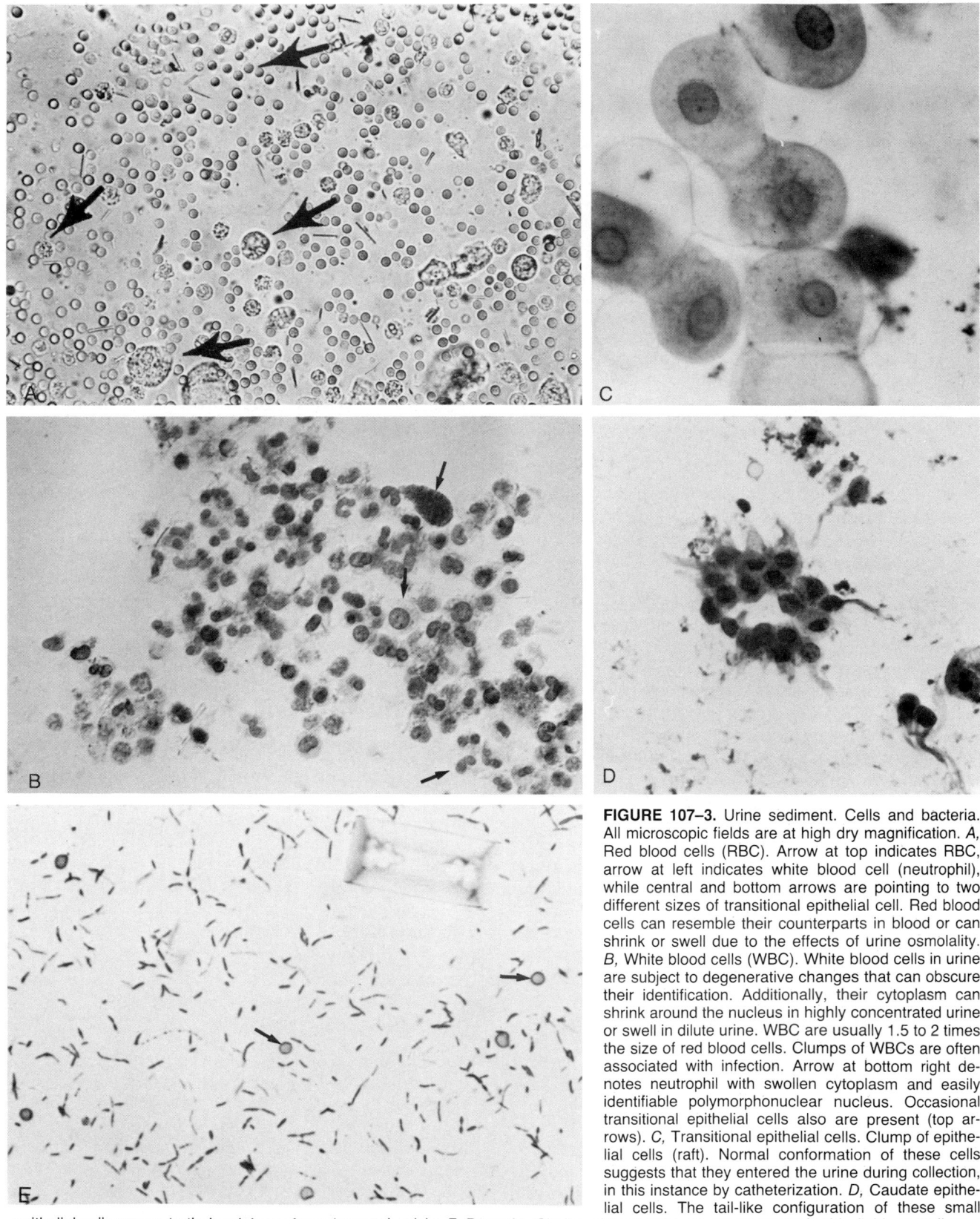

FIGURE 107–3. Urine sediment. Cells and bacteria. All microscopic fields are at high dry magnification. *A,* Red blood cells (RBC). Arrow at top indicates RBC, arrow at left indicates white blood cell (neutrophil), while central and bottom arrows are pointing to two different sizes of transitional epithelial cell. Red blood cells can resemble their counterparts in blood or can shrink or swell due to the effects of urine osmolality. *B,* White blood cells (WBC). White blood cells in urine are subject to degenerative changes that can obscure their identification. Additionally, their cytoplasm can shrink around the nucleus in highly concentrated urine or swell in dilute urine. WBC are usually 1.5 to 2 times the size of red blood cells. Clumps of WBCs are often associated with infection. Arrow at bottom right denotes neutrophil with swollen cytoplasm and easily identifiable polymorphonuclear nucleus. Occasional transitional epithelial cells also are present (top arrows). *C,* Transitional epithelial cells. Clump of epithelial cells (raft). Normal conformation of these cells suggests that they entered the urine during collection, in this instance by catheterization. *D,* Caudate epithelial cells. The tail-like configuration of these small epithelial cells suggests their origin as from the renal pelvis. *E,* Bacteria. Chains of bacterial rods are apparent in this field, as well as a few RBC (arrow) and a struvite crystal. Bacteria are most readily identified when they are rods and often are seen between WBC that are clumped together, or within WBC.

PHYSICAL PROPERTIES

Visual inspection of the sample and specific gravity are usually performed first, followed by chemical dipstrip measurements, and evaluation of the urine sediment. A standard amount of urine should be centrifuged, usually 5 to 8 ml, to allow semiquantitative comparison of abnormal findings among different samples.

Color, clarity, and specific gravity are physical parameters reported in the urinalysis. Color and clarity are very subjective and may be of little value, based on recent studies.[50] Normal canine and feline urine is said to be clear, but some cloudy samples were normal and clear ones abnormal in these studies. Urine is normally light yellow to amber, due to the presence of urochromes. Very concentrated samples may be dark, whereas dilute urine may be nearly colorless. In one study urine that was red, pink, or brown was always abnormal as determined by dipstrip chemical or microscopic evaluation.[50]

Specific gravity is the only parameter of renal function in the urinalysis. It is indirectly measured by the refraction of light, using a refractometer. The value of the USG as an indicator of tubular function is discussed above.

CHEMICAL PROPERTIES

Chemical properties of the urine are usually evaluated by semiquantitative colorimetric changes that develop in chemically impregnated pads on a dipstrip. Such pads are used for urine pH, protein, occult blood, glucose, ketone, and bilirubin determinations. The reading and reporting of such colorimetric reactions are subject to as much as 30 per cent variability among technicians.[50] Urine samples should be at room temperature during testing because some of the color reactions are temperature-dependent.

pH. Normal dogs and cats usually produce acidic urine over the course of 24 hours, due to the excretion of the acidic end products of protein catabolism. A wide range of urinary pH, however, can be considered normal (5.5 to 7.5),[51, 52] depending on the specific nature of the diet, the timing of urine collection in relation to eating (postprandial alkaline tide may increase urine pH for several hours), and systemic acid-base balance. Highly acidic urine (pH < 6.5) can be normal, or may be associated with metabolic or respiratory acidosis, acidifying drugs, increased protein catabolism, or paradoxical aciduria in metabolic alkalosis with chloride and potassium depletion. Urine pH > 7.5 may be associated with a vegetable-based diet, postprandial alkaline tide, urinary infection with a urease-producing organism, alkalinizing drugs, metabolic or respiratory alkalosis, or distal renal tubular acidosis. Urine pH > 7.5 was frequently associated with microscopic urinary sediment abnormalities in dogs and cats in a recent study.[53]

Protein. Trace to +1 (30 mg/dl) proteinuria in dogs and up to +2 (100 mg/dl) proteinuria in cats can be normal, particularly in concentrated urine samples. The dipstrip pad for chemical determination of protein is the most difficult one for technicians to accurately interpret because different protein concentrations are associated with subtle color differences.[54] The dipstrip methodology may overestimate proteinuria in cats when compared with alternate methods, possibly as a consequence of the high USG values observed in this species.[47] The assessment of proteinuria is discussed further in the section on glomerular disease.

Glucose. Glucose present in the glomerular filtrate is virtually completely reabsorbed in the proximal tubules of normal animals and should not be detected in urine when measured by dipstrip or tablet testing. Dipstrip methods use a glucose oxidase colorimetric reaction that is specific for glucose. Peroxide and hypochlorite contamination may result in false-positive results, and refrigerated urine, vitamin C, and formaldehyde may result in false-negative results. Tablets use copper reduction methods, which may measure reducing substances (e.g., fructose, lactose, galactose, vitamin C, penicillin, cephalosporins, salicylates, formaldehyde) other than glucose.[49]

Glucosuria (glycosuria) can be caused by any condition causing hyperglycemia to the extent that the renal tubular threshold for reabsorption of glucose is exceeded. The renal threshold for glucose (plasma concentration at which glucose first appears in the urine) is 180 mg/dl in the dog and in excess of 280 mg/dl for the cat.[55] Diabetes mellitus is the most common cause of glucosuria in dogs. Hyperadrenocorticism and severe stress with multiple hormonal interactions (e.g., epinephrine, cortisol, and ACTH) may also cause glucosuria. When glucosuria is present in the absence of hyperglycemia, proximal renal tubular disease is incriminated.

Glucosuria is more frequent in cats than in dogs, and transient glucosuria has been observed in cats after ketamine anesthesia.[53, 56] Approximately 20 per cent of cats with chronic renal failure had glucosuria in one study, and the majority of these had normal serum glucose concentrations.[1] As many as 33 per cent of cats with urethral obstruction have been reported to have glucosuria by dipstrip measurement.[56–59] Some of these cats had true glucosuria, but some had pseudoglucosuria, due to activation of the color reaction by an unidentified nonglucose substance.[58]

Glucosuria has been reported in nearly 20 per cent of dogs with renal amyloidosis and also has been observed in dogs with specific familial renal diseases.[60, 61] Primary renal glucosuria has been reported in Norwegian elkhounds and is a feature of Fanconi syndrome in the basenji.[62, 63] It can also be seen in nephrotoxic tubular injury caused by aminoglycosides, amphotericin B, and hypercalcemia.[64–66] Glucosuria can also occur after the infusion of glucose-containing fluids.

Ketones. Ketones (acetone, β hydroxybutyric acid, and acetoacetate) are absent from the urine in normal dogs and cats. Ketonuria indicates altered protein, carbohydrate, and fat metabolism and is most commonly observed in conjunction with glucosuria in diabetes mellitus with ketoacidosis. Other causes of ketonuria include starvation or prolonged fasting, persistent fever, noninsulin-mediated hypoglycemia, and possibly liver disease or a low carbohydrate diet.

Occult Blood. The occult blood reaction is negative in urine from healthy dogs and cats. The reagent pad measures either myoglobin or hemoglobin. It is more sensitive to free hemoglobin than that present in intact red blood cells. In some dipstrips one portion of the strip measures free hemoglobin and in another portion intact red blood cells are lysed and their hemoglobin detected. False-positive reactions can result from contamination with hypochlorite, iodides, bromides, and blood from flea feces.[49, 54] False-negative reactions may result from vitamin C and formaldehyde, as well as from failure to adequately mix samples in which intact red blood cells have settled. Positive occult blood reactions are usually due to the presence of intact red blood cells or those that have lysed *in vivo* in very dilute or alkaline urine.[49] Hemoglobinuria after intravascular hemolysis and myoglobinuria following rhabdomyolysis will result in positive occult blood reactions. It is necessary to compare the urinary sediment findings with positive occult blood reactions for proper interpretation.

Bilirubin. Bilirubin is absent from the urine of healthy cats, but can be present in trace to +1 amounts in normal dogs, especially males, with USG values > 1.040.[67] Bilirubinuria may indicate hemolysis, liver disease, or posthepatic obstruction. In dogs, bilirubinuria can also result from intravascular hemolysis because the canine kidney can metabolize filtered hemoglobin to conjugated bilirubin. This occurs predominantly in male dogs.[68] Bilirubinuria may precede hyperbilirubinemia in dogs because of the low renal threshold for conjugated bilirubin in this species.

Leukocyte Esterase. Esterase dipstrip reagent pads, designed to detect the presence of human white blood cells, are not reliable for the detection of white blood cells in dogs because of low sensitivity.[69] Studies in cats are not currently available. Consequently the routine use of this test is not recommended in either species.

Urine Specific Gravity by Dipstrip. Some dipstrips contain reagent pads for determination of specific gravity. There was poor correlation with USG as determined by refractometry when these pads were used to evaluate urine from various domestic species in our clinical laboratory. Thus it is recommended that USG be determined by refractometry rather than by dipstrip reaction.

MICROSCOPIC EVALUATION OF URINARY SEDIMENT

The presence of white blood cells (WBC), red blood cells (RBC), microorganisms, epithelial cells, casts, and crystals can be detected by microscopic evaluation of urinary sediment. Dipstrip evaluation alone failed to disclose any abnormalities in 11 to 16 per cent of canine and feline urine specimens that had abnormal urinary sediment findings.[50, 53] Urine samples containing WBC or bacteria were most likely to result in false-negative findings when examined by dipstrip reactions alone. These findings emphasize the value of a complete urinalysis.

Urinary sediment is evaluated microscopically after centrifugation to concentrate formed elements in higher numbers. Formed elements that require identification and quantification include RBC, WBC, epithelial cells, casts, crystals, and microorganisms. Urinary sediment from normal dogs and cats contains no bacteria and few

TABLE 107–3. NORMAL URINARY SEDIMENT

RBC	0–10 per HPF
WBC	0– 5 per HPF
Epithelial cells	
Transitional	0– 2 per HPF
Squamous	0– 1 per HPF
Caudate	0 per HPF
Bacteria	0 per HPF
Casts	
Hyaline	0– 2 per LPF
Granular	0– 1 per LPF
Waxy	0 per LPF
Cellular	0 per LPF

Normal values will vary among laboratories since centrifuged urine volume, centrifugal force, dilution from use of stain, size of sediment drop evaluated, and technical accuracy of estimates per microscopic field will vary. The greatest variability for normal values will occur for RBC, as their numbers can readily be increased during traumatic collection with catheters, expression, and cystocentesis. HPF = High-powered microscopic field (400 ×); LPF = low-powered microscopic field (100 ×).

cells or casts, but may contain certain crystals (see below). The method of collection must always be considered, since it influences the number and type of elements that can result from contamination or trauma. Table 107–3 summarizes findings in normal urinary sediment.

Cells. Up to 10 RBC and 5 WBC per high-power microscopic field (400 ×) may be normal when the urine sample has been obtained atraumatically. The number of RBC can greatly increase as a result of traumatic catheterization or small vessel trauma that can accompany cystocentesis when the bladder is minimally distended. The causes of excessive numbers of RBC (hematuria) and WBC (pyuria) are presented in Tables 107–4 and 107–5. See also Figure 107–3A and B for a morphologic description of RBC and WBC in urine.

The presence of occasional transitional epithelial cells is normal. The causes of abnormal numbers of transitional epithelial cells in urine sediment are presented in Table 107–6. Transitional epithelial cells vary widely in

TABLE 107–4. CAUSES OF HEMATURIA (> 10 RBC/HPF)

Urinary Tract Origin
Kidneys, ureters, bladder, and urethra

1. Traumatic collection
2. Trauma (blunt and sharp)
3. Inflammation
   a. Infection
   b. Urolithiasis
   c. Sterile
      Idiopathic (feline urinary syndrome)
      Immunologic renal
   d. Chemical (Cytoxan) [cyclophosphamide]
   e. Parasitic (Capillaria, Dioctophyma)
4. Neoplasia
5. Coagulopathy (warfarin, DIC, thrombocytopenia)
6. Renal infarction
7. Renal pelvic hematoma
8. "Benign" renal hematuria

Genital Tract Origin (contamination)
Uterus, vagina, vulva, prostate, prepuce, and penis
Inflammatory, traumatic, and neoplastic conditions, as listed above, must be considered, with the addition of estrus.

Excessive numbers of RBC in urine sediment necessitate consideration of all urinary and genital anatomic sites as possible portals for RBC entry. Localization of RBC origin is not possible by itself, unless RBC are incorporated into casts indicating renal origin. HPF = high-powered microscopic field (400×).

TABLE 107–5. CAUSES OF PYURIA (> 5 WBC/HPF)

Urinary Tract Origin
Kidneys, ureters, bladder, and urethra

Inflammation
  a. Infection
  b. Urolithiasis
  c. Sterile
     Idiopathic (mild in FUS)
     Immunologic renal
     Secondary to neoplasia
     Chemical (Cytoxan [cyclophosphamide])
     Post-traumatic

Genital Tract Origin (contamination)
Uterus, vagina, vulva, prostate, prepuce, and penis

Inflammatory and neoplastic conditions, as listed above, must be considered.

Excessive numbers of WBC in urine sediment necessitate consideration of all urinary and genital anatomic sites as possible portals for WBC entry. It is not possible to conclude what the origin of these WBC is, unless incorporated in casts which indicate renal origin. HPF = high-powered microscopic field (400×).

size. The kidney is only one source of small transitional epithelial cells; such cells also may originate from the lower urinary tract. Thus there is no localizing value to the detection of small transitional cells in the urine sediment. Small transitional epithelial cells with a tail-like configuration (caudate cells), occurring either in clumps or as isolated cells, are thought to arise from the renal pelvis and, consequently, may have localizing value. Squamous epithelial cells can be observed in voided specimens and are of no particular significance, as they arise from nonurinary tissue. The types of epithelial cells observed in urine sediment are depicted in Figure 107–3C and D.

Microorganisms. Bacteria are not seen in urine from normal dogs or cats. Both false-positive and false-negative findings are common.[47, 70] It is easier to detect rod-shaped bacteria in the urine sediment, since particulate debris and small crystals may resemble cocci when subjected to Brownian motion (see Figure 107–3E).

TABLE 107–6. CAUSES FOR EXCESSIVE EPITHELIAL CELLS

Squamous
  Contamination:
    distal urethral, vagina, prepuce, skin
Transitional
  Proximal urethra, bladder, ureter, renal pelvis
    Infection
    Sterile inflammation
    Neoplasia
    Trauma
     Catheterization
     Urolithiasis
    Parasites
Renal Tubular Epithelium
  Renal ischemia
  Nephrotoxicity
  Renal trauma
  Neoplasia

Excessive numbers of epithelial cells in urine sediment necessitate consideration of all urinary and genital anatomic sites as possible portals for entry. Squamous cells are easily identified and their origin limited to the lower urinary and genital tracts. Transitional and renal tubular epithelial cells cannot reliably be differentiated as to their origin from upper or lower sites since they can be the same size and appearance, unless epithelial cells are incorporated into casts indicating renal origin.

Specimens with reported bacteria should be gram-stained and quantitative urine culture performed to confirm the presence of bacterial organisms (see microbiology below).

Yeast and fungal hyphae are rarely encountered in urine sediment. These are most often contaminants from the environment or stain rather than pathogens. Bacterial rods can assume a filamentous shape in urine and cause them to be mistaken for hyphae.

Casts. Casts are cylindrical molds of proteins and cells that form in the lumen of the ascending limb of Henle's loop and distal tubule. They are rare in urine from normal dogs or cats. Casts form and persist more readily in highly acidic urine because acidic urine favors precipitation of the Tamm-Horsfall matrix mucoprotein.[71, 75] Tamm-Horsfall mucoprotein is normally secreted in low concentration in the loop of Henle and the distal tubule.[76-78] High urine concentration and low tubular flow rate favor aggregation of this matrix protein. The nature of matrix proteins and dynamics of cast formation as described in humans have not been characterized in the dog and cat.

The presence of excessive numbers of casts in urine (cylindruria) localizes a disease process to the kidney and indicates accelerated renal cell degeneration, protein leakage across glomeruli, hemorrhage, or exudation into tubular lumina. Renal ischemia, nephrotoxicity, nephritis, and renal trauma may result in cast formation.

Cellular casts consist of RBC, WBC, renal tubular epithelial cells, or combinations of these. Such casts are abnormal, regardless of their numbers. RBC casts are observed rarely in animals with glomerulonephritis and occur occasionally after severe renal trauma or biopsy. WBC casts (pus casts) indicate renal inflammation, often that caused by bacterial infection (pyelonephritis) (Figure 107–4A). Epithelial cell casts develop as the lining of the renal tubule sloughs after severe nephrotoxic or ischemic insult (Figure 107–4B). Cellular casts are fragile, and their presence may be easily missed if urine is not examined soon after collection.

Granular casts are observed more commonly in renal disease than are cellular casts. They usually are absent from the urine of normal dogs and cats, but as many as one granular cast per low-power microscopic field (100 ×) may be normal. Granular casts form as cellular casts undergo degeneration, according to the classic theory of Addis (see Figure 107–6).[79, 80] If this theory is correct, the activity of the disease process is lower at the time when many granular casts are observed as compared with that when cellular casts were abundant. It is also possible that granular casts represent cellular detritus after gradual degeneration of renal epithelial cells. A third possibility is that the granules within casts are precipitates of serum proteins that have been filtered and not reabsorbed in the proximal tubule. Whatever their origin, the presence of granular casts may indicate renal tubular damage resulting from ischemic or nephrotoxic injury and may also result from altered glomerular permeability or decreased proximal tubular reabsorption of protein. There is no actual significance to the observation of coarse as opposed to fine granular casts, although most laboratories make this distinction (Figure 107–4C and D).

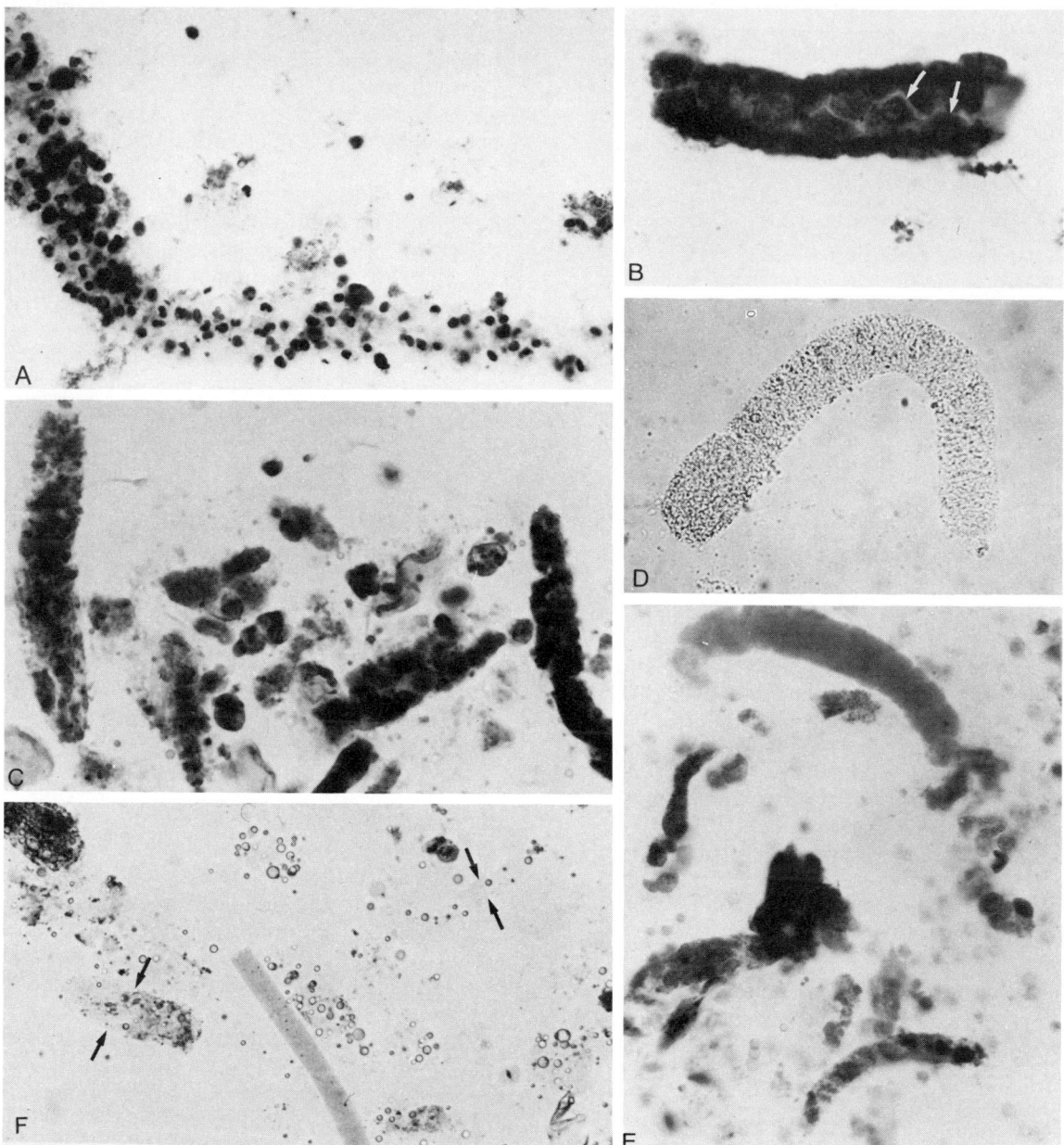

FIGURE 107–4. Urine sediment. Casts. *A,* White blood cell cast. Neutrophils can be seen contributing to the cellularity of this cast. Often their presence indicates renal bacterial infection but also can occur in a variety of renal inflammatory responses. It is not always possible to identify the nature of cells in a cast. *B,* Epithelial cell cast. Renal tubular epithelium has sloughed into this cast. Small mononuclear cells can readily be identified in this field (arrow). (Courtesy of Nancy Facklam.) *C,* Coarsely granular cast. A "shower" of casts is obvious in this field. The cast at the far left clearly illustrates coarse granules, while the cast on the far right illustrates a cellular cast undergoing degeneration. *D,* Finely granular cast. *E,* Waxy cast. The cast at the top is waxy, while the other casts are granular. Notice that this cast is translucent, compared with the transparent nature of hyaline casts. They often are brittle, with cracks and sharply broken ends. Red blood cells and occasional epithelial cells also are present. *F,* Hyaline cast. Notice the transparent nature of these casts (between arrows). It is easy to miss these casts, as their optical density is very low, necessitating low illumination for optimal visualization. The darker cast in the center of the field is waxy. Many lipid droplets are in the background.

Waxy casts represent the final degradation products of cellular casts, according to the theory of Addis (Figures 107–4*E* and 10–6). This type of cast, consequently, requires the longest intrarenal time for development, and the presence of waxy casts is thought to imply substantial stasis of tubular flow. Waxy casts are not found in the urine of healthy dogs or cats.

Hyaline casts are nearly pure precipitates of Tamm-Horsfall mucoprotein (Figure 107–4*F*), and their for-

mation is favored by the presence of serum proteins within tubular lumina. Severe dehydration, high urine concentration, and low tubular flow rate can result in hyaline cast formation by concentration of the small quantity of matrix mucoprotein that is normally present. Fever, strenuous exercise, and passive congestion of the kidney also can result in proteinuria from glomerular hemodynamic changes with consequent hyaline cast formation. Primary glomerular diseases such as glomerulonephritis (GN) and glomerular amyloidosis may result in prominent hyaline cast formation secondary to proteinuria.

Crystals. Crystals are commonly observed in urine sediment from normal dogs and cats and often are not of diagnostic significance (Figure 107–5). The magnitude of crystalluria depends on the presence of the particular crystalloid in the urine, its concentration, urine pH, and the temperature of the urine sample. Table 107–7 summarizes the types of crystalluria and their possible significance.

MICROBIOLOGY

The identification and quantification of bacteria isolated from urine or tissues of the urinary tract allow differentiation of sterile and infectious inflammatory conditions of the urinary tract. Urinary tract infections (UTI) are common in dogs. Nearly 14 per cent of dogs will develop UTI during their lives[81] and 5 to 10 per cent of hospitalized dogs have UTI,[82] regardless of the reason for their admission. Most dogs with UTI are asymptomatic.[81, 82] Although clinical signs and urinalysis

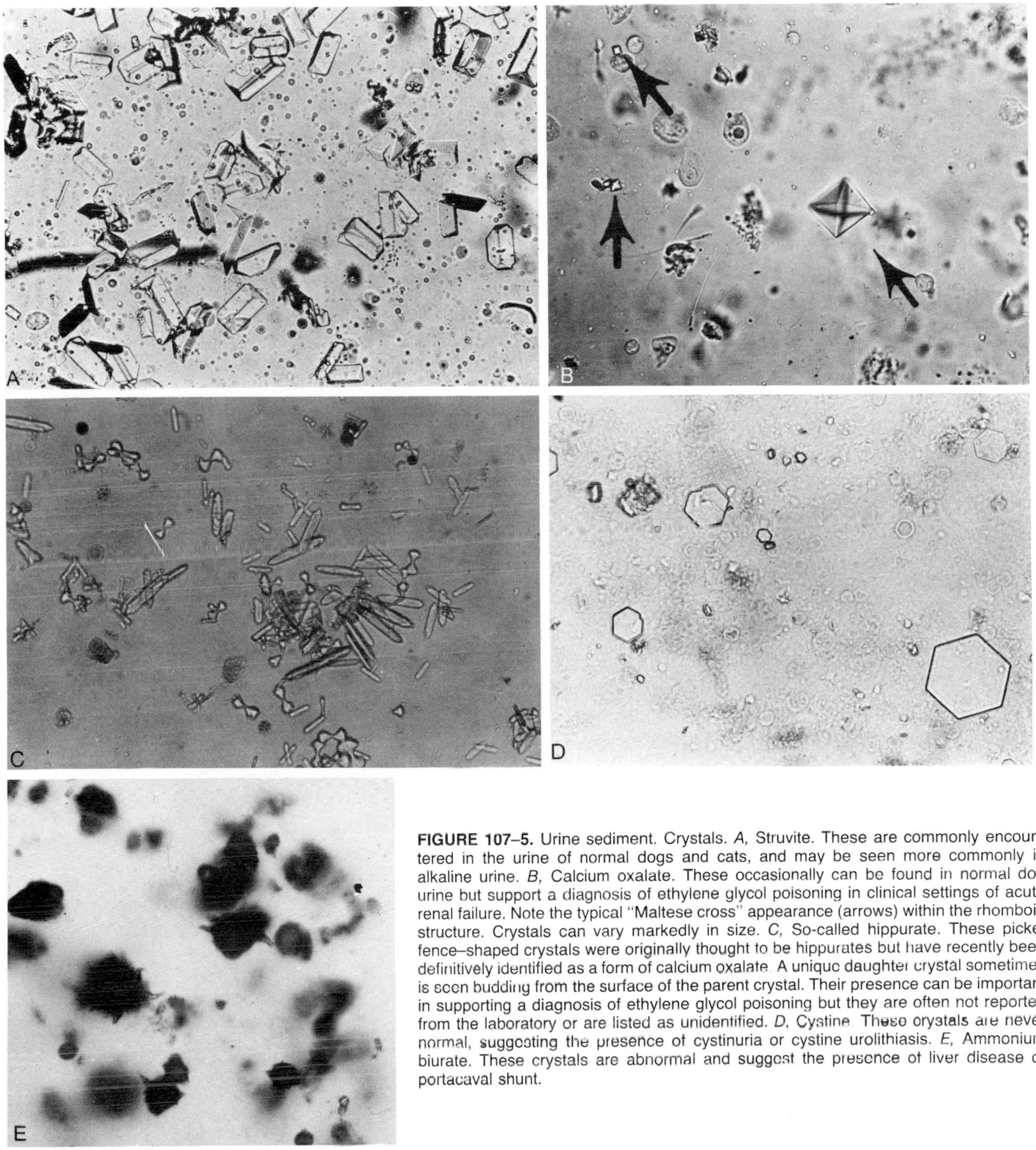

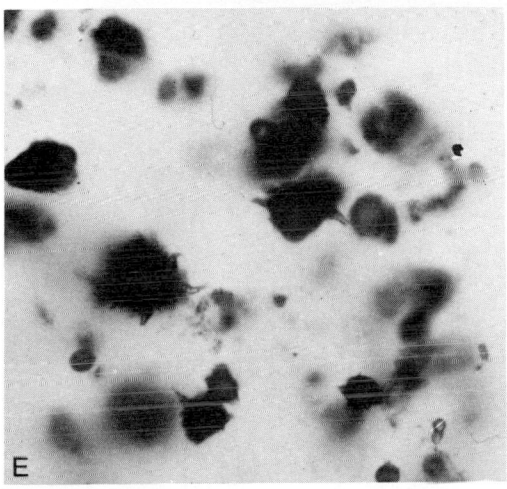

FIGURE 107–5. Urine sediment. Crystals. *A,* Struvite. These are commonly encountered in the urine of normal dogs and cats, and may be seen more commonly in alkaline urine. *B,* Calcium oxalate. These occasionally can be found in normal dog urine but support a diagnosis of ethylene glycol poisoning in clinical settings of acute renal failure. Note the typical "Maltese cross" appearance (arrows) within the rhomboid structure. Crystals can vary markedly in size. *C,* So-called hippurate. These picket fence–shaped crystals were originally thought to be hippurates but have recently been definitively identified as a form of calcium oxalate. A unique daughter crystal sometimes is seen budding from the surface of the parent crystal. Their presence can be important in supporting a diagnosis of ethylene glycol poisoning but they are often not reported from the laboratory or are listed as unidentified. *D,* Cystine. These crystals are never normal, suggesting the presence of cystinuria or cystine urolithiasis. *E,* Ammonium biurate. These crystals are abnormal and suggest the presence of liver disease or portacaval shunt.

TABLE 107–7. CRYSTALLURIA

Type	Associations
Alkaline Urine	
Struvite ("triple phosphate")	Normal, urolithiasis
Amorphous phosphate	Normal, urolithaisis
Calcium phosphate	Urolithiasis
Calcium carbonate	Urolithiasis
Ammonium biurate	Liver disease, portosystemic shunt
Acid Urine	
Uric acid	Urolithiasis, metabolic defect
Cystine	Urolithiasis, metabolic defect
Calcium oxalate	Normal, ethylene glycol poisoning
"Hippurates"	Ethylene glycol poisoning

Crystals often are normal in urine, particularly when the sample is highly concentrated (high urinary specific gravity), the sample has been refrigerated, and the urinary pH is favorable for precipitation. Reference to the urinary pH can be helpful when considering the likelihood of crystal identification. Medications can result in the appearance of difficult-to-identify crystals.

may provide a presumptive diagnosis, microbiology remains the standard method for documentation of UTI.

Antimicrobial susceptibility testing of organisms provides information useful in the selection of appropriate antibiotic therapy for UTI. Disc diffusion methods (Kirby-Bauer) have limited value, but determination of the minimum inhibitory concentration (MIC) allows selection of drugs based on urinary concentrations known to be achieved after standard dosages. Treatment of urinary infections is discussed in Chapters 108 and 112.

The renal parenchyma, renal pelvis, ureter, bladder, and proximal urethra of the normal dog and cat are sterile, whereas a normal bacterial flora populates the distal urethra, prepuce, and vagina. UTI occurs when microorganisms colonize areas that are normally sterile.[83]

Aerobic gram-negative bacteria account for about 70 to 75 per cent of all UTI in dogs and cats. Gram-positive organisms account for the remaining 25 per cent, and fungi or yeast accounts for less than 1 per cent.[83, 91]

Anaerobic bacteria are rarely isolated from the urine of dogs or cats with UTI except for occasional reports of clostridial infection with associated gas formation in the urinary tract.[85, 91–93] UTI usually is caused by one organism (monomicrobic), but infection with two or more organisms (polymicrobic) has been reported in as many as 18 per cent of cases in dogs,[81] and in 2 per cent of cases in cats.[85]

E. coli is most common, causing up to 40 per cent of UTI in dogs and cats treated at referral centers and up to 67 per cent of UTI in a random study of dogs at euthanasia.[83–90, 94] *Proteus, Staphylococcus aureus*, and *Streptococcus* are also commonly isolated, while *Enterobacter* spp., *Klebsiella*, and *Pseudomonas* are less frequent. In cats, *Pasteurella multocida* is second to *E. coli* in frequency, while *Staphylococcus aureus, Proteus* spp., and *Streptococcus* spp. are less frequent. *Enterobacter, Klebsiella*, and *Pseudomonas* are rarely encountered in cats.[83]

Attempts to isolate *Mycoplasma* spp. have not been undertaken routinely, but a study in dogs utilizing cystocentesis suggests that *Mycoplasma* spp. may cause monomicrobic UTI or occur in association with one or more other bacteria.[95] Many dogs from which pure cultures of *Mycoplasma* were obtained had clinical signs attributable to UTI, but the overall importance of mycoplasmal infections remains to be determined. Special media are required to isolate *Mycoplasma*, and their isolation is valuable only if obtained from a portion of the urinary tract that is normally sterile.

The method of urine collection affects the potential for bacterial contamination from the distal urethra, vagina, prepuce, or skin because these areas normally harbor bacteria. Urine that traverses the urethra and prepuce or vagina during voiding or manual compression of the bladder has the greatest opportunity for bacterial contamination, in the absence of actual UTI (false-positive results). Catheterization may inoculate the bladder with bacteria from the distal urethra. The extent of

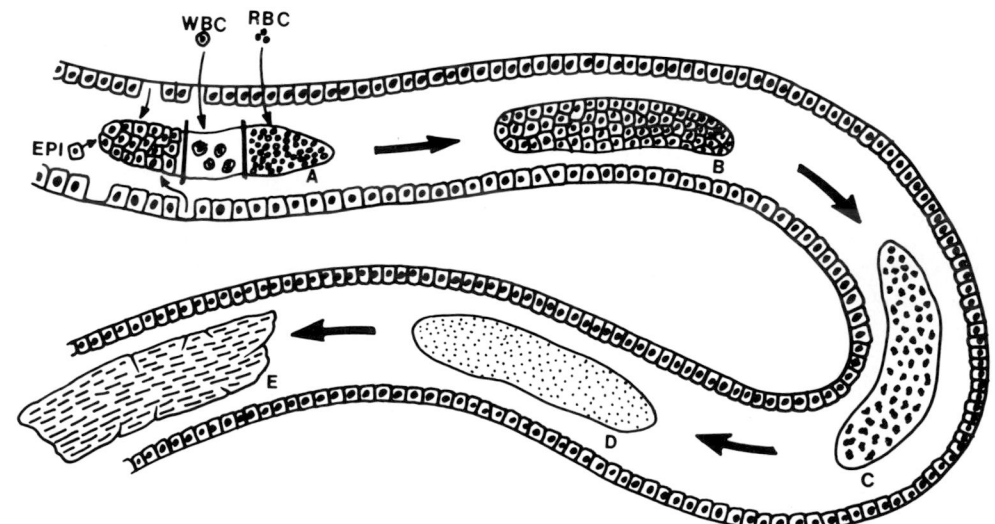

FIGURE 107–6. Addis theory of cast formation. According to this theory, granular casts result from the breakdown of cells and waxy casts from the further degeneration of granular casts. Cast A is a cellular cast from the conglomeration of red cells, white cells, or renal tubular epithelilal cells. Cast B is a degenerating cellular cast in which it is not possible to definitively identify the origin of the cells. Cast C is coarsely granular and cast D is finely granular. Cast E is waxy.

bacterial contamination resulting from catheterization is less than that which occurs during voiding or manual expression of urine. Cystocentesis effectively bypasses the normal flora of the distal urethra and vagina or prepuce, and urine collected by this method should be sterile in normal dogs and cats.

The normal flora of the distal urethra and prepuce or vagina has been established in the dog. *S. aureus* and *Mycoplasma* spp. were the aerobic organisms recovered most commonly in a study of the prepuce and distal urethra of normal male dogs, whereas *S. aureus* and *Streptococcus canis* were the most frequent isolates from intact and spayed female dogs.[96] A wide variety of organisms, however, was encountered. In another study, *E. coli* was commonly isolated from the vaginas of intact bitches.[97, 98] *Mycoplasma*, Bacteroidaceae (anaerobic), and *Pasteurella* were frequently encountered in yet another study.[99] Specimens obtained from the vagina, prepuce, or urethra often yielded more than one organism,[96, 97] and the number of isolates obtained from the prepuce was greater than that obtained from the urethra. Coagulase-positive staphylococci were isolated more commonly from the vagina of prepuberal bitches up to six months of age, and the magnitude of growth was greatest during estrus.[98, 99] Growth from the prepuce of normal dogs was greater than that obtained from the urethra and attained a magnitude of $> 10^5$ in 20 per

cent of the dogs, whereas growth from the urethra was $\leq 10^4$.[96] Generally, quantitative cultures from the urethra and prepuce grew $< 10^3$ organisms, while cultures from the vagina yielded $< 10^4$.[96] Because bacteria normally inhabit the distal urethra, vagina, and prepuce, contamination of urine samples can result in the laboratory isolation of bacteria, but true colonization of these portions of the genitourinary tract does not normally occur.

The number of bacterial colonies that grow from 1 ml of urine is determined by quantitative urine culture and is expressed as colony-forming units per milliliter (cfu/ml). The value of quantitative culture is based on the probability that low numbers of bacteria will signify contamination in a properly collected urine sample, while high numbers of bacteria will indicate the presence of UTI. The numbers of bacteria that indicate UTI rather than contamination will vary with the method of urine collection, species, and sex (see Table 107–8).

The number of organisms isolated from urine is critical to the diagnosis of UTI, and the specimen should be submitted for quantitative culture within 30 minutes of collection. If prompt culture is not possible, the sample should be refrigerated immediately to limit bacterial replication. The bacterial count may double every 20 to 40 minutes at room temperature.[70, 82, 100, 101] Storage of canine urine at room temperature for 24 hours resulted

TABLE 107–8. QUANTITATIVE URINE CULTURE IN NORMAL DOGS AND CATS

Method of Collection	Species	Sex	Cfu/ml	% of Normal Animals
Cystocentesis	Canine	Male	$>10^3$	0
	Canine	Female	$>10^3$	0
	Feline	Male	$>10^3$	0
	Feline	Female	$>10^3$	0
Catheterization	Canine	Male	$>0 <5 \times 10^2$	5
			0	95
	Canine	Female	$>10^5$	20
			$<10^2$	30
			0	50
	Feline	Male	$>10^1 <10^2$	25
			0	75
	Feline	Female	$>10^2 <10^3$	10
			0	90
Midstream Void	Canine	Male	$>10^6$	10
			$<5 \times 10^2$	65
			0	25
	Canine	Female	$>10^5$	45
			10^3 or less	45
			0	10
	Feline	Male	$>10^5$	10
			$>10^4 <10^5$	10
			$>10^3 <10^4$	35
			$10^2–10^3$	45
			0	0
	Feline	Female	$>10^5$	10
			$10^3–10^4$	30
			$10^2–10^3$	10
			$10^1–10^2$	10
			0	40

Diagnosis of UTI requires comparison of the degree of quantitative bacterial growth from patient urine to that expected (if any) from normal urine. Most normal urine samples have some growth when obtained by catheter or by midstream void. Samples for culture are best obtained by cystocentesis since no growth should occur, followed by catheterized samples, while voided samples are not recommended due to the high frequency of large quantitative growth from normal urine.

Data from Comer KM and Ling GL: Results of urinalysis and bacterial culture of canine urine obtained by antepubic cystocentesis, catheterization, and the midstream voided methods. JAVMA 179:891, 1981. Lees GE, et al.: Results of analyses and bacterial cultures of urine specimens obtained from clinically normal cats by three methods. JAVMA 184:449, 1984.

in significant bacterial growth that was not evident in fresh specimens. In the same study, significant loss of bacterial growth did not occur in infected specimens for up to six hours after refrigeration, and in only one specimen did a significant decline in growth occur after 24 hours (false-negative).[102] The addition of preservatives (boric acid–glycerol-sodium formate) to canine urine specimens in combination with refrigeration for 72 hours resulted in quantitative bacterial growth similar to that observed in freshly inoculated urine.[103] The use of preservatives may thus be helpful when samples must be mailed.

Culture of midstream voided urine from normal dogs results in some bacterial growth in 60 to 85 per cent of cases.[46, 104, 105] The magnitude of growth varies widely, with many samples yielding $< 10^3$,[46, 105] but some yielding $\geq 10^5$ cfu/ml.[46] Normal female dogs have bacteriuria more frequently than do males and display greater quantitative growth.[46] In urine samples with bacterial growth, two or more organisms frequently were isolated from both sexes.[46] Bacterial growth also frequently occurs in approximately 80 per cent of voided urine samples from normal cats, but the quantity obtained is less than in dogs, usually from 10^2 to 10^4 cfu/ml. As observed in dogs, cat specimens usually yielded two or more bacterial isolates. Unlike the situation in dogs, however, bacterial growth was more frequent in specimens obtained from males than in those obtained from females.[47]

In normal dogs and cats, bacteria are isolated less frequently and in lower numbers from specimens obtained by catheterization as compared with midstream voided specimens. Approximately 13 to 26 per cent of catheterized urine samples in dogs can be expected to yield some bacterial growth.[46, 104, 105] Usually catheterized samples yield $< 10^4$ cfu/ml, but in one study 10 per cent of the samples yielded $> 10^5$ cfu/ml.[46] There were striking differences in bacterial growth when samples were compared by sex, as only 1 of 16 samples from male dogs grew any bacteria, while those from females had growth in 7 of 14 instances.[46] *Streptococcus* spp., *E. coli*, *Staphylococcus* spp., *Proteus* and micrococci were isolated most frequently from these female dogs. Normal cat urine obtained by catheterization yielded growth in 17 per cent of the samples. The numbers of organisms obtained were smaller ($< 10^3$ cfu/ml) in both males and females as compared with dogs.[47] *E. coli* was the most common isolate from feline urine samples, followed by *Staphylococcus* spp., *Streptococcus* spp., *Corynebacterium* spp., *Pasteurella* spp., and *Flavobacterium*.[47]

Urine obtained by cystocentesis from normal dogs and cats should yield no growth, as would be expected of urine obtained by pyelocentesis or ureteral catheterization at the time of abdominal celiotomy. Because cystocentesis bypasses the normal bacterial flora, it is the standard against which culture results obtained by voiding or catheterization are compared. Because small numbers of organisms from the skin or environment may contaminate the sample during cystocentesis, growth of $< 10^3$ cfu/ml arbitrarily has been considered suggestive of contamination. Inadvertent penetration of the colon during specimen collection, however, can result in growth of large numbers of many different bacteria.

Based on the data described above, it is obvious that interpretation of bacterial growth from urine samples without regard to the number of organisms and method of collection can be confusing. In most cases, urine samples from dogs with UTI yield heavy bacterial growth ($\geq 10^5$ cfu/ml by catheter[87, 100] and $> 10^4$ cfu/ml by cystocentesis),[106] but 25 to 30 per cent of affected dog samples collected by cystocentesis may yield $< 10^4$ cfu/ml.[48, 82, 84] UTI caused by *Mycoplasma* result in isolation of $\geq 10^4$ cfu/ml from samples obtained by cystocentesis.[95] Samples collected by cystocentesis are highly preferred for ease and accuracy of interpretation, since any such specimen that results in $> 10^3$ cfu/ml signifies the presence of UTI. Isolation of bacteria from urinary tissues (bladder wall, renal biopsy) obtained during surgery is indicative of UTI, regardless of the number obtained.

Quantitative culture of urine obtained by urethral catheterization is less desirable, but such data still may be helpful in the diagnosis of UTI. The extent of growth indicative of UTI ("significant bacteriuria") for catheterized urine samples has not been determined. Most authorities have recommended $\geq 10^5$ cfu/ml as the number required to establish UTI in both dogs and cats of either sex. Because bacterial growth of this magnitude can occur in 20 per cent of urine samples collected by catheterization of normal female dogs,[46] a false-positive rate of 20 per cent can be expected in the diagnosis of UTI. Isolation of bacteria after urethral catheterization in normal male dogs is unusual.[46] Based on these results, significant bacteriuria in catheterized male dogs may be considered as $> 10^3$ cfu/ml, but our current recommendation is $> 10^4$ cfu/ml. Because of the large numbers of bacteria that can be isolated from some female dogs, a significant level of $\geq 10^5$ cfu/ml is recommended, with the knowledge that some false-positive results will occur. It appears that quantitative urine culture of catheterized specimens is valuable in male dogs but should be used in female dogs only to rule out UTI ($> 10^4$ cfu/ml). Because urine samples collected by catheterization from normal male and female cats apparently yield $< 10^3$ cfu/ml, significant bacteriuria is set at $\geq 10^3$ cfu/ml in this species.[47]

Voided urine samples are the least desirable for qualitative and quantitative culture in dogs and cats due to the frequency of contamination by bacteria from the normal genitourinary flora, and are not recommended. There is no level of significant bacteriuria in voided specimens that will establish a diagnosis of UTI, since marked bacterial contamination can occasionally occur in male and female dogs and cats. No growth or low counts can be helpful in excluding UTI, however.

Microscopic examination of Gram-stained urine samples can be helpful in the diagnosis of UTI in dogs.[70, 83, 103, 107, 108] By one method, a drop of fresh uncentrifuged urine is allowed to air-dry, unsmeared, on a slide. The slide is then fixed, stained, and examined under oil immersion, and the number of bacteria per field counted. Two or more organisms per oil immersion field were highly correlated with bacterial counts of $> 10^3$ cfu/

ml, while no organisms were visible in those specimens with $< 10^3$.[103] Bacteria were not visible under high-power dry field (400 ×) in a study of wet-mount urine sediment evaluations in cats, regardless of the extent of bacterial growth, but methods using Gram stain were not used.[47] Documentation of bacteriuria by Gram stain may be helpful when bacterial culture is unsuccessful but there is a high index of suspicion for UTI. It is also helpful to know whether UTI is the result of gram-positive or gram-negative organisms when prescribing treatment before definitive isolation and identification of the organism.

RADIOLOGY

Total renal mass may reflect renal function or stage of renal disease. For example, small kidneys often are associated with chronic renal disease, while normal or enlarged kidneys may be associated with acute renal disease. Radiography provides precise information about renal size, which frequently cannot be obtained from physical examination. Measurement of renal dimensions is of little value, since renal size varies widely in normal dogs[109] and cats,[110] even among those of similar size. In an effort to correct for variation in patient size and radiographic magnification, renal size is evaluated in reference to surrounding anatomic landmarks, usually the length of the second lumbar vertebra (excluding the intervertebral space).

SURVEY RADIOGRAPHS

Survey radiographs are frequently used in the initial evaluation of dogs and cats with suspected renal disease. The animal should be fasted and the colon evacuated to maximize visualization of the abdominal viscera. Both ventrodorsal and lateral views should be obtained. The right lateral view is preferred in dogs because it allows maximal separation of the right and left renal shadows, and also allows the left kidney to be seen more clearly.[111]

The kidneys should be evaluated for number, position, size, shape, contour, and radiodensity. The left kidney is normally well visualized in the dog, but the right kidney often cannot be seen as well, especially its cranial pole. Both kidneys should be identified in both dogs and cats; the ureters are not normally visible. In the dog, the left kidney is located near vertebrae L2 to L5, while the right kidney is located more cranially, near vertebrae T13 to L3. The location of kidneys in the cat is less predictable because they are more movable. Visualization of the kidneys depends on good radiographic technique, the amount of retroperitoneal fat, and the absence of obscuring abdominal fluid.

Renal length as compared with length of vertebra L2 is the most useful and widely used measurement of size on survey films. Normal dogs will have ventrodorsal ratios of 2.5 to 3.5 × L2,[109] whereas cats will have values of 2.0 to 3.0 (see Table 107–9).[110, 112] Unfortunately accurate measurement of the right kidney rarely can be made in the dog, and in only 50 per cent of dogs can the left kidney be adequately measured.[109] The

TABLE 107–9. RATIO OF KIDNEY MEASUREMENTS TO 2ND LUMBAR VERTEBRA

Survey Radiographs		Ref
Dog	2.98 ± 0.22 length of ventrodorsal left kidney/L2	109
	2.79 ± 0.23 length of lateral left kidney/L2	109
Cat	2.49 ± 0.25 length of kidney/L2	110
	1.76 ± 0.20 width of kidney/L2	110
Excretory Urography (Intravenous Pyelography-IVP)		
Dog	3.03 ± 0.25 length of ventrodorsal kidney/L2	109
	3.02 ± 0.26 length of kidney/L2	113
	1.98 ± 0.20 width of kidney/L2	113
Cat	2.4 to 3.0 length of ventrodorsal kidney/L2	112
	3.0 to 3.5 cm kidney width	112

Measurement of renal dimensions includes the maximum width or length. L2 length is that on ventrodorsal projection and does not include the disk space.

contour of the kidneys should be smooth, and they should have a homogenous fluid density. Occasionally, in obese cats, the renal pelvis and diverticula may be outlined if surrounded by sufficient fat.

EXCRETORY UROGRAPHY

Excretory urography (intravenous pyelography, IVP) is the term given to the positive contrast study obtained when a triiodinated organic contrast agent is excreted by the kidneys after intravenous administration. The time course of the appearance and disappearance of renal opacification can yield semiquantitative information about renal function, but this assessment is crude and primarily limited to comparison of one kidney with the other.[112] Excretory urography is best used for the anatomic evaluation of the urinary tract. The magnitude of renal measurements made during excretory urography exceeds those made on survey films, owing to the diuretic effect of the contrast agent.

Excretory urography is indicated when renal size, shape, and location cannot be adequately determined on survey radiographs studies and when additional information about the renal parenchyma and pelvis is required. It is the radiographic procedure of choice in the evaluation of rupture of the upper urinary tract because leakage of urine is easily visualized, and for evaluation of ectopic ureter. Excretory urography is also helpful in the diagnosis of obstructive nephropathy and hydronephrosis, and in the evaluation of renal enlargement.

Triiodinated contrast medium is rapidly administered at a dosage of 400 mg/lb of iodine by way of an indwelling venous catheter. Films are taken immediately and at 5, 20, and 40 minutes after injection.[113] Higher doses and delayed timing sequences may be necessary in animals with severe primary renal azotemia, and even using higher dosages, the kidneys may not become opacified. Renal opacification in laboratory dogs is not increased with dosages exceeding 800 mg/lb because contrast-induced diuresis supervenes.[114]

Arteriography, nephrography, pyelography, and visualization of the ureter and bladder constitute the four phases of excretory urography. The arteriographic phase is easily missed if films are not obtained within seven to ten seconds of contrast injection. The renal parenchyma is best evaluated immediately and at 5 minutes after injection, the renal pelvis at 20 and 40 minutes, the pelvic diverticula at 40 minutes, and the ureters at 5 and 20 minutes.[113] Accurate measurements of renal length can be readily determined for both kidneys when adequate dye excretion occurs. Normal values for the ratio of renal length to the length of vertebra L2 in dogs five minutes after dye injection were 3.02 ± .26 (2.54 to 3.73) in one study[113] and 3.03 ± .24 (2.58 to 3.74) in another study.[109] Both of these values slightly exceed those obtained on survey studies. Measurements of the renal pelvis, diverticula, and ureter also can be made, but usually these structures are assessed subjectively.[113] Dilatation of the pelvis and ureter can be encountered with acute or chronic pyelonephritis and with urinary tract obstruction. Diverticula can be dilated in chronic pyelonephritis but often lack filling in acute pyelonephritis. Table 107–9 summarizes radiographic measurements of normal kidneys.

The density of the nephrogram and pyelogram is determined by several factors, including GFR, plasma concentration of the contrast agent, concentration of dye in tubular fluid, tubular flow rate, volume of the collecting system, and resistance to outflow of urine.[115] The nephrogram should be homogeneous, except in the very earliest phase, when the cortex may be more dense than the medulla, referred to as the vascular phase or vascular nephrogram. The opacity of the renal pelvis during the pyelogram should be denser than the nephrogram in health.[112] When GFR is decreased, the filtered load of dye will also be reduced, resulting in less opacification. In general, poor renal opacification indicates poor renal function, but this is not specific, as solute or water diuresis will also reduce opacification. On the other hand, highly opacified kidneys are not necessarily normal either, as any condition that results in avid reabsorption of water and salt along the nephron (e.g., partial obstruction, dehydration, renal vein thrombosis) can increase opacification. Filling defects (nonhomogeneous filling) within the renal parenchyma (neoplasia, abscess, cyst) or renal pelvis (neoplasia, calculus, blood clot, exudate) can also be identified.

Excretory urography should not be performed in dehydrated patients or in those with known hypersensitivity to contrast media. Although excretory urography is normally safe in animals, decreased GFR can persist for several days after the administration of intravenous contrast agents even in normal dogs.[116] Intravenous contrast media can cause acute renal failure in humans, particularly in dehydrated patients and in those with multiple myeloma or diabetes mellitus. This complication has yet to be documented in veterinary medicine. There is controversy as to whether or not excretory urography is harmful in animals with primary renal failure. The success of excretory urography in animals with primary renal azotemia is unpredictable, and rigid guidelines for performance of excretory urography in azotemic animals should be avoided.

ULTRASONOGRAPHY

Diagnostic ultrasound has become increasingly available in veterinary medicine. Sonograms are useful in the evaluation of renal disease, often providing infor-

mation about renal structure that is not available from conventional radiographic techniques (Figure 107–7A and B). Ultrasonography has been considered a secondary investigative tool to be used in conjunction with excretory urography, but it can be used as the initial study in the presence of marked azotemia or if there is risk of contrast-induced toxicity.[117]

The main advantage of renal imaging by ultrasound is that the internal structure of the kidney can be studied regardless of the level of renal function. Furthermore, the imaging procedure is entirely noninvasive and there is no known hazard to the animal. Renal masses can be evaluated and biopsied or aspirated under ultrasound guidance.[118-121] The only disadvantage is that no semiquantitative information about the level of renal function is obtained.

Sonographic images that are obtained in the normal dog include the cortex, medulla, pelvis, pelvic diverticula, peripelvic fat, interlobar vessels, and renal capsule.[122] The echogenic patterns of the renal cortex and

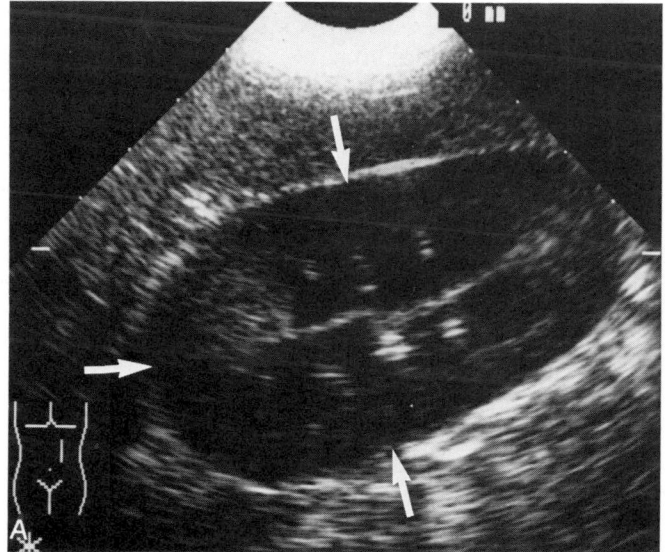

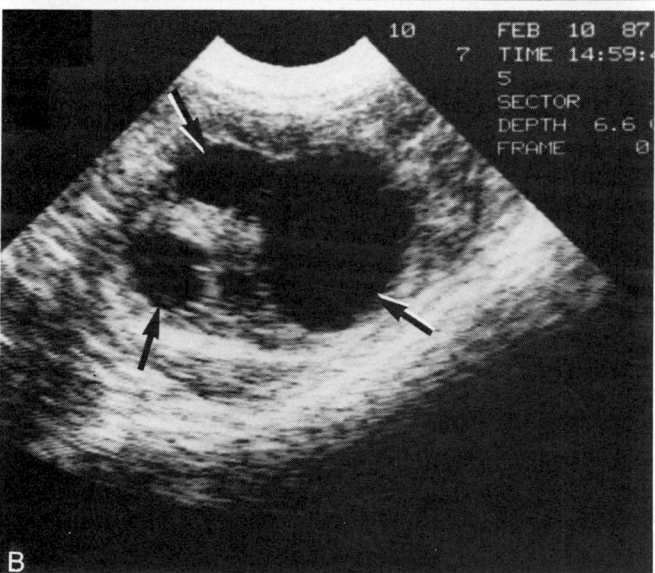

FIGURE 107–7. Renal ultrasound. *A*, Normal dog kidney. *B*, Polycystic kidneys. Arrows point to large cysts within renal parenchyma. (Courtesy of Dr. Bret Kantrowitz and Dr. David Biller.)

medulla are readily distinguished, with the medulla being anechoic to hypoechoic. The cortex is more echogenic than the medulla but less so than spleen, liver, or prostate. High-density echoes emanate from the renal sinus and diverticular areas, while the cavity of the renal pelvis is not normally observed, even during diuresis.[118, 122] The renal cortex, medulla, sinus, crest, and capsule can be consistently visualized during sagittal sonography of normal cats, but vessels and diverticula are not observed. Vessels can be readily detected, however, if high-frequency scanners are used. The echogenic patterns of the renal cortex and medulla are the same in cats as in dogs.[123]

Individual anatomic areas have characteristic acoustic patterns in health that can be disrupted in various disease states.[124] Abnormalities in renal architecture may be focal, multifocal, or diffuse, and may occur in the cortex, medulla, renal sinus, or perinephric regions. The echogenic pattern is described as normal, hypoechoic, hyperechoic, anechoic, or complex when a combination of these patterns exists.[118] Abnormal dimensions of the cortex, medulla, pelvis, and diverticula are noted. The sonographic patterns of several renal diseases in dogs and cats have been described,[118, 119, 124–126] including renal neoplasia, nephrolithiasis, nephrocalcinosis, hydronephrosis, cystic renal disease, acute tubular necrosis, glomerulonephritis, and chronic interstitial nephritis (end-stage renal disease).

Abnormal patterns are most helpful in the diagnosis of renal neoplasia and least specific for characterizing diffuse parenchymal disease.[118, 125] Although renal ultrasound is more sensitive than survey radiographs and excretory urography, a normal echo pattern does not rule out primary renal disease. In one study approximately 33 per cent of dogs had normal echogenic patterns despite the presence of histologically confirmed renal disease.[118]

Diagnosis of acute and chronic primary parenchymal renal disease can be supported by sonographic studies, but a specific morphologic diagnosis is not possible without biopsy. Changes in renal size, corticomedullary dimensions, and echodensity can be detected. Chronic renal diseases are associated with reduced cortical dimensions. Hyperechoic cortical patterns, loss of cortical homogeneity, and loss of distinct corticomedullary boundaries can occur in a variety of acute and chronic primary renal disorders, and the severity of the disease correlates with the extent of changes present. A prominent hypoechogenic renal medulla may be seen in animals with polyuric renal failure, while a hyperechogenic pattern of the medulla may indicate advanced fibrosis.[124]

ANGIOGRAPHY

Renal angiography is seldom used in veterinary medicine because it requires sophisticated and expensive equipment and is an invasive procedure requiring anesthesia and arterial catheterization. The need for angiography has been further reduced by the advent of ultrasonography. The main indication for renal angiography is the need to specifically evaluate the architecture of the renal vascular supply as in the case of congenital malformations or primary vascular disease (Figure 107–8).

Selective, semiselective, and nonselective angiographic techniques can be used after establishing vascular access, usually by surgical or percutaneous catheterization of the femoral artery. Selective renal artery catheterization is preferred, to provide a study of maximum quality.

Renal angiography consists of three phases: arterial, nephrographic, and venous. The arterial phase is visualized 0.5 to 3.0 seconds after injection and delineates the arterial system to the level of the arcuate arteries. The nephrogram is seen immediately after the arterial phase as homogeneous opacification of the renal parenchyma. During this stage, measurements are made for the corticomedullary ratio, with normal values ranging from 0.40 to 0.69 with a mean of 0.53. The venous phase is visualized two to four seconds after injection, during which time the intrarenal and renal veins are visualized. Maximal opacification of the renal vein usually occurs four to seven seconds after injection.[127] The caliber of intrarenal vessels, vascular morphology, cortical width, renal circulation time, and renal vein patency can be determined during renal angiography and may be helpful in selected cases.

Digital subtraction angiography can define the renal arterial system after a simple intravenous injection of contrast agent. This procedure, however, still requires general anesthesia because the animal must remain completely still.[128] Unfortunately, the equipment required is sophisticated and generally unavailable in veterinary practice.

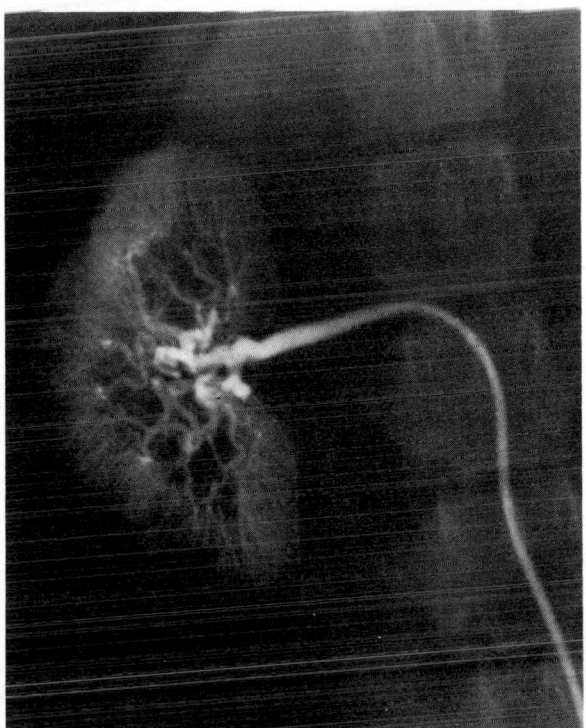

FIGURE 107–8. Renal angiography. Congenital anomaly (renal dysplasia). Notice the lack of vascular pattern within renal cortex.

NUCLEAR MEDICINE

Radioactive pharmaceuticals that are excreted predominantly by glomerular filtration can be used to determine GFR, using renal scintigraphy. ^{99m}Tc diethylenetriaminepentaacetic acid (DTPA) is filtered and concentrated in the kidneys. It is possible to quantify the accumulation and disappearance of renal radioactivity after injection of this compound. Comparison with plasma concentrations (time-activity curves) allows mathematical calculation of GFR. The advantage to this technique is that the GFR of each kidney can be determined individually without need for urine or blood samples.

Scintigraphy provides an image from which renal size can be estimated, but poor anatomic information is provided. Asymmetry of uptake suggests unilateral disease. An image can be obtained during acute renal failure, even if GFR is unmeasurable. Scintigraphy could be used in settings where classic clearance studies would be performed, such as in the early diagnosis of renal insufficiency. It may be particularly useful in the localization of unilateral hematuria after DTPA tagging to colloid, in which case radioactivity would provide an image only in the kidney experiencing active bleeding.[128, 129] Scintigraphy is a rapid procedure and poses no risk to the animal. Unfortunately it requires very sophisticated equipment and has largely been used for research purposes.

RENAL BIOPSY

Renal biopsy allows the clinician to establish a histologic diagnosis, and should be considered when the information obtained is likely to alter patient management. Examples of such situations include differentiation of protein-losing glomerular diseases, differentiation of acute renal failure from chronic renal failure, determination of the status of tubular basement membranes in acute renal failure, and establishing the response of the patient to therapy or the progression of previously documented renal disease. A renal biopsy should not be performed until thorough clinical and radiographic evaluation of the patient has been completed. The contraindications to renal biopsy are few and include pyonephrosis, perirenal abscess, hydronephrosis, renal cyst, or the presence of a confirmed coagulopathy. Relative contraindications to biopsy include a solitary kidney, extremely small kidneys, confirmed pyelonephritis, or renal neoplasia.

Methods. Several techniques for renal biopsy have been described, and consist of blind percutaneous, keyhole, open, and laparoscopic approaches. The reader is referred elsewhere for a complete description of these techniques.[130–132] The choice of technique largely depends on the experience and technical skill of the operator, the species to be biopsied, and the size of sample required. The blind percutaneous technique works well in cats because their kidneys can be readily palpated and immobilized per abdomen.[133] The keyhole approach is commonly used in dogs and is most useful when the operator is experienced with the technique.[131] If the operator is less familiar with renal biopsy or a larger sample is required, an open approach and wedge biopsy by means of laparotomy are recommended for dogs. The advantages of this procedure include the ability to visually inspect the kidneys and other abdominal organs, to choose the specific biopsy site, to take an adequately sized sample, and to observe the kidney for hemorrhage. Laparoscopy also allows direct visualization of the kidney and detection of hemorrhage but requires special equipment and expertise.[132] All techniques necessitate general anesthesia to provide adequate patient restraint and analgesia. Occasionally tissue architecture is less important (e.g., renal lymphosarcoma, feline infectious peritonitis), and aspiration of the kidney, using a 23- or 25-gauge needle, may provide useful material for cytology.

Technique. Before renal biopsy, an intravenous catheter should be placed and the patient's clotting ability evaluated by bleeding time and an estimation of platelet numbers. Although platelet function in uremia may be abnormal despite normal platelet numbers, renal biopsy has not been found to be more hazardous in uremic patients as compared with those without uremia.[130] The patient's hematocrit and total plasma proteins should be determined before biopsy but after adequate rehydration with parenteral fluids. These parameters may then be monitored after biopsy to detect hemorrhage.

The most commonly used biopsy instruments consist of the Franklin-modified Vim-Silverman needle and the Tru Cut biopsy needle. Excessive penetration of the kidney with the outer cannula of the Franklin-modified Vim-Silverman instrument should be avoided to prevent retrieval of an insufficient amount of renal cortex.[130] The potential for compression artifact in the biopsy sample also appears to be greater using this instrument.[134] Samples from dogs obtained with the Vim-Silverman needle averaged 25 glomeruli in one study, while samples from cats averaged 14 glomeruli in another study using the Tru Cut needle.[130, 133]

Care should be taken when directing the angle of the biopsy instrument so as to avoid the renal hilus and major vessels (Figure 107–9). Samples containing large amounts of medulla are more likely to contain large vessels and lead to infarction of renal tissue.[130, 133, 135] Therefore, it is recommended that the biopsy needle be directed along the long axis of the kidney, solely through cortical tissue. Because of the small size of feline kidneys, it is common to obtain relatively large amounts of medullary tissue, and this has been associated with infarction and fibrosis.[133] A modification of the Tru Cut biopsy needle for cats has been described that allows for collection of smaller sized samples.[136]

After biopsy, the kidney should be digitally compressed for five minutes and, after release, the abdomen inspected for hemorrhage. The biopsy sample may be dislodged from the biopsy instrument using a stream of sterile saline solution from a syringe or, alternatively, the biopsy instrument may be immersed directly in fixative. For routine histopathology, the sample should be fixed in buffered ten per cent formalin for three to four hours. For immunofluorescence studies, the sample may be snap-frozen in liquid nitrogen and isopentane ($-160°C$) or Dry Ice and acetone ($-90°C$). These freezing agents should not come into direct contact with the

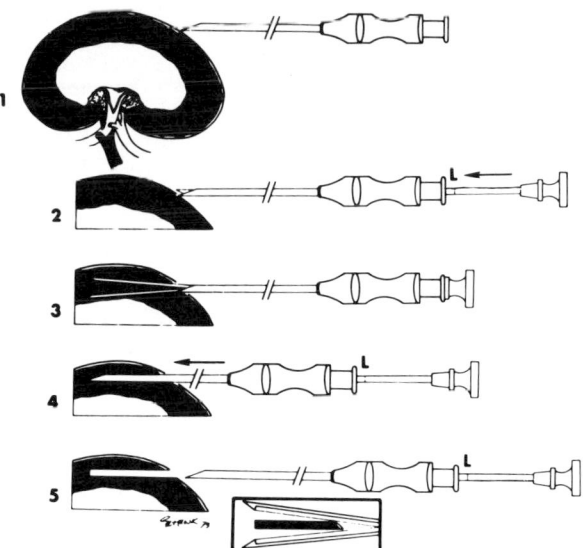

FIGURE 107–9. Demonstration of technique of renal biopsy and needle placement using a Franklin-modified Vim Silverman needle. (1) The tip of the outer cannula with stylet is in contact with the renal capsule. (2) The stylet is replaced by the cutting prong. (3) The cutting prongs are thrust into the renal cortex. (4) The outer cutting cannula is advanced over the cutting prongs. (5) The outer cannula and cutting prongs are removed from the kidney. (From Osborne CA: Kidney biopsy. Vet Clin North Am 4(2):351–365, 1974.)

biopsy sample. Alternatively, the sample can be preserved for immunofluorescence in Michel's transport medium.[137] Care should be taken that the vial is leakproof, completely full of fixative, and properly packaged for transport. Immunopathology studies also may be performed by a peroxidase-antiperoxidase method using formalin-fixed samples without need for special preservation of the sample.[138] If electron microscopy is required, one sample should be minced into one to two mm cubes and placed immediately into chilled two per cent glutaraldehyde.

After renal biopsy, a brisk fluid diuresis should be initiated to prevent potential clot formation in the renal pelvis.[130] The patient's hematocrit and total plasma proteins should be monitored at appropriate intervals over the next 12 to 24 hours to detect serious hemorrhage.

Complications. The most common complication of renal biopsy is hemorrhage. Subcapsular hemorrhage commonly occurs at the site of biopsy, and 80 per cent of patients experience microscopic hematuria during the first 48 hours after biopsy.[139] Macroscopic hematuria is less common, and has been reported in seven per cent of cases in one study.[130] Severe hemorrhage into the peritoneal cavity is rare and usually is associated with improper technique.[130, 139] Such hemorrhage must be treated aggressively by compression bandage of the abdomen, fresh whole blood transfusion, and exploratory surgery if necessary.

Linear infarcts in the path of the biopsy needle are commonly observed after renal biopsy in both dogs and cats.[133, 135, 140] These are small and superficial when the biopsy is limited to the renal cortex. If, however, an arcuate artery is damaged by passage of the biopsy needle through the corticomedullary junction, a wedge-shaped infarct may occur. This is more common in the

cat because of the small size of the kidneys in relation to the length of the biopsy needle.[133, 135]

Hydronephrosis occasionally complicates renal biopsy. If penetrated by the biopsy needle, bleeding into the renal pelvis and clot formation can occur, leading to obstruction and hydronephrosis.[130] This complication should be considered if the biopsy report indicates the presence of transitional epithelium at one end of the biopsy or if progressive renal enlargement is detected after renal biopsy. It is more likely in cats, in which penetration of the renal pelvis is more common because of the smaller size of feline kidneys. The risk of this complication is minimized by limiting the biopsy site to the renal cortex and instituting a fluid diuresis afterward.[130]

Renal infection, retention cysts caused by tubular obstruction and dilatation, urine fistula, and iatrogenic arteriovenous fistula are rare complications of renal biopsy.

Interpretation. The histologic components of the kidney include the glomeruli, interstitium, vessels, and tubules, and these components are interdependent so that damage to one frequently affects the others. The pathologist should consider the technique by which the sample was taken when evaluating the renal biopsy. Compression artifact and intraluminal desquamation of tubular epithelial cells have been observed in samples obtained by Vim-Silverman needle and are less likely in Tru Cut samples.[132, 134] Uniform tissue thickness is essential so that the pathologist becomes accustomed to normal cellularity. Mean nuclear counts of normal canine and feline glomeruli in one micron sections were 71 and 63, respectively, and these values are influenced by tissue thickness.[141, 142] Studies have shown an approximate 90 per cent concordance rate between biopsy diagnosis and necropsy diagnoses.[130, 139]

CHARACTERIZATION OF AZOTEMIA

The localization of azotemia as nonrenal, prerenal, primary intrarenal, or postrenal in origin is necessary to provide an accurate diagnosis, treatment, and prognosis, but no single test specifically allows this distinction to be made. Rather, integration of findings from the history, physical examination, laboratory evaluation, and radiographic studies is required to establish an accurate diagnosis.

The diagnosis of postrenal azotemia may be made after initial physical examination and radiographic studies. Physical examination may reveal an enlarged, painful bladder, abdominal mass, renal pain, or the source of urethral obstruction during abdominal and perineal palpation and rectal examination. Renal ultrasonography or excretory urography may be used to document the presence of urinary tract obstruction (hydroureter, pelvic and diverticular dilatation). Excretory urography may reveal a ruptured kidney or ureter as the cause for loss of retroperitoneal detail discovered on survey radiographs, while positive contrast cystourethrography is preferred in the initial evaluation of abdominal effusion due to a ruptured bladder or urethra. Comparison of

TABLE 107–10. DIFFERENTIATION OF PRERENAL, INTRINSIC RENAL, AND POSTRENAL AZOTEMIA

	Prerenal	Intrinsic-Renal Acute	Intrinsic-Renal Chronic	Postrenal Obstruction	Postrenal Uroperitoneum
BUN	↑	↑	↑	↑	↑
Serum creatinine	↑	↑	↑	↑	↑
Urine:					
SG	>1.030	<1.030	<1.030	variable	variable
Sediment	−	+, − Casts	−	RBC, WBC, epi	RBC, WBC, epi
Protein	−	+, −	+, −	+	+
Renal size	N	↑, or N	↓, or N	↑, or N	N
Hematocrit (anemia)	N	N (early)	↓, or N	N (early)	N
BUN/Scr after IV fluids	Rapid Decrease	Little Change	Little Change	Little Change	Little Change
pU/pD (long-standing)	−	−	+	− (acute)	−
Oliguria	+	+, or −	−, or + (terminal)	Variable	Variable
Hypothermia	−	+ if nephrosis	−	−	−
Renal pain	−	+, −	−	+, −	−, + if renal tear
Ischemic episode	+	+	−	−	+ (trauma)
Nephrotoxin exposure	−	+	−	−	−
Renal ultrasound	N	↑ Echo	↑ Echo/Calcinosis	↑ pelvis/diverticula	N
Contrast urography	N	Absent, or Delayed & Persistent Nephrogram	↓ Excretion	↑ pelvis/diverticula	Contrast leakage
Serum calcium	N	↓, or N	N, ↓, or ↑ (rarely)	N, or ↓	N, or ↓
Serum phosphorus	N, or ↑	↑	↑	↑	↑
Serum potassium	N	↑, or N	N, or ↓, or ↑ (terminal)	N, or ↑	N, or ↑
Metabolic acidosis	−	Moderate to Severe	Mild to Moderate	− early, + late	− early, + late
Abdominal fluid	None	+ (if overhydrated)	−	None	+
Blood pressure	↓, or N	N, or ↑	↑, or N	N, or ↑ (chronic)	N, or ↓
Renal biopsy	N	Abnormal	Abnormal	N, early	N

Findings from history, physical examination, serum biochemistry, urinalysis, hematology, radiography, renal histopathology, and special diagnostics may be necessary to distinguish conclusively the type of azotemia. Usually it is relatively easy to decide if azotemia is from postrenal causes after physical examination and routine abdominal radiography. Urinary specific gravity is the most important single test to differentiate prerenal and intrinsic renal azotemia. Urinary sediment, renal size, and hematocrit are also helpful. Results listed in this table are those prior to any drug, fluid, or surgical treatments. When two results are listed, the one noted first is most common. Findings will vary in severity according to the stage at which the disease process is investigated. N = normal, − = negative result, + = positive result, ↑ = value increased above normal, ↓ = value decreased below normal, pU/pD = polyuria and polydipsia.

urea nitrogen and creatinine concentrations in abdominal fluid with those in serum should show a gradient, with higher concentrations of urea nitrogen and creatinine in the abdominal fluid (see Chapter 112).

After postrenal causes have been excluded, urinalysis and radiographic evaluation of renal size provide the most important information for distinguishing prerenal from primary renal azotemia. Physical examination may reveal abnormalities compatible with the presence of renal disease, but their presence is not consistent (see section on physical examination). Dogs and cats with prerenal azotemia should produce highly concentrated urine if their kidneys are normal, although exceptions occur in disorders that selectively interfere with the renal concentrating mechanism. Although experimental renal failure in cats has been associated with USG values greater than 1.030,[20] clinical renal failure in cats most often is associated with USG in the isosthenuric range.[1] Animals with prerenal azotemia should have normal radiographic renal size, whereas those with primary renal azotemia may have small, normal, or enlarged kidneys. See Table 107–10 for a summary of diagnostic criteria differentiating prerenal, postrenal, and primary renal azotemia.

PATHOPHYSIOLOGY OF UREMIA

Uremia may be defined as the constellation of clinical signs and biochemical abnormalities associated with a critical loss of functioning nephrons.[143] It may be considered a pervasive intoxication caused by the combined effects of many metabolites retained as a result of loss of renal excretory function.[144, 145] The syndrome of uremia, however, also includes many metabolic and endocrine disturbances that arise from loss of renal homeostatic, synthetic, and catabolic functions as well as abnormalities that are consequences of renal compensatory mechanisms and therapeutic intervention. The presence of the extrarenal manifestations of advanced renal disease (e.g., hemorrhagic gastroenteritis, hemostatic defects, anemia, osteodystrophy) usually is implied when a patient is described as being uremic.

Uremic Toxins

The conceptual view of uremia as an intoxication and the observation that dialysis ameliorates many of its symptoms have led to a search for the responsible uremic toxin. It has become clear, however, that many compounds are involved in the pathogenesis of uremia and no single compound is likely to explain the diversity of uremic symptoms (see Table 107–11). The criteria for classification of a compound as a uremic toxin have been enumerated[144]: (1) it must be identified chemically and quantitated in biological fluids, (2) it must be present in higher concentration in biological fluids from uremic as compared with normal patients, (3) its concentration must be correlated with clinical symptoms, and (4) its toxic effects must be reproduced experimentally. To this may be added the condition that reduction in the plasma concentration of the uremic toxin should be accompanied by improvement in clinical symptoms. Few compounds qualify as uremic toxins if these criteria are rigidly applied.

Urea and creatinine are markers of decreased GFR and are unlikely to be important uremic toxins.[146, 147] High concentrations of urea, however, can lead to fatigue, nausea, vomiting, headache, glucose intolerance, and bleeding tendency.[148] Guanidine compounds (methylguanidine, guanidinoacetic acid, guanidinosuccinic acid) are products of nitrogen metabolism that accumulate in renal failure, and have been implicated in such abnormalities of the uremic state as weight loss and altered platelet factor 3 release.[149] The clinical relevance of these observations, however, remains uncertain.[150]

Uric acid accumulates in human patients with renal failure, but any pathogenetic role in domestic animals must take into consideration the fact that dogs other than Dalmatians metabolize uric acid to allantoin. Oxalates accumulate in the myocardium and kidney in uremia, but these deposits are unlikely to be of functional significance.

The aliphatic amines, dimethylamine and trimethylamine, result from the breakdown of choline by gastrointestinal bacteria and are increased in uremia.[151] These compounds may contribute to the "fishy" odor of uremic breath and may be associated with neurobehavioral alterations, based on improvement after therapy with nonabsorbable antibiotics. The polyamines, spermine and spermidine, accumulate in renal failure, and spermine has been suggested to inhibit erythropoiesis.[152] Other metabolites that are produced by the action of the bacterial flora of the gut and that have been considered possible uremic toxins include other polyamines (putrescine, cadaverine), phenols, aromatic amines, and indoles.

Myoinositol has been shown to decrease nerve conduction velocity and is toxic to dorsal root ganglion cells in tissue culture.[117] It has been considered as a possible toxic factor in uremic neuropathy. Cyclic adenosine monophosphate (cAMP) has been shown to decrease platelet aggregation, and ribonuclease to impair cellular proliferation and erythropoiesis.[144]

The observation that patients treated with peritoneal dialysis had better improvement in their neuropathy than those treated with hemodialysis led to the middle molecule hypothesis.[153] According to this hypothesis, toxic molecules in the range of 500 to 2000 daltons are present in uremic plasma and are removed by peritoneal dialysis, but not hemodialysis. Middle molecules have been suggested to be responsible for many uremic abnormalities, including defective erythropoiesis, peripheral neuropathy, defective immune function, decreased cellular proliferation, defective transepithelial sodium transport, defective platelet function, and altered cellular energy production.[154, 155] The major stumbling block to the middle molecule hypothesis has been the technical difficulty in identifying the chemical nature of these compounds with certainty. Although they clearly exist and are toxic in biological systems, the clinical relevance of middle molecules remains to be proved.[155]

Trace elements also have been considered to play a role in the pathogenesis of uremia.[146, 156] Aluminum intoxication from water used in dialysis and from oral phosphorus binding agents (e.g., $AlOH_3$) may contribute to osteodystrophy, defective erythropoiesis, and dialysis encephalopathy.[157, 158] Zinc deficiency may play a role in defective cell-mediated immunity.

Parathyroid hormone (PTH) is probably the only compound that fulfills all criteria for a uremic toxin.[150] It is increased not as a result of the loss of excretory function, but as a result of the renal compensatory response to phosphorus retention. PTH has been shown to cause decreased motor nerve conduction and electroencephalographic abnormalities in uremic patients.[159] It is not clear whether this is due to a primary toxic effect of PTH or to the accumulation of calcium in the brain and peripheral nerves. In addition to its neurotoxicity, PTH has been shown to contribute to the anemia of renal failure by impairment of erythropoiesis[160] and to result in myocardial toxicity, presumably by increasing the calcium content of the myocardium.[150] The role of

TABLE 107–11. SOME COMPOUNDS THAT ACCUMULATE IN UREMIA

Urea	Oxalic acid
Creatinine	Acetoin
Methylguanidine	2,3-butylene glycol
Guanidinosuccinic acid	Lipochromes
Uric acid	Glucagon
Pyridine derivatives	Parathyroid hormone
Cyclic AMP	Natriuretic hormone
Amino acids	Growth hormone
Aliphatic amines	Gastrin
Aromatic amines	Renin
Polyamines	Beta-2 microglobulin
Indoles	Lysozyme
Phenols	Retinol-binding protein
Myoinositol	Beta-2 glucoprotein
Mannitol	Ribonuclease
Glucuronic acid	Sulfates
Ammonia	Phosphates
Lactate	Guanidine
Pyruvate	Creatine
Monoamine oxidase	Guanidinoacetic acid
Insulin	Cyanate
Hippurate	Middle molecules

Modified from Bergstrom J and Furst P: Uremic toxins. Kidney Int 13:(Suppl 8):S9, 1978.

PTH in renal osteodystrophy is considered further in the section on chronic renal failure.

Hemostatic Defects in Uremia

Uremia is characterized by abnormal hemostasis, and patients with acute and chronic renal failure are predisposed to hemorrhage.[161] In dogs and cats, gastrointestinal bleeding is most common. The major hemostatic abnormality in uremia is a qualitative defect in platelet function.[162] Platelet numbers are usually normal, and defective hemostasis in uremia is manifested by prolongation of the bleeding time. In fact, the risk of hemorrhage in uremic patients is most closely correlated with abnormal bleeding time. In uremic patients, hemostasis is best evaluated by determination of bleeding time, which indirectly allows evaluation of vascular contractility, platelet numbers, platelet function, and factor VIII complex function.

The abnormalities of platelet function in uremia include abnormal platelet aggregability, abnormal platelet factor 3 release, abnormal binding of fibrinogen to platelets, abnormal platelet adhesiveness, decreased clot retraction, and abnormal platelet prostanoid metabolism.[161, 162] In uremia, there is decreased thromboxane ($TXA2$) production by platelets, due to a functional defect in cyclooxygenase. Also, there is increased production of prostacyclin ($PGI2$) by vascular endothelium in uremic patients, which further impairs platelet function.

The ultimate cause of the platelet defect in uremia is not known, but a uremic toxin is suspected because the defect is often corrected by dialysis, and incubation of uremic platelets with normal plasma leads to correction of the defect. Urea is not thought to be of major importance in the pathogenesis of the hemostatic defect because the bleeding tendency is poorly correlated with the severity of azotemia. Although both guanidinosuccinic and phenolic acids in concentrations similar to those found in uremic plasma impair platelet function *in vitro*, there is no direct evidence of their clinical importance.[162] Other studies have focused on the effects of PTH or PTH fragments in stimulating cAMP and impairing platelet function, but the clinical importance of these observations also is uncertain.

The functional defect in platelet cyclooxygenase activity and the metabolic abnormality of the uremic vascular endothelium have recently received much attention. Also, the role of abnormalities in factor VIII complex and its interaction with platelets and the vascular endothelium have been studied.[163] Lastly, the anemia of renal failure aggravates the hemostatic defect by altering blood flow, which in turn allows less interaction of platelets with the vascular endothelium.[162]

The Anemia of Renal Failure

Anemia in renal failure is common, but variable in severity. Morphologically, it is normochromic, normocytic, and nonregenerative. Echinocytes may be seen in blood smears and are the result of membrane alterations in red cells.

The pathogenesis of anemia in renal failure is multifactorial.[164–166] The major factor is inadequate production of erythropoietin by the diseased kidneys such that the uremic patient cannot meet the demand for new red cells necessitated by loss from hemolysis and hemorrhage. That this is true is evidenced by the correction of anemia in human patients with end-stage renal disease, using recombinant human erythropoietin.[167]

The life span of red cells in uremic patients is reduced to approximately half that observed in healthy individuals. Normal red cells have reduced life span when transfused into uremic patients, and the red cells of uremic patients have a normal life span in normal individuals, suggesting that an extracorpuscular factor is responsible for the reduced life span.

Erythropoiesis in uremia may be further impaired by factors in uremic plasma. Spermine and ribonuclease have been considered to play roles, but most data suggest a role for PTH.[160] There is some evidence that PTH inhibits red cell precursor proliferation in the bone marrow, but this is controversial and has not been borne out in culture.[168] Other potential effects of PTH include induction of bone marrow fibrosis, increased osmotic fragility of red cells caused by increased influx of calcium ions, and aggravation of bleeding by impairment of platelet aggregation.[160]

A further reason for impaired erythropoiesis is that increased plasma phosphate concentrations lead to increased erythrocyte 2,3-diphosphoglycerate, which causes a decrease in hemoglobin affinity for oxygen and enhanced tissue delivery of oxygen.[169] Thus, there is less tissue hypoxia to stimulate erythropoiesis, and anemia is better tolerated by uremic patients. The bleeding tendency of uremia resulting from platelet dysfunction defects also leads to blood loss and may result in iron deficiency.

Membrane Transport Defects

Red cell Na^+/K^+ ATPase activity is decreased in uremia, resulting in increased intracellular sodium content and decreased cellular potential difference.[150, 170] Many uremic toxins and metabolic derangements of uremia have been considered to play a role in this defect and it is improved by dialysis. The clinical significance of these findings is unknown.

Neutrophil Function and Cell-Mediated Immunity

Infection is a common cause of death in uremic patients, and therefore inflammatory cell and immunologic functions have been evaluated.[164] Neutrophilic leukocytosis with hypersegmentation of neutrophils may be seen in uremia, regardless of the presence of infection. Chemotaxis is impaired, possibly by inhibition of chemotactic complement fragments by uremic toxins. The data on phagocytosis are controversial, and bactericidal activity of neutrophils is normal.

Cell-mediated immunity is impaired to a greater extent than humoral immunity, and immunoglobulin concentrations usually are normal in uremic patients. The cause of the apparent defect in cell-mediated immunity is unknown and is not corrected by dialysis. Several of the toxins of uremia have been shown to interfere with DNA synthesis and cellular proliferation, and these may be factors in the impairment of cellular immunity. Lymphopenia is commonly observed, and although it is often attributed to the stress of chronic disease, it apparently is not associated with corticosteroids.[171] The circulating numbers of both B and T lymphocytes are decreased.

Neurologic Complications

The two major neurologic complications of uremia in humans are uremic encephalopathy and neuropathy.[172, 173] Uremic encephalopathy is a metabolic encephalopathy characterized by slowing of the electroencephalogram (EEG), and usually does not develop until GFR is reduced to approximately ten per cent of normal. Its severity is related to the rate of development of renal failure, and it is more severe in acute than in chronic renal failure.

There is no evidence of cerebral edema or intracellular acidosis, and although decreased oxygen consumption and alterations in the activity of Na^+/K^+ ATPase have been demonstrated, there is no clear evidence that these derangements contribute to the encephalopathy. Likewise, the brain content of aluminum is increased in humans and dogs with renal failure, but the role of increased brain aluminum in the pathogenesis of uremic encephalopathy is unclear. Increased brain osmolality has been observed, and is caused almost entirely by urea in acute renal failure, while in chronic renal failure about half of the increase is due to urea and the remainder is due to idiogenic osmoles. Whether these changes are detrimental also is unclear.

Increased concentrations of PTH in renal failure may lead to increased transport of calcium into the brain and cause EEG changes. Thus PTH has received much attention in the pathogenesis of uremic encephalopathy.[159] Increased brain content of calcium and typical EEG changes also have been observed experimentally in dogs with renal failure.[174] Recently the possibility has been considered that derangements in the amino acid content of plasma and cerebrospinal fluid caused by malnutrition or uremic toxins could lead to alteration of neurotransmitters and contribute to uremic encephalopathy.[175]

Uremic encephalopathy is uncommon in dogs with chronic renal failure; in dogs with acute renal failure it is often difficult to distinguish such a syndrome from the clinical manifestations of the severe acid-base and electrolyte disturbances that develop. Likewise, the neurologic manifestations of ethylene glycol intoxication may mimic uremic encephalopathy. Uremic encephalopathy, however, was reported in three young dogs with renal failure.[176] These dogs displayed such signs as facial twitching, head bobbing, abnormal behavior, tremors, and seizures. In one dog typical EEG changes consisted of slowing and paroxysms of increased voltage spikes.

Uremic neuropathy is an insidious, distal, symmetrical, mixed polyneuropathy suggestive of a dying back neuropathy, and is indistinguishable from other metabolic neuropathies.[172] It develops over a long period (over six months), does not occur until GFR is below 10 per cent of normal, and may be present (as characterized by decreased motor nerve conduction velocity) despite normal physical examination. Several of these features may explain why this complication has not been detected clinically in dogs with renal failure.

Many toxins and abnormalities of the uremic state have been investigated in studying the pathogenesis of this abnormality, including urea, creatinine, myoinositol, middle molecules, methylguanidine, decreased transketolase activity, and PTH. Although PTH seems to play an important role in uremic encephalopathy, there is no good evidence that it plays a major role in uremic neuropathy. In dogs with experimentally induced chronic renal failure of six months' duration, there was no change in motor nerve conduction velocity and no increase in peripheral nerve calcium content.[174] In another study, however, decreased nerve conduction velocity and increased peripheral nerve calcium content were found in acutely uremic dogs.[177] It is more likely that the neuropathy of uremia is caused by anatomic nerve damage due to the cumulative effects of multiple toxins over a period of years.[172]

Gastrointestinal Complications

The most important gastrointestinal complications of uremia in the dog and cat are stomatitis and hemorrhagic gastroenteritis. The oral lesions consist of erosions and ulcers of the buccal mucosa and tongue (see Figure 107–1A and B). These may result from increased excretion of urea into the oral cavity, degradation of urea to ammonia by bacterial urease, and consequent damage to the mucosa. Occasionally, tongue-tip necrosis is observed in uremic dogs. This may result from fibrinoid necrosis and arteritis with focal ischemia, necrosis, and ulceration. Uremic gastropathy has recently been described.[178] Lesions included glandular atrophy, edema of the lamina propria, mast cell infiltration, fibroplasia, mineralization, and submucosal arteritis.

Factors that may be involved in the development of uremic gastroenteritis include uremic alterations in mucus that could allow back-diffusion of acid, bleeding caused by platelet dysfunction, erosions caused by ammonia liberated from urea by bacterial urease, ischemia caused by vascular lesions, and increased concentrations of gastrin. Gastrin is excreted by glomerular filtration, and increased plasma concentrations occur when GFR is markedly reduced. In three dogs with end-stage renal disease, plasma gastrin concentrations were found to be increased,[179] but in humans, the consequences of increased plasma gastrin concentrations in uremia are uncertain.[180]

Vomiting is a common clinical sign of uremia in dogs but is less common in uremic cats.[181] It is thought to be due to stimulation of the chemoreceptor trigger zone in the medulla by an as yet unidentified uremic toxin. Methylguanidine, a bacterial degradation product of creatinine, and urea have been considered as possible toxins in the pathogenesis of vomiting in uremia.

Cardiopulmonary Complications

In humans, the cardiovascular complications of uremia include accelerated atherogenesis owing to hypertension and alterations in the triglyceride content of lipoprotein fractions, uremic cardiomyopathy, and uremic pericarditis.[150] There is increased deposition of oxalates and calcium in the myocardium in uremia. The increased calcium content of the myocardium may be mediated by increased PTH concentration, and has been reported in dogs with experimental uremia, but uremia does not appear to be associated with clinical heart disease in the dog.[182]

Pericarditis is a well-recognized complication of uremia and dialysis in humans. Azotemia and overhydration are factors that may play roles in the pathogenesis of uremic pericarditis.[183] In dogs, however, this complication is rare. One dog with renal failure, ascites, pleural effusion, and pericardial effusion has been reported.[184] In a series of dogs with pericardial disease, however, only one was considered to have uremic pericarditis.[185]

Hypertension is an important complication of renal disease in humans, the dog, and the cat. The causes are multifactorial, and include renal ischemia with activation of the renin-angiotensin system, plasma volume expansion, and activation of the sympathetic nervous system.[186–188] Hypertension has been reported in surveys of dogs with acute and chronic renal disease.[189, 190] It has been reported to occur in 60 per cent of all dogs with renal disease and in 80 per cent of those with glomerular disease.[5] These figures agree with those obtained in another study wherein 75 per cent of dogs with renal disease were reported to have hypertension.[191] Left ventricular hypertrophy and proliferation of the tunica media of vessels are observed at necropsy in dogs and cats with chronic renal disease and are suggestive of long-standing hypertension.[192] Calcification of the tunica media of vessels also may be observed.

The pulmonary complications of uremia include lesions ranging from mild pulmonary edema to a clinical disorder called uremic pneumonitis, which resembles adult respiratory distress syndrome. Pulmonary calcification also may lead to decreased pulmonary compliance and chronic obstructive pulmonary disease. These abnormalities have been described infrequently in dogs and cats with uremia. Recently, however, there has been a report of pulmonary complications in dogs with end-stage renal disease.[193] Some affected dogs had severe dyspnea and alveolar pulmonary infiltrates radiographically, while others had no clinical signs. Histologically, the lesions consisted of congestion of alveolar capillaries, variably thickened alveolar septa, moderate mononuclear infiltration, and fibrin-rich alveolar edema fluid.

Metabolic and Endocrine Complications

Many small polypeptides are normally filtered by the kidney, reabsorbed, and then degraded in the proximal tubular cells. Thus the kidney is responsible for the clearance of several important peptide hormones, and loss of this catabolic function can result in metabolic derangements caused by hormone excess.

Uremia is associated with peripheral insulin resistance and mild fasting hyperglycemia.[170, 194] Serum insulin concentrations are increased in response to peripheral insulin resistance and decreased clearance of insulin by the kidney. In some uremic patients there is also defective insulin secretion.[195] When GFR decreases to 10 to 20 per cent of normal, the metabolic clearance of insulin is decreased. A toxin of uremia may be present that contributes to decreased hepatic degradation of insulin. Deranged insulin metabolism may contribute to hyperlipemia in uremia. Increased plasma insulin concentrations may cause increased very low density lipoprotein (VLDL) synthesis by the liver, and adverse effects of insulin resistance on lipoprotein lipase (LPL) function may decrease clearance of triglycerides from the blood.

The kidney is the main site of glucagon catabolism, and in uremia there are increased plasma concentrations of glucagon and its prohormone that result from decreased metabolic clearance of these peptides. Increased glucagon concentrations may result in increased hepatic gluconeogenesis using alanine from muscle as substrate. This metabolic derangement may contribute to negative nitrogen balance and tissue catabolism in uremia. Other polypeptide hormones that may be increased in the plasma of uremic patients as a result of decreased metabolic clearance are growth hormone, prolactin, and luteinizing hormone.

Serum thyroxine (T_4) concentrations are normal or slightly low in uremia, but triiodothyronine (T_3) concentrations are decreased, owing to impairment of peripheral conversion of T_4 to T_3.[196] Cortisol and adrenocorticotropin concentrations in uremia are normal or slightly increased.

SPECIFIC RENAL SYNDROMES

Chronic Renal Failure

PATHOPHYSIOLOGY

As Homer Smith pointed out,[197] the kidneys are often thought of in terms of their final product, but it is more instructive to think of them in relation to their critical role in the control of extracellular fluid volume and composition. The pathophysiologic changes that occur during the course of progressive renal disease can be considered in light of three specific categories of renal function: excretory, regulatory, and endocrine.

Loss of excretory function leads to retention of solutes handled by glomerular filtration, such as urea and creatinine. Derangements in regulatory function result in the characteristic compensatory adaptations of the diseased kidney and, ultimately, in the disturbances in water, electrolyte, and acid-base balance, which complicate terminal uremia. Loss of endocrine or synthetic function results in deficient production of erythropoietin and contributes to the anemia of renal failure. Likewise, decreased hydroxylation of 25-hydroxycholecalciferol leads to decreased production of 1,25-dihydroxychole-calciferol (calcitriol or 1,25-dihydroxyvitamin D_3), and results in malabsorption of calcium by the gut, impaired effectiveness of PTH on bone, and aggravation of renal secondary hyperparathyroidism. Loss of metabolic functions such as degradation of polypeptides by proximal tubular cells leads to increased plasma concentrations of hormones such as gastrin, insulin, and glucagon and may contribute further to the endocrine disturbances of uremia.

Intact Nephron Hypothesis. The intact nephron hypothesis states that, even in the presence of a heterogeneity of morphologic changes in the nephrons of diseased kidneys, there is relative homogeneity of glomerulotubular balance.[198] That is, in damaged nephrons with decreased single-nephron GFR (SNGFR) there is a proportionate decrease in tubular reabsorptive rate, while in hypertrophied nephrons with increased SNGFR there is a proportionate increase in tubular reabsorptive rate. These changes may be mediated in part by alterations in postglomerular Starling forces.

Mechanisms of Adaptation in Residual Nephrons. Three major patterns of nephron adaptation occur in progressive renal disease.[199] A given solute may be classified as having *no regulation*, *regulation with limitation*, or *complete regulation*. These patterns are depicted in Figure 107–10. Solutes that are excreted by glomerular filtration follow the pattern of *no regulation* and are exemplified by urea and creatinine. Each 50 per cent decrement in GFR results in a doubling of the serum concentration of such solutes. As expected, the curve labeled no regulation is identical to a plot of BUN or S_{cr} against GFR (see Figure 107–2).

Solutes that experience *limited regulation* are handled by glomerular filtration and some combination of tubular reabsorption and secretion. Solutes regulated in this manner include urate and phosphate, and the adaptation of acid-base regulation during progressive renal disease also can be considered to fall into this category. In the case of phosphate, limited regulation is accomplished by a progressive decrease in the fractional reabsorption

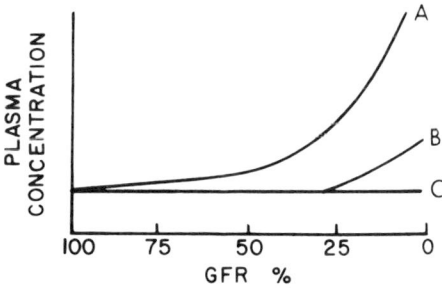

FIGURE 107–10. Renal regulation of solute balance. See text for explanation. (From Bricker NS and Fine LG: The renal response to progressive nephron loss. *In* Brenner BM and Rector FC: The Kidney, 2nd ed. Philadelphia, WB Saunders, 1981, p 1058.)

of filtered phosphate as GFR decreases in the face of constant phosphate intake. This adaptation is the result of progressive increases in the serum PTH concentration and results in the development of renal secondary hyperparathyroidism (Figure 107–11).

Solutes such as sodium and potassium are handled by glomerular filtration, tubular reabsorption, and tubular secretion, and experience *complete regulation*. Normal serum concentrations of sodium and potassium can be maintained even when GFR has decreased to less than five per cent of normal.[200] Despite the increasing fractional excretion of water that occurs as renal disease progresses, normal hydration is maintained by an intact thirst mechanism. Dehydration may develop rapidly, however, if an animal with chronic renal failure is denied access to water.

Sodium balance is maintained in chronic renal disease by a progressive increase in the fractional excretion of sodium by the kidneys.[201, 202] Even before the biochemical characterization of atrial natriuretic peptide (ANP), it was realized that increasing concentrations of such a substance could explain this effect.[203, 204] The biochemistry and physiologic effects of ANP have recently been elucidated and increased plasma concentrations have been found in patients with chronic renal failure.[205–207]

Although sodium balance can be maintained at a very

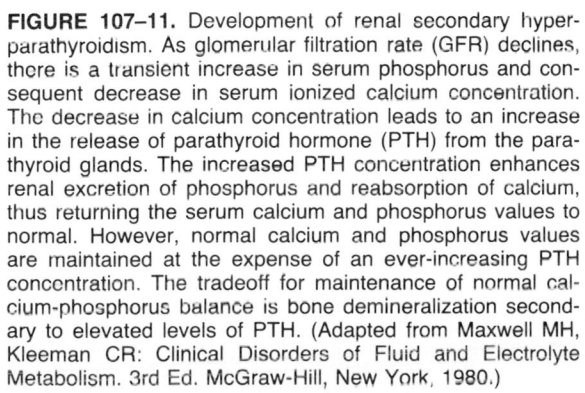

FIGURE 107–11. Development of renal secondary hyperparathyroidism. As glomerular filtration rate (GFR) declines, there is a transient increase in serum phosphorus and consequent decrease in serum ionized calcium concentration. The decrease in calcium concentration leads to an increase in the release of parathyroid hormone (PTH) from the parathyroid glands. The increased PTH concentration enhances renal excretion of phosphorus and reabsorption of calcium, thus returning the serum calcium and phosphorus values to normal. However, normal calcium and phosphorus values are maintained at the expense of an ever-increasing PTH concentration. The tradeoff for maintenance of normal calcium-phosphorus balance is bone demineralization secondary to elevated levels of PTH. (Adapted from Maxwell MH, Kleeman CR: Clinical Disorders of Fluid and Electrolyte Metabolism. 3rd Ed. McGraw-Hill, New York, 1980.)

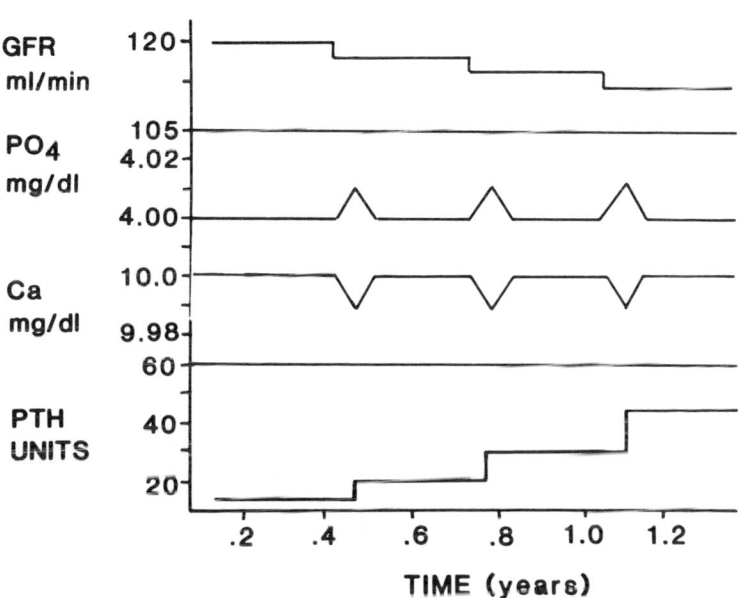

low GFR, patients with chronic renal failure are much less flexible in their response to changes in sodium intake and take longer to reestablish balance after an abrupt change in sodium intake.[202, 208] This may be the result of increased concentrations of ANP and the prevailing high rate of sodium excretion in remnant nephrons. The increased fractional excretion of sodium in progressive renal disease can be prevented experimentally by proportional reduction in sodium intake (Table 107–12).[209]

Similarly, serum potassium is maintained by a progressive increase in the fraction of filtered potassium that is excreted, and this is accomplished by increased tubular secretion of potassium in remnant nephrons. The increased fractional excretion of potassium in experimental renal disease also can be prevented by proportional reduction in potassium intake.[210]

The Trade-off Hypothesis. The "trade-off" hypothesis suggests that the biological price to be paid for maintaining external balance for a given solute as renal disease progresses is the induction of one or more of the abnormalities of the uremic state.[211, 212] In the case of phosphorus, the price paid for the maintenance of normal serum concentrations of calcium and phosphate is renal osteodystrophy. Thus in the increased concentrations that occur in advanced renal disease, regulatory hormones may be revealed to be uremic toxins.

Polyuria/Polydipsia and Defective Urinary Concentrating Ability. The patient in chronic renal failure maintains water balance by a progressive increase in the fraction of filtered water excreted as GFR declines with time. Diseased nephrons filter less and residual functional nephrons must filter more plasma and thus operate under conditions of osmotic diuresis. The high flow rate of fluid in these remnant nephrons is the major contributing factor to polyuria and defective concentrating ability in progressive renal disease and leads to restriction of the maximal urine osmolality that can be achieved.[199, 200] The origin of osmotic diuresis in remnant nephrons is demonstrated in Table 107–13.

TABLE 107–12. EFFECT OF NORMAL SODIUM INTAKE COMPARED TO PROPORTIONAL REDUCTION OF SODIUM INTAKE ON RENAL EXCRETION OF SODIUM DURING PROGRESSIVE DECLINE IN GLOMERULAR FILTRATION RATE

Normal Sodium Intake			
GFR (ml/min)	100	70	30
Na intake (mEq/day)	144	144	144
Serum Na (mEq/L)	140	140	140
Filtered Na (mEq/min)	14	9.8	4.2
Na excreted (mEq/day)	144	144	144
Na excreted (mEq/min)	0.1	0.1	0.1
Fraction filtered reabsorbed (%)	99.3	99.0	97.6
Fraction filtered excreted (%)	0.7	1.0	2.4
Proportional Reduction in Sodium Intake			
GFR (ml/min)	100	70	30
Na intake (mEq/day)	144	101	43
Serum Na (mEq/L)	140	140	140
Filtered Na (mEq/min)	14	9.8	4.2
Na excreted (mEq/day)	144	101	43
Na excreted (mEq/min)	0.1	0.07	0.03
Fraction filtered reabsorbed (%)	99.3	99.3	99.3
Fraction filtered excreted (%)	0.7	0.7	0.7

A state of balance is assumed.
Adapted from references 200 and 208.

TABLE 107–13. DEMONSTRATION OF OSMOTIC DIURESIS IN REMNANT NEPHRONS AND DEVELOPMENT OF POLYURIA IN CHRONIC RENAL FAILURE

In this example, the following assumptions are made:

1. 25 kg dog (0.85 square meters)
2. Normal GFR = 60 ml/min/square meter
3. Normal urine output = 33 ml/kg/day
4. Normal urine osmolality = 1000 mOsm/kg
5. Normal daily solute load for 25 kg dog = 825 mOsm
6. 75% loss of nephrons caused by progressive disease
7. Urine osmolality in presence of this amount of renal disease = 500 mOsm/kg
8. Urine output with this amount of renal disease and same daily solute load = 825 mOsm/500 mOsm/kg = 1650 ml = 66 ml/kg/day
9. Compensatory hypertrophy will increase GFR in diseased kidneys by 50% above that expected by loss of nephrons alone

	Normal	Diseased
Total no. nephrons	1,000,000	250,000
GFR (ml/min)	50	20
SNGFR (nl/min)	50	80
Urine output (ml/kg/day)	33	66
Urine output (ml/min)	0.6	1.1
Urine output/nephron (nl/min)	0.6	4.4
% filtered water absorbed	98.8%	94.5%
% filtered water excreted	1.2%	5.5%

The pathophysiology of defective concentrating ability in chronic renal failure is more complex, however, and other factors are likely to be involved.[112, 213] Anatomic alterations in the renal medulla caused by disease and a compensatory increase in medullary blood flow may diminish the magnitude of the potential osmotic gradient between collecting duct fluid and the medullary interstitium.[214] Impaired transport of sodium and chloride in the ascending limb of the loop of Henle in uremia may result from high concentrations of ANP and further limit concentrating capacity. Finally, decreased responsiveness of the collecting duct to the effects of ADH has been observed in uremia.[213, 215] The latter defect would allow diluting ability to remain relatively intact, and patients with chronic renal failure do maintain diluting ability as evaluated by free water clearance. Nonetheless, they typically excrete urine that is relatively isosmotic with plasma, presumably as a result of osmotic diuresis in residual functional nephrons. Isosthenuria usually is detected in chronic renal failure after approximately 67 per cent of the nephrons have become nonfunctional.

Regulation of Acid-Base Balance. The role of the kidney in regulation of acid-base balance entails reabsorption of bicarbonate, excretion of titratable acid (mainly phosphate), and ammonium ion excretion. Secretion of hydrogen ions that titrate filtered bicarbonate achieves reclamation of filtered bicarbonate but does not contribute to net acid excretion and generation of new bicarbonate. These latter processes result from the excretion of titratable acidity and ammonium ions.

In chronic renal failure the compensatory adaptation in acid-base balance can be considered as *regulation with limitation*.[199] The fractional reabsorption of bicarbonate is increased in dogs with experimentally induced renal disease despite increases in the fractional excretion of sodium and phosphate.[216–219] Arterial pH, serum bicarbonate, and PCO_2 are normal until GFR is decreased to approximately 20 per cent of normal, at which time serum bicarbonate concentration decreases and metabolic acidosis with respiratory compensation becomes evident.[200] The metabolic acidosis is not usually progressive, despite the development of a positive hydrogen ion balance, probably because of the chronic buffering effect of calcium carbonate released from bone.[220] In fact, compensation may remain adequate even when GFR is reduced to five per cent of normal.[199] Such patients, however, are in a precarious state of balance that may be easily disrupted by concurrent disease states (e.g., diarrhea). This effect represents another trade-off in that acid-base balance is maintained at the expense of bone demineralization.

The metabolic acidosis of chronic renal failure may be hyperchloremic (normal anion gap) or normochloremic (increased anion gap) if acid metabolites that titrate bicarbonate have accumulated as unmeasured anions (e.g., phosphate, sulfate).[221] Effects of the metabolic acidosis that are adaptive for the affected individual are preservation of serum ionized calcium concentration through the effects of acidosis on the charge of plasma proteins and shifting of the hemoglobin-oxygen saturation curve to the right, thus improving tissue delivery of oxygen and partially compensating for the anemia of chronic renal failure. The main cause of metabolic acidosis in progressive renal disease is a decrease in net acid excretion by the kidneys.[222] There is an adaptive increase in ammonia secretion by residual functional nephrons, but eventually these nephrons fail to keep pace with the continued destruction of nephrons caused by the presence of progressive renal disease, and net acid excretion declines. This occurs despite the fact that residual nephrons have the capacity to increase their rate of acid excretion by a factor of 4 to 8 by means of increased ammonia production from glutamine.[221]

Renal Secondary Hyperparathyroidism and Osteodystrophy.
Normal calcium and phosphorus homeostasis is maintained by the actions of three hormones (PTH, calcitriol, and calcitonin) on three body organs (kidney, gut, and bone).[223] The kidney plays a central role in these processes because it is the major source of 1-α-hydroxylase, the enzyme that converts 25-hydroxycholecalciferol to the active form of vitamin D_3, 1,25-dihydroxycholecalciferol (calcitriol), and an important site of metabolism and excretion of PTH.

The major effects of calcitriol are increased intestinal absorption of calcium, which is mediated by increased production of calcium-binding protein; a permissive effect on bone resorption in conjunction with PTH; and negative feedback control on the secretion of PTH by the parathyroid glands. The major stimulus for PTH release is decreased serum calcium concentration, and its primary effects are on the kidney and bone. In the kidney, PTH decreases proximal and distal tubular reabsorption of phosphate, resulting in an increase in the fractional excretion of phosphorus. It decreases proximal reabsorption of calcium and sodium while it increases distal reabsorption of calcium, so that there is a net decrease in the fractional excretion of calcium. The effects of PTH on bone result in bone remodeling and

resorption of calcium and phosphate. Calcitonin appears to play a relatively minor role in calcium and phosphorus homeostasis. It is released in response to increased serum calcium concentration and limits the tendency toward hypercalcemia caused by PTH release. Calcitonin acts by limiting osteoclastic bone resorption and by promoting urinary excretion of calcium and phosphorus.

The term renal osteodystrophy includes all skeletal disorders that may occur in renal failure.[223] Its diverse histologic features have become apparent in human patients whose lives have been prolonged by dialysis and transplantation. In fact, aluminum present in dialysate water has recently been shown to make an important contribution to bone disease in uremic patients. The shorter survival time of dogs and cats with renal failure is likely to limit the clinical detection of renal osteodystrophy in these species.

Renal secondary hyperparathyroidism is one of the earliest and most consistent findings in patients with progressive renal disease, and its development is directly related to decreased serum calcium concentration.[223, 224] The pathogenesis of relative hypocalcemia in renal failure is complex. Phosphorus retention results from declining GFR, and as a result of the mass law effect, there is a transient decrease in serum calcium concentration. This results in stimulation of the parathyroid glands to secrete PTH, thus returning serum phosphorus and calcium concentrations to normal through the effects of PTH on the kidney and bone. Thus calcium and phosphorus homeostasis is maintained by ever-increasing serum concentrations of PTH (see Figure 107–11). When GFR decreases to approximately 20 per cent of normal, this compensatory mechanism is exceeded and hyperphosphatemia develops. It has been shown that this pathophysiologic course of events can be prevented in dogs by proportionate reduction in the dietary intake in phosphorus as GFR decreases (Table 107–14).[225–227]

Altered vitamin D metabolism in renal failure also contributes to hypocalcemia and hyperparathyroidism. As GFR declines, reduced serum calcitriol concentrations occur as a result of inadequate renal hydroxylation of 25-hydroxycholecalciferol. The relative lack of calcitriol leads to impaired absorption of calcium from the gut and impairs the mobilization of calcium from bone in response to PTH.[228] Lastly, decreased calcitriol concentration results in decreased negative feedback to the parathyroid glands. All of these events further increase PTH secretion and aggravate secondary hyperparathyroidism. Decreased numbers and affinity of parathyroid gland receptors for calcitriol have recently been observed in patients with renal failure, and this deficiency further impairs negative feedback by calcitriol.[229, 230]

Other factors that may contribute to hyperparathyroidism are decreased degradation of PTH by the diseased kidney and an increase in the set point for response of the parathyroid glands to calcium. Alterations in the set point may result from the increased tissue mass of the hyperplastic parathyroid glands.[231] Thus a higher serum calcium concentration is required to shut off PTH secretion at a time when less calcium is available.

The increase in circulating PTH leads to bone demin-

TABLE 107–14. EFFECT OF NORMAL PHOSPHORUS INTAKE COMPARED TO PROPORTIONAL REDUCTION OF PHOSPHORUS INTAKE ON RENAL EXCRETION OF PHOSPHORUS DURING PROGRESSIVE DECLINE IN GLOMERULAR FILTRATION RATE

Normal Phosphorus Intake			
GFR (L/day)	180	130	90
Phosphorus intake (mmol/day)	20	20	20
Plasma phosphorus (mmol/L)	1.2	1.2	1.2
Filtered phosphorus (mmol/day)	216	156	108
Phosphorus reabsorbed (mmol/day)	196	136	88
Phosphorus excreted (mmol/day)	20	20	20
Fraction filtered reabsorbed (%)	91	87	82
Fraction filtered excreted (%)	9	13	18
Plasma PTH	Normal	Increased	Very Increased
Proportional Reduction in Phosphorus Intake			
GFR (L/day)	180	130	90
Phosphorus intake (mmol/day)	20	14	9.7
Plasma phosphorus (mmol/L)	1.2	1.2	1.2
Filtered phosphorus (mmol/day)	216	156	108
Phosphorus reabsorbed (mmol/day)	196	142	98.3
Phosphorus excreted (mmol/day)	20	14	9.7
Fraction filtered reabsorbed (%)	91	91	91
Fraction filtered excreted (%)	9	9	9
Plasma PTH	Normal	Normal	Normal

A state of balance is assumed.
Adapted from references 200 and 225.

eralization, which may be viewed as one of the trade-offs of progressive renal disease. In this instance, bone demineralization is the biologic price paid for maintenance of normal calcium and phosphorus homeostasis. Aluminum also may contribute to defective bone mineralization, and although the main source of aluminum in human patients is probably dialysate water, there is evidence that absorption of aluminum may occur after ingestion of binding gels such as $AlOH_3$.[232, 233] Because the kidney is the only organ that removes aluminum from the body, ingestion may represent another source of aluminum intoxication. Metabolic acidosis may contribute to bone demineralization in that bone carbonate may be a substantial source of buffer over long periods of time. This prevention of progressive systemic acidosis by release of calcium carbonate from bone may be viewed as another trade-off in uremia. The lack of calcitriol may aggravate bone mineralization further through lack of its beneficial effect in preparing bone collagen for mineralization.

Rarely, hypercalcemia is observed in renal failure patients.[234] Many factors may be operative in the pathogenesis of hypercalcemia. The increased set point for PTH suppression in hyperplastic parathyroid glands and autonomous hypersecretion of PTH by massively hyperplastic glands may be important factors. Increased complexed calcium, such as that bound to citrate, may be present in renal failure; there may be decreased degradation of PTH by the diseased kidney; and insufficient amounts of calcium may be excreted at very low GFR. Lastly, treatment with vitamin D compounds may cause hypercalcemia.

Progression of Renal Disease. Chronic renal disease typically progresses to end-stage renal disease after a critical number of nephrons have been damaged. In human patients, progression to end-stage renal disease usually occurs when GFR falls below 25 ml/min.[235–237] This progression occurs even when aggravating factors such as systemic hypertension and infection are controlled. The progression of chronic renal disease may be monitored in humans and dogs by plotting the reciprocal of the S_{cr} against time.[238–240] Typically, a linear decrease in this parameter is observed over time, and the slope is more dependent on the individual than on the underlying disease.

When renal mass is decreased by disease or experimental ablation, the decrease in total GFR is blunted by an increase in SNGFR in surviving nephrons. For example, after unilateral nephrectomy, GFR in the remaining kidney increases by approximately 40 per cent within two to four weeks so that GFR declines only to 70 per cent of the prenephrectomy value rather than to 50 per cent.[236] The beneficial effect of this adaptation is preservation of GFR, but there is evidence that this response ultimately is maladaptive.

The increase in SNGFR is mediated hemodynamically by afferent and efferent arteriolar vasodilatation. The afferent arteriole dilates more than the efferent arteriole, resulting in increased glomerular capillary plasma flow and increased transcapillary hydraulic pressure (Figure 107–12). These changes lead to the observed increase in SNGFR.[241] The magnitude of change is proportional to the amount of renal tissue that has been destroyed. In the diseased kidney there is a wide distribution of SNGFR values such that nephrons that are severely damaged and not working have subnormal values, while functional ones have supranormal values. Glomerulotubular balance is maintained in hyperfiltering glomeruli by increased tubular reabsorption presumably owing to changes in postglomerular Starling forces.[242]

There is evidence, however, that these physiologic changes ultimately lead to adverse functional and morphologic changes in remnant glomeruli,[241, 243] which may represent the final common pathway of renal parenchymal destruction in progressive renal disease, regardless

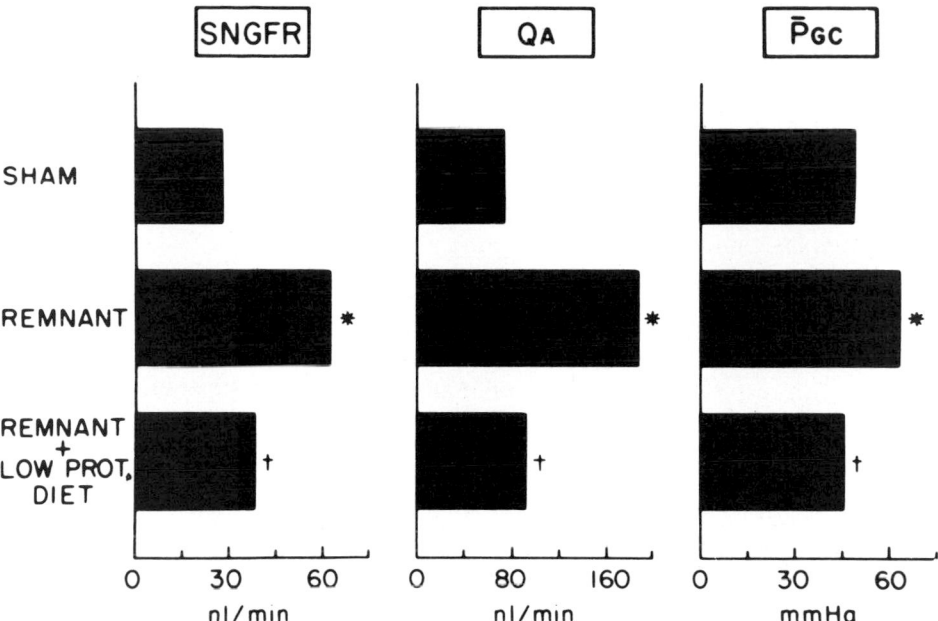

FIGURE 107–12. Roles of glomerular capillary flow and transcapillary hydrostatic pressure in the development of glomerular hyperfiltration. Average increases in SNGFR, Q_A, and P_{GC} in remnant glomeruli of rats undergoing 90 per cent nephrectomy 7 days previously *(middle row)* relative to values in sham-operated control rats *(top row)* and 90 per cent nephrectomy rats fed low (6 per cent) protein chow *(bottom row)*. Animals in top and middle rows were fed 24 per cent protein diets. (From Brenner BM: Nephron adaptation to renal injury or ablation. Am J Physiol 241:F324, 1985.)

of the initiating insult. Remnant glomeruli are less charge and size selective than normal glomeruli, and proteinuria develops.[243] Increased transglomerular movement of plasma proteins provokes ultrastructural changes in the remnant glomeruli that consist of detachment of endothelial and epithelial cells from the basement membrane and a progressive increase in mesangial matrix and cellularity.[243] These ultrastructural changes ultimately lead to glomerular sclerosis. This course of events can be considered another trade-off in that the price to be paid for minimizing the decline in total GFR is the ultimate sclerosis and failure of hyperfiltering glomeruli.

Restriction of dietary protein leads to abrogation of these adaptive functional responses and prevents the development of their morphologic counterparts (Figure 107–12).[241, 243, 244] It is unknown how decreased protein intake prevents these alterations in glomerular function, but a hormonal effect is suspected.[235, 242, 245] A recent study suggests that these hemodynamic changes are not due to growth hormone, but may be due to glucagon.[246] It has been hypothesized that glomerular hyperfiltration represents a normal response of the kidney to the protein challenge characteristic of intermittent feeding.[242, 245] The change in feeding from an intermittent to continuous pattern as has occurred with the civilization of humans and the domestication of animals may necessitate such hemodynamic changes on a regular basis. Such feeding patterns may contribute to the observed age-related decline in GFR and appearance of glomerular sclerosis in humans. The effects of dietary protein on glomerular hemodynamics have important consequences for the treatment of chronic renal disease as well.

It has been clearly shown that progressive glomerular sclerosis occurs in rats after renal ablation when rats are fed high-protein diets,[243, 247] but there has been debate about its occurrence in other species. Significant morphologic changes and progression were not observed in dogs with 75 per cent nephrectomy fed 19 per cent, 27

per cent, and 56 per cent protein and followed for four years, but there was a tendency for morphologic changes to be greatest in dogs fed the highest protein diet.[248, 249] In another study, dogs with experimentally induced renal failure were fed 8 per cent, 17 per cent, or 44 per cent protein diets. Mortality and urine protein excretion were highest in the dogs fed 44 per cent protein, but inulin clearance, although markedly reduced, remained stable in all three groups of dogs over a period of 40 weeks.[250] In a recent study, dogs with 87 per cent nephrectomy fed 26 per cent protein were studied for approximately three years, and there was evidence of proteinuria, mesangial hyperplasia, focal glomerular sclerosis, and, in some dogs, progressive decline in GFR.[251]

The role of dietary phosphorus in the progression of chronic renal disease also has been studied. Phosphorus restriction may prevent the progression of renal disease by blunting renal secondary hyperparathyroidism and preventing renal interstitial mineralization. In rats with experimentally induced chronic renal failure, detrimental histologic changes, such as interstitial mineralization, inflammation, and fibrosis, could be prevented and residual renal function maintained by restriction of dietary phosphorus.[252, 253] In cats with experimentally induced renal disease, histologic changes, but not functional changes, could be prevented by phosphorus restriction.[254] Rats fed a low-phosphorus diet, however, consume less food than controls, and it has been considered that reduced protein or caloric intake could have been responsible for the observed beneficial effect rather than decreased phosphorus intake.[255] In a recent study in rats with 80 per cent nephrectomy, diet was carefully controlled so that only phosphorus intake differed between groups and a beneficial effect of phosphorus restriction was clearly demonstrated with regard to mortality, proteinuria, histologic changes, creatinine clearance, and serum lipid concentrations over a period of 14 weeks.[256] Similar beneficial effects were observed in dogs with 90 per cent nephrectomy fed diets differing only in phosphorus content and followed for 12 months.[257] These recent studies reaffirm the original findings that phosphate restriction is beneficial in modifying the progression of renal disease.

DIAGNOSIS

Laboratory and Radiographic Evaluation. Blood and urine samples should be collected before fluid therapy to avoid later difficulty in interpretation of renal function data. Abnormal laboratory findings in chronic renal failure consist of normochromic, normocytic anemia, lymphopenia, azotemia, hyperphosphatemia, metabolic acidosis with respiratory compensation, and mild hyperglycemia. Serum calcium concentration may be slightly low, normal, or, occasionally, increased. Isosthenuria is typically observed on urinalysis, and the sediment should be evaluated for clues to any specific underlying renal disease (e.g., proteinuria in glomerular disease, pyuria or leukocyte casts and bacteriuria in pyelonephritis). Plain abdominal radiographs should be taken to evaluate kidney size.

Differentiation of Acute from Chronic Renal Failure

Differentiation of acute from chronic renal failure is based on evaluation of renal size, the presence or absence of polyuria and polydipsia, and the presence or absence of anemia. The presence of small kidneys and anemia in a patient with a long history of polyuria and polydipsia is strongly suggestive of chronic renal failure. Patients with acute renal failure are more frequently oliguric, hyperkalemic, and hypothermic, but these criteria are much less reliable because they may occur in terminal chronic renal failure, and dogs with acute renal failure may be polyuric. In some cases a renal biopsy will be required to establish the diagnosis (see Table 107–10 and Figure 107–13). Diseases associated with chronic renal failure in the dog and cat are listed in Table 107–15.

Acute Renal Failure

Acute renal failure (ARF) is characterized by an abrupt decline in renal function of sufficient magnitude to result in azotemia and inability to regulate solute and water balance.[258-265] ARF can be divided into prerenal, postrenal, and intrinsic renal failure (AIRF) categories, but the term acute renal failure is used most often to describe AIRF.[264] AIRF may occur in kidneys that were normal before insult, or in those with preexisting chronic renal disease. It should be noted that recent recognition of azotemia is not necessarily the same as recent onset of azotemia. Previous serum biochemistry values often are not available for comparison, and chronic renal failure may suddenly become symptomatic. Postrenal azotemia is discussed in Chapters 108 and 112 and in Characterization of Azotemia earlier in this chapter. Prerenal azotemia has been previously discussed in the diagnostic portion of this chapter but will be considered further in this section, since it often coexists with AIRF and the causes of ischemic AIRF are often extensions of those processes that cause prerenal azotemia.

AIRF can be caused by a wide variety of factors, including tubulointerstitial nephritis (Table 107–16), glomerular and vascular disease (Table 107–17), nephrotoxins (Table 107–18), and renal ischemia (Table 107–19). The definition of AIRF previously included oliguria as a necessary diagnostic finding, but more recently nonoliguric AIRF has assumed predominance in humans.[266-268] The frequency of nonoliguric AIRF is prob-

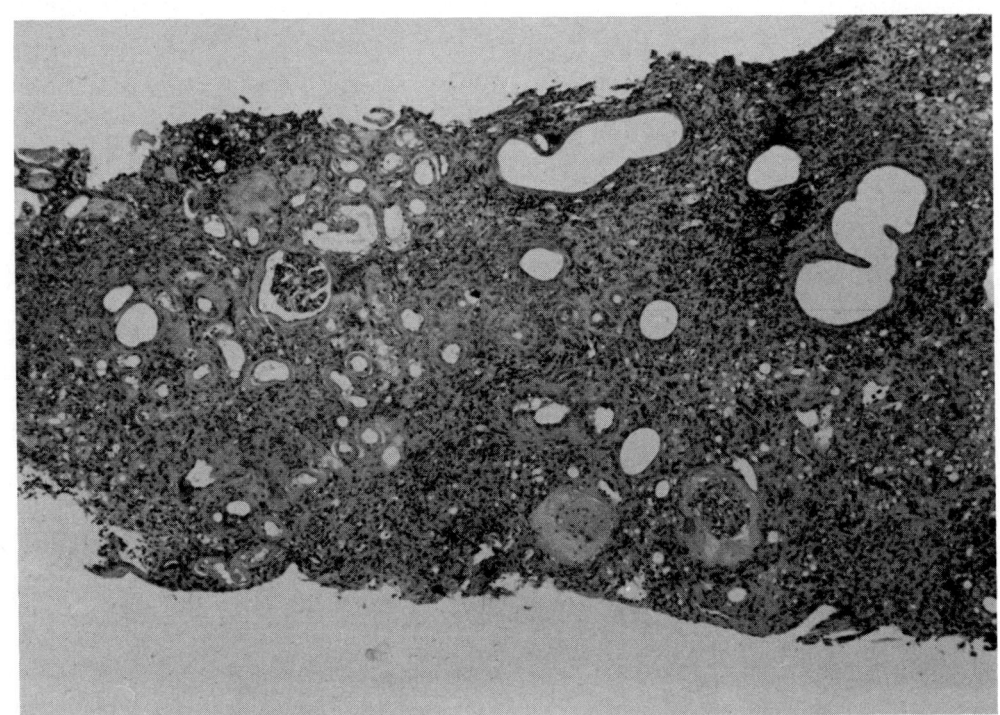

FIGURE 107–13. Routine low-power microscopic view of the lesions of end-stage renal disease in renal biopsy from a cat, showing interstitial fibrosis, tubular atrophy, tubular dilatation, and glomerular sclerosis.

TABLE 107–15. DISEASES ASSOCIATED WITH CHRONIC RENAL FAILURE IN THE DOG AND CAT

Causes of CRF in the Dog

I. Pyelonephritis
II. Chronic interstitial nephritis of unknown cause
III. Polycystic kidneys
IV. Familial renal disease
   A. Norwegian elkhound
   B. Lhasa apso
   C. Shih Tzu
   D. Samoyed
   E. Cocker spaniel
   F. Doberman pinscher
   G. Standard poodle
   H. Soft-coated Wheaton terrier
V. Amyloidosis
VI. Glomerulonephritis
VII. Leptospirosis
VIII. Healing of acute renal failure (ARF) by interstitial fibrosis
   A. Chemotherapeutic agents (e.g., aminoglycosides)
   B. Heavy metals (e.g., thiacetarsamide)
   C. Organic solvents (e.g., ethylene glycol)
IX. Hypercalcemia
X. Bilateral hydronephrosis

Causes of CRF in the Cat

I. Pyelonephritis
II. Chronic interstitial nephritis of unknown cause
III. Polycystic kidneys
   A. Congenital
   B. Acquired
IV. Amyloidosis
   A. Occurs sporadically in all breeds of cat
   B. Occurs as a familial disease in the Abyssinian cat
V. Glomerulonephritis
VI. Renal vascular disease (e.g., polyarteritis nodosa)
VII. Nephrotoxins
   A. Chemotherapeutic agents
   B. Heavy metals
   C. Organic solvents
VIII. Hypercalcemia
   A. Rare in cats
   B. May accompany lymphosarcoma
IX. Bilateral hydronephrosis
X. Renal lymphosarcoma
XI. Pyogranulomatous nephritis due to feline infectious peritonitis

From Chew DJ and DiBartola SP: Manual of Small Animal Nephrology and Urology. New York, Churchill Livingstone, 1986, pp 88–89.

ably underestimated in human and veterinary medicine.[267] The actual frequency of AIRF in small animals is unknown, and the relative proportions of oliguric or nonoliguric AIRF are, likewise, not documented. AIRF occurs, however, far less frequently in dogs and cats than does chronic renal failure. The tubulointerstitial disorders listed in Table 107–16 and the glomerular and

TABLE 107–16. AIRF ASSOCIATED WITH TUBULOINTERSTITIAL NEPHRITIS

Bacterial pyelonephritis
Embolic nephritis (septic or nonseptic)
Leptospirosis
Drug-induced (allergic)
   methicillin, cimetidine, penicillamine, others sporadically
Herpes canis
Papillary necrosis (also with chronic renal disease)
   Basenji dog with Fanconi syndrome
   Medullary renal amyloid (cats)
   Upper urinary tract infection
   Diabetes mellitus
Rejection of renal transplant

TABLE 107–17. AIRF ASSOCIATED WITH GLOMERULAR AND VASCULAR DISEASE

Acute glomerulonephritis
Vasculitis
Disseminated intravascular coagulation
Malignant hypertension/glomerulosclerosis
Bilateral renal vein obstruction
   Thrombosis
   Compression
Bilateral renal artery obstruction
   Thrombosis
   Embolization
   Vasculitis
   Atherosclerosis (hypothyroidism)

vascular disorders listed in Table 107–17 are uncommon causes of AIRF in small animals. Nephrotoxins account for most cases of AIRF in dogs and cats, while renal ischemia alone is an uncommon cause. This differs substantially from what has been observed in humans, in whom renal ischemia accounts for most cases of AIRF, followed by nephrotoxins.[267] The remainder of this section emphasizes the pathophysiology of nephrotoxins and renal ischemia in AIRF. Some of the same mechanisms, however, also may be operative in tubulointerstitial nephritis and renovascular occlusive disorders. Additional information regarding the diagnosis

TABLE 107–18. AIRF ASSOCIATED WITH NEPHROTOXINS

Glycols
   Ethylene glycol, diethylene glycol
Antimicrobials
   Aminoglycosides
   Amphotericin B
   Cephaloridine
   Sulfonamides
   Tetracyclines
   Polymyxin B
   Colistin
Cancer chemotherapeutic agents
   Cisplatin
   High-dose methotrexate
   High-dose doxorubicin
   High-dose cyclophosphamide
   Mithramycin
   Streptozotocin
Hypercalcemia/hypercalciuria
   Humoral hypercalcemia of malignancy
   Hypervitaminosis D (iatrogenic, new-generation rodenticide)
Heavy metals
   Arsenic, mercury, thallium, cadmium
Hydrocarbons
   Methanol
   Carbon tetrachloride—solvent
   Toluene—solvent
   Chlordane—insecticide
   Paraquat—herbicide
Intravenous radiocontrast agents
Fluorinated inhalational anesthetics
   Methoxyflurane/enflurane
Miscellaneous
   Thiacetarsamide (organic arsenical)
   Cyclosporin
   Elemental phosphorus—rodenticide
   EDTA
   Mushroom poisoning
   Mycotoxins
   Hemoglobinuria/myoglobinuria
   Snake bite/bee sting (may involve significant hypoperfusion also)

TABLE 107–19. AIRF ASSOCIATED WITH RENAL ISCHEMIA (HYPOPERFUSION)

Intravascular Volume Depletion
  Dehydration
    Vomiting
    Diarrhea
    Sequestration
  Blood loss
  Hypoalbuminemia
  Trauma
  Hypoadrenocorticism
  Hyponatremias (nondilutional)
Decreased Cardiac Output
  Congestive heart failure
  Low output without overt failure
    Restrictive pericardial disease
    Tamponade
    Arrhythmias
    Positive pressure ventilation
  Prolonged resuscitation following cardiac arrest
Altered Renal and Systemic Vascular Resistances
  Renal vasoconstriction
    Catecholamines (epinephrine, norepinephrine, ergotamine)
    Sympathetic nervous stimulation
    Vasopressin
    Angiotensin II
    Hypercalcemia
    Amphotericin B
    Hypothermia
    Myoglobinuria
    Hemoglobinuria
  Systemic vasodilation
    Arteriolar vasodilator treatment
    Anaphylaxis
    Inhalational anesthesia
    Sepsis
    Heatstroke
Increased Blood Viscosity
  Multiple myeloma
  Polycythemia (absolute or severe dehydration)
Interference with Renal Autoregulation During Hypotension
  Nonsteroidal antiinflammatory drugs
    Inhibition of renal prostaglandin synthesis
Following Renal Transplantation (warm or cold ischemia)

and treatment for specific causes of AIRF can be found in Chapter 108.

ACUTE INTRINSIC RENAL FAILURE CAUSED BY NEPHROSIS

The term nephrosis refers to degenerative or necrotic lesions of the renal tubules secondary to nephrotoxic or ischemic injury, with minimal interstitial inflammatory cell infiltrates (Figure 107–14A and B). Synonyms include lower nephron nephrosis, acute tubular necrosis, and acute tubular insufficiency. The kidneys may be enlarged or normal in size. Grossly, the renal capsule is not adherent, and the parenchyma may be pale and bulging on its cut surface.

Most attention has been focused on the effects of nephrotoxins and ischemia on the renal tubules because histopathologic lesions are more obvious in the tubules, but effects on glomerular function and ultrastructure also may occur.[269–274] There may be poor correlation between histopathology and renal function in clinical patients, and severe reductions in renal function can exist in the absence of demonstrable histologic renal lesions.[269, 275, 276] By contrast, histopathology in experi-

mentally induced AIRF usually is severe and diffuse, possibly as a result of a greater degree of renal insult in experimental settings.[276] Lesions in nephrotoxic AIRF affect the proximal tubule most severely, and there is preservation of tubular basement membranes; in ischemic AIRF there is a patchy distribution of lesions in the proximal and distal tubules with greater disruption of the tubular basement membranes.[275] In general, the more severe the renal insult, the more widespread the lesions, regardless of whether the initiating insult was nephrotoxic or ischemic.

Phases. There are many similarities in the pathophysiology of nephrotoxic and ischemic AIRF. Both forms of AIRF display gradients of sublethal to lethal cell injury, decreased cellular energy production, cellular swelling, and increased permeability of renal tubular cell membranes. Loss of concentrating ability is the most consistent early functional change in nephrotoxic or ischemic AIRF whether it is oliguric or nonoliguric.[267, 276] There are potentially three phases of AIRF caused by nephrosis (Figure 107–15).[258, 260, 265, 277–280]

The *induction phase* (early, latent, or incipient AIRF) is the time from the renal insult until the development of azotemia, defective concentrating ability, and oliguria or polyuria. Sublethal injury to tubular epithelial cells characterizes this phase initially, but progressively more cells sustain lethal injury if the insult continues. The induction phase is not commonly recognized unless the animal is closely observed because the initial changes in GFR and USG are not readily apparent. Clinical intervention at this stage (i.e., removal of nephrotoxic agents or correction of renal ischemia) prevents progression to the maintenance phase of AIRF. The induction phase is characterized by an early and progressive loss of concentrating ability, progressive azotemia, progressive increase in the numbers of renal tubular epithelial cells and casts in the urine sediment, and, occasionally, glucosuria.

The *maintenance phase* (fixed, established, or well-established AIRF) develops after a critical amount of nephron injury. Irreversible renal epithelial cell injury is crucial for the development of this phase.[281, 282] GFR and renal blood flow (RBF) are both decreased, but GFR is decreased much more than RBF.[268, 283, 284] Elimination of the inciting factor at this point does not result in rapid improvement in renal function, even when RBF returns to normal or above normal levels, because autoregulation of GFR and RBF has been severely disturbed.[268, 272] During this phase, reductions in RBF are more severe in the cortex than in the medulla in both nephrotoxic and ischemic forms of AIRF.[283] The maintenance phase is characterized by progression of azotemia to a new steady-state level. At this point, correction of all prerenal factors fails to result in any substantial decrease in BUN or S_{cr} concentrations.[277] There is no characteristic urine volume during this phase, and nonoliguric AIRF tends to result from less severe injury, whereas oliguric AIRF develops after more severe renal injury. The maintenance phase may last two to three weeks before normal renal function returns as renal lesions resolve. If the initial injury was severe, return of adequate renal function may not be possible because resolution of renal lesions may occur

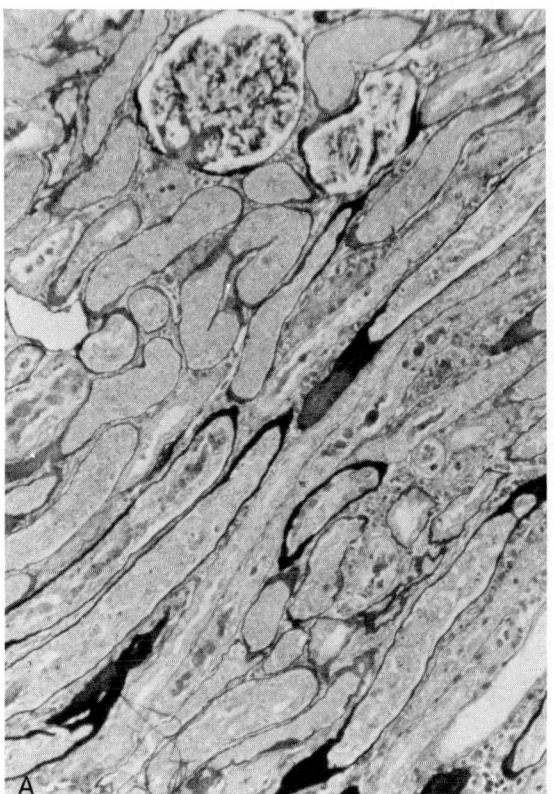

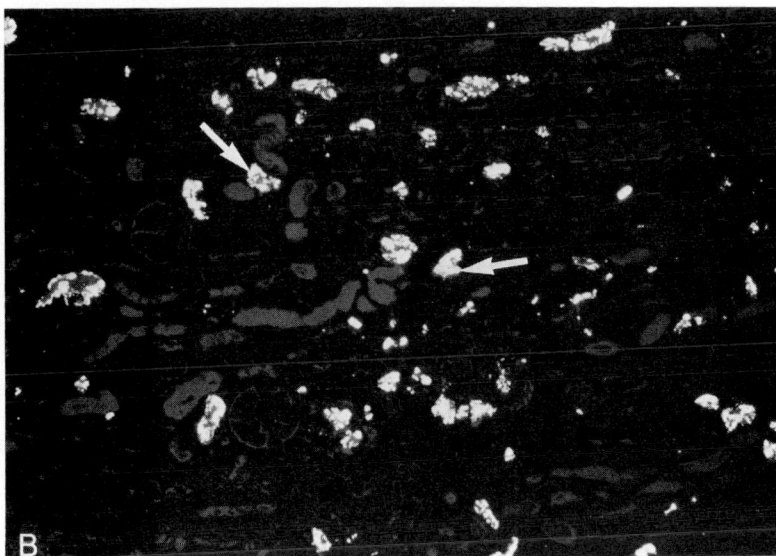

FIGURE 107–14. Typical histology of severe nephrosis. *A,* Aminoglycoside nephrotoxicity. Note severe loss of tubular detail and necrosis. Basement membrane is still intact and glomerulus is normal. (Periodic acid methenamine silver). (Courtesy of Dr. Kathy Harmon.) *B,* Ethylene glycol nephrotoxicity. Note presence of intratubular crystals typical of calcium oxalate under polarizing light. Some tubules are dilated, presumably due to intratubular obstruction from the crystals. Glomeruli are normal.

by nephron loss, interstitial fibrosis, and interstitial inflammation characteristic of chronic renal disease. Many animals with severe uremia due to AIRF die during the maintenance phase even when the renal lesions are potentially reversible, unless supported by dialysis treatments.

If sufficient renal healing occurs, the animal may enter the *recovery phase.* GFR can increase to the point that azotemia resolves, but GFR is still diminished when evaluated by clearance techniques. Urinary concentrating and acidifying abilities may be permanently impaired, but these deficits are not of major consequence to the patient.[264] In oliguric AIRF, entry into the recovery phase is heralded by the onset of a diuresis, but this development is not associated immediately with improvement in GFR. In nonoliguric AIRF, entry into the recovery phase is heralded by resolution of azotemia. The recovery phase may last for months, as an increase

FIGURE 107–15. Potential phases for development of acute intrinsic renal failure (AIRF) following exposure to ischemia or nephrotoxin. Prolonged reduction in GFR is encountered during the maintenance phase even if the ischemic event or nephrotoxin is removed. While many animals die from uremia before renal function improves, others enter the recovery phase as renal lesions resolve and renal function improves.

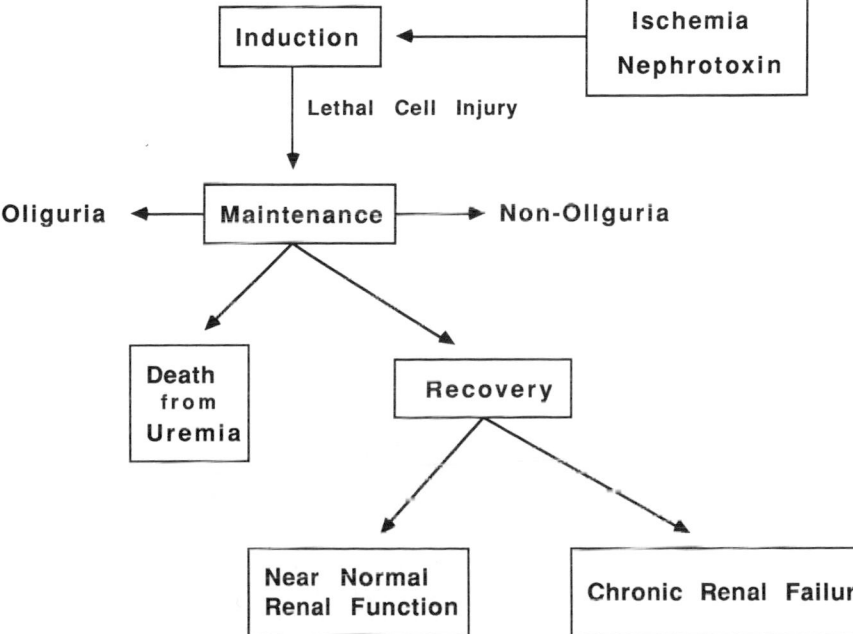

in single nephron GFR occurs as an adaptive response to permanent nephron loss after the nephrotoxic or ischemic insult.

MECHANISMS THAT CONTRIBUTE TO DECREASED GLOMERULAR FILTRATION RATE OR REDUCED URINE FLOW

Three mechanisms may contribute to decreased GFR or reduced tubular flow rate during AIRF: tubular obstruction, tubular backleak, and primary filtration failure (Figure 107–16).[262, 265, 272, 282, 285, 286] The mechanism that predominates in laboratory animal models depends on the model itself, the severity of the injury, and the phase of AIRF. Mechanisms that predominate during the induction phase of AIRF may be different from those responsible for the maintenance phase.[272, 286] Laboratory models emphasize one particular mechanism or another, but it seems likely that several mechanisms may be operative in clinical patients.

Intraluminal cast formation or extraluminal compression from swollen tubular cells can cause tubular obstruction.[264] Obstructing casts can arise from cellular debris as progressive cellular injury develops. Extensive loss of brush border membranes and reflux of intracellular organelles into the tubular lumens can contribute

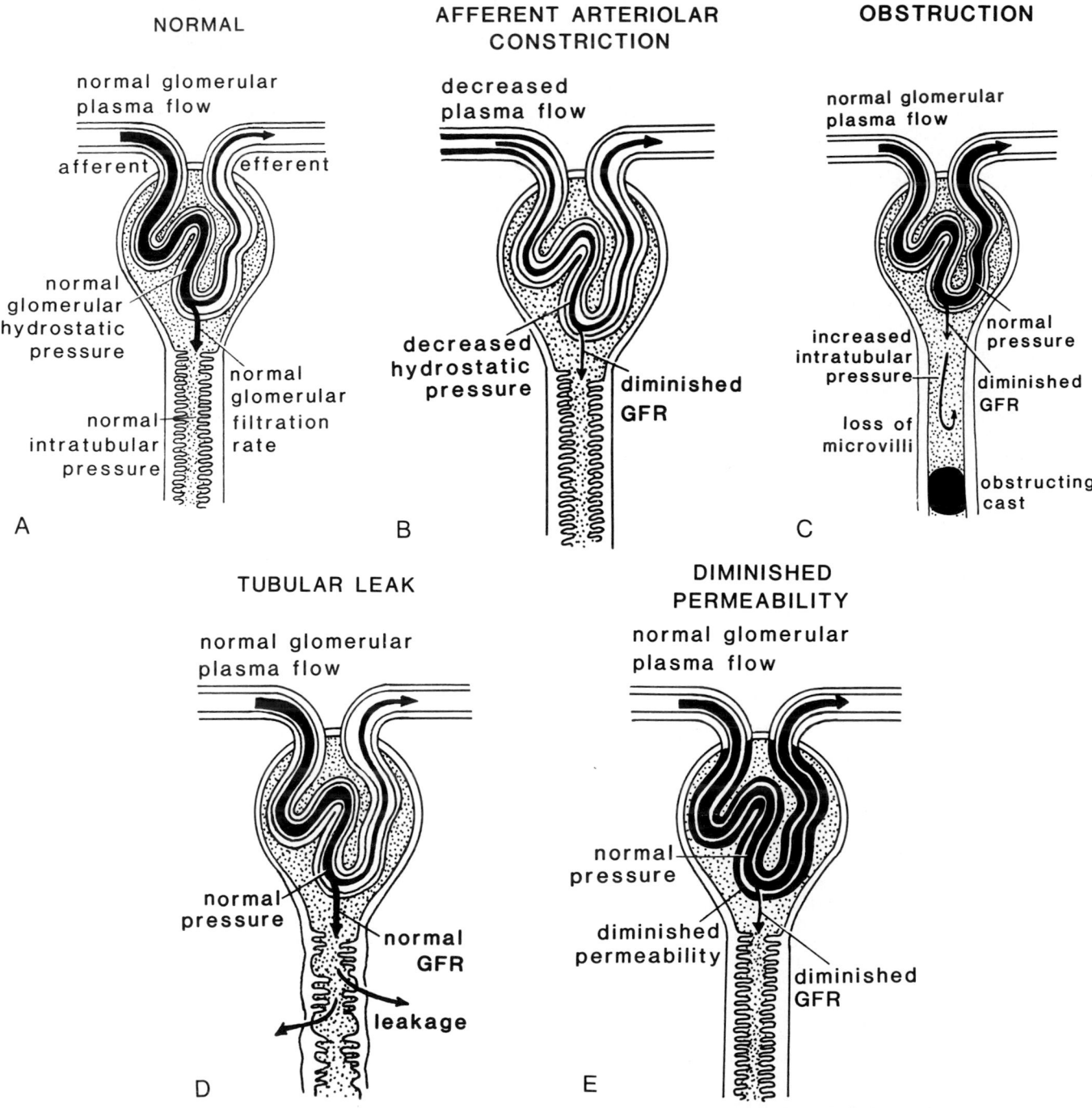

FIGURE 107–16. General mechanisms contributing to decreased GFR or oliguria in AIRF. *A–E,* Pathophysiology of decreased glomerular filtration rate (GFR) or oliguria during intrarenal acute renal failure (ARF). (Adapted from Schrier RW: Acute renal failure: Pathogenesis, diagnoses and management. Hosp Pract March, 93, 1981).

to the formation of casts that lodge in the distal nephron.[264, 287, 288] Myoglobin and hemoglobin in tubular fluid favor precipitation of matrix protein leading to cast formation if these pigments are present.[275] Intratubular pressure increases in some models of AIRF but not in others. Increased intratubular pressure reduces GFR by opposing glomerular capillary hydrostatic pressure, while reflex afferent arteriolar vasoconstriction in glomeruli of obstructed nephrons further contributes to reduced GFR.

Backleak of tubular fluid into the interstitium across damaged tubules can be demonstrated in some models of AIRF.[285] This mechanism appears to be operative in the severest forms of tubular injury and may contribute to oliguria. Glomerular filtration may be normal, but methods used to measure GFR will falsely indicate a decrease, since the concentration of marker solutes (e.g., inulin, creatinine) in tubular fluid is decreased by backleak after filtration. Backleak of tubular fluid can contribute to oliguria and apparent decreases in GFR only if glomerular ultrafiltrate continues to be formed. Backleak of tubular fluid is expected to occur to the greatest extent after severe tubular injury with cast formation and increased intratubular pressure. Backleak of tubular fluid can occur across damaged cells or through the intercellular space.

Primary filtration failure occurs when processes within the glomeruli reduce filtration. Intraglomerular control of filtration depends on glomerular plasma flow, the balance of tone between the afferent and efferent arterioles, and vascular permeability.[283] Afferent arteriolar constriction or efferent arteriolar dilatation, or both, will result in reduced glomerular capillary hydrostatic pressure and reduced GFR. Vasoconstriction of preglomerular vessels occurs in a variety of renal injuries, resulting in AIRF, and is sometimes referred to as vasomotor nephropathy.[283] The role of efferent vasodilatation has not been proved, yet a hypothesis supporting the role of this mechanism has been advanced.[283] Reduced glomerular permeability can account for reduced glomerular filtration even when glomerular plasma flow and glomerular capillary hydrostatic pressures are normal.[264, 270–272, 289, 290] Swollen podocytes, reduced number or diameter of endothelial fenestrae, and reduced surface area available for filtration have been demonstrated ultrastructurally in some models of AIRF and might account for reduced permeability. Contraction of mesangial cells in response to the local action of angiotensin II in the glomerulus may also reduce the surface area available for filtration.[291]

ACUTE INTRINSIC RENAL FAILURE CAUSED BY NEPHROTOXINS

Nephrotoxins are substances that are capable of directly inducing lethal renal tubular cell injury in the initial stages after exposure, and some additionally cause hypoperfusion from renal vasoconstriction.[282, 292, 293] Hypoperfusion can follow the initial nephrotoxic injury, however, and may be important in the maintenance phase of nephrotoxic AIRF (Figure 107–17). Experimental studies allow evaluation of the isolated effects of nephrotoxins, but many of the chemotherapeutic agents listed in Table 107–18 are likely to be encountered in a complex clinical setting in which the role of other nephrotoxins and renal ischemia must also be considered.

The kidneys are at high risk for injury after exposure to endogenous or exogenous toxins as a consequence of their excretory function. Despite their relatively small size, blood flow to the kidneys is larger than that of any other organ at approximately 25 per cent of cardiac output.[264, 282] High RBF ensures a large exposure to potential toxins, but development of toxicity depends on the dose of toxin, the duration of exposure, and the mechanism by which the toxin is excreted by the kidney. The intracellular or interstitial concentration of a toxin ultimately may determine its toxicity, but measurements of such concentrations are not widely available.[282] Tubular reabsorption and secretion of a toxin can increase its intracellular concentration, and the countercurrent mechanism potentially can increase its interstitial concentration. After filtration of a toxin by the glomeruli, the luminal membranes of the proximal tubular cells are exposed to progressively increasing concentrations of the toxin as water and sodium are isosmotically reabsorbed. The brush border of the proximal tubule provides a large surface area for interaction of the toxin with cell membranes.

A general scheme for the mechanisms of toxic injury in the kidney is presented in Figure 107–17. Attachment of the toxin to luminal, basolateral, or intracellular organelle membranes is the critical initial event.[282, 293] Increased tubular membrane permeability and loss of function can occur directly after toxin attachment, or after activation of phospholipase. Phospholipids are abundant in cell membranes, and their degradation appears to be central in initiating and perpetuating tubular cell injury. Cell swelling and reduced ability to generate adenosine triphosphate (ATP) lead to further compromise of function and possible lethal cell injury.[281, 282] The role of intracellular calcium in the initial stages of nephrotoxic injury is not clear, but redistribution of calcium within the cell may be important in the early activation of phospholipase.[281, 282] Mitochondria preferentially take up calcium at the expense of oxidative phosphorylation, and calcium-induced injury at this site may be crucial. Progressive cellular injury is associated with increasing influx of calcium, but whether this contributes to further injury or is a marker of the degree of injury is controversial.[281, 282, 291] The specific membrane interactions for toxins listed in Table 107–18 are not well known, with the exception of those for aminoglycosides, amphotericin B, and the heavy metals.

Nephrotoxicity is enhanced if animals are volume-depleted before the toxic insult.[264] This may reflect increased concentration of the toxin in tubular fluid as sodium and water are more avidly reabsorbed or, possibly, lower tubular flow rates could allow greater time for membrane-toxin interaction. Low tubular flow rate and high osmolality of tubular fluid also favor cast formation. Volume depletion also imposes an element of vasoconstriction that can enhance nephrotoxicity.

Exposure of animals with preexisting chronic renal disease to nephrotoxins results in enhanced nephrotoxicity.[294] Adaptive changes in remnant nephrons may

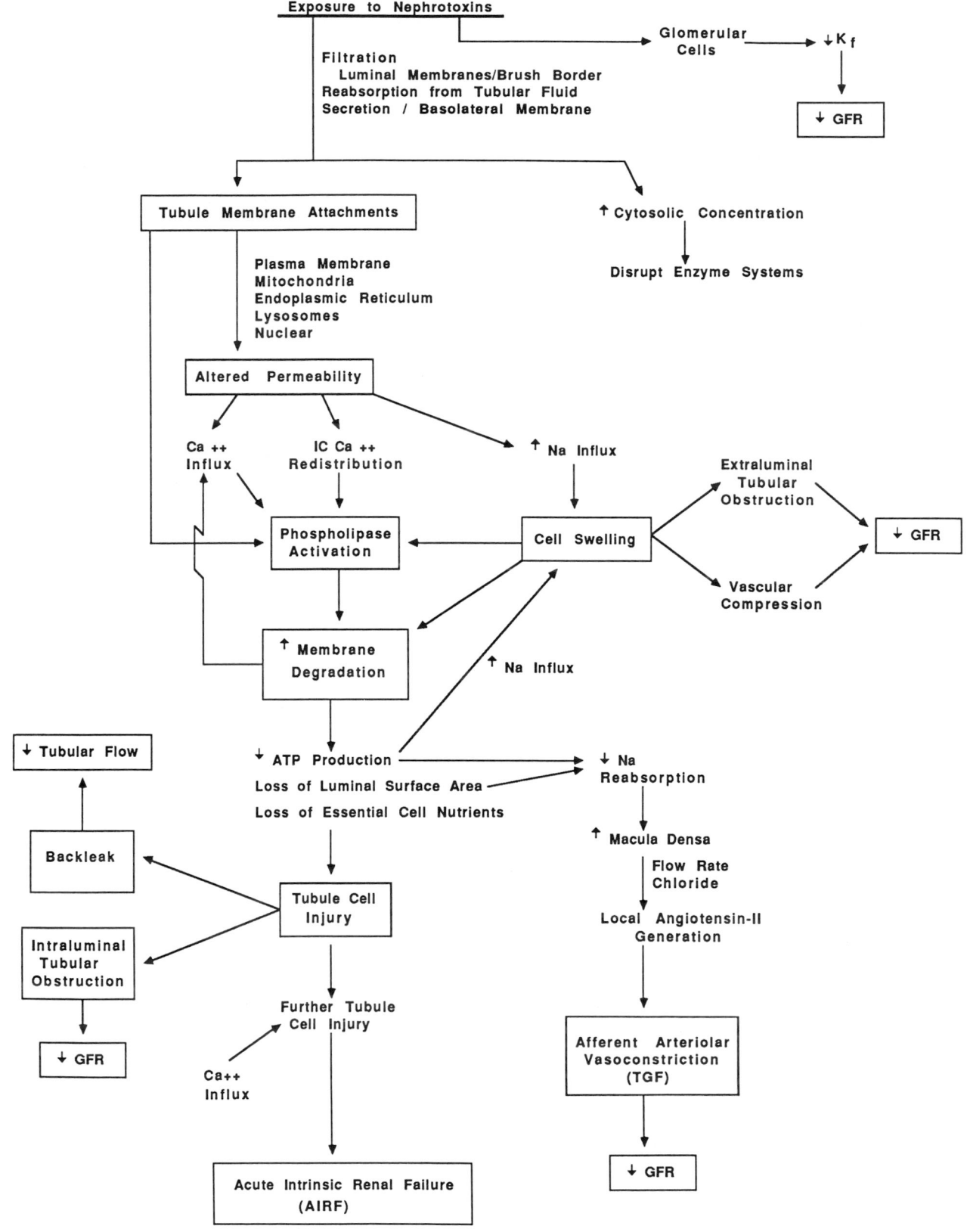

FIGURE 107–17. Potential pathways for nephrotoxicity to cause acute intrinsic renal failure (AIRF). Kf = glomerular ultrafiltration coefficient (permeability), Ca^{++} = calcium, IC = intracellular. (Adapted from Humes HD: Role of calcium in pathogenesis of acute renal failure. Am J Physiol 250:F579, 1986; Schrier RW et al: Cellular calcium in ischemic acute renal failure: role of calcium entry blockers. Kidney Int 32:313, 1987; Porter GA, Bennett WM: Nephrotoxin-induced acute renal failure. *In* Brenner BM and Rector FC: Acute Renal Failure. New York, Churchill Livingstone, 1980, p 123; Porter GA, Bennett WM: Toxic nephropathies. *In* Brenner BM and Rector FC: The Kidney. Philadelphia, WB Saunders, 1981, p 2045.)

explain this propensity, as increased single-nephron GFR exposes tubules to a higher filtered load of toxin per nephron. Additionally, hypertrophy of remaining tubules may provide increased surface area along the lumen for enhanced membrane-toxin interactions. Animals with chronic renal disease also may lack the ability to produce sufficient amounts of intrarenal vasodilatory prostaglandins that otherwise could counteract renal vasoconstriction.[295]

Specific Nephrotoxins. Ingestion of ethylene glycol, usually as antifreeze, is the most common cause for AIRF in dogs and cats. Ethylene glycol is not toxic until metabolized to glycolaldehyde, glyoxylic acid, glycolate, and oxalic acid.[296-306] Animals that enter the maintenance phase of ethylene glycol–induced AIRF usually are oliguric, and total anuria may occur. In ethylene glycol–induced AIRF, animals with severe oliguria or anuria during the maintenance phase rarely recover enough renal function to support life despite dialysis support.[307-309] Oliguria and azotemia have been attributed to tubular obstruction and cell necrosis caused by the deposition of calcium oxalate crystals in tubular lumens and in tubular cells themselves.[62, 308, 310-312] Infusion of ethylene glycol metabolites can cause AIRF without deposition of crystals, however, and the presence of crystals may only be a marker of early disease.[303, 306, 313-315] Crystal deposition may contribute to the maintenance phase by causing obstruction and backleak after damage to tubular cells (Figure 107–14B).

Many antibiotics may cause nephrotoxic AIRF, depending on dosage, route of administration, and clinical setting.[316-319] The aminoglycosides and the antifungal agent amphotericin B are the most important with regard to nephrotoxicity. Cephaloridine is the only cephalosporin associated with a significant nephrotoxicity, and for this reason other cephalosporins should be used.[320-323] Historically, sulfonamides have caused AIRF as a result of precipitation within tubular lumens and tubular obstruction. Modern sulfonamides are highly soluble, and nephrotoxic reactions are rarely recognized. Tetracyclines have a relatively narrow margin of safety with regard to nephrotoxicity when administered intravenously in dogs.[324]

Aminoglycoside nephrotoxicity is the second most common cause of AIRF in dogs and cats, and its frequency appears to be increasing.[258, 325-327] Aminoglycoside-induced AIRF is often non-oliguric.[328, 329] All aminoglycosides potentially are nephrotoxic (see Figure 107–14A).[330-334] Neomycin is the most nephrotoxic, streptomycin the least nephrotoxic, and the toxicity of kanamycin, gentamicin, amikacin, tobramycin, sosiamicin, and netilmicin is intermediate.[282, 293, 316, 335, 336] Netilmicin has been demonstrated to be less nephrotoxic than gentamicin in dogs, while it is uncertain whether amikacin and tobramycin are less nephrotoxic than gentamicin.[331, 332] Aminoglycosides are polycations that bind to the brush border of the proximal tubule initially, are taken into the cell by endocytosis, and accumulate within lysosomes (Figure 107–18).[337] Aminoglycosides apparently inhibit lysosomal phospholipase, causing accumulation of membrane material and drug and resulting in formation of myeloid bodies.[336-340] The presence of myeloid bodies cannot be correlated to development of

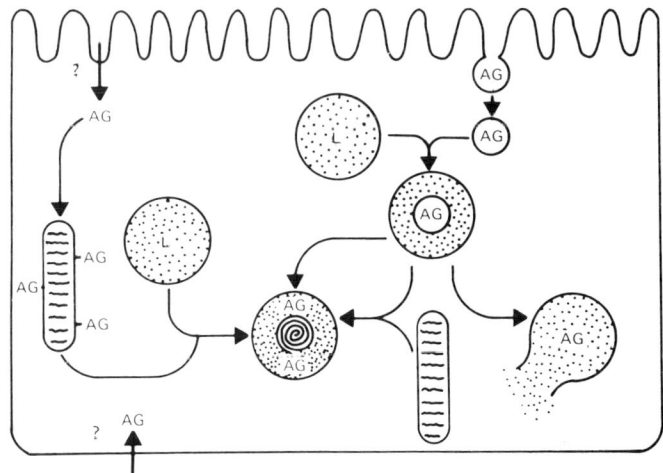

FIGURE 107–18. Pathways of aminoglycoside-induced cellular injury. On the right the aminoglycoside (AG) is shown entering the cell by pinocytosis and subsequently fusing with a primary lysosome (L). The aminoglycoside may interfere with normal lysosomal digestion, giving rise to myeloid body formation, and the aminoglycosides may labilize lysosomes, leading to the release of potent acid hydrolases into the cytosol. If aminoglycosides gained entry into the cell by other pathways as depicted on the left, then the aminoglycosides could cause direct injury to intracellular organelles. (From Kaloyanides GJ and Pastoriza-Munoz E: Aminoglycoside nephrotoxicity. Kidney Int 18:571, 1980.)

AIRF, however, because even single small doses can cause their formation. Aminoglycosides can reduce glomerular permeability during the induction phase of AIRF in rats, while reduction in diameter of endothelial fenestrae in glomeruli contributes to the maintenance of reduced GFR.[286, 337, 341, 342] Aminoglycosides accumulate in the renal cortex and may persist for months after administration.[332, 336] Azotemia often progresses despite discontinuation of drug therapy.[326, 336]

Nephrotoxicity after amphotericin B therapy is the third most frequent cause of AIRF in small animals. Binding of amphotericin to sterols in tubular cell membranes and vasoconstriction of afferent arterioles are important during the induction phase of AIRF.[282, 316, 343-346] Progression to the maintenance phase usually can be prevented by temporarily discontinuing drug therapy and decreasing the subsequent dosage. Treatment with intravenous fluids and diuretics may prevent the induction phase or limit progression to the maintenance phase.[347-349]

Aggressive cancer chemotherapy uncommonly can result in nephrotoxic AIRF. Therapeutic protocols using high-dose methotrexate, doxorubicin, or cyclophosphamide can be associated with nephrotoxicity not seen when using lower doses of these drugs.[350] Cisplatin can cause direct tubular cell injury, but protocols using cisplatin infusion over several hours after prior volume expansion have not resulted in AIRF in our experience.[350-353] Mithramycin and streptozotocin are rarely used highly nephrotoxic anticancer agents.[351]

Hypercalcemia occasionally results in AIRF, but it more commonly results in chronic renal failure.[354-358] The differential diagnosis of hypercalcemia is discussed in Chapter 94. Hypercalcemia may become more common as a cause of AIRF with the increasing use of rodenticides that contain vitamin D (cholecalciferol).

Serum calcium values in excess of 15 mg/dl result in severe reductions of GFR and RBF in conscious dogs.[359] Initially, there is preglomerular vasoconstriction and later there is intrinsic damage to renal tubular cells. Even small increases in serum ionized calcium may cause tubular mineralization at the ultrastructural level, but clinically detectable decreases in renal function and histologic lesions may not occur unless the calcium x phosphorus product exceeds 60.[355]

AIRF caused by poisoning with heavy metals or hydrocarbons is seldom encountered, but AIRF after thiacetarsamide has been reported.[282, 360, 361] Intravenous contrast agents may cause AIRF by direct toxicity to tubular cells and through hemodynamic changes, but

clinical cases in veterinary medicine have yet to be reported.[316] Apparently, AIRF after radiographic contrast administration in humans is much more likely to occur in the presence of diabetes mellitus, multiple myeloma, or dehydration.[282] Fluorinated inhalation anesthetics may result in fluoride metabolites that are nephrotoxic, but this also has not been reported in animals.[282, 316, 362] Myoglobinuria and hemoglobinuria can result in AIRF through nephrotoxic and ischemic mechanisms. Pure hemoglobin does not appear to be toxic, but after hemolysis other factors that contribute to toxicity may be released.[264] Myoglobin is nephrotoxic, particularly in the clinical setting of acidosis and dehydration.[264, 286, 363, 364] Myoglobin and hemoglobin nephro-

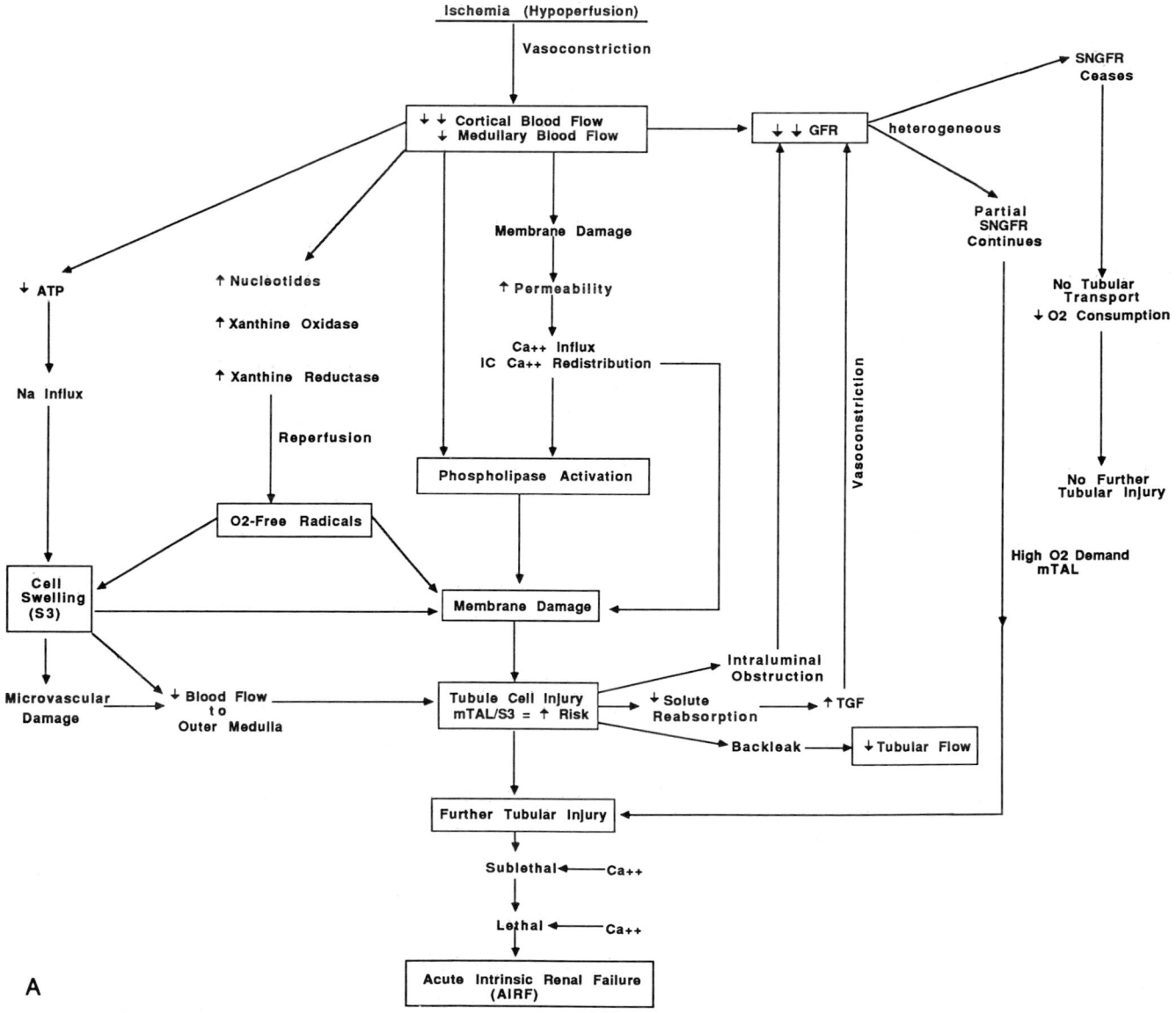

FIGURE 107–19. *A* and *B,* Potential pathways for ischemia to cause acute intrinsic renal failure (AIRF). *A* emphasizes the development of tubular lesions, while *B* emphasizes the initial development of vascular lesions that lead to persistent renal vasoconstriction. According to this scheme, the mTAL is central in the pathogenesis of tubular injury due to its unique location, energy requirements, and oxygen supply. See text for further detail. Ca++ = calcium, IC = intracellular, mTAL = medullary thick ascending limb of the loop of Henle, S3 = pars recta or straight portion of proximal tubule, SNGFR = single nephron glomerular filtration rate, TGF = tubulo-glomerular feedback, Kf = glomerular ultrafiltration coefficient (permeability). (Adapted from Brezis M et al: Renal ischemia: a new perspective. N Engl J Med 26:375, 1984; Humes HD: Role of calcium in pathogenesis of acute renal failure. Am J Physiol 250:F579, 1986; Schrier RW, et al: Cellular calcium in ischemic acute renal failure: role of calcium entry blockers. Kidney Int 32:313, 1987.)

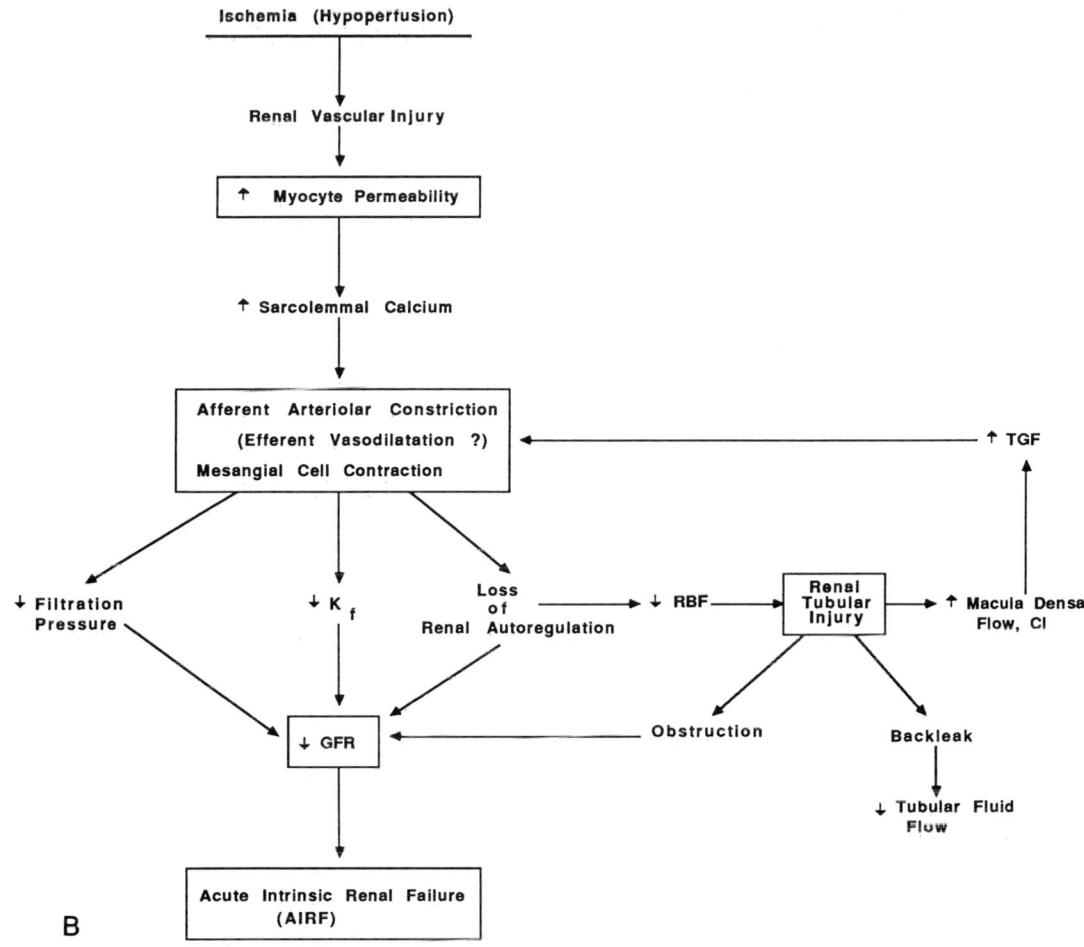

Figure 107–19 *Continued*

ACUTE INTRINSIC RENAL FAILURE CAUSED BY ISCHEMIA (HYPOPERFUSION)

The causes of ischemia that may result in AIRF are listed in Table 107–19. These same conditions may cause prerenal azotemia, and when they are more long-standing or severe, AIRF may develop. In an attempt to maintain systemic blood pressure during these conditions, increased vasopressor activity occurs as a result of increased activity of the sympathetic nervous system and increased systemic or intrarenal release of epinephrine, norepinephrine, angiotensin II, and vasopressin.[368-370] The renal vasculature also participates in vasoconstriction from stimulation of renal catecholamine and angiotensin receptors,[283, 368-374] but this effect is counterbalanced by the intrarenal production and action of vasodilatory prostaglandins in normal animals.[282, 295, 375] GFR and RBF are maintained at nearly normal levels during early ischemia in normal animals, but further renal vasoconstriction occurs as systemic hypotension progresses. Initially, efferent arteriolar constriction reduces RBF but maintains GFR. Later, afferent arteriolar vasoconstriction reduces both GFR and RBF.[368, 376] The normal kidney can maintain normal RBF and GFR until systemic blood pressure falls below 80 mmHg, but

some of the conditions listed in Table 107–19 may interfere with renal autoregulation, causing reductions in RBF and GFR to occur at higher systemic pressures.[368, 369] Ischemia initially causes prerenal azotemia without intrinsic renal lesions, but lethal cell injury can eventually follow and result in AIRF with tubular cell necrosis or cortical necrosis in extreme situations.

AIRF owing primarily to ischemia is uncommonly recognized in small animal medicine, but experimental studies in dogs and rats have contributed to our understanding of the pathophysiology of ischemic injury.[377] Experimental ischemia usually is created by complete renal artery clamping, intrarenal infusion of catecholamines, hemorrhagic hypotension, or intramuscular glycerol injection.[264, 276, 286] These forms of ischemic injury are far more severe than those likely to be encountered in clinical practice. Figure 107–19 summarizes the potential pathways by which ischemic insult can result in renal injury.

Renal vasoconstriction is central to the development of ischemic AIRF during the induction phase and can persist during the maintenance phase (Figure 107–19A). Ischemia may injure smooth muscle cells of the renal vessels, causing increased permeability to calcium.[291] Increased intracellular calcium may then increase myocyte contractility, resulting in vasoconstriction that could persist in the absence of vasopressors (Figure 107–19B). Additionally, mesangial cell contraction may re-

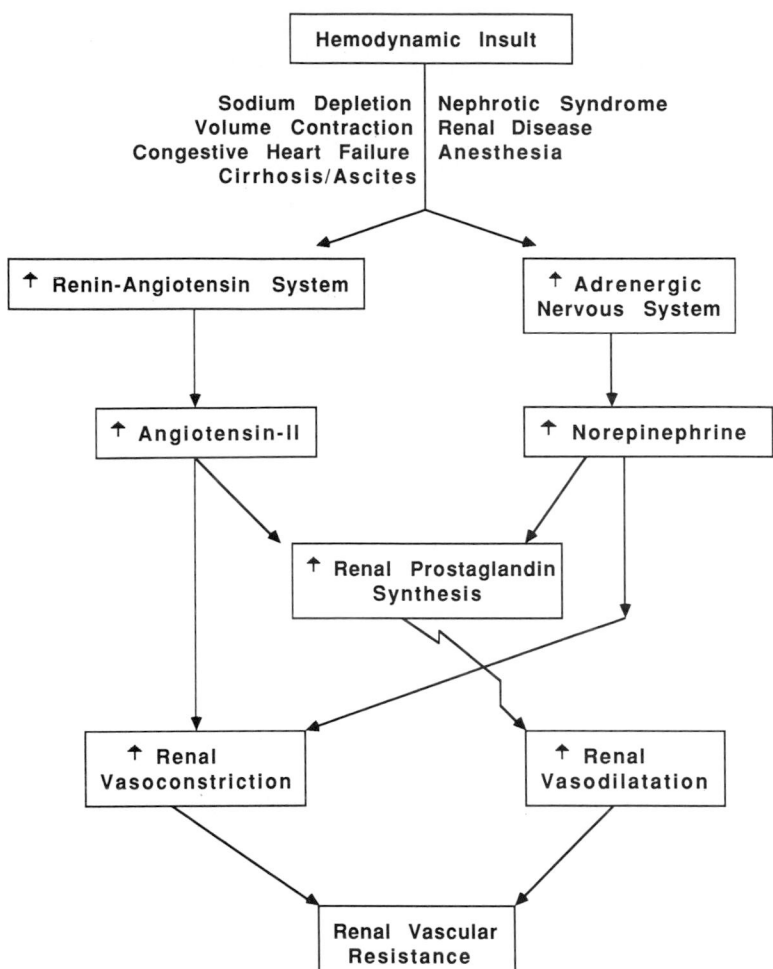

FIGURE 107–20. Normal renal vascular resistance and renal blood flow can be relatively well maintained during periods of high vasoconstrictor activity if countervailing renal vasodilators are synthesized. Blocking the synthesis of renal vasodilatory prostaglandins with nonsteroidal antiinflammatory drugs allows unopposed renal vasoconstriction during hemodynamic insult and possible progression to acute intrinsic renal failure (AIRF). (Adapted from Stoff JS, Clive DM: Role of prostaglandins and thromboxane in acute renal failure. *In* Brenner BM and Lazarus JM: Acute Renal Failure. Philadelphia, WB Saunders, 1983, p 157; Clive D and Stoff, JS: Renal syndromes associated with nonsteroidal antiinflammatory drugs. N Engl J Med 310(9):563–572, 1984; Humes HD and Weinberg JM: Toxic Nephropathies. *In* Brenner BM and Rector FC, The Kidney. 3rd. ed, Philadelphia, WB Saunders, 1986, p 1491.)

duce GFR by causing a decrease in the ultrafiltration coefficient (Kf). This type of renal vascular injury may explain the loss of autoregulation in postischemic kidneys.

Renal hypoperfusion can occur if nonsteroidal antiinflammatory drugs (antiprostaglandins) are administered in the setting of systemic hypotension and increased concentration of vasopressors.[295] The normal renal response in these instances is to increase the production of vasodilatory prostaglandins that counteract renal vasoconstriction (Figure 107–20), but this countervailing maneuver is blocked by antiprostaglandin therapy, resulting in unopposed renal vasoconstriction. Antiprostaglandins such as indomethacin do not influence RBF or GFR in normal dogs, but result in dramatic reductions in RBF and GFR during hemodynamic insult (e.g., hypotension, hemorrhage, salt depletion, general anesthesia, congestive heart failure).[295, 375] The development of AIRF during antiprostaglandin therapy has been observed in dogs, but often in a complex clinical setting in the presence of complicating factors (e.g., nephrotoxic drugs, hemodynamic compromise, sepsis).

Renal vasoconstriction after ischemia decreases RBF in both the cortex and the medulla, but this decrement is not equally shared, and greater reduction occurs in the cortex (see Figure 107–19A).[283] Swelling of proximal tubular cells (pars recta) located in the outer medulla reduces RBF by compression of blood vessels in this region, thus potentiating ischemic injury to the nearby thick ascending limb of Henle's loop. Relative preservation of blood flow to the medulla may be a protective mechanism to supply oxygen to the metabolically active tubular cells in the outer medulla.[264, 276] The degree of success in maintaining adequate oxygenation to this region of high oxygen demand may determine whether or not lethal cell injury follows ischemic insult.

Ischemic tubular injury is most likely to occur in regions of the kidney that are most metabolically active and that have relatively low oxygen availability.[276] Oxygen tension progressively decreases from renal cortex to outer and inner medulla, providing regions of relative hypoxia for tubular cells in the medulla.[276] The pars recta (straight portion of the proximal tubule, or S3) and the medullary thick ascending limb of Henle's loop are structures with high metabolic activity that are located in the outer medulla and are at high risk for ischemic injury according to this hypothesis. Indeed, the earliest lesions after ischemia can be demonstrated in the medullary thick ascending limb of Henle's loop.[276] Tubular cells most distant from the vascular bundles sustain greater injury, adding more credence to the role of relative hypoxia.[276] Tubular cell injury in this region parallels the metabolic demand for sodium reabsorption during the ischemic insult. Experimental manipulations to reduce sodium reabsorption and tubular energy consumption by pretreatment with ouabain or furosemide demonstrate less ischemic tubular cell injury.[276] Similar attenuation of tubular cell lesions is seen after hyperoncotic albumin infusion, which results in cessation of glomerular filtration and subsequent reduction in energy demand for sodium reabsorption. The importance of early tubular cell lesions in the outer medulla has long been unappreciated, since such lesions are difficult to recognize in routine histologic sections, and tissue from this region is not routinely included in clinical biopsy specimens.[276]

Initial injury to the medullary thick ascending limb of Henle's loop offers an attractive explanation for perpetuation of renal vasoconstriction if tubuloglomerular feedback is activated after detection of nonreabsorbed solute by the macula densa. Vasoconstriction of afferent arterioles in parent glomeruli then reduces GFR and the filtered load of sodium, thus conferring protection on tubular cells of these nephrons as less metabolic demand for sodium reabsorption occurs.[276] Some nephrons, however, may continue glomerular filtration, which will result in continued metabolic demand for sodium reabsorption in a state of hypoxia. In this setting additional cellular injury may occur as discussed earlier.

Early injury to cells of the medullary thick ascending limb of Henle's loop also may explain the early loss of concentrating ability observed after ischemic insult. This region of Henle's loop is critical in maintaining the maximal hyperosmolality of the renal interstitium required for urine concentration.[378] Disturbance of sodium and chloride reabsorption at this site could result in rapid dissipation of renal interstitial hyperosmolality and impairment of concentrating ability.

A spectrum of lesions, from focal to diffuse injury of the medullary thick ascending limb tubular cells to more widespread injury of all tubular cells along the nephron, may occur during severe injury. Injured tubular cells undergo swelling, reduction in ATP generation, and activation of membrane phospholipase, as described for nephrotoxic injury.[264, 276, 291] These changes result in altered cell membrane permeability and loss of normal cell function. Free oxygen radicals generated during the hypoxic phase can be liberated after reperfusion and may further contribute to cellular injury.[291] Increases in intracellular calcium that occurred during early ischemic cell injury may contribute to additional cell damage.[291] The sum of these effects will determine whether cell injury after ischemia and reperfusion is lethal or sublethal.

Cast formation and tubular obstruction can contribute to reduced GFR after ischemia, as the brush border of the proximal tubular cells sloughs into the tubular lumen. Backleak of tubular fluid across severely damaged tubules can further contribute to the perceived decrease in GFR, and Kf also may decrease after ischemic AIRF.

ACUTE INTRINSIC RENAL FAILURE CAUSED BY NEPHRITIS

Acute tubulointerstitial nephritis (see Table 107–16) is associated with inflammatory cell infiltrates consisting of neutrophils, eosinophils, lymphocytes, and/or plasma cells, depending on the specific cause, and with tubular cell and glomerular necrosis of varying severity. Reduc-

tions in GFR and RBF occur as a consequence of vascular compression from the inflammatory infiltrate and also after necrosis of tubular epithelium and subsequent tubular obstruction. Oliguria may occur as a consequence of tubular disruption, with backleak of tubular fluid into the interstitium. Toxic effects on tubular function from elements of the inflammatory response can result in decreased sodium reabsorption and possible activation of tubuloglomerular feedback, further decreasing GFR. The glomerular and vascular disorders listed in Table 107–17 can result in reduced GFR and RBF by physically restricting the flow of blood through the glomeruli or by altering Kf.

DIAGNOSIS OF ACUTE INTRINSIC RENAL FAILURE

Table 107–10 summarizes the clinical and laboratory data used to distinguish prerenal, intrinsic renal, and postrenal azotemia, while Chapter 108 details specific diagnoses of acute renal failure. In general, the diagnosis of AIRF is based on the clinical findings of an acute onset, absence of long-standing polyuria and polydipsia, normal or enlarged kidneys on abdominal palpation or radiographs, absence of anemia early in the course of disease, dilute urine before treatment, and abnormal urinary sediment (e.g., renal epithelial cells, cellular casts, granular casts). Renal biopsy occasionally will be necessary to distinguish AIRF from chronic renal disease. Renal biopsies from animals with AIRF should display tubular cell necrosis or degeneration with minimal fibrosis and mononuclear inflammation. Gradual resolution of azotemia after supportive fluid therapy or dialysis adds further support to a diagnosis of AIRF.

Pathophysiology of Glomerular Disease

The two major glomerular diseases of dogs and cats are immune complex glomerulonephritis and amyloidosis. Both diseases may lead to massive proteinuria and progressive loss of functional renal mass. Classically, the nephrotic syndrome has been considered to include proteinuria, hypoalbuminemia, hypercholesterolemia, and edema or ascites. More recently, however, patients that lose more than 3.5 gm of protein per 1.73 m² body surface area have been defined as having nephrotic syndrome.[379]

NORMAL GLOMERULAR STRUCTURE AND FUNCTION

The glomeruli function as filters across which an ultrafiltrate of plasma is created by the force of cardiac contraction. The filtration barrier is composed of three major components: the fenestrated endothelium of the glomerular capillary, the glomerular basement membrane, and the visceral epithelial cells (podocytes) (Figure 107–21). The interdigitating foot processes of the podocytes and the slit diaphragms between them are negatively charged due to the presence of acidic glycoproteins (glomerular polyanion). The basement membrane and endothelium also contain negatively charged glycoproteins.

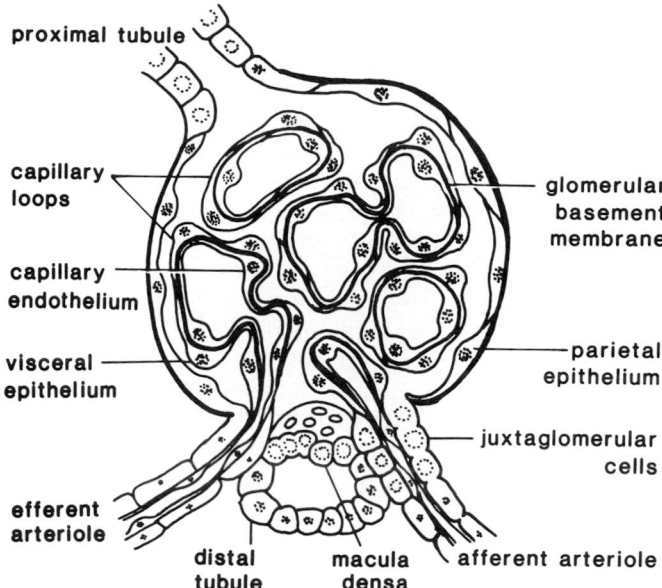

FIGURE 107–21. Normal glomerular morphology. (From Chew DJ and DiBartola SP: Manual of Small Animal Nephrology and Urology. New York, Churchill Livingstone, 1986, p 229.)

The normal glomerulus functions both as a size- and charge-selective filter.[380, 381] Its size-selective properties are thought to reside primarily in the basement membrane and are such that circulating macromolecules with radii greater than 34 Å or 3.4 nm are excluded from filtration. Serum albumin with a molecular weight of 69,000 and effective molecular radius of 36 Å or 3.6 nm is normally excluded from filtration. The presence of glomerular polyanion restricts filtration of circulating negatively charged macromolecules, and the fractional clearance of particles of similar size differs substantially, depending on their charge (Figure 107–22).

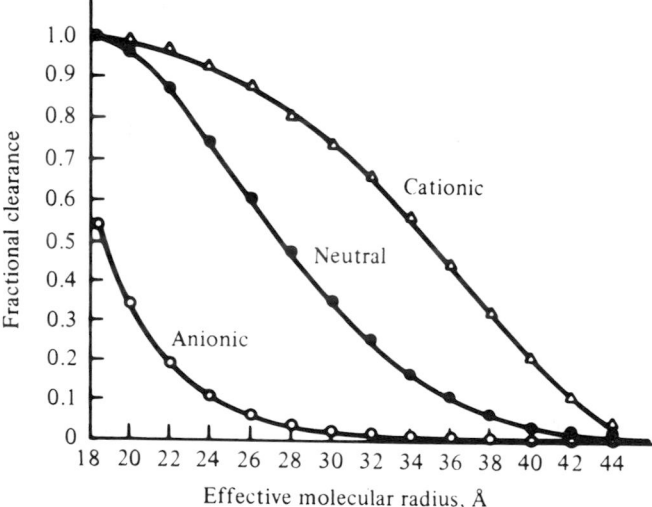

FIGURE 107–22. Charge selectivity of the glomerulus demonstrated by fractional clearance of anionic, neutral, and cationic dextrans. Fractional clearances (the ratio of the filtration of a substance to that of inulin, which is freely filtered) of anionic, neutral, and cationic dextrans as a function of effective molecular radius. Both molecular size and charge are important, as smaller or cationic molecules are more easily filtered. As a reference, the effective molecular radius of albumin is about 36 Å. (From Rose BD: Pathophysiology of Renal Disease. New York, McGraw-Hill, 1987, p 13).

MECHANISMS OF GLOMERULAR INJURY IN GLOMERULONEPHRITIS

Immune-mediated damage is largely responsible for glomerular injury in glomerulonephritis (Figure 107–23). For many years trapping of circulating soluble immune complexes in the glomeruli was thought to be the major determinant of glomerular injury. Experimentally, soluble complexes formed in antigen excess were observed to circulate and deposit in subepithelial locations. Despite demonstration of subepithelial localization of circulating immune complexes, glomerular disease resembling that seen clinically was not reliably produced.[382] Types of injury have recently been classified by the glomerular sites of immune complex deposition, and the importance of in situ reaction of antigen with antibody has been emphasized.[383–385]

Subepithelial immune complexes may be formed when circulating antibody reacts with fixed intrinsic glomerular antigens or, more commonly, nonglomerular antigens that have been planted in the glomerulus. Cationic antigens may bind to negative charges in the glomerular capillary wall and then bind circulating antibody. Cationic immunoglobulins such as IgG may bind to negative charges in glomeruli and subsequently bind anionic antigens such as deoxyribonucleic acid. Lastly, nonim-

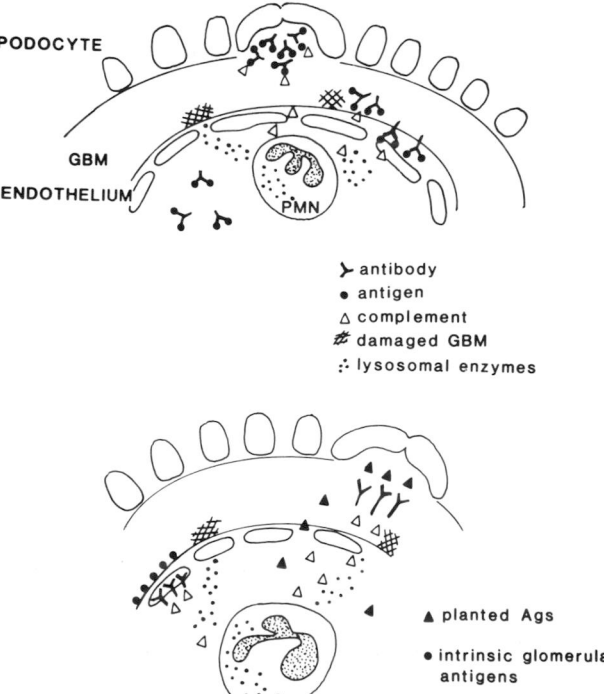

FIGURE 107–23. Immunologic mechanisms of glomerular injury. Schematic representation of the two major types of immunologically mediated glomerular injury. Circulating soluble immune complexes have become trapped in the glomerular filter and have fixed complement. Chemotactic complement components have attracted neutrophils to the area. The release of free oxygen radicals and lysosomal enzymes from the neutrophils has resulted in damage to the glomerulus (top). Damage may also result from attachment of autoantibodies directed against fixed intrinsic glomerular antigens (bottom, left). Finally, damage may result from attachment of antibodies directed against planted nonglomerular antigens (bottom, right). (From Chew DJ and DiBartola SP: Manual of Small Animal Nephrology and Urology. New York, Churchill Livingstone, 1986, p 232.)

mune cationic protein products of inflammatory cells or platelets may bind to negatively charged glomerular sites and then bind anionic antigens. The role of circulating immune complexes in the pathogenesis of glomerular injury currently is considered controversial.

There is no strong evidence that mesangial and subendothelial deposits result from in situ reaction of antibody with intrinsic glomerular antigens. Nonglomerular cationic antigens, however, may bind to the endothelium of the glomerular capillary wall, attract antibodies, and initiate an inflammatory response. The more marked histopathologic response to deposits in this site can be attributed to contact of the antigen with circulating antibodies and inflammatory cells. Subepithelial deposits, on the other hand, are less accessible to inflammatory cells and are more likely to cause increased glomerular permeability with minimal cellular infiltration and proliferation. Circulating immune complexes also may be trapped at subendothelial and mesangial sites.

The offending antigens in glomerulonephritis usually are not of glomerular origin, but their source is rarely determined. They may be endogenous (e.g., tumor antigens, nuclear antigens) or exogenous (e.g., infectious agents, drugs) in origin. Disease processes that may be associated with a continuous high level of antigenic exposure include chronic infections, neoplasia, and immune-mediated diseases (see Table 107–20).

The histopathologic lesions produced and the impairment of renal function in glomerulonephritis depend on the site of deposition of antigen and antibody as well as on the mediators of inflammation involved.[382, 385] There is evidence that antibody deposition alone can increase the permeability of the glomerulus without inflammation, presumably by loss of negative glomerular charge. Subepithelial deposition of complement alone can lead to glomerular damage by activation of the membrane attack complex (C5b-9).[382] Chemotactic and anaphylatoxic complement fragments (C3a, C5a, C567) may attract inflammatory cells (neutrophils, macrophages), which then damage the glomerulus by release of proteolytic enzymes and, more important, by production of reactive oxygen species. Cell-mediated injury to the glomerulus can occur without the presence of complement when inflammatory cells (neutrophils, macrophages) bind to the Fc portion of immunoglobulins (immune adherence). Platelets release cationic proteins that may induce immune complex formation and act as chemotaxins.[386] Platelets may adhere to damaged endothelium and activate the coagulation system, resulting in deposition of fibrin in glomeruli. Lastly, mesangial cells themselves can participate in the inflammatory process by release of chemical mediators. These cellular interactions are more likely to occur in subendothelial and mesangial sites than in subepithelial sites, which are less accessible to circulating inflammatory cells and complement.

Immunofluorescence studies demonstrate discontinuous granular deposition of immunoglobulins and complement in glomeruli, resulting in the so-called lumpy-bumpy pattern of fluorescence in immune complex glomerulonephritis (Figure 107–24B). In antiglomerular basement membrane disease, antibody attaches to intrinsic antigens along the glomerular basement membrane, and immunofluorescence studies demonstrate a continuous linear pattern of fluorescence (Figure 107–24A). Antiglomerular basement membrane disease is uncommon in humans (less than five per cent of cases of glomerulonephritis) and has not been documented in dogs and cats. A summary of pathologic findings on light microscopy, electron microscopy, and immunofluorescent microscopy in dogs with glomerulonephritis is listed in Table 107–21.

PATHOGENESIS OF AMYLOIDOSIS

Amyloidosis is not a single disease, but a group of diseases that have in common the extracellular deposition of fibrillar proteins with a specific biochemical conformation known as the β-pleated sheet. Amyloid deposits are characteristically green when stained with alkaline Congo red and viewed under polarized light, and this property is used in the clinical diagnosis of amyloidosis. The various amyloid syndromes in humans have been classified as reactive systemic, immunoglobulin-associated, heredofamilial, and localized.[387] Several different precursor proteins that may be deposited as amyloid have been identified (Table 107–22).[388]

Reactive systemic amyloidosis may be associated with chronic infectious, inflammatory, or neoplastic disease.[389] The amyloidogenic precursor is a serum protein that is increased in many inflammatory and neoplastic diseases by virtue of its behavior as an acute-phase reactant (Table 107–22). The source of this precursor, known as serum amyloid A protein (SAA), is the liver. In this type of amyloidosis, tissue deposits are composed of amino-terminal fragments of SAA and are called amyloid AA. Spontaneous amyloidosis in dogs and cats is an example of reactive systemic amyloidosis.[390, 391]

Although amyloid deposits may occur in many organs, deposits in the kidneys lead to progressive renal disease and death due to chronic renal failure in dogs and cats

TABLE 107–20. DISEASES ASSOCIATED WITH GLOMERULONEPHRITIS IN THE DOG AND CAT

Dogs	Cats
Infectious	
Canine adenovirus-1	Feline leukemia virus
Ehrlichiosis	Feline infectious peritonitis
Brucellosis	Polyarthritis (*Mycoplasma gateae*)
Leishmaniasis	Other
Bacterial endocarditis	
Pyometra	
Dirofilariasis	
Other	
Inflammatory	
Pancreatitis	Pancreatitis
Systemic lupus erythematosus	Systemic lupus erythematosus
Neoplastic	
Lymphosarcoma	Hemolymphatic neoplasia
Mastocytoma	Other
Other	
Idiopathic	
Many cases	Many cases
Familial	
Doberman pinschers (?)	Glomerulonephritis in sibling cats

From DiBartola SP and Chew DJ: Glomerular disease in the dog and cat. *In* Kirk RW (ed): Current Veterinary Therapy IX. Philadelphia, WB Saunders, 1986, pp 1132–1137.

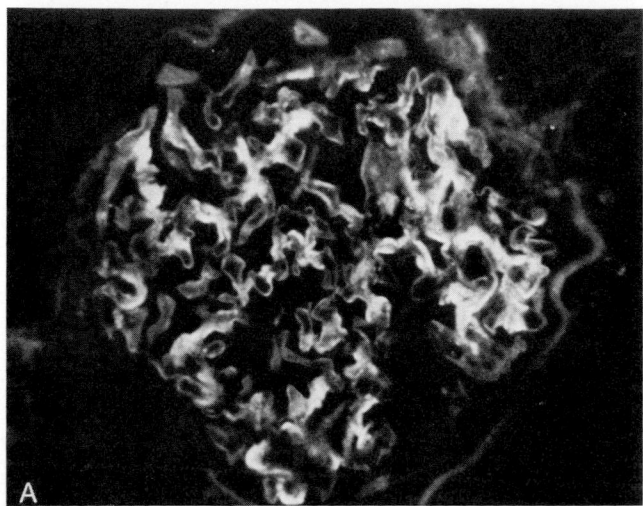

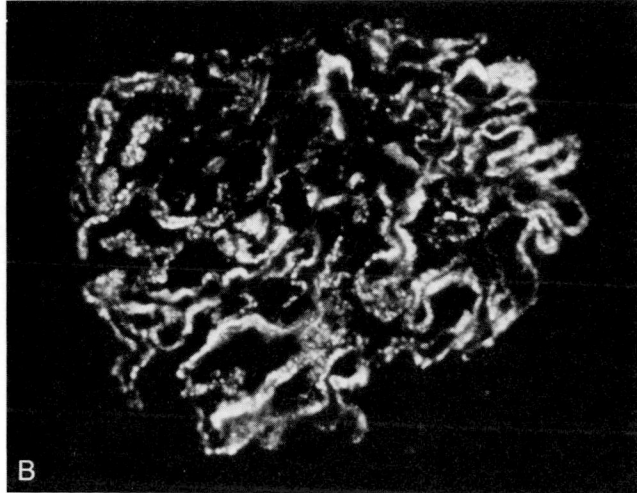

FIGURE 107–24. Immunofluorescent patterns of glomerular disease. *A,* Linear continuous immunofluorescence suggestive of anti-GBM glomerulonephritis. (Courtesy of RM Lewis and CA Smith.) *B,* Lumpy-bumpy discontinuous pattern of immunofluorescence characteristic of immune-complex glomerulonephritis. (Courtesy of R.M. Lewis and C.A. Smith.)

TABLE 107–21. PATHOLOGIC FINDINGS IN DOGS WITH GLOMERULONEPHRITIS

Reference	Light Microscopy	Immunofluorescence	Electron Microscopy
Murray 1971 (N = 1)	Mesangioproliferative	ND	Subepithelial deposits, foot process fusion
Osborne 1973 (N = 1)	Membranous	Discontinuous Igs; C	Subepithelial, subendothelial, and mesangial deposits; foot process fusion
Lewis 1976 (N = 50)	Proliferative; membranous	ND	ND
Rouse & Lewis 1975 (N = 15)	Proliferative; membranous	Discontinuous IgG; C[1]	ND
Kurtz 1972 (N = 8)	Mesangioproliferative	Discontinuous IgG; C	Mesangial and subendothelial deposits; foot process fusion[2]
Murray 1974 (N = 42)	Proliferative, membranous	IgG; C3	Subepithelial and membranous deposits
Muller-Peddinghaus 1977 (N = 94)	Membranous, membranoproliferative, mesangioproliferative, mesangiosclerosing	Discontinuous IgG; C3	Subepithelial, subendothelial, and mesangial deposits
Jaenke 1986 (N = 14)	Membranous	IgG, A	Subepithelial[3]
MacDougall 1986 (N = 40)	Focal, mesangioproliferative, endocapillary, mesangiocapillary, crescentic, sclerosing	IgG, M; C3	Mesangial, subepithelial, intramembranous, and subendothelial deposits[4]
Wright 1981 (N = 5)	Membranous	IgG; C3	Subepithelial, intramembranous, and mesangial deposits; foot process fusion[5]

ND: not determined.
[1]Negative elution studies.
[2]Subepithelial deposits not observed.
[3]Recovered or developed glomerular sclerosis.
[4]No membranous nephropathy and no minimal change disease observed.
[5]All cases were idiopathic.

TABLE 107–22. AMYLOIDOGENIC PROTEINS

Fibril Precursor	Fibril	Clinical Syndromes
Serum amyloid A protein	Amyloid A protein	Reactive amyloidosis
Immunoglobulin light chains	Immunoglobulin light chains	Primary amyloidosis; multiple myeloma; solitary amyloid nodules in skin, respiratory tract, and urogenital tracts
Prealbumin (transthyretin)	Prealbumin variants	Familial neuropathic and cardiomyopathic syndromes; senile cardiac amyloidosis
Beta-2 microglobulin	Beta-2 microglobulin	Hemodialysis-associated amyloidosis
Cystatin C (Gamma trace)	Cystatin C (Gamma trace)	Familial cerebrovascular amyloidosis
Procalcitonin	Procalcitonin	Medullary carcinoma of thyroid
Proinsulin?; Pancreatic neuropeptide?	Proinsulin?; Pancreatic neuropeptide?	Islet cell amyloidosis of pancreas
Keratin filaments	Altered keratin	Cutaneous amyloidosis
Unknown	Beta protein	Alzheimer's disease
Apolipoprotein A-II	AS_SAM	Amyloidosis in senescence-accelerated mouse
Atrial natriuretic peptide	Atrial natriuretic peptide	Atrial amyloidosis

with amyloidosis. In some cases the underlying inflammatory or neoplastic disease is detected, but in approximately 70 per cent of dogs with amyloidosis,[392] no predisposing disease can be found. Amyloidosis is uncommon in cats, and an underlying predisposing disease is rarely found.[393] In the Abyssinian cat, however, systemic amyloidosis characterized by the presence of amyloid protein AA is a familial disease.[394–396]

In immunoglobulin-associated amyloidosis such as that associated with multiple myeloma, the amyloid deposits contain amino-terminal fragments from the variable region of immunoglobulin light chains. These light chains originate from plasma cells, and such deposits are designated amyloid AL. Approximately 10 per cent of humans with multiple myeloma develop amyloidosis, but amyloidosis in dogs and cats with multiple myeloma appears to be rare.

Amyloidosis develops in only a few human patients with chronic inflammation, thus persistent elevation of SAA is not solely responsible for the disease. Other host-related factors are likely to be important in the pathogenesis of reactive systemic amyloidosis. For example, there are two predominant polymorphs of SAA, one of which appears to be more amyloidogenic. Also, genetically determined and acquired host factors may lead to defective proteolysis of SAA.[397, 398]

Heredofamilial neuropathic and cardiopathic syndromes of amyloidosis in humans have not been recognized in domestic animals. Localized amyloidosis, however, does occur in the pancreatic islets of older domestic cats.[399, 400]

PATHOPHYSIOLOGY AND COMPLICATIONS OF NEPHROTIC SYNDROME

Hyperlipemia. Hyperlipemia characterized by increases in the plasma concentrations of cholesterol, phospholipids, and triglycerides is characteristic of the nephrotic syndrome. There is an inverse relation between serum albumin and cholesterol concentrations. Decreased oncotic pressure and decreased albumin concentrations are correlated with increased total plasma cholesterol concentration, and may stimulate the synthesis of very low density lipoproteins by the liver.[401] Increasing the oncotic pressure of plasma by albumin infusion lowers the serum cholesterol concentration.

In addition, there is defective processing of lipoproteins in the nephrotic syndrome, which may be due to abnormal lipoprotein lipase (LPL) function. The defect in LPL function in turn may be related to a decrease in heparin sulfate, a cofactor for normal LPL function. The decrease in heparin sulfate may be related to loss of another glycosaminoglycan, urosomucoid, in the urine and diversion of necessary sugar intermediates as the liver attempts to replace the lost urosomucoid.[402]

Hypoalbuminemia. Factors that may contribute to decreased serum albumin concentration in the nephrotic syndrome are urinary loss of albumin and alterations in the synthesis and catabolism of albumin. The normal human liver can synthesize albumin at a rate of 8 to 14 gm/day, a rate that would be sufficient to offset similar daily urinary losses.[403] Likewise, human patients on chronic ambulatory peritoneal dialysis often have daily losses of albumin in excess of those observed in the nephrotic syndrome, yet progressive hypoalbuminemia does not occur.[404] Thus urinary loss of albumin alone cannot explain the hypoalbuminemia. Some catabolism of filtered albumin occurs in the proximal tubules of the kidney but to an extent unlikely to contribute to the hypoalbuminemia. In fact, the absolute rate of albumin catabolism in the nephrotic syndrome is decreased.[402] The liver is stimulated to increase albumin synthesis in the nephrotic syndrome but, for reasons that are unclear, does not respond sufficiently to restore serum albumin concentrations to normal.

Decreased serum albumin concentrations are not always associated with edema. Edema is not likely to occur until the serum albumin concentration falls below 1 gm/dl,[405] and ascites and edema are relatively uncommon findings in dogs with glomerular disease.[406, 407] The interstitial space normally demonstrates low compliance, which hinders loss of fluid from the intravascular space, and decreased permeability of the capillary wall to albumin may occur in the presence of hypoalbuminemia.[408] Probably the most important factor in preventing edema, however, is a dramatic increase in lymphatic flow, which occurs in response to loss of fluid from the vessel and carries protein back into the intravascular space.[402, 408] For these reasons other factors must be

Pathogenesis of ascites/edema formation in nephrotic syndrome:

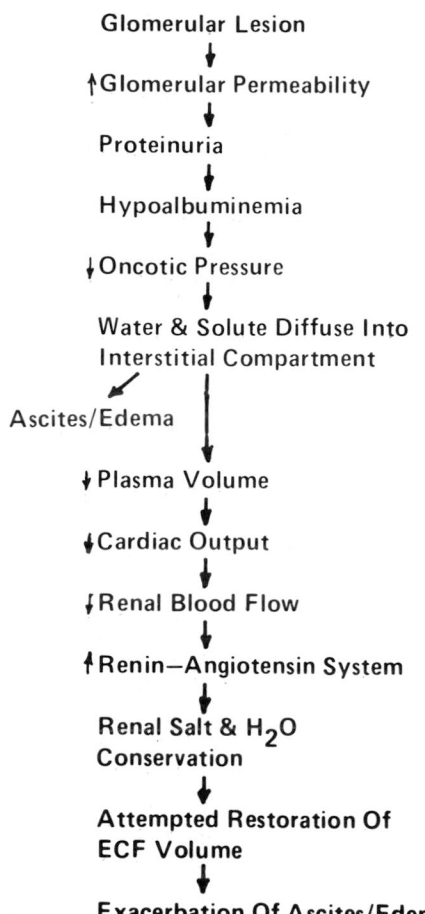

Glomerular Lesion

↓

↑Glomerular Permeability

↓

Proteinuria

↓

Hypoalbuminemia

↓

↓Oncotic Pressure

↓

Water & Solute Diffuse Into Interstitial Compartment

↓

Ascites/Edema

↓

↓Plasma Volume

↓

↓Cardiac Output

↓

↓Renal Blood Flow

↓

↑Renin—Angiotensin System

↓

Renal Salt & H$_2$O Conservation

↓

Attempted Restoration Of ECF Volume

↓

Exacerbation Of Ascites/Edema

FIGURE 107–25. Classical theory for the development of ascites and edema in nephrotic syndrome. (From Chew DJ and DiBartola SP: Manual of Small Animal Nephrology and Urology. New York, Churchill Livingstone, p 237, 1986.)

considered to explain the tendency toward edema in the nephrotic syndrome.

Sodium Retention, Hypertension, and Edema. Patients with nephrotic syndrome may retain sodium, contributing to ascites, edema, and hypertension. The classic explanation for the pathogenesis of ascites and edema formation in the nephrotic syndrome is based on altered Starling forces and activation of the renin-angiotensin system (Figure 107–25). Progressive loss of albumin in the urine leads to hypoalbuminemia, decreased oncotic pressure, and loss of water from the extracellular fluid space. Decreased effective circulating volume causes decreased RBF and activation of the renin-angiotensin system. This in turn leads to increased aldosterone production and consequent renal conservation of salt and water. This attempt to restore the extracellular fluid volume to normal is ineffective because hypoalbuminemia prevents retention of water in the vascular space. Recent evidence, however, suggests that this classic explanation is inadequate.[402, 405, 409, 410]

Studies have shown that approximately 50 per cent of nephrotic patients have increased blood volume and suppression of the renin-angiotensin system based on low or normal concentrations of renin and aldosterone.[409] Furthermore, blockade of the system by captopril, while leading to decreased aldosterone concentrations, did not prevent sodium retention,[411] and volume expansion by albumin infusions was, likewise, ineffective in reversing sodium retention.[409] When remission of the nephrotic syndrome occurs, natriuresis develops and plasma aldosterone concentrations increase, suggesting previous suppression by the sodium-retaining state.[413] These observations demonstrate that sodium retention in the nephrotic syndrome is probably due to a primary intrarenal mechanism.

In one study the intrarenal mechanism of sodium retention was localized to the distal nephron. In the model of nephrotic syndrome created by administration of puromycin aminonucleoside, Kf was decreased. The filtered load of sodium was decreased, but reabsorption of sodium in the proximal tubule and loop of Henle also was decreased so that there was no difference between control and affected kidneys in the amount of sodium reaching the distal nephron. Despite this, the affected kidneys retained sodium, thus leading to the conclusion that the intrarenal mechanism for sodium retention was in the distal nephron.[414] Others have observed a marked decrease in filtration fraction and Kf in nephrotic syndrome and emphasized the possibility of a glomerular defect in the filtration of sodium and water.[405, 415]

Some patients with nephrotic syndrome do have low blood volume as well as high plasma renin and aldosterone concentrations.[409] It is speculated that in these patients, marked hypoalbuminemia has led to volume depletion severe enough to activate the renin-angiotensin system despite the intrarenal mechanism for sodium retention.[409]

Hypercoagulability. The nephrotic syndrome is a hypercoagulable state and affected patients are predisposed to thromboembolism.[416] In dogs the pulmonary vessels are affected most commonly and sudden onset of dyspnea may be the major presenting clinical sign (Figure 107–26).[417, 418] Other vessels that may be involved include the coronary, splenic, renal, mesenteric, iliac, and brachial arteries or the portal vein.[417]

The pathogenesis of the hypercoagulable state in the nephrotic syndrome appears to be multifactorial. Alterations in the plasma concentration of many coagulation proteins have been described. In humans, clotting factors I (fibrinogen), II, V, VII, VIII, and X are increased, whereas factors IX, XI, and XII are decreased.[419, 420] The decrease in these latter factors presumably is due to urinary loss, since they have relatively low molecular weights. The observed increase in factors V and VIII is thought to be a consequence of increased hepatic protein synthesis, which occurs in response to hypoalbuminemia. In dogs with nephrotic syndrome increased plasma concentrations of fibrinogen and factor VIII have been demonstrated.[421] The increase in fibrinogen is most consistent and likely to play an important role in the hypercoagulability of the nephrotic syndrome.

Antithrombin III is an α-2 globulin with a molecular weight of 65,000 that acts as an inhibitor of coagulation factors. It is a serine protease that inactivates activated clotting factors, especially factor II but also factors IX, X, XI, and XII. Heparin acts as a cofactor for antithrom-

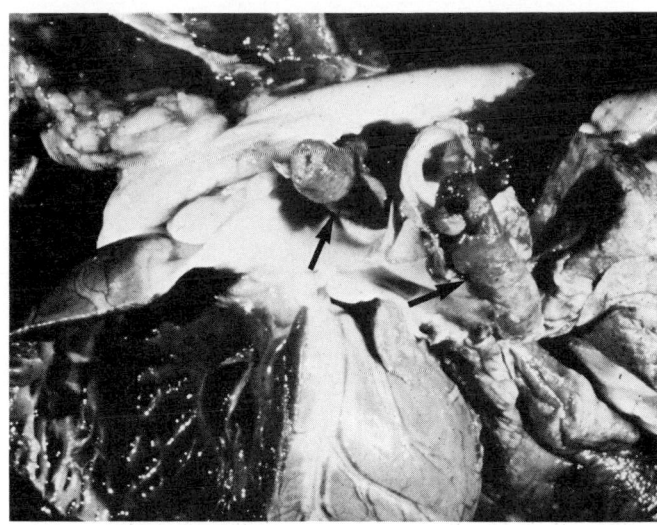

FIGURE 107–26. Thrombi in the pulmonary arteries of a dog with renal amyloidosis and pulmonary thromboembolism. (From Meuten DJ and DiBartola SP: Renal amyloidosis in two dogs presented for thromboembolic phenomena. JAAHA 16:129, 1980.)

bin III and increases its affinity for these clotting factors. The plasma concentration of antithrombin III may be markedly decreased in humans and dogs with nephrotic syndrome.[421–423] Antithrombin III is lost in the urine in the nephrotic syndrome to the extent that inactivation of activated clotting factors may be insufficient to prevent thromboembolism. In one study, dogs with antithrombin III concentrations less than 70 per cent of normal and fibrinogen concentrations greater than 300 mg/dl were considered at risk for thromboembolism.[421] On the other hand, increased concentrations of the acute phase reactant, α-2 macroglobulin, an inhibitor of thrombin, also have been reported in the nephrotic syndrome and may counterbalance the effect of decreased antithrombin III.[424]

Platelet hyperaggregability also appears to contribute to the hypercoagulable state.[425, 426] Increased fibrinogen concentration may be contributory, and the hyperaggregability of platelets is indirectly related to hypoalbuminemia. Albumin normally binds arachidonic acid, and the increased amount of arachidonic acid available for binding to platelets in hypoalbuminemic states may cause increased thromboxane A2 release from platelets, and hyperaggregability. Markedly increased platelet aggregation in response to adenosine diphosphate (ADP) was shown in platelets from dogs with nephrotic syndrome, and increasing the albumin concentration of the plasma decreased this tendency.[427] The hypercholesterolemia of the nephrotic syndrome also may contribute to platelet hyperaggregability by altering platelet membrane composition or affecting platelet adenylate cyclase response to prostaglandin E_1.[420] Impaired fibrinolysis may occur in the nephrotic syndrome due to decreased plasminogen concentrations and decreased concentrations of plasmin inhibitors.[420]

Diagnosis of Glomerular Disease

LABORATORY FINDINGS

Urinalysis. The presence of persistent proteinuria, despite unremarkable sediment findings, in urine samples collected by catheterization or cystocentesis is in-

dicative of glomerular disease. Other urinalysis findings that may be observed are cylindruria and lipiduria. Hyaline casts are often seen, but in a recent study of dogs with glomerulonephritis, granular casts were more common.[407] The presence of hematuria and red cell casts is strongly suggestive of acute glomerulonephritis in humans, but these findings are rarely observed in dogs and cats with glomerular disease.

Classification and Localization of Proteinuria. The hallmark of glomerular disease is proteinuria. Proteinuria can be classified as prerenal, renal, or postrenal in origin.[40] Prerenal proteinuria may occur when there has been excessive release of proteins that are normally bound in the plasma to other proteins or overproduction of proteins normally reabsorbed and degraded by the tubular epithelial cells. Examples are myoglobinuria and hemoglobinuria with saturation of transport proteins or Bence Jones proteinuria in multiple myeloma, owing to overproduction of immunoglobulin light chains. Postrenal proteinuria is caused by addition of protein to the urine as a result of secretions or diseases of the lower urinary tract or genital tract. Renal proteinuria includes benign transient proteinuria induced by stress, fever, exercise, or extremes of temperature as well as pathologic renal proteinuria. Pathologic renal proteinuria may result from increased transport of proteins across glomeruli or leakage of proteins from damaged tubular cells or parenchymal inflammation. Care must be taken by the clinician to localize proteinuria by careful consideration of the history, physical examination findings, method of urine collection, and urinary sediment findings.

Determination of Urine Protein Concentration. Urine protein determinations should be performed on the supernatant of the urine sample, and results should always be considered in light of the total urine solute concentration as reflected by the USG. For example, 500 mg of protein excreted in a urine volume of 500 ml (higher total solute concentration) would result in a urine protein concentration of 100 mg/dl (2+), while the same amount of protein excreted in a urine volume of 2000 ml (lower total solute concentration) would result in a urine protein concentration of only 25 mg/dl (1+).[428]

Routine screening for proteinuria is performed using dipstick reagent pads containing tetrabromphenol blue. This qualitative method is colorimetric and much more sensitive to albumin than to globulins. False-positive results can occur with alkaline urine or urine contaminated by benzalkonium chloride (Zephiran), while false-negative results can occur with very acidic or dilute urine. The sensitivity of this test is about 20 mg/dl.

If the presence of globulins is suspected, another screening test should be used, such as the turbidimetric sulfosalicylic acid test, which is only slightly more sensitive to albumin than to globulins. The sulfosalicylic acid test is somewhat more sensitive than the tetrabromphenol blue test (5 to 10 mg/dl), but radiographic contrast agents and several drugs (e.g., penicillins, cephalosporins, sulfisoxazole, tolbutamide) may cause false-positive results whereas very alkaline or dilute samples may cause false-negative results. If the sulfosalicylic acid test is positive but the tetrabromphenol blue test is negative, the heat test or, preferably, urine immunoelectrophoresis should be used to determine the presence of Bence Jones proteins.

Quantitative tests of proteinuria have a sensitivity of 2 mg/dl and are equally sensitive to albumin and globulins. The trichloroacetic acid–ponceau S and Coomassie brilliant blue tests are two such procedures that are used to quantitate proteinuria in the presence of suspected glomerular disease.

Estimation of Daily Urinary Protein Loss. Quantitation of proteinuria may be achieved by measuring the 24-hour urine protein excretion or evaluating a urine protein–urine creatinine ratio (U_p/U_{cr}). Reported values for 24-hour urine protein excretion in dogs, using quantitative techniques for protein determination (trichloroacetic acid–ponceau S or Coomassie brilliant blue), range from 2.3 ± 1.2 mg/kg/day to 13.9 ± 7.71 mg/kg/day.[40, 429–434] In the cat, a value of 17.4 ± 9.05 mg/kg/day was obtained.[41] Studies have shown that dogs with glomerular disease have markedly increased 24-hour urine protein excretion values, and those with amyloidosis generally have the highest 24-hour urine protein excretion values (Table 107–23).[406, 431–434]

The U_p/U_{cr} eliminates the necessity of a 24-hour urine collection and has been shown to be highly correlated with 24-hour values.[431–434] Its value lies in the fact that although both U_{cr} and U_p concentrations are affected by total urine solute concentration, their ratio is not. Reported mean U_p/U_{cr} values for normal dogs have ranged from 0.076 ± 0.044 to 0.28 ± 0.24.[431–434] In recent studies U_p/U_{cr} results were not significantly affected by differences in sex, method of urine collection, fasted versus fed states, or time of day of collection.[434, 435] Values were slightly higher in exercise-restricted (hospitalized) dogs as compared with those without exercise restriction (outpatients).[435] Dogs with proteinuria on screening urinalysis have been shown to have increased U_p/U_{cr} values.[431–434] In only one of these studies, however, were glomerular lesions documented by biopsy or necropsy. In that study, dogs with amyloidosis had the highest U_p/U_{cr} values.[433] There is, however, a high degree of overlap between dogs with glomerulonephritis and those with amyloidosis with regard to their 24-hour urine protein excretion and U_p/U_{cr} values.[406, 433] Thus renal biopsy remains the only reliable way to differentiate these two diseases.

Serum Chemistry Findings. Hypoalbuminemia and hypercholesterolemia are found in the majority of dogs with glomerular disease.[406, 407] Total serum protein concentrations, however, are usually normal or increased due to increases in the α, β, and gamma fractions, which may occur because of chronic inflammation often associated with glomerulonephritis or amyloidosis.[407] If glomerular disease has led to chronic renal failure, the remaining serum biochemical values will be consistent with that syndrome.

Histologic Findings. Renal biopsy is the only reliable way to differentiate glomerulonephritis from amyloidosis. The distinction is important because amyloidosis is a progressive disease with a poor prognosis, while the clinical course of glomerulonephritis appears to be more variable. Routine light microscopy using hematoxylin and eosin, Congo red, and thioflavine-T stains is sufficient for the diagnosis of amyloidosis. The diagnosis of glomerulonephritis, however, often requires immuno-

TABLE 107–23. EVALUATION OF PROTEINURIA

	Reference Number							
	429	431	432	40	430	433	434	435
24-hr value (mg/kg)	3.8; 7.0	4.8 ± 3.7	2.3 ± 1.2	13.9 ± 7.71	7.9 ± 5.6	2.45 ± 2.26	7.6 ± 5.47	NA
U_{PR}/U_{CR}	NA	0.17 ± 0.15	0.076 ± 0.044	NA	NA	0.09 ± 0.09	0.09 ± 0.08	0.153 to 0.401
Number normal	10	8	16	17	29	19	14	10
Number abnormal	0	10	14	0	0	38	9	0
R value 24 hr vs. U_{PR}/U_{CR}		0.86	0.975	NA	NA	0.8	NA	NA
Method	TCA CBB	TCA	CBB	TCA	TCA	TCA	NA	CBB
Comments	[1]					[2]	[3]	[4]

TCA: Trichloroacetic acid; CBB: Coomassie brilliant blue.
NA: not available.
[1] 10 kg body weight assumed; higher value for CBB method.
[2] Dogs with amyloidosis had the highest values.
[3] No difference between sexes or between day or night collection; higher values in hospitalized dogs compared with outpatients.
[4] No difference between fasted or fed state and no differences attributed to time of day of collection.

pathology and electron microscopy for adequate characterization of the lesions.

In humans, the various types of glomerulonephritis have been classified according to the types of immunoglobulins present, their location within glomeruli, and the pathologic response of the glomeruli to their presence. These histologic types of glomerulonephritis have been correlated with specific clinical syndromes. The histologic features of glomerulonephritis in dogs and cats have been well characterized, but there has been no correlation with specific clinical syndromes.

In dogs, light microscopy usually has resulted in the classification of glomerulonephritis as membranous, proliferative, or membranoproliferative (mesangiocapillary).[406, 407, 436–441] In a few studies, however, some dogs also had mesangioproliferative and mesangiosclerosing lesions.[438, 439, 442] Immunofluorescent studies have documented the presence of IgG and C3 in glomeruli more often than IgM and IgA.[407, 436–440] Deposits typically occur in a granular discontinuous pattern (see Figure 107–24B).[406, 407, 438–440] In one study IgA deposition was common.[430] Linear continuous fluorescence reminiscent of antiglomerular basement membrane disease has been observed in dogs, but elution studies to detect antibodies to glomerular antigens were negative (see Figure 107–24A).[406, 407] Ultrastructural studies have shown the presence of subepithelial, subendothelial, and mesangial deposits, as well as foot process fusion.[436–439, 442–446] In one study subepithelial deposits were conspicuously absent.[439] These findings are summarized in Table 107–21.

In cats, glomerulonephritis usually is characterized by diffuse thickening of the glomerular capillary wall without cellular proliferation (membranous nephropathy).[447] Immunopathologic studies have demonstrated the presence of IgG and C3 most commonly, followed by IgM, and IgA least commonly.[448, 449] Ultrastructurally, there are loss of foot processes and electron-dense deposits located in subepithelial or intramembranous locations.

In the kidney of the dog, amyloid deposits are first observed in the glomerular mesangium (Figure 107–27). Deposits eventually enlarge and obliterate the normal glomerular architecture so that glomeruli are hypocellular and occasionally enlarged. In the cat, glomerular deposits occur in about 75 per cent of affected animals,[396] and usually are located in mesangial and subendothelial locations.[395] Occasionally, however, these deposits can extend through the glomerular basement membrane to form densely packed, radially oriented bundles in subepithelial locations resembling immune complex deposits in periodic acid–methenamine–stained sections (Figure 107–28A and B). In most cats, however, the medullary deposition of amyloid is more striking.[393, 395, 396, 450] and has clinically important consequences, such as isosthenuria and papillary necrosis (Figure 107–29A and B).

Upper Urinary Tract Infection and Pyelonephritis

UTI occurs whenever organisms colonize urine or urinary tissue that is normally sterile, which includes all sites proximal to the urethra.[48, 59, 83, 106] The value of quantitative bacterial culture to document the presence of UTI is discussed in the diagnostic portion of this chapter. Isolation of significant numbers of bacteria, however, does not localize the site of infection in the urinary tract. It is not known how often UTI in dogs and cats occurs exclusively in the lower urinary tract (bladder and urethra) or upper urinary tract (renal parenchyma, renal pelvis, and ureter), and how often both are affected.[451–453] This uncertainty reflects the lack of reliable laboratory tests to verify the presence of upper UTI.[451, 454, 455] Furthermore, routine culture of renal pelvis, renal parenchyma, or ureter is not performed during necropsy. Techniques such as nephropyelocentesis and ureteral catheterization can be used to obtain samples for bacterial culture of the upper urinary tract but are not commonly used.[456] In addition, bacterial isolation from renal pelvic urine is not proof that invasion of the renal parenchyma has occurred. Organisms were isolated from samples obtained by nephropyelocentesis in approximately 50 per cent of female dogs with UTI on the basis of quantitative bacterial culture of samples obtained by cystocentesis.[457]

The prevalence of renal disease and impaired renal function resulting from naturally occurring UTI is unknown in dogs and cats. It is sometimes said that lower UTI poses substantial risk for upper UTI, pyelonephritis, impairment of renal function, and progression to end-stage renal disease, but these claims are unsubstantiated. In humans, it is thought that UTI rarely results in progression to end-stage renal disease in the absence of urinary obstruction or reflux.[458]

UPPER URINARY TRACT INFECTION AND PYELONEPHRITIS IN CLINICAL ANIMALS

The organisms causing upper UTI and pyelonephritis are similar to those responsible for lower UTI. *E. coli* is the most frequently isolated organism in dogs, while *Proteus, Staphylococcus, Streptococcus, Enterobacter,* and *Pseudomonas* occur sporadically. *Corynebacterium renale* and *Salmonella* occur rarely.[459, 460] The observation that upper UTI is associated with the same organisms that cause lower UTI suggests a role for the ascent of bacteria to the kidneys from the lower urinary tract.

The role of anaerobic bacteria, *Chlamydia,* and *Mycoplasma* in upper UTI or pyelonephritis has not yet been defined because the special media required for their isolation are not commonly used. *Mycoplasma* has been isolated from canine urine and may cause clinical signs, but localization of the infection to the lower or upper urinary tract has not been accomplished.[95] Studies in humans and rats indicate that *Mycoplasma* spp. can play a role in acute or chronic pyelonephritis.[461–463] *Mycoplasma* also has been isolated from the canine kidney, but not in association with renal disease.[101, 464–466] *Chlamydia* spp. are pathogenic in the human lower urinary tract, but their role in the upper urinary tract is unknown. Fungal organisms are isolated uncommonly from the upper urinary tract, but the kidneys can be involved in systemic mycoses. Acute renal infection by leptospires can occur after bacteremia,[467] but the clinical course is quite different from that associated with the common ascending uropatho-

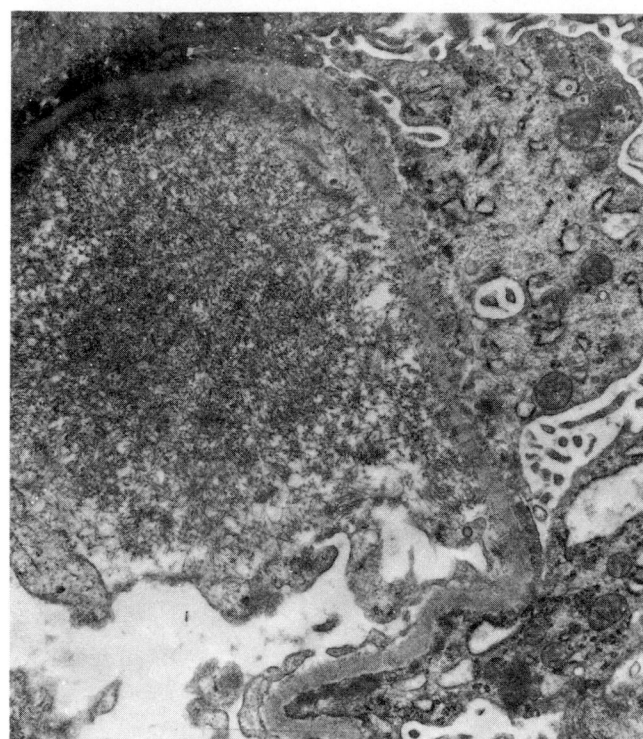

FIGURE 107–27. Transmission electron micrograph showing amyloid deposition in the glomerulus of a dog. (Courtesy of R. Minor.)

FIGURE 107–28. Glomerular amyloid deposition in a cat. High power light microscopic stained with PAMS (A) and transmission electron micrograph (B) to show radially oriented bundles resembling spiking. (A From Chew et al: JAVMA[394]; B From Boyce et al: Vet Pathol.[395])

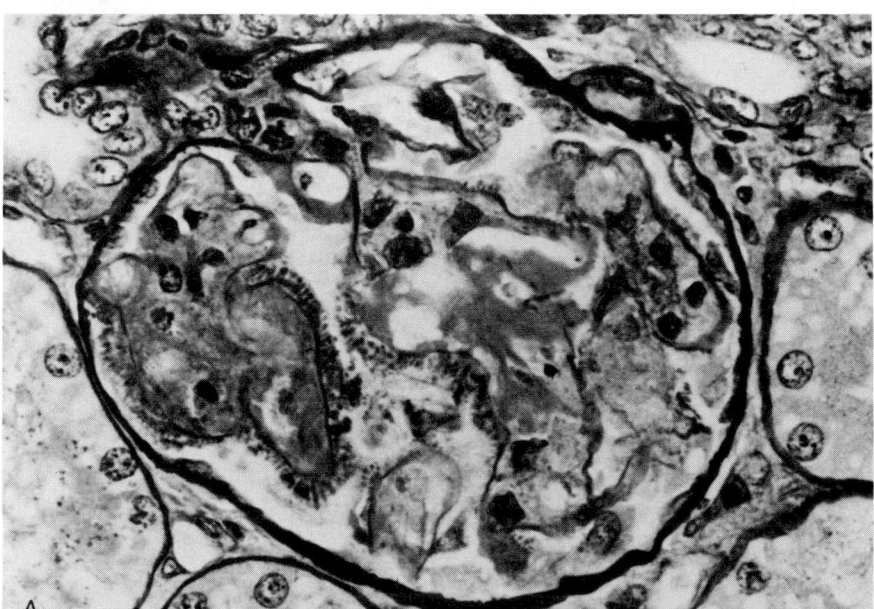

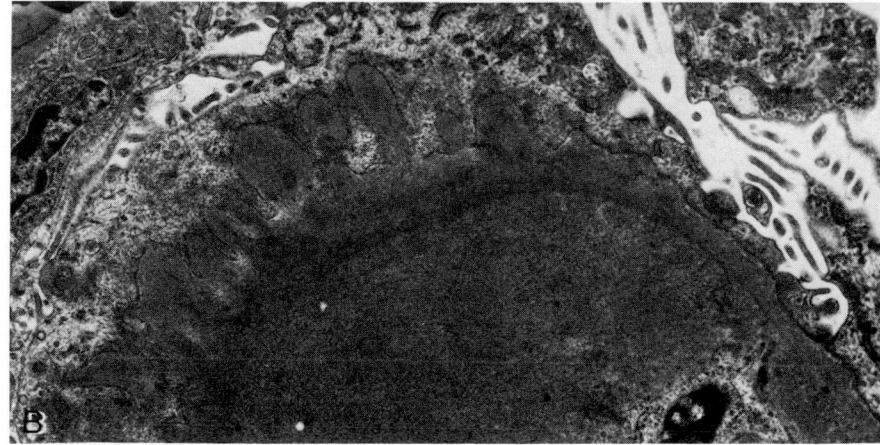

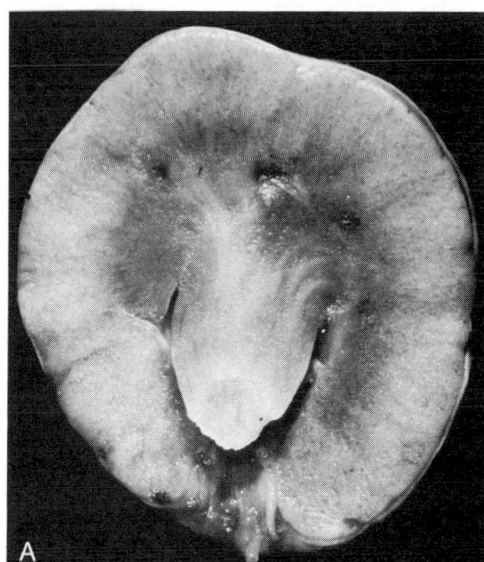

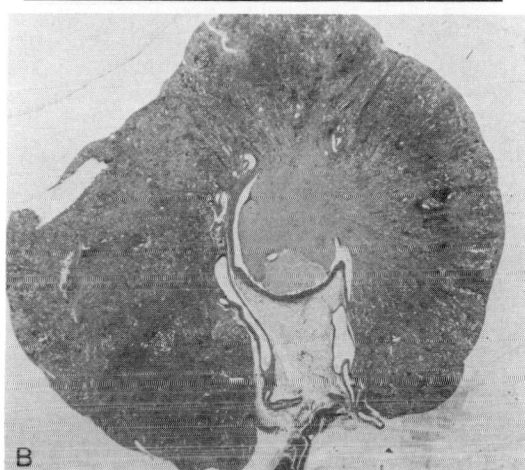

FIGURE 107–29. Medullary amyloid deposition in a cat leading to papillary necrosis (*A*, gross specimen; *B*, low power microscopic view.)

gens. Leptospiral organisms are difficult to isolate, and the special techniques required for their isolation are used infrequently.

Given their presence in the kidney, the role of bacteria in acute pyelonephritis is clearly important. Neutrophilic and mononuclear infiltration, as well as bacteria in the renal interstitium and tubular lumina, are observed in initial stages (Figure 107–30). Chronic pyelonephritis is characterized by pyelitis, mononuclear parenchymal inflammation, and a variable amount of fibrosis and deformity. These effects usually are attributed to bacteria, which may or may not be present at the time of diagnosis.[460, 468, 469] Tubulointerstitial disease with mononuclear cell infiltrates is a nonspecific reaction to a variety of renal insults, but bacteria appear to be an important factor when inflammation of the renal pelvis and medullary fibrosis also are present.[101] Intact bacteria often are not demonstrated histologically at this time and cultures are often negative.

Pyelitis or pyelonephritis was observed histologically in 2 per cent of normal beagles,[470] in 15 per cent[471] or 19 per cent[459] of apparently normal mixed breed dogs, and in 8 per cent of dogs with various types of nephri-

tis.[472] Chronic pyelitis and pyelonephritis have been described more frequently in the bitch, but in another study male dogs were affected more frequently.[459, 471] Bacteriuria has been observed more commonly in female dogs by some, which could place females at increased risk to develop pyelonephritis.[94, 471, 473] It also appears that older dogs have a greater risk of developing pyelitis than do younger dogs.[459] In a prospective necropsy study of cats bacteria were isolated from the kidneys in only one cat with chronic tubulointerstitial disease, but the author concluded that the histologic lesions in most cats were initiated by bacteria.[474] In a recent study the frequency of chronic pyelonephritis in cats with chronic renal disease was 9.5 per cent, but isolation of bacteria from renal tissue was not attempted.[1] Chronic pyelonephritis appears to be more common than acute pyelonephritis.

Urinary Tract Defenses

ANTIBACTERIAL PROPERTIES OF URINE

Is normal urine a good culture medium? The answer to this question depends both on the bacterial species and on the animal from which the urine is obtained. For example, *E. coli* grows readily in normal human urine but often is killed by normal canine urine, whereas *Staphylococcus* spp. grow well in the urine of both species.[475, 476] In general, urine will support the growth of common uropathogens over a pH range of 6.0 to 7.0 and an osmolality range of 300 to 600,[475] whereas anaer-

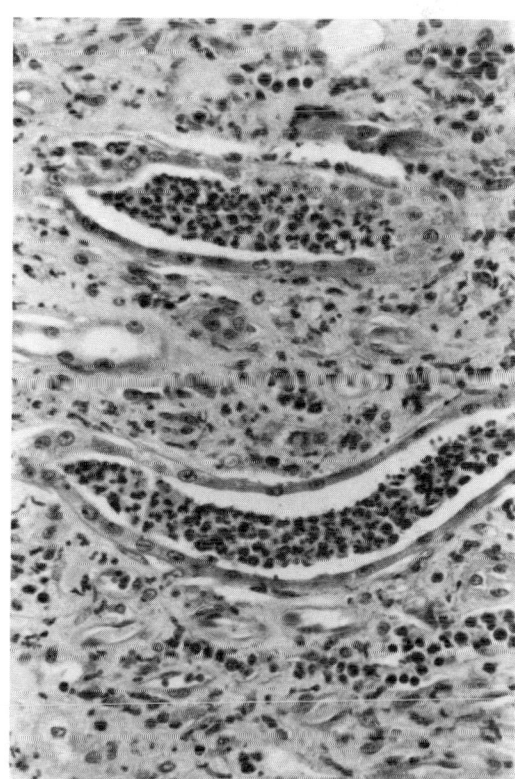

FIGURE 107–30. Chronic pyelonephritis histology. Note white blood cells in casts and in the interstitium, as well as mononuclear infiltrate, fibroplasia, and tubular dropout.

obic bacteria grow poorly under these circumstances. In general, broth media support bacterial growth much better than urine. The number of organisms inoculated into urine is also an important factor, since the bactericidal properties of normal urine are more effective when the inoculum is small.[475, 477] Urine is more inhibitory to bacterial growth *in vivo* than *in vitro* because bacterial numbers can double within 20 minutes *in vitro* compared with 50 minutes *in vivo*.[101] These effects may be due to a lack of exposure to air *in vivo*.

The inhibitory properties of normal urine on bacterial growth have been attributed to osmolality and pH as well as to the urea and ammonia present in urine. Of these factors, osmolality is the most important, followed by pH.[475] Urine osmolality may have a bacteriostatic or bactericidal effect, depending on its magnitude. Gram-positive bacteria are better able to survive in highly concentrated urine than are gram-negative organisms,[477, 478] an effect that may be particularly important in cats, in which high urine osmolality may explain the relative lack of bacterial UTI in this species.[475] Cats undergoing diuresis, however, become susceptible to UTI caused by gram-negative bacteria as a result of decreased urine osmolality.[479] High urine osmolality affects growth of gram-negative bacteria to a variable extent. For example, osmolality greater than 1200 mOsm/kg is bactericidal for *E. coli*, but similar inhibition of *Proteus* may require urine osmolality greater than 1700.[475]

The inhibitory effect of high urine osmolality on bacterial growth is operative in the lower urinary tract, but in the kidney, the situation is more complex. In the kidney, high urine osmolality can be deleterious to the host, as it can favor the survival of bacteria without cell walls and interfere with the renal medullary inflammatory response (see below).

Urine pH < 6.0 or > 7.0 is inhibitory to bacterial growth,[475] but the effect of acidic urine is greater. Furthermore, the alkaline pH required to significantly inhibit bacterial growth is beyond the physiologic range. Highly acidic urine increases the lag phase before bacterial replication and decreases the rate of replication, resulting in reduced quantitative growth.[475]

NORMAL VOIDING

Frequent and complete emptying of the urinary bladder mechanically flushes out small numbers of bacteria that ascend into the bladder (hydrokinetic washout).[83, 101, 475] This effect also maintains the number of bacteria in the urethra at a low level.[83] Although helpful, this mechanism cannot eliminate all bacteria when the inoculum is large.[83, 477] In addition, complete emptying of the bladder minimizes the residual urine volume available for bacterial replication, facilitates close contact of mucosal surface with remaining bacteria (intrinsic bactericidal factor), and maintains optimal blood flow to the mucosa of the bladder.[83, 477] Sterile urine entering the bladder from the ureters dilutes the small number of bacteria remaining in the bladder.[101]

The unidirectional flow of urine from renal pelvis to bladder by way of the ureters and from bladder to the exterior by way of the urethra is an important factor in preventing the ascent of bacteria.[83, 475] Retrograde flow is called reflux and can occur occasionally in normal animals when urine from the bladder enters the ureters (vesicoureteral reflux),[453, 480, 481] or when urine in the urethra enters the bladder during voiding.[101] Vesicoureteral reflux is prevented in most normal animals by compression of the intramural portion of the ureter in the bladder wall during bladder filling, but this effect depends on the ratio of ureteral length to width within the bladder wall.[480, 481] Ureteral peristalsis contributes to unidirectional flow of urine into the bladder and helps to prevent transmission of intraluminal bladder pressure to the kidney during voiding if vesicoureteral reflux is present.[482]

INITIATION AND MAINTENANCE OF URINARY TRACT INFECTION

The pathophysiology of naturally occurring acute or chronic pyelonephritis in dogs and cats has not been studied; consequently most knowledge about pyelonephritis in these species is derived from animals infected with *E. coli* experimentally. The normal kidney is very resistant to infection after intravenous injection of organisms or their inoculation into the bladder.[460] Prior renal damage facilitates bacterial colonization in the kidney possibly by decreasing RBF or increasing tissue pressure.[477] Such changes can occur after temporary ureteral obstruction, hypotension, renal arterial or venous clamping, renal thermocautery, massage of renal tissue, multiple needle punctures, ureteral meatotomy, or the placement of foreign bodies in the urinary tract.[101, 451, 477, 483, 484] The greater the number of bacterial organisms challenging the kidney, the more likely that renal colonization will occur by either the ascending or hematogenous route.[477] A summary of experimental ascending and hematogenous upper UTI and pyelonephritis in dogs has been tabulated in a recent review.[460]

The likelihood that UTI will become established largely depends on exposure to uropathogenic bacteria, the magnitude of that exposure, the presence of epithelial receptors for uropathogens, properties of the uroepithelium opposing bacterial adherence, antibacterial properties of urine, the pattern of voiding, the integrity of intrinsic mucosal defense mechanisms, and the presence of normal urinary tract anatomy.[83, 475] Defense mechanisms of the lower urinary tract are vital, since they constitute the first line of defense against UTI. The defense mechanisms of the lower urinary tract are discussed in greater detail in Chapter 112.

Exposure of the lower urinary tract to uropathogens is the initial step in the development of lower UTI (Figure 107–31*A* and *B*). The origin of bacteria causing UTI in dogs and cats has not been established. Based on studies in women, it is assumed that gram-negative organisms from the native bowel flora gain access to the urinary tract from the patient's perineum. Contamination from the skin, environment, vagina, or prepuce may be the source of gram-positive UTI. It is proposed that there is contamination and initial colonization of the perineum, followed by sequential ascent into the vagina or prepuce, urethra, bladder, ureter, renal pelvis, renal medulla, and renal cortex. As bacterial numbers

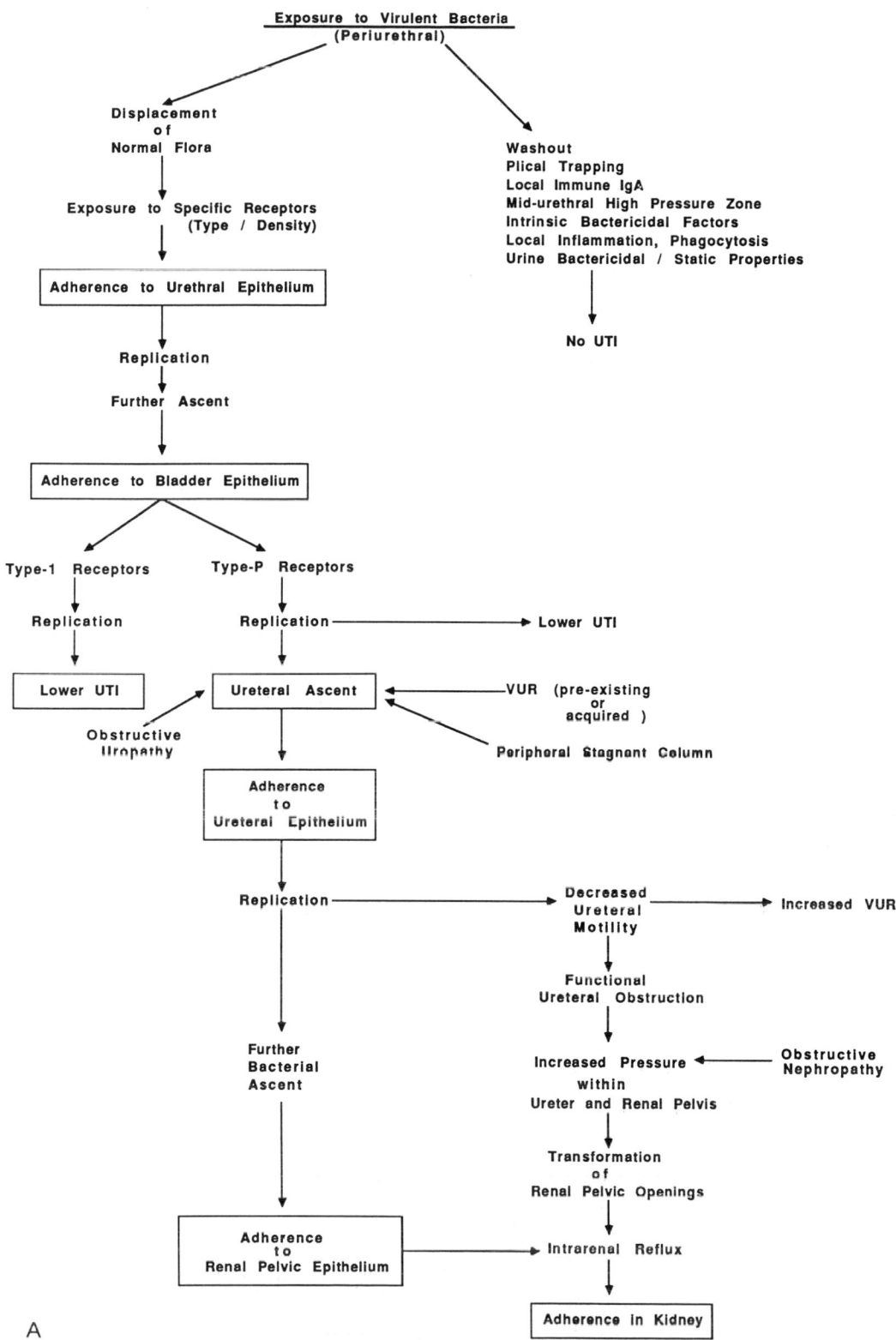

A

FIGURE 107–31. General schematic representation for initiation and establishment of urinary tract infection via the ascending route. Proposed pathways are not proven in all instances, and may vary by specific bacterial organism. A details possible events from initial exposure until entry into the kidney and B details potential pathways following bacterial entry into renal parenchyma. UTI = urinary tract infection; VUR = vesicoureteral reflux, THP = Tamm-Horsfall mucoprotein. (Adapted and modified from Roberts JA: Pathogenesis of pyelonephritis. J Urol 129:1102, 1983.)

Illustration continued on following page

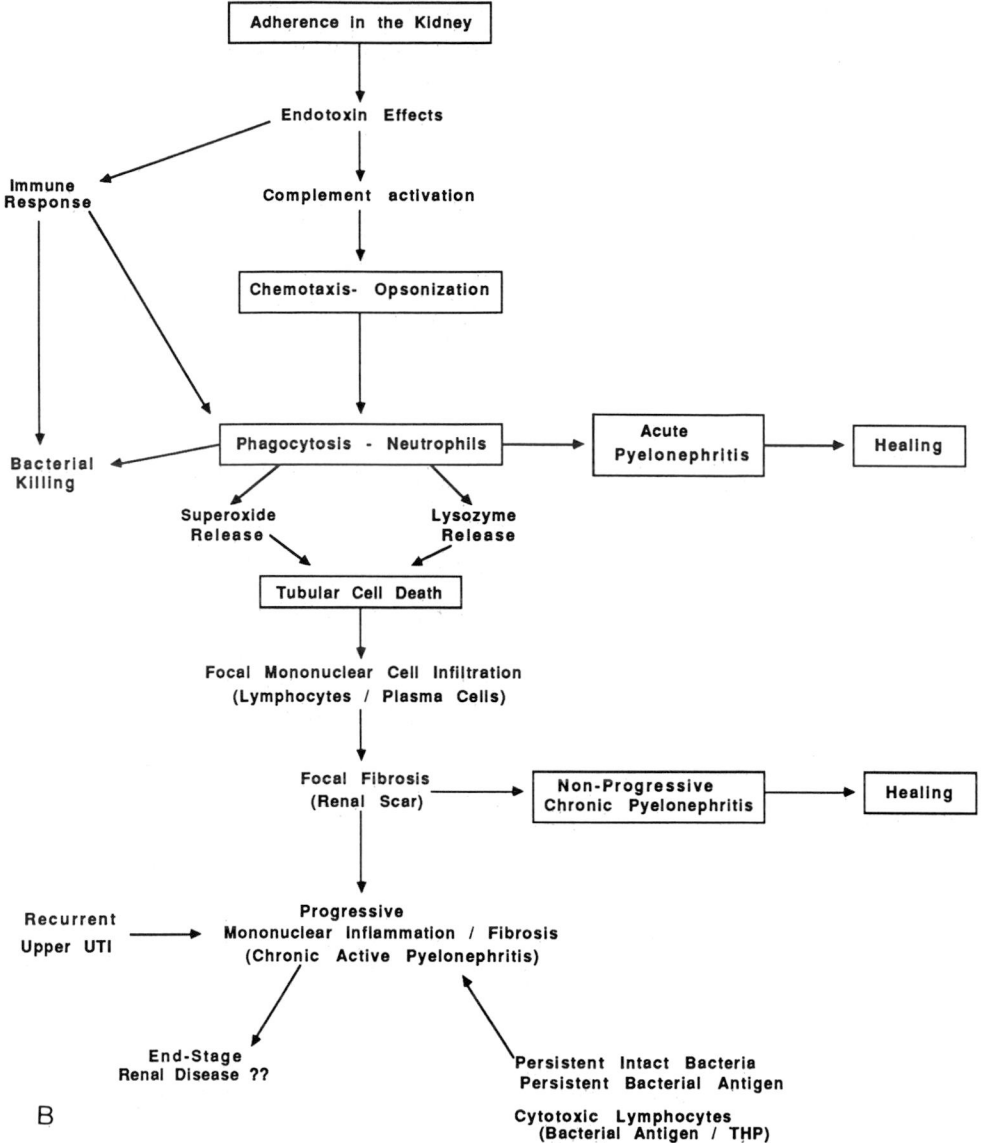

Figure 107–31 *Continued*

increase distally, colonization of more proximal sites can follow, if conditions are favorable. It is probable that upper UTI and pyelonephritis develop clinically only when obstruction to urinary flow is superimposed on bacterial infection of the lower urinary tract.[101, 105, 452, 460, 468, 469]

Hematogenous and lymphatic routes of invasion are also possible but are far less common than the ascending route.[83, 460, 485] This is supported by studies in humans that show no increased occurrence of upper UTI or pyelonephritis after bacteremia.[460] Another possible route is direct extension of organisms from an infected site near the urinary tract, as can occur in patients with perinephric abscesses, wounds, or infected surgical sites.

The ability of bacteria to establish upper UTI differs by species and strain. For example, specific strains of *E. coli* are more likely than others to produce UTI in humans, and only a few cause pyelonephritis (i.e., nephritogenic strains).[101, 460, 469] Many interacting factors determine the virulence of a specific microorganism, including surface antigens, capsule, pili, and motility.[83,]

[101, 453, 485] The ability to produce urease, β-lactamase, colicins, hemolysins, and R-plasmids, and to ferment dulcitol, in addition to other poorly characterized factors, may also contribute to virulence.[486] Bacterial surface antigens, such as the O and K antigens of *E. coli*, may be important in conferring virulence, while the density of K antigen is important in the development of pyelonephritis.[101] The virulence of *Pseudomonas* is enhanced by a heavy mucopolysaccharide capsule that inhibits phagocytosis,[101] and the motility of *Proteus* may facilitate ascension in the urinary tract.[83] *Proteus* and *Staphylococcus* may produce a urease that is directly toxic to renal tubules.[101] Bacterial virulence factors also are probably important in the development of UTI in dogs and cats,[457, 487] but whether specific nephritogenic strains exist is not known. In one study, *E. coli* strains from dogs with acute UTI had greater antibiotic resistance and R-plasmid transfer than did isolates from humans with acute infection.[486]

Exposure to uropathogenic bacteria alone usually is not sufficient for the development of UTI. Rather, cell receptors capable of binding pathogenic bacteria may be required to allow bacterial adherence and replication.[468, 469, 477, 485] In humans, individuals prone to UTI have uroepithelial cells that bind uropathogenic bacteria more easily than those of normal people.[477] Such differences could be a consequence of both the presence and the density of specific receptors.[469] Furthermore, occupation of receptor sites by the normal bacterial flora may be an important defense mechanism that prevents binding of uropathogenic bacteria,[232] or alternatively, the normal flora may utilize essential nutrients required by uropathogens.[485] In a study of experimentally induced *E. coli* UTI in dogs, prior infection with canine adenovirus greatly increased the frequency of lower and upper UTI,[488] possibly by induction of increased numbers or availability of receptors.[485]

Adhesins are proteins found on bacterial surfaces that facilitate binding to specific epithelial receptors.[453, 469, 485] They can be seen on electron microscopy as filamentous, rigid projections. These projections are called pili (fimbriae in gram-negative organisms and fibrillae in gram-positive organisms), and are present on most gram-negative bacteria and on some gram-positive ones.[485] A variety of adhesins may be present, and two have been characterized in *E. coli*: mannose-sensitive (type-1) and mannose-resistant (P-fimbria).[101, 468, 485] One or both of these may be present on the same organism. Mannose-sensitive receptors are present on mucin, Tamm-Horsfall mucoprotein (THP), epithelial cells of the bladder and urethra, and white blood cells.[469, 477] Binding to mucin receptors may represent a host defense mechanism as bound bacteria are swept away during voiding,[485] but binding to urothelial cells can favor colonization. P-fimbria receptors are present throughout the urinary tract but are particularly numerous in the renal tubules, and bacteria that possess these fimbriae are more able to establish upper UTI and pyelonephritis.[477] The number and type of fimbriae expressed by a uropathogen can change, thus affecting bacterial virulence. For example, *E. coli* may lose type-1 fimbriae after entry into the renal parenchyma, reducing the likelihood for phagocytosis by neutrophils.[477] In experimentally infected rats *Proteus* spp. with more numerous pili colonized the renal pelvis more readily; however, numerous pili were a liability for bacterial survival once within the renal parenchyma.[489] Densely fimbriated canine strains of *E. coli* with enhanced virulence for the lower urinary tract can develop *in vitro* after serial passage in broth.[457]

Defense mechanisms of the perineum, vagina, prepuce, and urethra have not been well characterized. Acidic pH and local immunoglobulin secretion (IgA) may be important in the vagina,[477] but the perineum and prepuce are largely unstudied. Ultrastructural studies of the canine urethra have demonstrated surface projections from cells of the distal urethra resembling those found in the vagina (microvilli), while projections from cells of the proximal urethra resemble those found in transitional cells of the bladder (microplicae).[453, 490] Microplicae may be important in trapping bacteria and preventing ascent. The normal urethra possesses a functional area of high pressure (midurethral high-pressure zone) that represents a barrier to bacterial ascent when organisms are inoculated distally.[491] UTI may be more

common in female dogs than in males. If so, the relatively wide and short urethra of the female and the presence of prostatic antibacterial secretions in the male may in part explain this predisposition.[83]

The normal bladder is inherently resistant to UTI because of the efficiency of hydrokinetic washout during voiding, the properties of urothelium that resist bacterial adhesion, the intrinsic bactericidal properties of the mucosal surface, and the access to circulating inflammatory cells.[83, 477, 485, 492] Transitional cells of the bladder secrete a mucopolysaccharide (glycosaminoglycan) layer that inhibits adherence of bacteria.[485, 493, 494] Experimental disruption of this layer results in a nonspecific increase in bacterial adherence.[451, 457, 477] The effectiveness of this layer may vary throughout the estrous cycle, since estrogen and progesterone can affect its synthesis and secretion. The increased susceptibility of ovariectomized rabbits to experimental UTI was attributed to a lack of estrogen on this protective layer. The frequency of UTI in spayed female dogs was greater than that in intact females in this same study, suggesting a possible role for an altered glycosaminoglycan layer.[494]

Lower UTI is established when bacterial adherence and replication exceed washout of organisms during voiding, antibacterial effects of urine, and the intrinsic bactericidal properties of the bladder. Maintenance of lower UTI, however, does not imply that bacteria will necessarily ascend to the ureters and kidney.

Inoculation of bacteria from the bladder into the ureters may occur when vesicoureteral reflux (VUR) is present. Highly virulent organisms in the lower urinary tract can cause upper UTI and pyelonephritis in the absence of detectable VUR,[101] but less virulent organisms require VUR. VUR is common in puppies less than two months of age and decreases in frequency with age.[400, 401] It still can be encountered in approximately ten per cent of normal dogs seven years of age or older.[480] VUR is considered to be physiologically normal in puppies, and normally is corrected as the length of intramural ureter continues to increase during growth. It may be that VUR in mature dogs is a result of inadequate development of the intramural ureter, but VUR also can be acquired after lower UTI, urinary calculi, neurogenic disorders of micturition, and urinary obstruction.[480, 495] The presence of cystic calculi in female dogs was frequently associated with VUR in one study, while male dogs with calculi exhibited VUR much less frequently.[495] VUR also can occur frequently in dogs with experimental UTI, particularly that caused by *Proteus*[483] and *E. coli*.[496] Successful treatment of UTI can result in the resolution of VUR in experimental dogs,[483] adding further credence that UTI can cause VUR. Presumably, UTI caused anatomic alterations in the bladder wall that changed the obliquity and ratio of length to width of the intramural ureter. High voiding pressures can occur during lower UTI and contribute to VUR in dogs, but VUR and UTI can also occur in the presence of low voiding pressure.[483] When present, VUR extended to the renal pelvis in more than 90 per cent of affected dogs in one study,[480] suggesting that VUR may provide an opportunity to inoculate the renal pelvic epithelium with organisms from the lower urinary tract. One investigator noted a close association between the presence of VUR and histologic evidence of pyelonephritis in a study of apparently normal dogs.[481] Similar studies in cats are not available.

Even in the absence of VUR, bacteria can ascend the ureters by gaining access to urine in the periphery of the ureter, where stagnant flow exists,[468, 469] by random Brownian motion or by active motility. The ureters possess receptors for P-fimbriae, which are important for the initial adherence and continued replication of bacteria in this region of the upper urinary tract.[469] Bacterial endotoxin can diminish ureteral peristalsis, thus facilitating further bacterial ascent.[497] Ureteral paralysis may also be important in the inoculation of bacteria into renal parenchyma by intrarenal reflux, since the adynamic ureter results in functional obstruction with increased intraluminal pressure within the ureter and renal pelvis.[468]

The renal pelvis and papillary openings are the last barriers to the ascent of bacteria into the renal parenchyma.[468] No properties that prevent adherence, similar to those found in the bladder, have been identified in the kidney.[477] Anatomic studies in humans and pigs have demonstrated refluxing and nonrefluxing types of papillary openings. The refluxing papillary openings dilate when intrapelvic pressure increases, allowing inoculation of bacteria into renal parenchyma. Whether such openings occur in dogs or cats is unknown. A gradual increase in pressure may convert some openings from the nonrefluxing to the refluxing conformation.[468] In theory, bacteria may be able to ascend from the renal pelvis into the renal parenchyma only if refluxing openings are present. Binding of bacteria to renal pelvic epithelium with subsequent replication probably precedes intrarenal reflux. The balance between binding, replication, hydrokinetic washout, and exfoliation[498] of organisms bound to renal pelvic epithelium may determine whether or not upper UTI becomes established at the level of the renal pelvis. A roughened, thickened renal pelvic epithelium may be observed at necropsy during early infection, while subepithelial aggregates of lymphocytes and some plasma cells are seen microscopically. As infection advances, ulceration of the renal pelvic epithelium may occur, sometimes in combination with dilatation of the renal pelvis.[460]

The extent of bacterial replication and colonization in renal tissue depends on the subsequent inflammatory and immune response. Once bacteria gain access to the renal parenchyma, an acute inflammatory reaction ensues, largely mediated by neutrophils.[460] The renal medulla is much more susceptible to the development of infection than is the renal cortex in both hematogenous and ascending infection. The hypertonic environment of the renal medulla interferes with the effectiveness of the inflammatory response because complement is inactivated, antigen-antibody binding is impaired, and phagocytosis by WBC is decreased as compared with the cortex. Additionally, RBF is much lower in the medulla than in the cortex.[101, 453, 460]

The inflammatory response can eliminate organisms from the renal parenchyma, but can also damage the surrounding tissue, possibly as a result of superoxide radical release with resultant tubular and glomerular necrosis.[227] The severity of tissue damage depends on the degree of neutrophilic infiltration, as has been demonstrated in rats after depletion of WBC by pretreatment with nitrogen mustard,[499] and by studies in which the early inflammatory response was decreased by antimicrobial treatments. Some mononuclear cell infiltration and fibroplasia will follow the initial neutrophilic infiltration.[460] Further progression will result in necrotizing inflammation of the renal pelvis and adjacent tissues with further fibroplasia, and influx of neutrophils with abscess formation. There is a pronounced demarcation between involved and uninvolved regions of the kidney.

Chronic pyelonephritis has been thought to result from recurrent bacterial infection in the kidney, but this is disputed, since renal disease can progress after a single infection, despite eradication of infection and subsequent inability to isolate bacteria from tissue or urine.[458] Lymphocytes predominate in the infiltrate at this stage, in association with smaller numbers of plasma cells and neutrophils. Immunofluorescence studies have demonstrated the presence of specific antibacterial antibody in the plasma cells of these infiltrates.[460] Bacterial antigen can persist in the area of mononuclear infiltrate or fibrosis for an extended period and could result in a delayed hypersensitivity reaction.[101, 468] An immunologic response against Tamm-Horsfall mucoprotein (THP) may be important in perpetuating renal injury after elimination of intact bacteria from the renal parenchyma, since THP has been identified in the interstitium of patients with chronic pyelonephritis.[458] Because THP shares some antigenic sites with uropathogenic bacteria, it is possible that bacteria sensitize cytotoxic lymphocytes against native THP.[458] Sensitization of cytotoxic lymphocytes against THP and subsequent mononuclear inflammation occur in laboratory animals immunized with THP and in those subjected to VUR, as THP regurgitates into the interstitium.[458] The precise role of cellular immunity, however, remains uncertain.[101]

DIAGNOSIS OF UPPER URINARY TRACT INFECTION AND PYELONEPHRITIS

The definitive diagnosis of upper urinary tract infection and pyelonephritis is difficult. Isolation of bacteria from ureteral or renal pelvic urine confirms that UUTI is present but does not conclusively demonstrate infection of renal tissue. Antibody coating of bacteria and bladder washout tests designed to determine the origin of bacteria from the upper or lower urinary tract are unreliable. Isolation of bacteria from the renal parenchyma alone provides conclusive evidence of renal infection.

The diagnosis of acute pyelonephritis is based on the clinical findings of acute onset, painful kidneys on abdominal palpation, normal or enlarged kidneys on abdominal palpation or radiographs, an abnormal intravenous pyelography (IVP), fever, leukocytosis with left shift, pyuria, bacteriuria, and cylindruria, especially with WBC casts. These clinical and laboratory findings may be transient, however, and may not be present at the time of clinical evaluation. Azotemia and dilute urine are variable findings.

The diagnosis of chronic pyelonephritis is even more difficult than the diagnosis of acute pyelonephritis because the offending bacteria may not be present at the time of clinical evaluation. Clinical signs in animals with chronic pyelonephritis may be absent, or clinical signs of uremia may be present. The diagnosis of chronic pyelonephritis is based on the clinical findings of normal-to small-sized, irregular-shaped kidneys on abdominal palpation or radiographs, an abnormal IVP, pyuria, bacteriuria, cylindruria, and dilute urine. Azotemia and nonregenerative anemia may be present if sufficient renal damage has occurred to cause loss of 75 per cent or more of nephrons. Renal biopsy shows patchy areas of mononuclear interstitial cellular infiltrates and interstitial fibrosis extending from the medulla into some areas of the cortex.

References

1. DiBartola, SP, et al.: Clinicopathologic findings associated with chronic renal failure in cats: 74 cases (1973–1984). JAVMA 190:1196, 1987.
2. Gwin, RM, et al.: Hypertensive retinopathy associated with hypothyroidism, hypercholesterolemia, and renal failure in a dog. JAAHA 14:200, 1978.
3. Barclay, SM and Riis, RC: Retinal detachment and reattachment associated with ethylene glycol intoxication in a cat. JAAHA 15:719, 1979.
4. Morgan, RV: Systemic hypertension in four cats: ocular and medical findings. JAAHA 22:615, 1986.
5. Cowgill, LD and Kallet, AJ: Recognition and management of hypertension in the dog. In Kirk, RW (ed): Current Veterinary Therapy VIII. Philadelphia, WB Saunders, 1983, p 1025.
6. Finco, DR and Duncan, JR: Evaluation of blood urea nitrogen and serum creatinine concentrations as indicators of renal dysfunction: A study of 111 cases and a review of related literature. JAVMA 168:593, 1976.
7. Watson, ADJ and Church, DB: Postprandial changes in plasma urea and creatinine concentrations in dogs. Am J Vet Res 42:1878, 1981.
8. Epstein, ME, et al.: Postprandial changes in plasma urea nitrogen and plasma creatinine concentrations in dogs fed commercial diets. JAAHA 20:779, 1984.
9. Finco, DR, et al.: Effect of immunosuppressive drug therapy on blood urea nitrogen concentrations in dogs with azotemia. JAVMA 185:664, 1984.
10. Rose, BD: Clinical assessment of renal function. In Rose, BD (ed): Pathophysiology of Renal Disease. New York, McGraw-Hill, 1987, p 1.
11. Robinson, T, et al.: Influence of reduced renal mass on tubular secretion of creatinine in the dog. Am J Vet Res 35:487, 1974.
12. Dubb, JW, et al.: Effect of cimetidine on renal function in normal man. Clin Pharmacol Therap 24:76, 1978.
13. Berglund, F, et al.: Effect of trimethoprim-sulfamethoxazole on the renal excretion of creatinine in man. J Urol 114:802, 1975.
14. Molitch, ME, et al.: Spurious serum creatinine elevations in ketoacidosis. Ann Intern Med 93:280, 1980.
15. Osbaldiston, GW and Fuhrman, W: The clearance of creatinine, inulin, para-aminohippurate and phenolsulfonphthalein in the cat. Can J Comp Med 34:138, 1970.
16. Finco, DR: Simultaneous determination of phenolsulfonphthalein excretion and endogenous creatinine clearance in the normal dog. JAVMA 159:336, 1971.
17. Bovee, KC and Joyce, T: Clinical evaluation of glomerular function: 24-hour creatinine clearance in dogs. JAVMA 174:488, 1979.
18. Finco, DR, et al.: Simple, accurate method for clinical estimation of glomerular filtration rate in the dog. Am J Vet Res 42:1874, 1981.
19. Finco, DR, et al.: Procedure for a simple method of measuring glomerular filtration rate in the dog. JAAHA 18:804, 1982.
20. Ross, LA and Finco, DR: Relationship of selected clinical renal function tests to glomerular filtration rate and renal blood flow in cats. Am J Vet Res 42:1704, 1981.
21. Carlson, GP and Kaneko, JJ: Simultaneous estimation of renal function in dogs using sodium sulfanilate and sodium iodohippurate-131I. JAVMA 158:1229, 1971.
22. Maddison, JE, et al.: Clinical evaluation of sodium sulfanilate clearance for the diagnosis of renal disease in dogs. JAVMA 185:961, 1984.
23. Fettman, MJ, et al.: Single-injection method for evaluation of renal function with 14C-inulin and 3H-tetraethylammonium bromide in dogs and cats. Am J Vet Res 46:482, 1985.
24. Mercer, HD, et al.: Bioavailability and pharmacokinetics of several dosage forms of ampicillin in the cat. Am J Vet Res 38:1353, 1977.
25. Powers, TE, et al.: Study of the double isotope single-injection method for estimating renal function in purebred beagle dogs. Am J Vet Res 38:1933, 1977.
26. van den Brom, WE and Biewenga, WJ: Assessment of glomerular filtration rate in normal dogs: analysis of the 51Cr-EDTA clearance and its relation to several endogenous parameters of glomerular filtration. Res Vet Sci 30:152, 1981.
27. Biewenga, WJ and van den Brom, WE: Assessment of glomerular filtration rate in dogs with renal insufficiency: analysis of the 51Cr-EDTA clearance and its relation to the plasma concentrations of urea and creatinine. Res Vet Sci 30:158, 1981.
28. Krawiec, DR, et al.: Evaluation of 99mTc-diethylenetriaminepentaacetic acid nuclear imaging for quantitative determination of glomerular filtration rate of dogs. Am J Vet Res 47:2175, 1986.
29. Rose, BD: Clinical Physiology of Acid Base and Electrolyte Disorders. McGraw-Hill Book Co., New York, 1977, p. 14.
30. Hendriks, HJ, et al.: The clinical refractometer: A useful tool for the determination of specific gravity and osmolality in canine urine. Tijdschr Diergeneesk 103:1065, 1978.
31. Bovee, KC: Urine osmolarity as a definitive indicator of renal concentrating capacity. JAVMA 155:30, 1969.
32. Feeney, DA, et al.: Effects of radiographic contrast media on results of urinalysis, with emphasis on alteration in specific gravity. JAVMA 176:1378, 1980.
33. Hardy, RM and Osborne, CA: Water deprivation test in the dog: Maximal normal values. JAVMA 174:479, 1979.
34. Mulnix, JA, et al.: Evaluation of a modified water-deprivation test for diagnosis of polyuric disorders in dogs. JAVMA 169:1327, 1976.
35. Lage, AL: Nephrogenic diabetes insipidus. In Kirk RW (ed): Current Veterinary Therapy VI. Philadelphia, WB Saunders, 1977, p 1102.
36. Hardy, RM and Osborne, CA: Aqueous vasopressin response test in clinically normal dogs undergoing water diuresis: Techniques and results. Am J Vet Res 43:1987, 1982.
37. Hardy, RM and Osborne, CA: Repositol vasopressin response test in clinically normal dogs undergoing water diuresis: Techniques and results. Am J Vet Res 43:1991, 1982.
38. Kaufmann, CF and Kirk, RW: The sixty-minute plasma phenolsulfonphthalein concentration as a test of renal function in the dog. JAAHA 9:66, 1973.
39. Brobst, DF, et al.: Plasma phenolsulfonphthalein determination as a measure of renal function in dogs. White Plains, New York, Gaines Veterinary Symposium, 1967, p 15.
40. DiBartola, SP, et al.: Quantitative urinalysis including 24-hour protein excretion in the dog. JAAHA 16:537, 1980.
41. Russo, EA, et al.: Evaluation of renal function in cats, using quantitative urinalysis. Am J Vet Res 47:1308, 1986.
42. Thornhill, JA: Renal tubular acidosis. In Kirk RW (ed): Current Veterinary Therapy VI. Philadelphia, WB Saunders, 1977, p 1087.
43. Feeney, DA, et al.: Vesicoureteral reflux induced by manual compression of the urinary bladder of dogs and cats. JAVMA 182:795, 1983.
44. Biertuempfel, PH, et al.: Urinary tract infection resulting from catheterization in healthy dogs. JAVMA 178:989, 1981.
45. Thomas, JE: Urinary tract infection induced by intermittent urethral catheterization in dogs. JAVMA 178:989, 1981.
46. Comer, KM and Ling, GL: Results of urinalysis and bacterial culture of canine urine obtained by antepubic cystocentesis, catheterization, and the midstream voided methods. JAVMA 179:891, 1981.

47. Lees, GE, et al.: Results of analyses and bacterial cultures of urine specimens obtained from clinically normal cats by three methods. JAVMA 184:449, 1984.

48. Ling, GV: Antepubic cystocentesis in the dog: An aseptic technique for routine collection of urine. Calif Vet 30:50, 1976.

49. Chew, DJ: Urinalysis. In Bovee, KC (ed): Canine Nephrology. Media, PA, Harwall Pub Co, 1984, p 235.

50. Fettman, MJ: Evaluation of the usefulness of routine microscopy in canine urinalysis. JAVMA 190:892, 1987.

51. Stevens, JB and Osborne, CA: Urinalysis: indications, methodology, and interpretation. Proc AAHA, 1974, p 359.

52. Finco, DR: Kidney function. In Kaneko, JJ (ed): Clinical Biochemistry of Domestic Animals, 3rd ed. Orlando, FL, Academic Press, 1980, p 337.

53. Barlough, JE, et al.: Canine and feline urinalysis: Value of macroscopic and microscopic examinations. JAVMA 178:61, 1981.

54. Barsanti, JE: Urine analysis. In Lorenz, MD and Cornelius, LM (eds): Small Animal Medical Diagnosis. Philadelphia, JB Lippincott, 1987, p 592.

55. Kruth, SA and Cowgill, LD: Renal glucose transport in the cat. Proc ACVIM, 1982, p 78.

56. Osborne, CA, et al.: Clinical significance of glucosuria. Minn Vet 20:16, 1980.

57. Rich, LJ and Kirk, BS: The relationship of struvite crystals to urethral obstruction in cats. JAVMA 154:153, 1969.

58. Loeb, WF: Glucosuria and pseudoglucosuria in cats with urethral obstruction. Mod Vet Pract 40, 1971.

59. Burrows, CF and Bovee, KC: Characterization and treatment of acid-base and renal defects due to urethral obstruction in cats. JAVMA 172:801, 1978.

60. DiBartola, SP and Tarr, MJ: Clinicopathologic findings in dogs with renal amyloidosis: 59 cases (1976-1986). JAVMA in review.

61. Davenport, DJ, et al.: Familial renal disease in the dog and cat. In Breitschwerdt, EB (ed): Contemporary Issues in Small Animal Practice. Nephrology and Urology. New York, Churchill Livingstone, 1986, p 137.

62. Cowgill, LD: Diseases of the kidney. In Ettinger, SJ: Textbook of Veterinary Internal Medicine. Philadelphia, WB Saunders, 1983, p 1793.

63. Bovee, KC, et al.: Characterization of renal defects in dogs with a syndrome similar to the Fanconi syndrome in man. JAVMA 174:1094, 1979.

64. Anning, ST, et al.: The toxic effects of calciferol. Q J Med 17:203, 1948.

65. Transbol, I and Halver, B: Relation of renal glycosuria and parathyroid function in hypercalcemic sarcoidosis. J Clin Endocrinol 27:1193, 1967.

66. Spangler, WL, et al.: Vitamin D intoxication and the pathogenesis of vitamin D nephropathy in the dog. Am J Vet Res 40:73, 1979.

67. Osborne, CA, et al.: Clinical significance of bilirubinuria. Comp Cont Ed 2:897, 1980.

68. DeSchepper, J: Degradation of haemoglobin to bilirubin in the kidney of the dog. Tijdschr Diergeneesk 99:699, 1974.

69. Vail, DM, et al.: Applicability of leukocyte esterase test strip detection of canine pyuria. JAVMA 189:1451, 1986.

70. Ling, GV and Kaneko, JJ: Microscopic examination of canine urine sediment. Calif Vet 30:14, 1976.

71. McQueen, EG and Engel, GB: Factors determining the aggregation of urinary mucoprotein. J Clin Pathol 19:392, 1966.

72. McQueen, EG: The nature of urinary casts. J Clin Pathol 15:367, 1962.

73. McQueen, EG: Composition of urinary casts. Lancet 1:397, 1966.

74. Rutecki, GJ, et al.: Characterization of proteins in urinary casts. N Engl J Med 284:1049, 1971.

75. Orita, Y, et al.: Immunofluorescent studies of urinary casts. Nephron 19:19, 1977.

76. Schenk, EA, et al.: Tamm-Horsfall mucoprotein. Localization in the kidney. Lab Invest 25:92, 1971.

77. McKenzie, JK and McQueen, EG: Immunofluorescent localization of Tamm-Horsfall mucoprotein in human kidney. J Clin Pathol 22:334, 1969.

78. Pollak, VE and Arbel, C: The distribution of Tamm-Horsfall mucoprotein (uromucoid) in the human nephron. Nephron 6:667, 1969.

79. Relman, AS and Levinsky, NG: Clinical examination of renal function. In Straus, MB and Welt, LG (eds): Disease of the Kidney, 2nd ed. Boston, Little, Brown, 1971, p 87.

80. Addis, T: Glomerular Nephritis. New York, Macmillan, 1948.

81. Ling, GV: Therapeutic strategies involving antimicrobial treatment of the canine urinary tract. JAVMA 185:1162, 1984.

82. Ling, GV: Treatment of urinary tract infections with antimicrobial agents. In Kirk, RW (ed): Current Veterinary Therapy VIII. Philadelphia, WB Saunders, 1983, p 1051.

83. Chew, DJ and Kowalski, JP: Urinary tract infection. In Bojrab, MJ (ed): Pathophysiology in Small Animal Surgery. Philadelphia, Lea & Febiger, 1981, p 255.

84. Ling, GV: The use of antimicrobial agents in the management of urinary tract infections. Proc 7th Kal Kan Symposium, Kal Kan Foods, 1984, p 101.

85. Wooley, RE and Blue, JL: Quantitative and bacteriological studies of urine specimens from canine and feline urinary tract infections. J Clin Microbiol 4:326, 1976.

86. Wooley, RE and Blue, JL: Bacterial isolations from canine and feline urine. Mod Vet Pract :535, 1976.

87. Klausner, JS, et al.: Clinical evaluation of commercial reagent strips for detection of significant bacteriuria in dogs and cats. Am J Vet Res 37:719, 1976.

88. Ling, GV and Gilmore, CJ: Penicillin G or ampicillin for oral treatment of canine urinary tract infections. JAVMA 171:358, 1977.

89. Ling, GV and Ruby, AL: Chloramphenicol for oral treatment of canine urinary tract infections. JAVMA 172:914, 1978.

90. Ling, GV and Ruby, AL: Trimethoprim in combination with a sulfonamide for oral treatment of canine urinary tract infections. JAVMA 174:1003, 1979.

91. Berg, JN and Folks, WH: Canine and feline anaerobic bacterial infections. Vet Scope, 1977.

92. Middleton, DJ and Comas, GR: Emphysematous cystitis due to *Clostridium perfringens* in a nondiabetic dog. J Sm Anim Pract 20:433, 1979.

93. Sherding, RG and Chew, DJ: Nondiabetic emphysematous cystitis in two dogs. JAVMA 174:1105, 1979.

94. Kivisto, AK, et al.: Canine bacteriuria. J Sm Anim Pract 18:707, 1977.

95. Jang, SJ, et al.: Mycoplasma as cause of canine urinary tract infection. JAVMA 185:45, 1984.

96. Ling, GV and Ruby, AL: Aerobic bacterial flora of the prepuce, urethra, and vagina of normal adult dogs. Am J Vet Res 39:695, 1978.

97. Hirsch, DC and Wiger, N: The bacterial flora of the normal canine vagina compared with that of vaginal exudates. J Sm Anim Pract 18:25, 1977.

98. Olson, PNS and Mather, EC: Canine vaginal and uterine bacterial flora. JAVMA 172:708, 1978.

99. Baba, E, et al.: Vaginal and uterine microflora of adult dogs. Am J Vet Res 44:606, 1983.

100. Klausner, JS, et al.: The interpretation and misinterpretation of bacteriuria. Minn Vet 15:43, 1975.

101. Rubin, RH, et al.: Urinary tract infection, pyelonephritis, and reflux nephropathy. In Brenner, BM and Rector, FC (eds): The Kidney. Philadelphia, WB Saunders, 1986, p 1085.

102. Padilla, J, et al.: Effects of storage time and temperature on quantitative culture of canine urine. JAVMA 178:1077, 1981.

103. Allen, TA, et al.: Microbiologic evaluation of canine urine: Direct microscopic examination and preservation of specimen quality for culture. JAVMA 190:1289, 1987.

104. Carter, JM, et al.: Comparison of collection techniques for quantitative urine culture in dogs. JAVMA 173:296, 1978.

105. Finco, DR and Kern, A: Pyelonephritis. In Kirk, RW (ed): Current Veterinary Therapy VI. Philadelphia, WB Saunders, 1977, p 1106.

106. Lees, GA and Rogers, KS: Diagnosis and localization of urinary tract infection. In Kirk, RW (ed): Current Veterinary Therapy IX. Philadelphia, WB Saunders, 1986, p 1118.

107. Ling, GV, et al.: Bacterial pathogens associated with urinary tract infections. Vet Clin North Am 9:617, 1979.

108. Barsanti, JA and Finco, DR: Laboratory findings in urinary tract infections. Vet Clin North Am 9:729, 1979.

109. Finco, DR, et al.: Radiologic estimation of kidney size of the dog. JAVMA 159:995, 1971.
110. Walter, PA, et al.: Feline renal ultrasonography: Quantitative analyses of image anatomy. Am J Vet Res 48:596, 1987.
111. Grandage, J: Some effects of posture on the radiographic appearance of the kidneys of the dog. JAVMA 166:165, 1975.
112. Feeney, DA and Johnston, GR: The kidneys and ureters.
113. Feeney, DA, et al.: Normal canine excretory urogram: Effects of dose, time, and individual dog variation. Am J Vet Res 40:1596, 1979.
114. Biery, DN: Upper urinary tract. In Radiographic Diagnosis of Abdominal Disorders in the Dog and Cat: Radiographic Interpretation, Clinical Signs, Pathophysiology. Philadelphia, WB Saunders, 1978, p 481.
115. Talner, B: Urographic contrast media in uremia. Radiol Clin North Am 10:421, 1972.
116. Feeney, DA, et al.: Effect of multiple excretory urograms on glomerular filtration of normal dogs: A preliminary report. Am J Vet Res 41:960, 1980.
117. Konde, LJ, et al.: Comparison of radiography and ultrasonography in the evaluation of renal lesions in the dog. JAVMA 188:1420, 1986.
118. Walter, PA, et al.: Ultrasonographic evaluation of renal parenchymal diseases in dogs: 32 cases (1981–1986). JAVMA 191:999, 1987.
119. Walter, PA, et al.: Applications of ultrasonography in the diagnosis of parenchymal kidney disease in cats: 24 cases (1981–1986). JAVMA 192:92, 1988.
120. Nyland, TG and Kantrowitz, BM: Ultrasound in diagnosis and staging of abdominal neoplasia. In Gorman, NT (ed): Oncology. New York, Churchill Livingstone, 1986, p 1.
121. Hager, DA, et al.: Ultrasound-guided biopsy of the canine liver, kidney, and prostate. Vet Rad 26:82, 1985.
122. Konde, LJ, et al.: Ultrasonographic anatomy of the normal canine kidney. Vet Rad 25:173, 1984.
123. Walker, PA, et al.: Renal ultrasonography in healthy cats. Am J Vet Res 48:600, 1987.
124. Konde, L: Sonography of the kidney. Vet Clin North Am 15:1149, 1985.
125. Konde, LJ, et al.: Sonographic appearance of renal neoplasia in the dog. Vet Rad 26:74, 1985.
126. Cartee, RE, et al.. Ultrasonographic diagnosis of renal disease in small animals. JAVMA 176:426, 1980.
127. Barber, DL: Renal angiography in veterinary medicine. Vet Rad 16:187, 1975.
128. Cowgill, LD and Hornof, WJ: Assessment of individual kidney function by quantitative renal scintigraphy. In Kirk, RW (ed): Current Veterinary Therapy IX. Philadelphia, WB Saunders, 1986, p 1108.
129. Cowgill, LD: ACVIM, San Diego, 1985.
130. Osborne, CA: Clinical evaluation of needle biopsy of the kidney and its complications in the dog and cat. JAVMA 158:1213, 1971.
131. Osborne, CA, et al.: Kidney biopsy. Vet Clin North Am 4(2):351, 1974.
132. Grauer, GF, et al.: Evaluation of laparoscopy for obtaining renal biopsy specimens. JAVMA 183:677, 1983.
133. Nash, AS, et al.: Renal biopsy in the normal cat: an examination of the effects of a single needle biopsy. Res Vet Sci 34:347, 1983.
134. Osborne, CA and Low, DG: Size, adequacy, and artifacts of canine renal biopsy samples. Am J Vet Res 32:1865, 1971.
135. Nash, AS, et al.: Renal biopsy in the normal cat: Examination of the effects of repeated needle biopsy. Res Vet Sci 40:112, 1986.
136. Nash, AS: Renal biopsy in the cat: Development of a modified disposable biopsy needle. Res Vet Sci 40:246, 1986.
137. Wolfe, MJ, et al.: Immunofluorescent staining of cutaneous and renal biopsy specimens: A comparison of preservation by quick-freezing with or without storage in transport medium of Michel. JAAHA 18:444, 1982.
138. Arthur, JE, et al.: An immunohistological study of feline glomerulonephritis using the peroxidase-antiperoxidase method. Res Vet Sci 37:12, 1984.
139. Jeraj, K, et al.: Evaluation of renal biopsy in 197 dogs and cats. JAVMA 181:367, 1982.
140. Sweet, EI, et al.: Complications of needle biopsy of the kidney in the dog. Radiology 92:849, 1969.
141. Crowell, WA, et al.: Canine glomeruli: Light and electron microscopic change in biopsy, perfused, and in situ autolyzed kidney from normal dogs. Am J Vet Res 35:889, 1974.
142. Crowell, WA and Leininger, JR: Feline glomeruli: morphologic comparisons of normal, autolytic, and diseased kidneys. Am J Vet Res 37:1075, 1976.
143. Bovee, KC: The uremic syndrome. JAAHA 12:189, 1976.
144. Bergstrom, J and Furst, P: Uremic toxins. Kidney Int 13:S9, 1978.
145. Bergstrom, J: Uremia is an intoxication. Kidney Int 28:S2, 1985.
146. Wills, MR: Uremic toxins and their effect on intermediary metabolism. Clin Chem 31:5, 1985.
147. Powell, D, et al.: Toxins and inhibitors in chronic renal failure. Am J Kid Dis 7:292, 1986.
148. Johnson, WJ, et al.: Effects of urea loading in patients with far-advanced renal failure. Mayo Clinic Proc 47:21, 1972.
149. Horowitz, HI, et al.: Further studies on the platelet-inhibitory effect of guanidinosuccinic acid and its role in uremic bleeding. Am J Med 49:336, 1970.
150. Mujais SK, et al.: Pathophysiology of the uremic syndrome. In Brenner BM and Rector FC: The Kidney, 3rd ed. Philadelphia, WB Saunders, 1986, p 1587.
151. Simenhoff, ML and Saukkonen, JJ: Importance of aliphatic amines in uremia. Kidney Int 13:S16, 1978.
152. Radtke, HW, et al.: Identification of spermine as an inhibitor of erythropoiesis in patients with chronic renal failure. J Clin Invest 67:1623, 1981.
153. Babb, AL, et al.: The genesis of the square-meter-hour hypothesis. Trans Am Soc Artif Internal Organs 17:81, 1971.
154. Navarro, J, et al.: Are "middle molecules" responsible for toxic phenomena in chronic renal failure? Nephron 32:301, 1982.
155. Brunner, H and Mann, H: What remains of the "middle molecule" hypothesis today? Contr Nephrol 44:14, 1985.
156. Tsukamato, Y, et al.: Disturbances of trace element concentrations in plasma of patients with chronic renal failure. Nephron 26:174, 1980.
157. Malluche, HH and Faugere, MC: Aluminum: Toxin or innocent bystander in renal osteodystrophy? Am J Kidney Dis 6:336, 1985.
158. Nebeker, HG and Coburn, JW: Aluminum and osteodystrophy. Ann Rev Med 37:79, 1986.
159. Massry, SG: Neurotoxicity of parathyroid hormone in uremia. Kidney Int 28:S5, 1985.
160. Massry, SG: Pathogenesis of the anemia in uremia: Role of secondary hyperparathyroidism. Kidney Int 24:S204, 1983.
161. Jubelirer, SJ: Hemostatic abnormalities in renal disease. Am J Kidney Dis 5:219, 1985.
162. Wooley, AC: Platelet dysfunction in uremia. The Kidney 19:15, 1987.
163. Deykin, D: Uremic bleeding. Kidney Int 24:698, 1983.
164. Anagnostou, A and Kurtzman, NA: Hematological consequence of renal failure. In Brenner BM and Rector FC: The Kidney, 3rd ed. Philadelphia, WB Saunders, 1986, p 1631.
165. Fisher, JW: Mechanism of the anemia of chronic renal failure. Nephron 25:106, 1980.
166. Eschbach, JW and Adamson, JW: Anemia of end-stage renal disease. Kidney Int 28:1, 1985.
167. Eschbach, JW, et al.: Correction of the anemia of end-stage renal disease with recombinant human erythropoietin: Results of a combined phase I and II clinical trial. N Engl J Med 316:73, 1987.
168. Delwiche, F, et al.: High levels of the circulating form of parathyroid hormone do not inhibit in vitro erythropoiesis. J Lab Clin Med 102:613, 1983.
169. Mitchell, TR and Pegrum, CD: The oxygen affinity of haemoglobin in chronic renal failure. Br J Haematol 21:263, 1971.
170. Bovee, KC: Metabolic disturbances of uremia. In Bovee KC: Canine Nephrology. Media, PA, Harwall Pub, 1984, p 555.
171. Salvin, R and Gallagher, MI: The lymphocyte in acute experimental uremia. J Lab Clin Med 76:992, 1970.
172. Arieff, AI: Neurological manifestations of uremia. In Brenner BR and Rector FC: The Kidney, 3rd ed. Philadelphia, WB Saunders, 1986, p 1731.

173. Raskin, NH and Fishman, RA: Neurologic disorders in renal failure. N Engl J Med 294:143, 1976.

174. Mahoney, CA and Arieff, AI: Central and peripheral nervous system effects of chronic renal failure. Kidney Int 24:170, 1983.

175. Biasioli, S, et al.: Uremic encephalopathy: An updating. Clin Nephrol 25:57, 1986.

176. Wolf, AM: Canine uremic encephalopathy. JAAHA 16:735, 1980.

177. Goldstein, DA, et al.: Effect of parathyroid hormone and uremia on peripheral nerve calcium and motor nerve conduction velocity. J Clin Invest 701:88, 1978.

178. Cheville, NF: Uremic gastropathy in the dog. Vet Pathol 16:292, 1979.

179. Thornhill, JA: Control of vomiting in the uremic patient. In Kirk RW: Current Veterinary Therapy VIII. Philadelphia, WB Saunders, 1983, p 1022.

180. Taylor, IL, et al.: Serum gastrin in patients with chronic renal failure. Gut 21:1062, 1980.

181. Lucke, VM: Renal disease in the cat. Vet Rec 102:301, 1978.

182. Kraikitpanitch, S, et al.: Effect of azotemia on the myocardial accumulation of calcium. Mineral Elect Metab 1:12, 1978.

183. Renfrew, R, et al.: Pericarditis and renal failure. Ann Rev Med 31:345, 1980.

184. Madewell, BR and Norrdin, RW: Renal failure associated with pericardial effusion in a dog. JAVMA 167:1091, 1975.

185. Berg, RJ and Wingfield, W: Pericardial effusion in the dog: A review of 42 cases. JAAHA 20:721, 1984.

186. Acosta, JH: Hypertension in chronic renal disease. Kidney Int 22:702, 1982.

187. Weidmann, P: Pathogenesis of hypertension associated with chronic renal failure. Contr Nephrol 41:47, 1984.

188. Blythe, WB: Natural history of hypertension in renal parenchymal disease. Am J Kidney Dis 5:A50, 1985.

189. Anderson, LJ and Fisher, EW: The blood pressure in canine interstitial nephritis. Res Vet Sci 9:304, 1968.

190. Valtonen, MH and Oksanen, A: Cardiovascular disease and nephritis in dogs. J Sm Anim Pract 13:687, 1972.

191. Weiser, MG, et al.: Blood pressure measurement in the dog. JAVMA 171:364, 1977.

192. Lucke, VM: Renal disease in the domestic cat. J Pathol Bacteriol 95:67, 1968.

193. Moon, ML, et al.: Uremic pneumonitis-like syndrome in ten dogs. JAAHA 22:687, 1986.

194. DeFronzo, RA, et al.: Carbohydrate metabolism in uremia: a review. Medicine 52:469, 1973.

195. DeFronzo, RA and Smith, JD: Is glucose intolerance harmful for the uremic patient? Kidney Int 28:S88, 1985.

196. Lim, VS, et al.: Thyroid dysfunction in chronic renal failure: a study of the pituitary thyroid axis and peripheral turnover kinetics of thyroxine and triiodothyronine. J Clin Invest 60:522, 1977.

197. Papper, S: Clinical Nephrology, 2nd ed. Boston, Little, Brown & Co, 1978, p 35.

198. Bricker, NS: On the meaning of the intact nephron hypothesis. Am J Med 46:1, 1969.

199. Bricker, NS and Fine, LG: The renal response to progressive nephron loss. In Brenner BM, Rector FC: The Kidney, 2nd ed. Philadelphia, WB Saunders, 1981, p 1056.

200. Valtin, H: Renal dysfunction: Mechanisms involved in fluid and solute imbalance. Boston, Little, Brown, & Co, 1979, p 266.

201. Slatopolsky, E, et al.: Studies on characterization of the control system governing sodium excretion in uremic man. J Clin Invest 47:521, 1968.

202. Bricker, NS: Sodium homeostasis in chronic renal disease. Kidney Int 21:886, 1982.

203. Bricker, NS, et al.: On the biology of sodium excretion: The search for a natriuretic hormone. Yale J Biol Med 48:293, 1975.

204. Bourgoignie, JJ, et al.: A natriuretic factor in the serum of patients with chronic uremia. J Clin Invest 51:1514, 1972.

205. Smith, S, et al.: Role of atrial natriuretic peptide in adaptation of sodium excretion with reduced renal mass. J Clin Invest 77:1395, 1986.

206. Hasegawa, K, et al.: Plasma levels of atrial natriuretic peptide in patients with chronic renal failure. J Clin Endocrinol Metabol 63:819, 1986.

207. Anderson, JV, et al.: Effect of hemodialysis on plasma concentrations of atrial natriuretic peptide in adult patients with chronic renal failure. J Endocrinol 110:193, 1986.

208. Bourgoignie, JJ, et al.: Sodium homeostasis in dogs with chronic renal insufficiency. Kidney Int 21:820, 1982.

209. Schmidt, RW, et al.: On the adaptation in sodium excretion in chronic uremia. The effects of "proportionate reduction" of sodium intake. J Clin Invest 53:1736, 1974.

210. Fine, LG, et al.: Functional profile of the isolated uremic nephron. Potassium adaptation in the rabbit cortical collecting duct. J Clin Invest 64:1033, 1979.

211. Bricker, NS: On the pathogenesis of the uremic state: an exposition of the "trade-off" hypothesis. N Engl J Med 286:1093, 1972.

212. Bricker, NS and Fine, LG: The trade-off hypothesis: Current status. Kidney Int 13:55, 1978.

213. Schrier, RW and Berl, T: Nonosmolar factors affecting renal water excretion. N Engl J Med 292:141, 1975.

214. Carriere, S, et al.: Redistribution of renal blood flow in acute and chronic reduction of renal mass. Kidney Int 3:364, 1973.

215. Tannen, RL, et al.: Vasopressin-resistant hyposthenuria in advanced chronic renal disease. N Engl J Med 280:1135, 1969.

216. Schmidt, RW, et al.: Bicarbonate reabsorption in the dog with experimental renal disease. Kidney Int 10:287, 1976.

217. Arruda, JAL, et al.: Bicarbonate reabsorption in chronic renal failure. Kidney Int 9:481, 1976.

218. Wong, NLM, et al.: Tubular handling of bicarbonate in dogs with experimental renal failure. Kidney Int 25:912, 1984.

219. Schmidt, RW and Gavellas, G: Bicarbonate reabsorption in experimental renal disease: Effects of proportional reduction of sodium or phosphate intake. Kidney Int 12:393, 1977.

220. Lehmann, J, et al.: The effects of chronic acid loads in normal man: Further evidence for the participation of bone mineral in the defense against chronic metabolic acidosis. J Clin Invest 45:1608, 1966.

221. Rose, BD: Clinical Physiology of Acid-Base and Electrolyte Disorders, 2nd ed. New York, McGraw-Hill, 1984, p 234.

222. Dorhout-Mees, EJ, et al.: The functional adaptation of the diseased kidney. III. Ammonium excretion. J Clin Invest 45:289, 1966.

223. Coburn, JW and Slatopolsky, E: Vitamin D, Parathyroid hormone, and renal osteodystrophy. In Brenner BM, Rector FC: The Kidney, 3rd ed. Philadelphia, WB Saunders, 1986, p 1657.

224. Slatopolsky, E, et al.: On the pathogenesis of hyperparathyroidism in chronic renal insufficiency in the dog. J Clin Invest 50:492, 1971.

225. Slatopolsky, E, et al.: On the prevention of secondary hyperparathyroidism in experimental chronic renal disease using "proportional reduction" of dietary phosphorus intake. Kidney Int 2:147, 1972.

226. Slatopolsky, E and Bricker, NS: The role of phosphorus restriction in the prevention of secondary hyperparathyroidism in chronic renal disease. Kidney Int 4:141, 1973.

227. Kaplan, MA, et al.: Reversal of hyperparathyroidism in response to dietary phosphorus restriction in the uremic dog. Kidney Int 15:43, 1979.

228. Jacob, AI, et al.: Calcemic and phosphaturic response to parathyroid hormone in normal and chronically uremic dogs. Kidney Int 22:21, 1982.

229. Korkor, AB: Reduced binding of 1,25-dihydroxyvitamin D_3 in the parathyroid glands of patients with renal failure. N Engl J Med 316:1573, 1987.

230. Merke, J, et al.: Diminished parathyroid 1,25$(OH)_2D_3$ receptors in experimental uremia. Kidney Int 32:350, 1987.

231. Brown, EM, et al.: Abnormal regulation of parathyroid hormone release by calcium in secondary hyperparathyroidism due to chronic renal failure. J Clin Endocrinol Metab 54:172, 1982.

232. Kaehny, WD, et al.: Gastrointestinal absorption of aluminum from aluminum-containing antacids. N Engl J Med 296:1389, 1977.

233. Andreoli, SP, et al.: Aluminum intoxication in nondialyzed azotemic children from aluminum containing phosphate binders. N Engl J Med 310:1079, 1984.

234. Finco, DR and Rowland, GN: Hypercalcemia secondary to chronic renal failure in the dog: A report of four cases. JAVMA 173:990, 1978.

235. Brenner, BM: Hemodynamically mediated glomerular injury and

the progressive nature of kidney disease. Kidney Int 23:647, 1983.

236. Anderson, S, et al.: The role of hemodynamic factors in the initiation and progression of renal disease. J Urol 133:363, 1985.

237. Hostetter, TH: Progressive glomerular injury: roles of dietary protein and compensatory hypertrophy. Pharm Rev 36:101S, 1984.

238. Mitch, WE, et al.: A simple method for estimating progression of chronic renal failure. Lancet 2:1326, 1976.

239. Rutherford, WE, et al.: Chronic progressive renal disease: Rate of change of serum creatinine concentration. Kidney Int 11:62, 1977.

240. Allen, TA, et al.: A technique for estimating progression of chronic renal failure in the dog. JAVMA 190:866, 1987.

241. Hostetter, TH, et al.: Hyperfiltration in remnant nephrons: A potentially adverse response to renal ablation. Am J Physiol 241:F85, 1981.

242. Brenner, BM: Nephron adaptation to renal injury or ablation. Am J Physiol 249:F324, 1985.

243. Olson, JL, et al.: Altered glomerular permselectivity and progressive sclerosis following extreme ablation of renal mass. Kidney Int 22:112, 1982.

244. Hostetter, TH, et al.: Chronic effects of dietary protein in the rat with intact and reduced renal mass. Kidney Int 30:509, 1986.

245. Brenner, BM, et al.: Dietary protein intake and the progressive nature of kidney disease: the role of hemodynamically mediated glomerular injury in the pathogenesis of progressive glomerular sclerosis in aging, renal ablation, and intrinsic renal disease. N Engl J Med 307:652, 1982.

246. Hirschberg, R and Kopple, JD: Role of growth hormone in the amino acid-induced acute rise in renal function in man. Kidney Int 32:382, 1987.

247. Kleinknecht, C, et al.: Effects of various protein diets on growth, renal function, and survival of uremic rats. Kidney Int 15:534, 1979.

248. Bovee, KC, et al.: Long-term measurement of renal function in partially nephrectomized dogs fed 56, 27, or 19 per cent protein. Invest Urol 16:378, 1979.

249. Robertson, JL, et al.: Long-term renal responses to high dietary protein in dogs with 75 per cent nephrectomy. Kidney Int 29:511, 1986.

250. Polzin, DJ, et al.: Influence of reduced protein diets on morbidity, mortality, and renal function in dogs with induced chronic renal failure. Am J Vet Res 45:506, 1984.

251. Bourgoignie, JJ, et al.: Glomerular function and morphology after renal mass reduction in dogs. J Lab Clin Med 109:380, 1987.

252. Ibels, LS, et al.: Preservation of function in experimental renal disease by dietary restriction of phosphate. N Engl J Med 298:122, 1978.

253. Karlinsky, ML, et al.: Preservation of renal function in experimental glomerulonephritis. Kidney Int 17:293, 1980.

254. Ross, LA, et al.: Effect of dietary phosphorus restriction on the kidneys of cats with reduced renal mass. Am J Vet Res 43:1023, 1982.

255. Laouari, D, et al.: Beneficial effect of low phosphorus diet in uremic rats: a reappraisal. Clin Sci 63:539, 1982.

256. Lumlertgul, D, et al.: Phosphate depletion arrests progression of chronic renal failure independent of protein intake. Kidney Int 29:658, 1986.

257. Brown, S, et al.: Beneficial effect of moderate phosphate restriction in partially nephrectomized dogs on a low protein diet. Kidney Int 31:380, 1987.

258. Chew, DJ: Acute renal failure. Proc 7th Kal Kan Symp, Kal Kan Foods, 1984, p 9.

259. Chew, DJ: Urogenital emergencies. In Sherding, RG (ed): Medical Emergencies. New York, Churchill Livingstone, 1985, p 187.

260. DiBartola, SP: Acute renal failure: Pathophysiology and management. Comp Cont Ed Pract Vet 2:952, 1980.

261. Cowgill, LD: Acute renal failure. In Bovee, KC (ed): Canine Nephrology. Media, PA, Harwall Pub, 1984, p 405.

262. English, PB: Acute renal failure in the dog and cat. Aust Vet J 50:384, 1974.

263. Senior, DF: Acute renal failure in the dog: A case report and literature review. JAAHA 19:837, 1983.

264. Brezis, M, et al.: Acute renal failure. In Brenner, BM and Rector, FC (eds): The Kidney, 3rd ed. Philadelphia, WB Saunders, 1986, p 735.

265. Schrier, RW: Acute renal failure: Pathogenesis, diagnosis, and management. Hosp Pract, Mar 1981, p 93.

266. Anderson, FJ, et al.: Nonoliguric acute renal failure. N Engl J Med 296:1134, 1977.

267. Dixon, BS and Anderson, RJ: Nonoliguric renal failure. Am J Kidney Dis 6:71, 1985.

268. Myers, BD and Morgan, SM: Hemodynamically mediated acute renal failure. N Engl J Med 314:97, 1986.

269. Kreisberg, JI, et al.: Morphologic factors in acute renal failure. In Brenner, BM and Lazarus, JM (ed): Acute Renal Failure. Philadelphia, WB Saunders, 1983, p 21.

270. Evan, AP, et al.: Glomerular filtration barrier in ischemic and nephrotoxic acute renal failure. In Solez, K and Whelton, A (eds): Acute Renal Failure: Correlations Between Morphology and Function. New York, Marcel Dekker, 1984, p 119.

271. Stein, JH and Sorkin, MI: Pathophysiology of a vasomotor and nephrotoxic model of acute renal failure in the dog. Kidney Int 10:S86, 1976.

272. Stein, JH, et al.: Current concepts on the pathophysiology of acute renal failure. Am J Physiol 234:F171, 1978.

273. Johnston, WH and Latta, H: Glomerular mesangial and endothelial cell swelling following temporary renal ischemia and its role in the no-reflow phenomenon. Am J Pathol 89:153, 1977.

274. Flores, J, et al.: The role of cell swelling in ischemic renal damage and the protective effect of hypertonic solute. J Clin Invest 51:118, 1972.

275. Venkatachalam, MA: Pathology of acute renal failure. In Brenner, BM and Stein, JH (eds): Acute Renal Failure. New York, Churchill Livingstone, 1980, p 79.

276. Brezis, M, et al.: Renal ischemia: A new perspective. N Engl J Med 26:375, 1984.

277. Ng, RCK and Suki, WN: Treatment of acute renal failure. In Brenner, BM and Stein, JH (eds): Acute Renal Failure. New York, Churchill Livingstone, 1980, p 229.

278. Finn, WF: Postischemic acute renal failure initiation, maintenance, and recovery. Invest Urol 17:427, 1980.

279. Levinsky, LNG, et al.: Acute renal failure. In Brenner, BM and Rector, FC (eds): The Kidney. Philadelphia, WB Saunders, 1981, p 1181.

280. Franklin, SS and Maxwell, MH: Acute renal failure. In Clinical Disorders of Fluid and Electrolyte Metabolism. New York, McGraw-Hill, 1980, p 745.

281. Humes, HD: Role of calcium in pathogenesis of acute renal failure. Am J Physiol 250:F579, 1986.

282. Humes, HD and Weinberg, JM: Toxic nephropathies. In Brenner, BM and Rector, FC (eds): The Kidney, 3rd ed. Philadelphia, WB Saunders, 1986, p 1491.

283. Oken, DE: Hemodynamic basis for human acute renal failure (vasomotor nephrology). Am J Med 76:702, 1984.

284. Franklin, SS and Maxwell, MH: Acute renal failure. In Clinical Disorders of Fluid and Electrolyte Metabolism. New York, McGraw-Hill, 1972, p 727.

285. Flamenbaum, W: Pathophysiology of acute renal failure. Arch Intern Med 131:911, 1973.

286. Hostetter, TH, et al.: Renal circulatory and nephron function in experimental acute renal failure. In Brenner, BM and Lazarus, JM (eds): Acute Renal Failure. Philadelphia, WB Saunders, 1983, p 99.

287. Arbeit, LA and Weinstein, SW: Acute tubular necrosis pathophysiology and management. Med Clin North Am 65:147, 1981.

288. Smolens, P and Stein, JH: Hemodynamic factors in acute renal failure: Pathophysiologic and therapeutic implications. In Brenner, BM and Stein, JH (eds): Acute Renal Failure. New York, Churchill Livingstone, 1980, p 180.

289. Racusen, LC and Solez, K: Podocyte changes in postischemic acute renal failure. In Solez, K and Whelton, A (eds): Acute Renal Failure: Correlations Between Morphology and Function. New York, Marcel Dekker, 1984, p 135.

290. Gattone, VH, et al.: The morphology of the renal microvascu-

lature in glycerol- and gentamicin-induced acute renal failure. J Lab Clin Med 101:183, 1983.

291. Schrier, RW, et al.: Cellular calcium in ischemic acute renal failure: Role of calcium entry blockers. Kidney Int 32:313, 1987.

292. Porter, GA and Bennett, WM: Nephrotoxin-induced acute renal failure. *In* Brenner, BM and Stein, JH (eds): Acute Renal Failure. New York, Churchill Livingstone, 1980, p 123.

293. Porter, GA and Bennett, WM: Toxic nephropathies. *In* Brenner, BM and Rector, FC (eds): The Kidney. Philadelphia, WB Saunders, 1981, p 2045.

294. Riviere, JE: A possible mechanism for increased susceptibility to aminoglycoside nephrotoxicity in chronic renal disease. N Engl J Med 307:252, 1982.

295. Clive, D and Stoff, JS: Renal syndromes associated with nonsteroidal anti-inflammatory drugs. N Engl J Med 310:563, 1984.

296. Beasly, VR and Buck, WB: Acute ethylene glycol toxicosis: A review. Vet Hum Toxicol 22:255, 1980.

297. Osweiler, GD, et al.: Ethylene glycol (antifreeze). *In* Clinical and Diagnostic Veterinary Toxicology. Dubuque, Kendall/Hunt Pub Co, p 398.

298. Thrall, MA, et al.: Clinicopathologic findings in dogs and cats with ethylene glycol intoxication. JAVMA 184:37, 1984.

299. Grauer, GF and Thrall, MA: Ethylene glycol (antifreeze) poisoning in the dog and cat. JAAHA 18:493, 1982.

300. Grauer, GF, et al.: Early clinicopathologic findings in dogs ingesting ethylene glycol. Am J Vet Res 45:2299, 1984.

301. Johnson, SE, et al.: Current status of ethylene glycol toxicity in dogs - a review. Minn Vet 19:32, 1979.

302. Sanyer, JL, et al.: Systematic treatment of ethylene glycol toxicosis in dogs. Am J Vet Res 34:527, 1973.

303. Nunamaker, DM, et al.: Treatment of ethylene glycol in the dog. JAVMA 159:310, 1971.

304. Murphy, MJ, et al.: 1,3 Butanediol treatment of ethylene glycol toxicosis in dogs. Am J Vet Res 45:2293, 1984.

305. DaRoza, R, et al.: Acute ethylene glycol poisoning. Crit Care Med 12:1003, 1984.

306. Parry, MF and Wallach, R: Ethylene glycol poisoning. Am J Med 57:143, 1974.

307. Rowland, J: Incidence of ethylene glycol intoxication in dogs and cats seen at Colorado State University veterinary teaching hospital. Vet Hum Toxicol 29:41, 1987.

308. Berg, P, et al.: Renal allograft in a dog poisoned with ethylene glycol. JAVMA 158:468, 1971.

309. DiBartola, SP, et al.: Hemodialysis of a dog with acute renal failure. JAVMA 186:3123, 1985.

310. Beckett, SD and Shields, RP: Treatment of acute ethylene glycol (antifreeze) toxicosis in the dog. JAVMA 158:472, 1971.

311. Cieciura, L, et al.: Ultrastructural appearances of nephron damage in acute poisoning with ethylene glycol. Proc EDTA 20:636, 1983.

312. Szabuniewicz, M, et al.: A new approach to the treatment of ethylene glycol poisoning in dogs. Southwest Vet 28:7, 1975.

313. Van Stee, EW, et al.: The treatment of ethylene glycol toxicosis with pyrazole. J Pharmacol Exp Ther 192:251, 1975.

314. Kersting, EJ and Nielsen, SW: Experimental ethylene glycol poisoning in the dog. Am J Vet Res 27:574, 1966.

315. Kersting, EJ and Nielsen, SW: Ethylene glycol poisoning in small animals. JAVMA 146:113, 1965.

316. Coggins, CH and Fang, LST: Acute renal failure associated with antibiotics, anesthetic agents, and radiographic contrast agents. *In* Brenner, BM and Lazarus, JM (eds): Acute Renal Failure. Philadelphia, WB Saunders, 1983, p 283.

317. Appel, GB and Neu, HC: The nephrotoxicity of antimicrobial agents. N Engl J Med 296:663, 1977.

318. Appel, GB and Neu, HC: The nephrotoxicity of antimicrobial agents. N Engl J Med 296:722, 1977.

319. Appel, GB and Neu, HC: The nephrotoxicity of antimicrobial agents. N Engl J Med 296:784, 1977.

320. Thompson, RL: The cephalosporins. Mayo Clin Proc 52:625, 1977.

321. Fried, JS and Hinthorn, DR: The cephalosporins. *In* Disease-A-Month. Chicago, Year Book Med Pub, 1985, p 1.

322. Moellering, RC and Swartz, MN: The newer cephalosporins. N Engl J Med 294:24, 1976.

323. Papich, MG: Clinical pharmacology of cephalosporin antibiotics. JAVMA 184:344, 1984.

324. Stevenson, S: Oxytetracycline nephrotoxicosis in two dogs. JAVMA 176:530, 1980.

325. Brown, SA, et al.: Fanconi syndrome and acute renal failure associated with gentamicin therapy in a dog. JAAHA 22:635, 1986.

326. Brown, SA, et al.: Gentamicin-associated acute renal failure in the dog. JAVMA 186:686, 1985.

327. Raisbeck, MF: Fatal nephrotoxicosis associated with furosemide and gentamicin therapy in a dog. JAVMA 183:892, 1983.

328. Greco, DS, et al.: Urinary gamma-glutamyl transpeptidase activity in dogs with gentamicin-induced nephrotoxicity. Am J Vet Res 46:2332, 1985.

329. McNeil, JS, et al.: The role of prostaglandins in gentamicin-induced nephrotoxicity in the dog. Nephron 33:202, 1983.

330. Adelman, RD, et al.: Furosemide enhancement of experimental gentamicin nephrotoxicity: Comparison of function and morphological correlations with urinary enzyme activities. J Infect Dis 140:342, 1979.

331. Adelman, RD, et al.: Comparative nephrotoxicity of gentamicin and netilmicin: Functional and morphological correlations with urinary enzyme activities. Curr Probl Clin Biochem 9:166, 1979.

332. Cronin, RE, et al.: Natural history of aminoglycoside nephrotoxicity in the dog. J Lab Clin Med 95:463, 1980.

333. Hardy, ML, et al.: The nephrotoxic potential of gentamicin in the cat: Enzymuria and alterations in urine concentrating capability. J Vet Pharmacol Ther 8:382, 1985.

334. Short, CR, et al.: The nephrotoxic potential of gentamicin in the cat: A pharmacokinetic and histopathologic investigation. J Vet Pharmacol Ther 9:325, 1986.

335. Burrows, GE: Aminocyclitol antibiotics. JAVMA 176:1280, 1980.

336. Humes, HD, et al.: Clinical and pathophysiologic aspects of aminoglycoside nephrotoxicity. Am J Kidney Dis 2:5, 1982.

337. Kaloyanides, GJ and Pastoriza-Munoz, E: Aminoglycoside nephrotoxicity. Kidney Int 18:571, 1980.

338. Morin, JP, et al.: Gentamicin-induced nephrotoxicity: A cell biology approach. Kidney Int 8:583, 1980.

339. Marche, P, et al.: Aminoglycoside-induced alterations of phosphoinositide metabolism. Kidney Int 31:59, 1987.

340. Bennett, WM: Aminoglycoside nephrotoxicity. Nephron 35:73, 1983.

341. Schor, N, et al.: Pathophysiology of altered glomerular function in aminoglycoside-treated rats. Kidney Int 9:288, 1981.

342. Gattone, VH, et al.: The morphology of the renal microvasculature in glycerol- and gentamicin-induced acute renal failure. J Lab Clin Med 101:183, 1983.

343. Pyle, L: Clinical pharmacology of amphotericin B. JAVMA 179:83, 1981.

344. Gerkens, JF, et al.: Effect of aminophylline on amphotericin B nephrotoxicity in the dog. J Pharmacol Exp Ther 224:609, 1983.

345. Reiner, NF and Thompson, WL: Dopamine and saralasin antagonism of renal vasoconstriction and oliguria caused by amphotericin B in dogs. J Infect Dis 140:564, 1979.

346. Cappasso, G, et al.: Amphotericin B and amphotericin B methylester: Effect on brush border membrane permeability. Kidney Int 30:311, 1985.

347. Gerkens, JF and Branch, RA: The influence of sodium status and furosemide on canine acute amphotericin B nephrotoxicity. J Pharmacol Exp Ther 214:306, 1980.

348. Bullock, WE, et al.: Can mannitol reduce amphotericin B nephrotoxicity? A double blind study and description of a new vascular lesion in kidneys. Antimicrob Agents Chemother 10:555, 1976.

349. Hellebusch, AA, et al.: The use of mannitol to reduce the nephrotoxicity of amphotericin B. Surg Gynecol Obstet 134:241, 1972.

350. Garnick, MB, et al.: Acute renal failure associated with cancer treatment. *In* Brenner, BM and Lazarus, JM (eds): Acute Renal Failure. Philadelphia, WB Saunders, 1983, p 527.

351. Lohrer, PJ and Einhorn, LH: Cisplatin. Ann Intern Med 100:704, 1984.

352. Ries, F and Klastersky, J: Nephrotoxicity induced by cancer chemotherapy with special emphasis on cisplatin toxicity. Am J Kidney Dis 8:368, 1986.

353. Safirstein, R, et al.: Cisplatin nephrotoxicity. Am J Kidney Dis 8:356, 1986.

354. Chew, DJ and Capen, CC: Hypercalcemic nephropathy and associated disorders. In Kirk, RW (ed): Current Veterinary Therapy VII. Philadelphia, WB Saunders, 1980, p 1067.

355. Chew, DJ and Meuten, DJ: Disorders of calcium and phosphorus metabolism. Vet Clin North Am 12(3):411, 1982.

356. Chew, DJ and Meuten, DJ: Primary hyperparathyroidism. In Kirk, RW (ed): Current Veterinary Therapy VIII. Philadelphia, WB Saunders, 1983, p 880.

357. Meuten, DJ: Hypercalcemia. Vet Clin North Am 14(4):891, 1984.

358. Kruger, JM, et al.: Treatment of hypercalcemia. In Kirk, RW (ed): Current Veterinary Therapy IX. Philadelphia, WB Saunders, 1986, p 75.

359. Lins, BE: Renal function in hypercalcemic dogs during hydropenia and during saline infusion. Acta Physiol Scan 106:177, 1979.

360. Tsukamotto, H, et al.: Nephrotoxicity of sodium arsenate in dogs. Am J Vet Res 44:2324, 1983.

361. Leib, MS, et al.: Acute renal failure associated with thiacetarsamide sodium treatment for adult heartworms in a dog. JAAHA 20:973, 1984.

362. Fleming, JT and Pedersoli, WM: Serum inorganic fluoride and renal function in dogs after methoxyflurane anesthesia, tetracycline treatment, and surgical manipulation. Am J Vet Res 41:2025, 1980.

363. Flamenbaum, W, et al.: Acute renal failure associated with myoglobinuria and hemoglobinuria. In Brenner, BM and Lazarus, JM (eds): Acute Renal Failure. Philadelphia, WB Saunders, 1983, p 269.

364. Rowland, LP and Penn, AS: Myoglobinuria. Med Clin North Am 1233, 1972.

365. Spangler, WL and Muggli, FM: Seizure-induced rhabdomyolysis accompanied by acute renal failure in a dog. JAVMA 172:1190, 1978.

366. Krum, SH and Osborne, CA: Heatstroke in the dog: A polysystemic disorder. JAVMA 170:531, 1977.

367. Gannon, JR: Exertional rhabdomyolysis (myoglobinuria) in the racing greyhound. In Kirk, RW (ed): Current Veterinary Therapy VII. Philadelphia, WB Saunders, 1980, p 783.

368. Rose, BD: Renal circulation and glomerular filtrate. In Rose, DD (ed): Clinical Physiology of Acid-Base and Electrolyte Disorders. New York, McGraw-Hill, 1984, p 53.

369. Koushanpour, E and Kriz, W: Regulation of renal blood flow and glomerular filtration rate. In Renal Physiology. New York, Springer-Verlag, 1986, p 73.

370. Adams, HR and Parker, JL: Pharmacologic management of circulatory shock: Cardiovascular drugs and corticosteroids. JAVMA 175:186, 1979.

371. Kopp, UC and DiBona, GF: The function of the renal nerves. Kidney 15:17, 1982.

372. Dimerstein, RJ, et al.: Histofluorescence techniques provide evidence for dopamine containing neuronal elements in canine kidney. Science 205:497, 1979.

373. Adam, WR: Aldosterone and dopamine receptors in the kidney: Sites for pharmacologic manipulation of renal function. Kidney Int 18:623, 1980.

374. Lucas, CE: The renal response to acute injury and sepsis. Surg Clin North Am 56:953, 1976.

375. Stoff, JS and Clive, DM: Role of prostaglandins and thromboxane in acute renal failure. In Brenner, BM and Lazarus, JM (eds): Acute Renal Failure. Philadelphia, WB Saunders, 1983, p 157.

376. Osswald, H, et al.: Glomerular dynamics in dogs at reduced renal artery pressure. Am J Physiol 236:F25, 1979.

377. Stone, EA, et al.: Renal function after prolonged hypotensive anesthesia and surgery in dogs with reduced renal mass. Am J Vet Res 42:1675, 1981.

378. Jamison, RL and Maffly, RH: The urinary concentrating mechanism. N Engl J Med 295:1059, 1976.

379. Rose, BD: Pathophysiology of Renal Disease, 2nd ed. New York, McGraw-Hill, 1987, p 159.

380. Brenner, BM, et al.: Molecular basis of proteinuria of glomerular origin. N Engl J Med 298:826, 1978.

381. Kanwar, YS: Biophysiology of glomerular filtration and proteinuria. Lab Invest 51:7, 1984.

382. Couser, WG: Mechanisms of glomerular injury in immune-complex disease. Kidney Int 28:569, 1985.

383. Couser, WG, et al.: Complement and the direct mediation of immune glomerular injury: a new perspective. Kidney Int 28:879, 1985.

384. Couser, WG and Salant, DJ: In situ immune complex formation and glomerular injury. Kidney Int 17:1, 1980.

385. Adler, S and Couser, W: Review: Immunologic mechanisms of renal disease. Am J Med Sci 289:55, 1985.

386. Cameron, JS: Platelets in glomerular disease. Ann Rev Med 35:175, 1984.

387. Glenner, GG: Amyloid deposits and amyloidosis: The β fibrilloses. N Engl J Med 302:1283, 1980.

388. Husby, G and Sletten, K: Chemical and clinical classification of amyloidosis. Scand J Immunol 23:253, 1986.

389. Maury, CPJ: Reactive (secondary) amyloidosis and its pathogenesis. Rheumatol Int 5:1, 1984.

390. DiBartola, SP, et al.: Isolation and characterization of amyloid protein AA in the Abyssinian cat. Lab Invest 52:485, 1985.

391. Benson, MD, et al.: Identification and characterization of amyloid protein AA in spontaneous canine amyloidosis. Lab Invest 52:448, 1985.

392. Slauson, DO, et al.: A clinicopathologic study of renal amyloidosis in dogs. J Comp Pathol 80:335, 1970.

393. Clark, LD and Seawright, AA: Generalized amyloidosis in seven cats. Path Vet 6:117, 1969.

394. Chew, DJ, et al.: Renal amyloidosis in related Abyssinian cats. JAVMA 181:139, 1982.

395. Boyce, JT, et al.: Familial renal amyloidosis in Abyssinian cats. Vet Pathol 21:33, 1984.

396. DiBartola, SP, et al.: Tissue distribution of amyloid deposits in Abyssinian cats with familial amyloidosis. J Comp Path 96:387, 1986.

397. Lavie, G, et al.: Degradation of serum amyloid A protein by surface-associated enzymes of human blood monocytes. J Exp Med 148:1020, 1978.

398. Maury, CPJ and Teppo, AM: Mechanism of reduced amyloid A-degrading activity in serum of patients with secondary amyloidosis. Lancet 2:234, 1982.

399. Yano, BL, et al.: Feline insular amyloid: Histochemical distinction from secondary systemic amyloid. Vet Pathol 18:181, 1981.

400. Johnson, KH, et al.: Feline insular amyloid: Immunohistochemical and immunochemical evidence that the amyloid is insulin-related. Vet Pathol 22:463, 1985.

401. Appel, GB, et al.: The hyperlipidemia of the nephrotic syndrome: Relation to plasma albumin concentration, oncotic pressure, and viscosity. N Engl J Med 312:1544, 1985.

402. Kaysen, GA, et al.: Mechanisms and consequences of proteinuria. Lab Invest 54:479, 1986.

403. Rothschild, MA, et al.: Albumin synthesis. N Engl J Med 286:748, 1972.

404. Kaysen, GA and Schoenfeld, PY: Albumin homeostasis in patients undergoing continuous ambulatory peritoneal dialysis. Kidney Int 25:107, 1984.

405. Dorhout Mees, EJ, et al.: Blood volume and sodium retention in the nephrotic syndrome: a controversial pathophysiological concept. Nephron 36:201, 1984.

406. DiBartola, SP, et al.: Urinary protein excretion and immunopathologic findings in dogs with glomerular disease. JAVMA 177:73, 1980.

407. Center, SA, et al.: Clinicopathologic, renal immunofluorescent, and light microscopic features of glomerulonephritis in the dog: 41 cases (1975-1985). JAVMA 190:81, 1987.

408. Brown, EA: The nephrotic syndrome. Postgrad Med J 61:1057, 1985.

409. Brown, E, et al.: Is the renin-angiotensin-aldosterone system involved in the sodium retention of the nephrotic syndrome? Nephron 32:102, 1982.

410. Dorhout Mees, EJ: Edema formation in the nephrotic syndrome. Contrib Nephrol 43:64, 1984.

411. Brown, EA, et al.: Lack of effect of captopril on the sodium retention of the nephrotic syndrome. Nephron 37:43, 1984.

412. Brown, EA, et al.: Evidence that some mechanism other than the renin system causes sodium retention in the nephrotic syndrome. Lancet 2:1237, 1982.

413. Brown, EA, et al.: Sodium retention in nephrotic syndrome is due to an intrarenal defect: evidence from steroid-induced remission. Nephron 39:290, 1985.

414. Ichikawa, I, et al.: Role for intrarenal mechanism in the impaired salt excretion of experimental nephrotic syndrome. J Clin Invest 71:91, 1983.

415. Geers, AB, et al.: Functional relationships in the nephrotic syndrome. Kidney Int 26:324, 1984.

416. Kendall, AG, et al.: Nephrotic syndrome: A hypercoagulable state. Arch Intern Med 127:1021, 1971.

417. Slauson, DO and Gribble, DH: Thrombosis complicating renal amyloidosis in dogs. Vet Pathol 8:352, 1971.

418. DiBartola, SP and Meuten, DJ: Renal amyloidosis in two dogs presented for thromboembolic phenomena. JAAHA 16:129, 1980.

419. Thomson, C and Forbes, CD, et al.: Changes in blood coagulation and fibrinolysis in the nephrotic syndrome. Q J Med 43:399, 1974.

420. Llach, F: Hypercoagulability, renal vein thrombosis, and other thrombotic complications of nephrotic syndrome. Kidney Int 28:429, 1985.

421. Green, RA and Kabel, AL: Hypercoagulable state in three dogs with nephrotic syndrome: role of acquired antithrombin III deficiency. JAVMA 181:914, 1982.

422. Kauffmann, RH, et al.: Acquired antithrombin III deficiency and thrombosis in the nephrotic syndrome. Am J Med 65:607, 1978.

423. Jorgensen, KA and Stoffersen, E: Antithrombin III and the nephrotic syndrome. Scand J Hematol 22:442, 1979.

424. Boneu, B, et al.: Comparison of progressive antithrombin activity and concentration of three thrombin inhibitors in nephrotic syndrome. Thromb Haemost 46:623, 1981.

425. Walter, E, et al.: Platelet hyperaggregability as a consequence of the nephrotic syndrome. Thrombosis Res 23:473, 1981.

426. Rasadee, A and Feldman, BF: Nephrotic syndrome: a platelet hyperaggregability state. Vet Res Comm 9:199, 1985.

427. Green, RA, et al.: Hypoalbuminemia-related platelet hypersensitivity in two dogs with nephrotic syndrome. JAVMA 186:485, 1985.

428. Rose, BD: Pathophysiology of Renal Disease, 2nd ed. New York, McGraw-Hill, 1987, p 15.

429. Barsanti, JA and Finco, DR: Protein concentration of urine of normal dogs. Am J Vet Res 40:1583, 1979.

430. Biewenga, WJ: Urinary protein loss in the dog: Nephrological study of 29 dogs without signs of renal disease. Res Vet Sci 33:366, 1982.

431. White, JV, et al.: Use of protein-to-creatinine ratio in a single urine specimen for quantitative estimation of canine proteinuria. JAVMA 185:882, 1984.

432. Grauer, GF, et al.: Estimation of quantitative proteinuria in the dog, using the urine protein-to-creatinine ratio from a random, voided sample. Am J Vet Res 46:2116, 1985.

433. Center, SA, et al.: 24-hour urine protein/creatinine ratio in dogs with protein-losing nephropathies. JAVMA 187:820, 1985.

434. McCaw, DL, et al.: Effect of collection time and exercise restriction on the prediction of urine protein excretion, using urine protein/creatinine ratio in dogs. Am J Vet Res 46:1665, 1985.

435. Jergens, AE, et al.: Effects of collection time and food consumption on the urine protein/creatinine ratio in the dog. Am J Vet Res 48:1106, 1987.

436. Jaenke, RS and Allen, TA: Membranous nephropathy in the dog. Vet Pathol 23:718, 1986.

437. Murray, M and Wright, NG: A morphologic study of canine glomerulonephritis. Lab Invest 30:213, 1974.

438. Muller-Peddinghaus, R and Trautwein, G: Spontaneous glomerulonephritis in dogs. Classification and immunopathology. Vet Pathol 14:1, 1977.

439. Kurtz, JM, et al.: Naturally occurring canine glomerulonephritis. Am J Pathol 67:471, 1972.

440. Rouse, BT and Lewis, RJ: Canine glomerulonephritis: Prevalence in dogs submitted at random for euthanasia. Can J Comp Med 39:365, 1975.

441. Lewis, RJ: Canine glomerulonephritis: Results from a microscopic evaluation of fifty cases. Can Vet J 17:171, 1976.

442. McDougall, DF, et al.: Canine chronic renal disease: Prevalence and types of glomerulonephritis in the dog. Kidney Int 29:1144, 1986.

443. Wright, NG, et al.: Membranous nephropathy in the cat and dog: A renal biopsy and follow-up study of sixteen cases. Kidney Int 45:269, 1981.

444. Osborne, CA and Vernier, RL: Glomerulonephritis in the dog and cat: a comparative review. JAAHA 9:101, 1973.

445. Osborne, CA, et al.: Membranous lupus glomerulonephritis in a dog. JAAHA 9:295, 1973.

446. Murray, M, et al.: Glomerulonephritis in a dog. A histological and electron microscopical study. Res Vet Sci 12:493, 1971.

447. Nash, AS, et al.: Membranous nephropathy in the cat: A clinical and pathological study. Vet Rec 105:71, 1979.

448. Arthur, JE, et al.: An immunohistological study of feline glomerulonephritis using the peroxidase-antiperoxidase method. Res Vet Sci 37:12, 1984.

449. Arthur, JE, et al.: The long-term prognosis of feline idiopathic membranous glomerulonephropathy. JAAHA 22:731, 1986.

450. Lucke, VM and Hunt, AC: Interstitial nephropathy and papillary necrosis in the domestic cat. J Pathol Bacteriol 89:723, 1965.

451. Finco, DR, et al.: Evaluation of methods for localization of urinary tract infection in the female dog. Am J Vet Res 40:707, 1979.

452. Finco, DR and Barsanti, JA: Bacterial pyelonephritis. Vet Clin North Am 645, 1979.

453. Allen, TA and Jaenke, RS: Pyelonephritis in dogs. Comp Cont Ed 7:421, 1985.

454. Ling, GV, et al.: Relation of antibody-coated urine bacteria to the site(s) of infection in experimental dogs. Am J Vet Res 41:686, 1980.

455. Ling, GV, et al.: Relationship of upper and lower urinary tract infection and bacterial invasion of uroepithelium to antibody-coated bacteria test results in female dogs. Am J Vet Res 46:499, 1985.

456. Ling, GV, et al.: Percutaneous nephropyelocentesis and nephropyelostomy in the dog: A description of the technique. Am J Vet Res 40:1605, 1979.

457. Ling, GV, et al.: Chronic urinary tract infection in dogs: Induction by inoculation with bacteria via percutaneous nephropyelostomy. Am J Vet Res 48:794, 1986.

458. Andriole, V: The role of Tamm-Horsfall protein in the pathogenesis of reflux nephropathy and chronic pyelonephritis. Yale J Biol Med 58:91, 1985.

459. Crowell, WA and Finco, DR: Frequency of pyelitis, pyelonephritis, renal perivasculitis, and renal infarction in dogs. Am J Vet Res 36:111, 1975.

460. Kelly, DF: Pyelonephritis and renal response to infection. In Bovee, KC (ed): Canine Nephrology. Media, PA, Harwall Pub, 1984, p 481.

461. Thomsen, AC: Mycoplasmas in human pyelonephritis: Demonstration of antibodies in serum and urine. J Clin Microbiol 8:197, 1978.

462. Thomsen, AC: Occurrence of mycoplasmas in urinary tracts of patients with acute pyelonephritis. J Clin Microbiol 8:84, 1978.

463. Thomsen, AC: The occurrence of mycoplasmas in the urinary tract of patients with chronic pyelonephritis. Acta Pathol Microbiol Scand (B) 83:10, 1975.

464. Koshimizu, K and Ogata, M: Characterization and differentiation of mycoplasmas of canine origin. Jpn J Vet Sci 36:391, 1974.

465. Stamm, WE, et al.: Causes of the acute urethral syndrome in women. N Engl J Med 303:409, 1980.

466. Komaroff, AL: Acute dysuria in women. N Engl J Med 310:368, 1984.

467. Green, CA, et al.: Quantitative estimation of Mycobacterium leprae in exhaled nasal breath. Lepr Rev 54:337, 1983.

468. Roberts, JA: Pathogenesis of pyelonephritis. J Urol 129:1102, 1983.

469. Roberts, JA: Urinary tract infections. Am J Kidney Dis 4:103, 1984.

470. Hottendorf, GH and Hirth, RS: Lesions of spontaneous subclinical disease in beagle dogs. Vet Pathol 11:240, 1974.

471. Christie, BA: The occurrence of vesicoureteral reflux and pyelonephritis in apparently normal dogs. Invest Urol 10:359, 1973.

472. Wettimuny, SG and De, S: Pyelonephritis in the dog. J Comp Pathol 77:193, 1967.

473. Bush, BM: A review of the etiology and consequences of urinary tract infections in the dog. Br Vet J 132:632, 1976.

474. Lucke, VM: Renal disease in the domestic cat. J Pathol Bacteriol 95:67, 1968.

475. Lees, G and Osborne, CA: Antibacterial properties of urine: A comparative review. JAAHA 5:125, 1979.

476. Davis, EG and Hain, RF: Urinary antisepsis: The antiseptic properties of normal dog urine. J Urol 2:309, 1918.

477. Sobel, JD and Kaye, D: Host factors in the pathogenesis of urinary tract infections. Am J Med 76:122, 1984.

478. Mulholland, SG, et al.: The antibacterial properties of urine. Invest Urol 6:569, 1969.

479. Lees, GA, et al.: Adverse effects of open indwelling urethral catheterization in clinically normal male cats. Am J Vet Res 42:825, 1981.

480. Christie, BA: Vesicoureteral reflux in dogs. JAVMA 162:772, 1973.

481. Lenaghan, D and Cussen, LJ: Vesicoureteral reflux in pups. Invest Urol 5:449, 1968.

482. King, LR and Sellards, HG: The effect of sterile vesicoureteral reflux on renal growth and development in puppies. Invest Urol 9:95, 1971.

483. Sommer, JL and Roberts, JA: Ureteral reflux in dogs resulting from chronic urinary infection. J Urol 95:502, 1966.

484. Rocha, H: Experimental pyelonephritis: Characteristics of the infection in dogs. Yale J Biol Med 36:183, 1963.

485. Senior, DF: Bacterial urinary tract infections: Invasion, host defenses, and new approaches to prevention. Comp Cont Ed Pract Vet 7:334, 1985.

486. Nolan, LK, et al.: Comparison of virulence factors and antibiotic resistance profiles of *Escherichia coli* strains from humans and dogs with urinary tract infections. J Vet Intern Med 1:152, 1987.

487. Kelly, DF, et al.: Experimental pyelonephritis in the cat. Gross and histologic changes. J Comp Pathol 89:125, 1979.

488. Ginder, DR: Urinary tract infection and pyelonephritis due to *Escherichia coli* in dogs infected with canine adenovirus. J Infect Dis 129:715, 1974.

489. Silverblatt, FJ and Ofek, I: Influence of pili on the virulence of *Proteus mirabilis* in experimental hematogenous pyelonephritis. J Infect Dis 138:664, 1978.

490. Mooney, JK and Hinman, F: Surface differences in cells of proximal and distal canine urethra. J Urol 111:495, 1974.

491. Hinman, F: Urethrovesical dysfunction and infection. Annu Rev Med 24:83, 1973.

492. Gillenwater, JY: Host antibacterial defenses of the lower urinary tract. *In* Bacteriuria and Urinary Tract Infections. New York, National Kidney Foundation, 1974, p 125.

493. Moorevill, M, et al.: Enhancement of the bladder defense mechanisms by an exogenous agent. J Urol 130:607, 1983.

494. Mulholland, SG, et al.: Effect of hormonal deprivation on the bladder defense mechanism. J Urol 127:1010, 1982.

495. Goulden, BE: Vesico-ureteral reflux in the dog. N Z Vet J 16:167, 1968.

496. Schoenberg, HW, et al.: Effect of lower urinary tract infection upon ureteral function. J Urol 92:107, 1964.

497. Grana, L, et al.: Effects of gram-negative bacteria on ureteral structure and function. J Urol 99:539, 1968.

498. Appleton, JA, et al.: Scanning electron microscopy of experimentally induced pyelonephritis in the rat. Am J Vet Res 42:351, 1981.

499. Shimamura, T: Mechanisms of renal tissue destruction in an experimental acute pyelonephritis. Exp Mol Pathol 34:34, 1981.

108 DISEASES OF THE KIDNEYS AND URETERS

DAVID POLZIN, CARL OSBORNE, and TIM O'BRIEN

SYNDROMES IN VETERINARY UROLOGY/NEPHROLOGY

Diseases of the urinary tract may be associated with a wide and sometimes confusing array of clinical manifestations. This diversity of clinical manifestations is made more manageable by the fact that most canine and feline urinary tract disorders can be categorized into ten primary clinical syndromes (Table 108–1). Detection of these syndromes is not difficult and can usually be accomplished on the basis of routine clinical and laboratory findings (Table 108–2). Categorizing clinical signs according to the correct syndrome is useful because it provides order and direction to subsequent diagnosis and therapy.

To identify these syndromes, a problem-specific urinary tract data base should be collected for all patients suspected of having urinary tract disease (Table 108–3). The defined urinary tract data base permits detection of nearly all cases of acute renal failure, chronic renal failure, nephrotic syndrome, dysuria/pollakiuria, and abnormal micturition. Many episodes of urinary tract infection, urinary obstruction, renal tubular defects, and "asymptomatic" urinary abnormalities can also be defined from this data base alone. Addition of urine cultures and survey abdominal radiography will enhance detection of urinary tract infection and urolithiasis. Some syndromes may require additional studies for verification (e.g., quantification of urine protein excre-

tion to confirm nephrotic syndrome; contrast radiography to identify some uroliths). Likewise, unusual or atypical features of a syndrome, coexistence of two or more syndromes, and/or overlapping of syndromes (e.g., urolithiasis and urinary obstruction) may require additional diagnostic studies.

The syndromes of acute renal failure, chronic renal failure, nephrotic syndrome, or renal tubular abnormalities localize clinical abnormalities to the kidneys. Asymptomatic urinary abnormalities, urolithiasis, urinary obstruction, or urinary tract infection may be associated with disease of the upper urinary (kidneys and ureters) and/or lower urinary (bladder and urethra) tract. Syndromes of dysuria/pollakiuria and abnormal micturition (abnormalities related to the storage and voiding phases of micturition, such as urinary incontinence or reflex dyssynergia) indicate involvement of the bladder and/or urethra. Aspects of syndromes related to the lower urinary tract are discussed in Chapters 110, 111, and 112.

ACUTE RENAL FAILURE

Definition and Clinical Characteristics

The term renal failure implies sufficient loss of organ function to alter homeostasis. Renal functions may be broadly subclassified into excretory, regulatory, and biosynthetic functions. Excretory function refers to elimination of waste products of body metabolism, toxins, and drugs. Azotemia is the common clinical marker of renal excretory failure. Regulatory function involves maintenance of body fluid and electrolyte balance. Renal regulatory function is usually assessed by determining urine concentrating ability during dehydration or azotemia, since concentration of urine is the principal means by which the kidneys regulate fluid balance. Biosynthetic function of the kidneys involves synthesis of hormones and autacoids (autacoids are physiologically active, endogenous substances that do not meet

TABLE 108–1. SYNDROMES OF VETERINARY CLINICAL UROLOGY/NEPHROLOGY

Acute renal failure (ARF)
Chronic renal failure (CRF)
Nephrotic syndrome (NS)
Tubular defects (TD)
Asymptomatic urinary abnormalities (AUA)
Urinary obstruction (UO)
Urolithiasis (ULT)
Urinary tract infection (UTI)
Dysuria/pollakiuria (D/P)
Abnormal micturition (AM)

TABLE 108–2. CLINICAL AND LABORATORY FINDINGS IN CLINICAL SYNDROMES

Clinical Findings	ARF	CRF	NS	TD	UTI	ULT	UO	AUA	D/P	AM
Polydipsia	O	O		O	O					
Polyuria	O	O		O	O					
Nocturia		O			O	O			O	
Oliguria/anuria	X						X			
Dysuria					O	O	O		S	
Pollakiuria					O	O			S	✓
Incontinence										S
Urinary retention							X			X
Slow urine stream							X			X
Urolith voided						S				
Malodorous urine					O	O				
Lumbar pain					O	O	O			
Tender bladder					O	O	O		O	
Renomegaly							O	O		
Azotemia	X	X					X			
Uremia	X	X					X			
Anemia		O								
Skeletal Dz		O								
Edema/ascites			X							
Hematuria					O	O			O	O
Proteinuria			X	O						
Pyuria					X	O			O	
Glucosuria				X						
Weight loss		X	O							
Bacteriuria					X	O			O	

This list of signs is not all encompassing of all possible signs for each syndrome. Only common or important signs that guide syndrome identification are listed. More than one syndrome may occur in any patient. O, occurs in the syndrome; X, important clue to the syndrome; S, sufficient to identify the syndrome.

the classic definition for hormones; e.g., angiotensin, prostaglandins), which regulate a variety of renal and nonrenal functions. Examples of hormones or autacoids produced or activated locally by the kidneys include erythropoietin, 1,25-dihydroxycholecalciferol, renin, and prostaglandins. Clinical assessment of renal biosynthetic function is less direct than assessment of renal regulatory or excretory function. For example, renal production of erythropoietin is usually evaluated by examining complete blood counts for evidence of nonregenerative anemia. Renal 1,25-dihydroxycholecalciferol production is evaluated by examining radiographs or bone biopsies for evidence of renal osteodystrophy.

In order for the kidneys to perform these excretory, regulatory, and biosynthetic functions four conditions must exist: (1) renal perfusion with blood must be maintained at a level that allows near normal rates of glomerular filtration and tubular ion and fluid transport; (2) intrinsic renal cell functions must be intact; (3) urine formed should freely pass through the excretory pathway; and (4) a sufficient number of viable, functioning nephrons must be present.[1]

Acute renal failure (ARF) is defined as rapid onset of azotemia over hours to days (at most two weeks), or pathologic oliguria that could not have been present for more than a few days.[1] Oliguria is defined as a urine production rate of less than 0.22 ml/lb/hr for dogs. This figure is based on the estimated minimum quantity of urine in which an average daily solute load can be excreted by kidneys with normal urine concentrating ability. Dogs producing less than this quantity of urine cannot excrete their daily solute load, and thus excretory failure must exist. Rapid onset of azotemia or oliguria indicates rapid deterioration or loss of renal function. The rapid deterioration of renal function characteristic of ARF contrasts with the indolent, inevitable progres-

sion of chronic renal failure (CRF) over months to years. Implicit in the diagnosis of ARF is the potential for reversibility as well as the threat of sudden or rapid deterioration in renal function.

Not all patients with ARF are oliguric. An estimated 30 per cent to 80 per cent of human patients with ARF have normal or increased urine output, a condition termed acute nonoliguric renal failure.[2] Although reliable statistics comparing the relative incidence of oliguric versus nonoliguric ARF have not been reported for dogs and cats, nonoliguric ARF is being recognized with increased frequency in these species.

Although ARF may not by itself constitute an emergency, its causes (e.g., hypovolemia, shock, urinary obstruction, sepsis) and consequences (e.g., hyperkalemia and metabolic acidosis) often are life-threatening. In addition, the potential for enhancing reversibility of renal lesions and return of renal function may be lost if therapeutic intervention is delayed. In contrast to CRF, rapid diagnosis and initiation of therapy may greatly enhance a favorable prognosis in ARF.

Causes

OVERVIEW

ARF may result from prerenal, postrenal, and/or primary renal causes (Table 108–4). Some classification schemes exclude prerenal and postrenal categories as causes of ARF. Because prerenal and postrenal azotemia is often recognized by oliguria and/or azotemia, and may be accompanied by clinical signs of uremia, the authors have included these categories in the syndrome of ARF in order to facilitate recognition of the syndrome, and to promote consideration of prerenal

TABLE 108–3. OUTLINE OF MINIMUM DATA BASE FOR URINARY DISORDERS

1. **Medical History Checklist**
   a. Diet: Type? Frequency of feeding? Supplements? Recent diet changes?
   b. Water consumption: Increased? Decreased? No change? Unknown? If changes noted, when?
   c. Duration of problem?
   d. Previous illness or injury?
   e. Past history of renal disease? Recent evaluation indicating adequate renal function?
   f. Other pets at home? Normal or abnormal?
   g. Exposure to other animals, possible nephrotoxins, drugs?
   h. Micturition
      (1) Character? Frequency? Quantity?
      (2) Pollakiuria (dysuria, tenesmus)?
      (3) Polyuria? If yes, duration?
      (4) Nocturia? If yes, duration?
      (5) Oliguria or anuria?
      (6) Change in urine color?
      (7) Uroliths voided during micturition?
      (8) Urinary incontinence?
      (9) Micturition in abnormal locations?
   i. Change in odor of urine?
   j. Association with other signs not directly related to the urinary tract
      (1) Vomiting?
      (2) Diarrhea?
      (3) Anorexia?
      (4) Weight loss? If yes, recent or chronic?
      (5) Evidence of cardiac disease?
      (6) Others?
   k. Are problems increasing in severity, decreasing in severity, or remaining the same?
   l. Medication history: Medications given? When given? Dosage? Response?
   m. Evidence of recent fluid loss, hypovolemia, or hypotension?
   n. Recent trauma, surgery, or anesthetic episode?
2. **Physical Examination Checklist**
   a. Temperature, pulse rate, and respiratory rate
   b. Hydration status (skin pliability, xerostomia, etc.)
   c. Body weight
   d. Mouth
      (1) Mucosal ulcers?
      (2) Discoloration of tongue?
      (3) Pallor of mucous membranes?
      (4) Evidence of vomitus?
      (5) Loose or missing teeth?
      (6) Enlargement of maxillary tissues?
   e. Cardiovascular system
      (1) Pulse rate and character?
      (2) Mucous membrane color?
      (3) Capillary refill time?
      (4) Heart sounds (murmur, gallop)?
      (5) Venous distention?
      (6) Arterial blood pressure (if available)?
   f. Kidneys
      (1) Both palpable? bilaterally symmetrical?
      (2) Position in abdominal cavity?
      (3) Size?
      (4) Shape, consistency, and contour?
      (5) Pain?
   g. Urinary bladder
      (1) Size, shape, and consistency?
      (2) Position?
      (3) Grating or nongrating masses with or adjacent to bladder lumen? If yes, constant or variable in location?
      (4) Pain?
      (5) Thickness of bladder wall?
   h. Prostate gland
      (1) Position?
      (2) Size, shape, and consistency?
      (3) Pain?
   i. Urethra
      (1) Examination of prepuce and penis in male dogs and cats; urethral or prepucial discharge?
      (2) Examination of perineal urethra in male dogs
      (3) Rectal examination of urethra for
         (a) Position?
         (b) Size, shape, and consistency?
         (c) Periurethral abnormalities?
   j. Ophthalmoscopic examination of fundus (seeking evidence of hypertensive vascular disease)
3. **Laboratory Data**
   a. Urinalysis
   b. Kidney function tests (serum urea nitrogen, serum creatinine concentration, or both)

Adapted from Klausner, JS and Osborne, CA: The urinary tract: Minimum and problem-specific data bases. Vet Clin North Am 11:523, 1981.

and postrenal causes in the diagnostic analysis of ARF. Prerenal and postrenal factors must not be overlooked as causes of ARF because they often are rapidly reversible and therefore are associated with favorable outcomes.

PRERENAL AZOTEMIA

Prerenal azotemia reflects reduction in glomerular filtration rate (GFR) resulting from renal hypoperfusion; it does not result from renal structural damage. It can be immediately reversed (over hours) by restoration of blood flow to the kidneys. However, if renal hypoperfusion is severe or prolonged, or if the patient is predisposed to renal damage, prerenal conditions may progress to acute primary renal failure. Renal hypoperfusion may result from a wide variety of conditions (Table 108–4), the most common of which are disorders that cause dehydration or hemorrhage and associated intravascular volume depletion. Although less common, "third-space" sequestration of fluids and the various causes of reduced "effective" blood volume and primary renal hemodynamic alterations may also cause prerenal azotemia. They may be overlooked as prerenal causes of ARF if evidence of their presence is not specifically sought.

Renal hypoperfusion activates a compensatory protective mechanism called renal autoregulation, designed to preserve GFR, excretory capacity, and restoration of adequate intravascular volume and renal perfusion. When successful, this protective mechanism enables the kidneys to sustain normal renal blood flow (RBF) and GFR despite marked changes in renal perfusion pressure. However, autoregulation preserves GFR more effectively than RBF by increasing the quantity of fluid extracted from blood perfusing the glomerulus to form glomerular filtrate (Chapter 107). If more fluid has been extracted from blood perfusing the glomerular capillaries, blood leaving the glomerulus to enter capillaries that surround the proximal tubules will have a higher protein concentration (little protein passes through the glomerular barrier, thus plasma protein concentration increases when fluid is extracted from blood to form glomerular filtrate). The increased protein concentration

TABLE 108–4. CAUSES OF ACUTE RENAL FAILURE

Prerenal Causes
Intravascular volume depletion
  Hemorrhage
  Dehydration owing to renal or gastrointestinal fluid losses
  "Third-space" sequestration of fluids—abdominal surgery,
    pancreatitis, trauma, peritonitis, burns
Decreased "effective" arterial blood volume
  Peripheral vasodilation—drugs (e.g., antihypertensives), sepsis
  Reduced cardiac output—heart failure, pericardial tamponade,
    arrhythmias, pulmonary embolus, pulmonary hypertension,
    positive-pressure mechanical ventilation
  Hypoalbuminemia—nephrotic syndrome, hepatic failure,
    malnutrition
Primary renal hemodynamic alterations
  Prostaglandin synthesis inhibitors
  Hypercalcemia
  Hepatorenal syndrome (?)
  Vasoconstrictor drugs (alpha-adrenergic agonists, angiotensin II)
  Vasodilation of efferent arteriole (captopril or other converting
    enzyme inhibiting agents)
Postrenal Causes
Obstruction to urine flow
  Upper urinary tract (renal pelvis and ureters)
    Intraluminal—blood clot, urolith, sloughed renal papilla
    Ureteral stricture—congenital, traumatic, postsurgical
    Extrinsic—neoplasm, retroperitoneal fibrosis, inadvertent
      surgical ligation, aberrant vessel, malposition
  Bladder
    Structural obstruction—urolith, neoplasm, malposition (e.g.,
      perineal hernia)
    Functional obstruction—impaired contractility owing to
      neurologic dysfunction or chronic outflow obstruction
  Urethra
    Intraluminal—urolith, blood clot
    Urethral wall—stricture, trauma, neoplasm
    Extraluminal—neoplasm, impingement by pelvic fractures,
      malposition
Reabsorption of urine into circulation
  Urine leakage into peritoneal cavity, retroperitoneal space, or
    periurethral tissues owing to rent anywhere in the urinary
    tract resulting from trauma, neoplasm, or inadequate surgical
    anastomosis
Primary Renal Causes
Tubular epithelium
  Acute tubular necrosis—nephrotoxins or ischemia
  Intratubular obstruction—oxalates, uric acid, myeloma proteins,
    methotrexate, others
Glomerular diseases
Interstitial diseases
  Pyelonephritis (infectious and noninfectious)
  Hypercalcemia
Vascular diseases
Vascular obstruction

in peritubular capillaries surrounding the proximal renal tubules causes increased reabsorption of salt and water (by Starling forces acting across peritubular capillary walls). Increased proximal tubular fluid reabsorption coupled with aldosterone-stimulated increased distal tubular sodium reabsorption results in marked reduction of urine sodium concentration. In addition, increased plasma vasopressin (ADH) levels caused by volume contraction or reduced cardiac output augment water reabsorption in the collecting tubules. All of these mechanisms result in physiologic oliguria characterized by formation of a reduced quantity of urine largely devoid of sodium.

POSTRENAL AZOTEMIA

Postrenal causes of azotemia include obstruction to urine flow (obstructive uropathy) and reabsorption of

urine into the circulation subsequent to loss from the excretory pathway (Table 108–4). Obstructive uropathy is defined as reduction in GFR secondary to resistance to low pressure urine flow anywhere in the excretory pathway. Outflow obstruction or loss of urine from kidneys and/or ureters may be bilateral or unilateral. Unilateral urinary obstruction or urine leakage will not cause azotemia or other major changes in body composition if the contralateral kidney is functioning normally. However, bilateral upper urinary tract and lower urinary tract obstruction or urine leakage causes progressive azotemia, and may result in life-threatening metabolic abnormalities.

Although findings obtained by history and physical examination often reveal obstruction or rupture of the lower urinary tract, renal and ureteral obstruction often requires radiographic or ultrasonographic studies for detection. Urinary obstruction that persists may cause irreversible renal damage. However, early recognition and correction of urinary obstruction may result in complete restoration of renal function.

PRIMARY RENAL FAILURE

Acute Tubular Necrosis. **DEFINITION.** While acute primary renal failure may result from diverse renal diseases and injuries (Table 108–4), the syndrome of acute tubular necrosis (ATN) accounts for the majority of cases. ATN is a syndrome of abrupt and sustained reduction in GFR resulting from an ischemic or toxic renal insult. Reduced GFR is thought to result from a combination of vascular and tubular effects (Table 108–5; see Chapter 107). Reduction in GFR is not immediately reversed when the initiating disturbance is eliminated; tubular cell damage is typical of this condition. Defining ATN in this manner excludes prerenal causes, postrenal causes, and other forms of acute primary renal failure (e.g., glomerulonephritis, pyelonephritis).

The term *acute tubular necrosis* is somewhat of a misnomer because histologic evidence of tubular cell necrosis is not always evident.[3] In addition, factors other than or in addition to tubular cell injury are usually responsible for the abrupt decline in renal function. Other names that have been proposed for this entity include "lower nephron nephrosis," "vasomotor nephropathy," "tubulointerstitial nephritis," and "functional renal failure." Although none of these terms is entirely desirable, ATN is the most commonly used term. From a pathophysiologic standpoint, the term *functional renal failure* may be the least misleading.

ISCHEMIC ACUTE TUBULAR NECROSIS. Conditions predisposing to hypotension, hypovolemia, circulatory collapse, or renal hypoperfusion may contribute to ini-

TABLE 108–5. FACTORS THAT MAY PROMOTE OLIGURIA AND REDUCED GLOMERULAR FILTRATION RATE IN ACUTE TUBULAR NECROSIS

Vascular Factors
  Reduced renal blood flow
  Reduced glomerular capillary ultrafiltration coefficient
Tubular Factors
  Renal tubular obstruction
  Renal transtubular backleak of glomerular filtrate

tiation of ATN. When transient, these factors may also cause prerenal azotemia (Table 108–4). In humans, major trauma, hemorrhage, myohemoglobinuria, cardiac arrest with resuscitation, and interruption of RBF during surgery are among the most commonly reported causes of ischemic ATN.

Varying degrees of renal hypoperfusion may be associated with varying degrees of renal parenchymal injury ranging from none in prerenal azotemia to frank renal cortical necrosis.[2] Mild renal hypoperfusion causes prerenal azotemia characterized by sufficient renal tubular function to adequately concentrate urine (Table 108–6). Prerenal azotemia may be almost completely reversed 12 to 24 hours after correction of the causative extrarenal factors (e.g., rehydration of a dehydrated patient).

If renal hypoperfusion persists or is more severe, there may be a transition from prerenal azotemia to ATN. A syndrome of mild to moderate renal damage that is reversible over several days has been termed "intermediate syndrome."[2] Other terms proposed for this condition include "polyuric prerenal failure," "incipient renal failure," and "partial acute tubular necrosis." The authors have observed the pattern of intermediate syndrome in several azotemic dogs and cats. The transition phase from prerenal azotemia to ATN may be recognized clinically when azotemia slowly improves (over several days) after correction of extrarenal causes of renal hypoperfusion. Because the degree of tubular damage is variable, urine concentrating ability and urine sodium concentration may be variably affected during transition from prerenal azotemia to ATN.

More severe renal ischemia may cause sustained loss of renal function manifested as oliguric or nonoliguric ATN. Extreme renal hypoperfusion may result in renal cortical necrosis. Nonoliguric ATN probably represents less severe renal parenchymal injury than does oliguric ATN.[2]

In humans, the magnitude of ischemia required to induce ATN is highly variable.[3] Surprisingly, profound systemic hypotension does not appear to be essential for development of ischemia-associated ATN.[2] For example, hypotension occurred in fewer than 50 per cent of cases of postsurgical ARF in one prospective study of human patients.[4] In some patients transient hypotension results in ATN, whereas in others, hours to days of renal ischemia fail to produce ATN. Similar variations probably exist in dogs and cats. Advanced age, preexisting renal disease, and certain drugs (e.g., nonsteroidal anti-inflammatory agents) may predispose to ischemic ATN and account for some of the variability in individual response to renal hypoperfusion. It is unclear whether dogs and cats are as susceptible to ischemia-induced ATN as humans.

NEPHROTOXIC ACUTE TUBULAR NECROSIS. Mechanisms of drug-induced nephrotoxicity have recently been reviewed.[5, 6] The high rate of blood flow, high rate of metabolic activity, and excretory function of the kidneys predispose them to toxic effects of drugs and other endogenous and exogenous toxins.[5] Because of active tubular secretion, reabsorption, and urine-concentrating mechanisms, renal tubular cells may be exposed to toxin concentrations many times greater than those of other body tissues.[2] It is therefore not surprising that renal tubule cells are often a site of direct toxicity for a wide variety of drugs, diagnostic reagents, chemical toxins, and heavy metals, as well as some endogenous products.[2] The clinical importance of recognizing nephrotoxic ARF

TABLE 108–6. DISCRIMINATION OF PRERENAL AZOTEMIA, POSTRENAL AZOTEMIA, ACUTE PRIMARY RENAL FAILURE, AND CHRONIC PRIMARY RENAL FAILURE

Data	Prerenal Azotemia	Acute Parenchymal Renal Failure	Chronic Parenchymal Renal Failure	Postrenal Azotemia
Blood urea nitrogen	↑	↑	↑	↑
Serum creatinine	↑	↑	↑	↑
Serum phosphorus	N, ↑	↑	↑	↑
Serum calcium	N	↓, N, ↑	↓, N, ↑	N
Serum sodium	N, (↑), (↓)	↓, N, ↑	N	N
Serum potassium	N	N, ↑	N	N, ↑
Serum chloride	N	↓, N, ↑	N, ↑	N
Blood bicarbonate	↓, N	↓, N	↓, N	↓, N
Urine specific gravity	>1.030** >1.035***	<1.030** <1.035***	<1.030** <1.035***	*
Urine sodium†	<10 mEq/L	>25 mEq/L	>25 mEq/L	*
FE$_{na}$†	<1.0	>1.0	>1.0	*
Ratio of urine creatine:serum creatine (U$_{cr}$:S$_{cr}$ ratio)	>20	<5	<5	*
Urine output	↓ (N)	↓, N, ↑	↑, (↓, N)	↓ (N, ↑)
Packed cell volume	N, ↑	N, ↑ (↓)	↓, (N)	N
Previous history of polyuria/ polydipsia	0	0	+ (0)	0(+)
Previous history of oliguria/ anuria	+ (0)	+ /0	+ (0)	+ (0)
Previous history of uremic symptoms	0	0	+ /0	0
Debilitation	0	0	+ /0	0
Renal osteodystrophy	0	0	+ /0	0
Kidney size	N	N, ↑	↓, N, ↑	N, ↑

↑, increased; N, normal range; ↓, decreased; ( ), uncommon; *, no specific values characteristic of the condition; 0, absent; +, present; **, canine; ***, feline; †, extrapolated from data in human beings.

is that further damage may be prevented if continued exposure to the toxin(s) is prevented.

As with ischemic renal injury, there is individual variation in functional and structural response to nephrotoxins. Factors that may influence the occurrence and extent of nephrotoxic injury include concentration of the toxin, duration of exposure, and occurrence of various predisposing factors (Table 108–7).[2] Specific risk factors for nephrotoxicity in humans may also apply to dogs and cats. Therefore, the need for administration of potentially nephrotoxic drugs to patients with one or more of these predisposing conditions should be carefully evaluated. If the drugs are deemed to be essential, patients should be monitored in order to detect evidence of ARF at an early stage. Monitoring of plasma drug concentrations may also be considered.

Toxins and drugs commonly associated with ATN in dogs and cats include ethylene glycol, amphotericin B, and aminoglycoside antibiotics.[7–13] Intravenously administered tetracyclines and iodinated radiocontrast agents and ingestion of zinc have also occasionally been associated with ATN.[14, 15] Nonsteroidal anti-inflammatory agents have been recognized as a frequent cause of renal failure in humans; increased use of these compounds may be associated with increased recognition of their role in ARF in dogs and cats.[16, 17] The list of compounds reported to cause ARF in dogs and cats is increasing. Many drugs and toxins are known to cause ARF in humans; this list is provided to prompt consideration of possible exposure to these compounds when evaluating dogs and cats with ARF (Table 108–8).

SEQUENTIAL PHASES OF OLIGURIC ACUTE TUBULAR NECROSIS. The clinical course of oliguric ATN may be characterized by three sequential phases: (1) initiation, (2) maintenance, and (3) diuresis (recovery). The initiation phase begins with onset of renal injury and continues through onset of oliguria. Because renal cell damage develops during the initiation phase, the greatest potential for preventing or reversing tubular damage and progression to overt renal failure exists during this phase. GFR may begin to fall immediately after the renal insult (as in the case of shock), or it may be delayed for hours to days (as is the case with exposure to most nephrotoxic drugs).[1]

Reduction in urine output below 0.22 ml/lb/hr (0.5 ml/kg/hr) marks the onset of the oliguric or maintenance phase of oliguric ATN in dogs. Onset of the oliguric phase typically occurs during the first 24 hours of ATN but may be delayed up to one week. Duration of the oliguric or maintenance phase is highly variable, but it usually persists for about one to two weeks. It may be

TABLE 108–7. RISK FACTORS THAT MAY PROMOTE NEPHROTOXICITY

Advanced age
Preexisting or active renal disease/failure
Volume depletion
Fever
Sepsis
Liver disease
Electrolyte disturbances (e.g., hypokalemia, acidosis)
Concomitant or recent administration of nephrotoxic drugs
Excessive dosages, prolonged or repeated treatment with nephrotoxic drugs

TABLE 108–8. DRUGS AND TOXINS ASSOCIATED WITH ACUTE RENAL FAILURE IN HUMANS

Antibiotics	Toxins
Aminoglycosides	Ethylene glycol
Amphotericin B	Heavy metals
Cephalosporins	Lead
Tetracyclines	Mercury
Polymyxin B and	Cadmium
colistimethate	Arsenic
Others	Bismuth
Endogenous Pigments	Zinc
Myoglobin (rhabdomyolysis)	Others
Hemoglobin (hemolysis)	Carbon tetrachloride
Radiographic Contrast Agents	Mushrooms
Diatrizoate	Insecticides
Iothalamate	Herbicides
Bunamiodyl	Toluene
Iopanoic acid	Gasoline
Other Drugs	Kerosene
Cimetidine	Turpentine
Dextrans	**Nonsteroidal Anti-Inflammatory**
EDTA	**Drugs**
Cis-platinum	Aspirin
Methotrexate	Indomethacin
D-Penicillamine	Phenylbutazone
Thiacetarsamide	Acetaminophen
Anesthetic Agents	Ibuprofen
Methoxyflurane	**Biotoxins**
Enflurane	Snake bites
	Bacterial toxins
	Insect stings

as short as hours, or it may last for several weeks. The oliguric phase is characterized by predictable fluid and electrolyte imbalances, including alterations in hydration, hyponatremia, hyperkalemia, high anion gap metabolic acidosis, hypocalcemia, and hyperphosphatemia. Even though oliguric patients are frequently dehydrated, their oliguric state predisposes them to overhydration. Hyponatremia may occur because oliguria limits renal water excretion. Hyperkalemia results from failure of the kidneys to excrete potassium. In absence of exogenous sources of potassium, hyperkalemia may result from release of potassium from tissues. High anion gap metabolic acidosis commonly occurs because the kidneys' ability to excrete hydrogen ions is impaired. Hyperkalemia and acidosis may be more severe in patients with hypercatabolism caused by trauma, surgery, or sepsis. Hypocalcemia and hyperphosphatemia may develop early in the course of ATN.

Clinical signs typically develop during the oliguric phase of ATN, including gastrointestinal, hematologic, and neurologic manifestations of renal failure. Gastrointestinal disorders are common, and include anorexia, vomiting, and mucosal ulcerations and hemorrhage (primarily gastric and colonic). Considerable gastrointestinal hemorrhage may initially escape clinical detection. However, massive gastrointestinal hemorrhage is a significant cause of death in humans with ATN. A hemorrhagic diathesis may contribute to gastrointestinal blood loss. It primarily results from defective platelet function, but may also be associated with thrombocytopenia, decreases in various coagulation factors, and defects in capillary function. Progressive anemia and neurologic disorders characterized by lethargy, depression, stupor, and coma may also occur during the oliguric phase. Delayed and inadequate wound healing and infection are frequent complications of ATN and may contribute substantially to mortality. Despite these severe alterations in homeostasis that occur during the oliguric phase of ATN, important (although clinically unapparent) repair and recovery of tubular structure and function may occur during this phase.

Transition from the oliguric to the diuretic phase heralds the onset of reestablishment of tubular continuity, dissolution and/or mobilization of intratubular casts, and return to near normal patterns of renal perfusion. Urine output may double each day as the diuretic phase begins. However, increased urine output may not be associated with restoration of normal GFR. The usual indices of GFR (serum urea nitrogen and creatinine concentrations) may continue to deteriorate during the first few days of the diuretic phase and then improve exponentially as renal function returns.

Tubular function, although improving, remains impaired during the diuretic phase. Diuresis persists because of impaired ability of tubules to reabsorb sodium and to respond to ADH. If fluid replacement is inadequate during this phase, diuresis may cause volume depletion. Appropriate monitoring of fluid and electrolyte intakes and losses during this phase is recommended to minimize imbalances.

Clinical manifestations observed during the oliguric phase often persist into the diuretic phase. In some patients infections and/or gastrointestinal bleeding may first become apparent during the diuretic phase. About 25 per cent of mortality in human patients with ATN occurs during the diuretic phase. Canine and feline patients may also die during this phase but appear more likely to recover.

The concomitant occurrence of ATN and rhabdomyolysis in humans has been associated with hypercalcemia during the diuretic phase. Apparently, massive release of phosphate from muscle during rhabdomyolysis leads to deposition of calcium in tissues during the oliguric phase. Subsequent reabsorption and release of calcium is thought to occur as phosphate concentrations decrease during the diuretic phase.

SEQUENTIAL PHASES OF NONOLIGURIC ACUTE TUBULAR NECROSIS. Nonoliguric ATN is not characterized by the distinct series of clinical phases observed with oliguric ATN. In patients with nonoliguric ATN, urine volume is initially fixed, typically within the normal range. However, the recovery phase of nonoliguric ATN is characterized by an abrupt increase in urine output as the magnitude of azotemia declines. Complications resulting from excretory and regulatory failure are generally less severe in patients with nonoliguric ATN, probably because urine output is adequate to support excretion of water, electrolytes, and some wastes.

Other Causes of Acute Primary Renal Failure. Although disorders that cause ATN appear to account for the majority of cases of acute intrinsic renal failure in dogs and cats, ARF may also result from diseases that affect glomeruli, renal vasculature, or renal interstitium (Table 108–4). Acute immune-mediated glomerulonephritis, thromboembolism of large renal vessels, malignant hypertension or inflammatory vasculitis that affects small renal vessels, and acute interstitial inflammation induced by drugs or infection are well recognized causes

of ARF in humans.[1] Acute pyelonephritis, leptospirosis, and glomerular amyloidosis are infrequent but recognized causes of ARF in dogs and cats.[18, 19] Hypercalcemia may cause acute, reversible azotemia through a direct effect of calcium on renal tubules and blood vessels, causing polyuria and solute losses.[20] However, prolonged hypercalcemia may cause slowly progressive nephrocalcinosis, which may culminate in CRF.[20]

Diagnosis

SYNDROME IDENTIFICATION

Early differentiation of ARF from CRF is important because rapid diagnostic and therapeutic intervention will maximize the potential for reversing renal damage. In order to categorize renal failure as acute or chronic, it is desirable to attempt to date the onset of renal failure. ARF may be recognized by an abrupt onset of azotemia or oliguria, rapidly progressive azotemia, or sudden onset of clinical signs of uremia in a previously healthy patient. Although azotemia, hyperphosphatemia, hyperkalemia, and metabolic acidosis may occur in patients with ARF or CRF, these values are often progressive in ARF and stable in CRF.[1] Methods of localizing causes of azotemia are summarized in Table 108–6.

A preliminary diagnosis of ARF is based on evidence gleaned from the medical history, previous data concerning renal function, and lack of physical evidence of CRF (e.g., chronic weight loss, poor haircoat condition, rubber jaw, growth retardation in puppies). Acute medical and/or surgical illness associated with an abrupt onset of azotemia in a patient known to have not previously been azotemic is unequivocal evidence of ARF. Unfortunately, affected patients often have established azotemia of undetermined duration; previous renal function is often unknown unless the patient was being monitored during nephrotoxic drug therapy, anesthesia, or surgery. A previous history of weight loss, polyuria, polydipsia, or laboratory abnormalities caused by renal dysfunction (e.g., repeatedly low urine specific gravity values, azotemia), support a diagnosis of underlying CRF. Physical examination of patients with ARF typically reveals good nutritional status and haircoat, whereas CRF is usually characterized by poor nutritional status and other changes suggestive of chronic illness. Even conclusive evidence of CRF does not rule out the possibility that ARF has occurred in the setting of CRF, and that some recovery of renal function may be possible (CRF may predispose to ARF).

SYNDROME ANALYSIS

Organization of Diagnostic Studies. Careful organization and prioritization of the initial diagnostic plan will foster formulation of efficient and effective medical therapy for patients with ARF. Diagnostic efforts should be sequentially directed toward (a) identifying life-threatening complications, (b) localizing the cause of ARF (i.e., prerenal, postrenal, or primary renal failure), (c) determining urine volume, (d) differentiating ARF

**TABLE 108–9. CHECKLIST OF DIAGNOSTICS
IN ACUTE RENAL FAILURE**

1. Assume azotemia results from ARF until proved otherwise (Table 108–6)
2. Identify life-threatening complications
   a. Hyperkalemia
   b. Metabolic acidosis
   c. Volume depletion
   d. Infection
   e. Underlying disease processes
3. Localize to prerenal, postrenal, or primary renal failure
   a. History and physical examination
   b. Assess urine-concentrating ability
   c. Urinalysis
   d. Serum urea nitrogen and creatinine concentrations
   e. Response to therapy
4. Determine urine production rate (oliguria versus nonoliguria)
5. Discriminate between ARF and CRF (or both)
6. Identify specific cause of primary renal failure

from CRF (if previously unresolved), (e) determining the cause of ARF, and (f) monitoring patient response to therapy (Table 108–9).

Because of the potentially life-threatening nature of many of the complications of ARF and diseases that precipitate ARF, diagnostic and therapeutic efforts are often performed simultaneously. However, the impact of therapy on results of diagnostic tests must be considered. The initial problem-specific data base should be obtained before initiating therapy in order to maximize the value of the data obtained. It is particularly important to obtain a urine sample for analysis and culture before initiating fluid therapy because fluid therapy may cause concentrated urine to become dilute, making diagnosis of prerenal azotemia difficult. In addition, fluid therapy may alter the urine sediment, causing erroneous interpretation.

Initial Problem-Specific Data Base. The purpose of the problem-specific data base (Table 108–10) is to provide data necessary to detect life-threatening complications of ARF, to localize the cause of ARF, and to

**TABLE 108–10. PROBLEM-SPECIFIC DATA BASE
FOR RENAL FAILURE**

1. Medical history and physical examination (Table 108–3)
2. Urinalysis
3. Urine culture (or screening urine culture)
4. Complete blood count
5. Serum urea nitrogen concentration
6. Serum creatinine concentration
7. Serum (or plasma) electrolyte and acid-base profile
   a. Sodium, potassium, and chloride concentrations
   b. Bicarbonate or total carbon dioxide concentrations
   c. Calcium and phosphorus concentrations
8. Kidney-bladder-urethra survey radiographs
   a. Kidneys—size, shape, location, number
   b. Uroliths or masses affecting ureters or urethra
   c. Urinary bladder—size, shape, location, uroliths
9. Consider
   a. Freezing aliquots of serum (or plasma) and urine for additional diagnostic determinations that may be desired later
   b. Renal ultrasound (to rule out urinary obstruction, renal uroliths, renal cystic disease, renal neoplasia)
   c. Intravenous urography (to rule out urinary obstruction, renal uroliths, pyelonephritis, renal cystic disease, renal neoplasia)
   d. Blood pressure determination (to rule out systemic hypertension)
   e. Renal biopsy (may provide etiologic diagnosis; primarily indicated when kidneys are normal size or enlarged)

provide baseline data for determining patient response to therapy. Information obtained should be entered into flow sheets or computer spreadsheets to permit rapid and easy detection of data trends. The trends indicated by the data may be more important than the values themselves. For example, the fact that serum creatinine concentration is increasing or decreasing is usually more important than the actual value for serum creatinine concentration.

Identification of Medical Emergencies in Acute Renal Failure. CAUSES OF MEDICAL EMERGENCIES. Several life-threatening complications may occur in patients with ARF, including hyperkalemia, metabolic acidosis, severe anemia, volume depletion, and sepsis. In addition, the disease process that caused ARF may be an important cause of morbidity and mortality.

HYPERKALEMIA. Hyperkalemia is a common complication of oliguric acute primary renal failure and urinary tract obstruction. It is less commonly associated with nonoliguric acute primary renal failure and is rarely associated with prerenal azotemia unless prerenal azotemia results from Addison's disease. Detection of bradycardia or other cardiac dysrhythmias should alert one to the possibility of hyperkalemia.

Hyperkalemia is confirmed by determination of serum potassium concentrations; however, electrocardiography provides a rapid means of detecting hyperkalemia (see Chapter 11). Typical electrocardiographic changes observed with mild to moderate hyperkalemia include tall, peaked T waves, slowing of the heart rate, flattening of P waves, and prolongation of the P-R interval and QRS complex. With more severe hyperkalemia, bradycardia, atrial standstill, prolongation of the Q-T interval, complete heart block, or cardiac arrest may occur. In the absence of serious cardiotoxicity, mild to moderate hyperkalemia usually does not require specific treatment. However, hyperkalemia associated with serious cardiac dysrhythmias is a potentially life-threatening condition that requires immediate therapy.

Patients with azotemia, hyperkalemia, and hyponatremia may have hypoadrenocorticism (Addison's disease). Dogs with hypoadrenocorticism often have impaired urine concentrating ability, making differentiation of acute primary renal failure and hypoadrenocorticism difficult. However, it is important to differentiate between these conditions because a combination of fluid therapy and hormone replacement therapy will rapidly and completely correct hypoadrenocorticism in most patients. Although rapid response to such therapy is indicative of hypoadrenocorticism, the diagnosis should be confirmed by an ACTH response test. The major disadvantage of administering hormone replacement therapy for ARF patients that do not have hypoadrenocorticism is that the catabolic effect of corticosteroid administration may increase the magnitude of azotemia.[21]

METABOLIC ACIDOSIS. Metabolic acidosis is a relatively common but inconsistent finding in ARF. The magnitude of renal dysfunction appears to be a poor predictor of metabolic acidosis. Acidosis may be more common in patients with oliguric ARF than in those with nonoliguric ARF, but not all patients with oliguric ARF have significant metabolic acidosis. Therefore, diagnosis of metabolic acidosis should be based on evaluation of blood bicarbonate (or total carbon dioxide) concentration and, if available, blood pH. Urine pH is an inconsistent guide to systemic acid-base status and should not be chosen as a definitive diagnostic tool.

Clinical effects of acidosis are usually minimal unless blood pH is less than 7.20.[22] However, when blood pH drops to less than 7.10, acidosis may (a) reduce cardiac contractility and the inotropic response to catecholamines, (b) predispose to ventricular arrhythmias, and (c) promote neurologic signs ranging from lethargy to coma.[22]

In rare instances metabolic alkalosis may develop subsequent to severe vomiting in patients with ARF. These patients may have gastric outflow obstruction in addition to renal failure as the cause for their vomiting. Some of these patients may have concurrent metabolic acidosis and metabolic alkalosis. Serum bicarbonate concentrations may be decreased, normal, or increased, depending on the predominant acid-base dysfunction. Diagnosis of combined metabolic acidosis and metabolic alkalosis is facilitated by determining the anion gap.[23] Increased anion gap most often indicates metabolic acidosis. When the anion gap is markedly elevated and serum bicarbonate concentration is near normal, combined metabolic acidosis and metabolic alkalosis is likely. Because alkalemia causes the anion gap to increase, interpretation of the anion gap may be misleading in patients with elevated serum bicarbonate concentrations.

VOLUME DEPLETION. At the time of diagnosis, most patients with ARF have some degree of volume depletion. Although volume depletion can usually be detected by physical examination, physical changes can be subtle, particularly when fluid loss has occurred quickly and recently. Detection and early correction of volume depletion is a critical part of initial therapy of ARF because continued volume depletion may promote additional renal injury. In addition, correction of volume depletion dramatically reduces the severity of azotemia and clinical signs in many patients with ARF, regardless of cause. Therefore, it is usually inadvisable to render a prognosis before the patient's response to volume repletion has been assessed. Detection of volume depletion is described in the section on prerenal azotemia.

INFECTION. Infection (acute pyelonephritis, often associated with obstruction) may be a cause or complication of ARF. Dilute urine, oliguria, anuria, and urinary obstruction predispose to urinary tract infection.[2, 24, 25] Furthermore, uremia is characterized by reduced immunocompetence.[26] Because of these factors, infection is an important cause of morbidity and mortality in uremic patients. It accounts for about 50 per cent of deaths in humans with ARF.[2, 26] Many infections are related to invasive diagnostic and therapeutic procedures such as vascular and, especially, urinary catheterization.[24, 25, 27] Careful attention to detail and intelligent decisions regarding application of use of catheters and invasive diagnostic and therapeutic procedures will dramatically reduce the incidence of infection-related mortality. Routine administration of antibiotics as a prophylactic procedure is an inappropriate and inadequate substitute for good technique and may provide a false sense of security.

Urinalysis, urine culture, and a complete blood cell count are indicated to rule out infection as a cause or complication of ARF. When pyrexia, physical examination, or laboratory findings indicate the probability of infection, its location and cause should be vigorously sought so that the most appropriate and least nephrotoxic antimicrobial therapy may be initiated.

UNDERLYING DISEASE PROCESSES. Patients may die of the disease process that initiated ARF (e.g., acute pancreatitis, sepsis, shock, hypercalcemia, ethylene glycol intoxication) rather than from ARF or its complications. Therefore, diagnosis and initiation of specific therapy for diseases that may have precipitated ARF should be a high priority.

Localization of Prerenal, Postrenal, and Primary Renal Failure.
IMPORTANCE OF LOCALIZATION. The history, physical examination, and urinalysis are usually sufficient to rule out prerenal and postrenal causes of azotemia. However, in some cases differentiation of ARF from CRF may require additional diagnostic studies (Table 108–6). A diligent search for these potentially reversible conditions is always indicated. It is emphasized that prerenal azotemia typically accompanies acute intrinsic renal failure and postrenal azotemia.

PRERENAL AZOTEMIA. Findings from the physical examination and urinalysis are often sufficient to permit classification of azotemia as prerenal. Volume depletion may be assessed by skin pliability, moisture of mucous membranes, temperature of the extremities, capillary refill time, pulse rate and character, and blood pressure. Because RBF may be reduced with hepatic failure or congestive heart failure, evidence of hepatic failure (e.g., hyperbilirubinemia, hypoalbuminemia, abnormal liver function tests) or congestive heart failure (e.g., elevated neck veins, rales, diastolic gallop, edema, and ascites) may also indicate prerenal azotemia. Abrupt changes in body weight usually indicate fluid shifts. Thus, a 7 per cent reduction in body weight over 24 hours probably indicates 7 per cent dehydration. Changes in body weight are most useful as an index of hydration if serial body weights have been determined. An accurate scale is one of the most important yet underutilized pieces of hospital equipment for management of critical patients.

Urine specific gravity values of 1.030 or greater in dogs and 1.035 or greater in cats are indicative of adequate intrinsic renal function and, therefore, support a diagnosis of prerenal azotemia. Because factors other than urine-concentrating ability may affect urine specific gravity (e.g., protein, glucose, and drugs), other diagnostic indices, including urine osmolality, urine sodium concentration, fractional excretion of sodium, and urine creatinine–to–serum creatinine ratio, have been recommended for differentiating prerenal azotemia from primary renal failure in humans (Table 108–6).[1, 28] Although these diagnostic tests may prove useful, further experience with them is needed in dogs and cats. Fortunately the greater intrinsic concentrating ability of dogs and cats as compared with humans probably enhances the value of urine specific gravity in discrimination of prerenal azotemia from primary renal failure in these species.

Response to therapy may be useful in differentiating

prerenal azotemia from acute primary renal failure. Rapid resolution of azotemia after elimination of a prerenal abnormality indicates that the major cause of azotemia is prerenal. In contrast, azotemia that is unresponsive to correction of prerenal conditions indicates primary renal failure. Azotemia that responds slowly (over several days) to correction of prerenal conditions may suggest the transition phase between prerenal and primary renal dysfunction (intermediate syndrome).

In humans a disproportionate increase in the ratio of serum urea nitrogen concentration to serum creatinine concentration (SUN:SC) is reported to indicate prerenal azotemia; however, this has not been confirmed in dogs.[29] Normal SUN:SC ratio in humans is about 10. In dogs this ratio is greatly influenced by dietary protein intake (a prerenal effect) and may vary from 10 to 30.[30] Although identification of an elevated SUN:SC ratio is not proof of prerenal azotemia, identification of a SUN:SC ratio approaching or exceeding 30 should prompt consideration of prerenal causes of azotemia, including diet, gastrointestinal hemorrhage, and hypercatabolism (Table 108–4).

POSTRENAL AZOTEMIA. Palpation, radiographic or ultrasonographic examinations of the urinary system, and observation of voiding will permit detection of most cases of urinary obstruction. Lower urinary tract obstruction is usually characterized by historical and physical findings of stranguria, and distention of the urinary bladder. Rectal examination and palpation of the perineum may reveal evidence of urethral lesions causing obstruction. An attempt should be made to observe the patient voiding. Persistent stranguria in a patient with a distended bladder, narrowing of the urine stream, or reduced urine flow velocity during micturition suggests urinary obstruction.

Upper urinary tract obstruction is more difficult to detect than lower urinary tract obstruction. If the contralateral kidney is functioning adequately, unilateral obstruction will not cause azotemia. Cranial abdominal pain, renomegaly, and detection of renoliths or ureteroliths may suggest renal or ureteral outflow obstruction. Acute ureteral obstruction by ureteroliths may cause vomiting. Large uroliths located at the neck of the bladder can obstruct both ureters as well as the urethra. Masses in or adjacent to the trigone can obstruct both ureters (e.g., spay granulomas, neoplasms). Upper urinary tract obstruction should be confirmed by contrast radiographic or ultrasonographic procedures.

Urine production rate may be helpful in detecting postrenal azotemia. Urinary obstruction rather than prerenal or primary renal azotemia should be particularly considered in the setting of complete anuria. Prerenal azotemia and ATN are often associated with oliguria; they are rarely associated with anuria. Large fluctuations in urine output (alternating between oliguria and polyuria) suggest the possibility of intermittent urinary obstruction.

An early consequence of acute urinary tract obstruction is prostaglandin-mediated renal vasodilation, an effect that helps to support GFR. However, continued production of urine despite obstruction causes increased pressure within the renal pelvis and collecting system. As a result, tubular flow rates decline. Initially, augmented reabsorption of sodium, water, and urea produces urine that is remarkably similar in composition to that observed during prerenal azotemia. However, persistent obstruction results in renal tubular cell dysfunction, reduced RBF, and reduced GFR. These changes result in impaired urine concentration and rapidly progressive azotemia, findings suggestive of primary renal damage.[1] Therefore, urinalysis findings alone will not differentiate postrenal azotemia from prerenal or primary renal causes of azotemia.

PRIMARY RENAL FAILURE. A diagnosis of primary renal failure encompasses elimination of prerenal and postrenal causes of azotemia. The diagnosis may be further supported by seeking a historical association between the onset of ARF and recent trauma, surgery, drugs, volume contraction (owing to any of the prerenal causes listed in Table 108–4), hypotension, sepsis, radiocontrast agents, systemic disease, or potentially nephrotoxic diagnostic or therapeutic maneuvers.[1]

Urinalysis findings are especially helpful in identifying patients with primary renal failure. However, to maximize its diagnostic value, collection of urine for analysis must be accomplished before initiation of therapy. Urinalysis findings in patients with prerenal azotemia are characterized by normal urine chemistries and an inactive urine sediment. Occasionally small numbers of hyaline or fine granular casts may be detected. Depending on the cause of obstruction, postrenal azotemia may be associated with crystalluria, hematuria, and/or pyuria. Large numbers of granular or cellular casts, inappropriate alkaluria or glucosuria, and moderate to severe proteinuria in the absence of inflammation or hematuria suggest primary renal disease.

Oliguria Versus Nonoliguria. Detecting oliguria early in the course of treatment of ARF is important because (a) overly aggressive fluid therapy may cause overhydration in oliguric patients, and (b) therapy to convert oliguria to nonoliguria is most likely to succeed when initiated early in the course of ARF.[1] However, because physiologic oliguria commonly occurs in dehydrated patients, urine production rate is best determined after patients have been rehydrated. If oliguria is resolved by fluid therapy alone, oliguria should be presumed to have been physiologic in origin, and additional therapy designed to enhance urine production (e.g., diuretics, vasodilators) usually are not warranted.

Acute primary renal failure has been classically associated with oliguria. However, in recent years nonoliguric ARF has been recognized with increased frequency in dogs and cats admitted to the University of Minnesota Veterinary Medical Teaching Hospital.[2] Thus finding a normal to increased urine production rate does not itself rule out ARF or suggest CRF rather than ARF. Nonoliguric ARF is thought to result from less severe renal injury than oliguric ARF.[1]

Urine output can be estimated using several methods, including: (a) serial collection of voided urine, (b) collection of urine in a metabolism cage, (c) serial collection of urine obtained by intermittent catheterization, or (d) collection of urine using an indwelling urinary catheter. When urine collection is not possible, serial palpation of bladder size or serial radiographic or ultrasonographic estimation of bladder size will provide a semiquantitative assessment of urine output. In patients able to void spontaneously, serial collection of voided samples or samples collected using a metabolism cage have the advantages of moderate quantitative accuracy and noninvasiveness. The major disadvantage of these techniques is a delay in accurately assessing urine output as a result of dependence on the patient's ability to void, and/or infrequent and erratic collection intervals. Serial palpation or radiographic or ultrasonographic evaluations of bladder size have the advantage of noninvasiveness but provide only crude estimates of urine production. These methods are of greatest value when the patient is producing large rather than small volumes of urine (e.g., patients that become polyuric after administration of rehydrating fluids).

Although urinary catheterization provides highly accurate quantitative results, it may be associated with an unacceptably high risk of iatrogenic urinary tract infection (UTI), especially when indwelling catheters are used.[25, 27, 31] Recall that formation of unconcentrated urine, decreased flow of urine caused by oliguria, and uremia are predispositions to UTI.[25] Catheter-induced infections are usually caused by hospital-acquired (nosocomial) microorganisms that are resistant to many antimicrobial drugs. The urinary tract has been reported to be one of the most common sites of origin of bacteremia in dogs.[32]

We avoid routine urinary catheterization of patients with ARF because of their predisposition to UTI. When catheterization is deemed essential for determining urine production rate, intermittent catheterization is preferred. However, if patients are difficult to catheterize, use of indwelling catheters may be necessary. Systemic antibiotic therapy is not a consistently effective means of preventing UTI in patients with indwelling urinary catheters and may promote development of resistant infections.[32] Therefore, in such cases, a sterilized, closed urine drainage system should be used to minimize risk of ascending UTI. Because development of UTI during indwelling catheterization may be related to duration of catheterization, indwelling catheters should be maintained only as long as necessary to determine urine production rate or to evaluate response to therapy designed to enhance urine production.[27, 31] Urine cultures should be performed after urinary catheters are removed, in order to detect and effectively treat iatrogenic UTI.

Serial determination of urine losses for the purpose of monitoring fluid therapy and hydration may require the use of an indwelling urinary catheter. However, in most cases this function can be accomplished by serial assessment of body weight (correcting for weight loss from inadequate calorie intake) and by estimating hydration on the basis of physical findings. Monitoring of fluid balance (in and out) can also be accomplished by measuring urine production in a metabolism cage or collecting voided urine. In cats urine production can be measured by weighing the litter pan before and after the cat voids (increased weight in grams is approximately equal to urine output in milliliters).

Acute Versus Chronic Renal Failure. ARF and CRF can often be differentiated on the basis of the medical history and physical examination (Table 108–6). How-ever, if the medical history is uncertain or contradictory, it becomes necessary to seek other evidence. Failure to rapidly differentiate ARF and CRF may lead to needless progression of ARF and formulation of an inappropriately poor long-term prognosis.

Radiographic examination of kidney size and skeletal integrity may be useful for differentiating ARF and CRF. Reduced kidney size indicates long-term renal damage and is evidence of CRF. However, kidney size may be normal or increased in either ARF or CRF. Radiographic or physical evidence of renal osteodystrophy indicates long-standing renal secondary hyperparathyroidism and is unequivocal evidence of CRF.

Although ARF and CRF cannot be differentiated on the basis of serum creatinine concentrations, serial determinations of serum creatinine concentration over several days typically reveal progressive, often rapidly increasing values in patients with ARF compared with relatively stable values in patients with CRF. Progressive azotemia or persistent oliguria imply a degree of renal dysfunction that could not have been present for more than a few days.[1] If evidence of progressive azotemia is detected in a patient with other evidence supporting CRF, the probability of ARF occurring in the setting of CRF should be considered.

Hypocalcemia, hyperphosphatemia, and mild nonregenerative anemia may occur with either ARF or CRF and are often not helpful in differentiating these two conditions, although the magnitudes of hyperphosphatemia and nonregenerative anemia may be more severe with CRF.

Detection of CRF does not rule out concurrent ARF, because CRF is a recognized predisposition to ARF. Development of ARF in a patient with CRF is not the same as terminal end-stage renal failure. Because ARF is potentially reversible, even in patients with underlying CRF, its correction may result in amelioration of clinical signs.

Determining the Cause of Primary Renal Failure. NONINVASIVE DIAGNOSTIC PROCEDURES. The etiology of ARF can often be ascertained without renal biopsy. Known recent exposure to recognized nephrotoxins (e.g., ethylene glycol, gentamicin) or ischemia (e.g., hypovolemia, shock) provides strong support for a diagnosis of ATN. Urinalysis findings may provide additional support for the diagnosis.[28] The urine sediment of humans with ATN typically contains pigmented (muddy brown) granular casts with amorphous debris and many RBCs, leukocytes, and renal tubular epithelial cells (localization of cell origin usually requires special cytologic techniques).[1, 28] However, urine sediment may be more scant with nonoliguric ARF than with oliguria. Glucosuria despite normoglycemia, and alkaline urine despite systemic acidosis may indicate proximal tubular damage typical of ATN.[28] Dogs with gentamicin-induced ATN were observed to have proteinuria (eight of eight dogs), hematuria (six of eight dogs), cylindruria (six of eight dogs), and glucosuria (one of eight dogs).[7]

ATN appears to be responsible for most cases of acute primary renal failure in dogs and cats. However, other possible causes of ARF should be considered when findings inconsistent with ATN are detected. Findings atypical of ATN include moderate to marked proteinuria, red blood cell (RBC) casts, clinical signs consistent with polysystemic disease other than uremia (e.g., polyarthritis, eosinophilia, rash), severe hypertension, or lack of an inciting cause for ATN.

Glomerulonephritis has rarely been recognized as a cause of ARF in dogs and cats. Human patients with acute glomerulonephritis typically manifest moderate to marked proteinuria, hematuria, RBC casts, hypertension, and extrarenal manifestations of disease.[1, 28] In humans, absence of significant proteinuria, hematuria, and RBC casts virtually excludes glomerulonephritis as a cause of ARF.[28] If a diagnosis of glomerulonephritis is being considered, additional supportive evidence may be obtained from immunologic studies (antinuclear antibody test, lupus erythematosus cell preparation, and serum complement levels). Small-vessel vasculitis, which is also frequently immune-mediated, has also been associated with RBC casts, inflammatory urine sediment, hypertension, and systemic signs of disease in humans.

Acute allergic renal interstitial inflammation occurs subsequent to administration of a variety of drugs to humans. It is characterized by fever, rash, eosinophilia, hematuria, eosinophiluria, proteinuria, and pyuria.[1, 28] These drug reactions are idiosyncratic; they resolve after withdrawal of the offending medication. Although it likely occurs, acute allergic interstitial nephritis has not been documented in dogs and cats.

Acute pyelonephritis usually causes only mild reductions in renal function, provided urine outflow is not impeded. Renal infections are more likely to result in ARF when they occur in patients with urinary outflow obstruction and sepsis. Pyelonephritis severe enough to cause ARF is typically associated with sepsis and polysystemic signs of illness. Urinalysis findings suggestive of acute pyelonephritis include pyuria, significant bacteriuria, and cellular casts. Leukocyte casts are especially significant but are uncommonly detected because white blood cells (WBC) rapidly disintegrate to form granular casts. Acute pyelonephritis is not typically associated with radiographically detectable changes.[33] (See section on Pyelonephritis).

RENAL BIOPSY. Renal biopsy may help to differentiate ARF from CRF. In addition, it may provide an etiologic diagnosis and allow assessment of the potential reversibility of renal injury. However, because renal biopsy is an invasive procedure that entails several risks, it should not be performed unless necessary. Not every patient with ARF requires renal biopsy.

Biopsy results are not usually needed as a guide for treatment in patients with well-defined clinical and laboratory evidence of ATN.[28] Prognosis and appropriate therapy for these patients may be determined on the basis of response to therapy. Biopsy should be considered if the clinical course of disease does not progress as expected or if more demanding forms of therapy (e.g., hemodialysis or peritoneal dialysis) become necessary. If the clinical course casts doubt on the reversibility of renal lesions, renal biopsy should be considered.[34]

Proposed criteria for performing renal biopsy in human patients with acute intrinsic renal failure include (a) absence of an obvious cause for ARF, (b) persistence of severe oliguria or anuria beyond two to three weeks, (c) extrarenal manifestations of a more diffuse disease (e.g., vasculitis), and (d) exclusion of acute interstitial nephritis in patients who require continued therapy with a drug possibly responsible for the renal failure.[28] Similar criteria are applicable for dogs and cats. In addition, biopsy should be considered for patients with proteinuria of sufficient magnitude to suggest glomerular disease.

Early Detection in High-Risk Patients. Patients that are predisposed to ARF because of disease or drug therapy should be monitored so that development of ARF may be detected as early as possible. The severity of renal damage may be minimized by withdrawal of the inciting cause of ARF and/or early use of renoprotective therapy. Such patients may be monitored by serial examinations of urinalyses, serum urea nitrogen or creatinine concentrations, and urine enzymes.[2, 7, 8]

Serial examination of urine for proteinuria, glucosuria, and cylindruria is likely to detect renal damage earlier than serial determinations of serum urea nitrogen or serum creatinine concentration.[7, 8] However, in one study in dogs, termination of aminoglycoside therapy before or at the time of detection of nephrotoxicity did not consistently prevent progression of renal injury to ATN.[7] Thus, although urinalysis appears superior to determination of serum urea nitrogen or serum creatinine concentration for early detection of developing ATN, these tests have failed to consistently detect tubular damage early enough to prevent development of ATN.

Because of the limited sensitivity of available methods for monitoring and detecting acute renal damage, urine enzymes and renal tubule epithelial antigen have been evaluated as early markers of nephrotoxicity.[2] Urinary gamma-glutamyl transpeptidase activity is a more sensitive indicator of gentamicin-induced renal injury in dogs than measurement of serum urea nitrogen or creatinine concentrations or endogenous creatinine clearance.[35] Ideally, enzymuria should be quantified on the basis of a 24-hour urine collection. One recent study revealed that the ratio of urinary gamma-glutamyl transpeptidase activity to urinary creatinine concentration correlated with 24-hour urine enzyme excretion.[36]

Prognosis

The prognosis for dogs and cats with acute primary renal failure has generally been poor. Poor survival rates reflect several factors, including the considerable time and effort required to manage affected patients, financial expenditures required of clients, the limited experience of many veterinarians in treating ARF, and a tendency to terminate treatment prematurely by setting unrealistic deadlines for response to therapy.

Ultimately prognosis is best determined by response to therapy. However, the outcome may not become apparent for days to weeks after diagnosis. Although it is often difficult to offer an accurate prognosis early in the course of acute primary renal failure, severe and progressive hyperkalemia, metabolic acidosis, and uremic symptoms are negative prognostic indicators. In the absence of these factors, patient treatment and monitoring should be continued, even if azotemia continues to increase.

A guarded to favorable prognosis is indicated for patients with nonoliguric ARF in which severe hyperkalemia, metabolic acidosis, and intractable uremia do not develop. Likewise, patients with oliguric ARF in which severe hyperkalemia, metabolic acidosis, and intractable uremia do not develop can survive the oliguric phase and recover when given proper treatment and sufficient time for recovery.

Other factors that may influence prognosis include urine output, age of the patient, underlying renal diseases, and the nature of the disease responsible for the episode of ARF (Table 108–6).[2, 7, 14, 37] Studies in humans and preliminary evidence in dogs indicate that the prognosis for nonoliguric ARF is generally better than the prognosis for oliguric ARF, perhaps suggesting a lesser magnitude of renal injury in nonoliguric ARF.[2, 14] Advanced age and underlying renal disease are negative prognostic indicators in humans.[2, 14] The cause of ARF is also important. In man, mortality rates for ATN resulting from surgery or trauma are at least twice that observed for aminoglycoside-induced ATN.[2]

Treatment

With carefully designed therapy, patients with ARF may regain sufficient renal function to maintain homeostasis without the need for long-term management. Restoration of adequate renal function may be enhanced by (a) elimination of underlying cause(s) so that renal lesions do not progress, and (b) sustaining the patient's life until body repair mechanisms result in restoration of renal functions (Table 108–11).

Although therapy designed to eliminate the cause(s) of ARF will not directly result in repair of renal lesions, it will minimize the severity and extent of renal damage. Symptomatic and supportive therapy designed to minimize deficits and excesses in fluid, electrolyte, acid-base, and nutritional balance will often allow life to be sus-

TABLE 108–11. PRINCIPLES OF THERAPY FOR ACUTE RENAL FAILURE

Eliminate Underlying Causes of Renal Injury
  Reversible renal and nonrenal disorders that promote renal injury should be detected and eliminated (Table 108–4).
  There is no therapy that will eliminate renal lesions; renal lesions must heal spontaneously.
  The potential reversibility of renal lesions should be evaluated with the knowledge that adequate renal function is not synonymous with total renal function.
Sustain the Patient's Life Until Renal Functions Recover
  Supportive and symptomatic therapy should be formulated to minimize alterations in fluid, electrolyte, acid-base, endocrine, and nutrient balance.
  Formulation of therapy should be based, in part, on whether the patient is oliguric or nonoliguric.
  Drugs should be administered only after considering their routes and rates of metabolism and elimination and their potential for inducing adverse drug reactions in patients with renal failure.
  Consider the potential for inducing iatrogenic infection when planning or performing diagnostics, therapeutics, and nursing care; use good technique in preference to prophylactic antibiotics to prevent infection.
  Avoid overtreatment.

TABLE 108–12. TREATMENT OF ACUTE RENAL FAILURE

1. Collect baseline data and initiate data flow sheet.
2. Place intravenous fluid line and rehydrate the patient.
3. Consider emergency therapy for life-threatening electrolyte and acid-base disturbances:
     Hyperkalemia
     Metabolic acidosis
4. Determine urine production after fluid therapy restores hydration:
     Diuretics and vasoactive drugs may be considered for patients with oliguria in order to convert them to nonoliguria
     Diuretics and vasoactive drugs are generally not indicated for patients with normal to increased urine production rates.
5. Continue nondialytic medical management during maintenance and recovery phases of ARF:
     Maintain fluid and electrolyte balance.
     Ameliorate uremic manifestations.
     Maintain adequate nutrition.
     Prevent infection and drug reactions.
     Continue to monitor renal function and response to therapy.

tained until the body can restore adequate renal structure and function.

Because many of the complications of ARF are medical emergencies, it is often necessary to initiate therapy before diagnostic evaluations can be completed. Furthermore, treatment of ARF should be modified according to patient response. Therefore, diagnostic and therapeutic efforts complement each other when performed in an organized fashion (Table 108–12).

BASELINE DATA COLLECTION AND PATIENT MONITORING

Response to therapy is assessed by comparing pretreatment and serial posttreatment data. Data should be entered into flow sheets to facilitate detection of data trends (Table 108–13). Additional parameters may be monitored as indicated by individual patient circumstances or concurrent disease.

Frequency of data collection should be individualized to patient needs. Patients with severe metabolic disturbances may require frequent laboratory and clinical evaluation, whereas patients with less severe disturbances generally require less frequent monitoring. Not every characteristic listed on the flow sheet need be evaluated at the same frequency. In general, clinical characteristics (e.g., body weight, hydration) are evaluated at least twice daily. Early in the course of ARF, when substantial changes are occurring, laboratory values are determined at least daily. In patients with marked hyperkalemia and metabolic acidosis, these parameters may be monitored several times daily until controlled. The frequency of monitoring is altered according to trends observed and the clinical condition of the patient. Although economic considerations cannot be ignored in monitoring patient response, inadequate patient monitoring may adversely affect the patient.

FLUID THERAPY

Initial Therapy. Most patients with ARF are volume depleted before initiation of therapy. However, the decision to administer fluid therapy should be based on clinical assessment of hydration. Fluid therapy is indi-

TABLE 108–13. FLOW SHEET FOR MONITORING PATIENTS WITH ACUTE RENAL FAILURE

Observation	Date/Time							
Pulse rate								
Pulse character								
Temperature								
Respiratory rate								
Mucous membrane color								
Capillary refill time								
Body weight								
Hydration								
Fluid intake								
Urine output								
Blood pressure								
Clinical observations								
Appetite								
Alertness								
Vomiting								
Stool								
Packed cell volume								
Total plasma proteins								
Serum urea nitrogen								
Serum creatinine								
Serum [Na$^+$]								
Serum [K$^+$]								
Serum [Cl$^-$1]								
Total CO$_2$								
Serum calcium								
Serum phosphate								
Serum albumin								
Drugs (dose/route)								

cated to correct volume depletion, regardless of urine volume. Replacement fluids should not be indiscriminantly administered to hydrated or overhydrated patients. Some patients appear to be normally hydrated but have historical findings consistent with fluid losses (e.g., vomiting, diarrhea, lack of water consumption). The authors usually assume such patients to be subclinically dehydrated (less than five per cent) and carefully administer fluids to them at the rate of one to three per cent of body weight on the premise that mild overhydration is less likely to have adverse effects than unrecognized volume depletion. Even mild volume depletion may promote renal injury in patients predisposed to ARF.[2–4]

Because hypovolemia and hypotension cause oliguria and may contribute to the genesis of ATN or predispose to further renal damage, volume depletion should be rapidly corrected. Patients should be rehydrated with a replacement fluid using an aseptically placed intravenous catheter. Selection of an appropriate replacement fluid is based on knowledge of deficits and excesses in water, electrolytes, and acid-base balance. In most cases, lactated Ringer's solution is satisfactory. Selection of replacement fluids is discussed in detail in Chapter 53.

The volume of fluid to be administered is based on the magnitude of dehydration (percentage of dehydration × body weight in pounds × 450 = milliliters of replacement fluid). The total fluid dose for rehydration should be administered over two to six hours unless the patient has known cardiac dysfunction, demonstrates intolerance to fluid administration, or becomes overhydrated (e.g., exhibits dyspnea, elevated neck veins, rales, diastolic gallop rhythm, pulmonary edema). Administration of fluid at this rate will help to rapidly restore adequate renal perfusion. In addition, in patients in which oliguria was physiologic in origin (i.e., prerenal azotemia), urine volume will increase. However, careful monitoring of the patient's response to fluid therapy is essential. If fluid overload occurs, the rate of fluid administration should be reduced or temporarily discontinued. Monitoring of central venous pressure may be necessary for patients with cardiac dysfunction or intolerance to fluid therapy.

Fluid Therapy During Maintenance and Recovery Phases. A favorable clinical response and normalization of blood pressure usually indicate successful restoration of normal hydration. Subsequent fluid therapy is directed toward maintaining fluid balance and preventing hypovolemia. Because even subclinical volume depletion may promote additional azotemia and renal damage, it may be desirable to induce a state of mild overhydration (one to three per cent of body weight) over the subsequent 6 to 12 hours in nonoliguric patients that have normal cardiopulmonary function. This mild state of overhydration assures adequate volume replacement and may serve as a buffer against subclinical dehydration. However, overt overhydration must be avoided in patients with persistent pathologic oliguria.

Urine volume and other contemporary losses (e.g., vomiting and diarrhea) greatly influence fluid requirements during the maintenance and recovery phases of ARF. Measurement of urine volume may provide a particularly useful guide to fluid therapy during the diuretic phase of ATN. Patients are predisposed to dehydration during this phase because involuntary urine losses are often great. In order to prevent dehydration, the volume of parenteral fluids administered and oral fluids consumed should equal the sum of (a) urine volume, (b) contemporary fluid losses (e.g., fluid lost through vomiting, diarrhea), and (c) insensible fluid losses. Insensible fluid losses have been estimated to be about 10 to 12 ml/lb/day (20 to 25 ml/kg/day), but may vary with body temperature, air temperature, and humidity.[18] Because estimation of contemporary and insensible fluid losses may be inaccurate, serial determinations of body weight are commonly used to guide fluid therapy. The quantity of maintenance fluids administered should be adjusted so that body weight remains stable. However, in patients that are not receiving sufficient calories, a weight loss of 0.05 to 0.15 lb (0.1 to 0.3 kg) should be allowed for each 1000 calories required daily.

Overly aggressive fluid therapy during the diuretic phase of ATN may promote continued polyuria. As urine volume stabilizes or begins to decline, the volume of fluids administered should be correspondingly reduced. Because dehydration may recur if fluid administration is reduced too rapidly, body weight and clinical assessment of hydration status should be carefully monitored as fluid therapy is reduced.

Selection of fluids for maintenance therapy should be based on the route of fluid loss. Insensible fluid losses related to the respiratory tract consists of electrolyte-free water and should be replaced by oral water or parenteral administration of dextrose five per cent in water. Urinary and gastrointestinal fluid and electrolyte losses can usually be replaced using balanced electrolyte solutions (e.g., lactated Ringer's solution).

Fluids should be modified according to changes in serum sodium concentrations. Progressive hypernatremia may develop in normally hydrated patients when inadequate quantities of electrolyte-free water are provided. In such patients more electrolyte-free water (e.g., dextrose five per cent in water) and less sodium-containing electrolyte solution (e.g., lactated Ringer's solution) should be administered. Progressive hyponatremia may indicate excessive administration or consumption of electrolyte-free water or excessive sodium losses. Hyponatremia in overhydrated patients may be treated by restricting administration or oral consumption of electrolyte-free water. In normally hydrated hyponatremic patients, administration or oral consumption of electrolyte-free water should be reduced in favor of sodium-containing fluids.

THERAPY OF POTASSIUM AND ACID-BASE IMBALANCES

Disorders of Potassium Homeostasis. HYPERKALEMIA. OVERVIEW. Hyperkalemia is commonly associated with oliguric ARF and may cause skeletal muscle weakness, reduce cardiac contractility, and cause a variety of cardiac conduction disturbances (including bradycardia, atrioventricular dissociation, asystole, and ventricular fibrillation). These effects occur because hyperkalemia reduces the neuromuscular resting membrane potential, causing it to be less negative, thereby lessening the rate of elevation of the action potential and slowing electrical conduction. Hyponatremia, hypocalcemia, and acidemia may exacerbate the clinical signs of hyperkalemia.[38] Hyperkalemia is less often a problem in nonoliguric patients because increased tubular secretion of potassium may partially or completely compensate for the decrease in GFR.[37, 39]

Serum potassium concentrations that do not exceed 6 to 8 mEq/L typically do not induce life-threatening cardiotoxicity. Hyperkalemia of this magnitude often responds to intravenous fluid therapy and elimination of extrarenal factors that promote hyperkalemia (Table 108–14).[40] However, if serum potassium concentrations exceed 8 mEq/L, or if serious cardiotoxicity occurs, therapy with sodium bicarbonate, glucose, glucose with insulin, or calcium gluconate should be considered. Of these drugs, sodium bicarbonate is commonly used first because many hyperkalemic patients also require this drug for treatment of concurrent metabolic acidosis. Administration of glucose and insulin or calcium gluconate is indicated primarily for rapid correction of severe hyperkalemic cardiotoxicity.

SODIUM BICARBONATE. Intravenous administration of sodium bicarbonate promotes intracellular movement of potassium, thereby lowering serum potassium concentration. The shift of potassium into cells enhances restoration of the normal transcellular gradient, and therefore, tends to correct hyperkalemic cardiotoxicity without altering total body potassium. In patients with metabolic acidosis, dosage of sodium bicarbonate may be based on the bicarbonate deficit (see the section on

TABLE 108–14. FACTORS THAT PROMOTE HYPERKALEMIA

1. Oral or parental potassium supplements
2. Enteral feeding solutions; excessive dietary potassium content
3. Drugs
   a. Potassium-containing drugs
   b. Digitalis
   c. Heparin
   d. Captopril
   e. Nonsteroidal anti-inflammatory drugs
   f. Potassium-sparing diuretics
   g. Beta blocking drugs (e.g., propranolol)
   h. Alpha-adrenergic agonists
   i. Others
4. Acidemia
5. Hypertonicity
   a. Hypernatremia
   b. Hyperglycemia
6. Hypoadrenocorticism
7. Insulin deficiency
8. Hypercatabolism
   a. Infection
   b. Pyrexia
   c. Burns
9. Rhabdomyolysis
10. Tumor lysis syndrome
11. Transfusion
12. Hyporeninemic hypoaldosteronism
13. Others

Treatment of Metabolic Acidosis in ARF). In patients that are not acidotic, sodium bicarbonate may still ameliorate hyperkalemia when administered intravenously at a dose of 0.22 to 0.44 mEq/lb (0.5 to 1.0 mEq/kg) body weight over 15 minutes.[41] The effect of sodium bicarbonate on serum potassium concentration occurs within minutes and may last for up to several hours. Sodium bicarbonate should be used cautiously in patients with pathologic oliguria or cardiac failure because it may induce fluid volume overload. It should also be used with caution in hypocalcemic patients because alkalinization promotes clinical signs of hypocalcemia by reducing plasma ionized calcium concentrations.

GLUCOSE AND INSULIN. Intravenous administration of glucose (20 per cent solution) at a dose of 0.22 to 0.44 gm/lb (0.5 to 1.0 gm/kg) body weight with or without insulin will induce transfer of extracellular potassium ions intracellularly.[41] If insulin is used, it should be added at a rate of 1 unit of regular insulin for each 3 gm of glucose administered. However, addition of insulin probably offers little additional benefit over the effects of glucose alone.[42] The effects of glucose therapy are rapid in onset and may last for several hours.

CALCIUM GLUCONATE. Because calcium acts as a direct antagonist to the cardiac effects of hyperkalemia, calcium gluconate (10 per cent solution) may be used to treat hyperkalemic cardiotoxicity. During electrocardiographic monitoring it should be administered intravenously over 10 to 15 minutes in a dose sufficient to correct life-threatening dysrhythmias. The total dose of calcium gluconate should not exceed 0.22 to 0.44 gm/lb (0.5 to 1.0 gm/kg) body weight.[38] If calcium gluconate causes progressive bradycardia, administration should be terminated. Although calcium gluconate infusion rapidly corrects hyperkalemic cardiotoxicity, its beneficial effects typically last for only 10 to 15 minutes. It does not lower serum potassium concentrations. Therefore, calcium therapy is intended only as a short-term measure to sustain the patient while other therapy to correct hyperkalemia can be initiated.

BETA-ADRENERGIC AGONISTS. Another potential therapy for hyperkalemia is administration of β_2-agonists. β-adrenergic agonists promote intracellular uptake of potassium through a mechanism that involves stimulation of β_2-adrenoreceptors.[43] This effect is independent of the effects of insulin or aldosterone. Intravenous administration of albuterol sulfate (a β_2-adrenergic agonist) has been shown to rapidly and effectively reduce serum potassium concentrations in humans with severe renal failure.[43] The intravenous form of this drug is not currently available in the United States.

TREATMENT OF HYPERKALEMIA DURING THE MAINTENANCE PHASE. Hyperkalemia may be minimized during the maintenance phase of ARF by (a) restricting potassium intake, (b) eliminating extrarenal factors that promote hyperkalemia (Table 108–14), (c) promoting urine output, (d) administering furosemide, and/or (e) orally administering cationic exchange resins. In most patients a combination of the first three of these therapeutic options will maintain serum potassium concentrations near or within normal limits. The authors have successfully used intermittent furosemide therapy to minimize hyperkalemia in some patients. However, furosemide may promote fluid and electrolyte imbalances.

Polystyrene sulfonate (Kayexalate) is a cationic exchange resin that promotes gastrointestinal potassium elimination. It may be administered orally or rectally. Each gram of resin binds 1 to 3 mEq of potassium after releasing an equivalent amount of sodium. Therefore, it may be useful for patients with persistent hyperkalemia. It should not be given concurrently with nonabsorbable cation-donating antacids.[38] Polystyrene sulfonate is given orally at a dose of 1 gm/lb (2 gm/kg) body weight/day in three divided doses (each gram should be suspended in at least 3 to 4 ml of water).[38] It may also be given as a retention enema at the rate of 15 gm in 100 ml of 1 per cent methylcellulose or 10 per cent dextrose. The rectal dose may be increased threefold to fourfold as needed to increase potassium exchange.[38] The solution should be retained within the colon for a minimum of 30 minutes. Because potassium is exchanged for sodium, this drug may promote overhydration and hypertension. Hypokalemia, hypomagnesemia, or hypocalcemia may also occur with chronic use. In addition, chronic administration may be associated with fecal impaction. Therefore, it is usually administered with a cathartic to prevent constipation.

HYPOKALEMIA. Hypokalemia may occur in some patients with nonoliguric ARF owing to renal potassium losses and inadequate potassium intake. It is most prevalent in association with gentamicin-induced ARF, the diuretic phase of ATN, and/or after therapeutically induced diuresis.[7] Clinical signs of hypokalemia may include extreme muscle weakness, vomiting, anorexia (associated with paralytic ileus and gastric distention), and cardiac dysrhythmias. Hypokalemia in cats is often manifested by inability to elevate the head. Treatment consists of oral or parenteral potassium supplementation, usually as potassium chloride. Therapy for hypokalemia has recently been reviewed[44] (see Chapter 53).

Metabolic Acidosis. The decision as to when to treat metabolic acidosis should be based on clinical and laboratory assessment of the patient. Metabolic acidosis typically has little immediate effect unless blood pH is below 7.10 (usually associated with blood bicarbonate or total carbon dioxide concentrations less than 10 to 12 mEq/L).[22] Therefore, not all patients with metabolic acidosis require immediate treatment of their acid-base disorder. Alkalinization therapy should be considered for patients with blood pH values less than 7.20. Immediate correction of metabolic acidosis is usually unnecessary when blood pH values exceed 7.20. Mild to moderate metabolic acidosis often improves after fluid therapy alone.

Metabolic acidosis is treated by administration of alkali. In most cases sodium bicarbonate is the drug of choice because it replaces lost bicarbonate. Sodium acetate, sodium lactate, and sodium citrate have also been used for treatment of acidosis, but appear to offer little clear advantage.[22] The major disadvantage of these alternative drugs is that they require hepatic metabolism for their alkalinizing effects. Initial sodium bicarbonate dosage in milliequivalents is calculated as 0.134 × body weight (lbs) × bicarbonate deficit (0.3 × body weight (kg) × bicarbonate deficit). One half of this dose should be administered as a slow intravenous injection. The remainder of the calculated dose is administered in intravenous fluids over the subsequent four to six hours. Initially, sodium bicarbonate administered intravenously is limited to the vascular space and induces large increases in blood bicarbonate concentration.[22] Bicarbonate equilibrates throughout the extracellular fluid within 15 minutes and then equilibrates with the extracellular buffers over the subsequent two to four hours.[22] After the initial calculated dose has been administered, the acid-base status of the patient should be reassessed (blood gas analysis, total CO_2, or CO_2 combining power). Subsequent therapy should be formulated on the basis of serial analysis of the patient's response to sodium bicarbonate therapy. Because intracellular buffers play an increasing role in severe metabolic acidosis, the quantity of sodium bicarbonate required by patients with severe metabolic acidosis may greatly exceed the calculated dose. Therefore, the total dose is best titrated by serially assessing response to treatment.

The goal of alkalinization therapy is not to normalize acid-base balance but to moderate significant acidosis. The initial therapeutic goal in patients with severe acidosis should be to increase blood pH values to about 7.20, a level likely to prevent adverse cardiac effects of acidosis. Only small increases in blood bicarbonate concentration are needed to correct life-threatening acidemia in most cases.[22] Blood bicarbonate concentration of 14 mEq/L or greater usually indicates adequate correction of metabolic acidosis in patients with normal respiratory compensation and no complicating factors.

Subsequent therapy of metabolic acidosis continuing through maintenance and recovery phases of ARF should be based on serial determination of acid-base status. Renal tubular damage in patients with ATN may rarely be associated with excessive urinary bicarbonate losses, resulting in persistent metabolic acidosis (type II renal tubular acidosis). Continued treatment of metabolic acidosis is usually indicated only if blood pH declines below 7.20. Sodium bicarbonate may be administered orally or added to intravenous fluids in a dose adequate to maintain blood pH above 7.20.

Sodium bicarbonate therapy may be associated with a variety of important adverse effects, including metabolic alkalosis, reduced blood ionized calcium concentration, sodium overload (particularly in oliguric patients), and hypertension. Calcium carbonate may be used as an alternative drug and may be less likely to result in volume overload and hypertension. However, administration of calcium carbonate to patients with hyperphosphatemia may cause deposition of calcium in soft tissues and additional renal damage. Therefore, it is uncommonly utilized.

CONVERTING OLIGURIA TO NONOLIGURIA

Indications for Therapy. Therapy specifically designed to convert oliguria to nonoliguria should be considered only for oliguric patients that are unresponsive to fluid volume replacement. If oliguria persists despite correction of fluid deficits, an attempt should be made to increase urine volume because clinical management of nonoliguric patients is easier and their prognosis appears to be better. Use of diuretics or vasodilators in nonoliguric patients is generally discouraged because

they are rarely needed and, therefore, unnecessarily expose the patient to risk of fluid and electrolyte depletion, additional renal injury, or adverse drug reactions.

Diuretics. OVERVIEW. Early recommendations for use of diuretics in treatment of ARF were based on studies of laboratory models in which various diuretics proved to be of benefit in minimizing or reversing acute oliguric renal failure.[14, 45] Diuretics appear to be particularly useful when administered before or immediately after experimentally induced renal injury. However, diuretics are of questionable efficacy in reversing established ARF. The clinical value of diuretic therapy for spontaneous canine and feline ARF must be determined by controlled clinical studies. Nonetheless, based on empirical clinical use, diuretics have a well-established role in treatment of oliguric ARF. In addition, diuretic therapy generally entails minimal risk if the patient's fluid volume and electrolyte status are carefully monitored.

Diuretics can increase urine flow in most humans with early ARF. In uncontrolled clinical studies, infusion of 12.5 to 25.0 gm of mannitol, sometimes repeated once or twice, reversed oliguria in about two of every three humans with oliguric ARF.[45] Use of loop diuretics, such as furosemide, was similarly successful.[45] Analyses of these studies were interpreted to suggest that patients with early ARF were more likely to survive if their urine output increased after administration of diuretics. However, improved survival of diuretic responders may indicate more than one possibility: (1) diuretics may alter the natural course of ARF, or (2) response to diuretics may occur in patients in which ARF is less severe.

Potential benefits of diuretic therapy include promotion of diuresis (i.e., correcting oliguria), inhibition or relieving of intratubular obstruction, and, in some cases, enhancement of renal function. Diuretics do not appear to limit tubular cell necrosis, accelerate cellular regeneration, or consistently enhance renal function. In addition, increased urine output per se is not a reliable index of improved renal function. In general, diuretics appear to have limited ability to prevent, reverse, or speed recovery from established ARF in humans.[45]

A therapeutic trial with at least one diuretic is indicated for most canine or feline patients with oliguric ARF. Furosemide and mannitol are the diuretics most commonly used. Patients that fail to respond to one of these diuretics may respond to the other or a combination of both. Alternatively, diuretics may be used in combination with vasodilators such as dopamine.

FUROSEMIDE. Furosemide has been the most commonly used diuretic in canine and feline patients with oliguric ARF because it is relatively safe, readily available, and familiar to most veterinarians. Initially it should be administered intravenously at a dose of 1 mg/lb (2 mg/kg) body weight. If no substantial diuresis develops within one hour after administration, the dose may be doubled (2 mg/lb or 4 mg/kg). If this dose also fails to induce diuresis, the dose may be further increased to 3 mg/lb (6 mg/kg) body weight. If diuresis still does not ensue, very large doses of furosemide, an alternative diuretic (e.g., mannitol), or the combination of furosemide and dopamine may be considered.

In humans with ARF, administration of very large doses of furosemide (500 to 2000 mg daily) has been successfully used to induce diuresis in patients unresponsive to more modest doses.[45] High dose therapy, however, has been associated with a variety of acute side-effects. Administration of furosemide at a dose of 22 mg/lb (50 mg/kg) has been associated with lowered blood pressure, apathy, and staggering in normal dogs. Administration of 4.4 mg/lb (10 mg/kg) of furosemide induced transient apathy and anorexia in normal cats. Because controlled studies documenting safety and efficacy of high-dose furosemide therapy have not been performed, it cannot be routinely recommended at this time.

If furosemide successfully induces diuresis, it may be administered every eight hours as needed to sustain diuresis and promote potassium excretion. However, the need for continued furosemide therapy must be considered in light of its potential adverse effects, including electrolyte depletion (particularly hypokalemia; sometimes hypocalcemia), dehydration, hypotension, gastrointestinal upsets, ototoxicity, hematologic reactions, restlessness, and weakness.[41] It has been suggested that furosemide should not be used in patients with suspected gentamicin-induced ATN because it may promote nephrotoxicity of gentamicin.[8]

MANNITOL. Mannitol is an osmotic diuretic commonly used to treat oliguric ARF. Mannitol has at least three theoretical advantages over furosemide: (1) it may enhance renal function by minimizing renal tubular cell swelling by means of its osmotic properties, (2) mannitol exerts its diuretic effects along the entire nephron and therefore may directly affect the proximal tubule; and (3) mannitol may expand the extracellular fluid volume. The major disadvantage of mannitol is the potential for vascular overload if oliguria persists. Therefore, mannitol should be avoided in overhydrated oliguric patients. Mannitol (20 per cent or 25 per cent solution) is administered intravenously over five to ten minutes at a dose of 0.1 to 0.22 gm/lb (0.25 to 0.5 gm/kg) body weight. If substantial diuresis ensues, administration of mannitol can be repeated every four to six hours, or it can be given as a maintenance infusion (8 to 10 per cent solution) during the initial 12 to 24 hours of treatment.

Vasodilators. Because reduced RBF may contribute to the pathogenesis of ARF (Table 108–5), vasodilators are a logical therapy for patients with ARF. Dopamine, a precursor of norepinephrine, has been suggested for patients that are unresponsive to osmotic and/or loop diuretics. Infusion of low doses of dopamine reduces renal vascular resistance and increases RBF, particularly to the inner renal cortex.[46] Unlike most other drugs that decrease renal vascular resistance, dopamine does not cause peripheral vascular resistance and systemic arterial pressure to decline when given in low doses intravenously.[17] These effects are mediated by stimulation of dopaminergic receptors in the renal vasculature. Studies of the effects of dopamine and furosemide on early uranyl nitrate–induced ARF in dogs suggest that combination therapy of dopamine with furosemide was more effective in inducing vasodilation and diuresis and preventing decline in GFR than either drug used alone.[48]

Dopamine should be administered by intravenous infusion at a rate of 1 to 2.2 μgm/lb/min (2 to 5 μgm/kg/min.). Dilution of 50 mg of dopamine in 500 ml of lactated Ringer's solution or dextrose 5 per cent in water will yield a solution containing 100 μgm/ml. This solution should be administered using an intravenous fluid administration pump or under close supervision to assure accurate fluid delivery rates. At higher dose rates dopamine may cause tachycardia and other cardiac arrhythmias and renal vasoconstriction. Therefore, electrocardiographic monitoring during dopamine administration may be advisable. Patients with moderate to severe hyperkalemia may be predisposed to cardiac dysrhythmias during administration of dopamine. Response to dopamine therapy is usually rapid. If urine flow does not increase within the first few hours of therapy, infusion of dopamine should be discontinued.

NONDIALYTIC MANAGEMENT DURING THE MAINTENANCE PHASE

Dialytic Versus Nondialytic Management. Nondialytic management is designed to sustain patients until adequate renal function to maintain homeostasis returns. It is most successful in patients with nonoliguric ARF, but the authors have successfully used this technique in patients with oliguric ARF. Clinical and laboratory findings that suggest that response to nondialytic therapy may be less satisfactory include severe metabolic acidosis, marked hyperkalemia (serum potassium concentration greater than approximately 8 mEq/L), severe gastrointestinal and neurologic complications of uremia, or disease processes likely to promote catabolism (e.g., sepsis, pyrexia). Dialysis may be required to effectively manage patients with these findings. Goals of nondialytic management are to (a) maintain fluid, electrolyte, and acid-base balance (described in the sections above); (b) ameliorate clinical signs of uremia; (c) maintain adequate nutrition; and (d) prevent or treat complications of ARF.

Amelioration of Uremic Manifestations. **DIETARY MANAGEMENT.** Clinical manifestations of uremia are ameliorated by a combination of dietary protein restriction and pharmacologic control of uremic gastritis and vomiting. Protein intake should be restricted regardless of whether the patient is receiving enteral or parenteral feeding. Adult dogs should receive approximately 8 to 12 per cent of their calories as protein. Adult cats have a higher daily protein requirement than dogs, and therefore should receive approximately 20 per cent of their diet calories as protein. Protein restriction minimizes production of nitrogenous waste products that may be responsible for many clinical signs of uremia. In addition, protein restriction may have a protective effect against additional ischemic or nephrotoxic renal injury.[49, 50] (Dietary treatment of renal failure is discussed in the CRF section of this chapter).

CONTROL OF UREMIC VOMITING. Uremic gastritis is a major cause of vomiting in patients with renal failure. Renal gastrin clearance is decreased in renal failure, resulting in hypergastrinemia. Hypergastrinemia in turn causes prolonged stimulation of histamine H_2-receptors located on gastric parietal cells, and thereby promotes gastric acid secretion and uremic gastritis (Figure 108–

1A). Mucosal irritation caused by gastric hyperacidity contributes to vomiting and anorexia. In addition, gastrointestinal hemorrhage associated with uremic gastritis may promote vomiting by increasing the magnitude of azotemia.

Cimetidine (Tagamet) has been recommended for control of uremic hemorrhagic gastritis because it blocks gastrin-stimulated gastric hyperacidity (Figure 108–1B).[51] For dogs in uremic crisis, cimetidine is given intravenously at an initial dose of 4.5 mg/lb (10 mg/kg) body weight. Thereafter it is given intravenously at 2.2 mg/lb (5 mg/kg) body weight every 12 hours. Once uremic gastritis has been controlled and oral medication can be tolerated, cimetidine may be administered orally at a dose of 2.2 mg/lb (5 mg/kg) body weight given every 12 hours for two to three weeks. The dosage is reduced to 2.2 mg/lb (5 mg/kg) given once daily for two to three weeks before being withdrawn. Dosage recommendations for cats are approximately one half of the canine

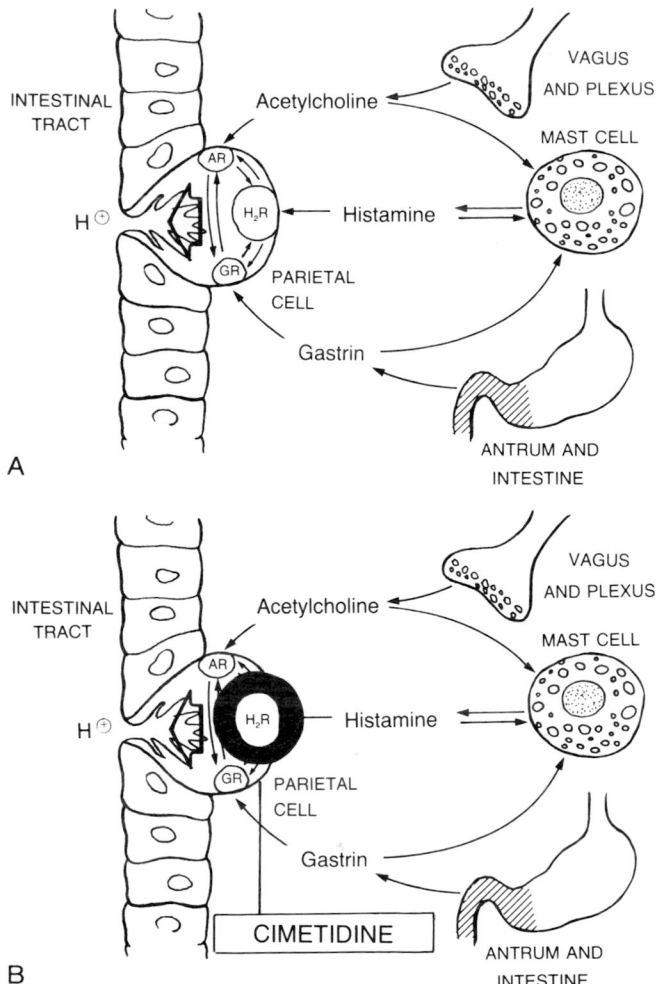

A

B

FIGURE 108–1. *A,* Relationship between parietal cell histamine H_2-receptors, gastrin, and acetylcholine receptors. Renal failure is characterized by hypergastrinemia, which causes prolonged stimulation of histamine H_2-receptors, thereby promoting gastric acid secretion and uremic gastritis. (From Thornhill, JA: Control of vomiting in the uremic patient. *In* Kirk, RW (ed): Current Veterinary Therapy VIII. Philadelphia, WB Saunders Co, 1983, pp. 1022–1025.) *B,* Cimetidine antagonism of the parietal cell H_2-receptors. (From Thornhill, JA: Control of vomiting in the uremic patient. *In* Kirk, RW (ed): Current Veterinary Therapy VIII. Philadelphia, WB Saunders Co., 1983, pp. 1022–1025.)

dose.[41] Adverse effects of cimetidine recognized in humans include: leukopenia, thrombocytopenia, aplastic anemia, pyrexia, interstitial nephritis, renal failure, hepatitis, pancreatitis, arthralgia, myalgia, somnolence, transient diarrhea, and drug interaction because of induction of hepatic enzymes.[41] Adverse effects associated with use of cimetidine have not yet been reported for dogs and cats.

Because uremic vomiting may also result from stimulation of the chemoreceptor trigger zone by poorly defined uremic toxins, intravenously administered centrally acting antiemetics may be useful in controlling vomiting. However, hypotension and sedation are potential pitfalls associated with antiemetic therapy. Chlorpromazine (0.22 mg/lb or 0.5 mg/kg), prochlorperazine (0.06 mg/lb q or 0.13 mg/kg q6h), and trimethobenzamide (1.4 mg/lb or 3 mg/kg q8h) are centrally acting antiemetics that may ameliorate nausea and vomiting in uremic patients.

Nutritional Management. Proper nutrition is an integral part of supportive care of ARF because many patients are hypercatabolic. Also, tissue catabolism may promote azotemia as body proteins are used for calories. Inadequate nutrition may result in suboptimal renal regeneration and tissue repair, thus slowing recovery from ARF. Unfortunately use of enteral nutrition is rarely feasible early in the course of ARF because of gastrointestinal dysfunction. Therefore, parenteral nutritional support and therapy with essential amino acids is the treatment of choice in patients with ARF. If parenteral hyperalimentation is not feasible because of economic or technical considerations, enteral hyperalimentation should be initiated as soon as the patient's condition permits.

Parenteral hyperalimentation may provide considerable benefit to patients with ARF. For example, amino acid administration augmented the rate of renal regeneration and tissue repair in experimental ARF.[52] Administration of hypertonic dextrose or combined hypertonic dextrose and essential amino acids doubled survival time in anephric dogs compared with dogs given either oral nutrition or parenteral administration of dextrose 5 per cent in water.[53] Although some studies indicate that parenteral hyperalimentation may enhance metabolic stability, and recovery of renal function and improve survival in humans with ARF, these findings are not universally accepted.[52] Controlled studies on the benefit of parenteral hyperalimentation in spontaneous canine and feline ARF have apparently not been performed (see Chapter 54).

Preventing Urinary Tract Infections and Adverse Drug Reactions. Major complications in patients with ARF are related to infection and drug therapy. As described earlier, urinary and vascular catheters are likely sites for introduction of infection. Therefore, urinary catheters should be used only when necessary, and serial urine cultures should be performed to detect UTI as early as possible. Treatment of UTI should be based on results of microbe susceptibility testing. In addition, success of treatment should be confirmed by performing urine cultures during as well as after treatment (see Chapter 112).

Great care must be used in selection of drugs for

patients with ARF. Nephrotoxic drugs should be avoided if possible. Dosages of drugs excreted by the kidneys often require adjustment (see section on CRF). Because of the risks associated with drug therapy in these patients, only drugs with clear indications and proven effectiveness should be administered.

Minimizing Hyperphosphatemia. Hyperphosphatemia, which results from renal retention of phosphorus, is not a medical emergency in patients with ARF. However, minimizing hyperphosphatemia during the maintenance phase of ARF may be desirable because hyperphosphatemia promotes hypocalcemia and soft-tissue mineralization, including nephrocalcinosis. Treatment of hyperphosphatemia includes minimizing phosphorus intake, and oral administration of intestinal phosphorus binding agents (see section on Therapy of Divalent Ion Imbalance in CRF).

DIALYSIS

Peritoneal dialysis and hemodialysis have been successfully used for treatment of dogs and cats with ARF.[54-56] Because of economic and technical considerations, hemodialysis is limited primarily to university teaching hospitals or large referral centers. Although peritoneal dialysis could be performed by most veterinary facilities, the technical and time demands of this procedure are great. In addition, peritonitis is a common complication of long-term peritoneal dialysis which has limited its use. Peritonitis has particularly been a problem when peritoneal dialysis is performed by individuals who are unfamiliar with the technique. For these reasons, conservative therapy is used when possible.

Some patients clearly require dialytic therapy. Indications for dialysis in dogs and cats with ARF include: (1) failure to respond adequately to nondialytic management, (2) the need to eliminate a nephrotoxic drug being retained because of ARF, (3) overhydration associated with oliguria, (4) severe, intractable hyperkalemia or acidosis, and (5) the need to minimize metabolic imbalances and azotemia in patients that require emergency surgery (e.g., for repair of urinary trauma or leakage). Cost and availability of dialysis facilities and personnel are also important factors that affect the decision to use dialysis. However, dialysis is probably most effective when initiated before the onset of severe uremic complications. Therefore, the decision to use dialysis should be made as early as possible. Methods for hemodialysis and peritoneal dialysis have been described in detail elsewhere.[54-56]

CHRONIC RENAL FAILURE

Definition and Clinical Significance

Chronic renal failure (CRF) is probably the most common of the syndromes that affect only the kidneys. It is defined as primary renal failure that has persisted for an extended period, usually months to years. Regardless of the cause(s) of nephron loss, CRF is characterized by irreversible renal structural lesions. After correcting reversible and/or prerenal or postrenal components of renal dysfunction, further improvement in renal function should not be expected in patients with CRF because maximum compensatory and adaptive changes designed to sustain renal function have already occurred. Likewise, unless an additional form of renal injury occurs, rapid deterioration of intrinsic renal function is also unusual. Therefore, renal function typically remains stable for weeks to months. Nonetheless, renal function progressively deteriorates over months to years in patients with CRF.[57, 58] Surprisingly, it is not necessary for the disease process responsible for the initial renal injury to persist for progressive dysfunction to occur. Thus, irrespective of underlying causes, CRF is an irreversible and a progressive disease.

Despite the poor long-term prognosis, patients with CRF often survive for many months to years with a good quality of life. Although no treatment can correct the irreversible renal lesions of CRF, the clinical and biochemical consequences of reduced renal function can be minimized by symptomatic and supportive therapy. In addition, recent advances in understanding of the spontaneously progressive nature of CRF have provided clues as to how this self-perpetuating deterioration of renal function may be slowed or stopped.

Clinical Characteristics

AFFECTED POPULATION

Although frequently considered a disease of older animals, CRF occurs with varying frequency in dogs and cats of all ages. In a survey of 170 canine and 36 feline patients with CRF, the mean age at diagnosis was 7.0 years for dogs and 7.4 years for cats.[18] In another study of 119 dogs with CRF, the mean age at diagnosis was 6.5 years.[59] Fifty-three per cent of affected cats were over seven years old in a recent review of feline CRF, but animals ranged in age from 9 months to 22 years.[60]

CRF occurs in immature and young dogs and cats primarily in association with acquired or congenital and familial renal diseases.[61] Although no obvious breed predilection has been observed for acquired CRF, there are several well recognized breed predilections for congenital and familial renal diseases (Table 108–15). The rate at which congenital or hereditary renal diseases progress to renal failure and uremia depends on the type and severity of renal lesions and the breed involved. Although some of these animals live only for weeks or months, a substantial number survive for many years. Congenital and hereditary renal diseases of dogs and cats have recently been reviewed.[61, 62]

CLINICAL AND LABORATORY FINDINGS

Most of the clinical signs of CRF result from the effects of loss of renal function rather than from renal lesions themselves. Therefore, the spectrum of clinical signs arising from CRF is very broad. In its earliest stages, CRF often remains clinically silent for extended periods. Mild to moderate polyuria, polydipsia, and nocturia are often among the earliest signs observed in

TABLE 108–15. CONGENITAL AND FAMILIAL RENAL DISEASES OF DOGS AND CATS

Breed	Renal Lesions	References
Abyssinian cat	Renal amyloidosis	243–245
Alaskan malamute	Renal cortical hypoplasia?	246
	Renal dysplasia	62
Basenji	Fanconi-like syndrome	63, 247–249
Beagle	Unilateral renal agenesis	250, 251
	Renal dysplasia	252
	Polycystic kidneys	253
Boxer	Renal dysplasia	254
Bulldog	Renal dysplasia	62
Cairn terrier	Polycystic kidney disease	255
Cocker spaniel	Renal cortical hypoplasia?	256, 257
Doberman pinscher	Glomerulopathy	62, 258, 259
	Unilateral agenesis	258, 259
Domestic longhair cat	Polycystic kidneys	260
Domestic shorthair cat	Unilateral renal agenesis	261
Great Dane	Renal dysplasia	62, 262
Great Pyrenees	Renal dysplasia	
Himalayan cat	Unilateral renal agenesis	261
	Polycystic kidney disease	261
Irish wolfhound	Renal dysplasia	
Keeshond	Renal cortical hypoplasia?	263
King Charles spaniel	Renal dysplasia	62
Lhasa apso	Renal dysplasia	62, 264
Miniature poodle	Polycystic kidneys	265
Norwegian elkhound	Tubulointerstitial nephropathy	266–268
	Fanconi-like syndrome	62
Persian cat	Renal dysplasia	261
Samoyed	Glomerulopathy	62, 269–271
	Renal dysplasia	62
Schnauzer	Fanconi-like syndrome	63
Shetland sheepdog	Fanconi-like syndrome	63
Shih Tzu	Renal dysplasia	62, 264
Soft-coated Wheaton terrier	Renal dysplasia	272, 273
Standard poodle	Renal dysplasia	274
Yorkshire terrier	Renal dysplasia	275

dogs with CRF. However, such evidence of altered fluid balance is typically not as prominent in cats with CRF. In contrast to findings in dogs, polyuria was reported in only 26 of 73 cats (35.6 per cent) with spontaneous CRF.[60] This finding may be related to poor owner attention to the micturition habits of their cats, or to the apparently greater intrinsic urine-concentrating ability of cats with CRF compared with dogs.[184] However, in the same study of feline CRF, urine specific gravity values were found to be less than 1.015 in 42 of 74 cats, and exceeded 1.025 in only 8 of 74 cats. Other common clinical findings that occur early in the course of canine and feline CRF include variable weight loss, poor haircoat (loss of sheen, increased shedding), lethargy, and selective appetite.

In more advanced states CRF is associated with uremia. Common manifestations of advanced CRF include anorexia, depression, severe weight loss, vomiting, diarrhea, dehydration, oral ulcerations, discoloration and necrosis of the tongue, hemorrhage (primarily gastrointestinal), pallor of the mucous membranes, and conjunctival and scleral injection. Vomiting apparently occurs less commonly in cats than in dogs with CRF.[60]

Abdominal palpation often reveals small, irregularly shaped kidneys, but kidney size can be normal or even increased, depending on the cause of CRF. Based on palpation alone, kidneys were found to be enlarged in 17 of 68 cats, and small and irregular in 17 of 68 cats with CRF.[60] Reduced kidney size typically reflects loss of nephrons and their subsequent replacement with connective tissue. Kidney size may be increased in patients with CRF because of polycystic kidney disease, chronic urinary obstruction, or renal neoplasia.

Relatively uncommon manifestations of moderate to advanced CRF include uremic pneumonitis, uremic pericarditis, congestive heart failure, neurologic signs (neuromuscular irritability, seizures, stupor, and coma), hypertensive retinopathy (hyphema, retinal detachments, dilated and tortuous retinal vessels), and clinically detectable renal osteodystrophy. While microscopic evidence of renal osteodystrophy may be found in most dogs with CRF, clinical signs related to skeletal disease are typically absent. However, clinical manifestations of severe renal osteodystrophy may include skeletal decalcification, pathologic fractures, proliferative and cystic bone lesions (Figure 108–2), bone pain, growth retardation, loose teeth, and *rubber jaw syndrome*.[64] Skeletal lesions caused by renal failure are often more severe in immature animals because growing bones are particularly vulnerable to the alterations in vitamin D metabolism and hyperparathyroidism. See Chapter 107 for additional information on the pathophysiology of renal osteodystrophy.

Common laboratory findings in dogs with CRF include azotemia, hyperphosphatemia, metabolic acidosis, hypermagnesemia, and normocytic, normochromic anemia. Azotemia, hyperphosphatemia, metabolic acidosis, and hypermagnesemia occur as a result of renal excretory failure. Anemia results primarily from reduced renal erythropoietin production, but increased hemolysis and blood loss may also be factors.

Urinalysis typically reveals an inappropriately low urine specific gravity, mild to moderate proteinuria, and inactive urine sediment in dogs and cats with CRF.

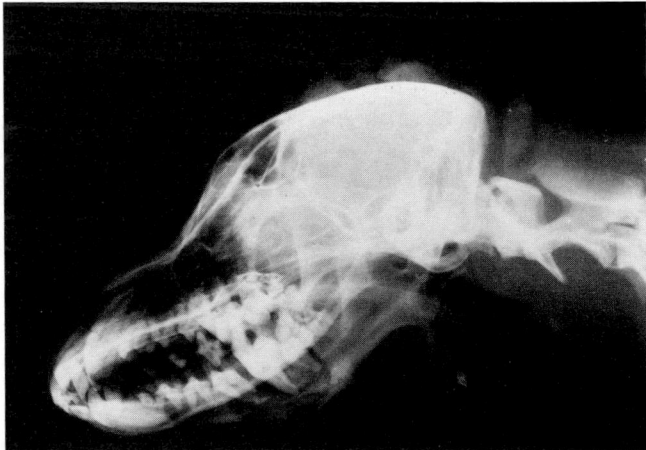

FIGURE 108–2. Radiograph of the skull and mandible of a dog with experimental renal failure. A large, noninflammatory cyst-like lesion has developed in the mandible after 48 weeks of renal failure. Lesions of this type are a rare manifestation of renal secondary hyperparathyroidism. They are often called brown tumors in humans because they are stained brown due to hemosiderin deposition.

Pyuria and bacteriuria are relatively uncommon in dogs and cats with CRF. When detected, they suggest pyelonephritis or secondary urinary tract infection (UTI). Other abnormalities in the urinalysis may suggest active urinary tract disease (e.g., hematuria may suggest urolithiasis, neoplasia, infection, or cystic disease), provide clues as to the cause of renal injury (e.g., glucosuria and alkaline urine pH may suggest Fanconi syndrome), or indicate systemic disease (e.g., glucosuria and ketonuria suggest diabetic ketoacidosis).

Serum calcium concentration is often normal but may be increased or decreased in patients with CRF.[65, 66] Hypocalcemia results from the combined effects of reduced renal production of 1,25-dihydroxycholecalciferol (biosynthetic failure), intestinal malabsorption of calcium, skeletal resistance to parathyroid hormone, and possibly a direct effect of hyperphosphatemia on reducing serum calcium concentrations. Mechanisms of hypercalcemia of CRF are unknown but may include decreased renal excretion of calcium, binding of calcium to retained organic anions (e.g., citrate), excess production of 25-dihydroxycholecalciferol, excess parathyroid hormone production, decreased renal degradation of parathyroid hormone, increased circulating concentrations of substances that enhance release of calcium from bone, hypervitaminosis A, dietary phosphate restriction, or increased intestinal absorption of calcium.[65, 66] However, hypercalcemia of CRF may not be associated with clinically significant increases in ionized calcium concentrations. In two dogs with CRF in which total serum calcium concentrations exceeded 13.5 mg/dl, the authors measured blood ionized calcium concentrations and found them to be within normal limits. Serum albumin concentrations were within normal limits in these dogs and, therefore, did not account for the increase in total serum calcium concentrations.

Because sodium and potassium regulatory capacity is retained until later stages of CRF, serum sodium and potassium concentrations typically remain normal in patients with CRF.[65, 67] However, hypokalemia occasionally develops even in early renal failure and may be manifested as profound muscle weakness.[60, 68, 69] The cause of hypokalemia in these patients is not known, but has been proposed to result from enhanced kaliuresis.[69]

Serum amylase and lipase activities are increased in a substantial percentage of patients with CRF.[70] In dogs with CRF, serum amylase activity reportedly increases approximately two and one-half fold over normal values, while serum lipase activity increases by a factor of two- to fourfold. Marked increases in serum amylase and/or lipase activities rarely develop solely as a result of renal failure. It appears likely that hyperamylasemia and hyperlipasemia of CRF results, at least in part, from reduced renal excretion or degradation of these enzymes.[70, 71] However, the magnitude of enzyme elevation does not appear to correlate well with the severity of renal dysfunction.

Acute pancreatitis occurs in some human patients with CRF,[72] but the incidence of acute pancreatitis in dogs with CRF is unknown. It has been hypothesized that renal failure may promote or induce development of uremic pancreatitis, but evidence supporting this hypothesis is lacking in dogs and cats. Nonetheless, marked elevations in serum amylase and lipase activity should prompt consideration of acute pancreatitis in dogs with CRF.[70] Because of the questionable value of serum pancreatic enzyme activities in patients with CRF, confirmation of acute pancreatitis should be supported by clinical, radiographic, and other laboratory findings.

Serum alkaline phosphatase activity may be increased in patients with severe renal osteodystrophy, particularly young animals, but typically remains within normal limits. Serum alanine aminotransferase, aspartate aminotransferase, and creatinine phosphokinase activities are usually normal in patients with CRF.

Diagnosis

SYNDROME IDENTIFICATION

Most cases of CRF can be detected by the defined minimum data base for urinary disorders (Table 108–3). Diagnosis of primary renal failure in azotemic patients is usually based on demonstrating concurrent azotemia and inadequate urine-concentrating ability.[73, 74] The chronicity of primary renal failure may be confirmed by evidence that primary renal failure has been present for an extended period (i.e., months to years). Evidence of chronicity should be sought from the medical history, physical examination, and laboratory, radiographic, or biopsy studies (Table 108–5). Renal osteodystrophy, reduced kidney size, and serial laboratory confirmation of persistent primary renal failure over several months provide unequivocal evidence of chronicity. (See section on ARF for additional information).

Although CRF is usually characterized by azotemia, some patients with early renal failure (sometimes called renal insufficiency) may be nonazotemic. Renal function in nonazotemic patients suspected of having renal disease must be determined by endogenous or exogenous clearance techniques (e.g., creatinine clearance; see Chapter 107).

EARLY DETECTION

CRF is often diagnosed at an advanced stage when uremia develops. By this time, irreversible, moderate to severe renal dysfunction has occurred, and treatment by conservative medical management may be less rewarding than would have been possible had renal dysfunction been detected and treatment initiated earlier in the course of disease. In addition, determining the initiating cause of renal dysfunction is often difficult or impossible once end-stage renal failure has developed. Therefore, specific therapy designed to eliminate or control the underlying cause of renal dysfunction may not be feasible.

Because clinical signs of incipient CRF are typically nonlocalizing and often subtle, early detection of CRF requires an index of suspicion. These signs include deterioration of haircoat quality (dull hair, increased shedding of hair), gradual loss of body weight, poor or selective appetite, and decreased activity. Signs that direct attention toward the urinary tract, including polyuria, nocturia, polydipsia, hematuria, dysuria, pollaki-uria, or urinary incontinence, are variable in patients with early renal failure. Polyuria and polydipsia in dogs and cats with CRF may be unexpectedly subtle (urine volumes one and one-half to two times normal) and are particularly difficult for owners to detect in multiple-pet households. Detection of clinical signs indicative of disease of the lower urinary tract (dysuria, pollakiuria, and urinary incontinence) should not be interpreted as conclusively ruling out involvement of the kidneys. For example, CRF predisposes to development of UTI, which may cause dysuria and pollakiuria. Polyuria resulting from CRF may promote urinary incontinence in dogs with hormone-responsive urinary incontinence.

Screening tests designed to rule out renal disease and renal failure should be considered for dogs with historical or physical findings consistent with CRF. Routine use of such screening tests may also be considered for geriatric dogs and cats. As a minimum, determination of urine specific gravity should be performed yearly on dogs and cats at risk for development of CRF. Urine concentrating ability is considered adequate when urine specific gravity equals or exceeds 1.030 in dogs and 1.035 in cats. Except in some patients with severe glomerular disease, in which adequate renal tubular function persists despite marked reduction in glomerular filtration rate (GFR) (a condition often called glomerular-tubular imbalance), detection of adequate urine-concentrating ability is usually a reliable index that CRF is not present. Patients with severe glomerular disease can be identified by concomitant measurement of urine protein concentrations.

If the urine specific gravity fails to confirm that urine-concentrating ability is adequate, CRF cannot be ruled out and additional evaluation is indicated. As a minimum evaluation, another urine specific gravity determination should be performed on a subsequently obtained urine sample. If urine specific gravity persistently remains below 1.030 in dogs or 1.035 in cats, a problem-specific urinary tract data base (Table 108–3) should be evaluated. This data base may confirm azotemic renal failure or direct the clinician to consider additional diagnostic tests to rule out renal and nonrenal causes of decreased urine-concentrating ability.[75]

Screening evaluation of urine specific gravity is an incomplete means of assessing the urinary tract for disease. This approach is proposed only as a simple, inexpensive means of detecting renal failure relatively early in the course of disease. Because of its simplicity and low cost, it could potentially be incorporated into routine physical examination and/or vaccination protocols. However, if clinical signs related to the urinary tract are present, a complete urinary tract minimum data base should be evaluated (Table 108–3).

SYNDROME ANALYSIS

Problem-Specific Data Base. The goals of syndrome analysis of CRF are summarized in Table 108–16. Syndrome analysis should be based on data provided by the defined problem-specific data base for patients with renal failure (Table 108–10). This approach to diagnostics in patients with CRF is designed to individualize

TABLE 108–16. GOALS OF SYNDROME ANALYSIS OF CHRONIC RENAL FAILURE

1. Identify complications of CRF that may require symptomatic or supportive therapy.
   a. Azotemia/uremia and associated clinical signs
   b. Polyuria/dehydration
   c. Metabolic acidosis
   d. Hypokalemia/hyperkalemia
   e. Hyponatremia/hypernatremia
   f. Hyperphosphatemia
   g. Hypocalcemia/hypercalcemia
   h. Renal osteodystrophy
   i. Nonregenerative anemia
2. Identify conditions that may exacerbate clinical signs of uremia or promote continued, progressive renal damage.
   a. Prerenal conditions (see Table 108–4)
   b. Urinary obstruction (see Table 108–4)
   c. Systemic hypertension
   d. Urinary tract infection
   e. Concurrent nonrenal diseases
3. Determine cause of primary renal failure in order to formulate specific therapy for renal disease.
4. Establish baseline laboratory values against which subsequent response to therapy or progression of disease may be compared.

therapy to the specific needs of the patient. In addition, it provides an organized framework for detecting complicating factors that may hamper success of treatment and/or promote progressive renal injury.

Determining Etiology. CRF may be congenital/familial (Table 108–15) or acquired in origin. Congenital and familial causes of CRF can often be suspected on the basis of breed and family history, age of onset of renal disease/failure, or radiographic and ultrasonographic findings (e.g., polycystic kidney disease). Acquired CRF may result from any disease process that injures renal glomeruli, tubules, interstitium, and/or vasculature and causes sufficient irreversible loss of functional nephrons to result in primary renal failure. However, in many patients with acquired CRF, determining the primary etiology responsible for renal injury may not be possible.[76] Inability to identify the inciting cause of renal failure derives from three important phenomena related to the evolution of progressive renal diseases: (1) various components of nephrons (glomeruli, tubules, peritubular capillaries, and interstitial tissue) are functionally interdependent, (2) morphologic and functional abnormalities of the kidneys can be manifested clinically in only a limited number of ways, irrespective of underlying cause, and (3) following maturation, new nephrons cannot be formed to replace others irreversibly destroyed by disease. If any portion of the nephron is irreversibly destroyed, the function of the remaining portions is also damaged. Progressive irreversible lesions initially localized to the renal vascular system, glomeruli, tubules, or interstitial tissue are eventually responsible for development of lesions in the remaining but initially unaffected portions of nephrons. For example, progressive lesions confined initially to glomeruli will decrease peritubular capillary perfusion of tubules, and thus induce tubular cell atrophy, degeneration, and necrosis. Nephron destruction initiated by progressive glomerular disease ultimately will stimulate repair by fibrosis. Likewise, generalized progressive pyelonephritis will damage or destroy tubules and glomeruli, and stimulate repair by fibrosis. If the majority of nephrons have been destroyed, these events will be associated with reduction in kidney size, capsular adhesions, and generalized pitting of the capsular surface of the cortex.

Because of structural and functional interdependence of various components of nephrons, antemortem and postmortem differentiation of various generalized, progressive renal diseases that have reached an advanced stage may be difficult. Varying types of functional and structural change prominent during earlier phases of progressive generalized renal diseases may permit identification of a specific cause and/or localization of the initial lesion to one or more components of the nephrons. With time, however, destructive changes of varying severity (atrophy, inflammation, fibrosis, and mineralization of diseased nephrons), which are superimposed on compensatory and adaptive changes (hypertrophy and hyperplasia) of partially and totally viable nephrons, provide a gross and microscopic similarity to these diseases. As a generality, the greater the degree of destruction of nephrons by irreversible progressive renal diseases, the less obvious are the differences in parameters of their functional capacity and in their gross and microscopic appearance. The important point is that primary irreversible, progressive diseases of glomeruli, tubules, vessels, and interstitial tissue may lead to chronic generalized nephropathy. The underlying cause of chronic generalized nephropathy may not be detected.

At one time, poor understanding of renal response to injury and lack of laboratory and biopsy techniques with which to detect antemortem lesions at an early stage of development led to the widespread but erroneous assumption that the vast majority of *chronic generalized nephropathy* was caused by a specific disease entity called *chronic interstitial nephritis* (so-called CIN). Because leptospirosis was a well documented cause of acute interstitial nephritis, the hypothesis was dogmatically advanced that leptospirosis was the most common cause of CIN. Primary irreversible, progressive diseases of the renal interstitium (CIN) can cause chronic generalized nephropathy characterized by reduction in renal size. Although it may occur elsewhere in the world, leptospirosis is apparently an extremely uncommon cause of CIN or chronic generalized nephropathy in the United States.

Interstitial nephritis, whether it be acute or chronic, is a valid descriptive term. When used as a morphologic diagnosis, however, it suggests that the underlying disorder is characterized by morphologic and functional abnormalities of interstitial tissue, which, if progressive, may induce changes in the renal tubules, glomeruli, and vessels. Interstitial nephritis is distinguished from other types of primary renal disease by changes that initially and predominantly affect interstitial tissue. Unfortunately, many chronic generalized diseases of the kidneys that originate in vessels, glomeruli, or tubules are associated with a marked degree of interstitial inflammation and fibrosis.

The term *end-stage kidney* implies the presence of renal diseases that are generalized, progressive, irreversible, and at an extremely advanced or end stage of development. End-stage kidneys are one step beyond chronic generalized nephropathy, and the term applies

to all cases in which the antecedent cause of renal destruction cannot be identified or localized to any particular portion of the nephron. In some cases disease processes initially responsible for renal damage are no longer present or active in these kidneys. The histopathologic appearance of such kidneys is consistently characterized by sclerotic glomeruli, abundant mononuclear tubulointerstitial infiltrate, dilated tubules, and simplified tubular epithelium.[76]

Despite the generalized nature of irreversible renal lesions, active renal disease may be present and contribute to progression of CRF. It is particularly important that active renal diseases that may be amenable to treatment be considered. Potentially treatable renal diseases that should be ruled out include bacterial pyelonephritis, chronic urinary obstruction, nephrolithiasis, renal lymphoma (particularly in cats), and immune-mediated renal diseases (Table 108–17).

Oxalate crystals may occur in the tubular lumina of cats with CRF. Detection of oxalate crystals should therefore not be interpreted as proof that ethylene glycol intoxication was the cause of renal injury. A diagnosis of ethylene glycol toxicity must be supported by other relevant findings.

Prognosis

Prognosis for patients with CRF is usually subcategorized according to the probability of immediate survival (short-term prognosis) and survival over the subsequent months to years (long term prognosis).[64] It should be offered in the context of recovery with and without treatment. A guarded prognosis indicates that the chances for recovery are unpredictable. Fair, good, or excellent prognoses indicate varying degrees of probable recovery, while poor or grave prognoses indicate that recovery is improbable or hopeless.[64] Loss of renal

TABLE 108–17. CAUSES OF CHRONIC RENAL FAILURE POTENTIALLY AMENABLE TO SPECIFIC THERAPY

Disease Process	Diagnostic Studies
Pyelonephritis	Quantitative urine culture
	Intravenous urography
	Renal biopsy (and culture)
Obstructive uropathy	Intravenous urography
	Renal ultrasonography
Nephrolithiasis	Survey abdominal radiographs
	Intravenous urography
	Renal ultrasonography
Immune-mediated diseases	Urine protein/creatinine ratio
	24-hour urine protein
	Immune panel
	Rule out dirofilariasis
	Renal biopsy (including light, immunofluorescent, and electron microscopic studies)
Hypertensive disease	Blood pressure determination
	Retinal examination
Renal neoplasia	Renal ultrasound
	Intravenous urography
	Renal angiography
	Renal biopsy
Hypercalcemic nephropathy	Serum calcium concentration
	Blood ionized calcium concentration (?)
	Renal biopsy

function is permanent in patients with CRF; recovery refers to improvement of biochemical deficits and excesses and amelioration of clinical signs, rather than to recovery of renal function.

Factors to be considered in establishing meaningful prognoses for patients with CRF include (1) severity of clinical signs and complications of uremia, (2) probability of improving renal function (reversibility, primarily of prerenal, postrenal, and newly acquired primary renal conditions), (3) severity of intrinsic renal functional impairment, (4) rate of progression of renal dysfunction with or without therapy, and (5) age of the patient.

Severity of uremic signs is often a relatively good predictor of short-term prognosis. Patients without clinical signs of uremia usually have a fair to good short-term prognosis. Patients with severe clinical signs of uremia typically have a guarded to poor short-term prognosis. However, it is best to determine whether renal function can be therapeutically improved in such cases before establishing the short-term prognosis. A uremic crisis often occurs in patients with CRF as a consequence of superimposed acute primary renal failure or prerenal or postrenal conditions. Although CRF is an irreversible condition, improvement of renal function is potentially possible when uremia results from the sum effects of CRF and a potentially reversible cause of azotemia. If treatment improves renal function and ameliorates clinical signs of uremia, the short-term prognosis may be guarded to good.

Severity of renal dysfunction as determined by serum creatinine concentration or endogenous creatinine clearance provides a less accurate means of assessing short-term prognosis than does the clinical condition of the patient. Short-term prognosis should not be established based solely on one measurement of the severity of renal dysfunction because: (1) the relationship between severity of renal dysfunction and clinical signs of uremia is highly variable, and (2) a single determination of renal function fails to assess the potential for improvement in renal function.

Severity of renal dysfunction is typically more useful in establishing long-term prognoses. In general, severe renal dysfunction is associated with shorter long-term survival and, often, a lower quality of life. In our experience, long-term prognosis for dogs and cats with serum creatinine concentrations of about 3 to 4 mg/dl or less is typically good. However, the prognosis should be established in light of the clinical condition of the patient, rate of progression of renal dysfunction, response to therapy, cause of the underlying renal disease (if known), and other complicating factors (e.g., UTI, nephrotic syndrome).

Treatment

CONSERVATIVE MEDICAL MANAGEMENT

Overview. Conservative medical management of CRF consists of supportive and symptomatic therapy designed to correct deficits and excesses in fluid, electrolyte, acid-base, endocrine, and nutritional balance, and thereby minimize the clinical and pathophysiologic consequences of reduced renal function (Table 108–18). It should not be expected to halt, reverse, or eliminate renal lesions responsible for CRF. Therefore, conservative medical management is most beneficial when combined with specific therapy directed at correcting the primary cause of renal disease.

Specific therapy of renal disease consists of therapy designed to slow or stop development of renal lesions by influencing the etiopathogenic processes responsible for the lesions. Examples of specific treatment include correction of hypercalcemia that has caused calcium nephropathy, administration of antibiotics to eliminate bacterial infections, administration of antimycotic agents to eliminate mycotic infections, removal of lesions causing obstructive uropathy (e.g., tumors or uroliths), and correction of abnormal renal perfusion that has caused ischemic renal lesions. While determining the initiating disease process in dogs and cats with CRF is frequently difficult or impossible, the value of formulating specific therapy based on an etiologic/pathologic diagnosis should not be overlooked. Because renal lesions responsible for CRF are irreversible, they cannot be completely reversed or eliminated by specific therapy. Nonetheless, progression of renal lesions, and thus failure, may be slowed or stopped by therapy designed to eliminate active renal diseases. Therefore, diagnostic efforts directed especially at detecting treatable renal diseases should be performed before formulating plans for conservative medical management (Table 108–17). In addition, nonrenal conditions that may aggravate or precipitate uremic crisis (e.g., prerenal and postrenal causes listed in Table 108–4) should be sought and corrected.

TABLE 108–18. CONSERVATIVE MEDICAL MANAGEMENT OF CHRONIC RENAL FAILURE IN DOGS AND CATS

Clinical or Laboratory Abnormality	Treatment Options
Progression of CRF	Diet therapy
	Modify phosphate intake
	Others (?)
Azotemia/uremia	Diet therapy
Polyuria and polydipsia	Avoid stress
	Free access to water
	Consider diet therapy
Dehydration (prophylaxis)	Avoid stress
	Free access to water
	Adequate dietary salt intake
	Supplemental fluid therapy (?)
Metabolic acidosis	Therapeutic alkalinization
Anemia of CRF	Androgen therapy
	Transfusion therapy
	Recombinant human erythropoietin
Hyperphosphatemia	Diet therapy
	Intestinal phosphate-binding agents
Hypocalcemia	Minimize hyperphosphatemia
	Oral calcium supplements
	Vitamin D therapy
Renal osteodystrophy (prophylaxis/treatment)	Minimize hyperphosphatemia
	Oral calcium supplements
	Vitamin D therapy
Systemic hypertension	Sodium restriction
	Antihypertensive drug therapy
Drug reactions/overdosage	Adjust drug dosages according to renal function
	Avoid nephrotoxic drugs
Urinary tract infection	Monitor for infection
	Antibiotic therapy

Hemodialysis, chronic ambulatory peritoneal dialysis, and renal transplantation are the mainstays of treatment of advanced CRF in humans. Although these methods have been used for treatment of renal failure in dogs and cats, routine application of these methods has been severely limited by their expense, technical difficulties, and limited experience on the part of most veterinarians.[53, 55, 77–81] The current status of these treatment methods in dogs and cats has been recently reviewed.[53, 55, 81]

Application and Goals. Conservative medical management is intended for patients with compensated CRF; it is not intended for patients that are unable to eat or accept oral medications because of severe uremia. Clinical signs and complications of uremia should be managed as described in the section on ARF before attempting conservative medical management.

The goals of conservative medical management of patients with chronic primary renal failure are to: (1) ameliorate clinical signs of uremia, (2) minimize disturbances associated with excesses or losses of electrolytes, vitamins, and minerals, (3) support adequate nutrition by supplying daily protein, calorie, and mineral requirements, and (4) modify progression of renal failure. These goals are best achieved when recommendations regarding conservative medical management are individualized to patient needs based on clinical and laboratory findings (Tables 108–16 and 108–18). Because CRF is progressive and dynamic, serial clinical and laboratory assessment of the patient, and modification of the therapy in response to changes in the patient's condition, is an integral part of conservative medical management (Table 108–19).

MODIFICATION OF PROGRESSION

The Progressive Nature of Renal Failure. It was first observed in rodents that loss of a critical mass of functional renal tissue invariably led to failure of the remaining nephrons. For example, removal of approximately three-quarters or more of the functional renal mass in rats by surgical resection, infarction, or a combination of these techniques, resulted in a syndrome of progressive azotemia, proteinuria, arterial hypertension, and, eventually, death due to uremia.[82, 83] Progression occurred despite the fact that remaining renal tissue was initially normal, albeit reduced in quantity.

Similarly, in humans with renal disease, renal insufficiency predictably progresses to renal failure, regardless of the initiating cause of renal damage.[83] Such progression occurs even when the initiating cause of renal dysfunction is no longer present or active. The predictability of this progression is emphasized by the fact that the inverse of serum creatinine concentration declines almost linearly with time for many patients with a wide variety of renal diseases.[57, 84, 85] The slope of this line, indicating the rate of deterioration of renal function, appears to remain constant for individual patients, regardless of the type of underlying renal disease.

In contrast to findings in rats and humans, the progressive nature of canine renal failure is controversial. Two long-term studies performed for the purpose of determining if reduced renal mass promotes progressive deterioration of renal function in dogs failed to detect progressive reduction in renal function during 40 weeks to 42 months of study.[30, 86] In the first study, dogs with

TABLE 108–19. MONITORING GUIDELINES FOR PATIENTS WITH CHRONIC RENAL FAILURE

Test	Purpose
History	To assess response to therapy; to ascertain compliance with recommendations and owner-perceived problems with therapy; to detect communication problems with the client; to detect new problems or complications
Physical examination	To detect new problems or complications; to assess hydration; to assess nutritional status and well-being of the animal
Body weight	To assess nutritional and hydration status
Serum creatinine concentration	To assess severity and progression of renal dysfunction; to detect concomitant prerenal and postrenal azotemia
Serum urea nitrogen concentration	To assess compliance with dietary recommendations; to detect concomitant prerenal and postrenal azotemia
Urinalysis	To detect urinary tract infection; to detect changes in urine sediment or urine chemistries that may suggest active or changing renal lesions that may warrant specific therapy or changes in therapy
Serum phosphorus concentration	To determine success of dietary phosphorus restriction and to adjust dosages of intestinal phosphate binders
Serum calcium concentration	To assess need for and to adjust dosage of calcium supplements and vitamin D
Serum albumin concentration	To assess nutritional status; important for monitoring impact of urinary protein loss in patients with glomerulopathies; necessary for interpretation of serum calcium values and assessment of influence on protein-bound drugs
Total carbon dioxide	To assess need for alkalinization therapy; necessary for adjusting dosage of alkalinization therapy
Packed cell volume or complete blood count	To assess response to therapy for anemia; may also be useful for assessing nutritional status
Urine culture	Indicated (a) if urinalysis supports possible UTI, (b) to confirm that previously detected and treated UTIs have been successfully eradicated, (c) as routine part of follow-up studies in patients with recurrent UTI and CRF

75 per cent reduction in renal mass were monitored for over 42 months.[86] Because the magnitude of renal dysfunction induced in this study was very mild, most dogs were not azotemic. GFR remained essentially stable in these dogs throughout the study. However, it is possible that the magnitude of renal dysfunction induced in this canine study was not sufficient to initiate self-perpetuating renal dysfunction. It has been suggested that detectable progressive deterioration of GFR in humans may not become obligatory until serum creatinine concentrations exceed 4 mg/dl.[87] In addition, progressive renal damage may not always be detected by serial assessment of GFR.

In a second long-term study, dogs with 11/12 reduction in renal mass were studied for 40 weeks.[30] Despite the more severe reduction in renal mass, renal function again remained stable for the duration of the study, suggesting that functional deterioration of the remaining renal tissue did not occur. However, progressive proteinuria and development of renal lesions indicative of destruction of functioning nephrons in residual renal tissue suggested that renal lesions were progressive, even though renal function did not decline. Similar findings have been reported in rats with induced renal failure; proteinuria and renal lesions were found to progress despite apparently stable renal function.[88]

More recent studies provide good evidence in support of the progressive nature of canine renal failure. Bourgoignie has shown that reduction of renal mass in dogs results in glomerulopathy and proteinuria, the severity of which appears to be proportional to the amount of renal mass ablated and that precedes decline in renal function.[89] During the 15 to 39 months of this study, renal function remained stable in 7 dogs and progressively declined in 3 dogs. In another study of induced canine CRF, progressive decline in renal function was observed in dogs fed a low protein, high phosphate diet, resulting in a mortality rate of 67 per cent during the first year of study.[90] The progressive nature of canine CRF is further suggested by the recently reported observation that the reciprocal of serum creatinine versus time may decline linearly in some dogs with spontaneous renal failure (Figure 108–3).[58] However, this clinical observation requires validation in large numbers of carefully studied dogs.

Although clinical impression suggests that feline CRF is also a spontaneously progressive disease, clinical or experimental evidence supporting progression in this species has not yet been reported.

Cause(s) of Progression. **OVERVIEW.** Progressive renal damage may result from: (1) persistence of the renal disease(s) responsible for initiating renal failure, (2) different or additional renal insults, and/or (3) a variety of complications and sequela of CRF, such as UTI, systemic hypertension, and intrarenal mineral deposition. In addition, it is now apparent that a variety of factors may promote spontaneous, self-perpetuating nephron damage in CRF.[91] Some factors that contribute to self-perpetuating renal dysfunction are compensatory phenomena that develop in an attempt to sustain renal function and homeostasis.[92, 93] Examples of such factors include glomerular capillary hypertension and hyperfiltration, renal growth (hypertrophy), increased renal

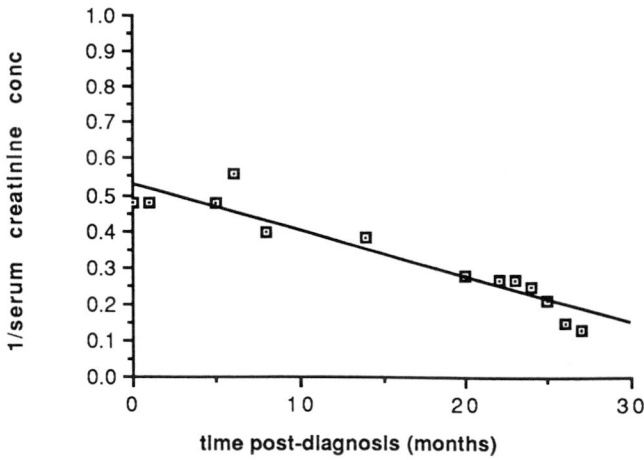

FIGURE 108–3. Graph of reciprocal of serum creatinine concentration (1/SC) versus time for a one-year-old female Shih Tzu dog with CRF caused by congenital renal dysplasia. The relatively steep linear decline in 1/SC indicates progressive deterioration of renal function with time.

oxygen consumption, and increased renal ammoniagenesis. Other nonadaptive factors may also be potentially injurious to surviving nephrons in CRF, including altered phosphate metabolism, altered lipid composition, and increased activity of the coagulation system. Recognition and therapeutic manipulation of these factors may retard progression of CRF.

GLOMERULAR CAPILLARY HYPERTENSION AND HYPERFILTRATION. Recent experimental evidence suggests that the glomerular hemodynamic response to widespread renal injury may be the initiating factor leading to progressive nephron damage.[83] Experimentally induced or naturally occurring reduction in renal mass results in increased glomerular capillary perfusion and glomerular capillary hypertension, which are in turn associated with increased GFR in individual remaining functional nephrons (often referred to as increased single-nephron glomerular filtration rate and abbreviated SNGFR).[92, 93] This increase in SNGFR is termed *glomerular hyperfiltration*. Although total GFR is still reduced following loss of renal mass, the increase in SNGFR that occurs in surviving nephrons causes total GFR to be greater than would have been predicted after reduction in renal mass. For example, total GFR is reduced by less than 50 per cent following removal of 75 per cent of the functional renal mass in dogs. Presumably, glomerular hyperfiltration evolved as a compensatory phenomenon designed to maximize GFR in failing kidneys. Although this compensatory adaptation appears to be initially beneficial, current evidence suggests that persistent hemodynamic changes resulting in glomerular capillary hypertension and glomerular hyperfiltration may eventually damage surviving nephrons and lead to progressive deterioration of renal function.[92, 94]

It has been known for over 50 years that marked reduction of renal mass in rats results in proteinuria, progressive glomerular sclerosis, and, ultimately, uremic death.[95] Focal, segmental glomerular sclerosis is the most prominent renal lesion observed after reduction in renal mass in rats, as well as in dogs (Figure 108–4).[89, 96, 97] With time, the prevalence (percentage of glomeruli

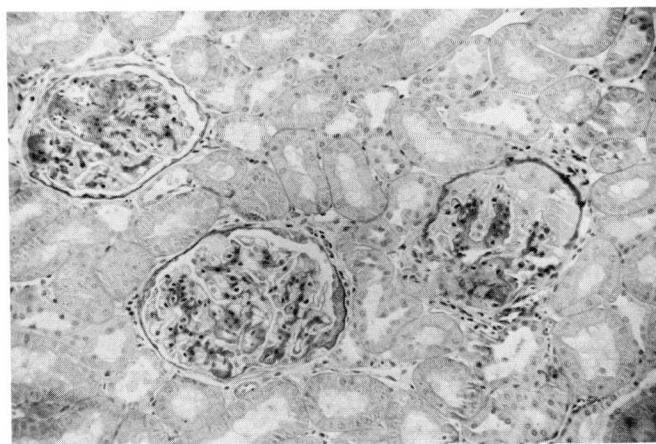

FIGURE 108–4. Photomicrograph of the viable portion of a kidney 20 weeks after removal of 11/12 of functional renal mass. Glomerular lesions are characterized by mild to moderate increases in mesangial matrix and cells. Changes in the renal tubules and interstitium are minimal. Two micron section; PAS stain; original magnification × 100.

involved) and extent (severity of individual glomerular damage) of glomerular involvement increases.[88] The rate of progression of these lesions appears to be proportional to the magnitude of loss of renal mass. The magnitude of increase in the hemodynamic changes previously described (i.e., glomerular hypertension and hyperfiltration) is also related to the extent to which renal mass has been reduced.

Dietary protein intake or parenteral administration of amino acids may profoundly influence renal hemodynamics. High protein intake enhances RBF and GFR, whereas dietary protein restriction minimizes these hemodynamic effects. The mechanism(s) by which dietary protein intake enhances renal hemodynamics is poorly understood but probably involves activation of some circulating or hormonal effector system. Proposed circulating or hormonal effectors of this phenomenon include glucagon, growth hormone, prostaglandins, the renin-angiotensin system, biogenic amines, and a hepatic-derived renal vasodilator known as glomerulopressin.[98–101] Amino acids may also have a direct effect on renal hemodynamics.[98]

Restricting dietary protein intake minimizes the hemodynamic changes that occur after reduction in renal mass.[92] Rats with induced CRF fed a diet containing 24 per cent protein had markedly increased glomerular capillary pressures and flows, whereas rats fed a diet containing 6 per cent protein had glomerular capillary pressures and flows comparable to those observed in normal rats fed a standard laboratory rat chow containing 24 per cent protein.[92] Normalization of hemodynamics by reduced protein feeding minimized development of proteinuria and glomerular sclerosis in this study.[92] Attenuation of glomerular hyperfiltration by dietary protein restriction has also been shown to minimize development of glomerular lesions and/or progression of renal dysfunction in a variety of other experimental models of renal disease, including post-salt hypertension, mineralocorticoid hypertension, and nephrotoxic serum nephritis in rats, and the mouse model of systemic lupus erythematosus.[83]

The hemodynamic effects of reducing renal mass may also be mitigated by antihypertensive drugs such as the angiotensin converting enzyme inhibitor enalapril.[102] Enalapril prevents systemic and glomerular hypertension and thereby mitigates proteinuria and glomerular injury in rats with reduced renal mass.[102] Antihypertensive therapy that normalizes glomerular capillary pressure affords virtually complete protection against progressive glomerular injury in rats with reduced renal mass.[103] However, antihypertensive therapy that minimizes systemic hypertension but not glomerular hypertension does not prevent proteinuria and glomerular injury.[104] Because of these observations, glomerular hypertension is currently held to be the primary hemodynamic factor responsible for development of progressive glomerular damage following loss of renal mass.[94, 102–107] Further evidence supporting this view is the observation that dietary protein restriction may reduce glomerular hypertension, proteinuria, and glomerular injury without altering systemic hypertension.[102]

Glomerular hyperfiltration and/or glomerular capillary hypertension has been hypothesized to be responsible for development of renal structural lesions (glomerular sclerosis) and proteinuria in rats with reduced renal mass, thereby serving as the link between high dietary protein intake and progression of renal failure.[29, 91, 93] It has been proposed that sustained hemodynamic changes associated with excessive protein consumption injure the glomerular vasculature, possibly as a result of direct mechanical injury to glomerular capillary walls.[98] Increased intraglomerular pressure may promote formation of microaneurysms and endothelial damage, which may in turn lead to deposition of platelets and platelet aggregation.[108]

Damage to the charge- and size-selective properties of the glomerular capillary walls also results in increased glomerular permeability to relatively small anionic and large plasma macromolecules.[91] Proteinuria is one result. In addition, damage to the glomerular vasculature results in increased movement of macromolecules through the glomerular mesangium. Accumulation of proteins in this region may stimulate increased mesangial cell proliferation and/or mesangial matrix formation.[91] It has also been proposed that resident macrophages and/or influx of platelets and monocytes derived from the systemic circulation may influence proliferation of mesangial cells.[108] Macrophages have been shown to induce proliferation of mesangial cells in tissue culture.[108, 109] Macrophages also release several growth factors and enzymes capable of modifying collagen, elastic tissue, and other tissues, which may cause destruction of basement membrane and lead to glomerular scarring. The eventual development of glomerular sclerosis exerts a positive feedback stimulus for compensatory changes in less affected glomeruli, contributing in turn to their eventual destruction.

In summary, glomerular hypertension may serve as the final common pathway for progression of CRF after a threshold loss of renal mass. As the functional contribution of sclerosing glomeruli is lost, less severely affected glomeruli undergo further compensatory hyperfiltration, leading to their injury and additional loss of nephrons and renal function. Reduced protein diets appear to protect against progression of renal failure by mitigating hemodynamic adaptations resulting from high protein consumption.[30, 91, 93] Antihypertensive drugs that limit glomerular hypertension may be similarly beneficial.

DIETARY PHOSPHATE AND RENAL MINERALIZATION. Altered calcium and phosphate metabolism causing secondary hyperparathyroidism result in deposition of calcium and phosphate in the renal parenchyma of animals with CRF.[110] Renal deposition of calcium and phosphate leads to inflammation, scarring, and subsequent loss of nephrons.[108, 110, 111] Studies of rats with experimentally induced CRF suggest that dietary phosphate restriction may prevent proteinuria, renal mineralization, renal histologic alterations, renal functional deterioration and death due to uremia, which occur when higher phosphate diets are fed.[111]

Dietary phosphate restriction also appears to slow progression and prolong survival in induced canine CRF.[90] Studies performed in cats with induced renal failure revealed that normal dietary phosphate consumption was associated with microscopic evidence of renal mineralization, fibrosis, and mononuclear cell infiltration.[112] Restriction of dietary phosphate prevented these abnormalities. However, evidence of progressive renal dysfunction was not detected in either normal or restricted phosphate groups in this study.

Studies on the effectiveness of phosphate restriction in preventing progression of CRF in humans have yielded conflicting results.[113–120] The extent to which phosphate was restricted in different studies may have been responsible for the apparent differences in effectiveness of phosphate restriction observed. In studies reporting a beneficial effect of phosphate restriction, plasma phosphate concentrations were maintained between 2 and 3 mg/dl.[113, 114] In contrast, when serum phosphate concentrations were simply maintained within the normal range, a beneficial effect of phosphate restriction was not detected.[121] Thus, normalizing serum phosphate may be insufficient to retard progression of CRF in humans. The extent to which phosphate must be restricted to prevent progressive renal injury in dogs and cats is as yet unknown. In addition, the dietary form of phosphate may influence renal mineralization.[116]

Hyperphosphatemia precedes development of soft-tissue mineralization of most organs in patients with CRF. In contrast, renal mineralization may precede hyperphosphatemia in humans, rats, and dogs.[90, 110, 117] It has been suggested that renal mineralization may result from intrarenal mechanisms related more to fractional excretion of phosphate than to serum phosphate concentration.[110]

Although the mechanism of phosphate-induced progressive renal dysfunction remains unclear, it appears likely that nephron loss is mediated, at least in part, through renal mineralization.[110, 117] Phosphate restriction may also retard progression of CRF by: (1) minimizing renal intracellular calcium concentrations, thus preventing calcium-mediated cellular injury, (2) inhibiting renal cell injury by reducing cellular energy metabolism, (3) influencing abnormalities of lipid metabolism associated with uremia, (4) suppressing immune responsiveness, or (5) influencing glomerular hypertension.[118, 119]

Chronic subcutaneous administration of verapamil, a calcium channel blocking agent, to rats with experimental renal failure also protected against progression of renal dysfunction, histologic damage, and nephrocalcinosis.[120] This beneficial effect was independent of any effect on systemic blood pressure. Thus, prevention of nephrocalcinosis may be one mechanism of the observed protective effect. However, verapamil may also protect against progressive renal damage by minimizing glomerular hypertension. The effects of chronic verapamil therapy on progression of canine and feline CRF have not been studied.

RENAL AMMONIAGENESIS. Spontaneous and induced CRF are characterized by widespread tubulointerstitial lesions of undetermined origin. It has been proposed that compensatory changes in tubular function that accompany reduction in renal mass may be injurious to the renal tubulointerstitium, and thereby promote progressive renal injury.[122] Reduction in renal mass is associated with compensatory hyperfunction of renal tubules, including increased renal ammoniagenesis. Increased renal ammoniagenesis is attended by a rise in renal tissue ammonia concentration. Local toxic and inflammatory effects of ammonia may include triggering of the alternative complement pathway by the reaction of ammonia with the third component of complement, culminating in deposition of complement proteins and initiation of complement-mediated cellular infiltration and tissue injury. These effects further impair tubular function and may promote a self-perpetuating cycle of adaptation and injury. In rats with induced renal failure, dietary supplementation with sodium bicarbonate has been shown to lower tissue ammonia concentrations, reduce peritubular deposition of complement components, and diminish functional and structural tubulointerstitial lesions.[122]

Chronic hypokalemia is also associated with development of renal tubulointerstitial lesions in rats.[123] Because hypokalemia enhances renal ammoniagenesis, it has been suggested that development of these lesions may be mediated by ammonia. The severity of renal tubulointerstitial lesions in hypokalemic rats may be ameliorated by oral sodium bicarbonate supplementation.[123] Sodium bicarbonate supplementation diminishes hypokalemia-induced renal ammonia production and renal tissue concentrations of ammonia, although the mechanisms involved have not been fully elucidated.

Renal ammoniagenesis may also be reduced by feeding reduced protein diets. However, it has not been determined if feeding reduced protein diets limits development of renal tubulointerstitial lesions and peritubular complement deposition.[124]

LIPIDS. Results of recent studies suggest a role for dietary lipids in modulating progression of experimental renal disease in rodents.[121, 125–129] The mechanisms may be related, in part, to renal prostaglandin synthesis. The composition of dietary lipids may influence systemic blood pressure, blood lipid composition, platelet aggregation, blood viscosity, the immunologic system, and fibrinolytic activity.[129] It has also been hypothesized that certain lipids may promote progressive damage to the glomerular basement membrane and mesangial structures.[130]

Diets rich in linoleic acid have been found to ameliorate progression of renal disease in rats with reduced renal mass.[125, 127] Feeding a diet high in linoleic acid to rats with subtotal renal ablation increased GFR and RBF, and reduced blood pressure, proteinuria, and glomerular lesions.[125] The beneficial effects of high linoleate intake appears to be additive with the beneficial effect of reduced protein diets in this model.[131] In contrast, dietary linoleic acid did not appear to affect the clinical course of mice with immune-mediated renal disease.[128] The mechanisms responsible for the beneficial effects of linoleic acid support a role for increased glomerular prostaglandin (PGE_2 - a vasodilator) production.[131]

Considerable attention has been drawn to the purported beneficial effects of dietary fish oil in preventing cardiovascular disease in humans.[121] Eicosapentaenoic acid (EPA) appears to be the active component responsible for many of the beneficial effects of fish oil. Increased dietary EPA inhibits production of arachidonic acid–derived cyclooxygenase metabolites, and thus may exert an antiplatelet effect, reduce production of biologically active thromboxane, and, perhaps, lower blood pressure.[126] However, impaired prostaglandin production may be detrimental because adequate production of renal prostaglandins, specifically PGE_2 and PGI_2, is important for maintaining glomerular filtration. Fish oil–enriched diets have been shown to be beneficial in reducing proteinuria in certain immune-mediated renal diseases in mice and humans.[126] However, fish oil diets appear to accelerate deterioration of renal function and structure in rats with non–immune-mediated renal disease induced by surgical ablation of renal tissue.[126]

The effects of altering dietary lipids on progression of spontaneous or experimental renal disease in dogs and cats are unknown. Dietary lipids may influence progression of different forms of renal disease in different ways, depending on the mechanism of renal injury. Generalizations concerning formulation of dietary lipids for patients with renal failure may not be possible. Until results of controlled studies on the impact of altering dietary lipids on progression of canine and feline CRF become available, specific recommendations concerning formulation of diet lipids are not possible.

ANTICOAGULANTS. Mechanical injury to the glomerular vasculature may lead to denudation of endothelial cells from the glomerular basement membrane. Endothelial damage may result in exposure of circulating plasma proteins to basement membrane constituents, precipitating intracapillary coagulation. Capillary thrombosis has been observed in glomeruli of rats with induced renal failure; heparin therapy has been shown to limit progression of this model of glomerular disease.[132–135] Drugs that inhibit thromboxane synthesis and impair platelet aggregation may also limit glomerular injury.[136] Heparin therapy is reported to be among the most effective means of slowing progression of experimentally induced renal failure in rats.[108, 133] However, in addition to its anticoagulant properties, heparin may: (1) modify systemic blood pressure by its diuretic properties, (2) prevent proliferation of smooth-muscle cells, and (3) abolish the effects of growth factors derived from mononuclear cells.[108] Recent data suggest that the protective effects of heparin on glomerular pathology and progression of renal failure most likely result from its anticoagulant and/or antiproliferative properties.[185]

Aspirin has been shown to prevent hyperfiltration and glomerular basement membrane thickening in rats with experimental diabetes mellitus.[137] The mechanism of aspirin in this model is not known, but may relate more to inhibition of prostaglandin synthesis than to aspirin's anticoagulant properties.

DIET THERAPY

Overview. Modification of diets to minimize deficits and excesses of metabolites associated with generalized renal dysfunction is not an all-or-none phenomenon. Best results are achieved when diet therapy is combined with other components of conservative medical management. Although diet therapy is of major value in controlling some of the polysystemic disturbances associated with uremia, it is not a panacea that can be expected to control or modify all dysfunctions associated with primary renal failure.

Rationale. Loss of renal function leads to accumulation of a wide variety of nitrogen-containing compounds (Table 108–20). Many waste products of protein catabolism are excreted primarily by glomerular filtration. Patients with primary renal failure have impaired ability to excrete proteinaceous catabolites because of marked reduction in GFR. Retention of metabolic waste may be further aggravated by impaired tubular secretion, and by extrarenal factors that promote renal hypoperfusion and increased catabolism of body tissues. Although accumulation of proteinaceous wastes is largely the result of decreased renal excretion or increased protein catabolism, production of some compounds may also be increased (e.g., guanidines).[138] Because these compounds are derived almost entirely from protein degradation, their production increases when dietary protein increases. Although a direct cause and effect relationship has not been proved, retained protein catabolites may contribute significantly to production of uremic signs and many of the laboratory abnormalities found in patients with renal failure.[138–142]

The rationale for restricting protein intake of patients with CRF is based on the premise that controlled reduction of nonessential proteins will result in decreased production of nitrogenous wastes with consequent amelioration of clinical signs. This hypothesis has been supported by results of studies in dogs with experimental renal failure.[30] By formulating diets that contain

TABLE 108–20. A PARTIAL LIST OF SUBSTANCES THAT HAVE BEEN INCRIMINATED AS POTENTIAL UREMIC TOXINS

Aromatic compounds	Polyamines
Phenolic acid	Conjugated amino acids
Hydroxyphenolic acid	Nucleotides
Aromatic amines	Peptides
Indoles	Middle molecules
Guanidine and its derivatives	Sulfates
Guanidinoacetic acid	Hydrogen ions
Guanidinosuccinic acid	Urea
Methylguanidine	Acetoin
	Aliphatic amines

a reduced quantity of high-quality protein and adequate nonprotein calories, many of the signs associated with uremia may be reduced in severity or eliminated, even though renal function remains essentially unchanged.

Effectiveness of Reduced Protein Diets. The efficacy of reduced protein diets in preventing progression of CRF in dogs is still under investigation. Studies of experimentally induced CRF in dogs have shown that low-protein diets reduce glomerular hyperfiltration and proteinuria compared with standard canine diets.[30, 143] In addition, high-protein diets and/or glomerular hyperfiltration appears to promote development of glomerular lesions similar to those observed in rats with induced CRF.[97] Although studies in our laboratory have thus far failed to demonstrate a consistent relation between protein intake and development of renal lesions, dogs with enhanced inulin clearance rates (indicating glomerular hyperfiltration) had significantly more severe renal lesions compared with dogs with lower clearance rates.[97] In a long-term study of dogs with 75 per cent reduction in renal mass, dogs fed a 56 per cent protein diet developed significantly more severe light microscopic renal lesions than dogs fed 27 or 19 per cent protein diets.[144] The results of this study were interpreted to suggest that significant differences in renal lesions due to these diets did not exist because ultrastructural renal studies failed to confirm findings obtained by light microscopy. Although the type of ultrastructural studies performed in the aforementioned study may permit a more specific evaluation of renal lesions, in our opinion they are an insensitive means of assessing the extent and severity of the lesions described by light microscopy. Therefore, de-emphasis of the more sensitive light microscopic findings in favor of the more specific ultrastructural studies is potentially misleading.

To determine if reduced renal mass promotes progressive deterioration of renal function in dogs, two long-term studies have been performed. In one study, dogs with 75 per cent reduction in renal mass were monitored for over 42 months.[86] The GFR remained stable in these dogs throughout the study. It is possible, however, that the magnitude of renal dysfunction induced may not have been sufficient to initiate self-perpetuating renal dysfunction. In another long-term study performed in our laboratory, dogs with 11/12 reduction in renal mass were evaluated for 40 weeks.[29] Despite the more severe reduction in renal mass, renal function remained stable for the duration of the study, suggesting that functional deterioration of the remaining renal tissue did not occur. Progressive proteinuria and development of renal lesions indicative of destruction of nephrons in residual renal tissue (Figure 108–5) suggested that renal lesions were progressive, even though renal function did not decline. Similar findings occur in rats with induced renal failure; proteinuria and renal lesions may progress despite apparently stable renal function.[88]

We hypothesize that failure of serial GFR measurements to detect progressive renal damage in the aforementioned studies may reflect a renal reserve that allows remaining intact nephrons to be recruited to replace the function of nephrons that are damaged and lost.[145] Development of hyperfiltration in these recruited neph-

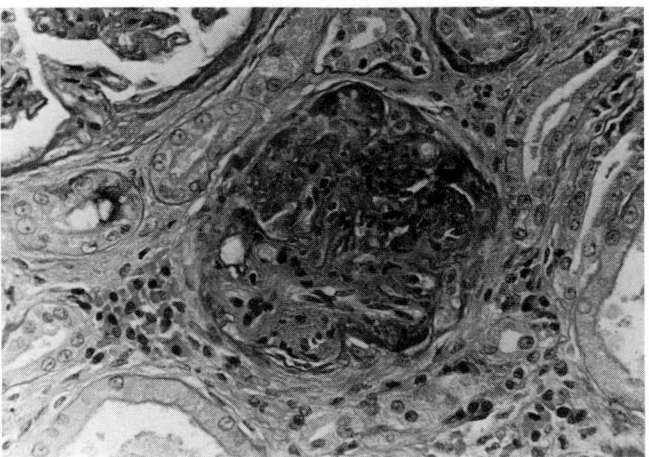

FIGURE 108–5. Photomicrograph of kidney 70 weeks after removal of 11/12 of functional renal mass. Glomerular sclerosis, tubular dilatation, and marked interstitial fibrosis are evident in the surviving portion of the kidney. This portion of the kidney was structurally normal before renal mass was reduced. Two micron section; PAS stain; original magnification × 170.

rons may eventually promote glomerular sclerosis, additional nephron loss, and ultimately depletion of the renal reserve. A measurable decline in GFR would be expected to occur at this time. In a study performed subsequent to the 40-week study described earlier, persistence of additional renal reserve was documented by a cross-over model using the same remnant kidney dogs that had been used in the 40-week study.[143] The GFR was found to increase when the high-protein diet was fed as compared with the reduced protein diets, indicating that GFR could be boosted by increasing dietary protein intake.

In summary, a preponderance of evidence supports a potential therapeutic role for dietary protein restriction in limiting progression of canine renal failure. Similar data are unavailable for cats, but are the subject of current studies in our laboratory.

Potential Benefits. Traditionally, the principal benefit ascribed to dietary protein restriction in patients with CRF has been amelioration of clinical signs of uremia due to reduced retention of nitrogenous waste products. However, protein restriction may also benefit renal failure patients in a variety of other ways.

Protein restriction may minimize spontaneous, progressive renal damage in patients with CRF by modifying renal hemodynamics.[83] Because proteinaceous foods contain phosphate, dietary protein restriction simultaneously reduces phosphate intake.[65, 124] Reducing phosphate intake may ameliorate hyperphosphatemia, renal secondary hyperparathyroidism, and renal osteodystrophy, as well as minimize progression of CRF.[65, 90]

Severity of polyuria and polydipsia is lessened when renal failure patients are fed reduced protein diets because less solute load is delivered to the kidneys in the form of proteinaceous waste products. Feeding diets restricted in both protein and salt content largely normalizes urine output and water consumption rates in dogs with mild to moderate CRF.[30, 143]

Moderate protein restriction may reduce the severity of anemia of CRF.[146] Protein restriction increases red blood cell mass in part by reducing retention of waste products that promote hemolysis and blood loss. Proteinaceous waste products promote blood loss by causing gastrointestinal ulcerations and impairing platelet function. In contrast, excessive dietary protein restriction may promote anemia as a by-product of protein malnutrition.[146]

Because hydrogen ions are a by-product of protein catabolism, protein restriction may minimize metabolic acidosis. However, studies in dogs indicate that some reduced protein diet formulations promote hyperchloremic metabolic acidosis, even in mild to moderate renal failure.[124] The diet-associated metabolic acidosis was readily amenable to alkalinization therapy.

Indications. There is little controversy as to the value of reduced protein diets in dogs that develop overt clinical signs of uremia when fed normal or high protein diets. Justification for reducing dietary protein intake in these individuals is based on the need to minimize retention of toxic waste products of protein catabolism that contribute to clinical signs of uremia.

In contrast, a consensus of opinion of the therapeutic value of recommending reduced-protein diets for dogs with early renal failure is just now emerging. Although the efficacy of dietary protein restriction in preventing progression of renal failure has not yet been conclusively proved, the preponderance of currently available evidence suggests that reducing protein intake early in the course of CRF may be beneficial in slowing progressive renal damage. There is no evidence to support the contention that moderate protein restriction early in the course of CRF is deleterious to the patient. Although excessive protein restriction may have adverse nutritional consequences, this complication may be prevented by proper diet formulation and monitoring the patient's response to therapy. Therefore, pending results of further experimental and clinical studies, reduced-protein diets should be recommended for dogs with early CRF because: (1) efficacy is likely, (2) there is no better therapeutic option available, and (3) potential benefits outweigh risks.

Protein Requirements for Dogs. The minimum requirement for high-biologic-value protein for normal dogs has been reported to be approximately 1.25 to 1.75 mg/kg/day.[147-149] Optimum protein and amino acid requirements have not been established for dogs with CRF. Based on the assumption that nonessential amino acids could be synthesized using ammonium derived from urea nitrogen in the intestines, it was once postulated that patients with CRF may have reduced protein requirements.[150, 151] However, current data suggest that intestinal urea nitrogen is not significantly utilized for protein synthesis in uremic humans.[152-156]

Current evidence derived from studies in humans and rats suggests that protein requirements for uremic individuals may be greater than those for normal individuals.[152, 157, 158] This is not surprising, since uremia is a catabolic state induced by a variety of endocrine and metabolic derangements.[159-161] Protein and amino acid requirements of uremic patients may be altered by a variety of pathophysiologic disturbances, including any combination of the following: (1) glucose intolerance, (2) impaired intestinal absorption of amino acids, (3) impaired renal tubular reabsorption of amino acids, (4)

decreased activities of intestinal dipeptidases and disaccharidases, which may result in impaired digestion of proteins and carbohydrates, and (5) elevated serum concentrations of some hormones, such as glucagon, somatotropin, and parathyroid hormone.[158] In addition, acidosis may be associated with enhanced urea production, and total body potassium depletion (which may occur especially in anorectic renal failure patients) may promote protein catabolism.[149] Protein requirements may also be increased by external losses of protein, including albuminuria, hematuria, and gastrointestinal hemorrhage.

Dogs with a moderate degree of CRF that were fed a diet containing the estimated minimum daily requirement of high-biologic-value protein for normal dogs (0.57 gm of cooked egg protein/lb/day or 1.25 gm/kg/day) for 40 weeks developed clinical and laboratory evidence of malnutrition characterized by hypoalbuminemia, anemia, weight loss, and reduced body tissue mass.[146] In this same study, dogs fed 1.7 gm of protein/lb/day or 3.6 gm/kg/day did not develop clinical or biochemical evidence of protein malnutrition. Studies performed in our laboratory have indicated that reduction of dietary protein intake from 0.9 to 0.32 gm/lb/day (2.0 to 0.7 gm/kg/day) may be associated with varying degrees of protein malnutrition, the severity of which is related to the degree of protein restriction. However, reduced consumption of dietary protein also consistently resulted in a proportional reduction of serum urea nitrogen concentrations. In a subsequent study, dogs with moderate CRF (mean serum creatinine concentration, 3.2 mg/dl) were fed 0.9 gm of protein/lb/day (2.0 gm of protein/kg/day) for 16 weeks without developing detectable evidence of protein malnutrition.

Because normal control dogs were not used in these studies, it is not possible to unequivocally conclude that dogs with CRF require more protein than normal dogs. However, results of this study emphasize that excessive dietary protein restriction may be associated with development of protein malnutrition. Furthermore, these studies have indicated that maximum protein restriction (i.e., 0.57 gm or less of high-biologic-value protein/lb/day) is not required for therapeutic efficacy in all dogs with CRF.

Recommendations. DIETARY PROTEIN INTAKE FOR DOGS. The authors currently recommend that dogs with mild to moderate CRF (mean serum creatinine concentration = 1.5 to approximately 4.5 mg/dl) be fed approximately 0.9 to 1.0 gm of high-biologic-value protein/lb/day (2.0 to 2.2 gm of high-biologic-value protein/kg/day). However, the authors emphasize the need to consider the intrinsic variability of protein requirements of normal dogs and the probable varied influence of uremia on protein requirements of uremic dogs. Therefore, dietary protein should be adjusted to meet individual needs of individual patients.

The extent to which protein intake must be restricted to minimize progressive renal damage is as yet unknown. Therefore, the goal of protein restriction should be to minimize progressive renal damage and clinical signs of uremia while maintaining adequate nutrition. This goal can be achieved only by monitoring the patient's response to diet therapy by means of serial assessment of renal function, clinical response, and nutritional status. If evidence of protein malnutrition occurs (hypoalbuminemia, anemia, weight loss, or loss of body tissue mass), dietary protein should gradually be increased until these abnormalities are corrected.

If diets designed to provide 0.9 gm of protein/lb/day (2.0 gm of protein/kg/day) do not result in amelioration of the clinical and biochemical manifestations of uremia, or if evidence of progressive renal dysfunction is detected (progressive reduction in GFR or progressive proteinuria), dietary protein intake may be cautiously reduced further. The decision to reduce dietary protein further must be based primarily on clinical assessment of the patient. Dietary protein should not be reduced for the sole purpose of attaining a prescribed reduction in serum urea nitrogen concentration! The clinician should strive to achieve the best attainable compromise between the impact of diet on the biochemical and clinical manifestations of uremia, renal function, and prevention of malnutrition.

DIETARY PROTEIN INTAKE FOR CATS. Cats have significantly higher dietary protein requirements compared with dogs. Dietary protein requirements for normal adult cats have been estimated to be approximately three times the protein requirement for adult dogs (12.5 per cent of diet calories as protein for cats versus 4 per cent of diet calories as protein for dogs).[162] The higher protein requirement for cats is not solely the result of a higher requirement for one or more essential amino acids. Rather, it appears to reflect reduced efficiency of anabolic utilization of dietary protein in cats compared with other species. A significant portion of the protein in their diets is used as a source of calories.

Dietary protein requirements of cats with CRF are not known; studies documenting the safety and efficacy of reduced protein diets in treatment of feline renal failure have not been reported. In absence of this data, the authors cautiously recommend that cats with CRF be fed diets containing approximately 20 per cent of calories as protein (equivalent to 1.5 to 1.6 gm/lb/day of high-biologic-value protein or 3.3 to 3.5 gm/kg/day when consuming 32 to 37 Kcal/lb/day or 70 to 80 Kcal/kg/day).[163] Protein intake should be individualized in cats with CRF as described above for dogs with CRF. However, caution is advised in reducing dietary protein intake below 20 per cent protein calories.

CALORIE INTAKE. Dietary energy is as important as dietary protein for maintenance of nitrogen balance and prevention of protein malnutrition. Modification of diets for treatment of chronic primary polyuric failure should encompass provision of adequate nonprotein calories in addition to reduction of protein. Caloric intake should be adjusted to optimize protein anabolism.

Minimum daily requirements for calories, carbohydrates, and fats have not been established for dogs and cats with CRF. Because this information is unavailable, it has been necessary to make the unproved assumption that minimum requirements for these nutrients are the same as those for normal dogs. Accordingly, most nephrologists have recommended that dogs receive 32 to 50 Kcal/lb/day (70 to 110 Kcal/kg/day), and cats receive 32 to 37 Kcal/lb/day (70 to 80 Kcal/kg/day). Since carbohydrate, fat, and caloric requirements may

be affected by metabolic disturbances characteristic of the uremic syndrome (including glucose intolerance, maldigestion, and elevated serum insulin and glucagon concentrations), these values should be used as guidelines. Determination of caloric requirements should be individualized to patient needs based on serial determinations of body weight. Unless the patient is markedly obese and weight reduction is deemed necessary, an attempt should be made to maintain stable body weight. If the patient is malnourished, caloric intake should be increased for an appropriate period.

WATER-SOLUBLE VITAMINS. Uremic humans have a tendency to develop deficiencies of water-soluble vitamins, especially folate, ascorbate, and pyridoxine.[164] The tendency to develop vitamin deficiencies is most apparent in patients with poor dietary intakes. Minimum daily requirements for water-soluble vitamins have not been established for dogs and cats with renal failure. However, based on results of studies in uremic humans, the possibility that vitamin deficiencies may develop in uremic dogs and cats must be considered. Because of this concern, the authors recommend that B complex and C vitamin supplements be administered to dogs and cats with CRF, particularly during periods of reduced food consumption.

VITAMIN D. Progressive loss of renal mass is associated with impaired conversion of vitamin D precursors to their most active form (1,25-vitamin D). Even though the need for oral or parenteral administration of 1,25-vitamin D increases as renal function decreases, oral or parenteral administration of vitamin D without consideration of serum and dietary concentrations of calcium and phosphate is extremely hazardous. Therapeutic elevation of subnormal plasma concentrations of calcium in patients with hyperphosphatemia may result in soft-tissue calcification and further deterioration of renal function. Therefore, supplementation of the diet with vitamin D must be carefully individualized to the patient (see sections on divalent ion imbalances).

VITAMIN A. Although the minimum daily requirement for vitamin A has not been determined for dogs with CRF, human patients with renal failure often develop an excess of vitamin A.[158] Excess vitamin A may directly or indirectly increase parathyroid hormone release, and thereby aggravate renal osteodystrophy and acidosis.[165] Supplementation of vitamin A beyond minimum daily requirements is thus not recommended.

Complications of Diet Therapy. **PROTEIN MALNUTRITION.** Inadequate protein nutrition is probably the most significant potential adverse effect associated with feeding low-protein diets. In our experience, protein malnutrition has not been a substantial problem when dogs with CRF are fed 0.9 gm or more (2.0 or more gm/kg/day) of high-biologic-value protein/lb/day. However, dogs fed less than this quantity of protein for long periods may develop clinical and laboratory evidence of protein deficiency. Signs of protein malnutrition include: (1) reduced muscle mass, (2) progressive loss of body weight, and (3) progressive reductions in packed cell volumes and/or serum albumin concentrations. Unfortunately, these signs may not be sensitive indicators of malnutrition, and malnutrition may be fairly advanced before abnormalities become apparent. If malnutrition is detected before or after initiating diet therapy, consideration should be given to increasing dietary protein intake. It may be necessary to seek a balance between the adverse nutritional effects and the beneficial clinical effects of protein restriction.

ANOREXIA. Anorexia and poor appetite are common impediments to successful conservative medical management of dogs with CRF. The pathogenesis of anorexia in uremic patients has not been fully elucidated; however, it appears to be related to retention of uremic toxins. The hypothesis that retained uremic toxins contribute to anorexia is supported by observations that modified protein diets and/or dialysis improve or correct anorexia. Studies in dogs indicate that anorexia may occur in association with stimulation of the medullary emetic chemoreceptor trigger zone by uremic toxins.[166] Ablation of this area in nephrectomized dogs suppressed the onset of anorexia. Altered taste perception may also contribute to anorexia. Treatment of anorexia may involve: (1) feeding several smaller meals throughout the day, (2) enhancing palatability of the diet, and/or (3) pharmacologic stimulation of appetite.

Feeding several small meals rather than a single large meal generally increases daily food consumption. In addition, the timing of feeding may influence consumption. Despite an initially good appetite, sometimes uremic humans experience nausea and anorexia after starting to eat breakfast. These same patients are often able to eat later in the day without developing nausea and anorexia. Some dogs appear to experience similar waxing and waning of appetite throughout the day. By offering fresh food several times each day, the probability of encountering an interval during which the appetite is good is enhanced. As noted earlier, observations in humans suggest that failure to consume a meal after showing initial interest should not necessarily be interpreted as a palatability problem; it may represent food-induced nausea or anorexia, which may not persist throughout the day.

A possible drawback to this method of enhancing food consumption is the recent observation in rats suggesting that ad libitum or frequent feeding may promote more sustained glomerular hyperperfusion and hyperfiltration compared with alternate-day feeding.[167] These observations suggest that frequent feeding may promote renal injury when compared with once daily or alternate-day feeding. In addition, alternate-day feeding has been shown to retard development of glomerulosclerosis and proteinuria in some rats.[168, 169] The significance of these observations in dogs and cats with CRF is currently unknown. Pending further studies, the authors recommend frequent feeding of multiple small daily meals only to those patients that fail to consume adequate calories when fed once or twice daily.

Reducing dietary protein and sodium content often reduces palatability. Palatability may be enhanced by warming foods (usually to about 37° C); however, the food should not be served hot. Food can also be flavored with small quantities of meat, animal fat, or other flavor enhancers. Poultry fat (especially turkey fat) is particularly effective for many cats. However, it is possible to create nutritional imbalances by adding excessive quantities of these substances (e.g., addition of too much

meat may increase dietary protein consumption, promoting uremia; excessive addition of fat may reduce dietary protein content, thereby promoting protein malnutrition). Sometimes palatability can be improved by formulating homemade diets based on known dietary preferences of the patient.

As a general rule, the authors prefer to attempt to stimulate eating by the methods described above before attempting pharmacologic management. Treatment with drugs designed to stimulate appetite is generally reserved for patients that fail to respond to more conservative forms of therapy, or for patients developing malnutrition as a result of chronic anorexia.

Diazepam and other benzodiazepines have been successfully used as appetite stimulants in a variety of animal species, including dogs and cats.[170] In uncontrolled clinical trials in uremic dogs and cats, the authors have used diazepam as an appetite stimulant with variable success. In some cases a dramatic improvement in food consumption has followed initiation of diazepam therapy. When given intravenously, onset of eating is rapid, but the duration of effect from an individual dose is brief. Given orally, onset of action is slower, but appetite stimulation is more prolonged, often leading to greater overall food consumption. Other benzodiazepines that may prove useful include oxazepam (Serax, 10 mg capsules) and flurazepam (Dalmane, 15 mg capsule). Oxazepam is administered orally at a dose of 0.1 mg/lb (0.2 mg/kg) given once daily. Flurazepam is given orally every four to seven days at a dose of 0.1 to 0.2 mg/lb (0.2 to 0.4 mg/kg). All of these drugs appear to be more effective in cats than in dogs.

Recommended dosages of diazepam in anorectic cats are 0.02 to 0.2 mg/lb (0.05 to 0.4 mg/kg) given orally, intravenously, or intramuscularly.[170] Dogs have been reported to require higher doses than cats.[171, 172] In cats, the authors have used doses of from 0.5 to 2 mg given orally one or two times daily. Diazepam is available in 2, 5, and 10 mg scored tablets. It may be used short-term to initiate eating, and then withdrawn if the patient continues to eat spontaneously. Sometimes the drug must be continued long-term to sustain adequate food consumption.

Diazepam is metabolized in the liver to activate metabolites that are excreted in urine. Diazepam and other benzodiazepines are usually well tolerated by humans and dogs with renal failure; when used for sedation, dosage is generally not reduced.[173] However, administration to patients with renal failure may lead to excessive sedation as well as other central nervous system side effects.[173] Sedation and ataxia have been noted in some of our patients. Because efficacy may be best at higher doses, and because renal failure patients may be more sensitive to the sedative effects of these drugs, it may be necessary to seek a balance between these effects based on patient response.

Although administered primarily for treatment of anemia of CRF, anabolic steroids have been advocated as appetite stimulants for dogs with renal failure. In a recent study designed to evaluate the efficacy of one anabolic steroid in treatment of dogs with experimental renal failure, the anabolic steroid tested did not appear to enhance food consumption.[174] Clinical studies designed to evaluate the effectiveness of this and other anabolic steroids in promoting appetite in dogs with spontaneous CRF have apparently not been performed.

In some patients, anorexia may be a manifestation of uremic gastroenteritis. In such cases, cimetidine or central-acting antiemetics may be beneficial in controlling nausea and promoting food intake (see section on ARF). Chlorpromazine (0.2 mg/lb or 0.5 mg/kg), prochlorperazine (0.06 mg/lb or 0.13 mg/kg q6h), or trimethobenzamide (1.4 mg/lb or 3 mg/kg q8h) may be used to control nausea and vomiting in uremic patients. Long-term therapy with these drugs should generally be restricted to animals that will not continue eating unless drug therapy is continued.

THERAPY FOR FLUID, ELECTROLYTE, AND ACID-BASE DISORDERS

Fluid. Patients with CRF typically have obligatory polyuria, which is induced, at least in part, by (1) impaired ability to maintain a hypertonic medullary interstitium and, therefore, a functional countercurrent system, and (2) excretion of abnormally large quantities of solute through viable nephrons as a result of generalized nephron destruction and retention of metabolic wastes. Fluid balance in patients with polyuric renal failure is maintained by compensatory polydipsia. If water consumption is insufficient to balance excessive water loss associated with polyuria, dehydration and renal hypoperfusion may precipitate a uremic crisis. If dehydration and decreased RBF persist, additional renal damage may occur. For these reasons, fresh, clean, unadulterated water should be available in adequate quantities at all times.

Cats with CRF may fail to consume sufficient water to prevent volume depletion. The authors have had some success using various flavored liquids, such as clam juice, to promote additional fluid consumption. Such fluids should generally be used to supplement fluid consumption, not as a substitute for water consumption. The impact of the mineral and electrolyte content of such supplemental fluids should be considered. For example, milk provides large quantities of phosphate, and broths may contain large quantities of sodium.

For patients in which voluntary fluid intake is inadequate to prevent dehydration, supplemental fluids may be administered subcutaneously at home by the owner. Composition of fluids selected for chronic parenteral administration should provide free water as well as electrolytes for maintenance (so-called maintenance fluids composed of approximately two-thirds dextrose five per cent in water and one-third balanced electrolyte solution such as lactated Ringer's solution, supplemented with potassium chloride). Unfortunately, fluids containing dextrose may be irritating when administered subcutaneously. Chronic administration of lactated Ringer's solution or normal saline solution as the principal maintenance fluid source may cause hypernatremia because they fail to provide sufficient electrolyte-free water.

In our experience, polyuric dogs with renal failure frequently consume inadequate quantities of fluid during periods of hospitalization. If insufficient thirst leads to

negative body water balance characterized by rapid loss in body weight, loss of skin pliability, and/or hemoconcentration, supplemental fluids should be given orally or parenterally.

Sodium. Sodium balance is maintained primarily by the kidneys. By altering the fraction of filtered sodium that is excreted, called fractional excretion of sodium (FE_{Na}), normal individuals can maintain normal sodium balance despite wide variations in dietary sodium intake. As GFR falls in patients with CRF, residual nephrons increase FE_{Na} to adapt to the increased sodium load delivered to each nephron. Sodium balance is maintained so long as FE_{Na} increases sufficiently to adjust for the reduction in GFR. Typically, sodium regulatory capacity is lost only in very advanced renal failure, but the kidneys' ability to adapt to varying sodium intake becomes narrowed as GFR continues to decline.

In the past, diets high in sodium chloride content were recommended for dogs with CRF because: (1) sodium-induced diuresis was hypothesized to minimize tubular reabsorption of potential uremic toxins, (2) pathologic sodium-wasting was thought to routinely accompany generalized renal dysfunction, mandating therapeutic sodium replacement, and (3) reduced sodium intake might promote metabolic acidosis in dogs with CRF by reducing renal tubular capacity to reabsorb bicarbonate. Results of preliminary studies performed in our laboratory support the concept that high sodium intakes (approximately 1200 mg of sodium/100 gm of dry weight) may enhance urinary excretion of nitrogenous waste products, and thereby decrease the magnitude of azotemia.

Urinary FE_{Na} is elevated in dogs with experimentally induced CRF that are fed standard canine maintenance diets.[175] It has been shown that this increase in FE_{Na} may be prevented by reducing sodium intake in proportion to the reduction which has occurred in renal function.[176] Thus, the increase in FE_{Na} appears to be an adaptive physiologic response to a high level of dietary sodium intake, rather than an obligatory pathologic loss of sodium resulting from renal dysfunction.[176] Whether or not such an adaptive phenomenon regularly occurs in dogs with all forms of spontaneously occurring renal failure is not known. However, certain forms of renal disease recognized in humans (especially diseases that primarily affect the renal medulla) may be associated with a true pathologic "sodium-wasting" tendency. Inability to adapt to varying sodium intakes may occur in certain forms of canine and feline renal disease. Patients that are unable to adapt to varying sodium intakes may be predisposed to volume depletion when fed diets containing reduced sodium content.

In humans, hypertension is an established cause of renal dysfunction. It may also aggravate the polysystemic signs of uremia, and may be among the most important factors that promote progression of CRF. It has recently been recognized that high sodium intake may contribute to hypertension in dogs with CRF.[177] The role of hypertension in development and progression of renal dysfunction in dogs is currently under investigation and is discussed in greater length in Chapter 109.

Because of the apparent link between sodium intake,

hypertension, and renal disease, and because of limited capacity of failing kidneys to adapt to wide fluctuations in sodium intake, the authors recommend that dogs with CRF be fed "normal" (as opposed to high) or "moderately restricted" sodium diets. For comparison, diets that contain about 800 mg of sodium/100 gm dry weight diet would be considered "normal sodium" diets; diets that contain about 250 mg of sodium/100 gm dry weight diet would be considered "moderately sodium restricted" diets. Severely restricted sodium diets (less than 200 mg of sodium/100 gm dry weight diet) may promote volume depletion in patients with CRF, and therefore should not be used routinely. Establishment of sodium requirements for dogs with polyuric CRF must be based on future controlled experimental and clinical studies designed to evaluate sodium balance and its impact on hypertension and hypertension-related complications. Until such data become available, dietary sodium should be individualized on the basis of knowledge of current disease processes (e.g., hypertension, congestive heart failure, hypoproteinemia, edema) and response to modification of dietary sodium intake.

Dietary sodium may be modified in an attempt to achieve the following goals: (1) minimize or prevent sodium-associated hypertension, (2) prevent negative sodium balance and volume depletion, and (3) avoid inducing metabolic acidosis. Changes in sodium should always be made gradually. Patients with CRF may adapt to a wide range of dietary consumption patterns; however, adaptation may occur only gradually. Abrupt changes in dietary sodium may be associated with transient imbalances between intake and urine loss. Sudden reduction in dietary sodium may reduce extracellular fluid volume, which in turn may lead to poor renal perfusion and further reduction in renal function. The authors recommend that changes in dietary sodium be made over at least a two-week period.

Response to adjustments in dietary sodium may be determined by monitoring body weight, hydration, renal function, and acid-base status during and for several weeks after reduction of dietary sodium. Progressive loss of body weight, progressive azotemia, and/or dehydration suggests that the patient may be unable to adapt to reduced sodium intake. In this event, a more gradual and smaller reduction of sodium intake may be considered.

It has been reported that renal tubular bicarbonate reabsorption may be decreased when sodium intake is restricted in dogs with CRF, thereby potentially promoting metabolic acidosis.[178] However, preliminary studies performed in our laboratory have not revealed substantial metabolic acidosis when diets containing 250 mg of sodium/100 gm of dry food were fed to dogs with moderate experimental CRF. Whether or not clinically significant metabolic acidosis would result from more profound dietary sodium restriction is unknown.

Although dietary sodium intake has generally been incriminated as a major causative or contributory factor in development of systemic hypertension, recent studies in humans and rats suggest that the anion with which sodium is associated greatly influences the propensity to promote hypertension.[179-181] Studies indicate that although sodium chloride may promote hypertension in humans with essential hypertension or CRF, other forms of sodium, such as sodium citrate or sodium bicarbonate, tend not to be retained to the same extent or promote systemic hypertension in these patients.[179-181] Perhaps not all forms of sodium need to be restricted in CRF.

Potassium. **OVERVIEW.** The kidneys maintain potassium homeostasis by renal modification of potassium excretion. The majority of potassium appears in urine as a result of distal renal tubular potassium secretion. In patients with CRF, the residual nephrons maintain potassium balance by increasing distal tubular secretion of potassium, thereby increasing fractional excretion of potassium.[182] Gastrointestinal secretion of potassium may also increase in CRF.[101] Because of these adaptations, most patients with CRF are able to tolerate normal dietary potassium intake (about 0.4 per cent of a diet that provides 4 Kcal of metabolizable energy/gm of food) until renal dysfunction is severe. However, the ability to rapidly excrete a potassium load may be impaired in CRF.[182]

HYPERKALEMIA. Hyperkalemia is unusual in dogs and cats with mild to moderate polyuric CRF. Specific treatment of mild to moderate hyperkalemia that is not associated with hyperkalemic cardiotoxicity is usually not necessary. However, persistent hyperkalemia should be minimized by eliminating the cause of hyperkalemia or controlling complicating factors that may promote hyperkalemia (Table 108-11). If these measures fail to normalize serum potassium concentrations, dietary potassium restriction or administration of sodium-potassium exchange resins may be necessary (see section on Treatment of Hyperkalemia in ARF).

Development of hyperkalemia in patients with mild to moderate renal failure may indicate reduced renal renin production (hyporeninemic hypoaldosteronism). In such cases, administration of a mineralocorticoid such as Florinef (fludrocortisone acetate) (0.1 to 0.2 mg/day) should correct the hyperkalemia. However, chronic mineralocorticoid therapy may promote sodium retention.

HYPOKALEMIA. Hypokalemia occurs occasionally in dogs and cats with CRF. Although the precise mechanism has not been determined, it appears to result when urinary loss exceeds dietary intake of potassium. Hypokalemic polymyopathy has been observed in cats in association with an apparent potassium-losing nephropathy.[68, 69, 183] The cardinal sign of hypokalemia, regardless of cause, is generalized muscle weakness. Cats with hypokalemia have been observed to have profound cervical ventroflexion and difficulty ambulating. The authors have observed generalized flaccid muscle weakness and mild cardiac rhythm disturbances (Figure 108-6) in hypokalemic dogs with CRF. In one dog, muscle weakness was severe enough to cause respiratory failure and death.

Muscle weakness usually resolves within one to five days after initiating parenteral or oral potassium supplementation.[44] Oral administration is the safest route of administration for potassium; parenteral therapy is generally reserved for patients that require emergency therapy. Potassium gluconate tablets may be given orally at the rate of 2.2 mEq of potassium/100 calories of required energy intake. Potassium gluconate elixir (Kaon Elixir) has also been recommended for dogs at a dosage of 5

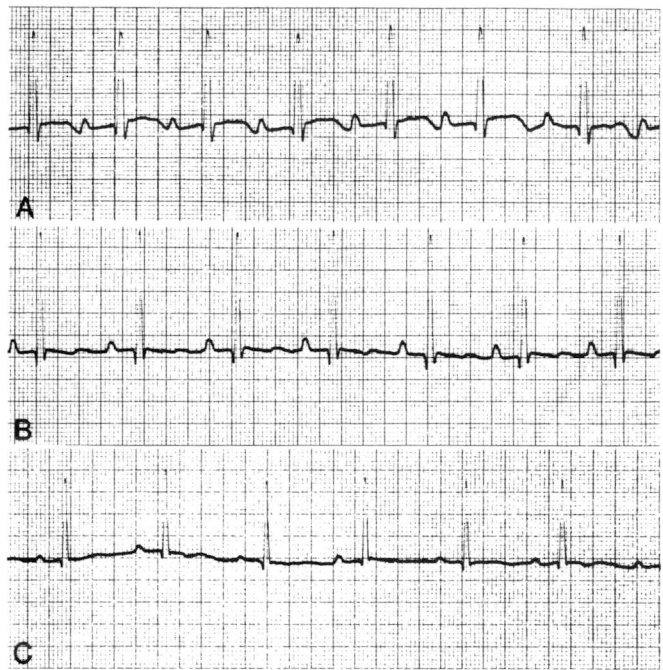

FIGURE 108–6. Electrocardiogram from a dog with hypokalemia and CRF. At a serum potassium concentration of 1.2 mEq/L *(A)*, ECG alterations included prolongation of the P and QRS complexes (0.055 sec and 0.065 sec, respectively) and P-R interval (0.16 sec). The ST segment was slightly elevated. Elevation of serum potassium concentration to 2.1 mEq/L by oral potassium supplementation was accompanied by reduced P and QRS duration, increased R wave voltage, normalization of the ST segment, and reduction of heart rate *(B)*. As serum potassium concentration approached normal (3.4 mEq/L), further reduction in P and QRS voltages and durations, reduction of heart rate, and shortening of the PR interval occurred *(C)*. The T wave was low in amplitude.

ml given q8 to 12h and for cats at a dosage of 2 to 4 mEq given q12h. Oral potassium chloride may be given to dogs at a dose of 1 to 3 gm/day and to cats at 0.2 gm/day. It has been suggested that cats do not tolerate potassium chloride as well as the potassium gluconate elixir.[68] Oral potassium supplements may cause gastrointestinal irritation, ulceration, nausea, and vomiting. They should be used with caution in older and debilitated patients (see Chapter 53). Treatment of hypokalemia has recently been reviewed.[44]

Dietary potassium supplementation may be required to prevent recurrent hypokalemia in patients that have developed hypokalemic polymyopathy.[60] Although dietary potassium deficiency is unlikely to be the sole cause of hypokalemia in these patients, inadequate potassium intake appears to be a contributing factor.

***Metabolic Acidosis.* PATHOPHYSIOLOGY.** The kidneys play a central role in maintenance of acid-base balance, since they continuously excrete metabolically derived nonvolatile acid. Metabolism of sulfur-containing amino acids in the diet is a major source of metabolic acid (hydrogen ions). Hydrogen ions are excreted in urine as titratable acid (usually a salt of phosphate) or as ammonium (hydrogen ions bound to ammonia).

Initially as renal function is lost, the kidneys are able to sustain their capacity to excrete hydrogen ions by increasing ammoniagenesis in surviving nephrons. However, the capacity of surviving nephrons to increase ammoniagenesis is limited. When this capacity is ex-

ceeded, metabolic acidosis occurs because the kidneys can no longer completely excrete the quantity of metabolic acid produced daily. Presumably this occurs when the population of surviving nephrons becomes too small to meet the demand for ammonia production. Reduced excretion of titratable acid resulting from reduced glomerular filtration of phosphate and other buffers, as well as increased urinary loss ("wasting") of bicarbonate may also contribute to acidosis of CRF, but their contribution appears to be relatively small.

Despite continued retention of hydrogen ions, metabolic acidosis is rarely progressive in patients with CRF.[22] Acidosis tends to remain stable, at least in part, because retained hydrogen ions are buffered by bone. Unfortunately, such bone buffering may adversely affect skeletal integrity. Detection of more severe or progressive acidosis should prompt consideration of complicating factors or additional contributing causes of metabolic acidosis, such as diarrhea.

TREATMENT. Therapy for metabolic acidosis may not be indicated for all patients with CRF. The limited fall in plasma HCO_3^- concentration plus respiratory compensation usually maintains blood pH at a level that poses no important physiologic risk to the patient (i.e., pH greater than 7.20). Alkalinization therapy is clearly indicated when plasma bicarbonate concentration is below about 12 mEq/L or blood pH is below approximately 7.20.

The need for therapy when plasma bicarbonate concentration is greater than 12 mEq/L or blood pH is greater than 7.20 is less clear. However, even mild to moderately reduced plasma bicarbonate concentrations may limit the patient's capacity to adapt to additional acid stress resulting from such factors as diarrhea, dehydration, or respiratory acidosis. Alkalinization therapy may improve the patient's ability to cope with these additional acid-base insults. In addition, minimizing acidosis may limit skeletal damage resulting from bone buffering. Alkalinization therapy may also minimize the potential adverse effects of increased renal ammoniagenesis on self-perpetuation of progressive renal failure.[122] Therefore, alkalinization therapy may be of benefit for patients with mild to moderate metabolic acidosis.

Oral sodium bicarbonate is the most commonly used alkalinizing agent for patients with metabolic acidosis of CRF. Because the effects of gastric acid on oral sodium bicarbonate are unpredictable, the dosage should be individualized for each patient. The suggested initial dose is 4 to 5 mg/lb (8 to 12 mg/kg) q8 to 12h. Alkalinizing agents should be given in several smaller doses rather than in a single large dose, to minimize fluctuations in blood pH. Blood bicarbonate concentration should be monitored at appropriate intervals to assess adequacy of therapy. Ideally, blood should be collected just prior to administration of the drug. The goal of therapy is to maintain plasma bicarbonate (or total CO_2) concentration between 18 and 24 mEq/L. Dosage should be adjusted according to changes in blood pH or plasma bicarbonate (or total CO_2) concentration. Urine pH is an insensitive means of assessing the need for or response to treatment and is not recommended for these purposes.

Despite its frequent use, sodium bicarbonate is not

an innocuous drug. It must be used judiciously to avoid inducing metabolic alkalosis. It may be advisable to minimize or avoid administration of sodium-containing drugs to patients with congestive heart failure, nephrotic syndrome, hypertension, oliguria, or volume overload. However, sodium bicarbonate may not promote fluid retention to the same extent as sodium chloride.[179-181] Nonetheless, calcium carbonate or calcium lactate may be considered for use in patients that may be intolerant of additional sodium intake.

In addition to alkalinization therapy, other therapeutic endeavors may also influence acid-base balance. Reducing dietary protein intake may limit the quantity of substrate available for renal ammonia production, thereby limiting renal ammoniagenesis and promoting metabolic acidosis.[124] However, this effect may be moderated by consumption of reduced quantities of protein-derived acid precursors. Because phosphate is the predominant buffer involved in excretion of hydrogen ions as urinary titratable acid, excessive dietary phosphate restriction and use of phosphate binding agents may promote metabolic acidosis by limiting urine phosphate excretion.[186] Dietary restriction of phosphate may enhance tubular reabsorption of HCO_3^- in dogs, whereas dietary restriction of sodium may inhibit tubular reabsorption of HCO_3^- in dogs.[178] The clinical importance of these possible effects for dogs with spontaneous CRF is unclear. However, they emphasize the need for monitoring response to treatment.

THERAPY OF DIVALENT ION IMBALANCES

Overview. Disturbances in calcium, phosphate, and magnesium metabolism begin early in the course of CRF and progress as renal function deteriorates. Therefore, patients with CRF are likely to have some clinical or laboratory abnormalities related to disordered divalent ion balance, regardless of the severity of their renal dysfunction (Table 108–21).[187, 188] In addition to the consequences of disordered divalent ion metabolism recognized in dogs and cats with CRF, pruritus, proximal myopathy, skin ulcerations, and soft-tissue necrosis have been reported to occur in affected humans.[187] The pathophysiology of these disorders is described in detail in Chapter 107.

Therapy designed to minimize divalent ion imbalances in dogs and cats with CRF includes: (1) dietary phos-

TABLE 108–21. MANIFESTATIONS OF ALTERED DIVALENT ION METABOLISM IN CHRONIC RENAL FAILURE

Hyperphosphatemia
Hypocalcemia
Hypercalcemia
Hypermagnesemia
Increased fractional excretion of phosphate
Renal secondary hyperparathyroidism
Elevated serum alkaline phosphatase activity
Defective intestinal absorption of calcium and phosphate
Relative or absolute deficiency of 1,25-dihydroxyvitamin D
Renal osteodystrophy (characterized by bone pain, increased endosteal fibrosis, defective mineralization, pathologic fractures, fibrocystic osteodystrophy)
Soft tissue calcification, including nephrocalcinosis

TABLE 108–22. GOALS OF THERAPY FOR DIVALENT ION IMBALANCES IN CHRONIC RENAL FAILURE

1. Normalize blood calcium and phosphate concentrations.
2. Minimize secondary hyperparathyroidism.
3. Prevent or reverse renal osteodystrophy.
4. Prevent or reverse soft tissue calcification.
5. Minimize progression of renal dysfunction.

phate restriction and use of intestinal phosphate binding agents, (2) oral supplementation of calcium, and (3) administration of vitamin D or its metabolites. Maintaining good hydration that facilitates GFR is also of value. The goals of therapy are summarized in Table 108–22. Blood calcium and phosphate concentrations are interdependent; excessive levels of either or both may promote soft-tissue calcification and renal injury and dysfunction. Therefore, the authors emphasize that calcium supplementation and administration of vitamin D are generally contraindicated in patients with hyperphosphatemia. If calcium and/or vitamin D is used, serum calcium and phosphate concentrations and renal function must be monitored throughout therapy to avoid iatrogenic renal injury or mineral imbalances. Because of the primary role of phosphate in the genesis of these mineral imbalances and the dire consequences of inducing hypercalcemia in hyperphosphatemic patients, normalization of serum phosphate concentration is always the first priority in management of divalent ion imbalances in CRF.

Dietary Phosphate Restriction and Use of Intestinal Phosphate Binding Agents. EFFECTS OF PHOSPHATE RETENTION. Phosphate retention and hyperphosphatemia play a primary role in the genesis and progression of renal secondary hyperparathyroidism and renal osteodystrophy.[187, 189-191] Although the precise mechanisms through which hyperphosphatemia induces secondary hyperparathyroidism are still being debated, by minimizing hyperphosphatemia, secondary hyperparathyroidism and its various effects can largely be prevented.[187, 189-193]

Phosphate influences parathyroid hormone (PTH) secretion by inducing reciprocal changes in serum concentrations of ionized calcium and 1,25-dihydroxyvitamin D.[192] Phosphorus regulates renal 1α-hydroxylase activity, the enzyme responsible for conversion of 25-hydroxycholecalciferol (25-hydroxyvitamin D) to its most metabolically active form, 1,25-dihydroxyvitamin D.[194] Hyperphosphatemia limits production of 1,25-dihydroxyvitamin D by inhibiting this enzyme. Because 1,25-dihydroxyvitamin D is important in regulation of intestinal absorption of calcium, hyperphosphatemia may impair intestinal absorption of calcium. Furthermore, 1,25-dihydroxyvitamin D normally decreases synthesis and secretion of PTH.[195] Parathyroid glands of patients with CRF and low blood 1,25-dihydroxyvitamin D levels require higher concentrations of calcium to suppress PTH release. The combination of hyperphosphatemia and low blood 1,25-dihydroxyvitamin D concentration causes skeletal resistance to PTH. Thus, more PTH is required to mobilize calcium from bone in an attempt to maintain normal serum calcium concentrations.[192]

Phosphate retention may also promote progression of CRF in some species. Although phosphate retention does not appear to promote progression of CRF in humans, results of recent studies in dogs and cats support a beneficial effect of phosphate restriction in slowing progression of renal failure and/or renal mineralization in these species.[90, 112] Clearly, minimizing hyperphosphatemia is important in canine and feline patients with CRF.

THERAPY. Meat and dairy products are important sources of dietary phosphate. Phosphate is absorbed from the gastrointestinal tract and excreted primarily by the kidneys via glomerular filtration. In patients with CRF, reduced GFR results in phosphate retention and subsequent hyperphosphatemia. It has been suggested that optimum control of hyperphosphatemia would be achieved by reducing dietary phosphate "in proportion" to the decrease in GFR.[190] Because proteinaceous foods are the major dietary sources for phosphate, dietary protein restriction results in reduced phosphate intake. Although the extent to which phosphate intake can be decreased by diet alone is limited, dietary restriction is an important and effective first step in controlling hyperphosphatemia, hyperparathyroidism, hypovitaminosis D, and renal osteodystrophy.[65, 187, 190, 196, 197]

The goal of therapy is normalization of serum phosphate concentrations (Table 108–22). However, in advanced renal failure, dietary protein restriction alone may fail to prevent hyperphosphatemia. When hyperphosphatemia occurs despite dietary protein/phosphate restriction, administration of intestinal phosphate binding agents should be considered. Aluminum-containing intestinal phosphate binding agents include antacid compounds, available over-the-counter (Table 108–23). These agents render ingested phosphate and the phosphate contained in saliva, bile, and intestinal juices unabsorbable.[187]

Because phosphate is present in the intestinal tract in greatest quantities in association with food consumption, administration of phosphate binding agents should be timed to coincide with feeding. These agents are best administered with or mixed into the food, or just before each meal. Dosage should be individualized so that serum phosphate concentrations are normalized. An initial dose of 15 to 40 mg/lb/day (30 to 90 mg/kg/day) has been recommended. The effect should be monitored by serial evaluation of serum phosphate concentrations at 10- to 14-day intervals. The dosage should be adjusted until normalization of serum phosphate concentration is achieved. Thereafter, serum calcium and phosphate concentration should be monitored monthly or as needed. Samples obtained for determinations of serum phosphate concentration should be collected after a 12-hour fast, to avoid postprandial effects. They should not be determined in hemolyzed samples since RBCs contain substantial quantities of phosphorus.

High dietary phosphate content may greatly limit the effectiveness of phosphate binding agents, or substantially increase the dosage required to achieve the desired therapeutic effect. Administration of 1500 to 2500 mg of aluminum carbonate to dogs with moderate CRF failed to consistently correct hyperphosphatemia when dogs were fed diets that contained greater than one per cent phosphate on a dry matter basis.[198] Phosphate binding agents are reported to be ineffective in controlling hyperphosphatemia when dietary phosphate intake exceeds 2 gm/day in humans.[187] In addition, capsules and tablets appear to be less effective than liquid gels in reducing serum phosphate concentrations in humans.[187, 199] Aluminum oxide has been found to bind phosphate more effectively than aluminum hydroxide or aluminum carbonate in dogs, but aluminum oxide is not currently available.[200]

The principal disadvantage of long-term use of aluminum-containing antacids in humans with CRF is development of aluminum toxicity. Aluminum contained in phosphate binding antacids may be absorbed from the intestinal tract and accumulate in various tissues of the body, such as bone and brain.[187] Encephalopathies and bone disease (particularly osteomalacia) related to aluminum toxicity have been extensively reported in humans patients treated with these drugs. The potential for toxicity of aluminum salts in dogs and cats with CRF is significant, but evidence of toxic accumulation of aluminum has not been reported in these species. Finco and colleagues examined the problem of aluminum toxicity in 6 dogs given 1500 mg of aluminum carbonate/day and 6 dogs given 2500 mg of aluminum carbonate/day.[198] After three months of antacid therapy, aluminum levels in kidney and brain tissue were nondetectable. However, parenteral administration of large quantities of aluminum to dogs has been shown to cause marked disturbances in calcium metabolism and renal function, and osteomalacia.[201, 202]

Because of concerns related to aluminum retention in patients with renal failure, calcium carbonate and calcium citrate have recently been recommended as alternatives to aluminum-containing phosphate binding

TABLE 108–23. ALUMINUM-CONTAINING INTESTINAL PHOSPHATE BINDING AGENTS

	Manufacturer	Al (OH)$_3$ mg/5 ml Liquid or mg/ Tablet or Capsule
Liquid Antacids		
Alternagel	Stuart Pharmaceutical	600
Amphojel suspension	Wyeth Laboratories	320
Basaljel extra-strength liquid	Wyeth Laboratories	1000*
Nephrox suspension	Fleming	320
Solid Antacids		
Alu-Cap	Riker	475
Alu-Tab	Riker	600
Amphojel tablets	Wyeth Laboratories	600
Basaljel capsules	Wyeth Laboratories	500*
Dialume capsules	Armour Pharmaceuticals	500

*Contains Al (CO)$_3$ rather than Al (OH)$_3$.

agents. These agents are effective in humans with renal secondary hyperparathyroidism.[192, 203] Calcium carbonate is effective in limiting intestinal absorption of phosphate in normal dogs and in dogs with induced renal failure.[204] Calcium-containing phosphate binding agents have the additional benefit of providing increased calcium intake. However, a major disadvantage of calcium carbonate is its potential for inducing hypercalcemia. This risk may be particularly great in patients with severe hyperphosphatemia. As a consequence, it has been recommended that use of calcium-containing phosphate binding agents be limited to patients with serum phosphate concentrations in the range of 6 to 7 mg/dl. Aluminum-containing antacids may be indicated for patients with more marked hyperphosphatemia. Once hyperphosphatemia has been reduced to 6 to 7 mg/dl, calcium carbonate or calcium citrate therapy may be initiated to maintain phosphate balance.

The human dosage of calcium carbonate is 1 to 2 gm given with each meal. The recommended dosage of calcium citrate is about 2 to 5 gm given with each meal. Dosage should be individualized according to response to treatment, with the goal being normalization of serum phosphate concentration (Table 108–22). Serum calcium concentrations should not exceed about 11 mg/dl. When calcium citrate is used, serum total CO_2 should be monitored to detect and avoid metabolic alkalosis. Some humans treated with calcium carbonate have developed gastrointestinal disturbances.[205] To minimize this effect, it has been suggested that calcium carbonate be administered with food and the dosage be adjusted according to the phosphate content consumed at each meal. Another alternative is to add an aluminum-containing antacid and reduce the dosage of calcium carbonate. The manufacturer claims that calcium citrate may be less likely to induce gastrointestinal disturbances. It has not yet been determined whether chronic calcium carbonate therapy is associated with soft-tissue calcification or other long-term adverse effects.

Some calcium carbonate preparations may not be effective because they fail to dissolve well in the gastrointestinal tract. Treatment failure with calcium carbonate may be investigated by examining the stool or radiographing the abdomen for evidence of undissolved tablets.

Polyuronic acid polymer is another aluminum-free intestinal phosphate binding agent that may become available soon.[205] This compound has been shown to be effective in limiting phosphate absorption in normal dogs.[206] Preliminary studies in humans indicate that this compound is likely to be effective in reducing serum phosphate concentrations in CRF.

Renal secondary hyperparathyroidism and renal osteodystrophy are known to develop early in the course of canine CRF, even though serum phosphate concentrations remain normal during this phase of CRF.[190] It has been suggested that when serum phosphate concentrations are found to be normal in patients with CRF, phosphate balance should be investigated further by measuring plasma PTH activities or fractional excretion of phosphate.[207] The fractional excretion of phosphate may serve as an indirect means of assessing plasma PTH activity.[207] Fractional excretion of phosphate in normal

dogs is 0.10 or less, and values of 0.30 or less are suggested as evidence of adequate phosphate restriction in dogs with renal failure.[207] The clinical effectiveness of defining normalization of plasma PTH activity or fractional excretion of phosphate as the therapeutic end point for phosphate restriction has not yet been ascertained. Until studies supporting safety and clinical benefit of this therapeutic end point become available, the authors continue to recommend normalization of serum phosphate concentration as the goal of dietary phosphate restriction for most patients.

Patients treated with both dietary phosphate restriction and intestinal phosphate binding agents should be carefully monitored to avoid inadvertent induction of hypophosphatemia. Severe hypophosphatemia and phosphate depletion may cause debility, weakness, and anorexia, which may be confused with signs of uremia. In addition, phosphate depletion may aggravate bone disease and even cause osteomalacia. Constipation is another commonly reported side effect of phosphate binding agents.

Oral Supplementation of Calcium. Intestinal malabsorption of calcium is common in patients with CRF, but calcium absorption can be improved or normalized when dietary calcium intake is increased.[187] Increasing calcium intake may increase serum calcium concentrations and prevent or ameliorate renal osteodystrophy. Early initiation of calcium supplementation may prevent renal osteodystrophy and other manifestations of renal secondary hyperparathyroidism. However, the optimum time during the course of CRF to initiate calcium therapy is not yet known. Indications for calcium supplementation include: (1) hypocalcemia, (2) clinical, radiographic, or histologic evidence of renal osteodystrophy, and (3) inadequate dietary calcium intake.

Hypercalcemia is the major side effect of calcium supplementation therapy, and has been reported to induce nausea, vomiting, mental confusion, lethargy, and hypertension in humans with CRF.[187] Hyperphosphatemia is an absolute contraindication to calcium therapy because administration of calcium to patients with hyperphosphatemia may promote soft-tissue calcification and renal injury. Hyperphosphatemia should be normalized before calcium supplementation is initiated. Gastrointestinal disturbances are also a common side effect of oral calcium supplements, particularly when administered in large doses.

Calcium carbonate may be the preferred calcium salt in many patients with CRF because of its alkalinizing properties. Initially, calcium carbonate should be administered at a dose of 45 mg/lb/day (100 mg/kg/day). Serum calcium and phosphate concentrations should be monitored every 10 to 14 days; the dosage of calcium carbonate should be individualized according to response. Administration of frequent, small doses is more likely to be effective and less likely to induce complications than fewer large doses.

Calcium may also be supplied as calcium lactate, calcium gluconate, or calcium glubionate. Calcium chloride should not be used for calcium supplementation in patients with CRF because of its acidifying properties.[187] Elemental calcium constitutes 40 per cent of calcium carbonate, 12 per cent of calcium lactate, 8 per cent of calcium gluconate, and 6 per cent of calcium glubionate.[187] Dosages of calcium preparations should be calculated based on supplying equimolar amounts of elemental calcium. Systemic acid-base balance should be considered when selecting the calcium salt to be used; calcium carbonate and calcium lactate may be useful in patients with metabolic acidosis but are undesirable in alkalemic patients.

Administration of Vitamin D or Its Metabolites. Relative or absolute deficiency of 1,25-dihydroxyvitamin D plays a pivotal role in development of renal secondary hyperparathyroidism and renal osteodystrophy.[187, 188] Inhibition of renal 1α-hydroxylase activity appears to be a major factor responsible for limiting renal production of 1,25-dihydroxyvitamin D in patients with CRF. Inhibition of renal 1α-hydroxylase activity may result, at least in part, from hyperphosphatemia and increased renal cytoplasmic calcium concentrations.[194, 208] In addition, recent evidence suggests that 1,25-dihydroxyvitamin D binding by parathyroid glands may be diminished in renal failure.[209, 210] This decreased binding may promote hyperparathyroidism through reduced 1,25-dihydroxyvitamin D-induced inhibition of PTH secretion. Intestinal sensitivity to 1,25-dihydroxyvitamin D-stimulated calcium absorption may be suppressed in renal failure, but this suppression may be overcome by increasing levels of vitamin D.[211] Thus, vitamin D therapy may improve intestinal malabsorption of calcium in patients with CRF. Administration of 25-hydroxyvitamin D in conjunction with proportional reduction in phosphate intake has been of benefit in controlling renal secondary hyperparathyroidism and its associated skeletal abnormalities in dogs with induced CRF.[188]

Hypercalcemia is a frequent and potentially serious complication of vitamin D therapy. Hypercalcemia has been reported to occur in 30 to 57 per cent of humans treated with 1,25-dihydroxycholecalciferol.[187] Vitamin D therapy does not have a direct adverse effect on renal function, but hypercalcemia can induce a reversible or irreversible reduction in GFR if sustained hypercalcemia develops during therapy.[187] Vitamin D therapy in patients with hyperphosphatemia may also promote renal calcification and injury. Therefore, serum phosphate concentration must be normalized before vitamin D therapy is initiated.

Because of the potential adverse consequences of vitamin D, selection of rapidly acting and rapidly metabolized agents that permit rapid correction of hypercalcemia is preferred. Vitamin D preparations that do not require 1α-hydroxylation may be more effective in patients with CRF because their of impaired 1α-hydroxylase activity.

A form of vitamin D that is chemically and clinically identical to naturally occurring 1,25-dihydroxyvitamin D is commercially available (Rocaltrol Capsules, 0.25 and 1.50 μg). This drug has rapid onset (one to four days) and short duration of action (half-life less than one day), permitting rapid control of unwanted hypercalcemia. It does not require renal activation for maximum efficacy. Dosage for 1,25-dihydroxyvitamin D has not yet been determined for dogs. The suggested dosage for humans is 0.014 to 0.025 μg/lb/day (0.03 to 0.06 μg/kg/day). It has been proposed that a similar dosage is likely to be

effective in dogs and cats.[212] Serum calcium concentrations were reported to remain within normal limits when this drug was administered to normal dogs at a dosage of 0.025 μg/lb/day (0.06 μg/kg/day) for four weeks, but hypercalcemia developed when a dosage of 0.05 μg/lb/day (0.12 μg/kg/day) was administered for four weeks.

Another vitamin D preparation suitable for use in patients with CRF is dihydrotachysterol (Hytakeral capsules or oral solution). Dihydrotachysterol requires hepatic 25-hydroxylation for maximum biologic activity, but it does not undergo and presumably does not require renal 1α-hydroxylation for maximal biologic activity. Its biologic activity lies between 25-hydroxyvitamin D and 1,25-dihydroxyvitamin D. The polarity and lower dosage requirements of dihydrotachysterol limit its storage in fat, making significant or prolonged vitamin D intoxication unlikely.[212] Recommended dosage of dihydrotachysterol is 0.005 mg/lb/day (0.01 mg/kg/day).[212]

Regardless of the vitamin D preparation selected, optimum dosage must be determined for each patient on the basis of serial evaluation of serum calcium and phosphate concentrations. If initially elevated, serum alkaline phosphatase activities may also provide some guidance as to the impact of therapy on skeletal lesions. Initially, serum calcium and phosphate concentrations should be evaluated at 24- to 48-hour intervals until an appropriate dosage is determined. Because the onset of hypercalcemia after initiation of vitamin D therapy is unpredictable, and may occur after days to months of treatment, continued monitoring of serum calcium, phosphate, and creatinine concentrations is necessary to detect hypercalcemia, hyperphosphatemia, or deteriorating renal function before irreversible renal damage ensues. If hypercalcemia develops, it is advisable to stop treatment completely rather than reduce the dose. Therapy may be reinstituted with a reduced dosage after serum calcium concentration returns to normal.[187] Administration of vitamin D is not recommended if serum calcium and phosphate concentrations cannot be monitored.

Chronic administration of verapamil, a calcium channel blocking agent, has been shown to improve duodenal calcium absorption and increase plasma 1,25-dihydroxyvitamin D levels in rats with experimental renal failure.[208] It was hypothesized that by minimizing renal calcium uptake and cytoplasmic calcium concentrations, verapamil promoted renal 1α-hydroxylase activity and increased renal production of 1,25-dihydroxyvitamin D. Increased plasma levels of 1,25-dihydroxyvitamin D were probably responsible for increasing duodenal calcium absorption. The effects of verapamil on calcium and vitamin D homeostasis have not been evaluated in canine and feline patients with CRF.

THERAPY OF NONREGENERATIVE ANEMIA

Anemia of CRF—Overview. A hypoproliferative anemia characterized by normocytic, normochromic RBCs is typical of CRF. In a recent study of feline CRF, nonregenerative anemia was detected in 30 of 73 (41.1 per cent) cats.[60] Although anemia is often mild with apparently minimal clinical impact, moderate to severe anemia may occur and promote lethargy, weakness, and anorexia. Patients with CRF may tolerate anemia better than patients with comparably severe anemia due to other causes, because of a reduced affinity of hemoglobin for oxygen that promotes more effective oxygen delivery to tissues.[213, 214] Unfortunately, reduced hemoglobin-oxygen affinity may further reduce the stimulus for renal erythropoietin production.[214]

Severity of anemia varies widely in dogs and cats with CRF. Correlations between severity of anemia, magnitude of renal dysfunction, and cause of renal failure have not been determined. In humans with CRF, severity of anemia tends to correlate directly with magnitude of renal dysfunction and erythropoietin production.[215, 216] Although the etiology of CRF typically does not influence severity of anemia in humans, anemia is often unexpectedly mild in patients with polycystic kidneys or systemic hypertension, and disproportionately more severe in patients with nephrotic syndrome.[214] If anemia is unexpectedly severe, complicating factors (Table 108 24) should be sought and corrected, if possible.

The genesis of anemia of CRF is multifactorial. Primary mechanisms include a relative decrease in erythropoietin production, shortened RBC survival, and uremic inhibitors of erythropoiesis.[214, 215, 217–220] Secondary complicating factors that may aggravate severity of anemia include gastrointestinal hemorrhage, malnutrition, and myelofibrosis associated with renal secondary hyperparathyroidism.[214, 217, 218, 221, 222]

Treatment of the anemia of CRF may encompass administration of androgens, transfusion therapy, and hormone replacement. The only satisfactory treatments for anemia of CRF in humans are renal transplantation or hormone replacement therapy with recombinant human erythropoietin.[223] Since hormone replacement therapy with recombinant human erythropoietin is expensive, and renal transplantation is not currently available for most canine and feline CRF patients, androgen therapy is often used. The efficacy of androgen therapy for anemia of CRF has not been critically evaluated in dogs and cats. Our impression is that response to androgen therapy is often poor. A therapeutic trial with androgens may be indicated for patients with moderate to severe anemia of CRF, since adverse side effects have not been recognized.

Androgens. Androgens stimulate erythropoiesis by: (1) direct effects on the pluripotential stem cells and erythroid progenitor cells, and (2) stimulating erythro-

TABLE 108–24. FACTORS THAT MAY PROMOTE ANEMIA IN CHRONIC RENAL FAILURE

Decreased erythropoietin production
  Infection
  Malnutrition
Enhanced hemolysis
  Oxidant substances or drugs
  Hypophosphatemia
  Microangiopathy
  Hypersplenism
  Uremic toxins
Nutritional factors
  Malnutrition
  Iron deficiency
  Folic acid deficiency
Hemorrhage
Myelofibrosis

poietin production, which further augments erythroid differentiation and proliferation.[224] Several weeks to months are required for substantial response to androgen therapy to become evident. Androgens may also increase concentrations of 2,3-DPG in RBCs. In addition to their potential benefit for treatment of uremic anemia, androgens have been hypothesized to stimulate appetite, promote anabolism, enhance skeletal calcium deposition, and promote intestinal absorption of calcium.[225] However, in dogs with acute uremia, 3-oxo-1,4 androstadiene-17β-ol-undecylenate (boldenone undecylenate), a testosterone derivative, failed to enhance appetite or promote anabolism.[174]

Usefulness of androgens in therapy for anemia of end-stage renal disease in humans has been confirmed by a number of studies.[224] When response to therapy does occur, it may be temporary or incomplete.[223] Androgens appear to be effective in about 50 per cent of human patients with CRF, but the hematocrit rarely returns to normal.[224] Androgens have not yet been proved safe or efficacious in treatment of anemia of CRF in dogs and cats, yet they constitute the mainstay of therapy for anemia of CRF in these species.

In humans, androgens appear to be more effective in stimulating RBC production when they are administered parenterally than when administered by other routes.[224] Reduced effectiveness of orally administered agents may be related to the fact that testosterone administered orally has only one sixth the potency of injected testosterone, probably because of hepatic inactivation following gastrointestinal absorption.[224] Specific androgens appear to vary considerably in their effectiveness in humans. Nandrolone decanoate has been documented to be effective in several human studies, whereas oxymethalone has been shown to be largely ineffective in treatment of anemia of CRF.[224, 226, 227] The relative effectiveness of various androgens in treatment of anemia of canine and feline CRF has not been determined.

Patients with moderate to severe anemia are candidates for androgen therapy, but caution is advised in use of these products because of the dearth of data validating their clinical efficacy, expense, inconvenience of administration, and potential side effects. Potential adverse effects of androgens include sodium and fluid retention, hepatotoxicity, recurrence and worsening of perianal adenoma, perineal herniation, premature epiphyseal closure, and prostatomegaly in males.[228, 229] Oral administration of methyltestosterone has been reported to induce hepatotoxicity in beagles.[230] Hepatotoxicity occurs primarily with oral androgens, whereas parenteral forms are generally considered nonhepatotoxic.[214] Serial monitoring of hepatic enzyme activities and serum albumin concentrations is recommended for dogs and cats receiving chronic oral androgen therapy. In humans, hepatotoxicity is generally reversible on termination of therapy.[231]

A variety of androgen products are available (Table 108 25).[232] The authors cautiously recommend parenteral therapy when necessary. Because response to treatment may be dose dependent, if the hematocrit has not increased by at least three volume per cent after three months of therapy, consideration should be given to doubling the dosage.[224] If after three more months of

TABLE 108–25. DOSAGES OF ANDROGENS USED FOR TREATMENT OF ANEMIA

Androgen Class	Trivial Name	Dosage	A:A Ratio
Testosterone esters	Testosterone propionate	1.0 mg/lb IM q7d	1:1
	Testosterone enanthate	1.8–3.2 mg/lb IM q7d	1:1
Norsteroids	Nandrolone decanoate	0.45 mg/lb IM q7d	1:2.5
	Nandrolone phenylpropionate	0.45 mg/lb IM biweekly	
17-alkylated compounds	Stanozolol	1–4.5 mg/lb IM q7d	1:3
		0.1–1.4 mg/lb PO q24h	
	Fluoxymesterone	0.1–0.45 mg/lb PO q24h	1:1

A:A ratio, androgen–anabolic activities.

therapy at this increased dosage the hematocrit has still not increased by at least three volume per cent, doubling the dosage a second time or switching to an agent of another class may be considered. Human patients who fail to respond to androgen therapy after nine months of treatment using this dosing schedule are generally unresponsive to androgen therapy.[224] It is advisable to monitor patients carefully for signs of toxicity or adverse drug reactions, particularly when increased drug doses are used.

Transfusion Therapy. RBC transfusion is an effective means of correcting the clinical signs of tissue hypoxia in patients with severe anemia.[217] However, response to transfusion therapy is only transiently effective and may risk exposure to infectious disease (e.g., feline leukemia virus infection, canine distemper) and transfusion reaction. In addition, erythroid marrow suppression may occur if excessive quantities of RBCs are administered. Repeated transfusions may further suppress erythrocyte production such that repeated transfusion therapy becomes mandatory (i.e., transfusion dependency).[217] Because of these concerns, transfusion therapy should be reserved for patients with severe anemia that have clinical signs referable to their anemia. When transfusion is deemed necessary, blood administered should probably be limited to that quantity required to increase the hematocrit to about 25 volume per cent. Blood should be obtained from A negative donors only because repeated transfusions may be necessary. Administration of freshly collected RBCs is preferred because stored RBCs generally have reduced content of 2,3-DPG, impairing their tendency to release oxygen to tissues.[213]

Recombinant Human Erythropoietin. Hormone replacement with recombinant human erythropoietin has been shown to correct anemia of CRF.[223] That this drug will correct uremic anemia in a uniform, dose-dependent, and predictable manner supports the view that the primary cause of anemia in patients with CRF is erythropoietin deficiency, and that hemolysis and inhibition of erythropoiesis are typically of lesser importance. When human CRF patients undergoing hemodialysis were given intravenous injections of recombinant human erythropoietin three times weekly, increased numbers of circulating reticulocytes were observed after two or three doses, and the hematocrit could be increased by as much as ten percentage points within three weeks.[223] Increases in hematocrit were associated with improved appetite, weight gain, activity, and cognition. The rise in hematocrit appeared to promote hypertension in some patients. With the exception of occasional seizures related to hypertension, no evidence of organ dysfunction,

toxic effects, allergic reactions, or antibody formation was noted. Although the efficacy of this product has not been evaluated in dogs and cats with anemia of CRF, it is a major technological advance that is likely to become a routine part of CRF management.

DRUG THERAPY

The kidneys are responsible for elimination of many drugs from the body. In patients with renal failure, renal drug clearance is reduced, causing the half-life of the drug to be prolonged. In addition, distribution, protein binding, and hepatic biotransformation of drugs may be altered in renal failure.[233] The sum effect of these changes is that drugs normally excreted by the kidneys tend to accumulate in patients with renal failure, promoting an increased rate of adverse drug reactions and nephrotoxicity. In addition, patients with preexisting renal disease and renal failure may be predisposed to nephrotoxicity. For these reasons, nephrotoxic drugs and drugs that require renal excretion should generally be avoided in patients with renal failure.

Because drug accumulation in patients with CRF is primarily a result of reduced renal drug clearance, dosage adjustments should be made according to changes in drug clearance.[233–235] Changes in renal drug clearance are usually assumed to parallel changes in GFR. Therefore, drug clearance may be estimated by measuring creatinine clearance (C_{cr}). Drug dosage may then be adjusted according to the percentage reduction in C_{cr} (i.e., the ratio of patient C_{cr} to normal C_{cr}), also known as the dose fraction (K_f):[233] K_f = (patient C_{cr}/ normal C_{cr}). Dosage regimens can be adjusted by decreasing the normal dose or increasing the normal dosage interval in direct proportion to K_f.[233] For drugs excreted 100 per cent unchanged by the kidneys, a precise increase in dosage interval may be calculated by dividing the normal dosing interval by K_f:[233, 235] modified dose interval = (normal dose interval/K_f). For example, if a drug is normally administered q8h and the patient's C_{cr} is 25 per cent of normal (i.e., K_f = 0.25), then the appropriate dosing interval is (8 hr ÷ 0.25) or 32 hours. Likewise, dose reduction may be determined by multiplying the normal dose by K_f:[233, 235] modified dose reduction = (normal dose × K_f). For example, if the normal dosage is 10 mg/lb given q8h and the patient's C_{cr} is 25 per cent of normal (i.e., K_f = 0.25), then the appropriate dosage is (10 mg/lb × 0.25) or 2.5 mg/lb given q8h. Even using the reduced dosage, normal interval method, the first dose of drug should be administered at the usual dosage to initiate therapeutic drug concentrations in tissues and blood.

Dosage of antimicrobial drugs may be modified according to three general patterns, depending on the fraction of the drug eliminated by the kidneys (Table 108–26): (1) doubling the dosing interval or halving the drug dosage in patients with severe reduction in renal function, (2) increasing the dosage interval according to ranges of creatinine clearance values, and (3) precise dosage modification as described above.[233] Drugs in the first category are relatively nontoxic. Drugs that require dosage modification according to C_{cr} values are more likely to be toxic. For drugs in this class, dosing interval is increased twofold when C_{cr} is between 1.0 and 0.5 ml/min/kg, threefold when C_{cr} is between 0.5 and 0.3 ml/min/kg, and fourfold when C_{cr} is less than 0.3 ml/min/kg. Some relatively toxic antimicrobial drugs that are excreted solely by glomerular filtration (particularly aminoglycoside antibiotics) require precise dosage modification according to K_f. For these drugs, increased interval, fixed dosage regimens appear to result in less nephrotoxicity than reduced dosage, fixed interval methods.[233] A combination of dosage reduction and interval extension has been recommended for animals with severe renal dysfunction (C_{cr} less than 0.7 ml/min/kg). A nomogram is available for calculating dosages and dosage intervals for these patients.[233]

As described earlier, C_{cr} is the preferred measure of

TABLE 108–26. DOSAGE MODIFICATIONS FOR PATIENTS WITH RENAL FAILURE

Drug	Route(s) of Excretion*	Nephrotoxic?	Dosage Adjustment in Renal Failure†
Amikacin	R	Yes	Pr
Amoxicillin	R	No	D/I
Amphotericin B	O	Yes	Pr
Ampicillin	R, (H)	No	D/I
Cephalexin	R	No	C_{cr}
Cephalothin	R, (H)	No (?)	C_{cr} or D/I
Clindamycin	H, (R)	No	N
Chloramphenicol	H, (R)	No	N, A
Corticosteroids	H	No	N
Cyclophosphamide	H, (R)	No	N
Dicloxacillin	R, (H)	No	N
Digoxin	R, (O)	No	Pr
Doxycycline	GI, (R)	?	N
Furosemide	R	No (?)	N
Gentamicin	R	Yes	Pr
Heparin	O	No	N
Kanamycin	R	Yes	Pr
Neomycin	R	Yes	C/I
Nitrofurantoin	R	No	C/I
Penicillin	R, (H)	No	D/I
Propranolol	H	No	N
Streptomycin	R	Yes	C_{cr}
Sulfisoxazole	R	Yes	C_{cr}
Tetracycline	R, (H)	Yes	C/I
Tobramycin	R	Yes	Pr
Trimethoprim/ sulfamethoxazole	R	Yes	C_{cr}, A

*Routes of excretion: R, renal; H, hepatic; GI, gastrointestinal; O, other (minor route in parentheses).

†Dosage modification: N, normal; D/I, half dose or double dosage interval (in severe renal dysfunction); C_{cr}, adjust according to C_{cr}; Pr, precise dosage modification (adjust according to K_f); C/I, contraindicated; A, avoid in advanced renal failure.

renal dysfunction for modifying drug therapy in CRF. However, serum creatinine concentration is a more universally available measure of renal dysfunction than C_{cr}. Although the relation between serum creatinine concentration and C_{cr} is not linear, the reciprocal of serum creatinine concentration may be used to approximate C_{cr} when serum creatinine concentration is less than 4 mg/dl.[233] This rule of thumb will overestimate C_{cr} when serum creatinine concentration exceeds 4 mg/dl. Serum urea nitrogen concentration is influenced by many extrarenal factors and does not provide an accurate basis for modifying drug dosage regimens. Despite increased expense and effort involved, the authors recommend using C_{cr} as the basis for modifying drug dosage schedules whenever possible. This recommendation is particularly relevant when a potentially nephrotoxic drug must be administered.

Another means of adjusting drug dosage in patients with CRF is to monitor plasma drug concentrations. Based on knowledge of specific therapeutic ranges and toxic levels of the drug, dosage may be adjusted according to measured plasma drug concentrations. Use of therapeutic drug concentrations for monitoring therapy is particularly advisable when toxic drugs such as aminoglycosides must be administered to patients with CRF. Clinical monitoring of drug concentrations in dogs and cats has recently been reviewed.[236]

The potential risks and benefits associated with use of nephrotoxic drugs and drugs that require renal excretion should always be considered before initiating therapy with such drugs in patients with CRF. Careful clinical and laboratory monitoring for toxicosis and pharmacologic effect (i.e., is the drug producing the desired effect?) is essential.

HYPERTENSION IN RENAL FAILURE PATIENTS

Systemic hypertension appears to be a relatively common complicating factor in dogs with CRF.[177, 237, 238] However, hypertension tends to be relatively mild in most dogs with CRF. It may be more severe in dogs with primary glomerular diseases. The incidence and severity of hypertension in cats with CRF is less well known but is likely to be similar to that in dogs. Dogs and cats do tend to develop minimal to mild hypertension when renal failure is induced by a combination of nephrectomy and renal arterial ligation. In contrast, certain strains of rats develop pronounced hypertension with this model of renal failure.

Hypertension may be easily overlooked because it is often clinically silent and inconvenient to measure. Diagnosis of systemic hypertension requires measurement of blood pressure using special equipment (see Chapter 109). Systemic hypertension is occasionally manifested clinically as retinal hemorrhages, dilated, tortuous retinal vessels, hyphema, and retinal detachment.[239] Occurrence of these ocular lesions should prompt consideration of systemic hypertension and renal failure.

Hypertension is significant in patients with CRF because it may cause and/or promote progressive renal injury. When systemic hypertension is transmitted to glomerular capillaries, glomerular damage is a likely result.[103] Therefore, therapy for hypertension must limit glomerular capillary hypertension to effectively limit hypertensive renal damage. The extent to which systemic hypertension is transmitted to glomerular capillaries may vary, depending on the cause of hypertension. The normal renal autoregulatory response to moderate hypertension is preglomerular vasoconstriction, which tends to protect the glomerular capillaries from barotrauma. However, renal autoregulation appears to be altered in rats with CRF that are fed high-protein diets.[240, 241] Disordered renal autoregulation may contribute to progressive renal injury in animals with CRF.

Controlled clinical studies documenting efficacy of antihypertensive therapy in modifying development or progression of canine or feline CRF have not yet been reported. Until such data are available, selective use of antihypertensive therapy (sodium restriction, diuretics, and various antihypertensive drugs) for affected patients should be considered. When selecting antihypertensive agents for dogs and cats with CRF, the effectiveness of these agents in limiting glomerular hypertension should be considered. Angiotensin converting enzyme inhibitors have been shown to be of particular value in this regard.

DETECTION AND MANAGEMENT OF URINARY TRACT INFECTION

Urinary tract infection (UTI) is a frequent complication in patients with CRF. Because uremic patients are often immunocompromised, UTI may initiate septicemia.[29, 31] Therefore, patients with CRF should be routinely examined for UTI. When UTI is detected, therapy should be carefully designed to eradicate infection with minimal risk of adverse drug reaction or therapeutic failure. The route of drug excretion and potential for nephrotoxicity should be considered when selecting an antimicrobial agent, but potential for nephrotoxicity alone is not an absolute contraindication. Urine should be cultured during and after treatment to assure that infection has been eradicated. Treatment of UTI in patients with CRF may be difficult because impaired filtration of the drug may result in suboptimal drug concentrations in urine. Standard urine antibiotic concentration values used for selecting antibiotics on the basis of minimum inhibitory concentrations may not be appropriate for CRF patients (see Chapter 107 and the section of this chapter on UTI).

PATIENT MONITORING

Response to Therapy. Response to treatment should be monitored at appropriate intervals so that treatment can be individualized to the specific, and often changing, needs of the patient. The problem-specific data base obtained before initiation of conservative medical management should be used as a baseline for comparison of the patient's progress. An outline of the minimum studies necessary for monitoring most patients with CRF is summarized in Table 108–19. This evaluation should be repeated at appropriate intervals; monthly evaluations are suggested for the first several months. The frequency of evaluation may vary, depending on severity of renal dysfunction, complications present in the patient, and response to treatment. For example, patients that require adjustment of therapy for metabolic acidosis or hyperphosphatemia should be examined every 10 to 14 days until satisfactory response is achieved.

Patient reevaluation at regular intervals is necessary to accurately assess response to therapy. Diet formulation and other forms of symptomatic and supportive therapy should be altered on the basis of these reevaluations to best meet individual patient needs.

Progression of Renal Failure. Serial assessment of renal function may be used to determine a more accurate prognosis and to assess the impact of therapy on renal failure. On the basis of this information, therapy may be modified to better achieve the important therapeutic goal of slowing or stopping progressive deterioration of renal function. Several methods for determining progression of renal dysfunction are available, but all have certain intrinsic disadvantages. Serial measurement of endogenous or exogenous C_{cr} provides a measure of GFR, but such studies are inconvenient and highly variable, and may be associated with the risk of catheter-induced UTI. In addition, incomplete urine collections may constitute an important error in clearance calculations.

Monitoring serial changes in the reciprocal ($1/S_{Cr}$) or logarithm ($\log S_{Cr}$) of the serum creatinine concentration are commonly used to provide an estimate of changes in renal function during long-term therapy of CRF in humans.[57, 242] However, this technique is useful only when serum creatinine concentrations exceed about 3 mg/dl. Serum or plasma creatinine concentration is used rather than serum urea nitrogen because the latter varies with dietary protein intake as well as with renal function. In humans with CRF, one of these two relations is typically found to be linear. In one study, $1/S_{Cr}$ was linear in 57.5 per cent of patients and $\log S_{Cr}$ was linear in 16.4 per cent of patients.[85] Linearity of $1/S_{Cr}$ suggests that renal function is lost at a constant rate (i.e., the same number of nephrons every day), whereas linearity of $\log S_{Cr}$ suggests loss of renal function at a constant fractional rate (i.e., the same fraction of nephrons every day).[84, 242] These techniques provide an assessment of the rate of loss of residual renal function, not a measure of residual GFR.[242] The initiating cause of renal dysfunction does not generally appear to influence the mode of progression.[85] Preliminary studies in dogs suggest that reciprocal of serum creatinine concentration versus time may be linear in this species as well.[58] It has been proposed that the effect of therapy on progression of disease may be assessed by comparing the slope determined before initiation of therapy with that measured during therapy.[85] However, recent data indicate that measuring the slope of the reciprocal of serum creatinine versus time does *not* permit an accurate assessment of the rate of progression of renal disease.

NEPHROTIC SYNDROME

Definition and Clinical Implications

The clinical constellation of proteinuria, hypoalbuminemia, hyperlipidemia, lipiduria, and edema is commonly called the nephrotic syndrome (NS).[276] However, there is a lack of consensus in both human and veterinary medicine as to which of these characteristics is essential for diagnosis of NS. Because massive urine loss of plasma proteins is ultimately responsible for the other constituents of the NS, proteinuria of large magnitude requires the same diagnostic inquiry as the NS. From a diagnostic, prognostic, and therapeutic point of view, entry of large quantities of plasma proteins into the urine through a defect in glomerular barrier function is, in essence, the NS.[277]

Diagnosis of NS indicates localization of renal disease to glomeruli and indicates that the magnitude of loss of plasma proteins in urine is sufficient to predispose the patient to edema, hypotension, malnutrition, hyperlipidemia, and thrombotic diathesis. In humans, massive or *nephrotic range proteinuria* has been defined as urine protein loss in excess of 3.5 gm/24 hr.[277] Proteinuria of this magnitude could result only from glomerular damage. A similar figure has not been established for dogs and cats. However, if proteinuria is of sufficient magnitude to cause hypoalbuminemia, it must be of glomerular origin. The best working definition for NS in dogs and cats is proteinuria of sufficient magnitude to cause clinically significant hypoalbuminemia.

Although NS indicates glomerular disease, most patients with glomerular disease do not develop NS. Canine and feline glomerular diseases may cause NS, CRF, asymptomatic proteinuria, or, in rare instances, ARF. The syndrome(s) that occurs as a result of glomerular disease depends on the severity of the lesions and the biologic behavior of the disease. Lesions that primarily affect selectivity of the filtration barrier are most likely to cause NS. If glomerular lesions are mild or early in the course of disease, or if the patient is able to accommodate large urinary losses of protein, persistent proteinuria may be the sole effect. This condition would be classified as an asymptomatic urinary abnormality. Renal lesions in such patients primarily affect the glomerular basement membranes and visceral epithelial cells and usually are not associated with large numbers of infiltrating or inflammatory cells. Lesions that impair glomerular filtration and/or blood flow through glomerular capillaries are likely to cause ARF or CRF, depending on the rate of progression of the disease process. Renal lesions in these patients are usually characterized by glomerular hypercellularity (so-called proliferative glomerular lesions) and an increase in mesangial matrix (so-called glomerular sclerosis). Some diseases initially affect primarily the filtration barrier, causing NS, and then progressively damage glomerular capillaries and the mesangium, resulting in CRF. Regardless of the syndrome identified, persistent proteinuria of sufficient magnitude to indicate glomerular disease should be pursued diagnostically in the fashion described here for the NS.

In humans, glomerulonephropathy (GN) may also be associated with at least two additional syndromes, acute nephritic syndrome (acute glomerulonephritis) and rapidly progressive glomerulonephritis, which have not as yet been well documented in dogs and cats.[276] Acute nephritic syndrome (NS) in humans is characterized by relatively abrupt onset of hematuria, red blood cell casts, abnormal proteinuria, reduced GFR, circulatory congestion, edema, and hypertension. It is most often associated with infectious diseases, particularly those caused by group A β-hemolytic streptococci. Rapidly progressive glomerulonephritis in humans is characterized by abrupt or insidious onset of hematuria and abnormal proteinuria, with rapidly progressive decline in GFR.

Clinical and Laboratory Characteristics

GN and NS occur in dogs and cats of all ages, but they particularly affect young adults.[278] In recent studies of idiopathic membranous GN, the mean age of cats at the time of diagnosis was 3.2 years,[279, 280] and the mean age of dogs at diagnosis was reported to be 4.5 and 6.5 years.[280, 281] The average age at diagnosis of feline renal amyloidosis has been reported to be 7.5 years (range, 1 to 17 years).[282] However, the mean age at diagnosis of Abyssinian cats with familial renal amyloidosis has been reported to be 3.3 years (range, 2 to 5.5 years). Inherited glomerulopathies have been reported in several breeds of dogs (Table 108—15). It has been suggested that certain cats may be genetically predisposed to GN, but this has not been proved.[283] Male dogs and cats may be affected more frequently than females.[284, 285]

Clinical findings in dogs and cats with NS are often nonspecific. In addition, when glomerular injury results from systemic infectious, inflammatory, or neoplastic diseases, clinical signs may primarily reflect these other disease processes. Common clinical findings in dogs and cats with NS include anorexia, weight loss, poor haircoat, lethargy, and depression that develop insidiously, preceding development of edema.

From a pathophysiologic viewpoint, transudative edema is typically a late clinical finding of the NS (if it occurs). In fact, most studies indicate that edema develops in only a minor percentage of dogs and cats with massive proteinuria and hypoalbuminemia. When edema occurs, it often affects the limbs and/or ventral midline. In severely affected cats, subcutaneous edema may extend to the forelimbs, neck, and even the head.[278] Ascites may occur with or without peripheral edema in both species.[279] Pleural and pericardial effusion may occur, but are less commonly recognized. Edema occasionally affects the intestinal tract, causing nutrient malabsorption, anorexia, and diarrhea.

The NS is associated with an increased tendency toward intravascular coagulation, predisposing nephrotic patients to thromboembolism. Thromboembolism appears to be especially common in dogs with renal amyloidosis.[286, 287] In one study, thrombosis occurred in 20 of 52 dogs with renal amyloidosis.[287] This enhanced thrombotic diathesis may be related to the observation that proteinuria is often more severe in dogs with renal amyloidosis than it is with most other types of GN.[286, 288] The probability of thromboembolic complications is enhanced as the magnitude of proteinuria increases, regardless of the renal lesion involved. The frequency with which thrombotic complications develop in cats with NS is unclear.

The pulmonary vessels are a predominant site of thromboembolic complications in dogs with NS.[286, 287]

Thromboemboli have also been reported to occur in portal veins, femoral arteries, coronary arteries, renal arteries and veins, splenic arteries, and mesenteric arteries.[282] Although renal vein thrombosis is the principal thrombotic phenomenon accompanying NS of humans, renal vein thrombosis appears to be relatively uncommon in dogs and cats with NS.[286, 287] Clinical signs of thromboembolism are related to the location and extent of vascular occlusion. Pulmonary thromboembolism may be recognized by sudden onset of dyspnea, tachypnea, and tachycardia. Thrombi located elsewhere in the body may be associated with acute or chronic intermittent pain; however, many are clinically silent. Acute mesenteric arterial thrombosis may cause sudden onset of abdominal pain, vomiting, and bowel evacuation.[289] Acute renal arterial thrombosis may cause sudden flank pain and hematuria.[289]

Clinical findings referable to the urinary tract are often lacking in patients with NS. During early stages of the disease, most patients retain considerable urine-concentrating ability, and therefore urine volumes are typically normal. Even after azotemic CRF develops, patients with GN may retain some degree of urine-concentrating ability. This discrepancy between reduced GFR and retained urine-concentrating ability (a renal tubular function) is called glomerular-tubular imbalance. During the time when edema is developing, humans with NS may have transient oliguria because of avid sodium and fluid retention. Similar transient, nonpathologic oliguria may occur in dogs or cats as well.

At the time of diagnosis, patients with NS may have concomitant CRF. In fact, GN in dogs is often not detected until signs of renal failure have developed.[278] Unless NS is present, CRF due to GN is typically indistinguishable clinically from CRF due to nonglomerular diseases, on the basis of clinical signs alone. In a prospective survey of 111 dogs with chronic renal disease, 52 per cent were reported to have glomerular disease.[290] In contrast, cats with GN appear more likely to be initially admitted because of edema due to proteinuria. They may ultimately develop CRF.[278] In a recent survey of 74 cats with chronic renal disease, only 6 cats were determined to have GN.[60]

As renal function deteriorates, the magnitude of proteinuria may decline because the quantity of protein cleared as glomerular filtrate decreases. As the quantity of plasma proteins lost into urine declines, clinical manifestations of NS may subside, whereas clinical signs of renal failure become predominant. In addition, patients with NS are predisposed to development of ARF (see sections on ARF and CRF).

Physical findings in patients with NS may be limited to edema and evidence of poor nutrition (e.g., thin, reduced muscle mass, poor haircoat), or they may be associated with characteristic signs of renal failure (when two syndromes coexist). Kidney size may be normal, increased, or decreased on palpation. Increased size may suggest renal amyloidosis or acute GN, whereas decreased size may suggest chronic GN or renal amyloidosis.

Canine and feline glomerular diseases are characterized by moderate to severe proteinuria without hematuria or pyuria. In most patients with NS, semiquantitative tests reveal 3+ or 4+ proteinuria. Urine devoid of protein excludes NS from consideration. Cylindruria is also a common finding in NS. Hyaline casts are thought to occur as plasma proteins bind with Tamm-Horsfall mucoprotein to form protein polymers. Granular casts may be associated with larger plasma proteins embedded in Tamm-Horsfall mucoprotein, or as a result of tubular epithelial cell death caused by progressive glomerular destruction. Microscopic hematuria, a common finding in humans with GN and NS, is unusual in dogs and cats with glomerular disease. Pyuria and other cellular sediment debris are typically absent. Because inflammation and hemorrhage from any location in the urinary tract may cause proteinuria, the possibility of multiple causes of proteinuria should be considered in patients with hypoalbuminemia, hematuria, and/or pyuria.

Hypoalbuminemia occurs in all patients with NS. The magnitude of reduction in serum albumin concentration is variable, but may decrease below 1 gm/dl in severe cases. Hypercholesterolemia and hypertriglyceridemia are also characteristic of NS. Serum α_2- and β_1-globulin concentrations have been reported to be increased in humans and dogs.[284, 292] Total serum globulin concentration may be increased, normal, or decreased. Hyperglobulinemia is probably the result of systemic inflammatory processes. Hypogammaglobulinemia may result from urinary losses of gamma globulin, and is often associated with enhanced risk of infection.[276]

Serum urea nitrogen and creatinine concentrations may be normal or increased, and endogenous creatinine clearance normal or decreased, depending on whether GFR has become substantially impaired. Thus diagnosis of renal disease cannot be excluded based solely on the results of a renal function test. Unless the patient is in renal failure, serum sodium, potassium, chloride, total CO_2, and phosphorus concentrations are typically within normal limits. The anion gap may be reduced because of decreased serum albumin concentration (albumin is an anionic protein). Blood ionized calcium concentration is usually normal; however, total serum calcium concentration may be reduced because approximately 40 to 50 per cent of calcium is bound to albumin.

Nonregenerative anemia occurs with variable frequency in dogs and cats with NS.[284, 285] Increased packed cell volumes may reflect hemoconcentration secondary to hyperproteinemia in some patients. Neutrophilic leukocytosis in patients with NS most often indicates a nonrenal inflammatory lesion or recent corticosteroid administration.[284] Platelet counts are usually normal, but may be decreased.

The macroscopic appearance of kidneys from dogs and cats with NS due to GN is often normal.[285] If GN has progressed to CRF, the kidneys may be reduced in size with finely granular capsular surfaces and narrowed cortices. Kidney size may be increased, normal, or decreased with renal amyloidosis. Kidneys from cats with glomerular and interstitial amyloidosis are often small, irregular, pale, and yellow.[283] They may be scarred, pitted, and firm. The cut surfaces often reveal an unevenly narrowed cortex and indistinct corticomedullary junction. Papillary necrosis may occur as a result of interstitial accumulations of amyloid, and is recognized by a blunt, irregular papillae with a small hemorrhagic zone where partial or complete separation of the renal pelvis from the medulla has occurred.

Causes

GLOMERULONEPHROPATHIES

Overview. The terms glomerulonephropathy and glomerulonephritis (GN), with various qualifying prefixes (Table 108–27), are commonly used to describe the variable responses of different cells and structures within glomeruli to injury. Because glomerular lesions in many patients are not associated with an obvious inflammatory response, the less specific term, glomerulonephropathy, may provide a more accurate collective description than glomerulonephritis. Because the etiopathogenesis of this disorder appears to be highly variable, a morphologic diagnosis of GN does not imply a specific diagnosis. GN is characterized by morphologic and functional abnormalities in glomeruli that, if progressive, may induce changes in renal tubules, interstitial tissue, and blood vessels. GNs are distinguished from other types of primary renal disease (i.e., tubular disease, pyelonephritis, interstitial disease) by changes that initially and predominantly affect glomeruli.

The term primary glomerulopathy is used when damage to the glomerulus results from a disease largely confined to this structure.[277] Glomerular damage that occurs in association with a variety of systemic and heredofamilial disorders is termed secondary GN. In these disorders, the underlying disease process damages not only the glomerulus, but other major organs as well. Examples of secondary GNs that may occur in dogs or cats include systemic amyloidosis, systemic lupus erythematosus, diabetic nephropathy, dirofilariasis, hyperadrenocorticism, mercury intoxication, and bacterial endocarditis.

Clinically significant glomerular diseases often result from immunologic injury to the glomerulus. These immunologic injuries are thought to result from the following two basic types of processes: (1) immune complex disease in which the immunologic reaction is directed against nonglomerular antigens (or altered glomerular antigens), and (2) anti-glomerular basement membrane (anti-GBM) disease, in which antibodies are directed against antigens in the GBM. These two forms of GN may be differentiated by immunofluorescence microscopy. Immune complex disorders are characterized by

TABLE 108–27. PRIMARY GLOMERULOPATHIES OF HUMANS—TYPICAL MORPHOLOGY

| Morphologic Diagnosis | Morphologic Lesions | | |
	Light Microscopy	Immunofluorescence Microscopy	Electron Microscopy
Minimal change	Normal	Negative	Loss of foot processes
Membranous	Thick capillary wall	Granular IgG and C3 in capillary loops	Subendothelial deposits*
Membranoproliferative			
Type I	Increased mesangial matrix, cellularity, and thick capillary wall	C3, variable Ig in capillary loops and mesangium	Subendothelial deposits, mesangial interposition
Type II	Same as Type I	C3 in capillary loops and mesangium	Intramembranous dense deposits
Mesangial proliferative	Mesangial proliferation	Negative or mesangial IgM	Mesangial deposits
Focal and segmental glomerulosclerosis	Focal and segmental glomerular sclerosis and/or hyalinization	Negative or segmental IgM and C3 in affected areas	Focal sclerosis, loss of foot processes, subendothelial deposits
Idiopathic crescentic			
Type I	Epithelial crescents	Linear anti-GBM, Ig and C3	No deposits
Type II	Same as Type I	Granular Ig and C3 in capillary loops	Capillary wall dense deposits
Type III	Same as Type I	Negative	No deposits
Acute poststreptococcal	Diffuse proliferation	Granular diffuse IgG and C3 in capillary loops and mesangium	Subepithelial "humps"
IgA nephropathy	Mesangial proliferation	Mesangial IgA and C3, also IgG and/or IgM, less intense than IgA	Mesangial deposits

| Morphologic Diagnosis | Recommended Treatment in Humans | Renal Prognosis for Humans | Occurs In Dogs and Cats? | |
			Dogs	Cats
Minimal change	Corticosteroids/cytotoxic agents	Excellent	?	?
Membranous	{ ?-Corticosteroids { ?-Cytotoxic agents	Fair	Yes	Yes
Membranoproliferative	{ ?-Corticosteroids { ?-Antiplatelet agents	Poor	Yes	Yes
Mesangial proliferative	?	?	Yes	?
Focal and segmental glomerulosclerosis	Supportive	Poor	Yes	Yes
Idiopathic crescentic	{ ?-Corticosteroids { ?-Cytotoxic agents { ?-Plasmapheresis { ?-Antiplatelet agents	Poor	Yes	?
Acute poststreptococcal	Supportive	Good	No	No
IgA nephropathy	Supportive	Good	?	?

*Dogs and cats are reported to have predominantly subepithelial deposits in membranous GN.
Adapted from The primary and secondary glomerulopathies. In: Brenner, BM, Coe, FL, and Rector, FC, eds.: Clinical Nephrology. Philadelphia, WB Saunders, 1987, pp. 73–160.

interrupted (granular) fluorescence (usually of IgG and complement) along glomerular capillary walls (Figure 108–7). In contrast, anti-GBM disorders are characterized by uninterrupted linear fluorescence along the GBM. However, presence of anti-GBM antibody has not yet been confirmed in dogs and cats in which a linear fluorescence pattern was detected.[284]

With few exceptions, spontaneous canine and feline GN have been of the immune complex type.[284, 285] Immune complex disease may result from deposition of circulating immune complexes or from local (*in situ*) formation of immune complexes.[293] *In situ* formation of immune complexes may involve antibody reacting locally against exogenous antigens that have been "planted" into glomeruli or against altered glomerular constituents.[294] Subepithelial (epimembranous) deposits of immune complexes are most likely to result from *in situ* immune complex formation, whereas mesangial and subendothelial deposits are typical of deposition of circulating immune complexes.[293] In either situation, immune complex deposition may injure glomeruli through activation of humoral and cell-mediated inflammatory processes. There is also evidence that glomerular injury in membranoproliferative GN and some forms of proliferative GN may result from activation of the alternative complement pathway independent of immune complex deposition.[295]

Although the majority of primary GNs appear to result from immunologic processes, GNs may also result from coagulation disturbances, metabolic/biochemical defects, toxic insults, or hemodynamic processes. Examples of diseases in which GN may occur as a result of these processes include hemolytic-uremic syndrome, diabetes mellitus, mercury toxicity, and hyperadrenocorticism (see Chapter 107).

Morphologic Forms of Glomerulonephropathy in

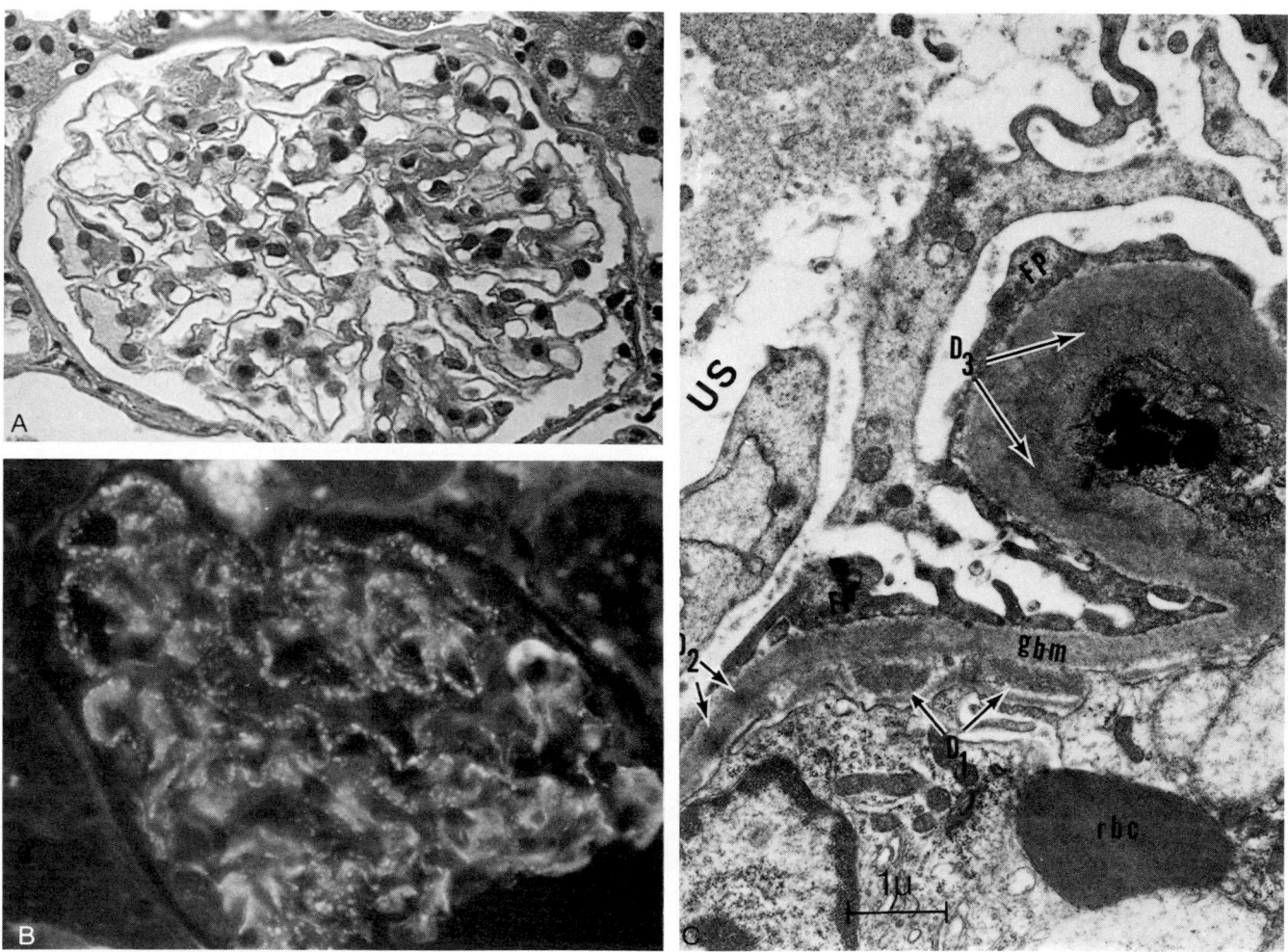

FIGURE 108–7. *A,* Photomicrograph of a renal biopsy specimen obtained from a four-year-old male Great Dane with a history of nephrotic syndrome. There is segmental thickening of the walls of glomerular capillaries. Two micron section; H & E stain; original magnification × 160. *B,* Fluorescent micrograph of a glomerulus contained in a renal biopsy sample from the same dog. Fluorescein-labeled antibody to canine complement (C_3) is localized in an interrupted granular pattern along glomerular capillary walls. A similar pattern was observed when the glomeruli were evaluated for immunoglobulin G. Original magnification × 170. *C,* Transmission electron micrograph of the renal biopsy sample depicted in *A.* Electron-dense deposits, presumably immune-complexes, are on the endothelial side (D_1) and within the glomerular basement membranes, (D_2). Foot processes (FP) of visceral epithelial cells adjacent to the electron-dense deposits are swollen. Electron-dense, subendothelial deposits (D3) are also evident in a tangentially sectioned portion of the capillary. gbm = glomerular basement membrane; us = urinary space; rbc = red blood cell. (From Osborne CA, et al: Natural remission of nephrotic syndrome in a dog with immune-complex glomerular disease. J Am Vet Med Assoc 168:129, 1976.)

Dogs and Cats. OVERVIEW. Classification of GNs should be based on an understanding of their etiopathogenesis. Because the cause of GN is often unknown, it is common practice to describe GN according to glomerular morphologic lesions. Knowledge of glomerular lesions is of great importance in human medicine because it traditionally has been used as the basis for formulating prognoses and planning therapy (Table 108–27). Similar correlations between glomerular morphology and prognosis and treatment have not been developed for dogs and cats. Because application of human classification schemes to canine and feline GNs has not been validated, a universal classification scheme for canine and feline GN has not been agreed on.

Glomerular lesions are described according to changes in glomerular capillary membrane thickness, changes in glomerular cellularity (number, type, and location of cells, if possible), and location and extent of lesions. Membrane thickening is generally described as *membranous GN*, while increased cellularity is described as *proliferative GN*. A combination of membrane thickening with increased cellularity is called *membranoproliferative GN*. Glomerular scarring associated with increases in mesangial matrix and sometimes cellularity is described as *glomerular sclerosis*. These reactions are further described as diffuse (i.e., involving all glomeruli), focal (i.e., involving only some glomeruli), generalized (i.e., involving all portions of affected glomeruli), or segmental (i.e., involving only portions of affected glomeruli).

MEMBRANOUS GLOMERULONEPHROPATHY. The light microscopic appearance of membranous GN is characterized by progressive thickening of glomerular capillary walls (basement membranes) with minimal cellular proliferation or infiltrate.[279, 281, 283] Early lesions may be only minimally discernible by light microscopy.[285] Immunofluorescence microscopy typically reveals diffuse granular deposition of IgG and C3. Other immunoglobulins may also be detected. When examined by electron microscopy, subepithelial (epimembranous) electron-dense deposits may be found along glomerular capillary basement membrane.[279, 281] The GBM is commonly thickened and irregular, presumably as a result of increased GBM synthesis. Proliferation and remodelling of the GBM may progressively encompass the epimembranous electron-dense deposits to form "spikes" that are unique to membranous GN. In advanced cases, these spikes may be seen by light microscopy if sections are stained with silver stains.

Membranous GN is the most common form of GN in cats, and often results in NS in this species. However, if lesions become more advanced, and if GFR begins to decline, many cats initially recognized as having NS ultimately develop CRF.[279] In a recent study of 24 cats with idiopathic membranous GN, all had proteinuria and hypoalbuminemia. Only six cats were also uremic.[279]

Membranous GN appears to be less common than the various proliferative forms of GN in dogs.[296] Many dogs with this condition are recognized after CRF has developed. In a recent study of canine membranous GN, 9 of 14 dogs were azotemic, although only 6 of the 14 had NS.[281] In another study, membranous GN was reported to be no more likely than proliferative forms of GN to result in NS.[284]

MEMBRANOPROLIFERATIVE (MESANGIOCAPILLARY) GLOMERULONEPHROPATHY. Membranoproliferative GN is characterized by diffuse and global expansion of the mesangium due to an increase of both cells and matrix.[297] These changes often accentuate the lobular appearance of the glomerulus. The peripheral capillary walls are thickened due to interposition of mesangium between the endothelial cell layer and the GBM proper, giving rise to an appearance of "splitting" or "reduplication" of the peripheral capillary walls. Electron microscopy typically reveals subendothelial and mesangial electron-dense deposits and the interposition of mesangial cytoplasm and matrix.

PROLIFERATIVE GLOMERULONEPHROPATHY. Proliferative GN encompasses all glomerular lesions that are characterized by a definite increase in the cellularity of individual glomeruli.[297] Morphologically, proliferative lesions may be divided into two broad groups: diffuse proliferative GN and focal proliferative GN. Individual glomeruli may be segmentally or globally affected. Furthermore, cellular proliferation may involve the glomerular capillary tufts themselves or be predominantly extracapillary.

Increased glomerular cellularity may result from proliferation of epithelial, endothelial, or mesangial cells, or from influx of mononuclear or polymorphonuclear leukocytes into (primarily) the mesangium or around the glomerulus. Thus, glomerular hypercellularity is not solely caused by cellular proliferation. Hypercellularity may be divided into three categories: (1) pure proliferative GN, in which hypercellularity is the result of increased number and rate of division of mesangial, endothelial, or epithelial cells, (2) pure exudative, in which hypercellularity is the result of infiltration with inflammatory cells, and (3) mixtures of combined proliferative and exudative lesions. Differentiation of infiltrating mononuclear cells from proliferating mesangial cells is difficult, and may require use of special staining techniques.

When examined by electron microscopy, proliferative GN is characterized by subendothelial, membranous, or mesangial electron-dense deposits. Immunofluorescence microscopy typically reveals interrupted granular deposits of IgG and C3 in the mesangium and along glomerular capillary walls. Proliferative GN may be slowly or rapidly progressive. It typically results in CRF without NS.

GLOMERULAR SCLEROSIS. Glomerular sclerosis is a nonspecific lesion characterized by increased mesangial matrix and limited mesangial cellular proliferation. This lesion is often seen in glomeruli of patients with CRF. Nonimmunologic processes that may be associated with glomerular sclerosis include aging, nonglomerular renal diseases, radiation nephrotoxicity, glomerular hypertension, and a variety of other causes. It may occur as a focal or generalized lesion, and may be segmental or diffuse.

Etiologic Factors Associated with Glomerulonephritis. A variety of etiologic factors incriminated in spontaneous and experimental GN should be investigated in dogs and cats with NS (Table 108–28).[276, 282, 298, 299] In one recent study, chronic extrarenal medical disorders were identified in 88 per cent of dogs with GN.[284] In

TABLE 108–28. CAUSATIVE FACTORS THAT MAY BE ASSOCIATED WITH GLOMERULONEPHROPATHIES IN DOGS AND CATS

Inflammatory—Infectious
  Canine adenovirus I infection
  Feline leukemia virus infection
  Feline infectious peritonitis
  Canine dirofilariasis
  Bacterial endocarditis
  Canine pyometra *(Escherichia coli)*
  Ehrlichiosis (dogs)
  Brucellosis (dogs)
  Leishmaniasis (dogs)
  Borelliosis (Lyme disease)
  Trypanosoma cruzi
  Chronic bacterial infections or abscessation
Inflammatory—Noninfectious
  Systemic lupus erythematosus (viral?)
  Chronic inflammatory skin disease
  Polyarthritis
  Pancreatitis
  Gastroenteritis
  Chronic active hepatitis/cirrhosis associated with *Corynebacterium parvum* immunotherapy
  Other immune-mediated diseases
Neoplasia
  Lymphomas
  Others
Metabolic/Toxic
  Corticosteroids
  Diabetes mellitus
  Cyanotic heart disease
  Ampicillin
  Mercury
  Others

addition to the infectious, inflammatory, and neoplastic processes commonly recognized as being associated with NS and GN, toxic and metabolic processes have also been implicated in glomerular injury, including hyperadrenocorticism, exogenous administration of corticosteroids, ampicillin, diabetes mellitus, mercury toxicity, and cyanotic heart disease.[284, 300–303] GNs associated with endogenous and exogenous corticosteroids, ampicillin, and diabetes mellitus are of uncertain clinical significance, but appear to be unlikely causes of NS. However, mercury intoxication and cyanotic heart disease have been reported to cause NS in cats and humans.[276, 302, 303] Additional agents reported to cause GN and NS in humans, and which should be considered potential etiologic factors in dogs and cats, include nonsteroidal anti-inflammatory agents, organic gold, D-penicillamine, probenecid, bismuth, bee stings, pollens, food allergies, contact dermatitis (poison oak and ivy), vesicoureteral reflux, renal arterial stenosis, malignant hypertension, and immunizations.[276, 292]

AMYLOIDOSIS

Overview. Amyloidosis is a heterogeneous group of diseases in animals and humans that have one major feature in common: the replacement of functional tissue by pathologic fibrillar protein. Amyloidosis is not a single disease, and amyloid is not a single chemical substance. Thus, amyloid has become a generic term for pathologic protein deposits that share certain morphologic, physical, and chemical characteristics. Regardless of the type, amyloid deposits in tissue sections may

be recognized by their characteristic affinity for Congo red dye, which is seen as orange-red staining with brightfield microscopy and green birefringence under polarized light. By electron microscopy, amyloid has the appearance of a felt-like array of linear, nonbranching fibrils, which are 7.5 to 10.0 nm in diameter and of indefinite length.[304] Biochemically, amyloid fibrils are formed by polymerization of repeated peptide segments.[304] An apparently constant feature of the repetitive protein segments in amyloid fibrils is the arrangement of amino acids in a so-called β-pleated sheet structure.[305, 306] This chemical configuration is thought to be due to the high proportion of hydrophobic amino acids in amyloid proteins, and accounts for their relative insolubility and stability.[304]

Over the last decade, the classification of amyloidosis has become increasingly complex as new amyloid fibril precursor proteins are identified. Nine different proteins are currently known to be amyloid fibril precursors. Current classification schemes incorporate both the protein precursors and the clinical syndrome.

Renal Amyloidosis. In humans, several forms of amyloidosis are known to cause renal disease, whereas in dogs and cats only reactive systemic amyloidosis (so-called secondary amyloidosis) has been definitely identified in the kidney.[307, 308] Reactive systemic amyloidosis is so named because of its association with a variety of chronic inflammatory diseases and some neoplasms. The amyloid fibril precursor in this form of amyloidosis is an acute phase reactant protein known as serum protein AA (SAA).[309] Thus the current designation for this type of amyloidosis is AA amyloidosis. SAA is manufactured in the liver and is known to dramatically increase in serum concentration within hours of injury or onset of various disease processes.[310, 311] The mechanisms by which some individuals with chronic inflammatory disease develop this form of amyloidosis while others do not are not known. In dogs, AA amyloid deposits are most frequently found in the glomeruli, where they are deposited in the glomerular capillary wall and mesangium. These deposits are often associated with marked proteinuria and NS. In contrast, the medullary interstitium is the most common site of amyloid deposition in cats, although it may occur throughout the kidneys, including glomeruli. Interstitial amyloid deposition is more likely to be recognized as CRF rather than NS because proteinuria may be minimal. Thus, renal amyloidosis in cats is most often recognized as CRF.

An inherited form of AA amyloidosis was described in Abyssinian cats.[243] Amyloid deposits in these cats were always found in renal medullary interstitium and were less commonly found in glomeruli.[244, 312] In addition, other organs, including small intestine, spleen, heart, adrenals, pancreas, liver, lymph nodes, and bladder, often had amyloid deposits in these cats. It is unclear as to why Abyssinians develop AA amyloidosis, since predisposing inflammatory diseases were not consistently found in affected cats.

The most common form of renal amyloidosis in humans is immunocyte dyscrasia associated amyloidosis (so-called primary amyloidosis). This form of amyloidosis is associated with diseases of B lymphocytes or plasma cells, such as multiple myeloma, monoclonal gammopathy, and Waldenstrom's macroglobulinemia.[304] The precursor protein is derived from the variable region of immunoglobulin light chains,[313] and therefore, this form of amyloidosis is referred to as AL amyloid. AL amyloid deposits occur in the kidneys in the same locations as AA amyloid. This form of amyloidosis has not been documented in the kidneys of dogs or cats.

Another form of amyloidosis, which may be found in human renal blood vessels, is senile amyloidosis (SSA).[314] This form of amyloidosis typically is found in the heart, lung, and blood vessels in many organs except the brain in the elderly. The amyloid fibril precursor protein to this form of amyloid is transthyretin (prealbumin), a circulating serum protein.[315] Both AA and AL amyloidosis may be deposited in renal arteries and veins. These deposits may partially occlude the vessels and produce tissue ischemia.

It was recognized that patients undergoing long-term hemodialysis for renal failure develop a peculiar form of amyloidosis in which the amyloid deposits occur predominantly in synovium and bone. The amyloid fibril precursor in this disease is β_2-microglobulin, which is normally present on the surfaces of nucleated cells in association with class I histocompatibility antigens.[316, 317] Rarely, urinary stones and tubular casts composed of this type of amyloid may form in uremic patients on hemodialysis.[318]

Etiologic Factors Associated with Amyloidosis. Amyloidosis may occur subsequent to a variety of chronic suppurative, granulomatous, neoplastic, or inflammatory diseases. It may also occur in patients without identifiable preexisting illnesses. More than 70 per cent of dogs and most cats with renal amyloidosis have been reported to have no obvious predisposing cause.[287] In Abyssinian cats, systemic amyloidosis associated with amyloid protein AA is a familial disease.[282]

Diagnosis

SYNDROME IDENTIFICATION

The NS should be considered whenever persistent proteinuria and hypoalbuminemia occur together. The syndrome is confirmed by determining that hypoalbuminemia results from renal loss of plasma proteins. This association is usually tested by determining if the magnitude of proteinuria is sufficiently great to have caused hypoalbuminemia. However, the correlation between the magnitude of proteinuria and development of hypoalbuminemia is approximate at best; the minimum quantity of proteinuria necessary to cause hypoalbuminemia in dogs and cats has not been determined. Therefore, when the association between proteinuria and hypoalbuminemia is in doubt, it may be necessary to rule out other causes of hypoalbuminemia, such as hepatic failure, protein-losing gastroenteropathy, and severe malnutrition.

As described earlier, urinalyses of patients with NS are characterized by persistent proteinuria without significant hematuria and pyuria. Care must be used in interpreting the significance of proteinuria, since it may be of renal or nonrenal origin. Mild and transient proteinuria may result from pyrexia, seizures, stress, exercise, exposure to extremes of temperature, or venous congestion. Although it has been reported that hematuria and pyuria do not significantly affect urine protein measurements, caution is advised in interpretation of proteinuria when hematuria and pyuria are present.[319, 319a] Marked hematuria, regardless of cause, may be associated with moderate to severe proteinuria because of concomitant plasma protein loss. Slight to large quantities of protein may also appear in urine in association with inflammatory exudate (pyuria, hematuria, and proteinuria) from any location in the genitourinary tract. In humans, certain types of GN may be associated with exudation of inflammatory cells, resulting in proteinuria, pyuria, and hematuria, that are difficult to distinguish from inflammatory lesions of the lower urinary tract. When inflammation or hematuria cloud interpretation of proteinuria, concomitant hypoalbuminemia may provide support for the conclusion that persistent proteinuria is of glomerular origin. In such instances the glomerular origin of proteinuria may be further supported by ruling out other causes of hypoalbuminemia.

Because semiquantitative tests for urine protein are greatly influenced by urine specific gravity, urinalysis findings should be confirmed by assessing the magnitude of proteinuria by means of measuring 24-hour urine protein excretion or determining the urine protein:creatinine ratio (UP:UC). Quantitation of 24-hour urine protein excretion is generally considered the benchmark test for determining the magnitude of proteinuria. The principal advantages of this test are that the quantity of protein lost in urine daily is precisely measured, and that GFR may be determined simultaneously by endogenous creatinine clearance. This information is not only of diagnostic significance, but may also be of value in formulating dietary therapy. The primary disadvantages of tests that require timed urine collections are that they are inconvenient to perform and are subject to error if urine collections are incomplete. If catheterization is required for urine collection, iatrogenic UTI may be introduced. Urinary catheterization should be avoided in patients with NS because they may have compromised immune systems.

Several researchers have published normal values for 24-hour urine protein excretion in dogs (Table 108–29). Urine protein excretion in excess of 13 mg/lb/day (29 mg/kg/day) has been suggested as evidence of glomerular disease in dogs.[284] In 24 normal cats evaluated in our laboratory, 24-hour urine protein excretion ranged from

TABLE 108–29. URINE PROTEIN EXCRETION FOR NORMAL DOGS

Protein (mg/day)		Method of Analysis	Reference
Range	Mean		
41–317	110	TCA-PS	319b
48–1,040	333	TCA-PS	319a
8–151	38	TCA-PS	363
24–197	70	CBB	363
Protein (mg/kg/day)			
2.7–23.2	6.6	TCA-PS	319b
4.55–28.3	13.9	TCA-PS	319a

CBB, Coomassie brilliant blue; TCA-PS, trichloroacetic acid Ponceau-S.

1.3 to 4.0 mg/lb/24 hr (3.0 to 8.9 mg/kg/24 hr) with a mean value of 2.2 mg/lb/24 hr (4.9 mg/kg/24 hr) (see Chapter 107).

To circumvent difficulties associated with collection of timed urine samples, the UP:UC ratio was devised as an alternative means of assessing urine protein losses. This test has the advantage of requiring only a random "spot" urine sample. Recent food consumption does not appear to influence results.[320] All that is required for this test is determination of urine creatinine and protein concentrations. The ratio is calculated by dividing the urine protein concentration (in mg/dl) by the urine creatinine concentration (in mg/dl). Several investigators have confirmed that this ratio has an excellent correlation with 24-hour urine protein excretion.[321–323] Values for normal dogs are typically less than 0.5.[321–323] In our laboratory normal UP:UC ratios for cats have been determined to average 0.13, with a range of from 0.07 to 0.24. For both dogs and cats, UP:UC values less than 1.0 are considered normal, and values between 1.0 and 2.0 are considered suspect. In the absence of pyuria and hematuria, a UP:UC ratio of greater than 2.0 is highly suggestive of glomerular proteinuria.

It is possible to estimate 24-hour urine protein losses from the UP:UC ratio.[323] When the Coomassie brilliant blue method is used to determine urine protein concentration in dogs, 24-hour protein values (mg/kg/day) can be estimated by the equation:[323]

$$\frac{(UP:UC) + (0.036)}{(0.05)}$$

Using the trichloroacetic acid–Ponceau S method for determining urine protein concentration in dogs, 24-hour protein values (mg/kg/day) can be estimated by the equation:[321]

$$\frac{(UP:UC) - (0.006)}{(0.033)}$$

While substantial proteinuria detected by either of these methods supports a diagnosis of glomerular injury, the degree of proteinuria is often poorly correlated with the severity and extent of glomerular morphologic lesions and renal dysfunction.[288] Although amyloidosis is often associated with the greater magnitude of proteinuria, the type of glomerular lesion present cannot be consistently predicted by the magnitude of proteinuria.

SYNDROME ANALYSIS

Problem-Specific Data Base. Syndrome analysis provides information relevant to formulation of prognosis, and specific and supportive therapy for patients with NS (Table 108–30). Knowledge of the etiopathogenesis of GN is necessary for optimum treatment of NS. Unfortunately, the etiopathogenesis of GN cannot be determined in many instances. Nonetheless, efforts to define the cause of GN and NS are indicated for all patients with these disorders. The problem-specific data base (PSDB) for NS (Table 108–31) provides organization and guidance for evaluating patients with NS and GN.

TABLE 108–30. GOALS OF SYNDROME ANALYSIS FOR THE NEPHROTIC SYNDROME

1. Determine etiology of GN in order to formulate specific therapy for renal disease responsible for NS (Table 108–28).
2. Identify complications that may develop with NS and GN:
   a. Proteinuria, hypoalbuminemia, and hypercholesterolemia
   b. Edema
   c. Thrombotic diathesis
   d. Reduced renal function
   e. Hypertension
   f. Malnutrition
   g. Anemia
3. In formulating an accurate prognosis, consider:
   a. Magnitude of proteinuria and hypoalbuminemia
   b. Renal function status
   c. Amyloid vs other causes of GN
   d. Renal morphology in GN
4. In planning specific therapy for GN and supportive therapy for NS, consider:
   a. Renal morphologic lesions
   b. Primary disease responsible for GN
   c. Magnitude of proteinuria
   d. Renal function
   e. Hypertension
   f. Fluid volume and electrolyte status
   g. Nonregenerative anemia

Selection of optional diagnostic tests from the PSDB should be based on probabilities determined in part from the medical history and findings obtained from the physical examination.

Caution is advised when interpreting immune studies such as antinuclear antibody titers and lupus erythematosus preparations. These tests are often nonspecific and insensitive indicators of immune-mediated disorders in dogs and cats.[324] Therefore, identification of an immunologic process should not be viewed as a diagnostic end point. Additional efforts should be directed toward identification of possible etiologic factors that may have initiated the immunologic process. Failure to pursue these additional diagnostic possibilities may lead to formulation of inappropriate therapy.

Renal Biopsy. INDICATIONS. Evaluation of NS in humans pivots about use of renal biopsy (Table 108–27).[298] In general, renal biopsy is always performed in humans with NS unless the cause of NS is known or strongly presumed, and details of the tissue abnormality will not affect treatment or influence prognosis.[277] Some veterinary internists have agreed that renal biopsy is indicated for dogs and cats with NS or those patients suspected of having GN based on proteinuria. A primary justification given in support of biopsy has been that renal biopsy is usually required to differentiate renal amyloidosis from glomerulonephritis. Differentiation of these two conditions may be important because they differ greatly in prognosis and recommended treatment.

Percutaneous renal biopsy is usually a safe procedure when performed by experienced individuals. Jeraj reported only eight serious complications in a retrospective study of percutaneous renal biopsies performed on 163 dogs and 34 cats.[325] There was a high degree of correlation between the occurrence of biopsy complications and lack of experience of the individuals performing the biopsy procedure. Percutaneous renal biopsy involves significant risk when performed by individuals unfamiliar with the technique. Severe hypertension may also in-

TABLE 108–31. PROBLEM-SPECIFIC DATA BASE FOR NEPHROTIC SYNDROME

1. Medical history and physical examination (Table 108–3)
2. Urinalysis
3. Quantitative measure of proteinuria
   a. 24-hour protein excretion
   b. Urine protein-creatinine ratio
4. Serum total protein, albumin, and globulin concentrations
5. Kidney function tests
   a. Serum urea nitrogen
   b. Serum creatinine concentration
   c. Consider endogenous C_{cr} for nonazotemic patients
6. Serum cholesterol concentration (triglycerides?)
7. Complete blood count (including cytologic examination of blood cells)
8. Serum (or plasma) electrolyte and acid-base profile
   a. Sodium, potassium, and chloride concentrations
   b. Bicarbonate or total carbon dioxide concentrations
   c. Calcium and phosphorus concentrations
9. Serum alanine aminotransferase, alkaline phosphatase, amylase, and lipase activities (R/O hepatic and pancreatic disease)
10. Blood pressure determination (R/O systemic hypertension)
11. Consider:
    a. Freezing aliquots of serum (or plasma) and urine for additional diagnostic determinations that may be desired later (e.g., titers against infectious agents, toxicologic studies, etc.)
    b. Survey radiographs of thorax and abdomen (to identify/localize infectious, inflammatory, or neoplastic processes)
    c. Knott's test, occult heartworm test—R/O dirofilariasis
    d. Immune panel—R/O immune-mediated diseases
       (1) Coombs' test
       (2) Antinuclear antibody test
       (3) Lupus erythematosus preparation
       (4) Joint taps?
       (5) Serum protein electrophoresis
       (6) Others?
    e. Fundic examination—R/O hypertensive lesions, infectious diseases
    f. Screening for infectious diseases
       (1) R/O feline leukemia virus—FeLv test
       (2) R/O bacterial endocarditis—blood cultures, echocardiogram
       (3) R/O borreliosis—specific antibody titers
       (4) R/O brucellosis—specific antibody titers
       (5) R/O ehrlichiosis—specific antibody titers
    g. Coagulation studies—particularly antithrombin III and fibrinogen levels
    h. Renal biopsy to identify morphologic lesion
       (1) Light microscopy
       (2) Immunofluorescence microscopy
       (3) Electron microscopy

R/O, rule out.

crease the risk of biopsy-related complications. Potential complications of renal biopsy include significant hemorrhage, urinary tract obstruction (hydronephrosis) subsequent to clot formation in the renal pelvis or ureters, anesthetic death, infarction of functional renal mass subsequent to vascular damage induced by the biopsy needle, and development of thromboembolic phenomenon following the procedure.

The value of renal biopsy in formulating therapy in humans has recently been questioned.[326–328] A decision analysis study of biopsy-tailored treatment versus empirical treatment indicated that a therapeutic trial with corticosteroids followed by antiplatelet therapy was equivalent to biopsy-tailored therapy in effectiveness in adult nephrotics.[326, 327] Preliminary data indicated that renal biopsy was of only marginal benefit in humans with systemic lupus erythematosus.[328] These researchers argued that expensive or invasive procedures such as biopsy cannot be justified solely on the basis that the procedure yields information, but rather that they should yield useful information that cannot be obtained by simpler and less hazardous means.[328] In the absence of clear guidelines relating biopsy findings to therapy, the need for routine biopsy of all cases of NS and GN in dogs and cats should be questioned. The decision to perform renal biopsy should be based on consideration of risks, the need for an accurate prognosis, and the therapeutic goals of the owner (i.e., will specific therapy be considered or is therapy to be limited to supportive therapy alone?).

METHODS. In dogs, needle biopsies obtained by the keyhole technique typically provide adequate samples for diagnosis with minimum risk of needle-induced hemorrhage. Canine biopsies may also be obtained surgically or with the aid of a laparoscope. In cats, renal biopsies may readily be obtained by percutaneous routes, provided the kidneys are not decreased in size. Ideally, samples should be collected for light, immunofluorescence, and electron microscopy. Specimens for light microscopy should be fixed in 10 per cent buffered formalin solution. Specimens for immunofluorescence microscopy may be placed in either Michel's solution (at room temperature) or isopentane, and "snap-frozen" in liquid nitrogen or a slurry of acetone and dry ice. Many clinicians prefer Michel's solution because it appears to preserve immunofluorescence characteristics well and can be handled at room temperature. Immunoperoxidase techniques that can be performed on formalin-fixed tissue provide an alternative means of evaluating the immunologic basis of renal disease.[329] Samples for electron microscopy should be minced into 1 mm cubes and placed in fresh cold 2 per cent glutaraldehyde. All tissues should be rapidly submitted for examination because storage of samples for processing later may cause artifactual changes to develop.

Complete evaluation of GN requires light, immunofluorescent, and electron microscopic analysis. Characteristic lesions of some of the common forms of GN in dogs and cats have been described earlier. Morphologic descriptions of lesions observed in various human glomerulonephritides are summarized in Table 108–27. However, appropriate caution is advised in extrapolating human classifications to lesions observed in dogs and cats with GN.

In most instances, renal amyloidosis can be identified by light microscopic techniques alone. Routine hematoxylin and eosin staining will provide a preliminary diagnosis of glomerular amyloid, but amyloidosis is best confirmed by use of special stains. Amyloid may be confirmed by its characteristic apple green color when stained with alkaline Congo red and viewed under polarized microscopy. Thioflavine-T will stain amyloid so that it appears yellow-green when viewed by fluorescence microscopy, but this phenomenon is not specific for amyloid. It may also be readily detected ultrastructurally by its appearance as clusters of haphazardly arranged sticks. A presumptive diagnosis of reactive amyloidosis (amyloid AA) may be made using permanganate oxidation techniques.[282] Deposits containing amyloid AA will no longer stain with Congo red after oxidation with permanganate.

Occasionally, gross examination of renal tissue stained by iodine followed by dilute sulfuric acid will provide a preliminary diagnosis of amyloidosis. Iodine stains amyloid red-brown. Using this technique, severely affected glomeruli may be grossly visible as brown "dots" (Figure 108–8).

Prognosis

GLOMERULONEPHRITIS

Although the majority of patients with GN ultimately die as a result of renal-related disease, long-term remissions are not uncommon. Spontaneous recovery may occur.[279, 330] Improvement in renal function and magnitude of proteinuria has been observed in dogs and cats with glomerulonephritis. Survivals of several years have been reported for both dogs and cats.[279, 284, 330] Thus the short-term prognosis (weeks to months) for dogs and cats with glomerulonephritis may be guarded to good, whereas the long-term (years) prognosis is typically guarded.

Factors that may influence prognosis of patients with glomerulonephropathy include: (1) severity of proteinuria, (2) nutritional status of the patient, (3) magnitude of renal dysfunction (and development of uremia), (4) subcutaneous edema, ascites, and hydrothorax, and (5) clinical evidence of thrombosis. Patients with mild to moderate proteinuria and hypoalbuminemia without severe malnutrition and edema often have a relatively good short-term prognosis; their long-term prognosis is guarded. Serial evaluation of such patients is the best means of assessing long-term prognosis. In our experience, the prognosis for dogs and cats with severe proteinuria, weight loss, and ascites is generally poor. The prognosis for azotemic or uremic nephrotic patients is, likewise, poor. However, the clinical condition, existence of prerenal factors, and other complicating factors should be considered[284, 285] (see section on CRF).

Prognosis for cats with membranous GN has been studied in detail.[279] Feline membranous GN may be associated with slow or rapid progression of renal disease, prolonged remissions, or complete recovery.[279] Arthur et al. reported that 8 of 18 cats with membranous GN and NS survived from 2.5 to 6 years; 7 cats recovered completely.[279] With the exception of uremia, clinical signs did not provide a reliable guide to prognosis; uremia heralded a poor prognosis. Although light microscopy provided little guidance as to the eventual outcome, the degree of immune complex deposition and the site of electron-dense deposits were useful prognostic indicators.[279] Cats that were long-term survivors typically had only IgG and/or C_3 deposits in glomerular capillary walls. In contrast, cats that were uremic or survived for only a short time after biopsy had IgM and/or IgA deposits in addition to IgG and C_3 deposits. Detection of intramembranous as well as subepithelial deposits by electron microscopy was associated with more advanced disease and a less favorable long-term prognosis.[279]

RENAL AMYLOIDOSIS

The long-term prognosis for dogs and cats with renal amyloidosis appears to be uniformly poor. Once NS or CRF has developed in patients with renal amyloidosis, the disease inexorably progresses to end-stage failure. Progression to end-stage failure may be rapid or relatively slow (months to years). Patients with amyloidosis are also at increased risk for potentially life-threatening thromboembolic complications that may contribute substantially to mortality.

Treatment

OVERVIEW

Therapy for NS may be subcategorized into specific therapy designed to alter or correct glomerular lesions responsible for development of NS and symptomatic and supportive therapy designed to ameliorate complications associated with NS. In most instances, specific therapy for canine and feline GN is limited by lack of understanding of the etiopathogenesis of glomerular lesions. The effectiveness of most forms of specific

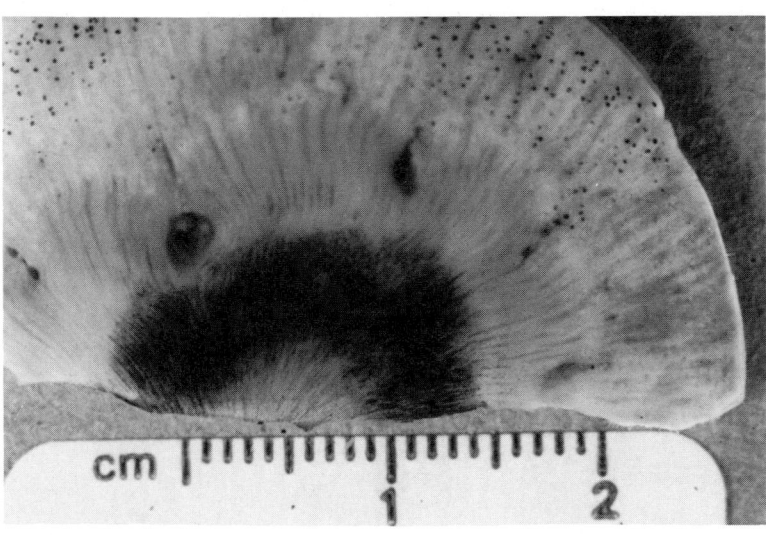

FIGURE 108–8. Kidney section from a four-year-old male Springer spaniel with systemic (AA) amyloidosis, nephrotic syndrome, and an abdominal foreign body. The kidney was stained with Lugol's iodine solution followed by dilute sulfuric acid to demonstrate glomerular (multiple dark round foci in cortex) and interstitial (dark staining regions in medulla) amyloid deposits. The amyloid deposits had strong immunoreactivity (peroxidase-anti-peroxidase stain) to antiserum against canine AA amyloid.

therapy for GN in humans remains controversial. The exceptions are a few select glomerulonephropathies that are not recognized in dogs and cats (e.g., minimal change disease). Studies designed to correlate therapeutic effectiveness with biopsy findings in dogs and cats with GN have apparently not been performed. The fact that even adult humans and children differ greatly in their responses to various forms of treatment emphasizes the caution needed in extrapolation of human therapies to dogs and cats.

Specific treatment of GN is based on identification and removal of antigens and modification of the pathologic processes responsible for glomerular injury. Therapies designed to ameliorate glomerular injury include: (1) immunosuppressive agents to reduce antibody formation, (2) steroidal and nonsteroidal anti-inflammatory agents to reduce the inflammatory effect of immune deposits, (3) anticoagulants to prevent glomerular fibrin deposition, and (4) antiplatelet agents to reduce platelet-mediated glomerular injury. Often, several of these therapies are used simultaneously (e.g., corticosteroids with antiplatelet agents).

Specific therapeutic measures for GN in dogs and cats have been empirical. Many are ineffective; some are potentially hazardous. Caution must be used in selecting potentially harmful drugs for treating patients with GN because the prognosis is not so uniformly poor in all animals that any type of treatment is warranted. Controlled therapeutic trials designed to evaluate the safety and efficacy of various treatment modalities in canine and feline GN are urgently needed. Until results of these trials become available, use of potentially harmful treatments should be recommended only after the owner has been thoroughly appraised of the potential risks and lack of proved efficacy of such treatments. When such therapies are used, the patient must be closely monitored for evidence of adverse effects or response to therapy. In addition, because some forms of GN may be characterized by spontaneous remissions and recovery, caution is advised in concluding that any clinical improvement is the result of the treatment administered.

SPECIFIC TREATMENT OF GLOMERULONEPHRITIS

Elimination of Causative Factors. Elimination of diseases responsible for development of immunologic disturbances and glomerular disease may halt progression of glomerular disease or induce its resolution. For this reason, it is important to attempt to identify infectious and noninfectious agents in dogs and cats suspected of having immune complex GN (Table 108–28). The authors have observed significant improvement in the severity of proteinuria and hypoalbuminemia in some glomerulonephritic dogs with dirofilariasis after elimination of adult parasites and microfilaria by medical therapy. Likewise, removal of the uterus from dogs with pyometra may be associated with improvement in the subclinical glomerular lesions occasionally associated with that disorder. Similar beneficial effects may occur in other forms of GN. Although elimination of antigens is the most logical and seemingly safest therapeutic approach to GN, it is limited in many instances by the obscurity of the antigenic source, the fact that more than one antigen may be involved, and/or identification of an antigenic source that is currently impossible to eliminate (e.g., feline leukemia virus).

Corticosteroid and Immunosuppressive Therapy. Corticosteroids and immunosuppressive drugs (particularly cyclophosphamide, chlorambucil, cyclosporine A, and others) have been used for treating patients with GN with the expectation that they will suppress formation of immune complexes and ameliorate the glomerular inflammatory reaction initiated by antigen-antibody-complement reactions. One theoretical basis for use of these drugs is the concept that patients with GN have a hyperactive immune system, leading to formation of immune complexes that otherwise would not have been formed. However, naturally occurring immune complex GN is not consistently associated with hyperactivity of the immune system. To the contrary, at least some patients with immune complex disease may have suppressed rather than hyperactive immune systems. Formation during moderate antigen excess (a condition most likely to occur with an impaired immune system) produces immune complexes of the size most likely to be deposited in glomeruli and initiate glomerular injury. Failure of the mononuclear phagocyte system to eliminate circulating immune complexes may also facilitate their glomerular deposition. Moderate antigen excess and failure of the mononuclear phagocyte system are consistent with an immunosuppressed condition. Therefore, administration of corticosteroids and cytotoxic agents to patients with GN that results from glomerular deposition of circulating immune complexes may be harmful rather than beneficial. However, this line of reasoning may not be valid when immune complexes are formed *in situ*, because glomerular injury does not result from deposition of circulating immune complexes or lack of their destruction by the mononuclear-phagocyte system.

Although corticosteroids appear an illogical choice for some patients with GN, they are of recognized benefit in treatment of minimal change disease in humans (Table 108–27). In addition, some recent studies indicate that corticosteroids and/or immunosuppressive agents (primarily alkylating agents) may be beneficial in treatment of human patients with membranous GN, membranoproliferative GN, and proliferative GN.[297, 331, 332] Other studies of the effectiveness of corticosteroids and immunosuppressive agents in treatment of membranous and proliferative GN in humans have provided conflicting results. Therefore their use to treat the aforementioned types of GN remains controversial.[294, 331, 333, 334] A major factor confounding interpretation of studies designed to evaluate effectiveness of these drugs in treatment of GN is the unpredictable course of many forms of GN. For example, the clinical outcome has been reported to be unfavorable in only 13 per cent of humans with membranous GN. Because the vast majority of patients with this disease do well without treatment, it is difficult to assess the value of empirical use of corticosteroids on the population as a whole.

Controlled studies of the effectiveness of corticosteroids and/or immunosuppressive agents in therapy of canine and feline GNs have not been reported. The fact that these drugs appear to be of value in treatment of GN in humans provides a rationale for their use in some dogs and cats. However, uncontrolled clinical observations fail to support the view that corticosteroids are beneficial in canine or feline GN.[279, 284, 335–337] Pending the results of controlled studies, the empirical use of corticosteroids and/or immunosuppressive therapy for canine and feline patients with GN must be considered in light of the balance between potential benefits and known adverse effects of such therapy.

Empirical use of corticosteroids to treat canine and feline GNs is not without risk. Corticosteroids may increase the magnitude of azotemia and promote development of uremia in glomerulonephritic patients with reduced GFR.[26] Because of this effect and the probability that corticosteroid therapy will be of no value in patients with GN once CRF has already developed, corticosteroids are not routinely recommended for patients with chronic GN.[298] The immunosuppressive effects of corticosteroids may also increase risk of infection and promote earlier glomerular deposition of circulating immune complexes. When GN results from neoplasia, corticosteroid therapy may increase the number of metastases and induce metastases in unusual locations.[294] Corticosteroids also appear to increase the risk of thromboembolism.[338]

Another major concern is the possibility that corticosteroids may promote proteinuria and additional glomerular injury. Recent studies in rats have shown that chronic administration of corticosteroids to rats with extensive ablation of renal mass is associated with striking acceleration of glomerular injury.[339] It has been hypothesized that glomerular injury results from glomerular hypertension in a manner similar to that which occurs with high-protein feeding after reduction in renal mass (see section on Diet Therapy of CRF). Glomerular hypertension appears to result from a renal vasodilatory effect of corticosteroids.[340] Corticosteroids are known to increase GFR in dogs, rats, and humans.[340] The clinical significance of this phenomenon is emphasized by the recent observation that 14 of 41 dogs with GN had spontaneous canine Cushing's syndrome or had been treated with corticosteroids.[284]

If empirical corticosteroid therapy is elected, the success of therapy may be influenced by several factors, including: (1) drug dosage, (2) route of administration, (3) duration of therapy, and (4) drug combination used.[297, 331, 333] Several recent reports in humans with GN indicate success using corticosteroid "pulse" therapy. Large intravenous doses of methylprednisolone were administered for several days followed by standard alternate-day oral therapy with prednisolone.[297, 334] It is noteworthy that corticosteroid "pulse" therapy has been reported to be effective in treatment of autoimmune skin disease in dogs.[341] The impact of corticosteroid pulse therapy on proteinuria and glomerular injury is unknown, but it has been suggested that low-dose corticosteroid therapy combined with immunosuppressive agents may be less likely to adversely affect the glomerulus. However, administration of immunosuppressive agents may be associated with a variety of nonglomerular toxicities and side effects, depending on the drug selected. Patients treated with corticosteroids should be closely monitored for development of the side effects described earlier as well as for gastrointestinal complications (see Chapter 52).

Anticoagulant and Anti-Platelet Therapy. Anticoagulant (heparin, coumadin) and antiplatelet (aspirin, indomethacin, dipyridamole, and others) therapies have been used for treatment of GN in humans because of the apparent role of the coagulation system in development of glomerular lesions. Intraglomerular coagulation and fibrin deposition appear to play a role in many glomerulonephritides, although the cause of glomerular fibrinogenesis remains unknown.[342, 342a] There is also evidence from both experimental GN and spontaneous human GN that platelets may be involved in mediating or amplifying glomerular injury by: (1) promoting proliferation of glomerular mesangial and endothelial cells, and (2) by increasing vascular permeability, thereby facilitating glomerular localization of circulating immune complexes.[343] Platelets may also promote proteinuria through glomerular localization of platelet-derived cationic secretory proteins, leading to loss of glomerular fixed anionic charge and enhanced glomerular capillary permeability.[297] Platelet-related antigens have been demonstrated in glomeruli of patients with GN.[343]

Platelets have been described as inflammatory cell fragments that can induce inflammation and release chemotactic and mitogenic substances.[344] Platelet turnover, an indicator of platelet activity, has been found to be increased in several forms of GN.[344] Furthermore, a positive correlation has been reported between intraglomerular cell proliferation and increased platelet consumption.[345] Evidence supporting a link between increased platelet destruction, proliferation of mesangial cells, and glomerular inflammation is based on observations that platelet-derived factors stimulate proliferation and migration of arteriolar smooth muscle cells and are chemotactic for monocytes and neutrophils.[345, 346] Such effects may be even more pronounced in patients with NS because platelets are hyperaggregable in nephrotics.

Anticoagulant and antiplatelet therapies have been used primarily for treatment of membranoproliferative GN in humans. Combination therapy with cyclophosphamide, dipyridamole, and warfarin sodium was found to have no beneficial effect on renal function and glomerular morphology in two randomized controlled trials of humans with membranoproliferative GN.[346, 347] In contrast, platelet-inhibitor therapy with dipyridamole and aspirin slowed progression of renal disease and retarded deterioration of renal function in humans with membranoproliferative GN.[346] However, proteinuria, hematuria, and levels of serum complement were not influenced by this treatment. It was proposed that platelet-inhibitor therapy slowed progressive glomerular injury as a result of reduced platelet-vascular wall interaction or platelet consumption, or reduced renal and platelet prostaglandin production (particularly thromboxane A_2). Thromboxane A_2 may act as an important mediator of glomerular injury by influencing renal vasoconstriction, platelet aggregation, and leukocyte adhesiveness.[346]

Therapy with the antiplatelet agents ticlopidine and dipyridamole significantly reduced urinary protein excretion in rats with nephrotoxic serum nephritis, but significant differences in glomerular morphology were not seen.[343] It was proposed that dipyridamole may have antiproteinuric effects other than inhibition of platelet aggregation. However, the precise mechanism of the antiproteinuric effect of these antiplatelet agents was not determined.

The efficacy and safety of antiplatelet agents and anticoagulants have not yet been evaluated in dogs and cats with GN. However, in humans, combination therapy with dipyridamole and aspirin was associated with hemorrhagic complications. Anticoagulant therapy may be associated with a substantial risk of hemorrhagic complications.[296, 347] In one study, 37 per cent of patients given the combination of cyclophosphamide, coumadin, and dipyridamole had significant hemorrhagic complications.[347] Pending results of controlled clinical trials documenting the safety and efficacy of these drugs in treatment of canine and feline GN, treatment with this class of drugs should probably be limited to administration of low doses of aspirin.

Other Modes of Therapy. A variety of other treatments have been used in an attempt to modify the course of GN, including administration of levamisole as an immunomodulating agent, and plasmapheresis in an attempt to remove circulating immune complexes and/or antigens.[348–350] Although experience with such treatments has been limited, preliminary results with plasmapheresis in treatment of canine GN have not been encouraging. The authors have no experience with levamisole therapy in canine or feline GN.

SPECIFIC TREATMENT OF AMYLOIDOSIS

Renal amyloidosis appears to be highly resistant to specific therapy; to date, no therapy has proved efficacious in slowing or eliminating renal or systemic amyloidosis. Patients with reactive systemic amyloidosis (amyloid AA) may respond to removal of the underlying disease process, including chronic inflammatory, granulomatous, or neoplastic diseases. Although such therapy may be of great benefit in early renal amyloidosis, there is little evidence that removal of an inciting cause will result in improvement or resolution of renal amyloidosis once sufficient renal damage has occurred to cause NS or renal failure. Nonetheless, treatment of the primary inciting cause is a rational and generally safe therapeutic approach.

Dimethyl-sulfoxide (DMSO) has been proposed as potential therapy for amyloidosis, but its effectiveness is highly controversial. It was reported to be ineffective in four dogs with spontaneous renal amyloidosis.[351] However, renal function was observed to improve in some human patients treated with DMSO.[282] It has also been reported to be beneficial in at least two dogs with renal amyloidosis.[18] In the first, 57 mg/lb (125 mg/kg) of DMSO was administered orally twice daily as a 10 per cent solution for nine months. Renal function and clinical condition were reported to improve, but the magnitude of proteinuria did not decline.[18] In the second dog, DMSO administered three times weekly at a dose of 36 mg/lb (80 mg/kg) reduced the magnitude of pro-

teinuria and corrected hypoalbuminemia during two years of therapy.[352] The drug was administered subcutaneously the first year and topically the second year. Improvement in proteinuria may have occurred subsequent to resolution of factors responsible for development of amyloidosis (rather than solely as an effect of DMSO therapy).

The mechanism(s) by which DMSO affects renal function and proteinuria in patients with renal amyloidosis is not completely understood. Dimethylsulfoxide may: (1) aid in solubilizing amyloid fibrils and removing amyloid subunit proteins, (2) decrease plasma concentrations of the amyloid precursor protein SAA, and (3) reduce inflammation and fibrosis in affected kidneys.[282] Despite evidence that DMSO improves renal function and proteinuria, it appears unlikely that DMSO reduces renal amyloid deposition.[352] It has been suggested that the beneficial effects of DMSO may result from its anti-inflammatory effects on any primary localized or systemic inflammatory conditions and on the intrarenal inflammatory and fibrotic response to amyloid deposition. Amyloid-induced renal inflammation and fibrosis may be a major cause of reduced renal function in renal amyloidosis.[352]

DMSO may be administered intravenously, subcutaneously, topically, or orally. It reportedly has low systemic toxicity. In one of the dogs described above, the only side effect observed during two years of treatment was the characteristic unpleasant odor of DMSO.[352] Potential side effects include perivascular inflammation and local thrombosis with use of undiluted DMSO, reversible hemolytic anemia subsequent to repeated intravenous administration of concentrated DMSO, and reversible reduced lucency of the lens cortex.[352] Considering the apparent low toxicity of DMSO, the progressive nature of renal amyloidosis, and the lack of effective alternative therapy, a therapeutic trial with DMSO may be justified for patients with renal amyloidosis.

Colchicine is another agent that has been used for certain forms of amyloidosis in humans. Colchicine acts by blocking hepatocyte secretion of SAA. There is evidence that it reduces the incidence of amyloidosis in human patients with familial Mediterranean fever.[282] However, colchicine therapy is probably of greater prophylactic benefit than of therapeutic benefit once amyloidosis has developed. It has not been critically evaluated in dogs and cats.

Because renal amyloidosis almost always progresses inexorably to renal failure, and there is no proven specific treatment for the disorder, it is tempting to consider any therapy that may alter its progression. Nonetheless, care should be used in formulating therapy for patients with renal amyloidosis because inappropriate therapy may accelerate deposition of amyloid or promote life-threatening complications. For example, corticosteroids and immunosuppressive agents appear to be of no proven benefit and may promote renal deposition of amyloid. Corticosteroids promoted amyloidosis in rats after intraperitoneal injection of casein, and may increase the risk for development of thromboembolism.[338, 353]

SYMPTOMATIC AND SUPPORTIVE TREATMENT

Renal Failure. As described earlier, GNs may be associated with ARF or CRF instead of or in addition to NS. Primary or secondary glomerular diseases may cause sufficient irreversible loss of nephrons to result in CRF. Patients with NS may be predisposed to ARF because of volume depletion associated with the NS, or because of the nature of their glomerulopathy (i.e., acute glomerular injury). Because specific therapy, such as corticosteroids or immunosuppressive agents, may be indicated for glomerulonephropathies associated with ARF but is generally not indicated for patients with CRF, it is important to determine if renal failure is acute or chronic in these patients (see sections on ARF and CRF).

Proteinuria and Hypoalbuminemia. OVERVIEW. Proteinuria, and particularly albuminuria, is central to the pathophysiology of NS. All of the principal complications of NS, including hypoalbuminemia, edema, hyperlipidemia, and hypercoagulability, can ultimately be attributed to excessive albuminuria. Hypoalbuminemia may also result in an increased incidence of drug toxicity because of reduced protein-binding of drugs and trace mineral (zinc, iron, and copper) deficiency due to urinary excretion of binding proteins.[276] Therefore, minimizing the magnitude of proteinuria, and particularly albuminuria, is an important therapeutic goal.

Proteinuria may result from dysfunction of either of two interdependent but discrete permeability functions of the glomerular capillaries: the charge-selective capillary barrier or the size-selective capillary barrier.[354] The charge-selective capillary barrier is based on the interaction between charges of circulating plasma protein molecules and anionic moieties (sulfated glycosoaminoglycans, sialoglycoproteins, and the free carboxyl groups of collagen) in glomerular capillary walls. Neutralization or alteration in the synthesis or catabolism of these molecular and cellular components of capillary walls and basement membranes will cause loss of the electrorepulsive action of similarly charged elements. Because albumin acts as a polyanion at normal blood pH and is of sufficiently small size to penetrate into the pores of the capillary wall, albuminuria is the principal clinical manifestation of such a disturbance in barrier charge structure. The size-selective capillary barrier is based on the observation that the glomerular capillary wall behaves as if it were penetrated by a series of cylindrical pores of similar dimensions (isosporous) having internal radii of approximately 4.7 to 5.0 nm.[354] With GNs, the density of pores decreases and the total filtration area is reduced, but a new population of pores emerges that has larger internal dimensions. This altered-pore population with large pores results in increased heteroporosity of the capillary wall and loss of larger molecules such as IgG (nonselective proteinuria). Protein loss through large pores may be further enhanced because these pores may have reduced charge selectivity as well. Thus albuminuria suggests disordered charge-selective barrier function, while gammaglobulinuria suggests disordered size-selective barrier function.

Although albuminuria is ultimately responsible for hypoalbuminemia in patients with NS, it is not the only factor that determines serum albumin concentration. Factors that influence development of hypoalbuminemia include (1) the magnitude of albuminuria, (2) dietary protein intake, (3) the rate of uptake and catabolism of filtered protein by the proximal renal tubules, (4) partitioning of albumin between intravascular and extravascular spaces, and (5) the rate of hepatic albumin synthesis.[298] Because serum albumin concentration may be influenced by these diverse factors, patients with similar magnitudes of proteinuria often have markedly dissimilar serum albumin concentrations.

In addition to albuminuria, nephrotic patients may have reduced plasma concentrations of a host of other important proteins due to exaggerated urinary losses, including IgG, factor B of the alternative complement pathway, calciferol-binding globulin, and transferrin.[298] Diminished concentrations of IgG and factor B may predispose nephrotic patients to infection. Deficiency of calciferol-binding globulin may cause vitamin D deficiency and promote hypocalcemia, secondary hyperparathyroidism, and renal osteodystrophy. Transferrin deficiency may result in microcytic, hypochromic anemia resistant to iron supplementation.

MODIFYING THE MAGNITUDE OF PROTEINURIA. Dietary protein supplements and high-protein diets have often been recommended for patients with NS on the assumption that hypoalbuminemia may be improved by increased protein intake. Surprisingly, recent studies have shown that high dietary protein intake may have an adverse effect on the magnitude of proteinuria and hypoalbuminemia.[355] Because consumption of high-protein diets is typically associated with glomerular hypertension, such diets may also promote progressive glomerular injury.[332] Nephrotic rats that were fed a high-protein diet had increased albuminuria and more severe hypoalbuminemia than rats fed a lower protein diet.[356] Preliminary studies in our hospital suggest that reducing dietary protein intake (from levels found in typical canine maintenance diets to approximately 14 per cent calories as protein) in dogs with NS markedly reduced their magnitude of proteinuria. Kaysen has shown that reducing dietary protein intake in humans with NS limits proteinuria without impairing protein nutrition.[355] In fact, total body albumin mass was preserved and plasma albumin concentrations increased when low-protein diets were fed. It was concluded that protein restriction may be beneficial in patients with NS. Changes in the magnitude of albuminuria were detected within 14 days of diet change in humans and dogs. However, the long-term consequences of protein restriction in humans, dogs, and cats with NS have not yet been conclusively determined.

Based on these findings, it is recommended that dogs with NS initially be fed diets formulated to contain approximately 12 to 14 per cent of their calories as protein (i.e., protein intake similar to that recommended for canine CRF). Cats with NS should be fed diets formulated to contain approximately 20 per cent of their calories as protein. Approximately two weeks after diet change, renal function, serum albumin concentration, and proteinuria (24-hour urinary protein quantitation or the UP:U_{Cr} ratio) should be reevaluated. If the reduction in protein intake has been effective in decreasing the magnitude of proteinuria, and has not adversely affected renal function or serum albumin concentration, dietary protein restriction may be continued. However, adverse nutritional effects of protein restriction may not become apparent for weeks or months. Therefore, continued monitoring of renal function, proteinuria, and serum albumin concentration is recommended. Because serum albumin concentration may be an insensitive indicator of protein nutrition, body weight and subjective assessments of protein nutrition such as muscle mass and haircoat condition should also be monitored.

It has been recommended that the quantity of protein lost daily in urine be replaced by supplementing the diet with the same quantity of protein, usually in the form of egg protein. The impact of such supplementation on the magnitude of proteinuria and the renal structure and function in dogs and cats with NS is unknown. However, if the magnitude of proteinuria is great, restricted protein diets may fail to provide sufficient protein. If protein replacement therapy is elected, the impact of such therapy on the magnitude of proteinuria should be assessed. Protein supplementation should be discontinued if proteinuria and/or hypoalbuminemia worsens.

Dietary lipids may also influence the magnitude of proteinuria and development of progressive glomerular injury. There is accumulating evidence of altered eicosanoid* synthesis in glomerular disease. Although the exact role of eicosanoids in glomerular disease is complex and not well understood, these compounds appear to play an important role in control of renal hemodynamics and the inflammatory response in glomerulonephropathies. There is also indirect evidence that eicosanoids mediate proteinuria, although their role in filtration of proteins and other macromolecules is yet to be established. Eicosanoid synthesis may be influenced by manipulation of dietary lipid formulation.[357] Diets high in eicosapentanoic acid or linoleic acid, or deficient in essential fatty acids have beneficial effects in various rodent models of glomerular disease.

Administration of angiotensin converting enzyme (ACE) inhibitors reduces the magnitude of proteinuria in humans with diabetic nephropathy, primary glomerular disease, and various other renal diseases.[358-360] Although the mechanism(s) by which ACE inhibitors reduce proteinuria is unknown, proposed mechanisms include: (1) reduced glomerular hypertension, (2) reduced glomerular hyperpermeability due to reduced angiotensin II formation, (3) anti-inflammatory effects, and (4) antiplatelet effects.[360] Reduction of systemic blood pressure alone does not account for the antiproteinuric effect because administration of other forms of antihypertensive medications fails to produce an equivalent reduction in the magnitude of proteinuria.[358] Infusion of angiotensin II enhances efferent arteriolar (postglomerular) vasoconstriction and promotes proteinuria in rats.[361] Recent studies suggest that the antipro-

teinuric effect of ACE inhibitors is most likely the result of amelioration of intraglomerular hypertension by postglomerular arteriolar vasodilation.[358]

Edema. OVERVIEW. Edema is a predictable consequence of hypoalbuminemia in patients with NS. Reduced serum albumin concentration diminishes plasma oncotic pressure, and thereby favors translocation of intravascular fluid into the interstitial fluid compartment. Serum albumin concentration usually decreases below approximately 1 gm/dl before this occurs, but this value may vary greatly. The resulting deficit in intravascular volume initiates a series of homeostatic adjustments involving the renin-angiotensin-aldosterone axis, sympathetic nervous system, antidiuretic hormone (ADH), atrial natriuretic peptide, and other factors. No single factor has been conclusively identified as being of primary importance. The net effect of these homeostatic alterations is to cause the kidneys to conserve salt and water in an attempt to restore plasma volume and circulatory stability. Avid renal retention of salt and water during development of edema may result in transient oliguria. Some retained fluid remains in the vascular space, but because of the alteration in capillary hemodynamics associated with hypoalbuminemia and the fact that sodium and water freely pass through capillary walls, most of the retained fluid enters the interstitial space and becomes manifest as edema. A new equilibrium is ultimately established in which high interstitial pressure offsets the loss of plasma oncotic pressure, and increased lymphatic flow may balance any residual excess net capillary filtration of water and salt, so that net loss of fluid into the tissues ceases. The sum effect is a markedly expanded total extracellular fluid volume with a plasma volume that may be reduced. Renal sodium and water retention in this setting is an appropriate compensation in that it restores the plasma volume, even though it also augments the degree of edema. Because of altered capillary hemodynamics, removal of edema fluid, by diuretics or other means, may reduce plasma volume and tissue perfusion, occasionally to clinically significant levels.

Some humans with NS have reduced GFR and increased rather than decreased intravascular volume.[362] Consistent with an increased intravascular volume, plasma renin and aldosterone values have been found to be low in these patients. The mechanism of edema formation in such patients is not understood, but is probably related to inability to maintain normal fluid balance at normal renal perfusion pressure. Because intravascular volume is increased, removal of edema fluid in such cases is unlikely to have adverse effects on fluid balance.

TREATMENT. Nephrotic edema rarely causes life-threatening complications unless pleural or pericardial effusion occurs. Therefore, therapy solely for the purpose of cosmetic effects of reducing edema is inadvisable. Treatment should be reserved for patients with moderate to severe edema that may result in complications such as respiratory embarrassment. Because retention of edema fluid is compensatory, removal of edema fluid will probably diminish the effective circulating volume. Nonetheless, in human patients with NS, removal of edema fluid often improves the patient's sense

*The term eicosanoids refers to all of the products of arachidonic acid synthesized by way of cyclooxygenase and lipoxygenase pathways. Eicosanoids derived from the cyclooxygenase pathway are prostaglandins and thromboxane, and are referred to as prostanoids. Lipoxygenase products are monohydroxylated and dihydroxylated eicosatetranoic acids and leukotrienes.

of well-being, despite induction of a mild degree of volume contraction.[22] Similar beneficial effects may occur in dogs and cats with NS; therefore, rigid guidelines concerning treatment of edema are not possible.

In patients with mild to moderate edema, conservative therapy consisting of cage rest and sodium restriction, combined with efforts to correct the primary glomerular disease and proteinuria, should be attempted before initiating diuretic therapy except when edema fluid must be rapidly eliminated (e.g., when edema impairs respiration). Often, several days of cage rest alone results in marked improvement or resolution of edema. Because renal sodium retention contributes to the pathogenesis of nephrotic edema, restricting dietary sodium intake will limit the quantity of fluid that can be retained.[280] Salt restriction may also be of value in limiting the systemic hypertension common in patients with GN. Initially, commercially available reduced sodium diets that contain approximately 250 mg of sodium/100 gm of dry food, or their homemade equivalent are recommended. Additional restriction of sodium intake may be necessary for optimum response. It may also be advisable to minimize the use of sodium-containing medications.

Diuretics are effective in treatment of nephrotic edema, but they may promote additional fluid volume contraction, hypotension, reduced renal function, and electrolyte disturbances (including metabolic alkalosis, hypokalemia, hyponatremia, or hypomagnesemia). Therefore, diuretics should be used sparingly in nephrotic patients. Loop diuretics such as furosemide are generally more effective than thiazide diuretics or aldosterone antagonists in correcting nephrotic edema. However, chronic use of loop diuretics is more likely to be associated with serious fluid and electrolyte disturbances. Such use may also contribute to mineralization of the renal parenchyma.

Furosemide (Lasix) is most commonly used for acute relief of edema associated with the NS. Furosemide should initially be administered at a dosage of 1 to 2 mg/lb (2 to 4 mg/kg) given orally, intravenously, or subcutaneously. This dosage may be given from one to four times daily until edema resolves. Nephrotic edema is rarely diuretic resistant, and excessive therapy should be avoided for the reasons described above. After therapeutic resolution of edema, the dosage of furosemide may be reduced to alternate day therapy. If alternate day therapy maintains the patient edema free for a trial period of one to two weeks, the dose may be further reduced to once every three days. If the patient remains edema free at this dosage, furosemide may be discontinued. In patients that require long-term diuretic therapy to control edema, the lowest dose that maintains the patient acceptably free of edema should be used. As already mentioned, overly aggressive diuretic therapy may cause fluid and electrolyte depletion and compromise renal function, but these effects can be prevented by proper management of diuretic dosage and replacement therapy with fluid and electrolytes when necessary.

Diuretics are usually sufficiently effective that removal of fluid by paracentesis is rarely required. Thoracentesis should be considered only if pleural fluid is impairing respiration. Repeated therapeutic paracentesis should be avoided if possible because it may deplete the patient of fluids and metabolites.

Intravenous administration of solutions containing protein is of potential value for patients in circulatory collapse caused by hypovolemia and for initiating diuresis in patients with refractory edema.[299] Salt-poor albumin infusions have been used in human nephrotics to increase plasma oncotic pressure and expand plasma volume, thus enhancing the effectiveness of diuretics administered. However, most of the albumin administered is lost into the urine within 24 to 48 hours, thus limiting the value of such therapy. In general, albumin infusion is reserved for patients with clinical evidence of severe intravascular volume depletion that requires surgery or invasive diagnostic procedures, or for patients that have life-threatening signs related to edema.[362]

Hypertension. Systemic hypertension has been reported to occur in a high percentage of dogs with GN.[363] It also occurs in some cats with glomerular disease. However, despite the reportedly high incidence of hypertension in dogs with glomerular disease, renal and vascular lesions typical of hypertension are not a prominent finding in such patients.[290] Hypertension commonly occurs in humans with chronic glomerulonephritis and represents a bad prognostic sign, since it is associated with a greater probability that renal function will deteriorate.[364] In humans, systemic hypertension may be the single most important factor leading to progressive renal morphologic and functional deterioration, and end-stage renal failure. Hypertension may cause fibrinoid degeneration and hyalinization of glomerular vessels, thereby aggravating glomerular damage.[282] Antihypertensive therapy that limits transmission of systemic hypertension to the glomerulus may minimize progressive glomerular injury. ACE inhibitors such as captopril and enalapril appear to limit glomerular hypertension, and thus may be the antihypertensive agents of choice in patients with renal disease (see Chapter 109).

Hyperlipidemia. Hypercholesterolemia and hypertriglyceridemia are characteristic of NS. This hyperlipidemia is related to the magnitude of proteinuria in nephrotic humans.[365] Furthermore, it is the urinary loss of protein rather than the ensuing rate of albumin synthesis that appears to be central to development of hyperlipidemia. Infusion of albumin or dextrans markedly reduces serum lipid concentrations.[366] Therefore, plasma oncotic pressure has been proposed as an important mediator of the hyperlipidemia of NS.

Indirect evidence suggests that hyperlipidemia may contribute to progression of glomerular disease and the thrombotic diathesis associated with NS. Although hypercholesterolemia may promote atherosclerotic heart disease in humans with NS, direct evidence that hyperlipidemia has a deleterious effect on canine and feline patients with NS is lacking. In absence of evidence that nephrotic hyperlipidemia adversely affects dogs and cats, specific therapy designed to reduce hyperlipidemia is probably not warranted. Because hyperlipidemia is primarily a consequence of glomerular proteinuria, therapy designed to minimize proteinuria and additional glomerular damage is likely to result in reduced serum cholesterol and triglyceride concentrations.

Thrombotic Diathesis. OVERVIEW. The thrombotic diathesis of NS is multifactorial in origin (Table 108–32).[367, 368] Although studies on the factors that promote thromboembolism in canine NS are limited, preliminary results indicate probable roles for antithrombin III deficiency, hyperfibrinogenemia, hypoalbuminemia-related platelet hypersensitivity, and corticosteroid therapy.[338, 369, 370] Studies on the mechanisms of thromboembolism in feline NS have not been reported.

Plasma antithrombin III (AT III) activity is often reduced in dogs and humans with NS because of urinary loss of this low-molecular-weight protein.[368–370] AT-III is a serine protease inhibitor that inactivates activated serine protease clotting factors (factors II, IX, X, XI, and XII). It therefore acts as an anticoagulant. Deficiency of AT-III is associated with diminished inhibition of fibrin formation and marked facilitation of thrombosis.[369] In a study of three dogs with NS, AT-III activity was mildly reduced (74 per cent of normal) in one dog and markedly reduced in two dogs (48 per cent and 32 per cent of normal).[369] Plasma fibrinogen concentrations were markedly increased in all three dogs.

Platelet aggregation may be enhanced in dogs with NS, thereby promoting thromboembolic complications.[370] Platelets from two dogs with NS were shown to have an increased tendency to aggregate when exposed to a low dose of adenosine diphosphate. This platelet hypersensitivity could be corrected by increasing plasma albumin concentration by adding purified dog albumin. Albumin is known to modulate the platelet release reaction by binding certain platelet products that would otherwise stimulate platelet aggregation. It therefore appears likely that platelet hypersensitivity in NS is directly related to hypoalbuminemia. In the aforementioned study of dogs with NS, increased platelet sensitivity to hypoalbuminemia persisted despite aspirin therapy.[370]

TABLE 108–32. FACTORS THAT PREDISPOSE TO THROMBOEMBOLISM IN HUMAN PATIENTS WITH NEPHROTIC SYNDROME[367, 368]

Primary Factors
Reduced activities of plasma anticoagulants
    Antithrombin III (heparin cofactor)
    Protein S (a component of the vitamin K–dependent protein C–protein S anticoagulant system)
Increased plasma clotting factor activities
    Fibrinogen (factor I)
    Factors V and VIII
Thrombocytosis and increased platelet adhesiveness and aggregability
Impaired fibrinolysis

Modulating Factors
Urinary loss of low-molecular-weight coagulation factors, particularly factors IX and XII
Inflammatory processes that may selectively enhance production of "acute phase" proteins leading to increased levels of fibrinogen and factor VIII
Consumptive coagulopathy
Increased blood viscosity (primarily caused by increased fibrinogen concentrations)
Uremic vasculitis
Hyperlipidemia
Dehydration
Vascular stasis associated with inactivity or edema
Drugs
    Corticosteroids
    Diuretics

TREATMENT. Prophylaxis and treatment of thromboembolism in patients with NS may encompass: (1) anticoagulation therapy, (2) efforts to ameliorate the magnitude of proteinuria, and (3) therapy of complicating factors that may promote thromboembolism (Table 108–32). Because the pathogenesis of thrombosis in nephrotic patients can largely be traced to urinary protein loss, it is logical to attempt to reduce the magnitude of proteinuria in patients with the thrombotic diathesis of NS. Although controlled studies on the efficacy of this approach are lacking, an additional advantage to this method is that it may be beneficial in ameliorating many of the complications of the NS without the risk of hemorrhage associated with anticoagulant therapy. Strategies for reducing the magnitude of proteinuria are described above. In addition to reducing the magnitude of proteinuria, efforts should be directed toward minimizing factors known to promote thrombosis in nephrotic patients (Table 108–32).

Anticoagulant therapy may be considered to prevent thromboembolism and/or to limit growth of thrombi and emboli that have already formed. However, because anticoagulant therapy may be associated with serious hemorrhage, the patient's clinical condition and coagulation system must be closely monitored. Even with careful monitoring, the risk of hemorrhagic complications persists. Therefore, the potential benefits of such therapy should be balanced against the likelihood of serious thromboembolic complications.

Prophylactic anticoagulants are not routinely recommended in humans with NS because the risk:benefit ratio is unclear.[276] An additional problem in dogs and cats is that a reliable means of identifying patients at high risk for developing thromboembolism has not yet been determined. It has been suggested that determinations of plasma AT-III activity and plasma fibrinogen concentration may be used as an index of thrombosis based on the ratio of fibrinogen to AT-III (per cent normal fibrinogen/per cent normal AT-III).[369] Normal values for this ratio are 0.5 to 1.5 in dogs.[369] Dogs with AT-III activities less than 70 per cent of normal and fibrinogen values greater than 300 mg/dl may be at increased risk for thromboembolic complications. Other tests that may suggest thrombotic diathesis include increased fibrin (and fibrinogen) degradation products, increased platelet adhesiveness, and shortened activated partial thromboplastin time, prothrombin time, or thrombin time.[289]

Treatment of thrombosis in dogs and cats has been recently reviewed.[289] Commonly used anticoagulants include heparin for short-term therapy and coumarin derivatives such as warfarin for long-term therapy. Because heparin acts by increasing the affinity of AT-III for clotting factors, AT-III deficiency is likely to impair the effectiveness of heparin as an anticoagulant. For this reason, heparin should be less effective than coumadin in patients with NS. In addition, heparin may increase AT-III turnover rate, which would further limit the role of AT-III in inhibiting further thrombus formation.[369] Pharmacologic inhibition of platelet function using aspirin or other antiplatelet drugs may provide an inexpensive and practical alternative for limiting thrombus formation and growth in patients with NS, but studies on the efficacy of such therapy in dogs and cats with NS have apparently not been reported.

Streptokinase and urokinase are thrombolytic agents that activate the plasminogen system. Because they stimulate lysis of clots throughout the body, administration of fibrinolytic drugs is associated with a considerable risk of hemorrhage. The authors have insufficient experience using anticoagulants or thrombolytic drugs in canine or feline patients with NS to recommend their use at this time.

TUBULAR DEFECTS

Definition and Identification

Tubular defects (TDs) encompass a diverse group of uncommonly recognized diseases which have in common anatomic or functional disorders of the renal tubules (Table 108–33). They may be congenital (e.g., Fanconi syndrome in Basenji dogs) or acquired (e.g., Fanconi syndrome associated with gentamicin nephrotoxicity). Anatomic TDs may be detected initially as asymptomatic urinary abnormalities (e.g., abnormal kidney size or shape, hematuria), CRF, or in association with UTI. Additional studies are generally required to confirm cysts of renal tubular origin as the cause of the disorder. Functional TDs result in altered urine composition, which may be reflected in plasma. For example, impaired distal tubular secretion of hydrogen ions, known as distal renal tubular acidosis, may be manifested as inappropriately alkaline urine and metabolic acidosis. Functional TDs may be initially detected as urolithiasis (cystinuria), CRF (Fanconi syndrome or renal tubular acidosis), unexpected urinalysis findings (glucosuria, inappropriate urine specific gravity), or polyuria (nephrogenic diabetes insipidus). However, in many instances, diagnostic studies beyond those included in the minimum data base for urinary disorders (Table 108–3) are required for detection and confirmation of TDs (e.g., plasma electrolyte and acid-base values). Because of the diverse nature of these disorders, each condition will be described independently.

Anatomic Tubular Defects

RENAL CYSTS AND POLYCYSTIC KIDNEYS

Cysts are cavities lined by epithelium and filled with liquid or semisolid material. Renal cysts are dilated

TABLE 108–33. RENAL TUBULAR DEFECTS OF DOGS AND CATS

Anatomic Defects
Solitary and multiple renal cysts
Polycystic kidneys
Acquired renal cysts
Feline perirenal cysts (pseudocysts)*
Functional Defects
Renal tubular acidosis
Fanconi syndrome
Cystinuria
Renal glucosuria
Nephrogenic diabetes insipidus

*Not of renal tubular origin, but listed here because it may be confused with other types of cystic disorders.

nephron segments that may involve the glomerular capsule or any portion of the renal tubules; they may be solitary or multiple. Polycystic simply means many cysts. Cysts may remain small and clinically unimportant, or they may enlarge and displace normal renal parenchyma. Renal cysts may result from genetic (familial), developmental, or acquired processes. Even in patients with cysts of genetic origin, cyst development may be influenced or caused by a variety of environmental factors, including microbes, diet, chemicals, and other undefined agents.[371]

Congenital solitary or multiple renal cysts have been reported in dogs and cats, but appear to be uncommon.[372] Polycystic disease suspected of being hereditary has also been reported (Table 108–15).[257, 262, 371] In long-haired cats and Cairn terriers, polycystic renal disease (Figure 108–9) is similar to autosomal recessive kidney disease of humans (also known as infantile polycystic kidney disease). Affected animals appeared normal at birth, but abdominal enlargement due to renomegaly developed by two to six weeks of age. Most kittens died because of uremia, but the puppies were euthanized before developing clinical signs. The condition is potentially lethal in affected individuals. In Cairn terriers, cystic alterations in the biliary tree have also been observed. Familial and other congenital renal cystic disorders in humans often affect nonurinary organs, including the liver, pancreas, and blood vessels (e.g., aneurysms of the circle of Willis).[373] Hepatomegaly may contribute to abdominal enlargement in such patients.

Multiple acquired renal cysts may develop in association with chronic generalized nephropathy of diverse origins. Acquired renal cystic disorders appear to be more common than hereditary polycystic disease, but nonetheless are recognized infrequently. Acquired cysts are characteristically associated with substantial tubulointerstitial inflammation and/or fibrosis, a feature which differentiates them from most congenital or inherited cysts.

Polycystic kidney disease is recognized in most adult cats because of abdominal masses detected by the owner, or because of clinical signs of uremia. Physical findings may include renomegaly, altered kidney shape, abdominal enlargement, and findings typical of CRF. Renal cysts can also cause pain because of rupture, hemorrhage, or infection. Hemorrhage may cause blood clots to form in the renal pelvis, which may lead to urinary obstruction. If infection develops, pyuria and hematuria may occur. However, if the affected cyst is not continuous with the excretory pathway, urinalysis findings may be normal. Cysts may also be detected incidentally during laparotomy, necropsy, or renal sonographic or radiographic examinations.

In most cases, the diagnosis can be confirmed by intravenous urography or renal ultrasound. Renal ultrasonography is particularly useful for differentiation of solitary cysts from renal neoplasms. Aspiration biopsy may also be useful to confirm the diagnosis of cystic disease. Renal tissue biopsy is seldom necessary for diagnosis of cystic disease, but may be useful in determining if the cysts are congenital or acquired. In addition, a family history and evidence of hepatic cysts (hepatic sonography or biopsy) should be sought to further define the origin of the cysts.

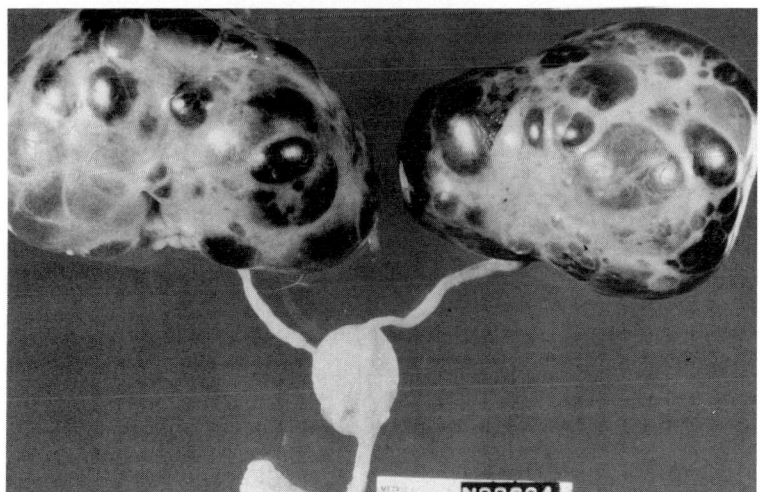

FIGURE 108–9. Adult polycystic kidney disease in an 11-year-old female domestic longhaired cat. Note bilateral, asymmetrical kidney enlargement and multiple large fluid-filled cysts replacing renal parenchyma.

Unless they become infected, solitary or multiple cysts that do not enlarge are of little clinical consequence. However, polycystic kidney disease is a progressive condition for which no specific treatment exists (see section on CRF). If the medical history suggests a possible hereditary origin, the genetic implications should be discussed with the owner if breeding animals are involved.

Infection is of particular concern in management of patients with renal cysts; iatrogenic infection (e.g., via urinary catheterization) should be assiduously avoided. When present, infection may involve one or more cysts and/or renal parenchyma (pyelonephritis). In diffuse pyelonephritis, urinalysis may reveal pyuria and bacteriuria, and microbes may be cultured from urine. However, infection of isolated cysts may not be detected by urinalysis or urine culture. In addition, penetration of antibiotics into cysts presents a substantial therapeutic problem.[374] Cysts are often sufficiently large that delivery of antibiotics into the cyst by glomerular filtration is insignificant. Therefore, it is necessary to rely on diffusion of antibiotics across the cyst wall to achieve effective therapeutic concentrations of antibiotics. In general, ampicillin and aminoglycosides penetrate cysts poorly. Lipid-soluble antibiotics such as chloramphenicol, clindamycin, erythromycin, tetracyclines, and trimethoprim penetrate cysts more readily.

FELINE PERIRENAL PSEUDOCYSTS

Perirenal pseudocysts (also called perinephric pseudocyst, renal capsular cyst, capsulogenic renal cyst, capsular hydronephrosis, pseudohydronephrosis, and retroperitoneal perirenal cyst) are accumulations of fluid which develop external to the renal parenchyma, between the renal parenchyma and renal capsule (with the renal capsule as the outer wall of the cyst), or between the renal capsule and a thin-walled fibrous sac attached to the capsule.[375, 376] They are termed pseudocysts rather than cysts because they are not lined by epithelium. Because only a limited number have been examined histologically, it is unknown whether all such perirenal fluid-filled structures are pseudocysts.[375] They are not true tubular disorders because they do not originate from the renal tubules.

The origin of perirenal pseudocysts is not known. Possible causes include: (1) chronic extravasation of urine into the perirenal tissues (due to trauma, urinary obstruction, or renal biopsy), resulting in inflammation, lysis of perinephric fat, and subsequent formation of a fibrous capsule surrounding the fluid, (2) resolution of perirenal hematomas, and (3) perirenal lymphocele formation. The fluid contained in these structures in cats has typically been a transudate, rather than urine or lymph.[375, 376]

Of five reported cases, all were intact or castrated male cats, eight years of age or older.[375] In three cats, both kidneys were affected, whereas in two cats only the left kidney was affected. Three cats were of mixed breeding and two were Persians. Clinical signs were typically characterized by progressive abdominal enlargement. Abdominal palpation reveals a large, firm, nonpainful mass located in the area of the kidneys. Renal function tests and urinalyses have typically been normal. However, mild azotemia has been reported. Excretory urography may reveal fluid accumulation exterior to the renal parenchyma; kidney size and shape are usually normal, but the cortical margins may be irregular in the area of the pseudocyst. The contour of the excretory pathway has often been normal, but on occasion was locally compressed by the cyst. Extravasation of intravenously administered radiopaque contrast material into the perirenal pseudocyst has not been reported. Renal sonography may provide an alternative means of confirming the diagnosis.

Short-term prognosis for cats with perirenal pseudocysts appears to be good. Long-term prognosis for these patients is not known because it is unclear if pseudocysts are in some way associated with underlying lesions in the renal parenchyma that may be progressive. Treatment has encompassed exploratory surgery to confirm the diagnosis, drainage of the cyst fluid, and resection of as much of the cyst wall as possible. To date, nonsurgical means of managing patients with perirenal pseudocysts have not been assessed. If azotemia or other evidence of additional renal disease/dysfunction is detected, additional studies are indicated to determine its cause, as perirenal pseudocysts are an unlikely explanation for its occurrence. Needle or wedge biopsy of the kidneys may be obtained at the time of surgery.

Functional Tubular Defects

RENAL TUBULAR ACIDOSIS

Renal tubular acidosis (RTA) refers to conditions in which metabolic acidosis results from diminished ability of the kidneys to secrete hydrogen ions.[377] Depending on the site of defective hydrogen ion secretion, RTA has been classified as proximal (type 2) or distal (type 1) RTA (Table 108–34). Proximal RTA is associated with inappropriate loss of bicarbonate in urine as a result of decreased proximal renal tubular bicarbonate reclamation (which requires hydrogen ion secretion); the ability to maximally acidify urine by the distal renal tubule is retained. Proximal RTA rarely occurs as an isolated defect, but rather in association with other renal tubular defects (see the next section on Fanconi syndrome).[249] In contrast, distal RTA is almost invariably associated with impaired ability to maximally acidify urine and often occurs as an isolated defect. In humans, it may occur either in a complete form, resulting in systemic acidosis, or in an incomplete form, in which systemic acidosis does not occur despite impaired hydrogen ion secretory ability.

RTAs may be congenital or acquired. However, these conditions have seldom been recognized in dogs and cats. Even when recognized, the etiopathogenesis of the tubular hydrogen ion secretory defect has not been determined. Proximal RTA has been reported to occur as part of an acquired proximal tubular functional defect (Fanconi syndrome) associated with gentamicin nephrotoxicity in dogs.[378] Distal RTA has been reported in a cat with pyelonephritis.[379] Distal RTA has also been reported in association with hepatic lipidosis in a cat, but the relation, if any, between hepatic dysfunction and RTA is unclear.[380] In humans, RTA may occur in association with hypercalciuric disorders, various renal diseases (pyelonephritis, obstructive nephropathy, amyloidosis), autoimmune disorders (e.g., hypergammaglobulinemias, systemic lupus erythematosus, chronic active hepatitis), genetically transmitted systemic diseases (e.g., Ehlers-Danlos syndrome), and drugs or toxins, including amphotericin B, outdated tetracyclines, lead, mercury, and other heavy metals.[381]

Clinical signs of RTA are often subtle. Chronic metabolic acidosis may be associated with muscle weakness, anorexia, nausea, weight loss, neurologic signs (varying from lethargy to coma), and growth retardation in young animals. Hypokalemia may accompany RTA and contribute to muscle weakness. Urolithiasis and its associated clinical signs may also develop in some patients with RTA.[381] Struvite uroliths have been reported in dogs with proximal and distal RTA, but calcium phosphate uroliths are typical of humans with distal RTA.[381]

Hyperchloremic (normal anion gap) metabolic acidosis is the hallmark that usually prompts consideration of RTA.[21, 381] RTA should also be considered in patients with radiographically evident nephrocalcinosis, calcium phosphate uroliths, hypokalemia, and other renal tubular dysfunctions, and in acidotic patients with urine pH values that are consistently greater than 6.0.

Proximal RTA is most often characterized by hyperchloremic metabolic acidosis; because distal acidification is intact, patients often have acid urine (pH values below 6.0). However, urine pH values will be alkaline during periods of substantial bicarbonaturia. Proximal RTA is rarely seen alone. Therefore, other proximal TDs (glucosuria, aminoaciduria, and phosphaturia) should be sought when this condition is suspected. The diagnosis of proximal RTA is usually based on reduced ability of the renal tubules to reabsorb filtered bicarbonate at normal blood bicarbonate concentrations.

Concurrent metabolic acidosis and inappropriately high urine pH values (greater than 6.0) are highly suggestive of complete distal RTA. The only condition other than distal RTA likely to cause this constellation of findings is proximal RTA or UTI with urea-splitting organisms in the face of another cause of metabolic acidosis. Quantitative urine culture will rule out bacterial UTI as the cause of inappropriately alkaline urine. Proximal RTA and distal RTA can be differentiated by infusing sodium bicarbonate at a rate sufficient to induce an increase in blood bicarbonate concentration of approximately 0.5 to 1.0 mEq/L/hr. With proximal RTA, increasing blood bicarbonate concentrations will increase urine pH and fractional excretion of bicarbonate. In humans with proximal RTA, fractional excretion of bicarbonate typically exceeds 15 per cent of filtered load. With distal RTA, increasing blood bicarbonate concentrations are usually not associated with marked increases in urine pH or bicarbonate excretion. In adult humans with distal RTA, fractional excretion of bicarbonate rarely exceeds 5 per cent of filtered load at serum bicarbonate concentrations of 20 mEq/L.[377]

When distal RTA is suspected in patients that are not acidemic (i.e., blood pH less than about 7.35), an acid load may be administered in an attempt to evaluate maximum urine acidification capacity. Ammonium chloride has usually been used for this purpose. The authors recommend oral administration of ammonium chloride at a dosage of 0.1 gm/lb (0.2 gm/kg) (given over one hour as six divided doses of a solution containing 40 mg/ml of ammonium chloride).[381] The bladder should be emptied and urine pH determined every one to two hours for at least six hours after administration of this acidifier in order to determine maximum urine acidification capacity. Urine pH must be determined immediately or collected under oil to prevent loss of CO_2,

TABLE 108–34. TYPES OF RENAL TUBULAR ACIDOSIS

Characteristics	Proximal RTA	Distal RTA	
		Complete	Incomplete
Metabolic acidosis	+	+	−
Hypokalemia	+/−	+/−	−
Aminoaciduria/glucosuria	+/−	−	−
Urine pH during acidemia (spontaneous or induced)	<6.0	>6.0	>6.0
Urine-concentrating defect	−	+	−
Hypercalciuria	−	+	+
Nephrocalcinosis	−	+	+
Urolithiasis	−	+	+

which will alter urine pH values. The authors have found that maximum reduction in urine pH values occurs about four to five hours after administration of a single dose of 0.2 mg/kg of ammonium chloride.[381] Failure to reduce urine pH to 6.0 or lower supports a diagnosis of distal RTA. Urine acidification studies should not be performed in patients that are spontaneously acidemic, since inability to acidify urine is apparent, and because administration of acid to a patient with acidosis is dangerous.

RTA is treated by: (1) identification and elimination of the underlying cause (if known), and (2) oral administration of alkalinizing drugs, primarily sodium bicarbonate. Orally administered sodium citrate has also been effective in this condition.[379] The dosage of sodium bicarbonate depends on the form of RTA present. Typical dosages for human patients with distal RTA are 0.5 to 1 mEq/lb/day (1 to 2 mEq/kg). Similar doses may be effective in dogs and cats. However, in patients with proximal RTA, normalizing plasma bicarbonate concentration dramatically increases bicarbonaturia; thus very large doses of sodium bicarbonate are often required. The appropriate dosage of sodium bicarbonate should be determined by response to therapy in both forms of RTA.

Sodium bicarbonate may be administered as tablets, powder (baking soda), or a solution. In order to minimize expense, it has been suggested that an 8-oz box of baking soda be added to 2.88 L of distilled water to produce a solution containing 1 mEq of bicarbonate per milliliter. This solution will remain stable for at least two months if kept capped and refrigerated.[377] The solution may be administered orally by syringe or mixed in a small quantity of food.

Potassium supplementation may be required in some patients with RTA. Potassium therapy may be especially important for patients that are hypokalemic before treatment because therapeutic alkalinization will promote hypokalemia by driving potassium from extracellular fluid into cells. Potassium therapy is also important for patients with proximal RTA because sodium bicarbonate may exacerbate potassium wasting and potassium loss. Potassium may be administered as the chloride salt or preferably as potassium bicarbonate or citrate. In patients with proximal RTA, potassium-sparing diuretics may be indicated to reduce kaliuresis.

FANCONI SYNDROME

Fanconi syndrome is characterized by a generalized dysfunction of the proximal renal tubules, which may lead to excessive urinary loss of glucose, amino acids, phosphate, bicarbonate (proximal RTA), potassium, sodium, calcium, magnesium, uric acid, and other organic acids.[382] Although glucosuria and aminoaciduria are not manifested by decremental changes in plasma concentrations of these constituents, hypophosphatemia, hypokalemia, hypouricemia, and metabolic acidosis may develop. In humans, Fanconi syndrome may be inherited or acquired. Conditions that have been associated with development of Fanconi syndrome include heavy metal poisoning (e.g., lead, cadmium, mercury), drugs (e.g., outdated tetracyclines, gentamicin,

cephalosporins), organic compounds (e.g., Lysol, nitrobenzines, streptozotocin), malignancies (e.g., myeloma, monoclonal gammopathies), nutritional deficiencies (e.g., vitamin D deficiency), and renal disease (e.g., nephrotic syndrome).[382]

An idiopathic proximal TD suspected of having a genetic origin and associated with impaired renal tubular reabsorption of amino acids, glucose, phosphate, sodium, potassium, and uric acid has been reported in basenjis, Norwegian elkhounds, Shetland sheepdogs, and schnauzers.[249, 383–385] This condition has been studied extensively in basenji dogs.[249, 383–385] In this breed, clinical signs developed between one and six years of age, and included polyuria, polydipsia, and weight loss. Typical urinalysis findings included glucosuria, proteinuria, and urine specific gravity values of 1.001 to 1.018. Although some dogs remained stable for several years after diagnosis, other dogs died within a few months after onset of clinical signs.[385] Death usually occurred in association with ARF and papillary necrosis. Severe metabolic acidosis, presumably the result of proximal RTA, preceded development of azotemia. Acquired Fanconi syndrome has been reported subsequent to gentamicin therapy in a dog.[378]

Diagnosis of Fanconi syndrome is based on serum and urine solute studies. Evidence of generalized proximal tubular dysfunction characterized by aminoaciduria, glucosuria, and electrolyte loss in urine, in addition to serum electrolyte abnormalities, establishes the diagnosis.

Treatment is based on correcting the primary cause, if possible (e.g., treatment for lead toxicity or withdrawal of a drug responsible for proximal tubular damage). Therapy designed to replace solutes lost via urine may also be of value (e.g., sodium, potassium, and bicarbonate).

CYSTINURIA

Cystinuria, abnormally increased urinary excretion of the amino acid cystine, results from an inherited defect in renal tubular transport of cystine and dibasic amino acids.[385] It has been reported in several breeds, but appears to be most common in dachshunds.[18] The low solubility of cystine in urine predisposes to formation of cystine urolithiasis. However, uroliths do not develop in all dogs with cystinuria. Urolithiasis is the only clinical significance of cystinuria (see Chapter 111).

RENAL GLUCOSURIA

Renal glucosuria is an inborn error of proximal renal tubular transport of glucose.[18] It has been recognized as an inherited defect in Norwegian elkhounds. It has also been observed in Scottish terriers and mongrels.[385] Renal glucosuria is diagnosed when abnormally large amounts of glucose are found in the urine of a patient with normal blood glucose concentration. Further, glucosuria is the only abnormal urinary finding, thus discriminating this entity from more generalized proximal RTDs. Patients with renal glucosuria are typically asymptomatic, but may have mild polyuria and polydipsia. By itself, renal glucosuria is a benign condition that does not require treatment. It is critical that this condition not be confused with diabetes mellitus, because administration of insulin to patients with renal glucosuria is potentially dangerous. Although it has been stated that glucosuria predisposes patients to UTIs, this association has not been confirmed.

NEPHROGENIC DIABETES INSIPIDUS

Nephrogenic diabetes insipidus (DI) refers to a large group of physiologic, pharmacologic, and pathologic conditions in which the kidneys fail to concentrate urine despite physiologic or supraphysiologic circulating concentrations of antidiuretic hormone (ADH).[386] It may be congenital or acquired, and may result from structural or functional abnormalities that alter ADH-induced cell membrane permeability to water in the distal renal tubules and collecting duct.[386–388] Acquired nephrogenic DI may result from conditions that diminish renal responsiveness to ADH, including CRF, renal diseases that primarily affect the renal tubules and collecting ducts (e.g., pyelonephritis, obstructive nephropathy), hypercalcemia, hypokalemia, hyperadrenocorticism, hypoadrenocorticism, hyperthyroidism, hepatic failure, pyometra, and drug toxicities. Diagnosis and treatment of these conditions are described elsewhere in this text (see Chapter 29).

Congenital nephrogenic DI is characterized by insatiable polydipsia, voluminous polyuria (often 5 to 20 times normal), and nocturia, which become apparent after weaning. Vomiting and abdominal distention due to chronic overdistention of the stomach, and growth retardation may also be noted. Physical examination typically reveals a greatly enlarged urinary bladder. Urine specific gravity values are often in the range of 1.001 to 1.003, and plasma osmolality values are typically slightly increased, indicating a mild degree of volume contraction due to the massive polyuria. The diagnosis of congenital nephrogenic DI is based on: (1) polyuria and polydipsia since immaturity, (2) hypotonic urine, (3) elimination of acquired causes of nephrogenic DI, and (4) failure to concentrate urine in response to water deprivation, partial water deprivation, saline loading, or ADH administration.

The only effective means of controlling polyuria of congenital nephrogenic DI is administration of chlorothiazide combined with a salt-restricted diet.[49] Such therapy may reduce polyuria by up to 85 per cent. Chlorothiazide produces a mild negative salt balance, thereby contracting extracellular fluid volume and stimulating enhanced proximal renal tubular reabsorption of sodium, chloride, and water. The net effect is to substantially reduce the volume of fluid delivered to the distal renal tubules and collecting ducts. Thus, less urine is available for elimination (even though it is still dilute and relatively large in volume). The recommended dose of chlorothiazide is 10 to 20 mg/lb (20 to 40 mg/kg) q12h. A low-sodium diet should be fed in concert with administration of chlorothiazide to optimize its effect.

ASYMPTOMATIC URINARY ABNORMALITIES

Definition and Identification

Hematuria, proteinuria, or casts detected by routine urinalysis in healthy patients that have no other evidence of urinary tract disease are the definition and description of asymptomatic urinary abnormalities (AUA). Radiographic (e.g., altered kidney size, shape, or location) or physical evidence of urinary disease (e.g., lesions visualized during surgery or laparoscopic examination) that is seemingly not associated with clinical signs of illness may also be considered as AUA. The goal in pursuing these problems is to detect diseases that would eventually lead to clinical signs, with the hope of eliminating them by treatment. However, because these patients are not sick, restraint should often be exercised in the extent of diagnostic evaluation of these abnormalities. They may require surveillance, but exhaustive investigation of their cause may not be necessary or productive. Before additional diagnostics are pursued, persistence of abnormal urine findings should be confirmed by repeating a urinalysis several days later. The decision as to the appropriate diagnostic course of action depends on the client's wishes and the likelihood that a potentially serious condition may exist. AUA typically resolve spontaneously, or progress until they can be classified as a more specific syndrome or disease.

Hematuria

OVERVIEW

An isolated instance of transient hematuria may not be of clinical importance. However, persistent or recurrent hematuria may indicate serious disease and should, therefore, be pursued. Hematuria may originate anywhere in the urinary tract (Table 108–35); therefore, the first step in diagnostic evaluation of persistent or recurrent hematuria is to localize its origin. Physical findings such as renomegaly, a palpable mass in the bladder, or prostatomegaly may prove helpful in localizing hematuria. Hematuria accompanied by dysuria or pollakiuria indicates lower urinary tract disease. Red blood cell (RBC) casts unequivocally localize hematuria to the kidneys. However, RBC casts are an uncommon finding, and their absence does not rule out a renal origin for hematuria. Determining when during voiding gross hematuria is most severe may be helpful in localizing its source. Persistent hematuria of renal origin is characterized by urine that contains blood throughout micturition. This pattern of hematuria may also occur with generalized bladder diseases, coagulopathies, severe prostatic disease, or proximal urethral diseases. Hematuria observed predominantly at the end of micturition suggests a focal lesion in the ventral or ventrolateral aspect of the urinary bladder. This pattern may also be seen in dogs with intermittent gross hematuria of renal origin. Hematuria that occurs independent of micturition usually indicates a urethral or genital (i.e.,

TABLE 108–35. CAUSES OF HEMATURIA IN DOGS AND CATS

Renal and Ureteral	Bladder and Urethra
Urinary tract infection	Urinary tract infection
Urolithiasis	Urolithiasis
Neoplasia	Idiopathic "FUS"
Renal cell carcinoma	Neoplasia
Transitional cell	Transitional cell
carcinoma	carcinoma
Hemangioma	Squamous cell carcinoma
Hemangiosarcoma	Adenocarcinomas
Others	Papillomas
Trauma	Others
Renal cystic diseases	Polypoid cystitis
Polycystic kidneys	Trauma
Isolated renal cysts	*Capillaria plica* or *feliscati*
Idiopathic renal hematuria	*Dioctophyma renale*
Glomerulonephropathy	Others
Dioctophyma renale	**Other Causes/Sources**
Capillaria plica	Coagulopathies
Telangiectasia	Iatrogenic contamination
Renal infarcts	Cystocentesis
Vascular abnormalities	Catheterization
Chronic passive congestion	Genital contamination
Strenuous exercise	Prostatic disease
Others	Estrus
	Others

prostate in males and vagina or uterus in females) origin. When findings obtained from the problem-specific urinary tract data base fail to localize the source of hematuria, additional diagnostics such as complete blood cell counts (to assess the effect of hematuria on hematocrit values, and to identify thrombocytopenia or evidence of systemic inflammatory disease), coagulation studies (to rule out coagulopathies), and contrast radiographic and/or ultrasonographic studies (to localize lesions in the urinary tract) should be considered. In rare instances, exploratory laparotomy and/or biopsy may be required to ascertain the source and cause of hemorrhage (see Chapters 32, 105, 110, 111, and 112).[389]

RENAL HEMATURIA

Overview. Although renal hematuria is uncommon in dogs and cats, it may result from a wide variety of conditions (Table 108–35). Findings obtained from the urinalysis or urine cytologic studies may be helpful in further defining the most likely cause of hematuria. For example, pyuria and bacteriuria suggest infection, while neoplastic cells indicate a probable neoplastic basis for hematuria. Contrast radiography (intravenous urography, renal arteriography), ultrasonography, renal biopsy, and/or exploratory surgery are required to identify most causes of renal hematuria. Pyelonephritis, renal cystic disorders, and glomerulopathies are described elsewhere in this chapter (see also Chapter 111).

Renal and Ureteral Neoplasia. Primary renal neoplasms are relatively uncommon in dogs and cats. They primarily occur in older animals. No breed or sex predilections have been detected for most renal neoplasms in dogs or cats; however, renal carcinomas and urothelial carcinomas occur more often in male dogs. The majority of renal neoplasms are malignant in both species.[14, 390] Clinical signs of renal neoplasia vary with their location, size, and duration. Renal cell carcinomas, transitional cell carcinomas, hemangiomas, and heman-

giosarcomas are the neoplasms most likely to cause hematuria.[389] Other clinical signs that may occur include renomegaly, abdominal distention, and various polysystemic signs, including anorexia, weight loss, anemia, and pyrexia. A presumptive diagnosis of renal neoplasia may be based on radiographic and ultrasonographic findings, but definitive diagnosis requires biopsy. Canine and feline renal neoplasia has recently been reviewed.[14, 390, 391]

Benign renal neoplasms are often clinically insignificant. However, renal hemangiomas, the most common benign renal neoplasm of dogs, are an exception to this generality.[14, 390] This neoplasm frequently causes constant or intermittent gross hematuria and varying degrees of renomegaly.[14]

Renal carcinomas (also called hypernephroma, renal adenocarcinoma, clear cell carcinoma, and malignant nephroma) are the most common primary malignant neoplasms of dogs and cats.[14, 390] These neoplasms are thought to develop from proximal tubular epithelial cells. Although hematuria and renomegaly may occur, clinical signs are often nonspecific and may not localize disease to the urinary tract. The natural history of renal carcinomas is unpredictable.[14] In general, they have a highly malignant potential. Their growth may be characterized by an explosive increase in size with widespread metastases, or it may be slow and asymptomatic. The most common sites of metastasis in dogs and cats include the lungs, lymph nodes, liver, brain, and bone. However, any organ may be affected, and metastases to unusual sites occur frequently. In some cases, these neoplasms are first recognized because of their metastases.

A syndrome characterized by bilateral, multifocal renal cystadenocarcinomas and nodular dermatofibrosis has been reported in German shepherd dogs.[392] Multiple uterine leiomyomas were also observed in 10 of 11 affected females. The multifocal and bilateral nature of renal cystadenocarcinomas in this syndrome contrasts with the unilateral, solitary nature characteristic of sporadic renal carcinomas. Renal cystadenocarcinomas in this syndrome have most commonly metastasized to lymph nodes, liver, and lungs. Pedigree analysis of affected dogs indicated that this syndrome was probably hereditary, and that the pattern of transmission was autosomal dominant. The mean age of affected dogs was 8.5 years.

Embryonal nephroma (also known as Wilms' tumor, nephroblastoma, or congenital mixed tumor) is considered a congenital neoplasm derived from the pleuripotential metanephric blastema.[14, 390] This neoplasm primarily occurs in young dogs and cats, although it has been observed in animals over four years of age. Embryonal nephromas are typically unilateral but may be bilateral. They may be microscopic or grow to an enormous size. Embryonal nephromas can cause hypertrophic osteoarthropathy. Local tissue invasion may occur if embryonal nephromas penetrate the renal capsule. Distant metastases also occur. The most common sites of metastasis include the lungs, liver, mesentery, and lymph nodes. Clinical signs of embryonal nephromas are similar to those of renal carcinoma.

Transitional cell carcinomas and squamous cell carcinomas of the renal pelvis are rare.[14] They may cause hematuria and obstruction of the upper urinary tract. Metastasis to distant sites may also occur, particularly involving regional lymph nodes, lungs, and liver. Renal sarcomas are less common than epithelial neoplasms or nephroblastomas. They frequently penetrate adjacent tissues and are associated with widespread metastases.[14]

Primary ureteral neoplasms are rare in dogs and cats. Transitional cell carcinoma, papillary carcinoma, leiomyoma, and leiomyosarcoma have been reported.[391] Clinical signs are often limited to hematuria and back pain unless the neoplasm becomes particularly large or causes ureteral obstruction, hydronephrosis, and hydroureter. The diagnosis may be suggested by excretory urography. Confirmation usually requires exploratory laparotomy and biopsy or resection.

Compared with primary renal neoplasia, metastatic neoplasms are commonly found in the kidneys. This difference may be related to the large blood volume perfusing the kidneys and the abundant number of renal capillaries. The most common metastatic neoplasms that affect canine kidneys have been osteosarcomas, hemangiosarcomas, lymphosarcomas, mast cell sarcomas, and malignant melanomas.[14] Focal accumulations of neoplastic cells within the kidneys usually do not produce clinical signs; most patients succumb as a result of neoplastic destruction of some other body organ or tissue before signs related to renal disease have time to develop.

Lymphosarcoma is the most common neoplasm that affects feline kidneys. The abdominal form of feline lymphosarcoma is commonly associated with extensive renal involvement, and the kidneys have been reported to be affected in up to 45 per cent of cats with lymphoma.[393] Even when renomegaly appears to affect only one kidney, both kidneys usually prove to be affected when examined microscopically.[393] Progressive weight loss, lethargy, anorexia, vomiting, diarrhea, anemia, abdominal distention, and renomegaly are characteristic findings in cats with renal lymphosarcoma. Renal failure, cachexia, fever, anemia, and secondary infections may complicate the terminal phases of the condition. Unlike in primary renal neoplasms, hematuria is not typical, and proteinuria is only occasionally observed.[393] A positive test for feline leukemia virus infection has been observed in about 50 per cent of cats with renal lymphoma. Cats with feline lymphoma have the potential for long-term survival with chemotherapy. In one study, the mean survival time for seven feline leukemia virus–negative cats that had a complete response to induction chemotherapy was 610+ days (median, 256 days).[393] One cat was still alive over seven years after diagnosis. Cats that were feline leukemia virus positive and had a complete response to induction chemotherapy had a mean survival time of 267+ days (median, 131 days). Moderate to severe azotemia appeared to have a negative effect on survival, but some azotemic cats had long survival times.

Prognosis for patients with primary renal neoplasia depends on the type, location, and extent of neoplastic involvement; presence and extent of metastases; and biologic behavior of the neoplasm.[14] If a unilateral primary neoplasm can be completely resected, the prog-

nosis may be good. In cases with bilateral renal involvement or known metastases, or when treatment is not provided, the prognosis is guarded to poor.

Treatment modalities that may be applied to renal neoplasms encompass chemotherapy, surgery, and radiation therapy (see Chapter 59).[14, 390, 391]

Idiopathic Renal Hematuria in Dogs. Idiopathic renal hematuria that resembles human benign essential hematuria has been reported in five dogs.[394, 395] This condition was characterized by gross hematuria and voiding of blood clots. Renal function and urine-concentrating ability were normal, although hydronephrosis and hydroureter were evident during intravenous urography in several dogs. The cause of hematuria was not determined. However, in each case the condition was unilateral, and hematuria resolved following surgical removal of the affected kidneys and ureters. In one dog, multiple well-demarcated, wedge-shaped, mature infarcts were identified in the renal cortex. Criteria for classification of humans as having benign essential hematuria include a negative history of hemorrhagic diathesis, renal surgery, radiation therapy, or trauma; a normal urinalysis except for hematuria; normal renal function; and a normal excretory urogram.[396]

Telangiectasia of Pembroke Welsh Corgis. A disorder characterized by multiple vascular lesions that involves the kidneys and various other organs has been reported in eight red Pembroke Welsh corgis.[396] Five males and three females were affected. The age of onset varied from two to eight years; the dogs were not known to be related. Seven of the eight dogs had intermittent gross hematuria, often with several months passing between episodes. Microscopic hematuria persisted even when gross hematuria remitted. UTI often accompanied episodes of hematuria. Other clinical signs included abdominal pain, whining, vomiting, and occasional dysuria. One dog had no clinical signs. Early in the disease, radiographic changes were absent, but intravenous pyelograms often revealed distortion of the renal pelvis with chronic involvement. Nephroliths or renal calcification often developed after several years.

Renal Parasites. *Dioctophyma renale* and *Capillaria* species are uncommon parasites that affect the urinary tract. Infections are often asymptomatic and are most often discovered by detection of parasite ova in urine sediment. They occasionally are discovered in association with microscopic or gross hematuria.

In dogs, *D. renale* primarily affects the peritoneal cavity and kidneys (especially the right kidney by a factor of 7:1 over the left kidney), although it may also occur in the urinary bladder, urethra, ovary, uterus, and pericardium.[397] Ingestion of raw fish or frogs containing encysted and infective larva appears to be the source for *D. renale* infections. Clinical signs are typically absent, but bilateral renal infections (about 3 per cent of *D. renale* infections) or unilateral infections in the absence of adequate function in the contralateral kidney can cause renal failure. Other possible clinical signs include ascites, hemoperitoneum, gross hematuria, dysuria due to passage of blood clots, and signs referable to involvement of an unusual location. Eosinophilia, basophilia, and hyperglobulinemia are typical. Diagnosis is often based on finding ova in urine sediment, but ova occur only when gravid females are present in the urinary tract (about 40 per cent of infections that involve the urinary tract).[397] Because of the high prevalence of peritoneal involvement (up to 75 per cent of infected cases), abdominocentesis and peritoneal lavage may be used to identify infection. Excretory urography is useful in localizing renal involvement and may suggest its cause. Nephrectomy or nephrotomy with surgical removal of the parasite are the only available treatments. Complete abdominal exploration and removal of parasites is indicated at the time of nephrectomy/nephrotomy.

Capillaria plica and *feliscati* are primarily parasites of the lower urinary tract of dogs (*C. plica*) and cats (*C. feliscati*). In dogs, *C. plica* may affect the urothelium of the ureter and renal pelvis (see Chapter 112).

Proteinuria

Proteinuria commonly accompanies hematuria and pyuria, but may also occur in absence of cellular elements (isolated proteinuria). When proteinuria occurs together with hematuria, causes of hematuria should be pursued as described earlier. Proteinuria with pyuria suggests inflammatory disease of the urogenital system (see section on UTI).

Finding isolated proteinuria gives rise to two important questions: (1) does the proteinuria reflect underlying renal disease, and, if so, (2) will the disease eventually cause morbidity or death?[398] Isolated proteinuria does not always indicate renal disease; strenuous exercise, extremes of heat or cold, stress, fever, seizures, and venous congestion have been reported as causes of isolated proteinuria. These causes are termed functional proteinuria. They are characteristically mild and transient, and therefore are considered nonpathologic. Proteinuria may also result from increased plasma concentrations of certain proteins (e.g., hemoglobin, myoglobin, or immunoglobulin light-chain monomers and dimers) that are small enough to pass through the glomerular barrier into urine. Because such proteins overwhelm tubular reabsorptive mechanisms, this condition is called overload proteinuria. Proteinuria resulting from immunoglobulin fragments should be suspected when protein is detected by turbidometric techniques for urine protein, but not by dipstick methods. However, radiographic contrast agents, penicillins, cephalosporins, or sulfonamide metabolites may cause false-positive reactions with turbidometric tests. Myoglobin and hemoglobin may be detected by tests for urine occult blood.

Because transient proteinuria is often of nonrenal origin, persistent proteinuria should be confirmed by repeating the urinalysis after several days. If the second urinalysis confirms proteinuria, further diagnostic inquiry is indicated because persistent proteinuria in absence of an active urine sediment is almost invariably a sign of renal structural disease even when other aspects of renal function are normal. The amount of protein excreted by such patients is of considerable diagnostic significance. Heavy proteinuria associated with hypoalbuminemia is NS and indicates generalized glomerular

disease. Urinary excretion of lesser quantities of protein may indicate either glomerular or nonglomerular renal diseases (proteinuria in nonglomerular diseases may result from glomerular hyperperfusion/hypertension or renal tubular dysfunction in which tubular reabsorption of filtered proteins is impaired). Urine protein:creatinine ratios may provide guidance in differentiating glomerular from nonglomerular disease. Ratios greater than two suggest (but do not conclusively prove) glomerular disease (see section on NS).

The clinical significance of mild persistent isolated proteinuria is uncertain in dogs and cats. Even when proteinuria does signal glomerular disease, it is not always progressive. Spontaneous remissions and even resolution of glomerular disease may occur in dogs and cats.[279, 330]

In humans, persistent, isolated proteinuria affects from 0.6 to 8.8 per cent of otherwise healthy young adults. Up to 70 per cent of these individuals have abnormal renal biopsies.[276] However, the renal lesions are highly variable and of uncertain clinical significance. About half of these patients continue to have proteinuria, but their prognosis is typically excellent. Some adult humans with isolated proteinuria have been followed for over 40 years without development of serious disease. Nonetheless, humans with persistent proteinuria appear to develop progressive renal failure more often than nonaffected individuals.[399]

A conservative approach to patients with isolated proteinuria is recommended. Although the ideal frequency of evaluation has not been established, the authors suggest evaluating these patients every three to six months to determine persistence or progression of proteinuria. As a minimum, urinalysis and renal function should be monitored; however, important additional information may be gleaned from serial evaluation of urine protein:creatinine ratios. Patients in which a pattern of persistent but stable proteinuria is established may require evaluation less often. Diagnostic inquiry into the various causes of secondary glomerular disease should be considered for patients in which glomerular proteinuria is suspected. NS or CRF may develop in some patients. Patients with evidence of progressive proteinuria should be evaluated as described in the section on NS.

Renal biopsy may be used to ascertain a precise morphologic diagnosis in patients with persistent proteinuria. However, data of therapeutic value may not be obtained, and serial assessment of proteinuria and renal function provides a more accurate prognosis. For these reasons, renal biopsy is not routinely recommended for most patients with asymptomatic persistent proteinuria.

Urinary Casts

Casts form when Tamm-Horsfall glycoprotein gels within renal tubular lumens. This event appears to be more likely in concentrated, acid urine. Casts may disappear in dilute, alkaline urine. Material within the tubular lumen at the time of cast formation may be incorporated into casts, including cells, free fat particles, cellular debris, pigments, or crystals. The net result is a variety of different types of casts, including hyaline, epithelial, granular, waxy, fatty, red blood cell (RBC), white blood cell (WBC), hemoglobin, bile-stained, and mixed casts. Although classification of casts in this manner reflects the character of the renal tubular lesion, cast morphology is rarely of specific diagnostic importance. Casts containing various cellular constituents are important in that they may localize hemorrhage (RBC casts), inflammation (WBC casts), or proteinuria (hyaline casts) to the kidneys.

Small numbers of hyaline and granular cats may be observed in urine of normal individuals. Fever, drugs (e.g., diuretics), and exercise can dramatically increase the number of hyaline casts present in human urine, perhaps due to increased glomerular protein loss.[399] In absence of these causes, large numbers of casts in urine indicate active renal injury, which is usually acute. However, the number of casts in urine is not a reliable index of the severity, duration, reversibility, or irreversibility of the underlying disease. This lack of correlation may result in part from the fact that casts appear to be discharged in intermittent showers from the renal tubules, resulting in varying numbers of casts in urine.[400]

In most instances, detection of large numbers of casts indicates the need for surveillance of renal function and urinalysis. In some patients, the medical history may reveal a potential cause of renal injury (e.g., administration of a nephrotoxic drug, renal ischemia). In the absence of an obvious cause of renal injury, the need for additional diagnostic studies should be based on evidence of persistent or progressive renal injury.

SYNDROME OF URINARY OBSTRUCTION

Definition and Clinical Significance of Urinary Obstruction

Urinary obstruction (UO) is defined as any impediment to low-pressure urine flow anywhere in the excretory pathway. The impediment to urine flow may be acute or chronic, partial or complete. It may result from lesions within or outside the excretory pathway, from the renal tubules to the urethral meatus. In dogs and cats, UO most often occurs at the level of the neck of the urinary bladder or urethra. Diseases that cause lower urinary tract obstruction are discussed in Chapters 110, 111, and 112. The most common causes of obstruction of the kidneys and ureters include uroliths, blood clots, neoplasms, trauma, inadvertent surgical ligation, and retroperitoneal disease. Bilateral upper urinary tract obstruction is rare, occurring primarily in association with diseases that affect the trigone area of the bladder (especially neoplasms). Intrarenal tubular obstruction leading to obstructive uropathy has been recognized in humans with uric acid nephropathy, polycystic kidneys, and myeloma casts.[401]

Obstruction to urine flow at any location in the urinary tract may result in temporary or permanent alterations in renal structure and function. Obstructive uropathy is a term used to describe the functional, structural, and biochemical alterations that occur as a consequence of urinary tract obstruction.[402] Sudden complete obstruction to urine outflow results in ARF; chronic partial obstruction to urine outflow may lead to progressive atrophy and destruction of nephrons and, if bilateral, CRF. Other possible complications and sequelae of urinary obstruction include: (1) urinary tract infection, (2) hypertension, (3) polyuria, (4) anuria, (5) urolithiasis, and (6) polycythemia.[401] The importance of recognizing UO is that early diagnosis and implementation of therapy may prevent or correct most adverse sequela.

Clinical Signs and Complications of Urinary Obstruction

CLINICAL SIGNS

Clinical manifestations of urinary tract obstruction are variable and may be influenced by the degree (partial or complete), duration, and location of obstruction, presence of obstruction, and whether obstruction is unilateral or bilateral.

Obstruction of the lower urinary tract (urinary bladder or urethra) may be associated with dysuria, pollakiuria, post-voiding dribbling, overflow incontinence, enlargement of the abdomen, reduction in the force and size of the urine stream, variations in urine output, and/or UTI. Abdominal palpation may reveal an enlarged and painful urinary bladder. Location of abnormalities that cause obstruction may be detected by abdominal and/or rectal palpation. Partial or intermittent UO may be associated with wide fluctuations in urine output. Chronic partial obstruction may result in polyuria and nocturia. Anuria is a cardinal sign of complete urinary tract obstruction (acute prerenal azotemia and primary renal failure are often associated with oliguria, but rarely cause total anuria). Obstruction to urine outflow should always be considered in patients with acute renal failure, especially when urine output changes rapidly or anuria occurs suddenly.[402]

Acute upper urinary tract obstructions (ureter and renal pelvis) may be associated with an acute onset of abdominal pain that is often severe, but difficult to localize. Pain results from distention of the collecting system and renal capsule, and may be associated with restlessness, depression, vomiting, tense abdomen, and resistance to abdominal palpation. The severity of pain is related to the rate of onset of obstruction; sudden onset of obstruction results in severe pain. In contrast, slowly progressive hydronephrosis may be associated with severe renal damage that is initially asymptomatic. Chronic obstruction may remain unrecognized until CRF ensues (partial bilateral obstruction), or until the hydronephrotic kidney is incidentally discovered by physical examination, abdominal radiography, or at necropsy (unilateral obstruction). Unilateral obstruction does not substantially affect renal function or urine volumes in patients with an adequately functioning contralateral kidney.

COMPLICATIONS

Obstructive uropathy may be associated with a variety of secondary complications, including: (1) UTI, (2) urolithiasis, (3) systemic hypertension, and (4) polycythemia.[401, 402] Patients with urinary tract obstruction are predisposed to UTI that may be difficult to eradicate.[401] Catheterization or other instrumentation of the urinary tract is a major source of infection.[401, 403] Infection associated with obstructive uropathy is particularly damaging because it may accelerate destruction of nephrons, and because it may aggravate the obstructive process. Infection may interfere with normal urodynamics by: (1) altering ureteral function, (2) stimulating local inflammation and edema, and (3) enhancing collagen and fibrous tissue deposition in ureteral and bladder walls.[404] In addition, struvite uroliths may rapidly develop as a result of urinary infection with urease-producing bacteria.[405] Urinary stasis encourages colonization and proliferation of microbes as well as formation of struvite crystals.[406]

In humans, acute and subacute unilateral ureteral obstruction may be associated with hypertension as a result of increased renin production by the obstructed kidney. However, chronic unilateral or bilateral obstruction in the absence of extracellular volume expansion or other forms of renal disease rarely results in hypertension.[406] An association between hypertension and spontaneously occurring urinary obstruction in dogs and cats has not been reported. However, experimentally induced acute elevations in renal pelvic pressure in dogs was associated with increased renin release from the obstructed kidney.[401]

Polycythemia is a rare complication of hydronephrosis in humans.[401] It has been postulated that hydronephrotic polycythemia results from increased erythropoietin production by hypoxic renal tissue.

EFFECT OF OBSTRUCTION ON RENAL FUNCTIONS

The effects of UO on renal functions are variable, being dependent on duration and completeness of obstruction, whether one or both kidneys are affected, and the rate of urine flow at the time of obstruction.[401, 402, 407] In general, urinary obstruction results in impairment of all renal functions except urine dilution (see Chapter 107 and references).[14, 404, 408, 409]

GFR progressively declines as long as urinary obstruction persists. However, reduced GFR does not necessarily indicate irreversible renal damage. The initial reduction in GFR is functional rather than structural, and is therefore potentially reversible. However, when obstruction persists for longer periods, irreversible structural damage ensues. Therefore, early identification and correction of urinary obstruction will optimize therapeutic response.

Impairment of urine-concentrating ability is an early and characteristic effect of bilateral urinary obstruction.[404] The magnitude of this defect is variable, but it can be marked.[402] Less consistent renal tubular dysfunctions that have been observed during or after relief of urinary obstruction include defects in: (1) urine acidification, (2) phosphate excretion, (3) calcium excretion, (4) magnesium excretion, (5) potassium excretion, (6) sodium reabsorption, (7) maximum tubular transport (Tm) of para-aminohippuric acid, and (8) Tm glucose.[402, 404, 410] These defects may result in acid-base and electrolyte disturbances, including hyperkalemic metabolic acidosis and volume depletion, which may require therapy.[404] The reversibility of these defects depends on the duration and severity of renal damage.

Diagnosis of Urinary Obstruction

UO suspected on the basis of clinical signs and physical examination should be confirmed by radiographic or ultrasonographic procedures. Physical or radiographic evidence of abnormal or inappropriate distention of the excretory pathway by urine is unequivocal evidence of UO. Additional diagnostic studies in patients with UO should encompass: (1) localization of the site(s) of obstruction, (2) identification of the obstructive lesion(s), (3) evaluation of renal function, and (4) identification of complications (such as UTI and urolithiasis).

The bladder, caudal abdomen, pelvic canal, and urethra should be palpated for evidence of intraluminal or extraluminal structures or masses that may be impinging on the urinary outflow tract. The prostate gland in males, vagina in females, and urethral meatus in both sexes should be examined. Anal sphincter tone, perineal reflex, and bulbourethral reflex should also be examined to assess neural control of voiding. In addition, the animal should be observed during voiding to assess: (1) initiation and maintenance of micturition, (2) stream size and force, and (3) completeness of voiding.

In addition to the problem-specific urinary tract data base, routine laboratory evaluation of patients suspected of having urinary tract obstruction should include quantitative urine culture, complete blood count, and radiographic studies. Urinalysis findings may provide clues to the cause of obstruction. Urine sediment examination often reveals hematuria, pyuria, and/or bacteriuria; however, urine sediment may be normal. Hematuria may be caused by urolithiasis, neoplasia, or inflammation. Pyuria and bacteriuria suggest UTI. However, bacterial UTI is more often a result than a cause of obstruction. Results of urine specific gravity, serum urea nitrogen (SUN), and S_{Cr} determinations may indicate the completeness and duration of obstruction, as well as the severity of renal dysfunction. Serum electrolyte concentrations should be determined in uremic patients with complete urinary tract obstruction, because hyperkalemia and metabolic acidosis may be correctable, life-threatening complications.

Radiographic procedures are the key to detection and localization of urinary tract obstruction. Survey radiographs are useful in detecting uroliths and in evaluating kidney and bladder size, shape, and location. Obstruction of the lower urinary tract may be demonstrated by intravenous urography, retrograde urethrocystography, antegrade cystourethrography, or voiding cystourethrography. Obstruction of the upper urinary tract is best detected by intravenous urography. In patients with renal failure, high-dose intravenous urograms should be considered. The urinary system proximal to the site of obstruction is characteristically dilated. However, dilatation of a portion of the urinary tract does not invariably indicate UO. Other findings characteristic of urinary tract obstruction include: (1) delayed appearance of the nephrogram, (2) prolonged nephrogram that becomes progressively more dense with time, (3) faint pyelogram, especially when the renal pelvis is markedly dilated, (4) renomegaly (acute obstruction), and (5) a rim sign representing the thin remnant of functional renal mass remaining in chronic hydronephrosis.[404, 406] The study should be continued until the site of obstruction has been determined or the contrast media has been excreted (by way of renal or nonrenal routes).

Ultrasonography is a noninvasive technique that may be used to detect renal structural alterations characteristic of obstruction. However, normal ultrasonic findings do not totally rule out obstructive disease, in part because lesser degrees of distention of the urinary tract may not be reliably detected.[411] Ultrasound is particularly useful in patients that may be predisposed to radiocontrast agent–induced ARF (e.g., patients with advanced renal disease, oliguric renal failure, or severe volume depletion).

Other diagnostic procedures that may be used to evaluate the upper urinary system for obstructive disease include diuresis urography or renography, renal arteriography, radioisotope renography, pressure/flow perfusion studies, retrograde ureteropyelography performed via cystoscopy, and antegrade pyeloureterography performed via percutaneous nephrostomy.[401, 404]

Prognosis

Recovery of renal function may occur after correction of unilateral or bilateral obstruction. Improvement in GFR, RBF, certain renal tubular functions, concentrating ability, and urinary acidification has been reported to occur.[404]

The potential for recovery of renal function after relief of obstruction depends on whether irreversible renal damage has occurred. Factors that may influence development of irreversible renal damage during obstruction include: (1) the degree of obstruction (complete or partial), (2) sites of obstruction (bilateral or unilateral), (3) duration of obstruction, and (4) presence of infection.[406] Complete obstruction with infection can result in total renal destruction within days.

Recovery of GFR occurred after seven days of complete unilateral ureteral obstruction in dogs.[412] One hour after release of obstruction, GFR was 25 per cent of preobstruction values. The GFR progressively increased and reached stable values 4 to 57 days later. At the time of maximum recovery, GFR was 68 per cent of normal. After contralateral nephrectomy, GFR in the previously obstructed kidney increased to values greater than those measured before obstruction.

Sequential studies in dogs with unilateral ureteral obstruction revealed that recovery of renal function is proportional to the duration of obstruction.[413] In the absence of infection, kidneys have a remarkable ability to recover function after relatively long periods of obstruction. Furthermore, the magnitude of functional recovery is markedly influenced by the presence of a contralateral kidney. After 28 days of complete unilateral obstruction, GFR was only 22 per cent of preobstruction GFR at the time of maximum recovery. However, after contralateral nephrectomy, GFR in the previously obstructed kidneys increased to 95 to 114 per cent of control values. The ability of previously obstructed kidneys to concentrate urine was impaired after relief of obstruction. However, the ability to dilute urine or to produce an alkaline or acid urine was not impaired.[413]

Prediction of reversibility of dysfunction prior to relief of obstruction is difficult. Means of assessing reversibility of renal dysfunction are: (1) use of temporary nephrostomy tubes to serially measure clearances, (2) renal biopsy, and (3) use of intravenous urograms to determine the width of the cortex and degree of dysfunction.[404] However, these tests provide only crude estimates of reversibility. In one study of dogs, excellent predictions of recovery were obtained by evaluating sodium iodohippurate ^{131}I renal scans.[404] The kidneys of dogs were obstructed for two, four, or six weeks. There was a 38.7 per cent recovery of renal function after 2 weeks of obstruction, 9.8 per cent recovery after 4 weeks of obstruction, and 2 per cent recovery after 6 weeks of obstruction. In all cases, the renogram accurately predicted long-term recovery of renal function.

Results of these experimental and clinical studies underscore the fact that varying degrees of reversibility of renal function may occur after elimination of the cause of obstruction. In human beings with UO of sufficient severity to cause marked reduction in the thickness of the renal cortex, elimination of obstruction may be associated with substantial improvement in GFR.[404] In the absence of conclusive evidence of irreversibility, efforts to decompress the urinary tract and eliminate the cause of obstruction should be considered, since at least partial restoration of renal function is likely.

Treatment

THERAPEUTIC GOALS AND PRIORITIES

The four primary goals of treatment of UO are to: (1) preserve renal function, (2) correct obstruction-induced uremia and metabolic abnormalities, (3) prevent or treat UTI, and (4) eliminate the underlying cause(s) of obstruction. Treatment of urinary obstruction may include therapy for uremia and metabolic abnormalities, elimination of UO, antimicrobial therapy directed at treatment and/or prevention of UTI and septicemia, and diagnostic and therapeutic efforts directed at prevention of recurrence of obstruction (e.g., urolithiasis).

Specific therapeutic plans for patients with UO should be determined after considering the metabolic status of the patient, presence of UTI or septicemia, and nature of the obstructive process (i.e., location, completeness, cause, and duration of obstruction). Correction of life-threatening metabolic and/or infectious complications is the priority in treatment of obstructed patients. These abnormalities may be corrected by a combination of conventional medical therapy or dialysis, antimicrobial therapy, and/or relief of UO. For details concerning management of postrenal uremia and associated fluid and electrolyte disturbances, see the section on ARF. After correcting life-threatening abnormalities and stabilizing the patient's condition, efforts should be directed toward minimizing irreversible loss of renal function. Renal function is best preserved by eliminating obstruction and infection as soon as possible.

RELIEF OF OBSTRUCTION

Three options are available to correct UO: (1) surgical intervention, (2) nonsurgical intervention, and (3) non-intervention with serial monitoring of renal functions and obstruction. Choice of therapeutic options and the timing of intervention should be based on the metabolic status of the patient, nature of the obstructive lesion (i.e., completeness, location, cause, and duration of obstruction), and the presence of UTI. It is emphasized that obstruction associated with infection mandates rapid relief of obstruction combined with antimicrobial therapy.[406]

In the absence of UTI, immediate surgical intervention is usually not essential. Even in patients with complete obstruction and uremia, nonsurgical therapy (e.g., hydropropulsion of urethral uroliths, repeated cystocentesis), fluid therapy, and/or peritoneal dialysis usually obviates need for immediate surgical intervention so that the patient's metabolic condition may be stabilized.

If obstruction is partial, the urine is sterile, and the cause of obstruction is likely to resolve spontaneously (e.g., trauma, inflammation, blood clots), the patient may be monitored for several weeks or even months. However, in cases of complete obstruction of the renal pelvis or ureter, intervention should be initiated within a few days. For example, surgical intervention is usually not recommended in humans when ureteral uroliths are causing partial obstruction unless the uroliths do not pass, or at least migrate, after four to eight weeks of observation.[401] However, uroliths that completely obstruct the renal pelvis or ureter and remain stationary are usually removed within two to three days.

When obstruction results from causes that may be treated medically (e.g., uroliths amenable to therapeutic dissolution, certain neoplasms, inflammation), guidelines similar to those outlined above are applicable. If obstruction is complete, the urine is sterile, and the cause of obstruction is potentially responsive to medical therapy, then medical therapy may be attempted to determine if complete obstruction can be converted to partial obstruction. If complete obstruction persists for longer than two or three days, surgical intervention should be considered. If partial obstruction exists, or if a patient with complete obstruction is converted to partial obstruction, the urine is sterile, and the metabolic status of the patient permits, the patient may be observed for several weeks or months. If there is evidence of progressive resolution of obstruction, the conservative approach to management should be continued. For

example, surgery may not be required for dogs with struvite uroliths treated by dietary dissolution as long as obstruction remains partial, progressive dissolution of the nephrolith can be demonstrated, and associated infection does not exacerbate renal dysfunction.

Urinary tract obstruction unlikely to resolve spontaneously or following medical treatment must be treated more aggressively. Surgical correction of partial UO is recommended for human patients with recurrent UTIs, urinary retention, progressive renal damage, recurrent hemorrhage, or persistent pain.[401, 406] Similar recommendations would appear prudent in dogs and cats.

ANTIMICROBIAL THERAPY

Patients with UTI and UO should be treated with antimicrobial agents chosen on the basis of results of quantitative urine culture and bacterial susceptibility tests. Because UO predisposes to UTI, prophylactic antimicrobial therapy should be considered when procedures likely to induce UTI are performed. Use of prophylactic antimicrobial therapy is not routinely indicated in noninfected patients that are being monitored for spontaneous resolution or response to medical therapy. However, these patients should be monitored for evidence of developing UTI.

POSTOBSTRUCTIVE DIURESIS

Substantial urinary losses of sodium and water may follow relief of complete bilateral UO. This phenomenon is known as *postobstructive diuresis*. Postobstructive diuresis does not occur after relief of unilateral obstruction, and only occurs in some patients after relief of bilateral UO. It may persist for several hours to a few days. Most human patients with bilateral UO either develop no significant natriuresis after relief of obstruction, or develop a physiologic diuresis to eliminate excess quantities of retained sodium and water.[407] Less commonly, an occasional patient develops large inappropriate losses of water and sodium.

The mechanism(s) responsible for development of postobstructive diuresis has not been fully elucidated. However, factors that may be involved include: (1) accumulation of excess extracellular fluid volume before relief of obstruction, (2) systemic accumulation of solutes (e.g., urea) during obstruction, (3) development of an intrinsic defect in renal tubular function during obstruction, and/or (4) accumulation of humoral agents during anuria that directly affect renal tubular water and sodium reabsorption.[402] Studies in rats with bilateral ureteral obstruction indicate that postobstructive diuresis is not a physiologic response to volume expansion or solute load.[401, 402] It is likely that impaired sodium and water reabsorption occurring during the postobstructive state is related to changes in the composition of plasma. Additional studies in rats have supported the concept that accumulation of natriuretic factors in blood during periods of anuria may contribute to postobstructive diuresis.[402]

Postobstructive diuresis may result in volume depletion and reduced renal function if it is not detected and treated appropriately. In animals with advanced bilateral obstruction, postobstructive diuresis should be evaluated by monitoring fluid balance. Diuresis that occurs after administration of excessive volumes of parenteral fluids may reflect appropriate elimination of fluid rather than postobstructive diuresis. Such diuresis will persist as long as excessive fluid administration is continued. After bilateral urinary tract obstruction is relieved, postobstructive diuresis may be associated with physiologic or inappropriate losses of sodium and water. Therefore, fluid intake, urine output, packed cell volume, total plasma protein concentration, body weight, and clinical assessment of hydration should be serially monitored during the postobstructive period. Fluid therapy should be administered if evidence of dehydration, prerenal azotemia, or excessive fluid losses is detected. In most cases, lactated Ringer's solution is the fluid of choice. Potassium chloride supplementation may be indicated in patients with marked kaliuresis.

Diuresis may be increased and/or prolonged by excessive fluid therapy. When diuresis results from excretion of retained sodium and water, fluid therapy should be withheld until fluid balance is normalized.

SYNDROME OF UROLITHIASIS

Urolithiasis is defined as the formation of one or more polycrystalline concretions within the urinary tract. Physical, radiographic, or ultrasonographic evidence of uroliths retained in the urinary system, or spontaneous voiding of uroliths is unequivocal evidence of urolithiasis. Urolithiasis is primarily a disorder of the lower urinary tract in dogs and cats. Nonetheless, renoliths and ureteroliths are occasionally observed, and may be associated with UO, UTI, ARF, and CRF. If uroliths are detected in the lower urinary tract, the entire urinary tract should be evaluated for additional stones (see Chapter 111).

SYNDROME OF URINARY TRACT INFECTION

Definition and Clinical Significance

Urinary tract infection (UTI) encompasses a variety of clinical entities whose common denominator is microbial invasion of any part of the urinary tract. Although pyelonephritis, cystitis, and urethritis are commonly used as generic terms, they refer to localized UTI that has the potential to spread to other parts of the urinary tract. The entire urinary tract is at risk of microbial invasion once any of its parts becomes colonized with bacteria. Although microbes can potentially invade the renal parenchyma by a blood-borne route, most UTIs occur as a consequence of ascending migration of microbes through the urethra and/or genital tract to the bladder. In the normal urinary tract, ascending infection above the bladder is impeded by unidirectional urine flow and the interference of the vesicoureteral junctions.

Unidirectional flow of urine from the ureters into the urinary bladder is important because it protects the kidneys from contamination with bladder urine. Retroflow of urine provides a means by which infection may spread from the bladder to the upper urinary tract. Depending on the integrity of these and other defense mechanisms, bladder infections may or may not ascend the ureters to affect the kidneys. Infections of the bladder and urethra are recognized more commonly than upper UTIs, because of associated hematuria and dysuria. The true incidence of renal and ureteral infections in dogs and cats is unknown because it is more difficult to identify involvement of these organs.

Although the microbial etiology of urinary infections is similar throughout the urinary system, the clinical features, response to treatment, complications, and ultimate prognosis are influenced by the sites of infection. This section focuses on bacterial infections of the kidneys. Herein, the term pyelonephritis is used synonymously with bacterial pyelonephritis (see Chapter 112).

The term pyelonephritis actually means inflammation of the kidney (i.e., tubulointerstitial inflammation) and its pelvis. A variety of etiologic factors can induce pathologic changes characterized by tubulointerstitial inflammation, including drug reactions, toxins, metabolic disturbances, immunologic disorders, and infections. However, by common usage, the term pyelonephritis has come to indicate bacterial infection of the kidneys. Nonetheless, tubulointerstitial inflammation detected by pathologic studies should not be assumed to be bacterial in origin unless confirmed by urine culture, as described in Chapter 112, or by direct culture of bacteria from kidney tissue. In humans, UTI is presumed to be the cause for tubulointerstitial inflammation and renal injury only when the pelvocalyceal system is affected.[414] Furthermore, it is held that urinary infection in the absence of an underlying urinary tract abnormality or vesicoureteral reflux rarely causes serious renal disease. Vesicoureteral reflux is the most common factor predisposing to pyelonephritic scarring in humans.[414]

Vesicoureteral Reflux and Pyelonephritis

Vesicoureteral reflux is regurgitation or retrograde flow of urine from the urinary bladder into the ureters and renal pelves through incompetent vesicoureteral junctions. On the basis of pathogenesis, it has been classified as primary or secondary. Primary vesicoureteral reflux indicates intrinsic maldevelopment of the ureterovesical junction(s), whereas secondary vesicoureteral reflux implies an acquired disorder of vesicoureteral function. Factors that affect the functional competency of the ureterovesical valve include (1) length of the intravesical segment of the ureter, (2) diameter of the intravesical ureter, (3) ratio of the length to the width of the intravesical ureter, (4) pliability of the roof of the intravesical portion of the distal ureter that functions as a flap valve, (5) integrity of the detrusor muscle, and (6) ureteral peristalsis.[14]

Primary vesicoureteral reflux has been reported in up to 50 per cent of otherwise normal dogs less than 6 months of age.[415] It usually disappears as the animal matures, occurring in less than 10 per cent of adult dogs.[415] It occurs more frequently in females than in males and is more often bilateral than unilateral. In the normal urinary tract, vesicoureteral reflux is prevented by the length of the intramural segment of the ureter. The ureter is obliquely inserted into a tunnel in the bladder wall so that the intravesical portion of the ureter is compressed by the bladder musculature during micturition. It has been hypothesized that vesicoureteral reflux in immature dogs is related to a disproportionate increase in diameter as compared with length during early development of the intramural portion of the ureter. Because the intramural portion of the ureter elongates with growth, it is less susceptible to reflux. Thus, primary vesicoureteral reflux progressively resolves during growth of immature dogs.

Secondary vesicoureteral reflux may occur as a result of inflammation of the vesicoureteral junction, UO distal to the bladder neck, neurogenic disease of the urinary bladder, surgical damage to the trigone, or ectopic ureters. It is unclear whether bladder infection can cause reflux. In one experimental study of dogs, bladder infection alone was not a significant cause of vesicoureteral reflux.[416] However, in another experimental study, reflux occurred in four of eight dogs infected with *E. coli*, and in 16 of 17 dogs infected with *Proteus* species.

Manual compression of the urinary bladder in an attempt to induce micturition may also induce vesicoureteral reflux.[417] The greater the pressure applied to the bladder, the more likely reflux is to occur. The mechanism of reflux was proposed to be related to lack of coordinated relaxation of the smooth muscle internal urethral sphincter and striated muscle external urethral sphincter which normally occurs during voiding. It is advisable to avoid manual compression of the bladder for urine collection in patients suspected of having UTI.

It is unclear whether vesicoureteral reflux causes renal damage in the absence of bacterial infection.[414] It has been postulated that renal parenchymal damage may be associated with the escape of antigenic proteins derived from the excretory pathway into the renal interstitium.[14] However, in a study in dogs, spontaneous and surgically induced vesicoureteral reflux in the absence of persistent bladder infection did not cause radiographic, gross, or microscopic changes in the kidneys or ureters.[418] When persistent urinary infection was induced by implanting a foreign body within the bladder lumen, pyelonephritis and renal dysfunction developed. Similar results have been reported by other investigators, but it was concluded that impaired ureteral peristalsis was an additional contributing factor.[419] Vesicoureteral reflux may also perpetuate lower UTI and increase susceptibility of patients to persistent or recurrent UTI as a result of post-voiding retention of urine within the ureters.

Vesicoureteral reflux may be diagnosed by contrast radiography. Procedures that permit its detection include voiding cystourethrography, retrograde urethrocystography, maximum distention cystourethrography, and compression cystourethrography. Our current recommendation is to use either voiding or maximum distention cystourethrography. Appropriate caution must be used because iatrogenic vesicoureteral reflux

may be induced in normal patients as a result of the type of anesthetic agent used, depth of anesthesia, patient positioning, and degree of distention of the urinary bladder.[14] Concomitant vesicoureteral reflux with proven bacterial UTI should prompt suspicion of pyelonephritis. However, vesicoureteral reflux may occur in the absence of pyelonephritis or renal damage.

Clinical and Laboratory Findings in Pyelonephritis

Pyelonephritis may be subclassified as acute (days to weeks) or chronic (months to years). Classic signs associated with acute pyelonephritis include pyrexia, tremors, lethargy, malaise, anorexia, vomiting, and renal pain. Caution is advised in ascribing cranial abdominal pain to the kidneys. In dogs with experimentally induced acute pyelonephritis, renal pain was either transient or absent.[420, 421] However, fever was transient in these dogs. Thus, clinical findings in patients with acute pyelonephritis vary from mild, nonspecific findings to profound clinical signs consistent with septicemia. Some patients may be asymptomatic. Concurrent lower urinary tract signs (dysuria and pollakiuria) may distract attention away from the kidneys. Because of difficulty in recognizing or confirming acute pyelonephritis in the absence of acute clinical signs (which are at best suggestive of pyelonephritis), the frequency with which it occurs as a mild or asymptomatic condition is unknown.

Clinical manifestations of chronic pyelonephritis are often subtle, but may be characterized by only polyuria and polydipsia. Loss of urine-concentrating ability appears to be a relatively early finding with chronic pyelonephritis.[420] A common test used to localize UTI to the kidneys in human patients involves testing maximum morning urine-concentrating ability. Polyuria and polydipsia may cease and urine concentration ability improve after eradication of infection. Recurrent UTI should prompt consideration of chronic pyelonephritis. Chronic pyelonephritis may be associated with recurrent asymptomatic bacteriuria, urethrocystitis, or episodes of acute pyelonephritis. Such recurrent infections are typically relapses rather than reinfections. Repeated relapse of UTI after appropriate treatment in female dogs is highly suggestive of chronic pyelonephritis.[422] In males, such relapses are more likely related to chronic prostatic infection, but may result from chronic pyelonephritis. Struvite nephroliths may develop in dogs and cats with chronic pyelonephritis resulting from urease-producing bacteria. More advanced pyelonephritis may result in CRF and its associated clinical and laboratory manifestations.

The hemogram of patients with acute pyelonephritis may be characterized by leukocytosis, whereas lower UTI typically does not alter the hemogram. An exception to this generality is acute prostatitis, which may be associated with UTI and leukocytosis. Absence of leukocytosis does not rule out pyelonephritis. In fact, chronic pyelonephritis is typically not associated with changes in the hemogram.

Evaluation of urine sediment of patients with pyelonephritis may reveal bacteriuria, pyuria, and casts. Finding WBC casts with bacteriuria is particularly significant and strongly suggests bacterial pyelonephritis. However, WBC casts were absent in dogs with experimental pyelonephritis.[420, 421] WBC casts are also an unusual finding in dogs with naturally occurring pyelonephritis. Because infection of the renal medulla frequently results in impairment of the countercurrent system, urine specific gravity values may be reduced. Unless the disease is generalized and chronic, isosthenuria is uncommon.[420, 421]

Quantitative urine culture is essential to the diagnosis of pyelonephritis. However, the numbers of bacteria present and the types of organisms identified from bladder urine do not help to localize infection (see Chapter 112).

Diagnosis of Pyelonephritis

Diagnosis of UTI is based on results of quantitative urine culture as described in Chapter 112. Clinical and laboratory findings may occasionally indicate pyelonephritis, but confirmation of the diagnosis is, at best, difficult. Numerous tests have been proposed for the purpose of localizing UTI in human patients (e.g., ureteral catheterization with differential urine cultures, bladder washout techniques, antibody on bacterial surfaces, relapse after therapy, and others), but a satisfactory sensitive, specific, and noninvasive method for identifying renal infection in dogs and cats is not currently available.[422, 423]

Intravenous pyelography may be considered to detect chronic pyelonephritis. Unfortunately, it is neither specific nor sensitive for diagnosis of bacterial pyelonephritis.[422] Radiographic findings consistent with bacterial pyelonephritis include renal pelvic and/or ureteral dilatation, decreased opacity of the vascular nephrogram, and decreased opacity of the contrast medium in the collecting system.[424] In dogs with experimentally induced renal infections, abnormal radiographic changes could be detected nine to ten days postinfection.[424] Kidney size progressively declined over 58 days of study in these dogs. However, kidney size may be increased during acute pyelonephritis.[422] Many dogs suspected of having spontaneous acute or chronic pyelonephritis have no radiographically detectable abnormalities. An additional complicating factor is that renal pelvic lesions may represent previous renal injury rather than the site of current infection.

Diagnosis of pyelonephritis is often tentative, since it must be based on supporting data derived primarily from clinical findings, radiographic studies, and nonspecific laboratory data. Pyelonephritis may be conclusively diagnosed if a positive culture can be obtained from ureteral or renal pelvic urine.[425] However, because pyelonephritis is a focal disease, random kidney biopsy often will not yield either pathologic or bacteriologic diagnosis.[423]

Prognosis of Pyelonephritis

The short-term prognosis for acute pyelonephritis depends on the underlying cause. Without treatment,

chronic pyelonephritis or septicemia may result. Acute renal infections associated with UO can lead to rapid destruction of renal tissue and septicemia and should be considered a medical emergency. The long-term prognosis for acute pyelonephritis after successful eradication of the predisposing cause and the infection is good.

If dogs and cats with chronic pyelonephritis do not have signs of systemic illness, their short-term prognosis is typically good with or without treatment. However, their long-term prognosis is unpredictable. In adult humans, chronic pyelonephritis, with or without persistent infection, is often benign in the absence of UO or underlying structural abnormalities of the urinary tract.[423] However, a small percentage of patients appear to be at risk of significant renal damage.

Treatment of Pyelonephritis

The goals of treatment of UTI are to eliminate the underlying cause(s), prevent or treat systemic sepsis, eradicate sequestered infection, relieve clinical signs, and prevent long-term sequelae.[414] Treatment of UTIs is described in Chapter 112. Selection of antimicrobial agents and dosage schedules for pyelonephritis are similar to those used for treating infections of the lower urinary tract. However, there are some important differences. For example, superficial mucosal infections (typical of bladder infections) can be eliminated by delivery of effective antimicrobial concentrations into the urine; serum antimicrobial levels are less important.[414] In pyelonephritis, effective serum concentrations appear to be advantageous, since such concentrations are more likely to reflect renal interstitial concentrations than are urine concentrations.

Intravenous antimicrobial therapy should be considered for patients with systemic sepsis. Parenteral therapy should generally be continued until the patient is afebrile, at which time oral therapy may be initiated. If UO is present, it should be rapidly corrected.[14]

Eradication of bacteria from the kidneys is generally considered to be more difficult than eradication of bacteria from the lower urinary tract. Therefore, antibiotic therapy is usually continued for a minimum of four to six weeks. Sterile cultures of urine collected by cystocentesis should be used as a guide to efficacy of therapy.

Because pyelonephritis may predispose to nephrotoxicity, nephrotoxic drugs should be avoided when possible. For example, the nephrotoxicity of gentamicin is increased in pyelonephritic rats.[426] Drug dosages for patients with reduced renal function may require adjustment (see section on CRF).

Long-term monitoring of response to therapy is important to detect and treat relapses. Urinalyses and urine cultures should be obtained by cystocentesis monthly for three months, and then every three months for one year. If relapse of infection occurs, therapy should be reinstituted as described. Long-term, low-dose antimicrobial therapy can be considered for patients that continue to relapse despite repeated attempts at therapy for pyelonephritis (see Chapter 112).

References

1. Brenner, BM, et al.: Acute Renal Failure. *In* Brenner, BM, et al., (eds): Clinical Nephrology. Philadelphia, WB Saunders, 1987, p 36.
2. Brezis, M, et al.: Acute Renal Failure. *In* Brenner, BM and Rector, FC (eds): The Kidney. Philadelphia, WB Saunders, 1986, p 735.
3. Wilkes, BM and Mailloux, LU: Acute renal failure, pathogenesis and prevention. Am J Med 80:1129, 1986.
4. Hou, SH, et al.: Hospital-acquired renal insufficiency: a prospective study. Am J Med 74:243, 1983.
5. Brown, SA and Engelhardt, JA: Drug-related nephropathies. Mechanisms, diagnosis, and management. Comp Cont Ed 9:148, 1987.
6. Engelhardt, JA and Brown, SA: Drug-related nephropathies: Commonly used drugs. Comp Cont Ed 9:281, 1987.
7. Brown, SA, et al.: Gentamicin-associated acute renal failure in the dog. JAVMA 186:686, 1985.
8. Brown, SA: Gentamicin nephrotoxicosis in the dog. *In* Kirk, RW (ed): Current Veterinary Therapy IX. Philadelphia, WB Saunders, 1986, p 1146.
9. Raisbeck, MF and Hewitt, WR: Fatal nephrotoxicosis associated with furosemide and gentamicin administration in a dog. JAVMA 183:892, 1983.
10. Burrows, GE: Topics in drug therapy: Gentamicin. JAVMA 177:301, 1979.
11. Grauer, GF, et al.: Early clinicopathologic findings in dogs ingesting ethylene glycol. Am J Vet Res 45:2299, 1984.
12. Thrall, MA, et al.: Clinicopathologic findings in dogs and cats with ethylene glycol intoxication. JAVMA 184:37, 1984.
13. Rubin, SI: Nephrotoxicity of Amphotericin B. *In* Kirk, RW (ed): Current Veterinary Therapy IX. Philadelphia, WB Saunders, 1986, p 1142.
14. Osborne, CA, et al.: The urinary system: Pathophysiology, diagnosis, treatment. *In* Gourley, IM and Vasseur, PB: General Small Animal Surgery. Philadelphia, JB Lippincott, 1985, p 479.
15. Breitschwerdt EB, et al.: Three cases of acute zinc toxicosis in dogs. Vet Hum Toxicol 28:109, 1986.
16. Spyridakis, LK, et al.: Ibuprofen toxicosis in a dog. JAVMA 189:918, 1986.
17. Rubin, SI: Nonsteroidal antiinflammatory drugs, prostaglandins, and the kidney. JAVMA 188:1065, 1986.
18. Cowgill, LD: Diseases of the Kidney. *In* Ettinger, SJ (ed): Textbook of Veterinary Internal Medicine, 2nd ed. Philadelphia, WB Saunders, 1983, p 1793.
19. Greene, CE: Leptospirosis. *In* Greene, CE, (ed): Clinical Microbiology and Infectious Diseases of the Dog and Cat. Philadelphia, WB Saunders, 1984, p 588.
20. Cotran, RS, et al.: Tubulointerstitial Diseases. *In* Brenner, BM and Rector, FC: The Kidney. Philadelphia, WB Saunders, 1986, p 1158.
21. Finco, DR, et al.: Effect of immunosuppressive drug therapy on blood urea nitrogen concentration in dogs with azotemia. JAVMA 185:664, 1984.
22. Rose, BD: Clinical Physiology of Acid-Base and Electrolyte Disorders. New York, McGraw-Hill, 1984, p 424.
23. Polzin, DJ, et al.: Clinical application of the anion gap in evaluation of acid-base disorders in dogs. Comp Cont Ed 4:1021, 1982.
24. Osborne, CA, et al.: Urinary tract infections: Normal and abnormal host defense mechanisms. Vet Clin North Am 9:587, 1979.
25. Lees, GE, et al.: Urine: A medium for bacterial growth. Vet Clin North Am 9:611, 1979.
26. Brigham, KL and Bernard, G: Pulmonary complications of chronic renal failure. Seminars in Nephrology 1:188, 1981.
27. Barsanti, JA, et al.: Urinary tract infection due to indwelling bladder catheters in dogs and cats. JAVMA 187:384, 1985.
28. Rudnick, MR, et al.: The differential diagnosis of acute renal failure. *In* Brenner, BM and Lazarus JM (eds): Acute Renal Failure. Philadelphia, WB Saunders, 1983, p 176.
29. Finco, DR and Duncan, JR: Evaluation of blood urea nitrogen and serum creatinine concentrations as indicators of renal dysfunction: A study of 111 cases and a review of related literature. JAVMA 168:593, 1976.
30. Polzin, DJ, et al.: Influence of reduced protein diets on morbidity, mortality, and renal function in dogs with induced chronic renal failure. Am J Vet Res 45:506, 1984.
31. Lees, GE: Risks of urinary catheterization. *In* Kirk, RW (ed): Current Veterinary Therapy IX. Philadelphia, WB Saunders, 1986, p 1127.
32. Calvert, CA and Greene, CE: Cardiovascular infections. *In* Greene CE (ed): Clinical Microbiology and Infectious Diseases of the Dog and Cat. Philadelphia, WB Saunders, 1984, p 220.
33. Finco, DR and Barsanti, JA: Bacterial pyelonephritis. Vet Clin North Am 9:645, 1979.
34. Richet, G: When should renal biopsy be done in acute uremia? Tomorrow could be too late. Kidney Intern 28, 17:S152, 1985.
35. Greco, DS, et al.: Urinary gamma-glutamyl transpeptidase activities in dogs with gentamicin-induced nephrotoxicity. Am J Vet Res 46:2332, 1985.
36. Gossett, KA: Evaluation of gamma-glutamyl transpeptidase-to-creatinine ratio from spot samples of urine supernatant, as an indicator of urinary enzyme excretion in dogs. Am J Vet Res 48:455, 1987.
37. Anderson, RJ, et al.: Nonoliguric acute renal failure. N Engl J Med 296:1134, 1977.
38. Willard, MD: Treatment of Hyperkalemia. *In* Kirk, RW (ed): Current Veterinary Therapy IX. Philadelphia, WB Saunders, 1986, p 94.
39. Kopple, JD: Nutritional therapy in kidney failure. Nutr Rev 39:193, 1981.
40. Schaer, M: Disorders of potassium metabolism. Vet Clin North Am 12:399, 1982.
41. Polzin, DJ and Osborne, CA: Diseases of the urinary tract. *In* Davis, L: Manual of Therapeutics in Small Animal Practice. New York, Churchill Livingstone, 1985, p 333.
42. Hiatt, N and Sheinkopf, JA: Treatment of experimental hyperkalemia with large doses of insulin. Surg Gynecol Obstet 133:833, 1971.
43. Montoliu, J, et al.: Potassium-lowering effect of Albuterol for hyperkalemia in renal failure. Arch Int Med 147:713, 1987.
44. Bell, FW and Osborne, CA: Treatment of hypokalemia. *In* Kirk, RW (ed): Current Veterinary Therapy IX. Philadelphia, WB Saunders, 1986, p 101.
45. Levinsky, NG, et al.: Mannitol and diuretics in acute renal failure. *In* Brenner BM and Lazarus JM: Acute Renal Failure. Philadelphia, WB Saunders, 1983, p 712.
46. Hardaker, WT and Wechsler, AS: Redistribution of renal intracortical blood flow during dopamine infusion in dogs. Circ Res 33:437, 1973.
47. McNay, JL, et al.: Direct renal vasodilation produced by dopamine in the dog. Circ Res 26:510, 1965.
48. Lindner, A, et al.: Synergism of dopamine plus furosemide in preventing acute renal failure in the dog. Kidney Intern 16:158, 1979.
49. Andrews, PM and Bates, SB: Dietary protein prior to renal ischemia dramatically affects postischemic kidney function. Kidney Intern 30:299, 1986.
50. Remuzzi, G, et al.: Low-protein diet prevents glomerular damage in adriamycin-treated rats. Kidney Intern 28:21, 1985.
51. Thornhill, JA: Control of vomiting in the uremic patient. *In* Kirk, RW (ed): Current Veterinary Therapy VIII. Philadelphia, WB Saunders, 1983, p 1022.
52. Takala, J: Nutrition in acute renal failure. Critical Care Clinics 3:155, 1987.
53. Van Buren, CT, et al.: Effects of intravenous essential L-amino acids and hypertonic dextrose on anephric beagles. Surg Forum 23:83, 1972.
54. Thornhill, JA: Peritoneal dialysis in the dog and cat: An update. Comp Cont Ed 3:20, 1981.
55. McCall-Kaufman, G: Peritoneal dialysis. Proc ACVIM, San Diego, 1987, p 4.
56. Merdan-Dhein, CR: Hemodialysis in the dog. Comp Cont Ed 3:1031, 1981.
57. Mitch, WE, et al.: A simple method for estimating progression of chronic renal failure. Lancet 2:1326, 1976.
58. Allen, TA, et al.: A technique for estimating progression of chronic renal failure in the dog. JAVMA 190:866, 1987.
59. Richards, MA and Hoe, CM: A long-term study of renal disease in the dog. Vet Rec 80:640, 1967.

60. DiBartola, SP, et al.: Clinicopathologic findings associated with chronic renal disease in cats: 74 cases (1973–1984). JAVMA 190:1196, 1987.
61. Davenport, DJ, et al.: Familial renal disease in the dog and cat. *In* Breitschwerdt, EB (ed): Nephrology and Urology. New York, Churchill Livingstone, 1986, p 137.
62. Picut, CA and Lewis, RM: Microscopic features of canine renal dysplasia. Vet Path 24:156, 1987.
63. Breitschwerdt, EB, et al.: Multiple endocrine abnormalities in basenji dogs with renal tubular dysfunction. JAVMA 182:1348, 1983.
64. Finco, DR, et al.: Physiology and pathophysiology of renal failure. *In* Ettinger, SJ (ed): Textbook of Veterinary Internal Medicine. Philadelphia, WB Saunders, 1975, p 1453.
65. Polzin, DJ, et al.: Influence of modified protein diets on electrolyte, acid-base, and divalent ion balance in dogs with experimentally induced chronic renal failure. Am J Vet Res 43:1978, 1982.
66. Finco, DR and Rowland, GN: Hypercalcemia secondary to chronic renal failure in the dog: A report of 4 cases. JAVMA 173:990, 1978.
67. Widmer, B, et al.: Serum electrolyte and acid-base composition. The influence of graded degrees of chronic renal failure. Arch Int Med 139:1099, 1979.
68. Dow, SW, et al.: Potassium depletion in cats: Hypokalemic polymyopathy. JAVMA 191:1563, 1987.
69. Dow, SW, et al.: Potassium depletion in cats: Renal and dietary influences. JAVMA 191:1569, 1987.
70. Polzin, DJ, et al.: Serum amylase and lipase activities in dogs with chronic primary renal failure. Am J Vet Res 44:404, 1983.
71. Hudson, EB and Strombeck, DR: Effects of functional nephrectomy on the disappearance rates of canine serum amylase and lipase. Am J Vet Res 39:1316, 1978.
72. Rutsky, EA, et al.: Acute pancreatitis in patients with end-stage renal disease without transplantation. Arch Intern Med 146:1741, 1986.
73. Polzin, DJ and Osborne, CA: Dietary management of chronic renal failure. *In* Breitschwerdt, EB (ed): Nephrology and Urology. New York, Churchill Livingstone, 1986, p 151.
74. Polzin, DJ and Osborne, CA: Conservative medical management of canine chronic polyuric renal failure. *In* Kirk, RW (ed): Current Veterinary Therapy VIII. Philadelphia, WB Saunders, 1983, p 997.
75. Hardy, RM: Disorders of water metabolism. Vet Clin North Am 12:353, 1982.
76. Hostetter, TH: Progressive renal disease: Is the slippery slope species specific? J Lab Clin Med 109:375, 1987.
77. Finco, DR, et al.: Kidney graft survival in transfused and nontransfused sibling beagle dogs. Am J Vet Res 46:2327, 1985.
78. Gregory, CR, et al.: Experience with cyclosporine A following renal allografting in two dogs. Vet Surg 15:441, 1986.
79. Gregory, CR, et al.: Preliminary results of clinical renal allograph transplantation in the dog and cat. J Vet Intern Med 1:53, 1987.
80. Finco, DR, et al.: Efficacy of azathioprine versus cyclosporine on kidney graft survival in transfused and nontransfused unmatched mongrel dogs. J Vet Intern Med 1:61, 1987.
81. Schall, WD, et al.: Editorial: Clinical transplantation in veterinary medicine. J Vet Intern Med 1:95, 1987.
82. Kleinknecht, C, et al.: Effect of various protein diets on growth, renal function, and survival of uremic rats. Kidney Int 15:534, 1979.
83. Hostetter, TH: The hyperfiltering glomerulus. Med Clin North Am 68:387, 1984.
84. Rutherford, WE, et al.: Chronic, progressive renal disease: Rate of change of serum creatinine. Kidney Int 13:62, 1977.
85. Oksa, H, et al.: Progression of chronic renal failure. Nephron 35:31, 1983.
86. Bovee, KC, et al.: Long-term measurement of renal function in partially nephrectomized dogs fed 56, 27, or 19 per cent protein. Invest Urol 16:378, 1979.
87. Dezie, C, et al.: The evolution of chronic renal failure. Kidney Int 29:317A, 1986.
88. Hostetter, TH, et al.: Chronic effects of dietary protein in the rat with intact and reduced renal mass. Kidney Int 30:509, 1986.
89. Bourgoignie, JJ, et al.: Glomerular function and morphology after renal mass reduction in dogs. J Lab Clin Med 109:380, 1987.
90. Brown, S, et al.: Beneficial effect of moderate phosphate restriction in partially nephrectomized dogs on a low protein diet. Kidney Intern 31:380(abstr), 1987.
91. Brenner, BM, et al.: Dietary protein intake and the progressive nature of kidney disease: The role of hemodynamically mediated glomerular injury in the pathogenesis of progressive glomerular sclerosis in aging, ablation, and intrinsic renal disease. N Engl J Med 307:652, 1982.
92. Hostetter, TH, et al.: Hyperfiltration in remnant nephrons: A potentially adverse response to renal ablation. Am J Physiol 241:F85, 1981.
93. Olson, JL, et al.: Altered glomerular permselectivity and progressive glomerular sclerosis following extreme ablation of renal mass. Kidney Int 22:112, 1982.
94. Anderson, S and Brenner, BM: The role of intraglomerular pressure in the initiation and progression of renal disease. J Hypertension 4(suppl 5):S236, 1986.
95. Chanutin, A and Ferris, EB: Experimental renal insufficiency produced by partial nephrectomy. I. Control diet. Arch Int Med 49:767, 1932.
96. Shimamura, T and Morrison, AB: A progressive glomerulosclerosis occurring in partial five-sixth nephrectomized rats. Am J Path 79:95, 1975.
97. Polzin, DJ, et al.: Development of renal lesions in dogs after 11/12 reduction of renal mass: Influences of dietary protein. Lab Invest 55:172, 1988.
98. Dunn, BR, et al.: The hemodynamic basis of progressive renal disease. Semin Nephrol 6:122, 1986.
99. Paller, MS and Hostetter, TH: Dietary protein increases plasma renin and reduces pressor reactivity to angiotensin II. Am J Physiol 251:F34, 1986.
100. Levine, MM, et al.: Effect of protein on glomerular filtration rate and prostanoid synthesis in normal and uremic rats. Am J Physiol 251:F653, 1986.
101. Hayes, CP, et al.: An extra-renal mechanism for the maintenance of potassium balance in severe CRF. Trans Assoc Amer Physicians 80:207, 1967.
102. Meyer, TW, et al.: Reversing glomerular hypertension stabilizes established glomerular injury. Kidney Intern 31:752, 1987.
103. Anderson, S and Brenner, BM: Role of glomerular hypertension in the initiation and progression of renal disease. *In* Kaplan, NM, et al. (eds): The Kidney in Hypertension. New York, Raven Press, 1987, p 67.
104. Anderson, S, et al.: Antihypertensive therapy must control glomerular hypertension to limit glomerular injury. J Hypertension 4(suppl 5):S242, 1986.
105. Meyer, TW, et al.: Reversing glomerular hypertension stabilizes established glomerular injury in renal ablation. J Hypertension 4(suppl 5):S239, 1986.
106. Anderson, S, et al.: Control of glomerular hypertension limits glomerular injury in rats with reduced renal mass. J Clin Invest 76:612, 1985.
107. Anderson, S, et al.: Therapeutic advantage of converting enzyme inhibitors in arresting progressive renal disease associated with systemic hypertension in the rat. J Clin Invest 77:1993. 1986.
108. Klahr, S, et al.: Factors that may retard the progression of renal disease. Kidney Intern 32:S35, 1987.
109. Lovett, DH, et al.: Stimulation of rat mesangial cell proliferation by macrophage interleukin I. J Immunol 131:2830, 1983.
110. Haut, LL, et al.: Renal toxicity of phosphate in rats. Kidney Intern 17:722, 1980.
111. Ibels, LS, et al.: Preservation of function in experimental renal disease by dietary restriction of phosphate. N Engl J Med 298:122, 1978.
112. Ross, LA, et al.: Effect of dietary phosphorus restriction on the kidneys of cats with reduced renal mass. Am J Vet Res 43:1023, 1982.
113. Walser, M, et al.: The effect of nutritional therapy on the course of chronic renal failure. Clin Nephrol 11:66, 1979.
114. Walser, M: Does dietary therapy have a role in the predialysis patient. Am J Clin Nutr 33:1629, 1980.
115. Barrientos, A, et al.: Role of phosphate in the progression of chronic renal failure. Mineral Electrolyte Metab 7:127, 1982.
116. Hitchman, AJ, et al.: Phosphate-induced renal calcification in the rat. Can J Physiol Pharmacol 57:92, 1979.

117. Gimenez, LF, et al.: Relation between renal calcium content and renal impairment in 246 human renal biopsies. Kidney Intern 31:93, 1987.

118. Lumlertgul, D, et al.: Phosphate arrests progression of chronic renal failure independent of protein intake. Kidney Intern 29:658, 1986.

119. Brenner, BM and Meyer, TW: Mechanisms of progression of renal disease. Proc 9th Intl Cong Nephrology, New York, Springer-Verlag, 1984, p 1233.

120. Harris, DCH, et al.: Verapamil protects against progression of experimental chronic renal failure. Kidney Intern 31:41, 1987.

121. Glomset, JA: Fish, fatty acids, and human health. N Engl J Med 312:1253, 1985.

122. Nath, KA, et al.: Pathophysiology of chronic tubulo-interstitial disease in rats. J Clin Invest 76:667, 1985.

123. Tolins, JP, et al.: Hypokalemic nephropathy in the rat. J Clin Invest 79:1447, 1987.

124. Polzin, DJ, et al.: The importance of egg protein in reduced protein diets designed for dogs with renal failure. J Vet Intern Med 2:15, 1988.

125. Heifets, M, et al.: Effect of dietary lipids on renal function in rats with subtotal nephrectomy. Kidney Intern 32:335, 1987.

126. Scharschmidt, LA, et al.: Effects of dietary fish oil on renal insufficiency in rats with subtotal nephrectomy. Kidney Intern 32:700, 1987.

127. Barcelli, UO, et al.: Effects of a dietary prostaglandin precursor on the progression of experimentally induced chronic renal failure. J Lab Clin Med 100:786, 1982.

128. Hurd, ER, et al.: Prevention of glomerulonephritis and prolonged survival in New Zealand black/New Zealand white F1 hybrid mice fed an essential fatty acid-deficient diet. J Clin Invest 67:476, 1981.

129. Barcelli, U and Pollak, VE: Is there a role for polyunsaturated fatty acids in the prevention of renal disease and renal failure? Nephron 41:209, 1985.

130. Moorehead, JF, et al.: Lipid nephrotoxicity in chronic progressive glomerular and tubulo-interstitial disease. Lancet 11:1309, 1982.

131. Ito, Y, et al.: A low protein–high linoleate diet increases glomerular PGE2 and protects renal function in rats with reduced renal mass. Prostaglandins, Leukotrienes, and Medicine 28:277, 1987.

132. Klahr, S, et al.: The influence of anticoagulation in the progression of experimental renal disease. In Mitch, W, Brenner, BM, and Stein, J (eds): Contemporary Issues in Nephrology, 14. New York, Churchill Livingstone, 1986, p 45.

133. Purkerson, ML, et al.: Pathogenesis of the glomerulopathy associated with renal infarction in rats. Kidney Int 9:407, 1976.

134. Purkerson, ML, et al.: Inhibition of anticoagulant drugs of the progressive hypertension and uremia associated with renal infarction in rats. Thrombosis Res 26:227, 1984.

135. Olson, JL: Role of heparin as a protective agent following reduction of renal mass. Kidney Intern 25:376, 1984.

136. Purkerson, ML, et al.: Inhibition of thromboxane synthesis prevents progressive renal disease in rats with 5/6 nephrectomy (abstract). Kidney Intern 25:251, 1984.

137. Moel, DI, et al.: Effect of aspirin on experimental diabetic nephropathy. J Lab Clin Med 110:300, 1987.

138. Kelly, RA and Mitch, WE: Creatinine, uric acid, and other nitrogenous waste products: Clinical implication of the imbalance between their production and elimination in uremia. Semin Nephrol 3:286, 1983.

139. Johnson, WJ: Does elevated blood urea participate in the pathogenesis of the uremic syndrome? Semin Nephrol 3:265, 1983.

140. Campbell, RA: Polyamines, uremia, and anemia. Semin Nephrol 3:273, 1983.

141. Massry, SG and Kopple, JD: Uremic toxins: What are they? How are they identified? Semin Nephrol 3:263, 1983.

142. Keshaviah, P and Kjellstrand, CM: Middle molecules: Do they exist? Are they toxic? Semin Nephrol 3:295, 1983.

143. Polzin, DJ, et al.: Effects of modified protein diets in dogs with chronic renal failure. JAVMA 183:980, 1983.

144. Robertson, JL, et al.: Long-term responses to high dietary protein in dogs with 75 per cent nephrectomy. Kidney Int 29:511, 1986.

145. Bosch, JP, et al.: Renal functional reserve in humans: Effect of protein intake on glomerular filtration rate. Am J Med 75:943, 1983.

146. Polzin, DJ, et al.: Influence of modified protein diets on the nutritional status of dogs with induced chronic renal failure. Am J Vet Res 44:1694, 1983.

147. Corbin, JE, et al.: Nutrient requirements of domestic animals: Nutritional requirements of dogs. No. 8, Washington, DC, National Academy of Sciences, National Research Council, 1972.

148. Morris, ML and Doering, GG: Dietary management of renal failure in dogs. Canine Pract 5:46, 1978.

149. Rice, EE, et al.: Nutrient requirements of domestic animals: Nutrient requirements of dogs, publication 989, Washington, DC, National Academy of Sciences, National Research Council, 1962.

150. Bovee, KC: The uremic syndrome: Patient evaluation and treatment. Comp Cont Ed 1:279, 1979.

151. Giordano, C: Use of exogenous and endogenous urea for protein synthesis in normal and uremic subjects. J Lab Clin Med 62:231, 1963.

152. Kopple, JD and Coburn, JW: Metabolic studies of low protein diets in uremia. I. Nitrogen and potassium. Medicine 52:583, 1973.

153. Mitch, WE, et al.: Effects of oral neomycin and kanamycin in chronic uremia patients: I. Urea metabolism. Kidney Int 11:116, 1977.

154. Pennisi, AJ, et al.: Effects of protein amino acid diets in chronically uremic and control rats. Kidney Int 13:472, 1978.

155. Varcoe, AR, et al.: Anabolic role of urea in renal failure. Am J Clin Nutr 31:1601, 1978.

156. Varcoe, AR, et al.: Efficiency of utilization of urea nitrogen for albumin synthesis by chronically uremic and normal man. Clin Sci & Molecular Med 48:379, 1975.

157. Delaporte, C, et al.: Variations in muscle cell protein of severely uremic children. Kidney Int 10:239, 1976.

158. Walser, M and Mitch, WE: Dietary management of renal failure. The Kidney 10:13, 1977.

159. Abitbol, CL and Holiday, MA: Effect of energy and nitrogen intake upon urea nitrogen production in children with uremia and undernutrition. Clin Nephrol 10:9, 1978.

160. Bagade, JD, et al.: Evidence for an accelerated adaptation to starvation in chronic uremia. Metabolism 26:1107, 1977.

161. Walser, M: The conservative management of the uremic patient. In Brenner, BM and Rector, FC: The Kidney. Philadelphia, WB Saunders, 1976, p 1613.

162. Burger, IH, et al.: The protein requirement of adult cats for maintenance. Feline Pract 14:8, 1984.

163. Osborne, CA and Polzin, DJ: Conservative medical management of feline chronic polyuric renal failure. In Kirk, RW (ed): Current Veterinary Therapy VIII. Philadelphia, WB Saunders, 1983, p 1008.

164. Kopple, JD: Chronic renal failure: Nutritional and nondialytic management. In Glassock, RJ (ed): Current Therapy in Nephrology and Hypertension, 1984-85. St. Louis, CV Mosby, 1984, p 252.

165. Avioli, LV and Tietelbaum, SL: The renal osteodystrophies. In Brenner, BM and Rector, FC: The Kidney. Philadelphia, WB Saunders, 1976, p 1542.

166. Borison, HL and Hebertson, LM: Role of medullary emetic chemoreceptor trigger zone in post-nephrectomy vomiting dogs. Am J Physiol 197:850, 1959.

167. Gehrig, JJ, et al.: Effect of intermittent feeding on renal hemodynamics in conscious rats. Am J Physiol 250:F566, 1986.

168. Everitt, AV, et al.: Effects of caloric intake and dietary composition on the development of proteinuria, age-associated renal disease and longevity in the male rat. Gerontology 28:168, 1982.

169. Tucker, SM, et al.: Influence of diet and feed restriction on kidney function of aging male rats. J Gerontology 31:264, 1976.

170. Macy, DW and Gasper, PW: Diazepam-induced eating in anorexic cats. JAAHA 21:17, 1985.

171. Della Fera, MA, et al.: Benzodiazepine-like chemicals and feeding behavior in puppies. The Physiologist 20:21, 1978.

172. Randall, LO: Pharmacology of methaminodiazepoxide. Dis Nerv Sys 21:7, 1960.

173. Anderson, RJ, et al.: Fate of drugs in renal failure. In Brenner, BM and Rector, FC (eds): The Kidney. Philadelphia, WB Saunders, 1981, p 2659.

174. Finco DR, et al.: Effects of an anabolic steroid on acute uremia in the dog. Am J Vet Res 45:2285, 1984.

175. Schultze, R, et al.: Studies on the control of sodium excretion in experimental uremia. J Clin Invest 48:869, 1969.

176. Schmidt, RW, et al.: On the adaptation in sodium excretion in chronic uremia: The effects of proportional reduction of sodium intake. J Clin Invest 53:1736, 1974.

177. Cowgill, LD and Kallet, AJ: Recognition and management of hypertension in the dog. In Kirk, RW, (ed): Current Veterinary Therapy VIII. Philadelphia, WB Saunders, 1983, p 1025.

178. Schmidt, RW and Gavellas, G: Bicarbonate reabsorption in experimental renal disease: Effects of proportional reduction of sodium or phosphate intake. Kidney Intern 12:393, 1977.

179. Weinberger, MH: Sodium chloride and blood pressure. N Engl J Med 317:1084, 1987.

180. Husted, FC, et al.: NaHCO$_3$ and NaCl tolerance in chronic renal failure. J Clin Invest 56:414, 1975.

181. Kurtz, TW, et al.: "Salt-sensitive" essential hypertension in men. Is the sodium ion alone important? N Engl J Med 317:1043, 1987.

182. Bourgoignie, JJ, et al.: Renal handling of potassium in dogs with chronic renal insufficiency. Kidney Int 20:482, 1981.

183. Dow, SW, et al.: Hypokalemic polymyopathy in 6 cats. Proc, 5th Ann Forum ACVIM. San Diego, CA, 1987, p 912.

184. Ross, LA, et al.: Relationship of selected clinical renal function tests to glomerular filtration rate and renal blood flow in cats. Am J Vet Res 42:1704, 1981.

185. Ichikawa, I, et al.: Effect of heparin on the glomerular structure and function of remnant nephrons. Kidney Intern 34:638, 1988.

186. Schwartz, WB, et al.: On the mechanism of acidosis in chronic renal disease. J Clin Invest 38:39, 1959.

187. Massry, SG: Prevention and treatment in divalent ion metabolism in renal failure. Semin Nephrol 6:114, 1986.

188. Rutherford, WE, et al.: Phosphate control and 25-hydroxycholecalciferol administration in preventing experimental renal osteodystrophy in the dog. J Clin Invest 60:332, 1977.

189. Slatopolsky, E, et al.: On the pathogenesis of hyperparathyroidism in chronic and experimental renal insufficiency in the dog. J Clin Invest 50:492, 1971.

190. Slatopolsky, E, et al.: On the prevention of secondary hyperparathyroidism in experimental chronic renal disease using "proportional reduction" of dietary phosphors intake. Kidney Intern 2:147, 1972.

191. Slatopolsky, E and Bricker, NS: The role of phosphorus restriction in the prevention of secondary hyperparathyroidism in chronic renal disease. Kidney Intern 4:141, 1973.

192. Slatopolsky, E, et al.: Calcium carbonate as a phosphate binder in patients with chronic renal failure undergoing dialysis. N Engl J Med 315:157, 1986.

193. Barsotti, G, et al.: Reversal of hyperparathyroidism in severe uremics following very low-protein and low-phosphorus diet. Nephron 30:310, 1982.

194. Tanaka, Y and DeLuca, HF: The control of 25-dihydroxyvitamin D metabolism by inorganic phosphorus. Arch Biochem Biophys 154:566, 1973.

195. Oldham, SB, et al.: The acute effects of 1,25-dihydroxycholecalciferol on serum immunoreactive parathyroid hormone in the dog. Endocrinology 104:248, 1979.

196. Tessitore, N, et al.: Relationship between serum vitamin D metabolites and dietary intake of phosphate in patients with early renal failure. Mineral Electrolyte Metab 13:38, 1987.

197. Sherwood, LM: Vitamin D, parathyroid hormone, and renal failure. N Engl J Med 316:1601, 1987.

198. Finco, DR, et al.: Effects of three diets on dogs with induced chronic renal failure. Am J Vet Res 46:646, 1985.

199. Balasa, RW, et al.: Phosphate-binding properties and electrolyte content of aluminum hydroxide antacids. Nephron 45:16, 1987.

200. Rutherford, WE, et al.: An evaluation of a new and effective phosphorus binding agent. Trans Am Soc Artif Intern Organs 19:446, 1973.

201. Henry, DA, et al.: Parenteral aluminum administration in the dog: II. Induction of osteomalacia and effect on vitamin D metabolism. Kidney Intern 25:36, 1984.

202. Goodman, WG, et al.: Parenteral aluminum administration in the dog: I. Plasma kinetics, tissue levels, calcium metabolism, and parathyroid hormone. Kidney Intern 25:362, 1984.

203. Slatopolsky, E, et al.: Alternative phosphate binders in dialysis patients: calcium carbonate. Semin Nephrol 6 (suppl. 1):3541, 1986.

204. Lopez, S, et al.: Evaluation of calcium carbonate as an effective phosphorus binder in the dog. Clin Res 32:452A, 1984.

205. Hercz, G and Coburn, JW: Prevention of phosphate retention and hyperphosphatemia in uremia. Kidney Intern 32(suppl 22): S215, 1987.

206. Nebeker, HG, et al.: A non-aluminum containing phosphate binder: Polyuronic acid. Kidney Intern 27:147, 1985.

207. Finco, DR: The role of phosphorus restriction in the management of chronic renal failure in the dog and cat. 7th Annual Kal Kan Symposium for the Treatment of Small Animal Diseases, Columbus, Ohio, 1983, p 131.

208. Goligorsky, MS, et al.: Verapamil improves defective duodenal calcium absorption in experimental chronic renal failure. Mineral Electrolyte Metab 12:363, 1986.

209. Korkor, AB: Reduced binding of [3H]1,25-dihydroxyvitamin D in the parathyroid glands of patients with renal failure. N Engl J Med 316:1573, 1987.

210. Merke, J, et al.: Diminished parathyroid 1,25(OH)2D3 receptors in experimental uremia. Kidney Intern 32:350, 1987.

211. Goldstein, DA, et al.: The duodenal mucosa in patients with renal failure: response to 1,25(OH)2D3. Kidney Intern 19:324, 1981.

212. Peterson, ME: Hypoparathyroidism. In Kirk, RW (ed): Current Veterinary Therapy XI. Philadelphia, WB Saunders, 1986, p 1039.

213. Miller, ME: Oxygen transport in uremia. Semin Nephrol 5:140, 1985.

214. Anagnostou, A and Kurtzman, NA: Hematological consequences of renal failure. In Brenner BM and Rector FC: The Kidney. Philadelphia, WB Saunders, 1986, p 1631.

215. McGonigle RJS, et al.: Erythropoietin deficiency and inhibition of erythropoiesis in renal insufficiency. Kidney Intern 25:437, 1984.

216. Pavlovic-Kentera, V, et al.: Erythropoietin and anemia in chronic renal failure. Exp Hematol 15:785, 1987.

217. Eschbach, JW and Adamson, JW: Anemia of end-stage renal disease. Kidney Intern 28:1, 1985.

218. Anagnostou, A and Kurtzman, NA: The anemia of chronic renal failure. Semin in Nephrology 5:115, 1985.

219. Caro, J and Erslev, AJ: Uremic inhibitors of erythropoiesis. Semin in Nephrology 5:128, 1985.

220. Eaton, JW and Leida, MN: Hemolysis in chronic renal failure. Semin Nephrol 5:133, 1985.

221. Zingraff, J, et al.: Anemia and secondary hyperparathyroidism. Arch Int Med 138:1650, 1978.

222. Weinberg SG, et al.: Myelofibrosis and renal osteodystrophy. Am J Med 63:755, 1977.

223. Eschbach, JW, et al.: Correction of the anemia of end-stage renal disease with recombinant human erythropoietin. N Engl J Med 316:73, 1987.

224. Dainiak, N: The role of androgens in the treatment of chronic renal failure. Semin Nephrol 5:147, 1985.

225. Osborne, CA and Polzin, DJ: Strategy in the diagnosis, prognosis, and management of renal disease, renal failure, and uremia. Proc 46th Ann Mtg, AAHA, New Orleans, LA, 1979, p 559.

226. Doane BD, et al.: Response of uremic patients to nandrolone decanoate. Arch Intern Med 135:972, 1975.

227. Hendler ED, et al.: Controlled study of androgen therapy in anemia of patients on maintenance hemodialysis. N Engl J Med 291:1046, 1974.

228. Chew DJ, et al.: Pharmacologic manipulation of urination. In Kirk, RW (ed): Current Veterinary Therapy IX. Philadelphia, WB Saunders, 1986, p 1207.

229. Polzin DJ, and Osborne CA: Update—Conservative medical management of chronic renal failure. In Kirk, RW (ed): Current Veterinary Therapy IX. Philadelphia, WB Saunders, 1986, p 1167.

230. Heywood R, et al.: Toxicity of methyl testosterone in the beagle dog. Toxicology 7:357, 1977.

231. Barsanti, JA: Treatment of aplastic anemia with androgens. Proc 46th Ann Mtg, AAHA, New Orleans, LA, 1979, p 233.

232. Schall, WD and Perman, V: Diseases of the red blood cells. In Ettinger SJ: Textbook of Veterinary Internal Medicine. Philadelphia, WB Saunders, 1975, p 1607.

233. Riviere, JE: Calculation of dosage regimens of antimicrobial drugs in animals with renal and hepatic dysfunction. JAVMA 185:1094, 1984.

234. Davis, LE: Drug therapy in renal disorders. In Kirk, RW (ed): Current Veterinary Therapy VII. Philadelphia, WB Saunders, 1980, p 1114.

235. Senior, DF: Drug therapy in renal failure. Vet Clin North Amer 9:805, 1979.

236. Neff-Davis, CA: Clinical monitoring of drug concentrations. In Davis, L: Manual of Therapeutics in Small Animal Practice. New York, Churchill Livingstone, 1985, p 633.

237. Spangler, WL, et al.: Canine hypertension: A review. JAVMA 170:995, 1977.

238. Weiser, MG and Spangler, WL: Blood pressure measurement in the dog. JAVMA 171:364, 1977.

239. Gwin, RM, et al.: Hypertensive retinopathy associated with hypothyroidism, hypercholesterolemia, and renal failure in a dog. JAAHA 14:200, 1978.

240. Bidani, AK, et al.: Renal autoregulation and vulnerability to hypertensive injury in remnant kidney. Am J Physiol 252:F1003, 1987.

241. Seney, FD, et al.: Modification of tubuloglomerular feedback signal by dietary protein. Am J Physiol 252:F83, 1987.

242. Mitch, WE: The influence of the diet on the progression of renal insufficiency. Ann Rev Med 35: 249, 1984.

243. Chew, DJ, et al.: Renal amyloidosis in related Abyssinian cats. JAVMA 181:139, 1982.

244. Boyce, JT, et al.: Familial renal amyloidosis in Abyssinian cats. Vet Path 21:33, 1984.

245. DiBartola, SP, et al.: Isolation and characterization of amyloid protein AA in the Abyssinian cat. Lab Invest 52:485, 1985.

246. Kaufman, CF, et al.: Renal cortical hypoplasia with secondary hyperparathyroidism in the dog. JAVMA 155:1679, 1969.

247. Easley, JR and Breitschwerdt, EB: Glucosuria associated with renal tubular dysfunction in three basenji dogs. JAVMA 168:938, 1978.

248. Bovee, KC, et al.: The Fanconi syndrome in basenji dogs: A new model for renal transport defects. Science 201:1129, 1978.

249. Bovee, KC, et al.: Characterization of renal defects in dogs with a syndrome similar to the Fanconi syndrome in man. JAVMA 174:1094, 1979.

250. Vymental, F: Case reports: Renal aplasia in beagles. Vet Rec 77:1344, 1965.

251. Robbins, CR: Unilateral renal agenesis in the beagle. Vet Rec 77:1345, 1965.

252. Murti, GS: Agenesis and dysgenesis of the canine kidneys. JAVMA 146:1120, 1965.

253. Fox, MW: Inherited polycystic mononephrosis in the dog. J Hered 55:29, 1964.

254. Lucke, VM, et al.: Chronic renal failure in young dogs—possible renal dysplasia. J Sm Anim Pract 21:169, 1980.

255. McKenna, SC and Carpenter, JL: Polycystic kidney disease of the kidney and liver in the Cairn Terrier. Vet Path 17:436, 1980.

256. Steward, AP and MacDougall, DF: Familial nephropathy in the cocker spaniel. J Sm Anim Pract 25:15, 1984.

257. English, PB and Winter, H: Renal cortical hypoplasia in a dog. Aust Vet J 55:181, 1979.

258. Wilcock, BP and Patterson, JM: Familial glomerulonephritis in Doberman pinscher dogs. Can Vet J 20:244, 1979.

259. Chew, DJ, et al.: Juvenile renal disease in Doberman pinscher dogs. JAVMA 182:481, 1983.

260. Crowell, WA and Hubbell, JJ: Polycystic renal disease in related cats. JAVMA 175:286, 1979.

261. Lulich, JP, et al.: Urologic disorders of immature cats. Vet Clin North Amer 17:663, 1987.

262. Norrdin, RW: Fibrous osteodystrophy with facial hyperostosis in a dog with renal cortical hypoplasia. Cornell Vet 65:173, 1975.

263. Klopfer, U, et al.: Renal cortical hypoplasia in a Keeshond litter. VM/SAC 70:1081, 1975.

264. O'Brien, TD, et al.: Clinicopathologic manifestations of progressive renal disease in Lhasa apso and Shih Tzu dogs. JAVMA 180:658, 1982.

265. McQueen, SD, et al.: Bilateral congenital polycystic kidneys with vague symptomatology in a dog (A case report). VM/SAC 70:1167, 1975.

266. Finco, DR, et al.: Familial renal disease in Norwegian elkhound dogs. JAVMA 156:747, 1970.

267. Finco, DR, et al.: Familial renal disease in Norwegian elkhound dogs: physiologic and biochemical examinations. Am J Vet Res 37:87, 1976.

268. Finco, DR, et al.: Familial renal disease in Norwegian elkhound dogs: morphologic examinations. Am J Vet Res 37:941, 1978.

269. Bernard, MA and Vali, VE: Familial renal disease in Samoyed dogs. Can Vet J 18:181, 1977.

270. Bloedow, AG: Familial renal disease in Samoyed dogs. Vet Rec 108:167, 1981.

271. Jansen, B, et al.: Samoyed hereditary glomerulopathy (SHG): Evolution of splitting of glomerular capillary basement membranes. Am J Pathol 125:536, 1986.

272. Nash, AS, et al.: Progressive renal disease in soft-coated Wheaton terriers: possible familial nephropathy. J Sm Anim Pract 25:479, 1984.

273. Eriksen, K and Grondalen J: Familial renal disease in softcoated Wheaton terriers. J Sm Anim Pract 25:489, 1984.

274. DiBartola, SP, et al.: Juvenile renal disease in related standard poodles. JAVMA 183:693, 1983.

275. Klopfer, U, et al.: A nephropathy similar to renal cortical hypoplasia in a Yorkshire Terrier. VM/SAC 73:327, 1978.

276. Hutt, MP and Kelleher, SP: Proteinuria and the nephrotic syndrome. In Schrier, RW (ed): Renal and Electrolyte Disorders, 3rd ed. Boston, Little, Brown and Co, 1986, p 565.

277. Brenner, BM: Clinical and laboratory assessment of patients with renal and urinary tract disease. In Brenner, BM, et al. (eds): Clinical Nephrology. Philadelphia, WB Saunders, 1987, p 1.

278. Wright, NG and Nash, AS: Glomerulonephritis in the dog and cat. Irish Vet J 37:4, 1983.

279. Arthur, JE, et al.: The long-term prognosis of feline idiopathic membranous glomerulonephropathy. JAAHA 22:731, 1986.

280. Wright, NG, et al.: Membranous nephropathy in the cat and dog. Lab Invest 45:269, 1981.

281. Jaenke, RS and Allen, TA: Membranous nephropathy in the dog. Vet Path 23:718, 1986.

282. DiBartola, SP and Chew, DJ: Glomerular disease in the dog and cat. In Kirk, RW (ed): Current Veterinary Therapy IX. Philadelphia, WB Saunders, 1986, p 1132.

283. August, JR and Lieb, MS: Primary renal diseases of the cat. Vet Clin North Am 14:1247, 1984.

284. Center, SA, et al.: Clinicopathologic, renal immunofluorescent, and light microscopic features of glomerulonephritis in the dog: 41 cases (1975-1985). JAVMA 190:81, 1987.

285. Lucke, VM: Glomerulonephritis in the cat. The Veterinary Annual 22:270, 1982.

286. DiBartola, SP and Meuten, DJ: Renal amyloidosis in two dogs presented for thromboembolic phenomena. JAAHA 16:129, 1980.

287. Slauson, DO and Gribble, DH: Thrombosis complicating renal amyloidosis in dogs. Vet Path 8:352, 1971.

288. DiBartola, SP, et al.: Urinary protein excretion and immunopathologic findings in dogs with glomerular disease. JAVMA 177:73, 1987.

289. Feldman, BF: Thrombosis-Diagnosis and treatment. In Kirk, RW (ed): Current Veterinary Therapy IX. Philadelphia, WB Saunders, 1986, p 505.

290. Macdougall, DF, et al.: Canine chronic renal disease: Prevalence and types of glomerulonephritis in the dog. Kidney Intern 29:1144, 1986.

291. Levey, AS, et al.: Serum creatinine and renal function. Ann Rev Med 39:465, 1988.

292. Schnaper, HW and Robson, AM: Nephrotic syndrome: Minimal change disease, focal glomerulosclerosis, and related disorders. In Schrier, RW and Gottschalk, CW (eds): Diseases of the Kidney, 4th ed. Boston, Little, Brown and Co, 1988, p 1949.

293. McClusky, RT: Immunopathogenic mechanisms in renal disease. Am J Kidney Disease 10:172, 1987.

294. Garattini, S, et al.: What is the basis for the use of steroids in the treatment of idiopathic membranous nephropathy? Nephron 45:1, 1987.

295. Robbins, SL, et al.: Pathologic basis of disease, 3rd ed. Philadelphia, WB Saunders, 1984, p 991.

296. Murray, M, et al.: A morphologic study of canine glomerulonephritis. Lab Invest 30:213, 1974.

297. Glassock, RJ: Natural history and treatment of primary proliferative glomerulonephritis: A review. Kidney Int 28 (suppl 17): S136, 1985.

298. The primary and secondary glomerulopathies. *In* Brenner, BM, et al. (eds): Clinical Nephrology. Philadelphia, WB Saunders, 1987, p 73.

299. Osborne, CA and Jeraj, K: Glomerulonephropathy and the nephrotic syndrome. *In* Kirk, RW (ed): Current Veterinary Therapy VII. Philadelphia, WB Saunders, 1980, p 1053.

300. Jeraj, K, et al.: Immunofluorescence studies of renal basement membranes in dogs with spontaneous diabetes. Am J Vet Res 45:1162, 1984.

301. Wright, NG and Nash, AS: Experimental ampicillin glomerulopathy. J Comp Path 94:357, 1984.

302. Shirtoh, K, et al.: Glomerulopathy in a cat with cyanotic congenital heart disease. Vet Path 24:280, 1987.

303. Shull, RM, et al.: Membranous glomerulopathy and nephrotic syndrome associated with iatrogenic metallic mercury poisoning in a cat. Vet Hum Toxicol 23:1, 1981.

304. Glenner, GG: Amyloid deposits and amyloidosis. The β-fibrilloses. N Engl J Med 302:1283, 1980.

305. Eanes, ED and Glenner, GG: X-ray diffraction studies of amyloid fibrils and immunoglobulin proteins. J Histochem Cytochem 16:673, 1968.

306. Termine, JD, et al.: Infrared spectroscopy of human amyloid fibrils and immunoglobulin proteins. Biopolymers 11:1103, 1972.

307. Westermark, P, et al.: AA-amyloidosis in dogs: Partial amino acid sequence of protein AA and immunohistochemical cross-reactivity with human and cow AA-amyloid. Comp Biochem Physiol 82:211, 1985.

308. Benson, MD, et al.: Identification and characterization of amyloid protein AA in spontaneous canine amyloidosis. J Exp Med 138:373, 1980.

309. Levin, M, et al.: The amino acid sequence of a major nonimmunoglobulin component of some amyloid fibrils. J Clin Invest 51:2773, 1972.

310. Sellinger, MJ, et al.: Monokine-induced synthesis of serum amyloid A protein by hepatocytes. Nature 285:498, 1980.

311. Benson, M and Kleiner, E: Synthesis and secretion of serum amyloid protein A (SAA) by hepatocytes in mice treated with casein. J Immunol 124:495, 1980.

312. DiBartola, SP, et al.: Tissue distribution of amyloid deposits in Abyssinian cats with familial amyloidosis. J Comp Path 96:387, 1986.

313. Glenner, GG, et al.: Amyloid fibril proteins: Proof of homology with immunoglobulin light chains by sequence analyses. Science 172:1150, 1971.

314. Pitkanen, P, et al.: Senile systemic amyloidosis. Am J Pathol 117:391, 1984.

315. Sletten, K, et al.: Senile cardiac amyloidosis is related to prealbumin. Scand J Immunol 12:503, 1980.

316. Gejyo, F, et al.: A new form of amyloid protein associated with chronic hemodialysis was identified as β$_2$-microglobulin. Biochem Biophys Res Comm 129:701, 1985.

317. Gorevic, PD, et al.: Polymerization of intact β$_2$-microglobulin in tissue causes amyloidosis in patients on chronic hemodialysis. Proc Natl Acad Sci USA 83:7908, 1986.

318. Linke, RP, et al.: Amyloid kidney stones of uremic patients consist of β$_2$-microglobulin fragments. Biochem Biophys Res Comm 136:665, 1986.

319. McCaw, DL, et al.: Effect of collection time and exercise restriction on the prediction of urine protein excretion, using urine protein/creatinine ratio in dogs. Am J Vet Res 46:1665, 1985.

319a. DiBartola, SP, et al.: Quantitative urinalysis including 24-hour protein excretion in the dog. JAAHA 16:537, 1980.

319b. Biewenga, WJ, et al.: Urinary protein loss in the dog: nephrological study of 29 dogs without signs of renal disease. Res Vet Sci 33:366, 1982.

320. Jergens, AE, et al.: Effects of collection time and food consumption on the urine protein/creatinine ratio in the dog. Am J Vet Res 48:1106, 1987.

321. White, JV, et al.: Use of protein-to-creatinine ratio in a single urine specimen for quantitative estimation of canine proteinuria. JAVMA 185:882, 1984.

322. Center, SA, et al.: 24-Hour urine protein/creatinine ratio in dogs with protein-losing nephropathies. JAVMA 187:820, 1985.

323. Grauer, GF, et al.: Estimation of quantitative proteinuria in the dog, using the urine protein-to-creatinine ratio from a random, voided sample. Am J Vet Res 46:2116, 1985.

324. Shull, RM, et al.: Investigation of the nature and specificity of antinuclear antibody in dogs. Am J Vet Res 44:2004, 1983.

325. Jeraj, K, et al.: Evaluation of renal biopsy in 97 dogs and cats. JAVMA 181:367, 1982.

326. Levey, AS, et al.: Idiopathic nephrotic syndrome: Puncturing the biopsy myth. Ann Int Med 107:697, 1987.

327. Kassier, JP: Is renal biopsy necessary for optimal management of the idiopathic nephrotic syndrome? Kidney Intern 24:561, 1983.

328. Fries, JF, et al.: Marginal benefit of renal biopsy in systemic lupus erythematosus. Arch Int Med 138:1386, 1978.

329. Arthur, JE, et al.: An immunohistological study of feline glomerulonephritis using the peroxidase-antiperoxidase method. Res Vet Sci 37:12, 1984.

330. Osborne, CA, et al.: Natural remission of nephrotic syndrome in a dog with immune-complex glomerular disease. JAVMA 168:129, 1976.

331. West, CD: Childhood membranoproliferative glomerulonephritis: An approach to management. Kidney Intern 29:1077, 1986.

332. Ponticelli, C: Prognosis and treatment of membranous nephropathy. Kidney Intern 29:927, 1986.

333. Ponticelli, C, et al.: Controlled trial of methylprednisolone and chlorambucil in idiopathic membranous nephropathy. N Engl J Med 310:946, 1984.

334. West, ML, et al.: A controlled trial of cyclophosphamide in patients with membranous glomerulonephritis. Kidney Intern 32:579, 1987.

335. Nash, AS, et al.: Membranous nephropathy in the cat: A clinical and pathological study. Vet Rec 105:71, 1979.

336. Wright, NG, et al.: Membranous nephropathy in the cat and dog: A renal biopsy and follow-up study of sixteen cases. Lab Invest 45:269, 1981.

337. Slauson, DO, et al.: Naturally-occurring immune-complex glomerulonephritis in the cat. J Pathol 103:131, 1971.

338. Burns, MG, et al.: Pulmonary artery thrombosis in three dogs with hyperadrenocorticism. JAVMA 178:388, 1981.

339. Garcia, DL, et al.: Chronic glucocorticoid therapy amplifies glomerular injury in rats with renal ablation. J Clin Invest 80:867, 1987.

340. Baylis, C and Brenner, BM: Mechanism of the glucocorticoid–induced increase in glomerular filtration rate. Am J Physiol 234:F166, 1978.

341. White, SD, et al.: Corticosteroid (methylprednisolone sodium succinate) pulse therapy in five dogs with autoimmune skin disease. JAVMA 191:1121, 1987.

342. Hancock, W and Atkins, R: Activation of coagulation pathways and fibrin deposition in human glomerulonephritis. Semin Nephrol 5:69, 1985.

342a. Barnes, JL and Venkatachalam, MA: The role of platelets and polycationic mediators in glomerular vascular injury. Semin Nephrol 5:57, 1985.

343. Izumino, K, et al.: Effect of antiplatelet agents ticlopidine and dipyridamole on nephrotoxic serum nephritis in rats. Nephron 45:306, 1987.

344. Cameron, JS: Platelets in glomerular disease. Ann Rev Med 35:175, 1984.

345. George, CRP, et al.: A kinetic evaluation of hemostasis in renal disease. N Engl J Med 291:1111, 1974.

346. Donadio, JV, et al.: Membranoproliferative glomerulonephritis: A prospective clinical trial of platelet inhibitor therapy. N Engl J Med 310:1421, 1984.

347. Cattran, DC, et al.: Results of a controlled drug trial in membranoproliferative glomerulonephritis. Kidney Intern 27:436, 1985.

348. Tanphaichitr, P, et al.: Treatment of nephrotic syndrome with levamisole. J Pediatrics 96:490, 1980.

349. Clark, WF, et al.: Monthly plasmapheresis for systemic lupus erythematosus with diffuse proliferative glomerulonephritis: a pilot study. Can Med Assoc J 125:171, 1981.

350. Kauffmann, RH, and Houwert, DA: Plasmapheresis in rapidly progressive Henoch-Schoenlein glomerulonephritis and the effect on circulating IgA immune complexes. Clin Nephrol 16:155, 1981.

351. Gruys, E, et al.: Dubious effect of dimethlysulphoxide (DMSO) therapy on amyloid deposits and amyloidosis. Vet Res Comm 5:21, 1981.

352. Spyridakis, L, et al.: Amyloidosis in a dog: Treatment with dimethylsulphoxide. JAVMA 189:690, 1986.

353. Osborne, CA, et al.: Renal amyloidosis in the dog. JAVMA 153:669, 1968.
354. Glassock, RJ: Clinical aspects of glomerular diseases. Am J Kidney Dis 10:181, 1987.
355. Kaysen, GA, et al.: Effect of dietary protein intake on albumin homeostasis in nephrotic patients. Kidney Intern 29:527, 1986.
356. Kaysen, GA, et al.: Albumin homeostasis in the nephrotic rat: nutritional considerations. Am J Physiol 247:F192, 1984.
357. Rahman, MA, et al.: The roles of eicosanoids in experimental glomerulonephritis. Kidney Intern 32 (suppl 22):S40, 1987.
358. Heeg, JE, et al.: Reduction of proteinuria by angiotensin converting enzyme inhibition. Kidney Intern 32:78, 1987.
359. Taguma, Y, et al.: Effect of captopril on heavy proteinuria in azotemic diabetics. N Engl J Med 313:1617, 1985.
360. Lagrue, G, et al.: Antiproteinuric effect of captopril in primary glomerular disease (letter). Nephron 46:99, 1987.
361. Bohrer, MP, et al.: Mechanism of angiotensin II-induced proteinuria in the rat. Am J Physiol 233:F13, 1977.
362. Brenner, BM: The primary and secondary glomerulopathies. In Brenner, BM, et al. (eds): Clinical Nephrology. Philadelphia, WB Saunders, 1987, p 93.
363. Barsanti, JA and Finco, DR: Protein concentration in urine of normal dogs. Am J Vet Res 40:1583, 1979.
364. Orofino, L, et al.: Hypertension in primary glomerulonephritis: Analysis of 288 biopsied patients. Nephron 45:22, 1987.
365. Kaysen, GA, et al.: Albumin synthesis, albuminuria, and hyperlipemia in nephrotic patients. Kidney Intern 31:1368, 1987.
366. Appel, GB, et al.: The hyperlipidemia of the nephrotic syndrome. N Engl J Med 312:1544, 1985.
367. Vigano-D'Angelo, S, et al.: Protein S deficiency occurs in the nephrotic syndrome. Ann Int Med 107:42, 1987.
368. Skorecki, KL, et al.: Renal and systemic manifestations of glomerular disease. In Brenner BM and Rector FC: The Kidney. Philadelphia, WB Saunders, 1986, p 891.
369. Green, RA and Kabel, AL: Hypercoagulable state in three dogs with nephrotic syndrome: Role of acquired antithrombin III deficiency. JAVMA 181:914, 1982.
370. Green, RA, et al.: Hypoalbuminemia-related platelet hypersensitivity in two dogs with nephrotic syndrome. JAVMA 186:485, 1985.
371. Lulich, JP, et al.: Feline idiopathic polycystic kidney disease. Comp Cont Ed 10:1030, 1988.
372. Crowell, WA: Polycystic renal disease. In Kirk, RW (ed): Current Veterinary Therapy IX. Philadelphia, WB Saunders, 1986, p 1138.
373. Brenner, BM: Tubulointerstitial nephropathies. In Brenner, BM, et al. (eds): Clinical Nephrology. Philadelphia, WB Saunders, 1987, p 161.
374. Grantham, JJ and Gabow, PA: Polycystic kidney disease. In Schreir, RW and Gottschalk, CW: Diseases of the Kidney, 4th ed. Boston, Little, Brown, 1988, p 583.
375. Brace, JJ: Perirenal cysts (pseudocysts) in the cat. In Kirk, RW (ed): Current Veterinary Therapy VIII. Philadelphia, WB Saunders, 1983, p 980.
376. Abdinoor, DJ: Perinephric pseudocysts in a cat. JAAHA 16:763, 1980.
377. Rose, BD: Clinical Physiology of Acid-Base and Electrolyte Disorders. New York, McGraw-Hill, 1984, p 394
378. Brown, SA, et al.: Fanconi syndrome and acute renal failure associated with gentamicin therapy in a dog. JAAHA 22:635, 1986.
379. Drazner, FH: Distal renal tubular acidosis associated with chronic pyelonephritis in a cat. Calif Vet 6:15, 1980.
380. Brown, SA, et al.: Distal renal tubular acidosis and hepatic lipidosis in a cat. JAVMA 189:1350, 1986.
381. Polzin, DJ, et al.: Distal renal tubular acidosis and urolithiasis. Vet Clin North Amer 16:241, 1986.
382. Friedman, AL and Chesney, RW: Isolated renal tubular disorders. In Schreir, RW and Gottschalk, CW: Diseases of the Kidney, 4th ed. Boston, Little, Brown, 1988, p 663.
383. Breitschwerdt, EB, et al.: Multiple endocrine abnormalities in Basenji dogs with renal tubular dysfunction. JAVMA 182:1348, 1983.
384. Bovee, KC, et al.: Spontaneous Fanconi syndrome in the dog. Metabolism 27:45, 1978.
385. Bovee, KC: Genetic and metabolic diseases of the kidney. In Bovee, KC (ed): Canine Nephrology. Philadelphia, Harwal Publishing, 1984, p 339.
386. Breitschwerdt, EB: Nephrogenic diabetes insipidus. In Kirk, RW (ed): Current Veterinary Therapy IX. Philadelphia, WB Saunders, 1986, p 1140.
387. Breitschwerdt, EB, et al.: Nephrogenic diabetes insipidus in three dogs. JAVMA 179:235, 1981.
388. Lage, AL: Nephrogenic diabetes insipidus in a dog. JAVMA 163:251, 1973.
389. Stone, EA: Renal hematuria in dogs. In Kirk, RW (ed): Current Veterinary Therapy IX. Philadelphia, WB Saunders, 1986, p 1130.
390. Caywood, DD, et al.: Neoplasms of the canine and feline urinary tract. In Kirk, RW (ed): Current Veterinary Therapy VII. Philadelphia, WB Saunders, 1980, p 1203.
391. Crow, SE: Urinary tract neoplasms in dogs and cats. Comp Cont Ed 7:607, 1985.
392. Hereditary multifocal renal cystadenocarcinomas and nodular dermatofibromatosis in the German shepherd dog: Macroscopic and histopathologic changes. Vet Path 22:447, 1985.
393. Mooney, SC, et al.: Renal lymphoma in cats: 28 cases (1977–1988). JAVMA 191:1473, 1987.
394. Stone, EA, et al.: Massive hematuria of non-traumatic renal origin in dogs. JAVMA 183:868, 1983.
395. Straw, RC, et al.: Idiopathic hematuria of unilateral renal origin in a dog. JAVMA 187:1371, 1985.
396. Moore, FM and Thornton, GW: Telangiectasia of Pembroke Welsh Corgi Dogs. Vet Path 20:203, 1983.
397. Brown, SA and Prestwood, AK: Parasites of the urinary tract. In Kirk, RW (ed): Current Veterinary Therapy IX. Philadelphia, WB Saunders, 1986, p 1153.
398. Robinson, RR: Isolated proteinuria in asymptomatic patients. Kidney Intern 18:395, 1980.
399. Kassier, JP and Harrington, JT: Laboratory evaluation of renal function. In Schreir, RW and Gottschalk, CW: Diseases of the Kidney, 4th ed. Boston, Little, Brown, 1988, p 393.
400. Osborne, CA and Stevens, JB: Handbook of canine and feline urinalysis. St. Louis, Ralston Purina, 1981, p 91.
401. Wright, FS and Howards, SS: Obstructive Injury. In Brenner, BM and Rector, FC (eds): The Kidney, 2nd ed. Philadelphia, WB Saunders, 1981, p 2008.
402. Klahr, S: Pathophysiology of obstructive nephropathy. Kidney Intern 23:414, 1983.
403. Lees, GE and Osborne, CA: Urinary tract infection associated with the use and misuse of urinary catheters. Vet Clin North Am 9:713, 1979.
404. Gillenwater, JY: Clinical aspects of urinary tract obstruction. Semin Nephrol 2:46, 1982.
405. Klausner, JS and Osborne, CA: Urinary tract infection and urolithiasis. Vet Clin North Am 9:701, 1979.
406. Brenner, BM, et al.: Urinary tract obstruction. In Petersdorf, RG, et al.: Harrison's Principles of Internal Medicine, 10th ed. New York, McGraw-Hill, 1983, p 1676.
407. Wright, FS: Effects of urinary tract obstruction on glomerular filtration rate and renal blood flow. Semin Nephrol 2:5, 1982.
408. Urinary tract obstruction. In Brenner, BM, et al.: Clinical Nephrology. Philadelphia, WB Saunders, 1987, p 180.
409. Wilson, DR: Urinary tract obstruction. In Schreir, RW and Gottschalk, CW: Diseases of the Kidney, 4th ed. Boston, Little, Brown, 1988, p 715.
410. Yarger, WE and Buerkert, J: Effect of urinary tract obstruction on renal tubular function. Semin Nephrol 2:17, 1982.
411. Beck, LH, et al.: Obstructive uropathy. In Early, LE and Gottschalk, CW (eds): Strauss and Wells' Diseases of the Kidney, 3rd ed. Boston, Little, Brown and Co, 1979, p 877.
412. Kerr, WS, Jr.: Effects of complete ureteral obstruction for one week on kidney function. J Appl Physiol 6:762, 1954.
413. Kerr, WS, Jr.: Effect of complete ureteral obstruction in dogs on kidney function. Am J Physiol 184:521, 1956.
414. Rubin, RH, et al.: Urinary tract infection, pyelonephritis, and reflux nephropathy. In Brenner BM and Rector FC: The Kidney. Philadelphia, WB Saunders, 1986, p 1085.
415. Christie, BA: Incidence and etiology of vesicoureteral reflux in apparently normal dogs. Invest Urol 10:184, 1971.
416. Harrison, L, et al.: Role of bladder infection in the etiology of vesicoureteral reflux in dogs. Invest Urol 12:123, 1974.
417. Feeney, DA, et al.: Vesicoureteral reflux induced by manual compression of the urinary bladder in dogs and cats. JAVMA 182:795, 1983.

418. Newman, L, et al.: Experimental production of reflux in the presence and absence of infected urine. Radiology 111:591, 1974.
419. Tsuchida, S, et al.: Ascending pyelonephritis in dogs induced by ureteral dysfunction. Invest Urol 10:450, 1973.
420. Finco, DR, and Barsanti, JA: Bacterial pyelonephritis. Vet Clin North Am 9:645, 1979.
421. Finco, DR, et al.: Evaluation of methods for localization of urinary tract infection in the dog. Am J Vet Res 40:707, 1979.
422. Lees, GE and Rogers, KS: Diagnosis and localization of urinary tract infection. In Kirk, RW (ed): Current Veterinary Therapy IX. Philadelphia, WB Saunders, 1986, p 1118.
423. Ronald, AR and Simonsen, N: Infections of the upper urinary tract. In Schreir, RW and Gottschalk, CW: Diseases of the Kidney, 4th ed. Boston, Little, Brown, 1988, p 1065.
424. Barber, DL and Finco, DR: Radiographic findings in induced bacterial pyelonephritis in dogs. JAVMA 175:1183, 1979.
425. Ling, GV, et al.: Percutaneous nephropyelocentesis and nephropyelostomy in the dog: A description of the technique. Am J Vet Res 40:1605, 1979.
426. Beauchamp, D, et al.: Increased nephrotoxicity of gentamicin in pyelonephritic rats. Kidney Intern 28:106, 1985.

DRUG INDEX

Generic	Trade	Dosage	Route	Frequency	Description
Aluminum hydroxide	See Table 108–23	30 to 90 mg/kg/day 15 to 40 mg/lb/day	Oral	With food	Intestinal phosphate binding agents
Androgens	. . . .	See Table 108–25	. . . .		Promote RBC production
Calcium carbonate	Equilet	1 to 2 g[a]	Oral	With food	Intestinal phosphate binding agent
Calcium carbonate	Equilet	100 mg/kg/day[b] 45 mg/lb/day[b]	Oral	With food	Oral calcium supplement
Calcium citrate	Citrical	2 to 5 g[a]	Oral	With food	Intestinal phosphate binding agent
Chlorpromazine		0.5 mg/kg 0.25 mg/lb	IV, IM	q 12 h[c]	Antiemetic
Chlorothiazide	Diuril	20 to 40 mg/kg 10 to 20 mg/kg	Oral	q 12 h	Diuretic
Cimetidine	Tagamet	10 mg/kg—1 dose, then 5 mg/kg[e, f] 5 mg/lb—1 dose, then 2.5 mg/lb[e, f]	IV	q 12 h	H$_2$ blocker, antiemetic
Diazepam	Valium	0.04 to 0.4 mg/kg 0.02 to 0.2 mg/lb	Oral[g]	q 8 to 24 h	Appetite stimulant
Dihydrotachysterol	Hytakeral	0.01 mg/kg[b] 0.0045 mg/lb[b]	Oral	q 24 h	Vitamin D supplement
1,25-dihydroxyvitamin D	Rocatrol	0.03 to 0.06 μg/kg 0.015 to 0.03 μg/lb	Oral	q 24 h	Vitamin D supplement
Dimethyl sulfoxide		125 mg/kg (10% soln) 55 mg/lb	Oral	q 12 h	Used to treat amyloidosis
		80 mg/kg 40 mg/lb	SQ, T[h]	3×/week	Used to treat amyloidosis
Dopamine	Intropin	2 to 5 μg/kg/min 1 to 2.5 μg/lb/min	IV	Continuous	Renal vasodilator
Flurazepam	Dalmane	0.2 to 0.4 mg/kg 0.1 to 0.2 mg/lb	Oral	q 4 to 7 d	Appetite stimulant
Furosemide	Lasix	2 mg/kg[i] 1 mg/lb[i]	IV	q 8 h	Diuretic
Mannitol		0.25 to 0.5 g/kg 0.11 to 0.25 g/lb	IV	q 4 to 6 h	Diuretic
Oxazepam	Serax	0.2 mg/kg 0.1 mg/lb	Oral	q 24 h	Appetite stimulant
Polystyrene sulfonate	Kayexalate	0.7 g/kg 0.32 g/lb	Oral	q 8 h	Intestinal potassium binding agent
Prochlorperazine	Compazine	0.13 mg/kg 0.06 mg/lb	IM	q 6 h[c]	Antiemetic
Trimethobenzamide	Tigan	3 mg/kg 1.4 mg/lb	IM	q 5 h[d]	Antiemetic

[a]Dosage recommended for humans. Dosage should be adjusted to effect (see text).
[b]Dosage adjusted to effect (see text).
[c]Double dosage interval for cats
[d]Dosage not established for cats
[e]Feline dose one-half canine dose
[f]Dosage gradually reduced with time (see text)
[g]May also be given IV or IM.
[h]T = topical application
[i]Dosage may be increased in refractory cases

109 HYPERTENSIVE DISEASE

LINDA A. ROSS

Hypertension has, until recently, received little attention in clinical veterinary medicine. The most important factor in its neglect appears to be the perception that it is difficult to measure blood pressure in dogs and cats, although techniques for measurement of blood pressure in dogs have been reported as early as 1930.[1] The presence of hypertension in a collie with spontaneous nephritis was noted in a 1923 paper.[2] Many investigators have reported techniques for indirect blood pressure measurements in dogs over the past 50 years.[1-15] Despite the fact that these studies describe simple, accurate methods, blood pressure measurement has not been accepted as a routine diagnostic tool by the veterinary community.

Whereas primary, or essential, hypertension has an incidence in people of as high as 15 per cent of the population,[16] several surveys of large numbers of clinically normal dogs have reported an incidence of hypertension of less than 1 per cent.[17-19] Secondary hypertension, on the other hand, has been documented in animals with a variety of diseases. Because hypertension can cause significant pathology in several organ systems, it behooves veterinarians to become familiar with its pathophysiology, diagnosis, and management.

NORMAL DETERMINANTS OF BLOOD PRESSURE

To understand hypertension, knowledge of the physical and physiologic factors that determine arterial pressure is necessary. Pressure is force per unit area, and the force is a function of the volume of fluid in the system. Arterial blood volume is a function of the rate at which blood enters the arterial system (left ventricular output) and the rate at which blood leaves the system. The physical equation expressing pressure is: mean arterial pressure = cardiac output times total peripheral resistance. Neuroendocrine factors regulate and control both cardiac output and total peripheral resistance, and therefore pressure.

The neural and endocrine factors involved can be subdivided into two systems: (1) a system that results in rapid changes in blood pressure (acting within one minute), which is primarily neural and (2) a system that is involved in long-term maintenance of blood pressure (requiring 30 minutes to several hours for action), which is primarily humoral.[20]

There are three major nervous control mechanisms involved in the maintenance of arterial blood pressure. The baroreceptor feedback system is probably the most important in adjusting to minute-to-minute changes in pressure. Sensory receptors (baroreceptors) are located in both the carotid sinus (the wall of each internal carotid artery just above the bifurcation) and the aortic arch. Afferent nerves from these receptors travel to the vasomotor center in the brain stem. The fibers from the carotid sinus are carried by way of Hering's nerve to the glossopharyngeal nerve; those from the aortic arch travel with the vagus nerve. A rise in arterial pressure causes an increase in the number of impulses transmitted to the vasomotor center. These impulses cause inhibition of the normal tonic activity of the vasomotor center, resulting in decreased sympathetic discharge, vasodilation, and decreased cardiac activity; a fall in blood pressure then occurs. A decrease in arterial pressure results in the opposite response.

Chemoreceptors, located in the carotid and aortic bodies, constitute the second nervous pressure control system. They have only a minor role in blood pressure control in the normal pressure range; however, the hypoxia that may occur in hypotensive states will cause an increase in impulses from the chemoreceptors to the vasomotor center. These impulses excite this center, increasing sympathetic tone and, therefore, blood pressure.

The central nervous ischemic response is the third major nervous control system. It is activated only when blood pressure and flow to the brain are sufficiently low to cause ischemia of the neurons of the vasomotor center. The ischemia results in a massive sympathetic discharge, resulting in profound elevations in blood pressure. The vasoconstriction can be severe enough to cause ischemia of other organs, such as the kidneys. It is, therefore, considered a "last-ditch" attempt by the body to maintain cerebral blood flow at the expense of other systems.

There are four known humoral mechanisms involved in rapid adjustments in arterial blood pressure. Increased sympathetic activity acts not only on the heart and blood vessels, but also stimulates the adrenal medulla to secrete epinephrine and norepinephrine. These catecholamines augment sympathetic activity by increasing heart rate and force of contraction and by causing vasoconstriction. Vasopressin is secreted by the pituitary gland in response to a fall in arterial blood pressure. Acute elevations of this hormone cause vasoconstriction; it also has the long-term effect of reducing water excretion by the kidney.

The renin-angiotensin-aldosterone system has both short- and long-term effects on the control of blood pressure. Renin is formed and stored in the juxtaglomerular (JG) apparatus located in proximity to the vascular pole of each glomerulus in the kidney. It is released into the circulation in response to a decrease in pressure in the glomerular afferent arteriole, as would occur with a drop in systemic arterial pressure, or a decrease in sodium or chloride load or transport at the macula densa. It is also released in response to an increase in sympathetic activity to the JG cells. Renin, in turn, cleaves a circulating polypeptide known as angiotensinogen (renin substrate) into angiotensin I. This hormone has no effect on blood pressure, but must first be converted to angiotensin II by a converting enzyme (ACE). This enzyme is found in high concentration in the lungs, where most of the reaction occurs. Angiotensin II is a potent arteriolar vasoconstrictor. It also plays a role in the long-term control of blood pressure,[20] as discussed later.

Atrial natriuretic hormone (ANH) is a recently characterized polypeptide hormone that is formed and stored in atrial myocytes. It is released into the circulation in response to atrial stretch, which in turn may be due to vascular volume overload or primary cardiac disease. It has been shown to have a variety of actions that can cause a reduction in blood pressure. It inhibits vascular smooth-muscle contraction, apparently mediated by cyclic guanosine monophosphate (GMP). It causes an increase in glomerular filtration rate without an increase in renal blood flow, due to glomerular efferent arteriolar vasoconstriction.[21–24] Natriuresis and an accompanying increase in water excretion occur, although the mechanism for this effect is not entirely clear. An increased filtration fraction occurs as the result of glomerular efferent arteriolar vasoconstriction; this in turn results in increased distal tubular delivery of sodium.[21–24] In addition, some investigators have found that ANH has a direct inhibitory effect on sodium chloride transport in the papillary collecting duct.[21, 24] It directly suppresses renin secretion as well as aldosterone synthesis.[21, 23] The precise role of ANH in controlling blood pressure in both the normal animal and in various disease states is currently under investigation.

Long-term control mechanisms are important in the maintenance of normal blood pressure over months to years, despite short-term variations. The most important of these is the renal-body fluid system, which causes a natriuresis and increased water excretion in response to a rise in arterial pressure. Although the kidneys obviously are vital to this response, it may be that ANH also plays a role in this mechanism. The renin-angiotensin-aldosterone system has two long-term effects on the maintenance of blood pressure. First, angiotensin causes

sodium and water retention by a direct effect on the kidneys. Second, angiotensin causes increased secretion of aldosterone by the adrenal cortex, which in turn decreases sodium and water excretion by the kidney. These mechanisms are important because the short-term mechanisms discussed earlier lose their sensitivity to sustained changes in blood pressure after several days. In addition, the short-term mechanisms may not return the blood pressure all the way to its resting level, whereas long-term mechanisms can completely restore normal pressure.[20]

PATHOPHYSIOLOGY

The term hypertension refers to elevation of arterial blood pressure above the level generally considered normal for the population of the species. The definition is therefore somewhat arbitrary.[25, 26] In addition, two components of blood pressure (systolic and diastolic) are usually measured. Hypertension is said to exist when one or both of these components are elevated. Elevations in diastolic blood pressure are felt to be more significant in the development of pathology and clinical signs associated with hypertension, however.[27] Surveys of clinically normal conscious dogs have reported mean systolic blood pressures ranging from 112 to 192 mmHg and mean diastolic pressures of 56 to 110 mmHg.[28–33] Blood pressures greater than 160/95 would seem to indicate hypertension, according to the normal values established by most studies. Few studies have been performed on cats. One investigator reported a mean systolic pressure of 171 ± 22 mmHg and a mean diastolic pressure of 123 ± 17 mmHg in 10 normal cats.[32] It is therefore difficult to recommend upper limits of normal blood pressure for cats. Extrapolating from the canine values would include all cats with hypertension, but might include some cats with normal blood pressure as well.

Hypertension can occur as the result of an abnormality in any of the mechanisms involved in the normal control of blood pressure. It may be classified by type (systolic or diastolic), by degree (malignant or benign); or by cause (primary or essential, or secondary) (Table 109–1).

Primary (Essential) Hypertension

Primary, or essential, hypertension is responsible for 95 per cent of the hypertension in human beings.[34] Despite extensive research, the pathophysiologic mechanisms that initiate and sustain the chronic increase in systemic blood pressure are not clear.[20, 25, 26] The most popular theories include chronic volume expansion owing to excess sodium intake in susceptible individuals, increased peripheral resistance owing to centrally mediated neurogenic input and/or stiffening of peripheral vessels from atherosclerotic changes, and increased activity of the renin-angiotensin-aldosterone system.[26] It may well be that essential hypertension represents not one disorder, but a heterogeneous group of disorders,

TABLE 109–1. CLASSIFICATION OF HYPERTENSION

By Kind
  Systolic
    1. Decreased arterial compliance (arteriosclerosis)
    2. Increased stroke volume
      a. Hyperthyroidism
      b. Severe anemia
      c. Aortic valvular regurgitation
      d. Patent ductus arteriosus (PDA)
      e. AV shunt
  Diastolic
By Degree
  Malignant
  Nonmalignant
By Cause
  Primary (essential)
  Secondary
    1. Renal
      a. Renal disease
        (1) Glomerulonephritis
        (2) Pyelonephritis
        (3) Interstitial nephritis
        (4) Congenital renal dysplasia
        (5) Obstructive uropathy
        (6) Polycystic kidney
        (7) Renin-producing tumor
      b. Renal arterial disease
        (1) Atherosclerosis
        (2) Thromboembolism
    2. Endocrine
      a. Hyperadrenocorticism
      b. Pheochromocytoma
      c. Hyperthyroidism
      d. Hypothyroidism
      e. Hyperparathyroidism
      f. Acromegaly
    3. Neurogenic

all of which result in elevation of blood pressure. It has been suggested that it may be analogous to fever in this respect; an obvious, easily quantifiable physiologic parameter with multiple possible etiologies but one that can be deleterious in and of itself.[35] Primary hypertension occurs in certain strains of laboratory rats,[26, 34, 36] which have been utilized in much of the research in this area. It has not been reported in cats and is apparently rare in dogs. Examination of some of the early studies on the incidence of hypertension in dogs reveals that some of the dogs reported as having primary hypertension had renal disease or adrenocortical adenomas at necropsy, both of which are associated with secondary hypertension.[9, 17, 19] An isolated case of primary hypertension was reported in a five-year-old Siberian husky presented for ocular lesions.[37] An inherited form of primary hypertension has recently been described in dogs; the mechanism for the hypertension and mode of inheritance remains under investigation.[38]

Secondary Hypertension

Secondary hypertension, in contrast to the primary form, is common in dogs and cats. Although the incidence of secondary hypertension has been reported only for dogs with renal disease[31, 32] and hyperadrenocorticism,[39] it has been seen in association with many of the diseases discussed below.

RENAL DISEASE

The incidence of hypertension in dogs with renal disease has been reported to range from 50 to 93 per cent.[31, 32] This range may be attributed to different types of renal disease, varying methods of measurement of blood pressure, and different definitions of hypertension by the investigators. Two studies of dogs with familial renal disease did not find a significant difference in blood pressure between affected and normal dogs,[40, 41] although seven of ten affected dogs in one study did have cardiac eccentric hypertrophy at necropsy.[41] Fifty-nine per cent of 34 dogs with renal disease studied by the author had hypertension. In addition, lesions identical to those resulting from hypertension are noted in a number of papers that review the pathologic lesions associated with both spontaneous and experimental renal failure in dogs, although blood pressure measurements were not reported.[33, 42–48] The lesions involved the cardiovascular system and included left ventricular hypertrophy and fibrinoid necrosis, hyalinosis, and hyperplasia of the smooth muscle of the tunica media of arteries and arterioles.

The incidence of hypertension in cats with renal disease has been noted only briefly. One paper found hypertension in four cats, all of which had mild to moderate elevations in serum creatinine concentration.[49] Eleven of 17 cats (65 per cent) with varying degrees of renal insufficiency studied by this author had hypertension.

The mechanism by which renal parenchymal disease produces hypertension is not clear,[16, 26, 50, 51] although a number of theories have been proposed. There is a higher incidence of hypertension in animals and people with glomerular diseases than in those with interstitial disease or pyelonephritis.[16, 31, 32] It has been postulated that the arteriolar lesions associated with glomerular disease result in reduced intrarenal blood flow and subsequent activation of the renin-angiotensin-aldosterone system.[16] Chronic volume expansion associated with high dietary sodium levels (and possibly concurrent activation of the renin-angiotensin-aldosterone system) could contribute to elevations in blood pressure. There is some evidence that such a mechanism may be involved in dogs with chronic failure. Dogs with chronic renal failure and hypertension fed a reduced sodium diet experienced reductions in blood pressure, implicating sodium and volume overload as a cause.[32] Increased cardiac output associated with the anemia of chronic renal failure has been suggested to contribute to elevations in blood pressure.[51] Decreased capacitance of the peripheral vascular system could also result in elevation of blood pressure. Reduced venous compliance has been noted in dogs with one form of experimental hypertension.[50] The mechanism for the reduction in compliance, or stiffening of the veins is not known; it could be the result of alterations in either the vessel wall or surrounding tissues. Secondary hyperparathyroidism is an inevitable consequence of chronic renal failure.[52] Elevated parathyroid hormone levels in primary hyperparathyroidism are associated with hypertension, although the mechanism is not clear.[53] The elevated parathyroid hormone levels associated with renal secondary hyperparathyroidism could also contribute to increases in blood pressure. Reduced levels of renal vasodepressor substances (possibly prostaglandins) have also been postulated to contribute to hypertension.[51, 54]

The renin-angiotensin-aldosterone system is involved in the pathogenesis of two specific types of kidney-associated hypertension. Renovascular hypertension is the result of stenosis of the renal artery or one of its branches, or, less commonly, a cortical infarct owing to an embolus or trauma. It does not necessarily result in nor must it be associated with parenchymal renal disease. Reduction of renal arterial blood flow results in activation of the renin-angiotensin-aldosterone system with subsequent elevations in blood pressure. Arteriosclerosis is usually responsible for the stenosis in humans.[26, 55] This form of hypertension has not yet been documented as a spontaneous disease in small animals, possibly because of the low incidence of arteriosclerosis. It is, however, the basis of the most common form of experimental hypertension in dogs and rats—the so-called Goldblatt kidney. In this model a clip is placed on one or both renal arteries to reduce renal blood flow; hypertension is consistently produced by the mechanism described above.[26, 55-57] Renin-secreting tumors of cells of the JG apparatus are a rare cause of hypertension in humans. Such tumors have not yet been described in small animals.[16, 26]

ENDOCRINE DISEASES

Hyperadrenocorticism is associated with hypertension in up to 84 per cent of affected human beings.[53] One study of dogs with spontaneous hyperadrenocorticism found that 9 of 11 animals (82 per cent) had elevations in both systolic and diastolic blood pressures; one additional dog had an elevated systolic pressure.[58] Another investigator reported an incidence of hypertension of 59 per cent (8 of 14 dogs with hyperadrenocorticism).[39] There appear to be several mechanisms by which hyperadrenocorticism causes hypertension. Elevated levels of glucocorticoids increase the production of angiotensinogen (plasma renin substrate), which leads to angiotensin-mediated vasoconstriction.[53, 59] They also increase the sensitivity of the cardiovascular system to catecholamines.[53] Volume expansion caused by increased renal sodium reabsorption and secondary water retention may contribute to elevations in blood pressure.[53, 60]

Pheochromocytomas are tumors of the chromaffin cells of the adrenal medulla that secrete catecholamines, and thereby cause elevations in blood pressure. They are rare in dogs and cats.[60-63] In humans, most pheochromocytomas produce norepinephrine (which causes predominantly vasoconstriction) or both norepinephrine and epinephrine (which cause increased cardiac output as well as increased peripheral resistance).[60, 62, 64] The patterns of catecholamine secretion in dogs and cats are not known. Hypertension occurs in 98 per cent of humans with pheochromocytomas, although it is paroxysmal in 50 per cent.[64] One study of dogs with pheochromocytomas found hypertension in 50 per cent of those animals in which blood pressure was determined.[62] Another report of 39 dogs with pheochromocytomas mentioned a similar incidence.[60]

Both hyperthyroidism and hypothyroidism have been associated with hypertension in humans.[53] Hyperthyroidism is probably the most common endocrine disorder in cats, in which it is usually caused by functioning adenomatous hyperplasia of the thyroid gland.[60, 65] It is uncommon in dogs but has been seen in association with thyroid tumors.[60] Approximately 50 per cent of humans with hyperthyroidism have hypertension, with the elevation usually occurring in the systolic phase.[65] The incidence of hypertension in cats and dogs with hyperthyroidism has not been reported. Hyperthyroid cats do exhibit a number of cardiac changes that are consistent with hypertension, including cardiomegaly and left ventricular hypertrophy.[65, 66] There are several mechanisms by which elevated circulating levels of thyroxine (T_4) and triiodothyronine (T_3) are believed to cause hypertension. Hearts from experimentally produced hyperthyroid animals have increased numbers of β-adrenergic receptors, which enhance cardiac response to catecholamines.[67] Increased levels of thyroid hormones also increase the activity of several enzymes, including myosin, calcium-stimulated, and sodium-potassium-stimulated adenosine triphosphatase (ATPase).[67] A direct inotropic and chronotropic effect of thyroid hormones appears to be mediated by a thyroid hormone specific adenylate cyclase-cyclic adenosine monophosphate (AMP) system.[53, 60, 67] These effects result in tachycardia and increased cardiac output and stroke volume, which account for the increase in systolic pressure; diastolic pressure is less commonly elevated because of a decrease in peripheral resistance.[53, 60, 67]

Approximately 50 per cent of humans with hypothyroidism have hypertension.[53] The mechanism for the increase in blood pressure is not clear; it may be related to the presence of myxedema or atherosclerosis, which results in decreased vascular compliance. The incidence of hypertension in dogs and cats with hypothyroidism has not been reported, although there is one clinical case report of a dog with hypertension and hypothyroidism.[68]

Hyperparathyroidism in humans is associated with hypertension in 33 to 70 per cent of patients,[53] although the exact mechanism is not clear. The associated increase in blood calcium concentration seems to be involved in the pathogenesis, as hypercalcemia alone will also induce increases in blood pressure.[53] Calcium is the second messenger for both angiotensin and adrenocorticotropin (ACTH). In addition, it initiates smooth muscle contraction by activating myosin kinase; elevated blood levels may therefore enhance vasoconstriction. Elevated levels of parathyroid hormone itself may affect plasma renin activity and sodium excretion.[53] The incidence of hypertension in animals with primary hyperparathyroidism has not been reported, although secondary hyperparathyroidism could be involved in the pathogenesis of hypertension in animals with renal disease, as discussed earlier.

Acromegaly is a condition that results from elevated circulating levels of growth hormone. Whereas overgrowth of connective tissue, bones, and viscera is the predominant clinical feature in humans, diabetes mellitus is the most common finding in dogs and cats.[60, 69] Hypertension has been diagnosed in 23 to 40 per cent of humans with acromegaly, and there appears to be a correlation between growth hormone levels and the degree of elevation of blood pressure. The mechanism by which hypertension is produced appears to be an increase in exchangeable sodium and extracellular fluid volume; vascular lesions from diabetes mellitus may also play a role.[53] The incidence of hypertension in animals with acromegaly has not yet been reported. The high incidence of cardiomyopathy and congestive heart failure in cats with acromegaly[69] could be related to hypertension.

Neurogenic hypertension occurs in humans with anxiety or stress as the result of chronic elevations in catecholamine and/or glucocorticoid levels. Increases in blood pressure have been noted in dogs that were stimulated while blood pressure was being measured, and in those stressed experimentally.[70, 71] It is not known whether dogs and cats in normal living situations experience this form of hypertension.

CLINICAL CONSEQUENCES

The clinical consequences of hypertension depend on both the severity and the duration of the increase in arterial pressure. Although many organ systems can be affected, the predominant effects are those on the heart, brain, eyes, and kidneys. Elevations in blood pressure cause vasoconstriction of peripheral arterioles as an autoregulatory phenomenon. Sustained hypertension results in pathologic lesions in small arteries and arterioles that consist of hypertrophy and hyperplasia of the tunica media, loss of the internal elastic lamina, and fibrinoid necrosis.[33, 42, 45, 72–74] It is therefore not surprising that the organs most affected are those that are involved in regulating blood flow (the heart) and those that contain extensive arteriolar or capillary networks. Because much of the work on experimental hypertension has been performed in dogs,[26, 36, 56, 57, 75] some of the data can be extrapolated to clinical situations.

Autoregulation within the brain results in vasoconstriction in response to an increase in blood pressure. Sustained increases in pressure may result in a shift of the set point to a pressure higher than normal. This may reduce the ability of the brain to compensate for decreases in blood pressure, such as that which might occur under general anesthesia. Clinical neurologic abnormalities, however, are usually the result of intracerebral hemorrhages. Such hemorrhages are apparently the result of weakening and eventual rupture of arterial or arteriolar walls as the result of the pathologic lesions described above.[76] The clinical signs will depend on the size and location of the hemorrhage, but can include seizures, dementia, various neurologic deficits, and death. The incidence of neurologic dysfunction in dogs and cats with hypertension is not known.

Hypertrophy of the left ventricle of the heart is a common consequence of arterial hypertension (Figure 109–1). The hypertrophy results in a decrease in myocardial wall tension. This enables the heart to overcome the increased afterload resulting from the increase in peripheral resistance. The mechanism by which the

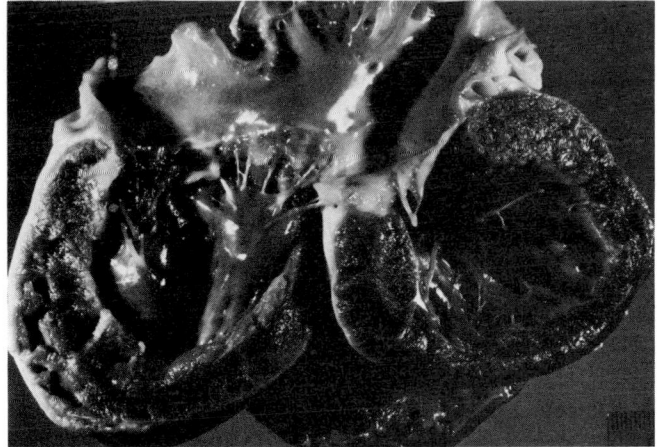

FIGURE 109–1. Left ventricular hypertrophy of the heart of an eight-year-old male golden retriever that had hypertension and chronic renal failure owing to glomerulonephritis.

hemodynamic stimulus of pressure overload results in ventricular hypertrophy is not clear.[77] It has been postulated that other factors may also influence the cardiac response in hypertension, including increased preload (volume overload) due to expansion of the vascular volume and increased myocardial contractility as the result of increased adrenergic stimulation.[77] The hypertrophied ventricle may be at greater risk for ischemia because of relative decreases in coronary artery blood flow.[78] Cardiac dysfunction and frank congestive heart failure can occur as the result of severe ventricular hypertrophy. Regression of the hypertrophy can occur with reduction of blood pressure to normal levels.

The ocular lesions that occur with hypertension have the particular advantage of being detectable by routine physical examination procedures. The characteristic lesions include straightening and narrowing of larger retinal arteries in association with mild hypertension, or dilated, tortuous vessels with more severe hypertension; "cotton-wool" spots on the retina; retinal hemorrhages, exudates, and detachments; and papilledema.[49, 79–83] Straightening and narrowing of the retinal vessels are thought to represent the autoregulatory process of vasoconstriction in response to the increase in blood pressure. The vasodilation that is seen with more severe hypertension may be due to autoregulatory failure or hypertension-induced vascular damage.[49, 80, 81] The "cotton-wool" spots have been shown to be due to ischemia of nerve fibers in the retina as the result of arterial vasoconstriction or vascular pathology. Mitochondria and other axonal organelles accumulate at the border of the lesion, which results in swelling and the grayish white appearance.[49, 79, 80, 82] Retinal hemorrhages and exudates may result from arterial wall damage with rupture and bleeding or exudation of plasma (Figure 109–2).[79, 80] Retinal detachments can occur as the result of exudation or edema.[49, 79, 80] The pathogenesis of papilledema is not clear, although it occurs only with severe hypertension. It has been postulated that it may represent transmission of increased intracranial pressure or intracellular swelling of nerve fibers.[49, 80–82] A grading system is used to classify human hypertensive retinal lesions; it has not yet been applied to small animals.[82] Ocular lesions result in loss of visual acuity (a phenom-

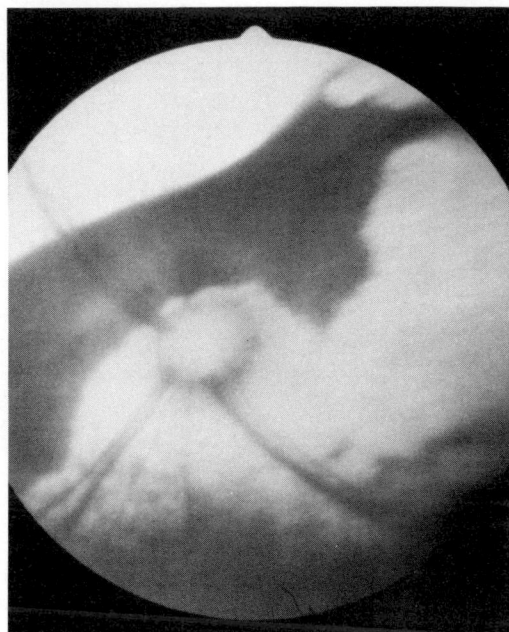

FIGURE 109–2. A large retinal hemorrhage dorsotemporal to the optic disc in the right eye of a cat with hypertension and renal disease. (JAAHA 22:616, 1986).

enon rarely detected in dogs or cats) or blindness. Loss of vision may be the presenting complaint in some animals with hypertension.[37, 49]

Hypertensive ocular changes have been reported in experimental hypertension in animals,[79, 80, 82, 83] as well as in clinical cases. Retinal hemorrhages and exudates and papilledema were seen in a nine-year-old fox terrier[83] and a five-year-old Siberian husky,[37] both of which were presumed to have essential hypertension. Similar changes, including retinal detachment, were noted in a 12-year-old miniature poodle with hypertension and renal disease,[83] and in an 11-year-old basenji with hypertension associated with hypothyroidism.[68] Retinal hemorrhages, detachments, hyphema, and vitreal hemorrhages were seen in four cats with hypertension and renal disease.[49]

The renal vascular lesions seen with hypertension are similar to those seen in other organs. Focal and segmental glomerular proliferation and glomerulosclerosis occur. Severe, untreated hypertension frequently leads to renal failure in humans,[16] although its effect in dogs is less clear. One study of dogs with experimental (Goldblatt one-kidney) hypertension was unable to document changes in glomerular filtration rate or renal plasma flow over a one-year period.[84] It has recently been proposed that systemic hypertension may contribute to glomerular hyperfiltration in animals and humans with renal insufficiency, hastening the rate of progression of renal failure[85–87] (see also Chapter 107). While dogs made experimentally uremic do exhibit glomerular lesions,[88, 89] it is not known whether the hypertension in dogs and cats with spontaneous renal disease contributes to progression of their disease. In fact, the observation originally made by Bright in 1827 still stands: "From the work done so far, it is not clear how important hypertension might be in causing spontaneous vascular disease in the dog or what part it might play in the pathogenesis of interstitial nephritis, particularly in the progression from the acute to the chronic stage."[42]

MEASUREMENT OF BLOOD PRESSURE

Arterial blood pressure can be measured by either direct or indirect methods. A number of studies have shown good correlation between the two methods as long as attention is paid to careful technique.[2, 6–10, 12, 13, 90] Although some investigators believe that only the direct method gives accurate results, the following statement by Allen in 1941 appears to be applicable to measurements in clinical settings. "Assuming, for argument, that errors may occur even greater than those reported, possibly to the extent of 10 or 15 mm deviation from the true intra-arterial pressure, the general conclusion remains that direct methods may be used for precise

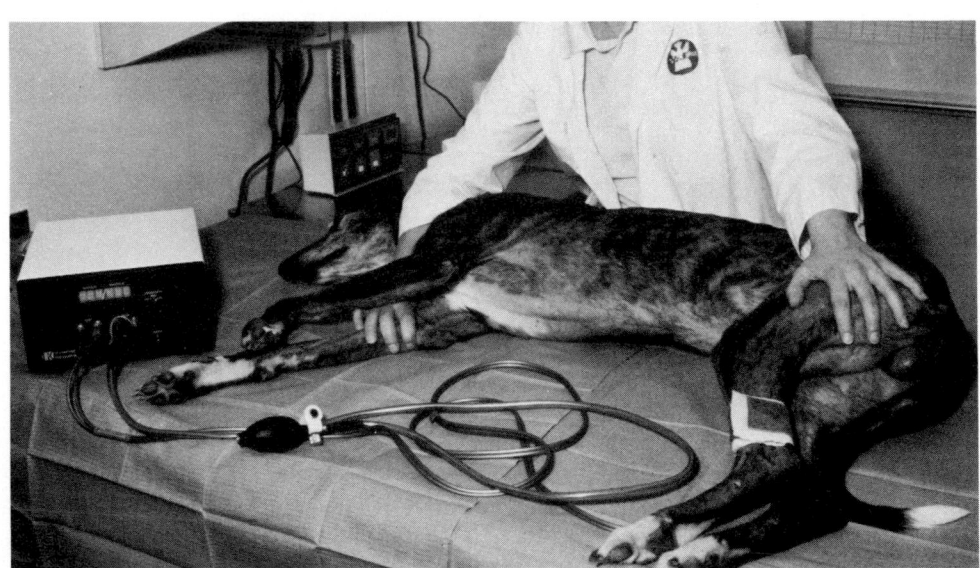

FIGURE 109–3. A dog positioned for an indirect blood pressure determination.

acute experiments or for occasional checks on the indirect readings. For chronic experiments the frequently repeated readings by the convenient auscultatory method give a better picture of the general condition than a smaller number of technically exact determinations, which are subject to the far greater variations in the animal from hour to hour or from day to day."[11]

Direct blood pressure measurement involves the placement of a needle or catheter into a peripheral artery, usually the femoral. Local anesthesia is used if necessary; most dogs and some cats tolerate the procedure with no apparent discomfort. The catheter is attached to a transducer and the pressure recorded.

Indirect blood pressure measurement can be performed by the palpatory, auscultatory, or oscillometric method (Figure 109–3). In each instance a peripheral artery is occluded by inflation of a cuff. The closing and opening of the artery are detected as the cuff is inflated and deflated. The cranial tibial artery is most commonly used for measurements (Figure 109–4), although the brachial artery may be used as well. The cuff should be approximately 40 per cent and the length 150 per cent of the circumference of the limb. Cuffs that are too small may give artifactually high readings and those that are too large, low readings. The cuff is inflated to a pressure 30 to 40 mmHg higher than that required to obliterate the pulse. The cuff is gradually deflated. As blood begins to flow through the artery, a series of sounds can be detected (Korotkoff sounds) (Table 109–2). The first appearance of the sound (phase I) indicates the initiation of blood flow through the artery and indicates the systolic pressure. It is recommended that the diastolic pressure be measured at Phase IV, although, practically, phases IV and V are usually quite close. It requires some practice to become familiar with the technique and to be able to reproduce accurate readings. There is a small amount of minute-to-minute variation in blood pressure because of respiration, move-

TABLE 109–2. KOROTKOFF SOUNDS USED FOR INDIRECT BLOOD PRESSURE DETERMINATION

Phase I:	Sudden appearance of a clear, sharp sound that grows louder
Phase II:	Sound softens and becomes prolonged into a murmur
Phase III:	Sound again becomes crisper and increases in intensity
Phase IV:	Distinct abrupt muffling of sound
Phase V:	Sound disappears

ment, and heart rate. For this reason it is suggested that at least three readings be taken at several-minute intervals and the results averaged.

THERAPY

Because most hypertension in dogs and cats is secondary in origin, identification and removal of the inciting cause are the most important steps in medical management. Various maneuvers may be tried to lower blood pressure in animals in which the cause of the hypertension cannot be determined (primary); the inciting cause cannot be removed (e.g., chronic renal failure); or the degree of blood pressure elevation is life-threatening.

Restriction of dietary sodium intake may be effective in lowering blood pressure in animals that are chronically volume expanded. Animals with hypertension associated with renal disease may fall into this category. Virtually all commercial dog foods contain high levels of sodium (0.5 to 1.0 per cent).[91] Clinical studies of dogs with hypertension and renal failure have shown that blood pressure can be significantly reduced by feeding a sodium-restricted diet.[32, 92] Comparable studies in cats have not been performed, but it is assumed that a similar situation exists. Current recommendations are to feed dogs with hypertension and renal failure a diet containing 0.1 per cent to 0.3 per cent sodium on a dry weight basis (5 to 20 mg/lb/day or 10 to 40 mg/kg/day).[32, 93] Recommended levels have not been formulated for cats, but it is suggested that a reduced sodium diet be fed (sodium 0.4 per cent on a dry weight basis; commercial canned cat foods contain 0.75 per cent sodium on the average).[93] Certain commercial diets are formulated to meet these recommendations. Implementation of these diets should be done gradually over a period of two to four weeks, because animals with renal disease cannot adapt to rapid changes in dietary sodium intake. Consequently, they will continue to excrete high levels of sodium in the urine for a period of time after sodium intake is lowered. Total body sodium and water depletion, hypovolemia, and subsequent reduction in renal blood flow could occur.

Pharmacologic management of hypertension should be attempted if sodium restriction fails to lower blood pressure. There are a variety of drugs of different classes and with different mechanisms of action that may be tried. Because the pathogenesis of the hypertension in any given animal will not be known, it is generally not possible to predict which drug or combination of drugs will be effective. Veterinary medicine has therefore

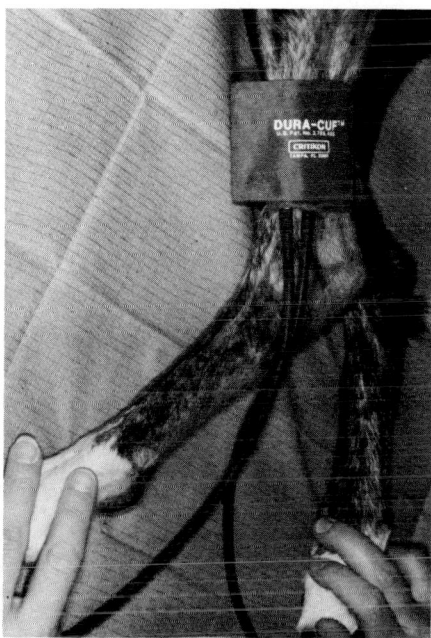

FIGURE 109–4. Correct placement of the inflatable cuff over the cranial tibial artery for indirect blood pressure determination.

adopted an approach similar to that used in humans. Antihypertensive drugs are administered in a logical order, beginning with those that have the mildest activity and fewest side effects. Each drug is administered for two to four weeks before it is determined that it is ineffective in lowering blood pressure. If a particular drug fails, a drug in the next class is selected rather than a different drug in the same class.[93] The order of drug administration is somewhat empiric and based on the clinician's experience; it is, however, important to be consistent. Pharmacologic management should not be attempted unless the clinician has access to blood pressure monitoring equipment to assess the efficacy of therapy.

Diuretics are the first class of antihypertensive agents to be administered. They act by inducing urinary sodium and water excretion, which results in a decrease in extracellular fluid volume.[93] Thiazide diuretics such as chlorothiazide or hydrochlorothiazide can be administered. Furosemide may be tried if thiazides are ineffective. Animals with renal failure are generally refractory to the action of thiazides,[32] and furosemide should probably be the first choice in these patients. It should be used cautiously because of the potential of producing excessive sodium and water loss, volume depletion, and decreased renal blood flow.

β-adrenergic antagonists constitute the second class of drugs. The mechanism by which these drugs reduce blood pressure is not entirely clear, but may involve reduction of cardiac output, inhibition of renin release, interference with central sympathetic activity, and/or presynaptic blockade of adrenergic neurons.[32, 93, 94] Propranolol is the most commonly used drug in this class and can also be administered in conjunction with diuretics. There is a relative contraindication to its use in animals with preexisting cardiac or pulmonary disease, since it can cause bradycardia, decreased cardiac output, and bronchospasm.[94]

Vasodilators represent the third class of antihypertensive drugs. They may be used as the sole pharmacologic agent or may be given in conjunction with diuretics and β-adrenergic antagonists. Hydralazine causes direct relaxation of arterioles and small arteries, and therefore reduces peripheral vascular resistance. However, it also stimulates reflex sympathetic increases in heart rate and cardiac output and enhances renin release. It is therefore best administered in conjunction with propranolol and a diuretic.[32, 95] Prazosin is an α-adrenergic receptor antagonist that causes dilation of both arterioles and veins. Because it activates only receptors on vascular walls, it does not cause reflex tachycardia or stimulate renin release. Prazosin may cause such a rapid decrease in blood pressure that severe weakness or even syncope may occur after the initial dose. This effect is short-lived and self-limiting, but it may be prudent to hospitalize animals for the first day or two of therapy. Prazosin appears to be fairly effective and consistent in lowering blood pressure in dogs;[95] experience in cats is minimal. Calcium channel blocking agents such as verapamil or nifedipine cause arteriolar dilation by inhibiting calcium transport through slow channels in smooth-muscle cell membranes. Verapamil is a negative inotrope and slows AV conduction time; it is probably best not to admin-ister it in conjunction with propranolol. Nifedipine produces more arterial dilation and has little effect on AV conduction time; it has a very short half-life in the dog, however, which may limit its clinical usefulness[96] (see also Chapters 73 and 76.)

Angiotensin converting enzyme (ACE) inhibitors (captopril, enalapril) represent a fourth class of pharmacologic agents. They act by inhibiting the conversion of angiotensin I to angiotensin II, resulting in arteriolar dilation and venodilation. Aldosterone secretion is also suppressed, which results in increased sodium excretion. In addition, ACE inhibitors cause vasodilation in association with increased concentrations of bradykinin and prostaglandin E_2 (PGE_2).[97] These agents can be used for hypertension that is refractory to all other drugs or may be substituted for class 3 drugs. There is some evidence in humans and rats with hypertension and renal failure that reduction of blood pressure with ACE inhibitors is more effective in preventing the progression of renal failure than reduction with other drugs.[98-101] Angiotensin II appears to have a greater vasoconstrictive effect on the glomerular efferent arteriole rather than the afferent arteriole. This effect increases the filtration fraction and may contribute to glomerular capillary hyperfiltration, suggesting a mechanism for the beneficial effect of ACE inhibitors.[64] On the other hand, proteinuria, glomerular disease, and frank renal failure have been seen in both humans and dogs treated with ACE inhibitors.[97] Captopril has been associated with both acute interstitial nephritis and membranous glomerulopathy in humans,[102, 103] and high doses of enalapril, with proximal tubular necrosis.[104]

Severe hypertension associated with clinical signs necessitates emergency therapy. Animals with pheochromocytomas or renal failure are most likely to fall into this category. Clinical signs can include retinal detachment, encephalopathy, or acute heart failure. Intravenous administration of small boluses of acepromazine can be tried. If this is unsuccessful in lowering blood pressure, an intravenous infusion of sodium nitroprusside or phentolamine may be necessary.[31] The precipitating cause of the hypertension should be treated; other pharmacologic agents (as discussed above) are used for long-term control.

References

1. Ferris, HW and Hynes, SF: Indirect blood pressure readings in dogs. Description of method and report of result. J Lab Clin Med 16:597, 1930.
2. Allen, FM: Auscultatory estimation of the blood pressure of dogs. J Metab Res 4:431, 1923.
3. Valtonen, MH and Eriksson, LM: The effect of cuff width on accuracy in indirect measurement of blood pressure in dogs. Res Vet Sci 11:358, 1970.
4. Coulter, DB and Keith, JC: Blood pressures obtained by indirect measurement in conscious dogs. JAVMA 184:1375, 1984.
5. Rule, C: A simple auscultatory technique for the estimation of the blood pressure of dogs. J Lab Clin Med 29:97, 1944.
6. Freundlich, JJ, et al.: Indirect blood pressure determination by the ultrasonic Doppler technique in dogs. Curr Therap Res 14:73, 1972.
7. Wessale, JL, et al.: Indirect auscultatory systolic and diastolic

pressures in the anesthetized dog. Am J Vet Res 46:2129, 1985.

8. Garner, HE, et al.: Indirect blood pressure measurement in the dog. Lab Anim Sci 25:197, 1975.

9. Weiser, MG et al.: Blood pressure measurement in the dog. JAVMA 171:364, 1977.

10. Wakerlin, GE: Normotension and hypertension in the dog. JAVMA 102:346, 1943.

11. Allen, FM: Auscultatory blood pressure methods for dogs. J Lab Clin Med 27:371, 1941.

12. Hamlin, RL, et al.: Noninvasive measurement of systemic arterial pressure in dogs by automatic sphygmomanometry. Am J Vet Res 43:1271, 1982.

13. McLeish, I: Doppler ultrasonic arterial pressure measurement in the cat. Vet Rec 100:290, 1977.

14. Wilhelmj, CM: Observations on canine blood pressure, normal and hypertensive. Small Anim Clin 3:334, 1963.

15. Shingatgeri, MK, et al.: A preliminary report on the use of a modified compression cuff to fit the sphygmomanometer in determining arterial blood pressure in dogs. Indian Vet J 40:770, 1963.

16. Kincaid-Smith, P: Parenchymatous diseases of the kidney and hypertension. In Genest, J (ed): Hypertension, 2nd ed. New York, McGraw-Hill, 1983, p 989.

17. Hamilton, WF, et al.: Blood pressure values in street dogs. Am J Physiol 128:233, 1939.

18. Katz, JI, et al.: Pathogenesis of spontaneous and pyelonephritic hypertension in the dog. Circ Res 5:137, 1957.

19. McCubbin, JW and Corcoran, AC: Arterial pressures in street dogs: Incidence and significance of hypertension. Proc Soc Exp Biol Med 84:121, 1953.

20. Guyton, AC: Textbook of Medical Physiology, 7th ed. Philadelphia, WB Saunders, 1986.

21. Zeidel, ML and Brenner, BM: Actions of atrial natriuretic peptides on the kidney. Seminars in Nephrology 7:91, 1987.

22. Laragh, SH: Atrial natriuretic hormone, the renin-aldosterone axis, and blood pressure-electrolyte homeostasis. N Engl J Med 313:1330, 1985.

23. Needleman, P and Greenwald, JE: Atriopeptin: A cardiac hormone intimately involved in fluid, electrolyte, and blood pressure homeostasis. N Engl J Med 314:828, 1986.

24. Ballermann, BJ, et al.: Renal actions of atrial natriuretic peptides. In Mulrow, PJ and Schuer, R (eds). Atrial Hormones and Other Natriuretic Factors. Bethesda, MD, American Physiological Society, 1987, p 83.

25. Pieart, WS: General review of hypertension. In Genest, J (ed): Hypertension, 2nd ed. New York, McGraw-Hill, 1983, p 3.

26. Page, IH: Hypertension Mechanisms. New York, Grune & Stratton, 1987.

27. Page, LB: Epidemiology of hypertension. In Genest, J (ed): Hypertension, 2nd ed. New York, McGraw-Hill, 1983, p 683.

28. Spangler, WL, et al.: Canine hypertension. A review. JAVMA 170:995, 1980.

29. Valtonen, MH and Oksanen, A: Cardiovascular disease and nephritis in dogs. J Sm Anim Pract 13:687, 1972.

30. Anderson, LJ and Fisher EW: The blood pressure in canine interstitial nephritis. Res Vet Sci 9:304, 1968.

31. Cowgill, LD and Kallet, AS: Recognition and management of hypertension in the dog. In Kirk, RW (ed): Current Veterinary Therapy VIII. Philadelphia, WB Saunders, 1983, p 1025.

32. Cowgill, LD and Kallet, AJ: Systemic hypertension. In Kirk, RW (ed): Current Veterinary Therapy IX. Philadelphia, WB Saunders, 1986, p 360.

33. Anderson, LJ: Arterial disease in canine interstitial nephritis. J Pathol Bacteriol 95:47, 1968.

34. Julius, S and Hansson, L: Classification of hypertension. In Genest, J (ed): Hypertension, 2nd ed. New York, McGraw-Hill, 1983, p 679.

35. Laragh, JH: Personal reviews on the mechanisms of hypertension. In Genest, J (ed): Hypertension, 2nd ed. New York, McGraw-Hill, 1983, p 615.

36. Bianchi, G and Ferian, P: Animal models for arterial hypertension. In Genest, J (ed): Hypertension, 2nd ed. New York, McGraw-Hill, 1983, p 534.

37. Blanchard, GL, et al.: Primary essential hypertension in a Siberian husky dog (abstr). Fed Proc 38:1350, 1979.

38. Bovée, KC, et al.: Essential hereditary hypertension in dogs: a new animal model (abstr). Proc 18th Annual Mtg Am Soc Nephrol, 1985, p 93A.

39. Kallet, A and Cowgill, LD: Hypertensive states in the dog. Proceed ACVIM, Salt Lake City, 1982, p 79.

40. Finco, DR: Familial renal disease in Norwegian Elkhound dogs: Physiologic and biochemical examinations. Am J Vet Res 37:87, 1976.

41. Piersson, F, et al.: Blood pressure in dogs with renal cortical hypoplasia. Acta Vet Scand 2:129, 1961.

42. Pirie, HM, et al.: The relationships between renal disease and arterial lesions in the dog. Ann NY Acad Sci 127:861, 1965.

43. Innes, JRM: Arteriosclerotic kidney (primary contracted type) and secondary contracted kidney in the dog. Vet Rec 10:698, 1930.

44. Dayton, H: Reliability of dogs as subjects for experimental nephritis. J Med Res 31:177, 1914.

45. Platt, H: Morphological changes in the cardiovascular system associated with nephritis in dogs. J Pathol Bact 64:539, 1952.

46. McIntyre, WIM and Montgomery, GL: Renal lesions in Leptospira canicola infection in dogs. J Pathol Bacteriology 64:145, 1952.

47. Montgomery, PO and Muirhead, EE: Similarities between the lesions in human malignant hypertension and in the hypertensive state of the nephrectomized dog. Am J Path 29:1147, 1953.

48. McGill, HC, et al.: Two forms of necrotizing arteritis in dogs related to diet and renal insufficiency. Arch Pathol 65:66, 1958.

49. Morgan, RV: Systemic hypertension in four cats: Ocular and medical findings. JAAHA 22:615, 1986.

50. Brod, J: Hypertension and renal parenchymal disease: Mechanisms and management. Cardiovasc Clin 9:137, 1978.

51. Linas, SL and Schrier, RW: The renin-angiotensin-aldosterone system and the etiology of hypertension in renal disease. In Brenner, BM and Rector, FC (eds): The Kidney, 2nd ed. Philadelphia, WB Saunders, 1981, p 2344.

52. Osborne, CA, et al.: Pathophysiology of renal disease, renal failure, and uremia. In Ettinger, SJ (ed): Textbook of Veterinary Internal Medicine, 2nd ed. Philadelphia, WB Saunders, 1983, p 1733.

53. Hamet, P: Endocrine hypertension: Cushing's syndrome, acromegaly, hyperparathyroidism, thyrotoxicosis, and hypothyroidism. In Genest, J (ed): Hypertension, 2nd ed. New York, McGraw-Hill, 1983, p 964.

54. Muirhead, EE, et al.: Renal medullary system of blood pressure control. J Hypertension 4(Suppl 4):S27, 1986.

55. Genest, J, et al.: Renovascular hypertension. In Genest, J (ed): Hypertension, 2nd ed. New York, McGraw-Hill, 1983, p 1007.

56. Goldblatt, H, et al.: Studies on experimental hypertension. I. The production of persistent elevation of systolic blood pressure by means of renal ischemia. J Exp Med 59:347, 1934.

57. Haas, E: Reminiscences and Reflections. J Hypertension 4(Suppl 4):S21, 1986.

58. Scott, DW: Hyperadrenocorticism (Hyperadrenocorticoidism, Hyperadrenocorticalism, Cushing's disease, Cushing syndrome). Vet Clin North Am 9:3, 1979.

59. Peterson, ME: Hyperadrenocorticism. Vet Clin North Am 14:731, 1984.

60. Feldman, EC and Nelson, RW: Canine and Feline Endocrinology and Reproduction. Philadelphia, WB Saunders, 1987.

61. Carpenter, JL, et al.: Tumors and tumor-like lesions. In Holzworth, J (ed): Diseases of the Cat. Philadelphia, WB Saunders, 1987, p 406.

62. Twedt, DC and Wheeler, SL: Pheochromocytoma in the dog. Vet Clin North Am 14:767, 1984.

63. Twedt, DC, et al.: Grand rounds conference: Pheochromocytoma in a canine. JAAHA 11:491, 1975.

64. Kuchel, O: Adrenal medulla: Pheochromocytoma. In Genest, J (ed): Hypertension, 2nd ed. New York, McGraw-Hill, 1983, p 947.

65. Peterson, ME: Feline hyperthyroidism. Vet Clin North Am 14:809, 1984.

66. Moise, NS and Dietze, AE: Echocardiographic, electrocardiographic, and radiographic detection of cardiomegaly in hyperthyroid cats. Am J Vet Res 47:1487, 1986.

67. Klein, I and Levey, GS: New perspectives on thyroid hormones, catecholamines and the heart. Am J Med 76:167, 1984.

68. Gwin, RM, et al.: Hypertensive retinopathy associated with hypothyroidism, hypercholesterolemia, and renal failure in a dog. JAAHA 14:200, 1978.
69. Peterson, ME, et al.: Spontaneous acromegaly in the cat (abstract). *In* Proceed Fourth Annual Veterinary Medical Forum, ACVIM, 1986, p 14–43.
70. Yinchang, J, et al.: Development of hypertension in dogs under intensified tension of higher nervous activities. Scientia Sinica 23:665, 1980.
71. Wilhelmj, CM, et al.: Emotional elevations of blood pressure in trained dogs. Psychosom Med 15:390, 1953.
72. Muirhead, EE, et al.: Hypertensive cardiovascular disease (nature and pathogenesis of the arteriolar sclerosis induced by bilateral nephrectomy as revealed by a study of its tinctorial characteristics). Arch Pathol 52:266, 1951.
73. Muirhead, EE, et al.: Cardiovascular lesions following bilateral nephrectomy dogs. Arch Intern Med 91:250, 1953.
74. Muirhead, EE: Hypertensive cardiovascular disease (an experimental study of tissue changes in bilaterally nephrectomized dogs). Arch Pathol 48:234, 1949.
75. Grollman, A: Experimental hypertension in the dog. Am J Physiol 147:647, 1946.
76. Sandok, BA and Whisnant, JP: Hypertension and the brain: Clinical Aspects. *In* Genest, J (ed): Hypertension, 2nd ed. New York, McGraw-Hill, 1983, p 777.
77. Frohlich, ED: The heart in hypertension. *In* Genest, J (ed): Hypertension, 2nd ed. New York, McGraw-Hill, 1983, p 791.
78. Mueller, TM, et al.: Effect of renal hypertension and left ventricular hypertrophy on the coronary circulation in dogs. Circ Res 42:543, 1978.
79. Editorial: Pathogenesis of hypertensive retinopathy. Br Med J 1:700, 1975.
80. Garner, A, et al.: Pathogenesis of hypertensive retinopathy: An experimental study in the monkey. Br J Ophthal 59:3, 1975.
81. Editorial: Pathogenesis of retinopathy in malignant hypertension. Br J Ophthal 59:1, 1975.
82. Dollery, CT: Hypertensive retinopathy. *In* Genest, J (ed): Hypertension, 2nd ed. New York, McGraw-Hill, 1983, p 723.
83. Rubin, LF: Atlas of Veterinary Ophthalmoscopy. Philadelphia, Lea & Febiger, 1974, pp 110, 132.
84. Stamler, J, et al.: Serial renal clearances in dogs with nephrogenic and spontaneous hypertension. J Exp Med 90:511, 1949.
85. Brenner, BW, et al.: Dietary protein intake and the progressive nature of kidney disease. N Engl J Med 307:642, 1982.
86. Hostetter, TH: The hyperfiltering glomerulus. Med Clin North Am 68:387, 1984.
87. Finco, DR: Progression of renal failure. *In* Proceed 2nd Annual Veterinary Medical Forum, ACVIM, 1984, p 139.
88. Hostetter, TH: Progressive renal disease: Is the slippery slope species specific? (Editorial). J Lab Clin Med 109:375, 1987.
89. Bourgoignie, JJ, et al.: Glomerular function and morphology after renal mass reduction in dogs. J Lab Clin Med 109:380, 1987.
90. Stegall, HF: Indirect measurement of arterial blood pressure by Doppler ultrasonic sphygmomanometry. J Applied Phys 25:793, 1968.
91. Lewis, L and Morris, ML, Jr: Small Animal Clinical Nutrition. Topeka KS, Mark Morris Associates, 1983.
92. Cowgill, LD: Diseases of the Kidney. *In* Ettinger, SJ (ed): Textbook of Veterinary Internal Medicine, 2nd ed. Philadelphia, WB Saunders, 1983, p 1793.
93. Allen, TA: The treatment of hypertension. *In* Proceed Fourth Annual Veterinary Medical Forum, ACVIM, 1986, p 3–105.
94. Muir, W: β-blocking therapy in dogs and cats. *In* Kirk, RW (ed): Current Veterinary Therapy IX. Philadelphia, WB Saunders, 1986, p 343.
95. Bonagura, JD and Muir, W: Vasodilator therapy. *In* Kirk, RW (ed): Current Veterinary Therapy IX. Philadelphia, WB Saunders, 1986, p 329.
96. Keene, BW and Hamlin, RL: Calcium antagonists. *In* Kirk, RW (ed): Current Veterinary Therapy IX. Philadelphia, WB Saunders, 1986, p 340.
97. Knowlen, GG and Kittleson, MD: Captopril therapy in dogs with heart failure. *In* Kirk, RW (ed): Current Veterinary Therapy IX. Philadelphia, WB Saunders, 1986, p 334.
98. Jackson, B, et al.: Progression of renal disease: Effects of different classes of antihypertensive therapy. J Hypertension 4 (suppl 5): S269, 1986.
99. Jackson, B, et al.: Preservation of renal function in the rat remnant kidney model of chronic renal failure by blood pressure reduction. Clin Exp Pharmacol Physiol 13:319, 1986.
100. Hall, RL, et al.: Captopril slows the progression of chronic renal disease in partially nephrectomized rats. Toxicol Appl Pharmacol 80:517, 1985.
101. Bauer, JH and Gaddy, P: Effects of enalapril alone, and in combination with hydrochlorothiazide, on renin-angiotensin-aldosterone, renal function, salt and water excretion, and body fluid composition. Am J Kidney Diseases 6:222, 1985.
102. Donker, AJM: Nephrotoxicity of angiotensin converting enzyme inhibition. Kidney Int 31(Suppl 20):S132, 1987.
103. Lewis, EJ: Glomerular abnormalities in patients receiving angiotensin converting enzyme inhibitor therapy. Kidney Int 31(Suppl 20):S138, 1987.
104. MacDonald, JS, et al.: Renal effects of enalapril in dogs. Kidney Int 31(Suppl 20):S148, 1987.

DRUG INDEX

Generic	Trade	Dosage	Route	Frequency	Brief Description
Chlorothiazide	Diuril	10–20 mg/lb	Orally	q12–24h	Diuretic
Hydrochlorothiazide	Hydrodiuril	1–2 mg/lb	Orally	q12–24h	Diuretic
Furosemide	Lasix	0.5–1 mg/lb	Orally	q8–12 h	Diuretic
Propranolol	Inderal	0.125–0.25 mg/lb	Orally	q8h	Beta-adrenergic antagonist
Hydralazine	Apresoline	1–1.5 mg/lb	Orally	q12h	Vasodilator
Prazosin	Minipress	0.25–2.0 mg	Orally	q8h	Vasodilator
Verapamil	Isoptin	0.5–1.5 mg/lb	Orally	q8h	Vasodilator–calcium channel blocker
Captopril	Capoten	0.5–1 mg/lb	Orally	q8–12h	Angiotensin-converting enzyme inhibitor

110 FELINE LOWER URINARY TRACT DISORDERS

CARL A. OSBORNE, JOHN M. KRUGER,
GARY R. JOHNSTON, and DAVID J. POLZIN

TERMINOLOGY

The term *feline urologic syndrome* and the acronym FUS have been commonly used by the veterinary profession as diagnostic terms to describe naturally occurring and experimentally induced disorders of domestic cats characterized by hematuria, dysuria, pollakiuria, and partial or complete urethral obstruction. However, with the exception of urinary incontinence, varying combinations of these signs may be associated with any cause of feline lower urinary tract disease. The similarity of clinical signs caused by diverse causes is not surprising since the feline urinary tract responds to various diseases in a limited and predictable fashion. It follows that FUS should be redefined as feline urologic *signs*. Since clinical signs of lower urinary tract disease may be produced by a variety of different etiologic mechanisms, FUS is a term of limited value.

Widespread use of FUS to refer to feline lower urinary tract disorders with different sites of involvement, different combinations of clinical signs, and fundamentally different underlying causes has led to the widespread misconception that FUS represents a single pathophysiological entity induced by the interaction of multiple factors. This in turn has resulted in frequent misinterpretation of data obtained from experimental models of feline lower urinary tract disease as being representative of almost all forms of naturally occurring lower urinary tract disease. In addition, it has led to a stereotyped approach to diagnosis, treatment, and prevention of lower urinary tract diseases, irrespective of cause.

The authors are advocates of the concept that feline urological syndrome is a poor synonym for a heterogeneous group of lower urinary tract diseases of cats that may result from fundamentally different causes. The causes may be single, multiple and interacting, or unrelated (Table 110–1).[1] This change in the perspective with which the authors view naturally occurring forms of FUS is of considerable clinical significance because it helps to eliminate the stereotyped approach to treatment

and prevention of FUS that is currently in vogue. The authors have suggested that the term feline urological syndrome be abandoned and substituted with descriptive terms pertaining to site (e.g., urethra, bladder), causes (e.g., bacteria, parasites, neoplasms, metabolic disturbances, idiopathic forms), morphologic changes (e.g., inflammation, neoplasia), and pathophysiologic mechanisms (e.g., obstructive uropathy, reflex dyssynergia) whenever possible. In this fashion, the same terminology and approach to diagnosis and treatment used for other species (such as dogs and humans) will be used for cats.

Some investigators have defended the use of the term feline urologic syndrome, provided it does not encompass bacterial urinary tract infections, various forms of urolithiasis, neoplasia, anomalies, and so on.[2] They have suggested an approach of what is not the cause of feline urologic syndrome rather than what is the cause of feline urologic syndrome. In this situation, FUS becomes an exclusion diagnosis. If used as an exclusion diagnosis (the cause of feline lower urinary tract disease cannot be identified after appropriate evaluation), the authors suggest it be called idiopathic FUS (IFUS). Idiopathic lower urologic complex (LUC) may be a better alternative since more than one etiologic agent or mechanism may be involved.

EPIDEMIOLOGIC STUDIES

Several dozen epidemiologic studies of FUS have been published.[2, 3] Although many contain useful data, almost all have utilized the FUS concept previously defined as the common denominator to group affected cats. Few populations selected for study were defined on the basis of standard or contemporary clinical diagnostic procedures. Thus, results of most of these studies must be interpreted in the context of a combination of all feline lower urinary tract diseases, rather than specific disorders.

INCIDENCE AND PROPORTIONAL MORBIDITY

The incidence of a disease is defined as the annual rate of appearance of new cases of disease among the

TABLE 110–1. EXAMPLES OF CONFIRMED CAUSES OF LOWER URINARY TRACT DISEASE IN DOMESTIC CATS

Metabolic Disorders (including nutritional)	**Anatomic abnormalities**	
Uroliths	Congenital	
Struvite	Urachal anomalies	Phimosis
Newberyite	Persistent uterus masculinus	Others?
Calcium phosphate	Acquired	
Calcium oxalate	Urethral strictures	Others?
Ammonium urate		
Uric acid	**Neoplastic**	
Cystine	Benign	
Mixed mineral composition	Cystadenoma (bladder)	Leiomyoma (bladder)
Matrix (e.g., mineralized blood clots)	Fibroma (bladder)	Papilloma (bladder)
Others?	Hemangioma (bladder)	
Urethral Plugs	Malignant	
Struvite crystals only	Transitional cell carcinoma (bladder and urethra)	
Matrix only	Squamous cell carcinoma (bladder)	
Inflammatory products	Adenocarcinoma (bladder)	
Sloughed tissue	Unclassified carcinoma (bladder)	
Blood clots	Hemangiosarcoma (bladder)	
Others?	Leiomyosarcoma (bladder)	
Matrix and struvite crystals	Lymphosarcoma (primary and metastatic in bladder)	
Matrix and other crystals	Myxosarcoma (bladder)	
(e.g., calcium oxalate, ammonium urate)	Prostatic adenocarcinoma (urethra)	
	Rhabdomyosarcoma (bladder)	
Inflammatory Disorders	Endometrial adenocarcinoma (extraurinary invading and compressing urethra)	
Infectious agents		
Viral (only experimental confirmed)		
Bacterial	**Neurogenic**	
Mycoplasma/Ureaplasma ? (confirmed in dogs, rats, and humans)	Reflex dyssynergia	
	Urethral spasm	
Mycotic	Hypotonic or atonic bladder (primary or secondary)	
Parasitic	Others	
Others		
Noninfectious	**Iatrogenic**	
Immune mediated ? (human)	Reverse flushing solutions	
Others	Urethral catheters (reverse flushing)	
	Indwelling urethral catheters	
Trauma	Postsurgical urethral catheters	
	Urethrostomy complications	
	Idiopathic	

Except when noted, all these causes have been identified in cats with naturally occurring urinary tract disorders.

entire population of individuals at risk for the disease.[3, 4] The incidence of hematuria, dysuria, and/or urethral obstruction in domestic cats in the United States and Great Britain has been reported to be approximately 0.5 to 1.0 per cent per year.[4–6]

The incidence of naturally occurring hematuria, dysuria, and/or urethral obstruction in domestic cats should not be confused with the frequency with which such cats are seen in veterinary hospitals (so-called proportional morbidity ratios).[4] Although the proportional morbidity ratio of cats with lower urinary tract disorders has been reported to be as high as 10 per cent,[7] the most commonly reported frequency is 1 to 6 per cent.[3, 4, 8] Proportional morbidity ratios for FUS are not a reliable index of FUS incidence, since they may be affected by factors such as local population economics, geography, season, type of veterinary practice, and the interest and training of veterinarians.[4]

RISK FACTORS

Many risk factors for FUS have been identified (Table 110–2), some of which appeared to be synergistic.[3, 4] This led to the hypothesis that FUS was a multifactorial disorder.[9] In fact, an FUS Profile was identified. Based on epidemiologic data, the typical FUS cat was depicted as a two- to four-year-old neutered overweight male that lived indoors and consumed primarily dry food.[10, 11]

When considered in light of the population characteristics of many epidemiologic studies, the hypothesis that FUS is a multifactorial disease is not surprising. Likewise, difficulty in identification of the specific mode(s) of interaction of identified risk factors is not unexpected. It is highly probable that the latter will not be accomplished until epidemiologic studies are repeated on subsets of cats with lower urinary tract diseases defined on the basis of specific diagnostic criteria.

INFECTIOUS AGENTS

VIRUSES

Experimental Studies. The first substantial observation that feline lower urinary tract disease might be causally linked to a virus was reported in 1969, when investigators at Cornell University produced urethral obstruction in susceptible cats by injecting pooled, filtered urine obtained from naturally obstructed cats into their urinary bladders.[12] Subsequent isolation of a picornavirus (calicivirus) from the urine of a naturally ob-

TABLE 110–2. SOME RISK FACTORS REPORTED IN CATS WITH LOWER URINARY TRACT DISEASE

Factor	Comment
Age	Uncommon in cats less than 1 year old; most common between 1 and 10 years of age, with peak occurrence between 2 and 6 years
Sex	Urethral obstruction occurs most commonly in males; males and females have a similar risk for nonobstructive forms of disease
Neutering	Increased risk of disease in neutered males and females, irrespective of age of neutering
Diet	Consumption of an increased proportion of dry food in the daily ration is associated with increased disease risk
Feeding frequency	Increased frequency of feeding associated with increased risk of disease, regardless of diet fed
Excessive weight	Obesity associated with increased risk of disease
Water consumption	Decreased daily water consumption associated with increased disease risk
Sedentary life style	Lazy cats have increased risk for disease
Spring or winter season	Seasonal variations has been implicated as a risk factor by some investigators but not by others
Indoor life style	Cats using indoor litterboxes for micturition and defecation have increased risk for disease

structed male Manx cat, and experimental induction of urethral obstruction in conventionally reared cats by inoculation of their urinary bladders with the Manx picornavirus, supported the causal role of viruses in the etiology of feline lower urinary tract disease.[12] Results of further investigations performed at Cornell were interpreted to indicate that the Manx picornavirus was not a primary etiologic agent but, rather, acted as an inciter of a latent virus, perhaps feline syncytium-forming virus.[13, 14] Yet another virus, a strongly cell-associated herpesvirus isolated from cell cultures established from kidney tissues obtained from normal kittens and kittens with lower urinary tract disease, was also implicated as a causal agent.[15, 16] Results of subsequent experimental studies of cell-associated herpesvirus, Manx picornavirus, and feline syncytium-forming virus have led these investigators to hypothesize that naturally occurring lower urinary tract disease is caused by a cell-associated herpesvirus. They have interpreted their experimental data to suggest that concomitant infection with a calicivirus (originally called the Manx picornavirus): (1) increases the susceptibility of male cats to the disorder, (2) reduces the duration of the preclinical stage of infection, and (3) augments the severity of clinical signs. This experimental virus model has many clinical features that are similar to some, but not all, forms of naturally occurring lower urinary tract disease in male cats.

Other investigators have been unsuccessful in attempts to experimentally induce disease by inoculating the urinary bladders of cats with urine obtained from cats with naturally occurring lower urinary tract disease.[19, 20, 21] While the reason for this disparity is unknown, it is important that all urine donors were selected solely on the basis of urethral obstruction. Little consideration was given to identifying other possible causes of obstructive uropathy unrelated to viral infectious agents. In addition, comparison of results of various inoculation studies is difficult owing to inconsistent methodologies in sample handling and recipient inoculation, and lack of comprehensive post inoculation follow-up studies.

In an effort to substantiate previous reports and further characterize the Cornell cell-associated herpesvirus (CAHV) model of virally induced feline lower urinary tract disease, the authors inoculated CAHV into the urinary bladder and peritoneal cavities of six conventionally reared adult cats. Three additional cats served as uninfected controls.[22] After 90 days, lower urinary tract signs were not observed in CAHV infected

or control cats. Similarly, attempts to isolate CAHV from urine were consistently negative. Multiple episodes of microscopic hematuria were observed in one infected male cat. Focal cystitis was present histologically in one infected male and one infected castrated male cat. CAHV was reisolated from autogenous urinary bladder explants in five of six CAHV infected cats. CAHV was not recovered from control cats. Following inoculation, low titers of CAHV serum neutralizing (SN) antibody were detected in five of six infected cats. All six CAHV infected cats seroconverted with high immunofluorescent (IFA) CAHV antibody titers ($\geq$ 1:2560). Control cats were consistently negative for CAHV antibody by SN and IFA methodologies. These results confirm that CAHV is able to produce a persistent subclinical infection in adult cats, which is not detectable by conventional laboratory diagnostic methods.

Clinical Studies. Although initial virus isolations and experimental studies by investigators at Cornell were encouraging, subsequent studies by other investigators yielded conflicting results concerning the causative role of CAHV and calicivirus in naturally occurring lower urinary tract disease. Attempts by other investigators have been uniformly unsuccessful in demonstrating the presence of CAHV or calicivirus in spontaneous forms of lower urinary tract disease serological methods or virus isolation techniques.[16, 19–25] Virus isolations have been attempted in over 160 naturally occurring cases of feline lower urinary tract disease. Interestingly, CAHV and feline calicivirus have only rarely been isolated from urinary tracts of affected cats. While these negative findings raise serious questions about the causative roles of CAHV and Manx calicivirus in natural forms of feline lower urinary tract disease, they may also reflect inappropriate or inconsistent selection of representative cases, failure to obtain suitable samples of tissue or fluids, or limited use of explantation/cocultivation techniques.

Serologic methods have also been used to evaluate the causative role of CAHV in naturally occurring feline lower urinary tract disease. In studies conducted at the University of Minnesota and Texas A and M University, more than 250 cats with clinical signs of lower urinary tract disease were evaluated for CAHV antibody by serum neutralization assay. The results were negative. Likewise, cats experimentally infected with CAHV typically produced low to undetectable CAHV serum neutralizing antibody titers. However, they produced very high CAHV immunofluorescent antibody titers.

Recently, the authors detected virus-like particles in urethral plugs obtained from male cats with naturally occurring urethral obstruction. The urethral plugs contained minerals (primarily magnesium ammonium phosphate) and matrix. Studies are in progress to verify the viral origin of these structures (Figure 110–1).

The role of viruses as causative agents in naturally occurring feline urologic syndrome remains unresolved. In light of the fact that a substantial number of male and female cats develop hematuria, dysuria, and/or urethral obstruction without demonstrable cause, and in light of the difficulty in routinely isolating viruses from naturally occurring cases, the search for viral pathogens must continue. It is noteworthy that polyomavirus, adenovirus type II, and herpes zoster have been incriminated as causes of hemorrhagic cystitis in humans.[26–28]

Diagnosis. Diagnostic criteria for viral infections include: (1) isolation and characterization of viral agents, (2) direct demonstration of virus particles, viral antigens, or viral nucleic acids in tissues or body fluids, and/or (3) detection and quantitation of specific viral antibodies.[29] Identification and localization of viruses to the lower urinary tract of cats is essential to document their etiopathogenic role in naturally occurring hematuria, dysuria, and/or urethral obstruction. Since not all cats with lower urinary tract disease are likely to have viral infections, exclusion of other known causes of these clinical signs by routine diagnostic techniques should precede attempts to establish a specific diagnosis of viral infection (Table 110–3).

Isolation and characterization of viruses from active or latent infections of the urinary tract often require specialized sampling, cultivation, and identification techniques. To date, use of standard cell culture inoculation techniques to isolate viral pathogens from the urine of cats with experimentally induced and naturally occurring lower urinary tract disease has been unrewarding.[17, 19–]

[21, 23] However, negative findings may be related to the cell-associated nature of some viruses, the virucidal characteristics of feline urine, inappropriate handling of samples, and/or improper selection of cases. Support for the latter statement is derived from the fact that cell-associated herpesvirus has been consistently isolated from the urinary bladders of experimentally infected cats by explantation-cocultivation techniques, even though viruses could not be isolated from their urine.[17] To date, very few cases of naturally occurring lower urinary tract disease have been evaluated by explantation-cocultivation methods.

Viral pathogens often can be classified on the basis of clinical findings, cytopathogenic effects observed in tissue culture, electron microscopic appearance, and hemadsorption-hemagglutination techniques. However, specific identification of viral pathogens requires serological procedures and/or use of DNA and/or RNA enzymes that allow viral nucleic acid "fingerprinting."[29] Herpesviruses recovered from cats experimentally infected with cell associated herpesvirus were readily identified by negative-stain electron microscopy and serological procedures.

Although virus isolation is currently the primary method of establishing a specific diagnosis of virus infection, expense, time, sample requirements, and the biological characteristics of some viruses limit its clinical applicability. Techniques designed to directly identify virus particles, viral antigens, or viral nucleic acids in tissues or body fluids provide an alternative means of virus identification and localization. Electron microscopy, immunofluorescence, immunohistochemistry, radioimmunoassay, enzyme-linked immunoabsorbent assay, and in situ DNA hybridization are procedures currently utilized for viral diagnosis.[29]

Detection and quantification of specific viral antibodies provide an indirect method of diagnosis of viral

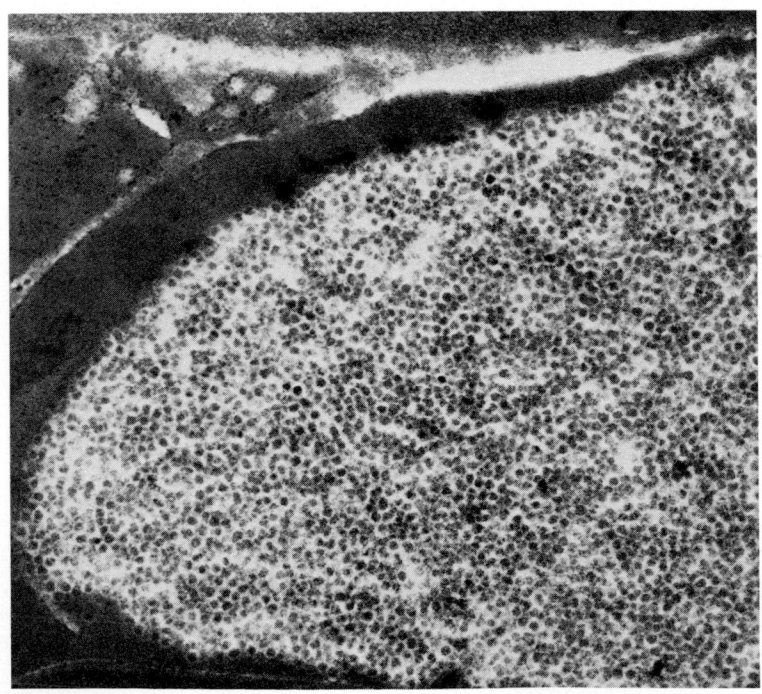

FIGURE 110–1. Transmission electron micrograph of a urethral plug obtained from a three-year-old male Abyssinian cat. The mineral component consisted of 80 per cent magnesium ammonium phosphate and 20 per cent calcium apatite. Note the viral particles contained within the nucleus of an unidentified cell. 64,000 $\times$ = original magnification.

TABLE 110–3. DIAGNOSTIC PLAN FOR FELINE DYSURIC HEMATURIA

Factor	With Urethral Obstruction		Without Urethral Obstruction	
	First or Infrequent Episodes	*Frequent or Persistent Episodes*	*First or Infrequent Episodes*	*Frequent or Persistent Episodes*
Defined history	+ + + +	+ + + + +	+ + + + +	+ + + + +
Defined physical examination	+ + + + +	+ + + + +	+ + + + +	+ + + + +
Urinalysis (with sediment)*	+ + + + +	+ + + + +	+ + + + +	+ + + + +
Screening, quantitative urine culture*	+ + +	+ + + +	+ + +	+ + + +
Serum chemistry profile (esp. SUN, creatinine, K^+, and $T\text{-}CO_2$)	+ + + + +	+ + + + +	+	+ +
Assess lesion(s), site(s), and cause(s)				
Palpation	+ + + + +	+ + + + +	+ + + + +	+ + + + +
Survey radiography	+ + +	+ + + + +	+ + +	+ + + + +
Contrast radiography (retrograde urethrocystography or antegrade cytourethrography)	+	+ + + + +	+	+ + + +
Analysis of urethral plug or urolith†	+ + + + +	+ + + + +	+ + + + +	+ + + + +
Urine urease activity	+	+ +	+	+ +
CBC count	+	+ + +	+	+ + +
Surgical biopsy	±	±	±	±
Urine electrolytes	±	±	±	+

*Urine sample preferably collected by cystocentesis; †if available, submit for quantitative analysis.

infections.[29] Ideally, serum samples obtained during the acute and convalescent phases of the disease should be evaluated for a rise in specific antibody titer. A single serum sample may be adequate if viral pathogens cause persistent or lifelong infections. However, because of the persistent and often asymptomatic nature of cell-associated herpesvirus and calicivirus infections in cats, and because of widespread use of calicivirus vaccines, caution must be used in establishing a diagnosis of viral infections on the basis of serological evidence alone.[30] Whereas indirect immunofluorescent (IFA) procedures appear to be a sensitive marker of feline cell-associated herpesvirus urinary tract infections, serum neutralizing antibody tests have been unreliable. Seroconversion for cell-associated herpesvirus detected by IFA reached its maximum three to six weeks following infection. Feline calicivirus serum neutralizing antibodies are readily detected 7 to 14 days following infection, and may persist for months to years at moderate titers in cats with persistent asymptomatic infections.[30, 31]

THERAPY

In recent years, interest in specific treatment of viral disorders has resulted in development of several chemotherapeutic and biologic agents with antiviral properties. To date, however, antiviral agents available for clinical use are relatively few in number, and are limited

in antiviral specificity.[29, 32, 33] None has been evaluated in cats with lower urinary tract disease.

Management of lower urinary tract disease in cats suspected to be caused by viral agents has been limited to supportive and symptomatic treatment given during the course of clinical signs. Remission of signs during the course of empirical therapy has frequently been interpreted as evidence of the benefits of such therapy. There is no doubt that those who have placed as much emphasis on empirical studies as on properly controlled studies have been responsible for the initiation and perpetuation of therapeutic myths.

In a prospective clinical study designed to detect causes of hematuria, dysuria, and/or urethral obstruction in 143 male and female cats with naturally occurring disease, preliminary evaluation of data indicated that a causative agent (infectious agents, uroliths, neoplasms, etc.) could not be detected in 77 (53 per cent) cases (Table 110–4). The authors were unable to identify pathogenic viruses from the urine of affected patients, although no attempt was made to explant urinary tract tissues for virus isolation. It is noteworthy that clinical signs of hematuria and dysuria in many nonobstructed cats with this idiopathic form of lower urinary tract disease spontaneously subsided approximately one week after diagnosis. Although this prospective study was not designed to study the cause and frequency of recurrence of lower urinary tract disease, a similar pattern of self

TABLE 110–4. FREQUENCY OF OCCURRENCE OF VARIOUS TYPES OF DISORDERS IN 143 CATS WITH HEMATURIA AND DYSURIA

Group	Idiopathic	Urethral Plug	Uroliths	Uroliths and UTI	UTI
Nonobstructed females (n=43)	25	0	17	1*	0
Nonobstructed males (n=47)	37	0	8	0	2‡a
Obstructed males (n=53)	15	32	5	1†	0

*Struvite urolith and pseudomonas UTI; †struvite urolith and staphylococcal and corynebacterium UTI; ‡staphylococcal UTI; ªEscherichia UTI

TABLE 110–5. INTERPRETATION OF QUANTITATIVE URINE CULTURES IN DOGS AND CATS*

Collection Method	Significant		Suspicious		Contaminant	
	Dog	Cat	Dog	Cat	Dog	Cat
Cystocentesis	≥ 1000	≥ 1000	100 to 1000	100 to 1000	≤ 100	≤ 100
Catheterization	≥ 10,000	≥ 1000	1000 to 10,000	100 to 1000	≤ 1000	≤ 100
Voluntary voiding	≥ 100,000†	≥ 10,000	10,000 to 90,000	1000 to 10,000	≤ 10,000	≤ 1000
Manual compression	≥ 100,000†	≥ 10,000	10,000 to 90,000	1000 to 10,000	≤ 10,000	≤ 1000

*These data represent generalities. On occasion, bacterial UTI may be detected in dogs and cats with fewer numbers of organisms (i.e., false-negative results).
†Cautions: Contamination of midstream samples may result in colony counts > 10,000/ml in some dogs (i.e., false-positive results).

limiting clinical disease was subsequently observed in several cats. The point to be emphasized is that the unpredictability with which signs of lower urinary tract disorders undergo remission and exacerbation mandates carefully designed and controlled clinical trials in patients known to have an identical disorder to prove efficacy of therapeutic and prophylactic regimens.[1]

Bacteria

ETIOPATHOGENESIS

Results of several clinical investigations of feline lower urinary tract disease indicate that the initial episode usually occurs in the absence of significant numbers of detectable bacteria.[23, 34] In a prospective diagnostic study of obstructed and nonobstructed cats at the University of Minnesota, bacterial UTI was identified in only 4 of 143 patients (2.8 per cent) (Table 110–4). In those instances where significant bacteria have been confirmed, it frequently (but not invariably) occurred as a secondary or complicating rather than a primary etiologic factor. Bacterial UTI is a common sequela to use of indwelling urinary catheters and perineal urethrostomy.[35–38] In a controlled prospective clinical study of prevention of recurrent urethral obstruction in male cats performed at the University of Minnesota, episodes of bacterial UTI occurred in 17 per cent of cats treated with perineal urethrostomies, 10 per cent of cats treated with perineal urethrostomies and dietary therapy, and none of the cats treated with dietary therapy alone. Results of this study emphasize the importance of the

TABLE 110–6. SUMMARY OF OBJECTIVES FOR TREATMENT OF URINARY TRACT INFECTIONS

1. The predisposing or complicating causes of the UTI should be identified and eliminated.
2. Causative pathogens are identified by qualitative and quantitative culture, and antimicrobials are selected on the basis of antimicrobial susceptibility tests. Ideally, the agent chosen should have the narrowest possible spectrum of antimicrobial activity.
3. Aggressive treatment with appropriate dosages of antimicrobials is indicated.
4. Although it is usually unnecessary, urine pH can be altered to enhance antimicrobial activity.
5. Urine should be recultured three to five days after initiation of therapy to check the efficacy of the antimicrobial agent in sterilizing the urine.
6. Antimicrobial therapy is continued until there is clinical and laboratory evidence of response. The patient's response is monitored by bacterial culture and urinalysis.
7. Because symptomatic or asymptomatic recurrences may be associated with progressive and potentially irreversible disease, they should be anticipated, prevented, and, if necessary, treated.

distal urethra in prevention of urinary tract infections in male cats.

The infrequency with which bacteria have been isolated from urine of cats during the early phases of lower urinary tract disease may be related to highly effective local host defense mechanisms in this species. Local host defense mechanisms that normally inhibit bacterial growth in the urinary tract include production of highly concentrated urine that is acid and that contains a large quantity of urea.[39] The fact that kidneys of cats are capable of producing highly concentrated urine (specific gravity up to approximately 1.080), and the fact that their carnivorous nature promotes the production of acid urine that is high in urea concentration, has prompted the hypothesis that they may be innately less susceptible to urinary tract infections with bacteria than are other species of animals.[40]

DIAGNOSIS

Caution must be used in the interpretation of confirmed bacteriuria in cats, because identification of bacteria in urine is not synonymous with bacterial urinary tract infection. The problem is related to the fact that a commensal population of bacteria inhabits the mucosal surface of the distal urinary tract. Therefore, urine that passes through the urethra may be contaminated with bacteria that are not of clinical significance. The problem of overinterpretation of bacteriuria has been largely circumvented by the concept of significant bacteriuria and quantitative urine cultures.[41] However, the problem of underinterpretation of bacteriuria is also deserving of consideration. Because cat urine is innately less likely to support the growth of bacterial pathogens than is dog or human urine, lower numbers of bacteria per milliliter are likely to be of greater clinical significance in cats than in dogs (Table 110–5).

Since bacterial urinary tract infection is an uncommon cause of lower urinary tract disease in cats, detection should arouse one's index of suspicion that an underlying cause is present (so-called complicated UTI). Further diagnostic procedures that may be considered include exfoliative cytology of urine sediment, survey and contrast radiography, ultrasonography, and biopsy (Table 110–3).

TREATMENT

The infrequency with which bacteria are isolated from male and female cats with diseases of the lower urinary tract prompts questions about the widespread, routine use of antimicrobial agents in treating this disorder. Results of a prospective double-blind study of the efficacy of chloramphenicol in treatment of ten male and female cats with "feline urologic syndrome" revealed no differences between the treated and control group (70 per cent complete remission of signs in both groups).[42] Caution must be used to prevent overtreatment.

Efforts to prevent iatrogenic UTI in patients should include: (1) avoiding indiscriminate use of urinary catheters, (2) use of closed systems if indwelling urinary catheters are deemed essential, (3) cautious use of indwelling urinary catheters in patients during therapeutic diuresis, (4) appropriate use of antimicrobial agents to prevent or control iatrogenic UTI, and (5) use of surgical techniques that minimize trauma and microbial contamination of the urinary tract.

It is important to recognize that urinary tract infections may be associated with transient reversible abnormalities in local host defenses. Such disorders are usually recognized as uncomplicated forms of UTI. In such patients, self repair of damaged host defenses may result in spontaneous resolution of UTI. However, it is emphasized that remission of clinical signs is not necessarily synonymous with eradication of infection.

The status of host defense mechanisms is an extremely important determinant in the pathogenesis of urinary tract infections. Although it is possible to induce UTI by overwhelming normal host defenses with a massive inoculum of pathogenic bacteria, such a phenomenon is uncommon in naturally occurring cases of UTI. Because bacteria can establish and propagate themselves when host defenses are inadequate, the underlying causes of complicated UTI must be eliminated or controlled if permanent eradication of pathogens is to be accomplished.

Although antimicrobial agents are the cornerstone of therapy for urinary tract infections, they should not be given haphazardly without follow-up (Table 110–6). The success or failure of therapy should not be solely based on elimination or persistence of clinical signs, but rather should be monitored by serial evaluation of urine cultures and urinalyses performed at appropriate intervals. Equally important is the necessity to anticipate, prevent and/or treat symptomatic or asymptomatic recurrences since they may be associated with progressive and potentially irreversible disease.

Mycoplasmas, Ureaplasmas, Mycotic Agents and Parasites

MYCOPLASMAS AND UREAPLASMAS

Mycoplasmas are known to cause urethritis in humans.[43, 44] Ureaplasmas (urease producing mycoplasmas) are known to cause struvite urolithiasis in humans, dogs, and rats.[45] Efforts to isolate mycoplasmas and ureaplasmas from urine of more than 143 cats with naturally occurring lower urinary tract disease have been unsuccessful at the University of Minnesota (Table 110–3). Other investigators have reported similar findings.[19, 23] Further studies are desirable, however, because ureaplasmas are fastidious and cell associated. Factors reported to limit growth of ureaplasmas in broth cultures

include pH > 7.5, osmotic activity > 600 mOsm/kg, and high ammonia concentrations.[45]

MYCOTIC AGENTS

Although very uncommon, urinary tract infections with *Candida* spp. and *Aspergillus fumigatus* have been reported in cats.[46–48] Typically host defenses have been severely compromised as a result of immunosuppression, diabetes mellitus, or indwelling catheterization coupled with antimicrobial therapy. The authors encountered a *Cephalosporium* spp. fungal urinary tract infection in an eight-year-old male domestic short hair cat with concomitant bacterial urinary tract infection, struvite urolithiasis and cardiomyopathy. The cat had a perineal urethrostomy. A tentative diagnosis of fungal UTI may be established by identification of yeasts or mycelia in urine or culture media. Confirmation of fungal UTI requires demonstration of fungal agents in tissue. Because of limited experience with fungal UTI in cats, generalizations regarding therapy cannot be made. Flucytosine may be considered for *Candida* spp. UTI.[47]

PARASITES

Although cats may develop infections with *Capillaria feliscati*, most (but not all) remain asymptomatic.[49] Lack of morbidity associated with these nematodes may be related to their superficial attachment to the bladder mucosa, and numbers present. Treatment is not necessary unless concomitant signs are present. In that instance, fenbendazole (12 mg/lb or 25 mg/kg given q12h for 3 to 10 days) may be considered.[49]

UROLITHIASIS

Terminology

The urinary system is designed to dispose of body wastes in liquid form. However, some waste products are sparingly soluble and occasionally precipitate out of solution. In the past, confusion has occurred as a result of various terms used to describe precipitates that form in urine. Depending on the size and consistency of the precipitates, they have been referred to as crystals, sand, sabulous plugs, gravel, pebbles, stones, rocks, uroliths, and/or calculi.

The word crystal is derived from the Greek word *krystallosus*, which means ice, and is used to refer to the solid phase of substances having a specific internal structure and enclosed by symmetrically arranged planar surfaces. The term sabulous is derived from the Latin word *sabulosus* meaning sand. The Latin word *calculus* means pebble. The Greek word *lithos* means stone, and -*uria* is a suffix derived from a Greek word (*ouron*) meaning urine. The preferred terminology for abnormal microscopic precipitates in urine is crystalluria, whereas macroscopic concretions are called uroliths (nephroliths, urocystoliths, and so on). Plugs are defined as objects of any composition that close or obstruct passageways or ducts. Pending further studies, urethral plugs should

TABLE 110–7. COMMON CHARACTERISTICS OF FELINE STRUVITE UROLITHS

1. Chemical name   Crystal name
   Magnesium ammonium phosphate hexahydrate   Struvite
2. Formula
   $Mg\,NH_4\,PO_4 \cdot 6H_2O$
3. Variations in mineral composition
   Struvite only (especially sterile struvite)
   Struvite mixed with lesser quantities of calcium apatite and/or ammonium acid urate (especially infection-induced struvite)
   Nucleus of a different mineral surrounded by variable layers composed primarily of struvite. Small quantities of calcium apatite and/or
      ammonium acid urate may also be present.
4. Physical characteristics
   a. *Color:* Struvite uroliths are usually white, cream, or light-brown in color. The surface of uroliths is commonly red because of
      concomitant hematuria.
   b. *Shape:* Sterile struvite uroliths obtained from the urinary bladder of cats commonly have a wafer or disc shape; they are thicker at the
      center than at the periphery. Sterile struvite uroliths may also have a rough, jagged, quartz-like appearance. Infection-induced feline
      struvite uroliths are often larger than sterile struvite uroliths, and tend to be more egg-shaped. They also contain more matrix than
      sterile struvite uroliths.
   c. *Nuclei and laminations:* Uncommon in sterile struvite uroliths. Infection-induced struvite may surround sterile struvite.
   d. *Matrix:* Sterile struvite uroliths contain little matrix and characteristically are very dense and brittle. Infection-induced struvite uroliths
      are somewhat softer because they contain more matrix.
   e. *Density:* Struvite is radiodense compared with nonskeletal tissue on survey radiographs.
   f. *Location:* Most occur in the urinary bladder; some may lodge in the urethra, especially of male cats. Struvite uroliths may affect the
      kidneys, but this location has been very uncommon.
   g. *Number:* Single or multiple.
   h. *Size:* Subvisual to a size limited by the capacity of structure (kidney and urinary bladder) in which they form.
5. Predisposing factors
   a. Sterile struvite
      (1) Tendency to form in alkaline or less acid urine
      (2) Supersaturation of urine with magnesium, ammonium, and/or phosphate
      (3) Excessive consumption of magnesium and perhaps other minerals
      (4) Formation of concentrated urine
      (5) Retention of urine
      (6) Unidentified factors
   b. Infection-induced struvite
      (1) Urinary tract infection with urease-producing microbes, especially staphylococci
      (2) Excretion of large quantities of urea in urine
6. Characteristics of affected patients
   a. May be detected at any age, but usually between 1 and 10 years of age.
   b. When uroliths occur in immature cats, they usually have been infection-induced struvite.
   c. No apparent sex predisposition.
   d. Obesity reflects excessive food consumption. Excessive calories are stored as fat. Minerals consumed with excessive food are excreted in
      urine and may predispose to urolith formation.

be described with terminology that reflects their approximate proportion and type of minerals and matrix.

There are physical and probable etiopathogenic differences between feline uroliths and urethral plugs (Tables 110–7 and 110–8). Therefore, these terms should not be used as synonyms. Uroliths are polycrystalline concretions composed primarily of minerals (organic and inorganic crystalloids) and smaller quantities of matrix.[45] In contrast, feline urethral plugs commonly are composed of large quantities of matrix mixed with minerals. However some urethral plugs are composed primarily of matrix, others are composed primarily of aggregates of crystalline minerals, and some consist of sloughed tissue, blood, and/or inflammatory reactants.[1]

A variety of different minerals have been identified in uroliths (Table 110–9; Figure 110–2) and urethral plugs (Table 110–10) of cats. The mineral composition of uroliths and urethral plugs should be used to describe them since most therapeutic regimens have been based on their mineral composition.

DIAGNOSIS

Uroliths are usually suspected on the basis of typical findings obtained by history and physical examination. Urinalyses, quantitative urine cultures, radiography, and ultrasonography may be required to differentiate uroliths from other causes of clinical signs such as urinary tract infections, inflammatory polyps, and neoplasia (Tables 110–1 and 110–3).

In a recent prospective diagnostic study of feline lower urinary tract disorders, uroliths were detected by radiography in more than 20 per cent of the patients (Table 110–12). In many instances the solitary nature and/or small size of the uroliths prevented their detection by palpation. From a diagnostic yield perspective, radiography of the abdomen of previously untreated cats with hematuria, dysuria, and/or urethral obstruction is more likely to yield positive information (> 20 per cent) than quantitative urine cultures (± 3 per cent).

Struvite Urolithiasis

As of mid-1987, the mineral composition of approximately 80 per cent of the naturally occurring uroliths submitted to the University of Minnesota by veterinarians in the USA and Canada was primarily struvite (Table 110–9; Figures 110–3 and 110–4). The 80 per cent frequency of naturally occurring struvite uroliths observed in 1987 represents approximately a 10 per cent decrease from the series the authors reported in 1984.[50]

TABLE 110–8. CHARACTERISTICS OF FELINE STRUVITE URETHRAL PLUGS

1. Chemical name   Crystal name
   Magnesium ammonium   Struvite
   phosphate hexahydrate
2. Formula
   $Mg\ NH_4\ PO_4 \cdot 6H_2O$
3. Variations in composition
   Struvite only
   Struvite mixed with relatively small quantities of calcium apatite
4. Physical characteristics
   Color: Struvite urethral plugs are typically white, cream, or light brown in color
   Shape: Often have a cylindrical shape; sometimes they form a shapeless gelatinous mass
   Nuclei and laminations: None grossly visible
   Matrix: Contain large quantities of matrix and therefore are very fragile
   Density: Soft and easily compressible
   Number: Usually single; occasionally multiple
   Size: Diameter conforms to diameter of urethra. Length varies from a few millimeters to several centimeters, and may be interrupted along length of urethra.
5. Predisposing factors
   Reduced diameter of the penile urethra
   Locally produced matrix?
   Factors affecting struvite crystalluria?
6. Characteristics of affected patients
   Mean age = 3.8 years (range, < 1 to > 12 yr)
   No obvious breed disposition
   Consistently (if not invariably) in males

TABLE 110–9. MINERAL COMPOSITION OF 748 FELINE UROLITHS ANALYZED BY QUANTITATIVE METHODS*

Predominant Mineral Type	Number of Uroliths	Percentage
Magnesium ammonium phosphate hexahydrate	590	78.9
100%	(452)	(60.4)
70–99%†	(138)	(18.5)
Magnesium hydrogen phosphate trihydrate		
70–99%	2	0.3
Calcium oxalate		
Calcium oxalate monohydrate	33	4.4
100%	(9)	(1.2)
70–99†	(14)	(1.9)
Calcium oxalate dihydrate		
70–99%†	(8)	(1.1)
Calcium oxalate monohydrate & dihydrate		
100%	(2)	(0.3)
Calcium phosphate		
Calcium phosphate	21	2.8
100%	(10)	(1.3)
70–99%†	(8)	(1.1)
Calcium hydrogen phosphate dihydrate		
100%	(2)	(0.3)
70–99%†	(1)	(0.1)
Uric acid and urates	31	4.1
Ammonium acid urate		
100%	(20)	(2.7)
70–99%†	(8)	(1.1)
Uric acid		
100%	(2)	(0.3)
70–99%†	(1)	(0.1)
Cystine	1	0.1
Silica	0	0
Mixed‡	36	4.8
Compound§	9	1.2
Matrix	25	3.3
Total	748	100%

*Analysis performed by optical crystallography and x-ray diffraction
†Urolith composed of 70–99% of mineral type listed; no nucleus or shell detected.
‡Uroliths did not contain at least 70% of mineral type listed; no nucleus and shell detected.
§Uroliths contained an identifiable nucleus and one or more surrounding layers of different mineral type.

As of mid-1987, the mineral composition of approximately 90 per cent of the naturally occurring urethral plugs submitted to the University of Minnesota was primarily struvite (Table 110–10). The 90 per cent frequency of naturally occurring struvite urethral plugs observed in 1987 represents approximately a 4 per cent decrease from the series the authors reported in 1984.[50]

The decline in appearance of naturally occurring struvite uroliths and urethral plugs during this three year period coincides with widespread use of a new calculolytic diet designed to dissolve struvite uroliths,[45] and modification of maintenance and prevention diets designed to minimize struvite crystalluria. It also appears to be associated with a trend toward an increase in the frequency of occurrence and detection of nonstruvite uroliths and urethral plugs, especially ammonium urate and calcium oxalate (Tables 110–9 and 110–10).[50]

Results of our clinical and experimental studies indicate that three distinct etiologic mechanisms may be responsible for development of clinically significant urinary tract precipitates containing large quantities of struvite.[1, 45] Formation of sterile struvite uroliths (perhaps in association with dietary factors) is *one* type. Formation of "infected" or "urease" struvite uroliths as a sequela to urinary tract infection with urease producing bacteria is a *second* type. A combination of a sterile struvite nidus that predisposes to urinary tract infection with urease-producing microbes may result in formation of an outer layer of infection-induced struvite. Formation of urethral plugs containing a large quantity of matrix in addition to varying quantities of struvite is a *third* form.

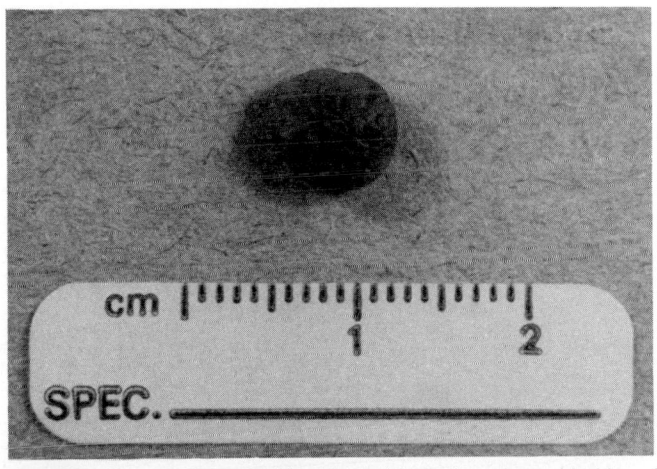

FIGURE 110–2. Solitary urolith removed from the urinary bladder of a four-year-old castrated male domestic shorthair cat. The mineral component of the urolith was 100 per cent magnesium ammonium phosphate.

TABLE 110–10. MINERAL COMPOSITION OF 374 FELINE URETHRAL PLUGS ANALYZED BY QUANTITATIVE METHODS*

Predominant Mineral Type	Number of Uroliths	Percentage
Magnesium ammonium phosphate hexahydrate	337	90.1
100%	(286)	(76.5)
70–99%†	(51)	(13.7)
Calcium oxalate	7	1.9
Calcium oxalate monohydrate		
100%	(2)	(0.5)
70–99%†	(4)	(1.1)
Calcium oxalate dihydrate		
100%	(1)	(0.3)
Calcium phosphate	7	1.9
Calcium apatite		
100%	(3)	(0.8)
70–99%†	(4)	(1.1)
Ammonium acid urate	5	1.3
100%	(5)	(1.3)
Mixed‡	1	0.3
Matrix	17	4.5
Total	374	100%

*Analysis performed by optical crystallography and x-ray diffraction.

†Urolith composed of 70–99% of mineral type listed; no nucleus or shell detected.

‡Uroliths did not contain at least 70% of mineral type listed; no nucleus and shell detected.

EXPERIMENTAL STUDIES OF STERILE STRUVITE UROLITHS

Results of experimental studies of cats indicate that sterile struvite uroliths may be initiated by altering dietary composition. Seven groups of investigators have reported convincing data concerning experimental production of magnesium phosphate and magnesium ammonium phosphate uroliths in previously normal cats consuming calculogenic diets containing 0.15 to 1.0 per cent dry weight magnesium.[45, 51–58] In the mid-1970's, canned cat foods commercially manufactured in the United States contained 0.03 to 0.15 per cent dry weight

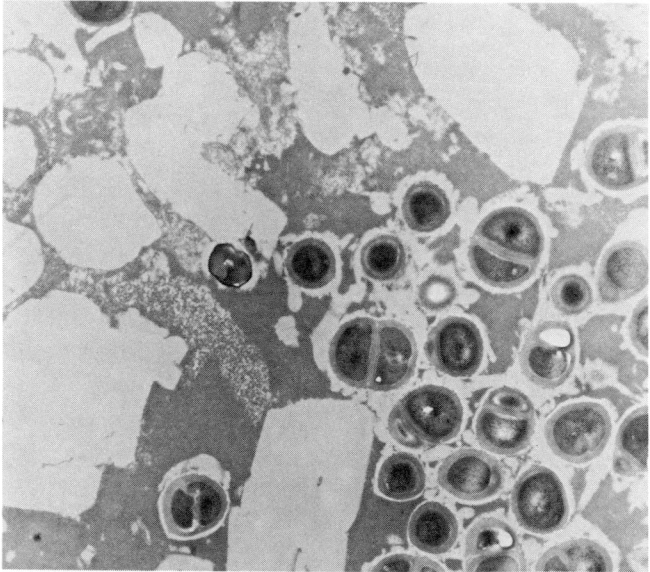

FIGURE 110–3. Transmission electron micrograph of the struvite urolith described in Figure 110–4. Note the bacterial cocci surrounded by matrix. 16,000 × = original magnification.

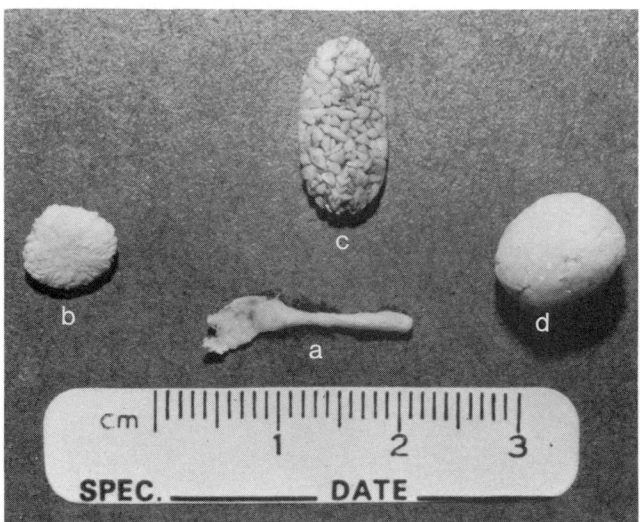

FIGURE 110–4. A struvite urethral plug *(A)*, two wafer-like sterile struvite uroliths *(B and C)*, and an infection-induced struvite urolith *(D)* removed from the lower urinary tracts of male cats. One end of the struvite urethral plug was crushed with an index finger to illustrate its friable nature. (From Minnesota Veterinarian, 22:33, 1982.)

magnesium; semimoist food contained 0.07 to 0.16 per cent, and dry food contained 0.15 to 0.16 per cent dry weight magnesium.[59, 60] Similar values have recently been reported, and stated to be 4 to 18 times higher than the amount needed to fulfill the cat's daily requirement of 0.016 per cent dry weight magnesium.[61] However, it has been emphasized that the percentage of magnesium in experimental diets (and also commercially manufactured diets) may be a misleading indication of dietary magnesium intake because of differences in caloric density, palatability, and digestibility.[57, 61] Calcium, phosphorus, and other dietary minerals may also influence the calculogenic potential of various diets containing magnesium.[62] Although consumption, absorption, and urinary excretion of comparatively large quantities of magnesium have been often incriminated as important features of calculogenic diets, recent studies indicate that other factors may also play a role.[57]

Uroliths experimentally produced in cats by one group of investigators were similar in gross appearance and mineral composition to naturally occurring sterile struvite uroliths commonly encountered in male and female cats.[45, 63] However, in all experimental studies of feline struvite calculogenesis reported to date, none has resulted in production of urethral plugs containing substantial quantities of matrix in addition to struvite crystals. When urethral obstruction has occurred, aggregates of crystalline material with very little if any matrix have been observed. These observations suggest that the aforementioned dietary models of struvite urolithiasis are not analogous to the naturally occurring form of feline urethral obstruction associated with matrix struvite plugs (Table 110–8).

Uroliths produced during early experimental studies were composed of magnesium phosphate (Figure 110–5), while those produced in subsequent studies were found to contain magnesium, ammonium, and phosphate.[51, 54, 57, 58, 62] Results of further studies indicate that the precise mineral composition of uroliths induced by

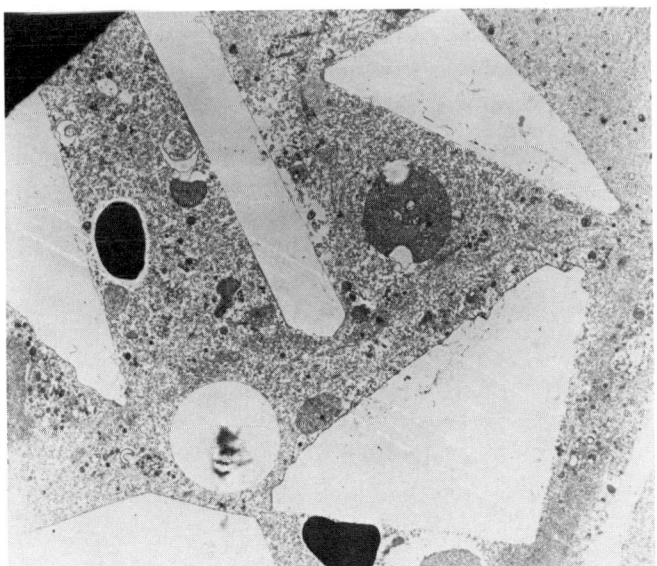

FIGURE 110–5. Transmission electron micrograph of a urethral plug obtained from an adult male neutered domestic shorthair cat. The crystalline component consisted of 100 per cent magnesium ammonium phosphate. Note the fragments of red cells entrapped in the matrix adjacent to the struvite crystals. 3300 × = original magnification.

dietary excess of magnesium may be influenced by urine pH.[64] Administration of a sufficient quantity of magnesium oxide alkalizes urine produced by cats. Uroliths formed in this situation often contain magnesium hydrogen phosphate trihydrate (newberyite).[45] They are nearly devoid of ammonium ion. However, if the composition of the diet is modified so that urine of neutral or slightly acid pH is produced, uroliths composed of magnesium ammonium phosphate may be induced.[57, 64] Subsequent studies further emphasized the importance of urine pH on the calculogenic potential of magnesium supplemented diets.[57] Consumption of diets supplemented with magnesium oxide may produce struvite uroliths in cats. However, consumption of diets with a similar quantity of magnesium in the form of magnesium chloride (a urine acidifying agent) did not result in struvite urolith formation because of sufficient urine acidification to prevent oversaturation of urine with struvite. Also, addition of a sufficient quantity of acidifier (ammonium chloride) to diets supplemented with potentially calculogenic quantities of magnesium oxide inhibited struvite urolith formation.[63]

The association of alkaline urine with formation of sterile struvite uroliths is in need of further study. As mentioned previously, magnesium hydrogen phosphate (newberyite) was produced in cats consuming canned food supplemented with up to 1 per cent magnesium in the form of magnesium oxide.[45, 51, 54, 62] Presumably, reduction of the need of the renal tubules to produce ammonia buffer because of formation of alkaline urine reduced the quantity of ammonium to combine with magnesium and phosphate. In a clinical study of 20 cats with naturally occurring struvite urocystoliths without detectable urinary tract infection, the mean urine pH at the time of diagnosis was 6.9 ± 6.4. The urine of affected cats was not persistently alkaline. This point is of clinical significance when attempting to modify urine

pH in an attempt to dissolve or prevent sterile struvite uroliths. Based on available data, one should strive to achieve a pH value of approximately 6.0 to 6.2 in an attempt to dissolve or prevent struvite uroliths.

In conclusion, data derived from cats with induced sterile struvite uroliths indicate that several dietary factors play a role in the etiopathogenesis of naturally occurring sterile struvite uroliths. Of these, factors affecting urine magnesium concentration and urine pH are of major therapeutic importance.[2, 45, 61]

The relationship of diets to formation of urethral plugs is not clear. Although dietary ingredients could contribute to the mineral component of urethral plugs, it is not known whether or not they contribute to the matrix component of urethral plugs. It is conceivable that formation of large quantities of crystalline material could stimulate production of matrix substances by tissues lining the urethral lumen. Hypercalciuria has been recently incriminated in the pathogenesis of hematuria in children.[65] However, further studies are necessary before meaningful conclusions can be formulated about the etiopathogenesis of naturally occurring urethral plugs in cats. Progress to date has been hindered by lack of a reproducible model of feline lower urinary tract disease characterized by urethral plug formation.

NATURALLY OCCURRING STERILE STRUVITE UROLITHS

As described in the preceding section on experimental study of sterile struvite uroliths, the mineral composition and physical characteristics of some experimentally induced and naturally occurring sterile struvite uroliths are almost identical (Tables 110–7 and 110–9). At this time, approximately 80 per cent of the naturally occurring uroliths removed from cats contain primarily struvite (Table 110–9). Although the exact percentage of sterile versus infection-induced struvite uroliths in this series could not be precisely determined, the authors estimate that at least 75 to 80 per cent were composed of sterile struvite. Sterile struvite uroliths contain less matrix than infection-induced struvite, and have other characteristic features (Table 110–7). Unlike infection-induced struvite uroliths, bacteria cannot be detected in their matrix by culture, light microscopy, or electron microscopy.

Of the 585 struvite uroliths summarized in Table 110–9, 268 occurred in males and 271 were encountered in females. Neutered males (n = 158) and neutered females (n = 175) were more commonly affected than intact males (n = 88) and intact females (n = 75) (in 43 affected cats, the gender was not recorded). The urinary bladder was the most common site of detection of struvite uroliths (n = 448), while the urethra (n = 35), bladder and urethra (n = 13), kidney (n = 3), kidney and ureters (n = 1), and kidney, ureters, and bladder (n = 1) were less common sites (the site of 82 struvite uroliths was not recorded).

There is need to repeat epidemiologic studies on cats known to have naturally occurring sterile struvite uroliths. Based on currently available information, several associations are predicted. For example, a decrease in urine volume and increase in urine specific gravity secondary to decreased water consumption would be a logical risk factor for urolith formation. Likewise, excessive consumption of food (perhaps associated with ad libitum feeding) would be expected to result in obesity and excretion of excess minerals (some of which could be calculogenic) in urine. It has been reported that cats maintain magnesium homeostasis by excreting excessive dietary magnesium in their urine.[57] Rather than link obesity as a risk factor for "FUS," it is logical that both obesity and urolithiasis may be linked to excessive food consumption. Finally, the infrequency with which immature cats develop sterile struvite uroliths may be associated with their tendency to form more acid urine than adults. It has been reported that the capacity to form significantly alkaline urine does not develop until cats are approximately one year of age.[65a] However, this factor does not protect immature cats from infection-induced struvite uroliths. In our experience, most uroliths encountered in immature male and female cats have been infection-induced struvite secondary to abnormalities in local host defense mechanisms.

NATURALLY OCCURRING INFECTION-INDUCED STRUVITE UROLITHS

Infection of the feline urinary tract with urease producing microbes (especially staphylococci) may result in the rapid production of magnesium ammonium phosphate uroliths in a fashion identical to that which occurs in dogs.[45] Rather than being linked to urinary excretion of excessive quantities of dietary minerals, the etiopathogenesis of infection-induced struvite is linked to microbial urease that hydrolyzes urea. The result is alkalinization of urine associated with large quantities of ammonia and phosphate ion. The difference in etiopathogenesis of infection-induced and sterile struvite uroliths is of great therapeutic significance.

Because cats are innately resistant to bacterial urinary tract infections, infection-induced struvite uroliths are far less commonly encountered than sterile struvite uroliths. However, when encountered, they usually affect cats whose local host defenses have been altered by persistent diseases (congenital anomalies, neoplasia, etc.), perineal urethrostomies, or indwelling urinary catheters.[1, 45, 66, 67]

Infection-induced struvite uroliths often contain a greater quantity of matrix than sterile struvite uroliths, presumably as a result of increased production of inflammatory reactants (Table 110–7).[45] They also tend to grow in size more rapidly, and frequently are larger in size. Urease producing microbes can readily be cultured from their inner portions, and can be detected by light and electron microscopy.

NATURALLY OCCURRING STRUVITE URETHRAL PLUGS

Naturally occurring urethral plugs in cats are typically cylindrical when observed by radiography or at necropsy. If forced through the distal urethral orifice by manual compression of the urinary bladder or forceful attempts to void, they may have the appearance and physical properties of toothpaste.[1]

The most commonly encountered form of naturally occurring urethral plugs contains relatively large quantities of matrix and struvite crystals (Tables 110–8 and 110–10). The authors presume that factors associated with formation of struvite crystals are the same as those associated with formation of sterile struvite or infection-induced struvite uroliths.

Light and electron microscopic studies of naturally occurring urethral plugs obtained from male cats have revealed that their matrix is morphologically heterogeneous. The matrix may surround red cells, white cells, sperm, bacteria and/or as yet unidentified structures, in addition to crystals. Some cells contained in plugs appear to contain virus particles. The point to be emphasized is that urethral plugs are not identical.

Which is more important, the crystals or the matrix? It is our impression that formation of matrix is an extremely important event leading to the occurrence of matrix-crystal urethral plugs. Unfortunately, the specific composition and origin (urine and/or tissue surrounding the urinary tract) of matrix in urethral plugs have not yet been identified. Nonetheless, the authors hypothesize that some abnormality (infectious agents?) stimulates formation of matrix, which if produced in sufficient quantity forms a gel in the urethral lumen. Hematuria and dysuria are events concomitant with matrix production. If an affected male cat has associated but etiologically unrelated struvite crystalluria, the combination of matrix (mortar) and crystals (bricks) results in formation of a plug that obstructs their normally small diameter urethral lumen. If a male cat does not have a significant degree of concomitant crystalluria, or if a female cat with or without crystalluria is affected, the matrix passes through the urethral lumen, and signs of hematuria and dysuria occur without urethral obstruction. This hypothesis provides a plausible explanation for different types of minerals, cells and microbes in urethral plugs, the expression of obstructive and nonobstructive forms of the disease in male cats, and sex differences in occurrence of urethral obstruction.

Results of a prospective clinical diagnostic study at the University of Minnesota have confirmed that obstructive urethropathy in male cats may be caused by one or more intraluminal, mural, or extramural abnormalities located at one or more sites (Table 110–11). Formation of matrix-struvite urethral plugs appears to be the most common, but not the only cause of urethral obstruction. Conceptual understanding of this phenomenon is of paramount diagnostic and therapeutic importance.

Ammonium Urate Uroliths

In our feline urolith series, ammonium urate and uric acid comprised approximately 4 per cent of the total (Table 110–9). All were located in the urethra and/or urinary bladder. However, ammonium urate and uric acid uroliths have been reported in the kidneys and ureters of cats.[68, 69] In our series, males were affected twice as often as females.

There have been isolated case reports of uric acid and ammonium urate uroliths in cats during the past 20

TABLE 110–11. POSSIBLE CAUSES OF URETHRAL OBSTRUCTION IN MALE CATS

Primary Causes	Perpetuating Causes	Iatrogenic Causes

I. Intraluminal
  A. Urethral plugs (matrix and/or crystals)
  B. Urethroliths
  C. Tissue sloughed from urinary bladder or urethra
II. Mural or Extramural
  A. Strictures
  B. Prostatic lesions
  C. Urethral neoplasms
  D. Anomalies
  E. Reflex dyssynergia
III. Combinations
IV. Others?
	I. Intraluminal
	  A. WBC, RBC, and fibrin
	  B. Sloughed tissue
	  C. Increased production of mucoprotein
	
	II. Mural
	  A. Inflammatory swelling
	  B. Muscular spasm (reflex dyssynergia?)
	  C. Strictures
	
	III. Combinations
	IV. Others
		I. Tissue Damage
		  A. Reverse flushing solutions
		  B. Catheter trauma
		  C. Catheter-induced foreign body reaction
		  D. Catheter-induced infection
		II. Postsurgical dysfunction

years.[50, 68–74] Although a renal tubular reabsorptive defect and portovascular anomalies have been incriminated as causes in a few cases, the cause of formation of most feline urate uroliths was not established.[72, 73] The authors have not been able to precisely determine the cause of feline urate uroliths in their stone series. However, formation of highly acid, highly concentrated urine associated with consumption of diets high in purine precursors (especially liver) appears to be involved in some cases.

Calcium Oxalate Uroliths

In our series, calcium oxalate uroliths comprised approximately 4 per cent of the total (Table 110–9). They were detected in the kidneys (n=6), urinary bladder (n=14), urethra (n=6), and urinary bladder and urethra (n=1) (the location of four calcium oxalate stones was not recorded). The detection of higher numbers of calcium oxalate uroliths in the upper urinary tract of cats coincides with findings of other investigators.[75] In our series, male cats were affected twice as frequently as females.

The underlying cause(s) of naturally occurring calcium oxalate urolithiasis in cats is unknown. Although experimentally induced vitamin B_6 deficiency resulted in oxalate nephrocalcinosis in kittens, a naturally occurring form of this syndrome has not been observed.[77] It is noteworthy that magnesium has been reported to be a calcium oxalate crystallization inhibitor in rats and humans.[78] For this reason, orally administered magnesium is sometimes recommended to prevent recurrence of calcium oxalate uroliths. It is also of interest that use of urine acidifiers and/or supplemental sodium (usually sodium chloride) has been associated with hypercalciuria in some species.[78] Since therapy of feline sterile struvite uroliths often encompasses restriction of magnesium, sodium chloride–induced diuresis, and acidification of urine, the relationship of these factors to feline calcium oxalate uroliths is deserving of further study.

CALCIUM PHOSPHATE UROLITHS

In our series, calcium phosphate accounted for approximately 3 per cent of the naturally occurring feline uroliths (Table 110–9). Most (n=9) were located in the kidneys, although the urinary bladder (n=7) and urethra (n=1) were also affected (the location of four uroliths was not recorded). Calcium phosphate uroliths occurred in males and females with equal frequency.

In some instances, calcium phosphate uroliths have occurred as a result of mineralization of blood clots that were formed and trapped in the urinary system. This phenomenon most commonly affected the diverticula of the renal pelves. Although calcium phosphate uroliths are often associated with primary hyperthyroidism in humans and dogs,[79] this association has not yet been made in cats.

MISCELLANEOUS UROLITHS

We encountered only one cystine urolith (in a six-year-old male Korat) in our series (Table 110–9). A xanthine urolith has also been reported.[74]

Compound stones (nucleus of one mineral type and shell of a different mineral type) occurred in 2.3 per cent of our series (Table 110–9). Examples include a nucleus of calcium oxalate surrounded by struvite, and a nucleus primarily composed of ammonium urate surrounded by a layer primarily composed of calcium phosphate.

BIOLOGICAL BEHAVIOR OF UROLITHS AND URETHRAL PLUGS

There have been few studies of the natural course of urolithiasis in cats. The authors have observed spontaneous dissolution of naturally occurring bladder uroliths presumed to be sterile struvite in two adult cats. In one, a five-year-old female domestic shorthair, uroliths spontaneously dissolved 18 days following their radiographic detection. Radiographic evidence of uroliths was not detected during seven monthly follow-up examinations. However, in the eighth month, multiple urocystoliths were detected but they dissolved spontaneously during the next three and a half months.

In two retrospective studies of uroliths, recurrence rates of 19 per cent and 37 per cent were reported.[74, 80] Unfortunately, the type of minerals in the recurrent uroliths was not specified. In our experience, sterile and infection-induced struvite uroliths have recurred within weeks to several months after elimination. Calcium oxalate, calcium phosphate (Brushite) and ammonium urate uroliths also have an unpredictable tendency to recur, typically within months (rather than weeks) following removal.

Small uroliths that form in the urinary bladder may pass into the urethra of male or female cats. Likewise small renoliths may pass into the ureters. Because of the tendency of uroliths to change in size and position, radiographic evaluation of the urinary system should be repeated if there has been a significant time lapse between diagnosis and surgery scheduled to remove them.

The biological behavior of any disorder is influenced by its cause. Future studies of the biologic behavior of obstructive uropathy in male cats must encompass efforts to detect and specify the nature of the obstruction (Table 110–11).

Of the various manifestations of feline lower urinary tract disease, the consequences of urethral obstruction and postrenal azotemia have received the greatest emphasis. There is general agreement that obstruction to urine outflow produces predictable clinical and biochemical abnormalities that vary with the duration and degree of obstruction. However, systemic abnormalities in fluid, acid-base, and electrolyte balance caused by urethral obstruction probably occur irrespective of specific cause (uroliths, plugs, strictures, etc.).

It is generally accepted that feline urethral plugs are associated with a frequent but unpredictable tendency to recur. However, this generality appears to be an overstatement since most investigators have considered urethral obstruction in male cats and struvite urethral plugs to be identical. Recent clinical studies, however, indicate that urethral obstruction in male cats may be initiated and maintained at one or more sites by one or a combination of primary, secondary, and/or iatrogenic causes (Table 110–11). Even in those instances in which recurrent obstruction is caused by urethral plugs, there have been no studies specifically designed to evaluate comparisons of the nature and composition of first-occurrence plugs and recurrent obstructing material.

Treatment and Prevention of Uroliths

Refer to Chapter 111 on canine urolithiasis for specific information about surgical versus medical management of uroliths, and details pertaining to indications for and objectives of medical dissolution of uroliths.

TABLE 110–12. RADIOGRAPHIC FINDINGS IN 143 CATS WITH NATURALLY OCCURRING HEMATURIA AND DYSURIA

Finding	Number	Percentage
No abnormalities	14	9.8
Radiodense urethral plug*	5	3.5
Uroliths (31) and sand (1)†	32	21.7
Vesicourachal diverticula	33	23.1
Irregular mucosa	64	44.8
Vesicoureteral reflux	32	22.4

*Detected by survey radiography.
†Excludes material identified by double-contrast cystography that could not be distinguished from blood clots or sand.

Formulation of therapy to reduce the composition of specific calculogenic crystalloids in urine is dependent on knowledge of the composition of uroliths. For example, use of magnesium restricted diets might enhance calcium oxalate urolith formation since magnesium is an inhibitor of calcium oxalate crystal formation. On the other hand, use of magnesium restricted diets might be beneficial in preventing recurrent magnesium ammonium phosphate urolith formation. In situations in which consideration is being given to medical therapy, but uroliths are not available for analysis, one may be forced to make an educated guess about their composition (Table 110–13).

STRUVITE UROLITHS

Experimental and clinical studies of feline sterile struvite uroliths have confirmed the feasibility of inducing their dissolution by medical therapy. Key components in inducing dissolution of most struvite uroliths in cats appear to be reduction of urine pH to approximately 6.0, and reduction of urine magnesium by consumption of magnesium-restricted diets (Table 110–14).

In a clinical study of 27 cats with 30 episodes of uroliths, 28 uroliths presumed to be composed of struvite dissolved in a mean of 38 ± 27.4 days (range = 14 to 141 days).[81] The cats were fed a high moisture (canned), high energy (640 kilocalories metabolizable energy per 15 ounces), calculolytic diet (Prescription Diet Feline S/D) containing 41.4 per cent dry weight protein. The diet was formulated to contain reduced quantities of magnesium (0.058 per cent dry weight) and to promote formation of acid urine (pH ± 6.0). The diet was also supplemented with sodium chloride (0.79 per cent of dry weight sodium) to stimulate thirst and promote diuresis.

Because of different etiopathogenic mechanisms involved in formation of sterile and infection-induced struvite uroliths, there are some important differences in dissolution protocols. In addition to diet therapy, it is advisable to utilize antimicrobics as long as infection-induced struvite uroliths can be radiographically detected. The reason is that viable calculogenic microbes tend to persist in inner portions of the uroliths, and may cause a relapse of infection (Table 110–14). Control of urease-positive infection in cats with infection-induced struvite uroliths is especially important since the calculolytic diet (Prescription Diet Feline S/D) is not protein restricted. Protein restriction has been avoided because cats normally have a relatively high protein requirement. The authors emphasize that the protein-restricted struvitolytic diet designed for use in dogs (Prescription Diet Canine S/D) is contraindicated for use in cats.

Differences in the causes and treatment of feline sterile and infection-induced struvite are associated with differences in their dissolution. In a prospective clinical trial performed at the University of Minnesota, the time required to induce dissolution of sterile struvite urocystoliths in 20 cats utilizing the protocol described in Table 110–14 was 36 days (range = 14 to 141 days). The time required to dissolve staphylococcus-induced struvite uroliths in 3 cats was 79 days (range = 64 to 92 days).[81]

Since the feline struvitolytic diet is supplemented with

**TABLE 110–13. CHECKLIST OF FACTORS THAT MAY AID IN "GUESSTIMATION"
OF MINERAL COMPOSITION OF UROLITHS**

1. Radiodensity and physical characteristics of uroliths
2. Urine pH
   a. Sterile struvite – usually 6.5 or higher
   b. Infected struvite – usually 7.5 or higher
   c. Calcium phosphate – presumed to be alkaline, except for Brushite, which is acid
   d. Ammonium urate – acid to neutral
   e. Uric acid – presumed to be acid
   f. Calcium oxalate – presumed to be variable
   g. Cystine – acid (in one case)
   h. Silica – not yet identified in cats
3. Identification of crystals in urine sediment
4. Type of bacteria, if any, isolated from urine
   a. Urease-producing bacteria, especially staphylococci, commonly associated with infection-induced struvite uroliths.
   b. Urinary tract infections often absent with sterile struvite uroliths and metabolic uroliths. When present they are associated with a variety of urease positive or urease negative bacteria.
   c. Sterile struvite and metabolic uroliths may predispose cats to UTI. If infections are caused by urease-producing microbes, infected struvite may precipitate around them.
5. Serum chemistry evaluation
   a. Hypercalcemia may be associated with calcium-containing uroliths (apparently uncommon in cats)
   b. Hyperuricemia may be associated with urate uroliths (apparently uncommon in cats)
   c. Hyperchloremia, hypokalemia, and acidemia may be associated with distal renal tubular acidosis and calcium phosphate uroliths (not yet documented in cats)
6. Urine chemistry evaluation
   a. Patient should be consuming a standardized diagnostic diet or the diet being consumed when uroliths formed.
   b. Although no controlled studies have been performed in cats, excessive quantities of one or more minerals contained in the urolith are expected.
7. Analysis of urolith fortuitously passed during micturition (especially female cats)

sodium chloride, and since it is formulated to produce aciduria, neither sodium chloride nor urine acidifiers should be concomitantly given with it. It should not be given to immature cats since they may develop metabolic acidosis, anorexia, and dehydration. Likewise, this diet should not be given to cats that are acidemic (post-renal azotemia, primary renal dysfunction, etc.), or to cats with positive fluid balance (cardiac dysfunction, hypertension, etc.).

Empirical clinical studies performed at the University of Minnesota indicate that acidification of urine to a pH of approximately 6.0 to 6.2 and consumption of low magnesium diets are effective in preventing recurrence of naturally occurring sterile struvite urocystoliths in male and female cats. No attempt was made to determine whether acidification of urine and/or low magnesium diets were the major factor(s) responsible for the beneficial results. If diets designed to promote formation of acid urine are used, additional urine acidifiers should be used with appropriate reason and caution. If non-acidifying diets are used, acidifiers such as methionine may be mixed with them. Alternatively, acidifiers in tablet form may be given at meal time. The goal is to reduce post-prandial alkalinization of urine. Therefore

TABLE 110–14. SUMMARY OF RECOMMENDATIONS FOR MEDICAL DISSOLUTION OF FELINE STRUVITE UROLITHS

1. Perform appropriate diagnostic studies including complete urinalyses, quantitative urine culture, and diagnostic radiography. "Guesstimate" urolith composition by evaluation of appropriate clinical data (Table 110–13).
2. Initiate dietary management designed to reduce the urine concentration of magnesium and create a pH of 6.0 or less. No other food should be fed to patients consuming calculolytic diets. Monitor urine pH four to eight hours after eating. Urine that is acid at this time is likely to be acid throughout the day.
3. Although attempts may be made to stimulate thirst-induced diuresis by addition of sodium chloride to the diet, it is not essential. Thirst-induced diuresis may be of benefit to patients with slowly dissolving uroliths
4. Antimicrobic therapy
   a. Sterile struvite
      Attempt to eradicate or control secondary urinary tract infections with antimicrobial agents.
      Although control of secondary UTI is not essential to induce sterile struvite urolith dissolution, it is warranted to prevent damage of tissues of the urinary tract by bacteria and their metabolites.
   b. Infection-induced struvite: Initiate antimicrobic therapy to eradicate or control urease positive UTI. Maintain therapy as long as uroliths can be detected by radiography.
5. Periodically (two to four week intervals) monitor the size of uroliths by survey radiography. Survey radiography is preferable to retrograde contrast radiography to monitor urolith dissolution since use of catheters during retrograde radiographic studies may result in iatrogenic urinary tract infection. Alternatively, intravenous urography may be considered.
6. Periodic evaluation of urine sediment for crystalluria may be considered. *In vivo* struvite crystals should not form if therapy has been effective in promoting formation of urine that is undersaturated with magnesium ammonium phosphate.
7. Continue calculolytic diet therapy for at least one month following radiographic disappearance of uroliths. The rationale is to provide therapy of adequate duration to dissolve small uroliths that cannot be detected by survey radiography.
8. If uroliths increase in size during dietary management or do not begin to decrease in size after approximately four to eight weeks of appropriate medical management, alternative methods should be considered. Difficulty in inducing complete dissolution of uroliths by creating urine that is undersaturated with the suspected calculogenic crystalloid should prompt consideration that: (1) the wrong mineral component was identified (Table 110–13), (2) the nucleus of the urolith is of different mineral composition than other portions of the urolith, and (3) the owner of the animal is not complying with medical recommendations.

the dosage of urine acidifiers should be monitored by evaluation of four to six hour post-prandial urine pH values. Adequate acidification to prevent sterile struvite uroliths has been achieved with methionine (approximately 1000 mg/cat/day) or ammonium chloride (approximately 800 mg/cat/day).[61, 63, 82–85] The authors prefer methionine since ammonium chloride occasionally causes gastrointestinal signs. Caution should be used to avoid toxic doses of methionine since it has been reported to cause Heinz-body anemia in cats.[86]

Prevention of infection-induced struvite uroliths in cats should be based on the same principles as those described for dogs (consult Chapter 111). The key to prevention of recurrence is eradication or control of infection.

AMMONIUM URATE UROLITHS

Medical protocols that will consistently promote dissolution of ammonium urate uroliths in cats have not yet been developed. Therefore surgical removal remains the most reliable method to remove them from the urinary tract. Prevention should encompass consumption of diets low in purine precursors (such as liver) and striving to produce less acid urine (pH = ± 7.0) that is not highly concentrated. There have been no studies of the efficacy or potential toxicity of allopurinol in cats.

CALCIUM OXALATE UROLITHS

Medical protocols that will promote dissolution of calcium oxalate uroliths in cats are as yet unavailable. Surgical removal remains as the only alternative for removal of clinically active calcium oxalate uroliths. However, some calcium oxalate uroliths, especially those located in the kidneys, may remain clinically silent for months to years. Because of the unavoidable destruction of nephrons during nephrotomy, this procedure is not recommended unless it can be established that the stones are a cause of clinically significant disease. Serially performed urinalyses, renal function tests, serum electrolyte evaluations, and/or radiographic studies may be indicated to evaluate the clinical activity of calcium oxalate uroliths.

No controlled studies designed to evaluate the efficacy of calcium oxalate urolith prevention protocols have been reported. Thus, procedures recommended for prevention of calcium oxalate uroliths in dogs should be considered (see Chapter 111). Use of magnesium-restricted diets is not recommended since magnesium is reported to be a calcium oxalate crystallization inhibitor in other species.

OTHER UROLITHS

Protocols designed to dissolve or prevent calcium phosphate and cystine uroliths in cats have not been studied. Therefore, surgical removal remains as the most reliable way to remove them from the urinary tract. The authors emphasize that surgery may be unnecessary for clinically inactive calcium phosphate uroliths. See Chapter 111 for additional details.

Treatment and Prevention of Urethral Plugs

MEDICAL TREATMENT

Irrespective of the cause(s) of urethral obstruction, predictable clinical and biochemical abnormalities subsequently develop. They are characterized by systemic deficits and/or excesses in fluid (dehydration), electrolyte (hypercalcemia, hyperphosphatemia, etc.), and acid-base (metabolic acidosis) balance, and retention of metabolic wastes (creatinine, urea, other protein catabolites). The magnitude of these systemic abnormalities varies with the degree and duration of obstruction.

Obstructive uropathy which persists longer than about 24 hours usually results in postrenal uremia. This occurs because increased back pressure induced by obstruction to outflow impairs glomerular filtration, renal blood flow, and tubular function. Following obstruction of the urethra of normal cats, death will occur in three to six days. Damage to the mucosal surface of the urinary bladder may shorten survival time. Despite the potentially catastrophic outcome of urethral obstruction, the biochemical consequences of this disorder are potentially reversible provided appropriate supportive and symptomatic parenteral therapy is given. Consult the chapter on Diagnosis and Treatment of Kidney Diseases for further details (Chapter 108). In severe cases, initiation of supportive therapy to correct hyperkalemia, metabolic acidosis, and volume depletion should begin immediately after decompression of the excretory pathway by cystocentesis (see the following section on reestablishing urethral patency for details).

The immediate need to remove urethral plugs within hours of their discovery precludes attempts to cause their dissolution over a period of days or weeks. However, it is often possible to repulse urethral plugs into the bladder lumen. Thus the question arises, can such plugs be dissolved by medical therapy? As previously described, urethral plugs contain a substantially greater quantity of matrix than do classical uroliths. Although it is probable that medical protocols effective in inducing sterile struvite urolith dissolution would also be effective in dissolving the struvite crystalline component of urethral plugs located in the bladder lumen, such therapy may not result in dissolution of plug matrix. It is also emphasized that calcium oxalate and ammonium urate crystals have been identified in a few naturally occurring feline urethral plugs (Table 110–8). These factors may account for lack of expected response to therapy in some patients.

Attempts to dissolve struvite crystals with urine acidifiers or diets designed to promote acid urine should not be initiated in cats with postrenal azotemia. Since severe metabolic acidosis is a common sequela to urethral obstruction, diets or drugs designed to acidify urine should not be utilized until the metabolic sequelae of urethral obstruction have been corrected.

REESTABLISHMENT OF URETHRAL PATENCY

Obstructive urethropathy may be caused by one or more intraluminal, mural, or extramural abnormalities located at one or more sites (Table 110–11). It follows that reverse flushing solutions may be very effective in dissolving urethral plugs, but would have no effect on obstructive lesions located in the urethral wall or periurethral tissue. Inability to restore patency by flushing the urethral lumen with a solution should arouse one's suspicion of a mural or periurethral lesion in addition to, or instead of, a firmly lodged urethral plug or urethrolith.

Restraint. Physical restraint alone, or in combination with topical anesthesia, may be sufficient for relief of urethral obstruction in patients that are particularly docile or severely depressed. Wrapping the cat in a bath towel may help to protect the patient and the assistant. If local anesthetics are used to anesthetize the urethral mucosa, they should be administered only in a quantity sufficient to accomplish this goal. The authors do not recommend use of local anesthetic agents as primary reverse flushing solutions since they may induce systemic toxicity if absorbed in sufficient quantity. Their absorption may be enhanced by damage to the urothelium, and their toxic potential may be enhanced by post renal uremia.

Because of an increased risk of adverse drug reactions associated with obstructive uropathy, pharmacologic restraint should be avoided when feasible. However, the risk of adverse drug reactions must be weighed against the possibility of iatrogenic trauma to the urethra in an uncooperative patient. If the disposition of the patient is such that attempts to dislodge the urethral obstruction are likely to be associated with additional damage to the urethra, or if there is a high risk of iatrogenic urinary tract infection, some form of pharmacologic restraint should be considered. Short acting barbiturates (thiamylal) that are metabolized by the liver and/or inhalant anesthetics may be considered if general anesthesia is required. Anesthetics must be given cautiously since dosages less than those recommended for patients with normal renal function are required in patients with post renal azotemia. If ketamine hydrochloride is used, similar caution must be used since it is excreted in active form by the kidneys. Low doses (0.5 to 1 mg/lb or 1 to 2 mg/kg given intravenously) have been successfully used by many clinicians. However, if difficulty is encountered in relieving outflow obstruction, it is generally inadvisable to administer additional quantities of ketamine.

Priority of Procedures. The authors recommend a step by step priority of procedures when attempting to restore urethral patency to an obstructed male cat.[89] In order of priority they are: (1) massage of distal urethra; (2) attempts to induce voiding by gentle palpation of urinary bladder; (3) cystocentesis; (4) retrograde urethral flushing; (5) combinations of 1 to 4; (6) diagnostic radiology to determine if the cause of urethral obstruction is intraluminal, mural, and/or extramural; (7) surgical procedures.

GENTLE MASSAGE. Gentle massage of the penis between the thumb and fingers may help to dislodge plugs located in the penile urethra. If necessary, the penis may be manipulated while it is retracted within the prepuce. Plugs located in the preprostatic (abdominal) or membranous (pelvic) urethra may occasionally be dislodged by massaging the urethra per rectum. Although these methods are often ineffective, their simplicity and occasional success make them worth trying prior to consideration of cystocentesis or catheterization. In addition, they may disrupt material in urethral plugs confined to the penile urethra to such a degree that subsequent palpation of the urinary bladder may dislodge them.

DIGITAL COMPRESSION. Inability of a cat to void urine spontaneously indicates that increasing intraurethral pressure by *digitally compressing the urinary bladder* is unlikely to be effective. However, if this technique is utilized *following* urethral massage, sufficient intraluminal pressure may be generated to dislodge fragments of urethral precipitates. Appropriate caution should be used to prevent iatrogenic damage to the urinary bladder. If urinary tract infection is likely, the consequence of inducing vesicoureteral reflux of urine during palpation should be considered since microbes may be forced into the upper urinary tract.

CYSTOCENTESIS. In general, cystocentesis should be performed if the aforementioned techniques are ineffective in re-establishing urethral patency.[87] The *advantages* of performing cystocentesis prior to attempts to remove urethral plugs by reverse flushing are: (1) a urine sample suitable for analysis and culture is obtained; (2) decompression of an overdistended urinary bladder by removing most (but not all) of the urine provides a mechanism to temporarily halt the continued adverse effects of obstructive urethropathy (irrespective of cause); (3) decompression of an overdistended urinary bladder and proximal urethra may facilitate repulsion of a urethral plug or urolith into the bladder lumen; and (4) the gross character of aspirated urine may provide valuable clues about the nature of the obstructive disorder (intraluminal precipitates of matrix and crystalline material versus extraluminal compression). Urine that contains large quantities of visible precipitates suggests a greater likelihood of re-obstruction following subsequent flushing of the urethral lumen.

The potential *disadvantages* of performing cystocentesis are that: (1) it may result in extravasation of urine into the bladder wall and/or peritoneal cavity, and (2) it may injure the bladder wall or surrounding structures. Although these complications could be severe in patients with a devitalized bladder wall, in our experience this has been the exception rather than the rule if the majority of the urine is removed from the bladder. Loss of a small quantity of urine into the peritoneal cavity is usually of little consequence, especially if it does not contain pathogens. The potential of trauma to the bladder and adjacent structures can be avoided by proper technique.

We are not advocating an always or never recommendation regarding diagnostic and therapeutic cystocentesis. Clinical judgment is required regarding its use in each patient. However, it is preferable to decompress the urinary bladder by cystocentesis (saving an aliquot for appropriate diagnostic tests) prior to use of reverse flushing procedures in patients likely to have adequate integrity of the bladder wall, and in which immediate overdistention of the bladder lumen is not allowed to recur.

The bladder should be emptied as completely as is

consistent with atraumatic technique. It is undesirable to attempt complete evacuation of the bladder lumen since this will allow the sharp point of the needle to damage the bladder wall.

The need for prophylactic antibacterial therapy following cystocentesis must be determined on the basis of the status of the patient and retrospective evaluation of technique. If subsequent restoration of urethral patency requires intermittent or indwelling catheterization, preventative antimicrobial therapy should be considered.

FLUSHING THE URETHRAL LUMEN. With sterilized solutions following urethral catheterization one may dislodge urethral plugs and uroliths. However, it is emphasized that urethral obstruction may be caused by a combination of intraluminal precipitates (uroliths or urethral plugs), swelling of the urethral wall, and/or spasm of urethral musculature (Table 110–11).

Reverse flushing solutions should be selected cautiously since accumulation and absorption of large quantities of acid or anesthetic solutions from an inflamed urinary bladder may cause systemic toxicity. In addition, they may damage the coating of glycosaminoglycans (GAGs) that lines the surface of the urothelium. Glycosaminoglycans normally minimize adherence of crystals and microbes to the urethral mucosa.[88] Adherence of crystals to the urothelium is most likely to occur if acidic solutions are utilized with the objective of dissolving struvite crystals. Pending results of further studies, the authors prefer physiological saline or lactated Ringer's solution because they are readily available, sterilized, nontoxic, nonirritating, and economical.

The general guidelines to be followed with reverse flushing feline urethras to re-establish patency are outlined in Table 110–15 and shown in Figure 110–6. Use of proper restraint, atraumatic urethral catheters, and nonirritating flushing solutions will greatly minimize damage to the urethral mucosa and surrounding structures.

INABILITY TO ESTABLISH ADEQUATE URETHRAL PATENCY. Inability to establish adequate urethral patency by use of catheters and reverse flushing should arouse a high index of suspicion that the underlying cause is not a urethral plug (Table 110–11). Appropriate *diagnostic procedures* should be considered (Table 110–3).[89] The authors do not recommend *surgical intervention* to correct obstructive urethropathy in uremic cats unless no reasonable alternative exists.

IMMEDIATE AFTERCARE

After urine flow has been re-established by nonsurgical techniques, most of the urine should be removed from the bladder lumen. It is unnecessary and inadvisable to remove all the urine from the bladder lumen since trauma associated with such efforts may aggravate the severity of bladder lesions. Manual compression may be used provided it does not require substantial pressure to induce voiding. Manual compression of the bladder is not necessarily the procedure of choice if an overdistended bladder has been recently decompressed by cystocentesis, since it may result in extravasation of urine into the bladder wall or peritoneal cavity. Alternative methods include the use of a catheter and syringe, or cystocentesis. Each of these procedures has advantages or disadvantages which must be considered in light of the status of the urinary bladder and urethra of each patient. If the gross appearance of voided or aspirated urine suggests that re-obstruction due to intraluminal debris is likely, removal of this material with saline or lactated Ringer's solution flushes of the bladder lumen

TABLE 110–15. GENERAL GUIDELINES FOR REVERSE FLUSHING MALE FELINE URETHRAS OBSTRUCTED WITH INTRALUMINAL MATERIALS

1. Make every effort to protect the patient from iatrogenic complications associated with catheterization of the urethra (especially trauma, and urinary tract infection with bacteria).
2. Strive to use meticulous aseptic "feather-touch" technique.
3. Use only sterile catheters.
4. Cleanse the penis and prepuce with warm water prior to catheterization.
5. Select the shortest Minnesota olive-tipped feline urethral catheter* for initial catheterization of the urethra.
6. Coat the olive tip with sterile aqueous lubricant.
7. Prior to insertion of the catheter into the external urethral orifice, the extended penis should be displaced dorsally until the long axis of the urethra is approximately parallel to the vertebral column.
8. Carefully advance the catheter to the site of obstruction. If necessary, replace the short olive-tipped Minnesota needle with a longer one. Record the site of suspected obstruction, since this information may be of value when considering use of muscle relaxants, and/or when considering urethral surgery to prevent recurrent obstruction. CAUTION: Do not mistake resistance induced by curvature of the feline male urethra for a site of obstruction. In addition never use excessive force when advancing the catheter.
9. Next, a large quantity of physiologic saline or lactated Ringer's solution (as much as several hundred ml) should be flushed into the urethral lumen and allowed to reflux out the external urethral orifice. When possible, the catheter may be advanced toward the bladder. As a result of this maneuver, the obstructed urethral plugs may be gradually dislodged and flushed around the catheter and out of the urethral lumen. Application of steady but gentle digital pressure to the bladder wall after the urethra has been flushed with physiologic saline or lactated Ringer's solution may result in expulsion of a urethral plug or urolith from the urethral lumen. Excessive pressure should not be used because it may result in: (1) trauma to the bladder, (2) reflux of potentially infected urine into the ureters and renal pelvis, and/or (3) rupture of the bladder wall.
10. If the technique outlined in step 9 is unsuccessful, it may be necessary to attempt repulsion of suspected urethral plugs or uroliths back into the bladder lumen by occluding the distal end of the urethra around the olive tip of the catheter before injecting fluid into the urethra. By preventing reflux of solutions out of the external urethral orifice, this maneuver will tend to dilate the urethral lumen. If the obstruction persists, an atempt may be made to gently advance the suspected plug or urolith toward the bladder. *Excessive force should not be used.*
11. On occasion it is advantageous to allow the reverse flushing solution to soften the obstructing urethral plugs (this technique is ineffective for most uroliths) before attempting to propel them back into the bladder. Allowing lapse of several hours between attempts to remove firmly lodged plugs by reverse flushing has been effective.

*Minnesota feline olive tipped urethral catheters are available from EJAY International, Inc., P.O. Box 1835, Glendora, California 91740.

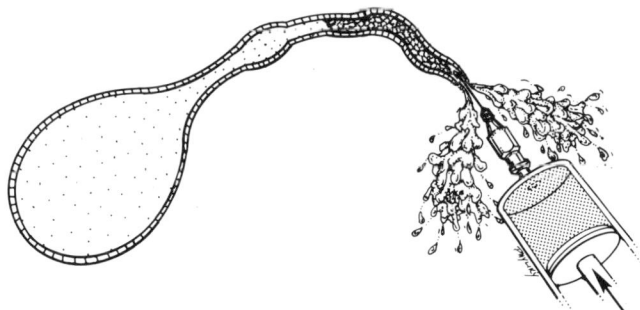

FIGURE 110–6. Schematic illustration of reverse flushing feline urethra obstructed with a urethral plug. After insertion of a Minnesota olive-tipped feline urethral catheter, a large quantity of saline is injected into the urethral lumen and allowed to reflux out of the distal urethra. Fifty to 200 ml of saline may be required to flush away all the obstructing material.

may be of value in minimizing re-obstruction. Local instillation of antimicrobial agents into the bladder lumen in attempt to prevent or treat urinary tract infection is of unproved value. Unless the bladder wall is hypotonic or atonic, the antimicrobial agent is likely to be voided soon after instillation. If circumstances dictate the need for antimicrobial agents, they should be given orally or parenterally to maximize their effectiveness.

The urinary bladder should be periodically evaluated following restoration of adequate urethral patency to ensure that urethral obstruction has not recurred and/or that the detrusor muscle is not hypotonic. Micturition induced by gentle digital compression of the bladder may facilitate evaluation of urethral patency.

Caution must be used when selecting various drugs for azotemic cats. Although glucocorticoid therapy has been advocated (but never proved) to minimize inflammatory swelling of the urethra, glucocorticoids may aggravate the severity of potentially life threatening uremia by inducing protein catabolism through gluconeogenesis. Likewise, administration of acidifying agents to azotemic cats may aggravate the severity of existing metabolic acidosis. Indiscriminate use of any drug in patients with renal dysfunction must be avoided because of potential adverse drug reactions associated with the uremic state.

Following relief of urethral obstruction, a transitory obligatory post-obstructive diuresis may develop. Even though polyuric cats may consume some water, it is often insufficient to maintain proper fluid balance. Therefore, it may be necessary to supplement water intake by parenteral administration of rehydrating or maintenance fluids.

INDWELLING URINARY CATHETERS

We do not recommend routine use of indwelling urinary catheters in cats following relief of urethral obstruction because they may induce further damage to the urinary tract.[90] Disruption of the glycosaminoglycan (GAG) coating of the urothelium as a result of indwelling urethral catheters may promote adherence of microbes and urinary tract infection. Disruption of the GAG coating may also facilitate adherence of crystals to the urothelium, facilitating their growth and/or aggregation.[88]

Indwelling urinary catheters may be indicated following relief of urethral obstruction to: (1) facilitate measurement of urine formation rate during intensive care of critically ill cats, (2) promote recovery of detrusor atony by maintaining an empty bladder, and (3) prevent recurrence of urethral obstruction caused by urine precipitates or mural abnormalities in high risk patients (Table 110–11). The likelihood of whether or not a cat will voluntarily resume micturition may be assessed by evaluation of: (1) the caliber of the urine stream during the voiding phase of micturition, (2) the abundance of material in urine with the potential to occlude the urethral lumen, and (3) the adequacy of detrusor tone immediately following relief of urethral obstruction.

When use of indwelling urinary catheters is deemed to be beneficial, several precautions will minimize catheter-induced complications.[90] Sterilized catheters composed of soft pliable material are preferred because they are less likely to cause trauma to the urinary tract. Catheters constructed of relatively inert material will minimize toxicity to adjacent tissues. To minimize injury to proximal portions of the urethra and especially the urinary bladder, insertion of an excessive length of catheter should be avoided. If the wall of the urinary bladder is not hypotonic, use of an open-ended catheter that does not extend into the bladder lumen is recommended. To minimize ascending urinary tract infection, the urethral catheter should be connected to a closed sterilized drainage system when possible.[90] Likewise, administration of a broad spectrum antimicrobial agent such as ampicillin is recommended. Since urinary tract infection by resistant microbes will develop in some patients during antimicrobial therapy, follow-up urine culture and susceptibility tests are essential to determine the need for, and the type of, additional antimicrobial therapy. Urethral catheters should be removed in as short a time span as possible (12 to 36 hours?) to minimize catheter-induced iatrogenic disease. The cat should then be observed for signs of re-obstruction during a 12 to 24 hour period before discharge from the hospital.

HYPOTONIC URINARY BLADDERS AND REFLEX DYSSYNERGIA

Severe and/or prolonged distention of the urinary bladder caused by obstruction to urine outflow may cause the detrusor muscle to become hypotonic. The underlying cause is thought to be related to disruption of specialized portions of bladder smooth muscle cells, the so-called tight junctions, that normally transmit neurogenic impulses from smooth muscle pacemaker cells.

Once urethral patency has been re-established, therapy designed to maintain relatively low pressure within the bladder lumen often results in restoration of a normal micturition reflex. One alternative consists of trial therapy with bethanechol, a parasympathomimetic agent. The recommended oral dosage for cats is 1.25 to 2.5 mg q8h.[91] Alternatively, an indwelling catheter whose tip is located within the bladder lumen may be utilized. Periodic attempts to induce voiding by manual compression of the urinary bladder may also be considered, provided they do not result in a marked increase in intraluminal pressure.

If an indwelling urinary catheter is utilized to minimize accumulation of urine within the bladder, the previously described precautions designed to prevent catheter-induced injury should be considered. In addition to orally administered antimicrobial agents, irrigation of the bladder lumen with antimicrobial solutions may be considered provided a sufficient quantity of the agent will remain in the bladder long enough to have a beneficial effect. Only sterilized solutions should be injected in volume sufficient to allow contact with all portions of the bladder mucosa.

Reflex dyssynergia may be a cause or complication of urethral outflow obstruction in male cats, and may co-exist with a hypotonic detrusor muscle (Table 110–11).[1, 92] This disorder is characterized by failure of the urethral sphincter to relax during the voiding phase of micturition. The suggested treatment of this complex of neuromuscular dysfunction is administration of an alpha-adrenergic blocking agent (phenoxybenzamine at an oral dosage of 2.5 up to 10.0 mg given once per day) for dyssynergia of the internal urethral smooth muscle sphincter.[92] If dyssynergia of the external urethral skeletal muscle sphincter is present, a skeletal muscle relaxant such as diazepam may be given. Simultaneously, the hypotonic detrusor muscle may be treated with bethanechol at the dosage described above.

PREVENTION

We emphasize that obstructive urethropathy may occur at different sites due to different causes (Table 110–11). Therefore the need for, and the type of, prophylactic therapy should be based on appropriate diagnostic information. The following discussion pertains to obstructive urethropathy associated with matrix-crystalline urethral plugs.

There is a significant but unpredictable potential for recurrence of urethral obstruction caused by matrix-crystalline plugs. Because of associated morbidity and mortality, many medical and surgical protocols have been advocated to deal with this problem. Unfortunately, lack of understanding of the diverse cause(s) of this disorder has resulted in recommendation of a variety of therapeutic maneuvers based on personal opinion and empirical clinical evidence rather than on studies of relevant experimental models and controlled clinical trials.[1, 82]

Medical Protocols. Since insoluble crystals appear to be an integral component of many matrix-crystalline urethral plugs, use of medical protocols to prevent crystal formation in affected patients is logical. Struvite has been the primary mineral component of most naturally occurring urethral plugs, although other mineral types have been encountered (Table 110–10). Consult the previous sections on medical prevention of various types of feline urethral stones for details. Successful prevention of recurrent urethral obstruction utilizing diets designed to reduce urine pH and urine magnesium and phosphorus concentration has been reported.[93]

Surgical Protocols. Perineal urethrostomies are an effective method to minimize recurrent obstruction of

the penile urethra of patients unresponsive to nonsurgical therapeutic and prophylactic management. However, contrast antegrade cystourethrography or retrograde urethrocystography should be performed to localize the site(s) of urethral obstruction before considering this technique.[89]

We emphasize that perineal urethrostomies may be associated with significant short-term and long-term complications. They include bacterial urinary tract infections, abnormal urethral pressure profiles, and urethral strictures.[38, 93–95] If staphylococcal urinary tract infections develop as a result of surgical removal of the penile urethra and associated local host defense mechanisms, infection-induced struvite urocystoliths may subsequently develop.[93, 94]

ANATOMIC ABNORMALITIES

As with other species, congenital and acquired abnormalities of the lower urinary tract may be associated with hematuria, dysuria, and/or urethral obstruction (Table 110–1; Figure 110–7). Consult the chapter entitled Diseases of the Bladder and Urethra for specific details (Chapter 112). Of these, recent knowledge about vesicourachal diverticula warrants additional explanation.

Vesicourachal Diverticula

FUNCTION AND DYSFUNCTION

The urachus is a fetal conduit that provides communication between the urinary bladder and the allantois (a portion of the placenta). The fetal urachus is continuous with the developing urinary bladder and the allantoic sac. This structure allows varying quantities of fetal urine to pass from the urinary bladder through the urachus to the placenta, where unwanted metabolites are presumably absorbed by maternal circulation and subsequently excreted in the mother's urine. During later stages of fetal development, the function of the

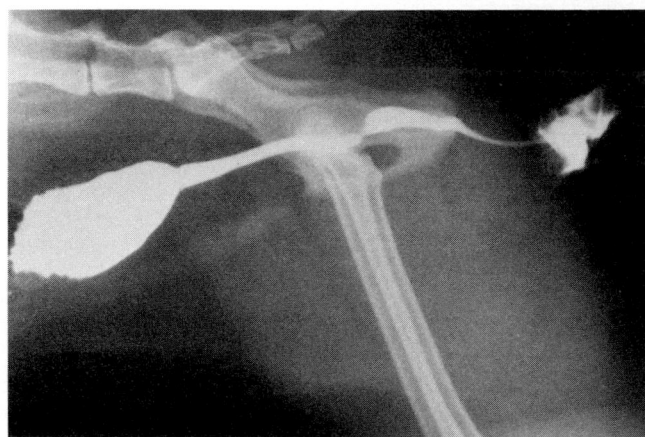

FIGURE 110–7. Positive contrast retrograde urethrocystogram of a three-year-old male domestic shorthair cat illustrating a stricture in the post-prostatic urethra.

urachus as a conduit for urine apparently declines, while that of the urethra increases. At the time of birth, the urachus is nonfunctional. Thus all of the urine that accumulates in the urinary bladder during the storage phase of micturition flows through the urethra during the voiding phase of micturition.

To date, the general consensus of opinion has been that vesicourachal diverticula (partially patent urachus) result if that portion of the urachus located at the bladder vertex fails to close. The result is a blind diverticulum of varying size that protrudes from the bladder vertex at the time of birth. This type of urachal anomaly has been linked to increased resistance to urine outflow through the urethra. However, there have been no definitive studies in cats to document this hypothesis. Recent evidence suggests that microscopic urachal remnants persisting in the vertex of the urinary bladder following birth may represent a risk factor for development of macroscopic diverticula of the urinary bladder in adult cats.[68] Abnormal and/or sustained increase of bladder intraluminal pressure associated with feline lower urinary tract disorders may lead to development of self-limiting macroscopic diverticula of varying size.

MICROSCOPIC DIVERTICULA

Studies of feline urinary bladders obtained from a variety of sources have revealed microscopic evidence of urachal remnants located in the vertex of the urinary bladder.[66, 96] From a two-dimensional light microscopic perspective, the abnormality is characterized by islands of transitional epithelium of varying size that occasionally contain microscopic lumens. The authors presume that the three-dimensional appearance of these structures would be tubular. These microscopic structures, thought to be remnants of the urachus, sometimes persist at the bladder vertex from the level of the submucosa to the subserosa.

Although it is well established that the urachus is nonfunctional at the time of birth, the mechanism(s) responsible for atrophy of the urachus apparently have not been defined. Part of the atrophy may be associated with disuse. Since the mechanism(s) of physiologic atro-

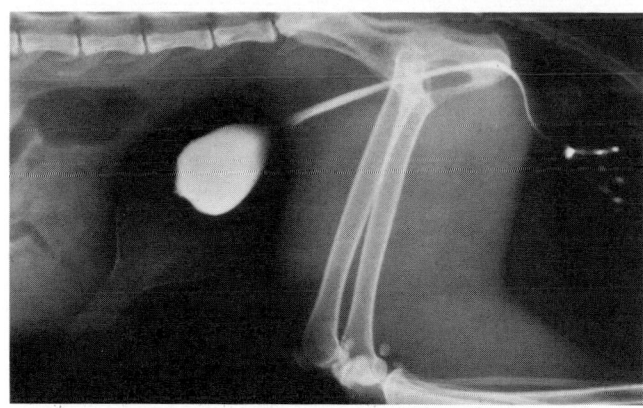

FIGURE 110–9. Positive contrast retrograde urethrocystogram of the cat described in Figure 110–8. This study was performed nine days later. Note reduction in size of the diverticulum.

phy are unknown to us, events that lead to persistence of microscopic urachal remnants in the bladder vertex are also unknown.

MACROSCOPIC DIVERTICULA

In one study, radiographically detectable diverticula affecting the vertex of the urinary bladder wall (Figure 110–8) were detected in almost one of four adult cats with hematuria, dysuria, and/or urethral obstruction (Table 110–12). They occurred twice as often in male (27 per cent) as female (14 per cent) cats.[66] A breed predisposition was not detected. The mean age of affected cats was 3.7 years (range = 1 to 11 years); clinical signs were not observed when the cats were younger than one year of age. The probable explanation of the higher frequency of occurrence in males is they are more likely to develop urethral outflow obstruction due to intraluminal precipitates and/or swelling or spasm of the urethral wall.

There appear to be two etiologically distinct forms of macroscopic vesicourachal diverticula. Congenital macroscopic vesicourachal diverticula, presumed to be caused by impaired urine outflow, probably develop prior to or soon after birth, and may persist for an indefinite period. In our experience, they have been

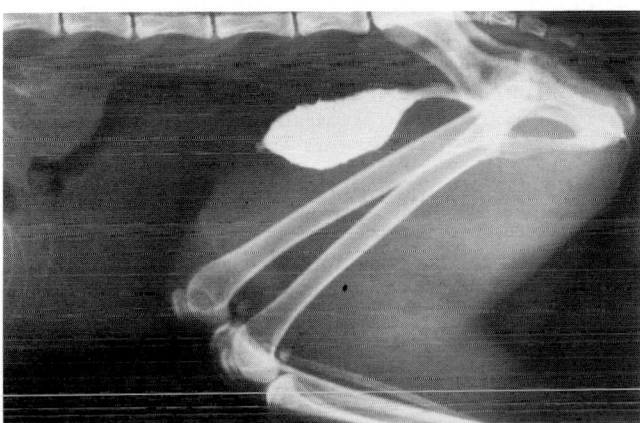

FIGURE 110–8. Positive contrast retrograde urethrocystogram of a two-year-old male domestic shorthair cat illustrating a diverticulum protruding from the vertex of the urinary bladder. The cat had an urinary outflow obstruction caused by a urethral plug.

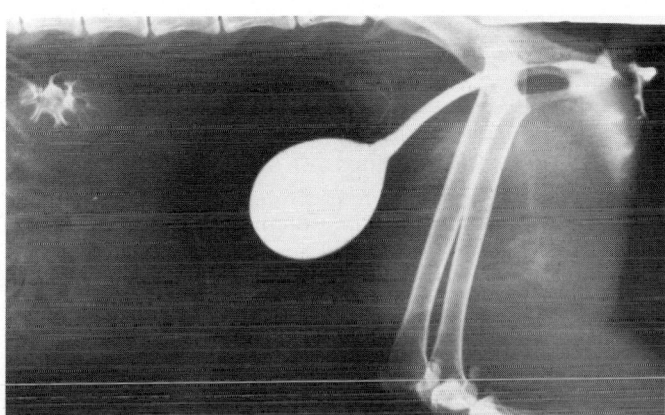

FIGURE 110–10. Positive contrast retrograde urethrocystogram of the cat shown in Figures 110–8 and 110–9. This study was performed 19 days following initial evaluation. A perineal urethrostomy was performed on day 15. There is no evidence of the bladder diverticulum.

uncommon. The most likely explanation of persistence of that portion of the urachal canal adjacent to the bladder wall in immature cats is pressure within the bladder lumen that is abnormally high and/or sustained. Possibilities include anatomic or functional (reflex dyssynergia) outflow obstruction of the lower urinary tract, disorders associated with detrusor hyperactivity, and/or abnormal production of a large volume of urine. Further studies are required to investigate these possibilities. Persistent congenital macroscopic diverticula may predispose to urinary tract infection. If infections are caused by urease-producing calculogenic microbes (especially staphylococci), infection-induced struvite uroliths may develop.

In the second and most common form, microscopic remnants of the urachus located at the bladder vertex of cats remain clinically silent until lower urinary tract disease associated with increased bladder lumen pressure develops. Our clinical studies suggest that radiographically detectable acquired vesicourachal diverticula may develop at the bladder vertex of cats with microscopic vesicourachal remnants following onset of acquired diseases associated with increased intraluminal pressure caused by urethral obstruction and/or detrusor hyperactivity induced by inflammation.

We have observed spontaneous resolution of acquired macroscopic diverticula in 15 of 15 adult male cats evaluated by serial radiography. The diverticula were initially identified at the time of radiographic evaluation of these patients for the underlying cause of hematuria, dysuria, and/or urethral obstruction. Subsequently these clinical signs resolved spontaneously or in conjunction with some form of therapy. Initially the time lapse between initial detection of diverticula and follow-up examination was often more than one year. However, in a two-year-old intact male with obstructive uropathy caused by a urethral plug, partial resolution of an extramural diverticulum was identified 9 days after initial detection, and complete resolution of the diverticulum occurred 19 days after initial evaluation.[66] It is probable that acquired diverticula heal within two to three weeks following elimination of the underlying cause of increased intraluminal pressure.

TREATMENT

Introduction. Contrary to the widely accepted view that urachal diverticula are a primary factor in development of feline lower urinary tract disease, our studies suggest that most macroscopic diverticula of the bladder vertex are a sequela of lower urinary tract dysfunction. Furthermore, at least some, and probably most, macroscopic diverticula may be self limiting if the urinary bladder and urethra return to a normal state of function.[66] Therefore, diverticulectomy is not always warranted.

Cats with Bacterial Urinary Tract Infection. If bacterial urinary tract infection is confirmed by quantitative culture of urine samples properly collected from a cat with a diverticulum of the bladder vertex, it should be treated with appropriate antimicrobics. If present, causes of unrelated diseases associated with increased bladder intraluminal pressure should also be eliminated

or controlled. If the bladder diverticulum is self-limiting, eradication of the urinary tract infection may result in elimination of lower urinary tract disease.

If bacterial urinary tract infection persists or recurs despite proper antimicrobic therapy, the status of the diverticulum should be reevaluated by contrast radiography. If a macroscopic diverticulum of the bladder vertex persists (for more than four to eight weeks?) in a patient with persistent or recurrent urinary tract infection, diverticulectomy should be considered.

Abacteriuric Cats Scheduled for Urethral Surgery. If a diverticulum of the bladder vertex is detected by contrast radiography in an abacteriuric male cat being evaluated for perineal urethrostomy, the client should be informed that removal of the penile urethra (which contributes to local host defenses) combined with the diverticulum (an abnormality of local host defenses) may result in bacterial urinary tract infection. If the infection is caused by urease-producing bacteria such as staphylococci, infection-induced struvite uroliths may develop. Rather than recommend a perineal urethrostomy and/or diverticulectomy, one should re-evaluate the indications for urethral surgery and serially evaluate the size of the diverticulum. If the diverticulum subsides, but a confirmed abnormality of the penile urethra predisposing to urethral obstruction persists, the risk of postsurgical urinary tract infection is reduced but not eliminated. If the diverticulum persists and an abnormality of the penile urethra predisposing to an unacceptable recurrence of urethral obstruction persists, a perineal urethrostomy may be considered. If urethral surgery is performed in a patient with a persistent bladder diverticulum, the cat should be periodically monitored for bacterial urinary tract infection. If frequently recurrent or persistent urinary tract infection occurs after perineal urethrostomy, diverticulectomy should then be considered.

Abacteriuric Cats with Hematuria and Dysuria. The concomitant occurrence of hematuria, dysuria, and urethral obstruction with a diverticulum of the bladder vertex is not an immediate indication for diverticulectomy. Contrast radiography performed two to three weeks after the initial evaluation may reveal varying degrees of resolution of the diverticulum. Therefore, the major focus of effort should be directed at detection and elimination of the underlying cause of the lower urinary tract inflammation and the increased pressure within the bladder lumen. If an underlying cause (metabolic uroliths, urethral plugs, urinary tract infection, infection-induced struvite uroliths, and so on) cannot be identified, resolution of the hematuria, dysuria, and bladder diverticulum may occur with or without symptomatic therapy.

Cats with Urocystoliths. Cats with acquired diverticula of the bladder vertex and sterile struvite– or infection-induced struvite urocystoliths may be successfully managed by medical therapy (consult the section on feline urolithiasis in this chapter).[96] Because effective protocols to induce medical dissolution of feline calcium oxalate, calcium phosphate, ammonium urate, and uric acid urocystoliths have not yet been developed, surgery remains the most reliable method for treating patients with metabolic urolithiasis and diverticula of the vertex of the urinary bladder.

IDIOPATHIC LOWER URINARY TRACT DISEASE

Current Status of Etiopathogenesis

The cause(s) of hematuria, dysuria, and/or urethral obstruction often cannot be detected in a substantial number of patients. In a prospective clinical study designed to detect causes of hematuria, dysuria, and/or urethral obstruction in 143 male and female cats with naturally occurring disease, preliminary evaluation of data indicates that a causative agent (infectious agents, uroliths, neoplasms, etc.) could not be detected in 77 (53 per cent) cases (Table 110–4).[97] Although the authors were unable to identify viruses in urine of affected patients, no attempt was made to explant tissues for virus isolation. This fact is noteworthy in light of our ability to identify herpesvirus from explanted tissue, but not urine, of cats with induced cell-associated herpesvirus urinary tract infection.[22] Likewise, inability to identify mycoplasma or ureaplasma from urine of cats in our series may represent technical difficulties in culturing these fastidious organisms from urine.

TREATMENT

The clinical signs of hematuria and dysuria in many untreated nonobstructed male and female cats with idiopathic lower urinary tract disease frequently subside within approximately one week.[1, 42, 97] These signs may recur after a variable period and again subside without treatment. In this situation, any form of therapy might appear to be beneficial, as long as it is not harmful. The self-limiting nature of some forms of idiopathic feline lower urinary tract disease underscores the need for controlled clinical trials in order to prove efficacy of various forms of therapy.

Antibacterial Agents. The infrequency with which bacteria have been identified at the onset of clinical signs of lower urinary tract disorders has been well established (Table 110–4).[23, 25] The uselessness of antimicrobial agents in the treatment of abacteriuric cats with lower urinary tract disease has also been documented.[42] Indiscriminate use of antimicrobial agents has undoubtedly been responsible, at least in part, for the emergence of the resistant strains of microbes that populate veterinary hospitals.

Urinary Tract Antiseptics. Urinary tract antiseptics are sometimes used as adjunctive agents in the treatment, control, and prevention of UTI in humans. Although their use is frequently acknowledged in treatment of bacterial UTI in dogs, and is occasionally mentioned for treatment of lower urinary tract disorders in cats, there have been no studies to substantiate their effectiveness in these species.

Methenamine is a cyclic hydrocarbon. In an acid environment (pH less than 6.0) methenamine hydrolyzes to form formaldehyde, an essential component of its antimicrobial activity. Because of the necessity of acid urine for formation of formaldehyde, methenamine is usually given in combination with acidifiers such as mandelic acid (methenamine mandelate) or hippuric acid (methenamine hippurate). Methenamine must remain in the urinary tract for a sufficient period to allow generation of effective concentrations of formaldehyde. However, once generated in sufficient concentration, formaldehyde is capable of killing microbes at any urine pH. In light of the hypothesis that some forms of lower urinary tract disorders in cats are caused by viruses, the unproved suggestion that methenamine may have virucidal action in urine is of interest. However, definitive proof that viruses are a cause of naturally occurring lower urinary tract disorders in cats, and further studies of the efficacy of methenamine in such patients, are required before recommendations can be formulated. At this time, use of methenamine to treat cats with feline urinary tract disorders represents no more than an idea.

Methylene blue (tetramethylthionine chloride) is a weak antiseptic agent that at one time was popularly used in combination products designed to treat lower urinary tract symptoms. Use of medications containing methylene blue is contraindicated in cats because methylene blue has the potential to cause Heinz bodies and severe anemia.[98]

Urinary Tract Analgesics. Phenazopyridine is an azo dye that is commonly used as a urinary tract analgesic in humans. Its use alone or in combination with sulfa drugs is contraindicated in cats because it has the potential to cause methemoglobinemia and irreversible oxidative changes in hemoglobin, resulting in formation of Heinz bodies and anemia. Cats have been very susceptible to dose-related toxicity of this agent.[99]

Smooth Muscle Antispasmodics. Many cats with inflammation of the lower urinary tract develop urge incontinence, which is an uncontrollable desire to void that results in involuntary loss of urine. Incontinence occurs soon after the sensation of bladder fullness. It is characterized by inability to control micturition between the time of urge to micturate and the actual time of voiding. Micturition usually occurs at a low volume of bladder filling. Apparently there is no damage to the urethral sphincter mechanisms, because continuous loss of urine is not observed.

Because the exact mechanism of urge incontinence is unknown, details about specific therapy are unavailable. It is logical to consider smooth muscle antispasmodics as symptomatic treatment of urge incontinence. Combination preparations designed to treat signs of lower urinary tract disorders frequently contain atropine, hyoscyamine, and/or scopolamine. The efficacy, if any, of these agents in cats with dysuria has not been established by properly controlled clinical trials.

Propantheline minimizes the force and frequency of uncontrolled detrusor contractions, but has negligible effect on urethral sphincter pressure. In a controlled clinical study of the efficacy of propantheline (7.5 mg given orally on one occasion) in the treatment of naturally occurring hematuria and dysuria in nonobstructed male and female cats, no difference in rate of recovery was observed between cats treated with propantheline and control groups.[42] This is not an unexpected finding, because propantheline represents a symptomatic form of therapy.

Propantheline may be considered to reduce the severity and frequency of urge incontinence in nonobstructed male and female cats. It has a rapid onset of action. However, care must be used to prevent urinary retention resulting from using excessive quantities in cats. Because the smallest tablet is 7.5 mg, the suggested dose is 7.5 mg given orally approximately every 72 hours. Further studies utilizing appropriate dosages and maintenance intervals are required to substantiate a beneficial symptomatic effect of propantheline in cats with urge incontinence.

Anti-Inflammatory Agents. It is reasonable to assume that most cats with hematuria and dysuria have an inflammatory lesion of the lower urinary tract. Hematuria is indicative of, but not pathognomonic of, inflammation; dysuria indicates involvement of the lower urinary tract. The cause of the inflammation in many cats is unknown. In many patients, however, it can be established what the cause is not.

Lack of specific therapy for abacteriuric cats with hematuria and dysuria has stimulated many to question the value of anti-inflammatory agents to reduce the severity of clinical signs. Success in minimizing the frequency of voiding would not only be beneficial to affected cats, it would eliminate owner frustration associated with the socially unacceptable problem of frequent voiding on floors, carpets, and furniture. Unfortunately, there have been no controlled clinical trials to study the short- and long-term effectiveness of anti-inflammatory agents in the symptomatic treatment of dysuria and hematuria in cats. The authors emphasize that hematuria and dysuria in abacteriuric cats without uroliths is often self-limiting.

GLUCOCORTICOIDS. Consideration of glucocorticoids to minimize persistent signs associated *with inflammation in cats with idiopathic dysuria* and hematuria is logical. Consideration of glucocorticoids to symptomatically treat signs associated with microbe-induced inflammation, urolith-induced inflammation, neoplasia-induced inflammation, and so on is illogical.

Because of their catabolic effect, glucocorticoids are generally contraindicated in cats with urethral obstruction and post-renal azotemia. They should not be considered in such patients until deficits and excesses in fluid, electrolyte, and acid-base balance have been corrected. Likewise, glucocorticoids are contraindicated in cats with bacterial UTI. Use of glucocorticoids in cats with indwelling catheters is especially apt to be hazardous.

DIMETHYLSULFOXIDE (DMSO). DMSO is an analgesic anti-inflammatory agent with weak antibacterial, antifungal, and antiviral activity. It has been reported to be effective in the treatment of a variety of genitourinary disorders of humans including interstitial cystitis, radiation cystitis, chronic prostatitis, and female chronic trigonitis.[100] Retrograde infusion of 50 per cent solutions of pyrogen-free DMSO into the bladder lumens of humans with interstitial cystitis has been reported to minimize associated clinical signs in more than 50 per cent of the patients.

DMSO has been used to treat lower urinary tract disease in cats, presumably because of its reported efficacy in humans with interstitial cystitis. However, it is not known whether any type of lower urinary tract disease in cats is morphologically similar to interstitial cystitis in humans. It is known that not all forms of lower urinary tract disease in cats are similar to interstitial cystitis in humans.

Appropriately controlled clinical trials that are designed to evaluate the effectiveness of local instillation of DMSO into the urinary bladders of cats with signs of lower urinary tract disease have not been reported. Dosages and frequency of administration have been entirely empirical.

Local instillation of varying quantities (up to 25 ml) of solutions containing 25 to 50 per cent DMSO into the urinary bladders of dogs weighing 15 to 40 kg every other week for up to six months revealed no detectable side effects. Use of solutions containing 100 per cent DMSO caused mucosal edema and hemorrhage. Licensed products available to veterinarians contain 90 per cent DMSO and are not pyrogen-free; licensed products available to physicians contain 50 per cent DMSO and are pyogen-free. Side effects of DMSO in cats have apparently not been evaluated. Pending further studies, the authors discourage its use to treat idiopathic feline lower urinary tract disorders.

OTHER AGENTS. A variety of other agents have been advocated to treat and prevent feline lower urinary tract disorders. None has been evaluated by appropriate selection of patients for study, nor by controlled clinical trials. Recommendations for testosterone, castor oil, progesterone, vitamin A, hyaluronidase, and various homeopathic preparations appear to be based on supposition rather than fact. The authors do not recommend them.

UROTHELIAL DEBRIDEMENT. Cystotomy to lavage and debride the bladder mucosa has been recommended by some to treat patients with cystitis, urethritis, and/or urethral obstruction. Although this procedure is still used by many veterinarians, there are no controlled experimental or clinical studies to indicate efficacy for the procedure. In fact, reports of clinical experiences suggest that the technique is of little benefit. This is not surprising since the urethra and urinary bladder are affected in many cats with dysuria, hematuria, and pollakiuria. If one assumes (and the authors do not) that debridement of the urothelium is of some therapeutic benefit, removal of the bladder mucosa would have no obvious beneficial effect on the urethra. Our recommendation is this: before considering surgical debridement of the mucosal surface of the urinary bladder to treat hematuria and dysuria in your patients, ask if on the basis of available information you would allow a similar procedure to be performed on yourself in an attempt to "cure" similar signs.

References

1. Osborne, CA, et al.: Redefinition of the feline urologic syndrome: Feline lower urinary tract disease with heterogeneous causes. Vet Clin North Am 14:409, 1984.
2. Barsanti, JA and Finco, DR: Feline urologic syndrome. *In* Breitschwerdt, EB (ed): Contemporary Issues in Small Animal Practice—Nephrology and Urology. New York, Churchill Livingstone, 1986.

3. Willeberg, P: Epidemiology of feline urological syndrome. Adv Vet Sc Comp Med 25:311, 1981.
4. Willeberg, P: Epidemiology of naturally occurring feline urologic syndrome. Vet Clin North Am 14:455, 1984.
5. Lawler, DF, et al.: Incidence rates of feline lower urinary tract disease in the United States. Fel Pract 15:13, 1985.
6. Fennell, C: Some demographic characteristics of the domestic cat population in Great Britain with particular reference to feeding habits and the incidence of feline urologic syndrome. J Sm Anim Pract 16:775, 1975.
7. Foster, SJ: The "urolithiasis" syndrome in male cats: a statistical analysis of the problems with clinical observations. J Sm Anim Pract 8:207, 1967.
8. Walker, AD, et al.: An epidemiological survey of feline urological syndrome. J Sm Anim Pract 18:283, 1977.
9. Willeberg, P: Interaction effects of epidemiologic factors in the feline urologic syndrome. Nord Vet Med 28:193, 1976.
10. Bovee, KC, et al.: Recurrence of feline urethral obstruction. JAVMA 174:93, 1979.
11. Reif, JS, et al.: Feline urethral obstruction: a case control study. JAVMA 170:1320, 1977.
12. Rich, LJ and Fabricant, CG: Urethral obstruction in male cats. Can J Comp Med 33:164, 1969.
13. Fabricant, CG: Urolithiasis: a review of recent viral studies. Fel Pract 3:22, 1973.
14. Fabricant, CG, et al.: Feline viruses XI. Isolation of a virus similar to myxovirus from cats in which urolithiasis was experimentally induced. Cornell Vet 59:667, 1969.
15. Fabricant, CG: Viruses associated with urinary tract disease. Vet Clin North Am 9:631, 1979.
16. Fabricant, CG and Gillespie, JH: Identification and characterization of a second feline herpesvirus. Infect Immun 9:460, 1974.
17. Fabricant, CG: Herpesvirus induces urolithiasis in specific pathogen-free male cats. Am J Vet Res 38:1837, 1977.
18. Fabricant, CG: Serologic responses to the cell associated herpes virus and the manx calicivirus of SPF male cats with herpesvirus-induced urolithiasis. Cornell Vet 71:59, 1981.
19. Barsanti, JA, et al.: Feline urologic syndrome: further investigation into etiology. JAAHA 18:391, 1982.
20. Gaskell, RM, et al.: Studies on a possible viral etiology for the feline urological syndrome. Vet Rec 105:243, 1979.
21. Jackson, OF: The case against a viral etiology in feline urolithiasis. Vet Rec 96:70, 1975.
22. Kruger, JM, et al.: Experimental induction of feline lower urinary tract disease in cats with cell associated herpes virus. Proc ACVIM, Washington, DC, 1986.
23. Martens, JG, et al.: The role of infectious agents in naturally occurring feline urologic syndrome. Vet Clin North Am 14:503, 1984.
24. Rich, LJ and Fabricant, CG: Urethral obstruction in male cats: transmission studies. Can J Comp Med 33:164, 1969.
25. Shroyer, EL and Shalaby, MR: Isolation of feline syncytia-forming virus from oropharyngeal swab samples and buffy coat cells. Am J Vet Res 39:555, 1978.
26. Arthur, RR, et al.: Association of BK viruria with hemorrhagic cystitis in recipients of bone marrow transplants. N Engl J Med 315:230, 1986.
27. Meyer, R, et al.: Herpes zoster involving the urinary bladder. N Engl J Med 260:1062, 1959.
28. Nurazaki, Y and Kumasaka, T: Further study on acute hemorrhagic cystitis due to adenovirus type 2. N Engl J Med 289:344, 1973.
29. Fenner, F, et al.: Veterinary Virology. New York, Academic Press, 1987.
30. Povey, RC, et al.: Feline picornavirus infection: the *in vivo* carrier state. Vet Rec 92:224, 1973.
31. Povey, RC: Feline respiratory infections: a clinical review. Can Vet J 17:93, 1976.
32. DeClerg, E: Present trends in the development of antiviral agents. *In* Peterson, PK, et al. (eds): Antimicrobial Agents Annual. Amsterdam, Elsevier Sci Pub, 1986, p 526.
33. Decter, RG and Khanderia, U: Recent advances in antiviral therapy. Clin Pharm 5:961, 1986.
34. Lees, GE: Epidemiology of naturally occurring feline bacterial urinary tract infections. Vet Clin North Am 14:471, 1984.
35. Lees, GE, et al.: Adverse effects of open indwelling urethral catheterization in normal male cats. Am J Vet Res 42:825, 1981.
36. Smith, CW, et al.: Effects of indwelling urinary catheters in male cats. JAAHA 17:427, 1981.
37. Barsanti, JA, et al.: Urinary tract infection due to indwelling bladder catheters in dogs and cats. JAVMA 187:384, 1985.
38. Gregory, CR and Vasseur, PB: Long-term examination of cats with perineal urethrostomy. Vet Surg 12:210, 1983.
39. Lees, GE and Osborne, CA: Antibacterial properties of urine: a comparative review. JAAHA 15:125, 1979.
40. Lees, GE, et al.: Antibacterial properties of urine: studies of feline urine specific gravity, osmolality, and pH. JAAHA 15:135, 1979.
41. Lees, GE and Osborne, CA: Feline urinary tract infections. *In* Kirk, RW (ed): Current Veterinary Therapy VIII. Philadelphia, WB Saunders, 1983.
42. Barsanti, JA, et al.: Feline urologic syndrome: further investigation into therapy. JAAHA 18:391, 1982.
43. Taylor-Robinson, D, et al.: Human intra-urethral inoculation of ureaplasmas. Quart J Med 46:309, 1977.
44. Taylor-Robinson, D: Mycoplasmal and mixed infections of the human male urogenital tract and their possible complications. *In* The Mycoplasmas. New York, Academic Press, 1985, p 27.
45. Osborne, CA, et al.: Struvite urolithiasis in animals and man: formation, detection, and dissolution. Adv Vet Sci Comp Med 29:1, 1985.
46. Barsanti, JA: Opportunistic fungal infections. *In* Greene, CE (ed): Clinical Microbiology and Infectious Diseases of the Dog and Cat. Philadelphia, WB Saunders, 1984, p 733.
47. Polzin, DJ and Jeraj, K: Urethritis, cystitis, and ureteritis. Vet Clin North Am 9:661, 1979.
48. Kirkpatrick, RM: Mycotic cystitis in a male cat. VM/SAC 77:1365, 1982.
49. Brown, SA and Prestwood, AK: Parasites of the urinary tract. *In* Kirk, RW (ed): Current Veterinary Therapy IX. Philadelphia, WB Saunders, 1986, p 1153.
50. Osborne, CA, et al.: Epidemiology of naturally occurring feline uroliths and urethral plugs. Vet Clin North Am 14:481, 1984.
51. Rich, LJ, et al.: Urethral obstruction in cats: experimental production by addition of magnesium and phosphate to diet. Fel Pract 4:44, 1974.
52. Jackson, OF: The dry cat food controversy. Urolithiasis in laboratory and domestic cats. Vet Rec 91:292, 1972.
53. Chow, FC, et al.: Effect of dietary additives on experimentally produced feline urolithiasis. Fel Pract 9:51, 1976.
54. Kallfelz, FA, et al.: Urethral obstruction in random source and SPF male cats induced by high levels of dietary magnesium or magnesium and phosphorus. Fel Pract 10:25, 1980.
55. Lewis, LD: Nutritional causes and management of feline urolithiasis. Sci Proc AAHA, Denver, 1981, p 273.
56. Lewis, LD: Feeding, and dissolving and preventing calculi. Sci Proc AAHA, Denver, 1983, p 314.
57. Finco, DR, et al.: Characterization of magnesium-induced urinary disease in the cat and comparison with feline urologic syndrome. Am J Vet Res 46:391, 1985.
58. Buffington, CA, et al.: Feline struvite urolithiasis: Magnesium effect depends on urinary pH. Fel Pract 15:29, 1985.
59. Feldman, BM, et al.: Dietary minerals and feline urologic syndrome. Fel Pract 7:39, 1977.
60. Chow, FC, et al.: Feline urolithiasis cat foods: concentration of calcium, magnesium, phosphate, and chloride in various cat foods and their relationship to feline urolithiasis. Fel Pract 5:15, 1975.
61. Lewis, LD, et al.: Small Animal Clinical Nutrition, 3rd ed. Topeka, Mark Morris Associates, 1987.
62. Lewis, LD, et al.: Effect of various dietary mineral concentrations on the occurrence of feline urolithiasis. JAVMA 172:559, 1978.
63. Taton, GF, et al.: Urinary acidification in the prevention and treatment of feline struvite urolithiasis. JAVMA 184:437, 1984.
64. Finco, DR and Barsanti, JA: Diet-induced feline urethral obstruction. Vet Clin North Am 14:529, 1984.
65. Stapleton, FB, et al.: Hypercalciuria in children with hematuria. N Engl J Med 310:1345, 1984.
65a. Buffington CAT: Effects of age and food deprivation on urinary pH in cats. Proceeding of 3rd Annual Symposium of European Society of Veterinary Nephrology and Urology, pp 60–72, Barcelona, 1988.

66. Osborne, CA, et al.: Etiopathogenesis and biological behavior of feline vesicourachal diverticula. Vet Clin North Am 17:697, 1987.

67. Osborne, CA, et al.: New insights into management of feline lower urinary tract disease. Proc 4th Ann Forum, ACVIM, 1986, p 4.

68. Ryan, CP and Smith, RA: Bilateral nephrolithiasis in a cat. JAVMA 158:1946, 1971.

69. Wolf, AM, et al.: Uric acid ureteral calculus and pararenal cyst in a cat. JAAHA 15:767, 1979.

70. Kirkpatrick, RM: Urate calculus in a male cat. VM/SAC 72:1171, 1977.

71. Ryan, CP and Wolfer, JJ: Cystic calculi in four cats. VM/SAC 73:1414, 1978.

72. Jackson, OF and Sutor, DJ: Ammonium acid urate calculus in a cat with a high uric acid excretion possibly due to a renal tubular reabsorption defect. Vet Rec 86:335, 1970.

73. Rothuizen, J, et al.: Congenital porto-systemic shunts in sixteen dogs and three cats. J Sm Anim Pract 23:67, 1982.

74. Hesse, A and Sanders, G: A survey of urolithiasis in cats. J Sm Anim Pract 26:465, 1985.

75. Lawler, DF and Evans, RH: Urinary tract disease in cats. Water balance studies, urolith and crystal analyses, and necropsy findings. Vet Clin North Am 14:537, 1984.

76. Ryan, CP: Nephrolithiasis in a cat. JAVMA 172:162, 1978.

77. Gershoff, SN, et al.: Vitamin B6 deficiency and oxalate nephrocalcinosis in the cat. Am J Med 27:72, 1959.

78. Osborne, CA, et al.: Etiopathogenesis, clinical manifestations, and management of canine calcium oxalate urolithiasis. Vet Clin North Am 16:133, 1986.

79. Klausner, JS and Osborne, CA: Canine calcium phosphate uroliths. Vet Clin North Am 16:171, 1986.

80. Bohonowych, RO, et al.: Features of cystic calculi in cats in a hospital population. JAVMA 173:301, 1978.

81. Osborne, CA, et al.: Medical dissolution of feline struvite urocystoliths: Prospective clinical trial of 30 cases. J Am Vet Med Assoc, In press.

82. Polzin, DJ and Osborne, CA: Medical prophylaxis of feline lower urinary tract disorders. Vet Clin North Am 14:661, 1984.

83. Senior, DF, et al.: Testing the effects of ammonium chloride and dl-methionine on the urinary pH of cats. Vet Med 81:88, 1986.

84. Lloyd, WE and Sullivan, DJ: Effects of orally administered ammonium chloride and methionine on feline urinary acidity. Vet Med 79:773, 1984.

85. Finco, DR, et al.: Ammonium chloride as a urinary acidifier in cats. Mod Vet Pract 67:537, 1986.

86. Maede, Y, et al.: Methionine toxicosis in cats. Am J Vet Res 48:289, 1987.

87. Osborne, CA, et al.: Immediate relief of feline urethral obstruction. Vet Clin North Am 14:585, 1984.

88. Khan, SR, et al.: Crystal retention by injured urothelium of the rat urinary bladder. J Urol 132:153, 1984.

89. Johnston, GR and Feeney, DA: Localization of feline urethral obstruction. Vet Clin North Am 14:555, 1984.

90. Lees, GE and Osborne, CA: Use and misuse of indwelling urinary catheters in cats. Vet Clin North Am 14:599, 1984.

91. Moreau, PM: Neurogenic disorders of micturition in the dog and cat. Comp Cont Ed 4:12, 1982.

92. Lees, GE and Moreau, PM: Management of hypotonic and atonic urinary bladders in cats. Vet Clin North Am 14:641, 1984.

93. Osborne, CA, et al.: New insights into the management of feline lower urinary tract disease. Proc 4th Ann ACVIM Forum, 1986, p 4.

94. Osborne, CA, et al.: Surgonomics of FUS. Proc 54th Ann Mtg AAHA, 1987, p 156.

95. Smith, CW and Schiller, AG: Perineal urethrostomy in the cat: a retrospective study of complications. JAAHA 14:225, 1978.

96. Wilson, GP, et al.: The relationship of urachal defects in the feline urinary bladder to feline urologic syndrome. Proc 7th Kal Kan Symposium, Kal Kan Foods, Vernon, CA, 1983, p 125.

97. Osborne, CA, et al.: New insights into the cause of FUS: the diagnosis that never was. Proc 54th Ann Mtg AAHA, 1987, p 146.

98. Schecter, RD, et al.: Heinz body hemolytic anemia associated with use of urinary antiseptics containing methylene blue in the cat. JAVMA 162:37, 1973.

99. Harvey, JW and Kornick, HP: Phenazopyridine toxicosis in the cat. JAVMA 169:327, 1976.

100. Shirley, JW, et al.: Dimethyl sulfoxide in treatment of inflammatory genitourinary disorders. Urology 11:215, 1975.

DRUG INDEX

Generic	Trade	Dosage	Route	Frequency	Description
Fenbendazole	Panacur	22.7 mg/lb	Oral	q 12 hr.	Anthelmintic
Propantheline	Probanthine	7.5 mg/cat	Oral	q 48 to 72 hr.	Anticholinergic
Bethanechol	Urecholine	1.25 to 2.5 mg/cat	Oral	q 8 hr.	Cholinergic
Phenoxybenzamine	Dibenzyline	2.5 to 10.0 mg/cat	Oral	q 24 hr.	Alpha-adrenergic blocker
Diazepam	Valium	1.25 to 2.5 mg/cat*	Oral	q 12–24 hr.	Skeletal muscle relaxation

*Dosage not well established in a suitable population of cats

111 CANINE UROLITHIASIS

CARL A. OSBORNE, DAVID J. POLZIN,
GARY R. JOHNSTON, and TIMOTHY D. O'BRIEN

CHEMICAL AND PHYSICAL CHARACTERISTICS

Uroliths are polycrystalline concretions that typically contain greater than 90 to 95 per cent organic or inorganic crystalloids, and less than five to ten organic matrices (weight versus weight ratio). They also may contain a number of minor constituents. A variety of different types of uroliths may occur in dogs (Table 111–1). Uroliths are not disorganized precipitates of crystalline material, but typically are comprised of organized crystal aggregates with a complex internal structure. Consult the chapter on Feline Lower Urinary Tract Disorders (Chapter 110) for details about urethral plugs. Cross sections of uroliths frequently reveal nuclei and laminations, and less frequently radial striations. The fact that the composition of urine that bathes uroliths varies in composition (and probably in degree of saturation with calculogenic crystalloids) from day to day and perhaps from hour to hour is of conceptual importance in trying to understand the physical characteristics of uroliths.

NAMES

Uroliths may be named according to mineral composition (Table 111–2), location (nephroliths, renoliths, ureteroliths, cystoliths, vesical calculi, urethroliths), or shape (smooth, faceted, pyramidal, laminated, mulberry, jackstone, staghorn or branched). Characteristic shapes of crystals and uroliths are influenced primarily by the internal structure of crystals and the environment in which they form. Crystals of calcium oxalate monohydrate tend to fuse, producing smoothly rounded or mamillated uroliths. Crystals of calcium oxalate dihydrate typically appear as sharp spiculated structures. Amorphous silica commonly produces stones that resemble small six-pronged metal pieces used in the children's game of jacks (and thus the name jackstone). Local factors that influence the size and shape of uroliths include: (1) number of uroliths present, (2) mobility or fixation of uroliths, (3) flow characteristics of urine, and (4) anatomical configuration of the structure in which uroliths grow.

MINERAL COMPOSITION

The most common mineral type found in uroliths of dogs is magnesium ammonium phosphate (Table 111–1). Ammonium acid urate, uric acid, calcium phosphate, and calcium oxalate (monohydrate and dihydrate) occur much less frequently. In contrast, calcium-containing uroliths (calcium oxalate and calcium phosphate) are most prevalent in humans living in developed countries of the world. Trace elements, including iron, copper, zinc, tin, lead, and aluminum, have been identified in human uroliths.[1] It is logical to suspect that they may also occur in canine uroliths. These elements appear to be incorporated into calculi by adsorption during growth; they do not appear to play an important role in initiation or growth of calculi.

Even though a particular mineral usually predominates, the mineral composition of many uroliths may be mixed (Table 111–1). On occasion, the center of a urolith may be composed of one type of crystalloid (for example, silica), whereas outer layers are composed of a different crystalloid (especially struvite). Detection, treatment, and/or prevention of the causes underlying urolithiasis are dependent on knowledge of the composition and structure of all portions of uroliths.

MATRIX COMPOSITION

The nondialyzable portion of uroliths that remains after crystalline components have been dissolved with mild solvents is organic matrix. Uroliths consistently contain variable quantities of organic matrix substances in addition to crystalloids.[2] Organic matrix substances identified in human uroliths and experimentally produced in animals include matrix substances A, Tamm-Horsfall mucoprotein, uromucoid, serum albumin, and alpha and gamma globulins.[3] Of these, matrix substances A, Tamm-Horsfall mucoprotein, and uromucoid appear to be quantitatively more significant than alpha and gamma globulins.[4]

The macromolecular complex of diverse mucoprotein compounds comprising matrix substances has been hypothesized by some to represent the skeleton of uroliths. In vitro studies utilizing human urine revealed that

TABLE 111–1. MINERAL COMPOSITION OF 1713 CANINE UROLITHS*

Predominant Mineral		Number	Percentage
Magnesium ammonium phosphate hexahydrate		1046	61.1
	100%	(593)	(34.6)
	70–99%†	(453)	(26.4)
Magnesium hydrogen phosphate trihydrate			
	70–99%	1	0.1
Calcium oxalate		232	13.5
Calcium oxalate monohydrate			
	100%	(42)	(2.5)
	70–99%	(73)	(4.3)
Calcium oxalate dihydrate			
	100%	(19)	(1.1)
	70–99%†	(30)	(1.8)
Calcium oxalate monohydrate and dihydrate			
	100%	(35)	(2.0)
	70–99%†	(33)	(1.9)
Calcium phosphate			
Calcium phosphate		34	2.0
	100%	(16)	(0.9)
	70–99%†	(9)	(0.1)
Calcium hydrogen phosphate dihydrate			
	100%	(5)	(0.3)
	70–99%†	(4)	(0.2)
Uric acid and urates		90	5.3
Ammonium acid urate			
	100%	(59)	(3.4)
	70–99%†	(24)	(1.4)
Sodium acid urate			
	100%	(2)	(0.1)
	70–99%†	(1)	(0.1)
Uric acid			
	100%	(3)	(0.2)
	70–99%†	(1)	(0.1)
Cystine		32	1.9
Silica		33	1.9
	100%	(26)	(1.5)
	70–99%†	(7)	(0.4)
Mixed‡		57	3.3
Compound§		178	10.4
Matrix		10	0.6
Total		1713	100%

*Analysis performed by optical crystallography and x-ray diffraction.
†Urolith composed of 70–99% of mineral type listed; no nucleus or shell detected.
‡Uroliths did not contain at least 70% of mineral type listed; no nucleus and shell detected.
§Uroliths contained an identifiable nucleus and one or more surrounding layers of different mineral type.

TABLE 111–2. GLOSSARY OF CRYSTALLINE SUBSTANCES THAT MAY BE DETECTED IN UROLITHS

Chemical Name	Crystal Name	Formula
Oxalates		
Calcium oxalate monohydrate	Whewellite	$CaC_2O_4 \cdot H_2O$
Calcium oxalate dihydrate	Weddellite	$CaC_2O_4 \cdot 2H_2O$
Phosphates		
B-tricalcium phosphate (calcium orthophosphate)	Whitlockite	$B\text{-}Ca_3(PO)_2$
Carbonate-apatite	Same	$Ca_{10}(PO_4CO_3OH)_6(OH)_2$
Calcium hydrogen phosphate dihydrate	Brushite	$CaHPO_4 \cdot 2H_2O$
Calcium phosphate	Hydroxyapatite	$Ca_{10}(PO_4)_6(OH)_2$
Magnesium ammonium phosphate hexahydrate	Struvite	$MgNH_4PO_4 \cdot 6H_2O$
Magnesium hydrogen phosphate trihydrate	Newberyite	$MgHPO_4 \cdot 3H_2O$
Uric Acid and Urates		
Anhydrous uric acid	Same	$C_5H_4N_4O_3$
Uric acid dihydrate	Same	$C_5H_4N_4O_3 2H_2O$
Ammonium acid urate	Same	$C_5H_3N_4O_3NH_4$
Sodium acid urate monohydrate	Same	$C_5H_3N_4O_3N_aH_2O$
Cystine	Same	$(SCH_2CHNH_2COOH)_2$
Silicone Dioxide	Same	SiO_2
Xanthine	Same	$C_5H_4N_4O_2$

Tamm-Horsfall protein is related to formation of calcium oxalate crystals.[5] Although the physical characteristics of uroliths suggest an organized relationship between the matrix skeleton and crystalline-building blocks, the role of each of these components in formation, retention, and growth of calculi is poorly understood.

In summary, organic matrix may affect urolith formation by one or more of several mechanisms including: (1) a site for heterogeneous nucleation; (2) a template for organizing and modifying growth of crystals; (3) a binding agent that cements calculus particles together and promotes retention of crystals; and/or (4) protective colloids that prevent further growth of calculi. Organic matrix could also be a passive substance with no effect on stone formation or growth.

Etiopathogenesis

The urinary system is designed to dispose of waste products in soluble form. However, some waste products are sparingly soluble and occasionally precipitate out of solution to form crystals. Urolithiasis may be conceptually defined as the formation of urinary stones from less soluble crystalloids of urine as a result of multiple congenital and/or acquired physiologic and pathologic processes. If such crystalloids become trapped in the urinary system, they may grow to sufficient size to cause clinical signs.

Urolithiasis should not be conceived of as a single disease, but rather as a sequela of one or more underlying abnormalities. The fact that urolith formation is often erratic and unpredictable indicates that several interrelated complex physiologic and pathologic factors are involved.

It is beyond the scope of this chapter to discuss the etiopathogenesis of urolith formation in detail. This information is described elsewhere.[5, 7, 8] The following is a conceptual overview of calculogenesis.

Initiation and Growth of Uroliths

Urolith formation is associated with two complementary but separate phases: initiation and growth. It appears that initiating events are not the same for all types of uroliths. In addition, factors that initiate urolith formation may be different from those that allow it to grow.

The initial step in formation of a urolith is formation of a crystal nidus (or crystal embryo). This phase of initiation of urolith formation, called nucleation, is dependent on supersaturation of urine with calculogenic crystalloids. The degree of urine supersaturation may be influenced by the magnitude of renal excretion of the crystalloid, urine pH, and/or the presence of crystallization inhibitors in urine. Noncrystalline proteinaceous matrix substances may also play a role in nucleation in some instances.

Further growth of the crystal nidus is dependent on the following: (1) its ability to remain in the lumen of the excretory pathway of the urinary system; (2) the degree and duration of supersaturation of urine with crystalloids identical or different from that in the nidus; and (3) physical characteristics of the crystal nidus. If they are compatible with other crystalloids some crystals may align themselves and grow on the surface of others.

Detection

Uroliths are usually suspected on the basis of typical findings obtained by history and physical examination. Urinalyses, urine culture, radiography, and ultrasonography may be required to differentiate uroliths from urinary tract infection, diverticula of the bladder, inflammatory polyps, blood clots, and neoplasia (Table 111–3).

A variety of methods have been used to evaluate the composition of uroliths including gross appearance, crystalluria, radiographic appearance, qualitative analysis, quantitative analysis, and urolith culture. Of these, quantitative analysis provides the most definitive diagnostic, prognostic, and therapeutic information. With the exception of qualitative chemical analysis, information gained by other methods of evaluation also may be of value in assessing the integrity of the urinary tract of patients with urolithiasis.

TABLE 111–3. PROBLEM-SPECIFIC DATA BASE FOR UROLITHIASIS

1. Obtain appropriate history and perform physical examination, including rectal examination of urethra.
2. Perform complete urinalysis; save aliquot for possible determination of mineral concentration.*
3. Perform complete blood cell count.
4. Freeze aliquot of serum collected at time of venipuncture to obtain complete blood cell count for possible determination of urea nitrogen, creatinine, calcium, and/or uric acid concentrations.
5. Obtain quantitative urine culture and determine urine urease activity; obtain antimicrobial susceptibility if bacterial pathogens are identified. Consider attempts to isolate ureaplasmas if urease positive urine is bacteriologically sterile.
6. Obtain radiographs
    a. Take survey radiographs of entire urinary system.
    b. Consider IV urography for patients with renal or ureteral uroliths.
    c. Consider IV urography or contrast cystography for patients with bladder uroliths.
    d. Consider contrast urethrography for patients with urethral uroliths.
    e. Ultrasonography is recommended if equipment is available.
7. Remove bladder or kidney biopsy specimens for microscopic examination during nephrotomy or cystotomy.
8. If anatomic defects are present, correct them during surgical procedure performed to remove uroliths.
9. Compare number of uroliths removed during surgery with number of uroliths identified by radiography; postsurgical radiographs should be obtained to evaluate completeness of urolith removal, if necessary.
10. Save all uroliths for qualitative or quantitative analysis.
11. Initiate therapy to promote dissolution or arrest of growth of uroliths, if necessary.
12. Initiate therapy to eradicate urinary tract infection.
13. Initiate therapy to prevent recurrence of uroliths.
14. Formulate follow-up protocol with clients.

*The patient should be consuming food utilized at time of urolith formation. Alternately, a standardized diet designed to promote reproducible excretion of minerals in the urine of normal animals may be used.

CRYSTALLURIA

Crystalluria, by definition, is the appearance of crystals in urine. Proper identification and interpretation of urine crystals are important in formulation of medical protocols to dissolve uroliths. Routine laboratory procedures for detection of crystalluria are qualitative, not quantitative. Caution must be used in interpreting the significance of crystalluria because crystal formation is influenced by several *in vivo* and *in vitro* variables.[9] *In vivo* variables include: (1) the concentration of crystallogenic substances in urine (which in turn is influenced by their rate of excretion and urine concentration of water); (2) urine pH; (3) the solubility of crystallogenic substances in urine; and (4) excretion of diagnostic agents (such as radiopaque contrast agents) and medications (such as sulfonamides and ampicillin).

In vitro variables include: (1) temperature; (2) evaporation; (3) pH; and (4) the technique of specimen preparation (i.e., centrifugation versus non-centrifugation, volume of urine examined, etc.). It is emphasized that significant *in vitro* changes which occur following urine collection may enhance formation or dissolution of crystals. When knowledge of *in vivo* urine crystal type and quantity is especially important, fresh specimens should be examined. Ideally they should be at body temperature. If this is not possible, they should be at room temperature, and not at refrigeration temperature.

Care must be used not to over-interpret or under-interpret the significance of crystalluria. Because crystals only occur in urine that is supersaturated with crystallogenic substances, it represents a risk factor for urolithiasis. However in most instances, crystalluria that occurs in association with an anatomically and functionally normal urinary tract is harmless. Identification of crystals in such patients does not justify therapy. On the other hand, detection of some types of crystals, or large aggregates of others, may be of diagnostic, prognostic and/or therapeutic importance. For example, ammonium urate crystalluria may be indicative of portal vascular anomalies or primary hepatic disorders. Calcium oxalate monohydrate and calcium oxalate dihydrate crystalluria may occur in dogs with ethylene glycol toxicity or hypercalcemia; cystine crystalluria is pathognomonic of cystinuria.

Identification of urine crystals should not be relied upon as definitive identification of the mineral composition of uroliths. The latter should be determined by quantitative urolith analysis.

The term "habit" is commonly used by mineralogists to refer to the characteristic shape or shapes of mineral crystals. The habit of crystals is widely used as an index of crystal composition. However, microscopic evaluation of the habits of urine crystals only represents a tentative identification of their composition because variable conditions associated with their formation, growth, and dissolution may alter their appearance. Therefore, definitive identification of crystal composition is dependent on optical crystallography, infrared spectrophotometry, thermal analysis, x-ray diffraction, and/or electron microprobe analysis.[9] In situations where confirmation of the composition of microscopic crystalluria is desirable, it may be of value to attempt to prepare a large pellet of crystals by centrifugation of an appropriate volume of urine in a conical tipped centrifuge tube. Evaluation of the pellet of sediment by quantitative methods designed for urolith analysis may provide meaningful information about crystalluria and urolith composition.

RADIOGRAPHY AND ULTRASONOGRAPHY

The primary objective of radiographic or ultrasonographic evaluation of patients suspected of having uroliths is to determine their site(s), number, density, and shape. Once urolithiasis has been confirmed, radiographic and/or ultrasonographic evaluation also is an important technique to detect predisposing abnormalities.

The radiographic and ultrasonographic appearance of uroliths is influenced by their size, number, location, and mineral composition. Most uroliths have varying degrees of radiodensity, and therefore can be detected by survey abdominal radiography (Table 111–4) or ultrasonography.[10] Very small uroliths may not be visualized by survey radiography or ultrasonography. Oxalate, phosphate, and silica uroliths are typically, but not invariably, more radiodense than cystine and urate uroliths. Urate uroliths may be radiolucent, but usually are radiodense. Because of significant variation, the radiodensity of uroliths is not a reliable index of mineral composition.

Uroliths must be differentiated from: (1) nephrocalcinosis associated with dystrophic or metastatic calcification of the renal parenchyma; (2) radiodense medications or ingesta in the gastrointestinal system; (3) calcified mesenteric lymph nodes; (4) osseous metaplasia of transitional epithelium or mineralization of a neoplasm; (5) radiodensities in the gallbladder (uncommon in dogs and cats); and (6) large nipples in female dogs. Calcifications of the renal parenchyma typically are in proximity of, but not within, the renal pelvis. Radiodense calculi within the excretory pathway may disap-

TABLE 111–4. TYPICAL RADIOGRAPHIC CHARACTERISTICS OF UROLITHS COMMONLY ENCOUNTERED OCCURRING IN DOGS

Mineral Type	Degree of Radiopacity	Shape
Cystine	+ to + +	Smooth; usually small; round to oval
Oxalate	+ + + +	Smooth or rough; round to oval
Magnesium ammonium phosphate (struvite)	+ to + + + +	Smooth; round or faceted; sometimes assume shape of renal pelvis, ureter, bladder, or urethra; sometimes laminated
Calcium phosphate (calcium apatite)	+ + + +	Smooth; round or faceted
Ammonium urate and uric acid	0 to + +	Smooth; round or oval
Silica	+ + to + + + +	Typically jackstone
Mixed	+ to + + + +	Varies with composition; may have detectable nucleus and shell
Matrix	0 to +	Usually round but may be influenced by location

pear or become radiolucent following excretion of radiopaque contrast agents. Radiodense objects outside the excretory pathway remain radiodense.

In the authors' experience, radiolucent uroliths are uncommon in dogs. Uric acid uroliths in human beings are typically radiolucent. However, in the authors' experience, many ammonium acid urate uroliths of dogs are radiodense. This may be related to a variable quantity of phosphates in urate uroliths of dogs. Matrix uroliths may be radiolucent or have some radiodensity. Blood clots are radiolucent and may be mistaken for radiolucent uroliths. Radiolucent uroliths may be readily distinguished from blood clots when evaluated by two-dimensional gray-scale ultrasonography. Uroliths usually produce sharply marginated shadows containing few echoes, and are associated with acoustic shadowing.

Uroliths which appear radiodense by survey radiography may appear to be radiolucent when evaluated by positive contrast radiography. This is related to the fact that many calculi are more radiodense than body tissue, but less radiodense than the contrast material. A diagnosis of radiolucent stones should be based on their radiodensity compared to soft tissues, and not their radiodensity compared to positive contrast material.

It is possible for a urolith to be larger than that depicted by its radiodensity if only a portion of it contains radiodense minerals. This phenomenon is most likely to occur with rapidly growing struvite uroliths.

ANALYSIS OF UROLITHS

The location of the uroliths removed from the urinary tract should be recorded, in addition to their size, shape, color, and consistency. All uroliths should be saved in a container (preferably a sterile one) for future analysis. Do not give uroliths to owners if they need to be analyzed. One or more uroliths may be placed into a container of 10 per cent buffered formalin if microscopic examination is desired.

Because many uroliths contain more than one mineral component, it is important to examine representative portions. The mineral composition of crystalline nuclei may be identical or different from the remainder of uroliths. The nuclei of uroliths should be analyzed separately from outer zones when possible, since the underlying cause of the urolith may be suggested by knowledge of the mineral composition of the nuclei.

The authors do not recommend analysis of uroliths by single qualitative chemical analysis. The major disadvantage of this procedure is that only some of the chemical radicals and ions can be detected. In addition, the proportion of the different chemical constituents in the urolith cannot be quantified.

In contrast to chemical methods of analysis, physical methods have proven to be far superior in identification of crystalline substances. They also permit differentiation of various subgroups of minerals (i.e., calcium oxalate monohydrate and calcium oxalate dihydrate, or uric acid and ammonium acid urate), and allow semi-quantitative determinations of various mineral components. Physical methods commonly used by laboratories which specialize in quantitative urolith analysis include a combination of polarizing light microscopy, x ray diffractometry, infrared spectroscopy, and thermogravimetry.[11, 12] Some laboratories also are equipped to perform elemental analysis with an energy dispersive x-ray microanalyzer (EDAX). On occasion, chemical methods of analysis and paper chromatography may be used to supplement information provided by the physical methods mentioned.

UROLITH CULTURE

Bacteria harbored inside uroliths are not always the same as those present in urine. Bacteria detected within uroliths probably represent those present at the time the stone was formed, and may serve as a source of recurrent urinary tract infection. Bacteria may remain viable within the uroliths for long periods. In a pilot study, the authors were able to culture viable staphylococci from struvite uroliths removed from a miniature schnauzer up to three months following surgery. When all the uroliths cannot be removed from the patient, knowledge of the type of associated bacterial pathogens and their antimicrobial susceptibility may be of therapeutic significance. Procedures for culture of microbes from the inner portions of uroliths have been developed.[11, 13]

"GUESSTIMATION" OF UROLITH COMPOSITION

Formulation of effective medical protocols for urolith dissolution is dependent on knowledge of the mineral composition of uroliths. The authors recommend a protocol that allows "guesstimation" of urolith composition with a high degree of success (Table 111–5). Formulation of medical therapy based on this protocol is usually associated with a high degree of success in dissolving uroliths, or arresting their growth. Attempts to induce dissolution of uroliths may be hampered if the uroliths are heterogeneous in composition. This has not been a significant problem in dogs with uroliths composed primarily of magnesium ammonium phosphate with lesser quantities of calcium apatite because the solubility characteristics of the two minerals are similar. However, the authors have encountered difficulty in dissolving uroliths composed primarily of struvite with an outer shell composed primarily of calcium apatite. Difficulty will also be encountered in attempting to induce complete dissolution of a urolith with a nucleus of calcium oxalate, calcium phosphate, ammonium urate, or silica and a shell of struvite, because the solubility characteristics of this combination of minerals are dissimilar. This phenomenon should be considered if medical therapy seems to be ineffective after initially reducing the size of a urolith.

STRUVITE UROLITHIASIS

MINERAL COMPOSITION

The most common type of mineral encountered in uroliths of dogs is magnesium ammonium phosphate

TABLE 111–5. CHECKLIST OF FACTORS THAT MAY AID IN "GUESSTIMATION" OF MINERAL COMPOSITION OF CANINE UROLITHS

1. Radiographic density and physical characteristics of uroliths
2. Urine pH
   a. Struvite and calcium apatite uroliths–usually alkaline
   b. Ammonium urate uroliths–acid to neutral
   c. Cystine uroliths–acid*
   d. Calcium oxalate–variable*
   e. Silica–acid to neutral*
3. Identification of crystals in uncontaminated fresh urine sediment, preferably at body temperature
4. Type of bacteria, if any, isolated from urine
   a. Urease-producing bacteria, especially staphylococci and less frequently Proteus spp, are typically associated with canine struvite uroliths. Ureaplasmas may cause struvite uroliths
   b. Urinary tract infections often are absent in patients with calcium oxalate, cystine, ammonium urate, and silica uroliths
   c. Calcium oxalate, cystine, ammonium urate, and silica uroliths may predispose patients to urinary tract infections; if infections are caused by urease-producing bacteria, struvite may precipitate around metabolic uroliths
5. Serum chemistry evaluation
   a. Hypercalcemia may be associated with calcium-containing uroliths
   b. Hyperuricemia may be associated with uric acid or urate uroliths
   c. Hyperchloremia, hypokalemia, and acidemia may be associated with distal renal tubular acidosis and calcium phosphate or struvite uroliths
6. Urine chemistry evaluation
   a. Patient should be consuming a standardized diagnostic diet, or the diet consumed when uroliths formed
   b. Excessive quantities of one or more minerals contained in the urolith are expected. The concentration of crystallization inhibitors may be decreased
7. Breed of dog and history of occurrence of uroliths in patient's ancestors or littermates
8. Quantitative analysis of uroliths fortuitously passed during micturition and collected

*Concomitant infection with urease-producing microbes may result in formation of an alkaline urine.

hexahydrate (MAP) or struvite. However, canine struvite uroliths are frequently impure, containing minor quantities of calcium phosphate (also called calcium apatite) and carbonate apatite.[6] Carbonate apatite may be a minor constituent in uroliths that form in patients with urinary tract infections caused by urease-producing microbes (especially staphylococci, *Proteus* spp., and ureaplasmas). Generation of carbonate ion (CO_3^{2-}) as a consequence of hydrolysis of urea by microbial urease is sometimes associated with displacement of some phosphate anions in calcium apatite molecules. Canine struvite uroliths may also contain small quantities of ammonium acid urate.

ETIOPATHOGENESIS

Urine must be supersaturated with magnesium ammonium phosphate for struvite uroliths to form. Supersaturation of urine with MAP may be associated with several factors including urinary tract infections with urease-producing microbes, alkaline urine, genetic predisposition, and diet.[6]

Infection-Induced Struvite. When urinary tract infection with urease-producing microbes (especially staphylococcus, *Proteus* spp., and ureaplasmas) occurs in dogs forming urine with a sufficient quantity of urea, the unique combination of concomitant elevation in the

concentrations of ammonium and carbonate (CO_3^{2-}) in an alkaline environment may develop. These conditions favor formation of uroliths containing struvite (Mg-$NH_4PO_4 \cdot 6H_2O$), calcium apatite [$Ca_{10}(PO_4)_6(OH)_2$], and carbonate-apatite [$Ca_{10}(PO_4)6CO_3$]. The following mechanisms are involved: (1) urease (a metallo-enzyme containing nickel) produced by bacteria or ureaplasma hydrolyzes urea to form two molecules of ammonia and a molecule of carbon dioxide. Since urease is not consumed during this reaction, a single urease molecule may catalyze the hydrolysis of multiple urea molecules; (2) the ammonia molecules react spontaneously with water to form ammonium and hydroxyl ions (pK of NH_3 = 9.03), which alkalinizes urine by reducing its hydrogen ion concentration. Ammonia also damages the glycosaminoglycan lining of the urothelium, increasing the ability of bacteria to adhere to mucosa. The solubility of struvite (and calcium apatite) decreases in alkaline urine. In addition to alkalinization of urine, the newly generated ammonium ion is available for formation of MAP crystals; (3) the newly generated molecule of carbon dioxide combines with water to form carbonic acid, which in turn dissociates to form bicarbonate (pK = 6.33) and hydrogen ion. In an extremely alkaline environment, bicarbonate may lose its proton to become carbonate (pK = 10.1). Anions of carbonate may displace anions of phosphate in calcium apatite crystals to form carbonate apatite crystals; (4) in the progressively alkaline environment induced by microbial hydrolysis of urea, dissociation of monobasic hydrogen phosphate (H_2PO_4) results in an increased concentration of dibasic hydrogen phosphate (HPO_4^{2-}) and anionic phosphate (PO_4^{3-}). Given a constant concentration of total phosphate, a change in pH from 6.80 to 7.40 increases the PO_4^{3-} concentration by a factor of approximately 6. Anionic phosphate is then available in increased quantities to combine with magnesium and ammonium to form struvite, or with calcium to form calcium-apatite; (5) ammonium ions may combine with urates to form ammonium acid urate.

The quantity of dietary protein catabolized for energy influences formation and dissolution of infection-induced struvite uroliths. Consumption of dietary protein in quantities that exceed daily protein requirements for anabolism results in the formation of urea from catabolism of amino acids. Hyperammonuria, hypercarbonaturia, and alkaluria mediated by microbial urease are dependent on the quantity of urea (the substrate of urease) in urine.

Abnormal urinary excretion of minerals as a result of enhanced glomerular filtration rate, reduced tubular reabsorption, and/or enhanced tubular secretion is not required for initiation and growth of infection-induced struvite uroliths. However, metabolic and anatomic abnormalities may indirectly induce struvite uroliths by predisposing to urinary tract infections.

Sterile Struvite. Clinical studies indicate that microbial urease is not involved in formation of struvite uroliths in some dogs.[6] Several observations suggest that dietary or metabolic factors may be involved in the genesis of sterile struvite uroliths in these species. Pilot studies of clinical cases of sterile struvites in dogs revealed a population of patients (9 of 20) whose urine was frequently alkaline, but did not contain identifiable bacteria, and did not contain detectable quantities of urease.[6] Microscopic examination of demineralized Gram-stained sections of some struvite uroliths removed from dogs with bacteriologically sterile urine revealed no Gram-positive bacteria. Whereas infection-induced human struvite uroliths frequently contain calcium apatite or carbonate apatite, a large number of the canine sterile uroliths were 100 per cent struvite.

Although struvite is less soluble in alkaline than acid urine, the mechanism(s) of sterile struvite urolith formation in dogs is not clear. Under physiologic conditions associated with alkaluria, urine contains low concentrations of ammonia (and thus ammonium ion). Thus alkaline urine formed in absence of ureolysis would not be expected to favor formation of crystals that contain ammonia ion (such as magnesium ammonium phosphate hexahydrate). Clinical studies of naturally occurring urolithiasis in human patients support this generality. Formation of persistently alkaline urine in absence of urease-mediated ureolysis may predispose to formation of uroliths containing hydroxyapatite $[Ca_{10}(PO_4)_6(OH)_2]$, but not carbonate-apatite.

In vitro studies consisting of addition of magnesium ($MgSO_4$), ammonium (NH_4Cl), or phosphate ($NH_4H_2PO_4$ or NaH_2PO_4) to sterile human urine ranging in pH from 5.0 to 9.6 revealed that struvite crystals could be induced in an acid or an alkaline environment.[14] High ammonia concentrations were not necessary for formation of struvite crystals provided the concentration of $[Mg] \times [NH_4] \times [PO_4]$ was of sufficient magnitude at a given pH. Corresponding *in vivo* studies in dogs have not yet been performed.

BIOLOGICAL BEHAVIOR

Clinical and experimental studies performed at the University of Minnesota revealed that struvite uroliths can form within two to eight weeks following infection with urease-producing staphylococci.[15, 16] Struvite uroliths associated with urinary tract infections caused by staphylococci or *Proteus* spp. have been detected in puppies as young as five weeks of age.[17] Retrospective analysis of clinical cases of urolithiasis in immature dogs indicates that struvite uroliths are more common than metabolic uroliths.

Although spontaneous dissolution of uroliths appears to be uncommon, it can occur. The authors have observed five cases (two renoliths and three cystic uroliths) of struvite urolithiasis in dogs in which uroliths underwent spontaneous dissolution.[18] Spontaneous dissolution of canine nephroliths has also been reported by others.[19] Bilateral renal uroliths were reported to exist for approximately four years in a miniature schnauzer before causing death from renal failure.[20]

Uroliths located in the urinary bladder commonly pass into the urethra. They commonly lodge behind the os penis in male dogs, but frequently are voided to the exterior by females. Although renoliths are much less common in dogs than in man,[21] when they form they may pass into the ureters. The rapid rate at which struvite uroliths form, and the potential they have to migrate to lower portions of the urinary tract, are of

clinical importance. If several days have elapsed between the date of diagnostic radiography and the date of surgery scheduled to remove uroliths, the number and location of stones should be reevaluated by radiography.

Struvite uroliths have a tendency to recur following surgical removal or medical dissolution.[22, 23] In a retrospective survey of 438 dogs with urolithiasis, 111 patients had 155 known recurrences.[22] Recurrence was observed in 17 per cent of dogs with urate uroliths, 47 per cent of dogs with cystine uroliths, and 25 per cent of dogs with oxalate uroliths. Recurrence was most commonly detected within the first year following surgery. Although the highest prevalence of struvite uroliths was observed in females, the highest rate of recurrent struvite uroliths was observed in males. The authors have evaluated miniature schnauzers with more than seven known recurrences following surgery. However, most instances of multiple recurrences have been associated with poor control of recurrent urinary tract infection caused by urease-producing microbes. With the advent of effective therapeutic and preventative antimicrobial protocols to control recurrent or persistent UTI, the frequency of recurrent struvite urolithiasis in dogs has declined.

To date, most clinical studies of recurrence of canine uroliths have been based on post-surgical evaluations. The rate of recurrence following medical dissolution of canine struvite uroliths has not yet been evaluated in a large population of patients. However, preliminary observations indicate that the rate of recurrence is less frequent than that associated with surgery. In addition, time lapse between recurrent episodes is longer following medical dissolution. The apparent higher rate of recurrence associated with surgical removal of uroliths may be associated with inability to remove all uroliths, especially those located in inaccessible places and/or those that are subvisual in size. The tendency for uroliths to recur following surgery may also be associated with persistence of an environment that favors initiation and growth of struvite at the time of removal.

Medical Treatment

Therapy of struvite urolithiasis encompasses: (1) relief of obstruction to urine outflow when necessary, (2) elimination of existing uroliths, (3) eradication or control of urinary tract infection, and (4) prevention of recurrence of uroliths. Detailed descriptions of nonsurgical and surgical methods of reestablishing urine outflow are beyond the scope of the discussion but are available elsewhere.[24, 25] Likewise, details pertaining to surgical removal of uroliths, endoscopic and percutaneous manipulation of uroliths, chemolysis via nephrostomy, disintegration of renal and ureteral uroliths via ultrasound, and shock wave lithotripsy have been reviewed.[24]

INDICATIONS

Surgery has been a time-honored approach for management of all types of urolithiasis in dogs. Although surgery has been an effective method that provides immediate elimination of uroliths, it is associated with several limitations. These include: (1) persistence of underlying causes and high rate of recurrence of uroliths despite surgery; (2) patient factors that enhance adverse consequences of general anesthesia or surgery; and (3) inability to remove all uroliths or fragments of uroliths during surgery. In addition, situations occasionally arise in which owners of companion animals will not consent to surgical therapy but will consider medical therapy. For these and other reasons (i.e., the urolith is asymptomatic), medical dissolution of struvite uroliths may be considered.

Despite the feasibility of dissolution of struvite uroliths, it is emphasized that this form of therapy is associated with potential hazards. Uroliths always represent a predisposing cause of urinary tract infection, and always are a predisposition to obstructive uropathy. Both risks and benefits of medical versus surgical and medical therapy must be considered for each patient.

OBJECTIVES

The objectives of medical management of uroliths are to arrest further urolith growth and/or to promote urolith dissolution by correcting or controlling underlying abnormalities. For therapy to be effective, it must induce undersaturation of urine with calculogenic crystalloids by: (1) increasing the solubility of crystalloids in urine, (2) increasing the volume of urine in which crystalloids are dissolved or suspended, and (3) reducing the quantity of calculogenic crystalloids in urine. For example, attempts to increase the solubility of crystalloids in urine often include administration of medications designed to change urine pH in order to create a less favorable environment for crystallization. Likewise, induction of diuresis is a method commonly used to increase the volume of urine in which crystalloids are dissolved or suspended. Change in diet is an example of a method to reduce the quantity of calculogenic crystalloids in urine.

These objectives may be hampered because uroliths are not homogeneous in composition. This has not been a significant problem in dogs with uroliths composed primarily of magnesium ammonium phosphate with lesser degrees of calcium phosphate because the solubility characteristics of the two minerals are similar. However, it is logical to expect difficulty in attempting to induce dissolution of a urolith with a nucleus of cystine or silica and a shell of struvite, because the solubility characteristics of these two minerals are dissimilar. This phenomenon should be considered if medical therapy seems to become ineffective after initially reducing the size of a urolith.

INFECTION-INDUCED STRUVITE UROLITHS

Current recommendations include: (1) eradication or control of urinary tract infections with appropriate antimicrobial agents, (2) use of calculolytic diets, and (3) administration of urease inhibitors (acetohydroxamic acid) to patients with *persistent* urinary tract infections caused by urease-producing microbes (Table 111–6).[6]

TABLE 111–6. SUMMARY OF RECOMMENDATIONS FOR MEDICAL DISSOLUTION OF CANINE STRUVITE UROLITHS

A. Adult dogs with urinary tract infection:
 1. Perform appropriate diagnostic studies including complete urinalyses, quantitative urine culture, and diagnostic radiography. Determine precise location, size, and number of uroliths. The size and number of uroliths are not a reliable index of probable efficacy of therapy.
 2. If available, determine mineral composition of uroliths. If unavailable, "guesstimate" their composition by evaluation of appropriate clinical data (Table 111–5).
 3. Consider surgical correction if uroliths are obstructing urine outflow, and/or if correctable abnormalities predisposing to recurrent urinary tract infection are identified by radiography or other means.
 4. Eradicate or control urinary tract infections with appropriate antimicrobial agents. Maintain antimicrobial therapy during, and for 3 to 4 weeks after, urolith dissolution.
 5. Initiate therapy with calculolytic diets. No other food or mineral supplements should be fed to the patient. Compliance with dietary recommendations is suggested by reduction in SUN concentration (usually ≤ 10 mg/dl).
 6. Feed patients calculolytic diet for one month following disappearance of uroliths as detected by survey radiography.
 7. If possible, avoid diagnostic follow-up studies requiring urinary catheterization.
 8. Consider administration of acetohydroxamic acid (25 mg/kg/day divided into 2 equal doses) to patients with persistent urease-producing urinary microbial agents despite use of antimicrobial agents and calculolytic diets.
 9. Devise a protocol for periodic follow-up including:
  a. Serial urinalyses. Urine pH, specific gravity, and microscopic examination of sediment or crystals are especially important. Remember, crystals formed in urine stored at room or refrigeration temperatures may represent artifacts.
  b. Serial radiography at monthly intervals to evaluate stone location(s), number, size, density, and shape.
  c. Quantitative urine culture where indicated.
B. Adult dogs with sterile urine:
 1. Follow the protocol described above, but do not administer antimicrobial agents or acetohydroxamic acid.
 2. Periodically culture urine specimens obtained by cystocentesis to detect secondary urinary tract infections. If UTI develops, initiate antimicrobial therapy.
C. Immature dogs:
 1. Use caution in consideration of use of protein-restricted diets in growing pups.
 2. Short-term therapy with calculolytic diets may be considered. If initiated, monitor the patient for evidence of nutritional deficiencies (especially protein malnutrition).
 3. Acetohydroxamic acid has not been evaluated in growing pups.
 4. Pending further studies, surgery remains the safest means of removing uroliths from immature dogs.

Indices of therapeutic responses are summarized in Table 111–7.

Eradication of UTI. The importance of urinary tract infections with urease-producing bacteria in the formation of most struvite uroliths in dogs emphasizes the importance of therapy to eradicate or control them. Because of the quantity of urease produced by bacterial pathogens, it may be impossible to acidify urine with urine acidifiers administered at dosages which prevent systemic acidosis. Therefore, sterilization of urine appears to be an important objective in creating a state of struvite undersaturation that may prevent further growth of uroliths or that promotes their dissolution.

Appropriate antimicrobial agents selected on the basis of susceptibility or minimum inhibitory concentration tests should be used at therapeutic dosages (consult

TABLE 111–7. CHARACTERISTIC CLINICAL FINDINGS BEFORE AND FOLLOWING INITIATION OF MEDICAL THERAPY* TO DISSOLVE STRUVITE UROLITHS IN NONAZOTEMIC DOGS

Factor	Pre-Rx	During Rx	Following Successful Rx†
Polyuria	±	+ to + + +	Negative
Pollakiuria	+ to + + + +	Transient ↑; Subsequent ↓	Negative
Gross hematuria	0 to + + + +	↓ by 5 to 10 days	Negative
Abnormal urine odor	0 to + + + +	↓ by 5 to 10 days	Negative
Small uroliths voided	±	Common in females	Negative
Urine specific gravity	Variable	± 1.004 to ± 1.014	Normal
Urine pH	≥ 7.0	Decreased (usually acid)	Variable
Urine protein	+ to + + + +	Decreased to absent	Negative
Urine RBC	+ to + + + +	Decreased to absent	Negative
Urine WBC	+ to + + + +	Decreased to absent	Negative
Struvite crystals	0 to + + + +	Usually absent	Variable
Other crystals	Variable	May persist	May persist
Bacteriuria	0 to + + + +	Decreased to absent	Negative
Quantitative bacterial urine culture	0 to + + + +	Decreased to absent	Negative
Serum urea nitrogen	≥ + 15 mg/dl	< ± 10 mg/dl	Dependent on diet
Serum creatinine	Normal	Normal	Normal
Serum alkaline phosphatase	Normal	↑ by 2 to 5×	Normal
Serum albumin	Normal	↓ by 0.5 to 1.0 gm/dl	Normal
Serum phosphorus	Normal	Slight decrease	Normal
Urolith size (radiographic)	Small-large	Progressive decrease	Negative
Hemogram	Normal	Normal	Normal

*For dogs with urinary tract infection, therapy consists of a calculolytic diet and antimicrobial agents; for dogs without urinary tract infection, therapy consists of calculolytic diet (Prescription Diet Canine s/d).
†All forms of therapy withdrawn.

Chapter 112). The fact that diuresis reduces the urine concentration of the antimicrobial agent should be considered when formulating antimicrobial dosages. Antimicrobial agents should be administered as long as the uroliths can be identified by survey radiography. This recommendation is based on the fact that bacterial pathogens harbored inside uroliths may be protected from antimicrobial agents. Whereas the urine and surface of calculi may be sterilized following appropriate antimicrobial therapy, the original infecting organisms may remain viable below the surface of the urolith. Discontinuation of antimicrobial therapy may result in relapse of bacteriuria and infection.

Although use of antimicrobial agents alone may result in dissolution of struvite uroliths in some patients, experimental studies in rats and dogs, and clinical studies in human beings, indicate that this phenomenon represents the exception rather than the rule.[6] In addition to the unpredictable response to this form of therapy, the time required to induce urolith dissolution with antimicrobial agents is usually measured in multiples of months rather than in multiples of weeks.

Calculolytic Diets. The goal of calculolytic diets is to reduce urine concentration of urea (the substrate of urease), phosphorus, and magnesium. A calculolytic diet (Prescription Diet Canine s/d) was formulated that contains a reduced quantity of high quality protein and reduced quantities of phosphorus and magnesium. The diet was supplemented with sodium chloride to stimulate thirst and induce compensatory polyuria. Reduction of hepatic production of urea from dietary protein reduces renal medullary urea concentration, and further contributes to diuresis.

The efficacy of the aforementioned diet in inducing infected-struvite urolith dissolution has been confirmed by controlled experimental and clinical studies in dogs.[6, 26, 27] When a combination of calculolytic diet and antimicrobial agents was given to 11 dogs with naturally occurring urease-positive urinary tract infections and urocystoliths presumed to be composed of struvite, urolith dissolution occurred. The mean time required to induce urocystolith dissolution was approximately three months (range was two weeks to seven months).[6]

Consumption of calculolytic diets by dogs with infection-induced struvite uroliths is typically associated with a marked reduction in the serum concentration of urea nitrogen and mild reductions in the serum concentrations of magnesium, phosphorus, and albumin.[6, 26, 27] A mild increase in the serum activity of hepatic alkaline phosphatase isoenzyme may also be observed. These alterations in serum chemistry values were of no detectable clinical consequence during six month experimental studies or during clinical studies. However, they underscore the fact that the diet is designed for short term (weeks to months) dissolution therapy rather than long term (months to years) prophylactic therapy. Changes in serum urea nitrogen concentrations may be used as one index of client and patient compliance with dietary recommendations.

Urease Inhibitors. Experimental and clinical studies in dogs have revealed that administration of microbial urease inhibitors in pharmacologic doses is capable of inhibiting struvite urolith growth and/or promoting struvite urolith dissolution. Acetohydroxamic acid (AHA) given orally to dogs at a dosage of 12 mg/lb (25 mg/kg) (divided into two daily subdoses) will reduce urease activity, struvite crystalluria, and urolith growth.[28] By reducing the pathogenicity of staphylococci, it may also result in less severe dysuria, bacteriuria, pyuria, hematuria, and proteinuria.

Although higher dosages of AHA may result in urolith dissolution, they are not recommended since they may cause a reversible hemolytic anemia and abnormalities in bilirubin metabolism.[28] Likewise AHA should not be administered to pregnant dogs since it is teratogenic.[29]

The authors have not routinely utilized AHA in promoting dissolution of infection-induced struvite uroliths in dogs because of efficacy of calculolytic diet and antimicrobial therapy. However, the authors have utilized this agent in combination with calculolytic diets and antimicrobial agents in patients that have recalcitrant urease-producing urinary tract infections.[6] If infection-induced struvite uroliths do not dissolve following an appropriate trial of therapy with diet modification and antimicrobial agents, AHA may be added to the therapeutic regimen.

STERILE STRUVITE UROLITHS

Current recommendations include: (1) use of calculolytic diets and (2) utilization of urine acidifiers (Table 111–6). Indices of therapeutic response are summarized in Table 111–7.

Calculolytic Diets. Controlled experimental and clinical studies have confirmed the efficacy of calculolytic diets (Prescription Diet Canine s/d) in inducing sterile struvite urolith dissolution.[26, 27] Unless secondary urinary tract infection develops, antibiotics and urease inhibitors are not required. The time required to induce dissolution of sterile struvite is usually shorter than that required for infection-induced struvite. When the calculolytic diet was given to nine dogs with naturally occurring sterile uroliths presumed to be composed of struvite, uroliths dissolved in a mean time of six weeks (range = one month to three months).

Urine Acidifiers. Preliminary studies indicate that protein restriction is not essential for dissolution of canine sterile struvite uroliths. Acidification of urine to approximately 6.0 has been effective in promoting sterile struvite urolith dissolution.[30] In this respect, they are similar to feline sterile struvite uroliths (consult Chapter 110). Studies are in progress to evaluate the efficacy of magnesium- and phosphorus-restricted acidifying diets in dissolving canine sterile struvite stones.

MONITORING RESPONSE TO THERAPY

The size of uroliths should be periodically monitored by survey radiography. The authors recommend radiography at monthly intervals. Survey radiography is usually preferable to retrograde contrast radiography since use of catheters during retrograde radiographic studies may result in iatrogenic urinary tract infection. Alternatively, intravenous urography may be considered.

Periodic evaluation of urine sediment for crystalluria also may be considered (consult the discussion about crystalluria in this chapter). Struvite crystals should not form if therapy has been effective in promoting formation of urine that is undersaturated with magnesium ammonium phosphate.

Urinary tract infection may persist despite antimicrobial therapy in patients with infection-induced struvite uroliths consuming the calculolytic diet. However, in most patients the magnitude of bacteriuria is usually reduced substantially (i.e., from $> 10^5$ bacteria/ml of urine to 10^2 or 10^3 bacteria/ml of urine), and the associated inflammatory response progressively subsides. Difficulty in eradication of infection while uroliths persist may be related to persistence of viable microbes harbored within the stones. Diet-induced diuresis should be considered when formulating dosages of antimicrobial agents that will achieve minimum inhibitory concentrations in urine. Despite persistent bacteriuria during antimicrobial and dietary treatment of infected patients with struvite uroliths, the authors have had excellent success in inducing urolith dissolution. Concomitant use of calculolytic diets, antimicrobial agents, and acetohydroxamic acid in this situation provided the most effective method of inducing urolith dissolution.

Since small uroliths may escape detection by survey radiography, the authors recommend that the calculolytic diet and (if necessary) antimicrobial agents be continued for at least one month following radiographic documentation of urolith dissolution. This maneuver is likely to prevent rapid recurrence of radiographically detectable uroliths and bacterial urinary tract infection following cessation of therapy.

If uroliths increase in size during therapy, or do not begin to decrease in size after approximately eight weeks of appropriate medical therapy, alternative methods of management should be considered. Small uroliths that become lodged in the urethra of male or female dogs during therapy may be readily returned to the urinary bladder lumen by urohydropropulsion. Complete obstruction of a ureter or renal pelvis, especially with concomitant urinary tract infection, is an absolute indication for surgical intervention.

Difficulty in inducing complete dissolution of uroliths by creating urine that is undersaturated with the suspected calculogenic crystalloid should prompt consideration that: (1) the wrong mineral component was identified, (2) the nucleus of the urolith is of different mineral composition than outer portions of the urolith, and (3) the owner is not complying with therapeutic recommendations.

PRECAUTIONS

The diet (Prescription Diet Canine s/d) designed to dissolve canine struvite uroliths is restricted in protein and supplemented with sodium chloride. Therefore it should not be given to patients with concomitant diseases associated with positive fluid balance (heart failure, nephrotic syndrome) or hypertension. Nonobstructing struvite nephroliths have been dissolved in patients with nonazotemic renal failure caused by ascending pyelonephritis.[6, 31] However, protein-restricted calculolytic diets should be used with caution in patients with azotemic primary renal failure. The diet could induce protein malnutrition if given for prolonged periods to dogs with moderate azotemic primary renal failure.[32]

Diuresis induced by augmenting water consumption appears to be a logical method to decrease the urine concentration of struvite and other calculogenic substances. However, additional salt is not recommended for dogs fed the calculolytic diet previously described because it has been formulated to contain supplemental sodium chloride. In addition, depletion of renal medullary urea as a consequence of dietary protein restriction is associated with an obligatory diuresis.[26]

The protein, phosphorus, and magnesium diet designed to promote dissolution of struvite uroliths will not dissolve calcium oxalate, calcium phosphate, silica, or cystine uroliths. Consult appropriate sections in this chapter for current recommendations about medical management of these forms of uroliths.

PREVENTION

Infection-Induced Struvite Uroliths. Eradication or control of infections of the urinary tract due to urease-producing bacteria is the most important factor in preventing recurrence of most infection-induced struvite uroliths. If recurrent urinary tract infection persists, indefinite therapy with prophylactic dosages of antimicrobial agents eliminated in high concentration in urine is indicated. These include nitrofurantoin and trimethoprim-sulfa.

In light of the effectiveness of diets in inducing dissolution of struvite uroliths, use of dietary modification to prevent recurrence of uroliths is logical and feasible. However, further studies must be performed to evaluate the long-term effects of low-protein calculolytic diets in dogs before reliable recommendations can be established. Because they induce polyuria, varying degrees of hypoalbuminemia, and mild alteration in hepatic enzymes and morphology, the authors recommend long-term use of severely protein-restricted calculolytic diets only if patients develop recurrent urolithiasis despite augmented fluid intake, urine acidification, and attempts to control infection.

Studies to evaluate the effectiveness of acetohydroxamic acid in the prevention of struvite urolithiasis in dogs with persistent urinary tract infection with urease-producing bacteria have been encouraging. Administration of 12 mg of AHA per lb (25 mg of AHA per kg) per day to dogs with urinary bladder foreign bodies (zinc discs) and experimentally induced urease-positive staphylococcal urinary tract infections has been effective in preventing formation of uroliths and minimizing the growth rate of uroliths.[33] Acetohydroxamic acid has also been reported to be effective in prevention of struvite uroliths in rats induced by urease-producing mycoplasmas.[34]

Studies are in progress to evaluate the preventative efficacy of mild to moderate restrictions in protein, magnesium, and phosphorus of acidifying diets. Caution must be used in deciding whether or not to induce prophylactic diuresis in patients with a history of struvite uroliths induced by recurrent urinary tract infections. Although formation of dilute urine tends to minimize supersaturation of urine with calculogenic crystalloids, it tends to counteract innate antimicrobial properties of urine. Experimental studies performed in rats and cats indicate that diuresis tends to minimize pyelonephritis but enhance lower urinary tract infections.[35]

Sterile Struvite Uroliths. When compared to patients with infection-induced struvite uroliths in which the UTI has been eradicated or controlled, sterile struvite uroliths have a greater tendency to recur. If the urine pH of patients with sterile struvite urolithiasis remains alkaline, administration of urine acidifiers should be considered. The prophylactic value of concomitant restriction of dietary phosphorus and magnesium is being investigated.

URIC ACID AND AMMONIUM URATE UROLITHS

MINERAL COMPOSITION

Uric acid is one of several biodegradation products of purine nucleotide metabolism. Ammonium acid urate (also known as ammonium urate and ammonium biurate) is the monobasic ammonium salt of uric acid. Sodium acid urate (sodium urate) is the monobasic sodium salt of uric acid.

Urate uroliths occur uncommonly in dogs, comprising approximately two to eight per cent of all canine uroliths.[30, 36–38] Canine urate uroliths are typically composed of one of several chemical forms of uric acid (Tables 111–1 and 111–2). Combinations of ammonium acid urate, sodium acid urate and/or uric acid in an individual urolith are apparently uncommon. Ammonium acid urate is found as the major constituent (greater than 70 per cent urolith mineral composition) in approximately 90 per cent of urate uroliths in both Dalmatian and non-Dalmatian dogs (Table 111–1). In contrast, uroliths composed of predominantly sodium acid urate or uric acid have been infrequently observed (Table 111–1).

Struvite is the most frequently observed minor crystalloid constituent of compound urate uroliths (less than 30 per cent of urolith mineral composition), especially those composed of ammonium acid urate.[39] Other minor mineral constituents less frequently associated with urate uroliths include calcium apatite, calcium oxalate monohydrate, and calcium oxalate dihydrate.

ETIOPATHOGENESIS

Dalmatians. Dalmatian dogs are traditionally recognized as being uniquely predisposed to urate uroliths due to heritable defects in uric acid metabolism. The ability of Dalmatians to oxidize uric acid to allantoin is intermediate between human beings and non-Dalmatian dogs.[40–42] Human beings have a serum uric acid concentration of approximately 3 to 7 mg/dl, and excrete approximately 500 to 700 mg of uric acid in their urine per day. Non-Dalmatian dogs have a serum uric acid concentration of less than 0.5 mg/dl, and excrete approximately 10 to 60 mg of uric acid in their urine per day. Dalmatians have a serum uric acid concentration that is two to four times that of non-Dalmatians, and excrete approximately 400 to 600 mg of uric acid in their urine per day.

Studies of the fate of uric acid in Dalmatians have revealed unique hepatic and renal pathways of metabolism. Of these two sites of unique purine metabolism, reciprocal allogenic renal and hepatic transplantations between Dalmatians and non-Dalmatians indicate that the hepatic mechanism is quantitatively the most significant.[43–45] The liver of Dalmatians does not completely oxidize available uric acid, even though it contains a sufficient concentration of uricase. Compared to non-Dalmatians, Dalmatians convert uric acid to allantoin at a reduced rate. It has been hypothesized that hepatic cellular membranes are partially impermeable to uric acid.

The proximal renal tubules of Dalmatians reabsorb less uric acid than non-Dalmatians; a small amount is secreted by the distal tubules. In non-Dalmatian dogs, 98 to 100 per cent of the uric acid in glomerular filtrate is reabsorbed by the proximal tubules and returned to the liver for further metabolism. Uric acid present in urine of non-Dalmatians is thought to be secreted by the distal tubules.[46]

The definitive cause of urate urolith formation in Dalmatian dogs remains unknown. Increased urate excretion is a predisposing rather than a primary cause. While all Dalmatians excrete relatively high quantities of urate in their urine, only a small percentage (especially males) form urate stones. At one time, it was thought that stone-forming Dalmatians did not excrete greater quantities of urate in their urine than non–stone-forming Dalmatians. However, recent studies indicate that insensitive methods of measurement of urine uric acid concentration were responsible for this conclusion. When steps are taken to ensure that urine uric acid remains in solution, differences in urine uric acid concentrations between non–stone-forming Dalmatians and stone-forming Dalmatians may be expected.[47]

Non-Dalmatian Dogs. Various breeds of dogs have been reported to be affected with urate urolithiasis. While urate uroliths are commonly encountered in Dalmatian dogs, approximately 30 to 60 per cent of all canine urate uroliths analyzed by quantitated methods are found in other breeds.[36, 38, 39] Although other non-Dalmatian breeds have not been reported to have a significantly higher incidence of urate urolithiasis based on quantitative analyses, the authors' observations suggest that bulldogs and Yorkshire terriers may have a high incidence of urate urolithiasis.[39]

Like Dalmatians, urate uroliths of non-Dalmatian dogs have been most frequently recognized in males. They have been detected throughout the life-span of affected dogs but are most frequently detected in dogs three to six years of age.[36, 39]

Extensive clinical and laboratory investigation has identified potential mechanisms of urate lithogenesis in Dalmatian dogs. However, comparatively little is known about urate lithogenesis in non-Dalmatian dogs that do not have portovascular anomalies. Potential predisposing factors to urate lithogenesis in dogs include: (1) increased renal excretion and urine concentration of uric acid, (2) increased renal excretion, renal production, or microbial urease production of ammonium ion, (3) low urine pH, and (4) presence of promoters or absence of inhibitors of urate urolith formation.[39]

Regardless of cause, severe hepatic dysfunction may predispose dogs to urate lithogenesis, especially ammonium urate uroliths. The authors' observations and evidence from other experimental models suggest that prolonged consumption of severely protein-restricted diets may be associated with formation of urate uroliths in dogs.[39] Biochemical and histological evaluations of these dogs suggest that chronic consumption of diets severely restricted in protein may induce hepatocellular dysfunction and concomitant hyperuricemia. Hepatic cirrhosis has also been reported to be associated with urate uroliths in dogs and other species.[48, 49] However, in the authors' experience, cirrhosis, severely restricted protein diets, and other causes of hepatic dysfunction have been uncommon causes of ammonium urate urolithiasis. Nonetheless, their significance relative to ammonium urate lithogenesis is deserving of further study.

Clinical evaluation of four male English Bulldogs with confirmed ammonium urate urocystoliths revealed mild elevations in serum uric acid concentration. The size of their livers was normal, as was serum concentration of hepatic enzymes, blood concentration of ammonia, and bromsulphalein retention.

PORTAL VASCULAR ANOMALIES

A high incidence of ammonium urate uroliths has been observed in dogs with portal vascular anomalies.[39, 49–51] They occur in both males and females, and usually are detected prior to three years of age.

Direct communication between the portal and systemic vasculature bypasses blood around the liver, resulting in severe hepatic atrophy and diminished hepatic function. Hepatic dysfunction in turn is associated with reduced hepatic conversion of uric acid to allantoin, and ammonia to urea. The predisposition of dogs with portal systemic shunts to urate urolithiasis is probably associated with concomitant hyperuricemia, hyperammonemia, hyperuricuria, and hyperammonuria.[39, 50] Serum uric acid concentrations in 15 dogs with portal systemic shunts evaluated at the University of Minnesota Veterinary Teaching Hospital were found to be increased (values ranged from 1.2 to 4.0 mg/dl).[50] Concurrent hyperuricuria, hyperammonuria, hyperuricemia, and hyperammonemia was observed in an 18 month old Bernese Mountain Dog with recurrent ammonium urate uroliths associated with a portal vascular anomaly.[39] In this dog, urine uric acid concentrations were ± 42 mg/kg/24 hr, and urine ammonia concentration was 3.2 mM/kg/24 hr, during consumption of a protein-restricted diet.

Not all dogs with portal systemic shunts develop concurrent ammonium urate urolithiasis. Definition and characterization of other factors responsible for promoting or inhibiting urate lithogenesis in affected dogs require further investigation.

BIOLOGICAL BEHAVIOR

The biological behavior of ammonium acid urate, sodium acid urate, or uric acid uroliths has not been carefully evaluated in Dalmatian and non-Dalmatian dogs. It is known that uroliths have the potential to undergo spontaneous dissolution, remain active (grow), or become inactive (remain unchanged). Although spontaneous dissolution of non–uric acid calculi has occasionally been observed, similar experiences with urate uroliths have not been well documented.

A relatively high incidence of recurrence following surgical removal is a unique characteristic of urate calculi in Dalmatian and non-Dalmatian dogs. In several studies utilizing qualitative urolith analysis, recurrence was observed in approximately 33 to 50 per cent of dogs with urate uroliths.[21, 22, 52] In these dogs, recurrences generally occurred within one year after diagnosis and treatment. Recurrence of urate uroliths may be influenced by several factors including: (1) persistence of underlying causes, (2) incomplete removal of all uroliths from the urinary tract at the time of surgery, (3) persistence or recurrence of bacterial urinary tract infections with urease (and thus ammonium)-producing bacteria, or (4) failure to comply with therapeutic or prophylactic recommendations.

MEDICAL MANAGEMENT

Dogs Without Portal Vascular Anomalies. The authors' current recommendations for medical dissolution of canine ammonium acid urate uroliths include a combination of: (1) calculolytic diets, (2) administration of xanthine oxidase inhibitors (allopurinol), (3) alkalinization of urine, and (4) eradication or control of urinary tract infections (Table 111–8). Although formation of an increased quantity of dilute urine may also be valuable, this may be accomplished by dietary modification.

CALCULOLYTIC DIETS. The goal of dietary modification for patients with uric acid or ammonium acid urate uroliths is to reduce urine concentration of uric acid, ammonium ion, and hydrogen ion. In the authors' initial clinical studies, the authors utilized the purine-restricted (low in kidney, liver, and other glandular organs) diet designed for dissolution of canine struvite uroliths. However, this diet has the disadvantage of tending to acidify urine, necessitating addition of alkalinizing drugs to the dissolution regimen.[53] In addition, it contains supplemental sodium, which is less than desirable if sodium bicarbonate is utilized as a urine alkalinizing agent. With recent modifications in the protein-restricted diet designed for moderate to severe renal insufficiency (Prescription Diet U/D), a purine-restricted nonacidifying diet that does not contain supplemental sodium is available.[30] These changes should make this diet superior to the struvitolytic diet (Prescription Diet Canine S/D) for management of canine ammonium urate uroliths. Clinical studies are in progress to test this hypothesis.

XANTHINE OXIDASE INHIBITORS. Allopurinol is a synthetic isomer of hypoxanthine.[54] It rapidly binds to and inhibits the action of xanthine oxidase, and thereby decreases production of uric acid by inhibiting the conversion of hypoxanthine to xanthine, and xanthine to uric acid. The result is a reduction in serum and urine uric acid concentration within approximately two days, and a concomitant but lesser degree of increase in the serum concentrations of hypoxanthine and xanthine.[46, 53] Although allopurinol has a short half-life in humans with normal renal function (approximately 90 minutes), its metabolic derivative oxypurinol is also a xanthine oxidase inhibitor and has a half-life of approximately 12 to 16 hours.[46] The biological half-life of allopurinol and oxypurinol in dogs is unknown to us.

The dosage of allopurinol that the authors have used

TABLE 111–8. SUMMARY OF RECOMMENDATIONS FOR MEDICAL DISSOLUTION OF CANINE AMMONIUM ACID URATE UROLITHS

1. Perform appropriate diagnostic studies including complete urinalyses, quantitative urine culture, and diagnostic radiography. Determine precise location, size, and number of uroliths. The size and number of uroliths are not a reliable index of probable efficacy of therapy.
2. If available, determine mineral composition of uroliths. If unavailable, "guesstimate" their composition by evaluation of appropriate clinical data (Table 111–5).
3. Consider surgical correction if uroliths are obstructing urine outflow.
4. Determine baseline pretreatment serum uric acid concentrations and (if possible) fractional excretion of urine uric acid.
5. Initiate therapy with calculolytic diet. No other food or mineral supplements should be fed to the patient. Compliance with dietary recommendation is suggested by reduction in SUN concentration (usually $\leq$ 10 mg/dl).
6. Initiate therapy with allopurinol at a dosage of 30 mg/kg/day divided into two equal subdoses (a lesser dose will be required in azotemic patients).
7. If necessary, administer sodium bicarbonate orally in order to eliminate aciduria. Strive for a urine pH of approximately 7.0.
8. If necessary, eradicate or control urinary tract infections with appropriate antimicrobial agents. Maintain antimicrobial therapy during, and for an appropriate period following, urate urolith dissolution.
9. Devise a protocol to monitor efficacy of therapy.
   a. Try to avoid diagnostic follow-up studies that require urinary catheterization. If they are required, give appropriate pericatheterization antimicrobial agents to prevent iatrogenic urinary tract infection.
   b. Evaluate serial urinalyses. Urine pH, specific gravity, and microscopic examination of sediment for urate crystals are especially important. Remember, crystals formed in urine stored at room or refrigeration temperatures may represent *in vitro* artifacts.
   c. Serially evaluate the serum uric acid concentrations and (if possible) fractional excretion of urine uric acid.
   d. Evaluate urolith(s) location(s), number, size, density, and shape at approximately monthly intervals. Intravenous urography may be utilized for radiolucent uroliths located in the kidneys, ureters, or urinary bladder. Retrograde contrast urethrocystography may be required for radiolucent uroliths located in the bladder and urethra.
   e. If necessary, perform quantitative urine cultures. They are especially important in patients that are infected prior to therapy, and in patients that are catheterized during therapy.
10. Continue calculolytic diet, allopurinol, and alkalinizing therapy for approximately one month following disappearance of uroliths as detected by radiography.

for dissolution of ammonium acid urate uroliths in dogs is 14 mg/lb/day (30 mg/kg/day) divided into two or three subdoses.[53] The authors have given this dosage to non-azotemic urate urolith–forming dogs for up to six months without detectable consequences. Formation of xanthine crystals around ammonium urate uroliths is a potential problem. According to the manufacturer, the drug has been given to normal dogs at this dosage for one year without causing significant abnormalities.[55]

Allopurinol uncommonly has caused adverse side reactions in humans. They include gastrointestinal complaints, skin rashes, leukopenia, thrombocytopenia, vasculitis, and hepatitis.[56–58] Adverse reactions to allopurinol in dogs and cats are apparently uncommon. The authors have not detected them and found no reports of their occurrence in dogs in the literature.

Because allopurinol and its metabolites are dependent on the kidneys for elimination, the dosage is commonly reduced in patients with renal dysfunction. Allopurinol has been reported to cause life-threatening erythematous desquamative skin rash, fever, hepatitis, eosinopenia, and further decline in renal function when given to human patients with renal insufficiency.[54] Pending further studies, appropriate precautions should be used when considering use of allopurinol in dogs with primary renal failure.

ALKALINIZATION OF URINE. Because ammonium ion and hydrogen ion appear to precipitate urates in dog urine, administration of alkalinizing agents, such as oral sodium bicarbonate or potassium citrate, appears to be of value in preventing acid metabolites from increasing renal tubular production of ammonia. Recall that under physiologic conditions associated with alkaluria, urine contains low concentrations of ammonia and ammonium ion.[59]

Dosage of urine alkalinizers should be individualized for each patient. Preliminary dosages of sodium bicarbonate vary from approximately 10 to 90 grains per day depending on the size of the patient and pretreatment urine pH values. Alternatively, potassium citrate in wax matrix tablets may be given (Urocit-K). Administration of divided doses is suggested to maintain a consistently nonacidic environment in the urinary tract.

The goal of treatment with urine alkalinizers is to maintain a urine pH of approximately 7.0. Higher values (> 7.5) should be avoided until it is determined whether or not they provide a significant risk factor for formation of calcium phosphate and/or calcium oxalate uroliths. Deposition of a layer of calcium phosphate crystals around existing urate uroliths could impede stone dissolution. Owners may participate in monitoring urine pH with pH paper.

ERADICATION OR CONTROL OF URINARY TRACT INFECTION. Clinical studies indicate that urinary tract infections in dogs with ammonium acid urate uroliths usually occur as a consequence of altered local host defenses. These alterations may be caused by urolith-induced trauma to the urothelium, or they may occur as a consequence of catheterization or other invasive diagnostic procedures. Every effort should be made to prevent, eradicate, or control them since they may cause problems of equal or greater severity as the uroliths.

Studies of ammonium acid urate uroliths in man have been interpreted to suggest that urinary tract infection caused by urease-producing microbes may be a causative factor.[60] In this circumstance, formation of ammonium ion as a consequence of urease-mediated hydrolysis of urea may result in formation of insoluble ammonium acid urate crystals. If a similar phenomenon occurs in dogs, eradication or control of potent urease-producing microbes (staphylococci, *Proteus* spp., and ureaplasmas) would be especially important.

Appropriate antimicrobial agents selected on the basis of susceptibility or minimum inhibitory concentration tests should be used at therapeutic dosages. The fact that diuresis reduces the urine concentration of the antimicrobial agent should be considered when formulating antimicrobial dosages.

AUGMENTING URINE VOLUME. Augmenting urine volume with the goal of decreasing urine uric acid and ammonium concentration, and enhancing urine flow

through the excretory pathway, appears to be a logical recommendation. Because the calculolytic diet designed for urate urolith dissolution impairs urine concentrating capacity by decreasing renal medullary urea concentration, additional diuretic agents are not required. Excessive dietary sodium should be avoided, particularly if the urine pH is high, since excessive sodium excretion may cause hypercalciuria. This event may in turn cause calcium phosphate crystals to form (consult the section on calcium oxalate urolithiasis).

It is of interest that oral sodium chloride given to normal human volunteers for ten days did not alter urine uric acid concentration.[3] Long term administration (up to three years) of hydrochlorothiazide to human patients with uroliths containing calcium salts resulted in a rise in serum and urine uric acid concentration.[61]

Dogs with Portovascular Anomalies. There apparently have been few studies of the biological behavior of ammonium acid urate uroliths in dogs with portovascular anomalies. It is logical to hypothesize that elimination of hyperuricuria and reduction of urine ammonium concentration following surgical correction of anomalous shunts would result in spontaneous dissolution of uroliths composed primarily of ammonium acid urate. Appropriate clinical studies are needed to prove or disprove this hypothesis. The authors observed a substantial reduction of urine uric acid concentration in a three-month-old female miniature schnauzer following surgical correction of an extrahepatic portacaval shunt.[39] Additional clinical studies are needed to evaluate the relative value of calculolytic diets, allopurinol, and/or alkalinization of urine in dissolving ammonium acid urate uroliths in dogs with portovascular anomalies. The efficacy of allopurinol may be altered in such dogs, since biotransformation of this drug, which has a very short half-life, to oxypurinol, which has a longer half-life, requires adequate hepatic function.[53]

MONITORING RESPONSE TO THERAPY

In the authors' experience, ammonium acid urate urocystoliths have a propensity to move into the urethra of dogs. This may be related to their small size, their round to ovoid shape, and their smooth surface. If small enough, they readily pass through the urethra. However, they often become lodged behind the os penis of males. Therefore owners should be informed of this likelihood, and given a written summary of associated clinical findings. In those circumstances where urethroliths cause clinical signs, they may be easily returned to the bladder lumen by urohydropropulsion.[62] Their physical characteristics which promote their passage into the urethra also facilitate their removal from the urethra.

The size of the uroliths should be periodically monitored by survey and (if necessary) double contrast radiography. It is more difficult to monitor changes in the size and number of uroliths that are radiolucent. However, the authors have successfully used retrograde double contrast urethrocystography to monitor dissolution of radiolucent urethrocystoliths without causing iatrogenic urinary tract infections. A balloon catheter does not need to be inserted beyond the distal urethra when utilizing this technique.[63]

Urine pH should be monitored at appropriate intervals. Periodic evaluation of urine sediment for crystalluria should also be considered. Ammonium acid urate crystals should not form in fresh urine if therapy has been effective in promoting formation of urine that is undersaturated with ammonia and uric acid. Likewise periodic evaluation of serum urea nitrogen concentration, serum uric acid concentration, and (if possible) urine uric acid concentration is recommended. Reduction of serum urea nitrogen concentration below pretreatment values (usually 10 mg/dl in previously nonazotemic patients) indicates owner compliance with recommendations to feed the calculolytic diet exclusively. Reductions in serum and urine uric acid concentrations also indicate compliance with recommendations for dietary and allopurinol therapy.

Since small uroliths may escape detection by survey and contrast radiography, the authors recommend that therapy be continued for approximately one month following documentation of urolith dissolution.

There is no rigid therapeutic time interval after which response to dissolution therapy is unlikely. The fact that current medical protocols are not designed to induce dissolution of urolith matrix may be a factor that influences dissolution rate. The time required to induce dissolution in the authors' clinical study has ranged from 8 to 11 weeks.[53] If uroliths increase in size during therapy, or do not begin to decrease in size after approximately eight weeks of appropriate medical therapy, reevaluation of the diagnosis and/or alternative methods of management should be considered.

PREVENTION

Prophylactic therapy should be considered for dogs at high risk for recurrent urate uroliths. As a first choice, diets that are restricted in purines and that promote formation of dilute alkaline urine should be considered. If urate crystalluria or hyperuricuria persists, serial evaluation of urine pH to ensure appropriate alkalinization is indicated. If necessary, alkalinizing agents may be added to the protocol. If difficulties persist, allopurinol (approximately 4.5 to 9 mg/lb or 10 to 20 mg/kg per day) may be given. Recent studies performed at the University of California indicate that prolonged administration of high doses (14 mg/lb or 30 mg/kg per day) of allopurinol may result in formation of xanthine uroliths.[61] Therefore appropriate caution in long term administration of this drug is indicated. Since it is possible to induce dissolution of recurrent ammonium urate uroliths, it is unnecessary to risk the use of prophylactic protocols that may cause disorders themselves.

CYSTINE UROLITHIASIS

MINERAL COMPOSITION

The prevalence of cystine uroliths in dogs varies with geographic location, being encountered in 2.4 to 3.3 per cent of the stones removed from dogs in the United States,[36-38] and as high as 39 per cent in some European stone centers.[65] Quantitative analysis of canine cystine uroliths has revealed that most are pure, but a few contain ammonium urate. Although uncommon, secondary urinary tract infections with urease-producing microbes may result in a nucleus of cystine surrounded by outer layers of struvite.

ETIOPATHOGENESIS

Cystinuria is an inborn error of metabolism characterized by abnormal transport of cystine (a nonessential sulfur-containing amino acid composed of two molecules of cystine) and other amino acids by the renal tubules. The name cystine was coined because this substance was first identified from urine removed from the urinary bladder (or urocyst), and therefore was thought to have originated from the bladder.[66]

Cystine is normally present in low concentrations in plasma. Normally, circulating cystine is freely filtered at the glomerulus and most is actively reabsorbed in the proximal tubules. The solubility of cystine in urine is pH dependent. It is relatively insoluble in acid urine but becomes more soluble in alkaline urine.

The exact mechanism of abnormal renal tubular transport of cystine in dogs is unknown. Plasma concentration of cystine in affected dogs is normal, indicating faulty tubular function rather than hyperexcretion.[8, 67] Plasma methionine has been found to be elevated in cystinuric dogs. Some studies in human beings suggest that tubular reabsorption of cysteine, the immediate precursor of cystine, may be normal.[68] The increase in urine cystine concentration may result from dimerization of two cysteine molecules in tubular urine.

CANINE CYSTINURIA

In dogs with cystinuria, the exact pattern of aminoaciduria reported by various investigators has been variable.[67, 69-71] Two populations of cystinuric dogs have been reported.[67] One group had cystinuria without loss of other amino acids. Another group had cystinuria and a lesser degree of lysinuria.

Unless protein intake is severely restricted, cystinuric dogs have no detectable abnormalities of amino acid loss with the exception of formation of cystine uroliths. This is related to the fact that cystine is sparingly soluble at the usual urine pH range of 5.5 to 7.0. Cystinuria would probably be a medical curiosity if cystine were not the least soluble naturally occurring amino acid. The major causes of morbidity and mortality associated with this disorder are the sequelae of urolith formation.

The exact mechanism(s) of cystine urolith formation is unknown. Since not all cystinuric dogs form uroliths, cystinuria is a predisposing rather than the primary cause of cystine urolith formation. In one study, 4 of 14 dogs with a history of cystine urolith formation had urine cystine concentrations that fell within the range of control dogs.[67] Many breeds of dogs have been reported to develop cystine uroliths, especially dachshunds.[72] The authors' empirical clinical observations indicate that English bulldogs also have an unexpectedly high prevalence of cystine uroliths.

With two exceptions, cystine uroliths have been reported only in male dogs.[37, 73] However, cystinuria has been observed in female dogs.[67] This observation suggests that lack of detection of cystine calculi in females may be related to the passage of small calculi through their relatively short, wide, and distensible urethra.

Cystine uroliths are usually detected in the bladder and/or urethra of affected males dogs. Although they are radiodense, they are typically less dense than calcium-containing and struvite uroliths (Table 111–4). Pure cystine uroliths are usually multiple, ovoid and smooth. They have a light-yellow color, and vary in size from 0.5 mm to several centimeters.

Detection of characteristic flat hexagonal cystine crystals provides strong support for a diagnosis of cystinuria. However, not all dogs with cystine uroliths have concomitant cystine crystalluria. Acidification, refrigeration, and centrifugation of urine may foster cystine crystal formation. If a sufficient quantity of cystine is present in urine (75 to 125 mg per gram of creatinine), the cyanide-nitroprusside test for cystine will be positive.[74] Ampicillin and sulfur-containing drugs have been reported to cause false positive reactions to this test.[75]

BIOLOGICAL BEHAVIOR

The precise genetic mode of inheritance of canine cystinuria is unknown; however, a sex-linked or autosomal recessive pattern has been suggested.[76, 77] Surprisingly, cystine uroliths often are not recognized until affected dogs reach maturity, the average age of detection being approximately three to five years.[76] Because cystinuria is an inherited defect, uroliths commonly recur to cause clinical signs in 6 to 12 months, unless prophylactic therapy has been initiated.

MEDICAL MANAGEMENT

Current recommendations for dissolution of cystine uroliths encompass reduction in the urine concentration of cystine and increasing the solubility of cystine in urine. This may be accomplished by dietary modification, alkalinization of urine, and administration of thiol-containing drugs.

Dietary Modification. Reduction of dietary protein has the potential of minimizing formation of cystine uroliths. By decreasing intake of methionine, a precursor of cystine, some decrease in urine cystine excretion might occur. An even more important indirect effect would be a reduction in renal medullary urea concentration and associated reduction in urine concentration. A protein-restricted alkalinizing diet (Prescription Diet Canine u/d) was observed to have a beneficial effect in promoting reduction in cystine urocystolith size in a three-year-old male dachshund.[30]

Alkalinization Of Urine. The solubility of cystine is pH dependent. In dogs, the solubility of cystine at a urine pH of 7.8 has been reported to be approximately double that at a urine pH of 5.0.[78] Changes in urine pH that remain in the acidic range have minimal effect on cystine solubility. Therefore a sufficient quantity of potassium citrate or sodium bicarbonate should be given orally in divided doses to sustain a urine pH of approximately 7.5. Recent data derived from studies in cystinuric humans suggest that dietary sodium may enhance cystinuria.[79, 80] Therefore, potassium citrate may be preferable to sodium bicarbonate as a urine alkalinizer. Further studies are required to evaluate the effect of dietary sodium on urine excretion of sodium in dogs.

Thiol-Containing Drugs. D-Penicillamine (dimethylcysteine) is a nonmetabolizable degradation product of penicillin that may combine with cysteine to form cystine-D-penicillamine disulfide.[75] This disulfide exchange reaction is facilitated by an alkaline pH. The resulting compound has been reported to be 50 times more soluble than free cystine.[81] The cysteine–D-penicillamine complex does not react with nitroprusside as does cystine, providing a mechanism to titrate dosage of the drug.[75]

The most commonly utilized dosage of D-penicillamine for dogs has been 14 mg/lb/day (30 mg/kg/day) given in two divided subdoses.[82] Higher dosages frequently cause vomiting, and may cause other undesirable side reactions. If nausea and vomiting occur with the aforementioned dosage, the drug may be mixed with food or given at mealtimes. In some instances, it may be necessary to prevent disturbances by initiating therapy with low dosages, and gradually increasing them until full dosage is reached.

D-Penicillamine has been associated with a variety of adverse reactions in man including immune-complex glomerulonephropathy, fever, lymphadenopathy, and skin hypersensitivity.[75] The authors have encountered fever and lymphadenopathy in a dachshund given D-penicillamine in a dosage of 14 mg/lb/day (30 mg/kg/day). The signs subsided following withdrawal of the drug and administration of glucocorticoids.

N-(2-mercaptopropionyl)-glycine (MPG) is a drug that decreases the concentration of cystine by a thiol disulfide exchange reaction similar to that of D-penicillamine.[75, 83] Studies in man indicate that the drug is highly effective in reducing urinary cystine concentration with less toxicity than D-penicillamine.[83] Oral administration of MPG to dogs with cystine uroliths has been reported by other investigators to be beneficial in inducing stone dissolution.[84] The authors were able to induce cystine urolith dissolution in a three-year-old male dachshund by a combination of diet (Prescription Diet Canine u/d), urine alkalinization (sodium bicarbonate), and MPG (14 mg/lb/day or 30 mg/kg/day divided into two equal subdoses) therapy.

PREVENTION

Because cystinuria is an inherited metabolic defect, and because cystine uroliths recur in a high percentage of stone-forming dogs within one year following surgical removal,[76] prophylactic therapy should be considered. A combination of dietary therapy combined with urine alkalinizing therapy may be initiated with the objective of minimizing cystine crystalluria and promoting a negative cyanide-nitroprusside test. If necessary, MPG (14 mg/lb/day or 30 mg/kg/day) or D-penicillamine (9 to 14 mg/lb/day or 20 to 30 mg/kg/day) may be added to the regimen.

CALCIUM OXALATE UROLITHIASIS

MINERAL COMPOSITION

Canine calcium oxalate uroliths have been encountered in approximately six to ten per cent of the dogs in the United States (Table 111–1).[36–38] Although different combinations of calcium oxalate salts have been identified in canine uroliths, the predominant form encountered in the authors' series has been calcium oxalate monohydrate (Table 111–1). Pure calcium oxalate monohydrate has been observed in dogs more frequently than pure calcium oxalate dihydrate uroliths. However, calcium oxalate dihydrate appears to occur more frequently in man than dogs.[85] The significance of this observation has not yet been determined, although it has been suggested that calcium oxalate dihydrate may form initially and then be converted to calcium oxalate monohydrate.[86–88]

The importance of differentiating calcium oxalate monohydrate from calcium oxalate dihydrate in canine uroliths remains to be established. In man, it has been suggested that detection of calcium oxalate dihydrate on the outside of a urolith is indicative of recent formation, whereas detection of external layers of calcium oxalate monohydrate indicates lack of recent urolith formation.[25] If valid, this hypothesis would be of great clinical significance since it would help to determine the activity of disorders leading to calcium oxalate urolith formation and therefore the need for continuous therapy to minimize urolith recurrence. In one study, human patients with calcium oxalate dihydrate uroliths had more urolith recurrences than patients with calcium oxalate monohydrate uroliths.[85] Comparable data have not yet been compiled for dogs.

Calcium oxalate uroliths may be detected anywhere in the urinary tract. They are very radiodense (Table 111–4), may be single or multiple, and vary in size from fractions of a millimeter to several centimeters. Calcium oxalate monohydrate uroliths are usually round or elliptical and have a smooth polished surface. On occasion, they may develop a jackstone shape.[89] Calcium oxalate dihydrate uroliths and mixed calcium oxalate monohydrate-calcium oxalate dihydrate uroliths are usually round to ovoid and have an irregular surface caused by protrusion of sharp edged crystals.

Calcium oxalate uroliths are more commonly encountered in males (approximately 70 per cent) than females (approximately 30 per cent); most are seen in older dogs (mean age = eight to nine years).[89] They have been most commonly observed in Dalmatians, Lhasa apsos, miniature schnauzers, poodles, Shih Tzus, and Yorkshire terriers, although any breed may be affected.[36, 39]

ETIOPATHOGENESIS

Current information about the etiopathogenesis of calcium oxalate uroliths has been primarily based on studies in man and laboratory animals.[89] Factors incriminated in the etiopathogenesis of calcium oxalate urolithiasis include hypercalciuria, hyperoxaluria, and hyperuricosuria. Although studies in humans may serve as valuable models, appropriate caution must be used in extrapolating this information for use in dogs.

Hypercalcemic Hypercalciuria. Excessive filtration and excretion of calcium in urine as a result of hypercalcemia alters the physiochemical composition of urine such that nucleation and growth of calcium salts (calcium phosphate and calcium oxalate) are favored. However, hypercalcemic hypercalciuria appears to be a relatively infrequent cause of calcium-containing uroliths in dogs.[89, 90] When uroliths form, they may be composed primarily of calcium phosphate with lesser quantities of calcium oxalate. Formation of uroliths primarily composed of calcium oxalate occurs less frequently.

Potential causes of hypercalcemia in dogs include primary hyperparathyroidism, pseudohyperparathyroidism, vitamin D intoxication, osteolytic neoplasia, and hyperthyroidism.[91] Although the authors encountered several calcium oxalate (and calcium phosphate) uroliths in dogs with primary hyperparathyroidism, they have not observed calcium-containing uroliths in dogs caused by pseudohyperparathyroidism, vitamin D intoxication, osteolytic neoplasia, or hyperthyroidism. The authors have observed a calcium apatite urolith in a dog with normocalcemic malignant lymphoma.[92]

Normocalcemic Hypercalciuria (Absorption and Renal Hypercalciuria). Normocalcemic hypercalciuria is a much more common finding in humans with calcium oxalate uroliths than hypercalcemic hypercalciuria.[93] Calcium oxalate uroliths have also been identified in normocalcemic hypercalciuric dogs.[92, 94]

In past years, normocalcemic hypercalciuric calcium oxalate urolith formers were usually placed in an etiologic group called "idiopathic hypercalciuria." However, recent studies in man suggest that idiopathic hypercalciuria is a heterogeneous group of diseases in which the underlying causes are related either to increased intestinal absorption of calcium (so-called absorptive hypercalciuria), or decreased renal tubular reabsorption of calcium (so-called renal-leak hypercalciuria).[93] Pilot studies indicate similar groups may exist in dogs.[94] Conceptual understanding of the mechanisms involved in the different types of normocalcemic hypercalciuria is of great therapeutic importance. Specific treatment to minimize intestinal absorption of calcium may be of benefit to patients with absorptive hypercalciuria, but is potentially deleterious to patients with renal-leak hypercalciuria since it may aggravate negative body calcium balance. Likewise, specific treatment designed to enhance renal tubular reabsorption of calcium could be beneficial to patients with renal-leak hypercalciuria, but could cause hypercalcemia in patients with absorptive hypercalciuria.

The basic defect in patients with *absorptive hypercalciuria* is intestinal hyperabsorption of calcium. The result is an increase in the quantity of calcium excreted in urine. Not only is there enhanced filtration of calcium, but decreased renal tubular reabsorption of filtered calcium occurs as a consequence of decreased parathormone secretion by the parathyroid glands. Hypercalciuria represents an appropriate compensatory response to excessive intestinal absorption of calcium in order to maintain serum calcium concentration within physiologic limits.

Humans with absorptive hypercalciuria have a normal or low serum parathormone concentration, normal or low urine cyclic AMP concentration, and normal fasting urine calcium concentration.[93] Preliminary studies of dogs with apparent absorptive hypercalciuria suggest similar findings.[94] Excessive skeletal mobilization of calcium (resorptive hypercalciuria) and renal-leak hypercalciuria are unlikely if fasting urine calcium concentration is normal or low.

The specific cause(s) of absorptive hypercalciuria is unknown. However, a vitamin-D dependent abnormality may be involved in some patients. In one study, approximately one third of the human patients with absorptive hypercalciuria had elevated serum concentrations of 1,25-vitamin D.[95] Serum vitamin D concentrations have apparently not yet been evaluated in dogs with absorptive hypercalciuria. The mechanism(s) involved in production of excessive serum concentrations of 1,25-vitamin D have not been completely elucidated. However, results of clinical studies in man suggest that a primary abnormality involving a renal tubular leak of phosphorus may lead to increased synthesis of 1,25-vitamin D and subsequent enhancement in intestinal absorption of calcium.[93] Recently, the role of vitamin D and its metabolites in human calcium oxalate urolithiasis has been challenged.[96]

The basic defect in patients with *renal-leak hypercalciuria* is impaired tubular reabsorption of calcium.[93] The resulting decline in serum calcium concentration results in secondary hyperparathyroidism, enhanced secretion of parathormone, and subsequent increased synthesis of 1,25-vitamin D. A secondary increase in intestinal calcium absorption may further contribute to hypercalciuria.

Human patients with renal-leak hypercalciuria have elevated serum parathormone concentrations, elevated urine cyclic-AMP concentrations, normocalcemia, and high fasting urine calcium concentrations.[93] The authors have observed one calcium oxalate–forming dog with this pattern.[94] Other findings include hypocitraturia, an exaggerated calciuric response to carbohydrate ingestion, an abnormal natriuretic response to thiazide, impaired maximum renal concentrating capacity, and normomagnesemic magnesuria.[93] It has been postulated that some of these abnormalities may occur as a consequence of urinary tract infections.[93]

Hyperuricuria and Hyperoxaluria. Hyperuricuria and hyperoxaluria are less common causes of calcium oxalate uroliths in man.[93, 97] They have not yet been documented in dogs with calcium oxalate uroliths.

BIOLOGICAL BEHAVIOR

The biological behavior of calcium oxalate uroliths in dogs is poorly understood. The authors' clinical experience with recurrent calcium oxalate uroliths suggests that they may grow from subvisual particles to uroliths of sufficient size to cause clinical signs within two to three months. Calcium oxalate renoliths were produced within four weeks in rats by supplementing their diet with ammonium oxalate.[98] Oxamide (the diamide of oxalic acid) deposits were reported to form on the renal papilla of dogs 3 to 5 days after oxamide was added to their diet.[99] It has been suggested that calcium oxalate monohydrate uroliths affecting humans grow at a slower rate than calcium oxalate dihydrate uroliths.[98] Comparable data are not available for dogs.

Canine calcium oxalate uroliths have a tendency to recur following surgical removal. In one study of dogs, calcium oxalate uroliths recurred in 25 per cent of the patients treated surgically.[22] It has been suggested that pure calcium oxalate dihydrate uroliths recur more frequently than calcium oxalate monohydrate uroliths in man.[85, 100]

MEDICAL TREATMENT AND PREVENTION

In contrast to struvite and urate uroliths, which readily dissolve when oversaturation of urine with calculogenic substances is abolished, attempts to dissolve calcium oxalate uroliths in dogs have been disappointing. In man, it has been suggested that inability to induce dissolution of calcium oxalate uroliths may be related to inability to effectively reduce urine concentration of calcium salts. In dogs, lack of effective protocols to induce dissolution of calcium oxalate uroliths is related to lack of knowledge about the etiopathogenesis of their formation and growth. Thus, there is insufficient information to formulate specific treatment that will reverse biologic derangements. However, enough observations have been made to suggest that there are similarities between calcium oxalate urolithiasis in man and dogs. Even though surgery remains the most effective method to remove canine calcium oxalate uroliths, some therapeutic modalities found to be effective in humans with calcium oxalate uroliths may be cautiously considered for use in dogs to prevent further growth of calcium oxalate uroliths, or to minimize their recurrence following removal (Table 111–9). In general, medical treatment should be formulated in step-wise fashion, with the initial goal of reducing the urine concentration of calculogenic substances. Medications that have the potential to induce a sustained alteration in body composition of metabolites in addition to urine concentration of metabolites should be reserved for patients with active or frequently recurrent calcium oxalate uroliths. Caution must be used so that side effects of treatment are not more detrimental than the effects of the uroliths.[89]

Dietary Considerations. Although reduction in dietary oxalate and/or calcium consumption appears to be a logical approach in formulating therapy for calcium oxalate uroliths, it is not necessarily a harmless maneuver. Reducing consumption of only one of these constituents (such as calcium) may be counterproductive because of an increase in the bioavailability of the other (such as oxalate) for absorption and excretion in urine. In general, therefore, reduction in dietary calcium should be accompanied by an appropriate reduction in dietary oxalate.

Humans with calcium oxalate uroliths are often cautioned to avoid milk and milk products because their carbohydrate component (lactose) may augment intestinal absorption of calcium from any dietary source.[101] Likewise, they are discouraged from consuming foods containing relatively high quantities of oxalate.

Although there is agreement that excessive consump-

**TABLE 111–9. SUMMARY OF RECOMMENDATIONS
FOR MEDICAL TREATMENT OF
CANINE CALCIUM OXALATE UROLITHS**

1. Perform appropriate diagnostic studies including complete urinalysis, quantitative urine culture, serum biochemical profile, and diagnostic radiography. Determine precise location, size, and number of uroliths.
2. If available, determine mineral composition of uroliths. If unavailable, "guesstimate" their composition by evaluation of appropriate clinical data (Tables 111–4 and 111–5).
3. Determine urine concentrations of appropriate metabolites (if possible), especially calcium, oxalate, magnesium, uric acid, and citrate.
4. Consider immediate surgical correction if uroliths thought to be composed of calcium oxalate are causing intolerable clinical signs.
5. If necessary, eradicate or control secondary urinary tract infections with appropriate antimicrobial agents.
6. Hypercalcemic hypercalciuric patients.
   a. Have high index of suspicion of primary hyperparathyroidism. If confirmed, surgically correct abnormality of parathyroid glands.
   b. If uroliths are symptomatic, consider surgical removal.
   c. Avoid thiazide diuretics since they may aggravate hypercalcemia.
   d. Induce polyuria (but avoid excessive dietary sodium supplements).
7. Normocalcemic patients with active calcium oxalate urolithiasis.
   a. Induce diuresis, but avoid excessive dietary supplementation with sodium.
   b. Consider oral administration of potassium citrate.
   c. Consider change to a diet that does not contain excessive calcium, oxalate, or protein.
   d. Consider therapy with thiazide diuretics. Strive to reduce hypercalciuria without causing significant elevations in serum calcium concentration.
   e. Avoid dietary or therapeutic supplements of ascorbic acid.

tion of calcium and oxalate should be avoided, the general consensus of urologists is that it is not advisable to restrict dietary calcium in calcium oxalate urolith formers unless it has been documented that they have absorptive hypercalciuria. Even then, only moderate restriction is advocated in order to prevent negative balances of calcium in the body.[102]

Because consumption of high levels of sodium may augment renal excretion of calcium, moderate dietary restriction of sodium is recommended for human calcium oxalate stone formers.[102] Pending further studies, a similar recommendation is made for dogs with active calcium oxalate urolithiasis.

Studies in laboratory animals, dogs, and man suggest that dietary phosphorus should not be restricted in patients with calcium oxalate urolithiasis because this action may contribute to urolith formation. Reduction in dietary phosphorus is known to augment hypercalciuria.[25, 102]

Although dietary magnesium may contribute to the formation of magnesium ammonium phosphate uroliths in some species (cats, ruminants, and so on), urine magnesium is thought to inhibit formation of calcium oxalate crystals.[89, 103] Therefore, magnesium should not be restricted from the diets of patients with calcium oxalate uroliths. In fact, supplemental magnesium has been used to minimize recurrence of calcium oxalate uroliths in man.[104]

Ingestion of foods that contain high quantities of animal protein (meat, poultry, and fish) may contribute to calcium oxalate urolithiasis in man by increasing urine

calcium concentration, increasing urine uric acid concentration, and decreasing urine citrate concentration.[102] Comparable studies have not been performed in dogs. Pending completion of such studies, the authors cautiously recommend that excessive dietary protein consumption be avoided in dogs with active calcium oxalate urolithiasis.

The canine calculolytic diet designed to induce struvite urolith dissolution (Prescription Diet Canine S/D), has been evaluated in three dogs with confirmed calcium oxalate uroliths. After periods of treatment ranging from 10 to 24 weeks, there was no formation, growth, or dissolution of urocystoliths.[89] These results are not surprising in light of the fact that the diet is not restricted in salt, but is restricted in phosphorus and magnesium. In addition, consumption of the diet is associated with mild hypercalciuria.[25] Lack of new urolith formation and lack of growth of existing uroliths may have resulted from the marked polyuria caused by consumption of the diet.

Pending further studies, a diet moderately restricted in protein, calcium, oxalate, and sodium may be considered to help prevent recurrence of calcium oxalate uroliths in dogs with active urolithiasis.

Thiazide Diuretics. Thiazide diuretics effectively decrease renal excretion of calcium provided excessive sodium is not present in glomerular filtrate.[97, 105, 106] Thiazides may reduce urine calcium excretion by reducing the filtered load of calcium. However, the primary mechanism is thought to be an indirect augmentation of tubular reabsorption of calcium.[97] Thiazide diuretics cause sodium loss in urine, leading to a mild contraction of extracellular fluid volume. The latter stimulates reabsorption of sodium and calcium (because of closely linked transport mechanisms). Thiazides may also potentiate the action of parathormone in enhancing renal tubular reabsorption of calcium.[107]

Thiazide diuretics have effectively reduced the rate of calcium oxalate urolith recurrence in human patients.[93, 97] Chlorothiazide has been shown to prevent formation of uroliths composed of calcium salts in rats fed diets supplemented with terephthalate.[108] Although thiazide diuretic therapy is ideally suited for patients with renal-leak hypercalciuria, it apparently has been used in patients with absorptive hypercalciuria without detectable abnormalities associated with excessive body calcium balance.[93, 97] Nonetheless, serum calcium and urine calcium concentration should be monitored during thiazide therapy since the risk of chronic calcium retention exists. Thiazide diuretics should not be given to hypercalcemic patients.

Unwanted side effects that may occur in human patients treated for recurrent calcium oxalate uroliths with thiazides include hypokalemia, hypocitraturia, and chronic calcium retention.[93, 97] Hypokalemia and hypocitraturia are commonly corrected by concomitant oral administration of potassium citrate.[109, 110]

Based on favorable results of thiazide therapy in humans with calcium oxalate urolithiasis, it has become popular to recommend thiazides in an attempt to prevent recurrence of calcium oxalate uroliths in dogs.[89] The authors have had limited clinical experience with use of thiazide diuretics to prevent recurrence of canine calcium oxalate urolithiasis. Oral administration of chlorothiazide at a dosage of 17 mg/lb (35 mg/kg) per day divided into two equal subdoses for four months to a three-year-old male miniature schnauzer with normocalcemic (serum calcium = 10.2 mg/dl) apparently normocalciuric (24-hour urine calcium = 2.21 mg/kg) calcium oxalate dihydrate urolithiasis resulted in a reduction in urine calcium concentration (24-hour urine calcium = 1.10 mg/kg).[89, 92] However, the serum calcium concentration gradually increased (11.2 mg/dl). Although no abnormalities were associated with the change in serum calcium concentration, the possibility of chronic calcium overload exists. This case experience emphasizes the need to monitor the effects of agents that have the capacity to adversely modify body metabolism.

Citrates. Citrates are calcium oxalate crystal inhibitors because of their ability to complex with calcium to form salts that are more soluble than calcium oxalate.[111] Several investigators have observed that some humans with calcium oxalate uroliths have abnormally low quantities of citrate in their urine.[89, 112] Therefore, oral administration of citrate has been commonly recommended to prevent recurrence of calcium oxalate uroliths in man.[102] During recent years, the most commonly recommended form of oral citrate has been potassium citrate. This agent is commonly given in conjunction with thiazide diuretics because it tends to minimize thiazide-induced hypokalemia and enhance citrate excretion in urine.

Recently, wax matrix tablets of potassium citrate have been developed to augment administration and to allow delayed absorption and excretion of citrate throughout the day. A dosage found to be effective in maintaining persistently high urine citrate concentration in humans was 60 mEq (3.78 grams) of Urocit-K per patient per day divided into two or three equal subdoses.[113]

There have been no studies of the efficacy of potassium citrate in dogs with calcium oxalate uroliths. However, preliminary studies indicate that not all dogs with calcium oxalate urolithiasis have hypocitraturia.[94] However, pilot studies suggest that potassium citrate is unlikely to be associated with serious side effects in dogs with calcium oxalate uroliths. Since citrates alkalinize urine, it is possible that potassium citrate might enhance formation or growth of calcium phosphate uroliths.

Other Agents. A variety of other agents have been suggested for management of calcium oxalate urolithiasis in man.[89] They include sodium cellulose phosphate to bind intestinal calcium, magnesium to inhibit calcium oxalate crystal formation, orthophosphates to minimize calcium excretion and calcium oxalate crystal formation, allopurinol to prevent uric acid–induced calcium oxalate urolith formation, and methylene blue to prevent calcium oxalate urolith recurrence. Consult references for details and applications to veterinary medicine.[89, 93, 97]

CALCIUM PHOSPHATE UROLITHIASIS

MINERAL COMPOSITION

Calcium phosphate uroliths are commonly called apatite uroliths (Table 111–2). The most common forms of calcium phosphate observed in canine uroliths are hydroxyapatite and carbonate-apatite (Table 111–1). The name carbonate-apatite is derived from the fact that carbonate ion may displace phosphate ion in some uroliths. Less common forms of calcium phosphate include brushite, whitlockite, and octacalcium phosphate.

Calcium phosphate is commonly found as a minor component of struvite and calcium oxalate uroliths (consult appropriate sections in this chapter for additional information). However, uroliths composed primarily of calcium phosphate are uncommon in dogs, accounting for about three per cent of those submitted to stone centers (Table 111–1).[36, 38, 114]

ETIOPATHOGENESIS

Pure calcium phosphate uroliths are infrequently encountered in dogs. When present, they usually occur in association with metabolic disorders such as primary hyperparathyroidism, renal tubular acidosis, and excessive dietary calcium and phosphorus. Refer to the section on calcium oxalate urolithiasis in this chapter, and to other chapters for additional information about these disorders.

With the exception of brushite, calcium phosphates are more insoluble in alkaline urine. Alkaline urine favors the dissociation of monobasic phosphate ($H_2PO_4^-$) to dibasic phosphate (HPO_4^{2-}) and phosphate ions (PO_4^{3-}). Brushite is the stable phase of calcium phosphate in acid urine.[115] In human beings with urine at a pH of greater than 6.9, brushite undergoes rapid transformation into calcium phosphates of a higher Ca/P ratio, such as calcium apatite (hydroxyapatite).[115] Although brushite stones have been observed in dogs, factors responsible for their formation have not yet been determined.

MEDICAL TREATMENT AND PREVENTION

The solubility of calcium phosphate in urine is dependent on hydrogen ion concentration, calcium ion concentration, and total inorganic phosphate ion concentration. Although use of effective acidifiers to reduce urine pH would be expected to be of value, this treatment alone has been ineffective in humans.[116] Likewise, use of acetohydroxamic acid in an *in vitro* study to promote urine acidification was not as effective in promoting calcium phosphate dissolution as it was in magnesium ammonium phosphate dissolution.[117] It has been suggested that administration of citric acid may increase the solubility of calcium phosphate by formation of soluble calcium complexes.[118] Refer to the section on medical dissolution of calcium oxalate uroliths for further information on proposed methods to reduce urine supersaturation with calcium.

Although use of calcium chelating agents has been reported to be of value in inducing dissolution of calcium phosphate uroliths in man,[116] there have been no controlled studies reported concerning the feasibility of medical dissolution of calcium phosphate uroliths in dogs. Since uroliths primarily composed of calcium phosphate are most likely to be encountered in dogs with diseases associated with hypercalcemia or renal tubular acidosis, it is tempting to speculate that correction of these metabolic abnormalities might be associated with formation of urine undersaturated with calcium phosphate crystalloids. If this hypothesis is accurate, calcium phosphate uroliths would be expected to dissolve. However, the authors did not observe dissolution of calcium phosphate uroliths in an eight-year-old female Welsh corgi dog with hypercalcemic hyperparathyroidism nine months following surgical removal of a parathyroid adenoma.[119]

SILICA UROLITHIASIS

MINERAL COMPOSITION

Silica accounts for approximately two to eight per cent of the uroliths submitted to stone centers in the United States since the mid 1970s.[36-38] The majority of silica uroliths have been composed almost entirely of amorphous silica.[130] However, minor quantities of struvite, calcium apatite, and calcium oxalate have been present in a few uroliths.

Most silica uroliths have a characteristic jackstone configuration. Although they may easily be differentiated from calcium oxalate uroliths by gross inspection, both silica and calcium oxalate may appear as jackstones when evaluated radiographically (Table 111–4).[120] Silica uroliths may be single or multiple, of variable size (less than one mm to more than three cm), and have been invariably found in the urinary bladder or urethra. They are radiodense.

ETIOPATHOGENESIS

Naturally occurring silica jackstones were first encountered in dogs in the mid-1970s.[120] At that time, they were confined to the United States and Canada. However, in 1985, canine silica jackstones were also recognized in Japan. Calcium magnesium aluminum silicate uroliths without a jackstone configuration were identified in dogs native to Kenya in 1977.[121]

Available clinical information provides a strong link between canine silica uroliths and dietary ingredients. Diets containing substantial quantities of corn gluten feed and/or soybean hulls are especially suspect.[30, 120]

For as yet unexplained reasons, more than 95 per cent of the canine silica uroliths have affected male dogs.[120] The authors hypothesize that the low rate of detection of silica uroliths in female dogs is related to voiding small uroliths during micturition before they induce clinical signs. Twenty-nine of the 107 (27 per cent) dogs affected by silica uroliths in the authors' series have been German shepherds, the remainder encompassed 32 other breeds.[120] The explanation of this apparently high prevalence of silica uroliths in German shepherd dogs is unknown, but may be related to their popularity as a large breed. Larger breeds of dogs are often fed dry foods containing relatively large quantities of plant ingredients (such as corn gluten feed). Soybean hulls are sometimes added to reducing diets as a non-nutritive ingredient.

BIOLOGICAL BEHAVIOR

The time required for naturally occurring silica uroliths to develop in susceptible dogs is unknown. Silica uroliths have been experimentally induced in dogs four months after being given diets containing large quantities of silicic acid.[122] They have been produced in rats within eight weeks following consumption of tetraethylorthosilicate.[123] Evaluation of case reports of human beings who have developed silica uroliths while consuming silicate-containing antacids suggests that the uroliths developed over a period of years.[120]

Because many of the silica uroliths evaluated in the authors' series were submitted for analysis by colleagues throughout the United States, long-term follow-up of the majority of affected dogs was not possible. However, silica uroliths have recurred in at least five dogs following surgical removal from the lower urinary tract.[120] In at least two dogs, struvite urocystoliths developed as a consequence of infection with urease-producing staphylococci following surgical removal of silica urocystoliths. Formation of struvite uroliths in this situation is not surprising since urease-producing staphylococci are known to be calculogenic in dogs.

MEDICAL MANAGEMENT AND PREVENTION

Effective medical protocols to induce dissolution of canine silica jackstones have not yet been developed. Calculolytic diets that do not contain vegetable proteins, and that induce diuresis, may prevent further growth of silica uroliths. However, surgery remains as the only viable alternative to remove them.

Because initiating and perpetuating causes of silica urolithiasis are unknown, only nonspecific measures to reduce the degree of supersaturation of urine with calculogenic substances can be recommended for prevention. At this time, the authors' recommendations include the following: change of diet, augmentation of urine volume, and consideration of altering urine pH (Table 111–10).[120]

Although the role of diet in the genesis of canine silica uroliths is speculative, it seems reasonable to recommend that the diet of affected patients be changed, especially if the problem is recurrent. Even though

---

TABLE 111–10. SUMMARY OF RECOMMENDATIONS FOR PREVENTION OF CANINE SILICA UROLITHS

1. Perform appropriate diagnostic studies including complete urinalyses, quantitative urine culture, and diagnostic radiography. Determine precise location, size, and number of uroliths.
2. If available, determine mineral composition of uroliths. If unavailable, determine their composition by evaluation of appropriate clinical data (Tables 111–4 and 111–5).
3. Consider surgical removal of uroliths causing clinical disease.
4. In order to prevent further growth of existing silica uroliths, or to prevent recurrence of surgically removed silica uroliths:
   a. Avoid use of diets containing substantial plant proteins, and especially avoid those containing soybean hulls or corn gluten feed.
   b. Enhance diuresis by adding moisture to the diet and/or stimulating thirst with supplemental sodium chloride.
   c. Avoid efforts to deliberately acidify urine.
5. If necessary, eradicate or control urinary tract infections with appropriate antimicrobial agents.

empirical, this maneuver is unlikely to be harmful and may be helpful. Based on the assumption that the primary source of excessive silica in diets is vegetable in origin (especially soybean hulls and corn gluten feed), selection of a diet with reduced quantities of vegetable protein and non-nutritive plant ingredients is recommended.

For dogs with recurrent silica uroliths, increasing the volume of urine produced by increasing water consumption will increase the volume of urine in which calculogenic substances are dissolved or suspended. Oral administration of sodium chloride has been a favored empirical method to induce diuresis in dogs with uroliths. Depending on the size of the dog, the quantity of urine produced prior to therapy, and the functional status of the cardiovascular system, the authors recommend oral administration of 0.5 to 10 gm of sodium chloride per day. A satisfactory response is suggested by reduction of a previously elevated specific gravity value to a range < 1.020 to 1.030. Provided that consumption of sodium chloride is effective in inducing formation of less concentrated urine and is tolerated by the patient, it may be continued.

Silica is less soluble in acid than alkaline water, and currently available information suggests that silica is less soluble in acid than alkaline biologic environments.[120] It is noteworthy that the urine pH of eight noninfected dogs with silica uroliths was acid to neutral at the time of diagnosis (mean = 6.0; range = 5.0 to 7.0).[120] Whether or not alkalinization of urine is of benefit in increasing the solubility of silica or silicates in urine is unknown. Likewise, the effects of orally administered alkalinizing agents (such as sodium bicarbonate) on the absorbability of silica from the gastrointestinal tract have not been evaluated. Nonetheless, it seems prudent to recommend that efforts to deliberately acidify the urine of dogs with recurrent silica uroliths be avoided. Mild alkalinization of the urine (but not of the digestive system) might be considered for dogs affected by silica uroliths that recur frequently. The authors emphasize, however, that we have had no experience with this form of therapy.

UNCOMMON UROLITHS

Uroliths uncommonly encountered in dogs include xanthine, calcium carbonate, and those composed of drug metabolites. Consult reference material for further details.[124]

INDICATIONS FOR SURGICAL MANAGEMENT

Detection of uroliths is not, in itself, an indication for surgery. However, along with medical management, surgical intervention has a vital role in therapy of urolithiasis. Surgical candidates include: (1) patients with urolith-induced obstruction to urine outflow that cannot be corrected by nonsurgical techniques, espe-

cially in patients with concomitant urinary tract infection; (2) patients with uroliths that are refractory to current methods of medical dissolution (e.g., silica, calcium oxalate and calcium phosphate uroliths); (3) patients with uroliths that are increasing in size and/or number despite medical therapy designed to inhibit their growth or cause their dissolution (especially if they are causing obstruction to urine outflow and/or progressive deterioration in renal function); (4) patients with nephroliths and renal dysfunction of such nature that the time required to induce medical dissolution is likely to be associated with more renal dysfunction than that associated with surgical procedures; (5) patients with anatomic defects of the urogenital tract that predispose to recurrent UTI and urolithiasis and are amenable to surgical correction at the time uroliths are removed; and (6) patients unable to respond to medical management because of poor client compliance with therapeutic recommendations.

Complete obstruction to urine outflow caused by uroliths in patients with concomitant urinary tract infection should be regarded as a surgical emergency. In this situation, rapid spread of infection and associated damage to the urinary tract, especially the kidneys, are likely to induce septicemia and peracute renal failure caused by a combination of obstruction and pyelonephritis.

Unilateral renoliths and/or ureteroliths that have caused outflow obstruction and substantial impairment of function of the associated kidney should be managed by surgical intervention or (if possible) percutaneous nephropyelonephrostomy. Medical therapy designed to induce urolith dissolution during a period of several weeks in patients with poorly draining kidneys is unlikely to be effective since the urolith(s) will not be continually bathed with newly formed urine modified to induce litholysis. The same concept applies to urethroliths that cannot be removed by nonsurgical methods.

Combined use of surgical removal of struvite uroliths followed by medical calculolytic protocols may be of value in some patients. Examples include patients in which uroliths or fragments of uroliths remain following surgery, and patients with struvite crystalluria of a character and magnitude that indicate rapid recurrence is likely. In this circumstance, meticulous procedure should be utilized in repairing surgical incisions in dogs since canine calculolytic diets are protein restricted.

References

1. Meyer, JL and Angino, EE: The role of trace elements in calcium lithiasis. Invest Urol 14:347, 1977.
2. Osborne, CA and Clinton, CW: Urolithiasis: terms and concepts. Vet Clin North Am 16:3, 1986.
3. Breslau, NA and Pak, CYC: Lack of effect of salt intake on urinary uric acid excretion. J Urol 129:531, 1983.
4. Sutor, DJ, et al.: Isolation and identification of some urinary inhibitors of calcium phosphate formation. Clin Chem Acta 89:273, 1978.
5. Rose, AG and Sulaimans: Tamm-Horsfall mucoproteins promote calcium oxalate crystal formation in urine. J Urol 127:177, 1982.
6. Osborne, CA, et al.: Struvite urolithiasis in animals and man:

formation, detection and dissolution. Adv Vet Sci Comp Med 29:1, 1985.

6a. Senior, DF and Finlayson, B: Initiation and growth of uroliths. Vet Clin North Am 16:19, 1986.

7. Bovee, KC: Urolithiasis. *In* Bovee, KC (ed): Canine Nephrology. Media, PA, Harwal Pub Co, 1984, p 355.

8. Osborne, CA, et al.: Crystalluria. Observations, interpretations, and misinterpretations. Vet Clin North Am 16:45, 1986.

9. Johnston, GR, et al.: Radiographic and ultrasonographic features of uroliths and urinary tract filling defects. Vet Clin North Am 16:261, 1986.

10. Osborne, CA, et al.: Analysis of canine and feline uroliths. *In* Kirk, RW (ed): Current Veterinary Therapy. Philadelphia, WB Saunders, 1983, p 1061.

11. Ruby, AL and Ling, GV: Methods of analysis of canine uroliths. Vet Clin North Am 16:293, 1986.

12. Ruby, AL and Ling, GV: Bacterial culture of uroliths: techniques and interpretation of results. Vet Clin North Am 16:325, 1986.

13. Boistelle, R, et al.: Growth and stability of magnesium ammonium phosphate in acidic sterile urine. Urol Res 12:79, 1984.

14. Klausner, JS, et al.: Struvite urolithiasis in a litter of miniature schnauzer dogs. Am J Vet Res 40:712, 1980.

15. Klausner, JS, et al.: Experimental induction of struvite uroliths in miniature schnauzer and beagle dogs. Invest Urol 18:127, 1980.

16. Hardy, RM, et al.: Urolithiasis in immature dogs. VM/SAC 67:1205, 1972.

17. Klausner, JS and Osborne, CA: Dissolution of a struvite nephrolith in a dog. JAVMA 174:1100, 1979.

18. Kirby, R, et al.: Dissolution of a nephrolith in a dog. JAVMA 178:827, 1983.

19. Pollack, S and Wagner, BM: Renal calculi in a dog. A four year clinical picture. VM/SAC 71:1693, 1976.

20. Finco, DR, et al.: Canine urolithiasis: a review of 133 clinical and 23 necropsy cases. JAVMA 157:1225, 1970.

21. Brown, NO, et al.: Recurrence of canine urolithiasis. JAVMA 170:419, 1977.

22. Clark, WT: The distribution of canine urinary calculi and their recurrence following treatment. J Sm Anim Pract 15:437, 1974

23. Osborne, CA, et al.: Pathophysiology, diagnosis, and treatment of surgical disorders of the urinary system. *In* Gourley, IM and Vasseur, PB (eds): A Textbook of Small Animal Surgery. Philadelphia, JB Lippincott, 1985, p 574.

24. Stone, EA: Surgical therapy for urolithiasis. Vet Clin North Am 14:77, 1984.

25. Abdullahi, SU, et al.: Evaluation of a calculolytic diet in female dogs with induced struvite urolithiasis. Am J Vet Res 45:1508, 1984.

26. Osborne, CA, et al.: Medical dissolution and prevention of canine struvite uroliths. *In* Kirk, RW (ed): Current Veterinary Therapy IX. Philadelphia, WB Saunders, 1986, p 1177.

27. Krawiec, DR, et al.: Effect of acetohydroxamic acid on dissolution of canine uroliths. Am J Vet Res 45:1266, 1984.

28. Bailie, NC, et al.: Teratogenic effect of acetohydroxamic acid in clinically normal beagles. Am J Vet Res 47:2604, 1986.

29. Osborne, CA: Unpublished data. University of Minnesota, St. Paul, 1987.

30. Osborne, CA, et al.: Medical management of canine uroliths with special emphasis on dietary modification. Comp Anim Pract 1:72, 1987.

31. Osborne, CA, et al.: Medical dissolution of canine struvite uroliths. Vet Clin North Am 16:349, 1986.

32. Polzin, DJ, et al.: Effects of modified protein diets in dogs with chronic renal failure. JAVMA 183:980, 1983.

33. Krawiec, DR, et al.: Effect of acetohydroxamic acid on prevention of canine struvite uroliths. Am J Vet Res 45:1276, 1984.

34. Lamm, DL, et al.: Medical therapy of experimental infection stones. Urol 10:418, 1977.

35. Lees, FE, et al.: Adverse effects of open indwelling urethral catheterization in clinically normal male cats. Am J Vet Res 42:825, 1981.

36. Osborne, CA, et al.: Prevalence of canine uroliths: Minnesota Urolith Center. Vet Clin North Am 16:27, 1986.

37. Ling, GV and Ruby, AL: Canine uroliths: analysis of data derived from 813 specimens. Vet Clin North Am 16:303, 1986.

38. Bovee, KC and McGuire, T: Qualitative and quantitative analysis of uroliths in dogs. Definitive determination of chemical type. JAVMA 185:983, 1984.

39. Kruger, JM and Osborne, CA: Etiopathogenesis of uric acid and ammonium urate uroliths in nonDalmatian dogs. Vet Clin North Am 16:87, 1986.

40. Duncan, H, et al.: The effects of intravenous administration of uric acid on its concentration in plasma and urine of Dalmatian and non-Dalmatian dogs. J Lab Clin Med 58:876, 1961.

41. Duncan, H and Curtiss, AS: Observations on uric acid transport in man, the Dalmatian, and the non-Dalmatian dog. Henry Ford Hosp Med J 19:105, 1971.

42. Friedman, M and Byers, SO: Observations concerning the causes of excess excretion of uric acid in the Dalmatian dog. J Biol Chem 175:727, 1948.

43. Appleman, RM, et al.: Effect of reciprocal allogeneic renal transplantation between Dalmatian and non-Dalmatian dogs on urinary excretion of uric acid. Proc Soc Exp Biol Med 121:1094, 1966.

44. Cohn, R, et al.: Renal allotransplantation and allantoin excretion of Dalmatians. Arch Surg 91:911, 1965.

45. Kuster, G, et al.: Uric acid metabolism in Dalmatians and other dogs. Arch Int Med 129:492, 1972.

46. Foreman, JW: Renal handling of urate and other organic acids. *In* Bovee, KC (ed): Canine Nephrology. Media, PA, Harwal Pub, 1984, p 144.

47. Schaible, RH: Genetic predisposition to purine uroliths in Dalmatian dogs. Vet Clin North Am 16:127, 1986.

48. Rothuizen, J, et al.: Congenital porto-systemic shunts in sixteen dogs and three cats. J Sm Anim Pract 23:67, 1982.

49. Ungar, H and Ungar, R: Further studies on the pathogenesis of urate calculi in the urinary tract of white rats. Am J Path 28:291, 1952.

50. Hardy, RM and Klausner, JS: Urate calculi associated with portal vascular anomalies. *In* Kirk, RW (ed): Current Veterinary Therapy VIII. Philadelphia, WB Saunders, 1983, p 1073.

51. Marretta, SM, et al.: Urinary calculi associated with porto-systemic shunts in six dogs. JAVMA 178:133, 1981.

52. Weaver, AD: Canine urolithiasis: chemical composition and outcome of 100 cases. J Sm Anim Pract 11:93, 1970.

53. Osborne, CA, et al.: Dissolution of canine ammonium urate uroliths. Vet Clin North Am 16:375, 1986.

54. Hande, K, et al.: Allopurinol Kinetics. Clin Pharm Ther 23:598, 1978.

55. Zoprim, Product Insert. Burroughs Wellcome, North Carolina, November 1981.

56. Al Kawas, FH, et al.: Allopurinol hepatotoxicity. Ann Int Med 95:588, 1981.

57. Medline, A, et al.: Liver granulomas and allopurinol. Br Med J 1:1320, 1978.

58. O'Sullivan, WJ: Metabolic side-effects of allopurinol. Prog Biochem Pharm 9:174, 1974.

59. Tannen, RL: Ammonia and acid-base homeostasis. Med Clin North Am 67:781, 1983.

60. Garcia del Pena, E and Cifuentes Dellatte, L: Forms of ammonium urate presentation in urinary calculi of noninfectious and infectious origin. *In* Smith, LH, et al. (eds): Urolithiasis: Clinical and Basic Research. New York, Plenum Press, 1981, p 935.

61. Pak, CYC, et al.: Enhancement of renal excretion of uric acid during long-term thiazide therapy. Invest Urol 16:191, 1978.

62. Osborne, CA and Polzin, DJ: Nonsurgical management of canine obstructive urolithopathy. Vet Clin North Am 16:333, 1986.

63. Johnston, GR, et al.: Retrograde contrast urethrography. *In* Kirk, RW (ed): Current Veterinary Therapy, 6th ed. Philadelphia, WB Saunders, 1977, p 1189.

64. Ling, GV: Unpublished data. Department of Medicine, School of Veterinary Medicine, University of California, 1987.

65. Hicking, W, et al.: Investigation with polarizing microscopy for the classification of urinary stones from humans and dogs. *In* Smith, LH, et al.: Urolithiasis: Clinical and Basic Research. New York, Plenum Press, 1981, p 901.

66. Segal, S and Thier, SO: Cystinuria. *In* Stanbury, JB, et al.: The Metabolic Basis for Inherited Disease, 5th ed. New York, McGraw-Hill, 1983, p 1774.

67. Bovee, KC: Genetic and metabolic diseases of the kidney. *In* Bovee, KC (ed): Canine Nephrology. Media, PA, Harwal Pub, 1984, p 339.

68. Bartter, FC, et al.: Cystinuria. Ann Int Med 62:796, 1965.

69. Clark, WT and Cuddeford, D: A study of amino acids in urine from dogs with cystine urolithiasis. Vet Rec 88:414, 1971.

70. Cornelius, CE, et al.: A quantitative study of amino aciduria in dachshunds with a history of cystine urolithiasis. Cornell Vet 57:177, 1967.

71. Crane, CW and Turner, AW: Amino acid patterns of urine and blood plasma in a cystinuric labrador dog. Nature 177:237, 1956.

72. Osborne, CA and Klausner, JS: War on urolithiasis: problems and their solutions. Sci Proc AAHA, Denver, Colorado, 1978, p 569.

73. Brown, NO, et al.: Canine urolithiasis: retrospective analysis of 438 cases. JAVMA 170:415, 1977.

74. Kachmar, JF: Proteins and amino acids. *In* Tietz, NW (ed): Fundamentals of Clinical Chemistry. Philadelphia, WB Saunders, 1970, p 248.

75. Pahira, JJ: Management of the patient with cystinuria. Urol Clin North Amer 14:339, 1987.

76. Bovee, KC: Canine cystine urolithiasis. Vet Clin North Am 16:211, 1986.

77. Brand, E, et al.: Canine cystinuria. V. Family history of two Irish terriers and cystine determinations in dog urine. J Biol Chem 133:431, 1940.

78. Treacher, RJ: Urolithiasis in the dog. Biochemical aspects. J Sm Anim Pract 7:537, 1966.

79. Jaeger, P, et al.: Anticystinuric effects of glutamine and of dietary sodium restriction. N Engl J Med 315:1120, 1986.

80. Anon: Cystinuria is reduced by low-sodium diets. Nutr Rev 45:79, 1987.

81. Lotz, M, et al.: D-penicillamine therapy in cystinuria. J Urol 95:257, 1966.

82. Frimpter, GW, et al.: Penicillamine in canine cystinuria. JAVMA 151:1084, 1967.

83. Pak, CYC, et al.: Management of cystine nephrolithiasis with α-mercaptopropionyl glycine. J Urol 136:1003, 1986.

84. Hoppe, A, et al.: Unpublished data. Department of Medicine Swedish University of Agricultural Sciences, Uppsala, Sweden, 1986.

85. Koide, T, et al.: Clinical manifestations of calcium oxalate monohydrate and dihydrate urolithiasis. J Urol 127:1067, 1982.

86. Leusmann, DB, et al.: Scanning electron microscopy of urinary calculi. Scan Elect Microscopy 3:1427, 1984.

87. Otnes, B: Urinary stone analysis: Methods, materials, and value. Scan J Urol Nephrol (Suppl) 71:7, 1983.

88. Schubert, G, and Brian, G: Crystallographic investigations of urinary calcium oxalate calculi. Int Urol Nephrol 13:249, 1981.

89. Osborne, CA, et al.: Etiopathogenesis, clinical manifestations, and management of canine calcium oxalate urolithiasis. Vet Clin N Am 16:133, 1986.

90. Klausner, JS, et al.: Canine primary hyperparathyroidism and its association with urolithiasis. Vet Clin N Am 16:227, 1986.

91. Kruger, JM, et al.: Treatment of hypercalcemia. *In* Kirk, RW (ed): Current Veterinary Therapy, Ed 9. Philadelphia, WB Saunders, 1986, p 75.

92. Osborne, CA, et al.: Canine calcium oxalate urolithiasis. *In* Proc Amer Coll Vet Int Med Ann Forum, Vol 1, pp 4–23, 1986.

93. Pak, CYC: Pathophysiology of calcium nephrolithiasis. *In* Seldin, DW, et al (eds): The Kidney: Physiology and Pathophysiology. Vol 2. New York, Raven Press, 1985, p 1365.

94. Lulich, JP, and Osborne, CA: Unpublished data. Department of Small Animal Clin Sci, College Vet Medicine, University of Minnesota, 1987.

95. Kaplan, RA, et al.: The role of 1-alpha 25-dihydroxy-vitamin D in the mediation of intestinal hyperabsorption of calcium in primary hyperparathyroidism and absorptive hypercalciuria. J Clin Invest 59:756, 1977.

96. Netelenbos, JC, et al.: Vitamin D status in urinary calcium stone formation. Arch Int Med 145:681, 1985.

97. Coe, FL, and Favus, MJ: Disorders of stone formation. *In* Brenner, BM, and Rector, FC (eds): The Kidney. Vol 2, 2nd ed. Philadelphia, WB Saunders Co, 1981, p 1950.

98. Gregory, JG, et al: Effect of alkalinizing agents on calcium oxalate stone formation in a rat model. Urol Res 12:48, 1984.

99. Borden, TA, and Vermeulen, CW: The renal papilla in calculogenesis of oxamide stones. Invest Urol 4:125, 1966.

100. Berenyl, M, et al.: Theoretical and clinical importance of the differentiation between the two types of calcium oxalate hydrate. Int Urol Nephrol 4:341, 1972.

101. Vermeulen, CW, and Roberts, JA: Milk and milk constituents as calculogenic agents in rat urolithiasis. Invest Urol 1:2, 1963.

102. Pak, CYC, et al.: Dietary management of idiopathic calcium urolithiasis. J Urol 133:123, 1984.

103. Li, MK, et al.: Effects of magnesium on calcium oxalate crystallization. J Urol 133:123, 1985.

104. Johansson, G, et al.: Effects of magnesium hydroxide in renal stone disease. J Am Coll Nutr 1:179, 1982.

105. Constanzo, LS, and Windhager, EE: Calcium and sodium transport by the distal convoluted tubule of the rat. Am J Physiol 235:F492, 1978.

106. Suki, WN, et al.: Mechanism of the effect of thiazide diuretics on calcium and uric acid. Clin Res 15:78, 1967.

107. Maggio, AJ, et al.: The role of vitamin D in idiopathic hypercalciuria. J Urol 122:147, 1979.

108. Wolkowski-Tyl, R, et al.: Chemically induced urolithiasis in weanling rats. Am J Path 107:419, 1982.

109. Sakhaee, K, et al.: Contrasting effects of potassium citrate and sodium citrate therapies on urine chemistries and crystallization of stone-forming salts. Kidney Int 24:348, 1983.

110. Pak, CYC: Medical management of nephrolithiasis. J Urol 128:1157, 1982.

111. Meyer, JL, and Smith, LH: Growth of calcium oxalate crystals. II. Inhibitors by natural urinary crystal growth inhibitors. Invest Urol 13:36, 1975.

112. Menon, M, and Mahle, CJ: Urinary citrate excretion in patients with renal calculi. J Urol 129:1158, 1983.

113. Pak, CYC, et al.: Augmentation of renal citrate excretion by oral potassium administration: Time, course, dose frequency schedule, and dose-response relationship. J Clin Pharmacol 24:19, 1984.

114. Klausner, JS, and Osborne, CA: Canine calcium phosphate uroliths. Vet Clin N Am 16:171, 1986.

115. Pak, CYC: Calcium urolithiasis. Pathogenesis, diagnosis and management. New York, Plenum Medical Book Co, 1978, p 25.

116. Sheldonn, CA, and Smith, AD: Chemolysis of calculi. Urol Clin N Am 9:121, 1982.

117. Griffith, DP, et al.: Dissolution of struvite urinary stones. Experimental studies in vitro. Invest Urol 13:351, 1976.

118. Elliott, JS: Calcium phosphate solubility in urine. J Urol 77:269, 1957.

119. Klausner, JS, et al.: Calcium urolithiasis in two dogs with parathyroid adenomas. J Am Vet Med Assoc 191:1423, 1987.

120. Osborne, CA, et al.: Etiopathogenesis, clinical manifestations, and management of canine silica urolithiasis. Vet Clin N Am 16:185, 1986.

121. Brodey, RS, et al.: Silicate renal calculi in Kenyan dogs. J Small Animal Pract 18:523, 1977.

122. McCullagh, KG, and Eberhard, LA: Silica urolithiasis in laboratory dogs fed semisynthetic diets. J Am Vet Med Assoc 164:712, 1974.

123. Emerick, RJ: Chloride and phosphate as impediments to silica urinary calculi in rats fed tetraethyl orthosilicate. J Nutr 114:733, 1984.

124. Osborne CA, et al.: Etiopathogenesis of uncommon canine uroliths: Xanthine, carbonate, drugs, and drug metabolites. Vet Clin N Am 16:217, 1986.

DRUG INDEX

Generic	Trade	Dosage	Route	Frequency	Description
Acetohydroxamic acid	Lithostat	12.5 mg/kg	Oral	q12h	Urease inhibitor
Allopurinol	Zyloprim	15 mg/kg	Oral	q12h	Xanthine oxidase inhibitor
Potassium citrate	Urocit-K	To effect for alkalinization of urine (12.5 mg/kg?)*	Oral	q12h	Urine alkalinizer; increases urine calcium solubility
D-penicillamine	Cupramine	15 mg/kg	Oral	q12h	Reduces urine cystine concentration
N-(2-mercaptopropionyl)-glycine	Thiola	15 mg/kg	Oral	q12h	Reduces urine cystine concentration
Chlorthiazide	Diuril	17.5 mg/kg	Oral	q12h	Diuretic; reduces urine calcium excretion

*Optimum dosage to increase urine calcium solubility not yet established for dogs.

112 DISEASES OF THE BLADDER AND URETHRA

SCOTT A. BROWN and JEANNE A. BARSANTI

ANATOMY AND PHYSIOLOGY

The lower urinary tract is a storage reservoir (urinary bladder) and a conduit (urethra) for urine and seminal fluid (male). The bladder consists of a neck (vesicourethral junction, which is elongated in the cat), body, and apex (vertex). Reflections of the peritoneal covering of the bladder form the two lateral ligaments and the single median ligament ventrally, loosely attaching the bladder to the abdominal wall.[1,2] The bladder trigone is a triangular area near the neck of the bladder, formed by the urethral and two ureteral orifices.[1] The segment of the ureter lying within the bladder wall forms the vesicoureteral valve, preventing reflux of urine.[3]

The urethra of the male consists of prostatic, pelvic (membranous), and penile (cavernous) portions.[1,2,4] The prostate (see Chapter 105) encompasses the proximal urethra in the male dog and cat. The membranous urethra extends from the prostate to the bulb of the penis (bulbourethral gland in the cat) and is surrounded by striated muscle.[1,2] The penile portion extends to the urethral orifice at the tip of the penis.[1] The smooth muscle of the urethra is continuous with that of the bladder wall (detrusor). There are generally three layers of smooth muscle throughout the length of the urethra, which are gradually replaced by striated muscle at the level of the pelvic urethra.[5] The female urethra is considerably shorter than the male (7 to 10 cm versus 10 to 35 cm in the dog) and is analogous to the prostatic portion with skeletal replacing smooth muscle prior to the urethral meatus, which is approximately 0.5 centimeter caudal to the vaginovestibular junction.[1,2] Transitional epithelium (urothelium) lines the urinary tract of both species from the renal pelvis to the midurethra, where it gradually becomes stratified columnar or cuboidal, to be replaced by stratified squamous at the external orifice.[1,5–8] The lone exception is in the female cat, where the mucosa remains stratified columnar to the external orifice.[8] Mucous glands (urethral glands of Littre) are present throughout the male cat urethra, and distally in the female cat.[5,8] Marked distensibility char-

acterizes the entire lower urinary tract, except at the level of the prominent ventral groove of the os penis in the male dog, which accounts for the frequent occurrence of urolithiasis at this site. Because of the orientation of its penis, the urethra of the male cat lies dorsal to its less well developed os penis.

Innervation, blood supply, and physiology of micturition are discussed elsewhere (see Chapters 30 through 32).[1,9–17]

CLINICAL SIGNS OF LOWER URINARY TRACT DISEASE

Characteristic clinical signs of lower urinary tract disease include dysuria, hematuria, stranguria, pollakiuria, and urinary incontinence (see Chapters 30 through 32). While these signs may suggest localization of a disease process they do not suggest a cause.

Some lower urinary tract diseases may have systemic consequences due to extension of the primary disease process, for example septicemia from bacterial urinary tract infection or metastasis of lower urinary tract neoplasia. Polyuria or uremia may be present in cases of lower urinary tract obstruction (see Chapters 31 and 108) or when a disease process concurrently affects the lower and upper urinary tract.

DIAGNOSTIC TECHNIQUES FOR LOWER URINARY TRACT DISEASE

Reliable diagnosis of lower urinary tract disease requires careful integration of history and physical examination, which includes careful abdominal palpation and observation of micturition. Special diagnostic techniques are indicated on the basis of information obtained from the history and physical examination.

HEMATOLOGY/BLOOD CHEMISTRY VALUES

These tests are seldom beneficial in the initial diagnostic evaluation of a patient with lower urinary tract disease, except to assess the possibility of obstruction, leak, or disease processes in other organs. Azotemia is not expected in simple lower urinary tract disease.

URINALYSIS

A complete urinalysis is an inexpensive, specific, sensitive test for lower urinary tract disorders. A urinalysis includes gross observation, dipstick evaluation of chemical constituents, and a sediment examination.

Used alone, macroscopic examination of urine results in false negative results nearly 20 per cent of the time.[18] In contrast to dipstick methods, examination of urine sediment is a reliable method to detect the presence of pyuria and bacteriuria.[18–23]

Because of the anatomy of the lower urinary tract, the method of collection of a urine specimen is important in interpretation of results. Urine may be collected by cystocentesis, catheterization, or voiding. To evaluate diseases involving the urinary bladder or upper urinary tract, a cystocentesis sample is preferred. In contrast, urethral diseases may best be evaluated with a voided specimen, or by comparison of voided and cystocentesis samples.

Cystocentesis can be performed with the animal standing, suspended by its forelimbs or hindlimbs, or lying on its side or back (Figures 112–1, 112–2, and 112–3). The bladder is palpated, a small area is clipped and scrubbed, and the bladder is immobilized with the palpating hand. It is ill-advised to perform a cystocentesis through hair or unprepared skin, since both are bacteria laden and the cystocentesis needle will enter both peritoneal cavity and urinary bladder. A 22-gauge

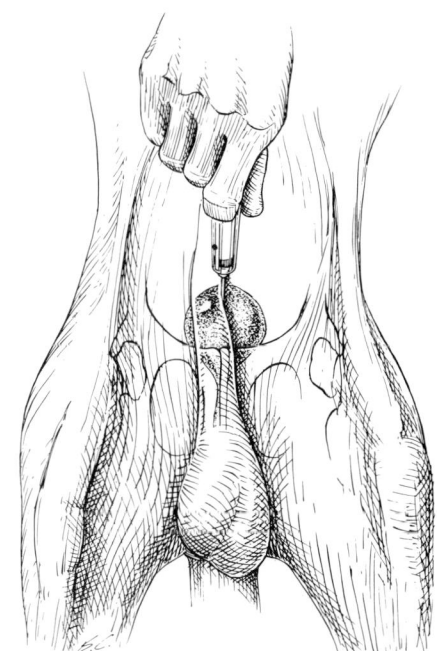

FIGURE 112–2. Cystocentesis with the dog in dorsal recumbency or suspended by the front limbs. Cystocentesis using the blind technique is demonstrated: the needle is inserted perpendicular to the body wall, 1 to 2 inches cranial to the cranial edge of the pubic bone. (From Barsanti JA: Genitourinary tract infections. *In* Greene CE (ed): Clinical Microbiology and Infectious Diseases of the Dog and Cat. Philadelphia, WB Saunders, 1984, p 274.)

(or smaller) one or one and a half inch needle is inserted into the bladder and urine is aspirated. The presence of bacteria on sediment examination of urine obtained by cystocentesis is unequivocal evidence of a bacterial urinary tract infection. If bowel penetration is suspected (more common with techniques not relying upon bladder palpation) urine sediment may reveal fecal debris and multiple bacterial species with minimal pyuria. Leakage is uncommon, though it may occur at the puncture site in dogs and cats with distended bladders who are unable to urinate because of urethral obstruction or detrusor dysfunction.

Because of the normal microflora of the distal urethra, vagina, and prepuce,[21] catheterization requires special care to avoid contamination of the specimen and/or induction of a urinary tract infection. In the male, the prepuce is retracted, the penis cleansed, and a sterile lubricated catheter inserted with the aid of a sterile instrument. In the female the vulva should be cleansed and a sterile speculum used to pass a sterile lubricated catheter. Catheterization allows collection of urine at the control of the veterinary clinician, but in female dogs frequently induces contamination (50 per cent incidence) or urinary tract infection (UTI) (20 per cent incidence).[24, 25] Urethral catheterization in the cat generally requires sedation or anesthesia and may still be traumatic.[26]

A urine specimen obtained during midstream voiding or manual expression is useful in evaluation of urethral or prostatic diseases or urine concentrating ability. However, because of the prevalence of contamination from normal urethral or genital microflora this technique is not useful for urine culture. Manual expression may

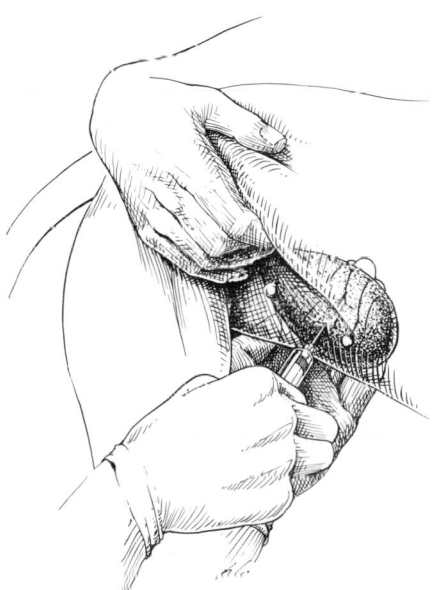

FIGURE 112–1. Cystocentesis with the dog standing. The thumb of the palpating hand can be placed along the cranial border of the bladder to push the bladder toward the pelvis and further immobilize it. (From Barsanti JA: Genitourinary tract infections. *In* Greene CE (ed): Clinical Microbiology and Infectious Diseases of the Dog and Cat. Philadelphia, WB Saunders, 1984, p 273.)

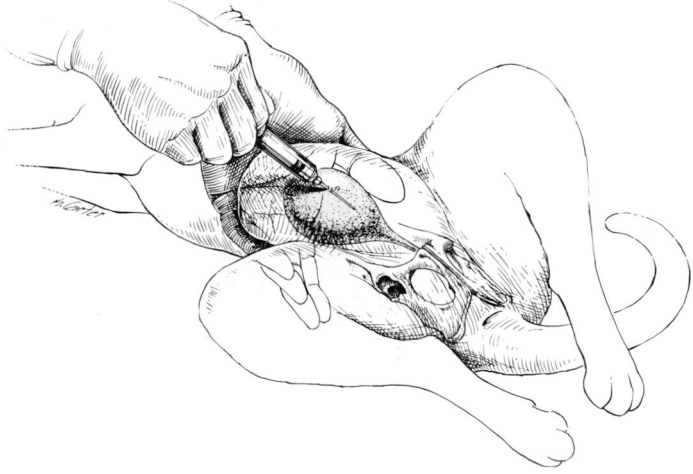

FIGURE 112–3. Cystocentesis with the cat in dorsal recumbency. The bladder is stabilized by abdominal compression applied cranially. (From Barsanti JA: Genitourinary tract infections. *In* Greene CE (ed): Clinical Microbiology and Infectious Diseases of the Dog and Cat. Philadelphia, WB Saunders, 1984, p 274.)

enhance the risk of extension of lower urinary tract infection to the upper tract through vesicoureteral reflux.[27] Replacement of litter with plastic beads will allow collection of voided urine in cats, but uncontaminated voided specimens are difficult to obtain in this species.

CYTOLOGY

Evaluation of urethral discharge, aspirate of a bladder mass, or bladder wash cytology may be beneficial, especially in cases of suspected neoplasia. A bladder wash is performed by infusion of 50–100 ml of sterile saline (or other isotonic electrolyte solution) into the bladder through a urinary catheter. Use of bladder washes to obtain cytologic specimens will avoid cellular distortion induced by long-term storage in urine.

URINE CULTURE

Although a recent study indicated that urine sediment examination was a sensitive and specific method for detection of bacteriuria, generally 10,000 or more bacteria/ml must be present to be seen on urine sediment exam, with cocci more difficult to visualize.[28-30] Failure to demonstrate bacteria by sediment examination does not rule out bacteriuria. The ideal method to evaluate for the presence of UTI is quantitative urine culture. Quantitative culture is required for catheterized and voided, and preferred for cystocentesis samples. To obtain quantitative urine cultures, the clinician may submit the sample to a commercial laboratory or use bacteriologic loops (0.01 and 0.001 ml) or pipettes to inoculate Blood and MacConkey's Agar for overnight incubation at 37°C to allow quantitation and preliminary identification of bacterial species (Table 112–1).[21, 31]

In both dogs and cats, the number of organisms present and the method of urine collection are more important considerations in diagnosing infection than the type of organism found.[32] Normal distal urethral, vaginal, and preputial microflora will result in contamination of urine specimens obtained by catheterization or voiding. Properly performed catheterization of male dogs results in occasional contamination with small numbers of bacteria (less than 10^3 in one of 16 dogs[24]).

Catheterization of female dogs induces contamination 50 per cent of the time.[24] Urine obtained by voiding is least useful in the diagnosis and management of UTI, since contamination from distal urethral flora may result in bacterial counts greater than 10^5 in voided samples. The term "significant bacteriuria" has been used to define the quantity of bacteria present necessary to distinguish contamination from true infection (Table 112–2). This is based on the premise that bacteria present in urine of an animal with UTI will exceed 100,000 bacteria/ml because of bacterial proliferation in urine.[33] This premise, valid in human urine which serves as a good medium for bacterial growth, does not always hold for canine and particularly feline urine, with extremes of urine osmolality and pH less favorable to bacterial replication.[33] Nor does this premise hold in animals recently receiving antimicrobial therapy. Consequently, UTI may be present in the cat (and dog) with colony counts less than 100,000/ml.[29, 33-35] Only urine obtained by cystocentesis will reliably identify UTI in such patients.

Even very low numbers of contaminating organisms will be detrimental in the management of dogs with UTI. Although urethral contaminants are frequently gram positive organisms, the clinician managing a patient with UTI will be unable to reliably separate the infecting organism from the contaminant, and accordingly may use inappropriate antimicrobial therapy.

Urine for quantitative culture should be processed as soon as possible. False negative and positive results have been reported with storage at room temperature for as little as two to three hours.[36] If not cultured within 30 minutes, urine should be refrigerated (39°F, 4°C), preferably for six hours or less.[36] False negative samples may result if the sample is frozen or kept in the refrigerator over 24 hours.[36, 37] If longer periods are required, support medium should be used, after quantitative culture with calibrated loops (0.01 or 0.001 ml). A storage medium may allow storage of urine for quantitative culture in the refrigerator for up to 72 hours.[28, 38]

Urine for culture may also be obtained at surgery by cystocentesis or pyelocentesis or ureteral catheterization. Percutaneous nephropyelocentesis, a technique wherein an arterial or catheter needle is inserted into

TABLE 112–1. IDENTIFICATION OF COMMON UROPATHOGENS[21, 31]

Organism (Prevalence %)	Gram Stain	Blood Agar	MacConkey's Agar
E. coli (38%)	Negative rods	Gray, opaque, smooth colonies, may be hemolytic	Red colonies
Klebsiella spp. (8%)	Negative rods	Mucoid, gray-white colonies	Red-tinged, often slimy colonies
Proteus spp. (16%)	Negative rods	Confluent swarming colonies	Colorless colonies
Pseudomonas spp. (3%)	Negative rods	Gray or green colonies with metallic sheen, fruity or ammonia odor, often hemolytic	Colorless colonies
Streptococcus (alpha) (10%)	Positive cocci	Tiny pinpoint colonies, partial hemolysis (green)	No growth
Staphylococcus (14%)	Positive cocci	White or yellow opaque colonies, frequently hemolytic	No growth

the renal pelvis visualized by use of excretory urography and fluoroscopy, represents an alternative for demonstrating upper UTI.[39] This technique may be enhanced if the renal pelvis is dilated by an abdominal compression band. Cultures of renal or bladder mucosal biopsies or the center of a urolith represent alternatives for documentation of UTI.

For a discussion of antibiotic sensitivity testing, see the section on UTI.

RADIOGRAPHY

With the noted exceptions of emphysematous cystitis and radiopaque calculi, contrast radiographs are required to identify most urinary tract abnormalities.[23, 40, 41] Positive, negative, and double contrast cystography will aid in the identification of mucosal irregularities, changes in bladder wall thickness, diverticula, leakage or rupture, and luminal filling defects (Figure 112–4). To avoid fatal air embolization, carbon dioxide is preferable to air for negative contrast.[42–44] Overdistention of the bladder during retrograde urethrocystography may be associated with vesicoureteral reflux, or hemorrhagic cystitis and development of urinary tract infection.[45, 46] Retrograde positive contrast urethrography or voiding cystourethrography will allow visualization of urethral luminal filling defects, anatomic abnormalities, and leaks. In interpretation of urethrograms it is difficult to distinguish between urethral spasms and anatomic strictures.[23, 47] Excretory urography is useful in assessing diseases of the bladder trigone.

Positive contrast vagino-urethrography involves placement of a Foley catheter in the female dog's vestibule for injection of positive contrast material (approximately 0.3 to 0.5 ml/lb or 0.6 to 1.0 ml/kg).[48] It is generally

TABLE 112–2. NUMBER OF BACTERIA PER MILLILITER CONSIDERED SIGNIFICANT ACCORDING TO METHOD OF URINE COLLECTION IN DOGS[21] AND CATS[339]

Method of Collection	Dog	Cat
Cystocentesis	>0*	>0*
Catheterization	>100,000	>1000
Voided	†	>10,000

*Reliability of low colony counts (<1000) is dependent upon good cystocentesis technique.

†A colony count >100,000 is suspicious in a voided specimen, although this occurs in 35% of samples from normal dogs.

performed with the aid of sedation or anesthesia and usefulness may be enhanced with fluoroscopy. This technique outlines the vagina, urethra, and ectopic ureters if they communicate with the vagina.

Since hypertonic radiographic contrast media will falsely increase urine specific gravity, cause cell shrinkage and fragmentation, and may produce false positive reactions for protein and glucose in urine,[49] urinalysis and urine cytology should be performed prior to radiographic contrast studies.

ULTRASONOGRAPHY

Real-time ultrasonography complements radiography in evaluation of the urinary bladder, particularly in cases involving luminal filling defects (Figure 112–5).[41, 50] It has the added advantage of not requiring invasive catheterization or contrast injection.

BLADDER/URETHRAL ENDOSCOPY

Urethral diameter and length have been limiting factors in application of endoscopy to the lower urinary tract of dogs and cats. The mucosal surface of the urethra and bladder can be visualized and biopsied with standard cystoscopy in medium to large female dogs.[51, 52] An arthroscope may be used in some smaller female dogs.

A recent study reported results of diagnostic cystoscopy and urethroscopy in 38 clinical canine cases.[53] Use of a 3.6 mm diameter flexible fiberoptic pediatric bronchoscope was possible in 13/21 (62 per cent) of male dogs ranging in size from 20 to 55 lb (9.5 to 25 kg).[53] The os penis was the limiting factor in eight dogs, many of which were medium or large breed dogs. In 25 of 27 female dogs (weight ranging from 13 to 33 lb), a 10 to 13 French sized rigid pediatric cystoscope or resectoscope was used. The two female dogs in which passage of the endoscope was not possible had urethral tumors.

Prepubic percutaneous cystoscopy utilizing a laparoscope or arthroscope has been described in cats and dogs.[54]

Vaginoscopy may be used to visualize the urethral meatus in the female dog.

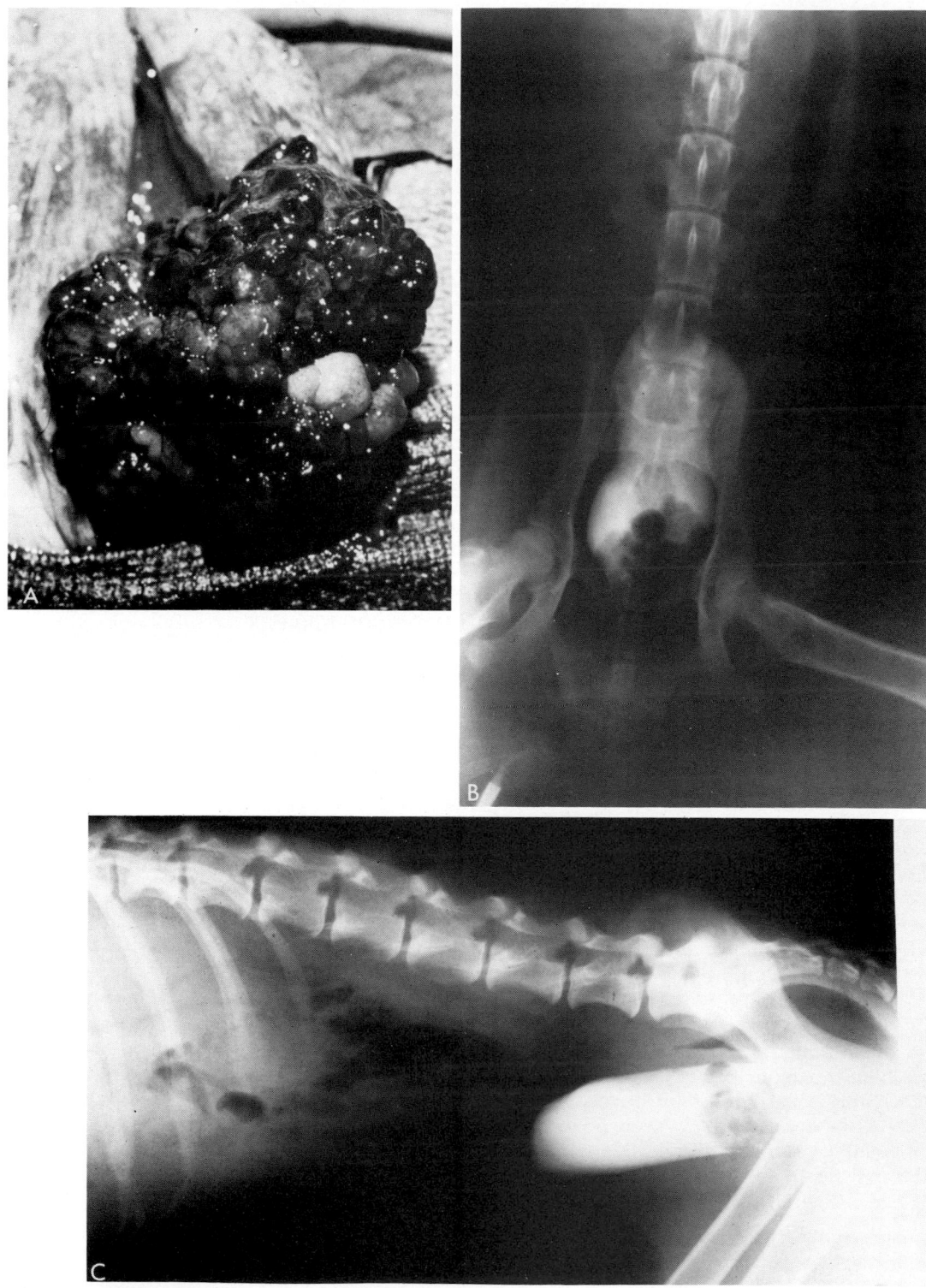

FIGURE 112–4. Malignant tumor of the bladder. *A,* Embryonal rhabdomyosarcoma of the urinary bladder in a nine-month-old Doberman pinscher. *B,* Ventrodorsal and *C,* lateral views, using positive-contrast radiography and showing the mass in the trigone area. (From Greene RW, Scott RC: Diseases of the bladder and urethra. *In* Ettinger SJ (ed): Textbook of Veterinary Internal Medicine. Philadelphia, WB Saunders Co, 1983, p 1910.)

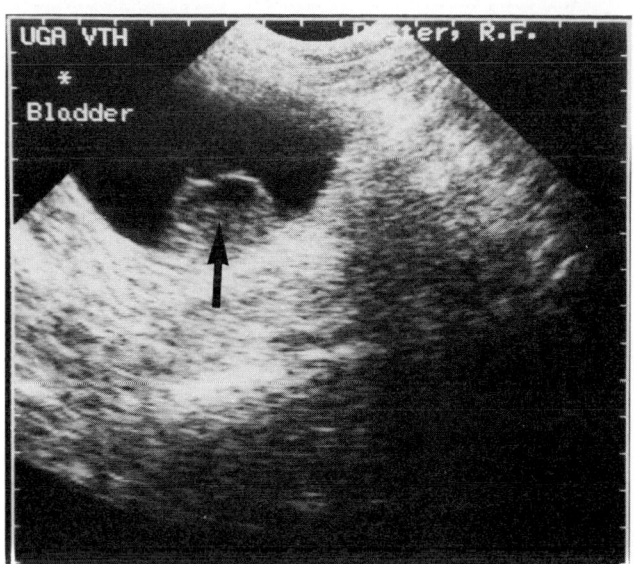

FIGURE 112–5. Real time ultrasonography of a bladder transitional cell carcinoma (arrow) in a nine-year-old female mixed breed.

BLADDER/URETHRAL BIOPSY

A catheter biopsy technique for the lower urinary tract has been described.[55] With this technique a urinary catheter is positioned at the suspected lesion site by palpation or radiography, negative pressure is applied with a 12-ml syringe containing a small amount of saline, and the catheter is moved back and forth over the lesion. Following slow release of the negative pressure, the catheter is removed and the sample evaluated cytologically and histologically if large enough.

Surgery and cystoscopy/urethroscopy are alternative methods of visualizing and obtaining a biopsy of lesions of the lower urinary tract.

CYSTOMETRY AND URETHRAL PROFILOMETRY

Cystometry is the recording of changes in intravesicular pressure during filling and contraction of the bladder (see Chapter 30).[23, 56] During controlled infusion of carbon dioxide, relaxation of the normal bladder results in no rise in pressure until detrusor contraction. This technique may detect failure of the detrusor to contract, changes in bladder capacity, changes in bladder wall compliance, and heightened reactivity of the bladder (spasticity).

Urethral profilometry is used to evaluate urethral function in incontinent dogs (see Chapter 30). This technique measures pressure exerted by the urethral musculature during controlled infusion of saline.[23, 56, 57] Frequently an electromyogram of the striated urethral musculature is obtained simultaneously by means of a modified catheter. This technique may detect reductions or localized increases in urethral pressure or reduction in functional urethral length.

Simultaneous cystometry and uroflowmetry in dogs involves percutaneous antepubic placement of a urinary bladder catheter for measurement of vesicular pressure simultaneously with measurement of urine flow during micturition. This technique is useful in assessment of incontinent animals, particularly those with functional outflow obstruction, as it allows study of both storage and voiding phases of micturition.[58, 59]

ANATOMIC DEFECTS OF THE BLADDER

Urinary bladder duplication, dysplasia, hypoplasia, agenesis, and exstrophy (absence of ventral bladder and abdominal wall) have been reported, often in association with other urinary tract defects.[3, 60-66] Diagnosis is by physical examination, observation of micturition, and contrast radiography. Clinical signs and therapy are dependent upon the type of defect present, and may include surgery or urinary diversion procedures.

PARASITES OF THE LOWER URINARY TRACT

Three nematode parasites, *Capillaria plica*, *Capillaria feliscati*, and *Dioctophyma renale*, infect the lower urinary tract of domesticated small animals.[67-75]

CAPILLARIA PLICA

C. plica uncommonly infects the urinary tract of the dog.[30, 31, 39] The adults are yellow thread-like nematodes reaching lengths of 60 mm, barely visible grossly. The prevalence of infection in the dog is low compared to the fox (23.5 per cent prevalence in wild foxes in Netherlands) and raccoon (> 50 per cent prevalence in raccoons in the southeastern United States) which likely represent the natural definitive hosts.[76, 77] However, high prevalence of infection may develop in kennels where soil or grass surfaces are employed.[68]

Bipolar ova are passed in the urine and subsequently embryonate. Ova containing the first stage larva are ingested by earthworms and develop to the infective stage. Other intermediate hosts have not been identified. Following ingestion of the infected earthworm patent infection develops in dogs in 61 to 88 days.[68] Adults invade the mucosa of the urinary bladder, ureter, and renal pelvis, producing a mild superficial inflammatory response.[68]

While dysuria and hematuria may be present in heavy infections, clinical signs are usually absent in dogs and cats infected with *Capillaria* spp.[68, 70, 71]

Diagnosis depends on demonstration of the characteristic ova in the urine sediment of affected dogs. There is no information on the prevalence of occult infection.

Treatment of individual dogs is usually not necessary since affected animals often develop negative ovum counts within 12 weeks.[68] Successful treatment has been reported with fenbendazole (23 mg/lb or 50 mg/kg daily for 3 to 10 days).[78] Albendazole (23 mg/lb or 50 mg/kg q12h for 10 to 14 days) is effective, but frequently causes anorexia at this dose.[68]

CAPILLARIA FELISCATI

C. feliscati is a trichurid nematode that infects the urinary bladder of the domestic cat. For unknown reasons the prevalence is high in Australia, reportedly 18 to 34 per cent.[69-72] There are few reports of the parasite in the United States.[79, 80,]

Life cycle details are unknown. Bipolar ova are reportedly present in the urine of all infected cats and are similar morphologically to those of *C. plica*, measuring 50 to 68 μm long by 22 to 32 μm wide. Urine contamination of feces have apparently resulted in spurious reports of feline whipworm infection.[79]

Treatment is not necessary unless clinical signs are present. Successful treatment has been reported with methyridine (90 mg/lb or 200 mg/kg orally, single dose), which is unavailable in the United States.[70, 81] Levamisole is reportedly effective, but toxicity limits its usefulness in cats.[81] Fenbendazole (11 mg/lb or 25 mg/kg q12h for 10 days) has been recommended.[75] One case of feline urinary capillariasis treated with fenbendazole had negative ova counts by day 7, remained negative at day 21, but was again shedding ova 2 months later.[82] Whether this represented treatment failure or reinfection could not be determined.

DIOCTOPHYMA RENALE

D. renale parasitizes dogs, cats, and other mammals.[73, 74] Although the adult generally is in the abdominal cavity or kidney, it has been reported in the urethra and urinary bladder of the dog.[74] Diagnosis is by demonstration of the characteristic ova in urine or abdominal fluid.

BACTERIAL URINARY TRACT INFECTION

DEFINITIONS

Cystitis is inflammation of the urinary bladder. The most common cause in the dog is bacterial infection; most cases in the cat are idiopathic (see Chapter 110).[83] Other causes of urinary tract infection may include viruses, fungi, algae, and yeast.[3, 84-88] Noninfectious causes of bladder inflammation include urolithiasis (see Chapters 110 and 111), neoplasia, chemicals, trauma, and primary inflammatory conditions.

Bacterial urinary tract infection (UTI) is the invasion of the urinary tract by bacteria, which reportedly occurs at some time in the life of 14 per cent of all dogs.[31] Surveys of the canine population have reported the prevalence of significant bacteriuria to be 5 to 27 per cent, with prevalence in females generally higher.[21, 89, 90]

Bacterial urethritis, cystitis, ureteritis, and pyelonephritis refer to bacterial invasion of the kidney(s), ureter(s), bladder, and urethra respectively. Occasionally bacterial invasion is limited to the urine only (bacteriuria). Since bacteriuria is an abnormal condition which can not be distinguished from tissue invasion clinically, the clinician should assume the identification of significant bacteriuria (see Table 112–2) is synonymous with invasion of the urinary tract (UTI).

Gram-negative fecal flora are the predominant uropathogens in the dog, with gram-positive organisms accounting for approximately 25 per cent of naturally occurring UTI.[29, 91] The most commonly isolated causes of UTI in dogs are *Escherichia coli*, *Staphylococcus* spp., *Proteus* spp., *Klebsiella* spp., and *Streptococcus* spp.[29, 32, 37, 91-94] Although *Proteus* was the most prevalent bacterial isolate in female dogs in one study, most have identified *E. coli* as the most common isolate.[29, 32, 37, 91, 95] The organisms most frequently associated with bacterial UTI in cats have been *E. coli*, *Pasteurella* spp., *Proteus* spp., *Staphylococcus* spp., and *Streptococcus* spp.[32, 91]

Polymicrobic (multiple isolates) infections are uncommon (7.9 per cent in the dog and 1.9 per cent in the cat), although a prevalence rate as high as 18 per cent has been reported for the dog.[91, 96] Anaerobic UTI is rare.[95, 97]

CONSEQUENCES OF UTI

Sequelae to UTI include septicemia, discospondylitis, urolithiasis, incontinence, prostatitis, pyelonephritis, renal failure, and potentially bladder neoplasia.[31, 98-100] In humans, over 50 per cent of gram-negative septicemias originate from the genitourinary tract.[98] The combination of UTI and diagnostic/therapeutic instrumentation of the urinary tract (endoscopy or urethral catheterization) enhances the risk, particularly in immunocompromised patients.[31] UTI with urease-positive organisms (especially *Staphylococcus aureus* and *S. intermedius* and *Proteus* spp.) is a causative factor in the development and recurrence of struvite calculi (see Chapter 111). Urinary incontinence may result from interference with smooth muscle function causing urethral incompetence or inflammation causing detrusor hyperactivity (see Chapter 30).[37, 101] Chronic renal infection may result in scarring and renal failure.[31, 102, 103] Commonly, infection will spread to the prostate gland in the male and possibly spermatic cord and testicles, leading to bacterial prostatitis and infertility. Finally, byproducts of chronic inflammation may be carcinogenic.[104]

NORMAL DEFENSE MECHANISMS OF THE LOWER URINARY TRACT

"It is generally accepted that . . . UTI will develop only if compromised host defenses allow entrance and proliferation of opportunistic microbes."[105] Bacteria may reach the normally sterile areas of the urinary tract from several routes: ascending, hematogenous, lymphogenous, or extension from adjacent tissue.[22] Ascending is the most common path.[21, 22, 37] Consequently the host defenses of most importance are those preventing ascent of bacteria. The importance of normal host defense mechanisms is pointed out by studies indicating that instillation of bacteria into the bladder of normal dogs will cause bacterial cystitis only when compromise of normal host defense mechanisms is present.[106]

Normal host defenses consist of anatomic, physical, microbiologic, chemical, and immunologic barriers to colonization of the urinary tract. The possibility of the presence of abnormal host defense mechanisms should be suspected in any animal developing a UTI. Sometimes identification of a UTI is the only clinical clue to the presence of a serious polysystemic disease in a patient. The veterinarian must be alert to the fact that certain therapeutic or diagnostic manipulations compromise host resistance.

ANATOMIC BARRIERS—NORMAL

The length and diameter of the urethra, particularly in the male dog, reduces the potential for colonization of the urinary tract by uropathogens. The increased tone of the midurethra and the vesicourethral junction act to localize the initial battlefield to the distal urethra, where normal flora can readily colonize and may potentially ascend the urethra by inherent mobility and progressive growth.[107]

The intact urothelium serves as a mechanical barrier to bacterial colonization. A direct antibacterial effect of urothelium has been proposed.[105, 107] The surface of the proximal urethral epithelium contains folds termed microplicae which may be responsible for the lack of normal flora in the proximal urethra.[108] Bacterial adherence to the mucosal surfaces of the lower urinary tract is achieved by molecular binding of the adhesin portions of bacterial surface fimbriae/fibrillae to surface receptors of the urothelium.[107] Glycosaminoglycans, secreted by the mucosa, play a vital role in prevention of UTI by serving as a surface layer which reduces bacterial adherence.[107, 109]

ANATOMIC BARRIERS—ABNORMAL

In the female, an anatomically shorter urethra and proximity of the external orifice to the rectal flora may predispose to UTI.

Mechanical disruption of the normal urothelial surface, such as occurs with urolithiasis, urethral catheterization, or neoplasia, will alter this defense against uropathogens. Some anatomic abnormalities (e.g., ectopic ureters, urethral incompetence, urethrorectal fistula, bladder exstrophy) or therapeutic manipulations (e.g., catheterization, cystoscopy) may bypass the host defense inherent in normal anatomy, increasing the likelihood of UTI. Other anatomic abnormalities (e.g., bladder diverticulum) may allow the sequestration of bacteria.

The surface glycosaminoglycan layer can be disrupted by acid or povidone iodine, allowing bacterial adherence to urothelium.[107, 110] As production of this protective layer is under hormonal control in rabbits,[107] its reduction may predispose ovariohysterectomized pets to UTI. Alternatively, some *E. coli* are nephritogenic, their adherence fimbriae allowing them to ascend the urinary tract of normal people.[111]

PHYSICAL FLOW OF URINE—NORMAL

The unidirectional flow of urine acts to mechanically remove bacteria.[105, 107] This effect occurs at all levels of the urinary tract, though its importance in preventing UTI is most significant in the ureters and lower urinary tract. This effect is dependent upon unidirectional flow and complete emptying of the urinary bladder.

PHYSICAL FLOW OF URINE—ABNORMAL

Foreign bodies (e.g., urethral catheter), urine retention (e.g., bladder atony, neurogenic bladder dysfunction, bladder diverticula), partial or complete urethral obstruction (e.g., urethral tumor or urolith), or anatomic anomalies creating turbulent or static flow (e.g., urethral stenosis) all predispose to UTI by altering this mechanical clearing of bacteria.

Vesicoureteral reflux (see Chapter 108) appears to represent a primary method for extension of lower urinary tract infection to the upper urinary tract.[27, 112] Young age (less than six months old) and manual bladder expression are known predisposing factors in dogs.[27]

MICROBIOLOGIC FLORA—NORMAL

While bacteria are not normally found in the proximal urethra, the canine vulva, vagina, prepuce, and distal urethra are colonized by commensal organisms (predominantly gram positive).[32] The most commonly identified organisms are *Staphyloccus aureus*, *Streptococcus canis*, *Corynebacterium* spp., and *E. coli*.[26, 113, 116]

The importance of bacterial interference from normal flora in prevention of UTI is controversial.[117, 118] However, to be a successful lower urinary tract inhabitant, a bacterium must compete for nutrients in a limited environment with many other species.[107] Consequently, the normal flora of the distal urethra, vagina, and prepuce act as competitive inhibitors of urinary tract pathogens.[118] To avoid mechanical removal by urine flow, a pathogen must bind to the urothelium by way of bacterial adhesin–urothelial receptor interaction. Normal flora may occupy these urothelial binding sites, preventing establishment of uropathogens. Finally, byproducts of normal floral metabolism may be toxic to other bacteria (bacteriocins).[107, 117]

MICROBIOLOGIC FLORA—ABNORMAL

Alterations in lower urogenital tract flora may play a role in development of UTI. Uropathogen colonization (altered flora) of the vulva and/or urethra may precede development of UTI and be associated with recurrent UTI in women.[119, 120]

CHEMICAL DEFENSE—NORMAL

Although the antibacterial properties of urine are relatively unimportant in human beings, high osmolality and pH extremes frequently present in dog and cat urine are unfavorable for growth of many bacterial species, particularly rods.[33, 105, 121]

Prostatic and vaginal secretions may be antibacterial.[101, 122] The role of these secretions in reducing the prevalence of urinary tract infections in the dog and cat remains to be verified. The absence of prostatic antibacterial factor may contribute to the apparent increased incidence of UTI in female dogs.[89, 101]

CHEMICAL DEFENSE—ABNORMAL

Polyuric states (e.g., polyuric renal failure, diabetes mellitus, hypercortisolism) will result in reduced urine osmolality, favoring bacterial growth.[101, 105, 123] Although polyuric states enhance mechanical bacterial clearance, alterations in chemical composition associated with polyuria (reduced osmolality) apparently override this beneficial effect in the lower urinary tract.[33, 101, 105] Additionally, urine retention in polyuric animals may result in bladder distention with reduction in mucosal antibacterial effects (reduced mucosal blood flow and reduced bladder surface area to volume ratio).[37] Hyperglycemia or primary renal glucosuria may enhance bacterial growth (see Emphysematous Cystitis below).[124]

IMMUNOLOGY—NORMAL

Although opsonization and complement-mediated lysis are unlikely to play an important role in defense against uropathogens, secretory immunoglobulins in vaginal mucus and urine may block bacterial adherence, reducing migration of bacteria from the distal urethra to the bladder.[101, 107] Other roles for systemic and local immunity in preventing infection appear to be minor.

IMMUNOLOGY—ABNORMAL

Some women with recurrent infections have reduced levels of secretory IgA in urine and/or mucosal secretions.[120, 125] The role of the secretory immune system in naturally occurring canine and feline UTI has not been evaluated, although recurrent UTI represents a significant problem.[31]

COMPROMISE OF HOST DEFENSE

Some disease states or therapeutic manipulations have been associated with an increased risk for development of UTI in dogs and cats, including hypercortisolism, diabetes mellitus, and urinary catheterization.

EXCESS GLUCOCORTICOIDS

Long-term administration of glucocorticoids was associated with the development of UTI (defined by urine culture) in 39 per cent of 71 dogs undergoing therapy for dermatologic disease.[94] There were no differences in prevalence of UTI with regards to method of dosing (alternate day versus daily administration), steroid dosage, or duration of therapy. Females and castrated males had a significantly greater frequency of infection. In dogs on steroid therapy that developed UTI, clinical signs of UTI were identified in less than 40 per cent of dogs and pyuria was present in only 54 per cent of cases. A high prevalence (50 to 69 per cent) of UTI and a lack of concurrent pyuria in dogs with spontaneous hyperadrenocorticism have been noted previously.[126, 127]

Hypothesized reasons for the high prevalence of UTI include reduced urine osmolality (reduced urine antibacterial effect) and reduced immunocompetence.[94] The antiinflammatory effects of glucocorticoids may explain the frequent lack of clinical signs and pyuria. These results indicate that all dogs with hypercortisolism (spontaneous or therapeutic) are at risk for the development of UTI, and routine urine culture (at least every three months) is indicated, regardless of results of urinalysis or clinical evaluation.

DIABETES MELLITUS

Several authors have indicated diabetic dogs and cats may be at an increased risk for the development of UTI.[94, 101, 128] However, controlled studies have not evaluated this issue. In one large study, bacteriuria was frequently identified in diabetic dogs, but method of collection and quantitation of bacteriuria were not reported.[128] Urinary tract infection was documented in 18 per cent of dogs on follow-up examination.[128] Whether this prevalence rate is greater than nondiabetic age matched controls subjected to similar diagnostic and therapeutic maneuvers is unknown (prevalence of bacteriuria in clinically asymptomatic female dogs is reportedly as high as 26.6 per cent).[89] Once an infection becomes established in a diabetic human or animal, the potential for serious sequelae is present. In the setting of immunocompromise and glucosuria, pyelonephritis or emphysematous cystitis may develop.[124, 129–131]

CATHETERIZATION

Procedures involving the genitourinary tract (e.g., urethral catheterization, cystoscopy, vaginoscopy) will increase the likelihood of UTI by bacterial contamination, alteration of normal flora, and compromise of normal host defense mechanisms (urothelial interruption).

Intermittent catheterization induced UTI in 20 per cent of adult female dogs.[25] Repeated intermittent catheterization of male dogs led to UTI.[132] Indwelling closed (continuous sterile drainage system closed to environmental contamination) catheterization in clinical management of cats and dogs resulted in the development of UTI in 52 per cent of animals.[133] The risk of infection increased with duration of catheterization. Infection was noted in 8/12 normal male cats within three days of open (collection system open to environment) catheterization.[35, 134] Bacteriuria developed after five days of open catheterization in 4/8 healthy male cats, and 7/12 male cats with perineal urethrostomies.[34] The risk to cats of indwelling catheters in the management of feline lower urinary tract disease (including obstructive urolithiasis) is probably enhanced by the presence of inflammatory lesions of the bladder mucosa.

While catheter-induced bacteriuria may spontaneously resolve in normal animals, 60 per cent of cats with perineal urethrostomy remained infected 85 days following catheter-induced UTI.[34] In a prospective clinical trial, antibiotic therapy during indwelling catheterization reduced occurrence of UTI, but contributed to infection with resistant *Pseudomonas* spp. or *Proteus* spp.[133] Similarly, treatment of healthy cats with open indwelling catheters tended to increase development of UTI by antibiotic resistant gram-negative rods.[35] The reduction in bacteriuria from systemic antibiotic therapy is probably not worth the attendant risk of development of resistant UTI.[35, 133, 135]

In contrast to the case with indwelling urinary catheters, systemic antibiotic therapy may be of value in single diagnostic catheterizations.[136] The goal is to sterilize the urine before tissue invasion is achieved. Ampicillin, amoxicillin, or penicillin may be effective in short course or single dose therapy, because of rapid urinary excretion.[136]

Indwelling catheters should be used only when indicated, such as in the management of critically ill patients or in postobstructive management of patients with persistent urethral stenosis or bladder atony.[116] While both frequent intermittent catheterization and indwelling catheterization are associated with an increased risk for the development of UTI compared to a single diagnostic catheterization, intermittent catheterization may be preferable.[136]

Catheters may introduce bacteria into the urinary bladder by three routes: transport of bacteria into the bladder with the catheter, retrograde flow of contaminated urine from the collection system, and movement of bacteria along the mucous layer between the outside of the catheter and the urethral mucosa.[135] Use of careful aseptic technique will minimize but not eliminate the first.[136] A closed urine drainage system will minimize the second.[133, 135] The third mechanism is probably the most significant in properly managed closed drainage systems. Clinical trials in human beings have indicated that infecting organisms often colonize the urethral meatus prior to ascent into the lower urinary tract.[135]

Appropriate indwelling catheter care includes aseptic placement of an adequately lubricated soft sterile catheter, use of a closed catheter drainage system, positioning of the drainage bag below the level of the patient, addition of antiseptic to the drainage bag (60 ml of 1:500 chlorhexidine or 30 ml of three per cent hydrogen peroxide per liter), aseptic catheter care with minimal manipulation, avoiding obstruction and use of retrograde flush, avoiding disconnection and resultant contamination at catheter ports, washing hands between patients, withholding antimicrobial therapy until after catheter removal, and urine culture and sensitivity following removal of the catheter.

Since even a single intermittent catheterization may induce bacteriuria in normal dogs, urine culture and sensitivity is appropriate following any catheterization. Because of the high prevalence of UTI in animals with indwelling catheters, urine culture and sensitivity should be performed following removal. Alternatively, if the animal was not on antibiotic therapy during catheterization, culture may be performed following a 14 day course of ampicillin or trimethoprim-sulfa therapy.

Diagnosis of UTI

CLINICAL SIGNS

Clinical signs characteristic of lower urinary tract infection include hematuria, stranguria, dysuria, pollakiuria, and inappropriate urination (see Chapters 30 through 32). These clinical signs are not specific for UTI, since such diverse diseases as urolithiasis, neoplasia, and trauma cause similar signs. Signs of systemic illness, such as fever and vomiting, are not associated with lower UTI. If present, disease of other organs should be considered. Veterinary patients with urinary tract infection may have no clinical signs.[21, 94] Since the sequelae of UTI occur independently of clinical signs, a finding of significant bacteriuria warrants therapy, regardless of the presence or absence of clinical signs.[31]

PHYSICAL EXAMINATION

The bladder may be contracted and painful on abdominal palpation. Cystic calculi or bladder wall thickening (usually diffuse in bacterial cystitis) may be noted.

LABORATORY FINDINGS

The hemogram and clinical chemistries are usually normal in simple lower urinary tract infection. Abnormalities indicative of systemic disease may be present in complicated UTI.

RADIOGRAPHIC FINDINGS

Radiographic or other imaging studies may be of value in assessment of UTI, to determine localization of infection or identify the presence of complicating factors. Thickened bladder wall, anatomic anomalies, urolithiasis, or bladder masses (neoplastic or inflammatory) may be identified as supportive evidence. However, radiographs are not useful in establishing the diagnosis of UTI.

URINALYSIS

The diagnosis of bacterial cystitis relies upon results of urinalysis and urine culture (see section on diagnostic techniques). A complete urinalysis is the cheapest, most rapid method for identification of UTI. Hematuria, pyuria, proteinuria, and bacteriuria are findings characteristic of UTI.

The urine may be cloudy and hemorrhagic with a foul odor. Foul odor from formation of ammonia or the presence of byproducts of enteric bacterial metabolism or red discoloration from hematuria or hemoglobinuria may be present as supportive evidence of UTI.[21] Although urine specific gravity may be reduced in bacterial pyelonephritis, it can be any value in UTI. Alkalinuria, which can also be a normal finding, may result from infection by urea-splitting bacteria (usually *Staphylococcus* spp. or *Proteus* spp.).

Proteinuria is generally present in UTI and is due to leakage of plasma proteins (measured in gm/dl) across the inflamed bladder mucosa into the urine (measured in mg/dl).

Hematuria (> 5 RBC per HPF) and pyuria (> 5 to 8 WBC per HPF in midstream voided and > 3 WBC per HPF in cystocentesis samples)[21] are supportive of urinary tract inflammation, especially in the presence of proteinuria. The presence of white blood cell casts, red blood cell casts, or increased numbers of granular casts is supportive of a finding of renal inflammation. These findings, while supportive of inflammation, do not establish the etiology.[37]

Alternatively, UTI may exist with no urinalysis abnormalities, particularly in dogs with spontaneous or therapeutic hypercortisolism.[21, 94, 126]

URINE CULTURE

The laboratory findings of proteinuria, hematuria, and pyuria are generally indicative of urinary tract inflammation or hemorrhage. Identification of bacteriuria is the only reliable evidence of UTI. Quantitative urine culture is used to establish the diagnosis of UTI; qualitative urine culture is used to identify the infecting organism and select the appropriate antibiotic.

Antibiotic Sensitivity Testing. Therapeutic studies have demonstrated the reliability of *in vitro* testing in demonstrating the efficacy of antibiotic treatment of UTI *in vivo.*[137–146] Determination of bacterial sensitivity to antimicrobials is generally done by one of two in vitro techniques, the disc diffusion method and the determination of the minimum inhibitory concentration (MIC). With the exception of nitrofurantoin which is tested at urine concentrations, the Kirby-Bauer (disc diffusion) method is based on the susceptibility of microbes to levels of antimicrobials normally present in the serum. Since the concentration of antimicrobial is generally 10 to 100 times greater in urine than serum, this method is a reliable predictor of bacterial sensitivity but not resistance (i.e., bacteria sensitive to an antimicrobial at serum concentrations would be expected to be sensitive to the high levels normally present in the urine). A disc diffusion prediction of resistance is not a reliable result. A preferable method of sensitivity testing is based upon concentrations of antimicrobials that will inhibit the growth of the microorganism, the minimum inhibitory concentration (MIC). This method allows one to base therapeutic choice on the concentration of antimicrobial present in the urine. A ratio of expected urine antibiotic concentration (see Table 112–6) to MIC greater than four will yield an expected efficacy of about 95 per cent.[31, 147, 148]

All tests are performed *in vitro* and consequently do not take into account factors that may alter antimicrobial effectiveness, factors related to the patient (e.g., reduced renal excretion of antimicrobial in renal dysfunction, effect of polyuric states on antibiotic concentration, urinary catheterization, or immunoincompetence) or factors related to the drug (e.g., method of administration, dosage form, dose, bio-availability, metabolism and excretion rates, and intestinal absorption).[146]

Recommendations for antibiotic therapy will vary depending upon location of infection within the urinary tract. The possible presence of pyelonephritis (see Chapter 108) or prostatitis (see Chapter 105) points out the necessity of considering localization of UTI when making therapeutic decisions.

LOCALIZATION OF URINARY TRACT INFECTIONS

Localization of infection is the process of identifying which anatomic areas of the urinary tract are involved once bacterial UTI is proven. Implicit in the process of localization are three things. First, it is necessary to prove the existence of UTI. Second, identifying UTI is not equivalent to a diagnosis of cystitis, pyelonephritis, or prostatitis and the presence of infection at one site does not eliminate other sites from involvement. Third, localization offers the veterinary clinician and patient advantages in determining prognosis and selecting therapy.

Bacterial infection of different areas of the urinary tract does not carry the same consequences. Bacterial infections of the bladder are seldom associated with the serious consequences of systemic illness and/or progressive renal dysfunction that may occur with pyelonephritis (see Chapter 108).[92, 149] Therapy varies with location of infection, since penetration of antibiotics and degree of tissue invasion by bacteria are often different between upper and lower tract.[92, 149]

Various clinical tools have been utilized to localize UTI. In practice, the lower urinary tract is generally assumed to be involved in all cases of UTI. The key question of localization is whether the infection involves the prostate (see Chapter 105) and/or upper tract (see Chapter 108).

Clinical Signs. Clinical signs characteristic of lower UTI have been described. These are based on various lines of evidence, including clinical impression, isolated autopsy studies, and extrapolation of information from disease in human beings.[92]

Bacterial cystitis/urethritis is usually characterized by dysuria, hematuria, stranguria, inappropriate urination, and/or pollakiuria. Although discomfort may be marked, systemic signs are usually not apparent.

Acute bacterial prostatitis is characterized by abdominal and prostatic pain, fever, and bloody or purulent urethral discharge. Chronic bacterial prostatitis may be manifested as urethral discharge only.

Acute pyelonephritis is associated with fever and lumbar pain, whereas both may be absent in chronic renal infection.

Laboratory Findings. Few laboratory findings are specific for localization. Some findings are supportive of renal involvement, such as the presence of azotemia, leukocytosis, low urine specific gravity, and cylindruria.[92, 149] However, all of these findings may be present in dogs with infection localized to the urinary bladder and in dogs with no UTI. Absence of these laboratory findings does not eliminate pyelonephritis.

Radiography and Other Imaging Modalities. Anatomic changes may provide circumstantial evidence of localization. Without better methods of localization anatomic alterations are presumed evidence of involvement.[92] Diffuse or focal thickening of the bladder wall are consistent with bacterial cystitis. Adequate evaluation of the upper urinary tract frequently requires excretory urography.[92, 150] Lesions demonstrated in dogs with experimental pyelonephritis include slight increase or decrease in kidney size, dilation of the pelvis, and dilation of the ureter within ten days of infection.[144, 186] Changes were not present in all dogs, and renal lesions may be absent radiographically and at gross postmortem examination in acute infections.[92, 150] Alterations in pelvic diverticula or radiodense renoliths may be supportive of renal involvement. Changes associated with feline pyelonephritis have not been as well characterized; however, recent reports and extrapolation from other species would support similar inferences to those outlined above for the dog.[102, 103]

Therapeutic Findings. Resolution of UTI in response to a single dose of an antimicrobial is an empirical method for identification of lower urinary tract infection in human beings.[151, 152] Experimental and clinical trials indicate this method would be unreliable in the dogs.[153, 154]

Special Techniques. Methods for evaluation of prostatic involvement include evaluation of ejaculate or prostatic massage, imaging modalities, and/or biopsy (see Chapter 105). In male dogs with UTI, because of the high prevalence of prostatic involvement, bacterial prostatitis is assumed to be present unless proven otherwise.

Ureteral catheterization allows separation of unilateral from bilateral pyelonephritis and upper from lower UTI, although it risks extension of urinary tract infection to the upper tract in cases where it is not already present. This technique is restricted to patients subjected to surgery or endoscopy.

Nephropyelostomy is a method for localization of infection to the kidney.[39] The technique provides direct evidence of unilateral/bilateral renal infection by obtaining a sample of urine from the renal pelvis; however, it requires sedation/anesthesia and fluoroscopy for reliable collection.

Bladder washout techniques consist of urethral catheterization and instillation of a solution of antibiotic and enzymes (streptokinase, fibrinolysin) into the bladder to kill bacteria.[92, 149, 155] The rapid recurrence of bacteriuria in cases of upper tract infection distinguishes it from lower tract infection where bacteriuria recurs more slowly. Although useful in human infections, its utility was poor in experimental canine UTI.[149]

Antibody-coated bacteria tests are based on the assumption that local production of antibody occurs in renal and/or deep tissue infections but not superficial lower UTI.[93, 149] Bacteria present in urinary sediment are examined with fluorescein-stained anti-globulin.[92, 93, 149] The test is unreliable in the dog, with false positive and false negative test results reported.[93, 149]

In bacterial pyelonephritis, renal damage may result in release of brush border and cytoplasmic enzymes or proximal tubular antigens into the urine.[156–158] Although urinary enzymes or proteins have been employed as an index of renal damage in canine experimental acute renal failure, their clinical usefulness in canine and feline UTI remains to be established.[159, 160]

Tissue biopsy/culture may be diagnostic aids in localization of UTI, particularly in cases of prostatitis or generalized pyelonephritis. Utility is limited by risk of these invasive procedures and the focal medullary location of pyelonephritis which may be missed by a biopsy. Renal cortical tissue is inferior to pelvic or ureteral urine for diagnostic cultures.

Therapy of UTI—General Principles

Successful treatment of UTI requires that the veterinarian adequately characterize the patient's condition and carefully monitor the response to therapy. Although identification of UTI and administration of antibiotic therapy are frequently curative, the clinician should be concerned that unidentified compromise of host defense mechanisms may predispose to recurrence of UTI or development of serious sequelae.

To establish a prognosis and therapeutic plan, it is useful to further subdivide the problem of urinary tract infection in terms of localization (upper or lower), time course (acute or recurrent) and as to the presence or absence of predisposing factors (simple or complicated). Therapy of upper urinary tract infection is discussed elsewhere (see Chapter 108). Acute infections are those not previously treated, characterized by sudden onset of hematuria and dysuria coincident with significant bacteriuria. Complicated infections are present when identifiable abnormalities of the normal host defense mechanism are present, e.g., urolithiasis or ectopic ureters. Because prostatic infection represents a complicating factor which commonly occurs in male dogs, UTI in a male dog is always considered complicated. *Recurrent UTIs* are those recurring following cessation of therapy and are due to either *persistent infections* (relapse or recurrence of same bacterium) or *reinfections* (different microorganism). While recurrent infections may be uncomplicated in theory, they should be assumed complicated until carefully evaluated. With this classification scheme, infections in dogs and cats can be categorized for therapy as either *simple acute, complicated acute,* or *recurrent.*

In general, treatment of UTI is based on identity of the organism rather than antibiotic sensitivity testing. This scheme is based on retrospective analysis of antimicrobial susceptibility patterns of urinary tract pathogens (Table 112–3).[137–146]

Owners should be carefully instructed on the importance of correct administration of medication. Dogs should be encouraged to urinate only immediately prior to the time the owners are due to give the next dose of medication.[31]

In complicated or recurrent UTI, verification of successful therapeutic response is recommended, based

TABLE 112–3. ANTIMICROBIAL SELECTION FOR COMMON UROPATHOGENS

Microbe(s)	Antimicrobial Recommended
Staphylococcus	Penicillins,* Trimethoprim,† Nitrofurantoin, Cephalexin, or Chloramphenicol
Streptococcus	Penicillins* or Trimethoprim†
E. coli	Trimethoprim, Nitrofurantoin, or Cephalexin
Proteus	Penicillins,* Trimethoprim,† or Cephalexin
Pseudomonas	Tetracycline
Klebsiella	Cephalexin or Trimethoprim†
Polymicrobic UTI:	
Staph plus Strep	Penicillins*
Staph/Strep plus *E. coli/Proteus*	Trimethoprim†
Any combination of *E. coli, Proteus, Klebsiella*	Trimethoprim† or Cephalexin
Pseudomonas plus any other microbe	Treat other microbe first, then Tetracycline

*Penicillin, Ampicillin, or Amoxicillin.
†Trimethoprim-Sulfonamide combinations.

upon negative urine culture (cystocentesis sample) three to five days following institution of therapy. Urine culture is superior to urinalysis since as many as 10^4 (rods) to 10^5 (cocci) bacteria per ml may not be detected on sediment examination.[96] If bacteriuria is present during therapy, alternate antimicrobial selections should be considered. Clinical response to therapy is not adequate justification for assuming eradication of infection, since small reductions in number of bacteria may result in remission of signs. Follow-up examination (urine culture and sensitivity) is recommended five to seven days following discontinuation of antibiotic therapy. If therapeutic failure is identified, a reason must be ascertained.

SIMPLE ACUTE UTI

Clinical signs and urinalysis results consistent with simple acute UTI should be evaluated with a urinalysis collected by cystocentesis. Although these infections can be treated empirically with a broad spectrum antibiotic for 10 to 14 days, a urine culture is recommended. Bacterial culture will allow proper choice of antibiotic on the basis of infecting organism (Table 112–3) and knowledge of infecting organism is valuable information in cases of therapeutic failure or recurrence.

COMPLICATED ACUTE UTI

Acute complicated infections are generally associated with prostatic infection (assumed in male dogs), abnormal bladder or urethral function, urinary tract trauma, catheterization, neoplasia, renal infection or failure, urolithiasis, diabetes mellitus, hyperadrenocorticism, prolonged steroid administration, or toxicity (e.g., cyclophosphamide).

A complete urinalysis and quantitative culture of a cystocentesis sample is recommended. Antibiotic sensitivity testing is desirable if previous antibiotic therapy has been administered for any reason. Complete evaluation of the complicating factor(s) is essential. Since prostatic infections are difficult to cure, all male dogs with UTI should be evaluated by cytology and quantitative culture of an ejaculate or a prostatic massage sample (see Chapter 105).

Therapy in male dogs should be maintained for at least 21 days, with careful follow-up. An antimicrobial agent with prostatic penetrance (e.g., chloramphenicol, trimethoprim, carbenicillin, or macrolides) is recommended, depending upon the organism's sensitivity.

Therapy for other complicated infections is dependent upon successful treatment of the underlying complicating factor. If the underlying factor cannot be controlled, successful treatment of UTI may not be possible. With temporary complicating factors (e.g., catheterization or abnormal bladder function), antimicrobial therapy should be withheld until the complicating factor is removed to avoid infection with a resistant organism. Methenamine may be used during this time. Methenamine is generally administered with mandelic or hippuric acid, since methenamine is hydrolyzed to the antibacterial formaldehyde only in the presence of acidic urine.[37] Urine pH (goal <6.0) should be monitored if methenamine is relied upon for ancillary therapy, since additional urinary acidifiers are often required to maintain aciduria.

Therapy for complicated infections requires weeks or months depending on the underlying cause. Urinalysis and urine culture should be performed during therapy, one week and one month after therapy to detect recurrence.

RECURRENT UTI

Recurrent infections may be detected as recurrence of clinical signs or a positive urine culture following discontinuation of antimicrobial therapy. They are either relapsing infections (same microorganism) or reinfections (different microorganism). With some common microorganisms (e.g., *E. coli*), it may be difficult to distinguish between these two, although serotyping or comparison of antimicrobial sensitivity patterns may be of help.

Reinfections. Reinfections actually represent multiple bouts of simple acute UTI, generally attributed to undetectable abnormalities of host defense (e.g., vaginal epithelial abnormalities in women). Management is the same as for simple acute UTI, unless frequent bouts occur. When a high rate of recurrence of UTI is documented (> three per year), low dose (one-third to one-half the normal daily dose) continuous suppressive therapy has been associated with a marked reduction in incidence of reinfection.[31, 96, 145] Underlying complicating factors (e.g., urolithiasis, inflammatory or neoplastic mass, urachal diverticulum, or abnormal bladder function) must be eliminated by careful clinical and radiographic assessment prior to institution of this method of therapy.

Trimethoprim-sulfa, cephalexin, or nitrofurantoin are recommended for dogs with recurrent gram-negative or mixed infections and penicillin G or ampicillin for dogs with gram-positive or *Proteus* UTI.[31, 37, 96, 145] Trimethoprim-sulfa has the added advantage of increased concentration in the secretions of the vagina and urethra.[161] One-half (trimethoprim-sulfa combinations) to one-third the normal daily dose should be administered once daily, at night, with urination prevented for several hours. This method will result in several hours of therapeutic concentrations of antimicrobial and additional contact of microbe to "subtherapeutic" concentrations which may reduce bacterial adherence.[107, 145] The reduced dose schedule should be continued for six months, with monthly culture of cystocentesis samples. If infection is documented on follow-up examination, appropriate antibiotics are administered at standard dosage schedules for 10 to 14 days, with follow-up urine culture at the end of this regimen. If the urine culture is again negative, the once daily regimen is resumed. Following six consecutive months of negative cultures, the low dose suppressive antibiotic therapy may be discontinued. Long-term administration of antibiotics is not risk free; nontoxic antibiotics should be selected. Long-term side effects, such as the occurrence of keratoconjunctivitis sicca or folate deficiency anemia with trimethoprim/sulfa combinations, should be considered. Patients treated with trimethoprim-sulfa for longer than six weeks should receive dietary supplementation with folate.

Persistent or Relapsing UTI. These are infections which do not respond to appropriate therapy or that recur with the same microorganism within a few weeks of discontinuing antimicrobial therapy. Relapses occur because of therapeutic factors such as inappropriate antimicrobial, inadequate dose or length of administration, failure of owner to administer medication, patient factors including predisposing conditions not eliminated, or microbial factors with development of resistance to a previously appropriate antibiotic.

The diagnostic plan must include a careful search for underlying complicating factors. This includes semen cytology and quantitative culture in male dogs, survey radiography, excretory urography, contrast cystography, and ultrasonography (if available). Retrograde urethrography and contrast vaginography are useful in selected cases. Treatment includes resolution of complicating factors if possible. If no underlying factors are identified, chronic infection of the urinary tract should be assumed and localized (e.g., chronic pyelonephritis, chronic cystitis, and/or chronic prostatitis).

Antibiotic sensitivity testing should be performed, with treatment based upon sensitivity and antibiotic penetrance into identified affected organs. MIC determination is preferable, with susceptibility anticipated only if the MIC is < 25 per cent of the mean urine concentration (see Table 112–6). MIC determination is desirable for highly resistant bacteria and complicated or recurrent infections. If the microorganism is highly resistant, urinary antiseptics such as methenamine or nitrofurantoin may be tried. However, with the exception of nitrofurantoin in renal infections, antiseptics are useful only for infections localized to the bladder and urethra.

Antimicrobial therapy should be continued for six to eight weeks. Urinalysis and urine culture should be performed one week after initiation of therapy and immediately prior to discontinuation of therapy. Follow-up urinalysis and urine cultures should be performed one week, one month and two months later.

If the infection relapses again, diagnostic consideration of underlying factors should be reconsidered and therapy reinstituted for four to six months, with cultures repeated as above. Some relapsing infections cannot be cured. As with multiple bouts of simple acute infections (reinfections), continuous nightly administration of reduced dose antimicrobials is the best remaining therapeutic alternative.

Therapeutic Failures. Immediate therapeutic failures are identified during therapy or at reculture five to seven days following discontinuation of therapy. They are generally due to either failure of the drug to reach the pathogen in adequate concentration or failure of the drug to kill the pathogen, despite adequate delivery.[31] Inadequate dose or duration of antimicrobial or failure of the owner to administer the drug could result in failure of drug to reach the pathogen. Although acute infections are generally managed by 10 to 14 days of therapy, chronic infections, particularly those involving the prostate or kidney, may require four to six weeks or longer of therapy. Altered pharmacokinetics, such as

interaction of the drug with food or another drug, failure of drug absorption, or inadequate urinary concentration in renal insufficiency could result in inadequate drug concentrations. The presence of an unidentified nidus for infection (e.g., urolith, deep tissue infection, bladder diverticulum, urinary neoplastic mass) could prevent the drug from reaching the organism. Adequate concentrations of drug may fail to eradicate the UTI in cases of polymicrobic infections, or if the organism was originally or subsequently became resistant to the antimicrobial. While *Staphylococcus* spp., *Streptococcus* spp., *Proteus* spp., and *Pseudomonas* spp. are less likely to acquire resistance during therapy, gram-negative enterics (*E. coli*, *Klebsiella* spp., and *Enterobacter* spp.) rapidly change susceptibility to antimicrobials through acquisition of extrachromosomal DNA (resistance plasmids) which code for resistance.[31] If antibiotic therapy is not effective with two or three appropriate choices, MIC determination should be used as the basis of therapy in these cases. Ninety-five per cent efficacy of therapy is expected when the MIC is < 25 per cent of the mean urine concentration of the antimicrobial (see Table 112–6).

Newer penicillins (e.g., ticarcillin, piperacillin, azlocillin), third generation cephalosporins (e.g., moxalactam, cefotaxime), or quinolones (e.g., ciprofloxacin) may be effective in therapy of highly resistant UTI without the toxicity of the aminoglycosides.[151, 162, 163] Quinolones are nalidixic acid derivatives which do not select for resistance plasmids, spare protective enteric flora, and are effective against β-lactam- and aminoglycoside-resistant microbes.[163] However, quinolones cannot be recommended until there is adequate evaluation of toxicity and pharmacokinetics in the veterinary species.

ANCILLARY THERAPY

A single dose of antibiotic often eradicates lower urinary tract infection in human beings.[151, 152] Single dose therapy is not effective in experimental or clinical canine trials.[153, 154]

Use of alkalinuria to monitor success of therapy or recurrence of infection may be of value in cases of urea-splitting organisms (generally *Staphylococcus* spp. or *Proteus* spp.).[21, 64] Manipulation of urine pH by alkalinization (sodium bicarbonate) or acidification (ammonium chloride) may enhance the activity of antimicrobials.[37] The activity of chloramphenicol, the aminoglycosides, and erythromycin may be enhanced at alkaline pH, while acidification of urine may increase the activity of nitrofurantoin, tetracycline, penicillin, ampicillin, and carbenicillin.[22, 37, 165] Adjustment of urine pH outside of the 5.0 to 7.5 range may enhance its antibacterial effect, although this effect is probably not of great consequence.[165]

Urinary bladder lavage with 3.22 mM EDTA disodium salt–50 mM Tris lavage has been recommended for resistant UTI on the basis of its *in vitro* lysis of *Pseudomonas* spp.[166–168] EDTA-Tris also inhibits the growth of *Staphylococcus aureus* and *Streptococcus* spp. and enhances the uptake of various antimicrobials by *E. coli* and *Proteus vulgaris*.[167, 168] Although an attractive alternative in resistant lower UTI, it requires local instillation (urethral catheterization) and consequently may induce infection with other bacteria. If used, it should be instilled two to three times daily by aseptic intermittent catheterization, left in place for at least 60 minutes, and combined with systemic antibiotic therapy chosen on the basis of MIC. It is worthless for cases with prostatic or renal involvement.

The addition of clavulanic acid (β-lactamase inhibitor) reduced the MIC of amoxicillin for *E. coli* and *Proteus mirabilis in vitro*.[169, 170] Although the anticipated enhancement was not tested *in vivo*, improved efficacy of amoxicillin is expected on the basis of MIC susceptibilities.

Nalidixic acid and methylene blue are urinary antiseptics, antibacterial agents with local rather than systemic effects.[171] They are not commonly used because of toxicities. Nalidixic acid is both neurotoxic and hepatotoxic and methylene blue is associated with oxidative injury to red blood cells, especially in cats.[171, 172]

Cranberry juice (containing quinic acid) and vitamin C (ascorbic acid) have some inherent antibacterial properties aside from their urinary acidifying effect.[101] Their efficacy remains to be established.

Phenazopyridine is an azo dye which when used as a urinary analgesic causes orange discoloration of urine. Its value in canine and feline cystitis has not been substantiated, and it may cause Heinz body hemolytic anemia in cats and acute keratoconjunctivitis sicca in dogs.[173, 174]

Propantheline is a parasympatholytic drug that may reduce urinary incontinence due to spastic detrusor activity associated with bacterial cystitis. Agents with similar effects include butyl hyoscine and aminopromazine (see Chapter 30).

Induction of polyuria with the addition of sodium chloride to the diet has been advocated.[37] This practice will enhance mechanical removal of bacteria. However, it will reduce the antibacterial effect of urine, reduce the concentration of antimicrobials in the urine, and may cause bladder distention with resultant reductions in blood flow and mucosal antimicrobial effect. Reduction of urine specific gravity may be beneficial for infections of the upper urinary tract by reducing medullary hypertonicity and enhancing local host protective mechanisms.[101] Some benefit to forced diuresis has been inferred from studies of acute urethrocystitis in women; however, extrapolations from this disease syndrome to UTI in dogs and cats may not be valid.[152] With the high prevalence of UTI in polyuric states, induction of polyuria cannot be recommended unless its benefit can be verified by experimental or controlled clinical trials.[32, 33, 94, 128]

Emphysematous Cystitis

Occasionally, bacterial metabolism results in accumulation of gas within the wall (emphysematous cystitis) and/or lumen (pneumaturia) of the bladder.[97, 124, 175] This condition has most frequently been reported in diabetic dogs and cats.[124] The increased prevalence in glucosuric diabetic animals has been attributed to gas production by glucose-metabolizing aerobic and anaerobic enteric bacteria.[97, 124] The condition has been reported in nonglucosuric and glucosuric, nondiabetic dogs.[97, 175] Clinical signs are characteristic of lower urinary tract disease, although they may be absent.[124] The condition must be differentiated from other causes of gas within the urinary bladder, such as air introduction associated with urinary catheterization. Diagnosis is based upon the demonstration of gas in the wall of the bladder (more common) or free within the lumen. The patient should be evaluated for glucosuria (see Chapter 108). Treatment is similar to other forms of bacterial cystitis. Response to therapy is usually good, with resolution of emphysema reported with improved regulation of serum glucose alone.[124] The presence of emphysematous cystitis should alert the clinician to the possible presence of glucosuria/diabetes mellitus, with bacterial fermentation of glucose potentially confounding the diagnosis of glucosuria.[124] The presence of emphysematous cystitis should be suspected in difficult to regulate diabetics since elevations of plasma concentrations of glucose counterregulatory hormones (growth hormone, glucagon, cortisol, and epinephrine) are expected in diabetic patients with bacterial infection.[176]

Proliferative Cystitis

Chronic bacterial cystitis in the dog may be associated with submucosal lymphoid proliferation, resulting in a grossly visible irregular mucosal surface, termed follicular cystitis.[3]

Polypoid cystitis is an inflammatory condition of the bladder mucosa, with a variable number of inflammatory polyps protruding from the mucosa into the lumen.[177, 178] It is generally associated with chronic UTI, frequently with multiple therapeutic failures.[177, 178] Whether inflammation associated with UTI leads to polyp formation or vice versa has not been determined. Hematuria, dysuria, and pollakiuria are reported clinically, with pyuria, bacteriuria, and marked hematuria generally found on urinalysis. Diagnosis is by contrast radiography, with small lesions best seen by double contrast cystography (see Figure 112–6). Clinical, radiographic, and labora-

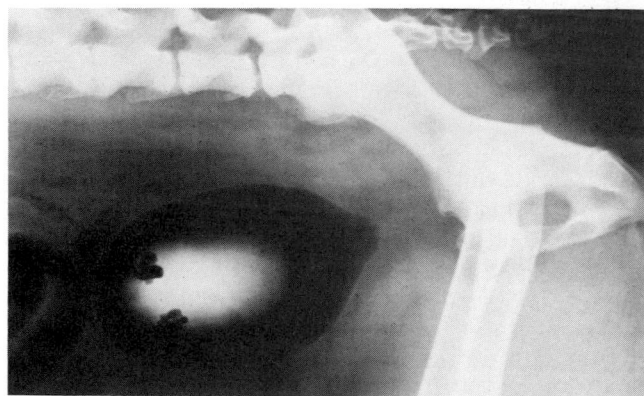

FIGURE 112–6. Double contrast cystography of inflammatory bladder polyps in a three-year-old female chow chow. The polyps were associated with chronic bacterial UTI and multiple therapeutic failures prior to surgical resection.

tory findings are frequently identical to those of urinary bladder neoplasia.[177] Distinguishing features which may help to identify bladder neoplasia include frequent involvement of the trigone, lung metastasis, and/or anaplastic cells in the urine sediment. However, a biopsy is usually required. Therapy of polypoid cystitis is surgical removal and long-term antibiotic therapy (six to eight weeks).

Mycoplasmal UTI

Mycoplasma has previously been isolated from genital tracts of healthy dogs.[113, 179] A role for mycoplasma in UTI has been suggested.[180] *Mycoplasma*, principally *M. canis*, was isolated from cystocentesis samples from dogs. Clinical signs present in the sampled population included pollakiuria, hematuria, stranguria, polyuria, polydipsia, urinary incontinence, and fever.[180] Thirty-two per cent of dogs had a mixed mycoplasmal-bacterial infection. Although many dogs with clinical signs had pure mycoplasmal cultures, the absence of concomitant urinary tract disease potentially responsible for these signs was not documented and 11 of 31 dogs with positive urine mycoplasmal cultures had no clinical signs. Negative cultures were reported following treatment with tylosine (9/9), tetracycline (1/2), and cephalexin (1/1). Although this report documents the presence of mycoplasmal UTI, its clinical significance remains to be established.

Candidal UTI

Urinary tract candidiasis is rare in veterinary medicine.[37, 88] In one report the isolation of *Candida albicans* was reported in 0.6 per cent of urine specimens, although associated clinical signs were not described.[91] Candida are ubiquitous normal gastrointestinal inhabitants. The method of infection is unknown, although compromised host defense is the rule. Urinary tract candidiasis has been associated with indwelling urinary tract catheters, long-term antibiotic or glucocorticoid therapy, and diabetes mellitus.[22, 37, 88]

Diagnosis of candiduria depends on urine sediment examination or culture (Sabouraud's agar or blood agar without cycloheximide). The presence of candiduria is occasionally noted in asymptomatic patients. Treatment is centered on restoration of normal host defenses (e.g., removal of urethral catheter, discontinuation of chronic steroid or broad-spectrum antibiotic therapy, or improved glucose regulation in the diabetic dog or cat). Alkalinization of the urine and ketoconazole therapy have been recommended, but are unlikely to be effective if host defense mechanisms are not restored.

Cyclophosphamide Cystitis

Cyclophosphamide is an alkylating agent frequently used in the management of neoplastic and immune-mediated disorders. Cystitis may result from the presence of its toxic activated metabolites in the urine, which cause urothelial ulceration, necrosis of underlying smooth muscle and vasculature, edema, and hemorrhage.[181] The renal pelves may be similarly affected. Clinical signs which include hematuria, dysuria, stranguria, and pollakiuria are frequently severe. The reported prevalence rate is 6.4 per cent, occurring after a mean duration of cyclophosphamide therapy of 22 weeks.[181] Long-term therapy with intermittent high doses, dehydration during therapy, and concurrent UTI may enhance toxicity.[181] Potential sequelae include development of UTI, since generalized damage to the urothelium and immunosuppression may increase susceptibility to uropathogens.[181, 182] Repair of damage from short-term injury is generally complete within 14 to 21 days; however, long-term sequelae include bladder fibrosis and development of transitional cell carcinoma.[6, 183, 184] Treatment consists of induction of diuresis, withdrawal of cyclophosphamide, and chemical cautery. Methenamine mandelate (4.5 mg/lb or 10 mg/kg orally q6h) may be effective in mild cases.[185] In severe cases local instillation of 1 to 4 per cent formalin (0.4 to 1.5 per cent formaldehyde) may control hematuria of bladder origin.[185–187] (Histologic grade formalin is generally 10 per cent formalin which is 3.7 per cent formaldehyde.) This form of therapy is not risk free, as metabolic acidosis, bladder fibrosis, detrusor spasticity, vesicoureteral reflux, and ureteral stenosis with hydronephrosis all are potential sequelae, especially at higher concentrations of formalin.[187]

Measures to reduce the prevalence of this complication are aimed at minimizing the concentration of toxic metabolites in the urine (e.g., adequate fresh water available at all times and administration of low doses of thiazide or furosemide diuretics or addition of sodium chloride to the diet) and minimizing contact time of metabolites with urine mucosa (e.g., frequent opportunities to void). Frequent small doses (daily versus weekly dosing) and concurrent administration of corticosteroids may reduce toxicity.[181]

Cyclophosphamide has been implicated in the development of transitional cell carcinoma in dogs.[6, 183, 184] Chronic inflammation and immunosuppression are factors that may contribute to Cytoxan tumorigenesis. However, clinical signs of cystitis may be absent in dogs developing transitional cell carcinoma secondary to Cytoxan. Although tumors generally develop after long-term cyclophosphamide therapy (mean duration of therapy of 30 weeks), this complication has been reported after as little as 6 weeks of therapy.[183, 184]

URINARY BLADDER NEOPLASIA

Neoplasms of the lower urinary tract are infrequent, presenting diagnostic dilemmas when present. Because of the nonspecific clinical signs, they are often managed inappropriately as UTI for prolonged periods of time. Consequently, early diagnosis and treatment of lower urinary tract neoplasia is infrequent. This limits the therapeutic options and worsens the prognosis. Veterinary patients with lower urinary tract disease nonresponsive to therapy should be thoroughly evaluated.

Biologic Behavior and Tumor Types

Urinary bladder neoplasia is uncommon in the dog, comprising 0.5 to 1.0 per cent of all canine neoplasia.[188–190] Bladder neoplasia is reportedly rare in the cat, although the prevalence in one study was similar to that for the dog.[188, 191] Most bladder neoplasia in the dog and cat is malignant and primary (Table 112–4).[6, 185, 188–196] Secondary neoplasia, which may metastasize to the bladder from the urethra, prostate, kidney, mammary gland, bowel, ovary, ureter, and bone, comprised 4.6 per cent of canine urinary neoplasia in one study.[188, 190, 196, 197] Secondary tumors include hemangiosarcoma, transitional cell carcinoma, malignant lymphoma, and osteosarcoma.[188, 193, 198] A urinary bladder tumor may occur concurrently with other histologic tumor types present in the bladder or at distant sites.[190] Primary bladder neoplasia usually is locally invasive, with metastasis reported in 27 per cent of canine cases.[188] Local invasion and lymph node metastasis predominate over distant metastasis in clinical disease.[188, 193] The most prevalent tumor of the urinary bladder of both dogs and cats is transitional cell carcinoma.[6, 185, 188, 189, 195–197]

With the exception of embryonal or botryoid rhabdomyosarcoma which occurs in young dogs (mean age 1.7 years, range 1 to 5 years), most bladder tumors occur in older animals (mean age 8.3 years, range 1 to 15 years in dogs; mean age 9.3 years, range 0.33 to 15 years in cats).[193] Other surveys have reported similar results.[188, 189, 196] Female dogs may have a greater relative risk.[185, 189, 190, 193] Sex predilection in cats is unclear.[189, 193, 196] While sex hormones are not implicated directly, some have suggested the reduced prevalence in male dogs may be related to the presence of prostatic secretions or frequent elimination behavior, with reduced contact time of carcinogens to the bladder mucosa.[189, 199, 200] There is a reported increased prevalence in terriers (Cairn, West Highland white, Scottish, and Airedale) in one study and a breed predisposition for Scottish terriers, Shetland sheepdogs, beagles, and collies was suggested in another.[189, 190] Others have reported finding no breed or sex predisposition.[188, 195]

Epithelial Tumors

BENIGN

Papillomas comprised 18 per cent of primary tumors in one study, compared to a 60 per cent prevalence of carcinomas.[188] Papillomas may be single or multiple and may be difficult to distinguish from polyps present in polypoid cystitis.[177, 178] Carcinogenesis studies indicate that papillomas may transform into carcinomas.[188, 197]

MALIGNANT

Although other malignant epithelial tumors have been reported, transitional cell carcinoma is the most prevalent canine and feline bladder tumor (see Table 112–4). The gross appearance of a transitional cell carcinoma may vary from a single papillary growth to a large, ulcerated mass. Reports of bladder tumors show that this tumor type predominates, and characterization of biologic behavior of bladder neoplasia in the dog and cat is generally identical to that of the transitional cell carcinoma. This tumor is locally invasive, frequently involves the trigone of the bladder, and metastases have been identified approximately 50 per cent of the time.[196, 210] Metastasis most frequently occurred to the regional lymph nodes (41 per cent of cases) and lungs (36.4 per cent of cases).[188] Spread was often by local invasion of the prostate, urethra, ureters, rectum, vagina, and uterus.[202] Although distant metastases may occur to essentially any organ, they have been most often reported to the distant lymph nodes, prostate, kidney, brain, uterus, spleen, bone, and liver.[188, 190]

In contrast, metastasis is considerably less frequent with the second most prevalent canine malignant epithelial tumor, the squamous cell carcinoma, reported to occur in < 10 per cent of cases.[201]

Nonepithelial Tumors

BENIGN

Although bladder fibromas are uncommon, a large series of these tumors has been reported.[204] Gross or

TABLE 112–4. HISTOLOGIC TYPES OF PRIMARY URINARY BLADDER NEOPLASMS

	Dog		Cat
Neoplasm	*Osborne et al.*[188]	*Burnie and Weaver*[190]	*Schwarz et al.*[196]
Epithelial			
Transitional cell carcinoma	43	44	8
Adenocarcinoma	6	3	3
Squamous cell carcinoma	11	—	4
Papilloma	22	8	—
Unclassified carcinoma	15	—	—
Nonepithelial			
Fibroma	5	—	1
Fibrosarcoma	4	—	—
Unclassified sarcoma	4	1	—
Leiomyoma	5	3	3
Fibroleiomyoma (sarcoma)	3	1	—
Leiomyosarcoma	4	—	2
Embryonal rhabdomyosarcoma	1	—	1
Hemangioma	1	2	1
Hemangiosarcoma	—	—	2
Total	124	62	25

microscopic hematuria was present in 96 per cent of cases. Bladder calculi and UTI were commonly reported.[204, 205] Leiomyomas originate in the smooth muscle of the bladder and form smooth nodules frequently interfering with trigonal outflow.[3]

MALIGNANT

With the exception of one five-year-old dog, all reported cases of embryonal rhabdomyosarcoma (RMS) have been in dogs 12 to 18 months of age.[185, 188, 193, 206–211] Large or giant breeds are more frequently affected. The appearance of the tumor in the bladder resembles grape clusters, hence the term botryoid, and frequently the tumor invasively involves the trigone.[206] The tumor is believed to originate from embryonic myoblasts or pluripotential mesodermal cells arising from the embryonic urogenital ridge.[208, 209] Metastasis occurs in approximately 20 per cent of reported cases. The invasive nature of the tumor mandates a poor prognosis. Although little is known about its behavior in the cat, RMS has been reported.[196]

Leiomyosarcoma has been reported in the dog and cat.[188, 196, 212] They reportedly do not frequently metastasize, although this is inconsistent.[3, 212]

Unusual mesenchymal tumors include chemodectoma and neurofibrosarcoma.[213–215]

Etiology

In dogs, neoplasms of the urinary tract most commonly involve the lower urinary tract, possibly due to prolonged contact with carcinogenic substances excreted in the urine.[6, 185, 188, 197, 216] The prevalence of canine bladder cancer has been linked to the level of environmental industrial activity.[217] Experimental studies have indicated the importance of chemical carcinogenesis in the development of canine bladder tumors, and veterinarians should be aware of the possibility of the dog as a sentinel for environmental carcinogens.[188, 216, 217] Cyclophosphamide has been implicated in the development of transitional cell carcinoma in dogs.[183, 184] The role of bacterial UTI in carcinogenesis is unknown, but our emerging understanding of the role of chronic inflammation in carcinogenesis may indicate that the simultaneous occurrence of chronic bacterial infection and neoplasia in the lower urinary tract is a more difficult cause-effect question than previously appreciated.

The reduced prevalence of bladder neoplasms in the cat may be due to altered metabolism of certain compounds, such as marked reduction in urinary concentrations of potentially carcinogenic tryptophan metabolites.[188, 218] Feline lower urinary tract tumors are also apparently not correlated with FeLV infection.[196]

Diagnosis and Clinical Staging

Diagnosis is dependent upon integration of history, clinical signs, and laboratory and radiographic findings. Definitive diagnosis requires histologic confirmation, although a reliable diagnosis can be made in many cases without surgical biopsy.

The biologic behavior of urinary tract neoplasia is characterized by slow, invasive growth. Consequently the history is often chronic and progressive. However, in some cases clinical signs are intermittent or appear to occur suddenly, with rapid progression.[201]

Clinical signs of lower urinary tract neoplasia are typical of the signs apparent in all diseases of the lower tract; signs of inflammation (e.g., hematuria, dysuria, stranguria, pollakiuria) and/or incontinence (e.g., dribbling, stranguria) are most common. Some cases may have no associated clinical signs, and the identity of a urinary tract tumor may be an incidental finding. Hematuria, the most prominent clinical sign in the dog and cat, may be intermittent, but is often progressive.[196, 197, 219] Dysuria may be present, particularly with masses located in the urethra or trigone.[196] Incontinence may develop from detrusor atony, reduced bladder capacity, increased bladder irritability, obstruction to outflow, and urethral incompetence or partial obstruction from tumor extension (see Chapter 30). Signs of uremia (e.g., vomiting, lethargy, depression, anorexia, and dehydration) may be apparent if urethral or ureteral obstruction or bladder rupture are present.[197, 200] Some dogs with urinary tract neoplasia have psychogenic polydipsia.[197, 201] Other clinical signs of systemic illness are generally absent and animals frequently maintain appetite and body weight, even in the advanced stages of the tumor, except in cases with signs referable to metastatic disease, or in cases of the paraneoplastic syndrome, hypertrophic osteopathy (HPO).[190] Clinical signs of HPO include firm, often painful, swellings due to periosteal proliferation of long bones of the extremities.[185] Hypertrophic osteopathy has been observed in cases of transitional cell carcinoma, embryonal rhabdomyosarcoma, and neurofibrosarcoma.[190, 203, 207, 211, 214, 220] In HPO associated with bladder tumors, pulmonary involvement may be absent or radiographically inapparent.[203, 207, 214, 220] The prevalence of HPO may be as high as 50 per cent for embryonal RMS, frequently without pulmonary involvement.

Physical examination may be unremarkable. A thickened bladder wall, evidence of a bladder mass, or cystic calculi may be noted on careful abdominal or rectal palpation.[197] Clinical findings suggestive of a vaginal or vestibular mass may be present, including a palpable mass or hematocolpos, in which case digital vaginal examination is useful.[221]

Hematologic and biochemical findings are generally normal unless intercurrent disease or azotemia due to obstruction are present. Urinalysis may indicate the presence of hematuria, pyuria, and proteinuria. The diagnosis may be confounded by the concurrent presence of UTI or urolithiasis. Bladder and urethral neoplasia predispose to UTI by compromising host defenses. The tumor may serve as a nidus for calculus formation.[190, 207, 211, 220]

Urine sediment or bladder wash cytology is useful in the diagnosis of bladder neoplasia, especially transitional cell carcinoma. Evaluation of bladder wash (see section on diagnostic techniques) will enhance recovery and morphology of cells.[201] Urinary cytology must be performed prior to positive contrast radiography to avoid distortion of cells by hypertonic media. Urine cytology may contain clusters of anaplastic epithelial cells in cases of transitional cell carcinoma.[6, 185, 197, 210, 216, 222–224] Unfortunately similar appearing cells may occasionally be observed in cases of inflammatory bladder disease.[185, 197] In carcinomas, the presence of clusters of large pleomorphic cells with prominent nuclear membranes and nucleoli and variable nuclear size (high nuclear to cytoplasmic ratio) is supportive of a diagnosis of neoplasia (Figure 112–7). Cytology in embryonal RMS is predominantly indicative of inflammation, although small tumor cells with eccentric nuclei and minimal cytoplasm are generally present.[206] Unfortunately, the presence of abnormal cells is not a consistent finding in neoplastic diseases of the lower urinary tract and repeated urine sediment examinations or bladder washes are recommended.[190, 193, 201] In one study, seven of ten dogs with urinary bladder tumors had tumor cells in the urine sediment.[190] One large study in human patients indicated a false-negative urine cytology in 26 per cent of cases with known bladder cancer, and a low incidence (7 per cent) of false positives where inflammatory lesions were mistaken for neoplasia.[224] Use of an isotonic bladder wash and integration of cytology results with other findings would be expected to reduce the false negative and false positive results respectively. Cytologic evaluation of vaginal mucosal scraping or a fine needle aspirate of a mass or thickened bladder wall may provide further supportive evidence for the diagnosis of neoplasia.

Radiographic studies are important in distinguishing among the various causes of lower urinary tract inflammation. Space occupying lesions are more easily diagnosed than diffusely infiltrating tumors. It is important to note that both are consistent with malignant, benign, and inflammatory conditions.[177, 178, 196] Pyogranulomatous masses, polypoid cystitis, cystitis cystica, or benign tumors may present with radiographic findings identical to those for malignant neoplasia.[177, 178, 225, 226]

Contrast radiography should include an excretory urogram to identify the presence and extent of ureteral involvement/obstruction and contrast or double contrast cystography to delineate diffuse or focal thickening of the bladder wall, irregular mucosal margin, or space occupying masses, particularly at the area of the trigone (Figure 112–4).[185, 201] CO_2 is preferred to air for negative contrast because of the potential for air embolization through ulcerated bladder surfaces.[42–44]

Tumor location is quite variable. Trigonal location, particularly for transitional cell carcinomas and embryonal rhabdomyosarcomas, is prevalent.[190, 201] Canine leiomyosarcomas are frequently multicentric in the dog.[201] The ventral bladder wall, trigone, and diffuse involvement are most frequently reported in the cat.[196]

Other radiographic findings consistent with lower tract neoplasia include sublumbar lymphadenopathy or osteolysis/osteoproliferation of the sublumbar vertebral bodies or pelvis.[185]

Thoracic radiographs are required to adequately characterize the extent of metastasis. Findings consistent with thoracic metastasis of lower urinary tract neoplasia include multiple well-defined interstitial nodules, diffuse increase in interstitial density, lobar interstitial or alveolar infiltrates, subpleural thickening, or no abnormalities.[203, 227] Diffuse nonstructured interstitial opacity may be confused with age changes.[227]

Other diagnostic imaging tests that may have utility include ultrasound, computer assisted tomography scan, arteriography, and magnetic resonance imaging.[201] Diagnostic ultrasound may yield information similar to contrast radiographs without invasion of the urinary tract (Figure 112–5).

Cystoscopy is the best alternative to cytology for establishing a definitive diagnosis. It has the advantage of allowing direct visualization, brush cytology, and biopsy (see section on diagnostic techniques). Laparoscopy or urinary catheter biopsy may provide alternatives for histologic diagnosis without surgery.

The combination of history, clinical signs, and cytologic and radiographic findings frequently establishes a diagnosis of bladder neoplasia. Definitive diagnosis prior to surgery will allow definitive therapy during surgery.[185] Ideally treatment is based upon this information, rather than subjecting the animal to the stress of surgery and general anesthesia for a diagnosis.[6, 228] In some cases definitive diagnosis and clinical staging may require a biopsy obtained by surgical exploration or cystoscopy. The importance of accurate diagnosis is evident, since some benign bladder conditions may be difficult to separate from neoplasia on the basis of the historical, clinical, radiographic, and cytologic findings.

Information obtained in diagnostic evaluation or at the time of definitive therapy should allow clinical staging according to World Health Organization recommendations (Table 112–5).[6, 185, 229] Use of clinical staging in diagnosis and management of veterinary neoplasia will allow categorization of disease for prognostication and selection of treatment regimens. It is important for the clinician to know the degree of local invasion and extent of metastases to regional and distant sites.

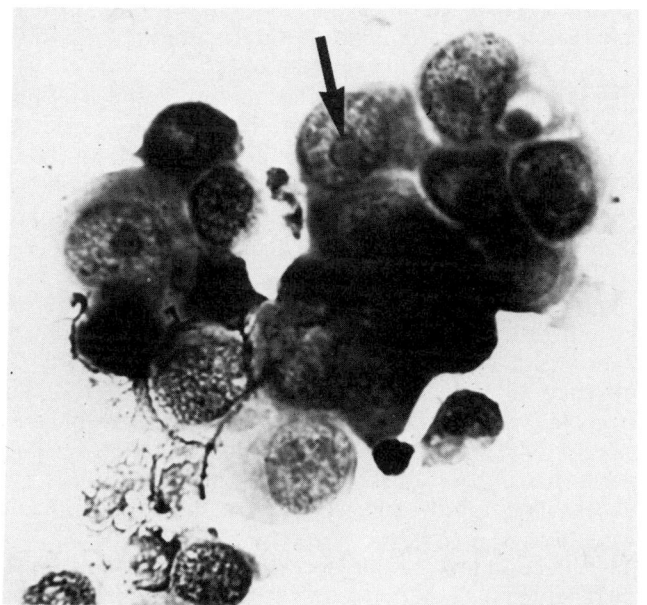

FIGURE 112–7. Urinary cytology of a transitional cell carcinoma. Clumps of anaplastic cells with prominent nucleoli (arrow) and variable nuclear-to-cytoplasm ratio were evident.

TABLE 112–5. CLINICAL STAGES OF BLADDER TUMORS[6, 185, 229]

Category	Designation	Description	Diagnostic Tests
Primary tumor	T0	No evidence of tumor	Clinical examination
	T1S	Carcinoma in situ	Urinary cytology
	T1	Superficial papillary tumor	Contrast cystography
	T2	Tumor invading bladder wall with induration	Excretory urography
	T3	Tumor invading neighboring organs (prostate, uterus, vagina, anal canal)	Cystoscopy Laparotomy
Regional lymph nodes	N0	No involvement	Laparotomy
	N1	Regional* nodes involved	Laparoscopy
	N2	Regional and juxtaregional† nodes involved	
Distant metastasis	M0	No evidence of metastasis	Clinical examination
	M1	Distant metastasis present (specify sites)	Thoracic radiographs Laparotomy Laparoscopy

*Internal and external iliac lymph nodes.
†Lumbar lymph nodes.

In humans, prognosis and likelihood of metastasis are related to depth of invasion of the bladder wall, with invasion of muscle and fat invariably associated with metastasis.[6, 197, 201, 230] Although extrapolation is probably valid, correlation has not yet been firmly established in veterinary medicine. At this time, it seems reasonable to conclude that tumors invading beyond the lamina propria are malignant and likely to be metastatic.[6, 197] However, noninvasive neoplastic growths are not assumed to be benign.

Treatment of Urinary Bladder Neoplasia

The best method of therapy for lower urinary tract neoplasia is unknown.[6, 185, 193, 201, 202, 228] Major limitations to therapy include frequent late diagnoses due to lack of pathognomonic clinical signs, expense of therapy, local invasiveness (especially trigonal), relatively high prevalence of metastasis, lack of a satisfactory urinary diversion procedure, and low prevalence of disease which limits accumulation of information on treatment modalities. Most commonly, therapy is palliative, consisting of partial cystectomy or intravesicular chemotherapy.

Although adequate data to make predictions of life expectancy are not available, it is apparent that prognosis varies with histologic diagnosis and clinical stage of the disease but is generally poor. Findings supportive of a poor prognosis include histologic evidence of deep invasion of the bladder wall, trigonal involvement, obstructive hydroureter or hydronephrosis, and pelvic lymphadenopathy or other evidence of metastasis. Of 70 dogs for which survival data following surgical diagnosis of bladder cancer were reported, 44 dogs survived less than one week, 11 additional dogs died within 4 months, 4 dogs survived 4 to 6 months, and 11 survived 6 months to 5 years.[190] All dogs surviving greater than 6 months had histologically benign tumors. Of 22 cats with bladder tumors, 11 were euthanatized at or soon after surgical diagnosis, 7 additional cats were euthanatized within 6 months, and 4 (including 2 with malignant lesions) survived for greater than 6 months.[196]

Reports of therapy have appeared in the veterinary literature.[196, 197, 201, 204, 205, 215, 228, 231–234] Surgical resection of

bladder fibromas resulted in a good prognosis for short-term recovery, although long term follow-up was not well characterized.[204] Successful therapy of neurofibrosarcoma with no histologic evidence of tumor recurrence at six months was reported with segmental resection, intravesicular thiotepa, and systemic cyclophosphamide.[215] However, at this time cure is not a reasonable goal for most lower urinary tract neoplastic disease. Survival rates for human beings with advanced transitional cell carcinoma of the bladder may be as low as 20 to 40 per cent.[235] The goal of therapy is to control local disease (hematuria, urinary incontinence, and obstruction) and to prevent development of metastasis.[185] Specific goals of local therapy are to prevent urinary obstruction, incontinence, and discomfort.

Adequate management of UTI, urolithiasis, and hematuria are important. Control of hematuria may be necessary in some cases. Aseptic instillation of methenamine or dilute formalin may be effective (see section on cyclophosphamide cystitis).[185]

Treatment of UTI, if present, is based on quantitative urine culture and sensitivity and follow-up urine cultures. The importance of prompt aggressive therapy for concurrent UTI is based on the presence of the neoplastic mass which acts as a nidus for localization of infection, disrupts normal mucosal defense mechanisms, and serves as an ulcerative surface for the development of urosepsis.

Definitive therapy includes surgery and/or adjuvant therapy (immuno-, chemo-, and radiation therapy). Surgical options include segmental resection, total cystectomy, and radical cystectomy. A high incidence of recurrence is expected with segmental resection, and because of the high prevalence of trigonal involvement segmental resection does not generally preserve vesicoureteral communication. Total cystectomy involves removal of the bladder, urethra, and prostate (male). Radical cystectomy also includes removal of local lymph nodes. Care must be taken in manipulation of tumor, since seeding of the abdominal cavity or incision may occur,[203, 211, 235, 236] which may be more prevalent with embryonal RMS.

Cystectomy and frequently segmental resection require urinary diversion procedures. Diversion of urine into the gastrointestinal tract (ureteral or trigonal colostomy) or use of an isolated segment of bowel as a conduit for urine to the exterior (ureteroileostomy or gastrocystoplasty) have been utilized.[6, 60, 185, 237, 238]

All of the currently utilized techniques have a high prevalence of significant patient morbidity. Gastric cystoplasty involves use of a section of the gastric wall for urine storage, with an isolated ileal segment as a conduit to the exterior (flank).[6] This technique is difficult and requires a great deal of care on the part of the owners. With ureteroileostomy the ureters are implanted into an isolated ileal loop which is subsequently drawn through the pelvic canal and external anal sphincter.[6, 238] Perineal urine scalding, incontinence, and UTI are frequent complications. This technique, unless further modified, is not suitable for clinical use. Variable results have been reported with ureteral and trigonal colostomies.[6, 185, 232, 237] Associated problems reported with a variable prevalence include azotemia, diarrhea, pyelonephritis, and hyperchloremic acidosis.[6, 60, 185, 232, 237] The most acceptable procedures appear to be the trigonal or ureteral colostomy. However, trigonal invasion by the neoplastic mass often precludes use of the trigonal colonic anastomosis. A variation of jejunal cystoplasty may offer an alternative in select cases.[239]

Chemotherapy (local or systemic) of lower urinary tract neoplasia in the dog and cat has not been extensively studied. Agents with some demonstrated efficacy include mycophenolic acid, cyclophosphamide (Cytoxan), doxorubicin hydrochloride (Adriamycin), cisplatin, 5-fluorouracil, vincristine, actinomycin D, and triethylenethiophosphoramide (Thiotepa).[197, 201, 228, 235, 236, 240–243, 342]

Radiation therapy has been recommended.[6, 185, 228, 244] Problems encountered include the presence of metastasis (frequently unidentifiable) and complications associated with radiation therapy (bladder fibrosis). Preoperative external cobalt beam irradiation may be associated with excessive scatter,[185, 228] but reductions in size of the bladder tumor facilitate surgery in 7 to 10 days.[6] Preoperative radiation therapy may be beneficial by sealing lymphatics, altering tumor cell viability to prevent seeding during surgery, and destroying tumor foci in local lymph nodes. Hemorrhage is the main complication. Alternatively, intraoperative plus postoperative radiation therapy will allow a definitive biopsy diagnosis, accurate clinical staging, and irradiation of involved lymph nodes at the time of surgery.[6] Although partial regression of tumor size has been noted with this technique,[228] it has been associated with a high prevalence of urinary incontinence due to bladder fibrosis.[6] The advantages of intraoperative radiation therapy include skin sparing, increased accuracy of dose delivery, reduced damage to normal tissue, and use of a single dose.[244] Disadvantages are the attendant risk of surgery including the possibility of tumor implantation, special radiotherapy requirements, delayed healing of surgical incisions, and tumor manipulation.[244]

Even less is known about therapy of bladder neoplasia in the cat. Surgical resection may be palliative in malignant or curative in benign lesions.[196, 233]

Transurethral photodynamic therapy (laser therapy of photosensitized tumor via cystoscopy), interstitial implants (cesium and radon), immunotherapy, and local hyperthermia may represent alternative effective therapies.[228, 245, 246]

PATIENT FOLLOW-UP

Use of radiography, urinalysis, and urinary cytology, rather than return of clinical signs, should be relied upon for patient follow-up. Management of recurrence, which depends on clinical stage of the disease, is generally symptomatic.

TREATMENT OF TRANSITIONAL CELL CARCINOMA

Although not a great deal is known about treatment of lower urinary tract neoplasia, the therapy of transitional cell carcinoma has been most well studied (Table 112–6).[6, 185, 193, 201, 228, 232, 241, 242, 247, 342]

Superficial papillary tumors without metastasis are treated with a combination of surgical resection and radiation therapy and/or chemotherapy.

Locally invasive tumors with evidence of distant metastasis may be managed by a combination of surgery, chemotherapy and/or radiation therapy.

A preoperative external cobalt beam and intraoperative radiation therapy protocol has been described.[6, 247] Intraoperative plus postoperative radiation therapy,[6] or surgical reduction in tumor mass followed 28 days later by intraoperative radiation therapy, represent alternatives.[6, 228, 247]

Combination chemotherapy (intravesicular and systemic), including cisplatin chemotherapy (alone or in combination protocols) have been recommended for transitional cell carcinoma in the dog (Table 112–6).[201, 228, 241, 342] Intravesicular chemotherapy may be of most value for control of local complications in nonresectable trigonal masses.

TREATMENT OF RHABDOMYOSARCOMA

Because of the difficulty in establishing a cytologic diagnosis of RMS, biopsy may be necessary. It is particularly critical to avoid implantation of this tumor into the body or bladder wall incisions or abdominal cavity. Alternatives to establish a diagnosis include bladder wash cytology or a biopsy via cystoscope or catheter. As tumors frequently extensively involve the trigone, biopsy may be the only surgical alternative. Systemic chemotherapy utilizing dactinomycin, vincristine, and cyclophosphamide may be an effective mode of therapy (Table 112–6).[241, 247]

URETHRAL NEOPLASIA

Urethral neoplasia is uncommon in the dog and rare in the cat.[7, 185, 193, 248–257] The most frequently identified tumors in the dog are transitional cell carcinoma, squamous cell carcinoma, and adenocarcinoma. While tumors of the proximal urethra occur in both male and female dogs, tumors of the distal urethra have been reported most frequently in the female.[248, 255] Urethral

TABLE 112–6. RECOMMENDED THERAPY[*31, 185, 228, 340, 341, 342]

Generic (Trade)	Dosage	Route	Frequency	Description (Mean Urine Concentration, μg/ml)†
Penicillin G	17,000 U/lb	Oral	TID	Antimicrobial (294)
Penicillin V	12 mg/lb	Oral	TID	Antimicrobial (148)
Ampicillin	12 mg/lb	Oral	TID	Antimicrobial (309)
Amoxicillin	5 mg/lb	Oral	TID	Antimicrobial (202)
Tetracycline	8 mg/lb	Oral	TID	Antimicrobial (138)
Chloramphenicol	15 mg/lb	Oral	TID	Antimicrobial (124)
Sulfisoxazole	10 mg/lb	Oral	TID	Antimicrobial (1466)
Cephalexin	8 mg/lb	Oral	TID	Antimicrobial (805)
Nitrofurantoin	2.5 mg/lb	Oral	TID	Antimicrobial (100)
Trimethoprim/sulfa	6 mg/lb	Oral	BID	Antimicrobial (55)
Amikacin	2.5 mg/lb	SQ	TID	Antimicrobial (342)
Gentamicin	1 mg/lb	SQ	TID	Antimicrobial (107)
Kanamycin	1.7 mg/lb	SQ	TID	Antimicrobial (530)
Tobramycin	0.5 mg/lb	SQ	TID	Antimicrobial (66)
Ticarcillin	18 mg/lb	Oral	QID	Antimicrobial
Cyclophosphamide (Cytoxan)	50–75 mg/m^2	Oral	4× weekly	Chemotherapy
	200–300 mg/m^2	IV	Weekly	Chemotherapy
Doxorubicin (Adriamycin)	30 mg/m^2	IV	Q 21 days	Chemotherapy
5-fluorouracil	200 mg/m^2	IV	Weekly	Chemotherapy
	300 mg/m^2	intravesicular	Weekly	Chemotherapy
Triethylenethio-phosphoramide (Thiotepa)	15–30 mg/m^2	intravesicular	Q 7–14 days	Chemotherapy
Vincristine (Oncovin)	0.5–0.75 mg/m^2	IV	1–2×/week	Chemotherapy
Actinomycin D (Cosmegen)	1.5 mg/m^2	IV	Q 7 days	Chemotherapy
CisPlatinum (Platinol)	50–70 mg/m^2	IV‡	Variable	Chemotherapy

*Consult references on therapy for consideration of toxicities, interactions, and dosage adjustments for cats.
†Mean urine concentrations based on listed canine dosages.
‡Special requirements for therapy, including pretreatment with saline and antiemetics. Concurrent administration of saline and mannitol recommended.

neoplasia generally occurs in older dogs (mean age 10.4 years, range 3 to 14 years).[7] RMS of the canine urethra may be more prevalent in young dogs.[7, 249] Secondary tumors generally spread by local invasion from primary bladder, prostatic, or vaginal tumors.[221, 255] Mesenchymal tumors also occur in the urethra.[7, 193, 248] Female dogs have approximately a 10-fold increase in relative risk, perhaps because of the presence of prostatic secretions in the male urethra which dilute urinary carcinogens or because of an increased susceptibility of the female urethra to carcinogens.[7, 185, 193, 248] A breed predilection has been reported for beagles.[248] Malignant urethral neoplasia frequently metastasizes to local lymph nodes, lumbosacral vertebral bodies, pelvic bones, and the lungs.[7, 185, 193, 248, 257] Lymph node metastasis is reported in 33 per cent of cases on post mortem examination.[7] Ocular, myocardial, and adrenal metastasis have also been reported.[256] Extension of tumor to involve both urethra and bladder is common, occurring approximately one-third of the time.[248] In the cat, urethral tumors are rare; TCC is reported most frequently.

Diagnosis

Clinical signs are characteristic of urethral disease, and include stranguria, hematuria, urinary incontinence, and urethral discharge.[7, 248, 251-254] The clinical picture of urethral neoplasia may mimic chronic prostatitis (see Chapter 105).[252] Clinical signs of uremia may be present if urethral obstruction is present, with signs referable to metastasis in advanced cases.[185]

Careful palpation, including rectal examination, may identify a urethral mass. Although tumors may be localized or diffuse, they are frequently extensive by the time of diagnosis, involving a large segment of the urethra. Cytologic evaluation of voided urine or urethral discharge may confirm the presence of anaplastic cells.[7] Contrast urethrography (retrograde or voiding) is the most useful and consistently accurate diagnostic technique (Figure 112-8).[185] Characteristic findings of a positive contrast retrograde urethrogram include a space occupying mass, leakage of contrast material, irregular mucosal margins giving a moth-eaten appearance, and urethral stenosis.[7, 257] Cystography will determine degree of involvement of the bladder. Thoracic and abdominal radiographs are required to adequately characterize the extent of metastasis.

Although cytology or evaluation of a biopsy obtained via cystoscope or catheter may be diagnostic, definitive diagnosis is usually by exploratory surgery. Abdominal exploratory surgery will document the extent of metastasis to regional lymph nodes and urinary bladder, and allow visualization of the proximal urethra.[7, 202] Frequently a pubic osteotomy is required to determine the extent of the tumor.[202] Previously unidentified involvement of the bladder and/or prostate may be apparent at the time of surgery.[248]

As with malignant bladder tumors, prognosis is generally poor. Surgical resection is dependent upon stage

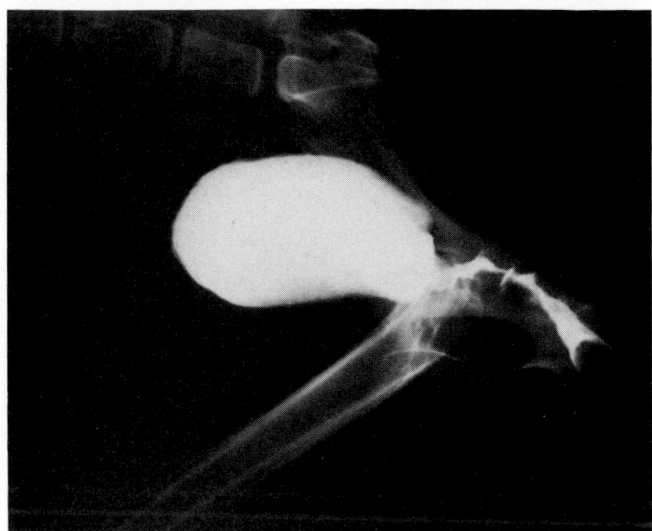

FIGURE 112–8. Positive contrast cystogram-urethrogram of a dog with a urethral adenocarcinoma. Note the irregular mucosal margins of the urethra.

of the tumor. Localized tumors may allow urethrectomy and prepubic urethrostomy.[185] Advanced cases may require urethrocystectomy and urinary diversion procedures. Anastomosis of the bladder neck to the abdominal wall or anastomosis of the proximal and penile urethra may provide alternatives in select cases.[202, 254, 258–260] Adjuvant chemotherapy or radiation therapy is dependent upon the histologic type and extent and stage of the tumor (see section on bladder neoplasia).[185]

URINARY TRACT TRAUMA

Traumatic injury to the urinary tact may occur as a consequence of either blunt or penetrating injuries.[161–265] Further, it is important to recognize that injuries characteristic of trauma (e.g., ruptured bladder or urethra) may be caused by disease processes other than trauma (e.g., neoplasia, traumatic palpation or catheterization).[200, 261, 262, 266] Ruptured urinary bladder, kidney, urethra, ureter, and perirenal hematoma represent the most frequent traumatic urinary tract injuries in decreasing order of prevalence.[267, 268]

The actual incidence of urinary tract injury in traumatized patients is largely unknown and may depend upon the criteria of the search. Urinary tract traumatic injuries were identified in the clinical evaluation of 2.5 per cent of 600 dogs involved in motor vehicle accidents.[264] In another study, critical radiographic evaluation of 100 consecutive dogs with traumatically induced pelvic fractures revealed a 39 per cent incidence of urinary tract injuries.[269] The low incidence of reported injury in clinical diagnosis of urinary tract injury may indicate that some radiographically identifiable injuries are not of apparent clinical significance.

DIAGNOSIS

Scant information is available to suggest which urinary tract injuries require intervention, nor is it apparent which clinical signs are suggestive of significant injuries. However, all animals with evidence of external abdominal trauma, spinal or pelvic injury, or injury to other intrabdominal organs should be carefully evaluated for urinary tract trauma.[268] Female dogs with pelvic fractures may be more likely to have significant urinary tract injuries than males.[269] Failure to identify urinary tract injury until late probably leads to a higher incidence of mortality.[261, 262, 270]

CLINICAL SIGNS

Clinical signs are neither specific for urinary tract injury nor does their absence eliminate urinary tract trauma.[269] Clinical signs of urinary tract injury may not be apparent for 24 to 48 hours and are dependent upon the area of the tract injured and the degree of injury. Hypovolemic shock may be a consequence of renal parenchymal/pedicle injuries (see Chapter 108). Leakage of urine from a ruptured bladder may result in signs of chemical peritonitis (painful abdomen, vomiting, and splinting), abdominal distention, or uremia one to three days after initial presentation.[261, 262] Injury to the urethra may result in bladder distention due to lack of urethral patency, swelling in the perineal region due to subcutaneous urine leakage, or signs of uremia.[261, 263] Hematuria was the most frequent clinical sign of urinary tract trauma in one study.[269] Discomfort on abdominal palpation, vomiting, and CNS depression are generally apparent less than 24 hours following bladder rupture.[262]

Urinary tract rupture may present as unexplained patient deterioration one to three days after trauma. Although mean time to death in experimental canine bladder rupture is 2.5 days, a slow or intermittent leak may allow significantly more time before clinical signs of uremia develop.[262] Urinary tract rupture may be suspected when abdominal fluid accumulates rapidly in an animal that is receiving parenteral fluid therapy.

PHYSICAL EXAMINATION

Physical examination may be unrewarding in the detection of urinary tract injury. No clinical evidence of urinary tract injury was present in 13/39 dogs with radiographic evidence of urinary tract trauma in one study.[269] However, astute observation of urination, careful abdominal and rectal palpation, and passage of a urethral catheter in selected cases are essential for successful diagnostic evaluation of traumatized patients. Aseptic technique is particularly critical in passage of a urethral catheter in patients suspected of having a urinary tract leak, since contamination may lead to bacterial peritonitis or retroperitonitis.[265] Neither successful passage of a urethral catheter with collection of urine nor observation of spontaneous urination eliminates the possibility of an avulsed ureter, ruptured bladder or lacerated urethra. However, these evaluations are fruitful if properly performed.

Within the first 6 to 12 hours, the only useful laboratory evaluation is a urinalysis, with particular attention paid to the presence of proteinuria and hematuria. In cases of significant urine leak, azotemia and other biochemical changes may be apparent in 12 to 36 hours.[262]

Hemoconcentration, hyponatremia, hypochloremia, hyperphosphatemia, hyperkalemia and metabolic acidosis may result.[262, 268] Protracted vomition may alter acid-base and electrolyte status, leading to metabolic alkalosis and hypokalemia in some cases.[270] Urine specific gravity may be any value. Preexisting renal failure may complicate the diagnosis.

FURTHER DIAGNOSTIC TESTS

The selection of patients for further diagnostic evaluation of the urinary tract is a difficult decision. The presence of dysuria, hematuria, abdominal or perineal swelling or discoloration, palpable mass in the sublumbar region, vomiting, or unexplained deterioration in a patient's condition 24 to 72 hours subsequent to trauma are indications for careful evaluation of the urinary tract. However, the presence of hematuria does not absolutely indicate that an injury requiring intervention has occurred, nor does it indicate the level of the injury.[269]

Abdominal paracentesis with a syringe and 22-gauge needle may provide evidence of intrabdominal urine leakage. Such abdominal fluid is generally classified as a modified transudate, which may appear blood tinged and turbid with reactive mesothelial cells present. In patients with a preexisting UTI, bacteria may be present in the abdominal effusion. Intra- or retroperitoneal accumulation of hypertonic feline or canine urine causes a shift of plasma fluid, sodium, and chloride into the abdomen. If a urinary tract infection is present, the combination of chemical, osmotic, and microbial toxins will have dire consequences for the animal. The presence of abdominal fluid urea or creatinine in excess of plasma levels is indicative of urine leakage into the abdomen. Because of the small molecular size and rapid transperitoneal equilibration of urea, it is less reliable than creatinine in evaluation of uroperitoneum.[262] The use of a peritoneal dialysis catheter has been recommended to facilitate detection of abdominal fluid.[261, 271] Following radiographic studies, infusion of 10 ml of warmed sterile saline per pound body weight for diagnostic peritoneal lavage is indicated if urine leakage is suspected but not detected by abdominocentesis.[272, 273] Injuries to the kidneys, ureters, urethra, and urinary bladder occasionally result in urine leakage into the retroperitoneal or subcutaneous space, which will not be detected by these techniques.

Radiographic studies will be necessary in cases where there is inadequate abdominal fluid accumulation or retroperitoneal fluid accumulation. Survey radiographic studies are useful diagnostic techniques.[267, 269] Careful clinical evaluation combined with survey radiographic studies are the best screen for evaluation of patients with pelvic fractures, since as many as 16 per cent of dogs with pelvic fractures had urinary tract injuries which warranted surgical therapy (i.e., avulsed ureter, ruptured bladder, or ruptured urethra).[269] The presence of intrabdominal effusion (lack of contrast), retroperitoneal density changes (increased density with mottling or streaking of retroperitoneal space, and absent or asymmetrical renal shadows), intestinal ileus, hernia, or absence of a visible bladder may be indicative of significant urinary tract injury.[261, 262, 269, 274] Retroperitoneal

space effusion was the most useful survey radiographic finding in one study, and was best identified on lateral views.[269] Other studies have suggested that displacement or asymmetry of the kidneys, loss of renal shadow, reduction in size or absence of the bladder, or abdominal fluid are indications for more thorough evaluation of the urinary tract.[261, 267, 274]

Survey radiographs may be nondiagnostic (36 per cent false negative in one study).[269] If clinical, laboratory, or survey radiographic findings are suspicious, contrast radiographic studies represent the most reliable method of establishing the site and extent of urinary tract trauma. This may include an excretory urogram to document renal and ureteral injuries, positive contrast cystography to assess bladder integrity, and positive contrast urethrography to diagnose urethral injuries. Failure to fully distend the bladder during contrast cystography may result in false-negative results with small tears. Negative contrast is less useful for evaluation of traumatic injuries, with the exception of the location and definition of the extent of blood clots. Fifty to one hundred ml of air injected into a urinary catheter will usually produce an audible sound upon escaping through a rent in the bladder wall.[262] CO_2 is preferable to room air for instillation into the urinary bladder to avoid air embolism.[42–44]

EMERGENCY TREATMENT

Generally traumatic injuries of the lower urinary tract are not emergencies. An identified urine leakage should be managed but not to the detriment of other emergency care of the patient. The principal exceptions are severe hemorrhage, total obstruction to urine flow, and internal leakage of infected urine. Significant hemorrhage of urinary tract origin is generally associated with renal parenchymal lacerations, fractures, or pedicle injuries.[261] These may necessitate emergency surgical intervention, with care in the management of anesthesia of unstable patients (see Chapter 108).[275] Because of the anatomic structure of the urinary tract, surgical exploration without adequate preoperative documentation of the integrity of the urinary tract is frequently unrewarding.

Obstruction to urine flow will result in marked distention of the bladder and obstructive damage to the detrusor wall and the kidney (see Chapters 31 and 108). If micturition is absent and the bladder is not distended, a ruptured bladder, bilateral ureteral disruption, or oliguric renal disease should be suspected. Aggressive fluid therapy coupled with urethral catheterization and/or excretory urography should allow differentiation of these conditions. If disruption of the lower urinary tract prevents passage of urine, and careful attempts to pass a catheter are unsuccessful, the bladder should be decompressed. Repeated cystocenteses, cystostomy catheter, or marsupialization of the bladder are acceptable management techniques. Repeated cystocenteses are technically easy, and do not require anesthesia, but run the risk of urine leakage through bladder wall puncture sites, particularly if used for more than 24 hours. In some unstable patients, this method is preferable for initial management. If required, cystostomy with a balloon tipped catheter (placed through a purse-string suture on the cranioventral aspect of the bladder) will provide antisepsis and adequate urine drainage throughout management of the primary obstructive problem.[261]

Ruptured Bladder. Ruptured urinary bladder is the most frequently diagnosed traumatic injury of the urinary tract.[267] The reported mortality rate in dogs and cats with a ruptured urinary bladder is over 40 per cent.[262] Bladder rupture may be more likely when there is a sudden increase in intravesicular pressure, such as may occur with blunt abdominal trauma with a full bladder.[264, 265] While motor vehicle accidents are the most frequent cause, traumatic bladder rupture may also occur from a kick, fall, traumatic palpation, catheterization, penetrating abdominal injuries, or with no identifiable cause.[261, 265, 268, 270, 274, 276] Spontaneous rupture may occur with urolithiasis, neoplasia, necrotizing cystitis, or atony.[200, 266, 270] The reported increased prevalence in males has been questioned.[262, 264, 265, 269, 276]

Ruptured bladder usually leads to peritoneal urine leak in the dog and cat, although retroperitoneal or perineal, subcutaneous leak may occur.[277]

Classically, a history of recent abdominal trauma, abnormal micturition of small volumes of bloody urine, ascites, inability to palpate the bladder, progressive depression and vomition, and ready demonstration of a leak with a properly performed contrast cystogram are expected with a ruptured bladder.[265, 270] However, this condition may represent one of the most challenging diagnoses in clinical medicine. Nearly one-fourth of clinical diagnoses are not made until necropsy.[262] All of the following findings are consistent with a ruptured bladder and may confound the diagnosis: absence of hematuria, presence of normal micturition, successful catheterization with urine present in the bladder, no history of trauma, no physical or radiographic evidence of abdominal fluid accumulation, and urine specific gravity of any value. A normal properly performed positive contrast cystogram is not consistent with a ruptured bladder.

Initial management of bladder rupture is dependent upon the status of the patient. If the problem has been identified prior to the onset of metabolic alterations (i.e., azotemia, metabolic acidosis, hyponatremia, hypokalemia) definitive surgical therapy is indicated. However, since hypersensitivity to anesthetic agents may be present in traumatized patients or those with metabolic derangements, initial stabilization is required. Establishing adequate urine drainage should be attempted with a closed system continuous drainage urethral catheter with the catheter tip near the bladder trigone.[270, 275] Soft urethral catheters are preferred and should be used with care to avoid excessive length intraabdominally.[278, 279] In some situations peritoneal dialysis may be required.

Diuresis should be established with isotonic fluid therapy, with a balanced electrolyte solution (3 to 5 ml/pound/hour intravenously). Antibiotic therapy is indicated in cases with a history of UTI, devitalized tissue, or septic abdominal effusion. A patient can be managed in this manner for several days if necessary. Once metabolic, fluid, and electrolyte control is achieved, a routine midventral surgical approach, surgical debridement, closure of bladder lacerations, and copious lavage of the peritoneal cavity with 1 to 2 liters of warmed

isotonic electrolyte solution represent appropriate definitive therapy. Tears frequently occur in the fundus or ventral bladder wall but a thorough evaluation of the bladder is mandatory.[276] Abdominal drains are not indicated.[270]

Ruptured Urethra. Traumatic injuries of the urethra occur predominantly in male dogs and cats and are frequently associated with pelvic fractures.[269, 274] A ruptured urethra may occur in association with pelvic fractures, bite wounds, poor catheterization technique, urolithiasis, and os penis fractures.[265, 266, 268] Rupture of the urethra most frequently occurs near the junction with the bladder and may cause retroperitoneal, perineal, or subcutaneous abdominal urine accumulation.[267, 277] This may not be apparent for several hours (up to 72 hours in some cases). Positive contrast urethrography is the best diagnostic test. Successful passage of a urinary catheter is frequently still possible in cases of incomplete disruption of the urethra. Periurethral extravasation of urine may cause inflammation of periurethral tissues leading to obstruction. Although urine may be sterile initially, the presence of normal urethral flora and devitalized tissue may result in contamination at the leakage sites, resulting in marked leukocytosis in such cases of localized infection. Secondary fistula formation may occur.

Small urethral lacerations may heal over an appropriately sized catheter left in place 7 to 21 days, with stricture formation more likely if the catheter distends the urethra.[268, 280] Primary urethral repair, extrapelvic anastomosis of the bladder to the urethra (male dogs), antepubic urethrostomy, or urinary diversion procedures represent alternatives for surgical management of major urethral injury.[259–261, 263, 280] Pelvic urethral tears require surgical exploration. Urethral stricture and urinary incontinence (see Chapters 30 and 31) represent frequent complications following urethral injuries, particularly where prostatectomy is involved.[259, 263, 281]

A fracture of the os penis may occur, causing immediate disruption of the penile urethra secondary to fragment displacement or callus formation leading to stenosis and obstruction several weeks to several months later.[282] If a catheter can be passed, the fracture may heal satisfactorily.[261, 280] Initial catheterization (24 to 48 hours) may avoid obstruction from acute swelling. If the fragment is displaced, surgery to remove or realign the fragment may be required.[282] A prescrotal urethrotomy for catheter placement or a prescrotal urethrostomy may be required to relieve obstruction.[261] Total ostectomy may hinder ability to breed and hence a partial ostectomy with removal of one wall of the urethral groove of the os penis or internal fixation has been recommended.[282, 283]

DISEASES ASSOCIATED PRIMARILY WITH URINARY INCONTINENCE

Many of the diseases discussed in this chapter may present initially for evaluation of urinary incontinence. The physiology, diagnosis, and management of urinary incontinence are discussed elsewhere (see Chapter 30).

Diseases in which urinary incontinence may be the only or primary manifestation include pelvic bladder, urachal remnant, idiopathic urinary incontinence in dogs and cats, and ectopic ureters.

Pelvic Bladder. Caudal displacement of a portion of the bladder into the pelvic canal, referred to as pelvic bladder, has been cited as a cause of urinary incontinence.[284-286] Incontinence has been attributed to the presence of an abnormal vesicourethral junction or urethral incompetence due to shortened functional length.[284-286] With a pelvic bladder, any increase in intraabdominal pressure may be transmitted to the bladder but not the shortened urethra, resulting in incontinence, particularly in an animal with a marginally competent urethra. Most male and some female dogs with bladders lying within the pelvic canal do not have incontinence, so other factors must be involved.[284, 287] Associated urologic abnormalities include congenital anomalies (urachal diverticula and ectopic ureters) and UTI.[284, 286] Although surgical intervention for urethral incompetence has been described, thorough diagnostic and therapeutic management of identified clinical problems is most appropriate.[66, 288]

Urachal Remnant. The urachus is a remnant of the embryological communication between the urinary bladder and the allantoic sac, which atrophies after birth to form a fibrous scar at the bladder vertex.[289, 290] Occasionally, a fibrous cord extending from the vertex to the umbilicus persists.[289-291]

Several types of congenital anomalies resulting from incomplete closure of the urachus have been described:[289, 290] patent urachus, urachal diverticulum, umbilical urachal sinus, and intraabdominal urachal cyst. A prevalence as high as 25 per cent has been described in cats.[291] An association between urachal anomalies and feline urologic disease has been hypothesized, although recent evidence suggests urachal diverticula may be caused by bladder distention in cats (see Chapter 110).[291-295]

Clinical signs and appropriate therapy are dependent upon the type of anomaly present. With complete urachal patency, continuous urinary incontinence, urine scalding of the ventrum, and development of bacterial urinary tract infections may be noted (UTI).[290-295] Diverticula predispose to UTI by serving as a nidus for bacteria.[296] Definitive diagnosis of both is by positive contrast cystography. When indicated, treatment consists of surgical resection, bacterial culture and sensitivity of urine, and 2 to 4 weeks of appropriate antibiotic therapy. Surgical resection of an infected urachal sinus is generally curative. A urachal cyst may become distended with fluid secreted by the epithelial lining, necessitating removal.[290]

Canine Idiopathic Urethral Incompetence. Urinary incontinence in dogs is frequently associated with reduced urethral resistance to urine flow during the storage phase of micturition.[9-17, 58, 59, 66, 288] This urethral incompetence is associated with normal bladder function and pressures, occurs most commonly in the female, and is often idiopathic. Incontinence may be continuous, but usually occurs when the animal is sleeping. Owners may complain of urine staining of the dog's bed or resting place. The diagnosis and management of this condition are discussed elsewhere (see Chapter 30).

Idiopathic Feline Incontinence. Incontinence in cats may be caused by any disease process interfering with normal urinary tract function (ectopic ureter, UTI, neoplasia, or neurologic dysfunction).[297-301] Idiopathic urinary incontinence has been associated with feline leukemia virus infection, often coincident with anisocoria.[297] In some cases, the urinary incontinence has been attributed to detrusor spasticity.[301] Diagnostic evaluation and management are similar to those for other forms of incontinence (see Chapter 30).

Ectopic Ureters. The most common cause of non-neurogenic urinary incontinence in young female dogs is ectopic ureter, in which there is an extravesicular termination of one or both ureters.[64, 302-312] Although ectopic ureters occur in male dogs, the prevalence is approximately 20 times higher in females.[61, 303, 305, 306, 308-310] The longer functional urethral length in the male may prevent urinary incontinence in some cases, resulting in an underestimation of the actual incidence in the male.[61, 308-311, 313] The ureter will generally empty into the urethra, the uterus, the vagina, or the vas deferens.[309, 313] Unilateral involvement is equivalent between right and left sides, and bilateral involvement occurs in approximately 25 per cent of cases.[61, 309] Ectopic ureters have been uncommonly reported in cats.[314-320]

While acquired ureterovaginal fistulas have been reported in the dog and cat, this condition generally occurs as a result of disruption of development of the mesonephric and metanephric duct systems.[64, 320, 321] Vitamin A or folic acid deficiency may induce this congenital defect in the offspring of pregnant rats,[304] but the cause is generally unknown in veterinary patients. A genetic component is suspected on the basis of epidemiologic evidence identifying high-risk breeds (Siberian husky, West Highland white terrier, fox terrier, and miniature and toy poodles) and familial occurrence in Siberian huskies and Labrador retrievers.[61, 304, 309]

DIAGNOSIS

Clinical signs consist of urinary incontinence and/or urine soilage of the perineum. Although generally identified in young animals, some cases will present in adults. Urinary incontinence associated with ectopic ureters may be continuous or intermittent if urine pooling occurs, and animals will usually have normal micturition. In some cases of bilateral involvement, urine does not flow retrograde into the bladder and normal micturition does not occur. A urinalysis may reveal the presence of a UTI, since bladder and possibly urethral defense mechanisms will be bypassed by the ectopic ureter(s). An excretory urogram is the most useful diagnostic technique, although false negative studies do occur (see Figure 112–9). Ectopic ureters may present a diagnostic challenge, and are frequently not identified on radiographic studies.[309] The presence of hydroureter in a young incontinent animal is strong supportive evidence, justifying cystotomy if careful patient evaluation has eliminated other possibilities. Other diagnostic tests that may be of value include vaginoscopy with or without new methylene blue dye administration (dogs only) and positive contrast vaginography, vaginourethrography or retrograde urethrography.[309] A suspected ectopic ure-

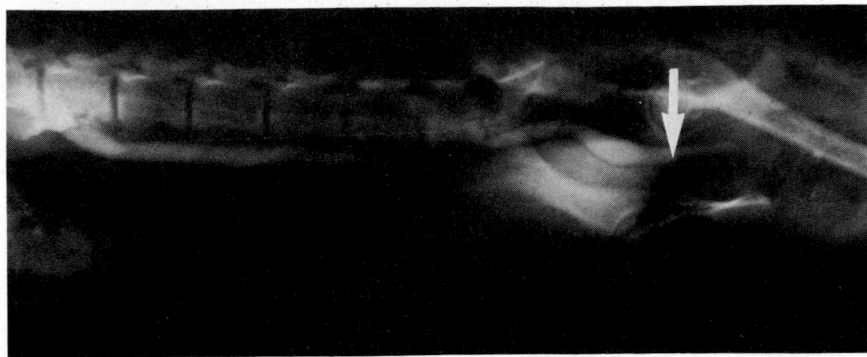

FIGURE 112–9. Oblique view of an excretory urogram of an ectopic ureter in a three-month-old female dog. The ectopic ureter (arrow) was not evident on lateral or ventrodorsal views.

teral orifice visualized by vaginoscopy may be identified by retrograde positive contrast ureterography.

Reduced bladder size has been documented in some cases of ectopic ureters, probably secondary to reduced urine delivery to the bladder. Hydroureter and hydronephrosis are frequently present, possibly due to distal ureteral stenosis, interference with ureteral peristalsis from infection, or ureteral developmental anomalies.[61, 313] Hypoplasia of the bladder and kidneys, ureterocele, persistent hymen, urethral abnormalities, and partial or complete ureteral duplication have also been reported in dogs in conjunction with ectopic ureters.[61, 64] In cats, hydronephrosis, hydroureter, renal aplasia, and phimosis have been associated.[312, 315]

TREATMENT

In surgical management of ectopic ureters, it is important to recognize that bilateral ectopia is present in approximately 25 per cent of canine cases.[61] Most ectopic ureters enter the serosa of the bladder in a normal position and bypass the bladder via a submucosal extension into the urethra.[313] Consequently, the identification of one ectopic ureter and apparent normal entry site of the other may be misleading.[309, 313] Ventral cystotomy with careful exploration of the trigone is essential to document a normal ureteral orifice. Ureteral implantation represents the surgical therapy of choice.[66, 311–313] Occasionally a new ureteral orifice may be created by incising over the ectopic ureter along its submucosal path, in which case ligation of the distal aspect of the ureter is essential.[311–313] Postoperative hydroureter does not necessitate a poor prognosis.[303, 309]

Unilateral nephrectomy is not indicated unless severe unilateral renal disease with concurrent bacterial infection and adequate contralateral renal function have been documented. Dye excretion during an excretory urogram may provide adequate evidence about unilateral renal function, although complete characterization of unilateral glomerular filtration rate requires nuclear scintigraphy or selective ureteral catheterization (see Chapter 108). Resection of a kidney on the basis of morphological, rather than functional, criteria may result in the unexpected demise of an animal due to uremia.

Following surgical correction, urinary incontinence may remain for several months or permanently. This may be due to urethral neuromuscular dysfunction, urine pooling in an abnormally developed vagina (vestibulovaginal stenosis), or the presence of previously undetected ectopic or branched ureters.[61, 303, 309]

URETHRAL DISEASE

Any disease of the urethra will produce characteristic clinical signs, including dysuria, stranguria, hematuria, pollakiuria, and urethral discharge.[22] Urethral discharge independent of micturition may originate from the urethra, prostate, or vagina. Urethral disease frequently induces urinary incontinence (see Chapter 30) or obstruction (see Chapter 31). Disease of the urethra often occurs in conjunction with disease of other areas of the urogenital tract (prostate, urinary bladder, or vagina).

Diagnosis

Diagnosis of urethral disease is based upon identification of characteristic clinical signs and/or urethral discharge. The minimum data base should include careful physical examination (including rectal examination), cytology of urethral discharge, and urinalysis (comparison of voided and cystocentesis sample preferred). Collection of urethral discharge for cytologic evaluation should be preceded by careful cleansing of the urethral meatus to allow for collection of urethral rather than preputial or vaginal discharge. Culture of urethral discharge is difficult to interpret, and should not be relied upon for the diagnosis of bacterial urethritis or urethrocystitis. If bacterial urethritis is suspected on the basis of other clinical findings, culture of urethral discharge can be used to estimate an effective antibiotic. The presence of gram-negative rods (predominantly uropathogens) rather than gram-positive cocci (frequently normal flora of distal urethra) may be a distinguishing feature. Evaluation of the prostate by collection of ejaculate or prostatic massage in the male and vaginoscopy for visualization of the urethral meatus and vaginal mucosa and collection of a sample for vaginal cytology are further diagnostic tests. Use of adjunctive diagnostic testing (urethrography) is dependent upon results. Radiography (survey and contrast) may provide evidence of a neoplastic mass, urolithiasis, stricture, or structural mucosal alterations due to inflammation or trauma.

CONGENITAL/HEREDITARY URETHRAL DISEASES

Although uncommon, congenital/hereditary diseases of the urethra have been reported to include urethral agenesis, imperforate urethra, hypospadias, epispadias (in combination with bladder exstrophy), urethral duplication, urethral diverticula, urethrorectal fistula, and urethral stenosis.[65, 66, 290, 322–328] Other anomalies may occur in association with hermaphroditism and pseudohermaphroditism (see Chapters 101 and 106).[290, 329]

Hypospadias. Hypospadias is a developmental defect due to failure of the urethral grooves to fuse during elongation of the phallus.[280, 290, 313, 328] The urethral opening is ventral and caudal to the tip of the penis. The urethral meatus may be classified on the basis of anatomic localization as glandular, penile, scrotal, perineal, or anal.[313, 328] The penis or scrotum may be underdeveloped as well.

Clinical signs, which are dependent on the site of the urethral meatus, include cutaneous urine scalding and complications of increased susceptibility to UTI. Surgical correction is dependent upon the site of the urethral meatus, although most will be amenable to a modification of the prescrotal urethrostomy.[313] Urinalysis and contrast radiography of the lower urinary tract will delineate concurrent abnormalities prior to surgery.

Urethral Fistulas. Although potentially of acquired origin, urinary fistulas most commonly develop in the dog as a congenital defect.[277, 324–326] Clinical signs are dependent upon the type of fistula present. Diagnosis is generally accomplished by contrast radiographic studies, usually retrograde urethrography.

Urethrorectal fistulas appear to be more prevalent in the English bulldog, possibly as a congenital defect due to abnormal separation of the embryonal cloaca into the urethra and rectum.[290, 377] Clinical signs include hematuria and dysuria secondary to UTI.[324, 325] Simultaneous passage of urine from the anus and urethra during micturition may be noted.[325] Surgical correction and concurrent management of UTI constitute appropriate therapy.

ACQUIRED URETHRAL DISEASES

Possible etiologies of acquired urethral diseases include inflammation (infectious or noninfectious), urolithiasis (see Chapters 110 and 111), neoplasia (see section on urethral tumors), and trauma (see section on urinary tract trauma).

Urethritis/Urethrocystitis. Urethritis may be caused by trauma such as excessive licking or masturbation, bite wounds, catheterization, or infectious agents, or it may be primary inflammatory with no identifiable cause.

Traumatic urethritis is treated symptomatically. Excessive masturbation, apparently more common in brachycephalic males, may respond to castration. Histologic evidence of catheter induced urethritis is expected with indwelling urinary catheters in dogs and cats.[134, 330] Minimizing the duration of catheterization, atraumatic placement, use of soft catheters, and careful management of indwelling catheters where required will reduce this sequela.

Bacterial urethritis frequently occurs in conjunction with cystitis and is difficult to separate clinically. Since *Staphylococcus* spp. and *Mycoplasma* spp. predominate in the distal urethra of normal dogs, interpretation of microbiologic cultures of the urethra is difficult.[113] Factors predisposing to bacterial urethritis are similar to those discussed under bacterial UTI.

Granulomatous urethritis of unknown cause has been described in the dog.[290] Recommended therapy includes prednisone at a dosage of 1 mg/lb daily for seven days, with gradual reduction to none over four weeks. Recurrence is treated by reinitiation of therapy at the highest dose. Urinary diversion or urethral bypass procedures may be required in nonresponsive cases.

Cases of urethral inflammation where the cause has not been identified have been termed nonspecific urethritis.[290]

Therapy of Urethritis. Bacterial urethritis is generally associated with bacterial infection of other areas of the urogenital tract, and therapy aimed at control of infection in the primary area will generally eradicate the urethral component.

Since the urethra is normally not sterile, antibacterial therapy has been recommended in all cases of confirmed urethral inflammation (urethritis). Trimethoprim-sulfa or erythromycin has been recommended over ampicillin on the basis of increased concentrations in the canine urethral and vaginal mucosa, and a broader spectrum of activity against gram-negative enteric flora.[161] It is preferable to withhold antibiotic therapy in cases of catheter-induced urethritis until after the removal of the catheter.

Antispasmodic or anti-inflammatory therapy may be indicated in cases of severe urethritis to relieve urethral spasms and associated stranguria and obstruction.[22, 331] If obstruction occurs secondary to urethral disease, urethral catheterization may be necessary, although this may exacerbate urethral inflammation.

Urethral Stricture or Stenosis. Physiologic urethral stenosis is referred to as reflex dyssynergia (see Chapter 30). Morphologic urethral stricture or stenosis may occur following previous urethral surgery, trauma, removal of urethroliths, inflammatory urethral disease, foreign bodies, or ureterocele or as a congenital condition (see Chapter 31).[4, 86, 322, 323, 332–334] Urethral stricture due to granulomatous reaction may occur secondary to urethral prostheses in male cats.[280, 335] Use of these shunts is not recommended. Although uncommon, bladder distention, hydroureter, and hydronephrosis may occur secondary to urethral stenosis.[322] Clinical signs include dysuria, stranguria, hematuria, and urinary incontinence (see Chapters 30 through 32).[263, 322] Urine stasis may predispose to the development of bacterial UTI. Urinary incontinence is due to partial urethral obstruction.

Surgical repair of urethral strictures may be necessary.[263, 280] Since urethral strictures are frequently caudal to the scrotum in the dog, prescrotal urethrostomy may be effective therapy. In the male cat, perineal urethrostomy may be necessary in cases of urethral stricture secondary to urolithiasis, traumatic catheterization, or previous unsuccessful urethrostomy. Replacement of urethra with artificial materials, vaginal tissue grafts, skin grafts, and venous patches has been attempted but is not yet clinically useful.[238] In cases of stenosis of the proximal urethra, urinary diversion procedures may be necessary.[60, 238]

Urethral Prolapse. Urethral mucosal prolapse may cause dysuria and hemorrhage from the tip of the penis of the male dog. It appears to have an increased prevalence in young English bulldogs and Boston terriers.[263, 336-338] Resection of affected urethral mucosa may be curative.[263, 280] Postoperative hemorrhage is minimized by tranquilization of excitable dogs to reduce the incidence of erections and placement of an Elizabethan collar or a side brace to prevent self-inflicted wound trauma. Prevalence of recurrence is unknown.

References

1. Christensen, GC: The urogenital system and mammary glands. *In* Miller, MM (ed): Anatomy of the Dog. Philadelphia, WB Saunders, 1964, p 741.
2. Christie, BA: Anatomy of the urinary tract. *In* Slatter, DH (ed): Textbook of Small Animal Surgery. Philadelphia, WB Saunders, 1985, p 1706.
3. Maxie, MG: The urinary system. *In* Jubb, KVF, et al. (eds): Pathology of Domestic Animals. Orlando, Academic Press, 1985, p 343.
4. Waldron, DR, et al.: The canine urethra: A comparison of first and second intention healing. Vet Surg 14:213, 1985.
5. Banks, WJ: Urinary system. *In* Applied Veterinary Histology. Baltimore, Williams and Wilkins, 1986, p 431.
6. Bojrab, MJ, et al.: Transitional cell carcinomas of the canine bladder: diagnosis and management. Comp Cont Ed 8:495, 1986.
7. Tarvin, G, et al.: Primary urethral tumors in dogs. JAVMA 172:931, 1978.
8. Bharadwaj, MB and Calhoun, ML: Histology of the urethral epithelium of domestic animals. Am J Vet Res 20:841, 1959.
9. Oliver, JE and Osborne, CA: Neurogenic urinary incontinence. *In* Kirk, RW (ed): Current Veterinary Therapy VII. Philadelphia, WB Saunders, 1980, p 1122.
10. Rosin, AE and Ross, L: Diagnosis and pharmacologic management of disorders of urinary continence in the dog. Comp Cont Ed 183:601, 1981.
11. Rosin, AE and Barsanti, JA: Diagnosis of urinary incontinence in dogs: role of the urethral pressure profile. JAVMA 178:814, 1981.
12. Barsanti, JA, et al.: Testosterone responsive urinary incontinence in a castrated male dog. JAAHA 17:117, 1981.
13. Barsanti, JA and Finco, DR: Hormonal responses to urinary incontinence. *In* Kirk, RW (ed): Current Veterinary Therapy VIII. Philadelphia, WB Saunders, 1983, p 1086.
14. Creed, KE: Effect of hormones on urethral sensitivity to phenylephrine in normal and incontinent dogs. Res Vet Sci 34:177, 1983.
15. Barsanti, JA and Downey, R: Urinary incontinence in cats. JAAHA 20:979, 1984.
16. Holt, PE: Urinary incontinence in the bitch due to sphincter mechanism incompetence: prevalence of referred dogs and retrospective analysis of sixty cases. J Sm Anim Pract 26:181, 1985.
17. Richter, KP and Ling, GV: Clinical response and urethral pressure profile changes after phenylpropanolamine in dogs with primary sphincter incompetence. JAVMA 187:605, 1985.
18. Barlough, JE, et al.: Canine and feline urinalysis: value of macroscopic and microscopic examinations. JAVMA 178:61, 1980.
19. Klausner, JS, et al.: Clinical evaluation of commercial reagent strips for detection of significant bacteriuria in dogs and cats. Am J Vet Res 37:719, 1976.
20. Vail, DM, et al.: Applicability of leukocyte esterase test strip in detection of canine pyuria. JAVMA 189:1451, 1986.
21. Barsanti, JA and Finco, DR: Laboratory findings in urinary tract infections. Vet Clin North Am 9:729, 1979.
22. Polzin, DJ and Jeraj, K: Urethritis, cystitis, and ureteritis. Vet Clin North Am 9:661, 1979.
23. Barsanti, JA: Diagnostic procedures in urology. Vet Clin North Am 14:3, 1984.
24. Comer, KM and Ling, GV: Results of urinalysis and bacterial culture of canine urine obtained by antepubic cystocentesis, catheterization, and the midstream voided methods. JAVMA 179:891, 1981.
25. Biertuempfel, PH, et al.: Urinary tract infection resulting from catheterization in healthy dogs. JAVMA 178:989, 1981.
26. Lees, GE, et al.: Results of analyses and bacterial cultures of urine specimens obtained from clinically normal cats by three methods. JAVMA 184:449, 1984.
27. Klausner, JS and Feeney, DA: Vesicoureteral reflux. *In* Kirk, RW (ed): Current Veterinary Therapy VIII. Philadelphia, WB Saunders, 1983, p 1041.
28. Allen, TA, et al.: Microscopic evaluation of canine urine: Direct microscopic examination and preservation of specimen quality for culture. JAVMA 190:1289, 1987.
29. Ling, GV, et al.: Bacterial pathogens associated with urinary tract infections. Vet Clin North Am 9:617, 1979.
30. Duncan, JR and Prasse, KW: Clinical examination of the urine. Vet Clin North Am 6:647, 1976.
31. Ling, GV: Therapeutic strategies involving antimicrobial treatment of the canine urinary tract. JAVMA 185:1162, 1984.
32. Barsanti, JA: Genitourinary tract infections. *In* Greene, CE (ed): Clinical Microbiology and Infectious Diseases of the Dog and Cat. Philadelphia, WB Saunders, 1984, p 269.
33. Lees, GE, et al.: Urine: A medium for bacterial growth. Vet Clin North Am 9:611, 1979.
34. Smith, CW, et al.: Effects of indwelling urinary catheters in male cats. JAAHA 17:427, 1981.
35. Lees, GE, et al.: Adverse effects of open indwelling urethral catheterization in clinically normal male cats. Am J Vet Res 42:825, 1981.
36. Padilla, J, et al.: Effects of storage time and temperature on quantitative culture of canine urine. JAVMA 178:1077, 1981.
37. Allen, TA: Urinary Tract Infections. *In* Breitschwerdt, EB (ed): Nephrology and Urology. New York, Churchill Livingstone, 1986, p 89.
38. B-D Urine Culture Kit, Becton-Dickinson, Rutherford, NJ.
39. Ling, GV, et al.: Percutaneous nephropyelocentesis and nephropyelostomy in the dog: A description of the technique. Am J Vet Res 40:1605, 1979.
40. Feeney, DA, et al.: The excretory urogram. Interpretation of abnormal findings. Comp Cont Ed 4:321, 1982.
41. Feeney, DA and Johnston, GR: Urogenital imaging: A practical update. Seminars in Vet Med and Surg (Small Anim) 1:144, 1986.
42. Ackerman, N, et al.: Fatal air embolism associated with pneumourethrography and pneumocystography in a dog. JAVMA 160:1616, 1972.
43. Zontine, WJ and Andres, LK: Fatal air embolism as a complication of pneumocystography in 2 cats. J Am Vet Radiol Soc 19:8, 1978.
44. Thayer, GW, et al.: Fatal venous air embolism associated with pneumocystography in a cat. JAVMA 176:643, 1980.
45. Feeney, DA, et al.: Maximum distension retrograde urethrocystography in healthy male dogs: Occurrence of vesicoureteral reflux. Am J Vet Res 48:953, 1984.
46. Barsanti, JA, et al.: Complications of bladder distension during retrograde urethrography. Am J Vet Res 42:819, 1981.
47. Johnston, GR, et al.: Radiographic findings in urinary tract infection. Vet Clin North Am 9:749, 1979.
48. Holt, PE, et al.: An evaluation of positive contrast vaginourethrography as a diagnostic aid in the bitch. J Sm Anim Pract 25:531, 1984.
49. Feeney, DA, et al.: Effects of radiographic contrast media on results of urinalysis, with emphasis on alteration in specific gravity. JAVMA 176:1378, 1980.
50. Feeney, DA and Johnston, GR: Comparative organ imaging: Lower urinary tract. Vet Rad 25:146, 1984.
51. Ensor, et al.: Cystoscopy and ureteral catheterization in the dog. JAVMA 149:1067, 1966.
52. Cooper, JE, et al.: Cystoscopic examination of male and female dogs. Vet Rec 115:571, 1984.
53. Brearley, MJ and Cooper, JE: The diagnosis of bladder disease in dogs by cystoscopy. J Sm Anim Pract 28:75, 1987.

54. McCarthy, TC and McDermaid, SL: Prepubic cystoscopy in the dog and cat. JAAHA 22:213, 1986.

55. Melhoff, T and Osborne, CA: Catheter biopsy of the urethra, urinary bladder, and prostate gland. *In* Kirk, RW (ed): Current Veterinary Therapy VI. Philadelphia, WB Saunders, 1977, p 1173.

56. Gregory, CR, et al.: Electromyographic and urethral pressure profilometry: Assessment of urethral function before and after perineal urethrostomy in cats. Am J Vet Res 45:2062, 1984.

57. Rosin, A, et al.: Canine urethral pressure profile. Am J Vet Res 41:1113, 1980.

58. Moreau, PM, et al.: Simultaneous cystometry and uroflowmetry (micturition study) for evaluation of the caudal part of the urinary tract in dogs: Studies of the technique. Am J Vet Res 44:1769, 1983.

59. Moreau, PM, et al.: Simultaneous cystometry and uroflowmetry for evaluation of micturition in two dogs. JAVMA 183:1084, 1987.

60. Bovee, KC, et al.: Trigonal colonic anastomosis: A urinary diversion procedure in dogs. JAVMA 174:184, 1979.

61. Smith, CW, et al.: Ectopic ureter in the dog: A review of cases. JAAHA 17:245, 1981.

62. Archibald, J and Owen, RR: Urinary system. *In* Archibald, J (ed): Canine Surgery. Santa Barbara, CA, 1974, p 629.

63. Osborne, CA, et al.: Canine and Feline Urology. Philadelphia, WB Saunders, 1972, p 330.

64. Owen, R, et al.: Canine ureteral ectopia: A review. Embryology and aetiology. J Sm Anim Pract 14:407, 1973.

65. Hobson, HP and Ader, PL: Exstrophy of the bladder in a dog. JAAHA 15:103, 1979.

66. Hobson, HP and Bushby, P: Surgery of the bladder. *In* Slatter, DH (ed): Textbook of Small Animal Surgery. Philadelphia, WB Saunders, 1985, p 1786.

67. Medway, W and Skelley, JF: *Capillaria plica* infection in a dog. JAVMA 139:907, 1961.

68. Senior, DF, et al.: *Capillaria plica* infection in dogs. JAVMA 176:901, 1980.

69. Waddell, AH: *Capillaria feliscati* in the bladder of cats in Australia. Austr Vet J 43:297, 1967.

70. Waddell, AH: Further observations on *Capillaria feliscati* infections in the cat. Austr Vet J 44:33, 1968.

71. Wilson-Hanson, S and Prescott, CW: Capillaria in the bladder of the domestic cat. Austr Vet J 59:190, 1982.

72. Wilson-Hanson, SL and Prescott, CW: A survey for parasites in cats. Austr Vet J 59:195, 1982.

73. Ehrenford, FA and Snodgrass, TB: Incidence of canine dioctophymiasis (giant kidney worm infection) with a summary of cases in North America. JAVMA 126:415, 1955.

74. Osborne, CA, et al.: *Dioctophyma renale* in the dog. JAVMA 155:605, 1969.

75. Brown, SA and Prestwood, AK: Parasites of the urinary tract. *In* Kirk, RW (ed): Current Veterinary Therapy IX. Philadelphia, WB Saunders, 1986, p 1153.

76. Borgsteede, FHM: Helminth parasites of wild foxes in the Netherlands. Z Parasitenkd 70:281, 1984.

77. Prestwood, AK: Personal communication, 1986.

78. Gillespie, D: Successful treatment of canine *Capillaria plica* cystitis. VM/SAC 78:681, 1983.

79. Enzie, FD: Do whipworms occur in domestic cats in North America? JAVMA 119:210, 1951.

80. Harris, LT: Feline bladderworm. VM/SAC 76:844, 1981.

81. Georgi, JR: Parasitology for Veterinarians. Philadelphia, WB Saunders, 1980, p 334.

82. Brown, SA: Unpublished observations, 1986.

83. Finco, DR: Medical management of feline urologic syndrome. *In* Kirk, RW (ed): Current Veterinary Therapy VI. Philadelphia, WB Saunders, 1977, p 1184.

84. Fabricant, CG: Viruses associated with diseases of the urinary tract. Vet Clin North Am 9:631, 1979.

85. Barsanti, JA: Opportunistic fungal infections. *In* Greene, CE (ed): Clinical Microbiology and Infectious Diseases of the Dog and Cat. Philadelphia, WB Saunders, 1984, p 728.

86. Doster, AR, et al.: Trichosporonosis in two cats. JAVMA 190:1184, 1987.

87. Tyler, DE: Protothecosis. *In* Greene, CE (ed): Clinical Microbiology and Infectious Diseases of the Dog and Cat. Philadelphia, WB Saunders, 1984, p 747.

88. Polzin, DJ and Klausner, JS: Treatment of urinary tract candidiasis. *In* Kirk, RW (ed): Current Veterinary Therapy VIII. Philadelphia, WB Saunders, 1983, p 1055.

89. Kivisto, AK, et al.: Canine bacteriuria. J Sm Anim Pract 18:707, 1977.

90. Bush, BM: A review of the etiology and consequences of urinary tract infections in the dog. Br Vet J 132:632, 1976.

91. Wooley, RE and Blue, JL: Quantitative and bacteriological studies of urine specimens from canine and feline urinary tract infections. J Clin Micro 4:326, 1976.

92. Finco, DR and Barsanti, JA: Localization of urinary tract infections in the dog. Vet Clin North Am 9:775, 1979.

93. Ling, GV, et al.: Relationship of upper and lower urinary tract infection and bacterial invasion of uroepithelium to antibody-coated bacteria test results in female dogs. Am J Vet Res 46:499, 1985.

94. Ihrke, PJ, et al.: Urinary tract infection associated with long-term corticosteroid administration in dogs with chronic skin diseases. JAVMA 186:43, 1985.

95. Oxenford, CJ, et al.: Bacteriuria in the dog. J Sm Anim Pract 25:83, 1984.

96. Ling, GV: Treatment of urinary tract infections. Vet Clin North Am 9:795, 1979.

97. Middleton, DJ and Lomas, GR: Emphysematous cystitis due to *Clostridium perfringens* in a non-diabetic dog. J Sm Anim Pract 20:433, 1979.

98. Carter, JM, et al.: Comparison of collection techniques for quantitative urine culture in dogs. JAVMA 173:296, 1978.

99. Barsanti, JA: Bacteremia of urinary tract origin (urosepsis). *In* Kirk, RW (ed): Current Veterinary Therapy IX. Philadelphia, WB Saunders, 1986, p 1150.

100. Warren, JW, et al.: Sequelae and management of urinary infection in the patient requiring chronic catheterization. J Urol 125:1, 1981.

101. Osborne, CA, et al.: Urinary tract infections: Normal and abnormal host defense mechanisms. Vet Clin North Am 9:587, 1979.

102. Dibartola, SP, et al.: Clinicopathologic findings associated with chronic renal disease in cats: 74 cases (1973–1984). JAVMA 190:1196, 1987.

103. Kelly, DF, et al.: Experimental pyelonephritis in the cat. Gross and histologic findings. J Comp Pathol 89:125, 1979.

104. Cerutti, PA: Prooxidant states and tumor production. Science 227:375, 1985.

105. Lees, GE and Osborne, CA: Antibacterial properties of urine: A comparative review. JAAHA 15:125, 1979.

106. Gregory, JG, et al.: Bladder resistance to infection. J Urol 105:220, 1971.

107. Senior, DF: Bacterial urinary tract infections: Invasion, host defenses, and new approaches to prevention. Comp Cont Ed 7:334, 1985.

108. Mooney, JK and Hinman, F: Surface differences in cells of proximal and distal canine urethra. J Urol 111:495, 1974.

109. Parsons, CL, et al.: Bladder-surface glycosaminoglycans: An efficient mechanism of environmental adaptation. Science 208:605, 1980.

110. Chang, SY, et al.: Povidone-iodine bladder injury in rats and protection with heparin. J Urol 130:382, 1983.

111. Tolkoff-Rubin, NE and Rubin, RH: New approaches to the treatment of urinary tract infection. Am J Med 82:S270, 1987.

112. Christie, BA: Incidence of vesicoureteral reflux in apparently normal dogs. Invest Urol 10:184, 1971.

113. Ling, GV and Ruby, AL: Aerobic bacterial flora of the prepuce, urethra, and vagina of normal adult dogs. Am J Vet Res 39:695, 1978.

114. Allen, WE and Dagnall, GJR: Some observations on the aerobic bacterial flora of the genital tract of the dog and bitch. J Sm Anim Pract 23:325, 1982.

115. Hinman, F: Meatal colonization in bitches. Trans Am Assoc Genitourinary Surg 68:73, 1977.

116. Lees, GE: Risks of urinary catheterization. *In* Kirk, RW (ed): Current Veterinary Therapy IX. Philadelphia, WB Saunders, 1986, p 1127.

117. Fowler, et al.: Studies of introital colonization in women with recurrent urinary tract infections. The role of bacterial interference. J Urol 118:296, 1977.

118. Chan, CYR, et al.: Adherence of cervical, vaginal and distal

urethral normal microbial flora to human epithelial cells and inhibition of adherence of gram negative uropathogens by competitive exclusion. J Urol 131:596, 1984.

119. Stamey, TA, et al.: Recurrent urinary infections in adult women. The role of introital enterobacteria. Calif Med 115:1, 1971.

120. Stamey, TA, et al.: The immunologic basis of recurrent bacteriuria: Role of cervicovaginal antibody in enterobacterial colonization of the introital mucosa. Medicine 57:47, 1978.

121. Lees, GE, et al.: Antibacterial properties of urine: Studies of feline urine, specific gravity, osmolality, and urine pH. JAAHA 15:135, 1979.

122. Stamey, TA, et al.: Antibacterial nature of prostatic fluid. Nature 218:444, 1968.

123. Freedman, LR: Experimental pyelonephritis. 13. On the ability of water diuresis to induce susceptibility to E. coli bacteriuria in the normal rat. Yale J Biol Med 39:255, 1967.

124. Root, CR and Scott, RC: Emphysematous cystitis and other radiographic manifestations of diabetes mellitus in dogs and cats. JAVMA 158:721, 1971.

125. Reidasch, G, et al.: Does low urinary sIgA predispose to urinary tract infection? Kidney Int 23:759, 1983.

126. Ling, GV, et al.: Canine hyperadrenocorticism: Pretreatment clinical and laboratory evaluation of 17 cases. JAVMA 174:1211, 1979.

127. Lorenz, MD: Diagnosis and medical management of canine Cushing's syndrome: a study of 57 consecutive cases. JAAHA 18:707, 1982.

128. Ling, GV, et al.: Diabetes mellitus in dogs: A review of initial evaluation, immediate and long-term management, and outcome. JAVMA 170:521, 1977.

129. Latimer, KS and Mahaffey, EA: Neutrophil adherence and movement in poorly and well-controlled diabetic dogs. Am J Vet Res 45:1498, 1984.

130. Stickle, JE, et al.: Adherence of neutrophils from dogs with diabetes mellitus. Am J Vet Res 47:541, 1986.

131. Cotran, RS and Pennington, JE: Urinary tract infection, pyelonephritis, and reflux nephropathy. In Brenner, BM and Rector, FC (eds): The Kidney. Philadelphia, WB Saunders, 1981, p 1571.

132. Thomas, JE: Urinary tract infection induced by intermittent urethral catheterization in dogs. JAVMA 174:705, 1979.

133. Barsanti, JA, et al.: Urinary tract infection due to indwelling bladder catheters in dogs and cats. JAVMA 187:384, 1985.

134. Lees, GE, et al.: Adverse effects caused by polypropylene and polyvinyl feline urinary catheters. Am J Vet Res 41:1836, 1980.

135. Stamm, WE: Prevention of urinary tract infections. Am J Med:148, 1984.

136. Lees, GE and Osborne, CA: Urinary tract infections associated with the use and misuse of urinary catheters. Vet Clin North Am 9:713, 1979.

137. Ling, GV and Gilmore, CJ: Penicillin G or ampicillin for oral treatment of canine urinary tract infections. JAVMA 171:358, 1977.

138. Ling, GV and Ruby, AL: Chloramphenicol for oral treatment of canine urinary tract infections. JAVMA 172:914, 1978.

139. Ling, GV and Ruby, AL: Trimethoprim in combination with a sulfonamide for oral treatment of canine urinary tract infections. JAVMA 174:1003, 1979.

140. Ling, GV and Ruby, AL: Gentamicin for treatment of resistant urinary tract infections in dogs. JAVMA 175:480, 1979.

141. Ling, GV, et al.: Tetracycline for the oral treatment of canine urinary tract infection caused by Pseudomonas aeruginosa. JAVMA 179:578, 1981.

142. Ling, GV and Ruby, AL: Cephalexin for oral treatment of canine urinary tract infection caused by Klebsiella pneumoniae. JAVMA 182:1346, 1983.

143. Ling, GV and Hirsch, DC: Antimicrobial susceptibility tests for urinary tract pathogens. In Kirk, RW (ed): Current Veterinary Therapy VIII. Philadelphia, WB Saunders, 1983, p 1048.

144. Ling, GV: Treatment of urinary tract infections with antimicrobial agents. In Kirk, RW (ed): Current Veterinary Therapy VIII. Philadelphia, WB Saunders, 1983, p 1051.

145. Ling, GV, et al.: Canine urinary tract infections: a comparison of in vitro antimicrobial susceptibility test results and response to oral therapy with ampicillin or with trimethoprim-sulfa. JAVMA 185:277, 1984.

146. Ling, GV: Management of urinary tract infections. In Kirk, RW (ed): Current Veterinary Therapy IX. Philadelphia, WB Saunders, 1986, p 1174.

147. Stamey, TA, et al.: Serum versus urinary antimicrobial concentrations in cure of urinary-tract infections. N Engl J Med 291:1159, 1974.

148. Rohrich, PJ, et al.: In vitro susceptibilities of canine urinary tract bacteria to selected antimicrobial agents. JAVMA 183:863, 1983.

149. Finco, DR, et al.: Evaluation of methods for localization of urinary tract infection in the female dog. Am J Vet Res 40:707, 1979.

150. Barber, DL and Finco, DR: Radiographic findings in induced bacterial pyelonephritis in dogs. JAVMA 175:1183, 1979.

151. Ronald, AR, et al.: Bacteriuria: localization and response to single-dose therapy in women. JAMA 235:1854, 1976.

152. Sheehan, G, et al.: Advances in the treatment of urinary tract infection. Am J Med 76(5A):141, 1984.

153. Rogers, KS, et al.: Efficacy of short-course antibiotic therapy in experimentally induced E. coli urinary tract infection in dogs. ACVIM Proc 4:14, 1986.

154. Leesm GE, et al.: Efficacy of single-dose amikacin treatment of urinary tract infections in dogs.: A clinical trial. ACVIM Proc 5:895, 1987.

155. Fairley, KF, et al.: Simple test to determine the site of urinary tract infection. Lancet 2:427, 1967.

156. Carvajah, HF, et al.: Urinary lactic dehydrogenase isoenzyme 5 in the differential diagnosis of kidney and bladder infections. Kidney Int 8:176, 1975.

157. Vigano, J, et al.: N-acetyl-β-D-glucosaminidase (NAG) and NAG isoenzymes in children with upper and lower urinary infection. Clin Chem Acta 130:297, 1983.

158. Tolkoff-Rubin, NE: Monoclonal antibodies in the diagnosis of renal disease: a preliminary report. Kidney Int 29:142, 1986.

159. Spangler, WL, et al.: Gentamicin nephrotoxicity in the dog: sequential light and electron microscopy. Vet Pathol 17:206, 1980.

160. Greco, DS, et al.: Urinary gamma-glutamyl transpeptidase activity in dogs with gentamicin-induced nephrotoxicity. Am J Vet Res 46:2332, 1985.

161. Hoyme, U, et al.: Antibiotic excretion in canine vaginal and urethral secretion. Invest Urol 16:35, 1978.

162. Gillenwater, JY: Use of β-lactam antibiotics in urinary tract infections. J Urology 129:457, 1983.

163. Neu, HC: Ciprofloxacin: An overview and prospective appraisal. Am J Med 82:S395, 1987.

164. Finco, DR and Barsanti, JA: Bacterial pyelonephritis. Vet Clin North Am 9:645, 1979.

165. Finco, DR and Barsanti, JA: Urinary acidifiers. In Kirk, RW (ed): Current Veterinary Therapy VIII. Philadelphia, WB Saunders, 1983, p 1095.

166. Eastman Kodak Company, Rochester, NY.

167. Wooley, RE and Jones, MS: Action of EDTA-Tris and antimicrobial agent combinations on selected pathogenic bacteria. Vet Micro 8:271, 1983.

168. Wooley, RE, et al.: Uptake of antibiotics in gram-negative bacteria exposed to EDTA-Tris. Vet Micro 10:57, 1984.

169. Senior, DF, et al.: Amoxycillin and clavulanic acid combination in the treatment of experimentally induced bacterial cystitis in cats. Res Vet Sci 39:42, 1985.

170. Senior, DF, et al.: Amoxicillin and clavulanic acid combination in the treatment of experimentally induced bacterial cystitis in dogs. JAAHA 22:227, 1986.

171. Lees, GE and Rogers, KS: Treatment of urinary tract infections in dogs and cats. JAVMA 189:648, 1986.

172. Schecte, RD, et al.: Heinz body hemolytic anemia associated with the use of urinary antiseptics containing methylene blue in the cat. JAVMA 162:37, 1973.

173. Harvey, HJ and Kornick, HP: Phenazopyridine toxicosis in the cat. JAVMA 169:327, 1976.

174. Christie, BA: Principles of urinary tract surgery. In Slatter, DG (ed): Textbook of Small Animal Surgery. Philadelphia, WB Saunders, 1985, p 1754.

175. Sherding, RG and Chew, DJ: Nondiabetic emphysematous cystitis in two dogs. JAVMA 174:1105, 1979.

176. Rayfield, EJ, et al.: Infection and diabetes: The case for glucose control. Am J Med 72:439, 1982.

177. Johnston, SD, et al.: Canine Polypoid cystitis. JAVMA 166.1155, 1975.

178. Johnston, SD, et al.: Canine polypoid cystitis. *In* Kirk, RW (ed): Current Veterinary Therapy VII. Philadelphia, WB Saunders, 1980, p 1137.

179. Bruchim, A, et al.: Isolation of mycoplasmas from the canine genital tract: A survey of 80 healthy dogs. Am J Vet Res 39:695, 1978.

180. Jang, SS, et al.: Mycoplasma as a cause of canine urinary tract infection. JAVMA 185:45, 1984.

181. Crow, SE, et al.: Cyclophosphamide-induced cystitis in the dog and cat. JAVMA 171:259, 1977.

182. Masih, BK and Hinman, F: Voiding and intrinsic defenses of the lower urinary tract in the female dog. Effect of immunosuppressive drugs on canine urethral and vaginal flora. Invest Urol 8:494, 1971.

183. Weller, RE, et al.: Transitional cell carcinoma of the bladder associated with cyclophosphamide therapy in a dog. JAAHA 15:733, 1979.

184. Macy, DW, et al.: Transitional cell carcinoma of the bladder associated with cyclophosphamide administration. JAAHA 19:965, 1983.

185. Crow, SE: Urinary tract neoplasms in dog and cats. Comp Cont Ed 7:607, 1985.

186. Weller, RE: Intravesical instillation of dilute formalin for treatment of cyclophosphamide-induced hemorrhagic cystitis in two dogs. JAVMA 172:1206, 1978.

187. Godec, CJ and Gleich, P: Intractable hematuria and formalin. J Urol 130:688, 1983.

188. Osborne, CA, et al.: Neoplasms of the canine and feline urinary bladder: Incidence, etiologic factors, occurrence and pathologic features. Am J Vet Res 29:2041, 1968.

189. Hayes, HM: Canine bladder cancer: Epidemiologic features. Am J Epidemiology 104:673, 1976.

190. Burnie, AG and Weaver, D: Urinary bladder neoplasia in the dog: A review of seventy cases. J Sm Anim Pract 24:129, 1983.

191. Wimberly, HC and Lewis, RM: Transitional cell carcinoma in the domestic cat. Vet Pathol 16:223, 1979.

192. Engle, GC and Brodey, RS: A retrospective study of 395 feline neoplasms. JAAHA 5:21, 1969.

193. Caywood, DD, et al.: *In* Kirk, RW (ed): Current Veterinary Therapy VII. Philadelphia, WB Saunders, 1980, p 1203.

194. Brearley, MJ, et al.: Three cases of transitional cell carcinoma in the cat and a review of the literature. Vet Rec 110:91, 1906.

195. Strafuss, AC and Dean, MJ: Neoplasms of the canine urinary bladder. JAVMA 166:1161, 1975.

196. Schwarz, PD, et al.: Urinary bladder tumors in the cat: A review of 27 cases. JAAHA 21:237, 1985.

197. Osborne, CA, et al.: Neoplasms of the canine and feline urinary bladder: Clinical findings, diagnosis, and treatment. JAVMA 152:247, 1968.

198. Paul, R, et al.: Metastasis of osteosarcoma to the bladder in a Finnish harrier: A case report. J Sm Anim Pract 25:639, 1984.

199. Marshall, VF, et al.: Hormonal influences on the experimental production of bladder tumors in dogs. Cancer 9:622, 1956.

200. Grognet, J: Transitional cell carcinoma and subsequent rupture of the canine bladder: A case report and review of the literature. Can Vet J 24:338, 1983.

201. Madewell, BR and Theilen, GH: Tumors of the urinary tract. *In* Theilen, GH and Madewell, BR (eds): Veterinary Cancer Medicine. Philadelphia, Lea & Febiger, 1987, p 567.

202. Stone, EA: Urogenital tumors. Vet Clin North Am 15:597, 1985.

203. Brodey, RS, et al.: Hypertrophic pulmonary osteopathy in a dog with carcinoma of the urinary bladder. JAVMA 162:474, 1973.

204. Esplin, DG: Urinary bladder fibromas in dogs: 51 cases. JAVMA 190:440, 1987.

205. Birchard, SJ, et al.: Fibroma of the urinary bladder of a dog. JAAHA 18:63, 1982.

206. Roszel, JF: Cytology of urine from dogs with botryoid sarcoma of the bladder. Acta Cytologica 16:443, 1972.

207. Halliwell, WH and Ackerman, N: Botryoid rhabdomyosarcoma of the urinary bladder and hypertrophic osteoarthropathy in a young dog. JAVMA 165:911, 1974.

208. Pletcher, JM and Dalton, L: Botryoid rhabdomyosarcoma in the urinary bladder of a dog. Vet Path 18:695, 1981.

209. Kelly, DF: Rhabdomyosarcoma of the urinary bladder in dogs. Vet Path 10:375, 1973.

210. Stamps, P and Haris, DL: Botryoid rhabdomyosarcoma of the urinary bladder of a dog. JAVMA 153:1064, 1968.

211. Teunissen, GHB and Misdorp, W: Rhabdomyosarcoma of the urinary bladder and fibromatosis of the extremities in a young dog. Zbl Vet Med [A] 15:81, 1968.

212. Seely, JC, et al.: Leiomyosarcoma of the canine urinary bladder, with metastasis. JAVMA 172:1427, 1978.

213. Patnaik, AK, et al.: Chemodectoma of the urinary bladder in a dog. JAVMA 164:797, 1974.

214. Mandel, M: Hypertrophic osteoarthropathy secondary to neurofibrosarcoma of the urinary bladder in a cocker spaniel. VM/SAC 70:1307, 1975.

215. Hawe, RS and Montali, RJ: Treatment of a neurofibrosarcoma of the urinary bladder in a dog. JAAHA 18:47, 1982.

216. Okajima, E, et al.: Urinary bladder tumors induced by N-butyl-N-(4-hydroxybutyl) nitrosamine in dogs. Cancer Res 41:1958, 1981.

217. Hayes, HM, et al.: Bladder cancer in pet dogs: A sentinel for environmental cancer? Am J Epidemiology 114:229, 1981.

218. Brown, RR and Price, JM: Quantitative studies on metabolites of tryptophan in the urine of the dog, cat, rat, and man. J Biol Chem 219:985, 1956.

219. Dill, GS, et al.: Transitional cell carcinoma of the urinary bladder in a cat. JAVMA 160:743, 1972.

220. Brodey, RS: Hypertrophic osteoarthropathy in the dog: A clinicopathologic survey of 60 cases. JAVMA 159:1242, 1971.

221. Magne, ML, et al.: Urinary tract carcinomas involving the canine vagina and vestibule. JAAHA 21:767, 1985.

222. Alroy, J: Ultrastructure of canine urinary bladder carcinoma. Vet Pathol 16:693, 1979.

223. Rozengurt, N, et al.: Urinary cytology of a canine bladder carcinoma. J Comp Path 96:581, 1986.

224. Wiggishoff, CC and McDonald, JH: Urinary exfoliative cytology in the diagnosis of bladder tumors. Acta Cytologica 16:139, 1972.

225. Moldoff, DL and Gordon, RP: Pyogranuloma of a canine urinary bladder. JAAHA 12:507, 1976.

226. Zachary, JF: Cystitis cystica, cystitis glandularis, and Brunn's nests in a feline urinary bladder. Vet Path 18:113, 1981.

227. Walter, PA, et al.: Radiographic appearance of pulmonary metastases from transitional cell carcinoma of the bladder and urethra of the dog. JAVMA 185:411, 1984.

228. Crow, SE: Management of transitional cell carcinoma of the urinary bladder. *In* Kirk, RW (ed): Current Veterinary Therapy VIII. Philadelphia, WB Saunders, 1983, p 1119.

229. Owen, LN: TNM Classification of tumours in domestic animals. World Health Organization (Geneva), 1980, p 34.

230. Koss, LG: Tumors of the Urinary Bladder. Washington DC, Armed Forces Institute of Pathology, 1975, p 38.

231. MacEwen, EG, et al.: Urinary tract tumors. *In* Kirk, RW (ed): Current Veterinary Therapy VI. Philadelphia, WB Saunders, 1977, p 1204.

232. Montgomery, RD and Hankes, GH: Ureterocolonic anastomosis in a dog with transitional cell carcinoma of the urinary bladder. JAVMA 190:1427, 1987.

233. Patnaik, AK and Greene, RW: Intravenous leiomyoma of the bladder in a cat. JAVMA 175:381, 1979.

234. Osborne, CA: Neoplasms of the urinary system. *In* Kirk, RW (ed): Current Veterinary Therapy V. Philadelphia, WB Saunders, 1974, p 878.

235. Prout, GR, et al.: The bladder. *In* Holland, JF and Frei, E (eds): Cancer Medicine. Philadelphia, Lea & Febiger, 1982, p 1896.

236. Theilen, GH and Madewell, BR: Tumors of the urogenital tract. *In* Theilen, GH and Madewell, BR (eds): Veterinary Cancer Medicine. Philadelphia, Lea & Febiger, 1979, p 357.

237. Beamer, RJ: Ureterocolostomy for relief of urinary stenosis in the domestic cat. JAVMA 134:201, 1959.

238. Bjorling, DE, et al.: Bilateral ureteroileostomy and perineal urinary diversion in dogs. Vet Surg 14:204, 1985.

239. Crowe, DT and Calvert, C: Personal communication, 1987.

240. Bush, H, et al.: Chemotherapy in the management of invasive bladder cancer. Cancer Chemother Pharmacol 3.87, 1979.

241. Theilen, GH, et al.: Chemotherapy. *In* Theilen, GH and Madewell, BR (eds): Veterinary Cancer Medicine. Philadelphia, Lea & Febiger, 1987, p 157.

242. Brewer, WG and Theilen, GH: Cancer chemotherapy. *In* Gour-

ley, IM and Vaseur, PB (eds): General Small Animal Surgery. Philadelphia, JB Lippincott, 1985, p 961.

243. Caywood, DD and Osborne, CA: Urinary system. *In* Slatter, DH (ed): Textbook of Small Animal Surgery. Philadelphia, WB Saunders, 1985, p 2561.

244. Craig, JA, et al.: Effects of intraoperative irradiation on gastric and urinary bladder incisions in the dog. Am J Vet Res 46:1647, 1985.

245. Dewhirst, MW, et al.: New methods of therapy. *In* Theilen, GH and Madewell, BR (eds): Veterinary Cancer Medicine. Philadelphia, Lea & Febiger, 1987, p 197.

246. Nseyo, UO, et al.: Experimental photodynamic treatment of canine bladder. J Urology 133:311, 1985.

247. Barton, C: Management of Bladder Neoplasia. *In* Kirk, RW (ed): Current Veterinary Therapy X. Philadelphia, WB Saunders, 1989.

248. Wilson, GP, et al.: Canine urethral cancer. JAAHA 15:741, 1979.

249. Clark, WT, et al.: Rhabdomyosarcoma of the urethra in a dog. J Sm Anim Pract 25:203, 1984.

250. Barrett, RE and Nobel, TA: Transitional cell carcinoma of the urethra in a cat. Cornell Vet 66:14, 1976.

251. Al-Zubaidy, AJ: Canine prostatic and urethral neoplasms: A clinico-pathological study. Can Vet J 16:71, 1982.

252. Gorman, NT, et al.: A case of transitional cell carcinoma of the canine urethra. JAAHA 20:817, 1984.

253. Ryan, CP and Holshuh, HJ: Urethral adenocarcinoma in a dog. VM/SAC 76:1315, 1981.

254. Pollock, S: Urethral carcinoma in the dog: A case report. J Am Rad Soc 9:95, 1968.

255. Alexander, JW, et al.: Transitional cell carcinoma of the canine urethra: Case report and review of the literature. Vet Surg 7:90, 1978.

256. Szymanski, C, et al.: Transitional cell carcinoma of the urethra metastatic to the eyes in a dog. JAVMA 185:1003, 1984.

257. Ticer, JW, et al.: Transitional cell carcinoma of the urethra in four female dogs: Its urethrographic appearance. Vet Rad 21:12, 1980.

258. Hoffer, RE: Transplantation of the neck of the bladder to the abdominal wall. Small Anim Clin 2:129, 1962.

259. Yoshioka, MM and Carb, A: Antepubic urethrostomy in the dog. JAAHA 18:290, 1982.

260. Knecht, CD and Slusher, R: Extrapelvic anastomosis of the bladder and penile urethra in a dog. JAAHA 6:247, 1970.

261. Bjorling, DE: Traumatic injuries of the urogenital system. Vet Clin North Am 14:61, 1984.

262. Burrows, CA and Bovee, KC: Metabolic changes due to experimentally induced rupture of the canine urinary bladder. Am J Vet Res 35:1083, 1974.

263. Rawlings, CA and Wingfield, WE: Urethral reconstruction in dogs and cats. JAAHA 12:850, 1976.

264. Kolata, RJ and Johnston, DE: Motor vehicle accidents in urban dogs: A study of 600 cases. JAVMA 167:938, 1975.

265. Osborne, CA, et al.: Canine and Feline Urology. Philadelphia, WB Saunders, 1972, p 338.

266. Hill, BL and Postlewaite, RC: Urethral rupture in a bitch with urolithiasis. JAVMA 174:170, 1979.

267. Kleine, LJ and Thornton, GW: Radiographic diagnosis of urinary tract trauma. JAAHA 7:318, 1971.

268. Morgan, RV: Urogenital emergencies. Comp Cont Ed 11:908, 1982.

269. Selcer, BA: Urinary tract trauma associated with pelvic trauma. JAAHA 19:785, 1982.

270. Burrows, CF and Kolata, RJ: Rupture of the canine urinary bladder. *In* Kirk, RW (ed): Current Veterinary Therapy VII. 1980, p 1139.

271. Trocath, McGraw Laboratories, American Hospital Supply Corporation, Norcross, GA.

272. Bjorling, DE, et al.: Penetrating abdominal wounds in dogs and cats. JAAHA 18:742, 1982.

273. Crowe, DT and Crane, SW: Diagnostic paracentesis and lavage in the evaluation of abdominal injuries in dogs and cats: Clinical and experimental investigations. JAVMA 168:700, 1976.

274. Pechman, RD: Urinary trauma in dogs and cats: A review. JAAHA 18:33, 1982.

275. Trim, C: Anesthesia and the kidney. Comp Cont Ed 11:843, 1979.

276. Meynard, J: Traumatic rupture of the bladder in the dog: A clinical study of nine cases. J Sm Anim Pract 2:131, 1961.

277. Rawlings, CA: Extraperitoneal urinary bladder rupture and urinary fistula in a dog. JAVMA 115:123, 1969.

278. Sovereign Feeding Tube, Sherwood Medical Industries Inc, St Louis, MO.

279. Argyle Suction Catheter, Sherwood Medical Industries Inc, St Louis, MO.

280. Smith, CW: Surgical diseases of the urethra. *In* Slatter, DH (ed): Textbook of Small Animal Surgery. Philadelphia, WB Saunders, 1985, p 1799.

281. Hardie, EM, et al.: Complications of prostatic surgery. JAAHA 20:50, 1984.

282. Bradley, RL: Complete urethral obstruction secondary to fracture of the os penis. Comp Cont Ed 7:759, 1985.

283. Johnston, DE and Archibald, J: Male genital system. *In* Archibald, J and Catcott, EJ (eds): Canine and Feline Surgery. Santa Barbara, American Veterinary Publications Inc, 1984, p 293.

284. Adams, WM and Dibartola, SP: Radiographic and clinical features of pelvic bladder in the dog. JAVMA 182:1212, 1983.

285. Holt, PE: Importance of urethral length, bladder neck position and vestibulovaginal stenosis in the incontinent bitch. Res Vet Sci 39:364, 1985.

286. Dibartola, SP and Adams, WWM: Urinary incontinence associated with malposition of the urinary bladder. *In* Kirk, RW (ed): Current Veterinary Therapy VIII. Philadelphia, WB Saunders, 1983, p 1089.

287. Mahaffey, MB, et al.: Pelvic bladder in dogs without urinary incontinence. JAVMA 184:1477, 1984.

288. Holt, PE: Urinary incontinence in the bitch due to sphincter mechanism incompetence: surgical treatment. J Sm Anim Pract 26:237, 1985.

289. Osborne, CA, et al.: Patent urachus in the dog. Anim Hosp 2:245, 1966.

290. Greene, RW and Scott, RC: Diseases of the bladder and urethra. *In* Ettinger, SJ (ed): Textbook of Veterinary Internal Medicine. Philadelphia, WB Saunders, 1983, p 1890.

291. Hansen, JS: Urachal remnant in the cat: occurrence and relationship to the feline urological syndrome. VM/SAC 72:1735, 1977.

292. Gotthelf, LN: Persistent urinary tract infection and urolithiasis in a cat with a urachal diverticulum. VM/SAC 76:1745, 1981.

293. Greene, RW and Bohning, RH: Patent persistent urachus associated with urolithiasis in a cat. JAVMA 158:489, 1971.

294. Glennon, JC and Orsher, RJ: Urachal diverticulum in a cat with signs of lower urinary tract disease. Comp Cont Ed 8:310, 1986.

295. Osborne, CA, et al.: Etiopathogenesis and biological behavior of feline vesicourachal diverticula. Vet Clin North Am, 1987.

296. Wilson, JW, et al.: Canine vesicourachal diverticula. Vet Surg 8:63, 1979.

297. Barsanti, JA and Downey, R: Urinary incontinence in cats. JAAHA 20:979, 1984.

298. Rochlitz, I: Feline dysautonomia (the Key Gaskell or dilated pupil syndrome): a preliminary review. J Sm Anim Pract 25:587, 1984.

299. Sharp, NJH, et al.: Feline dysautonomia (the Key Gaskell syndrome): a clinical and pathological study of forty cases. J Sm Anim Pract 25:599, 1984.

300. Barsanti, JA: Feline urinary incontinence. *In* Kirk, RW (ed): Current Veterinary Therapy IX. Philadelphia, WB Saunders, 1986, p 1159.

301. Lappin, MR and Barsanti, JA: Urinary incontinence secondary to idiopathic detrusor instability: Cystometrographic diagnosis and pharmacologic management in two dogs and a cat. JAVMA 191:1439, 1987.

302. Lane, JG: Canine ectopic ureter: Two case reports. J Sm Anim Pract 14:555, 1973.

303. Owen, RR: Canine ureteral ectopia: A review. 2. Incidence, diagnosis, and treatment. J Sm Anim Pract 14:419, 1973.

304. Johnston, GR, et al.: Familial ureteral ectopia in the dog. JAAHA 13:168, 1977.

304a. Barton, C: Personal communication, 1987.

305. Lennox, JS: A case report of unilateral ectopic ureter in a male Siberian husky. JAAHA 14:331, 1978.

306. Smith, CW, et al.: Bilateral ectopic ureter in a male dog with urinary incontinence. JAVMA 177:1022, 1980.

307. Holt, P: Ectopic ureter in the bitch. Vet Rec 98:299, 1976.
308. Osborne, CA, et al.: Urinary incontinence due to ectopic ureter in a male dog. JAVMA 166:273, 1969.
309. Holt, PE, et al.: Canine ectopic ureter—a review of twenty-nine cases. J Sm Anim Pract 23:195, 1982.
310. Martin, RA, et al.: Bilateral ectopic ureters in a male dog: A case report. JAAHA 21:80, 1985.
311. Tangner, CH: A review of ectopic ureters and methods of surgical correction. Southwestern Vet 34:113, 1981.
312. Christie, BA: Ureters. In Slatter, DH (ed): Textbook of Small Animal Surgery. Philadelphia, WB Saunders, 1985, p 1777.
313. Rawlings, CA: Correction of congenital defects of the urogenital system. Vet Clin North Am 14:49, 1984.
314. Rutgers, C, et al.: Bilateral ectopic ureters in a female cat without urinary incontinence. JAVMA 184:1394, 1984
315. Bebko, RL, et al.: Ectopic ureters in a male cat. JAVMA 171:738, 1977.
316. Biewanga, WJ, et al.: Ectopic ureters in the cat: A report of two cases. J Sm Anim Pract 19:531, 1977.
317. Reis, RH: Renal aplasia, ectopic ureter and vascular anomalies in a domestic cat. Anat Rec 135:105, 1959.
318. Smith, CW, et al.: Bilateral ureteral ectopia in a male cat with urinary incontinence. JAVMA 182:172, 1983.
319. Grauer GF, et al.: Urinary incontinence associated with an ectopic ureter in a female cat. JAVMA 182:707, 1983.
320. Allen, WE and Webbon, PM: Two cases of urinary incontinence in cats associated with acquired vaginoureteral fistula. J Sm Anim Pract 21:367, 1980.
321. Pearson, H and Gibbs, C: Urinary incontinence in the dog due to accidental vagino-ureteral fistulation during hysterectomy. J Sm Anim Pract 21:287, 1980.
322. Breitschwerdt, EB, et al.: Bilateral hydronephrosis and hydroureter in a dog associated with congenital urethral stricture. JAAHA 18:799, 1982.
323. Scott, RC, et al.: Unilateral ureterocele associated with hydronephrosis in a dog. JAAHA 10:126, 1974.
324. Miller, CF: Urethrorectal fistula with concurrent urolithiasis in a dog. VM/SAC 75:73, 1980.
325. Osborne, CA, et al.: Congenital urethrorectal fistula in two dogs. JAVMA 166:999, 1975.
326. Goulden, B, et al.: Canine urethrorectal fistula. J Sm Anim Pract 14:143, 1973.
327. Lipowitz, AJ: Diseases of the canine urethra. In Kirk, RW (ed): Current Veterinary Therapy. VIII. Philadelphia, WB Saunders, 1983, p 1114.
328. Adler, PL and Hobson, HP: Hypospadias: A review of the veterinary literature and a report of three cases in the dog. JAAHA 14:721, 1978.
329. Holt, PE, et al.: Disorders of urination associated with canine intersexuality. J Sm Anim Pract 24:475, 1983.
330. Englebart, RH, et al.: Urethral reaction to catheter materials in dogs. Invest Urol 16:55, 1978.
331. Osborne, CA, et al.: Ancillary therapy of urinary tract infections. In Kirk, RW (ed): Current Veterinary Therapy VII. Philadelphia, WB Saunders, 1980, p 1164.
332. Stowater, JL and Springer, AL: Ureterocele in a dog. VM/SAC 74:1753, 1979.
333. Reavley, G: Urethral ballistics. Vet Rec 114:364, 1984.
334. Morshead, D: Submucosal urethral calculus secondary to foxtail awn migration in a dog. JAVMA 182:1247, 1983.
335. Taylor, RA: Reconstructive surgery after use of a urethral prosthesis in a castrated cat. VM/SAC 75:437, 1980.
336. Firestone, WM: Prolapse of the male urethra. JAVMA 99:135, 1941.
337. Hobson, HP and Heller, RA: Prolapse of the male urethra. VM/SAC 66:1177, 1971.
338. Sinibaldi, KR and Green, RW: Surgical correction of prolapse of the male urethra in three English bulldogs. JAAHA 9:450, 1973.
339. Lees, GE and Rogers, KS: Diagnosis and localization of urinary tract infection. In Kirk, RW (ed): Current Veterinary Therapy IX. Philadelphia, WB Saunders, 1986, p 1118.
340. Tilmant, L, et al.: Pharmacokinetics of ticarcillin in the dog. Am J Vet Res 46:479, 1985.
341. Page, R: Cisplatin, a new antineoplastic drug in veterinary medicine. JAVMA 186:288, 1985.
342. Shapiro, W, et al.: Cisplatin for treatment of transitional cell and squamous cell carcinomas in dogs. JAVMA 193:1530, 1988.

DISEASES OF BLOOD CELLS, LYMPH NODES, AND SPLEEN

113 ERYTHROCYTES AND ASSOCIATED DISORDERS

M. G. WEISER

ERYTHROPOIESIS

The bone marrow, spleen, liver, and lymph nodes comprise the potential hematopoietic organs that may support erythropoiesis. In the adult, erythropoiesis is confined to marrow spaces, principally in the axial skeleton and ends of long bones. When there is increased demand for cell production, such as in blood loss or hemolytic disease, erythropoiesis expands in marrow and may expand to the above organs. The latter expansion is referred to as extramedullary hematopoiesis.

The normal animal may produce several billion erythrocytes/kg/day. The cellular components involved in erythropoiesis can be divided into a series of functional hematopoietic compartments and their supportive surroundings known as the hematopoietic inductive microenvironment. Much of our knowledge about erythropoiesis has come from research on murine hematopoietic systems.

A population of pluripotential stem cells supports production of megakaryocytes, granulocytes, monocytes, and erythrocytes. These cells have properties of self-renewal, proliferation, and differentiation. Dependent on need for erythropoietic cells, a proportion of this population makes entry into a compartment of progenitor cells committed to erythropoiesis. When marrow cells are cultured and appropriately stimulated, at least two subsets of progenitor cells that give rise to mature erythrocytes can be identified. These are referred to as erythroid burst forming units (BFU-E) and erythroid colony forming units (CFU-E). While it is not clear what stimulates uncommitted cells to enter the committed BFU-E compartment, it is likely that factors released from local mononuclear cells, collectively known as burst promoting activity, regulate entry and stimulate formation of erythropoietin receptors. Erythropoietin activity, produced by the kidney, is a regulatory hormone system for determining rate of effective erythrocyte production. Erythropoietin stimulates BFU-E to differentiate into CFU-E. CFU-E, also erythropoietin sensitive, in turn differentiate into the rubriblast, the first morphologically recognizable erythroid precursor (Figure 113–1).

Techniques for culturing these cell populations are important for *in vitro* investigation of various factors in the pathogenesis of injury to erythropoiesis.[1, 3] Ultimately, treatment of a number of hematologic diseases may involve manipulation of stem cell populations as we gain improved understanding of their function and responses to injury. More detailed reviews on hematopoietic stem cells are available.[4, 5]

Morphologically recognizable erythroid precursors in marrow are the result of three to four divisions by each rubriblast, giving rise to 8 to 16 cells that undergo progressive maturation (Figure 113–1). This process of transit from the rubriblast to erythrocyte requires four to seven days in the normal animal but may be accelerated to about two days under conditions of erythroid marrow stimulation. Events visualized during erythroid maturation include progressively decreasing size, nuclear chromatin condensation, and hemoglobinization. The denucleated polychromatophilic cell continues to synthesize hemoglobin and shed organelles before becoming a mature erythrocyte, as observed on the Wright's stained blood film. Morphologic features of this process are very important to the microscopist for evaluation of erythropoietic pathology.

TECHNOLOGICAL CONSIDERATIONS IN VETERINARY HEMATOLOGY

There are a number of technical aspects of veterinary hematology which deserve brief review here. Knowledge about these factors in the laboratory is essential to generation of accurate or meaningful hematologic data. When interfacing with a human laboratory, it will generally be the responsibility of the veterinarian to provide this information to the laboratorians. Additionally, information provided here may be useful to some veterinary laboratories.

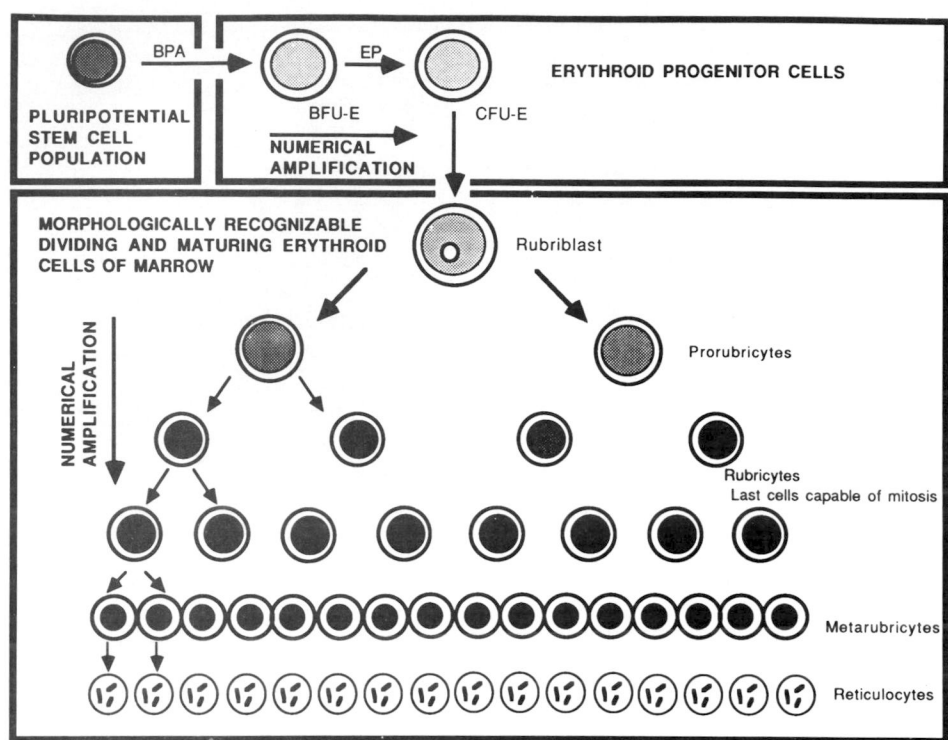

FIGURE 113–1. Model of erythropoiesis showing stem cell compartments and morphologically recognizable maturation compartment. Numerical amplification of cell production is important at indicated points. BPA = burst promoting activity, EP = erythropoietin activity, BFU-E = erythroid burst forming unit, CFU-E = erythroid colony forming unit.

The availability of automation in human hematology has stimulated adaptation in veterinary hematology to automated systems. The objectives of utilizing this technology in centralized laboratories have been to maintain low relative cost, provide more complete analyses, and improve reliability of data. Instrument modification and recalibration are required for successful use of these systems for veterinary applications. Widespread use of this instrumentation has resulted in an experience base that has contributed to reliable use in most settings.

SIZING OF ERYTHROCYTES AND LIMITATIONS OF AUTOMATED CELL COUNTING

Automated cell counting systems not only count individual cells but also measure individual cell volume. Some systems measure hematocrit by summing erythrocyte volumes in a fixed volume of blood. Mean cell volume (MCV) is then calculated from the erythrocyte count and hematocrit. This same technology in an affordable, less automated form is becoming available to larger veterinary hospital settings. On more sophisticated systems, a histogram or volume distribution curve of the erythrocyte population is generated (Figure 113–2). Normal erythrocyte size distribution has been characterized for dogs, cats, horses, and cows.[6]

The MCV is directly determined from analysis of the volume distribution and the hematocrit is then calculated by multiplying the MCV by the erythrocyte concentration. An additional value, the red cell distribution width, is provided by analysis of the histogram. This value is an expression of volume anisocytosis or heterogeneity. It is of use to the laboratorian as an adjunct to evaluation of erythrocyte pathology on blood films. By itself, it will have little value to the clinician.

Automated erythrocyte analysis is reliable for canine blood on instruments in human laboratories.[7, 8] However, erythrocytes of cats and other common domestic species are too small to be properly analyzed on these systems without electronic modifications. This is only done on instruments used solely for veterinary applications. Therefore, human medical laboratories should use microhematocrit centrifugation for measuring hematocrit values in cats.

The same counting and sizing functions exist for counting platelets on some advanced systems. Systems are designed with a threshold system to separate platelets and erythrocytes by volume. Analysis of erythrocytes and platelets is very reliable for canine blood. For cats, there is considerable overlap between erythrocyte

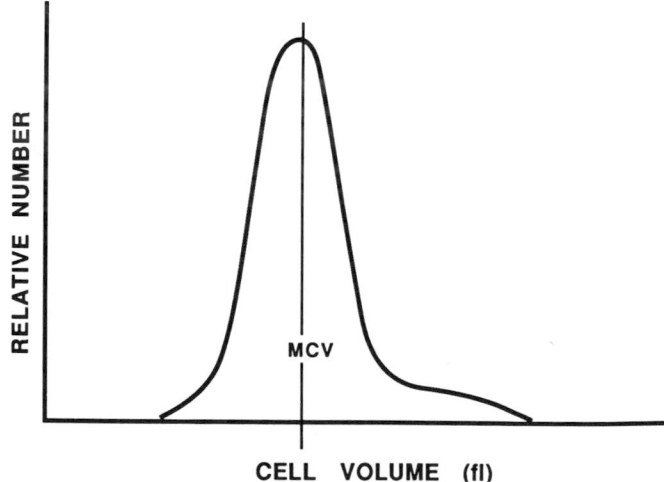

FIGURE 113–2. Erythrocyte volume distribution curve generated by an electronic cell counter with attached particle size analyzer. The mean cell volume (MCV) is indicated by the vertical bar.

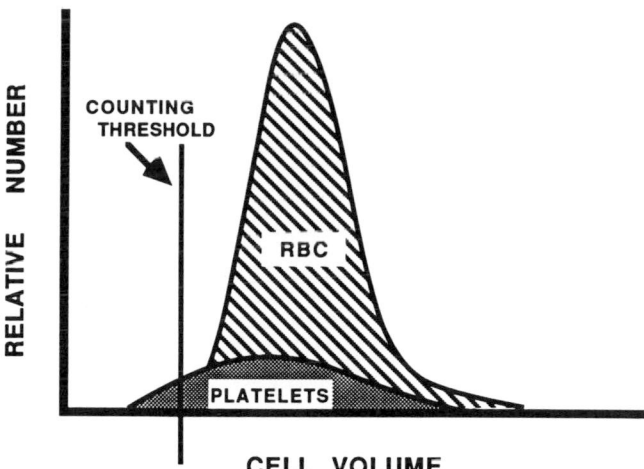

FIGURE 113–3. Feline erythrocyte/platelet size distribution curves illustrating potential overlap in volume of these two cell populations. The overlap complicates resolution of the two populations with respect to counting thresholds on an electronic cell counter, as explained in text.

and platelet volume (Figure 113–3). This means that cell counting systems cannot resolve the cells into two distinct populations. This has several implications for the feline hemogram. First, whole blood platelet counts are not feasible on automated cell counters.[7] Platelets must be enumerated manually by hemocytometer or electronically on platelet-rich plasma in which the erythrocytes have been removed by differential centrifugation.[9, 10] Second, a large but variable proportion of platelets are included in the erythrocyte count. Thus, platelet mass is included in the determination of the hematocrit. This is rarely a problem, since the concentration of platelets is usually small compared to the concentration of erythrocytes. In severely anemic cats with a concurrent high platelet count, the hematocrit may be overestimated by one to four per cent. However, due to size similarity, platelets do not appreciably interfere with electronic determination of the MCV. Third, when using single channel cell counters, such as the Coulter Z series instruments, inclusion of platelets in the erythrocyte count may cause considerable error in traditional MCV values calculated from the erythrocyte count and packed cell volume determined by microhematocrit centrifugation. This phenomenon has likely contributed to the relatively high upper reference range limit for calculated MCV values and has impaired detection of macrocytosis associated with regenerative anemia, as well as FeLV-associated anemia.[11–13] It is suggested that with the availability of current technology, traditional calculated MCV values are not worth doing, especially for feline hemograms. More detail on this technology may be obtained elsewhere.[6–8]

ERYTHROCYTE MORPHOLOGY ON WRIGHT'S STAINED BLOOD FILMS

The number and subtlety of morphologic abnormalities on stained blood films used in contributing to diagnoses have steadily increased.[11–15] Many of the distinctions made are dependent upon an intact chain of events starting from an optimally prepared and stained blood film and ending with the experience of the microscopist. A defect in any point in the chain compromises the information gained from the hematologic examination. In most veterinary medical settings, this job should be delegated to the veterinary pathology laboratory. Only veterinarians with an enthusiastic interest in microscopy should attempt to learn to make the morphologic interpretations utilized in characterizing hematologic disease today. Clinicians performing their own hematologic work should recognize when second opinion is needed from the external laboratory and obtain it without hesitation.

Normal erythrocytes have a degree of uniformity that must be appreciated by the microscopist in order to detect the presence of erythrocyte pathology (Figure 113–4). Increased anisocytosis is present when the normal diameter uniformity is altered. This is due to the presence of abnormally large cells, small cells, or both. Anisocytosis means little to the clinician; its proposed importance is that it indicates to the laboratorian that one or more specific morphologic changes is present.

Polychromatophilic Cells. Polychromatophilic cells represent newly released erythrocytes still undergoing maturation. They have a blue-gray tint compared to more acidophilic mature cells (Figure 113–5). An increase of these cells, subjectively recognized as greater than one per oil immersion field in a monolayer, is interpreted as evidence for accelerated erythrocyte regeneration. When produced under conditions of erythroid marrow stimulation, these cells are somewhat larger than normal in diameter, their volume is increased, and they therefore contribute to increasing the MCV value observed in regenerative anemia. Macrocytosis associated with regenerative anemia is generally much more prominent in cats than in dogs. With maximally stimulated erythroid marrow, cats will release cells with approximately twice normal volume whereas dogs usually release cells with only about 1.2 to 1.5 times the normal volume.

Nucleated Erythrocytes. Nucleated erythrocytes or metarubricytosis may accompany reticulocytosis in blood during regenerative anemia (Figure 113–5). They may also be observed in myeloproliferative disease (particularly involving the erythroid series), dysmyelopoiesis, and extramedullary hematopoiesis. In the instances of marrow disease, the nucleated erythrocytes are usually present in the face of non-regenerative anemia and reticulocytopenia.

Basophilic Stippling. Basophilic stippling is spontaneous aggregation of ribosomes and other organelles into small, homogeneously dispersed, basophilic granules during erythrocyte maturation (Figure 113–6). In dogs, basophilic stippling may occur rarely during active erythrocyte regeneration. If observed in conjunction with unexplained erythrocyte regeneration and/or metarubricytosis, the suspicion of lead toxicity should be raised. It is occasionally observed in cats during active erythrocyte regeneration. It should not be interpreted as indicating lead poisoning in the cat.

Heinz Bodies. Heinz bodies are frequently observed on Wright's stained blood films as round bodies that may protrude to varying degrees from the cell contour (Figures 113–7 and 113–16). They are observed fre-

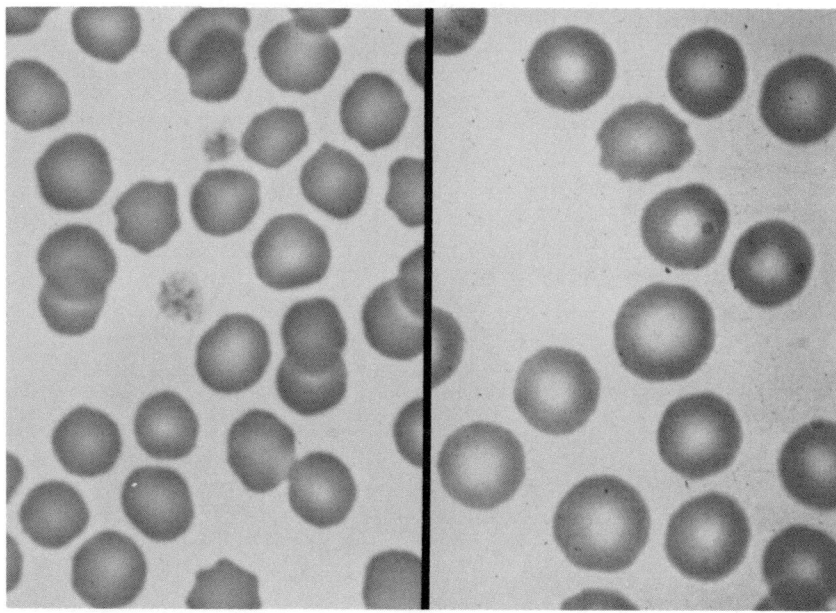

FIGURE 113–4. Normal uniformity and central pallor for canine (left of split field) and feline (right of split field) erythrocytes. Wright-Giemsa stain.

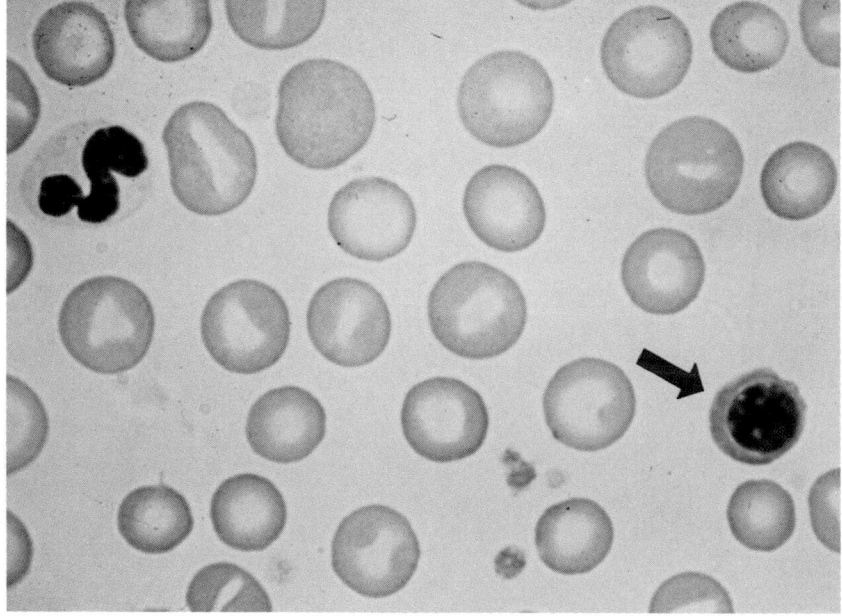

FIGURE 113–5. Polychromatophilic erythrocytes and nucleated erythrocyte (arrow). Polychromatophilic erythrocytes are recognized by their blue-gray cytoplasmic tint. Wright-Giemsa stain.

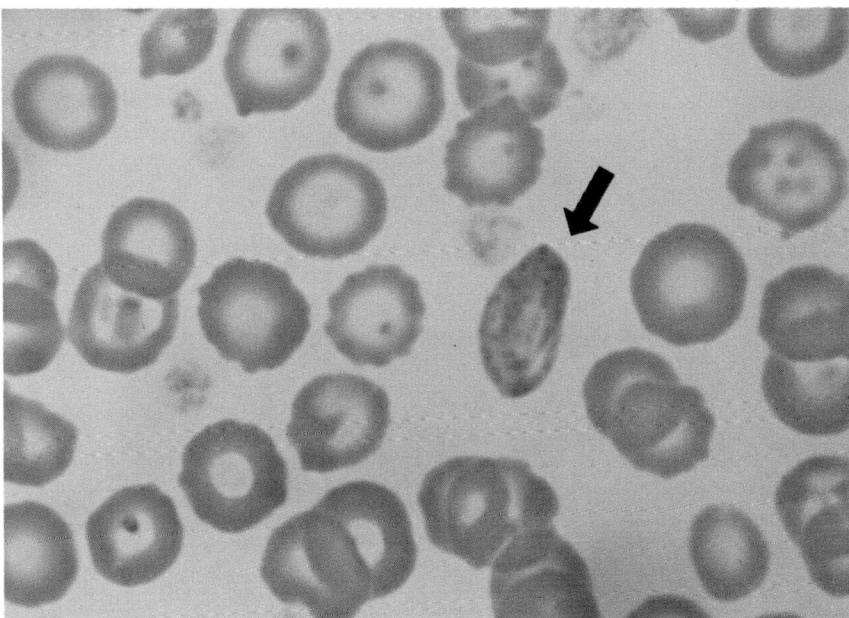

FIGURE 113–6. Basophilic stippling (arrow), canine blood. Wright-Giemsa stain.

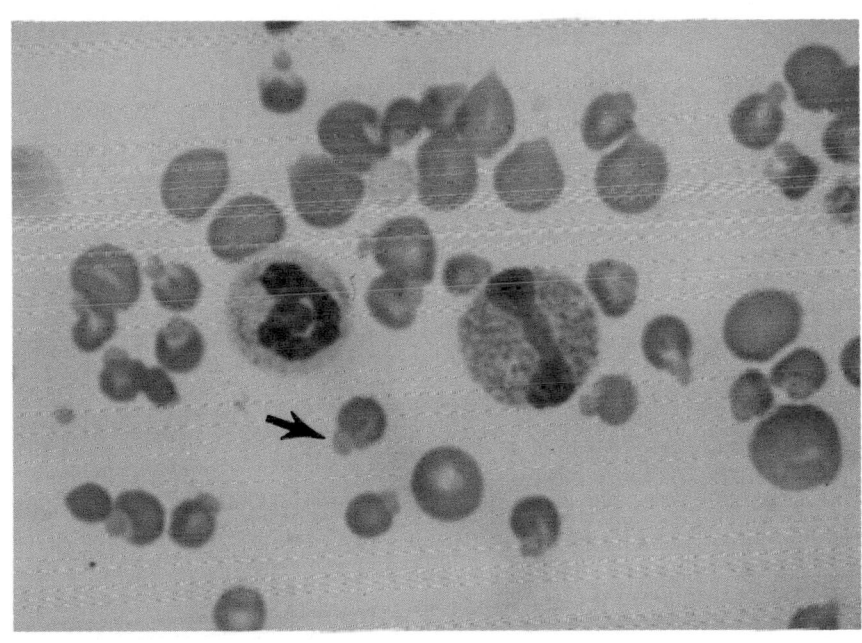

FIGURE 113–7. Heinz bodies in feline blood. The majority of cells have a single Heinz body recognizable as a protrusion from the membrane contour. The Heinz bodies stain the same color as surrounding hemoglobin, but are slightly lighter. Wright-Giemsa stain.

quently in cats and usually occur as a single body per cell. They have been regarded as normal in the cat when present in small numbers. An alternative interpretation is that they represent true erythrocyte injury, which is often not of clinical importance. Heinz body–bearing cells likely have shortened survival, but the associated hemolysis is not clinically detectable. Heinz bodies stain blue and are much easier to visualize with one of the reticulocyte stains. In dogs, Heinz bodies are more subtle and are very difficult to visualize with Wright's stain. The reason is that Heinz bodies in dogs are usually multiple small bodies per cell and tend not to protrude from the membrane. Heinz body formation in the dog is most frequently associated with onion ingestion.

Eccentrocytes. Eccentrocytes are associated with Heinz body oxidative injury in dogs (Figure 113–8). Features include shifting of hemoglobin to one side of the cell, loss of normal central pallor, and a clear zone outlined by membrane. The observation of eccentrocytes should prompt the laboratorian to examine a reticulocyte preparation for the presence of Heinz bodies.

Spherocytes. Spherocytes are a hallmark morphologic change of immune-mediated hemolytic anemia (Figure 113–9). When comprising a large proportion of cells and confirmed by an experienced microscopist, spherocytes may be regarded as diagnostic for immunohemolytic anemia in dogs. Occasionally, sphere formation is incomplete; cells have a dimple of remnant central pallor making the interpretation uncertain. Spherocytes are difficult if not impossible to identify in the cat due to the normal lack of central pallor. It is recommended that the suspicion of sphere-injured cells be confirmed with the saline fragility assay when morphologic assessment is uncertain.

Immune-Mediated Agglutination. Immune-mediated agglutination may be observed with immunohemolytic anemia. Agglutination results in irregular spherical clumps both in saline wet mounts and on Wright's stained films (Figure 113–10). Prominent agglutination may be observed grossly (Figure 113–11). Refrigerating the blood for 10 to 15 minutes will maximize the agglutination. Agglutination should be confirmed by microscopy to distinguish it from prominent rouleaux formation (Figure 113–12). With moderate to marked agglutination, this can be done by examining the thick portion of the blood film with low magnification (see Figure 113–10). Otherwise, a fresh wet mount, made by the addition of a very small amount of blood to a drop of saline, should be examined (see Figure 113–10). It is important to examine an area of the wet mount having a dispersed monolayer. The technique of examining a 1:1 mixture of blood and saline is not recommended because high erythrocyte concentration on the preparation makes interpretation difficult.

Rouleaux Formation. Rouleaux formation is the spontaneous association of erythrocytes in linear chains. Its appearance has been described as similar to "stacking of coins" (see Figure 113–12). This is a normal finding in dogs and cats, but is enhanced by increases in plasma high molecular weight proteins such as fibrinogen and immunoglobulins. When prominent, rouleaux may appear grossly indistinguishable from mild agglutination—

when allowed to flow down the inside of an inverted blood tube.

Erythrocyte Fragmentation. Fragmentation of erythrocytes into smaller, irregularly shaped pieces indicates shearing by intravascular trauma (Figure 113–13). This may be observed with disseminated intravascular coagulation, vascular neoplasms, myelofibrosis, and iron deficiency. To dispel a common myth, fragmentation is not an artifact of blood film preparation.

Howell-Jolly Bodies. Howell-Jolly bodies are nuclear fragments that may occur in the newly released erythrocyte and are not particularly important. They are small, round, basophilic inclusions, which usually occur singly. They are a normal finding in small numbers and are more likely to be observed during regenerative anemia. Their accumulation is enhanced by splenectomy or by use of drugs that suppress splenic phagocytic functions.

Hypochromic Cells. Hypochromic cells are characteristic of iron deficiency anemia in dogs (see Figure 113–13). The diameter of hypochromic cells is not appreciably altered but the volume is reduced. As a result, the cell thickness is reduced, giving rise to an exaggerated area of central pallor and overall pale staining appearance. Hypochromic cells are not observed in cats.

Acanthocyte-like Cells. Acanthocyte-like cells have irregular projections from the cell contour (Figure 113–14). In humans, these cells have defined biochemical abnormalities that result in the shape change. In severe human hepatic failure, there are increased membrane cholesterol, decreased deformability, and shortened erythrocyte survival. They also occur in other rare abnormalities of lipid metabolism. The association of these cells with liver disease in dogs is not convincing. Cells with acanthocytic change are commonly observed in dogs with hemangiosarcoma. The best interpretation for these cells in dogs is that they should raise suspicion of the presence of hemangiosarcoma and alternatively may be associated with severe chronic hepatic insufficiency. The genesis of the shape change in hemangiosarcoma is not known; membrane biochemistry has not been characterized. It is possible that these cells represent part of an unusual fragmentation process associated with passage through abnormal vascular passages of the neoplasm. They are observed in cats with severe hepatic lipidosis.

Leptocytosis, Punched Out Cells, and Crenation. Relatively unimportant morphologic changes include leptocytosis (target cells and folded cells), punched out cells, and crenation (echinocyte change). They are mentioned to help avoid both existing common overinterpretation of their significance and their morphologic misinterpretation. Leptocytosis has been associated with a number of chronic diseases. Cells are apparently produced with an increased membrane to volume ratio, resulting in extra contours added to the biconcave shape. The change should be regarded as nonspecific. Additionally, leptocytosis can be artifactually induced in dog blood by excess EDTA associated with incomplete filling of blood tubes. Punched out cells are probably an artifactual shape change resulting in an exaggerated, sharp demarcation between the hemoglobinized area and central pallor. The inexperienced microscopist may

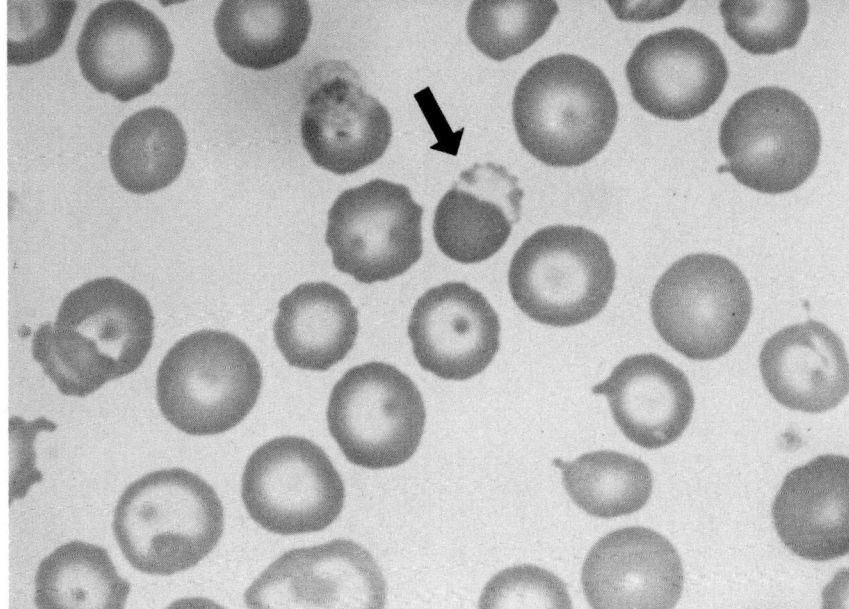

FIGURE 113–8. Eccentrocyte in canine blood (arrow). Eccentrocyte formation is associated with oxidative Heinz body formation in dogs. Wright-Giemsa stain.

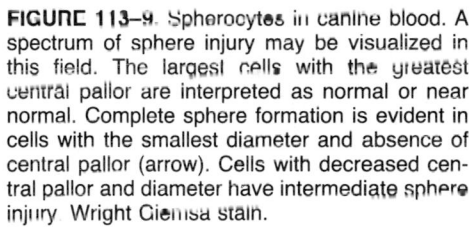

FIGURE 113–9. Spherocytes in canine blood. A spectrum of sphere injury may be visualized in this field. The largest cells with the greatest central pallor are interpreted as normal or near normal. Complete sphere formation is evident in cells with the smallest diameter and absence of central pallor (arrow). Cells with decreased central pallor and diameter have intermediate sphere injury. Wright-Giemsa stain.

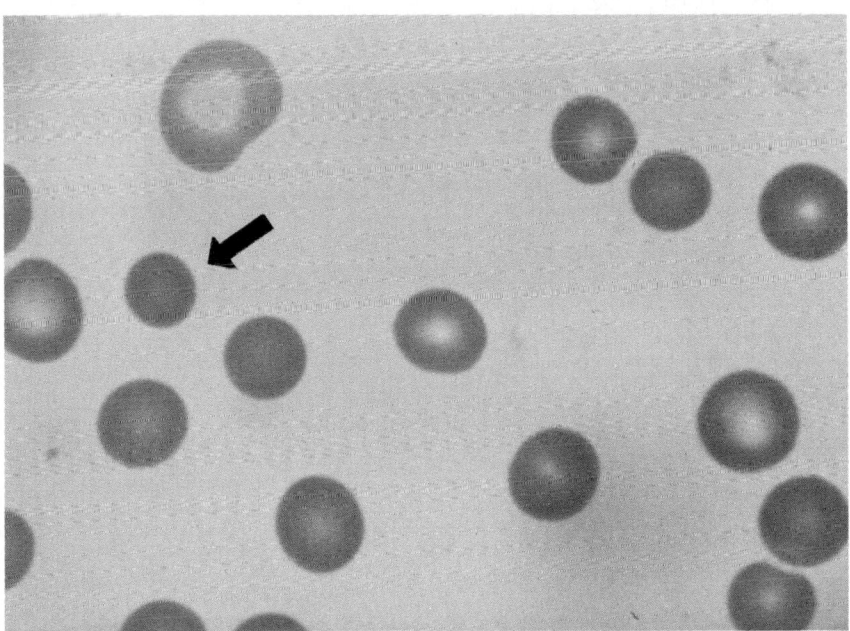

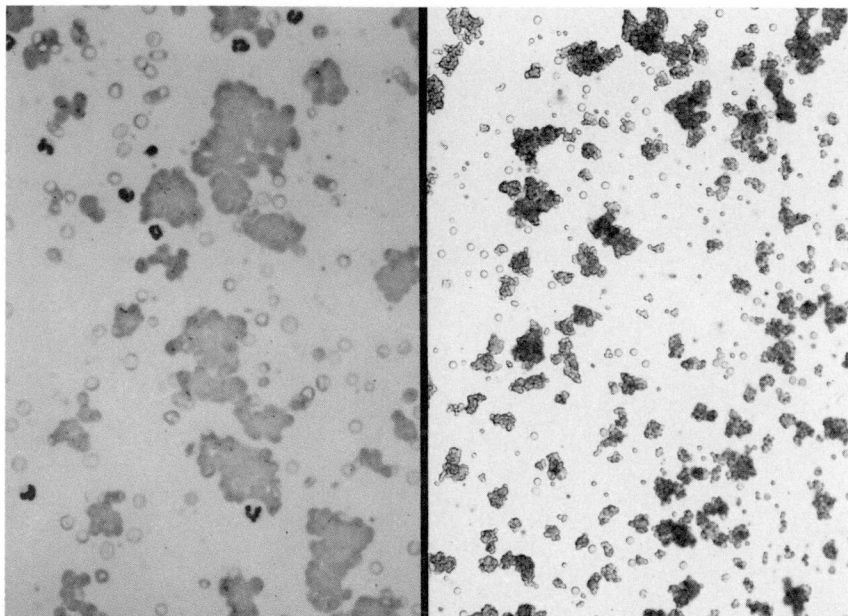

FIGURE 113–10. Left split field is a low magnification view of immune-mediated agglutination of canine erythrocytes on a Wright-Giemsa stained blood film. The right split field is a low magnification view of immune-mediated agglutination on an unstained wet mount.

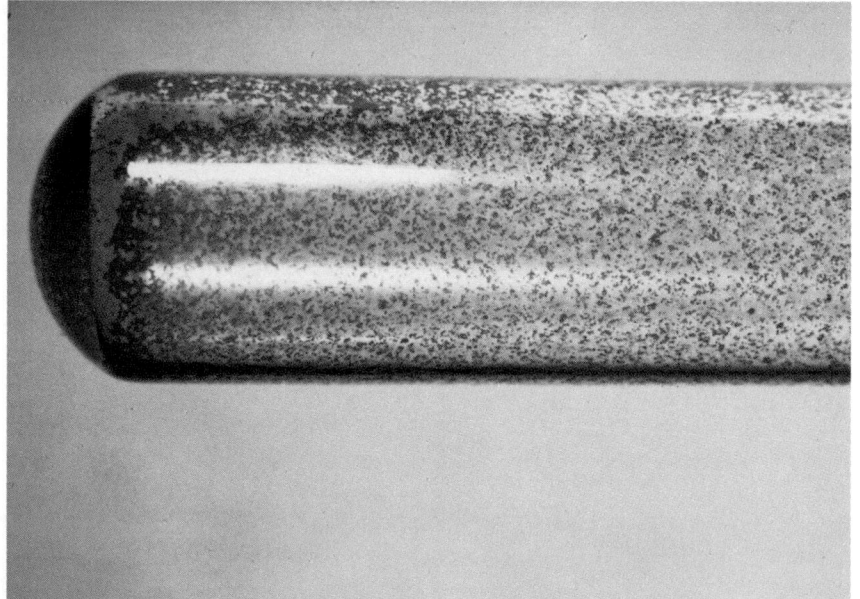

FIGURE 113–11. Gross appearance of immune-mediated agglutination on the wall of a blood tube from a dog with immunohemolytic anemia.

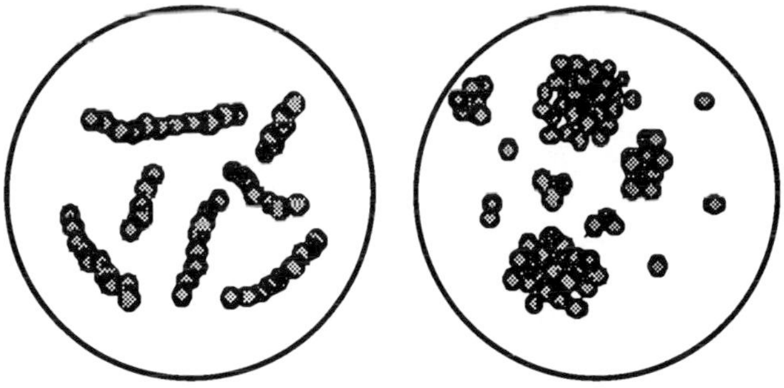

ROULEAUX FORMATION **AGGLUTINATION**

FIGURE 113–12. Schematic diagram depicting low magnification difference in appearance of agglutination and rouleaux formation on Wright's stained blood films. In saline wet mounts, rouleaux will disperse while agglutination will either not disperse or may slowly dissociate.

methylene blue has been the traditional stain used. Brilliant cresyl blue is available in a convenient packaged form which consists of stain dried to the bottom of disposable tubes (Retic-Set, Curtin Matheson Scientific Co). This product has the advantages of being relatively free of precipitate and not requiring preparation and filtering of solutions. It comes with simple instructions for preparing reticulocyte films. The count is performed by differentiating 1000 consecutive erythrocytes as either reticulocytes or nonreticulocytes. The resultant percentage of reticulocytes may be multiplied by the erythrocyte count to yield reticulocytes per µl of blood. This eliminates the need to interpret a reticulocyte percentage relative to the hematocrit or erythrocyte concentration.

Canine reticulocytes almost always have aggregated condensation of the organelles, making counting a relatively simple process. The cat is unique in producing at least two forms of reticulocytes, which have quite different interpretations and contribute to confusion in doing the reticulocyte count. While various terminology has been applied to differentiating feline reticulocytes, the author suggests that the simple aggregate and punctate designations are most easy to relate to reticulocyte morphology (Figures 113–15 and 113–16). The aggregate reticulocyte has clumped organelles that coalesce into aggregates. These cells correspond to polychromatophilic cells on Wright's stained films.[16] Following a short maturation time of about 12 hours, the aggregate form becomes a punctate form.[17, 18] The punctate form has variable numbers of individual dots, which do not coalesce, and has a maturation time as long as 10 to 12 days.[17, 19] As a result, very high punctate reticulocyte counts may develop with responsive blood repopulation. The interpretation is that the aggregate form represents *active* regeneration, while the punctate form represents fairly recent *cumulative* regeneration. For this reason, it is best to include only the aggregate form in a reticulocyte count and at most record a subjective statement about the presence of punctate forms. This is important

misinterpret the change as hypochromia. Crenation is the presence of many regular membrane projections involving most or all of the cells. It is usually an artifact of slow drying of the blood film during preparation. The high pH of the glass surface can induce the shape change in the fluid phase. The change may also rarely occur with very severe renal failure complicated by severe electrolyte disturbances.

RETICULOCYTE COUNTING

Reticulocytes are visualized by staining blood with a vital stain, which induces ribosomes and other organelles of the immature erythrocyte to clump into visible granules. Counting reticulocytes is the preferred method of quantitating the regenerative response. While a subjective assessment of regeneration can be made by examining for polychromatophilic cells on Wright's stained films, error in interpretation may be encountered with inappropriately prepared or maintained stains. New

FIGURE 113–13. Erythrocyte fragmentation and hypochromia in a dog with iron deficiency anemia. Note that a few cells have increased central pallor compared to normal. A small fragment is indicated by the arrow. In addition, several oxidative membrane fusions which appear like vacuoles are present. These may subsequently rupture, leading to membrane protrusions in an oxidative fragmentation process recognized in iron deficiency anemia. For more detail, see Figure 113–21 and related text under discussion of iron deficiency.

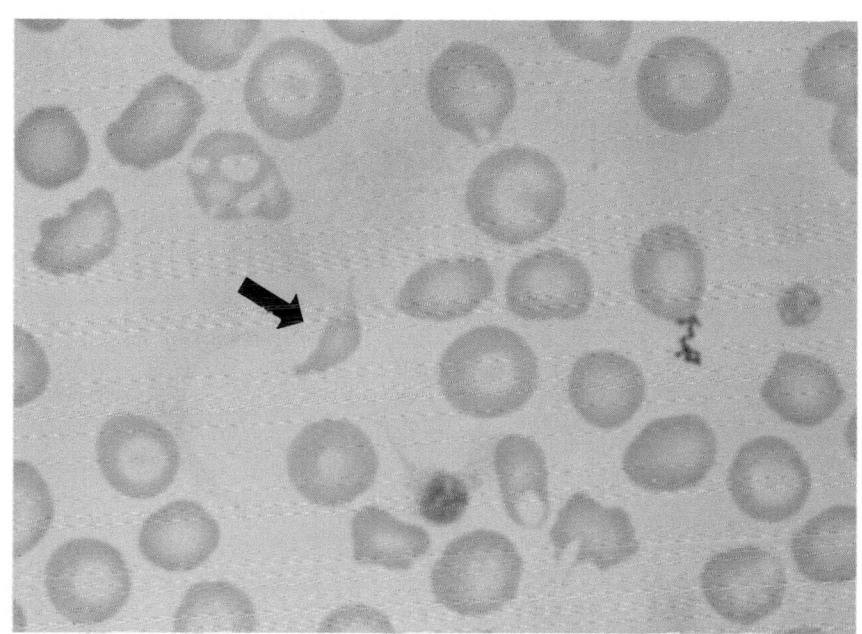

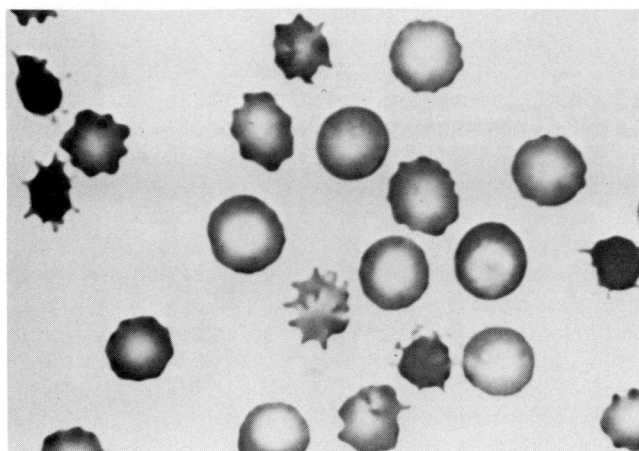

FIGURE 113–14. Canine acanthocyte-like cells. This interpretation is applied to the several cells present with irregular projections.

in cats because anemias, which are initially regenerative and then become nonregenerative, may have a large number of punctate forms and an absence of aggregate forms.[19]

DETECTION OF IMMUNOGLOBULIN AND/OR COMPLEMENT ON ERYTHROCYTES

The antiglobulin or Coombs' test requires use of species-specific serum prepared against these molecules and properly adsorbed with normal erythrocytes. The test should be performed in the veterinary laboratory using the appropriate reagents. The current use and interpretation of Coombs' testing in dogs and cats is probably at best in a state of confusion. In short, information in human hematology has been superficially extrapolated to veterinary hematology. There are a few surveys of Coombs' positive reactions in dogs and cats.[20–23] Two of these specifically examined cats with FeLV-associated anemia, one examined 20 cats with a variety of anemias, and one examined a large number of dogs with a variety of disorders including dogs without anemia.[20–23] Several things are clear. First, positive Coombs' tests alone are not diagnostic of immunohemolytic disease, and therefore results are not simple to interpret. Positive reactions may occur with a variety of anemias and in conditions without accompanying anemia.[22, 23] There is documented association of Coombs'-positive reactions with FeLV infection. However, there

has been no convincing correlation of this observation with hemolytic disease. In summary, other hematologic evidence is necessary to support a diagnosis of immunohemolytic disease. Second, a variety of technical problems result in false-negative Coombs' reactions when overt immunohemolytic disease is present.[24] Third, Coombs' tests done at 39°F (4°C) are overutilized and overinterpreted in veterinary medicine. Cold-reacting antibodies may be a normal finding in dogs and cats. The same occurs in humans. In some human infectious diseases, high levels of cold-reacting antibodies develop without the occurrence of hemolytic disease. There has been a tendency to do these assays only in animals suspected of having a specific hemolytic disease. We know little about incidence of positive reactions in non-hemolytic diseases and as a result have little basis for specificity of their interpretation. Currently, the most appropriate interpretation for positive Coombs' tests is that there is detectable immunoglobulin and/or complement bound or adsorbed to erythrocyte membranes.

In both animals and humans, existing techniques need methodical study, and new techniques for detecting erythrocyte immunoinjury need to be developed. A new generation of immunohematologic technology is required to enhance our understanding of disease mechanisms in erythrocyte immunoinjury and improve diagnostic tests. Techniques are needed that will allow quantitation of specific immunoglobulin types and complement on erythrocytes to be correlated with measurable erythrocyte immunoinjury. Pertinent erythrocyte injury assessments include erythrocyte survival time, deformability, susceptibility to lysis in hypotonic saline, and perhaps assays on interaction with phagocytic cells having complement and immunoglobulin Fc receptors. An additional impediment is difficulty in experimentally inducing immunohemolytic disease in a form suitable for study.

ERYTHROCYTE FRAGILITY AND DEFORMABILITY

A variety of techniques for detecting erythrocyte injury based on measuring either fragility or deformability have been used in human hematology. These have been reviewed.[25] Of these, the saline fragility test has been evaluated in veterinary hematology.[26] This assay measures erythrocyte resistance to lysis in decreasing concentrations of saline. It may be performed in a variety of commercial and human laboratory settings.

PROGRESSION OF FELINE RETICULOCYTE MATURATION

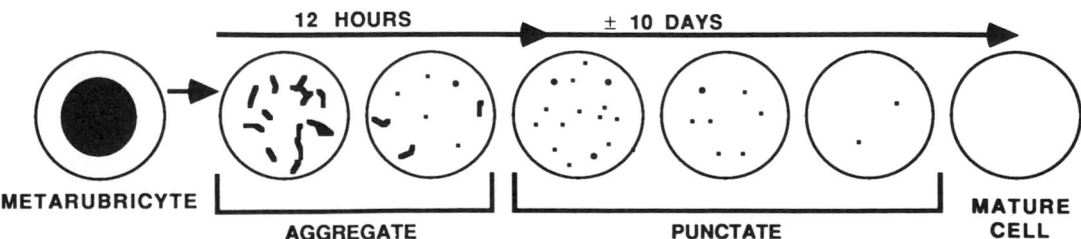

FIGURE 113–15. Diagram of sequential reticulocyte maturation and associated maturation times. Morphology of sequence is depicted as visualized by a reticulocyte stain (new methylene blue or brilliant cresyl blue).

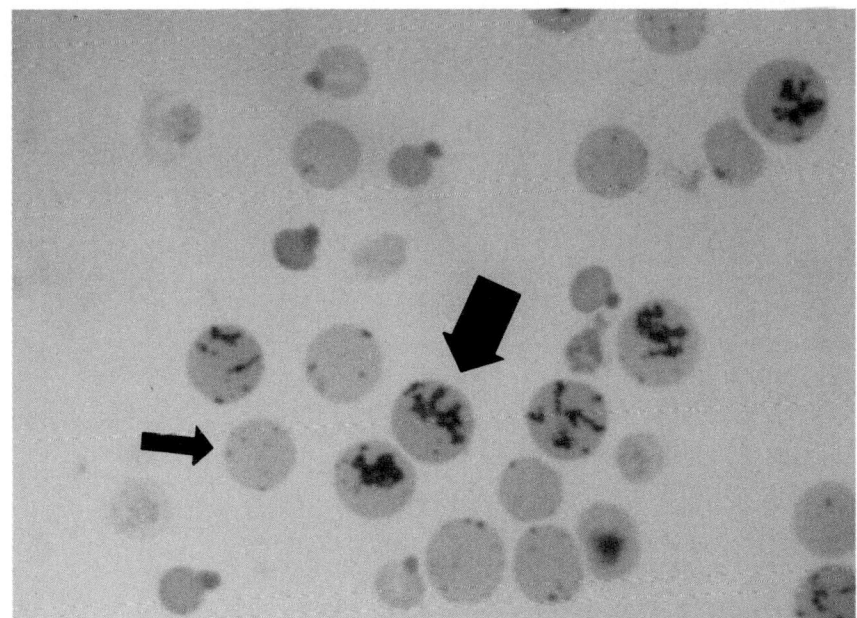

FIGURE 113–16. Feline reticulocytes and Heinz bodies as visualized with brilliant cresyl blue stain. Round, homogeneous Heinz bodies stain medium blue with this stain; most protrude from the membrane contour in this field. Several aggregate reticulocytes (large arrow) and punctate reticulocytes (small arrow) are present. The reticulum stains dark blue compared to Heinz bodies.

Results are easier to interpret if a graph is prepared of per cent hemolysis versus saline concentration (Figure 113–17).

The reference ranges of saline concentrations resulting in 50 per cent hemolysis in dogs and cats are 0.36 to 0.48 (mean 0.43) and 0.46 to 0.64 (mean 0.54), respectively.[26] The assay results are stable for blood stored at 39°F (4°C) for three to four days.[26, 27] The assay is probably most specific for detecting sphere formation involved in immune-mediated removal of erythrocyte membrane in animals. It is useful for documenting immune-mediated erythrocyte injury in dogs when sphere formation is morphologically imperfect and is currently the best assay to detect erythrocyte immunoinjury in the cat. Since sphere formation is difficult if not impossible to detect morphologically in the cat, this underutilized assay should receive more consideration in evaluation of feline hemolytic anemias. With sphere injury in immunohemolytic disease, the curve will shift to the left and the 50 per cent hemolysis point will be increased above 0.50 and 0.65 per cent saline for dogs and cats, respectively. The assay's specificity for immunoinjury should be subjected to more complete evaluation in a variety of erythrocyte injuries resulting in anemia. In addition, new technology for measuring fragility or deformability would be valuable in studying erythrocyte injury. These will undoubtedly appear in the future.

Other causes of increased fragility in humans, such as sickle cell anemia, have not been observed in the dog and cat. Results are not altered by the presence of Heinz bodies in cats. Some hemolytic anemias, for example pyruvate kinase deficiency of dogs, may be associated with decreased fragility. This is attributed to blood repopulation with new cells and a high proportion of reticulocytes. These cells are larger and have a greater

FIGURE 113–17. Erythrocyte fragilogram used for plotting saline fragility curves of per cent hemolysis versus per cent saline. The canine reference range is indicated by the shaded area, with mean 50 per cent hemolysis occurring in about 0.43 per cent saline. The upper limit of acceptable fragility for cats is indicated by the curve marked "FELINE." Increased fragility in hypotonic saline, indicating sphere injury, is detected by a shift in the curve to the left of the limit accepted as normal for the species being tested.

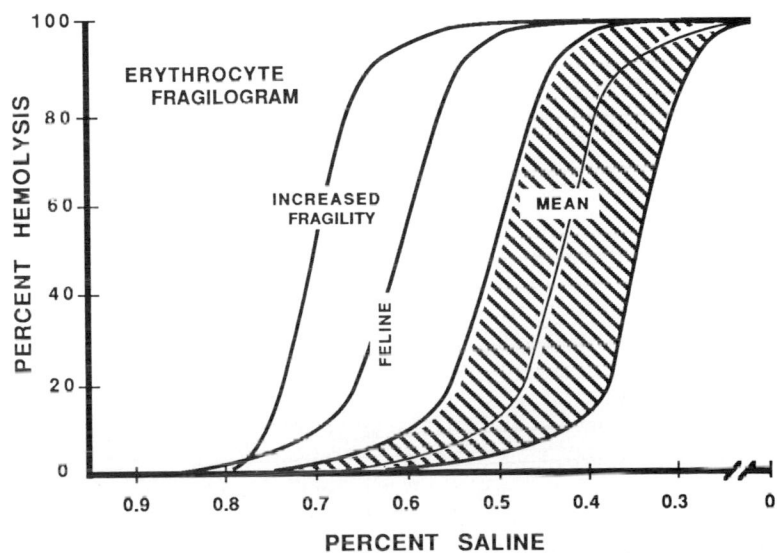

membrane surface area to volume ratio, providing a greater capacity to swell. Decreased fragility associated with postregenerative macrocytosis has not been studied in the cat.

REFERENCE VALUES FOR CLINICAL EVALUATION OF ERYTHROCYTES

In this section, reference value guidelines and some interpretive perspective are given as a supplement to reference values provided in Chapter 3. It is assumed that most veterinarians utilize an external laboratory for routine hemograms. The data provided by the laboratory are generally more complete than what is required for clinical interpretations, but are necessarily generated when using automated cell counting systems. For hemograms generated within the veterinary hospital by manual procedures, evaluation of erythrocytes should be kept simple. This includes packed cell volume determined by microhematocrit centrifugation, blood film examination of erythrocyte morphology, and reticulocyte counts in anemic patients. As mentioned, it is not desirable to count erythrocytes and calculate the MCV value by manual techniques within the veterinary hospital laboratory, but these may be useful values when provided by the automated laboratory.

Existing published studies on reference values in veterinary hematology suffer from several factors including establishment of a normal population, multiplicity of breeds, lack of detail related to age, and data collections pre-dating modern technology. Living with these acknowledged limitations, we must work with what exists. Interpretation of hemograms should ideally be done with respect to reference values determined by the laboratory employed. However, most values related to the erythron are fairly uniform between laboratories.

Hematocrit values cover a considerably wide range, posing some interpretive problems. While some normal cats and dogs may have hematocrit values as low as 25 and 36 per cent, respectively, these and slightly greater values are difficult to interpret since there is a reasonable probability this may represent anemia in many individuals. Some breeds of dogs, notably the basenji, beagle, boxer, Chihuahua, German shepherd, and poodle, can be expected to have hematocrit values in excess of 50 per cent. One solution to this problem would be to establish the patient's reference hematocrit in a database during a routine examination.

The MCV value should be determined by a direct technique employed in a cell counter. The ranges of 60 to 72 fl for dogs and 37 to 49 fl for cats are appropriate for interpretation of directly measured MCV values.[6] Two breeds of dogs present exceptions. Akitas usually have MCV values ranging from 52 to 60 fl. Some poodles may have MCV values ranging from 80 to 100 fl, a peculiarity referred to as poodle macrocytosis. While there are subtle megaloblastic changes in myeloid and erythroid marrow cells, affected poodles do not have impaired hematopoiesis and their hematocrit values are normal. The condition is not related to vitamin B_{12} or folate deficiency and is regarded as an incidental finding.

In the presence of anemia, macrocytosis is usually interpreted as reflecting either current or recent accelerated erythrocyte regeneration. The increase in volume of newly released erythrocytes is proportional to the severity of anemia or erythroid marrow stimulation. When erythroid marrow is maximally stimulated, cells with about twice the normal volume may be produced in most species, with dogs being an exception. Markedly regenerative anemias in dogs are usually accompanied by modest increases in MCV, whereas in cats the MCV may almost double. Once released as a macrocyte, the cell undergoes very gradual size reduction, but will remain larger than normal for most or all of its lifespan. As a result, markedly regenerative anemia with complete blood repopulation can establish macrocytosis, which will persist for several weeks after the reticulocyte count and hematocrit return to normal. In cats, this has been referred to as postregenerative macrocytosis.[19] Prominent macrocytosis may be observed in FeLV-associated anemias whether regenerative or not.[13] This may reflect residual macrocytosis from a regenerative response occurring before bone marrow failure and arrival for veterinary care related to severe anemia. Macrocytosis related to vitamin deficiencies, as occurs in humans and ruminants, probably does not occur in dogs and cats.

Microcytosis is a feature of iron deficiency anemia in dogs.[28] It has not been observed in the adult cat. It has been observed in kittens with neonatal iron deficiency and theoretically could occur with marked erythrocyte fragmentation.[29]

The "normal" reticulocyte count is for animals with a normal hematocrit. In the face of anemia, normal must be somewhat greater than 60,000/μl for an interpretation of regenerative anemia. The magnitude of reticulocytosis ($> 60,000/\mu l$) is proportional to the degree of bone marrow stimulation and depends on the time of sampling during response to anemia.

Hemoglobin, erythrocyte count, mean corpuscular hemoglobin, and mean corpuscular hemoglobin concentration are redundant values and therefore have little interpretive use. On automated systems, the erythrocyte count is used to calculate hematocrit, and the hemoglobin value is used to calculate the mean corpuscular hemoglobin concentration (MCHC). The MCHC may become decreased in markedly regenerative anemia. This value is important for use by the laboratory to help identify problems in automated instrumentation. For example, malfunctions of either diluter or counting subsystems usually manifest as error in the MCHC generated by an automated system. Any factor interfering with light transmittance in the hemoglobinometer will give a falsely high MCHC. Lipemia and large numbers of Heinz bodies are the usual causes. Immune-mediated agglutination can also result in a falsely high MCHC because of improper determination of hematocrit. It is the job of the laboratorian to recognize these problems and correct the data.

NEONATAL AND JUVENILE VALUES

Reference values for puppies and kittens deserve some mention. Dogs are born with large erythrocytes

(95–100 fl) and relatively high hematocrit values. These cells are progressively replaced by cells with normal volume, and the MCV value becomes normal by two to three months of age. Hematocrit values decline to a nadir of about 30 per cent by four to six weeks. Hematocrit values then progressively increase into the adult reference range by four to six months. Individuals attain their normal adult hematocrit values between 6 and 12 months of age.[30–32] The physiologic anemia is regarded as a balance between fetal erythrocyte destruction, modest production, and rapid body growth rate. A general interpretive guideline is that pups between one and four months of age with hematocrit values in the low 30s are not anemic if the erythron is otherwise normal.

Kittens are born with mean hematocrit values of about 35 per cent.[29, 33, 34] Mean hematocrit values then decline to a nadir of 25 per cent by three to four weeks. Mean hematocrit values then slowly increase to adult values of 35 per cent by 16 weeks. Kittens are born with relatively macrocytic erythrocytes (MCV 60 to 69 fl), which are rapidly replaced by four to five weeks of age. The transient anemia is likely related to a combination of rapid blood repopulation and rapid growth rate occurring during the first few weeks. Iron availability may result in more severe anemia and microcytosis between four and eight weeks of age in some kittens.[29]

ERYTHROCYTE KINETICS

Erythrocyte Survival. Erythrocyte lifespan in dogs ranges from 110 to 120 days.[35] Half survival time of canine erythrocytes using ^{51}Cr is 21 to 30 days. The cat has considerably shorter erythrocyte lifespan compared to other common domestic species. The reason for relatively short erythrocyte survival in the cat is not known but could be related to oxidative injury to which cat hemoglobin is sensitive. Erythrocyte lifespan measured with incorporation labels is 76 ± 0.9 days with diisopropyl fluorophosphate-32 (DF^{32}P), 77 days with glycine-^{15}N, 73 days with glycine-2-^{14}C, and 78 ± 4 days with ^{14}C-cyanate.[36–39] Erythrocyte half survival times, determined with ^{51}Cr, have been reported to be 10.7 days, 6 days, and 13.7 days.[19, 40, 41] Elution of chromium from labelled erythrocytes during circulation, estimated at 2.4 to 6 per cent per day, likely accounts for the variation in this procedure. Elution may be minimized by using low quantities of high specific activity ^{51}Cr when labelling cells.

Chromium-determined half survival time is probably the most convenient method of estimating erythrocyte survival. Owing to variable elution, it is stressed that control animals be used when doing erythrocyte survival experiments. The ^{14}C-cyanate technique appears useful in that elution is minimal.[39]

Erythrocyte Senescence. About 0.9 and 1.3 per cent of the erythrocytes are removed daily from the circulation of normal adult dogs and cats, respectively. Most of these are removed by the mononuclear phagocyte system. A small proportion may lyse in the circulation. In this instance, hemoglobin is bound by haptoglobin, a plasma protein that complexes with hemoglobin and is

extracted from plasma by the mononuclear phagocyte system. Hemoglobin is rapidly degraded to constituent iron, amino acids, and bilirubin. Bilirubin formed in macrophages is released to plasma where it is bound to albumin and transported to the liver. Hepatocytes take up and conjugate bilirubin. Most conjugated bilirubin is excreted in the bile, but some is regurgitated to the plasma where it is then excreted in the urine.

In hemolytic disease and internal hemorrhage these mechanisms are accelerated. With extravascular hemolysis there is accelerated phagocytosis of injured erythrocytes. With internal hemorrhage, there is a mononuclear infiltrate that phagocytoses erythrocytes. When hemolysis is moderate to severe or internal hemorrhage is severe in multiple sites, the rate of bilirubin formation may exceed the hepatic clearance rate, resulting in hyperbilirubinemia. Refer to Chapter 24 for additional discussion of pathogenesis of hyperbilirubinemia.

With intravascular hemolysis, haptoglobin may bind only relatively small amounts of free hemoglobin. If the rate of hemoglobin release exceeds the haptoglobin binding capacity, free hemoglobin will be increased in plasma and be filtered in the urine, giving rise to hemoglobinemia and hemoglobinuria, respectively. Measurement of serum haptoglobin has been proposed to detect more subtle forms of hemolysis. A reference range of 31 to 126 mg/dl has been reported for the cat.[42] Decreased haptoglobin values are interpreted as evidence of ongoing hemolysis. Following cessation of hemoglobin release, haptoglobin will return to normal concentrations within 48 hours. Haptoglobin may increase with inflammatory disease. Stimulation of haptoglobin synthesis could mask a decrease in haptoglobin associated with minor hemolysis.

Kinetics of Marrow Response to Anemia. Knowledge of marrow response kinetics is important for clinical assessment of anemia. This allows informed detection of subtle marrow disease and monitoring of recovery in selected disorders.

When marrow response mechanisms are intact, reticulocytosis will develop within two days of the onset of anemia and will peak at four to seven days. A burst of metarubricytosis may be associated with the early phase of this response and may persist in decreasing numbers throughout the response. The reticulocyte count will return to normal as the hematocrit normalizes. The dog probably can produce up to 300,000 erythrocytes/μl/day under conditions of maximal marrow stimulation. Since the reticulocyte maturation time is about two days with maximal marrow stimulation, peak reticulocyte counts as high as 600,000/μl may be observed.

Near the end of the regenerative response, many punctate reticulocytes may be observed in cats.[17–19] The short aggregate maturation time has caused confusion about feline erythrocyte regenerative responses. Aggregate counts did not achieve very high numbers in studies on experimental blood loss.[17] This has led to an interpretation that the feline bone marrow is relatively slow in responding to anemia. Actually, the opposite is true. In common domestic species, the potential rate of erythrocyte regeneration is greatest in the cat. It has been estimated that the cat may produce up to 600,000 erythrocytes/μl/day.[19] The cat may achieve a maximum aggregate reticulocyte count in the range of 300,000 to 500,000 per μl in experimental hemolytic disease.[19] The relatively short maturation time does not allow accumulation of large numbers reflecting the regenerative rate. Blood repopulation and recovery from anemia are rapid enough that high reticulocyte counts are easily missed if sampling does not coincide with peak reticulocytosis. With only modest marrow stimulus, such as anemia which may occur with hemorrhage, the reticulocyte count may be below 60,000/μl. In cats, caution must be used in making an interpretation of non-regenerative anemia unless reticulocytes are absent. In these instances of a count of about 60,000/μl, an increasing number of punctate reticulocytes or rising hematocrit over a period of several days may be a better indicator that regeneration has occurred.

ERYTHROCYTE BIOCHEMISTRY

Hemoglobins. The dog has a relatively simple hemoglobin system. Embryonic, fetal, and adult hemoglobins are indistinguishable. Canine hemoglobin has a high oxygen affinity, which is modulated principally by binding 2,3-diphosphoglycerate and possibly other unknown metabolites. Canine erythrocytes contain relatively high concentrations of 2,3-diphosphoglycerate, but this metabolite apparently does not increase in response to anemia induced by phlebotomy.[43] While not well characterized in the dog, increased binding of these metabolites to hemoglobin under conditions of anemia or hypoxemia decreases the affinity of hemoglobin for oxygen, resulting in a greater fraction of oxygen release at pO_2 levels encountered at tissues sites. This is one of the physiologic adaptations to anemia that contributes to survival until blood repopulation can occur.

Cats have unique intrinsic hemoglobin oxygen affinity and modulation of oxygen affinity by hemoglobin interaction with metabolites such as 2,3-diphosphoglycerate. There are two hemoglobin types in normal cat blood, designated HbA and HbB. These hemoglobins have identical α chains but differ by several amino acid substitutions in β chains.[44] Feline hemoglobins have a relatively high concentration of oxidizable sulfhydryl groups, which is thought to account for increased susceptibility to oxidative denaturation.[45] Compared to hemoglobins of other species, feline hemoglobins have relatively low oxygen affinity, which facilitates oxygen delivery at pO_2 levels encountered at the tissue site. Normal cats have relatively low concentrations of erythrocyte 2,3-diphosphoglycerate. This metabolite imposes change in HbA oxygen affinity, but has no effect on HbB.[44, 46] There are also small quantities of closely related hemoglobin B subtypes, designated HbB_1, HbB_2, and HbB_3. These have very high oxygen affinities. During experimental hemolytic anemia, erythrocytes produced under conditions of marrow stimulation have unchanged levels of HbA, decreased HbB, and increased quantities of HbB subtype hemoglobins. The paradoxically high oxygen affinity of B subtype hemoglobins would appear to be disadvantageous in anemia. However, this is compensated for by considerable increases in 2,3-diphosphoglycerate and adenosine triphosphate, which sterically interact with hemoglobin A to decrease oxygen affinity.[47] The cat is unique in that during anemia this spectrum of hemoglobin oxygen affinity exists and the affinity difference between oxygenated and deoxygenated blood is relatively small. The reason for having a complicated response in anemia is not clear, but having a mixture of hemoglobins with different oxygen affinities at different pO_2 levels may improve adaptation to a wider range of oxygenation conditions.

Metabolism. Review of mechanisms for protecting against oxidative injury and associated energy metabolism is useful for understanding related diseases. Since most disorders involving metabolic pathways result in hemolysis, associated diseases will be covered under hemolytic anemias. A simplified diagram of metabolism is present in Figure 113–18.

The principal energy source is metabolism of glucose via an anaerobic glycolytic pathway. Glucose is actively taken up by energy-dependent membrane transfer, which is independent of insulin. The majority of glucose is metabolized to pyruvate or lactate via glycolysis.

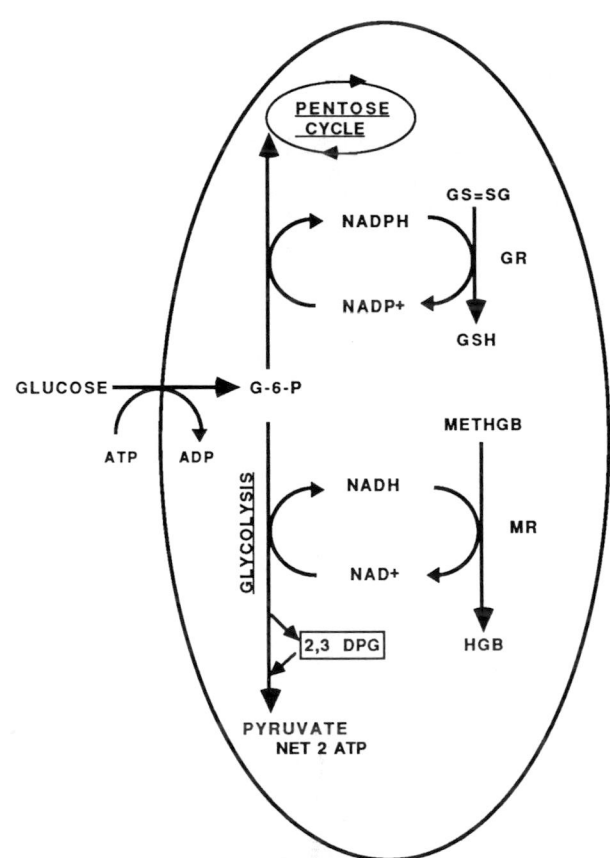

FIGURE 113–18. Diagram summarizing energy metabolism pathways important in erythrocyte maintenance and protection from oxidative injury. GS=SG = oxidized glutathione, GSH = reduced glutathione, GR = glutathione reductase, NADPH = reduced nicotinamide-adenine dinucleotide phosphate, NADP+ = nicotinamide-adenine dinucleotide phosphate, G-6-P = glucose 6-phosphate, ATP = adenosine triphosphate, ADP = adenosine diphosphate, METHGB = methemoglobin, HGB = hemoglobin, MR = methemoglobin reductase, NADH = reduced nicotinamide-adenine dinucleotide, NAD+ = nicotinamide-adenine dinucleotide, DPG = diphosphoglycerate.

Important energy intermediates obtained are ATP and reduction of NAD^+ to NADH. ATP is essential for a variety of metabolic activities related to maintenance of transmembrane electrolyte gradients and cell shape. NADH is utilized in methemoglobin reduction. A branch of the glycolytic pathway gives rise to 2,3-diphosphoglycerate. Another proportion of glucose is metabolized via the hexose monophosphate shunt or pentose cycle. This pathway results in intermediates that join the glycolytic pathway and in the process result in reduction of $NADP^+$ to NADPH. NADPH is an important energy intermediate necessary for reduction of oxidized glutathione and glutathione containing disulfides. Detailed information on enzymology of these pathways is available.[48]

Glutathione (GSH) is a tripeptide that is synthesized in erythrocytes and is regenerated from oxidized glutathione (GSSG). The tripeptide is:

γ-glutamyl-cysteinyl-glycine

GSH is oxidized by endogenous peroxides and a variety of drugs by forming a disulfide linkage between the cysteine sulfhydryl groups of two molecules of GSH or between one molecule of GSH and a sulfhydryl group of erythrocyte proteins. GSH protects hemoglobin and other erythrocyte components from oxidative injury. Regeneration of GSH is important in maintaining its presence for this protection. This is accomplished by the enzyme glutathione reductase, which utilizes NADPH made available from the pentose cycle.

Iron in hemoglobin is normally present in the reduced (Fe^{++}) or ferrous state. Methemoglobin is formed when a variety of endogenous and exogenous compounds oxidize hemoglobin iron to the ferric (Fe^{+++}) state. This continually occurs to a small degree so that normally there is one or two per cent methemoglobin present. Methemoglobin is non-functional in that it is incapable of binding oxygen. A variety of oxidants may result in marked methemoglobinemia with clinical signs and even death related to impaired oxygen transport. Hemoglobin maintenance and the therapeutic rationale in oxidant toxicities are dependent on methemoglobin reduction. The erythrocyte enzyme system that accomplishes this is methemoglobin reductase. It utilizes the energy intermediate NADH made available by the glycolytic pathway.

Most oxidative injuries to protein sulfhydryl groups are reversible. Many drugs with oxidant potential may also result in oxidative denaturation of hemoglobin resulting in Heinz bodies. As stated, feline hemoglobins are quite susceptible to this injury. This is an irreversible change that may result in hemolysis.

ANEMIA

Anemia is one of the most important and frequent laboratory abnormalities encountered in veterinary medicine. An overview of anemia and description of associated clinical findings are given in Chapter 20. This very important clinical condition is logically approached

as a secondary disorder. The causes of anemia are numerous. One objective of this section is to establish that characterization of anemia contributes to making a diagnosis of many primary diseases. Because treatment of anemia usually defaults to correction of the primary problem, discussion of treatment has been deleted for many of the anemias. The reader is referred to other chapters related to the primary disease in these instances.

An orderly approach to anemia is a very helpful diagnostic tool in the complicated medical patient. A systematic approach to anemia should include a thorough history and physical examination, a complete hemogram, reticulocyte count, plasma protein value, and ability to have the blood film pathology reviewed. In the history, duration of illness will help differentiate chronic, non-regenerative anemias from acute hemolytic disease or obscure hemorrhage. Size of the spleen and lymph nodes, presence of icterus, pattern of visible hemorrhages, and pigmentations of urine and feces are useful items in the physical examination. Specific helpful items in the physical examination will be given under each major category of anemia in the sections that follow.

This information should be used in concert with the hematologic data to rapidly classify the anemia into one of four categories: hemorrhage, hemolysis, extra-marrow disease (erythropoietic depression by disease outside the marrow), and intra-marrow disease (hematopoietic disturbance by disease in the marrow space).

The first step is to determine if the anemia is regenerative or not based on reticulocyte concentration. If regenerative, the anemia must be due to either hemorrhage or hemolysis. The plasma protein value is then useful in distinguishing between these. Plasma protein values greater than 6.5 gm/dl are most likely associated with hemolysis. With hemorrhage, plasma proteins are lost proportionally with erythrocytes, and values will usually decrease below 6.0 gm/dl. If the anemia is nonregenerative, other components of the hemogram need to be evaluated. If leukocytes and platelets are normal or responding in an orderly fashion, there is selective depression of erythropoiesis. This is usually due to disease outside the marrow. Examples include anemia associated with renal failure, endocrine failure, chronic disease, and simple erythroid hypoplasia associated with FeLV infection in cats. If there is failure to produce adequate numbers of leukocytes and/or platelets or there are abnormal circulating cells, then there is evidence of disturbed production of more than one cell line. This is usually due to disease within the marrow. Examples include myeloaplasia, myelodysplasia, myeloproliferative disease, other neoplastic infiltrates, and myelofibrosis. Figure 113–19 summarizes this approach in a flowchart.

This approach greatly simplifies the final list of differential diagnoses and selection of further case work-up. While these guidelines work for most cases, some exceptions will be encountered. However, the logic and simplicity afforded by this approach is of major help to young clinicians. Exceptions to the guidelines are infrequent and are too complicated to be reviewed in detail. They are best dealt with by experience.

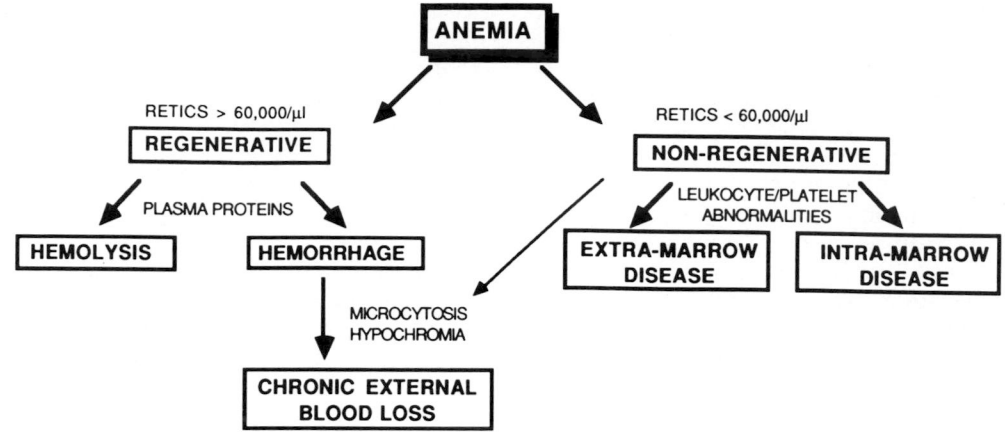

FIGURE 113–19. Overview flowchart of approach to anemia. The clinician should develop this flowchart as a mental reflex for rapid placement of anemia into one of several categories for further, focused characterization.

HEMORRHAGE

The most frequent cause of hemorrhage is trauma. When hemorrhage occurs either spontaneously or disproportionately to injury, then a disorder of platelets, clotting biochemistry, or vasculature must be considered.

The physical examination yields important information in the approach to hemorrhage. Hemorrhage at one body site suggests a local problem, while hemorrhage at multiple sites indicates a defect in coagulation. The physical appearance of hemorrhages is also important. Pinpoint or petechial hemorrhages visible on skin and/or mucous membranes suggest thrombocytopenia. Hematomas, large subcutaneous hemorrhages, or bleeding into body cavities suggest a defect in clotting biochemistry. Either fresh blood or dark, tarry discoloration of feces is indicative of gastrointestinal bleeding.

Trauma/Lacerations. These are the most common cause of hemorrhage and are the most obvious to diagnose. With very acute blood loss the hematocrit does not reflect the severity of the process. Of greatest concern is development of shock when 30 to 50 per cent of the circulating volume is lost. Over a period of hours following onset of blood loss, compensatory fluid shift to the vascular space decreases the hematocrit and plasma proteins. Treatment should consist of careful monitoring for shock and administration of a balanced electrolyte fluid to replace estimated blood loss. A target volume range of 10 to 20 ml/lb is recommended. Transfusions are generally not required unless hemorrhage has occurred continuously in the face of volume replacement, resulting in hematocrits below 15 or 20 per cent.

Thrombocytopenia. Decreased platelet mass accounts for most of the generalized bleeding disorders in small animals. The probability of thrombocytopenia being associated with hemorrhage increases considerably as the count decreases below 50,000/μl. Cats are less likely than other species to have hemorrhage associated with thrombocytopenia. Often no hemorrhage is observed clinically with counts as low as 10,000/μl, although microscopic and gastrointestinal hemorrhage will likely be present.

A common misconception is that hemorrhage from other causes may result in thrombocytopenia. This has resulted from overinterpretation of statements in literature. In response to hemorrhage, compensatory platelet release from the bone marrow megakaryocyte reserve occurs rapidly. There is also a considerable concentration of platelets existing in a splenic reserve, which may be released during acute hemorrhage. Almost all cases of hemorrhage not attributable to thrombocytopenia will have platelet counts in excess of 200,000/μl. It is extremely unlikely for the count to drop below 150,000/μl.

The clinician should try to determine if thrombocytopenia is due to decreased survival or decreased production. Analogous to anemia, a platelet regenerative response usually occurs with decreased survival. Increased numbers of megakaryocytes visible on marrow aspirate films and large circulating platelet forms are morphologic features that suggest accelerated platelet production. When platelets reproducibly approach or exceed the size of erythrocytes, the interpretation of large or "shift" platelets can be made. In severe thrombocytopenia, too few platelets will be present to make this morphologic evaluation. Also, this interpretation cannot be made in cats because large platelet forms may be observed in almost any hematologic disturbance. Morphologic features of decreased production include absence or rarity of megakaryocytes on marrow aspirate films and a uniform population of normal-sized platelets on the blood film.

Immune-mediated thrombocytopenia is probably the most common form of thrombocytopenia in dogs. This is discussed in Chapter 119. Thrombocytopenia may occur in association with bone marrow failures discussed later in this chapter and in Chapter 117. Thrombocytopenia associated with myeloaplasia and myeloproliferative disease is accompanied by other hematologic manifestations of those disorders. The expected regenerative response to hemorrhage does not occur.

Treatment of thrombocytopenia consists of steroids, minimizing trauma, and platelet or fresh blood transfusions as a last measure. If related to bone marrow disease, the cause of marrow failure must be corrected, if possible. Immunosuppressive doses of steroids are indicated in immune-mediated thrombocytopenia to inhibit mononuclear-phagocyte system platelet clearance. Steroids may also be of value in minimizing hemorrhage associated with other causes of thrombocytopenia. The rationale is that a steroid-mediated increase in vascular endothelial integrity reduces diapedesis of erythrocytes. Since platelets have a relatively short half-life, especially in immune-mediated thrombocytopenia, platelet transfusion is performed as a last resort. A fresh platelet-containing whole blood transfusion is necessary when bleeding has been severe and cannot be stopped by any other measure. This may result in temporary control of the bleeding.

Defects in Coagulation Biochemistry. The reader is referred to Chapter 116 for discussion of coagulation biochemistry abnormalities resulting in hemorrhage. Other reviews are also available.[49–51]

Iron Deficiency Anemia. This anemia is considered as a special form of hemorrhage. Iron deficiency per se is not a serious medical problem. It is important to recognize the presence of iron deficiency anemia because it is a clear indication in adult dogs that chronic external blood loss has been occurring. Chronic external blood loss is often not obvious, particularly when it occurs in the gastrointestinal tract. Additionally, iron deficiency may suggest that known hemorrhage has been more severe or protracted than suspected. Some of the more common causes of blood loss leading to iron deficiency anemia include severe flea infestation, hookworm disease in young dogs, and bleeding gastrointestinal neoplasms.[28, 52] Overused blood donors frequently develop the most severe iron deficiency. While it is theoretically possible to develop iron deficiency anemia as a result of poor diet or malabsorption, this is simply not encountered in adult dogs. Dietary related iron deficiency, which is relatively common in man, is not recognized in adult animals fed commercial diets.

Since most of the body iron is in hemoglobin, external hemorrhage may rapidly deplete body iron stores as iron is mobilized in compensatory hemoglobin synthesis. Compounding this situation is a limited ability to increase intestinal iron absorption. The following example of iron bookkeeping helps visualize development of deficiency. Consider that a healthy medium sized dog has 200 mg of storage iron, intestinal iron absorption may increase from a normal level of about 0.5 up to about 2 mg/day, and a gram of hemoglobin contains 3.4 mg of iron. Assuming 5 mg of iron in 10 ml of blood (3.4 mg iron/gm hemoglobin × 1.5 gm hemoglobin/10 ml), blood loss averaging as little as 10 ml per day may deplete iron stores at the rate of 3 mg/day. Features of iron deficiency anemia will begin to develop within 60 to 70 days.

With continued hemoglobin (iron) loss, a sequence of events takes place until complete features of iron deficiency anemia are established (Figure 113–20). Achievement of a critical hemoglobin concentration appears to trigger nuclear degeneration in maturing rubricytes. When iron availability is moderately decreased, hemoglobin synthetic rate becomes decreased in rubricytes. The result is that nuclear degeneration is delayed and extra mitoses may occur. This leads to smaller daughter cells and contributes to development of microcytosis.

A number of alterations are present in cells finally released to the blood. Although cells are reduced in volume, their diameters are normal or near normal.

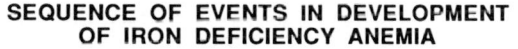

SEQUENCE OF EVENTS IN DEVELOPMENT OF IRON DEFICIENCY ANEMIA

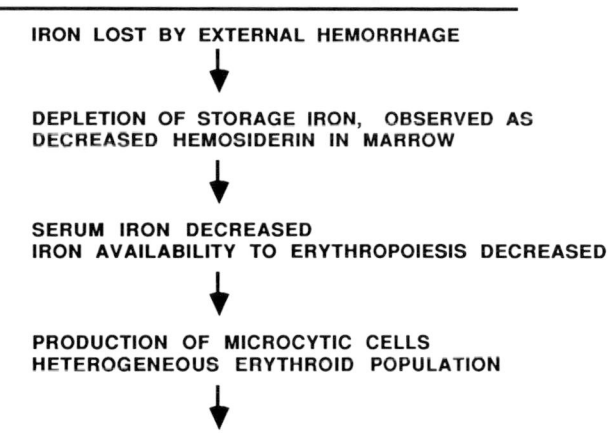

IRON LOST BY EXTERNAL HEMORRHAGE

↓

DEPLETION OF STORAGE IRON, OBSERVED AS DECREASED HEMOSIDERIN IN MARROW

↓

SERUM IRON DECREASED
IRON AVAILABILITY TO ERYTHROPOIESIS DECREASED

↓

PRODUCTION OF MICROCYTIC CELLS
HETEROGENEOUS ERYTHROID POPULATION

↓

HOMOGENEOUS POPULATION OF MICROCYTIC CELLS

FIGURE 113–20. Progressive sequence of events leading to development of erythroid features characteristic of iron deficiency anemia.

This is due to a decreased cell thickness to diameter ratio, which contributes to their pale staining character on the blood film. Increased membrane stiffness and decreased deformability have been documented in rat and human erythrocytes produced under conditions of iron deficiency.[53] This has been attributed to oxidative cross-linking injury to membrane proteins. Enzymes related to protection of erythrocytes from oxidative injury may be reduced in iron deficiency. Prominent erythrocyte fragmentation may be related to increased membrane stiffness, resulting in increased mechanical fragility when exposed to normal intravascular trauma (Figure 113–21).

Hematologic features of iron deficiency anemia include those of hemorrhage and erythrocyte microcytosis. Hematocrit values vary widely, from as low as 10 to 40 per cent. The maintenance of erythrocyte mass should be viewed as a balance between rates of erythrocyte loss, survival, and production. The anemia is usually regenerative, although puppies with severe hookworm infestation may have severe non-regenerative anemia. Reticulocyte counts as high as 500,000/μl may be ob-

OXIDATIVE INJURY LEADING TO MEMBRANE LESIONS INTERPRETED AS A SPECTRUM OF CELL FRAGMENTATION

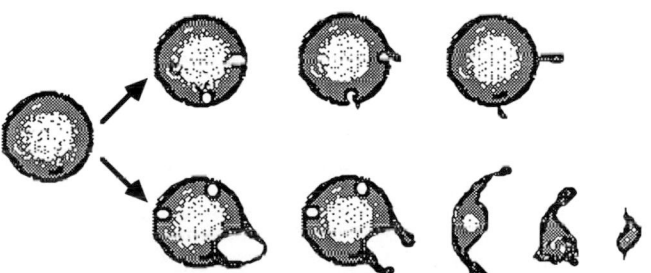

FIGURE 113–21. Proposed sequence of events leading to morphologic changes in iron deficiency anemia collectively interpreted as a fragmentation process. Clear areas are thought to represent oxidative membrane fusions which exclude hemoglobin. These may then break open to result in variously shaped membrane projections. Shearing into more conventional small erythrocyte fragments may also occur.

served. Plasma proteins are decreased when the rate of blood loss is relatively high, but may be low normal with repeated loss of small blood volumes. In the laboratory, erythrocyte histograms are useful for identifying relatively early iron deficiency anemia. Early in iron deficiency anemia, cells of decreased volume result in increased volume anisocytosis, but the MCV may still be normal. This change is detectable on erythrocyte histograms as widening of the distribution toward smaller volume (Figure 113–22A). As blood repopulation with microcytes continues, the MCV becomes decreased until a homogeneous population of small erythrocytes is finally present (Figure 113–22B). The above volume changes are difficult to visualize by microscopy because one is assessing diameters. Hypochromia and fragmentation are usually seen on the blood film,[28] but obviously increased central pallor and decreased staining intensity are detectable by microscopy

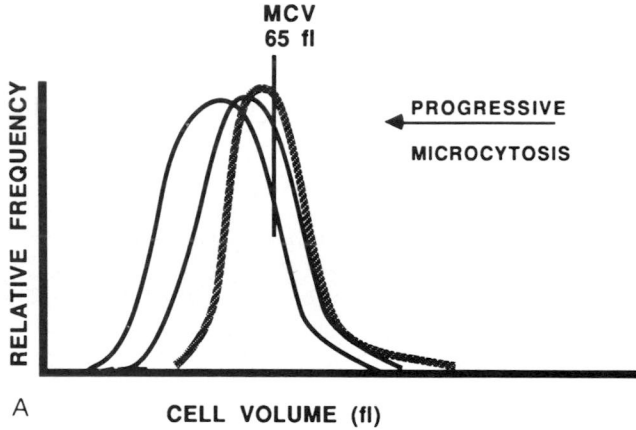

A

relatively late in the disease. Decreased erythrocyte deformability results in decreased erythrocyte packing during traditional microhematocrit centrifugation. The associated plasma trapping results in falsely high hematocrit values. Subsequent calculation of erythrocytic indices yields a falsely high MCV and a falsely low mean corpuscular hemoglobin concentration (MCHC). The traditional low MCHC value in iron deficiency anemia was a useful artifact. Automated, direct determination of erythrocyte volume and calculation of hematocrit eliminate the artifact of trapped plasma. MCHC values determined by automated techniques are either normal or mildly decreased. Thrombocytosis with large platelets is a regular occurrence. Platelet counts may exceed $1 \times 10^6/\mu l$. Too little is known about regulation of thrombopoiesis to suggest a specific mechanism for this observation, but it intuitively appears to be related to stimulation of thrombopoiesis by chronic blood loss.

Serum iron values are useful for documenting iron deficiency unless the animal has been transfused or given iron. Animals that have been treated or are undergoing spontaneous recovery from iron deficiency may have normal serum iron, but may still have morphologic abnormalities in erythrocytes. Serum iron values of less than 60 μg/dl and transferrin saturation values of less than 15 per cent are guidelines for documenting iron deficiency (see Chapter 3). Dogs with severe iron deficiency may have serum iron values as low as 15 μg/dl and transferrin saturation values as low as 5 per cent. Total iron binding capacity values are not increased in dogs with iron deficiency as is commonly extrapolated from human literature. When marrow is examined either histologically or cytologically there is an absence of hemosiderin.

Treatment of iron deficiency should first involve correction of the cause of blood loss. This is followed by oral supplementation of iron for 30 to 60 days. Methods for giving oral iron include ferrous sulfate (100 to 300 mg/day), ferrous gluconate tablets, and Visorbin (1 to 3 teaspoons per day; also contains multiple vitamins). Injectable iron is an alternative to consider in dogs with severe long-standing iron deficiency. A single injection of 5 to 10 mg/lb (10 to 20 mg/kg) of iron dextran (Imferon) should be followed by the oral supplement. Young dogs with severe anemia related to hookworm infestation may require a transfusion. With successful treatment, the hematocrit may normalize within two to four weeks. However, it is expected to take 60 to 120 days or longer for the animal to reestablish normal erythrocyte morphology and erythrocyte volume distribution. This is dependent on establishing normal iron-dependent erythropoiesis and removal of cells produced under conditions of iron deficiency.

Dogs with portacaval shunts often have microcytosis, but the cause is not documented. Serum iron values are usually normal. It is suspected that at an early age, before veterinary care is sought, gastrointestinal blood loss associated with pica and rapid growth rate establishes conditions for producing erythrocytes under conditions of iron deficiency. Later iron repletion may occur, but microcytosis may persist for one to two months as blood repopulates with normocytic cells. At this time, serum iron values may be normal.

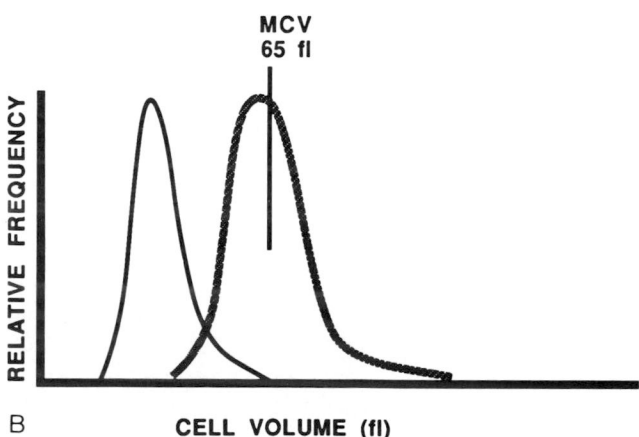

B

FIGURE 113–22. Erythrocyte volume distribution curves in iron deficiency anemia. A: Early in iron deficiency anemia there is heterogeneous erythrocyte volume due to progressive repopulation of blood with microcytes and a decreasing proportion of normal cells. As the repopulation process continues, the mean cell volume (MCV) progressively decreases. The cell volume changes occur in the opposite direction during recovery from long-standing iron deficiency. A normal, homogeneous volume distribution is indicated by the heavy, broken-line curve. B: A homogeneous population of microcytes indicates long-standing iron deficiency anemia. This is a result of complete blood repopulation with microcytes. A normal, homogeneous volume distribution is indicated by the heavy, broken-line curve.

Iron deficiency has not been recognized in the adult cat. The reason for this is not clear. It is possible that the cat has a much greater capacity for gastrointestinal iron absorption than man or dogs and is able to compensate for blood loss. Alternatively, iron deficiency may occur but is not detected since changes in central pallor of small mammalian erythrocytes may not be observable. Increased central pallor is not observed in kittens with documented iron deficiency anemia. Microcytosis correlated with iron deficiency in kittens has not been observed in adults, further suggesting that this process may not occur. Study of this aspect of feline hematology would be helpful.

Iron deficiency has been recognized in kittens at weaning age.[29] This appears to be related to the age when individual kittens start taking in solid food. As mentioned, kittens repopulate blood in the first few weeks of life. In one study, kittens that had normal serum iron by three weeks of age repopulated the blood with normal-sized erythrocytes by five weeks of age. Kittens that had decreased serum iron in the first few weeks repopulated the blood with microcytic cells. MCV values were observed as low as 24 fl. Some of these kittens were anemic, with hematocrit values ranging from 12 to 30 per cent.[29] Prominent erythrocyte fragmentation, similar to that observed in dogs, was frequently observed. Following intake of dietary iron, these kittens again repopulated blood with normal-sized cells by ten weeks of age. These changes, characterized as transient neonatal iron deficiency, may be prevented by giving a 50 mg iron dextran injection at 18 days of age. The efficacy of routinely giving iron to kittens has not been determined. Since anemia can be quite severe in a small proportion of kittens, it is conceivable that neonatal iron deficiency anemia may contribute to the unexplained death of young kittens.

HEMOLYSIS

Most forms of hemolytic disease in companion animals are extravascular, that is, they are a result of accelerated phagocytic erythrocyte destruction by the mononuclear phagocyte system. As a result, splenomegaly may be observed. If the rate of erythrocyte destruction is rapid, the rate of bilirubin formation may exceed the rate of hepatic clearance leading to hyperbilirubinemia, clinically visible icterus, and increased fecal excretion of bile pigments. Combined hemoglobinemia and hemoglobinuria indicate intravascular hemolysis.

Immune-mediated Hemolytic Anemias. **IMMUNO-HEMOLYTIC ANEMIA.** A number of mechanisms may result in immunoglobulin and/or complement-mediated decreased erythrocyte survival. These immune components may be attached either directly or indirectly to erythrocyte membranes. In most instances, there is likely indirect attachment of immunoglobulin to an antigen, which is adsorbed on the erythrocyte membrane. Examples include drug-associated immunohemolysis, and perhaps both canine and feline hemobartonellosis. Antigens associated with inflammatory disease or infections possibly act in this fashion in what we most commonly recognize as immunohemolytic disease of uncertain genesis. Alternatively, formed immune complexes may be adsorbed to the erythrocyte membrane. Neonatal isoerythrolysis is an example of direct immunoglobulin attachment to a known erythrocyte membrane antigen.

Regardless of the attachment mechanism, the final common pathway of erythrocyte injury usually results from interaction with phagocytic cells.[54] Macrophages have receptors for complement and the Fc portion of immunoglobulin, which allow attachment to the coated erythrocyte. Once attached, the interaction may result in either complete phagocytosis or removal of a portion of the membrane. The latter results in sphere injury (Figure 113–23). The sphere is considerably less deformable and highly susceptible to splenic entrapment where further interactions with phagocytic cells result in phagocytosis. Thus, most forms of immunohemolytic disease occur by extravascular hemolysis. In some instances, such as neonatal isoerythrolysis, a component of intravascular hemolysis may occur. This is likely due to cytolysis associated with fixation of complement to completion.

Immunohemolytic anemia is the most frequent and important cause of hemolytic disease in dogs. The tra-

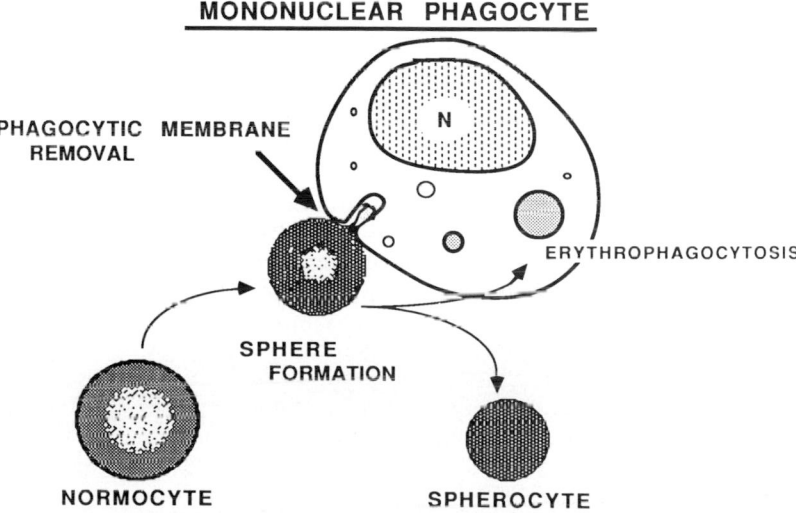

FIGURE 113–23. Diagram depicting pathogenesis of sphere formation in immunohemolytic anemia. Phagocytic cells attach to erythrocytes and remove membrane as described in text. Alternatively, phagocytic cells may phagocytose the injured erythrocyte. N = nucleus.

ditionally extrapolated discussion of classification of antibody type and whether the disease is primary or secondary is not particularly important or useful in dogs. Tools for accurately making these distinctions are not perfected and this information does not currently influence therapeutic approach. Reviews of possible mechanisms of this anemia in veterinary literature patterned after human hematology texts are available.[20, 55] The attempt to classify the disease as either warm- or cold-reacting antibody type is particularly artificial. It is likely that variable combinations of IgG, IgM, and complement are involved in most or all canine cases of immunohemolytic anemia. Surveys for each of these components, using specific Coombs' test antisera, are not conclusive because relatively large concentrations of specific molecules are required for Coombs' test detection, and immunoglobulins are frequently eluted during erythrocyte washing procedures. Due to the usually transient disease course, it is suspected that immunohemolytic anemia in most cases is an epiphenomenon of an immunologic response related to an underlying inflammatory lesion. When the process is chronic or is associated with other non-hematologic immunologically mediated lesions, the possibility of multi-system immune-mediated disease, more in the realm of true autoimmunity, should be considered (see systemic lupus erythematosus in Chapter 119).

Because hemolysis and development of anemia usually occur rapidly, features of acute anemia including sudden onset of exercise intolerance, pale mucous membranes, tachycardia, and hyperpnea may be present. Fever and icterus may occur. Hemoglobinuria associated with an intravascular hemolytic component is uncommon.

Hematologic features usually include moderate to severe anemia, marked reticulocytosis, spherocytosis, and some degree of agglutination when blood cools to room temperature. A striking morphologic feature on the blood film is extreme variation in erythrocyte size, due to the presence of spheres with decreased diameter and polychromatophilic cells with increased diameter. The MCV may be increased if a high proportion of newly released cells are present. However, the volume of spheres is normal. On automated systems, the presence of agglutination may cause a false high MCV and false low hematocrit values. The laboratorian detects this by a false high error in the MCHC. When this occurs, an accurate hematocrit should be determined by microhematocrit centrifugation. Variable degrees of neutrophilic leukocytosis with a left shift and monocytosis are expected. The neutrophilia has been attributed to non-specific marrow stimulation by acute anemia. When moderate to marked, the neutrophilia indicates the presence of an underlying inflammatory lesion, which frequently is associated with immunohemolytic anemia. Immune-mediated thrombocytopenia often occurs in conjunction with immunohemolytic anemia.

It is important to put the numerous hematologic features into priority of importance for establishing a diagnosis of immunohemolytic anemia. Spherocytosis observed by a competent microscopist is the most definitive and reliable feature of immunohemolytic anemia. Immune-mediated agglutination is the next most con-

vincing evidence for this disease. When sphere formation is incomplete or otherwise not convincing, the saline fragility test is helpful for documenting sphere injury. A positive Coombs' test is regarded as supportive of the diagnosis when other essential features are present. A common misconception is that a positive Coombs' test is required to make a diagnosis. On the contrary, when convincing spherocytosis is present, a Coombs' test is not required. This misconception has frequently resulted in the interpretation of a false negative Coombs' test as ruling out immunohemolytic anemia in the face of the above hallmark features. As discussed under technology, the Coombs' test has several limitations related to making a diagnosis of immunohemolytic anemia. One of the most common causes of false negative reactions is elution of immunoglobulin during washing of red cells in preparation for the test. One piece of evidence for this is that spontaneous agglutination usually disappears while washing the cells.

A nonregenerative form of immunohemolytic anemia is characterized by the usual hematologic features except that a complete absence of reticulocytes exists.[56, 57] Reticulocytopenia appears to be a result of immune-mediated consumption of developing erythroid precursors in marrow. There are several important features of this form. First, the clinician usually does not think of hemolytic disease when reticulocytes are absent. Second, a transfusion is more likely to be required early in treatment. Third, a much longer period is required for hematologic improvement. It can be expected that two to three weeks may be required for reticulocytosis and an increasing hematocrit to develop. To diagnose this form, it is exceedingly important to recognize sphere formation. This is often difficult for the inexperienced microscopist because of the uniform appearance of erythrocytes in the absence of polychromatophilic cells.

Marrow aspirate examination may be helpful for characterizing the non-regenerative form. There is usually a distinct maturation block at one stage anywhere from the rubriblast to the metarubricyte. The stages that are present are hyperplastic. Polychromatophilic cells are not present. Phagocytosis of mature erythrocytes and nucleated forms may be reproducibly observed.

Pure red cell aplasia may represent a special case of an immune-mediated injury to erythroid stem cells. This is based on observations of occasional response to immunosuppressive therapy, mostly in man. There is an absence of erythroid cells in marrow, presumably due to destruction of committed stem cells. Antigens involved are theoretically present on stem cells, but not on more differentiated cells because injury to mature erythrocytes is not recognized.

Immunohemolytic anemia is not recognized in cats as frequently as in dogs. Of cats with immunohemolytic anemia reported in the literature, features have been quite variable but are similar to those of the dog.[20, 21] Hemobartonellosis may be regarded as a form of immunohemolytic anemia since immunoglobulin can be detected on erythrocytes and agglutination has been observed in this disease. It is likely that some cats with hemobartonellosis may be diagnosed as having immunohemolytic anemia if organisms are not detected on the blood film examination. Since recognition of spherocytosis is difficult in the cat, the saline fragility test should be used to help detect erythrocyte sphere injury. The diagnosis depends on the presence of the following in decreasing order of importance: evidence of hemolytic anemia, increased fragility in hypotonic saline, agglutination, and a positive Coombs' test. Blood films from more than one bleeding should be scrutinized for hemobartonellosis.

A small number of reported cases of immunohemolytic disease diagnosed in FeLV-positive cats with positive Coombs' tests has led to speculation that FeLV infection may result in immunohemolytic disease.[21, 58, 59] A relatively high frequency of positive Coombs' tests has also been observed in FeLV-positive cats without evidence of hemolytic disease.[22] The interpretation of this finding is not clear. Immunohemolysis strictly related to FeLV infection is not conclusively documented and has not been reproduced to date in specific pathogen-free cats inoculated with various strains of the virus. Uncharacterized hemolytic disease has been reported in kittens inoculated with the A strain of virus.[60] Again, in cats with naturally occurring disease, the possibility that some have undetected hemobartonellosis-associated Coombs' positive tests cannot be excluded. Further, investigation is required to document hemolytic disease in some forms of FeLV infection.

Treatment of immunohemolytic anemia includes steroid suppression of erythrophagocytosis and supportive therapy including a transfusion if essential. Any underlying inflammatory or systemic disorder should be treated as indicated. If there is any doubt about the presence of hemobartonellosis, appropriate antibiotic therapy should be utilized. Prednisone or prednisolone at 1 to 2 mg/lb (2 to 4 mg/kg) per day is recommended. Some persons prefer to administer this dosage divided twice daily. There is uncertainty about how long steroids should be given. Generally, they should be given until an increasing hematocrit is established and it is clear that newly produced cells are not involved in immune-mediated injury. This requires a minimum of two to three weeks. The dosage is decreased in step-wise fashion to cessation over a 7 to 14 day period with monitoring for recurrence of hemolytic disease. The guidelines for giving a transfusion are no different than for other forms of anemia. When the hematocrit falls to a life-threatening value, a transfusion of 5 to 10 ml/lb (10 to 20 ml/kg) should be given using the same precautions employed with any anemic patient. This is more likely to be required in the nonregenerative form. The only basis for the statement that transfusions are contraindicated in this disease is repetition from one textbook to the next.

There is popular usage of more potent cytotoxic and immunosuppressive drugs in this anemia in small animal medicine. However, this may represent overtreatment, and use of these drugs may induce myelosuppressive toxicity in severely anemic animals, which may have altered drug metabolism. Proclaimed efficacy of these drugs is based solely on subjective clinical impressions and similar proclamations from human medicine. The effectiveness of these drugs and the rate of inducing undesirable side effects in immunohemolytic anemia has not been appropriately documented in animals. Appropriately controlled studies comparing different treatments are needed. Drugs commonly utilized for more potent immunosuppressive therapy include cyclophosphamide at 50 mg/m² given orally for four consecutive days per week or azathioprine at 1 mg/lb (2 mg/kg) given orally once per day.

Criteria for evaluating response to treatment are not well developed. Most clinicians use rising hematocrit as an indication of response. This may be misleading in a number of cases. One should consider that recovery involves a variable balance between kinetics of at least two populations of cells. The existing sphere-injured cells have shortened survival. Repopulation of blood from marrow occurs at variable rates. If the rate of egress and entry occurring in these two populations remains somewhat equal, it is possible for the hematocrit to remain unchanged for as long as 7 to 14 days. An example is a dog with an erythrocyte count of 2×10^6/µl and matched destruction and production rates of 200,000 cells/µl/day. Therapy in this example may be totally adequate. Only cases with a maximal regenerative response established at the beginning of treatment will have an increasing hematocrit as soon as two to three days. When the hematocrit does not increase in four to five days, the misinterpretation of ineffective therapy is made too often. The decision is then made to institute more aggressive immunosuppressive therapy. When the hematocrit finally begins to increase several days later, success is proclaimed for the more aggressive therapy. It is recommended here that more aggressive therapy not be used until it becomes clear that the immunologic injury involves newly produced cells.

The predicted outcome for dealing with immunohemolytic anemia in dogs is reasonably good, but individual cases must be given a guarded prognosis when first diagnosed. Most cases respond favorably without recurrence of disease. Sudden death may occur as a result of acute anemia leading to cardiopulmonary failure. In retrospect, these are probably preventable by blood transfusion. A small proportion of cases may have protracted hemolytic disease that eventuates in death due to other complications. The prognosis should be more guarded in cats because of the limited experience base and the reasonable probability that investigation will lead to a more severe underlying disease such as FeLV infection sequelae.

DRUG RELATED. Drug-associated immunohemolytic anemia is a relatively common occurrence in man. This occurs rarely if ever in the dog; however, it is difficult to document. Suspected levamisole-induced immunohemolysis has been reported in dogs.[61] An eight per cent prevalence of immunohemolytic anemia and thrombocytopenia has been reported in cats with hyperthyroidism given propylthiouracil.[62] Cats were Coombs' test positive, had petechial hemorrhages, and had severe anemia. The mechanism of toxicity is not known but may involve anti-drug antibody production, which then binds to drug adsorbed on platelet and erythrocyte membranes. Some of the cats developed increased antinuclear antibody titers. It is recommended that cats receiving propylthiouracil therapy be hematologically monitored once weekly. Treatment of this toxicity includes cessation of drug therapy and supportive care.

The anemia and thrombocytopenia resolve fairly rapidly and immunologic test results return to normal within two weeks.

COLD-AGGLUTININ DISEASE. Cold-agglutinin disease occurs rarely in dogs.[63] Presence of abnormally high titers of immunoglobulin capable of binding to erythrocytes with optimal activity below 98.6° F (37° C) may cause intravascular agglutination. This may occur in ear tips, tail tip, and feet upon exposure to cold environmental temperatures. Extremities are susceptible to local temperature decreases, which can result in *in vivo* erythrocyte agglutination in the presence of pathologic cold-agglutinating antibodies of the IgM class. The agglutination in vasculature obliterates blood supply, which in turn causes gangrenous necrosis. Diagnosis is dependent on determining that the animal was exposed to low environmental temperature and demonstrating cold-induced agglutination *in vitro*. This is simply done by examining a blood sample for agglutination at room temperature or exaggerating it at 39.2° F (4° C). If no agglutination can be induced *in vitro*, it is inconceivable for it to occur *in vivo* in extremities. The term cold-agglutinin disease is occasionally used inappropriately to describe immunohemolytic anemia having *in vitro* agglutination. However, conventional immunohemolytic anemia may accompany cold agglutinin disease.

Cold agglutinin disease has been reported in a cat based on a positive Coombs' test and the ability of serially diluted patient serum to macroscopically agglutinate donor erythrocytes at 39.2° F (4° C).[64] The cat had gangrenous necrosis of ear tips, tail tip, and front paws. Hemolytic anemia was not a feature.

NEONATAL ISOERYTHROLYSIS. Hemolysis due to antibody passage to the newborn, recognized best in humans and horses, is rare in dogs and cats. The disease may be experimentally induced in offspring of bitches sensitized by transfusion of CEA-l or 2 type blood. In one feline report, sudden death of kittens at one to two days of age prevented collection of blood to conclusively document neonatal isoerythrolysis, but serologic studies on queens and other circumstantial evidence was highly supportive of this diagnosis.[65] The queens were primiparous and had anti-A antibodies. A high proportion of cats with type-B erythrocytes have anti-A antibodies. (See discussion of erythrocyte antigens in the section on transfusions.) This disorder may occur more frequently than is appreciated, but is likely limited to geographical regions with a high proportion of blood type B in the cat population. It should be considered in situations of neonatal death. If recognized in advance, foster nursing prevents neonatal isoerythrolysis in kittens.

Hemolytic Anemias Due to Erythroparasitic Organisms. **HEMOBARTONELLOSIS.** *Hemobartonella felis*, an organism in the order Rickettsiales, is the causative agent of feline infectious anemia. It is an epicellular organism firmly attached to the erythrocyte membrane. Events preceding development of anemia in natural disease are poorly understood. Transmission is thought to involve blood transfer. Blood-sucking arthropods may serve as natural vectors. Carrier cats likely serve as a reservoir of infection. The disease has been experimentally induced by injection of infected blood and frozen hemolysate from infected cats.[66] The time from experimental inoculation and development of parasitemic cycles varies from 2 to 17 days. Parasitemic cycles lasted three to eight weeks during which organism proliferation resulted in moderate to severe hemolytic anemia. Since hematocrits did not normalize during this interval, multiple hemolytic episodes of variable severity occurred.

After recovery, the cat may remain a carrier for years. In this stage, the organism can be intermittently found in small numbers on blood films and be associated with subclinical anemia.[66] There is evidence that the organism is harbored in splenic macrophages.[67] It has been generally thought that stress and other primary diseases result in exacerbation of organism proliferation and overt hemolytic anemia. This is derived from clinical observations that feline infectious anemia is often accompanied by other disease such as cat fight abscesses or FeLV-related disease. However, attempts to induce such exacerbation in experimental cats have not been successful.[66] An alternative explanation is that concurrent infection and other disease results in greater probability of the cat being taken to a veterinarian compared to either disease alone. It is likely that anemia associated with small numbers of organisms may be interpreted as active disease, when in fact it may represent the carrier state in combination with other superimposed causes of anemia such as FeLV infection. This aspect of hemobartonellosis requires further study and reinterpretation.

Diagnosis currently depends on finding organisms on erythrocytes using Wright's stained blood films. Ring forms and rod forms are the two general shapes recognized. Ring forms appear superimposed on the cell. They consist of a fine basophilic ring with a hollow center. Rod shapes are observed on the periphery of the cell contour. The proportion of numbers of each form varies markedly between cases (Figure 113–24). Experience is required to distinguish organisms from precipitated stain. The latter may adhere to the cell contour, but is irregular in size and shape and appears relatively refractile when focusing up and down. The number and detectability of organisms may fluctuate markedly. A diagnosis may require examination of blood films over several days. It is extremely unlikely to find organisms if the cat is receiving tetracycline. Other clinical signs that occur variably include weight loss, intermittent anorexia, hyperbilirubinemia, spleno-

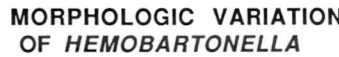

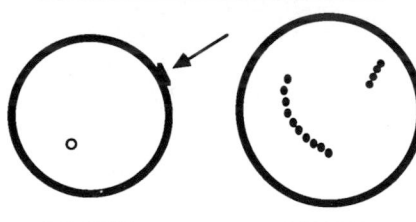

FIGURE 113–24. Schematic representation of morphology of canine and feline *Hemobartonella* organisms on erythrocytes. In cats, the rod shaped organism at the perimeter of the cell diameter (arrow) is the traditionally described morphology. A delicate, basophilic ring form superimposed on the cell may also be seen. In dogs, the organisms occur in chains across the cell surface.

megaly, and fever. Diagnostic tests for detecting active disease in between parasitemic cycles and for distinguishing the carrier state from active disease are of value in studying the relationship of hemobartonellosis to other disease.

The mechanism of hemolysis is not completely understood. It does not cause intravascular cell lysis to any appreciable degree. It has been demonstrated that organisms are removed principally in the spleen by two processes.[67] Most parasitized erythrocytes are phagocytosed by splenic cordal macrophages, while others have the organism stripped from the membrane by the macrophage, a process referred to as pitting. Observations of agglutination, increased fragility in hypotonic saline, and positive Coombs' tests are highly suggestive of immunohemolysis as a mechanism for clearing parasitized cells. Such a mechanism is compatible with ultrastructural studies that demonstrate macrophage interaction with parasitized erythrocytes. It is not known whether an attached organism is required for erythrocyte destruction. It is possible that an erythrocyte that has had an organism removed still has attached antigens of the organism and undergoes sphere injury. This view is compatible with observations of immunoinjury when the organisms have decreased in numbers during peak hemolysis. This component of the disease requires further study.

Treatment should consist of oral tetracycline (26 mg/lb or 60 mg/kg q8h) for two to three weeks. Steroids have been advocated since an immune-mediated hemolytic component is likely. Supportive therapy and specific therapy for any concurrent disease are intuitive. Transfusion may be required in the more severe cases and in those that do not have erythrocyte regeneration for some underlying reason.

Hemobartonellosis is of less importance in dogs since it is rare and usually occurs only in splenectomized dogs. It may occur rarely in severely debilitated or immunosuppressed dogs that have a spleen. There is concurrent sphere formation and the anemia may be Coombs' positive.[69] These items indicate that immunoglobulin directed at the organism results in sphere injury and that immunohemolytic disease is an important component in canine hemobartonellosis. The process is more morphologically evident in dogs than in cats. During active hemolytic disease, organisms are readily identified. Their morphology is somewhat different from the cat in that they usually occur in chains across the surface (see Figure 113–24). Treatment of canine hemobartonellosis should consist of tetracycline using the same regimen as for the cat. Steroids may be used as in treatment for immunohemolytic anemia if judgment indicates there is prominent hemolysis attributable to spherocytosis.

BABESIOSIS. This protozoal disease of dogs may be caused by two organisms, *Babesia canis* and *Babesia gibsoni*. Both produce similar hemolytic disease and are transmitted principally by the brown dog tick *Rhipicephalus sanguineus*. The clinical manifestations are highly variable. An acute, severe form characterized by intravascular hemolysis indicated by hemoglobinuria, hyperbilirubinemia, dehydration, severe acidosis, fever, anorexia, depression, and collapse tends to occur in younger

dogs. Subacute or chronic forms are characterized by fever, anorexia, depression, and mild to moderate anemia. The chronic form is more difficult to diagnose because of more non-specific signs and low level of parasitemia. The anemias are regenerative. In one survey, a high proportion of dogs with hemolytic anemia had positive Coombs' tests, suggesting an immune-mediated component.[70] The diagnosis is made by examination of stained blood films for intraerythrocytic pyriform bodies. *B. canis* organisms are larger and usually occur in pairs. *B. gibsoni* organisms are smaller but vary considerably in size and shape (Figure 113–25). A serologic test exists for establishing a diagnosis when organisms are difficult to find. Because the brown dog tick is the principal vector, concurrent infection with *Ehrlichia canis* has been recognized in dogs with babesiosis. It has been recommended that a serologic test for ehrlichiosis be done as part of evaluation for babesiosis.

Treatment involves anti-parasite drugs and appropriate supportive therapy. Drugs that rapidly eliminate the organism are not available. The objective is to control the organism until the dog's immunity controls the disease. Recovered dogs remain inapparent carriers. The two most commonly recommended drugs, diminazine aceturate and imidocarb diproprionate, are not approved for use in the United States. These drugs have relatively narrow margins of safety and toxicity related to reversible central nervous system disturbances. The use of these drugs in other countries has been outlined.[71] Considering the difficulty in obtaining these drugs, it is recommended that tetracycline be used as described for hemobartonellosis. In addition to the above, treatment of the acute form may require a blood transfusion, fluid therapy, and sodium bicarbonate to correct severe acidosis.

Feline babesiosis exists, but has not been identified in North America.[72, 73] A detailed review of babesiosis is available.[74]

CYTAUXZOONOSIS. This is a protozoal disease which occurs principally in southern states, extending from Oklahoma and Texas to Florida.[75–77] The causative agent is *Cytauxzoon felis*. It is a consistently fatal disease in domestic cats with death occurring a few days after development of clinical signs. The extraerythrocytic form of the organism proliferates in macrophages associated with vasculature and results in fatal blood stasis and vascular occlusion. Published information has concentrated on pathologic description of this component of the disease. Refer to Chapter 46 for discussion of the macrophage form that produces systemic disease.

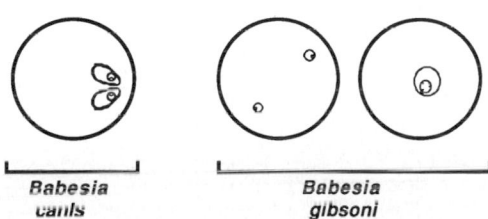

FIGURE 113–25. Schematic representation of *Babesia* organism morphology on canine erythrocytes. *Babesia gibsoni* piroplasms are considerably more pleomorphic than those of *Babesia canis*.

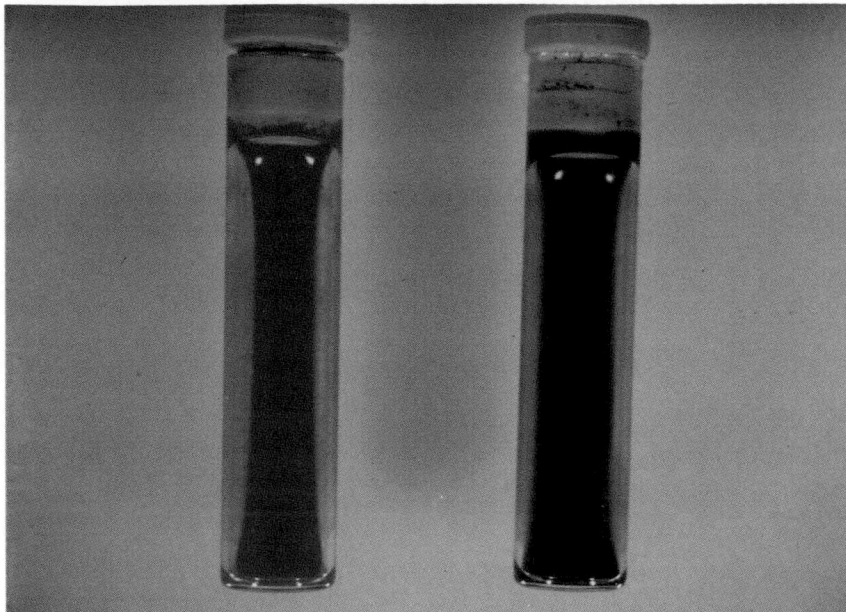

FIGURE 113–26. Blood from a dog with methemoglobinemia with characteristic chocolate brown discoloration (tube on right) compared to normal oxygenated canine blood (tube on left).

The organism's intraerythrocytic form is observed in affected cats, but the associated anemia has not been well characterized. Since prominent splenic erythrophagocytosis is observed, mild to moderate hemolysis most likely accounts for development of anemia. A component of hemorrhage contributes to the anemia in that petechial hemorrhages are observed in body cavities. The genesis of petechial hemorrhages is also not characterized but is likely related to vasculitis. The status of platelets in the disease has not been reported. In erythrocytes, the organism is usually singular but up to four may be present per cell. They are usually ring forms from 0.5 to 1.5 μm in diameter with a small basophilic nucleus, but some may be up to 2.5 μm in diameter or be elongated and bipolar. The organism and anemia have been confused with hemobartonellosis in some clinical cases. When clinical signs first appear, a small proportion of the cells (usually less than five per cent) contain organisms, making diagnosis on blood films difficult, but the erythroparasitemia increases terminally. Studies focusing on hematologic components of the disease are required.

Oxidative Injury to Erythrocytes—Hemolysis and Methemoglobinemia.
Erythrocyte oxidative injury may take at least three forms including oxidation of heme iron resulting in methemoglobinemia, and oxidative denaturation of hemoglobin resulting in Heinz body formation. Oxidative injury to membrane proteins is more subtle in that it is often not detectable morphologically. These injuries usually occur after depletion of biochemical protective mechanisms, such as glutathione within erythrocytes. However, some intoxicants may cause Heinz body formation without altering antioxidant biochemistry.

Methemoglobinemia is a reversible injury in which affected hemoglobin is incapable of carrying oxygen. It may develop within an hour or two upon exposure to oxidants. Clinical signs related to acute hypoxia occur when 20 to 40 per cent of the hemoglobin has been converted to methemoglobin. Severe respiratory distress and lateral recumbency occur with 50 to 70 per cent methemoglobin, and death is expected with greater than 70 per cent methemoglobin. Methemoglobinemia imparts a characteristic chocolate brown discoloration to blood (Figure 113–26). This, in conjunction with poor tissue oxygenation, imparts a cyanotic-brownish color to mucous membranes. Methemoglobin concentration can be readily determined at most human medical laboratories.

Membrane injury and Heinz body formation are irreversible changes. These injuries result in altered erythrocyte deformability, which contributes to shortened erythrocyte survival. Heinz bodies usually appear within 24 hours of exposure to an intoxicant and take several days to eventuate in hemolysis. Because of slower development and a lesser proportion of hemoglobin involvement, clinical signs of anemia are usually minimal. Heinz body hemolytic disease is principally an extravascular process, but an appreciable intravascular component may occur simultaneously.

CANINE DISEASE. The most common cause of Heinz body hemolysis in dogs is related to ingestion of onions. Their toxic effect appears to be equal whether raw, cooked, or dehydrated.[78–81] While the toxicity has been known for over 50 years, animal owners still unknowingly feed onions to dogs, usually as part of table scraps. The hemolytic episode may be difficult to correlate with onion ingestion because it occurs several days later. Clinical signs are related to moderate anemia. Experimental onion toxicity has recently been characterized using a single dose of dehydrated onions.[81] Heinz body formation occurred within one day followed by hemolysis, which resulted in hematocrit nadirs by day five. The hemolysis was mostly extravascular, but an intravascular component occurred as evidenced by transient hemoglobinemia. Minimal, unimportant increases in methemoglobin concentration are associated with onion toxicity. The hemolysis is associated with a prominent regenerative response.

Heinz bodies are more difficult to recognize in dogs compared to cats because they tend to be small and multiple per cell, although single large bodies may be observed. They tend to be membrane associated, so when large they may protrude from the cell contour. Often, the most obvious finding on Wright's stained blood films are eccentrocytes. Seeing these is an indication to carefully examine a blood film stained for reticulocyte counting. The clear zone likely represents membrane oxidative injury resulting in adherence of the upper and lower membranes and consequent compression of hemoglobin to the opposite side of the cell (Figure 113–27). Eccentrocytes undoubtedly have decreased deformability and therefore are involved in hemolysis.

Acetaminophen toxicity may occur accidentally in dogs having access to improperly stored drug containers. The recommended dose of up to 22 mg/lb (45 mg/kg) per day causes no toxicity in the dog. Moderate and severe toxic doses are in the range of 90–110 mg/lb and 200–500 mg/kg, respectively.[82] Toxicity results in severe methemoglobinemia and hepatocellular necrosis, which may result in death. It is likely that Heinz body formation also occurs, but in reports to date it appears that this aspect has not been examined.

Benzocaine-containing topical products have been reported to produce methemoglobinemia as high as 51 per cent and mild Heinz body hemolysis in dogs with ulcerated skin lesions.[83] It was postulated that ulceration was required for absorption of toxic amounts of benzocaine.

Methemoglobin reductase deficiency has been described as a rare disorder of dogs. Methemoglobin concentrations were chronically increased and there was predisposition to development of severe methemoglobinemia.[84–86]

FELINE DISEASE. Unusual metabolism and unique hemoglobin structure in cats result in increased sensitivity to oxidative injury. These injuries are therefore more frequent and important in feline medicine. Feline hemoglobin may be oxidized to methemoglobin by a variety of oxidants at a rate comparable to other species.[45] However, feline hemoglobin is considerably more susceptible to oxidative denaturation.[45] This has been attributed to eight to ten sulfhydryl groups per molecule compared to two to four per molecule in other species.[87, 88] This may explain the high prevalence of spontaneous Heinz body formation and clinical recognition that a variety of chemical agents result in Heinz body formation in cats.[27] Normal cats have a high prevalence of Heinz body formation and the proportion of erythrocytes involved has varied from 0 to 96 per cent.[27, 89] Heinz body clearance appears to be independent of the spleen in cats.[27]

A variety of chemical agents and drugs may induce Heinz body formation and severe hemolysis. Methylene blue–induced Heinz body hemolysis has been characterized extensively in the cat. This was first recognized in cats given urinary antiseptic drugs containing methylene blue.[90] Injectable methylene blue has been suitable for inducing experimental Heinz body hemolysis to study feline erythroid responses.[19, 91] In experimental Heinz body hemolysis, the cat may completely replace its circulating erythrocyte mass within about 14 days.[19] During acute hemolysis, all Heinz body–bearing cells may be removed within seven days with mean hematocrit values remaining above 20 per cent, with minimal to no clinical signs of anemia. This observation is explained by the marked regenerative capacity of the cat to produce macrocytes.[19] This suggests the need for reinterpretation of spontaneous Heinz body formation in cats. Since anemia is often not observed, it has been interpreted that Heinz body–bearing cells may have relatively normal survival. However, considering the capacity of feline marrow to regenerate erythrocytes and that prominent aggregate reticulocytosis may not be observed in mild anemia, it is possible that mild Heinz body hemolysis in normal cats may not be recognized. While the relationship between spontaneous Heinz body formation and hemolysis is not clear, clinical cases of regenerative hemolytic anemia attributable to Heinz bodies of unknown origin do occur.[14] The cause of spontaneous Heinz body formation in cats is not understood.

Diagnosis of overt Heinz body hemolysis depends on observing relatively large Heinz bodies in an appreciable

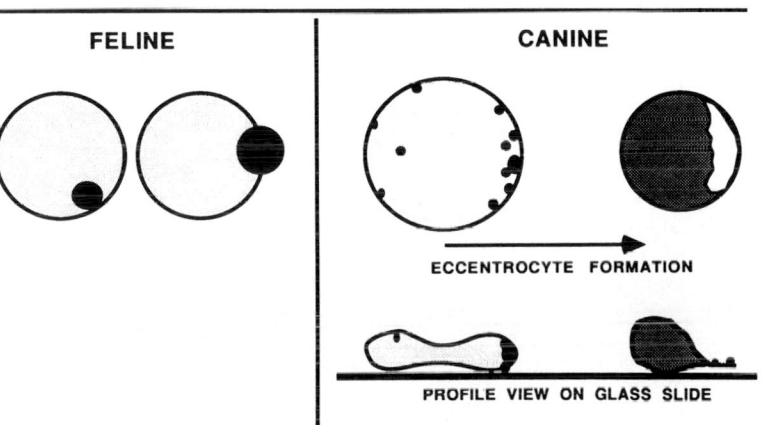

FIGURE 113–27. Comparison of feline and canine Heinz body morphology. The precipitates usually occur singly in the feline cell. The larger Heinz bodies which protrude from the membrane contour may be easily visualized on Wright's stained blood films. In the canine cell, Heinz bodies are usually small and occur in multiples, making recognition on Wright's stained blood films very difficult. Eccentrocyte formation often accompanies Heinz body formation in dogs. Eccentrocyte formation may represent oxidative membrane fusion as depicted on the profile view. This could account for the appearance of the clear, non-hemoglobinized area seen by transmitted light.

MORPHOLOGY RELATED TO HEINZ BODIES

FELINE | **CANINE**

ECCENTROCYTE FORMATION

PROFILE VIEW ON GLASS SLIDE

proportion of erythrocytes in conjunction with a hemolysis pattern to the hemogram. Heinz bodies are usually singular and may project from the membrane in feline erythrocytes. Large Heinz bodies may be observed on Wright's stained blood films, but are best visualized with one of the reticulocyte stains. On these preparations the bodies stain blue and all sizes are visible (see Figure 113–16). The observation of small Heinz bodies with a normal hematocrit is interpreted as either normal or subclinical disease of little importance.

Acetaminophen toxicity results in a combination of methemoglobinemia and Heinz body hemolytic anemia. The best characterized aspects of acetaminophen toxicity include the clinical signs, drug metabolism, methemoglobinemia, and antidote evaluation of the acute toxicity.[92] The toxicity has occurred commonly, since animal owners may unknowingly administer the compound in toxic doses.[92, 93] Cats develop toxicity at doses considerably lower than for other species;[82, 94] as little as one-half tablet (163 mg) has been reported to cause toxicity.[92] This may be related to differences in drug metabolism. Most species excrete the majority of acetaminophen as a glucuronide conjugate. The cat excretes the majority of acetaminophen as a sulfate conjugate and this pathway is saturated at relatively low drug concentrations.[82] Within a few hours of receiving the drug, erythrocyte glutathione is markedly decreased and methemoglobinemia occurs. A dose of 27 mg/lb (60 mg/kg) may result in methemoglobin levels in excess of 20 per cent. At a higher dose of 55 mg/lb (120 mg/kg), 45 per cent methemoglobin was observed.[82] Clinical signs include labored respiration and increased heart rate associated with reduced oxygen carrying capacity, depression, hematuria, and hemoglobinuria. At the higher doses, salivation and facial edema may be observed. Markedly regenerative anemia may occur with a hematocrit nadir and reticulocyte peak occurring about one week after drug administration.[82, 94] The anemia and hemoglobinuria have been attributed to a component of intravascular hemolysis and are associated with Heinz body formation.[82, 94] It is likely that there is also generalized oxidation of erythrocyte membranes, which results in both intravascular and extravascular hemolysis.

Important hepatocellular injury associated with acute acetaminophen toxicity in other species is not observed in the cat. This is probably due to the fact that cats develop oxidative toxicity at much lower doses than those required for hepatotoxicity in other species. Cats with acute toxicity may lack hepatic micropathology, but may have variable increases in serum alanine aminotransferase.[96, 97] Chronic administration of low doses of acetaminophen has caused hepatic necrosis and fibrosis in cats.[98]

Other recognized causes of methemoglobinemia in cats include phenazopyridine, benzocaine, phenacetin, and DL-methionine. Phenazopyridine, a urinary analgesic drug, has caused methemoglobinemia and Heinz body hemolysis.[99] A laryngeal local anesthetic spray containing benzocaine (Cetacaine), used to facilitate intubation, has been associated with development of methemoglobinemia.[100] Peak methemoglobinemia ranging from 2 to 30 per cent occurred in seven experimental cats 20 to 30 minutes after benzocaine application and persisted for 1 to 3 hours. Heinz body formation was not observed. The more severely affected cats became cyanotic and had rapid respiration. Methemoglobinemia complicates anesthetic risk, especially in anemic or debilitated cats. Benzocaine-containing laryngeal spray should be avoided in the cat; lidocaine appears to be a suitable alternative. Phenacetin, contained in some analgesic mixtures, is metabolized to acetaminophen. DL-methionine administered to cats in high doses as a urinary acidifier may cause Heinz body hemolysis and mild methemoglobinemia.[101] Doses of 0.2 to 0.4 gm/lb (0.5 to 1 gm/kg) produce toxicity. A metabolite of methionine appears to be the oxidizing agent.

TREATMENT OF OXIDATIVE INJURIES. Treatment of Heinz body hemolysis involves cessation of any identifiable offending drug and simple supportive care. With an intact marrow response, blood repopulation is expected to occur rapidly enough to avoid severe anemia. The reticulocyte count is useful in monitoring this response when the hematocrit decreases below 20 per cent. Transfusions are not likely to be required unless the marrow response is impaired due to other concurrent disease. There is no treatment indicated for Heinz body formation in cats without anemia.

Severe methemoglobinemia should be treated vigorously. Methylene blue (0.45 mg/lb or 1 mg/kg given once IV) will accelerate reduction of methemoglobin back to the functional state. Methylene blue acts as an electron donor for an alternate, normally non-functional methemoglobin reductase. The drug should not be given repeatedly or in higher doses because it will cause Heinz body formation in both dogs and cats. A blood transfusion may provide a lifesaving fraction of functional hemoglobin until methemoglobin can be reduced. Oxygen therapy has been advocated, but it is probably of little benefit because functional hemoglobin fraction is already virtually 100 per cent saturated with oxygen at the lung.

Treatment of acetaminophen toxicity should include the above approach to methemoglobinemia. Other measures are useful in addition to any obvious supportive care.[95–97] If ingestion has occurred within two hours, vomition should be induced with activated charcoal. Either oral or intravenous N-acetylcysteine (65 mg/lb or 140 mg/kg q8h) and intravenous sodium sulfate (22 mg/lb or 50 mg/kg q8h) result in considerable improvement by increasing acetaminophen clearance rate and contributing to methemoglobin reduction.[82] N-Acetylcysteine likely acts by increasing sulfate availability for acetaminophen biotransformation and by restoring blood and hepatic reduced glutathione concentrations.

Hemolytic Disease Associated with Inherited Metabolic Disorders. Several inherited enzyme deficiencies that result in variably shortened erythrocyte survival have been recognized. These disorders are unlikely to be encountered because they are rare. In addition, most carrier and affected animals have been removed from the breeding population. A few may be maintained in breeding colonies for study. There currently is no specific treatment for these disorders.

PYRUVATE KINASE (PK) DEFICIENCY. This glycolytic enzyme deficiency has been recognized in basenjis and beagles.[102–106] It is inherited as an autosomal recessive trait. It is characterized by chronic, severe hemolysis with fairly stable kinetics. Extremely shortened erythrocyte survival is attributable to impaired generation of the energy intermediate ATP. Reticulocytes have high pyruvate kinase activity, but the enzyme is not stable and activity rapidly declines in mature erythrocytes. The very high reticulocyte counts makes the disorder difficult to document by enzyme assays. The enzymopathy is easier to detect in the carrier parent dogs because, although not affected by disease, they have reduced erythrocyte pyruvate kinase activity. Carrier dogs obviously should not be used for breeding stock.

The hematocrit is usually 15 to 30 per cent when the disease is first recognized at about three to six months of age. Thereafter, it slowly declines over the next one to three years until the affected animal becomes terminally ill. During this time there are marked alterations, which are very stable from month to month. These include marked macrocytosis (MCV of 85 to 105 fl) and very high reticulocyte fractions (25 to 60 per cent). There is prominent splenomegaly as a result of intense extramedullary hematopoiesis. A diagnosis is presumed based on the very stable kinetics of the anemia and lack of other known hemolytic defects. A pathology laboratory may be contacted to investigate availability of enzyme assays to document the disease. Terminal myelofibrosis may develop. Demands for erythrocyte production can no longer be met and the animal develops terminal anemia.

PHOSPHOFRUCTOKINASE (PFK) DEFICIENCY. This deficiency has been reported in two English springer spaniel dogs.[107] It is less severe than PK deficiency. There is mild to moderate chronic hemolysis with more severe superimposed hemolytic episodes. The hemolytic episodes are precipitated by vigorous exercise or panting associated with overheating. This is a result of exquisite erythrocyte sensitivity to alkaline pH–induced hemolysis. Hemolytic episodes are intravascular in nature. *In vivo* and *in vitro* studies on erythrocytes from PFK deficient dogs may be reviewed.[107]

FELINE PORPHYRIA. Congenital erythropoietic porphyria, a rare disorder in cats,[108] has an autosomal dominant mode of inheritance. The underlying enzymatic abnormality has not been characterized but is likely a partial deficiency of uroporphyrinogen III cosynthetase as in cows and humans. As a result, the dead-end metabolic isomeric products uroporphyrinogen I and coproporphyrinogen I accumulate in tissues and are excreted in urine and feces in increased quantities. Porphyrin metabolism may be reviewed in more detail elsewhere.[109]

The tissue accumulation results in visible brown to reddish discoloration of teeth and bones. The pigments fluoresce when exposed to ultraviolet light. The degree of pigmentation, occurrence of photosensitization, and development of anemia were variable between two reported porphyric families. In a family of domestic short-hair cats, photosensitization was not present and anemia was not present or was minimal.[108] Porphyria described in a family of Siamese cats was associated with prominent pigmentation of mineralized tissues and viscera, photosensitization, and severe anemia.[110] The anemia was described as hemolytic based on extramed-

ullary hematopoiesis, hemosiderosis, and erythrocyte macrocytosis. Reticulocyte counts or evaluations of degree of polychromatophilia were not done. The mechanism of hemolysis is not known, but the severity of shortened erythrocyte survival in porphyric cows is related to concentrations of porphyrins in erythrocytes. Porphyrin concentrations were markedly increased in cats with anemia. An unusual feature in the Siamese cats was renal injury and failure characterized by mesangial proliferation, tubular degeneration, and necrosis.

Miscellaneous Causes of Hemolysis. **MICROANGIOPATHIC HEMOLYTIC DISEASE.** Microangiopathic hemolytic disease is due to mechanical fragmentation of erythrocytes. Erythrocytes may be sheared by strands of fibrin deposition in small vessel lumina. Sheared erythrocytes release small quantities of hemoglobin before spontaneous membrane resealing. Ordinarily, the rate of hemolysis is subclinical and hemoglobinemia does not develop. Occasionally, more overt hemolysis may develop. Hemoglobinemia and hemoglobinuria may develop as a result of summation of erythrocyte shearing. Postcaval syndrome associated with heartworm disease (see Chapter 80) and splenic torsion are examples of overt microangiopathic hemolysis.

COPPER TOXICITY. Intravascular hemolysis has been observed in copper-associated hepatitis in Bedlington terriers (see Chapter 89). This is associated with hepatic necrosis, which results in massive release of copper to the circulation. The mechanism of copper-associated hemolysis is not well understood, but it may be related to acute oxidative damage and inhibition of glycolytic enzymes.[111]

EXTRA-MARROW DISEASE—SELECTIVE ERYTHROPOIETIC DEPRESSION

As implied by the term extra-marrow disease, this non-regenerative anemia is the result of a group of major systemic disorders. Categories of selective depression of erythropoiesis, which are well documented in dogs and humans, include chronic renal disease, anemia of chronic disease, and endocrine failures. Again, characterization of the anemia is useful for elucidating the underlying condition in the patient with complications. Clinical features of anemia are usually overshadowed by signs of the primary disease. It is usually detected only after hematologic examination. Because the development of anemia is slow enough for physiologic adaptations to occur, animal owners usually do not detect changes in exercise tolerance related to anemia.

Hematologic findings include reticulocyte counts ranging from 0 to about 20,000/µl, normocytic/normochromic indices, and unremarkable morphology. Unimportant, non-specific morphologic changes such as leptocytosis may be observed on blood films. Plasma protein values are reflective of the underlying disorder.

Anemia of Chronic Disease. This is probably the most common form of nonregenerative anemia in man and dogs.[112-115] The pathogenesis is also the least understood. It develops in association with many infectious, noninfectious, and neoplastic disorders. It is assumed that anemias observed in this wide range of disorders are related, because they share common features such as normocytic/normochromic erythrocytes, decreased erythrocyte survival, decreased serum iron and iron binding capacity, increased tissue iron stores, and apparent bone marrow hyporesponsiveness.[116–118] Our current knowledge is that the pathogenesis of anemia involves a combination of iron sequestration by the mononuclear-phagocyte system, shortened erythrocyte survival, and lack of appropriate marrow responsiveness to erythropoietin.[119–125] Much of the investigative attention has been directed toward iron kinetics. While considerable iron is sequestered by the mononuclear phagocyte system and serum iron is modestly decreased, the anemia does not have usual features of iron deficiency such as microcytosis, hypochromia, or responsiveness to iron administration. This disorder requires a new approach to elucidate its pathogenesis.

Hematocrit values are usually only mildly decreased, ranging from 25 to 35 per cent, unless complicated by blood loss. As a result, the anemia is rarely treated. Correction of the primary lesion is expected to result in resolution of the anemia.

Anemia of Renal Failure. Chronic renal failure with azotemia is regularly associated with non-regenerative anemia of mild to moderate magnitude. The anemia has been attributed to a combination of failure to release adequate erythropoietin, impaired hematopoietic cell response to erythropoietin, and shortening of erythrocyte survival perhaps related to metabolic injury. Use of alkylated anabolic steroids (oxymetholone, 0.45 mg/lb or 1 mg/kg q24h) has been advocated in anemia of renal failure. This is based on observations that these drugs increase erythrocyte mass in normal animals and in humans with chronic renal failure. If this therapy is to have any benefit, it requires a minimum of a month or longer to be evident. The benefit is not convincingly established in animals. The decision to use this drug should weigh the effort of administration against the overall condition of the patient and the benefit expected.

Endocrine Failures. Mild anemia is associated with hypothyroidism and hypoadrenocorticism. Both respective hormones have a facilitatory effect on erythropoietin stimulation of marrow. In hypothyroidism, it is possible that the reduction in hematocrit is a physiologic adaptation to reduced oxygen consumption. The anemia is expected to slowly resolve with appropriate hormone replacement therapy.

Anemias associated with these disorders in cats are not well characterized; this is likely related to their relative prevalence compared to FeLV-associated anemia. Our understanding of these anemias in cats is therefore extrapolated from what is known in other species. Mild to moderate anemia may be observed in about 40 per cent of cats with end stage renal disease and chronic azotemia.[126] Severe dehydration likely masked the presence of anemia in a number of cats in this series. More important examples of anemia of chronic disease in cats include feline infectious peritonitis, pyothorax, and malignant neoplasms. Hypothyroidism and associated anemia have not been documented in the cat.

Feline Leukemia Virus-Associated Nonregenerative Anemia. It is impressive that a large proportion of cats with anemia have disease referable to one of the many direct or indirect manifestations of FeLV infection. Indeed, overt or underlying FeLV infection should be a first suspicion when evaluating a cat with anemia. It has been reported that as many as 70 per cent of cats with anemia will be positive for the presence of feline leukemia virus.[13, 127] Thus, evaluation of any cat with anemia that is not immediately explainable should include testing for FeLV infection.

The hematologic findings in FeLV-associated anemia are extremely varied. The best guideline is that virtually any combination of hematologic alterations may be observed. While not all of the associated anemias are due to simple selective erythropoietic depression, it seems appropriate here to provide brief overview of major categories of anemia occurring in association with FeLV infection. Figure 113–28 may help the reader conceptualize the variety of hematologic responses that occur. Simple non-regenerative anemia refers to selective depression of erythrogenesis, while platelet and leukocyte production remain apparently normal. Primary bone marrow disease such as myeloproliferative disorders and dysplastic hematopoiesis are frequently observed in association with anemia. These may result in other cytopenias such as neutropenia and/or thrombocytopenia. Development of overt leukemia may be observed in cases of myeloproliferative disease. Associated hemolytic disorders may include spontaneous Heinz body hemolysis, hemobartonellosis, and immunohemolytic anemia. The relationship between these hemolytic diseases and the virus is not clear. One hypothesis that remains unproven is that bone marrow hyperplasia associated with hemolytic disease helps provide conditions that allow the virus to cause advanced injury. The rationale is that presence of virus in rapidly proliferating bone marrow cells would increase the chances of whatever viral-host cell interactions are involved in the pathogenesis of stem cell injury. This would be compatible with the long but variable incubation period between viral infection and development of

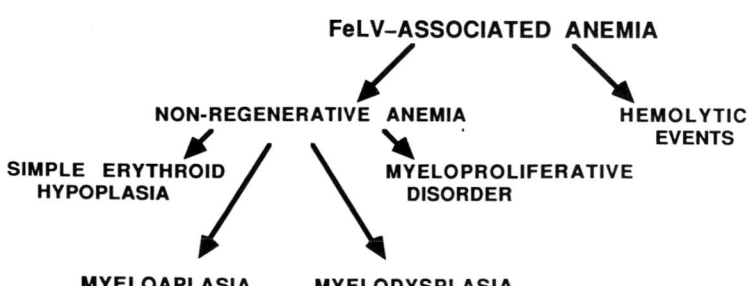

FIGURE 113–28. Diagram depicting the variety of events which may result in anemia in association with feline leukemia virus (FeLV) infection.

hematologic disease. The anemias due to hemolysis and bone marrow failures are covered in respective sections of this chapter.

The distinction between intra- and extra-marrow disease in FeLV-associated anemia should be deemphasized in the reader's mind. The presentation here is kept consistent with the approach to anemia presented earlier. The clinician should not labor over subclassification of FeLV-associated anemia. The distinctions are perhaps artificial, in many cases are not clear, and are highly dependent on subtle morphologic features in blood and bone marrow. For example, many cases with simple non-regenerative anemia summarized in the literature and encountered by veterinarians would likely have myelodysplastic change if blood and marrow were carefully examined. However, description of observed variation serves to provide appreciation of the intricate manifestations of interaction between FeLV and the feline hematopoietic system.

Simple nonregenerative anemia has been one of the more frequently recognized forms of FeLV-associated anemia. Examination of bone marrow aspirate films reveals non-specific erythroid hypoplasia. The anemia has been characterized as normocytic, normochromic based on lack of reticulocytosis.[127] However, when erythrocyte volume is measured directly, many cases of this anemia are macrocytic.[13, 14, 128] Furthermore, most FeLV positive cats, whether anemic or not, have increased erythrocyte volume and volume heterogeneity.[13] It is not clear why macrocytosis develops, but it may be related to accelerated erythrocyte regeneration occurring before development of bone marrow failure. Macrocytosis may reflect residual macrocytes from a regenerative response occurring within the previous two months.[19] Regenerative anemia may be recognized in about 20 per cent of cats before development of erythroid hypoplasia.[13, 127] An alternative explanation would be that a high proportion of cats infected with FeLV have dysplastic erythropoiesis giving rise to release of macrocytes of varying volume. However, this would have to establish macrocytosis before development of bone marrow hypocellularity. Most likely, a combination of post-regenerative macrocytosis and myelodysplasia accounts for macrocytosis. The change is not likely due to vitamin B_{12} or folate deficiency. Cats on a folate deficient diet had megaloblastic changes in marrow but did not develop erythrocyte macrocytosis or anemia.[129] Furthermore, serum concentrations of vitamin B_{12} and folate were not significantly altered in several cats with FeLV-associated macrocytosis and megaloblastic changes in erythroid precursors.[130] Naturally occurring

B_{12} or folate deficiency probably does not occur in the cat.

Erythroid hypoplasia is the most simple of the FeLV-associated anemias to reproduce experimentally. In experimental studies, bone marrow erythroid hypoplasia or aplasia has been directly associated with FeLV subgroup C infection or a viral mixture containing subgroup C.[1–3, 60, 131] While the mechanism of injury to the stem cell populations remains unknown, the injury appears to occur at the level of the BFU-E. Viral mediated injury could be a result of direct effects on either erythroid stem cells or cells that regulate erythroid stem cells. Following experimental inoculation with this strain of virus into susceptible kittens, anemia begins to develop within four weeks and reaches fatal severity by eight weeks. There are profound decreases in BFU-E and CFU-E from marrow cultures preceding development of the anemia.[1–3] From *in vitro* studies on marrow cells exposed to viral components, it has been suggested that viral envelope proteins may selectively inhibit erythropoiesis.[132] Erythropoietin levels are increased as hypoplastic anemia develops, further indicating there is failure of a population of cells to respond to normal hematopoietic signals.[133]

INTRA-MARROW DISEASE—GENERALIZED HEMATOPOIETIC DISTURBANCE

Myeloaplasia, myelodysplasia, and myeloproliferative diseases are disorders that result from injury to stem cell populations. Damage may be either to the microenvironment necessary for supporting hematopoiesis or to stem cells directly. Mechanisms of stem cell injury are multiple, but details at the level of the stem cell are poorly understood in specific, naturally occurring diseases. Known forms of injury are categorized into marrow microenvironmental damage and various direct stem cell injuries induced by irradiation, chemicals or drugs, immune-mediated mechanism, and viruses. Extensive reviews of evidence for these mechanisms in man and experimental animals are available.[134–136] The final common manifestations of stem cell injuries are either generalized failure of hematopoiesis (aplasia) or ineffective hematopoiesis associated with disturbed proliferative responses ranging from dysplasia to overt neoplasia (Figure 113–29). While important in all domestic species, they are most important in the cat because of the frequency of FeLV infection and its ability to cause stem cell injury.

Myeloaplasia (Aplastic Anemia). Myeloaplasia is characterized by severe marrow depopulation and blood

FIGURE 113–29. Diagram depicting various manifestations of irreversible stem cell injury. Note that dysplastic cell production may progress to overt neoplastic cell production.

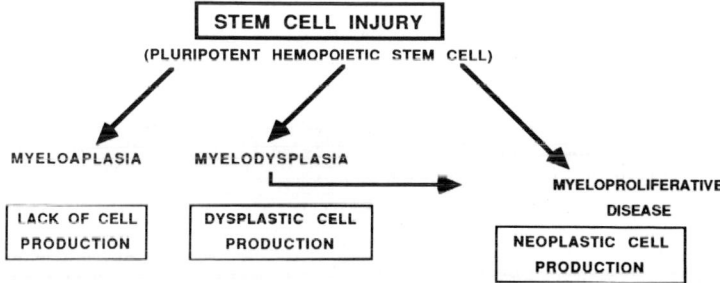

cytopenias including nonregenerative anemia, neutropenia, and thrombocytopenia. Examination of marrow aspirates reveals severely reduced numbers or absence of normal hematopoietic elements. Aspirate findings include fat, remnant lymphocytes, plasma cells, mast cells, and supportive cells. If fat particles are obtained they will appear markedly hypocellular. Because aspirates are frequently hemodiluted and difficult to interpret, a histologic section of marrow is often required to conclusively establish marrow hypoplasia or aplasia. The architecture is as described earlier for fat particles. Following are reproducible examples of aplastic anemia.

FELINE LEUKEMIA VIRUS INFECTION. This virus may induce aplastic anemia as one of its many sequelae in cats.

ESTROGEN TOXICITY. Either large, repeated doses of diethylstilbestrol or single injections of the potent, long-acting estrogen estradiol cyclopentylpropionate may cause severe marrow suppression in dogs.[12, 133, 134] Most toxicities have been related to injections to prevent pregnancy following unwanted matings. The mechanism of estrogen-induced aplasia is unknown, but recent *in vitro* studies suggest injury to cell populations regulating stem cell population proliferative capacity.[139] An alternative is that an *in vivo* metabolite of estrogen mediates a more direct stem cell injury.

Hematologic effects of estrogen toxicity are delayed and timing is variable. An unusual feature of estrogen toxicity is that a transient, marked granulocytic hyperplasia and leukocytosis occur early in the disease. At this time thrombocytopenia develops and the marrow is devoid of megakaryocytes and erythroid precursors. These changes occur in about 10 to 20 days following estrogen administration. Granulocytosis lasts a few days and is followed by extreme marrow hypocellularity and neutropenia. In this relatively short time span anemia develops only as a result of hemorrhage. There is no regenerative response to blood loss.

Endogenous estrogen toxicity may occur in dogs with estrogen-secreting Sertoli cell tumors and in ferrets with prolonged estrus.[140, 141] Cats are apparently resistant to development of estrogen toxicity.

PHENYLBUTAZONE TOXICITY. Severe marrow suppression has been reported in humans and dogs receiving phenylbutazone.[142] Hematologic cytopenias with thrombocytopenic hemorrhage similar to estrogen toxicity may occur. It is recommended that if phenylbutazone is used in dogs, it should be cautiously given and the blood count monitored regularly.

CHEMOTHERAPY. Use of myelosuppressive drugs in treatment of hematopoietic as well as other types of neoplasia is associated with frequent generalized hematopoietic suppression. Toxicity studies done in normal animals have resulted in dosage guidelines. However, animals with hematopoietic neoplasia likely have impaired drug metabolism, especially when parenchymal organs are infiltrated or severe anemia is present. For this reason, toxicity must be anticipated even when recommended dosages are used. See Chapter 59 for discussion of chemotherapy.

CANINE EHRLICHIOSIS. This is a rickettsial disease with complex hematologic manifestations. The recurring cytopenias may result from several mechanisms. In the acute form of disease there is marrow hypercellularity in the face of blood cytopenias. The cytopenias may be the result of immune-mediated injury to well-differentiated cells of all three cell lines. Marrow hypocellularity with features of aplastic anemia may develop in the chronic form of the disease. Whether this is progression of immune-mediated injury or some other direct injury mediated by the organism is not clear. See Chapter 46 for specific discussion of ehrlichiosis.

UNKNOWN CAUSE. The cause is unknown for occasional dogs with aplastic anemia. There is no known history of drug treatment. Upon scrutiny, the history may reveal exposure to household chemicals such as cleaners or paint thinners, but a conclusive cause cannot be established. A long list of organic chemicals is established in humans and experimental animals as being capable of causing aplastic anemia.[136]

TREATMENT OF APLASTIC ANEMIA. There currently is no specific treatment that results in stem cell repopulation. Bone marrow transplantation will become an increasingly utilized therapy for restoring hematopoiesis until more effective measures become available. Until these advances become routine, only symptomatic and supportive therapy can be utilized to provide time and opportunity for stem cell repopulation to occur. Death in aplastic anemia may be related to development of overwhelming infection, hemorrhage due to thrombocytopenia, or severe anemia. Broad-spectrum antibiotics and transfusions should be utilized as indicated. If platelets are required to control hemorrhage, a fresh transfusion containing platelets should be given. Steroids may be utilized to reduce thrombocytopenic hemorrhage. Commonly advocated use of anabolic steroids and hematinics probably represents wishful thinking.

It is possible for stem cell repopulations to occur if the animal is sustained from intervening complications. With intensive therapy, dogs with estrogen toxicity, phenylbutazone toxicity, and chronic ehrlichiosis have recovered within a few weeks. Most injuries related to chemotherapy are reversible. Early signs of recovery are best documented by emergence of blood reticulocytes or prominently increasing platelet and/or neutrophil counts.

Occasional cats with FeLV-related marrow suppression may make spontaneous improvement in association with steroids and other symptomatic treatment. These improvements usually yield to recurrence or development of myeloproliferative disease.

Myelodysplasia. In myelodysplasia, also referred to as dysmyelopoiesis, cytopenias may occur in the face of a relatively normal appearing quantity of hematopoietic activity in marrow. Since the marrow often has adequate or increased cellularity, the cytopenias are attributed to ineffective erythropoiesis. This suggests that, for some unknown reason, cells are being produced but do not survive through maturation and entry into blood in a manner sufficient to maintain normal blood cellularity. The process is most frequently recognized as involving erythrocyte production. Myelodysplasia is best recognized in the cat. It may, but does not always, progress to overt leukemia in humans. This progression has also

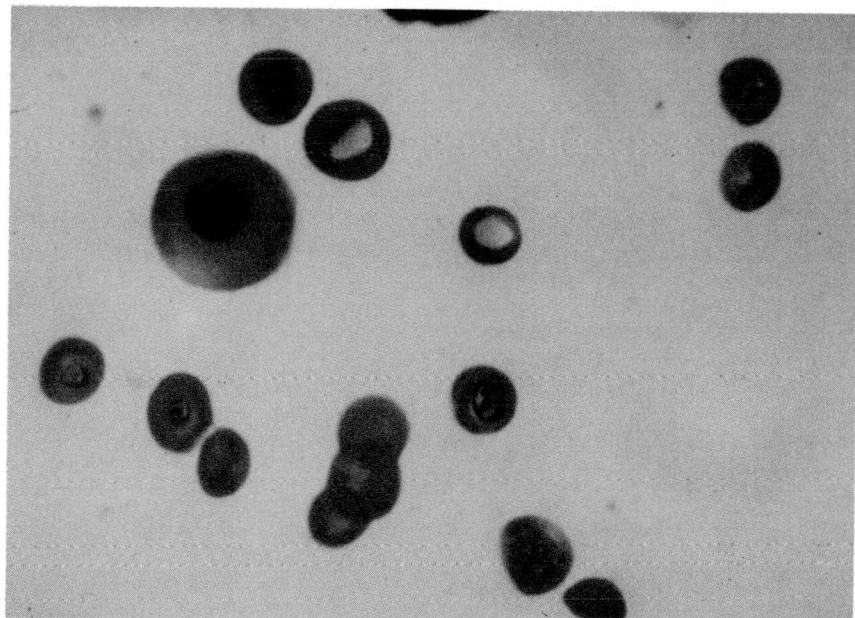

FIGURE 113–30. Disturbed erythroid maturation in myelodysplasia. Note that the nucleated cell is unusually large, has complete hemoglobinization as evidenced by lack of polychromatophilic staining, and has a retained pyknotic nucleus.

been documented in cats.[143-145] The natural history is difficult to study because most cats are not available for sequential observations for one reason or another.

Blood findings may include any combination of nonregenerative anemia, nucleated erythrocytes without reticulocytosis, increased erythrocyte volume heterogeneity, erythrocyte macrocytosis, neutropenia, hypersegmented or unusually large neutrophils, monocytosis, extremely large platelets, and thrombocytopenia. In blood and marrow, subtle morphologic changes observed in erythroid series cells may include megaloblastosis, altered synchrony of nuclear/cytoplasmic maturation, and nuclear fragmentation. Maturation defects are most easily observed in nucleated erythroid cells but these and nuclear abnormalities may also occur in granulocytic and megakaryocytic cells.[143] The most common example of disturbed erythroid maturation synchrony is advanced cell hemoglobinization and incomplete nuclear maturation (Figure 113–30). A disproportionately increased number of blasts may be observed in the marrow. This latter observation results in difficulty distinguishing myelodysplasia from neoplastic marrow disease.

Myeloproliferative Disorders. The term myeloproliferative disorder denotes purposeless, neoplastic proliferation. They are observed most commonly in cats, but also are well defined in dogs. They are diagnosed when the blood and marrow cytologic findings are indicative of an overt neoplastic process involving one or more cell lines. Myelodysplasia and myeloproliferative disorders are best considered to be a continuum of stem cell disease. The separation between dysplastic and neoplastic hemopoiesis is difficult and is perhaps artificial. Either process may involve one or more marrow cell lines. In addition, it is established that myelodysplastic change may progress to overt neoplastic change within individuals. Considerable attention given to subclassification of these disorders in humans[146] is not reflected here. The pathogenesis of myeloproliferative disease is

thought to involve stem cell injury leading to clonal emergence of a stem cell population with varying degrees of impaired capacity for cell differentiation and maturation. This is manifested in ineffective production of the involved cells and the presence of morphologic changes utilized in making a cytologic diagnosis.

The proliferation of abnormal cells at the expense of normal hematopoiesis is poorly understood. Proliferation and differentiation of normal stem cells do not occur or are severely reduced. Elaboration of inhibitory factors by abnormal cells or deficiency of normal humoral stimulators may be involved. Physical space occupation by abnormal cells does not appear to be a factor. Depression of hematopoiesis can be observed before marked marrow hypercellularity. Also, remaining hematopoietic supportive tissue is present in most cases.

Generally, marrow cytologic features include absence of severely reduced production of normal cellular elements, increased cellularity with predominance of the neoplastic cell type, and an apparent maturation arrest of the proliferating cell type (Figure 113–31). Cytologic features of myelodysplasia may also be observed. In blood, there is severe nonregenerative anemia with hematocrits in the 5 to 15 per cent range, combinations of other cytopenias, and leukemia may be present. (Polycythemia vera is an exception in that there is functional erythrocyte production in excess. Polycythemia is covered in detail in Chapter 22.) Hemorrhage may be a component of the anemia when thrombocytopenia is present. Blasts present in blood are usually similar to those predominating in marrow and may vary markedly in concentration. Classification of specific myeloproliferative disorders is dependent on morphologic features of the predominant cell type (see Chapter 114). Erythremic myelosis is a specific myeloproliferative disorder comprised of neoplastic proliferation of the erythroid cell line. Since there is an apparent maturation arrest between the rubriblast and rubricyte stages, retic-

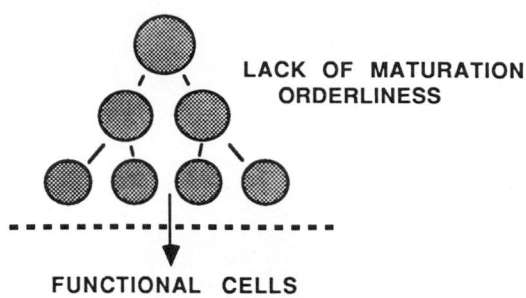

LACK OF MATURATION ORDERLINESS

FUNCTIONAL CELLS

APPARENT LOSS OF CAPACITY FOR DIFFERENTIATION

FIGURE 113–31. Production disturbance of neoplastic cell population in myeloproliferative disease. Proliferation of cells early in the maturation sequence lacks orderly progression of increasing numbers of more mature cells of the series. The inability to mature into functional cells may result in cytopenia of cell line.

ulocytes are usually not present. More clinical detail on myeloproliferative disorders involving other cell types and their treatment is considered in Chapters 59 and 114.

Treatment of myeloproliferative disorders is discouraging. Advanced marrow displacement and organ infiltrate usually are not reversible with chemotherapeutic agents currently in use. Transfusions and other supportive therapy as described for aplastic anemia may provide symptomatic improvement. See Chapter 113 for chemotherapeutic approaches that may be attempted.

Other Forms of Marrow Injury. MYELOFIBROSIS AND OSTEOSCLEROSIS. These lesions have been considered myeloproliferative diseases and may occur as terminal lesions in myeloproliferative disorders involving another cell type. However, the failure to identify clonal proliferation of fibroblasts suggests myelofibrosis is a response to injury, which might be similar to postinjury fibrosis recognized in many other tissues. In any event, the proliferation of either fibrous or osseous elements injures the marrow space to the point that it will not support hematopoiesis. The nature of injury required to induce these lesions or their progression from other proliferative abnormalities is unknown. With osteosclerosis there is cortical thickening and increased irregular medullary bone density on radiographic examination of long bones. These lesions should be suspected when there is failure to obtain marrow on aspiration. They are confirmed by histologic examination of a marrow section. Extramedullary hematopoiesis is a prominent feature representing an attempt to populate blood.

Osteosclerosis has been observed in anemic cats experimentally infected with FeLV and in naturally occurring cases with either nonregenerative anemia or myeloproliferative disease.[147, 148] Myelofibrosis is occasionally recognized in dogs following marrow injury or necrosis of uncertain genesis.[149] As already mentioned, it is also a sequela of pyruvate kinase deficiency.

LYMPHOPROLIFERATIVE DISORDERS. Lymphoma that involves marrow space, referred to as lymphocytic leukemia, may have an influence on erythropoiesis that is similar to myeloproliferative disorders. Well-differentiated lymphocytic leukemia (termed chronic lymphocytic leukemia by some) is associated with mild to moderate anemia.[150] The anemia may be regenerative

and there is reason to believe that low-grade immunohemolytic disease occurs frequently in lymphoproliferative disorders. With myeloma, neoplastic marrow infiltrates are usually focal and coexist with normal or near normal hematopoietic activity. Mild nonregenerative anemia may be observed. With poorly differentiated lymphocytic leukemia, the proliferation of lymphoid blast elements may predominate in the marrow space, while erythroid and other normal marrow cells become markedly reduced in number. Severe nonregenerative anemia and other cytopenias may occur. See Chapter 115 for detail on lymphoproliferative disorders.

CHLORAMPHENICOL TOXICITY. As occurs in a number of species, chloramphenicol may cause hematologic injury in dogs and cats.[151] Severe, idiosyncratic bone marrow aplasia associated with chloramphenicol administration in some humans has not been observed in animals. Reversible bone marrow suppression may occur in dogs receiving doses in the range of 100 to 120 mg/lb/day (225 to 275 mg/kg/day). Cats are relatively susceptible to dose-dependent toxicity; this may be related to species differences in drug metabolism. Dose ranges of 12 to 55 mg/lb/day (25 to 120 mg/kg/day) have been studied. Marrow features include vacuolation of early myeloid and erythroid precursors, apparent maturation arrest, and reduction in cellularity. The mechanism of vacuolar injury to marrow cells is not known. Some cats develop neutropenia, and decreases in platelet concentration occur within the normal range. Anemia has not been observed in toxicity studies. However, in these studies drug administration was limited to three weeks. Furthermore, observed dehydration may have masked early development of anemia. Based on changes observed in marrow, anemia is expected to develop if the drug is given for longer periods. Nonhematologic signs of toxicity in cats include anorexia, vomiting, diarrhea, dehydration, and CNS depression.

A dose rate of 12 to 20 mg/lb/day (25 to 40 mg/kg/day) minimizes toxicity although morphologic changes may still be observed in marrow.[152] The efficacy of relatively low dosages has not been determined. Consistency of administration may be an important factor in toxicity; in one study, a dose of 10 to 45 mg/lb/day (25 to 100 mg/kg/day) for 5 days per week for 30 days was not associated with toxicity.[153] It is currently recommended that, if used at all in the cat, chloramphenicol be limited to the smallest dose and shortest duration possible. The toxicity observed is reversible when administration of the drug is ceased. It should not be used in dogs or cats with nonregenerative anemia.

PRINCIPLES OF BLOOD TRANSFUSION

There are no strict guidelines for transfusion administration relative to hematocrit value; it is a matter of judgment in individual cases. Generally, a transfusion is given when the hematocrit decreases below 10 to 15 per cent. Some animals may tolerate a hematocrit of 10 to 12 per cent for days without difficulty. Increasing heart and respiratory rates related to a low hematocrit are a clear indication that a transfusion is needed.

Acutely developing anemia may require a transfusion at a higher hematocrit than chronically developing anemia. When anemia develops in association with massive hemorrhage, a transfusion or fluid replacement is a major benefit to prevent shock and support circulatory volume regardless of the hematocrit.

Laboratory techniques related to blood transfusion should be performed by the veterinary laboratory. The laboratory should be able to locate institutions performing blood typing for selection of permanent blood donors. Simple canine crossmatches may also be performed by the human medical laboratory. The rare crossmatch should not be performed in the veterinary hospital. If the veterinary hospital utilizes crossmatches frequently enough to maintain the technical expertise, it may be desirable to perform them on site. Techniques are available in any standard textbooks of veterinary hematology or clinical pathology.[12]

CANINE TRANSFUSIONS

The canine unit of blood is approximately 500 ml, of which about 50 to 60 ml is citrate anticoagulant solution (either acid-citrate-dextrose or citrate-phosphate-dextrose-adenine). A variety of commercially prepared plastic bags or vacuum bottles containing anticoagulant are available for blood collection and storage. Canine blood may be stored for 21 days without major loss of erythrocyte viability upon transfusion. An alternate "storage medium for blood" has been shown to increase storage time of canine blood to six weeks.[154]

The recommended quantity of transfused blood usually involves giving a unit for most sizes of dogs. The target of 5 to 10 ml/lb (10 to 20 ml/kg) accomplishes the objective of improving oxygen carrying capacity to a tolerable level. For small or large dogs, the unit of blood should be substituted by the above target dose range. More complicated formulas used to arrive at a desired hematocrit in the transfused patient are not necessary.

The ideal canine "resident" blood donor is negative for erythrocyte antigens CEA-1, CEA-2, and CEA-7; free of blood-borne infectious diseases; greater than 50 lb (25 kg) in weight; bled less than once per month to prevent iron deficiency; well nourished; and supplemented with oral iron. Achievement of this perfection is balanced against existing time, resources, and need for blood. Because naturally occurring antibodies against canine erythrocyte antigens do not exist, the first transfusion may be given without regard to donor blood type or a crossmatch. However, the risk of "blind" transfusion is that the recipient may become sensitized to the relatively immunogenic antigens mentioned above. This may result in shortened survival of the transfused cells on the first transfusion and predispose the dog to severe transfusion reaction on subsequent transfusions. Donors for multiple transfusions should be selected on the basis of compatibility documented by crossmatch.

FELINE TRANSFUSIONS

A satisfactory approach to the feline "unit" of blood is to collect about 40 ml of blood into a 60 ml syringe containing 10 ml of commercial acid-citrate-dextrose or citrate-phosphate-dextrose-adenine anticoagulant. This may be collected by either cardiac puncture or jugular venipuncture. Viability of feline erythrocytes is stable for at least 30 days in blood refrigerated in acid-citrate-dextrose solution.[155] The whole unit is generally given to adult cats. This will yield a transfusion of 5 to 10 ml/lb (10 to 20 ml/kg) for most cats. Kittens or adults weighing considerably less than 4 lb (2 kg) should be given a proportionately smaller volume. A suitable vein should be used for administering the transfusion. It also is very satisfactory to inject blood into the femoral marrow space, especially if a marrow aspirate is being performed at the same time.

Current practice used by most clinicians is that initial transfusions are given without consideration of the donor blood type or the need for a crossmatch. Donor cats should be negative for FeLV infection. When transfused multiple times, it is recommended that the donor be selected based on an agglutination crossmatch. The blood group system of cats includes group A, group B, and group AB. Very few cats have group AB.[156] In Australia, most group B cats have high titers of anti-A antibodies; thus there is potential for major transfusion reaction when giving A blood to group B cats or B blood (plasma) to group A cats. Group A cats have a low prevalence of low titers of anti-B antibodies. Severe reactions are observed in approximately 50 per cent of group B cats transfused with group A cells.[157] Blood typing surveys of cats in Australia, England, and France have shown considerable geographic variation in the proportion of type B cats in the population.

The prevalences of various blood groups in feline populations of the United States are not known. Of 64 cats blood typed in California, all were A-positive, suggesting a very low incidence of cats with type B erythrocytes.[65] The extremely low incidence of transfusion reactions in cats in the United States suggests a low proportion of type B cats in the population. Alternatively, transfusion reactions may not be appropriately recognized or the prevalence of isoantibodies is much lower.

Survival of transfused cells has been studied in cats. Cells transfused into cats of the same group have nearly normal half survival time of 30 days, whereas if cells of one group are transfused into a cat of another group the half survival is reduced to about 10 to 14 days. For cats transfused multiple times with cells of a different group, the half survival time is reduced to five days.[39] Clearly, transfusions in cats are most efficacious if donor and recipient are of the same blood type.

Transfusion reactions are documented in cats. Signs of shock were observed in experimental, anesthetized group B cats given one ml of a 50 per cent suspension of group A cells. Signs included transient severe hypotension, apnea, and sometimes atrioventricular block.[158] Hemolytic transfusion reactions, which would be easier to recognize as a transfusion reaction than shock, have not been reported in the cat. Potential forms of transfusion reaction have been reviewed elsewhere.[159, 160] (Also see Chapter 119.)

It has been advocated in other countries that feline donors and recipients be routinely blood typed or that at least donor selection be made by crossmatch.[158, 159] Prevalence of blood groups and isoantibodies needs to be evaluated in detail in the United States. If the vast majority of cats in the United States are group A or if there is a prevalence of isoantibodies much different than reported, the need for a conservative approach to first transfusion donor selection may not be warranted. Since information published on blood groups and isoantibodies is not compatible with current practices, it is clear that feline immunohematology needs further study and clarification on a geographic basis. This information is necessary to formulate appropriate guidelines for donor selection and recipient considerations.

In the meantime, we should increase our surveillance for transfusion reactions.

References

1. Testa, NG, et al.: Haemopoietic colony formation (BFU-E, GM-CFC) during the development of pure red cell hypoplasia induced in the cat by feline leukemia virus. Leukemia Res 7:103, 1983.
2. Boyce, JT, et al.: Feline leukemia virus-induced erythroid aplasia: *In vitro* hemopoietic culture studies. Exp Hematol 9:990, 1981.
3. Gasper, PW and Hoover, EA: Feline leukemia virus strain specific abatement of erythroid burst forming units (BFU-E). Leukemia Reviews International 1:71, 1983.
4. Quesenberry, P and Levitt, L: Hematopoietic stem cells. New Engl J Med 301:755, 1979.
5. Weiss, L: Haemopoiesis in mammalian bone marrow. *In* Microenviroments in Haemopoietic and Lymphoid Differentiation. (Ciba Foundation symposium 84). London, Pitman Medical, 1981, p 5.
6. Weiser, MG: Erythrocyte volume distribution analysis in healthy dogs, cats, horses, and dairy cows. Am J Vet Res 43:163, 1982.
7. Weiser, MG: Comparison of two automated multi-channel blood cell counting systems for analysis of blood of common domestic animals. Vet Clin Pathol 12:25, 1983.
8. Weiser, MG: Modification and evaluation of a multichannel blood cell counting system for blood analysis in veterinary hematology. JAVMA 190:411, 1987.
9. Greene, CE, et al.: Microtechnique for quantitative platelet isolation from blood enabling electronic counting and sizing of animal and human platelets. Am J Vet Res 46:2648, 1985.
10. Weiser, MG and Kociba, GJ: Platelet concentration and platelet volume distribution in healthy cats. Am J Vet Res 45:518, 1984.
11. Schalm, OW, et al.: Veterinary Hematology, 3rd ed. Philadelphia, Lea and Febiger, 1975.
12. Jain, NC: Schalm's Veterinary Hematology, 4th ed. Philadelphia, Lea and Febiger, 1986.
13. Weiser, MG and Kociba, GJ: Erythrocyte macrocytosis in feline leukemia virus associated anemia. Vet Pathol 20:548, 1983.
14. Schalm, OW: Manual of Canine and Feline Hematology. Santa Barbara, CA, Veterinary Practice Publishing, 1980.
15. Rich, LJ: The Morphology of Canine and Feline Blood Cells. St. Louis, Ralston Purina, 1976.
16. Alsaker, RD, et al.: A comparison of polychromasia and reticulocyte counts in assessing erythrocytic regenerative response in the cat. JAVMA 170:39, 1977.
17. Cramer, DV and Lewis, RM: Reticulocyte response in the cat. JAVMA 160:61, 1972.
18. Fan, LC, et al.: Reticulocyte response and maturation in experimental acute blood loss anemia in the cat. JAAHA 14:219, 1978.
19. Weiser, MG and Kociba, GJ: Persistent macrocytosis assessed by erythrocyte subpopulation analysis following erythrocyte regeneration in cats. Blood 60:295, 1982.
20. Werner, LL: Coombs' positive anemias in the dog and cat. Comp Cont Ed 2:96, 1980.
21. Scott, DW, et al.: Autoimmune hemolytic anemia in the cat. JAAHA 9:530, 1973.
22. Dunn, JK, et al.: The diagnostic significance of a positive direct antiglobulin test in anemic cats. Can J Comp Med 48:349, 1984.
23. Slappendal, RJ: The diagnostic significance of the direct antiglobulin test (DAT) in anemic dogs. Vet Immunol Immunopathol 1:49, 1979.
24. Gilliland, BC: Coombs-negative immune hemolytic anemia. Sem Hematol 13:267, 1976.
25. Mohandas, N: Red cell deformability and hemolytic anemias. Sem Hematol 16:95, 1979.
26. Jain, NC: Osmotic fragility of erythrocytes of dogs and cats in health and in certain hematologic disorders. Cornell Vet 63:411, 1973.
27. Jain, NC: Studies on the occurrence and persistence of Heinz bodies in erythrocytes of the cat. Folia Haematol 99:28, 1973.
28. Weiser, MG and O'Grady, M: Erythrocyte volume distribution analysis and hematologic changes in dogs with iron deficiency anemia. Vet Pathol 20:230, 1983.
29. Weiser, MG and Kociba, GJ: Sequential changes in erythrocyte volume distribution and microcytosis associated with iron deficiency in kittens. Vet Pathol 20:1, 1983.
30. Ewing, GO, et al.: Hematologic values of normal Basenji dogs. JAVMA 161:1661, 1972.
31. Bulgin, MS, et al.: Hematologic changes to 4 1/2 years of age in clinically normal Beagles. JAVMA 157:1064, 1970.
32. Anderson, AC and Gee, W: Normal blood values in the Beagle. Vet Med 53:135, 1958.
33. Anderson, L, et al.: Haematological values in normal cats from four weeks to one year of age. Res Vet Sci 12:579, 1971.
34. Meyers-Wallen, VN: Hematologic values in healthy neonatal, weanling, and juvenile kittens. Am J Vet Res 45:1322, 1984.
35. Spurling, N: The hematology of the dog. *In* Archer, RK and Jeffcott, LB (eds): Comparative Clinical Haematology. Oxford, Blackwell Scient Pub, 1977.
36. Kreier, JP, et al.: Erythrocyte life span and label elution in monkeys (Macaca mulatta) and cats (Felis catus) determined with chromium-51 and diisopropyl fluorophosphatc-32. Am J Vet Res 31:1429, 1970.
37. Valentine, WN, et al.: Heme synthesis and erythrocyte life span in the cat. Proc Soc Exp Biol Med 77:244, 1951.
38. Kaneko, JJ, et al.: Erythrocyte survival in the cat as determined by glycine-2-C[14]. Proc Soc Exp Biol Med 77:783, 1966.
39. Marion, RS and Smith, JE: Survival of erythrocytes after autologous and allogeneic transfusion in cats. JAVMA 183:1437, 1983.
40. Spink, RR, et al.: Determination of erythrocyte half life and blood volume in cats. Am J Vet Res 27:1041, 1966.
41. Madewell, BR, et al.: Ferrokinetic and erythrocyte survival studies in healthy and anemic cats. Am J Vet Res 44:424, 1983.
42. Harvey, JW and Gaskin, JM: Feline haptoglobin. Am J Vet Res 39:549, 1978.
43. Smith, JE and Agar, NS: The effect of phlebotomy on canine erythrocyte metabolism. Res Vet Sci 18:231, 1975.
44. Taketa, F, et al.: β-chain amino termini of the cat hemoglobins and the response to 2,3-diphosphoglycerate and adenosine triphosphate. J Biol Chem 246:4471, 1971.
45. Harvey, JW and Kaneko, JJ: Oxidation of human and animal haemoglobins with ascorbate, acetylphenylhydrazine, nitrite, and hydrogen peroxide. Br J Haematol 32:193, 1976.
46. Bunn, HF: Evolution of mammalian hemoglobin function. Blood 58:189, 1981.
47. Mauk, AG, et al.: Anemia in domestic cats: Effect on hemoglobin components and whole blood oxygenation. Science 185:447, 1974.
48. Beutler, E: Energy metabolism and maintenance of erythrocytes. *In* Williams, W, et al (eds): Hematology, 3rd ed. New York, McGraw-Hill, 1983, p 339.
49. Kociba, GJ: The diagnosis of hemostatic disorders. Vet Clin North Am 6(4):609, 1976.
50. Green, RA: Hemostasis and disorders of coagulation. Vet Clin North Am 11(2):289, 1981.
51. Dodds, WJ: Hemostasis and Coagulation. *In* Kaneko, JJ (ed):

Clinical Biochemistry of Domestic Animals, 3rd ed. New York, 1980.

52. Harvey, JW, et al.: Chronic iron deficiency anemia in dogs. JAAHA 18:946, 1982.
53. Yip, R, et al.: Red cell membrane stiffness in iron deficiency. Blood 62:99, 1983.
54. Logue, G and Rosse, W: Immunologic mechanisms in autoimmune hemolytic disease. Sem Hematol 13:277, 1976.
55. Dodds, WJ: Autoimmune hemolytic disease and other causes of immune-mediated anemia: An overview. JAAHA 13:437, 1977.
56. Jonas, LD, et al.: Nonregenerative form of immune-mediated hemolytic anemia in dogs. JAAHA 23:201, 1987.
57. Stockham, SL, et al.: Canine autoimmune hemolytic disease with a delayed erythroid regeneration. JAAHA 16:927, 1980.
58. Madewell, BR and Feldman, BF: Characterization of anemias associated with neoplasia in small animals. JAVMA 176:419, 1980.
59. Maggio, L: Anemia in the cat. Comp Cont Ed 1:114, 1979.
60. Mackey, L, et al.: Anemia associated with feline leukemia virus in cats. J Natl Cancer Inst 54:209, 1975.
61. Atwell, RB, et al.: Haemolytic anaemia in two dogs suspected to have been induced by levamisole. Aust Vet J 55:292, 1979.
62. Peterson, ME, et al.: Propylthiouracil-associated hemolytic anemia, thrombocytopenia, and antinuclear antibodies in cats with hyperthyroidism. JAVMA 184:806, 1984.
63. Greene, CE, et al.: Cold hemagglutinin disease in a dog. JAVMA 170:505, 1977.
64. Schrader, LA and Hurvitz, AI: Cold agglutinin disease in a cat. JAVMA 183:121, 1983.
65. Cain, GR and Suzuki, Y: Presumptive neonatal isoerythrolysis in cats. JAVMA 187:46, 1985.
66. Harvey, JW and Gaskin, JM: Experimental feline haemobartonellosis. JAAHA 13:28, 1977.
67. Maede, Y: Sequestration and phagocytosis of Haemobartonella felis in the spleen. Am J Vet Res 40:691, 1979.
68. Harvey, JW and Gaskin, JM: Feline haemobartonellosis: attempts to induce relapses of clinical disease in chronically infected cats. JAAHA 14:453, 1978.
69. Bellamy, JE, et al.: Cold-agglutinin hemolytic anemia and Haemobartonella canis infection in a dog. JAVMA 173:397, 1978.
70. Farwell, GE, et al.: Clinical observations on Babesia gibsoni and Babesia canis infections in dogs. JAVMA 180:507, 1982.
71. Abdullahi, SU and Sannusi, A: Canine babesiosis. In Kirk, RW (ed): Current Veterinary Therapy, 9th ed. Philadelphia, WB Saunders, 1986, p 1096.
72. Futter, GJ and Belonje, PC: Studies on feline babesiosis: 1. Historical review. J S Afr Vet Assoc 50:105, 1980.
73. Futter, GJ and Belonje, PC: Studies on feline babesiosis: 2. Clinical observations. J S Afr Vet Assoc 51:143, 1980.
74. Breitschwerdt, E: Babesiosis. In Green, CE (ed): Clinical Microbiology and Infectious Diseases of the Dog and Cat. Philadelphia, WB Saunders, 1984, p 796.
75. Wagner, JE: A fatal cytauxzoonosis-like disease in cats. JAVMA 168:585, 1976.
76. Wightman, SR, et al.: Feline cytauxzoonosis: clinical features of a newly described blood parasite disease. Fel Prac 7:23, 1977.
77. Glenn, BL and Stair, EL: Cytauxzoonosis in domestic cats: Report of two cases in Oklahoma, with a review and discussion of the disease. JAVMA 184:822, 1984.
78. Farkas, MC and Farkas, JN: Hemolytic anemia due to ingestion of onions in a dog. JAAHA 10:65, 1974.
79. Lees, GE, et al.: Idiopathic Heinz body hemolytic anemia in three dogs. JAAHA 15:143, 1979.
80. Spice, RN: Hemolytic anemia associated with ingestion of onions in a dog. Can Vet J 17:181, 1976.
81. Harvey, JW and Rackear, D: Experimental onion-induced hemolytic anemia in dogs. Vet Pathol 22:387, 1985.
82. Savides, MC, et al.: The toxicity and biotransformation of single doses of acetaminophen in dogs and cats. Toxicol Appl Pharmacol 74:26, 1984.
83. Harvey, JW, et al.: Benzocaine-induced methemoglobinemia in dogs. JAVMA 175:1171, 1979.
84. Harvey, JW, et al.: Methemoglobin reductase deficiency in a dog. JAVMA 164:1030, 1974.
85. Atkins, CE, et al.: Methemoglobin reductase deficiency and methemoglobinemia in a dog. JAAHA 17:829, 1981.
86. Letchworth, GJ, et al.: Cyanosis and methemoglobinemia in two dogs due to a NADH methemoglobin reductase deficiency. JAAHA 13:75, 1977.
87. Taketa, F, et al.: Hemoglobin heterogeneity in the cat. Biochem Biophys Res Commun 30:219, 1968.
88. Hamilton, MN and Edelstein, SJ: Cat hemoglobin. pH dependence of cooperativity and ligand binding. J Biol Chem 249:1323, 1974.
89. Beritic, T: Studies on Schmauch bodies. The incidence in normal cats (Felis domestica) and the morphologic relationship to Heinz bodies. Blood 25:999, 1965.
90. Schecter, RD, et al.: Heinz body hemolytic anemia associated with the use of urinary antiseptics containing methylene blue in the cat. JAVMA 162:37, 1973.
91. Harvey, JW and Kaneko, JJ: Interactions between methylene blue and erythrocytes of several mammalian species, in vitro. Proc Soc Exp Biol Med 147:245, 1974.
92. Cullison, RF: Acetaminophen toxicosis in small animals: clinical signs, mode of action, and treatment. Comp Cont Ed Pract Vet 6:315, 1984.
93. Finco, DR, et al.: Acetaminophen toxicosis in the cat. JAVMA 166:469, 1975.
94. Hjelle, JJ and Grauer, GF: Acetaminophen-induced toxicosis in dogs and cats. JAVMA 188:742, 1986.
95. Savides, MC, et al.: Effects of various antidotal treatments on acetaminophen toxicosis and biotransformation in cats. Am J Vet Res 46:1485, 1985.
96. Gaunt, SD, et al.: Clinicopathologic evaluation of N-acetylcysteine therapy in acetaminophen toxicosis in the cat. Am J Vet Res 42:1982, 1981.
97. St Omer, VV and McKnight, ED: Acetylcysteine for treatment of acetaminophen toxicosis in the cat. JAVMA 176:911, 1980.
98. Eder, H: Chronic toxicity studies on phenacetin, N acetyl p aminophenol (NAPA) and acetylsalicylic acid on cats. Acta Pharmacol Toxicol 21:197, 1964.
99. Harvey, JW and Kornick, HP: Phenazopyridine toxicosis in the cat. JAVMA 169:327, 1976.
100. Krake, AC, et al.: Cetacaine-induced methemoglobinemia in domestic cats. JAAHA 21:527, 1985.
101. Maede, Y, et al.: Methionine toxicosis in cats. Am J Vet Res 48:289, 1987.
102. Ewing, GO: Familial nonspherocytic hemolytic anemia of Basenji dogs. JAVMA 154:503, 1969.
103. Tasker, JB, et al.: Familial anemia in the basenji dog. JAVMA 154:158, 1969.
104. Searcy, GP, et al.: Congenital hemolytic anemia in the basenji dog due to erythrocyte pyruvate kinase deficiency. Can J Comp Med 35:67, 1971.
105. Harvey, JW, et al.: Erythrocyte pyruvate kinase deficiency in a Beagle dog. Vet Clin Pathol 6:13, 1977.
106. Prasse, KW, et al.: Pyruvate kinase deficiency anemia with terminal myelofibrosis and osteosclerosis in a Beagle. JAVMA 166:1170, 1975.
107. Giger, U, et al.: Inherited phosphofructokinase deficiency in dogs with hyperventilation-induced hemolysis: Increased in vitro and in vivo alkaline fragility of erythrocytes. Blood 65:345, 1985.
108. Glenn, BL, et al.: Congenital porphyria in the domestic cat (Felis catus): Preliminary investigations on inheritance pattern. Am J Vet Res 29:1653, 1968.
109. Kaneko, JJ (ed): Clinical Biochemistry of Domestic Animals, 3rd ed. New York, Academic Press, 1980, p 165.
110. Giddens, WE, et al.: Feline congenital erythropoietic porphyria associated with severe anemia and renal disease. Am J Pathol 80:367, 1975.
111. Boulard, M, et al.: The effect of copper on red cell enzyme activities. J Clin Invest 51:459, 1972.
112. Hansen, NE: The anaemia of chronic disorders—a bag of unsolved questions. Scand J Haematol 31:397, 1983.
113. Lee, GR: The anemia of chronic disorders. Semin Hematol 20:61, 1983.
114. Bently, DP: Anaemia and chronic disease. Clin Haematol 11:465, 1982.

115. Samson, D: The anaemia of chronic disorders. Postgrad Med J 59:543, 1983.
116. Erslev, AJ: Anemia of chronic disorders. *In* Williams, W, et al. (eds): Hematology, 3rd ed. New York, McGraw-Hill, 1983, p 522.
117. Feldman, BF, et al.: Anemia of inflammatory disease in the dog: clinical characterization. Am J Vet Res 42:1109, 1981.
118. Douglas, SW and Adamson, JW: The anemia of chronic disorders: studies of marrow regulation and iron metabolism. Blood 45:55, 1975.
119. Haurani, FI, et al.: Defective reutilization of iron in the anemia of inflammation. J Lab Clin Med 65:560, 1984.
120. Feldman, BF, et al.: Anemia of inflammatory disease in the dog: Ferrokinetics of adjuvant-induced anemia. Am J Vet Res 42:583, 1981.
121. Weiss, DJ and Krehbiel, JD: Studies of the pathogenesis of anemia of inflammation. Am J Vet Res 44:1830, 1983.
122. Rigsby, PG, et al.: Studies in the anemia of inflammatory states. Erythrocyte survival in dogs with acute and chronic turpentine abscesses. J Lab Clin Med 59:244, 1962.
123. Lukens, JN, et al.: Anemia in adjuvant-induced inflammation in rats. Proc Soc Exp Biol Med 126:346, 1967.
124. Mikolajew, M, et al.: Haematological changes in adjuvant disease in the rat. Ann Rheum Dis 28:172, 1969.
125. Werts, ED, et al.: Chronic inflammation suppresses bone marrow stromal cells and medullary erythropoiesis. J Lab Clin Med 93:995, 1979.
126. DiBartola, SP, et al.: Clinicopathologic findings associated with chronic renal disease in cats: 74 cases (1973–1984). JAVMA 190:1196, 1987.
127. Cotter, SM: Anemia associated with feline leukemia virus infection. JAVMA 175:1191, 1979.
128. Hirsch, V and Dunn, J: Megaloblastic anemia in the cat. JAAHA 19:873, 1983.
129. Thenen, SW and Rasmussen, KM: Megaloblastic erythropoiesis and tissue depletion of folic acid in the cat. Am J Vet Res 39:1205, 1978.
130. Dunn, JK, et al.: Serum folate and vitamin B_{12} levels in anemic cats. JAAHA 20:999, 1984.
131. Hoover, EA, et al.: Erythroid hypoplasia in cats inoculated with feline leukemia virus. J Natl Cancer Inst 53:1271, 1974.
132. Wellman, ML, et al.: Inhibition of erythroid colony-forming cells by an M,15,000 protein of feline leukemia virus. Cancer Res 44:1527, 1984.
133. Kociba, GJ, et al.: Serum erythropoietin changes in cats with feline leukemia virus-induced erythroid aplasia. Vet Pathol 20:548, 1983.
134. Camitta, BM, et al.: Aplastic anemia. New Engl J Med 306:645, 1982.
135. Boggs, DR and Boggs, SS: Possible pathogenic mechanisms in aplastic anemia. Transplantation Proceedings 10:125, 1978.
136. Williams, WJ, et al.: Hematology, 3rd ed. New York, McGraw-Hill, 1983.
137. van Kruiningen, HJ and Friedland, TB: Responsive estrogen-induced aplastic anemia in a dog. JAVMA 191:91, 1987.
138. Legendre, AM: Estrogen-induced bone marrow hypoplasia in a dog. JAAHA 12:525, 1976.
139. Gaunt, SD and Pierce, KR: Effects of estradiol on hematopoietic and marrow adherent cells of dogs. Am J Vet Res 47:906, 1986.
140. Sherding, RG, et al.: Bone marrow hypoplasia in eight dogs with Sertoli cell tumor. JAVMA 178:497, 1981.
141. Kociba, GJ and Caputo, CA: Aplastic anemia associated with estrus in pet ferrets. JAVMA 178:1293, 1981.
142. Schalm, OW: Phenylbutazone toxicity in two dogs. *In* Schalm, OW (ed): Manual of Canine and Feline Hematology. Santa Barbara, Veterinary Practice Publishing, 1980.
143. Raskin, RE and Krehbiel, JD: Myelodysplastic changes in a cat with myelomonocytic leukemia. JAVMA 187:171, 1985.
144. Madewell, BR, et al.: Hematologic abnormalities preceding myeloid leukemia in three cats. Vet Pathol 16:510, 1979.
145. Maggio, L, et al.: Feline preleukemia: an animal model of human disease. Yale J Biol Med 51:469, 1978.
146. Bennett, JM, et al.: Proposals for the classification of the myelodysplastic syndromes. Br J Haematol 51:189, 1982.
147. Hoover, EA and Kociba, GJ: Bone lesions in cats with anemia induced by feline leukemia virus. J Natl Cancer Inst 53:1277, 1974.
148. Flecknell, PA, et al.: Myelosclerosis in a cat. J Comp Pathol 88:627, 1978.
149. Weiss, DJ and Armstrong, PJ: Secondary myelofibrosis in three dogs. JAVMA 187:423, 1985.
150. Leifer, CE and Matus, RE: Chronic lymphocytic leukemia in the dog: 22 cases (1974–1984). JAVMA 189:214, 1986.
151. Watson, ADJ and Middleton, DJ: Chloramphenicol toxicosis in cats. Am J Vet Res 39:1199, 1978.
152. Watson, ADJ: Further observations on chloramphenicol toxicosis in cats. Am J Vet Res 41:293, 1980.
153. Teske, RH and Mercer, HD: Subchronic effects of chloramphenicol on the hemopoietic system of cats. Can Vet J 17:19, 1976.
154. Smith, JE, et al.: A new storage medium for canine blood. JAVMA 172:701, 1978.
155. Marion, RS and Smith, JE: Posttransfusion viability of feline erythrocytes stored in acid-citrate-dextrose solution. JAVMA 183:1459, 1983.
156. Auer, L and Bell, K: The AB blood group system of cats. Anim Blood Groups Biochem Genet 12:287, 1981.
157. Auer, L and Bell, K: Transfusion reactions in cats due to type AB blood group incompatibility. Res Vet Sci 35:145, 1983.
158. Auer, L, et al.: Blood transfusion reactions in the cat. JAVMA 180:729, 1978.
159. Killingsworth, CR: Use of blood and blood components for feline and canine patients. JAVMA 185:1452, 1984.
160. Weisz-Carrington, P: Principles of Clinical Immunohematology. Chicago, Year Book Med Pub, 1986.

114 LEUKOCYTES IN HEALTH AND DISEASE

KENNETH S. LATIMER and DENNIS J. MEYER

Leukocytes participate in host defense against pathogens and in surveillance and removal of non-self antigens.[1] Although considerable cell turnover occurs in health, blood leukocyte numbers and morphology remain relatively constant. In disease, however, both leukocyte numbers and morphology may change dramatically. These changes constitute the leukocyte response which is monitored clinically by performing the total and differential white blood cell counts (with calculation of absolute cell numbers per microliter of blood) and by examining leukocyte morphology.[2] These data comprise the leukogram, which is a portion of the complete blood count. Although the leukogram is seldom pathognomonic for a given disease, valuable clinical information can be obtained to construct a differential diagnosis, evaluate the severity of a disease, determine the efficacy of treatment, and provide a prognosis. Occasionally, interpretation of the leukogram is facilitated by cytological examination of bone marrow, lymph nodes, exudates, body fluids, or other solid tissues.[2] Knowledge of leukocyte production, distribution, and pathophysiology is essential for meaningful interpretation of the leukogram. In addition, the clinician should understand the methodologies and inherent limitations of common laboratory tests used to acquire leukocyte data.

Hematology Techniques

Blood Sample Collection. In adult dogs and cats, blood samples preferably are collected by jugular venipuncture whereby the sample may be procured rapidly, conveniently, and with less chance for clotting. Alternate collection sites include the cephalic, femoral, or lateral saphenous veins of conscious animals, and the sublingual vein of anesthetized dogs.[3] When drawing blood samples from catheters used for intravenous fluid administration, precautions should be taken to prevent obtaining a diluted sample resulting in pseudoleukopenia and factitious anemia. Blood samples should be mixed with dipotassium or disodium ethylenediaminetetraacetate (1 to 2 mg EDTA /ml blood) which prevents blood coagulation by chelating calcium. This anticoagulant preserves cellular morphology and allows excellent staining detail with Romanowsky stains.[4]

The blood sample should be processed as soon as possible following collection because changes in leukocyte morphology develop within hours. The earliest alterations in leukocyte morphology include vacuole formation in monocytes and swelling of lymphocytes which may be mistaken as immaturity. Vacuolation of the neutrophil cytoplasm can occur following several hours exposure to EDTA,[5] and may be mistaken for toxic change. If a delay in sample processing is anticipated, air-dried smears should be made when the blood specimen is drawn. These smears will reflect the leukocyte morphology at the time the sample was procured. The remaining blood (not the blood smears) should be refrigerated and will produce an acceptable leukocyte count for 24 hours.[6]

Small blood samples can be obtained from the marginal ear vein of kittens and puppies by coating the haired skin with petroleum jelly and puncturing the blood vessel with a lancet. A toenail clipped into the quick is an alternative site. Enough blood can be obtained to perform manual leukocyte counts with a hemacytometer and to make blood smears for differential counts. The blood is collected into anticoagulant coated-glass capillary tubes or pediatric microcontainers for the white cell count. Capillary tubes usually are coated with heparin to delay clotting by accelerating the action of antithrombin III. However, heparin distorts the size and shape of leukocytes and interferes with Romanowsky staining of blood smears.[4] If blood is collected in heparin

Editor's Note: There are extensive specific references in the tables to disease entities. These have been omitted for purposes of clarity and page space conservation. Interested readers may contact Drs. Latimer and Meyer for additional reference information.

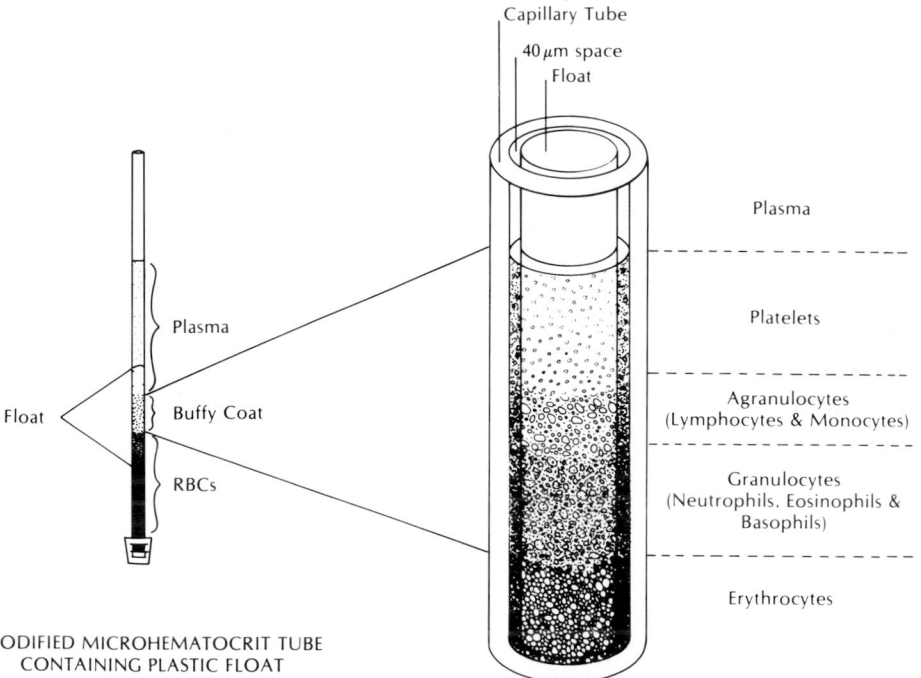

Capillary Tube

40 μm space
Float

Plasma

Platelets

Agranulocytes
(Lymphocytes & Monocytes)

Granulocytes
(Neutrophils, Eosinophils &
Basophils)

Erythrocytes

Plasma

Float

Buffy Coat

RBCs

MODIFIED MICROHEMATOCRIT TUBE
CONTAINING PLASTIC FLOAT

FIGURE 114–1. Schematic diagram of a quantitative buffy coat analysis tube after centrifugation showing an enlarged view of the buffy coat. The buffy coat has been expanded by localization of a plastic float and the various blood components (platelets, leukocytes, and erythrocytes) are layered according to density. Cell counts are calculated from predictive algorithms after measuring the thicknesses of the various layers. (Brown, SA and Barsanti, JA: Quantitative buffy coat analysis for hematologic measurements of canine, feline, and equine blood samples and for the detection of microfilaremia in dogs. Am J Vet Res 49:321, 1988.)

for the leukocyte count, we suggest making smears for the differential count from a drop of fresh blood without heparin.

Estimation of the Leukocyte Count

In emergency situations, the leukocyte count can be estimated from a stained blood smear. The estimate is made by examining the area of the smear used for the differential count. Using the 40-45× high-dry or 50× oil immersion objective, the average number of leukocytes in ten fields of view is determined. A semiquantitative estimate of the white blood cell (WBC) count per microliter (/μl) is calculated by multiplying the average number of leukocytes per field of view by 1,500 or 2,000, respectively. Estimation of leukocyte numbers also may be learned by estimating the white cell counts on smears from blood samples with known leukocyte counts. The estimated leukocyte count, furthermore, provides a crude verification of the accuracy of automated leukocyte counts where the laboratory result does not "fit" the patient. We must stress, however, that an estimated leukocyte count is no substitute for a properly performed quantitative count.

Quantitative Leukocyte Counts

Manual Counts. Manual counts are done with a Neubauer-ruled hemacytometer, calibrated coverglass, disposable capillary pipette, and plastic reservoir chamber containing a premeasured volume of diluent (Unopette

System test #5855; Becton, Dickinson and Company, Rutherford, NJ). With this system, both total leukocyte and platelet counts can be determined on a 20 μl blood sample. Although the reproducibility error of manual white cell counts for experienced technicians is approximately 16 per cent, these counts are acceptable for routine clinical use.[7]

Electronic Particle Counters. Electronic particle counters and automated diluting techniques reduce the error of the leukocyte count to approximately 4 per cent.[7] These instruments, originally designed for use with human blood samples, can be adapted for dog and cat leukocyte counting with minor adjustments in the instrument thresholds.[8, 9] Failure to perform threshold adjustment may result in leukocyte counts that are 14 per cent lower than expected in dogs.[9] With careful technique to avoid bubbles or cell contamination ("carry-over") from previous samples, electronic particle counters can produce accurate leukocyte counts on profoundly leukopenic human samples.[10] Caution should be exercised, however, when performing leukocyte counts on markedly leukopenic cats. Feline platelets are considerably larger than platelets from other species[11] and this size variation can be accentuated further in disease.[12] Macroplatelets may be counted as leukocytes, resulting in a falsely high leukocyte count. In one study, interfering particles, presumably platelets, resulted in inaccurate leukocyte counts in 8 per cent of the feline blood samples analyzed with an electronic particle counter commonly used in commercial laboratories.[9] Extremely high leukocyte counts that exceed the counting capacity of the instrument may be counted accurately by diluting the sample.[7, 9] When using electronic particle counters, one must remember that air bubbles, fat globules (lipemia), trash, and detritus also may be counted as leukocytes, so careful attention to cleanliness is mandatory.

Quantitative Buffy Coat Analysis. The quantitative buffy coat analysis system is based upon the principle that erythrocytes, leukocytes, and platelets will layer according to density upon centrifugation. The various layers are expanded by a plastic float (Figure 114–1) and are identified by their acridine orange staining patterns as observed under blue-violet light.[13] The widths of the various layers or bands are measured, and these values are inserted into a predictive algorithm. The total leukocyte count, the relative percentage and absolute mononuclear and granulocyte counts, the platelet count, and the packed cell volume subsequently are calculated.[13] Initial studies in dogs and cats indicate that leukocyte counts derived by quantitative buffy coat analysis correlate very well with values derived using hemacytometers[14] or electronic particle counters.[15] Occasionally, the granulocyte and erythrocyte layers will not separate clearly and the leukocyte count cannot be determined. This effect has been observed with 27 per cent of the blood samples from hospitalized dogs and 3 per cent of the blood samples from hospitalized cats.[15] Additional clinical experience with this instrument will ultimately decide the accuracy of this device for quantitating leukocyte parameters in sick dogs and cats.

The Differential Count

The differential count is performed to determine the percentages of various leukocyte types in stained blood smears. The absolute leukocyte counts are calculated subsequently. In routine differential counts usually 100 or 200 consecutive leukocytes are classified according to accepted criteria for cell identification (Table 114–1). Several sources of error may be associated with the differential count and, therefore, affect both the absolute cell counts and interpretation of the leukogram.[2, 16, 17] The greatest identification error involves distinguishing segmenter from band neutrophils by technicians experienced with human blood, but not with canine and feline blood. The common error is to identify too many bands.[2, 16] Despite attempts to standardize identification by defining bands as having an S- or U-shaped nucleus with parallel sides and no indentation exceeding 50 per cent of the width of the nucleus,[6] individual variations still exist between technicians in identifying these cells. Therefore, it is not unusual to see a marginal left shift appear, disappear, and reappear over the course of several days of hematologic study if the differential counts are done by different technicians. Medical technicians in human laboratories also have difficulty in identifying cat basophils. In Romanowsky-stained blood smears, feline basophils are larger than neutrophils and filled with round to oval, gray to mauve colored granules. Occasionally, feline basophils will retain a few metachromatic granules which facilitates identification.[2] Other difficulties involving cell identification in blood smears of sick animals include distinguishing toxic swollen neutrophil bands and metamyelocytes from mono-cytes, distinguishing lymphocytes from nucleated erythrocytes,[17] and identifying degranulated eosinophils.

Correction of the Leukocyte Count for the Presence of Nucleated Erythrocytes

When performing a total leukocyte count manually or with a semiautomated device, neither the technician nor the machine can distinguish a nucleated erythrocyte from a leukocyte. This distinction is made on the differential count where the number of nucleated erythrocytes per 100 leukocytes counted is determined. The correction is made when 5 or more nucleated erythrocytes are present per 100 leukocytes. The white blood cell count is corrected by the formula $(100 \div [100 + \#nRBC]) \times$ WBC count = corrected WBC count.

Use of Absolute Cell Counts to Interpret Leukograms

Absolute cell counts for the various leukocyte types are calculated by multiplying the relative percentages obtained from the differential count times the (corrected) leukocyte count. These "absolute" cell counts provide a clinically useful measure of the leukocyte response in most instances and are associated with fewer leukogram interpretation errors than relying on relative percentages alone.[6] Eosinophils and basophils are often present in small numbers, and if precise information is needed concerning their concentration in the blood alternative hematology methods must be used.[7] In this instance a special stain-based diluent and a hemacytometer are used to perform the count. For example, absolute eosinophil counts are done to monitor the response of canine hyperadrenocorticism to op'DDD treatment.

Bone Marrow Examination

Bone marrow biopsy is a valuable adjunct in evaluating diseases of the hematopoietic tissues. Indications for bone marrow examination associated with disorders of leukocytes include: persistent pancytopenia or neutropenia of unknown cause, suspected hematopoietic malignancy or myeloproliferative disease, leukocyte cytoplasmic and/or nuclear maturation abnormalities, assessment of lymphoproliferative disorders including documentation of multiple myeloma, and suspicion of infiltrative marrow disease secondary to neoplasia, infectious agents, or stromal proliferation.[6, 18–22]

Techniques for bone marrow biopsy have been detailed and illustrated.[22–24] The biopsy specimen may be obtained as an aspirate using Illinois sternal or Rosenthal needles or as a tissue core using a Jamshidi needle. Several excellent illustrated reviews are available for identification of myeloid and erythroid cells in cytological preparations of bone marrow,[6, 19, 21, 23] and primary identifying features of these cells are in Table 114–2.

When bone marrow biopsies are taken, several points should be emphasized. First, every marrow biopsy

TABLE 114–1. IDENTIFYING FEATURES OF NUCLEATED CELLS IN DOG AND CAT ROMANOWSKY-STAINED BLOOD SMEARS

Cell Category/Type	Nuclear Morphology	Cytoplasmic Morphology	Comments
Leukocytes			
Segmented neutrophil	Lobulated nucleus; coarse, condensed chromatin; sex chromatin body occasionally present (2 to 7% of PMNs)	Nonstaining (neutral) cytoplasm	Toxic change may be present in infection*
Band neutrophil	S or U shaped nucleus; parallel sides	Cytoplasm unstained or slightly blue	Toxic change may be present in infection
Lymphocyte	Slightly indented nucleus; coarse, aggregated chromatin; nucleus almost fills cytoplasm	Thin rim of light blue cytoplasm; few azurophilic granules may be present at nuclear indentation	Larger than RBC, but smaller than PMN; cells swell if sample stands
Immunocyte	Scalloped nuclear margin; moderately condensed chromatin; nucleolar ring may be present	Dark blue cytoplasm; Golgi zone may be present	Low numbers on smear; tabulated as lymphocytes
Monocyte	Oval, bilobed, or trilobed nucleus; lacy chromatin (less condensed)	Abundant gray cytoplasm; fine, pink lysosomal granules; pseudopodia usually present; vacuoles may be present	Largest leukocyte in blood; small monocyte in dog blood resembles segmented PMN; more vacuoles if sample stands
Eosinophil	Nucleus may be lobulated or band shaped; sex chromatin body rare in female	Orange-red cytoplasmic granules; round granules in dogs; rod-shaped granules in cats	Partially degranulated eosinophils in greyhounds
Basophil	Nucleus poorly lobulated or resembles a twisted ribbon	Few round, purple, scattered granules in dogs; numerous grayish to mauve granules in cats	Cat basophils generally lack metachromasia; mast cells have round to oval nuclei and numerous purple granules; basophil larger than neutrophil
Erythrocytes			
Nucleated erythrocytes	Small, round, central to eccentric nucleus; very condensed chromatin	Abundant blue-gray to gray-orange cytoplasm	Cell size same as small lymphocyte; small nucleus and relatively abundant cytoplasm

*Toxic change is discussed under neutrophils.

TABLE 114–2. IDENTIFYING FEATURES OF COMMON NUCLEATED CELLS IN DOG AND CAT ROMANOWSKY-STAINED BONE MARROW SMEARS

Cell Series/Type	Nuclear Morphology	Cytoplasmic Morphology
Myeloid (granulocytic series)		
Myeloblast	Round to oval nucleus, finely stippled chromatin, one or more nucleoli or nucleolar rings	Light blue cytoplasm, no granules present
Promyelocyte (Progranulocyte)	Round nucleus, finely stippled chromatin, rare nucleoli or nucleolar rings	Light blue cytoplasm, fine reddish azurophilic granules
Myelocytes	Round to oval nuclei, fine chromatin	Specific granules present Neutrophil granules unstained Eosinophil granules red-orange Basophil granules chunky and purple
Metamyelocytes	Indented nuclei with bulbous ends, fine chromatin	Specific granules present (see above)
Bands	S or U shaped nuclei with parallel sides, fine to slightly condensed chromatin	Specific granules present (see above)
Segmenters	Lobulated nucleus, condensed chromatin	Specific granules present (see above); cat basophils show loss of metachromatic staining
Erythroid series		
Rubriblast	Round nucleus, finely stippled chromatin, nucleoli or nucleolar rings present	Narrow rim of dark blue cytoplasm
Prorubricyte	Round nucleus, minimal condensation of chromatin, no nucleoli or nucleolar rings	Dark blue cytoplasm; Golgi zone may be present
Rubricytes	Round nucleus; nucleus decreases in size and chromatin condensation increases with maturity	Cell decreases in size with maturity and cytoplasmic color changes from blue to gray-orange as hemoglobin produced
Metarubricyte	Solid black or pyknotic, eccentric nucleus	Cytoplasm gray to orange depending upon amount of hemoglobin produced
Other cells		
Megakaryocyte	Nuclei fused into single irregular mass	Very large cells (> 100 μm), granular blue (immature) to pink (mature) cytoplasm
Lymphocytes/stem cells	Round slightly indented nuclei with condensed chromatin	Thin rim of light blue cytoplasm
Plasma cells	Round eccentric nucleus, patchy chromatin	Abundant dark blue cytoplasm with Golgi zone
Monocytes/macrophages	Oval to lobated nucleus, lacy chromatin	Abundant gray cytoplasm, occasional pseudopodia, phagocytosed debris
Mitotic figures	Chromosomes apparent	Distinct cell margins, bluish cytoplasm

should be interpreted with knowledge of the peripheral blood data obtained at the time of marrow biopsy.[18, 21] Second, failure to aspirate marrow ("dry tap") is usually the result of faulty technique.[18] Third, focal marrow disease such as a plasma cell myeloma may be missed on a random marrow biopsy sample. The chances of correctly identifying the disease, however, may be increased substantially if skeletal survey radiographs are taken, sites of bone lysis are identified, and the involved sites are biopsied.[21] Fourth, marrow aspirates provide only a subjective estimate of overall cellularity while core biopsies provide definitive information concerning marrow cellularity.[18, 20, 21] Fifth, myelophthisis and metastatic marrow disease are best detected by core biopsy.[18-22]

Buffy Coat Smears

Indications for buffy coat smear examination include: concentration of suspected neoplastic cells that may be present in low numbers in the blood and concentration of leukocytes to search for fungal organisms (Histoplasma capsulatum), rickettsial morulae (Ehrlichia canis), parasites (Hepatozoon canis, Toxoplasma gondii), and viral inclusions (canine distemper) or antigen (fluorescent antibody testing for feline leukemia virus). In addition, buffy coat smears are prepared as the final step in the LE (lupus erythematosus) cell test to concentrate these cells for identification.

The buffy coat is prepared by centrifuging anticoagulated blood in a disposable glass Wintrobe tube. The buffy coat is identified as the grayish white layer between the plasma and the red cell column.[6] This layer is composed of platelets, leukocytes, and nucleated erythrocytes. Occasionally, moderate numbers of reticulocytes and leptocytes are present and give the buffy coat a reddish cast. Using a Pasteur pipette, the plasma is discarded, and the buffy coat and upper portion of the red cell column are collected. Small drops of this material are placed on clean glass slides and conventional smears are made, air-dried, and stained.

As a result of leukocyte concentration, basophils may appear to be more obvious, and very low numbers of plasma cells and mast cells may be noted in health. Increased numbers of mast cells may be found in both blood smears[24] and buffy coat preparations from dogs with acute inflammatory diseases. When mast cells are identified, the important differential diagnosis is mastocytemia associated with disseminated mast cell neoplasia in dogs or splenic mastocytosis in cats. Neoplasia may be differentiated based upon physical findings of skin tumors in dogs or hepatosplenomegaly in cats, cytologic evidence of a mast cell tumor, or the presence of a leukemic blood picture on routine blood smears.

Leukocyte and Bone Marrow Reference Intervals for Dogs and Cats

The reference intervals used for interpretation of leukocyte and bone marrow data in our laboratories are presented in Tables 114–3 and 114–4. These intervals

TABLE 114–3. BLOOD AND BONE MARROW REFERENCE INTERVALS FOR DOGS

Blood Values

Cell Type	Distribution Range (%)	Absolute Range (cells/μl)
Leukocytes	—	6,000–17,000
Neutrophils		
Segmenters	60–77	3,000–11,400
Bands	0–3	0–300
Lymphocytes	12–30	1,000–4,800
Monocytes	3–10	150–1,350
Eosinophils	2–10	100–750
Basophils	0–2	0–200

Bone Marrow Values

Cell Type	Range (%)	Mean (%)
Myeloid (Granulocytic) series		
Myeloblasts	0.7–1.1	0.9
Promyelocytes	1.7–2.5	2.1
Neutrophil		
Myelocytes	5.3–7.3	6.3
Bands	9.1–13.5	11.3
Segmenters	22.2–24.8	23.5
Eosinophil		
Myelocytes	0.4–0.8	0.6
Metamyelocytes	0.4–1.0	0.7
Bands	0.8–1.6	1.2
Segmenters	0.3–1.3	0.8
Basophilic cells	0.0–0.06	0.02
Total Myeloid Cells	49.3–61.1	55.2
Erythrocytic series		
Rubriblasts, prorubricytes	6.1–6.9	6.5
Rubricytes, metarubricytes	23.2–32.0	27.6
Total Erythroid Cells	29.4–38.8	34.1
M:E Ratio	1.3–2.1	1.7
Other Cells		
Lymphocytes	5.5–10.9	8.2
Plasma cells	0.4–1.0	0.7
Monocytes	0.2–5.2	1.2
Macrophages	0.2–0.6	0.4
Mitotic figures	1.1–1.7	1.4

have been obtained from the literature and modified slightly by data accumulated within our laboratories.[6, 25-28] We believe these values should be reasonably accurate using modified electronic particle counters and accepted criteria for leukocyte identification. These reference intervals, although not applicable to all practice settings, may serve as rough guidelines for interpretation of laboratory data. When using reference intervals established for a diverse population of dogs or cats, cell count data are more variable to account for the effects of sex, age, activity, breed, and geographical location (which reflects the effects of climate, prevalence of parasitism, and so on).[6] Subtle alterations in cell counts due to these factors may not always be discerned in health except for age-related changes in the hemogram.

Age-related changes in cell counts do exist in health and may alter the interpretation of the leukogram slightly. Hematologic studies of beagle puppies have shown that the average leukocyte count is high at birth (16,500 cells/μl), declines during the early phase of nursing (10,500 cells/μl), increases abruptly during weaning, and peaks at two to three months of age (17,858 cells/μl).[29-31] Neutrophil counts parallel the total leukocyte counts. Blood smears from puppies generally contain segmented neutrophils except in the early neonatal period where low numbers of bands or metamye-

TABLE 114–4. BLOOD AND BONE MARROW REFERENCE INTERVALS FOR CATS

Blood Values

Cell Type	Distribution Range (%)	Absolute Range (cells/µl)
Leukocytes	—	5,500–19,500
Neutrophils		
Segmenters	35–75	2,500–12,500
Bands	0–3	0–300
Lymphocytes	20–55	1,500–7,000
Monocytes	1–4	0–850
Eosinophils	2–12	0–750
Basophils	0–2	0–200

Bone Marrow Values

Cell Type	Range (%)	Mean (%)
Myeloid (Granulocytic) series		
Myeloblasts	0.0–1.8	0.4
Promyelocytes	0.6–3.8	1.2
Neutrophils		
Myelocytes	0.4–5.4	2.2
Metamyelocytes	0.6–9.6	4.2
Bands	5.0–19.4	11.0
Segmenters	17.8–38.6	27.8
Eosinophil series	0.6–7.2	3.0
Basophil series	0.0–0.4	0.2
Total Myeloid Cells	39.4–64.4	52.0
Erythrocytic series		
Rubriblasts	0.0–1.6	0.6
Prorubricytes, rubricytes	—	12.4
Metarubricytes	15.6–32.2	23.6
Total Erythroid Cells	24.0–48.8	36.6
M:E Ratio	0.9–2.5	1.5
Other Cells		
Lymphocytes	3.2–22.6	11.4
Plasma cells	0.0–1.2	0.2
Mitotic cells	0.0–2.0	1.0

locytes may be observed.[29, 30, 32] Absolute numbers of lymphocytes increase after birth from an average 2,529 cells/µl to 4,142 cells/µl, and peak at approximately 5,700 to 6,100 cells/µl at 1.5 to 2 months of age.[29–31] After two to three months of age, the total leukocyte, neutrophil, and lymphocyte counts decrease to adult values by six months of age, and then decline very slowly through ten years of age.[29, 31, 33] The mild decline in the leukocyte count with age is attributed to decreased numbers of lymphocytes in the blood.[31, 33, 34]

Total leukocyte, neutrophil, and lymphocyte counts in cats are highly variable[35, 36] which accounts for the wider reference intervals in cats than in dogs. In kittens, the average total leukocyte counts have been shown to increase from 9,670 cells/µl in the postnatal period to a peak of 23,680 cells/µl by eight to nine weeks of age.[37] This latter time period approximates weaning age, and the increased neutrophil and lymphocyte counts suggest that the changes observed are the result of physiologic leukocytosis, an epinephrine-induced change.[6, 38] Review of data collected from hematologic studies of young cats suggests that physiologic leukocytosis is almost invariably present.[6, 35–37] Physiologic leukocytosis causes a more dramatic increase in the absolute neutrophil count in cats than in dogs because a larger marginal neutrophil pool is mobilized.[39] The absolute lymphocyte count may overshadow changes in the absolute neutrophil count. Occasionally, physiologic leukocytosis in cats may be characterized by marked lymphocytosis exceeding 24,000 lymphocytes/µl.[6]

Overview of Hematopoiesis

Blood cell development begins in early embryogenesis within the yolk sac where primitive mesenchymal cells produce the yolk sac stem cells.[40] The yolk sac stem cells, in turn, seed the fetal liver, spleen, lymph nodes, and thymus thereby expanding the sites of blood cell formation. By the first one-third of gestation, the fetal liver has assumed a major role in blood cell production. By mid gestation, medullary cavities have formed within the bones and hematopoiesis follows rapidly. The bone marrow has become the major site of blood cell development by late gestation,[40] and produces granulocytes, monocytes, erythrocytes, megakaryocytes, and some lymphocytes. The majority of the lymphocytes, however, are produced in extramedullary sites including the thymus, spleen, lymph nodes, tonsils, gut-associated lymphoid tissue (GALT), and bronchial-associated lymphoid tissue (BALT).

Almost all bones of the body are engaged in blood cell production at birth,[40] but as adulthood approaches active hematopoiesis continues primarily within the vertebrae, ribs, sternebrae, pelvis, and proximal long bones.[41] Active hematopoiesis may resume within the diaphyses of the long bones, the spleen, and the liver secondary to profoundly increased blood cell demand or unregulated blood cell proliferation.[40]

Studies of transfused, lethally irradiated animals in vivo and of bone marrow cultures in vitro have indicated that all blood cells, including leukocytes, erythrocytes, and platelet-producing megakaryocytes, are derived from a common pluripotential stem cell (Figure 114–2) that has the morphological appearance of a small lymphocyte.[42, 43] Stem cells are present within the bone marrow and blood, and can self-replicate and/or differentiate in a favorable hematopoietic-inductive microenvironment under the influence of growth factors.[44–46] Following severe bone marrow insult such as radiation-induced damage, cell destruction by parvovirus, or drug toxicity, viable stem cells can effect repopulation of the bone marrow accompanied by normal blood leukocyte counts within 7 to 14 days.[47–53] Except for lymphocytes, blood cells generally have a limited lifespan and are incapable of self-renewal; therefore, viable stem cells are a prerequisite for blood cell replacement.[54] The proliferative capacity of stem cells has been demonstrated to decline with age.[55, 56] This fact could have important clinical implications in recovery from bone marrow damage in older animals. A practical example of this age-associated decrease in marrow repopulating potential can be seen in estrogen-induced bone marrow toxicity in dogs wherein younger dogs recover faster than older dogs.[57] Further remarks concerning development of specific cell lines and diseases associated with altered hematopoiesis will be made in the following sections.

NEUTROPHILS

Neutrophils provide one of the first lines of host defense against invading pathogens, especially bacte-

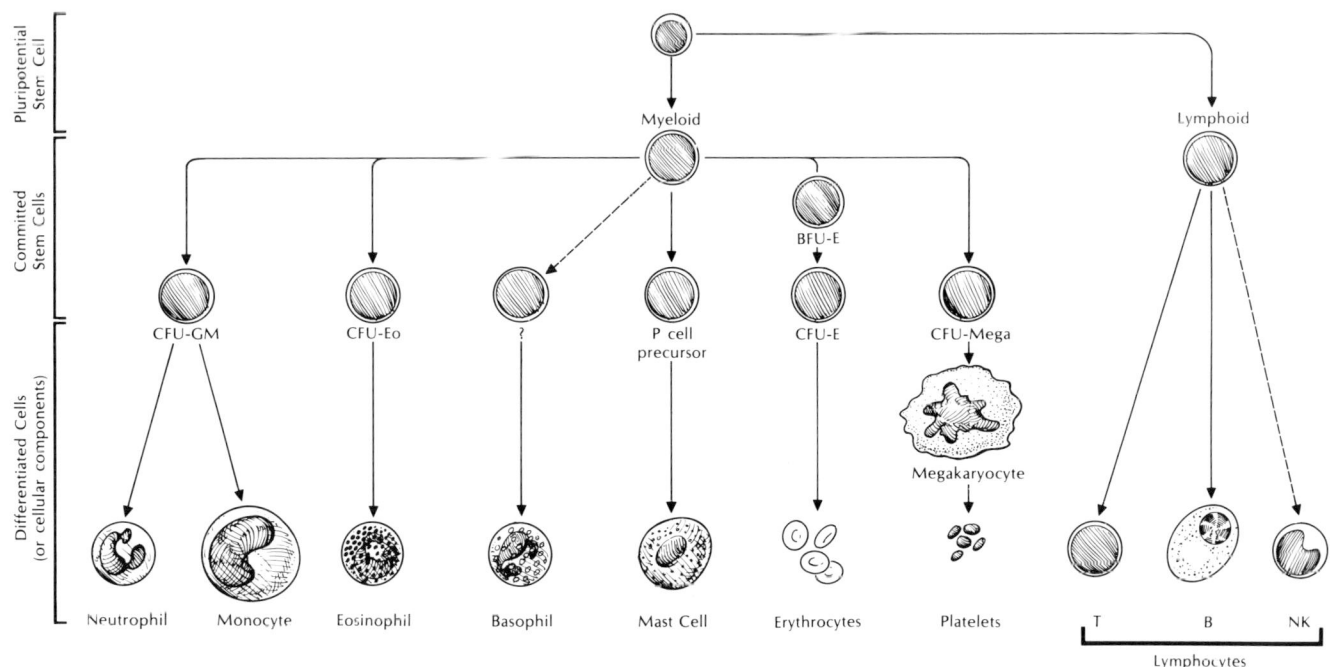

FIGURE 114–2. Diagram depicting the interrelated development of differentiated blood cells or cellular components. CFU-GM = granulocyte-macrophage colony-forming unit; CFU-Eo = eosinophil colony-forming unit; P cell = persisting cell precursor; BFU-E = erythroid burst-forming unit; CFU-E = erythroid colony-forming unit; CFU-Mega = megakaryocyte colony-forming unit. Basophil and natural killer (NK) cell lineages have not been established definitively.

ria.[58–60] In addition, neutrophils also have the ability to kill or inactivate fungi, yeast, algae (*Prototheca* sp.), parasites, and viruses as determined by in vitro testing.[58–63] Destruction of these organisms by neutrophils in vivo may be more difficult because of host pathogen interactions on other cellular systems that may, in turn, modulate neutrophil activity. Other functions ascribed to neutrophils include elimination of infected and transformed cells, amplification and modulation of acute inflammatory reactions, enhancement of immunocompetent cell function, and regulation of granulopoiesis.[58, 60, 64, 65]

MORPHOLOGY

In Romanowsky-stained blood smears, mature neutrophils of dogs and cats contain a segmented nucleus with two to four lobes of coarse chromatin. Filament formation between nuclear lobes is present occasionally, but the lobes usually are separated by narrow constrictions. The presence of five or more nuclear lobes indicates hypersegmentation.[6] An oval to teardrop-shaped chromatin appendage that is attached to the nucleus by a single filament may be observed within neutrophils from females. This appendage is called the sex chromatin body (drumstick appendage, Barr body) and is present in 2 to 7 per cent of the neutrophils from bitches and 4 to 11 per cent of the neutrophils from queens.[6, 66–68] Sex chromatin bodies also are present in 2 to 4 per cent of the neutrophils from male calico cats with chromosomal mosaicism (Kleinfelter's syndrome).[68, 69] The cytoplasm of Romanowsky-stained neutrophils from

healthy dogs and cats appears clear to faint gray or may have a diffuse but indistinct pink granulation.[6] Although numerous primary and secondary granules may be observed in electron microscopic preparations,[70] the granules generally remain unstained or neutral in health.

Nuclear Morphologic Variations in Health

Pelger-Huët Anomaly. Pelger-Huët anomaly is an hereditary disorder of leukocyte development in which neutrophils as well as other granulocytes and monocytes have hyposegmented nuclei in the presence of a mature, coarse chromatin pattern (Figure 114–3). Circulating granulocytes from healthy females lack sex chromatin bodies. Megakaryocyte nuclei also are hypolobulated, suggesting a stem cell defect in the nuclear segmentation or lobulation process.[71]

Pelger-Huët anomaly is uncommon, but has been described in both dogs and cats.[6, 71–74] Geographical clustering of cases may be expected due to the hereditary nature of the anomaly. Pelger-Huët anomaly presumably is transmitted as an autosomal dominant trait in dogs and cats.[74, 75] Most of the clinical cases described are the heterozygous state of the anomaly where the affected animal inherits one Pelger-Huët gene. This phenotype resembles a persistent left shift and most neutrophils have band-shaped or bilobed nuclei (Figure 114–3A). The homozygous form of the anomaly, where the animal inherits two Pelger-Huët genes (one from each parent) is extremely rare, but has been described in one stillborn kitten. Most of the circulating granulocytes and monocytes in this kitten had round to oval nuclei (Figure 114–3B).[76]

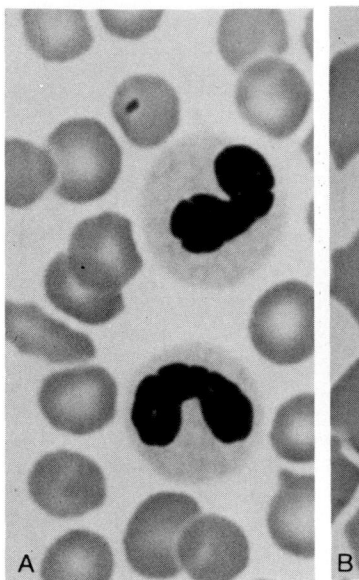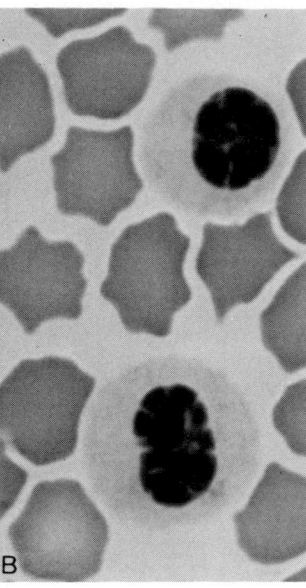

FIGURE 114–3. Neutrophils from cats with Pelger-Hüet anomaly. *A,* Heterozygous form of the anomaly showing band-shaped nuclei with coarse, mature chromatin pattern. *B,* Homozygous form of the anomaly with round to oval nuclei and extremely coarse chromatin pattern. (All blood smears are Romanowsky-stained and photographed at 960 × magnification unless indicated otherwise.)

The presence of Pelger-Hüet anomaly may be a serendipitous finding in a healthy animal. More often the anomaly is encountered in sick animals and is mistaken for severe bacterial infection, developing leukemia, or a drug-induced change in nuclear morphology.[74] The anomaly is suspected by documenting a persistent left shift without associated infection, marrow-associated neoplasia, or drug exposure. An hereditary basis for the anomaly can be documented clinically by finding Pelger-Hüet cells in stained blood smears from the parents and littermates, or by prospective breeding trials if related animals cannot be located for blood smear examination.[74] Recognition of the anomaly is important to avoid unnecessary and expensive diagnostic tests, and to prevent inappropriate drug therapy.

Recent studies in dogs and cats indicate that the heterozygous form of the anomaly is benign as no predisposition to infection exists.[72, 76, 77] In contrast to a previous study in dogs with Pelger-Hüet anomaly,[72] neutrophil adherence, chemotaxis, phagocytosis, and bactericidal activity are unimpaired.[77] In addition, the immune system is intact.[77] The homozygous form of the anomaly, however, may have medical consequences including fetal death and resorption in utero, stillbirth, and possible skeletal deformities.[76]

Cytoplasmic Morphologic Variations in Health

Birman Cat Neutrophil Granulation Anomaly. An inherited anomaly of neutrophil granulation has been reported in Birman cats from several Canadian catteries.[78] The anomaly is inherited as an autosomal recessive trait. Neutrophils from affected cats contain fine eosinophilic intracytoplasmic granules in Romanowsky-stained blood smears, presumably due to an increased affinity of lysosomal granules for eosin dye (Figure 114–4). In bone marrow aspirates, affected granules stain similarly to the primary (azurophilic) granules of promyelocytes but persist throughout neutrophil maturation. The neutrophil granules are not metachromatic following toluidine blue staining, and other granulocytic cell lines are uninvolved.

Clinically, Birman cats with the neutrophil granulation anomaly are not predisposed to bacterial infection. Examination of neutrophil integrity in one cat indicated normal ultrastructure, cytochemistry, phagocytosis, oxidative metabolism, and bactericidal activity.[78] Although clinical and experimental evidence indicates that the Birman cat neutrophil anomaly is of little consequence, it must be differentiated from toxic granulation and mucopolysaccharidosis type VI (Maroteaux-Lamy syndrome). Toxic granulation usually is associated with clinical evidence of infection and a left shift, and disappears with resolution of the disease state. Cats with mucopolysaccharidosis may have clinical evidence of facial dysmorphia, and the persistent intracytoplasmic inclusions observed in Romanowsky-stained neutrophils are intensely metachromatic when stained with toluidine blue dye.[79]

Nuclear Morphologic Variations in Disease

Nuclear Hyposegmentation. Nuclear hyposegmentation may indicate either immaturity of the neutrophil series or inability, on the part of a mature cell, to properly segment. Immaturity of the neutrophil series is recognized by the presence of bands and juveniles (metamyelocytes and earlier forms) in the blood (Tables 114–1 and 114–2). These various immature neutrophil stages have finely stippled chromatin (Figure 114–5), and when present in sufficient numbers constitute a clinically important left shift. If the neutrophil count is within the reference interval or increased, a significant left shift is indicated by the presence of 1,000 or more bands/μl of blood. If neutropenia exists, a significant left shift is present if bands and/or juveniles constitute

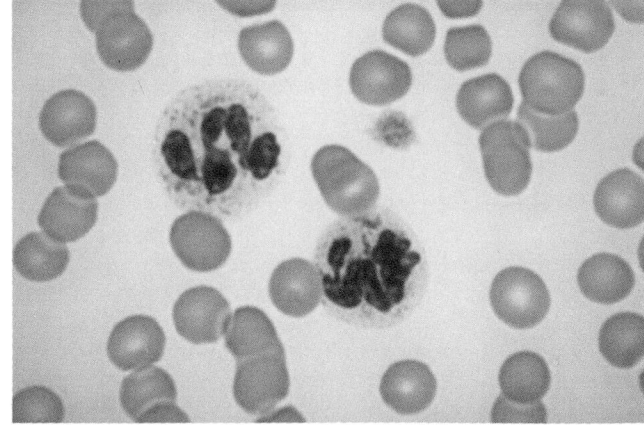

FIGURE 114–4. Birman cat hereditary granulation anomaly showing intensely stained primary granules. (Courtesy of Dr. Gene P. Searcy, Western College of Veterinary Medicine, University of Saskatchewan, Saskatoon, Saskatchewan, Canada.)

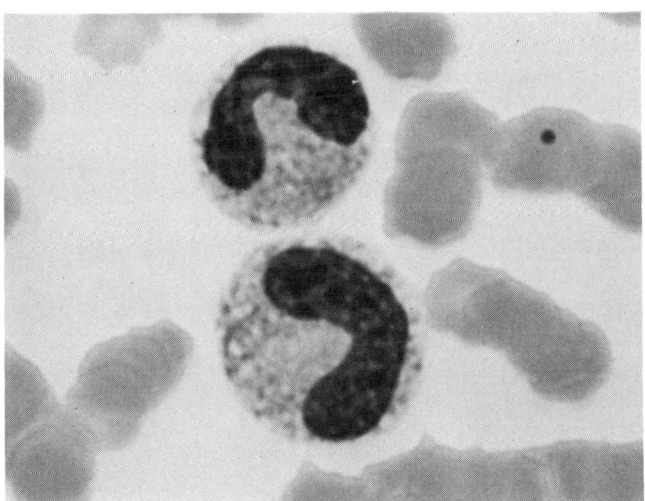

FIGURE 114–5. Feline neutrophil bands with finely stippled chromatin and toxic change (cytoplasmic basophilia and vacuolation).

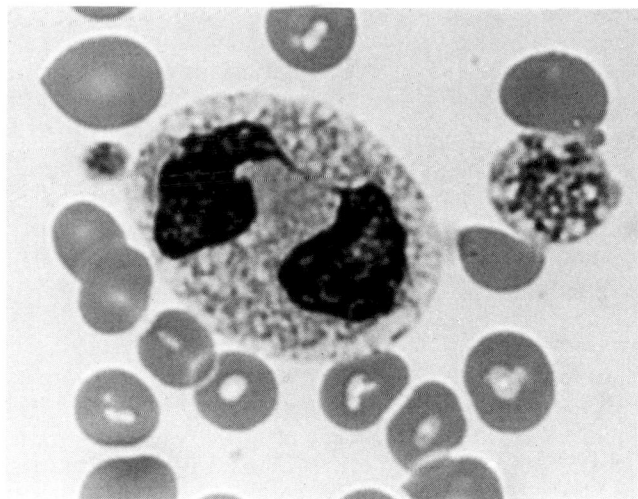

FIGURE 114–6. Enlarged, toxic neutrophil from a cat with a severe bacterial infection. Asynchronous nuclear maturation is evident where two lobes of fine chromatin are connected by a delicate filament.

10 per cent or more of the neutrophil population. Severe or "degenerative" left shifts exist when the number of immature neutrophils approaches, equals, or exceeds the number of segmented neutrophils in the blood regardless of the total leukocyte count.[26]

Mature hyposegmented neutrophils are cells that have an immaturely shaped nucleus (band-shaped or earlier forms) but, paradoxically, have a coarse, mature chromatin pattern. In healthy animals, this change is exemplified by Pelger-Huët anomaly. In disease, this change is designated as pseudo-Pelger-Huët anomaly. Pseudo-Pelger-Huët anomaly occurs secondary to chronic infection, drug administration, myeloid metaplasia, and primary or metastatic neoplasia of the marrow cavity in humans.[80] Nuclear hyposegmentation may disappear with successful treatment of the underlying disease, but may recur with exacerbation of the disease process. Pseudo-Pelger-Huët anomaly has been associated with drug administration in a dog, but recent evidence suggests that this dog may have had the true congenital anomaly.[71, 81] Feline leukemia virus-induced myeloid leukemia in cats also is associated with the presence of pseudo-Pelger-Huët neutrophils in the blood.[82] In pseudo-Pelger-Huët anomaly fewer neutrophils are hyposegmented than in the true congenital anomaly although exceptions do exist.

Asynchronous Nuclear Maturation. Asynchronous nuclear maturation occurs most commonly in cats during periods of intense granulopoietic activity associated with severe bacterial infection or recovery from infectious panleukopenia, but also may be a feature of myeloid leukemia. Affected cells have finely stippled chromatin in nuclei which are bizarrely coiled or have enlarged lobes that are connected by delicate filaments (Figure 114–6).[6, 83] Occasionally, the nuclei assume ring (donut) configurations with a regular or irregular nuclear contour.[84] Neutrophils with asynchronous maturation often are swollen and have cytoplasmic toxic change.[83]

Nuclear Hypersegmentation. Canine and feline neutrophils with five or more nuclear lobes are hypersegmented (Figure 114–7).[6] In human hematology, a presumptive diagnosis of hypersegmentation is made if three or more neutrophils with five or more lobes are seen during performance of the differential count.[7] In veterinary hematology, this nonspecific change in neutrophil morphology is reported infrequently and only if enough abnormal cells are present to impress the medical technologist. Neutrophil hypersegmentation in blood smears from dogs and cats usually is secondary to an endogenous (prolonged stress, hyperadrenocorticism) or exogenous (iatrogenic) corticosteroid effect that prolongs the circulating half-life of neutrophils in the blood.[2, 6] These hypersegmented neutrophils are of normal size and are scattered throughout the blood smear in low numbers. Hypersegmented neutrophils also may be observed in granulocytic and myelomonocytic leukemia, where 42 to 72 per cent of the neutrophils may be involved and affected cells may appear as enlarged segmenters (macropolycytes).[6, 85] Low numbers of normal-sized to enlarged, hypersegmented neutrophils also are seen in blood smears from miniature and toy poodles with erythrocyte macrocytosis. This condition is recognized from the hemogram by observing a marked in-

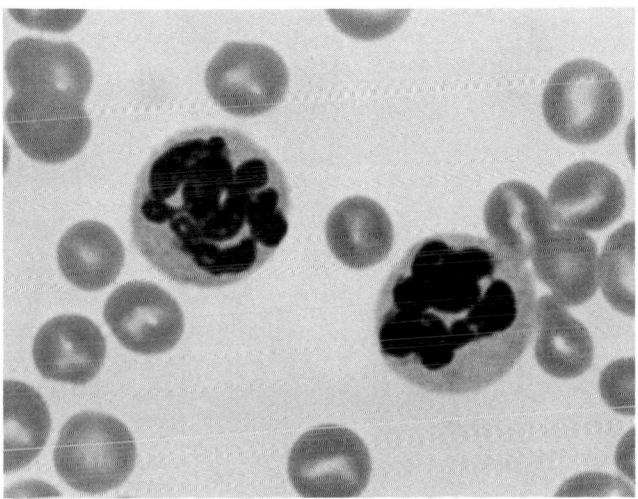

FIGURE 114–7. Hypersegmented neutrophils in the blood of a cat with chronic suppurative inflammation.

crease in the erythrocytic mean corpuscular volume (85 to 107 fl) in the absence of anemia (PCV 41 to 53 per cent) or evidence of red cell regeneration (polychromasia).[6, 86] The erythrocyte count is at the low end of the reference interval. This condition is thought to be of genetic origin, is usually an incidental finding, and does not appear to affect the dog's health adversely.[6]

Cytoplasmic Morphologic Alterations in Disease

Toxic Change. The most common disease-induced cytoplasmic changes in neutrophil morphology are designated collectively as "toxic change" (Figure 114–5).[87, 88] These changes usually are associated with severe localized or systemic infections (septicemia), but also may occur with sterile inflammation and drug toxicity.[6, 87–90] A guarded prognosis is indicated when most neutrophils in the blood smear have toxic change.[6, 87, 88] The various types of toxic change include cytoplasmic basophilia and vacuolation, the presence of Döhle (Doehle) bodies, and/or intensely stained primary granules (toxic granulation).[87]

Toxic vacuolation and cytoplasmic basophilia are observed commonly in blood smears from dogs and cats with severe infection. These changes result from disturbed cellular maturation in the bone marrow resulting in a loss of both granule and membrane integrity (vacuolation) and in persistence of ribosomes (basophilia).[87, 89, 91] Following appropriate treatment, cytoplasmic vacuolation may resolve within 12 to 24 hours,[91] but cytoplasmic basophilia persists for a longer period of time.

By light microscopy, Döhle bodies are 0.5 to 2.0 μm angular blue-gray particles that usually are located in the periphery of the cytoplasm (Figure 114–8). Ultrastructurally, these particles consist of lamellar aggregates of rough endoplasmic reticulum.[87] Döhle bodies are seen more frequently in blood smears from cats than from dogs.

Toxic granulation is observed infrequently in canine and feline neutrophils. This type of toxic change results from increased primary granule membrane permeability to Romanowsky stains and disappears with resolution of the disease process.[87, 88] Toxic granulation should be distinguished from mucopolysaccharidosis in cats and dogs and from the hereditary granulation anomaly in Birman cats.[78, 79, 92]

Intracytoplasmic Inclusions in Specific Infectious Diseases. Occasionally, neutrophil inclusions may be observed in the course of a routine differential count that provide a very specific disease diagnosis. These inclusions may be associated with viral, rickettsial, fungal, or protozoal infections.

Canine distemper inclusions are round to irregularly shaped magenta structures within leukocytes and/or erythrocytes on Romanowsky- or Diff-Quik–stained blood smears (Figure 114–9A).[93–95] Although these inclusions are reported to occur in dogs shortly after vaccination,[2] they are most often observed in early stages of naturally occurring viral infections.[93, 94] In instances of dual infection with canine parvovirus and canine distemper virus, we have observed viral inclusions within lymphocytes when neutropenia exists.

Rickettsial inclusions are found within various leukocyte types. In the dog, the etiological agents include *Ehrlichia canis* and *Ehrlichia equi*, and the morulae appear as intracytoplasmic, deep magenta to grayish-staining, mulberry structures (Figure 114–9B).[96, 97] Buffy coat smear examination may facilitate identification of morulae within leukocytes; however, inclusions are transient and infrequently observed. Rickettsial diseases, therefore, are best diagnosed by determination of acute and convalescent antibody titers which will identify the specific agent(s) involved.

Histoplasma capsulatum yeasts appear as intracytoplasmic "clusters of grapes" within neutrophils and/or monocytes (Figure 114–9C).[98] These organisms arc approximately two μm in diameter and have a thin cell wall. On rare occasions, yeasts may be seen within cells on routine blood smears, but the organisms usually are found more readily by examining buffy coat smears. Buffy coat smears should be examined in dogs and cats with fevers of unknown origin when fungal infection is suspected.

Hepatozoon canis gametocytes may be observed within neutrophils and/or monocytes upon examination of stained blood smears (Figure 114–9D).[99, 100] Although these agents may be discovered serendipitously within a single blood smear, extensive examination of several blood smears may be necessary to demonstrate the organism. Blood smears, however, must be made without delay because the organism may escape from infected leukocytes, leaving a nonstaining capsule that may easily be overlooked.[100] The gametocytes are oval, measure approximately 5 × 10 μm, and stain ice-blue on Romanowsky-stained smears. Parasitemia, if detected, usually involves only one or two cells per 1,000 leukocytes.[100] In cases where organisms are not observed within leukocytes, the clinician may be alerted to the possibility of hepatozoonosis by the presence of neutrophilic leukocytosis (20,000 to 200,000 cells/μl), occasional eosinophilia, and radiographic signs of periosteal bone proliferation. Definitive diagnosis of canine hepatozoonosis may require histological examination of skel-

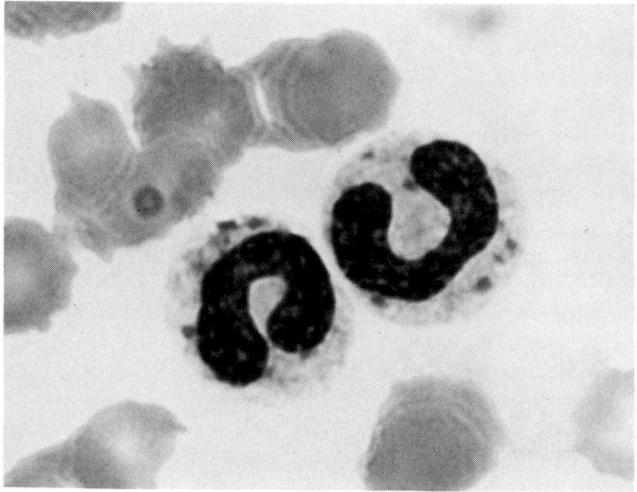

FIGURE 114–8. Döhle bodies in the peripheral cytoplasm of band neutrophils from a dog with sepsis.

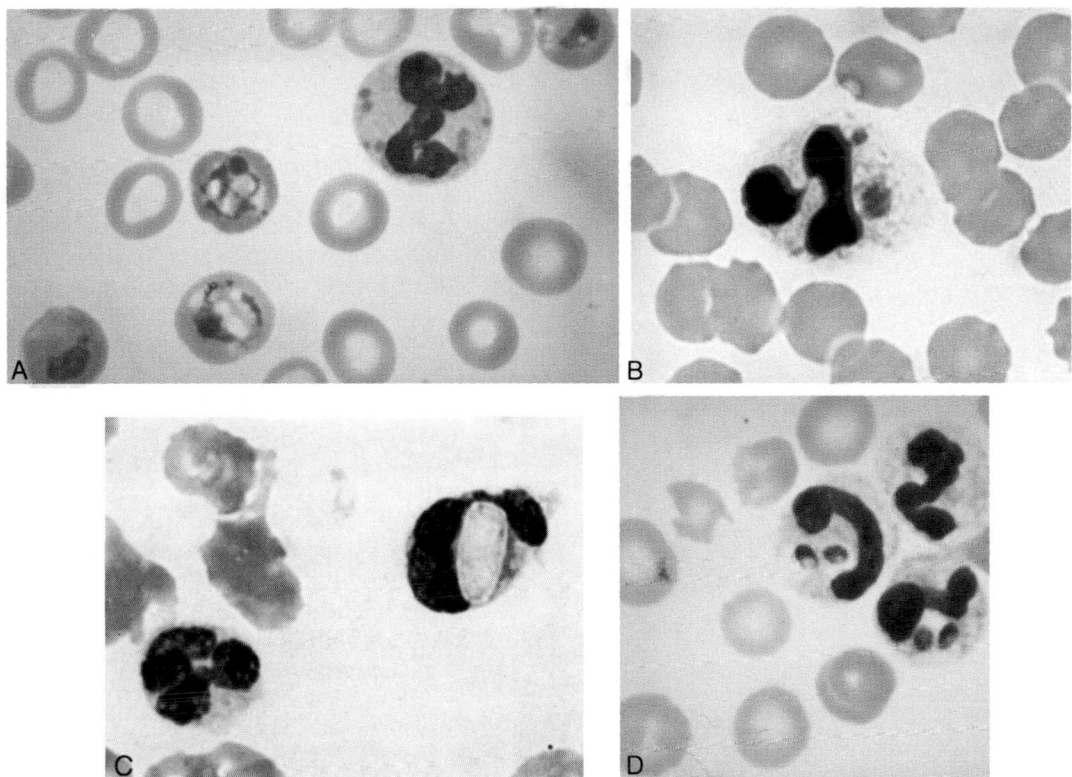

FIGURE 114–9. Intracytoplasmic inclusions in blood cells from dogs with various infectious diseases. *A,* Canine distemper viral inclusions in a neutrophil and erythrocytes. *B, Ehrlichia canis* morulae in a neutrophil. *C, Hepatozoon canis* gametocyte within a neutrophil. (Courtesy of Dr. Claudia A. Barton, College of Veterinary Medicine, Texas A&M University, College Station, Texas.) *D, Histoplasma capsulatum* within peripheral blood neutrophils. (Courtesy of Dr. Jan VanSteenhouse, College of Veterinary Medicine, Colorado State University, Fort Collins, Colorado.)

etal muscle biopsies for the presence of developing macroschizonts.[99, 100]

Cytoplasmic Inclusions in Congenital Diseases. Congenital diseases characterized by neutrophil or leukocyte inclusions include some forms of mucopolysaccharidosis and Chediak-Higashi syndrome. Although a presumptive diagnosis of mucopolysaccharidosis is based upon finding characteristic inclusions within neutrophils, definitive diagnosis of the specific enzymatic deficiency or defect requires biochemical testing.

The mucopolysaccharidoses are a group of lysosomal storage diseases that usually are inherited in an autosomal recessive pattern. These diseases are accompanied by a lack of specific enzyme production or function that is essential to degrade large, complex molecules. In the absence of enzyme activity, intermediate degradation products of these molecules accumulate within cellular lysosomes compromising both cellular and organ function.[101, 102] In mucopolysaccharidosis type VI in cats and in mucopolysaccharidosis type VII in dogs, inclusions may be found within neutrophils that stain pinkish-purple with Romanowsky stains and metachromatically with 1 per cent toluidine blue dye.[79, 92, 103, 104]

Mucopolysaccharidosis type VI (Maroteaux-Lamy syndrome) occurs in Siamese cats as a result of arylsulfatase B deficiency.[79, 103, 104] Approximately 90 per cent to 100 per cent of the circulating neutrophils contain a few to numerous coarse pinkish-purple granules on Romanowsky-stained blood smears (Figure 114–10A),

and these granules stain metachromatically with toluidine blue dye.[79, 103, 104] Basophil granules also may be enlarged and metachromatic.[103] Clinical features of the disease, first apparent by six weeks of age, include broad flattened facial bones, small ears, large forepaws, pectus excavatum, and diffuse corneal clouding.[79] Affected cats have progressive skeletal disease with secondary neurologic deficits.[79, 103, 104] Arylsulfatase activity of homozygous cats is 6 per cent of control values, and heterozygotes have a level of enzyme activity that is intermediate between homozygous and normal cats.[79] Treatment of affected cats has been attempted experimentally by bone marrow transplantation.[105, 106] Normal restoration of arylsulfatase B activity was accomplished in one cat with subsequent improvement of facial dysmorphia and ambulation, as well as resolution of the corneal opacity.[105]

Mucopolysaccharidosis VII has been described in a dog with progressive rear limb weakness, severe skeletal disease, and corneal granularities.[92] Beta-glucuronidase activity was less than 2 per cent of control values and neutrophil intracytoplasmic inclusions were similar to those described for the cats above.

Chediak-Higashi syndrome occurs in Persian cats with a diluted blue smoke haircoat color and yellow-green, as opposed to normal copper-colored, irises.[107, 108] The syndrome is inherited in an autosomal recessive manner, and is characterized by enlarged intracytoplasmic granules in circulating leukocytes and in melanocytes.[107–109]

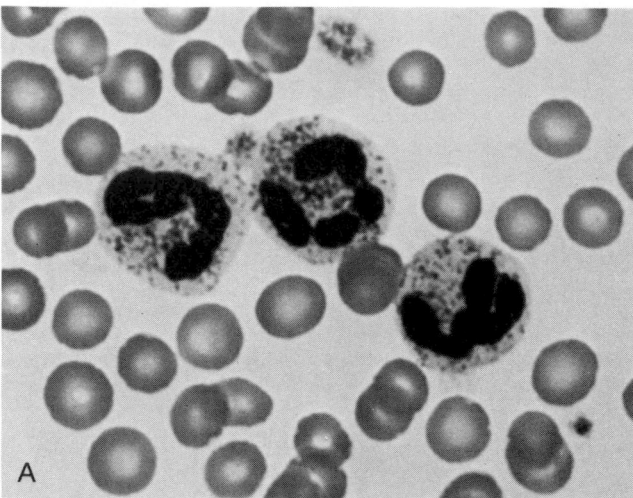

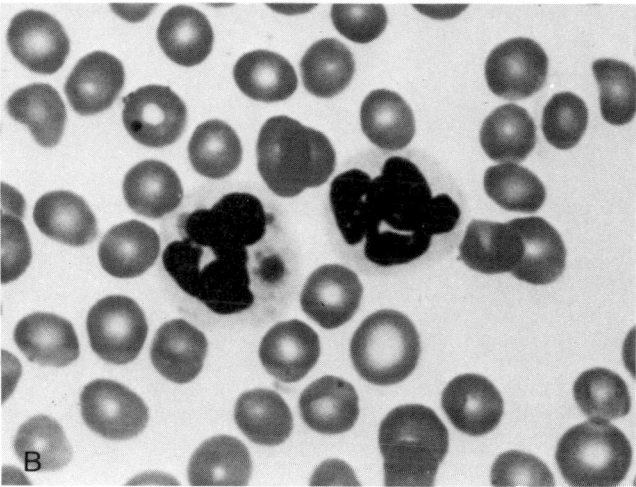

FIGURE 114–10. Intracytoplasmic inclusions in congenital diseases of cats. *A,* Intracytoplasmic inclusions in neutrophils from a cat with mucopolysaccharidosis type VI. (Courtesy of Dr. Mark E. Haskins, School of Veterinary Medicine, University of Pennsylvania, Philadelphia, Pennsylvania.) *B,* Giant lysosomes within the cytoplasm of a neutrophil (left) from a cat with Chediak-Higashi syndrome. (Courtesy of Dr. John W. Kramer, College of Veterinary Medicine, Washington State University, Pullman, Washington.)

The enlarged granules result from fusion of more normally sized preexisting lysosomes[110] and are recognized readily within leukocytes on Romanowsky-stained blood smears. The intracytoplasmic inclusions are pink to magenta, 2 μm or greater in diameter, and may be single or multiple (Figure 114–10*B*).[107, 108] Eosinophil granules also may appear plump or enlarged.[107]

People with Chediak-Higashi syndrome are predisposed to infection and bleeding.[107] Infection is attributed to delayed fusion of the enlarged lysosomes with the phagosome resulting in retarded neutrophil bactericidal activity.[110] An increased incidence of infection in affected cats has not been observed even though defective neutrophil chemotaxis exists in vitro.[107, 111] In both humans and cats, bleeding is secondary to abnormal platelet function. In cats with Chediak-Higashi syndrome, impaired platelet aggregation results from a deficient storage pool of adenine nucleotides, an absence of serotonin, and decreased concentrations of magnesium.[112] From a clinical standpoint, it is important to identify cats with Chediak-Higashi syndrome because

they bleed longer and more profusely than normal cats following venipuncture and minor surgery.[2, 107] Presumptive diagnosis may be based upon breed, haircoat color, iris color, presence of photophobia, and a red fundic reflex, and supported by finding the characteristic inclusions within leukocytes.[107–109]

Neutrophil Cytoplasmic Changes and Inclusions in Miscellaneous Diseases. Vacuolation of the neutrophil cytoplasm occurs with drug toxicity in cats, especially after high dosages of chloramphenicol (50 mg/kg/day IM or 120 mg/kg/day PO) and phenylbutazone (44 mg/kg day PO).[90, 113, 114] Drug-induced changes in neutrophil morphology resemble "toxic changes." Vacuolation may be apparent in blood leukocytes and in erythroid and myeloid precursor cells in bone marrow aspirates.[90, 113, 114] Döhle bodies also may be observed within neutrophils.[90] Changes in cellular morphology may be accompanied by decreased marrow cellularity and leukopenia.[90, 113, 114]

Intracytoplasmic hemosiderin granules may be seen in neutrophils and monocytes from dogs with immune-mediated hemolytic anemia following whole blood transfusion.[115] On Romanowsky-stained smears, the granules are 1 to 4 μm in diameter and have a brownish coloration. Multiple granules are present within some neutrophils, and these inclusions stain positively for iron by the Prussian blue method. Although the precise mechanism for formation of these sideroleukocytes is unknown, iron may be scavenged within splenic, hepatic, and bone marrow sinusoids by circulating leukocytes.[115] In rare instances of hemolytic disease with severe jaundice, bilirubin (hematoidin) crystals may be observed within neutrophils (Figure 114–11).[116]

Lupus erythematosus (LE) cells are leukocytes, usually neutrophils, that have phagocytosed antinuclear antibody-coated DNA. The resulting intracytoplasmic inclusion is round, homogeneous, magenta, and displaces the nucleus to the periphery of the cell.[117] LE cells must be distinguished from tart cells which are leukocytes that have phagocytosed nuclear debris. The intracytoplasmic inclusions of tart cells are round but

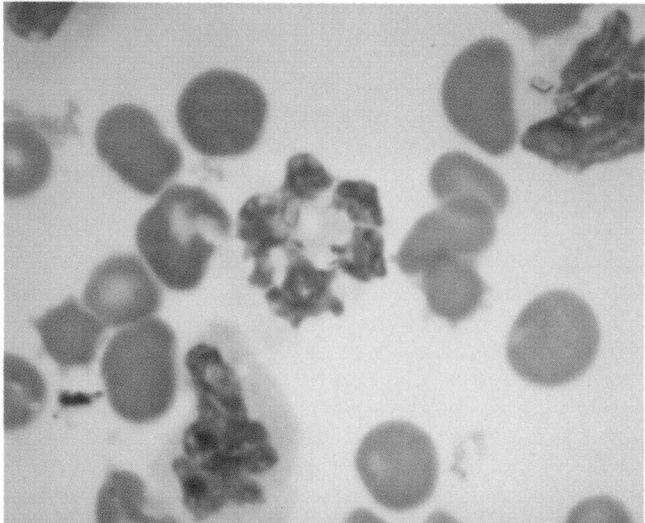

FIGURE 114–11. Blood neutrophil with intracytoplasmic bilirubin (hematoidin) crystals from a cat with severe hemolytic anemia and hyperbilirubinemia. (Courtesy of Dr. Edward A. Mahaffey, College of Veterinary Medicine, University of Georgia, Athens, Georgia.)

retain a normal chromatin pattern and stain deep purple. Although LE cells usually are observed after laboratory processing of clotted blood samples, they are observed infrequently in fresh bone marrow specimens from cats with myeloproliferative disease[6, 118] and in fresh synovial fluid and body cavity fluid smears from dogs with immune-mediated diseases. The LE cell phenomenon, when observed, is highly specific for systemic lupus erythematosus but the sensitivity of the test is low. Approximately 40 per cent of dogs with systemic lupus erythematosus have negative LE cell tests.[119]

PRODUCTION AND KINETICS

Neutrophils are produced in the bone marrow from committed bipotential stem cells that can produce either neutrophils or monocytes. Under the influence of increased concentrations of granulocyte-macrophage colony stimulating factor (a glycoprotein produced by macrophages, stimulated T-lymphocytes, fibroblasts, and endothelial cells), the stem cell will proliferate favoring neutrophil production and differentiation.[120, 121] Feedback inhibition of granulopoiesis is mediated by lactoferrin release from neutrophil secondary (specific) granules.[65, 120]

In health, a steady state exists where neutrophil production in the bone marrow is roughly equivalent to neutrophil uptake by the tissues. This daily expenditure of cells is called the neutrophil turnover rate and is expressed as the number of neutrophils consumed per pound of body weight per day. The neutrophil turnover rate is tremendous and approximates 1½ billion and 3 billion neutrophils/lb/day for dogs and cats, respectively.[39, 122]

Bone Marrow Pools and Compartments. Neutrophil production in the bone marrow represents an orderly proliferation and maturation sequence whereby cells progress through the following stages: myeloblast, promyelocyte (progranulocyte), myelocyte, metamyelocyte, band, and segmenter. Figuratively, the bone marrow can be divided into two pools based upon the mitotic capabilities of the various cells within the neutrophil series.[1] The mitotic pool, also designated as the proliferation and maturation compartment, consists of cells that are capable of mitosis and includes myeloblasts, promyelocytes, and myelocytes. The non-mitotic pool, also designated as the storage and maturation compartment, consists of cells that are incapable of division and includes metamyelocytes, bands, and segmenters.

Neutrophil precursors within the mitotic pool undergo a finite number of divisions and some degree of maturation. Radioisotope studies have estimated that myeloblasts and promyelocytes each divide once while myelocytes divide two or three times.[7, 123, 124] Following five doubling divisions, 32 metamyelocytes are produced. In dogs, however, myelocyte attrition from intramarrow cell death results in a 20 per cent rate of ineffective granulopoiesis termed the "myelocyte sink."[123] This phenomenon is species specific for dogs and does not occur in cats.[124] Metamyelocytes emerge as the product of the final myelocyte divisions. The transit time through the

mitotic pool resulting in metamyelocyte formation is approximately two days.[123, 124]

The postmitotic pool acts as a buffer between the mitotic cell pool and neutrophil release into the blood. Within the postmitotic pool, metamyelocytes pass through the band stage before maturing into segmenters. The transit time through the postmitotic pool approximates two days.[123, 124] Because neutrophil segmenters may be stored within the bone marrow for a variable period of time averaging another two days,[125] the transit time will fluctuate. In health, the total marrow transit time from the onset of stem cell or myeloblast division until segmented neutrophils are released into the blood is roughly 3.5 to 6 days.[123–126] Neutrophils are released from the bone marrow into the blood in an age-ordered manner (segmenters > bands > juveniles).[123] The precise mechanism regulating leukocyte release from the bone marrow is unknown, but involves soluble plasma factors such as leukocytosis-inducing factor, neutrophil-releasing factor, and complement fragments (C3e).[127–129]

An increased tissue demand for neutrophils alters bone marrow granulocyte kinetics considerably. Increasing concentrations of granulocyte-macrophage colony stimulating factor recruit more resting bipotential stem cells into active cell division and shorten the granulocytic doubling time. Increased numbers of neutrophils are produced at a faster rate.[120, 130] In the dog, decreased attrition of neutrophils within the myelocyte sink may immediately increase neutrophil production.[123] Facilitated bone marrow release by plasma factors results in an accelerated age-ordered release of granulocytes.[127–130] As the storage pool is depleted of segmenters, increased numbers of bands and then juveniles are released into the blood, reflecting a left shift.[130–132]

Blood Neutrophil Pools. The total blood neutrophil pool contains approximately one-half billion and one and one half billion neutrophils/lb of body weight in dogs and cats, respectively.[39, 122] Within the blood, radioisotope studies indicate that neutrophils are unevenly distributed and leave in a random fashion.[133, 134] The total blood neutrophil pool is divided into two dynamic subpools, the circulating and the marginal neutrophil pools, respectively.[134] The circulating neutrophil pool consists of cells within the axial circulation and are the cells quantitated by the total and differential leukocyte counts (Figure 114–12). The marginal neutrophil pool consists of cells that move slowly along the endothelial lining of capillaries and venules where reduced blood flow favors cell margination. Rapid changes in the distribution of cell numbers between the circulating and marginal neutrophil cell pools may occur, and these changes are reflected in the leukogram as neutrophilia or neutropenia.

In healthy dogs, the total blood neutrophil pool is almost equally divided between the circulating neutrophil pool and the marginal neutrophil pool, producing a 1:1 ratio.[122] In healthy cats the circulating neutrophil pool is smaller than the marginal neutrophil pool, producing a 1:3 ratio.[39] The neutrophil circulating half life within the blood averages 5.6 and 7.4 hours in healthy dogs and cats, respectively.[39, 122] Cell margination and emigration into the tissues is unidirectional; the neutrophils do not return to the circulation.[135] Neutrophils can

BLOOD

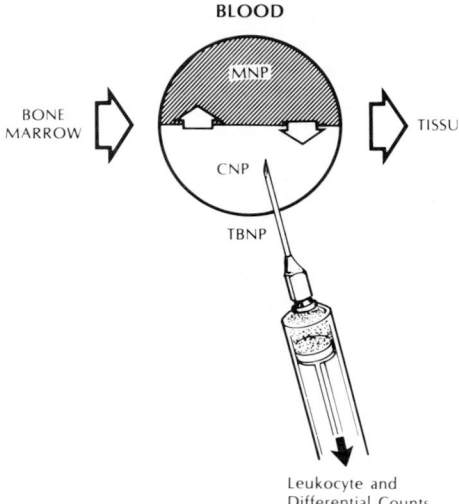

FIGURE 114–12. The total blood neutrophil pool (TBNP) is distributed between the marginal neutrophil pool (MNP) and the circulating neutrophil pool (CNP). When blood samples are drawn for the leukocyte and differential counts, the specimens only reflect the status of the circulating neutrophil pool.

function within the tissues for one or two days, and subsequently are phagocytized by the monocyte-macrophage system or are lost from mucosal surfaces following transmigration through the epithelium.[58]

Three factors govern the blood neutrophil concentration as determined by the leukocyte and differential counts. These factors include: the rate of neutrophil release from the bone marrow into the blood, the distribution of the blood neutrophil numbers between the circulating and marginal neutrophil pools, and the rate of neutrophil emigration from the blood vessels into the tissues.[1] One or a combination of these parameters may be altered by various physiologic or disease-associated states.

NEUTROPHIL RESPONSE PATTERNS

Neutrophilia

Neutrophilia is defined as the presence of greater than 11,400 neutrophils/μl of blood in dogs and greater than 12,500 neutrophils/μl of blood in cats. In most instances, neutrophilia can be classified as physiologic neutrophilia (pseudoneutrophilia), corticosteroid-associated neutrophilia, or neutrophilia in response to tissue inflammation or infection.[136, 137] Some causes of neutrophilia are listed in Table 114–5.

Physiologic Neutrophilia (Pseudoneutrophilia). Physiologic neutrophilia occurs with fear, excitement, strenuous exercise (including struggling during restraint for venipuncture), or after epinephrine injection.[2, 6, 35, 134, 138] There is a transient shift of neutrophils from the marginal neutrophil pool into the circulating neutrophil pool without a left shift. The decreased neutrophil adherence presumably is mediated by a plasma factor that increases intracellular cAMP concentration and by increased

TABLE 114–5. CAUSES OF NEUTROPHILIA AND NEUTROPENIA IN DOGS AND CATS

Neutrophilia	
Physiologic response (excitement, fear)	dog, cat
Infection	
Bacteria (various species)	dog, cat
Rickettsia	
Rocky Mountain spotted fever	dog
Viruses	
Canine distemper	dog
Feline rhinotracheitis	cat
Fungi (various species)	dog, cat
Parasites	
Toxoplasmosis	dog, cat
Hepatozoonosis	dog
Immune-mediated diseases	dog, cat
Autoimmune hemolytic anemia	
Lupus erythematosus	
Polymyositis	
Polyserositis	
Rheumatoid arthritis	
Tissue necrosis	dog, cat
Thrombosis and infarction	
Burns	
Malignancy	
Uremia	
Drug administration	
Corticosteroids	dog, cat
Epinephrine	dog
Estrogen (early)	dog
Paraneoplastic syndrome	
Fibrosarcoma	dog
Renal tubular carcinoma	dog
Miscellaneous	dog, cat
Acute severe stress (any cause)	
Sterile foreign body	
Hemolytic disease	
Hemorrhage	
Neutropenia	
Infection	
Bacteria (septicemia, endotoxemia)	dog, cat
Rickettsia	
Ehrlichia canis	dog
Viruses	
Parvoviral enteritis	dog
Feline panleukopenia	cat
Feline leukemia virus	cat
Feline T-lymphotropic lentivirus	cat
Fungi	
Histoplasmosis (disseminated)	cat
Drug administration	
Relatively predictable	
Estrogen (overdose)	dog
Chemotherapy agents	dog, cat
Chloramphenicol	cat
Idiosyncratic	
Cephalosporins	dog, cat
Phenylbutazone	dog
Thiacetarsamide	dog
Noxema ingestion	dog
Bone marrow necrosis	dog
Myelofibrosis and osteopetrosis	dog
Neoplastic and myelodysplastic disease	
Acute granulocytic leukemia	dog
Acute lymphoblastic leukemia	dog
Acute myelomonocytic leukemia	dog
Erythremic myelosis	cat
Large granular lymphoma	cat
Megakaryocytic myelosis/leukemia	dog, cat
Multicentric lymphosarcoma	dog
Myelodysplastic syndromes	dog
Cyclic hematopoiesis	
Gray collies (congenital)	dog
Miscellaneous dog breeds	
(unknown origin)	dog
Cyclophosphamide administration	dog
Feline leukemia virus-associated	cat
Immune-mediated mechanisms?	dog, cat
Radiation	dog, cat

blood flow through the microvasculature.[138][139] In the dog, the majority of neutrophil mobilization occurs from the pulmonary circulation.[137] The bone marrow release rate, neutrophil circulating half life, and size of the total blood neutrophil pool remain unchanged (Figure 114–13).[136]

Physiologic neutrophilia occurs very rapidly and cell counts usually peak at 15,000 neutrophils/μl.[2] Epinephrine-associated changes in the neutrophil count are of greater magnitude in young animals, and are more pronounced in the cat than in the dog.[2] These effects are transient and diminish within 10 to 20 minutes. Physiologic neutrophilia is accompanied by other characteristic changes in the leukogram that collectively are

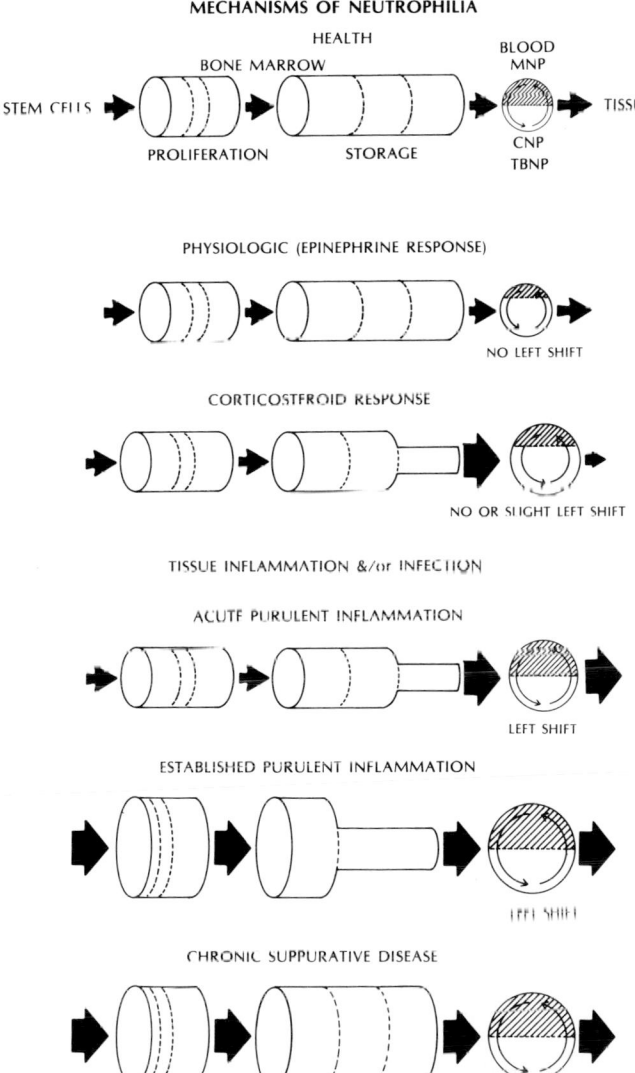

FIGURE 114–13. Mechanisms of neutrophilia. The sizes of the arrows represent rates of movement of neutrophils through the mitotic (proliferation) and non-mitotic (storage) bone marrow pools and the blood. The sizes of the cylinders and circles indicate the sizes of the bone marrow pools and total blood neutrophil pool (TBNP), respectively. Within the circles, the shaded and clear areas represent the sizes of the marginal neutrophil pool (MNP) and circulating neutrophil pool (CNP), respectively. (Adapted from Prasse KW. White blood cell disorders. In Ettinger, SJ (ed): Textbook of Veterinary Internal Medicine; Diseases of the Dog and Cat. 2nd ed. Philadelphia, WB Saunders, 1983.)

designated "physiologic leukocytosis." Physiologic leukocytosis is identified by observing leukocytosis, neutrophilia without a left shift, lymphocytosis, and monocyte and eosinophil counts that are unaffected or elevated slightly.[2] The lymphocytosis is frequently of greater magnitude than the neutrophilia, especially in the cat.[6]

Corticosteroid-Associated Neutrophilia. Either endogenous release of cortisol from the adrenal cortex or exogenous administration of corticosteroids or ACTH can cause neutrophilia. Although diurnal variations in endogenous cortisol production and leukocyte counts exist, these changes are clinically insignificant and difficult to verify in hospitalized animals.[29, 140, 141] Severe stress or acute disease must be present before endogenous cortisol release is sufficient to cause overt changes in the leukogram.

Neutrophilia follows corticosteroid administration in dogs and cats, and the magnitude depends upon the type, dosage, and route of drug administration.[2, 6, 135, 142, 143] Studies in dogs and humans demonstrate that corticosteroid administration increases the bone marrow release rate of neutrophils by 3 to 7.5 fold, which is the primary reason for expansion of the total blood neutrophil pool (Figure 114–13).[134, 135, 144] A secondary effect includes decreased neutrophil adherence with a shift of neutrophils from the marginal to the circulating neutrophil pool and slight prolongation of the neutrophil circulating half life.[134, 135, 144]

Following a single dose of 20 mg of prednisolone in dogs and 5 mg of prednisolone in cats, peak neutrophilia occurs within four to six hours, with a two- to threefold increase in the neutrophil count.[142, 143] A left shift will not be observed unless the bone marrow storage pool is depleted. Baseline values are regained 12 to 24 hours later. The magnitude of the response diminishes with continuous corticosteroid treatment or release. Clinically, dogs on long-term corticosteroid treatment or with hyperadrenocorticism have moderate increases in the neutrophil count.[6, 145] The neutrophil counts return to baseline values 48 to 96 hours following drug withdrawal.[6, 142, 143]

Characteristic corticosteroid-induced changes in the leukogram include leukocytosis with neutrophilia, monocytosis, lymphopenia, and eosinopenia.[6, 142, 143] Prolonged corticosteroid usage decreases neutrophil adherence which reduces cell mobilization into the tissues and predisposes the patient to infection. The probability of developing an infection can be reduced by the use of alternate-day drug therapy. Neutrophil counts, circulating half life, and response to inflammation are unimpaired on the "off" day.[146, 147]

Neutrophilia Associated with Inflammation and/or Infection. Suspicion of inflammation or infection is the foremost reason for performing total and differential leukocyte counts. Once detected, both the clinical course and resolution of these processes can be monitored by repetitive leukograms.[2] Generally, the magnitude of the total neutrophil response is a reflection of the intensity of the disease process, whereas the degree of the left shift is suggestive of the severity of the disease.[148] Much of the scientific basis for clinical interpretation of leukograms in human medicine is derived from experimental studies in dogs in which the hematologic responses to killed *Salmonella* spp., purified endotoxin, spontaneous infections, and experimentally induced pneumococcal and staphylococcal pneumonias were determined.[130–132, 135]

Neutrophilia with a left shift is considered the clinical hallmark of purulent inflammation, but most of these leukograms are from patients with established disease and sustained neutrophilia (Figure 114–13). Leukocyte changes in early infection or inflammation may be quite different. Exposure to endotoxin, for example, is associated with a rapidly developing but transient neutropenia occurring over one to three hours.[130] The neutropenia lasts for two to three hours and is the result of a shortened neutrophil circulating half life, increased cell margination within blood vessels, and enhanced cell emigration into the tissues. Accelerated bone marrow release of neutrophils occurs and a rebound neutrophilia follows rapidly with cell counts peaking two- to three-fold above baseline values within six to eight hours.[130] In contrast, early gram positive bacterial infection, exemplified by pneumonia, is accompanied by accelerated release of neutrophils from the bone marrow, expanded total blood neutrophil and marginal neutrophil pools, and a decreased neutrophil circulating half life, but the neutrophil count is within the reference interval. These changes collectively constitute a "masked" neutrophilia because the expanded marginal neutrophil pool is not detected by the leukocyte count.[132]

Once infection or inflammation is established, sustained neutrophilia occurs if the bone marrow release rate of neutrophils exceeds the rate of neutrophil emigration into the tissues.[137] In this relative steady state, the total blood neutrophil pool is expanded and the neutrophil circulating half life is normal to prolonged.[132, 136, 137] Neutrophilic leukocytosis is observed frequently in clinical practice and accounts for approximately 30 per cent of the leukocyte abnormalities in dogs and cats.[149] With elevated counts, total leukocyte numbers ranging from 20,000 to 30,000 cells/µl occur most commonly while total leukocyte counts in excess of 50,000 cells/µl are uncommon.[149] Generally, the magnitude of the neutrophilia is greater with localized inflammation or abscesses than with generalized inflammatory diseases, and pyogenic bacteria produce more intense neutrophilia than other etiological agents.[2]

The presence and severity of neutrophilia-associated left shifts will depend upon the number of maturing neutrophils within the bone marrow storage pool, the magnitude of increase in the bone marrow release rate in response to tissue demands, and the rapidity with which neutrophil precursors in the proliferation compartment can replenish cell numbers in the maturation and storage compartment. Mild, clinically insignificant left shifts (300 to 1,000 bands/µl) are associated with inflammatory disorders such as hemorrhagic cystitis, seborrheic dermatitis, tracheobronchitis, catarrhal or hemorrhagic enteritis, and granulomatous diseases in which the neutrophil is a minimal component of the exudate and/or tissue demand for neutrophils is very mild.[2, 150] Significant left shifts ($\geq$ 1,000 bands/µl) accompany pyoderma, pleuritis, peritonitis, pyometra, and abscess formation.[150, 151] These shifts are related to purulent exudative processes involving pyogenic bacteria,

fungi, foreign bodies, or necrotic tissue.[150] These sites of tissue damage usually can be identified with a combination of a thorough physical examination and radiographs. In some instances, however, the site of tissue injury may remain elusive in the face of dramatic neutrophilia, and generalized exudate loss from the skin or into the gastrointestinal tract,[2] genitourinary tract, joints, and tissue planes should be considered. This type of insensible neutrophil loss may be detected with cytology or biopsy preparations. Additionally, obscure loss of neutrophils is associated with hemorrhagic and hemolytic anemias, especially immune-mediated hemolytic anemia.[2] Degenerative left shifts imply an intense suppurative disease and a guarded prognosis.

As bone marrow production of neutrophils replenishes the postmitotic pool, the magnitude of the left shift diminishes.[2] Convalescence is associated with the appearance of hypersegmented neutrophils in the blood, the so-called "right shift."[2, 7] In clinical practice, however, right shifts rarely are observed during a routine differential count. The persistence of neutrophilic leukocytosis with a diminishing or minimal left shift in the presence of continued clinical illness denotes a chronic suppurative disease (Figure 114–13).[2]

Leukemoid Reactions and Extreme Neutrophilic Leukocytosis. The term "leukemoid reaction" refers to a granulocytic leukemia-like blood picture, but implies a benign disease process. Originally, this term was used for decreased, normal, or increased white cell counts with many bands and juveniles or with an extreme number of mature neutrophils.[152] In veterinary medicine, the term leukemoid reaction suggests a total leukocyte count exceeding 75,000 cells/µl with a severe left shift that may extend to myeloblasts.[26] The term "extreme neutrophilic leukocytosis" implies a neutrophil count exceeding 100,000 cells/µl with a mild left shift and no evidence of myeloid neoplasia. In human medicine, granulocytic leukemia and leukemoid reactions may be distinguished readily by cytochemical staining (decreased neutrophil alkaline phosphatase activity in leukemia), karyotype analysis (Philadelphia chromosome positive in leukemia), and the presence of anemia and thrombocytopenia.[1, 7] Distinguishing leukemoid reactions from granulocytic leukemia is more difficult in dogs and cats. Canine and feline chromosomal markers analogous to the Philadelphia chromosome of humans have yet to be described. Hepatosplenomegaly, anemia, and thrombocytopenia may arouse suspicion of granulocytic leukemia but do not confirm the diagnosis.[6, 82, 153–156] Although neutrophil precursors in both leukemoid reactions and granulocytic leukemia exhibit cytoplasmic basophilia, the additional presence of toxic vacuolation and Döhle bodies would favor a diagnosis of infection and leukemoid response. Alkaline phosphatase cytochemical staining may provide a method to distinguish leukemoid reactions from granulocytic leukemia in dogs and cats. Dog and cat neutrophils are devoid of alkaline phosphatase activity in health and in states of infection characterized by neutrophilia and leukemoid reactions.[157–160] In naturally occurring cases of granulocytic leukemia in dogs and cats, neutrophils are reported to show a variable degree of staining with the alkaline phosphatase technique, but scientific documentation of these assertions is limited.[6, 161, 162] As cytochemical staining is more widely applied in canine and feline leukemias, alkaline phosphatase positivity may prove to be a definitive marker for granulocytic leukemia in these species.

Until definitive markers are found, distinguishing granulocytic leukemia from a leukemoid response in dogs and cats is easier said than done. Frequently, multiple leukograms must be evaluated over a period of days. Favorable prognostic signs associated with a resolving leukemoid reaction include a decreasing leukocyte count with a diminishing left shift and resolution of toxic change. These responses are observed sometimes following empirical antibiotic therapy.

Extreme neutrophilic leukocytosis usually results from severe, localized pyogenic infections, especially pyometra in dogs and abscesses in cats.[148, 149] Cases of suspected or documented[163–165] neutrophil dysfunction with secondary bacterial infection also are associated with extreme leukocytosis. In a dog with canine granulocytopathy syndrome and in a dog with neutrophil glycoprotein deficiency, peak neutrophil counts were 194,000 and 188,000 cells/μl, respectively.[164, 165] Other associations with extreme neutrophilic leukocytosis in dogs include *Hepatozoon canis* infection (173,300 PMN/μl), immune-mediated hemolytic anemia, and paraneoplastic syndromes secondary to metastatic fibrosarcoma (121,800 PMN/μl) and renal tubular carcinoma (238,800 PMN/μl).[166–168] Because extreme neutrophilic leukocytosis is the result of tremendously increased granulopoiesis, intensification of the neutrophilia may transiently follow surgical or medical treatment of the underlying disease. Examples include abrupt removal of the tissue demand for neutrophils by ovariohysterectomy in cases of pyometra, and augmented release of neutrophils from the bone marrow following corticosteroid treatment of immune-mediated hemolytic anemia. These changes in the leukogram are expected and do not indicate surgical complications or infection. The neutrophil counts will begin to fall toward baseline within 48 to 96 hours.

Neutropenia

Neutropenia is defined as less than 3,000 neutrophils/μl of blood in dogs and less than 2,500 neutrophils/μl of blood in cats. Because neutrophils are the predominant circulating leukocyte type in these species, neutropenia almost always produces leukopenia. Neutropenia results from one or a combination of three mechanisms including deficient neutrophil production within the bone marrow, shifts in neutrophils from the circulating neutrophil pool into the marginal neutrophil pool, and emigration of neutrophils from the blood into the tissues at a rate that exceeds the release of neutrophils from the bone marrow into the blood (Figure 114–14).[169] Mechanisms of neutropenia are defined clearly in human medicine, but have received much less attention in veterinary medicine. Conditions associated with neutropenia in dogs and cats are listed in Table 114–5.

The major clinical consequence of neutropenia is infection, and a rough correlation exists between the degree of neutropenia and risk of bacterial infection.

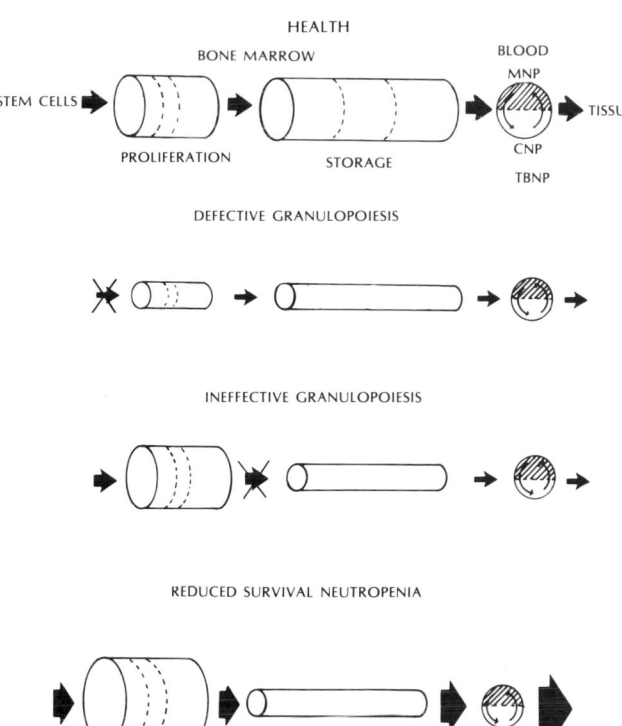

FIGURE 114–14. Mechanisms of neutropenia. The size of the arrows represents the rates of movement of neutrophils through the mitotic (proliferation) and non-mitotic (storage) bone marrow pools. The sizes of the cylinders and circles represent the sizes of the bone marrow pools and the total blood neutrophil pool (TBNP), respectively. Within the circles, the shaded and clear areas represent the sizes of the marginal neutrophil pool (MNP) and circulating neutrophil pool (CNP), respectively. (Adapted from Prasse KW: White blood cell disorders. *In* Ettinger, SJ (ed): Textbook of Veterinary Internal Medicine; Diseases of the Dog and Cat. 2nd ed. Philadelphia, WB Saunders, 1983.)

Compensatory monocytosis, if present, reduces the risk of infection considerably even though the bactericidal capabilities of monocytes are inferior to those of neutrophils.[169]

Defective Neutrophil Production

Mechanisms responsible for defective neutrophil production include: hematopoietic stem cell death from ionizing radiation, drug exposure, or infectious agents (most notably viruses and rickettsia); reduced hematopoietic space secondary to myelophthisis; cyclic stem cell proliferation; and T-lymphocyte–mediated suppression of granulopoiesis. Although these mechanisms may be associated with neutropenia alone, they also may present as pancytopenia. Bone marrow aspirates may be hypocellular to hypercellular, but the post-mitotic pool is depleted of more mature neutrophils. The total blood neutrophil pool is diminished and the small size of the circulating neutrophil pool is reflected as a neutropenia with or without a left shift (Figure 114–14).[137]

Hematopoietic Stem Cell Death

Radiation Effects. A single total body irradiation dosage of 12 Grays in dogs and 6.5 to 7 Grays in cats produces profound neutropenia in ten days and six days, respectively.[47, 105, 106, 170] These dosages of radiation usually are lethal unless the hematopoietic stem cell population is returned by transfusion or by bone marrow transplantation.[47, 170] Ionizing radiation is the method of choice to precondition dogs and cats for bone marrow transplantation as a treatment for mucopolysaccharidosis, cyclic hematopoiesis, pyruvate kinase deficiency, and lymphosarcoma.[105, 106, 171–177]

Chemotherapy Drugs. Drugs such as cyclophosphamide, daunomycin, dimethyl myleran, doxorubicin, and 6-thioguanine induce predictable myelosuppression in dogs and cats.[53, 106, 178, 179] The nadir of leukopenia occurs within 4 to 7 days and hematologic recovery may occur within 20 to 40 days.[53, 178, 179] Potential complications of drug administration include thrombocytopenia with subsequent hemorrhage, irreversible myelosuppression, and overwhelming sepsis.[178–180]

Estrogen Toxicity in Dogs. Exogenously administered or endogenously produced estrogen compounds can cause myelotoxicosis in dogs.[57, 181–186] Both diethylstilbestrol and estradiol cyclopentylpropionate administration can produce myelosuppression, but the latter drug is more effective.[182] Individual or idiosyncratic sensitivity to estrogens probably is involved because bone marrow suppression may be produced in some dogs with dosages of estradiol cyclopentylpropionate as low as 0.07 to 0.30 mg/lb (0.16 to 0.70 mg/kg) of body weight.[57, 183] Historically, estrogen toxicosis is related to treatment of bitches for mismating, infertility, or urinary (spay) incontinence and of male dogs for perianal adenomas.[182–183] Estrogen-induced myelotoxicity also occurs as a paraneoplastic syndrome of male dogs with Sertoli cell tumors.[185, 186] Clinical signs of estrogen toxicosis include exercise intolerance, pale mucous membranes, petechiation, hemorrhage, and fever, a reflection of the pancytopenia.[182, 183, 185, 186] In dogs with Sertoli cell tumors, additional signs of endocrine alopecia and feminization (attraction of other male dogs, gynecomastia, and pendulous prepuce) also may be present.[185, 186] Pancytopenia occurs relatively late in the estrogen toxicity syndrome, and earlier changes in the hemogram may be quite different.

Following estrogen overdosage, thrombocytosis develops and peaks within five to seven days post-injection. A precipitous decline in the platelet count follows and thrombocytopenia (less than 50,000 platelets/μl) is evident 13 days post-injection.[57, 184] Bone marrow aspirates from days five to seven display suppression of megakaryocytopoiesis and erythropoiesis, and stimulation of granulopoiesis. The M/E ratio is increased.[57, 184] By post-injection day ten, bone marrow aspirates show complete cessation of megakaryocytopoiesis and erythropoiesis. Although neutrophil maturation continues, neutrophil precursors are depleted.[57]

Leukocytosis occurs immediately after estrogen injection and peaks between post-injection days 17 and 23 with leukocyte counts ranging from 29,000 to 50,000 cells/μl.[57, 181, 184] The leukocyte counts begin to decline and leukopenia develops rapidly. Bone marrow aspirates obtained on post-injection day 20 demonstrate resumption of megakaryocytopoiesis and erythropoiesis, but granulopoiesis ceases. If total hematopoietic recovery

occurs, younger dogs recover more quickly than older dogs.[57] Hematologic recovery in clinical cases of estrogen toxicity occurs within three months.[182]

Initial experimental studies of estrogen toxicity in dogs suggest that these compounds inhibit the proliferation of pluripotential stem cells while concurrently stimulating the differentiation and maturation of committed stem cells.[57] More recent studies, using bone marrow culture techniques, indicate that both granulocyte-macrophage and fibroblast colony-forming units are decreased following estrogen injection, but fibroblast colony-forming units from estradiol-treated dogs can still support granulocyte-macrophage colony formation in vitro.[184] These observations suggest that the hematopoietic inductive microenvironment is partially intact. Additionally, the mean numbers of fibroblast and granulocyte-macrophage colony-forming units from control dogs, when cultured in the presence of estradiol, are not significantly different from control cultures without estradiol.[184] Parent estrogen compounds, therefore, may not result in cytotoxic injury to stem cells and the ultimate marrow suppression seen clinically may be the effect of estrogen metabolites. However, estrogen-related stem cell death cannot be discounted, especially in animals dying from irreversible hematopoietic suppression.

Chloramphenicol Toxicity in Cats. Chloramphenicol administration at daily dosages as low as 22 mg/lb (50 mg/kg) can produce bone marrow hypocellularity and leukopenia in cats within 14 to 21 days.[113] Associated clinical signs include depression, dehydration, anorexia, soft feces or diarrhea, and vomiting.[90, 113] Higher daily dosages (30 to 55 mg/lb or 60 to 120 mg/kg daily) of chloramphenicol can produce leukopenia within one week, and neutrophils may contain Döhle bodies.[90] In some instances, hypocellular bone marrows have an increased M/E ratio with giant metamyelocytes and vacuolated neutrophil precursors suggesting defective maturation. Hematologic and bone marrow parameters return to baseline within one week of drug withdrawal.[90] The toxic effects of chloramphenicol in cats are attributed to the nitrobenzene structure of the drug molecule[113] and the inability of cats to conjugate such molecules with glucuronic acid.[90] Clinical dosages of chloramphenicol up to 22 mg/lb (50 mg/kg) TID have been recommended in cats with bacterial infections. Because experimental studies indicate that leukopenia may be a predictable effect of chloramphenicol administration, drug-induced myelosuppression should be considered in the differential diagnosis of persistent neutropenia in cats receiving this drug.

Phenylbutazone Toxicosis in Dogs. Most reported cases of phenylbutazone toxicity in dogs appear to be idiosyncratic drug reactions presenting as pancytopenia.[187–190] Leukopenia may be severe (less than 200 cells/μl) and neutropenia may occur with or without toxic change and a left shift.[187–190] Bone marrow aspirates, when taken, are hypoplastic. Incriminated drug dosages generally range from 200 to 600 mg daily in divided doses and commonly are given for prolonged periods of time ranging from one to four months.[187–190] However, leukopenia has been associated with drug administration for only eight days.[188] Clinical signs of phenylbutazone toxicity include depression, anorexia, vomiting (sometimes containing blood), fever, petechiation, and hemorrhage. Following drug withdrawal, hematologic recovery occurs within two days to greater than five months.[188]

Cephalosporin Antibiotics. Cephalosporin compounds are used commonly to treat bacterial infections in humans and animals, and neutropenia is reported as an idiosyncratic drug reaction in both species.[169, 191] In an experimental study in dogs, high dosage cefazedone administration (250 to 400 mg/lb or 540 to 840 mg/kg daily IV) produced neutropenia in 8 of 14 animals after 6 to 10 weeks of treatment. Neutropenia was associated with a reduction of granulocyte-macrophage colony-forming units in bone marrow cultures and ultrastructural evidence of mitochondrial damage. Following drug withdrawal, hematologic recovery occurred within one week.[191] Neutropenia secondary to cefadroxil treatment has been observed in one dog at the University of Georgia Veterinary Medical Teaching Hospital. This dog received cefadroxil (14 mg/lb or 30 mg/kg body weight daily PO) for approximately 12 days before neutropenia developed. The neutropenia resolved within five days following drug withdrawal. At the University of Florida Veterinary Medical Teaching Hospital neutropenia also has been observed in one cat receiving cephalosporin. This neutropenia also resolved following drug withdrawal.

Miscellaneous Drugs. Idiosyncratic drug reactions in dogs characterized by pancytopenia or neutropenia also have been observed with thiacetarsamide administration and ingestion of medicated skin cream (Noxzema).[192-193] In the latter case, benzene-related components including menthol, camphor, clove oil, eucalyptus oil, and/or phenol probably were responsible for myelotoxicity.

Parvovirus Infection of Dogs (Parvoviral Enteritis) and Cats (Feline Panleukopenia). Parvoviruses have a predilection for tissues in active mitosis including gastrointestinal crypt epithelium, lymphoid tissue, and hematopoietic tissue.[48, 50, 52, 194-200] Infection of young dogs and cats typically is associated with acute gastroenteritis accompanied at some time period by profound leukopenia.[50, 194, 195, 200] An incubation period of four to seven days precedes the development of clinical signs which include anorexia, depression, vomiting, diarrhea (frequently bloody), dehydration, fever, and abdominal tenderness.[51, 52, 194, 195, 197-200] Leukopenia is most severe approximately five to eight days post-infection, and usually is accompanied by a left shift to juveniles and toxic change.[51, 194-196, 200] Laboratory detection of leukopenia depends upon the stage of disease. If a single blood sample is analyzed from dogs with suspected parvoviral enteritis at the time of hospital admission, approximately 34 per cent will be leukopenic. If at least three serial blood counts are done, approximately 86 per cent of the diseased dogs will exhibit leukopenia.[50] Mean leukocyte counts approximate 938 to 2,800 cells/μl.[50-52, 194, 196] With supportive care, hematologic recovery begins within one to six days and the rapidly rising leukocyte count is characterized by a rebound leukocytosis in both dogs (25,000 to 60,000 cells/μl) and cats (15,700 to 42,700 cells/μl).[50, 51, 194, 198] A continued left shift may be present during recovery.[50, 195]

The mechanism of neutropenia in parvovirus infection is multifaceted. Evidence exists that parvovirus is cytotoxic for hematopoietic cells, and stem cell destruction is inferred as a cause of neutropenia and bone marrow hypocellularity.[48, 50, 194-196, 198, 199] However, cytologic aspirates and histological sections of bone marrow confirm neutrophil depletion of the maturation and storage pool, suggesting increased bone marrow release of neutrophils in response to gastrointestinal tissue damage and/or to endotoxemia.[194-196, 198, 199] Endotoxemia also causes a shift of blood neutrophils from the circulating to the marginal pool which may potentiate neutropenia.[136, 137] Furthermore, phagocytosis of neutrophils by macrophages in some bone marrow smears from parvovirus-infected dogs[199] may indicate increased ineffective hematopoiesis (Figure 114–14). In contrast, canine coronavirus-induced gastrointestinal disturbances commonly are associated with lymphopenia, but neutropenia and, consequently, leukopenia generally do not occur.[201]

Feline Leukemia Virus Infection. Feline leukemia virus readily infects hematopoietic tissue, and viral antigen can be detected in the bone marrow 7 to 21 days after infection.[202] Feline leukemia virus usually is not cytopathic, but certain viral subgroups (FeLV$_A$) may produce neutropenia.[202, 203] Development of protracted neutropenia may occur from 21 to 56 days post-infection and coincides with the release of virus-infected cells from the bone marrow.[202] Clinically, cats with infections and neutropenia are frequently feline leukemia virus–test positive. However, a negative test result does not eliminate entirely the possibility of feline leukemia virus infection because latent viral infections do exist. Latent viral infections in nonviremic cats may be demonstrated by bone marrow culture.[204]

Neutropenia is apparent in approximately 50 per cent of feline leukemia virus–infected cats presented for illness.[205] Examination of blood and bone marrow data indicates that three patterns of neutropenia exist. The most frequent pattern is mild neutropenia with relatively normal granulopoiesis. The second pattern is moderate neutropenia with granulopoietic hypoplasia, referred to as the "panleukopenia-like syndrome." Gastrointestinal signs, however, may not be present.[206] The third pattern consists of severe, persistent, insidious neutropenia with marked granulopoietic hyperplasia previously designated as subleukemic granulocytic leukemia, preleukemia, or hemopoietic dysplasia.[25, 207] In each of the three patterns left shifts (sometimes severe) with toxic neutrophils may be found.[205] Presumably, neutropenia results from viral destruction of hematopoietic precursors, from retardation of cellular maturation, or from tissue consumption of neutrophils secondary to infection. Bone marrow culture studies indicate that feline leukemia virus infection suppresses the growth of fibroblast colony-forming units,[208] suggesting that the bone marrow hematopoietic inductive microenvironment also may be disturbed. Granulocytic hyperplasia in the face of persistent neutropenia (termed ineffective granulopoiesis) suggests a prolonged neutrophil transit time through or impaired release of neutrophils from the bone marrow, but radiotracer studies have not been performed to confirm these hypotheses. Such changes also could represent a myelodysplastic syndrome characterized by disturbed cellular maturation.[82]

Lentivirus Infection of Cats. Feline T-lymphotropic lentivirus (abbreviated FTLV) is the newest retrovirus isolated from feline leukemia virus–test negative cats with various immunodeficiency syndromes.[209] Inoculation of susceptible kittens with FTLV produces leukopenia (neutropenia) accompanied by fever, peripheral lymphadenopathy, and secondary bacterial infection. Leukopenia develops within two weeks of viral inoculation and persists for two to four weeks.[209] In addition, abnormalities in the neutrophil maturation sequence may be apparent (Personal communication: Dr. Niels C. Pedersen, University of California, Davis, CA, 95616). Feline leukemia virus test–negative cats with leukopenia and immunodeficiency syndromes are seen occasionally in clinical practice. These animals probably are good candidates for lentivirus testing.

Canine Ehrlichiosis. Canine ehrlichiosis is a rickettsial disease caused by *Ehrlichia canis* and transmitted by the brown dog tick. Clinical signs of disease include fever, lethargy, anorexia, weight loss, edema of the limbs and scrotum, and hemorrhage (petechial to ecchymotic hemorrhages of the skin and mucous membranes, hyphema, and occasionally dramatic epistaxis).[210–213] Clinical laboratory abnormalities vary and may include transient leukopenia, pancytopenia, chronic thrombocytopenia, and hyperglobulinemia that occasionally appears as a monoclonal gammopathy with electrophoresis.[210, 213–217] Pancytopenia is presumed to result from bone marrow hypoplasia, and bacterial infection secondary to neutropenia is common.[210–212] Transient leukopenia is associated with early rickettsial infection and may be related to endothelial cell damage.[214] Although canine ehrlichiosis has classically been described as an acute disease, subclinical or chronic forms of the disease are being recognized with increased frequency.[215–217] These forms of the disease may last for years and have fewer instances of pancytopenia, thrombocytopenia, or bleeding disorders.[215, 216] Neutropenia is present in 18 to 30 per cent of dogs with chronic ehrlichiosis.[215, 216] The presence of increased numbers of plasma cells within bone marrow aspirates[215] suggests that neutropenia may result from immune-mediated mechanisms. Canine ehrlichiosis is best diagnosed by acute and convalescent antibody titers which remain elevated in chronic disease states.[216, 217]

Reduced Hematopoietic Space

Neutropenia secondary to reduced hematopoietic space is unusual but may occur with bone marrow necrosis or myelophthisic disease. In most instances, bone marrow aspiration and core biopsies will be necessary for a definitive diagnosis.

Bone Marrow Necrosis. Bone marrow necrosis–associated neutropenia has been reported in one dog.[218] The precise cause of necrosis was undetermined, but sepsis may have been involved. Neutropenia secondary to severe bacterial sepsis occurs in humans, presumably from bacterial and/or endotoxin–induced damage of neutrophil precursors. *Staphylococcus*, *Pneumococcus*, and *Klebsiella* spp. are involved most often.[219] We have seen two or three cases of suspected bone marrow

necrosis, indicating that this entity may occur more frequently than is recognized currently.

Myelofibrosis and Osteopetrosis. Neutropenia also may be secondary myelophthisis (obliteration of the marrow space). Both myelofibrosis and osteopetrosis reduce effective hematopoietic space by deposition of fibrous connective tissue and bone, respectively. Myelofibrosis usually is secondary to bone marrow necrosis or neoplasia,[220, 221] and may be suspected upon finding abnormally shaped erythrocytes (elliptocytes, schizocytes, keratocytes, dacryocytes) within the blood smear. Osteopetrosis-associated pancytopenia has been reported in one dog.[222] Osteopetrosis is suspected when increased long bone density is observed on survey skeletal radiographs. Moderate to severe osteopetrosis can be produced experimentally in cats following feline leukemia virus inoculation, but neutropenia is not observed.[223]

Neoplastic and Myelodysplastic Diseases. Myelophthisis secondary to neoplastic involvement of the marrow cavity produces neutropenia sporadically. A variety of neoplastic or preneoplastic diseases may be involved including erythremic myelosis, large granular lymphoma, and megakaryocytic myelosis in cats as well as acute granulocytic leukemia, acute myelomonocytic leukemia, megakaryoblastic leukemia, myelodysplastic syndromes, acute lymphoblastic leukemia, and lymphosarcoma in dogs.[221, 224–233] In one study, neoplastic cells infiltrated the marrow cavity in 36 per cent of dogs with multicentric lymphosarcoma, but neutropenia was present in only 11 per cent of these animals.[233] However, approximately 85 per cent of the dogs with marrow infiltration will have some type of cytopenia.[233] A presumptive diagnosis of hematologic neoplasia is suggested by finding increased numbers of blast cells in the blood. The tentative diagnosis of neoplasia may be confirmed morphologically by bone marrow aspiration and/or core biopsy, but identification of the specific blast cell line may require cytochemical staining of blood and bone marrow smears. Myelodysplastic syndromes, on the other hand, are characterized by disturbed cellular maturation with or without an increase in blast cells.[234]

Disseminated Granulomatous Disease. Neutropenia or pancytopenia secondary to generalized granulomatous disease is rare, but has been associated with histoplasmosis infection in cats. Pancytopenia is secondary to advanced systemic disease with obliteration of normal marrow architecture by the inflammatory cell infiltrate.

Cyclic Stem Cell Input or Proliferation

Cyclic stem cell input is responsible for periodic failures of granulopoiesis or hematopoiesis in dogs and cats. The most profound laboratory abnormality is neutropenia and the most serious clinical consequence is development of infections during the nadir of neutropenia.

Canine Cyclic Hematopoiesis. Cyclic hematopoiesis is an hereditary stem cell disease of gray collie dogs.[235] Affected collies have a diluted haircoat color (silver-gray, beige, or charcoal) and usually die prematurely.[235] Without supportive care, the mortality rate of gray collie puppies is 67 per cent within the first week of life, with only 2 per cent of the puppies surviving for one year.[236] The syndrome is transmitted in an autosomal recessive manner and the gene has pleiotropic effects that influence both haircoat color and hematopoiesis.[235-237] Clinical signs are related to profound, cyclic neutropenia with subsequent development of recurrent, severe, life threatening infections.[235, 238-241] Predisposition to infection is enhanced by abnormalities in neutrophil bactericidal activity.[242] A 100 per cent incidence of amyloidosis exists in gray collies surviving 24 weeks or longer, and amyloid deposition is assumed to be secondary to repeated infections.[240] Amyloid is deposited in many tissues and may cause organ failure, most notably involving the kidney and liver, resulting in renal disease and coagulopathies.[239-241]

Hematologic findings in gray collies with inherited cyclic hematopoiesis are quite characteristic and begin within the first week of life.[243] Cyclic fluctuations of leukocytes (neutrophils, monocytes, lymphocytes, and eosinophils), reticulocytes, and platelets occur approximately every 11.5 days with cycle lengths ranging from 10 to 12.4 days.[235, 244, 245] The cycle length varies slightly between dogs, but is constant for all cellular elements in a given individual.[244]

Hematologic changes are most dramatic with respect to the neutrophil count, and profound neutropenia may be manifested by a total absence of circulating neutrophils.[235] Neutropenia lasts for two to four days, during which time the platelet, reticulocyte, and eosinophil counts peak successively.[235, 246] Monocytes, because of their short marrow transit time, reappear in the blood before neutrophils. Monocytosis develops rapidly, often "rebounding" above the reference interval with absolute counts approximating 20,000 monocytes/μl.[239] The neutrophil count also "rebounds" with absolute cell counts reaching 65,000 neutrophils/μl.[239, 246] The similar cycle length for leukocytes, reticulocytes, and platelets probably results from increased recruitment of pluripotential stem cells for a given cell line in time of need.[245] Stem cell recruitment for proliferation and differentiation undoubtedly is mediated through growth factors such as granulocyte-macrophage colony stimulating factor and erythropoietin which cycle in an inverse relationship to the neutrophil and reticulocyte counts, respectively.[247-249]

Hereditary canine cyclic hematopoiesis is a stem cell defect that can be reproduced or abrogated by bone marrow transplantation.[172, 248, 250] The molecular basis of the syndrome is unknown but may involve a derangement of purine and pyrimidine synthesis with increased intracellular production of deoxyribosylthymine triphosphate which may inhibit DNA synthesis and stem cell proliferation.[235, 251]

Clinical treatment of gray collies with cyclic hematopoiesis is unrewarding. With intensive antibiotic therapy and supportive care, affected dogs survive less than three years.[235] Both endotoxin injections and lithium carbonate administration (10 to 13 mg/lb or 21 to 26 mg/kg of body weight/day PO) will eliminate cyclic neutropenia.[235, 252-254] However, endotoxin has undesirable side effects including fever, chills, pain, and induction of shock, while lithium is highly toxic and must be monitored carefully. Bone marrow transplants are curative, but only have been done experimentally.[172]

Cyclic hematopoiesis may not be unique to gray collies and crossbred research dogs.[255] Cyclic hematopoiesis also has been observed in a cocker spaniel at the University of Georgia Veterinary Medical Teaching Hospital and in a Pomeranian.[256] The cocker spaniel had cyclic fluctuation of hematopoietic elements every 11 days. The Pomeranian had variable cycle lengths ranging from 10 to 29 days.[256] The hereditary nature of the cyclic hematopoiesis in these dogs was undetermined.

Cyclophosphamide-Induced Cyclic Neutropenia. Cyclic neutropenia can be produced in dogs following cyclophosphamide administration (0.7 to 1.7 mg/lb or 1.5 to 3.7 mg/kg of body weight/day PO).[257] Oscillation of the neutrophil count is apparent after the overall neutrophil count is depressed from one-third to one-half the normal count. The cycle length ranges from 11 to 13 days, and oscillation of the platelet count also may be observed.[257]

Feline Leukemia Virus Infection. Cyclic neutropenia has been observed in four feline leukemia virus–infected cats.[258, 259] Most of these cats presented with infections secondary to neutropenia. Neutrophil cycle lengths ranged from 8 to 16 days. In one cat, cycling of neutrophils, platelets, reticulocytes, and eosinophils was documented, while in another cat cycling of neutrophils, monocytes, reticulocytes, and platelets was noted.[258, 259] Oral prednisolone stopped the neutrophil cycling in two cats and was eventually decreased or withdrawn.[258, 259] Another cat stopped cycling spontaneously.[259] These reports suggest that cyclic neutropenia in feline leukemia virus–infected cats is the result of exaggerated oscillations of the negative feedback mechanism similar to cyclophosphamide-induced effects in dogs.[257]

Immune Suppression of Granulopoiesis

T-lymphocyte–mediated suppression of granulopoiesis exists in some people with neutropenia, and the success of clinical response to corticosteroid treatment can be predicted using *in vitro* bone marrow cultures.[260, 261] Although immune suppression of granulopoiesis has not been documented in animals, reports of steroid responsive neutropenias in dogs and cats suggest that this entity exists.[262, 263] As dog and cat bone marrow culture techniques become more routine, cases of idiopathic neutropenia may be shown to have an immune basis, and the ability to screen drugs singly and in combination *in vitro* should improve the probability of response to treatment.

Reduced Survival Neutropenia

Reduced survival neutropenia implies a shortened neutrophil lifespan. The shortened lifespan generally is associated with massive emigration of neutrophils from the blood vessels into the tissues, but may result from intravascular or intrasinusoidal sequestration or destruction of neutrophils. Neutrophil production and release from the bone marrow occur at a normal to accelerated rate, and the total blood neutrophil pool is decreased (Figure 114–14).[136, 137]

Increased Tissue Demand for Neutrophils. Neutropenia usually results from sudden, massive tissue utilization of neutrophils at a rate exceeding neutrophil replacement in the blood by the bone marrow.[2] Clinically, neutropenia is usually secondary to localized bacterial infections of the body cavities, lung, uterus, gastrointestinal tract, or secondary to generalized septicemia.[2, 6, 25, 26, 131, 150, 264, 265] Neutropenia in bacterial diseases such as salmonellosis partially results from endotoxemia which causes an immediate shift in neutrophils from the circulating to marginal neutrophil pool even though the total blood neutrophil pool may be unchanged initially.[130, 135–137, 264, 265] This pool shift of neutrophils is sometimes called "pseudoneutropenia."[136] Endotoxin also has the ability to activate the complement cascade, generating a fragment of the fifth component of complement (C5a) that promotes neutrophil aggregation. Cell sequestration occurs, especially in the pulmonary microvasculature, as leukoemboli lodge within capillaries or diminished blood flow favors neutrophil margination.[266–268] In addition, increased tissue uptake of neutrophils probably potentiates and intensifies the neutropenia of parvovirus, feline leukemia virus, and lentivirus infections. Severe infections are associated with severe, frequently degenerative, left shifts and toxic changes.

Immune-Mediated Neutropenia. The hematologic picture of immune-mediated leukopenia is persistent, profound neutropenia with a compensatory monocytosis. Other hematologic elements are unaffected, and bone marrow aspirates may range from hypocellular to hypercellular with an increased M:E ratio and depletion of mature neutrophils from the bone marrow storage pool.[269] In dogs and cats, a presumptive diagnosis of immune-mediated neutropenia may be made from characteristic hematologic findings, but confirmation of the diagnosis requires demonstration of antineutrophil antibodies in the serum or on neutrophils.[269] Demonstration of antineutrophil antibodies may be done by leukoagglutination or immunofluorescent techniques, with the latter test being more sensitive.[270] Antineutrophil antibodies generally are of the IgG class, may be complement dependent or independent, and usually act as leukoagglutinins. Following opsonization of the neutrophil cell membrane, the cells may be sequestered in the microvasculature and phagocytosed by macrophages in the spleen, liver, and lymph nodes.[269]

Clinical cases of immune-mediated neutropenia have yet to be documented in dogs and cats, although one dog with suspected leukoagglutination and partially steroid-responsive neutropenia has been reported.[262, 269] No attempt was made to demonstrate antineutrophil antibodies in this dog. Immune-mediated neutropenia has been produced experimentally to study the pathogenesis of urate crystal–induced joint disease and gingivitis in dogs and to study the effects of heterologous antineutrophil antibody administration in cats.[271–273] As antineutrophil antibody testing becomes more routine, reports of immune-mediated neutropenia in dogs and cats should be forthcoming.

Prognosis of Neutrophil Response Patterns

Certain neutrophil response patterns imply a guarded prognosis until a definitive diagnosis is established and/or an appropriate response to treatment is observed. Response patterns that initially warrant a guarded prognosis include: any form of neutropenia, a degenerative left shift with or without toxic change or maturation abnormalities, and a leukemoid response or extreme neutrophilic leukocytosis. A favorable response to medical or surgical treatment is indicated by return of the neutrophil count to the reference interval with concomitant resolution of left shifts, toxic change, and disturbed cellular maturation.

Neutrophil Functional Abnormalities

The ability of neutrophils to protect the body from infection by bacteria requires a complex, carefully orchestrated series of events involving both humoral factors and neutrophils (Figure 114–15).[274] When pathogenic bacteria invade the body and damage tissues, an interaction with plasma proteins and cells generates an array of chemotactic factors including complement products (C5a, C567), arachidonic acid metabolites (leukotriene B), kinin system derivatives (kallikrein), and fibrin split products (fibrinopeptide B).[274] Neutrophils

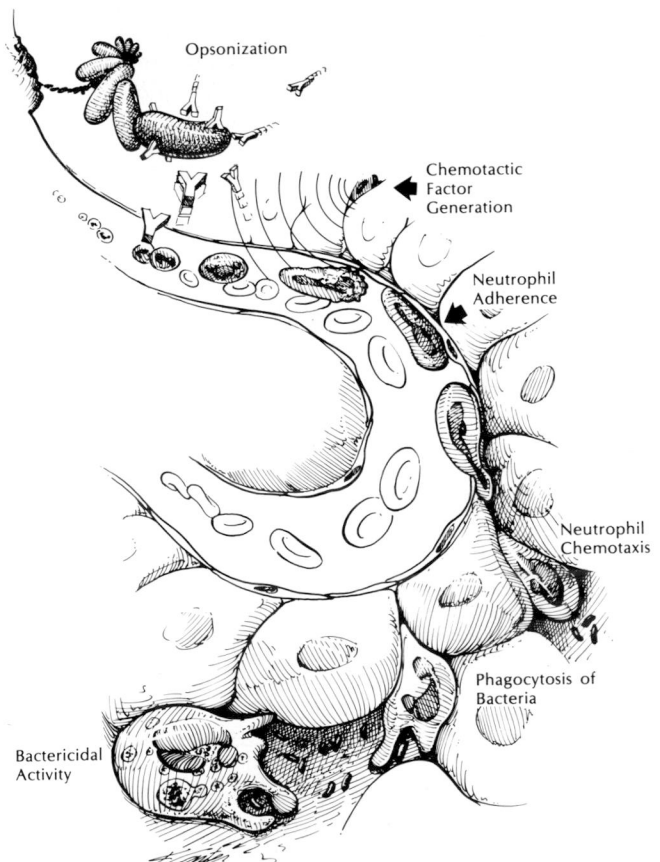

FIGURE 114–15. Schematic drawing illustrating the role of humoral factors and neutrophils in host defense against bacterial infection. Invading bacteria are opsonized with antibody and complement. Generation of chemotactic factor gradients promotes neutrophil adherence within and emigration from blood vessels. Neutrophils exhibit directional movement (chemotaxis) toward the source of the gradient and encounter bacteria which are phagocytosed and killed.

respond by adhering to the vascular endothelium and emigrating into the tissues.[58, 59, 274] Within the tissues, neutrophils exhibit chemotaxis or directional movement toward the source of the chemotactic milieu where opsonized (IgG and/or C3b-coated) bacteria are recognized and are phagocytosed.[58, 59, 274] During the phagocytic process there is an increase in oxygen consumption called the respiratory burst.[275, 276] The phagocytosed bacteria are contained within phagosomes (inverted membranous sacs) that fuse with the primary and secondary lysosomal granules to form phagolysosomes.[274] Granule constituents are expelled into the phagolysosomes and oxygen is reduced to form bactericidal toxic radicals. In the presence of adequate granule constituents and toxic radicals, bacterial killing and digestion occur rapidly.[274–276]

Abnormalities in chemotactic factor generation or in neutrophil adherence, chemotaxis, phagocytosis, or bacterial killing can predispose an animal to infection. Congenital abnormalities in neutrophil function should be suspected in any neonate that experiences severe, recurrent bacterial infections in the presence of a normal to markedly increased neutrophil count. Acquired deficiencies of neutrophil function also may occur in adults. Numerous instances of neutrophil dysfunction are described in human medicine,[59] but similar conditions are reported infrequently in dogs and cats (Table 114–6).[72, 77, 81, 111, 164, 165, 242, 277–291]

Major problems in documenting defective neutrophil function in animals include a lack of awareness of these problems and a lack of adequate laboratory facilities to test cell function in vitro. Limited neutrophil studies in dogs and cats usually have concentrated on one or two aspects of cellular function. More definitive information can be obtained by screening all major aspects of chemotactic factor generation and neutrophil function (adherence, chemotaxis, phagocytosis, and bacterial killing), and then performing refined testing to characterize specific abnormalities. Using this approach, multiple abnormalities of neutrophil function have been discerned in hyperalimentation-induced hypophosphatemia in dogs and in feline leukemia virus–infected cats.[282, 284] In addition, the specific molecular basis of defective neutrophil adherence and chemotaxis was established in one dog where deficiency of membrane glycoproteins was observed.[165]

Unfortunately, many bioassays of cell function are subject to great variability and may not detect subtle impairments in cell function.[292–294] The variations observed may be intensified by inflammation or infection and may be modified by drug administration.[292, 295] To minimize these effects, it is preferable to examine neutrophil function on the patient during periods of disease remission.[280] In addition, defective neutrophil function also may occur in myelodysplastic disorders.[296] Although specific therapy for basic defects in neutrophil function is rarely possible, diagnosis of neutrophil functional disorders allows the clinician to anticipate infections and plan the medical management of these complications in advance.[292]

The chemotactic properties of neutrophils also can be exploited clinically to identify sites of localized, acute inflammation such as abdominal abscesses. Neutrophils

TABLE 114–6. CONDITIONS ASSOCIATED WITH DEFECTIVE NEUTROPHIL FUNCTION IN DOGS AND CATS

Adherence	
Intrinsic cell defects	
Membrane glycoprotein deficiency	dog
Metabolic or nutritional disease	
Diabetes mellitus (poorly regulated)	dog
Chemotaxis	
Abnormal chemotactic factor generation	
Complement deficiency (C3)	dog
Cellular or chemotactic factor-directed inhibitors?	
Protothecosis	dog
Intrinsic cellular defects	
Pelger-Huët anomaly*	dog
Chediak-Higashi syndrome	cat
Membrane glycoprotein deficiency	dog
Infectious diseases	
Bacterial pyoderma	dog
Feline leukemia virus infection	cat
Metabolic or nutritional disease	
Hyperalimentation-induced hypophosphatemia	dog
Phagocytosis	
Intrinsic or opsonic defects	
Complement deficiency (C3)	dog
Metabolic or nutritional disease	
Hyperalimentation-induced hypophosphatemia	dog
Miscellaneous conditions	
Filtration leukopheresis-collected neutrophils	dog
Bacterial killing	
Intrinsic cellular defects	
Canine granulocytopathy syndrome	dog
Cyclic neutropenia	dog
Doberman pinschers	dog
Infectious diseases	
Feline leukemia virus infection	cat
Toxic diseases	
Lead intoxication	dog
Turpentine-induced toxic neutrophils	dog
Metabolic or nutritional disease	
Hyperalimentation-induced hypophosphatemia	dog

*Chemotactic deficits probably do not occur in canine Pelger-Huët anomaly.

are separated from blood, labeled with a gamma-emitting radioisotope (^{111}In-oxine), and reinfused into the patient. After allowing the neutrophils a suitable time period to localize within the lesions, abscesses are identified by gamma camera imaging.[297]

MONOCYTES

The monocyte-macrophage system is comprised of bipotential stem cells, monoblasts, and promonocytes in the bone marrow; monocytes in the bone marrow and blood; and macrophages in the tissues.[298] Blood monocytes can be envisioned as adolescent members of the monocyte-macrophage system which provide a replacement pool for various wandering and fixed tissue macrophages.[2] Cells of the monocyte-macrophage system have diverse functions including defense against infectious agents (bacteria, fungi, protozoa, and viruses), phagocytic removal of damaged or aged cells, elimination of virus-infected and tumor cells, and remodeling of tissues during growth and healing.[298] The secretory capabilities of macrophages are surpassed only by hepatocytes. Macrophage-derived secretory proteins include integral components or regulators of the complement, kinin, and hemostasis/fibrinolysis cascades. In addition, macrophages secrete interleukins that are involved in granulopoiesis, in immunomodulation by stimulating T-lymphocyte proliferation, and in production of fever.[65, 299, 300]

Morphology

Monocytes are the largest leukocytes in the blood of dogs and cats in health.[2] In dog blood smears, a smaller monocyte with a segmented-appearing nucleus occasionally may be observed. This cell closely resembles a neutrophil except for the presence of gray cytoplasm and pseudopodia.[6] The appearance of monocytes in Romanowsky-stained blood and bone marrow smears is somewhat variable, but common identifying features are presented in Table 114–1. Generally, mature monocytes have lobated, indented, or twisted nuclei, while less mature promonocytes have round to oval nuclei.[301]

Cytoplasmic vacuolation, consistently mentioned as an identifying feature of monocytes, is primarily an artifact of sample handling. If blood smears are prepared immediately, few vacuoles are observed within monocytes. Vacuoles are frequently observed in monocytes if the blood sample stands for several hours before smears are prepared.[2] Monocyte vacuolation, however, may be a feature of certain diseases such as sphingomyelinosis (Niemann-Pick disease) of Siamese cats and autoimmune hemolytic anemia of dogs wherein monocytic vacuolation may be associated with erythrophagia (Figure 114–16).[115, 302]

Intracytoplasmic inclusions of monocytes, similar to those described for neutrophils, may be observed in various diseases including canine distemper, canine ehrlichiosis, histoplasmosis, canine hepatozoonosis, and in transfused dogs with autoimmune hemolytic anemia (hemosiderin granules). Buffy coat smears may facilitate demonstration of some of these infectious agents.

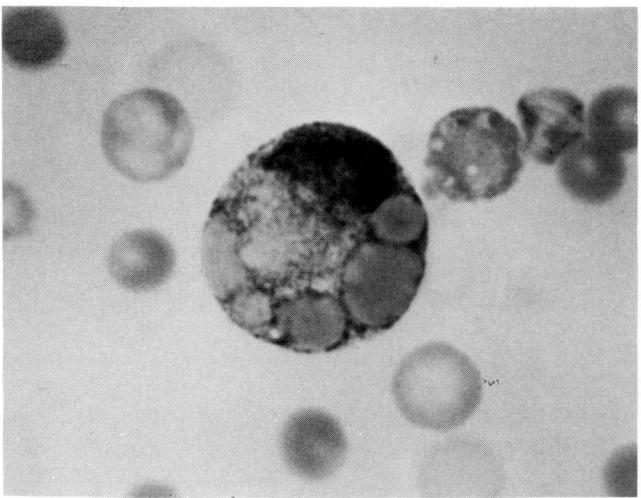

FIGURE 114–16. Monocyte with phagocytosed erythrocytes in a blood smear from a dog with autoimmune hemolytic anemia.

Production and Kinetics

Specific information concerning monocyte production and kinetics in dogs and cats is lacking. Drawing corollaries from other mammalian studies, monocytes share a committed bipotential stem cell with neutrophils (Figure 114–2).[42, 43] Low concentrations of granulocyte-macrophage colony stimulating factor favor production of monocytes by the bipotential stem cell.[120]

Approximately two to four mitoses occur between the monoblast and monocyte stages of development.[301] Monocytes have a very short marrow transit time of 1 to 2.5 days before entering the blood resulting in no appreciable marrow storage pool.[298, 301] At the time of bone marrow release, newly formed monocytes are equivalent in cell maturation to a neutrophil metamyelocyte.[2, 123] Despite the lack of a marrow storage pool, the monocyte proliferative capacity of the bone marrow is used only partially in health and may expand rapidly in disease.[301]

Monocytes rarely are identified in Romanowsky-stained bone marrow aspirates in health because of their rapid release into the circulation. In addition, early monocytes may be difficult to distinguish from granulocyte precursors in Romanowsky-stained marrow smears.[303] However, in diseases such as neutropenia with compensatory monocytosis, monocytic cells may be identified more easily in the bone marrow.

Monocytes are unevenly distributed in the blood. Similarly to neutrophils, the total blood monocyte pool can be divided into a circulating monocyte pool and a marginal monocyte pool. Cell distribution between the circulating and marginal pools in humans is in a 1:3.5 ratio, and, in contrast to neutrophils, this association is consistent in both health and disease.[304] Monocytes have a circulating half life of 8.4 hours, randomly leave the blood, and do not return to the circulation.[298, 304] In tissues, monocytes undergo a remarkable metamorphosis into macrophages, exemplified by changes in their ultrastructure, cell receptors and/or metabolism.[298, 305, 306] These macrophages may have an extended lifespan which ranges from days to months.[298]

Initial demands for monocytes in infection may be met partially by immediate release of monocytes and promonocytes from the bone marrow mitotic cell pool.[301] In addition to a shortened maturation time, more resting bipotential stem cells are recruited for monocyte production. As these cells proliferate, the cell cycle time is reduced by 44 per cent.[301] The end result is that many more monocytes are produced at a faster rate. Sustained monocytosis may be observed on the leukogram as the total blood monocyte pool is expanded. These blood monocytes are recruited to sites of tissue infection where they markedly increase macrophage numbers. Macrophages may undergo limited mitosis in situ, but local proliferation contributes minimally to the tissue macrophage pool.[298]

MONOCYTE RESPONSE PATTERNS

Monocytosis

The presence of greater than 1,350 monocytes/μl of blood in dogs and greater than 850 monocytes/μl of blood in cats is defined as monocytosis. Monocytosis is a common laboratory finding and is observed in approximately 31 per cent of the routine leukograms from hospitalized dogs and in approximately 11 per cent of the leukograms from hospitalized cats (Table 114–7).[2] Both acute and chronic diseases result in monocytosis, and most of the acute conditions are trauma-related injuries.[2] Disorders associated with suppuration, necrosis, malignancy, hemolysis, internal hemorrhage, pyogranulomatous inflammation, and immune-mediated diseases are accompanied by neutrophilia and concomitant monocytosis.[2, 148, 149] Monocytosis also occurs following corticosteroid injection, but is the least characteristic change in the leukogram.[2, 142, 143] The mechanism producing monocytosis following corticosteroid administration is unknown, but decreased cellular adherence with mobilization of the marginal monocyte pool is likely.[2] Recovery from leukopenia or cyclic neutropenia frequently is heralded by monocytosis because of the short marrow transit time.[239, 259] Rebound cell counts may peak at greater than 20,000 monocytes/μl in dogs with cyclic hematopoiesis, which could be mistaken for monocytic leukemia on the basis of one blood sample, especially if the dog is not a gray collie.[154, 239] Monocytosis commonly is accompanied by neutrophilia except in some unusual presentations of bacterial endocarditis and/or bacteremia in dogs wherein monocytosis may be the only or predominant change in the leukogram.[307, 308]

Monocytopenia

Because of the large range in monocyte counts, persistent monocytopenia is infrequently documented and clinically unimportant. In cases of pancytopenia, neutropenia has more severe clinical consequences and little attention is given to the alterations in monocyte numbers.

Disorders of the Monocyte-Macrophage System

Disorders of the monocyte-macrophage system include reactive monocytosis or granulomatous disease,

TABLE 114–7. DISEASES ASSOCIATED WITH MONOCYTOSIS* IN DOGS AND CATS

Infectious	
Bacterial endocarditis	dog
Bacteremia	dog
Suppuration, necrosis	dog, cat
Pyogranulomatous inflammation	dog, cat
Feline leukemia virus (cyclic)	cat
Acquired, noninfectious, nonneoplastic diseases	dog, cat
Hemorrhage, hemolysis	dog, cat
Immune-mediated diseases	dog, cat
Corticosteroid treatment	dog, cat
Trauma	dog, cat
Neutropenia w/ compensatory monocytosis	dog, cat
Congenital diseases	
Cyclic hematopoiesis	dog
Neoplastic diseases	
Nonspecific malignancies	dog
Monocytic leukemia	dog, cat
Myelomonocytic leukemia	dog, cat

*Monocytosis occurs in both acute and chronic diseases.

inborn errors of metabolism or lysosomal storage disease, and (myelo)monocytic leukemia.[309] Monocyte functional abnormalities also occur in people; however, the concomitant neutrophil functional abnormalities are more serious clinically.[310]

Hereditary disturbances of the monocyte-macrophage system in Bernese mountain dogs may present as a benign systemic histiocytosis or malignant histiocytosis.[311, 312] Malignant histiocytosis also has been described in other breeds of dogs, but the hereditary nature of the disease is undetermined.[313] These disease states are unaccompanied by specific changes in the leukogram although anemia may occur.[313, 314]

Inborn errors of metabolism are associated with cell or organ dysfunction secondary to lysosomal retention of intermediate metabolites that cannot be degraded. The leukogram is unchanged although rare changes in monocyte morphology may be apparent.[302]

Myelomonocytic and monocytic leukemia are described infrequently in dogs and cats, but the presence of extremely high cell counts and blasts in the blood make the diagnosis obvious.[154, 315] These neoplastic conditions are discussed under leukemias.

LYMPHOCYTES

Lymphocytes are the second most numerous leukocyte in the blood of dogs and cats in health.[6] These cells are essential in host defense and are major components of the immune system. Although lymphocytes may have a similar morphologic appearance on Romanowsky-stained preparations, their cellular functions may be quite diverse and are involved in both humoral and cell-mediated immune responses.[1, 40] Blood lymphocyte numbers are altered frequently and dramatically secondary to physiological states, various diseases, and drug administration.[35–37, 142, 143, 149, 150, 232, 233, 315] Diseases involving lymphocytes per se may have minimal effects on circulating lymphocyte numbers, but alterations in cell function may be profound. These unusual diseases are manifested by decreased resistance to infection by common environmental pathogens (immunodeficiency disorders) or by increased reactivity against self antigens (immune-mediated disorders).[316, 317]

Blood lymphocytes also are unique in that they recirculate and retain the ability to mitose.[1, 2, 6] Recirculation allows for recruitment of blood lymphocytes into the tissues in response to penetrating antigen and redistribution of sensitized lymphocytes throughout the body resulting in a generalized, logarithmic amplification of the immune response as lymphocytes proliferate following local antigen exposure.[318]

Morphology

Identifying features of blood lymphocytes are in Table 114–1. Although small, medium, and large lymphocytes can be observed on stained blood smears, cell size is more of a continuum than trimodal.[2, 6, 25, 40, 319] Variation in cell size relates to both the metabolic activity and the degree of flattening of the cells on the blood smear.[2, 25] In addition, lymphocytes will swell if blood smear preparation is delayed for a few hours after the sample is drawn.

Generally, T- and B-lymphocytes in the peripheral blood cannot be differentiated by routine light microscopy. Identification of lymphocyte subpopulations requires demonstration of cell-associated immunoglobulin, cell membrane receptors or antigens, and assays of cell function. In Romanowsky-stained smears lymphocytes appear relatively homogeneous in health. Antigenically stimulated lymphocytes termed immunocytes (atypical lymphocytes, plasmacytoid cells) occasionally may be observed in low numbers within the blood smear in health. These cells are recognized readily by their large size and vivid royal blue cytoplasm (Table 114–1; Figure 114–17) and are classified as lymphocytes on the differential count. Increased numbers of these cells may be observed following routine immunizations, infection, or other instances of antigenic stimulation.[2, 6, 320–322]

Rarely, two specific lymphocyte subtypes may be observed in blood and buffy coat smears in health. These cells are plasma cells, the ultimate expression of a B-lymphocyte, and large granular lymphocytes or natural killer cells, which are null cells. Plasma cells may be found more readily in buffy coat smears than in routine blood smears, and are identified by their eccentric nucleus with coarse clumped chromatin and abundant dark blue cytoplasm that sometimes has a pale-staining Golgi zone. Natural killer cells have distinctive azurophilic granules that often are clustered at the nuclear indentation.[323]

Morphologic changes of lymphocytes may be apparent in some diseases. Intracytoplasmic inclusions may be present within lymphocytes in canine distemper virus infection or in canine ehrlichiosis (see neutrophils). In sphingomyelinosis (Niemann-Pick disease) of Siamese cats, lymphocytes may appear vacuolated.[302] Lymphoblasts are large lymphocytes with finely stippled chromatin, multiple nucleolar rings, and an obvious rim of dark blue cytoplasm. These cells, rarely observed in health, should arouse suspicion of lymphoid neoplasia

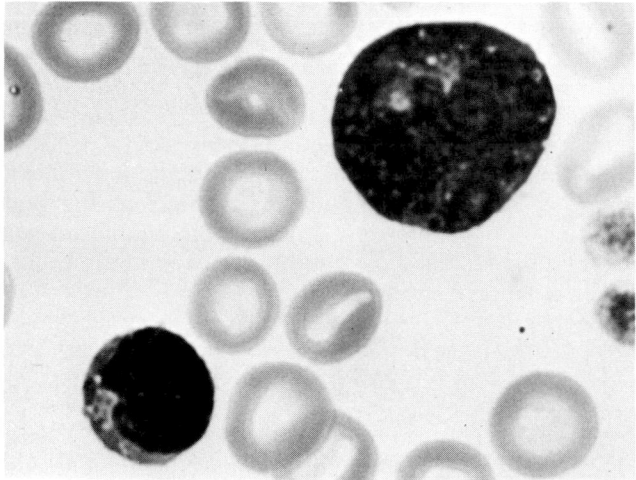

FIGURE 114–17. A small lymphocyte and immunocyte in the blood smear from a dog following recent vaccination. The immunocyte is larger and has a scalloped nuclear margin and dark cytoplasm.

when present in increased numbers on the blood smear.[319]

Production, Recirculation, and Kinetics

Lymphopoiesis. Development of the lymphoid (immune) system begins during early fetal development and is essentially complete in puppies and kittens at birth.[324, 325] The lymphoid system is complex and diverse, with the total body lymphocyte pool distributed among the bone marrow, thymus, lymph nodes, spleen, GALT (tonsils and Peyer's patches), BALT, and blood.[26, 318] The blood, a transit system for lymphocyte distribution and recirculation, contains less than five per cent of the total body lymphocyte pool in health.[1]

Continued lymphopoiesis in neonates and adults is dependent upon pluripotential stem cells within the bone marrow and, to a lesser extent, the blood.[44] Within the bone marrow, lymphoid stem cells diverge from pluripotential stem cells at an early stage of development (Figure 114–2).[42, 43] Progeny of the proliferating lymphoid stem cells are predestined to become T-lymphocytes, B-lymphocytes, and probably null cells (non-T, non-B lymphocytes).[43]

Pre-T-lymphocytes migrate from the bone marrow to the thymus in the blood (Figure 114–18). Within the thymus, a central lymphoid organ, these unsensitized lymphocytes proliferate and mature to T-lymphocytes under the influence of epithelial cell-derived hormones such as thymosin.[326] Following initial maturation, T-cells migrate from the thymus to peripheral lymphoid organs (lymph nodes, spleen, GALT, and BALT) localizing in the splenic periarteriolar lymphatic sheaths and paracortical areas of various lymphoid tissues. Further T-lymphocyte migration in the blood allows these cells to infiltrate virtually all tissues to which lymphocytes have access.[318]

T-lymphocytes are a heterogeneous population of cells defined by specific effector or memory functions. Effector functions are triggered by exposure to antigen and are accomplished by direct cell-cell interactions or indirect cell-cell interactions mediated by T-lymphocyte secretory products called lymphokines.[326] T-lymphocyte effector functions include a helper activity on induction of B-lymphocyte proliferation, differentiation, and antibody synthesis in response to thymus-dependent antigens; helper/inducer activities on other T-lymphocytes, macrophages, and hematopoietic cells mediated by lymphokines; cytolytic activity against infected cells (bacteria, viruses, protozoa, and fungi), transformed (neoplastic) cells, or transplanted cells; modulation of immune reactions as suppressor cells that diminish T- and B-lymphocyte activities; and production of memory cells for future response to specific antigens.[1, 326, 327] These various T-lymphocyte effector functions collectively are termed cell-mediated immune responses.

Pre-B-lymphocytes mature to B-lymphocytes within the bone marrow (Figure 114–18). In mammals the bone marrow acts as a central lymphoid tissue for B-lymphocyte production and maturation analogous to the bursa of Fabricius in birds. Mature B-lymphocytes migrate in the blood from the bone marrow to the peripheral

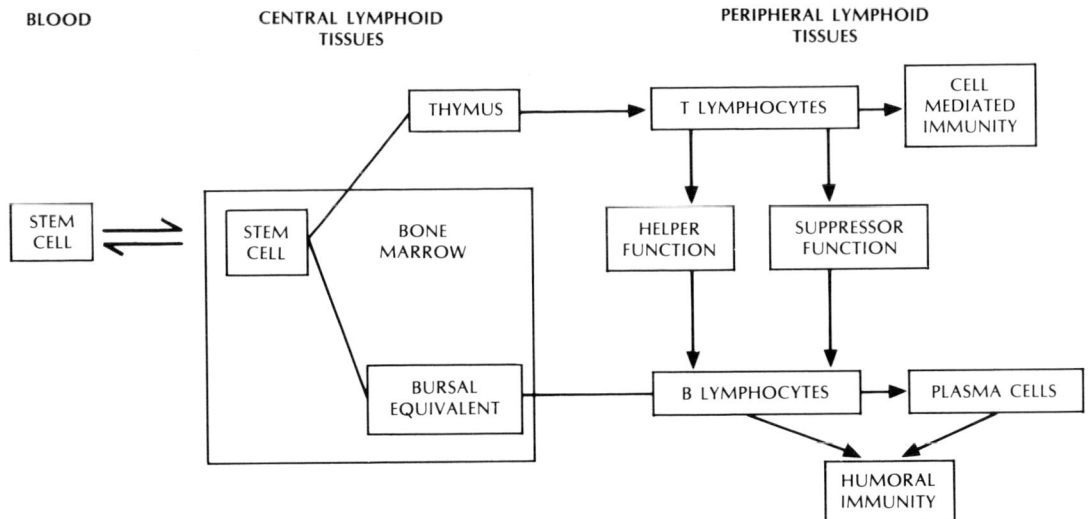

FIGURE 114–18. Schematic diagram depicting the development of the lymphoid system and the interaction of T- and B-lymphocytes. (Modified from Boggs, DR and Winkelstein, A: White Cell Manual, 4th ed. Philadelphia, FA Davis, 1983.)

lymphoid tissues and populate the subcapsular sinuses, germinal centers, and medullary cords of these tissues and lymphoid follicles throughout the body.[318] Antigen exposure triggers B-lymphocyte proliferation and differentiation into functional plasma cells and antigen-specific memory cells. Plasma cells are found primarily within the secondary lymphoid tissues and, to a lesser extent, in skin and other diseased tissues.[318] Plasma cells manufacture and secrete antibodies which are classified collectively by type as immunoglobulins.[1] Immunoglobulins function in humoral immunity to neutralize viruses and toxins, opsonize encapsulated bacteria for subsequent phagocytic removal, and hyperacute rejection of transplanted tissues.[1]

Null cells are presumed to be of lymphoid lineage and include precursor cells, natural killer cells (large granular lymphocytes), and killer cells. Recent evidence suggests that natural killer and killer cells are similar or identical. These cells function in cytolytic reactions by spontaneous lysis of target cells or by antibody-dependent cellular cytotoxicity.[1, 323]

Lymphocyte Lifespan. Because lymphocytes retain the ability to transform and divide, the cell lifespan may be defined as the intermitotic interval or the timespan from the last mitosis until cell death.[7] Generally, B-lymphocytes have a short lifespan ranging from days to weeks while T-lymphocytes have a lifespan of months to years. However, both B- and T-lymphocyte memory cells have a prolonged lifespan. The total body lymphocyte pool remains relatively constant in health because most of the lymphocytes produced are short-lived.[318, 328]

Blood Lymphocytes. Although some lymphocytes are released into the circulation from the thymus and bone marrow, most of the blood lymphocytes originate from the peripheral lymphoid organs.[21, 326] Blood lymphocytes can generally be described as small-sized, recirculating, long-lived, memory T- lymphocytes.[1, 318, 328, 329] The distribution of blood lymphocyte populations in dogs and cats is 50 to 74 per cent T-lymphocytes, 18 to 34 per cent B-lymphocytes, and 8 to 16 per cent null cells.[329, 330]

Recirculation and Kinetics. The recirculating lymphocyte population is composed of small long-lived T- and B-lymphocytes contained within the blood, lymphatics, and peripheral lymphoid tissues.[7] Recirculation generally is non-random in that lymphocytes return preferentially to the tissues from which they were derived. This "homing" response is probably mediated by receptors on both lymphocytes and endothelial cells that promote cell adhesion and extravasation.[331] Both the lymphocyte subtype and tissue affect the recirculation time. Generally, B-lymphocytes recirculate more slowly than T-lymphocytes, and cell migration through the lymph nodes is much slower (15 to 20 hours) than cell migration through the spleen (5 to 6 hours).[7, 332] The major lymphocyte recirculation route begins as blood lymphocytes migrate from the venules into the lymphoid tissues. After a variable period of time within the tissues, the lymphocytes enter the efferent lymphatics, the thoracic duct, and reenter the blood.[7, 318, 331, 332] Evidence also exists for lymphocyte recirculation from blood into lymph nodes with direct reentry into the blood. This recirculation route may be more important in disease states where increased numbers of lymphocytes enter the lymph nodes through the afferent lymphatics.[331] The usual recirculation pattern of lymphocytes also may be altered in various disease states.

LYMPHOCYTE RESPONSE PATTERNS

Lymphocytosis

Lymphocytosis is the presence of greater than 4,800 lymphocytes/μl of blood in dogs and greater than 7,000 lymphocytes/μl of blood in cats. Causes of lymphocytosis are listed in Table 114–8.

Physiologic Lymphocytosis. Transient lymphocytosis, a feature of physiologic leukocytosis in dogs and cats, occurs more frequently in young animals and is more dramatic in the cat. In this species, elevations in

TABLE 114–8. CONDITIONS ASSOCIATED WITH LYMPHOCYTOSIS AND LYMPHOPENIA IN DOGS AND CATS

Lymphocytosis

Physiologic (epinephrine response)	dog, cat
Antigenic stimulation (various etiologies)	
Blastomycosis	dog
Chronic canine ehrlichiosis	dog
Chronic Rocky Mountain spotted fever	dog
Feline leukemia virus infection	cat
Lymphoid neoplasia	
Lymphosarcoma	dog, cat
Lymphocytic leukemia (acute and chronic)	dog, cat
Thymoma	dog, cat
Hypoadrenocorticism (Addison's disease)	dog

Lymphopenia

Immunosuppressive drugs and/or radiation	dog, cat
Corticosteroid-induced	
Exogenous corticosteroids or ACTH	dog, cat
Endogenous corticosteroid release	
Acute stress	dog, cat
Hyperadrenocorticism (Cushing's disease)	dog, cat
Acute systemic infection (various etiologies)	
Canine parvovirus	dog
Canine coronavirus	dog
Canine distemper	dog
Infectious canine hepatitis	dog
Feline panleukopenia	cat
Septicemia/endotoxemia	dog, cat
Loss of lymphocyte-rich lymph	
Chylothorax (ruptured thoracic duct)	dog, cat
Effusion of cardiac disease	cat
Protein losing enteropathy	dog
Lymphangiectasia	dog
Ulcerative enteritis	dog, cat
Granulomatous enteritis	dog, cat
Alimentary lymphosarcoma	dog, cat
Enteric neoplasms	dog, cat
Disruption of lymph node architecture	
Multicentric lymphosarcoma	dog, cat
Generalized granulomatous disease	dog, cat
T-lymphocyte deficiency	
Acquired (neonatal infection)	
Canine distemper	dog
Feline leukemia virus infection (fading kitten syndrome)	cat
Congenital	dog
Combined immunodeficiency (Basset hound)	

the lymphocyte count occasionally may be profound and exceed 24,000 lymphocytes/μl.[6] The precise mechanism resulting in lymphocytosis is unknown but probably involves epinephrine release. Possible explanations for the abrupt increase in lymphocyte numbers include facilitated release of recirculating lymphocytes from the thoracic duct and/or impaired recirculation secondary to alterations in cell receptor sites on lymphocytes and endothelial cells. Physiologic lymphocytosis may be avoided if dogs and cats are not forcibly restrained or frightened during venipuncture, or if the animals are acclimated to the procedure.[2, 6, 38] In clinical practice, resolution of physiologic lymphocytosis usually can be demonstrated by resampling the calmed or tranquilized patient six to eight hours later. Resampling, therefore, provides an easy method to distinguish marked lymphocytosis resulting from physiologic responses (transient lymphocytosis) and lymphocytic leukemia (persistent lymphocytosis).

Lymphocytosis Secondary to Chronic Antigenic Stimulation. Lymphocytosis occasionally is seen in dogs and cats with chronic infectious diseases or inflammatory lesions. Persistent antigen induces lymphocyte proliferation with expansion of the blood lymphocyte pool in some instances. Examples of persistent antigen-associated lymphocytosis include blastomycosis, chronic ehrlichiosis, and chronic Rocky Mountain spotted fever in dogs and feline leukemia virus–associated peripheral lymph node hyperplasia in cats.[217, 333–335] In some mature dogs with chronic canine ehrlichiosis, the absolute lymphocyte counts reach 10,200 cells/μl, suggesting a possible diagnosis of lymphocytic leukemia.[217] This lymphocytosis secondary to antigenic stimulation may coexist with hypergammaglobulinemia. Serum protein electrophoresis usually demonstrates a polyclonal gammopathy; however, monoclonal gammopathy also may occur.[217]

Lymphoid Neoplasia. Lymphoid neoplasia in dogs and cats may cause lymphocytosis. Lymphosarcoma, a proliferation of solid tissue masses, is the most frequent neoplasm with lymphocytosis. Approximately 11 per cent of dogs and 27 per cent of cats with lymphosarcoma will have lymphocytosis characterized by immature or atypical lymphocytes on the blood smear.[233, 336] Lymphoid leukemia, an initial proliferation of neoplastic cells in the bone marrow and blood, is observed less frequently. In leukemia, however, leukocytosis may be profound with cell counts reaching 54,000 cells/μl. In acute lymphoblastic leukemia the blood lymphocytes may appear immature, while in chronic lymphocytic leukemia the lymphocytes may appear small and well differentiated.[232, 337] In the latter instance, extremely high lymphocyte counts (23,000 to greater than 100,000 cells/μl) suggest a diagnosis of chronic lymphocytic leukemia.[337] The diagnosis is confirmed by bone marrow biopsy.

Hypoadrenocorticism. Lymphocytosis, reportedly a consistent feature of hypoadrenocorticism (Addison's disease) in dogs, is present in only 11 to 20 per cent of diseased dogs.[338, 339] However, the lack of lymphopenia in a stressed animal would increase the suspicion of glucocorticoid deficiency.[339]

Lymphopenia

Lymphopenia is designated as less than 1,000 lymphocytes/μl of blood in dogs and less than 1,500 lymphocytes/μl of blood in cats. Causes of lymphopenia are listed in Table 114–8.

Corticosteroid-Associated Lymphopenia. Both exogenous administration of corticosteroids or ACTH and endogenous corticosteroid release will cause transient, predictable lymphopenia in dogs and cats. Short-term corticosteroid exposure produces a rapid lymphopenia by redistributing circulating lymphocytes to the bone marrow or other body compartments.[147, 340] Lymphocyte redistribution involves primarily T-lymphocytes (the major type of recirculating lymphocyte), but is not selective for T-lymphocyte subtypes.[340, 341]

Following a single dose of corticosteroids or ACTH, lymphopenia is observed within four to six hours and cell counts return to baseline within 24 hours.[6, 142, 143, 340] Similar changes occur with alternate-day corticosteroid administration.[342] With daily corticosteroid treatment, the lymphocyte count may remain depressed until drug withdrawal, after which cell counts return to baseline within 48 to 72 hours.[142] This situation is analogous to severe stress with acute diseases except that recovery from disease is heralded by a rising lymphocyte count. Although changes in the neutrophil count may diminish with long-term corticosteroid exposure, lymphopenia will almost always be a feature of the leukogram as can be observed in dogs with hyperadrenocorticism.[145] Lymphopenia due to corticosteroid-induced lysis of lymphocytes or depletion of lymphoid tissues occurs only with high drug doses over a prolonged period of time.[343]

Lymphopenia in Acute Infection. Several mechanisms may be involved in producing lymphopenia during an acute infection. Stress-associated endogenous corticosteroid release promotes redistribution of lymphocytes.[340] The presence of antigen (infectious agents) may cause trapping of cells within lymphoid tissues. Following antigen exposure, blood flow to the lymph nodes increases, resulting in increased emigration or recruitment of circulating lymphocytes into these tissues. Temporary obstruction of efferent lymph outflow blocks lymphocyte recirculation, resulting in lymphopenia.[331, 332] Lastly, infectious agents such as canine distemper, feline leukemia virus, and parvovirus can result in atrophy and/or destruction of lymphoid tissue.[200, 344, 345]

Loss, Sequestration, or Blockage of Lymphocyte-Rich Lymph. Lymphopenia also may occur secondary to reduction of the recirculating lymphocyte population. Loss of lymphocyte-rich afferent lymph into the intestinal lumen occurs in some instances of protein-losing enteropathy.[346] In chylothorax, recirculating lymphocytes in efferent lymph can be sequestered in the thoracic cavity.[347, 348] Lastly, blockage of afferent and/or efferent lymph flow may occur with lymphangiectasia, disseminated granulomatous inflammation, or neoplasia.[26, 349, 350] In these instances, lymphatic channels either fail to form (lymphangiectasia) or are occluded by inflammatory cell infiltration or tumor cell emboli.

EOSINOPHILS

Eosinophils are recognized by their bright red-orange granules in Romanowsky-stained blood and bone marrow smears. Although eosinophils are present in relatively low numbers within the blood, these cells are important components of the host defense system within the tissues. Primary functions of eosinophils include destruction of parasites and modulation of hypersensitivity reactions; however, these two functions are not always clearly separable.[351–353]

Both helminth parasites and other particulate antigens can provoke hypersensitivity reactions. Exposure to these antigens can induce plasma cells to produce IgE, and this cytophilic antibody attaches to mast cell membrane receptors in various tissues. Re-exposure to the sensitizing antigen can cause mast cell perturbation and degranulation with the release of chemotactic substances for eosinophils. Eosinophils subsequently are recruited from the blood into the tissues in response to the hypersensitivity reaction.[352]

Parasite killing by eosinophils is enhanced by opsonization with antibody (IgG) and/or complement.[354] The eosinophils attach to opsonized organisms and degranulate, releasing major basic protein and peroxidase. Major basic protein damages the surface of the parasite, and peroxidase generates toxic oxygen products which probably assist in the killing process.[352]

Evidence for eosinophil modulation of immune reactions is derived from *in vitro* studies demonstrating that these cells can dampen the effects of mast cells. Specifically, eosinophils can: phagocytose extruded mast cell granules, inactivate the slow reacting substance of anaphylaxis (leukotrienes C4, D4, and E4) with arylsulfatase B, degrade histamine with histaminase, inactivate platelet activating factor with phospholipase D, and neutralize heparin with major basic protein.[351–353] Indiscriminate tissue damage by eosinophils may occur in various hypersensitivity reactions as major basic protein and peroxidase are released. Resulting tissue damage may be localized as in allergic pneumonitis or widespread as in idiopathic hypereosinophilia.[351–353, 355, 356]

Morphology

Eosinophils are first recognized in the bone marrow at the myelocyte stage of development when red-orange specific granules may be observed in Romanowsky-stained preparations. In blood and bone marrow smears the intracytoplasmic granules are bright red-orange, but in tissue aspirates the granules may have a dull, muddy, red-brown appearance. Dog eosinophils have a moderate number of variably sized round granules while cat eosinophils have numerous rod-shaped granules. Greyhounds occasionally have "moth-eaten," vacuolated, or degranulated eosinophils in health.[6] Degranulated eosinophils, although rare, are seen more commonly in disease, especially in dirofilariasis, allergic reactions, and hypereosinophilic syndromes (Figure 114–19E).[357] In

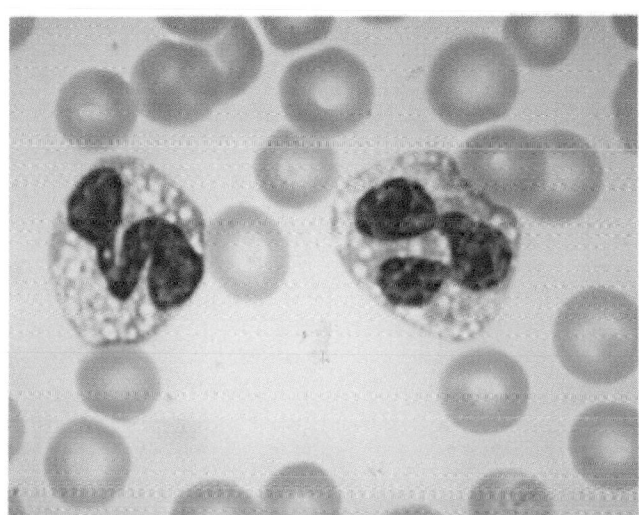

FIGURE 114–19. A pair of degranulated eosinophils from a dog with heartworm disease.

Persian cats with Chediak-Higashi syndrome, eosinophil granules may appear plump or enlarged.[107]

Production and Kinetics

Eosinophils are produced in the bone marrow from eosinophil colony-forming units under the influence of eosinophilopoietin, a T-lymphocyte lymphokine.[351, 353] The total marrow transit time for eosinophil production in humans is approximately three days,[353] but the transit times for dogs and cats are unknown. Development of eosinophils and neutrophils is similar, including the presence of a bone marrow storage pool.[353]

Eosinophil release from the bone marrow is facilitated by a humoral substance called eosinophil releasing factor. Within the blood, eosinophils may be unevenly distributed in circulating and marginal pools, and evidence exists that a minor degree of cell recirculation may occur. The eosinophil circulating half-life in humans is variable, ranging from 2 to 12 hours in various studies, and cells leave the blood in a random manner.[353] A similar situation is presumed to exist in dogs and cats, but precise figures are undetermined. Although the canine eosinophil circulating half-life has been quoted as being 30 minutes,[6] this value probably is inaccurate. This figure was obtained from a single cross transfusion experiment between two dogs using Pelger-Huët cells as a biological tracer and has not been corroborated.[358]

Following a brief sojourn in the blood, eosinophils migrate into the tissues and localize primarily in subepithelial sites in the skin, respiratory tract, gastrointestinal tract, and genitourinary tract.[353] An increased influx of these cells may be present in the female genitourinary tract depending upon the stage of the reproductive cycle. This effect is mediated by estrogen receptors. Eosinophils may function for several days within the tissues after which they may be removed by the monocyte-macrophage system or lost from the body following epithelial transmigration.[353]

EOSINOPHIL RESPONSE PATTERNS

Eosinophilia

Eosinophilia is defined as greater than 750 eosinophils /μl of blood in dogs and cats. Some causes of eosinophilia in these species are presented in Table 114–9.

Parasitism. Eosinophilia is associated frequently with parasitism, especially with nematodes that undergo tissue migration. T-lymphocytes play an important role in the production and maintenance of sustained eosinophilia. This lymphocyte-eosinophil interaction is analogous to the generation of an immune response in that a delayed onset of eosinophilia occurs with the first exposure to antigen. The second exposure to the same antigen produces a more dramatic and rapid eosinophilia, an antigen-specific memory response.[351, 353]

Inflammation and/or Hypersensitivity Reactions. Inflammatory lesions of the skin, gastrointestinal tract, lungs, and genitourinary tract can result in eosinophilia

presumably because of mast cell degranulation and subsequent chemoattraction of eosinophils. A paradox exists, however, in that local lesions may have massive eosinophil infiltration in the absence of peripheral blood eosinophilia. Tissue eosinophilia may result from basophil or mast cell degranulation, complement-derived chemotactic factors, lymphokine and vasoactive amine synthesis and/or release, and deposition of immune complexes within the tissues.[353]

Hypereosinophilic Syndromes and Tumor-Associated Eosinophilia. Idiopathic hypereosinophilic syndromes are characterized by persistent eosinophilia, an unknown etiology, and cellular infiltration of various tissues.[359] These syndromes are seen most frequently in cats and are difficult, if not impossible, to distinguish from eosinophilic leukemia.[360–365] Both diseases are associated with profound eosinophilia and extensive tissue infiltration. Fatal hypereosinophilic syndromes in humans are associated with infiltrative organ dysfunction.[359]

Tumor-associated eosinophilia in humans is most often associated with carcinomas arising from mucin-secreting epithelium (bronchus, gut, pancreas, or uterus), but also may accompany sarcomas, lymphomas, and leukemias.[353, 366–368] Waxing and waning of the eosinophilia may accompany periods of tumor relapse and remission during surgical or chemotherapy treatments.[366, 367] Mechanisms of tumor-associated eosinophilia have not been studied extensively. A tumor-derived eosinophilopoietic polypeptide was isolated from one human patient with an anaplastic pulmonary large-cell carcinoma.[367] Also, the association between lymphoid neoplasms and eosinophilia in people and cats suggests that these neoplasms may elaborate lymphokines.[2, 366]

Eosinopenia

Eosinopenia is best defined by experience in a clinical setting when using reference intervals, and usually presents as one component of a stress leukogram (neutrophilia, lymphopenia, eosinopenia, and monocytosis). To obtain precise data on cell numbers in eosinopenic states, absolute eosinophil counts should be done with a hemacytometer and an eosin-based diluent. This procedure is used most frequently in dogs with hyperadrenocorticism to monitor the response to op'DDD treatment.[6]

Corticosteroid-Associated Eosinopenia. Exogenous corticosteroid or ACTH administration produces rapid eosinopenia. With a single dose of corticosteroids or ACTH, eosinopenia will occur within one to six hours depending upon the drug dosage and route of administration. Cell counts subsequently return to baseline within 12 to 24 hours.[6, 142, 143] Eosinophils are not destroyed by these drugs but are sequestered in the vascular bed, probably within the marginal cell pool.[369]

Bone marrow effects of corticosteroid administration depend upon the dosage and duration of drug treatment. Brief drug exposure produces no visible effect on eosinophilopoiesis. Short-term corticosteroid administration (1.5 to 12 days) is associated with increased numbers of

TABLE 114–9. SOME CONDITIONS ASSOCIATED WITH EOSINOPHILIA AND EOSINOPENIA IN DOGS AND CATS

Eosinophilia		*Spirocerca lupi*	dog
Hypersensitivity and/or inflammatory lesions		*Trichinella spiralis*	cat
Alimentary tract		*Trichuris vulpis*	dog
Oral granulomas	dog	Trematodes	
Gastroenteritis (ulcerative)	dog, cat	*Heterobilharzia americana*	dog
Intestinal eosinophilic granulomas	dog	*Paragonimus kellicotti*	cat
Genitourinary tract		*Platynosomum concinnum*	cat
Pyometra	dog	Insects	
Musculoskeletal system		Fleas	dog, cat
Myositis (poorly documented)	dog	Trombiculosis	cat
Panosteitis (rare)	dog	Protozoa	
Respiratory tract		*Hepatozoon canis*	dog
Pulmonary granulomas (heartworm-related ?)	dog	Feline leukemia virus–associated	
Pulmonary infiltrates with eosinophilia	dog	Cyclic hematopoiesis	cat
Skin and special senses		Leukemoid reaction	cat
Atopy	cat	Neoplasia-associated	
Canine eosinophilic granuloma	dog	Eosinophilic leukemia/hypereosinophilic syndrome	cat
Eosinophilic keratitis	cat	Paraneoplastic syndrome	
Feline eosinophilic granuloma complex	cat	Fibrosarcoma	dog
Flea allergy dermatitis	dog, cat	Lymphosarcoma	cat
Food hypersensitivity	cat	Mammary carcinoma	dog
Sterile eosinophilic pustulosis	dog	Mast cell neoplasia (disseminated)	dog
Parasites		Miscellaneous conditions	
Nematodes		Hypoadrenocorticism (unpredictable)	dog
Aelurostrongylus abstrusus	cat	**Eosinopenia**	
Ascarids	dog	Acute infection	dog, cat
Dipetalonema reconditum	dog	Endogenous corticosteroid release	
Dirofilaria immitis	dog, cat	Acute stress (various causes)	dog, cat
Hookworms	dog	Hyperadrenocorticism	dog, cat
Ollulanus tricuspis?	cat	Drug administration	
Oslerus (Filaroides) osleri	dog	ACTH	dog, cat
Pentastoma	dog	Corticosteroids	dog, cat
Physaloptera sp	dog		

eosinophils in the bone marrow secondary to delayed marrow release of these cells. With prolonged high-dose corticosteroid treatment, eosinophil production is decreased.[369] Eosinopenia associated with corticosteroid therapy may, therefore, be a combination of vascular sequestration and impaired bone marrow release of these cells.[250]

Eosinopenia also may be observed with endogenous corticosteroid release which occurs with acute stress or hyperadrenocorticism.[2, 6, 145, 370, 371] Hematologic changes may be identical to those produced by drug administration.

Eosinopenia of Acute Infection. Classically, the eosinopenia of acute infection has been attributed to endogenous corticosteroid release, but this assumption has not been supported by determination of blood steroid levels. The precise mechanism of eosinopenia remains unknown, but cell margination within blood vessels or emigration into the tissues is postulated.[369]

BASOPHILS

Basophils are the least numerous leukocyte in the blood of healthy dogs and cats but, nonetheless, have important functions in host defense. These functions include: participation in immune-mediated inflammatory reactions such as anaphylaxis and cutaneous hypersensitivity; both prevention (heparin release) and promotion (basophil kallikrein-like activity) of hemostasis; involvement in plasma lipolysis (heparin activates lipoprotein lipase); rejection of parasites, especially ticks;

and possible tumor cytotoxicity.[372–381] Basophil activity may be mediated by T-lymphocytes, especially in hypersensitivity reactions.[373, 382]

Basophils are infrequently observed in blood smears from dogs and cats in health, and account for less than two per cent of the leukocyte differential count when present. Generally, only sustained, overt basophilia can be detected by routine hematologic methods wherein basophils constitute at least three to six per cent of the differential count.[381] Precise determination of basophil numbers in human medicine requires an absolute basophil count using a hemacytometer and alcohol-based toluidine blue stain.[376] With this technique, the limits of basophilia (greater than 80 cells/µl) and basopenia (less than 10 cells/µl) have been defined clearly.[383] Similar studies have not been done in dogs and cats.

Morphology

In dogs, basophils are slightly larger than neutrophils and have a lobulated or "twisted ribbon" appearance of the nucleus. Cytoplasmic granules are rounded, variably sized, and widely scattered (Figure 114–20*A*). Cat basophils also are larger than neutrophils and have a nuclear morphology as described for dogs. Cytoplasmic granules are numerous, round, and uniformly sized. On Romanowsky-stained blood smears, feline basophil granules usually lack metachromasia and stain a grayish to mauve color (Figure 114–20*B*). Medical technicians in human hospital laboratories fail to recognize normal cat basophils during the differential count because of their unique tinctorial property. Metachromatic gran-

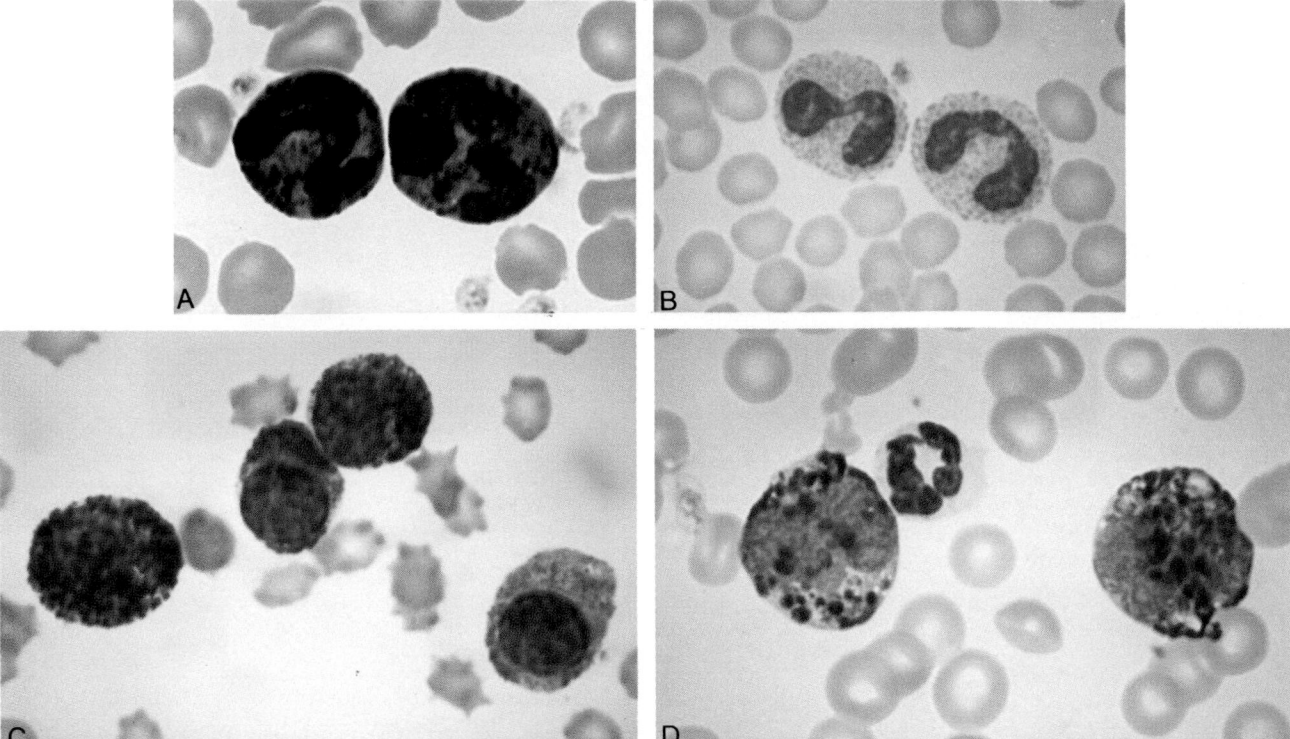

FIGURE 114–20. Differentiation of mast cells and basophils in dog and cat blood smears. *A,* A pair of canine basophils with small, scattered specific (metachromatic) granules. *B,* A pair of basophils from a cat with Pelger-Huët anomaly showing nuclear hyposegmentation. The specific granules are numerous, round, and lightly staining (lack metachromasia). *C,* Mast cell leukemia in a cat. The neoplastic cells contain round to oval nuclei and few to numerous, fine darkly staining (metachromatic) granules. *D,* Basophilic leukemia in a dog. The neoplastic cell is larger than the neutrophil, contains chunky dark-staining specific granules, and has an indented nucleus.

ules, when present, facilitate cell identification, and usually more metachromatic granules are apparent in bone marrow than in blood basophils. Enlarged, metachromatic granules also may be present in blood basophils of cats with mucopolysaccharidosis.[103]

Mast cells can be differentiated from basophils by the presence of a round to oval nucleus and numerous small, round, metachromatic, intracytoplasmic granules that may obscure nuclear detail (Figure 114–20C). This distinction is consistent in health and disseminated, well-differentiated mast cell neoplasia, but may present difficulty in rare cases of basophilic leukemia where more immature (less segmented) cells are present (Figure 114–20D).[384]

Production and Kinetics

Both basophils and mast cells originate in the bone marrow. Although the immediate stem cell of mast cells has been identified and designated as the "P" (persisting) cell, a similar stem cell for the basophil has yet to be described.[43, 385] Kinetic data for dog and cat basophils have not been determined.

Basophilia

Basophilia is defined arbitrarily as a sustained elevation in the basophil count exceeding two per cent of the differential leukocyte count or a routinely calculated cell count exceeding 200 basophils/μl. This definition of basophilia is crude at best, but may be revised as techniques for absolute basophil counts are applied to dogs and cats in various disease situations. Generally, basophilia occurs concomitantly with eosinophilia in dogs and cats, but may be of sufficient magnitude to overshadow changes in the eosinophil count. Some causes of basophilia in dogs and cats are listed in Table 114–10. The most frequent clinical cause of basophilia in dogs and cats is heartworm infestation, especially in cases of occult disease.[386–389] Although basophilia is stated to occur in instances of persistent lipemia accompanying hyperadrenocorticism, chronic liver disease, ne-

TABLE 114–10. CAUSES OF BASOPHILIA IN DOGS AND CATS

Hypersensitivity and/or inflammatory lesions	
Allergic respiratory disorders	dog, cat
Canine cutaneous eosinophilic granuloma	dog
Feline eosinophilic granuloma complex	cat
Pulmonary eosinophilic granuloma	dog
Parasitic diseases	
Dirofilaria immitis	dog, cat
Dipetalonema reconditum	dog
Neoplasia	
Basophilic leukemia	dog, cat
Mast cell neoplasia (disseminated)	dog
Polycythemia vera?	cat
Drug administration	
Heparin	dog
Penicillin	dog

phrotic syndrome, and diabetes mellitus,[2, 6] these assertions are unproven in most clinical reports. If basophilia does occur in these situations, absolute basophil counts probably will be necessary to detect subtle increases in cell numbers.

Leukemias and Myeloproliferative Syndromes

Terminology and Classification. Leukemia is defined as a neoplastic proliferation of hematopoietic cells within the bone marrow and other tissues. In a general context, the term leukemia encompasses neoplasia of all hematopoietic cell lines (Figure 114–2) including granulocytes, monocytes, lymphocytes, mast cells, erythrocytes, and megakaryocytes. Unregulated proliferation of these cell lines may occur singly or in combination. A diagnosis of leukemia may be further qualified by descriptive adjectives that designate the time course of the disease, the cell lineage, and/or the presence or absence of neoplastic cells in the blood.[1, 7]

The time course of the disease process, classified as acute or chronic, implies the rapidity of onset of disease, the degree of differentiation of the neoplastic cell line, and the expected lifespan in the absence of chemotherapy. Acute leukemia implies a relatively short clinical presentation, variable numbers of immature (poorly differentiated or undifferentiated) cells in the blood and bone marrow, and short life expectancy. The antithesis, chronic leukemia, suggests a prolonged clinical course, an increased number of mature (well-differentiated) cells on blood and bone marrow smears, and a longer life expectancy. These classifications are arbitrary, however, because patients with acute leukemia may have greater longevity than patients with chronic leukemia following effective chemotherapy, and chronic leukemia may terminate acutely in a "blast crisis" characterized by many immature cells in the blood and bone marrow.[1, 7]

Classification of the leukemia by the predominant cell type is accomplished using Romanowsky-stained blood and bone marrow smears, a battery of cytochemical stains, and electron microscopy. For convenience, the types of leukemia are broadly divided into myeloproliferative and lymphoproliferative disorders (Table 114–11). Myeloproliferative leukemias include neoplastic proliferation of granulocytes, monocytes, erythrocytes, megakaryocytes, and mast cells, while lymphoproliferative disorders are limited to neoplastic proliferation of lymphocytes and plasma cells. In addition, multiple cell lines may be involved in the neoplastic process. Common examples are myelomonocytic leukemia where the bipotential stem cell produces both neutrophils and monocytes (Figure 114–2), and erythroleukemia wherein both erythrocytes and granulocytes are formed.[6]

Romanowsky-stained specimens allow diagnosis of well-differentiated leukemias with recognizable cellular morphology, but cannot distinguish one immature or blast cell line from another. Cytochemistry, which detects characteristic staining patterns, usually allows classification of blast cells within a specific cell lineage.[6, 154, 156, 161, 390–392] Although batteries of stains identify leukemic

TABLE 114–11. A SIMPLIFIED CLASSIFICATION OF LEUKEMIAS IN DOGS AND CATS

Myeloproliferative Disorders
Granulocytes
  Granulocytic (myeloid, neutrophilic) leukemia
  Eosinophilic leukemia
  Basophilic leukemia
Monocytes
  Monocytic leukemia
Erythrocytes
  Erythremic myelosis
  Polycythemia vera
Megakaryocytes
  Megakaryocytic leukemia (myelosis)
Mixed cell lines
  Myelomonocytic leukemia (neutrophils and monocytes)
  Erythroleukemia (erythrocytes and granulocytes)
Miscellaneous
  Mast cell leukemia
  Undifferentiated leukemia
Lymphoproliferative Disorders
Lymphocytes
  Acute lymphoblastic leukemia
  Chronic lymphocytic leukemia
Plasma cells
  Plasma cell leukemia

cell lines with more certainty (Table 114–12), cytochemistry is not perfect. Irregularity and heterogeneity of cytochemical staining patterns in some undifferentiated leukemias may make it difficult to identify the cell lineage precisely.[6] When weak or equivocal cytochemical staining exists, ultrastructural examination of the neoplastic cells may be beneficial. Electron microscopy can be used to demonstrate certain cytochemical reactions ultrastructurally or to reveal characteristic features that may identify the neoplastic cell line.[6, 154, 393, 394] Immunochemical markers are available for the diagnosis of some human leukemias, but similar products are not available commercially for specific use in dogs and cats. Clinically, definitive diagnosis of the neoplastic cell line is important in choosing an effective chemotherapy protocol.[390, 395]

The use of cytochemistry and immunochemical markers to classify human leukemias indicates that some instances of leukemia may involve multiple cell clones. Furthermore, a leukemia characterized by the expression of markers reflecting a particular cell line at the initial diagnosis may relapse with a leukemia expressing a different phenotype. This apparent change in cell type is referred to as a "lineage switch."[396] Evidence of lineage switching has been observed in Romanowsky-stained preparations from a cat with myeloproliferative disease.[397]

Lastly, leukemias may be classified according to the presence (leukemic, subleukemic) or absence (aleukemic) of neoplastic cells in the blood. These adjectives not only refer to the presence or absence of immature cells in the blood but also infer changes in the total leukocyte count. "Leukemic" suggests an increased leukocyte count with the presence of many neoplastic cells in the blood. "Subleukemic" implies a leukocyte count that is within the reference interval or decreased with few neoplastic cells in the blood. "Aleukemic" suggests a leukocyte count that is within the reference interval or decreased and neoplastic cells are not present in the blood.[1, 7]

TABLE 114–12. EXPECTED CYTOCHEMICAL STAINING PATTERNS OF LEUKEMIC CELLS IN DOGS AND CATS

Cytochemical Stain	Leukemia Type			
	Granulocytic	Myelomonocytic	Monocytic	Lymphocytic
Naphthol AS-D chloroacetate esterase	+	+	−	−
Peroxidase	+	+	±	−
Sudan black B	+	+	±	−
Alpha naphthyl acetate esterase*	−	+	+	±

+ positive staining reaction
− negative staining reaction
± weak-to-negative staining reaction
*Focal intracytoplasmic staining of T-lymphocytes resists fluoride inhibition, but diffuse intracytoplasmic staining of monocytes is fluoride sensitive.

In addition to leukemias, hematologic dyscrasias exist with cytopenias of one or more blood cell lines and no evidence of overt neoplasia in either the blood or bone marrow. Cellular maturation abnormalities, however, may exist.[221, 228, 230, 231, 398, 399] These dyscrasias are termed myeloproliferative syndromes and are characterized by an irreversible derangement in the development of hematopoietic cell lines resulting from progressive impairment of precursor cell maturation and ineffective hematopoiesis.[400] Leukemia may develop in the terminal stage of disease. The diagnosis of myeloproliferative syndromes is challenging and often a definitive diagnosis is made retrospectively after leukemia has developed. In this situation the terms myeloproliferative disease or preleukemia may be used.[221, 228, 399, 401]

Incidence and Etiology

The annual incidence rate for leukemias in dogs and cats is approximately 31 and 224 cases per 100,000 animals, respectively.[402] Lymphoid malignancies, including lymphosarcoma, are responsible for 87.4 per cent of all leukemias in dogs and 68.9 per cent of all leukemias in cats. Cats, as compared to dogs, have a 6.1 times greater incidence of lymphosarcoma and a 15.7 times greater incidence of myeloproliferative disease. In dogs, the incidence of leukemia increases with age. In the cat, a bimodal age pattern exists for leukemias and lymphosarcoma with more cases being recorded for young and older animals. Myeloproliferative disease, however, is seen in younger cats.[402]

In cats, leukemias are almost invariably associated with feline leukemia virus infection, and experimental inoculation of cats with virus isolates has produced both granulocytic and eosinophilic leukemias.[82, 336, 403, 404] The etiology of canine leukemias is undetermined, although evidence of viral infection has been demonstrated.[399] Additionally, genetic factors, environmental factors, radiation, and chemical exposure should be considered.

Clinical Signs and Physical Findings. The clinical signs associated with leukemias are variable and vague, including lethargy, anorexia, rapid weight loss, shifting limb lameness, persistent fever, dyspnea, vomiting, and diarrhea. Physical findings frequently include splenomegaly, hepatomegaly, enlargement of the lymph nodes and/or tonsils, pallor of mucous membranes, fever, and emaciation.[154, 155] In some instances, clinical signs may be specifically related to organ or tissue dysfunction secondary to neoplastic cell infiltration. These signs, often unique in presentation, may be misleading until a complete blood count is performed as part of a routine procedure to assess the patient's health status.[6, 405, 406] The suggestion of leukemia on the complete blood count may be confirmed by a bone marrow biopsy.

General Remarks. Leukemias originate in the bone marrow and, unless aleukemic in nature, will eventually infiltrate various tissues of the body. Although myelomonocytic leukemia is cited as having more extensive tissue infiltration than other forms of leukemia,[2] the degree of tissue invasion generally depends upon the diligence with which lesions are sought at necropsy. In rare instances, greenish sarcomatous tissue masses may be apparent in granulocytic leukemia and myelomonocytic leukemia. These masses are called chloromas, a descriptive term referring to the greenish color imparted by neutrophil myeloperoxidase.[2, 6]

Animals with leukemia may die as a consequence of infection, severe anemia, hemorrhage, or organ dysfunction secondary to neoplastic cell infiltration and proliferation. The frequency of secondary infections may be related to defective neutrophil function and bactericidal capabilities as well as suppression of normal antibody production by paraprotein in lymphoproliferative disorders.[296, 407, 408] Following chemotherapy, patients are at even greater risk of infection.

The following discussion will include a brief overview of leukemias. Additional information concerning lymphoproliferative disorders, mast cell neoplasia, erythroid neoplasia, and megakaryocytic neoplasia can be found elsewhere. Chemotherapy has been omitted purposely.

FIGURE 114–21. Photomicrographs of leukemic blood cells from dogs and cats. *A,* Acute granulocytic leukemia in a cat showing poorly differentiated neutrophil precursors. *B,* Granular staining pattern of neutrophil precursors following application of the peroxidase technique. (*A* and *B* courtesy of Dr. John W. Harvey, College of Veterinary Medicine, University of Florida, Gainesville, Florida.) *C,* Acute monocytic leukemia in a dog showing various developmental stages of monocytes. *D,* Diffuse intracytoplasmic staining of monoblasts by the alpha naphthyl acetate esterase technique. *E,* Acute lymphoblastic leukemia in a dog showing large, immature lymphocytes with finely stippled chromatin, nucleolar rings, and a rim of dark cytoplasm. *F,* Chronic lymphocytic leukemia in a dog showing small, well-differentiated lymphocytes with coarsely aggregated chromatin, no nucleoli, and only a thin rim of cytoplasm. *G,* "Flaming" plasma cell in the blood of a dog with multiple myeloma. The dark peripheral cytoplasm corresponds to a deep pink color on Romanowsky-stained preparations.

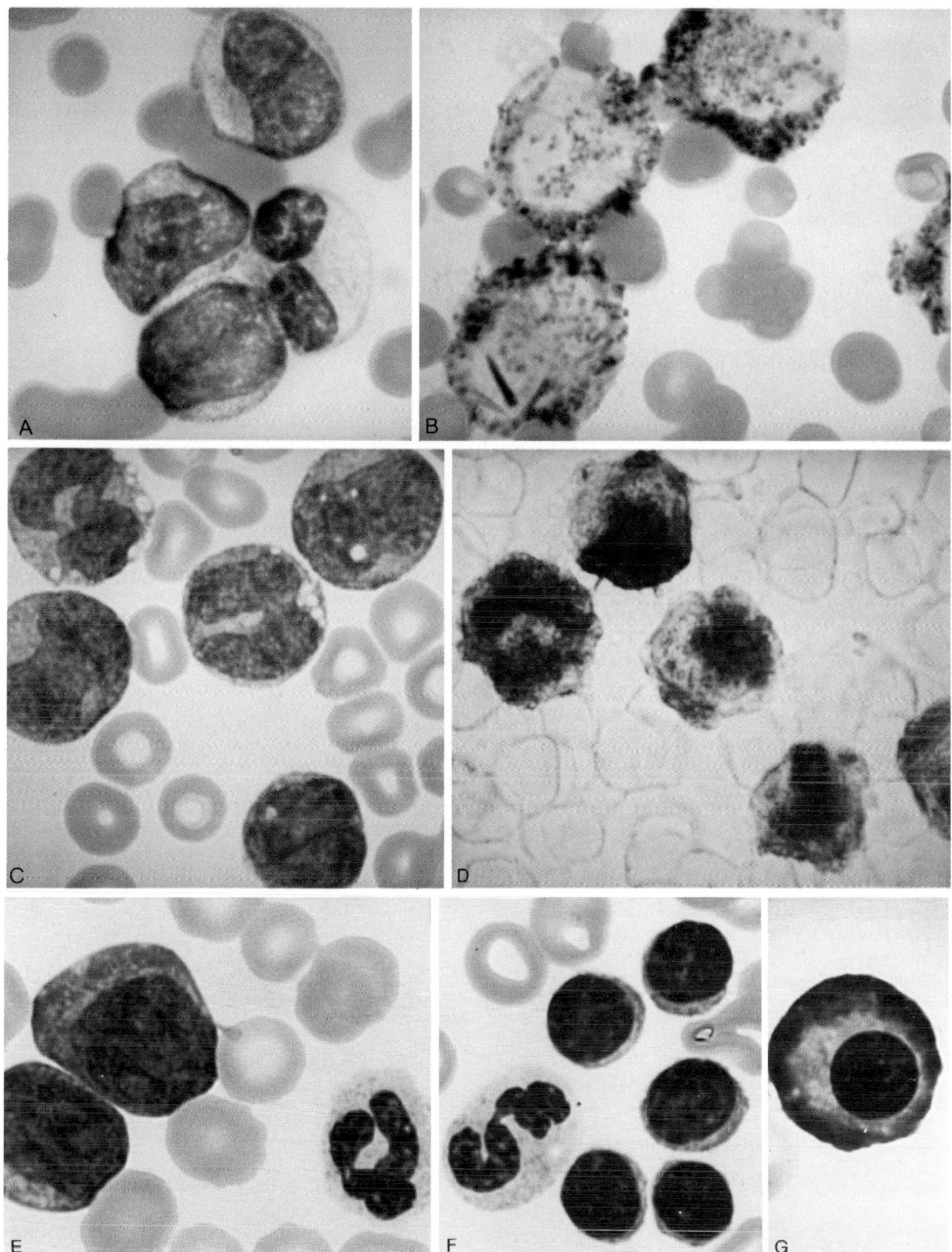

Figure 114–21 *See legend on opposite page*

Other than lymphoproliferative disorders, leukemias are relatively uncommon and treatment, where attempted, has been given on an individual basis. More effective chemotherapy protocols inevitably will be developed as refined diagnostic techniques are introduced and used to rapidly diagnose the various leukemias. Until that time, practitioners are encouraged to study the current literature and consult veterinary oncologists about individual patient management.

Myeloproliferative Disorders

Granulocytic (Myeloid, Neutrophilic) Leukemia. Granulocytic leukemia has been reported in both the dog and the cat.[6, 153, 155, 156, 161, 162, 226, 391–393, 398, 405, 409–426] The total leukocyte count is variable, ranging from leukopenia to marked leukocytosis. Anemia usually is severe and may be related to the longer neutrophil transit time compared to monocytes. Chronic granulocytic leukemia may present with increased numbers of more differentiated neutrophils, and must be distinguished from a leukemoid response secondary to infection (see neutrophilia; leukemoid reactions and extreme neutrophilia).[2] The diagnosis of leukemia is more obvious in acute granulocytic leukemia or in chronic granulocytic leukemia terminating in a blast crisis; however, cytochemistry is often necessary to positively identify the cell line (Figure 114–21 A, B).

Myelomonocytic Leukemia. Myelomonocytic leukemia results from unregulated production of both neutrophils and monocytes by the bipotential stem cell. Myelomonocytic leukemia is one of the more common myeloproliferative diseases in dogs and also has been reported in cats.[6, 85, 155, 156, 161, 162, 207, 227, 228, 390, 392–395, 406, 427–431] The mixture of monocytes and neutrophils may change during progression of the disease, and both cell lines may be identified with cytochemical staining in the acute form of the disease. The severity of anemia generally is moderate.

Monocytic Leukemia. Monocytic leukemia is uncommon in the dog and in the cat (Figure 114–21C, D).[6, 154–156, 162, 391, 392, 394, 412, 425, 432–437] When observed, this form of leukemia generally is accompanied by a mild to moderate degree of anemia even with leukocyte counts reaching 800,000 cells/μl.[433] The relatively mild anemia presumably is the result of a short marrow transit time and the absence of a prominent bone marrow monocyte storage pool.[298, 301]

Eosinophilic Leukemia. Eosinophilic leukemia has only been reported in the cat, and is difficult, if not impossible, to distinguish from hypereosinophilic syndromes.[6, 360, 365] In cats, both eosinophilic leukemoid reactions and eosinophilic leukemia have been produced experimentally with feline leukemia virus inoculation.[404] However, naturally occurring cases of eosinophilic leukemia in cats also have been feline leukemia virus–test negative or free of viral particles on ultrastructural examination.[6, 336, 360, 361, 438] In all reported cases of leukemia the cells were well differentiated and diagnosis was made by the presence of characteristic specific granules.

Basophilic Leukemia. Basophilic leukemia is ex-

tremely rare in both the cat and dog.[336, 384, 409, 437, 439–443] Basophilic leukemia may be difficult to distinguish from mast cell leukemia and the authenticity of some reports in dogs has been questioned.[6] In cases of canine basophilic leukemia, nuclear hyposegmentation is expected and granule ultrastructure is equivocal in confirming the diagnosis (Figure 114–20D). Cytochemistry, however, may be helpful in establishing a diagnosis.[384] The etiology of canine basophilic leukemia is unknown, but all cases of basophilic leukemia in cats have been feline leukemia virus–test positive.[315]

Mast Cell Leukemia. Mast cell leukemia usually is associated with splenic enlargement in cats and with primary cutaneous mast cell tumors in dogs.[315, 444] Mast cell neoplasia should be the first consideration in cats with large round cells containing numerous purple granules on the stained blood smear (Figure 114–20C). Systemic mast cell neoplasia in the absence of cutaneous tumors may be difficult to distinguish from basophilic leukemia in the dog although the latter is extremely rare. Cytochemical staining may be helpful.[161, 384]

Erythremic Myelosis. Erythroid malignancies are relatively common in cats with numerous reports in the literature; however, this form of leukemia is rare in the dog.[2, 6, 221, 315, 391, 445–448] In cats, erythremic myelosis usually is accompanied by a very severe anemia. Although numerous nucleated erythrocytes may be present on the blood smear, the anemia is nonregenerative with aggregate reticulocyte counts of less than one per cent. In acute erythremic myelosis more blast cells are present. These primitive cells are round to oval, 10 to 15 μm in diameter, and have an eccentric nucleus. The nuclear chromatin is finely stippled and a single, prominent nucleolus is present. The cytoplasm is moderately abundant, blue, and may contain scattered purple granules. Broad pseudopodia also may be observed.[2, 6, 445, 446] In chronic erythremic myelosis, large numbers of rubricytes and metarubricytes are present on the stained blood smear without evidence of polychromasia. Changes in erythroid cell morphology may occur with termination in a blast crisis.[397, 449]

Erythroleukemia. Erythroleukemia is the neoplastic proliferation of erythrocytes and leukocytes, usually granulocytes. This form of leukemia has been reported in cats.[6, 23, 162, 391, 393, 450] Erythroleukemia may be one stage in the progression of myeloproliferative disease wherein erythremic myelosis evolves into erythroleukemia and terminates in myeloblastic leukemia.[6, 397]

Polycythemia Vera (Polycythemia Rubra Vera, Primary Erythrocytosis). Polycythemia vera has been reported in the dog and cat.[451, 452] A diagnosis of polycythemia is suggested by finding brick-red mucous membranes, splenomegaly, and an increased packed cell volume. Documentation of polycythemia vera requires demonstration of an expanded red cell mass in the presence of a normal P_aO_2 and a decreased serum erythropoietin concentration. The diagnostic workup also should eliminate the possibility of tumors that may produce polycythemia secondarily.[451, 453–455]

Megakaryocytic Leukemia (Myelosis). Megakaryocytic leukemia has been reported in both the cat and the dog.[225, 229, 336, 456–460] Both leukocyte and platelet counts are variable, but megakaryoblasts may be found in the blood.[225, 229, 336, 456, 457, 460] Diagnosis may depend upon cytochemical staining (periodic acid-Schiff, alpha naphthyl acetate esterase, acetylcholinesterase, and factor VIII positive) and electron microscopy (alpha dense granules and internal membrane systems).[229, 457, 460-462] Myeloproliferative diseases also have been described that are characterized by the proliferation of megakaryocytes alone, or in conjunction with proliferating neutrophils or erythroid precursors.[463-466] Megakaryocyte precursors in the blood may mimic lymphocytes and are designated micromegakaryocytes.[461, 464] Cats with megakaryocytic leukemia may be feline leukemia virus–test negative.[225, 457]

Lymphoproliferative Disorders

Lymphocytic Leukemias. Lymphocytic leukemia is one of the most common forms of leukemia in dogs and cats.[6, 155, 161, 232, 315, 337, 391-394, 467] Sarcomatous masses are not present in true leukemia, but are expected with lymphosarcoma. This is an important differentiating feature as approximately 11 per cent of dogs and 27 per cent of cats with lymphosarcoma will present with a leukemic blood picture.[233, 336] Acute lymphoblastic leukemia is characterized by immature cells in the blood, and cytochemistry may be needed to identify the cell lineage (Figure 114–21E). In chronic lymphocytic leukemia, the lymphocytes are small and well differentiated (Figure 114–21F). This form of leukemia must be distinguished from physiologic lymphocytosis, especially in cats,[6] and from antigenic stimulation-induced lymphocytosis as in chronic canine ehrlichiosis.[217] Retrospective studies in dogs indicate that the mean survival time is longer with chronic lymphocytic leukemia (452 days) than with acute lymphoblastic leukemia (68 days) following diagnosis and chemotherapy.[232, 337]

Plasma Cell Leukemia. Plasma cell myelomas have four diagnostic features including: a monoclonal gammopathy, the presence of greater than 20 per cent plasma cells within bone marrow aspirates, Bence Jones proteinuria, and radiographic evidence of osteolysis. Two of these four features are considered essential to diagnose a plasma cell myeloma.[408] Despite sporadic reports of plasma cell myeloma in dogs and cats, plasma cell leukemia is rare.[468-470] Neoplastic plasma cells may appear normal to slightly aberrant (plasmacytoid) on Romanowsky-stained blood smears (Figure 114–21G). In one dog, flaming plasma cells were characterized by a peripheral rim of pink cytoplasm juxtaposed to the usual blue cytoplasm.[470]

References

1. Boggs, DR and Winkelstein, A: White Cell Manual, 4th ed. Philadelphia, FA Davis, 1983.
2. Prasse, KW: White blood cell disorders. In Ettinger, SJ (ed): Textbook of Veterinary Internal Medicine, 2nd ed. Philadelphia, WB Saunders, 1983, p 2001.
3. Bentick-Smith, J: Hematology. In Medway, W, et al. (eds): Textbook of Veterinary Clinical Pathology. Baltimore, Williams and Wilkins, 1969, p 205.
4. Schmidt, CH, et al.: A new anticoagulant for routine laboratory procedures: A comparative study. US Armed Forces Med J 4:1556, 1953.
5. Gossett, KA and Carakostas, MC: Effect of EDTA on morphology of neutrophils of healthy dogs and dogs with inflammation. Vet Clin Pathol 13:22, 1984.
6. Jain, NC: Schalm's Veterinary Hematology, 4th ed. Philadelphia, Lea & Febiger, 1986.
7. Wintrobe, MM: Clinical Hematology, 8th ed. Philadelphia, Lea & Febiger, 1981.
8. Weiser, MG: Comparison of two automated multi-channel blood cell counting systems for analysis of blood of common domestic animals. Vet Clin Pathol 12:25, 1983.
9. Weiser, MG: Modification and evaluation of a multichannel blood cell counting system for blood analysis in veterinary hematology. JAVMA 190:411, 1987.
10. Hurd, KE, et al.: A comparative study for the enumeration of peripheral blood white cell counts below 2.0 × 10⁹/l using counting chambers and the Coulter counter model 'S'. J Clin Pathol 30:1005, 1977.
11. Weiser, MG and Kociba, GJ: Platelet concentration and platelet volume distribution in healthy cats. Am J Vet Res 45:518, 1984.
12. Boyce, JT, et al.: Feline leukemia virus-induced thrombocytopenia and macrothrombosis in cats. Vet Pathol 23:16, 1986.
13. Wardlaw, SC and Levine, RA: Quantitative buffy coat analysis: A new laboratory tool functioning as a screening complete blood cell count. JAMA 249:617, 1983.
14. Levine, RA, et al.: Quantitative buffy coat analysis of blood collected from dogs, cats, and horses. JAVMA 189:670, 1986.
15. Brown, SA and Barsanti, JA: Quantitative buffy coat analysis for hematologic measurements of canine, feline, and equine blood samples and for the detection of microfilaremia in dogs. Am J Vet Res 49:321, 1988.
16. Koepke, JA: A delineation of performance criteria for the differentiation of leukocytes. Am J Clin Pathol 68:202, 1977.
17. Rich, LJ: The Morphology of Canine & Feline Blood Cells Including Equine References. St. Louis, Ralston Purina, 1976.
18. Perman, V, et al.: Bone marrow biopsy. Vet Clin North Am 4:293, 1974.
19. Lewis, HB and Rebar, AH: Bone Marrow Evaluation in Veterinary Practice. St. Louis, Ralston Purina, 1979.
20. Meyer, DJ: Bone marrow. In Bojrab, MJ, et al. (eds): Current Techniques in Small Animal Surgery, 2nd ed. Philadelphia, Lea & Febiger, 1983, p 491.
21. Harvey, JW: Canine bone marrow: Normal hematopoiesis, biopsy techniques, and cell identification and evaluation. Comp Cont Ed 6:909, 1984.
22. Hoff, B, et al.: An appraisal of bone marrow biopsy in assessment of sick dogs. Can J Comp Med 49:34, 1985.
23. Schalm, OW: Manual of Feline and Canine Hematology. Santa Barbara, Veterinary Practice Pub, 1980.
24. Stockham, SL, et al.: Mastocytemia in dogs with acute inflammatory diseases. Vet Clin Pathol 15:16, 1986.
25. Prasse, KW and Mahaffey, EA: Hematology of normal cats and characteristic responses to disease. In Holzworth, J (ed): Diseases of the Cat: Medicine and Surgery. Philadelphia, WB Saunders, 1987, p 739.
26. Duncan, JR and Prasse, KW: Veterinary Laboratory Medicine: Clinical Pathology, 2nd ed. Ames, Iowa State University Press, 1986.
27. Melveger, BE, et al.: Sternal bone marrow biopsy in the dog. Lab Anim Care 19:866, 1969.
28. Bloom, F and Meyer, LM: The morphology of the bone marrow cells in normal dogs. Cornell Vet 34:13, 1944.
29. Andersen, AC and Gee, W: Normal blood values in the beagle. Vet Med 53:135, 1958.
30. Shifrine, M, et al.: Hematologic changes to 60 days of age in clinically normal beagles. Lab Anim Sci 23:894, 1973.
31. Bulgin, MS, et al.: Hematologic changes to four and one-half years of age in clinically normal beagles. JAVMA 157:1064, 1970.
32. Earl, FL, et al.: The hemogram and bone marrow profile of normal neonatal and weanling beagle dogs. Lab Anim Sci 23:690, 1973.
33. Dougherty, JH and Rosenblatt, LS: Changes in the hemogram of the beagle with age. J Gerontol 20:131, 1965.

34. Michaelson, SM, et al.: The blood of the normal beagle. JAVMA 148:532, 1966.
35. Johnson, KH and Perman, V: Normal values for jugular blood in the cat. Vet Med 63:851, 1968.
36. Anderson, L, et al.: Haematological values in normal cats from four weeks to one year of age. Res Vet Sci 12:579, 1971.
37. Meyers-Wallen, VN, et al.: Hematologic values in healthy neonatal, weanling, and juvenile kittens. Am J Vet Res 45:1322, 1984.
38. Schalm, OW and Hughes, JP: Some observations on physiologic leukocytosis in the cat and horse. Calif Vet 18:23, 1964.
39. Prasse, KW, et al.: Blood neutrophilic granulocyte kinetics in cats. Am J Vet Res 34:1021, 1973.
40. Beck, WS: Leukocytes I. Physiology. In Beck, WS (ed): Hematology, 3rd ed. Cambridge, MIT Press, 1981, p 253.
41. Greenberg, ML, et al.: Erythropoietic and reticuloendothelial function in dogs. Science 152:526, 1966.
42. Quesenberry, P and Levitt, L: Hematopoietic stem cells. N Engl J Med 301:755, 819, 868, 1979.
43. Schrader, JW: Bone marrow differentiation in vitro. CRC Crit Rev Immunol 4:196, 1984.
44. Raghavachar, A, et al.: Stem cells from peripheral blood and bone marrow: A comparative evaluation of the hemopoietic potential in the dog. Int J Cell Cloning 1:191, 1983.
45. Golde, DW and Takaku, F (eds): Hematopoietic Stem Cells. New York, Marcel Dekker, 1985.
46. Metcalf, D: The Hematopoietic Colony Stimulating Factors. New York, Elsevier, 1984.
47. Calvo, W, et al.: Regeneration of blood-forming organs after autologous leukocyte transfusion in lethally irradiated dogs. Distribution and cellularity of the marrow in irradiated and transfused animals. Blood 47:593, 1976.
48. Young, N and Mortimer, P: Viruses and bone marrow failure. Blood 63:729, 1984.
49. Theilen, GH and Madewell, BR (eds): Veterinary Cancer Medicine. Philadelphia, Lea & Febiger, 1979.
50. Jacobs, RM, et al.: Clinicopathologic features of canine parvoviral enteritis. JAAHA 16:809, 1980.
51. Riser, WH: The behavior of the peripheral blood elements in panleucopenia (agranulocytosis) of the domestic cat. Am J Vet Res 8:82, 1947.
52. Rohovsky, MW and Griesemer, RA: Experimental feline infectious enteritis in the germfree cat. Pathol Vet 4:391, 1967.
53. Henness, AM, et al.: Clinical investigation of doxorubicin, daunomycin, and 6-thioguanine in normal cats. Am J Vet Res 38:521, 1977.
54. Ogawa, M, et al.: Renewal and commitment to differentiation of hemopoietic stem cells (an interpretive review). Blood 61:823, 1983.
55. Mauch, P, et al.: Decline in bone marrow proliferative capacity as a function of age. Blood 60:245, 1982.
56. Lipschitz, DA, et al.: Effect of age on hematopoiesis in man. Blood 63:502, 1984.
57. Chiu, T: Studies on estrogen-induced proliferative disorders of hemopoietic tissue in dogs. Ph.D. Dissertation, University of Minnesota, Minneapolis, 1974.
58. Wade, BH and Mandell, GL: Polymorphonuclear leukocytes: Dedicated professional phagocytes. Am J Med 74:686, 1983.
59. Smith, GS and Lumsden, JH: Review of neutrophil adherence, chemotaxis, phagocytosis and killing. Vet Immunol Immunopathol 4:177, 1983.
60. Wright, DG: The neutrophil as a secretory defense organ. In Gallin, JI and Fauci, AS (eds): Advances in Host Defense Mechanisms. New York, Raven Press, 1982, p 75.
61. Phair, JP and et. al: Phagocytosis and algicidal activity of human polymorphonuclear neutrophils against Prototheca wickerhamii. J Infect Dis 144:72, 1981.
62. Wilson, CB and Remington, JS: Activity of human blood leukocytes against Toxoplasma gondii. J Infect Dis 140:890, 1979.
63. Pearson, RD and Steigbigel, RT: Phagocytosis and killing of the protozoan Leishmania donovani by human polymorphonuclear leukocytes. J Immunol 127:1438, 1981.
64. Kooistra, L, et al.: Identification of feline monocytes and neutrophils as effector cells in antibody-dependent cellular cytotoxicity: Sequential analysis, using light microscopy, histochemistry, and scanning electron microscopy. Am J Vet Res 46:2626, 1985.
65. Bagby, GC, et al.: Regulation of colony-stimulating activity production: Interactions of fibroblasts, mononuclear phagocytes, and lactoferrin. J Clin Invest 71:340, 1983.
66. Porter, KA: A sex difference in morphology of neutrophils in the dog. Nature 179:784, 1957.
67. Irfan, M: Studies on the peripheral blood picture of the dog and cat in health and disease with special reference to lymphatic leukosis, together with observations on the pathology and drug therapy of lymphatic leukosis in dogs. Irish Vet J 15:65, 1961.
68. Loughman, WD, et al.: XY/XXY bone marrow mosaicism in three male tricolor cats. Am J Vet Res 31:307, 1970.
69. Jones, TC: Sex chromosome anomaly, Kleinfelter's syndrome. Comp Pathol Bull 1:5, 1969.
70. Bertram, TA: Neutrophilic leukocyte structure and function in domestic animals. Adv Vet Sci Comp Med 30:91, 1985.
71. Latimer, KS, et al.: Nuclear segmentation, ultrastructure, and cytochemistry of blood cells from dogs with Pelger-Huët anomaly. J Comp Pathol 97:61, 1987.
72. Bowles, CA, et al.: Studies of the Pelger-Huët anomaly in foxhounds. Am J Pathol 96:237, 1979.
73. Weber, SE, et al.: Pelger-Huët anomaly of granulocytic leukocytes in two feline littermates. Feline Pract 11:44, 1981.
74. Latimer, KS, et al.: Pelger-Huët anomaly in cats. Vet Pathol 22:370, 1985.
75. Pace, EM: Pelger-Huët anomaly transmission. Canine Pract 4:33, 1977.
76. Latimer, KS, et al.: Homozygous Pelger-Huët anomaly and chondrodysplasia in a stillborn kitten. Vet Pathol 25:325, 1988.
77. Latimer, KS, et al.: Leukocyte function in Pelger-Huët anomaly of dogs. J Leukocyte Biol (in press).
78. Hirsch, VM and Cunningham, TA: Hereditary anomaly of neutrophil granulation in Birman cats. Am J Vet Res 45:2170, 1984.
79. Haskins, ME, et al.: Mucopolysaccharidosis VI Maroteaux-Lamy syndrome: Arylsulfatase B-deficient mucopolysaccharidosis in the Siamese cat. Am J Pathol 105:191, 1981.
80. Brunning, RD: Morphologic alterations in nucleated blood and marrow cells in genetic disorders. Human Pathol 1:99, 1970.
81. Shull, RM and Powell, D: Acquired hyposegmentation of granulocytes (pseudo-Pelger-Huët anomaly) in a dog. Cornell Vet 69:241, 1979.
82. Toth, SR, et al.: Histopathological and hematological findings in myeloid leukemia induced by a new feline leukemia virus isolate. Vet Pathol 23:462, 1986.
83. Schalm, OW and Smith, R: Signs of defective neutrophil maturation in the cat. Calif Vet 17:33, 1963.
84. Langenhuijsen, MMAC: Neutrophils with ring-shaped nuclei in myeloproliferative disease. Br J Hematol 58:227, 1985.
85. Raskin, RE and Krehbiel, JD: Myelodysplastic changes in a cat with myelomonocytic leukemia. JAVMA 187:171, 1985.
86. Schalm, OW: Erythrocyte macrocytosis in miniature and toy poodles. Canine Pract 3:55, 1976.
87. McCall, CE, et al.: Lysosomal and ultrastructural changes in human "toxic" neutrophils during bacterial infection. J Exp Med 129:267, 1969.
88. Sutro, CJ: Cytoplasmic changes in circulating leukocytes in infection. Arch Int Med 51:747, 1933.
89. Gossett, KA and MacWilliams, PS: Ultrastructure of canine toxic neutrophils. Am J Vet Res 43:1634, 1982.
90. Watson, ADJ and Middleton, DJ: Chloramphenicol toxicosis in cats. Am J Vet Res 39:1199, 1978.
91. Zieve, PD, et al.: Vacuolization of the neutrophil: An aid to the diagnosis of septicemia. Arch Int Med 118:356, 1966.
92. Haskins, ME, et al.: Beta-glucuronidase deficiency in a dog: A model of human mucopolysaccharidosis VII. Pediatr Res 18:980, 1984.
93. Gossett, KA and MacWilliams, PS: Viral inclusions in hematopoietic precursors in a dog with distemper. JAVMA 181:387, 1982.
94. McLaughlin, BG, et al.: Canine distemper viral inclusions in blood cells of four vaccinated dogs. Can Vet J 26:368, 1985.
95. Harvey, JW: Hematology tip - stains for distemper inclusions. Vet Clin Pathol 11:12, 1982.
96. Troy, GC, et al.: Canine ehrlichiosis: A retrospective study of 30 naturally occurring cases. JAAHA 16:181, 1980.
97. Madewell, BR and Gribble, DH: Infection in two dogs with an agent resembling Ehrlichia equi. JAVMA 180:512, 1982.

98. Van Steenhouse, JL and DeNovo, RC: Atypical Histoplasma capsulatum infection in a dog. JAVMA 188:527, 1986.
99. Barton, CL, et al.: Canine hepatozoonosis: A retrospective study of 15 naturally occurring cases. JAAHA 21:125, 1985.
100. Craig, TM: Hepatozoonosis. In Greene, CE (ed): Clinical Microbiology and Infectious Diseases of the Dog and Cat. Philadelphia, WB Saunders, 1984, p 771.
101. Kolodny, EH: Current concepts in genetics: Lysosomal storage diseases. N Engl J Med 294:1217, 1976.
102. Glew, RH, et al.: Biology of disease: Lysosomal storage diseases. Lab Invest 53:250, 1985.
103. Cowell, KR, et al.: Mucopolysaccharidosis in a cat. JAVMA 169:334, 1976.
104. Haskins, ME, et al.: Spinal cord compression and hindlimb paresis in cats with mucopolysaccharidosis VI. JAVMA 182:983, 1983.
105. Gasper, PW, et al.: Correction of feline arylsulphatase B deficiency (mucopolysaccharidosis VI) by bone marrow transplantation. Nature 312:467, 1984.
106. Haskins, ME, et al.: Bone marrow transplantation in the cat. Transplantation 37:634, 1984.
107. Kramer, JW, et al.: The Chediak-Higashi syndrome of cats. Lab Invest 36:554, 1977.
108. Prieur, DJ, et al.: The diagnosis of feline Chediak-Higashi syndrome. Feline Pract 9:26, 1979.
109. Prieur, DJ and Collier, LL: Inheritance of the Chediak-Higashi syndrome in cats. J Hered 72:175, 1981.
110. Mills, EL and Quie, PG: Congenital disorders of the functions of polymorphonuclear neutrophils. Rev Infect Dis 2:505, 1980.
111. Brickman, TJ, et al.: In vitro demonstration of defective neutrophil chemotaxis in Chediak-Higashi affected cats. Fed Proc 43:390, 1984.
112. Meyers, KM, et al.: Evaluation of the platelet storage pool deficiency in the feline counterpart of the Chediak-Higashi syndrome. Am J Hematol 11:241, 1981.
113. Penny, RHC, et al.: Effects of chloramphenicol on the haemopoietic system of the cat. Br Vet J 123:145, 1967.
114. Carlisle, CH, et al.: Toxic effects of phenylbutazone on the cat. Br Vet J 124:560, 1968.
115. Gaunt, SD and Baker, DC: Hemosiderin in leukocytes of dogs with immune-mediated hemolytic anemia. Vet Clin Pathol 15:8, 1986.
116. Sen Gupta, PC, et al.: Bilirubin crystals in neutrophils of jaundiced neonates and infants. Acta Haematol 70:69, 1983.
117. Medleau, L and Miller, WH: Immunodiagnostic tests for small animal practice. Comp Cont Ed 5:705, 1983.
118. Schalm, OW and Ling, GV: The LE cell phenomenon in the dog. Calif Vet 24:20, 1970.
119. Schultz, RD and Adams, LS: Immunologic methods for the detection of humoral and cellular immunity. Vet Clin North Am 8:721, 1978.
120. Burgess, AW and Metcalf, D: The nature and action of granulocyte-macrophage colony stimulating factors. Blood 56:947, 1980.
121. Baserga, R: The cell cycle. N Engl J Med 304:453, 1981.
122. Raab, SO, et al: Granulokinetics in normal dogs. Am J Physiol 206:83, 1964.
123. Patt, HM and Maloney, MA: A model of granulocyte kinetics. Ann NY Acad Sci 113:515, 1964.
124. Prasse, KW, et al.: A model of granulopoiesis in cats. Lab Invest 28:292, 1973.
125. Maloney, MA and Patt, HM: Granulocyte transit from bone marrow to blood. Blood 31:195, 1968.
126. Deubelbeiss, KA, et al.: Neutrophil kinetics in the dog. J Clin Invest 55:833, 1975.
127. Gordon, AS, et al.: Plasma factors influencing leukocyte release in rats. Ann NY Acad Sci 113:766, 1964.
128. Boggs, DR, et al.: Neutrophil-releasing activity in plasma of dogs injected with endotoxin. J Lab Clin Med 72:177, 1968.
129. Ghebrehiwet, B: The release of lysosomal enzymes from human polymorphonuclear leukocytes by human C3e. Clin Immunol Immunopathol 30:321, 1984.
130. Perry, S, et al.: The combined use of typhoid vaccine and P32 labeling to assess myelopoiesis. Blood 12:549, 1957.
131. Christensen, RD, et al.: The leukocyte left shift in clinical and experimental neonatal sepsis. J Pediatr 98:101, 1981.
132. Marsh, JC, et al.: Neutrophil kinetics in acute infection. J Clin Invest 46:1943, 1967.
133. Mauer, AM, et al.: Leukokinetic studies. II. A method for labeling granulocytes in vitro with radioactive diisopropyl flurophosphate (DFP32). J Clin Invest 39:1481, 1960.
134. Athens, JW, et al.: Leukokinetic studies. IV. The total blood, circulating and marginal granulocyte pools and the granulocyte turnover rate in normal subjects. J Clin Invest 40:989, 1961.
135. Boggs, DR, et al.: Leukokinetic studies. IX. Experimental evaluation of a model of granulopoiesis. J Clin Invest 44:643, 1965.
136. Boggs, DR: The kinetics of neurophilic [sic] leukocytes in health and in disease. Semin Hematol 4:359, 1967.
137. Walker, RI and Willemze, R: Neutrophil kinetics and the regulation of granulopoiesis. Rev Infect Dis 2:282, 1980.
138. Ambrus, CM and Ambrus, JL: Regulation of the leukocyte level. Ann NY Acad Sci 77:445, 1959.
139. MacGregor, RR: Granulocyte adherence changes induced by hemodialysis, endotoxin, epinephrine, and glucocorticoids. Ann Intern Med 86:35, 1977.
140. Rijnberk, A, et al.: Investigation on the adrenocortical function of normal dogs. J Endocrinol 41:387, 1968.
141. Johnston, SD and Mather, EC: Canine plasma cortisol (hydrocortisone) measured by radioimmunoassay: Clinical absence of diurnal variation and results of ACTH stimulation and dexamethasone suppression tests. Am J Vet Res 39:1766, 1978.
142. Jasper, DE and Jain, NC: The influence of adrenocorticotrophic hormone and prednisolone upon marrow and circulating leukocytes in the dog. Am J Vet Res 26:844, 1965.
143. Jain, NC and Schalm, OW: Influence of corticosteroids on total and differential blood leukocyte counts. Calif Vet 20:28, 1966.
144. Bishop, CR, et al.: Leukokinetic studies XIII. A non-steady-state kinetic evaluation of the mechanisms of cortisone-induced granulocytosis. J Clin Invest 47:249, 1968.
145. Ling, GV, et al.: Canine hyperadrenocorticism: Pretreatment clinical and laboratory evaluation of 117 cases. JAVMA 174:1211, 1979.
146. Dale, DC, et al.: Alternate-day prednisone: Leukocyte kinetics and susceptibility to infections. N Engl J Med 291:1154, 1974.
147. Fauci, AS, et al.: NIH conference: Glucocorticosteroid therapy: Mechanism of action and clinical considerations. Ann Intern Med 84:304, 1976.
148. Schalm, OW: Interpretation of leukocyte responses in the dog. JAVMA 142:147, 1963.
149. Schalm, OW: Leukocyte responses to disease in various domestic animals. JAVMA 140:557, 1962.
150. Prasse, KW and Duncan, JR: Clinical interpretation of leukocyte abnormalities. Vet Clin N Am 6:581, 1976.
151. De Schepper, J, et al.: Anaemia and leukocytosis in one hundred and twelve dogs with pyometra. J Sm Anim Pract 28:137, 1987.
152. Hilts, SV and Shaw, CC: Leukemoid blood reactions. N Engl J Med 249:434, 1953.
153. Leifer, CE, et al.: Chronic myelogenous leukemia in the dog. JAVMA 183:686, 1983.
154. Latimer, KS and Dykstra, MJ: Acute monocytic leukemia in a dog. JAVMA 184:852, 1984.
155. Couto, CG: Clinicopathologic aspects of acute leukemias in the dog. JAVMA 186:681, 1985.
156. Grindem, CB, et al.: Morphological classification and clinical and pathological characteristics of spontaneous leukemia in 17 dogs. JAAHA 21:219, 1985.
157. Atwal, OS and McFarland, LZ: Histochemical study of the distribution of alkaline phosphatase in leukocytes of the horse, cow, sheep, dog, and cat. Am J Vet Res 28:971, 1967.
158. Jain, NC: Alkaline phosphatase activity in leukocytes of some animal species. Acta Haematol (Basel) 39:51, 1968.
159. Willson, JE and Brown, DE: Leukemoid reaction resembling myelogenous leukemia in a dog. Failure of the leukocyte alkaline phosphatase test to aid in the differential diagnosis. Cornell Vet 55:55, 1965.
160. Jain, NC: Alkaline phosphatase activity in the canine and feline granulocytes. Vet Rec 81:266, 1967.
161. Facklam, NR and Kociba, GJ: Cytochemical characterization of leukemic cells from 20 dogs. Vet Pathol 22:363, 1985.
162. Grindem, CB, et al.: Morphological classification and clinical and pathological characteristics of spontaneous leukemia in ten cats. JAAHA 21:227, 1985.

163. Edwards, DF: Transient diabetes mellitus and ketoacidosis in a dog. JAVMA 180:68, 1982.

164. Renshaw, HW, et al.: Canine granulocytopathy syndrome: Neutrophil dysfunction in a dog with recurrent infections. JAVMA 166:443, 1975.

165. Giger, U, et al.: Deficiency of leukocyte surface glycoproteins Mo1, LFA-1, and Leu M5 in a dog with recurrent bacterial infections: An animal model. Blood 69:1622, 1987.

166. Gaunt, PS, et al.: Extreme neutrophilic leukocytosis in a dog with hepatozoonosis. JAVMA 182:409, 1983.

167. Chinn, DR, et al.: Neutrophilic leukocytosis associated with metastatic fibrosarcoma in a dog. JAVMA 186:806, 1985.

168. Lappin, MR and Latimer, KS: Hematuria and extreme neutrophilic leukocytosis in a dog with renal tubular carcinoma. JAVMA 192:1289, 1988.

169. Finch, SC: Neutropenia. In Williams, WJ, et al. (eds). Hematology, 3rd ed. New York, McGraw-Hill, 1983, p 773.

170. Storb, R, et al.: Studies of marrow transplantation in dogs. Transplant Proc 8:545, 1976.

171. Dale, DC and Graw, RG: Transplantation of allogenic bone marrow in canine cyclic neutropenia. Science 183:83, 1974.

172. Jones, JB, et al.: Canine cyclic haematopoiesis: Marrow transplant between littermates. Br J Haematol 30:215, 1975.

173. Weiden, PL, et al.: Severe hereditary haemolytic anemia in dogs treated by marrow transplantation. Br J Haematol 33:357, 1976.

174. Weiden, PL, et al.: Prolonged disease free survival in dogs with lymphoma after total body irradiation and autologous marrow transplantation: Consolidation of combination chemotherapy-induced remission. Blood 54:1039, 1979.

175. Appelbaum, FR, et al.: Marrow transplant studies in dogs with malignant lymphoma. Transplantation 39:499, 1985.

176. Deeg, HJ, et al.: Autologous marrow transplantation as consolidation therapy for canine lymphoma: Efficacy and toxicity of various regimens of total body irradiation. Am J Vet Res 46:2016, 1985.

177. Appelbaum, FR, et al.: Cure of malignant lymphoma in dogs with peripheral blood stem cell transplantation. Transplantation 42:19, 1986.

178. Storb, R, et al.: Allogenic canine bone marrow transplantation following cyclophosphamide. Transplantation 7:378, 1969.

179. Kolb, HJ, et al.: Immunologic, toxicologic and marrow transplantation studies in dogs given dimethyl myleran. Biomedicine 20:341, 1974.

180. Harris, CK, et al.: Bone marrow transplantation in the dog. Comp Cont Ed 8:337, 1986.

181. Crafts, RC: The effects of estrogens on the bone marrow of adult female dogs. Blood 3:276, 1948.

182. Lowenstein, LJ, et al.: Exogenous estrogen toxicity in the dog. Calif Vet 26:14, 1972.

183. Schalm, OW: Exogenous estrogen toxicity in the dog. Canine Pract 5:57, 1978.

184. Gaunt, SD and Pierce, KR: Effects of estradiol on hematopoietic and marrow adherent cells of dogs. Am J Vet Res 47:906, 1986.

185. Edwards, DF: Bone marrow hypoplasia in a feminized dog with a Sertoli cell tumor. JAVMA 178:494, 1981.

186. Sherding, RG, et al.: Bone marrow hypoplasia in eight dogs with Sertoli cell tumor. JAVMA 178:497, 1981.

187. Miller, RM and Kind, RE: Phenylbutazone toxicity in a dog. Mod Vet Pract 43:69, 1962.

188. Schalm, OW: Phenylbutazone toxicity in two dogs. Canine Pract 6:47, 1979.

189. Watson, ADJ, et al.: Phenylbutazone-induced blood dyscrasias suspected in three dogs. Vet Rec 107:239, 1980.

190. Badame, FG, et al.: Reversible phenylbutazone-induced pancytopenia in a dog. Can Vet J 25:269, 1984.

191. Deldar, A, et al.: Investigation of pathogenetic mechanisms of a cephalosporin-induced blood disorder in dogs. Proceedings 37th Ann Mtg Am Coll Vet Pathol and 21st Ann Meet of Am Soc for Vet Clin Pathol, New Orleans, 1986, p 10.

192. Watson, ADJ: Bone marrow failure in a dog. J Sm Anim Pract 20:681, 1979.

193. Searcy, GP: The differential diagnosis of anemia. Vet Clin North Am 6:567, 1976.

194. Hammon, WD and Enders, JF: A virus disease of cats, principally characterized by aleucocytosis, enteric lesions and the presence of intranuclear inclusion bodies. J Exp Med 69:327, 1939.

195. Lawrence, JS, et al.: Infectious feline agranulocytosis. Am J Pathol 16:333, 1940.

196. Ichijo, S, et al.: Clinical and hematological findings and myelograms on feline panleukopenia. Jpn J Vet Sci 38:197, 1976.

197. Kramer, JM, et al.: Canine parvovirus update. VM/SAC 75:1541, 1980.

198. Potgieter, LND, et al.: Experimental parvovirus infection in dogs. Can J Comp Med 45:212, 1981.

199. Boonsinger, TR, et al: Bone marrow alterations associated with canine parvoviral enteritis. Vet Pathol 19:558, 1982.

200. Pollock, RVH: The parvoviruses. Part II. Canine parvovirus. Comp Cont Ed 6:653, 1984.

201. Appel, M, et al.: Canine viral enteritis. Canine Pract 7:22, 1980.

202. Rojko, JL and Olsen, RG: The immunobiology of the feline leukemia virus. Vet Immunol Immunopathol 6:107, 1984.

203. Onions, D, et al.: Growth of FeLV in haemopoietic cells in vitro. Develop Cancer Res 4:513, 1980.

204. Madewell, BR and Jarrett, O: Recovery of feline leukaemia virus from non-viremic cats. Vet Rec 112:339, 1983.

205. Prasse, KW: Clinical, hematological and postmortem findings in feline leukovirus infected cats: A retrospective study of 95 naturally occurring cases. Proc 31st Ann Meet Am Coll Vet Pathol, New Orleans, 1980, p 42.

206. Reinacher, M: Feline leukemia virus-associated enteritis—A condition with features of feline panleukopenia. Vet Pathol 24:1, 1987.

207. Madewell, BR, et al.: Hematologic abnormalities preceding myeloid leukemia in three cats. Vet Pathol 16:510, 1979.

208. Wellman, ML, et al: Suppression of feline bone marrow fibroblast colony-forming units by feline leukemia virus. Am J Vet Res 49:227, 1988.

209. Pedersen, NC, et al.: Isolation of a T-lymphotropic virus from domestic cats with an immunodeficiency-like syndrome. Science 235:790, 1987.

210. Walker, JS, et al.: Clinical and clinicopathologic findings in tropical canine pancytopenia. JAVMA 157:43, 1970.

211. Huxsoll, DL, et al.: Tropical canine pancytopenia. JAVMA 157:1627, 1970.

212. Hildebrandt, PK, et al.: Pathology of canine ehrlichiosis (tropical canine pancytopenia). Am J Vet Res 34:1309, 1973.

213. Buhles, WC, et al.: Tropical canine pancytopenia: Clinical, hematologic, and serologic response of dogs to Ehrlichia canis infection, tetracycline therapy, and challenge inoculation. J Infect Dis 130:357, 1974.

214. Reardon, MJ and Pierce, KR: Acute experimental canine ehrlichiosis. I. Sequential reaction of the hemic and lymphoreticular systems. Vet Pathol 18:48, 1981.

215. Kuehn, NF and Gaunt, SD: Clinical and hematologic findings in canine ehrlichiosis. JAVMA 186:355, 1985.

216. Codner, EC and Farris-Smith, LL: Characterization of the subclinical phase of ehrlichiosis in dogs. JAVMA 189:47, 1986.

217. Breitschwerdt, EB, et al.: Monoclonal gammopathy associated with naturally occurring canine ehrlichiosis. J Vet Intern Med 1:2, 1987.

218. Weiss, DJ, et al.: Bone marrow necrosis in the dog. JAVMA 187:54, 1985.

219. Murdoch, JM and Smith, CC: Hematological aspects of systemic disease. Infect Clin Haematol 1:619, 1972.

220. Weiss, DJ and Armstrong, PJ: Secondary myelofibrosis in three dogs. JAVMA 187:423, 1985.

221. Ward, JM, et al.: Myeloproliferative disease and abnormal erythrogenesis in the cat. JAVMA 155:879, 1969.

222. O'Brien, SE, et al.: Osteopetrosis in an adult dog. JAAHA 23:213, 1987.

223. Hoover, EA and Kociba, GJ: Bone lesions in cats with anemia induced by feline leukemia virus. J Nat Cancer Inst 53:1277, 1974.

224. Franks, PT, et al.: Feline large granular lymphoma. Vet Pathol 23:200, 1986.

225. Schmidt, RE, et al.: Megakaryocytic myelosis in cats: Review and case report. J Sm Anim Pract 24:759, 1983.

226. Roscher, AA, et al.: Acute myelogenous leukemia with histopathologic studies, following total body irradiation of a dog. JAVMA 136:491, 1960.

227. Ragan, HA, et al.: Acute myelomonocytic leukemia manifested as myelophthisic anemia in a dog. JAVMA 169:421, 1976.

228. Couto, CG and Kallet, AJ: Preleukemic syndrome in a dog. JAVMA 184:1389, 1984.

229. Shull, RM, et al.: Megakaryoblastic leukemia in a dog. Vet Pathol 23:533, 1986.

230. Hirsch, VM and Mitcham, SA: Multiple cytopenias associated with monocytic proliferation in a dog. Vet Clin Pathol 13:16, 1984.

231. Weiss, DJ, et al.: Myelodysplastic syndrome in two dogs. JAVMA 187:1038, 1985.

232. Matus, RE, et al.: Acute lymphoblastic leukemia in the dog: A review of 30 cases. JAVMA 183:859, 1983.

233. Madewell, BR: Hematological and bone marrow cytological abnormalities in 75 dogs with malignant lymphoma. JAAHA 22:235, 1986.

234. Bennett, JM, et al.: Proposals for the classification of the myelodysplastic syndromes. Br J Haematol 51:189, 1982.

235. Campbell, KL: Canine cyclic hematopoiesis. Comp Cont Ed 7:57, 1985.

236. Ford, L: Hereditary aspects of human and canine cyclic neutropenia. J Hered 60:293, 1969.

237. Lund, JE, et al.: Additional evidence on the inheritance of cyclic neutropenia in the dog. J Hered 61:47, 1970.

238. Lund, JE, et al.: Cyclic neutropenia in grey collie dogs. Blood 29:452, 1967.

239. Cheville, NF: The gray collie syndrome. JAVMA 152:620, 1968.

240. Machado, EA, et al.: The cyclic hematopoietic dog: A model for spontaneous secondary amyloidosis. Am J Pathol 92:23, 1978.

241. DiGiacomo, RF, et al.: Clinical and pathologic features of cyclic hematopoiesis in grey collie dogs. Am J Pathol 111:224, 1983.

242. Chusid, MJ, et al.: Defective polymorphonuclear leukocyte metabolism and function in canine cyclic neutropenia. Blood 46:921, 1975.

243. Jones, JB, et al.: Early-life hematologic values of dogs affected with cyclic neutropenia. Am J Vet Res 35:849, 1974.

244. Dale, DC, et al.: Cyclic hematopoiesis: The mechanism of cyclic neutropenia in grey collie dogs. J Clin Invest 51:2197, 1972.

245. Patt, HM, et al.: Cyclic hematopoiesis in grey collie dogs: A stem-cell problem. Blood 42:873, 1973.

246. Dale, DC, et al.: Studies of neutrophil production and turnover in grey collie dogs with cyclic neutropenia. J Clin Invest 51:2190, 1972.

247. Yang, TJ, et al.: Serum colony-stimulating activity of dogs with cyclic neutropenia. Blood 44:41, 1974.

248. Jones, JB, et al.: Canine cyclic neutropenia: Erythropoietin and platelet cycles after bone marrow transplantation. Blood 45:213, 1975.

249. Dunn, CDR, et al.: Progenitor cells in canine cyclic hematopoiesis. Blood 50:1111, 1977.

250. Weiden, PL, et al.: Canine cyclic neutropenia: A stem cell defect. J Clin Invest 53:950, 1974.

251. Osborne, WAR, et al.: Canine cyclic hematopoiesis is associated with abnormal purine and pyrimidine metabolism. J Clin Invest 71:1348, 1983.

252. Hammond, WP, et al.: Cyclic hematopoiesis: Effects of endotoxin on colony-forming cells and colony-stimulating activity in grey collie dogs. J Clin Invest 63:785, 1979.

253. Hammond, WP and Dale, DC: Lithium therapy of canine cyclic hematopoiesis. Blood 55:26, 1980.

254. Hammond, WP and Dale, DC: Cyclic hematopoiesis: Effects of lithium on colony-forming cells and colony-stimulating activity in grey collie dogs. Blood 59:179, 1982.

255. Jones, JB, et al.: Cyclic hematopoiesis in a colony of dogs. JAVMA 166:365, 1975.

256. Alexander, JW, et al.: Recurrent neutropenia in a pomeranian: A case report. JAAHA 17:841, 1981.

257. Morley, A and Stohlman, F: Cyclophosphamide-induced cyclical neutropenia. N Engl J Med 282:643, 1970.

258. Gabbert, NH: Cyclic neutropenia in a feline leukemia-positive cat: A case report. JAAHA 20:343, 1984.

259. Swenson, CL, et al.: Cyclic hematopoiesis associated with feline leukemia virus infection in two cats. JAVMA 191:93, 1987.

260. Bagby, GC, et al.: T-lymphocyte-mediated granulopoietic failure. N Engl J Med 309:1073, 1983.

261. Chan, WC, et al.: T-cell imbalance in neutropenia of uncertain etiology. Am J Clin Pathol 81:54, 1984.

262. Maddison, JE, et al.: Steroid responsive neutropenia in a dog. JAAHA 19:881, 1983.

263. Willard, MD: Corticosteroid-responsive leukopenia and neutropenia associated with FeLV infection in 2 cats. Mod Vet Pract 66:719, 1985.

264. Timoney, JF, et al.: Salmonellosis: A nosocomial outbreak and experimental studies. Cornell Vet 68:211, 1978.

265. Calvert, CA: Salmonella infections in hospitalized dogs: Epizootiology, diagnosis, and prognosis. Comp Cont Ed 21:499, 1985.

266. Jacob, HS, et al.: Complement-induced granulocyte aggregation: An unsuspected mechanism of disease. N Engl J Med 302:789, 1980.

267. Hammerschmidt, DE, et al.: Complement-induced granulocyte aggregation in vivo. Am J Pathol 102:146, 1981.

268. Thommasen, HV, et al.: Effect of pulmonary blood flow on leukocyte uptake and release by dog lung. J Appl Physiol: Respirat Environ Exercise Physiol 56:966, 1984.

269. Chickering, WR and Prasse, KW: Immune neutropenia in man and animals: A review. Vet Clin Pathol 10:6, 1981.

270. Chickering, WR, et al.: Development and clinical application of methods for detection of antineutrophil antibody in serum of the cat. Am J Vet Res 46:1809, 1985.

271. Chang, Y and Gralla, EJ: Suppression of urate crystal-induced canine joint inflammation by heterologous antipolymorphonuclear leukocyte serum. Arth Rheum 11:145, 1968.

272. Attström, R, et al.: Effect of experimental neutropenia on initial gingivitis in dogs. Scand J Dent Res 87:7, 1979.

273. Chickering, WR, et al.: Effects of heterologous antineutrophil antibody in the cat. Am J Vet Res 46:1815, 1985.

274. Stossel, TP and Boxer, LA: Functions of neutrophils. In Williams, WJ, et al. (eds): Hematology, 3rd ed. New York, McGraw-Hill, 1983, p 744.

275. Bender, HS and Chickering, WR: Superoxide, superoxide dismutase and the respiratory burst. Vet Clin Pathol 12:7, 1983.

276. Babior, BM: Oxidants from phagocytes: Agents of defense and destruction. Blood 64:959, 1984.

277. Latimer, KS and Mahaffey, EA: Neutrophil adherence and movement in poorly and well-controlled diabetic dogs. Am J Vet Res 45:1498, 1984.

278. Winkelstein, JA, et al.: Genetically determined deficiency of the third component of complement in the dog: In vitro studies on the complement system and complement-mediated serum activities. J Immunol 129:2598, 1982.

279. Rakich, PM and Latimer, KS: Altered immune function in a dog with disseminated protothecosis. JAVMA 185:681, 1984.

280. Latimer, KS, et al.: A transient deficit in neutrophilic chemotaxis in a dog with recurrent staphylococcal pyoderma. Vet Pathol 19:223, 1982.

281. Latimer, KS, et al.: Neutrophil movement in selected canine skin diseases. Am J Vet Res 44:601, 1983.

282. Swenson, CL, et al.: Neutrophil function in cats with feline leukemia virus. Proc 31st Ann Meet Am Coll Vet Pathol and 21st Ann Meet Am Soc Vet Clin Pathol, New Orleans, 1986, p 17.

283. Kiehl, AR, et al.: Effects of feline leukemia virus infection on neutrophil chemotaxis in vitro. Am J Vet Res 48:76, 1987.

284. Craddock, PR, et al.: Acquired phagocyte dysfunction: A complication of the hypophosphatemia of parenteral hyperalimentation. N Engl J Med 290:1403, 1974.

285. Cook, LO, et al.: In vitro functional capabilities of canine polymorphonuclear neutrophils collected simultaneously by continuous-flow centrifugation and continuous-flow filtration leukopheresis. Am J Hematol 4:225, 1978.

286. Renshaw, HW, et al.: Canine granulocytopathy syndrome: Defective bactericidal capacity of neutrophils from a dog with recurrent infections. Clin Immunol Immunopathol 8:384, 1977.

287. Renshaw, HW and Davis, WC: Canine granulocytopathy syndrome: An inherited disorder of leukocyte function. Am J Pathol 95:731, 1979.

288. Breitschwerdt, EB, et al.: Rhinitis, pneumonia, and defective neutrophil function in the Doberman pinscher. Am J Vet Res 48:1054, 1987.

289. Caldwell, KC, et al.: Induction of myeloperoxidase deficiency in granulocytes in lead-intoxicated dogs. Blood 53:588, 1979.

290. Gossett, KA, et al.: In vitro function of canine neutrophils during experimental inflammatory disease. Vet Immunol Immunopathol 5:151, 1983.

291. Latimer, KS and Prasse, KW: Neutrophilic movement of a

basenji with Pelger-Huët anomaly. Am J Vet Res 43:525, 1982.

292. Boxer, LA and Stossel, TP: Qualitative abnormalities of neutrophils. *In* Williams, WJ (ed.): Hematology, 3rd ed. New York, McGraw-Hill, 1983, p 802.
293. Latimer, KS, et al.: Quantitative evaluation of neutrophilic chemotaxis in beagles. Am J Vet Res 42:1254, 1981.
294. Gallin, JI: Human neutrophil heterogeneity exists, but is it meaningful? Blood 63:977, 1984.
295. Yourtee, EL and Root, RK: Antibiotic-neutrophil interactions in microbial killing. *In* Gallin, JI and Fauci, AS (eds): Advances in Host Defense Mechanisms, Vol. 1. New York, Raven Press, 1982, p 187.
296. Martin, S, et al.: Defective neutrophil function and microbiocidal mechanisms in the myelodysplastic disorders. J Clin Pathol 36:1120, 1983.
297. McAfee, JG, et al.: Distribution of leukocytes labeled with In-111 oxine in dogs with acute inflammatory lesions. J Nucl Med 21:1059, 1980.
298. Lasser, A: The mononuclear phagocytic system: A review. Human Pathol 14:108, 1983.
299. Nathan, CF, et al.: The macrophage as an effector cell. N Engl J Med 303:622, 1980.
300. McMillan, FD: Fever: Pathophysiology and rational therapy. Comp Cont Ed 7:845, 1985.
301. Meuret, G, et al.: Kinetics of human monocytopoiesis. Blood 44:801, 1974.
302. Snyder, SP, et al.: Niemann-Pick disease; sphingomyelinosis of siamese cats. Am J Pathol 108:252, 1982.
303. Mackey, L: Haematology of the cat. *In* Archer, RK and Jeffcott, LB (eds): Comparative Clinical Haematology. Oxford, Blackwell Scientific Publications, 1977, p 441.
304. Meuret, G and Hoffman, G: Monocyte kinetic studies in normal and disease states. Br J Haematol 24:275, 1973.
305. Hocking, WG and Golde, DW: The pulmonary-alveolar macrophage. N Engl J Med 301:580, 639, 1979.
306. Shaw, SE and Anderson, NV: Isolation and functional analysis of normal canine blood monocytes and resident alveolar macrophages. Am J Vet Res 45:87, 1984.
307. Calvert, CA: Valvular bacterial endocarditis in the dog. JAVMA 180:1080, 1982.
308. Calvert, CA and Greene, CE: Bacteremia in dogs: Diagnosis, treatment, and prognosis. Comp Cont Ed 8:179, 1986.
309. Groopman, JE and Golde, DW: The histiocytic disorders: A pathophysiologic analysis. Ann Int Med 94:95, 1981.
310. Van der Valk, P and Herman, CJ: Leukocyte functions. Lab Invest 57:127, 1987.
311. Moore, PF: Systemic histiocytosis of Bernese Mountain Dogs. Vet Pathol 21:554, 1984.
312. Moore, PF: Malignant histiocytosis of Bernese Mountain Dogs. Vet Pathol 23:1, 1986.
313. Wellman, ML, et al.: Malignant histiocytosis in four dogs. JAVMA 187:919, 1985.
314. Rosin, A, et al.: Malignant histiocytosis in Bernese Mountain Dogs. JAVMA 188:1041, 1986.
315. Cotter, SM and Holzworth, J: Disorders of the hematopoietic system. *In* Holzworth, J (ed): Diseases of the Cat: Medicine and Surgery. Philadelphia, WB Saunders, 1987, p 755.
316. Degen, MA and Breitschwerdt, EB: Canine and feline immunodeficiency. Comp Cont Ed 8:313, 379, 1986.
317. Gorman, NT and Werner, LL: Immune-mediated diseases of the dog and cat. Br Vet J 142:395, 403, 491, 498, 1986.
318. Craddock, CG, et al.: Lymphocytes and the immune response. N Engl J Med 285:324, 378, 1971.
319. Wilkins, RJ: Morphologic features of feline peripheral blood lymphocytes. JAAHA 10:362, 1974.
320. Wierup, M, et al.: Evaluation of a killed feline panleukopenia virus vaccine against canine parvoviral enteritis in dogs. Am J Vet Res 43:2183, 1982.
321. Schalm, OW: Leukocyte counts and lymph node cytology in salmon poisoning of dogs. Canine Pract 5:59, 1978.
322. Schalm, OW: Special characteristics of lymphocytes and monocytes in infectious canine hepatitis. Canine Pract 6:51, 1979.
323. Trinchieri, G and Perussia, B: Human natural killer cells: Biologic and pathologic aspects. Lab Invest 50:489, 1984.
324. Kelly, WD: The thymus and lymphoid morphogenesis in the dog. Fed Proc 22:600, 1963.

325. Ackerman, GA: Developmental relationship between the appearance of lymphocytes and lymphopoietic activity in the thymus and lymph nodes of the fetal cat. Anat Rec 158:387, 1967.
326. Parks, ED and Chisari, FV: Production and distribution of lymphocytes and plasma cells. *In* Williams, WJ, et al. (eds): Hematology, 3rd ed. New York, McGraw-Hill, 1983, p 923.
327. Moretta, A, et al.: Recent advances in the phenotypic and functional analysis of human T lymphocytes. Semin Hematol 21:257, 1984.
328. Röpke, C, et al.: Long-lived T and B lymphocytes in the bone marrow and thoracic duct lymph of the mouse. Cell Immunol 15:82, 1975.
329. Rojko, JL, et al.: Characterization and mitogenesis of feline lymphocyte populations. Int Arch Allergy Appl Immunol 68:226, 1982.
330. Chandler, JP and Yang, TJ: Identification of canine lymphocyte populations by immunofluorescence surface marker analysis. Int Arch Allergy Appl Immunol 65:62, 1981.
331. Hopkins, J and McConnell, I: Immunological aspects of lymphocyte recirculation. Vet Immunol Immunopathol 6:3, 1984.
332. Ford, WL and Gowans, JL: The traffic of lymphocytes. Semin Hematol 6:67, 1969.
333. Legendre, AM, et al.: Canine blastomycosis: A review of 47 clinical cases. JAVMA 178:1163, 1981.
334. Breitschwerdt, EB, et al.: Canine Rocky Mountain spotted fever: A kennel epizootic. Am J Vet Res 46:2124, 1985.
335. Moore, FM, et al.: Distinctive peripheral lymph node hyperplasia of young cats. Vet Pathol 23:386, 1986.
336. Hardy, WD: Hematopoietic tumors of cats. JAAHA 17:921, 1981.
337. Leifer, CE and Matus, RE: Chronic lymphocytic leukemia in the dog: 22 cases (1974–1984). JAVMA 189:214, 1986.
338. Willard, MD, et al.: Canine hypoadrenocorticism: Report of 37 cases and review of 39 previously reported cases. JAVMA 180:59, 1982.
339. Rakich, PM and Lorenz, MD: Clinical signs and laboratory abnormalities in 23 dogs with spontaneous hypoadrenocorticism. JAAHA 20:647, 1984.
340. Fauci, AS: Mechanisms of corticosteroid action on lymphocyte subpopulations: I. Redistribution of circulating T and B lymphocytes to the bone marrow. Immunology 28:669, 1975.
341. Schuyler, MR, et al.: Prednisone and T-cell subpopulations. Arch Intern Med 144:973, 1984.
342. Fauci, AS and Dale, DC: Alternate-day prednisone therapy and human lymphocyte subpopulations. J Clin Invest 55:22, 1975.
343. Dillon, AR, et al.: Prednisolone induced hematologic, biochemical, and histologic changes in the dog. JAAHA 16:831, 1980.
344. Krakowa, S, et al.: Canine distemper virus: Review of structural and functional modulations in lymphoid tissue. Am J Vet Res 41:284, 1980.
345. Anderson, LJ, et al.: Feline leukemia virus infection of kittens: Mortality associated with atrophy of the thymus and lymphoid depletion. J Nat Cancer Inst 47:807, 1971.
346. Breitschwerdt, EB, et al.: A hereditary diarrhetic syndrome in the basenji characterized by malabsorption, protein losing enteropathy and hypergammaglobulinemia. JAAHA 16:551, 1980.
347. Berg, JN: Chylothorax in the dog and cat. Comp Cont Ed 4:986, 1982.
348. Fossum, TW, et al.: Chylothorax in 34 dogs. JAVMA 188:1315, 1986.
349. Burns, MG: Intestinal lymphangiectasia in the dog: A case report and review. JAAHA 18:97, 1982.
350. Meschter, CL, et al.: Intestinal lymphangiectasia with lipogranulomatous lymphangitis in a dog. JAVMA 190:427, 1987.
351. Weller, PF and Goetzl, EJ: The human eosinophil: Roles in host defense and tissue injury. Am J Pathol 100:793, 1980.
352. Butterworth, AE and David, JR: Eosinophil function. N Engl J Med 304:154, 1981.
353. Tavassoli, M: Eosinophil, eosinophilia, and eosinophilic disorders. CRC Crit Rev Lab Sci 16:35, 1981.
354. Kay, AB: The role of the eosinophil. J Allergy Clin Immunol 64:90, 1979.
355. Fauci, AS, et al.: The idiopathic hypereosinophilic syndrome: Clinical, pathophysiologic, and therapeutic considerations. Ann Intern Med 97:78, 1982.

356. Schatz, M, et al.: The eosinophil and the lung. Arch Intern Med 142:1515, 1982.
357. Tai, PC and Spry, CJF: The mechanisms which produce vacuolated and degranulated eosinophils. Br J Haematol 49:219, 1981.
358. Carper, HA and Hoffman, PL: The intravascular survival of transfused canine Pelger-Huët neutrophils and eosinophils. Blood 27:739, 1966.
359. Zucker-Franklin, D: Eosinopenia and eosinophilia. In Williams, WJ, et al. (eds): Hematology, 3rd ed. New York, McGraw-Hill, 1983, p 825.
360. Hendrick, M: A spectrum of hypereosinophilic syndromes exemplified by six cats with eosinophilic enteritis. Vet Pathol 18:188, 1981.
361. McEwen, SA, et al.: Hypereosinophilic syndrome in cats: A report of 3 cases. Can J Comp Med 49:248, 1985.
362. Simon, N and Holzworth, J: Eosinophilic leukemia in a cat. Cornell Vet 57:579, 1967.
363. Silverman, J: Eosinophilic leukaemia in a cat. JAVMA 158:199, 1971.
364. Schalm, OW: The feline leukemia complex: Less common forms of leukemic leukemia. Fel Pract 6:36, 1976.
365. Finlay, D: Eosinophilic leukaemia in the cat: A case report. Vet Rec 116:567, 1985.
366. Catovsky, D, et al.: The association of eosinophilia with lymphoblastic leukaemia or lymphoma: A study of seven patients. Br J Haematol 45:523, 1980.
367. Slungaard, A, et al.: Pulmonary carcinoma with eosinophilia: Demonstration of a tumor-derived eosinophilopoietic factor. N Engl J Med 309:778, 1983.
368. Beeson, PB: Cancer and eosinophilia. N Engl J Med 309:792, 1983.
369. Mahmoud, AAF and Austen, KF: The Eosinophil in Health and Disease. New York, Grune & Stratton, 1980.
370. Zerbe, CA, et al.: Hyperadrenocorticism in a cat. JAVMA 190:559, 1987.
371. Peterson, ME and Steele, P: Pituitary-dependent hyperadrenocorticism in a cat. JAVMA 189:680, 1986.
372. Dvorak, AM and Dvorak, HF: The basophil: Its morphology, biochemistry, motility, release reactions, recovery, and role in the inflammatory responses of IgE-mediated and cell-mediated origin. Arch Pathol Lab Med 103:551, 1979.
373. Askenase, PW: Mechanisms of hypersensitivity: Cellular interactions. Basophil arrival and function in tissue hypersensitivity reactions. J Allergy Clin Immunol 64:79, 1979.
374. Halliwell, REW and Schemmer, KR: The role of basophils in the immunopathogenesis of hypersensitivity to fleas (Ctenocephalides felis) in dogs. Vet Immunol Immunopathol 15:203, 1987.
375. Newball, HH, et al.: Basophil mediators and their release, with emphasis on BK-A. J Invest Dermatol 74:344, 1980.
376. Parwaresch, MR: The Human Blood Basophil: Morphology, Origin, Kinetics, Function and Pathology. New York, Springer-Verlag, 1976.
377. Jasper, DE and Jain, NC: Postprandial lipemia in dogs. Calif Vet 18:27, 1964.
378. Brown, SJ and Askenase, PW: Immune rejection of ectoparasites (ticks) by T cell and IgG₁ antibody recruitment of basophils and eosinophils. Fed Proc 42:1744, 1983.
379. Dvorak, HF, et al.: Immunologic rejection of diethylnitrosamine-induced hepatomas in strain 2 guinea pigs. J Exp Med 137:751, 1973.
380. Anthony, HM: Blood basophils in lung cancer. Br J Cancer 45:209, 1982.
381. May, ME and Waddell, CC: Basophils in peripheral blood and bone marrow: A retrospective review. Am J Med 76:509, 1984.
382. Goetzl, EJ, et al.: A basophil-activating factor from human T lymphocytes. Immunology 53:227, 1984.
383. Zucker-Franklin, D: Basophilopenia, basophilia, and mastocytosis. In Williams, WJ, et al. (eds): Hematology, 3rd ed. New York, McGraw-Hill, 1983, p 828.
384. Mahaffey, EA, et al.: Basophilic leukaemia in a dog. J Comp Pathol 97:393, 1987.
385. Hayashi, C, et al.: Bone marrow origin of mast cell precursors in mesenteric lymph nodes of mice. Exp Hematol 11:772, 1983.
386. Rawlings, CA, et al.: Eosinophilia and basophilia in Dirofilaria immitis and Dipetalonema reconditum infections. JAAHA 16:699, 1980.
387. Calvert, CA and Rawlings, CA: Diagnosis and management of canine heartworm disease. In Kirk, RW (ed): Current Veterinary Therapy VIII. Philadelphia, WB Saunders, 1983, p 348.
388. Dillon, R, et al.: Indirect immunofluorescence testing for the diagnosis of occult Dirofilaria immitis infection in three cats. JAVMA 180:80, 1982.
389. Calvert, CA and Mandell, CP: Diagnosis and management of feline heartworm disease. JAVMA 180:550, 1982.
390. Jain, NC, et al.: Clinical-pathological findings and cytochemical characterization of myelomonocytic leukaemia in 5 dogs. J Comp Pathol 91:17, 1981.
391. Facklam, NR and Kociba, GJ: Cytochemical characterization of feline leukemic cells. Vet Pathol 23:155, 1986.
392. Grindem, CB, et al.: Cytochemical reactions in cells from leukemic dogs. Vet Pathol 23:103, 1986.
393. Grindem, CB: Ultrastructural morphology of leukemic cells in the cat. Vet Pathol 22:147, 1985.
394. Grindem, CB: Ultrastructural morphology of leukemic cells from 14 dogs. Vet Pathol 22:456, 1985.
395. Rohrig, KE: Acute myelomonocytic leukemia in a dog. JAVMA 182:137, 1983.
396. Stass, S, et al.: Lineage switch in acute leukemia. Blood 64:701, 1984.
397. Engelman, RW, et al.: Changing manifestations of a chronic feline haematopoietic proliferative disease during immunotherapy with staphylococcal protein A. J Comp Pathol 96:177, 1986.
398. Harvey, JW: Myeloproliferative disorders in dogs and cats. Vet Clin North Am 11:349, 1981.
399. Sykes, GP, et al.: Retrovirus-like particles associated with myeloproliferative disease in the dog. J Comp Pathol 95:559, 1985.
400. Delacretaz, F, et al.: Histopathology of myelodysplastic syndromes. The FAB classification (proposals) applied to bone marrow biopsy. Am J Clin Pathol 87:180, 1987.
401. Maggio, L, et al.: Feline preleukemia: An animal model of human disease. Yale J Biol Med 51:469, 1978.
402. Schneider, R: Comparison of age- and sex-specific incidence rate patterns of the leukemia complex in the cat and the dog. J Natl Cancer Inst 70:971, 1983.
403. Jarrett, WHF, et al.: Myeloid leukaemia in a cat produced experimentally by feline leukaemia virus. Res Vet Sci 12:385, 1971.
404. Lewis, MG: Retroviral-associated eosinophilic leukemia in the cat. Am J Vet Res 46:1066, 1985.
405. Theilen, GH and Schalm, OW: Myeloproliferative disease in the dog. A case report of granulocytic leukemia. Calif Vet 24:10, 1970.
406. Christopher, MM, et al.: Acute myelomonocytic leukemia with neurologic manifestations in the dog. Vet Pathol 23:140, 1986.
407. Williams, DA: Gammopathies. Comp Cont Ed 3:815, 1981.
408. Campbell, KL and Latimer, KS: Polysystemic manifestations of plasma cell myeloma in the dog: A case report and review. JAAHA 21:59, 1985.
409. Henness, AM and Crow, SE: Treatment of feline myelogenous leukemia: Four case reports. JAVMA 171:263, 1977.
410. Meier, H: Neoplastic diseases of the hematopoietic system (so-called leukosis-complex) in the dog. Zentralbl Veterinaermed 4:633, 1957.
411. Medway, W and Rapp, JP: A case of chronic granulocytic leukemia with thrombocytopenic purpura in a dog. Cornell Vet 52:242, 1962.
412. Lucke, VM and Sumner-Smith, G: A case of myeloid leukaemia in the dog. J Sm Anim Pract 7:23, 1963.
413. Skelley, JF: Clinico-pathologic conference from the School of Veterinary Medicine, University of Pennsylvania. JAVMA 142:646, 1963.
414. Rouse, BT, et al.: Acute granulocytic leukaemia in a bitch. Vet Rec 80:408, 1967.
415. Cameron, TP, et al.: Irradiation of a dog with myelogenous leukemia. JAVMA 154:279, 1969.
416. Cooper, BJ and Watson, ADJ: Myeloid neoplasia in a dog. Aust Vet J 51:150, 1975.
417. Schalm, OW: Granulocytic (myelogenous) leukemia in the dog. Canine Pract 3:22, 1976.

418. Joiner, GN, et al.: A case of chronic granulocytic leukemia in a dog. Can J Comp Med 40:153, 1976.

419. Pollet, L, et al.: Blastic crisis in chronic myelogenous leukaemia in a dog. J Sm Anim Pract 19:469, 1978.

420. Weller, RE, et al.: Myeloblastic leukemia and leukemic meningitis in a dog. Mod Vet Pract 61:42, 1980.

421. Sutton, RH and Wilkins, S: A case of canine myeloid neoplasia. J Sm Anim Pract 22:139, 1981.

422. Keller, P, et al.: Acute myeloblastic leukaemia in a dog. J Comp Pathol 95:619, 1985.

423. Eyestone, WH: Myelogenous leukemia in the cat. J Natl Cancer Inst 12:599, 1951.

424. Meier, H and Patterson, DF: Myelogenous leukemia in a cat. JAVMA 128:211, 1956.

425. Holzworth, J: Leukemia and related neoplasms in the cat. II. Malignancies other than lymphoid. JAVMA 136:107, 1960.

426. Fraser, CJ, et al.: Acute granulocytic leukemia in cats. JAVMA 165:355, 1974.

427. Barthel, CH: Acute myelomonocytic leukemia in a dog. Vet Pathol 11:79, 1974.

428. Green, RA and Barton, CL: Acute myelomonocytic leukemia in a dog. JAAHA 13:708, 1977.

429. Linnabary, RD, et al.: Acute myelomonocytic leukemia in a dog. JAAHA 14:71, 1978.

430. Loeb, WF, et al.: Myelomonocytic leukemia in a cat. Vet Pathol 12:464, 1975.

431. Stann, SE: Myelomonocytic leukemia in a cat. JAVMA 174:722, 1979.

432. Loeb, WF, et al.: Monocytic leukemia in a dog. *In* Clark, WJ, et al. (eds): Myeloproliferative Disorders of Animals and Man. US Atomic Energy Commission, Division of Technical Information, 1970, p 687.

433. Mackey, LJ, et al.: Monocytic leukaemia in the dog. Vet Rec 96:27, 1975.

434. Schalm, OW: Acute monocytic leukemia. Reticulum cell sarcoma. Canine Pract 3:19, 1976.

435. Henness, AM, et al.: Monocytic leukemia in three cats. JAVMA 170:1325, 1977.

436. Tsujimoto, H, et al.: Monocytic leukemia in a cat. Jpn J Vet Sci 43:957, 1981.

437. Saar, C and Reichel, C: Einige besondere Leukoseformen bei der Katze. Prakt Tierarzt 5:443, 1983.

438. Toth, S, et al.: Chronic eosinophilic leukaemia in blast crisis in a cat negative for feline leukaemia virus. Vet Rec 117:471, 1985.

439. Romanelli, V: Sopra la leucemia basofila leucemica del cane. Arch Vet Ital 4:499, 1953.

440. Rampichini, L and Coluzzi, G: Contributo allo studio della leucemia basofila negli animali domestici. Descrizione di un caso fiscontrato in un cane. Atti Soc Ital Sci Vet 16:271, 1962.

441. Kammermann-Leuscher, VB: Blutbasophilen-leukose beim Hund gewebsbasophilen-reticulose bei der katze. Berl Münch Tierarztl Wschr 79:459, 1966.

442. Alroy, J: Basophilic leukemia in a dog. Vet Pathol 9:90, 1972.

443. MacEwen, EG, et al.: Treatment of basophilic leukemia in a dog. JAVMA 166:376, 1975.

444. O'Keefe, DA, et al.: Systemic mastocytosis in 16 dogs. J Vet Intern Med 1:75, 1987.

445. Gilmore, CE, et al.: Reticuloendotheliosis, a myeloproliferative disorder of cats: A comparison with lymphocytic leukemia. Pathol Vet 1:161, 1964.

446. Crow, SE, et al.: Feline reticuloendotheliosis: A report of 4 cases. JAVMA 170:1329, 1977.

447. Liu, SK and Carb, AV: Erythroblastic leukemia in a dog. JAVMA 152:1511, 1968.

448. Thompson, JC and Johnstone, AC: Myelofibrosis in the dog: Three case reports. J Sm Anim Pract 24:589, 1983.

449. Harvey, JW, et al.: Feline myeloproliferative disease: Changing manifestations in the peripheral blood. Vet Pathol 15:437, 1978.

450. Zawidzka, ZZ, et al.: Erythremic myelosis in a cat: A case resembling Di Guglielmo's syndrome in man. Pathol Vet 1:530, 1964.

451. Peterson, ME and Randolph, JF: Diagnosis of canine primary polycythemia and management with hydroxyurea. JAVMA 180:415, 1982.

452. Reed, C, et al.: Polycythemia vera in a cat. JAVMA 157:85, 1970.

453. Brodsky, I: The differential diagnosis of polycythemia. Ann Clin Lab Med 10:311, 1980.

454. Peterson, ME: Inappropriate erythropoietin production from a renal carcinoma in a dog with polycythemia. JAVMA 179:995, 1981.

455. Nelson, RW, et al.: Renal lymphosarcoma with inappropriate erythropoietin production in a dog. JAVMA 182:1396, 1983.

456. Michel, RL, et al.: Megakaryocytic myelosis in a cat. JAVMA 168:1021, 1976.

457. Holscher, MA, et al.: Megakaryocytic leukemia in a cat. Feline Pract 13:8, 1983.

458. Nielsen, SW: Myeloproliferative disorders in animals. *In* Clark, WJ, et al. (eds): Myeloproliferative Disorders of Animals and Man. US Atomic Energy Commission, Division of Technical Information, 1970, p 297.

459. Rudolph, R and Hübner, C: Megakaryocyte leukosis in a dog. Kleintierpraxis 17:9, 1972.

460. Holscher, MA, et al.: Megakaryocytic leukemia in a dog. Vet Pathol 15:562, 1978.

461. Tolle, DV, et al.: Circulating micromegakaryocytes preceding leukemia in three dogs exposed to 2.5 R/day gamma radiation. Vet Pathol 20:111, 1983.

462. Cain, GR, et al: Radiation-induced megakaryoblastic leukemia in a dog. Vet Pathol 22:641, 1985.

463. Harvey, JW, et al.: Myeloprolifcrative disease with megakaryocytic predominance in a dog with occult dirofilariasis. Vet Clin Pathol 11:5, 1982.

464. Canfield, PJ, et al.: Myeloproliferative disorder in four dogs involving derangements of erythropoiesis, myelopoiesis, and megakaryopoiesis. J Sm Anim Pract 27:7, 1986.

465. Sutton, RH, et al.: Myeloproliferative disease in the cat: A granulocytic and megakaryocytic disorder. NZ Vet J 26:273, 1978.

466. Saar, C: Erythro-Megakaryozythämie bei einer Katze. Berl Münch Tierärztl Wochenschr 83:70, 1970.

467. Hodgkins, EM, et al.: Chronic lymphocytic leukemia in the dog. JAVMA 177:704, 1980.

468. Braund, KG, et al.: Neurologic complications of IgA multiple myeloma associated with cryoglobulinemia in a dog. JAVMA 174:1321, 1979.

469. Couto, CG, et al.: Plasma cell leukemia and monoclonal (IgG) gammopathy in a dog. JAVMA 184:90, 1984.

470. Zinkl, JG, et al.: "Flaming" plasma cells in a dog with IgA multiple myeloma. Vet Clin Pathol 12:15, 1983.

115 DISEASES OF THE LYMPH NODES AND THE SPLEEN

C. GUILLERMO COUTO

The lymph nodes and the spleen constitute the major source of reticuloendothelial and immunologic cells in the body. Due to their dynamic state, they constantly reshape and change in size in response to a variety of stimuli. The majority of the tissue changes within these structures result in organ enlargement. This organomegaly oftentimes represents the only physical abnormality in an otherwise healthy patient, and alerts the clinician to an ongoing disease process.

LYMPH NODES

Anatomy, Histology, and Physiology

The lymph nodes are ovoid encapsulated structures whose primary functions are to filter lymph and to participate in immunologic reactions.[1, 2] In the dog and cat, they are well-developed and have a convex shape with an indentation, the hilus, through which lymphatic vessels leave the node and blood vessels enter. Afferent lymphatics penetrate the node through the convex surface of the capsule.[1]

Histologically, a lymph node is composed of a capsule, subcapsular spaces, a cortical area, a paracortical area, and a medulla (Figure 115–1). The connective tissue *capsule* surrounds all the other structures. The *subcapsular spaces* contain the reticuloendothelium responsible for filtering particles that arrive to the node through the afferent lymphatics; these areas are also referred to as subcapsulary sinuses. Macrophages within this area also play an important role in presenting antigen to the lymphoid cells. The cortical area is composed primarily of B lymphocytes arranged in round or oval lymphatic nodules, referred to as *lymphoid follicles*. Follicles composed of tightly packed small lymphocytes are referred to as *primary follicles*, while those with a central zone of larger, immature lymphocytes and macrophages are termed *secondary follicles*; the pale central areas are referred to as *germinal centers*. The paracortical area is composed mostly of T cells. The medulla is similar to

the subcapsular area in that it is rich in reticuloendothelium; lymph flows from this area to the efferent lymphatics in the hilar region.[1] Another important component of the lymph node structure is the blood vessels, since it is through these vascular structures that recirculation of lymphocytes occurs (see below).

The two main functions of the lymph nodes are filtration of lymph and recirculation of lymphocytes. Filtration of particulate matter occurs as the lymph percolates through the node; also, during this process some products of phagocytic degradation become immunogenic. Lymphocytes in peripheral blood recirculate through the lymph node; they do so by exiting the blood through the postcapillary venules, unique anatomic structures found in the cortical area and composed of elongated endothelial cells. This recirculating lymphocyte pool is composed primarily of T cells.[2] It should be kept in mind that these physiologic changes occur constantly, and can therefore result in significant changes in lymph node size, shape, and consistency that will oftentimes clue the clinician to the presence of an underlying disease process.

From the clinical standpoint, it is important to become familiar with the characteristics of palpable lymph nodes in normal animals, so that subtle changes will be easily detected. Palpable lymph nodes in the dog and cat are depicted in Figure 115–2. They are the mandibulars, prescapulars (or superficial cervicals), axillaries, superficial inguinal, and popliteal. Other lymph nodes become palpable only when enlarged; these include the facial, retropharyngeal, and iliac (or sublumbar) nodes (Figure 115–2).[3–5]

Lymphadenopathy

DEFINITIONS

In the context of this chapter, the term lymphadenopathy refers to lymph node enlargement. Solitary or isolated lymphadenopathy refers to enlargement of a single lymph node. Regional lymphadenopathy de-

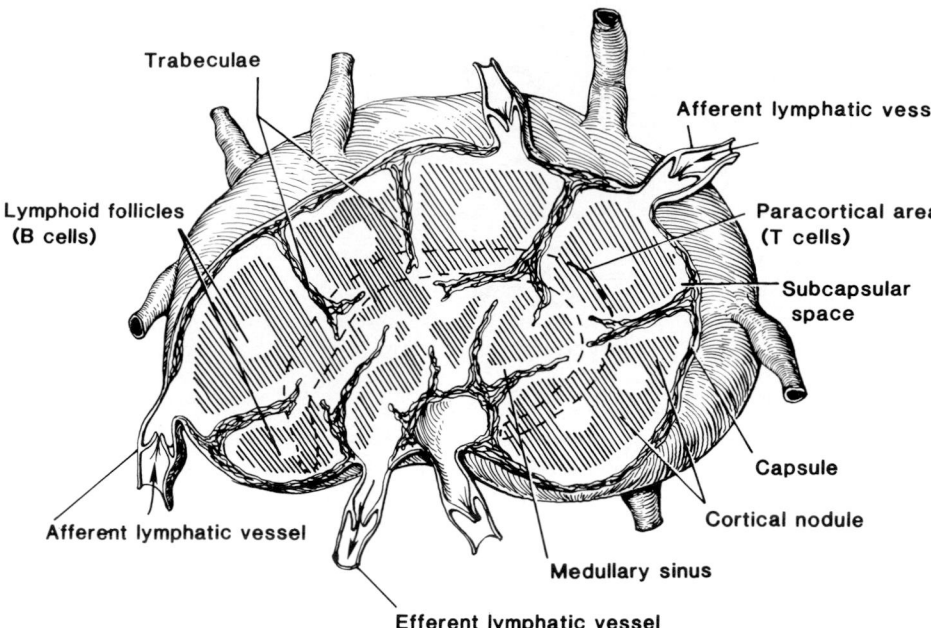

FIGURE 115–1. Microscopic anatomy of a canine or feline lymph node. For a detailed discussion, please refer to the text.

scribes the enlargement of more than one lymph node draining a given anatomic area; these nodes are usually interconnected. Generalized lymphadenopathy refers to multicentric lymph node enlargement affecting more than one anatomic area. Lymphadenopathies can also be classified as superficial or deep, according to their anatomical location.

PATHOGENESIS

As discussed above, lymph nodes are in a dynamic state; this results in constant reshaping. Lymph node enlargement usually occurs as a consequence of proliferation of normal cells or infiltration with normal or abnormal cells. When normal cells proliferate within a node, the term *reactive lymphadenopathy* is used. Proliferation of normal lymphoid or reticuloendothelial cells occurs in response to various stimuli, mainly infectious and immunologic, although occasionally the clinician will face a dog or cat with reactive lymphadenopathy in which an etiologic agent cannot be identified (idiopathic reactive lymphadenopathy). When polymorphonuclear leukocytes or inflammatory macrophages predominate in the lymph node infiltrate, the term *lymphadenitis* is used; this is usually secondary to infectious processes. If neutrophils predominate, the lymphadenitis is considered to be suppurative; if macrophages are the predominant cell, then the inflammation is granulomatous; if macrophages and neutrophils occur, the term pyogranulomatous lymphadenitis is preferred.

Infiltrative lymphadenopathies result from displacement of normal lymph node tissue by neoplastic or inflammatory cells. Neoplasms involving the lymph nodes can be either primary hematopoietic tumors or secondary (metastatic) neoplasms. To the author's knowledge, infiltrative lymphadenopathies in association with lysosomal storage diseases (Gaucher's disease) have not been reported in the dog or cat.

Table 115–1 lists a classification of lymphadenopathies in dogs and cats. Since most of the diseases listed in this table have been discussed elsewhere in this book, only certain specific lymphadenopathies and hemolymphatic neoplasms will be addressed in this chapter.

EVALUATION OF THE PATIENT WITH LYMPHADENOPATHY

History and Physical Findings. Several important clues of diagnostic value can be obtained from the history. A detailed travel history should be obtained in dogs presented for evaluation of generalized lymphadenopathy, since certain diseases (e.g., leishmaniasis, salmon poisoning, some systemic mycoses) have a defi-

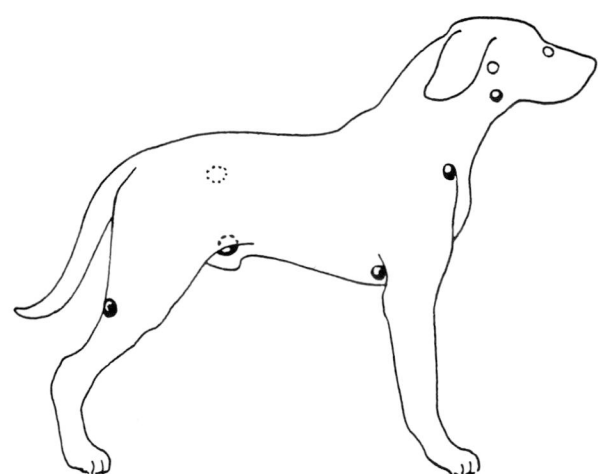

FIGURE 115–2. Palpable lymph nodes in the dog. In open circles are nodes that are not palpable unless enlarged; they include (from cranial to caudal): facial, retropharyngeal, and iliacs (in dotted line). The dark circles depict the lymph nodes that are commonly palpable, even when normal in size. They include (from cranial to caudal): mandibulars, prescapulars, axillaries, superficial inguinals, and popliteals.

TABLE 115–1. CLASSIFICATION OF LYMPHADENOPATHIES IN DOGS AND CATS

Type	Species
Proliferative Lymphadenopathies	
Infectious	
Bacterial	
Streptococci	C, D
Corynebacterium	C
Brucella	D
Mycobacteria	C, D
Actinomyces spp.	C, D
Nocardia spp.	C, D
Septicemia	C, D
Localized bacterial infection	C, D
Rickettsial	
Ehrlichiosis	D
Rocky Mountain spotted fever	D
Salmon poisoning	D
Fungal	
Histoplasmosis	C, D
Blastomycosis	C, D
Cryptococcosis	C, D
Coccidioidomycosis	C, D
Aspergillosis	C, D
Sporotrichosis	C?, D
Phaeohyphomycosis	C?, D
Phycomycosis	C?, D
Algal	
Protothecosis	C?, D
Parasitic	
Demodicosis	C, D
Trypanosomiasis	D
Leishmaniasis	D
Hepatozoonosis	D
Babesiosis	D
Toxoplasmosis	C, D
Viral	
Infectious canine hepatitis	D
Canine herpesvirus	D
Canine viral enteritides	D
Feline leukemia virus	C
Feline infectious peritonitis	C
Noninfectious	
Postvaccinal	C, D
Immune-mediated disorders	
Systemic lupus erythematosus	D
Rheumatoid arthritis	D
Immune-mediated polyarthritides	C, D
Localized inflammation	C, D
Idiopathic	C, D
Infiltrative Lymphadenopathies	
Neoplastic	
Primary Hematopoietic Neoplasms	
Lymphomas (lymphosarcomas)	C, D
Malignant histiocytosis	D
Leukemias	C, D
Multiple myeloma	C, D
Systemic mast cell disease	C, D
Metastatic Neoplasms	
Carcinomas	C, D
Sarcomas	C, D
Mast cell tumors	C, D
Malignant melanomas	D
Non-neoplastic	
Mast cell infiltration (non-neoplastic)	C, D
Eosinophilic granuloma complex	C, D?

C: cats; D: dogs, ?: questionable

nite geographical distribution. Other diseases associated with lymphadenopathy have a seasonal distribution (Rocky Mountain spotted fever [RMSF] cases occur predominantly during the spring and summer months). The presence or absence of systemic clinical signs is also helpful in guiding the clinician to a diagnosis in dogs or cats with generalized lymphadenopathy, since severe systemic signs are more common in certain diseases (e.g., systemic mycoses, salmon poisoning, RMSF, leishmaniasis, acute leukemias) than in others (lymphoma, chronic leukemia). A vaccination history should also be obtained, since it is not uncommon to observe generalized reactive lymphadenopathy shortly following vaccination.

The distribution of the lymphadenopathy is of diagnostic significance. When evaluating a patient with solitary or regional lymphadenopathy, the clinician should focus attention on the area drained by those lymph nodes, since with almost certainty that is where the primary lesion will be found. For example, it is not unusual to make a diagnosis of neoplasia after tumor cells are found in a needle aspirate from a single enlarged lymph node (see below); when the area drained by that node is carefully examined, the primary neoplasm can oftentimes be detected. In the author's experience, most cases of superficial solitary or regional lymphadenopathy in dogs and cats are the result of localized inflammatory (or infectious) processes or of metastatic neoplasia, while most cases of deep (intraabdominal, intrathoracic) solitary or regional lymphadenopathy are due to metastatic neoplasia or systemic infectious diseases (systemic mycoses). On the contrary, most cases of generalized lymphadenopathy are due to systemic fungal or rickettsial infections, or to hemopoietic neoplasia (Table 115–2).

The palpable characteristics of the nodes are also important. In most dogs and cats with lymphadenopathy, regardless of whether it is solitary, regional, or generalized, the lymph nodes are firmer than usual, are irregular, painless, have normal temperature to the touch (cold lymphadenopathies), and do not adhere to the surrounding tissues. The main exception to this rule occurs in patients with lymphadenitis, in which the nodes may be softer than usual, are tender and warmer than normal, and adhere to surrounding structures (fixed lymphadenopathy). Metastatic lesions and lymphomas with extracapsular invasion also may present as fixed lymphadenopathies.

From the clinical standpoint, the size of the affected lymph nodes is also important. In the author's experience, marked lymphadenopathy (lymph node size 5 to

TABLE 115–2. CORRELATION BETWEEN CLINICAL PRESENTATION AND ETIOLOGY IN DOGS AND CATS WITH LYMPHADENOPATHY (IN RELATIVE ORDER OF IMPORTANCE IN THE MIDWEST)

Generalized	Solitary/Regional	
	Superficial	*Intracavitary*
Lymphomas	Abscess	Histoplasmosis
Histoplasmosis	Periodontal disease	Blastomycosis
Blastomycosis	Paronychia	Perianal gland aCA[1]
Postvaccinal	Deep pyoderma	Apocrine gland aCA
Canine ehrlichiosis	Demodicosis	Primary lung tumors
Leukemias	MCT[2]	Lymphoma
Brucellosis	Malignant melanoma	MCT
SMCD[3]	EGC[4]	
Multiple myeloma	Lymphoma	
Malignant histiocytosis		
SLE[5]		
Other		

[1]Adenocarcinoma
[2]Mast cell tumor
[3]Systemic mast cell disease
[4]Eosinophilic granuloma complex
[5]Systemic lupus erythematosus

10 times normal) occurs almost exclusively with lymphadenitis (lymph node abscessation) and with lymphomas. Occasionally, metastatic lymph nodes will show this degree of lymph node enlargement. Dogs with salmon poisoning may also present with marked generalized lymphadenopathy and bloody diarrhea.[6, 7] Mild lymph node enlargement (two to four times normal size) occurs mostly in a variety of reactive lymphadenopathies (ehrlichiosis, RMSF, systemic mycoses) and in leukemias.[8–13]

As already mentioned, a thorough examination of the area(s) draining the enlarged lymph node/s should always be performed, paying particular attention to the skin and subcutis. Also, in patients with generalized lymphadenopathy it is important to evaluate other hemolymphatic organs, including the spleen, liver, and bone marrow (see below).

Hematologic and Serum Biochemical Findings. Obtaining a complete blood count (CBC) and serum biochemical parameters is of importance, particularly when evaluating patients with generalized lymphadenopathy. Changes in the CBC may suggest a systemic inflammatory process (leukocytosis due to neutrophilia, left shift, and monocytosis) or suggest a diagnosis of hematopoietic neoplasia (presence of circulating blasts, or marked lymphocytosis suggestive of chronic lymphocytic leukemia). Occasionally, the etiologic agent may be identified by examining a blood smear (ehrlichiosis, histoplasmosis, trypanosomiasis, babesiosis).

Anemia in patients with lymphadenopathy can occur due to a wide variety of reasons (see below for specific disorders). Briefly, anemia of chronic disease can be seen in inflammatory, infectious, or neoplastic disorders; hemolytic anemia is usually present in patients with hemoparasitic lymphadenopathies; severe nonregenerative anemia may be seen in dogs with chronic ehrlichiosis, in cats with feline leukemia virus (FeLV)-related disorders, and in dogs and cats with primary bone marrow neoplasms (leukemias).

Thrombocytopenia is a common finding in patients with ehrlichiosis, RMSF, sepsis, lymphoma, leukemias, multiple myeloma, systemic mastocytosis, malignant histiocytosis, and some immune-mediated disorders.[8, 9, 12, 14–18] Pancytopenia is common in dogs with chronic ehrlichiosis, malignant histiocytosis, and systemic immune-mediated disorders; in dogs and cats with lymphoma and leukemia; and in cats with FeLV-related disorders.[8, 12, 14, 17–20]

Two major serum biochemical abnormalities are of diagnostic value in dogs and cats with lymphadenopathy; these are hypercalcemia and hyperglobulinemia. Hypercalcemia is a paraneoplastic syndrome that occurs in approximately 10 to 20 per cent of dogs with lymphoma and multiple myeloma; it has also been documented in dogs with blastomycosis.[14, 15, 21] Monoclonal hyperglobulinemia commonly occurs in dogs and cats with multiple myeloma, and occasionally in dogs with lymphoma and ehrlichiosis.[14, 15, 22, 23] Polyclonal hyperglobulinemia commonly occurs in dogs and cats with systemic mycoses, in cats with FIP, and in dogs with ehrlichiosis and lymphoma.[8, 13, 14, 23, 24]

Radiographic and Ultrasonographic Abnormalities. Radiographic abnormalities in dogs with lymphadenop-

athy vary with the primary disorder. In general, plain radiographs are beneficial in cases of deep regional lymphadenopathy involving the thoracic and abdominal cavities. Contrast studies (lymphangiograms) may be beneficial in evaluating lymph nodes draining highly metastatic primary neoplasms (e.g., apocrine gland adenocarcinoma). However, due to the technical difficulties involved in performing lymphangiograms, this technique is rarely used in small animal patients.

In this author's experience, ultrasonography is the noninvasive procedure that provides the greatest benefit in evaluating intraabdominal lymphadenopathy. With this technique, lymph nodes can be accurately imaged and measured, so that therapeutic progress can be monitored.[25] Moreover, ultrasound-guided biopsies can be performed in these patients with minimal complications.[26]

Bone Marrow Evaluation. Evaluation of bone marrow aspirates or core biopsies may be beneficial in patients with generalized lymphadenopathy due to hematopoietic neoplasia. In this regard, acute or chronic leukemia in dogs may be difficult to diagnose on the basis of a lymph node aspirate for cytology.[18] However, the combination of hematologic findings and bone marrow evaluation is usually diagnostic.

Lymph Node Aspirate. Cytologic evaluation of lymph node aspirates provides the clinician with a wealth of information and is usually the definitive diagnostic procedure in patients with lymphadenopathy. Superficial lymph nodes can be aspirated with minimal difficulty; however, the successful aspiration of intrathoracic or intraabdominal lymph nodes requires some expertise. To obtain a fine needle aspirate (FNA) of a superficial node the area does not need to be surgically prepared. Aspiration of intrathoracic and intraabdominal structures requires surgical preparation of the area and adequate restraint of the patient. Ultrasonographic guidance may be beneficial in obtaining the desired specimen. Certain intraabdominal lymph nodes (markedly enlarged mesenteric or iliac nodes) are easily aspirated transabdominally using manual isolation of the mass. Iliac lymph nodes can be aspirated transrectally using a two to three inch needle.

When evaluating a patient with generalized lymphadenopathy the clinician must decide which node to aspirate. It is important to aspirate a node in which the tissue changes are representative of the ongoing disease process. For example, it is advisable not to obtain a specimen from the largest lymph node, since central necrosis usually results in obtaining a nondiagnostic sample. Moreover, because clinical or subclinical gingivitis is common in older dogs and cats, submandibular lymph nodes should not be aspirated routinely since they are usually reactive and they may obscure the primary diagnosis.

Using a 22 to 25 gauge (1 to 1.5 inch) hypodermic needle coupled to a 12 ml to 20 ml syringe, the needle is inserted into the mass, and suction is applied to the plunger. In order to obtain enough cells for a cytologic diagnosis, at least 6 to 8 ml of suction is necessary. The needle is then redirected within the mass, and the procedure is repeated two or three times. The suction should be released prior to withdrawing the needle from the tissue in order to prevent aspirating the material inside the barrel of the syringe, where it is usually irretrievable. The amount of cells contained within the hub of the needle is usually sufficient to make two to six coverslip smears. The slides are air dried and stained with Wright or Giemsa stains. Diff-Quick stain is fast, practical, and convenient for in-office use. Samples obtained by fine needle aspiration can also be used for microbiologic evaluation and for ultrastructural studies.

Several reviews of cytologic evaluation of lymphoid tissues have appeared in the veterinary literature.[27–32] Briefly, *normal lymph nodes* are composed primarily of small lymphocytes (80 to 90 per cent of all cells); a low number of macrophages, medium or large lymphocytes, plasma cells, and mast cells can also be found. *Reactive lymph nodes* are characterized by variable numbers of lymphoid cells in different stages of development (small, medium, and large lymphocytes; immunoblasts; plasma cells). The cytologic features of *lymphadenitis* vary with the etiologic agent and the type of reaction elicited (neutrophils in suppurative inflammation; macrophages in granulomatous reactions; an admixture of both in pyogranulomatous reactions). Etiologic agents can usually be identified in cytologic specimens obtained from nodes with lymphadenitis.[32] *Metastatic neoplasms* have a different cytologic picture depending upon the degree of involvement and the cell type. Carcinomas, adenocarcinomas, melanomas, and mast cell tumors are easily diagnosed on cytology; cytologic diagnosis of sarcomas may be difficult, since their cells do not exfoliate easily. *Primary lymphoid neoplasms* (lymphomas) are characterized by a monomorphic population of lymphoid cells, which are usually immature (high nuclear:cytoplasmic ratio, presence of one or more nucleoli, basophilic cytoplasm, vacuolation) (Figure 115–3).

Lymph Node Biopsy. When cytologic examination of an enlarged lymph node does not provide a definitive diagnosis, excision of the affected node for histopathologic examination is indicated. In this regard, it is preferable to excise the whole node, since core biopsies are difficult to interpret because the lymph node architecture is not well preserved. Care should be exerted in handling the node during surgical manipulation, since trauma may induce considerable artifact and preclude interpretation of the specimen. The popliteal lymph nodes are easily accessible, and are the ones usually excised in dogs and cats with generalized lymphadenopathy.

Once a node is excised, it should be sectioned in half lengthwise, impression smears made for cytology, and the node fixed in 10 per cent buffered formalin, at a rate of one part of tissue to nine parts of fixative. The specimen is then ready to be referred to a laboratory for evaluation. It is always advisable to make several impression smears of the excised lymph node for cytologic evaluation prior to fixation.

SELECTED DISORDERS ASSOCIATED WITH LYMPHADENOPATHY IN DOGS AND CATS

As mentioned above, a variety of infectious and noninfectious diseases are commonly associated with lymphadenopathy in small animals. Since the majority

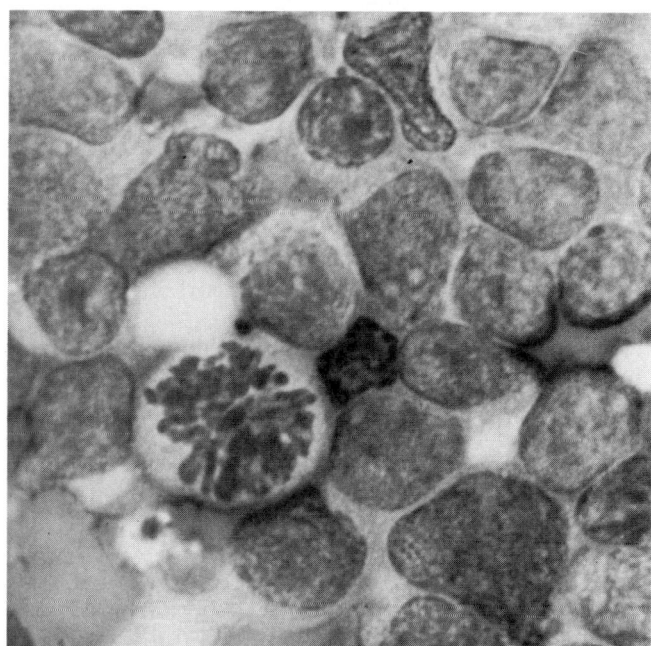

FIGURE 115–3. Fine needle aspirate from an enlarged lymph node in a dog with generalized lymphadenopathy. The presence of a monomorphic population of large cells (2.5 to 3 times the size of RBCs), with large nuclei, clumped chromatin, and presence of nucleoli are highly suggestive of lymphoma. A mitotic figure can be seen (Wright Giemsa, 960 X).

of them have already been discussed in this book, only a limited number of disease processes that present with lymph node enlargement will be addressed in this chapter.

Bacterial Lymphadenitis. Two syndromes presumptively associated with pyogenic bacterial infections and lymphadenitis, *contagious streptococcal lymphadenitis of cats* and *puppy strangles*, have been described in small animals.[33–36] In addition, localized streptococcal and staphylococcal infections may also result in solitary or regional lymphadenopathy in these species.

CONTAGIOUS STREPTOCOCCAL LYMPHADENITIS. Contagious streptococcal lymphadenitis was described in several kittens in a cat colony.[33, 34] The kittens developed diarrhea and fever at four weeks of age, followed by cervical lymphadenopathy two weeks later. The lymph nodes in these cats were markedly enlarged, and developed draining purulent lesions. An adult unrelated cat housed with these kittens also developed similar signs and lesions, and the disease could be transmitted orally by administration of lymph node material from the affected cats.[33, 34] All the cats were negative for circulating feline leukemia virus (FeLV) p27 antigen. Lancefield group G β-hemolytic streptococci were isolated from the abscessed lymph nodes and from heart blood in one of the kittens that died of septicemia. Most cats responded to treatment with penicillin.[33]

PUPPY STRANGLES. Puppy strangles is a disorder associated with cutaneous cellulitis of the head and neck, and cervical lymphadenopathy in 4- to 12-week-old dogs.[35, 36] Pups usually present with fever, deep facial pyoderma, and cervical lymphadenopathy; more than one pup in the litter are commonly affected. Fine needle aspiration of affected lymph nodes reveals purulent lymphadenitis, and staphylococcal or streptococcal organisms may be cultured. However, due to the lack of response to antibiotic therapy in a high proportion of cases, the absence of bacteria in most cultures obtained from affected areas, and the subsequent response to immunosuppressive doses of corticosteroids, a hypersensitivity reaction to bacterial antigens is suspected.[35]

In addition to the above, a case of *Corynebacterium equi* lymphadenitis resulting in generalized lymphadenopathy simulating lymphoma was reported in an FeLV-negative cat.[37]

Idiopathic Lymphadenopathies. Three recent reports describe the occurrence of idiopathic lymphadenopathy in cats.[38–40] In one report, 14 cats with generalized lymphadenopathy ranging in ages from five months to two years were evaluated.[38] The term distinctive peripheral lymph node hyperplasia (DPLH) was chosen by the authors for this condition. Eight cats were clinically normal on initial physical examination, except for the presence of lymphadenopathy; clinical signs in the other six cats included fever (five cats), lethargy (three cats), anorexia (three cats), pallor, hematuria, eczema, vomiting, and mastitis (one cat each).[38] Nine of the 14 cats for which CBCs were available had anemia; one cat had neutrophilia and lymphocytosis; and three cats had neutropenia. Six of nine cats evaluated for FeLV antigen in peripheral blood were positive. Therapy in affected cats included antibiotics, corticosteroids, and fluids. In six cats the lymphadenopathy resolved within two weeks to four months; one of these cats subsequently developed intrathoracic lymphoma and died; one additional cat had recurrence of the lymphadenopathy over five years and was euthanized; three cats had persistent lymphadenopathy and were also euthanized within a month of the initial diagnosis; four cats were lost to follow-up.[38] Histologic changes in the affected nodes included distortion of the architecture; proliferation of histiocytes, lymphocytes, plasma cells and immunoblasts in the paracortical regions; and numerous prominent postcapillary venules.[38] These changes were similar to the ones observed in seven cats with experimental FeLV infection.[38] Based on this and on the fact that six of the nine cats evaluated were FeLV-positive, the authors postulated that this syndrome is secondary to this retroviral infection.

Mooney et al. recently described six young cats with marked generalized lymphadenopathy resembling lymphoma.[39] The cats ranged in age from one to four years, and three of them were Maine Coon cats. Most peripheral nodes were two to three cm in diameter and firm. Four cats had leukocytosis and one had leukopenia. One of the cats was anemic and atypical lymphocytes were seen in the blood smear. Five cats evaluated for FeLV viremia were negative. Serum protein electrophoresis in five cats revealed the presence of polyclonal gammopathies; one cat was hypercalcemic. Most histopathologic features were suggestive of lymphoma and included loss of normal lymph node architecture, presence of a uniform population of lymphoid cells in the paracortical areas, capsular and perinodal infiltration, and presence of large follicular structures without germinal center. However, other features were not compatible with malignancy, including abundant vascularity;

lymphoid follicles with active germinal centers; and presence of a mixed population of lymphoid cells, plasma cells, histiocytes, and granulocytes in the sinuses.[39] One of the cats was euthanized on presentation; the remaining five cats were not treated. Resolution of the lymphadenopathy was seen in all cats within 5 to 120 days; all cats were alive 12 to 84 months after initial diagnosis.[39]

A clinical syndrome characterized by solitary cervical or inguinal lymphadenopathy in cats ranging in ages from 3 to 14 years, and referred to as plexiform vascularization of lymph nodes was recently described.[40] The lesions were unilateral in seven of nine cases studied. Most cats were asymptomatic and the FeLV status was not reported. Surgical removal of the affected nodes resulted in uneventful recovery in most cats; however, postoperative edema occurred in two of the cats. Histologically, the nodes showed replacement of the interfollicular pulp by a plexiform proliferation of small capillary-sized vascular channels and lymphoid atrophy. The pathogenesis of this syndrome has not yet been elucidated.[40]

FELINE LYMPHOMA

The term lymphoma (malignant lymphoma or lymphosarcoma) refers to a lymphoid neoplasm that originates in solid hematopoietic organs such as the lymph nodes, liver, or spleen.[41] Lymphomas represent the most common hemolymphatic tumor in cats, accounting for 60 to 90 per cent of all hemolymphatic tumors in this species.[41] It is currently accepted that the majority of lymphomas in the cat are induced by FeLV.

According to the anatomic distribution of the lesions, lymphomas can be classified as mediastinal, alimentary, multicentric, leukemic, and miscellaneous.[42–44] The frequency of presentation of the different anatomic forms varies geographically; this may reflect a different prevalence of FeLV strains, differences in the genetic make-up of cats, or different criteria used for classification.[42, 44] The therapeutic approaches to dogs and cats with lymphoma will be discussed at the end of this section.

Mediastinal Form. This form is also referred to as thymic, although the term mediastinal is more appropriate, since the anterior and posterior mediastinal lymph nodes, rather than the thymus, are commonly affected. Its prevalence varies in different areas of the world, comprising between 18 and 48 per cent of the cases reported by different investigators.[42–45] The average age of cats with mediastinal lymphoma is two to three years and approximately 80 per cent of cats with mediastinal lymphoma are FeLV-positive.[44]

Clinical signs in cats with this anatomic form are usually acute in onset and include dyspnea, tachypnea, regurgitation, coughing, anorexia, depression, and weight loss. Physical findings include dyspnea, cyanosis, non-compressible anterior mediastinum, displacement of cardiac sounds dorsocaudally, absence of normal bronchovesicular sounds on the cranioventral aspect of the lungs, and dull sound on thoracic percussion. In most cats with mediastinal lymphoma thoracocentesis reveals the presence of a serohemorrhagic to frankly hemorrhagic effusion with abundance of vacuolated neoplastic lymphoid cells. Chylothorax due to tumor erosion of the thoracic duct occasionally occurs. In most cats with mediastinal forms, tumor involvement of other organs, with the possible exception of the bone marrow, is rare.

Plain thoracic radiographs are extremely helpful in establishing a diagnosis. Although other neoplasms may occupy the anterior or posterior mediastinum in cats (e.g., thymoma; ectopic thyroid adenocarcinoma), they usually occur in older animals. The presence of a mediastinal mass in a young cat should be strongly suggestive of lymphoma. A confirmatory diagnosis can be obtained through cytologic examination of the pleural fluid or of percutaneous fine needle aspirates of the mass(es). In this regard, mediastinal masses can be easily and safely aspirated with a 25 to 23 gauge needle, using a lateral intercostal approach.

Alimentary Form. The alimentary form is characterized by neoplastic involvement of the gastrointestinal tract and/or mesenteric lymph nodes. Its prevalence ranged from 15 to 45 per cent of the cases reported in several studies.[42, 44] The average age of cats with alimentary lymphoma is higher than in other anatomic forms (eight years versus two to five years).[44] Cats with alimentary lymphoma are FeLV-positive only in 30 per cent of the cases, and therefore, they are rarely anemic.[44] The low prevalence of FeLV infection in cats with alimentary lymphomas is not surprising, since most of these tumors originate from B-lymphocytes in the gut-associated lymphoid tissue. It is generally accepted that the majority of FeLV-induced neoplasms are of T-cell origin.[44] Clinical signs and physical findings in cats with alimentary lymphoma are discussed in Chapter 86.

If a presumptive diagnosis of alimentary lymphoma is made, a cytologic specimen obtained from an enlarged mesenteric lymph node or from an intraabdominal mass by percutaneous fine needle aspiration is usually confirmatory. Endoscopic biopsies of upper or lower gastrointestinal lesions are generally diagnostic. However, caution should be exerted when interpreting biopsy results in which a diagnosis of lymphoplasmacytic gastroenteritis has been made, since the majority of early lymphomatous lesions are submucosal, and can be surrounded by areas of lymphoplasmacytic inflammation.[18]

Multicentric Form. Considerable confusion arises when classifying cats within the multicentric form, since some investigators include in this category cats with true lymphoid leukemia and cats with extranodal involvement.[42–44] The author prefers to reserve the term multicentric for cats with solid hemolymphatic organ involvement, including deep and superficial lymph nodes, liver, spleen, and/or bone marrow. Bone marrow and/or extranodal involvement in these cases is usually secondary. Cats with primary bone marrow involvement should be classified as having lymphoid leukemia.

The prevalence of the multicentric form ranged from 18 to 43 per cent of all cases reported by several investigators.[42–44] However, in one study cats with primary bone marrow involvement were also classified within this category.[44] The majority (80 per cent) of cats with the multicentric form are FeLV positive and display the FOCMA on the surface of the tumor cells.[44] The average age of presentation for cats with this form is four years.[44]

Clinical signs and physical findings in cats with the multicentric form are variable, and are directly related to tumor volume and location. A high percentage of cats with this form of lymphoma are asymptomatic. In others, nonspecific signs such as anorexia, lethargy, and weight loss are noticed. Generalized, painless lymphadenopathy is usually detected by the owner during routine grooming. Physical abnormalities include superficial or deep lymphadenopathy, more than two lymph nodes being commonly affected. The lymph nodes are considerably enlarged (four to ten times the normal size), to the point that some of them are visible upon inspection. The nodes are usually firm, unattached to the surrounding tissues, and painless. Hepatomegaly, splenomegaly, and tonsillar enlargement are also common findings. Extranodal involvement is relatively common with this anatomic form; therefore, common sites of extranodal involvement such as the eyes, kidneys, and central nervous system should be thoroughly evaluated in these cases.

As with other anatomic forms, a confirmatory diagnosis is usually obtained through cytologic examination of an enlarged lymph node, of liver, or of splenic aspirate; surgical biopsies are rarely needed. Cytologic specimens usually reveal a monomorphic population of immature lymphocytes. However, in cats with lymphocytic, well-differentiated lymphoma, establishing a diagnosis can be difficult since the cells are morphologically indistinguishable from normal lymphocytes.

Since the majority of cats with the multicentric form are FeLV-positive, the prevalence of anemia in this group is high. As with the other anatomic forms, cats with advanced disease appear to have a poorer prognosis.

Leukemic Form. This form of presentation is discussed in Chapter 114.

Miscellaneous Forms. Most miscellaneous forms involve extranodal, nonlymphoid tissue, so that the term extranodal lymphomas is preferred.[46] This form of presentation develops when tissue lymphoid cells are affected by an oncogenic stimulus or stimuli. In this regard, it should be remembered that extranodal lymphomas can arise from a single lymphocyte; therefore, they can affect any organ or tissue in the body. Extranodal forms account for less than 10 per cent of all lymphomas.[42] Common extranodal sites in the cat include the eyes, kidneys, skin, central and peripheral nervous system, and upper respiratory tract.[41] These forms of presentation will be discussed in their respective chapters.

Therapy for Feline Lymphomas. Since lymphomas are usually systemic in nature, chemotherapy is the preferred treatment modality (see Oncology chapters). However, in selected cases, other therapeutic approaches (surgery, radiotherapy, and blood component therapy) have been successfully used.

Client education constitutes one of the most important aspects of the successful treatment of cats with lymphoma. Owners should understand that, with few exceptions, a cure is not the goal of therapy. Therapeutic success consists of inducing prolonged remissions (either complete or partial) while attaining minimal toxicity and side effects. This aspect is extremely important, since owners generally find it difficult to cope with cats that exhibit signs of toxicity from chemotherapy. The clinician should explain to the owner the biologic behavior of the tumor, the probabilities of successfully inducing remission, the probabilities of causing side effects or toxicities, and the life expectancy with and without therapy. The author has found that offering the owners the possibility of initiating therapy, conditioned to the response and side effects observed within the first two or three weeks of therapy, usually helps them reach a decision in favor of treatment.

Different anticancer drugs and drug combinations have been used successfully in the treatment of cats with different anatomic forms of lymphoma. However, to this author's knowledge, only two controlled studies have been published.[47, 48] In general, multiple drug combinations are favored over single agent chemotherapy (see Oncology chapters).

The chemotherapeutic strategy used to treat cats with lymphoma can be divided into 4 different phases: *induction of remission, intensification, maintenance,* and *reinduction of remission* (or rescue) (Table 115–3). During the initial phase (induction of remission) a multiple drug combination is used in an attempt to significantly reduce the tumor mass; the goal in this phase is to induce complete remission (CR). Induction chemotherapy is moderately "intensive" when compared with maintenance protocols, and it requires frequent visits to the veterinarian. A multitude of protocols can be used for induction of remission (see below). If the patient does not achieve CR (complete disappearance of the tumor mass(es), the following phase is intensification. During this phase, agents such as L-asparaginase or doxorubicin are used in an attempt to consolidate CR. If the patient

TABLE 115–3. CHEMOTHERAPY PROTOCOLS FOR FELINE LYMPHOMA USED AT THE OHIO STATE UNIVERSITY VETERINARY TEACHING HOSPITAL

Induction of remission
COAP Protocol:
- Cyclophosphamide (Cytoxan) 50 mg/m²BSA, PO, 4 days a week (or every other day)
- Vincristine (Oncovin) 0.5 mg/m²BSA, IV, once a week
- Cytosine arabinoside (Cytosar-U) 100 mg/m²BAS/day, IV drip or SQ, for only 2 days
- Prednisone 40 mg/m²BSA, PO, s.i.d. for a week; then 20 mg/m²BSA PO, every other day

(This protocol is used for 6 weeks; at the end of the induction phase, the patient is started on maintenance therapy.)
Intensification
L-Asparaginase (Elspar) 10,000–20,000 IU/m² BSA, SQ (one dose)
Maintenance
LMP:
- Chlorambucil (Leukeran) 2 mg/m² BSA, PO, every other day, or 20 mg/m² BSA, PO, every other week
- Methotrexate (Methotrexate) 2.5 mg/m² BSA, PO, 2 to 3 times per week
- Prednisone 20 mg/m², PO, every other day
COAP:
- Use as above every other week for 6 treatments, then every third week for additional 6 treatments, and try to maintain the patient on 1 treatment every 4th week.
Rescue
1st relapse: COAP
2nd relapse:
- Doxorubicin hydrochloride (Adriamycin) 30 mg/m² BSA, IV, once every 3 weeks

has achieved CR during the induction phase, maintenance chemotherapy should be initiated. This phase is characterized by a moderately aggressive protocol, usually combining three or more drugs. The author uses a combination of oral chlorambucil (Leukeran), methotrexate (Methotrexate), and prednisone (Table 115–3). The use of oral maintenance chemotherapy minimizes expenses and visits to the veterinarian. During this phase, cats are usually examined every four to six weeks, at which time a CBC is obtained and the patient is thoroughly evaluated. On the average, cats remain in remission for two to four months while on maintenance therapy. If the patient shows progressive disease (PD), reinduction of remission should be attempted. If the patient responded to the initial induction protocol with complete, sustained remission, the same drug combination should be used for the first relapse. If the response to the initial induction was not complete or sustained, or if the patient relapses for a second or third time, drug combinations including doxorubicin (Adriamycin) are preferred. At the present time it is not known if achievement of CR is necessary in order to experience long term survivals. The author has treated a limited number of patients that never experienced CR but had prolonged survivals (in excess of ten months). Therefore, if CR cannot be obtained, the same treatment should be continued unless there is evidence of tumor progression. In a controlled study, however, Cotter found that cats with PR (partial remission) seldom maintained this response for more than four to six weeks.[47]

Cotter treated 53 cats with different anatomic forms of lymphoma and acute lymphoblastic leukemia using the COP protocol, a combination of cyclophosphamide (Cytoxan; 300 mg/m², PO, on days 1 and 22), vincristine (Oncovin; 0.75 mg/m², IV, on days 1, 8, 15, and 22), and prednisone (1 mg/lb or 2 mg/kg, q24h).[47] Overall, 64 per cent of the cats attained CR and 22 per cent PR, with a median duration of remission of five months (range 1 to 42+ months). However, when the cats were stratified as having either lymphoma or lymphoid leukemia, the remission rates were 79 per cent for the former and 27 per cent for the latter, indicating that the prognosis for cats with lymphoma is significantly better than for cats with acute lymphoid leukemia. Moreover, when the cats were subdivided according to the anatomic form of presentation, it was apparent that cats with nodal lymphomas had a higher percentage of CR than cats with extranodal forms. Poor prognostic indicators, in addition to leukemia, were anemia, neutropenia, sepsis, and large or widely disseminated tumors. Survival times were not recorded in this study, since, as the author stated ". . . survival times may vary with persistence of owners or veterinarians. . . ."[47] However, since several of the cats in the study were treated with other drug combinations after relapse, most survival times would have been conceivably longer than the duration of remission.[47]

In another report, Jeglum et al. evaluated 75 cats with different forms of lymphoma treated with a combination of vincristine (Oncovin; 0.01 mg/lb or 0.025 mg/kg, IV, on weeks 1 and 3), cyclophosphamide (Cytoxan; 4.5 mg/lb or 10 mg/kg, IV, on week 2), and methotrexate (0.35

mg/lb or 0.8 mg/kg, IV or PO, on week 4), with or without prednisolone (5 mg per cat, sid), and L-asparaginase (Elspar; 180 IU/lb or 400 IU/kg, IV or IP).[48] The response rates varied according to the anatomic forms of presentation. Cats with multicentric lymphoma had a 68 per cent response rate and a median survival of 21.5 months; cats with alimentary forms had a response rate of 50 per cent and a median survival of 11.3 months; cats with renal forms had a response rate of 16 per cent and a median survival of 4.8 months; and cats with mediastinal form had a response rate of 45 per cent and a median survival of 2.6 months.[48] The low response rate and short survival times reported for cats with mediastinal lymphoma in this study are in contrast with those reported by Cotter and observed by the author.[47] This may have been due to a high frequency of tumor-related deaths early in the course of chemotherapy.[48]

In this author's experience, the results obtained in cats with different anatomic forms of lymphoma using a combination of cyclophosphamide (Cytoxan), vincristine (Oncovin), cytosine arabinoside (Cytosar), and prednisone (see Table 115–3) are comparable to those previously reported.

Radiotherapy is also effective in treating localized lymphomas, solitary extranodal masses, or lymphomatous masses that mechanically compress vital structures or organs (e.g., epidural or mediastinal masses). Most lymphoma cells are exquisitely radiosensitive, and a total dose of 10 to 15 Gy usually results in CR. Radiation is best delivered by external beam irradiation, using 300 to 400 cGy per fraction; these fractions are delivered on a Monday, Wednesday, and Friday basis to the affected tissue. This approach has been used successfully to treat neural, renal, and mediastinal lymphomas by the author and others.[10, 49]

Results of immunotherapeutic trials in cats with hemolymphatic neoplasia are discussed in Chapter 59.

CANINE LYMPHOMA

In contrast to cats, in which different anatomic forms have significantly different prevalences according to their geographic location, the multicentric form is by far the most common form of presentation in dogs, comprising approximately 80 per cent of all cases.[42] In one study, the alimentary form was the second most common, followed by mediastinal, and extranodal (and other miscellaneous forms).[42] Another contrasting feature of canine lymphomas is that most cases occur in older dogs, while in cats there is a bimodal age of presentation.[14, 44] In addition, there is a definitive breed predisposition for lymphoma, with Boxers, basset hounds, Saint Bernards, and Scottish terriers being at increased risk.[50]

Clinical signs and physical findings in dogs with lymphoma are similar to those of affected cats and will not be discussed herein. Different chemotherapeutic protocols used in the treatment of canine lymphoma are listed in Table 115–4. The author uses the protocols listed in Table 115–3 in dogs, with only slight modifications. These modifications include mainly the use of cytosine arabinoside for four days rather than two, and the induction phase consisting of eight weeks rather than

TABLE 115–4. COMBINATION CHEMOTHERAPY AND CHEMOIMMUNOTHERAPY PROTOCOLS FOR CANINE LYMPHOMA (REVIEWED IN REFERENCE 14)

Protocol	Drugs and Dosages
VCP-6MP	V:* 0.014 mg/lb (0.030 mg/kg), IV, days 1 & 8 C: 2.8 mg/lb (5.0 mg/kg) day, PO days 15–21 P: 0.9 mg/lb (2.0 mg/kg) day, PO, days 1–8; then 1.0 mg/kg/day, PO, days 9–21 6-MP: 0.45 mg/lb (5.0 mg/kg) day, PO, days 15–21 (Repeat protocol every 30 days)
Madewell	*Induction of remission* V: 0.5 mg/m² BSA, IV, single dose C: 50.0 mg/m² BSA, PO, 4 days a week P: 10.0 mg/m² BSA, PO, BID for 7 days QOD thereafter *Maintenance A* C: 50.0 mg/m² BSA, PO, 4 days a week 6-MP: 50.0 mg/m² BSA, PO, SID MTX: 2.5 mg/m² BSA, PO, BID once a week *Maintenance B* P: 10.0 mg/m² BSA, BID, QOD C: 50.0 mg/m² BSA, 4 days a week
COAP-L	C: 50.0 mg/m² BSA, PO, SID, 4 times a week for 8 weeks V: 0.5 mg/m² BSA, IV, once a week for 8 weeks A: 100 mg/m² BSA, IV, SID, first 4 days of therapy P: 20 mg/m² BSA, PO, BID, for 7 days; then 10 mg/m² BSA, BID, QOD for 7 weeks L: 20,000 IU/m² BSA, IP, once on weeks 9 and 10
COAP-L + Autologous Vaccine	Same as above plus autologous tumor vaccine on weeks 10, 11, 12, 14, and 16.
AMC	V: 0.011 mg/lb (0.025 mg/kg), IV days 1 and 14 L: 181 mg/lb (400 IU/kg), IP days 1, 7, 14, and 21 C: 4.5 mg/lb (10 mg/kg), IV day 7 MTX: 0.36 mg/lb (0.8 mg/kg), IV day 21
AMC + Levamisole	As above plus Lz Lz: 2.3 mg/lb (5 mg/kg), PO, Monday, Wednesday, & Friday
COP	C: 300 mg/m² BSA, PO day 1 V: 0.75 mg/m² BSA, IV days 1, 8, and 15 P: 0.45 mg/lb (1 mg/kg), PO, SID for 22 days; then every other day

*V: Vincristine (Oncovin, Eli Lilly)
C: Cyclophosphamide (Cytoxan, Mead)
P: Prednisone or prednisolone
6-MP: 6-Mercaptopurine (Purinthethol, Burroughs)
MTX: Methotrexate (Methotrexate, Lederle)
A: Cytosine arabinoside (Cytosar-U, Upjohn)
L: L-asparaginase (Elspar, Merck)
Lz: Levamisole

six weeks. Survival times achieved with different protocols are listed in Table 115–5.

SPLEEN

"The spleen, Galen's organ of mystery, its function especially mystifying as it could apparently be removed without obvious untoward effects, and with so complex an anatomical structure, has been reluctant to give up all its secrets. Only now are we beginning to appreciate the full extent of its functional complexity. To para-

TABLE 115–5. SURVIVAL TIMES IN DOGS WITH LYMPHOMA (REVIEWED IN REFERENCE 14)

Therapy	Mean Objective Remission (days)	Mean Survival (days)	Median Survival (days)
No therapy	NR†	30	NR
Prednisolone	NR	75	NR
Chlorambucil	NR	105	NR
Cyclophosphamide	NR	135	NR
Prednisolone + Chlorambucil	NR	69	NR
VCP-6MP	136	NR	NR
VCP, C, 6-MP, MTX, P	104.8	211.5	NR
COAP-L	31	198	196
COAP-L + autologous tumor vaccine	202	414	336
V, L, C, MTX	132*	NR	219
COP	180*	NR	NR
V, L, C, MTX LZ	NR	NR	273

*Median objective remission
†NR = Not recorded

phrase a saying, the spleen has been all things to all men. It intrigued the ancient physicians and philosophers. More recently, it has become a common meeting ground for physician, surgeon, haematologist, histopathologist, oncologist, physicist and physiologist." (SM Lewis: The Spleen. Clin Haematol 12(2):361, 1983).

The spleen constitutes the single largest component of the reticuloendothelial system, and is directly interposed between the portal and the systemic circulation. Its unique anatomical and functional features make it prone to undergo pathologic changes in a wide variety of disease processes.

Anatomy and Histology

The spleen is located in the left anterior quadrant of the abdomen in a dorsoventral orientation and weighs approximately 50 grams in a medium sized dog.[3] It is a flattened red organ with a somehow falciform shape. Its dorsal end is relatively fixed near the midline, caudal to the last rib. The rest of the spleen (the body and the distal end or tip) is freely movable, and its location varies with the animal's body configuration (deep-chested versus flat-chested) and with the degree of fullness of the stomach (the spleen is easily palpable postprandially since its contour conforms to the greater curvature of the stomach so that it lies parallel to the last rib). The spleen is attached to the greater omentum along a ridge (the hilus) that runs longitudinally along its visceral surface. The parietal surface is convex and lies mostly against the left flank. The splenic artery and sympathetic nerves enter the spleen through the hilus, while the splenic vein and the efferent lymphatic vessels leave the spleen through this region. The spleen has no afferent lymphatics.[3]

During a routine physical examination, the normal spleen is easily palpable in pups and in cats as a flat structure oriented dorsoventrally in the left anterior abdominal quadrant. In some deep-chested dogs (Irish setters, German shepherds, greyhounds) and in some miniature breeds (schnauzers) the normal spleen is also easily palpable during routine examination in the ventral mid-abdomen or in the left anterior quadrant.

The splenic pulp in dogs and cats is enclosed in a fibromuscular capsule that branches to form trabeculae.[51] The large amount of smooth muscle contained in the capsule enables the canine and feline spleen to contract; it is also responsible for the splenomegaly observed after administration of barbiturates or tranquilizers that result in relaxation of the smooth muscle fibers. Smooth muscle fibers contract in response to endogenous or exogenous catecholamines.[51, 52]

Histologically, the spleen consists of four main components: white pulp, marginal zone, red pulp, and fibromuscular capsule and trabeculae.[51] The latter were previously discussed. The *white pulp* consists primarily of lymphocytes and reticuloendothelial cells distributed along the course of arterial vessels; these are cylindrical structures that surround the arteries after they leave the trabeculae and are referred to as periarterial lymphatic sheaths (PALS). Zones rich in T and B lymphocytes can be found within the white pulp (lymphoid nodules).[2, 51]

The *marginal zone* separates the white pulp from the surrounding red pulp; in dogs and cats it is poorly developed. In other species, it is populated with macrophages and receives blood from the arteries, so that blood filtration and phagocytosis occur.[51, 53]

The *red pulp* consists primarily of arterial capillaries, small venous vessels, a reticulum filled with macrophages, and blood.[51, 54, 55] The central arteries of the white pulp terminate in arterial capillaries that deliver blood into the red pulp reticulum. Once the arteries enter the red pulp, they loose the PALS and become surrounded by a dense sheath of reticulum and macrophages (the *periarteriolar macrophage sheath* [PAMS], also referred to as the ellipsoid). Endothelial cells in the terminal arterial capillaries are separated by gaps through which particles, cells, and plasma pass into the spaces of the PAMS.[54] The PAMS is well-developed in dogs and cats and constitutes the major clearing site of blood-borne particles.[51]

The vascular arrangements in dog and cat spleen are anatomically open and communicate freely with pulp spaces (red pulp reticulum) in the meshwork after leaving the PAMS (see below).[54] These red pulp spaces, that are not lined by endothelium, constitute vascular channels of an intermediate circulation interposed between the arterial and venous vessels.[52]

The major anatomical and functional difference between canine and feline spleens is the structure of the venous vessels in the red pulp. In dogs, these vessels consist of an anastomosing system of venous sinuses composed of long, rod-shaped endothelial cells that lie parallel to one another and to the longitudinal axis of the vessels.[51, 52] These endothelial structures are incompletely covered by rings of basement membrane and reticular cells. The sinuses are closed and blunt at their origins and terminate by converging to form major veins that drain into the trabecular veins. To leave the spleen, blood cells need to squeeze between adjacent endothelial cells and enter the sinus lumen (see below).[51, 52] The canine spleen is therefore considered to be a sinusal spleen.

In contrast, venous vessels in the cats' splenic red pulp, termed pulp venules, are thin-walled and lined by flat squamous-shaped endothelium. Contiguous endothelial cells are pulled apart at various points to form large apertures through which blood cells can escape into the lumen without changing shape. Moreover, pulp venules are open-ended at their origins. Like sinuses, pulp venules drain into trabecular veins. Cat spleens are therefore considered to be nonsinusal (see below).[51-55]

Physiology

The spleen has multiple functions, including those of hematopoiesis; filtration and phagocytosis; blood reservoir; and immunologic. In addition, some miscellaneous functions have been recently identified (see below). All these functions are equally important in maintaining homeostasis.

HEMATOPOIESIS

The spleen is one of the major hematopoietic organs during fetal development. This activity diminishes before or shortly after birth and the normal adult canine and feline spleens have no hematopoietic activity.[56] However, the spleen retains its ability to initiate extramedullary hematopoiesis (EMH) in most adult animals. This occurs with infiltrative diseases of the bone marrow (leukemia, lymphoma, bone marrow hypoplasia, and myelofibrosis) or the spleen (splenitis, splenic hyperplasia, neoplasia), or when the bone marrow demands are significantly increased by peripheral blood cell destruction or consumption (immune hemolytic anemia; leukocytosis in pyometra). A wide variety of disorders associated with splenic EMH in dogs have been observed by the author, including splenic and extrasplenic hemangiosarcoma (HSA), splenic and extrasplenic lymphomas, multiple myeloma, leukemias, immune hemolytic anemia, eosinophilic gastroenteritis, estrogen-induced bone marrow hypoplasia, pyometra and other septic processes, and ehrlichiosis, among others.[18] In the author's opinion, EMH does not appear to be as common in cats as it is in dogs; the author observed splenic EMH in association with FeLV-related red cell aplasia, hemobartonellosis, lympho- and myeloproliferative disorders, and systemic mast cell disease in a limited number of cats. It should be mentioned here that EMH may result in splenomegaly. The hemograms of dogs and cats with EMH are characterized primarily by a leukoerythroblastic reaction (presence of immature red cell and white cell precursors); this is probably because the factors inhibiting the release of immature cells from the bone marrow are not operative at extramedullary sites.[57]

The role of the spleen in regulation of marrow hematopoiesis in small animals is still to be determined. In rats, splenectomy results in a sustained leukocytosis.[58] In humans, the total leukocyte, neutrophil, lymphocyte, and monocyte counts increase significantly three months or more after splenectomy.[59] However, minimal changes in the white blood cell count following splenic removal could be documented in a group of splenectomized dogs evaluated for 15 weeks.[60] In the same study, there was a significant elevation in the platelet count, reaching maximum values of 740,000/µl by the third postoperative week (from 320,000/µl preoperatively).[60]

In the dog, erythropoiesis is also influenced by the spleen. In the same study cited above, the hematocrit decreased to 78 per cent of that of the control group by six to eight weeks post splenectomy; the mean hematocrit remained at least 15 per cent below the control values throughout the six months post splenectomy.[60] At the same time, the blood volume decreased by 30 per cent, and the plasma volume by 18 per cent; there was no change in the red cell life span throughout the study. The RBC iron turnover decreased approximately 35 per cent, indicating a decrease in erythropoiesis. Moreover, the total number of circulating reticulocytes increased 67 per cent, and the intravascular reticulocyte maturation time was increased from 0.4 to 0.9 day.[60] These changes indicate that splenectomy in the dog causes a significant reduction in the circulating RBC volume with decreased RBC production but normal RBC life span. This could be due to either the removal of a splenic RBC reservoir (see below) or the removal of an organ that normally produces a humoral factor controlling erythropoiesis. The 125 per cent increase in the intravascular life span of the reticulocytes observed in this study may have been due to the premature release of these cells from the bone marrow, slower maturation of the reticulocytes once released into peripheral circulation, or the loss of the organ that normally sequesters and "pits" the RBC of intracytoplasmic inclusions (see below).

The spleen is also involved in iron metabolism. Following splenectomy in dogs, the plasma iron turnover decreases approximately 32 per cent, while the RBC iron turnover decreases by approximately 37 per cent.[60] As discussed above, this is considered to be a reflection of decreased RBC production. Despite the fact that iron turnover decreases, because of the spleen's role in recycling iron to the bone marrow for erythropoiesis, serum iron concentrations after splenectomy tend to be low for considerable time.[57]

FILTRATION, PHAGOCYTOSIS, AND RESERVOIR FUNCTION

The spleen has a unique vascular structure through which the blood circulates in close contact with the reticuloendothelium, allowing for ample biologic filtration of cells and particles (see above). The spleens of dogs and cats normally maintain a reservoir of RBCs stored as a slowly exchanging pool.[55] Using kinetic analyses of RBC washout from perfused isolated spleens it was determined that the blood flow in canine and feline spleen is composed of three functional compartments: a fast compartment receiving 90 per cent of the total splenic blood flow through which the RBCs circulate in 30 seconds, comparable to the transit of RBCs through conventional capillaries in skeletal muscle; an intermediate compartment receiving nine per cent of the blood flow, but containing 56 per cent of the RBCs in the spleen because of a longer transit time of eight minutes; and a slow compartment receiving approximately one per cent of the splenic blood flow and containing reticulocytes, with a transit time of one hour.[55] Contraction of the spleen expels the stored RBCs and almost eliminates the intermediate compartment; in a contracted spleen, 98 per cent of the blood flow is in the rapid compartment, similar to the physiologic situation occurring in normal human spleens.[55, 61] The blood flow through sinusal spleens (dog) does not appear to differ from that of non-sinusal spleens (cat).[55]

A major difference exists between sinusal and nonsinusal spleens in their ability to "pit" cytoplasmic inclusions. As discussed above, the passage of normal RBCs through the slits separating the endothelial cells in sinusal spleens is facilitated by their pliancy and deformability. The presence of rigid cytoplasmic inclusions (Heinz bodies, hemoparasites, nuclear remnants) allows for the pliant portion of the erythrocyte to pass through the slit, but the portion containing the inclusion is "severed" and retained in the red pulp spaces where it is phagocytized.[55, 61, 62] If the whole cell is undeformable (spherocytes, acanthocytes, senescent RBCs, IgG-coated RBCs) it is retained in the splenic red pulp spaces and subsequently phagocytized.[55, 56, 61, 62] The spleen also removes excessive membrane from the reticulocytes, therefore accelerating their maturation; it is due to this function that the spleen has been referred to as a reticulocyte "training camp."[62, 63] Moreover, the spleen reduces the membrane surface area of the RBCs by one third, converting them from targets into biconcave disks; it also removes surface RBC craters.[61]

In animals with splenomegaly, this filtering capability is significantly enhanced. Splenomegaly is generally associated with an increased splenic red cell volume, with most of the RBCs being located in the red pulp. The hematocrit in the spleen increases considerably, and the RBCs have to compete with the metabolically active leukocytes and macrophages. The increased hematocrit of the splenic blood results in sluggish circulation and increased transit time (shift of RBCs to the intermediate and slow pools). This results in an adverse metabolic environment for the RBCs due to decrease in the glucose concentration and blood pH that in turn cause instability of the RBC membrane due to lack of ATP. These cells with unstable membranes may continue to circulate or are removed from circulation by the reticuloendothelium.[61, 64]

The spleen is also a critical line of defense against blood-borne bacteria (see Immunologic Functions). In this regard, intravenous inoculation of radiolabeled *Salmonella* spp., *E coli*, and pneumococci has shown that the liver clears the bulk of the well-opsonized bacteria, but that the spleen is approximately 60 times more effective in removing poorly opsonized bacteria.[61, 62, 65]

The canine and feline spleens have a great capacity to store blood.[52, 56, 66, 67] The spleen in these species may store between 10 and 20 per cent of the total blood volume. Moreover, due to the smooth muscle relaxation of the splenic capsule induced by tranquilizers and barbiturates, pooling of blood in an enlarged spleen may represent 30 per cent of the total blood volume.[56] Although it has been stated that the blood storage capacity of the spleen is related to the abundance of venous sinuses (the canine spleen has a greater reservoir capacity than its feline counterpart), recent evidence suggests that the blood storage capacity of the feline spleen is similar to that of the dog.[56, 66] In this regard, the blood volume in awake nonsplenectomized cats was approximately 26 ml/lb (56 ml/kg) of body weight, while that of splenectomized cats was approximately 20 ml/lb (44 ml/kg), indicating that the feline spleen is an RBC storage organ.[66] In cats anesthetized with barbiturates, the PCV decreased significantly from 26.4 per cent to 21.5 per cent; administration of epinephrine or splenic massage resulted in the PCV increasing significantly to 32.3 per cent. After splenectomy, the mean PCV increased to 36.1 per cent.[67]

The reservoir function of the spleen serves several roles. First, due to splenic contraction, the RBCs stored within the spleen are released during strenuous exercise, thus adding a sufficient volume of RBCs to prevent hypoperfusion of the kidneys and other organs.[68] This mass of RBCs is also readily available in case of acute blood loss or hemolysis. In this regard, an appreciable decrease in the PCV after hemorrhage may not occur for several hours due to the RBC mass contributed to the blood volume by splenic contraction.[66]

Platelets are also pooled in the spleen.[69] It is estimated that approximately 30 per cent of the total platelet mass is in the spleen at any given time, where they circulate slowly.[69] In humans with splenomegaly, up to 70 per cent of the total circulating platelet pool may be sequestered in the spleen.[70] As discussed above, as a consequence of this platelet storage function, splenectomy in the dog results in significant elevations of the platelet count.[60]

IMMUNOLOGIC FUNCTION

Some of the immunologic functions of the spleen have been discussed under Filtration, Phagocytosis, and Reservoir Function. In addition to the phagocytic function, the spleen is primarily involved in the synthesis of IgM, tuftsin, and properdin.[61] IgM is one of the major immunoglobulins involved in the primary antibody response. Tuftsin is a tetrapeptide that coats blood neutrophils to promote phagocytosis; properdin is a vital component of the alternate pathway of complement activation.[71, 72] Serum concentrations of IgM, tuftsin, and properdin decrease in humans following splenectomy.[61]

Fulminant bacteremia is a relatively common complication of hyposplenism and splenectomy in humans, particularly in children.[61, 62, 73, 74] Sepsis following splenectomy or hyposplenism appears to be rare in the dog and cat. In a published report, a ten-year-old male Scottish terrier with splenic lymphosarcoma and secondary bacterial splenitis developed fatal septicemia due to *Bacteroides fragilis* and *Proteus mirabilis*.[75] Of a total of 131 splenectomies in dogs and cats reported in the literature or reviewed by the author, mortality due to fulminant sepsis was observed in only four dogs splenectomized for immune hemolytic anemia; these dogs were undergoing aggressive immunosuppressive therapy at the time of surgery.[18, 76, 77]

One of the important immunologic functions of the canine and feline spleens appears to be the protection from parasitemia in animals with hemoparasitic infections such as hemobartonellosis and babesiosis.[78, 79] The protective function of the spleen in dogs and cats with intraerythrocytic parasites is apparently related to its "pitting" function. However, the spleen has no effect on the incubation period, frequency or degree of parasitemia, or survival in dogs experimentally infected with *Trypanosoma brucei*.[80]

Based on the above information, it appears that the immunologic function of the spleen in dogs and cats is not as important as in man, since although the prevalence of postsplenectomy sepsis appears to be similar in both species,[81] only dogs undergoing immunosuppressive therapy were affected.

From the human health standpoint, dog bite wounds in splenectomized humans can lead to fulminant sepsis with a microorganism designated DF-2.[82–84]

OTHER FUNCTIONS

Other less understood functions of the spleen include: (a) storage and activation of factor VIII coagulant activity and factor VIII antigen (von Willebrand's factor); (b) regulation of the formation, liberation, or degradation of angiotensin-converting enzyme; and (c) modulation of plasma norepinephrine levels and/or renal PGE2 activity (splenectomy protects from epinephrine-induced acute tubular nephrosis and myocardial infarction).[62]

Splenic Masses

DEFINITIONS AND NOMENCLATURE

The term splenic mass (or localized splenomegaly) is used in this context to define a localized palpable enlargement of the spleen. Most splenic masses are round and irregular, and can be found in the left anterior or middle abdominal quadrant.

It appears that splenic masses are more common than diffuse splenomegalies in dogs, while the opposite appears to occur in cats. Fifty-nine per cent of 69 canine splenectomies reported in the literature and performed at the VTH-OSU were due to splenic masses.[18, 76] In another series of cases reported, a distinction between diffuse splenomegaly and splenic masses was not made.[77] In an additional report of 82 splenectomies performed in dogs, the author states that "about 50 per cent were neoplasms and 20 per cent rupture/hematoma types."[85]

Splenic masses can be classified as neoplastic or non-neoplastic. Neoplastic splenic masses are represented mainly by hemangiomas and hemangiosarcomas (HA/HSA); other neoplasms that oftentimes present as splenic masses are fibrosarcomas, leiomyosarcomas, leiomyomas, myelolipomas, and occasionally lymphomas (primarily in dogs).[18, 76, 77, 86–88] Non-neoplastic splenic masses include primarily hematomas and abscesses.

Hemangiomas/Hemangiosarcomas. Vascular tumors of the spleen appear to be extremely common in dogs and are rare in cats.[76, 77, 89–95] According to several authors, HA/HSA constitute the most common splenic neoplasm in splenic tissues collected during splenectomy in dogs.[77, 86]

These neoplasms occur predominately in older, large breed dogs, and there is an apparent predilection for males and for German shepherds.[86, 89, 90, 96] Clinical signs and physical findings in dogs with splenic HA/HSA are usually vague and nonspecific, and include anorexia, weight loss, abdominal distention, weakness, pallor, and vomiting.[18, 89, 90, 96] A large majority of cases are examined because of rupture of the primary tumor or its metastases.[90]

Despite the fact that hemangiomas can be quite large, surgical excision usually results in the cure of the patient. Hemangiosarcomas, however, have an aggressive biologic behavior, and as many as 50 per cent of the dogs have gross evidence of metastatic disease on initial presentation.[90] Metastatic lesions are usually found in the liver, omentum, peritoneum, kidneys, heart, and lungs. A presumptive diagnosis of HA/HSA is usually made on the basis of clinical signs, physical findings (cranial or midabdominal mass), radiographic and ultrasonographic findings (see below), and hematologic abnormalities.

Hematologic findings in dogs with HSA have recently been reviewed.[96] The following abnormalities were detected in ten dogs with splenic or hepatic HSA for which complete blood counts were available: anemia (eight dogs), which was regenerative in five dogs; presence of nucleated RBCs in the blood smear (seven dogs); poikilocytosis (nine dogs); presence of acanthocytes (nine dogs) and schistocytes (eight dogs); presence of Howell-Jolly bodies (six dogs); thrombocytopenia (nine dogs); and neutrophilia (seven dogs).[96] Two of the dogs with thrombocytopenia had detectable fibrin degradation products in circulation.[96] The fragmentation anemia and thrombocytopenia are probably due to microangiopathic changes in the tumor vascular bed, although disseminated intravascular coagulation is also common in dogs with HSA.[18, 97, 98] A correlation between HSA and acanthocytosis has also been established.[99] Some of the hematologic changes may be due to hyposplenism (see below).

Surgical resection has been the mainstay of therapy in dogs with splenic hemangiosarcoma. In one study, splenectomy in dogs with HSA resulted in a median survival of 65 days (mean, 80 days); when surgery was followed by adjuvant immunotherapy using mixed bacterial vaccine the median survival was 91 days (mean, 143 days); when adjuvant postoperative immunotherapy and chemotherapy utilizing vincristine (0.006 mg/lb or 0.0125 mg/kg, IV, once weekly), cyclophosphamide (0.45 mg/lb or 1 mg/kg, PO, q24h), and methotrexate (0.18 to 0.28 mg/lb or 0.4 to 0.6 mg/kg, IV, once weekly) were used, the median survival was 117 days (mean, 148 days).[90] Therefore, from this study it can be concluded that chemo- or immunotherapy is of no benefit in dogs with HSA.

The median survival in nine dogs with HSA treated by the author using a combination of vincristine (0.75 mg/m2, IV, on days 8 and 15 of a 21 day cycle), doxorubicin (30 mg/m2, IV, on day 1 of the cycle), and cyclophosphamide (100–200 mg/m2, IV, on day 1 of the cycle) following surgical excision was 187 days (mean,

213 days), with objective remissions being observed in 8 of the 9 dogs (disappearance or over 50 per cent reduction in the size of the lesions). Due to the severe myelosuppression associated with this protocol, the dogs were maintained on sulfadiazine-trimethoprim (Tribrissen, 7 mg/lb, PO, bid).[18]

Hematomas. Splenic hematomas represented the most common splenic mass in 42 dogs splenectomized at the VTH-OSU, comprising 36 per cent of the lesions. Of a total of 131 dogs splenectomized, hematomas were found in 15 per cent of the cases.[18, 76, 77] In the majority of the cases, no underlying causes predisposing to intrasplenic hemorrhage could be found. However, spontaneous hematomas occurred in two dogs with splenic lymphoma observed by the author. This may be due to vascular erosion from the tumor or to distortion of the splenic architecture by the neoplastic cells.

Neither the size nor the gross appearance of splenic masses can be used as a guide to determine their biologic behavior. It is not uncommon to observe extremely large splenic hematomas (the author has observed a 12.6 pound splenic hematoma in a 41.6 lb dog), while HSAs may be quite small. Moreover, hepatic EMH or regenerative hyperplasia may result in the appearance of hepatic masses that mimic metastatic lesions, even in dogs with splenic hematomas. This is extremely important when counseling owners on performing euthanasia of their pet while under anesthesia. Ultrasonographic changes in splenic hematomas may mimic those seen in splenic neoplasia (see below). In addition, since vascular neoplasms of the spleen oftentimes result in intrasplenic hematoma formation, tissue samples from several areas should be submitted for histopathology to rule out the presence of a HSA.

Splenomegaly

DEFINITIONS

The term splenomegaly will be used in this context to refer to diffuse enlargement of the spleen. On the contrary, asymmetric or solitary enlargements of this organ are referred to as splenic masses (see above), since that is usually the clinical impression obtained by the clinician upon performing a physical examination.

PATHOGENESIS OF SPLENOMEGALY

Four major categories of splenomegaly exist when one considers the pathogenetic mechanisms involved. Similarly to what occurs with the lymph nodes, splenic enlargement can result from inflammatory changes (splenitis), lymphoreticular hyperplasia, congestion, or infiltration with abnormal cells or substances (amyloidosis) (Table 115–6). It should be emphasized that palpably enlarged spleens are not always abnormal, and that enlarged spleens are not always palpable.[61]

Inflammatory Splenomegaly. Inflammatory changes within the spleen usually result in localized or diffuse enlargement of this organ. Most disorders associated with splenitis are infectious or granulomatous in nature. In addition to lymphoreticular hyperplasia (see below),

TABLE 115–6. CLASSIFICATION OF SPLENOMEGALY IN DOGS AND CATS

Type	Species
Inflammatory Splenomegaly	
Suppurative Splenitis	
Penetrating abdominal wounds	C, D
Migrating foreign bodies	C, D
Bacterial endocarditis	C, D
Septicemia	C, D
Splenic torsion	D
Toxoplasmosis	C, D
Infectious canine hepatitis (acute)	D
Necrotizing Splenitis	
Splenic torsion	D
Splenic neoplasia	D
Infectious canine hepatitis (acute)	D
Salmonellosis	D, C
Eosinophilic Splenitis	
Eosinophilic gastroenteritis	D, C?
Hypereosinophilic syndrome	C
Lymphoplasmacytic Splenitis	
Infectious canine hepatitis (chronic)	D
Ehrlichiosis (chronic)	D
Pyometra	D, C
Brucellosis	D
Hemobartonellosis	D, C
Granulomatous Splenitis	
Histoplasmosis	D, C
Mycobacteriosis	D, C
Leishmaniasis	D
Pyogranulomatous Splenitis	
Blastomycosis	D, C?
Sporotrichosis	D
Feline infectious peritonitis	C
Hyperplastic Splenomegaly	
Bacterial endocarditis	D
Brucellosis	D
Diskospondylitis	D
Systemic lupus erythematosus	D
Hemolytic disorders (see text)	D, C
Congestive Splenomegaly	
Pharmacologic (tranquilizers, anticonvulsants)	D, C
Portal hypertension	D, C
Splenic torsion	D
Infiltrative Splenomegaly	
Neoplastic	
Acute and chronic leukemias	D, C
Systemic mastocytosis	D, C
Malignant histiocytosis	D
Lymphoma	D, C
Multiple myeloma	D, C
Metastatic neoplasia	D, C
Non-neoplastic	
Extramedullary hematopoiesis	D, C?
Hypereosinophilic syndrome	C
Amyloidosis	D

splenic changes in splenitis include hematogenous infiltration with inflammatory cells (e.g., polymorphonuclear leukocytes). According to the course of the disease splenitides can be classified as either acute, subacute, or chronic; according to the predominant cell type they can be classified as suppurative (when the predominant cell type is the neutrophil), necrotizing (when necrosis predominates), eosinophilic (when eosinophils predominate), lymphoplasmacytic (when lymphocytes and plasma cells predominate), granulomatous (when the predominant cell types are macrophages, epithelioid cells, lymphocytes, or multinucleated giant cells), and pyogranulomatous (when both granulomatous changes and neutrophilic infiltration are present). It is important to classify the splenitis according to the predominant cell type, since different etiologic agents are associated with different pathologic forms.

The majority of disorders associated with splenitis have been discussed elsewhere in this book; therefore, emphasis will be placed on the pathogenesis and tissue changes in splenitis.

Suppurative splenitides are usually acute or subacute, although chronic suppurative changes of the spleen can also occur. When discrete cavitated lesions filled with pus occur in the spleen, the term splenic abscess is preferred. Diseases associated with suppurative splenitis include penetrating wounds to the abdomen, migrating foreign bodies (e.g., plant awns), hematogenous dissemination of bacterial infections (e.g., subacute bacterial endocarditis, septicemia with pyogenic organisms), bacterial infections secondary to splenic torsion (see below), protozoal infections (e.g., toxoplasmosis), and certain viral diseases (e.g., acute canine infectious hepatitis), among others (Table 115–6).[18, 33, 34, 100–103]

Necrotizing splenitis caused by gas-forming anaerobes has been reported in the dog in association with splenic torsion and splenic lymphoma and observed by the author in dogs with isolated splenic torsion and gastric dilatation-volvulus complex involving the spleen, and in a dog with splenic hemangiosarcoma.[18, 75, 100] In dogs, focal accumulations of gas in the splenic region can be detected on plain radiographic and ultrasonographic examination of the abdomen. Coagulation necrosis of the spleen with associated inflammation can also be seen in dogs with infectious canine hepatitis and in dogs and cats with salmonellosis.[18, 101, 104]

Eosinophilic infiltrates in the spleen have been observed in association with the hypereosinophilic syndrome in cats and with eosinophilic gastroenteritis in dogs.[18, 105] However, since these proliferative changes may not be inflammatory in nature, they will be discussed under Infiltrative Splenomegaly.

Lymphoplasmacytic splenitis commonly occurs in association with subacute or chronic infectious disorders such as canine infectious hepatitis, canine ehrlichiosis, pyometra, brucellosis, and hemobartonellosis, among others (Table 115–6).[7, 9, 18, 79, 101, 102, 106] In these cases, the splenic changes are characterized by lymphoplasmacytic hyperplasia with significant plasma cell infiltration.

Granulomatous splenitis occurs in some systemic mycoses (e.g., histoplasmosis) and mycobacterial infections; pyogranulomatous splenitis also occurs in association with systemic mycoses such as blastomycosis and sporotrichosis, in tuberculosis, and in some viral infections such as feline infectious peritonitis (Table 115–6).[13, 18, 24, 107–109]

Hyperplastic Splenomegaly. The spleen commonly reacts to blood-borne antigens and to red cell destruction with hyperplasia of the reticuloendothelial and lymphoid components. This hyperplasia has been referred to as work hypertrophy, since it usually results in varying degrees of splenic enlargement.[61]

Hyperplastic splenomegaly appears to be common in dogs with subacute bacterial endocarditis and chronic bacteriemic disorders such as diskospondylitis and brucellosis.[102, 106] In addition, it has been seen in association with systemic lupus erythematosus, even when hemolytic anemia is not an important component of the syndrome.[18]

It has been recognized for some time that red blood cell phagocytosis by the splenic reticuloendothelium in man leads to hyperplasia of this cell population, resulting in splenomegaly.[61, 64, 110] The same seems to occur in dogs and cats with certain hemolytic disorders including immune hemolytic anemia, drug-induced hemolysis, pyruvate kinase deficiency anemia, phosphofructokinase deficiency anemia, familial nonspherocytic hemolysis in poodles, Heinz body hemolysis, and hemobartonellosis, among others.[18, 79, 111–114]

Congestive Splenomegaly. The canine and feline spleen has a great capacity to store blood, and under normal circumstances it stores between 10 and 20 per cent of the total blood volume (see above). Although, as discussed above, it has been stated that the blood storage capacity of this organ is related to the abundance of venous sinuses and that therefore the blood storage capacity of the canine spleen is considerably higher than its feline counterpart, recent evidence contradicts this theory.[56, 66, 67]

Owing to the smooth muscle relaxation of the splenic capsule, tranquilizers and barbiturates increase blood pooling; pooling of blood in an enlarged spleen can account for up to 30 per cent of the total blood volume.[56] For example, in cats anesthetized with barbiturates, the PCV decreased significantly from a mean of 26.4 per cent to 21.5 per cent ($p < 0.05$), or 18 per cent.[67] Other anesthetics such as halothane also result in significant decreases in the PCV and plasma protein (PP) concentration. In a study of dogs and monkeys anesthetized with halothane, Steffey et al. found that this drug caused significant decreases in the PCV (15 to 20 per cent) and plasma protein concentration (10 to 20 per cent) that remained decreased throughout the duration of the anesthesia.[115] Splenectomized dogs experienced a smaller reduction in the PCV (5 to 10 per cent), but no changes in the plasma protein concentration.[115] This suggests that although halothane causes some splenic blood sequestration, other mechanisms such as intravascular volume expansion with fluid shifts between the extravascular and intravascular compartments may be responsible for some of these changes.[115] These findings are of significance when evaluating red blood cell parameters in blood obtained from anesthetized or tranquilized patients, since the PCV and/or PP concentration may be artificially low.

Portal hypertension can also lead to congestive splenomegaly; however, splenic congestion secondary to portal hypertension does not appear to be as common in dogs and cats as it is in humans.[116] This may be due to the development of velar-omental veins that decompress the spleen by shunting blood to the left renal vein in both species.[116, 117] Causes of portal hypertension that may lead to splenomegaly in small animals are listed in Table 115–6. Of these, right-sided congestive heart failure, obstruction of the caudal vena cava (e.g., due to congenital anomalies, neoplasia or heartworm disease), and intrahepatic obstruction appear to be more common.[116, 117] Compression of the caudal vena cava resulting in posthepatic portal hypertension with or without splenomegaly has been observed in dogs with right atrial hemangiosarcomas by this author.[18] Ultrasonographic evaluation of the spleen in these patients usually reveals markedly distended splenic, portal, and/or hepatic veins.

A relatively common cause of congestive splenomegaly in the dog is splenic torsion. Torsion of the spleen, either isolated or associated with the gastric dilatation-volvulus (GDV) syndrome commonly results in significant splenomegaly due to congestion.[118–126] Splenic torsion is commonly a component of the GDV syndrome, to the point that palpation of a markedly enlarged spleen in a dog with severe abdominal distention of acute onset is helpful in determining that the patient has GDV.[126] For a detailed discussion of GDV syndrome please refer to Chapter 84. Splenic torsion can also occur independently of the GDV syndrome. Most affected dogs are of large, deep chested breeds, primarily Great Danes and German shepherds.[118–125] Clinical signs can be either acute or chronic in nature; dogs with acute splenic torsion usually present with acute abdominal pain and distention, vomiting, depression, and anorexia. Dogs with chronic splenic torsion display a wide variety of clinical signs including anorexia, weight loss, intermittent vomiting, abdominal distention, polyuria and polydipsia, pigmenturia (due to hemoglobinuria), and abdominal pain. Physical examination usually reveals marked splenomegaly. Ultrasonographic evaluation of these patients may reveal the presence of greatly distended splenic veins. Hematologic abnormalities include anemia, presence of target cells, leukocytosis due to regenerative left shift, and leukoerythroblastosis (presence of red blood cell and white blood cell precursors in circulation).[18, 118, 119, 124] Disseminated intravascular coagulation appears to be a common complication in dogs with torsion of the spleen.[18, 118] A high percentage of dogs with splenic torsion have hemoglobinuria, possibly as a consequence of intravascular or intrasplenic hemolysis.[18, 118, 119] The treatment of choice for dogs with splenic torsion is splenectomy (see below).

Infiltrative Splenomegaly. Infiltration of the spleen with neoplastic cells constitutes one of the most common causes of splenomegaly in small animals.[127] Marked splenomegaly is a common finding in dogs and cats with acute and chronic leukemias, although it appears to be more common in the former;[10–12, 41] this splenic infiltration is considered to be primarily hematogenous, although neoplastic EMH is also thought to play a role. Marked splenomegaly is also a common feature of systemic mastocytosis in dogs and cats and of some forms of malignant histiocytosis in dogs.[16, 17, 128–131] In addition, neoplastic infiltration of the spleen may occur in dogs and cats with malignant lymphoma and multiple myeloma.[14, 15, 22] Splenomegaly due to metastatic splenic infiltration from non-hematologic neoplasms is rare in dogs and cats; the author has seen a limited number of dogs and cats with splenic metastases from mammary adenocarcinomas and from intraabdominal undifferentiated carcinomas and sarcomas.[18]

Non-neoplastic causes of infiltrative splenomegaly are less common than neoplastic ones. Splenic extramedullary hematopoiesis (EMH) resulting in splenomegaly appears to be common in dogs.[132] As discussed earlier in this chapter, the spleen retains its fetal hematopoietic

potential during adult life; a variety of stimuli (red blood cell destruction, severe splenic or extrasplenic inflammation, neoplastic infiltration of the spleen, bone marrow hypoplasia, and splenic congestion) may result in the spleen retaking its fetal hematopoietic function and producing red blood cells, white blood cells, and platelets. In a series of 28 dogs and 5 cats with splenomegaly or splenic masses in which fine needle aspiration cytology was utilized for diagnosis, EMH was found in 8 dogs (28 per cent) but in none of the cats.[132] The author has also observed splenic EMH in dogs with pyometra, immune-mediated hemolysis, immune-mediated thrombocytopenia, several infectious diseases, and a variety of malignant neoplasms.[18]

Another disorder that commonly results in prominent splenomegaly is the hypereosinophilic syndrome (HES) of cats, a disease characterized by peripheral blood eosinophilia, bone marrow hyperplasia of the eosinophil precursors, and multiple organ infiltration by mature eosinophils.[105, 133, 134] Clinical signs and physical findings in cats with HES include diarrhea, vomiting, anorexia and weight loss, lethargy, hepatomegaly, splenomegaly, emaciation, thickened bowel loops, presence of intraabdominal masses, and occasional cutaneous lesions. Laboratory abnormalities include marked eosinophilia (range: 2100 to 41,000/μl) and hyperplasia of eosinophil precursors in the bone marrow. Histopathologic changes consist mainly of infiltration of various tissues with mature eosinophils. Therapy with immunosuppressive doses of corticosteroids in 6 of 7 cats reported in the literature resulted in variable response and survival times ranging from one week to 22 months; survival in cats with multisystemic involvement ranged from one to 16 weeks.[105, 133, 134] Finally, splenic amyloidosis resulting in splenomegaly appears to be rare.

EVALUATION OF THE PATIENT WITH SPLENOMEGALY

History and Physical Findings. Clinical signs in dogs and cats with splenomegaly are usually vague and nonspecific, and in general are related to the primary disease rather than to the splenic enlargement per se.[127] Disorders in which the clinical signs are primarily related to the splenic enlargement are splenic torsion and primary splenic hyperplasia. Signs in dogs with splenomegaly include anorexia, weight loss, weakness, abdominal distension, vomiting, diarrhea, and polyuria/polydipsia (PU/PD). The latter appears to occur commonly in dogs with marked splenomegaly, particularly in those with splenic torsion.[118, 119] Although the pathogenesis of these signs is unclear, psychogenic polydipsia due to abdominal pain or distention of splenic stretch receptors may be a contributory mechanism. Splenectomy in these patients usually results in prompt resolution of the signs.[18] Other signs associated with splenomegaly are those resulting from the hematologic consequences of the splenic enlargement (see below) and include spontaneous bleeding, pallor, and fever.

Physical findings in these patients are also variable. Patients with hematologic abnormalities secondary to splenomegaly may have pallor, petechiae, or ecchymoses. As discussed above, not all enlarged spleens are palpable and not every palpable spleen is abnormal. In this author's experience, the spleen is easily palpable, to the point of being prominent, in thin cats, deep-chested dogs, and in some small breeds of dogs such as miniature schnauzers, particularly after eating. The clinician can usually estimate the degree of splenomegaly during abdominal palpation. The palpable characteristics of the spleen are variable. In most cats with marked splenomegaly, the surface of the organ is smooth; in dogs, an enlarged spleen can be either smooth or irregular (i.e., "lumpy-bumpy"). Localized splenic enlargements are also common in the dogs and they were discussed under Splenic Masses. In patients with hemolymphatic neoplasms or with posthepatic portal hypertension, hepatomegaly may also be a prominent feature.

Hematologic and Serum Biochemical Findings. The spleen exerts a marked influence in the hemogram. Two patterns of hematologic changes are recognized in dogs and cats with splenomegaly: hypersplenism and hyposplenism (or asplenia). The former results from increased reticuloendothelial activity and is rare; the latter is more common, and results in hematologic changes similar to the ones seen in splenectomized patients. The hematologic abnormalities in patients with splenomegaly are summarized in Table 115–7.

Bone marrow evaluation should always be conducted prior to splenectomy in patients with cytopenias. It is not uncommon for the spleen to take over the primary hematopoietic function in patients with primary bone marrow disorders such as hypoplasia or aplasia. Splenectomy in these patients usually removes the sole source of circulating blood cells, leading to death. However, a recent report describes a dog with bone marrow hypoplasia that responded to splenectomy with resolution of the hematologic abnormalities.[135]

Serum biochemical abnormalities associated with splenomegaly are rare. Hemoglobinemia resulting in hemoglobinuria is a relatively common finding in dogs with splenic torsion.[118] Biochemical abnormalities associated with local or systemic diseases that result in splenomegaly will not be discussed.

Splenic Imaging. The spleen is normally well visualized on plain abdominal radiographs, but there is a wide variation in its appearance. On dorsoventral (DV) or ventrodorsal (VD) views, the spleen is visualized between the gastric fundus and the left kidney. The length of the gastrosplenic ligament and the degree of gastric distention affect the portion of the spleen that is visualized. The size and location of the spleen are more variable on lateral radiographs than on VD or DV projections. However, the body and tail of the spleen are visualized in the ventral abdomen as far craniad as

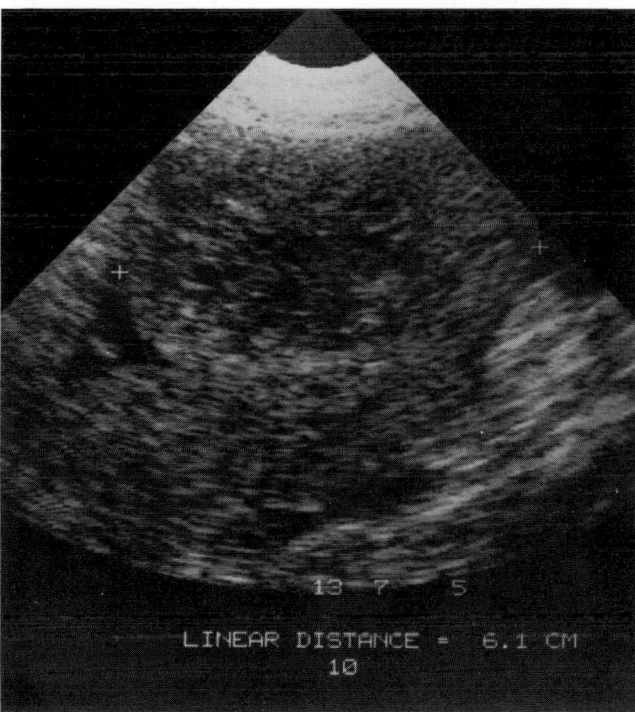

FIGURE 115–4. Splenic ultrasonogram of a dog presented with acute onset of depression, anemia, and a midabdominal mass. A spherical mass with an admixture of hyperechoic and hypoechoic areas is visualized. The +'s indicate the outer limits of the mass. The histopathologic diagnosis was splenic hemangiosarcoma.

the infrasternal fossa or as caudad as the umbilical region.[136] Large splenic masses usually appear in the caudal or midabdomen on survey radiographs. It should be remembered that tranquilization or anesthesia usually results in congestive splenomegaly, making interpretation of splenic size on plain radiographs extremely difficult.

Two-dimensional gray scale ultrasonography is extremely helpful in evaluating patients with splenomegaly or splenic masses.[137, 138] In addition, ultrasound-guided fine-needle aspirates or biopsies can be easily performed.[26] The spleen should be evaluated ultrasonographically for location, size, and parenchymal appearance. The normal splenic contour should be smooth, and its size must be subjectively considered to be similar to that of the liver. The parenchyma should appear uniform in appearance, with a finer and slightly more dense stromal pattern than the liver. The splenic vein and its branches can be identified near the hilus.[137] Two main ultrasonographic patterns can be identified: normal to decreased echogenicity without parenchymal abnormalities, seen in congestive splenomegaly and diffuse infiltrative disorders; and focal parenchymal abnormalities, such as cysts, hematomas, abscesses, or neoplasia (Figure 115–4). Focal hypoechoic lesions can also occur in dogs with splenic lymphoma.[18, 137] Distention of the splenic veins may be visualized in dogs with splenic torsion. In patients with posthepatic portal hypertension, dilatation of the portal vessels is commonly seen. Ultrasonographic evaluation of the liver and perisplenic structures should also be conducted to evaluate for the presence of metastatic lesions.

Radionuclide imaging using technetium-99m (^{99m}Tc)

TABLE 115–7. HEMATOLOGIC ABNORMALITIES IN DOGS AND CATS WITH SPLENOMEGALY

Hypersplenism	Hyposplenism/Asplenia
Regenerative anemia	Target cells
Neutropenia	Acanthocytes
Thrombocytopenia	Howell-Jolly bodies
Bicytopenias	Nucleated RBCs
Pancytopenia	Increased percentage of reticulocytes
	Thrombocytosis

or Indium-111m (^{111m}In) is widely used in humans with splenic disorders;[139] however, its use in animals is limited. ^{99}Tc^m is considered ideal for splenic imaging since it has a short half-life (six hours) and low associated radiation effects. The ^{99}Tc^m sulfur colloid scan has become an accepted method of splenic imaging in humans.[62] It utilizes 1 μm diameter sulfur colloid particles of which 10 per cent are normally phagocytized by the spleen and 90 per cent by the liver. This technique only measures the spleen's ability to clear particulate matter. In addition, computerized tomography (CT) and magnetic resonance imaging (MRI) can also be used to visualize the spleen.

Splenic Aspiration. Transabdominal fine-needle aspiration (FNA) of the spleen constitutes a safe and reliable method to evaluate patients with splenomegaly.[132, 140] These aspirates are obtained with the patient in right lateral or dorsal recumbency, using manual restraint or mild sedation. It should be remembered that performing transabdominal splenic FNA in patients chemically restrained with phenothiazine tranquilizers or barbiturates usually results in blood-diluted specimens due to splenic congestion. The area to be aspirated is identified and surgically prepared, and the spleen is manually isolated. Using a 12 ml or 20 ml disposable plastic syringe attached to a 23 or 25 gauge 1 to 1.5 inch needle, the abdominal wall is penetrated and the needle advanced into the splenic parenchyma. The use of an aspiration gun (Aspir Gun) facilitates this procedure, since it provides a better control of the tip of the needle. After suction is applied to the syringe three or four times, the needle and syringe are quickly removed. The suction is released before the needle is withdrawn from the splenic parenchyma to prevent aspiration of the material into the syringe. The specimens are then placed on coverslips and pull smears are made. These are air-dried and stained with Wright-Giemsa or Diff-Quick stain (Diffco). The patients are then observed for three to six hours for bleeding.[132]

This procedure is safe, reliable, and provides results within 15 minutes. In a recent series of 28 dogs and 5 cats that had transabdominal FNAs performed for evaluation of splenomegaly or splenic masses, no complications were detected, even in patients with thrombocytopenia or other coagulopathies.[132] Histopathologic evaluation of the spleen was done in 14 patients; all cytologic diagnoses in these animals correlated with their final histopathologic diagnoses. The most common cytologic diagnoses were EMH (24 per cent) and hematopoietic neoplasia (24 per cent); other diagnoses included lymphoreticular hyperplasia, hemorrhage, and neoplasia of unknown cell type.[132] No abnormalities were found in six cases (18 per cent) and hepatic tissue was obtained in two dogs.[132]

Splenic Surgery. When a diagnostic tissue specimen cannot be obtained through transabdominal FNA, the clinician must face the decision of performing an exploratory celiotomy.[127, 141] Exploratory celiotomies provide considerable information regarding the gross morphology of the spleen and adjacent organs and tissues. However, direct visualization of these structures may be misleading, since it may be impossible to differentiate some benign splenic masses (i.e., hematoma, heman-

gioma) from their malignant counterpart (i.e., hemangiosarcoma) on the basis of gross morphology alone. For example, the surgeon may recommend to the owners that the animal be euthanized on the table because he/she has a splenic mass and nodules in the liver, when indeed those hepatic nodules may represent nodular hyperplasia or EMH, while the primary mass was benign.

A discussion of the techniques used during splenectomy is beyond the scope of this chapter. However, the indications and contraindications of splenectomy will be briefly discussed. Splenectomy is indicated in the following situations: (a) splenic torsion; (b) splenic rupture; (c) symptomatic splenomegaly (regardless of the cause); and (d) splenic masses. The value of splenectomy is questionable in: (a) dogs with immune-mediated blood disorders (although a recent report suggests its beneficial value);[142] (b) dogs and cats with splenomegaly due to lymphoma in which chemotherapy failed to induce splenic remission; and (c) dogs and cats with leukemias. Splenectomy is generally contraindicated in patients with bone marrow hypoplasia in which the spleen is the main hematopoietic site.

A review of 131 splenectomies performed in small animals published in the literature or performed at the VTH-OSU revealed that 130 cases were in dogs and only one in a cat.[18, 76, 77] The histopathologic findings in the excised spleens were as follows: 36 per cent were hemangiomas and hemangiosarcomas (no distinction between these two neoplasms was made in one of the series); 18 per cent non-vascular neoplasms, 61 per cent of which were hematopoietic malignancies (i.e., lymphomas, leukemias, systemic mast cell disease, multiple myeloma); 15 per cent were hematomas; 7 per cent were splenic ruptures (including the only cat in these series); 6 per cent were torsions; and 16 per cent were miscellaneous disorders, including lymphoreticular hyperplasia (mainly in dogs with immune-hemolytic anemia), splenomegaly of unknown pathogenesis, and splenitis. Therefore, it appears that over half of the splenectomies are performed because of splenic neoplasia. Only four fatal complications due to sepsis were observed among the 131 patients (3 per cent); they all occurred in dogs splenectomized at the VTH-OSU for refractory immune hemolytic anemia. All dogs were undergoing severe immunosuppressive therapy at the time of surgery.[18]

On the basis of these data, the overall risk of developing septic complications following splenectomy in dogs is approximately 3 per cent; this is similar to what occurs in humans, where the risk of complications ranges from 2.5 to 4 per cent.[81] However, it should be remembered that all the dogs that developed postsplenectomy sepsis were undergoing immunosuppressive therapy at the time of surgery. When those four dogs are excluded from the series, no complications were detected among 127 cases. The risk of developing postsplenectomy sepsis in man is greatest during the first year of life.[81] In the series reviewed by the author this risk could not be identified.

References

1. Weiss, L: Lymphatic vessels and lymph nodes. *In* Weiss, L (ed): Histology Cell and Tissue Biology, 5th ed. New York, Elsevier Medical, 1983, p 527.

2. Bellanti, JA and Kadlec, JV: General Immunobiology. *In* Bellanti, JA (ed): Immunology III. Philadelphia, WB Saunders, 1985, p 16.
3. Saar, LI and Getty, R: Carnivore lymphatic system. *In* Getty, R (ed): Sisson and Grossman's The Anatomy of the Domestic Animals. Philadelphia, WB Saunders, 1975, p 1652.
4. Shelton, ME and Forsythe, WB: Buccal lymph nodes in the dog. Am J Vet Res 40:1638, 1979.
5. Rumph, PF, et al.: Facial lymph nodes in dogs. JAVMA 176:342, 1980.
6. Gorham, JR and Foreyt, WJ: Salmon poisoning disease. *In* Greene, CE (ed): Clinical Microbiology and Infectious Diseases of the Dog and Cat. Philadelphia, WB Saunders, 1984, p 538.
7. Hibler, SC, et al.: Rickettsial infections in dogs. Part III. Salmon disease complex and hemobartonellosis. Comp Cont Ed 8:251, 1986.
8. Hibler, SC, et al.: Rickettsial infections in dogs. Part I. Rocky Mountain spotted fever and coxiella infections. Comp Cont Ed 7:856, 1985.
9. Hibler, SC, et al.: Rickettsial infections in dogs. Part II. Ehrlichiosis and infectious cyclic thrombocytopenia. Comp Cont Ed 8:106, 1986.
10. Leifer, CE and Matus, RE: Chronic lymphocytic leukemia in the dog: 22 cases (1974–1984). JAVMA 189:214, 1986.
11. Leifer, CE, et al.: Chronic myelogenous leukemia in the dog. JAVMA 183:686, 1983.
12. Couto, CG: Clinicopathologic aspects of acute leukemia in the dog. JAVMA 186:681, 1985.
13. Attleberger, MH: Systemic mycoses. *In* Kirk, RW (ed): Current Veterinary Therapy VIII. Philadelphia, WB Saunders, 1983, p 1180.
14. Couto, CG: Canine lymphomas: Something old, something new. Comp Cont Ed 7:291, 1985.
15. Matus, RE, et al.: Prognostic factors for multiple myeloma in the dog. JAVMA 188:1288, 1986.
16. O'Keefe, DA, et al.: Systemic mastocytosis in 16 dogs. J Vet Int Med 1:75, 1987.
17. Wellman, ML, et al.: Malignant histiocytosis in 4 dogs. JAVMA 187:919, 1985.
18. Couto, CG: Unpublished observation, 1987.
19. Scott, DW, et al.: Lymphoreticular neoplasia in a dog resembling malignant histiocytosis (histiocytic medullary reticulosis) in man. Cornell Vet 69:176, 1979.
20. Cotter, SM: Feline viral neoplasia. *In* Greene, CE (ed): Clinical Microbiology and Infectious Diseases of the Dog and Cat. Philadelphia, WB Saunders, 1984, p 490.
21. Dow, SW, et al.: Hypercalcemia associated with blastomycosis in dogs. JAVMA 188:706, 1986.
22. Drazner, FH: Multiple myeloma in the cat. Comp Cont Ed 4:206, 1982.
23. Breitschwerdt, EB, et al.: Monoclonal gammopathy associated with naturally occurring canine ehrlichiosis. J Vet Intern Med 1:2, 1987.
24. Pedersen, NC: Feline coronavirus infections. *In* Greene, CE (ed): Clinical Microbiology and Infectious Diseases of the Dog and Cat. Philadelphia, WB Saunders, 1984, p 514.
25. Nyland, TG and Kantrowitz, BM: Ultrasound in diagnosis and staging of abdominal neoplasia. *In* Gorman, NT (ed): Oncology. Churchill Livingstone, 1986, p 1.
26. Smith, S: Ultrasound-guided biopsy. Vet Clin North Am 15:1249, 1985.
27. Zinkl, JG and Keeton, KS: Lymph node cytology. California Vet 33(1):9, 1979.
28. Zinkl, JG and Keeton, KS: Lymph node cytology—II. California Vet 33(4):6, 1979.
29. Zinkl, JG and Keeton, KS: Lymph node cytology—III. Neoplasia. California Vet 35(5):19, 1980.
30. Barrett, RP: Lymph node cytology. VM/SAC 73:768, 1978.
31. Mills, JN: Diagnoses from lymph node fine-aspiration cytology. Austr Vet Pract 14:14, 1984.
32. Thrall, MA: Cytology of lymphoid tissues. Comp Cont Ed 9:104, 1987.
33. Swindle, MM, et al.: Contagious streptococcal lymphadenitis in cats. JAVMA 177:829, 1980.
34. Swindle, MM, et al.: Pathogenesis of contagious streptococcal lymphadenitis in cats. JAVMA 179:1208, 1981.
35. Muller, GH, et al.: Animal Dermatology. Philadelphia, WB Saunders, 1983, p 237.
36. Chapman, WL: Diseases of the lymph nodes and spleen. *In* Ettinger, S (ed): Textbook of Veterinary Internal Medicine, 1st ed. Philadelphia, WB Saunders, 1975, p 1664.
37. Jang, SS, et al.: A cat with *Corynebacterium equi* lymphadenitis clinically simulating lymphosarcoma. Cornell Vet 65:232, 1975.
38. Moore, FM, et al.: Distinctive peripheral lymph node hyperplasia of young cats. Vet Pathol 23:386, 1986.
39. Mooney, SC, et al.: Generalized lymphadenopathy resembling lymphoma in cats: six cases (1972–1976). JAVMA 190:897, 1987.
40. Lucke, YM, et al.: Plexiform vascularization of lymph nodes: An unusual but distinctive lymphadenopathy in cats. J Comp Path 97:109, 1987.
41. Couto, CG: Oncology. *In* Sherding, RG (ed): The Cat: Diseases and Management. New York, Churchill Livingstone, 1988, p 589.
42. Theilen, GH and Madewell, BR: Leukemia-sarcoma disease complex. *In* Theilen, GH and Madewell, BR (eds): Veterinary Cancer Medicine, 1st ed. Philadelphia, Lea and Febiger, 1979, p 204.
43. Mackey, LY and Jarrett, WFH: Pathogenesis of lymphoid neoplasia in cats and its relationship to immunologic cell pathways. Morphologic aspects. J Nat Cancer Inst 49:853, 1972.
44. Hardy, WD: Hematopoietic tumors of cats. JAAHA 17:921, 1981.
45. Gruffydd-Jones, TJ, et al.: Clinical and radiological features of anterior mediastinal lymphosarcoma in the cat: A review of 30 cases. Vet Rec 104:304, 1979.
46. Couto, CG: Canine extranodal lymphomas. *In* Kirk, RW (ed): Current Veterinary Therapy IX. Philadelphia, WB Saunders, 1986, p 473.
47. Cotter, SM: Treatment of lymphoma and leukemia with cyclophosphamide, vincristine, and prednisone. Treatment of cats. JAAHA 19:166, 1983.
48. Jeglum, AK, et al.: Chemotherapy for lymphoma in 75 cats. JAVMA 190:174, 1987.
49. Turrel, JM: Radiation therapy and hyperthermia. *In* Holzworth, J (ed): Diseases of the Cat—Medicine and Surgery. Philadelphia, WB Saunders, 1987, p 606.
50. Priester, WA: The occurrence of tumors in domestic animals. J Natl Cancer Inst Monograph 54, 1980, p 166.
51. Weiss, L: The spleen. *In* Weiss, L (ed): Histology. Cell and Tissue Biology (5th ed). New York, Elsevier Medical, 1983, p 544.
52. Lipowitz, AJ, et al.: The spleen. *In* Slatter, DH (ed): Textbook of Small Animal Surgery. Philadelphia, WB Saunders, 1985, p 1204.
53. Blue, J and Weiss, L: Species variation in the structure and function of the marginal zone—An electron microscope study of cat spleen. Am J Anat 161:169, 1981.
54. Blue, J and Weiss, L: Electron microscopy of the red pulp of the dog spleen including vascular arrangements, periarterial macrophage sheaths (ellipsoids), and the contractile, innervated reticular meshwork. Am J Anat 151:189, 1981.
55. Blue, J and Weiss, L: Vascular pathways in nonsinusal red pulp—an electron microscope study of the cat spleen. Am J Anat 161:135, 1981.
56. Barton, CL: The spleen: Pathophysiology of disease. *In* Bojrab, MJ (ed): Pathophysiology in Small Animal Surgery. Philadelphia, Lea and Febiger, 1981, p 502.
57. Wintrobe, MM, et al.: Clinical Hematology, 8th ed. Philadelphia, Lea and Febiger, 1981.
58. Palmer, JG: Studies on the effect of splenectomy on the total leukocyte count in the albino rat. Blood 6:3, 1951.
59. McBride, JA, et al.: The effect of splenectomy on the leukocyte count. Br J Haematol 14:225, 1968.
60. Walderman, TA, et al.: The effect of splenectomy on erythropoiesis in the dog. Blood 15:873, 1960.
61. Eichner, ER: Splenic function: Normal, too much and too little. Am J Med 66:311, 1979.
62. Sills, RH: Splenic function: Physiology and splenic hypofunction. CRC Critical Reviews Oncol/Hematol 7:1, 1987.
63. Crosby, WH: Splenic remodelling of red cell surfaces. Blood 50:643, 1977.
64. Ferrant, A: The role of the spleen in haemolysis. Clin Haematol 12:489, 1983.

65. Schulkind, ML, et al.: Effect of antibody upon clearance of I^{125}-labelled pneumococci by the spleen and liver. Pediatr Res 1:178, 1967.
66. Breznock, EM and Strack, D: Blood volume of nonsplenectomized and splenectomized cats before and after hemorrhage. Am J Vet Res 43:1811, 1982.
67. Breznock, EM and Strack, D: Effects of the spleen, epinephrine, and splenectomy on determination of blood volume in cats. Am J Vet Res 43:2062, 1982.
68. Vatner, SF, et al.: Role of the spleen in the peripheral vascular response to severe exercise in untethered dogs. Cardiovasc Res 8:276, 1974.
69. Aster, RH: Pooling of platelets in the spleen: role in the pathogenesis of hypersplenic thrombocytopenia. J Clin Invest 45:645, 1966.
70. Hill-Zobel, RL, et al.: Organ distribution and fate of human platelets: Studies of asplenic and splenomegalic patients. Am J Hematol 23:231, 1986.
71. Spirer, Z, et al.: Decreased tuftsin concentrations in patients who have undergone splenectomy. Br Med J 2:1574, 1977.
72. Carlisle, HN and Saslaw, S: Properdin levels in splenectomized persons. Proc Soc Exp Biol Med 102:150, 1959.
73. Eraklis, AJ, et al.: Hazard of overwhelming infection after splenectomy in childhood. N Engl J Med 276:1225, 1967.
74. Gopal, V and Bisno, AL: Fulminant pneumococcal infections in "normal" asplenic hosts. Arch Intern Med 173:1526, 1977.
75. Ridgway, RL, et al.: Hematogenous *Bacteroides fragilis* and *Proteus mirabilis* infection in a dog with lymphocytic lymphoma of the spleen. JAVMA 172:711, 1978.
76. Hosgood, G: Splenectomy in the dog: A retrospective study of 31 cases. JAAHA 23:275, 1987.
77. Frey, AJ and Betts, CW: A retrospective survey of splenectomy in the dog. JAAHA 13:730, 1977.
78. Breitschwerdt, E: Babesiosis. In Greene, CE (ed): Clinical Microbiology and Infectious Diseases of the Dog and Cat. Philadelphia, WB Saunders, 1984, p 796.
79. Harvey, JW: Hemobartonellosis. In Greene, CE (ed): Clinical Microbiology and Infectious Diseases of the Dog and Cat. Philadelphia, WB Saunders, 1984, p 576.
80. Kaggwa, E, et al.: The role of the spleen in *Trypanosoma brucei* infection in dogs. Zbl Vet Med B 31:470, 1984.
81. Cooper, MJ and Williamson, RCN: Splenectomy: Indications, hazards, and alternatives. Br J Surg 71:173, 1984.
82. Kalb, R, et al.: Cutaneous infection at dog bite wounds associated with fulminant DF-2 septicemia. Am J Med 78:687, 1985.
83. Waters, ML, et al.: Dysgonic fermenter - 2 septicemia. Pathol 18:162, 1986.
84. Scully, RE, et al.: Case records of the Massachusetts General Hospital. N Engl J Med 315:241, 1986.
85. Bartels, P: Indications for splenectomy and the post-operative survival rate. J Sm Anim Pract 10:781, 1970.
86. Brodey, RS: Vascular tumors of the canine spleen. Mod Vet Pract 45:39, 1964.
87. Sander, CH and Langham, RF: Myelolipoma of the spleen in a cat. JAVMA 160:1101, 1972.
88. Zimmer, MA and Stair, EL: Splenic myelolipomas in two dogs. Vet Pathol 20:637, 1983.
89. Fees, DL and Withrow, SJ: Canine hemangiosarcoma. Comp Cont Ed 3:1047, 1981.
90. Brown, NO, et al.: Canine hemangiosarcoma: Retrospective analysis of 104 cases. JAVMA 186:56, 1985.
91. Oksanen, A: Hemangiosarcoma in dogs. J Comp Path 88:585, 1978.
92. Pearson, GR and Head, KW: Malignant hemangioendothelioma (angiosarcoma) in the dog. J Sm Anim Pract 17:737, 1976.
93. Waller, T and Rubarth, S: Hemangioendothelioma in domestic animals. Acta Vet Scand 8:234, 1967.
94. Patnaik, AK and Liu, SK: Angiosarcoma in cats. J Sm Anim Pract 18:191, 1977.
95. Scavelli, TD, et al.: Hemangiosarcoma in the cat: retrospective evaluation of 31 surgical cases. JAVMA 187:817, 1985.
96. Ng, CY and Mills, JN: Clinical and haematological features of hemangiosarcoma in dogs. Aust Vet J 62:1, 1985.
97. Rebar, AH, et al.: Microangiopathic hemolytic anemia associated with radiation-induced hemangiosarcoma. Vet Pathol 17:443, 1980.
98. Antman, KA, et al.: Microangiopathic hemolytic anemia and cancer: A review. Medicine 58:377, 1979.
99. Hirsch, VM, et al.: A retrospective study of canine hemangiosarcoma and its association with acanthocytosis. Can Vet J 22:152, 1981.
100. Wong, PL: Pneumoperitoneum associated with splenic necrosis and clostridial peritonitis. JAAHA 17:463, 1981.
101. Greene, CE: Infectious canine hepatitis. In Greene, CE (ed): Clinical Microbiology and Infectious Diseases of the Dog and Cat. Philadelphia, WB Saunders, 1984, p 406.
102. Calvert, CA and Greene, CE: Cardiovascular infections. In Greene, CE (ed): Clinical Microbiology and Infectious Diseases of the Dog and Cat. Philadelphia, WB Saunders, 1984, p 220.
103. Greene, CE and Prestwood, AK: Coccidial infections. In Greene, CE (ed): Clinical Microbiology and Infectious Diseases of the Dog and Cat. Philadelphia, WB Saunders, 1984, p 824.
104. Greene, CE: Enteric bacterial infections. In Greene, CE (ed): Clinical Microbiology and Infectious Diseases of the Dog and Cat. Philadelphia, WB Saunders, 1984, p 617.
105. Hendrick, M: A spectrum of eosinophilic syndrome exemplified by six cats with eosinophilic enteritis. Vet Pathol 18:188, 1981.
106. Greene, CE and George, LW: Canine brucellosis. In Greene, CE (ed): Clinical Microbiology and Infectious Diseases of the Dog and Cat. Philadelphia, WB Saunders, 1984, p 646.
107. Woodward, DC: Splenic sporotrichosis in a dog. VM/SAC 75:1011, 1980.
108. Clinkenbeard, KD, et al.: Disseminated histoplasmosis in cats: 12 cases (1981, 1986). JAVMA 190:1445, 1987.
109. Johnson, JD and Raff, MJ: Fungal splenic abscess. Arch Intern Med 144:1987, 1984.
110. Bowdler, AJ: The spleen in haemolytic disorders. Clin Haematol 4:231, 1975.
111. Jackson, ML and Kruth, SA: Immune-mediated hemolytic anemia and thrombocytopenia in the dog: A retrospective study of 55 cases diagnosed from 1969 through 1983 at the Western College of Veterinary Medicine. Can Vet J 26:245, 1985.
112. Randolph, JF, et al.: Familial nonspherocytic hemolytic anemia in poodles. Am J Vet Res 47:687, 1986.
113. Ewin, GO: Familial nonspherocytic hemolytic anemia of Basenji dogs. JAVMA 154:503, 1969.
114. Giger, U, et al.: Inherited phosphofructokinase deficiency in dogs with hyperventilation-induced hemolysis: Increased in vitro and in vivo alkaline fragility of erythrocytes. Blood 65:345, 1985.
115. Steffey, ED, et al.: Effects of halothane and halothane–nitrous oxide on hematocrit and plasma protein concentration in dog and monkey. Am J Vet Res 37:959, 1976.
116. Johnson, SE: Portal hypertension. Pathophysiology and clinical consequences. Comp Cont Ed 9:741, 1987.
117. Johnson, SE: Portal hypertension. Clinical assessment and treatment. Comp Cont Ed 9:917, 1987.
118. Stevenson, S, et al.: Torsion of the splenic pedicle in the dog: A review. JAAHA 17:239, 1981.
119. Maxie, MG, et al.: Splenic torsion in three Great Danes. Can Vet J 11:249, 1970.
120. Stead, AK, et al.: Splenic torsion in dogs. J Sm Anim Pract 24:549, 1983.
121. Brodie, JD: Splenic torsion in the dog. Vet Rec 94:322, 1974.
122. Iverson, WO: Torsion of the splenic pedicle and complete splenic separation in a St. Bernard. VM/SAC 71:1565, 1978.
123. Orman, ME and Lorenz, MD: Torsion of the splenic pedicle in a dog. JAVMA 160:1099, 1972.
124. Lipowitz, AJ, et al.: Clinicopathologic conference. JAVMA 170:65, 1977.
125. O'Neill, JA: Managing an unusual case of splenic torsion. Vet Med 80:35, 1985.
126. Twedt, DC and Wingfield, WE: Diseases of the stomach. In Ettinger, SJ (ed): Textbook of Veterinary Internal Medicine, 2nd ed. Philadelphia, WB Saunders, 1983, p 1233.
127. Couto, CG: Splenomegaly. Proc 52nd AAHA, 1985, p 342.
128. Liska, WD, et al.: Feline systemic mastocytosis: A review of results of splenectomy. JAAHA 15:589, 1979.
129. Rosin, A, et al.: Malignant histiocytosis in Bernese mountain dogs. JAVMA 188:1041, 1986.
130. Moore, PF: Systemic histiocytosis of Bernese mountain dogs. Vet Pathol 21:554, 1984.
131. Moore, PF and Rosin, A: Malignant histiocytosis of Bernese mountain dogs. Vet Pathol 23:1, 1986.

132. O'Keefe, DA and Couto, CG: Fine-needle aspiration of the spleen as an aid in the diagnosis of splenomegaly. J Vet Int Med 1:102, 1987.

133. Center, SA: Feline Diseases. Proceed 52nd AAHA, 1985, p 199.

134. Scott, DW, et al.: Hypereosinophilic syndrome in a cat. Fel Pract 15:22, 1985.

135. Kuehn, NF and Gaunt, SD: Hypocellular marrow and extramedullary hematopoiesis in a dog: Hematologic recovery after splenectomy. JAVMA 188:1313, 1986.

136. Ackerman, N and Silverman, S: Splenic disease. Mod Vet Pract 59:53, 1978.

137. Nyland, TG and Hager, DA: Sonography of the liver, gallbladder, and spleen. Vet Clin North Am 15:1123, 1985.

138. Feeney, DA, et al.: Two-dimensional, gray-scale ultrasonography for assessment of hepatic and splenic neoplasia in the dog and cat. JAVMA 184:68, 1984.

139. Myers, MJ: Spleen imaging. Clin Haematol 12:395, 1983.

140. Swisher, SN and Dale, WA: Splenic aspiration biopsy in the dog. Blood 10:812, 1965.

141. Hermann, RE, et al.: Splenectomy for the diagnosis of splenomegaly. Ann Surg 168:896, 1968.

142. Feldman, BF, et al.: Splenectomy as adjunctive therapy for immune-mediated thrombocytopenia and hemolytic anemia in the dog. JAVMA 187:617, 1985.

116 HEMOSTATIC DISORDERS: COAGULOPATHIES AND THROMBOTIC DISORDERS

ROBERT A. GREEN

INTRODUCTION

Hemostasis involves dynamic interactions between the vasculature, coagulation factors, platelets, and blood flow. Extensive investigation into the thrombotic and bleeding disorders of both domestic animals and man has continued to expand our understanding of acquired and hereditary hemostatic disorders. Recent insight into the role of several natural hemostatic inhibitors (antithrombin III (ATIII), protein C, and α-2-macroglobulin) has elucidated the importance of modulating the hemostatic plug reaction in thrombotic diseases.[1, 2] New concepts have emerged concerning interactions between the coagulation factors of the intrinsic coagulation cascade, particularly with respect to differences between *in vivo* and *in vitro* coagulation reactions. Earlier coagulation studies identified the important factors involved in the intrinsic cascade, whereas more recent kinetic studies have indicated the importance of their amplification and modulation.[3] Why do some animals with severe intrinsic deficiencies not bleed? The newly identified alternate extrinsic coagulation pathway partially explains this paradox.[4, 5] However, many poorly understood hemostatic relationships remain to be elucidated, making hemostasis an exciting area for future clinical research. Unfortunately, these developments have also made aspects of hemostasis very specialized and consultation with coagulation specialists is often required to clarify a patient's status. This discussion will focus on the pathophysiology of hemostasis and laboratory evaluation of the common coagulopathies encountered in small animal practice.

PHYSIOLOGY OF HEMOSTASIS

A thorough understanding of hemostatic plug formation remains essential to evaluate bleeding disorders. Following vascular injury, activation of the hemostatic mechanism results in formation of the initial platelet plug (Figure 116–1). This reaction represents an interaction between platelets, von Willebrand's factor (VWF), and subendothelium which sustains reflex vaso-

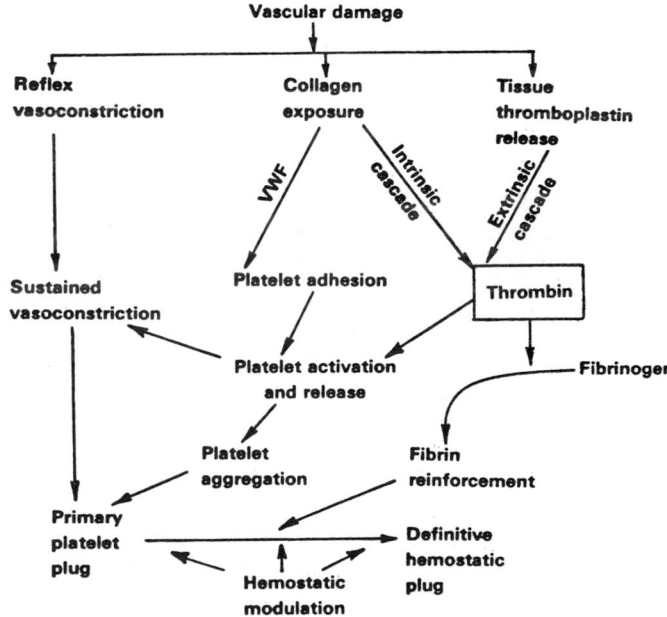

FIGURE 116–1. Factors influencing formation of the hemostatic plug.

constriction and covers the injured area with a mass of interlinked platelets (the primary platelet plug).

The initial vascular injury exposes subendothelial collagen and tissue factor to flowing blood. Subsequent platelet activation results in exposure of specific surface receptors for VWF and fibrinogen. The VWF-mediated binding of platelets to subendothelial collagen serves to localize the reaction to the area of injury. Further interplatelet stabilization is provided by platelet-platelet fibrinogen linkages. Thrombin generation by the coagulation cascade promotes the platelet release reaction.[6] Thromboxane A_2 release from activated platelets causes marked platelet aggregation and vasoconstriction.[7] Soluble fibrin monomer, generated by the activated coagulation cascade, interacts with VWF to facilitate further platelet incorporation into the growing platelet plug.[8] These initial reactions are monitored by the bleeding time test and are usually sufficient to stop bleeding from minor injuries.

The second stage of hemostatic plug formation centers on reinforcement of the primary platelet plug with an interlocked network of polymerized fibrin. Fibrin generation results from activation of two interconnected enzymatic pathways, the intrinsic and extrinsic coagulation cascades (Figure 116–2). These classical pathways represent widely accepted views of coagulation, but oversimplify the importance of alternate pathways and secondary amplification reactions. Initial activation of the intrinsic cascade follows binding of FXII to collagen, while activation of the extrinsic coagulation cascade occurs when "tissue factor" is released from damaged cells and forms a calcium-dependent complex with FVII. Platelet activation *in vivo* may mask deficiencies in the contact activation of the intrinsic pathway.[9] Following initial cascade activation, further sequential activation of circulating coagulation factors occurs on the surface of collagen-bound platelets.[10]

The coagulation factors circulate as inactive zymogens, with the possible exception of FVII which has some enzymatic activity in its basal state. Factors XII, XI, X, IX, VII, and thrombin have the amino acid serine at their active site and therefore are known as serine proteases. Factors V and FVIII:C form complexes with calcium and platelet phospholipid and act as cofactors in amplifying coagulation cascade activity. Both pathways merge at the point of FX activation to form a common pathway that ultimately results in fibrin formation. The reader is referred elsewhere for an in-depth review of the complex surface chemistry reactions underlying fibrin formation.[10] The cascade reactions shown in Figure 116–2 represent a vast oversimplification of the cyclic interactions that occur during normal hemo-

FIGURE 116–2. Simplified scheme of fibrin formation by the extrinsic and intrinsic coagulation cascades. Factors followed by "a" indicates the factor's activated form.

*Thrombin increases fibrin production at low concentrations, but decreases fibrin production at high concentration. HMWK = high molecular weight kininogen, PK = prekallikrein.

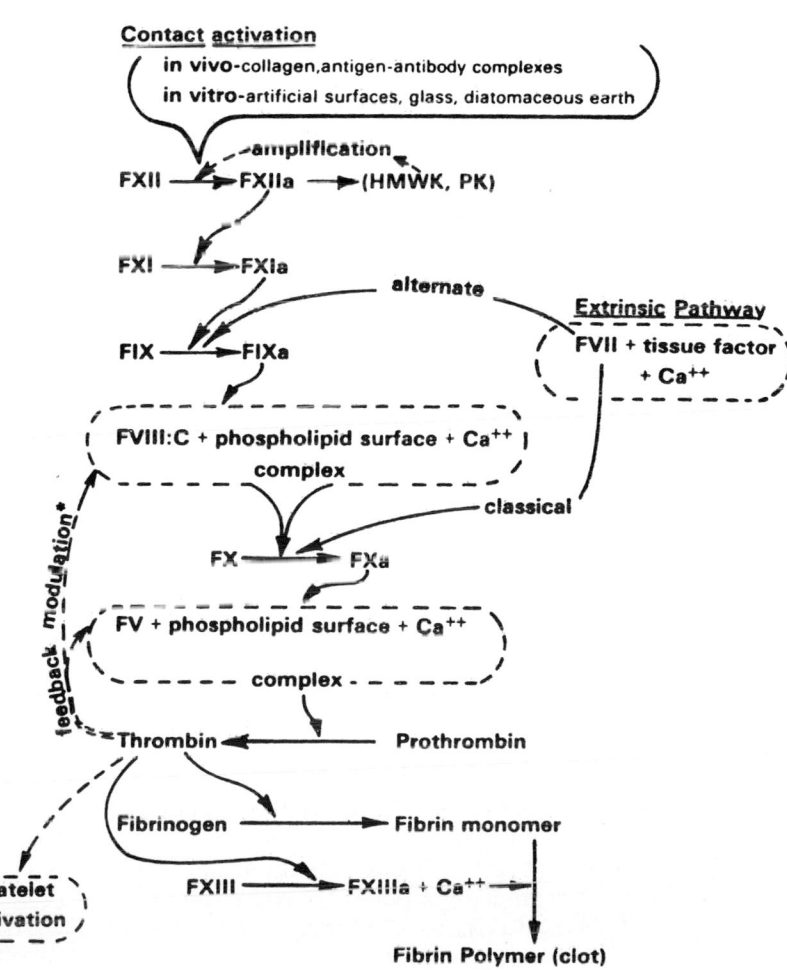

stasis; however, this scheme provides an acceptable basis for relating abnormalities of the screening coagulation tests to the common hemostatic defects.

Recent identification of an important alternative extrinsic pathway emphasizes the complexity of the classical cascade pathways.[4] Activation of FVII was found to activate not only FX but also FIX.[5] Indeed, kinetic studies indicate that as much FXa is generated indirectly through FIX activation by FVII as by the direct action on FX by FVII. Therefore, activation of both the intrinsic and extrinsic pathways occurs following activation of FVII with considerable feedback reamplification of factor activity which promotes the overall efficiency of FXa generation. Failure of these amplification mechanisms in FVIII and FIX deficiency explains why these defects cause serious bleeding disorders. In contrast, individuals affected with deficiencies of "contact factors" do not bleed because these factors are less important in feedback loops or suitable biologic alternatives exist.

Thrombin plays a key role in stimulating both platelet and coagulation reactions, and therefore its concentration must be controlled to prevent inappropriate hemostatic responses.[6, 11] At low concentration, thrombin activates FVIII:C and FV; but at higher concentration, thrombin causes inactivation of FVa and FVIII:Ca (through the protein C mechanism discussed below). Thus, thrombin initially increases its own production and later decreases it. This important regulatory role prevents thrombosis by limiting potent thrombin-mediated hemostatic reactions.

Optimal fibrin formation depends not only on adequate activation of the circulating coagulation factors, but also on their binding to specific receptor sites on platelet surfaces that were incorporated into the hemostatic plug. The platelet's binding of the activated forms of FV and FVIII:C, FVa and FVIII:Ca, in addition to previously bound factor VWF and fibrinogen, is critical to amplification of the cascade's generation of fibrin. The binding of activated serine proteases to the platelet surface also protects them from ATIII-mediated neutralization (see below).[12] As vasoconstriction in the injured area diminishes, the fibrin-reinforced hemostatic plug is able to withstand the stress of reperfusion. Failure of fibrin reinforcement may lead to rebleeding several hours after the initial bleeding ceases as the initial hemostatic reactions diminish. Delayed bleeding is commonly found in patients with poor hemostatic plug formation caused by hereditary coagulation factor deficiencies.[13]

HEMOSTATIC MODULATION

The healthy endothelium surrounding the area of vascular injury is antithrombogenic and is strategically placed to limit the extension of the hemostatic plug.[14] Part of the natural repulsion between platelets and healthy endothelium is attributed to the similar negative charges on their surfaces. Altered arachidonic acid metabolism in endothelial cells produces prostacyclin, a potent prostaglandin that causes vasodilation and opposes the platelet aggregating effect of thromboxane.[15] Thus, the physiologic functions of normal endothelium promote increased blood flow to the injured area which

removes excess activated coagulation factors and increases their interaction with natural plasma inhibitors.

The most important plasma inhibitor of coagulation is ATIII, accounting for about 80 per cent of the naturally occurring plasma inhibitory activity (Figure 116-3).[16] The inhibitory action of ATIII is markedly enhanced by heparin (or heparin-like groups on the endothelial surface), particularly against FXa and thrombin.[17] It forms irreversible complexes with all serine proteases, which are subsequently swept away from the areas of injury and are cleared by the liver. This effect is limited during platelet activation by the release of platelet factor IV (antiheparin factor) which binds to membrane-associated heparin groups and interferes with maximal ATIII activation.[18] The fibrin-generating potential of thrombin is also limited by the inhibitory effects of fibrin-degradation products (FDP) and fibrin-mediated thrombin adsorption.

The important roles of the nonserine protease cofactors, FVIII:Ca and FVa, in augmenting thrombin generation are modulated by a vitamin K–dependent plasma inhibitor called protein C.[19] Interestingly, excessive thrombin binds to an endothelial receptor, thrombomodulin, and this complex converts protein C to its active form, protein Ca. Protein Ca rapidly inactivates FVa and FVIII:Ca, which markedly diminishes thrombin production by the intrinsic cascade. Another recently identified vitamin K–dependent protein, protein S, serves as a cofactor in this reaction by promoting the inhibitory action of protein Ca. Overall, the protein C mechanism limits hemostatic plug growth by tying up thrombin in the thrombomodulin complex, inactivating FVa and FVIII:Ca, and enhancing fibrinolysis.

DISSOLUTION OF THE PLATELET PLUG (FIBRINOLYSIS)

The fibrinolytic mechanism accounts for the gradual dissolution of the fibrin clot. This is accomplished by generation of the proteolytic enzyme, plasmin, within the hemostatic plug.[20] Plasmin generation is modulated by a complex system of activators and inhibitors (Figure 116-4).[21] The plasma protein precursor of plasmin, plasminogen, has a high affinity for fibrin and is incorporated into the hemostatic plug as fibrin is generated. Damaged endothelial cells release a substance called tissue plasminogen activator (tPA) which has a high affinity for bound plasminogen and promotes plasmin generation. Release of tPA from endothelium is promoted by thrombin.[22] Tissue plasminogen activator is transiently inhibited by a specific inhibitor released from activated platelets which prevents premature clot lysis by the fibrinolytic mechanism.[23] Activated protein C appears to stimulate fibrinolysis by neutralizing a plasminogen activator inhibitor.[24] Generation of plasmin is strongly inhibited in plasma by antiplasmins, particularly α-2-antiplasmin. In addition to fibrin, other potential substrates for plasmin include fibrinogen, FV, FVIII:C, and the platelet receptor for fibrinogen. These substrates may become deficient in primary fibrinolysis, which is associated with marked hyperplasminemia. The action of plasmin on fibrin or fibrinogen results in the formation

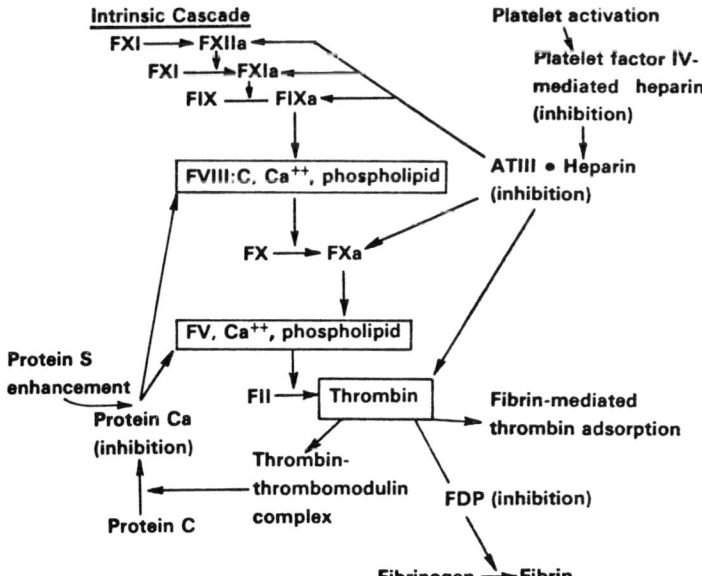

FIGURE 116–3. Scheme of hemostatic modulation. Note the inhibitory roles of ATIII and Protein C on fibrin production by the intrinsic coagulation cascade.

of FDP which interfere with normal platelet function and the action of thrombin.

LABORATORY EVALUATION OF HEMOSTASIS

QUALITY CONTROL AND SAMPLE COLLECTION

Precise quality control is necessary to detect the subtle differences between normal individuals and those with mild hemostatic defects. At the outset it is conceded

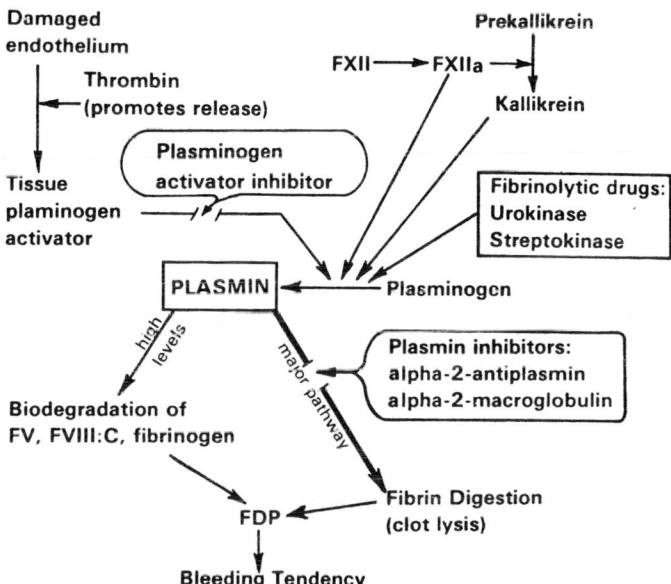

FIGURE 116–4. Factors influencing the fibrinolytic activity of plasmin. High levels of plasmin activity increase FDP levels and reduce availability of fibrin precursors, which results in the bleeding tendency associated with primary fibrinolysis.

that certain screening tests are only qualitative. For example, prolongation of activated partial thromboplastin time (APTT) is minimal until coagulation factor levels approach 30 per cent of normal. Clotting studies are enzymatic reactions that can be influenced by improper sample handling and various laboratory errors. Such factors must be carefully controlled if identification of individuals with mild bleeding diatheses is required.

Improper blood collection technique commonly causes erratic laboratory results. The sample should be collected with minimum excitement, as this can increase platelet count, platelet aggregation, and the levels of several coagulation factors (e.g., FV, FVIII:C, VWF, fibrinogen). Ideally, the sample should be obtained with minimal probing for the vessel and minimal venous stasis. As animals with coagulopathies may exhibit excessive bleeding from venipuncture sites, blood samples should be collected from cephalic or saphenous veins because excessive bleeding is easier to control at these sites. Blood samples for hemostatic testing should not be collected through catheters that have been used for heparin therapy. Indeed, blood collection through any type of long catheter may activate hemostatic components due to blood-surface interactions. It is important that the surface of any collection, holding, or transfer containers be consistent (all plastic or all siliconized), particularly with reference to platelet function studies. Nonsiliconized glass containers should not be used for collecting or storing blood or plasma samples for coagulation testing because glass activation of the intrinsic cascade will alter subsequent test results.[25]

The preferred anticoagulant for most coagulation tests is 3.8 per cent sodium citrate, owing to its superior preservation of hemostatic components. The ratio of anticoagulant to blood is 1:9 for most procedures. The sample should be collected in new plastic syringes containing the correct amount of anticoagulant for the volume of blood aspirated. Deviation from the above citrate to blood ratio can limit calcium availability in the test systems and cause erratic results. This is particularly a problem in polycythemic animals when the routine 1:9

2250 SECTION XIII—Diseases of Blood Cells, Lymph Nodes, and Spleen

ratio yields plasma that is overcitrated. The excess citrate results in artificial coagulation test prolongation by lowering calcium levels which subsequently delay formation of the fibrin clot. If blood samples are collected using citrated Vacutainer tubes, a similar excess of citrate occurs when the tube is filled to less than two-thirds of the required volume. The formula to correct the amount of citrate for variation in hematocrit is as follows:

$$C = 0.00185 \text{ V} (100 - \text{HCT})$$

where C = ml of 3.8 per cent sodium citrate, HCT = hematocrit (%), and V = ml of blood to be collected. For example, 9 ml of blood from a dog with a hematocrit of 80 would only require 0.33 ml of 3.8 per cent sodium citrate. Similarly, "routine" collection of (undercitrated) samples from markedly anemic animals may mask the presence of mild coagulopathies by artifactual shortening of clotting times.

Errors induced by variation in technique, sample transportation or storage are not uncommon when citrated samples are submitted to outside clinical laboratories for evaluation. Although FV and FVIII:C are particularly labile, losses are reduced considerably by immediately placing the sample in an ice bath. The sample should be centrifuged and the plasma removed within 30 minutes of blood collection. The plasma is stored in an ice bath and capped to prevent pH changes. If these precautions are followed, the sample should be stable for about four hours.

When freezing samples for mailing it to an outside laboratory, the following recommendations should be followed. The blood sample should be centrifuged at high speed (2500 to 3500 rpm) for 15 minutes and the plasma removed with a plastic pipette. Then the plasma should be rapidly frozen (preferably in alcohol and dry ice) in small aliquots (1 ml) to prevent ice crystal formation. Slow freezing or thawing of samples induces cryoprecipitation of coagulation factors, particularly FVIII:C, and can be a source of erratic coagulation test results. The sample should subsequently be stored or transported at −20°C or lower. Packing specimens with a large amount of dry ice (10 to 12 pounds) in a styrofoam container is necessary to maintain this temperature requirement. Submission of blood from a normal individual of the same species provides a valuable control to rule out artifacts induced during sample processing and transportation. This recommendation is particularly critical if the coagulation laboratory analyzing the sample is not familiar with veterinary samples. Minor variation in laboratory technique or reagents can create major difficulties in final interpretation of test results.

Most coagulation tests are enzymatic, and therefore, factors known to influence rates must be controlled. These factors include ion concentrations, pH, incubation times, and reagent stability. Failure to prewarm reaction tubes to 37°C or variation in the temperature of an incubator is a common cause of aberrant clotting tests. The ability of different technicians to detect the fibrin endpoint varies; however, variation in final results is minimal when controls are assayed by the same techni-

cian. Duplicate test determinations should always be performed and tolerance limits for each test should be established. When duplicate clotting times agree within 5 per cent (usually variation is less than one second in normal animals), the average result is reported for both the patient and control sample. A graph of laboratory results performed on control samples should be maintained so that shifts or trends are easily recognized. Any changes in reagents, instrumentation, or technical modifications of procedures necessitate that the normal range be reestablished. When abnormalities in a control sample are encountered, the sample should be redrawn from an alternative donor. Small laboratories may choose to prepare stable reference control samples from freshly frozen citrated plasma samples from a pool of normal animals (usually five or more). These samples are stable for six months when stored below −50°C. Commercially prepared lyophilized control samples and borderline abnormal control samples are available to check the coagulation test's capacity to detect mild coagulopathies.

The Common Coagulation Tests

It is beyond the scope of this discussion to consider all aspects of coagulation tests. The reader is referred to an excellent manual by D.A. Tripplett and C.S. Harms, *Procedures for Coagulation Laboratory* available from the American Society of Clinical Pathologists, Chicago. The following comments concern an overview of the principles of the more common coagulation tests used in veterinary medicine and their interpretation.

ACTIVATED COAGULATION TIME AND PARTIAL THROMBOPLASTIN TIME

The two tests commonly used to evaluate the intrinsic coagulation system are the activated coagulation time (ACT) and the activated partial thromboplastin time (APTT). The ACT test is similar to other whole blood clotting time methods but uses diatomaceous earth as an inert surface-activating agent to shorten clotting times. The ACT has better sensitivity than older inaccurate whole blood clotting time methods, i.e., the Lee White and capillary tube methods, which are no longer recommended. In performing the ACT test on canine samples, two ml of whole blood is injected into a prewarmed ACT tube, mixed by inversion five times, placed in a 37°C incubator or water bath for one minute and then observed at five-second intervals for the first evidence of clotting. In cats, observation for clotting should begin after the blood sample has incubated for only 45 seconds because their clotting times are shorter. Normally, the entire two ml blood sample clots abruptly. In abnormal samples only tiny clots may form at the end point. The inexpensiveness and simplicity of the ACT test make it useful as a presurgical or prebiopsy screening test for veterinary practice. Inexperienced personnel can rapidly achieve high precision with ACT. After a diagnosis has been confirmed, ACT also provides a convenient test for monitoring the patient's response to specific therapy.

Normal ACT values in dogs range from 60 to 90

seconds, with a mean of 75 seconds. Normal ACT values in cats are less than 65 seconds. Patients with severe nonresponding thrombocytopenia (platelet counts under 10,000/μl) may have prolonged ACT tests, owing to reduced platelet phospholipid availability. Some qualitative platelet function defects such as thrombocytopathy of uremia, also cause prolonged ACT. Severe hypofibrinogenemia is associated with either poor clot quality or formation of only a few small clots. In determining the ACT of heparinized patients, the blood must be carefully observed for the first evidence of coagulation, since the normal abrupt production of fibrin is inhibited.

The APTT test is more versatile and accurate than the ACT test in detection of mild abnormalities of the intrinsic coagulation pathway, but does require more technical expertise to obtain uniform results. In the APTT test, citrated plasma is incubated with an activator of factor XII (kaolin or celite) and cephaloplastins, which substitute for platelet phospholipid requirements. After addition of ionic calcium, the time required to form fibrin is exactly determined. The mean clotting time for dog plasma using different commercial APTT reagents varies significantly (11 to 19 seconds), but the normal range is more uniform when the same reagent is used (our laboratory range is 12 to 16 seconds). The APTT of normal cats (our laboratory range is 14 to 20 seconds) is slightly longer. Variation is often encountered in cat samples due to difficulties in sample collection. Avoid prolonged storage of uncapped plasma samples, particularly at room temperature, which causes variation in APTT results.[16]

Acquired and hereditary coagulation disorders are characterized by reduction in one or more factors in the intrinsic coagulation cascade. Usually the activity of a single factor must be reduced below 30 per cent of normal before the APTT test is prolonged. Therefore, APTT is normal in most heterozygous carriers of coagulation factor deficiencies (usually having 40 to 60 per cent reduction in coagulation factor activity). Increased FVIII:C levels accompany various diseases and may shorten APTT slightly. Determination of the specific factor deficiency in the intrinsic pathway can be obtained by performing APTT on 1:1 mixtures of patient plasma and known factor deficient plasmas. When the factors that are deficient are different (for example, combining plasma from a patient deficient in FXII with plasma having known FIX deficiency), the two deficient plasmas mutually correct their respective deficiencies and the APTT of the mixture is normal. In contrast, when the same defect is present in both plasma samples, the APTT fails to correct and the identity of the deficient factor is established. Factor deficiencies may also be differentiated from effects of inhibitor (heparin) by repeating the APTT following dilution of the abnormal plasma 1:1 with normal plasma. Correction of the APTT suggests a factor deficiency, whereas failure to correct suggests the presence of an inhibitor. When the APTT returns to normal after increasing the incubation time with APTT activator (before adding calcium), deficiencies of prekallikrein, and high molecular weight kininogen should be suspected (these defects are clinically asymptomatic).[26]

ONE-STAGE PROTHROMBIN TIME

The status of the extrinsic coagulation cascade is evaluated by the one-stage prothrombin time (OSPT). Citrated plasma is added to a thromboplastin-calcium mixture, and the length of time required to form fibrin is exactly determined. Phospholipids contained in the thromboplastin mixture make the test independent of platelet function. High concentration of thromboplastin in some reagents can shorten OSPT markedly and interfere with detection of mild defects in the extrinsic cascade.[27] If this test is performed by a local clinical laboratory, the patient's sample and the control sample should be transported in an ice bath and assayed within four hours of collection. The normal range for most OSPT methods is seven to ten seconds in dogs and 9 to 13 seconds in cats. Duplicate determinations should agree within one second.

Abnormalities of OSPT are associated with liver disease, disseminated intravascular coagulation (DIC), and hereditary or acquired deficiencies of any factors in the extrinsic cascade. Owing to the short half-life of factor VII, the test is very sensitive to vitamin K deficiency or antagonism (rodenticide toxicosis). The OSPT is less sensitive to heparin than APTT and therefore is not preferred in monitoring heparin therapy.

THROMBIN TIME

The thrombin time (TT) measures the reactivity of fibrinogen to exogenous thrombin. This important functional assay of fibrinogen is independent of other factors in the intrinsic and extrinsic coagulation cascades. Commercial bovine thrombin is diluted with saline to a concentration that produces a TT of 6.0 to 9.0 seconds, when 0.1 ml thrombin is added to 0.2 ml normal canine plasma. Prolonged TT is associated with severe hypofibrinogenemia (< 100 mg/dl) and dysfibrinogenemia. Thrombin inhibitors, such as heparin or fibrinogen degradation products (FDP), may also prolong TT. For these reasons, it is particularly useful in monitoring patients with abnormalities of fibrinolysis or hepatic function.

FIBRINOGEN ASSAYS

Fibrinogen has the highest concentration of any of the coagulation factors and is the only factor whose concentration is determined routinely. Fibrinogen concentration is measured by various semiquantitative techniques based on heat precipitation, thrombin time, or ammonium sulfate precipitation. Quantitative fibrinogen determination is performed by converting fibrinogen to fibrin with thrombin. The fibrin clot is dissolved in alkali and a phenol reagent is added, which reacts with tyrosine moieties in the fibrinogen molecule. Subsequent determination of optical density and comparison with a standard curve allows the fibrinogen concentration to be determined. The most common fibrinogen assay is based on the selective heat precipitation of fibrinogen after incubating plasma at 56° C for three to eight minutes. Then the fibrinogen level is determined by measuring the difference in plasma protein level both before and after heating with a refractometer. This approach is often variable and unsatisfactory in measuring the fibrinogen levels of hypofibrinogenemic patients. The accuracy of this technique is improved through use of an ocular micrometer instead of the more common refractometric method.[28] Discrepancies between methods may be induced by high levels of FDP, which do not clot with thrombin but which can be precipitated by heat. Fibrinogen concentration ranges from 150 to 300 mg/dl in normal dogs and cats, using this technique. Our laboratory routinely utilizes a modified thrombin time (Fibriquik) method to determine fibrinogen levels of patients with bleeding disorders.

Hypofibrinogenemia may be associated with either decreased production (in the late stages of liver failure) or increased consumption (in acute DIC). In chronic DIC syndromes, increased hepatic fibrinogen production may maintain fibrinogen levels within or above the normal range, despite considerable fibrinogen consumption. Hereditary hypofibrinogenemia has been reported in dogs, but is very rare. Acquired dysfibrinogenemia may occur secondary to hyperplasminemia or liver disease.

FIBRIN(OGEN) DEGRADATION PRODUCTS (FDP) ASSAY

A variety of techniques are available for detecting FDP. The most commonly used method is the Thrombo-Wellco test. This test uses antisera to human fibrinogen fragments D and E (which also crossreact with the FDP of other species). The specific antibodies are absorbed to latex particles and their concentration is adjusted so that macroscopic agglutination occurs when FDP exceed two μg/ml. By performing the test using different dilutions of the patient's plasma, an approximate concentration of FDP is determined. False elevation of FDP may occur when fibrinogen is not clotted by thrombin in the collection tube and remains in solution. This may occur in patients that are on heparin therapy because thrombin inhibition permits fibrinogen to remain in solution[29] or in patients with dysfibrinogenemia because fibrinogen fails to clot and remains in solution.[30] Obviously, the antigens of fibrinogen are recognized by the antibodies and agglutination occurs.

The action of plasmin on fibrin or fibrinogen results in an accumulation of FDP in the plasma. The half-life of circulating FDP is about 9 to 12 hours, although clearance may be prolonged by impaired reticuloendothelial cell function. The presence of FDP induces hemostatic abnormalities by impairing thrombin-mediated fibrin formation, fibrin polymerization, and perhaps most importantly, hemostatic plug formation.[31]

CHROMOGENIC SUBSTRATES IN COAGULATION ASSAYS

Perhaps the most interesting recent development in coagulation testing has been the synthesis of chromogenic substrates with high specificity for certain coagulation-related factors and inhibitors. These spectrophotometric tests are easily performed by many modern chemistry analyzers used routinely in larger clinical pathology laboratories. The chromogenic substrate consists of a small peptide linked to a chromophore, usually p-nitroaniline. The specificity of these synthetic peptides permits functional evaluation of either the coagulation factor activity or its inhibition. The subsequent release of the chromophore is measured under controlled spectrophotometric conditions and is proportional to the enzymatic activity of the coagulation factor reaction being assayed. Some of the hemostasis-related chromogenic methods include assays for heparin, antithrombin III, antiplasmin, plasminogen, FX, FVIII:C, and thrombin.

For example, antithrombin III is easily measured using a chromogenic substrate.[32] In this reaction the patient's plasma is incubated with an excess of thrombin and heparin. The patient's antithrombin III neutralizes some of the thrombin and the residual thrombin is then reacted with a thrombin-specific chromogenic substrate. The chromophore release from the latter reaction is inversely proportional to the patient's antithrombin III levels.

VON WILLEBRAND'S FACTOR ASSAY

The most common test for the diagnosis of von Willebrand's disease (VWD) is based on determining the patient's level of FVIIIR:Ag by rocket immunoelectrophoresis.[33] In this technique the patient's plasma containing VWF is electrophoresed in agarose gel containing canine-specific FVIII antibody. A rocket-shaped precipitin pattern develops along the axis of migration; the height of which is proportional to the amount of FVIIIR:Ag in the patient's plasma. The patient's per cent of FVIIIR:Ag is determined by comparing the rocket height of serial dilutions of the patient's plasma with those of normal canine pooled plasma. Normal FVIIIR:Ag levels in dogs range from 60 to 172 per cent. Reduced FVIIIR:Ag is noted in VWD (see Table 116–1). Sufficient cross reactivity between canine FVIII and commercial rabbit antihuman FVIII makes the latter useful as a source of antibody for the immunoelectrophoretic technique; however, it is more expensive and homologous antisera is preferred.[34] A rapid qualitative technique for detection of VWD, based on venom coagglutinin-induced platelet aggregation, is also satisfactory in dogs; however, a platelet aggregometer is required.[35]

THE COAGULOPATHIES

Vitamin K Deficiency and Antagonism

PATHOPHYSIOLOGY

Vitamin K is required for the postribosomal carboxylation of glutamyl residues of FII, FVII, FIX, and FX. Vitamin K is also required for synthesis of protein C, the specific inhibitor of FV and FVIII. In vitamin K deficiency or antagonism, the liver produces inactive proteins antigenically similar to FII, FVII, FIX and FX.[36] These are known as proteins induced by vitamin

TABLE 116–1. GUIDELINES FOR INTERPRETATION OF FVIIIR:R:AG LEVELS IN DOGS WITH VON WILLEBRAND'S DISEASE†

Bleeding Time	FVIIIR:Ag (%)	Interpretation
Normal	60–172	Normal range for dogs
Normal	>200	Indicates increased release of FVIIIR:Ag from storage sites, possibly related to stress; retest for true FVIIIR:Ag level
Prolonged	>60	Check for platelet or vascular dysfunctions
Normal to prolonged	50–59	Borderline abnormality; dog should be retested or only bred to higher testing mates and all progeny tested for VWD
Normal (may develop subsequent bleeding problems)	<50	Asymptomatic heterozygous carrier of VWD; Dog should be bred only to higher testing mates and all progeny tested for VWD
Prolonged	<50	Clinically affected heterozygous carrier of type 1 VWD; do not use for breeding
Normal or prolonged	<7%	Severe (penetrant) heterozygous form of type 1 VWD.* Do not use for breeding

*If the dog is a Scottish terrier or a Chesapeake Bay retriever, the dog has the homozygous form of type III VWD (with 0%FVIIIR:Ag) and is the product of mating two asymptomatic heterozygous parents.
†Courtesy W. J. Dodds.

K antagonism (PIVKA) and methods to detect their presence in animal samples have been described.[37] The functional forms of FII, FVII, FIX and FX disappear in accordance with their half-lives of 41, 6, 14, and 16.5 hours, respectively. Their synthesis remains inhibited until the antagonist is metabolized and excreted. The duration of the antagonism is variable, usually lasting from several days to a month following a single ingestion of rodenticide. The half-lives of common anticoagulants are as follows: warfarin, one-half day; diphacinone, four and one-half days; brodifacoum, six days.[38] Repeated low doses of rodenticide may produce toxicity with a lower total dose than that associated with a massive single exposure. Circulating PIVKA are rapidly converted to their functional forms following vitamin K administration.

Dietary deficiency of vitamin K is virtually nonexistent in dogs and cats fed modern commercial diets. Only limited amounts of vitamin K are required to maintain sufficient levels of vitamin K–dependent coagulation factors to prevent bleeding diatheses. Transient deficiency of vitamin K–dependent coagulation factors has occasionally been suspected in neonatal puppies, although inadequacy of hepatic protein synthesis in the immature puppy or malnutrition of the bitch during gestation may also be involved. A major source of vitamin K is K_1 which is found in green leafy vegetables and is absorbed via the lymphatics in the upper portions of the small intestine. An additional source is bacterial synthesis of vitamin K_2 which occurs in the small intestine and is similarly absorbed via the lymphatics. Synthetic vitamin K_3 is absorbed by capillaries of the colon. Patients with chronic malabsorptive disorders characterized by abnormal fat assimilation or its lymphatic transport may eventually develop mild vitamin K deficiency,

particularly if bacterial synthesis of vitamin K is also inhibited by oral antibiotics. Vitamin K deficiency was suspected recently in two cats with malabsorption (lymphocytic-plasmacytic enteritis) that eventually developed bleeding problems.[38a] Periodic supplementation with parenteral vitamin K_1 appears warranted in long-standing cases maintained on fat restricted diets or those having marked fat malassimilation. When bleeding is encountered in these patients, other contributing causes should also be considered, e.g., underlying liver disease or endotoxemia.

Vitamin K antagonism due to accidental ingestion of anticoagulant rodenticide is a common cause of coagulopathy in dogs. Both commercial exterminators and laymen often place anticoagulant rodenticides in locations that are accessible to pets. Progressive resistance of the rodent population to the older (first generation) anticoagulant rodenticides has stimulated development of newer (second generation) anticoagulant rodenticides with much higher toxicity to pets. The first generation of anticoagulants (coumadins) had fairly low toxicity for non-target species and generally required repeated ingestion of the rodenticide to produce lethal effects (so-called multiple feeding anticoagulants). Warfarin, pindone, and indandione are examples of this form of anticoagulant. In the 1960s the more potent (second generation) rodenticides were introduced that were lethal to rodents after a single feeding. Bromadiolone and brodifacoum are examples of second generation anticoagulant rodenticides. Newer rodenticides also have much longer biologic half-lives than warfarin and now create the possibility of secondary intoxication in a pet after eating a poisoned rodent. The obvious implication in treatment of animals poisoned with second generation anticoagulants is that vitamin K therapy should be extended for at least a month to prevent recurrent anticoagulant effects in the host during the period of slow rodenticide excretion. The coccidiostat sulfaquinoxaline is also a potent vitamin K antagonist that occasionally produces fatal coagulopathy in dogs. Several factors influence the severity of the induced coagulopathy. They include the bioavailability of vitamin K, the amount of rodenticide ingested and its rate of metabolism, disappearance rates of vitamin K–dependent coagulation factors, alteration in hepatic receptor affinity for the antagonist, and other coexisting hemostatic abnormalities. Whenever possible the rodenticide should be specifically identified so that the approximate duration of therapy can be determined.

CLINICAL SIGNS

The spectrum of clinical signs encountered in anticoagulant toxicoses is broad and is generally related to organ dysfunction induced by hypovolemia or hemorrhage into organ parenchyma, surrounding tissues, or body cavities. The first clinical signs are seen about three days following ingestion of the anticoagulant. Acute death, without previous signs of illness, may follow sudden hemorrhage into the brain, pericardial sac, or thoracic cavity. Poisoned dogs often have marked dyspnea associated with acute hypovolemia and bleeding into the pleural space, both of which restrict respiratory compensation. Anemia, weakness, pallor, hematemesis, epistaxis, or bloody feces are commonly seen in less acutely affected animals. Extensive, external hematomas may occur in areas of trauma or at venipuncture sites. Bleeding into joint spaces can lead to acute lameness or hemarthrosis. Neurologic signs may predominate following hemorrhage into brain, spinal cord, or subdural space. A recent survey of 158 cases of warfarin or "warfarin-like" poisoning of dogs treated at United States veterinary institutions indicated that 35 (22 per cent) died.[39] Decreased levels of vitamin K–dependent factors are manifested by abnormalities in laboratory tests of both intrinsic and extrinsic pathways. In early warfarin toxicosis the rapid disappearance of FVII causes prolongation of only the OSPT. After three days of toxicosis, APTT is also prolonged and bleeding problems become more frequent as deficiencies of FIX, FX, and FII occur. Therefore, when an intoxicated patient is presented to the veterinarian, the typical laboratory findings include marked prolongation of OSPT with moderate prolongation of APTT or ACT.[40] Platelet count, AT III, fibrinogen, and thrombin time usually remain within normal limits. Mildly increased FDP levels have been observed in occasional cases and may cause additional hemostatic impairment.[41]

THERAPY

The three major treatment priorities are to correct the hypovolemia; correct the coagulopathy; and minimize organ dysfunction induced by accumulation of extravascular blood. As in other acute hemorrhagic anemias, the patient's packed cell volume may not reflect the true severity of hypovolemia. Patients in shock should be handled with extreme care. Transfusion of fresh whole blood at 10 ml/lb (20 ml/kg) intravenously may be critical to survival in severe cases. Usually, 50 per cent of this dose is administered rapidly and the remainder slowly by intravenous drip. Oxygen therapy is indicated, if available. Correction of the coagulopathy is accomplished by subcutaneous administration of vitamin K_1 (Aquamephyton). Vitamin K_1 should not be given intravenously, as anaphylaxis may occur. In warfarin toxicosis, vitamin K should be administered at an initial loading dose of 1.3 mg/lb (3 mg/kg) (use several sites) followed by a daily parenteral oral dose of 0.45 mg/lb (1 mg/kg) for one week. In the case of the longer acting rodenticides vitamin K therapy needs to be extended for three to six weeks. The usual recommendation is to continue daily vitamin K at 0.2 mg/lb (0.5 mg/kg) during the second week, and 0.1 mg/lb (0.25 mg/kg) for the third and fourth weeks. If screening coagulation tests (OSPT, ACT) are within normal limits and remain stable for four days following cessation of therapy, then the anticoagulant has been excreted and further therapy is not required. The primary complication of vitamin K therapy at high levels (2.3 mg/lb or 5 mg/kg) is Heinz body anemia.[42] In uncomplicated cases, vitamin K therapy alone results in rapid improvement in both clinical signs and laboratory tests within 12 hours. Vitamin K_3 (menadione) is not recommended in treatment of toxicoses, as patient responses are considerably slower than those to vitamin K_1. Hematomas and most hemorrhagic

pleural effusions in convalescent animals resolve without further medical intervention. Reabsorption of erythrocytes from body cavities (autotransfusion) may dramatically increase the packed cell volume in some cases. Thoracic radiography of patients with severe dyspnea may reveal hemorrhagic effusions. After transfusion of such patients to restore normal clotting potential, careful thoracentesis to remove excess blood may ease respiratory difficulties. Caution is indicated, however, as this procedure may only reinitiate thoracic bleeding and exaggerate the hypovolemia. Unless blood obtained from body cavities is carefully filtered, it should not be readministered to the patient because small clots or platelet aggregates in effusions may initiate thromboembolization. A useful pamphlet entitled *The Professional's Guide to Managing Poisoning by Anticoagulant Rodenticides* is available from Chempar, 660 Madison Avenue, New York, NY 10021.

Disseminated Intravascular Coagulation (DIC)

PATHOPHYSIOLOGY

DIC, also known as consumption coagulopathy and defibrination syndrome, is one of the most common coagulopathies encountered in veterinary medicine and occurs secondary to many diseases.[43] In DIC, simultaneous activation of the coagulation and fibrinolytic system results in microvascular thrombosis or bleeding tendencies as factors and platelets are depleted. Examples of the activating triggers for DIC include vascular damage, bacterial endotoxins, and release of tissue thromboplastin from necrotic or malignant tissues. Any disease producing vascular stasis or vascular endothelial injury favors induction of DIC. The intimal damage associated with severe dirofilariasis in dogs commonly induces DIC. Alternatively, decreased clearance of procoagulants due to impaired reticuloendothelial function augments DIC in certain diseases, particularly those associated with hepatic failure.

Whether DIC is manifested as an acute or chronic process depends on the triggering mechanism, its rate of release, duration of exposure, and, most important, the ability of the liver and bone marrow to replace consumed factors and platelets. Chronic DIC produced experimentally in the dog by infusions of brain thromboplastin revealed varying compensatory ability of the liver and marrow.[44] In general, the liver's capacity to increase synthesis of coagulation factors was greater than the marrow's ability to increase platelet production. In some cases overcompensation of hepatic production led to elevated levels of fibrinogen and FV when infusions were continued for longer than one week. Chronic compensated DIC may be characterized solely by elevated FDP and is difficult to differentiate from other coagulopathies.

CLINICAL SIGNS

The clinical manifestations of DIC are twofold. Fibrin deposition in microvasculature, particularly in the kidney and lung, leads to ischemia and variable organ failure. Simultaneously, the depletion of coagulation factors and platelets in the presence of the anticoagulant effects of FDP, leads to a bleeding tendency. Antithrombin III (ATIII) complexes with and neutralizes excessive generation of activated serine proteases (Figure 116–5). Markedly reduced ATIII levels in DIC patients enhance thromboembolization due to inadequate modulation of platelet plug formation. Of course, the predominant clinical signs may relate to the primary disease problem causing DIC.[45] Frequently, clinical signs of DIC become more obvious during the terminal stages of a disease. As an animal's compensatory mechanisms fail, hypoperfusion and shock cause exacerbation of the underlying coagulopathy. The important role of secondary fibrinolysis in minimizing intravascular thrombosis can not be overemphasized, and therapeutic attempts to inhibit fibrinolysis in DIC cases are contraindicated.

LABORATORY EVALUATION

DIC can be suspected when the following laboratory findings are present: thrombocytopenia, hypofibrinogenemia, elevated FDP, and prolongation of screening coagulation tests (APTT or ACT).[46] The patient's ATIII levels decrease in proportion to serine protease activation and are valuable in establishing prognosis. Retrospective studies found ATIII levels had the highest rate of abnormality (85 per cent) of any laboratory tests commonly utilized in DIC.[47] The author has found ATIII levels in dogs with DIC range from 80 per cent of normal in mildly affected cases to 50 per cent of normal in moderately severe cases. Dogs with severe DIC often have ATIII levels below 50 per cent and a poor prognosis.

Occasional patients with DIC have altered coagulation factor levels, but minimal clinical information is obtained by assaying for specific factor levels. Indeed, erroneous results may occur when using standard APTT-derived assay techniques with substrates deficient in clotting factors due to preactivation of circulating coagulation factors in DIC. For example, short clotting times in a FVIII:C assay (due to high circulating FXa levels)

would indicate increased FVIII:C levels, when reduced levels were actually present.[48] The most common factors found to be reduced in spontaneous cases of DIC in dogs are fibrinogen, FV, and FVIII:C. Other factors may be reduced, depending in part on liver function and the nature of the initiating cause. Intravascular fibrin deposition and intimal proliferation of arterioles may cause fragmentation of erythrocytes that can be detected as schistocytes on peripheral blood films. The rapid generation of soluble fibrin monomer can be confirmed by the protamine sulfate or ethanol gelation tests. The latter tests are usually negative in primary fibrinolysis.

Few cases of DIC have been reported in cats. Experimentally induced feline infectious peritonitis was characterized by a chronic DIC syndrome that featured elevated fibrinogen and FDP levels, thrombocytopenia, and lowered levels of FVII, FVIII:C, FX, FXI, and FXII.[49]

Favorable therapeutic response is indicated by increasing ATIII and fibrinogen levels with decreasing FDP levels and shortening of clotting tests (APTT, ACT). Platelet count is usually the slowest parameter to recover after satisfactory therapy is initiated. The prognostic usefulness of serial ATIII determinations was recently demonstrated in monitoring the clinical course of horses with DIC secondary to torsion of the large colon.[50]

THERAPY

The therapy of DIC centers on resolving the inciting cause, administration of fluids and electrolytes to maintain tissue perfusion, and limited anticoagulant therapy.[51] Since acute DIC is often secondary to severe diseases, the added deleterious effects of DIC create a high mortality regardless of treatment. The primary focus of therapy must be on the underlying disease if satisfactory results are to be obtained. Adequate supportive treatment for shock, fluid imbalance, acidosis, systemic infection, or renal failure is often critical to survival. In DIC patients that are actively hemorrhaging, whole blood should be administered to maintain perfusion, platelet counts and fibrinogen levels.

During the past decade, the use of heparin in DIC patients has been debated.[18] Commercial heparin preparations consist of mixtures of anionic polysaccharides having molecular weights ranging from 3000 to 40,000 daltons. Although heparin enhances ATIII activity and reduces thrombotic complications of DIC, its side effects are of increasing concern during therapy. Low molecular weight heparin preparations (available in Europe) have increased ATIII-mediated inhibitory effect on FXa and decreased inhibitory effect on thrombin, but data on their safety are still in question.[52] Heparin-mediated complications include thrombocytopenia, reduced ATIII levels, hemorrhage, and hypersensitivity reactions.[53] Heparin administration to normal dogs at 100 units/lb (200 units/kg) q6h for ten days caused a 40 per cent reduction in ATIII levels.[54] This implies that abrupt cessation of heparin therapy might predispose patients to thrombotic complications. Other conservative approaches may be as effective, particularly in patients that can not be monitored for potential heparin-induced

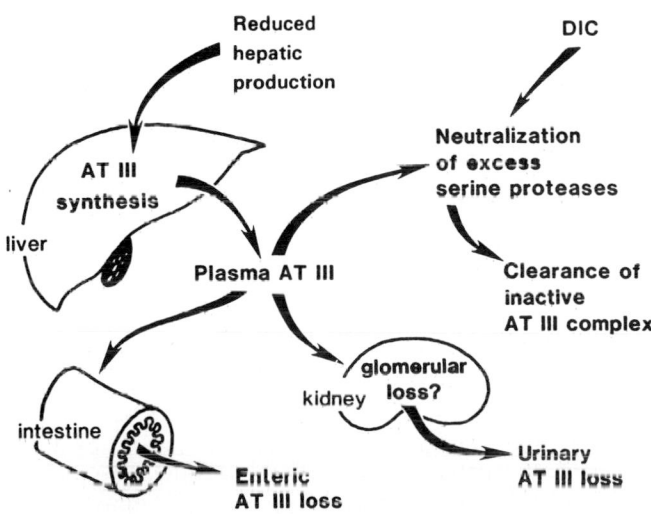

FIGURE 116–5. Pathophysiology of ATIII deficiency.

complications. Indeed, preliminary studies of a DIC model in dogs indicated that supplementing ATIII alone had equal efficacy and fewer complications than heparin (alone) or combined heparin-ATIII therapy.[55] Optimal anticoagulant therapy may not depend on maximal ATIII activation by exogenous heparin, but on providing sufficient ATIII for endogenous activation at required sites.[56]

Heparin should not be given to actively bleeding patients that have severe factor depletion and thrombocytopenia, as fatal hemorrhage may result. Heparin is also ineffective when ATIII levels are below 40 per cent of normal or when platelet antiheparin factor is excessive. For these reasons the author's approach has been to provide sufficient fresh whole blood to maintain platelet counts over $30,000/\mu l$ and fibrinogen levels over 50 mg/dl before administering heparin. Then heparin is administered subcutaneously at a low dose ranging from 20 to 45 units/lb (50 to 100 units/kg) q6h. Alternatively, sufficient heparin should be administered to prolong the APTT to 1.5- to 2-fold normal. Maintaining a constant level of anticoagulation with heparin appears more effective than administering a fixed dose in patients prone to thromboembolization.[57]

Difficulty in monitoring patients on heparin therapy is not uncommon. Normal dogs vary considerably with respect to the dose of heparin required to produce a given level of anticoagulation. Further variation is encountered in DIC because the patients' ability to synthesize coagulation factors and to metabolize heparin changes during illness. This problem is partially resolved through *in vitro* use of heparin-neutralizing agents, such as Polybrene.[58] By determining the APTT both before and after Polybrene, heparin-induced APTT prolongation can be separated from prolongation due to changes in the patient's basal coagulation factor status. Polybrene can also be useful in confirming heparin as a cause of APTT prolongation due to inadvertent sample contamination, often noted when heparin is used as a flush solution to maintain patency of intravenous catheters. By eliminating the heparin-related effect on APTT, the clinician's ability to monitor the patient's baseline coagulation status and response to therapy is improved.

Primary (Pathologic) Fibrinolysis

Pathologic fibrinolysis results when either excess activators or decreased plasma inhibitors induce hyperplasminemia. The resultant digestion of fibrinogen modifies the molecule so that it binds thrombin but does not clot, and thereby generates a circulating anticoagulant. Further enzymatic digestion of plasmin substrates leads to reduced levels of fibrinogen, FV, and FVIII:C accompanied by increased FDP levels (Figure 116–4). These changes result in a clinical disorder characterized by a bleeding tendency and rapid digestion of blood clots. It most frequently accompanies DIC, in which it is an appropriate physiologic response to formation of microthrombi throughout the vascular system (called secondary fibrinolysis). On rare occasions it may occur as a sequel to severe liver disease, when defective synthesis of antiplasmin or reduced clearance of activators leads

to hyperplasminemia (called primary fibrinolysis). Other conditions can also lead to primary fibrinolysis by excessive production of plasminogen activators. These include heat stroke, malignancy, genitourinary tract surgery, and progranulocytic leukemia. The existence of primary fibrinolysis as a discrete entity is debated by some, and it may only represent an atypical form of chronic, partially compensated DIC with high fibrinolytic activity.

The laboratory differentiation of primary fibrinolysis from the secondary fibrinolysis of DIC is difficult. DIC tends to have thrombocytopenia, hypofibrinogenemia, schistocytosis, and relatively low fibrinolytic activity. In contrast, primary fibrinolysis tends to have more normal platelet counts, no schistocytosis, less severe hypofibrinogenemia, and marked fibrinolytic activity. The relative fibrinolytic activity can easily be obtained by comparing the dilute whole blood clot lysis test in the patient with a control. Occasionally technicians may note the rapid lysis of blood clots in test tubes submitted for other laboratory tests. Other tests used occasionally to distinguish fibrinolytic states include the euglobulin clot lysis time and paracoagulation tests.

The treatment of primary fibrinolysis tends to be conservative. While epsilonamino caproic acid (EACA) is an effective inhibitor of fibrinolysis, there is often uncertainty about whether fibrinolysis is primary or secondary. Certainly in second fibrinolysis, one would not want to enhance thrombosis by inhibiting fibrinolysis. Therefore, patients are often given plasma to replace hemostatic deficiencies and heparin to inhibit consumption of coagulation factors. Dosages for plasma and heparin are similar to those used in DIC.

Liver Disease

PATHOPHYSIOLOGY

The liver is the site of synthesis of most plasma coagulation proteins and their respective inhibitors. Hepatocellular damage results in variable deficiencies of hemostatic proteins because their synthesis is impaired and their half-lives are often shortened by increased consumption.[59] Rapid hepatocyte regeneration usually maintains hemostasis within reasonable limits, although sudden decompensation may occur following involved surgical procedures or acute exacerbations of chronic disease processes. Bleeding problems associated with hepatic diseases of dogs and cats are relatively uncommon, with the exception of fulminating hepatic failure. In 32 dogs with hepatopathies, no bleeding tendencies were found despite laboratory detection of underlying coagulation abnormalities in two thirds of the population studied.[60] In contrast, bleeding was marked in the severe hepatopathy associated with naturally occurring cases of aflatoxicosis.[61]

In acute fulminating hepatopathies, sudden loss of over 70 per cent of the hepatocellular mass severely limits hepatic capacity to maintain normal levels of coagulation factors, particularly those with shorter half-lives. In addition, localized liver necrosis may trigger increased coagulation factor and platelet consumption (due to DIC) and secondary fibrinolysis. Levels of FVIIIR:Ag are often increased due to release from vascular storage sites. Synthesis of dysfunctional coagulation factors is occasionally noted in acute hepatopathies in man.[62] In more chronic hepatopathies, a gradual loss of hepatocytes leads to generalized reduction in coagulation factors regardless of coagulation factor half-life.

CLINICAL ASPECTS

Development of various hemostatic complications is not uncommon in severe hepatopathy in dogs and cats. When hepatic synthetic or clearance mechanisms fail, the patient may manifest thrombotic, fibrinolytic, or hemorrhagic complications, depending on interrelationships between the plasma half-lives of hemostasis-related proteins and their respective inhibitors. The reduced synthesis of inhibitors of fibrinolysis or reduced clearance of plasminogen activators may enhance the rate of fibrinolysis.[63] Enhanced plasmin generation in liver disease promotes activation of kinins that cause hypotension, shock, and end-organ damage, in addition to plasmin's well-known biodegradation effect on clotting factors.[64] On the other hand, reduced synthesis of ATIII and reduced clearance of activated coagulation factors provide a stimulus for thrombosis in liver disease. Secondary renal or pulmonary thrombosis can be a life-threatening sequel of liver disease and must always be considered when a patient's clinical condition suddenly deteriorates. Secondary factors, such as hypotension, sepsis, vasculitis or hypovolemia, play important synergistic roles in the development of pansystemic thrombotic sequelae. This delicate hemostatic balance between coagulation activators and inhibitors may be difficult to reestablish in a decompensated patient with severe liver disease. Certainly, providing judicious fluid therapy to maintain normal microvascular tissue perfusion is warranted in hepatic disease.

LABORATORY ASPECTS

The ultimate usefulness of a laboratory test is its reliability in guiding the clinician toward accurate patient management decisions. Coagulation tests, by estimating the severity of deficiency of coagulation factors, provide an accurate prognostic index in patients with acute liver failure. Decreased albumin levels are commonly noted in hepatic disease and reflect reduced hepatic protein synthesis. Coagulation factors, having much shorter half-lives than albumin, are particularly useful in detecting the severity of acute hepatic disease. In addition to reduced synthesis of most coagulation factors, increased consumption of selected coagulation factors may also result from DIC associated with fulminating hepatic disease.[65]

Evaluation of liver disease with routine coagulation tests can be misleading, especially with respect to partially compensated forms of liver disease.[66, 67] The routine coagulation tests (OSPT and APTT) may not detect mild to moderate deficiencies (coagulation factor levels above 30 per cent of normal) frequently associated with mild hepatopathies. Also, moderate ATIII deficiency

may shorten coagulation times and mask moderate deficiencies of coagulation factors. The suggestion that coagulation tests more readily disclosed mild defects when performed on diluted plasmas from animals with liver disease appears to depend on the methodology being used.[60] Coagulation tests on diluted plasma detects borderline deficiencies when using visual tilt tube methodology, but not when using techniques highly sensitive to the early generation of fibrin, e.g., electro-optical timing techniques.[68] In addition, some hemostatic defects are not detected with routine coagulation tests, e.g., abnormalities of fibrinolysis or platelet function. These factors must be carefully considered before subjecting animals with known hepatopathies to extensive surgical procedures that may cause hemostatic decompensation. Generally, severe acute canine hepatopathies tend to prolong both OSPT and APTT, whereas chronic partially compensated canine hepatopathies cause slight APTT prolongation and OSPT remains within normal limits.

Determination of relative deficiencies of individual coagulation factors in canine hepatopathies is rarely attempted, with the exception of fibrinogen. When DIC can be excluded, low fibrinogen levels confer an unfavorable prognosis in hepatic disease. In 28 dogs with naturally occurring hepatic disease, assays of specific factor deficiencies (FVII, FVIII:C, FVIII:RA, FIX, FX, FXI) or thrombin time indicated that measurement of individual coagulation tests was more sensitive than levels of hepatic enzymes (ALT, ALP), or routine coagulation tests (OSPT, APTT, or FDP levels) in detection of the major types of hepatic disease.[69] As FVII has a half-life of six hours, it decreases rapidly when synthesis is reduced by severe hepatic disease. In screening the coagulation defects of people with acute liver failure, FVII levels had high prognostic significance.[70] Similar studies in dogs with acute hepatopathy due to experimental aflatoxicosis revealed that FVII levels remained within normal limits in mildly affected dogs, while those that were severely affected had levels under ten per cent by day four.[71]

While liver disease is associated with deficiencies in coagulation factors, most patients incur clinical bleeding only when concurrent platelet dysfunction exists. Both quantitative and qualitative platelet functions may be altered in hepatic disease. Reduced platelet function due to thrombocytopenia may be related to increased splenic sequestration of platelets, reduced megakaryocyte production of platelets or increased platelet consumption (usually related to DIC). The variable nature of the thrombocytopenia accompanying liver disease makes it a poor laboratory parameter to utilize in differentiating DIC from the primary fibrinolysis accompanying certain forms of chronic liver disease. Qualitative defects in platelet function have also been noted in recent experimental studies of cholestatic liver disease in dogs.[72] Such defects are infrequently evaluated in hepatopathics, and may explain the bleeding tendency in some patients having normal coagulation tests and platelet counts. The diminished ability of the diseased liver to clear FDP, in addition to increased production of FDP (due to excessive fibrinolysis), may also interfere with platelet function. The clot retraction test is not sufficiently sensitive to detect mild platelet abnormalities. Prolonged bleeding time may indicate abnormal platelet function when other causes can be excluded. Platelet aggregation, when available, is the test of choice in evaluating qualitative platelet dysfunctions (see Chapter 117).

Less commonly requested coagulation tests give additional insight into the hemostatic defects of liver disease. Thrombin time provides a useful screening test in hepatopathy, since it can be prolonged by hypofibrinogenemia, dysfibrinogenemia, and increased FDP. It may also be shortened (particularly in dogs with cirrhosis and hepatic neoplasia). Increased FDP values were found in about 50 per cent of dogs with hepatic neoplasia.[69] Some evidence suggests that increased FDP levels in hepatic disease may reflect the presence of unclottable fibrinogen (dysfibrinogenemia) and not true products of fibrinolysis (see methodology section). This has provided further controversy concerning the role of increased fibrinolysis as a component of hepatopathies. When the fibrinolytic component of hepatic disease is poorly controlled, marked deficiency of fibrinogen, FV, and FVIII:C may result from hyperplasminemia.

Deficiency of ATIII in hepatic diseases of domestic animals is poorly documented at present (Figure 116–5); however, ATIII measurement is being advocated in human medicine as an index of the severity of the hepatic problem.[73] Limited clinical studies in dogs with severe hepatic disease also suggest that ATIII levels decrease in proportion to severity and are useful in establishing a prognosis. In the author's survey of dogs with severe ATIII deficiency (ATIII levels less than 50 per cent of normal) due to hepatic disease, only 20 per cent survive. This group also has severe prolongation of coagulation tests. In experimental studies with aflatoxicosis in dogs, extremely low levels of ATIII (14 per cent of normal) developed in dogs that were severely affected (mortality rate of 60 per cent), while those that maintained ATIII levels within normal limits had no deaths.[71] The present cost of determining individual coagulation factors by manual methods as opposed to the ease of automated ATIII measurement, makes serial ATIII measurement promising with respect to evaluating the prognosis and therapeutic response of patients with hepatic disease. The ATIII levels of frozen samples are very stable and so can accurately be determined when samples are shipped to reference laboratories.

TREATMENT

Although bleeding is usually not severe in hepatic disease, acute exacerbations of chronic processes may occur, leading to hemorrhage. Since the hemostatic defect is usually multifactorial, fresh whole blood or platelet-rich plasma is the treatment of choice for animals with active bleeding. Often the additional stress and trauma of exploratory surgical procedures may be sufficient to cause decompensation with delayed bleeding resulting in a dangerous postsurgical problem. If laboratory tests detect hemostatic abnormalities, these should always be corrected with whole blood or plasma transfusion prior to biopsy procedures. Some hepatopathies are accompanied by increased consumption of

coagulation factors; however, the severity of DIC is usually not sufficient to warrant heparin therapy. Correcting underlying ATIII deficiency can slow coagulation factor turnover and appears adequate to reverse the smoldering hemostatic abnormalities of patients with either acute or chronic hepatic disease.[74] Supportive fluid therapy, with particular emphasis on treatment of hypotension and shock, is important in prevention of thrombotic disease in patients with liver disease.

Secondary abnormalities associated with hepatic disease may require treatment. As blood is readily converted to ammonia in the gastrointestinal tract, gastrointestinal bleeding can contribute markedly to the production of hyperammonemia and hepatic encephalopathy.[75] This usually occurs in the terminal stages of hepatic disease and requires appropriate treatment. Also, because fresh blood has a lower ammonia content than stored blood, animals with liver disease should always be transfused with fresh or fresh frozen blood products to avoid hyperammonemic complications. Ammonia contents of stored human blood have been estimated at 170, 330, and 900 μg/dl on days 1, 4, and 21 respectively.[76]

Diminished absorption of fat-soluble vitamin K may be associated with chronic biliary obstruction and may reduce synthesis of the vitamin K–dependent coagulation factors, particularly in animals given oral antibiotics. Progressive anemia due to gastrointestinal bleeding developed rapidly (within two weeks) following total extrahepatic bile duct obstruction in cats.[77] Bleeding was attributed to deficiency of vitamin K–dependent factors, although duodenal ulcerations and platelet function defects may have contributed to the hemostatic defect. For this reason all icteric patients with prolonged OSPT should be given vitamin K and its effect assayed the following day. Generalized decrease in hepatic protein synthesis is the most likely cause of OSPT prolongation when the patient is unresponsive to vitamin K administration.

Hereditary Coagulopathies

PATHOPHYSIOLOGY

The hereditary coagulopathies are deficiencies of specific coagulation factors, usually noted in purebred dogs (Table 116–2) that are inbred or linebred.[78] Occasional cases are reported in mongrels, cats, and other species. The severity of the bleeding defect depends on the importance of the factor's role in hemostatic plug formation. Bleeding problems in animals with mild to moderate factor deficiencies are infrequent and generally occur when additional stress is placed on the hemostatic mechanism by coexisting diseases or major trauma. Bleeding problems in animals with severe deficiencies are more frequent and occur spontaneously.

Hereditary coagulopathies are rare with the exception of von Willebrand's disease (VWD). A high prevalence (65 per cent) of the gene for VWD in Doberman pinschers and this breed's current popularity makes knowledge of this disease essential in small animal practice.[79] Other breeds with high incidence rates include

TABLE 116-2. FEATURES OF HEREDITARY COAGULATION DISORDERS IN DOGS AND CATS

Disease	Factor Deficient	Inheritance Pattern	Severity of Bleeding Diathesis	Affected Breeds	Coagulation Screening Tests			Definitive Tests
					OSPT	APTT	ACT	
Hemophilia A (classic hemophilia)	FVIII:C	Sex-linked recessive	Variable	Reported in most dog breeds, and mongrels and cats	N	ABN	ABN	Low FVIII:C activity; normal to increased FVIIIR:Ag
Hemophilia B (Christmas disease)	FIX	Sex-linked recessive	Often severe	Cairn terrier, Alaskan malamute, Saint Bernard, cocker spaniel, French bulldog (10 other breeds affected to date); British shorthair (cat)	N	ABN	ABN	Low FIX activity
Plasma thromboplastin antecedent (PTA) deficiency	FXI	Autosomal	Mild*	Springer spaniel, Great Pyrenees, Kerry blue terrier	N	ABN	ABN	Low FXI activity
Hageman trait (Hageman factor deficiency)	FXII	Autosomal	Normal hemastatic mechanism†	Mixed-breed cat, poodle	N	ABN	ABN	Low FXII activity
Hypopro-convertinemia	FVII	Autosomal incomplete dominance	Subclinical to mild†	Beagle, Alaskan malamute	ABN	N	N	Low FVII
Stuart factor deficiency	FX	Autosomal	Severe in neonates	Cocker spaniel, mongrel	ABN	ABN	ABN	Low FX activity
von Willebrand's disease	vWF	Autosomal incomplete dominance (occasionally autosomal recessive)	Mild*	Golden retriever, miniature schnauzer, German shepherd, Doberman pinscher, Scottish terrier (49 other breeds affected to date)	N	V	V	Low FVIII:C activity; Low FVIIIR:Ag

*Severe bleeding may occur following major surgical procedures or trauma.
†Usually discovered fortuitously by presurgical screening tests.
Abbreviations: N = Normal, ABN = Abnormal, V = Variable.

the standard Manchester terrier (46 per cent), Pembroke Welsh corgi (30 per cent), miniature schnauzer (19 per cent), Scottish terrier (16 per cent), toy Manchester terrier (11 per cent), golden retriever (9 per cent), Shetland sheepdogs (12 to 20 per cent), and standard poodle (2 to 20 per cent).[80]

VWD is quite variable with respect to its bleeding manifestations. Recent studies have disclosed an important relationship between the severity of bleeding and the role of higher molecular weight forms (multimers) of FVIIIR:Ag.[81] The higher molecular weight forms are more hemostatically effective than lower molecular weight forms and subsequently, multimeric analysis of FVIIIR:Ag has served as a basis for classifying VWD in man.[82] Type I VWD has generalized deficiency of all multimers, type II VWD has deficiency of the higher molecular weight multimers, and type III VWD has a total absence of FVIIIR:Ag. This system is also being used to classify VWD in dogs.

The most common form of VWD in dogs is an autosomal (type I) form with incomplete dominant expression characterized by generalized deficiency of all FVIIIR:Ag multimers. This form of disease has been recognized in 51 breeds to date and should be considered in any breed with appropriate clinical signs.[78] Both

heterozygous and homozygous individuals have a bleeding tendency, although homozygosity is usually lethal. A less common form of VWD, autosomal recessive (type III), occurs in Scottish terriers and Chesapeake Bay retrievers in which the homozygous individuals have undetectable (zero) levels of FVIIIR:Ag and frequent bleeding problems.[83] Their heterozygous parents are clinically unaffected but have reduced levels of FVIIIR:Ag (under 50 per cent). Undetectable FVIIIR:Ag level related to VWD was also found in a Himalayan cat that bled excessively after a routine tooth extraction.[84] A form of VWD with reduced high molecular weight multimers (similar to type II VWD) was recently found in German short-haired pointers. Active testing and restricted breeding programs are required to rid purebred lines of undesirable hemorrhagic traits.

CLINICAL SIGNS

The clinical signs exhibited by animals with hereditary coagulopathies are influenced by many factors. These include the severity of the deficiency and the relative importance of the deficient factor in normal hemostasis. Delayed oozing of blood from poorly reinforced hemostatic plugs produces hematomas and may eventually lead to life-threatening hypovolemia. Clinical signs largely depend on the impact of hemorrhage into body cavities or organs and the related impairment of physiologic functions. Severe factor deficiencies may be manifested by obvious bleeding abnormalities following tail docking, cosmetic otoplasty, or loss of teeth during early life. In some instances the coagulopathy may cause a high neonatal death rate. Lameness due to bleeding into joint spaces (hemarthrosis) is common in larger frisky breeds. Blood loss tends to become more severe when minimal tissue pressure is generated by extravascular bleeding, e.g., mucous membranes and body cavities. Alternatively, bleeding into organs, such as the brain, may cause sudden death with minimal change in hematocrit. Bleeding around airways or nerve trunks may impair their physiologic functions.

Clinical signs of dogs with VWD are an exception to the above and hematoma formation is rare. Their clinical signs are more similar to those noted in platelet dysfunctions and are caused by insufficient VWF-mediated platelet adherence during initial formation of the primary platelet plug. Typical clinical signs of VWD are epistaxis, hematuria, and melena due to persistent bleeding from mucous membranes. In dogs with VWD the correlation between FVIIIR:Ag deficiency and clinical bleeding is only approximate. Following cosmetic otoplasty performed on VWD-affected Doberman pups, increased bleeding was not found if their FVIIIR:Ag levels were above 30 per cent.[85] It is estimated that one-third of the Doberman population has sufficiently low FVIIIR:Ag levels to have an increased bleeding risk. Increased bleeding in VWD dogs is often due to the presence of concurrent disease impacting on platelet function, e.g., ehrlichiosis, neoplasia, bacterial cystitis, hypothyroidism. Indeed, hypothyroidism (alone) may produce an acquired VWD-like defect with reduced platelet adhesion and prolonged bleeding times.[86]

LABORATORY ASPECTS

In patients with suspected hereditary coagulopathies, the global screening tests, APTT and OSPT, facilitate localization of the deficiency within the intrinsic, extrinsic, or common pathways (Table 116–2). If OSPT is prolonged and APTT is normal, FVII deficiency is suggested; if OSPT is normal and APTT is prolonged, FXII, FXI, FIX, or FVIII:C deficiency is suggested; and if both OSPT and APTT are prolonged, FX, FV, FII (prothrombin), or fibrinogen deficiency is suggested. APTT may be prolonged due to deficiency of FVIII:C in VWD, but normal APTT results are more common. The strong binding between FVIII:C and all multimers of VWF serves to prolong the plasma half-life of FVIII:C in normal animals. In VWD lack of VWF (carrier protein) results in reduced plasma survival of FVIII:C and causes modest FVIII:C deficiency. Determination of FVIIIR:Ag is necessary to differentiate between VWD (characterized by reduced levels) and hemophilia A (characterized by normal to increased levels). In some instances, mixing studies with specific factor deficiency plasmas are required to confirm the severity of a specific factor deficiency.

Many human hospitals have the expertise and necessary reagents to identify the common defects. Species-specific reagents are not required to identify defects. Careful attention to accurate sample collection and processing for mailing is essential if meaningful results are desired.

Perhaps the most difficult decisions posed to clinicians concern advice to owners of carrier animals. In general the normal ranges of coagulation factor activity are quite broad, ranging from 50 to 150 per cent of normal. Except for VWD, the coagulation factor levels in carriers are low-normal, usually ranging from 40 to 60 per cent of normal. As previously discussed, small errors in sample collection, processing, or shipment can make retesting of animals with borderline test results necessary, particularly with respect to the more labile coagulation factors. These factors make accurate identification of carriers difficult as well as recommendations concerning their suitability for breeding. In FVIII:C deficiency (hemophilia A), carriers are identified by a ratio of FVIII:C to FVIIIR:Ag of 0.5 or less.[80] This method is 90 per cent accurate in identifying FVIII:C carriers in man and animals. Similar approaches for identifying carriers of other animal coagulopathies are not presently available, although most carriers have reduced clotting factor activity. Testing of animals for VWD should be done at an early age since the disorder often diminishes with age, causing false-negative test results in older animals. Refer to Table 116–1 for interpretation of FVIIIR:Ag test results in VWD.

Animals with FXII deficiency may present diagnostic dilemmas. This usually occurs when a coagulation profile reveals a marked abnormality in the presence of diseases with potential impact on the hemostatic mechanism, e.g., thrombocytopenia or feline hepatic lipidosis. As FXII is not required for normal hemostasis, even severely affected animals do not have bleeding problems. Interestingly, FXII is absent in normal birds, reptiles, and marine mammals. FXII deficiency is most common in cats and recently was reported in a family of miniature poodles.[87]

THERAPY

Management of animals with severe coagulation defects is largely restricted to periodic transfusion with whole blood or plasma during bleeding episodes. The bleeding patient should be confined to a small quiet environment with minimal excitement to allow the patient optimal opportunity to reinforce platelet plugs with fibrin. The short half-life of transfused coagulation factors means that frequent retreatment is often necessary to maintain hemostatic competence. Blood should be obtained from a universal donor or carefully cross-matched to avoid transfusion incompatibility during subsequent treatments.

Moderately affected animals with VWD often appear clinically normal, but life-threatening bleeding may follow major surgical procedures. If the VWD status of a patient requiring major surgery is unknown, the cuticle bleeding time should be performed prior to surgery.[88] If the cuticle bleeding time is normal (less than six minutes), then significant bleeding during surgery is unlikely. Presurgical treatment with homologous plasma (three to five ml/lb) corrects bleeding tendencies for about four hours. The cuticle bleeding time is also used to approximate adequacy of therapy when more definitive tests are unavailable. Hypothyroidism may increase the bleeding tendency of VWD and testing to exclude its presence is important in all VWD suspects.[79]

New drugs are presently being evaluated that transiently increase VWF levels in people with VWD as alternatives to augmenting VWF by transfusion. Ideally, the increase in VWF would be sufficient to permit minor surgical procedures without risk of hemorrhage. Administration of the vasopressin analog, desmopressin (DDAVP), doubled FVIIIR:Ag levels both in normal dogs (from 87 per cent to 198 per cent) and in dogs with VWD (from 15 per cent to 30 per cent).[89] Unfortunately in the VWD dogs, the FVIIIR:Ag response was inconsistent and remained at the lower limit necessary to normalize hemostasis. Levels of FVIIIR:Ag can be increased in blood collected from donors pretreated with DDAVP, which would benefit VWD patients. Another innovative approach is to administer thyroid hormone which increases FVIIIR:Ag levels and often has normalized hemostasis within 24 to 48 hours in dogs with VWD.[79] Further developments in this area may provide reasonable treatment alternatives in bleeding disorders.

THROMBOSIS

Thrombosis is an ischemic condition resulting from intravascular deposition of a fibrin-platelet mass.[53] Fragmentation of the thrombus produces emboli that may cause blockage and ischemia at remote sites in the vascular tree. The etiology of thrombosis centers on Virchow's triad: a variable interaction between endothelial damage, abnormalities of blood flow, and hypersensitivity of the hemostatic mechanism.[90] Thrombi undergo constant structural evolution during their development and dissolution. Various factors interact to determine the rates of thrombogenesis and thrombus dissolution. Blood flow is a major factor influencing the relative incorporation of fibrin and platelets into a propagating thrombus. Arterial thrombi (white thrombi) consist primarily of platelets with minimal fibrin, while venous thrombi (red thrombi) are primarily composed of erythrocytes and fibrin with fewer platelets. Deficient fibrinolysis and reduced prostacyclin production have also been implicated as factors that also influence thromboembolization in certain diseases.[15]

The natural plasma inhibitors play major roles in modulating hemostasis and preventing thrombogenesis following major vascular damage.[1, 2] A high concentration of heparin-like groups on the endothelial surface of veins increases ATIII activity and permits efficient neutralization of activated serine proteases despite reduced blood flow rates.[91] Other factors influencing the kinetics of thrombus propagation include rates of fibrinolysis, embolization of thrombus particles, and phagocytosis of fibrin by leukocytes.

Most thrombotic conditions of small animals are due to vascular endothelial injuries caused directly or indirectly by infectious agents, e.g., dirofilariasis, bacterial endocarditis, or vascular immune complex deposition.[92] The mechanisms underlying embolization of the terminal aorta in cats with cardiomyopathy remain poorly understood; however, sluggish atrial blood flow and endocardial damage present an ideal environment for propagation of emboli.[93] In dogs with nephrotic syndrome, high urinary loss of low molecular weight plasma proteins causes ATIII deficiency (Figure 116–5) and generates a hypercoagulable state.[94] Thrombosis is a common terminal problem in proteinuric dogs with nephrotic syndrome, particularly those with the marked proteinuria of renal amyloidosis.[95, 96] In people with nephrotic syndrome, the risk of thromboembolic complications is among the highest encountered in medicine.[97] Thrombotic problems in small animals also occur in a variety of miscellaneous diseases including diabetes mellitus, hyperadrenocorticism, neoplasia, and myeloproliferative diseases; however, factors influencing the underlying pathogenesis of thrombosis in these disorders are poorly defined.[92, 98, 99]

CLINICAL SIGNS

The clinical signs of thrombosis depend on the various physiologic functions of the ischemic organ and the ability of collateral circulation to maintain adequate perfusion. The most prominent clinical sign of pulmonary thrombosis is dyspnea. Occasional patients may develop hemoptysis associated with pulmonary embolization. Hematuria and sudden flank pain are often associated with renal embolization and infarction. Embolization of the central nervous system causes a variety of locomotor disturbances and can result in sudden death. Emboli commonly lodge in the aortic trifurcation of cats and the affected limb(s) becomes painful, cool, pulseless, paretic, and pale.[93] Ischemic muscular contraction causes the limb to be held in rigid extension. Visceral arterial embolization causes sudden abdominal pain, vomiting, and bowel evacuation. Bowel sounds progress from initial hyperactivity to hypoactivity after ischemia of several hours' duration.

DIAGNOSTICS

Thromboembolization is difficult to confirm without sophisticated techniques that are generally available only at veterinary centers, such as nuclear medicine imaging, ultrasonography, and contrast angiography. Laboratory tests are helpful, but are not specific for the presence of thromboembolization. Patients with thrombosis are frequently thought to have a hypercoagulable state, although screening coagulation tests are usually normal. In selected thrombotic patients a hypercoagulable state is suggested by modest shortening of coagulation test times (OSPT, APTT, and TT). These alterations are induced partially by increased levels of selected coagulation factors and partially by reduced inhibition of the natural plasma inhibitors, particularly ATIII. As previously noted, varying degrees of ATIII deficiency may be acquired in hepatopathies, glomerulonephropathies, and DIC. In humans, ATIII levels between 50 and 75 per cent of normal are associated with a moderately increased risk of thrombosis, while ATIII levels below

50 per cent of normal are associated with a markedly increased risk of thrombosis.[32]

Platelet hypersensitivity is noted in some thrombotic disorders and is usually documented by finding increased responsiveness to platelet agonists using aggregation techniques or measuring increased plasma levels of substances released during platelet activation, e.g., β-thromboglobulin, thromboxane. Albumin is thought to bind certain substances released during platelet activation, such as thromboxane, and thereby modulate (dampen) subsequent platelet activation. It follows that patients with marked hypoalbuminemia may have increased platelet aggregation responses because of the increased availability of thromboxane. In dogs with nephrotic syndrome, platelet reactivity is enhanced by an interaction between both ATIII and albumin deficiency which may account for the increased incidence of thrombotic sequelae.[100]

Other laboratory tests may be of value in selected thrombotic patients. These include measurement of plasma viscosity in myeloma, platelet adhesiveness, or other plasma inhibitors (protein C, protein S, α-2-antiplasmin). FDP levels may be elevated secondary to increased plasmin-mediated thrombolytic activity. Tests evaluating the patient's hydration are useful in managing fluid balance abnormalities.

THERAPY

The major goal of thrombotic therapy is to encourage thrombolysis and to diminish further thrombogenesis. Certainly, every effort should be made to correct underlying prothrombotic factors, e.g., sepsis, dehydration, ATIII deficiency. Therapy to reduce the patient's pain or dyspnea during acute thrombotic attacks is obviously important. Vasodilator drugs appear particularly useful in increasing collateral circulation in cats with aortic saddle embolization.[93] Despite recent improvements in the thrombogenic nature of intravenous catheters, their use in patients with hypercoagulability must be closely monitored to prevent further thrombotic complications. Thrombi often form on the tips of catheters or adjacent vessel wall and are dislodged into circulation as the catheter is removed. Catheter patency can be extended by frequent flushing with heparinized saline (100 to 200 U heparin per 100 ml saline).

The therapeutic approaches that diminish thrombogenesis include the use of short-term anticoagulants (heparin), long-term anticoagulants (coumadins), and antiplatelet drugs (aspirin or dipyridamole). These drugs primarily limit thrombogenesis and depend on natural fibrinolytic activity to reduce the size of existing thrombi. Both heparin and coumadin-type drugs have significant effects on the hemostatic mechanism but the dosages producing thrombolysis are close to those causing hemorrhagic complications. Critical monitoring of hypocoagulability is required for effective anticoagulant therapy; however, this is difficult in most veterinary practices. For these reasons therapeutic management of most thrombotic patients involves antiplatelet drugs and short term low-dose heparin therapy. Aspirin therapy must be balanced to minimize inhibition of endothelial prostacyclin production, while maximizing inhibition of platelet thromboxane production. Aspirin is given at a dose of 12 mg/lb (25 mg/kg) every third day for prophylactic treatment of cats affected by recurrent aortic thrombosis.[101] In human membranoproliferative glomerulonephritis, prophylactic use of aspirin and dypyridamole significantly slowed platelet consumption and the progression of renal disease.[102] Similar prospective clinical studies using platelet inhibitors to prevent thrombosis and the progression of renal disease also appear warranted in glomerular diseases in dogs.

Direct thrombolytic therapy using urokinase and streptokinase has been widely used to lyse existing thrombi in people. These drugs stimulate increased plasmin formation within the thrombus and thereby promote digestion of its fibrin component. Thrombolytic therapy is more successful when initiated within hours of thrombus formation and less successful when initiated on older well-organized thrombi.[103] Unfortunately, these drugs also create a systemic lytic state which may result in uncontrolled bleeding due to interference in formation of normal hemostatic plugs. For these reasons, critical monitoring of fibrinolysis is essential to maximize plasmin's thrombolytic effects but to minimize its systemic effects. Thrombin time may be useful in detecting the hypofibrinogenemia and increased FDP levels associated with accelerated fibrinolysis. Preliminary thrombolytic studies with streptokinase support its efficacy in dogs and cats; however, further clinical studies will be required to establish therapeutic guidelines for its administration in common thrombotic diseases. Modern biotechnology has recently produced additional fibrinolytic agents that appear promising in dogs with respect to their selective action on thrombi with reduced systemic side effects. These agents include tPA, recombinant urokinase, and acetylated streptokinase-plasminogen complexes.[21]

Acknowledgement: The author thanks Dr. W.J. Dodds and her staff at Griffin Laboratory, New York State Department of Health, for constructive criticism and generous support during preparation of this chapter. The author extends special thanks to Christine Tanner for typing assistance and to Philomena Sculco for preparing illustrations.

References

1. Messmore, HL: Natural inhibitors of the coagulation system. Sem Thromb Hemost 8:267, 1982.
2. Rosenberg, RD and Bauer, KA: New insights into hypercoagulable states. Hosp Prac 21:131, 1986.
3. Mertens, K, et al.: The role of factor VIII in the activation of human blood coagulation factor X by activated factor IX. Thromb Haemost 54:654, 1985.
4. Marlar, RA, et al.: An alternate extrinsic pathway of human blood coagulation. Blood 60:1353, 1982.
5. Nemerson, Y.: Regulation of the initiation of coagulation by factor VIII. Haemostas 13:150, 1983.
6. Harmon, JT and Jameison, GA: Platelet activation by α-thrombin is a receptor-mediated event. Ann NY Acad Sci 485:387, 1986.
7. Bennett, JS, et al.: A role for prostaglandins and thromboxanes in the exposure of platelet fibrinogen receptors. J Clin Invest 68:981, 1981.
8. Loscalzo, J, et al.: von Willebrand protein facilitates platelet incorporation in polymerizing fibrin. J Clin Invest 78:1112, 1986.

9. Walsh, PN: Platelet-mediated trigger mechanisms in the contact phase of blood coagulation. Semin Thromb Hemost 13:86, 1987.

10. Mann, KG: The assembly of blood clotting complexes on membranes. Trends in Biochem Sci 122:229, 1987.

11. Bennett, JS: Blood coagulation and coagulation tests. Med Clin North Am 68:557, 1984.

12. Walsh, PN: Platelets and coagulation proteins. Fed Proc 40:2086, 1981.

13. Sixma, JJ and Van Den Berg, A: The hemostatic plug in hemophilia A: a morphologic study of hemostatic plug formation in bleeding time skin wounds of patients with severe hemophilia A. Br J Hematol 58:741, 1984.

14. Nawroth, P, et al.: The role of endothelium in the homeostatic balance of hemostasis. Clin Hematol 14:531, 1985.

15. Wu, KK: Microvascular thrombosis: Pathophysiology and new strategies. Hosp Prac 20:47, 1985.

16. Noren, I, et al.: Vacutainer sampling for blood coagulation assays. Scan J Clin Lab Invest 38:63, 1978.

17. Wessler, S: Small doses of heparin and a new concept of hypercoagulability. Thromb Diath Haemorrh 33:81, 1975.

18. MacHarg, MA and Becht, JL: The pharmacology of heparin prophylaxis. JAVMA 183:129, 1983.

19. Clouse, LH and Comp, PC: The regulation of hemostasis: The protein C system. N Engl J Med 314:1298, 1986.

20. Castellino, FJ: Biochemistry of human plasminogen. Semin Thromb Hemost 10:18, 1984.

21. Verstraete, M and Collen, D: Thrombolytic therapy in the eighties. Blood 67:1529, 1986.

22. Bachmann, F and Kruithof, EKO: Tissue plasminogen activator: Chemical and physiological aspects. Semin Thromb Hemost 10:6, 1984.

23. Sprengers, ED and Kluft, C: Plasminogen activator inhibitors. Blood 69:381, 1987.

24. Van Hinsbergh, VWM, et al.: Activated protein C decreases plasminogen activator-inhibitor activity in endothelial cell-conditioned medium. Blood 65:444, 1985.

25. Rappaport, SI, et al.: The effect of glass upon the activity of the various plasma clotting factors. J Clin Invest 34:9, 1955.

26. Chinn, DR, et al.: Prekallikrein deficiency in a dog. JAVMA 188:69, 1986.

27. Mazzucconi, MG, et al.: Evaluation of the nature of mildly prolonged prothrombin times. Am J Hematol 24:37, 1987.

28. Blaisdell, FS and Dodds, WJ: Evaluation of two microhematocrit methods for quantitating plasma fibrinogen. JAVMA 171:340, 1977.

29. Connaghan, GD, et al.: Prevalence and clinical implications of heparin-associated false positive tests for serum fibrin (Ogen) degradation products. Am J Clin Pathol 86:304, 1986.

30. VanDeWater, L, et al.: Analysis of elevated fibrin (Ogen) degradation product levels in patients with liver disease. Blood 67:1468, 1986.

31. Bick, RL: The clinical significance of fibrinogen degradation products. Semin Thromb Hemost 8:302, 1982.

32. McGann, MA and Triplett, DA: Interpretation of antithrombin III activity. Lab Med 13:742, 1982.

33. Benson, RE, et al.: Efficiency and precision of electroimmunoassay for canine factor VIII-related antigen. Am J Vet Res 44:399, 1983.

34. Johnstone, IB and Crane, S: Determination of canine factor VIII-related antigen using commercial antihuman FVIII serum. Vet Clin Path 9:31, 1980.

35. Johnson, GS, et al.: Detection of von Willebrand's disease in dogs with a rapid qualitative test, based on venom-coagglutinin-induced platelet aggregation. Vet Clin Path 14:11, 1985.

36. Mount, ME, et al.: Vitamin K and its therapeutic importance. JAVMA 180:1354, 1982.

37. Mount, ME: Proteins induced by vitamin K absence or antagonists ("PIVKA"). In Kirk, RW (ed): Current Veterinary Therapy IX. Philadelphia, WB Saunders, 1986, p 513.

38. Mount, ME, et al.: The anticoagulant rodenticides. In Kirk, RW (ed): Current Veterinary Therapy IX. Philadelphia, WB Saunders, 1986, p 156.

38a. Edwards, DF and Russell, RG: Probable vitamin K–deficient bleeding in two cats with malabsorption syndrome secondary to lymphocytic-plasmacytic enteritis. J Vet Int Med 1:97–101, 1987.

39. Frantz, SC, et al.: A study of accidents, illnesses and deaths resulting from the use of commensal rodenticides. EPA Public Hearings on Rodenticide Bait Stations, Sacramento, CA, March 5, 1984.

40. Green, RA, et al.: Laboratory evaluation of coagulopathies due to vitamin K antagonism in the dog: Three case reports. JAAHA 15:691, 1979.

41. McCaw, DL, et al.: Effect of internal hemorrhage on fibrin (Ogen) degradation products in canine blood. Am J Vet Res 47:1620, 1986.

42. Fernandez, FR, et al.: Vitamin K-induced Heinz body formation in dogs. JAVMA 20:711, 1984.

43. Feldman, BF: Disseminated intravascular coagulation. Comp Cont Ed Prac Vet 3:46, 1981.

44. Owen, CA, et al.: Turnover of fibrinogen and platelets in dogs undergoing induced intravascular coagulation. Thromb Res 2:251, 1973.

45. Drazner, FH: Clinical implications of disseminated intravascular coagulation. Comp Cont Ed Prac Vet 4:974, 1982.

46. Ockelford, PA and Carter, CJ: Disseminated intravascular coagulation: The application and utility of diagnostic tests. Sem Thromb Hemostas 8:198, 1982.

47. Feldman, BF, et al.: Disseminated intravascular coagulation: Antithrombin, plasminogen, and coagulation abnormalities in 41 dogs. JAVMA 179:151, 1981.

48. Bick, RL: Disorders of Hemostasis and Thrombosis. Principles of Clinical Practice. Thieme, Inc, New York, 1985, p 176.

49. Weiss, RC, et al.: Disseminated intravascular coagulation in experimentally-induced feline infectious peritonitis. Am J Vet Res 41:663, 1980.

50. Holland, M, et al.: Antithrombin III activity in horses with large colon torsion. Am J Vet Res 47:897, 1986.

51. Reuhl, W, et al.: Rational therapy in disseminated intravascular coagulation. JAVMA 181:76, 1982.

52. Thomas, DP: Current status of low molecular weight heparin. Thromb Haemostas 56:241, 1986.

53. Feldman, BF: Thrombosis—diagnosis and treatment. In Kirk, RW (ed): Current Veterinary Therapy IX. Philadelphia, WB Saunders, 1986, p 505.

54. Hellebrekers, LJ, et al.: Effect of sodium heparin and antithrombin III concentration on activated partial thromboplastin time in the dog. Am J Vet Res 46:1460, 1985.

55. Mammen, EF, et al.: Human antithrombin concentrates and experimental disseminated intravascular coagulation. Semin Thromb Hemostas 121:373, 1985.

56. Hellgren, M, et al.: Antithrombin III concentrate as adjuvant in DIC treatment. A pilot study in 9 severely ill patients. Thromb Res 35:459, 1984.

57. Leyvraz, PF, et al.: Adjusted versus fixed dose subcutaneous heparin therapy in the prevention of deep-vein thrombosis after total hip replacement. N Engl J Med 309:954, 1983.

58. Green, RA, et al.: Use of hexadimethrine bromide (Polybrene) as a heparin-neutralizing agent in canine plasma. Am J Vet Res 48:496, 1987.

59. Stein, SF and Harker, LA: Kinetic and functional studies of platelets, fibrinogen and plasminogen in patients with hepatic cirrhosis. J Lab Clin Med 99:217, 1982.

60. Badylak, SF and Van Vleet, JF: Alterations of prothrombin time and activated partial thromboplastin time in dogs with hepatic disease. Am J Vet Res 42:2053, 1981.

61. Greene, CE, et al.: Disseminated intravascular coagulation complicating aflatoxicosis in dogs. Cornell Vet 67:29, 1977.

62. Francis, JL and Armstrong, DJ: Acquired dysfibrinogenemia in liver disease. J Clin Pathol 35:667, 1982.

63. Hersch, SL, et al.: The pathogenesis of accelerated fibrinolysis in liver cirrhosis: A critical role for tissue plasminogen activator inhibitor. Blood 69:1315, 1987.

64. Kaplan, AP and Silverberg, M: The coagulation-kinin pathway of human plasma. Blood 70:1, 1987.

65. Wigton, DH, et al.: Infectious canine hepatitis: Animal model for viral-induced disseminated intravascular coagulation. Blood 47:287, 1976.

66. Mannucci, PM: Diagnosis and assessment of bleeding tendency in chronic liver failure using three coagulation tests. Scan J Hematol 7:361, 1970.

67. Rock, WA: Laboratory assessment of coagulation disorders in liver disease. Clin Lab Med 4:419, 1984.

68. Johnstone, IB: The activated partial thromboplastin time of diluted plasma: Variability due to the method of fibrin detection. Can J Comp Med 48:198, 1984.

69. Badylak, SF, et al.: Plasma coagulation factor abnormalities in dogs with naturally occurring hepatic disease. Am J Vet Res 44:2336, 1983.

70. Dymock, IW, et al.: Coagulation studies as a prognostic index in acute liver failure. Br J Hematol 29:385, 1975.

71. Green, RA: Clinical implications of antithrombin III deficiency in animal diseases. Comp Cont Ed Prac Vet 6:537, 1984.

72. Meyer, DJ and Chiapella, AM: Cholestasis. Vet Clin North Am 15:215, 1985.

73. Rodzynek, JR, et al.: Diagnostic value of antithrombin III and aminopyrine breath test in liver disease. Arch Int Med 146:677, 1986.

74. Schipper, HG and Ten Cate, JW: Antithrombin III transfusion in patients with hepatic cirrhosis. Br J Hematol 52:25, 1982.

75. Twedt, DC: Jaundice, hepatic trauma, and hepatic encephalopathy. Vet Clin North Am 11:121, 1981.

76. Schenker, S: Hepatic encephalopathy. Gastroenterology 66:121, 1974.

77. Center, SA, et al.: Hematologic and biochemical abnormalities associated with induced extrahepatic bile duct obstruction in the cat. Am J Vet Res 44:1822, 1983.

78. Dodds, WJ: Bleeding disorders. *In* Morgan, RV (ed): Handbook of Small Animal Practice. New York, Churchill Livingstone, 1987.

79. Dodds, WJ: von Willebrand's disease in dogs. Mod Vet Prac 65:681, 1984.

80. Dodds, WJ: Genetic screening for hereditary bleeding disorders. Kal Kan Forum 1:52, 1982.

81. Mannucci, PM, et al.: Correction of the bleeding time in treatment patients with severe von Willebrand disease is not solely dependent on the normal multimer structure of plasma von Willebrand factor. Am J Hematol 25:55, 1987.

82. Ruggeri, ZM and Zimmerman, TS: Platelets and von Willebrand disease. Semin Hematol 22:203, 1985.

83. Johnson, GS, et al.: A bleeding disease (von Willebrand's disease) in a Chesapeake Bay retriever. JAVMA 176:1261, 1980.

84. French, TW, et al.: A bleeding disorder (von Willebrand's disease) in a Himalayan cat. JAVMA 190:437, 1987.

85. Johnson, GS, et al.: Hemorrhage from the cosmetic otoplasty of Doberman pinschers with von Willebrand's disease. Am J Vet Res 46:1335, 1985.

86. Edson, RJ, et al.: Low platelet adhesiveness and other hemostatic abnormalities in hypothyroidism. Ann Intern Med 82:342, 1975.

87. Randolph, JF, et al.: Factor XII deficiency and von Willebrand's disease in a family of miniature poodle dogs. Cornell Vet 76:3, 1986.

88. Giles, AR, et al.: A canine model of hemophilic (factor VIII:C deficiency) bleeding. Blood 60:727, 1982.

89. Johnstone, IB and Crane, S: The effects of desmopressin on plasma factor VIII/von Willebrand factor activity in dogs with von Willebrand's disease. Can J Vet Res 51:189, 1987.

90. Kitchens, CS: Concept of hypercoagulability: A review of its development, clinical application, and recent progress. Sem Thromb Hemostas 11:293, 1985.

91. Marcum, JA, et al.: Acceleration of thrombin-antithrombin complex formation in rat hindquarters via heparin like molecules bound to endothelium. J Clin Invest 74:341, 1984.

92. Migaki, G and Casey, HW: Conditions associated with thrombosis in animals. *In* Animal Models of Thrombosis and Hemorrhagic Diseases. Bethesda, MD, National Academy of Sciences and National Institutes of Health, 1975, p 55.

93. Flanders, JA: Feline aortic thromboembolism. Comp Cont Ed Prac Vet 8:473, 1986.

94. Green, RA and Kable, AL: Hypercoagulable state in three dogs with nephrotic syndrome: Role of antithrombin III deficiency. JAVMA 181:914, 1982.

95. DiBartola, SP, et al.: Urinary protein excretion and immunopathologic findings in dogs with glomerular disease. JAVMA 177:73, 1980.

96. Slauson, DO and Gribble, DH: Thrombosis complicating renal amyloidosis in dogs. Vet Pathol 8:352, 1971.

97. Llach, F: Hypercoagulability, renal vein thrombosis, and other thrombotic complications of nephrotic syndrome. Kidney Int 28:429, 1985.

98. Burns, MG, et al.: Pulmonary artery thrombosis in three dogs with hyperadrenocorticism. JAVMA 178:388, 1981.

99. Hargis, AM, et al.: Relationship of hypothyroidism to diabetes mellitus, renal amyloidosis, and thrombosis in purebred beagles. Am J Vet Res 42:1077, 1981.

100. Green, RA, et al.: Hypoalbuminemia-related platelet hypersensitivity in two dogs with nephrotic syndrome. JAVMA 186:485, 1985.

101. Greene, CE: Effect of aspirin and propranolol on feline platelet aggregation. Am J Vet Res 46:1820, 1985.

102. Donadio, JV, et al.: Membranoproliferative glomerulonephritis: A prospective trial with platelet-inhibitor therapy. N Engl J Med 310:1421, 1984.

103. Curl, GR, et al.: Efficacy of tissue plasminogen activator and urokinase in a canine model of prosthetic graft thrombosis. Arch Surg 121:782, 1986.

117 PLATELET DYSFUNCTION

BERNARD F. FELDMAN

Blood platelets and the coagulation mechanism act in concert to form a complex homeostatic system designed to prevent and arrest hemorrhage. The interaction of platelets and the blood vessel wall (adhesion) with other platelets (aggregation), along with the facilitating role of platelets in thrombin generation, are required for normal hemostasis since both qualitative and quantitative defects in these functions may result in hemorrhage.[1]

To best facilitate understanding platelet qualitative dysfunction, basic concepts of anatomy, biochemistry, and physiology will be examined before specific dysfunctions are considered.

NORMAL PLATELET FUNCTION

ANATOMY AND BIOCHEMISTRY

Platelets circulate as variably sized disc-shaped, anucleate cell fragments. On Romanovsky-stained peripheral blood smears, the platelets are the smallest formed elements, less than one-third the size of red blood cells (RBC), and usually exhibit purplish granules. On scanning electron microscopy, their surface contains numerous indentations thought to represent the openings of an elaborate system of tubules called the open canalicular system, which extends throughout the interior of the platelet. On transmission electron microscopy a peripheral zone composed of the plasma membrane, exterior coat, and the submembrane, a sol-gel zone, and an organelle zone may be identified.[2]

PERIPHERAL ZONE

The external membrane mediates all of the platelet's interactions with its environment. It is composed of a double layer of phospholipids in which glycoproteins, cholesterol, and proteins are embedded. Some of the negatively charged membrane phospholipids such as phosphatidylinositol, phosphatidylserine, and phosphatidylethanolamine, distributed on the inner surface of membrane, may move to the outer layer of the membrane when the platelet is activated, thus accounting for the increased clot-promoting effect of activated plate-

lets.[3] It is likely that the electrostatic repulsion between platelets results from their normally negative surface charge.

The interior of the platelet membrane is viewed as a sea of fluid lipid. Increasing the cholesterol content of the membrane tends to decrease overall membrane fluidity, and cholesterol-rich platelets have been found by some investigators to be especially sensitive to stimuli.[4] In hypercholesterolemic diseases such as hyperadrenalcorticism, diabetes mellitus, and nephrotic syndrome, membrane fluidity may be an important factor in determining platelet responsiveness.

The platelet membrane glycoproteins include glycoproteins Ia,b (GPIa,b), which have been implicated in several functional activities: as receptors for von Willebrand factor when platelets are stimulated with the platelet aggregating agent ristocetin, as a receptor for thrombin, as a receptor for drug-dependent antibodies, and as being in close proximity to the receptor for immune complexes.[5-7] Congenital absence of GPIa,b results in the Bernard-Soulier syndrome (see below).

Glycoproteins IIb and IIIa (GPIIb and GPIIIa) are associated as a calcium-dependent membrane complex.[8] These proteins are involved with the platelet receptor for fibrinogen, as a receptor for von Willebrand factor when platelets are stimulated by adenosine diphosphate (ADP) and thrombin, but not ristocetin.[9-11] Deficiency in GPIIb and IIIa is associated with thrombasthenia (see below).[12]

SOL-GEL ZONE

Platelets have the unusual ability to alter shape from a smooth disc to a spiny sphere with spike-like filopodia extending far out from its body.[13] Resting disc shape and shape change are thought to be controlled by the platelet's cytoskeleton composed of the contractile proteins actin and myosin (and other associated proteins) and proteins involved with microtubule formation, tubulin and its associated proteins. The microtubules are a circumferential band within the sol-gel zone. There may be only a single microtubule, which winds around the platelet several times, helping to give the platelet structure.[14]

ORGANELLE ZONE

The platelet contains a large number of granules that have been subdivided into alpha granules, dense bodies, and lysosomes (Table 117–1). The alpha granules are the most numerous and contain a large number of proteins, which can be released when the platelet is stimulated. Platelet factor 4 (PF4), beta thromboglobulin, and platelet basic protein are a few of the proteins associated with the alpha granules, and all, especially PF4, can neutralize heparin's anticoagulant effect. This phenomenon allows hemostasis to be localized. The release of PF4 also appears to cause neutrophil and monocyte migration to the area of injury, acting as a chemotactic agent for these cells.[15]

The alpha granules also contain fibrinogen and von Willebrand factor and fibronectin, proteins involved with adhesion of several cell types to different surfaces.[16]

The platelet contains lysosomes, rich in hydrolytic enzymes, that are bound by membranes. Dense bodies contain high concentrations of adenosine diphosphate (ADP), adenosine triphosphate (ATP), serotonin, calcium, histamine, and catecholamines.[1]

BIOCHEMISTRY

With very low concentrations of ribonucleic acid (RNA) and without a nucleus to direct the synthesis of more RNA, the central biochemical feature of the platelet is its minimal ability to synthesize protein. This is an important consideration when loss of enzymatic activity, as for example with irreversible aspirin-induced inhibition of the enzyme cyclooxygenase, cannot be thus compensated for by new synthesis of protein.

Energy Metabolism. Platelets contain enzymes for glycolysis, oxidative phosphorylation, and fatty acid

TABLE 117–1. A PARTIAL LIST OF PLATELET GRANULE CONTENTS

Alpha-granules
Low molecular weight platelet specific proteins
1. Platelet factor 4 (PF-4)
2. Beta-thromboglobulin
3. Platelet basic protein
High molecular weight glycoproteins
1. Fibronectin
2. Fibrinogen
3. von Willebrand factor (vWf)
4. Factor V
Albumin
Mitogenic Factors
Other granule contents
1. Collagenase
2. Vascular permeability factors
3. Proelastase and elastase
4. Antiplasmin
5. α-2-macroglobulin
6. α-1-protease inhibitor
Dense bodies
1. ADP
2. ATP
3. Calcium
4. Serotonin
Lysosomal enzymes
1. Acid phosphatase
2. Aryl sulfatase
3. Others

oxidation. The platelet can synthesize glucose and has a hexose monophosphate shunt, which is involved in the reduction of glutathione.

Lipids. Platelets can synthesize fatty acids and phospholipids. This is central in forming cyclooxygenase and prostaglandin intermediates, eventually leading to the production of thromboxane A_2 (TXA_2), a labile but potent aggregating agent. Platelets lack the enzyme prostacyclin synthetase (unlike endothelial cells) and thus prostacyclin (PGI2), a potent inhibitor of platelet aggregation, cannot be produced. Knowledge of this fact is utilized in platelet inhibitory therapy.[1]

A unique phospholipid originally called platelet activating factor but now identified as acetyl glyceryl ether phosphorylcholine (AGEPC) is synthesized in the platelet. It is also a potent aggregating agent.[17]

Adenine Nucleotides. Two separate pools of adenine nucleotides, one in the platelet cytoplasm (metabolic pool) and the other in dense granules (storage pool), are the sources of platelet ADP and ATP. These nucleotides are involved in recruitment of other platelets in aggregation.

PHYSIOLOGY

Within seconds of a blood vessel injury, platelets adhere to the site of injury and aggregate shortly thereafter by first attaching themselves to platelets adhering to the vessel wall. Then they adhere to platelets which lie on top of adherent platelets, and then finally degranulate, affecting the platelets associated with the vessel wall most and adherent but distal platelets the least. In time, the platelets pack together more tightly and fibrin strands are laid down enmeshing the platelets in their network. Adhesion, aggregation, release of granule contents, and association with coagulation will be briefly considered. The entire platelet response and its control will then be considered.

ADHESION

Platelets adhere rapidly to a variety of surfaces, especially subendothelial collagen. Variously involved are exogenous von Willebrand factor, the platelet receptor for von Willebrand factor, fibrinogen, and calcium. The degree and extent to which these molecules are involved depends on the surface and the shear rate.[18]

AGGREGATION

The platelet aggregometer permits the simple quantitative assessment of platelet aggregation. With newer knowledge of platelet anatomy and biochemistry and the use of various aggregating agonists and their association with specific platelet membrane receptors, specific lesions may be defined (Table 117–2).

Shape change is an energy-requiring event in which spike-like filopodia appear and there is a rapid increase in the platelet surface area resulting from externalization of the open canalicular system. This permits a greater area for potential contact, and reduction of the electrostatic charges tending to keep platelets apart.[19]

Exposure of fibrinogen receptors and von Willebrand

TABLE 117–2. PLATELET RESPONSE TO VARIOUS AGONISTS

ADP–Platelet shape change, fibrinogen receptor exposure, von Willebrand factor receptor exposure (?)

Epinephrine–Fibrinogen receptor exposure

Thrombin–Platelet shape change, fibrinogen receptor exposure, arachidonic acid release, release reaction, von Willebrand factor receptor exposure (?)

Collagen–Arachidonic acid release, release reaction

Ristocetin–von Willebrand factor receptor exposure

Snake venoms (Bothrops spp)–von Willebrand factor receptor exposure

Arachidonic acid–Obviates need for arachidonic acid release but requires cyclooxygenase

Platelet-Activating factor–Platelet shape change, fibrinogen receptor exposure (?)

---

factor receptors follows shape change, adhesion, and aggregation. The release of arachidonic acid results in the generation of TXA_2, instrumental in the release reaction. As ADP is one of the agents released and is a strong aggregating agent, a potential feedback loop is generated. Moreover, TXA_2 also induces shape change and aggregation, another feedback loop. Two aggregating agents, thrombin and collagen, stimulate both arachidonic acid release and metabolism and stimulate the platelet release reaction by a pathway independent of TXA_2 production. This allows the use of thrombin to subdivide patients with similar aggregation abnormalities into those with arachidonic acid release or metabolism abnormalities and those that lack adequate stores of ADP (and thus have abnormal release of ADP).

Primary aggregation occurs with agents that directly expose fibrinogen or von Willebrand factor receptors (Table 117–2) producing aggregation even when TXA_2 and the release reaction cannot take place. Secondary aggregation is induced by appropriate concentrations of ADP, thrombin, or epinephrine, and requires an intact release reaction and/or arachidonic acid metabolism. There is significant variation in aggregation with different agonists. Platelet aggregation *in vitro* is performed on citrated, platelet-rich plasma in which the concentration of ionized calcium is very low. Some responses may be artifactual because of the number of reagents involved in the procedure.

RELEASE REACTION

The release reaction is probably induced by an increase in cytosolic calcium. The increased calcium may initiate release by activating the contractile mechanism and by promoting the fusion of granule membranes with the plasma membranes of the open canalicular system or cell surface.

Increases in platelet cyclic adenosine monophosphate (cAMP) are associated with inhibition of the release reaction and thus platelet function. Intraplatelet cAMP is controlled by the enzyme adenylate cyclase which converts ATP into cAMP.[20] Adenylate cyclase is stimulated by exogenous PGI2 and other prostaglandins. The inhibitory effect of cAMP on the release reaction is, in part, due to the increased sequestration of calcium in the tubular system, decreased arachidonic acid from phospholipids, and inhibition of myosin activating enzymes.[21]

PLATELETS AND COAGULATION

Coagulation is catalyzed by platelet membrane phospholipids or phospholipoproteins called *platelet factor 3* (PF3). This factor interacts with factor V, calcium, and factor X in the production of thrombin through the activation of factor II (prothrombin). The result of this activation is the production of fibrin strands in intimate association with enmeshed platelets. The retraction of the clot is also associated with an intact platelet actinomyosin contractile mechanism. Clot retraction is abnormal with thrombasthenia (see below).[22]

CONTROL OF PLATELET FUNCTION

The ability of an activated platelet to produce arachidonic acid metabolites such as TXA_2 and to release aggregating agents such as ADP constitutes a positive feedback mechanism amplifying the initial response. Opposing, negative feedback systems are necessary for inherent stability.[1] Unfortunately, little is known about these mechanisms which must be in effect. Otherwise, platelets would be continually recruited until all platelets circulating would be involved.

Blood flow is probably the single most important factor limiting the platelet's contribution to hemostasis, determining the number of platelets passing a given point in a blood vessel at a given time, the length of time a platelet will have to adhere to the vessel wall or to aggregate with another platelet before being carried downstream, and the force with which a platelet will collide with either the vessel wall or another platelet.[1, 23] Platelets adhere to many types of surfaces but, uniquely, do not adhere to normal endothelial cells. The discovery that endothelial cells, unlike platelets, have enzymes to synthesize PGI2, the most potent known inhibitor of platelet adhesion and aggregation, has shifted attention to the activities of endothelial cells. The endothelial cell may be involved in limiting the platelet response by taking up released ADP, binding and removing thrombin, and, increasing PGI2 production in the presence of thrombin.[24] There is now evidence that endothelial cells may utilize platelet-produced cyclic endoperoxides, when platelets are stimulated, and convert them to PGI2.[25]

QUALITATIVE PLATELET DISORDERS

Qualitative platelet disorders, disorders of platelet function, or thrombocytopathias were, for many years, regarded as rare causes of hemorrhage. Because of the development of simple instruments in the 1960s to measure platelet aggregation, information concerning qualitative abnormalities of platelets has accumulated at an unprecedented rate (Table 117–3). A prolonged bleeding time in a patient with a normal platelet count suggests abnormal function. Tests of platelet function are now used in veterinary medicine to investigate suspected qualitative disorders (see below). Qualitative platelet abnormalities which involve one or more specific

TABLE 117–3. MAJOR PLATELET FUNCTIONAL DISORDERS

Hereditary

Defective platelet adhesion
1. Von Willebrand's disease
2. Bernard-Soulier syndrome
3. Canine thrombasthenic-thrombopathia (similar to 2 above)

Deficient release reaction
1. Storage pool disease
2. Gray platelet syndrome
3. Chediak-Higashi syndrome
4. Deficiencies of thromboxane synthetase, cyclooxygenase

Deficient platelet aggregation
1. Thrombasthenia
2. Canine thrombopathia
3. Canine thrombasthenic-thrombopathia (see defective platelet adhesion above)
4. Hypofibrinogenemia

Miscellaneous
1. Platelet factor 3 deficiency
2. May-Hegglin anomaly
3. Heritable connective tissue disorders
4. Mucopolysaccharidoses

Acquired

Drugs (see Table 117–6)
Uremia
Hematologic disorders
1. Dysproteinemias
2. Myelofibrosis
3. Polycythemia rubra vera
4. Myeloproliferative diseases
5. Thrombocythemia

Miscellaneous
1. Hepatic disease
2. Various hypercoagulable states—nephrotic syndrome, diabetes mellitus, hyperadrenalcorticism
3. In association with increased fibrin(ogen) degradation products

platelet functions have been described in a variety of hereditary and acquired conditions. The more common platelet dysfunctions, both hereditary and acquired, will be discussed. As with most platelet related disorders, hemorrhage is usually not severe unless aggravated by combined disorders. Commonly petechiae and ecchymoses are associated with the vascular-platelet phase of primary hemostasis. Deep bleeding, hematomas, and hemarthroses are associated with abnormalities of coagulation factors.

Hereditary Thrombocytopathies— Adhesion Defects

VON WILLEBRAND'S DISEASE

Von Willebrand's disease (VWD) is a hemorrhagic diathesis caused by a deficiency of von Willebrand factor (vWf), a plasma glycoprotein required for normal platelet adhesion during primary hemostasis. The disease is considered to be the most common heritable bleeding disorder of man. A severe form of VWD has been well documented in a family of swine and a less severe form has been reported in rabbits.[26–28] The disease, particularly common among dogs, has been detected in more than 30 breeds (Table 117–4), and is suspected to occur in cats.[29–30]

The vWf glycoprotein is thought to be a polymeric assemblage of identical single-chain polypeptide sub-

units, each with a molecular weight of approximately 270,000 which includes 19 per cent carbohydrate.[31] Disulfide bonds fasten subunits together into multimers of varying molecular weight.[31]

At least two cell types, endothelial cells and megakaryocytes, are able to synthesize vWf.[32] Platelets carry a substantial proportion of the circulating vWf in people.[33, 34] In contrast, canine platelets contain very little vWf.[33, 35] The platelet vWf is thought to be of megakaryocyte origin while plasma vWf is thought to be derived from endothelial cells.[34] Von Willebrand factor is necessary for the normal adhesion of platelets to exposed subendothelium of injured vessels, particularly when high shear forces exist in the microvasculature. Additionally, vWf may participate in platelet to platelet attachments in growing platelet plugs.[33, 36] A second function of vWf is to stabilize factor VIII, the coagulation factor (protein) deficient in hemophilia A.[33, 37]

Concentrations of vWf are modulated in plasma. In humans, illness, parturition, strenuous exercise, thyroxine, and estrogen cause long-lasting increased levels of vWf. Vasopressin and epinephrine induce transient decreases.[33, 38, 39] In dogs strenuous exercise does not seem to increase vWf. Increases in canine plasma have been seen at parturition, during liver disease, and in response to endotoxin infusion.[33]

Laboratory Evaluation of von Willebrand Factor. Several approaches to the laboratory diagnosis of VWD may be utilized. These include antigenic assays and the rate of vWf-dependent platelet aggregation. If measured antigenically, vWf is referred to by the abbreviation vWf:Ag (Table 117–5).[33] When platelet agglutination

TABLE 117–4. DOG BREEDS IN WHICH VON WILLEBRAND'S DISEASE HAS BEEN DIAGNOSED

Afghan hound
Airedale terrier
Basset hound
Boxer
Cairn terrier
Chesapeake Bay retriever
Doberman pinscher
English cocker spaniel
English springer spaniel
German shepherd
German shorthaired pointer
Golden retriever
Great Dane
Irish setter
Lakeland terrier
Labrador retriever
Lhasa Apso
Miniature dachshund
Miniature poodle
Miniature schnauzer
Papillon
Pembroke Welsh Corgi
Rottweiler
Scottish terrier
Shetland sheepdog
Soft-coated Wheaton
Standard dachshund
Standard Manchester terrier
Tibetan terrier
Vizsla

*Modified from Johnson, GS, et al.: Canine von Willebrand's disease: A heterogeneous group of bleeding disorders. Vet Clin North Am Vol 18, Jan 1988.

TABLE 117–5. PROPOSED ABBREVIATIONS FOR FACTOR VIII AND VON WILLEBRAND FACTOR*

	Abbreviation	
	Outmoded	Proposed
Factor VIII		
Protein	VIII:C	VIII
Antigen	VIIIC:Ag	VIII:Ag
Function	—	VIII:C
von Willebrand factor		
Protein	VIIIR:Ag	vWf
Antigen	VIIIR:Ag	vWf:Ag
Function	VIII:RCo; VIIIR:vWf	—

*Modified from Marder, VJ et al: Standard nomenclature for factor VIII and von Willebrand factor: A recommendation by the International Committee of Thrombosis and Haemostasis. Thromb Haemostas 54:871, 1985.

assays are utilized, vWf is considered a cofactor for the agglutination-inducing agent and the agent used to induce aggregation is named, such as ristocetin cofactor.[33] For convenience the vWf:Ag concentration in a canine pool of plasma is usually reported as 100 per cent or 1 unit/ml; however, the absolute vWf concentration in a plasma pool from healthy dogs has been measured at 6 μ/ml, within the range of concentration found in normal people.[33, 40] The cofactor and antigenic assays may not agree due, partially, to the multimeric nature of the vWf. The vWf:Ag concentrations are considered indicative of the amount of vWf in the sample without regard to its biological activity.[33] The platelet-agglutination cofactor activities reflect the platelet's ability to participate in platelet-plug formation.[33] The aggregation assays are not always reliable indicators of the hemostatic capacity of VWD patients and various cofactor assays are not always in agreement with each other.[33, 41, 42] The bleeding time assay is the best indicator of the platelet-vessel hemostatic status in VWD patients. The assay is quite crude and fraught with error. Other conditions than VWD can prolong the bleeding time by interfering with primary hemostasis. A buccal mucosa bleeding time for dogs has recently been described which appears to be accurate in detecting patients with defective primary hemostasis.[43] Other types of bleeding times are considered by this author to be inconsistent.

Another indirect assay for VWD (the bleeding time is the other) is the activated partial thromboplastin time (APTT). Few dogs with VWD have markedly lowered factor VIII:coagulant (VIII:C) activities. Activities of VIII:C less than 20 per cent of normal are required to prolong the APTT, obviating its value as a screening test.

The electroimmunoassay for vWf:Ag is the most commonly used assay for vWf and is available through research institutes, veterinary colleges and universities, and private veterinary laboratories. The adaptation to canine plasma has been described.[44, 45] This procedure utilizes citrated plasma which is placed in a well in agarose gel and electrophoresed against rabbit, anticanine vWf antibody. The result is a rocket-shaped precipitin line which is compared to control standard dilutions.[46] Recently, there has been a complete description and discussion of this test and other tests including crossed immunoelectrophoresis of vWf:Ag, multimeric analysis, platelet aggregation and agglutination assays for vWf, ristocetin cofactor, Polybrene cofactor, and

botrocetin cofactor.[33] A commercial plate-agglutination kit has been evaluated and at present has questionable value as previously marketed.[47]

Human von Willebrand's Disease. Human VWD is a heterogeneous disease. A number of subclassifications of the human disease have been proposed without universal acceptance. One convenient classification divides human VWD into three major categories. There are subcategories within each of the three major categories. As described, multimeric analysis of plasma from individuals with type I VWD reveals the presence of all vWf multimers found in normal plasma.[33] With type II VWD, the largest multimers cannot be detected in plasma.[33] Individuals with type III VWD have only a trace or no detectable vWf in their plasma. This latter form is the most severe form of the human disease with evidence for inheritance from both parents. Human type II VWD has subclassifications from type IIA through and including type IIF. Human type I also has numerous subclassifications.[33]

Canine von Willebrand's Disease. Canine VWD often presents with mucosal or cutaneous hemorrhage. Heterogeneity in the canine form of VWD may be similar to human VWD: counterparts of the three major types have been recognized in dogs, but systems for subtyping canine VWD have not been adapted for the dog, and species differences in vWf content of platelets suggest that use of the human subtyping system may be premature in dogs until specific etiologies in the dog have been examined.[33]

Information on several breeds of dogs has been accumulated. Von Willebrand's disease was first described in Scottish terriers in 1972.[48] Both homozygous (deficient) and heterozygous (carrier) animals have been found with bleeding tendencies associated with the homozygous animals and subtle bleeding tendencies associated with the heterozygous state.[33] Von Willebrand's disease in Scottish terriers resembles type III human VWD. Incidence of VWD in this breed currently approximates 18 per cent.[49]

Chesapeake Bay retrievers also appear to have type III VWD. Clinical cases have had protracted gingival hemorrhage, slight thrombocytopenia, normal prothrombin times (PT) and APTT, and slightly prolonged bleeding times. The vWf:Ag was found to be nondetectable with the various cofactor activities.[33, 50] The prevalence of VWD among Chesapeake Bay retrievers has not been determined and may be very low.[33] German shepherds were the first dogs in which VWD was described. The diagnosis was based upon bleeding tendencies, prolonged bleeding times, and abnormal platelet function tests.[33, 51] Subsequent studies revealed moderately reduced plasma concentrations of vWf:Ag. The high incidence of stillbirths from the two affected parents led to the suggestion that both dogs were heterozygotes and that homozygote progeny had severe VWD, though most died in utero.[33, 51] Prolonged bleeding times in these German shepherds were normalized by transfusion with purified human vWf.[33, 52]

Doberman pinschers with subnormal concentrations of vWf:Ag are commonly encountered. Despite the high prevalence of VWD in this breed, bleeding episodes are relatively uncommon, though reports of abnormal bleeding associated with this breed have appeared in the veterinary literature.[53–56] In a double blind study, Doberman puppies with vWf:Ag concentrations below 22 per cent bled more during otoplasty than did Doberman puppies above 38 per cent.[57] Dobermans had consistently prolonged buccal mucosal bleeding times with vWf:Ag concentrations less than 20 per cent, while normal dogs including Dobermans with vWf:Ag concentrations above 50 per cent have had normal buccal mucosal bleeding times.[47] Hypothyroidism, common among Doberman pinschers, may exacerbate the bleeding tendencies of dogs with VWD.[33, 49] Most or all Doberman pinschers with VWD have a form of the disease similar to type I human VWD.[33]

Airedale terriers also have an increased incidence of VWD similar to Type I human VWD.[33] German shorthair pointers appear to have VWD similar to human type II VWD.[58]

In addition to the breeds discussed above, many other breeds have been found to have increased incidence of VWD. Recently, in a random survey of a group of Danish golden retrievers, 18 per cent of the dogs had subnormal concentrations of vWf:Ag.[59]

To avoid confusion and to facilitate the distinction between clinically significant and subclinical forms of canine VWD, the term "canine von Willebrand's trait" has been suggested to refer to families of dogs in which the abnormal findings are restricted to laboratory test results.[33] The term "canine von Willebrand's disease" should be restricted to dogs in which the disease has been shown to adversely affect their health.[33] In breeds with a low prevalence of VWD, the occurrence of unexplained abnormal hemorrhage in one or a few dogs with subnormal vWf:Ag concentrations is unlikely to be coincidence and should be considered strong evidence that the breed has clinically significant VWD.[33] However, with breeds that include a high fraction of dogs testing abnormally, the incidence of hemorrhagic episodes in the abnormal population should be considered. In this population, rare bleeding episodes are to be expected from a variety of causes other than VWD.[33] In order to prove that VWD is clinically significant in those breeds, it may be necessary to demonstrate that hemorrhagic episodes have occurred more frequently in dogs with laboratory evidence for abnormal vWf.[33] The consistent demonstration of prolonged bleeding times in dogs with abnormal vWf-related laboratory test results should also be considered evidence that the dogs have VWD rather than von Willebrand's trait.[33]

CLINICAL SIGNS. Bleeding is exacerbated by physical, emotional, and physiologic stress, hormonal imbalances such as hypothyroidism, and by concomitant diseases such as parasitic, viral, and bacterial infections. Signs include mucosal bleeding, stillbirths or neonatal deaths ("fading puppies"), prolonged estrus or postpartum bleeding, lameness that mimics eosinophilic panosteitis, and severe parvoviral disease among VWD dogs.[49, 60]

Recently, VWD, factor XII deficiency, and familial nonspherocytic hemolytic anemia were described in a family of miniature poodles.[61]

TESTING. The laboratory should be consulted concerning handling and preparation of samples. Tests with borderline findings between normal and suspect should be repeated. Dogs which are unhealthy, receiving any type of medication, having had a vaccination within the preceding two weeks, or in estrus should not be tested. Test results for vWf:Ag concentrations are reported as a percentage relative to pooled canine plasma arbitrarily considered to be 100 per cent. Patients with vWf:Ag concentrations greater than 60 per cent are considered normal. Patients with concentrations less than 40 per cent are considered vWf:Ag deficient. Patients between 40 and 60 per cent are considered carriers.[49]

MEDICAL MANAGEMENT OF VON WILLEBRAND'S DISEASE. Cryoprecipitate is an enriched form of fibrinogen, hemophilic factors, and vWf. It is produced by freezing and then dissolving plasma. The cryoprecipitate is slow to redissolve and is easily aspirated from the plasma fraction. This is the preferred therapeutic agent but often is not readily available.

Transfusion with matched fresh plasma or whole blood is also satisfactory. Pretreatment of donor dogs with desamino-8-D-arginine vasopressin (desmopressin acetate; DDAVP-0.5 µg/lb body weight, subcutaneously) 30 minutes before obtaining donor blood will increase the vWf:Ag concentrations of the donors 30 to 40 per cent.[62] Ideally the vWf of the recipient should be increased to approximately 40 per cent of normal. Calculation of the amount of donor product to be delivered may be accomplished with knowledge of the recipient vWf concentration, canine blood volume (approximately 36 ml/lb or 80 ml/kg), the volume of the donor product, and the assumption that the donor product contains 100 per cent vWf:Ag concentration.

In hypothyroid dogs with VWD, recurrent hemorrhagic problems have been successfully alleviated, at least in part, by the use of hypothyroid-therapeutic doses of thyroxine.[49] Some dogs do not respond to thyroxine therapy and some dogs which initially respond become refractory to prolonged or repeated thyroxine therapy.

GENETICS AND RECOMMENDATIONS TO BREEDERS. If a normal dog, free of the VWD gene, is mated to a carrier or deficient, about one-half of the offspring will be carriers or deficients and the other one-half will be normal. If two carriers or deficients are bred, approximately three-quarters of the offspring will have the VWD gene. One-quarter will be severely affected or carriers like the parents and the remaining one-quarter will be normal. The more severely affected the parent, either carrier or deficient, the more likely affected puppies will be produced. More complete discussion of the philosophy and nuances of genetic counseling have been described.[33, 49]

THE BERNARD-SOULIER SYNDROME

This rare disorder of humans, similar, in part, to canine thrombasthenic-thrombopathia, is characterized by mild thrombocytopenia, giant platelets, deficient platelet adhesion, and specific abnormalities of membrane GPIa and b. The disorder is manifested by mild to moderate bleeding and is inherited as an autosomal recessive trait. The abnormality in GPIb is important because it is the major determinant of the vWf:Ag binding site on the platelet. In the absence of GPIb, platelet adhesion to subendothelium is impaired and, in man, ristocetin-induced platelet aggregation is deficient, both abnormalities being attributable to the failure of vWf:Ag to bind to platelets. Other glycoproteins may also be involved in this disorder.[63] The giant platelets may be more than twice normal size. Bleeding time is prolonged but clot retraction is normal.

CANINE THROMBASTHENIC-THROMBOPATHIA

Though primarily a platelet aggregation defect, canine thrombasthenic-thrombopathia will be discussed here because of similarity to the Bernard-Soulier syndrome. The autosomally inherited disorder occurring in Otterhounds has features in common with both the Bernard-Soulier syndrome (see above) and Glanzmann's thromboasthenia (see below).[60, 64] Platelets from affected dogs do not aggregate with appropriate physiologic stimuli and do not support clot retraction.[60] The characteristics of thrombasthenia are due to reduction in heterozygotes or absence in homozygotes of GPIIb and GPIIIa, membrane glycoproteins responsible for fibrinogen binding, platelet aggregation and clot retraction, and morphologic features of platelets in the Bernard-Soulier syndrome.[65]

Clinical signs are primarily associated with mucosal surface bleeding and are exacerbated by surgery, trauma, or stress. The defect is uniquely expressed in quantitative clot retraction tests.[60] A variant from the original platelet function defect due, perhaps to a new mutation or a self-selected variant, has been recognized.[60] The new expression of the platelet disorder may be cyclical with bleeding episodes triggered by stress (vaccination, illness, injury, surgery, and hormonal imbalance or change such as hypothyroidism or estrus) or occurring in regular rhythm somewhat like that of cyclic neutropenia (Gray Collie syndrome).[60] The original Otterhound platelet disorder involved two populations of circulating platelets, one normal and the other abnormal, the proportion of each varying in relation to the severity of the clinical signs.[60] This new variant could indicate proportionally more normal cells. Stress induces a bleeding episode and subsequently causes the bone marrow to produce even more normally functioning cells, temporarily correcting the functional defect during the stimulatory event.[60]

Hereditary Thrombocytopathies—Deficiencies of the Release Reaction

A variety of platelet defects may be associated with functional aberrations in secretory phenomena that comprise the release reaction. These abnormalities may be associated with structural abnormalities of platelet organelles that contain storage sites for various constituents. *Storage pool disease* has deficiencies of dense bodies. The ADP content of resting platelets and the amount of ADP released when platelets are stimulated are greatly reduced, similar to the effect that occurs with aspirin. This disorder seems to be inherited as an autosomal dominant trait in most kindreds and has been associated with albinism. *Chediak-Higashi* syndrome is

a form of storage pool disease.[66] The *Gray platelet syndrome* is characterized by decreases in the numbers and content of alpha granules. Morphologically these platelets and megakaryocytes are virtually agranular and are vacuolated.[1] In *cyclooxygenase deficiency*, the conversion of arachidonic acid to cyclic endoperoxides is deficient. In *thromboxane synthetase deficiency*, thromboxane A_2 is not formed though the precursor reaction, the conversion of arachidonate to labile endoperoxides, does not appear to be affected.[1] Both cyclooxygenase and thromboxane synthetase deficiencies are inherited as autosomal dominant traits.

Hereditary Thrombocytopathies—Deficiencies of Platelet Aggregation

THROMBASTHENIA

Thrombasthenia is a rare hereditary trait manifested by deficient platelet aggregation, impaired clot retraction, and moderately severe mucosal hemorrhage. This autosomal recessive trait is also known as Glanzmann's disease. The basic defect in thrombasthenia is the deficiency or aberration of membrane glycoproteins IIb and IIIa. The absence of these glycoproteins impairs the ability of both resting and activated platelets to bind fibrinogen and, as a consequence, platelet aggregation induced by ADP and most other platelet agonists is severely impaired. The failure of these platelets to interact with fibrinogen and fibrin may explain the clot retraction abnormalities. Thrombasthenia is one of the few forms of platelet dysfunction in which hemorrhage is severe. Bleeding of all types, including epistaxis, ecchymoses and hematomas, and gastrointestinal and urinary hemorrhage have been reported.[67] Petechiae are rare. Posttraumatic and postsurgical bleeding is profuse. Treatment of thrombasthenia is difficult. Both corticoids and platelet transfusions have been used without impressive results.[68]

CANINE THROMBASTHENIC—THROMBOPATHIA

This disorder of platelet aggregation was discussed under the section entitled Qualitative Platelet Disorders above because of its similarity to Bernard-Soulier syndrome.

CANINE THROMBOPATHIA

Clinical bleeding is the result of platelet dysfunction in this disease of Basset hounds. It is an autosomal defect attributable to abnormal cAMP metabolism and the consequent failure of thrombopathic platelets to aggregate and secrete in response to most stimuli.[60, 69, 70] The disorder is widespread in Basset hound breeding stock in North America.[60] Clinical signs are similar to those of canine thrombasthenic thrombopathia, although auricular hematomas are common in the Basset breed.[60]

Platelet morphology, clot retraction, and platelet aggregation with thrombin are normal, but platelet aggregation is abnormal with other agonists.[60] Affected platelets are able to undergo the normal shape change reaction. Analyses of surface and internal platelet constituents are also normal.[71–75] The result of the abnormal cAMP metabolism is a clinically significant bleeding disorder.[60, 71]

No definitive conclusions have been made about inheritance of the trait, although clinical and laboratory evidence suggest variable penetrance and expression.[60] Identification of the asymptomatic carrier state is based on platelet function testing although a test to screen for the trait has been developed and appears to detect at least some animals with mild thrombopathia or borderline platelet function.[60] The use of topical thrombin to control posttraumatic hemorrhage is suggested as the thrombopathic platelets are thrombin-responsive.

HEREDITARY HYPOFIBRINOGENEMIA

In patients with this poorly understood platelet dysfunction, bleeding time is prolonged and ADP-induced platelet aggregation is deficient. This appears to be consistent with evidence that fibrinogen is necessary for normal platelet aggregation.[76] Clinical signs are variable but may be severe, with muscle and joint bleeding seen in addition to mucosal bleeding. Therapy for bleeding episodes consists of fibrinogen replacement with cryoprecipitate. Hemostasis is usually adequate with fibrinogen concentrations of 50 to 100 mg/dl.[76]

Hereditary Thrombocytopathies— Miscellaneous Hereditary Platelet Functional Disorders

A number of heritable platelet functional disorders, described in people, include isolated platelet factor 3 (PF3) deficiency, May-Hegglin anomaly, Ehlers-Danlos syndrome, and the mucopolysaccharidoses. In PF3 deficiency, platelets are normal in most respects but are unable to accelerate the generation of thrombin, a function of the factor.

Acquired Thrombocytopathies— Secondary to Disease

UREMIA

The major cause of bleeding associated with uremia is platelet dysfunction but the etiology is multifactorial. Bleeding associated with uremia includes epistaxis, bleeding into fascial planes, serous cavities, and the gastrointestinal tract. Bleeding time is often prolonged, and platelet aggregation studies reveal evidence of deficient release reaction and abnormal PF3 activity. Primary ADP-induced aggregation is also reduced. The biochemical abnormalities are consistent with deficient thromboxane production due to functional cyclooxygenase deficiency.[77]

Several metabolites known to accumulate in uremia have been proposed as platelet toxins. These include urea, guanidinosuccinic acid, phenol, phenolic acids and

"middle molecules."[78] Acquired storage pool disease due to microangiopathic interactions of platelets with roughened vascular surfaces may be present.[78] Severe anemia per se may prolong the bleeding time in uremic patients but the cause of this phenomenon is obscure.[79] Uremic blood vessels apparently secrete abnormally large amounts of PGI2 which could further inhibit platelet function.[80] Hemodialysis reverses platelet dysfunction in some uremic patients but the response is not immediate or complete.[81] Aspirin and other inhibitors of platelet function should be avoided.

Cryoprecipitate and DDAVP shorten the bleeding time in uremic patients. Although the concentrations of hemophilic A factor (factor VIII:C) and vWf:Ag are usually elevated in uremia, as measured by usual methods, preliminary evidence indicates that factor VIII multimers are unusually small, a finding similar to some variants of VWD. It is theorized that this abnormality may be corrected by administration of cryoprecipitate, and that DDAVP produces a similar effect endogenously by inducing the endothelial synthesis of large factor VIII multimers. Both of these agents have been used in the treatment of uremic bleeding with some success, although the responses were transitory. The nature of the factor VIII abnormality in uremia and the rationale for these therapeutic modalities remain poorly understood.[82]

DYSPROTEINEMIA

Although hypergammaglobulinemia is known to produce abnormalities in clot formation as the result of its effect on the conversion of fibrinogen to fibrin, it appears as if a bleeding diathesis due to abnormal platelet function is present in some patients with myeloma. Prolongation of bleeding time and decreased platelet adhesion, along with variable abnormalities in platelet aggregation, are the most characteristic findings.[1, 83] There is reasonably good correlation between the plasma concentration of the myeloma protein and the degree of platelet dysfunction. Patients with IgA myeloma may have a disproportionately high risk of having platelet abnormalities. When the immunoglobulin concentration is reduced to normal, the platelet function defects tend to disappear. Protein coating of the surface of the platelet has been proposed to explain these phenomena and, in fact, it has recently been shown that there is an increase in firmly bound platelet associated IgG whenever the plasma concentration of IgG is increased, even in diseases such as systemic lupus erythematosus and rheumatoid arthritis. This last observation has significant implications for the interpretation of increased concentrations of platelet associated IgG as evidence of an immune platelet disorder in these dysproteinemic or hypergammaglobulinemic states.[83]

HEPATIC DISEASE

The effects of hepatic disease are multifactorial. Severe diffuse hepatic disease often results in hypersplenism due to shunting of hepatic blood to splenic vessels, splenic engorgement, and trapping of increased numbers of circulating platelets in the splenic pool (approximately one-third of the platelet mass is in the splenic pool at any given time normally). Severe diffuse liver disease is associated with defective coagulation protein synthesis as well. There is also evidence that low grade disseminated intravascular coagulation (DIC) occurs continually in severe liver disease. Impaired clearance of plasminogen activators, which substantially increase the circulating concentrations of the fibrinolytic enzyme plasmin, may further contribute to high concentrations of fibrin(ogen) degradation products. These products interfere with platelet function and their concentration correlates with clinical hemorrhage in severe hepatic cirrhosis. Reduced amounts of platelet membrane GPIb in hepatic disease may cause defects in platelet adhesion. Any attempt at therapy must be directed at the primary disease.[84]

MYELOPROLIFERATIVE DISEASES

Platelet function abnormalities occur in myeloproliferative diseases: chronic myeloid leukemia, polycythemia rubra vera, essential thrombocythemia, acute leukemias, and myelofibrosis. The platelet counts in these disorders are often elevated, but the bleeding time may be prolonged, and clinical bleeding may appear as mucosal hemorrhage and hematomas. The abnormality resembles storage pool disease. Megakaryocytes are often abnormal with separated nuclei; the peripheral platelets may be large and poorly granulated. Management of acute hemorrhage consists, ideally, of transfusion of normal platelets. Fresh blood may contribute enough platelets to stimulate the patient's defective platelets to undergo the release reaction, presumably by supplying enough ADP to induce aggregation of patient platelets.[84–86]

PANCREATITIS

Experimentally induced acute necrotizing pancreatitis and associated DIC are characterized by erythrocyte fragmentation, increased platelet turnover as indicated by megathrombocytes, and increased fibrin(ogen) degradation products. Platelet aggregation in the presence of arachidonic acid, ADP, and collagen is decreased. Plasma TXA_2 and prostaglandin E2 are unchanged. Defects in platelet function are thought to be the result of fibrin(ogen) degradation products and platelet exhaustion.[87]

CANINE EHRLICHIOSIS

Experimentally induced canine ehrlichiosis resulted in modest thrombocytopenia and significant decreases in mean platelet adhesiveness.[88] There was no correlation between platelet numbers and adhesiveness in dogs that were decomplemented.[88] However, there was a correlation between platelet numbers and adhesiveness in dogs with normal complement concentrations.[88] Dogs with normal complement concentrations also had more severe thrombocytopenia.[88] As heparin is known to reduce complement concentrations, therapy with this drug may be helpful in moderating the degree of thrombocytopenia and platelet dysfunction in these patients, and in patients with immune thrombocytopenia.

THROMBOCYTHEMIA

An elevated platelet count, a count beyond the reference interval, can result from various clinical disorders and is referred to as reactive thrombocytosis. In reactive thrombocytosis, tests of platelet function including bleeding time and measurements of platelet adhesion and aggregation are generally normal, and patients do not suffer from clinical hemorrhage or thrombosis. In contrast, the platelet count can be elevated autonomously in myeloproliferative disorders: chronic myeloid leukemia, myeloid metaplasia, myelofibrosis, polycythemia rubra vera, and essential thrombocythemia.[84, 89] In these situations, tests of platelet function are frequently abnormal and there is some propensity towards hemorrhage and thrombosis. There does not seem to be a correlation between the platelet number and clinical manifestations. However, the poorly functioning platelets evidently predispose to hemorrhage and, paradoxically, to thrombosis. Neither the platelet number nor platelet function measurement predict the degree of thrombosis or hemorrhage. Platelet lipoxygenase activity is always normal in patients with reactive thrombocytosis but is reduced or deficient in some patients with thrombocythemia of myeloproliferative disease. Curiously, patients were more likely to have bleeding complications (67 per cent) than thrombotic events (13 per cent).[85, 90, 91]

Clinically, the hemorrhagic signs include mucosal and particularly gastrointestinal bleeding, hematomas, and ecchymoses. Splenic, portal, and mesenteric vein thrombosis have been reported without pulmonary embolism.[90, 91]

In thrombocythemia, defective platelet function appears to be the main problem. Chemotherapy may depress the more dysplastic megakaryocytic clones and allow the more normally differentiated clones to deliver platelets. Alkylating agents such as melphelan (in increasing doses up to 4.0 mg/square meter) should be administered cautiously in an attempt to reduce platelet numbers. Hydroxyurea at a dose of 590 mg/square meter has been used successfully in dogs. This drug may cause severe megaloblastic anemia. Cycles of two weeks on therapy followed by two weeks off therapy will minimize this complication. Intravenous administration of serial doses of radioactive phosphorus to a total of 9.8 microcuries/square meter may also be used.[92] An ultralow dose aspirin (0.2 mg/lb or 0.5 mg/kg q12h) has proven to be most effective in inhibiting platelet aggregation if thrombosis is suspected of becoming a potential complicating factor.[93] Considering the number of patients with hemorrhagic diatheses rather than thrombosis, the use of aspirin or other nonsteroidal antiinflammatory agents requires some thought.

MISCELLANEOUS

In *systemic lupus erythematosus* and *chronic idiopathic thrombocytopenic purpura*, both diseases associated with antiplatelet antibodies, there are platelet functional de-

TABLE 117–6. DRUGS ASSOCIATED WITH PLATELET DYSFUNCTION

Anesthetics–local and general‡
Antibiotics–ampicillin, carbenicillin, cephalosporin, penicillin G, tetracycline‡
Antihistamines–chlorpheniramine maleate, diphenhydramine‡
Chemotherapeutic agents–daunorubicin
Diethylcarbamazine
Nonsteroidal antiinflammatory agents–aspirin, phenylbutazone, sulfinpyrazone, ibuprofen, indomethacin, tolbutamide*
Heparin
Macromolecules–dextran
Nitrofurantoin
Phenothiazines–chlorpromazine
Propanolol
Pyrimidine compounds–dipyrimadole†
Sulfasalazine
Vinca alkaloids

*Inhibitors of prostaglandin synthesis
†Elevate cyclic AMP
‡Membrane-active drugs

fects due to decreased granular content ATP. Platelet adhesive dysfunction in *hypothyroidism* may be due to decreased membrane concentrations of the factor VIII complex. In *cardiomyopathy* there is increased platelet sensitivity to ADP as an agonist. The mechanism is unknown.[60, 118]

Acquired Thrombocytopathies—Drug-Induced Disorders (Table 117–6)

SALICYLATES

Salicylates are salts or esters of salicylic acid used commonly by humans to medicate animals. Salicylates are available as over-the-counter preparations (Table 117–7). The principal site of salicylate metabolism is the liver, where it is conjugated with glucuronic acid. Glucuronyl transferase is the enzyme responsible for this reaction and is present in the hepatic microsomal system of mammals. Cats and neonates of most species have low concentrations of this enzyme. This is thought to be

TABLE 117–7. OVER-THE-COUNTER PREPARATIONS CONTAINING SALICYLATES*

Pain Relievers
Anacin (Whitehall)
Ben-Gay (Leeming)
Bufferin (Bristol-Myers)
Doan's Pills (Jeffrey Martin)
Excedrin (Bristol-Myers)
Ecotrin (Menley & James)
Momentum (Whitehall)
Antiinflammatory Agents
Ascriptin (Rorer)
Di-Gesic (Central)
Verin (Verex)
Cold Medicines
Alka-Seltzer Plus (Miles)
Bayer Children's Cold Tablets (Glenbrook)
Coricidin "D" Decongestant Tablets (Schering)
4-way Cold Tablets (Bristol-Myers)
Antidiarrheal
Pepto-Bismol (Proctor & Gamble)

*Modified from Handagama P: Salicylate toxicity. *In* Kirk RW (ed): Current Veterinary Therapy IX. Philadelphia, WB Saunders, 1986, p 523.

the reason for the inability of these individuals to metabolize salicylates rapidly, functionally prolonging the metabolic half-life of the compound. Salicylates as aspirin are largely excreted by the kidney through a combination of glomerular filtration and proximal tubular secretion. Excretion is influenced by the rate of urine flow and the pH of the urine.

Ingestion of aspirin affects all circulating platelets irreversibly. Cyclic endoperoxides and TXA_2 are potent inducers of platelet release and aggregation. Aspirin acetylates and inhibits cyclooxygenase that catalyzes synthesis of endoperoxides.[84, 94] Platelets, unlike cells that have nuclei, are unable to regenerate enzymes such as cyclooxygenase. After acetylation and inhibition of this enzyme the platelet is permanently impaired. Bleeding time is prolonged as aspirin, through these processes, is a potent inhibitor of platelet aggregation. In the presence of another hemostatic defect such as VWD, a disease where platelet adherence is impaired, the combined poor adherence and aggregation could lead to serious hemorrhage. Animals with renal or hepatic disease and marginal hemostatic systems may also be affected by aspirin therapy. Some apparently normal subjects display marked sensitivity to the action of aspirin, so that their bleeding times are prolonged and clinical hemorrhage may occur after surgery or trauma. These patients may have a mild form of storage pool disease.

Endothelial cells have nuclei and can rapidly regenerate inactivated enzymes. As a result the synthesis of arachidonate and the production of PGI2 is less susceptible than platelets to aspirin inhibition. Thus the absence of platelet aggregatory TXA_2 and the presence of a potent platelet antiaggregating agent PGI2 is another potential complication. This antiplatelet effect has been utilized in clinical situations in which thrombus formation is a potential problem.[94]

If a patient requires analgesia, acetaminophen may be used in dogs because it does not prolong the bleeding time. If salicylate therapy is required, the sodium salt appears to modify platelets only slightly.[84]

OTHER NONSTEROIDAL ANTIINFLAMMATORY AGENTS

These include indomethacin, phenylbutazone, naproxen, and ibuprofen. All of these agents produce inhibition of the platelet release reaction, although, unlike aspirin, the effect seems to last only as long as the drug is in the circulation. Platelet aggregation with arachidonic acid or collagen, but not ADP, as agonists detected phenylbutazone-induced platelet aggregation inhibition as early as 1.5 hours after administration in the dog.[95] Much less information is available about the clinical risks with the use of these drugs, but it is prudent to avoid them in patients at risk for excessive hemorrhage.[1]

DEXTRANS

The 40,000 dalton form of dextran is readily excreted but the 70,000 dalton form may persist in circulation for three days and interfere with platelet surface action. In addition to prolonging the bleeding time, there is evidence of red blood cell aggregation. Management involves support until the dextran is excreted. Transfused platelets are affected by dextrans in plasma.

ANTIBIOTICS

Carbenicillin and penicillin can inhibit platelet aggregation. Massive doses of penicillin prolong the bleeding time and impair collagen and ristocetin-induced platelet aggregation. Similar effects are seen with ticarcillin and ampicillin.

Moxalactam, a β-lactam antibiotic with a structure similar to that of carbenicillin, can cause hemorrhage by several apparently different mechanisms.[96, 97] It can cause a platelet functional defect after three to five days of therapy at a dosage greater than 4 gm per day. This disorder is characterized by a long bleeding time with a normal platelet count. Moxalactam apparently binds to a site on the platelet membrane that interferes with the development of the ADP-lectin required for platelet aggregation. If bleeding associated with this or other antibiotics is noted, the drug should be stopped. The use of moxalactam with nonsteroidal antiinflammatory agents that inhibit platelet cyclooxygenase should be avoided because these two classes of inhibitors may have additive and potentially disastrous effects on platelet function.

Moxalactam also inhibits the growth of gut flora, thereby blocking the endogenous production of vitamin K.

MISCELLANEOUS DRUGS

A wide variety of other agents can modify platelet function but it is not entirely clear that these agents cause clinical hemorrhage. Heparin may prolong the bleeding time slightly, but does not produce abnormal bleeding in normal subjects. Antihistamines and anesthetics may inhibit the platelet release reaction by stabilizing the membranes of mitochondria and other platelet organelles.[98]

Acquired Thrombocytopathies—Disorders Associated with Hypercoagulation

Hypercoagulability has been proposed to explain the increased incidence of thrombosis encountered in certain clinical states associated with thrombotic diatheses. Hypercoagulability has been defined as "an altered state of circulating blood that requires a smaller quantity of clot-promoting substances to induce intravascular coagulation than is required to produce comparable thrombosis in a normal subject."[99]

Hypercholesterolemia has two biologic effects, damage of the vascular endothelium and induction of platelet hyperfunction. Platelet hyperfunction is associated with hypercoagulability. The effect on platelet function has been extensively investigated.[100] Increased *in vitro* platelet aggregation by various aggregating agents occurs in Type II hyperlipoproteinemia. Enhanced platelet function is probably related to the incorporation of choles-

terol into membrane phospholipids, which leads to increased synthesis of TXA_2 via the cyclooxygenase pathway.[101] Hypercholesterolemia induces degenerative changes in the endothelium with a concurrent proliferation of smooth muscle cells. Moreover, hypercholesterolemic enhancement of platelet function increases the chance for platelets to interact with both the damaged vascular wall, to form mural thrombi, and with each other to form circulating platelet aggregates.[102] Several common hypercholesterolemic states will be briefly discussed because of the propensity of these problems towards thrombotic disease.

NEPHROTIC SYNDROME

The nephrotic syndrome can best be described as a complex of protein-wasting kidney diseases. It is caused by increased permeability to plasma proteins which results in increased filtration of proteins, especially albumin, into the renal tubules. This increased loss of plasma proteins leads to a decline in albumin concentration.

Nephrotic syndrome characterized by hypoalbuminemia and hyperlipidemia is associated with increased incidence of thrombotic disease and platelet hyperaggregability. Although plasma coagulation proteins are also abnormal, changes are too consistent to attribute thrombotic phenomena to the coagulation cascade alone. Antithrombin III has been shown to be deficient in nephrotic syndrome. The urinary loss of this endogenous serine protease inhibitor removes a natural barrier to hypercoagulation.[103, 104]

It is known that platelet-to-platelet interactions require exposure of platelet fibrinogen receptors, platelet crossbridging, and subsequent platelet aggregation. Hyperlipidemia and hypoalbuminemia in nephrotic syndrome increases the availability of TXA_2 by increasing the availability of precursor metabolites and the removal of TXA_2 inhibitors. Thromboxane A_2 is a known inducer of platelet aggregation partially through the exposure of platelet fibrinogen receptors.[103–106]

Platelet aggregation studies on dogs with nephrosis disclosed increased platelet sensitivity to ADP. Subsequent studies with isolated platelets and plasma indicated that a plasma factor was primarily responsible for inducing platelet hypersensitivity. The increased platelet aggregation response was corrected by increasing the albumin content of the plasma. The study suggested an important role for albumin in modulating platelet aggregation and may partially explain the tendency toward thrombosis noted in hypoalbuminemic dogs with renal disease.[106]

A complex *in vitro* effect of low albumin on platelet arachidonic acid metabolism has been described wherein there is an accelerated conversion of arachidonic acid to TXA_2.[101]

Management of nephrotic syndrome requires treatment of the underlying glomerular disease. Supportive care requires a diet that is normal in protein of good biologic value and provides essential vitamins. An ultra-low dose of aspirin (0.2 gm/lb or 0.5 gm/kg q12h) is suggested to inhibit platelet aggregation and potential thrombosis.[93]

DIABETES MELLITUS

Platelet aggregability in response to aggregating agents is enhanced in diabetes mellitus.[107, 108] Circulating platelet aggregates and plasma concentrations of β-thromboglobulin are also increased.[109] There is a correlation between platelet hyperfunction and vascular complications. Enhancement of platelet function appears to be related to alteration in platelet arachidonic acid metabolism. Thromboxane A_2 formation in response to platelet stimuli is increased in diabetics as compared to normal patients (see Nephrotic Syndrome above).[108] Platelet hyperfunction probably contributes to the occlusion of small arteries. However, mechanisms by which diabetes mellitus enhances atherogenesis are unclear.

HYPERADRENALCORTICISM

Thromboembolic complications have been reported in people and dogs with spontaneous hyperadrenalcorticism. A hypercoagulable state has been suggested in this syndrome and is characterized by impaired fibrinolysis, increased concentrations of coagulation factors, and platelet hypersensitivity.[109]

Because of the commonality of hypercholesterolemia in this and the preceding discussions, it seems clear that platelet hyperfunction in this disease is induced by similar metabolic pathways.[110–111]

PLATELET FUNCTION ASSESSMENT

It is generally agreed that the hemostatic system is composed of three separate but intimately related systems, that is, the vascular component, the contribution of platelets, and finally the coagulation of specific plasma proteins to form the blood clot. The vascular component is difficult to assess and few specific tests are available. The clinical assessment of the patient can add much to this aspect of the bleeding patient. Coagulation assessment is discussed elsewhere in this book.[112]

This section briefly focuses upon tests available for the evaluation of adequacy of platelet function. While newer information is coming from research laboratories, there are a number of platelet function procedures, used for some time, in which there is confidence. How these fit with the patient having a platelet problem is a clinical challenge.[112, 113]

PLATELET COUNTING

Platelet counting is the logical first step in the assessment of a platelet disorder. If the platelet count is known, the functions expected from the platelet component of the hemostatic process can be deduced. In thrombocytopenia, platelet function is obviously reduced even though individual platelets function normally. Conversely, normal numbers of functionally deficient platelets will result in problems for the patient.[112]

BLEEDING TIME

This relatively unsophisticated test is probably the easiest and best single test of platelet function. The test is fraught with iatrogenic problems. Most of these will normalize the test. In essence, practically everything in the test performed incorrectly will make a potentially abnormal test normal. However, a prolonged test in this milieu becomes quite significant. The test is uncomfortable for patients, requires close attention to detail, and is frequently invalidated by patient medications, chiefly nonsteroidal antiinflammatory agents.

The buccal mucosal bleeding time as previously described under the section in this chapter entitled Von Willebrand's Disease, is the most reproducible.[43] In this procedure the patient is held in lateral recumbency and a strip of 5 cm wide gauze is positioned around the maxilla to fold the upper lip upwards. The gauze should be just tight enough to slightly impede venous return causing modest engorgement of the mucosal surface. A spring loaded device (Simplate II: Organon Teknika Corp.) is use to make two parallel 5 mm by 1 mm deep incisions in the mucosal surface. Incision sites are chosen which are devoid of visible blood vessels and inclined so that shed blood should flow with gravity towards the dog's mouth. At the exact time the incisions are made a stopwatch is engaged. Shed blood should be blotted at approximately five second intervals with circles of filter paper gently placed against the mucosal surface 1 to 2 mm below the incisions. Care must be taken to prevent direct disturbance of the incision sites. The bleeding time endpoint is the time from incision until the filter paper fails to acquire a red crescent when positioned near the incision sites. With this technique, bleeding times for normal dogs range from 1.7 to 4.2 minutes with a mean of 2.6 minutes.[43]

For patients with platelet count above 75,000/μl, the bleeding time correlates well with platelet function. Below that platelet concentration, the bleeding time is progressively prolonged with decreasing platelet counts, in general being inversely correlated with the bleeding time. Nonsteroidal antiinflammatory agents will interfere with platelet function, and aspirin will interfere with platelet function for as long as one week. Therefore, drug history is mandatory for the interpretation of this study.[114]

CLOT RETRACTION

This simple test requires a test tube of whole blood. The tube is placed in a rack at room temperature and is observed for 24 hours. Normal clot retraction results in a small clot which is tightly adherent to a small section of the test tube. The clot has a smooth surface and is surrounded by clear serum. Clot retraction is dependent upon platelet numbers and the functional capacity of the platelets, the quantity of fibrinogen, and the packed cell volume. Retraction and expression of serum from the clot are poor in thrombocytopenia. The clot is small and red cell fallout is increased with hypofibrinogenemia and abnormalities in fibrinogen. An increased packed cell volume usually results in increased red cell fallout, as in polycythemia.[115]

PLATELET AGGREGATION

Platelet aggregation refers to the ability of the platelets to stick to one another. While ADP is the physiological agent usually responsible for *in vivo* aggregation, a variety of different substances are used in the laboratory for aggregation studies. These include epinephrine, collagen, thrombin, arachidonic acid, and ristocetin as well as ADP. The pattern of reactions provides the diagnostic information of use in evaluating platelet function. Because there is some variability in commercial reagents each laboratory must develop and utilize normal controls, normal patterns, and their own normal aggregation curves.

When blood is suspended in 0.1 M citrate, platelets can react with the aggregating agonists. The test requires differential centrifugation to obtain platelet rich plasma. This procedure can take as long as 30 minutes. As platelet viability and reactivity are markedly reduced within minutes, it is both ideal and critical to obtain fresh blood and immediately begin the platelet separation in preparation for the aggregation studies.

An aggregometer is an optical device in which a suspension of platelets is monitored for relative clarity. The platelets are maintained at 37°C in a uniform suspension by a magnetically driven ersatz flea. A suspension of single platelets is turbid, whereas aggregating platelets clear the suspension that is being monitored by a light path. A variety of aggregating agents are added to the platelet suspension and a record of relative turbidity with time is produced. Meticulous attention to details, including the provision of fresh samples and the adjustment of the platelet suspension to a standard concentration of platelets, is required for accurate testing.

PLATELET ADHESION

Platelet adhesion, in contrast to platelet aggregation, is defined as the irreversible sticking of platelets to any nonplatelet surface. It is dependent upon factors such as shear rate, platelet membrane glycoproteins, and red cell concentration.[112] *In vivo* adhesion is further influenced by the characteristics of the vascular endothelium as well as plasma concentrations of vWf. It is the relationship to VWD that initially spurred interest in *in vivo* testing for disorders of adhesion. While there are a number of techniques for the measurement of adhesion including glass bead columns, newer tests for VWD have largely replaced the less specific adhesion tests.

TESTING FOR HYPERCOAGULABILITY

There is a need for a battery of tests which will effectively screen for thrombotic milieu. A number of

TABLE 117–8. TESTS FOR HYPERCOAGULABILITY

Routinely performed tests
Increased fibrin(ogen) degradation products
Decreased thrombin time
Decreased activated partial thromboplastin time
Decreased prothrombin time
Decreased fibrinogen concentration
Variable platelet counts above or below reference intervals
More specific tests
Decreased concentrations of antithrombin III
Decreased concentrations of Protein C
Less specific tests
Increased "hyperaggregable" platelets
Increased platelet adhesiveness
Increased blood viscosity

nonspecific tests have been described (Table 117–8) but, as yet, there are no tests which have withstood intensive scrutiny.[116] Antithrombin III (ATIII) deficient patients are predisposed to thrombosis. The thrombotic risk of patients having ATIII deficiency is considered moderate when ATIII concentrations are between 50 and 75 per cent of normal and are marked when ATIII concentrations are less than 50 per cent. Antithrombin III deficiencies in nephrotic syndrome, DIC, and hepatic disease are associated with thrombotic manifestations. Measurement of ATIII is indicated in animals with these diseases and in patients with other causes of recurrent thrombosis. These concentrations are also the logical basis for improving patient management and prognostic decisions.[117]

References

1. Coller, BS: Disorders of platelets. *In* Ratnoff, OD and Forbes, CD (eds): Disorders of hemostasis. New York, Grune & Stratton, 1984, p 73.
2. White, JG, et al.: Platelet ultrastructure. *In* Bloom, AL and Thomas, DP (eds): Haemostasis and Thrombosis. Edinburgh, Churchill Livingstone, 1981, p 22.
3. Zwall, RFA, et al.: Topological and kinetic aspects of phospholipids in blood coagulation. *In* Mann, KG and Taylor, FB, Jr (eds): The Regulation of Coagulation. New York, Elsevier North-Holland, 1980, p 95.
4. Shattil, SJ and Bennett, JS: Platelets and their membranes in hemostasis: Physiology and pathophysiology. Ann Intern Med 94:108, 1980.
5. Phillips, DR: An evaluation of membrane glycoproteins in platelet adhesion and aggregation. *In* Spaet, TH (ed): Progress in Hemostasis and Thrombosis. New York, Grune & Stratton, 1980, p 81.
6. Kunicki, TJ, et al,: Further studies of the human platelet receptor for quinine- and quinidine-dependent antibodies. J Immunol 126:398, 1981.
7. Moore, A, et al.: Interaction of platelet membrane receptors with von Willebrand factor, ristocetin, and the Fc region of immunoglobin G. J Clin Invest 62:1053, 1978.
8. Kunicki, TJ, et al.: The formation of Ca++-dependent complexes of platelet membrane glycoproteins IIB and IIIa in solution as determined by crossed immunoelectrophoresis. Blood 58:268, 1981.
9. Bennett, JS and Vilaire, G: Exposure of platelet fibrinogen receptors by ADP and epinephrine. J Clin Invest 64:1393, 1979.
10. Coller, BS: Interaction of normal, thrombasthenic, and Bernard-Soulier platelets with immobilized fibrinogen: defective platelet-fibrinogen interaction in thrombasthenia. Blood 55:169, 1980.
11. Lee, et al.: Relationship between fibrinogen binding and the platelet glycoprotein deficiencies in Glanzmann's thrombasthenia Type I and Type II. Br J Haematol 48:47, 1981.
12. Coller, BS: Preliminary characterization of hybridoma antibodies that inhibit fibrinogen-platelet interactions. Blood 58:191a, 1981.
13. Handagama, PJ, et al.: Scanning electron microscopic study of platelet release by canine megakaryocytes in vitro. Am J Vet Res 48:1003, 1987.
14. Nachmias, VT, et al.: Observations on the "cytoskeleton" of human platelets. Thromb Haemost 42:1661, 1979.
15. Deuel, TF, et al.: Platelet factor 4 is chemotactic for neutrophils and monocytes. Proc Natl Acad Sci USA 78:4587, 1981.
16. Niewiarowski, S: Platelet release reaction and secreted platelet proteins. *In* Bloom, AL and Thomas, DP (eds): Haemostasis and Thrombosis. Edinburgh, Churchill Livingstone, 1981, p 73.
17. Vargaftig, BB, et al.: Background and present status of research

on platelet-activating factor (PAF-acether). Ann NY Acad Sci 370:119, 1981.

18. Fauvel, F, et al.: Interaction of blood platelets with a microfibrillar extract form adult bovine aorta: Requirement for von Willebrand factor. Proc Natl Acad Sci USA 80:551, 1983.

19. Pethica, BA: The physical chemistry of cell adhesion. Exp Cell Res 8(suppl):123, 1961.

20. Feinstein, MB, et al.: Cyclic AMP and calcium in platelet function. In Gordon, JL (ed): Platelets in Biology and Pathology. Amsterdam, Elsevier/North-Holland, 1981, p 437.

21. Coller, BS: Inhibition of von Willebrand factor-dependent platelet function by increased platelet cyclic AMP and its prevention by cytoskeleton-disrupting agents. Blood 57:846, 1981.

22. Harris, HE and Weeds, AG: Platelet actin: sub-cellular distribution and association with profilin. FEBS Lett 90:84, 1978.

23. Dormandy, JA: Haemorheology and thrombosis. In Bloom, AL and Thomas, DP (eds): Haemostasis and Thrombosis. Edinburgh, Churchill Livingstone, 1981, p 610.

24. Lollar, P and Owen, WG: Active-site-dependent, thrombin-induced release of adenine nucleotides from cultured human endothelial cells. Ann NY Acad Sci 370:51, 1981.

25. Marcus, et al.: Synthesis of prostacyclin from platelet-derived endoperoxides by cultured human endothelial cells. J Clin Invest 66:979, 1980.

26. Dodds, WJ: Second international registry of animal models of thrombosis and hemorrhagic diseases. ILAR News 24:1, 1981.

27. Bowie, DJW, et al.: Tests of hemostasis in swine: normal values and values in pigs affected with von Willebrand's disease. Am J Vet Res 34:1405, 1973.

28. Benson, RE and Dodds, WJ: Autosomal factor VIII deficiency in rabbits: size variations of rabbit factor VIII. Thromb Haemostas 38:380, 1977.

29. Dodds, WJ: Bleeding diseases of small animals. Vet Ref Lab Newslet 8:1, 1984.

30. Johnson, GS: University of Missouri, College of Veterinary Medicine. Personal communication, 1987.

31. Chopek, MW, et al.: Human von Willebrand factor: a multivalent protein composed of identical subunits. Biochemistry 25:3146, 1986.

32. Jaffe, EA, et al.: Synthesis of antihemophilic factor antigen by cultured human endothelial cells. J Clin Invest 52:2757, 1973.

33. Johnson, GS, et al.: Canine von Willebrand's disease: a heterogeneous group of bleeding disorders. Vet Clin North Am Vol 18, Jan 1988.

34. Zucker, MB, et al.: Factor VIII-related antigen in human blood platelets: localization and release by thrombin and collagen. J Lab Clin Med 94:675, 1979.

35. Bowie, EJW, et al.: Transplantation of normal bone marrow into a pig with severe von Willebrand's disease. J Clin Invest 78:26, 1986.

36. Turitto, VT, et al.: Platelet interaction with rabbit subendothelium in von Willebrand's disease: altered thrombus formation distinct from defective platelet adhesion. J Clin Invest 74:1730, 1984.

37. Weiss, HJ, et al.: Stabilization of factor VIII in plasma by the von Willebrand factor: studies on posttransfusion and dissociated factor VIII and in patients with von Willebrand's disease. J Clin Invest 60:390, 1977.

38. Rogers, JS and Shane, SR: Factor VIII activity in normal volunteers receiving oral thyroid hormone. J Lab Clin Med 102:444, 1983.

39. Prentice, CRM, et al.: Rise of factor VIII after exercise and adrenaline infusion, measured by immunological and biological techniques. Thromb Res 1:493, 1972.

40. Hoyer, LW: The factor VIII complex: structure and function. Blood 58:1, 1981.

41. Marder, VJ, et al.: Standard nomenclature for factor VIII and von Willebrand factor: a recommendation by the International Committee of Thrombosis and Haemostasis. Thromb Haemostas 54:871, 1985.

42. Howard, MA, et al.: Variant von Willebrand's disease type B - revisited. Blood 60:1420, 1982.

43. Jergens, AE, et al.: Buccal mucosa bleeding times of healthy dogs and dogs in various pathologic states including thrombocytopenia, uremia, and von Willebrand's disease. Am J Vet Res 48:1337, 1986.

44. Benson, RE and Dodds, WJ: Immunologic characterization of canine factor VIII. Blood 48:521, 1976.

45. Benson, RE, et al.: Efficiency and precision of electroimmunoassay for canine factor VIII-related antigen. Am J Vet Res 44:399, 1983.

46. Benson, RE, et al.: A practical technique for preparation of antiserum to canine factor VIII-related antigen. Vet Immunol Immunopath 7:337, 1984.

47. Walker, DB, et al.: Evaluation of a kit for "in clinic" diagnosis of vWd. Vet Clin Path 15:4, 1986.

48. Meyers, LJ, et al.: Hemorrhagic diathesis resembling pseudo-hemophilia in a dog. JAVMA 161:1028, 1972.

49. Dodds, WJ: Von Willebrand's disease in dogs. Mod Vet Pract 65:681, 1984.

50. Johnson, GS, et al.: A bleeding disease (von Willebrand's disease) in a Chesapeake Bay retriever. JAVMA 176:1261, 1980.

51. Dodds, WJ: Further studies of canine von Willebrand's disease. Blood 45:221, 1975.

52. Bouma, BN, et al.: Infusion of human and canine VIII in dogs with von Willebrand's disease: studies of the von Willebrand and factor VIII synthesis stimulating factors. Scand J Haematol 17:263, 1976.

53. Hamilton, H, et al.: Von Willebrand's disease manifested by hemorrhage from the reproductive tract: two case reports. JAAHA 21:637, 1985.

54. Jolly, RD, et al.: Screening for genetic diseases: principles and practice. Adv Vet Sci Comp Med 25:245, 1981.

55. Johnstone, IB and Crane, S: Von Willebrand's disease in two families of Doberman pinschers. Can Vet J 22:239, 1981.

56. Romatowski, J: Intercurrent hypothyroidism, autoimmune anemia, and a coagulation deficiency (von Willebrand's disease) in a dog. JAVMA 185:309, 1984.

57. Johnson, GS, et al.: Hemorrhagic from the cosmetic otoplasty of Doberman pinschers with von Willebrand's disease. Am J Vet Res 46:1335, 1985.

58. Johnson, GS, et al.: Type II von Willebrands's disease in German shorthair pointers. Vet Clin Path, in press.

59. Feldman, BF and Brummerstedt, E: Von Willebrand's factor deficiency in a random population of Danish golden retrievers. Nord Vet-Med 38:378, 1986.

60. Catalfamo, JL and Dodds, WJ: Inherited and acquired thrombopathias. Vet Clin North Am Vol 18, Jan 1988.

61. Randolph, JF, et al.: Factor XII deficiency and von Willebrand's disease in a family of miniature poodles. Cornell Vet 76:3, 1986.

62. Johnson, GS, et al.: DDAVP-induced increases in coagulation factor VIII and von Willebrand factor in the plasma of conscious dogs. J Vet Pharm Ther 9:370, 1986.

63. Dodds, WJ: Inherited bleeding disorders. Canine Pract 5:49, 1978.

64. Dodds, WJ: Familial canine thrombocytopathy. Thromb Diath Haemorrh 26:241, 1967.

65. George, JN, et al.: Molecular defects in interactions of platelets with the vessel wall. N Engl J Med 311:1084, 1984.

66. Meyers, KM: Pathobiology of animal platelets. Adv Vet Sci Comp Med 30:131, 1985.

67. Norden, AT and Caen, JP: The different glycoprotein abnormalities in thrombasthenic and Bernard-Soulier platelets. Semin Hematol 16:234, 1979.

68. Weiss, HJ: Platelet physiology and abnormalities of platelet function. N Engl J Med 293:580, 1975.

69. Johnstone, IB and Lotz, F: An inherited platelet function defect in basset hounds. Con Vet J 20:211, 1979.

70. Boudreaux, MK, et al.: Elevated cyclic AMP levels in canine thrombopathia. Thromb Haemostas 54:278, 1980.

71. Boudreaux, MK, et al.: Impaired cAMP metabolism associated with abnormal function of thrombopathic canine platelets. Biochem Biophys Res Comm 140:595, 1986.

72. Boudreaux, MK: Evidence for regulatory control of canine platelet phosphodiesterase. Biochem Biophys Res Comm 140:589, 1986.

73. Dodds, WJ: Bleeding disorders. In Morgan, RV (ed): Handbook of Small Animal Practice. New York, Churchill Livingstone (in press).

74. Catalfamo, JL, et al.: Defective platelet-fibrinogen interaction in hereditary canine thrombopathia. Blood 67:1568, 1986.

75. Bell, TG, et al.: Platelet function in Basset hound hereditary thrombopathia. Fed Proc 41:101, 1982 (abstract).

76. Gralnick, HR: Congenital disorders of fibrinogen. *In* Williams, WJ, et al. (eds): Hematology. 2nd ed. New York, McGraw-Hill, 1977, p 1423.

77. Deykin, D: Uremic bleeding. Kidney Int 24:678, 1983.

78. Gallice, P, et al.: In vitro inhibition of platelet aggregation by uremic middle molecules. Biomedicine (Paris) 33:185, 1980.

79. Livio, M, et al.: Uraemic bleeding: role of anemia and beneficial effect of red cell transfusions. Lancet 2:1013, 1982.

80. Swartz, RD: Hemorrhage during high risk hemodialysis using controlled heparinization. Nephron 28:65, 1981.

81. Rabiner, SF: Bleeding in uremia. Med Clin North Am 56:221, 1972.

82. Manucci, PM, et al.: Desamino-8-D-arginine vasopressin shortens bleeding time in uremia. N Engl J Med 308:8, 1983.

83. McGrath, KM, et al.: Correlation between serum IgG, platelet membrane IgG and platelet function in hypergamma globulinemic states. Br J Haematol 42:585, 1979.

84. Schrier, S: Disorders of hemostasis and coagulation. *In* Rubenstein, E and Federman, DD (eds): Scientific American Medicine. New York, Scientific American Inc, 1987, p VI:1-45.

85. Keenan, JP, et al.: Defective platelet lipid peroxidation in myeloproliferative disorders, a possible defect of prostaglandin synthesis. Br J Haematol 35:275, 1977.

86. Canfield, PJ, et al.: Myeloproliferative disorder in four dogs involving derangements of erythropoiesis, myelopoiesis and megakaryopoiesis. J Sm Anim Pract 27:7, 1986.

87. Jacobs, RM, et al.: Platelet function in experimentally induced pancreatitis in the dog. Throm Haemosta 55:197, 1986.

88. Lovering, SL, et al.: Serum complement and blood platelet adhesiveness in acute canine ehrlichiosis. Am J Vet Res 41:1260, 1980.

89. Silverstein, MN: Primary or hemorrhagic thrombocythemia. Arch Int Med 123:18, 1968.

90. Schafer, AI: Deficiency of platelet lipoxygenase activity in myeloproliferative disorders. N Engl J Med 306:381, 1982.

91. Hirsch, J: Hypercoagulability. Semin Hematol 14:409, 1977.

92. Degen, MA: Essential thrombocythemia in a dog: a myeloproliferative disorder. Personal communication.

93. Rackear, D, et al.: The effect of three different dosages of acetylsalicylic acid on canine platelet aggregation. JAAHA 24:23, 1988.

94. Handagama, P: Salicylate toxicity. *In* Kirk, RW (ed): Current Veterinary Therapy IX. Philadelphia, WB Saunders, 1986, p 523.

95. Jackson, ML, et al.: The effect of oral phenylbutazone on whole blood aggregation in the dog. Can J Comp Med 49:271, 1985.

96. Weitekamp, MR and Aber, RC: Prolonged bleeding times and bleeding diathesis associated with moxalactam administration. JAMA 249:69, 1983.

97. Antimicrobials and haemostasis (editorial). Lancet 1:510, 1983.

98. Jain, MK, et al.: Correlation of inhibition of platelet aggregation by phenothiazine and local anesthetics with their effects on a phospholipid bilayer. Thromb Res 13:1067, 1978.

99. Wall, RT and Harker, LH: The endothelium and thrombosis. Ann Rev Med 31:361, 1980.

100. Carvalho, ACH, et al.: Platelet function in hyperlipoproteinemia. N Engl J Med 290:434, 1974.

101. Stuart, MJ, et al.: Effect of cholesterol on production of thromboxane B_2 by platelets in vitro. N Engl J Med 302:6, 1980.

102. Tremoli, E, et al.: Platelet thromboxanes and serum cholesterol. Lancet 1, 8107:107, 1979.

103. Rasedee, A and Feldman, BF: Nephrotic syndrome: a platelet hyperaggregability state. Vet Res Comm 9:199, 1985.

104. Rasedee, A, et al.: Naturally occurring canine nephrotic syndrome is a potentially hypercoagulable state. Acta Vet Scand 27:369, 1986.

105. Green, RA and Kabel, AL: Hypercoagulable state in three dogs with nephrotic syndrome. Role of antithrombin III deficiency. JAVMA 181:914, 1982.

106. Green, RA, et al.: Hypoalbuminemia-related platelet hypersensitivity in two dogs with nephrotic syndrome. JAVMA 186:485, 1985.

107. Suehiro, A, et al.: The role of platelet hyperfunction in thrombus formation in hyperlipidemia. Thromb Res 25:331, 1982.

108. Halushka, PV, et al.: Increased platelet thromboxane synthesis in diabetes mellitus. J Lab Clin Med 97:87, 1981.

109. Preston, FE, et al.: Elevated β-thromboglobulin levels and circulating platelet aggregates in diabetic microangiopathy. Lancet 1:238, 1978.

110. Halushka, PV, et al.: Increased synthesis of prostaglandin-E-like material by platelets from patients with diabetes mellitus. N Engl J Med 297:1306, 1977.

111. Feldman, BF and Rasedee, A: Haemostatic abnormalities in canine Cushing's syndrome. Res Vet Sci 41:228, 1986.

112. Koepke, JA: Coagulation testing systems. *In* Koepke, JA (ed): Laboratory Hematology. Vol. 2. New York, Churchill Livingstone, 1984, p 1113.

113. Vermylen, J, et al.: Normal mechanisms of platelet function in platelet disorders. Clin Haematol 12:1, 1983.

114. Huesbach, CA and Harker, LA: Disorders of platelet function—mechanisms, diagnosis and management. West J Med 134:109, 1981.

115. Sirridge, MS and Shannon, R: General principles of testing. *In* Laboratory Evaluation of Hemostasis and Thrombosis. Philadelphia, Lea & Febiger, 1983, p 58.

116. Feldman, BF: Thrombosis—diagnosis and treatment. *In* Kirk, RW (ed): Current Veterinary Therapy IX. Philadelphia, WB Saunders, 1986, p 505.

117. Green, RA: Pathophysiology of antithrombin III deficiency. Vet Clin North Am, Vol 18, Jan 1988.

118. Helenski, CA and Ross, JN: Platelet aggregation in feline cardiomyopathy. J Vet Intern Med 1:24, 1987.

THE
IMMUNOLOGIC
SYSTEM

118 PRINCIPLES OF IMMUNOLOGY

GEOFFREY SUNSHINE

SCOPE OF MODERN IMMUNOLOGY

Contemporary immunology is an exciting multifaceted discipline. It grew out of the descriptive sciences of medicine, pathology and microbiology and now includes chemistry, cell biology, genetics and molecular biology. All of these areas have contributed to our understanding of the fundamental mechanisms underlying the immune system.

Many of the studies in immunology over the last two decades have been performed with cells from rodents and humans. Basic immunologic studies in veterinary animals are not at such an advanced stage. Nonetheless, it is apparent that the central features of the immune response occur in all mammalian species. The purpose of this chapter is to outline how immunologic reactions occur, how such reactions may fail in some cases, and to describe how the reactions may be manipulated to benefit the patient.

CHARACTERISTICS OF THE IMMUNE RESPONSE

THE NATURE OF ANTIGEN

The term immunity refers to all those mechanisms used by an organism to protect itself from the potentially deleterious effects of an *antigen* or more strictly an *immunogen* (any agent able to evoke an immune response). Of necessity, the immune system must be able to deal with a highly diverse array of environmental agents. All types of chemical structure (organic and inorganic) can be immunogenic: proteins, nucleic acids, lipids and polysaccharides can all act as immunogens. Many factors influence whether or not a molecule is immunogenic. One consideration is the degree of foreignness of the material; thus, canine serum albumin evokes an immune response in the human but not in the canine. In general, high molecular weight chemically complex molecules are better immunogens than low molecular weight compounds. This is because a large molecule such as a protein comprises multiple regions—known as *antigenic determinants*—with different confor-

mations and amino acid sequences that are recognized as foreign by the immune system. A single antigenic determinant—the smallest unit able to evoke an immune response—is roughly eight amino acid or six saccharide units in length. Smaller molecules can, however, elicit a response if linked to larger molecules *(carriers)*. Responses to such small molecules *(haptens)* can be of clinical significance: the low molecular weight drug penicillin, for example, provokes an immune response in certain individuals after binding to circulating lymphoid cells, which act as carriers.

FEATURES OF THE IMMUNE SYSTEM

The first line of defense that the individual maintains against an invading organism involves physical barriers such as the skin and mucous membranes. If the pathogen does enter the body, internal defenses are brought into play. These include a variety of serum proteins such as lysozyme, polyamines and β-lysin as well as the complement, kinin and clotting systems. Phagocytic cells such as the blood monocyte and the polymorphonuclear leukocyte (PMN) ingest and attempt to degrade and destroy the potential pathogen. If, however, these defenses cannot contain the spread of the invading agent, the cells and products of the immune system are mobilized.

DIVISION OF LABOR IN THE IMMUNE SYSTEM

The immune system forms one of the most complex networks in the body. Many different cell types are involved and these cells interact in either a negative or positive manner. Furthermore, cellular elements of the immune system are found almost ubiquitously throughout the body.

The key cellular components of the immune response system are *lymphocytes,* which are in turn divided into two major sets: B and T. The role of B lymphocytes is to secrete *antibodies,* which bind to the foreign antigens. The binding of antibody to antigen triggers a number of the host's *effector* systems, eventually leading to the elimination of the invading agent. Because antibodies circulate freely in blood and lymph this limb of the immune response is referred to as *humoral*. Humoral immunity is very effective at dealing with extracellular pathogens. Once the pathogen is taken up by a cell, however, as in the case of bacteria growing inside a macrophage, antibody is not effective and T cell mediated immunity plays the predominant if not exclusive role in destroying the pathogen.

T lymphocytes in contrast do not produce antibodies. They may exert their effect by cell-cell contact, but predominantly they act by secreting a plethora of mediators called *lymphokines,* which affect the activity of many different cell types. T lymphocytes have three major functions. They may act as *helpers* or *inducers* for different cell types. They can for example help B cells make antibody and induce macrophages to kill facultative intracellular pathogens. T cells can also act as *killer* or *cytotoxic* cells. Such killing is important in removing virally infected cells from the body. Finally T cells may also act as *regulators* or *suppressors* of both B and T lymphocyte function and hence act as important controls on the immune response. T cells and their products can be completely independent of B cells in dealing with foreign agents. The responses mediated by T cells alone are referred to as *cell-mediated immunity* (CMI).

MEMORY AND SPECIFICITY

Figure 118–1 illustrates the characteristic features of a typical humoral immune response. After immunizing with antigen A, antibodies reactive to A are detected in serum after a lag of several days. Antibody levels then fall to baseline within days. This is known as a *primary response*. If the animal is subsequently reinjected with antigen A, however, antibody synthesis occurs after a much shorter lag phase. The levels of antibody produced are much higher in this *secondary response* and these levels are sustained for a longer period. Generally the affinity and avidity (the tightness) with which antibody binds to the antigen are higher in the secondary as compared to the primary response.

The archetypal pattern depicted in Figure 118–1 shows two major features of the immune response. The first is

memory, a characteristic unique to the immune and nervous systems. After initial exposure to A, subsequent challenge results in a much more rapid and effective immune response to A. The second feature of the immune response illustrated in Figure 118–1 is *specificity*. Secondary challenge with A results in a memory response only to A and not to B or any other unrelated antigen (the response to B, injected at the same time as the secondary challenge to A, is a primary).

A further critical feature of the immune response is that not only must the immune system be able to recognize and respond to any foreign substance, it must also *not* mount a response to the individual's own components. This property is known as *self–non-self discrimination*. How this discrimination is achieved is still unclear. Whatever the mechanism of self–non-self discrimination it is vital to the integrity of the individual. Failure to distinguish between self and non-self can result in pathological problems (autoimmunity) that will be discussed subsequently.

RECOGNITION IN THE IMMUNE RESPONSE

As described above in Figure 118–1, for the archetypal humoral immune response an individual's immune system must be able to respond in a specific manner to a highly diverse assortment of potential antigens—even those waiting to be synthesized in today's laboratories! At the same time the individual must not respond to self-components. The same general characteristics are also true of the cell mediated immune response to antigen.

A key implication of these findings is that the basis of the immune response is a highly specific *recognition* system. This is accomplished by having many different *clones* of lymphocytes. Each lymphocyte bears on its surface a single type of receptor with specificity for a unique or very limited range of antigenic determinants. Lymphocytes bearing receptors for all conceivable antigenic specificities thus exist *prior* to contact with antigen. Antigen activates only a small fraction of cells, which bears a complementary receptor structure. These cells proliferate and differentiate. Some cells in the

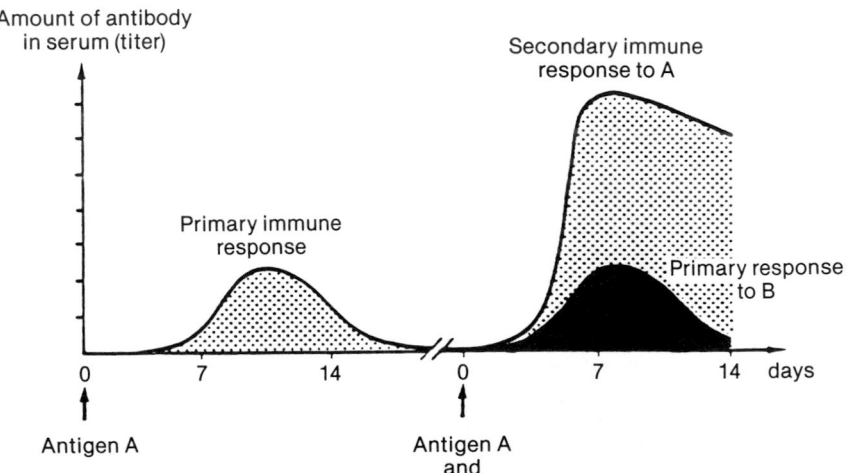

FIGURE 118–1. Characteristics of the humoral immune response. A primary response to antigen A is detected by the appearance in serum of antibodies specific for A after a lag of several days. Immunization at a later time with antigen A and an unrelated antigen B demonstrates the specificity of immunologic memory; the secondary response to A is both faster and greater than the primary response. The response to B is primary. (Modified from Tizard, IR: An Introduction to Veterinary Immunology, 3rd ed. Philadelphia, WB Saunders, 1987, p 4.)

expanded clone differentiate into *memory* cells, which may persist for years in some cases.

B and T lymphocytes have different antigen-specific receptors on their cell surface. The B lymphocyte antigen receptor is a glycoprotein *immunoglobulin* (Ig). The end result of antigen activation of a B cell with a complementary Ig receptor is the synthesis and secretion of Ig of identical specificity—this is the antibody that circulates freely in blood and lymph. The T cell receptor (TCR) is a non-Ig glycoprotein. Unlike the B cell receptor the TCR is not secreted after antigen activation of T cells. A further crucial difference between B and T cell recognition of antigen is that B cell recognition is directed at sites all over the surface of the native antigen; the three-dimensional conformation of the antigen is thus extremely critical in the antibody response. In contrast T cell recognition is limited to a small number of *immunodominant* sites, which are generally linear peptide sequences in the primary structure.

Since most antigens consist of more than one antigenic determinant more than one clone of antigen-specific lymphocytes (both B and T) is generally activated in an immune response. In other words, the response to a complex antigen is oligo- or poly-clonal. In the last few years, however, methods have been developed to study the responses of individual lymphocyte clones. The pioneering work of Kohler and Milstein immortalized individual antibody-producing B cells by fusing them with a B cell tumor.[1] By using this technique plus appropriate selection methods *monoclonal antibodies* of high specificity and uniformity can be produced. The use of monoclonal antibodies has revolutionized areas such as cellular analysis, disease diagnosis and indeed disease treatment. Monoclonal T cell lines have been generated in similar fashion; in this case antigen activated T cells are fused with a thymoma.[2] These T cell hybridomas have proved extremely useful for identifying precisely the nature of the antigenic determinant able to trigger the immune response.[3]

LYMPHOCYTE DIFFERENTIATION

Lymphocytes like other blood cells arise from a precursor *stem cell*. In adult mammals the bone marrow appears to be the only site that contains significant numbers of precursor cells. Lymphoid differentiation occurs along two different pathways in distinct *primary lymphoid organs*. T lymphocytes develop in the thymus and B lymphocytes, at least in birds, in the bursa of Fabricius. Mammals appear to have no bursa, and B cell differentiation occurs in either bone marrow or in sites of immune response, the *secondary lymphoid organs* such as the peripheral lymph nodes. Cells leaving the primary lymphoid organs migrate to T or B cell specific areas of secondary lymphoid organs or circulate throughout the body (Figure 118–2).

The steps in intrathymic differentiation have been intensely studied. Many issues remain unresolved, including the fundamental questions of how some precursor cells "commit" to the lymphoid as opposed to any other lineage and why some precursors migrate into the thymus. What is apparent though is that within the thymus a complex series of events occurs during which

each T cell acquires a unique antigen-specific receptor as well as a protein (or really a set of polypeptides) referred to as CD3, which is always found tightly associated with the TCR at the cell surface.[4] CD3, unlike the TCR, shows no cell to cell variability.

The thymus is also the organ in which the crucial feature of the immune system, self–non-self discrimination, is learned. Many studies have indicated that an individual's ability to recognize self is dictated by the thymus in which the T cell precursors mature.[5] A sense of "self" is thus not an inherent genetic quality of the cells. In other words, if T lymphocyte precursors from individual A are allowed to differentiate in the thymus of individual B, the mature T cells that arise learn to recognize B, and not A, as self.[6] Interaction of T cell precursors with structural elements of the thymus— either the thymic epithelium and/or thymic macrophages influences what is recognized as self.[7]

As they differentiate, T cells also acquire a set of cell surface glycoproteins known as *differentiation markers*. The two major markers—apart from CD3 and the TCR —are called CD4 and CD8. CD4 was formerly known as L3T4 in the mouse and T4 in the human. Similarly, CD8 was formerly known as Lyt 2 in the mouse and T8 in the human. Since it is now recognized that the murine and human proteins are highly homologous and that very similar molecules exist on the T cells of other species they have been given new generic names. Both CD4 and CD8 have homologies to Ig and the TCR, suggesting that they too may act as some type of receptor molecule.

CD4 and CD8 glycoproteins have been the focus of much interest. Indeed, the identification of these and other differentiation markers and the characterization of the cells on which they are expressed have been highly significant in understanding the processes of the immune response. Cells expressing unique surface structures can be separated by appropriate cell selection techniques such as fluorescence activated cell sorting, allowing their function to be studied in isolation. Cells with different patterns of cell surface markers have different functions. This has been particularly relevant to the study of T lymphocytes, because T cells expressing CD4 and not CD8 were believed to have helper or inducing functions whereas T cells expressing CD8 and not CD4 were believed to have cytotoxic and/or suppressor function.[8] Evidence has now accumulated to challenge this view of function correlating with phenotype[9] (*vide infra*, under "MHC restriction"). Nonetheless, it is apparent that CD4 and CD8 play key roles in cellular interactions in the immune response. It is also apparent that the identification of cell surface markers will be a powerful tool for aiding the characterization of any new cell described. Finally, it is worth noting that the human (but not murine) CD4 binds human immunodeficiency virus, allowing the virus to enter and destroy CD4+ cells, resulting in AIDS.[10]

Structure and Function of Antigen-Specific Receptors

B LYMPHOCYTES

As we have previously described, the antigen specific receptor on resting B lymphocytes is immunoglobulin

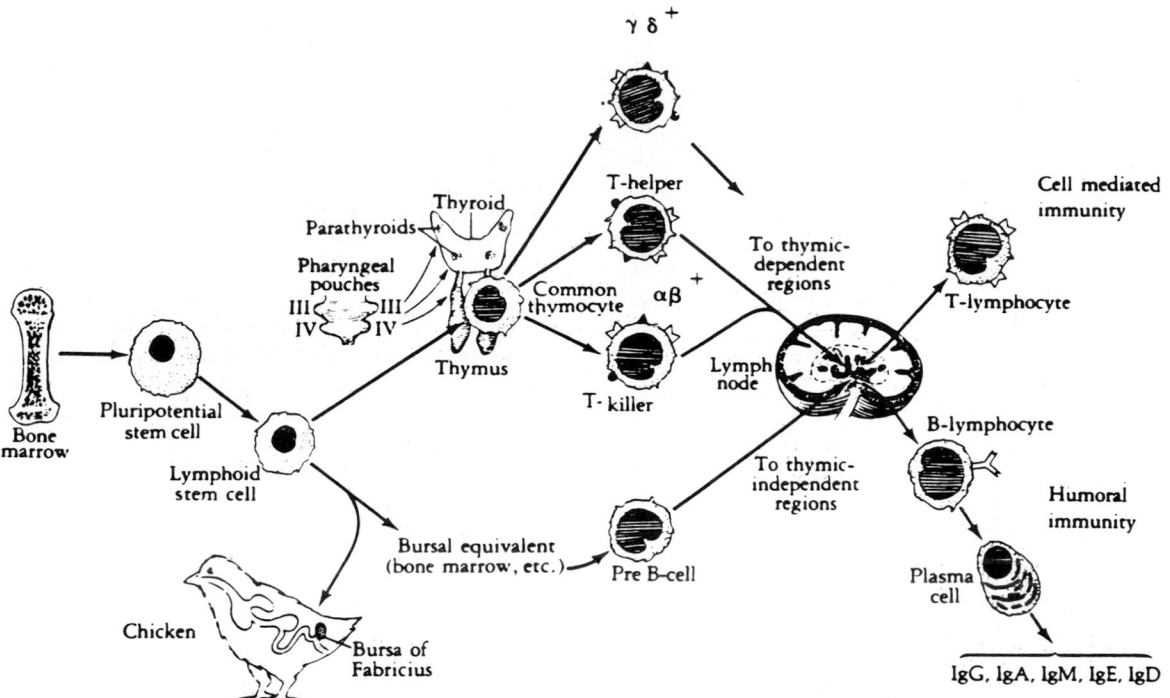

FIGURE 118–2. Differentiation of lymphocytes. Lymphoid precursor cells migrate to distinct primary lymphoid organs. Differentiation in the bursa of Fabricius, or an analogous organ in mammals, gives rise to the B lymphocyte series. Differentiation in the thymus results in the generation of subsets of T lymphocytes: cells expressing an α,β antigen-specific receptor may have helper, killer or suppressor function. The function of the small subset of T lymphocytes bearing a distinct antigen receptor γ, δ—is not clear. Antigen interacts with mature B and T lymphocytes in secondary lymphoid organs. (Modified from Bellanti, JA: Immunology III, Philadelphia, WB Saunders, 1985, p 48.)

(Ig), which is also the major secreted product of the fully differentiated B cell after antigenic stimulation. Secreted Ig can also bind to antigen, and such antigen-antibody complexes are able to interact with other cells and products of the immune system, leading to the removal of the antigen in the effector phase of the response. Ig has a number of structural features that make it an ideal bifunctional molecule: one end of the molecule binds antigen and the other end interacts with the effectors of the immune response. Although there are millions of different immunoglobulin structures they are all variations on the same theme. There are five major *isotypes* or *classes* of Ig: IgM, IgD, IgG, IgA and IgE. The secreted form of one isotype IgG has the prototypical structure shown in Figure 118–3. It is a four chain structure composed of two identical heavy (H) chains and two identical light (L) chains that form a disulfide bonded Y-shaped molecule. The L chains can be either kappa or lambda (but not a combination). The H chains of IgG are known as gamma. (The H chains of other isotypes are referred to as mu, delta, alpha, or epsilon). A small stretch of the heavy chain acts as a hinge allowing flexibility of the arms of the Y. Intrachain disulfide bonds pinch both H and L chains into loops that align to form tight globular structures or *domains* of approximately 110 amino acids. Papain digestion splits the IgG molecule at the hinge region into three fragments: 2 Fab and 1 Fc fragment. The crucial features are that each Fab fragment has one antigen binding site but no effector function; the Fc fragment—the tail of the Y—cannot bind antigen but is absolutely required for the effector function of the Ig molecule.

There are at least two H chain domains in the Fc fragment, and each domain is responsible for a different effector function. One Fc domain binds to and hence activates the first components of the serum *complement* cascade; activated complement components play a major role in removing antigen by enhancing the activity of phagocytic cells and by promoting the inflammatory response. Another Fc domain binds directly to cells bearing specific receptors (FcR); such FcR+ cells as

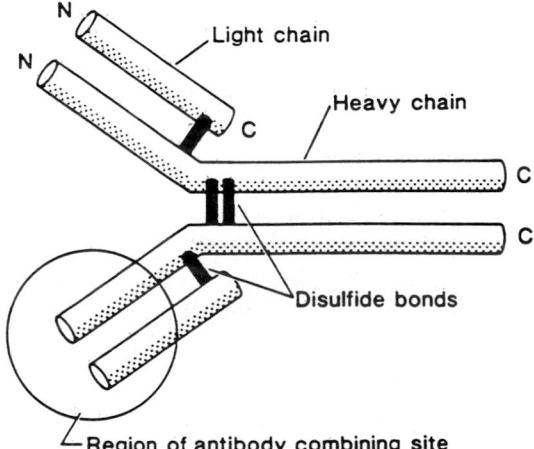

FIGURE 118–3. A prototypical IgG molecule illustrating the four chain structure and the antibody combining site. In the three dimensional structure the combining site forms a groove or cleft that fits antigenic determinants with the correct conformation. (From Tizard, IR: An Introduction to Veterinary Immunology, 3rd ed. Philadelphia, WB Saunders, 1987, p 36.)

macrophages and PMN are also vital in removing antigen complexed to antibody from the immune system.

FUNCTION OF Ig ISOTYPES

Each immunoglobulin may exist as a receptor on the surface of a B cell. In this form as a membrane receptor Ig has the basic polypeptide structure (2H and 2L) described above. When secreted by the activated B cell, however, the physical structure as well as the functions of the Ig may be quite distinct. The important point is that differences in biological function are attributable solely to the H chains of Ig. IgM-bearing cells are extremely important in the ontogeny of the immune response because IgM-bearing cells appear to be the precursor cells for all other isotypes. Thus IgM$^+$ cells are the first to appear in ontogeny; and if IgM is lost or modulated off the surface of these early cells, the cells are rendered nonfunctional and the other Ig isotypes do not appear in the animal. IgM-bearing cells form the vast majority of the resting mature B cell population in the normal adult. In these resting B cells, however, both IgM and IgD (of identical antigenic specificity) are expressed on the same cell. In contrast to the cells expressing only IgM, modulation of the surface Ig of IgM and IgD expressing cells results in activation rather than inactivation. It has thus been suggested that the major role of IgD (since it is not secreted in significant amounts) is to prevent the turning off of Ig$^+$ lymphocytes but how this may be accomplished is not clear.

IgM is the major product of primary responses and of responses to antigens known as "thymus independent." These latter are antigens with a repeating unit structure such as bacterial lipopolysaccharide that do not require help from T cells and that do not generally give rise to memory responses. Secreted IgM consists of five copies of the four chain unit and contains in addition an extra protein known as J chain required for the polymerization of the pentameric structure. In this form IgM thus has ten identical binding sites for antigen. This makes IgM extremely efficient at *cross linking* antigen, with the result that antigen-antibody complexes may form large lattices, which precipitate out of solution. This is the basis for hemagglutination reactions. IgM is also extremely efficient at activating the complement cascade.

In contrast to IgM, IgG is produced in greater amounts in the secondary response than the primary. It is also the major isotype found in blood. In species where maternal and fetal circulations are linked, IgG may cross the placenta and hence provide protection to the neonate. IgG too activates complement.

IgA is found in greatest abundance in secretions such as milk, and relatively little is found in blood. IgA in secretions consists of two copies of the basic four chain structure, J chain (as found in IgM) and *secretory component*, which is synthesized by epithelial cells. Secretory component appears to protect the IgA from proteolysis. In contrast to both IgM and IgG, IgA does not activate complement by what is known as the classical pathway but can activate the alternative pathway.

IgE exists at very low levels but is involved in two major responses: type I hypersensitivity reactions (q.v.) and the response to parasites, particularly worms. The Fc region of IgE binds to receptors on mast cells and basophils. When antigen binds to the mast cell that has bound IgE the cells degranulate, releasing a vast number of biologically active molecules including histamine and serotonin, which are important in the inflammatory response.

T LYMPHOCYTES

The antigen binding receptor of the T cell (TCR) is a two chain structure known as α and β. The α, β heterodimer shows some homology to the prototypic Ig structure and it is now generally accepted that Ig and the TCR, as well as a number of other surface molecules, evolved from a common ancestral gene. Thus Ig and the TCR as well as the CD4 and CD8 differentiation markers described previously are all included in an "Ig supergene family."[11]

Once antigen is bound by the α, β dimer it is believed that activating signals to the T cell are transmitted through the closely associated CD3 complex of polypeptides. Current models suggest that calcium mobilization and phosphatidyl inositol turnover are among the earliest intracellular events that follow engagement of the T cell receptor.[12] The end result of T cell activation does not result in secretion of the receptor as is the case in B cell activation.

FINE SPECIFICITY OF IG AND THE TCR

When many different purified Ig heavy and light chains were sequenced it became obvious that the carboxy half of the different Ig molecules was very similar. The amino termini, however, were quite distinct. Thus, the Ig molecule was divided into a constant (C) and variable (V) region. Closer analysis revealed that within the V region differences in primary amino acid sequence between molecules were confined to three or four *hypervariable* regions. We now know from x-ray crystallographic studies that these hypervariable regions of Ig heavy and light chains are brought together in the three dimensional configuration of the molecule. This creates a groove or pocket into which an antigenic determinant fits.[13] Thus the variety in antigen binding sites of immunoglobulins arises from the different amino acid combinations and hence three dimensional shapes of the hypervariable regions.

Studies of the structure of the TCR are not so advanced since the TCR has not been obtained in a highly purified form suitable for crystallography. It is known, however, that both α and β chains are similarly made up of variable and constant regions, with hypervariable regions at the amino terminus.[14]

Mechanism for the Generation of Diversity

The immune system's ability to respond to a highly diverse array of antigens is provided for by having a vast number of lymphocytes whose antigen-specific receptors differ in the shape and sequence of their binding sites. About 10^9 different receptors are required to accommodate the universe of antigens—how are all these distinct receptors coded for in the genome without overwhelming the genetic information available? The mechanisms used are striking and unique, and are best illustrated by considering the construction of an Ig kappa chain. Two basic themes are involved; first, that the variable and constant regions of the same Ig are encoded by *different* genes, and second, that the variable region, the antigen binding region, is itself constructed from two relatively small pools of gene segments—known as V_K and J_K (J for joining).[15] The J_K segment codes for a few amino acids in the third hypervariable region.

In the genome of an undifferentiated mouse cell such as a liver cell (germ line DNA) there are approximately 200 different murine V_K genes and five different J_K genes, and these are widely separated from each other and from the gene coding for the constant region, C_K (Figure 118–4). During the differentiation of an individual B cell, and before its encounter with antigen, one of the 200 V genes (say number 2, or V_{K2}) is translocated or *rearranged* so that it is apposed to one of the J genes (say J_{k3}). The intervening DNA (from V_3 to J_2 in Figure 118–4) is thought to be deleted. The DNA is then transcribed, resulting in a single mRNA, which is then translated into the complete kappa gene product. The variable regions of heavy chains are somewhat similarly constructed (Figure 118–5); in this case, however, the variable region is constructed from three gene pools, known as V_H, D_H (for diversity) and J_H that currently are thought to contain 200, 10 and 4 different members respectively.[16] The D_H segment encodes about 10 amino acids.

Formation of a $V_H D_H J_H$ thus requires two genetic rearrangements (D-J followed by V-DJ). In Figure 118–5, the selected VDJ is thus brought near to the mu chain constant region gene C_{mu}. Transcription and translation result in the formation of a complete mu chain. In this way IgM is the first isotype produced by any B cell. As the B cell differentiates during the response to antigen, however, it may switch isotypes, producing IgA for example or any of the other isotypes.[17] To produce IgA a third genetic rearrangement occurs, which brings the VDJ gene unit adjacent to the C_{alpha} gene (Figure

118–5). The cell now produces a complete α chain. Since the intervening genetic information is deleted (C_{mu} through $C_{epsilon}$) this cell cannot switch back. In summary, an individual B cell may switch isotypes (mu to alpha in this case) but retain its antigenic specificity since the specificity is coded for by the same VDJ unit.

If any one of the 200 possible V_K genes can associate with any one of the five J_K genes then there would be 1000 (200×5) different possible VJ combinations able to code for the antigen binding regions of the kappa chains. Similarly, random association of any V_H, D_H and J_H would generate 8000 heavy chain variable regions. Since the antigen-binding site is made up of variable regions from both heavy and light chains then approximately eight million different combinations of H and L chains could be made using less than 1000 genes (for kappa, lambda, and heavy chain).

Apart from the random combinations just described, two other mechanisms are also involved in generating diversity in the antibody repertoire. The first is what is known as *junctional diversity*. This is the result of imprecise joining of V and J or V, D and J genes after rearrangement. A second mechanism is *somatic mutation*—point mutations in the variable region genes of a cell after it has been activated. Such mutation results in antibody with greater affinity for the antigen. These additional mechanisms probably increase the diversity of antibodies up to 100-fold. Thus using only approximately 1000 genes, 10^9 different antigen-specific receptors can be generated, which are sufficient to deal with all antigenic determinants.

The T cell receptor universe is similarly constructed. In fact, the genes coding for the TCR were found only recently by looking for genes that rearranged specifically in T cells.[18] Thus, the variable regions of TCR α and β chains are constructed from the random association of VJ and VDJ gene segments respectively. Junctional diversity, as described for Ig, is important in further increasing the number of potential TCR. Thus, the number of potential TCR appears more than adequate to accommodate the number of determinants that activate T cells.

It is also noteworthy that during the study of rearranged genes in T cells one further rearranged gene,

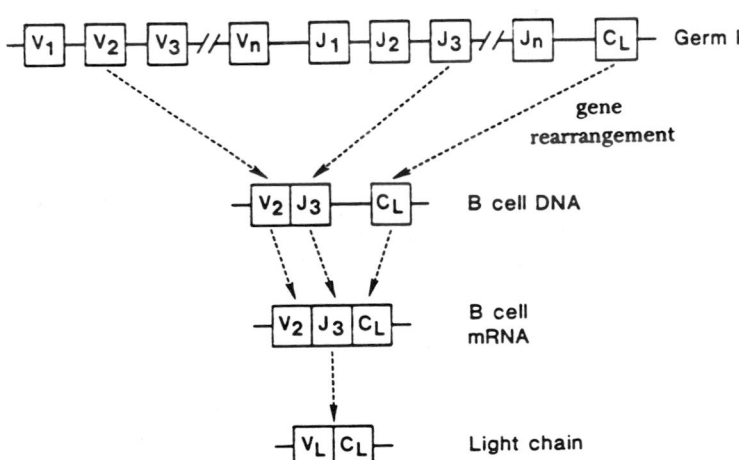

FIGURE 118–4. The production of an immunoglobulin kappa light chain. The variable region of a kappa chain is coded for by two gene segments, V and J. The constant region is coded for by one gene C_{kappa}. A number of different V and J gene segments exist in the genome of all cells (germline DNA) and these are widely separated from each other and the C_{kappa}. When a B cell commits to synthesizing kappa, its DNA rearranges so that one V and one J segment are brought together, close to the C_{kappa}. The VJC unit is then transcribed into mRNA and translated into a kappa light chain. (From Tizard, IR: An Introduction to Veterinary Immunology, 3rd ed. Philadelphia, WB Saunders, 1987, p 77.)

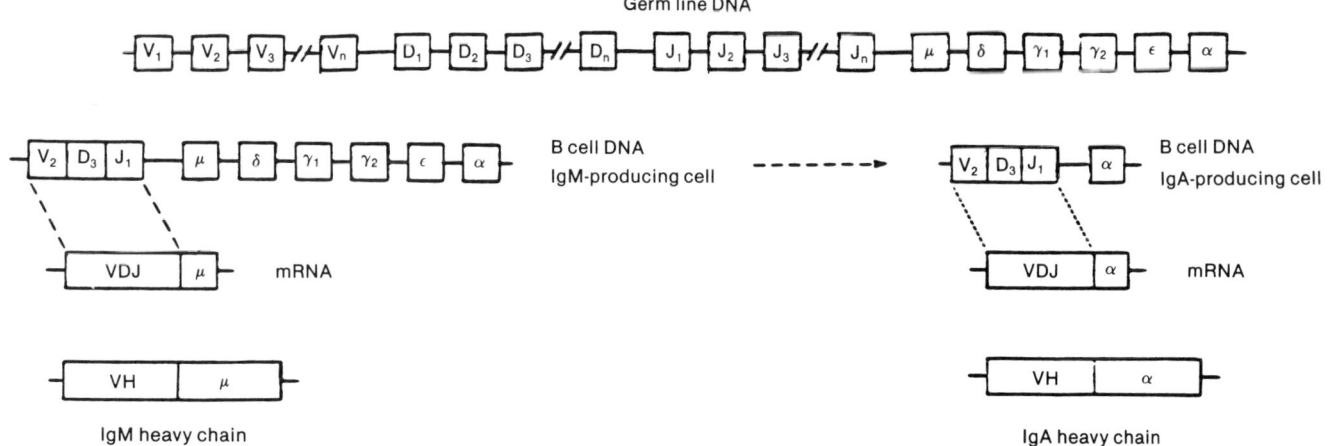

FIGURE 118–5. The production of IgM and IgA heavy chains. The variable region of a heavy chain is coded for by three gene segments, V, D, and J. When a B cell commits to synthesizing a particular variable region one of each of the V, D, and J gene segments rearranges so that the VDJ unit is formed, which is brought near to the gene for the mu constant region. A complete mu chain may then be transcribed and translated. Following antigenic stimulation this same B cell may move the VDJ unit in front of the C_{alpha} gene, resulting in the production of an α chain. In this way the B cell may switch isotypes but not antigenic specificity. (Modified from Tizard, IR: An Introduction to Veterinary Immunology, 3rd ed. Philadelphia, WB Saunders, 1987, pp 78 and 79.)

known as gamma, was found.[19] The gamma gene product has been recently found to be expressed in association with a molecule known as delta on the surface of a small subset of T cells, which does not express an α, β TCR[20] (illustrated at the top of Figure 118–2). Gamma, delta—like alpha,beta—is closely associated with the CD3 complex. Cells expressing gamma,delta arise earlier in ontogeny than α, β⁺ T cells.[21] Few gamma,delta⁺ cells express the CD4 or CD8 markers generally found on the conventional α, β⁺ cells. The function of the gamma,delta subset of T cells and whether gamma,delta acts as an antigen-specific receptor remain to be determined.

CLINICAL SIGNIFICANCE

We now understand at least some of the rules that govern how antigen-specific receptors are generated. With the advent of recombinant DNA technology we also have the ability to construct "tailormade" receptors with unique and defined specificity. This has been attempted thus far with immunoglobulins, to take advantage of their ability to bind specifically to antigens that could be expressed on the surface of a cell such as a tumor cell. Many ingenious approaches have been taken to generate modified antibodies with therapeutic potential and we will touch briefly only on some of them. One approach involves using a "magic bullet"; antibody is conjugated to a cell toxin such as ricin, which becomes active only after the antibody binds to its cellular target thus destroying the cell.[22] Another approach has been to make *chimeric* antibodies, in which the variable regions are derived from one species and the constant regions from another species.[23] This may reduce the immunogenicity of an injected immunoglobulin, since it is well known that immunoglobulin molecules from another species are highly immunogenic. Time will tell whether such constructed molecules have a significant role in treating diseases in veterinary animals.

CELLULAR INTERACTIONS IN THE IMMUNE RESPONSE

Role of Major Histocompatibility Complex (MHC) Gene Products in the Immune Response

B and T lymphocytes recognize antigen by distinct mechanisms. B cells may be triggered directly by intact or native antigen whereas T cells are not. To activate T cells antigen must first undergo limited degradation or *processing* in a cell known as an antigen-presenting cell (APC). This processing may take the form of a controlled intracellular proteolysis or of an unfolding of the molecule.[24] Within any individual one antigen will be processed into a limited number of fragments so that T cell clones with different TCR will be activated.

We now recognize that many different cell types with different characteristics can serve as APCs for helper or CD4⁺ T lymphocytes. APCs include such cells as macrophages, dendritic cells, endothelial cells and B lymphocytes.[25] The common characteristic of all APCs is their ability to express on their cell surface molecules referred to as *major histocompatibility complex (MHC) class II gene products*, which are also known as *Ia antigens*. Few cells, it should be noted, express Ia antigens constitutively—only the B lymphocyte and the spleen dendritic cell have so far been identified[26]—but many others, such as the macrophage and epithelial cell, can be *induced* to express Ia antigens in response to agents such as gamma-interferon (IFN_{gamma}).[27] Once a cell has been induced to express Ia it may now participate in the immune response by activating T cells. After processing, the fragments of antigen associate with Ia antigens on the surface of the APC and this combination of antigen plus Ia is then *presented* to CD4⁺ T cells (Figure 118–6).

Thus, MHC genes and their products play a crucial

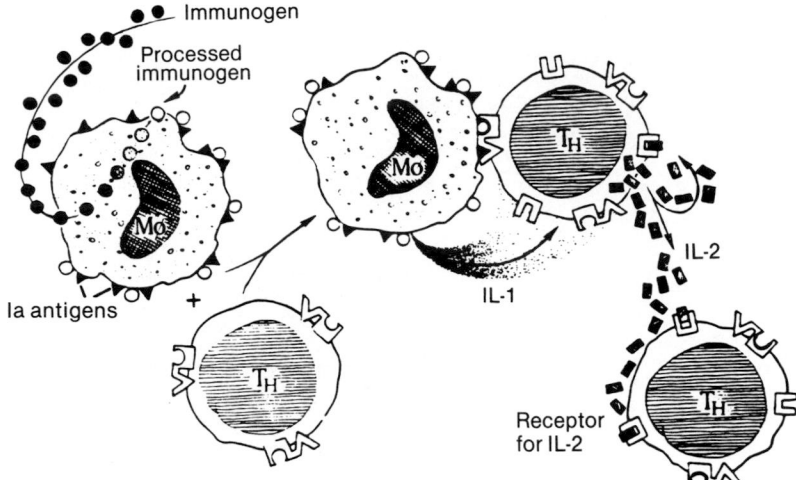

FIGURE 118–6. The cellular events in antigen processing and T cell activation. Immunogen is processed by an antigen-presenting cell such as a macrophage. Fragments of processed antigen associate with Ia antigens (MHC class II products) on the surface of the presenting cell. The complex of antigen plus Ia activates a CD4+ T helper cell with an appropriate α,β receptor. As a consequence of activation the antigen presenting cell secretes interleukin 1 (IL1) and the T cell a host of mediators including interleukin 2 (IL-2). (Modified from Bellanti, JA: Immunology III, Philadelphia, WB Saunders, 1985, p 146.)

role in antigen recognition by T cells. What are these MHC genes and products? All mammals have some type of MHC, a tightly linked series of genes divided into three categories—I, II, and III. MHC class I and II genes each code (in the human) for three sets of cell surface glycoproteins, which can be found on many different nucleated cells. MHC class III genes encode secreted complement components.

MHC genes were originally defined by the dominant role they played in the allograft or transplantation response, a response known to be mediated by T cells and their products. The role that the MHC plays in the everyday immune responses within an individual was recognized only recently. It is now believed that the essential functions of MHC class I and II gene products are to bind processed antigens and to present processed antigen to the appropriate T cells.[28] Within an individual there are differences in the nature of antigens that associate with MHC class I as opposed to MHC class II products. Generally, but not exclusively, processed viral antigens associate with MHC class I products whereas processed bacterial and other polypeptide antigens, such as ovalbumin, associate with MHC class II products.[29]

There is also an important correlation between the ability of an MHC product to bind to a particular peptide sequence and T cell activation.[30] A unique feature of the MHC gene system is its high *polymorphism*: the number of different forms or alleles of each class I or class II gene that exists stably in the population ranges from 10 to 50. Individuals may be high or low responders to a specific peptide depending on how well or how poorly the peptide interacts with an individual's MHC gene products; thus, as a consequence of different individuals within a species expressing different MHC gene products, any one antigenic determinant is unlikely to evoke an immune response in *all* the members of the species.

A further key feature of the MHC is that MHC gene products direct antigens to specific sets of T cells.[31] We say that T cell responses are *MHC restricted* (Figure 118–7). Cells that have antigen associated on the cell surface with MHC class I products activate CD8+ T lymphocytes (mainly T killer cells), whereas antigen associated with MHC class II products activates CD4+

T lymphocytes (mainly T helper cells). We do not currently know if CD4 and CD8 are physically associated with the TCR.

As a consequence of MHC restriction, T cells from individual A recognize antigens only in association with the MHC of individual A but *not* in association with the MHC of a different individual B. In other words, the constellation of MHC genes and products expressed by an individual defines "self" and "nonself." As we have stated previously this notion of "self" is not absolute— it is learned in the thymus.[5] As T cell precursors differentiate they interact with structural cells of the thymus,

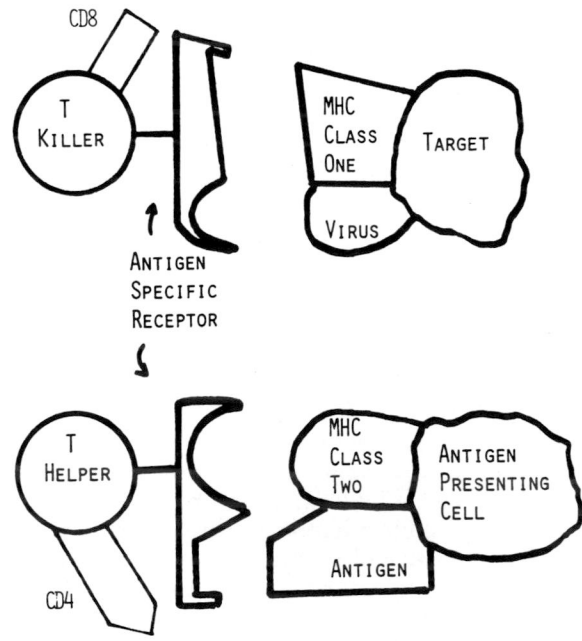

FIGURE 118–7. MHC restriction of the immune response. Certain antigens such as viral determinants associate with MHC class I products on the surface of a target cell. The complex of antigen plus MHC class I product is recognized by the antigen-specific receptor of a CD8+ T cell, which is generally a T killer cell. Other antigens such as bacterial products associate with MHC class II gene products and activate the antigen-specific receptor of a CD4+ T cell, which is generally a T helper cell.

which express MHC class II products. The MHC restriction and self tolerance patterns of mature T cells are thus determined by the allelic form of the MHC class II products, which the precursor cells encounter in the thymus.[7]

We should add that the allograft response—in which helper and CTL respond to foreign MHC products—does not transgress the rules of MHC restriction of T cell responses. Many clones of T cells can be isolated that respond both to a foreign MHC as well as to an antigen plus self MHC.[32] Since the clone has only one α, β receptor it is believed that the foreign MHC activates the TCR by mimicking the shape of antigen plus self MHC.

T CELL ACTIVATION

The MHC-restricted interaction of antigen, APCs and CD4$^+$ T cells depicted in Figure 118–6 results in the secretion of a plethora of molecules known as *cytokines,* released by both the APC and the T cell, which influence a variety of cell types. The key feature is that the triggering of the T cell is antigen specific; the products of T cell activation are not. Some of these molecules have been purified and sequenced; others have been synthesized using recombinant DNA technology. Thus we are now in a position to evaluate the clinical and therapeutic effects of highly purified molecules as modulators of the immune response.

As a concomitant of activation, macrophages release interleukin-1 (IL-1), which has many biologic activities including a variety of effects on different lymphoid cells. For instance, IL-1 acts at early stages of stem cell differentiation.[33] It also activates T cells both to synthesize and to respond to interleukin-2 (IL-2) by inducing the expression of IL-2 receptors; this is illustrated in Figure 118–6. Additionally, IL-1 causes fever and has a major influence on the inflammatory response.[34]

Once activated, the T cell releases an array of lymphokines. Activated T cells produce IL-2 and respond to it by increased proliferation. Furthermore, IL-2 is a differentiation factor for natural killer (NK) and T cytotoxic cell (CTL) precursors.[34] Activated T cells also release IFN$_{gamma}$ that up regulates Ia antigen expression, has antiviral properties and activates macrophages to kill intracellular parasites.[35] T cell products other than IFN$_{gamma}$ may also activate macrophages in sites of inflammation. At least two other molecules—IL-4 and IL-5—required for inducing B cell proliferation, differentiation and class switching are also secreted by activated T cells.[36] Like IL-1, the T cell product IL-3 may act at early stages of stem cell differentiation.[33, 37] Lymphotoxin and tumor necrosis factor—factors cytotoxic for virally infected and tumor cells—are also produced by activated T cells.[38] Currently many other T cell products are defined simply by their function such as "activatory" or "inhibitory" factor. Clearly, studies over the next few years will yield further insights into the effects of all these molecules and those yet to be isolated from activated T cells.

T cells may also be triggered other than directly through their α, β TCR, even at times without requiring an APC. Such responses are not antigen specific; all T cells may be activated by such plant-derived proteins as concanavalin A and phytohemagglutinin. Triggering can also be by antibodies specific for cell surface proteins; anti CD3 and anti CD2 (recognizing the molecule characterized as the sheep red blood cell receptor on human T cells) are both capable of T cell activation.[39] Such polyclonal activation results in the secretion of the set of T cell derived factors described above.

T-B CELL COOPERATION

The production of antibody generally requires MHC restricted cooperation between T and B lymphocytes. It appears that close contact between the T and B cells as well as the generation of the factors described above are optimally required to synthesize antibody and to induce isotype switching. It has become apparent that the B cell generation of antibody can occur by two different pathways.[40, 41] The first is the route described above where antigen is presented by macrophages to T cells, and the activated T cell in turn interacts with B cells in the presence of antigen.[40] A two cell pathway also exists. The initial event is antigen binding to antigen-specific B cells via Ig on their surface. The B cell then processes and presents degraded antigen to T cells in association with MHC class II molecules on the surface of the B cell. The T cell becomes activated and in turn activates the B cell to synthesize antibody.[41] Since B cells appear to be able to process and present very low concentrations of antigen, this second pathway may be favored at times when antigen is limiting.

T-T INTERACTIONS

Cytotoxic T Lymphocytes. IL-2 produced by activated helper T cells induces the differentiation of antigen specific cytotoxic T cells (CTL). Once activated, the CTLs kill target cells, which express the priming antigen on their cell surface. The α, β TCR of the CTL recognizes antigen when associated with the appropriate MHC gene product; thus, CD4$^+$ CTL kill targets expressing antigen associated with MHC class II gene products and CD8$^+$ CTL kill targets expressing antigen in association with MHC class I gene products.[42] The cytotoxic mechanism generally involves CTL-target contact, but there is also evidence for T cell factors playing a role in target cell killing.[43]

The generation of CTLs is generally not a major pathway in responses to protein antigens or in responses to bacteria that grow inside cells. CTLs do play an important role *in vivo* in removing virally infected cells, tumor cells and allografted tissue.

Suppressor Cells. The phenomenon of T cell mediated suppression—one set of T cells acting on another to prevent a response—has gained general acceptance since its description in 1971.[44] Since then many different types of antigen-specific T suppressor cells, as well as the factors that they produce, have been described. It has been suggested that T suppressor cell interactions with targets are MHC restricted by a region known as I-J in analogous fashion to the MHC restriction of T helper and cytotoxic cells described above.[45]

Nonetheless, several problems have emerged in the

study of T suppressor cells. Thus far, no gene product of the I-J region has been described. Furthermore I-J appears unique to the mouse. Finally cloned murine T suppressor cells do not have a conventional α, β TCR so it is not clear how they interact with antigen or with other antigen-specific cells.[46] Thus it is currently difficult to evaluate fully the role of populations of suppressor T cells in the immune response.

OTHER CELLS INVOLVED IN THE CELL MEDIATED IMMUNE RESPONSE

Natural Killer Cells. In addition to the B and T lymphocytes described above there are other cells with some but not all lymphocyte characteristics. These have been classified by the functions that they mediate and so are referred to as *natural killer* (NK) and *killer* (K) cells, although the two are considered to be overlapping populations. NK cells are capable of killing a number of virally infected as well as transformed cells. Most if not all NK activity has been found to be associated with a population of cells termed large granular lymphocytes (LGL), which can be activated by IL-2 and IFN_{gamma}.[47] LGL do not have an α, β T cell receptor, clearly distinguishing them from CTLs. LGL killing is thought to be mediated by a protein called perforin, which is released from the granules on target cell contact. The target structure recognized by LGL, however, is currently not identified.

K cells kill bacteria and some target cells that have been coated with antibody. K cells express receptors for the Fc portion of antibody (FcR). In the presence of antibody, K cells kill target cells in a process known as antibody-dependent cytotoxicity (ADCC).

Macrophages. We have already touched on two distinct roles of macrophages in the immune response, their ability to ingest and degrade potential pathogens and their ability to activate antigen-specific T cells. Macrophages that have been activated by T cell factors (IFN_{gamma} especially) also play a role in the effector arm of the immune response. Once activated they have tumoricidal and anti-viral effects, releasing agents such as a tumor necrosis factor as well as α and β interferons.[38, 48] Activated macrophages also are able to kill facultative intracellular parasites such as *Listeria*. T cell derived factors such as macrophage activating factor, inhibitory factor and chemotactic factor are thought to be important *in vivo* in drawing macrophages to the sites of inflammation and preventing their migration out of the site.

REGULATION OF THE IMMUNE SYSTEM

The induction and effector phases of the immune response to antigen are not simple on and off switches; rather, like other complex networks such as the nervous system, the immune system is tightly regulated and exhibits multiple levels of control.

One of the most conspicuous ways of controlling the immune response is by removing the triggering antigen. The binding of antibody to free antigen results in immune complexes, which are cleared by phagocytic cells such as macrophages and PMN. Immune complexes also activate the complement cascade of serum proteins. Complexes are even more readily removed by phagocytic cells coated by some of the activated complement components.

The route and method of immunization are critical parameters in the induction of an immune response. Thus subcutaneous or intraperitoneal injections strongly favor the induction of an immune response whereas intravenous injection favors the development of tolerance or suppression (see below). This may be due to the presence of different antigen presenting cells in these different compartments since the type of APC that antigen first encounters may possibly influence the set of lymphocytes that is activated.[49] Furthermore, antigen administered along with adjuvants such as alum or Freund's complete adjuvant induces an immune response whereas antigen injected in aqueous solutions favors the induction of non-responsiveness.

The initial concentration of antigen is also significant. Too much or too little antigen can lead to the induction of a state of *acquired tolerance* in which antigen-specific cells are not able to respond. (Intermediate ranges of antigen concentration are generally required to induce an immune response—what this appropriate range is has to be ascertained for each antigen.) This state of tolerance can be induced in both B and T lymphocytes.[50] As with the induction of self-tolerance, the precise cellular and molecular mechanisms involved in acquired tolerance are not clear but may involve the down-regulation of the antigen-specific receptor preventing triggering.[51] T suppressor cells may also play a role in the phenomenon—many complicated circuits of interacting suppressor and helper type T cells have been described as regulating the immune response.[52]

Once antibody has been produced it may exert a "feedback" control on immune induction by preventing the triggering of antigen-specific cells. Again the mechanisms involved in this phenomenon are not well understood. It is of some practical importance because in many species it is difficult to vaccinate successfully while large amounts of maternally derived antibody are still circulating in the neonate.

A further level of control is through the *idiotype network*. Antibodies with many distinct antigen-binding sites are generated in the response to a single antigen and it has been suggested that the antigen-binding sites of these antibodies may be immunogenic in the same individual; in other words any antibody molecule may also act as an antigen.[53] Antigenic determinants expressed by the binding site of antibodies are known as *idiotypic determinants*. Since these determinants are clone specific, the idiotype of an antibody may evoke an immune response within the same individual, thus producing anti-idiotypic antibody. This in turn could induce anti-anti-idiotypic antibody and so on *ad infinitum*. From this perspective the immune response may be regarded as a series of oscillating waves, dampened down by regulatory interactions at each phase. Since T cell receptors express unique antigen-specific receptors it is possible that they too may participate in the network. Indeed, recognition between sets of T suppressor cells has been described to occur via idiotype–anti-idiotype interactions.[52] In some cases where anti-idiotypic antibodies have been isolated the sequence and structure of the binding site of the anti-idiotypic antibody resemble the structure and sequence of the priming antigen. This suggests that animals could potentially be vaccinated with anti-idiotypic antibody rather than antigen itself.[54]

Immunologic Diseases

Many specific immunological diseases will be covered in other chapters. In this section we will discuss only the fundamental immunological principles underlying disease states.

HYPERSENSITIVITY RESPONSES

When the consequences of a secondary response to antigen result in a pathological state we talk of a hypersensitivity reaction. Figure 118–8 describes the four types of hypersensitivity reactions that have been defined. *Type I* or *immediate hypersensitivity* occurs within minutes of re-exposure to an antigen. The trigger for the response is antigen cross-linking IgE bound via its Fc region to specific receptors on the surface of mast cells or basophils. As a result the cell releases a number of mediators stored in cytoplasmic granules, and synthesizes products that draw eosinophils into the area of the response. The factors released by mast cell degranulation, of which histamine is a prime component, are highly vasoactive and can have systemic as well as local effects. In some extreme cases the effects of the vasoactive products can even be fatal. Nonetheless, this IgE-eosinophil interaction is not always deleterious—it also plays a beneficial role in the host's immune response to parasitic infestations.[55]

In *type II hypersensitivity* the antibody response directed at a cellular antigen results in the lysis of the cell on which the antigen is expressed. A prototypical type II response follows transfusion of red cells from a donor with unmatched blood groups. The antibodies synthesized as a result of this untoward priming bind to the red cells expressing the antigen. Complement is activated and the target cells may be lysed either by the direct action of complement or via NK-mediated antibody-dependent cellular cytotoxic mechanisms.

In *type III hypersensitivity* responses, in contrast, immune complex formation is not directly cytotoxic. Rather, immune complexes are deposited in filtering organs such as kidney glomeruli. Complement is thus activated at the site of deposition of the complexes and activated complement components draw in neutrophils to the area. The accumulation of neutrophils, however, may lead to tissue destruction at the site of complex deposition. These responses occur within 6 to 12 hours of antigen challenge.

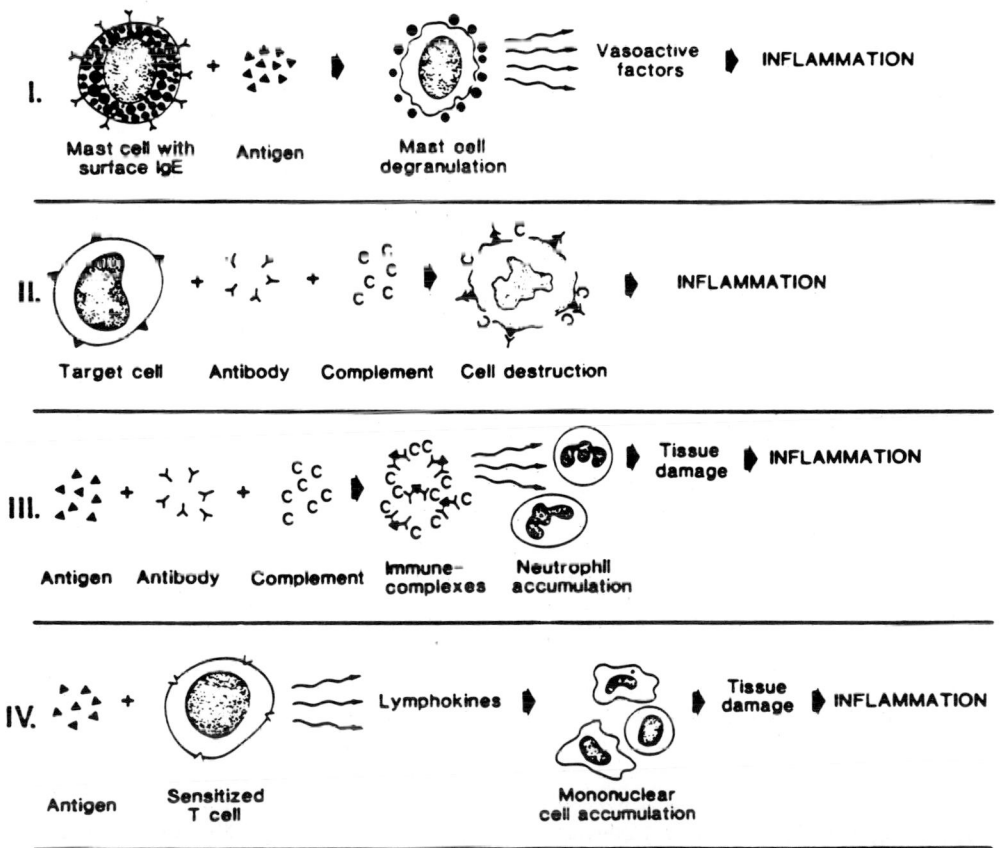

FIGURE 118–8. The four types of hypersensitivity response. The key cells and soluble mediators are illustrated. For further details see text. (From Tizard, IR: An Introduction to Veterinary Immunology, 3rd ed. Philadelphia, WB Saunders, 1987, p 274.)

Type IV hypersensitivity—delayed type hypersensitivity (DTH)—occurs 24 to 48 hours after antigenic stimulation. Antigen-primed T cells enter tissues following the early increases in vascular permeability. As a consequence of restimulation the T cells release the array of lymphokines described previously, resulting in the attraction of monocytes to the site where they interact with the T cells. Although categorized in these four distinct ways hypersensitivity responses to any one antigen frequently involve all the different reactivity patterns.

AUTOIMMUNITY

Autoimmunity is the result of a breakdown in the fundamental distinction between self and non-self. As a consequence the individual produces antibodies reactive to self-components. In examples such as systemic lupus erythematosus (SLE) the autoantibody generated reacts with a variety of cell types and cellular components whereas in diseases like Hashimoto's thyroiditis the autoantibodies are much more restricted in their specificity. The result in either case is tissue damage, which may take the form of any of the types of hypersensitivity responses described above.

What are the events that trigger such a breakdown? Several theories have been proposed but as yet it remains difficult to identify the triggering event with certainty. One possibility is that a self-component that was previously sequestered subsequently becomes exposed to cells of the immune system. Any agent such as a virus that modifies either the cellular location or indeed the physical structure of a self-component may induce an autoimmune response. One recent theory to explain autoimmune thyroiditis suggests that as a result of immune stimuli MHC class II antigens are induced on thyroid epithelial cells. As a consequence other surface components of the thyroid cell may be presented to T cells, resulting in autoimmunity.[56] A further possibility is that a breakdown in the function of regulator cells allows the emergence of "forbidden clones"—those that are self-reactive. A genetic component may also have a role; many diseases have been found to correlate with the expression of specific MHC alleles. This is particularly noted for certain MHC class II genes and autoimmunity in the human. (Few comparable data are available in species other than the mouse and human.) Sequencing of one human MHC class II gene product, DQ_{beta}, from normal and insulin-dependent diabetes mellitus (IDDM) patients indicates that the presence or absence of a single amino acid at one position in the molecule determines the level of susceptibility or resistance to IDDM.[57] Despite this fine analysis, however, the triggering events as well as the immunological mechanisms in IDDM and other autoimmune diseases are still incompletely understood.

IMMUNODEFICIENCY

Any cell in the immune system may become aberrant in its function or simply fail to develop. Either of these conditions results in a deficiency of the immune response. Immunodeficiencies have been most intensely

studied in humans but it is apparent that they are observed in many different species. Two broad categories of deficiencies can be described, congenital or acquired. Congenital deficiencies are most serious when they affect precursor cells—the most devastating being a total defect in stem cells for all hematopoietic development (reticular dysgenesis) or for all lymphoid development (combined immune deficiency). These can be treated only by giving genetically matched precursor cells from normal individuals. A further congenital condition of significance occurs when the thymus fails to develop properly (DiGeorge's syndrome in the human); in this case the lymphoid precursors are normal but the T cell compartment fails to develop. Thymus grafting may be the only suitable treatment.

Acquired or secondary immune deficiencies arise under many conditions, for example as concomitants of tumors, suppressive drug treatments or malnutrition. There are many examples of viruses inducing immunodeficient states either directly by destroying lymphoid tissue or indirectly by affecting immunoregulation. Much attention is currently focused on the human disease acquired immune deficiency syndrome (AIDS) and analogous animal syndromes in which retroviruses cause massive destruction of lymphocytes. The human AIDS virus (HIV-1) binds to the CD4 molecule expressed on T cells (and some brain cells).[10] The $CD4^+$ cells may then be killed directly or by the fusion of normal $CD4^+$ cells to infected cells. Since, as we have described, $CD4^+$ T cells play a key role in the interaction with other cells of the immune system the elimination of $CD4^+$ cells is devastating.

Manipulation of the Immune Response

VACCINATION

In immunological terms, the concept of vaccination is to use the memory response to antigen to eliminate a pathogen before it can cause disease. The fundamental practical principle in the production of a suitable vaccine is to reduce the pathogenicity of the material while retaining its immunological integrity. The success or failure of potential vaccines therefore follows from our general discussion of immune reactivity. Thus it is important to know at the outset whether humoral and/or cell mediated immunity plays the dominant role in the response to the pathogen. Such factors as the site of application of the vaccine and the immunological status of the host play major roles in determining what type of response (IgA rather than IgG antibodies for example) or indeed whether any immune response results. Furthermore, depending on the lifetime of memory cells specific for a particular antigen an animal may have to be repeatedly immunized or boostered.

Many procedures have been followed to produce successful vaccines, in particular by using killed or inactivated viral and bacterial pathogens. The drastic procedures required to inactivate a pathogen, however, can alter its antigenic determinants. To avoid this problem, attenuated viruses whose pathogenicity has been reduced by passage through different hosts, and naturally occurring nonvirulent viruses, which have similar or identical determinants to pathogenic viruses, have been used to vaccinate in some diseases.

Recent advances in technology as well as increased knowledge of the different pathways of immune response and of the structure of viruses and bacteria have played major roles in the design of new vaccines. The potential use of anti-idiotypic antibody as a vaccine was referred to in a previous section.[54] Another possibility is to prevent the entry of pathogens into target cells. Recent studies indicate that soluble forms of the CD4 molecule, the receptor for human immunodeficiency virus, may block the infectivity of the virus by preventing the initial entry of the virus into CD4+ cells.[58] A major approach is to modify the genetic organization of the pathogen, for example, by removing from bacteria the genes coding for the toxins they produce—in the case of viruses the genes encoding enzymes required in viral reproduction. These genetically manipulated bacteria or viruses can then be used to generate an immune response.

A different approach has been to identify and sequence the precise antigenic determinants, which are recognized by T and B cells following infection. Attempts are also under way to predict the structure of immunodominant T cell determinants by analyzing the amino acid sequence of protein antigens.[59] The notion is to vaccinate with small synthetic peptides; such peptides must be linked to "carrier" molecules to generate an immune response.[60] Because of MHC differences between individuals one antigenic determinant may not elicit an immune response in the whole population. It may therefore be essential to inject a potpourri of antigenic determinants in a potential vaccine to ensure protection in all or at least most of the individuals in the population at risk.

MODIFICATION OF THE HOST

As the preceding sections have demonstrated there has been a great deal of progress in the last few years in unraveling the complex pathways that constitute the immune response. The clinical application of this increased knowledge is in the use of cellular products to manipulate the immune response to the benefit of the patient; the intention is to move away from generalized immunostimulatory or immunosuppressive treatments that affect multiple sets of cells and towards the manipulation of individual sets or even individual clones of cells. Given the complexity of the cells and products of the immune system this task may not be straightforward. It is apparent, nonetheless, that treatments of animals with interleukins and other lymphokines and with monoclonal anti-idiotypic antibodies are valid attempts to treat clinical conditions.

One further possibility is the introduction of genes into animals—thus far this approach has been limited to the construction of transgenic animals in which a gene, such as human growth hormone, has been injected into fertilized embryos of swine. Similarly, it may be possible to introduce genes conferring disease resistance into the embryos of different species. All these studies are in their earliest stages. Time will tell which of these approaches will be successful in preventing and treating disease in veterinary animals.

References

1. Kohler, G and Milstein, C: Continuous cultures of fused cells secreting antibody of predefined specificity. Nature 256:495, 1975.
2. Kappler, JW, et al.: Antigen-inducible, H-2 restricted, Interleukin-2 producing T cell hybridomas. J Exp Med 153:1198, 1981.
3. Shimonkevitz, R, et al.: Antigen recognition by H2 restricted T cells. I. Cell free antigen processing. J Exp Med 158:303, 1984.
4. Weiss, A, et al.: The role of the T3/antigen receptor complex in T-cell activation. Ann Rev Immunol 4:593, 1986.
5. Zinkernagel, RM, et al.: On the thymus in the differentiation of H-2 self recognition by T cells: evidence for dual recognition? J Exp Med 147:822, 1978.
6. Singer, A, et al.: Self recognition in allogeneic radiation bone marrow chimeras. J Exp Med 153:1286, 1981.
7. Lo, D and Sprent, J: Identity of cells that imprint H-2 restricted T-cell specificity in the thymus. Nature 319:672, 1986.
8. Cantor, H and Boyse, EA: Functional classes of T lymphocytes bearing different Ly antigens. I. The generation of functionally distinct T cell subclasses is a differentiative process independent of antigen. J Exp Med 141:1375, 1975.
9. Swain, S: T cell subsets and the recognition of MHC class. Immunol Rev 74:129, 1983.
10. Dalgleish, AG, et al.: The CD4 (T4) antigen is an essential component of the receptor for the AIDS retrovirus. Nature 312:763, 1984.
11. Williams, AF: A year in the life of the immunoglobulin superfamily. Immunol Today 8:298, 1987.
12. Imboden, JB and Stobo, JD: Transmembrane signalling by the T cell antigen receptor. J Exp Med 161:446, 1985.
13. Inbar, D, et al.: Location of antibody binding sites within the variable portions of heavy and light chains. Proc Natl Acad Sci USA 69:2659, 1972.
14. Gascoigne, NRJ, et al.: Genomic organization and sequence of T-cell receptor β-chain constant and joining-region genes. Nature 310:387, 1984.
15. Cory, S, et al.: Sets of immunoglobulin V$_K$ genes homologous to ten cloned V$_K$ sequences: implications for the number of germline V$_K$ genes. J Mol Appl Genet 1:103, 1981.
16. Honjo, T: Immunoglobulin genes. Ann Rev Immunol 1:499, 1983.
17. Yamawaki-Kataoka, Y, et al.: Complete nucleotide sequence of Ig gamma 2b chain gene cloned from newborn mouse DNA. Nature 283:786, 1980.
18. Hedrick, SM, et al.: Isolation of cDNA clones encoding T cell-specific membrane-associated proteins. Nature 308:149, 1984.
19. Saito, H, et al.: Complete primary structure of a heterodimeric T-cell receptor deduced from cDNA sequences. Nature 309:757, 1984.
20. Brenner, MB, et al.: Identification of a putative second T-cell receptor. Nature 322:145, 1986.
21. Allison, JP and Lanier, LL: The T-cell antigen receptor gamma gene: rearrangement and lineages. Immunol Today 8:293, 1987.
22. Vitetta, ES, et al.: Redesigning nature's poisons to create anti-tumor reagents. Science 238:1098, 1987.
23. Aguila, HL, et al.: The production of more useful monoclonal antibodies. Immunol Today 7:380, 1986.
24. Streicher, HZ, et al.: Antigen conformation determines processing requirements for T cell activation. Proc Natl Acad Sci USA 81:6831, 1984.
25. Sunshine, GH, et al.: Heterogeneity of stimulator cells in the murine mixed leukocyte response. Eur J Immunol 12:9, 1982.
26. Sunshine, GH and Mitchell, TJ: Antigen presentation by spleen dendritic cells. J Invest Dermatol 85.110s, 1985.
27. Halloran, PF, et al.: The regulation of expression of major histocompatibility complex products. Transplantation 41:413, 1986.
28. Babbitt, B, et al.: Binding of immunogenic peptides to Ia histocompatibility molecules. Nature 317:359, 1985.

29. Germain, RN: The ins and outs of antigen processing and presentation. Nature 322:687, 1986.

30. Buus, S, et al.: The relationship between MHC restriction and the capacity of Ia to bind immunogenic peptides. Science 235:1353, 1987.

31. Morrison, LA, et al.: Differences in antigen presentation to MHC class I- and class II-restricted influenza virus specific cytolytic T lymphocyte clones. J Exp Med 163:903, 1986.

32. Sredni, B and Schwartz, RH: Alloreactivity of an antigen-specific T-cell clone. Nature 287:855, 1980.

33. Mochizuki, DY, et al.: IL-1 regulates hematopoietic activity, a role previously ascribed to hemopoietin 1. Proc Natl Acad Sci USA 84:5267, 1987.

34. Oppenheim, JJ, et al.: There is more than one interleukin 1. Immunol Today 7:45, 1986.

35. Toy, JL: The interferons. Clin Exp Immunol 54:1, 1983.

36. Vitetta, ES: T cell derived lymphokines that induce IgM and IgG secretion in activated murine B cells. Immunol Rev 78:137, 1984.

37. Stanley, ER, et al.: Regulation of very primitive multipotential hematopoietic cells by hemopoietin-1. Cell 45:667, 1986.

38. Ruddle, NH: Tumor necrosis factor and related cytotoxins. Immunol Today 8:129, 1987.

39. Nisbet-Brown, ER, et al.: Antigen-specific and nonspecific mitogenic signals in the activation of human T cell clones. J Immunol 138:3713, 1987.

40. Ramila, G, et al.: Evaluation of accessory cell heterogeneity. Eur J Immunol 15:189, 1985.

41. Lanzavecchia, A: Antigen-specific interaction between T and B cells. Nature 314:357, 1985.

42. Braakman, E, et al.: Are MHC class II-restricted cytotoxic T lymphocytes important? Immunol Today 8:265, 1987.

43. Podack, ER: The molecular mechanism of lymphocyte mediated tumor cell lysis. Immunol Today 6:21, 1985.

44. Gershon, RK and Kondo, K: Infectious immunological tolerance. Immunology 21:903, 1971.

45. Lowy, A, et al.: Identification of an I-J antigen-presenting cell required for third order suppressor cell activation. J Exp Med 157:353, 1983.

46. Hedrick, SM, et al.: Rearrangement and transcription of a T-cell receptor chain gene in different T-cell subsets. Proc Natl Acad Sci USA 82:531, 1985.

47. Ochoa, AC, et al.: Long-term growth of lymphokine-activated (LAK) cells. J Immunol 138:2728, 1987.

48. Robb, RJ: Interleukin 2: the molecule and its function. Immunol Today 6:156, 1984.

49. Usui, M, et al.: A role for macrophages in suppressor cell induction. J Immunol 132:1728, 1984.

50. Chiller, J, et al.: Kinetic differences in unresponsiveness of thymus and bone marrow cells. Science 171:813, 1971.

51. Zanders, ED, et al.: Tolerance of T-cell clones is associated with membrane antigen changes. Nature 303:625, 1983.

52. Green, DR, et al.: Immunoregulatory T-cell pathways. Ann Rev Immunol 1:439, 1983.

53. Jerne, N: Towards a network theory of the immune system. Ann Immunol 125:373, 1974.

54. Grzych, JM, et al.: An anti-idiotype vaccine against experimental schistosomiasis. Nature 316:74, 1985.

55. Capron, A, et al.: Immunity to schistosomes: progress toward vaccine. Science 238:1065, 1987.

56. Bottazzo, GF, et al.: Role of aberrant HLA-DR expression and antigen presentation in induction of endocrine autoimmunity. Lancet 11:1115, 1983.

57. Todd, JA, et al.: HLA-DQB gene contributes to susceptibility and resistance to insulin-dependent diabetes mellitus. Nature 329:599, 1987.

58. Weiss, RA: Receptor molecule blocks HIV. Nature 331:15, 1988.

59. Berzofsky, JA, et al.: Protein antigenic structures recognized by T cells: potential applications to vaccine design. Immunol Rev 98:9, 1987.

60. Francis, MJ, et al.: Non-responsiveness to a foot-and-mouth disease virus peptide overcome by foreign helper T-cell determinants. Nature 330:168, 1987.

119 IMMUNOLOGIC DISEASES

JAMES P. THOMPSON

Immune-mediated diseases are the result of immune responses directed at a variety of antigens that directly or indirectly lead to damage of host tissue. There are two major categories of immune-mediated diseases: primary (autoimmune) immune-mediated disease and secondary immune-mediated disease.

Primary (autoimmune) immune-mediated disease constitutes a variety of diseases in which self antigens are specifically recognized and destroyed by an immune response. The development of specific antibodies or T lymphocytes that exhibit reactivity against self antigens represents a failure of the immunoregulatory mechanisms of the immune system, which normally function to limit the production of immune responses. Critical in the regulation of host immune responses is the establishment of tolerance, a state of immunologic unresponsiveness, to self antigens. The expression of autoimmune disease is thus the result of regulation failure and escape from immune tolerance. Several hypotheses exist to explain the failure of the immune system to maintain strict immunologic tolerance. These hypotheses include (1) the forbidden clone, (2) exposure of hidden antigens, (3) cross-reacting antigens, (4) alteration of self antigens, and (5) failure of immunoregulation.

The Forbidden Clone. This hypothesis is based on the observation that during the early development of the immune system, deletion of autoreactive T and B lymphocytes occurs, which limits the numbers of forbidden T and B lymphocyte clones with the capacity to recognize self antigens. This mechanism is dependent on early exposure of autoreactive lymphocytes to self antigen. The deletion of autoreactive lymphocytes is not perfect, however, and many lymphocytes escape the deletion process and maintain the potential to initiate autoimmune disease. Strict regulatory control of these lymphocytes that have escaped deletion is essential to prevent their expansion and subsequent expression of autoimmune disease.

Exposure of Hidden Antigens. During the maturation of the immune system and the subsequent deletion of autoreactive lymphocytes described above, certain body tissues and their associated antigens are not exposed to the immune system (e.g., lens tissue). As a result, those autoreactive lymphocytes that express receptors for these hidden tissue antigens are not deleted. Consequently, exposure of the immune system to these anti-gens later in life, secondary to either a traumatic or an inflammatory event, may lead to the generation of an immune response to these previously hidden antigens and the development of an autoimmune disease.

Cross-Reacting Antigens. Antigens present on infectious agents, biologicals, or chemicals may share common structural properties (epitopes) present on self tissue. Immune responses directed against these foreign antigens may then cross-react significantly with self antigens and result in tissue damage.

Alteration of Self Antigens. The binding of chemicals or infectious agents to self antigens may cause a slight but significant alteration in the structure of the self antigen. The change in antigenic structure may stimulate an immune response, which recognizes both the altered and the unaltered self antigen and lead to the expression of autoimmune disease.

Failure of Immunoregulation. The proliferation of B lymphocytes and the production of autoantibodies are inhibited by specific immunoregulatory mechanisms. These regulatory mechanisms are established through interactions of B lymphocytes with T lymphocytes. There are two major classes of regulatory T lymphocytes: those T lymphocytes that induce or stimulate antibody production (T-helper lymphocytes) and those that inhibit or suppress antibody production (T-suppressor lymphocytes). Abnormalities within specific T-helper or T-suppressor lymphocytes or immune responses that bypass these regulatory cells may lead to the expression of an autoimmune disease. Within the general scheme of immunoregulation there are basically four methods in which the immune system may fail and result in autoimmune disease. These four methods are (1) increased T-helper lymphocyte activity, (2) decreased T-suppressor lymphocyte activity, (3) bypass of regulation requirement for T-helper or T-suppressor lymphocyte function, and (4) generation of anti-idiotypic antibodies. An excellent, in depth review of these immunoregulatory mechanisms has been recently written.[1]

Secondary immune-mediated diseases represent immune responses directed at antigens that lead to inadvertent damage of host tissue. This type of immune-mediated disease is not the result of an autoimmune process, but can be observed in numerous pathological processes including neoplasia, infection with parasites, viruses, bacteriae, rickettsiae, and fungal agents, and the administration of pharmaceutical agents. Treatment of a secondary immune-mediated disease should focus on the elimination of the underlying disease process.

There are classically four types of immunopathologic mechanisms active in the production of immune-mediated disease and virtually any organ system may be damaged. The four immunopathologic mechanisms are (1) immediate hypersensitivity, (2) cytotoxic hypersensitivity, (3) immune complex hypersensitivity, and (4) delayed hypersensitivity (Table 119–1). Each of these mechanisms will be discussed specifically in relation to the expression of immune-mediated disease within the various sections of this chapter.

IMMUNODEFICIENCY DISEASES

A deficiency in either the cells of the nonspecific immune system (monocytes, macrophages, and neutrophils) or components of the specific immune system (T and B lymphocytes) results in the expression of an immunodeficiency disorder.[2, 3] The clinical manifestations of immunodeficiency are typically associated with an increased frequency and severity of infection. Infectious processes that are chronic, fail to respond to conventional treatment, or are secondary to nonpathogenic organisms suggest the possibility of an underlying immunodeficiency disease.

Deficiencies of the immune system are either congenital (primary immunodeficiency) or acquired (secondary immunodeficiency). Specific immunodeficiencies may stem from a deficiency in either the humoral or the cellular immune system, or both. Animals that exhibit humoral immunodeficiencies generally show increased susceptibility to bacterial infections. Deficiencies in the cell-mediated immune system result more commonly in recurrent or persistent fungal, viral, or protozoal disease processes. Abnormalities of the nonspecific immune system (monocytes, macrophages, and neutrophils) are associated with defective phagocytosis (engulfment of microorganisms, cells, or foreign particles) and are generally associated with recurrent skin infections or systemic pyrogenic bacterial infections; the reader is referred to Chapter 114 for an in-depth discussion of abnormalities of these leukocytes.

Primary (Congenital) Immunodeficiencies

COMBINED IMMUNODEFICIENCY

Clinical Signs. Combined immunodeficiency is characterized by deficiencies of both B and T lymphocytes,

lymphoid hypoplasia, and thymic dysplasia. Combined immunodeficiency is probably the most severe of the congenital immunodeficiency diseases.[4] Documented cases of combined immunodeficiency in small animal medicine are limited to basset hound puppies.[5] The onset of disease occurs near three weeks of age and presenting complaints may include a failure to thrive, pyoderma, otitis, gingivitis, and stomatitis. The disease is transmitted as an X-linked recessive trait and affected male dogs should exhibit signs of disease.

Diagnosis. The diagnosis of combined immunodeficiency should be considered in young male basset hound puppies that exhibit persistent otitis, gingivostomatitis, pyodermatitis, and decreased growth rate. Definitive diagnosis requires microscopic demonstration of lymphoid hypoplasia, documentation of hypoglobulinemia (IgG and IgA deficiencies; IgM concentrations are variable), identification of persistent peripheral blood lymphopenia, and a lack of T lymphocyte responsiveness. Other dog and cat breeds that exhibit a similar type of clinical disease presentation should also be evaluated in an identical manner to rule out a combined immunodeficiency disease.

Treatment and Prognosis. No documented life-saving therapy currently exists for these puppies. Ideally, these patients should be given an allogeneic bone marrow transplant, but this procedure is not generally available and in these patients would likely be associated with a severe and possibly fatal graft versus host reaction. Modified live vaccines should not be administered, as the vaccine may induce fatal infection. The prognosis for these puppies is grave. All reported patients have died before reaching four months of age.[5]

SELECTED IGA DEFICIENCY

Clinical Signs. Selective IgA deficiency is characterized by decreased or absent serum concentrations of IgA. Although the precise etiology is not known, the immunologic defect probably lies in the maturation or differentiation of B lymphocytes destined to secrete IgA. The depressed levels of serum IgA predispose patients to increased incidences of infections involving mucosal surfaces. Increased infection rates of the mucosal surfaces are the direct result of decreased antibody in IgA present at these surfaces; the major function of IgA is to provide local mucosal immunity.

Recurrent upper respiratory and gastrointestinal tract infections, otitis, and dermatitis occur. Immunoglobulin A deficiencies have been described in the German shepherd, beagle, and Shar Pei,[4, 6–8] but documented cases of feline IgA deficiency are currently lacking.

Diagnosis. The diagnosis of IgA deficiency requires documentation of absent or markedly decreased serum concentrations of IgA; the comparison of serum IgA concentration with age matched normal control patients is critical.

Treatment and Prognosis. Specific treatments to effectively increase serum concentrations of IgA antibody are unknown and intranasal vaccination against *Bordetella bronchiseptica* and canine parainfluenza appears to be ineffective. Current recommendations include supportive antibiotic therapy and decreased exposure to

TABLE 119–1. IMMUNOPATHOLOGIC MECHANISMS OF IMMUNE-MEDIATED DISEASES

General Classification	Type-specific Classification	Effector Mechanisms
Immediate hypersensitivity	Type I hypersensitivity	IgE antibody, mast cells, basophils
Cytotoxic hypersensitivity	Type II hypersensitivity	IgG, M, A antibody and complement
Immune complex hypersensitivity	Type III hypersensitivity	IgG, M, A antibody and complement
Delayed hypersensitivity	Type IV hypersensitivity	T lymphocytes

infectious agents. In addition, an environment with reduced chances of induced systemic stress should promote improved general immune function. Infections are generally not life-threatening and the possibility exists that some dogs may outgrow their tendency to develop recurrent infections.[4]

TRANSIENT HYPOGAMMAGLOBULINEMIA OF INFANCY

Clinical Signs. This disorder is characterized by decreased serum concentrations of immunoglobulins and becomes readily apparent early in life as the decline in passively acquired maternal antibodies occurs. Puppies with this congenital immunodeficiency disorder may present with the primary complaints of respiratory tract infection and/or dermatitis, which typically begins about two to three months of age.[4]

Diagnosis. Diagnosis depends on the documentation of low immunoglobulin concentrations as compared to appropriately matched control dogs. Other laboratory tests are not contributory to a definitive diagnosis.

Treatment and Prognosis. This disease process is self-limiting and typically the puppies synthesize normal amounts of immunoglobulin by five to six months of age. Supportive antibiotic therapy and a clean environment are recommended for case management.

The prognosis must remain guarded until a documented rise in serum immunoglobulin concentration is observed. The documented increase in serum immunoglobulin should correlate with a good prognosis.

Secondary (Acquired) Immunodeficiencies

Secondary (acquired) immunodeficiencies are more common than primary (congenital) immunodeficiencies. The acquired immunodeficiencies may be secondary to numerous underlying disease processes, environmental factors, and endogenous substances. Agents responsible for inducing acquired immune deficiencies include infectious organisms, pharmacologic substances, endogenous hormones, splenectomy, aging, malnutrition, neoplasia, and radiation exposure.[2]

Infectious Organisms. Canine distemper virus, canine parvovirus, feline panleukopenia virus, and feline leukemia virus have each been shown to induce marked depression of the cell-mediated immune response. It has long been recognized that the leukemogenic nature of feline leukemia virus is less significant than the associated profound immunosuppression; most cats die of secondary infection related to feline leukemia virus rather than of lymphoma or of leukemia. Nonviral diseases such as demodecosis, ehrlichiosis, and systemic fungal disease are also closely associated with profound immunosuppression. It is unclear, however, whether infection with these organisms results in immunosuppression or whether an underlying immune defect is permissive for extensive infection.

Pharmacologic Substances. Corticosteroids and the various antineoplastic agents are probably the most commonly used pharmacologic agents that effectively induce immunosuppression; their mechanism of action

and use in modulating immune-mediated disease will be discussed later in this chapter. Drug agents not specifically utilized for direct immunosuppression, but that have been associated with this abnormality, include chloramphenicol, sulfamethoxypyridazine, clindamycin, dapsone, lincomycin, griseofulvin, and nalidixic acid.[2]

Endogenous Hormones. Hyperadrenocorticism, growth hormone deficiency, diabetes mellitus, and hyperestrogenism have each been associated with acquired immunodeficiency disease. Hyperadrenocorticism appears to inhibit immune function secondary to increased glucocorticoids, while growth hormone deficiency induces immunodeficiency by interfering with T lymphocyte maturation secondary to depressed thymic development. Patients with diabetes mellitus exhibit a predisposition to develop cutaneous, systemic, and urinary tract infections that may be related directly to decreased serum insulin concentrations or to hyperglycemia.[2] Immunosuppressive effects of hyperestrogenism are directly related to leukopenia.

Treatment and Prognosis. Treatment schemes for acquired immunodeficiencies focus on the underlying disease process believed to be responsible for the depressed immune system. Supportive patient care is also essential to ensure optimal patient response to treatment. The prognosis for acquired immunodeficiency diseases is variable. In some instances (e.g., profound hyperestrogenism) the immune defect may be so severe that despite aggressive and repeated efforts the patient may succumb. In other cases (e.g., diabetes mellitus) control of serum insulin and glucose concentrations results in a near natural life.

IMMUNOHEMATOLOGIC DISEASES

Immune-mediated hemolytic anemia and immune-mediated thrombocytopenia are frequently encountered immunohematologic diseases. Although not well documented in veterinary medicine, each cell type within the hematopoietic system (neutrophils, eosinophils, etc.) may potentially be the target of a primary or secondary cytotoxic hypersensitivity (Type II hypersensitivity) immune response.

IMMUNE-MEDIATED HEMOLYTIC ANEMIA

Immune-mediated hemolytic anemia (IHA) is characterized by an accelerated destruction of erythrocytes due to the presence of antibody attached to the surface of the erythrocyte membrane. The antibody may bind to unaltered endogenous erythrocyte membrane antigens (primary autoimmune hemolytic anemia) or to exogenous antigens such as drugs or microorganisms adherent to erythrocyte membranes (secondary immune-mediated hemolytic anemia). Regardless of whether the anemia is the result of a primary autoimmune disease or a secondary immune-mediated disease, the pathophysiology is related to the physical and chemical properties of the antibodies adherent to the surface of the erythrocyte.

Pathophysiology. The immunoglobulin (Ig) classes

most often identified in canine IHA are IgG and in some cases both IgG and IgM; rarely IgM antibodies alone have been identified.[9] In the cat, IgM antierythrocyte antibodies are more prominent and cats with antibody in IgG alone are noted in only approximately 25 per cent of reported cases.[10] The adherence of antibody onto the erythrocyte surface may activate the complement system and result in the deposition of complement proteins onto the erythrocyte surface membrane. Because of the pentameric structure of IgM, a single antibody molecule attached to the erythrocyte surface may activate the classical complement cascade. Antibodies in IgG may also activate the classical complement cascade; however, the erythrocyte surface must be covered with sufficient IgG molecules such that two molecules are in close enough proximity to allow the initial complement-activating protein (Clq) to bind to the Fc region of the two adjacent antibody molecules.

Antibodies active in IHA have traditionally been subclassified into one of five separate categories based on the clinical presentation of the hemolytic disease and the results of laboratory tests documenting conditions under which the antibodies bind to erythrocytes.

IN-SALINE ACTING AUTOAGGLUTININS. This category is represented by antibodies that agglutinate erythrocytes *in vitro* at 37° C and presumably may result in intravascular hemagglutination in the patient. Agglutination is best observed by placing a drop of blood on a glass microscope slide (Figure 119–1). Agglutination must, however, be differentiated from rouleau formation. The differentiation between agglutination and rouleaux is accomplished by mixing an equal volume of isotonic saline with the blood on the microscope slide and observing for the presence or absence of erythrocyte clumping; rouleau formation will disperse, but immune-mediated agglutination will persist. The demonstration of erythrocyte agglutination is diagnostic for immune-mediated hemolytic anemia and a Coombs' test would only be indicated to define the specific antibody class responsible for the hemagglutination.

INTRAVASCULAR HEMOLYSINS. This category is represented by antibodies that activate sufficient quantities of complement to induce intravascular hemolysis. It is important to note that numerous individual sites of complement activation on the erythrocyte surface are needed before the membrane damage will be sufficient to result in cell lysis.

INCOMPLETE ANTIBODY CLASS. This category consists of those antibodies that bind to the erythrocyte membrane in insufficient quantity to cause intravascular hemolysis or agglutination. This category represents the most common form of IHA. Erythrocyte destruction occurs following erythrophagocytosis within the reticuloendothelial system of the spleen, liver, and bone marrow.

COLD HEMAGGLUTININS. This category is represented by antibodies that are capable of agglutinating erythrocytes, but only at temperatures below 32° C. Care must be taken to identify a specific titer of cold hemagglutinins, as normal animals may contain up to 1:8 titers of cold hemagglutinins. The demonstration of cold hemagglutinins in titers greater than 1:8 is diagnostic for cryopathic immune-mediated hemolytic anemia.

COLD-ACTING NONAGGLUTININS. This category consists of antibodies that bind erythrocytes at low temperatures, but do not cause agglutination. Presumably these erythrocytes are destroyed by the reticuloendothelial system in cold climates, but the clinical significance of this disease is not known.

These five categories of antibody and erythrocyte interaction result in only three common clinical syndromes associated with immune-mediated hemolytic anemia. Each of these clinical syndromes represents a cytotoxic hypersensitivity reaction (Type II hypersensitivity). The three clinical syndromes are (1) immune-mediated extravascular hemolysis, (2) immune-mediated intravascular hemolysis, and (3) cryopathic immune-mediated hemolytic anemia.

IMMUNE-MEDIATED EXTRAVASCULAR HEMOLYSIS. Most often in IHA there is sufficient antibody adherent

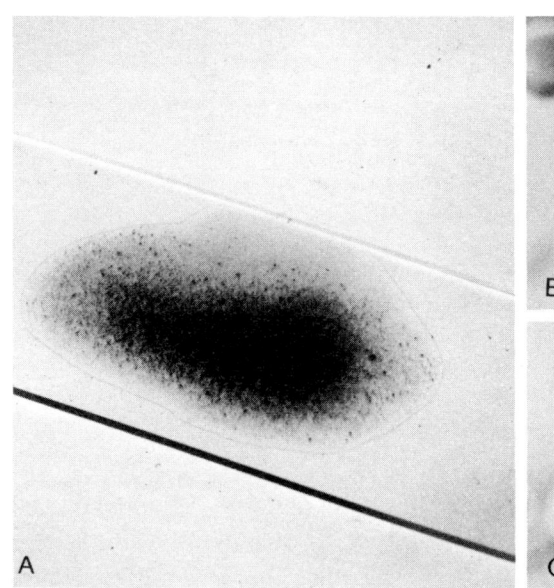

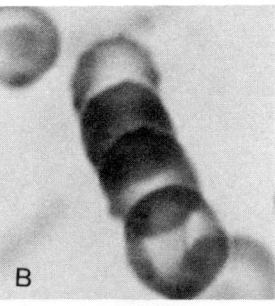

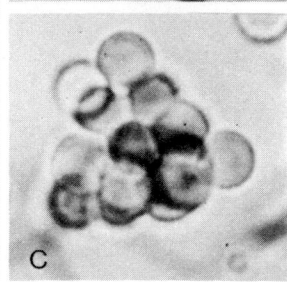

FIGURE 119–1. *A,* Direct macroscopic erythrocyte agglutination. One drop of peripheral blood collected in EDTA mixed with one drop of 0.9 per cent saline at room temperature. *B,* Microscopic wet preparation of canine blood demonstrating rouleau formation. Rouleau must be distinguished from autoagglutination. (Courtesy of Dr. Dennis J. Meyer.) *C,* Microscopic wet preparation of canine blood exhibiting autoagglutination. Note the clumping of erythrocytes typical of agglutination. (Courtesy of Dr. Dennis J. Meyer.)

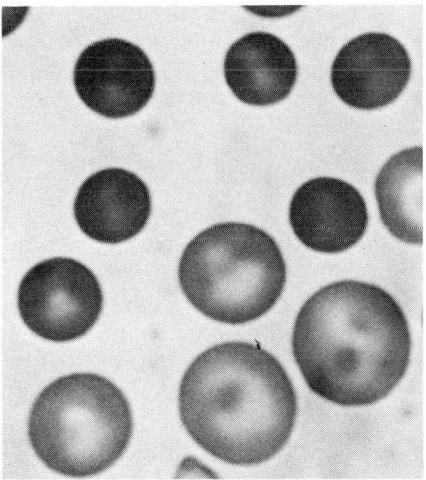

FIGURE 119–2. Peripheral blood smear demonstrating marked anisocytosis due to the presence of numerous small, round, spherocytes. (Courtesy of Dr. Dennis J. Meyer.)

to the erythrocyte surface to induce some complement system activation, but not enough complement activation to cause lysis of the erythrocyte. However, the adherent antibody and complement proteins cause significant erythrocyte membrane damage and induce decreased deformability of the erythrocyte. The erythrocytes characteristically become spherical and lose their central pallor and discoid shape. This type of erythrocyte is termed a spherocyte (Figure 119–2) and when present is highly suggestive of IHA; other disease processes in which spherocytes may be observed include those that cause fragmentation anemia such as microangiopathic hemolytic anemia seen in disseminated intravascular coagulation and the vena cava syndrome seen in dirofilariasis. The antibody coated erythrocytes are removed from the circulation by macrophages of the reticuloendothelial system within the spleen, liver, and bone marrow. The macrophages have specific receptors that recognize the Fc portion of adherent IgG antibody molecules and the complement split-protein C3b, which binds to membrane surfaces following the activation of the complement system. The engulfment of erythrocytes is termed erythrophagocytosis and can be observed in Figure 119–3. Within the macrophages the erythrocytes are lysed, the globulin portion of hemoglobin is degraded into its component amino acids, the iron molecule is removed from the heme molecule, and the heme

is converted to bilirubin and released into the blood stream as unconjugated (indirect acting) bilirubin, which is noncovalently bound to albumin.

IMMUNE-MEDIATED INTRAVASCULAR HEMOLYSIS. Intravascular hemolysis of antibody coated erythrocytes is due to extensive complement activation and erythrocyte lysis. The intravascular hemolysis of circulating erythrocytes results in hemoglobinemia. Circulating hemoglobin is rapidly bound by serum haptoglobin, and the resulting complex is too large to be filtered through the glomerulus of the kidney. If the intravascular hemolysis is severe, then the available haptoglobin will be saturated and free hemoglobin will filter through the renal glomerulus and hemoglobinuria will be present. The severity of intravascular hemolysis may lead to extensive glomerulonephritis and acute renal failure secondary to erythrocyte membrane antigen-antibody complex deposition and complement activation; in addition, free hemoglobin has been suggested to be toxic to renal tubular cells.

CRYOPATHIC IMMUNE-MEDIATED HEMOLYTIC ANEMIA. Cryopathic IHA has been described in the dog and cat.[11, 12] The disease has been associated with an IgM antibody response directed against erythrocyte membrane antigens, which bind only at temperatures below 32° C. Drugs or microorganisms have not been associated with this disease and presumably reported cases represent a primary autoimmune disease process. The end result is the agglutination of erythrocytes in the cooler, peripheral vascular beds, which can lead to obstruction of small vessels, acrocyanosis, and gangrenous necrosis of the feet, ear or tail tips, and nose (Figure 119–4). Hemolysis is rarely observed in humans and occurs only in patients with excessive antibody titers.

Diagnosis. The owners generally present their animal for the primary complaint of either anorexia, listlessness,

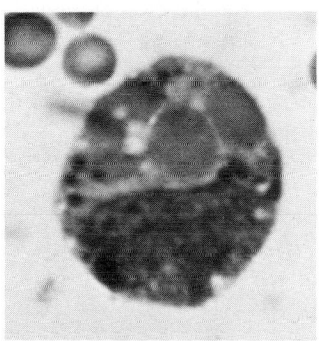

FIGURE 119–3. Photomicrograph depicting marked erythrophagocytosis. (Courtesy of Dr. Dennis J. Meyer.)

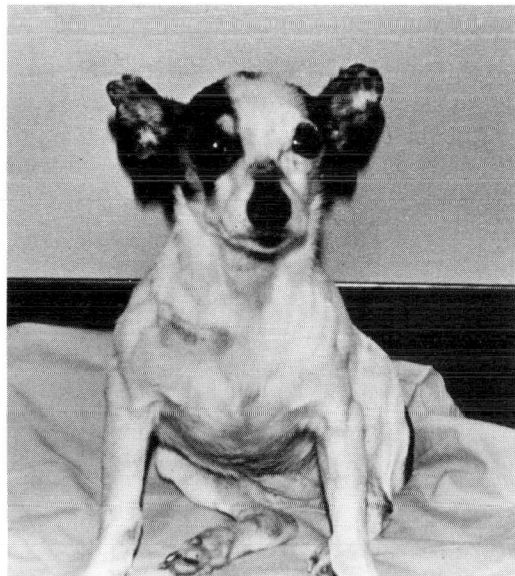

FIGURE 119–4. Distal extremity lesions involving the pinnae, planum nasale, tail tip and digits of an eleven-year-old female Fox terrier with cold agglutinin disease accompanying a lymphoproliferative disorder. Direct hemagglutination and a positive Coombs' test for IgM (both occurring at 4° C but not at 37° C) were significant diagnostic findings. (Courtesy of Dr. Linda L. Werner.)

weakness or depression. Physical examination typically reveals pale mucous membranes and tachycardia. Tachypnea may or may not be present. Depending on the extent of the anemia a mild heart murmur may be auscultated due to decreased blood viscosity. If extravascular hemolysis is the prominent mechanism of accelerated erythrocyte destruction then splenomegaly or hepatomegaly may be obvious. If intravascular hemolysis is present and extensive, then icterus, fever, and vomiting may be observed. Dogs and cats with cryopathic immune-mediated hemolytic anemia will exhibit distal extremity lesions of the ears, tail, or feet; these lesions should be considered in the context of the environmental temperature.

The complete blood cell count generally demonstrates a leukocytosis, often greater than 25,000/mm^3 blood, with an absolute neutrophilia and a significant left shift; total leukocytes greater than 60,000 with a left shift to 4000 metamyelocytes without toxic cytoplasm have been seen. The most common finding on the hemogram is a regenerative anemia typified by macrocytosis, polychromasia, anisocytosis, hypochromasia, and nucleated erythrocytes with occasional Howell-Jolly bodies. The presence of spherocytes on a peripheral blood smear is strongly suggestive of immune-mediated hemolytic anemia. The fibrinogen may be elevated and icterus or hemolysis observed; caution must be used to rule out lipemia-induced or sampling technique–induced *in vitro* hemolysis.

The serum chemistry profile may show elevated lactic dehydrogenase activity secondary to enzyme release from damaged erythrocytes. The hepatic enzymes (alanine and aspartate aminotransferases and alkaline phosphatase) may be mildly elevated. If intravascular hemolysis is present, the serum haptoglobin concentration may be decreased; quantitating haptoglobin concentration may be helpful in differentiating intravascular from extravascular hemolysis. In extensive intravascular and extravascular hemolysis, hyperbilirubinemia may be present.

The urinalysis may show hemoglobinuria if intravascular hemolysis is marked. The most common abnormalities identified in the urinalysis are increased urobilinogen and bilirubinuria. If extensive intravascular hemolysis is present then proteinuria and cylindruria may be present indicating glomerular and tubular nephritis. If an active urine sediment is present attention must be directed to insure adequate fluid intake and urine excretion.

DIRECT COOMBS' TEST. The diagnostic test of choice is the direct antiglobin or Coombs' test.[9] This test quantitates the amount of antibodies or complement bound to erythrocyte surface membranes. The Coombs' reagent must be species-specific and recognize IgG, IgM and C3b (the membrane bound protein split product deposited on the erythrocyte surface from the third component of the complement cascade). The patient's blood is collected in heparin or ethylenediaminetetraacetic acid (EDTA) and the erythrocytes washed three times in phosphate buffered saline. A two percent suspension of the red blood cells in phosphate buffered saline is prepared and added to serial two-fold dilutions of the Coombs' reagent to identify the amount of antibody (IgM or IgG) or complement (C3b) adherent to the erythrocyte membrane. After incubation at the appropriate temperature (37° C or 4° C depending upon the suspected pathophysiology of the immune-mediated anemia), the erythrocytes are observed for macroscopic and microscopic agglutination.

OSMOTIC FRAGILITY TEST. Another useful test to document abnormal erythrocyte membrane structure is the osmotic fragility test. This test is based on the known stability of normal canine erythrocytes in a 0.54 per cent saline solution. Erythrocytes damaged by the binding of antibody and complement to membrane antigens exhibit decreased membrane stability and will lyse when exposed to a 0.54 per cent hypotonic saline solution. The test is simple and is performed by placing 5 drops of blood in a centrifuge tube containing 3 ml of 0.9 per cent saline and 2 ml of water; a control test should be concurrently performed and consists of 5 ml of 0.9 per cent saline to which 5 drops of blood are added. Both centrifuge tubes are incubated at room temperature for five minutes and following incubation the tubes are centrifuged and the supernatants examined. Close inspection of the control tube supernatant should reveal no evidence of hemolysis, while a pink-tinged supernatant in the hypotonic saline solution indicates fragile erythrocytes and supports a diagnosis of immune-mediated hemolytic disease. An abnormal osmotic fragility test can be expected in approximately 85 per cent of canine cases of immune-mediated hemolytic anemia.

Feline erythrocytes are more sensitive to osmotic pressure, but may be similarly tested in a 0.64 per cent saline solution. The test is accomplished by placing 5 drops of blood in a centrifuge tube containing 5 ml of 0.9 per cent saline and 2 ml of water; a control test consisting of 7 ml of 0.9 per cent saline and 5 drops of blood should also be performed.

In a reported study approximately 40 per cent of 77 cases diagnosed as IHA were also associated with immune-mediated thrombocytopenia (20 per cent), systemic lupus erythematosus (17 per cent) or both IMT and SLE (3 per cent).[13] This finding demonstrates the necessity to perform an absolute platelet count and either an indirect fluorescence antinuclear antibody test or lupus erythematosus cell preparation in all cases of diagnosed IHA. Another consideration may be a coagulogram to rule out consumption coagulopathy as an underlying etiology for a thrombocytopenia associated with IHA.

Treatment. The therapeutic goal in the management of immune-mediated hemolytic anemia is the maintenance of tissue oxygenation and not necessarily the elevation of the packed cell volume to base-line normal values; a packed cell volume of 25 per cent may be compatible with a reasonably normal existence. A general treatment plan can be found in Table 119–2. Treatment with prednisone or prednisolone at 0.5 to 1 mg/lb (1 to 2 mg/kg) PO q12h is usually effective.[10] The aim of the glucocorticoid therapy is to decrease erythrocyte phagocytosis and is generally most effective in hemolytic anemias secondary to extravascular hemolysis. In addition the corticosteroids will decrease antibody production somewhat and consequently may help decrease erythrocyte opsonization. The dosage is maintained until

TABLE 119–2. TREATMENT PLAN FOR IMMUNE-MEDIATED HEMOLYTIC ANEMIA

I. Assess patient's demand for increased oxygen delivery
  A. Provide blood only if indicated (cross-matched preferred)
  B. Supplemental oxygen unlikely to benefit patient
  C. If blood is administered and neutrophil count > 2000/mm³, begin cyclophosphamide 1 mg/lb (50 mg/m²) PO or IV daily for 4 days
II. Assess patient's hydration status
  A. Rehydrate if indicated
  B. Provide at least maintenance fluid therapy PO, IV, or SQ
III. Assess type of hemolytic disease
  A. Extravascular
    (1) Begin prednisone 0.5–1.0 mg/lb (1–2 mg/kg) PO q12h
    (2) Assess PCV daily
  B. Intravascular
    (1) Begin prednisone 0.5–1.0 mg/lb (1–2 mg/kg) PO q12h
    (2) If neutrophil count > 2000/mm³, begin cyclophosphamide 1 mg/lb (50 mg/m²) PO or IV daily for 4 days
    (3) Monitor UA and renal status closely
    (4) Assess PCV q12h
  C. Cryopathic
    (1) Provide warm environment
    (2) Short course prednisone 0.5–1.0 mg/lb (1–2 mg/kg) PO q12h

the packed cell volume demonstrates significant improvement and then the dosage is gradually decreased. In some cases it may be possible to discontinue the glucocorticoid therapy two to three months after the packed cell volume returns to normal. If the packed cell volume fails to increase to normal, then low dose therapy with prednisone or prednisolone at 0.25 to 0.5 mg/lb (0.5 to 1 mg/kg) PO q48h may be required indefinitely.

If glucocorticoid therapy is unsuccessful in the initial management of the disease, then more potent immunosuppressive medication such as cyclophosphamide at 1 mg/lb (50 mg/m²) PO or IV q24h for four consecutive days of each week would be indicated along with prednisone or prednisolone at 0.5 to 1 mg/lb (1 to 2 mg/kg) PO q12h.[14] When the packed cell volume increases significantly the cyclophosphamide should be discontinued and the prednisone or prednisolone gradually reduced and discontinued if possible. Concern always exists that the cyclophosphamide may inhibit erythrocyte production and may therefore be contraindicated. However, as long as the leukocyte, platelet, and reticulocyte counts are appropriate, then aggressive therapy with cyclophosphamide should be continued. It should also be noted that therapy with cyclophosphamide may be necessary for 10 to 20 days before a significant improvement in packed cell volume is observed because the mechanism of cyclophosphamide-induced immunosuppression is due to a decrease in antibody synthesis and to a decrease in the numbers of plasma cells; antibody already present in the systemic circulation will have to be removed via adsorption to erythrocytes or normal catabolism.

Immediate initiation of cyclophosphamide and prednisone together has been previously suggested for those cases of IHA where intravascular hemolysis is marked or where autoagglutination occurs at body temperature. This recommendation appears appropriate based on the observation that a general response to glucocorticoid therapy alone is poor.[15]

Blood transfusions should be avoided and used only if absolutely necessary; blood transfusions may precipitate or accelerate a hemolytic crisis. When a blood transfusion is given to avert a life-threatening crisis, an immunosuppressant such as cyclophosphamide at 1 mg/lb (50 mg/m²) PO or IV q24h for four consecutive days should be considered to decrease any potential humoral immune response to the transfusion. Dogs and cats that present in hypoxemic shock require a blood transfusion, intravenous lactated Ringer's solution, and probably sodium bicarbonate to counteract a lactic acidosis likely associated with the hypoxemia.

Other forms of therapy may include plasmapheresis to decrease the amount of circulating antibody and splenectomy if other forms of therapy are unsuccessful.[16, 17] Splenectomy not only removes a major organ involved in erythrocyte phagocytosis, but also may remove an extensive source of antibody-producing lymphocytes. Caution must be observed in splenectomy as infection with *Haemobartonella canis* and secondary severe anemia have been reported in one splenectomized dog.[18] Although only palliative, the lowering of serum antibody concentrations with plasmapheresis may offer the potential of altering the rate of antibody-mediated erythrocyte destruction in acute IHA.

Prognosis. In a study of 45 cases of canine IHA, 33 per cent of the dogs died; males may have had a slightly higher death rate.[13] The prognosis is guarded when the hemolytic anemia is associated with severe hepatic and renal diseases and more guarded when associated with immune-mediated thrombocytopenia or systemic lupus erythematosus. Dogs with agglutinating antibody or intravascular hemolysis have the poorest prognosis and highest death rate.

IMMUNE-MEDIATED THROMBOCYTOPENIA

Immune-mediated thrombocytopenia (IMT) may occur alone or in association with other immune-mediated disorders such as immune-mediated hemolytic anemia (Evans's syndrome), systemic lupus erythematosus, and rheumatoid arthritis. Immune-mediated thrombocytopenia is a common disease in the dog, but has been rarely reported in the cat.[19, 20] The disease is associated with an absolute thrombocytopenia (< 200,000 thrombocytes/mm³), but clinical signs related to bleeding associated with the thrombocytopenia are rarely observed until the platelet count drops below 30,000 thrombocytes/mm³ blood.[21] The onset of bleeding may relate not only to the absolute numbers of platelets, but to the rapidity of the platelet decrease, to the stability of the capillary endothelial membrane, and to the incidence of traumatic events. Dogs with platelet counts of 8,000/mm³ may show no evidence of bleeding, while others with counts of 32,000/mm³ may bleed extensively (Figure 119–5).

Pathophysiology. The pathogenesis of decreased circulating platelet numbers is presumed to be secondary to either an increased antibody- and complement-mediated platelet phagocytosis within the spleen, bone marrow and liver (locations where the reticuloendothelial system exists) or to a decreased production of platelets secondary to an antibody- and/or complement-

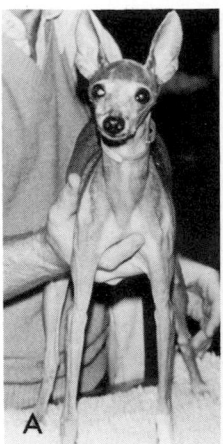
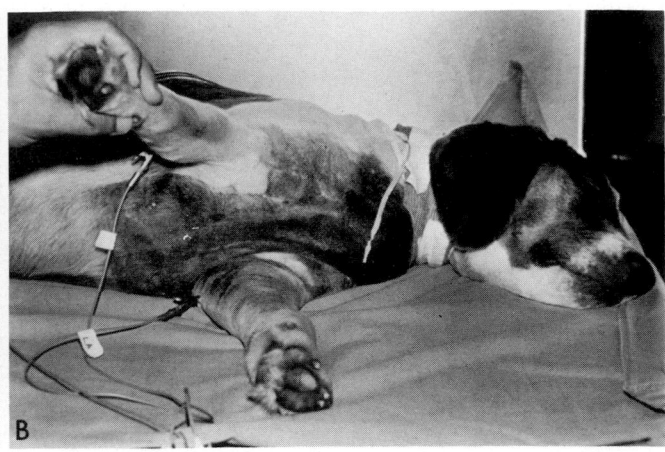

FIGURE 119–5. *A*, A ten-year-old Italian greyhound with a platelet count of 8,000/mm³ showed no evidence of hemorrhage except for jugular hematomas following venipuncture. In contrast, *B* shows a four-year-old male beagle with a 32,000/mm³ platelet count that presented semicomatose with massive ventral cutaneous ecchymoses, cardiac rhythm disturbance, and neurologic deficits suggestive of internal hemorrhage. Both dogs showed a positive platelet factor 3 test and responded to treatment for IMT. The beagle required fresh blood transfusion to control progressive hemorrhage. (Courtesy of Dr. Linda L. Werner.)

mediated destruction of megakaryocytes within the bone marrow.[22]

Diagnosis. The patient may be presented for a variety of complaints, which include epistaxis, lethargy, weakness, hematuria, hematochezia, hematemesis, melena, and dermal petechiation and ecchymosis. The physical examination most commonly reveals mucous membrane petechiation and other signs related to a bleeding disorder.

The complete blood cell count characteristically shows a thrombocytopenia and, if bleeding has occurred, an anemia and possibly low plasma proteins associated with the bleeding. If the bleeding has been a relatively recent event, then a normocytic normochromic anemia without signs of regeneration may be present. If the bleeding episode occurred more than 3 or 4 days prior to presentation then a regenerative anemia with macrocytosis, hypochromasia, polychromasia, and reticulocytosis may be evident. If the bleeding has been extensive and prolonged, then a blood loss–induced, iron deficient microcytic hypochromic anemia will likely be present. Concern must be directed in the bleeding patient to perform a complete coagulogram in order to exclude intrinsic and extrinsic coagulation system defects as a cause of the excessive bleeding with a general consumption of peripheral platelets.

The serum chemistry profile is usually normal. The urinalysis may reveal hematuria, but more common would be proteinuria secondary to antigen-antibody complex deposition within the glomerulus and a complement-induced glomerulonephritis.

The diagnostic tests of choice include a platelet factor-3 test and direct immunofluorescence of a bone marrow aspirate to identify antibody coated megakaryocytes.

PLATELET FACTOR-3 TEST. The platelet factor-3 (PF-3) test to detect antiplatelet antibody rests on the physiologic basis that the platelet specific antibody binds to platelets inducing membrane-associated platelet phospholipid release and that the coagulation cascade is accelerated in the presence of platelet phospholipid.[23] Briefly, platelets are collected from a normal dog by slow speed centrifugation of blood (platelet rich plasma; PRP), activated clotting factors XI and XII are added, and serum from the patient is added; a control test is also performed concurrently and consists of normal dog serum, clotting factors XI and XII, and the PRP. In the presence of antiplatelet antibody and subsequent PF-3 release, the coagulation process (activated by adding 0.025 M CaCl₂ to the test samples) is enhanced with a subsequent decrease in the clotting time. The patient serum is considered to have antiplatelet antibody if the coagulation time is decreased more than two standard deviations of normal serum coagulation time, generally 10 to 12 seconds shorter than the control test sample.

Many cases of suspected IMT do not exhibit positive PF-3 tests. In four separate studies the per cent positive tests ranged from 29 per cent of 31 dogs to nearly 70 per cent in more than 200 dogs.[23–26] Despite a negative PF-3 test a presumptive diagnosis of IMT may be justified in the presence of a response to treatment. A major drawback to the PF-3 test is the assumption that the antigen (or epitope) that the antibody molecules are recognizing will be present on the platelets obtained from a normal dog. This may not be necessarily true and may explain many of the negative results obtained in highly suspected cases of IMT. Another problem that arises is that when a drug is suspected as the underlying cause of the IMT the PF-3 test must be performed with the drug included in the test serum. Even this may prove not helpful as some drugs are structurally altered *in vivo* and the active component may not be present in the *in vitro* test procedure.

DIRECT IMMUNOFLUORESCENCE TEST. A more sensitive test to detect antiplatelet antibodies utilizes the direct immunofluorescence test to demonstrate antiplatelet antibodies bound to megakaryocytes. The technique is accomplished by preparing bone marrow aspirates on glass microscope slides, fixing the smears in absolute ethanol, and staining the smear with an anti-canine globulin conjugated with fluorescein isothiocyanate. The bone marrow smear is then examined under a fluorescent microscope for the presence of green fluorescence of megakaryocytes, which is diagnostic for an immune-mediated platelet destruction.[24] The disadvantage may be related to a marrow potentially devoid of adequate megakaryocytes to appropriately assess the test results.

Treatment. The treatment objective of immune-mediated thrombocytopenia is the resolution of bleeding tendencies and not necessarily restoration of the platelet count to normal. In secondary IMT this can be accomplished by the removal or elimination of any suspected microbial infection or offending drug. Usually, however, the IMT has an unexplained etiology, and a diagnosis of primary autoimmune thrombocytopenia is made. Conventional therapy has been oral prednisone or prednisolone at 0.5 to 1 mg/lb (1 to 2 mg/kg) q12h and tapering the dose over one to three months to 0.25 to 0.5 mg/lb (0.5 to 1 mg/kg) q48h. The glucocorticoid therapy functions to decrease macrophage ingestion of antibody and/or complement coated platelets and to decrease antibody production. The response to treatment is usually good and platelet counts can return to normal in less than one week. Some clinicians feel that dexamethasone may be more effective in the treatment of IMT.[27, 28] The dosage regimen for dexamethasone is 0.05 to 0.1 mg/lb (0.1 to 0.2 mg/kg) PO or IV q12h for five to seven days and then a gradual reduction over two weeks to a maintenance dose of 0.05 mg/lb (0.1 mg/kg) PO q48h or as needed.[32]

If the platelet count remains low despite adequate glucocorticoid therapy for one to two weeks then additional therapy with vincristine at 0.01 to 0.015 mg/lb (0.75 mg/m²) IV once each week should be instituted. After one to two weeks of combination treatment with glucocorticoid and vincristine and if the platelet counts are normal the vincristine should be discontinued and the glucocorticoid continued for an additional one to two months.

Another form of therapy that may be valuable, but that should be reserved for nonresponsive patients, is vincristine-loaded platelet therapy.[29] This technique uses 100 ml of allogeneic platelet-rich plasma (PRP) isolated by slow centrifugation of 500 ml of cross-matched canine blood collected in citrated-phosphate-dextrose solution. Three milligrams of vincristine are added to the PRP and the cells incubated at 37° C for one hour in the dark. Following incubation the platelets are gently packed by centrifugation and the excess plasma discarded leaving 35 ml of PRP. The platelets are then given by IV injection over approximately 30 minutes. The rationale for using vincristine-loaded platelets is based on the fact that the vincristine binds to tubulin within the platelet cytoplasm, and when the platelets are phagocytized by macrophages of the reticuloendothelial system, the large quantities of vincristine lead to dysfunction or death of those macrophages that have phagocytized the injected platelets. This therapy results in macrophage destruction and subsequent alleviation of the endogenous platelet destruction.

Another form of therapy in refractory cases of IMT involves splenectomy.[30] Splenectomy may achieve two objectives, removal of a large source of antibody-producing cells that may be manufacturing platelet-specific antibody and removal of macrophages responsible for platelet ingestion. Although splenectomy may accomplish these two objectives and although patients have been shown to benefit from this therapeutic approach, it should be noted that many patients suffer relapse following splenectomy, and increased susceptibility to pathogens may be observed.[29–31]

Prognosis. The prognosis for IMT is good, and with periodic monitoring cases with a tendency to relapse

can be identified. It probably is not necessary to restore the platelet count to baseline levels of 200,000 thrombocytes/mm³ blood since the majority of animals do not exhibit bleeding tendencies below 50,000 thrombocytes/mm³ blood. Some authors suggest that environmental stress and or hormonal imbalances may precipitate thrombocytopenic relapses, and ovariohysterectomy of intact females may be advisable once platelet counts and bleeding disorders have been corrected.

PARAPROTEINEMIAS

A paraprotein or monoclonal gammopathy is defined as an immunoglobulin produced by the clonal expansion of a single plasma cell. Paraproteins derived from any single patient are of a single immunoglobulin class and subclass and exhibit only one light chain (kappa or lambda) type. On serum electrophoresis a paraproteinemia is normally demonstrable as a sharply localized band (Figure 119–6). Paraproteinemias have been documented to be present in cases of multiple myeloma, chronic lymphocytic leukemia, plasma cell leukemia, primary (Waldenstrom's) macroglobulinemia, amyloidosis, benign (idiopathic) monoclonal gammopathy, and lymphoma.[33–41] The incidence of paraproteinemias varies with clinical disease. Approximately 6 per cent of canine lymphomas exhibit a paraproteinemia, whereas greater than 50 per cent of chronic lymphocytic leukemias express a monoclonal gammopathy. It has been estimated that nearly eight per cent of canine hematopoietic tumors are cases of multiple myeloma and about four per cent of canine bone tumors are the result of a plasma cell neoplasia based on histologic examination.

Occasionally a chronic infectious disease such as chrlichiosis may stimulate the production of large amounts of a single subclass of immunoglobulin, which on serum electrophoresis exhibits a sharply defined band.[42, 43] These have been considered a monoclonal gammopathy secondary to chronic infection, and treatment of the

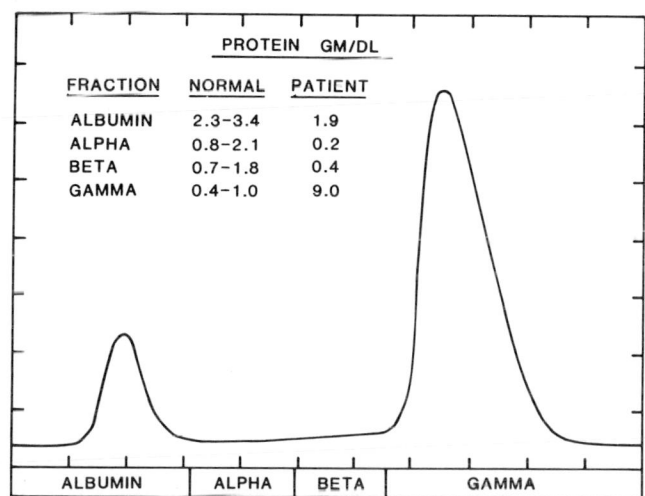

PROTEIN GM/DL		
FRACTION	**NORMAL**	**PATIENT**
ALBUMIN	2.3–3.4	1.9
ALPHA	0.8–2.1	0.2
BETA	0.7–1.8	0.4
GAMMA	0.4–1.0	9.0

| ALBUMIN | ALPHA | BETA | GAMMA |

FIGURE 119–6. Serum electrophoretic profile from a dog exhibiting hypoalbuminemia, hypoalphaproteinemia, hypobetaproteinemia, and hypergammaglobulinemia. The gammaglobulin peak demonstrates a restricted electrophoretic migratory pattern and is compatible with a diagnosis of paraproteinemia or monoclonal gammopathy.

underlying disease results in decreased concentrations of circulating immunoglobulin.

Clinical Manifestations of Paraproteinemias

The presence of a paraproteinemia may result in a hyperviscosity syndrome, in the formation of erythrocyte rouleaux and increased erythrocyte sedimentation rate, in a Coombs' positive anemia, and in bleeding diatheses.

Bleeding Disorders. A bleeding disorder is the typical reason for the animal presenting to the veterinary clinic and signs include ecchymoses or petechiae, epistaxis, bleeding from gingival surfaces, and possible intermittent gastrointestinal bleeding. These bleeding diatheses are considered specifically related to the coating of platelets with the paraprotein, subsequent poor platelet aggregation, and a failure of platelets to release platelet factor III. Paraproteinemias that are reported to occur most commonly in association with bleeding abnormalities are IgM and IgA monoclonal gammopathies. Probably the large molecular weight of IgM and the tendency of IgA to form polymers are underlying factors in the prevalence of these immunoglobulin classes in those cases with bleeding problems.

In addition, paraproteinemias have been associated with prolongation of the intrinsic and extrinsic coagulation systems. These prolongations are believed to be secondary to direct interaction of the paraproteins with coagulation cascade proteins; however, the exact mechanism is not known. No specific factor deficiency was reported in one well-studied canine case.[44]

Hyperviscosity Syndrome. The hyperviscosity syndrome impacts on the cardiovascular, neurologic, hemostatic, and renal systems and is the result of elevated concentrations of serum immunoglobulin, particularly IgM and polymers of IgG or IgA.[21, 41] The increased protein content within the vascular spaces results directly in increased oncotic pressure and secondary hypervolemia. This increase in vascular volume leads to increased perfusion pressure and a subsequent increase in cardiac work load. Because vascular perfusion is generally poor, myocardial hypoxia may develop. With the increased cardiac work load and myocardial hypoxia a vicious cycle can be established, which results in cardiac failure.

Profound central nervous system depression, which may be characterized by coma, dementia, and ataxia, can also be observed in patients with hyperviscosity syndrome. The CNS depression is directly related to cerebral hypoxia as a result of poor vascular perfusion.

Renal damage is another potential concern in patients with paraproteinemia. Along with possible renal hypoxemia induced by decreased vascular perfusion, the high serum concentrations of protein may result in the degeneration of renal tubules as the consequence of high protein content in the glomerular filtrate. In addition, the increased concentration of tubular protein may result in the direct development of proteinaceous casts.

Clinical Diseases Associated with Paraproteinemias

Discussion of clinical diseases associated with paraproteinemias will be limited to multiple myeloma, pri-

mary (Waldenstrom's) macroglobulinemia, benign (idiopathic) monoclonal gammopathy, and α-chain disease; the reader is referred to other excellent reviews regarding chronic lymphocyte leukemia, plasma cell leukemia, and lymphoma as disease processes frequently associated with secretion of paraproteins.[36, 41, 45]

MULTIPLE MYELOMA

Multiple myeloma is a neoplastic disease involving lymphocytes that have differentiated into plasma cells. The plasma cells have been reported to secrete either IgG or IgA;[46] paraproteinemias associated with the production of IgD or IgE have not been described in the dog or cat. Although plasma cells are found throughout the body, the neoplastic proliferation of plasma cells typically occurs within the bone marrow. Reports of plasma cell tumors have documented tumors within the gastrointestinal tract, upper respiratory tract, and in the skin.

Clinical Signs. Clinical signs may be attributable to either the effects of the tumor cells directly on surrounding tissues or to the proteins that the plasma cell tumor secretes. Signs attributed to the tumor mass may include bone pain and spinal cord compression with secondary pain and/or neurologic signs.[47] Clinical signs produced as a result of high levels of paraprotein are largely due to serum hyperviscosity.[35, 36, 42]

Diagnosis. The diagnosis of multiple myeloma requires the demonstration of two of the following four criteria:[42] (1) osteolytic lesion on radiographic analysis, (2) monoclonal gammopathy, (3) plasma cells present on cytologic examination of a bone marrow aspirate (Figure 119–7), and (4) presence of Bence Jones proteinuria. The diagnostic tests include radiographs, serum electrophoresis, bone marrow aspiration, and a heat precipitation or urine electrophoresis to detect Bence Jones proteins.

Clinical Management. Clinical management of patients with multiple myeloma can be very rewarding.

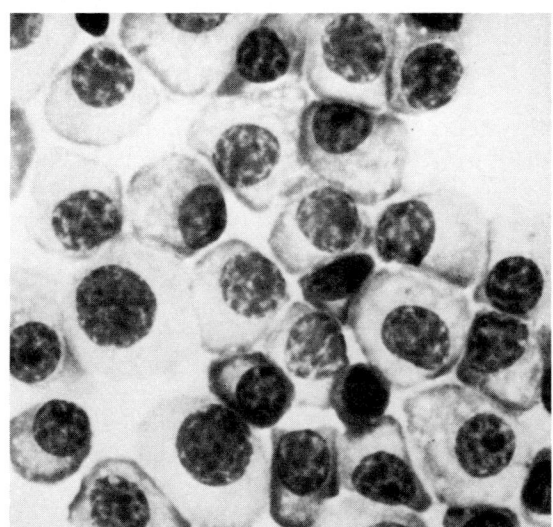

FIGURE 119–7. Bone marrow cytology demonstrating a profound accumulation of plasma cells in a sheet-like arrangement. Note the eccentrically placed nucleus and negative-staining Golgi apparatus typical of plasma cells.

Because numerous organ systems may be affected, several laboratory tests are usually obtained to accurately assess the patient and stage the neoplastic disease (Table 119–3). The laboratory tests that should be assessed include a complete blood cell count, platelet count, serum chemistry profile, urinalysis, bleeding time or platelet function test, activated partial thromboplastin time, prothrombin time, immunoelectrophoresis, and immunoglobulin quantitation. Serum viscosity should also be measured and an ophthalmologic examination performed to determine the presence or absence of evidence to support hyperviscosity, which is a serious complication of multiple myeloma. Ophthalmic examination findings that would support a diagnosis of serum hyperviscosity include dilated, tortuous, retinal vessels with the appearance of sausage shaped dilations and the presence of focal retinal hemorrhages.

Interpretation of the complete blood cell count should be considered in the context of whether hemorrhage has recently occurred, whether an infectious process is present, and to what extent the plasma cell tumor has infiltrated the bone marrow. If the animal has exhibited a recent onset of hemorrhage, then a regenerative anemia may be present. If a regenerative anemia is present in the absence of a recent loss of blood, then careful attention to possible gastrointestinal blood loss or a concurrent Coombs' positive hemolytic disease process should be considered. A nonregenerative anemia may be observed in patients with acute blood loss (less than three days), in patients with severe bone marrow infiltration of plasmacytes, in patients with ehrlichiosis, or in those patients with underlying chronic renal failure with reduced levels of serum erythropoietin. Elevated leukocyte counts may be observed with concurrent bacterial infections or with a generalized increased bone marrow response associated with recent blood loss. Decreased leukocytes and/or thrombocytes should signify the possibility of severe bone marrow infiltration with tumor cells. Plasma protein concentrations should reflect an elevation secondary to increased immunoglobulin levels.

The serum chemistry profile is a valuable means to assess the extent of organ involvement. The BUN and creatinine may be elevated secondary to decreased perfusion or tubular damage secondary to protein accumulation. Increased serum concentrations of alanine aminotransferase and aspartate aminotransferase can be seen in hepatic infiltration or due to poor vascular perfusion. Hypoalbuminemia is common and usually is related to urinary protein loss; other causes could relate to decreased hepatic production secondary to liver failure or a compensatory mechanism to decrease the extent of serum oncotic pressure. Particular attention should be paid to the serum globulin concentration. The serum globulins are usually increased and the albumin to globulin ratio typically is less than 0.6. Serum calcium concentrations should be assessed, as they are used to stage the neoplastic disease process (Table 119–3).

Urinalysis may reveal proteinuria, isosthenuria, cylindruria, pyuria, hematuria, and bacteriuria. Interpretation of the urine specific gravity must be made within the context of the serum creatinine concentration. In addition to dipstick analysis of the urine protein concentration (measures only albumin content of urine), a Bence Jones heat precipitation test and/or a urine electrophoresis should be performed to assess the presence or absence of immunoglobulin light chains in the urine. Quantitations of urine content of immunoglobulin light chains may be of value in monitoring the patient's response to therapy. In addition, a urine protein to creatinine ratio or 24-hour urine protein quantitation could be performed to assess the extent of urinary protein loss.

Following the recognition of a hyperglobulinemia, the diagnostic test of choice is a serum electrophoresis to determine whether the hyperglobulinemia is secondary to a polyclonal or suggestive of a monoclonal gammopathy. If, after examination of the serum electrophoresis a monoclonal gammopathy is suspected, immunoelectrophoresis is performed to identify the specific immunoglobulin class being secreted by the tumor. In some instances an elevated globulin fraction will not be present despite the establishment of two or more criteria indicative of a plasma cell tumor. In these uncommon cases, a serum electrophoresis should also be performed, as a monoclonal spike may be observed in the absence of hyperglobulinemia.

In some cases of multiple myeloma a distinct absence of a monoclonal protein is apparent.[48–50] This may be due to an inability of the tumor cells to secrete immunoglobulin or may be related to the neoplastic cell secreting only light chains of the immunoglobulin molecule. In addition, some cases of multiple myeloma appear to be producing a polyclonal immunoglobulin response on serum electrophoresis. This may be merely an artifact, as many times a monoclonal immunoglobulin response may form polymers consisting of two or greater numbers of immunoglobulin molecules. As a direct result of increased molecular size the molecules migrate more slowly through the electrophoretic field, resulting in what appears to be a polyclonal gammopathy.

The final laboratory test should be the quantitation of each serum immunoglobulin class concentration. This will allow for absolute documentation of the decrease in paraproteinemia following treatment and for reas-

TABLE 119–3. CLINICAL STAGE CLASSIFICATION OF CANINE MULTIPLE MYELOMA

Stage I   Low tumor volume
- PCV > 37%
- Serum calcium < 11.5 mg/dl
- No osteolytic lesions
- Total immunoglobulin < 3 g/dl

Stage II   Intermediate tumor volume
- Fits neither Stages I nor III

Stage III   High tumor volume
- PCV < 25%
- Serum calcium > 11.5 mg/dl —Osteolytic lesions present
- Total immunoglobulin < 5 g/dl

Each stage may be subclassified according to signs of systemic illness.
- a. Without systemic signs
- b. With systemic signs
  - Coagulopathy
  - CNS signs
  - Azotemia

Modified from Matus, RE, et al.: Prognostic factors for multiple myeloma in the dog. JAVMA 188:1288, 1986.

sessment of how the remaining immunoglobulin classes respond to therapy.

Treatment. Treatment of multiple myeloma should be aimed at (1) decreasing the serum viscosity if it is sufficiently elevated at the time of diagnosis to cause signs attributable to hyperviscosity,[51] (2) reducing serum hypercalcemia if present, (3) supporting the patient with fluid therapy if hyperviscosity is absent and renal insufficiency is present, (4) providing a blood transfusion if a concurrent anemia is sufficient to induce clinical signs, and (5) providing antimicrobial support if signs of infection are present.

Specific treatment is focused on reducing the numbers of neoplastic cells secreting immunoglobulin. Melphalan has been and continues to be the antineoplastic drug of choice. The recommended dose, according to the author, is 0.05 mg/lb (0.1 mg/kg) PO q24h for 7 days at which time the drug is either discontinued if the neutrophil count is less than 3000/mm³ blood or decreased to 0.025 to 0.05 mg/lb (0.05 to 0.1 mg/kg) PO q48h if the neutrophil count is greater than 3000/mm³ blood. During the first month of treatment a complete blood cell count, platelet count, and total plasma protein concentration should be performed weekly and the dose of melphalan adjusted to maintain the neutrophil count between 4000 and 10,000 cells/mm³ blood. If the neutrophil count drops below 3000, the melphalan should be discontinued for one week and the dose subsequently adjusted. A serum chemistry profile should be performed periodically to assess the electrolytes, creatinine concentration, and hepatic enzyme activities.

Prognosis. The prognosis for patients with multiple myeloma is guarded.[52] Patients with increased serum calcium concentrations, increased creatinine, elevated globulins, and extensive areas of bony lysis have the poorest prognosis. Although some dogs can be managed successfully for several years, the prognosis must remain guarded.

PRIMARY (WALDENSTROM'S) MACROGLOBULINEMIA

This paraproteinemic disorder is characterized by a neoplastic proliferation of plasma cells associated with the secretion of an IgM monoclonal gammopathy in the absence of chronic lymphoid leukemia; chronic lymphocytic leukemia may be associated with a monoclonal IgM gammopathy, and differentiation from a primary (Waldenstrom's) macroglobulinemia may be difficult. Although not a commonly diagnosed disorder, primary macroglobulinemia probably represents about 10 per cent of diagnosed paraproteinemias.

Clinical Signs. Clinical signs are generally attributable to the proliferation of neoplastic cells or the secretion of the monoclonal immunoglobulin. Patients with primary macroglobulinemia classically exhibit signs referable to the serum hyperviscosity syndrome. The signs include cerebral dysfunction (coma, dementia, and ataxia), bleeding diathesis, congestive heart failure, and renal insufficiency. Clinical manifestations related to neoplastic cell proliferation may include lameness, paresis, and pathologic fractures, but are seen less frequently in cases of primary macroglobulinemia than in cases of multiple myeloma.

Diagnosis. The diagnosis of primary macroglobulinemia requires the documentation of an IgM monoclonal gammopathy, absence of chronic lymphoid leukemia, and the presence of either osteolytic lesions on radiographic analysis, bone marrow plasma cellular infiltration, or Bence Jones proteinuria.

Treatment and Prognosis. Major treatment efforts should focus on eliminating or reducing serum hyperviscosity if the patient is demonstrating clinical signs, decreasing the amount of macroglobulin produced, reducing the numbers of neoplastic plasma cells, and providing symptomatic therapy for any associated major organ system failure. The syndrome of serum hyperviscosity created by IgM can be controlled effectively by plasmapheresis[51] due to the primary intravascular location of this particular immunoglobulin class; approximately 80 per cent of IgM is located intravascularly as a result of the large molecular weight of this immunoglobulin molecule. Another potential method for the control of life-threatening serum hyperviscosity is exchange blood transfusion. Although serum hyperviscosity can be life-threatening, rarely is plasmapheresis or exchange blood transfusion required due to a rapid decline in total serum paraproteinemia typically associated with chemotherapy administration. The chemotherapy protocol for primary macroglobulinemia is identical to that described for multiple myeloma. Although longevity in many cases can extend up to several years, the prognosis must remain guarded.

BENIGN (IDIOPATHIC) MONOCLONAL GAMMOPATHY

Clinical Signs. Benign (idiopathic) monoclonal gammopathy is an asymptomatic plasma cell dyscrasia characterized by the presence of a serum elevation of a homogeneous population of immunoglobulin molecules. The immunoglobulin molecules are monoclonal in all respects based on serum electrophoresis, immunoelectrophoresis, and immunochemistry analysis. The clinical presentation is benign and by definition no clinical signs of disease are associated with this incidental finding of monoclonal gammopathy. Whether cases of benign monoclonal gammopathy progress to develop classical signs of multiple myeloma is not known in small animal medicine; however, in humans many of these cases do indeed progress to exhibit signs of malignant proliferation of plasma cells.

Diagnosis. The diagnosis is usually made based on an incidental finding of hyperproteinemia on a routine hemogram, which is then followed up by serum electrophoresis. Careful attention must be given to rule out other causes of paraproteinemia, which necessitates a complete blood cell count, serum chemistry profile, urinalysis to include a search for Bence Jones proteins, bone marrow cytology or histology, a serum titer for ehrlichiosis, and radiographic analysis.

Treatment and Prognosis. No treatment is generally recommended due to the absence of clinical signs; however, case management should include repeated physical examinations and serum electrophoresis profiles to accurately monitor the progression or resolution of the monoclonal gammopathy. Clinical cases are too few to render an accurate prognosis.

ALPHA-CHAIN DISEASE

Clinical Signs. Immunoglobulin molecules are composed of heavy and light chains of amino acids and it is therefore possible that a malignant plasma cell may fail to secrete intact immunoglobulin molecules, but rather secrete only one type of amino acid chain. A case of canine multiple myeloma associated with the secretion of only heavy chains of IgA has been described.[53] The dog exhibited a watery and bloody diarrhea, vomiting, anorexia, lethargy, and polydipsia. Although intestinal biopsies were not performed, the clinical presentation was very similar to IgA heavy chain disease in man. The syndrome in humans is characterized by lymphoid and/or plasmacytoid proliferation within the intestine, production of monoclonal α-chains, and the presence of nausea, vomiting, weight loss, abdominal pain, and diarrhea.

Diagnosis. The diagnosis of α-chain disease requires the documentation of high serum concentrations of α-chains without associated kappa or lambda light chains. Because α-chain disease may be associated with intestinal infiltration of lymphoid and/or plasmacytoid cells an intestinal biopsy to further document the natural history of this disease process should be considered.

Treatment and Prognosis. The treatment of α-chain and other heavy chain diseases is directed along the same lines as that for multiple myeloma. The prognosis is unknown, although a clinical case report[53] responded dramatically to initial treatment; long term follow-up was unavailable.

RHEUMATOID DISEASES

Rheumatoid diseases are characterized by a variety of disorders marked by inflammation, degeneration, or metabolic derangement of the connective tissue structures of the body. This section will focus on lupus erythematosus and rheumatoid arthritis as examples of rheumatoid diseases.

SYSTEMIC LUPUS ERYTHEMATOSUS

Systemic lupus erythematosus (SLE) is a polysystemic immune-mediated disease of unknown etiology. The disease was recognized to affect dogs in 1965 and case reports describing SLE in cats also exist.[54-56] The disease has been called the great imitator as numerous organ systems can be affected, resulting in a wide variety of clinical presentations.

Clinical Signs. Clinical signs associated with SLE may be sudden or insidious in onset. Often the signs of disease wax and wane and considerable time may elapse before the patient is presented for examination. Probably the most common clinical manifestation of SLE is a gait abnormality—a stilted gait or a shifting leg lameness.[57, 58] Physical examination may or may not reveal

joint distention secondary to a sterile, nonerosive polyarthritis or a diffuse polymyositis. The polymyositis generally is associated with muscle pain on palpation or diffuse muscle wasting. Cutaneous manifestations of SLE constitute another major clinical sign. Similar to the polysystemic nature of SLE, the dermatologic changes associated with this disease are many. Reported skin changes include a symmetrical to focal distribution of lesions affecting the limbs, body, head, ears, face, mucocutaneous junctions, and oral cavity.[57-60] The skin lesions may reveal ulceration, erythema, crusting, oozing, and alopecia. In addition, cellulitis, furunculosis, scarring and leukoderma have been reported. Nonspecific clinical signs that may be present include malaise, anorexia, and weakness.

Pathophysiology. The immunopathology of SLE is related to the presence of circulating antigen-antibody complexes and/or the presence of antibody molecules with specificity for hematopoietic cells (erythrocytes, leukocytes, or thrombocytes). The tissue inflammatory lesions created by circulating immune complexes (Type III immunologic injury) are non–organ-specific and can result in glomerulonephritis, arthritis, and vasculitis.[21] The extent and phase of immune complex formation are critical in the development of clinical signs of disease (Figure 119–8). If the immune complexes are large and precipitate on vascular endothelium, then very little damage results due to rapid phagocytosis of the deposited complexes. If, however, the immune complexes are soluble, then the complexes may diffuse deep into vascular endothelial channels, activate the complement cascade, and stimulate the migration of lymphocytes and neutrophils into the vascular tree, resulting in a marked amount of perivascular inflammation. This inflammation can lead to an acute necrotizing vasculitis that may progress to fibrinoid deposition and sclerosis. Immune complex deposition in the glomerulus of the kidney (Figure 119–9) typically results in thickening of the glomerular basement membrane (membranous glomerulonephritis). In severe cases glomerular basement membrane thickening may progress to mesangioproliferative glomerulonephritis; accumulation of neutrophils and endothelial swelling can be extensive.

Diagnosis. Because SLE mimics a great variety of disease processes, several diagnostic tests are likely to be evaluated during the management and diagnosis of the case. The hemogram may exhibit evidence of immune-mediated anemia, leukopenia, or thrombocytopenia. Depending on the target cell of the autoantibody the anemia may be regenerative or nonregenerative. If a regenerative anemia is present without evidence of detectable blood loss or autoagglutination, a direct Coombs' test should be performed. In the presence of a nonregenerative anemia a bone marrow aspirate is the diagnostic test of choice. Those hemograms that exhibit leukopenia or thrombocytopenia should also receive a bone marrow aspirate or core bone marrow sample for histologic examination. Ehrlichiosis is a disease process that may also induce a leukopenia, anemia, or thrombocytopenia and as such, a serum sample for an *Ehrlichia canis* titer is appropriate if a nonregenerative bone marrow sample is observed on cytologic review of the bone marrow aspirate. In the absence of an immune-

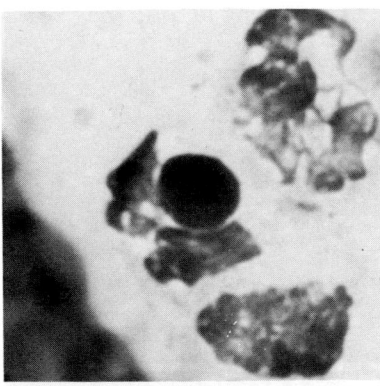

FIGURE 119–11. Photomicrograph of a neutrophil that has phagocytized an intact nucleus from a damaged cell. This cellular complex is termed a "tart cell" and must be distinguished from a lupus erythematosus cell. (Courtesy of Dr. Dennis J. Meyer.)

have bound to the mouse liver nuclei will the reagent remain on the slide; otherwise during the second rinsing cycle the fluorescein-labeled rabbit antidog immunoglobulin reagent will wash off. The advantage of the indirect immunofluorescence ANA test is that a higher percentage of patients with SLE are recognized when compared to the LE cell test. In addition, the indirect fluorescent ANA test is less transitory and steroid therapy tends not to influence the test results if the steroids have only recently been initiated. The major disadvantages include the absolute requirement for species-specific reagents and the necessary use of expensive laboratory equipment. Also, as in the LE cell test, some unrelated inflammatory diseases can be associated with antinuclear antibodies, which necessitates that serial dilutions of patient's serum be analyzed to record a specific titer of antinuclear antibodies present.

Treatment. The objectives of treatment are to reduce the concentration of ANA present in the serum, to decrease the ongoing inflammatory disease process, and to manage associated organ failure. Critical in the management of patients with SLE is the avoidance of bacterial infections. The presence of an infection warrants the exact identification of the bacteria present and the sensitivity of the organism to antibiotics. The infection must be treated specifically and aggressively, as infection is probably the most significant cause of death in patients with SLE.

The most widely used therapy for the treatment of SLE is prednisone or prednisolone. These glucocorticoids should be administered at a dose of 0.5 to 1.5 mg/lb (1 to 3 mg/kg) PO q12h until the patient exhibits signs of substantial clinical improvement. If no signs of improvement are noted within ten days after the start of therapy, then more potent immunosuppressive agents used in combination with glucocorticoids are required. Initially the use of azathioprine at 1 mg/lb (2 mg/kg) PO q24h with prednisone dosed at 0.5 to 1.5 mg/lb (1 to 3 mg/kg) PO q12h should be tried. If no clinical improvement is observed after another ten days, then the addition of cyclophosphamide at 1 mg/lb (50 mg/m²) PO q24h for four consecutive days each week should be initiated along with the prednisone at 0.5 mg/lb (1 mg/kg) PO q24h, and azathioprine at 1 mg/lb (2 mg/kg) PO q48h. Once the clinical remission has been achieved,

the cyclophosphamide should be reduced to 0.5 mg/lb (1 mg/kg) PO q24h for four consecutive days each week for an additional two weeks and then discontinued. If the disease remains in clinical remission then the prednisone should be decreased to an every other day dosage given on the days that azathioprine is not given. Eventually over the course of four to six weeks the prednisone dosage should be decreased to 0.25 to 0.5 mg/lb (0.5 to 1 mg/kg) PO q48h and the azathioprine dose dropped to 0.5 mg/lb (1 mg/kg) PO q48h. If at any time the disease recrudesces then the dosages should be increased.

Additional symptomatic therapy can utilize aspirin as a nonsteroidal anti-inflammatory analgesic. It is important to remember that the nonsteroidal anti-inflammatory drugs do not alter the underlying immunopathology or the natural progression of the disease. In addition, the use of aspirin is contraindicated in the presence of thrombocytopenia or gastrointestinal hemorrhage. Although the nonsteroidal anti-inflammatory analgesics do not alter the progression of SLE, they are useful in providing analgesic, antipyretic, and anti-inflammatory relief from the disease process.

Prognosis. The prognosis for SLE is guarded. Every effort must be made to avoid infections and if an infection is diagnosed, then aggressive treatment is indicated. Severe organ dysfunction at the time of diagnosis makes the prognosis worse and the presence of severe infection warrants a grave prognosis. Prior to initiating immunosuppressive therapy, the author recommends routine thoracic radiographs to rule out the possibility of an underlying pneumonia, which may be exacerbated by the initiation of immunosuppressive drugs.

CUTANEOUS (DISCOID) LUPUS ERYTHEMATOSUS

The relationship between cutaneous lupus erythematosus and systemic lupus erythematosus is not clear; however, cutaneous lupus erythematosus is generally considered to be a mild or benign form of systemic lupus erythematosus;[62] cutaneous lupus erythematosus lacks systemic involvement, and antinuclear antibody tests are usually negative. The most common sign associated with cutaneous lupus erythematosus is nasal dermatitis, which is seen in greater than 90 per cent of clinical cases. The nasal dermatitis is characterized by varying degrees of depigmentation, erythema, ulceration, and erosions. The extent of pruritus is variable; however, scaling and crusting of the nasal planum and nostrils are common. Crusting and scaling lesions of the pinnae, periorbital skin, and lip are observed in approximately 10 to 25 per cent of cases. In addition, the feet may exhibit erythema, scaling, or hyperkeratosis, and oral ulcerations may be observed. The duration of clinical signs may vary from weeks to years. Collies, German shepherds, Siberian huskies, and Shetland sheepdogs may be predisposed. In addition, a possible female predilection has been reported.[62]

Pathology. Routine histopathologic examination of affected skin is characterized by hyperkeratosis of the epidermis and associated hair follicles (Figure 119–12).

matosus focuses on immunosuppressive therapy with glucocorticoids (prednisone or prednisolone) at 0.5 mg/lb (1 mg/kg) PO q12h until signs of clinical remission are observed. Gradually the prednisone or prednisolone is decreased to the dosage that when administered on an alternate day schedule will maintain the disease process in remission. Oral administration of vitamin E at 400 IU q12h in the acetate or succinate form two hours before or after meals has also been successful in controlling disease signs. A lag period of 30 to 60 days has been reported before clinical signs of vitamin E efficacy have been observed and as such vitamin E as the sole inducer of clinical remission is generally not recommended. In very mild cases, topical betamethasone, topical sunscreen, and avoidance of sunlight may be adequate to control clinical manifestations of disease.[62] In addition, topical therapy and avoidance of ultraviolet light are recommended for those animals that exhibit severe depigmentation of the nose.

Prognosis. The prognosis for most patients is good and therapy with oral corticosteroids and/or vitamin E is effective and generally associated with long-term remission.

RHEUMATOID ARTHRITIS

Rheumatoid arthritis is a crippling joint disease with a poorly understood etiology. The disease is considered immune-mediated due to the identification of antibody (rheumatoid factor) reactive against immunoglobulin G (IgG) in many, but not all, cases of rheumatoid arthritis. Rheumatoid factor (RF) is not reactive against normal canine IgG, but expresses reactivity against antibody in IgG that has bound antigen and has undergone a conformational change to expose hidden epitopes (antigenic sites) within the IgG molecule.[63]

Pathophysiology. The exact pathophysiology of rheumatoid arthritis is not known; however, a hypothesis of the immunologic events that may result in the development of rheumatoid arthritis has been proposed. Initially an antigen-antibody interaction occurs within a joint with resultant exposure of hidden epitopes on the antibody molecule. The epitopes are then recognized by the immune system and local production of rheumatoid factor ensues. The rheumatoid factor complexes with the altered antibody molecules, which results in the induction of complement activation. The end result of complement activation is the influx of neutrophils in response to the complement split product C5a. The neutrophils then engulf the immune complexes and release lysosomal enzymes that induce cartilage damage. The damaged cartilage cells may then be the focus of an additional immune response to the possible exposure of hidden antigens on cartilage cells.[63]

Clinical Signs. The clinical signs of rheumatoid arthritis generally relate to morning stiffness, stiff legged gait, pain on manipulation of one or more joints, reluctance to exercise, and swelling of affected joints. Currently, there is no information regarding breed, sex, or age predilections. The extent of joint involvement may be so severe that animals may not be able to walk. The peripheral joints appear to be most often affected,

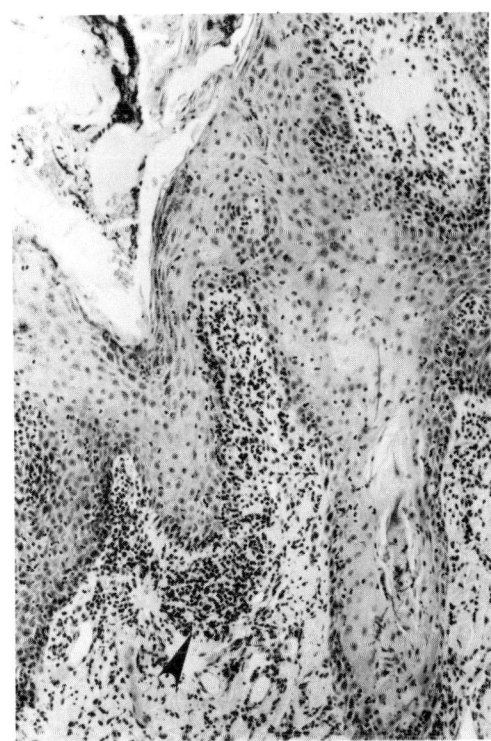

FIGURE 119–12. Cutaneous ("discoid") lupus erythematosus. Bandlike subepidermal lymphocytic infiltrate (arrow) with penetration of the overlying acanthotic epidermis. (Courtesy of Dr. James D. Conroy.)

The basement membrane zone is typically thickened and necrosis of basal cells in discrete focal distributions and the formation of civatte bodies (dyskeratotic basilar epidermal cells) may he evident. In addition, dermal edema, band-like subepidermal mononuclear inflammatory cell infiltrates (predominantly mononuclear and plasmacytic), and subepidermal vesicles can be seen. Perifollicular inflammation and pigment incontinence may also be observed.

Direct immunofluorescence of affected skin reveals the deposition of immunoglobulin (IgG, IgA, IgM) and/or complement (C3) along the basement membrane zone (lupus band) in a dense granular pattern. The frequency of observed lupus bands in cases of canine cutaneous lupus erythematosus has been reported to vary between 67 and 100 per cent of clinical cases.[54, 62]

Diagnosis. The diagnosis of cutaneous lupus erythematosus depends on a careful physical examination, dermatohistopathology and direct immunofluorescence tests. The differential diagnoses may include collie nose, trauma, neoplasia, pemphigus foliaceous and pemphigus vegetans. The diagnostic tests of choice include routine histopathology and direct immunofluorescence. If the histology and direct immunofluorescent tests are compatible with cutaneous lupus erythematosus, then an antinuclear antibody test, hemogram, serum chemistry profile, and urinalysis should be performed to rule out systemic lupus erythematosus as a cause for the disease presentation. In cutaneous lupus erythematosus the hemogram, urinalysis, and serum chemistry profile are typically normal and only rarely is a positive antinuclear antibody test observed.

Treatment. The treatment of cutaneous lupus erythe-

and variable amounts of pain, heat, and swelling may be present.

Diagnosis. The diagnosis of rheumatoid arthritis should be based on a number of criteria. Although all criteria need not be present, the criteria that should be evaluated include morning stiffness, pain on motion of at least one joint, swelling of the soft tissues around the joints, polyarthropathy, radiographic evidence of an erosive arthritis, positive rheumatoid factor test, nonseptic arthritis on arthrocentesis, and histological evidence of a proliferative synovitis with accumulation of plasma cells and lymphocytes adjacent to hypertrophic synovial epithelium. Examination of the synovial surface should demonstrate synovial villous projections extending into the joint space. In addition to changes observed on the synovial lining, perivascular inflammation consisting of plasma cell infiltrates with necrotizing arteritis may be noted.

The serologic diagnosis of rheumatoid arthritis is based on the demonstration of serum antibody reactive with IgG molecules bound to antigen. There are basically two tests that are utilized in veterinary medicine. One test utilizes rabbit IgG antibody bound to sheep erythrocytes (Rose-Waaler test) and the other test uses canine IgG bound to latex particles.[63] The specific laboratory methods used to perform these test are not important for discussion here, but it is important to know that a positive test result is based on the demonstration of agglutination of the IgG-coated sheep erythrocytes or latex particles. In addition, normal dog serum may contain small amounts of antibody reactive with the IgG used to coat the erythrocytes or latex particles and it is important to know those titers that are necessary to reach before the test result is significant. In the Rose-Waaler test a titer of 1:8 or less is generally considered nonsignificant.

Animals suspected of having rheumatoid arthritis should also be tested for the presence of antinuclear antibody, as it is important to differentiate the polyarthritis of systemic lupus erythematosus from that of rheumatoid arthritis.

Treatment. Treatment of rheumatoid arthritis generally is associated with aspirin as an analgesic and anti-inflammatory agent and the use of corticosteroids to decrease the amount of joint inflammation and to attempt to decrease the production of rheumatoid factor. Other immunosuppressive agents such as azathioprine or cyclophosphamide may be valuable as well. Although corticosteroids may markedly decrease the clinical signs of disease, these agents may actually contribute to disease progression due to their effect on cartilage.[63]

Prognosis. The prognosis for canine rheumatoid arthritis is guarded. Occasional cases will respond to treatment and signs will abate. It is reasonable to attempt to discontinue medication in these cases. On the other hand, many cases exhibit extensive joint deterioration despite aggressive treatment.

IMMUNE-MEDIATED DERMATOLOGIC DISEASES

Immune-mediated diseases that are manifested primarily by skin disorders have been recognized for more than a decade. Within the category of immune-mediated dermatologic diseases are those caused by an autoimmune disease process (pemphigus and pemphigoid) and those caused by an immune-mediated hypersensitivity (allergic) response to environmental antigens. In addition, there are some dermatologic diseases (e.g., canine dermatomyositis, canine herpetiform dermatitis, and alopecia areata) suspected of being caused by an immunopathologic mechanism, but definitive classifications of the pathophysiology or immunopathogenesis are currently lacking.

ATOPY

Atopy, also known as allergic inhalant dermatitis, atopic dermatitis, allergic dermatitis, and allergic eczema, is an inherited trait characterized by the production of IgE (reaginic) antibodies with specificity for environmental allergens and to express signs of clinical allergy.[64] Dogs afflicted with atopy typically exhibit severe pruritus manifested by foot licking, face rubbing, and axillary scratching. The onset of pruritus is generally noted between one and three years of age with only rare dogs developing atopy after seven years of age. Clinical signs of pruritus may be expressed seasonally or perennially; nearly all breeds are affected with canine atopic dermatitis. Dog breeds generally considered predisposed to develop atopy include the West Highland white; Cairn, Scottish, and wirehaired fox terriers; the English and Irish setters; the golden and Labrador retrievers; and the Dalmatian, Lhasa apso, miniature schnauzer, English bulldog, and beagle. Female dogs appear to be affected more often than male dogs. Those canine breeds considered to be at a decreased risk of expressing signs of atopy include the standard and toy poodles, cocker spaniel, dachshund, and German short-haired pointer. Skin changes associated with atopy include erythema, hyperpigmentation, lichenification, excoriation, papules, wheals, and alopecia. Initial lesions characteristically are found on the face, ears, paws, and ventrum. Seborrhea, otitis externa, and pyoderma may also be observed.[65]

Pathophysiology. Although atopy has also been termed allergic inhalant dermatitis, the offending antigen may enter through the gastrointestinal tract and skin, as well as through the respiratory system. Once in the systemic circulation the antigen complexes with IgE antibody fixed to skin mast cells, which induces mast cell degranulation. The degranulation of mast cells (Type I hypersensitivity) results in the release of numerous vasoactive amines, of which histamine appears particularly important. The release of histamine leads to tissue erythema and edema secondary to vasodilatation and increased capillary permeability, respectively. In addition, mast cell granules contain an eosinophil chemotactic factor that leads to local accumulation of eosinophils within the skin. These events lead to the characteristic histopathology associated with atopy (Figure 119–13): superficial edema associated with increased vascularity and congestion and the presence of tissue mast cells and eosinophils with or without the presence of plasma cells and neutrophils.[66] The reason for the skin being so extensively associated with the manifesta-

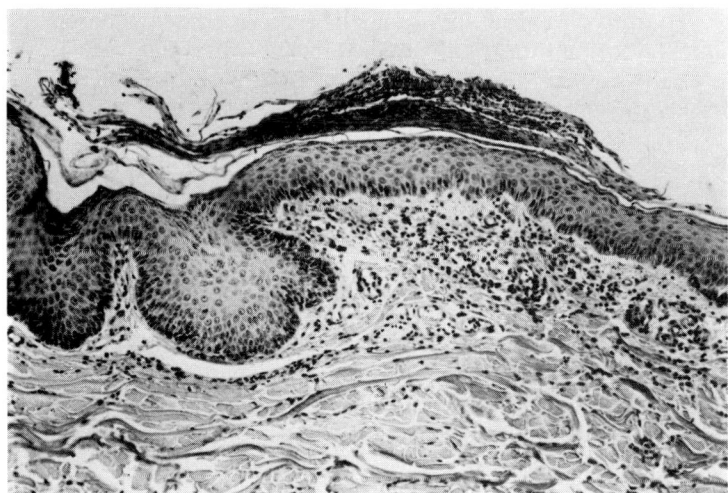

FIGURE 119–13. Canine atopy. Parakeratotic scale-crust with entrapped leukocytes associated with moderate acanthosis and a patchy superficial perivascular infiltrate. (Courtesy of Dr. James D. Conroy.)

tion of atopy is unclear, but probably relates to the preponderance of mast cells located along vessels in the dermis.

The allergens (antigens that stimulate the production of specific immune responses resulting in the expression of allergic diseases) responsible for inducing canine atopy are generally airborne. An airborne allergen (aeroallergen) must be buoyant, present in sufficient amount, and allergenic in order to be clinically significant.[67] Aeroallergens capable of inducing atopy include the pollens of grasses, trees, and weeds; mold spores; house dust; and animal or human epidermals. Of clinical importance is the documented regional differences in aeroallergens due to regional differences in flora and fauna.[64] Recognizing regional differences in the distribution of aeroallergens is important as it mandates that appropriate choices of allergenic extracts be made to accurately identify those allergens potentially involved in the expression of canine atopy.

A final concept critical in understanding the pathophysiology of canine atopy is that each atopic dog likely has a threshold for the induction of pruritus secondary to allergen stimulation.[68] Some animals may be capable of tolerating a moderate allergen exposure, while others may exhibit a very low threshold for even minute amounts of antigen. This threshold is probably influenced by genetic, immunologic, climatic, and physiologic factors. As a result, changes in the nutritional status, concurrent infectious diseases, external parasites, and environmental conditions may influence the degree of animal sensitivity to express clinical signs of atopy. Treatment plans for patients should take these factors into consideration.

Diagnosis. The diagnosis of canine atopy requires a careful history, physical examination, intradermal skin tests, and knowledge of the aeroallergens present in the environment during the time when the disease is clinically expressed. Critical in the diagnostic plan should be the careful ruling out of external parasites (fleas, scabies, and demodecosis), flea allergic dermatitis, food allergy and pelodera dermatitis. Appropriate diagnostic tests include examination for fleas, skin scraping, intradermal skin testing, skin biopsy for routine histopathology, and a restricted diet to exclude food allergy as the underlying etiology. In addition, it should be considered that the patient may also be exhibiting concurrent skin disease related to other underlying etiologies such as superficial pyoderma or hypothyroidism.

INTRADERMAL SKIN TEST. The only accepted *in vivo* method to diagnose atopy is by an intradermal injection of the suspected allergen and the documentation of an immediate type hypersensitivity reaction (wheal and flare).[64] The skin test should be performed without the use of tranquilizers, sedatives, or anesthesia; however, xylazine (Rompun) has been reported not to interfere with skin test responses to injected allergens.[65] The recommended injection volume of test allergen ranges from 0.02 ml to 0.1 ml and the skin test response is generally evaluated 15 to 20 minutes following intradermal injection. The intradermal skin test can be graded subjectively by visual inspection and palpation and subsequently scored as 0 (if the test reaction is the same size as the saline-negative control) through 4 (if the test reaction is the same size as the histamine-positive control). Factors that influence the grade of the skin test reaction include wheal diameter and elevation from the surrounding normal skin, erythema, turgidity, and pseudopodium formation; a light source held parallel to the skin test site in a dark room is commonly used to accentuate the visualization of the wheals. A false negative test result may occur in animals concurrently medicated with corticosteroids or antihistamines, in animals tested during estrus or during pseudopregnancy, if outdated antigens or excessively diluted antigens are used, if the test antigen is injected subcutaneously or if air is injected without antigen, and if the intradermal test is performed during the nonallergic season when IgE antibody may not be present. False positive test results may be observed if antigens are too concentrated and irritating to the skin, if bacterial products contaminate the antigenic extract, and if an excessive volume of test antigen is injected. Although a positive skin test does identify that the patient has IgE antibody on the surface of the skin mast cells with specificity for the allergen, it does not necessarily document that the patient's presenting skin disease is the result of atopy to that particular antigen.

Treatment. There are basically three methods available to treat the atopic patient: (1) avoidance of the offending allergen, (2) hyposensitization, and (3) medical therapy.[68]

AVOIDANCE. Avoidance of the inciting allergen is the most definitive method to halt the expression of atopic disease, but in many cases this is not possible. Every attempt should be made, however, to eliminate the inciting allergen. If complete avoidance is not possible, decreased exposure may be sufficient to reduce the allergenic load below the patient's threshold level for expression of clinical disease. If exposure to the allergen cannot be controlled, then the next therapeutic modality is to attempt control by hyposensitization.

HYPOSENSITIZATION. Hyposensitization is the parenteral administration of allergens in an attempt to induce an immunologic response that will lead to a decreased expression of clinical signs of allergy. The specific immunologic mechanisms responsible for the diminished signs of allergy are incompletely understood; however, the most widely accepted hypothesis is that hyposensitization induces the production of IgG antibodies with specificity for the allergen. The observed decrease in clinical allergic signs is believed to be secondary to the binding of the allergen with IgG, which renders the allergen unavailable to complex with mast cells sensitized with IgE antibodies. This mechanism then prevents mast cell degranulation and eliminates the clinical signs of atopy due to the prevented release of the biologic mediators of immediate type hypersensitivity. Another possible mechanism is that hyposensitization actually induces increased numbers of suppressor T lymphocytes, which prevent the induction of plasma cells that secrete IgE antibody with specificity for the allergen.

Hyposensitization has been reported to benefit about three-fourths of those dogs with a diagnosis of atopy.[68] About 50 per cent of atopic dogs treated with a hyposensitization protocol require no corticosteroids to control clinical signs and approximately 25 per cent of atopic dogs demonstrate a marked decrease in corticosteroid dosage to adequately control clinical signs; the remaining 25 per cent of animals do not respond to treatment as judged by both the attending veterinarian and client. The fewer the number of offending allergens in the disease process, the better the chance for control.[59] The three major methods used to induce hyposensitization are (1) aqueous antigenic extracts given weekly or biweekly for six months to three years for maximum effect, (2) alum precipitated antigenic extracts given as 8 to 12 injections over a 3 to 6 month time span for maximum effect, and (3) propylene glycol or glycerin emulsions of aqueous antigenic extracts given as four to eight injections over two to four months for maximum effect.

MEDICAL THERAPY. If both avoidance of the allergen and hyposensitization fail then the third treatment modality is corticosteroid and/or antihistamine therapy. Only short-acting oral corticosteroids should be used and alternate day therapy is recommended. Initial glucocorticoid dosage (prednisone or prednisolone) should be 0.5 mg/lb (1 mg/kg) PO q12 to 24h for one week to break the itch-scratch cycle. Following this period of time the dosage should be reduced to the lowest dosage possible that will control the signs of disease given on an alternate day regimen.

Long-acting corticosteroids such as methylprednisolone acetate administered at a dose of 0.5 mg/lb (1 mg/kg) IM should only be used in patients that exhibit a short seasonal presentation of clinical signs and when only one to two injections will effectively control the pruritus for the entire year.[68] Topical corticosteroids are considered effective for the symptomatic relief of focal pruritic lesions, but should not be used to control generalized pruritus. Antihistamines appear to be of minimal value in controlling clinical signs of atopy in the dog, but a therapeutic trial should be attempted.

Prognosis. Atopy is considered a treatable disease; however, because the pruritus is often severe and because the disease may be lifelong, difficulty may be encountered in controlling the disease process. If the owners are aware that considerable time, effort, and expense may be required to establish disease control, they are more likely to be satisfied with the outcome. Some dogs, however, fail to respond to treatment despite aggressive efforts by the veterinarian and client, and the disease process can be devastating. For these patients the prognosis is poor as the animal is plagued by unrelenting pruritus.

ALLERGIC CONTACT DERMATITIS

Clinical Signs. Allergic contact dermatitis has been reported to occur in 1 to 10 per cent of canine dermatology cases depending on the criteria for diagnosis, geographical area, and type of veterinary practice.[69] Very few cases have been definitively documented although numerous substances have been incriminated as allergens responsible for inducing allergic contact dermatitis.[59] Animals with this type of allergy present with a dermatitis confined to those body areas that make intimate contact with the offending allergen. Allergic contact dermatitis requires direct contact with the allergen and, in general, haired areas of the body are not affected. In most cases the cutaneous lesions are limited to the abdomen, medial thighs, axillae, ventral tail, chin, medial aspect of the ears, the feet, and the perineal area. Skin changes may range from mild erythema only to severely pruritic, papulovesicular lesions with secondary pigmentary changes. No age or sex predilections have been reported; however, poodles, Scottish terriers, West Highland white terriers, and yellow Labrador retrievers may be predisposed.[59]

Pathophysiology. Allergic contact dermatitis is initiated by contact of simple chemicals with the intact skin. The percutaneous application of these simple chemicals to the intact epidermis is, however, only the first criterion for the induction of clinical allergy. Before these chemical haptens can be recognized by the immune system and an allergic contact dermatitis can develop, the chemical hapten must form a covalent bond with protein molecules located within the skin. After a covalent bond is formed a primary (sensitizing) immune response occurs, which requires approximately four to ten days. This period of time allows for the development of a clone of memory lymphocytes with specificity for the allergen-protein complex. Following a second exposurc to the chemical allergen a dramatic and intense T lymphocyte–mediated (Type IV hypersensitivity or delayed-type hypersensitivity) immune response is generated. The T lymphocytes recognize the allergen-protein complex, proliferate to markedly increase cell numbers, and release a variety of lymphokines that attract other nonallergen-specific lymphocytes and macrophages to the cutaneous site. Histologically the cutaneous lesion is characterized by a massive accumulation of mononuclear cells with peak cell numbers present between 24 and 72 hours after allergen contact. Epidermal spongiosis can be frequently observed and may become so severe that vesicles form within the epidermis. Clinically the affected skin develops an erythematous plaque, which may be quite pruritic and exhibit an oozing, crusting, and papulovesicular appearance. If the offending allergen is removed, the lesions should subside in approximately ten days.

Diagnosis. The diagnosis of allergic contact dermatitis should be made by obtaining a careful history, performing a complete physical examination, evaluating patch test results, and examining skin biopsies from affected areas. It is important during historical questioning that information be obtained regarding any new additions of items into the immediate environment of the pet. Characterization of a seasonal or nonseasonal occurrence of clinical signs may be helpful in identifying the offending allergen. It should be emphasized, however, that allergies may develop to existing environmental antigens at any time and more than half of reported cases of allergic contact dermatitis may occur in response to antigens present in the environment for more than 2 years.[70]

The differential diagnostic considerations generally include flea bite or flea allergic dermatitis, sarcoptic mange, food allergy, atopy, pelodera dermatitis, and dermatophytosis. Because allergic contact dermatitis is relatively uncommon, initial diagnostic tests should focus on skin scraping, fungal culture, intradermal skin tests to investigate the potential of atopy or flea allergic dermatitis, and skin biopsy for routine histology. A food elimination diet should also be considered. If results of these diagnostic tests suggest a strong likelihood of allergic contact dermatitis, then patch testing should be performed.

Patch Skin Test. The definitive diagnosis of allergic contact dermatitis requires patch testing, skin biopsy, and the concurrent use of a control animal to rule out chemical or mechanical irritation as the cause of an observed positive patch test result. Briefly, the haircoat on the patient and a normal control dog should be clipped; one day later the suspected allergen is applied to the clipped area and an occlusive bandage applied directly over the allergen. The patch test site should be examined at 6, 24, 48, and 72 hours. If an erythematous plaque appears, then a punch biopsy of the skin test site should be obtained for histologic examination; the patch test site on the normal control dog should be concurrently biopsied. Erythematous skin lesions that appear within 6 hours and that dissipate within 24 hours are more likely secondary to irritation rather than an allergen specific Type IV hypersensitivity response.[59, 69]

Treatment. Therapy should focus on removing the allergen from the immediate environment of the pet. If this is not possible, then every attempt should be made to reduce the incidence of contact and the animal should be treated with prednisone or prednisolone at 0.25 to 0.5 mg/lb (0.5 to 1 mg/kg) PO q12 to 24h for seven days. The dosage of corticosteroids should then be gradually reduced to the lowest dose possible, given on an alternate day schedule, which effectively controls the expression of clinical disease signs. Although immune modulation may be possible, there does not currently exist a documented, efficacious hyposensitization protocol for allergic contact dermatitis. Until an effective protocol is developed, corticosteroids will remain the mainstay of therapy.

Prognosis. The prognosis is excellent if the offending allergen can be identified and removed from the environment. However, if the contact allergen cannot be removed, the pet may have to be relocated to an environment devoid of the allergic substance. In cases where the separation of the pet from the allergen cannot be achieved, then the prognosis is guarded as some dogs may continue to develop clinical signs even while being medically managed with oral corticosteroids. In addition, the possibility of multiple agents inducing the dermatitis cannot be excluded and therapy may be difficult to design. Critical in the overall prognosis is the establishment of good client relations and compliance by the owners.

CANINE DERMATOMYOSITIS

Canine dermatomyositis is a disease currently limited to juvenile Collies and Shetland sheepdogs and is characterized by dermatitis and myositis.[71-75] The etiology is unknown in the dog, but may relate to an immune-mediated disease process. The disease is inherited apparently as an autosomal dominant trait. Signs of dermatitis occur between 7 and 11 weeks of age, but expression of the disease is variable. Mildly affected dogs spontaneously resolve the dermatitis and exhibit minimal signs of muscular disease. Moderately and severely affected dogs demonstrate some dermatologic improvement, but the dermatitis persists. Clinical, electrodiagnostic, and histologic evidence of polymyositis is easily detected in dogs that exhibit moderate and severe signs of dermatitis.

The dermatitis is observed on the ears, face, lips, tip of the tail, and over bony prominences of the limbs.[72-74] The skin lesions are secondary to the formation of intraepidermal and subepidermal vesicles or pustules with a leukocytic intradermal infiltrate. Whether the skin pathology is caused by the documented increase in circulating immune complexes, the product of other immunopathologic mechanisms, or unrelated to an immune-mediated disease process remains to be answered.

The myositis is characterized by bilaterally symmetrical muscle atrophy of the head, neck, trunk, and extremities. In addition, facial palsy, decreased jaw tone, and a stiff gait with hyperreflexia may be noted in severely affected dogs.[71-73] Histologic examination of muscle tissue typically reveals myositis, fibrosis, and evidence of myofiber degeneration, atrophy, and regeneration. The motor nerve conduction in affected muscle is normal; however, needle electromyograms are abnormal. The abnormal electromyograms are characterized by the presence of fibrillation potentials, positive sharp waves, and bizarre high-frequency discharges.

Clinical Signs. Dermatitis is usually noted at three to six months of age. No obvious sex, coat, or color is predisposed to develop clinical signs.[71, 73] Cutaneous lesions initially occur on the face in approximately 80 per cent of case presentations; however, lesions on the tips of the ears and tail are very common. Least common are lesions on the extremities; however, they will develop later in the course of the disease.

Early skin lesions consist of small pustules, vesicles, papules, or nodules, which may progress to alopecic or crusted areas of skin. In some pups, lesions can also be seen on the mucous membranes and mucocutaneous junctions. These lesions spontaneously regress as the pups mature. The pustular stage of the disease may last from 3 to 21 days and in most instances is followed by focal crusting and scarring. The lesions are nonpruritic in greater than 70 per cent of cases. The disease course generally waxes and wanes over weeks to months.

Diagnosis. A young Collie or Shetland sheepdog presented for the primary complaint of facial dermatitis with involvement of the tips of the ears, tail, and/or extremities should be suspected of having dermatomyositis. Critical in the diagnostic approach is the ruling out of dermatophytosis and demodecosis, which is accomplished by fungal culture and skin scraping, respectively. Other diagnostic considerations include immunologic, metabolic, and infectious skin disorders as well as epidermolysis bullosa. Biopsies of skin and muscle along with electromyographic analysis are required to confirm a diagnosis of dermatomyositis.

ELECTROMYOGRAPHY. Changes observed on electromyographic analysis may include positive sharp waves and fibrillation potentials most prominent in the temporalis and masseter muscles, the tongue, the laryngeal muscles, distal extremities and tail.[71] Nerve conduction studies are typically normal. Serum chemistry profiles and serum creatinine phosphokinase activities are normal. Antinuclear antibody tests are negative. Clinical signs of myositis may consist of temporal and masseter muscle atrophy; difficulty drinking, chewing, and swallowing; and exercise intolerance.

HISTOLOGY. Follicular atrophy and perifollicular inflammation (approximately 80 per cent of dogs) are consistent and dramatic features of dermatohistopathology associated with canine dermatomyositis.[76] In addition, dermal fibrosis and dermatitis characterized by infiltrates of mononuclear cells, neutrophils, and occasionally eosinophils are commonly noted. Intraepidermal pustules are observed in less than 10 per cent of presented cases.

Prognosis. Most dogs spontaneously resolve their disease by about one year of age. Milder cases resolve faster than more severely affected cases. Very severely affected puppies exhibit a dermatitis that waxes and wanes over the dog's lifetime. These particular patients often exhibit extensive ulcerated, crusted lesions over all pressure points as well as the tail, ears and face. In general the more severe the initial course of the disease, the poorer the prognosis.

CANINE HERPETIFORM DERMATITIS

Dermatitis herpetiformis is an immune-mediated disease in humans that is characterized by a pruritic dermatitis associated with IgA deposition in dermal papillae and the formation of subepidermal bullae. The disease in humans is also associated with a gluten enteropathy and responds well to treatment with dapsone. There is a similar type of disease present in dogs,[77] but definitive documentation that the canine and human diseases are analogous does not exist. Specifically, the disease in humans is diagnosed based on (1) the granular deposition of IgA in dermal papillae, (2) a gluten-sensitive enteropathy, and (3) an association with specific histocompatibility antigens. None of these identified parameters has been documented in canine cases suspected to be dermatitis herpetiformis.[77]

Clinical Signs. The disease in dogs is only suspected on rare occasion in those patients that exhibit a papular, pruritic eruption of the trunk, head, ears and feet. Other diagnostic considerations include superficial staphylococcal hypersensitivity, subcorneal pustular dermatosis, bacterial folliculitis, drug eruption, SLE, and inhalant or food hypersensitivities.

Pathology. Histologic examination of skin obtained from dogs with canine herpetiform dermatitis closely resembles inflammatory changes seen in man. The progression of skin lesions in the dog is characterized initially by an accumulation of neutrophils in the dermal papillae, followed by eosinophils. The accumulation of inflammatory cells progresses to form a microabscess. The fusion of adjacent microabscesses results in the development of the subepidermal pustules.[78]

Treatment. Treatment of dermatitis herpetiformis in humans is with dapsone along with a gluten-free diet. Dapsone probably functions by interfering with the myeloperoxidase–hydrogen peroxidase–iodine system within neutrophils[79] and as such is effective in a variety of diseases where the neutrophil is a prominent cell in the inflammatory response. Because dapsone is effective in a variety of diseases, it should not be considered definitive evidence of dermatitis herpetiformis in dogs if the therapy results in substantial clinical improvement.[78]

Pemphigus

The term pemphigus is derived from the Greek word for blister and is the name given to a group of dermatological diseases caused by an autoimmune disease process.[80] The pemphigus skin diseases are characterized immunologically by the presence of autoantibodies that react with an antigen present in the intercellular spaces between epidermal cells. There are currently four variants of pemphigus recognized: foliaceous, erythematosus, vulgaris and vegetans. Although the pemphigus skin disorders are classified as bullous dermatoses, the clinical presentation of skin lesions is varied and includes vesiculobullous eruptions, cutaneous ulcerations, exfoliative lesions, and verrucous proliferations of the skin. Each pemphigus disease is characterized by the deposition of immunoglobulin within the intercellular spaces of the epidermis, the formation of acanthocytes, and cleft formation.

both are anaphylatoxins and are capable of inducing localized degranulation of mast cells, which results in the release of vasoactive amines and eosinophil chemotactic factor. The release of vasoactive amines results in increased capillary permeability and edema, while the eosinophil chemotactic factor leads to the focal accumulation of eosinophils. Together these events are generally believed to be responsible for the development of the intraepithelial pustules containing either neutrophils or eosinophils.

Diagnosis. The diagnosis of pemphigus skin diseases is generally based on histologic and immunofluorescence examinations of skin biopsies (Table 119–4). Because the vesiculopustules typical of pemphigus are extremely transient, frequent skin inspection and multiple biopsy specimens of early lesions are critical to establish a definitive diagnosis. Surgical preparation of the skin for biopsy is generally not recommended, as crusts may contain degenerated acanthocytes and lend support to a diagnosis of pemphigus. Direct immunofluorescence examination of biopsied skin should demonstrate the presence of immunoglobulin and/or complement within the intercellular spaces of the epidermis.[81, 82] The deposition of immunoglobulin within the epidermis may be extremely focal, and examination of many serial sections of tissue is often necessary to diagnose the presence of immunoglobulin and/or complement. Care must be taken in interpreting the direct immunofluorescence report, as a negative test result does not exclude the possibility of an existing disease process.

PEMPHIGUS FOLIACEOUS

Pemphigus foliaceous is one of the more common immune-mediated bullous skin diseases of dogs and has been most frequently reported to occur between the ages of two and seven years.[83] The disease is gradually progressive in approximately 75 per cent of cases and more rapid (developing in less than three months) in about 25 per cent of case presentations. Although pemphigus foliaceous is categorized as a bullous disease, pustules are recognized more frequently. Intact vesicles or bullae are rare, likely due to the extremely thin canine epidermis. In addition, an early neutrophilic infiltration frequently increases the difficulty in identifying intact vesicles or bullae due to the rapid development of a pustular appearance.

Clinical Signs. Pemphigus foliaceous may be gener-

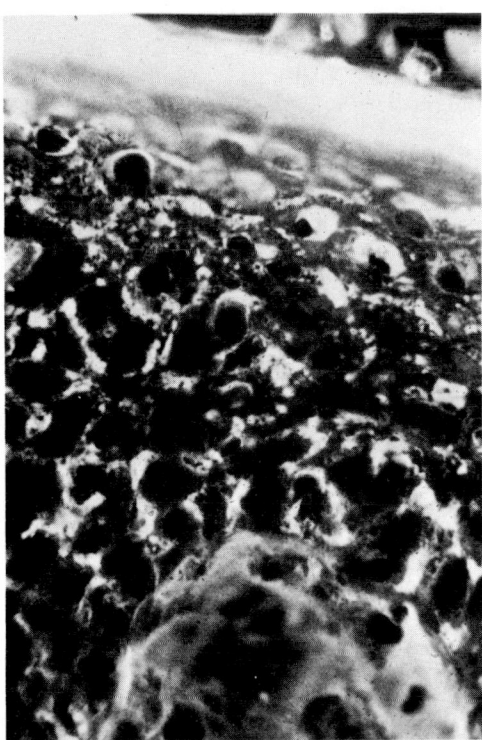

FIGURE 119–14. Pemphigus variety, direct immunofluorescence. Epidermis showing positive test with an intercellular pattern characteristic of the pemphigus group. (Courtesy of Dr. James D. Conroy.)

Pathophysiology. The etiology of the pemphigus skin diseases is considered to be related to an inappropriate secretion of autoantibodies that exhibit specificity for an intercellular epidermal antigen.[63] The definitive antigen to which the autoantibodies are directed is unknown, but it appears that the antigen is located in or near the cytoplasmic membrane of the epidermal cells (Figure 119–14). The binding of antibodies with the intercellular epidermal substance purportedly leads to acantholysis (the loss of cohesiveness between epidermal cells and their subsequent rounded up appearance) and complement activation. During the cascade reaction associated with complement activation, numerous complement split products are generated, and among these products, C3a and C5a appear to be most important. The complement split product C5a is chemotactic for neutrophils and results in the accumulation of neutrophils within the epidermis. The complement split products C3a and C5a

TABLE 119–4. DIAGNOSTIC PARAMETERS FOR AUTOIMMUNE SKIN DISEASES

Disease	Common Distribution	Epidermal Direct Immunofluorescence	Cleft Formation	Antinuclear Antibody	Systemic Disease
Pemphigus foliaceus	Nasal dermatitis and generalized	Intercellular	Subcorneal	–	+/–
Pemphigus erythematosus	Nasal dermatitis	Intercellular and basement membrane zone		Low titer	–
Pemphigus vulgaris	Mucocutaneous junctions and oral cavity	Intercellular	Suprabasilar	–	+/–
Pemphigus vegetans	Face and trunk	Intercellular		–	–
Bullous pemphigoid	Mucocutaneous junction, oral cavity, and generalized	Basement membrane zone	Subepidermal	–	+/–
Systemic lupus erythematosus	Mucocutaneous junction, oral cavity, and generalized	Basement membrane zone		+	+
Cutaneous lupus erythematosus	Nasal dermatitis	Basement membrane zone		Rare	–

alized, patchy, facial or pedal[84] in appearance; facial lesions are observed first in more than 80 per cent of dogs, and in greater than 50 per cent of dogs the initial site of involvement is the dorsal aspect of the muzzle.[83] The skin lesions appear similar in most dogs and are characterized by crusting, scaling, and alopecia; crusts frequently adhere to underlying skin and hair. Skin erosions and ulcerations are most frequently noted during episodes of disease exacerbation or secondary to self-inflicted trauma. Pruritus is manifested in less than 50 per cent of the dogs. Erythema and exudation are frequently seen in severely affected areas, and target lesions exhibiting peripheral collarettes are common. Although pemphigus foliaceous can affect virtually all breeds of dogs, the bearded collie, Newfoundland, akita, and schipperke appear to be at a significantly elevated risk.

Diagnosis. The diagnosis of pemphigus foliaceous generally rests on routine dermatohistology (Figure 119–15) and direct immunofluorescence skin tests. The most characteristic histologic alteration of the epidermis in pemphigus foliaceous consists of vesiculopustules or microabscesses in association with large numbers of acantholytic keratinocytes.[83] The vesiculopustules are most frequently found directly beneath the stratum corneum (subcorneal) or in an intraepidermal location. Microabscesses are generally observed within the external root sheath or within hair follicle lumens. Depending on the duration of acantholysis, the keratinocytes may exhibit a vesicular nucleus, a prominent nucleolus, and no cytologic signs of cytoplasmic degeneration; degenerated acanthocytes generally exhibit nuclear pyknosis and an eosinophilic cytoplasm. The acantholytic keratinocytes may be observed as single cells or as clusters of cells either adherent to the overlying stratum corneum or within the lumen of the vesiculopustule.

Direct immunofluorescence of the skin should exhibit an intercellular epidermal staining pattern. The epidermal staining pattern may be localized to the upper half of the epidermis or diffuse throughout the intercellular spaces of the epidermis. Approximately 75 per cent of dogs that exhibit histologic evidence of pemphigus foliaceous also demonstrate direct immunofluorescence in an intercellular pattern. Immunofluorescence with IgG is seen in nearly all cases, and deposition of C3 (the third component of the complement proteins) in a intercellular location is observed in about 80 per cent of those skin samples that demonstrate IgG deposition.[83] Antibody in IgM with reactivity against the intercellular substance of the epidermis is rarely seen, likely owing to the large molecular weight of the immunoglobulin class and its poor ability to diffuse into an intercellular location within the epidermis. Although some reports indicate that indirect immunofluorescence is unreliable in canine pemphigus foliaceous,[59, 85] other reports suggest that indirect immunofluorescence may be of some diagnostic value.[83] Another test that may be of value is a Tzanck preparation (Figure 119–16) from intact pustules or vesicles to cytologically assess the cellular components of the bulla. The appearance of acanthocytes, nontoxic neutrophils, and eosinophils within a pustule smear is highly suggestive of pemphigus foliaceous.

Nondermatologic signs that may be associated with pemphigus foliaceous include generalized lymphadenopathy, leukocytosis secondary to a mature neutrophilia, and a normocytic, normochromic anemia. In addition, some dogs may exhibit iridocyclitis and photophobia related to antigen-antibody complexes present within the anterior chamber of the eye.[83]

PEMPHIGUS ERYTHEMATOSUS

Clinical Signs. Pemphigus erythematosus is believed to be an abortive form or an initial stage of pemphigus foliaceous or a cross over between pemphigus and lupus erythematosus.[86, 87] The skin changes are typically confined to the face and are characterized by erythema, oozing, crusting, scaling, and alopecia. The specific sites of facial dermatitis appear to be the nose, periocular areas, and pinna. Oral ulceration is not considered to be associated with pemphigus erythematosus. At present no age, sex, or breed predilections are obvious based on the limited number of canine and feline documented cases.

Diagnosis. The list of diagnostic considerations for facial dermatitis includes bacterial folliculitis, fungal

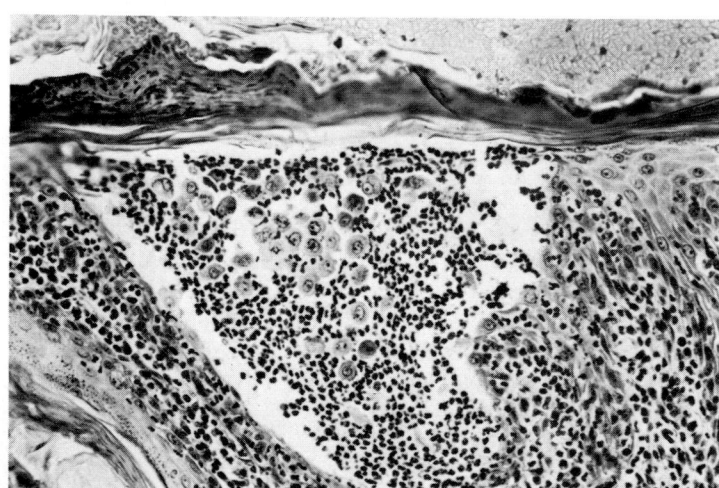

FIGURE 119–15. Pemphigus foliaceous. Subgranular intraepidermal vesicle pustule containing numerous acantholytic keratinocytes and granulocytes (neutrophils and eosinophils). (Courtesy of Dr. James D. Conroy.)

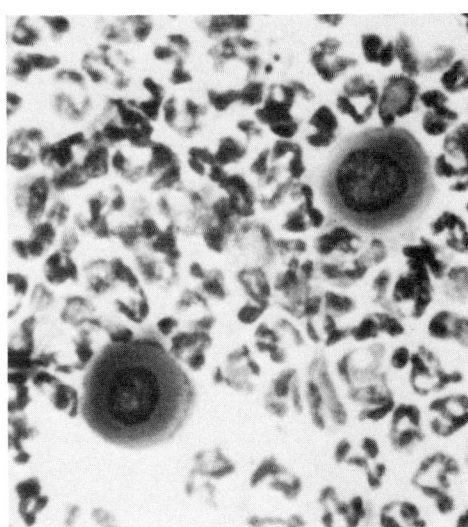

FIGURE 119–16. Aspiration cytology (Tzanck preparation) of a pustular dermatosis compatible with a diagnosis of pemphigus disease complex. Note the predominance of nontoxic neutrophils, lack of identifiable bacteria, and presence of acantholytic keratinocytes. (Courtesy of Dr. Dennis J. Meyer.)

dermatitis, solar dermatitis, contact dermatitis, atopy, food allergy, demodecosis, seborrheic dermatitis, subcorneal pustular dermatosis, pemphigus foliaceous, pemphigus erythematosus, systemic and cutaneous lupus erythematosus, zinc responsive dermatitis, and epidermolysis bullosa.[88] Because the list of potential diagnoses for facial dermatitis is long a systematic diagnostic plan should be followed to correctly diagnose the disease process: skin scrape, fungal culture, antinuclear antibody test, direct immunofluorescence, and routine histopathology.

Because both pemphigus erythematosus and pemphigus foliaceous generally begin on the face, and because the gross and histopathologic presentations are identical (subcorneal or intraepidermal abscess formation with prominent acantholytic keratinocytes), the distinction between the two diseases must rely on the basis of disease progression and immunologic test results. Pemphigus foliaceous generally progresses to diffuse cutaneous involvement, while pemphigus erythematosus remains localized to the face.

Immunologic tests to differentiate pemphigus erythematosus from pemphigus foliaceous include an antinuclear antibody test and direct immunofluorescence of affected skin. The antinuclear antibody test in pemphigus erythematosus typically reveals a low titer of circulating antibody to nuclear material, and the direct immunofluorescence test shows deposition of immunoglobulin and/or complement at the basement membrane zone and within the intercellular spaces of the epidermis.

PEMPHIGUS VULGARIS

Clinical Signs. Pemphigus vulgaris is characterized by epidermal ulceration with a predilection for the oral mucosa and the mucocutaneous junction.[89] Nail beds may be affected and secondary paronychia may result in sloughing of the nail. In rare cases the disease process may become generalized. The onset may be acute or insidious. The disease can be associated with pain and pruritus of affected skin. Animals may be systemically ill. Approximately 90 per cent of cases exhibit oral involvement consisting of ulcerative stomatitis, gingivitis, or glossitis, which may be the initial manifestation of the disease.[59] Insufficient cases have been documented to accurately define breed, sex, or age predilections.

Diagnosis. The differential diagnosis for clinical cases presented for ulcerative stomatitis and/or mucocutaneous ulcerations includes pemphigus vulgaris, mucocutaneous candidiasis, chemical induced stomatitis, idiopathic ulcerative stomatitis, and bullous pemphigoid. Histopathologic examination of affected epidermal tissues should demonstrate a suprabasilar cleft (Figure 119–17) and the formation of acanthocytes;[89–91] care must be taken to use a sharp instrument in the procurement of the skin biopsy to insure that the histopathology is not confused by iatrogenic damage of the epidermis.

PEMPHIGUS VEGETANS

Clinical Signs. Pemphigus vegetans is believed to be a variant of pemphigus vulgaris and is thought to represent a more benign disease process. The major difference lies in the healing of ulcerated skin lesions. In pemphigus vegetans, ulcerated epidermal surfaces exhibit characteristic healing with verrucous vegetations and papillomatous proliferations rather than a normal epidermal layer.[92]

Diagnosis. The diagnosis requires routine histopathology (Figure 119–18) and immunofluorescence testing. The histology should demonstrate papillomatosis and the accumulation of eosinophils within intraepidermal abscesses.[80, 92, 93] The direct immunofluorescence should show the presence of immunoglobulin within the intercellular spaces of the epidermal cells.

TREATMENT AND PROGNOSIS OF PEMPHIGUS

Approximately 40 per cent of dogs can be effectively treated with corticosteroids without the development of unacceptable side effects;[83] side effects associated with the use of prednisone include polydipsia, polyuria, weight gain, lethargy, weakness, pyoderma, and recurrent bacterial urinary tract infections. Initial dosages of oral corticosteroid (prednisone or prednisolone) should vary between 1 and 1.5 mg/lb (2 to 3 mg/kg) PO q12h. If substantial improvement is noted within 10 days, gradual reduction of the prednisone or prednisolone dose to 0.5 mg/lb (1 mg/kg) PO q48h should be attempted over a four week period. If no substantial improvement is noted during the first 10 days or if a reduction in glucocorticoid therapy cannot be achieved without disease recrudescence, then combination immunosuppression is recommended. Definitive evidence of the best combination drug schedule for effective immunosuppression in the treatment of pemphigus diseases is not available; however, three basic approaches have been used.

In the first approach, and probably the widest used, prednisone and azathioprine are given in combination. The dosages for the combined use of prednisone and

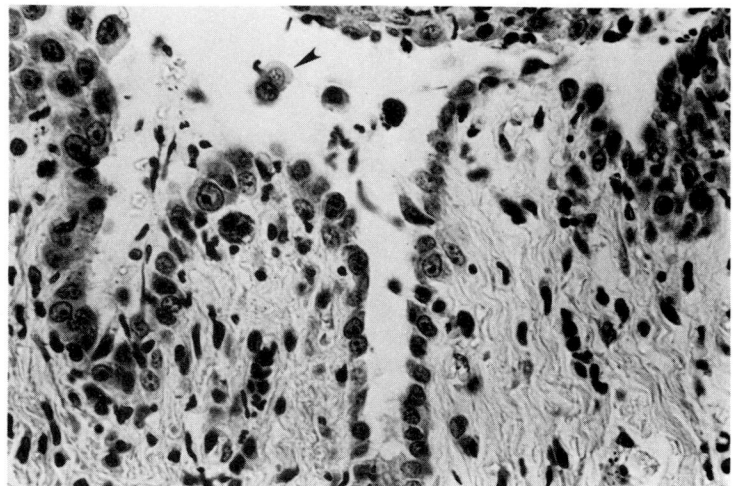

FIGURE 119–17. Pemphigus vulgaris. Suprabasal vesicle with intact basal cells showing the "tombstone" effect and several acantholytic keratinocytes (example at arrow) floating free in the vesicle. (Courtesy of Dr. James D. Conroy.)

azathioprine are 0.5 mg/lb (1 mg/kg) PO q12h and 1 mg/lb (2 mg/kg) PO q24h, respectively. If the disease responds to treatment over a 10 to 14 day period, then the medication is begun on an alternate day schedule (i.e., prednisone at 0.5 mg/lb (1 mg/kg) PO on one day followed by azathioprine 1 mg/lb (2 mg/kg) PO the following day). Following the establishment of continued remission, the prednisone and azathioprine dosages are gradually reduced to 0.5 mg/lb (1 mg/kg) PO given on alternate days.

The second combination immunosuppressive drug schedule utilizes prednisone and cyclophosphamide. Prednisone at 0.5 mg/lb (1 mg/kg) PO q12h and cyclo-

phosphamide at 1 mg/lb (50 mg/m²) PO q24h for four consecutive days each week are administered for 14 to 21 days to determine if disease remission will develop. Following the establishment of continued remission the dosages of prednisone and cyclophosphamide are each gradually reduced to 0.5 mg/lb (1 mg/kg) PO given together on an every other day basis.

The third immunosuppressive chemotherapy scheme for the treatment of pemphigus skin disorders utilizes prednisone at 0.5 mg/lb (1 mg/kg) PO q48h and aurothioglucose at 0.5 mg/lb (1 mg/kg) IM once weekly.

Approximately 50 per cent of dogs with pemphigus foliaceous can be successfully managed if the owner is willing and capable of supporting the financial commitment necessary for repeated examinations and laboratory evaluations.[83] Dogs that survive the first year of treatment can generally be maintained in disease remission throughout the remainder of their lives.

Although only a limited number of canine cases of pemphigus erythematosus have been documented, response to therapy is generally successful; therefore the prognosis should be good. A potential complication in canine pemphigus erythematosus is localized leukoderma of affected skin. The leukoderma results in increased susceptibility to photodermatitis, which must be managed by avoidance of sunlight or topical sunscreen application. If pigmented epithelium does not return, and sunburning is a recurrent problem, then tattooing of the affected area may prove beneficial.[87] Too few cases of pemphigus erythematosus exist in the cat to make a generalized prognostic statement; however, high dosages of prednisone or prednisolone at 2 mg/lb (4 mg/kg) PO q12h failed to induce remission in one case report.[87]

The prognosis for pemphigus vulgaris without therapy is poor to grave, with 95 per cent of cases being fatal due to progressive debilitation and terminal septicemia.[59] The prognosis for treated patients must remain guarded and the owner informed that therapy will very likely be life long.

Too few cases of pemphigus vegetans have been recorded to define a precise prognosis.

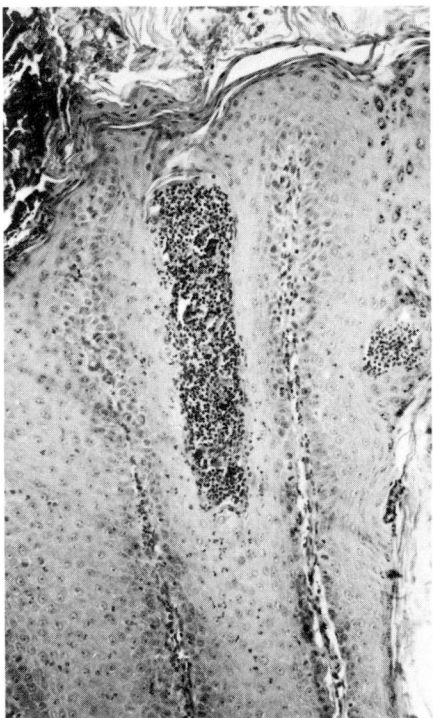

FIGURE 119–18. Pemphigus vegetans. Marked hyperplasia of the epidermis and hair follicle epithelium associated with deep granulocytic vesicopustules. (Courtesy of Dr. James D. Conroy.)

Pemphigoid

The name pemphigoid is given to a specific group of dermatological syndromes similar to but clearly distinguishable from those clinical syndromes of the pemphigus disease complex. The first tentative diagnosis of bullous pemphigoid in the dog was made in 1976 by Austin and Maiback.[94, 95] Although bullous pemphigoid is not a common skin disorder, it appears to be one of the more frequently diagnosed varieties of bullous autoimmune skin diseases.

BULLOUS PEMPHIGOID

Clinical Signs. Bullous pemphigoid is a vesiculobullous disease characterized by lesions affecting the oral cavity (approximately 80 per cent of cases), mucocutaneous junctions, footpads, and the skin of the trunk, groin, axillae, and abdomen.[89, 96, 97] The dermatologic manifestations of disease include blisters, crusts, epidermal collarettes, ulcerations, and erosions.[89, 97] The differential diagnosis for patients presenting with oral lesions should include mucocutaneous candidiasis, chemical irritant stomatitis, idiopathic ulcerative stomatitis, drug eruption, systemic lupus erythematosus, and pemphigus vulgaris. Diagnostic considerations for cutaneous lesions without oral lesions including pemphigus foliaceous, toxic epidermal necrolysis, cutaneous T-cell–like lymphoma, lymphoreticular neoplasia, cutaneous lupus erythematosus, and hidradenitis suppurativa.[97] No breed, sex, or age predilections have been definitively documented; however, collies, Shetland sheepdogs, and perhaps Doberman pinschers may be overrepresented.[97] Bullous pemphigoid has been speculated to occur in cats,[98] but definitive documentation is lacking.

Pathophysiology. Although the exact etiology of bullous pemphigoid is unknown, antibodies with specificity for the lamina lucida of the basement membrane zone are suspected to play a major role in the pathogenesis of the cutaneous lesions;[81, 97] it should be clearly stated that the specific antigen within the lamina lucida is not known and that definitive documentation of bullous pemphigoid as a canine or feline autoimmune disease is lacking. The binding of antibodies (IgG, IgA, and/or IgM) to the lamina lucida of the basement membrane zone[81] may result in the activation of the complement cascade and release those complement split-protein products that are anaphylatoxic (C3a and C5a) and chemotactic for neutrophils (C5a). The release of anaphylatoxins may result directly in tissue mast cell degranulation and subsequent release of vasoactive amines and eosinophil chemotactic factor, and induce the generation of an acute inflammatory cell infiltrate consisting of neutrophils and/or eosinophils. The associated increased capillary permeability (secondary to release of the vasoactive amines) may be a critical factor in the formation of the subepidermal vesicles, or alternatively the release of lysozymes from the accumulated inflammatory cells may lead to a loss of dermal-epidermal adherence and subsequent vesicle formation. Other immunopathogenic mechanisms are possible and until further definitive investigations are performed, the exact pathophysiology of the formation of vesicles and cutaneous lesions will remain speculative.

Diagnosis. The diagnosis of bullous pemphigoid depends on histologic and immunofluorescence tests.

HISTOPATHOLOGY. Routine histopathology of affected skin should demonstrate a cleft between the epidermis and dermis (subepidermal), and close examination of microscopic sections should fail to demonstrate acanthocytes (Figure 119–19). Strict attention must be insured when examining skin areas exhibiting epithelial regeneration, as a false impression of the presence of intraepidermal bullae may be perceived. Examination of bulla contents may reveal proteinaceous material, neutrophils, eosinophils, and monocytes. Within the surrounding connective tissue the dermis may exhibit mild inflammation with the presence of neutrophils and eosinophils, or an intense subepidermal band of inflammatory cells may be present.

DIRECT IMMUNOFLUORESCENCE. Direct immunofluorescence of affected skin should demonstrate a linear or globular deposition of immunoglobulin and/or complement within the basement membrane zone (junction of the epidermis and dermis) of the epidermis. Other disease processes that may show immunoglobulin deposition in the basement membrane zone include systemic lupus erythematosus, cutaneous lupus erythematosus, linear IgA disease, and dermatitis herpetiformis. Because the deposition of immunoglobulins in bullous pemphigoid is confined to the lamina lucida of the basement membrane zone, immunoelectron microscopy and double immunofluorescence microscopy can be used to differentiate bullous pemphigoid from the other disease processes that deposit immunoglobulin in the basement membrane zone;[89] in addition, bullous pemphigoid lacks the antinuclear antibodies commonly observed in systemic lupus erythematosus.

In summary, the requirements for a definitive diagnosis of bullous pemphigoid include (1) the demonstration of a subepidermal bulla with eosinophil and/or neutrophil infiltration, (2) the documentation of immunoglobulin and/or complement deposition in the lamina lucida of the basement membrane zone of the epidermis, and (3) the demonstration of circulating antibasement membrane zone antibodies.

Treatment. Corticosteroids (prednisone or prednisolone) are the preferred initial drugs for the treatment of bullous pemphigoid. These oral glucocorticoids have a rapid onset of action and induce immunosuppression by (1) reducing the numbers of immunocompetent cells at the inflammatory sites, (2) decreasing the function of cytotoxic effector cells, and (3) decreasing the quantity of antibody production.[89] The initial dosage ranges from 0.5 to 1.5 mg/lb (1 to 3 mg/kg) PO q12h. Prednisone and prednisolone will, however, fail to achieve disease remission or may induce undesirable side effects in more than 50 per cent of treated animals.[81] If the disease does not respond to corticosteroids over a ten day course, then consideration should be given to altering the treatment schedule to include the addition of more potent immunosuppressive agents. Azathioprine, cyclophosphamide, and aurothioglucose are potent immunosuppressive drugs that are commonly used in combination with prednisone or prednisolone to increase the efficacy

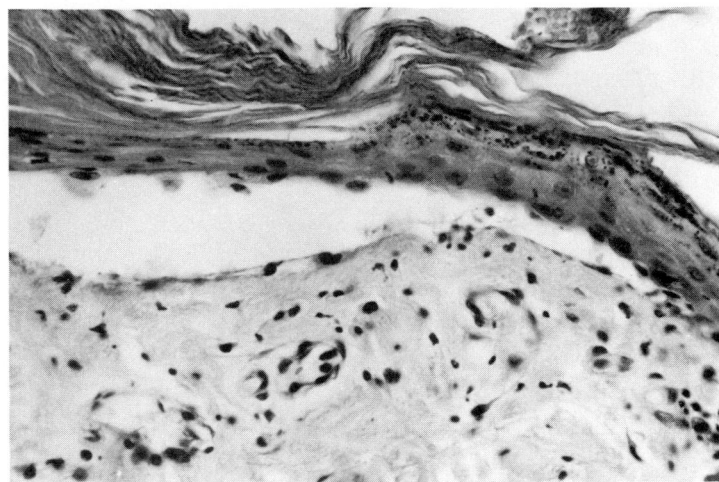

FIGURE 119–19. Bullous pemphigoid. Subepidermal vesicle with viable epithelium, no acantholysis and minimal inflammatory response. (Courtesy of Dr. James D. Conroy.)

of inducing disease remission and to decrease the undesirable side effects sometimes associated with the use of corticosteroids.

Azathioprine is an antimetabolite that functions as a competitive enzyme inhibitor in the synthesis of DNA molecules. When used in combination with prednisone, the prednisone and azathioprine dosages should be 0.5 mg/lb (1 mg/kg) PO q12h and 1 mg/lb (2 mg/kg) PO q24h, respectively, for the initial ten days of combination treatment. At the end of the first ten days the prednisone and azathioprine dosages should be scheduled on alternate days. Azathioprine should not be utilized as the initial sole inducer of immunosuppression, as a three to five week lag period has been reported before its effects are noted.[99, 100] Azathioprine may induce bone marrow suppression, skin eruptions, pyrexia, hepatic dysfunction, and gastrointestinal disturbances.[99, 101] These toxic effects are usually reversible when the drug is discontinued.

Cyclophosphamide is an alkylating agent that cross-links DNA and results in defective cellular replication and synthesis of proteins. Prednisone and cyclophosphamide are commonly used together and the initial recommended dosages are 0.5 mg/lb (1 mg/kg) PO q12h and 1 mg/lb (50 mg/m^2) PO q24h for four consecutive days each week, respectively. Following disease remission the dosages of prednisone and cyclophosphamide should be reduced to 0.5 mg/lb (1 mg/kg) PO given together every other day. Toxic side effects of cyclophosphamide include leukopenia, thrombocytopenia, gastrointestinal disturbances, nephrotoxicity, hepatoxicity, carcinogenicity, hemorrhagic cystitis, and alopecia.[97] Patients should be monitored weekly during the initial treatment schedule and the cyclophosphamide therapy discontinued if granulocytopenia (< 2,000 neutrophils/mm^3) or thrombocytopenia (< 100,000 platelets/mm^3) is observed. Cyclophosphamide-induced hemorrhagic cystitis is an absolute contraindication to continue cyclophosphamide therapy. Chlorambucil is another commonly used alkylating agent that may be substituted for cyclophosphamide. The dosage should be 0.05 mg/lb (0.1 mg/kg) PO q48h. Toxic side effects are fewer than those observed with cyclophosphamide, but include leukopenia and thrombocytopenia.

Aurothioglucose is a water-soluble gold compound suspended in oil. The mechanism of induced immunosuppression is unknown, but decreased immunoglobulin and prostaglandin synthesis, decreased activity of lysosomal enzymes containing sulfhydryl groups, anticomplement activity, inhibition of neutrophil and macrophage chemotaxis, and inhibition of T-cell function have been reported.[89, 99] Aurothioglucose therapy (chrysotherapy) is initiated by administering two IM test doses one week apart. Animals less than 22 lbs (10 kg) receive 1 mg followed by 2 mg injections, while larger patients receive 5 mg followed by 10 mg injections. If toxic signs are not observed (dermatitis, stomatitis, nephrotic syndrome, blood dyscrasia, thrombocytopenia, or allergic reactions), then therapy is continued at 0.5 mg/lb (1 mg/kg) IM weekly. Following the establishment of disease remission the aurothioglucose is gradually tapered to alternate weeks and then once monthly. Initial treatment should include concurrent therapy with prednisone at 0.5 to 1 mg/lb (1 to 2 mg/kg) PO q12 to 48h due to the observed several weeks of delay in the onset of aurothioglucose activity. A hemogram and urinalysis should be performed immediately prior to each injection of aurothioglucose. A documented development of peripheral blood eosinophilia may precede toxic side effects and consideration should be given to discontinuation of the aurothioglucose.[102]

Prognosis. The prognosis for bullous pemphigoid is guarded. Some patients readily respond to corticosteroid therapy and may be maintained in complete remission. Other clinical cases may be uncontrolled despite aggressive therapeutic measures. Critical in the management scheme is early recognition that corticosteroids alone are ineffective so that early induction of a combination immunosuppressive drug schedule can be implemented.

DRUG HYPERSENSITIVITIES

Drug hypersensitivities are defined as any adverse effect of a drug based on an antibody-drug or T lymphocyte–drug interaction. These immunologic reactions (allergic hypersensitivities) within an individual patient generally cannot be anticipated; exceptions to this rule are those patients with a known hypersensitivity to a particular drug. Drug hypersensitivity responses are not dose-related and minute quantities of drug may elicit severe allergic reactions. Although drug hypersensitivities account for six to ten per cent of all human drug reactions, the prevalence of drug hypersensitivities in veterinary medicine is unknown.[103]

Pathophysiology. Many drugs[104–107] have the potential to induce an immune hypersensitivity response (Table 119–5); however, before a drug may become immunogenic, it must form a covalent bond with either a host protein, polysaccharide, or polynucleotide. Following the binding of the drug to a host macromolecule, the drug may be recognized by T lymphocytes and macrophages as being foreign. The drug-macromolecule complex is then presented to the appropriate B lymphocyte, which differentiates into memory B lymphocytes and plasma cells. The plasma cells immediately begin to secrete antibody. Depending on the class of antibody secreted, the presence or absence of effector T lymphocytes, and the nature of the drug-macromolecule complex, one of four hypersensitivity reactions may occur. These allergic immune reactions include (1) immediate hypersensitivity, (2) cytotoxic hypersensitivity, (3) immune complex hypersensitivity, and (4) delayed hypersensitivity.

IMMEDIATE HYPERSENSITIVITY. Immediate hypersensitivity (also known as *Type I hypersensitivity and anaphylaxis*) is caused by the interaction of the drug-macromolecule complex with IgE antibody bound to tissue mast cells or basophils. Initial drug exposure typically induces an IgE antibody response with specificity for the drug-macromolecule complex, but by the time enough IgE antibodies have been produced (seven to ten days, generally), the drug has been eliminated from the body via normal drug metabolism. On the second exposure, however, the drug-macromolecule complex initiates cross-linking of IgE antibodies on the surface of tissue mast cells, leading directly to changes in the mast cell cytoplasmic membrane, which results in degranulation. The release of mast cell granules containing histamine, slow reacting substance of anaphylaxis, and eosinophil chemotactic factor initiates the classic signs associated with immediate hypersensitivity. These signs may include hypotension, bronchospasm, angioedema (Figure 119–20), urticaria, erythema, pruritus, pharyngeal and/or laryngeal edema, cardiac arrhythmias, vomiting, diarrhea, and hyperperistalsis.

TABLE 119–5. DRUGS AND BIOLOGICALS ASSOCIATED WITH IMMUNE HYPERSENSITIVITIES

Drugs and Biologicals	Classification of Immune Hypersensitivity
Foreign antisera, blood products, vaccines, L-asparaginase, penicillin	Immediate hypersensitivity
Penicillamine, α-methyldopa, sulfadiazine, propylthiouracil	Cytotoxic hypersensitivity
Sulfadiazine, propylthiouracil, hydralazine, procainamide, isoniazid	Immune complex hypersensitivity
Heavy metals, aniline dyes, organophosphate insecticides, neomycin	Delayed hypersensitivity

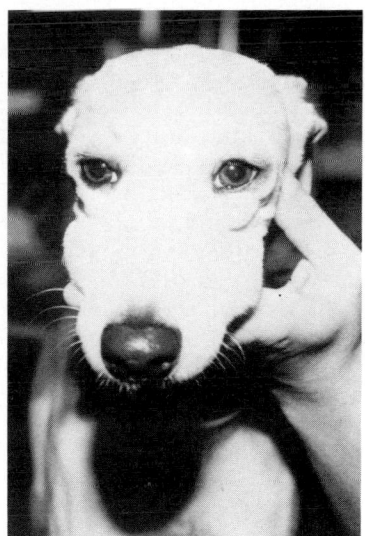

FIGURE 119–20. Canine patient exhibiting angioedema following a platelet-rich plasma transfusion to correct a thrombocytopathia prior to surgery. (Courtesy of Dr. Michael Schaer.)

CYTOTOXIC HYPERSENSITIVITY. Cytotoxic hypersensitivities (also known as *Type II hypersensitivities*) are seen most often with drug/antibody-induced damage of erythrocytes, thrombocytes, and possibly leukocytes. There are basically three mechanisms through which a drug may induce the cytotoxic hypersensitivity reaction resulting in direct damage to the target cell. These three mechanisms are (1) direct drug binding, (2) drug-induced antigenic modification, and (3) the innocent bystander phenomenon.

DIRECT DRUG BINDING. In this immunopathologic mechanism, the drug or a reactive metabolite of the drug binds covalently to the target cell (e.g., erythrocyte, thrombocyte, or granulocyte). The binding of the drug to the target cell stimulates the production of antibody molecules with specificity for the drug/cell complex. The binding of antibody may then result in an immune-mediated hemolytic anemia, thrombocytopenia, or granulocytopenia depending on the original cell type bound by the drug.

DRUG-INDUCED ANTIGENIC MODIFICATION. If the drug induces extensive membrane damage to circulating erythrocytes, thrombocytes, or leukocytes, the damage may render the circulating cells immunogenic. The modification of these existing cell-surface antigens permits the generation of an immune response directed against these neoantigens. The end result is an immune-mediated cytotoxicity.

THE INNOCENT BYSTANDER PHENOMENON. The interaction of drug with a circulating serum protein may elicit the production of a humoral immune response and the generation of circulating drug-protein antibody complexes. These circulating immune complexes may be absorbed nonspecifically onto the surface membranes of circulating erythrocytes, thrombocytes, and leukocytes and result in complement activation with subsequent cell lysis or phagocytosis.

IMMUNE COMPLEX HYPERSENSITIVITY. Immune complex hypersensitivity (also referred to as *Type III hypersensitivity*) is characterized by fever, lymphadenopathy, splenomegaly, erythematous and urticarial rashes, and polyarthritis. The pathogenesis of drug-induced immune complex hypersensitivity appears to be associated with an IgG antibody response directed against circulating drug or a drug metabolite bound to an unidentified serum protein. The IgG antibodies bind to the drug-protein complex and activate the classical complement cascade system. The net effect is decreased serum complement concentration and increased vascular permeability. If the drug-protein antibody complexes are in slight antigen excess, then the immune complexes will be able to diffuse through the vascular endothelium into the blood vessel wall. The subsequent fixation of complement deep within the vessel wall attracts neutrophils into these areas. As the neutrophils begin to phagocytize the immune complexes, lysosomal enzymes are released, which leads to increased vasculitis. Approximately two to four days after the drug has been discontinued the inflammation subsides. Numerous organs can be affected by this immunopathogenic process; however, the kidney is at greatest risk due to the extensive amount of blood flow and the complex renal vascular patterns.

DELAYED HYPERSENSITIVITY. This hypersensitivity disorder (also called *Type IV hypersensitivity*) is the result of a T lymphocyte–mediated immune response to the offending allergen. The classic allergic reaction in this category of hypersensitivity disorders is allergic contact dermatitis; the immunopathology of this disorder was reviewed earlier in the chapter. No specific drug has been described in small animal internal medicine that results in a systemic delayed hypersensitivity disease.

Diagnosis. A clinical diagnosis of drug hypersensitivity is tenable if the following criteria are met:[108] (1) the reaction does not resemble the documented pharmacologic actions of the drug; (2) the reaction can be elicited by small amounts of drug; (3) the observed reaction occurs no sooner than five to seven days following initial drug exposure; (4) observed signs are typical of an allergic type of disease process (anaphylaxis, urticaria, immune complex disease, etc.); (5) the reaction occurs promptly following re-exposure to minute amounts of the drug.

Therapy. Therapy for drug-induced hypersensitivity must be directed at the target organs affected and the suspected underlying immunopathologic process. Drug-induced immune-mediated hemolytic anemia should be treated with corticosteroids, fluid therapy to insure adequate urine output, and a blood transfusion depending on the severity of the hemolytic disease. In general, however, discontinuing the drug and placing the animal on prednisone or prednisolone 0.25 mg/lb (0.5 mg/kg) PO q12h for three to four days should be sufficient. Antihistamines may be of value if there is continued degranulation of mast cells; however, as soon as the medication is withdrawn mast cell degranulation should cease and antihistamine would offer no benefit. The best time to give antihistamines is when an immediate hypersensitivity response is suspected to be eminent.

Prognosis. The prognosis for recovery is excellent. Care must be made to record the suspected offending drug in the patient record so that the medication is avoided if at all possible in the future.

References

1. Gorman, NT and Werner, LL: Diagnosis of immune-mediated diseases and interpretation of immunologic tests. *In* Kirk, RW (ed): Current Veterinary Therapy, 9th ed. Philadelphia, WB Saunders, 1986, p 427.
2. Degen, MA and Breitschwerdt, EB: Canine and feline immunodeficiency. Part I. Comp Cont Ed 8:313, 1986.
3. Degen, MA and Breitschwerdt, EB: Canine and feline immunodeficiency. Part II. Comp Cont Ed 8:379, 1986.
4. Felsburg, PJ: Immunodeficiency. *In* Kirk, RW (ed): Current Veterinary Therapy, 9th ed. Philadelphia, WB Saunders, 1986, p 439.
5. Felsburg, PJ, et al.: A canine model for variable, combined immunodeficiency. Clin Res 30:347, 1982.
6. Moroff, SD, et al.: IgA deficiency in shar-pei dogs. J Vet Immunol Immunopathol 13:181, 1986.
7. Felsburg, PJ, et al.: Selective IgA deficiency in the dog. Clin Immunol Immunopathol 36:297, 1985.
8. Whitbread, TJ, et al.: Relative deficiency of serum IgA in the German shepherd dog: a breed abnormality. Res Vet Sci 37:350, 1984.
9. Slappendel, RJ: The diagnostic significance of the direct antiglobulin test (DAT) in anemic dogs. J Vet Immunol Immunopathol 1:49, 1979.
10. Werner, LL and Gorman, NT: Immune-mediated disorders of cats. Vet Clin North Am 14:1039, 1984.
11. Green, CE, et al.: Cold hemagglutinin disease in a dog. JAVMA 170:505, 1977.
12. Schrader, LA and Hurvitz, AI: Cold agglutinin disease in a cat. JAVMA 183:121, 1983.
13. Switzer, JW and Jain, NC: Autoimmune hemolytic anemia in dogs and cats. Vet Clin North Am 11:405, 1981.
14. Pederson, NC: Immunosuppressive drugs and their role in the treatment of immunologic disease of the dog. Proc 28th Gaines Vet Symposium, Tuskegee Institute, Alabama, 1978, p 13.
15. Werner, LL: Coombs' positive anemia in the dog and cat. Comp Cont Ed 2:96, 1980.
16. Matus, RE, et al.: Plasmapheresis as adjuvant therapy for autoimmune hemolytic anemia in two dogs. JAVMA 186:691, 1985.
17. Feldman, BF, et al.: Splenectomy as adjunctive therapy for immune-mediated thrombocytopenia and hemolytic anemia in the dog. JAVMA 187:617, 1985.
18. Middleton, DJ, et al.: Haemobartonellosis in a dog. Aust Vet J 59:29, 1982.
19. Davenport, DJ, et al.: Platelet disorders in the dog and cat. Part II. Diagnosis and management. Comp Cont Ed 4:788, 1982.
20. Jain, NC and Switzer, JW: Autoimmune thrombocytopenia in dogs and cats. Vet Clin North Am 11:421, 1981.
21. Werner, LL: Immunologic diseases affecting internal organ systems. *In* Ettinger, SJ (ed): Textbook of Veterinary Internal Medicine, 2nd ed. Philadelphia, WB Saunders, 1983, p 2158.
22. Murtaugh, RJ and Jacobs, RM: Suspected immune-mediated megakaryocytic hypoplasia or aplasia in a dog. JAVMA 186:1313, 1985.
23. Jain, NC and Kono, CS: The platelet factor-3 test for the detection of canine antiplatelet antibody. Vet Clin Pathol 9:10, 1980.
24. Joshi, BC and Jain, NC: Detection of antiplatelet antibody in serum and on megakaryocytes of dogs with autoimmune thrombocytopenia. Am J Vet Res 37:681, 1976.
25. Dodds, WJ and Wilkins, RJ: Canine and equine immune-mediated thrombocytopenia and idiopathic thrombocytopenic purpura. Am J Path 86:489, 1977.
26. Wilkins, RJ, et al.: Immunologically mediated thrombocytopenia in the dog. JAVMA 163:277, 1973.
27. Dodds, WJ: Immune-mediated blood diseases in dogs. Mod Vet Pract 64:375, 1983.
28. Dodds, WJ: Immune-mediated blood diseases in dogs. Part II. Management and treatment. Mod Vet Pract 64:453, 1983.
29. Helfand, SC, et al.: Vincristine-loaded platelet therapy for idiopathic thrombocytopenia in a dog. JAVMA 185:224, 1984.
30. Feldman, BF, et al.: Splenectomy as adjunctive therapy for immune-mediated thrombocytopenia and hemolytic anemia in the dog. JAVMA 187:617, 1985.

31. Helfand, SC: Splenectomy: An old issue of current controversy. JAVMA 188:461, 1986.

32. Williams, DA and Maggio-Price, L: Canine idiopathic thrombocytopenia: Clinical observations and long-term follow-up in 54 cases. JAVMA 185:660, 1984.

33. Williams, DA: Gammopathies. Comp Cont Ed 3:815, 1985.

34. Campbell, KL and Latimer, KS: Polysystemic manifestations of plasma cell myeloma in the dog: a case report and review. JAAHA 21:59, 1985.

35. Braund, KG, et al.: Neurologic complications of IgA multiple myeloma associated with cryoglobulinemia in a dog. JAVMA 174:1321, 1979.

36. Braund, KG, et al.: Neurologic manifestations of monoclonal IgM gammopathy associated with lymphocytic leukemia in a dog. JAVMA 172:1407, 1978.

37. Schwartzman, RM: Cutaneous amyloidosis associated with a monoclonal gammopathy in a dog. JAVMA 185:102, 1984.

38. Hurvitz, AI, et al.: Monoclonal cryoglobulinemia with macroglobulinemia in a dog. JAVMA 170:511, 1977.

39. MacEwen, EG and Hurvitz, AI: Diagnosis and management of monoclonal gammopathies. Vet Clin North Am 7:119, 1977.

40. Dewhirst, MW, et al.: Idiopathic monoclonal IgA gammopathy in a dog. JAVMA 170:1313, 1977.

41. Matus, RE and Leifer, CE: Immunoglobulin-producing tumors. Vet Clin North Am 15:741, 1985.

42. Breitschwerdt, EB, et al.: Monoclonal gammopathy associated with naturally occurring canine ehrlichiosis. J Vet Int Med 1:2, 1987.

43. Hoskins, JD, et al.: Serum hyperviscosity syndrome associated with *Ehrlichia canis* infection in a dog. JAVMA 183:1011, 1983.

44. Sheppard, VJ, et al.: Gamma-A myeloma in a dog with defective hemostasis. JAVMA 160:1121, 1972.

45. Couto, CG, et al.: Plasma cell leukemia and monoclonal (IgG) gammopathy in a dog. JAVMA 184:90, 1984.

46. Hawkins, EC, et al.: Immunoglobulin Λ myeloma in a cat with pleural effusion and serum hyperviscosity. JAVMA 188:876, 1986.

47. van Bree, H, et al.: Cervical cord compression as a neurologic complication in an IgG multiple myeloma in a dog. JAAHA 19:317, 1983.

48. MacEwen, EG, et al.: Extramedullary plasmacytoma of the gastrointestinal tract in two dogs. JAVMA 184:1396, 1984.

49. MacEwen, EG, et al.: Nonsecretory multiple myeloma in two dogs. JAVMA 184:1283, 1984.

50. Morton, LD, et al.: Oral extramedullary plasmacytomas in two dogs. Vet Pathol 23:637, 1986.

51. Matus, RE, et al.: Plasmapheresis and chemotherapy of hyperviscosity syndrome associated with monoclonal gammopathy in the dog. JAVMA 183:215, 1983.

52. Matus, RE, et al.: Prognostic factors for multiple myeloma in the dog. JAVMA 188:1288, 1986.

53. Hoenig, M: Multiple myeloma associated with the heavy chains of immunoglobuin A in a dog. JAVMA 190:1191, 1987.

54. Lewis, RM, et al.: Canine lupus erythematosus. Blood 55:143, 1965.

55. Heise, SC, et al.: Lupus erythematosus with hemolytic anemia in a cat. Feline Pract 3:14, 1973.

56. Scott, DW, et al.: A glucocorticoid responsive dermatitis in cats, resembling systemic lupus erythematosus in man. JAAHA 15:157, 1979.

57. Scott, DW, et al.: Canine lupus erythematosus. Systemic lupus erythematosus. JAAHA 19:461, 1983.

58. Grindem, CB and Johnson, KH: Systemic lupus erythematosus: Literature review and report of 42 new cases. JAAHA 19:489, 1983.

59. Scott, DW: Immunologic skin disorders in the dog and cat. Vet Clin North Am 8:641, 1978.

60. Conroy, JD: Immune-mediated diseases of skin and mucous membranes. *In* Ettinger, SJ (ed): Textbook of Veterinary Internal Medicine, 2nd ed. Philadelphia, WB Saunders, 1983, p 2140.

61. Halliwell, REW: Autoimmune disease in the dog. Adv Vet Sci Comp Med 22:221, 1978.

62. Scott, DW, et al.: Canine lupus erythematosus. Discoid lupus erythematosus. JAAHA 19:481, 1983.

63. Halliwell, REW: Skin diseases associated with autoimmunity. Vet Clin North Am 9:57, 1979.

64. Schick, RO and Fadok, VA: Responses of atopic dogs to regional allergens: 268 cases (1981–1984). JAVMA 189:1493, 1986.

65. Nesbitt, GH, et al.: Canine atopy: Part I. Etiology and diagnosis. Comp Cont Ed 6:73, 1984.

66. Conroy, JD: Dermatopathologic signs of internal causation. Symposium on the skin and internal disease. Vet Clin North Am 9:133, 1979.

67. Nesbitt, GH, et al.: Aeroallergens. Comp Cont Ed 6:63, 1984.

68. Nesbitt, GH, et al.: Canine atopy. Part II. Management. Comp Cont Ed 6:264, 1984.

69. Kunkle, GA and Gross, TL: Allergic contact dermatitis to *Tradescantia fluminensis* (Wandering Jew) in a dog—a case report. Comp Cont Ed 5:925, 1983.

70. Walton, GS: Allergic contact dermatitis. *In* Kirk, RW (ed): Current Veterinary Therapy, 6th ed. Philadelphia, WB Saunders, 1977, p 571.

71. Haupt, KH, et al.: Familial canine dermatomyositis: Clinical, electrodiagnostic, and genetic studies. Am J Vet Res 46:1861, 1985.

72. Haupt, KH, et al.: Familial canine dermatomyositis: clinicopathologic, immunologic, and serologic studies. Am J Vet Res 46:1870, 1985.

73. Kunkle, GA, et al.: Dermatomyositis in collie dogs. Comp Cont Ed 7:185, 1985.

74. Hargis, AM, et al.: A skin disorder in three shetland sheepdogs: Comparison with familial canine dermatomyositis of collies. Comp Cont Ed 7:306, 1985.

75. Hargis, AM, et al.: Post-mortem findings in a shetland sheepdog with dermatomyositis. Vet Pathol 23:509, 1986.

76. Gross, TL and Kunkle, GA: The cutaneous histology of dermatomyositis in collie dogs. Vet Pathol 24:11, 1987.

77. Halliwell, REW, et al.: Dapsone for treatment of pruritic dermatitis (dermatitis herpetiformis and subcorneal pustular dermatosis) in dogs. JAVMA 170:697, 1977.

78. Ackerman, L: Dermatitis herpetiformis—Does it exist? JAVMA 185:633, 1984.

79. Baranco, VP: Dapsone—Other indications. Int J Dermatol 21:513, 1982.

80. Ackerman, LJ: Canine and feline pemphigus and pemphigoid. Part I. Pemphigus. Comp Cont Ed 7:89, 1985.

81. Scott, DW, et al.: Observations on the immunopathology and therapy of canine pemphigus and pemphigoid. JAVMA 180:48, 1982.

82. Suter, MM, et al.: Pemphigus in the dog: Comparison of immunofluorescence and immunoperoxidase method to demonstrate intercellular immunoglobulins in the epidermis. Am J Vet Res 45:367, 1984.

83. Ihrke, PJ, et al.: Pemphigus foliaceous in dogs: A review of 37 cases. JAVMA 186:59, 1985.

84. Ihrke, PJ, et al.: Pemphigus foliaceous of the footpads in three dogs. JAVMA 186:67, 1985.

85. Medleau, L, et al.: Complement immunofluorescence in sera of dogs with pemphigus foliaceous. Am J Vet Res 48:486, 1987.

86. Ackerman, LJ: Pemphigus and pemphigoid in domestic animals. Can Vet J 26:185, 1985.

87. Scott, DW, et al.: Pemphigus erythematosus in the dog and cat. JAAHA 16:815, 1980.

88. Scott, DW: The differential diagnosis of facial dermatitis. *In* Kirk, RW (ed): Current Veterinary Therapy, 7th ed. Philadelphia, WB Saunders, 1980, p 436.

89. Halliwell, REW: Skin diseases associated with autoimmunity. The bullous autoimmune skin diseases. Comp Cont Ed 2:911, 1980.

90. Stannard, AA, et al.: A mucocutaneous disease in the dog, resembling pemphigus vulgaris in man. JAVMA 166:575, 1975.

91. Hurvitz, AI and Feldman, E: A disease in dogs resembling human pemphigus vulgaris: Case reports. JAVMA 166:585, 1975.

92. Scott, DW: Pemphigus vegetans in a dog. Cornell Vet 67:374, 1977.

93. Schultz, KT and Goldschmidt, M: Pemphigus vegetans in a dog: A case report. JAAHA 16:579, 1980.

94. Austin, AH: Bullous pemphigoid-like disease in a dog. Proc AAHA 43:138, 1976.

95. Austin, AH and Maiback, HI: Immunofluorescence testing in a bullous skin disease of a dog. JAVMA 168:322, 1976.

96. Mason, KV: Subepidermal bullous drug eruption resembling bullous pemphigoid in a dog. JAVMA 190:881, 1987.

97. Ackerman, LJ: Canine and feline pemphigus and pemphigoid. Part II. Pemphigoid. Comp Cont Ed 7:281, 1985.

98. Medleau, L, et al.: Ulcerative pododermatitis in a cat: immunofluorescent finding and response to chrysotherapy. JAAHA 18:449, 1982.

99. Manning, TO, et al.: Three cases of canine pemphigus foliaceous and observations on chrysotherapy. JAAHA 16:189, 1980.

100. Roenisk, HH and Doedhar, S: Pemphigus treatment with azathioprine. Arch Dermatol 107:353, 1973.

101. Dantzig, PI: Immunosuppressive and cytotoxic drugs in dermatology. Arch Dermatol 110:393, 1974.

102. Fadok, VA and Janney, EH: Thrombocytopenia and hemorrhage associated with gold salt therapy for bullous pemphigoid in a dog. JAVMA 181:261, 1982.

103. Wilcke, JR: Allergic drug reactions. *In* Kirk, RW (ed): Current Veterinary Therapy, 9th ed. Philadelphia, WB Saunders, 1986, p 444.

104. Von Hees, J, et al.: Levamisole-induced drug eruptions in the dog. JAAHA 21:255, 1985.

105. Giger, U, et al.: Sulfadiazine-induced allergy in six Doberman pinschers. JAVMA 186:479, 1985.

106. Davis, LE: Hypersensitivity reactions induced by antimicrobial drugs. JAVMA 185:1131, 1984.

107. Peterson, ME, et al.: Propylthiouracil-associated hemolytic anemia, thrombocytopenia, and antinuclear antibodies in cats with hyperthyroidism. JAVMA 184:806, 1984.

108. Werner, LL and Bright, JM: Drug-induced immune hypersensitivity disorders in two dogs treated with trimethoprim sulfadiazine: Case reports and drug challenge studies. JAAHA 19:783, 1983.

DRUG INDEX

Generic Name	Trade Name	Dosage Dog	Dosage Cat	Route	Frequency	Brief Description
Acetylsalicylic acid	Bayer Aspirin	5 mg/lb	5 mg/lb	PO	Dog: q 12–24 h Cat: q 52–72 h	Analgesia and anti-inflammation
Aurothioglucose	Solganal	1–5 mg first wk, 2–10 mg second wk, then 0.5 mg/lb	1 mg first wk, 2 mg second wk, then 0.5 mg/lb	IM	Once weekly, decreasing to once monthly	Maintenance immunosuppression
Azathioprine	Imuran	1 mg/lb	0.5 mg/lb	PO	q 24–48 h	General immunosuppression and antineoplasia
Chlorambucil	Leukeran	0.05 mg/lb	0.05 mg/lb	PO	q 48 h	General immunosuppression and antineoplasia
Cyclophosphamide	Cytoxan	1 mg/lb	1 mg/lb	PO, IV	Once daily for 3–4 days each wk	General immunosuppression and antineoplasia
Dapsone	Avlosulfon	0.5 mg/lb		PO	q 8 h, decreasing after remission	Decrease neutrophil function
Dexamethazone	Azium	0.05–0.2 mg/lb	0.05–0.2 mg/lb	PO, IV	q 12–48 h	General immunosuppression, anti-inflammation and decrease phagocytosis
Melphalan	Alkeran	0.05 mg/lb	0.05 mg/lb	PO	q 24–48 h	General immunosuppression and antineoplasia
Methylprednisolone acetate	Depo-medrol	0.5 mg/lb	1–2 mg/lb	IM	Once or twice yearly	General immunosuppression, anti-inflammation and decrease phagocytosis
Prednisone/Prednisolone		0.5–1.0 mg/lb	0.5–1.5 mg/lb	PO	q 12 h, decreasing after remission	General immunosuppression, anti-inflammation, and decrease phagocytosis
Vincristine	Oncovin	0.01–0.015 mg/lb	0.015 mg/lb	IV	q 7–14 d	General immunosuppression and antineoplasia
Vitamin E		400 IU		PO	q 12 h	Decrease inflammation

JOINT
AND
SKELETAL
DISORDERS

120 JOINT DISEASES OF DOGS AND CATS

NIELS C. PEDERSEN, ALIDA WIND,
JOE P. MORGAN, and ROY R. POOL

Disorders involving joints are etiologically diverse, as shown by Table 120–1. The outline of joint disease presented in this table will be used as a basis for the following discussion.

NONINFLAMMATORY JOINT DISEASE

Noninflammatory joint disorders are characterized by normal or near normal synovial fluid, and no systemic signs of illness such as depression, malaise, anorexia, fever, leukocytosis, hyperfibrinogenemia, or elevated erythrocyte sedimentation rate. Included in this group of disorders are degenerative joint disease (primary or secondary), traumatic joint disease, luxations and subluxations, meniscal disorders, sesamoid bone disorders, neuropathic arthropathies, developmental arthropathies, arthropathies secondary to inborn errors of metabolism, dietary arthropathies, and neoplasms involving the joints.

Degenerative Joint Disease (Osteoarthritis, Osteoarthrosis)

The term degenerative joint disease has gradually replaced the term osteoarthritis in common usage.[1] The name osteoarthritis implies that the condition is inflammatory in nature, however, degenerative changes occur initially in the cartilage in the absence of inflammation. The term osteoarthrosis, which is widely used in Europe, recognizes the noninflammatory nature of the disorder, yet retains the concept that it is a disease that ultimately involves both cartilage and associated bone.

Degenerative joint disease is the most common noninflammatory arthropathy of man and animals. It is particularly frequent in dogs,[2] but also occurs in many older cats. This disorder is more likely, however, to be clinically manifested in the dog than the cat. It is mainly a disorder of movable joints and is characterized grossly by fragmentation and loss of articular cartilage, and radiographically by narrowing of the joint space, sclerosis of subchondral bone, and osteophyte production at the joint margins.[1]

PRIMARY DEGENERATIVE JOINT DISEASE

The term "primary" implies that this is a specific disease syndrome that develops in the joints for no precise reason. In this sense, idiopathic degenerative joint disease might be a more correct term, because it is assumed that all cases are due to one or more unrecognized factors. Nevertheless, the term is ingrained in usage and in the literature, and it will be used here to describe degenerative joint disease that occurs without readily identifiable cause.

Primary degenerative joint disease becomes increasingly more prevalent with age, usually in dogs and cats aged ten years or older. It is due ultimately to the limited ability of cartilage to regenerate and maintain itself in the face of the cumulative effects of aging, wear and trauma, genetic predisposition, and other unknown factors. Primary degenerative joint disease is not always clinically apparent; discoloration and fibrillation of articular cartilage with lipping are also commonly identified in older dogs and cats even though signs of lameness may not be noticeable. One study of primary degenerative joint disease of the shoulder involved 149 aged colony-reared beagles (mean age 13.8 ± 3.21 years).[3] Radiographs and clinical histories taken periodically through the lifetimes of these dogs revealed no abnormalities during the first few years. Nevertheless, normal shoulder joint development was followed by eventual subchondral sclerosis, remodeling of joint contour, formation of periarticular osteophytes, and formation of enthesophytes (ossification of soft tissue attachments). These changes progressed with age and were typical of degenerative joint disease. Bilateral shoulder joint involvement was common. Evaluation of necropsy specimens revealed roughening and fissuring of the damaged articular cartilage. Total cartilage loss with polishing of the exposed subchondral bone was seen in severe cases. Joint capsule thickening, synovitis, pannus formation, and synovial chondroma formation were evident. In a second study, 20 per cent of randomly selected dogs had degenerative joint disease of the stifle joint at autopsy;

TABLE 120–1. CLASSIFICATION OF JOINT DISORDERS OF THE DOG AND CAT

I. Noninflammatory Joint Disease
  A. Degenerative joint disease
    1. Primary
    2. Secondary
  B. Traumatic joint disease
    1. Damage to articular cartilage
    2. Damage to soft tissue supporting the joint
      a. Sprains
      b. Tendon contractures
  C. Luxations and subluxations
    1. Shoulder joint
    2. Elbow joint
    3. Carpal joint
    4. Tarsal joint
    5. Hip joint
    6. Stifle joint
      a. Total luxation
      b. Rupture of cranial cruciate ligament
      c. Valgoid instability of stifle joint
    7. Temporomandibular instabilities
      a. Temporomandibular dislocations
      b. Temporomandibular luxations
    8. Instabilities of the spinal articulations
      a. Axial-atlantal-occipital malformations
      b. Caudal cervical instabilities
      c. Lumbosacral joint instability
  D. Meniscal disorders
    1. Meniscal tears
    2. Meniscal calcification
    3. Discoid meniscus
  E. Sesamoid bone disorders
  F. Neuropathic arthropathies
  G. Developmental arthropathies
    1. Conformational abnormalities
    2. Chondrodystrophy
    3. Physeal disorders
    4. Epiphysiolysis
    5. Limb shortening
    6. Osteochondrosis
    7. Elbow dysplasia (incongruity)
      a. Ununited anconeal process in nonchondrodystrophic breeds
      b. Fragmented medial coronoid process
      c. Osteochondritis dissecans of medial condyle distal humerus
    8. Ununited anconeal process in chondrodystrophic breeds
    9. Hypoplasia of the coronoid process
    10. Ectopic ossification centers
    11. Hip dysplasia
    12. Shoulder dysplasia
    13. Patellar luxations
    14. Aseptic necrosis
  H. Arthropathies due to inborn errors of metabolism
    1. Hemophilia A
    2. Panosteitis
    3. Mucopolysaccharidosis
    4. Multicentric periarticular calcinosis
  I. Dietary arthropathies
    1. Nutritional secondary hyperparathyroidism
    2. Hypervitaminosis A
  J. Neoplastic arthropathies
    1. Primary
      a. Synovioma
      b. Osteogenic sarcoma
      c. Villonodular synovitis
    2. Metastatic
      a. Lymphosarcoma
II. Inflammatory Joint Disease
  A. Infectious arthritis
    1. Bacterial
    2. Bacterial L-forms
    3. Mycoplasmal arthritis
    4. Rickettsial arthritis
    5. Spirochetal arthritis
    6. Viral arthritis
    7. Fungal arthritis
    8. Protozoal arthritis
  B. Noninfectious arthritis
    1. Immunologic
      a. Deforming or erosive arthritis
        (1) Rheumatoid arthritis of dogs
        (2) Polyarthritis of greyhounds
        (3) Feline chronic progressive polyarthritis (rheumatoid form)
      b. Periosteal proliferative arthritis
        (1) Feline chronic progressive polyarthritis (Reiter's form)
      c. Nondeforming or nonerosive arthritis
        (1) Idiopathic nondeforming arthritis
        (2) Nondeforming arthritis associated with chronic infectious diseases
        (3) Systemic lupus erythematosus
        (4) Nondeforming arthritis associated with neoplasia
        (5) Enteropathic arthritis
        (6) Plasmacytic-lymphocytic synovitis
        (7) Drug-induced arthritides
        (8) Periarteritis nodosa
    2. Crystal-induced arthropathies
      a. Gout
      b. Pseudogout

61 per cent of this group had no identifiable predisposing cause.[4] Two additional studies also concluded that primary degenerative joint disease was a common entity, often involving the shoulder joint of old dogs, both large and small in stature.[4, 5] A similar, but less frequent, disorder has been observed in the elbow joint of dogs.[5] The authors have also seen dogs and cats examined because of stiffness or lameness that appeared insidiously with age, tended to involve large weight-bearing joints, and had radiographic signs characteristic of degenerative joint disease. These animals did not have clinical, anatomic, or radiographic evidence of predisposing problems.

Degenerative joint disease involving multiple joints has also been extensively studied in colony maintained Labrador retrievers and in household pets.[6] The retrievers were genetically selected for hip dysplasia, and 82 per cent of the dogs had radiographic evidence of hip disease by one year of age.[6] An even greater percentage had hip lesions upon necropsy. Surprisingly, there was also a high incidence of degenerative joint disease in joints other than the hips. In a group of 92 dogs between 3 and 11 months of age, 71 per cent had hip joint involvement, 38 per cent shoulder joint involvement, 22 per cent stifle joint involvement, and 40 per cent had disease of multiple joints.[6] A similar pattern of degenerative joint disease involving multiple joints was seen in 100 adult household dogs that were necropsied for various reasons other than degenerative joint disease.[6] This study indicated a strong relationship between hip dysplasia and degenerative joint disease of other joints. Degeneration of dysplastic hips is thought to result from joint instability. Instability has not been previously associated with primary types of degenerative joint disease in other joints, however. The gross, histologic, and biochemical abnormalities seen in dysplastic hips in this study were identical to those seen in other degenerative joints of the same animals.[6] This led the authors to conclude that degeneration in nonhip joints was due to instability, or that both hip dysplasia and degenerative joint disease in other joints were associated with yet undetermined abnormalities.[6]

SECONDARY DEGENERATIVE JOINT DISEASE

Secondary degenerative joint disease is a more common cause of clinical lameness in dogs and cats than the primary form. In man, it has been recognized that degenerative changes can result basically from either abnormal force on normal joints or from normal force on abnormal joints.[7] With this in mind, Mitchell and Cruess classified the causes of degenerative joint disease in man, and this classification can be modified somewhat and applied to dogs and cats (Table 120–2).[7] Although oversimplified, such a classification has the advantage of emphasizing the basic pathophysiology of the disease.

TABLE 120–2. CONDITIONS THAT PREDISPOSE TO DEGENERATIVE JOINT DISEASE

I. Abnormal Concentration or Direction of Force on Normal Articulation
  A. Malalignment (intra-articular cause)
    1. Epiphyseal malformation
      a. Post-traumatic
      b. Congenital
    2. Elbow joint incongruity
    3. Hip dysplasia
    4. Ligamentous
      a. Ruptured cruciate ligament
      b. Ruptured teres ligament
  B. Malalignment (extra-articular cause)
    1. Inequality of leg length (acquired, congenital)
    2. Achondroplasia
    3. Congenital valgus or varus deformities
    4. Fractures with healing in a malaligned position
    5. Premature epiphyseal closures, e.g., radius curvus
    6. Acquired carpal and tarsal subluxations and luxations
  C. Loss of protective sensory reflexes
    1. Neuroarthropathy
    2. Repeated intra-articular injections of steroids or use of analgesic drugs
  D. Miscellaneous
    1. Obesity
    2. Excessive activity (working dogs, e.g., cattle or sheep dogs, hunting dogs, racing dogs, sled dogs)
II. Normal Concentration of Force on Abnormal Articulation
  A. Normal concentration of force on abnormal cartilage
    1. Osteochondrosis
    2. Transchondral fractures
    3. Meniscal tears, discoid menisci, meniscal calcification
    4. Loose bodies in joint
    5. Preexisting arthritis (septic, immunologic, chronic hemarthrosis)
    6. Metabolic abnormalities (chondrocalcinosis, mucopolysaccharidosis, hypervitaminosis A)
  B. Normal concentration of force on normal cartilage supported by weakened subchondral bone
    1. Osteonecrosis (aseptic necrosis, osteomyelitis)
    2. Osteoporosis
    3. Osteomalacia
    4. Osteitis fibrosa (primary or secondary hyperparathyroidism, pseudohyperparathyroidism)
  C. Normal concentration of force on normal cartilage supported by stiffened subchondral bone

The net result of the various disorders listed in Table 120–2 is to hasten the rate of cartilage loss, stimulate marginal bone production, and damage the synovial lining. Because many of these predisposing conditions can themselves be manifested as lameness or gait abnormalities in the early stages before degenerative changes occur, they will be covered in more detail as separate entities.

CLINICAL SIGNS OF DEGENERATIVE JOINT DISEASE

The clinical signs of degenerative joint disease in dogs and cats are similar, regardless of whether the disorder is primary or secondary. In cases that are secondary to some predisposing causes, lameness and/or gait abnormalities may precede signs referable to the degenerative joint disease by months or years. The earliest sign is a reluctance of the animal to perform certain tasks or maneuvers, without more obvious signs of stiffness or lameness. In the next stage, lameness and stiffness may occur following periods of sustained activity or after brief overexertion. After several days of rest, the clinical signs often disappear. As the degeneration becomes more severe, stiffness may be most pronounced following periods of rest, and with movement the animals appear to warm out of their lameness or stiffness. Cold and damp weather often increase the severity of clinical signs. Stiffness and lameness are fairly constant features in the final stages of the disease, although the severity of signs may still be influenced by environmental factors. Dogs may show signs of increased irritability and reclusiveness, and may snap or bite when approached or touched. Unfortunately, this type of behavior may often be directed against children. The owners may not appreciate that the continuous pain caused by the joint disease is responsible for the abnormal behavior.

Marked gross deformities of the joints are uncommon in primary degenerative joint disease. In contrast, animals with predisposing congenital or acquired deformities often develop pronounced gross joint abnormalities. Gross deformities consist of an increase in the dimensions of the joint due to the marginal new bone formation and thickening of the joint capsule and destruction of articular surfaces. Subluxation or luxation may occur in larger joints, especially the hip and stifle. Loss of range of motion leading to periarticular ankylosis of the joint is noted in severely affected joints. Palpable swelling of the joints due to effusions can occur in larger dogs with severe involvement, but is uncommon in smaller dogs and cats. Redness and heat in the area of the joint are not present. Restrictions in the range of motion of the joint can occur, and crepitus can be frequently detected in advanced cases.

RADIOGRAPHIC SIGNS OF DEGENERATIVE JOINT DISEASE

Joints with primary degenerative changes have normal morphologic features with superimposed periarticular osteophyte formation, subchondral sclerosis with superimposed bone remodeling, and changes in the contour of articular surfaces (Figure 120–1). These changes are

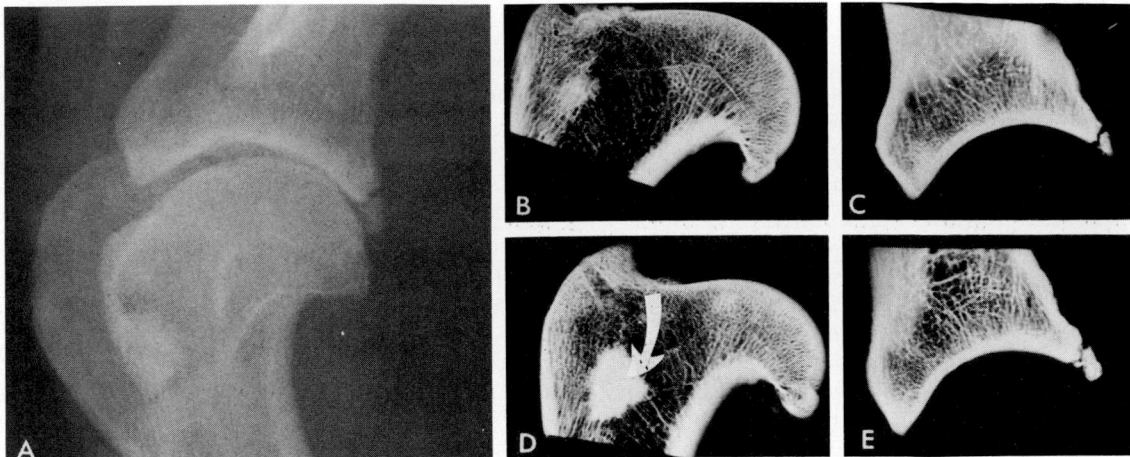

FIGURE 120–1. Lateral radiograph of shoulder obtained after death and radiographs of thin sections of the right humeral head and distal portion of the scapula of an 11-year-old female beagle with primary joint disease. Notice the dense periarticular lipping along the caudal margin of the humeral head and a similar process on the caudal margin of the glenoid cavity. The process on the glenoid cavity has a separate fragment of bone within it. The bony ridge with a prominent mass along the lesser tubercle is an enthesophyte. The denser area of bone within the humeral head (arrow) is not related to the joint disease but to the normal structure of the humerus.

usually bilaterally symmetrical. Because of the advanced age of most patients with primary joint disease, bone growth into sites of soft tissue attachments may be an additional radiographic change. These enthesophytes are often deeply embedded within soft tissue attachments and may be grossly inapparent. They are easily noted on radiographs, however. Their location and appearance are dependent on the sites of capsular, ligamentous and tendinous attachments (Figure 120–1).

Radiographic changes in dogs with secondary degenerative joint disease are usually much more severe than those occurring in dogs with primary degenerative joint disease and often occur at a younger age. Unlike the primary degenerative joint. which is morphologically intact, joints with secondary degenerative joint disease have the superimposed structural, functional, and anatomical abnormalities characteristics of the predisposing condition. For instance, degenerative changes in a hip joint occurring secondary to hip dysplasia (instability) or femoral head necrosis (collapse off the underlying bony matrix) will have distinctive radiographic features from each other and from a hip joint that is undergoing primary degenerative changes.

Regardless of etiology, however, the characteristic radiographic features of degenerative joint disease are rather stereotyped. They include eburnation of the subchondral bone, subchondral bone cysts, periarticular lipping, joint laxity, attrition or wearing away of subchondral bone, remodeling of adjacent bones, and intra- or peri-articular calcification or ossification, including formation of synovial osteochondromas (Figure 120–2).[8] New bone formation at soft tissue attachments (enthesophyte formation) is uncommon unless the patient is older (Figure 120–1).

The manner of presentation of the radiographic changes is dependent on the joint involved. The hip joint is a ball and socket that is easily positioned for radiographic examination, and changes involving the femoral head, acetabulum, and joint space are easily seen. Because of changes in weight-bearing, the femoral

neck undergoes remodeling due to change in stress lines early in the disease process. In contrast, the radial-carpal joint has motion in only one plane and manifests only limited radiographic changes; the width of the joint space is difficult to evaluate, and changes in the subchondral bone may be minimal. Likewise, other joints

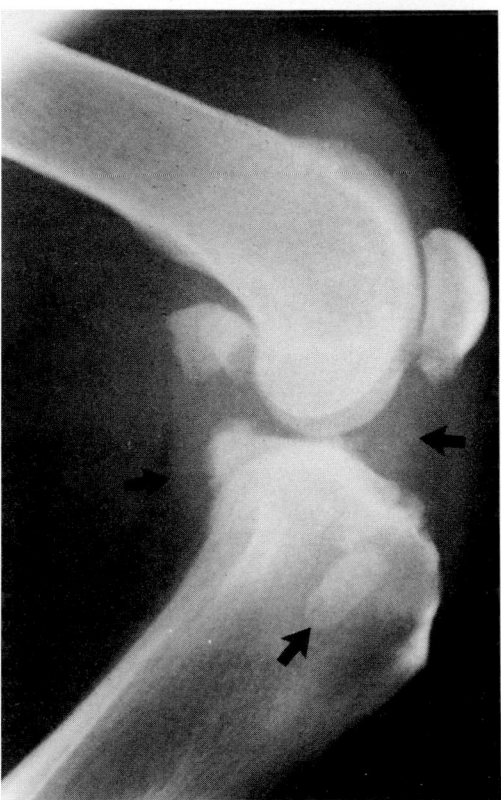

FIGURE 120–2. A lateral radiograph of the stifle joint of an older dog with secondary joint disease. Radiograph signs seen most clearly are thickening of the joint capsule (arrow) with joint effusion in the area of the fat pad just caudal to the patellar ligament (arrow). Periarticular new bone is noted on the distal patella and tibial plateau. Soft tissue calcification is noted lateral to the proximal tibia (arrow). Subchondral sclerosis is present but difficult to evaluate in this single projection.

have specific patterns of presentation of changes associated with degenerative joint disease. Eburnation, or increased density of subchondral bone, is a prominent finding of degenerative joint disease and indicates that articular cartilage is wearing thin. The subchondral bone assumes stress that had previously been absorbed by the cartilage. This change can be visualized irrespective of positioning for the radiographic study, and may be uniform in distribution or limited to one part of the subchondral bone.

Narrowing of the joint space is a second finding of importance. Unless the degree of change is severe, however, narrowing may only be noted in dogs on weight-bearing or simulated weight-bearing studies. The joint space may narrow equally throughout the joint or narrow more prominently on one side of the joint than the other. The degree of narrowing can become so severe that there is actual contact between the two opposing surfaces of subchondral bone, with no interposed cartilage present.

Another characteristic feature of degenerative joint disease is new bone formation. This may be in the form of periarticular lipping (periarticular osteophytes) or new bone formation at soft tissue attachments. There is not always a close relationship between the degree of this new bone formation and articular cartilage damage. Both forms of new bone suggest a response to joint instability. It is sometimes possible, however, to have periarticular osteophyte formation following ligamentous injury and preceding any major changes in joint cartilage or subchondral bone.[9]

Another feature of degenerative joint disease, particularly noted in the stifle joint of dogs, is subluxation or joint instability. The degree of instability or subluxation is much more obvious in weight-bearing than in non–weight-bearing studies. Different degrees of subluxation can be present. Most obvious is craniad displacement of the tibia resulting from injury to the anterior cruciate ligament. Another type is a lateral or medial shifting of the bone with formation of a reactive periarticular bone spur in an effort to provide stabilization to the joint. It has been suggested that instability is the initiating factor in osteophyte formation. In addition to a simple lateral or medial displacement, a degree of rotation is often noted. These findings in the stifle joint may be related to concomitant injury to the ligaments or menisci.

Attrition or wearing away of subchondral bone can be seen on the weight-bearing surface in cases of severe disease. Attrition of bone is a radiographic finding indicative of severe degenerative joint disease. Attrition can become so extensive that it is referred to as remodeling. This results from severe alterations in the lines of stress through the bones and is often associated with an increase in the width of both subchondral and cortical bone on one side. The shadow of the cortical bone on the opposite side is thinner than usual, indicating a decrease in the lines of stress imposed through that part of the bone.

Calcification is a common finding associated with longstanding degenerative joint disease. It may be intraarticular, within the synovial membrane, or in the joint capsule. Most calcified nodules represent foci of cartilaginous metaplasia in the synovium that undergo en-

dochondral ossification to form synovial osteochondromas. Others may begin as fragments of cartilage or bone. Calcified tissues without other radiographic findings of degenerative joint disease usually occur early in the course of joint disease.

Subchondral cysts are frequently noted in degenerative joint disease in horses and other large animals but are infrequently noted in small animals. The cysts vary in size but may reach a centimeter in diameter. The cysts have a very sharp border, and the surrounding subchondral bone is normal in appearance. Frequently the cysts appear to open into the joint space, while in other cases there appears to be a thin layer of subchondral bone between the cyst and the joint space.

In cases of advanced degenerative joint disease, especially involving the hip joint of the dog, radiographic changes are so extensive that the original cause of the joint disease, such as hip dysplasia, aseptic necrosis, or acetabular fracture, is difficult to determine.

PATHOLOGIC FINDINGS

The earliest lesions seen in an affected joint consist of an area of dullness in the articular cartilage accompanied by a color change from the normal flat-white of mature cartilage to a mottled gray-white or yellow hue. Irregular fissure lines (Figure 120–3) or a velvety disruption (Figure 120–4) of the articular surface may be grossly visible. As the articular cartilage deteriorates, the mechanical forces of weight bearing and movement are transferred directly to the underlying subchondral bone and it reacts by becoming thicker and denser (sclerosis) (Figure 120–5).

Changes in the joint capsule of dogs and cats with degenerative joint disease are stereotyped. There is a generalized increase in fibrous connective tissue in the synovium. Condensations of collagen occur immediately beneath the surface layer of the synovium, and there is collagenization of the adventitia of the small caliber vessels that form the superficial plexus in the synovium. Hyalinization of the subsynovial connective tissue with chondroid metaplasia and dystrophic calcification are sometimes present. These changes are not necessarily accompanying features of degenerative joint disease;

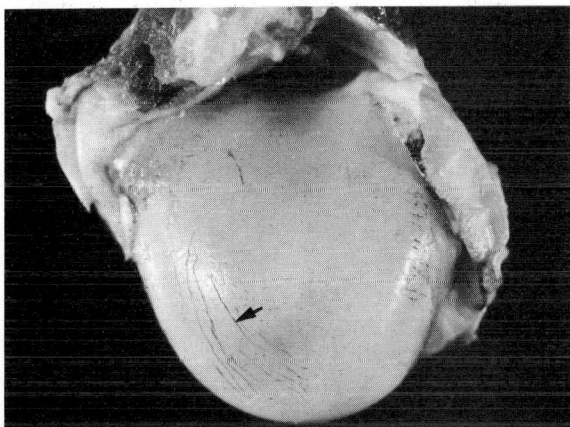

FIGURE 120–3. Proximal humerus of an older dog with primary degenerative joint disease. Fissures (arrow) in the surface were emphasized by rubbing the articular cartilage with carbon.

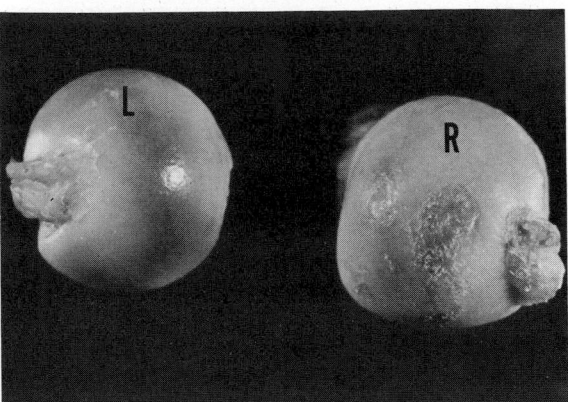

FIGURE 120–4. Femoral heads of a six-month-old dog two months following fracture of the right acetabulum. The left femoral head (L) is normal. The right femoral head (R) shows effects of secondary degenerative joint disease. Note the alteration in shape and size. Several areas of the articular surface are discolored and have a velvety appearance.

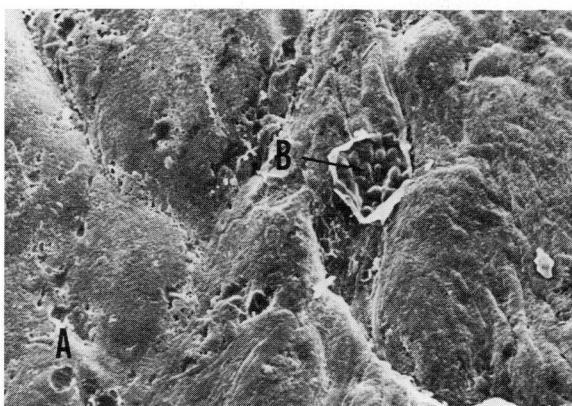

FIGURE 120–6. Scanning electron micrograph of early changes in a degenerating articular surface. The entire surface shows roughening and irregularity. Microscopic ulcerations (A) may be of sufficient depth to expose chondrocytes (B) of the tangential zone to the joint surface.

identical changes can also be seen in the joint capsule of aging animals without changes in the joint surfaces. Villous hypertrophy occurs more commonly in larger dogs and mainly in more severely affected proximal joints. Inflammation in the synovium is absent or mild. Mild chronic inflammatory changes can be centered around cartilaginous debris in the synovial recesses. Hemorrhage into the deeper tissue, probably resulting from joint instability and microtrauma, can lead to hemosiderosis and a sparse lymphocyte-plasmacyte infiltrate. Joint instability and microtrauma can also lead to sustained edema in the fibrous layer of the joint capsule and increased fibroplasia. This results in a permanent thickening of the joint capsule and contributes to a reduction in range of motion of the joint.

The earliest microscopic change seen in the degenerating articular cartilage is a roughening of the surface fiber layer, followed by the exposure and loss of underlying chondrocytes (Figure 120–6). Chondrocytes in these areas appear to have undergone degeneration and death, and there is a generalized loss of normal staining

properties of proteoglycan in the surrounding cartilage matrix.

As the degenerative process becomes more severe, the most superficial layer of cartilage is worn away, exposing the deeper layer of chondrocytes in the transitional zone. In an attempt at repair, chondrocytes in the area proliferate but are unable to separate and differentiate in the firm chondroid matrix of mature cartilage (Figure 120–7). These clones of newly formed chondrocytes produce a soft, imperfect matrix that wears more quickly than normal matrix. Fissures develop in the damaged cartilage, and may extend through to the subchondral bone (Figure 120–8). Chondrocytes immediately adjacent to the fissure lines make an abortive attempt at repair (Figure 120–9). When fissures reach the subchondral bone, a separation of the osteochondral junction occurs along with varying amounts of hemorrhage and necrosis. The resulting osteochondral defect heals with granulation tissue and fibrocartilage, and is visible radiographically as subchondral irregularities or cysts. On occasion, subchondral bone cysts filled with myxoid tissue may be found beneath degenerative articular surfaces. Such cystic changes are uncommon in dogs and cats and are most apt to be seen in larger joints in giant breeds of dogs. With continued cartilage loss, the

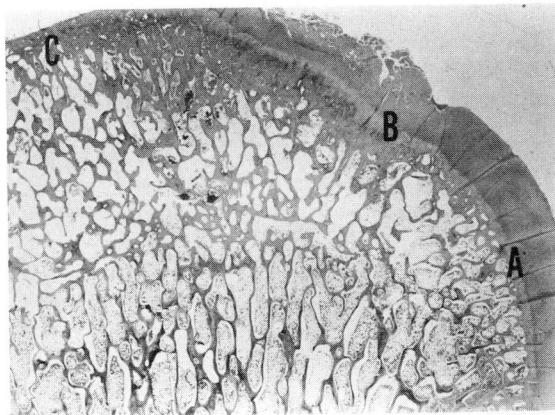

FIGURE 120–5. Microscopic changes in degenerative joint disease. Observe the loss of normal structure of the joint, beginning at the junction (A) of the normal cartilage and subchondral bone with the area (B) of cartilage degeneration and subchondral bone sclerosis, which becomes progressively more severe until the surface is eburnated (C).

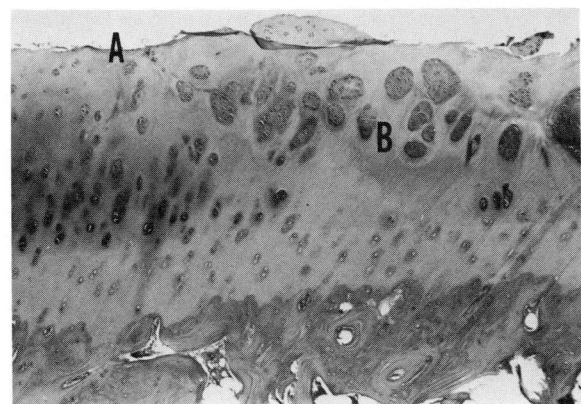

FIGURE 120–7. Loss of the superficial layer (A) and proliferation of nests of chondrocytes in the transitional and radial zones (B) in an ineffectual attempt at repair.

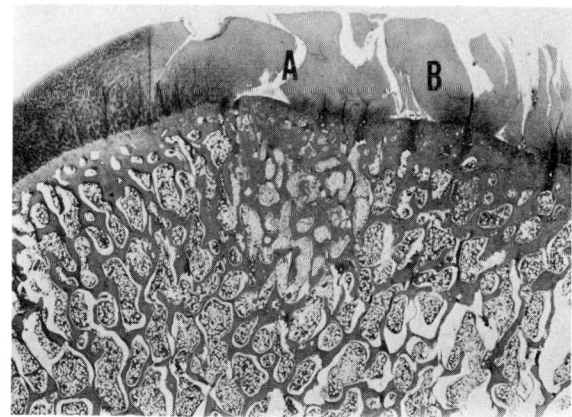

FIGURE 120–8. Fissures (A) extend completely through the layer of degenerative cartilage (B) and reach the subchondral bone.

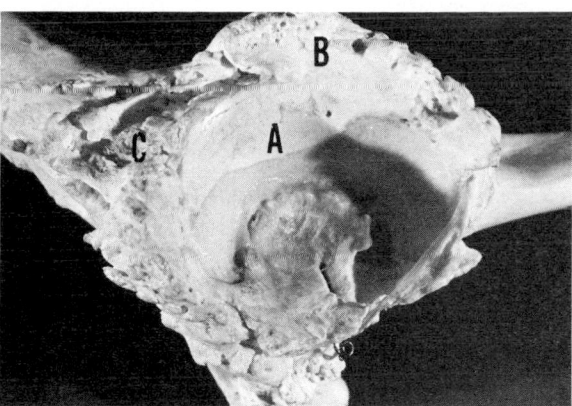

FIGURE 120–10. Severe secondary degenerative joint disease following chronic luxation of the hip. (A) Eburnated (polished) rim of the acetabulum. Osteophytic bone production is seen at the joint margin (B) and along the joint capsule insertion (C).

sclerotic subchondral bone becomes progressively exposed and is polished by the opposing articular surface, a process called eburnation.

Changes in the articular cartilage and subchondral bone lead to loss of normal contour of the articular surfaces, and this predisposes the joint to further abnormal movement. In an attempt to respond to these new stresses and to contain the abnormal motion, the borders of the articular surfaces undergo remodeling and extend the articular surface area (Figure 120–10). Typically, this is accompanied by bone proliferation manifested as osteophytes on the periarticular bone surfaces adjacent to or within the insertion line of the joint capsule (Figure 120–11).

The quantity of synovial fluid found in degenerating joints ranges from normal to copious. Copious effusions are seen mainly in larger joints, particularly the elbow and stifle. Such outpourings of synovial fluid can be more or less persistent, or they can become apparent after a period of overexertion or vigorous exercise. In cases in which the synovial fluid is increased in quantity, it is often thin or watery owing to dilution with edema fluid. The mucin quality remains normal, however, since there is no depolymerization of the hyaluronic acid. Debris from degenerative cartilage matrix and microhemorrhage in soft tissue initiates a sterile synovitis that leads to increased numbers of macrophages in the fluid, although total cell counts rarely exceed 4000 cells/μl. Polymorphonuclear neutrophils are not generally seen in numbers exceeding five per cent. Synovial fluid from degenerative joints is often yellow-tinged, mainly be-

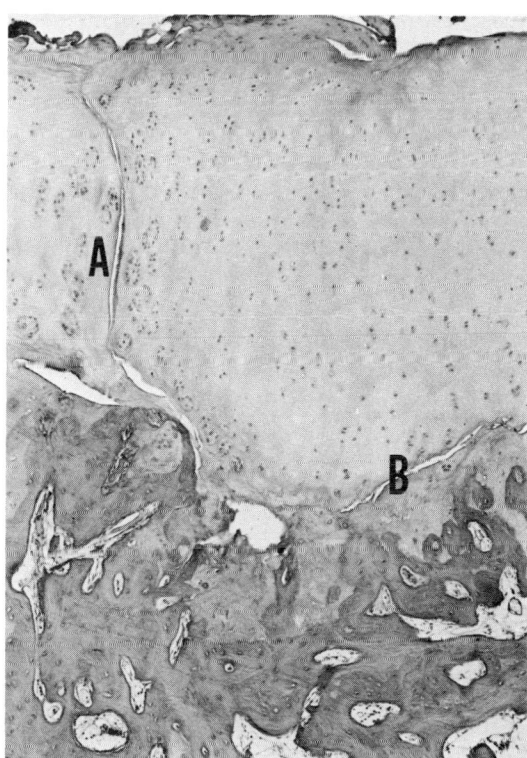

FIGURE 120–9. Chondrocytes adjacent to fissure lines proliferate (A) in an abortive attempt at repair. Note the continuation of the fissure line with the line of osteochondral separation (B).

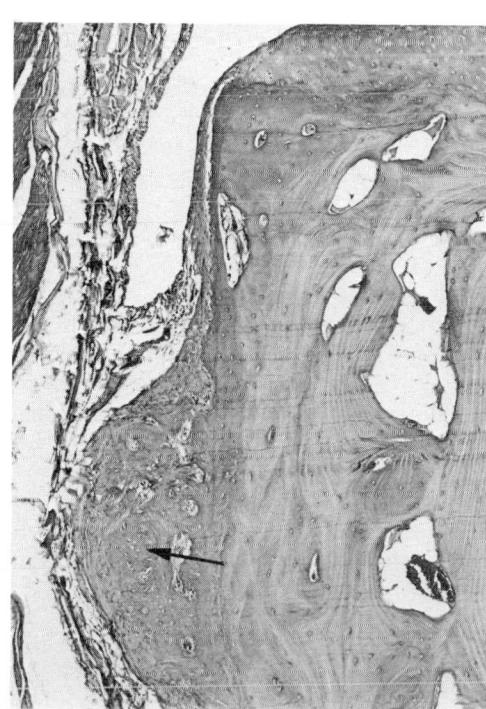

FIGURE 120–11. Formation of a periarticular osteophyte (arrow).

cause of hemosiderin pigments originating from microhemorrhage in the deeper layers of the synovium.

TREATMENT

The treatment of degenerative joint disease involves the following steps: (1) adequate daily periods of rest, (2) avoidance of overexertion of affected joints, (3) reduction of weight if the animal is obese, (4) properly administered exercise, (5) relief of pain by analgesic and anti-inflammatory drugs, and (6) orthopedic operative procedures to relieve pain, regain motion, or correct stressful deformities or instabilities.

Adequate rest of animals with degenerative joint disease is important for several reasons; excessive use of damaged joints can aggravate clinical signs, and more importantly, it can accelerate the joint destruction. Dogs with severe joint disease cannot be expected to function in the same manner as they did before developing the problem. Unfortunately, the amount of rest or exercise that an animal can tolerate is difficult to assess. Many dogs are so eager to please their masters that they will overexert themselves. In addition, some dogs will forego any considerations of pain because of sheer enjoyment of the activity, e.g., hunting, jogging, playing, or hiking with the owner or working with livestock. As a rule, any activity that causes the animal to become acutely lame for a period afterward is probably excessive and should be curtailed or cut back.

Although dogs with advanced degenerative joint disease should receive adequate rest and avoid strenuous exercise, they should not be allowed to become complete invalids. Properly administered and controlled exercise is important in maintaining muscle tone and keeping joints limber. Controlled exercise can consist of defined periods of walking with the owner, interspaced with short periods of rest or other controlled periods of play, swimming, or similar activities. As the disease becomes more advanced and less activity is tolerated, the amount of exercise should be reduced.

Analgesic and anti-inflammatory drugs are often necessary to control pain in severely affected dogs. Since cats do not often manifest the disease to the same extent as dogs, drug therapy is usually not needed. Buffered types of aspirin, at the dose of 12 to 25 mg/lb (25 to 50 mg/kg) body weight divided into two or three daily doses for dogs, and 12 mg/lb (25 mg/kg) once a day for cats, are usually well tolerated[10] and can afford some relief. Gastric ulceration, sometimes severe, is an uncommon side effect in dogs. Aspirin should be discontinued immediately in such animals and not used again.

A large number of other nonsteroidal, analgesic, and anti-inflammatory drugs have been developed for the treatment of degenerative joint disease in humans. Controlled studies in humans have shown them to be somewhat more efficacious than aspirin, but the degree of superiority does not always justify the added cost or side effects. Although they are often advertised as having no aspirin side effects, they are not without their own toxicity. Although they are usually mildly gastrotoxic to humans, they are usually much more gastrotoxic than aspirin for dogs.[11] The use of nonsteroidal analgesics such as naproxen and ibuprofen has been associated

with severe gastric ulceration in dogs.[12, 13] Indomethacin is also considerably more gastrotoxic to dogs than humans. A caution has been reported regarding the use of the anti-inflammatory agent diclofenac in dogs.[14] Because of the experience with nonaspirin analgesics in dogs, it is prudent for veterinarians not to use them until toxicity studies are completed. The toxicity of nonsteroidal analgesics other than aspirin for cats has not been determined.

Phenylbutazone is widely used by veterinarians to treat dogs with degenerative joint disease, based on the mistaken belief that it is much more effective than aspirin and does not have any side effects. For chronic use in dogs, the dosage is 20 mg/lb (40 mg/kg) divided three times a day for the first 48 hours, then decreased to the lowest effective amount.[10] The total daily dosage should not exceed 800 mg, regardless of the size of the animal. Bone marrow suppression can be a side effect of prolonged high level usage of the drug.

Prednisolone or prednisone is given at an initial dosage of 1 mg/lb (2 mg/kg) once daily for several days to either dogs or cats, followed by a chronic maintenance dose that should not exceed 0.5 mg/lb (1 mg/kg) every other day. There is evidence that corticosteroids may actually hasten the degenerative process, so what is gained in the short term may be lost, and more, in the long term. For this reason they should be restricted to advanced cases that are totally unresponsive to more conservative therapy, especially if the patient is in the terminal phase of life. Intra-articular injections of steroids should be avoided. When instigating chronic drug therapy, owners should be made aware of the fact that the control of signs is only partial and can never be complete.

Surgery should be used very selectively. Fusion of joints such as the elbow, carpus, or hock is occasionally warranted to help relieve pain and restore some use to the limb. Femoral head ostectomy or the insertion of a prosthetic joint can be effective in selected animals with painful and badly diseased hip joints. Some types of joint instability resulting from ligament damage or rupture can be corrected surgically. Obviously this must be done before secondary degenerative changes become too extensive. In situations wherein pieces of cartilage or osteophytic bone have become free within the joint cavity, surgical intervention is necessary for their removal. Reactive new bone should not be excised, except where it breaks into the joint cavity or impinges on tendons or nerves. Surgery should be avoided in situations other than the ones mentioned, because surgery without clear objectives and without an understanding of the pathophysiology of the disease can actually add to the joint insult and accelerate degenerative changes.

Traumatic Joint Disease

Joint trauma in dogs and cats is usually accidental, resulting from contact with larger animals or man and his machines. In certain instances, however, distinct types of trauma can be associated with various activities, e.g., skull, limb, and scapular fractures in working cattle dogs and various fractures and sprains of the limbs of racing greyhounds.[15, 16] Joint trauma can result from fractures of surrounding bones, damage to cartilage, or damage to soft tissue structures supporting the joints. Of these injuries, bone fractures are the easiest to diagnose, while damage to cartilage and soft tissue is more difficult to localize.

DAMAGE TO ARTICULAR CARTILAGE

Damage to the articular cartilage can occur as a result of acute or chronic trauma to the joint. In small animals such as the dog and cat, the trauma is usually acutely sustained. The most frequent causes include being hit by automobiles, gunshot wounds,[17, 18] fights with larger animals, or abuse from humans. In such instances cartilage damage frequently accompanies bone fractures or luxations. Because the cartilage damage cannot be assessed on radiographs, it may go undetected or be minimized in importance. Even with good bony reconstruction, degenerative joint disease or more appropriately termed, post-traumatic joint disease, frequently occurs months or years later (Figure 120–12).

The term canine spavin has been used to describe an exercise-related hock lesion of racing greyhounds.[19, 20] The disorder is basically a severe degenerative joint disease unassociated with grossly apparent fractures. The term spavin was applied to this condition because of its anatomic, radiographic, and pathologic similarity to the disorder of horses and cattle.

DAMAGE TO SOFT TISSUE SUPPORTING THE JOINT

Injuries of this sort, usually of traumatic origin, have been termed sprains. Sprains result from microtrauma to vascular (hemorrhage, edema), ligamentous (separations, tears), bursal, and synovial structures. They are relatively common in dogs, and it is often quite a diagnostic challenge to differentiate them from more serious entities. Careful physical and radiographic analysis to rule out other entities, coupled with time and rest, usually suffice to differentiate sprains from more serious problems.

Tendon contractures are a sequelae of direct damage to associated muscles, or to the blood supply or enervation of those muscles. This results in atrophy and fibrous replacement of the involved muscles and contracture of the associated tendon or tendons. Tendon contractures can result in gross stiffening of the involved limbs and immobilization of joints in severe cases. In milder forms, gait abnormalities and/or lameness may be the main presenting signs. Semitendinosus and infraspinatus tendon contractures are the most common disorders of the latter type. They tend to occur most often in German shepherds and Doberman pinschers, and in dogs used for work more than in nonworking animals. Semitendinosus tendon contracture resembles stringhalt of horses in etiology and clinical manifestations. Most tendon contractures are probably traumatic in origin, although the initial trauma often goes unnoticed. A characteristic halting gait anomaly of the involved hindlimb is the most noticeable feature of the disorder. Sectioning of the contracted tendon is often unsuccessful in correcting the abnormality in the case of semitendinosus tendon contractures and helpful in the case of intraspinatus tendon contractures.

Contracture of the tendons closing the lower jaw may be a sequela of the temporal and mandibular myopathies (eosinophilic, plasmacytic-lymphocytic, and idiopathic) of canines. Affected dogs have a progressive closing of the jaw to the point where they cannot open their mouths to eat. The prognosis for recovery of adequate lower jaw function is good with the use of long-term corticosteroid therapy.

LUXATIONS AND SUBLUXATIONS

Luxations and subluxations can involve virtually any joint of the appendicular and axial skeleton. They can be caused by acute trauma, or by developmental or acquired problems that affect the stability of the joint. It is important also to consider whether the luxation or subluxation was primary or secondary to preexisting joint disease.

The diagnosis of complete luxation is clinically and radiographically quite easy. Subluxations are most difficult to diagnose and require a knowledge of normal radiographic anatomy. For instance, the most obvious radiographic change in a dislocation is the failure of two or more opposing articular surfaces to interface normally. It must be remembered, however, that certain normal joints show considerable laxity without pathologic changes. In addition to a determination of whether or not a luxation has occurred, it is important to note the presence of small fragments originating from the articular surface or periarticular margin. Small avulsion or chip fractures frequently accompany luxations or subluxations of certain joints such as the hip or elbow of the dog and make reduction difficult.

The duration of a dislocation can only be estimated radiographically. Obvious osteoporosis, muscle atrophy, or bony remodeling leading to formation of pseudoar-

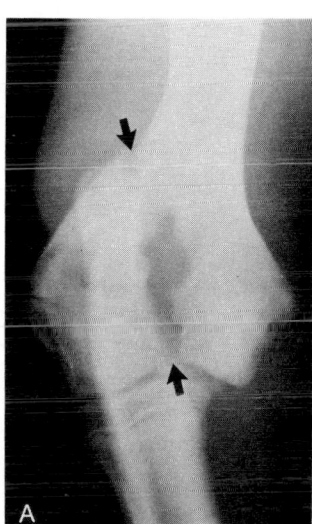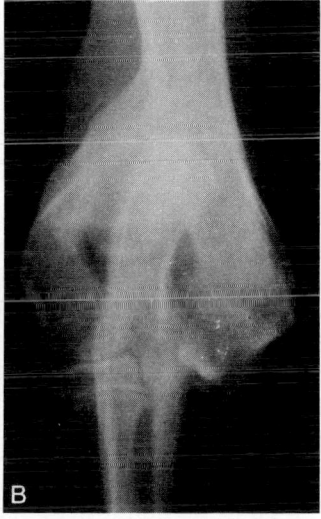

FIGURE 120–12. Craniocaudal radiographs of the elbow joint of a young dog at the time of intra-articular fracture of the distal humerus (A) (arrows) and later following bony healing (B). Malalignment of the bony fragments is easily seen radiographically along with the new bone formation. The damage to the articular cartilage must be evaluated indirectly.

throsis suggests a duration in excess of several weeks. A unique change occurs in luxation of the hip, following which the depth of the acetabulum often decreases as it is filled first with soft tissue and later with bone. Any evidence of secondary joint disease, such as periosteal lipping or remodeling, also suggests chronicity. The problem is often in deciding which came first, the luxation or the secondary joint disease. Luxation or subluxation due to a congenital anomaly is an important consideration in evaluation of what might otherwise appear to be a simple traumatic event. In these cases the subchondral bone is less dense and the contour of the articular portions of the bone is abnormal. Comparison studies of the opposite leg may be of value in such cases.

Subluxations are more difficult to diagnose than luxations and generally require that the radiographs be taken in weight-bearing, in simulated weight-bearing, or in flexed and extended positions. Joints that require such positions include the carpus, tarsus, stifle joint, and hip joint of animals with hip dysplasia.

Special views can be used to evaluate joint stability in certain joints. Partial luxation of the patella in the dog is best evaluated by a special skyline view that determines both the degree of patellar luxation and the depth of the trochlear groove.

Shoulder Joint. Luxations or subluxations of the shoulder joint are uncommon in both dogs and cats. In miniature breeds, medial luxations can be associated with medial joint capsule laxity and under-development of the medial labrum of the glenoid. In most instances, however, trauma is the predominant cause. Lateral luxations are associated with tearing of the infraspinatus tendon, lateral joint capsule and lateral glenohumeral ligament. They tend to occur in small and miniature breeds. Treatment can be conservative or surgical. In acute lateral luxation, conservative treatment consists of reduction and placement of the limb in a non–weight-bearing sling or spica splint for two to three weeks. In acute medial luxation, conservative treatment consists of reduction and placement of the limb in a Velpeau-type bandage for two to three weeks. This type of bandage forces the humeral head laterally. The most common surgical treatment for medial and lateral luxations involves the transplantation of the biceps tendon either laterally or medially.[21, 22]

Elbow Joint. The close fit of the bones forming the elbow joint, especially between the ulnar trochlear notch and the humeral trochlea, makes this an inherently stable joint. Its supporting structures are the radial collateral, ulnar collateral, oblique and olecranon ligaments.

Luxations or subluxations of the elbow joint can be associated with trauma[23] (Figure 120–13). In some cases, however, they can occur in otherwise normal dogs following fairly routine activity.[24] The luxating forces usually involve flexion of the elbow joint and rotation of the lower limb with disengagement of the anconeal process of the ulna from the olecranon fossa. Because of the greater caudal extension of the medial epicondylar crest of the humerus, the radius and ulna are usually luxated laterally rather than medially, except when associated with fractures.

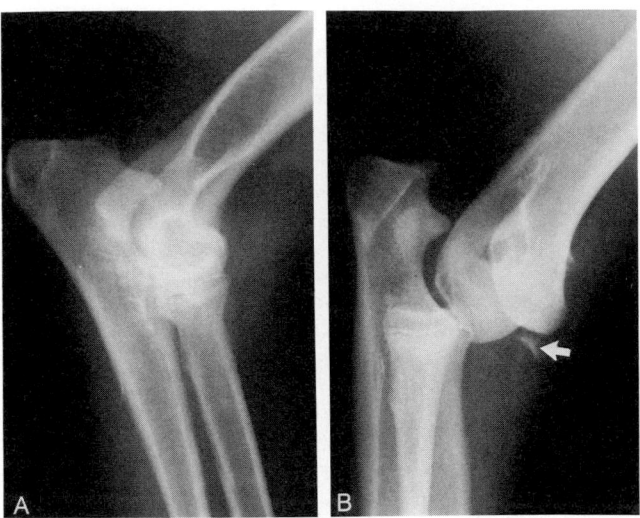

FIGURE 120–13. Lateral *(A)* and oblique *(B)* radiographs of the elbow of an immature dog show a luxation of the elbow joint. The lateral projection shows the bones almost perfectly positioned, and the lesion might be missed. The oblique projection clearly shows the completeness of the luxation and also permits evaluation of a chip or avulsion fragment (arrow) that probably originates from the lateral ulna at the attachment of the lateral collateral ligament.

Recent elbow luxations can be reduced without surgical invasion of the joint, but general anesthesia and good muscle relaxation are required. Following reduction, the leg is splinted with the elbow in moderate extension for two to three weeks. If closed reduction cannot be achieved, or the joint is extremely unstable following reduction, an open reduction is necessary with suturing or replacement of one or both collateral ligaments. Total elbow joint replacement with a silicone elastomer prosthesis has been reported in a cocker spaniel.[25]

Subluxations at the elbow joint may be associated with growth plate injuries of the radius and/or ulna in the young cat or dog. Distal or downward displacement of the proximal ulna is common in premature closure of the distal ulnar physis (resulting in radius curvus) and may cause a fracture of the anconeal process. Proximal or upward displacement of the proximal ulna is common in premature closure of the distal radial physis (less often the proximal radial physis) and may be associated with a fracture of the medial coronoid process of the ulna.

Downward displacement of the proximal ulna is also seen in the chondrodystrophic breeds and is due to a lagging ulnar growth rate. In the larger of these breeds (basset hound, English bulldog), fracture of the anconeal process may occur and cause lameness.

Another form of subluxation is associated with the three main developmental diseases of the elbow joint, ununited anconeal process, fragmented medial coronoid process and osteochondritis dissecans of the medial aspect of the humeral condyle. These are probably caused by an abnormal development of the ulnar trochlear notch. (See developmental diseases of the elbow.)

Congenital luxation of the elbow joint has been seen in puppies (Figure 120–14). In one case the luxation was corrected by closed reduction and the joint temporarily transfixed with a small Steinmann pin.[26]

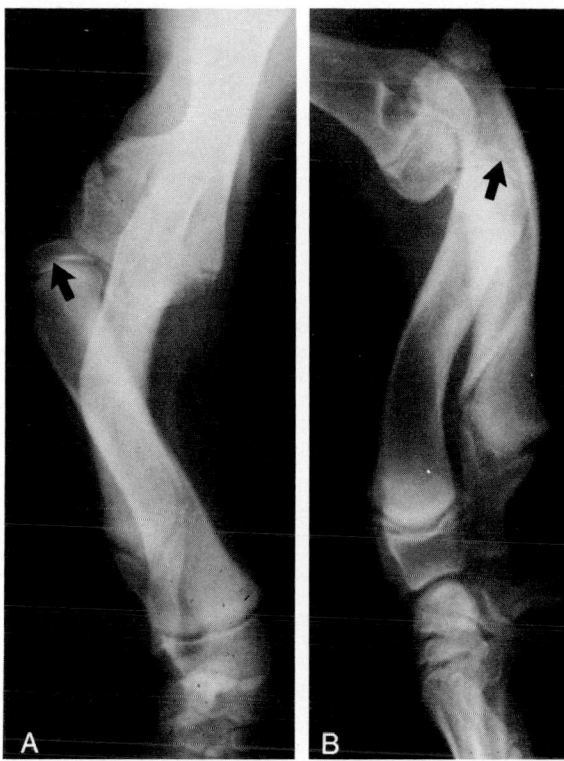

FIGURE 120–14. Craniocaudal and lateral radiographs of the foreleg of a three-month-old puppy with a congenital luxation of the elbow. The radial head is luxated laterally and caudally (arrows). Note the bowing of the ulna secondary to the luxation. The lucent line within the ulnar diaphysis results from a physeal dysplasia due to abnormal biomechanical forces on the dorsomedial edge of the physeal plate.

Carpal Joint. Severe carpal sprains usually lead to ligament damage. The most common carpal sprain is associated with forced hyperextension due to falls from heights or having the foot caught while running. Forced hyperextension causes rupture of the palmar ligaments and joint capsule (fibrocartilage), leading in turn to a clinical plantigrade subluxation or luxation once the animal begins bearing weight. When acute, the presenting complaint is a sudden non–weight-bearing lameness of one or both of the front legs. Some swelling may be present in the palmar region. The animal will usually not allow hyperextension of the joint due to the pain. It will mask the sprain by splinting the digital flexor tendons. Proper physical and radiographic examinations can only be done under anesthesia.

Stress radiographs of the carpus, i.e., lateral radiographs with the carpus in forced hyperextension, are necessary to pinpoint the area of ligament and joint capsule rupture. The ligaments and joint capsule of the middle carpal or carpometacarpal joints are more frequently involved than those of the antebrachiocarpal joint.

Complete acute carpal luxation occurs infrequently. In animals under 30 pounds, early reduction and casting in slight flexion can result in a pain-free fibrous ankylosis. Conservative therapy in the form of casting in slight flexion is rarely successful in animals over 40 pounds. Instead, a pancarpal or partial carpal arthrodesis is advised.[27–29]

Medial or lateral carpal instability may be caused by rupture of the radial or ulnar collateral ligament. Casting with the paw in the direction of the injury and the carpus in slight flexion usually suffices for animals presented with a single acute injury.

A carpal weakness is sometimes noted in puppies shortly after they are weaned and have gone to their new owners. This condition has also been reported in a group of two-month-old colony-reared puppies.[30] Carpal laxities have also been reported in Doberman pinschers, Great Danes, golden retrievers, German shepherds, black and tan hounds, and Chinese sharpeis.[31] Carpal weakness in puppies may express itself in hyperextension (knuckling over) and trembling of the front limbs. They may also walk on the medial or lateral aspect of their paw. The cause of carpal hyperextension in puppies is often related to rearing on hard surfaces in small enclosures that allow only limited exercise.[31] Moderately increasing exercise and food intake will allow gradual strengthening of the supporting structures of the carpus without altering the shape of the developing carpal bones. Splinting or casting of the carpus is contraindicated, since it removes the necessary strengthening stresses on the tendons and ligaments. Recovery may vary from a couple of days to several months.

A gradual weakening of the supporting structures of the carpus in old and obese dogs may result in hyperextension and varus deviation of the paw. Poor carpal configuration and chronic orthopedic problems of the hind limbs may be contributing factors. Breeds apparently predisposed to this condition are the Doberman, collie, Shetland sheepdog, Samoyed, and Labrador retriever.

Tarsal Joint. An extensive review of tarsal subluxations has been compiled by Campbell and co-workers, and others.[32–38]

INTERTARSAL. In the report by Campbell and co-workers,[32] only 11 of 44 intertarsal subluxations occurred because of trauma. In most cases the problem was apparently associated with degeneration of the plantar ligaments, borne out by the finding that it occurred most often in dogs over six years of age, in obese individuals, and in Shetland sheepdogs, collies, and Samoyeds. The condition was unilateral in all but five dogs; bilateral involvement was most likely to occur in Shetland sheepdogs.

Clinical signs of intertarsal joint subluxations include a moderate to severe semi–weight bearing lameness, abnormal dorsiflexion of the affected tarsal joint, and, in chronically affected dogs, a thickening of the joint capsule. Pain cannot be elicited in most dogs by manipulation of the joint. Radiographic findings are minimal early in the disorder, but if the condition is left uncorrected, there is a progressive development of degenerative joint disease (Figure 120–15).

TARSOMETATARSAL. Tarsometatarsal subluxations are less common than intertarsal subluxations.[32, 35] Unlike intertarsal subluxations, most tarsometatarsal subluxations are traumatic in origin. Separation of the tarsometatarsal joint capsule and overlying plantar attachments is usually associated with the subluxation. The clinical appearance, except for the frequent signs of accompanying trauma, resembles that of intertarsal joint subluxations.

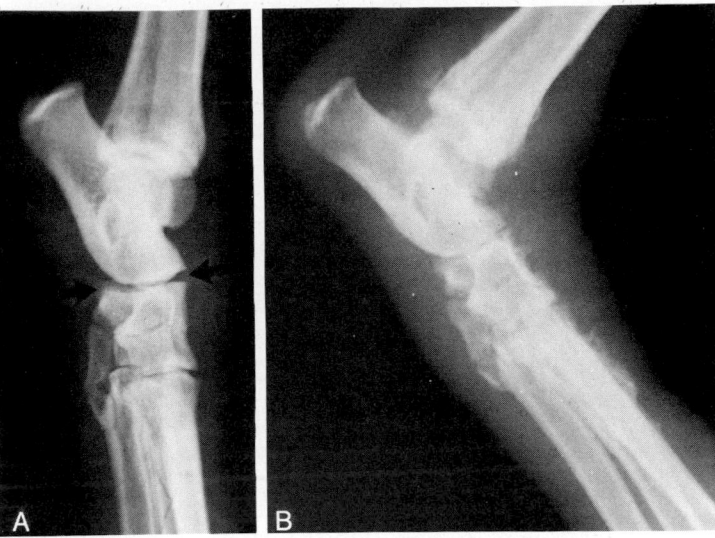

FIGURE 120–15. Lateral radiographs of the tarsus made at the time of injury *(A)* and 60 days later *(B)*. The subluxation at the proximal intertarsal joint is seen on the first study (arrows). The second study was made after providing support for the foot for two months. Post-traumatic periosteal new bone is noted from the level of the distal tibia to the level of the proximal metatarsal bone. Soft tissue swelling is prominent, and disuse osteoporosis is noted. Radiographic changes involving the joint spaces are difficult to identify, and the degree of cartilage destruction can be estimated only clinically. The foot at the time of the second study was not abnormally warm, the soft tissue walling was firm, and the foot was without pain. The differential diagnosis radiographically is that of an infectious arthritis.

TIBIOTARSAL. Tibiotarsal subluxations are slightly more common than tarsometatarsal subluxations in dogs. They may or may not involve malleolar fractures and are generally the result of severe trauma.[35]

Tarsal instabilities resulting from degeneration of supporting ligaments are almost always treated with tarsal arthrodesis. The procedure has been described by Campbell and associates, and by Dieterich.[32, 39] Tarsal instabilities of traumatic origin can be treated by reduction associated with wiring or temporary intraarticular pinning to maintain the joint in position. Tarsal arthrodesis is required when this proves unsuccessful.

HYPEREXTENSION. Hyperextension of the tarsal joint is frequently seen in association with hip dysplasia and is considered a compensatory mechanism. It allows for a limitation of extension of the hip joint without diminishing the length of the stride. It is seen especially in dogs with a rather loose conformation such as chow chows, Saint Bernards, and Newfoundlands. Treatment should be directed toward the hip dysplasia rather than the hyperextension of the tarsal joint.

Hyperextension of the tarsal joint without associated hip dysplasia has been seen as a developmental problem in some puppies. If left untreated, the tarsal joint can be severely traumatized. Smith treated such problems by shortening the Achilles tendon.[40]

Stifle and tibiotarsal hyperextension with lateral patellar luxation has been reported in a five-week-old Boston terrier puppy.[41] The animal presented with a stiff and hyperextended left hind limb that had been present since birth. The condition was successfully corrected by a combination of open reduction with correction of the luxated patella, trochlear grooving, and transarticular pinning of the stifle and tibiotarsal joints. The animal was maintained in a splint for two weeks, at which time the pins were removed. The limb was essentially normal one year later.

Hip Joint. The main stabilizing structures of this joint are the configuration of the acetabulum and the head of the femur. Traumatic luxation of the normal hip joint involves rupture of the teres ligament and the joint capsule. The luxating forces, usually abduction with external rotation or strong adduction, force the head craniodorsally. The altered appearance of the pelvic region and the apparent discrepancy in leg length may make the diagnosis obvious. Radiographs are often necessary to elucidate the underlying cause, however. The usual underlying cause is hip dysplasia. Other causative factors include avulsion fracture of the ligament of the head of the femur and a fractured dorsal rim of the acetabulum.

Treatment of a luxated hip is often accomplished by a closed reduction associated with the use of a non–weight-bearing sling that holds the leg in slight inward rotation and abduction.[42] This sling should be left on for about 14 days. If the closed reduction is unstable, an open reduction is necessary to clean out the acetabulum and to suture the dorsal joint capsule. If the acetabular or femoral joint capsule insertions are torn, screws or bone tunnels can be used to reattach the joint capsule. If the dorsal joint capsule cannot be reconstructed, an artificial one may be made with the use of a deVita pin (Figure 120–16). Other methods are transarticular pinning and toggle-pin fixation.[43–45]

In a review of 160 dogs treated for hip dislocation, 83 were replaced manually and 15 of these reluxated.[46] Open reduction with insertion of a Kirschner pin was done in 35 cases, open reduction with stitching the joint capsule in 9 cases, and femoral head excision in 5 cases. Dislocation occurred in 30 per cent of conservatively and 10 per cent of surgically treated animals.

If the predisposing cause of the luxation is hip dysplasia, the above methods are usually insufficient to result in a stable joint. Other modes of treatment such as femoral head ostectomy, triple pelvic ostectomy, and total hip replacement may be necessary to obtain a functional limb. These procedures will be covered in more detail in the section on hip dysplasia.

Stifle Joint.

TOTAL LUXATION. Total luxation of the stifle joint[47] is extremely rare, possibly due to the many and various ligaments and muscles which cross the joint. It is, however, the joint other than the dysplastic hip that is most likely to subluxate.

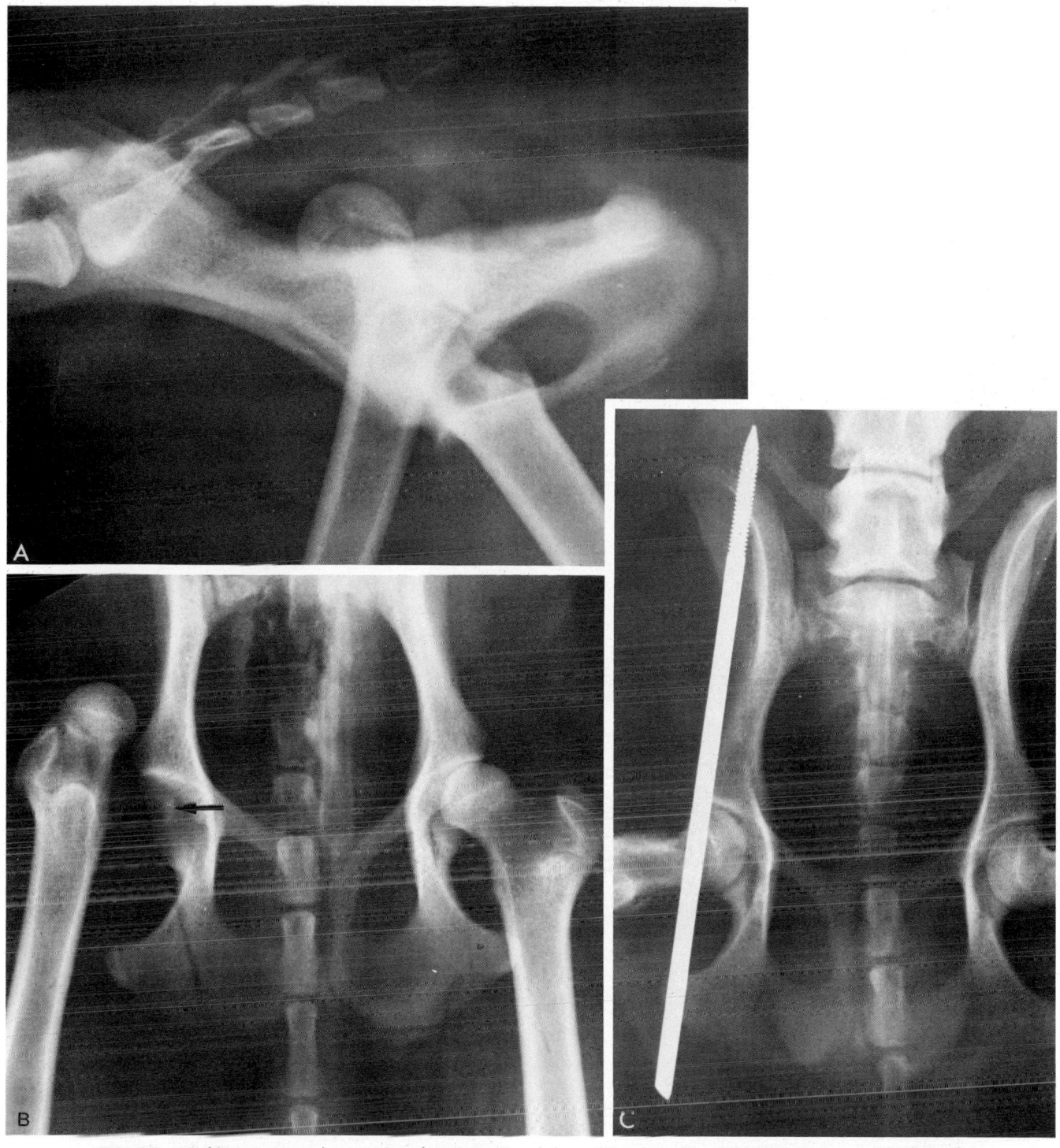

FIGURE 120–16. Lateral and ventrodorsal radiographs of the pelvis of an immature dog show a femoral head luxation wtih a free bony fragment within the acetabulum (arrow) that probably represents an avulsion of the attachment on the femoral head of the ligamentum teres. The reduction is stabilized by a deVita pin.

RUPTURE OF ANTERIOR CRUCIATE LIGAMENT. Rupture of the anterior cruciate ligament is the most common predisposing cause of stifle subluxations. This problem is most frequently seen in the middle aged and older dog, especially in overweight house pets. Although the rupture is acute, it is usually precipitated by only minor stress. There is usually a progressive degeneration of the ligament preceding the rupture.[48–50] The rupture usually occurs at the center of the ligament. Further

clinical evidence for a progressive deterioration is the tendency for the opposite ligament to rupture within a year or so of the first. Sometimes both ligaments rupture simultaneously and the resulting condition may be erroneously diagnosed as acute posterior paralysis.

Rupture of the anterior cruciate ligament in younger dogs is usually the result of trauma caused by a sudden forced hyperextension of the stifle, or by a combination of flexion and sudden forced inward rotation of the tibia.

This may cause rupture of the ligament from its center or avulsion of its bony attachments. The injuring force may simultaneously damage other joint components, especially the medial collateral ligament and the medial meniscus. Partial ruptures of the anterior collateral ligament may also occur in the eager hunting and field-trial dog. These partial ruptures do not heal, and will eventually become total.

A gradual relaxation of the ligaments of the stifle, associated with anterior drawer movement, is often an accompanying feature of plasmacytic lymphocytic synovitis of the dog (see following section). Such a relationship between cruciate ligament rupture and lymphocytic synovitis has been mentioned in passing by Tirgari,[48] although no cause and effect relationship was noted. Upon surgical exploration, the cruciate ligaments are either ruptured or intact but badly stretched. There is an obvious inflammatory synovitis accompanying the cruciate damage. This disorder can be seen in as many as 10 per cent of the dogs operated on for anterior cruciate rupture. For this reason, surgeons should be aware of its existence. If the cruciate is repaired without regard for the underlying disease, the surgery will be unsuccessful.

Rupture of the anterior cruciate ligament in dogs usually causes lameness. The involved leg is initially carried off the ground, but after a few days to a month or more, the dog will gradually put more and more weight on it. Some degree of lameness often persists, however, and is characterized by a decrease in the range of motion of the stifle joint. The tibia can be displaced cranially in relation to the femur on physical examination, the so-called anterior or cranial drawer sign. The drawer sign can best be elicited with the animal lying on its unaffected side. Standing behind the animal, the thumb and index finger of one hand are used to grasp the caudal aspect of the lateral fabella and the patella on the distal femur. The thumb and index finger of the other hand grasp the caudal aspect of the head of the fibula and the tibial crest on the proximal tibia. The stifle is slightly flexed and the femur is held steady while the tibia is pushed cranially and caudally. Only minimal cranial-caudal movement can be elicited in the normal adult canine or feline stifle. A greater amount of cranial-caudal movement is normal in younger animals. When the stifle is very painful or the animal apprehensive, sedation or anesthesia is necessary to properly assess the stability of the stifle joint.

Another method of diagnosing anterior cruciate rupture is the tibial compression test.[51] The metatarsus is grasped with one hand and the palm of the other hand is placed over the cranial aspect of the stifle with one finger over and down the tibial tuberosity. When the hock is flexed, tightening of the gastrocnemius muscle compresses the tibia and the femur. If the anterior cruciate is ruptured, the tibial tuberosity will slide cranially.

Joint instability caused by rupture of the anterior cruciate ligament eventually leads to degenerative joint disease and damage to the medial collateral ligament and medial meniscus.[48] The rate at which degenerative changes occur will be proportional to the weight and the activity of the animal. Degenerative changes often occur slowly in very small dogs and in cats.

The earliest signs of secondary degenerative joint disease are an increase in the volume of joint fluid and a thickening of the joint capsule. Thickening of the joint capsule is first noticed along the medial aspect of the joint in the region where the medial collateral ligament attaches to the medial meniscus. Thickening of the joint capsule and increased amounts of joint fluid cause a bulge of the joint capsule medial and lateral to the patellar tendon. Since these signs can be subtle, it is best to simultaneously palpate the normal and abnormal stifle.

Although one-half of dogs with ruptured anterior cruciate ligaments may regain adequate use of the leg without surgery,[52] spontaneous recovery should not always be relied upon. In very small dogs, a rest period of 12 to 16 weeks may be sufficient to resolve most cases. If lameness persists, however, surgery is advisable. Larger dogs should probably have surgery at the earliest time. Surgery to remove damaged tissue and stabilize the joint will not prevent subsequent secondary degenerative joint disease. It will slow its progression, however, and lessen its severity. The actual surgical technique that is selected probably has less relationship to success than the surgery itself, i.e., removal of debris, damaged menisci, tightening of the joint capsule, and stimulation of fibrous tissue.

Surgical treatment of anterior ligament ruptures involves one of many different approaches. Two basic types of reconstructive surgeries are used: static transfer and dynamic transfer.[53] In static transfer procedures, tendons or prosthetic materials are used. Dynamic transfer procedures utilize functioning muscles to replace the damaged ligament. The first surgical treatment for anterior cruciate ruptures was of the static type as described originally by Paatsama.[54] Numerous static and dynamic transfer surgeries have been developed since this time, each having its proponents and opponents. Reviews of various surgical procedures have been presented.[53, 55, 56, 58–60] The over the top technique is currently one of the more popular of the various techniques that have been developed.[57] Replacement of the anterior cruciate ligament with a carbon fiber prosthesis has had limited success.[61]

Rupture of the anterior cruciate ligament has also been described in cats.[62–66] Sixteen per cent of cats with ruptured anterior cruciate ligaments were traumatized just prior to admission. The cause of the remaining ligament ruptures could not be determined.[66] Among 18 cats with anterior cruciate ligament rupture in one study, 17 had unilateral disease, usually of the right hind limb.[66] Similar to small dogs, anterior cruciate ligament rupture in cats is usually treated conservatively. When owners were asked to confine their cats and to reduce the weight of obese animals, complete restoration of normal gait occurred within 1 to 16 weeks (mean 4.8 weeks).[66] The cats remained clinically normal for an observation period of 6 to 63 months. Periarticular thickening and radiographic changes of chronic stifle instability were observed in most cats at this time. Although most cats do regain normal limb function without surgery, a very low percentage of cats may still be lame after 16 weeks. These cats should have the affected joint opened, cleaned out, and the cruciate repaired by whatever procedure the surgeon prefers.

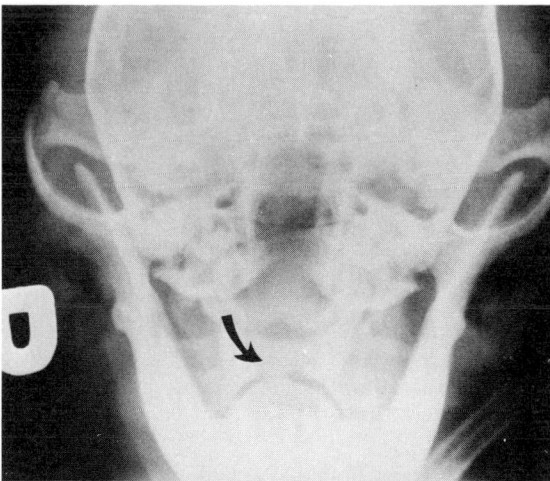

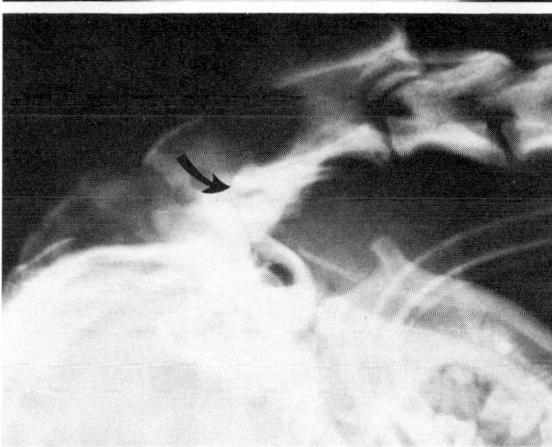

FIGURE 120–17. Flexed lateral and open-mouth ventrodorsal radiographs of a one-year-old female Japanese spaniel that fell from a four foot high fence two weeks prior to presentation. The patient remained stiff in the neck after treatment of corticosteroids. Instability at the atlanto-axial joint due to a hypoplastic odontoid process (arrows) caused the spinal cord injury. The history is typical with no clinical signs until minimal trauma results in injury to the spinal cord.

RUPTURE OF CAUDAL CRUCIATE LIGAMENT. Rupture of the caudal cruciate ligament is much less common, but has been reported in both cats and dogs.[56, 67, 68] Its main physical sign is the presence of a posterior or caudal drawer sign. Although less important for stifle stability than the anterior cruciate ligament, rupture of the caudal cruciate ligament leads to instability and degenerative joint disease. Because caudal cruciate rupture is usually due to severe trauma, it is frequently associated with other ligamentous injuries, and the reestablishment of functional joint stability can be a surgical challenge. Procedures for the correction of posterior cruciate ligament rupture have been described by Knecht[56] and by deAngelis and Betts.[69]

VALGOID INSTABILITY OF STIFLE JOINT. A valgoid instability of the stifle has been described in dogs.[70] It usually is seen in the recovery stage following repairs of femoral fractures or hip luxations, and involves atrophy of the quadriceps muscle, swelling of the anterior cruciate ligament, and weakness of the medial collateral ligaments. The valgoid position of the distal limb can be accentuated by medially directed pressure on the stifle joint, and the distal limb can be excessively rotated by twisting the lower leg while holding the femur in place.

The condition responds to cruciate ligament repair procedures.

TEMPOROMANDIBULAR INSTABILITIES

Traumatic Temporomandibular Dislocations. Temporomandibular dislocations occur in both dogs and cats.[71] They are usually traumatic in origin and are often associated with fractures.[72]

Nontraumatic Temporomandibular Luxations. Temporomandibular luxations unassociated with trauma can be of two types. In one type described by White,[73] there is a rostral movement of the mandible. This is manifested by malocclusion of the jaw and some interference with mouth opening. The second type, which is more common, is associated with open-mouth locking occurring after hyperextension of the jaw, and lasting for several seconds or persisting until manually reduced. Reduction can be achieved by hyperextending the jaw further while placing inward pressure on the displaced mandibular condyle. The condition has been described mainly in young basset hounds but has also been seen in Irish setters, weimaraners, dalmatians, and boxers.[72, 74–76] Prevention of jaw-locking in these dogs is accomplished by excising part of the zygomatic arch on the side of the lock-up. This surgery is based on the rationale that jaw-locking occurs because the condyloid process of the mandible is more oblique than is normal, thus allowing for lateral subluxation of the mandible. This allows the coronoid process on the side opposite the most involved joint to slip out of the coronoid fossa and engage the zygomatic arch. Dogs with this type of dislocation have a pronounced facial protuberance caused by the proximal end of the laterally shifted coronoid process on the locked side. The contralateral temporomandibular joint space is usually widened when visualized radiographically.[72] The developmental or genetic basis of the underlying deformity is unknown.

Two dogs with temporomandibular dysplasia unassociated with lateral displacement of the coronoid process of the mandible and impingement on the zygomatic arch have also been described.[77] Excision arthroplasty (mandibular condylectomy) was successful in preventing open-mouth jaw-locking and temporomandibular pain in these animals.

INSTABILITIES OF THE SPINAL ARTICULATIONS

Axial-atlantal-occipital Malformations. Malformations of the articulations of the axis, atlas, and occipital bone occur from time to time, most often in small toy breeds of dogs, but occasionally in large dogs as well (Figure 120–17).[78] Such instabilities are usually manifested by chronic cord compression associated with overextension or flexion of these articulations. Traumatic atlanto-occipital luxations are uncommon due to the structure of the joint and strength of supporting muscles and ligaments. A case of traumatic atlanto-occipital luxation has been described in a cat.[79]

Caudal Cervical Instabilities. Caudal cervical insta-

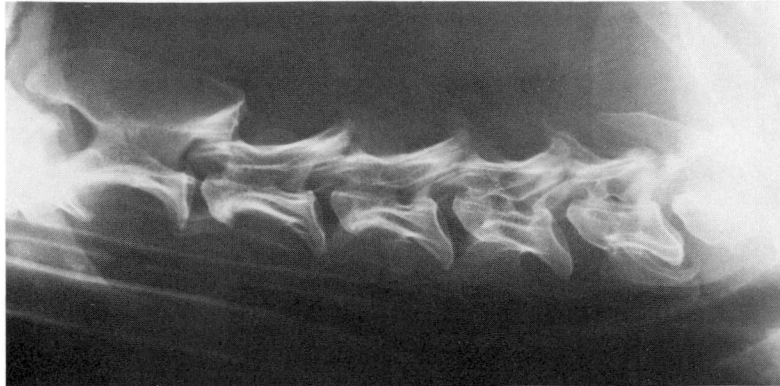

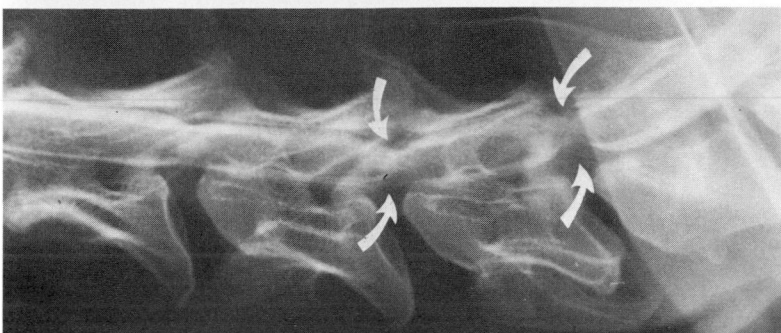

FIGURE 120–18. Lateral noncontrast and enlarged myelogram of an eight-year-old male Doberman pinscher with severe cervical pain and inability to walk. The noncontrast study shows only minimal narrowing of the C6–7 disk space and minimal new-bone production ventrally on the body of C7. The myelogram, however, clearly demonstrates the severity of the cord compression both dorsally and ventrally at both C5–6 and C6–7 (arrows). This patient clearly demonstrates the requirement to perform myelography prior to predicting a prognosis or attempting treatment in cases of this type.

bility (cervical vertebral instability, or CVI) has been described in Great Dane and Doberman pinscher dogs.[80, 81] but can be seen in many other large and giant breeds as well (Figure 120–18). The instability may involve the intervertebral disk, vertebral body, pedicles, or articular facets. Secondary bony and soft tissue changes lead to stenosis of the spinal canal and cord compression. Soft tissue changes include hypertrophy of the ligamentum flavum and dorsal longitudinal ligament, joint capsular thickening, or dorsal protrusion of the annulus fibrosus of the associated intervertebral disc. The net result of these changes is to cause chronic spinal cord compression. Even though instability is a major part of the disorder, the clinical signs are mainly neurologic and referable to damage of the spine at the level of the caudal cervical vertebrae. Surgical treatment, which generally involves reduction of cord compression and stabilization of the spine, has been described by Trotter and coworkers.[81]

Lumbosacral Joint. Degenerative disease of the lumbosacral articulation is a frequent occurrence in large, usually aged, dogs (Figure 120–19).[82] It is not clear whether this is due to an inherent instability of the true articulation, or to degeneration of the underlying disc.[83] Although often clinically inapparent, disease of this articulation can cause mild to moderately severe lower back pain.[82] These signs can mimic those caused by hip lameness. Unlike dogs with degenerative hips, dogs with clinically apparent lumbosacral instabilities often walk with their tails down. Forceful palpation of the lower spine and base of the tail, coupled with hyperflexion and hyperextension of the lumbosacral joint, can often help in localizing the lesion.

Meniscal Disorders

MENISCAL TEARS

A tear in the medial meniscus accompanies anterior cruciate ligament rupture in over one-half of dogs operated on for this condition.[84] Failure to remove all or part of the damaged meniscus can cause the lameness to persist after cruciate ligament surgery.[84–85] Meniscal tears are often manifested by a click during walking or on passive flexion and extension of the stifle joint.

Damage to the medial meniscus occurs infrequently as an isolated injury but is seen in athletic dogs of the larger breeds. It is usually associated with some damage to the medial collateral ligament and medial joint capsule. Genu valgum may be a predisposing factor. Considerable joint effusion may occur, especially following vigorous exercise. There is thickening of the medial aspect of the stifle joint with time and radiographic signs of degenerative joint disease.

MENISCAL CALCIFICATION

Degenerative joint disease associated with calcification of the medial menisci has been seen uncommonly in the stifle joints of dogs. Intrameniscal calcification and ossification have been reported in three cats.[86] The cats were 2, 7½, and 16 years of age; 2 were females and 1 was a male. All three cats presented with signs of acute lameness. The meniscal calcification and ossification in these three cats were thought to be incidental findings and not the cause of lameness. One of the cats had a septic osteomyelitis and synovitis, one had a

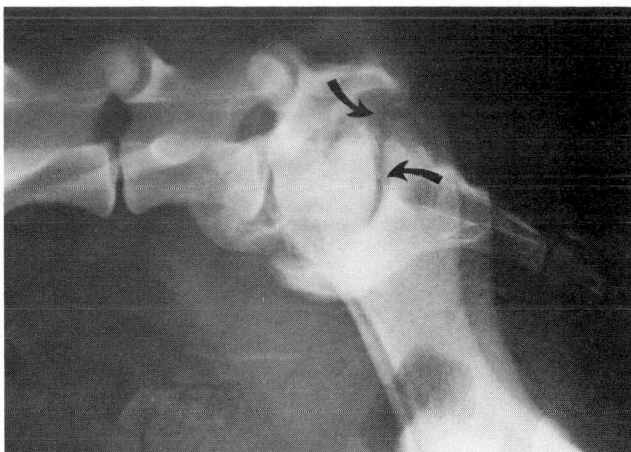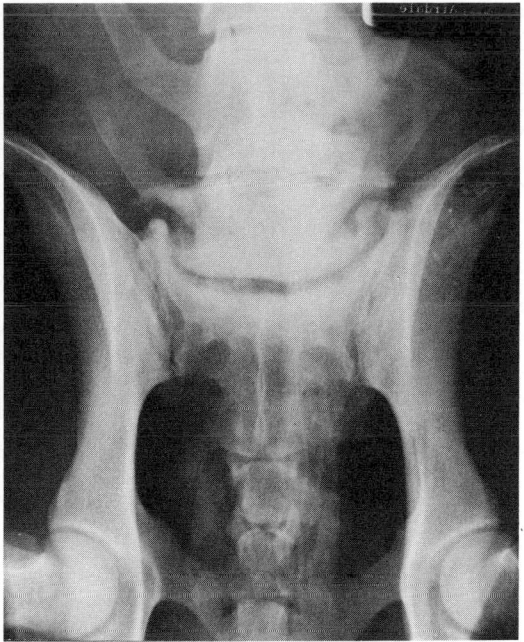

FIGURE 120–19. Lateral and ventrodorsal radiographs of the lumbo-sacral region of a five-year-old male Airedale terrier that was kicked in the back when young and now has had loss of both urinary and fecal control for the past three months. The severe changes that involve the lumbosacral articulation include marked ventral displacement of the sacrum, destruction with narrowing of the lumbo-sacral disk, reactive new bone laterally and ventrally at both L6–7 and lumbosacral articulation. Compression of the spinal canal is evident at the lumbosacral articulation (arrows). The significance of the luxation of the dorsal vertebral joints is not fully understood. The clinical history is suggestive of a trauma as the inciting event; however, the possibility of the lesion originating with disk degeneration must still be considered. Stress radiography, discography, or epidurography is necessary to completely evaluate the cause of the cauda equina syndrome.

ruptured cruciate ligament, and one had a lameness that resolved spontaneously in several days without treatment. Although the calcified meniscus in one of the cats may have been secondary to long-standing anterior cruciate ligament rupture, the meniscal changes bore a strong resemblance to the ossicles found in normal mature rodents and as vestigial structures in some humans.

DISCOID MENISCUS

A discoid meniscus is broad and disc-like in appearance, compared with the normal semilunar configuration. The condition occurs in as many as 2.7 per cent of humans.[87] In man it is not known whether it is congenital or acquired. The problem most frequently involves the lateral meniscus, and affected humans develop clinical symptoms similar to those produced by meniscal tears. This condition has been identified at necropsy in a dog.[88] The frequency of this problem in dogs and its clinical significance are both unknown at this time.

Sesamoid Bone Disorders

Degenerative disease of the volar sesamoid bones (usually the 2nd and 7th) of the metacarpophalangeal and metatarsophalangeal joints has been recently recognized in young dogs of larger breeds.[89] The disorder can be asymptomatic or associated with lameness. Since many young dogs of larger breeds have concurrent joint disorders, it is often difficult to determine what contribution, if any, the sesamoid disease has to the overall clinical picture. Sesamoid degeneration is associated with changes in the articular cartilage and calcification within ligamentous attachments. The etiology of the condition is unknown. Treatment is by surgical dissection of the affected sesamoids from its ligamentous attachments to the bone.

Fractures of the sesamoid bones, in particular those of the metacarpophalangeal joint, are a common problem in racing greyhounds.[90] This is a traumatic lesion, however, and is not due to degenerative changes.

Neuropathic Arthropathy

Neuropathic arthropathy occurs secondary to conditions that diminish normal pain, stretch, and proprioceptive reflexes. These changes result in a relaxation of supporting structures, chronic hyperextension and hyperflexion, and loss of neuromuscular and tendon reflexes that prevent the limb from being placed too forcefully on the ground. Although this type of disease is commonly associated with chronic neurologic diseases of man, it is very rare in the dog and cat. This is probably due to the fact that humans continue to use neurologically impaired limbs and that humans also live longer, thus providing time for destructive changes to occur. A good model for neuropathic arthropathy might be provided by horses with navicular disease that are denervated to diminish pain. If these horses are kept in vigorous use, the net effect is an acceleration of degenerative changes of the navicular bone and associated joint. In the case of such horses, however, there is both an anatomical (navicular disease) and a neurogenic (nerve severing) defect. The degenerative joint disease resulting from navicular disease is only accelerated by the posterior digital nerve sectioning. Neurogenic acceleration of degenerative joint disease has been experimentally induced in dogs.[91] Dogs that were subjected to unilateral dorsal-root gangliotomy (L_4 to S_1) failed to develop any clinical, gross, biochemical or histological signs of degenerative joint disease in the ipsilateral femoral condylar cartilage after a period of 16 months. In contrast, dogs that were subjected to transection of the anterior cruciate ligament two weeks after gangliotomy showed severe degenerative joint disease in the ipsilateral stifle joints after three weeks.

Clinical and experimental observations support the view that neurogenic arthropathy in dogs and cats is not easily induced by neurogenic deficits alone. If there is pre-existing joint disease, it will be accelerated by diminished pain and by neuromuscular, neurotendinous, and proprioceptive deficits.

Although not quite analogous, there is a relationship between the use of anti-pain and anti-inflammatory drugs and the rate of progression of degenerative joint disease. Chronic steroid injection into a degenerative joint may lead to diminished pain and inflammation and increased use of the damaged joint. The rate of degeneration of cartilage in the knees of dogs undergoing anterior cruciate ligament resection was also greater nine weeks later in dogs that were given aspirin daily than in nontreated dogs.[92]

Developmental Arthropathies

CONFORMATIONAL ABNORMALITIES

The importance of proper limb conformation, and its influence on soundness, is repeatedly stressed in equine orthopedics but is largely neglected in discussions of small animals. Abnormalities in the angulation of bones of the limbs can put great stress on joints. This stress cannot be normally dissipated by the joint, and the result can be degenerative joint disease and ligamentous degeneration. Conformational abnormalities are also common in small animals and can cause problems, although to a lesser extent than in cattle or horses. Conformational abnormalities can be acquired or congenital. If they are congenital, the anomaly may be noticeable at birth and as the animal grows. Straight stifle conformation and valgus and varus deformities of the elbow, stifles, tarsus, and carpus all occur in dogs, and to a much lesser extent in cats. Excessive plantigrade positions of the distal fore- or hindlimbs are also occasionally seen in both species. Nunamaker and Newton[93] have described three types of conformational abnormalities that affect only the femoral head and neck: (1) coxa valga, (2) coxa vara, and (3) increased anteversion. Coxa valga can lead to subluxation of the hip, while increased anteversion is associated with gait abnormalities, joint laxity, and pain. Increased anteversion is most often seen in giant breeds such as Saint Bernards, Newfoundlands, and Irish wolfhounds. These hip disorders can be corrected surgically.[93, 94]

CHONDRODYSTROPHY

Chondrodystrophy is inherent in bulldogs, pugs, Pekingese, basset hounds, dachshunds, and similar breeds. In these breeds the conformational abnormalities associated with chondrodystrophy are considered to be normal. Chondrodystrophy in some breeds, such as the Alaskan malamute, is considered highly undesirable, probably because enchondral ossification defects in this breed are also associated with defects in other organ systems.[95] Chondrodystrophic dwarfism has also been seen in a German shepherd dog.[96]

Chondrodystrophic animals, like chondrodystrophic human dwarfs, demonstrate angular deformities of the limb joints, and the cartilage surfaces vary greatly in structure.[97] These changes predispose the joints to degenerative changes. Fortunately, most chondrodystrophic breeds of dogs are not working animals and often lead rather sedate lives, which slows the progression of joint disease.

PHYSEAL (GROWTH PLATE) DISORDERS

Conformational abnormalities of the limbs can result from damage to the physes of immature animals. Such damage usually results in the cessation of longitudinal bone growth normally contributed by the injured growth plate. As summarized by Llewellyn,[97] the ultimate outcome is dependent on (1) the particular growth plate involved and its contribution to the total growth of the bone; (2) the age and breed of the animal, which will determine how much the growth will be affected; (3) the method of surgical reduction (if damaged by fracture); (4) the type of injury that caused the damage; and (5) the involvement of infection as a complicating factor.

Growth plate disorders are particularly common in dogs; they often result from trauma and usually involve the radius and ulna.[98] The manus is vulnerable because it receives a disproportionate amount of stress, its growth comes from several physes, and it is made up of two parallel bones. Growth plate injuries in other bones of the limbs are not usually of clinical significance. The mean age at the time of identifiable trauma is four months, and the angular deformities become apparent five to seven weeks later.[98]

Radioulnar Physeal Disorders. Rudy[99] described three possible deformities of the radioulnar segment that can result from growth plate disorders: (1) retarded or arrested growth of the distal ulnar physis, (2) retarded or arrested growth of the distal radial physis and (3) eccentric lateral premature closure of the proximal radial physis. Closure of epiphyses at three months of age will cause greater deformities than will closures at six to seven months of age, by which time most growth has taken place. Physeal injury may result in complete cessation of growth or only arrested growth and involve the entire physeal plate or only a portion of the physis.

Arrested growth of distal ulnar physis is the most common physeal disorder to occur in young dogs. The condition may or may not result from an identifiable trauma.[98–100] It is usually unilateral but can involve both forelimbs in about 15 per cent of the cases.[99] Because the distal ulnar physis accounts for 70 to 85 per cent of the ulnar growth,[101] premature closure of this physis can lead to severe problems. The shortened ulna can act as a restraining string in the bow formed by the more normally growing radius. This leads to a curving of the radius and a lateral angulation of the distal limb with outward rotation of the paw.[99–102] In addition, deformities often occur in the elbow joint, leading rapidly to a degree of subluxation and eventually to degenerative joint disease.[101]

Symmetric closure of the distal radial physis is infrequent, generally unilateral, and often associated with trauma.[99] The condition leads to a medial deformation of the distal limb, accompanied by a slight inward rotation of the paw and deformation of the elbow joint leading to subluxation.[99, 103, 104]

Eccentric lateral premature closure of the distal radial physis can occur, leaving the medial portion to continue to grow. This causes mainly an angular deformity of the radial articular surface, manifested by an outward rotation of the paw and carpal valgus deformity (Figure 120–20).[99, 103] Treatment is surgical.[103]

Premature closure of the proximal radial physis is uncommon. It leads to substantial deformities in the elbow joint.[99]

The treatment of abnormalities resulting from premature growth plate closures requires considerable surgical skill and a knowledge of the normal anatomic relationships. Premature closures of the distal ulnar physis can be treated by segmental ostectomies of the ulna if they are detected early enough. This, in effect, cuts the string of the bow, allowing the radius to grow unimpeded. Because the ostectomies can close rapidly, they may need to be repeated before growth ceases. A surgical technique whereby the distal styloid process of the ulna is resected and transposed may circumvent the problem of premature closures of the transected ulna.[105] In most cases, the condition is not detected until considerable growth abnormalities have occurred and physeal growth has essentially ceased. Surgery done at this point must be directed at reestablishment of normal angulation and rotational alignment, while maintaining as much of the normal limb length as possible.[99] Loss of too much limb length can create the "longleg-shortleg" syndrome, and predispose the joints of the forelimb to degenerative joint disease. Attention also must be paid to deformities of the elbow joint, which must be surgically corrected.[106]

EPIPHYSIOLYSIS. Spontaneous lysis of the apophysis of the supraglenoid tuberosity of the humeri has been observed over an eight-month period in a young German wire-haired pointer.[107] This resulted in nonunited supraglenoid processes and radiographic signs of degenerative joint disease in the shoulder joints. This condition has also been recognized in the proximal femur with spontaneous bilateral separation of the femoral heads.

LIMB SHORTENING

Fractures with overriding of fragments, if not properly treated, can result in a shortening of the limb upon healing. To compensate for the limb shortening, the angulations of the pelvic or thoracic girdle and distal and proximal joints are altered, which in turn predisposes these joints to degenerative changes. If fractures are repaired so that rotation of the distal segment occurs

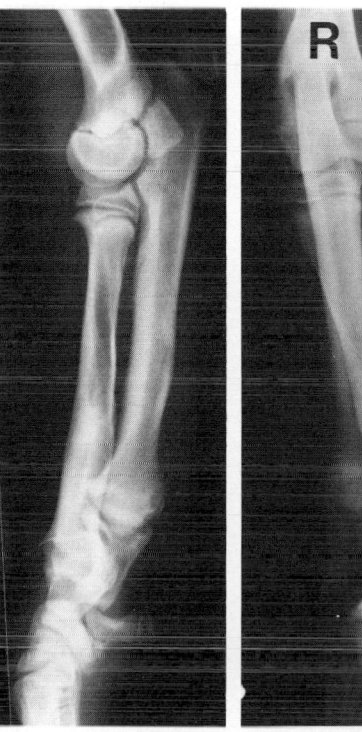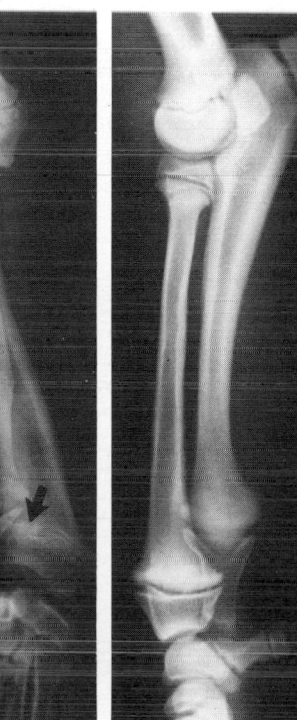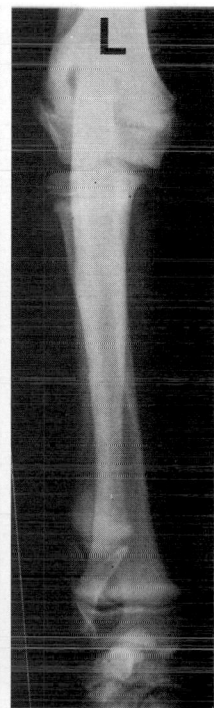

FIGURE 120–20. Craniocaudal and lateral radiographs of both forelegs of an immature dog with eccentric lateral premature closure of the distal radial physis on the right, leaving the medial portion of the physis continuing to grow. The left foreleg is normal by comparison.

upon healing, degenerative changes can occur in distal and proximal joints because of abnormal stresses imposed by the resulting malformation.

OSTEOCHONDROSIS (OSTEOCHONDRITIS)

Osteochondrosis is an important cause of both transient and permanent lameness in dogs.[108] It is not a problem in cats. Osteochondrosis can be clinically silent, apparent only histologically, or evident upon gross or radiographic examination of the joint. When osteochondrosis is associated with clinical signs, it means that the articular cartilage overlying the area of osteochondrosis has cracked and a loose cartilage flap has developed. This allows joint fluid to come in contact with subchondral bone. The exposure of subchondral bone to joint fluid is apparently painful and causes lameness. When a cartilage flap develops, the condition is usually referred to as *osteochondritis dissecans.*

The clinical, radiographic, etiologic, and pathologic features of osteochondrosis and osteochondritis dissecans have been extensively reviewed. Osteochondrosis was originally identified in shoulder joints of dogs, where the lesion occurs on the caudal aspect of the humeral head.[109–111] Osteochondrosis affects a number of joints, however, particularly the lateral and medial femoral condyles of the stifle (Figure 120–21), the medial condyle of the humerus, femoral trochlea, and the medial ridge of the talus.[112–120] It has also been reported to affect the lateral trochlear ridge of the talus.[121] Regardless of the anatomic location, the condition can be bilateral in one third or more of cases, although the lesion in one limb may clinically predominate.

Osteochondrosis in the dog is grossly or microscopically apparent at six to nine months of age. It may cause clinical signs of lameness or subtle gait abnormalities, or it may remain inapparent. Clinical signs persist for weeks or months. Permanent lameness may develop over a longer period of time as a result of secondary degenerative joint disease. There is tendency for the condition to occur more frequently in strains or breeds of dogs that are genetically selected for large size and rapid growth. Whitacre and Harrison[122] showed that

there was a close relationship between size and incidence, with most cases being in dogs over 60 lbs in weight. Males, which tend to grow faster than females, and animals on rapid growth-promoting diets are more often affected. There are exceptions, however, such as the high incidence in Brittany spaniels and some families of bull terriers, border collies, and greyhounds.[114, 123, 124]

Osteochondrosis is believed to be caused by disturbances in normal enchondral ossification.[108] In osteochondrosis, the articular cartilage in affected sites becomes thicker than normal because enchondral ossification does not keep pace with cartilage growth. Although the etiology is uncertain, the initial lesion is necrosis of chondrocytes in the deeper layers of the articular cartilage. One idea is that the necrosis is due to an inability of these deeply situated chondrocytes to receive adequate nutrients by diffusion from the synovial fluid or subchondral capillaries. This cartilage death tends to occur in areas of the joint receiving the greatest stress. The weight of the animal, congruity or incongruity of opposing articular surfaces, and type of activity may also be involved in the process. Following death of these deeply situated chondrocytes, the surrounding cartilage matrix fails to mineralize. Blood vessels from the subchondral bone will not invade the area of unmineralized articular cartilage as they normally would. Consequently, the osteogenic mesenchyme that accompanies these vessels does not penetrate the cartilage and normal ossification fails to occur.

All changes in the osteochondrotic lesion subsequent to the development of the area of chondromalacia are secondary events. At one extreme in this morphologic spectrum are those animals that are able to resolve the lesion spontaneously. The subchondral capillary bed is able to surround, bridge over, and bypass the area of chondromalacia and reestablish normal enchondral ossification superficial to the lesion. The result is a delay in the modeling of the developing articular surface, seen radiographically as a flattening of the subchondral bone. Grossly, the early lesion in the humoral head is outlined by a discoloration of the cartilage in the affected area (Figure 120–22). Percussion of the area is normal and indicates that there has been no separation of the

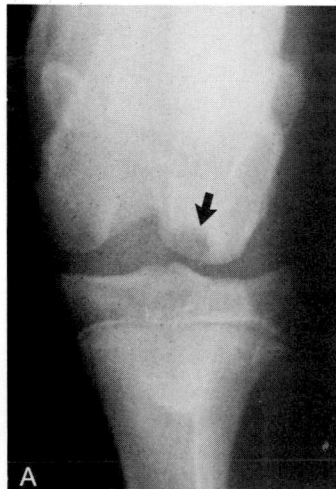
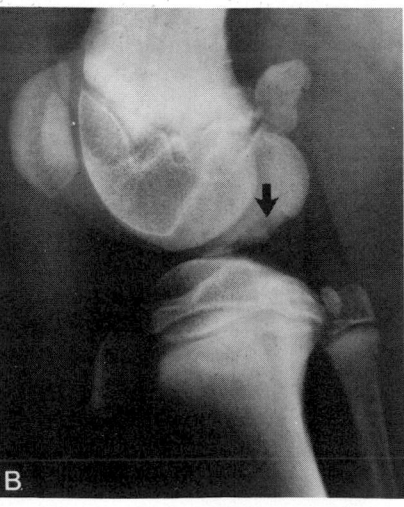

FIGURE 120–21. Caudocranial and lateral projections of the stifle joint of an immature dog with a large lucent lesion in the lateral condyle of the femur that is characteristic for osteochondrosis in this region.

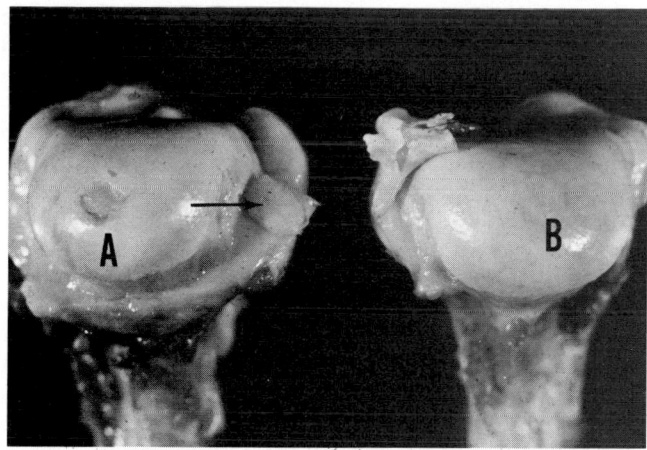

FIGURE 120–22. Osteochondrosis of the humoral head. Advanced lesion *(A)* shows a defect that has partially filled with fibrocartilage. Note that the detached piece of cartilage (arrow) has grown to be larger than the original defect. Early lesion *(B)* has a smooth articular surface but is outlined by discoloration of the cartilage.

cartilage from the subchondral bone. In the advanced lesion, a loosened area of cartilage usually tears partially away from the defective osteochondral junction and forms a flap. Complete separation can occur; in such a case, the detached piece of cartilage becomes a joint body (Figure 120–21). In either event, the animal is apt to show clinical signs of lameness. Healing of the defect occurs by granulation tissue arising from the subchondral bone, which eventually becomes fibrocartilage.

Synovial fluid from dogs with osteochondrosis resembles that of dogs with degenerative joint disease. If there is a great deal of necrotic cartilage debris, the number of phagocytic synovial mononuclear cells will be increased, and there may be an occasional neutrophil.

The lesion is demonstrated radiographically by an irregularly appearing subchondral surface, a focal defect in the subchondral bone, and varying degrees of increased bone density surrounding the defect (Figure 120–21). The defect may not have a distinct zone of increased density surrounding, or it may have a zone of 1 to 3 mm in thickness. The subchondral defect may have a small distinct opening at the surface of the joint or may appear as a large crater-like lesion. Free fragments are sometimes identified on survey radiographs. Cartilage flaps are more commonly noted on arthrograms. Secondary degenerative joint disease with an abnormally shaped epiphysis is seen in the chronic stages of the clinical disorder.

Since radiographic evidence of an osteochondrosis lesion does not automatically imply that it is clinically significant, i.e., an osteochondritis dissecans, the presenting clinical signs and radiographic findings must be compatible. If the clinical signs are equivocal, as might occur when an osteochondrosis lesion of the humerus occurs with panosteitis of the same humerus, an arthrogram may be advisable to outline the presence of a loose

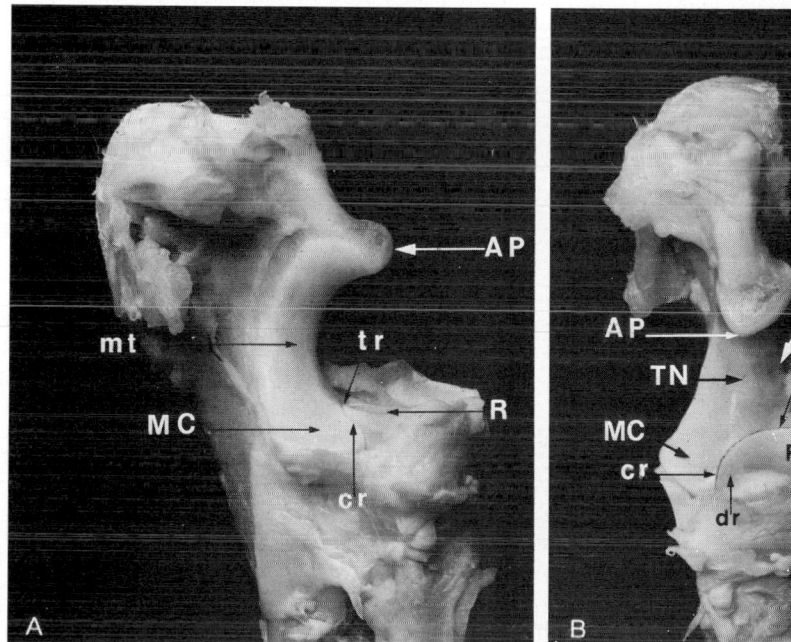

FIGURE 120–23. *A,* Gross morphology of normal left elbow joint, medial view. AP = anconeal process; R = radius; MC = medial coronoid process; mt = medial flange of trochlear notch; tr = articulation between central ridge of trochlear notch and radius (note the smooth transition from ulnar cartilage to radial cartilage); cr = articulation between downward sloping part of the radius and the medial coronoid process (note the smooth transition from radius to coronoid). *B,* Gross morphology of normal left elbow joint, cranial view; AP = anconeal process; TN = central ridge of trochlear notch with medial and lateral caudad sloping flanges. Central lateral flange has small area of cartilage atrophy (white arrow); R = radius; MC = medial coronoid process; LC = lateral coronoid process with marginal cartilage atrophy covered with synovium; dr = downward slope of the radius; tr = articulation between trochlear notch and radius (note the smooth transition from ulna to radius); cr = articulation between downward slope of radius and medial coronoid process, the process extending the length of the downward slope of the radius. (From Wind, AP: Elbow incongruity and developmental elbow diseases in the dog. JAAHA 22:711, 1986.)

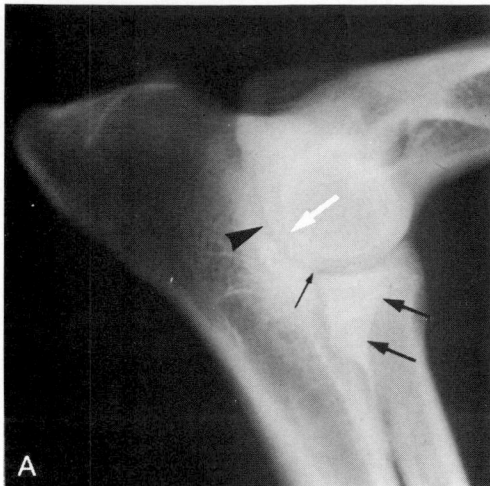

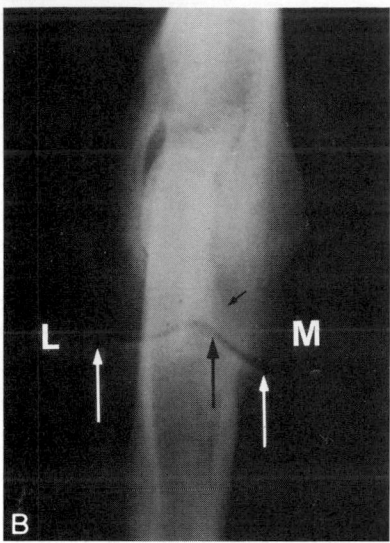

FIGURE 120–24. *A,* Radiograph of normal elbow joint, lateral view. White arrow points to joint space between central ridge of ulnar trochlear notch and humeral trochlea. Black arrow head points to joint space between the flanges of the trochlear notch and the humeral condyle. Small black arrow points to lateral coronoid process. Paired black arrows point to outline of medial coronoid process. Note the narrow uniform widths of the joint spaces. *B,* Radiograph of normal elbow joint, craniocaudal view. L = lateral aspect; M = medial aspect. Large black arrow and lateral white arrow point to joint space between humerus and radius. Large black arrow and medial white arrow point to joint space between humerus and medial coronoid process. Small black arrow points to medial flange of trochlear notch of the ulna. Note again the narrow uniform widths of the joint spaces. (From Wind, AP: Elbow incongruity and developmental elbow diseases in the dog. JAAHA 22:711, 1986.)

cartilage flap. If the radiographic lesion is an incidental finding, it may be advisable to slow the dog's growth rate by diet control and limit exercise to prevent the development of a loose cartilage flap.

The clinical findings of osteochondritis dissecans include lameness, an altered gait (if bilateral), a decrease in the range of motion of the affected joint, and pain on hyperextension and hyperflexion. Crepitation may be evident upon manipulation of the joint. There may or may not be muscle atrophy, depending on the duration of the lameness. If the humeral head is affected, the infraspinatus and the supraspinatus muscles are often atrophied. Joint effusion and joint capsule thickening along the affected side are early signs of elbow, stifle and hock joint involvement. They are not palpable in the shoulder joint, because of the heavy muscle cover. A special complication of osteochondritis dissecans occurs when a piece of fragmented cartilage enters the synovial tendon sheath of the biceps muscle (shoulder), the long digital extensor or popliteus muscles (stifle), or the flexor hallucis longus muscle (tibial-tarsal joint). This may lead to a severe and painful tenosynovitis.

Loose cartilage flaps gradually fragment and may become completely absorbed, or may be nourished by the joint fluid and become loose cartilage bodies (joint mice). Some cartilage fragments attach themselves to the synovium, where they can become vascularized and ossified. The defect in the articular cartilage will fill in with granulation tissue, which will change into a form of fibrocartilage with use. The joint contour can be re-established grossly in this manner, although not always radiographically. The ingrowth of granulation tissue is inhibited as long as the cartilage flap remains. In order to hasten the filling of the defect with granulation tissue and to minimize secondary degenerative changes, surgical removal of the flap and curettage of the defect are often advisable.[109, 125–127] This is especially true for animals that have an early onset of clinical signs (four to six months of age), or animals with large radiographic lesions. If the onset of clinical signs is late (seven and one-half to nine months), and the radiographic lesions are small, no surgery is usually necessary. It is advisable to give the animal a moderate amount of exercise to aid in the natural removal of the flap. Rest as a therapy is a waste of time because the loose cartilage flap will not heal without pressure from the opposing surface.

ELBOW DYSPLASIA

The term elbow dysplasia has been previously applied to a poorly understood disorder of the elbow joint that led to acute pain and dysfunction and/or chronic progressive degenerative joint disease. Ununited anconeal process was a common lesion in some, but not all, of such joints. Osteochondrosis of the medial condyle of the distal humerus was also a lesion that was sometimes seen in dysplastic elbow joints. More recently, the importance of fragmentation of the medial coronoid process in elbow dysplasia has been elucidated. As in all such processes, a unifying etiology was sought to explain all of the abnormalities that occurred in various combinations in the dysplastic elbow. All of these lesions were thought by some to be secondary manifestations of osteochondrosis.[108] The importance of rapid growth and genetic predisposition was also appreciated.[128, 129] Clinical descriptions of the various disorders that can make up the dysplastic elbow joint have been reported by a number of authors.[129–134]

Recent work on developmental anomalies of the elbow joint has discounted the primary role of osteochondrosis in the development of the lesions.[135–138] In this newest theory, all three developmental lesions of the elbow are themselves secondary to anatomic abnormalities in the developing elbow joint. Before this theory can be explained, it is important to understand the development of the normal elbow joint.

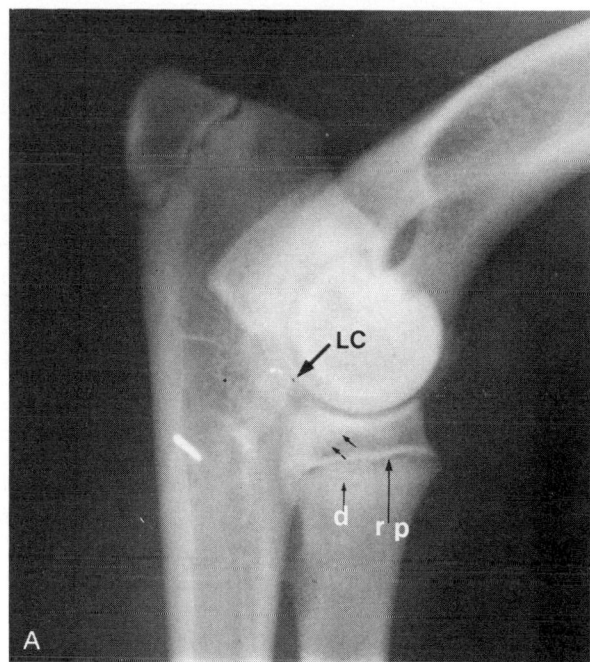

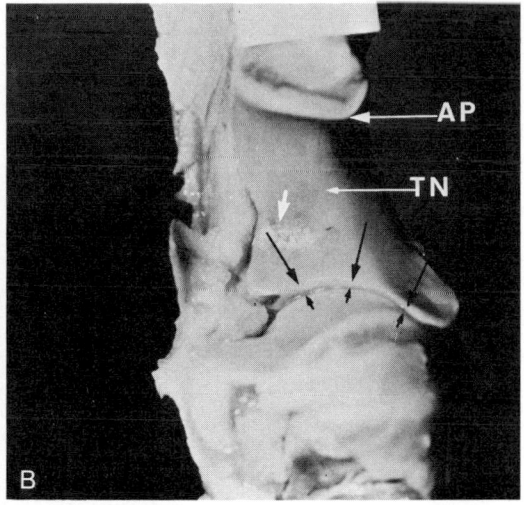

FIGURE 120–25. *A,* Radiograph of right elbow joint of 24-week-old Bernese mountain dog from parents with fragmented coronoid process. No evidence of fragmentation, but signs of minor incongruity. Lateral view. LC = lateral coronoid process; rp = physis of horizontal part of the radius; d = physis of downward slope of the radius. Small black arrows point to outline of the medial coronoid process. Note the increased distance between LC and the radius, and the increased joint spaces between the humerus and the radius. The humerus lies slightly cranial to the center of the radial articulation. *B,* Gross morphology of right elbow joint of dog in Figure 120–25*A,* cranial view. Moderate incongruity is present, but medial coronoid process is intact. AP = anconeal process. TN = central ridge of the trochlear notch. White arrow points to area of cartilage atrophy on the lateral flange of the notch. The articulation between the ulna and the radius is indicated by the large and small black arrows. Note that the distal edge of the trochlear notch with the medial and lateral coronoid processes lies above the level of the radius, creating a vertical step between the ulna and the radius. (From Wind, AP: Elbow incongruity and developmental elbow diseases in the dog. JAAHA 22:711, 1986.)

The gross appearance of the normal elbow joint, after disarticulation from the humerus, is characterized by a smooth transition between the articular surfaces of the trochlear notch of the ulna, the proximal radius, and the medial coronoid process of the ulna (Figures 120–23*A* and 23*B*). The articular cartilage of the trochlear notch extends medially and laterally to its attachment onto the joint capsule. In some joints, there is a slight thinning of the cartilage along the lateral aspect of the trochlear notch proximal to the lateral coronoid process.

The normal intact elbow joint is highly congruous, with narrow uniform spaces between the ulnar trochlear notch and the humeral trochlea (lateral view), and between the humeral condyle, radius, and the medial coronoid process of the ulna (craniocaudal view) (Figures 120–24*A* and 24*B*). The joint spaces between the trochlear notch and the humeral trochlea, and between the lateral humeral condyle and the radius, appear to lie on a continuous arc.

The unifying theory of the development of elbow dysplasia states that all three lesions (ununited anconeal process, fragmented medial coronoid process, and osteochondritis dissecans of the distal humerus) result from faulty development of the trochlear notch of the ulna. This faulty development results in a slightly elliptical articular surface of the trochlear notch and an arc of curvature on the radius that is too small to encompass the trochlea. This creates an incongruity between the articular surfaces of the proximal ulna and the distal humerus (Figures 120–25*A* and *B*). The incongruity results in too much contact in the areas of the anconeal and medial coronoid processes, and too little contact between the center of the trochlear notch and the humeral trochlea (Figures 120–26*A* and *B*).

The existence of joint incongruity can best be demonstrated by straight lateral and craniocaudal views, with the elbow in slight flexion (Figures 120–25*A* and B). Although special views may be better for demonstrating a fragmented coronoid process, an ununited anconeal process, or osteochondritis of the distal humerus,[133, 134] these views may be inadequate for assessing incongruity.

Fragmented Medial Coronoid Process. The fragmented coronoid process is the most frequent developmental disease of the canine elbow.[137] A genetic predisposition is present in large and intermediate sized breeds such as the German shepherd, rottweiler, Saint Bernard, and Bernese mountain dog.[139] Fragmented medial coronoid process has also been observed in the Shetland sheepdog, but whether this is due to joint incongruity has not been documented. Over 50 per cent of affected animals have bilateral involvement, and fragmented medial coronoid process may accompany ununited anconeal process and/or osteochondrosis of the distal humerus in the elbow.

Fragmentation of the process occurs usually between the age of four and six months. Depending on the degree of faulty development of the ulnar trochlear notch (see introduction), fragmentation may occur on the lateral portion of the process immediately adjacent to the radius (most common) or involve the entire cranial half (Figure 120–26*B*). Fragmentation of the distal edge of the trochlear notch may occur in some animals (Figures 120–27*A* and *B*). The joint incongruity

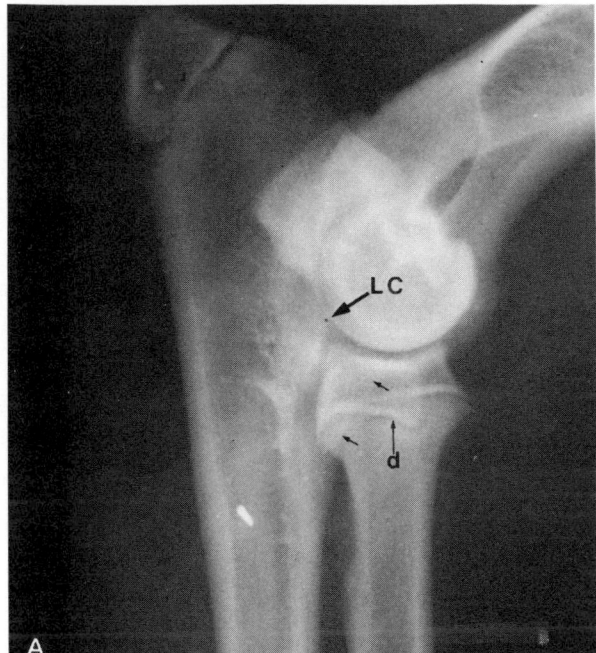

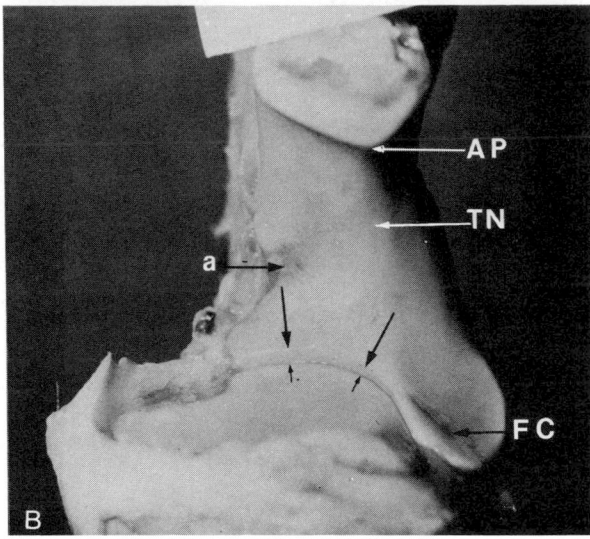

FIGURE 120–26. *A,* Radiograph of right elbow of littermate of dog in Figures 120–25A and 120–25B, also 24 weeks old. Lateral view. LC = lateral coronoid process; d = physis of downward slope of the radius. Small black arrows point to outline of medial coronoid process. Note step between LC and radius, and the increased humeroulnar and humeroradial joint spaces. The humerus lies cranially to the center of the radial articulation. *B,* Gross morphology of the right elbow joint of dog in Figure 120–26A, cranial view. AP = anconeal process; TN = central ridge of the trochlear notch; a = area of cartilage atrophy. Large and small black arrows point to radioulnar articulation. Note that the distal edge of the trochlear notch with the coronoid processes lies above the radius and that the medial coronoid process is fragmented. (FC). (From Wind, AP: Elbow incongruity and developmental elbow diseases in the dog. JAAHA 22:711, 1986.)

resulting from the faulty development of the trochlear notch may not be of sufficient magnitude to cause fragmentation, but may result in damage only to the articular cartilage. The fragmented coronoid process usually causes a kissing lesion on the opposite medial aspect of the humeral condyle (Figure 120–27B).

The clinical findings of fragmented medial coronoid process are lameness, an abnormal gait (if bilateral), and a subtle to moderate resistance to passive flexion

and extension of the elbow. This is infrequently accompanied by crepitation. In chronic cases, there is also thickening of the joint capsule, joint effusion and muscle atrophy. The lameness or abnormal gait is often characterized by excessive supination of the front paws. The animal may also hold the elbows bowed out or tucked inward. In severe cases, the owner may notice that the animal wants to sit or lie down a lot, plays less than other dogs its age, or can barely walk around the block.

Radiographic findings include joint incongruity, progressive secondary degenerative joint disease and, infrequently, a fracture through the medial coronoid process. On a lateral view, the abnormal elliptical shape and decreased curvature of the trochlear notch are evidenced by an increase in humeroulnar joint space in the central area of the trochlear notch, by a general increase of the humeroradial joint space, and a break in the normal continuous arc between the trochlear notch and radial

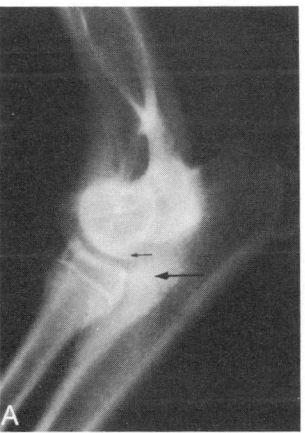

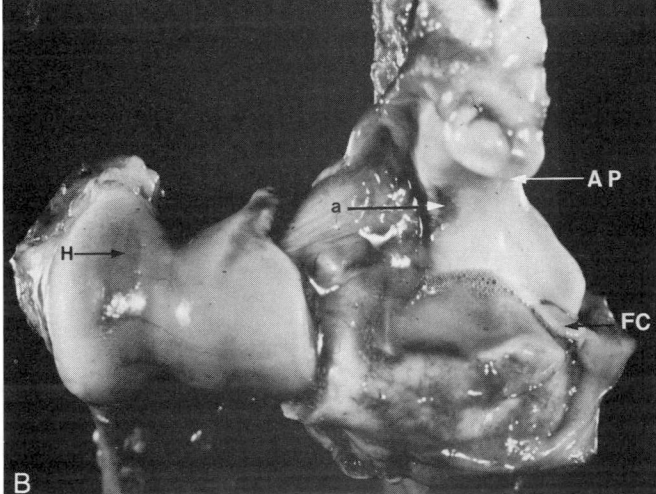

FIGURE 120–27. *A,* Radiograph of the right elbow joint of a six-month-old golden retriever with bilateral fragmented coronoid processes. Lateral view. Small arrow points to lateral coronoid process. Large arrow points to area of subchondral bone sclerosis of the trochlear notch. Note the increased joint spaces and the deformed anconeal process. *B,* Gross morphology of the right elbow joint of dog in Figure 120–27A, cranial view. FC = fragmented medial coronoid process; H = erosion of humeral cartilage opposite FC; a = area of cartilage erosion in center of lateral flange of trochlear notch. No corresponding lesion is present on the opposite cartilage of the humeral trochlea. Note that the distal edge of the trochlear notch and the medial coronoid process lie above the level of the adjoining radial articular cartilage. (From Wind, AP: Elbow incongruity and developmental elbow diseases in the dog. JAAHA 22:711, 1986.)

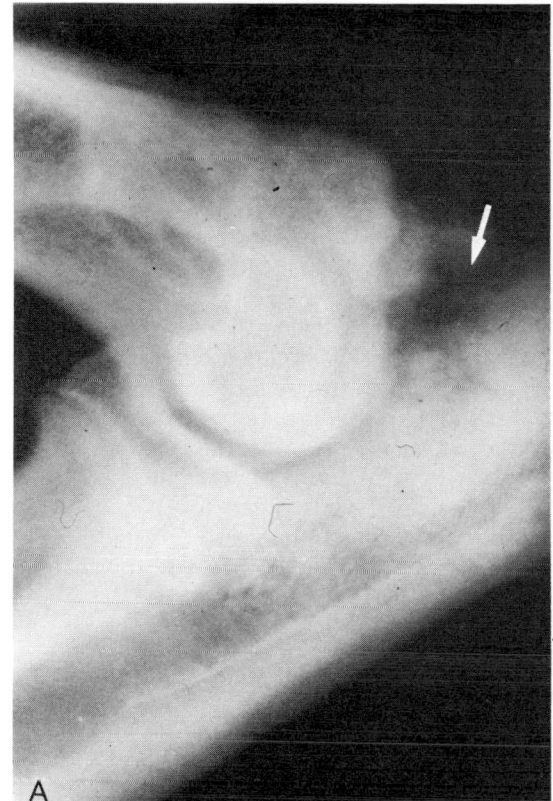

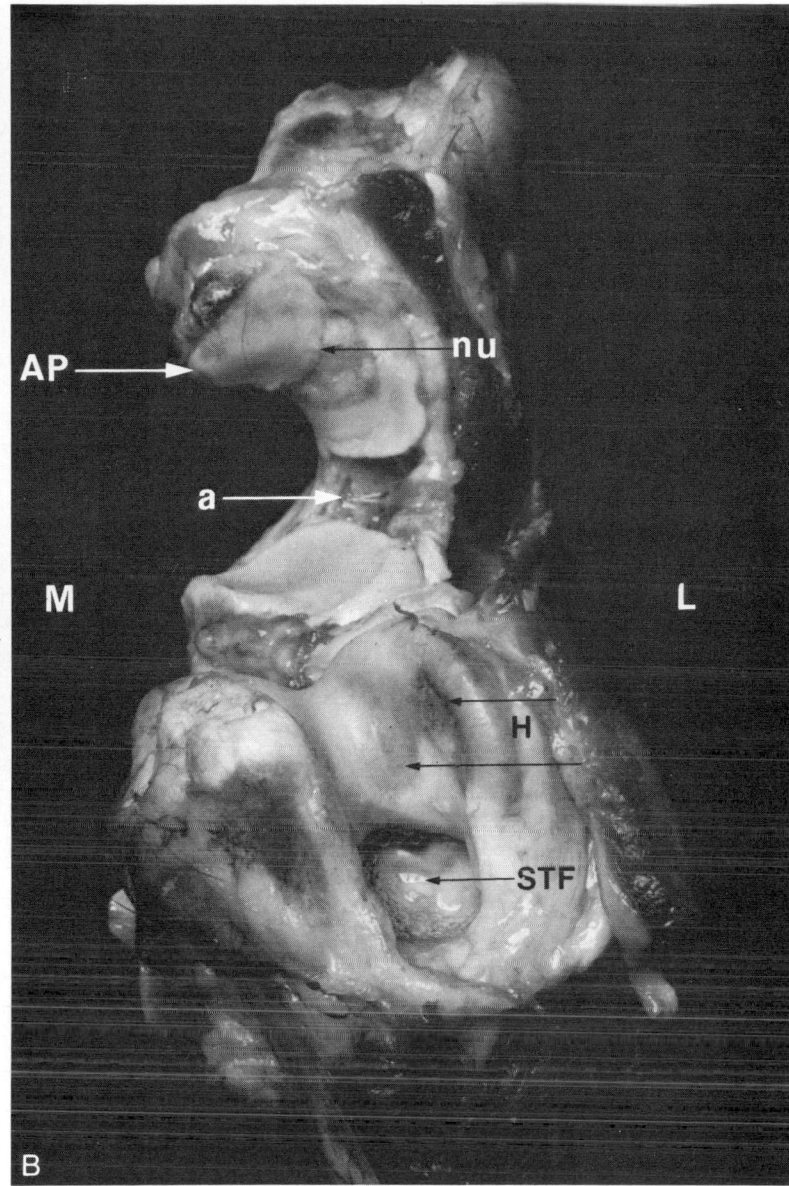

FIGURE 120-28. *A,* Radiograph of the left elbow joint of an eight-month-old Labrador with bilateral trochlear notch erosion and unilateral ununited anconeal process. Later view. Arrow points to the area of nonunion of the anconeal process. The trochlear notch is outlined poorly, and the lateral coronoid process is invisible. Note the increased humeroradial joint space. *B,* Gross morphology of left elbow of dog in Figure 120-28*A,* craniolateral view. nu = area of nonunion of the anconeal process with adjoining area of cartilage erosion. a = area of cartilage erosion involving the distal lateral flange of the trochlear notch and the lateral coronoid process. H = arrows point to cartilage damage to the olecranon fossa and lateral condylar ridge opposite the ununited anconeal process. Humeral trochlear cartilage opposite area "a" is normal grossly. STF = supratrochlear foramen. (From Wind, AP: Elbow incongruity and developmental diseases in the dog. JAAHA 22:711, 1986.)

articulation. This creates a step between the lateral coronoid process and the radius, and a cranial displacement of the humerus on the radius (Figures 120-25*A* and 120-26*A*).

Additional radiographic abnormalities may include subchondral bone sclerosis of the trochlear notch and a deformed anconeal process (Figure 120-27*A*). These changes reflect the increased pressure being borne by these areas in an incongruous elbow joint. Although cartilage erosion is usually associated with subchondral bone sclerosis on the trochlear notch, corresponding lesions may be absent from the opposing articular cartilage of the humeral trochlea (Figure 120-27*B*).

Direct radiographic visualization of the fragmented coronoid process is in most cases not possible. The fragmented piece commonly lies between the main part of the coronoid process and the radius and thus is obscured by the overlying shadows of these bones. The early diagnosis of fragmented coronoid process is usually based on age, breed, clinical findings and indirect radiographic signs.

The acute pain exhibited by dogs with fragmentation of the medial coronoid process is most likely caused by joint fluid entering the subchondral bone following fracture of the process. The fractured piece usually remains wedged between the radius and the main part of the coronoid process that is attached to the joint capsule. Acute pain can be alleviated by surgical removal of the fragment. Although surgery is advisable to lessen pain and to remove a potentially damaging piece of loose bone, the underlying cause of the fragmentation will still be present and the joint will gradually become degenerative. The rate of progression of the degenerative changes is dependent on the degree of joint incongruity. Weight control and the animal's natural inclination to limit its exercise will allow the animal to cope with the problem as much as possible.

Ununited Anconeal Process in Nonchondrodys-

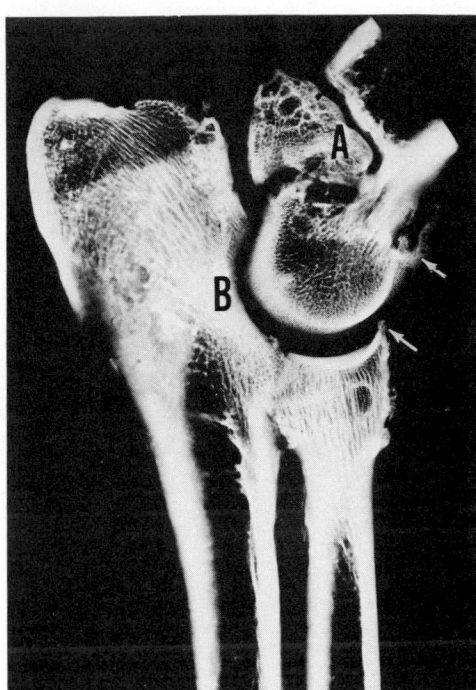

FIGURE 120–29. Ununited anconeal process (A) is lodged in the olecranon fossa. Secondary degenerative joint disease of the elbow is characterized by subchondral bone sclerosis in the trochlear notch of the ulna (B) and the formation of periarticular osteophytes (arrows).

trophic Breeds. Ununited anconeal process in nonchondrodystrophic breeds tends to occur between the ages of four and six months, at which time the bones are incompletely ossified. It tends to occur in breeds and individuals that have a separate center of ossification for the anconeal process. German shepherds, and some individuals of other breeds may have such separate ossification centers. Bony fusion of the anconeal process with the proximal ulna usually takes place between the age of five and six months. Bony union does not always occur, especially in the German shepherd. Instead, a cleavage line develops in the anconeal physis, separating the anconeal process from the ulna (Figure 120–28). Interestingly, ununited anconeal processes are practically unheard of in greyhounds, even though they tend to have a separate ossification center.[138] This observation supports the theory that joint incongruity is the main reason for the ununited anconeal process seen in breeds such as the German shepherd. Incongruity of the elbow joint is not seen in greyhounds. If an animal has a separate site of ossification, and an incongruous elbow joint surface, stresses caused by the abnormally tight fit between the anconeal process and the opposing trochlea may cause movement of the cartilage plates separating the center of anconeal ossification from the ulna. Such a separation will disrupt normal enchondral ossification and result in a nonunion of the anconeal process with the ulna.

The presenting signs of ununited anconeal processes include a variable degree of lameness of one or both front limbs, or an altered gait. There is often lateral positioning of the elbow and paw by the affected animal. Crepitation and pain may be evident upon flexion and extension of the elbow joint and on deep palpation of the olecranon fossa. There is joint capsule thickening, joint effusion and muscle atrophy of the limb in dogs with chronic secondary degenerative joint disease.

Radiographic examination reveals the presence of a radiolucent line between the anconeal process and the ulna (Figure 120–28A and B). In breeds that also have elbow joint incongruities, the ununited anconeal process may be associated with other anomalies, in particular a fragmented medial coronoid process. In dogs less than five months of age, the normal anconeal physis may appear ununited. This is of no significance unless accompanied by compatible clinical signs. Signs of joint incongruity similar to those seen in cases with a fragmented medial coronoid process may be seen in some individuals. Severe joint incongruity is seen in cases where distal displacement of the trochlear notch has occurred due to the mobility of the anconeal process. The progression of degenerative changes is similar to that described under fragmented medial coronoid process, but the first sign of sclerosis may be in the area of the anconeal process (Figure 120–29).

Removal of the loose process will lessen chronic irritation within the joint and a degree of lameness. Surgery will not alter the joint instability that the nonunited anconeal process has created. It will also not change the basic underlying incongruity of the joint. Reattachment of the loose anconeal process with a lagscrew is therefore of doubtful value and may even be contraindicated.

Osteochondritis Dissecans of the Medial Condyle of the Humerus. This is the final lesion associated with the syndrome of elbow incongruity.[137, 138, 140] It is probably due to an increased pressure exerted by the medial coronoid process on the opposing trochlear cartilage. This pressure can interfere with normal endochondral ossification, and exposes the more deeply and poorly fed chondrocytes to undue stress. Lateral radiographs show a flattening of the outline of the humeral condyle (Figure 120–30A). The actual defect is best localized on a craniocaudal view (Figure 120–30B). The lesion on the medial trochlea of the distal humerus is readily seen on gross inspection of the joint (Figure 120–30C).

Treatment of osteochondritis dissecans consists of curettage of the lesion. The prognosis depends on the size of the lesion and the degree of faulty development of the ulnar trochlear notch. In general, a progressive osteoarthrosis is expected.

UNUNITED ANCONEAL PROCESS IN CHONDRODYSTROPHIC BREEDS

A loose anconeal process can also be found in some of the larger chondrodystrophic breeds, primarily the basset hound and the English bulldog. However, this is not an ununited process, but a true fracture of the process caused by the distal (downward) subluxation of the anconeal process as the result of lagging longitudinal growth of the distal ulnar physis in these breeds. Healing of this fracture can occur at four to five months of age following cutting of the radioulnar ligament and freeing of the ulna from the distal pull of the radius. This procedure may not be successful in older dogs and removal of the process is recommended.[141, 142]

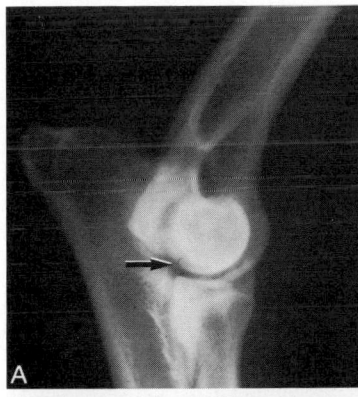
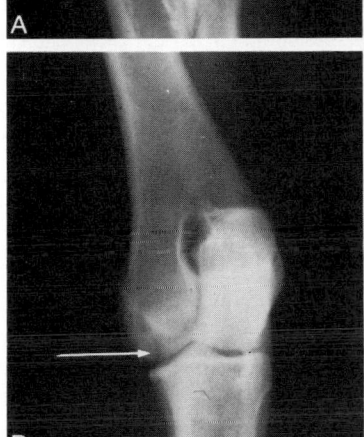
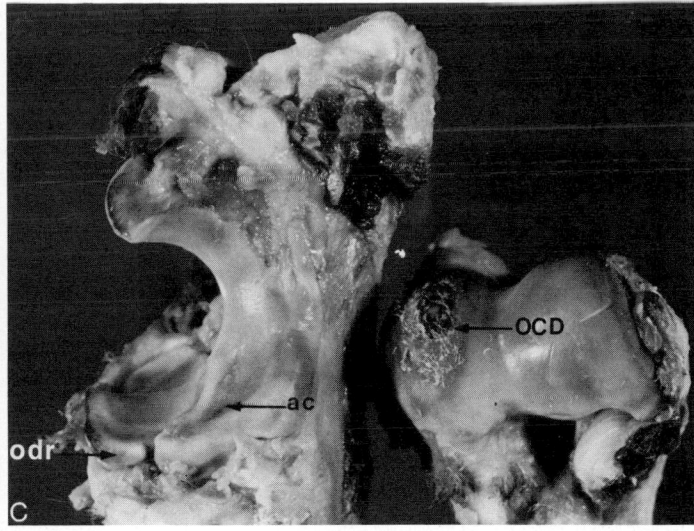

FIGURE 120–30. *A,* Lateral radiograph of elbow joint of a ten-month-old golden retriever with bilateral osteochondritis dissecans. Note the wide joint spaces. Arrow points to area of flattening of the outline of the humeral condyle. Also present are anconeal osteophytes, subchondral bone sclerosis of the trochlear notch, and cranial lipping of the radius. *B,* Note that the medial coronoid process lies above the level of the radius. Arrow points to area of radiolucency on the medial aspect of the humeral condyle. *C,* Gross morphology of the left elbow joint of the dog in Figure 120–30*A,* mediocranial view. OCD = OCD lesion on the medial aspect of the humeral condyle; ac = erosion of the cartilage of medial coronoid process; odr = lipping of the downward slope of the radial articulation. The distal edge of the trochlear notch and the medial coronoid process lie above the adjoining radial articular cartilage. (From Wind, AP: Elbow incongruity and developmental elbow diseases in the dog. JAAHA 22:711, 1986.)

HYPOPLASIA OF THE CORONOID PROCESS

Hypoplasia of the coronoid process of the dog is an uncommon clinical disorder. Hypoplasia may result from trauma, loss of contact with the trochlea of the humerus, or sustained pressure to the developing coronoid process. The entire thickness of the articular cartilage over the coronoid process is necrotic, and no germinativa cells remain to reinitiate the growth of the process (Figure 120–31). Radiographically, the lack of development of the coronoid process is readily apparent.

ECTOPIC OSSIFICATION CENTERS

An ectopic ossification center resembling a sesamoid bone has been observed medial to the head of the radius in the joint capsule of the elbow (Figures 120–32 and 120–33). It is considered an incidental radiographic finding and of no clinical significance. A similar ectopic ossification center can occasionally be seen over the dorsocranial aspect of the acetabulum of dogs (Figure 120–34); this condition also does not produce clinical signs.

HIP DYSPLASIA

Hip dysplasia is a developmental disease identified in most breeds of dogs. It tends to occur more frequently, however, in larger, well-fed, faster growing breeds.[143, 144] The development of hip dysplasia is strongly influenced by complex genetic factors[145–147] and affects both sexes of dogs with equal frequency. It has also been described in cats.[148–151] In cats, purebreds are much more likely to be affected than domestics.

The clinical progression of the disorder has been best documented in the canine, but the evolution of the changes in both dogs and cats appears to be rather stereotyped. Dysplastic dogs are born with normal hip joints that subsequently undergo progressive structural alterations. The following structural anomalies are identified either pathologically or radiographically: joint laxity; shallow acetabular cavities; subluxation; swelling, fraying, and rupture of the round ligament of the femoral head; erosion of the articular cartilage, with eburnation of the subchondral bone; remodeling of the acetabular rim and flattening of the femoral head; and periarticular osteophyte production (Figures 120–35 and 120–36).[152–154] The diagnosis of hip dysplasia by performing measurements on pelvic radiographs has always tempted radiologists. A recent study suggested that pelvic inlet measurements were valid in determining the status of the hip joints.[155] In another study of bone specimens, angles of femoral head inclination and anteversion were not found to play a role in the development of hip dysplasia.[156] There are considerable variations in the severity of the clinical signs, time of onset of structural changes, age at which clinical signs appear, rate of disease progression, and degree of pain and

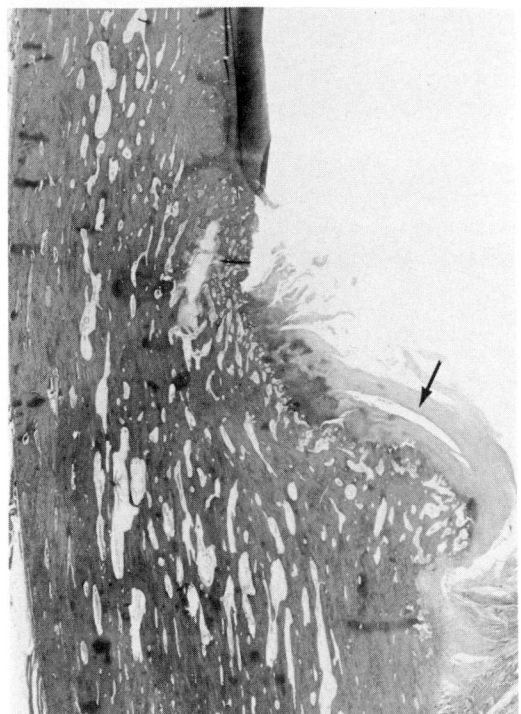

FIGURE 120–31. Hypoplasia of the coronoid process. Necrosis and fibrillation of the entire layer of articular cartilage (arrow).

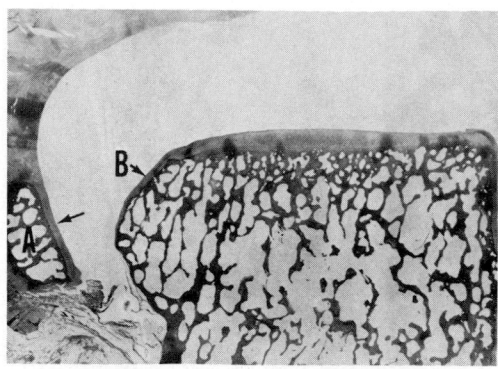

FIGURE 120–33. Radiograph of a 1-cm thick bone section that shows an ectopic ossification center (A) in the lateral joint capsule of a canine elbow (same case as in Figure 120–32). This small ossicle has a body of spongy bone that is covered by hyaline cartilage (arrow), which articulates with the head of the radius (B).

impaired mobility. Since joint laxity is the earliest sign of hip dysplasia,[157] gait abnormalities without overt lameness or stiffness may precede degenerative joint disease by many months. Degenerative joint disease may occur within the first year of life, but many animals show no clinical or radiographic signs until two to six years of age. There may be a poor correlation between clinical and radiographic signs. The changes noted radiographically are asymmetric in their presentation in over one-fourth of the patients examined.[158]

Young dogs with unstable hips are prone to bouts of acute lameness following exercise or strenuous activity. This does not mean that degenerative changes have occurred at this stage. Rest and analgesics for several days, will often be sufficient to treat the condition. It is mentioned only because there is a temptation on such occasions to assume the worst and to initiate more drastic therapeutic measures.

The precise etiology of hip dysplasia in the dog remains in question. As mentioned earlier, genetic factors are important. Environmental and nutritional factors, however, are involved in the expression of the abnormal phenotype.[143–147, 159] There is debate as to whether the fundamental cause is intrinsic or extrinsic to the hip joint. Proponents of an intrinsic cause believe that the primary change occurs in the development of the coxofemoral joint itself.[143, 160] One suggestion is that such structural abnormalities are due to osteochondrosis.[108] Proponents of an extrinsic cause believe that the hip abnormalities occur secondary to physical anomalies or inadequacies in the muscles that support the coxofemoral joint during development.[161–163] There are also breed factors governing the nature of the pelvic attachment and this influences the manner in which the dysplasia develops.[164] Whatever the cause, the end result is a joint that is unstable and predisposed to degeneration.

The treatment of hip dysplasia is mainly palliative and varies with the stage of the disease. In the early stages when there is considerable pain and minimal degenerative changes, rest, restriction of activities that put stress on the hips, and analgesic drugs may prove adequate. In dogs with more advanced disease, restricted activity and analgesics may not be sufficient to provide relief of

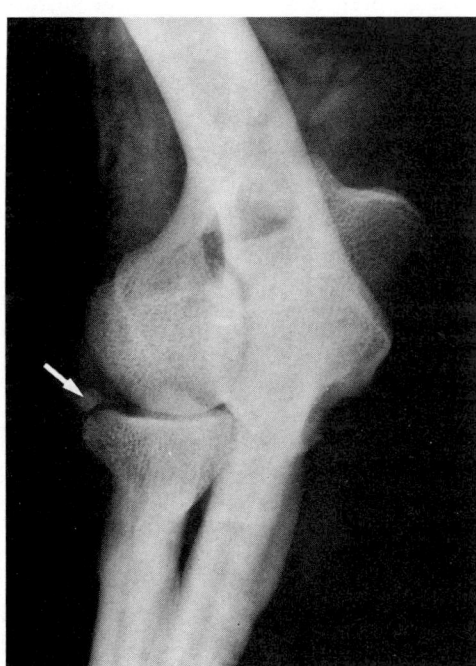

FIGURE 120–32. Oblique radiograph of the elbow joint of a mature dog with an ectopic ossification center that is craniolateral in location (arrow).

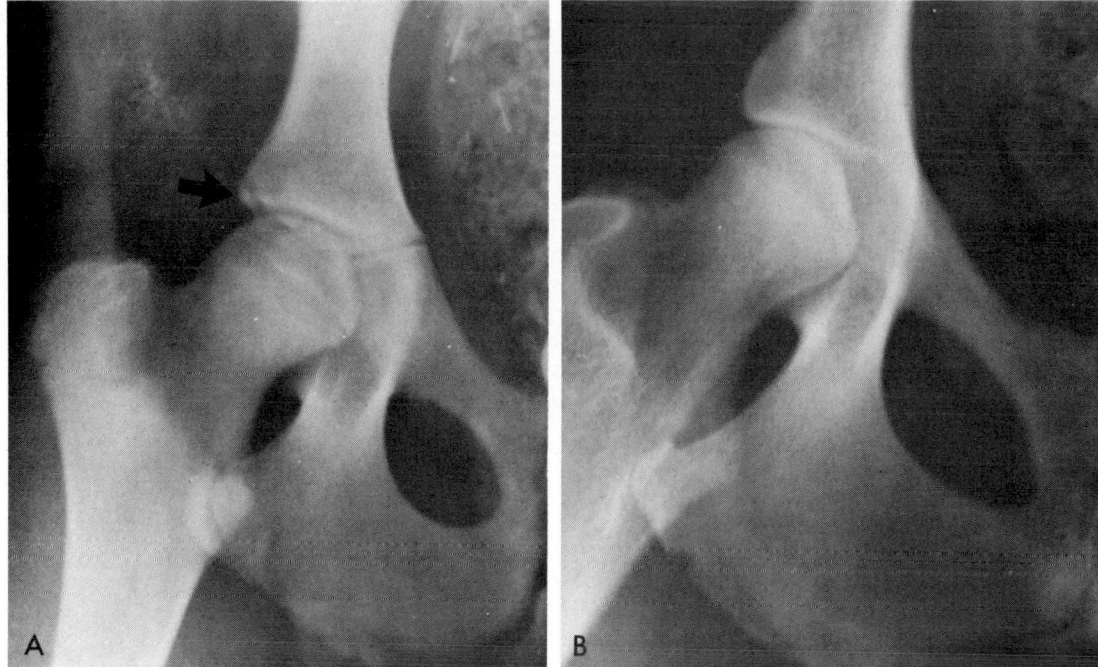

FIGURE 120–34. Ventrodorsal projections of a hip joint of a Great Dane at six months *(A)* and two years of age *(B)* with an ectopic ossification center (arrow) noted on the earlier study. The hip joint at two years of age is believed to be within normal limits.

pain. At this point, most dogs will show radiographic signs of degenerative joint disease. Sectioning of the pectineus muscle or tendon may afford relief from pain for periods of six months or more.[165] The procedure does not prevent the progression of degenerative changes but rather releases painful pressure (and perhaps severs sensory nerves that carry pain sensation) on the capsule of the hip joints. The procedure is not without controversy, and while some individual investigators advocate its use wholeheartedly, others are more reserved.[93, 165, 166] Some orthopedic surgeons believe that simultaneous sectioning of the adductor magnus muscle

gives more relief than if the pectineus muscle alone is sectioned.[93] Pectineal myotomy or tenonectomy has also been used with apparent benefit in cats with hip dysplasia.[150, 151]

Surgical repositioning of the acetabulum by pelvic osteotomy has been advocated in young animals with subluxating hips but without signs of joint disease.[167] This procedure requires considerable surgical skill and has seen limited application in practice. It does not prevent all subluxation, nor does it prevent eventual degenerative joint disease. It will, however, decrease the rate of progression and severity of such changes. A

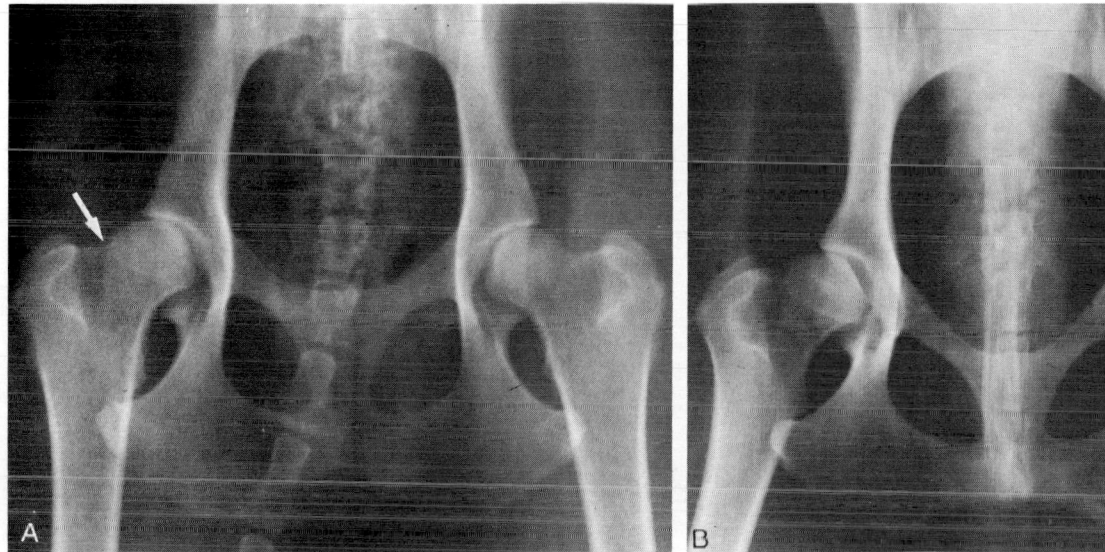

FIGURE 120–35. Ventrodorsal radiographs of the pelves of two dogs with minimal remodeling of the femoral neck (arrow) *(A)*, lipping of the acetabular rim (arrow) *(B)*, filling of the depths of the acetabulum with bone (black arrow), and subluxation that are characteristic of hip dysplasia.

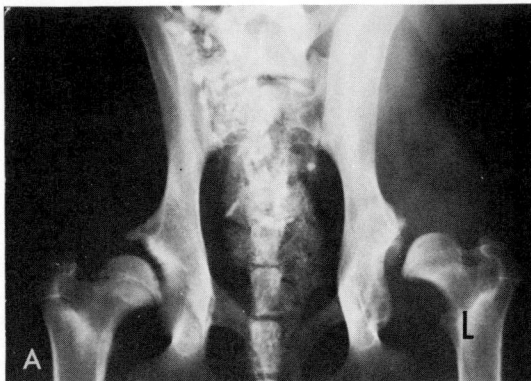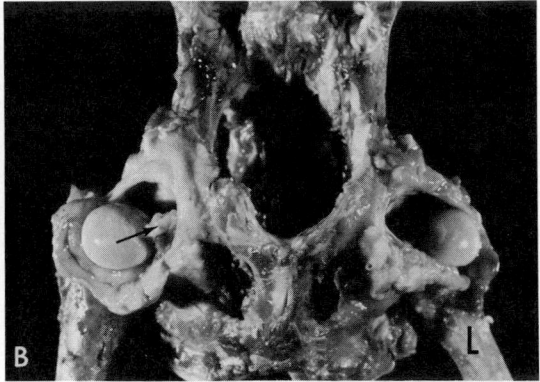

FIGURE 120–36. *A,* Radiograph of a dog with severe bilateral hip dysplasia, as evidenced by lesions characteristic of chronic secondary degenerative joint disease. Severe subluxation of the left hip (L) with an abnormally shallow acetabulum is demonstrated. Note the abnormal contours of the femoral heads and periarticular new bone formation. *B,* Gross tissue demonstrates the thickened joint capsules. The ligament of the head of the right femur was thickened and frayed, while the ligament of the left femur (L) was ruptured. Note that the left head has an abnormal shape and that the articular surface is irregular.

simpler procedure for acetabular repositioning has been described by Schrader.[168] Operated hip joints were followed for 1 to 5.5 years (mean 2.7 years).[169] Functional ability was satisfactory in 51/55 operated joints, although a few dogs had gait abnormalities. Eighty-two per cent of the joints had little or no radiographic evidence of degenerative joint disease. When evaluated functionally, physically, and radiographically, 73 per cent of the hips were sound. A 61 to 69 per cent success rate has been reported for a similar procedure done by other veterinarians.[170] With the high success rate of this surgery, there are no clinical reasons not to recommend it for young dogs with dysplastic hips. In addition to triple osteotomy, Chiari's technique for the treatment of human dysplastic hips has been applied to dogs.[171] The technique creates a new acetabulum by osteotomy.

The treatment of advanced hip dysplasia is essentially directed toward the degenerative joint disease. As such, the treatments listed in the discussion of degenerative joint disease are applicable. Femoral head ostectomies can be very effective in some dogs.[172–174] Dogs with intractable hip pain, but without significant disease in other joints or neurologic problems, are the best candidates. Although smaller dogs form more functional false joints, even large dogs can benefit from the surgery.[174] For dogs more than 38 to 45 lbs (18–20 kg), excision arthroplasty of the femoral head can be combined with the creation of a biceps femoris muscle sling.[175] Holt describes a cat with hip dysplasia that responded favorably to excision arthroplasty after a pectineus myotomy failed to give relief.[149]

The most attractive treatment for advanced hip dysplasia is total hip replacement.[176–180] Although this procedure is becoming practical from a technical aspect, the cost of the surgery has limited its use. The most common complication has been displacement of the prosthesis, while the most serious has been infection.

The ultimate control of hip dysplasia in dog populations has been by genetic selection of dogs for radiographically appearing normal hips. The Orthopedic Foundation for Animals evaluated [143, 181] hip radiographs from 151 breeds between 1974 and 1984.[182] The frequency of dysplasia varied from 0.6 per cent for borzois to 46.9 per cent for Saint Bernards. During this ten year period, a reduction in dysplasia was recorded for 27 breeds, no change in incidence in ten breeds, and an increased incidence in one breed (German shorthaired pointers). Among five popular breeds that showed significant reductions in hip dysplasia from base frequency (1966–1973), German shepherds had a reduction to 17.5 per cent, Old English sheepdogs to 23.1 per cent, rottweilers to 9.1 per cent, golden retrievers to 10.1 per cent, and Labrador retrievers to 6.8 per cent.[183]

SHOULDER DYSPLASIA

A condition resembling hip dysplasia has been described in the shoulder joints of dachshunds.[181, 183] The original report concerned 174 dachshunds with forelimb lameness and dysplastic changes in the scapula consisting of hypoplasia of the joint ends, flattening of the acetabula, and disturbances in the ossification of fusion centers in the supraglenoid tubercle and acetabular wall apophysis. The heads of the humeri were flattened, smaller than normal, and sloped caudoventrally. Luxation varied from partial to complete and degenerative joint disease was often quite severe and developed early in the course of the lameness. Post-mortem changes in 30 animals 5 months to 13 years of age showed disturbances in the fusion and ossification of the supraglenoid tubercle and the caudal acetabular apophysis and cartilage defects in the caudolateral joint surface.[183] These changes led to the formation of cartilage covered rims on the glenoid cavity and loose binding of the caudal acetabular apophysis to the joint surface by connective tissue. The humeral heads were deformed with overhanging calotte edges and cartilage erosions.

PATELLAR LUXATION

Patellar luxation is an orthopedic problem of varied etiology.[184] In cases of extreme valgus or varus deformities of the stifles, pressure by the quadriceps tendon is directed medially or laterally, depending on the character of the deformity. This maldirected tensile force will gradually pull the patella out of the trochlear groove. Such valgus or varus deformities can be congenital or can be acquired by virtue of femoral fractures that have healed with improper alignment. Traumatic luxations of the patella have also been described.[185]

The most common problem, however, is medial congenital patellar luxation occurring in small toy breeds of dogs.[184] This condition is infrequently seen in cats.[186, 187] The basic cause of congenital patellar luxation in small dogs is unknown. The trochlear ridge of the distal femur, which forms the patellar groove, appears unusually flattened. In addition. many of these dogs appear to have a degree of genu valgum. The disorder occurs as a spectrum, depending on the severity of the basic deformities,[184] and the deformities will often progress with time (Figure 120–37). In the mildest form the patella can be luxated with some difficulty by extending the stifle and pushing the patella medially while the pull of the quadriceps tendon remains nearly parallel to the trochlear groove. These dogs will become acutely lame when the patella luxates, but this lameness often lasts for only a few seconds or minutes, until the patella falls back into place. In more severe cases, the patella is pulled progressively more medially, the medial ridge of the trochlear groove becomes flattened, and the pull of the quadriceps tendon is directed more medially. To establish a straight line of motion between the quadriceps tendon and the tibial crest, and to keep the foot in a relatively normal position, the femur and tibia assume an S-shaped deformity. In the most severe cases the patella lies completely medial to the hypoplastic trochlear groove, the tibial crest is displaced medially, and there is prominent deformation of the distal femur and proximal tibia (Figure 120–38).

The treatment of patellar luxation depends mainly on the severity of the condition.[184] Many toy breeds with patellas that dislocate only occasionally can be treated with surgical procedures designed to reinforce the lateral ligamentous attachments to patella. In more severe cases this is accompanied by surgically deepening the trochlear groove. Repositioning of the tibial crest is also done in more severe cases. Osteotomies of the femur and tibia may also be needed to help correct malalignments in extreme cases.

ASEPTIC NECROSIS OF THE FEMORAL HEAD

Aseptic necrosis of the femoral head (Legg-Calvé-Perthes disease) frequently occurs without an apparent predisposing cause in adolescent dogs of toy and small breeds.[188] In breeds such as toy poodles, genetic factors may be involved in disease expression.[189] For some undetermined reason, a major portion of the blood supply to the capital epiphysis of the femur is compromised, and the ischemic portion undergoes necrosis (Figure 120–39). Aseptic necrosis can also occur following intracapsular fractures through the femoral neck or physis.

Following disruption of the blood supply to the femoral head, for whatever reason, the affected area of epiphyseal spongiosa undergoes necrosis while the overlying cartilage, which receives its nutrition from the synovial fluid, remains viable. The body tries to repair the defect with granulation tissue and new cancellous bone arising from the resulting fibro-osseous response (Figure 120–40). Unfortunately, the amount of bony repair is often insignificant or occurs too late to prevent collapse of the unsupported articular cartilage. Collapse of the femoral head affects the congruity of the articular surfaces and predisposes the joint to secondary joint disease.

Necrosis of the femoral head is manifested by slight to severe lameness. Since there is little likelihood of spontaneous resolution, femoral head ostectomy is the accepted treatment.[174, 190, 191]

An aseptic necrosis of the humeral head has been observed in a toy poodle.[192] The condition resembled its counterpart in the femoral head.

Arthropathies Due to Inborn Errors of Metabolism

HEMOPHILIA A

Lameness is one of the most common complaints of humans and dogs with congenital coagulation defects. In fact, factor 8 deficiency, or hemophilia A, of the dog can lead to an arthropathy indistinguishable from that occurring in hemophiliac humans.[193] Hemophilia A also occurs in cats, but much less is known about associated joint disease in this species.

The arthropathy of hemophilia A is caused by chronic hemorrhage into the joint, which is induced by clinical or subclinical trauma. Obviously, therefore, larger

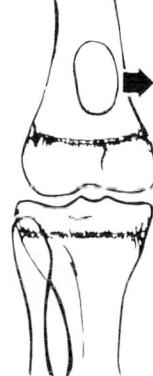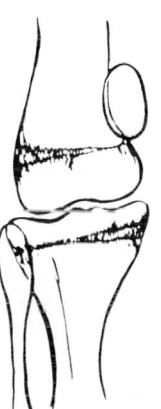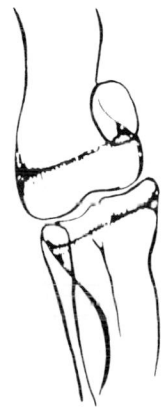

FIGURE 120–37. Medial patellar luxation in the dog. Medial patellar luxation in the puppy leads to abnormal growth in the physis on either side of the joint. The joint space is more angulated and secondary joint disease with cruciate and collateral ligament damage can result.

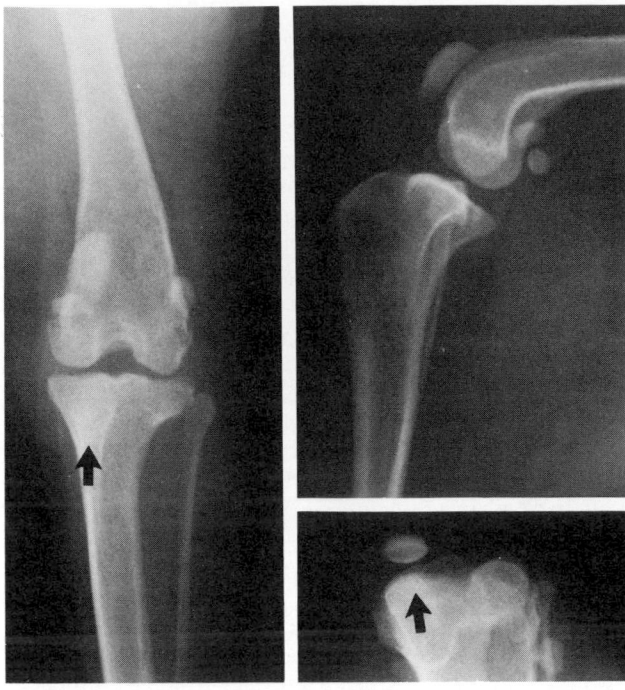

FIGURE 120–38. Caudocranial, lateral, and "skyline" projections of the stifle joint that show the medial displacement of the attachment on the tibia of the patellar ligament. The lateral and skyline projections show the failure of the trochlea to form normally.

weight-bearing joints such as the elbows and stifles are more likely to be involved, and larger and more active dogs will have more problems than smaller, less active dogs. The effusion of blood into the joint cavity resulting from synovial or subsynovial hemorrhage provokes an acute inflammatory reaction. The synovial membrane thickens and undergoes villous hypertrophy, and there is hyperplasia of the intimal layer and infiltration of lymphocytes, macrophages, and plasma cells. The reaction subsides after several days to weeks, but each subsequent hemorrhagic episode leads to further synovial fibrosis and hemosiderosis. However, the most significant sites of injury are the articular cartilage and subchondral bone. Injury to the articular cartilage is caused by granulation tissue covering the articular cartilage that arises from the synovium and from the subchondral bone. Synovial fluid may be frankly bloody during bouts of hemorrhage or xanthochromic with excess numbers of macrophages at other times.

PANOSTEITIS

Panosteitis is covered in detail in Chapter 121 and is mentioned here only because it is important in the differential diagnosis of lameness in adolescent dogs. Panosteitis is a disorder of endosteal ossification in the shafts of long bones.[194] It tends to occur in the same breeds and in the same age group as osteochondrosis, ununited anconeal and coronoid processes, and hip dysplasia. It is particularly common in German shepherd dogs and Doberman pinschers.

Panosteitis often occurs in dogs with von Willebrand's disease, a blood coagulation defect caused by a deficiency of functional factor 8 and abnormalities in platelet

aggregation. This association was first described by Dodds,[195] and a majority of the cases of panosteitis seen by the authors have shown the same relationship. Von Willebrand's disease in dogs is present in 5 to 20 per cent of dogs in some breeds and is often subclinical. The abnormal factor 8 and platelet aggregation persists through life although clinical signs tend to disappear with age.[195]

MUCOPOLYSACCHARIDOSIS

Arylsulfatase B enzyme deficiency (Maroteaux-Lamy syndrome) has been identified as an autosomal recessive trait in Siamese cats.[196] Hurler's syndrome, caused by a deficiency of α-L-iduronidase enzyme, has also been identified in a cat.[197] A dog with Morquio's syndrome (β-glucuronidase deficiency) has also been reported.[198] Animals with these disorders have in common an inability to properly metabolize aminoglycans, such as heparan, chondroitin and keratan sulfates. As such, they will often manifest abnormalities in tissues rich in such substances, e.g., cartilage, connective tissue, cornea.

MULTICENTRIC PERIARTICULAR CALCINOSIS

Ellison and Norrdin described a twelve-week-old Vizsla puppy with progressive lameness and periarticular

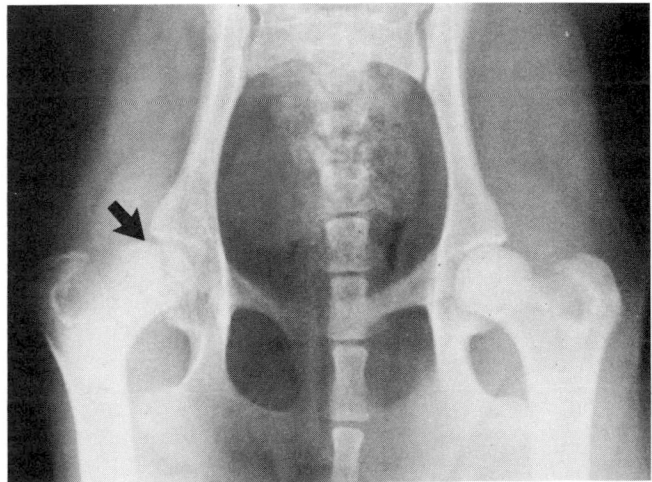

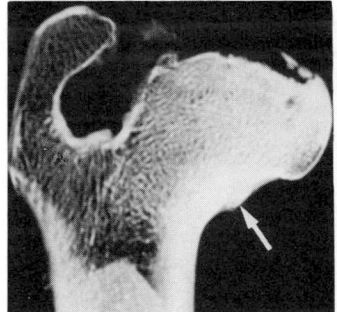
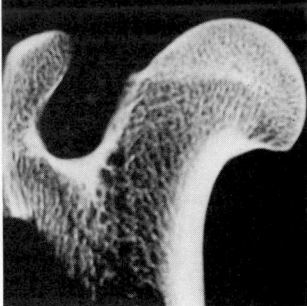

FIGURE 120–39. Ventrodorsal radiograph of tne pèlvis shows the fragmentation within the femoral head typical of aseptic necrosis of the femoral head or Legg-Calve-Perthe's disease (black arrow). Radiographs of thin bone sections show the fragmentation and collapse of the affected femoral head and the compensatory thickening of the femoral neck (white arrow). The figure on the lower right shows the normal opposite hip.

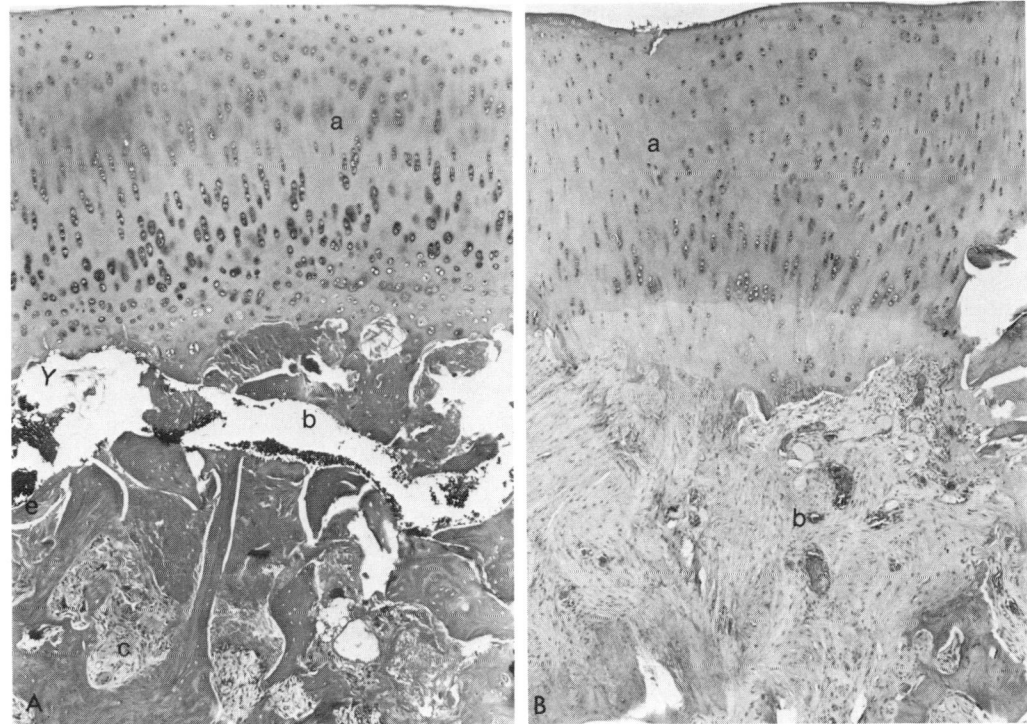

FIGURE 120–40. Aseptic necrosis of the femoral head. *A,* Acute lesion shows normal articular cartilage (a), necrosis and hemorrhage in the subchondral bone and adjacent epiphyseal spongiosa (b). Granulation tissue (c) arises in the marrow spaces along the border of the infarct. Healing lesion *(B)* shows abnormal articular cartilage (a), maturing granulation tissue replacing the area of bone necrosis (b), and attempts at the intramembranous bone formation in the fibrous connective tissue response.

calcinosis of all diarthrodial joints.[199] Although no definitive data were available, it was suggested that the disorder was due to a renal tubular defect (presumably in calcium-phosphorus transport). A Vizsla with a similar syndrome, and with a proven tubular defect in phosphorus transport, has been seen by the authors.

Dietary Arthropathies

NUTRITIONAL SECONDARY HYPERPARATHYROIDISM

Secondary hyperparathyroidism and a rickets-like syndrome has been seen in cats fed diets composed mainly of beef heart.[200, 201] Besides other skeletal lesions, major limb joints may undergo ankylosis of opposing joint surfaces.

HYPERVITAMINOSIS A

Hypervitaminosis A, a condition caused by consuming large amounts of raw liver, has been described as a naturally occurring entity of cats.[202] It is characterized by a bridging exostosis of the cervical and thoracic vertebrae and periarticular ankylosis of limb joints, especially the elbows. It is mentioned here because this disorder is frequently misdiagnosed in cats that actually have degenerative joint disease.

Neoplastic Arthropathies

PRIMARY NEOPLASTIC ARTHROPATHIES

Synovial Cell Sarcoma. Synovial cell sarcoma, or synovioma, is by far the most common primary joint tumor in animals. These tumors occur most frequently in middle-aged dogs (six to eight years old).[203–205] A slow growing synovial sarcoma has been diagnosed in a two and one-half-year-old dog with lameness of two years' duration.[206] Synoviomas also occur in cats.[207] Synovial cell sarcomas in dogs and cats typically involve a major limb joint, usually the stifle or the elbow joint. They present early as a lameness, at which time radiographic changes may be absent.[206] With time, however, bone surrounding the joint becomes quite lytic. Four dogs with blastomas of the stifle were treated initially for ruptured anterior cruciate ligaments.[208] Synovial sarcomas are characterized microscopically by the presence of varying proportions of two intermingled cellular components, a pleomorphic synovioblastic or epithelioid component and a spindle-cell or fibroblastic cellular component. Synovial sarcomas associated with tendon sheaths are probably just as common but are usually diagnosed as undifferentiated sarcomas of the deeper soft tissue.

Synovial cell sarcomas tend to grow rapidly and spread slowly by metastases to local lymph nodes. They tend to spread aggressively at the site of origin, and the accepted treatment is limb amputation. Tilmant and associates reported the successful treatment of a synovial cell sarcoma in a six-year-old chow chow with 20 mg of doxorubicin HCl IV every three weeks for seven administrations combined with cyclophosphamide orally at a dosage of 50 mg/m² for four consecutive days of each week for seven weeks.[204]

Osteogenic Sarcoma. The osteogenic sarcoma, or osteosarcoma, is a frequent cause of lameness in large and giant breeds of dogs and rarely invades through subchondral bone into the adjacent joint. It is important in the differential diagnosis of lameness in giant breeds of dogs. Osteosarcomas are discussed further in Chapter 121.

Villonodular Synovitis. Villonodular synovitis is a quasi-neoplastic or inflammatory disorder (possibly secondary to chronic hemorrhage and trauma) that has been most commonly observed in humans. A suspected case of villonodular synovitis has been reported in an eight-year-old male Labrador retriever.[209] The dog was examined because of recurring hip pain in the right hind limb. Radiography revealed osteolytic cysts of the right acetabulum and femoral head and neck. An excision arthroplasty was performed; the synovial membrane appeared yellow, thickened, and proliferative. The synovial fluid showed a mild inflammatory exudation. Villous hyperplasia of the synovium was pronounced, and the underlying tissues contained many hemosiderin deposits. A mild inflammatory infiltrate consisting of plasma cells and polymorphonuclear neutrophils was present. Six months later a similar lytic lesion appeared in the left hip joint, necessitating a second excision arthroplasty of the femoral head and neck. Similar synovial fluid, gross, and histologic changes were found. The only feature of etiologic significance was that the dog had been treated for hip dysplasia with bilateral pectineus muscle tenectomies twelve months prior to the time that the first hip became involved.

METASTATIC NEOPLASTIC ARTHROPATHIES

Lymphosarcoma. Tumors rarely metastasize to the joint, except for the arthropathy that occurs in some cats with lymphosarcoma.[210]

INFLAMMATORY JOINT DISEASE

This major form of joint disease is characterized by inflammatory changes in the synovial membrane and synovial fluid, and by systemic signs of illness such as fever, leukocytosis, malaise, anorexia, and hyperfibrinogenemia. The etiology of inflammatory joint disease of animals is diverse and includes both infectious and noninfectious causes.

Infectious Arthritis

BACTERIAL ARTHRITIS

Bacteria may gain entrance to the joint through penetrating wounds,[211] from contiguous sites of infection in bone or soft tissue, or from the bloodstream. Surgical contamination and non-sterile injections into the synovial cavity are other sources of sepsis. Infection via penetrating wounds is much more frequent in large animals than in dogs and cats. Grass awns, especially from foxtail barley, may penetrate the skin and subcutaneous tissue and enter the joint.

Bacteria may also gain entrance to the joints from infectious foci within the blood vascular system itself, e.g., heart valves or the umbilical vein. Omphalophlebitis, or umbilical vein infection, is common in both puppies and kittens. In many cases, this infection will spread via the bloodstream and is carried to the synovial lining, which has a rich blood supply and contains phagocytic cells that trap the bacteria. Omphalophlebitis in kittens often results when the queen chews off the umbilical cord flush with the abdominal wall. Normally, the umbilical cord is left several centimeters long and dries to form an impenetrable barrier. If it is chewed off too short, infection with direct access to the bloodstream occurs in the umbilical remnant. In kittens, the usual offending organism is *Pasteurella*, which normally inhabits the queen's oral cavity.

Bacterial septicemias are seen in puppies and kittens from sources other than omphalophlebitis. Streptococcal pharyngitis with abscessation of the retropharyngeal lymph nodes and septicemia occurs in some puppies during the first two weeks of life. Queens or bitches with post-parturient uterine or mammary gland infections can infect their young shortly after birth. If this leads to a systemic infection, joint abscessation may occur.

Subacute bacterial endocarditis occurs in both dogs and cats and is occasionally associated with a septic arthritis.[212-213] It is more common in dogs, probably because dogs have a higher incidence of predisposing congenital or acquired heart problems. Dogs also have a higher incidence of oral, genitourinary, and skin infections, which are frequent sources of bacteria.

Bacterial septicemias are common in older dogs, but uncommon in cats. Such systemic infections are frequently associated with septic arthritis. In older animals, the most common source of infection is the genitourinary tract, followed by the skin, oral cavity, and respiratory tract. Cystitis, pyelonephritis, prostatitis, pneumonia, pyodermas, and tooth infections can all be accompanied by septicemia at times. In dogs, infection of the disc spaces (discospondylitis) is often associated with septic arthritis, bacteremia, and bacteriuria. Systemic spread of infection may be potentiated in older animals by situations brought about by debilitating cancers, immunosuppressive drug therapy, neutropenias, or loss of bowel integrity during fulminating gastrointestinal infection.

Organisms commonly involved in joint infection include staphylococci, streptococci, *Erysipelothrix*, *Corynebacteria*, coliforms and *Pasteurella*, *Salmonella*, and occasionally *Brucella*.[212, 214, 215] The type of organism involved in the joint infection has some clinical significance. *Staphylococci* and some coliforms will cause rapid destruction of articular cartilage, whereas organisms such as *Erysipelothrix* and streptococci may be present in the joint without causing significant cartilage damage. As a rule, organisms that cause severe cartilage damage also cause toxic or degenerative changes in neutrophils present in the synovial fluid.

Septic arthritis, regardless of cause, is more apt to occur in giant or sporting breeds than in smaller dogs and males more frequently than females. The pattern of joint disease is more likely to be monarticular or pauciarticular (two to five joints) than polyarticular, and larger joints (shoulders, elbows, hips, and stifles) are more apt to be involved than smaller joints. Infection is more likely to localize in joints previously damaged by some other disease process such as degenerative joint disease. Septic arthritis will often be painful on palpation, and redness and swelling of the overlying skin and soft tissue may be present.

Synovial fluid from septic joints is frequently bloody, which differentiates it from most noninfectious joint disorders. The fluid contains large numbers of neutrophils, but the absolute count, although high, will overlap with the neutrophil counts in synovial fluid from nonseptic, inflamed joints. The presence of toxic, ruptured, and degranulated neutrophils should make one suspicious of a bacterial infection. As mentioned previously, however, not all types of bacteria are equally proficient at inducing such toxic changes.

The earliest radiographic findings of bacterial arthritis are often missed because of delay in presenting the animal for radiographic examination. These early findings are thickened synovial membrane, distended joint capsule with a displacement of adjacent fascial planes, and a slight widening of the joint space due to joint effusion. Radiolucent intra-articular shadows due to intra-articular fat pads may disappear, owing to the accumulation of exudate within the joints. Although radiographic changes such as this are often present in the early stages, the diagnosis should not be discarded when radiographic changes are not detected. If clinical signs are suggestive, a joint tap should be performed.

A radiographic finding more commonly noted in the later stages is a fine, faintly identifiable, periosteal proliferation on the bones adjacent to the joint space. This type of reactive periostitis is not to be confused with the prominent, better-defined, periarticular bony spurs that develop in degenerative joint disease or following trauma. Aspiration of the joint at this time is still necessary to reach a positive diagnosis. Following the period of early soft tissue swelling and inflammation, and dependent on the organism involved, the process expands with destruction of the articular cartilage and resulting loss of width of the joint space. Narrowing of the joint space is often unappreciated, because of the unwillingness of the animal to bear weight on the leg. If the disease is not controlled, it quickly leads to an osteomyelitis in the adjacent bones and a widening of the joint space as it fills with debris and exudate. It is difficult to attach time intervals from the time of onset for the various stages of bacterial arthritis. This is because of differences in the pathogenicity of the organisms, the manner of inoculation, host immunity, and the type of superimposed treatment that may delay (inappropriate or inadequate antibiotic therapy) or hasten (immunosuppressive drugs) the development of the pathologic process.

Complications of infectious arthritis include osteomyelitis, fibrous or bony ankylosis, and secondary joint disease. An osteomyelitis is present as soon as the articular plate is breached and the infectious process enters the subchondral bone (Figure 120–41). This compounds the severity of the disease and makes the prognosis more guarded. If the articular cartilage has been damaged, fibrotic or bony ankylosis can follow. This is a logical consequence, because the destruction of the cartilage exposes the subchondral bone and simulates a condition like that of a fracture. An abscess frequently forms within the exudate and debris, preventing bony fusion from occurring across the joint space. In these cases, reactive bone bridges the joint, leaving a radiolucent cavity around the abscess.

Dependent on the severity of the arthritis, a certain amount of articular damage is present at the time the infection is brought under control. The rate at which a secondary joint disease develops subsequently depends on the severity of the destructive process, the degree of use of the joint, and other factors such as the weight or conformation of the animal.

The treatment of bacterial arthritis is dependent on the isolation and identification of the organism, and on the determination of antibiotic sensitivities. If bacteria cannot be cultured from the joint, positive isolation from the blood or urine should be considered representative of the infection in the joints. Whenever possible, bactericidal antibiotics should be used. Most antibiotics will penetrate the vascular bed of an inflamed joint, so systemic treatment is usually effective. Local infusions of antibiotics can be used when a single joint is involved. In this situation, antibiotics are most effective if they are infused almost continuously and associated with drainage. Generally, antibiotics are given for periods of two weeks or more after the signs of infection have disappeared. In the case of bacterial endocarditis, antibiotic treatment may have to be continued longer.

BACTERIAL L-FORMS

L-forms are cell-wall–deficient bacteria. They are differentiated from *Mycoplasma* by their ability to revert to their parent cell-wall state with time in culture. The formation of L-forms is aided by the use of cell-wall directed antibiotics or host immune responses. Although they have been cultured from a wide range of disease processes in both man and animals, it has not usually been possible to fulfill Koch's postulates. An L-form of *Nocardia asteroides* was isolated from a dog with long standing immunosuppressive drug and antibiotic unresponsive polyarthritis.[216] A bacterial L-form has been associated with a distinct disease syndrome of cats. This disease is usually manifested by fistulating subcutaneous wounds, which sometimes spread to joints hematogenously or by extension. The source of infection is often from the bites of other cats. It is virtually impossible to isolate the causative agent, although it can be seen by electron microscopy and serially passaged in a pure form from cat to cat. It is sensitive to the antibiotic tetracycline.

MYCOPLASMAL ARTHRITIS

A mycoplasmal arthritis can result from the systemic spread of organisms from localized sites of inapparent

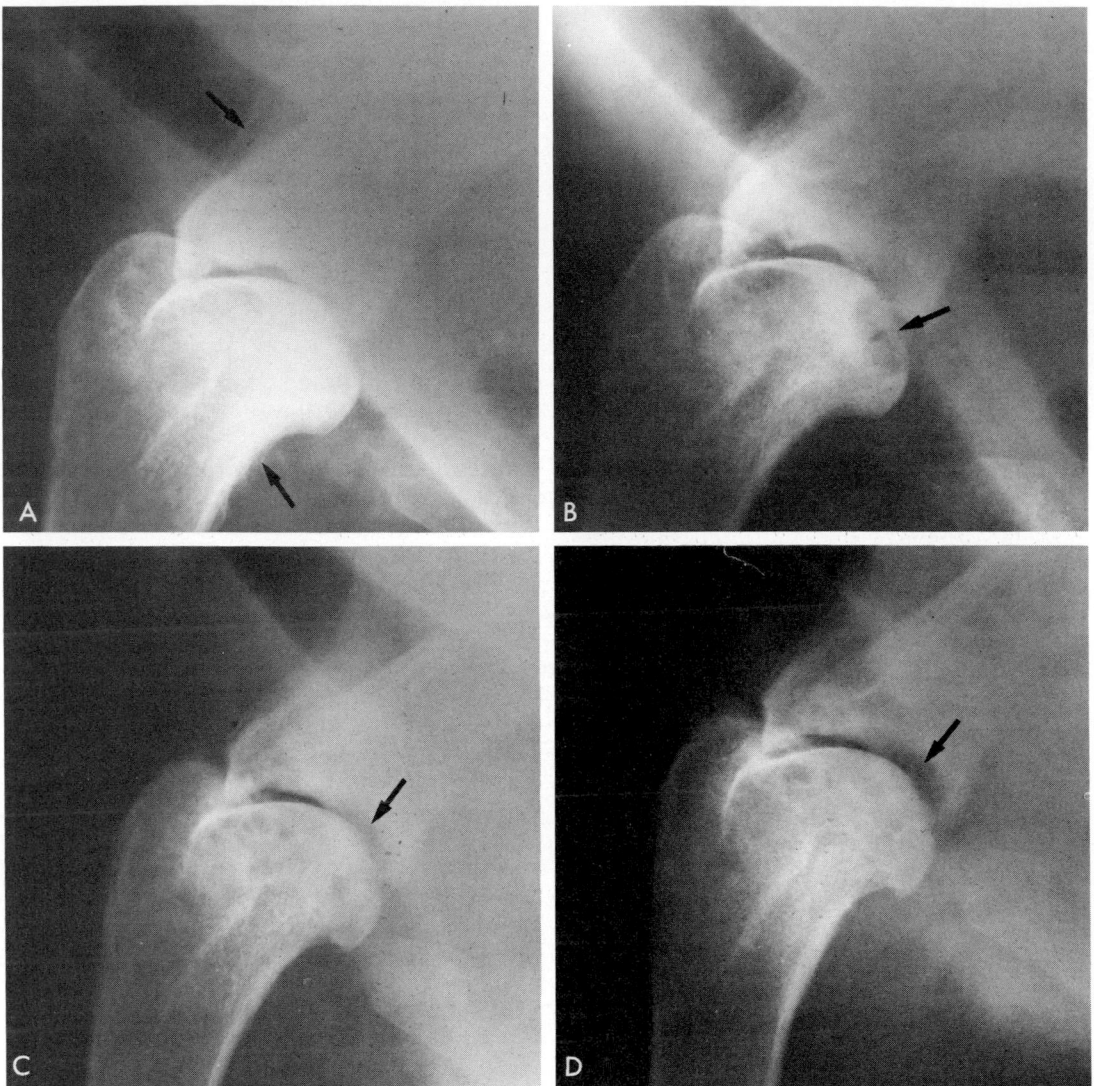

FIGURE 120–41. Lateral radiographs of the shoulder joint of an eight-year-old male German shepherd dog with progressive infectious arthritis and osteomyelitis, characterized by periosteal new bone response (arrow) and destructive lesions within the humeral head (arrow) and glenoid cavity. Radiographs are made (A) on the day of the first examination, (B) two months, (C) one year, and (D) 16 months after the first examination.

infection in the respiratory passages, oropharynx, conjunctival membranes, or urogenital tract. Although common in food animals, systemic spread of *Mycoplasma* leading to arthritis is uncommon in both the dog and cat. The authors have seen only three such cases in dogs and cats. A generalized mycoplasmal polyarthritis was observed in a dog undergoing chemotherapy for lymphosarcoma. A generalized mycoplasmal polyarthritis was also observed in two aged cats being treated for severely disseminated cancer. A mycoplasmal polyarthritis has also been reported in two older immunocompromised cats.[217, 218] *Mycoplasma* has also been isolated from a five month old greyhound that developed polyarthritis one month before death.[219]

RICKETTSIAL ARTHRITIS

Rickettsia and *Rickettsia*-like organisms have been increasingly associated with a nonerosive type polyarthritis in dogs. Perhaps the most severe of these diseases is Rocky Mountain spotted fever, a disorder mainly of the wooded regions extending through the middle of the United States from Colorado to the eastern seaboard.[220] The disease is caused by *R. rickettsii*, and is harbored and transmitted mainly by the ticks *Dermacentor andersoni* and *D. variabilis*. Related species of *Rickettsia* and appropriate tick vectors are also found in many similar regions of the world. The disease is associated with rapid dissemination of *Rickettsia* from the site of the tick bite to reticuloendothelial tissues throughout the body, causing vascular destruction. Early clinical signs include fever and edema of the lips, sheath, scrotum, and ears. This is followed by petechial and ecchymotic hemorrhage of ocular, oral, and genital mucous membranes in one-fifth of the cases. Dogs surviving the acute stages of illness may develop generalized central nervous system signs, uveitis, necrosis of previously edematous tissues, and polyarthritis.

A polyarthritis has been an important clinical manifestation of ehrlichiosis infection in dogs in Missouri and Tennessee.[221, 222] Unlike typical *E. canis* infections, inclusion bodies were seen in neutrophils. Serology for *E.*

canis was positive, however. Antibody titers to other ehrlichial agents such as *E. equi*, *E. risticii*, and *E. sennetsu* were negative in those dogs that were tested. In one group of dogs the polyarthritis was acute in onset, while in another animal it was chronic.[221, 222] Thrombocytopenia was observed in one animal,[222] and all responded to tetracycline therapy.

SPIROCHETAL ARTHRITIS

Lyme disease, a spirochetal infection of man and animals caused by *Borrelia burgdorferi*, has been reported in dogs in a number of regions of the world.[223, 224] It is most common in wooded mountainous and hilly areas where the vector tick *Ixodes dammini* is found. The infection is often chronic in humans and is not unlike persistent low-grade syphilis, with vague joint and neurologic signs being the most common clinical symptoms. The infection in dogs is often asymptomatic, as evidenced by a high rate of seropositivity in endemic areas.[224] Dogs usually present with a transient monarticular or pauciarticular arthritis.[223] Joint fluid contains high numbers of polymorphonuclear neutrophils. Most dogs are between one and four years of age and present in the fall to spring season of the year.[223] Spirochetes are difficult to culture or identify in synovial fluid. The diagnosis is usually made by demonstrating antibody titers of 1:512 or greater.[223] The presence of ticks on the animals, geographic areas, and age at onset are also helpful clues. Care must be taken in interpreting titers, however, because there is considerable overlap in titers between asymptomatic and diseased dogs from the same areas.[223] Indeed, the failure to identify the organism in a large percentage of suspected cases in one study indicates the difficulty in differentiating dogs with Lyme arthritis from those that may have been immunologically mediated.[224]

Because of the difficulty in differentiating some rickettsial and spirochetal arthritides from immune-mediated joint disorders, some clinicians will treat animals with bacterially sterile polyarthritis with tetracycline for five to seven days prior to switching them to immunosuppressive drug regimens. Even though rickettsial and spirochetal arthritides are relatively uncommon compared to immune-mediated joint disorders, this practice has some merit in endemic areas. If the animals begin to respond to tetracycline during the initial treatment course, tetracycline is continued for as long as improvement continues. If there is no response to tetracycline therapy, or if the disease only responds temporarily (immune-mediated diseases are often cyclical), then immunosuppressive drug therapy can be initiated with some confidence.

VIRAL ARTHRITIS

A fleeting and sometimes persistent arthropathy is a symptom of many acute viral diseases of man. It usually occurs in the postconvalescent period following mumps, coxsackie virus, or adenovirus infections.[225] Because animals show signs of pain only when the joint inflammation is relatively severe, the degree to which arthropathy complicates acute viral diseases in animals is unknown.

A sterile, usually generalized inflammatory joint disorder is seen commonly in younger dogs from six to ten months of age. The dogs are stiff, lame, and febrile. The arthritis may last for several days or persist for up to a month or more. The pattern and age of disease resemble human postviral arthritides. Synovial fluid from these dogs is thin, cloudy, and often yellow-tinged, and contains large numbers of normal appearing neutrophils. It is sterile for microorganisms. If the condition persists for more than several days, a week or two on corticosteroids will usually hasten its disappearance.

A fleeting stiffness, soreness, and lameness with high fever has been recognized by the authors in kittens 6 to 12 weeks of age.[226] The kittens will be sick for two to four days and then will recover, and may demonstrate pain when muscles and joints are manipulated. The condition is caused by two or more strains of calicivirus, which can be recovered readily from the blood during the acute phase of illness.[226] At least one strain that has been studied was not neutralized by antibodies produced by the more commonly used vaccine strains. It can also occur following vaccination with live calicivirus vaccines. Synovial fluid from kittens with this disease will contain an elevated number of macrophages, many of which contain phagocytosed neutrophils.

A transient, sometimes protracted, sterile inflammatory polyarthritis occurs as an uncommon sequela to vaccination in both dogs and cats. This postvaccinal reaction has been usually associated with live virus vaccines. It has not been possible to say which component of the multivalent vaccines generally used was responsible for reaction. Postvaccinal arthritis has been described as a rare complication of measles and smallpox immunizations of humans.[227] The arthritis is not usually treated unless it persists for more than five days, in which case corticosteroid therapy is instituted.

A mild to moderately severe synovitis has been observed by the author in cats with the effusive form of feline infectious peritonitis (FIP). In one instance, a cat presented with fever, lameness, and inflammatory joint fluid. It developed classical peritoneal effusions several days later. Synovial fluid from a number of cats with feline infectious peritonitis has been somewhat yellow and cloudy and contained increased numbers of polymorphonuclear neutrophils. Although the synovial inflammation appears to be relatively severe in some cats with FIP, most show no symptoms of lameness or stiffness.

FUNGAL ARTHRITIS

Fungal arthritis is infrequent in dogs and cats. It can occur as an extension of a fungal osteomyelitis or as a primary granulomatous synovitis, with the former occurring more commonly. *Coccidioides immitis*, *Blastomyces dermatitidis*, and *Filobasidiella (Cryptococcus) neoformans* are the most frequently encountered organisms. Desert rheumatism, an arthropathy that accompanies the primary respiratory stage of coccidioidomycosis of man, has also been seen in dogs. An arthritis caused by *Sporothrix schenckii* has been observed in a dog with a tibiotarsal swelling.[228] *Aspergillus fumigatus* has been isolated from an arthritis and osteomyelitis in a dog.[229] Aspergillosis in its visceral or nasal forms is particularly common in German shepherds.

PROTOZOAL ARTHRITIS

Visceral leishmaniasis, caused by *Leishmania donovani*, is a chronic systemic reticuloendothelial proliferative disease of man and some species of animals. The dog is a principal reservoir for the organism in many of the endemic areas in the Mediterranean, Africa, Asia, and South America.[230] The predominant presenting signs of the disease in dogs are fever, malaise, weight loss, dermatopathy, and polyarthritis.[230] Generalized lymphadenopathy and hepatosplenomegaly are also seen. The synovial membrane is infiltrated by large numbers of macrophages filled with leishmanial bodies.

Noninfectious Arthritis

The noninfectious arthritides of animals can be classified into several groups depending on the nature and etiology of the disorder.

ARTHRITIS OF APPARENT IMMUNOLOGIC CAUSE

Deforming or Erosive Arthritis. RHEUMATOID ARTHRITIS OF DOGS. Canine rheumatoid arthritis is a well-documented clinical entity.[231–234] It is an uncommon condition, occurring at an incidence of approximately two per 25,000 dogs examined at the authors' hospital. This disorder occurs mainly in small or toy breeds of dogs as young as eight months and as old as eight years of age.

Canine rheumatoid arthritis is manifested initially as a shifting lameness with soft tissue swelling around involved joints. Within several weeks or months, the disease localizes in particular joints and characteristic radiographic signs develop. Joint involvement is more severe in the carpal and tarsal joints, although in individual dogs, the elbow, stifle, shoulder, and hip joints may show similar radiographic signs. Involvement of the apophyseal joints and costovertebral articulations rarely progresses to the point of causing radiographic changes. In exceptional cases, however, involvement of the vertebral articulations only can occur. The disease is often accompanied by fever, malaise, anorexia, and lymphadenopathy in the earlier stages.

The earliest radiographic changes consist of soft tissue swelling and loss of trabecular bone density in the area of the joint. Lucent cyst-like areas are frequently seen in the subchondral bone. The prominent lesion is a progressive destruction of subchondral bone in the more central areas as well as marginally at the attachment of the synovium.[234, 235] Both narrowing and widening of the joint spaces are identified radiographically as a result of cartilage erosion and destruction of subchondral bone (Figure 120–42). Subluxation, luxation, and deformation occur most frequently in the carpal, tarsal, and phalangeal joints and occasionally in the elbow and stifle joints.

Fibrous ankylosis can occur in advanced cases, particularly in the intercarpal and intertarsal joint spaces. Soft tissue calcification and atrophy accompany disuse osteoporosis and other radiographic findings.

Hemograms are either normal or reflect the generalized inflammatory process with a leukocytosis, neutrophilia, and hyperfibrinogenemia.[234] Serum electrophoresis will often show hypoalbuminemia and variable elevation in α-2 and gamma globulins. Unlike the situation in humans, serologic abnormalities in canine rheumatoid arthritis are often absent. Rheumatoid factor is present in comparatively low titer in only about one quarter of the cases.[234] Moreover, they may be present in a number of other disease conditions totally unrelated to rheumatoid arthritis. LE-cell preparations and fluorescent antinuclear antibody tests are usually negative.

Synovial fluid changes are indicative of an inflammatory synovitis, with an elevated total cell count, a high proportion of neutrophils in the synovial fluid cell population, and a variable decrease in the quality of the mucin clot. Ragocytes (neutrophils that have ingested immune complexes), as described in human rheumatoid arthritis, are not usually seen. A characteristic finding of canine rheumatoid arthritis is the presence in synovial fluid of mononuclear cells containing IgG, with only occasional cells containing C3 protein.[234] These mononuclear cells may be producing the immunoglobulin or ingesting it from the synovial fluid.

The characteristic pathologic lesions consist of a villous hyperplasia of the synovial membrane, lymphoid and plasma cell infiltrates in the synovium, and erosion of articular cartilage at the margins of the joint (Figure 120–43A). The dense lymphoid and plasma cell infiltrate in the synovium (Figure 120–43B) and the subchondral erosions differentiate this disease from the synovitis seen in the nonerosive types of arthritis, which will be discussed in the following section. The erosion of the articular cartilage at the margins of affected joints occurs as a result of two pathologic processes, i.e., granulation tissue from an inflamed synovium either extends across the articular surface as a pannus or undermines the cartilage and subchondral bone. In the central regions of the joint, cartilage destruction is caused by a pannus arising from granulation tissue in the underlying marrow cavity (Figure 120–43C). Ankylosis in advanced lesions is not uncommon in the intercarpal and intertarsal joints (Figure 120–43D).

The pathogenesis of this disease in the dog is unknown. It is considered to be immunologic in nature because bacteria, viruses, *Mycoplasma,* or *Chlamydia* cannot be cultured from the affected joints, and because it responds to immunosuppressive drug therapy. Whether the etiology of the canine disease is identical to that of human rheumatoid arthritis remains to be established.

Canine rheumatoid arthritis responds only temporarily to systemic corticosteroids. There is an initial response, but this cannot be sustained even with high dosages. Aspirin has no appreciable therapeutic benefits in the authors' hands, probably because the disease is much more severe and rapidly progressive in dogs than in man. If the condition is recognized before severe joint damage occurs, it can usually be arrested with

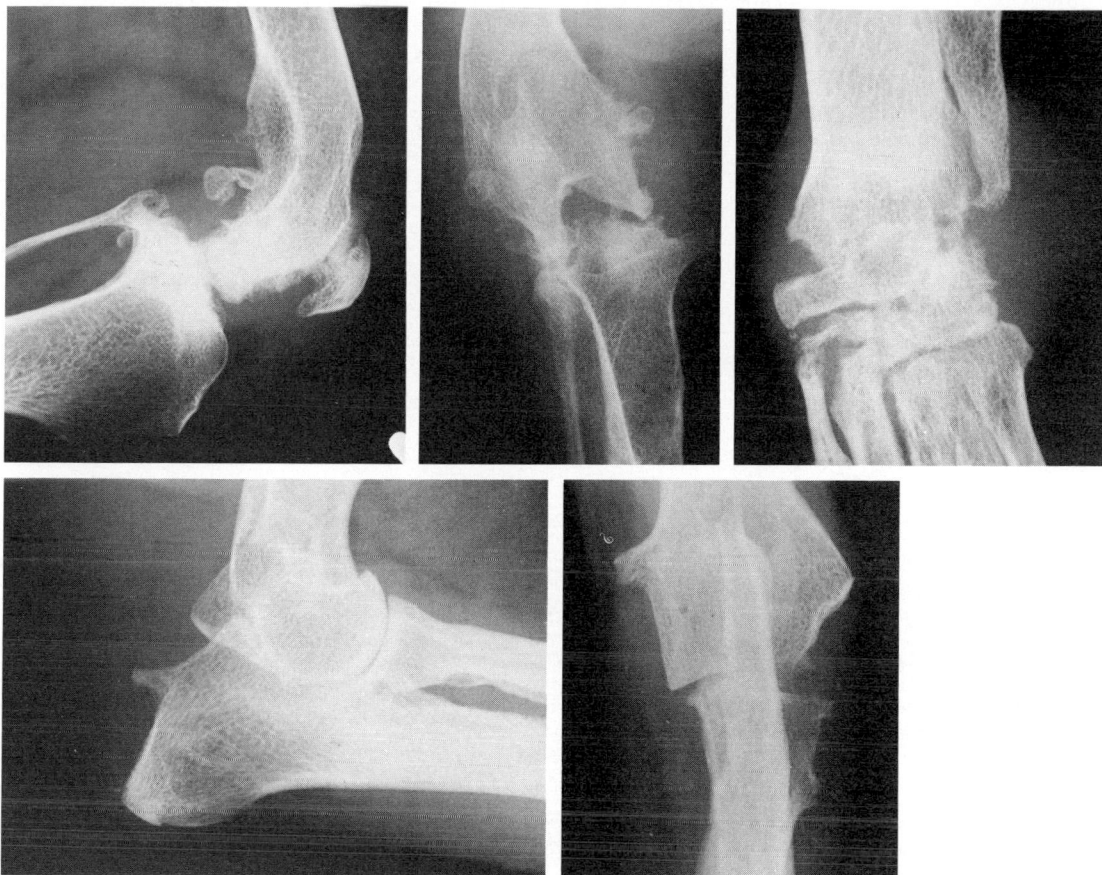

FIGURE 120–42. Radiographs of multiple joints of a female Welsh Corgi with a one-year history of lameness. The soft tissue swelling, periarticular subchondral erosions, formation of cystlike subchondral lucencies and subluxation and deformity of the joints are typical for noninfectious erosive (rheumatoid) arthritis of the dog.

cyclophosphamide and prednisolone given in combination. This type of therapy will be covered in detail in the discussion of drug therapy of immune-mediated arthritides. In dogs with advanced deformities, immunosuppressive drug therapy may have to be combined with arthrodesis of selected joints. Arthrodesis is not warranted if the disease process cannot first be successfully halted with drug therapy.

POLYARTHRITIS OF GREYHOUNDS. An erosive polyarthritis of the greyhound has been described in different parts of the world.[236, 237] The disease appears in animals from 3 to 30 months of age and most frequently attacks the proximal interphalangeal, carpal, tarsal, elbow, and stifle joints. The shoulder, hip, and atlanto-occipital joints are less frequently involved. A tenosynovitis may be an accompanying feature. The synovial membrane is edematous and hyperemic in the early course of the disease, and may be covered with a fine layer of fibrin. The synovial fluid is cloudy and yellowish, and often contains fibrin tags. In later stages, a lymphocyte and plasma cell infiltrate is seen in the synovial lining. Peripheral lymph nodes are enlarged and hyperactive. Pannus formation and marginal subchondral erosions are seen to a limited extent. Destruction of articular cartilage is accelerating in some joints but often is not associated with pannus formation. Gross deformities and radiographic changes are not as apparent as those seen in canine rheumatoid arthritis but appear more

pronounced than those described for nonerosive joint disease.

Mycoplasmal and bacterial isolations have usually been unsuccessful and dogs are serologically negative for *Erysipelothrix* and *Chlamydia*. Recently, however, *Mycoplasma spumans* was isolated from a young greyhound with polyarthritis.[219] The significance of this single isolate from a polyarthritis of greyhounds remains to be determined. Although no detailed discussion is available on therapy, this polyarthritis should be treated in the same manner as idiopathic nonerosive polyarthritis of dogs, which it most closely resembles.

FELINE PROGRESSIVE POLYARTHRITIS (EROSIVE FORM)

One form of feline chronic progressive polyarthritis is an erosive deforming arthritis that appears similar to canine and human rheumatoid arthritis.[238] Like the canine disease, the incidence is relatively low. This form of the disease is a less common variant of feline chronic progressive polyarthritis, which will be discussed in the next section.

The disease is insidious in onset, and the first abnormalities noted are often deformities of the carpal, metacarpophalangeal, metatarsophalangeal, and interphalangeal joints. Radiographic signs of erosion of the margins and central parts of the subchondral bone in these joints

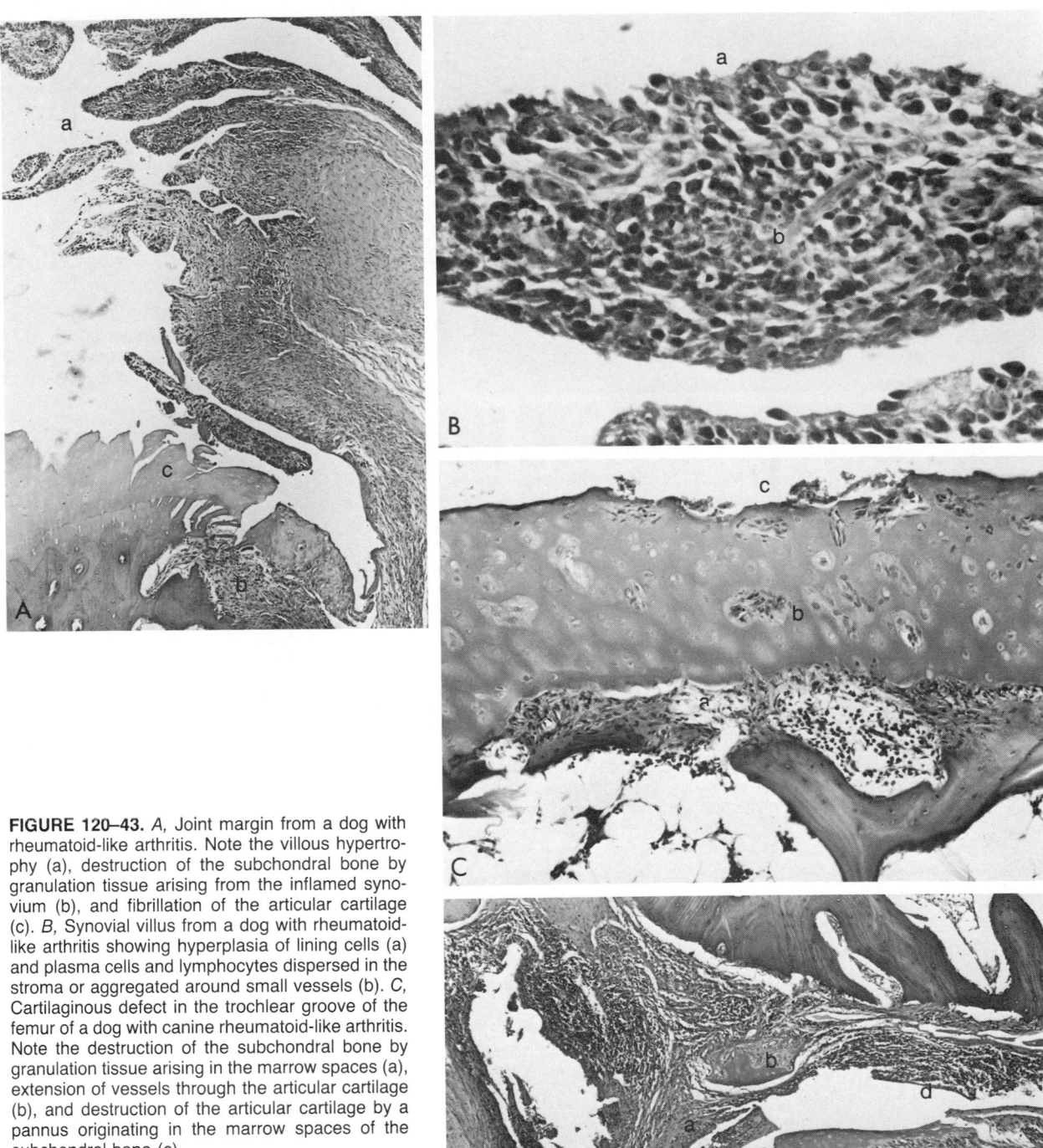

FIGURE 120–43. *A,* Joint margin from a dog with rheumatoid-like arthritis. Note the villous hypertrophy (a), destruction of the subchondral bone by granulation tissue arising from the inflamed synovium (b), and fibrillation of the articular cartilage (c). *B,* Synovial villus from a dog with rheumatoid-like arthritis showing hyperplasia of lining cells (a) and plasma cells and lymphocytes dispersed in the stroma or aggregated around small vessels (b). *C,* Cartilaginous defect in the trochlear groove of the femur of a dog with canine rheumatoid-like arthritis. Note the destruction of the subchondral bone by granulation tissue arising in the marrow spaces (a), extension of vessels through the articular cartilage (b), and destruction of the articular cartilage by a pannus originating in the marrow spaces of the subchondral bone (c).

precede joint instability and deformities. Proliferation of bone adjacent to affected joints can be identified, but proliferative bony findings are minor in degree, while destructive signs are excessive.

Synovial fluid from involved joints is abnormal and demonstrates a slight to moderate elevation of white cells. Neutrophils, lymphocytes, and synovial macrophages are present in varying proportions. There is very little experience with the treatment of this form of arthritis in cats. It appears to respond to immunosuppressive drugs, however. Immunosuppressive drug therapy can be complicated by the presence of an underlying feline leukemia virus infection that seems to be present in one half or so of the cases.[238]

Periosteal Proliferative Arthritis. FELINE CHRONIC PROGRESSIVE POLYARTHRITIS (PERIOSTEAL PROLIFERATIVE FORM).

This disorder occurs exclusively in male cats, with the common age at onset of one and one-half to four and one-half years.[238] Histopathologic abnormalities are similar to those occurring in both chronic Reiter's arthritis and rheumatoid arthritis of man.

The disease occurs suddenly with high fever, severe joint pain, and stiffness that usually starts in the tarsal and carpal joints, and lymphadenopathy that is regional to the inflamed joints. Radiographic signs progressing from osteoporosis, periosteal new bone formation, and ankylosis ensue over the next two to eight weeks or so. After the first few weeks, the fever tends to subside, and the disease takes a more chronic progressive course. This is manifested by severe generalized stiffness, emaciation, and gross bony enlargements in the area of the joints. This sequence differs considerably from the erosive or rheumatoid form, which does not begin with any noticeable signs, and tends to progress insidiously over a period of many months.

Chronic progressive polyarthritis of cats is not caused by identifiable bacteria or *Mycoplasma*, but it is etiologically linked to feline leukemia (FeLV) and feline syncytium-forming virus (FeSFV) infections.[238] Feline syncytium-forming virus can be isolated from the blood or detected by serologic means in all of the cats with the disease, while FeLV is isolated from one-half or less of the animals. The incidence of FeSFV infection in diseased cats is two to four times greater than age- and sex-matched normal cats living in the same geographic area, while the incidence of FeLV infection is six to ten times greater than expected. The arthritis cannot be reproduced with infectious material from diseased cats, however. It has been postulated, therefore, that the arthritis is an uncommon disease manifestation of FeSFV and FeLV infection that occurs in certain male cats and potentiated by FeLV.[238] The actual joint disease is probably immunologically mediated, as evidenced by the dense lymphocytic and plasmacytic synovial infiltrate.

Synovial fluid contains a greatly increased number of neutrophils. The fluid is usually yellow-tinged and very cloudy in appearance. The hemogram is variable, with leukocytosis predominating. Leukopenia and anemia, when present, are usually associated with cats that have an underlying FeLV infection. Immunosuppressive drugs, usually corticosteroids and cyclophosphamide, are used to treat the disease. Corticosteroids alone will lessen the severity of the disease and slow the course, but will rarely halt its progression. Combination immunosuppressive drug therapy has been successful in achieving a temporary remission in about half of the cats treated, but recurrences and drug refractiveness are common. Because of underlying FeLV-associated bone marrow suppression, cytotoxic drugs cannot be used to full effectiveness in some animals.

Nondeforming or Nonerosive Arthritis.

A noncrosive arthritis is identified in the dog and cat, and though etiologically diverse, it is probably mediated by similar immunopathologic mechanisms.[239, 239a] The presenting clinical signs of this type of arthritis are similar, whether it is idiopathic in origin or associated with secondary infectious disease, SLE, neoplasia, inflammatory bowel disease, or drug hypersensitivity. The joint disease tends to be cyclic in nature, has a predisposition for smaller distal joints, the carpus and tarsus in particular, and can occur in monarticular, pauciarticular, or polyarticular forms. Radiographic changes, even after many months of joint disease, tend to be minimal or nonexistent. Biopsies of the synovial membranes show a sparse mononuclear cell infiltrate, with moderate to severe superficial inflammation characterized by polymorphonuclear cell infiltrates and fibrin exudation. Villous hyperplasia, marginal erosions, and pannus formation are not prominent features in these diseases. Regardless of the overlying or underlying disease processes that lead to the arthritis, the joint disease is believed to be due to deposition of immune complexes in the synovial membrane with resultant immune-mediated inflammatory reactions. In idiopathic nondeforming arthritis, the origin and nature of the antigen in the complex are unknown; in systemic lupus erythematosus, the antigen is in part nucleic acid; in enteropathic arthritis, the antigen probably originates from the bowel contents; and in arthritis secondary to chronic infectious disease or neoplasia, the antigen originates from the microorganism that is causing the infection or from the tumor.

IDIOPATHIC NONDEFORMING ARTHRITIS.

Idiopathic nondeforming arthritis is by far the most common disorder of dogs manifesting immune-mediated arthritis.[239] It is termed idiopathic because there is no evidence of primary chronic infectious disease process, serologic abnormalities of SLE are absent, and joint disease is often the sole manifestation of the condition. This disorder occurs most commonly in large breeds of dogs, particularly German shepherd dogs, Doberman pinschers, and various breeds of retrievers, spaniels, and pointers. When seen in toy breeds, it most frequently occurs in toy poodles, Lhasa apsos, Yorkshire terriers, and Chihuahuas, and in mixes of these breeds. A similar condition has been less commonly recognized in cats.

The initial presenting history is one of a cyclic fever, during which malaise, anorexia, lameness, or generalized stiffness is noted. The fever is most pronounced in dogs with polyarticular disease and least pronounced in animals with monarticular involvement. In severely affected dogs, periods of remission are usually incomplete, in which case the disease can be very debilitating. Generalized muscle atrophy and disproportionate atrophy of the temporal and masseter muscles are frequently seen. This atrophy is due in part to disuse, but in many cases the disease process also involves the muscles or nerves.

During the most severe stages of the disease, swelling and heat in distal joints are sometimes detected. Generalized lymphadenopathy is often present in varying degrees. During attacks the dogs run a high fever and demonstrate leukocytosis with neutrophilia and hyperfibrinogenemia. The joint disease can be manifested as a single limb lameness in cases of monarticular or pauciarticular involvement. When the disease is monarticular in presentation, the elbow joint is often involved. Polyarticular involvement is the most common presentation, with the dogs showing generalized stiffness and reluctance to move their spine, tail, or limbs. Toy breeds, which often have severe generalized arthritis, can become virtually immobile, making it difficult to tell whether the joints are the source of the problem, or whether the immobility is due solely to depression.

Radiographic abnormalities are usually not present, except for an increase in the amount of periarticular soft tissue due to inflammation or fibrosis. If the disease is present for many months without treatment, however, some mild degenerative changes can occur in the joints. Persistent hyperemia of the synovium can lead to severe periarticular periosteal bone proliferation in rare individuals. These radiographic abnormalities can lead to a mistaken diagnosis of primary degenerative joint disease or degenerative joint disease secondary to some other problem. Obviously, this will greatly influence the type of therapy selected. It is important, therefore, to always take a sample of synovial fluid from dogs with periosteal proliferative changes without obvious disorders that would predispose to degenerative joint disease.

Diagnosis is made by consideration of the clinical history of an antibiotic-unresponsive cyclic fever, malaise, and anorexia, upon which is superimposed stiffness or lameness. Because of the cyclic nature of the fever and clinical signs, it is often difficult to ascertain whether the condition is responsive to antibiotics or not. Animals will be started on antibiotics when the fever appears and taken off when it disappears. The apparent improvement will frequently be attributed to the antibiotics rather than to the natural cycle of illness. When the fever and signs reappear, veterinarians will often change antibiotics, and the new antibiotics will also appear to work. After numerous cycles of antibiotic therapy using different drugs, it is finally realized that antibiotics are not really effective after all.

Synovial fluid contains from 5000 to 100,000 or more white cells per μl. The predominant cells in the fluid are the neutrophils; these cells appear nontoxic and with normal granulation. The fluid is sterile for bacteria, viruses, *Mycoplasma*, and *Chlamydia*. Serologic abnormalities such as the LE cell phenomenon, antinuclear antibody, and rheumatoid factor are absent. Blood cultures are negative for bacteria, and there are no signs of primary infectious processes in other areas of the body.

The treatment of the disorder involves the use of glucocorticoids alone or in combination with more potent immunosuppressive drugs (see following section). A complete remission of signs can usually be achieved. From 30 to 50 per cent of the dogs will have recurrences of illness after the drug therapy is discontinued.

An idiopathic polyarthritis, identical in nature to that seen in dogs, has been seen in cats. It is less frequent, however. Unlike the dog, cats are less likely to exhibit high fever, malaise, and inappetence. The lameness, as is the case of most lameness in cats, is subtle and difficult to recognize.

NONDEFORMING ARTHRITIS ASSOCIATED WITH CHRONIC INFECTIOUS DISEASES. A nondeforming arthritis associated with chronic infectious diseases has been described in dogs.[239, 239a] This type of arthritis has been associated with subacute bacterial endocarditis;

pyometra; vaginitis; chronic *Acitinomyces* infections in the chest, abdomen, or paravertebral musculature; chronic salmonellosis; heartworm disease; urinary tract infections or severe periodontitis. Since these infections are often difficult to pinpoint, the arthritis may be the main or sole presenting complaint. It is important, therefore, to make a thorough search for secondary infections every time a nonerosive type of arthritis is found in an ANA negative animal. This is especially important because immunosuppressive drugs will usually be used to treat cases in which infection is unrecognized.

Joint involvement in this type of disorder is usually monarticular or pauciarticular, and has a predisposition for the carpal and tarsal joints. Since the organisms involved in the primary disease process cannot be identified in the synovial membrane, it is likely that the joint disease is also of immune complex origin. A similar relationship between a sterile arthritis and chronic infections in other parts of the body was recognized much earlier in man.[240]

SYSTEMIC LUPUS ERYTHEMATOSUS. Canine systemic lupus erythematosus (SLE) was initially defined as the triad of glomerulonephritis, thrombocytopenia, and hemolytic anemia associated with a salicylate-responsive arthralgia in some cases.[241] It is apparent, however, that canine SLE is similar in its presentation to SLE of man; that is, articular, dermatologic, renal, and neuromuscular problems seem to be more common than hematologic abnormalities.[239, 242–244] Hematologic abnormalities in the dog, such as thrombocytopenia or hemolytic anemia, occur in only 10 to 20 per cent of the total cases of SLE that the authors have seen. We have seen a similar type of polyarthritis in two cats with SLE. From what we have seen of SLE in cats, it also resembles SLE in dogs and man. A more detailed description of SLE is given in Chapters 119 and 121.

The arthritis of canine and feline SLE is similar in every detail to that seen in cases of idiopathic nonerosive arthritis. In fact, both conditions predominate in the same breeds, and in these cases, serologic abnormalities such as antinuclear antibodies are the sole basis for classifying the conditions as SLE. In cases wherein other systemic manifestations of SLE are present with arthritis, the diagnosis is more easily made. The joint disease is usually polyarticular and, less commonly, pauciarticular.

The arthritis is seen in subacute bacterial endocarditis (SBE), and indeed the entire syndrome of SBE can mimic SLE. Two dogs described by Bennett and coworkers[212] best document this point. Chronic bacterial endocarditis can lead to continuous low-grade damage to parenchymal organs, high levels of circulating immune complexes, and a heightened responsiveness of the host's immune system. In man and animals this may result in the production of numerous autoantibodies, including antinuclear antibody and rheumatoid factors. Antinuclear antibodies result from chronic nucleoprotein release and heightened immunologic responsiveness, and rheumatoid factors are made in response to persistent immune-complex production. This phenomenon is important, because if such animals are mistakenly diagnosed as having SLE or rheumatoid arthritis, they will be treated with immunosuppressive drugs, with potentially serious consequences.

NONDEFORMING POLYARTHRITIS ASSOCIATED WITH NEOPLASIA. A sterile polyarthritis has been observed in some dogs and cats with overt or latent neoplastic processes in other parts of the body.[239, 239a] As such, the signs of polyarthritis may precede the signs of cancer or may be a minor to major component of the overall disease syndrome.

ENTEROPATHIC ARTHRITIS. Enteropathic arthritis is frequently associated with diseases like ulcerative colitis and regional enteritis of man. The cause of arthritis is unknown, but it is thought that either the bowel and joint disease share a common etiology, or antigenic products released into the blood from the inflamed bowel have some effect on the synovium. Hepatopathic arthropathy, which has been seen in several dogs with chronic active hepatitis and cirrhosis, is also a type of enteropathic arthritis. In this disease, antigenic material from the bowel probably gains access to the general bloodstream, because it is not being removed from the portal blood by the reticuloendothelial tissue of the liver.

Polyarthritis in dogs with ulcerative colitis and more fulminating enterocolitis has been recognized.[239] In addition, a small percentage of the dogs with idiopathic polyarthritis have problems with flatulence, occasional vomiting, and eventual gastric torsion; the latter indicates some degree of preexisting motility problem.

PLASMACYTIC-LYMPHOCYTIC SYNOVITIS. This is a condition that is seen most frequently in the stifle joints of small and medium-sized breeds of dogs. The condition is probably a variant of canine rheumatoid arthritis. It leads to pronounced joint laxity and instability, often manifested by cruciate ligament damage and drawer motion (see also the discussion on ruptured anterior cruciate ligaments). Except for hindlimb lameness, which can be pronounced, the dogs are often not systemically ill. The hemograms, however, many show leukocytosis, elevated gamma globulins, and hyperfibrinogenemia. Many of these dogs will go to surgery for cruciate repairs, and if the abnormal synovium and synovial fluid are not noticed at surgery, an apparently unsuccessful cruciate ligament repair will be the result.

The synovium is grossly thickened and edematous and has a reddish-yellowish tint. The synovial fluid is cloudy, often thin, and yellow-tinged. It contains from 5000 to 20,000 white cells per μl, with only 10 to 40 per cent of these being neutrophils. Unlike other inflammatory joint diseases, the predominant cell is often a small mononuclear cell, probably a lymphocyte. The fluid is sterile for known microorganisms.

Radiographic changes, when present, are minimal and include soft tissue swelling and periosteal proliferative changes. Erosive changes are absent or slight. Synovial biopsies show an intense lymphocytic-plasmacytic infiltrate and synovial hypertrophy that is sometimes villous. Subchondral erosions are minimal or absent. The condition can be successfully controlled with immunosuppressive drugs (see the following discussion).

DRUG-INDUCED ARTHRITIDES. Drug induced vasculitides are becoming increasingly more common in dogs. They are basically hypersensitivity reactions involving the deposition of drug-antibody complexes around blood vessels in different areas of the body. The drug may act directly as an antigen or may combine with host proteins as haptens to form neoantigens. Polyarthritis is only one feature of the disease syndrome; fever, lymphadenopathy, and various types of macular-papular or bullous type hemorrhagic rashes frequently accompany the disease. The most common offending drugs are antibiotics, particularly sulfa drugs, lincomycin, erythromycin, cephalosporins, and penicillins. Giger and associates[245] described sulfadiazine-induced (associated with trimethoprim-sulfa therapy) allergies in six Doberman pinschers, suggesting that this breed is more likely to become sensitized to sulfa drugs than others. The first sign of the allergic reaction occurred 10 to 21 days after initial trimethoprim-sulfa treatment. The disease could be recreated within 1 to 10 hours after reexposure to the sulfa component. The clinical signs included acute fever, polyarthritis, lymphadenopathy, polymyositis, anemia, glomerulonephritis, focal retinitis, skin rash, leukopenia, and thrombocytopenia. The authors have also recognized a similar syndrome in several larger mix-breed dogs being treated with antibiotics for primary pyodermas or flea-allergic dermatitis associated with secondary bacterial infections. The primary skin conditions responded well to treatment, but clinical signs began to recur after one to two weeks. Since skin lesions were prominent in the drug reactions, the veterinarians assumed that they were a recurrence of the primary problem and antibiotics were either continued or the dosage increased. The animals presented to the clinic with severe skin and joint inflammations, depression, fever, and varying degrees of emaciation. These signs disappeared two to seven days after drug therapy was halted. The diagnosis is readily apparent only if the clinician is astute enough to observe the appearance or worsening of clinical signs while on chronic drug treatment, the appearance of a diffuse maculopapular or bullous type skin eruption, often of a hemorrhagic nature, and the appearance of joint pain and stiffness associated with a sterile inflammatory polyarthritis and greatly increased number of non-degenerating polymorphonuclear neutrophils in the synovial fluids.

PERIARTERITIS NODOSA. Periarteritis nodosa is an inflammatory condition of small arteries, often of a granulomatous nature. It is a well-defined disease entity of humans, but whether or not it exists in a similar form in animals is uncertain. Nevertheless, reports of a similar disease in dogs and cats[246-248] have been made. The condition in dogs usually manifests itself as meningitis; polyarthritis or pauciarthritis being an accompanying feature in some individuals. The classical form of the disease occurs in young beagles, boxers, and German short-haired pointers. The disease is manifested by cyclical attacks of fever, depression, and extreme neck pain lasting for three to seven days, interspaced with periods of normalcy lasting a few days to several weeks. After several cycles of disease, the attacks become milder and longer spaced. Self-cure usually occurs in several weeks or months. Inflammation of one or more distal joints may accompany each attack, although signs of joint disease are usually overshadowed by the neck pain. A more severe form of this disease is seen in Bernese mountain dogs. The meningitis is more severe than in the other breeds, and chronic forms are more frequent.

7. Mitchell, NS and Cruess, RL: Classification of degenerative arthritis. Can Med Assoc J 117(7):763, 1977.

8. Morgan, JP: Radiological pathology and diagnosis of degenerative joint disease in stifle joint of the dog. J Sm Anim Pract 10:541, 1969.

9. Marshall, J: Periarticular osteophytes: Initiation and formation in the knee of the dog. Clin Orthop 62:37, 1969.

10. Booth, NH: Non-narcotic analgesics. In Jones, LM, et al. (eds): Veterinary Pharmacology and Therapeutics, 4th ed. Iowa State University Press, Ames, 1977, p 351.

11. Romatowski, J: Comparative therapeutics of canine and human rheumatoid arthritis. JAVMA 185:558, 1984.

12. Daehler, MH: Transmural pyloric perforation associated with naproxen administration in a dog. JAVMA 189:694, 1986.

13. Spyridakis, LK, et al.: Ibuprofen toxicosis in a dog. JAVMA 188:918, 1986.

14. Rupp, C and Suter, PF: Kurmitteilung an Tierarzte betreffend moglicher Nebenwirkungen von Diclofenac (voltaren) bei hunden. Schweiz Arch Tierheilkunde 127:660, 1985.

15. Hickman, J: Greyhound injuries. J Sm Anim Pract 16:455, 1976.

16. Prole, JHB: Greyhound injuries. Correspondence. J Sm Anim Pract 17:197, 1976.

17. Rendoano, VT and Abdinoor, D: Management of intra- and extra-articular extremity gunshot wounds. JAAHA 13:577, 1977.

18. Renegar, WR and Stoll, SG: Gunshot wounds involving the canine carpus: Surgical management. JAAHA 16:233, 1980.

19. Salazar, I, et al.: Spavin: a proposed term for a non-fracture associated canine hock lesion. Vet Rec 115:541, 1984.

20. Prole, JHB: Canine spavin (correspondence). Vet Rec 115:607, 1984.

21. Hohn, RB, et al.: Surgical stabilization of recurrent shoulder luxation. Vet Clin North Am 1:537, 1971.

22. deAngelis, MP: Luxations of the shoulder joint. In Bojrab, MJ (ed): Current Techniques in Small Animal Surgery. Philadelphia, Lea and Febiger, 1975.

23. Stoyac, JM: The elbow: Dislocation of the elbow. In Bojrab, MJ (ed): Current techniques in small animal surgery. Philadelphia, Lea and Febiger, 1975, p 523.

24. Lowry, EC and Betts, CW: Subluxation of the elbow in three dogs. JAAHA 9:458, 1973.

25. McCormick, DN: An important new variation of implant arthroplasty. Vet Med 81:406, 1986.

26. Withrow, SJ: Management of a congenital elbow luxation by temporary transarticular pinning. VM/SAC 72:1597, 1977.

27. Wind, A: Surgical diseases of the carpal joint and methods of treatment. In Bojrab, MJ (ed): Current techniques in small animal surgery. Philadelphia, Lea and Febiger, 1975, p 542.

28. Parker, RB, et al.: Pancarpal arthrodesis in the dog. A review of 45 cases. Vet Surg 10:35, 1981.

29. Slocum, B and Devine, T: Partial carpal fusion in the dog. JAVMA 180:1204, 1982.

30. Shires, PK, et al.: Carpal hyperextension in two-month-old pups. JAVMA 186:49, 1985.

31. Alexander, JW and Earley, TD: A carpal laxity syndrome in young dogs. J Vet Orthoped 3:22, 1984.

32. Campbell, JR, et al.: Intertarsal and tarsometatarsal subluxation in the dog. J Sm Anim Pract 17:427, 1976.

33. Arwedsson, G.: Arthrodesis in traumatic plantar subluxation of the metatarsal bones of the dog. JAVMA 120:21, 1954.

34. Clayton-Jones, DG: Hindleg lameness in the dog. In Gunsell, CSG and Hill, FWG (eds): Veterinary Annual, 14th edition. Bristol, UK, John Wright and Sons Ltd, 1974, p 167.

35. Holt, PE: Ligamentous injuries to the canine neck. J Sm Anim Pract 15:457, 1974.

36. Lawson, DD: Intertarsal subluxation in the dog. J Sm Anim Pract 1:179, 1961.

37. Meutstege, FJ: Die behandlung der intertarsalen subluxation beim hund durch gedeckte arthrodesis von Os tarsi fibulare und Os tarsal IV. Kleintierpraxis 16:12, 1971.

38. Pettit, GD: In Canine Surgery. 2nd Archibald Edition. Santa Barbara, CA, American Veterinary Publications, 1974.

39. Dieterich, HF: Arthrodesis of the proximal intertarsal joint for repair of rupture of proximal plantar intertarsal ligaments. VM/SAC 69:995, 1974.

40. Smith, KW: Achilles tendon surgery for correction of hyperextension of the hock joint. JAAHA 12:848, 1976.

41. Egger, EL and Freeman, L: Transarticular pinning and external splintage for treatment of congenital hyperextension of the stifle and tibiotarsal joint: A case report. JAAHA 21:663, 1985.

42. Robinson, GR and McCoy, L: In Bojrab, MJ (ed): Current Techniques in Small Animal Surgery. Philadelphia, Lea and Febiger, 1975, p 567.

43. Bennett, D and Duff, SR: Transarticular pinning as a treatment for hip luxation in the dog and cat. J Sm Anim Pract 21:373, 1980.

44. Hunt, CA and Henry, WB, Jr: Transarticular pinning for repair of hip dislocation in the dog: a retrospective study of 40 cases. JAVMA 187:828, 1985.

45. Brinker, WO, et al.: Handbook of Small Animal Orthopedics and Fracture Treatment. Philadelphia, WB Saunders, 1983, p 273.

46. Brass, W, et al.: Luxatio femoris beim hund-vergleich unterschiedlicher behandlungsverfahren. Kleintierpraxis 30(3):125, 1985.

47. Santi, A: Lateral external luxation of the knee in a dog. Folia Vet Lat 4:581, 1974.

48. Tirgari, M: Changes in the canine stifle joint following rupture of the anterior cruciate ligament. J Sm Anim Pract 19:17, 1978.

49. Zahm, H: Die ligamenta decessata in gesunden und arthroptischen kniegelenk des hundes. Kleintierpraxis 10:38, 1965.

50. Vasseur, PB, et al.: Correlative biomechanical and histologic study of the cranial cruciate ligament in dogs. Am J Vet Res 46:1842, 1985.

51. Henderson, RA and Milton, JL: The tibial compression mechanism: A diagnostic aid in stifle injuries. JAAHA 14:474, 1978.

52. Strande, A: Repair of the ruptured cranial cruciate ligament in the dog. Baltimore, Williams and Wilkins, 1967.

53. Adelaar, RS, et al.: Dynamic musculotendinous transfer to replace the anterior cruciate ligament in the dog. J Bone Joint Surg 65B:650, 1983.

54. Paatsama, S: Ligament injuries of the canine stifle joint: a clinical and experimental study. Thesis, University of Helsinki, Finland, 1952.

55. Hohn, RB and Newton, CD: Surgical repairs of ligamentous structures of the stifle joint. In Bojrab, MD (ed): Current Techniques in Small Animal Surgery. Philadelphia, Lea and Febiger, 1975, p 470.

56. Knecht, CD: Evolution of surgical techniques for cruciate ligament rupture in animals. JAAHA 12:717, 1976.

57. Arnoczky, SP, et al.: The over-the-top procedure: a technique for anterior cruciate ligament substitution in the dog. JAAHA 15:283, 1979.

58. Dickinson, CR and Nunamaker, DM: Repair of ruptured anterior cruciate ligament in the dog: Experience of 101 cases using a modified fascia strip technique. JAVMA 170:827, 1977.

59. Hulse, DA, et al.: A technique for reconstruction of the anterior cruciate ligament in the dog: preliminary report. Vet Surg 9:135, 1980.

60. Smith, GK and Torg, JS: Fibular head transposition for the repair of cruciate-deficient stifle in the dog. JAVMA 187(4):375, 1985.

61. Barclay, SM and Barclay, WP: Filamentous carbon fiber prosthesis for cranial cruciate ligament replacement in the dog—a pilot study. Cornell Vet 74:3, 1984.

62. Alexander, JW, et al.: Anterior cruciate rupture. Fel Pract 7:38, 1977.

63. Cucuel, JPE and Frye, FL: Anterior cruciate ligament repair in a cat. A case report. VM/SAC 65:38, 1970.

64. Matis, U and Kostlin, R: Cruciate ligament rupture in the cat. Prakt Tierarzt 59:582, 1978.

65. McManus, JL and Nimmons, GB: Ruptured anterior cruciate ligament in a cat. Can Vet J 7:264, 1967.

66. Scavelli, TD and Schrader, SC: Nonsurgical management of rupture of the cranial cruciate ligament in 18 cats. JAAHA 23:337, 1987.

67. Dalton, JR: Rupture of the posterior cruciate ligament in a cat. Vet Rec 104:319, 1979.

68. Johnson, KA: Posterior cruciate ligament rupture in a cat: A case report. JAAHA 14:480, 1978.

69. deAngelis, MP and Betts, CW: Posterior cruciate ligament rupture. JAAHA 9:447, 1973.

70. Cheli, R, et al.: Valgoid syndrome resulting from distension of the anterior cruciate ligament in the dog. Folia Vet Lat 4:638, 1974.

71. Ticer, JW and Spencer, CP: Injury of the feline temporomandibular joint: Radiographic signs. J Am Vet Radiol Soc 19:146, 1978.

72. Lantz, GC and Cantwell HD: Intermittent open-mouth lower jaw locking in five dogs. JAVMA 188:1403, 1986.

73. White, CA: Bilateral forward mandibular luxation in a dog. North Am Vet 50:777, 1949.

74. Robins, G and Grandage, J: Temporomandibular joint dysplasia and open-mouth jaw locking in the dog. JAVMA 171:1072, 1977.

75. Thomas, RE: Temporomandibular joint dysplasia and open-mouth jaw locking in a basset hound: a case report. J Sm Anim Pract 20:697, 1979.

76. Stewart, WC, et al.: Temporomandibular subluxation in the dog: a case report. J Sm Anim Pract 16:345, 1975.

77. Bennett, D and Prymak, C: Excision arthroplasty as a treatment for temporomandibular dysplasia. J Sm Anim Pract 27:361, 1986.

78. Watson, AG: Congenital occipitoatlanto-axial malformation (OAAM) in a dog. Anat Histol Embryol 8:187, 1979.

79. Lappin, MR and Dow, S: Traumatic atlanto-occipital luxation in a cat. Vet Surg 12:30, 1983.

80. Denny, HR, et al.: Cervical spondylopathy in the dog. A review of thirty-five cases. J Sm Anim Pract 18:117, 1977.

81. Trotter, EJ, et al.: Caudal cervical vertebral malformation-malarticulation in Great Danes and Doberman pinschers. JAVMA 168:917, 1976.

82. Wright, JA: Spondylosis deformans of the lumbosacral joint in dogs. J Sm Anim Pract 21:45, 1980.

83. Morgan, JP: Spondylosis deformans in the dog. Acta Orthop Scand Suppl 96, 1967.

84. Flo, GL and DeYoung, D: Meniscal injuries and medial meniscectomy in the canine stifle. JAAHA 14:683, 1978.

85. Clamen, C: Lesions meniscales associees aux ruptures du ligament croise anterieur et menisectomie. L'Animal de Compagne 14:311, 1979.

86. Whiting, PG and Pool, RR: Intrameniscal calcification and ossification in the stifle joints of three domestic cats. JAAHA 21:579, 1985.

87. Resnick, D: Arthrography, tenography and bursography. In Resnick, D and Niwayama, G (eds): Diagnosis of Bone and Joint Disorders, Vol 1. Philadelphia, WB Saunders, 1981, p 579.

88. Arnoczky, SP and Marshall, JL: Discoid meniscus in the dog: a case report. JAAHA 13:569, 1977.

89. Bennett, D and Kelly, DF: Sesamoid disease as a cause of lameness in young dogs. J Sm Anim Pract 26:567, 1985.

90. Bateman, JK: Fractured sesamoids in the Greyhound. Vet Rec 71:101, 1959.

91. Smith, MM, et al.: Neurogenic acceleration of degenerative joint lesions. J Bone Joint Surg 67A:562, 1985.

92. Palmoski, MJ and Brandt, KD: In vivo effect of aspirin on canine osteoarthritic cartilage. Arthr Rheum 26:994, 1983.

93. Nunamaker, DM and Newton, CD: Canine hip disorders. In Bojrab, MJ (ed): Current Techniques in Small Animal Surgery. Philadelphia, Lea and Febiger, 1975, p 437.

94. Nunamaker, DM: Surgical correction of large femoral anteversion angles in the dog. JAVMA 165:1061, 1974.

95. Fletch, SM, et al.: The Alaskan Malamute chondrodysplasia (dwarfism-anemia) syndrome in review. JAAHA 11:353, 1975.

96. Roberg, JW: Dwarfism in the German shepherd. Canine Pract 6(1):42, 1979.

97. Llewellyn, HR: Growth plate injuries—diagnosis, prognosis and treatment. JAAHA 12:77, 1976.

98. O'Brien, TR, et al.: Epiphyseal plate injuries in the dog: A radiographic study of growth disturbance in the forelimbs. J Sm Anim Pract 12:19, 1971.

99. Rudy, RL: Correction of growth deformity of the radius and ulna. In Bojrab, MJ (ed): Current Techniques in Small Animal Surgery. Philadelphia, Lea and Febiger, 1975, p 535.

100. Ramadan, RO and Vaughan, LC: Premature closure of the distal ulnar growth plate in dogs. A review of 58 cases. J Sm Anim Pract 19:647, 1978.

101. Carrig, CB and Morgan, JP: Asynchronous growth of the canine radius and ulna. Early radiographic changes following experimental retardation of longitudinal growth of the ulna. J Am Vet Rad Soc 16:121, 1975.

102. Skaggs, S, et al.: Deformities due to premature closure of the distal ulna in fourteen dogs. A radiographic evaluation. JAAHA 9:496, 1973.

103. Olson, NC, et al.: Premature closure of the distal radial physis in two dogs. JAVMA 176:906, 1980.

104. Wolff, EF: Ununited coronoid process in the dog: a review with two case reports. VM/SAC 74:1299, 1979.

105. Egger, EL and Stolls, G: Ulnar styloid transportation as an experimental treatment for premature closure of the distal ulnar physis. JAAHA 14:690, 1979.

106. Mason, TA and Baker, MJ: The surgical management of elbow joint deformity associated with premature growth plate closure in dogs. J Sm Anim Pract 19:639, 1978.

107. Mayrhofer, E: Epiphyseolysis of supraglenoid tuberosity in the dog. Wien Tierarzt Monatsschr 64:54, 1977.

108. Olsson, SE: Osteochondrosis. A growing problem to dog breeders. Gaines Dog Research Progress. Summer, 1976.

109. Smith, CW and Stowater, JL: Osteochondritis dissecans of the canine shoulder joint: a review of 35 cases. JAAHA 11:658, 1975.

110. Bras, W: Osteochondritis in the dog. Tierartzliche Umschau 2:200, 1956.

111. Pobisch, R: Aseptische nekrose des humeruskopfes-eine lahmheitsursache bei junghunden. Wien Tierarzt Monatsschr 49:571, 1962.

112. Punzet, G, et al.: Osteochondritis of the stifle joint in the dog. Kleintierpraxis 20:88, 1975.

113. Robins, GM: A case of osteochondritis dissecans of the stifle joints in a bitch. J Sm Anim Pract 11:813, 1970.

114. Johnson, KA and Davis, PE: Osteochondritis in the canine stifle joint (case report). Aust Vet Pract 9(4):201, 1977.

115. Mason, TA, et al.: Osteochondrosis of the elbow joint in young dogs. J Sm Anim Pract 21:641, 1980.

116. Wood, AKW, et al.: Osteochondritis dissecans of the distal humerus in a dog. Vet Rec 96:489, 1975.

117. Alexander, JW: Osteochondritis dissecans of the hock in the dog. Calif Vet 34:9, 1980.

118. Johnson, KA, et al.: Osteochondrosis in the hock joints in dogs. JAAHA 16:103, 1980.

119. Mason, TA and Lavelle, RB: Osteochondritis of the tibial tarsal bone in dogs. J Sm Anim Pract 20:423, 1979.

120. Olson, NC, et al.: Osteochondritis dissecans of the tarsocrural joint in three canine siblings. JAVMA 176:635, 1980.

121. Aron, DN, et al.: Free chondral fragment involving the lateral trochlear ridge of the talus in a dog. JAVMA 186:1095, 1985.

122. Whitacre, R and Harrison, JW: Osteochondritis dissecans: A clinical study of morbidity and incidence. The Speculum 23:14, 1972.

123. Woodard, DC: Osteochondritis dissecans in a family of bull terriers. VM/SAC 74:936, 1979.

124. Knecht, CD, et al.: Osteochondrosis of the shoulder and stifle in 3 of 5 Border Collie littermates. JAVMA 170:58, 1977.

125. Berzon, JL: Osteochondritis dissecans in the dog: diagnosis and therapy. JAVMA 175:796, 1979.

126. Clayton-Jones, DG: Osteochondritis of the canine stifle joint. Kleintierpraxis 25:441, 1980.

127. Wissler, J and Sumner-Smith, G: Osteochondrosis of the elbow joint of the dog. JAAHA 13:349, 1977.

128. Battershell, D: Ununited anconeal process. JAVMA 155:35, 1969.

129. Corley, EA, et al.: Genetic aspects of canine elbow dysplasia. JAVMA 153:543, 1968.

130. Corley, EA: Elbow dysplasia in the German Shepherd dog. Dissertation, Colorado State University, 1966.

131. Stevens, DR and Sander, RD: An elbow dysplasia syndrome in the dog. JAVMA 165:1065, 1974.

132. Grondalen, J: Arthrosis with special reference to the elbow joint of young rapidly growing dogs, II. Nord Vet Med 31:69, 1979.

133. Berzon, JL and Quick, CB: Fragmented coronoid process: Anatomical, clinical and radiographic considerations with case analyses. JAAHA 16:241, 1980.

134. Olsson, S: The early diagnosis of fragmented coronoid process and osteochondritis dissecans of the canine elbow joint. JAAHA 19:616, 1983.

135. Weis, M: Knochenwachstumsuntersuchungen mittels fluoreszen-mikroskopischer, mikroradiographischer und phasenkontrast-mikroskopischer techniken am elbogengelenk sowie distal an radius und ulna beim jungen hund. Dissertation, University of Zurich, 1983.

136. Wind, AP: Incidence and radiographic appearance of fragmented coronoid process (in the Bernese Mountain Dog). California Vet 6:19, 1982.

137. Wind, AP: Elbow incongruity and developmental elbow diseases in the dog. JAAHA 22:711, 1986.

138. Wind, AP and Packard, ME: Elbow incongruity and developmental elbow diseases in the dog. JAAHA 22:725, 1986.

139. Bienz, HA: Klinische und radiologische untersuchungen uber den fragmentierten processus coronoideus medialis im elbogengelenk des Berner Sennenhundes und der anderen Sennenhunde-rassen. Dissertation, University of Zurich, 1985.

140. Walde, I and Hutter, H: Osteochondrosis dissecans des medialen condylus humeri (Osteochondrosis dissecans cubiti-O.C.D.). Kleintierpraxis 29:173, 1984.

141. Hitz, D: Ulnadysplasie beim Bassethound. Schweiz Arch Tierheilk 116:285, 1974.

142. Henschel, E and Grull, F: Zur therapie der distractio cubiti beim Bassethound. Kleintierpraxis 20:267, 1975.

143. Lust, G: Pathogenesis of degenerative hip joint disease in young dogs. *In* Proceed Twenty-Third Annu Gaines Veterinary Symposium, Pullman, Washington, 1973, p 11.

144. Lust, G, et al.: Development of hip dysplasia in dogs. Am J Vet Res 34:87, 1973.

145. Hedhammer, A, et al.: Overnutrition and skeletal disease. An experimental study in growing Great Dane dogs. Cornell Vet 64(Suppl 5): 5, 1974.

146. Fisher, TM: The inheritance of canine hip dysplasia. Mod Vet Pract 60:897, 1979.

147. Leighton, EA, et al.: A genetic study of canine hip dysplasia. Am J Vet Res 38:241, 1977.

148. Hayes, HM, Jr, et al.: Feline hip dysplasia. JAAHA 14:447, 1979.

149. Holt, PE: Hip dysplasia in a cat. J Sm Anim Pract 19:273, 1978.

150. Kolde, DL: Pectineus tenectomy for treatment of hip dysplasia in a domestic cat: A case report. JAAHA 10:564, 1974.

151. Peiffer, RL, Jr and Blevins, WE: Hip dysplasia and pectineus resection in a cat. Feline Pract 4(3):40, 1974.

152. Morgan, JP: Hip dysplasia in the beagle: A radiographic survey. JAVMA 164:496, 1969.

153. Pharr, JW and Morgan, JP: Hip dysplasia in Australian shepherd dogs. JAAHA 12:439, 1976.

154. Morgan, JP and Stephens, M: Radiographic diagnosis and control of canine hip dysplasia. Iowa State University Press, 1986.

155. Morgan, JP and Rosenblatt, L: Canine hip dysplasia, the pelvic inlet parameter in diagnosis. Cal Vet, May/June 1986, p 15.

156. Hauptman, J, et al.: Angles of inclination and anteversion in hip dysplasia in the dog. Am J Vet Res 46:2033, 1985.

157. Wright, PJ and Mason, TA: Usefulness of palpation of joint laxity in puppies as a predictor of hip dysplasia in a guide dog breeding programme. J Sm Anim Pract 18:513, 1977.

158. Morgan, JP: Canine hip dysplasia: Asymmetry of change. Cal Vet, Mar/Apr, 1986, p 17.

159. Kasstrom, H: Nutrition, weight gain, and development of hip dysplasia. An experimental investigation in growing dogs with special reference to the effect of feeding intensity. Acta Radiol Suppl 344:136, 1975.

160. Larsen, JS: Symposium workshop panel reports in canine hip dysplasia. *In* Proceed Canine Hip Dysplasia Symposium and Workshop. St Louis, Missouri, 1973, p 153.

161. Cardinet, GH, III, et al.: Correlates of histochemical and physiologic properties in normal and hypertrophic pectineus muscles of the dog. Lab Invest 27:32, 1972.

162. Riser, WH and Shirer, JF: Correlation between canine hip dysplasia and pelvic muscle mass: A study of 95 dogs. Am J Vet Res 28:769, 1967.

163. Ihemelandu, EC, et al.: Canine hip dysplasia: Differences in pectineal muscles of healthy and dysplastic German shepherd dogs when two months old. Am J Vet Res 44:411, 1983.

164. Morgan, JP and Rosenblatt, L: Canine hip dysplasia: Significance of pelvic and sacral attachment. Cal Vet, Jan/Feb, 1987, p 12.

165. Wallace, LJ, et al.: Pectineus tendon or muscle surgery for treatment of clinical hip dysplasia in the dog. *In* Bojrab, MJ (ed): Current Techniques in Small Animal Surgery. Philadelphia, Lea and Febiger, 175, p 443.

166. Rubin, LD, et al.: Panel report. Hip dysplasia in dogs. Mod Vet Pract 60:255, 1979.

167. Hohn, RB and Janes, JM: Pelvic osteotomy in the treatment of canine hip dysplasia. Clin Orthop 62:70, 1969.

168. Schrader, SC: Triple osteotomy of the pelvis as a treatment for canine hip dysplasia. JAVMA 178:39, 1981.

169. Schrader, SC: Triple osteotomy of the pelvis and trochanteric osteotomy as a treatment for hip dysplasia in immature dogs: The surgical technique and results in 77 consecutive operations. JAVMA 188:659, 1986.

170. David, T: Dreifache beckenosteotomie mit pfannendachschwenkung (nach Thomas David, Wien). Prak Tier 67:325, 1986.

171. Bohler, N, et al.: Chiari's pelvic osteotomy as method of treating hip dysplasia in dogs. Wien Tierarzt Monatsschr 72(4):140, 1985.

172. Bonneau, NH and Breton, L: Excision arthroplasty of the femoral head. Canine Pract 8(2):13, 1981.

173. Duff, R and Campbell, JR: Long-term results of excision arthroplasty of canine hip. Vet Rec 101:181, 1977.

174. Gendreau, C and Cawley, AJ: Excision of the femoral head and neck: The long-term results of 35 operations. JAAHA 13:605, 1977.

175. Lippincott, CL: Excision arthroplasty of the femoral head and neck utilizing a biceps femoris muscle sling. The caudal pass. JAAHA 20:377, 1984.

176. Leighton, RL: The Richard's II canine total hip prosthesis. JAAHA 15:73, 1979.

177. Olmstead, ML and Holn, RB: Total hip replacement in 103 clinical cases at the Ohio State University. Kleintierpraxis 25:407, 1980.

178. Oloff, S and Kusswetter, W: Bie behandlung der coxarthrose bei diensthunden mit dem totalen huftgelenksersatz (Fruhergebnisse). Prak Tier 64:408, 1983.

179. Perot, F: Totale huftgelenkprosthese mit retinierender kunstoffpfanne beim hund. Kleintierpraxis 30:227, 1985.

180. Hohn, RB, et al.: Der huftgelenkersatz beim hund. Tier Praxis 14:377, 1986.

181. Mayrhofer, E and Koppel, E: Schultergelenkdysplasie beim Dachshund. I. Klinik und Rontgenbefunde. Zentralbl Veterinarmed A 32:202, 1985.

182. Corley, EA and Hogan, PM: Trends in hip dysplasia control: Analysis of radiographs submitted to the orthopedic foundation for animals, 1974 to 1984. JAVMA 187:805, 1985.

183. Koppel, E, et al.: Schultergelenkdysplasie beim Dachshund. Ergebnisse der pathoanatomischen und pathohistologischen untersuchung, schlussfolgerungen fur rassestandard und zucht. Zentralbl Veterinarmed A 32:214, 1985.

184. Harrison, JW: Patellar Dislocation. *In* Bojrab, MJ (ed): Current Techniques in Small Animal Surgery. Philadelphia, Lea and Febiger, 1975, p 479.

185. Irving, GW: What is your diagnosis? Medial luxation of the right patella. JAVMA 175:845, 1979.

186. Flecknell, PA and Gruffydd-Jones, TJ: Congenital luxation of the patella in the cat. Feline Pract 9(3):18, 1979.

187. Leighton, RL: Repair of a bilateral medial patellar luxation in a cat. Feline Pract 8(2):23, 1978.

188. Alexander, JW: Legg-Calvé-Perthe's-like disease in the dog. Canine Pract 7(1):32, 1980.

189. Pidduck, H and Webbon, PM: The genetic control of Perthe's disease in toy poodles. A working hypothesis. J Sm Anim Pract 19:729, 1978.

190. Lee, RM and Fry, PD: Some observations on the occurrence of Legg-Calve-Perthe's disease (coxa plana) in the dog and an evaluation of excision arthroplasty as a method of treatment. J Sm Anim Pract 10:309, 1969.

191. Ljunggren, GL: A comparative study of conservative and surgical treatment of Legg-Perthe's disease in the dog. Anim Hosp 2:6, 1966.

192. Gutbrod, F and Langguth, B: Aseptiche humeruskopfnekrose bei einem Kleinpudel. Kleintierpraxis 31:295, 1986.

193. Swanton, MC: The pathology of hemarthrosis in hemophilia. *In* Brinkhaus, KM (ed): Hemophilia and Hemophiloid Diseases. University of Carolina Press, Chapel Hill, NC, 1957, p 219.

194. Bone, DL: Canine panosteitis. Canine Pract 7(4):61, 1980.

195. Dodds, WJ: Inherited bleeding disorders. Canine Pract 6(5):49, 1978.

196. Jezyk, PF, et al.: Mucopolysaccharidosis in a cat with arylsulfatase B deficiency. A model of Maroteaux-Lamy syndrome. Science 198:834, 1977.

197. Haskins, ME, et al.: Mucopolysaccharidosis in a domestic short-haired—a disease distinct from that seen in the Siamese cat. JAVMA 175:384, 1979.

198. Haskins, ME, et al.: Betaglucuronidase deficiency in a dog. A model of human mucopolysaccharidosis VII. Pediatr Res 18:980, 1984.

199. Ellison, GW and Norrdin, RW: Multicentric periarticular calcinosis in a pup. JAVMA 177:542, 1980.

200. Riser, WH: Juvenile osteoporosis (osteogenesis imperfecta) in the dog and cat. J Am Vet Radiol Soc 3:50, 1962.

201. Scott, PP, et al.: The nature of osteogenesis imperfecta in the cat. J Bone Joint Surg 45:125, 1963.

202. Seawright, AH, et al.: Hypervitaminosis A of the cat. Adv Vet Sci Comp Med 14:1, 1970.

203. Lipowitz, AJ, et al.: Synovial sarcoma of the dog. JAVMA 174:76, 1969.

204. Tilmant, LL, et al.: Chemotherapy of synovial cell sarcoma in a dog. JAVMA 198:530, 1986.

205. Madewell, BR and Pool, R: Neoplasms of joints and related structures. Vet Clin North Am 8:511, 1978.

206. Bellah, JR and Patton, CS: Non-weight-bearing lameness secondary to synovial sarcoma in a young dog. JAVMA 198:730, 1986.

207. Gresti, A: Occurrence of bilateral articular synoviomas in two cats. Clin Vet 98:156, 1975.

208. Kammermeir, C, et al.: Blastom als differential-diagnose zur kreubandruptur beim hund. Kleintierpraxis 30:133, 1985.

209. Kusba, JK, et al.: Suspected villonodular synovitis in a dog. JAVMA 182:390, 1983.

210. Barclay, SM: Lymphosarcoma in tarsi of a cat. JAVMA 175:582, 1979.

211. Alexander, JW: Septic arthritis in the dog. Canine Pract 5(6):43, 1978.

212. Bennett, D, et al.: Bacterial endocarditis with polyarthritis in two dogs associated with circulating autoantibodies. J Sm Anim Pract 19:185, 1978.

213. Caywood, DD, et al.: Septic polyarthritis associated with bacterial endocarditis in two dogs. JAVMA 171:549, 1977.

214. Goudswarrd, J, et al.: *Erysipelothrix rhusiopathiae* Strain 7, a causative agent of endocarditis and arthritis in the dog. Tijdschr Diergeneeskd 98:416, 1973.

215. Clegg, FG and Rorrison, JM: *Brucella abortus* infection in the dog: A case of polyarthritis. Res Vet Sci 9:183, 1968.

216. Buchanan, AM, et al.: *Nocardia asteroides* recovery from a dog with steroid- and antibiotic-unresponsive idiopathic polyarthritis. J Clin Micro 18:702, 1983.

217. Moise, NS, et al.: *Mycoplasma gatae* arthritis and tenosynovitis in cats: case report and experimental reproduction of the disease. Am J Vet Res 44:16, 1983.

218. Hopper, PT, et al.: Mycoplasma polyarthritis in a cat with probable severe immune deficiency. Aust Vet J 62:352, 1985.

219. Barton, MD, et al.: Isolation of *Mycoplasma spumans* from polyarthritis in a Greyhound. Aust Vet J 62:206, 1985.

220. Greene, CG and Philip, RN: Rocky mountain spotted fever. *In* Green, CG (ed): Clinical Microbiology and Infectious. Diseases of the Dog and Cat. Philadelphia, WB Saunders, 1984, p 562.

221. Stockham, SL, et al.: Canine granulocytic ehrlichiosis in dogs from Central Missouri: a possible cause of polyarthritis. Vet Med Rev 6(2/4):3, 1985.

222. Bellah, JR, et al.: *Ehrlichia canis*-related polyarthritis in a dog. JAVMA 189:922, 1986.

223. Kornblatt, AN, et al.: Arthritis caused by *Borrelia burgdorferi* in dogs. JAVMA 186:960, 1985.

224. Lissman, BA, et al.: Spirochete-associated arthritis (Lyme disease) in a dog. JAVMA 185:219, 1984.

225. Bayer, AS: Arthritis associated with common viral infections.

226. Pedersen, NC, et al.: A transient febrile limping syndrome of kittens caused by two different strains of feline calicivirus. Feline Pract 13:26, 1983.

227. Steere, AC and Malawista, SE: Viral Arthritis. *In* McCarthy, DJ (ed): Arthritis and Allied Conditions. Philadelphia, Lea and Febiger, 1979, p 1391.

228. Goad, DL and Goad, MEP: Osteoarticular sporotrichosis in a dog. JAVMA 189:1326, 1986.

229. Oxenford, CJ and Middleton, DJ: Osteomyelitis and arthritis associated with *Aspergillus fumigatus* in a dog. Aust Vet J 63:59, 1986.

230. Chapman, WL, Jr, and Hanson, WL: Leishmaniasis. *In* Greene, CE (ed): Clinical Microbiology and Infectious Diseases of the Dog and Cat. Philadelphia, WB Saunders, 1984, p 764.

231. Halliwell, RE, et al.: Canine rheumatoid arthritis. A review and a case report. J Sm Anim Pract 13:239, 1972.

232. Liu, SK, et al.: Rheumatoid arthritis in a dog. JAVMA 154:495, 1969.

233. Newton, CD, et al.: Rheumatoid arthritis in dogs. JAVMA 169:113, 1976.

234. Pedersen, NC, et al.: Noninfectious canine arthritis: Rheumatoid arthritis. JAVMA 169:295, 1976.

235. Biery, DN and Newton, CD: Radiographic appearance of rheumatoid arthritis in the dog. JAAHA 11:607, 1975.

236. Castelli, MJ: Acute periarthritis in a kennel of Greyhounds. Vet Rec 84:652, 1969.

237. Huztable, CR and Davis, PE: The pathology of polyarthritis in young Greyhounds. J Comp Pathol 86:11, 1976.

238. Pedersen, NC, et al.: Feline chronic progressive polyarthritis. Am J Vet Res 41:522, 1980.

239. Pedersen, NC, et al.: Noninfectious canine arthritis: The inflammatory, nonerosive arthritides. JAVMA 169:304, 1976.

239a. Bennett, D: Naturally occurring models of inflammatory polyarthritis in the domestic dog and cat. Br J Clin Pract 43:3–12, 1986.

240. Coggeshall, HC, et al.: Synovial fluid and synovial membrane abnormalities resulting from varying grades of systemic inflammation and edema. Am J Med Sci 202:486, 1941.

241. Lewis, RM, et al.: Canine systemic lupus erythematosus. Blood 25:143, 1965.

242. Krum, SH, et al.: Polymyositis and polyarthritis associated with systemic lupus erythematosus in a dog. JAVMA 170:61, 1977.

243. Monier, JC, et al.: Antibody to soluble nuclear antigens in dogs (German shepherd) with a lupus-like syndrome. Develop Comp Immun 2:161, 1978.

244. Slappendel, RJ, et al.: Canine systemic lupus erythematosus treated with prednisone. Zentralbl Veterinaermed A 19:23, 1972.

245. Giger, U, et al.: Sulfadiazine-induced allergy in six Doberman Pinschers. JAVMA 186:479, 1985.

246. Altera, KP and Bonasch, H: Periarteritis nodosa in a cat. JAVMA 149:1307, 1966.

247. Lewis, RM, et al.: Autoimmune diseases in domestic animals. Ann NY Acad Sci 124.178, 1965.

248. Wilkinson, GT and Robins, GM: Polyarthritis in a young cat. J Sm Anim Pract 20:293, 1979.

249. Newton, CD, et al.: Gold salt therapy for rheumatoid arthritis in dogs. JAVMA 174:1308, 1979.

250. Carlson, RP, et al.: Questionable role of leukotriene B4 in monosodium urate (MSU)-induced synovitis in the dog. Prostaglandins 32:579, 1986.

251. Okuda, et al.: Arthritis induced in a cat by sodium urate: a possible animal model for tonic pain. Pain 18:287, 1984.

252. Miller, RM and Kind, RE: A gout-like syndrome in a dog. VM/SAC 61:236, 1966.

253. Gibson, JP and Roenigk, WJ: Pseudogout in a dog. JAVMA 161:912, 1972.

121 SKELETAL DISEASES

CHARLES D. NEWTON and DARRYL N. BIERY

DISEASES OF INFLAMMATION

An infectious or suppurative inflammation of bone marrow and adjacent bone called osteomyelitis is the most common inflammatory osseous disease in dogs and cats.[1, 2] While osteomyelitis is usually caused by suppurative organisms, nonsuppurative osteomyelitis also occurs. Nonsuppurative osteomyelitis results from granulomatous organisms or from metalosis. Normal bone union following fracture is also an inflammatory process of bone.

Suppurative Osteomyelitis

Pathogenesis. Suppurative osteomyelitis occurs when bacteria infect bone. Bacteria may reach bone by hematogenous routes, by extension of soft tissue infection into bone, or by direct contact with bone (i.e., open fracture or open surgery). Regardless of the source of contamination, once bacteria are present, bone mounts an inflammatory response that is similar to that of soft tissue.

Bone inflammation results in the infiltration and localization of granulocytic leukocytes. Many of the infiltrating cells are destroyed by the bacteria and release proteolytic enzymes into the bone. Tissue necrosis ensues, and bacteria and the lytic products of necrosis, pus cells and debris, are mingled to form a focus of suppuration.[3]

The severity of osteomyelitis depends on factors such as the occurrence of the process in cortical or metaphyseal bone, the contribution of other disease to bone abnormality, and the animal's age and general health. If the inflammatory process is successful, the osteomyelitis may be contained. If, however, the infection proves overwhelming to the inflammatory process, osteomyelitis will disseminate within the bone (Figure 121–1).

Infection in metaphyseal bone may break through the thin cortex and spread subperiosteally to most of the diaphysis. Infection in diaphyseal cortical bone spreads through the haversian canals. As infection spreads, vascular thrombosis occurs, resulting in localized areas of cortical bone ischemia. If ischemia is incomplete, the bone may respond by producing new bone around the area of infection. If ischemia is severe, bone death may result. Complete bone death results in cell death, and

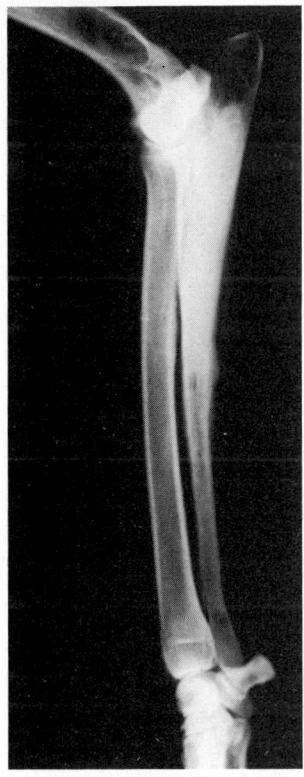

FIGURE 121–1. Acute bacterial osteomyelitis of the ulna secondary to a dog bite wound.

the resulting area is thus composed only of collagen and mineral. Such dead bone may be slowly revascularized and undergo lysis and subsequent new bone formation, or it may be sloughed. Dead bone is called a sequestrum; it often sits within a granulation tissue–filled bony depression (involucrum) (Figure 121–2).

Acute osteomyelitis occurs when the early changes herein described are recognized and appropriate treatment is initiated promptly. Chronic osteomyelitis occurs when the process continues for an extended period of time and results in disseminated infection within the bone and the inflammation fails to contain the infection. Chronic infection will usually result in disseminated infection, bone death, and evidence of aborted attempts at containment, i.e., involucrum and suppurating exudate, or pus that drains to the skin.[4]

Diagnosis. Acute or chronic suppurative osteomyelitis usually presents with pain, local swelling, and

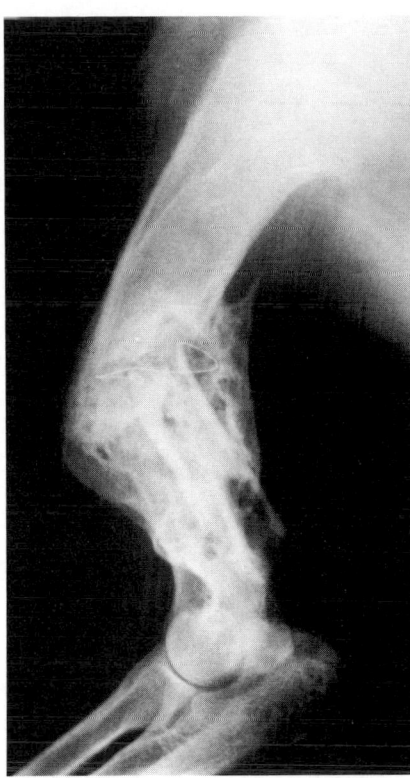

FIGURE 121–2. Chronic bacterial osteomyelitis of the humerus secondary to fracture repair in a two-year-old male German shepherd dog. Note the bony sequestrum.

pyrexia.[5, 6] With chronicity, obvious tracts and drainage may also be present. Most animals do not demonstrate significant hematologic alterations; moderate leukocytosis with a left shift was occasionally found in one study.[5]

On radiography, bone change associated with suppurative infection is limited to bony lysis, areas of periosteal new bone, or presence of a sequestrum, a nonvascularized fragment of bone, which is relatively more opaque than adjacent bone. Typical lytic and periosteal bone changes are not evident for 10 to 14 days following onset of infection.[7] Soft tissue changes are visible within 24 hours; such changes include soft tissue swelling and loss of fascial planes, and sometimes a fistulous tract.[8]

Bacteriologically, the most frequent organism isolated in the dog and cat with osteomyelitis is *Staphylococcus aureus*. *S. aureus* represented 60 per cent of the cases in one study,[9] 75 per cent of cases in a second study,[5] and 54 per cent in a third study.[10] Streptococcal infections follow *S. aureus* in frequency. Of equal importance is the prevalence of mixed infections: 47 per cent of the dogs in one study had two or more organisms present simultaneously.[5]

Treatment. The treatment method depends on the type of osteomyelitis, acute or chronic. In acute osteomyelitis, if fluid is present, the first step is to decompress and provide drainage from the area. The drainage should be protected against contamination from its surroundings with a bandage or a Robert Jones dressing.

Systemic antibiotics are used at this time, and although many antibiotics may be considered, a bactericidal drug should be chosen. If fluid is available it is submitted for culture, identification, and sensitivity tests. Systemic antibiotics are used in the interim before the results of the culture are known. The choice of antibiotic is important, since the first few days of treatment may determine the course of the infection. The author's experience has shown that penicillin with streptomycin or chloramphenicol is often not of value. Most forms of gram-positive cocci and bacilli along with gram-negative cocci respond well to amoxicillin, oxacillin or cephradine. The remaining gram-negative organisms usually respond to gentamicin or kanamycin. The author prefers cephradine or amoxicillin empirically until culture and sensitivity results are available, followed by use of one or a combination of the five previously mentioned drugs, as determined by sensitivity. Dosage depends on circulation: higher levels of antibiotics are needed when blood perfusion is poor, such as in cases of sequestered bone fragments or soft tissue edema and stasis around the fracture.[11]

Immobilization of the limb by bandage or cast may be indicated to prevent swelling, but it should be checked and changed daily. Radiography at ten day intervals is helpful to evaluate the extent and course of infection.

The treatment of chronic osteomyelitis may be similar to that of acute osteomyelitis; however, areas of dead bone or sequestra must be surgically removed. Following surgical removal, curettage of dead bone back to healthy bleeding bone is performed. The instillation of drains is often necessary to facilitate removal of blood or other postoperative debris. Culture of the deep wound or bone determines the organism(s) present and their drug sensitivities.

Chronic osteomyelitis is a difficult disease to cure and may persist despite extensive treatment.

Nonsuppurative Osteomyelitis

SYSTEMIC MYCOSES

Mycotic infections producing systemic disease often have bony manifestations. A nonsuppurative osteomyelitis is the most common bony change. Systemic mycotic infections are discussed at length in Chapter 49.

Coccidioidomycosis. *Coccidioides immitis* is a regional mycotic infection that occurs in the southwestern United States. Infection is acquired by inhalation of dust containing arthrospores of the fungus. There are three highly infective areas in the southwest: south Texas, south central Arizona, and the San Joaquin valley of California.

The literature describes the disease as being chronic in nature, with a two to five month course being typical. The disease begins as a respiratory infection. A chronic cough, typically dry and nonproductive, may be the first sign. The distribution of lesions produced by coccidioidal infections involves many organs. Although the lungs and thoracic lymph nodes appear to be the sites most commonly affected, approximately 50 per cent of the dogs will have bone involvement. Bone enlargement and soft tissue enlargement over the bone associated with lameness are common findings (Figure 121–3). While dogs

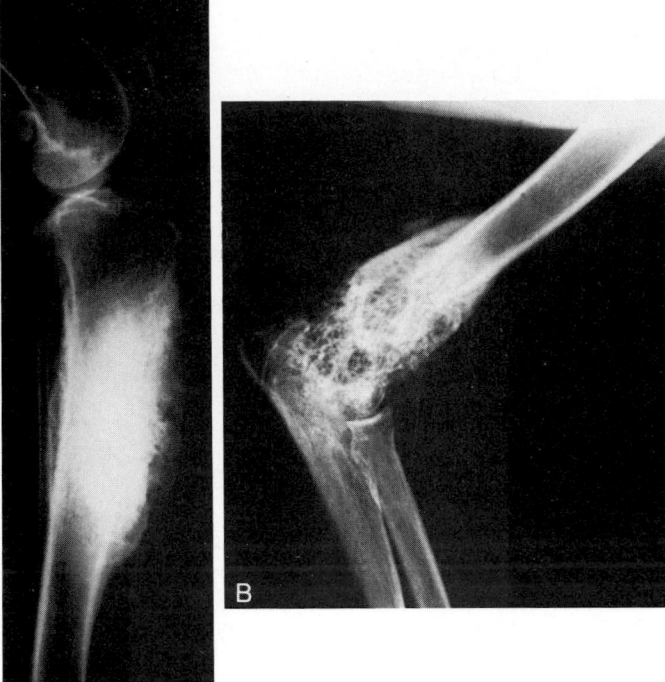

FIGURE 121–3. *Coccidioides immitis* osteomyelitis in the proximal tibia *(A)* and distal humerus *(B)* of two dogs. A blastic response is seen in the tibia *(A)* and a lytic and blastic response is seen in the distal humerus *(B)*. Differential diagnosis would include a tumor. (From Brodey, RS, et al.: Disseminated coccidioidomycosis in a dog. JAVMA 157:926, 1970.)

with respiratory infections may have constant elevated body temperatures, animals with bone or joint involvement may have only intermittent temperature elevations.[12–14] Most bony lesions occur late in the course of infection and are characterized by a combination of an increased radiopacity to bone, areas of bony lysis, and elevation of the periosteum, which looks proliferative.[15, 16] The radiographic appearance of osteomyelitis can mimic neoplasia of the bone.

Diagnosis is not always easy. Biopsy procedures for histopathology and culture are useful in differentiating bony lesions from bony neoplasms, but may also fail to prove coccidioidomycosis even after repeated attempts. The combination of the proper environment, presence of early respiratory disease, and a long chronic course of disease associated with bone lesions helps make a diagnosis by exclusion when other diagnostic tests are not conclusive.

Treatment of coccidioidomycosis seems to be limited to the use of amphotericin B.[17] There is a paucity of survival data in the literature. Ketaconazole has also been successfully used in this disorder (see Chapter 49).

Blastomycosis. *Blastomyces dermatitidis* causes a chronic systemic or cutaneous infection in dogs and cats.[18, 19] It has been confined to the United States (endemically in a zone reaching from Wisconsin south to Louisiana and across Kentucky to the Carolinas) and Canada and appears to be one of the most important systemic fungal infections in animals. It is characterized by suppurative granulomatous lesions of the skin, bone,

and lungs. Skeletal lesions may develop via hematogenous spread or by extension from a subcutaneous nodule. Edema, pain, and occasional draining tracts are found in the affected area.[20]

The radiographic features of blastomycosis are similar to those of any chronic pyogenic infection of bone. There is usually marked evidence of bone destruction with resulting periosteal bony reaction. The diagnosis relies on the direct microscopic examination of pus or other secretions. Identification is best confirmed by culture. The organism can usually be found in bone biopsy material. The differential diagnosis has to include suppurative osteomyelitis and bony neoplasia.

Treatment is usually confined to local excision of local lesions or treatment of the systemic disease with amphotericin B or ketoconazole.[17] The prognosis of systemic disease is poor.[21]

Histoplasmosis. *Histoplasma capsulatum* is a granulomatous disease affecting the reticuloendothelial system that produces respiratory and gastrointestinal disease most typically resulting in dyspnea and diarrhea.[22] The organism is endemic to the Ohio and Mississippi River valleys but has been seen throughout the world. Bone lesions in the reported cases have been confined to the tarsus and metatarsal bones;[23, 24] however, the disease may affect joints as well.[25] The radiographic signs seen in the reported cases include bony proliferation as well as focal areas of bone destruction. It is very difficult radiographically to differentiate the lesions from those of coccidioidomycosis, cryptococcosis, or blastomycosis.

The diagnosis can only be confirmed through histoplasmin tests or direct culture of the organism. Treatment is limited to the use of amphotericin B and ketaconazole.[17]

Cryptococcosis. *Cryptococcus neoformans* causes an upper respiratory disease seen primarily in cats. The most common signs include sinusitis and nasopharyngeal and pulmonary granulomas. Lesions of the bones usually result in osteolytic changes of the skull and sinuses or the diaphyses and metaphyses of the long bones.[22, 26, 27]

Treatment recommendations suggest the use of 5-fluorocytosine plus amphotericin B or ketaconzazole.[17]

Actinomycosis. *Actinomyces bovis* is a normal inhabitant of the mouth of most dogs and cats.[22, 28, 29] Penetrating wounds of the mouth may result in the organism being deposited into the soft tissues or bony parts of the mouth, with a resulting infection. The more common orthopedic manifestation is an osteomyelitis of the mandible. The lesion initially is characterized by bone destruction without new bone formation. As the osteomyelitis progresses, a very large bony reaction may be a prominent sign. Clinically a thick, mucoid pus may drain from any opening in the area, through the skin or into the mouth. *Sulfur granules* may be found in the pus.[2] Direct culture of the pus or bone lesion is necessary for a definitive diagnosis.

Treatment requires surgical opening of the lesion, curettage, and the use of local inorganic iodides and systemic antibiotics such as streptomycin.[17]

Nocardiosis. *Nocardia asteroides* causes a respiratory infection in dogs and cats, which can infect the skeletal system via hematogenous spread. The bones usually involved include long bones and the vertebral bodies of the spine. Lesions tend to mimic suppurative osteomyelitis when seen radiographically.[22, 30–32]

The diagnosis can only be confirmed by direct culture of the bone lesion or pus. Successful treatment of the disease has been reported with large doses of penicillin and streptomycin. Trimethoprim-sulfadiazine, sulfonamides, or penicillin-sulfonamide combinations have also been recommended.[17] Treatment should continue over at least a 6 to 12 week period.

Aspergillosis. *Aspergillus fumigatus* usually results in infection of the nasal passages of the dog.[33, 34] This is a result of infection of the lining tissues of the nasal turbinates as well as osteomyelitis of the nasal turbinates. Chronic nasal discharge is the cardinal sign of the disease. Radiographically, nasofungal infection may show loss of turbinate detail with large radiolucent spaces as well as areas of increased radiopacity. It is frequently very difficult to radiographically differentiate the fungal infection from a likely diagnosis of nasal neoplasia.

Treatment usually requires the surgical removal of the nasal turbinates as well as systemic treatment with ketoconazole or amphotericin B.[17]

Other Mycoses. Bony lesions have also been reported to be associated with adiaspiromycosis,[35] paecilomycosis,[2] Cephalosporium,[2] and Streptomyces.[36]

METALLOSIS

A noninfectious, nonsuppurative osteomyelitis often occurs around metal implants, which may result from metal corrosion, use of dissimilar metals, or animal allergy to an implant. Metallosis usually manifests itself clinically by lameness or draining tracts. The tract effluent will be serous and will not grow bacteria. Animals are not febrile and do not have marked hematologic abnormalities. Radiographic evidence of metallosis is bony lysis around the implant. A "halo" effect will be present around a portion or around the entire implant. Treatment will be unsuccessful unless the implant is removed. Following removal recovery is uneventful and antibiotics are unnecessary.[1, 2]

FRACTURE HEALING

Fracture healing is an inflammatory process by which a fractured bone heals. After fracture, the bone is damaged, as well as all of the surrounding soft tissues. Because of torn blood vessels within the bone and surrounding soft tissues, a hematoma forms within and around the fracture. Osteocytes at the fracture ends are deprived of normal nutrition and die. Depending on the amount of trauma associated with the fracture, periosteum and other surrounding soft tissues will also contain dead and necrotic material.[37]

The presence of necrotic bone and soft tissue elicits a rapid and intense acute inflammatory response. Acute inflammatory cells migrate to the region, as well as polymorphonuclear leukocytes and altered macrophages. Following the inflammatory phase of healing the fracture will go through a reparative phase and finally the remodeling phase.[37]

Bone fracture healing is an inflammatory process. It

is critical to remember that fact when analyzing early inflammatory lesions of dogs or cats. The early phase of fracture healing will look very similar to the early radiographic evidence of osteomyelitis (Figure 121–4).

METABOLIC BONE DISEASE

The term "metabolic bone disease" is at best confusing. The term is used to describe a wide range of medical diseases that result in osteoporosis. The diseases most commonly grouped as metabolic include primary hyperthyroidism, secondary renal hyperthyroidism, nutritional hyperthyroidism, and hyperadrenocorticism. All four of these diseases are discussed more completely in Chapters 94 and 97.

RENAL HYPERPARATHYROIDISM

A complication of chronic renal failure, renal hyperparathyroidism results in a metabolic state characterized by an excessive, but not autonomous, rate of parathyroid hormone (PTH) secretion. This is seen commonly in dogs but less frequently in cats. PTH increases osteoclastic resorption and bone remodeling, resulting in release of stored calcium from bone. The long standing increase in bone resorption that attempts to return serum calcium levels to normal eventually results in the

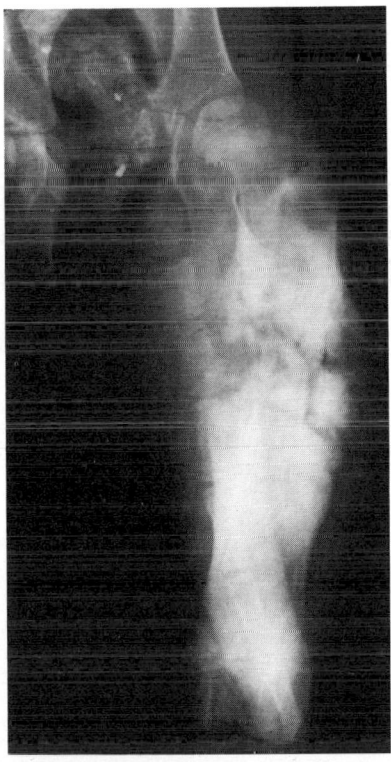

FIGURE 121–4. Radiographic appearance of a fractured femoral diaphysis in a four-month-old mixed breed dog. This documents three weeks of healing. The inflammatory appearance of the callus can easily be confused with osteomyelitis. (From Newton, CD: Fracture of the Femur. *In* Newton, CD and Nunamaker, DM (eds): Textbook of Small Animal Orthopaedics. Philadelphia, JB Lippincott, 1985, p 422.)

metabolic bone disease associated with chronic renal insufficiency.[38]

The bony osteoporosis that results is generalized but does not affect the skull, spine, and extremities uniformly. A commonly seen area for osteoporosis is the cancellous bones of the skull. The bone loss from the skull accentuates the decreased opacity to the mandible and maxilla and the teeth. This condition is commonly referred to as "rubber jaw."[38] Diffuse soft tissue swelling is usually present due to replacement of the bone by fibrous tissue.[39] Pathologic fractures may occur.

NUTRITIONAL HYPERPARATHYROIDISM

This metabolic disease is the direct result of nutritional imbalances that cause a compensatory increase in PTH levels. The diet that results in this disease will have a low content of calcium, excessive phosphorus with normal or low calcium, or inadequate amounts of cholecalciferol (vitamin D_3). The end result is hypocalcemia and parathyroid stimulation releasing PTH.

This metabolic bone disease is seen primarily in immature dogs or cats fed a diet predominantly of meat.[38]

The result of the metabolic imbalance is bony resorption resulting in osteoporosis. Cortical bone becomes uniformly thinner, and pathologic fracture is common (Figure 121–5). Fractures of the spine can result in pain and/or neurologic deficit, long bone fracture causes pain and skeletal deformity, and pelvic fracture can result in decreased lumen to the pelvic canal and inability to have normal parturition or defecation.[38]

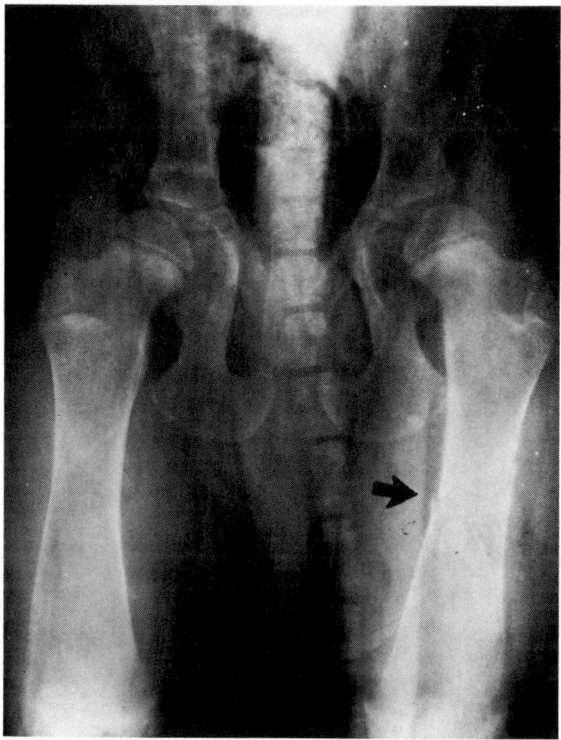

FIGURE 121–5. Generalized osteoporosis of the pelvis and femur is present in a young dog with nutritional hyperparathyroidism. Note the pathologic fracture of the femur (solid arrow) and compression type fracture of the left ilium (open arrow). (From Biery, DN: Orthopaedic Radiography. *In* Newton, CD and Nunamaker, DM (eds): Textbook of Small Animal Orthopaedics. Philadelphia, JB Lippincott, 1985, p 136.)

PRIMARY HYPERPARATHYROIDISM

In primary hyperparathyroidism a functional lesion of the parathyroid gland results in a higher than normal level of PTH. This is an uncommon disease, seen infrequently in the older dog.[39–42] The increased levels of PTH result in an accelerated osteocytic and osteoclastic bone resorption. Mineral is removed from the skeleton and replaced by immature fibrous connective tissue. The lesion is generalized throughout the entire skeleton but is more easily identified in the cancellous bones of the skull. Weakened vertebral bodies may undergo pathologic fracture, resulting in pain and/or neurologic dysfunction. Osteoporotic long bones fracture pathologically with minor trauma.[38]

HYPERADRENOCORTICISM

Hyperadrenocorticism refers to the presence of Cushing's disease or a chronic excessive administration of glucocorticoids.[1] The glucocorticoids inhibit absorption of calcium from the gut through an antagonistic effect on vitamin D. The steroids also increase urinary excretion of calcium, although the blood calcium levels are often normal. The development of osteoporosis is believed to be a primary result of the catabolic effect of the glucocorticoid on protein. The protein catabolic effect results in abnormal production of bone matrix. The glucocorticoids also decrease proliferation and differentiation of fibroblasts and osteoblasts, thus affecting the elaboration of collagen and bone matrix. Osteoporosis associated with this disease is usually prominent in the spine and long bones of the dog.[43] Hyperadrenocorticism is discussed in detail in Chapter 97.

OSTEOPOROSIS

Osteoporosis is a reduction in bone mass due to subnormal osteoid production, subnormal osteoid mineralization, or an excessive rate of deossification. Primary osteoporosis has not been reported in the dog or the cat. In man, primary osteoporosis is a disease of unknown etiology seen in elderly women and men. This is the only type of reduction in bone mass that is properly called osteoporosis, and the term osteoporosis properly refers to no other bone disease.[44] A reduction in bone mass results from certain anticonvulsive drugs and can be seen in primary hyperparathyroidism, nutritional hyperparathyroidism, secondary renal hyperparathyroidism, pseudohyperparathyroidism, hyperthyroidism, acromegaly, hepatic toxicities, disuse due to immobilization of a limb, long-term tetraplegia, multiple myeloma, and hyperadrenocorticism. None of these is a primary osteoporosis; therefore, osteoporosis in the dog and cat should be referred to as secondary osteoporosis.[1]

The clinical signs of secondary osteoporosis are pathological fractures of the long bones and compression fractures of the vertebrae. A limb immobilized for two to three weeks can develop disuse osteoporosis owing to the lack of stress of the bone.[45] Remineralization occurs after use begins; however, the bone can easily fracture during this remineralization time. Radiographically, a generalized decrease in bone opacity is seen.

There is resorption of the cortices and folding fractures of the long bones. Compression fractures of vertebral bodies can also occur.

Histologically, the normal architecture of the bone is preserved; however, there is a decrease in the amount of osteoid present.

The prognosis of osteoporosis depends entirely upon the underlying cause. The prognosis of secondary renal hyperparathyroidism is considerably worse than disuse osteoporosis.

GENETIC DISEASE OF BONE

Osteochondrodysplasias

Osteochondrodysplasias are abnormalities of cartilage or bone growth and development or both.

CHONDRODYSPLASIA PUNCTATA

Stippled epiphyses can occur in a variety of disorders not classified as primary chondrodysplasia punctata. A multiple epiphyseal dysplasia has been reported in beagles that was characterized by stippled epiphyses.[46] This condition has been referred to as chondrodysplasia punctata, but whether it truly belongs to this category or to multiple epiphyseal dysplasia is not clear. Poodles with pseudoachondroplasia also have stippling of the epiphyses radiographically.

ACHONDROPLASIA

The bony abnormalities observed include limb shortening and flared metaphyses, a depressed nasal bridge, and a shortened maxilla. Several breeds of dogs have characteristic features similar to those outlined for humans with achondroplasia. These include the bulldogs, the Boston terrier, the pug, the Pekingese, the Japanese spaniel, and the Shih Tzu. In the bulldogs, there are often wedge or hemivertebrae. Elbow luxations and medial patellar luxations occur and are probably associated with increased joint laxity. Achondroplasia appears to be an incompletely dominant autosomal trait in the dog.[47]

HYPOCHONDROPLASIA

Hypochondroplastic-type changes, characterized by limb shortening and a normal skull, are commonly seen in many breeds of dog. Among these are dachshunds, Welsh corgis, Dandie Dinmont terriers, Scottish terriers, Silky terriers, basset hounds, and beagles.[48] Major problems associated with these changes are intervertebral disc disease and the elbow dysplasias.

DYSCHONDROSTEOSIS

Deformities similar to those of dyschondrosteosis have been reported in dogs. Specifically, the autosomal recessive dwarfism in malamutes associated with spherocytosis and membrane abnormalities has many similarities.[49] The condition of ocular dysplasia and forelimb deformities described in Labrador retrievers also has similarities,[50] as does a syndrome in Samoyeds that involves ocular abnormalities and limb deformities much like those in the Labradors.[51] In the Samoyed syndrome, which is inherited as an autosomal recessive trait, the females are often more severely affected than the males. The syndromes in the Labradors and the Samoyeds also have features in common with hereditary arthro-ophthalmopathy.[52]

PSEUDOACHONDROPLASIA

An autosomal recessive form of this disorder has been reported in miniature poodles.[53-58] It is characterized by dwarfism and difficulties in locomotion due to the limb deformities, which consist of enlarged, stiff joints. Radiographically, there are stippling and patchy densities of the epiphyses in immature animals. In older animals, the bones are fully ossified but are short and severely malformed. Histologically, there is abnormal hyaline cartilage with an associated delay of ossification.

SPONDYLOEPIPHYSEAL DYSPLASIA TARDA

This is a rare disease described as mimicking the human disease and producing a "short spine" deformity in the dog.[59]

MULTIPLE CARTILAGINOUS EXOSTOSES

MCE is a benign, proliferative disease of bone and cartilage seen predominantly in young dogs,[60] and has been reported in cats as well.[61, 62] The disease is also referred to as osteochondromatosis, diaphyseal aclasis, and hereditary multiple exostoses. It is considered a benign bone tumor.

Animals are presented for examination with obvious bony enlargements or musculoskeletal or neurologic dysfunction. The dysfunction results from muscular realignment or compressive neurologic disease. Animals tend to be immature, as the disease occurs during the normal period of enchondral bone formation. Pain is generally not a part of the clinical disease unless neurologic compression occurs. Radiographically, bony exostotic lesions may be seen on any bone except the skull. Lesions tend to have radiopaque bony areas interspersed with more radiolucent areas of cartilage. If lesions originate from long bones, the metaphyseal region is usually involved (Figure 121–6).

The etiology of MCE is unknown though it probably is both a genetic disease as well as a neoplastic disease. The disease is hereditary in man, characterized by autosomal dominance with full penetrance.[63] Hereditary aspects of the canine disease have been reported,[64, 65] but have not been established. In the cat, feline leukemia virus has been associated with osteochondromas.[66]

While the pathogenesis is not entirely known, many aspects of the disease are understood. It is apparent that this is a disease of abnormal chondrocyte differentiation. It has been postulated that chondrocytes in the normal epiphyseal plate are forced out of the plate into surrounding metaphyseal bone.[67] Rather than differentiat-

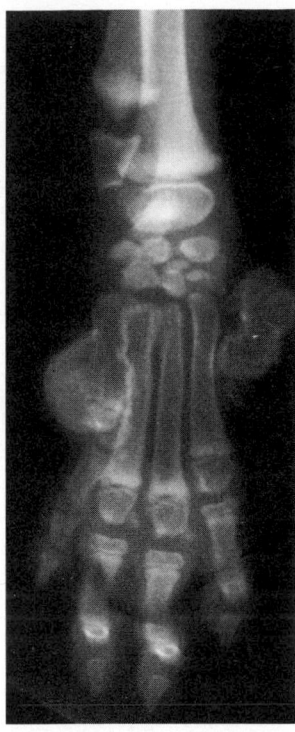

FIGURE 121–6. Multiple cartilaginous exostoses of metacarpal bones I and V in a four-month-old female mixed-breed dog.

ing into osteoblasts, the cells proliferate and continue to produce large islands of cartilage. Eventually the enlarged cartilage islands produce bone, which causes the exostosis.

Histologically, tissue from an exostosis resembles the epiphysis and metaphysis of growing bone. Normal cortical and cancellous bone is present, usually capped with a layer of hyaline cartilage.[68] Since the exostoses enlarge by endochondral bone formation, the cartilage cap resembles a normal physis.[60]

Treatment or physical limitation is usually minimal or unnecessary unless neurologic deficit is present. Without complications most exostoses mature and remain unchanged. Transformation of cartilaginous exostoses into osteosarcoma[69] and into chondrosarcoma[70, 71] has been reported.

Dysostoses

Malformations of individual bones, singly or in combination, are called dysostoses.

VERTEBRAL SEGMENTATION DEFECTS

The predominant feature of these disorders is involvement of the vertebral column, although the shoulder girdle and ribs are sometimes involved, and there may be soft tissue anomalies. In animals this grouping is represented predominantly by hemivertebrae and block vertebrae.

APODIA

Congenital absence of a forelimb has been described in the cat. It is likely that this is a relatively common dog or cat problem, but most of the affected individuals are destroyed at birth.[72]

ECTRODACTYLY SYNDROME

Maldevelopment of the central rays of the limbs may result in longitudinal splitting of the extremity. Autosomal dominant and recessive forms of this disorder can produce a "lobster claw" deformity. Usually this is the result of a splitting between the first and second metacarpal bones of the forepaw.[73]

POLYDACTYLY

The presence of one or more extra digits is termed polydactyly. In dogs and cats, preaxial polydactyly is by far the most common form of the disorder.[74, 75, 76] In cats, it is inherited as an autosomal dominant trait with variable expressivity.[74] A similar inheritance pattern appears to apply to the occurrence of multiple dewclaws in the dog.

SYNDACTYLY

This condition involves bony and/or soft tissue union of two or more digits. The condition has been reported in both the dog and cat though since it rarely causes clinical problems, it is assumed to be much more common than reflected in the literature.[72]

Chromosomal Aberrations

In the dog and cat, primary metabolic abnormalities affecting bone are characterized by the mucopolysaccharidoses. Mucopolysaccharidosis in man has been known as a distinct class of inherited metabolic diseases for 60 years.[48] At least seven specific forms are now recognized, each due to a defect in a different lysosomal enzyme concerned with the degradation of glycosaminoglycans, a general category of lysosomal storage diseases. Prominent features in man include multiple skeletal, neurologic, and ocular abnormalities, usually associated with dwarfism.[77]

MUCOPOLYSACCHARIDOSIS, TYPE I (MPS I; α-L-IDURONIDASE DEFICIENCY)

Mucopolysaccharidosis I has been recognized in both cats and dogs. The feline disease was first recognized in domestic short-haired cats and is characterized by facial dysmorphia with a large head, short ears, wide-spaced eyes and a broad nose, and larger than normal body size. Diffuse corneal clouding is present, and mitral insufficiency is common. Excessive urinary excretion of dermatan and heparan sulfates occurs, and α-L-iduronidase is deficient in all tissues tested, including peripheral white blood cells. Leukocytes are routinely used to identify affected and carrier animals. Radiographic features include joint anomalies including bilateral coxofemoral subluxation, fusion and widening of cervical vertebrae, and mild pectus excavatum. Affected animals have hindlimb gait abnormalities and appear to have some joint pain associated with the disorder. The disease is transmitted as an autosomal recessive trait and is most similar to the Hurler-Scheie syndrome in humans.[78, 79]

The canine form of MPS I was recognized in a family of Plott hounds. The affected dogs were dwarfed and had progressive motor and visual defects. Joints were swollen and painful. Glossoptosis and corneal clouding were present. Radiographically, there was epiphyseal dysgenesis and periarticular bony proliferation. The femoral diaphyses were also enlarged. Increased granulation of lymphocytes was noted. Fibroblasts had deficient α-L-iduronidase activity, and excessive amounts of dermatan and heparan sulfates were excreted in the urine. Pedigree analysis indicated an autosomal recessive mode of inheritance.[80, 81]

MUCOPOLYSACCHARIDOSIS, TYPE VI (MPS VI; ARYL-SULFATASE B DEFICIENCY)

Mucopolysaccharidosis, Type VI is a disease primarily of Siamese cats,[82, 83] although three dachshund pups have been reported with the disease.[84] MPS, Type VI was first recognized in a female Siamese cat in 1976.[82] The cat exhibited dwarfism, facial abnormalities, severe skeletal deformities, multifocal neurologic deficits, and retinal atrophy. Further study revealed metachromatic inclusion bodies in circulating leukocytes and very high urine concentrations of mucopolysaccharide. Subsequent breeding of the affected animal produced kittens with MPS, as well as confirmation of the autosomal recessive transmission of the disease.

Urine samples of the affected cats have high levels of dermatan sulfate. In many animals the level is 90 times that in normal cat urine.[83] Hematologic studies reveal MPS granules in lymphocytes and neutrophils. MPS granules in lymphocytes tend to be larger and to stain more darkly than azurophilic granules.[84] In many cases a clear space or "halo" may surround the granule.

Radiographic evidence of the disease is often confused with hypervitaminosis A. Cats often have severe bony bridging of cervical vertebral bodies with prolonged disease; the thoracic or lumbar spine may fuse. Bony changes in long bone epiphyses occur, resulting in broad irregular epiphyses. Bony proliferation around joints may become severe, resulting in ankylosis as the disease progresses (Figure 121–7).

This disease is caused by an inheritable defect that specifically results in a deficiency of arylsulfatase B. Treatment of affected animals is nonspecific, but the aim is toward alleviating symptoms. These animals may live comfortably as pets if the disease is treated.

MUCOPOLYSACCHARIDOSIS, TYPE VII (β-GLUCURONIDASE DEFICIENCY)

This is an extremely rare disorder only recently described in a family of mixed breed dogs. The affected dogs have large heads with a shortening of the maxilla and a protruding mandible. Typically animals show a progressive hindlimb paresis that progresses to complete hindlimb dysfunction by six months of age.[85]

Radiographic abnormalities seen include platyspondyly, caudal breaking of vertebrae, and a generalized epiphyseal dysplasia. Bilateral hip subluxation was also present.

BONE ABNORMALITIES SECONDARY TO DISTURBANCES OF EXTRASKELETAL SYSTEMS

PANHYPOPITUITARISM OR GROWTH HORMONE DEFICIENCY

This produces retardation of skeletal maturation and a short stature. An autosomal recessive form of the disorder occurs in the German shepherd.[86] These dogs are normal but for the uniform shortening of their forelimbs and hindlimbs.

CONGENITAL HYPOTHYROIDISM

This condition is known as *cretinism* in children. In the dog the condition has been described in the boxer. The dogs are dwarfed, with disproportionately short limbs and a broad skull with myxedematous facial features. Dogs are generally apathetic and lethargic, and have a juvenile hair coat. Marked epiphyseal dysgenesis has been seen in all but the older dogs. Long bones are typically short and wider than normal, with metaphyseal flaring that is most noticeable in the distal femur. Thoracolumbar kyphosis is commonly seen.

Dogs seem to respond well to L-thyroxine supplementation. Their apathy and state of mental depression (mental retardation?) seem to be reversible. Obviously the bony abnormalities remain for life.[72]

NUTRITIONAL DISEASES OF BONE

Nutritional disease of bone implies diseases induced by malnutrition involving calcium, phosphorus, and vitamin D; however, vitamin A, zinc, and possibly vitamin C have been implicated as well. Be aware that diet may potentiate some genetic diseases or play a role in metabolic disease (nutritional hyperparathyroidism).

HYPERVITAMINOSIS D

Hypervitaminosis D is a rare disorder caused by excessive intake of vitamin D, which results in high serum calcium levels and eventual deossification of the skeleton. The latter usually occurs without symptoms; however, prolonged high calcium levels produce signs referable to its effect on peripheral nerves, muscles (both skeletal and visceral), and possibly the brain. Metastatic calcification of numerous tissues, particularly the kidneys, may occur.[87]

The disease is rarely seen because of general awareness of the toxicity of vitamin D in high levels. When the disease is encountered, it usually results from a high dietary intake of cod liver oil or dietary vitamin supplements. Radiographically, generalized osteoporosis is noted in conjunction with hypervitaminosis D. Serum

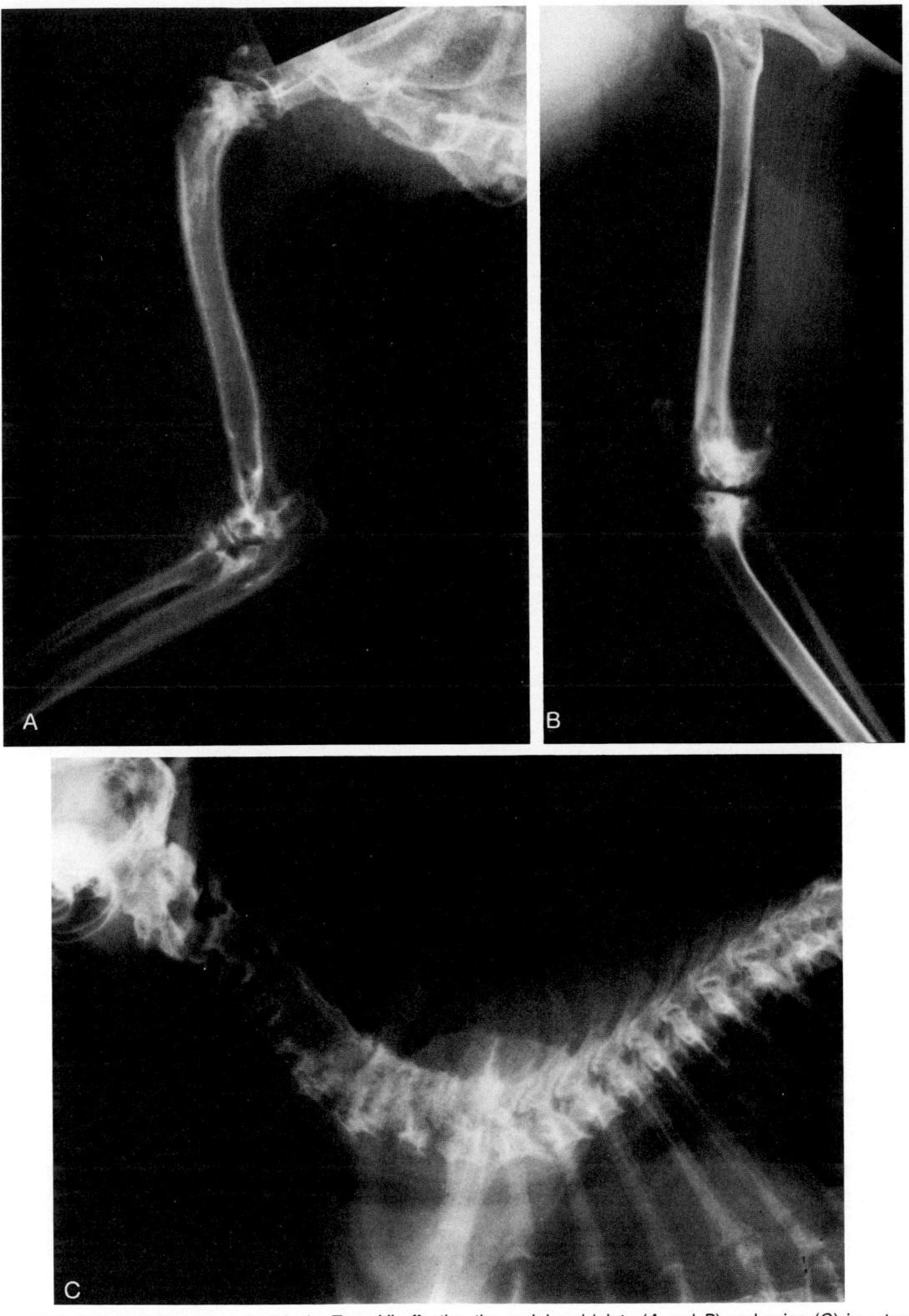

FIGURE 121–7. Mucopolysaccharidosis, Type VI affecting the peripheral joints (*A* and *B*) and spine (*C*) in a two-year-old female Siamese cat.

calcium levels will be elevated, while phosphorus levels are often normal or only slightly elevated.

The pathogenesis of the disease is unknown; however, it is postulated that vitamin D possesses a parahormone-like action that acts directly on bone, causing deossification.[87]

Proper dietary volumes of vitamin D, calcium, and phosphorus reverse the bony problems.

HYPOVITAMINOSIS D

Hypovitaminosis D is a rare problem seen in dogs or cats suffering from malabsorption of vitamin D due to excessive chronic administration of oral mineral oil. If linked with a diet of inadequate calcium and phosphorus, osteoporosis can result.[88] The problem is reversible with an appropriately balanced diet and cessation of the administration of mineral oil.

HYPERVITAMINOSIS A

Hypervitaminosis A is caused by the consumption of liver as a consistent diet rich in vitamin A or by the excessive intake of vitamin A concentrates. The disease affects primarily cats,[89, 90] although this condition has been experimentally produced in dogs.[91]

Clinical signs seen in cats with hypervitaminosis A include lethargy, hyperemia and edema of the gums, anorexia, abdominal distention, lameness, neck stiffness, and evidence of spinal exostoses.[90] In young animals, bone growth may be severely or permanently retarded, while bony exostoses are predominant lesions in mature animals. Dogs are usually lame but without fractures.

Radiographically, confluent exostoses are visible bridging cervical vertebral bodies often over an area as large as C1–T2. In chronic disease, vertebral fusion may occur at other spinal locations. Proliferative bony exostoses are visible on bone metaphyses or surrounding joints. Bony arthrodesis of joints may be seen radiographically if bone proliferation is extensive.

Hypervitaminosis A is the result of excessive vitamin A levels; relative proportions of calcium and phosphorus in the diet have little or no influence in the development of exostoses in chronic hypervitaminosis A.[89] Vitamin A is essential for the normal production, growth, and maturation of epiphyseal chondroblasts, and in enchondral bone growth. It is also a factor in the remodeling of bone, stimulating osteoblastic activity in areas where changes in conformation of bone mass are occurring.[87] It is apparent, however, that an excess of vitamin A causes an abnormal subperiosteal bone proliferation, one of the principal findings in chronic vitamin A toxicity.[87, 89, 90] It has been suggested that chronic ingestion of vitamin A greatly increases the sensitivity of periosteum to the effects of trauma.[90] Treatment necessitates removal of the source of vitamin A. Young animals will show permanent retardation of long bone length; however, appositional bone formation will return to normal. Mature cats show clinical improvement and reversal of most signs except those relating to bony arthrodesis. An increased incidence of primary bone tumors appears to be present in mature older cats with

hypervitaminosis A. Although plasma concentrations of vitamin A fall to normal limits within a few weeks of dietary change, the liver stores of vitamin A may remain elevated for years.[92]

HYPOVITAMINOSIS A

Hypovitaminosis A is a rarely seen disease, as vitamin A is generally abundant in all commercial pet foods. Affected dogs and cats are usually lame; long bones are radiographically bulky and ill-shaped.[88, 93]

Treatment requires replacement of daily oral vitamin A (100 IU/lb or 200 IU/kg). This should be added to a balanced diet that already contains 2,500 to 5,000 IU vitamin A/lb dry matter.[94, 95]

ZINC-RESPONSIVE CHONDRODYSTROPHY

Zinc-responsive chondrodystrophy is a form of dwarfism seen most often in Alaskan malamutes. The legs, primarily the forelegs, become short and bowed. Elevations in serum alkaline phosphatase activity and urinary acid mucopolysaccharide concentration suggest defective bone maturation.[96]

Affected dogs require supplementary zinc throughout life. The correct dose can be provided by giving 200 to 300 mg zinc sulfate or zinc gluconate.[88]

HYPOVITAMINOSIS C

Vitamin C is not required in the diet of dogs or cats. While the literature is filled with reports linking hypovitaminosis C to various skeletal and joint diseases, no absolute proof has been shown. In fact the NRC[95] disposes of the clinical observations as equivocal reports and concludes "that there is no adequate evidence to justify recommendation of routine vitamin C additions to the diet of the normal dog. . . ."

OVERNUTRITION OF THE GROWING DOG

A collection of bone abnormalities was induced in Great Dane pups by feeding a highly palatable diet ad libitum.[97] No abnormalities were seen in the control group fed the same diet at a rate restricted to twice maintenance. The skeletal abnormalities seen included coxa valga, panosteitis, hip dysplasia, hypertrophic osteodystrophy-like syndrome, osteochondritis dissecans, and wobblers syndrome. Control pups demonstrated none of the diseases.

This study has been interpreted to suggest that the supersupplementation of any growing pup may result in orthopedic disease. Pups should be fed the appropriate amount of food and never allowed ad libitum consumption of food.

NEOPLASTIC BONE DISEASE

Malignant and Benign Bone Tumors of the Dog

OSTEOSARCOMA

Osteosarcoma is a malignant primary tumor of bone consisting of malignant osteoid, bone, and/or cartilage formation.[98]

Osteosarcoma is the most common bone tumor in the dog. The frequency in comparison to other types of bone tumors has been reported as high as 80 per cent.[99] The average age of onset is about 7.5 years with a range of 1 to 15 years. Males represent 53 per cent of the cases and females 47 per cent.[100]

The breed of dog is an important factor in the diagnosis of osteosarcoma. In a study of 1215 dog osteosarcomas, the German shepherd had the highest incidence, followed by the Great Dane, Saint Bernard, boxer, Irish setter, Labrador retriever, Doberman pinscher, and collie.[99, 100] However, if the data are compared with the relative risk of a dog of any breed developing osteosarcoma then the greatest risk is to the Saint Bernard, followed by the Great Dane, golden retriever, Irish setter, Doberman pinscher, and German shepherd.[101]

A majority of the osteosarcomas (75 per cent) originate in long bones and 23 per cent arise in flat bones. The appendicular to axial ratio is 4:1. The fore limb to hind limb ratio is 1.7:1. Approximately 75 per cent of the tumors will arise in the metaphysis of the affected bone. Osteosarcoma is most prevalent away from the elbow (i.e., in the distal radius and proximal humerus) and around the knee (in the distal femur and proximal tibia) (Figure 121–8).[1]

Clinical signs include rapid onset of lameness over a two to five day period, localized swelling around the lesion, and occasionally fever and anorexia. Pathologic fracture is not uncommon.[99] Metastases occur to the lungs in 80 per cent of the cases by six months after the original diagnosis. The lungs are also the most common site for metastases:[102] 90 per cent of metastatic lesions are found in the lungs, the remaining 10 per cent are in other organs or in other bones.[103]

Radiographs reveal solitary lesions in the bones with either aggressive lytic or blastic areas, or both. A periosteal reaction is present in about 95 per cent of the lesions, with 33 per cent having a sunburst periosteal reaction (Figure 121–9). An eroded cortex and poorly demarcated lesion margins are common with neoplastic

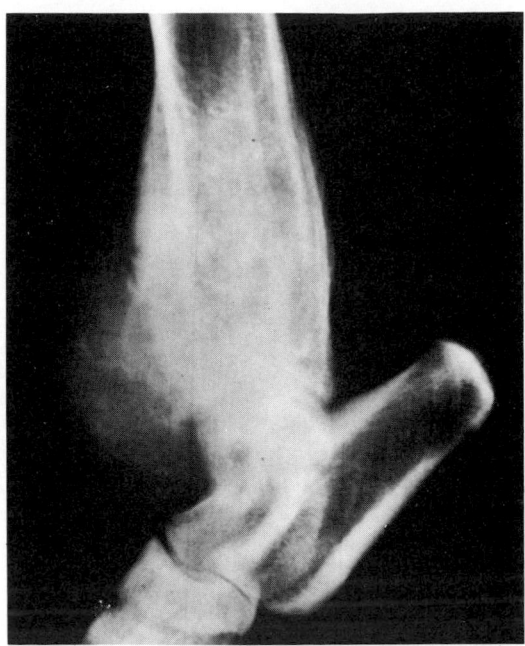

FIGURE 121–9. Osteogenic sarcoma in the distal tibia of an eight-year-old Irish setter. This tumor demonstrates primarily a blastic bony response. (From Biery, DN: Orthopaedic Radiography. *In* Newton, CD and Nunamaker, DM (eds): Textbook of Small Animal Orthopaedics. Philadelphia, JB Lippincott, 1985, p. 140.)

bone extending beyond the cortex. Growth rate of the tumor is rapid, with a large amount of soft tissue swelling usually present. Pathologic fracture may be present. Pulmonary metastases may not easily be recognized in the early stages of the tumor.[104]

Diagnosis of osteosarcoma is confirmed by biopsy of the lesion. Care must be taken to sample several sites; specifically, the margins of the tumor will be more likely to give an accurate diagnosis. Radiography following biopsy is helpful to confirm that the appropriate sites have in fact been biopsied. In lieu of biopsy, clinical signs, age, breed, location of the lesion, and radiography may be used to make a tentative diagnosis.

Treatment of osteosarcoma continues to be an area of ongoing research. While the results of research continue to offer hope, the reality is that only 10 to 15 per cent of dogs survive longer than nine months following diagnosis or amputation.[102] Amputation of the involved limb will alleviate pain, although as a clinical impression, it does not necessarily prolong the life of the dog unless it is coupled with an aggressive program of other modalities such as chemotherapy, immunotherapy, and radiotherapy. The most promising information available today indicates that amputation coupled with the administration of cisplatin has resulted in mean survival times of 47.5 weeks in a group of 12 dogs.[105] This is encouraging, as all of the animals in the amputation with no treatment studies have a mean survival time of only 18 weeks.[102, 105]

Histologically, osteosarcoma presents with a wide range of morphologic patterns. This includes a broad range of matrix patterns aligned in a haphazard way with osteonecrosis and/or new bone production.[106]

The prognosis for survival with osteosarcoma is very poor. Occasional dogs do survive for years following

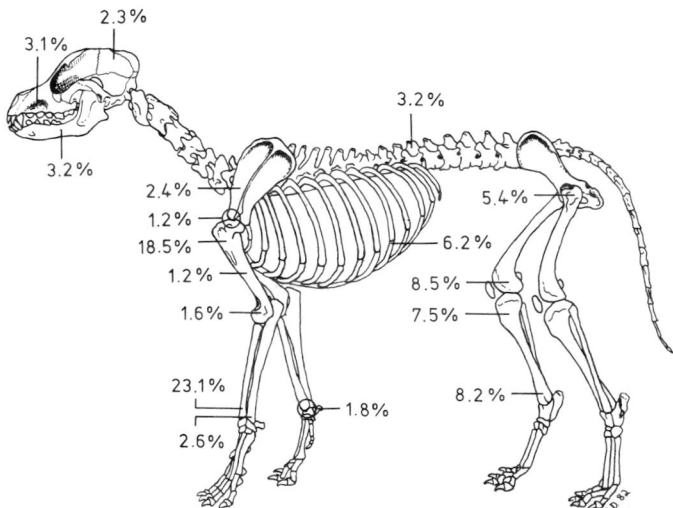

FIGURE 121–8. Site of origin of 1215 primary osteosarcomas in the dog. (From Goldschmidt, MH and Thrall, DE: Malignant Bone Tumors in the Dog. *In* Newton, CD and Nunamaker, DM (eds): Textbook of Small Animal Orthopaedics. Philadelphia, JB Lippincott, 1985, p 888.)

diagnosis; however, they are the very rare exception. Most dogs die within nine months following the diagnosis regardless of the modality of treatment.[102]

CHONDROSARCOMA

Chondrosarcoma is a malignant tumor in which the cells produce a neoplastic chondroid and fibrillar matrix but never directly produce neoplastic osteoid or bone. If neoplastic osteoid or bone is produced, then the tumor is classified as an osteosarcoma.[99]

Canine chondrosarcoma is the second most common bone tumor, comprising 10 per cent of all canine bone tumors.[106, 107, 108] A review of chondrosarcomas reveals the median age of affected dogs to be six years; there is no sex predilection. The age of dogs affected ranges from 1 to 12 years,[106] with an even distribution throughout. Major sites of origin are the ribs, nasal bones, and the pelvis.[107]

Clinical signs are related to the location of the lesion: rib involvement—large, hard, painless swelling at the costochondral junction; pelvis—lameness; and nasal cavity—sneezing, epistaxis, and nasal swelling.[1]

Radiographically, chondrosarcoma can produce osteolysis, osteoblastic or reactive periosteum with mineralization of the chondrosarcoma, or all of these (Figure 121–10).

Although frequently difficult, treatment is best accomplished by surgical removal of the tumor. The prognosis is good to guarded if complete excision of the tumor is accomplished. Metastasis to the lungs via a hematogenous route occurs in 10 per cent of all chondrosarcomas. Radiotherapy with or without surgery appears effective for treating nasal chondrosarcoma.

FIBROSARCOMA

Fibrosarcoma arises from malignant fibrous connective tissue elements that produce a collagenous matrix but no neoplastic cartilage or bone.[99]

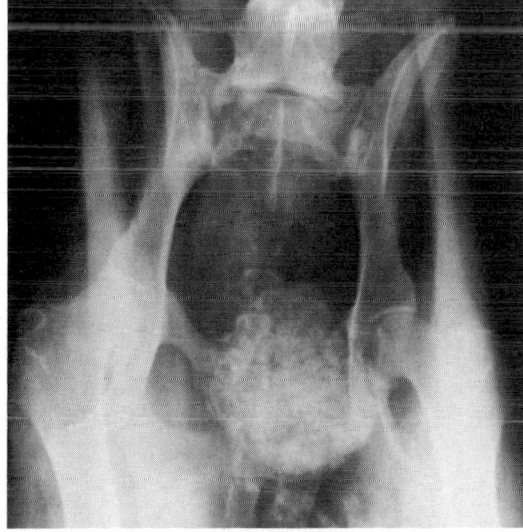

FIGURE 121–10. Ventrodorsal radiograph of the pelvis in which a chondrosarcoma can be seen. The pubic portion of the tumor is osteoblastic and the ischial portion osteolytic. (From Thrall, DE and Goldschmidt, MH: Radiography and Biopsy of Bony Neoplasia. *In* Newton, CD and Nunamaker, DM (eds): Textbook of Small Animal Orthopaedics. Philadelphia, JB Lippincott, 1985, p 882.)

Fibrosarcoma of bone is rare in the dog.[109] Fibrosarcomas and hemangiosarcomas account for seven per cent of all long bone tumors in the dog. These bony tumors occur primarily in medium to large sized male dogs. The tumors arise primarily in the metaphyseal area of the long bones. In our experience this is very commonly the distal femoral metaphysis.

Clinical signs are often masked for a period of time when the tumor is growing under a sizable muscle mass. Lameness or obvious swelling usually brings the animal to the veterinarian. Radiography can be helpful but it is almost impossible to differentiate between the primary and metastatic tumors of bone. Periosteal proliferation is seen early, and is followed by erosion of the bone adjacent to the tumor. Soft tissue swelling is more apparent early in the course of the disease.

Treatment requires surgical excision of the tumor mass. It is often helpful to also use local radiation therapy following the amputation. It is our experience that fibrosarcomas, though slow growing, will recur and can result in pulmonary metastasis as long as one year following amputation.[99]

BENIGN BONE TUMORS

Osteomas. Osteomas are protruding tumor masses composed of abnormally dense but otherwise normal bone formed in the periosteum.[98] These are rare in the dog. These tumors are most commonly seen on the skull and face. Clinical signs are referable only to the structures that they may impinge upon. Surgical removal is recommended only if tumor growth compromises another structure or if the tumor is cosmetically unacceptable.

Chondromas. Chondromas are benign tumors of cartilage origin. These rarely seen tumors are usually of flat bones and if clinical signs are seen, these are referable to the structures that are being pushed upon. Surgical excision is only necessary if the clinical signs suggest compromise of a vital system in the dog.

Mineralizing Hematomas. Mineralizing hematomas can occur at many sites but are commonly seen on the dorsum of the skull in rapidly growing giant breed pups. They are the result of striking the top of the skull on the underside of a table or other piece of furniture. The trauma results in a small bleed and formation of a hematoma on top of the skull. Since the trauma also breaks the periosteum, the hematoma mineralizes as does a fracture hematoma. While these masses can be very cosmetically displeasing to the owner, they are very difficult to remove, as the surgery commonly results in more trauma and the formation of another hematoma.

Osteochondromas. Osteochondromas are cartilage-capped bony projections that may arise in any bone. They are considered a benign bone tumor. The more common name is multiple cartilaginous exostoses (MCE). Since it is also considered a genetic disease of bone, it has already been discussed in that section of this chapter.

Malignant and Benign Bone Tumors in the Cat

Malignant and benign bone tumors are less common in the cat than in the dog. Few detailed reports of these tumors are available. The clinical, radiographic, and pathologic appearance of bone tumors in the cat is similar to that in the dog.

OSTEOSARCOMA

Osteosarcoma is the most common bone tumor seen in the cat. It is seen most commonly associated with the appendicular bones (15 of 22 cats in one study).[110] Axial tumors have been documented in the skull, vertebrae, and pelvis. Cats with osteosarcomas present with an age range of one year to twenty years, with a mean age of ten years.[66]

Presenting signs are usually associated with lameness or neurologic dysfunction in the case of spinal involvement. Radiographically, 80 per cent of the appendicular tumors appeared primarily as aggressive lytic lesions. There was a marked absence of new bone and periosteal proliferations. Axial tumors were primarily characterized by proliferative new bone formation.[110]

Treatment, using amputation of appendicular tumors without the addition of chemotherapy or immunotherapy, has had surprisingly good results. In one small study of twelve cats, five cats died with a mean survival time of 49.2 months, six cats were still alive at 64 months, and one cat was lost to follow up. Cats with axial tumors who were treated with various chemotherapeutic agents all died, with a mean survival time of only 5.5 months.[110]

Metastasis is less common than in the dog.[66] When it does occur, it is by hematogenous route usually to the lungs or other internal organs.[111] While the prognosis for this tumor is still very guarded, the outcome appears to be better than the same tumor in the dog.[110]

PAROSTEAL OSTEOSARCOMA

Parosteal osteosarcoma is the second most common bone tumor in the cat.[66, 112] This tumor is found immediately adjacent to the bone and arises on the outer surface of the cortex. It arises from fusiform cells, which produce chondroid and osseous foci.

The tumor is seen affecting long bones (primarily the humerus and femur) and the frontal bones and ramus of the mandible. Affected animals range in age from 1 to 14 years old with a mean age of 6.6 years.[66]

This is a very slow growing tumor that usually results in lameness due to expansion into surrounding muscles. In very chronic cases the tumor may erode through the cortex and extend into the medullary cavity. Metastasis to the lungs is possible but appears very rare. As a rule, amputation of the affected limb or area of tumor will be curative.[111]

LYMPHORETICULAR TUMORS

Lymphoreticular tumors arising as primary tumors in the bone are rare in the cat. However, replacement of the hematopoietic tissue by neoplastic lymphoid cells, without destruction of the cortical or medullary bone as evidenced radiographically or histologically, is common.[111]

BENIGN BONE TUMORS

Osteomas. Osteomas are rarely seen in the cat. They affect primarily flat bones of the head and face.[66] The clinical, gross, and histologic appearance of this tumor type is identical to its counterpart in the dog.

Osteochondromas. Osteochondromas can present as either solitary or multiple tumors. Solitary tumors are very rare and are seen only affecting the axial skeleton (Figure 121–11).[66]

Multiple osteochondromas, also known as multiple cartilaginous exostoses, are the most often recognized form of this tumor type. This tumor forms the perichondrium of flat bones and primarily affects mature cats, the age range being 1.3 years to 8 years. With advancing age, the tumors become larger. Clinical signs are referable to the structures being pushed upon.

Osteochondromas are thought to be caused by a virus, as C-type viral particles are seen within the chondrocytes of these cats. All cats with osteochondromas that have been tested have been positive for feline leukemia virus (FeLV).[66]

Metastatic Tumors of Bone in the Dog and Cat

Metastatic tumors of bone occur in both the dog and cat. These tumors include carcinomas, melanomas, nephroblastomas, aortic body tumors, sarcomas, fibromas, lymphosarcomas, hemangiosarcomas, reticulum cell sarcomas, and meningiomas.[1]

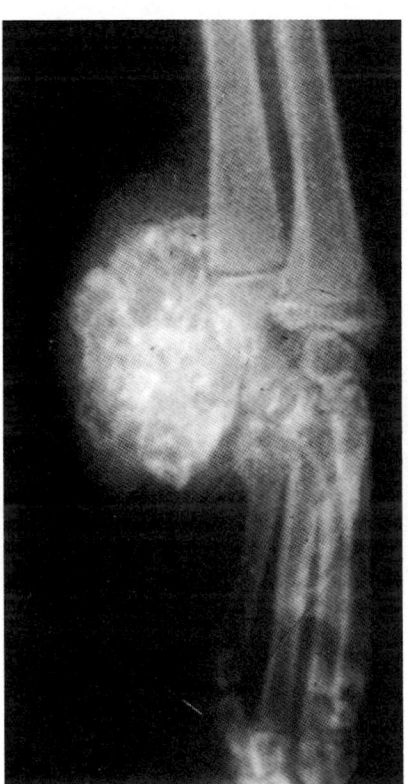

FIGURE 121–11. An osteochondroma is present arising from the caudal distal aspect of the ulna.

DISEASES OF UNDETERMINED ETIOLOGY

PANOSTEITIS

Panosteitis is a self-limiting inflammatory disease of the long bones that usually occurs in young large breed dogs. German shepherds have the highest breed incidence, with a ratio of 80 per cent male to 20 per cent female. The bones most commonly affected are the humerus, radius, ulna, femur, and tibia.[113, 114, 115]

Dogs with panosteitis commonly present clinically with an acute onset of lameness unrelated to trauma. The lameness may undergo spontaneous remission, only to reappear in a different limb. The age of onset is between 5 and 12 months in most dogs; however, dogs as young as 2 months and as old as 7 years may present with the disease. Physical examination is usually unremarkable except for pain on deep palpation of an affected bone.

Clinical pathologic findings in populations of dogs with panosteitis do not vary significantly from normal animals, although eosinophilia may be present.[116] Serum values for calcium, phosphorus, and alkaline phosphatase are also normal.

Radiography usually confirms the presumptive clinical diagnosis; however, the radiographic appearance may lag behind the clinical signs. Bone scintigrams using technetium 99m–labeled polyphosphate may be more sensitive in localizing early lesions not visible on radiographs.[117]

One or a combination of radiographic abnormalities may be seen in panosteitis. The most common abnormality is an increased radiopacity to the medullary cavity, usually most prominent at the nutrient canal. The increased opacity produces a patchy or mottled appearance and loss of the normal trabecular pattern. Occasionally the lesions may coalesce to fill the entire medullary cavity. Additional radiographic abnormalities that may be present with or without the medullary opacity include endosteal thickening and a periosteal reaction. The periosteal reaction is usually smooth (Figure 121–12).[113]

The least common radiographic finding seen is an increased radiolucency to the medullary portion of the bone.

During and following recovery, which is usual, the affected bones usually become radiographically normal.

Late in the disease, most previously mentioned radiographic changes disappear. The residual may be a coarser trabecular pattern or a cortical thickening. Following complete remission of the disease, most long bones will be radiographically normal.

The etiology of panosteitis is unknown; however, theories have been brought forth incriminating bacteria,[118] stress, hyperestrogenism,[119] and hereditary[114] and viral etiologies. None of these theories has been proven as the etiology for panosteitis.

Canine panosteitis, a disease of the adipose bone marrow, is often cyclic, and each episode is characterized by degeneration of medullary adipocytes followed by stromal cell proliferation, intramembranous ossifica-

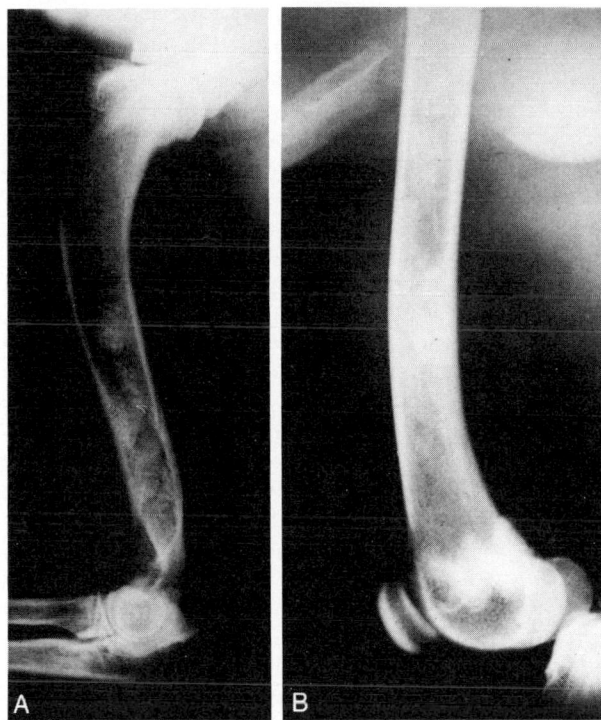

FIGURE 121–12. Panosteitis. Note the increased radiopacity occupying the medullary cavity of the humerus *(A)* and femur *(B)* in a six-month-old male German shorthaired pointer.

tion, removal of the medullary trabecular bone, and regeneration of the adipose bone marrow.[115]

Histologically, marked accentuation of osteoblastic and fibroblastic activity is found throughout the periosteum, endosteum, and marrow cavity. The overall pattern is uniform, and the abundance of osteoblasts and osteoclasts indicates an active bone turnover.[113] The processes involved in producing this disease affect periosteal, endosteal, or medullary cells, stimulating them to undergo osteoblastic or fibroblastic differentiation and activity.[116] The periosteal changes are secondary to the medullary changes.[115]

Treatment is symptomatic, with analgesics serving the primary role. Often anti-inflammatory drugs and corticosteroids may have the beneficial effect of relieving pain and decreasing lameness. Limitation of activity during the active disease may also be beneficial. The prognosis is excellent, with complete return to normal usually within several weeks to several months. The disease may disappear from one bone, only to reappear in another.

HYPERTROPHIC OSTEODYSTROPHY

Hypertrophic osteodystrophy (HOD) is usually a self limiting and bilateral bony disease affecting primarily young, rapidly growing large and giant breed dogs. The disease is also known as skeletal scurvy, Moeller-Barlow disease, osteodystrophy II, and metaphyseal osteopathy. The etiology remains uncertain.[120]

Dogs with hypertrophic osteodystrophy present clinically with mild to moderate painful swelling at the metaphyses, particularly of the distal radius and ulna, and tibia. Lameness or reluctance to move, fever, lethargy, and anorexia are often present. Fever may rise as high as 106°F and cycle, or remain high for prolonged periods. At onset of signs, most dogs are between three and seven months of age, and males are more frequently affected than females.[121] Dogs may have spontaneous remission of the disease or may progress to more severe forms of the disease, which can include bony deformity or death due to prolonged hyperthermia.

Radiographically, early HOD is diagnosed by the presence of an abnormal radiolucent line or bands within the metaphysis of the long bones and occasionally the costochondral junctions (Figure 121–13). Periosteal proliferation involving the mandible may also occur.

The abnormalities are most obvious in the distal ulna and radius and occasionally the tibia owing to the more rapid rate of bone growth in these areas. As the disease progresses, periosteal new bone forms around the metaphysis, which may eventually extend to involve the entire diaphysis (Figure 121–14). The physis and epiphysis are not usually involved. Soft tissue swelling over the area of proliferative bone may also be seen radiographically. As the disease regresses, in most cases residue bone scar or thickening of the metaphysis may be seen adjacent to normal new bone in the metaphysis. In severe and chronic cases, extensive periosteal and abnormal bone remodeling result in limb growth deformities.[122]

Clinical chemistries and hemograms do not reveal a consistent picture of this disease. Results include elevated sedimentation rates and elevated leukocyte counts as high as 19,000/mm³ (although most will be in the

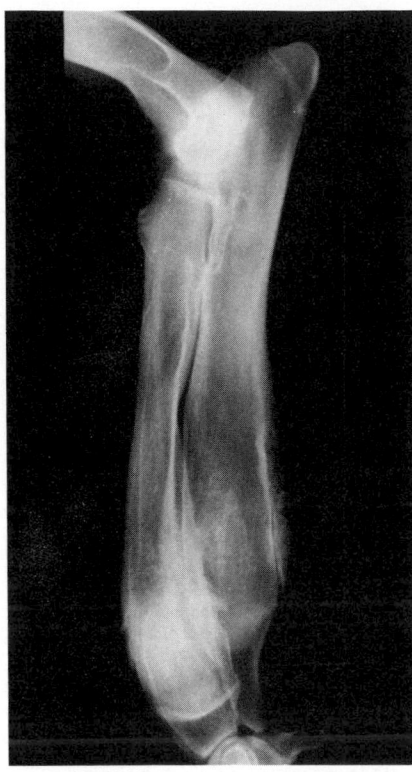

FIGURE 121–14. Chronic hypertrophic osteodystrophy. Note the periosteal new bone around the metaphysis.

normal range), with calcium, phosphorus, alkaline phosphatase, and serum ascorbic acid levels generally within normal limits.[121]

Histologically, the areas of abnormality reveal periosteal new bone formation at the perimeter of the lesion. The radiolucent band consists of necrotic bone infiltrated with polymorphonuclear leukocytes and lymphocytes. The necrotic bone band seems to initiate bony resorption by osteoclasts, which is at least temporarily replaced by fibrous tissue. During the course of the disease, rarefaction occurs followed by periosteal new bone formation along the metaphysis. The periosteal new bone appears to form as a sequela to reinforce bone that is weakened by the necrotic band. If the disease regresses and the dog grows, the band of necrosis and/or fibrous tissue is replaced by bone.[122]

The etiology of HOD is undetermined despite hypotheses of a nutritional disorder,[97] hypovitaminosis C,[123, 124] vitamin and mineral oversupplementation,[125] and other factors. The claim of hypovitaminosis C as the etiologic factor is substantiated by documenting levels that are slightly lower than normal during clinical disease.[126] Such lowered levels can simply be due to pain and stress during the disease. Recovery from HOD has had no relation to the levels of ascorbic acid.[121, 126]

Treatment of HOD is directed toward controlling fever and reducing pain. Rest and analgesics are usually sufficient; corticosteroids are reserved for severe cases. Most dogs show a spontaneous remission, regardless of treatment modality within several days to several weeks. In cases of severe disease, the dog may be left with permanent bony deformation or may succumb to the disease owing to hyperthermia. Relapses are rare.[120]

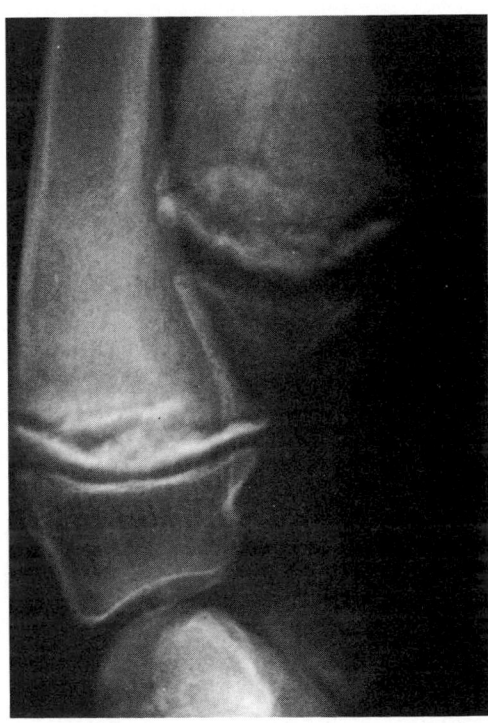

FIGURE 121–13. Radiolucent or lytic areas in the distal metaphysis of the radius and ulna represent the earliest and one of several radiographic abnormalities seen in hypertrophic osteodystrophy. (From Biery, DN: Orthopaedic Radiography. *In* Newton, CD and Nunamaker, DM (eds): Textbook of Small Animal Orthopaedics. Philadelphia, JB Lippincott, 1985, p 136.)

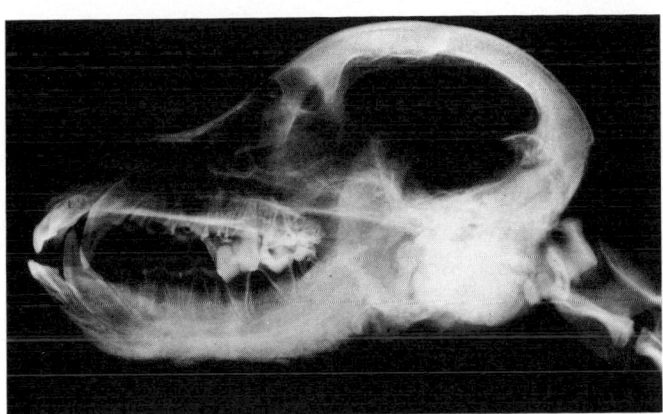

FIGURE 121–15. Craniomandibular osteopathy in an eight-month-old West Highland terrier. (From Riser, WH, et al.: Canine craniomandibular osteopathy. J Am Vet Radiol Soc 8:23, 1967.)

CRANIOMANDIBULAR OSTEOPATHY

Craniomandibular osteopathy (CMO) is a bony disease of young dogs characterized as a non-neoplastic proliferative disease. The disease predominates in Scottish terriers, West Highland white terriers, and Cairn terriers; however, boxers, Boston terriers, Labrador retrievers, Great Danes and Doberman pinschers may be affected. The disease primarily affects the mandibles, but occasionally the frontal and temporal bones of the skull and rarely a long bone of an extremity are involved. The disease may also involve the temporomandibular joints.[127]

Age at onset of the disease is usually between four and ten months. Clinically affected dogs may have mandibular swelling, drooling, inability to open the mouth, or pain on manipulation of the mouth.

On physical examination, symmetric soft tissue swelling and/or bony proliferation of the horizontal and occasionally vertical rami of the mandible are usually present. Dogs may be febrile during the period of bony proliferation.[128] Pain may be present on direct palpation of the bony swelling or when the dog's mouth is opened. In advanced disease, the mouth may not open more than 1 to 2 cm.

On radiography, symmetric bony enlargement of the mandible caudal to the middle mental foramen is usually present (Figure 121–15). The tympanic bullae and cranium may be sclerotic and thickened. The bony proliferation appears woven or as callus bone without a definitive cortex.[129] Rarely the disease may also simultaneously involve a long bone of an extremity.

The etiology of CMO is unknown. Recently, however, a recessive mode of inheritance has been described.[130] Osteoclastic resorption of mandibular lamellar bone occurs primarily, followed by production of woven bone. The woven bone is sufficiently proliferative to push beyond the normal periosteum. Similar new bone production may fill the medullary cavity. According to Pool and Leighton, these "irregular episodes of bone resorption and osteoblastic proliferation result in a characteristic histologic picture of new fibrous bone deposition separated by blue lines representing stages of metabolic rest from areas of incomplete destruction of older more mature bone."[131] The end result may be maturation of the fibrous bone that remains permanently. Rarely the dog may show a spontaneous reversal of the disease that returns the bone to its normal condition.

Treatment is symptomatic, with aspirin and corticosteroids used primarily to make the dog more comfortable. Although the bony changes are reversible when the disease disappears, many dogs will have some impaired mouth function but remain capable of maintaining normal nutritional status. Surgical intervention to reduce bony mass or to increase temporomandibular joint range of motion has not resulted in improvement.[128]

OTHER BONE DISEASES

BONE CYSTS

Bone cysts are benign lesions of unknown etiology. They are not commonly found in the dog or cat.[132] Bone cysts can occur at any age and may be monostotic or polyostotic. Most bone cysts do not produce clinical signs until they reach a fairly large size or develop a pathologic fracture. When signs occur, pain, swelling, and lameness may be noted, particularly if a pathologic fracture of the cyst has occurred.

Polyostotic bone cysts associated with fibrous dysplasia have been reported, most commonly in Doberman pinschers, in which the disease is thought to be inherited.[133]

The radiographic appearance is considered characteristic and in most cases enables the correct diagnosis to be made without biopsy. The radiographic findings are a nonaggressive, expansile, cystic (radiolucent) area (Figure 121–16). The cysts are usually in a long bone and involve the metaphysis near to but usually not affecting the physis and epiphysis.[134] The cyst may also

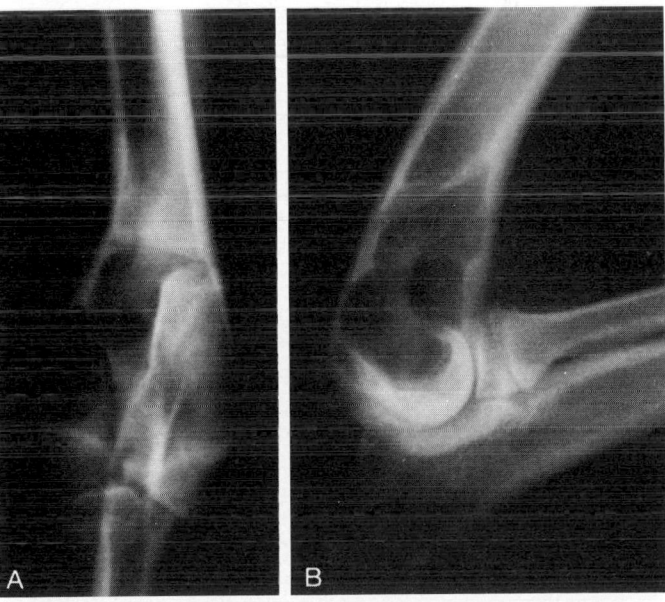

FIGURE 121–16. Radiographs of the distal humerus of a seven-month-old female Saluki. A well-demarcated multitrabeculated bone cyst is present. (From Biery, DN, et al.: Bone cysts in the dog. J Am Vet Radiol Soc 17:202, 1976.)

contain bony septa, cause cortical thinning, and have a pathologic fracture.

When trauma to the cyst has occurred followed by a pathologic fracture, a periosteal reaction of the callus and possibly additional fractures may produce an active-appearing lesion.

Although the radiographic signs are rather definitive, a differential diagnosis in the dog should include malignant bone and cartilage neoplasms, enchondroma, bone abscess, nonossifying fibroma, and fibrocystic osseous disease.[1]

On histology a poor to well defined inner lining of endothelial origin, an intermediate region of thin osseous trabeculae and/or unmineralized osseous tissue, and an outer fibrous subperiosteal layer are present. Normal compact bone is absent.

Blood pigment may be present in the lining. In areas of injury, both osteoblastic and osteoclastic activity will be evident. Callus will be laid down at the sites of pathological fracture.

Numerous theories of bone cyst pathogenesis have been proposed.[135] No definitive evidence of exact cause is known to date. The popular theory is that a bone cyst results from encapsulation and alteration of a focus of intramedullary hemorrhage. After encapsulation the affected area becomes distended by the transudation of fluid. Pressure from the cyst causes stagnation of the blood and lymph around it, erosion of the adjacent bone, and finally, expansion of the overlying cortex. Numerous other theories exist regarding the origin of bone cysts, including local disturbance in bone growth.

The four types of treatment depend on the clinical and radiographic signs and are benign neglect, splinting, curettage and bone graft, and en bloc surgical resection of the cyst.

Some solitary bone cysts in young dogs can heal spontaneously, possibly following a micro fracture. Surgical intervention usually expedites healing if fracture has not occurred, and may prevent future deformity of the bone owing to enlargement of the cyst or pathologic fracture.

Other types of bone cysts are extremely rare. One type called *aneurysmal bone cyst* is a neoplasm.[136] These cystic tumors are located within the metaphysis and have an aggressive appearance to the lytic or periosteal reaction.

Histologically an aneurysmal bone cyst has a remarkable lytic property, because the overlying compact bone is resorbed before it expands. The periosteum is pushed outward and reacts by laying down a thin shell of bone that is continuously replaced as the inner layer is eroded away. A bulky structure soon protrudes beyond the original surface of the uninvolved cortex, pushes soft tissue before it, and erodes other bones on contact.

The pathogenesis of aneurysmal bone cysts is unknown. Evidence from human disease suggests that it is an aggregate of arteriovenous communications that arises consequent to developmental fault or hemorrhage from hemangioma, spontaneous idiopathic hemorrhages in cancellous bone, or secondary to bone injury. Treatment is surgical excision or irradiation. Even partial curettage with no attempt to remove all the vascular tissue has resulted in cure.[136] Malignant transformation

as reported in man has not been described in the dog or cat.

BONE INFARCT

Bone infarction usually occurs in conjunction with osteosarcoma[137, 138, 139] and occasionally fibrosarcoma[140] in the dog. There are no clinical signs associated with bone infarcts. Occasionally the infarcts are truly coincident to the purpose of the radiograph. The infarcts occur more commonly in multiple long bones of the appendicular skeleton, but may involve any bone including the skull.

Bone infarcts have been reported in dogs from 6 to 13 years of age, have an equal sex distribution and affect mixed breeds as well as purebreeds (especially miniature schnauzers).[138]

Radiographically, bone infarcts appear as multiple irregularly demarcated areas of increased radiopacity within the medullary cavity of one or multiple bones. There are variable amounts of medullary obliteration by the infarcts (Figure 121–17). [139]

Histologically, bone infarcts demonstrate proliferation of new bone deposited on the endosteum and medullary trabeculae.

The pathogenesis of bone infarction in the dog is unknown. It is possible that metastatic showers of tumor are responsible for such bony necrosis; however, tumor cells have not been found in the infarcted areas. Although not found to date, it is also possible that other disease processes (e.g., lipid abnormalities, infection,

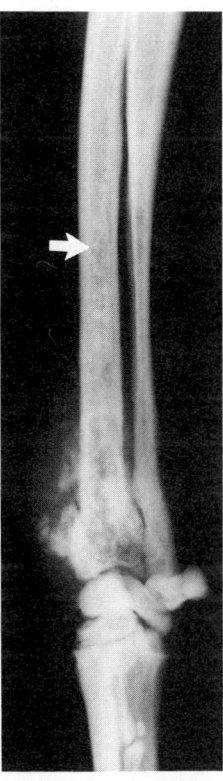

FIGURE 121–17. Radiograph of the left radius and ulna shows osteosarcoma of the distal radius. Infarcts are visible in the medullary cavity of the radius (arrow). (From Dubielzig, RR, et al.: Bone sarcomas associated with multifocal medullary bone infarction in dogs. JAVMA 179:64, 1981).

trauma) may cause the multifocal bony necrosis, and tumor results from such focus. It is known that sarcoma in man can develop secondary to necrosis and other underlying bony diseases.[140]

Clinical treatment of bone infarction is impossible. When infarction is diagnosed, one should look for the presence of a primary bone tumor.

HYPERTROPHIC OSTEOPATHY

Hypertrophic osteopathy (HO), also called hypertrophic pulmonary osteoarthropathy, is a bony disease of dogs and cats that produces a generalized symmetrical swelling and periosteal reaction.[141] The disease commonly produces lameness with other signs of bilateral tenderness and swelling of the legs, particularly the distal limbs. In most cases the disease is associated with intrathoracic disease,[142] usually a lung tumor, but the disease has been reported in association with bladder,[143] liver, and ovarian tumors without thoracic disease.

Many dogs with HO have warm distal limbs, are reluctant to move, and may exhibit pulsatile swellings rather than edematous limbs. There is no breed or sex predisposition and most dogs are middle-aged or older at the onset of the disease.[142]

Radiographically, bilateral symmetrical periosteal proliferations occur (Figure 121–18). The periosteal changes may be smooth or irregular and may be oriented parallel or perpendicular to the cortex. As the disease progresses, soft tissue swelling and the periosteal proliferation become more extensive. Gradual regression of the bony proliferation occurs after successful treatment of the primary disease. The periosteal changes usually affect the distal portions of the limbs first and more severely, particularly the abaxial surfaces of the second and fifth metacarpal and metatarsal bones. The disease can involve the proximal bones of the legs and occasionally the pelvis and vertebra.

Gross and histologic examination of affected limbs demonstrated several distinctive features: bone, tendons, and joints are surrounded by highly vascularized connective tissue, and diaphyses of affected bone are covered by irregular osteophytes. Histologically, the vascular connective tissue is composed of many thick-walled arteries. Bony changes are characterized as hypertrophic new bone production from the periosteum.

The lung or thoracic disease may be the result of metastatic lung disease, primary tumors of the lung, or esophageal sarcoma following *Spirocerca lupi* infection or thoracic lesions secondary to infections.[142, 144, 145] In a study of 180 dogs, 98 per cent had HO in association with intrathoracic disease. Of these, 92 per cent had either metastatic lung neoplasia or primary tumors of the esophagus or the lung. Only four cases had no intrathoracic involvement.[142]

The etiology of HO is unknown. A circulatory disturbance has been postulated for increased limb blood flow, or a nervous reflex that results in an increased peripheral blood flow.[141]

Treatment is aimed at the thoracic disease. While lobectomy or tumor resection is the primary method of treatment, unilateral intrathoracic vagotomy may aid in reversal of HO. Analgesics may make the animal with bone lesions more comfortable.

RETAINED ENCHONDRAL CARTILAGE CORES

Retained enchondral cartilage cores occur bilaterally in the distal ulnar metaphysis of young large and giant breed dogs. The retained enchondral cartilage is seen radiographically as a radiolucent inverted cone in the distal ulnar metaphysis (Figure 121–19). The persistence of the retained cartilage can cause disproportionate shortening of the ulna compared to the radius and result in a forelimb deformity including valgus, external rotation, or cranial bowing. Fortunately most cases of retained enchondral cartilage do not persist long enough to produce a deformity.[1]

The etiology is unknown but may relate to the vasculature of the metaphysis. It is postulated that there is an absence of vascular tissue that would normally penetrate hypertrophied cartilage cells prior to mineralization.[146] As a result of improper mineralization, the ulna does not lengthen as rapidly as the radius; thus deformity results.

Similarly, retained enchondral cartilage plays a role in the bony deformity of hindlimbs in giant breed dogs called genu valgum.[147] This deformity produces femoral shafts that bow medially ("knock-knees") and lateral patellar luxation. Retained enchondral cartilage can be seen radiographically and histologically in the lateral femoral condyles. The slowed growth of the lateral femoral condyle appears to have a primary role in the resultant deformity. The etiology of the retained femoral

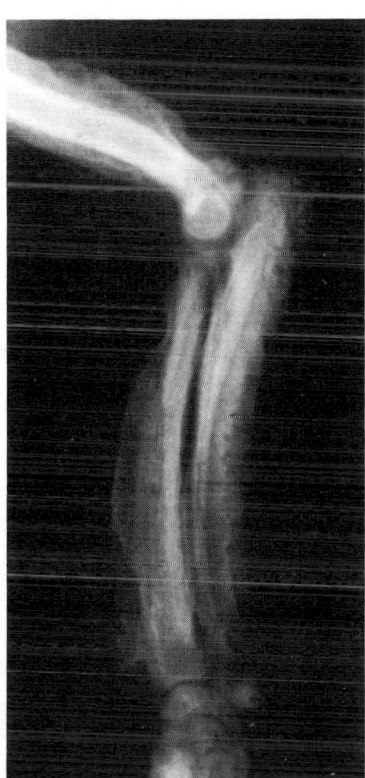

FIGURE 121–18. Hypertrophic osteopathy of the forelimb in a nine-year-old female Chihuahua with a primary bladder tumor and pulmonary metastasis.

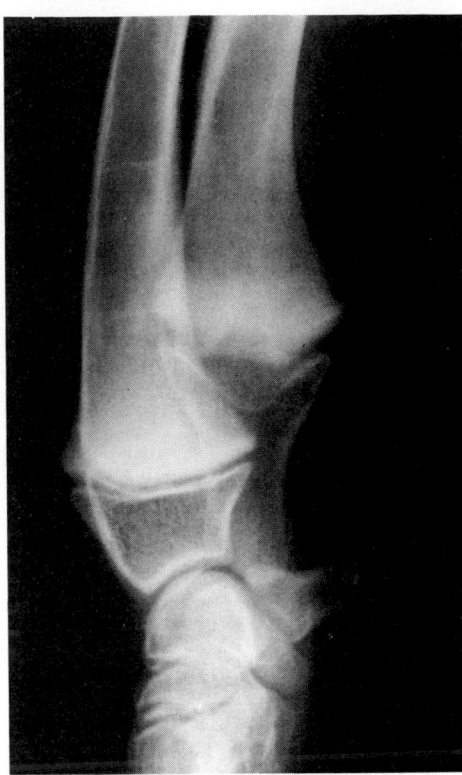

FIGURE 121–19. Retained enchondral cartilage core in the distal ulna of a three-month-old Saint Bernard.

cartilage is presumed similar to the one occurring in the ulna.

The growth deformities that result from retained enchondral cartilage are best handled surgically. Radial and ulnar deformities may be corrected and result in near normal animals; genu valgum may be corrected surgically, but the results are less gratifying.

DISUSE OSTEOPOROSIS

Disuse osteoporosis is a loss in mass of an individual bone or limb, or the entire skeleton, caused by lack of normal bony stress. In veterinary medicine, it usually relates to the bone beneath a rigid plate or to the bones immobilized within an external cast.[45]

Radiographically, affected bones become more radiolucent than normal with thinning cortices. Care must be taken in such animals to prevent pathologic fractures through the osteoporotic bones.

Animals with this disease usually have elevated serum calcium and phosphorus levels and may be excreting abnormally large quantities of urinary calcium.[148] The etiology and pathogenesis of disuse osteoporosis are known. With the lack of normal stresses, bones are remodeled by osteoclasts and new bone is not formed to replace it, resulting in bony loss. The process is reversible, and normal bone will be replaced when normal stress is reapplied to the affected bones.

LEAD POISONING

Lead poisoning is a disease of dogs caused by the ingestion of lead paint, linoleum, or other lead-containing materials. Lead toxicity may result in gastrointestinal, neurologic, and hematologic abnormalities.[149]

There are no clinical signs specifically referable to the skeletal system occurring following lead toxicity. Bony changes can occasionally be seen radiographically.

Radiographically, lead lines are dense sclerotic bands two to four mm wide, and when present are usually in the metaphysis of long bones of immature dogs. If present, they will be visible in all long bones; however, they are seen best in the distal radius and ulna, the sites of most active bone growth.

The origin of the bony lesion is presumed to be lead that is deposited with calcium during endochondral ossification. The lead incorporation stimulates new bone formation, which is seen histologically and radiographically as lead lines. Histologically, the lead lines in the metaphyseal areas are composed of longitudinally oriented trabeculae of new bone on cartilaginous cores containing increased amounts of mineralized cartilage.[150] Chronic toxicity of vitamin D, phosphorus, or bismuth can cause a similar histologic and radiographic lesion.[151]

ABNORMAL ESTROGEN METABOLISM

The target structures for estrogen in the growing skeleton are the articular cartilage and the osteoblasts. Estrogen arrests the proliferation of cartilage in endochondral ossification and apparently stimulates osteoblastic activity.[152] Generally, these compounds will decrease the growth of young animals by producing earlier union of the epiphyses with their shafts. The estrogens will promote a rapid maturation of the skeletal system, although the total bone length may be shorter than normal.[43]

References

1. Newton, CD and Siemering, G: Skeletal diseases. *In* Ettinger, SJ (ed): Textbook of Veterinary Internal Medicine. Philadelphia, WB Saunders, 1983, p 2236.
2. Nunamaker, DM: Osteomyelitis. *In* Newton, CD and Nunamaker, DM (eds): Textbook of Small Animal Orthopaedics. Philadelphia, JB Lippincott, 1985, p 499.
3. Aegerter, E and Kirkpatrick, JA (eds): Infectious diseases of bone. *In* Orthopaedic Disease. Philadelphia, WB Saunders, 1968, p 280.
4. Owen, LN: The pathology of bone infection. *In* Sumner-Smith, G (ed): Bone in Clinical Orthopaedics. Philadelphia, WB Saunders, 1982, p 261.
5. Caywood, DD, et al.: Osteomyelitis in the Dog: A review of 67 cases. JAVMA 172:943, 1978.
6. Smith, CW, et al.: Osteomyelitis in the dog: A retrospective study. JAAHA 14:589, 1978.
7. Boland, AL: Acute hematogenous osteomyelitis. Orthoped Clin North Am 3:225, 1972.
8. Walker, MA, et al.: Radiographic signs of bone infection in small animals. JAVMA 166:908, 1975.
9. Hirsch, DC and Smith, TM: Osteomyelitis in the dog: Microorganisms isolated and susceptibility to antimicrobial agents. J Sm Anim Pract 19:679, 1978.
10. Smith, GK: Unpublished Data. University of Pennsylvania, 1980.
11. Nunamaker, DM: Management of infected fractures. Vet Clin North Am 5:259, 1975.
12. Brodey, RS, et al.: Disseminated coccidioidomycosis in a dog. JAVMA 157:926, 1970.

13. Maddy, KT: Disseminated coccidioidomycosis of the dog. JAVMA 132:483, 1958.

14. Reed, RE: Diagnosis of disseminated canine coccidioidomycosis. JAVMA 128:196, 1956.

15. Ackerman, N and Spencer, CP: Radiographic aspects of mycotic diseases. Vet Clin North Am 12:175, 1982.

16. Millman, TM, et al.: Coccidioidomycosis in the dog: Its radiographic diagnosis. Vet Radiol 20:50, 1979.

17. Penwick, RC: Bone—Dog, Cat, Horse, Cow. In The Bristol Veterinary Handbook of Antimicrobial Therapy. Syracuse, New York, Bristol Laboratories 1982, p 46.

18. Dunn, TJ: Blastomycosis in a dog. Vet Med 72:1443, 1977.

19. Horne, RD: Feline systemic mycoses. Mod Vet Prac 45:45, 1964.

20. Roberts, RE: Osteomyelitis associated with disseminated blastomycosis in nine dogs. Vet Radiol 20:124, 1979.

21. Seabury, JH and Dascomb, HE: Results of treatment of systemic mycoses. JAVMA 188:590, 1964.

22. Small, E: Systemic mycoses. JAVMA 155:2002, 1969.

23. Burk, RL and Jones, BD: Disseminated histoplasmosis with osseous involvement in a dog. JAVMA 172:1416, 1978.

24. Lau, RE, et al.: Histoplasma capsulatum infection in a metatarsal of a dog. JAVMA 172:1414, 1978.

25. Mahaffey, E, et al.: Disseminated histoplasmosis in three cats. JAAHA 13:46, 1977.

26. Barron, CN: Cryptococcosis in animals. JAVMA 127:125, 1955.

27. Rutman, MA and Chandler, FW: Feline cryptococcosis. Feline Pract 5:36, 1975.

28. Horne, RD: Feline systemic mycoses: An up to date review. Mod Vet Pract 45:45, 1964.

29. Libke, KG and Walton, AM: Adenomycosis-like infection in the mandible of a cat. Mod Vet Pract 55:201, 1974.

30. Ditchfield, J: Nocardiosis in the dog. Mod Vet Pract 42:43, 1961.

31. Mitten, RW: Nocardial osteomyelitis in dogs. Mod Vet Pract 56:338, 1975.

32. Skelley, JF and Sauer, R: Cutaneous nocardiosis. Mod Vet Pract 46:78, 1965.

33. Harvey, CE, et al.: Radiographic diagnosis of chronic nasal disease. Vet Radiol 20:91, 1979.

34. Lang, JG, et al.: The diagnosis and successful treatment of Aspergillus fumigatus infection of the frontal sinuses and nasal chambers of the dog. J Sm Anim Pract 15:79, 1974.

35. Al-Doory, Y: Adiaspiromycosis in a dog. JAVMA 159:87, 1971.

36. Lewis, GE, et al.: Mycetoma in a cat. JAVMA 161:500, 1972.

37. Cruess, RL and Dumont, J: Healing of bone. In Newton, CD and Nunamaker, DM (eds). Textbook of Small Animal Orthopaedics. Philadelphia, JB Lippincott, 1985, p 35.

38. Capen, CC: Calcium-regulating hormones and metabolic bone disease. In Newton, CD and Nunamaker, DM (eds): Textbook of Small Animal Orthopaedics. Philadelphia, JB Lippincott, 1985, p 673.

39. Krook, L: Spontaneous hyperparathyroidism in the dog: A pathologic-anatomical study. Acta Pathol Microbiol Scand 41(Suppl 122): 1, 1957.

40. Carillo, JM, et al.: Primary hyperparathyroidism in a dog. JAVMA 174:67, 1979.

41. Legendre, AM, et al.: Primary hyperparathyroidism in a dog. JAVMA 168:694, 1976.

42. Pearson, PT, et al.: Primary hyperparathyroidism in a beagle. JAVMA 147:1201, 1965.

43. Siegel, ET: Effects of hormones on bone. Cornell Vet Suppl 58:95, 1968.

44. Aegerter, E and Kirkpatrick, JA (eds): Osteoporosis. In Orthopaedic Diseases. Philadelphia, WB Saunders, 1968, p 420.

45. Fetter, AW, et al.: Osteoporosis and osteopetrosis. In Newton, CD and Nunamaker, DM (eds): Textbook of Small Animal Orthopaedics. Philadelphia, JB Lippincott, 1985, p 627.

46. Rasmussen, PG: Multiple epiphyseal dysplasia in a litter of beagle puppies. J Sm Anim Pract 12:91, 1971.

47. Stockard, CR: The genetic and endocrine basis for differences in form and behavior as elucidated by studies of contrasted pure-line dogs and hybrids. Philadelphia, Wistar Institute, 1941.

48. McCusick, VA: Heritable Disorders of Connective Tissue. St. Louis, CV Mosby, 1972.

49. Fletch, SM, et al.: Clinical and pathologic features of chondrodysplasia (dwarfism) in the Alaskan malamute. JAVMA 162:357, 1973.

50. Carrig, CB, et al.: Retinal dysplasia associated with skeletal abnormalities in Labrador retrievers. JAVMA 170:49, 1977.

51. Meyers, VN, et al.: Short-limbed dwarfism and ocular defects in the Samoyed dog. JAVMA 183:975, 1983.

52. Stickler, GB, et al.: Hereditary progressive arthroophthalmopathy. Mayo Clin Proc 40:433, 1965.

53. Bruno, WJ and Janik, TA: What's your diagnosis? JAVMA 170:1097, 1977.

54. Cotchin, E and Dyce, KM: A case of epiphyseal dysplasia in a dog. Vet Rec 68:427, 1956.

55. Gardner, DL: Familial canine chondrodysplasia faetalis (achondroplasia). J Pathol Bateriol 77:243, 1959.

56. Hanlon, GF: Normal and abnormal bone growth in the dog. J Am Vet Radiol Soc 3:13, 1962.

57. Lodge, D: Two cases of epiphyseal dysplasia. Vet Rec 79:136, 1966.

58. Riser, WH, et al.: Pseudoachondroplastic dysplasia in miniature poodles: Clinical, radiographic and pathologic features. JAVMA 176:335, 1980.

59. Hansen, HJ: Historical evidence of an unusual deformity in dogs ("short-spine dog"). J Sm Anim Pract 9:103, 1968.

60. Gambardella, PC, et al.: Multiple cartilaginous exostoses in the dog. JAVMA 166:761, 1975.

61. Pool, RR and Carrig, CB: Multiple cartilaginous exostoses in a cat. Vet Path 9:350, 1972.

62. Riddle, WE and Leighton, RL: Osteochondromatosis in a cat. JAVMA 156:1428, 1970.

63. Solomon, L: Hereditary multiple exostoses. Am J Hum Genet 16:351, 1964.

64. Gee, BR and Doige, CE: Multiple cartilaginous exostoses in a litter of dogs. JAVMA 156:53, 1970.

65. Chester, DK: Multiple cartilaginous exostoses in two generations of dogs. JAVMA 159:895, 1971.

66. Turrell, JM and Pool, RR: Primary bone tumors in the cat: A retrospective study of 15 cats and a literature review. Vet Radiol 23:152, 1982.

67. Langenskiold, A: The stages of development of the cartilaginous foci in dyschondroplasia (Olliers Disease). Acta Ortho Scand 38:174, 1967.

68. Alexander, JW: Solitary and multiple cartilaginous exostoses in the dog. Canine Pract 5:43, 1978.

69. Owen, LN and Bostock, DE: Multiple cartilaginous exostoses with development of a metastasizing osteosarcoma in a Shetland sheepdog. J Sm Anim Pract 12:507, 1971.

70. Banks, WC and Bridges, CH: Multiple cartilaginous exostoses in a dog. JAVMA 129:131, 1956.

71. Doige, CE, et al.: Chondrosarcoma arising in multiple cartilaginous exostoses in a dog. JAAHA 14:605, 1978.

72. Jezyk, PF: Constitutional disorders of the skeleton in dogs and cats. In Newton, CD and Nunamaker, DM (eds): Textbook of Small Animal Orthopaedics. Philadelphia, JB Lippincott, 1985, p 637.

73. Carrig, CB, et al.: Ectrodactyly (split-hand deformity) in the dog. Vet Radiol 22:123, 1981.

74. Danforth, CH: Heredity of polydactyly in the cat. J Heredity 38:107, 1947.

75. Danforth, CH: Morphology of the feet of polydactyl cats. Am J Anat 80:143, 1947.

76. Sis, RF and Getty, R: Polydactylism in cats. VM/SAC 63:948, 1968.

77. Pennock, CA and Barnes, IC: The mucopolysaccharidoses. J Med Genet Biol 13:169, 1976.

78. Haskins, ME, et al.: Mucopolysaccharidosis in a domestic shorthaired cat: A disease distinct from that seen in the Siamese cat. JAVMA 175:384, 1979.

79. Haskins, ME, et al.: α-L-iduronidase deficiency in a cat. A model of mucopolysaccharidosis I. Pediatr Res 13:1294, 1979.

80. Skull, RM, et al.: Canine α-L-iduronidase deficiency: A model of mucopolysaccharidosis I. Anim J Path 109.244, 1982.

81. Spellacy, E, et al.: A canine model of human α-L-iduronidase deficiency. Proc Natl Acad Sci USA 80:6091, 1983.

82. Cowell, KR, et al.: Mucopolysaccharidosis in a cat. JAVMA 169:334, 1976.

83. Jezyk, PF, et al.: Mucopolysaccharidosis in a cat with arylsulfatase-B deficiency: A model of Maroteaux-Lamy syndrome. Science 198:834, 1977.

84. Schalm, OW: Mucopolysaccharidosis. Canine Prac 12:29, 1977.

85. Haskins, ME, et al.: β-glucuronidase deficiency in a dog: A model of human mucopolysaccharidosis VII. Ped Res 18:980, 1984.

86. Andresen, E and Willeberg, P: Pituitary dwarfism in German shepherd dogs: Additional evidence of simple autosomal recessive inheritance. Nord Vet Med 28:481, 1976.

87. Aegerter, E and Kirkpatrick, JA (eds): Hypervitaminosis D. *In* Orthopaedic Diseases. Philadelphia, WB Saunders, 1968, p 503.

88. Kronfeld, DS: Nutrition in orthopaedics. *In* Newton, CD and Nunamaker, DM (eds): Textbook of Small Animal Orthopaedics. Philadelphia, JB Lippincott, 1985, p 655.

89. Clark, L, et al.: Exostoses in hypervitaminotic A cats with optimal calcium/phosphorus intake. J Sm Anim Prac 11:553, 1970.

90. Seawright, A and English, P: Spondylosis in cats attributed to hypervitaminosis A. J Comp Path 77:35, 1967.

91. Cho, DY, et al.: Hypervitaminosis A in the dog. Am J Vet Res 36:1597, 1975.

92. English, PB: Clinical communication: A case of hyperostosis due to hypervitaminosis A in a cat. J Sm Anim Pract 10:207, 1969.

93. Bennett, D: Nutrition and bone disease in the dog and cat. Vet Rec 98:313, 1976.

94. Nutrient Requirements of Cats. Washington, DC, National Research Council, National Academy of Sciences, 1978.

95. Nutrient Requirements of Dogs. Washington, DC, National Research Council, National Academy of Sciences, 1974.

96. Brown, RG, et al.: Alaskan malamute chondrodysplasia V: Decreased gut zinc absorption. Growth 42:1, 1978.

97. Hedhammer, A, et al.: Overnutrition and skeletal disease: An experimental study in growing Great Dane dogs. Cornell Vet 64(suppl 5):1, 1974.

98. Spjut, HL, et al.: Tumors of bone and cartilage. *In* Atlas of Tumor Pathology, 2nd series, fascicle 5. Washington, DC, Armed Forces Institute of Pathology, 1971.

99. Goldschmidt, MH and Thrall, DE: Malignant bone tumors in the dog. *In* Newton, CD and Nunamaker, DM (eds): Textbook of Small Animal Orthopaedics. Philadelphia, JB Lippincott, 1985, p 887.

100. Kistler, KR: Canine osteosarcoma: 1462 cases reviewed to uncover patterns of height, weight, breed, sex, age, and site of involvement. Phi Zeta Awards. University of Pennsylvania School of Veterinary Medicine, 1981.

101. Priester, WA and McKay, FW: The occurrence of tumors in domestic animals. Natl Cancer Inst Monogr 54:169, 1980.

102. Brodey, RS and Abt, DA: Results of surgical treatment in 65 dogs with osteosarcoma. JAVMA 168:1032, 1976.

103. Helfand, SC: Cisplatin chemotherapy for canine osteosarcoma. Classroom handout, University of Pennsylvania School of Veterinary Medicine, 1987.

104. Weben, PM and Clayton-Jones, DG: Bone tumors. J Sm Anim Prac 19:251, 1978.

105. Shapiro, W, et al.: Use of cisplatin for treatment of appendicular osteosarcoma in dogs. JAVMA 192:507, 1988.

106. Ling, GV, et al.: Primary bone tumors in the dog: A combined clinical, radiographic and histologic approach to early diagnosis. JAVMA 165:55, 1974.

107. Brodey, R.S. et al.: Canine skeletal chondrosarcoma: A clinicopathologic study of 35 cases. JAVMA 165:68, 1974.

108. Brodey, RS, et al.: Canine bone neoplasms. JAVMA 143:471, 1963.

109. Peiffer, RL and Rebar, A: Fibrosarcoma involving the skeleton of the dog. VM/SAC 69:1143, 1974.

110. Bitetto, WV, et al.: Osteosarcoma in cats: 22 cases (1974–1984). JAVMA 190:91, 1987.

111. Goldschmidt, MH and Thrall, DE: Primary and secondary bone tumors in the cat. *In* Newton, CD and Nunamaker, DM (eds): Textbook of Small Animal Orthopaedics. Philadelphia, JB Lippincott, 1985, p 911.

112. Liu, SK, et al.: Primary and secondary bone tumors in the cat. J Sm Anim Prac 15:141, 1974.

113. Bohning, RH, et al.: Clinical and radiological survey of canine panosteitis. JAVMA 156:870, 1970.

114. Burt, JK and Wilson, GP: A study of eosinophilic panosteitis (enostosis) in German shepherd dogs. Acta Radiol Suppl 319:7, 1972.

115. Lenehan, TM, et al.: Canine panosteitis. *In* Newton, CD and Nunamaker, DM (eds): Textbook of Small Animal Orthopaedics. Philadelphia, JB Lippincott, 1985, p 591.

116. Cotter, SM, et al.: Enostosis of young dogs. JAVMA 153:401, 1968.

117. Turnier, JC and Silverman, S: A case study of canine panosteitis: Comparison of radiographic and radioisotopic studies. Am J Vet Res 30:1550, 1978.

118. Evers, WH: Enostosis in a dog. JAVMA 154:799, 1969.

119. Sprinkle, TA and Korak, L: Hip dysplasia, elbow dysplasia and eosinophilic panosteitis: Three clinical manifestations of hyperestrinism in the dog? Cornell Vet 60:476, 1970.

120. Lenehan, TM and Fetter, AW: Hypertrophic osteodystrophy. *In* Newton, CD and Nunamaker, DM (eds): Textbook of Small Animal Orthopaedics. Philadelphia, JB Lippincott, 1985, p 597.

121. Grondalen, J: Metaphyseal HOD in growing dogs: a clinical study. J Sm Anim Prac 17:721, 1976.

122. Olsson, SE: Radiology in veterinary pathology. A review with special reference to HOD and secondary hyperparathyroidism in the dog. Acta Radiol Supp 319:255, 1972.

123. Holmes, JR: Suspected skeletal scurvy in the dog. Vet Rec 74:801, 1962.

124. Vaananen, M and Wikman, L: Scurvy as a cause of osteodystrophy. J Sm Anim Prac 20:491, 1979.

125. Bennett, D: Nutrition and bone disease in the dog and cat. Vet Rec 98:313, 1976.

126. Teare, JA, et al.: Ascorbic acid deficiency and hypertrophic osteodystrophy in the dog: A rebuttal. Cornell Vet 69:384, 1979.

127. Riser, WH and Newton, CD: Craniomandibular osteopathy. *In* Newton, CD and Nunamaker, DM (eds): Textbook of Small Animal Orthopaedics. Philadelphia, JB Lippincott, 1985, p 621.

128. Alexander, JW: Craniomandibular osteopathy. Canine Pract 5:31, 1978.

129. Riser, WH, et al.: Canine craniomandibular osteopathy. J Amer Vet Rad Soc 8:23, 1967.

130. Padgett, GA and Mostosky, UV: Animal Model: The mode of inheritance of craniomandibular osteopathy in West Highland white terrier dogs. Am J Med Genetics 25:9, 1986.

131. Pool, RR and Leighton, RL: Craniomandibular osteopathy in a dog. JAVMA 154:657, 1969.

132. Goldschmidt, MH and Biery, DN: Bone cysts in the dog. *In* Newton, CD and Nunamaker, DM (eds): Textbook of Small Animal Orthopaedics. Philadelphia, JB Lippincott, 1985, p 611.

133. Carrig, CB and Seawright, AA: A familial canine polyostotic fibrous dysplasia with subperiosteal cortical defects. J Sm Anim Prac 10:397, 1969.

134. Biery, DN, et al.: Bone cysts in the dog. J Am Vet Radiol Soc 17:202, 1976.

135. Jaffe, HL and Lichtenstein, L: Solitary unicameral bone cyst. Arch Surg 44:1004, 1942.

136. Renegar, WR, et al.: Aneurysmal bone cyst in the dog: A case report. JAAHA 15:191, 1979.

137. Dubielzig, RR: Medullary bone infarction in dogs. *In* Newton, CD and Nunamaker DM (eds): Textbook of Small Animal Orthopaedics. Philadelphia, JB Lippincott, 1985, p 615.

138. Dubielzig, RR, et al.: Bone sarcomas associated with multifocal bone infarction in dogs. JAVMA 179:64, 1981.

139. Riser, WH, et al.: Bone infarctions associated with malignant bone tumors in dogs. JAVMA 160:411, 1972.

140. Furney, JG, et al.: Fibrosarcoma arising at the site of bone infarcts. J Bone Joint Surg 42A:802, 1960.

141. Lenehan, TM and Fetter, AW: Hypertrophic osteopathy. *In* Newton, CD and Nunamaker, DM (eds): Textbook of Small Animal Orthopaedics. Philadelphia, JB Lippincott, 1985, p 603.

142. Brodey, RS: Hypertrophic osteoarthropathy. *In* Spontaneous Animal Models of Human Disease. New York, Academic Press, 1979, p 241.

143. Halliwell, WH and Ackerman, N: Botryoid rhabdomyosarcoma of the urinary bladder and hyperosteoarthropathy in a young dog. JAVMA 165:911, 1974.

144. Brodey, RS, et al.: Hypertrophic osteoarthropathy in a dog with

pulmonary metastasis from a renal adenocarcinoma. JAVMA 132:231, 1958.

145. Leighton, RL and Olson, S: Hypertrophic osteoarthropathy in a dog with pulmonary abscess. JAVMA 150:1516, 1967.

146. Riser, WH and Shirer, JF: Normal and abnormal growth of the distal foreleg in large and giant dogs. J Am Vet Rad Soc 6:50, 1965.

147. Riser, WH, et al.: Genu valgum: a stifle deformity of giant dogs. J Am Vet Rad Soc 10:28, 1969.

148. Whittick, WG: Osteopenia due to a stress deficiency. *In* Canine Orthopaedics. Philadelphia, Lea & Febiger, 1974, p 41.

149. Zook, BC, et al.: Lead poisoning in dogs. JAVMA 155:1329, 1969.

150. Schunk, KL: Lead poisoning in dogs. Small Animal Veterinary Medical Update series 8:1, 1978.

151. Zook, BC: The pathologic anatomy of lead poisoning. Vet Path 9:310, 1973.

152. Krook, L: Metabolic bone disease in dogs and cats. Proc 38th Mtg AAHA, 1971.

153. Page, R: Cisplatin, a new antineoplastic drug in veterinary medicine. JAVMA 186:288, 1985.

DRUG INDEX

Generic	Trade	Dosage	Route	Frequency	Brief Description
Penicillin	Oxacillin	10 mg/lb	PO	t.i.d.	Antibiotic
		5 mg/lb	IV, IM	b.i.d.–t.i.d.	
Penicillin	Amoxicillin	5 mg/lb	PO	b.i.d.	Antibiotic
		5 mg/lb	IM, SQ	b.i.d.	
Cephradine Sodium	Velosef	9 mg/lb	PO	b.i.d.–t.i.d.	Antibiotic
Gentamicin	Gentocin	2 mg/lb	IM for one day, then IM	b.i.d. s.i.d.	Antibiotic
Kanamycin Sulfate	Kanamycin	3 mg/lb	IM	b.i.d.	Antibiotic
Amphotericin B.	Fungizone	0.1 mg/lb	IV	s.i.d.	Antifungal
Ketoconazole	Nizoral	9 mg/lb	PO	s.i.d. for 6 weeks	Antifungal
Streptomycin	Streptomycin	5–10 mg/lb	IM	t.i.d.	Antibiotic
Sulfonamides	Tribrissen	14 mg/lb	PO, IM, SQ	s.i.d.	Antibiotic
L-thyroxine	Synthroid	0.01 mg/lb	PO	b.i.d.	Hormone
Acetylsalicylic Acid	Bayer Bufferin	Dog 12 mg/lb Cat 18 mg/lb	PO PO	b.i.d.–t.i.d. q 72 hrs.	Analgesic, anti-inflammatory
Prednisolone Prednisone	Orasone	0.1 mg/lb	PO	s.i.d.–b.i.d.	Anti-inflammatory
Cisplatin	Platinol	50 mg/M^2	IV	Infusion over a 6-hour period diluted with NaCl and 5% dextrose [153]	Antineoplastic

INDEX

Note: Page numbers in *italics* refer to illustrations; page numbers followed by the letter t refer to tables.